AMA
AMERICAN MEDICAL ASSOCIATION



# ICD-10-CM 2027

## The Complete Official Codebook

AMA publications fund initiatives that drive improvements in patient health, practice innovation and medical education.

## Publisher's Notice



## Our Commitment to Accuracy

The AMA is committed to producing accurate and reliable materials. To report corrections, please call the AMA Unified Service Center at (800) 621-8335. To purchase additional copies, visit the AMA store at amastore.com. Refer to product number OP201427.

## Acknowledgments

Marianne Randall, CPC, *Senior Product Manager*
Anita Schmidt, BS, RHIA, AHIMA-approved ICD-10-CM/PCS Trainer, *Subject Matter Expert*
Leanne Patterson, CPC, *Subject Matter Expert*
Laura M. Anderson, RN, BSN, CCDS, *Subject Matter Expert*
Tara Rose, CPC, CPC-I, CPMA, RHIA, *Subject Matter Expert*
Stacy Perry, *Manager, Desktop Publishing*
Hope M. Dunn, *Senior Desktop Publishing Specialist*
Katie Russell, *Senior Desktop Publishing Specialist*
Lynn Speirs, *Editor*

## Copyright



Made in the USA
OP201427
BQ49:09/26

## Leanne Patterson, CPC

Ms. Patterson has more than 20 years of experience in the healthcare profession. She has an extensive background in professional component coding, with proven expertise in assignment of E/M codes, general surgery coding, medical record documentation improvement, and HIPAA compliance. Her experience includes serving as Director of Compliance, conducting chart-to-claim audits, and physician education. She has been responsible for coding and denial management in large multi-specialty physician practices, and most recently has been part of a team developing content for products related to ICD-10-CM. Ms. Patterson is credentialed by and is a member of the AAPC.

## Anita Schmidt, BS, RHIA, AHIMA-approved ICD-10-CM/PCS Trainer

Anita Schmidt has expertise in ICD-10-CM/PCS, DRG, and CPT with more than 20 years' experience in coding in multiple settings, including inpatient, observation, and same-day surgery. Her experience includes analysis of medical record documentation, assignment of ICD-10-CM and PCS codes, and DRG validation. She has collaborated with clinical documentation specialists to identify documentation needs and potential areas for physician education. Most recently she has been developing content for resource and educational products related to ICD-10-CM, ICD-10-PCS, DRG, and CPT. Anita is an AHIMA-approved ICD-10-CM/PCS trainer and is an active member of the American Health Information Management Association (AHIMA) and the Minnesota Health Information Management Association (MHIMA).

# Contents

# How to Use ICD-10-CM: The Complete Official Codebook 2027

## Introduction

*ICD-10-CM: The Complete Official Codebook* 2027 is your definitive coding resource, combining the work of the National Center for Health Statistics (NCHS), Centers for Medicare and Medicaid Services (CMS), American Hospital Association (AHA), and Publisher experts to provide the information you need for coding accuracy.

The International Classification of Diseases, 10th Revision, Clinical Modification (ICD-10-CM), is an adaptation of ICD-10, copyrighted by the World Health Organization (WHO). The development and maintenance of this clinical modification (CM) is the responsibility of the NCHS as authorized by WHO. Any new concepts added to ICD-10-CM are based on an established update process through the collaboration of WHO's Update and Revision Committee and the ICD-10-CM Coordination and Maintenance Committee.

In addition to the ICD-10-CM classification, other official government source information has been included in this manual. Depending on the source, updates to information may be annual or quarterly. This manual provides the most current information that was available at the time of publication. For updates to the source documents that may have occurred after this manual was published, please refer to the following:

- **NCHS, International Classification of Diseases, Tenth Revision, Clinical Modification (ICD-10-CM)**
  https://www.cms.gov/medicare/coding-billing/icd-10-codes
- **CMS Integrated Outpatient Code Editor (IOCE), version 27.2**
  https://www.cms.gov/Medicare/Coding/OutpatientCodeEdit/OCEQtrReleaseSpecs.html
- **CMS-HCC Risk Adjustment Model, version 28**
- **CMS ESRD-HCC Risk Adjustment Model, version 24**
- **CMS RxHCC Risk Adjustment Model, version 08**
  https://www.cms.gov/Medicare/Health-Plans/MedicareAdvtgSpecRateStats/Risk-Adjustors.html
- **HHS-HCC Commercial Risk Adjustment Model, version 08**
  https://www.cms.gov/CCIIO/Resources/Regulations-and-Guidance
- **CMS Quality Payment Program (QPP)**
  https://qpp.cms.gov/mips/explore-measures
- **AHA Coding Clinics**
  https://www.codingclinicadvisor.com/

The official NCHS ICD-10-CM classification includes three main sections: the guidelines, the indexes, and the tabular list, all of which make up the bulk of this coding manual. To complement the classification, Optum's coding experts have incorporated Medicare-related coding edits and proprietary features, such as supplementary notations, coding tools, and appendixes, into a comprehensive and easy-to-use reference. This publication is organized as follows:

## What's New for 2027

This section provides a high-level overview of the code changes made for fiscal 2027. The list of codes provided identifies new, revised, and deleted codes. Asterisked codes identify prior midyear changes that were made to the classification, effective April 1, 2026. All changes are based on official addenda, provided by the NCHS.

## Conversion Table

The conversion table was developed by NCHS to help facilitate data retrieval as new codes are added to the ICD-10-CM classification. This table provides a crosswalk from each fiscal 2027 new code to the equivalent code(s) assigned, prior to October 1, 2026, for that diagnosis or condition. Asterisked codes identify prior midyear additions, effective April 1, 2026. For the full conversion table, refer to the Conversion Table zip file at https://www.cms.gov/medicare/coding-billing/icd-10-codes.

## 10 Steps to Correct Coding

This step-by-step tutorial walks the coder through the process of finding the correct code — from locating the code in the official indexes to verifying the code in the tabular section — while following applicable conventions, guidelines, and instructional notes. Specific examples are provided with detailed explanations of each coding step along with advice for proper sequencing.

## Official ICD-10-CM Guidelines for Coding and Reporting

This section provides the full official conventions and guidelines regulating the appropriate assignment and reporting of ICD-10-CM codes. These conventions and guidelines are published by the U.S. Department of Health and Human Services (DHHS) and approved by the cooperating parties (American Health Information Management Association [AHIMA], NCHS, Centers for Disease Control and Prevention [CDC], and the American Hospital Association [AHA]).

## Indexes

### Index to Diseases and Injuries

The Index to Diseases and Injuries is arranged in alphabetic order by terms specific to a disease, condition, illness, injury, eponym, or abbreviation as well as terms that describe circumstances other than a disease or injury that may require attention from a health care professional.

### Neoplasm Table

The Neoplasm Table is arranged in alphabetic order by anatomical site. Codes are then listed in individual columns based upon the histological behavior (malignant, in situ, benign, uncertain, or unspecified) of the neoplasm.

### Table of Drugs and Chemicals

The Table of Drugs and Chemicals is arranged in alphabetic order by the specific drug or chemical name. Codes are listed in individual columns based upon the associated intent (poisoning, adverse effect, or underdosing). Drugs with an asterisk identify substances added to the table by Optum subject matter experts.

### External Causes Index

The External Causes Index is arranged in alphabetic order by main terms that describe the cause, the intent, the place of occurrence, the activity, and the status of the patient at the time the injury occurred or health condition arose.

## Index Notations

### With

The word "with" or "in" should be interpreted to mean "associated with" or "due to." The classification presumes a causal relationship between the two conditions linked by these terms in the index. These conditions should be coded as related even in the absence of provider documentation explicitly linking them unless the documentation clearly states the conditions are unrelated or when another guideline specifically requires a documented linkage between two conditions (e.g., the sepsis guideline for "acute organ dysfunction that is not clearly associated with the sepsis"). For conditions not specifically linked by these relational terms in the classification or when a guideline requires explicit documentation of a linkage between two conditions, provider documentation must link the conditions to code them as related.

The word "with" in the index is sequenced immediately following the main term, not in alphabetical order.

> **Dermatopolymyositis** M33.9Ø
> with
> myopathy M33.92
> respiratory involvement M33.91
> specified organ involvement NEC M33.99
> amyopathic M33.93

### See

When the instruction "see" follows a term in the index, it indicates that another term must be referenced to locate the correct code.

> **Hematoperitoneum** — *see* Hemoperitoneum

### See Also

The instructional note "see also" simply provides alternative terms the coder may reference that may be useful in determining the correct code but are not necessary to follow if the main term supplies the appropriate code.

> **Hematinuria** — *see also* Hemaglobinuria
> malarial B5Ø.8

### Default Codes

In the index, the default code is the code listed next to the main term and represents the condition most commonly associated with that main term. This code may be assigned when documentation does not support reporting a more specific code. Alternatively, it may provide an unspecified code for the condition.

> **Hemiatrophy** R68.89
> cerebellar G31.9
> face, facial, progressive (Romberg) G51.8
> tongue K14.8

### Parentheses

Parentheses in the indexes enclose nonessential modifiers, supplementary words that may be present or absent in the statement of a disease without affecting the code.

> **Pseudomeningocele** (cerebral) (infective) (post-traumatic) G96.198
> postprocedural (spinal) G97.82

### Brackets

ICD-10-CM has a coding convention addressing code assignment for manifestations that occur as a result of an underlying condition. This convention requires the underlying condition to be sequenced first, followed by the code or codes for the associated manifestation. In the index, italicized codes in brackets identify manifestation codes.

> **Polyneuropathy** (peripheral) G62.9
> alcoholic G62.1
> amyloid (Portuguese) E85.1 *[G63]*
> transthyretin-related (ATTR) familial E85.1 *[G63]*

### Shaded Guides

Exclusive vertical shaded guides in the Index to Diseases and Injuries and External Causes Index help the user easily follow the indent levels for the subentries under a main term. Sequencing rules may apply depending on the level of indent for separate subentries.

> **Hemicrania**
> congenital malformation QØØ.Ø
> continua G44.51
> meaning migraine — *see also* Migraine G43.9Ø9
> paroxysmal G44.Ø39
> chronic G44.Ø49
> intractable G44.Ø41
> not intractable G44.Ø49
> episodic G44.Ø39
> intractable G44.Ø31
> not intractable G44.Ø39
> intractable G44.Ø31
> not intractable G44.Ø39

### *Following* References

The Index to Diseases and Injuries includes "following" references to assist in locating out-of-sequence codes in the tabular list. Out-of-sequence codes contain an alphabetic character (letter) in the third- or fourth-character position. These codes are placed according to the classification rules — according to condition — not according to alphabetic or numeric sequencing rules.

> **Carcinoma** (malignant) — *see also* Neoplasm, by site, malignant
> neuroendocrine — *see also* Tumor, neuroendocrine
> high grade, any site C7A.1 (*following* C75)
> poorly differentiated, any site C7A.1 (*following* C75)

### Additional Character Required

The Index to Diseases and Injuries, Neoplasm Table, and External Causes Index provide an icon after certain codes to signify to the user that additional characters are required to make the code valid. The tabular list should be consulted for appropriate character selection.

> **Fall, falling** (accidental) W19 ☑
> building W2Ø.1 ☑

# Tabular List of Diseases

ICD-10-CM codes and descriptions are arranged numerically within the tabular list of diseases with 19 separate chapters providing codes associated with a particular body system or nature of injury or disease. There is also a chapter providing codes for external causes of an injury or health conditions, a chapter for codes that address encounters with healthcare facilities for circumstances other than a disease or injury, and finally, a chapter for codes that capture special circumstances such as new diseases of uncertain etiology or emergency use codes.

## Code and Code Descriptions

ICD-10-CM is an alphanumeric classification system that contains categories, subcategories, and valid codes. The first character is always a letter with any additional characters represented by either a letter or number. A three-character category without further subclassification is equivalent to a valid three-character code. Valid codes may be three, four, five, six, or seven characters in length, with each level of subdivision after a three-character category representing a subcategory. The final level of subdivision is a valid code.

### Boldface

**Boldface** type is used for all codes and descriptions in the tabular list.

### Italics

*Italicized* type is used to identify manifestation codes, those codes that should not be reported as first-listed diagnoses.

### Deleted Text

~~Strikethrough~~ on a code and code description indicates a deletion from the classification for the current year.

### Key Word

Green font is used throughout the Tabular List of Diseases to differentiate the key words that appear in similar code descriptions in a given category or subcategory. The key word convention is used only in those categories in which there are multiple codes with very similar descriptions with only a few words that differentiate them.

For example, refer to the list of codes below from category H55:

- ✓4th **H55 Nystagmus and other irregular eye movements**
  - ✓5th **H55.Ø Nystagmus**
    - **H55.ØØ Unspecified nystagmus**
    - **H55.Ø1 Congenital nystagmus**
    - **H55.Ø2 Latent nystagmus**
    - **H55.Ø3 Visual deprivation nystagmus**
    - **H55.Ø4 Dissociated nystagmus**
    - **H55.Ø9 Other forms of nystagmus**

The portion of the code description that appears in **green font** in the tabular list helps the coder quickly identify the key terms and the correct code. This convention is especially useful when the codes describe laterality, such as the following codes from subcategory H4Ø.22:

- ✓6th **H4Ø.22 Chronic angle-closure glaucoma**
  - Chronic primary angle closure glaucoma
  - ✓7th **H4Ø.221 Chronic angle-closure glaucoma, right eye** Rx
  - ✓7th **H4Ø.222 Chronic angle-closure glaucoma, left eye** Rx
  - ✓7th **H4Ø.223 Chronic angle-closure glaucoma, bilateral** Rx
  - ✓7th **H4Ø.229 Chronic angle-closure glaucoma, unspecified eye** Rx

## Tabular Notations

Official parenthetical notes as well as Optum's supplementary notations are provided at the chapter, code block, category, subcategory, and individual code level to help the user assign proper codes. The information in the notation can apply to one or more codes depending on where the citation is placed.

## Official Notations

### Includes Notes

The word INCLUDES appears immediately under certain categories to further define, clarify, or give examples of the content of a code category.

### Inclusion Terms

Lists of inclusion terms are included under certain codes. These terms indicate some of the conditions for which that code number may be used. Inclusion terms may be synonyms with the code title, or, in the case of "other specified" codes, the terms may also provide a list of various conditions included within a classification code. The inclusion terms are not exhaustive. The index may provide additional terms that may also be assigned to a given code.

### Excludes Notes

ICD-10-CM has two types of excludes notes. Each note has a different definition for use. However, they are similar in that they both indicate that codes excluded from each other are independent of each other.

#### Excludes 1

An EXCLUDES 1 note is a "pure" excludes. It means "NOT CODED HERE!" An Excludes 1 note indicates mutually exclusive codes: two conditions that cannot be reported together. An Excludes1 note indicates that the code excluded should never be used at the same time as the code above the Excludes1 note. An Excludes1 is used when two conditions cannot occur together, such as a congenital form versus an acquired form of the same condition.

An exception to the Excludes 1 definition is when the two conditions are unrelated to each other. If it is not clear whether the two conditions involving an Excludes 1 note are related or not, query the provider. For example, code F45.8 Other somatoform disorders, has an Excludes 1 note for "sleep related teeth grinding (G47.63)" because "teeth grinding" is an inclusion term under F45.8. Only one of these two codes should be assigned for teeth grinding. However psychogenic dysmenorrhea is also an inclusion term under F45.8, and a patient could have both this condition and sleep-related teeth grinding. In this case, the two conditions are clearly unrelated to each other, so it would be appropriate to report F45.8 and G47.63 together.

#### Excludes 2

An EXCLUDES 2 note means "NOT INCLUDED HERE." An Excludes 2 note indicates that although the excluded condition is not part of the condition it is excluded from, a patient may have both conditions at the same time. Therefore, when an Excludes 2 note appears under a code, it may be acceptable to use both the code and the excluded code together if supported by the medical documentation.

### Note

The term "NOTE" appears as an icon and precedes the instructional information. These notes function as alerts to highlight coding instructions within the text.

### Code First/Use additional code

These instructional notes provide sequencing instruction. They may appear independently of each other or to designate certain etiology/manifestation paired codes. These instructions signal the coder that an additional code should be reported to provide a more complete picture of that diagnosis.

In etiology/manifestation coding, ICD-10-CM requires the underlying condition to be sequenced first, followed by the manifestation. In these situations, codes with "In diseases classified elsewhere" in the code description are never permitted as a first-listed or principal diagnosis code and must be sequenced following the underlying condition code.

## Code Also

A "code also" note alerts the coder that more than one code may be required to fully describe the condition. The sequencing depends on the circumstances of the encounter. Factors that may determine sequencing include severity and reason for the encounter.

## Revised Text

The revised text ▶◀ "bow ties" alert the user to changes in official notations for the current year. Revised text may include the following:

- A change in a current parenthetical description
- A change in the code(s) associated with a current parenthetical note
- A change in how a current parenthetical note is classified (e.g., an Excludes 1 note that changed to an Excludes 2 note)
- Addition of a new parenthetical note(s) to a code

## Deleted Text

~~Strikethrough~~ on official notations indicate a deletion from the classification for the current year.

# Publisher Notations

### *AHA Coding Clinic* Citations

*Coding Clinics* are official American Hospital Association (AHA) publications that provide coding advice specific to ICD-10-CM and ICD-10-PCS.

*Coding Clinic* citations included in this manual are current up to the second quarter of 2026.

These citations identify the year, quarter, and page number of one or more Coding Clinic publications that may have coding advice relevant to a particular code or group of codes. With the most current citation listed first, these notations are preceded by the symbol **AHA:** and appear in purple type.

> **I15.1 Hypertension secondary to other renal disorders** Rx
> **AHA:** 2016, 3Q, 22

### Definitions

Definitions explain a specific term, condition, or disease process in layman's terms. These notations are preceded by the symbol **DEF:** and appear in purple type.

> √5th **M51.4 Schmorl's nodes**
> **DEF:** Irregular bone defect in the margin of the vertebral body that causes herniation into the end plate of the vertebral body.

### Coding Tips

The tips in the tabular list offer coding advice that is not readily available within the ICD-10-CM classification. It may relate official coding guidelines, indexing nuances, or advice from *AHA's Coding Clinic for ICD-10-CM/PCS*. These notations are preceded by the symbol **TIP:** and appear in brown type.

> √5th **M11.2 Other chondrocalcinosis**
> Chondrocalcinosis NOS
> **AHA:** 2018,3Q,20
> **TIP:** Pseudogout is captured with codes in this subcategory.

# Icons

**Note:** The following icons are placed to the left of the code.

Changes to ICD-10-CM codes since the last published edition of this manual are highlighted in two ways:

The following green icons identify new or revised codes effective April 1, 2026:

- ● **New Code — Midyear**
- ▲ **Revised Code — Midyear**

The following black icons identify new or revised codes effective October 1, 2026:

- ● **New Code**
- ▲ **Revised Code**
- √ **Additional Characters Required**
  - √4th This symbol indicates that the code requires a 4th character.
  - √5th This symbol indicates that the code requires a 5th character.
  - √6th This symbol indicates that the code requires a 6th character.
  - √7th This symbol indicates that the code requires a 7th character.

> √5th **H60.3 Other infective otitis externa**
> √6th **H60.31 Diffuse otitis externa**
> **H60.311 Diffuse otitis externa, right ear**
> **H60.312 Diffuse otitis externa, left ear**
> **H60.313 Diffuse otitis externa, bilateral**
> **H60.319 Diffuse otitis externa, unspecified ear**

√x7th **Placeholder Alert**

This symbol indicates that the code requires a 7th character following the placeholder "X". Codes with fewer than six characters that require a 7th character must contain placeholder "X" to fill in the empty character(s).

> √x7th **T16.1 Foreign body in right ear**

This manual provides the most current information that was available at the time of publication. Except where otherwise noted, the icons and/or color bars reflect edits provided in the Integrated Outpatient Code Editor (IOCE) quarterly files utilized under the outpatient prospective payment system (OPPS). Because the October 2026 quarterly files were not available at the time this book was printed, the edits in this manual are based on the July 2026 quarterly files.

The following is a list of IOCE edits specifically identified in this manual:

- Age
- Manifestation
- Unacceptable principal diagnosis

**Note:** The following icons are placed at the end of the code description.

### Age Edits

N **Newborn Age: 0**
These diagnoses are intended for newborns and neonates and the patient's age must be 0 years.

| | |
|---|---|
| **N47.0 Adherent prepuce, newborn** | N |

P **Pediatric Age: 0-17**
These diagnoses are intended for children and the patient's age must be between 0 and 17 years.

| | |
|---|---|
| **L21.1 Seborrheic infantile dermatitis** | P |

M **Maternity Age: 9-64**
These diagnoses are intended for childbearing patients between the age of 9 and 64 years.

| | |
|---|---|
| **O02.9 Abnormal product of conception, unspecified** | COM M |

A **Adult Age: 15-124**
These diagnoses are intended for patients between the age of 15 and 124 years.

**R54 Age-related physical debility** A
Frailty
Old age
Senescence
Senile asthenia
Senile debility
EXCLUDES 1 *age-related cognitive decline (R41.81)*
*sarcopenia (M62.84)*
*senile psychosis (F03.-)*
*senility NOS (R41.81)*

UPD **Unacceptable Principal Diagnosis**
This icon identifies codes that are not appropriate as a first-listed code for *outpatient* encounters. These codes describe circumstances that influence an individual's health status but are not a current illness or injury, or that are not specifically manifestations but may be due to an underlying cause.

| | |
|---|---|
| ✓7th **T48.5X5 Adverse effect of other anti-common-cold drugs** | UPD |

HCC **CMS-HCC Condition**
This icon identifies codes that are considered a CMS-HCC (hierarchical condition category) diagnosis.

The HCC codes represented in this manual have been updated to reflect the 2026 Initial ICD-10-CM Mappings for CMS-HCC Model v28. Midyear final mappings were not available at the time this publication went to print; refer to the following CMS website for final mappings: https://www.cms.gov/Medicare/Health-Plans/MedicareAdvtgSpecRateStats/Risk-Adjustors.html.

**P12.2 Epicranial subaponeurotic hemorrhage due to birth injury** HCC
Subgaleal hemorrhage

Rx **Rx-HCC Condition**
This icon identifies codes that are included in the Rx-HCC risk-adjustment model, which covers the Part D (prescription drug) benefit.

The Rx-HCC codes represented in this manual have been updated to reflect the 2027 Initial ICD-10-CM Mappings for CMS Rx-HCC Model v08. Midyear final mappings were not available at the time this publication went to print; refer to the following CMS website for final mappings: https://www.cms.gov/Medicare/Health-Plans/MedicareAdvtgSpecRateStats/Risk-Adjustors.html.

| | |
|---|---|
| **Z21 Asymptomatic human immunodeficiency virus [HIV] infection status** | HCC Rx ESR COM |

ESR **ESRD HCC Condition**
This icon identifies codes that are included in the end-stage renal disease (ESRD) HCC risk-adjustment model.

The ESRD HCC codes represented in this manual have been updated to reflect the 2027 Initial ICD-10-CM Mappings for CMS ESRD HCC Model v24. Midyear final mappings were not available at the time this publication went to print; refer to the following CMS website for final mappings: https://www.cms.gov/Medicare/Health-Plans/MedicareAdvtgSpecRateStats/Risk-Adjustors.html.

| | |
|---|---|
| **Z21 Asymptomatic human immunodeficiency virus [HIV] infection status** | HCC Rx ESR COM |

COM **Commercial HCC Condition**
This icon identifies codes that are included in the commercial HHS-HCC risk-adjustment model.

The commercial HCC codes represented in this manual are based on the commercial HCC Model v08. These mappings can be found at the following: https://www.cms.gov/CCIIO/Resources/Regulations-and-Guidance.

| | |
|---|---|
| **Z21 Asymptomatic human immunodeficiency virus [HIV] infection status** | HCC Rx ESR COM |

Q **QPP Condition**
This icon identifies codes recognized as a quality measure for claims-based reporting under CMS's Merit-based Incentive Payment System (MIPS) Claims Single Source v6.0.

**K22.70 Barrett's esophagus without dysplasia** Q
Barrett's esophagus NOS

PDx **Z-code as First-Listed Diagnosis**
Section IV of the official guidelines states that the term "first-listed diagnosis" is used instead of principal diagnosis in the outpatient setting and represents the diagnosis that is chiefly responsible for the services provided during the encounter. This icon identifies Z codes that, in general, may be reported only as a first-listed diagnosis. According to guideline I.C.21.c.15, these are the only Z codes that are specifically meant to be utilized as a first-listed diagnosis; all other Z codes may be either first-listed or secondary diagnoses, depending upon the circumstances of the encounter, coding instructions, and guidelines.

**Note:** The codes identified with this icon may be used as a secondary diagnosis if the patient has multiple encounters on the same day and those medical records are combined.

A comprehensive list of all Z codes primarily used as first-listed diagnoses appears in appendix D, at the back of this book.

| | |
|---|---|
| **Z52.21 Bone donor, autologous** | PDx |

## Color Bars

### Manifestation Code

Codes defined as manifestation codes appear in italic type, with a blue color bar over the code description. A manifestation cannot be reported as a first-listed code; it is sequenced as a secondary diagnosis with the underlying disease code listed first.

***G32.89 Other specified degenerative disorders of nervous system in diseases classified elsewhere***
Degenerative encephalopathy in diseases classified elsewhere

**Unspecified Diagnosis**

Codes that appear with a gray color bar over the alphanumeric code identify unspecified diagnoses. These codes should be used in limited circumstances, when neither the diagnostic statement nor the documentation provides enough information to assign a more specific diagnosis code. The abbreviation NOS, "not otherwise specified," in the tabular list may be interpreted as "unspecified."

| | | |
|---|---|---|
| G03.9 | **Meningitis, unspecified**<br>Arachnoiditis (spinal) NOS | COM |

## Chapter-Level Notations

**Chapter-specific Guidelines with Coding Examples**

Each chapter begins with the Official Guidelines for Coding and Reporting specific to that chapter, where provided. Coding examples specific to outpatient care settings have been provided to illustrate the coding and/or sequencing guidance in these guidelines.

**Muscle and Tendon Table**

ICD-10-CM categorizes certain muscles and tendons in the upper and lower extremities by their action (e.g., extension or flexion) as well as their anatomical location. The Muscle/Tendon table is provided at the beginning of chapter 13 and chapter 19 to help users when code selection depends on the action of the muscle and/or tendon.

**Note:** This table is not all-inclusive, and proper code assignment should be based on the provider's documentation.

## Appendixes

The additional resources described below have been included as appendixes for this book. These resources further instruct the professional coder on the appropriate application of the ICD-10-CM code set.

**Appendix A: Valid 3-character ICD-10-CM Codes**

The user may consult this table to confirm that no further specificity, such as the use of 4th, 5th, 6th, or 7th characters or placeholders (X), is necessary. All ICD-10-CM codes that are valid at the three-character level are listed.

**Appendix B: Pharmacology List 2027**

This reference is a comprehensive but not all-inclusive list of pharmacological agents used to treat acute and/or chronic conditions. Drugs are listed in alphabetical order by their brand and/or generic names along with their drug action and indications for which they may commonly be prescribed. Some drugs have also been mapped to their appropriate Z code for long-term drug use.

**Appendix C: Z Codes for Long-Term Drug Use with Associated Drugs**

This resource correlates Z codes that are used to identify current long-term drug use with a list of drugs that are typically categorized to that class of drug.

**Note:** These tables are not all-inclusive but list some of the more commonly used drugs.

**Appendix D: Z Codes Only as Principal/First-Listed Diagnosis**

This resource provides a comprehensive list of Z codes that are primarily used as first-listed diagnoses for outpatient encounters.

**Appendix E: Centers for Medicare & Medicaid Services Hierarchical Condition Categories (CMS-HCC)**

This resource provides the framework behind the Centers for Medicare and Medicaid Services' (CMS) Medicare Advantage (MA) program, a risk-adjustment model developed as a means of compensating health care plans with large numbers of Medicare Part C beneficiaries. It includes a brief synopsis of the evolution of the program from its inception and insight into the various elements needed to predict risk, including the principles used to develop the hierarchical condition categories (HCCs), which make up one of the fundamental components of the risk-adjustment model. This appendix also outlines the audit process used to ensure the accuracy of payments made to MA plans.

**Appendix F: Centers for Medicare & Medicaid Services Quality Payment Program**

This resource provides an overview of the Medicare Access and CHIP Reauthorization Act (MACRA), which replaced Medicare's sustainable growth rate (SGR) methodology with the Quality Payment Program (QPP). It summarizes the Merit-based Incentive Payment System (MIPS) track used by those who opt to participate in traditional Medicare and not an advanced alternative payment model (APM). This includes eligibility requirements and an overview of the four performance categories that combine to make up the MIPS.

## Illustrations

This section includes illustrations of normal anatomy with ICD-10-CM-specific terminology.

# What's New for 2027



## Official Updates

A summary of changes to the official ICD-10-CM code set is provided below, identifying changes made for fiscal 2027, effective October 1, 2026, to September 30, 2027. Asterisked codes identify prior midyear changes that were made to the classification, effective April 1, 2026. All code changes were made by the agency charged with maintaining and updating the ICD-10-CM code set, the National Center for Health Statistics (NCHS), a section of the Centers for Disease Control and Prevention (CDC).

### 190 New Codes

| | | | | |
|---|---|---|---|---|
| C78.31 | C78.32 | C79.83 | D69.11 | D69.19 |
| E89.83Ø | E89.838 | F64.A | I42.ØØ | I42.Ø1 |
| I42.Ø9 | I42.81 | I42.89 | I47.22 | I49.81 |
| I49.82 | I49.89 | J34.83Ø | J34.831 | J34.832 |
| J34.833 | J34.839 | J4B | K31.B | K6A.Ø1 |
| K6A.Ø9 | K6A.8 | K74.ØA | K76.83 | LØ2.237 |
| MØ4.3 | M67.AØ1 | M67.AØ2 | M67.AØ9 | M72.2Ø |
| M72.21 | M72.22 | M86.8X11 | M86.8X12 | M86.8X19 |
| M86.8X21 | M86.8X22 | M86.8X29 | M86.8X31 | M86.8X32 |
| M86.8X39 | M86.8X41 | M86.8X42 | M86.8X49 | M86.8X51 |
| M86.8X52 | M86.8X59 | M86.8X61 | M86.8X62 | M86.8X69 |
| M86.8X71 | M86.8X72 | M86.8X79 | M86.8X8Ø | M86.8X81 |
| M86.8X89 | N99.86Ø | N99.861 | OØØ.121 | OØØ.122 |
| OØØ.129 | OØØ.131 | OØØ.132 | OØØ.139 | OØØ.31 |
| OØØ.32 | OØØ.41 | OØØ.42 | OØØ.511 | OØØ.512 |
| OØØ.519 | OØØ.521 | OØØ.522 | OØØ.529 | O31.4ØXØ |
| O31.4ØX1 | O31.4ØX2 | O31.4ØX3 | O31.4ØX4 | O31.4ØX5 |
| O31.4ØX9 | O31.41XØ | O31.41X1 | O31.41X2 | O31.41X3 |
| O31.41X4 | O31.41X5 | O31.41X9 | O31.42XØ | O31.42X1 |
| O31.42X2 | O31.42X3 | O31.42X4 | O31.42X5 | O31.42X9 |
| O31.43XØ | O31.43X1 | O31.43X2 | O31.43X3 | O31.43X4 |
| O31.43X5 | O31.43X9 | Q87.A | QA1.71 | QA1.79Ø |
| QA1.791 | QA1.792 | QA1.798 | R78.72 | T52.811A |
| T52.811D | T52.811S | T52.812A | T52.812D | T52.812S |
| T52.813A | T52.813D | T52.813S | T52.814A | T52.814D |
| T52.814S | T52.821A | T52.821D | T52.821S | T52.822A |
| T52.822D | T52.822S | T52.823A | T52.823D | T52.823S |
| T52.824A | T52.824D | T52.824S | T52.891A | T52.891D |
| T52.891S | T52.892A | T52.892D | T52.892S | T52.893A |
| T52.893D | T52.893S | T52.894A | T52.894D | T52.894S |
| T59.821A | T59.821D | T59.821S | T59.822A | T59.822D |
| T59.822S | T59.823A | T59.823D | T59.823S | T59.824A |
| T59.824D | T59.824S | T65.851A | T65.851D | T65.851S |
| T65.852A | T65.852D | T65.852S | T65.853A | T65.853D |
| T65.853S | T65.854A | T65.854D | T65.854S | Z68.18 |
| Z68.19 | Z77.Ø13 | Z77.32 | Z77.33 | Z77.4Ø |
| Z77.41 | Z77.42 | Z77.49 | Z86.17 | Z87.89Ø1 |
| Z87.89Ø2 | Z87.89Ø3 | Z87.89Ø4 | Z87.89Ø9 | Z87.893 |

### 4 Revised Codes

**Note:** Each code is listed with its revised description only.

| | |
|---|---|
| LØ2.232 | Carbuncle of back [any part, except buttock and flank] |
| LØ3.312 | Cellulitis of back [any part except buttock and flank] |
| LØ3.322 | Acute lymphangitis of back [any part except buttock and flank] |
| Z29.14 | Encounter for prophylactic rabies immune globulin |

### 15 Deleted Codes

| | |
|---|---|
| S23.42ØA | Sprain of sternoclavicular (joint) (ligament), initial encounter |
| S23.42ØD | Sprain of sternoclavicular (joint) (ligament), subsequent encounter |
| S23.42ØS | Sprain of sternoclavicular (joint) (ligament), sequela |
| T52.8X1A | Toxic effect of other organic solvents, accidental (unintentional), initial encounter |
| T52.8X1D | Toxic effect of other organic solvents, accidental (unintentional), subsequent encounter |
| T52.8X1S | Toxic effect of other organic solvents, accidental (unintentional), sequela |
| T52.8X2A | Toxic effect of other organic solvents, intentional self-harm, initial encounter |
| T52.8X2D | Toxic effect of other organic solvents, intentional self-harm, subsequent encounter |
| T52.8X2S | Toxic effect of other organic solvents, intentional self-harm, sequela |
| T52.8X3A | Toxic effect of other organic solvents, assault, initial encounter |
| T52.8X3D | Toxic effect of other organic solvents, assault, subsequent encounter |
| T52.8X3S | Toxic effect of other organic solvents, assault, sequela |
| T52.8X4A | Toxic effect of other organic solvents, undetermined, initial encounter |
| T52.8X4D | Toxic effect of other organic solvents, undetermined, subsequent encounter |
| T52.8X4S | Toxic effect of other organic solvents, undetermined, sequela |

## Proprietary Updates

The following proprietary features have also been added:

- New definitions that describe, in lay terms, a specific condition or disease process
- New coding tips that provide coding advice beyond the code classification
- Updated *AHA Coding Clinic* references through second quarter 2026

# Conversion Table of ICD-10-CM Codes

The FY 2027 (October 1, 2026–September 30, 2027) Conversion Table for new ICD-10-CM codes is provided to assist users in data retrieval. For each new code, the table shows its previously assigned code equivalent. Asterisks identify new codes added to the classification April 1, 2026.

| Code Assignment Beginning 10/1/2026 | Previous Code(s) Assignment |
|---|---|
| C78.31 | C78.39 |
| C78.32 | C78.39 |
| C79.83 | C79.89 |
| D69.11 | D69.1 |
| D69.19 | D69.1 |
| E89.83Ø | E89.89 |
| E89.838 | E89.89 |
| F64.A | F64.9 |
| I42.ØØ | I42.Ø |
| I42.Ø1 | I42.Ø |
| I42.Ø9 | I42.Ø |
| I42.81 | I42.8 |
| I42.89 | I42.8 |
| I47.22 | I47.29 |
| I49.81 | I49.8 |
| I49.82 | I49.8 |
| I49.89 | I49.8 |
| J34.83Ø | J34.89 |
| J34.831 | J34.89 |
| J34.832 | J34.89 |
| J34.833 | J34.89 |
| J34.839 | J34.89 |
| J4B | B47.- and J98.8, B37.1, B38.Ø, B38.1, B38.2, B44.1 |
| K31.B | Q4Ø.Ø |
| K6A.Ø1 | K68.19 |
| K6A.Ø9 | K68.19 and K65.1 |
| K6A.8 | K92.89, N39.8, N5Ø.89, N94.89, R68.89 |
| K74.ØA | K74.Ø1 |
| K76.83 | K9Ø.83 |
| LØ2.237 | LØ2.232 |
| MØ4.3 | MØ4.8 |
| M67.AØ1 | M72.2 |
| M67.AØ2 | M72.2 |
| M67.AØ9 | M72.2 |

| Code Assignment Beginning 10/1/2026 | Previous Code(s) Assignment |
|---|---|
| M72.2Ø | M72.2 |
| M72.21 | M72.2 |
| M72.22 | M72.2 |
| M86.8X11 | M86.8X1 |
| M86.8X12 | M86.8X1 |
| M86.8X19 | M86.8X1 |
| M86.8X21 | M86.8X2 |
| M86.8X22 | M86.8X2 |
| M86.8X29 | M86.8X2 |
| M86.8X31 | M86.8X3 |
| M86.8X32 | M86.8X3 |
| M86.8X39 | M86.8X3 |
| M86.8X41 | M86.8X4 |
| M86.8X42 | M86.8X4 |
| M86.8X49 | M86.8X4 |
| M86.8X51 | M86.8X5 |
| M86.8X52 | M86.8X5 |
| M86.8X59 | M86.8X5 |
| M86.8X61 | M86.8X6 |
| M86.8X62 | M86.8X6 |
| M86.8X69 | M86.8X6 |
| M86.8X71 | M86.8X7 |
| M86.8X72 | M86.8X7 |
| M86.8X79 | M86.8X7 |
| M86.8X8Ø | M86.8X8 |
| M86.8X81 | M86.8X8 |
| M86.8X89 | M86.8X8 |
| N99.86Ø | N99.89 |
| N99.861 | N99.89 |
| OØØ.121 | OØØ.1Ø1 |
| OØØ.122 | OØØ.1Ø2 |
| OØØ.129 | OØØ.1Ø9 |
| OØØ.131 | OØØ.111 |
| OØØ.132 | OØØ.112 |
| OØØ.139 | OØØ.119 |
| OØØ.31 | OØØ.8Ø |
| OØØ.32 | OØØ.81 |
| OØØ.41 | OØØ.8Ø |
| OØØ.42 | OØØ.81 |
| OØØ.511 | OØØ.8Ø |

| Code Assignment Beginning 10/1/2026 | Previous Code(s) Assignment |
|---|---|
| OØØ.512 | OØØ.8Ø |
| OØØ.519 | OØØ.8Ø |
| OØØ.521 | OØØ.81 |
| OØØ.522 | OØØ.81 |
| OØØ.529 | OØØ.81 |
| O31.4ØXØ | O31.8X9Ø |
| O31.4ØX1 | O31.8X91 |
| O31.4ØX2 | O31.8X92 |
| O31.4ØX3 | O31.8X93 |
| O31.4ØX4 | O31.8X94 |
| O31.4ØX5 | O31.8X95 |
| O31.4ØX9 | O31.8X99 |
| O31.41XØ | O31.8X1Ø |
| O31.41X1 | O31.8X11 |
| O31.41X2 | O31.8X12 |
| O31.41X3 | O31.8X13 |
| O31.41X4 | O31.8X14 |
| O31.41X5 | O31.8X15 |
| O31.41X9 | O31.8X19 |
| O31.42XØ | O31.8X2Ø |
| O31.42X1 | O31.8X21 |
| O31.42X2 | O31.8X22 |
| O31.42X3 | O31.8X23 |
| O31.42X4 | O31.8X24 |
| O31.42X5 | O31.8X25 |
| O31.42X9 | O31.8X29 |
| O31.43XØ | O31.8X3Ø |
| O31.43X1 | O31.8X31 |
| O31.43X2 | O31.8X32 |
| O31.43X3 | O31.8X33 |
| O31.43X4 | O31.8X34 |
| O31.43X5 | O31.8X35 |
| O31.43X9 | O31.8X39 |
| Q87.A | Q87.89 |
| QA1.71 | Z15.Ø9 |
| QA1.79Ø | Z15.Ø9 |
| QA1.791 | Z15.Ø9 |
| QA1.792 | Z15.Ø9 |
| QA1.798 | Z15.Ø9 |
| R78.72 | R78.79 |

| Code Assignment Beginning 10/1/2026 | Previous Code(s) Assignment |
|---|---|
| T52.811A | T52.8X1A |
| T52.811D | T52.8X1D |
| T52.811S | T52.8X1S |
| T52.812A | T52.8X2A |
| T52.812D | T52.8X2D |
| T52.812S | T52.8X2S |
| T52.813A | T52.8X3A |
| T52.813D | T52.8X3D |
| T52.813S | T52.8X3S |
| T52.814A | T52.8X4A |
| T52.814D | T52.8X4D |
| T52.814S | T52.8X4S |
| T52.821A | T52.8X1A |
| T52.821D | T52.8X1D |
| T52.821S | T52.8X1S |
| T52.822A | T52.8X2A |
| T52.822D | T52.8X2D |
| T52.822S | T52.8X2S |
| T52.823A | T52.8X3A |
| T52.823D | T52.8X3D |
| T52.823S | T52.8X3S |
| T52.824A | T52.8X4A |
| T52.824D | T52.8X4D |
| T52.824S | T52.8X4S |
| T52.891A | T52.8X1A |
| T52.891D | T52.8X1D |
| T52.891S | T52.8X1S |
| T52.892A | T52.8X2A |
| T52.892D | T52.8X2D |
| T52.892S | T52.8X2S |
| T52.893A | T52.8X3A |
| T52.893D | T52.8X3D |
| T52.893S | T52.8X3S |
| T52.894A | T52.8X4A |
| T52.894D | T52.8X4D |
| T52.894S | T52.8X4S |
| T59.821A | T59.891A |
| T59.821D | T59.891D |
| T59.821S | T59.891S |
| T59.822A | T59.892A |

| Code Assignment Beginning 10/1/2026 | Previous Code(s) Assignment |
|---|---|
| T59.822D | T59.892D |
| T59.822S | T59.892S |
| T59.823A | T59.893A |
| T59.823D | T59.893D |
| T59.823S | T59.893S |
| T59.824A | T59.894A |
| T59.824D | T59.894D |
| T59.824S | T59.894S |
| T65.851A | T65.891A |
| T65.851D | T65.891D |
| T65.851S | T65.891S |
| T65.852A | T65.892A |
| T65.852D | T65.892D |
| T65.852S | T65.892S |
| T65.853A | T65.893A |
| T65.853D | T65.893D |
| T65.853S | T65.893S |
| T65.854A | T65.894A |
| T65.854D | T65.894D |
| T65.854S | T65.894S |
| Z68.18 | Z68.1 |
| Z68.19 | Z68.1 |
| Z77.Ø13 | Z77.Ø18 |
| Z77.32 | Z77.39 |
| Z77.33 | Z77.39 |
| Z77.4Ø | Z77.9 |
| Z77.41 | Z77.9 |
| Z77.42 | Z77.9 |
| Z77.49 | Z77.9 |
| Z86.17 | Z86.19 |
| Z87.89Ø1 | Z87.89Ø |
| Z87.89Ø2 | Z87.89Ø |
| Z87.89Ø3 | Z87.89Ø |
| Z87.89Ø4 | Z87.89Ø |
| Z87.89Ø9 | Z87.89Ø |
| Z87.893 | Z87.898 |

# 10 Steps to Correct Coding

Follow the 10 steps below to correctly code encounters for health care services.

### Step 1: Identify the reason for the visit or encounter (i.e., a sign, symptom, diagnosis and/or condition).

The medical record documentation should accurately reflect the patient's condition, using terminology that includes specific diagnoses and symptoms or clearly states the reasons for the encounter.

Choosing the main term that best describes the reason chiefly responsible for the service provided is the most important step in coding. If symptoms are present and documented but a definitive diagnosis has not yet been determined, code the symptoms. *For outpatient cases, do not code conditions that are referred to as "rule out," "suspected," "probable," or "questionable."* Diagnoses often are not established at the time of the initial encounter/visit and may require two or more visits to be established. Code only what is documented in the available outpatient records and only to the highest degree of certainty known at the time of the patient's visit. For inpatient medical records, uncertain diagnoses may be reported if documented at the time of discharge.

### Step 2: After selecting the reason for the encounter, consult the alphabetic index.

The most critical rule is to begin code selection in the alphabetic index. Never turn first to the tabular list. The index provides cross-references, essential and nonessential modifiers, and other instructional notations that may not be found in the tabular list.

### Step 3: Locate the main term entry.

The alphabetic index lists conditions, which may be expressed as nouns or eponyms, with critical use of adjectives. Some conditions known by several names have multiple main entries. Reasons for encounters may be located under general terms such as admission, encounter, and examination. Other general terms such as history, status (post), or presence (of) can be used to locate other factors influencing health.

### Step 4: Scan subterm entries.

Scan the subterm entries, as appropriate, being sure to review continued lines and additional subterms that may appear in the next column or on the next page. Shaded vertical guidelines in the index indicate the indentation level for each subterm in relation to the main terms.

### Step 5: Pay close attention to index instructions.

- Parentheses ( ) enclose nonessential modifiers, terms that are supplementary words or explanatory information that may or may not appear in the diagnostic statement and do not affect code selection.
- Brackets [ ] enclose manifestation codes that can be used only as secondary codes to the underlying condition code immediately preceding it. If used, manifestation codes must be reported with the appropriate etiology codes.
- Default codes are listed next to the main term and represent the condition most commonly associated with the main term or the unspecified code for the main term.
- "*See*" cross-references, identified by italicized type and "code by" cross-references indicate that another term *must be referenced* to locate the correct code.
- "*See also*" cross-references, identified by italicized type, provide alternative terms that may be useful to look up but *are not mandatory*.
- "Omit code" cross-references identify instances when a code is not applicable depending on the condition being coded.
- "With" subterms are listed out of alphabetic order and identify a presumed causal relationship between the two conditions they link.
- "Due to" subterms identify a relationship between the two conditions they link.
- "NEC," abbreviation for "not elsewhere classified," follows some main terms or subterms and indicates that there is no specific code for the condition even though the medical documentation may be very specific.
- "NOS," abbreviation for "not otherwise specified," follows some main terms or subterms and is the equivalent of unspecified; NOS signifies that the information in the medical record is insufficient for assigning a more specific code.
- *Following* references help coders locate alphanumeric codes that are out of sequence in the tabular section.
- Check-additional-character symbols flag codes that require additional characters to make the code valid; the characters available to complete the code should be verified in the tabular section.

### Step 6: Choose a potential code and locate it in the tabular list.

To prevent coding errors, always use both the alphabetic index (to identify a code) and the tabular list (to verify a code), as the index does not include the important instructional notes found in the tabular list. An added benefit of using the tabular list, which groups like things together, is that while looking at one code in the list, a coder might see a more specific one that would have been missed had the coder relied solely on the alphabetic index. Additionally, many of the codes require a fourth, fifth, sixth, or seventh character to be valid, and many of these characters can be found only in the tabular list.

### Step 7: Read all instructional material in the tabular section.

The coder must follow any Includes, Excludes 1 and Excludes 2 notes, and other instructional notes, such as "Code first" and "Use additional code," listed in the tabular list for the chapter, category, subcategory, and subclassification levels of code selection that direct the coder to use a different or additional code. Any codes in the tabular range A00.0–T88.9, Z00–Z99.8, and U00–U85 may be used to identify the diagnostic reason for the encounter. The tabular list encompasses many codes describing disease and injury classifications (e.g., infectious and parasitic diseases, neoplasms, symptoms, nervous and circulatory system, etc.).

Codes that describe symptoms and signs, as opposed to definitive diagnoses, should be reported when an established diagnosis has not been made (confirmed) by the physician. Chapter 18 of the ICD-10-CM code book, "Symptoms, Signs, and Abnormal Clinical and Laboratory Findings, Not Elsewhere Classified" (codes RØØ–R99), contains many, but not all, codes for symptoms.

ICD-10-CM classifies encounters with health care providers for circumstances other than a disease or injury in chapter 21, "Factors Influencing Health Status and Contact with Health Services" (codes ZØØ–Z99). Circumstances other than a disease or injury often are recorded as chiefly responsible for the encounter.

A code is invalid if it does not include the full number of characters (greatest level of specificity) required. Codes in ICD-10-CM can contain from three to seven alphanumeric characters. A three-character code is to be used only if the category is not further subdivided into four-, five-, six-, or seven-character codes. Placeholder character X is used as part of an alphanumeric code to allow for future expansion and as a placeholder for empty characters in a code that requires a seventh character but has no fourth, fifth, or sixth character. Note that certain categories require seventh characters that apply to all codes in that category. Always check the category level for applicable seventh characters for that category.

### Step 8: Consult the official ICD-10-CM conventions and guidelines.

The *ICD-10-CM Official Guidelines for Coding and Reporting* govern the use of certain codes. These guidelines provide both general and chapter-specific coding guidance.

### Step 9: Confirm and assign the code.

Having reviewed all relevant information concerning the possible code choices, assign the code that most completely describes the condition.

Repeat steps 1 through 9 for all additional documented conditions that meet the following criteria:

- They exist at the time of the visit *AND*
- They require or affect patient care, treatment, or management

### Step 10: Sequence codes correctly.

Sequencing is the order in which the codes are listed on the claim. List first the ICD-10-CM code for the diagnosis, condition, problem, or other reason for the encounter/visit that is shown in the medical record to be chiefly responsible for the services provided. List additional codes that describe any coexisting conditions. Follow the official coding guidelines (see the guidelines, section II, "Selection of Principal Diagnosis"; section III, "Reporting Additional Diagnoses"; and section IV, "Diagnostic Coding and Reporting Guidelines for Outpatient Services") on proper sequencing of codes.

## Coding Examples

**Diagnosis: Anorexia**

**Step 1:** The reason for the encounter was the condition, anorexia.

**Step 2:** Consult the alphabetic index.

**Step 3:** Locate the main term "Anorexia."

**Step 4:** Two possible subterms are available, "hysterical" and "nervosa." Neither is documented in this instance, however, so they cannot be used in code selection.

**Step 5:** The code listed next to the main term is called the default code selection. Because the two subentries (essential modifiers) do not apply in this instance, the default code (R63.Ø) should be used.

**Step 6:** Turn to code R63.Ø in the tabular list and read all instructional notes.

**Step 7:** The Excludes 1 note at code R63.Ø indicates that anorexia nervosa and loss of appetite determined to be of nonorganic origin should be reported with a code from chapter 5. The diagnostic statement does not describe the condition as anorexia nervosa, however, and does not indicate that the anorexia is of a nonorganic origin. There is no further division of the category past the fourth-character subcategory. Therefore, code R63.Ø is at the highest level of specificity.

**Step 8:** Review of official guideline I.C.18 indicates that a symptom code is appropriate when a more definitive diagnosis is not documented.

**Step 9:** The default code, R63.Ø Anorexia, is the correct code selection.

Repeat steps 1 through 9 for any concomitant diagnoses.

**Step 10:** Since anorexia is listed as the chief reason for the health care encounter, the first-listed, or principal, diagnosis is R63.Ø. Note that this is a chapter 18 symptom code but can be assigned for both inpatient and outpatient records since the provider did not establish a more definitive diagnosis, according to sections II.A and IV.D.

**Diagnosis: Acute bronchitis**

**Step 1:** The reason for the encounter was the condition, acute bronchitis.

**Step 2:** Consult the alphabetic index.

**Step 3:** Locate the main term "Bronchitis."

**Step 4:** There is a subterm for "acute or subacute." Additional subterms are not included in the diagnostic statement.

**Step 5:** Nonessential modifiers (with bronchospasm or obstruction) are terms that do not affect code assignment. Since no other subterms indented under "acute" apply here, the code listed next to this subentry—in this case J2Ø.9—should be chosen.

**Step 6:** Turn to code J2Ø.9 in the tabular list and read all instructional notes.

**Step 7:** The Includes note under category J2Ø lists alternative terms for acute bronchitis. Note that the list is not exhaustive but is only a representative selection of diagnoses that are included in the subcategory. The Excludes 1 note refers to category J4Ø for bronchitis and tracheobronchitis NOS. There are several conditions in the Excludes 2 notes that, if applicable, can be coded in addition to this code.

Note that the codes included in J2Ø represent acute bronchitis due to various infectious organisms that could be selected if identified in the documentation. In this case, the organism was not identified and there is no further division of the category past the fourth character subcategory. Therefore, code J2Ø.9 is at the highest level of specificity.

**Step 8:** Review of official guideline I.C.10 provides no additional information affecting the code selected.

**Step 9:** Assign code J2Ø.9 Acute bronchitis, unspecified.

Repeat steps 1 through 9 for any concomitant diagnoses.

**Step 10:** In the absence of additional diagnoses that may affect sequencing, code J2Ø.9 should be sequenced as the first-listed, or principal, diagnosis.

**Diagnosis: Cerebellar ataxia in myxedema**

**Step 1:** The reason for the encounter was the condition, cerebellar ataxia.

**Step 2:** Consult the alphabetic index.

**Step 3:** Locate the main term "Ataxia."

**Step 4:** Available subterms include "cerebellar (hereditary)," with additional indented subterms for "in" and "myxedema," all essential modifiers that are included in the diagnostic statement. Two codes are provided: EØ3.9 and G13.2, the latter of which is in brackets.

**Step 5:** Note the nonessential modifier (in parentheses) after the subterm cerebellar includes the term "hereditary." Because it is in parentheses, this term is not required in the diagnostic statement for this subentry to apply. The brackets around G13.2 identify this code as a manifestation of the condition described by code EØ3.9 and indicate that the two must be reported together and sequencing rules apply.

**Step 6:** Locate codes EØ3.9 and G13.2 in the tabular list, and read all instructional notes.

**Step 7:** For code EØ3.9, there are no instructional notes in the tabular list at the category EØ3 or code level that indicate that this condition should be coded elsewhere in the classification or that additional codes are required. Without further information from the diagnostic statement, myxedema, not otherwise specified (NOS), is appropriately reported with code EØ3.9 Hypothyroidism, unspecified, according to the inclusion term at this code.

Code G13.2 in the tabular list has an instructional note to "Code first underlying disease," which includes conditions found in category EØ3.-. Based on this note, codes EØ3.9 and G13.2 are to be coded together, with G13.2 listed only as a secondary diagnosis. This correlates with what the alphabetic index indicated. As there is no further division of codes in category G13 beyond the fourth character, G13.2 is at the highest level of specificity.

**Step 8:** Although there are some general conventions, such as how to interpret brackets in the alphabetic index, no chapter-specific guidelines apply to this coding scenario.

**Step 9:** Assign codes EØ3.9 Hypothyroidism, unspecified, and G13.2 Systemic atrophy primarily affecting the central nervous system in myxedema.

Repeat steps 1 through 9 for any concomitant diagnoses.

**Step 10:** Based on the alphabetic index and tabular instructional notations, code EØ3.9 should be sequenced as the first-listed, or principal, diagnosis followed by G13.2 as a secondary diagnosis.

**Diagnosis: Decubitus ulcer of right elbow with skin loss and necrosis of subcutaneous tissue**

**Step 1:** The reason for the encounter was the condition, decubitus ulcer.

**Step 2:** Consult the alphabetic index.

**Step 3:** Locate the main term "Ulcer."

**Step 4:** For the subterm "decubitus," there is no code provided or additional subterms indented, but a cross-reference is listed.

**Step 5:** The italicized cross-reference instructs the coder to "*see* Ulcer, pressure, by site."

Repeat steps 3 through 5 for the cross-reference:

**Step 3:** Locate the main term "Ulcer."

**Step 4:** Review the subentries for the subterm "pressure." The next level of indent lists either the site of the ulcer or the specific stage of the ulcer (stage 1–4, unstageable, and unspecified stages). The diagnostic statement provides the site, right elbow, and the extent of tissue damage (skin loss and necrosis of subcutaneous tissue) but does not specifically state that the ulcer is stage 1, stage 2, etc. Nonessential modifiers (in parentheses) at each stage include a description of the typical extent of damage at each stage. For example, stage 1 describes "pre-ulcer skin changes limited to persistent focal edema." Based on the documentation in the record, the coder can correlate the documentation to the nonessential modifiers and choose the specific stage from the index. The coder can also go directly to the body site, choosing the stage of the ulcer after reviewing the code options and instructional notations in the tabular list.

The diagnostic statement indicates that the extent of the damage to the elbow includes skin loss and necrosis of subcutaneous tissue, coinciding with the nonessential modifier next to the subentry "stage 3." The body site of elbow (L89.Ø-) is listed as another level of indent with other body sites.

**Step 5:** Note that code L89.Ø is followed by a dash and an additional-character-required icon, which indicate that more characters are needed to complete the code. From here, the tabular listing for L89.Ø- can be consulted.

**Step 6:** Locate code L89.Ø- in the tabular list and read all instructional notes.

**Step 7:** The tabular listing at category L89 has an Includes note for "decubitus ulcer," which confirms that category L89 is the appropriate category to represent what is documented in the diagnostic statement.

Several Excludes 2 notes are also listed at the category level. Excludes 2 notes represent conditions that can occur concomitantly with the decubitus ulcer and can be coded in addition to code L89, if supported by the documentation.

The subcategory codes under L89.Ø indicate that the fifth character describes laterality. Locate the right elbow at subcategory L89.Ø1. See that an additional sixth character to specify the stage of the ulcer is now needed to complete the code. The stage can be determined either by the specific documentation of the stage (e.g., stage 1, stage 2) or, in this case, a description that matches one of the inclusion terms that follow each stage code. For example, the diagnostic description in this case of "skin loss and necrosis of the subcutaneous tissue" matches the inclusion term under L89.Ø13 Pressure ulcer of right elbow, stage 3. No additional characters are required because code L89.Ø13 is at its highest level of specificity.

**Step 8:** The official guidelines contain quite a bit of information relating to pressure ulcers in chapter-specific guideline I.C.12 as well as information in general guideline I.B.14. These and any other pertinent guidelines should be reviewed to ensure appropriate code assignment.

**Step 9:** Assign code L89.Ø13 Pressure ulcer of right elbow, stage 3.

Repeat steps 1 through 9 for any concomitant diagnoses.

**Step 10:** Since the decubitus ulcer is listed as the chief reason for the health care encounter, the first-listed, or principal, diagnosis is L89.Ø13. However, according to the code first instructional note at the L89 category level, gangrene (I96) would be sequenced before the pressure ulcer if it were documented.

**Diagnosis: Emergency department visit for bimalleolar fracture of the right ankle due to trauma**

**Step 1:** The reason for the encounter was the condition, bimalleolar fracture.

**Step 2:** Consult the alphabetic index.

**Step 3:** Locate the main term "Fracture." Note that many main terms represent fractures: "Fracture, burst," "Fracture, chronic," "Fracture, insufficiency," "Fracture, nontraumatic NEC," "Fracture, pathological," and "Fracture, traumatic." Since the diagnostic statement specifically states that this fracture was the result of trauma, the main term "Fracture, traumatic" should be used.

**Step 4:** Subterms that should be referenced are "ankle" and "bimalleolar (displaced)," which lists code S82.84-.

**Step 5:** A nonessential modifier (in parentheses) next to the term bimalleolar for "displaced" indicates that S82.84- is the default category unless the fracture is specifically identified as "nondisplaced."

Note that code S82.84- is followed by a dash and an additional-character icon, both of which indicate that more characters are required. From here, the tabular list can be consulted.

**Step 6:** Locate code S82.84- in the tabular list and read all instructional notes.

**Step 7:** The instructional notes at category S82 indicate that fractures not specified as displaced or nondisplaced default to displaced and that fractures not designated as open or closed default to closed. Additional instructional notes can be found at the category level but none pertain to the current scenario.

Read through the subcategory codes under S82.84, and note that the sixth character specifies displaced or nondisplaced and laterality. Based on the index nonessential modifier (displaced) and the code note at category S82, code selection should identify a displaced fracture of the right side. A displaced bimalleolar fracture of the right lower leg is coded to S82.841.

To complete the code, a seventh character must be assigned to identify the type of encounter (initial, subsequent, or sequela) and whether the fracture is open or closed. Most of the codes in category S82 require a seventh character represented in the list at the category level. However, it is important to note that some subcategories have their own specific set of seventh characters. In this instance, subcategory S82.84- does not have a unique set of seventh characters and the list provided at the category level should be used. Without documentation of the fracture being open, the tabular notation indicates that the default is closed. Character A, representing "initial encounter for closed fracture," listed in the box at the category level is the most appropriate option.

**Step 8:** Assign code S82.841A Displaced bimalleolar fracture of right lower leg, initial encounter for closed fracture.

**Step 9:** Review chapter-specific guideline I.C.19. and any other official conventions or guidelines to ensure appropriate code assignment.

Repeat steps 1 through 9 for any concomitant diagnoses.

**Step 10:** Additional codes can be applied to relate the specific cause of the injury, the place of occurrence, the activity of the patient at the time of the injury, and the patient's status, when this information is available in the record. However, coding this information is voluntary and reporting requirements depend on state mandates and/or facility-specific reporting requirements. If assigned, the external cause codes should be reported as secondary diagnoses only with the injury (fracture) sequenced first. Most codes in chapter 20, "External Causes of Morbidity," require a seventh character to identify the type of encounter. The seventh character assigned to an external cause code should match the seventh character of the code assigned for the associated injury or condition for the encounter.

# 2027 ICD-10-CM Official Guidelines for Coding and Reporting



Narrative changes effective October 1, 2026 appear in **bold** text

Narrative changes effective April 1, 2026 appear in shaded text

Items underlined have been moved within the guidelines since the April 2026, FY 2026 version

*Italics* are used to indicate revisions to heading changes

The Centers for Medicare and Medicaid Services (CMS) and the National Center for Health Statistics (NCHS), two departments within the U.S. Federal Government's Department of Health and Human Services (DHHS) provide the following guidelines for coding and reporting using the International Classification of Diseases, 10th Revision, Clinical Modification (ICD-10-CM). These guidelines should be used as a companion document to the official version of the ICD-10-CM as published on the NCHS website. The ICD-10-CM is a morbidity classification published by the United States for classifying diagnoses and reason for visits in all health care settings. The ICD-10-CM is based on the ICD-10, the statistical classification of disease published by the World Health Organization (WHO).

These guidelines have been approved by the four organizations that make up the Cooperating Parties for the ICD-10-CM: the American Hospital Association (AHA), the American Health Information Management Association (AHIMA), CMS, and NCHS.

These guidelines are a set of rules that have been developed to accompany and complement the official conventions and instructions provided within the ICD-10-CM itself. The instructions and conventions of the classification take precedence over guidelines. These guidelines are based on the coding and sequencing instructions in the Tabular List and Alphabetic Index of ICD-10-CM, but provide additional instruction. Adherence to these guidelines when assigning ICD-10-CM diagnosis codes is required under the Health Insurance Portability and Accountability Act (HIPAA). The diagnosis codes (Tabular List and Alphabetic Index) have been adopted under HIPAA for all healthcare settings. A joint effort between the healthcare provider and the coder is essential to achieve complete and accurate documentation, code assignment, and reporting of diagnoses and procedures. These guidelines have been developed to assist both the healthcare provider and the coder in identifying those diagnoses that are to be reported. The importance of consistent, complete documentation in the medical record cannot be overemphasized. Without such documentation accurate coding cannot be achieved. The entire record should be reviewed to determine the specific reason for the encounter and the conditions treated.

The term encounter is used for all settings, including hospital admissions. In the context of these guidelines, the term provider is used throughout the guidelines to mean physician or any qualified health care practitioner who is legally accountable for establishing the patient's diagnosis. Only this set of guidelines, approved by the Cooperating Parties, is official.

The guidelines are organized into sections. Section I includes the structure and conventions of the classification and general guidelines that apply to the entire classification, and chapter-specific guidelines that correspond to the chapters as they are arranged in the classification. Section II includes guidelines for selection of principal diagnosis for non-outpatient settings. Section III includes guidelines for reporting additional diagnoses in non-outpatient settings. Section IV is for outpatient coding and reporting. It is necessary to review all sections of the guidelines to fully understand all of the rules and instructions needed to code properly.

# Section I. Conventions, general coding guidelines and chapter specific guidelines

The conventions, general guidelines and chapter-specific guidelines are applicable to all health care settings unless otherwise indicated. The conventions and instructions of the classification take precedence over guidelines.

## A. Conventions for the ICD-10-CM

The conventions for the ICD-10-CM are the general rules for use of the classification independent of the guidelines. These conventions are incorporated within the Alphabetic Index and Tabular List of the ICD-10-CM as instructional notes.

1. **The Alphabetic Index and Tabular List**
   The ICD-10-CM is divided into the Alphabetic Index, an alphabetical list of terms and their corresponding code, and the Tabular List, a structured list of codes divided into chapters based on body system or condition. The Alphabetic Index consists of the following parts: the Index of Diseases and Injury, the Index of External Causes of Injury, the Table of Neoplasms and the Table of Drugs and Chemicals.

   *See Section I.C.2. Neoplasms*

   *See Section I.C.19. Adverse effects, poisoning, underdosing and toxic effects*

2. **Format and Structure:**
   The ICD-10-CM Tabular List contains categories, subcategories and codes. Characters for categories, subcategories and codes may be either a letter or a number. All categories are 3 characters. A three-character category that has no further subdivision is equivalent to a code. Subcategories are either 4 or 5 characters. Codes may be 3, 4, 5, 6 or 7 characters. That is, each level of subdivision after a category is a subcategory. The final level of subdivision is a code. Codes that have applicable 7th characters are still referred to as codes, not subcategories. A code that has an applicable 7th character is considered invalid without the 7th character.

   The ICD-10-CM uses an indented format for ease in reference.

3. **Use of codes for reporting purposes**
   For reporting purposes only codes are permissible, not categories or subcategories, and any applicable 7th character is required.

4. **Placeholder character**
   The ICD-10-CM utilizes a placeholder character "X". The "X" is used as a placeholder at certain codes to allow for future expansion. An example of this is at the poisoning, adverse effect and underdosing codes, categories T36-T5Ø. Where a placeholder exists, the X must be used in order for the code to be considered a valid code.

5. **7th Characters**
   Certain ICD-10-CM categories have applicable 7th characters. The applicable 7th character is required for all codes within the category, or as the notes in the Tabular List instruct. The 7th character must always be the 7th character in the data field. If a code that requires a 7th character is not 6 characters, a placeholder X must be used to fill in the empty characters.

6. **Abbreviations**
   a. **Alphabetic Index abbreviations**
      NEC "Not elsewhere classifiable"

      This abbreviation in the Alphabetic Index represents "other specified." When a specific code is not available for a condition, the Alphabetic Index directs the coder to the "other specified" code in the Tabular List.

      NOS "Not otherwise specified"

      This abbreviation is the equivalent of unspecified.

   b. **Tabular List abbreviations**
      NEC "Not elsewhere classifiable"

      This abbreviation in the Tabular List represents "other specified". When a specific code is not available for a condition, the Tabular List includes an NEC entry under a code to identify the code as the "other specified" code.

      NOS "Not otherwise specified"

      This abbreviation is the equivalent of unspecified.

7. **Punctuation**
   [ ] Brackets are used in the Tabular List to enclose synonyms, alternative wording or explanatory phrases. Brackets are used in the Alphabetic Index to identify manifestation codes.

   ( ) Parentheses are used in both the Alphabetic Index and Tabular List to enclose supplementary words that may be present or absent in the statement of a disease or procedure without affecting the code number to which it is assigned. The terms within the parentheses are referred to as nonessential modifiers. The nonessential modifiers in the Alphabetic Index to Diseases apply to subterms following a main term except when a nonessential modifier and a subentry are mutually exclusive, the subentry takes precedence. For example, in the ICD-10-CM Alphabetic Index under the main term Enteritis, "acute" is a nonessential modifier and "chronic" is a subentry. In this case, the nonessential modifier "acute" does not apply to the subentry "chronic".

   : Colons are used in the Tabular List after an incomplete term which needs one or more of the modifiers following the colon to make it assignable to a given category.

   , Commas are used in the Alphabetic Index and have different meanings based on the context of the Index entry, including alternate verbiage, modifier (essential and nonessential), or alternative for "and/or."

8. **Use of "and".**
   *See Section I.A.14. Use of the term "And"*

9. **Other and Unspecified codes**
   a. **"Other" codes**
      Codes titled "other" or "other specified" are for use when the information in the medical record provides detail for which a specific code does not exist. Alphabetic Index entries with NEC in the line designate "other" codes in the Tabular List. These Alphabetic Index entries represent specific disease entities for which no specific code exists, so the term is included within an "other" code.

   b. **"Unspecified" codes**
      Codes titled "unspecified" are for use when the information in the medical record is insufficient to assign a more specific code. For those categories for 7

      which an unspecified code is not provided, the "other specified" code may represent both other and unspecified.

      *See Section I.B.18. Use of Signs/Symptom/Unspecified Codes*

10. **Includes Notes**
    This note appears immediately under a three-character code title to further define, or give examples of, the content of the category.

11. **Inclusion terms**
    List of terms is included under some codes. These terms are the conditions for which that code is to be used. The terms may be synonyms of the code title, or, in the case of "other specified" codes, the terms are a list of the various conditions assigned to that code. The inclusion terms are not necessarily exhaustive. Additional terms found only in the Alphabetic Index may also be assigned to a code.

12. **Excludes Notes**
    The ICD-10-CM has two types of excludes notes. Each type of note has a different definition for use, but they are all similar in that they indicate that codes excluded from each other are independent of each other.

    a. **Excludes1**
       A type 1 Excludes note is a pure excludes note. It means "NOT CODED HERE!" An Excludes1 note indicates that the code excluded should never be used at the same time as the code above the Excludes1 note. An Excludes1 is used when two conditions cannot occur together, such as a congenital form versus an acquired form of the same condition.

       An exception to the Excludes1 definition is the circumstance when the two conditions are unrelated to each other. If it is not clear whether the two conditions involving an Excludes1 note are related or not, query the provider. For example, code F45.8, Other somatoform disorders, has an Excludes1 note for "sleep related teeth grinding (G47.63)," because "teeth grinding" is an inclusion term under F45.8. Only one of these two codes should be assigned for teeth grinding. However psychogenic dysmenorrhea is also an inclusion term under F45.8, and a patient could have both this condition and sleep related teeth grinding. In this case, the two conditions are clearly unrelated to each other, and so it would be appropriate to report F45.8 and G47.63 together.

    b. **Excludes2**
       A type 2 Excludes note represents "Not included here." An excludes2 note indicates that the condition excluded is not part of the condition represented by the code, but a patient may have both conditions at the same time. When an Excludes2 note appears under a code, it is acceptable to use both the code and the excluded code together, when appropriate.

13. **Etiology/manifestation convention ("code first", "use additional code" and "in diseases classified elsewhere" notes)**
    Certain conditions have both an underlying etiology and multiple body system manifestations due to the underlying etiology. For such conditions, the ICD-10-CM has a coding convention that requires the underlying condition be sequenced first, if applicable, followed by the manifestation. Wherever such a combination exists, there is a "use additional code" note at the etiology code, and a "code first" note at the manifestation code. These instructional notes indicate the proper sequencing order of the codes, etiology followed by manifestation.

    In most cases the manifestation codes will have in the code title, "in diseases classified elsewhere." Codes with this title are a component of the etiology/manifestation convention. The code title indicates that it is a manifestation code. "In diseases classified elsewhere" codes are never permitted to be used as first listed or principal diagnosis codes. They must be used in conjunction with an underlying condition code and they must be listed following the underlying condition. See category FØ2, Dementia in other diseases classified elsewhere, for an example of this convention.

    There are manifestation codes that do not have "in diseases classified elsewhere" in the title. For such codes, there is a "use additional code" note at the etiology code and a "code first" note at the manifestation code, and the rules for sequencing apply.

In addition to the notes in the Tabular List, these conditions also have a specific Alphabetic Index entry structure. In the Alphabetic Index both conditions are listed together with the etiology code first followed by the manifestation codes in brackets. The code in brackets is always to be sequenced second.

An example of the etiology/manifestation convention is dementia with Parkinson's disease. In the Alphabetic Index, a code from category G20 is listed first, followed by code FØ2.8Ø or FØ2.81- in brackets. A code from category G2Ø-represents the underlying etiology, Parkinson's disease, and must be sequenced first, whereas codes FØ2.8Ø and FØ2.81- represent the manifestation of dementia in diseases classified elsewhere, with or without behavioral disturbance.

"Code first" and "Use additional code" notes are also used as sequencing rules in the classification for certain codes that are not part of an etiology/ manifestation combination.

*See Section I.B.7. Multiple coding for a single condition.*

**14. "And"**
The word "and" should be interpreted to mean either "and" or "or" when it appears in a title.

For example, cases of "tuberculosis of bones", "tuberculosis of joints" and "tuberculosis of bones and joints" are classified to subcategory A18.Ø, Tuberculosis of bones and joints.

**15. "With"**
The word "with" or "in" should be interpreted to mean "associated with" or "due to" when it appears in a code title, the Alphabetic Index (either under a main term or subterm), or an instructional note in the Tabular List. The classification presumes a causal relationship between the two conditions linked by these terms in the Alphabetic Index or Tabular List. These conditions should be coded as related even in the absence of provider documentation explicitly linking them, unless the documentation clearly states the conditions are unrelated or when another guideline exists that specifically requires a documented linkage between two conditions (e.g., sepsis guideline for "acute organ dysfunction that is not clearly associated with the sepsis").

For conditions not specifically linked by these relational terms in the classification or when a guideline requires that a linkage between two conditions be explicitly documented, provider documentation must link the conditions in order to code them as related.

The word "with" in the Alphabetic Index is sequenced immediately following the main term or subterm, not in alphabetical order.

**16. "See" and "See Also"**
The "see" instruction following a main term in the Alphabetic Index indicates that another term should be referenced. It is necessary to go to the main term referenced with the "see" note to locate the correct code.

A "see also" instruction following a main term in the Alphabetic Index instructs that there is another main term that may also be referenced that may provide additional Alphabetic Index entries that may be useful. It is not necessary to follow the "see also" note when the original main term provides the necessary code.

**17. "Code also" note**
A "code also" note instructs that two codes may be required to fully describe a condition, but this note does not provide sequencing direction. The sequencing depends on the circumstances of the encounter.

**18. Default codes**
A code listed next to a main term in the ICD-10-CM Alphabetic Index is referred to as a default code. The default code represents that condition that is most commonly associated with the main term or is the unspecified code for the condition. If a condition is documented in a medical record (for example, appendicitis) without any additional information, such as acute or chronic, the default code should be assigned.

**19. Code assignment and Clinical Criteria**
The assignment of a diagnosis code is based on the provider's diagnostic statement that the condition exists. The provider's statement that the patient has a particular condition is sufficient. Code assignment is not based on clinical criteria used by the provider to establish the diagnosis. If there is conflicting medical record documentation, query the provider.

# B. General Coding Guidelines

**1. Locating a code in the ICD-10-CM**
To select a code in the classification that corresponds to a diagnosis or reason for visit documented in a medical record, first locate the term in the Alphabetic Index, and then verify the code in the Tabular List. Read and be guided by instructional notations that appear in both the Alphabetic Index and the Tabular List.

It is essential to use both the Alphabetic Index and Tabular List when locating and assigning a code. The Alphabetic Index does not always provide the full code. Selection of the full code, including laterality and any applicable 7th character can only be done in the Tabular List. A dash (-) at the end of an Alphabetic Index entry indicates that additional characters are required. Even if a dash is not included at the Alphabetic Index entry, it is necessary to refer to the Tabular List to verify that no 7th character is required.

**2. Level of Detail in Coding**
Diagnosis codes are to be used and reported at their highest number of characters available and to the highest level of specificity documented in the medical record.

ICD-10-CM diagnosis codes are composed of codes with 3, 4, 5, 6 or 7 characters. Codes with three characters are included in ICD-10-CM as the heading of a category of codes that may be further subdivided by the use of fourth and/or fifth characters and/or sixth characters, which provide greater detail.

A three-character code is to be used only if it is not further subdivided. A code is invalid if it has not been coded to the full number of characters required for that code, including the 7th character, if applicable.

**3. Code or codes from AØØ.Ø through T88.9, ZØØ-Z99.8, UØØ-U85**
The appropriate code or codes from AØØ.Ø through T88.9, ZØØ-Z99.8, and UØØ-U85 must be used to identify diagnoses, symptoms, conditions, problems, complaints or other reason(s) for the encounter/visit.

**4. Signs and symptoms**
Codes that describe symptoms and signs, as opposed to diagnoses, are acceptable for reporting purposes when a related definitive diagnosis has not been established (confirmed) by the provider. Chapter 18 of ICD-10-CM, Symptoms, Signs, and Abnormal Clinical and Laboratory Findings, Not Elsewhere Classified (codes RØØ.Ø-R99) contains many, but not all, codes for symptoms.

*See Section I.B.18. Use of Signs/Symptom/Unspecified Codes*

**5. Conditions that are an integral part of a disease process**
Signs and symptoms that are associated routinely with a disease process should not be assigned as additional codes, unless otherwise instructed by the classification.

**6. Conditions that are not an integral part of a disease process**
Additional signs and symptoms that may not be associated routinely with a disease process should be coded when present.

**7. Multiple coding for a single condition**
In addition to the etiology/manifestation convention that requires two codes to fully describe a single condition that affects multiple body systems, there are other single conditions that also require more than one code. "Use additional code" notes are found in the Tabular List at codes that are not part of an etiology/manifestation pair where a secondary code is useful to fully describe a condition. The sequencing rule is the same as the etiology/manifestation pair, "use additional code" indicates that a secondary code should be added, if known.

For example, for bacterial infections that are not included in chapter 1, a secondary code from category B95, Streptococcus, Staphylococcus, and Enterococcus, as the cause of diseases classified elsewhere, or B96, Other bacterial agents as the cause of diseases classified elsewhere, may be required to identify the bacterial organism causing the infection. A "use additional code" note will normally be found at the infectious disease code, indicating a need for the organism code to be added as a secondary code.

"Code first" notes are also under certain codes that are not specifically manifestation codes but may be due to an underlying cause. When there is a "code first" note and an underlying condition is present, the underlying condition should be sequenced first, if known.

"Code, if applicable, any causal condition first" notes indicate that this code may be assigned as a principal diagnosis when the causal condition is unknown or not applicable. If a causal condition is known, then the code for that condition should be sequenced as the principal or first-listed diagnosis.

Multiple codes may be needed for sequela, complication codes and obstetric codes to more fully describe a condition. See the specific guidelines for these conditions for further instruction.

**8. Acute and Chronic Conditions**
If the same condition is described as both acute (subacute) and chronic, and separate subentries exist in the Alphabetic Index at the same indentation level, code both and sequence the acute (subacute) code first.

**9. Combination Code**
A combination code is a single code used to classify:

Two diagnoses, or

A diagnosis with an associated secondary process (manifestation)

A diagnosis with an associated complication

Combination codes are identified by referring to subterm entries in the Alphabetic Index and by reading the inclusion and exclusion notes in the Tabular List.

Assign only the combination code when that code fully identifies the diagnostic conditions involved or when the Alphabetic Index so directs. Multiple coding should not be used when the classification provides a combination code that clearly identifies all of the elements documented in the diagnosis. When the combination code lacks necessary specificity in describing the manifestation or complication, an additional code should be used as a secondary code.

**10. Sequela (Late Effects)**
A sequela is the residual effect (condition produced) after the acute phase of an illness or injury has terminated. There is no time limit on when a sequela code can be used. The residual may be apparent early, such as in cerebral infarction, or it may occur months or years later, such as that due to a previous injury. Examples of sequela include: scar formation resulting from a burn, deviated septum due to a nasal fracture, and infertility due to tubal occlusion from old tuberculosis. Coding of sequela generally requires two codes sequenced in the following order: the condition or nature of the sequela is sequenced first. The sequela code is sequenced second.

An exception to the above guidelines are those instances where the code for the sequela is followed by a manifestation code identified in the Tabular List and title, or the sequela code has been expanded (at the fourth, fifth or sixth character levels) to include the manifestation(s). The code for the acute phase of an illness or injury that led to the sequela is never used with a code for the late effect.

*See Section I.C.9. Sequelae of cerebrovascular disease*

*See Section I.C.15. Sequelae of complication of pregnancy, childbirth and the puerperium*

*See Section I.C.19. Application of 7th characters for Chapter 19*

**11. Impending or Threatened Condition**

Code any condition described at the time of discharge as "impending" or "threatened" as follows:

If it did occur, code as confirmed diagnosis.

If it did not occur, reference the Alphabetic Index to determine if the condition has a subentry term for "impending" or "threatened" and also reference main term entries for "Impending" and for "Threatened."

If the subterms are listed, assign the given code.

If the subterms are not listed, code the existing underlying condition(s) and not the condition described as impending or threatened.

**12. Reporting Same Diagnosis Code More than Once**

Each unique ICD-10-CM diagnosis code may be reported only once for an encounter. This applies to bilateral conditions when there are no distinct codes identifying laterality or two different conditions classified to the same ICD-10-CM diagnosis code.

**13. Laterality**

Some ICD-10-CM codes indicate laterality, specifying whether the condition occurs on the left, right or is bilateral. If no bilateral code is provided and the condition is bilateral, assign separate codes for both the left and right side. If the side is not identified in the medical record, assign the code for the unspecified side.

When a patient has a bilateral condition and each side is treated during separate encounters, assign the "bilateral" code (as the condition still exists on both sides), including for the encounter to treat the first side. For the second encounter for treatment after one side has previously been treated and the condition no longer exists on that side, assign the appropriate unilateral code for the side where the condition still exists (e.g., cataract surgery performed on each eye in separate encounters). The bilateral code would not be assigned for the subsequent encounter, as the patient no longer has the condition in the previously-treated site. If the treatment on the first side did not completely resolve the condition, then the bilateral code would still be appropriate.

When laterality is not documented by the patient's provider, code assignment for the affected side may be based on medical record documentation from other clinicians. If there is conflicting medical record documentation regarding the affected side, the patient's provider should be queried for clarification. Codes for "unspecified" side should rarely be used, such as when the documentation in the record is insufficient to determine the affected side and it is not possible to obtain clarification.

**14. Documentation by Clinicians Other than the Patient's Provider**

Code assignment is based on the documentation by the patient's provider (i.e., physician or other qualified healthcare practitioner legally accountable for establishing the patient's diagnosis). There are a few exceptions when code assignment may be based on medical record documentation from clinicians who are not the patient's provider (i.e., physician or other qualified healthcare practitioner legally accountable for establishing the patient's diagnosis). In this context, "clinicians" other than the patient's provider refer to healthcare professionals permitted, based on regulatory or accreditation requirements or internal hospital policies, to document in a patient's official medical record.

These exceptions include codes for:

- Body Mass Index (BMI)
- Depth of non-pressure chronic ulcers
- Pressure ulcer stage
- Coma scale
- NIH stroke scale (NIHSS)
- Social determinants of health (SDOH) classified to Chapter 21
- Laterality
- Blood alcohol level
- Underimmunization status
- Firearm injury intent

This information is typically, or may be, documented by other clinicians involved in the care of the patient (e.g., a dietitian often documents the BMI, a nurse often documents the pressure ulcer stages, and an emergency medical technician often documents the coma scale). However, the associated diagnosis (such as overweight, obesity, acute stroke, pressure ulcer, or a condition classifiable to category F1Ø, Alcohol related disorders) must be documented by the patient's provider. If there is conflicting medical record documentation, either from the same clinician or different clinicians, the patient's provider should be queried for clarification.

The BMI, coma scale, NIHSS, blood alcohol level codes, codes for social determinants of health and underimmunization status should only be reported as secondary diagnoses.

*See Section I.C.21.c.17. for additional information regarding coding social determinants of health.*

**15. Syndromes**

Follow the Alphabetic Index guidance when coding syndromes. In the absence of Alphabetic Index guidance, assign codes for the documented manifestations of the syndrome. Additional codes for manifestations that are not an integral part of the disease process may also be assigned when the condition does not have a unique code.

**16. Documentation of Complications of Care**

Code assignment is based on the provider's documentation of the relationship between the condition and the care or procedure, unless otherwise instructed by the classification. The guideline extends to any complications of care, regardless of the chapter the code is located in. It is important to note that not all conditions that occur during or following medical care or surgery are classified as complications. There must be a cause-and-effect relationship between the care provided and the condition, and the documentation must support that the condition is clinically significant. It is not necessary for the provider to explicitly document the term "complication." For example, if the condition alters the course of the surgery as documented in the operative report, then it would be appropriate to report a complication code. Query the provider for clarification if the documentation is not clear as to the relationship between the condition and the care or procedure.

**17. Borderline Diagnosis**

If the provider documents a "borderline" diagnosis at the time of discharge, the diagnosis is coded as confirmed, unless the classification provides a specific entry (e.g., borderline diabetes). If a borderline condition has a specific index entry in ICD-10-CM, it should be coded as such. Since borderline conditions are not uncertain diagnoses, no distinction is made between the care setting (inpatient versus outpatient). Whenever the documentation is unclear regarding a borderline condition, coders are encouraged to query for clarification.

**18. Use of Sign/Symptom/Unspecified Codes**

Sign/symptom and "unspecified" codes have acceptable, even necessary, uses. While specific diagnosis codes should be reported when they are supported by the available medical record documentation and clinical knowledge of the patient's health condition, there are instances when signs/symptoms or unspecified codes are the best choices for accurately reflecting the healthcare encounter. Each healthcare encounter should be coded to the level of certainty known for that encounter.

As stated in the introductory section of these official coding guidelines, a joint effort between the healthcare provider and the coder is essential to achieve complete and accurate documentation, code assignment, and reporting of diagnoses and procedures. The importance of consistent, complete documentation in the medical record cannot be overemphasized. Without such documentation accurate coding cannot be achieved. The entire record should be reviewed to determine the specific reason for the encounter and the conditions treated.

If a definitive diagnosis has not been established by the end of the encounter, it is appropriate to report codes for sign(s) and/or symptom(s) in lieu of a definitive diagnosis. When sufficient clinical information isn't known or available about a particular health condition to assign a more specific code, it is acceptable to report the appropriate "unspecified" code (e.g., a diagnosis of pneumonia has been determined, but not the specific type). Unspecified codes should be reported when they are the codes that most accurately reflect what is known about the patient's condition at the time of that particular encounter. It would be inappropriate to select a specific code that is not supported by the medical record documentation or conduct medically unnecessary diagnostic testing in order to determine a more specific code.

**19. Coding for Healthcare Encounters in Hurricane Aftermath**

**a. Use of External Cause of Morbidity Codes**

An external cause of morbidity code should be assigned to identify the cause of the injury(ies) incurred as a result of the hurricane. The use of external cause of morbidity codes is supplemental to the application of ICD-10-CM codes. External cause of morbidity codes are never to be recorded as a principal diagnosis (first-listed in non-inpatient settings). The appropriate injury code should be sequenced before any external cause codes. The external cause of morbidity codes capture how the injury or health condition happened (cause), the intent (unintentional or accidental; or intentional, such as suicide or assault), the place where the event occurred, the activity of the patient at the time of the event, and the person's status (e.g., civilian, military). They should not be assigned for encounters to treat hurricane victims' medical conditions when no injury, adverse effect or poisoning is involved. External cause of morbidity codes should be assigned for each encounter for care and treatment of the injury. External cause of morbidity codes may be assigned in all health care settings. For the purpose of capturing complete and accurate ICD-10-CM data in the aftermath of the hurricane, a healthcare setting should be considered as any location where medical care is provided by licensed healthcare professionals.

**b. Sequencing of External Causes of Morbidity Codes**

Codes for cataclysmic events, such as a hurricane, take priority over all other external cause codes except child and adult abuse and terrorism and should be sequenced before other external cause of injury codes. Assign as many external cause of morbidity codes as necessary to fully explain each cause. For example, if an injury occurs as a result of a building collapse during the hurricane, external cause codes for both the hurricane and the building collapse should be assigned, with the external causes code for hurricane being sequenced as the first external cause code. For injuries incurred as a direct result of the hurricane, assign the appropriate code(s) for the injuries, followed by the code X37.Ø-, Hurricane (with the appropriate 7th character), and any other applicable external cause of injury codes. Code X37.Ø- also should be assigned when an injury is incurred as a result of flooding caused by a levee breaking related to the hurricane. Code X38.-, Flood (with the appropriate 7th character), should be assigned when an injury is from flooding resulting directly from the storm. Code X36.Ø.-, Collapse of dam or man-made structure, should not be assigned when the cause of the collapse is due to the hurricane. Use of code X36.Ø- is limited to collapses of man-made structures due to earth surface movements, not due to storm surges directly from a hurricane.

**c. Other External Causes of Morbidity Code Issues**

For injuries that are not a direct result of the hurricane, such as an evacuee that has incurred an injury as a result of a motor vehicle accident, assign the appropriate external cause of morbidity code(s) to describe the cause of the injury, but do not assign code X37.Ø-, Hurricane. If it is not clear whether the injury was a direct result of the hurricane, assume the injury is due to the hurricane and assign code X37.Ø-, Hurricane, as well as any other applicable external cause of morbidity codes. In addition to code X37.Ø-, Hurricane, other possible applicable external cause of morbidity codes include:

X3Ø-, Exposure to excessive natural heat
X31-, Exposure to excessive natural cold
X38-, Flood

**d. Use of Z codes**

Z codes (other reasons for healthcare encounters) may be assigned as appropriate to further explain the reasons for presenting for healthcare services, including transfers between healthcare facilities, or provide additional information relevant to a patient encounter. The ICD-10-CM Official Guidelines for Coding and Reporting identify which codes maybe assigned as principal or first-listed diagnosis only, secondary diagnosis only, or principal/first-listed or secondary (depending on the circumstances). Possible applicable Z codes include:

Z59.Ø-, Homelessness
Z59.1, Inadequate housing
Z59.5, Extreme poverty
Z75.1, Person awaiting admission to adequate facility elsewhere
Z75.3, Unavailability and inaccessibility of health-care facilities
Z75.4, Unavailability and inaccessibility of other helping agencies
Z76.2, Encounter for health supervision and care of other healthy infant and child
Z99.12, Encounter for respirator [ventilator] dependence during power failure

The external cause of morbidity codes and the Z codes listed above are not an all-inclusive list. Other codes may be applicable to the encounter based upon the documentation. Assign as many codes as necessary to fully explain each healthcare encounter. Since patient history information may be very limited, use any available documentation to assign the appropriate external cause of morbidity and Z codes.

**20. Multiple Sites Coding**

The classification defines "multiple" as involving two or more sites. Follow chapter-specific guidelines for assigning codes for "multiple sites." In the absence of chapter-specific guidelines, assign codes describing specified sites individually when documented. When the specified site(s) are not documented, assign the appropriate code for "multiple sites."

## C. Chapter-Specific Coding Guidelines

In addition to general coding guidelines, there are guidelines for specific diagnoses and/or conditions in the classification. Unless otherwise indicated, these guidelines apply to all health care settings. Please refer to Section II for guidelines on the selection of principal diagnosis.

**1. Chapter 1: Certain Infectious and Parasitic Diseases (AØØ-B99), UØ7.1, UØ9.9**

**a. Human Immunodeficiency Virus (HIV) Infections**

**1) Code only confirmed cases**

Code only confirmed cases of HIV infection/illness. This is an exception to the hospital inpatient guideline Section II, H.

In this context, "confirmation" does not require documentation of positive serology or culture for HIV; the provider's diagnostic statement that the patient is HIV positive or has an HIV-related illness is sufficient.

**2) Selection and sequencing of HIV codes**

**(a) HIV disease**

If the term "AIDS" or "HIV disease" is documented or if the patient is treated for any HIV-related illness or is described as having any condition(s) resulting from the patient's HIV positive status; code B2Ø, Human immunodeficiency virus [HIV] disease, should be assigned.

**(b) Patient admitted for HIV-related condition**

If a patient is admitted for an HIV-related condition, the principal diagnosis should be B2Ø, Human immunodeficiency virus [HIV] disease followed by additional diagnosis codes for all reported HIV-related conditions.

An exception to this guideline is if the reason for admission is hemolytic-uremic syndrome associated with HIV disease. Assign code D59.31, Infection- associated hemolytic-uremic syndrome, followed by code B2Ø, Human immunodeficiency virus [HIV] disease.

**(c) Patient with HIV disease admitted for unrelated condition**

If a patient with HIV disease is admitted for an unrelated condition (such as a traumatic injury), the code for the unrelated condition (e.g., the nature of injury code) should be the principal diagnosis. Code B2Ø would be reported as a secondary diagnosis. Codes for other documented conditions should also be reported as secondary diagnoses.

**(d) Patient newly diagnosed with HIV disease**

Whether the patient is newly diagnosed or has had previous admissions/encounters for HIV conditions is irrelevant to the sequencing decision.

**(e) Asymptomatic human immunodeficiency virus**

When "HIV positive," "HIV test positive," or similar terminology is documented, and there is no documentation of symptoms or HIV-related illness, code Z21, Asymptomatic human immunodeficiency virus [HIV] infection status, should be assigned.

**(f) Inconclusive HIV serology**

Patients with documentation of inconclusive HIV serology, may be assigned code R75, Inconclusive laboratory evidence of human immunodeficiency virus [HIV].

**(g) Previously diagnosed HIV-related illness**

Patients with documentation of a prior diagnosis of an HIV-related illness should be coded to B2Ø. Once an HIV-related illness has developed, code B2Ø should always be assigned on every subsequent admission/encounter. Patients previously diagnosed with any HIV illness (B2Ø) should never be assigned to R75, Inconclusive laboratory evidence of human immunodeficiency virus [HIV] or Z21, Asymptomatic human immunodeficiency virus [HIV] infection status.

**(h) HIV Infection in Pregnancy, Childbirth and the Puerperium**

When a patient presents during pregnancy, childbirth or the puerperium with documented symptomatic HIV disease or an HIV related illness, assign a code from subcategory O98.7, Human immunodeficiency [HIV] disease complicating pregnancy, childbirth and the puerperium, followed by code B2Ø and additional code(s) for any HIV-related illness(es). Codes from Chapter 15 always take sequencing priority.

When a patient presents during pregnancy, childbirth or the puerperium with documented asymptomatic HIV infection status or is HIV-positive, assign a code from subcategory O98.7 followed by code Z21.

**(i) Encounters for HIV testing**

If a patient without signs or symptoms is tested for HIV, assign code Z11.4, Encounter for screening for human immunodeficiency virus [HIV]. Use additional codes for any associated high-risk behavior, if applicable.

If a patient with signs or symptoms of HIV presents for HIV testing, code the signs and symptoms. An additional counseling code Z71.7, Human immunodeficiency virus [HIV] counseling, may be assigned if counseling is provided during the encounter for the test. Code Z11.4, Encounter for screening for human immunodeficiency virus [HIV], should not be assigned if HIV signs or symptoms are present.

When a patient presents for follow up regarding their HIV test results and the test result is negative, assign code Z71.7, Human immunodeficiency virus [HIV] counseling.

If the results are positive, see previous guidelines and assign codes as appropriate.

**(j) HIV disease or HIV positive status managed by antiretroviral medication**

If a patient with documented HIV disease, HIV-related illness or AIDS is currently managed on antiretroviral medications, assign code B2Ø, Human immunodeficiency virus [HIV] disease.

If a patient with documented HIV positive status is currently managed on antiretroviral medication, assign code Z21, Asymptomatic human immunodeficiency virus [HIV] infection status, in the absence of any additional documentation of HIV disease, HIV-related illness or AIDS.

Code Z79.899, Other long term (current) drug therapy, may be assigned as an additional code to identify the long-term (current) use of antiretroviral medications.

**(k) Encounter for HIV Prophylaxis Measures**
When a patient is seen for administration of pre-exposure prophylaxis medication for HIV, assign code Z29.81, Encounter for HIV pre-exposure prophylaxis. Pre-exposure prophylaxis (PrEP) is intended to prevent infection in people who are at risk for getting HIV through sex or injection drug use. Any risk factors for HIV should also be coded.

**b. Infectious agents as the cause of diseases classified to other chapters**
Certain infections are classified in chapters other than Chapter 1 and no organism is identified as part of the infection code. In these instances, it is necessary to use an additional code from Chapter 1 to identify the organism. A code from category B95, Streptococcus, Staphylococcus, and Enterococcus as the cause of diseases classified to other chapters, B96, Other bacterial agents as the cause of diseases classified to other chapters, or B97, Viral agents as the cause of diseases classified to other chapters, is to be used as an additional code to identify the organism. An instructional note will be found at the infection code advising that an additional organism code is required.

**c. Infections resistant to antibiotics**
Many bacterial infections are resistant to current antibiotics. It is necessary to identify all infections documented as antibiotic resistant. Assign a code from category Z16, Resistance to antimicrobial drugs, following the infection code only if the infection code does not identify drug resistance.

**d. Sepsis, Severe Sepsis, and Septic Shock**

**1) Coding of Sepsis and Severe Sepsis**

**(a) Sepsis**
For a diagnosis of sepsis, assign the appropriate code for the underlying systemic infection. If the type of infection or causal organism is not further specified, assign code A41.9, Sepsis, unspecified organism.

A code from subcategory R65.2, Severe sepsis, should not be assigned unless severe sepsis or an associated acute organ dysfunction is documented.

**(i) Negative or inconclusive blood cultures and sepsis**
Negative or inconclusive blood cultures do not preclude a diagnosis of sepsis in patients with clinical evidence of the condition; however, the provider should be queried.

**(ii) Urosepsis**
The term urosepsis is a nonspecific term. It is not to be considered synonymous with sepsis. It has no default code in the Alphabetic Index. Should a provider use this term, he/she must be queried for clarification.

**(iii) Sepsis with organ dysfunction**
If a patient has sepsis and associated acute organ dysfunction or multiple organ dysfunction (MOD), follow the instructions for coding severe sepsis.

**(iv) Acute organ dysfunction that is not clearly associated with the sepsis**
If a patient has sepsis and an acute organ dysfunction, but the medical record documentation indicates that the acute organ dysfunction is related to a medical condition other than the sepsis, do not assign a code from subcategory R65.2, Severe sepsis. An acute organ dysfunction must be associated with the sepsis in order to assign the severe sepsis code. If the documentation is not clear as to whether an acute organ dysfunction is related to the sepsis or another medical condition, query the provider.

**(b) Severe sepsis**
The coding of severe sepsis requires a minimum of 2 codes: first a code for the underlying systemic infection, followed by a code from subcategory R65.2, Severe sepsis. If the causal organism is not documented, assign code A41.9, Sepsis, unspecified organism, for the infection. Additional code(s) for the associated acute organ dysfunction are also required.

Due to the complex nature of severe sepsis, some cases may require querying the provider prior to assignment of the codes.

**2) Septic shock**
Septic shock generally refers to circulatory failure associated with severe sepsis, and therefore, it represents a type of acute organ dysfunction.

For cases of septic shock, the code for the systemic infection should be sequenced first, followed by code R65.21, Severe sepsis with septic shock or code T81.12, Postprocedural septic shock.

Any additional codes for the other acute organ dysfunctions should also be assigned. As noted in the sequencing instructions in the Tabular List, the code for septic shock cannot be assigned as a principal diagnosis.

**3) Sequencing of severe sepsis**
If severe sepsis is present on admission, and meets the definition of principal diagnosis, the underlying systemic infection should be assigned as principal diagnosis followed by the appropriate code from subcategory R65.2 as required by the sequencing rules in the Tabular List. A code from subcategory R65.2 can never be assigned as a principal diagnosis.

When severe sepsis develops during an encounter (it was not present on admission), the underlying systemic infection and the appropriate code from subcategory R65.2 should be assigned as secondary diagnoses.

Severe sepsis may be present on admission, but the diagnosis may not be confirmed until sometime after admission. If the documentation is not clear whether severe sepsis was present on admission, the provider should be queried.

*For infection-associated hemolytic-uremic syndrome with severe sepsis, see guideline I.C.1.d.9.*

**4) Sepsis or severe sepsis with a localized infection**
If the reason for admission is sepsis or severe sepsis and a localized infection, such as pneumonia or cellulitis, a code(s) for the underlying systemic infection should be assigned first and the code for the localized infection should be assigned as a secondary diagnosis. If the patient has severe sepsis, a code from subcategory R65.2 should also be assigned as a secondary diagnosis. If the patient is admitted with a localized infection, such as pneumonia, and sepsis/severe sepsis doesn't develop until after admission, the localized infection should be assigned first, followed by the appropriate sepsis/severe sepsis codes.

*For hemolytic-uremic syndrome associated with sepsis, see guideline I. C.1.d.9.*

**5) Sepsis due to a postprocedural infection**

**(a) Documentation of causal relationship**
As with all postprocedural complications, code assignment is based on the provider's documentation of the relationship between the infection and the procedure.

**(b) Sepsis due to a postprocedural infection**
For sepsis following a postprocedural wound (surgical site) infection, a code from T81.41 to T81.43, Infection following a procedure, T81.49, Infection following a procedure, other surgical site, or a code from O86.00 to O86.03, Infection of obstetric surgical wound, or code O86.09, Infection of obstetric surgical wound, other surgical site, that identifies the site of the infection should be sequenced first, if known. Assign an additional code for sepsis following a procedure (T81.44) or sepsis following an obstetrical procedure (O86.04). Use an additional code to identify the infectious agent. If the patient has severe sepsis, the appropriate code from subcategory R65.2 should also be assigned with the additional code(s) for any acute organ dysfunction.

For infections following infusion, transfusion, therapeutic injection, or immunization, a code from subcategory T80.2, Infections following infusion, transfusion, and therapeutic injection, or code T88.0-, Infection following immunization, should be coded first, followed by the code for the specific infection. If the patient has severe sepsis, the appropriate code from subcategory R65.2 should also be assigned, with the additional codes(s) for any acute organ dysfunction.

**(c) Postprocedural infection and postprocedural septic shock**
If a postprocedural infection has resulted in postprocedural septic shock, assign the codes indicated above for sepsis due to a postprocedural infection, followed by code T81.12-, Postprocedural septic shock. Do not assign code R65.21, Severe sepsis with septic shock. Additional code(s) should be assigned for any acute organ dysfunction.

**6) Sepsis and severe sepsis associated with a noninfectious process (condition)**
In some cases, a noninfectious process (condition) such as trauma, may lead to an infection which can result in sepsis or severe sepsis. If sepsis or severe sepsis is documented as associated with a noninfectious condition, such as a burn or serious injury, and this condition meets the definition for principal diagnosis, the code for the noninfectious condition should be sequenced first, followed by the code for the resulting infection. If severe sepsis is present, a code from subcategory R65.2 should also be assigned with any associated organ dysfunction(s) codes. It is not necessary to assign a code from subcategory R65.1, Systemic inflammatory response syndrome (SIRS) of non-infectious origin, for these cases.

If the infection meets the definition of principal diagnosis, it should be sequenced before the non-infectious condition. When both the associated non-infectious condition and the infection meet the definition of principal diagnosis, either may be assigned as principal diagnosis.

Only one code from category R65, Symptoms and signs specifically associated with systemic inflammation and infection, should be assigned. Therefore, when a non-infectious condition leads to an infection resulting in severe sepsis, assign the appropriate code from subcategory R65.2, Severe sepsis. Do not additionally assign a code from subcategory R65.1, Systemic inflammatory response syndrome (SIRS) of non-infectious origin.

*See Section I.C.18. SIRS due to non-infectious process*

**7) Sepsis and septic shock complicating abortion, pregnancy, childbirth, and the puerperium**

*See Section I.C.15. Sepsis and septic shock complicating abortion, pregnancy, childbirth and the puerperium*

**8) Newborn sepsis**

*See Section I.C.16. f. Bacterial sepsis of Newborn*

**9) Hemolytic-uremic syndrome associated with sepsis**

If the reason for admission is hemolytic-uremic syndrome that is associated with sepsis, assign code D59.31, Infection-associated hemolytic-uremic syndrome, as the principal diagnosis. Codes for the underlying systemic infection and any other conditions (such as severe sepsis) should be assigned as secondary diagnoses.

**e. Methicillin Resistant Staphylococcus aureus (MRSA) Conditions**

**1) Selection and sequencing of MRSA codes**

**(a) Combination codes for MRSA infection**

When a patient is diagnosed with an infection that is due to methicillin resistant *Staphylococcus aureus* (MRSA), and that infection has a combination code that includes the causal organism (e.g., sepsis, pneumonia) assign the appropriate combination code for the condition (e.g., code A41.Ø2, Sepsis due to Methicillin resistant Staphylococcus aureus or code J15.212, Pneumonia due to Methicillin resistant Staphylococcus aureus). Do not assign code B95.62, Methicillin resistant Staphylococcus aureus infection as the cause of diseases classified elsewhere, as an additional code, because the combination code includes the type of infection and the MRSA organism. Do not assign a code from subcategory Z16.11, Resistance to penicillins, as an additional diagnosis.

*See Section C.1. for instructions on coding and sequencing of sepsis and severe sepsis.*

**(b) Other codes for MRSA infection**

When there is documentation of a current infection (e.g., wound infection, stitch abscess, urinary tract infection) due to MRSA, and that infection does not have a combination code that includes the causal organism, assign the appropriate code to identify the condition along with code B95.62, Methicillin resistant Staphylococcus aureus infection as the cause of diseases classified elsewhere for the MRSA infection. Do not assign a code from subcategory Z16.11, Resistance to penicillins.

**(c) Methicillin susceptible Staphylococcus aureus (MSSA) and MRSA colonization**

The condition or state of being colonized or carrying MSSA or MRSA is called colonization or carriage, while an individual person is described as being colonized or being a carrier.

Colonization means that MSSA or MSRA is present on or in the body without necessarily causing illness. A positive MRSA colonization test might be documented by the provider as "MRSA screen positive" or "MRSA nasal swab positive".

Assign code Z22.322, Carrier or suspected carrier of Methicillin resistant Staphylococcus aureus, for patients documented as having MRSA colonization. Assign code Z22.321, Carrier or suspected carrier of Methicillin susceptible Staphylococcus aureus, for patients documented as having MSSA colonization. Colonization is not necessarily indicative of a disease process or as the cause of a specific condition the patient may have unless documented as such by the provider.

**(d) MRSA colonization and infection**

If a patient is documented as having both MRSA colonization and infection during a hospital admission, code Z22.322, Carrier or suspected carrier of Methicillin resistant Staphylococcus aureus, and a code for the MRSA infection may both be assigned.

**f. Zika virus infections**

**1) Code only confirmed cases**

Code only a confirmed diagnosis of Zika virus (A92.5, Zika virus disease) as documented by the provider. This is an exception to the hospital inpatient guideline Section II, H. In this context, "confirmation" does not require documentation of the type of test performed; the provider's diagnostic statement that the condition is confirmed is sufficient. This code should be assigned regardless of the stated mode of transmission.

If the provider documents "suspected", "possible" or "probable" Zika, do not assign code A92.5. Assign a code(s) explaining the reason for encounter (such as fever, rash, or joint pain) or Z2Ø.821, Contact with and (suspected) exposure to Zika virus.

**g. Coronavirus infections**

**1) COVID-19 infection (infection due to SARS-CoV-2)**

**(a) Code only confirmed cases**

Code only a confirmed diagnosis of the 2019 novel coronavirus disease (COVID-19) as documented by the provider. For a confirmed diagnosis, assign code UØ7.1, COVID-19. This is an exception to the hospital inpatient guideline Section II, H. In this context, "confirmation" does not require documentation of a positive test result for COVID-19; the provider's documentation that the individual has COVID-19 is sufficient.

If the provider documents "suspected," "possible," "probable," or "inconclusive" COVID-19, do not assign code UØ7.1. Instead, code the signs and symptoms reported. See guideline I.C.1.g.1.g.

**(b) Sequencing of codes**

When COVID-19 meets the definition of principal diagnosis, code UØ7.1, COVID-19, should be sequenced first, followed by the appropriate codes for associated manifestations, except when another guideline requires that certain codes be sequenced first, such as obstetrics, sepsis, or transplant complications.

*For a COVID-19 infection that progresses to sepsis, see Section I.C.1.d. Sepsis, Severe Sepsis, and Septic Shock*

*See Section I.C.15.s. for COVID-19 infection in pregnancy, childbirth, and the puerperium*

*See Section I.C.16.h. for COVID-19 infection in newborn*

*For a COVID-19 infection in a lung transplant patient, see Section I.C.19.g.3.a. Transplant complications other than kidney.*

**(c) Acute respiratory manifestations of COVID-19**

When the reason for the encounter/admission is a respiratory manifestation of COVID-19, assign code UØ7.1, COVID-19, as the principal/first-listed diagnosis and assign code(s) for the respiratory manifestation(s) as additional diagnoses.

The following conditions are examples of common respiratory manifestations of COVID-19.

**(i) Pneumonia**

For a patient with pneumonia confirmed as due to COVID-19, assign codes UØ7.1, COVID-19, and J12.82, Pneumonia due to coronavirus disease 2019.

**(ii) Acute bronchitis**

For a patient with acute bronchitis confirmed as due to COVID-19, assign codes UØ7.1, and J2Ø.8, Acute bronchitis due to other specified organisms.

Bronchitis not otherwise specified (NOS) due to COVID-19 should be coded using code UØ7.1 and J4Ø, Bronchitis, not specified as acute or chronic.

**(iii) Lower respiratory infection**

If the COVID-19 is documented as being associated with a lower respiratory infection, not otherwise specified (NOS), or an acute respiratory infection, NOS, codes UØ7.1 and J22, Unspecified acute lower respiratory infection, should be assigned.

If the COVID-19 is documented as being associated with a respiratory infection, NOS, codes UØ7.1 and J98.8, Other specified respiratory disorders, should be assigned.

**(iv) Acute respiratory distress syndrome**

For acute respiratory distress syndrome (ARDS) due to COVID-19, assign codes UØ7.1, and J8Ø, Acute respiratory distress syndrome.

**(v) Acute respiratory failure**

For acute respiratory failure due to COVID-19, assign code UØ7.1, and code J96.Ø-, Acute respiratory failure.

**(d) Non-respiratory manifestations of COVID-19**

When the reason for the encounter/admission is a non-respiratory manifestation (e.g., viral enteritis) of COVID-19, assign code UØ7.1, COVID-19, as the principal/first-listed diagnosis and assign code(s) for the manifestation(s) as additional diagnoses.

**(e) Exposure to COVID-19**

For asymptomatic individuals with actual or suspected exposure to COVID-19, assign code Z2Ø.822, Contact with and (suspected) exposure to COVID-19.

For symptomatic individuals with actual or suspected exposure to COVID-19 and the infection has been ruled out, or test results are inconclusive or unknown, assign code Z2Ø.822, Contact with and (suspected) exposure to COVID-19. See guideline I.C.21.c.1, Contact/Exposure, for additional guidance regarding the use of category Z2Ø codes.

If COVID-19 is confirmed, see guideline I.C.1.g.1.a.

**(f) Screening for COVID-19**

For screening for COVID-19, including preoperative testing, assign code Z11.52, Encounter for screening for COVID-19.

**(g) Signs and symptoms without definitive diagnosis of COVID-19**

For patients presenting with any signs/symptoms associated with COVID-19 (such as fever, etc.) but a definitive diagnosis has not been established, assign the appropriate code(s) for each of the presenting signs and symptoms such as:

- RØ5.1, Acute cough, or RØ5.9, Cough, unspecified
- RØ6.Ø2, Shortness of breath
- R5Ø.9, Fever, unspecified

If a patient with signs/symptoms associated with COVID-19 also has an actual or suspected contact with or exposure to COVID-19, assign Z2Ø.822, Contact with and (suspected) exposure to COVID-19, as an additional code.

**(h) Asymptomatic individuals who test positive for COVID-19**
For asymptomatic individuals who test positive for COVID-19 and there is no provider documentation of a diagnosis of COVID-19, query the provider as to whether or not the individual has COVID-19. A false positive laboratory test is possible, and it is the provider's responsibility to confirm the diagnosis and document accordingly.

**(i) Personal history of COVID-19**
For patients with a history of COVID-19, assign code Z86.16, Personal history of COVID-19.

**(j) Follow-up visits after COVID-19 infection has resolved**
For individuals who previously had COVID-19, without residual symptom(s) or condition(s), and are being seen for follow-up evaluation, and COVID-19 test results are negative, assign codes ZØ9, Encounter for follow-up examination after completed treatment for conditions other than malignant neoplasm, and Z86.16, Personal history of COVID-19.

For follow-up visits for individuals with symptom(s) or condition(s) related to a previous COVID-19 infection, see guideline I.C.1.g.1.m.

*See Section I.C.21.c.8, Factors influencing health states and contact with health services, Follow-up*

**(k) Encounter for antibody testing**
For an encounter for antibody testing that is not being performed to confirm a current COVID-19 infection, nor is a follow-up test after resolution of COVID-19, assign ZØ1.84, Encounter for antibody response examination.

Follow the applicable guidelines above if the individual is being tested to confirm a current COVID-19 infection.

For follow-up testing after a COVID-19 infection, see guideline I.C.1.g.1.j.

**(l) Multisystem Inflammatory Syndrome**
For individuals with multisystem inflammatory syndrome (MIS) and COVID-19, assign code UØ7.1, COVID-19, as the principal/first-listed diagnosis and assign code M35.81, Multisystem inflammatory syndrome, as an additional diagnosis.

If an individual with a history of COVID-19 develops MIS, assign codes M35.81, Multisystem inflammatory syndrome, and UØ9.9, Post COVID-19 condition, unspecified.

If an individual with a known or suspected exposure to COVID-19, and no current COVID-19 infection or history of COVID-19, develops MIS, assign codes M35.81, Multisystem inflammatory syndrome, and Z2Ø.822, Contact with and (suspected) exposure to COVID-19.

Additional codes should be assigned for any associated complications of MIS.

**(m) Post COVID-19 Condition**
For sequela of COVID-19, or associated symptoms or conditions that develop following a previous COVID-19 infection, assign a code(s) for the specific symptom(s) or condition(s) related to the previous COVID-19 infection, if known, and code UØ9.9, Post COVID-19 condition, unspecified.

Code UØ9.9 should not be assigned for manifestations of an active (current) COVID-19 infection.

If a patient has a condition(s) associated with a previous COVID-19 infection and develops a new active (current) COVID-19 infection, code UØ9.9 may be assigned in conjunction with code UØ7.1, COVID-19, to identify that the patient also has a condition(s) associated with a previous COVID-19 infection. Code(s) for the specific condition(s) associated with the previous COVID-19 infection and code(s) for manifestation(s) of the new active (current) COVID-19 infection should also be assigned.

**(n) Underimmunization for COVID-19 Status**
Code Z28.31Ø, Unvaccinated for COVID-19, may be assigned when the patient has not received a COVID-19 vaccine of any type. Code Z28.311, Partially vaccinated for COVID-19, may be assigned when the patient has been partially vaccinated for COVID-19 as per the recommendations of the Centers for Disease Control and Prevention (CDC) in place at the time of the encounter. For information, visit the CDC's website https://www.cdc.gov/covidschedule.

*See Section I.B.14. for underimmunization documentation by clinicians other than patient's provider.*

**2. Chapter 2: Neoplasms (CØØ-D49)**
**General Guidelines**

Chapter 2 of the ICD-10-CM contains the codes for most benign and all malignant neoplasms. Certain benign neoplasms, such as prostatic adenomas, may be found in the specific body system chapters. To properly code a neoplasm, it is necessary to determine from the record if the neoplasm is benign, in-situ, malignant, or of uncertain histologic behavior. If malignant, any secondary (metastatic) sites should also be determined.

Primary malignant neoplasms overlapping site boundaries

A primary malignant neoplasm that overlaps two or more contiguous (next to each other) sites should be classified to the subcategory/code .8 ('overlapping lesion'), unless the combination is specifically indexed elsewhere. For multiple neoplasms of the same site that are not contiguous such as tumors in different quadrants of the same breast, codes for each site should be assigned.

Malignant neoplasm of ectopic tissue

Malignant neoplasms of ectopic tissue are to be coded to the site of origin mentioned, e.g., ectopic pancreatic malignant neoplasms involving the stomach are coded to malignant neoplasm of pancreas, unspecified (C25.9).

The neoplasm table in the Alphabetic Index should be referenced first. However, if the histological term is documented, that term should be referenced first, rather than going immediately to the Neoplasm Table, in order to determine which column in the Neoplasm Table is appropriate. For example, if the documentation indicates "adenoma," refer to the term in the Alphabetic Index to review the entries under this term and the instructional note to "see also neoplasm, by site, benign." The table provides the proper code based on the type of neoplasm and the site. It is important to select the proper column in the table that corresponds to the type of neoplasm. The Tabular List should then be referenced to verify that the correct code has been selected from the table and that a more specific site code does not exist.

*See Section I.C.21. Factors influencing health status and contact with health services, Status, for information regarding Z15.Ø, codes for genetic susceptibility to cancer.*

**a. Admission/Encounter for treatment of primary site**
If the malignancy is chiefly responsible for occasioning the patient admission/encounter and treatment is directed at the primary site, designate the primary malignancy as the principal/first-listed diagnosis.

The only exception to this guideline is if the administration of chemotherapy, immunotherapy or external beam radiation therapy is chiefly responsible for occasioning the admission/encounter. In that case, assign the appropriate Z51.-- code as the first-listed or principal diagnosis, and the underlying diagnosis or problem for which the service is being performed as a secondary diagnosis.

**b. Admission/Encounter for treatment of secondary site**
When a patient is admitted because of a primary neoplasm with metastasis and treatment is directed toward the secondary site only, the secondary neoplasm is designated as the principal diagnosis even though the primary malignancy is still present.

**c. Coding and sequencing of complications**
Coding and sequencing of complications associated with the malignancies or with the therapy thereof are subject to the following guidelines:

**1) Anemia associated with malignancy**
When admission/encounter is for management of an anemia associated with the malignancy, and the treatment is only for anemia, the appropriate code for the malignancy is sequenced as the principal or first-listed diagnosis followed by the appropriate code for the anemia (such as code D63.Ø, Anemia in neoplastic disease).

**2) Anemia associated with chemotherapy, immunotherapy and radiation therapy**
When the admission/encounter is for management of an anemia associated with an adverse effect of the administration of chemotherapy or immunotherapy and the only treatment is for the anemia, the anemia code is sequenced first followed by the appropriate codes for the neoplasm and the adverse effect (T45.1X5-, Adverse effect of antineoplastic and immunosuppressive drugs).

When the admission/encounter is for management of an anemia associated with an adverse effect of radiotherapy, the anemia code should be sequenced first, followed by the appropriate neoplasm code and code Y84.2, Radiological procedure and radiotherapy as the cause of abnormal reaction of the patient, or of later complication, without mention of misadventure at the time of the procedure.

**3) Management of dehydration due to the malignancy**
When the admission/encounter is for management of dehydration due to the malignancy and only the dehydration is being treated (intravenous rehydration), the dehydration is sequenced first, followed by the code(s) for the malignancy.

**4) Treatment of a complication resulting from a surgical procedure**
When the admission/encounter is for treatment of a complication resulting from a surgical procedure, designate the complication as the principal or first-listed diagnosis if treatment is directed at resolving the complication.

**d. Primary malignancy previously excised**
When a primary malignancy has been previously excised or eradicated from its site and there is no further treatment directed to that site and there is no evidence of any existing primary malignancy at that site, a code from category Z85, Personal history of malignant neoplasm, should be used to indicate the former site of the malignancy. Any mention of extension, invasion, or metastasis to another site is coded as a secondary malignant neoplasm to that site. The secondary site may be the principal or first-listed diagnosis with the Z85 code used as a secondary code.

*See section I.C.2.t. Secondary malignant neoplasm of lymphoid tissue.*

**e. Admissions/Encounters involving antineoplastic chemotherapy, immunotherapy and radiation therapy**

**1) Episode of care involves surgical removal of neoplasm**
When an episode of care involves the surgical removal of a neoplasm, primary or secondary site, followed by adjunct chemotherapy or radiation treatment during the same episode of care, the code for the neoplasm should be assigned as principal or first-listed diagnosis.

**2) Patient admission/encounter chiefly for administration of antineoplastic chemotherapy, immunotherapy and radiation therapy**
If a patient admission/encounter is chiefly for the administration of chemotherapy, immunotherapy or external beam radiation therapy for the treatment of a neoplasm, assign code Z51.Ø, Encounter for antineoplastic radiation therapy, or Z51.11, Encounter for antineoplastic chemotherapy, or Z51.12, Encounter for antineoplastic immunotherapy as the first-listed or principal diagnosis. If the reason for the encounter is more than one type of antineoplastic therapy, code Z51.Ø and codes from subcategory Z51.1 may be assigned together, in which case one of these codes would be reported as a secondary diagnosis.

The malignancy for which the therapy is being administered should be assigned as a secondary diagnosis.

If a patient admission/encounter is for the insertion or implantation of radioactive elements (e.g., brachytherapy) the appropriate code for the malignancy is sequenced as the principal or first-listed diagnosis. Code Z51.Ø should not be assigned.

**3) Patient admitted for radiation therapy, chemotherapy or immunotherapy and develops complications**
When a patient is admitted for the purpose of external beam radiotherapy, immunotherapy or chemotherapy and develops complications such as uncontrolled nausea and vomiting or dehydration, the principal or first-listed diagnosis is Z51.Ø, Encounter for antineoplastic radiation therapy, or Z51.11, Encounter for antineoplastic chemotherapy, or Z51.12, Encounter for antineoplastic immunotherapy followed by any codes for the complications.

When a patient is admitted for the purpose of insertion or implantation of radioactive elements (e.g., brachytherapy) and develops complications such as uncontrolled nausea and vomiting or dehydration, the principal or first-listed diagnosis is the appropriate code for the malignancy followed by any codes for the complications.

**f. Admission/encounter to determine extent of malignancy**
When the reason for admission/encounter is to determine the extent of the malignancy, or for a procedure such as paracentesis or thoracentesis, the primary malignancy or appropriate metastatic site is designated as the principal or first-listed diagnosis, even though chemotherapy or radiotherapy is administered.

**g. Symptoms, signs, and abnormal findings listed in Chapter 18 associated with neoplasms**
Symptoms, signs, and ill-defined conditions listed in Chapter 18 characteristic of, or associated with, an existing primary or secondary site malignancy cannot be used to replace the malignancy as principal or first-listed diagnosis, regardless of the number of admissions or encounters for treatment and care of the neoplasm.

*See section I.C.21. Factors influencing health status and contact with health services, Encounter for prophylactic organ removal.*

**h. Admission/encounter for pain control/management**
*See Section I.C.6. for information on coding admission/encounter for pain control/management.*

**i. Malignancy in two or more noncontiguous sites**
A patient may have more than one malignant tumor in the same organ. These tumors may represent different primaries or metastatic disease, depending on the site. Should the documentation be unclear, the provider should be queried as to the status of each tumor so that the correct codes can be assigned.

**j. Disseminated malignant neoplasm, unspecified**
Code C8Ø.Ø, Disseminated malignant neoplasm, unspecified, is for use only in those cases where the patient has advanced metastatic disease and no known primary or secondary sites are specified. It should not be used in place of assigning codes for the primary site and all known secondary sites.

**k. Malignant neoplasm without specification of site**
Code C8Ø.1, Malignant (primary) neoplasm, unspecified, equates to Cancer, unspecified. This code should only be used when no determination can be made as to the primary site of a malignancy. This code should rarely be used in the inpatient setting.

**l. Sequencing of neoplasm codes**

**1) Encounter for treatment of primary malignancy**
If the reason for the encounter is for treatment of a primary malignancy, assign the malignancy as the principal/first-listed diagnosis. The primary site is to be sequenced first, followed by any metastatic sites.

**2) Encounter for treatment of secondary malignancy**
When an encounter is for a primary malignancy with metastasis and treatment is directed toward the metastatic (secondary) site(s) only, the metastatic site(s) is designated as the principal/first-listed diagnosis. The primary malignancy is coded as an additional code.

**3) Malignant neoplasm in a pregnant patient**
When a pregnant patient has a malignant neoplasm, a code from subcategory O9A.1-, Malignant neoplasm complicating pregnancy, childbirth, and the puerperium, should be sequenced first, followed by the appropriate code from Chapter 2 to indicate the type of neoplasm.

**4) Encounter for complication associated with a neoplasm**
When an encounter is for management of a complication associated with a neoplasm, such as dehydration, and the treatment is only for the complication, the complication is coded first, followed by the appropriate code(s) for the neoplasm.

The exception to this guideline is anemia. When the admission/encounter is for management of an anemia associated with the malignancy, and the treatment is only for anemia, the appropriate code for the malignancy is sequenced as the principal or first-listed diagnosis followed by code D63.Ø, Anemia in neoplastic disease.

**5) Complication from surgical procedure for treatment of a neoplasm**
When an encounter is for treatment of a complication resulting from a surgical procedure performed for the treatment of the neoplasm, designate the complication as the principal/first-listed diagnosis. See the guideline regarding the coding of a current malignancy versus personal history to determine if the code for the neoplasm should also be assigned.

**6) Pathologic fracture due to a neoplasm**
When an encounter is for a pathological fracture due to a neoplasm, and the focus of treatment is the fracture, a code from subcategory M84.5, Pathological fracture in neoplastic disease, should be sequenced first, followed by the code for the neoplasm.

If the focus of treatment is the neoplasm with an associated pathological fracture, the neoplasm code should be sequenced first, followed by a code from M84.5 for the pathological fracture.

**m. Current malignancy versus personal history of malignancy**
When a primary malignancy has been excised but further treatment, such as an additional surgery for the malignancy, radiation therapy or chemotherapy is directed to that site, the primary malignancy code should be used until treatment is completed.

When a primary malignancy has been previously excised or eradicated from its site, there is no further treatment (of the malignancy) directed to that site, and there is no evidence of any existing primary malignancy at that site, a code from category Z85, Personal history of malignant neoplasm, should be used to indicate the former site of the malignancy.

Codes from subcategories Z85.Ø – Z85.85 should only be assigned for the former site of a primary malignancy, not the site of a secondary malignancy. Code Z85.89 may be assigned for the former site(s) of either a primary or secondary malignancy.

*See Section I.C.21. Factors influencing health status and contact with health services, History (of)*

**n. Leukemia, Multiple Myeloma, and Malignant Plasma Cell Neoplasms in remission versus personal history**
The categories for leukemia, and category C9Ø, Multiple myeloma and malignant plasma cell neoplasms, have codes indicating whether or not the leukemia has achieved remission. There are also codes Z85.6, Personal history of leukemia, and Z85.79, Personal history of other malignant neoplasms of lymphoid, hematopoietic and related tissues. If the documentation is unclear as to whether the leukemia has achieved remission, the provider should be queried.

*See Section I.C.21. Factors influencing health status and contact with health services, History (of)*

**o. Aftercare following surgery for neoplasm**
*See Section I.C.21. Factors influencing health status and contact with health services, Aftercare*

**p. Follow-up care for completed treatment of a malignancy**
*See Section I.C.21. Factors influencing health status and contact with health services, Follow-up*

**q. Prophylactic organ removal for prevention of malignancy**
*See Section I.C. 21, Factors influencing health status and contact with health services, Prophylactic organ removal*

**r. Malignant neoplasm associated with transplanted organ**
A malignant neoplasm of a transplanted organ should be coded as a transplant complication. Assign first the appropriate code from category T86.-, Complications of transplanted organs and tissue, followed by code C8Ø.2, Malignant neoplasm associated with transplanted organ. Use an additional code for the specific malignancy.

**s. Breast Implant Associated Anaplastic Large Cell Lymphoma**
Breast implant associated anaplastic large cell lymphoma (BIA-ALCL) is a type of lymphoma that can develop around breast implants. Assign code C84.7A, Anaplastic large cell lymphoma, ALK-negative, breast, for BIA-ALCL or C84.7B, Anaplastic large cell lymphoma, ALK-negative, in remission, for BIA-ALCL in remission. Do not assign a complication code from chapter 19.

**t. Secondary malignant neoplasm of lymphoid tissue**
When a malignant neoplasm of lymphoid tissue metastasizes beyond the lymph nodes, a code from categories C81-C85 with a final character identifying "extranodal and solid organ sites" should be assigned rather than a code for the secondary neoplasm of the affected solid organ. For example, for metastasis of diffuse large B-cell lymphoma to the lung, brain and left adrenal gland, assign code C83.398, Diffuse large B-cell lymphoma of other extranodal and solid organ sites.

**3. Chapter 3: Diseases of the blood and blood-forming organs and certain disorders involving the immune mechanism (D5Ø-D89)**
Reserved for future guideline expansion

**4. Chapter 4: Endocrine, Nutritional, and Metabolic Diseases (EØØ-E89)**

**a. Diabetes mellitus**
The diabetes mellitus codes are combination codes that include the type of diabetes mellitus, the body system affected, and the complications affecting that body system. As many codes within a particular category as are necessary to describe all of the complications of the disease may be used. They should be sequenced based on the reason for a particular encounter. Assign as many codes from categories EØ8 – E13 as needed to identify all of the associated conditions that the patient has.

**1) Type of diabetes**
The age of a patient is not the sole determining factor, though most type 1 diabetics develop the condition before reaching puberty. For this reason, type 1 diabetes mellitus is also referred to as juvenile diabetes.

**(a) Presymptomatic Type 1 Diabetes Mellitus**
Codes E1Ø.A-, Type 1 diabetes mellitus, presymptomatic, are assigned for early-stage type 1 diabetes that predates the onset of symptoms.

**(b) Type 2 diabetes mellitus in remission**
Code E11.A, Type 2 diabetes mellitus without complications in remission, is assigned based on provider documentation that the diabetes mellitus is in remission. If the documentation is unclear as to whether the Type 2 diabetes mellitus has achieved remission, the provider should be queried. For example, the term "resolved" is not synonymous with remission.

**2) Type of diabetes mellitus not documented**
If the type of diabetes mellitus is not documented in the medical record the default is E11.-, Type 2 diabetes mellitus.

**3) Diabetes mellitus and the use of insulin, oral hypoglycemics, and injectable non-insulin drugs**
If the documentation in a medical record does not indicate the type of diabetes but does indicate that the patient uses insulin, code E11-, Type 2 diabetes mellitus, should be assigned. Additional code(s) should be assigned from category Z79 to identify the long-term (current) use of insulin, oral hypoglycemic drugs, or injectable non-insulin antidiabetic, as follows:

If the patient is treated with both oral hypoglycemic drugs and insulin, both code Z79.4, Long term (current) use of insulin, and code Z79.84, Long term (current) use of oral hypoglycemic drugs, should be assigned.

If the patient is treated with both insulin and an injectable non-insulin antidiabetic drug, assign codes Z79.4, Long term (current) use of insulin, and Z79.85, Long-term (current) use of injectable non-insulin antidiabetic drugs.

If the patient is treated with both oral hypoglycemic drugs and an injectable non-insulin antidiabetic drug, assign codes Z79.84, Long term (current) use of oral hypoglycemic drugs, and Z79.85, Long-term (current) use of injectable non-insulin antidiabetic drugs.

Code Z79.4 should not be assigned if insulin is given temporarily to bring a type 2 patient's blood sugar under control during an encounter.

**4) Diabetes mellitus in pregnancy and gestational diabetes**
*See Section I.C.15. Diabetes mellitus in pregnancy.*

*See Section I.C.15. Gestational (pregnancy induced) diabetes*

**5) Complications due to insulin pump malfunction**

**(a) Underdose of insulin due to insulin pump failure**
An underdose of insulin due to an insulin pump failure should be assigned to a code from subcategory T85.6, Mechanical complication of other specified internal and external prosthetic devices, implants and grafts, that specifies the type of pump malfunction, as the principal or first-listed code, followed by code T38.3X6-, Underdosing of insulin and oral hypoglycemic [antidiabetic] drugs. Additional codes for the type of diabetes mellitus and any associated complications due to the underdosing should also be assigned.

**(b) Overdose of insulin due to insulin pump failure**
The principal or first-listed code for an encounter due to an insulin pump malfunction resulting in an overdose of insulin, should also be T85.6-, Mechanical complication of other specified internal and external prosthetic devices, implants and grafts, followed by code T38.3X1-, Poisoning by insulin and oral hypoglycemic [antidiabetic] drugs, accidental (unintentional).

**6) Secondary diabetes mellitus**
Codes under categories EØ8, Diabetes mellitus due to underlying condition, EØ9, Drug or chemical induced diabetes mellitus, and E13, Other specified diabetes mellitus, identify complications/manifestations associated with secondary diabetes mellitus. Secondary diabetes is always caused by another condition or event (e.g., cystic fibrosis, malignant neoplasm of pancreas, pancreatectomy, adverse effect of drug, or poisoning).

**(a) Secondary diabetes mellitus and the use of insulin, oral hypoglycemic drugs, or injectable non-insulin drugs**
For patients with secondary diabetes mellitus who routinely use insulin, oral hypoglycemic drugs, or injectable non-insulin drugs, additional code(s) from category Z79 should be assigned to identify the long-term (current) use of insulin, oral hypoglycemic drugs, or non-injectable non-insulin drugs as follows:

If the patient is treated with both oral hypoglycemic drugs and insulin, both code Z79.4, Long term (current) use of insulin, and code Z79.84, Long term (current) use of oral hypoglycemic drugs, should be assigned.

If the patient is treated with both insulin and an injectable non-insulin antidiabetic drug, assign codes Z79.4, Long-term (current) use of insulin, and Z79.85, Long-term (current) use of injectable non-insulin antidiabetic drugs.

If the patient is treated with both oral hypoglycemic drugs and an injectable non-insulin antidiabetic drug, assign codes Z79.84, Long-term (current) use of oral hypoglycemic drugs, and Z79.85, Long-term (current) use of injectable non-insulin antidiabetic drugs.

Code Z79.4 should not be assigned if insulin is given temporarily to bring a secondary diabetic patient's blood sugar under control during an encounter.

**(b) Assigning and sequencing secondary diabetes codes and its causes**
The sequencing of the secondary diabetes codes in relationship to codes for the cause of the diabetes is based on the Tabular List instructions for categories EØ8, EØ9 and E13.

**(i) Secondary diabetes mellitus due to pancreatectomy**
For postpancreatectomy diabetes mellitus (lack of insulin due to the surgical removal of all or part of the pancreas), assign code E89.1, Postprocedural hypoinsulinemia.

Assign a code from category E13 as the principal or first-listed diagnosis and a code from subcategory Z9Ø.41, Acquired absence of pancreas, as an additional code.

**(ii) Secondary diabetes due to drugs**
Secondary diabetes may be caused by an adverse effect of correctly administered medications, poisoning or sequela of poisoning.

*See section I.C.19.e. for coding of adverse effects and poisoning, and section I.C.20 for external cause code reporting.*

**b. Obesity**
The obesity codes in category E66, Overweight and obesity, include codes related to the cause of obesity, such as drug-induced obesity (E66.1), and codes related to effects of obesity, such as code E66.2, Morbid (severe) obesity with alveolar hypoventilation. There are other codes related to obesity in other categories of the classification, such as E88.82, Obesity due to disruption of MC4R pathway; and codes in fifth character subcategory O99.21, Obesity complicating pregnancy, childbirth, and the puerperium.

**1) Obesity class**
The obesity class codes in subcategory E66.81, Obesity class, require a fifth character to convey the severity of obesity. The obesity class should be documented in the medical record by the provider for these codes to be assigned. The obesity class codes can

be reported with other obesity codes in the classification found in Chapters 4 and 15 to fully describe the condition. However, if both class 3 obesity and morbid obesity are documented, only a code for class 3 obesity should be assigned as it is more specific.

**5. Chapter 5: Mental, Behavioral and Neurodevelopmental disorders (FØ1-F99)**

**a. Pain disorders related to psychological factors**

Assign code F45.41, for pain that is exclusively related to psychological disorders. As indicated by the Excludes 1 note under category G89, a code from category G89 should not be assigned with code F45.41.

Code F45.42, Pain disorders with related psychological factors, should be used with a code from category G89, Pain, not elsewhere classified, if there is documentation of a psychological component for a patient with acute or chronic pain.

*See Section I.C.6. Pain*

**b. Mental and behavioral disorders due to psychoactive substance use**

**1) In Remission**

Selection of codes describing "in remission" for categories F1Ø-F19, Mental and behavioral disorders due to psychoactive substance use (categories F1Ø-F19 with -.11, -.21, -.91) requires the provider's clinical judgment and are assigned only on the basis of provider documentation (as defined in the Official Guidelines for Coding and Reporting), unless otherwise instructed by the classification.

Mild substance use disorders in early or sustained remission are classified to the appropriate codes for substance abuse in remission, and moderate or severe substance use disorders in early or sustained remission are classified to the appropriate codes for substance dependence in remission.

**2) Psychoactive Substance Use, Abuse and Dependence**

When the provider documentation refers to use, abuse and dependence of the same substance (e.g. alcohol, opioid, cannabis, etc.), only one code should be assigned to identify the pattern of use based on the following hierarchy:

- If both use and abuse are documented, assign only the code for abuse
- If both abuse and dependence are documented, assign only the code for dependence
- If use, abuse and dependence are all documented, assign only the code for dependence
- If both use and dependence are documented, assign only the code for dependence.

**3) Psychoactive Substance Use, Unspecified**

As with all other unspecified diagnoses, the codes for unspecified psychoactive substance use (F1Ø.9-, F11.9-, F12.9-, F13.9-, F14.9-, F15.9-, F16.9-, F18.9-, F19.9-) should only be assigned based on provider documentation and when they meet the definition of a reportable diagnosis (see Section III, Reporting Additional Diagnoses). These codes are to be used only when the psychoactive substance use is associated with a substance related disorder (chapter 5 disorders such as sexual dysfunction, sleep disorder, or a mental or behavioral disorder) or medical condition, and such a relationship is documented by the provider.

**4) Medical Conditions Due to Psychoactive Substance Use, Abuse and Dependence**

Medical conditions due to substance use, abuse, and dependence are not classified as substance-induced disorders. Assign the diagnosis code for the medical condition as directed by the Alphabetical Index along with the appropriate psychoactive substance use, abuse or dependence code. For example, for alcoholic pancreatitis due to alcohol dependence, assign the appropriate code from subcategory K85.2, Alcohol induced acute pancreatitis, and the appropriate code from subcategory F1Ø.2, such as code F1Ø.2Ø, Alcohol dependence, uncomplicated. It would not be appropriate to assign code F1Ø.288, Alcohol dependence with other alcohol-induced disorder.

**5) Blood Alcohol Level**

A code from category Y9Ø, Evidence of alcohol involvement determined by blood alcohol level, may be assigned when this information is documented and the patient's provider has documented a condition classifiable to category F1Ø, Alcohol related disorders. The blood alcohol level does not need to be documented by the patient's provider in order for it to be coded.

*See Section I.B.14. for blood alcohol level documentation by clinicians other than patient's provider.*

**c. Factitious Disorder**

Factitious disorder imposed on self or Munchausen's syndrome is a disorder in which a person falsely reports or causes his or her own physical or psychological signs or symptoms. For patients with documented factitious disorder on self or Munchausen's syndrome, assign the appropriate code from subcategory F68.1-, Factitious disorder imposed on self.

Munchausen's syndrome by proxy (MSBP) is a disorder in which a caregiver (perpetrator) falsely reports or causes an illness or injury in another person (victim) under his or her care, such as a child, an elderly adult, or a person who has a disability. The condition is also referred to as "factitious disorder imposed on another" or "factitious disorder by proxy." The perpetrator, not the victim, receives this diagnosis. Assign code F68.A, Factitious disorder imposed on another, to the perpetrator's record. For the victim of a patient suffering from MSBP, assign the appropriate code from categories T74, Adult and child abuse, neglect and other maltreatment, confirmed, or T76, Adult and child abuse, neglect and other maltreatment, suspected.

*See Section I.C.19.f. Adult and child abuse, neglect and other maltreatment*

**d. Dementia**

The ICD-10-CM classifies dementia (categories FØ1, FØ2, and FØ3) on the basis of the etiology and severity (unspecified, mild, moderate or severe). Selection of the appropriate severity level requires the provider's clinical judgment and codes should be assigned only on the basis of provider documentation (as defined in the *Official Guidelines for Coding and Reporting*), unless otherwise instructed by the classification. If the documentation does not provide information about the severity of the dementia, assign the appropriate code for unspecified severity.

If a patient is admitted to an inpatient acute care hospital or other inpatient facility setting with dementia at one severity level and it progresses to a higher severity level, assign one code for the highest severity level reported during the stay.

**6. Chapter 6: Diseases of the Nervous System (GØØ-G99)**

**a. Dominant/nondominant side**

Codes from category G81, Hemiplegia and hemiparesis, and subcategories G83.1, Monoplegia of lower limb, G83.2, Monoplegia of upper limb, and G83.3, Monoplegia, unspecified, identify whether the dominant or nondominant side is affected. Should the affected side be documented, but not specified as dominant or nondominant, and the classification system does not indicate a default, code selection is as follows:

- For ambidextrous patients, the default should be dominant.
- If the left side is affected, the default is non-dominant.
- If the right side is affected, the default is dominant.

**b. Pain - Category G89**

**1) General coding information**

Codes in category G89, Pain, not elsewhere classified, may be used in conjunction with codes from other categories and chapters to provide more detail about acute or chronic pain and neoplasm-related pain, unless otherwise indicated below.

If the pain is not specified as acute or chronic, post-thoracotomy, postprocedural, or neoplasm-related, do not assign codes from category G89.

A code from category G89 should not be assigned if the underlying (definitive) diagnosis is known, unless the reason for the encounter is pain control/ management and not management of the underlying condition.

When an admission or encounter is for a procedure aimed at treating the underlying condition (e.g., spinal fusion, kyphoplasty), a code for the underlying condition (e.g., vertebral fracture, spinal stenosis) should be assigned as the principal diagnosis. No code from category G89 should be assigned.

**(a) Category G89 Codes as Principal or First-Listed Diagnosis**

Category G89 codes are acceptable as principal diagnosis or the first-listed code:

- When pain control or pain management is the reason for the admission/encounter (e.g., a patient with displaced intervertebral disc, nerve impingement and severe back pain presents for injection of steroid into the spinal canal). The underlying cause of the pain should be reported as an additional diagnosis, if known.
- When a patient is admitted for the insertion of a neurostimulator for pain control, assign the appropriate pain code as the principal or first-listed diagnosis. When an admission or encounter is for a procedure aimed at treating the underlying condition and a neurostimulator is inserted for pain control during the same admission/encounter, a code for the underlying condition should be assigned as the principal diagnosis and the appropriate pain code should be assigned as a secondary diagnosis.

**(b) Use of Category G89 Codes in Conjunction with Site Specific Pain Codes**

**(i) Assigning Category G89 and Site-Specific Pain Codes**

Codes from category G89 may be used in conjunction with codes that identify the site of pain (including codes from chapter 18) if the category G89 code provides additional information. For example, if the code describes the site of the pain, but does not fully describe whether the pain is acute or chronic, then both codes should be assigned.

(ii) **Sequencing of Category G89 Codes with Site-Specific Pain Codes**
The sequencing of category G89 codes with site-specific pain codes (including chapter 18 codes), is dependent on the circumstances of the encounter/admission as follows:

- If the encounter is for pain control or pain management, assign the code from category G89 followed by the code identifying the specific site of pain (e.g., encounter for pain management for acute neck pain from trauma is assigned code G89.11, Acute pain due to trauma, followed by code M54.2, Cervicalgia, to identify the site of pain).
- If the encounter is for any other reason except pain control or pain management, and a related definitive diagnosis has not been established (confirmed) by the provider, assign the code for the specific site of pain first, followed by the appropriate code from category G89.

2) **Pain due to devices, implants and grafts**
*See Section I.C.19. Pain due to medical devices*

3) **Postoperative Pain**
The provider's documentation should be used to guide the coding of postoperative pain, as well as *Section III. Reporting Additional Diagnoses* and *Section IV. Diagnostic Coding and Reporting in the Outpatient Setting.*

The default for post-thoracotomy and other postoperative pain not specified as acute or chronic is the code for the acute form.

Routine or expected postoperative pain immediately after surgery should not be coded.

(a) **Postoperative pain not associated with specific postoperative complication**
Postoperative pain not associated with a specific postoperative complication is assigned to the appropriate postoperative pain code in category G89.

(b) **Postoperative pain associated with specific postoperative complication**
Postoperative pain associated with a specific postoperative complication (such as painful wire sutures) is assigned to the appropriate code(s) found in Chapter 19, Injury, poisoning, and certain other consequences of external causes. If appropriate, use additional code(s) from category G89 to identify acute or chronic pain (G89.18 or G89.28).

4) **Chronic pain**
Chronic pain is classified to subcategory G89.2. There is no time frame defining when pain becomes chronic pain. The provider's documentation should be used to guide use of these codes.

5) **Neoplasm Related Pain**
Code G89.3 is assigned to pain documented as being related, associated or due to cancer, primary or secondary malignancy, or tumor. This code is assigned regardless of whether the pain is acute or chronic.

This code may be assigned as the principal or first-listed code when the stated reason for the admission/encounter is documented as pain control/pain management. The underlying neoplasm should be reported as an additional diagnosis.

When the reason for the admission/encounter is management of the neoplasm and the pain associated with the neoplasm is also documented, code G89.3 may be assigned as an additional diagnosis. It is not necessary to assign an additional code for the site of the pain.

*See Section I.C.2. for instructions on the sequencing of neoplasms for all other stated reasons for the admission/encounter (except for pain control/pain management).*

6) **Chronic pain syndrome**
Central pain syndrome (G89.0) and chronic pain syndrome (G89.4) are different than the term "chronic pain," and therefore codes should only be used when the provider has specifically documented this condition.

*See Section I.C.5. Pain disorders related to psychological factors*

## 7. Chapter 7: Diseases of the Eye and Adnexa (H00-H59)

### a. Glaucoma

1) **Assigning Glaucoma Codes**
Assign as many codes from category H40, Glaucoma, as needed to identify the type of glaucoma, the affected eye, and the glaucoma stage.

2) **Bilateral glaucoma with same type and stage**
When a patient has bilateral glaucoma and both eyes are documented as being the same type and stage, and there is a code for bilateral glaucoma, report only the code for the type of glaucoma, bilateral, with the seventh character for the stage.

When a patient has bilateral glaucoma and both eyes are documented as being the same type and stage, and the classification does not provide a code for bilateral glaucoma (i.e. subcategories H40.10, and H40.20) report only one code for the type of glaucoma with the appropriate seventh character for the stage.

3) **Bilateral glaucoma stage with different types or stages**
When a patient has bilateral glaucoma and each eye is documented as having a different type or stage, and the classification distinguishes laterality, assign the appropriate code for each eye rather than the code for bilateral glaucoma.

When a patient has bilateral glaucoma and each eye is documented as having a different type, and the classification does not distinguish laterality (i.e., subcategories H40.10, and H40.20), assign one code for each type of glaucoma with the appropriate seventh character for the stage.

When a patient has bilateral glaucoma and each eye is documented as having the same type, but different stage, and the classification does not distinguish laterality (i.e., subcategories H40.10 and H40.20), assign a code for the type of glaucoma for each eye with the seventh character for the specific glaucoma stage documented for each eye.

4) **Patient admitted with glaucoma and stage evolves during the admission**
If a patient is admitted with glaucoma and the stage progresses during the admission, assign the code for highest stage documented.

5) **Indeterminate stage glaucoma**
Assignment of the seventh character "4" for "indeterminate stage" should be based on the clinical documentation. The seventh character "4" is used for glaucomas whose stage cannot be clinically determined. This seventh character should not be confused with the seventh character "0", unspecified, which should be assigned when there is no documentation regarding the stage of the glaucoma.

### b. Blindness
If "blindness" or "low vision" of both eyes is documented but the visual impairment category is not documented, assign code H54.3, Unqualified visual loss, both eyes. If "blindness" or "low vision" in one eye is documented but the visual impairment category is not documented, assign a code from H54.6-, Unqualified visual loss, one eye. If "blindness" or "visual loss" is documented without any information about whether one or both eyes are affected, assign code H54.7, Unspecified visual loss.

## 8. Chapter 8: Diseases of the Ear and Mastoid Process (H60-H95)
Reserved for future guideline expansion

## 9. Chapter 9: Diseases of the Circulatory System (I00-I99)

### a. Hypertension
The classification presumes a causal relationship between hypertension and heart involvement and between hypertension and kidney involvement, as the two conditions are linked by the term "with" in the Alphabetic Index. These conditions should be coded as related even in the absence of provider documentation explicitly linking them, unless the documentation clearly states the conditions are unrelated.

For hypertension and conditions not specifically linked by relational terms such as "with," "associated with" or "due to" in the classification, provider documentation must link the conditions in order to code them as related.

1) **Hypertension with Heart Disease**
Hypertension with one or more heart conditions classified to I50.-, Heart failure, I51.4, Myocarditis, unspecified, I51.89, Other ill-defined heart diseases, or I51.9, Heart disease, unspecified, is assigned to a code from category I11, Hypertensive heart disease. Use additional code(s) from category I50, Heart failure, or I51, Complications and ill-defined descriptions of heart disease, to identify the heart condition.

Hypertension with one or more heart conditions classified to I51.5, Myocardial degeneration, or I51.7, Cardiomegaly, is assigned to a code from category I11, Hypertensive heart disease. No additional code is assigned to identify the specific heart condition.

The same heart conditions (I50.-, I51.4-I51.7, I51.89, I51.9) with hypertension are coded separately if the provider has documented they are unrelated to the hypertension. The applicable hypertension code I10, Essential (primary) hypertension, or a code from category I15, Secondary hypertension, should be assigned. Sequence according to the circumstances of the admission/encounter.

2) **Hypertensive Chronic Kidney Disease**
Assign codes from category I12, Hypertensive chronic kidney disease, when both hypertension and a condition classifiable to category N18, Chronic kidney disease (CKD), are present. CKD should not be coded as hypertensive if the provider indicates the CKD is not related to the hypertension.

The appropriate code from category N18 should be used as a secondary code with a code from category I12 to identify the stage of chronic kidney disease.

*See Section I.C.14. Chronic kidney disease.*

If a patient has hypertensive chronic kidney disease and acute renal failure, the acute renal failure should also be coded. Sequence according to the circumstances of the admission/encounter.

3) **Hypertensive Heart and Chronic Kidney Disease**
The codes in category I13, Hypertensive heart and chronic kidney disease, are combination codes that include hypertension, heart disease

and chronic kidney disease. Assign codes from combination category I13, Hypertensive heart and chronic kidney disease, when there is hypertension with both heart and chronic kidney disease. If heart failure is present, assign an additional code from category I5Ø to identify the type of heart failure.

The appropriate code from category N18, Chronic kidney disease, should be used as a secondary code with a code from category I13 to identify the stage of chronic kidney disease.

*See Section I.C.14. Chronic kidney disease.*

The Includes note at I13 specifies that the conditions included at I11 and I12 are included together in I13. If a patient has hypertension, heart disease and chronic kidney disease, then a code from I13 should be used, not codes from I11 or I12.

For patients with both acute renal failure and chronic kidney disease, the acute renal failure should also be coded. Sequence according to the circumstances of the admission/encounter.

**4) Hypertensive Cerebrovascular Disease**
For hypertensive cerebrovascular disease, first assign the appropriate code from categories I6Ø-I69, followed by the appropriate hypertension code.

**5) Hypertensive Retinopathy**
Subcategory H35.Ø, Background retinopathy and retinal vascular changes, should be used along with a code from categories I1Ø-I15, in the Hypertensive diseases section, to include the systemic hypertension. The sequencing is based on the reason for the encounter.

**6) Hypertension, Secondary**
Secondary hypertension is due to an underlying condition. Two codes are required: one to identify the underlying etiology and one from category I15 to identify the hypertension. Sequencing of codes is determined by the reason for admission/encounter.

**7) Hypertension, Transient**
Assign code RØ3.Ø, Elevated blood pressure reading without diagnosis of hypertension, unless patient has an established diagnosis of hypertension. Assign code O13.-, Gestational [pregnancy-induced] hypertension without significant proteinuria, or O14.-, Pre-eclampsia, for transient hypertension of pregnancy.

**8) Hypertension, Controlled**
This diagnostic statement usually refers to an existing state of hypertension under control by therapy. Assign the appropriate code from categories I1Ø-I15, Hypertensive diseases.

**9) Hypertension, Uncontrolled**
Uncontrolled hypertension may refer to untreated hypertension or hypertension not responding to current therapeutic regimen. In either case, assign the appropriate code from categories I1Ø-I15, Hypertensive diseases.

**10) Hypertensive Crisis**
Assign a code from category I16, Hypertensive crisis, for documented hypertensive urgency, hypertensive emergency or unspecified hypertensive crisis. Code also any identified hypertensive disease (I1Ø-I15, **I1A**). The sequencing is based on the reason for the encounter.

**11) Pulmonary Hypertension**
Pulmonary hypertension is classified to category I27, Other pulmonary heart diseases. For secondary pulmonary hypertension (I27.1, I27.2-), code also any associated conditions or adverse effects of drugs or toxins.

The sequencing is based on the reason for the encounter, except for adverse effects of drugs (See Section I.C.19.e.).

**12) Hypertension, Resistant**
Resistant hypertension refers to blood pressure of a patient with hypertension that remains above goal in spite of the use of antihypertensive medications. Assign code I1A.Ø, Resistant hypertension, as an additional code when apparent treatment resistant hypertension, treatment resistant hypertension, or true resistant hypertension is documented by the provider. A code for the specific type of existing hypertension is sequenced first, if known.

**b. Atherosclerotic Coronary Artery Disease and Angina**
ICD-10-CM has combination codes for atherosclerotic heart disease with angina pectoris. The subcategories for these codes are I25.11, Atherosclerotic heart disease of native coronary artery with angina pectoris and I25.7, Atherosclerosis of coronary artery bypass graft(s) and coronary artery of transplanted heart with angina pectoris.

When using one of these combination codes it is not necessary to use an additional code for angina pectoris. A causal relationship can be assumed in a patient with both atherosclerosis and angina pectoris, unless the documentation indicates the angina is due to something other than the atherosclerosis.

If a patient with coronary artery disease is admitted due to an acute myocardial infarction (AMI), the AMI should be sequenced before the coronary artery disease.

*See Section I.C.9. Acute myocardial infarction (AMI)*

**c. Intraoperative and Postprocedural Cerebrovascular Accident**
Medical record documentation should clearly specify the cause- and-effect relationship between the medical intervention and the cerebrovascular accident in order to assign a code for intraoperative or postprocedural cerebrovascular accident.

Proper code assignment depends on whether it was an infarction or hemorrhage and whether it occurred intraoperatively or postoperatively. If it was a cerebral hemorrhage, code assignment depends on the type of procedure performed.

**d. Sequelae of Cerebrovascular Disease**

**1) Category I69, Sequelae of Cerebrovascular disease**
Category I69 is used to indicate conditions classifiable to categories I6Ø-I67 as the causes of sequela (neurologic deficits), themselves classified elsewhere. These "late effects" include neurologic deficits that persist after initial onset of conditions classifiable to categories I6Ø-I67. The neurologic deficits caused by cerebrovascular disease may be present from the onset or may arise at any time after the onset of the condition classifiable to categories I6Ø-I67.

Codes from category I69, Sequelae of cerebrovascular disease, that specify hemiplegia, hemiparesis and monoplegia identify whether the dominant or nondominant side is affected. Should the affected side be documented, but not specified as dominant or nondominant, and the classification system does not indicate a default, code selection is as follows:

- For ambidextrous patients, the default should be dominant.
- If the left side is affected, the default is non-dominant.
- If the right side is affected, the default is dominant.

**2) Codes from category I69 with codes from I6Ø-I67**
Codes from category I69 may be assigned on a health care record with codes from I6Ø-I67, if the patient has a current cerebrovascular disease and deficits from an old cerebrovascular disease.

**3) Codes from category I69 and Personal history of transient ischemic attack (TIA) and cerebral infarction (Z86.73)**
Codes from category I69 should not be assigned if the patient does not have neurologic deficits.

*See Section I.C.21.4. History (of) for use of personal history codes*

**e. Acute myocardial infarction (AMI)**

**1) Type 1 ST elevation myocardial infarction (STEMI) and non-ST elevation myocardial infarction (NSTEMI)**
The ICD-10-CM codes for type 1 acute myocardial infarction (AMI) identify the site, such as anterolateral wall or true posterior wall. Subcategories I21.Ø-I21.2 and code I21.3 are used for type 1 ST elevation myocardial infarction (STEMI). Code I21.4, Non-ST elevation (NSTEMI) myocardial infarction, is used for type 1 non-ST elevation myocardial infarction (NSTEMI) and nontransmural MIs.

If a type 1 NSTEMI evolves to STEMI, assign the STEMI code. If a type 1 STEMI converts to NSTEMI due to thrombolytic therapy, it is still coded as STEMI.

For encounters occurring while the myocardial infarction is equal to, or less than, four weeks old, including transfers to another acute setting or a postacute setting, and the myocardial infarction meets the definition for "other diagnoses" (see Section III, Reporting Additional Diagnoses), codes from category I21 may continue to be reported. For encounters after the 4-week time frame and the patient is still receiving care related to the myocardial infarction, the appropriate aftercare code should be assigned, rather than a code from category I21. For old or healed myocardial infarctions not requiring further care, code I25.2, Old myocardial infarction, may be assigned.

**2) Acute myocardial infarction, unspecified**
Code I21.9, Acute myocardial infarction, unspecified, is the default for unspecified acute myocardial infarction or unspecified type. If only type 1 STEMI or transmural MI without the site is documented, assign code I21.3, ST elevation (STEMI) myocardial infarction of unspecified site.

**3) AMI documented as nontransmural or subendocardial but site provided**
If an AMI is documented as nontransmural or subendocardial, but the site is provided, it is still coded as a subendocardial AMI.

*See Section I.C.21.3. for information on coding status post administration of tPA in a different facility within the last 24 hours.*

**4) Subsequent acute myocardial infarction**
A code from category I22, Subsequent ST elevation (STEMI) and non-ST elevation (NSTEMI) myocardial infarction, is to be used when a patient who has suffered a type 1 or unspecified AMI has a new AMI within the 4 week time frame of the initial AMI. A code from category I22 must be used in conjunction with a code from category I21. The sequencing of the I22 and I21 codes depends on the circumstances of the encounter.

Do not assign code I22 for subsequent myocardial infarctions other than type 1 or unspecified. For subsequent type 2 AMI assign only code I21.A1. For subsequent type 4 or type 5 AMI, assign only code I21.A9.

If a subsequent myocardial infarction of one type occurs within 4 weeks of a myocardial infarction of a different type, assign the appropriate codes from category I21 to identify each type. Do not assign a code from I22. Codes from category I22 should only be assigned if both the initial and subsequent myocardial infarctions are type 1 or unspecified.

**5) Other Types of Myocardial Infarction**
The ICD-10-CM provides codes for different types of myocardial infarction. Type 1 myocardial infarctions are assigned to codes I21.Ø-I21.4.

Type 2 myocardial infarction (myocardial infarction due to demand ischemia or secondary to ischemic imbalance) is assigned to code I21.A1, Myocardial infarction type 2 with the underlying cause coded first, if applicable. Do not assign code I24.89, Other forms of acute ischemic heart disease, for the demand ischemia. If a type 2 AMI is described as NSTEMI or STEMI, only assign code I21.A1. Codes I21.Ø1-I21.4 should only be assigned for type 1 AMIs.

Acute myocardial infarctions type 3, 4a, 4b, 4c and 5 are assigned to code I21.A9, Other myocardial infarction type.

The "Code also" and "Code first" notes should be followed related to complications, and for coding of postprocedural myocardial infarctions during or following cardiac surgery.

**6) Myocardial Infarction with Coronary Microvascular Dysfunction**
Coronary microvascular dysfunction (CMD) is a condition that impacts the microvasculature by restricting microvascular flow and increasing microvascular resistance. Code I21.B, Myocardial infarction with coronary microvascular dysfunction, is assigned for myocardial infarction with coronary microvascular disease, myocardial infarction with coronary microvascular dysfunction, and myocardial infarction with non-obstructive coronary arteries (MINOCA) with microvascular disease.

## 10. Chapter 10: Diseases of the Respiratory System (JØØ-J99), UØ7.Ø

### a. Chronic Obstructive Pulmonary Disease [COPD] and Asthma

**1) Acute exacerbation of chronic obstructive bronchitis and asthma**
The codes in categories J44 and J45 distinguish between uncomplicated cases and those in acute exacerbation. An acute exacerbation is a worsening or a decompensation of a chronic condition. An acute exacerbation is not equivalent to an infection superimposed on a chronic condition, though an exacerbation may be triggered by an infection.

### b. Acute Respiratory Failure

**1) Acute respiratory failure as principal diagnosis**
A code from subcategory J96.Ø, Acute respiratory failure, or subcategory J96.2, Acute and chronic respiratory failure, may be assigned as a principal diagnosis when it is the condition established after study to be chiefly responsible for occasioning the admission to the hospital, and the selection is supported by the Alphabetic Index and Tabular List. However, chapter-specific coding guidelines (such as obstetrics, poisoning, HIV, newborn) that provide sequencing direction take precedence.

**2) Acute respiratory failure as secondary diagnosis**
Respiratory failure may be listed as a secondary diagnosis if it occurs after admission, or if it is present on admission, but does not meet the definition of principal diagnosis.

**3) Sequencing of acute respiratory failure and another acute condition**
When a patient is admitted with respiratory failure and another acute condition, (e.g., myocardial infarction, cerebrovascular accident, aspiration pneumonia), the principal diagnosis will not be the same in every situation. This applies whether the other acute condition is a respiratory or nonrespiratory condition. Selection of the principal diagnosis will be dependent on the circumstances of admission. If both the respiratory failure and the other acute condition are equally responsible for occasioning the admission to the hospital, and there are no chapter-specific sequencing rules, the guideline regarding two or more diagnoses that equally meet the definition for principal diagnosis (Section II, C.) may be applied in these situations.

If the documentation is not clear as to whether acute respiratory failure and another condition are equally responsible for occasioning the admission, query the provider for clarification.

### c. Influenza due to certain identified influenza viruses

Code only confirmed cases of influenza due to certain identified influenza viruses (category JØ9), and due to other identified influenza virus (category J1Ø). This is an exception to the hospital inpatient guideline Section II, H. (Uncertain Diagnosis).

In this context, "confirmation" does not require documentation of positive laboratory testing specific for avian or other novel influenza A or other identified influenza virus. However, coding should be based on the provider's diagnostic statement that the patient has avian influenza, or other novel influenza A, for category JØ9, or has another particular identified strain of influenza, such as H1N1 or H3N2, but not identified as novel or variant, for category J1Ø.

If the provider records "suspected" or "possible" or "probable" avian influenza, or novel influenza, or other identified influenza, then the appropriate influenza code from category J11, Influenza due to unidentified influenza virus, should be assigned. A code from category JØ9, Influenza due to certain identified influenza viruses, should not be assigned nor should a code from category J1Ø, Influenza due to other identified influenza virus.

### d. Ventilator associated Pneumonia

**1) Documentation of Ventilator associated Pneumonia**
As with all procedural or postprocedural complications, code assignment is based on the provider's documentation of the relationship between the condition and the procedure.

Code J95.851, Ventilator associated pneumonia, should be assigned only when the provider has documented ventilator associated pneumonia (VAP). An additional code to identify the organism (e.g., Pseudomonas aeruginosa, code B96.5) should also be assigned. Do not assign an additional code from categories J12-J18 to identify the type of pneumonia.

Code J95.851 should not be assigned for cases where the patient has pneumonia and is on a mechanical ventilator and the provider has not specifically stated that the pneumonia is ventilator-associated pneumonia. If the documentation is unclear as to whether the patient has a pneumonia that is a complication attributable to the mechanical ventilator, query the provider.

**2) Ventilator associated Pneumonia Develops after Admission**
A patient may be admitted with one type of pneumonia (e.g., code J13, Pneumonia due to Streptococcus pneumonia) and subsequently develop VAP. In this instance, the principal diagnosis would be the appropriate code from categories J12-J18 for the pneumonia diagnosed at the time of admission. Code J95.851, Ventilator associated pneumonia, would be assigned as an additional diagnosis when the provider has also documented the presence of ventilator associated pneumonia.

### e. Vaping-related disorders

For patients presenting with condition(s) related to vaping, assign code UØ7.Ø, Vaping-related disorder, as the principal diagnosis. For lung injury due to vaping, assign only code UØ7.Ø. Assign additional codes for other manifestations, such as acute respiratory failure (subcategory J96.Ø-) or pneumonitis (code J68.Ø).

Associated respiratory signs and symptoms due to vaping, such as cough, shortness of breath, etc., are not coded separately, when a definitive diagnosis has been established. However, it would be appropriate to code separately any gastrointestinal symptoms, such as diarrhea and abdominal pain.

*See Section I.C.1.g.1.c.i. for Pneumonia confirmed as due to COVID-19*

## 11. Chapter 11: Diseases of the Digestive System (KØØ-K95)

Reserved for future guideline expansion

## 12. Chapter 12: Diseases of the Skin and Subcutaneous Tissue (LØØ-L99)

### a. Pressure ulcer stage codes

**1) Pressure ulcer stages**
Codes in category L89, Pressure ulcer, identify the site and stage of the pressure ulcer.

The ICD-10-CM classifies pressure ulcer stages based on severity, which is designated by stages 1-4, deep tissue pressure injury, unspecified stage, and unstageable.

Assign as many codes from category L89 as needed to identify all the pressure ulcers the patient has, if applicable.

*See Section I.B.14. for pressure ulcer stage documentation by clinicians other than patient's provider.*

**2) Unstageable pressure ulcers**
Assignment of the code for unstageable pressure ulcer (L89.--Ø) should be based on the clinical documentation. These codes are used for pressure ulcers whose stage cannot be clinically determined (e.g., the ulcer is covered by eschar or has been treated with a skin or muscle graft). This code should not be confused with the codes for unspecified stage (L89.--9). When there is no documentation regarding the stage of the pressure ulcer, assign the appropriate code for unspecified stage (L89.-- 9).

If during an encounter, the stage of an unstageable pressure ulcer is revealed after debridement, assign only the code for the stage revealed following debridement.

**3) Documented pressure ulcer stage**
Assignment of the pressure ulcer stage code should be guided by clinical documentation of the stage or documentation of the terms found in the Alphabetic Index. For clinical terms describing the stage that are not found in the Alphabetic Index, and there is no documentation of the stage, the provider should be queried.

**4) Patients admitted with pressure ulcers documented as healed**
No code is assigned if the documentation states that the pressure ulcer is completely healed at the time of admission.

**5) Pressure ulcers documented as healing**
Pressure ulcers described as healing should be assigned the appropriate pressure ulcer stage code based on the documentation in the medical record. If the documentation does not provide information about the stage of the healing pressure ulcer, assign the appropriate code for unspecified stage.

If the documentation is unclear as to whether the patient has a current (new) pressure ulcer or if the patient is being treated for a healing pressure ulcer, query the provider.

For ulcers that were present on admission but healed at the time of discharge, assign the code for the site and stage of the pressure ulcer at the time of admission.

**6) Patient admitted with pressure ulcer evolving into another stage during the admission**
If a patient is admitted to an inpatient hospital with a pressure ulcer at one stage and it progresses to a higher stage, two separate codes should be assigned: one code for the site and stage of the ulcer on admission and a second code for the same ulcer site and the highest stage reported during the stay.

**7) Pressure-induced deep tissue damage**
For pressure-induced deep tissue damage or deep tissue pressure injury, assign only the appropriate code for pressure-induced deep tissue damage (L89.--6).

**b. Non-Pressure Chronic Ulcers**

**1) Patients admitted with non-pressure ulcers documented as healed**
No code is assigned if the documentation states that the non-pressure ulcer is completely healed at the time of admission.

**2) Non-pressure ulcers documented as healing**
Non-pressure ulcers described as healing should be assigned the appropriate non-pressure ulcer code based on the documentation in the medical record. If the documentation does not provide information about the severity of the healing non-pressure ulcer, assign the appropriate code for unspecified severity.

If the documentation is unclear as to whether the patient has a current (new) non-pressure ulcer or if the patient is being treated for a healing non-pressure ulcer, query the provider.

For ulcers that were present on admission but healed at the time of discharge, assign the code for the site and severity of the non-pressure ulcer at the time of admission.

**3) Patient admitted with non-pressure ulcer that progresses to another severity level during the admission**
If a patient is admitted to an inpatient hospital with a non-pressure ulcer at one severity level and it progresses to a higher severity level, two separate codes should be assigned: one code for the site and severity level of the ulcer on admission and a second code for the same ulcer site and the highest severity level reported during the stay.

*See Section I.B.14. for pressure ulcer stage documentation by clinicians other than patient's provider*

**13. Chapter 13: Diseases of the Musculoskeletal System and Connective Tissue (M00-M99)**

**a. Site and laterality**
Most of the codes within Chapter 13 have site and laterality designations. The site represents the bone, joint or the muscle involved.

**1) Bone versus joint**
For certain conditions, the bone may be affected at the upper or lower end, (e.g., avascular necrosis of bone, M87, Osteoporosis, M80, M81). Though the portion of the bone affected may be at the joint, the site designation will be the bone, not the joint.

**2) Multiple sites**
Codes describing specified sites are assigned individually by site when documented. When the specified site(s) are not documented, assign the appropriate code for "multiple sites."

**b. Acute traumatic versus chronic or recurrent musculoskeletal conditions**
Many musculoskeletal conditions are a result of previous injury or trauma to a site, or are recurrent conditions. Bone, joint or muscle conditions that are the result of a healed injury are usually found in chapter 13. Recurrent bone, joint or muscle conditions are also usually found in chapter 13. Any current, acute injury should be coded to the appropriate injury code from chapter 19. Chronic or recurrent conditions should generally be coded with a code from chapter 13. If it is difficult to determine from the documentation in the record which code is best to describe a condition, query the provider.

**c. Coding of Pathologic Fractures**
7th character A is for use as long as the patient is receiving active treatment for the fracture. While the patient may be seen by a new or different provider over the course of treatment for a pathological fracture, assignment of the 7th character is based on whether the patient is undergoing active treatment and not whether the provider is seeing the patient for the first time.

7th character D is to be used for encounters after the patient has completed active treatment for the fracture and is receiving routine care for the fracture during the healing or recovery phase. The other 7th characters, listed under each subcategory in the Tabular List, are to be used for subsequent encounters for treatment of problems associated with the healing, such as malunions, nonunions, and sequelae.

Care for complications of surgical treatment for fracture repairs during the healing or recovery phase should be coded with the appropriate complication codes.

*See Section I.C.19. Coding of traumatic fractures.*

**d. Osteoporosis**
Osteoporosis is a systemic condition, meaning that all bones of the musculoskeletal system are affected. Therefore, site is not a component of the codes under category M81, Osteoporosis without current pathological fracture. The site codes under category M80, Osteoporosis with current pathological fracture, identify the site of the fracture, not the osteoporosis.

**1) Osteoporosis without pathological fracture**
Category M81, Osteoporosis without current pathological fracture, is for use for patients with osteoporosis who do not currently have a pathologic fracture due to the osteoporosis, even if they have had a fracture in the past. For patients with a history of osteoporosis fractures, status code Z87.310, Personal history of (healed) osteoporosis fracture, should follow the code from M81.

**2) Osteoporosis with current pathological fracture**
Category M80, Osteoporosis with current pathological fracture, is for patients who have a current pathologic fracture at the time of an encounter. The codes under M80 identify the site of the fracture. A code from category M80, not a traumatic fracture code, should be used for any patient with known osteoporosis who suffers a fracture, even if the patient had a minor fall or trauma, if that fall or trauma would not usually break a normal, healthy bone.

**e. Multisystem Inflammatory Syndrome**
*See Section I.C.1.g.1.l. for Multisystem Inflammatory Syndrome*

**14. Chapter 14: Diseases of Genitourinary System (N00-N99)**

**a. Chronic kidney disease**

**1) Stages of chronic kidney disease (CKD)**
The ICD-10-CM classifies CKD based on severity. The severity of CKD is designated by stages 1-5. Stage 2, code N18.2, equates to mild CKD; stage 3, codes N18.30-N18.32, equate to moderate CKD; and stage 4, code N18.4, equates to severe CKD. Code N18.6, End stage renal disease (ESRD), is assigned when the provider has documented end-stage renal disease (ESRD).

If both a stage of CKD and ESRD are documented, assign code N18.6 only.

**2) Chronic kidney disease and kidney transplant status**
Patients who have undergone kidney transplant may still have some form of chronic kidney disease (CKD) because the kidney transplant may not fully restore kidney function. Therefore, the presence of CKD alone does not constitute a transplant complication. Assign the appropriate N18 code for the patient's stage of CKD and code Z94.0, Kidney transplant status. If a transplant complication such as failure or rejection or other transplant complication is documented, see section I.C.19.g for information on coding complications of a kidney transplant. If the documentation is unclear as to whether the patient has a complication of the transplant, query the provider.

**3) Chronic kidney disease with other conditions**
Patients with CKD may also suffer from other serious conditions, most commonly diabetes mellitus and hypertension. The sequencing of the CKD code in relationship to codes for other contributing conditions is based on the conventions in the Tabular List.

*See I.C.9. Hypertensive chronic kidney disease.*

*See I.C.19. Chronic kidney disease and kidney transplant complications.*

**15. Chapter 15: Pregnancy, Childbirth, and the Puerperium (O00-O9A)**

**a. General Rules for Obstetric Cases**

**1) Codes from chapter 15 and sequencing priority**
Obstetric cases require codes from chapter 15, codes in the range O00-O9A, Pregnancy, Childbirth, and the Puerperium. Chapter 15 codes have sequencing priority over codes from other chapters. Additional codes from other chapters may be used in conjunction with chapter 15 codes to further specify conditions. Should the provider document that the pregnancy is incidental to the encounter, then code Z33.1, Pregnant state, incidental, should be used in place of any chapter 15 codes. It is the provider's responsibility to state that the condition being treated is not affecting the pregnancy.

**2) Chapter 15 codes used only on the maternal record**
Chapter 15 codes are to be used only on the maternal record, never on the record of the newborn.

**3) Final character for trimester**
The majority of codes in Chapter 15 have a final character indicating the trimester of pregnancy. The timeframes for the trimesters are indicated at the beginning of the chapter. If trimester is not a component of a

code, it is because the condition always occurs in a specific trimester, or the concept of trimester of pregnancy is not applicable. Certain codes have characters for only certain trimesters because the condition does not occur in all trimesters, but it may occur in more than just one.

Assignment of the final character for trimester should be based on the provider's documentation of the trimester (or number of weeks) for the current admission/encounter. This applies to the assignment of trimester for pre-existing conditions as well as those that develop during or are due to the pregnancy. The provider's documentation of the number of weeks may be used to assign the appropriate code identifying the trimester.

Whenever delivery occurs during the current admission, and there is an "in childbirth" option for the obstetric complication being coded, the "in childbirth" code should be assigned. When the classification does not provide an obstetric code with an "in childbirth" option, it is appropriate to assign a code describing the current trimester.

**4) Selection of trimester for inpatient admissions that encompass more than one trimester**

In instances when a patient is admitted to a hospital for complications of pregnancy during one trimester and remains in the hospital into a subsequent trimester, the trimester character for the antepartum complication code should be assigned on the basis of the trimester when the complication developed, not the trimester of the discharge. If the condition developed prior to the current admission/encounter or represents a pre-existing condition, the trimester character for the trimester at the time of the admission/encounter should be assigned.

**5) Unspecified trimester**

Each category that includes codes for trimester has a code for "unspecified trimester." The "unspecified trimester" code should rarely be used, such as when the documentation in the record is insufficient to determine the trimester and it is not possible to obtain clarification.

**6) 7th character for fetus identification**

Where applicable, a 7th character is to be assigned for certain categories (O31, O32, O33.3-O33.6, O35, O36, O4Ø, O41, O6Ø.1, O6Ø.2, O64, and O69) to identify the fetus for which the complication code applies.

Assign 7th character "Ø":

- For single gestations
- When the documentation in the record is insufficient to determine the fetus affected and it is not possible to obtain clarification.
- When it is not possible to clinically determine which fetus is affected.

**7) Completed weeks of gestation**

In ICD-10-CM, "completed" weeks of gestation refers to full weeks. For example, if the provider documents gestation at 39 weeks and 6 days, the code for 39 weeks of gestation should be assigned, as the patient has not yet reached 40 completed weeks.

**b. Selection of OB Principal or First-listed Diagnosis**

**1) Routine outpatient prenatal visits**

For routine outpatient prenatal visits when no complications are present, a code from category Z34, Encounter for supervision of normal pregnancy, should be used as the first-listed diagnosis. These codes should not be used in conjunction with chapter 15 codes.

**2) Supervision of High-Risk Pregnancy**

Codes from category OØ9, Supervision of high-risk pregnancy, are intended for use only during the prenatal period. For complications during the labor or delivery episode as a result of a high-risk pregnancy, assign the applicable complication codes from Chapter 15. If there are no complications during the labor or delivery episode, assign code O8Ø, Encounter for full-term uncomplicated delivery.

For routine prenatal outpatient visits for patients with high-risk pregnancies, a code from category OØ9, Supervision of high-risk pregnancy, should be used as the first-listed diagnosis. Secondary chapter 15 codes may be used in conjunction with these codes if appropriate.

**3) Episodes when no delivery occurs**

In episodes when no delivery occurs, the principal diagnosis should correspond to the principal complication of the pregnancy which necessitated the encounter. Should more than one complication exist, all of which are treated or monitored, any of the complication codes may be sequenced first.

**4) When a delivery occurs**

When an obstetric patient is admitted and delivers during that admission, the condition that prompted the admission should be sequenced as the principal diagnosis. If multiple conditions prompted the admission, sequence the one most related to the delivery as the principal diagnosis. A code for any complication of the delivery should be assigned as an additional diagnosis. In cases of cesarean delivery, if the patient was admitted with a condition that resulted in the performance of a cesarean procedure, that condition should be selected as the principal diagnosis. If the reason for the admission was unrelated to the condition resulting in the cesarean delivery, the condition related to the reason for the admission should be selected as the principal diagnosis.

**5) Outcome of delivery**

A code from category Z37, Outcome of delivery, should be included on every maternal record when a delivery has occurred. These codes are not to be used on subsequent records or on the newborn record.

**c. Pre-existing conditions versus conditions due to the pregnancy**

Certain categories in Chapter 15 distinguish between conditions of the mother that existed prior to pregnancy (pre-existing) and those that are a direct result of pregnancy. When assigning codes from Chapter 15, it is important to assess if a condition was pre-existing prior to pregnancy or developed during or due to the pregnancy in order to assign the correct code.

Categories that do not distinguish between pre-existing and pregnancy-related conditions may be used for either. It is acceptable to use codes specifically for the puerperium with codes complicating pregnancy and childbirth if a condition arises postpartum during the delivery encounter.

**d. Pre-existing hypertension in pregnancy**

Category O1Ø, Pre-existing hypertension complicating pregnancy, childbirth and the puerperium, includes codes for hypertensive heart and hypertensive chronic kidney disease. When assigning one of the O1Ø codes that includes hypertensive heart disease or hypertensive chronic kidney disease, it is necessary to add a secondary code from the appropriate hypertension category to specify the type of heart failure or chronic kidney disease.

*See Section I.C.9. Hypertension.*

**e. Fetal Conditions Affecting the Management of the Mother**

**1) Codes from categories O35 and O36**

Codes from categories O35, Maternal care for known or suspected fetal abnormality and damage, and O36, Maternal care for other fetal problems, are assigned only when the fetal condition is actually responsible for modifying the management of the mother, i.e., by requiring diagnostic studies, additional observation, special care, or termination of pregnancy. The fact that the fetal condition exists does not justify assigning a code from this series to the mother's record.

**2) In utero surgery**

In cases when surgery is performed on the fetus, a diagnosis code from category O35, Maternal care for known or suspected fetal abnormality and damage, should be assigned identifying the fetal condition. Assign the appropriate procedure code for the procedure performed.

No code from Chapter 16, the perinatal codes, should be used on the mother's record to identify fetal conditions. Surgery performed in utero on a fetus is still to be coded as an obstetric encounter.

**f. HIV Infection in Pregnancy, Childbirth and the Puerperium**

During pregnancy, childbirth or the puerperium, a patient admitted because of an HIV-related illness should receive a principal diagnosis from subcategory O98.7-, Human immunodeficiency [HIV] disease complicating pregnancy, childbirth and the puerperium, followed by the code(s) for the HIV-related illness(es).

Patients with asymptomatic HIV infection status admitted during pregnancy, childbirth, or the puerperium should receive codes of O98.7- and Z21, Asymptomatic human immunodeficiency virus [HIV] infection status.

**g. Diabetes mellitus in pregnancy**

Diabetes mellitus is a significant complicating factor in pregnancy. Pregnant patients who are diabetic should be assigned a code from category O24, Diabetes mellitus in pregnancy, childbirth, and the puerperium, first, followed by the appropriate diabetes code(s) (EØ8-E13) from Chapter 4.

**h. Long term use of insulin and oral hypoglycemics**

*See section I.C.4.a.3 for information on the long-term use of insulin and oral hypoglycemics.*

**i. Gestational (pregnancy induced) diabetes**

Gestational (pregnancy induced) diabetes can occur during the second and third trimester of pregnancy in patients who were not diabetic prior to pregnancy. Gestational diabetes can cause complications in the pregnancy similar to those of pre-existing diabetes mellitus. It also puts the patient at greater risk of developing diabetes after the pregnancy.

Codes for gestational diabetes are in subcategory O24.4, Gestational diabetes mellitus. No other code from category O24, Diabetes mellitus in pregnancy, childbirth, and the puerperium, should be used with a code from O24.4.

The codes under subcategory O24.4 include diet controlled, insulin controlled, and controlled by oral hypoglycemic drugs. If a patient with gestational diabetes is treated with both diet and insulin, only the code for insulin-controlled is required. If a patient with gestational diabetes is treated with both diet and oral hypoglycemic medications, only the code for "controlled by oral hypoglycemic drugs" is required. Codes Z79.4, Long-term (current) use of insulin, Z79.84, Long-term (current) use of oral hypoglycemic drugs, and Z79.85, Long-term (current) use of injectable non-insulin antidiabetic drugs, should not be assigned with codes from subcategory O24.4.

An abnormal glucose tolerance in pregnancy is assigned a code from subcategory O99.81, Abnormal glucose complicating pregnancy, childbirth, and the puerperium.

**j. Sepsis and septic shock complicating abortion, pregnancy, childbirth and the puerperium**

When assigning a chapter 15 code for sepsis complicating abortion, pregnancy, childbirth, and the puerperium, a code for the specific type of infection should be assigned as an additional diagnosis. If severe sepsis is present, a code from subcategory R65.2, Severe sepsis, and code(s) for associated organ dysfunction(s) should also be assigned as additional diagnoses.

**k. Puerperal sepsis**

Code O85, Puerperal sepsis, should be assigned with a secondary code to identify the causal organism (e.g., for a bacterial infection, assign a code from category B95-B96, Bacterial infections in conditions classified elsewhere). A code from category A4Ø, Streptococcal sepsis, or A41, Other sepsis, should not be used for puerperal sepsis. If applicable, use additional codes to identify severe sepsis (R65.2-) and any associated acute organ dysfunction.

Code O85 should not be assigned for sepsis following an obstetrical procedure (See Section I.C.1.d.5.b., Sepsis due to a postprocedural infection).

**l. Alcohol, tobacco and drug use during pregnancy, childbirth and the puerperium**

**1) Alcohol use during pregnancy, childbirth and the puerperium**

Codes under subcategory O99.31, Alcohol use complicating pregnancy, childbirth, and the puerperium, should be assigned for any pregnancy case when a patient uses alcohol during the pregnancy or postpartum. A secondary code from category F1Ø, Alcohol related disorders, should also be assigned to identify manifestations of the alcohol use.

**2) Tobacco use during pregnancy, childbirth and the puerperium**

Codes under subcategory O99.33, Smoking (tobacco) complicating pregnancy, childbirth, and the puerperium, should be assigned for any pregnancy case when a patient uses any type of tobacco product during the pregnancy or postpartum.

A secondary code from category F17, Nicotine dependence, should also be assigned to identify the type of nicotine dependence.

**3) Drug use during pregnancy, childbirth and the puerperium**

Codes under subcategory O99.32, Drug use complicating pregnancy, childbirth, and the puerperium, should be assigned for any pregnancy case when a patient uses drugs during the pregnancy or postpartum. This can involve illegal drugs, or inappropriate use or abuse of prescription drugs. Secondary code(s) from categories F11-F16 and F18-F19 should also be assigned to identify manifestations of the drug use.

**m. Poisoning, toxic effects, adverse effects and underdosing in a pregnant patient**

A code from subcategory O9A.2, Injury, poisoning and certain other consequences of external causes complicating pregnancy, childbirth, and the puerperium, should be sequenced first, followed by the appropriate injury, poisoning, toxic effect, adverse effect or underdosing code, and then the additional code(s) that specifies the condition caused by the poisoning, toxic effect, adverse effect or underdosing.

*See Section I.C.19. Adverse effects, poisoning, underdosing and toxic effects.*

**n. Normal Delivery, Code O8Ø**

**1) Encounter for full term uncomplicated delivery**

Code O8Ø should be assigned when a patient is admitted for a full-term normal delivery and delivers a single, healthy infant without any complications antepartum, during the delivery, or postpartum during the delivery episode. Code O8Ø is always a principal diagnosis. It is not to be used if any other code from chapter 15 is needed to describe a current complication of the antenatal, delivery, or postnatal period. Additional codes from other chapters may be used with code O8Ø if they are not related to or are in any way complicating the pregnancy.

**2) Uncomplicated delivery with resolved antepartum complication**

Code O8Ø may be used if the patient had a complication at some point during the pregnancy, but the complication is not present at the time of the admission for delivery.

**3) Outcome of delivery for O8Ø**

Z37.Ø, Single live birth, is the only outcome of delivery code appropriate for use with O8Ø.

**o. The Peripartum and Postpartum Periods**

**1) Peripartum and Postpartum periods**

The postpartum period begins immediately after delivery and continues for six weeks following delivery. The peripartum period is defined as the last month of pregnancy to five months postpartum.

**2) Peripartum and postpartum complication**

A postpartum complication is any complication occurring within the six-week period.

**3) Pregnancy-related complications after 6-week period**

Chapter 15 codes may also be used to describe pregnancy-related complications after the peripartum or postpartum period if the provider documents that a condition is pregnancy related.

**4) Admission for routine postpartum care following delivery outside hospital**

When the mother delivers outside the hospital prior to admission and is admitted for routine postpartum care and no complications are noted, code Z39.Ø, Encounter for care and examination of mother immediately after delivery, should be assigned as the principal diagnosis.

**5) Pregnancy associated cardiomyopathy**

Pregnancy associated cardiomyopathy, code O9Ø.3, is unique in that it may be diagnosed in the third trimester of pregnancy but may continue to progress months after delivery. For this reason, it is referred to as peripartum cardiomyopathy. Code O9Ø.3 is only for use when the cardiomyopathy develops as a result of pregnancy in a patient who did not have pre-existing heart disease.

**p. Code O94, Sequelae of complication of pregnancy, childbirth, and the puerperium**

**1) Code O94**

Code O94, Sequelae of complication of pregnancy, childbirth, and the puerperium, is for use in those cases when an initial complication of a pregnancy develops a sequela or sequelae requiring care or treatment at a future date.

**2) After the initial postpartum period**

This code may be used at any time after the initial postpartum period.

**3) Sequencing of Code O94**

This code, like all sequela codes, is to be sequenced following the code describing the sequelae of the complication.

**q. Termination of Pregnancy and Spontaneous abortions**

**1) Abortion with Liveborn Fetus**

When an attempted termination of pregnancy results in a liveborn fetus, assign code Z33.2, Encounter for elective termination of pregnancy and a code from category Z37, Outcome of Delivery.

**2) Retained Products of Conception following an abortion**

Subsequent encounters for retained products of conception following a spontaneous abortion or elective termination of pregnancy, without complications are assigned OØ3.4, Incomplete spontaneous abortion without complication, or code OØ7.4, Failed attempted termination of pregnancy without complication. This advice is appropriate even when the patient was discharged previously with a discharge diagnosis of complete abortion. If the patient has a specific complication associated with the spontaneous abortion or elective termination of pregnancy in addition to retained products of conception, assign the appropriate complication code (e.g., OØ3.-, OØ4.-, OØ7.-) instead of code OØ3.4 or OØ7.4.

**3) Complications leading to abortion**

Codes from Chapter 15 may be used as additional codes to identify any documented complications of the pregnancy in conjunction with codes in categories in OØ4, OØ7 and OØ8.

**4) Hemorrhage following elective abortion**

For hemorrhage post elective abortion, assign code OØ4.6, Delayed or excessive hemorrhage following (induced) termination of pregnancy. Do not assign code O72.1, Other immediate postpartum hemorrhage, as this code should not be assigned for post abortion conditions.

**r. Abuse in a pregnant patient**

For suspected or confirmed cases of abuse of a pregnant patient, a code(s) from subcategories O9A.3, Physical abuse complicating pregnancy, childbirth, and the puerperium, O9A.4, Sexual abuse complicating pregnancy, childbirth, and the puerperium, and O9A.5, Psychological abuse complicating pregnancy, childbirth, and the puerperium, should be sequenced first, followed by the appropriate codes (if applicable) to identify any associated current injury due to physical abuse, sexual abuse, and the perpetrator of abuse.

*See Section I.C.19. Adult and child abuse, neglect and other maltreatment.*

**s. COVID-19 infection in pregnancy, childbirth, and the puerperium**

During pregnancy, childbirth or the puerperium, when COVID-19 is the reason for admission/encounter , code O98.5-, Other viral diseases complicating pregnancy, childbirth and the puerperium, should be sequenced as the principal/first-listed diagnosis, and code UØ7.1, COVID-19, and the appropriate codes for associated manifestation(s) should be assigned as additional diagnoses. Codes from Chapter 15 always take sequencing priority.

If the reason for admission/encounter is unrelated to COVID-19 but the patient has been diagnosed with COVID-19 during the admission/encounter, the appropriate code for the reason for admission/encounter should be sequenced as the principal/first-listed diagnosis, and codes O98.5- and UØ7.1, as well as the appropriate codes for associated COVID-19 manifestations, should be assigned as additional diagnoses.

**16. Chapter 16: Certain Conditions Originating in the Perinatal Period (PØØ-P96)**

For coding and reporting purposes the perinatal period is defined as before birth through the 28th day following birth. The following guidelines are provided for reporting purposes.

**a. General Perinatal Rules**

**1) Use of Chapter 16 Codes**
Codes in this chapter are never for use on the maternal record. Codes from Chapter 15, the obstetric chapter, are never permitted on the newborn record. Chapter 16 codes may be used throughout the life of the patient if the condition is still present.

**2) Principal Diagnosis for Birth Record**
When coding the birth episode in a newborn record, assign a code from category Z38, Liveborn infants according to place of birth and type of delivery, as the principal diagnosis. A code from category Z38 is assigned only once, to a newborn at the time of birth. If a newborn is transferred to another institution, a code from category Z38 should not be used at the receiving hospital.

A code from category Z38 is used only on the newborn record, not on the mother's record.

**3) Use of Codes from other Chapters with Codes from Chapter 16**
Codes from other chapters may be used with codes from chapter 16 if the codes from the other chapters provide more specific detail. Codes for signs and symptoms may be assigned when a definitive diagnosis has not been established. If the reason for the encounter is a perinatal condition, the code from chapter 16 should be sequenced first.

**4) Use of Chapter 16 Codes after the Perinatal Period**
Should a condition originate in the perinatal period, and continue throughout the life of the patient, the perinatal code should continue to be used regardless of the patient's age.

**5) Birth process or community acquired conditions**
If a newborn has a condition that may be either due to the birth process or community acquired and the documentation does not indicate which it is, the default is due to the birth process and the code from Chapter 16 should be used. If the condition is community-acquired, a code from Chapter 16 should not be assigned.

*For COVID-19 infection in a newborn, see guideline I.C.16.h.*

**6) Code all clinically significant conditions**
All clinically significant conditions noted on routine newborn examination should be coded. A condition is clinically significant if it requires:

- clinical evaluation; or
- therapeutic treatment; or
- diagnostic procedures; or
- extended length of hospital stay; or
- increased nursing care and/or monitoring; or
- has implications for future health care needs

Note: The perinatal guidelines listed above are the same as the general coding guidelines for "additional diagnoses," except for the final point regarding implications for future health care needs. Codes should be assigned for conditions that have been specified by the provider as having implications for future health care needs.

**b. Observation and Evaluation of Newborns for Suspected Conditions not Found**

**1) Use of Z05 codes**
Assign a code from category Z05, Observation and evaluation of newborn for suspected diseases and conditions ruled out, to identify those instances when a healthy newborn is evaluated for a suspected condition/disease that is determined after study not to be present. Do not use a code from category Z05 when the patient is documented to have signs or symptoms of a suspected problem; in such cases code the sign or symptom.

**2) Z05 on other than the birth record**
A code from categofry Z05 may also be assigned as a principal or first-listed code for readmissions or encounters when the code from category Z38 no longer applies. Codes from category Z05 are for use only for healthy newborns and infants for which no condition **is found to be present after study**.

**3) Z05 on a birth record**
A code from category Z05 is to be used as a secondary code after the code from category Z38, Liveborn infants according to place of birth and type of delivery.

**c. Coding Additional Perinatal Diagnoses**

**1) Assigning codes for conditions that require treatment**
Assign codes for conditions that require treatment or further investigation, prolong the length of stay, or require resource utilization.

**2) Codes for conditions specified as having implications for future health care needs**
Assign codes for conditions that have been specified by the provider as having implications for future health care needs.

Note: This guideline should not be used for adult patients.

**d. Prematurity and Fetal Growth Retardation**
Providers utilize different criteria in determining prematurity. A code for prematurity should not be assigned unless it is documented. Assignment of codes in categories P05, Disorders of newborn related to slow fetal growth and fetal malnutrition, and P07, Disorders of newborn related to short gestation and low birth weight, not elsewhere classified, should be based on the recorded birth weight and estimated gestational age.

When both birth weight and gestational age are available, two codes from category P07 should be assigned, with the code for birth weight sequenced before the code for gestational age.

**e. Low birth weight and immaturity status**
Codes from category P07, Disorders of newborn related to short gestation and low birth weight, not elsewhere classified, are for use for a child or adult who was premature or had a low birth weight as a newborn and this is affecting the patient's current health status.

*See Section I.C.21. Factors influencing health status and contact with health services, Status.*

**f. Bacterial Sepsis of Newborn**
Category P36, Bacterial sepsis of newborn, includes congenital sepsis. If a perinate is documented as having sepsis without documentation of congenital or community acquired, the default is congenital and a code from category P36 should be assigned. If the P36 code includes the causal organism, an additional code from category B95, Streptococcus, Staphylococcus, and Enterococcus as the cause of diseases classified elsewhere, or B96, Other bacterial agents as the cause of diseases classified elsewhere, should not be assigned. If the P36 code does not include the causal organism, assign an additional code from category B96. If applicable, use additional codes to identify severe sepsis (R65.2-) and any associated acute organ dysfunction.

**g. Stillbirth**
Code P95, Stillbirth, is only for use in institutions that maintain separate records for stillbirths. No other code should be used with P95. Code P95 should not be used on the mother's record.

**h. COVID-19 Infection in Newborn**
For a newborn that tests positive for COVID-19, assign code U07.1, COVID-19, and the appropriate codes for associated manifestation(s) in neonates/newborns in the absence of documentation indicating a specific type of transmission. For a newborn that tests positive for COVID-19 and the provider documents the condition was contracted in utero or during the birth process, assign codes P35.8, Other congenital viral diseases, and U07.1, COVID-19. When coding the birth episode in a newborn record, the appropriate code from category Z38, Liveborn infants according to place of birth and type of delivery, should be assigned as the principal diagnosis.

**17. Chapter 17: Congenital malformations, deformations, chromosomal abnormalities, *and genetic disorders* (Q00-*QA1*)**
Assign an appropriate code(s) from categories Q00-**QA1**, Congenital malformations, deformations, chromosomal abnormalities, **or genetic disorders** when a malformation/deformation, chromosomal abnormality, **or genetic disorder** is documented. A malformation/deformation/chromosomal abnormality, **or genetic disorder** may be the principal/first-listed diagnosis or secondary diagnosis on a record.

When a malformation/deformation, chromosomal abnormality, **or genetic disorder** does not have a unique code assignment, assign additional code(s) for any manifestations that may be present.

When the code assignment specifically identifies the malformation/deformation, chromosomal abnormality, **or genetic disorder,** manifestations that are an inherent component of the anomaly should not be coded separately. Additional codes should be assigned for manifestations that are not an inherent component.

Codes from Chapter 17 may be used throughout the life of the patient. If a congenital malformation or deformity has been corrected, a personal history code should be used to identify the history of the malformation or deformity. Although present at birth, a malformation/deformation, chromosomal abnormality, **or genetic disorder** may not be identified until later in life. Whenever the condition is diagnosed by the provider, it is appropriate to assign a code from categories Q00-**QA1**. For the birth admission, the appropriate code from category Z38, Liveborn infants, according to place of birth and type of delivery, should be sequenced as the principal diagnosis, followed by any congenital anomaly codes in categories Q00-**QA1**.

**18. Chapter 18: Symptoms, signs, and abnormal clinical and laboratory findings, not elsewhere classified (R00-R99)**
Chapter 18 includes symptoms, signs, abnormal results of clinical or other investigative procedures, and ill-defined conditions which no diagnosis classifiable elsewhere is recorded. Signs and symptoms that point to a specific diagnosis have been assigned to a category in other chapters of the classification.

**a. Use of symptom codes**
Codes that describe symptoms and signs are acceptable for reporting purposes when a related definitive diagnosis has not been established (confirmed) by the provider.

**b. Use of a symptom code with a definitive diagnosis code**
Codes for signs and symptoms may be reported in addition to a related definitive diagnosis when the sign or symptom is not routinely associated with that diagnosis, such as the various signs and symptoms associated with complex syndromes. The definitive diagnosis code should be sequenced before the symptom code.

Signs or symptoms that are associated routinely with a disease process should not be assigned as additional codes, unless otherwise instructed by the classification.

**c. Combination codes that include symptoms**
ICD-10-CM contains a number of combination codes that identify both the definitive diagnosis and common symptoms of that diagnosis. When using one of these combination codes, an additional code should not be assigned for the symptom.

**d. Repeated falls**
Code R29.6, Repeated falls, is for use for encounters when a patient has recently fallen and the reason for the fall is being investigated.

Code Z91.81, History of falling, is for use when a patient has fallen in the past and is at risk for future falls. When appropriate, both codes R29.6 and Z91.81 may be assigned together.

**e. Coma**
Code R4Ø.2Ø, Unspecified coma, should be assigned when the underlying cause of the coma is not known, or the cause is a traumatic brain injury and the coma scale is not documented in the medical record.

Do not report codes for unspecified coma, individual or total Glasgow coma scale scores for a patient with a medically induced coma or a sedated patient.

**1) Coma Scale**
The coma scale codes (R4Ø.21- to R4Ø.24-) can be used in conjunction with traumatic brain injury codes. These codes cannot be used with code R4Ø.2A, Nontraumatic coma due to underlying condition. They are primarily for use by trauma registries, but they may be used in any setting where this information is collected. The coma scale codes should be sequenced after the diagnosis code(s).

These codes, one from each subcategory, are needed to complete the scale. The 7th character indicates when the scale was recorded. The 7th character should match for all three codes.

At a minimum, report the initial score documented on presentation at your facility. This may be a score from the emergency medicine technician (EMT) or in the emergency department. If desired, a facility may choose to capture multiple coma scale scores.

Assign code R4Ø.24-, Glasgow coma scale, total score, when only the total score is documented in the medical record and not the individual score(s).

If multiple coma scores are captured within the first 24 hours after hospital admission, assign only the code for the score at the time of admission. ICD-10-CM does not classify coma scores that are reported after admission but less than 24 hours later.

*See Section I.B.14. for coma scale documentation by clinicians other than patient's provider*

**f. Functional quadriplegia**
GUIDELINE HAS BEEN DELETED EFFECTIVE OCTOBER 1, 2017

**g. SIRS due to Non-Infectious Process**
The systemic inflammatory response syndrome (SIRS) can develop as a result of certain non-infectious disease processes, such as trauma, malignant neoplasm, or pancreatitis. When SIRS is documented with a noninfectious condition, and no subsequent infection is documented, the code for the underlying condition, such as an injury, should be assigned, followed by code R65.1Ø, Systemic inflammatory response syndrome (SIRS) of non-infectious origin without acute organ dysfunction, or code R65.11, Systemic inflammatory response syndrome (SIRS) of non-infectious origin with acute organ dysfunction. If an associated acute organ dysfunction is documented, the appropriate code(s) for the specific type of organ dysfunction(s) should be assigned in addition to code R65.11. If acute organ dysfunction is documented, but it cannot be determined if the acute organ dysfunction is associated with SIRS or due to another condition (e.g., directly due to the trauma), the provider should be queried.

**h. Death NOS**
Code R99, Ill-defined and unknown cause of mortality, is only for use in the very limited circumstance when a patient who has already died is brought into an emergency department or other healthcare facility and is pronounced dead upon arrival. It does not represent the discharge disposition of death.

**i. NIHSS Stroke Scale**
The NIH stroke scale (NIHSS) codes (R29.7- -) can be used in conjunction with acute stroke codes (I6Ø–I63) to identify the patient's neurological status and the severity of the stroke. The stroke scale codes should be sequenced after the acute stroke diagnosis code(s).

At a minimum, report the initial score documented. If desired, a facility may choose to capture multiple stroke scale scores.

*See Section I.B.14. for NIHSS stroke scale documentation by clinicians other than patient's provider*

**19. Chapter 19: Injury, poisoning, and certain other consequences of external causes (SØØ-T88)**

**a. Application of 7th Characters in Chapter 19**
Most categories in chapter 19 have a 7th character requirement for each applicable code. Most categories in this chapter have three 7th character values (with the exception of fractures): A, initial encounter, D, subsequent encounter and S, sequela. Categories for traumatic fractures have additional 7th character values. While the patient may be seen by a new or different provider over the course of treatment for an injury, assignment of the 7th character is based on whether the patient is undergoing active treatment and not whether the provider is seeing the patient for the first time.

For complication codes, active treatment refers to treatment for the condition described by the code, even though it may be related to an earlier precipitating problem. For example, code T84.5ØXA, Infection and inflammatory reaction due to unspecified internal joint prosthesis, initial encounter, is used when active treatment is provided for the infection, even though the condition relates to the prosthetic device, implant or graft that was placed at a previous encounter.

7th character "A", initial encounter is used for each encounter where the patient is receiving active treatment for the condition.

7th character "D" subsequent encounter is used for encounters after the patient has completed active treatment of the condition and is receiving routine care for the condition during the healing or recovery phase.

The aftercare Z codes should not be used for aftercare for conditions such as injuries or poisonings, where 7th characters are provided to identify subsequent care. For example, for aftercare of an injury, assign the acute injury code with the 7th character "D" (subsequent encounter).

7th character "S", sequela, is for use for complications or conditions that arise as a direct result of a condition, such as scar formation after a burn. The scars are sequelae of the burn. When using 7th character "S", it is necessary to use both the injury code that precipitated the sequela and the code for the sequela itself. The "S" is added only to the injury code, not the sequela code. The 7th character "S" identifies the injury responsible for the sequela. The specific type of sequela (e.g. scar) is sequenced first, followed by the injury code.

*See Section I.B.10. Sequelae, (Late Effects)*

**b. Coding of Injuries**
When coding injuries, assign separate codes for each injury unless a combination code is provided, in which case the combination code is assigned. Codes from category TØ7, Unspecified multiple injuries should not be assigned in the inpatient setting unless information for a more specific code is not available. Traumatic injury codes (SØØ-T14.9) are not to be used for normal, healing surgical wounds or to identify complications of surgical wounds.

The code for the most serious injury, as determined by the provider and the focus of treatment, is sequenced first.

**1) Superficial injuries**
Superficial injuries such as abrasions or contusions are not coded when associated with more severe injuries of the same site.

**2) Primary injury with damage to nerves/blood vessels**
When a primary injury results in minor damage to peripheral nerves or blood vessels, the primary injury is sequenced first with additional code(s) for injuries to nerves and spinal cord (such as category SØ4), and/or injury to blood vessels (such as category S15). When the primary injury is to the blood vessels or nerves, that injury should be sequenced first.

**3) Iatrogenic injuries**
Injury codes from Chapter 19 should not be assigned for injuries that occur during, or as a result of, a medical intervention. Assign the appropriate complication code(s).

**c. Coding of Traumatic Fractures**
The principles of multiple coding of injuries should be followed in coding fractures. Fractures of specified sites are coded individually by site in accordance with both the provisions within categories SØ2, S12, S22, S32, S42, S49, S52, S59, S62, S72, S79, S82, S89, S92 and the level of detail furnished by medical record content.

A fracture not indicated as open or closed should be coded to closed. A fracture not indicated whether displaced or not displaced should be coded to displaced.

More specific guidelines are as follows:

**1) Initial vs. subsequent encounter for fractures**
Traumatic fractures are coded using the appropriate 7th character for initial encounter (A, B, C) for each encounter where the patient is receiving active treatment for the fracture. The appropriate 7th character for initial encounter should also be assigned for a patient who delayed seeking treatment for the fracture or nonunion.

Fractures are coded using the appropriate 7th character for subsequent care for encounters after the patient has completed active treatment of the fracture and is receiving routine care for the fracture during the healing or recovery phase.

Care for complications of surgical treatment for fracture repairs during the healing or recovery phase should be coded with the appropriate complication codes.

Care of complications of fractures, such as malunion and nonunion, should be reported with the appropriate 7th character for subsequent care with nonunion (K, M, N,) or subsequent care with malunion (P, Q, R).

Malunion/nonunion: The appropriate 7th character for initial encounter should also be assigned for a patient who delayed seeking treatment for the fracture or nonunion.

The open fracture designations in the assignment of the 7th character for fractures of the forearm, femur and lower leg, including ankle are based on the Gustilo open fracture classification. When the Gustilo classification type is not specified for an open fracture, the 7th character for open fracture type I or II should be assigned (B, E, H, M, Q).

A code from category M8Ø, not a traumatic fracture code, should be used for any patient with known osteoporosis who suffers a fracture, even if the patient had a minor fall or trauma, if that fall or trauma would not usually break a normal, healthy bone.

*See Section I.C.13. Osteoporosis.*

The aftercare Z codes should not be used for aftercare for traumatic fractures. For aftercare of a traumatic fracture, assign the acute fracture code with the appropriate 7th character.

**2) Multiple fractures sequencing**
Multiple fractures are sequenced in accordance with the severity of the fracture.

**3) Physeal fractures**
For physeal fractures, assign only the code identifying the type of physeal fracture. Do not assign a separate code to identify the specific bone that is fractured.

**d. Coding of Burns and Corrosions**
The ICD-10-CM makes a distinction between burns and corrosions. The burn codes are for thermal burns, except sunburns, that come from a heat source, such as a fire or hot appliance. The burn codes are also for burns resulting from electricity and radiation. Corrosions are burns due to chemicals. The guidelines are the same for burns and corrosions.

Current burns (T2Ø-T25) are classified by depth, extent and by agent (X code). Burns are classified by depth as first degree (erythema), second degree (blistering), and third degree (full-thickness involvement). Burns of the eye and internal organs (T26-T28) are classified by site, but not by degree.

**1) Sequencing of burn and related condition codes**
Sequence first the code that reflects the highest degree of burn when more than one burn is present.

a. When the reason for the admission or encounter is for treatment of external multiple burns, sequence first the code that reflects the burn of the highest degree.
b. When a patient has both internal and external burns, the circumstances of admission govern the selection of the principal diagnosis or first-listed diagnosis.
c. When a patient is admitted for burn injuries and other related conditions such as smoke inhalation and/or respiratory failure, the circumstances of admission govern the selection of the principal or first-listed diagnosis.

**2) Burns of the same anatomic site**
Classify burns of the same anatomic site and on the same side but of different degrees to the subcategory identifying the highest degree recorded in the diagnosis (e.g., for second and third degree burns of right thigh, assign only code T24.311-).

**3) Non-healing burns**
Non-healing burns are coded as acute burns.

Necrosis of burned skin should be coded as a non-healed burn.

**4) Infected burn**
For any documented infected burn site, use an additional code for the infection.

**5) Assign separate codes for each burn site**
When coding burns, assign separate codes for each burn site. Category T3Ø, Burn and corrosion, body region unspecified is extremely vague and should rarely be used.

Codes for burns of "multiple sites" should only be assigned when the medical record documentation does not specify the individual sites.

**6) Burns and corrosions classified according to extent of body surface involved**
Assign codes from category T31, Burns classified according to extent of body surface involved, or T32, Corrosions classified according to extent of body surface involved, for acute burns or corrosions when the site of the burn or corrosion is not specified or when there is a need for additional data. It is advisable to use category T31 as additional coding when needed to provide data for evaluating burn mortality, such as that needed by burn units. It is also advisable to use category T31 as an additional code for reporting purposes when there is mention of a third-degree burn involving 20 percent or more of the body surface. Codes from categories T31 and T32 should not be used for sequelae of burns or corrosions.

Categories T31 and T32 are based on the classic "rule of nines" in estimating body surface involved: head and neck are assigned nine percent, each arm nine percent, each leg 18 percent, the anterior trunk 18 percent, posterior trunk 18 percent, and genitalia one percent. Providers may change these percentage assignments where necessary to accommodate infants and children who have proportionately larger heads than adults, and patients who have large buttocks, thighs, or abdomen that involve burns.

**7) Encounters for treatment of sequela of burns**
Encounters for the treatment of the late effects of burns or corrosions (i.e., scars or joint contractures) should be coded with a burn or corrosion code with the 7th character "S" for sequela.

**8) Sequelae with a late effect code and current burn**
When appropriate, both a code for a current burn or corrosion with 7th character "A" or "D" and a burn or corrosion code with 7th character "S" may be assigned on the same record (when both a current burn and sequelae of an old burn exist). Burns and corrosions do not heal at the same rate and a current healing wound may still exist with sequela of a healed burn or corrosion.

*See Section I.B.10. Sequela (Late Effects)*

**9) Use of an external cause code with burns and corrosions**
An external cause code should be used with burns and corrosions to identify the source and intent of the burn, as well as the place where it occurred.

**e. Adverse Effects, Poisoning, Underdosing and Toxic Effects**
Codes in categories T36-T65 are combination codes that include the substance that was taken as well as the intent. No additional external cause code is required for poisonings, toxic effects, adverse effects and underdosing codes.

**1) Do not code directly from the Table of Drugs**
Do not code directly from the Table of Drugs and Chemicals. Always refer back to the Tabular List.

**2) Use as many codes as necessary to describe**
Use as many codes as necessary to describe completely all drugs, medicinal or biological substances.

**3) If the same code would describe the causative agent**
If the same code would describe the causative agent for more than one adverse reaction, poisoning, toxic effect or underdosing, assign the code only once.

**4) If two or more drugs, medicinal or biological substances**
If two or more drugs, medicinal or biological substances are taken, code each individually unless a combination code is listed in the Table of Drugs and Chemicals.

If multiple unspecified drugs, medicinal or biological substances were taken, assign the appropriate code from subcategory T5Ø.91, Poisoning by, adverse effect of and underdosing of multiple unspecified drugs, medicaments and biological substances.

**5) The occurrence of drug toxicity is classified in ICD-10-CM as follows:**

**(a) Adverse Effect**
When coding an adverse effect of a drug that has been correctly prescribed and properly administered, assign the appropriate code for the nature of the adverse effect followed by the appropriate code for the adverse effect of the drug (T36-T5Ø). The code for the drug should have a 5th or 6th character "5" (for example T36.ØX5-) Examples of the nature of an adverse effect are tachycardia, delirium, gastrointestinal hemorrhaging, vomiting, hypokalemia, hepatitis, renal failure, or respiratory failure.

**(b) Poisoning**
When coding a poisoning or reaction to the improper use of a medication (e.g., overdose, wrong substance given or taken in error, wrong route of administration), first assign the appropriate code from categories T36-T5Ø. The poisoning codes have an associated intent as their 5th or 6th character (accidental, intentional self-harm, assault and undetermined). If the intent of the poisoning is unknown or unspecified, code the intent as accidental intent. The undetermined intent is only for use if the documentation in the record specifies that the intent cannot be determined. Use additional code(s) for all manifestations of poisonings.

If there is also a diagnosis of abuse or dependence of the substance, the abuse or dependence is assigned as an additional code.

Examples of poisoning include:

(i) Error was made in drug prescription
Errors made in drug prescription or in the administration of the drug by provider, nurse, patient, or other person.

(ii) Overdose of a drug intentionally taken
If an overdose of a drug was intentionally taken or administered and resulted in drug toxicity, it would be coded as a poisoning.

(iii) Nonprescribed drug taken with correctly prescribed and properly administered drug
If a nonprescribed drug or medicinal agent was taken in combination with a correctly prescribed and properly administered drug, any drug toxicity or other reaction resulting from the interaction of the two drugs would be classified as a poisoning.

(iv) Interaction of drug(s) and alcohol
When a reaction results from the interaction of a drug(s) and alcohol, this would be classified as poisoning.

*See Section I.C.4. if poisoning is the result of insulin pump malfunctions.*

*For Sequela (Late Effects) see Section I.B.10.*

**(c) Underdosing**
Underdosing refers to taking less of a medication than is prescribed by a provider or a manufacturer's instruction. Discontinuing the use of a prescribed medication on the patient's own initiative (not directed by the patient's provider) is also classified as an underdosing. For underdosing, assign the code from categories T36-T5Ø (fifth or sixth character "6"). Documentation of a change in the patient's condition is not required in order to assign an underdosing code. Documentation that the patient is taking less of a medication than is prescribed or discontinued the prescribed medication is sufficient for code assignment.

Codes for underdosing should never be assigned as principal or first-listed codes. If a patient has a relapse or exacerbation of the medical condition for which the drug is prescribed because of the reduction in dose, then the medical condition itself should be coded.

Noncompliance (Z91.12-, Z91.13-, Z91.14- and Z91.A4-) or complication of care (Y63.6-Y63.9) codes are to be used with an underdosing code to indicate intent, if known.

**(d) Toxic Effects**
When a harmful substance is ingested or comes in contact with a person, this is classified as a toxic effect. The toxic effect codes are in categories T51-T65. When coding a toxic effect, assign the toxic effect code first, followed by codes for all associated manifestations of the toxic effect.

Toxic effect codes have an associated intent: accidental, intentional self-harm, assault and undetermined.

*For Sequela (Late Effects) see Section I.B.10. Sequela*

**f. Adult and child abuse, neglect and other maltreatment**
Sequence first the appropriate code from categories T74, Adult and child abuse, neglect and other maltreatment, confirmed, or T76, Adult and child abuse, neglect and other maltreatment, suspected, for abuse, neglect and other maltreatment, followed by any accompanying mental health or injury code(s).

If the documentation in the medical record states abuse or neglect, it is coded as confirmed (T74.-). It is coded as suspected if it is documented as suspected (T76.-).

For cases of confirmed abuse or neglect an external cause code from the assault section (X92-YØ9) should be added to identify the cause of any physical injuries. A perpetrator code (YØ7) should be added when the perpetrator of the abuse is known. For suspected cases of abuse or neglect, do not report external cause or perpetrator code.

If a suspected case of abuse, neglect or mistreatment is ruled out during an encounter code ZØ4.71, Encounter for examination and observation following alleged physical adult abuse, ruled out, or code ZØ4.72, Encounter for examination and observation following alleged child physical abuse, ruled out, should be used, not a code from T76.

If a suspected case of alleged rape or sexual abuse is ruled out during an encounter code ZØ4.41, Encounter for examination and observation following alleged adult rape or code ZØ4.42, Encounter for examination and observation following alleged child rape, should be used, not a code from T76.

If a suspected case of forced sexual exploitation or forced labor exploitation is ruled out during an encounter, code ZØ4.81, Encounter for examination and observation of victim following forced sexual exploitation, or code ZØ4.82, Encounter for examination and observation of victim following forced labor exploitation, should be used, not a code from T76.

*See Section I.C.15. Abuse in a pregnant patient.*

**g. Complications of care**

**1) General guidelines for complications of care**

**(a) Documentation of complications of care**
*See Section I.B.16. for information on documentation of complications of care.*

**2) Pain due to medical devices**
Pain associated with devices, implants or grafts left in a surgical site (for example painful hip prosthesis) is assigned to the appropriate code(s) found in Chapter 19, Injury, poisoning, and certain other consequences of external causes. Specific codes for pain due to medical devices are found in the T code section of the ICD-10-CM. Use additional code(s) from category G89 to identify acute or chronic pain due to presence of the device, implant or graft (G89.18 or G89.28).

**3) Transplant complications**

**(a) Transplant complications other than kidney**
Codes under category T86, Complications of transplanted organs and tissues, are for use for both complications and rejection of transplanted organs. A transplant complication code is only assigned if the complication affects the function of the transplanted organ. Two codes are required to fully describe a transplant complication: the appropriate code from category T86 and a secondary code that identifies the complication.

Pre-existing conditions or conditions that develop after the transplant are not coded as complications unless they affect the function of the transplanted organs.

*See I.C.21. for transplant organ removal status*

*See I.C.2. for malignant neoplasm associated with transplanted organ.*

*See I.C.1.d.4. for sequencing of sepsis due to infection in transplanted organ*

**(b) Kidney transplant complications**
Patients who have undergone kidney transplant may still have some form of chronic kidney disease (CKD) because the kidney transplant may not fully restore kidney function. Code T86.1- should be assigned for documented complications of a kidney transplant, such as transplant failure or rejection or other transplant complication. Code T86.1- should not be assigned for post kidney transplant patients who have chronic kidney (CKD) unless a transplant complication such as transplant failure or rejection is documented. If the documentation is unclear as to whether the patient has a complication of the transplant, query the provider.

Conditions that affect the function of the transplanted kidney, other than CKD, should be assigned a code from subcategory T86.1, Complications of transplanted organ, Kidney, and a secondary code that identifies the complication.

For patients with CKD following a kidney transplant, but who do not have a complication such as failure or rejection, *see section I.C.14. Chronic kidney disease and kidney transplant status.*

*See I.C.1.d.4. for sequencing of sepsis due to infection in transplanted organ*

**4) Complication codes that include the external cause**
As with certain other T codes, some of the complications of care codes have the external cause included in the code. The code includes the nature of the complication as well as the type of procedure that caused the complication. No external cause code indicating the type of procedure is necessary for these codes.

**5) Complications of care codes within the body system chapters**
Intraoperative and postprocedural complication codes are found within the body system chapters with codes specific to the organs and structures of that body system. These codes should be sequenced first, followed by a code(s) for the specific complication, if applicable.

Complication codes from the body system chapters should be assigned for intraoperative and postprocedural complications (e.g., the appropriate complication code from chapter 9 would be assigned for a vascular intraoperative or postprocedural complication) unless the complication is specifically indexed to a T code in chapter 19.

**20. Chapter 20: External Causes of Morbidity (VØØ-Y99)**
The external causes of morbidity codes should never be sequenced as the first-listed or principal diagnosis.

External cause codes are intended to provide data for injury research and evaluation of injury prevention strategies. These codes capture how the injury or health condition happened (cause), the intent (unintentional or accidental; or intentional, such as suicide or assault), the place where the event occurred the activity of the patient at the time of the event, and the person's status (e.g., civilian, military).

There is no national requirement for mandatory ICD-10-CM external cause code reporting. Unless a provider is subject to a state-based external cause code reporting mandate or these codes are required by a particular payer, reporting of ICD-10-CM codes in Chapter 20, External Causes of Morbidity, is not required. In the absence of a mandatory reporting requirement, providers are encouraged to voluntarily report external cause codes, as they provide valuable data for injury research and evaluation of injury prevention strategies.

**a. General External Cause Coding Guidelines**

**1) Used with any code in the range of AØØ.Ø-T88.9, ZØØ-Z99**
An external cause code may be used with any code in the range of AØØ.Ø-T88.9, ZØØ-Z99, classification that represents a health condition due to an external cause. Though they are most applicable to injuries, they are also valid for use with such things as infections or diseases due

to an external source, and other health conditions, such as a heart attack that occurs during strenuous physical activity.

**2) External cause code used for length of treatment**
Assign the external cause code, with the appropriate 7th character (initial encounter, subsequent encounter or sequela) for each encounter for which the injury or condition is being treated.

Most categories in chapter 20 have a 7th character requirement for each applicable code. Most categories in this chapter have three 7th character values: A, initial encounter, D, subsequent encounter and S, sequela. While the patient may be seen by a new or different provider over the course of treatment for an injury or condition, assignment of the 7th character for external cause should match the 7th character of the code assigned for the associated injury or condition for the encounter.

**3) Use the full range of external cause codes**
Use the full range of external cause codes to completely describe the cause, the intent, the place of occurrence, and if applicable, the activity of the patient at the time of the event, and the patient's status, for all injuries, and other health conditions due to an external cause.

**4) Assign as many external cause codes as necessary**
Assign as many external cause codes as necessary to fully explain each cause. If only one external code can be recorded, assign the code most related to the principal diagnosis.

**5) The selection of the appropriate external cause code**
The selection of the appropriate external cause code is guided by the Alphabetic Index of External Causes and by Inclusion and Exclusion notes in the Tabular List.

**6) External cause code can never be a principal diagnosis**
An external cause code can never be a principal (first-listed) diagnosis.

**7) Combination external cause codes**
Certain of the external cause codes are combination codes that identify sequential events that result in an injury, such as a fall which results in striking against an object. The injury may be due to either event or both. The combination external cause code used should correspond to the sequence of events regardless of which caused the most serious injury.

**8) No external cause code needed in certain circumstances**
No external cause code from Chapter 20 is needed if the external cause and intent are included in a code from another chapter (e.g., T36.ØX1-, Poisoning by penicillins, accidental (unintentional)).

**b. Place of Occurrence Guideline**
Codes from category Y92, Place of occurrence of the external cause, are secondary codes for use after other external cause codes to identify the location of the patient at the time of injury or other condition.

Generally, a place of occurrence code is assigned only once, at the initial encounter for treatment. However, in the rare instance that a new injury occurs during hospitalization, an additional place of occurrence code may be assigned. No 7th characters are used for Y92.

Do not use place of occurrence code Y92.9 if the place is not stated or is not applicable.

**c. Activity Code**
Assign a code from category Y93, Activity code, to describe the activity of the patient at the time the injury or other health condition occurred.

An activity code is used only once, at the initial encounter for treatment. Only one code from Y93 should be recorded on a medical record.

The activity codes are not applicable to poisonings, adverse effects, misadventures or sequela.

Do not assign Y93.9, Unspecified activity, if the activity is not stated.

A code from category Y93 is appropriate for use with external cause and intent codes if identifying the activity provides additional information about the event.

**d. Place of Occurrence, Activity, and Status Codes Used with other External Cause Code**
When applicable, place of occurrence, activity, and external cause status codes are sequenced after the main external cause code(s). Regardless of the number of external cause codes assigned, generally there should be only one place of occurrence code, one activity code, and one external cause status code assigned to an encounter. However, in the rare instance that a new injury occurs during hospitalization, an additional place of occurrence code may be assigned.

**e. If the Reporting Format Limits the Number of External Cause Codes**
If the reporting format limits the number of external cause codes that can be used in reporting clinical data, report the code for the cause/intent most related to the principal diagnosis. If the format permits capture of additional external cause codes, the cause/intent, including medical misadventures, of the additional events should be reported rather than the codes for place, activity, or external status.

**f. Multiple External Cause Coding Guidelines**
More than one external cause code is required to fully describe the external cause of an illness or injury. The assignment of external cause codes should be sequenced in the following priority:

If two or more events cause separate injuries, an external cause code should be assigned for each cause. The first-listed external cause code will be selected in the following order:

External codes for child and adult abuse take priority over all other external cause codes.

*See Section I.C.19., Child and Adult abuse guidelines.*

External cause codes for terrorism events take priority over all other external cause codes except child and adult abuse.

External cause codes for cataclysmic events take priority over all other external cause codes except child and adult abuse and terrorism.

External cause codes for transport accidents take priority over all other external cause codes except cataclysmic events, child and adult abuse and terrorism.

Activity and external cause status codes are assigned following all causal (intent) external cause codes.

The first-listed external cause code should correspond to the cause of the most serious diagnosis due to an assault, accident, or self-harm, following the order of hierarchy listed above.

**g. Child and Adult Abuse Guideline**
Adult and child abuse, neglect and maltreatment are classified as assault. Any of the assault codes may be used to indicate the external cause of any injury resulting from the confirmed abuse.

For confirmed cases of abuse, neglect and maltreatment, when the perpetrator is known, a code from YØ7, Perpetrator of maltreatment and neglect, should accompany any other assault codes.

*See Section I.C.19. Adult and child abuse, neglect and other maltreatment*

**h. Unknown or Undetermined Intent Guideline**
If the intent (accident, self-harm, assault) of the cause of an injury or other condition is unknown or unspecified, code the intent as accidental intent. All transport accident categories assume accidental intent.

**1) Use of undetermined intent**
External cause codes for events of undetermined intent are only for use if the documentation in the record specifies that the intent cannot be determined.

**i. Sequelae (Late Effects) of External Cause Guidelines**

**1) Sequelae external cause codes**
Sequela are reported using the external cause code with the 7th character "S" for sequela. These codes should be used with any report of a late effect or sequela resulting from a previous injury.

*See Section I.B.10: Sequela (Late Effects)*

**2) Sequela external cause code with a related current injury**
A sequela external cause code should never be used with a related current nature of injury code.

**3) Use of sequela external cause codes for subsequent visits**
Use a late effect external cause code for subsequent visits when a late effect of the initial injury is being treated. Do not use a late effect external cause code for subsequent visits for follow-up care (e.g., to assess healing, to receive rehabilitative therapy) of the injury when no late effect of the injury has been documented.

**j. Terrorism Guidelines**

**1) Cause of injury identified by the Federal Government (FBI) as terrorism**
When the cause of an injury is identified by the Federal Government (FBI) as terrorism, the first-listed external cause code should be a code from category Y38, Terrorism. The definition of terrorism employed by the FBI is found at the inclusion note at the beginning of category Y38. Use additional code for place of occurrence (Y92.-). More than one Y38 code may be assigned if the injury is the result of more than one mechanism of terrorism.

**2) Cause of an injury is suspected to be the result of terrorism**
When the cause of an injury is suspected to be the result of terrorism a code from category Y38 should not be assigned. Suspected cases should be classified as assault.

**3) Code Y38.9, Terrorism, secondary effects**
Assign code Y38.9, Terrorism, secondary effects, for conditions occurring subsequent to the terrorist event. This code should not be assigned for conditions that are due to the initial terrorist act.

It is acceptable to assign code Y38.9 with another code from Y38 if there is an injury due to the initial terrorist event and an injury that is a subsequent result of the terrorist event.

**k. External Cause Status**
A code from category Y99, External cause status, should be assigned whenever any other external cause code is assigned for an encounter, including an Activity code, except for the events noted below. Assign a code from category Y99, External cause status, to indicate the work status of the person at the time the event occurred. The status code indicates whether the event occurred during military activity, whether a non-military person was at

work, whether an individual including a student or volunteer was involved in a non-work activity at the time of the causal event.

A code from Y99, External cause status, should be assigned, when applicable, with other external cause codes, such as transport accidents and falls. The external cause status codes are not applicable to poisonings, adverse effects, misadventures or late effects.

Do not assign a code from category Y99 if no other external cause codes (cause, activity) are applicable for the encounter.

An external cause status code is used only once, at the initial encounter for treatment. Only one code from Y99 should be recorded on a medical record.

Do not assign code Y99.9, Unspecified external cause status, if the status is not stated.

**21. Chapter 21: Factors influencing health status and contact with health services (Z00-Z99)**

**Note:** The chapter specific guidelines provide additional information about the use of Z codes for specified encounters.

**a. Use of Z Codes in Any Healthcare Setting**

Z codes are for use in any healthcare setting. Z codes may be used as either a first-listed (principal diagnosis code in the inpatient setting) or secondary code, depending on the circumstances of the encounter. Certain Z codes may only be used as first-listed or principal diagnosis.

**b. Z Codes Indicate a Reason for an Encounter or Provide Additional Information about a Patient Encounter**

Z codes are not procedure codes. A corresponding procedure code must accompany a Z code to describe any procedure performed.

**c. Categories of Z Codes**

**1) Contact/Exposure**

Category Z20 indicates contact with, and suspected exposure to, communicable diseases. These codes are for patients who are suspected to have been exposed to a disease by close personal contact with an infected individual or are in an area where a disease is epidemic.

Category Z77, Other contact with and (suspected) exposures hazardous to health, indicates contact with and suspected exposures hazardous to health.

Contact/exposure codes may be used as a first-listed code to explain an encounter for testing, or, more commonly, as a secondary code to identify a potential risk.

**2) Inoculations and vaccinations**

Code Z23 is for encounters for inoculations and vaccinations. It indicates that a patient is being seen to receive a prophylactic inoculation against a disease. Procedure codes are required to identify the actual administration of the injection and the type(s) of immunizations given. Code Z23 may be used as a secondary code if the inoculation is given as a routine part of preventive health care, such as a well-baby visit.

**3) Status**

Status codes indicate that a patient is either a carrier of a disease or has the sequelae or residual of a past disease or condition. This includes such things as the presence of prosthetic or mechanical devices resulting from past treatment. A status code is informative, because the status may affect the course of treatment and its outcome. A status code is distinct from a history code. The history code indicates that the patient no longer has the condition.

A status code should not be used with a diagnosis code from one of the body system chapters, if the diagnosis code includes the information provided by the status code. For example, code Z94.1, Heart transplant status, should not be used with a code from subcategory T86.2, Complications of heart transplant. The status code does not provide additional information. The complication code indicates that the patient is a heart transplant patient.

For encounters for weaning from a mechanical ventilator, assign a code from subcategory J96.1, Chronic respiratory failure, followed by code Z99.11, Dependence on respirator [ventilator] status.

The status Z codes/categories are:

Z14 Genetic carrier
Genetic carrier status indicates that a person carries a gene, associated with a particular disease, which may be passed to offspring who may develop that disease. The person does not have the disease and is not at risk of developing the disease.

Z15 Genetic susceptibility to disease
Genetic susceptibility indicates that a person has a gene that increases the risk of that person developing the disease.
Codes from category Z15 should generally not be used as principal or first-listed codes. If the patient has the condition to which he/she is susceptible, and that condition is the reason for the encounter, the code for the current condition should be sequenced first. If the patient is being seen for follow-up after completed treatment for this condition, and the condition no longer exists, a follow-up code should be sequenced first, followed by the appropriate personal history and genetic susceptibility codes. If the purpose of the encounter is genetic counseling associated with procreative management, code Z31.5, Encounter for genetic counseling, should be assigned as the first-listed code, followed by a code from category Z15. Additional codes should be assigned for any applicable family or personal history.

Z16 Resistance to antimicrobial drugs
This category indicates that a patient has a condition that is resistant to antimicrobial drug treatment. Sequence the infection code first.

Z17 Estrogen, and other hormones and factors receptor status

Z18 Retained foreign body fragments

Z19 Hormone sensitivity malignancy status

Z21 Asymptomatic HIV infection status
This code indicates that a patient has tested positive for HIV but has manifested no signs or symptoms of the disease.

Z22 Carrier of infectious disease
Carrier status indicates that a person harbors the specific organisms of a disease without manifest symptoms and is capable of transmitting the infection.

Z28.3 Underimmunization status
*See Section I.B.14. for underimmunization documentation by clinicians other than the patient's provider.*

Z33.1 Pregnant state, incidental
This code is a secondary code only for use when the pregnancy is in no way complicating the reason for visit. Otherwise, a code from the obstetric chapter is required.

Z66 Do not resuscitate
This code may be used when it is documented by the provider that a patient is on do not resuscitate status at any time during the stay.

Z67 Blood type

Z68 Body mass index (BMI)
BMI codes should only be assigned when there is an associated, reportable diagnosis (such as obesity or anorexia) documented by the patient's provider.
Do not assign BMI codes during pregnancy. When the documentation reflects fluctuating BMI values during the current encounter for an associated reportable condition, assign a code for the most severe value.
*See Section I.B.14. for BMI documentation by clinicians other than the patient's provider.*

Z74.01 Bed confinement status

Z76.82 Awaiting organ transplant status

Z78 Other specified health status
Code Z78.1, Physical restraint status, may be used when it is documented by the provider that a patient has been put in restraints during the current encounter. Please note that this code should not be reported when it is documented by the provider that a patient is temporarily restrained during a procedure.

Z79 Long-term (current) drug therapy
Codes from this category indicate a patient's continuous use of a prescribed drug (including such things as aspirin therapy) for the long-term treatment of a condition or for prophylactic use. It is not for use for patients who have addictions to drugs. This subcategory is not for use of medications for detoxification or maintenance programs to prevent withdrawal symptoms (e.g., methadone maintenance for opiate dependence). Assign the appropriate code for the drug use, abuse, or dependence instead.
Assign a code from Z79 if the patient is receiving a medication for an extended period as a prophylactic measure (such as for the prevention of deep vein thrombosis) or as treatment of a chronic condition (such as arthritis) or a disease requiring a lengthy course of treatment (such as cancer). Do not assign a code from category Z79 for medication being administered for a brief period of time to treat an acute illness or injury (such as a course of antibiotics to treat acute bronchitis).

Z88 Allergy status to drugs, medicaments and biological substances
Except: Z88.9, Allergy status to unspecified drugs, medicaments and biological substances status

Z89 Acquired absence of limb

Z90 Acquired absence of organs, not elsewhere classified

Z91.0- Allergy status, other than to drugs and biological substances

Z92.82 Status post administration of tPA (rtPA) in a different facility within the last 24 hours prior to admission to a current facility
Assign code Z92.82, Status post administration of tPA (rtPA) in a different facility within the last 24 hours prior to admission to current facility, as a secondary diagnosis when a patient is received by transfer into a facility and documentation indicates they were administered tissue plasminogen activator (tPA) within the last 24 hours prior to admission to the current facility. This guideline applies even if the patient is still receiving the tPA at the time they are received into the current facility.

The appropriate code for the condition for which the tPA was administered (such as cerebrovascular disease or myocardial infarction) should be assigned first.
Code Z92.82 is only applicable to the receiving facility record and not to the transferring facility record.

Z93 Artificial opening status
Z94 Transplanted organ and tissue status
Z95 Presence of cardiac and vascular implants and grafts
Z96 Presence of other functional implants
Z97 Presence of other devices
Z98 Other postprocedural states
Assign code Z98.85, Transplanted organ removal status, to indicate that a transplanted organ has been previously removed. This code should not be assigned for the encounter in which the transplanted organ is removed. The complication necessitating removal of the transplant organ should be assigned for that encounter.
*See section I.C.19. for information on the coding of organ transplant complications.*
Z99 Dependence on enabling machines and devices, not elsewhere classified
Note: Categories Z89-Z9Ø and Z93-Z99 are for use only if there are no complications or malfunctions of the organ or tissue replaced, the amputation site or the equipment on which the patient is dependent.

**4) History (of)**

There are two types of history Z codes, personal and family. Personal history codes explain a patient's past medical condition that no longer exists and is not receiving any treatment, but that has the potential for recurrence, and therefore may require continued monitoring.

Family history codes are for use when a patient has a family member(s) who has had a particular disease that causes the patient to be at higher risk of also contracting the disease.

Personal history codes may be used in conjunction with follow-up codes and family history codes may be used in conjunction with screening codes to explain the need for a test or procedure. History codes are also acceptable on any medical record regardless of the reason for visit. A history of an illness, even if no longer present, is important information that may alter the type of treatment ordered.

The reason for the encounter (for example, screening or counseling) should be sequenced first and the appropriate personal and/or family history code(s) should be assigned as additional diagnos(es).

The history Z code categories are:

Z8Ø Family history of primary malignant neoplasm
Z81 Family history of mental and behavioral disorders
Z82 Family history of certain disabilities and chronic diseases (leading to disablement)
Z83 Family history of other specific disorders
Z84 Family history of other conditions
**Z84.A Family history of exposure to diethylstilbestrol**
**Note: Code Z84.A, Family history of exposure to diethylstilbestrol (DES), is assigned when the patient has a family member that was exposed to DES that could cause the patient to be at a higher risk for a condition related to the exposure. This code is used, for example, when the patient's maternal grandmother was exposed to DES**
Z85 Personal history of malignant neoplasm
Z86 Personal history of certain other diseases
Z87 Personal history of other diseases and conditions
Z91.4- Personal history of psychological trauma, not elsewhere classified
Z91.5- Personal history of self-harm
Z91.81 History of falling
Z91.82 Personal history of military deployment
Z91.85 Personal history of military service
Z92 Personal history of medical treatment
Except: Z92.Ø, Personal history of contraception
Except: Z92.82, Status post administration of tPA (rtPA) in a different facility within the last 24 hours prior to admission to a current facility

**5) Screening**

Screening is the testing for disease or disease precursors in seemingly well individuals so that early detection and treatment can be provided for those who test positive for the disease (e.g., screening mammogram).

The testing of a person to rule out or confirm a suspected diagnosis because the patient has some sign or symptom is a diagnostic examination, not a screening. In these cases, the sign or symptom is used to explain the reason for the test.

A screening code may be a first-listed code if the reason for the visit is specifically the screening exam. It may also be used as an additional code if the screening is done during an office visit for other health problems. A screening code is not necessary if the screening is inherent to a routine examination, such as a pap smear done during a routine pelvic examination.

Should a condition be discovered during the screening then the code for the condition may be assigned as an additional diagnosis.

The Z code indicates that a screening exam is planned. A procedure code is required to confirm that the screening was performed.

The screening Z codes/categories:

Z11 Encounter for screening for infectious and parasitic diseases
Z12 Encounter for screening for malignant neoplasms
Z13 Encounter for screening for other diseases and disorders Except: Z13.9, Encounter for screening, unspecified
Z36 Encounter for antenatal screening for mother

**6) Observation**

There are three observation Z code categories. They are for use in very limited circumstances when a person is being observed for a suspected condition that is ruled out. The observation codes are not for use if an injury or illness or any signs or symptoms related to the suspected condition are present. In such cases the diagnosis/symptom code is used with the corresponding external cause code.

The observation codes are primarily to be used as a principal/first-listed diagnosis. An observation code may be assigned as a secondary diagnosis code when the patient is being observed for a condition that is ruled out and is unrelated to the principal/first-listed diagnosis. Also, when the principal diagnosis is required to be a code from category Z38, Liveborn infants according to place of birth and type of delivery, then a code from category ZØ5, Encounter for observation and evaluation of newborn for suspected diseases and conditions ruled out, is sequenced after the Z38 code. Additional codes may be used in addition to the observation code, but only if they are unrelated to the suspected condition being observed.

Codes from subcategory ZØ3.7, Encounter for suspected maternal and fetal conditions ruled out, may either be used as a first-listed or as an additional code assignment depending on the case. They are for use in very limited circumstances on a maternal record when an encounter is for a suspected maternal or fetal condition that is ruled out during that encounter (for example, a maternal or fetal condition may be suspected due to an abnormal test result). These codes should not be used when the condition is confirmed. In those cases, the confirmed condition should be coded. In addition, these codes are not for use if an illness or any signs or symptoms related to the suspected condition or problem are present. In such cases the diagnosis/symptom code is used.

Additional codes may be used in addition to the code from subcategory ZØ3.7, but only if they are unrelated to the suspected condition being evaluated.

Codes from subcategory ZØ3.7 may not be used for encounters for antenatal screening of mother. *See Section I.C.21. Screening.*

For encounters for suspected fetal condition that are inconclusive following testing and evaluation, assign the appropriate code from category O35, O36, O4Ø or O41.

The observation Z code categories:

ZØ3 Encounter for medical observation for suspected diseases and conditions ruled out
ZØ4 Encounter for examination and observation for other reasons Except: ZØ4.9, Encounter for examination and observation for unspecified reason
ZØ5 Encounter for observation and evaluation of newborn for suspected diseases and conditions ruled out

**7) Aftercare**

Aftercare visit codes cover situations when the initial treatment of a disease has been performed and the patient requires continued care during the healing or recovery phase, or for the long-term consequences of the disease. The aftercare Z code should not be used if treatment is directed at a current, acute disease. The diagnosis code is to be used in these cases.

The aftercare Z codes should also not be used for aftercare for injuries. For aftercare of an injury, assign the acute injury code with the appropriate 7th character (for subsequent encounter).

The aftercare codes are generally first listed to explain the specific reason for the encounter. An aftercare code may be reported as an additional code when a specific type of aftercare is provided in addition to the reason for the encounter. An example of this would be the closure of a colostomy during an encounter for treatment of another condition.

Aftercare codes should be used in conjunction with other aftercare codes or diagnosis codes to provide better detail on the specifics of an aftercare encounter visit, unless otherwise directed by the classification. The sequencing of multiple aftercare codes depends on the circumstances of the encounter.

Certain aftercare Z code categories need a secondary diagnosis code to describe the resolving condition or sequelae. For others, the condition is included in the code title.

2027 ICD-10-CM Official Guidelines for Coding and Reporting

Additional Z code aftercare category terms include fitting and adjustment, and attention to artificial openings.

Status Z codes may be used with aftercare Z codes to indicate the nature of the aftercare. For example, code Z95.1, Presence of aortocoronary bypass graft, may be used with code Z48.812, Encounter for surgical aftercare following surgery on the circulatory system, to indicate the surgery for which the aftercare is being performed. A status code should not be used when the aftercare code indicates the type of status, such as using Z43.Ø, Encounter for attention to tracheostomy, with Z93.Ø, Tracheostomy status.

The aftercare codes are generally found in the following categories:

| | |
|---|---|
| Z42 | Encounter for plastic and reconstructive surgery following medical procedure or healed injury |
| Z43 | Encounter for attention to artificial openings |
| Z44 | Encounter for fitting and adjustment of external prosthetic device |
| Z45 | Encounter for adjustment and management of implanted device |
| Z46 | Encounter for fitting and adjustment of other devices |
| Z47 | Orthopedic aftercare |
| Z48 | Encounter for other postprocedural aftercare |
| Z49 | Encounter for care involving renal dialysis |
| Z51 | Encounter for other aftercare and medical care |

**8) Follow-up**

The follow-up codes are used to explain continuing surveillance following completed treatment of a disease, condition, or injury. They imply that the condition has been fully treated and no longer exists. They should not be confused with aftercare codes, or injury codes with a 7th character for subsequent encounter, that explain ongoing care of a healing condition or its sequelae. Follow-up codes may be used in conjunction with history codes to provide the full picture of the healed condition and its treatment. The follow-up code is sequenced first, followed by the history code.

A follow-up code may be used to explain multiple visits. Should a condition be found to have recurred on the follow-up visit, then the diagnosis code for the condition should be assigned in place of the follow-up code.

The follow-up Z codes/categories:

| | |
|---|---|
| ZØ8 | Encounter for follow-up examination after completed treatment for malignant neoplasm |
| ZØ9 | Encounter for follow-up examination after completed treatment for conditions other than malignant neoplasm |

Codes ZØ8, Encounter for follow-up examination after completed treatment for malignant neoplasm, and ZØ9, Encounter for follow up examination after completed treatment for conditions other than malignant neoplasm, may be assigned following any type of completed treatment modality (including both medical and surgical treatments).

Z39 Encounter for maternal postpartum care and examination

**9) Donor**

Codes in category Z52, Donors of organs and tissues, are used for living individuals who are donating blood or other body tissue. These codes are for individuals donating for others, as well as for self-donations. They are not used to identify cadaveric donations.

**10) Counseling**

Counseling Z codes are used when a patient or family member receives assistance in the aftermath of an illness or injury, or when support is required in coping with family or social problems.

The counseling Z codes/categories:

| | |
|---|---|
| Z3Ø.Ø- | Encounter for general counseling and advice on contraception |
| Z31.5 | Encounter for procreative genetic counseling |
| Z31.6- | Encounter for general counseling and advice on procreation |
| Z32.2 | Encounter for childbirth instruction |
| Z32.3 | Encounter for childcare instruction |
| Z69 | Encounter for mental health services for victim and perpetrator of abuse |
| Z7Ø | Counseling related to sexual attitude, behavior and orientation |
| Z71 | Persons encountering health services for other counseling and medical advice, not elsewhere classified<br>Note: Code Z71.84, Encounter for health counseling related to travel, is to be used for health risk and safety counseling for future travel purposes.<br>Code Z71.85, Encounter for immunization safety counseling, is to be used for counseling of the patient or caregiver regarding the safety of a vaccine. This code should not be used for the provision of general information regarding risks and potential side effects during routine encounters for the administration of vaccines.<br>Code Z71.87, Encounter for pediatric-to-adult transition counseling, should be assigned when pediatric-to-adult transition counseling is the sole reason for the encounter or when this counseling is provided in addition to other services, such as treatment of a chronic condition. If both transition counseling and treatment of a medical condition are provided during the same encounter, the code(s) for the medical condition(s) treated and code Z71.87 should be assigned, with sequencing depending on the circumstances of the encounter. |
| Z76.81 | Expectant mother prebirth pediatrician visit |

**11) Encounters for Obstetrical and Reproductive Services**

*See Section I.C.15. Pregnancy, Childbirth, and the Puerperium, for further instruction on the use of these codes.*

Z codes for pregnancy are for use in those circumstances when none of the problems or complications included in the codes from the Obstetrics chapter exist (a routine prenatal visit or postpartum care). Codes in category Z34, Encounter for supervision of normal pregnancy, are always first listed and are not to be used with any other code from the OB chapter.

Codes in category Z3A, Weeks of gestation, may be assigned to provide additional information about the pregnancy. Category Z3A codes should not be assigned for pregnancies with abortive outcomes (categories OØØ-OØ8), elective termination of pregnancy (code Z33.2), nor for postpartum conditions, as category Z3A is not applicable to these conditions. The date of the admission should be used to determine weeks of gestation for inpatient admissions that encompass more than one gestational week.

The outcome of delivery, category Z37, should be included on all maternal delivery records. It is always a secondary code.

Codes in category Z37 should not be used on the newborn record.

Z codes for family planning (contraceptive) or procreative management and counseling should be included on an obstetric record either during the pregnancy or the postpartum stage, if applicable.

Z codes/categories for obstetrical and reproductive services:

| | |
|---|---|
| Z3Ø | Encounter for contraceptive management |
| Z31 | Encounter for procreative management |
| Z32.2 | Encounter for childbirth instruction |
| Z32.3 | Encounter for childcare instruction |
| Z33 | Pregnant state |
| Z34 | Encounter for supervision of normal pregnancy |
| Z36 | Encounter for antenatal screening of mother |
| Z3A | Weeks of gestation |
| Z37 | Outcome of delivery |
| Z39 | Encounter for maternal postpartum care and examination |
| Z76.81 | Expectant mother prebirth pediatrician visit |

**12) Routine and Administrative Examinations**

The Z codes allow for the description of encounters for routine examinations, such as, a general check-up, or, examinations for administrative purposes, such as, a pre-employment physical. The codes are not to be used if the examination is for diagnosis of a suspected condition or for treatment purposes. In such cases the diagnosis code is used. During a routine exam, should a diagnosis or condition be discovered, it should be coded as an additional code. Pre-existing and chronic conditions and history codes may also be included as additional codes as long as the examination is for administrative purposes and not focused on any particular condition.

Some of the codes for routine health examinations distinguish between "with" and "without" abnormal findings. Code assignment depends on the information that is known at the time the encounter is being coded. For example, if no abnormal findings were found during the examination, but the encounter is being coded before test results are back, it is acceptable to assign the code for "without abnormal findings." When assigning a code for "with abnormal findings," additional code(s) should be assigned to identify the specific abnormal finding(s).

Pre-operative examination and pre-procedural laboratory examination Z codes are for use only in those situations when a patient is being cleared for a procedure or surgery and no treatment is given.

The Z codes/categories for routine and administrative examinations:

| | |
|---|---|
| ZØØ | Encounter for general examination without complaint, suspected or reported diagnosis |
| ZØ1 | Encounter for other special examination without complaint, suspected or reported diagnosis |
| ZØ2 | Encounter for administrative examination<br>Except: ZØ2.9, Encounter for administrative examinations, unspecified |
| Z32.Ø- | Encounter for pregnancy test |

**13) Miscellaneous Z Codes**

The miscellaneous Z codes capture a number of other health care encounters that do not fall into one of the other categories. Some of these codes identify the reason for the encounter; others are for use as additional codes that provide useful information on circumstances that may affect a patient's care and treatment.

**Prophylactic Organ Removal**

For encounters specifically for prophylactic removal of an organ (such as prophylactic removal of breasts due to a genetic susceptibility to cancer or a family history of cancer), the principal or first-listed code should be a code from category Z4Ø, Encounter for prophylactic surgery for risk factors related to malignant neoplasms, or subcategory Z4Ø.8, Encounter for other prophylactic surgery. If applicable, assign additional code(s) to identify any associated risk factor (such as genetic susceptibility or family history).

If the patient has a malignancy of one site and is having prophylactic removal at another site to prevent either a new primary malignancy or metastatic disease, a code for the malignancy should also be assigned in addition to a code from subcategory Z4Ø.Ø, Encounter for prophylactic surgery for risk factors related to malignant neoplasms. A Z4Ø.Ø code should not be assigned if the patient is having organ removal for treatment of a malignancy, such as the removal of the testes for the treatment of prostate cancer.

Miscellaneous Z codes/subcategories/categories:

| | |
|---|---|
| Z28 | Immunization not carried out<br>Except: Z28.3-, Underimmunization status |
| Z29 | Encounter for other prophylactic measures |
| Z4Ø | Encounter for prophylactic surgery |
| Z41 | Encounter for procedures for purposes other than remedying health state<br>Except: Z41.9, Encounter for procedure for purposes other than remedying health state, unspecified |
| Z53 | Persons encountering health services for specific procedures and treatment, not carried out |
| Z72 | Problems related to lifestyle<br>Note: These codes should be assigned only when the documentation specifies that the patient has an associated problem |
| Z73 | Problems related to life management difficulty<br>Note: These codes should be assigned only when the documentation specifies that the patient has an associated problem. |
| Z74 | Problems related to care provider dependency<br>Except: Z74.Ø1, Bed confinement status |
| Z75 | Problems related to medical facilities and other health care |
| Z76.Ø | Encounter for issue of repeat prescription |
| Z76.3 | Healthy person accompanying sick person |
| Z76.4 | Other boarder to healthcare facility |
| Z76.5 | Malingerer [conscious simulation] |
| Z91.1- | Patient's noncompliance with medical treatment and regimen |
| Z91.A- | Caregiver's noncompliance with patient's medical treatment and regimen |
| Z91.B | Personal risk factor of exposure to diethylstilbestrol<br>**Note: This code is assigned to show the patient was directly exposed to DES in utero (e.g., when the patient's mother was exposed to DES while the patient was in utero).** |
| Z91.83 | Wandering in diseases classified elsewhere |
| Z91.84- | Oral health risk factors |
| Z91.89 | Other specified personal risk factors, not elsewhere classified |

*See Section I.B.14. for Z55-Z65 Persons with potential health hazards related to socioeconomic and psychosocial circumstances, documentation by clinicians other than the patient's provider*

**14) Nonspecific Z Codes**

Certain Z codes are so non-specific, or potentially redundant with other codes in the classification, that there can be little justification for their use in the inpatient setting. Their use in the outpatient setting should be limited to those instances when there is no further documentation to permit more precise coding. Otherwise, any sign or symptom or any other reason for visit that is captured in another code should be used.

Nonspecific Z codes/categories:

| | |
|---|---|
| ZØ2.9 | Encounter for administrative examinations, unspecified |
| ZØ4.9 | Encounter for examination and observation for unspecified reason |
| Z13.9 | Encounter for screening, unspecified |
| Z41.9 | Encounter for procedure for purposes other than remedying health state, unspecified |
| Z52.9 | Donor of unspecified organ or tissue |
| Z86.59 | Personal history of other mental and behavioral disorders |
| Z88.9 | Allergy status to unspecified drugs, medicaments and biological substances status |
| Z92.Ø | Personal history of contraception |

**15) Z Codes That May Only be Principal/First-Listed Diagnosis**

The following Z codes/subcategories/categories may only be reported as the principal/first-listed diagnosis, except when there are multiple encounters on the same day and the medical records for the encounters are combined:

| | |
|---|---|
| ZØØ | Encounter for general examination without complaint, suspected or reported diagnosis<br>Except: ZØØ.6 |
| ZØ1 | Encounter for other special examination without complaint, suspected or reported diagnosis |
| ZØ2 | Encounter for administrative examination |
| ZØ4 | Encounter for examination and observation for other reasons |
| Z33.2 | Encounter for elective termination of pregnancy |
| Z31.81 | Encounter for male factor infertility in female patient |
| Z31.83 | Encounter for assisted reproductive fertility procedure cycle |
| Z31.84 | Encounter for fertility preservation procedure |
| Z34 | Encounter for supervision of normal pregnancy |
| Z39 | Encounter for maternal postpartum care and examination |
| Z38 | Liveborn infants according to place of birth and type of delivery |
| Z4Ø | Encounter for prophylactic surgery |
| Z42 | Encounter for plastic and reconstructive surgery following medical procedure or healed injury |
| Z51.Ø | Encounter for antineoplastic radiation therapy |
| Z51.1- | Encounter for antineoplastic chemotherapy and immunotherapy |
| Z52 | Donors of organs and tissues<br>Except: Z52.9, Donor of unspecified organ or tissue |
| Z76.1 | Encounter for health supervision and care of foundling |
| Z76.2 | Encounter for health supervision and care of other healthy infant and child |
| Z99.12 | Encounter for respirator [ventilator] dependence during power failure |

**16) Newborns and Infants**

*See Section I.C.16. Newborn (Perinatal) Guidelines, for further instruction on the use of these codes.*

Newborn Z codes/subcategories/categories:

| | |
|---|---|
| Z76.1 | Encounter for health supervision and care of foundling |
| ZØØ.1- | Encounter for routine child health examination |
| Z38 | Liveborn infants according to place of birth and type of delivery |

**17) Social Determinants of Health**

Social determinants of health (SDOH) codes describing social problems, conditions, or risk factors that influence a patient's health should be assigned when this information is documented in the patient's medical record. Assign as many SDOH codes as are necessary to describe all of the social problems, conditions, or risk factors documented during the current episode of care. For example, a patient who lives alone may suffer an acute injury temporarily impacting their ability to perform routine activities of daily living. When documented as such, this would support assignment of code Z6Ø.2, Problems related to living alone. However, merely living alone, without documentation of a risk or unmet need for assistance at home, would not support assignment of code Z6Ø.2. Documentation by a clinician (or patient-reported information that is signed off by a clinician) that the patient expressed concerns with access and availability of food would support assignment of code Z59.41, Food insecurity. Similarly, medical record documentation indicating the patient is experiencing homelessness would support assignment of a code from subcategory Z59.Ø-, Homelessness.

For social determinants of health classified to chapter 21, such as information found in categories Z55-Z65, Persons with potential health hazards related to socioeconomic and psychosocial circumstances, code assignment may be based on medical record documentation from clinicians involved in the care of the patient who are not the patient's provider since this information represents social information, rather than medical diagnoses. For example, coding professionals may utilize documentation of social information from social workers, community health workers, case managers, or nurses, if their documentation is included in the official medical record.

Patient self-reported documentation may be used to assign codes for social determinants of health, as long as the patient self-reported information is signed-off by and incorporated into the medical record by either a clinician or provider.

Social determinants of health codes are located primarily in these Z code categories:

| | |
|---|---|
| Z55 | Problems related to education and literacy |
| Z56 | Problems related to employment and unemployment |
| Z57 | Occupational exposure to risk factors |
| Z58 | Problems related to physical environment |
| Z59 | Problems related to housing and economic circumstances |
| Z6Ø | Problems related to social environment |
| Z62 | Problems related to upbringing |
| Z63 | Other problems related to primary support group, including family circumstances |
| Z64 | Problems related to certain psychosocial circumstances |
| Z65 | Problems related to other psychosocial circumstances |

*See Section I.B.14. Documentation by Clinicians Other than the Patient's Provider.*

**22. Chapter 22: Codes for Special Purposes (UØØ-U85)**

| | |
|---|---|
| UØ7.Ø | Vaping-related disorder (see Section I.C.1Ø.e., Vaping-related disorders) |
| UØ7.1 | COVID-19 (see Section I.C.1.g.1., COVID-19 infection) |
| UØ9.9 | Post COVID-19 condition, unspecified (see Section I.C.1.g.1.m.) |

# Section II. Selection of Principal Diagnosis

The circumstances of inpatient admission always govern the selection of principal diagnosis. The principal diagnosis is defined in the Uniform Hospital Discharge Data Set (UHDDS) as "that condition established after study to be chiefly responsible for occasioning the admission of the patient to the hospital for care."

The UHDDS definitions are used by hospitals to report inpatient data elements in a standardized manner. These data elements and their definitions can be found in the July 31, 1985, Federal Register (Vol. 50, No, 147), pp. 31038-40.

Since that time, the application of the UHDDS definitions has been expanded to include all non-outpatient settings (acute care, short term, long term care and psychiatric hospitals; home health agencies; rehab facilities; nursing homes, etc.). The UHDDS definitions also apply to hospice services (all levels of care).

In determining principal diagnosis, coding conventions in the ICD-10-CM, the Tabular List and Alphabetic Index take precedence over these official coding guidelines.

*(See Section I.A., Conventions for the ICD-10-CM)*

The importance of consistent, complete documentation in the medical record cannot be overemphasized. Without such documentation the application of all coding guidelines is a difficult, if not impossible, task.

**A. Codes for symptoms, signs, and ill-defined conditions**

Codes for symptoms, signs, and ill-defined conditions from Chapter 18 are not to be used as principal diagnosis when a related definitive diagnosis has been established.

**B. Two or more interrelated conditions, each potentially meeting the definition for principal diagnosis.**

When there are two or more interrelated conditions (such as diseases in the same ICD-10-CM chapter or manifestations characteristically associated with a certain disease) potentially meeting the definition of principal diagnosis, either condition may be sequenced first, unless the circumstances of the admission, the therapy provided, the Tabular List, or the Alphabetic Index indicate otherwise.

**C. Two or more diagnoses that equally meet the definition for principal diagnosis**

In the unusual instance when two or more diagnoses equally meet the criteria for principal diagnosis as determined by the circumstances of admission, diagnostic workup and/or therapy provided, and the Alphabetic Index, Tabular List, or another coding guidelines does not provide sequencing direction, any one of the diagnoses may be sequenced first.

**D. Two or more comparative or contrasting conditions**

In those rare instances when two or more contrasting or comparative diagnoses are documented as "either/or" (or similar terminology), they are coded as if the diagnoses were confirmed and the diagnoses are sequenced according to the circumstances of the admission. If no further determination can be made as to which diagnosis should be principal, either diagnosis may be sequenced first.

**E. A symptom(s) followed by contrasting/comparative diagnoses**

GUIDELINE HAS BEEN DELETED EFFECTIVE OCTOBER 1, 2014

**F. Original treatment plan not carried out**

Sequence as the principal diagnosis the condition, which after study occasioned the admission to the hospital, even though treatment may not have been carried out due to unforeseen circumstances.

**G. Complications of surgery and other medical care**

When the admission is for treatment of a complication resulting from surgery or other medical care, the complication code is sequenced as the principal diagnosis. If the complication is classified to the T8Ø-T88 series and the code lacks the necessary specificity in describing the complication, an additional code for the specific complication should be assigned.

**H. Uncertain Diagnosis**

If the diagnosis documented at the time of discharge is qualified as "probable," "suspected," "likely," "questionable," "possible," or "still to be ruled out," "compatible with," "consistent with," or other similar terms indicating uncertainty, code the condition as if it existed or was established. The bases for these guidelines are the diagnostic workup, arrangements for further workup or observation, and initial therapeutic approach that correspond most closely with the established diagnosis.

**Note:** This guideline is applicable only to inpatient admissions to short-term, acute, long-term care and psychiatric hospitals.

**I. Admission from Observation Unit**

**1. Admission Following Medical Observation**

When a patient is admitted to an observation unit for a medical condition, which either worsens or does not improve, and is subsequently admitted as an inpatient of the same hospital for this same medical condition, the principal diagnosis would be the medical condition which led to the hospital admission.

**2. Admission Following Post-Operative Observation**

When a patient is admitted to an observation unit to monitor a condition (or complication) that develops following outpatient surgery, and then is subsequently admitted as an inpatient of the same hospital, hospitals should apply the Uniform Hospital Discharge Data Set (UHDDS) definition of principal diagnosis as "that condition established after study to be chiefly responsible for occasioning the admission of the patient to the hospital for care."

**J. Admission from Outpatient Surgery**

When a patient receives surgery in the hospital's outpatient surgery department and is subsequently admitted for continuing inpatient care at the same hospital, the following guidelines should be followed in selecting the principal diagnosis for the inpatient admission:

- If the reason for the inpatient admission is a complication, assign the complication as the principal diagnosis.
- If no complication, or other condition, is documented as the reason for the inpatient admission, assign the reason for the outpatient surgery as the principal diagnosis.
- If the reason for the inpatient admission is another condition unrelated to the surgery, assign the unrelated condition as the principal diagnosis.

**K. Admissions/Encounters for Rehabilitation**

When the purpose for the admission/encounter is rehabilitation, sequence first the code for the condition for which the service is being performed. For example, for an admission/encounter for rehabilitation for right-sided dominant hemiplegia following a cerebrovascular infarction, report code I69.351, Hemiplegia and hemiparesis following cerebral infarction affecting right dominant side, as the first-listed or principal diagnosis.

If the condition for which the rehabilitation service is being provided is no longer present, report the appropriate aftercare code as the first-listed or principal diagnosis, unless the rehabilitation service is being provided following an injury. For rehabilitation services following active treatment of an injury, assign the injury code with the appropriate seventh character for subsequent encounter as the first-listed or principal diagnosis. For example, if a patient with severe degenerative osteoarthritis of the hip, underwent hip replacement and the current encounter/admission is for rehabilitation, report code Z47.1, Aftercare following joint replacement surgery, as the first-listed or principal diagnosis. If the patient requires rehabilitation post hip replacement for right intertrochanteric femur fracture, report code S72.141D, Displaced intertrochanteric fracture of right femur, subsequent encounter for closed fracture with routine healing, as the first-listed or principal diagnosis.

*See Section I.C.21.c.7., Factors influencing health states and contact with health services, Aftercare.*

*See Section I.C.19.a., for additional information about the use of 7th characters for injury codes.*

# Section III. Reporting Additional Diagnoses

GENERAL RULES FOR OTHER (ADDITIONAL) DIAGNOSES

For reporting purposes, the definition for "other diagnoses" is interpreted as additional clinically significant conditions that affect patient care in terms of requiring:

clinical evaluation; or

therapeutic treatment; or

diagnostic procedures; or

extended length of hospital stay; or

increased nursing care and/or monitoring.

The UHDDS item #11-b defines Other Diagnoses as "all conditions that coexist at the time of admission, that develop subsequently, or that affect the treatment received and/or the length of stay. Diagnoses that relate to an earlier episode which have no bearing on the current hospital stay are to be excluded." UHDDS definitions apply to inpatients in acute care, short-term, long term care and psychiatric hospital setting. The UHDDS definitions are used by acute care short-term hospitals to report inpatient data elements in a standardized manner. These data elements and their definitions can be found in the July 31, 1985, Federal Register (Vol. 50, No, 147), pp. 31038-40.

Since that time, the application of the UHDDS definitions has been expanded to include all non-outpatient settings (acute care, short term, long term care and psychiatric hospitals; home health agencies; rehab facilities; nursing homes, etc.). The UHDDS definitions also apply to hospice services (all levels of care).

The following guidelines are to be applied in designating "other diagnoses" when neither the Alphabetic Index nor the Tabular List in ICD-10-CM provide direction. The listing of the diagnoses in the patient record is the responsibility of the provider.

**A. Previous conditions**

If the provider has included a diagnosis in the final diagnostic statement, such as the discharge summary or the face sheet, it should ordinarily be coded. Some providers include in the diagnostic statement resolved conditions or diagnoses and status-post procedures from previous admissions that have no bearing on the current stay. Such conditions are not to be reported and are coded only if required by hospital policy.

However, history codes (categories Z8Ø-Z87) may be used as secondary codes if the historical condition or family history has an impact on current care or influences treatment.

**B. Abnormal findings**

Abnormal findings (laboratory, x-ray, pathologic, and other diagnostic results) are not coded and reported unless the provider indicates their clinical significance. If the findings are outside the normal range and the provider has ordered other tests to evaluate the condition or prescribed treatment, it is appropriate to ask the provider whether the abnormal finding should be added.

**Please note:** This differs from the coding practices in the outpatient setting for coding encounters for diagnostic tests that have been interpreted by a provider.

**C. Uncertain Diagnosis**
If the diagnosis documented at the time of discharge is qualified as "probable," "suspected," "likely," "questionable," "possible," or "still to be ruled out," "compatible with," "consistent with," or other similar terms indicating uncertainty, code the condition as if it existed or was established. The bases for these guidelines are the diagnostic workup, arrangements for further workup or observation, and initial therapeutic approach that correspond most closely with the established diagnosis.

**Note:** This guideline is applicable only to inpatient admissions to short-term, acute, long-term care and psychiatric hospitals.

# Section IV. Diagnostic Coding and Reporting Guidelines for Outpatient Services

These coding guidelines for outpatient diagnoses have been approved for use by hospitals/ providers in coding and reporting hospital-based outpatient services and provider-based office visits. Guidelines in Section I, Conventions, general coding guidelines and chapter-specific guidelines, should also be applied for outpatient services and office visits.

Information about the use of certain abbreviations, punctuation, symbols, and other conventions used in the ICD-10-CM Tabular List (code numbers and titles), can be found in Section IA of these guidelines, under "Conventions Used in the Tabular List." Section I.B. contains general guidelines that apply to the entire classification. Section I.C. contains chapter-specific guidelines that correspond to the chapters as they are arranged in the classification. Information about the correct sequence to use in finding a code is also described in Section I.

The terms encounter and visit are often used interchangeably in describing outpatient service contacts and, therefore, appear together in these guidelines without distinguishing one from the other.

Though the conventions and general guidelines apply to all settings, coding guidelines for outpatient and provider reporting of diagnoses will vary in a number of instances from those for inpatient diagnoses, recognizing that:

The Uniform Hospital Discharge Data Set (UHDDS) definition of principal diagnosis does not apply to hospital-based outpatient services and provider-based office visits.

Coding guidelines for inconclusive diagnoses (probable, suspected, rule out, etc.) were developed for inpatient reporting and do not apply to outpatients.

**A. Selection of first-listed condition**
In the outpatient setting, the term first-listed diagnosis is used in lieu of principal diagnosis.

In determining the first-listed diagnosis the coding conventions of ICD-10-CM, as well as the general and disease specific guidelines take precedence over the outpatient guidelines.

Diagnoses often are not established at the time of the initial encounter/visit. It may take two or more visits before the diagnosis is confirmed.

The most critical rule involves beginning the search for the correct code assignment through the Alphabetic Index. Never begin searching initially in the Tabular List as this will lead to coding errors.

1. **Outpatient Surgery**
When a patient presents for outpatient surgery (same day surgery), code the reason for the surgery as the first-listed diagnosis (reason for the encounter), even if the surgery is not performed due to a contraindication.

2. **Observation Stay**
When a patient is admitted for observation for a medical condition, assign a code for the medical condition as the first-listed diagnosis.

When a patient presents for outpatient surgery and develops complications requiring admission to observation, code the reason for the surgery as the first reported diagnosis (reason for the encounter), followed by codes for the complications as secondary diagnoses.

**B. Codes from AØØ.Ø through T88.9, ZØØ-Z99, UØØ-U85**
The appropriate code(s) from AØØ.Ø through T88.9, ZØØ-Z99 and UØØ-U85 must be used to identify diagnoses, symptoms, conditions, problems, complaints, or other reason(s) for the encounter/visit.

**C. Accurate reporting of ICD-10-CM diagnosis codes**
For accurate reporting of ICD-10-CM diagnosis codes, the documentation should describe the patient's condition, using terminology which includes specific diagnoses as well as symptoms, problems, or reasons for the encounter. There are ICD-10-CM codes to describe all of these.

**D. Codes that describe symptoms and signs**
Codes that describe symptoms and signs, as opposed to diagnoses, are acceptable for reporting purposes when a diagnosis has not been established (confirmed) by the provider. Chapter 18 of ICD-10-CM, Symptoms, Signs, and Abnormal Clinical and Laboratory Findings Not Elsewhere Classified (codes RØØ-R99) contain many, but not all codes for symptoms.

**E. Encounters for circumstances other than a disease or injury**
ICD-10-CM provides codes to deal with encounters for circumstances other than a disease or injury. The Factors Influencing Health Status and Contact with Health Services codes (ZØØ-Z99) are provided to deal with occasions when circumstances other than a disease or injury are recorded as diagnosis or problems.

*See Section I.C.21. Factors influencing health status and contact with health services.*

**F. Level of Detail in Coding**

1. **ICD-10-CM codes with 3, 4, 5, 6 or 7 characters**
ICD-10-CM is composed of codes with 3, 4, 5, 6 or 7 characters. Codes with three characters are included in ICD-10-CM as the heading of a category of codes that may be further subdivided by the use of fourth, fifth, sixth or seventh characters to provide greater specificity.

2. **Use of full number of characters required for a code**
A three-character code is to be used only if it is not further subdivided. A code is invalid if it has not been coded to the full number of characters required for that code, including the 7th character, if applicable.

3. **Highest level of specificity**
Code to the highest level of specificity when supported by the medical record documentation.

**G. ICD-10-CM code for the diagnosis, condition, problem, or other reason for encounter/visit**
List first the ICD-10-CM code for the diagnosis, condition, problem, or other reason for encounter/visit shown in the medical record to be chiefly responsible for the services provided. List additional codes that describe any coexisting conditions. In some cases, the first-listed diagnosis may be a symptom when a diagnosis has not been established (confirmed) by the provider.

**H. Uncertain diagnosis**
Do not code diagnoses documented as "probable", "suspected," "questionable," "rule out," "compatible with," "consistent with," or "working diagnosis" or other similar terms indicating uncertainty. Rather, code the condition(s) to the highest degree of certainty for that encounter/visit, such as symptoms, signs, abnormal test results, or other reason for the visit.

**Please note:** This differs from the coding practices used by short-term, acute care, long-term care and psychiatric hospitals.

**I. Chronic diseases**
Chronic diseases treated on an ongoing basis may be coded and reported as many times as the patient receives treatment and care for the condition(s).

**J. Code all documented conditions that coexist**
Code all documented conditions that coexist at the time of the encounter/visit and that require or affect patient care, treatment or management. Do not code conditions that were previously treated and no longer exist. However, history codes (categories Z8Ø-Z87) may be used as secondary codes if the historical condition or family history has an impact on current care or influences treatment.

**K. Patients receiving diagnostic services only**
For patients receiving diagnostic services only during an encounter/visit, sequence first the diagnosis, condition, problem, or other reason for encounter/visit shown in the medical record to be chiefly responsible for the outpatient services provided during the encounter/visit. Codes for other diagnoses (e.g., chronic conditions) may be sequenced as additional diagnoses.

For encounters for routine laboratory/radiology testing in the absence of any signs, symptoms, or associated diagnosis, assign ZØ1.89, Encounter for other specified special examinations. If routine testing is performed during the same encounter as a test to evaluate a sign, symptom, or diagnosis, it is appropriate to assign both the Z code and the code describing the reason for the non-routine test.

For outpatient encounters for diagnostic tests that have been interpreted by a physician, and the final report is available at the time of coding, code any confirmed or definitive diagnosis(es) documented in the interpretation. Do not code related signs and symptoms as additional diagnoses.

**Please note:** This differs from the coding practice in the hospital inpatient setting regarding abnormal findings on test results.

**L. Patients receiving therapeutic services only**
For patients receiving therapeutic services only during an encounter/visit, sequence first the diagnosis, condition, problem, or other reason for encounter/visit shown in the medical record to be chiefly responsible for the outpatient services provided during the encounter/visit. Codes for other diagnoses (e.g., chronic conditions) may be sequenced as additional diagnoses.

The only exception to this rule is that when the primary reason for the admission/encounter is chemotherapy or radiation therapy, the appropriate Z code for the service is listed first, and the diagnosis or problem for which the service is being performed listed second.

**M. Patients receiving preoperative evaluations only**
For patients receiving preoperative evaluations only, sequence first a code from subcategory ZØ1.81, Encounter for pre-procedural examinations, to describe the pre-op consultations. Assign a code for the condition to describe the reason for the surgery as an additional diagnosis. Code also any findings related to the pre-op evaluation.

**N. Ambulatory surgery**
For ambulatory surgery, code the diagnosis for which the surgery was performed. If the postoperative diagnosis is known to be different from the preoperative diagnosis at the time the diagnosis is confirmed, select the postoperative diagnosis for coding, since it is the most definitive.

**O. Routine outpatient prenatal visits**
*See Section I.C.15. Routine outpatient prenatal visits.*

**P. Encounters for general medical examinations with abnormal findings**
The subcategories for encounters for general medical examinations, Z00.0- and encounter for routine child health examination, Z00.12-, provide codes for with and without abnormal findings. Should a general medical examination result in an abnormal finding, the code for general medical examination with abnormal finding should be assigned as the first-listed diagnosis. An examination with abnormal findings refers to a condition/diagnosis that is newly identified or a change in severity of a chronic condition (such as uncontrolled hypertension, or an acute exacerbation of chronic obstructive pulmonary disease) during a routine physical examination. A secondary code for the abnormal finding should also be coded.

**Q. Encounters for routine health screenings**
*See Section I.C.21. Factors influencing health status and contact with health services, Screening*

# Appendix I. Present on Admission Reporting Guidelines

## Introduction

These guidelines are to be used as a supplement to the *ICD-10-CM Official Guidelines for Coding and Reporting* to facilitate the assignment of the Present on Admission (POA) indicator for each diagnosis and external cause of injury code reported on claim forms (UB-04 and 837 Institutional).

These guidelines are not intended to replace any guidelines in the main body of the *ICD-10-CM Official Guidelines for Coding and Reporting*. The POA guidelines are not intended to provide guidance on when a condition should be coded, but rather, how to apply the POA indicator to the final set of diagnosis codes that have been assigned in accordance with Sections I, II, and III of the official coding guidelines. Subsequent to the assignment of the ICD-10-CM codes, the POA indicator should then be assigned to those conditions that have been coded.

As stated in the Introduction to the *ICD-10-CM Official Guidelines for Coding and Reporting*, a joint effort between the healthcare provider and the coder is essential to achieve complete and accurate documentation, code assignment, and reporting of diagnoses and procedures. The importance of consistent, complete documentation in the medical record cannot be overemphasized. Medical record documentation from any provider involved in the care and treatment of the patient may be used to support the determination of whether a condition was present on admission or not. In the context of the official coding guidelines, the term "provider" means a physician or any qualified healthcare practitioner who is legally accountable for establishing the patient's diagnosis.

These guidelines are not a substitute for the provider's clinical judgment as to the determination of whether a condition was/was not present on admission. The provider should be queried regarding issues related to the linking of signs/symptoms, timing of test results, and the timing of findings.

Please see the CDC website for the detailed list of ICD-10-CM codes that do not require the reporting of a POA indicator (https://www.cdc.gov/nchs/icd/icd-10-cm/files.html). The codes and categories on this exempt list are for circumstances regarding the healthcare encounter or factors influencing health status that do not represent a current disease or injury or that describe conditions that are always present on admission.

## General Reporting Requirements

All claims involving inpatient admissions to general acute care hospitals or other facilities that are subject to a law or regulation mandating collection of present on admission information.

Present on admission is defined as present at the time the order for inpatient admission occurs -- conditions that develop during an outpatient encounter, including emergency department, observation, or outpatient surgery, are considered as present on admission.

A POA indicator is assigned to the principal and secondary diagnoses (as defined in Section II of the Official Guidelines for Coding and Reporting) and the external cause of injury codes.

Issues related to inconsistent, missing, conflicting or unclear documentation must still be resolved by the provider.

If a condition would not be coded and reported based on UHDDS definitions and current official coding guidelines, then the POA indicator would not be reported.

Reporting Options

Y – Yes

N – No

U – Unknown

W – Clinically undetermined

Unreported/Not used – (Exempt from POA reporting)

Reporting Definitions

Y = present at the time of inpatient admission

N = not present at the time of inpatient admission

U = documentation is insufficient to determine if condition **was** present on admission

W = provider is unable to clinically determine whether condition was present on admission or not

## Timeframe for POA Identification and Documentation

There is no required timeframe as to when a provider (per the definition of "provider" used in these guidelines) must identify or document a condition to be present on admission. In some clinical situations, it may not be possible for a provider to make a definitive diagnosis (or a condition may not be recognized or reported by the patient) for a period of time after admission. In some cases, it may be several days before the provider arrives at a definitive diagnosis. This does not mean that the condition was not present on admission. Determination of whether the condition was present on admission or not will be based on the applicable POA guideline as identified in this document, or on the provider's best clinical judgment.

If at the time of code assignment the documentation is unclear as to whether a condition was present on admission or not, it is appropriate to query the provider for clarification.

## Assigning the POA Indicator

Condition is on the "Exempt from Reporting" list

Leave the "present on admission" field blank if the condition is on the list of ICD-10-CM codes for which **the POA indicator** is not applicable. This is the only circumstance in which the field may be left blank.

POA Explicitly Documented

Assign Y for any condition the provider explicitly documents as being present on admission.

Assign N for any condition the provider explicitly documents as not present at the time of admission.

Conditions diagnosed prior to inpatient admission

Assign "Y" for conditions that were diagnosed prior to admission (example: hypertension, diabetes mellitus, asthma)

Conditions diagnosed during the admission but clearly present before admission

Assign "Y" for conditions diagnosed during the admission that were clearly present but not diagnosed until after admission occurred.

Diagnoses subsequently confirmed after admission are considered present on admission if at the time of admission they are documented as suspected, possible, rule out, differential diagnosis, or constitute an underlying cause of a symptom that is present at the time of admission.

Condition develops during outpatient encounter prior to inpatient admission

Assign Y for any condition that develops during an outpatient encounter prior to a written order for inpatient admission.

Documentation does not indicate whether condition was present on admission

Assign "U" when the medical record documentation is unclear as to whether the condition was present on admission. "U" should not be routinely assigned and used only in very limited circumstances. Coders are encouraged to query the providers when the documentation is unclear.

Documentation states that it cannot be determined whether the condition was or was not present on admission

Assign "W" when the medical record documentation indicates that it cannot be clinically determined whether or not the condition was present on admission.

Chronic condition with acute exacerbation during the admission

If a single code identifies both the chronic condition and the acute exacerbation, see POA guidelines pertaining to codes that contain multiple clinical concepts.

If a single code only identifies the chronic condition and not the acute exacerbation (e.g., acute exacerbation of chronic leukemia), assign "Y."

Conditions documented as possible, probable, suspected, or rule out at the time of discharge

If the final diagnosis contains a possible, probable, suspected, or rule out diagnosis, and this diagnosis was based on signs, symptoms or clinical findings suspected at the time of inpatient admission, assign "Y."

If the final diagnosis contains a possible, probable, suspected, or rule out diagnosis, and this diagnosis was based on signs, symptoms or clinical findings that were not present on admission, assign "N".

Conditions documented as impending or threatened at the time of discharge

If the final diagnosis contains an impending or threatened diagnosis, and this diagnosis is based on symptoms or clinical findings that were present on admission, assign "Y".

If the final diagnosis contains an impending or threatened diagnosis, and this diagnosis is based on symptoms or clinical findings that were not present on admission, assign "N".

Acute and Chronic Conditions

Assign "Y" for acute conditions that are present at time of admission and N for acute conditions that are not present at time of admission.

Assign "Y" for chronic conditions, even though the condition may not be diagnosed until after admission.

If a single code identifies both an acute and chronic condition, see the POA guidelines for codes that contain multiple clinical concepts.

Codes That Contain Multiple Clinical Concepts

Assign "N" if at least one of the clinical concepts included in the code was not present on admission (e.g., COPD with acute exacerbation and the exacerbation was not present on admission; gastric ulcer that does not start bleeding until after admission; asthma patient develops status asthmaticus after admission).

Assign "Y" if all of the clinical concepts included in the code were present on admission (e.g., duodenal ulcer that perforates prior to admission).

For infection codes that include the causal organism, assign "Y" if the infection (or signs of the infection) were present on admission, even though the culture results may not be known until after admission (e.g., patient is admitted with pneumonia and the provider documents Pseudomonas as the causal organism a few days later).

Same Diagnosis Code for Two or More Conditions

When the same ICD-10-CM diagnosis code applies to two or more conditions during the same encounter (e.g., two separate conditions classified to the same ICD-10-CM diagnosis code):

Assign "Y" if all conditions represented by the single ICD-10-CM code were present on admission (e.g. bilateral unspecified age-related cataracts).

Assign "N" if any of the conditions represented by the single ICD-10-CM code was not present on admission (e.g., traumatic secondary and recurrent hemorrhage and seroma is assigned to a single code T79.2, but only one of the conditions was present on admission).

Obstetrical conditions

Whether or not the patient delivers during the current hospitalization does not affect assignment of the POA indicator. The determining factor for POA assignment is whether the pregnancy complication or obstetrical condition described by the code was present at the time of admission or not.

If the pregnancy complication or obstetrical condition was present on admission (e.g., patient admitted in preterm labor), assign "Y".

If the pregnancy complication or obstetrical condition was not present on admission (e.g., 2nd degree laceration during delivery, postpartum hemorrhage that occurred during current hospitalization, fetal distress develops after admission), assign "N".

If the obstetrical code includes more than one diagnosis and any of the diagnoses identified by the code were not present on admission assign "N". (e.g., Category O11, Pre-existing hypertension with pre-eclampsia)

Perinatal conditions

Newborns are not considered to be admitted until after birth. Therefore, any condition present at birth or that developed in utero is considered present at admission and should be assigned "Y". This includes conditions that occur during delivery (e.g., injury during delivery, meconium aspiration, exposure to streptococcus B in the vaginal canal).

Congenital conditions and anomalies

Assign "Y" for congenital conditions and anomalies except for categories Q00-Q99, Congenital anomalies, which are on the exempt list. Congenital conditions are always considered present on admission.

External cause of injury codes

Assign "Y" for any external cause code representing an external cause of morbidity that occurred prior to inpatient admission (e.g., patient fell out of bed at home, patient fell out of bed in emergency room prior to admission)

Assign "N" for any external cause code representing an external cause of morbidity that occurred during inpatient hospitalization (e.g., patient fell out of hospital bed during hospital stay, patient experienced an adverse reaction to a medication administered after inpatient admission).

# ICD-10-CM Index to Diseases and Injuries

## A

- **Aarskog's syndrome** Q87.19
- **Abandonment** — *see* Maltreatment
- **Abasia** (-astasia) (hysterical) F44.4
- **Abderhalden-Kaufmann-Lignac syndrome** (cystinosis) E72.Ø4
- **Abdomen, abdominal** — *see also* condition
  - acute R1Ø.Ø
  - angina K55.1
  - muscle deficiency syndrome Q79.4
- **Abdominalgia** — *see* Pain, abdominal
- **Abduction contracture, hip or other joint** — *see* Contraction, joint
- **Aberrant** (congenital) — *see also* Malposition, congenital
  - adrenal gland Q89.1
  - artery (peripheral) Q27.8
    - basilar NEC Q28.1
    - cerebral Q28.3
    - coronary Q24.5
    - digestive system Q27.8
    - eye Q15.8
    - lower limb Q27.8
    - precerebral Q28.1
    - pulmonary Q25.79
    - renal Q27.2
    - retina Q14.1
    - specified site NEC Q27.8
    - subclavian Q27.8
    - upper limb Q27.8
    - vertebral Q28.1
  - breast Q83.8
  - endocrine gland NEC Q89.2
  - hepatic duct Q44.5
  - pancreas Q45.3
  - parathyroid gland Q89.2
  - pituitary gland Q89.2
  - sebaceous glands, mucous membrane, mouth, congenital Q38.6
  - spleen Q89.Ø9
  - subclavian artery Q27.8
  - thymus (gland) Q89.2
  - thyroid gland Q89.2
  - vein (peripheral) NEC Q27.8
    - cerebral Q28.3
    - digestive system Q27.8
    - lower limb Q27.8
    - precerebral Q28.1
    - specified site NEC Q27.8
    - upper limb Q27.8
- **Aberration**
  - distantial — *see* Disturbance, visual
  - mental F99
- **Abetalipoproteinemia** E78.6
- **Abiotrophy** R68.89
- **Ablatio, ablation**
  - retinae — *see* Detachment, retina
- **Ablepharia, ablepharon** Q1Ø.3
- **Abnormal, abnormality, abnormalities** — *see also* Anomaly
  - acid-base balance (mixed) E87.4
  - albumin R77.Ø
  - alphafetoprotein R77.2
  - alveolar ridge KØ8.9
  - anatomical relationship Q89.9
  - anti-CCP (cyclic citrullinated protein) R76.81
  - anti-cyclic citrullinated protein antibody and rheumatoid factor R76.81
  - apertures, congenital, diaphragm Q79.1
  - atrial septal, specified NEC Q21.19
  - auditory perception H93.29- ☑
    - diplacusis — *see* Diplacusis
    - hyperacusis — *see* Hyperacusis
    - recruitment — *see* Recruitment, auditory
    - threshold shift — *see* Shift, auditory threshold
  - autosomes Q99.9
    - fragile site Q95.5
  - basal metabolic rate R94.8
  - biosynthesis, testicular androgen E29.1
  - bleeding time R79.1
  - blood amino-acid level R79.83
  - blood-gas level R79.81

**Abnormal, abnormality, abnormalities** — *continued*

  - blood level (of)
    - cobalt R79.Ø
    - copper R79.Ø
    - iron R79.Ø
    - lithium R78.89
    - magnesium R79.Ø
    - mineral NEC R79.Ø
    - zinc R79.Ø
  - blood pressure
    - elevated RØ3.Ø
    - low reading (nonspecific) RØ3.1
  - blood sugar R73.Ø9
  - bowel sounds R19.15
    - absent R19.11
    - hyperactive R19.12
  - brain scan R94.Ø2
  - breathing RØ6.9
  - caloric test R94.138
  - cerebrospinal fluid R83.9
    - cytology R83.6
    - drug level R83.2
    - enzyme level R83.Ø
    - hormones R83.1
    - immunology R83.4
    - microbiology R83.5
    - nonmedicinal level R83.3
    - specified type NEC R83.8
  - chemistry, blood R79.9
    - C-reactive protein R79.82
    - drugs — *see* Findings, abnormal, in blood
    - gas level R79.81
    - minerals R79.Ø
    - pancytopenia D61.818
    - PTT R79.1
    - specified NEC R79.89
    - toxins — *see* Findings, abnormal, in blood
  - chest sounds (friction) (rales) RØ9.89
  - chromosome, chromosomal Q99.9
    - with more than three X chromosomes, female Q97.1
    - analysis result R89.8
      - bronchial washings R84.8
      - cerebrospinal fluid R83.8
      - cervix uteri NEC R87.89
      - nasal secretions R84.8
      - nipple discharge R89.8
      - peritoneal fluid R85.89
      - pleural fluid R84.8
      - prostatic secretions R86.8
      - saliva R85.89
      - seminal fluid R86.8
      - sputum R84.8
      - synovial fluid R89.8
      - throat scrapings R84.8
      - vagina R87.89
      - vulva R87.89
      - wound secretions R89.8
    - dicentric replacement Q93.2
    - ring replacement Q93.2
    - sex Q99.8- ☑
      - female phenotype Q97.9
        - specified NEC Q97.8
      - male phenotype Q98.9
        - specified NEC Q98.8
      - structural male Q98.6
    - specified NEC Q99.8- ☑
  - clinical findings NEC R68.89
  - coagulation D68.9
    - newborn, transient P61.6
    - profile R79.1
    - time R79.1
  - communication — *see* Fistula
  - conjunctiva, vascular H11.41- ☑
  - coronary artery Q24.5
  - cortisol-binding globulin E27.8
  - course, eustachian tube Q17.8
  - creatinine clearance R94.4
  - cytology
    - anus R85.619
      - atypical squamous cells cannot exclude high grade squamous intraepithelial lesion (ASC-H) R85.611

**Abnormal, abnormality, abnormalities** — *continued*

  - cytology — *continued*
    - anus — *continued*
      - atypical squamous cells of undetermined significance (ASC-US) R85.61Ø
      - cytologic evidence of malignancy R85.614
      - high grade squamous intraepithelial lesion (HGSIL) R85.613
      - human papillomavirus (HPV) DNA test
        - high risk positive R85.81
        - low risk positive R85.82
      - inadequate smear R85.615
      - low grade squamous intraepithelial lesion (LGSIL) R85.612
      - satisfactory anal smear but lacking transformation zone R85.616
      - specified NEC R85.618
      - unsatisfactory smear R85.615
    - female genital organs — *see* Abnormal, Papanicolaou (smear)
  - dark adaptation curve H53.61
  - dentofacial NEC — *see* Anomaly, dentofacial
  - development, developmental Q89.9
    - central nervous system QØ7.9
  - diagnostic imaging
    - abdomen, abdominal region NEC R93.5
    - biliary tract R93.2
    - bladder R93.41
    - breast R92.8
    - central nervous system NEC R9Ø.89
    - cerebrovascular NEC R9Ø.89
    - coronary circulation R93.1
    - digestive tract NEC R93.3
    - gastrointestinal (tract) R93.3
    - genitourinary organs R93.89
    - head R93.Ø
    - heart R93.1
    - intrathoracic organ NEC R93.89
    - kidney R93.42- ☑
    - limbs R93.6
    - liver R93.2
    - lung (field) R91.8
    - musculoskeletal system NEC R93.7
    - renal pelvis R93.41
    - retroperitoneum R93.5
    - site specified NEC R93.89
    - skin and subcutaneous tissue R93.89
    - skull R93.Ø
    - testis R93.81- ☑
    - ureter R93.41
    - urinary organs specified NEC R93.49
  - direction, teeth, fully erupted M26.3Ø
  - ear ossicles, acquired NEC H74.39- ☑
    - ankylosis — *see* Ankylosis, ear ossicles
    - discontinuity — *see* Discontinuity, ossicles, ear
    - partial loss — *see* Loss, ossicles, ear (partial)
  - Ebstein Q22.5
  - echocardiogram R93.1
  - echoencephalogram R9Ø.81
  - echogram — *see* Abnormal, diagnostic imaging
  - electro-oculogram [EOG] R94.11Ø
  - electrocardiogram [ECG] [EKG] R94.31
  - electroencephalogram [EEG] R94.Ø1
  - electrolyte — *see* Imbalance, electrolyte
  - electromyogram [EMG] R94.131
  - electrophysiological intracardiac studies R94.39
  - electroretinogram [ERG] R94.111
  - erythrocytes
    - congenital, with perinatal jaundice D58.9
  - feces (color) (contents) (mucus) R19.5
  - finding — *see* Findings, abnormal, without diagnosis
  - fluid
    - amniotic — *see* Abnormal, specimen, specified
    - cerebrospinal — *see* Abnormal, cerebrospinal fluid
    - peritoneal — *see* Abnormal, specimen, digestive organs
    - pleural — *see* Abnormal, specimen, respiratory organs
    - synovial — *see* Abnormal, specimen, specified
    - thorax (bronchial washings) (pleural fluid) — *see* Abnormal, specimen, respiratory organs
    - vaginal — *see* Abnormal, specimen, female genital organs

☑ **Additional Character Required — Refer to the Tabular List for Character Selection**

- **Abrasion** — *continued*
  - breast S2Ø.11- ☑
  - brow SØØ.81- ☑
  - buttock S3Ø.81Ø- ☑
  - calf — *see* Abrasion, leg
  - canthus — *see* Abrasion, eyelid
  - cheek SØØ.81- ☑
    - internal SØØ.512- ☑
  - chest wall — *see* Abrasion, thorax
  - chin SØØ.81- ☑
  - clitoris S3Ø.814- ☑
  - cornea SØ5.Ø- ☑
  - costal region — *see* Abrasion, thorax
  - dental KØ3.1
  - digit(s)
    - foot — *see* Abrasion, toe
    - hand — *see* Abrasion, finger
  - ear SØØ.41- ☑
  - elbow S5Ø.31- ☑
  - epididymis S3Ø.813- ☑
  - epigastric region S3Ø.811- ☑
  - epiglottis S1Ø.11- ☑
  - esophagus (thoracic) S27.818- ☑
    - cervical S1Ø.11- ☑
  - eyebrow — *see* Abrasion, eyelid
  - eyelid SØØ.21- ☑
  - face SØØ.81- ☑
  - finger(s) S6Ø.41- ☑
    - index S6Ø.41- ☑
    - little S6Ø.41- ☑
    - middle S6Ø.41- ☑
    - ring S6Ø.41- ☑
  - flank S3Ø.81A- ☑
  - foot (except toe(s) alone) S9Ø.81- ☑
    - toe — *see* Abrasion, toe
  - forearm S5Ø.81- ☑
    - elbow only — *see* Abrasion, elbow
  - forehead SØØ.81- ☑
  - genital organs, external
    - female S3Ø.816- ☑
    - male S3Ø.815- ☑
  - groin S3Ø.811- ☑
  - gum SØØ.512- ☑
  - hand S6Ø.51- ☑
  - head SØØ.91- ☑
    - ear — *see* Abrasion, ear
    - eyelid — *see* Abrasion, eyelid
    - lip SØØ.511- ☑
    - nose SØØ.31- ☑
    - oral cavity SØØ.512- ☑
    - scalp SØØ.Ø1- ☑
    - specified site NEC SØØ.81- ☑
  - heel — *see* Abrasion, foot
  - hip S7Ø.21- ☑
  - inguinal region S3Ø.811- ☑
  - interscapular region S2Ø.419- ☑
  - jaw SØØ.81- ☑
  - knee S8Ø.21- ☑
  - labium (majus) (minus) S3Ø.814- ☑
  - larynx S1Ø.11- ☑
  - leg (lower) S8Ø.81- ☑
    - knee — *see* Abrasion, knee
    - upper — *see* Abrasion, thigh
  - lip SØØ.511- ☑
  - lower back S3Ø.81Ø- ☑
  - lumbar region S3Ø.81Ø- ☑
  - malar region SØØ.81- ☑
  - mammary — *see* Abrasion, breast
  - mastoid region SØØ.81- ☑
  - mouth SØØ.512- ☑
  - nail
    - finger — *see* Abrasion, finger
    - toe — *see* Abrasion, toe
  - nape S1Ø.81- ☑
  - nasal SØØ.31- ☑
  - neck S1Ø.91- ☑
    - specified site NEC S1Ø.81- ☑
    - throat S1Ø.11- ☑
  - nose SØØ.31- ☑
  - occipital region SØØ.Ø1- ☑
  - oral cavity SØØ.512- ☑
  - orbital region — *see* Abrasion, eyelid
  - palate SØØ.512- ☑
  - palm — *see* Abrasion, hand
  - parietal region SØØ.Ø1- ☑
  - pelvis S3Ø.81Ø- ☑
  - penis S3Ø.812- ☑
  - perineum
    - female S3Ø.814- ☑
    - male S3Ø.81Ø- ☑
  - periocular area — *see* Abrasion, eyelid
  - phalanges
    - finger — *see* Abrasion, finger
    - toe — *see* Abrasion, toe
  - pharynx S1Ø.11- ☑
  - pinna — *see* Abrasion, ear
  - popliteal space — *see* Abrasion, knee
  - prepuce S3Ø.812- ☑
  - pubic region S3Ø.81Ø- ☑
  - pudendum
    - female S3Ø.816- ☑
    - male S3Ø.815- ☑
  - sacral region S3Ø.81Ø- ☑
  - scalp SØØ.Ø1- ☑
  - scapular region — *see* Abrasion, shoulder
  - scrotum S3Ø.813- ☑
  - shin — *see* Abrasion, leg
  - shoulder S4Ø.21- ☑
  - skin NEC T14.8- ☑
  - sternal region S2Ø.319- ☑
  - submaxillary region SØØ.81- ☑
  - submental region SØØ.81- ☑
  - subungual
    - finger(s) — *see* Abrasion, finger
    - toe(s) — *see* Abrasion, toe
  - supraclavicular fossa S1Ø.81- ☑
  - supraorbital SØØ.81- ☑
  - temple SØØ.81- ☑
  - temporal region SØØ.81- ☑
  - testis S3Ø.813- ☑
  - thigh S7Ø.31- ☑
  - thorax, thoracic (wall) S2Ø.91- ☑
    - back S2Ø.41- ☑
    - front S2Ø.31- ☑
  - throat S1Ø.11- ☑
  - thumb S6Ø.31- ☑
  - toe(s) (lesser) S9Ø.416- ☑
    - great S9Ø.41- ☑
  - tongue SØØ.512- ☑
  - tooth, teeth (dentifrice) (habitual) (hard tissues) (occupational) (ritual) (traditional) KØ3.1
  - trachea S1Ø.11- ☑
  - tunica vaginalis S3Ø.813- ☑
  - tympanum, tympanic membrane — *see* Abrasion, ear
  - uvula SØØ.512- ☑
  - vagina S3Ø.814- ☑
  - vocal cords S1Ø.11- ☑
  - vulva S3Ø.814- ☑
  - wrist S6Ø.81- ☑
- **Abrism** — *see* Poisoning, food, noxious, plant
- **Abruptio placentae** O45.9- ☑
  - with
    - afibrinogenemia O45.Ø1- ☑
    - coagulation defect O45.ØØ- ☑
      - specified NEC O45.Ø9- ☑
    - disseminated intravascular coagulation O45.Ø2- ☑
    - hypofibrinogenemia O45.Ø1- ☑
  - specified NEC O45.8- ☑
- **Abruption, placenta** — *see* Abruptio placentae
- **Abscess** (connective tissue) (embolic) (fistulous) (infective) (metastatic) (multiple) (pernicious) (pyogenic) (septic) LØ2.91
  - with
    - diverticular disease (intestine) K57.8Ø
      - with bleeding K57.81
      - large intestine K57.2Ø
        - with
          - bleeding K57.21
          - small intestine K57.4Ø
            - with bleeding K57.41
      - small intestine K57.ØØ
        - with
          - bleeding K57.Ø1
          - large intestine K57.4Ø
            - with bleeding K57.41
    - lymphangitis — *code by* site under Abscess
  - abdomen, abdominal
    - cavity K65.1
    - wall LØ2.211
  - abdominopelvic K65.1
  - accessory sinus — *see* Sinusitis
  - adrenal (capsule) (gland) E27.8
- **Abscess** — *continued*
  - alveolar KØ4.7
    - with sinus KØ4.6
  - amebic AØ6.4
    - brain (and liver or lung abscess) AØ6.6
    - genitourinary tract AØ6.82
    - liver (without mention of brain or lung abscess) AØ6.4
    - lung (and liver) (without mention of brain abscess) AØ6.5
    - specified site NEC AØ6.89
    - spleen AØ6.89
  - anerobic A48.Ø
  - ankle — *see* Abscess, lower limb
  - anorectal K61.2
  - antecubital space — *see* Abscess, upper limb
  - antrum (chronic) (Highmore) — *see* Sinusitis, maxillary
  - anus K61.Ø
  - apical (tooth) KØ4.7
    - with sinus (alveolar) KØ4.6
  - appendix K35.33
  - areola (acute) (chronic) (nonpuerperal) N61.1
    - puerperal, postpartum or gestational — *see* Infection, nipple
  - arm (any part) — *see* Abscess, upper limb
  - artery (wall) I77.89
  - atheromatous I77.2
  - auricle, ear — *see* Abscess, ear, external
  - axilla (region) LØ2.41- ☑
    - lymph gland or node LØ4.2
  - back (any part, except buttock and flank) LØ2.212
  - Bartholin's gland N75.1
    - with
      - abortion — *see* Abortion, by type complicated by, sepsis
      - ectopic or molar pregnancy OØ8.Ø
    - following ectopic or molar pregnancy OØ8.Ø
  - Bezold's — *see* Mastoiditis, acute
  - bilharziasis B65.1
  - bladder (wall) — *see* Cystitis, specified type NEC
  - bone (subperiosteal) — *see also* Osteomyelitis, specified type NEC
    - accessory sinus (chronic) — *see* Sinusitis
    - chronic or old — *see* Osteomyelitis, chronic
    - jaw (lower) (upper) M27.2
    - mastoid — *see* Mastoiditis, acute, subperiosteal
    - petrous — *see* Petrositis
    - spinal (tuberculous) A18.Ø1
      - nontuberculous — *see* Osteomyelitis, vertebra
  - bowel K63.Ø
  - brain (any part) (cystic) (otogenic) GØ6.Ø
    - amebic (with abscess of any other site) AØ6.6
    - gonococcal A54.82
    - pheomycotic (chromomycotic) B43.1
    - tuberculous A17.81
  - breast (acute) (chronic) (nonpuerperal) N61.1
    - newborn P39.Ø
    - puerperal, postpartum, gestational — *see* Mastitis, obstetric, purulent
  - broad ligament N73.2
    - acute N73.Ø
    - chronic N73.1
  - Brodie's (localized) (chronic) M86.8X- ☑
  - bronchi J98.Ø9
  - buccal cavity K12.2
  - bulbourethral gland N34.Ø
  - bursa M71.ØØ
    - ankle M71.Ø7- ☑
    - elbow M71.Ø2- ☑
    - foot M71.Ø7- ☑
    - hand M71.Ø4- ☑
    - hip M71.Ø5- ☑
    - knee M71.Ø6- ☑
    - multiple sites M71.Ø9
    - pharyngeal J39.1
    - shoulder M71.Ø1- ☑
    - specified site NEC M71.Ø8
    - wrist M71.Ø3- ☑
  - buttock LØ2.31
  - canthus — *see* Blepharoconjunctivitis
  - cartilage — *see* Disorder, cartilage, specified type NEC
  - cecum K35.33
  - cerebellum, cerebellar GØ6.Ø
    - sequelae GØ9
  - cerebral (embolic) GØ6.Ø
    - sequelae GØ9
  - cervical (meaning neck) LØ2.11
    - lymph gland or node LØ4.Ø
  - cervix (stump) (uteri) — *see* Cervicitis



☑ **Additional Character Required — Refer to the Tabular List for Character Selection**

**Abscess** — *continued*
- cheek (external) LØ2.Ø1
  - inner K12.2
- chest J86.9
  - with fistula J86.Ø
  - wall LØ2.213
- chin LØ2.Ø1
- choroid — *see* Inflammation, chorioretinal
- circumtonsillar J36
- cold (lung) (tuberculous) — *see also* Tuberculosis, abscess, lung
  - articular — *see* Tuberculosis, joint
- colon (wall) K63.Ø
- colostomy K94.Ø2
- conjunctiva — *see* Conjunctivitis, acute
- cornea H16.31- ☑
- corpus
  - cavernosum N48.21
  - luteum — *see* Oophoritis
- Cowper's gland N34.Ø
- cranium GØ6.Ø
- cul-de-sac (Douglas') (posterior) — *see* Abscess, pelvic, female, peritoneal
- cutaneous — *see* Abscess, by site
- dental KØ4.7
  - with sinus (alveolar) KØ4.6
- dentoalveolar KØ4.7
  - with sinus KØ4.6
- diaphragm, diaphragmatic K65.1
- Douglas' cul-de-sac or pouch — *see* Abscess, pelvic, female, peritoneal
- Dubois A5Ø.59
- ear (middle) — *see also* Otitis, media, suppurative
  - acute — *see* Otitis, media, suppurative, acute
  - external H6Ø.Ø- ☑
- entamebic — *see* Abscess, amebic
- enterostomy K94.12
- epididymis N45.4
- epidural GØ6.2
  - brain GØ6.Ø
  - spinal cord GØ6.1
- epiglottis J38.7
- epiploon, epiploic K65.1
- erysipelatous — *see* Erysipelas
- esophagus K2Ø.8Ø
- ethmoid (bone) (chronic) (sinus) J32.2
- external auditory canal — *see* Abscess, ear, external
- extradural GØ6.2
  - brain GØ6.Ø
    - sequelae GØ9
  - spinal cord GØ6.1
- extraperitoneal K68.19
  - meaning pelvic — *see* Abscess, pelvic
- eye — *see* Endophthalmitis, purulent
- eyelid HØØ.Ø3- ☑
- face (any part, except ear, eye and nose) LØ2.Ø1
- fallopian tube — *see* Salpingitis
- fascia M72.8
- fauces J39.1
- fecal K63.Ø
- femoral (region) — *see* Abscess, lower limb
- filaria, filarial — *see* Infestation, filarial
- finger (any) — *see also* Abscess, hand
  - nail — *see* Cellulitis, finger
- flank LØ2.217
- foot LØ2.61- ☑
- forehead LØ2.Ø1
- frontal sinus (chronic) J32.1
- gallbladder K81.Ø
- genital organ or tract
  - female (external) N76.4
  - male N49.9
    - multiple sites N49.8
    - specified NEC N49.8
- gestational mammary O91.11- ☑
- gestational subareolar O91.11- ☑
- gingival
  - aggressive KØ5.2Ø
    - generalized KØ5.229
      - moderate KØ5.222
      - severe KØ5.223
      - slight KØ5.221
    - localized KØ5.219
      - moderate KØ5.212
      - severe KØ5.213
      - slight KØ5.211
- gland, glandular (lymph) (acute) — *see* Lymphadenitis, acute

**Abscess** — *continued*
- gluteal (region) LØ2.31
- gonorrheal — *see* Gonococcus
- groin LØ2.214
- gum
  - aggressive KØ5.2Ø
    - generalized KØ5.229
      - moderate KØ5.222
      - severe KØ5.223
      - slight KØ5.221
    - localized KØ5.219
      - moderate KØ5.212
      - severe KØ5.213
      - slight KØ5.211
- hand LØ2.51- ☑
- head NEC LØ2.811
  - face (any part, except ear, eye and nose) LØ2.Ø1
- heart — *see* Carditis
- heel — *see* Abscess, foot
- helminthic — *see* Infestation, helminth
- hepatic (cholangitic) (hematogenic) (lymphogenic) (pylephlebitic) K75.Ø
  - amebic AØ6.4
- hip (region) — *see* Abscess, lower limb
- horseshoe K61.31
- ileocecal K35.33
- ileostomy (bud) K94.12
- iliac (region) LØ2.214
  - fossa K35.33
- infraclavicular (fossa) — *see* Abscess, upper limb
- inguinal (region) LØ2.214
  - lymph gland or node LØ4.1
- intersphincteric K61.4
- intestine, intestinal NEC K63.Ø
  - rectal K61.1
- intra-abdominal — *see also* Abscess, peritoneum K65.1
  - following procedure T81.43- ☑
    - obstetrical O86.Ø3
  - postprocedural T81.43- ☑
    - retroperitoneal K68.11
- intracranial GØ6.Ø
- intramammary — *see* Abscess, breast
- intramuscular, following procedure T81.42- ☑
  - obstetrical O86.Ø2
- intraorbital — *see* Abscess, orbit
- intraperitoneal K65.1
- intrasphincteric (anus) K61.4
- intraspinal GØ6.1
- intratonsillar J36
- ischiorectal (fossa) (specified NEC) K61.39
- jaw (bone) (lower) (upper) M27.2
- joint — *see* Arthritis, pyogenic or pyemic
  - spine (tuberculous) A18.Ø1
    - nontuberculous — *see* Spondylopathy, infective
- kidney N15.1
  - with calculus N2Ø.Ø
    - with hydronephrosis N13.6
  - puerperal (postpartum) O86.21
- knee — *see also* Abscess, lower limb
  - joint MØØ.9
- labium (majus) (minus) N76.4
- lacrimal
  - caruncle — *see* Inflammation, lacrimal, passages, acute
  - gland — *see* Dacryoadenitis
  - passages (duct) (sac) — *see* Inflammation, lacrimal, passages, acute
- lacunar N34.Ø
- larynx J38.7
- lateral (alveolar) KØ4.7
  - with sinus KØ4.6
- leg (any part) — *see* Abscess, lower limb
- lens H27.8
- lingual K14.Ø
  - tonsil J36
- lip K13.Ø
- Littre's gland N34.Ø
- liver (cholangitic) (hematogenic) (lymphogenic) (pylephlebitic) (pyogenic) K75.Ø
  - amebic (due to Entamoeba histolytica) (dysenteric) (tropical) AØ6.4
    - with
      - brain abscess (and liver or lung abscess) AØ6.6
      - lung abscess AØ6.5
- loin (region) LØ2.211
- lower limb LØ2.41- ☑
- lumbar (tuberculous) A18.Ø1
  - nontuberculous LØ2.212

**Abscess** — *continued*
- lung (miliary) (putrid) J85.2
  - with pneumonia J85.1
    - due to specified organism — *see* Pneumonia, in (due to)
  - amebic (with liver abscess) AØ6.5
    - with
      - brain abscess AØ6.6
      - pneumonia AØ6.5
- lymph, lymphatic, gland or node (acute) — *see also* Lymphadenitis, acute
  - mesentery I88.Ø
- malar M27.2
- mammary gland — *see* Abscess, breast
- marginal, anus K61.Ø
- mastoid — *see* Mastoiditis, acute
- maxilla, maxillary M27.2
  - molar (tooth) KØ4.7
    - with sinus KØ4.6
  - premolar KØ4.7
  - sinus (chronic) J32.Ø
- mediastinum J85.3
- meibomian gland — *see* Hordeolum
- meninges GØ6.2
- mesentery, mesenteric K65.1
- mesosalpinx — *see* Salpingitis
- mons pubis LØ2.215
- mouth (floor) K12.2
- muscle — *see* Myositis, infective
- myocardium I4Ø.Ø
- nabothian (follicle) — *see* Cervicitis
- nasal J32.9
- nasopharyngeal J39.1
- navel LØ2.216
  - newborn P38.9
    - with mild hemorrhage P38.1
    - without hemorrhage P38.9
- neck (region) LØ2.11
  - lymph gland or node LØ4.Ø
- nephritic — *see* Abscess, kidney
- nipple N61.1
  - associated with
    - lactation — *see* Pregnancy, complicated by
    - pregnancy — *see* Pregnancy, complicated by
- nose (external) (fossa) (septum) J34.Ø
  - sinus (chronic) — *see* Sinusitis
- omentum K65.1
- operative wound T81.49- ☑
- orbit, orbital — *see* Cellulitis, orbit
- otogenic GØ6.Ø
- ovary, ovarian (corpus luteum) — *see* Oophoritis
- oviduct — *see* Oophoritis
- palate (soft) K12.2
  - hard M27.2
- palmar (space) — *see* Abscess, hand
- pancreas (duct) — *see* Pancreatitis, acute
- parafrenal N48.21
- parametric, parametrium N73.2
  - acute N73.Ø
  - chronic N73.1
- paranephric N15.1
- parapancreatic — *see* Pancreatitis, acute
- parapharyngeal J39.Ø
- pararectal K61.1
- parasinus — *see* Sinusitis
- parauterine — *see also* Disease, pelvis, inflammatory N73.2
- paravaginal — *see* Vaginitis
- parietal region (scalp) LØ2.811
- parodontal — *see* Periodontitis, aggressive, localized
- parotid (duct) (gland) K11.3
  - region K12.2
- pectoral (region) LØ2.213
- pelvis, pelvic K6A.Ø9
  - female — *see also* Disease, pelvis, inflammatory K6A.Ø9
    - peritoneal — *see also* Peritonitis, pelvic, female K65.1
  - male K6A.Ø9
    - peritoneal K65.1
  - specified NEC K6A.Ø9
- penis N48.21
  - gonococcal (accessory gland) (periurethral) A54.1
- perianal K61.Ø
- periapical KØ4.7
  - with sinus (alveolar) KØ4.6
- periappendicular K35.33
- pericardial I3Ø.1
- pericecal K35.33

**Abscess** — *continued*
- pericemental — *see* Periodontitis, aggressive, localized
- pericholecystic — *see* Cholecystitis, acute
- pericoronal — *see* Periodontitis, aggressive, localized
- peridental — *see* Periodontitis, aggressive, localized
- perimetric — *see also* Disease, pelvis, inflammatory N73.2
- perinephric, perinephritic — *see* Abscess, kidney
- perineum, perineal (superficial) LØ2.215
  - urethra N34.Ø
- periodontal (parietal) — *see* Periodontitis, aggressive, localized
  - apical KØ4.7
- periosteum, periosteal — *see also* Osteomyelitis, specified type NEC
  - with osteomyelitis — *see also* Osteomyelitis, specified type NEC
    - acute — *see* Osteomyelitis, acute
    - chronic — *see* Osteomyelitis, chronic
- peripharyngeal J39.Ø
- peripleuritic J86.9
  - with fistula J86.Ø
- periprostatic N41.2
- perirectal K61.1
- perirenal (tissue) — *see* Abscess, kidney
- perisinuous (nose) — *see* Sinusitis
- peritoneum, peritoneal (perforated) (ruptured) K65.1
  - with appendicitis — *see also* Appendicitis K35.33
  - pelvic
    - female — *see* Peritonitis, pelvic, female
    - male K65.1
  - postoperative T81.43- ☑
  - puerperal, postpartum, childbirth O85
  - tuberculous A18.31
- peritonsillar J36
- perityphlic K35.33
- periureteral N28.89
- periurethral N34.Ø
  - gonococcal (accessory gland) (periurethral) A54.1
- periuterine — *see also* Disease, pelvis, inflammatory N73.2
- perivesical — *see* Cystitis, specified type NEC
- petrous bone — *see* Petrositis
- phagedenic NOS LØ2.91
  - chancroid A57
- pharynx, pharyngeal (lateral) J39.1
- pilonidal LØ5.Ø1
- pituitary (gland) E23.6
- pleura J86.9
  - with fistula J86.Ø
- popliteal — *see* Abscess, lower limb
- postcecal K35.33
- postlaryngeal J38.7
- postnasal J34.Ø
- postoperative (any site) — *see also* Infection, postoperative wound T81.49- ☑
  - retroperitoneal K68.11
- postpharyngeal J39.Ø
- posttonsillar J36
- post-typhoid AØ1.Ø9
- pouch of Douglas — *see* Abscess, pelvic, female, peritoneal
- premammary — *see* Abscess, breast
- prepatellar — *see* Abscess, lower limb
- presacral K68.19
- prevesical K6A.Ø1
- prostate N41.2
  - gonococcal (acute) (chronic) A54.22
- psoas muscle K68.12
- puerperal — *code by* site under Puerperal, abscess
- pulmonary — *see* Abscess, lung
- pulp, pulpal (dental) KØ4.Ø1
  - irreversible KØ4.Ø2
  - reversible KØ4.Ø1
- rectovaginal septum K63.Ø
- rectovesical — *see* Cystitis, specified type NEC
- rectum K61.1
- renal — *see* Abscess, kidney
- retina — *see* Inflammation, chorioretinal
- retrobulbar — *see* Abscess, orbit
- retrocecal K65.1
- retrolaryngeal J38.7
- retromammary — *see* Abscess, breast
- retroperitoneal NEC K68.19
  - postprocedural K68.11
- retropharyngeal J39.Ø
- retropubic K6A.Ø1
- retrouterine — *see* Peritonitis, pelvic, female
- retrovesical — *see* Cystitis, specified type NEC
- root, tooth KØ4.7

**Abscess** — *continued*
- root, tooth — *continued*
  - with sinus (alveolar) KØ4.6
- round ligament — *see also* Disease, pelvis, inflammatory N73.2
- rupture (spontaneous) NOS LØ2.91
- sacrum (tuberculous) A18.Ø1
  - nontuberculous M46.28
- salivary (duct) (gland) K11.3
- scalp (any part) LØ2.811
- scapular — *see* Osteomyelitis, specified type NEC
- sclera — *see* Scleritis
- scrofulous (tuberculous) A18.2
- scrotum N49.2
- seminal vesicle N49.Ø
- septal, dental KØ4.7
  - with sinus (alveolar) KØ4.6
- serous — *see* Periostitis
- shoulder (region) — *see* Abscess, upper limb
- sigmoid K63.Ø
- sinus (accessory) (chronic) (nasal) — *see also* Sinusitis
  - intracranial venous (any) GØ6.Ø
- Skene's duct or gland N34.Ø
- skin — *see* Abscess, by site
- specified site NEC LØ2.818
- spermatic cord N49.1
- sphenoidal (sinus) (chronic) J32.3
- spinal cord (any part) (staphylococcal) GØ6.1
  - tuberculous A17.81
- spine (column) (tuberculous) A18.Ø1
  - epidural GØ6.1
  - nontuberculous — *see* Osteomyelitis, vertebra
- spleen D73.3
  - amebic AØ6.89
- stitch T81.41- ☑
  - following an obstetrical procedure O86.Ø1
- sub-fascial, following an obstetrical procedure O86.Ø2
- subarachnoid GØ6.2
  - brain GØ6.Ø
  - spinal cord GØ6.1
- subareolar — *see* Abscess, breast
- subcecal K35.33
- subcutaneous — *see also* Abscess, by site
  - following procedure T81.41- ☑
    - obstetrical O86.Ø1
  - pheomycotic (chromomycotic) B43.2
- subdiaphragmatic K65.1
- subdural GØ6.2
  - brain GØ6.Ø
    - sequelae GØ9
  - spinal cord GØ6.1
- subgaleal LØ2.811
- subhepatic K65.1
- sublingual K12.2
  - gland K11.3
- submammary — *see* Abscess, breast
- submandibular (region) (space) (triangle) K12.2
  - gland K11.3
- submaxillary (region) LØ2.Ø1
  - gland K11.3
- submental LØ2.Ø1
  - gland K11.3
- subperiosteal — *see* Osteomyelitis, specified type NEC
- subphrenic K65.1
  - following an obstetrical procedure O86.Ø3
  - postoperative T81.43- ☑
- suburethral N34.Ø
- sudoriparous L75.8
- supraclavicular (fossa) — *see* Abscess, upper limb
- supralevator K61.5
- suprapelvic, acute N73.Ø
- suprarenal (capsule) (gland) E27.8
- sweat gland L74.8
- tear duct — *see* Inflammation, lacrimal, passages, acute
- temple LØ2.Ø1
- temporal region LØ2.Ø1
- temporosphenoidal GØ6.Ø
- tendon (sheath) M65.ØØ
  - ankle M65.Ø7- ☑
  - foot M65.Ø7- ☑
  - forearm M65.Ø3- ☑
  - hand M65.Ø4- ☑
  - lower leg M65.Ø6- ☑
  - pelvic region M65.Ø5- ☑
  - shoulder region M65.Ø1- ☑
  - specified site NEC M65.Ø8
  - thigh M65.Ø5- ☑
  - upper arm M65.Ø2- ☑

**Abscess** — *continued*
- testis N45.4
- thigh — *see* Abscess, lower limb
- thorax J86.9
  - with fistula J86.Ø
- throat J39.1
- thumb — *see also* Abscess, hand
  - nail — *see* Cellulitis, finger
- thymus (gland) E32.1
- thyroid (gland) EØ6.Ø
- toe (any) — *see also* Abscess, foot
  - nail — *see* Cellulitis, toe
- tongue (staphylococcal) K14.Ø
- tonsil(s) (lingual) J36
- tonsillopharyngeal J36
- tooth, teeth (root) KØ4.7
  - with sinus (alveolar) KØ4.6
  - supporting structures NEC — *see* Periodontitis, aggressive, localized
- trachea J39.8
- trunk LØ2.219
  - abdominal wall LØ2.211
  - back LØ2.212
  - chest wall LØ2.213
  - groin LØ2.214
  - perineum LØ2.215
  - umbilicus LØ2.216
- tubal — *see* Salpingitis
- tuberculous — *see* Tuberculosis, abscess
- tubo-ovarian — *see* Salpingo-oophoritis
- tunica vaginalis N49.1
- umbilicus LØ2.216
- upper
  - limb LØ2.41- ☑
  - respiratory J39.8
- urethral (gland) N34.Ø
- urinary N34.Ø
- uterus, uterine (wall) — *see also* Endometritis
  - ligament — *see also* Disease, pelvis, inflammatory N73.2
  - neck — *see* Cervicitis
- uvula K12.2
- vagina (wall) — *see* Vaginitis
- vaginorectal — *see* Vaginitis
- vas deferens N49.1
- vermiform appendix K35.33
- vertebra (column) (tuberculous) A18.Ø1
  - nontuberculous — *see* Osteomyelitis, vertebra
- vesical — *see* Cystitis, specified type NEC
- vesico-uterine pouch — *see* Peritonitis, pelvic, female
- vitreous (humor) — *see* Endophthalmitis, purulent
- vocal cord J38.3
- von Bezold's — *see* Mastoiditis, acute
- vulva N76.4
- vulvovaginal gland N75.1
- web space — *see* Abscess, hand
- wound T81.49- ☑
- wrist — *see* Abscess, upper limb

**Absence** (of) (organ or part) (complete or partial)
- adrenal (gland) (congenital) Q89.1
  - acquired E89.6
- albumin in blood E88.Ø9
- alimentary tract (congenital) Q45.8
  - upper Q4Ø.8
- alveolar process (acquired) — *see* Anomaly, alveolar
- ankle (acquired) Z89.44- ☑
- anus (congenital) Q42.3
  - with fistula Q42.2
- aorta (congenital) Q25.41
- appendix, congenital Q42.8
- arm (acquired) Z89.2Ø- ☑
  - above elbow Z89.22- ☑
    - congenital (with hand present) — *see* Agenesis, arm, with hand present
      - and hand — *see* Agenesis, forearm, and hand
  - below elbow Z89.21- ☑
    - congenital (with hand present) — *see* Agenesis, arm, with hand present
      - and hand — *see* Agenesis, forearm, and hand
  - congenital — *see* Defect, reduction, upper limb
  - shoulder (following explantation of shoulder joint prosthesis) (joint) (with or without presence of antibiotic-impregnated cement spacer) Z89.23- ☑
    - congenital (with hand present) — *see* Agenesis, arm, with hand present
- artery (congenital) (peripheral) Q27.8
  - brain Q28.3





☑ **Additional Character Required — Refer to the Tabular List for Character Selection**

- **Absence** — *continued*
  - teeth, tooth — *continued*
    - acquired — *continued*
      - due to — *continued*
        - specified — *continued*
          - class III K08.193
          - class IV K08.194
        - trauma K08.119
          - class I K08.111
          - class II K08.112
          - class III K08.113
          - class IV K08.114
      - partial K08.409
        - class I K08.401
        - class II K08.402
        - class III K08.403
        - class IV K08.404
        - due to
          - caries K08.439
            - class I K08.431
            - class II K08.432
            - class III K08.433
            - class IV K08.434
          - periodontal disease K08.429
            - class I K08.421
            - class II K08.422
            - class III K08.423
            - class IV K08.424
          - specified NEC K08.499
            - class I K08.491
            - class II K08.492
            - class III K08.493
            - class IV K08.494
          - trauma K08.419
            - class I K08.411
            - class II K08.412
            - class III K08.413
            - class IV K08.414
  - tendon (congenital) Q79.8
  - testis (congenital) Q55.0
    - acquired Z90.79
  - thumb (acquired) Z89.01- ☑
    - congenital — *see* Agenesis, hand
  - thymus gland Q89.2
  - thyroid (gland) (acquired) E89.0
    - cartilage, congenital Q31.8
    - congenital E03.1
  - toe(s) (acquired) Z89.42- ☑
    - with foot — *see* Absence, foot and ankle
    - congenital — *see* Agenesis, foot
    - great Z89.41- ☑
  - tongue, congenital Q38.3
  - trachea (cartilage), congenital Q32.1
  - transverse aortic arch, congenital Q25.49
  - tricuspid valve Q22.4
  - umbilical artery, congenital Q27.0
  - upper arm and forearm with hand present, congenital — *see* Agenesis, arm, with hand present
  - ureter (congenital) Q62.4
    - acquired Z90.6
  - urethra, congenital Q64.5
  - uterus (acquired) Z90.710
    - with cervix Z90.710
    - with remaining cervical stump Z90.711
    - congenital Q51.0
  - uvula, congenital Q38.5
  - vagina, congenital Q52.0
  - vas deferens (congenital) Q55.4
    - acquired Z90.79
  - vein (peripheral) congenital NEC Q27.8
    - cerebral Q28.3
    - digestive system Q27.8
    - great Q26.8
    - lower limb Q27.8
    - portal Q26.5
    - precerebral Q28.1
    - specified site NEC Q27.8
    - upper limb Q27.8
  - vena cava (inferior) (superior), congenital Q26.8
  - ventricular septum Q20.4
  - vertebra, congenital Q76.49
  - von Willebrand factor, complete (near) — *see also* Disease, von Willebrand D68.03
  - vulva, congenital Q52.71
  - wrist (acquired) Z89.12- ☑
- **Absorbent system disease** I87.8
- **Absorption**
  - carbohydrate, disturbance K90.49
  - chemical — *see* Table of Drugs and Chemicals
- **Absorption** — *continued*
  - chemical — *see* Table of Drugs and Chemicals — *continued*
    - through placenta (newborn) P04.9
      - environmental substance P04.6
      - nutritional substance P04.5
      - obstetric anesthetic or analgesic drug P04.0
  - drug NEC — *see* Table of Drugs and Chemicals
    - addictive
      - through placenta (newborn) — *see also* Newborn, affected by, maternal, use of P04.40
        - cocaine P04.41
        - hallucinogens P04.42
        - specified drug NEC P04.49
    - medicinal
      - through placenta (newborn) P04.19
    - through placenta (newborn) P04.19
      - obstetric anesthetic or analgesic drug P04.0
  - fat, disturbance K90.49
    - pancreatic K90.3
  - noxious substance — *see* Table of Drugs and Chemicals
  - protein, disturbance K90.49
  - starch, disturbance K90.49
  - toxic substance — *see* Table of Drugs and Chemicals
  - uremic — *see* Uremia
- **Abstinence symptoms, syndrome**
  - alcohol F10.239
    - with delirium F10.231
  - cocaine F14.23
  - neonatal P96.1
  - nicotine — *see* Dependence, drug, nicotine, with, withdrawal
  - opioid F11.93
    - with dependence F11.23
  - psychoactive NEC F19.939
    - with
      - delirium F19.931
      - dependence F19.239
        - with
          - delirium F19.231
          - perceptual disturbance F19.232
        - uncomplicated F19.230
      - perceptual disturbance F19.932
    - uncomplicated F19.930
  - sedative F13.939
    - with
      - delirium F13.931
      - dependence F13.239
        - with
          - delirium F13.231
          - perceptual disturbance F13.232
        - uncomplicated F13.230
      - perceptual disturbance F13.932
    - uncomplicated F13.930
  - stimulant NEC F15.93
    - with dependence F15.23
- **Abulia** R68.89
- **Abulomania** F60.7
- **Abuse**
  - adult — *see* Maltreatment, adult
    - as reason for
      - couple seeking advice (including offender) Z63.0
  - alcohol (non-dependent) F10.10
    - with
      - anxiety disorder F10.180
      - intoxication F10.129
        - with delirium F10.121
        - uncomplicated F10.120
      - mood disorder F10.14
      - other specified disorder F10.188
      - psychosis F10.159
        - delusions F10.150
        - hallucinations F10.151
      - sexual dysfunction F10.181
      - sleep disorder F10.182
      - unspecified disorder F10.19
      - withdrawal F10.139
        - with
          - perceptual disturbance F10.132
        - delirium F10.131
        - uncomplicated F10.130
    - counseling and surveillance Z71.41
    - in remission (early) (sustained) F10.11
  - amphetamine (or related substance) — *see also* Abuse, drug, stimulant NEC
    - stimulant NEC F15.10
      - with
        - anxiety disorder F15.180
        - intoxication F15.129
- **Abuse** — *continued*
  - amphetamine — *see also* Abuse, drug, stimulant — *continued*
    - stimulant — *continued*
      - with — *continued*
        - intoxication — *continued*
          - with
            - delirium F15.121
            - perceptual disturbance F15.122
        - withdrawal F15.13
  - analgesics (non-prescribed) (over the counter) F55.8
  - antacids F55.0
  - antidepressants — *see* Abuse, drug, psychoactive NEC
  - anxiolytic — *see* Abuse, drug, sedative
  - barbiturates — *see* Abuse, drug, sedative
  - caffeine — *see* Abuse, drug, stimulant NEC
  - cannabis, cannabinoids — *see* Abuse, drug, cannabis
  - child — *see* Maltreatment, child
  - cocaine — *see* Abuse, drug, cocaine
  - drug NEC (non-dependent) F19.10
    - with sleep disorder F19.182
    - amphetamine type — *see* Abuse, drug, stimulant NEC
    - analgesics (non-prescribed) (over the counter) F55.8
    - antacids F55.0
    - antidepressants — *see* Abuse, drug, psychoactive NEC
    - anxiolytics — *see* Abuse, drug, sedative
    - barbiturates — *see* Abuse, drug, sedative
    - caffeine — *see* Abuse, drug, stimulant NEC
    - cannabis F12.10
      - with
        - anxiety disorder F12.180
        - intoxication F12.129
          - with
            - delirium F12.121
            - perceptual disturbance F12.122
          - uncomplicated F12.120
        - other specified disorder F12.188
        - psychosis F12.159
          - delusions F12.150
          - hallucinations F12.151
        - unspecified disorder F12.19
        - withdrawal F12.13
      - in remission (early) (sustained) F12.11
    - cocaine F14.10
      - with
        - anxiety disorder F14.180
        - intoxication F14.129
          - with
            - delirium F14.121
            - perceptual disturbance F14.122
          - uncomplicated F14.120
        - mood disorder F14.14
        - other specified disorder F14.188
        - psychosis F14.159
          - delusions F14.150
          - hallucinations F14.151
        - sexual dysfunction F14.181
        - sleep disorder F14.182
        - unspecified disorder F14.19
        - withdrawal F14.13
      - in remission (early) (sustained) F14.11
    - counseling and surveillance Z71.51
    - hallucinogen F16.10
      - with
        - anxiety disorder F16.180
        - flashbacks F16.183
        - intoxication F16.129
          - with
            - delirium F16.121
            - perceptual disturbance F16.122
          - uncomplicated F16.120
        - mood disorder F16.14
        - other specified disorder F16.188
        - perception disorder, persisting F16.183
        - psychosis F16.159
          - delusions F16.150
          - hallucinations F16.151
        - unspecified disorder F16.19
      - in remission (early) (sustained) F16.11
    - hashish — *see* Abuse, drug, cannabis
    - herbal or folk remedies F55.1
    - hormones F55.3
    - hypnotics — *see* Abuse, drug, sedative
    - in remission (early) (sustained) F19.11
    - inhalant F18.10
      - with
        - anxiety disorder F18.180
        - dementia, persisting F18.17
        - intoxication F18.129

**Abuse** — *continued*
  drug — *continued*
    inhalant — *continued*
      with — *continued*
        intoxication — *continued*
          with delirium F18.121
          uncomplicated F18.12Ø
        mood disorder F18.14
        other specified disorder F18.188
        psychosis F18.159
          delusions F18.15Ø
          hallucinations F18.151
        unspecified disorder F18.19
      in remission (early) (sustained) F18.11
    laxatives F55.2
    LSD — *see* Abuse, drug, hallucinogen
    marihuana — *see* Abuse, drug, cannabis
    morphine type (opioids) — *see* Abuse, drug, opioid
    opioid F11.1Ø
      with
        intoxication F11.129
          with
            delirium F11.121
            perceptual disturbance F11.122
          uncomplicated F11.12Ø
        mood disorder F11.14
        opioid-associated amnestic syndrome F11.188
        other specified disorder F11.188
        psychosis F11.159
          delusions F11.15Ø
          hallucinations F11.151
        sexual dysfunction F11.181
        sleep disorder F11.182
        unspecified disorder F11.19
        withdrawal F11.13
      in remission (early) (sustained) F11.11
    PCP (phencyclidine) (or related substance) — *see* Abuse, drug, hallucinogen
    psychoactive NEC F19.1Ø
      with
        amnestic disorder F19.16
        anxiety disorder F19.18Ø
        dementia F19.17
        intoxication F19.129
          with
            delirium F19.121
            perceptual disturbance F19.122
          uncomplicated F19.12Ø
        mood disorder F19.14
        other specified disorder F19.188
        psychosis F19.159
          delusions F19.15Ø
          hallucinations F19.151
        sexual dysfunction F19.181
        sleep disorder F19.182
        unspecified disorder F19.19
        withdrawal F19.139
          with
            perceptual disturbance F19.132
          delirium F19.131
          uncomplicated F19.13Ø
    sedative, hypnotic or anxiolytic F13.1Ø
      with
        anxiety disorder F13.18Ø
        intoxication F13.129
          with delirium F13.121
          uncomplicated F13.12Ø
        mood disorder F13.14
        other specified disorder F13.188
        psychosis F13.159
          delusions F13.15Ø
          hallucinations F13.151
        sexual dysfunction F13.181
        sleep disorder F13.182
        unspecified disorder F13.19
        withdrawal F13.139
          with
            perceptual disturbance F13.132
          delirium F13.131
          uncomplicated F13.13Ø
      in remission (early) (sustained) F13.11
    solvent — *see* Abuse, drug, inhalant
    steroids F55.3
    stimulant NEC F15.1Ø
      with
        anxiety disorder F15.18Ø
        intoxication F15.129
          with
            delirium F15.121

**Abuse** — *continued*
  drug — *continued*
    stimulant — *continued*
      with — *continued*
        intoxication — *continued*
          with — *continued*
            perceptual disturbance F15.122
          uncomplicated F15.12Ø
        mood disorder F15.14
        other specified disorder F15.188
        psychosis F15.159
          delusions F15.15Ø
          hallucinations F15.151
        sexual dysfunction F15.181
        sleep disorder F15.182
        unspecified disorder F15.19
        withdrawal F15.13
      in remission (early) (sustained) F15.11
    tranquilizers — *see* Abuse, drug, sedative
    vitamins F55.4
  hallucinogens — *see* Abuse, drug, hallucinogen
  hashish — *see* Abuse, drug, cannabis
  herbal or folk remedies F55.1
  hormones F55.3
  hypnotic — *see* Abuse, drug, sedative
  inhalant — *see* Abuse, drug, inhalant
  laxatives F55.2
  LSD — *see* Abuse, drug, hallucinogen
  marihuana — *see* Abuse, drug, cannabis
  morphine type (opioids) — *see* Abuse, drug, opioid
  non-psychoactive substance NEC F55.8
    antacids F55.Ø
    folk remedies F55.1
    herbal remedies F55.1
    hormones F55.3
    laxatives F55.2
    steroids F55.3
    vitamins F55.4
  opioids — *see* Abuse, drug, opioid
  PCP (phencyclidine) (or related substance) — *see* Abuse, drug, hallucinogen
  physical (adult) (child) — *see* Maltreatment
  psychoactive substance — *see* Abuse, drug, psychoactive NEC
  psychological (adult) (child) — *see* Maltreatment
  sedative — *see* Abuse, drug, sedative
  sexual — *see* Maltreatment
  solvent — *see* Abuse, drug, inhalant
  steroids F55.3
  vitamins F55.4
**Acalculia** R48.8
  developmental F81.2
**Acanthamebiasis** (with) B6Ø.1Ø
  conjunctiva B6Ø.12
  keratoconjunctivitis B6Ø.13
  meningoencephalitis B6Ø.11
  other specified B6Ø.19
**Acanthocephaliasis** B83.8
**Acanthocheilonemiasis** B74.4
**Acanthocytosis** E78.6
**Acantholysis** L11.9
**Acanthosis** (acquired) (nigricans) L83
  benign Q82.8
  congenital Q82.8
  seborrheic L82.1
    inflamed L82.Ø
  tongue K14.3
**Acapnia** E87.3
**Acarbia** E87.29
**Acardia, acardius** Q89.89
**Acardiacus amorphus** Q89.89
**Acardiotrophia** I51.4
**Acariasis** B88.Ø9
  scabies B86
**Acarodermatitis** (urticarioides) B88.Ø9
**Acarophobia** F4Ø.218
**Acatalasemia, acatalasia** E8Ø.3
**Acathisia** (drug induced) G25.71
**Accelerated atrioventricular conduction** I45.6
**Accentuation of personality traits** (type A) Z73.1
**Accessory** (congenital)
  adrenal gland Q89.1
  anus Q43.4
  appendix Q43.4
  atrioventricular conduction I45.6
  auditory ossicles Q16.3
  auricle (ear) Q17.Ø
  biliary duct or passage Q44.5
  bladder Q64.79

**Accessory** — *continued*
  blood vessels NEC Q27.9
    coronary Q24.5
  bone NEC Q79.8
  breast tissue, axilla Q83.1
  carpal bones Q74.Ø
  cecum Q43.4
  chromosome(s) NEC (nonsex) Q92.9
    with complex rearrangements NEC Q92.5
      seen only at prometaphase Q92.8
    13 — *see* Trisomy, 13
    18 — *see* Trisomy, 18
    21 — *see* Trisomy, 21
    partial Q92.9
    sex
      female phenotype Q97.8
  coronary artery Q24.5
  cusp(s), heart valve NEC Q24.8
    pulmonary Q22.3
  cystic duct Q44.5
  digit(s) Q69.9
  ear (auricle) (lobe) Q17.Ø
  endocrine gland NEC Q89.2
  eye muscle Q1Ø.3
  eyelid Q1Ø.3
  face bone(s) Q75.8
  fallopian tube (fimbria) (ostium) Q5Ø.6
  finger(s) Q69.Ø
  foreskin N47.8
  frontonasal process Q75.8
  gallbladder Q44.1
  genital organ(s)
    female Q52.8
      external Q52.79
      internal NEC Q52.8
    male Q55.8
  genitourinary organs NEC Q89.89
    female Q52.8
    male Q55.8
  hallux Q69.2
  heart Q24.8
    valve NEC Q24.8
      pulmonary Q22.3
  hepatic ducts Q44.5
  hymen Q52.4
  intestine (large) (small) Q43.4
  kidney Q63.Ø
  lacrimal canal Q1Ø.6
  leaflet, heart valve NEC Q24.8
  ligament, broad Q5Ø.6
  liver Q44.79
    duct Q44.5
  lobule (ear) Q17.Ø
  lung (lobe) Q33.1
  muscle Q79.8
  navicular of carpus Q74.Ø
  nervous system, part NEC QØ7.8
  nipple Q83.3
  nose Q3Ø.8
  organ or site not listed — *see* Anomaly, by site
  ovary Q5Ø.31
  oviduct Q5Ø.6
  pancreas Q45.3
  parathyroid gland Q89.2
  parotid gland (and duct) Q38.4
  pituitary gland Q89.2
  preauricular appendage Q17.Ø
  prepuce N47.8
  renal arteries (multiple) Q27.2
  rib Q76.6
    cervical Q76.5
  roots (teeth) KØØ.2
  salivary gland Q38.4
  sesamoid bones Q74.8
    foot Q74.2
    hand Q74.Ø
  skin tags Q82.8
  spleen Q89.Ø9
  sternum Q76.7
  submaxillary gland Q38.4
  tarsal bones Q74.2
  teeth, tooth KØØ.1
  tendon Q79.8
  thumb Q69.1
  thymus gland Q89.2
  thyroid gland Q89.2
  toes Q69.2
  tongue Q38.3
  tooth, teeth KØØ.1

**Accessory** — *continued*
- tragus Q17.Ø
- ureter Q62.5
- urethra Q64.79
- urinary organ or tract NEC Q64.8
- uterus Q51.28
- vagina Q52.1Ø
- valve, heart NEC Q24.8
  - pulmonary Q22.3
- vertebra Q76.49
- vocal cords Q31.8
- vulva Q52.79

**Accident**
- birth — *see* Birth, injury
- cardiac — *see* Infarct, myocardium
- cerebrovascular (ischemic) I63.9
  - aborted I63.9
  - chronic (old) (remote) (imaging) (without sequelae) Z86.73
    - with residual defects — *see* Sequelae, disease, cerebrovascular
  - embolic I63.- ☑
  - hemorrhagic — *see* Hemorrhage, intracranial, intracerebral
  - old (without sequelae) Z86.73
    - with sequelae (of) — *see* Sequelae, infarction, cerebral
  - thrombotic I63.- ☑
- coronary — *see* Infarct, myocardium
- craniovascular I63.9
- vascular, brain I63.9

**Accidental** — *see* condition

**Accommodation** (disorder) — *see also* condition
- hysterical paralysis of F44.89
- insufficiency of H52.4
- paresis — *see* Paresis, of accommodation
- spasm — *see* Spasm, of accommodation

**Accouchement** — *see* Delivery

**Accreta placenta** O43.21- ☑

**Accretio cordis** (nonrheumatic) I31.Ø

**Accretions, tooth, teeth** KØ3.6

**Acculturation difficulty** Z6Ø.3

**Accumulation secretion, prostate** N42.89

**Acephalia, acephalism, acephalus, acephaly** QØØ.Ø

**Acephalobrachia monster** Q89.89

**Acephalochirus monster** Q89.89

**Acephalogaster** Q89.89

**Acephalostomus monster** Q89.89

**Acephalothorax** Q89.89

**Acerophobia** F4Ø.298

**Acetonemia** R79.89
- in Type 1 diabetes E1Ø.1Ø
  - with coma E1Ø.11

**Acetonuria** R82.4

**Achalasia** (cardia) (esophagus) K22.Ø
- congenital Q39.5
- pylorus Q4Ø.Ø
- sphincteral NEC K59.89

**Ache**(s) — *see* Pain

**Acheilia** Q38.6

**Achillobursitis** — *see* Tendinitis, Achilles

**Achillodynia** — *see* Tendinitis, Achilles

**Achlorhydria, achlorhydric** (neurogenic) K31.83
- anemia D5Ø.8
- diarrhea K31.83
- psychogenic F45.8
- secondary to vagotomy K91.1

**Achluophobia** F4Ø.228

**Acholia** K82.8

**Acholuric jaundice** (familial) (splenomegalic) — *see also* Spherocytosis
- acquired D59.8

**Achondrogenesis** Q77.Ø

**Achondroplasia** (osteosclerosis congenita) Q77.4

**Achroma, cutis** L8Ø

**Achromat** (ism), achromatopsia (acquired) (congenital) H53.51

**Achromia, congenital** — *see* Albinism

**Achromia parasitica** B36.Ø

**Achylia gastrica** K31.89
- psychogenic F45.8

**Acid**
- burn — *see* Corrosion
- deficiency
  - amide nicotinic E52
  - ascorbic E54
  - folic E53.8
  - nicotinic E52
  - pantothenic E53.8

**Acid** — *continued*
- intoxication — *see also* Acidosis E87.29
- peptic disease K3Ø
- phosphatase deficiency E83.39
- stomach K3Ø
  - psychogenic F45.8

**Acidemia** — *see also* Acidosis E87.2Ø
- argininosuccinic E72.22
- isovaleric E71.11Ø
- metabolic — *see also* Acidosis, metabolic
  - newborn P19.9
    - first noted before onset of labor P19.Ø
    - first noted during labor P19.1
    - noted at birth P19.2
- methylmalonic E71.12Ø
- pipecolic E72.3
- propionic E71.121

**Acidity, gastric** (high) K3Ø
- psychogenic F45.8

**Acidocytopenia** — *see* Agranulocytosis

**Acidocytosis** D72.1Ø

**Acidopenia** — *see* Agranulocytosis

**Acidosis** (lactic) E87.2Ø
- in Type 1 diabetes E1Ø.1Ø
  - with coma E1Ø.11
- kidney, tubular N25.89
- lactic E87.2Ø
  - acute E87.21
  - chronic E87.22
- metabolic NEC E87.2Ø
  - with respiratory acidosis E87.4
  - acute E87.21
  - chronic E87.22
  - hyperchloremic, of newborn P74.421
  - late, of newborn P74.Ø
- mixed metabolic and respiratory, newborn P84
- newborn P84
- renal (hyperchloremic) (tubular) N25.89
- respiratory E87.29
  - acute J96.Ø2
  - chronic J96.12
  - complicated by
    - metabolic
      - acidosis E87.4
      - alkalosis E87.4
- specified NEC E87.29

**Aciduria**
- 4-hydroxybutyric E72.81
- argininosuccinic E72.22
- gamma-hydroxybutyric E72.81
- glutaric (type I) E72.3
  - type II E71.313
  - type III E71.5- ☑
- orotic (congenital) (hereditary) (pyrimidine deficiency) E79.89
  - anemia D53.Ø

**Acladiosis** (skin) B36.Ø

**Aclasis, diaphyseal** Q78.6

**Acleistocardia** Q21.19

**Aclusion** — *see* Anomaly, dentofacial, malocclusion

**Acne** L7Ø.9
- artificialis L7Ø.8
- atrophica L7Ø.2
- cachecticorum (Hebra) L7Ø.8
- conglobata L7Ø.1
- cystic L7Ø.Ø
- decalvans L66.2
- excoriee (des jeunes filles) L7Ø.5
- frontalis L7Ø.2
- indurata L7Ø.Ø
- infantile L7Ø.4
- keloid L73.Ø
- lupoid L7Ø.2
- necrotic, necrotica (miliaris) L7Ø.2
- neonatal L7Ø.4
- nodular L7Ø.Ø
- occupational L7Ø.8
- picker's L7Ø.5
- pustular L7Ø.Ø
- rodens L7Ø.2
- rosacea L71.9
- specified NEC L7Ø.8
- tropica L7Ø.3
- varioliformis L7Ø.2
- vulgaris L7Ø.Ø

**Acnitis** (primary) A18.4

**Acosta's disease** T7Ø.29- ☑

**Acoustic** — *see* condition

**Acousticophobia** F4Ø.298

**ACPO** (acute colonic pseudo-obstruction) K59.81

**Acquired** — *see also* condition
- immunodeficiency syndrome (AIDS) B2Ø

**Acrania** QØØ.Ø

**Acroangiodermatitis** I78.9

**Acroasphyxia, chronic** I73.89

**Acrobystitis** N47.7

**Acrocephalopolysyndactyly** Q87.Ø

**Acrocephalosyndactyly** Q87.Ø

**Acrocephaly** Q75.ØØ9

**Acrochondrohyperplasia** — *see* Syndrome, Marfan

**Acrocyanosis** I73.89
- newborn P28.2
  - meaning transient blue hands and feet — *omit code*

**Acrodermatitis** L3Ø.8
- atrophicans (chronica) L9Ø.4
- continua (Hallopeau) L4Ø.2
- enteropathica (hereditary) E83.2
- Hallopeau's L4Ø.2
- infantile papular L44.4
- perstans L4Ø.2
- pustulosa continua L4Ø.2
- recalcitrant pustular L4Ø.2

**Acrodynia** — *see* Poisoning, mercury

**Acromegaly, acromegalia** E22.Ø

**Acromelalgia** I73.81

**Acromicria, acromikria** Q79.8

**Acronyx** L6Ø.Ø

**Acropachy, thyroid** — *see* Thyrotoxicosis

**Acroparesthesia** (simple) (vasomotor) I73.89

**Acropathy, thyroid** — *see* Thyrotoxicosis

**Acrophobia** F4Ø.241

**Acroposthitis** N47.7

**Acroscleriasis, acroscleroderma, acrosclerosis** — *see* Sclerosis, systemic

**Acrosphacelus** I96

**Acrospiroma, eccrine** — *see* Neoplasm, skin, benign

**Acrostealgia** — *see* Osteochondropathy

**Acrotrophodynia** — *see* Immersion

**ACTH ectopic syndrome** E24.3

**Actinic** — *see* condition

**Actinobacillosis, actinobacillus** A28.8
- mallei A24.Ø
- muris A25.1

**Actinomyces israelii** (infection) — *see* Actinomycosis

**Actinomycetoma** (foot) B47.1

**Actinomycosis, actinomycotic** A42.9
- with pneumonia A42.Ø
- abdominal A42.1
- cervicofacial A42.2
- cutaneous A42.89
- gastrointestinal A42.1
- pulmonary A42.Ø
- sepsis A42.7
- specified site NEC A42.89

**Actinoneuritis** G62.82

**Action, heart**
- disorder I49.9
- irregular I49.9
  - psychogenic F45.8

**Activated protein C resistance** D68.51

**Activation**
- mast cell (disorder) (syndrome) D89.4Ø
  - idiopathic D89.42
  - monoclonal D89.41
  - secondary D89.43
  - specified type NEC D89.49

**Active** — *see* condition

**Acute** — *see also* condition
- abdomen R1Ø.Ø
- gallbladder — *see* Cholecystitis, acute

**Acyanotic heart disease** (congenital) Q24.9

**Acystia** Q64.5

**Adair-Dighton syndrome** (brittle bones and blue sclera, deafness) Q78.Ø

**Adamantinoblastoma** — *see* Ameloblastoma

**Adamantinoma** — *see also* Cyst, calcifying odontogenic
- long bones C4Ø.9Ø
  - lower limb C4Ø.2- ☑
  - upper limb C4Ø.Ø- ☑
- malignant C41.1
  - jaw (bone) (lower) C41.1
    - upper C41.Ø
- tibial C4Ø.2- ☑

**Adamantoblastoma** — *see* Ameloblastoma

**Adams-Stokes** (-Morgagni) **disease or syndrome** I45.9

**Adaption reaction** — *see* Disorder, adjustment

**Addiction** — *see also* Dependence F19.2Ø

- **Addiction** — *continued*
  - alcohol, alcoholic (ethyl) (methyl) (wood) (without remission) F1Ø.2Ø
    - with remission F1Ø.21
  - drug — *see* Dependence, drug
  - ethyl alcohol (without remission) F1Ø.2Ø
    - with remission F1Ø.21
  - heroin — *see* Dependence, drug, opioid
  - methyl alcohol (without remission) F1Ø.2Ø
    - with remission F1Ø.21
  - methylated spirit (without remission) F1Ø.2Ø
    - with remission F1Ø.21
  - morphine (-like substances) — *see* Dependence, drug, opioid
  - nicotine — *see* Dependence, drug, nicotine
  - opium and opioids — *see* Dependence, drug, opioid
  - tobacco — *see* Dependence, drug, nicotine
- **Addison-Biermer anemia** (pernicious) D51.Ø
- **Addison-Schilder complex** E71.528
- **Addisonian crisis** E27.2
- **Addison's**
  - anemia (pernicious) D51.Ø
  - disease (bronze) or syndrome E27.1
    - tuberculous A18.7
  - keloid L94.Ø
- **Additional** — *see also* Accessory
  - chromosome(s) — *see also* Trisomy Q99.8- ☑
    - 21 — *see* Trisomy, 21
    - marker — *see* Extra, marker chromosomes
    - sex — *see* Abnormal, chromosome, sex
- **Adduction contracture, hip or other joint** — *see* Contraction, joint
- **Adenitis** — *see also* Lymphadenitis
  - acute, unspecified site L04.9
  - axillary I88.9
    - acute L04.2
    - chronic or subacute I88.1
  - Bartholin's gland N75.8
  - bulbourethral gland — *see* Urethritis
  - cervical I88.9
    - acute L04.Ø
    - chronic or subacute I88.1
  - chancroid (Hemophilus ducreyi) A57
  - chronic, unspecified site I88.1
  - Cowper's gland — *see* Urethritis
  - due to Pasteurella multocida (P. septica) A28.Ø
  - epidemic, acute B27.Ø9
  - gangrenous L04.9
  - gonorrheal NEC A54.89
  - groin I88.9
    - acute L04.1
    - chronic or subacute I88.1
  - infectious (acute) (epidemic) B27.Ø9
  - inguinal I88.9
    - acute L04.1
    - chronic or subacute I88.1
  - lymph gland or node, except mesenteric I88.9
    - acute — *see* Lymphadenitis, acute
    - chronic or subacute I88.1
  - mesenteric (acute) (chronic) (nonspecific) (subacute) I88.Ø
  - parotid gland (suppurative) — *see* Sialoadenitis
  - salivary gland (any) (suppurative) — *see* Sialoadenitis
  - scrofulous (tuberculous) A18.2
  - Skene's duct or gland — *see* Urethritis
  - strumous, tuberculous A18.2
  - subacute, unspecified site I88.1
  - sublingual gland (suppurative) — *see* Sialoadenitis
  - submandibular gland (suppurative) — *see* Sialoadenitis
  - submaxillary gland (suppurative) — *see* Sialoadenitis
  - tuberculous — *see* Tuberculosis, lymph gland
  - urethral gland — *see* Urethritis
  - Wharton's duct (suppurative) — *see* Sialoadenitis
- **Adenoacanthoma** — *see* Neoplasm, malignant, by site
- **Adenoameloblastoma** — *see* Cyst, calcifying odontogenic
- **Adenocarcinoid** (tumor) — *see* Neoplasm, malignant, by site
- **Adenocarcinoma** — *see also* Neoplasm, malignant, by site
  - acidophil
    - specified site — *see* Neoplasm, malignant, by site
    - unspecified site C75.1
  - adrenal cortical C74.Ø- ☑
  - alveolar — *see* Neoplasm, lung, malignant
  - apocrine
    - breast — *see* Neoplasm, breast, malignant
    - in situ
      - breast DØ5.8- ☑
      - specified site NEC — *see* Neoplasm, skin, in situ
      - unspecified site DØ4.9

- **Adenocarcinoma** — *continued*
  - apocrine — *continued*
    - specified site NEC — *see* Neoplasm, skin, malignant
    - unspecified site C44.99
  - basal cell
    - specified site — *see* Neoplasm, skin, malignant
    - unspecified site CØ8.9
  - basophil
    - specified site — *see* Neoplasm, malignant, by site
    - unspecified site C75.1
  - bile duct type C22.1
    - liver C22.1
    - specified site NEC — *see* Neoplasm, malignant, by site
    - unspecified site C22.1
  - bronchiolar — *see* Neoplasm, lung, malignant
  - bronchioloalveolar — *see* Neoplasm, lung, malignant
  - ceruminous C44.29- ☑
  - cervix, in situ — *see also* Carcinoma, cervix uteri, in situ DØ6.9
  - chromophobe
    - specified site — *see* Neoplasm, malignant, by site
    - unspecified site C75.1
  - diffuse type
    - specified site — *see* Neoplasm, malignant, by site
    - unspecified site C16.9
  - duct
    - infiltrating
      - with Paget's disease — *see* Neoplasm, breast, malignant
      - specified site — *see* Neoplasm, malignant, by site
      - unspecified site (female) C5Ø.91- ☑
        - male C5Ø.92- ☑
    - specified site — *see* Neoplasm, malignant, by site
    - unspecified site
      - female C56.9
      - male C61
  - eosinophil
    - specified site — *see* Neoplasm, malignant, by site
    - unspecified site C75.1
  - follicular
    - with papillary C73
    - moderately differentiated C73
    - specified site — *see* Neoplasm, malignant, by site
    - trabecular C73
    - unspecified site C73
    - well differentiated C73
  - Hurthle cell C73
  - in
    - adenomatous
      - polyposis coli C18.9
  - infiltrating duct
    - with Paget's disease — *see* Neoplasm, breast, malignant
    - specified site — *see* Neoplasm, by site, malignant
    - unspecified site (female) C5Ø.91- ☑
      - male C5Ø.92- ☑
  - inflammatory
    - specified site — *see* Neoplasm, by site, malignant
    - unspecified site (female) C5Ø.91- ☑
      - male C5Ø.92- ☑
  - intestinal type
    - specified site — *see* Neoplasm, by site, malignant
    - unspecified site C16.9
  - intracystic papillary
  - intraductal
    - breast DØ5.1- ☑
    - noninfiltrating
      - breast DØ5.1- ☑
      - papillary
        - with invasion
          - specified site — *see* Neoplasm, by site, malignant
          - unspecified site (female) C5Ø.91- ☑
            - male C5Ø.92- ☑
        - breast DØ5.1- ☑
        - specified site NEC — *see* Neoplasm, in situ, by site
        - unspecified site DØ5.1- ☑
      - specified site NEC — *see* Neoplasm, in situ, by site
      - unspecified site DØ5.1- ☑
    - papillary
      - with invasion
        - specified site — *see* Neoplasm, malignant, by site
        - unspecified site (female) C5Ø.91- ☑
          - male C5Ø.92- ☑
      - breast DØ5.1- ☑

- **Adenocarcinoma** — *continued*
  - intraductal — *continued*
    - papillary — *continued*
      - specified site — *see* Neoplasm, in situ, by site
      - unspecified site DØ5.1- ☑
    - specified site NEC — *see* Neoplasm, in situ, by site
    - unspecified site DØ5.1- ☑
  - islet cell
    - with exocrine, mixed
      - specified site — *see* Neoplasm, malignant, by site
      - unspecified site C25.9
    - pancreas C25.4
    - specified site NEC — *see* Neoplasm, malignant, by site
    - unspecified site C25.4
  - lobular
    - in situ
      - breast DØ5.Ø- ☑
      - specified site NEC — *see* Neoplasm, in situ, by site
      - unspecified site DØ5.Ø- ☑
    - specified site — *see* Neoplasm, malignant, by site
    - unspecified site (female) C5Ø.91- ☑
      - male C5Ø.92- ☑
  - mucoid — *see also* Neoplasm, malignant, by site
    - cell
      - specified site — *see* Neoplasm, malignant, by site
      - unspecified site C75.1
  - nonencapsulated sclerosing C73
  - papillary
    - with follicular C73
    - follicular variant C73
    - intraductal (noninfiltrating)
      - with invasion
        - specified site — *see* Neoplasm, malignant, by site
        - unspecified site (female) C5Ø.91- ☑
          - male C5Ø.92- ☑
      - breast DØ5.1- ☑
      - specified site NEC — *see* Neoplasm, in situ, by site
      - unspecified site DØ5.1- ☑
    - serous
      - specified site — *see* Neoplasm, malignant, by site
      - unspecified site C56.9
  - papillocystic
    - specified site — *see* Neoplasm, malignant, by site
    - unspecified site C56.9
  - pseudomucinous
    - specified site — *see* Neoplasm, malignant, by site
    - unspecified site C56.9
  - renal cell C64.- ☑
  - sebaceous — *see* Neoplasm, skin, malignant
  - serous — *see also* Neoplasm, malignant, by site
    - papillary
      - specified site — *see* Neoplasm, malignant, by site
      - unspecified site C56.9
  - sweat gland — *see* Neoplasm, skin, malignant
  - water-clear cell C75.Ø
- **Adenocarcinoma-in-situ** — *see also* Neoplasm, in situ, by site
  - breast DØ5.9- ☑
- **Adenofibroma**
  - clear cell — *see* Neoplasm, benign, by site
  - endometrioid D27.9
    - borderline malignancy D39.1Ø
    - malignant C56.- ☑
  - mucinous
    - specified site — *see* Neoplasm, benign, by site
    - unspecified site D27.9
  - papillary
    - specified site — *see* Neoplasm, benign, by site
    - unspecified site D27.9
  - prostate — *see* Enlargement, enlarged, prostate
  - serous
    - specified site — *see* Neoplasm, benign, by site
    - unspecified site D27.9
  - specified site — *see* Neoplasm, benign, by site
  - unspecified site D27.9
- **Adenofibrosis**
  - breast — *see* Fibroadenosis, breast
  - endometrioid N8Ø.ØØ
- **Adenoiditis** (chronic) J35.Ø2
  - with tonsillitis J35.Ø3
  - acute JØ3.9Ø
    - recurrent JØ3.91
    - specified organism NEC JØ3.8Ø
      - recurrent JØ3.81
    - staphylococcal JØ3.8Ø
      - recurrent JØ3.81

**Admission** — *continued*
- examination at health care facility — *see also* Examination — *continued*
  - clinical research investigation (control) (normal comparison) (participant) ZØØ.6
  - dental ZØ1.2Ø
    - with abnormal findings ZØ1.21
  - donor (potential) ZØØ.5
  - ear ZØ1.1Ø
    - with abnormal findings NEC ZØ1.118
  - eye ZØ1.ØØ
    - with abnormal findings ZØ1.Ø1
    - following failed vision screening ZØ1.Ø2Ø
      - with abnormal findings ZØ1.Ø21
  - general, specified reason NEC ZØØ.8
  - hearing ZØ1.1Ø
    - with abnormal findings NEC ZØ1.118
    - infant or child (over 28 days old) ZØØ.129
      - with abnormal findings ZØØ.121
  - postpartum checkup Z39.2
  - psychiatric (general) ZØØ.8
    - requested by authority ZØ4.6
  - vision ZØ1.ØØ
    - with abnormal findings ZØ1.Ø1
    - following failed vision screening ZØ1.Ø2Ø
      - with abnormal findings ZØ1.Ø21
    - infant or child (over 28 days old) ZØØ.129
      - with abnormal findings ZØØ.121
- fitting (of)
  - artificial
    - arm — *see* Admission, adjustment, artificial, arm
    - eye Z44.2- ☑
    - leg — *see* Admission, adjustment, artificial, leg
  - brain neuropacemaker Z46.2
    - implanted Z45.42
  - breast prosthesis (external) Z44.3- ☑
  - colostomy belt Z46.89
  - contact lenses Z46.Ø
  - cystostomy device Z46.6
  - dental prosthesis Z46.3
  - dentures Z46.3
  - device NEC
    - abdominal Z46.89
    - nervous system Z46.2
      - implanted — *see* Admission, adjustment, device, implanted, nervous system
    - orthodontic Z46.4
    - prosthetic Z44.9
      - breast Z44.3- ☑
      - dental Z46.3
      - eye Z44.2- ☑
    - substitution
      - auditory Z46.2
        - implanted — *see* Admission, adjustment, device, implanted, hearing device
      - nervous system Z46.2
        - implanted — *see* Admission, adjustment, device, implanted, nervous system
      - visual Z46.2
        - implanted Z45.31
  - hearing aid Z46.1
  - ileostomy device Z46.89
  - intestinal appliance or device NEC Z46.89
  - neuropacemaker (brain) (peripheral nerve) (spinal cord) Z46.2
    - implanted Z45.42
  - orthodontic device Z46.4
  - orthopedic device (brace) (cast) (shoes) Z46.89
  - prosthesis Z44.9
    - arm — *see* Admission, adjustment, artificial, arm
    - breast Z44.3- ☑
    - dental Z46.3
    - eye Z44.2- ☑
    - leg — *see* Admission, adjustment, artificial, leg
    - specified type NEC Z44.8
  - spectacles Z46.Ø
- follow-up examination ZØ9
- intrauterine device management Z3Ø.431
  - initial prescription Z3Ø.Ø14
- mental health evaluation ZØØ.8
  - requested by authority ZØ4.6
- observation — *see* Observation
- Papanicolaou smear, cervix Z12.4
  - for suspected malignant neoplasm Z12.4
- plastic and reconstructive surgery following medical procedure or healed injury NEC Z42.8
- plastic surgery, cosmetic NEC Z41.1

**Admission** — *continued*
- postpartum observation
  - immediately after delivery Z39.Ø
  - routine follow-up Z39.2
- poststerilization (for restoration) Z31.Ø
  - aftercare Z31.42
- procreative management Z31.9
- prophylactic (measure) — *see also* Encounter, prophylactic measures
  - oophorectomy for persons without known genetic/familial risk factors Z4Ø.81
  - organ removal Z4Ø.ØØ
    - breast Z4Ø.Ø1
    - fallopian tube(s) Z4Ø.Ø3
      - for persons without known genetic/familial risk factors Z4Ø.82
    - ovary(s) Z4Ø.Ø2
      - for persons without known genetic/familial risk factors Z4Ø.81
    - specified organ NEC Z4Ø.Ø9
    - testes Z4Ø.Ø9
  - salpingectomy for persons without known genetic/familial risk factors Z4Ø.82
  - vaccination Z23
- psychiatric examination (general) ZØØ.8
  - requested by authority ZØ4.6
- radiation therapy (antineoplastic) Z51.Ø
- reconstructive surgery following medical procedure or healed injury NEC Z42.8
- removal of
  - cystostomy catheter Z43.5
  - drains Z48.Ø3
  - dressing (nonsurgical) Z48.ØØ
  - implantable subdermal contraceptive Z3Ø.46
  - intrauterine contraceptive device Z3Ø.432
  - neuropacemaker (brain) (peripheral nerve) (spinal cord) Z46.2
    - implanted Z45.42
  - staples Z48.Ø2
  - surgical dressing Z48.Ø1
  - sutures Z48.Ø2
  - ureteral stent Z46.6
- respirator [ventilator] use during power failure Z99.12
- restoration of organ continuity (poststerilization) Z31.Ø
  - aftercare Z31.42
- sensitivity test — *see also* Test, skin
  - allergy NEC ZØ1.82
  - Mantoux Z11.1
- tuboplasty following previous sterilization Z31.Ø
  - aftercare Z31.42
- vasoplasty following previous sterilization Z31.Ø
  - aftercare Z31.42
- vision examination ZØ1.ØØ
  - with abnormal findings ZØ1.Ø1
  - following failed vision screening ZØ1.Ø2Ø
    - with abnormal findings ZØ1.Ø21
  - infant or child (over 28 days old) ZØØ.129
    - with abnormal findings ZØØ.121
- waiting period for admission to other facility Z75.1

**Adnexitis** (suppurative) — *see* Salpingo-oophoritis

**Adolescent X-linked adrenoleukodystrophy** E71.521

**Adrenal** (gland) — *see* condition

**Adrenalism, tuberculous** A18.7

**Adrenalitis, adrenitis** E27.8
- autoimmune E27.1
- meningococcal, hemorrhagic A39.1

**Adrenarche, premature** E27.Ø

**Adrenocortical syndrome** — *see* Cushing's, syndrome

**Adrenogenital syndrome** E25.9
- acquired E25.8
- congenital E25.Ø
- salt loss E25.Ø

**Adrenogenitalism, congenital** E25.Ø

**Adrenoleukodystrophy** E71.529
- neonatal E71.511
- X-linked E71.529
  - Addison only phenotype E71.528
  - Addison-Schilder E71.528
  - adolescent E71.521
  - adrenomyeloneuropathy E71.522
  - childhood cerebral E71.52Ø
  - other specified E71.528

**Adrenomyeloneuropathy** E71.522

**Adventitious bursa** — *see* Bursopathy, specified type NEC

**Adverse effect** — *see* Table of Drugs and Chemicals, categories T36-T5Ø, with 6th character 5

**Advice** — *see* Counseling

**Adynamia** (episodica) (hereditary) (periodic) G72.3

**Aeration lung imperfect, newborn** — *see* Atelectasis

**Aero-otitis media** T7Ø.Ø- ☑

**Aerobullosis** T7Ø.3- ☑

**Aerocele** — *see* Embolism, air

**Aerodermectasia**
- subcutaneous (traumatic) T79.7- ☑

**Aerodontalgia** T7Ø.29- ☑

**Aeroembolism** T7Ø.3- ☑

**Aerogenes capsulatus infection** A48.Ø

**Aerophagy, aerophagia** (psychogenic) F45.8

**Aerophobia** F4Ø.228

**Aerosinusitis** T7Ø.1- ☑

**Aerotitis** T7Ø.Ø- ☑

**Affection** — *see* Disease

**Afibrinogenemia** — *see also* Defect, coagulation D68.8
- acquired D65
- congenital D68.2
- following ectopic or molar pregnancy OØ8.1
- in abortion — *see* Abortion, by type, complicated by, afibrinogenemia
- puerperal O72.3

**African**
- sleeping sickness B56.9
- tick fever A68.1
- trypanosomiasis B56.9
  - gambian B56.Ø
  - rhodesian B56.1

**After-cataract** — *see* Cataract, secondary

**Aftercare** — *see also* Care Z51.89
- following surgery (for) (on)
  - amputation Z47.81
  - attention to
    - drains Z48.Ø3
    - dressings (nonsurgical) Z48.ØØ
      - surgical Z48.Ø1
    - sutures Z48.Ø2
  - circulatory system Z48.812
  - delayed (planned) wound closure Z48.1
  - digestive system Z48.815
  - explantation of joint prosthesis (staged procedure)
    - hip Z47.32
    - knee Z47.33
    - shoulder Z47.31
  - genitourinary system Z48.816
  - joint replacement Z47.1
  - neoplasm Z48.3
  - nervous system Z48.811
  - oral cavity Z48.814
  - organ transplant
    - bone marrow Z48.29Ø
    - heart Z48.21
    - heart-lung Z48.28Ø
    - kidney Z48.22
    - liver Z48.23
    - lung Z48.24
    - multiple organs NEC Z48.288
    - specified NEC Z48.298
  - orthopedic NEC Z47.89
  - planned wound closure Z48.1
  - removal of internal fixation device Z47.2
  - respiratory system Z48.813
  - scoliosis Z47.82
  - sense organs Z48.81Ø
  - skin and subcutaneous tissue Z48.817
  - specified body system
    - circulatory Z48.812
    - digestive Z48.815
    - genitourinary Z48.816
    - nervous Z48.811
    - oral cavity Z48.814
    - respiratory Z48.813
    - sense organs Z48.81Ø
    - skin and subcutaneous tissue Z48.817
    - teeth Z48.814
  - specified NEC Z48.89
  - spinal Z47.89
  - teeth Z48.814
- fracture — *code to* fracture with seventh character D
- involving
  - removal of
    - drains Z48.Ø3
    - dressings (nonsurgical) Z48.ØØ
    - staples Z48.Ø2
    - surgical dressings Z48.Ø1
    - sutures Z48.Ø2
  - neuropacemaker (brain) (peripheral nerve) (spinal cord) Z46.2
    - implanted Z45.42
  - orthopedic NEC Z47.89

- **Agraphia** (absolute) R48.8
  - with alexia R48.Ø
  - developmental F81.81
- **Ague** (dumb) — *see* Malaria
- **Agyria** QØ4.3
- **Ahumada-del Castillo syndrome** E23.Ø
- **Aichomophobia** F4Ø.298
- **AIDS** (related complex) B2Ø
- **Ailment heart** — *see* Disease, heart
- **Ailurophobia** F4Ø.218
- **AIN** — *see* Neoplasia, intraepithelial, anal
- **Ainhum** (disease) L94.6
- **AIPHI** (acute idiopathic pulmonary hemorrhage in infants (over 28 days old)) RØ4.81
- **Air**
  - anterior mediastinum J98.2
  - compressed, disease T7Ø.3- ☑
  - conditioner lung or pneumonitis J67.7
  - embolism (artery) (cerebral) (any site) T79.Ø- ☑
    - with ectopic or molar pregnancy OØ8.2
    - due to implanted device NEC — *see* Complications, by site and type, specified NEC
    - following
      - abortion — *see* Abortion by type, complicated by, embolism
      - ectopic or molar pregnancy OØ8.2
      - infusion, therapeutic injection or transfusion T8Ø.Ø- ☑
    - in pregnancy, childbirth or puerperium — *see* Embolism, obstetric
    - traumatic T79.Ø- ☑
  - hunger, psychogenic F45.8
  - rarefied, effects of — *see* Effect, adverse, high altitude
  - sickness T75.3- ☑
- **Airplane sickness** T75.3- ☑
- **Akathisia** (drug-induced) (treatment-induced) G25.71
  - neuroleptic induced (acute) G25.71
  - tardive G25.71
- **Akinesia** R29.898
- **Akinetic mutism** R41.89
- **Akureyri's disease** G93.39
- **Alactasia, congenital** E73.Ø
- **Alagille (-Watson) syndrome** Q44.71
- **Alastrim** BØ3
- **Albers-Schonberg syndrome** Q78.2
- **Albert's syndrome** — *see* Tendinitis, Achilles
- **Albinism, albino** E7Ø.3Ø
  - with hematologic abnormality E7Ø.339
    - Chediak-Higashi syndrome E7Ø.33Ø
    - Hermansky-Pudlak syndrome E7Ø.331
    - other specified E7Ø.338
  - I E7Ø.32Ø
  - II E7Ø.321
  - ocular E7Ø.319
    - autosomal recessive E7Ø.311
    - other specified E7Ø.318
    - X-linked E7Ø.31Ø
  - oculocutaneous E7Ø.329
    - other specified E7Ø.328
    - tyrosinase (ty) negative E7Ø.32Ø
    - tyrosinase (ty) positive E7Ø.321
  - other specified E7Ø.39
- **Albinismus** E7Ø.3Ø
- **Albright** (-McCune)(-Sternberg) syndrome Q78.1
- **Albuminous** — *see* condition
- **Albuminuria, albuminuric** (acute) (chronic) (subacute) — *see also* Proteinuria R8Ø.9
  - complicating pregnancy — *see* Proteinuria, gestational
    - with
      - gestational hypertension — *see* Pre-eclampsia
      - pre-existing hypertension — *see* Hypertension, complicating pregnancy, pre-existing, with, pre-eclampsia
  - gestational — *see* Proteinuria, gestational
    - with
      - gestational hypertension — *see* Pre-eclampsia
      - pre-existing hypertension — *see* Hypertension, complicating pregnancy, pre-existing, with, pre-eclampsia
  - orthostatic R8Ø.2
  - postural R8Ø.2
  - pre-eclamptic — *see* Pre-eclampsia
  - scarlatinal A38.8
- **Albuminurophobia** F4Ø.298
- **Alcaptonuria** E7Ø.29
- **Alcohol, alcoholic, alcohol-induced**
  - addiction (without remission) F1Ø.2Ø
    - with remission F1Ø.21

- **Alcohol, alcoholic, alcohol-induced** — *continued*
  - amnestic disorder, persisting F1Ø.96
    - with dependence F1Ø.26
  - anxiety disorder F1Ø.98Ø
  - bipolar and related disorder F1Ø.94
  - brain syndrome, chronic F1Ø.97
    - with dependence F1Ø.27
  - cardiopathy I42.6
  - counseling and surveillance Z71.41
    - family member Z71.42
  - delirium (acute) (tremens) (withdrawal) F1Ø.921
    - with intoxication F1Ø.921
      - in
        - abuse F1Ø.121
        - dependence F1Ø.221
    - abuse F1Ø.131
      - with intoxication F1Ø.121
    - dependence (acute) (tremens) (withdrawal) F1Ø.231
      - with intoxication F1Ø.221
    - use, unspecified F1Ø.931
      - with intoxication F1Ø.921
  - dementia F1Ø.97
    - with dependence F1Ø.27
  - depressive disorder F1Ø.94
  - deterioration F1Ø.97
    - with dependence F1Ø.27
  - hallucinosis (acute) F1Ø.951
    - in
      - abuse F1Ø.151
      - dependence F1Ø.251
  - insanity F1Ø.959
  - intoxication (acute) (without dependence) F1Ø.129
    - with
      - delirium F1Ø.121
      - dependence F1Ø.229
        - with delirium F1Ø.221
        - uncomplicated F1Ø.22Ø
    - uncomplicated F1Ø.12Ø
  - jealousy F1Ø.988
  - Korsakoff's, Korsakov's, Korsakow's F1Ø.26
  - liver K7Ø.9
    - acute — *see* Disease, liver, alcoholic, hepatitis
  - major neurocognitive disorder, amnestic-confabulatory type F1Ø.96
  - major neurocognitive disorder, nonamnestic-confabulatory type F1Ø.97
  - mania (acute) (chronic) F1Ø.959
  - mild neurocognitive disorder F1Ø.988
  - paranoia, paranoid (type) psychosis F1Ø.95Ø
  - pellagra E52
  - poisoning, accidental (acute) NEC — *see* Table of Drugs and Chemicals, alcohol, poisoning
  - psychosis — *see* Psychosis, alcoholic
  - psychotic disorder F1Ø.959
  - sexual dysfunction F1Ø.981
  - sleep disorder F1Ø.982
  - withdrawal (without convulsions) F1Ø.239
    - with delirium F1Ø.231
- **Alcoholism** (chronic) (without remission) F1Ø.2Ø
  - with
    - psychosis — *see* Psychosis, alcoholic
    - remission F1Ø.21
  - Korsakov's F1Ø.96
    - with dependence F1Ø.26
- **Alder** (-Reilly) **anomaly or syndrome** (leukocyte granulation) D72.Ø
- **Aldosteronism** E26.9
  - familial (type I) E26.Ø2
  - glucocorticoid-remediable E26.Ø2
  - primary (due to (bilateral) adrenal hyperplasia) E26.Ø9
  - primary NEC E26.Ø9
  - secondary E26.1
  - specified NEC E26.89
- **Aldosteronoma** D44.1Ø
- **Aldrich** (-Wiskott) **syndrome** (eczema-thrombocytopenia) D82.Ø
- **Alektorophobia** F4Ø.218
- **Aleppo boil** B55.1
- **Aleukemic** — *see* condition
- **Aleukia**
  - congenital D7Ø.Ø
  - hemorrhagica D61.9
    - congenital D61.Ø9
  - splenica D73.1
- **Alexia** R48.Ø
  - developmental F81.Ø
  - secondary to organic lesion R48.Ø
- **Algoneurodystrophy** M89.ØØ
  - ankle M89.Ø7- ☑

- **Algoneurodystrophy** — *continued*
  - foot M89.Ø7- ☑
  - forearm M89.Ø3- ☑
  - hand M89.Ø4- ☑
  - lower leg M89.Ø6- ☑
  - multiple sites M89.Ø9
  - shoulder M89.Ø1- ☑
  - specified site NEC M89.Ø8
  - thigh M89.Ø5- ☑
  - upper arm M89.Ø2- ☑
- **Algophobia** F4Ø.298
- **Alienation, mental** — *see* Psychosis
- **Alkalemia** E87.3
- **Alkalosis** E87.3
  - metabolic E87.3
    - with respiratory acidosis E87.4
    - of newborn P74.41
  - respiratory E87.3
- **Alkaptonuria** E7Ø.29
- **Allen-Masters syndrome** N83.8
- **Allergy, allergic** (reaction) (to) T78.4Ø- ☑
  - air-borne substance NEC (rhinitis) J3Ø.89
  - alveolitis (extrinsic) J67.9
    - due to
      - Aspergillus clavatus J67.4
      - Cryptostroma corticale J67.6
      - organisms (fungal, thermophilic actinomycete) growing in ventilation (air conditioning) systems J67.7
    - specified type NEC J67.8
  - anaphylactic reaction or shock T78.2- ☑
  - angioneurotic edema T78.3- ☑
  - animal (dander) (epidermal) (hair) (rhinitis) J3Ø.81
  - bee sting (anaphylactic shock) T63.44- ☑
  - biological — *see* Allergy, drug
  - colitis — *see also* Colitis, allergic K52.29
  - dairy products T78.119- ☑
    - with
      - reactivity to baked milk T78.111- ☑
      - tolerance to baked milk T78.11Ø- ☑
    - anaphylactic reaction T78.Ø79- ☑
      - with T78.Ø79- ☑
        - reactivity to baked milk T78.Ø71- ☑
        - tolerance to baked milk T78.Ø7Ø- ☑
  - dander (animal) (rhinitis) J3Ø.81
  - dandruff (rhinitis) J3Ø.81
  - dental restorative material (existing) KØ8.55
  - dermatitis — *see* Dermatitis, contact, allergic
  - diathesis — *see* History, allergy
  - drug, medicament & biological (any) (external) (internal) T78.4Ø- ☑
    - correct substance properly administered — *see* Table of Drugs and Chemicals, by drug, adverse effect
    - wrong substance given or taken NEC (by accident) — *see* Table of Drugs and Chemicals, by drug, poisoning
  - due to pollen J3Ø.1
  - dust (house) (stock) (rhinitis) J3Ø.89
    - with asthma — *see* Asthma, allergic extrinsic
  - eczema — *see* Dermatitis, contact, allergic
  - eggs T78.4Ø- ☑
    - adverse reaction NEC T78.129- ☑
      - with
        - reactivity to baked egg T78.121- ☑
        - tolerance to baked egg T78.12Ø- ☑
    - anaphylactic reaction T78.Ø89- ☑
      - with
        - reactivity to baked egg T78.Ø81- ☑
        - tolerance to baked egg T78.Ø8Ø- ☑
  - epidermal (animal) (rhinitis) J3Ø.81
  - feathers (rhinitis) J3Ø.89
  - food (any) (ingested) NEC T78.19- ☑
    - anaphylactic shock — *see* Shock, anaphylactic, due to food
    - dermatitis — *see* Dermatitis, due to, food
    - dietary counseling and surveillance Z71.3
    - in contact with skin L23.6
    - rhinitis J3Ø.5
    - status (without reaction) Z91.Ø18
      - beef Z91.Ø14
      - eggs Z91.Ø12Ø
        - with
          - reactivity to baked egg Z91.Ø122
          - tolerance to baked egg Z91.Ø121
      - lamb Z91.Ø14
      - mammalian meats Z91.Ø14
      - milk products Z91.Ø11Ø

Index

Agraphia — Allergy, allergic

- **Allergy, allergic** — *continued*
  - food — *continued*
    - status — *continued*
      - milk products — *continued*
        - with
          - reactivity to baked milk Z91.Ø112
          - tolerance to baked milk Z91.Ø111
      - peanuts Z91.Ø1Ø
      - pork Z91.Ø14
      - red meats Z91.Ø14
      - seafood Z91.Ø13
      - specified NEC Z91.Ø18
  - gastrointestinal — *see also* specific type of allergic reaction
    - meaning colitis — *see also* Colitis, allergic K52.29
    - meaning gastroenteritis — *see also* Gastroenteritis, allergic K52.29
    - meaning other adverse food reaction not elsewhere classified T78.19- ☑
  - grain J3Ø.1
  - grass (hay fever) (pollen) J3Ø.1
    - asthma — *see* Asthma, allergic extrinsic
  - hair (animal) (rhinitis) J3Ø.81
  - history (of) — *see* History, allergy
  - horse serum — *see* Allergy, serum
  - inhalant (rhinitis) J3Ø.89
    - pollen J3Ø.1
  - kapok (rhinitis) J3Ø.89
  - medicine — *see* Allergy, drug
  - milk protein — *see also* Allergy, food Z91.Ø11Ø
    - with
      - reactivity to baked milk Z91.Ø112
      - tolerance to baked milk Z91.Ø111
    - adverse reaction NEC T78.119- ☑
      - with
        - reactivity to baked milk T78.111- ☑
        - tolerance to baked milk T78.11Ø- ☑
    - anaphylactic reaction T78.Ø79- ☑
      - with
        - reactivity to baked milk T78.Ø71- ☑
        - tolerance to baked milk T78.Ø7Ø- ☑
    - dermatitis L27.2
    - enterocolitis syndrome K52.21
    - enteropathy K52.22
    - gastroenteritis K52.29
    - gastroesophageal reflux — *see also* Reaction, adverse, food K21.9
      - with esophagitis (without bleeding) K21.ØØ
        - with bleeding K21.Ø1
    - proctocolitis K52.29
  - nasal, seasonal due to pollen J3Ø.1
  - pneumonia J82.89
  - pollen (any) (hay fever) J3Ø.1
    - asthma — *see* Asthma, allergic extrinsic
  - primrose J3Ø.1
  - primula J3Ø.1
  - proctocolitis K52.29
  - purpura D69.Ø
  - ragweed (hay fever) (pollen) J3Ø.1
    - asthma — *see* Asthma, allergic extrinsic
  - rose (pollen) J3Ø.1
  - seasonal NEC J3Ø.2
  - Senecio jacobae (pollen) J3Ø.1
  - serum — *see also* Reaction, serum T8Ø.69- ☑
    - anaphylactic shock T8Ø.59- ☑
  - shock (anaphylactic) T78.2- ☑
    - due to
      - administration of blood and blood products T8Ø.51- ☑
      - adverse effect of correct medicinal substance properly administered T88.6- ☑
      - immunization T8Ø.52- ☑
      - serum NEC T8Ø.59- ☑
      - vaccination T8Ø.52- ☑
  - specific NEC T78.49- ☑
  - tree (any) (hay fever) (pollen) J3Ø.1
    - asthma — *see* Asthma, allergic extrinsic
  - upper respiratory J3Ø.9
  - urticaria L5Ø.Ø
  - vaccine — *see* Allergy, serum
  - wheat — *see* Allergy, food
- **Allescheriasis** B48.2
- **Alligator skin disease** Q8Ø.9
- **Allocheiria, allochiria** R2Ø.8
- **Almeida's disease** — *see* Paracoccidioidomycosis
- **Alopecia** (hereditaria) (seborrheica) L65.9
  - androgenic L64.9
    - drug-induced L64.Ø
- **Alopecia** — *continued*
  - androgenic — *continued*
    - specified NEC L64.8
  - areata L63.9
    - ophiasis L63.2
    - specified NEC L63.8
    - totalis L63.Ø
    - universalis L63.1
  - cicatricial L66.9
    - central centrifugal L66.81
    - specified NEC L66.89
  - circumscripta L63.9
  - congenital, congenitalis Q84.Ø
  - due to cytotoxic drugs NEC L65.8
  - frontal fibrosing L66.12
  - mucinosa L65.2
  - postinfective NEC L65.8
  - postpartum L65.Ø
  - premature L64.8
  - specific (syphilitic) A51.32
  - specified NEC L65.8
  - syphilitic (secondary) A51.32
  - totalis (capitis) L63.Ø
  - universalis (entire body) L63.1
  - X-ray L58.1
- **Alpers' disease** G31.81
- **Alpine sickness** T7Ø.29- ☑
- **Alport syndrome** Q87.81
- **ALTE** (apparent life threatening event) **in newborn and infant** R68.13
- **Alteration** (of), **Altered**
  - awareness
    - transient R4Ø.4
    - unintended under general anesthesia, during procedure T88.53- ☑
  - mental status R41.82
  - pattern of family relationships affecting child Z62.898
  - sensation
    - following
      - cerebrovascular disease I69.998
        - cerebral infarction I69.398
        - intracerebral hemorrhage I69.198
        - nontraumatic intracranial hemorrhage NEC I69.298
        - specified disease NEC I69.898
        - subarachnoid hemorrhage I69.Ø98
- **Alternating** — *see* condition
- **Altitude, high** (effects) — *see* Effect, adverse, high altitude
- **Aluminosis** (of lung) J63.Ø
- **Alveolitis**
  - allergic (extrinsic) — *see* Pneumonitis, hypersensitivity
  - due to
    - Aspergillus clavatus J67.4
    - Cryptostroma corticale J67.6
  - fibrosing (cryptogenic) (idiopathic) J84.112
  - jaw M27.3
  - sicca dolorosa M27.3
- **Alveolus, alveolar** — *see* condition
- **Alymphocytosis** D72.81Ø
  - thymic (with immunodeficiency) D82.1
- **Alymphoplasia, thymic** D82.1
- **Alzheimer's disease or sclerosis** — *see* Disease, Alzheimer's
- **Amastia** (with nipple present) Q83.8
  - with absent nipple Q83.Ø
- **Amathophobia** F4Ø.228
- **Amaurosis** (acquired) (congenital) — *see also* Blindness
  - fugax G45.3
  - hysterical F44.6
  - Leber's congenital H35.5Ø
  - uremic — *see* Uremia
- **Amaurotic idiocy** (infantile) (juvenile) (late) E75.4
- **Amaxophobia** F4Ø.248
- **Ambiguous genitalia** Q56.4
- **Amblyopia** (congenital) (ex anopsia) (partial) (suppression) H53.ØØ- ☑
  - anisometropic — *see* Amblyopia, refractive
  - deprivation H53.Ø1- ☑
  - hysterical F44.6
  - nocturnal — *see also* Blindness, night
    - vitamin A deficiency E5Ø.5
  - refractive H53.Ø2- ☑
  - strabismic H53.Ø3- ☑
  - suspect H53.Ø4- ☑
  - tobacco H53.8
  - toxic NEC H53.8
  - uremic — *see* Uremia
- **Ameba, amebic** (histolytica) — *see also* Amebiasis
- **Ameba, amebic** — *continued*
  - abscess (liver) AØ6.4
- **Amebiasis** AØ6.9
  - with abscess — *see* Abscess, amebic
  - acute AØ6.Ø
  - chronic (intestine) AØ6.1
    - with abscess — *see* Abscess, amebic
  - cutaneous AØ6.7
  - cutis AØ6.7
  - cystitis AØ6.81
  - genitourinary tract NEC AØ6.82
  - hepatic — *see* Abscess, liver, amebic
  - intestine AØ6.Ø
  - nondysenteric colitis AØ6.2
  - skin AØ6.7
  - specified site NEC AØ6.89
- **Ameboma** (of intestine) AØ6.3
- **Amelia** Q73.Ø
  - lower limb — *see* Agenesis, leg
  - upper limb — *see* Agenesis, arm
- **Ameloblastoma** — *see also* Cyst, calcifying odontogenic
  - long bones C4Ø.9- ☑
    - lower limb C4Ø.2- ☑
    - upper limb C4Ø.Ø- ☑
  - malignant C41.1
    - jaw (bone) (lower) C41.1
      - upper C41.Ø
  - tibial C4Ø.2- ☑
- **Amelogenesis imperfecta** KØØ.5
  - nonhereditaria (segmentalis) KØØ.4
- **Amenorrhea** N91.2
  - hyperhormonal E28.8
  - primary N91.Ø
  - secondary N91.1
- **Amentia** — *see* Disability, intellectual
  - Meynert's (nonalcoholic) FØ4
- **American**
  - leishmaniasis B55.2
  - mountain tick fever A93.2
- **Ametropia** — *see* Disorder, refraction
- **AMH** (asymptomatic microscopic hematuria) R31.21
- **Amianthosis** J61
- **Amimia** R48.8
- **Amino-acid disorder** E72.9
  - anemia D53.Ø
- **Aminoacidopathy** E72.9
- **Aminoaciduria** E72.9
- **AMKD** (APOL1-mediated kidney disease) (with glomerulonephritis) (with glomerulosclerosis) NØ7.B
- **Amnesia** R41.3
  - anterograde R41.1
  - auditory R48.8
  - dissociative F44.Ø
    - with dissociative fugue F44.1
  - hysterical F44.Ø
  - postictal in epilepsy — *see* Epilepsy
  - psychogenic F44.Ø
  - retrograde R41.2
  - transient global G45.4
- **Amnes(t)ic syndrome** (post-traumatic) FØ4
  - induced by
    - alcohol F1Ø.96
      - with dependence F1Ø.26
    - psychoactive NEC F19.96
      - with
        - abuse F19.16
        - dependence F19.26
    - sedative F13.96
      - with dependence F13.26
- **Amnion, amniotic** — *see* condition
- **Amnionitis** — *see* Pregnancy, complicated by
- **Amok** F68.8
- **Amoral traits** F6Ø.89
- **Amphetamine** (or other stimulant) **-induced**
  - anxiety disorder F15.98Ø
  - bipolar and related disorder F15.94
  - delirium F15.921
  - depressive disorder F15.94
  - obsessive-compulsive and related disorder F15.988
  - psychotic disorder F15.959
  - sexual dysfunction F15.981
  - sleep disorder F15.982
  - stimulant withdrawal F15.23
- **Ampulla**
  - lower esophagus K22.89
  - phrenic K22.89
- **Amputation** — *see also* Absence, by site, acquired
  - neuroma (postoperative) (traumatic) — *see* Complications, amputation stump, neuroma

**Anemia** — *continued*
- aplastic — *continued*
  - due to — *continued*
    - radiation D61.2
  - idiopathic D61.3
  - red cell (pure) D6Ø.9
    - chronic D6Ø.Ø
    - congenital D61.Ø1
    - specified type NEC D6Ø.8
    - transient D6Ø.1
  - specified type NEC D61.89
  - toxic D61.2
- aregenerative
  - congenital D61.Ø9
- asiderotic D5Ø.9
- atypical (primary) D64.9
- Baghdad spring D55.Ø
- Balantidium coli AØ7.Ø
- Biermer's (pernicious) D51.Ø
- blood loss (chronic) D5Ø.Ø
  - acute D62
- bothriocephalus B7Ø.Ø *[D63.8]*
- brickmaker's B76.9 *[D63.8]*
- cerebral I67.89
- childhood D58.9
- chlorotic D5Ø.8
- chronic
  - blood loss D5Ø.Ø
  - hemolytic D58.9
    - idiopathic D59.9
  - simple D53.9
- chronica congenita aregenerativa D61.Ø9
- combined system disease NEC D51.Ø *[G32.Ø]*
  - due to dietary vitamin B12 deficiency D51.3 *[G32.Ø]*
- complicating pregnancy, childbirth or puerperium — *see* Pregnancy, complicated by (management affected by), anemia
- congenital P61.4
  - aplastic D61.Ø9
  - due to isoimmunization NOS P55.9
  - dyserythropoietic, dyshematopoietic D64.4
  - following fetal blood loss P61.3
  - Heinz body D58.2
  - hereditary hemolytic NOS D58.9
  - pernicious D51.Ø
  - spherocytic D58.Ø
- Cooley's (erythroblastic) D56.1
- cytogenic D51.Ø
- deficiency D53.9
  - 2, 3 diphosphoglycurate mutase D55.29
  - 2, 3 PG D55.29
  - 6-PGD D55.1
  - 6 phosphogluconate dehydrogenase D55.1
  - amino-acid D53.Ø
  - combined B12 and folate D53.1
  - enzyme D55.9
    - drug-induced (hemolytic) D59.2
    - glucose-6-phosphate dehydrogenase (G6PD) D55.Ø
    - glycolytic D55.29
    - nucleotide metabolism D55.3
    - related to hexose monophosphate (HMP) shunt pathway NEC D55.1
    - specified type NEC D55.8
  - erythrocytic glutathione D55.1
  - folate D52.9
    - dietary D52.Ø
    - drug-induced D52.1
  - folic acid D52.9
    - dietary D52.Ø
    - drug-induced D52.1
  - G SH D55.1
  - G6PD D55.Ø
  - GGS-R D55.1
  - glucose-6-phosphate dehydrogenase D55.Ø
  - glutathione reductase D55.1
  - glyceraldehyde phosphate dehydrogenase D55.29
  - hexokinase D55.29
  - iron D5Ø.9
    - secondary to blood loss (chronic) D5Ø.Ø
  - nutritional D53.9
    - with
      - poor iron absorption D5Ø.8
      - specified deficiency NEC D53.8
  - phosphofructo-aldolase D55.29
  - phosphoglycerate kinase D55.29
  - PK D55.21
  - protein D53.Ø
  - pyruvate kinase D55.21

**Anemia** — *continued*
- deficiency — *continued*
  - transcobalamin II D51.2
  - triose-phosphate isomerase D55.29
  - vitamin B12 NOS D51.9
    - dietary D51.3
    - due to
      - intrinsic factor deficiency D51.Ø
      - selective vitamin B12 malabsorption with proteinuria D51.1
    - pernicious D51.Ø
    - specified type NEC D51.8
- Diamond-Blackfan (congenital hypoplastic) D61.Ø1
- dibothriocephalus B7Ø.Ø *[D63.8]*
- dimorphic D53.1
- diphasic D53.1
- Diphyllobothrium (Dibothriocephalus) B7Ø.Ø *[D63.8]*
- due to (in) (with)
  - antineoplastic chemotherapy D64.81
  - blood loss (chronic) D5Ø.Ø
    - acute D62
  - chemotherapy, antineoplastic D64.81
  - chronic disease classified elsewhere NEC D63.8
  - chronic kidney disease D63.1
  - deficiency
    - amino-acid D53.Ø
    - copper D53.8
    - folate (folic acid) D52.9
      - dietary D52.Ø
      - drug-induced D52.1
    - molybdenum D53.8
    - protein D53.Ø
    - zinc D53.8
  - dietary vitamin B12 deficiency D51.3
  - disorder of
    - glutathione metabolism D55.1
    - nucleotide metabolism D55.3
  - drug — *see* Anemia, by type — *see also* Table of Drugs and Chemicals
  - end stage renal disease D63.1
  - enzyme disorder D55.9
  - fetal blood loss P61.3
  - fish tapeworm (D. latum) infestation B7Ø.Ø *[D63.8]*
  - hemorrhage (chronic) D5Ø.Ø
    - acute D62
  - impaired absorption D5Ø.9
  - loss of blood (chronic) D5Ø.Ø
    - acute D62
  - myxedema EØ3.9 *[D63.8]*
  - Necator americanus B76.1 *[D63.8]*
  - prematurity P61.2
  - selective vitamin B12 malabsorption with proteinuria D51.1
  - transcobalamin II deficiency D51.2
- Dyke-Young type (secondary) (symptomatic) D59.19
- dyserythropoietic (congenital) D64.4
- dyshematopoietic (congenital) D64.4
- Egyptian B76.9 *[D63.8]*
- elliptocytosis — *see* Elliptocytosis
- enzyme-deficiency, drug-induced D59.2
- epidemic — *see also* Ancylostomiasis B76.9 *[D63.8]*
- erythroblastic
  - familial D56.1
  - newborn — *see also* Disease, hemolytic P55.9
  - of childhood D56.1
- erythrocytic glutathione deficiency D55.1
- erythropoietin-resistant anemia (EPO resistant anemia) D63.1
- Faber's (achlorhydric anemia) D5Ø.9
- factitious (self-induced blood letting) D5Ø.Ø
- familial erythroblastic D56.1
- Fanconi ('s) D61.Ø3
- favism D55.Ø
- fish tapeworm (D. latum) infestation B7Ø.Ø *[D63.8]*
- folate (folic acid) deficiency D52.9
- glucose-6-phosphate dehydrogenase (G6PD) deficiency D55.Ø
- glutathione-reductase deficiency D55.1
- goat's milk D52.Ø
- granulocytic — *see* Agranulocytosis
- Heinz body, congenital D58.2
- hemolytic D58.9
  - acquired D59.9
    - with hemoglobinuria NEC D59.6
    - autoimmune NEC D59.19
    - infectious D59.4
    - specified type NEC D59.8
    - toxic D59.4
  - acute D59.9

**Anemia** — *continued*
- hemolytic — *continued*
  - acute — *continued*
    - due to enzyme deficiency specified type NEC D55.8
    - Lederer's D59.19
  - autoimmune D59.1Ø
    - cold D59.12
    - drug-induced D59.Ø
    - mixed D59.13
    - warm D59.11
  - chronic D58.9
    - idiopathic D59.9
  - cold type (primary) (secondary) (symptomatic) D59.12
  - congenital (spherocytic) — *see* Spherocytosis
  - due to
    - cardiac conditions D59.4
    - drugs (nonautoimmune) D59.2
      - autoimmune D59.Ø
    - enzyme disorder D55.9
      - drug-induced D59.2
    - presence of shunt or other internal prosthetic device D59.4
  - familial D58.9
  - hereditary D58.9
    - due to enzyme disorder D55.9
      - specified type NEC D55.8
    - specified type NEC D58.8
  - idiopathic (chronic) D59.9
  - mechanical D59.4
  - microangiopathic D59.4
  - mixed type (primary) (secondary) (symptomatic) D59.13
  - nonautoimmune D59.4
    - drug-induced D59.2
  - nonspherocytic
    - congenital or hereditary NEC D55.8
      - glucose-6-phosphate dehydrogenase deficiency D55.Ø
      - pyruvate kinase deficiency D55.21
      - type
        - I D55.1
        - II D55.29
    - type
      - I D55.1
      - II D55.29
  - primary
    - autoimmune
      - cold type D59.12
      - mixed type D59.13
      - warm type D59.11
  - secondary D59.4
    - autoimmune
      - cold type D59.12
      - mixed type D59.13
      - warm type D59.11
  - specified (hereditary) type NEC D58.8
  - Stransky-Regala type — *see also* Hemoglobinopathy D58.8
  - symptomatic D59.4
    - autoimmune
      - cold type D59.12
      - mixed type D59.13
      - warm type D59.11
  - toxic D59.4
  - warm type (primary) (secondary) (symptomatic) D59.11
- hemorrhagic (chronic) D5Ø.Ø
  - acute D62
- Herrick's D57.1
- hexokinase deficiency D55.29
- hookworm B76.9 *[D63.8]*
- hypochromic (idiopathic) (microcytic) (normoblastic) D5Ø.9
  - due to blood loss (chronic) D5Ø.Ø
    - acute D62
  - familial sex-linked D64.Ø
  - pyridoxine-responsive D64.3
  - sideroblastic, sex-linked D64.Ø
- hypoplasia, red blood cells D61.9
  - congenital or familial D61.Ø1
- hypoplastic (idiopathic) D61.9
  - congenital or familial (of childhood) D61.Ø1
- hypoproliferative (refractive) D61.9
- idiopathic D64.9
  - aplastic D61.3
  - hemolytic, chronic D59.9
- in (due to) (with)
  - chronic kidney disease D63.1
  - end stage renal disease D63.1

- **Anemia** — *continued*
  - in — *continued*
    - failure, kidney (renal) D63.1
    - neoplastic disease — *see also* Neoplasm D63.0
  - intertropical — *see also* Ancylostomiasis D63.8
  - iron deficiency D50.9
    - secondary to blood loss (chronic) D50.0
      - acute D62
    - specified type NEC D50.8
  - Joseph-Diamond-Blackfan (congenital hypoplastic) D61.01
  - Lederer's (hemolytic) D59.19
  - leukoerythroblastic D61.82
  - macrocytic D53.9
    - nutritional D52.0
    - tropical D52.8
  - malarial — *see also* Malaria B54 *[D63.8]*
  - malignant (progressive) D51.0
  - malnutrition D53.9
  - marsh — *see also* Malaria B54 *[D63.8]*
  - Mediterranean (with other hemoglobinopathy) D56.9
  - megaloblastic D53.1
    - combined B12 and folate deficiency D53.1
    - hereditary D51.1
    - nutritional D52.0
    - orotic aciduria D53.0
    - refractory D53.1
    - specified type NEC D53.1
  - megalocytic D53.1
  - microcytic (hypochromic) D50.9
    - due to blood loss (chronic) D50.0
      - acute D62
    - familial D56.8
  - microdrepanocytosis D57.40
  - microelliptopoikilocytic (Rietti-Greppi- Micheli) D56.9
  - miner's B76.9 *[D63.8]*
  - myelodysplastic D46.9
  - myelofibrosis D75.81
  - myelogenous D64.89
  - myelopathic D64.89
  - myelophthisic D61.82
  - myeloproliferative D47.Z9 (*following* D47.4)
  - newborn P61.4
    - due to
      - ABO (antibodies, isoimmunization, maternal/fetal incompatibility) P55.1
      - Rh (antibodies, isoimmunization, maternal/fetal incompatibility) P55.0
    - following fetal blood loss P61.3
    - posthemorrhagic (fetal) P61.3
  - nonspherocytic hemolytic — *see* Anemia, hemolytic, nonspherocytic
  - normocytic (infectional) D64.9
    - due to blood loss (chronic) D50.0
      - acute D62
    - myelophthisic D61.82
  - nutritional (deficiency) D53.9
    - with
      - poor iron absorption D50.8
      - specified deficiency NEC D53.8
    - megaloblastic D52.0
  - of prematurity P61.2
  - orotaciduric (congenital) (hereditary) D53.0
  - osteosclerotic D64.89
  - ovalocytosis (hereditary) — *see* Elliptocytosis
  - paludal — *see also* Malaria B54 *[D63.8]*
  - pernicious (congenital) (malignant) (progressive) D51.0
  - pleochromic D64.89
    - of sprue D52.8
  - posthemorrhagic (chronic) D50.0
    - acute D62
    - newborn P61.3
  - postoperative (postprocedural)
    - due to (acute) blood loss D62
      - chronic blood loss D50.0
    - specified NEC D64.89
  - postpartum O90.81
  - pressure D64.89
  - progressive D64.9
    - malignant D51.0
    - pernicious D51.0
  - protein-deficiency D53.0
  - pseudoleukemica infantum D64.89
  - pure red cell D60.9
    - congenital D61.01
  - pyridoxine-responsive D64.3
  - pyruvate kinase deficiency D55.21
  - refractory D46.4

- **Anemia** — *continued*
  - refractory — *continued*
    - with
      - excess of blasts D46.20
        - 1 (RAEB 1) D46.21
        - 2 (RAEB 2) D46.22
        - in transformation (RAEB T) — *see* Leukemia, acute myeloblastic
      - hemochromatosis D46.1
      - sideroblasts (ring) (RARS) D46.1
    - megaloblastic D53.1
    - sideroblastic D46.1
    - sideropenic D50.9
    - without ring sideroblasts, so stated D46.0
    - without sideroblasts without excess of blasts D46.0
  - Rietti-Greppi-Micheli D56.9
  - scorbutic D53.2
  - secondary to
    - blood loss (chronic) D50.0
      - acute D62
    - hemorrhage (chronic) D50.0
      - acute D62
  - semiplastic D61.89
  - sickle-cell — *see* Disease, sickle-cell
  - sideroblastic D64.3
    - hereditary D64.0
    - hypochromic, sex-linked D64.0
    - pyridoxine-responsive NEC D64.3
    - refractory D46.1
    - secondary (due to)
      - disease D64.1
      - drugs and toxins D64.2
    - specified type NEC D64.3
  - sideropenic (refractory) D50.9
    - due to blood loss (chronic) D50.0
      - acute D62
  - simple chronic D53.9
  - specified type NEC D64.89
  - spherocytic (hereditary) — *see* Spherocytosis
  - splenic D64.89
  - splenomegalic D64.89
  - stomatocytosis D58.8
  - syphilitic (acquired) (late) A52.79 *[D63.8]*
  - target cell D64.89
  - thalassemia D56.9
  - thrombocytopenic — *see* Thrombocytopenia
  - toxic D61.2
  - tropical B76.9 *[D63.8]*
    - macrocytic D52.8
  - tuberculous A18.89 *[D63.8]*
  - vegan D51.3
  - vitamin
    - B6-responsive D64.3
    - B12 deficiency (dietary) pernicious D51.0
  - von Jaksch's D64.89
  - Witts' (achlorhydric anemia) D50.8
- **Anemophobia** F40.228
- **Anencephalus, anencephaly** Q00.0
- **Anergasia** — *see* Psychosis, organic
- **Anesthesia, anesthetic** R20.0
  - complication or reaction NEC — *see also* Complications, anesthesia T88.59- ☑
    - due to
      - correct substance properly administered — *see* Table of Drugs and Chemicals, by drug, adverse effect
      - overdose or wrong substance given — *see* Table of Drugs and Chemicals, by drug, poisoning
    - unintended awareness under general anesthesia during procedure T88.53- ☑
      - personal history of Z92.84
  - cornea H18.81- ☑
  - dissociative F44.6
  - functional (hysterical) F44.6
  - hyperesthetic, thalamic G89.0
  - hysterical F44.6
  - local skin lesion R20.0
  - sexual (psychogenic) F52.1
  - shock (due to) T88.2- ☑
  - skin R20.0
  - testicular N50.9
- **Anetoderma** (maculosum) (of) L90.8
  - Jadassohn-Pellizzari L90.2
  - Schweninger-Buzzi L90.1
- **Aneurin deficiency** E51.9
- **Aneurysm** (anastomotic) (artery) (cirsoid) (diffuse) (false) (fusiform) (multiple) (saccular) I72.9
  - abdominal (aorta) I71.40
    - infrarenal I71.43

- **Aneurysm** — *continued*
  - abdominal — *continued*
    - infrarenal — *continued*
      - ruptured I71.33
    - juxtarenal I71.42
      - ruptured I71.32
    - pararenal I71.41
      - ruptured I71.31
    - ruptured I71.30
    - syphilitic A52.01
  - aorta, aortic (nonsyphilitic) I71.9
    - abdominal I71.40
      - dissecting — *see* Dissection, aorta, abdominal
      - ruptured I71.30
    - arch I71.22
      - ruptured I71.12
    - arteriosclerotic I71.9
      - ruptured I71.8
    - ascending I71.21
      - ruptured I71.11
    - congenital Q25.43
    - descending I71.9
      - abdominal I71.40
        - ruptured I71.30
      - ruptured I71.8
      - thoracic I71.23
        - ruptured I71.13
    - dissecting — *see* Dissection, aorta
    - root Q25.43
    - ruptured I71.8
    - sinus, congenital Q25.43
    - syphilitic A52.01
    - thoracic I71.20
      - ruptured I71.10
    - thoracoabdominal I71.60
      - paravisceral I71.62
        - ruptured I71.52
      - ruptured I71.50
      - supraceliac I71.61
        - ruptured I71.51
    - thorax, thoracic I71.20
      - arch I71.22
        - ruptured I71.12
      - ascending I71.21
        - ruptured I71.11
      - descending I71.23
        - ruptured I71.13
      - ruptured I71.10
        - arch I71.12
        - ascending I71.11
        - descending I71.13
    - transverse I71.22
      - ruptured I71.12
    - valve (heart) — *see also* Endocarditis, aortic I35.8
  - arteriosclerotic I72.9
    - cerebral I67.1
      - ruptured — *see* Hemorrhage, intracranial, subarachnoid
  - arteriovenous (congenital) — *see also* Malformation, arteriovenous
    - acquired I77.0
      - brain I67.1
        - ruptured — *see* Aneurysm, arteriovenous, brain, ruptured
      - coronary I25.41
      - pulmonary I28.0
    - brain Q28.2
      - ruptured I60.8
        - intracerebral I61.8
        - intraparenchymal I61.8
        - intraventricular I61.5
        - subarachnoid I60.8
    - peripheral — *see* Malformation, arteriovenous, peripheral
    - precerebral vessels Q28.0
    - specified site NEC — *see also* Malformation, arteriovenous
      - acquired I77.0
  - basal — *see* Aneurysm, brain
  - basilar (trunk) I72.5
  - berry (congenital) (nonruptured) I67.1
    - ruptured I60.7
  - brain I67.1
    - arteriosclerotic I67.1
      - ruptured — *see* Hemorrhage, intracranial, subarachnoid
    - arteriovenous (congenital) (nonruptured) Q28.2
      - acquired I67.1

Index

Anomaly, anomalous — Anomaly, anomalous

**Anomaly, anomalous** — *continued*
- vena cava (inferior) (superior) Q26.9
- venous — *see* Anomaly, vein(s)
- venous return Q26.8
- ventricular
  - bands or folds Q24.8
  - septa Q21.0
- vertebra Q76.49
  - kyphosis — *see* Kyphosis, congenital
  - lordosis — *see* Lordosis, congenital
- vesicourethral orifice Q64.79
- vessel(s) Q27.9
  - optic papilla Q14.2
  - precerebral Q28.1
- vitelline duct Q43.0
- vitreous body or humor Q14.0
- vulva Q52.70
- wrist (joint) Q74.0

**Anomia** R48.8

**Anonychia** (congenital) Q84.3
- acquired L60.8

**Anophthalmos, anophthalmus** (congenital) (globe) Q11.1
- acquired Z90.01

**Anopia, anopsia** H53.46- ☑
- quadrant H53.46- ☑

**Anorchia, anorchism, anorchidism** Q55.0

**Anorexia** R63.0
- hysterical F44.89
- nervosa F50.00
  - atypical F50.9
  - binge-eating type F50.2- ☑
    - with purging F50.02- ☑
  - restricting type F50.01- ☑

**Anorgasmy, psychogenic** (female) F52.31
- male F52.32

**Anosmia** R43.0
- hysterical F44.6
- postinfectional J39.8

**Anosognosia** R41.85

**Anosteoplasia** Q78.9

**Anovulatory cycle** N97.0

**Anoxemia** R09.02
- newborn P84

**Anoxia** (pathological) R09.02
- altitude T70.29- ☑
- cerebral G93.1
  - complicating
    - anesthesia (general) (local) or other sedation T88.59- ☑
      - in labor and delivery O74.3
      - in pregnancy O29.21- ☑
      - postpartum, puerperal O89.2
    - delivery (cesarean) (instrumental) O75.4
  - during a procedure G97.81
  - newborn P84
  - resulting from a procedure G97.82
- due to
  - drowning T75.1- ☑
  - high altitude T70.29- ☑
- heart — *see* Insufficiency, coronary
- intrauterine P84
- myocardial — *see* Insufficiency, coronary
- newborn P84
- spinal cord G95.11
- systemic (by suffocation) (low content in atmosphere) — *see* Asphyxia, traumatic

**Anteflexion** — *see* Anteversion

**Antenatal**
- care (normal pregnancy) Z34.90
- screening (encounter for) of mother — *see also* Encounter, antenatal screening Z36.9

**Antepartum** — *see* condition

**Anterior** — *see* condition

**Antero-occlusion** M26.220

**Anteversion**
- cervix — *see* Anteversion, uterus
- femur (neck), congenital Q65.89
- uterus, uterine (cervix) (postinfectional) (postpartal, old) N85.4
  - congenital Q51.818
  - in pregnancy or childbirth — *see* Pregnancy, complicated by

**Anthophobia** F40.228

**Anthracosilicosis** J60

**Anthracosis** (lung) (occupational) J60
- lingua K14.3

**Anthrax** A22.9
- with pneumonia A22.1

**Anthrax** — *continued*
- cerebral A22.8
- colitis A22.2
- cutaneous A22.0
- gastrointestinal A22.2
- inhalation A22.1
- intestinal A22.2
- meningitis A22.8
- pulmonary A22.1
- respiratory A22.1
- sepsis A22.7
- specified manifestation NEC A22.8

**Anthropoid pelvis** Q74.2
- with disproportion (fetopelvic) O33.0

**Anthropophobia** F40.10
- generalized F40.11

**Antibodies, maternal** (blood group) — *see* Isoimmunization, affecting management of pregnancy
- anti-D — *see* Isoimmunization, affecting management of pregnancy, Rh
  - newborn P55.0

**Antibody**
- anticardiolipin R76.0
  - with
    - hemorrhagic disorder D68.312
    - hypercoagulable state D68.61
- antiphosphatidylglycerol R76.0
  - with
    - hemorrhagic disorder D68.312
    - hypercoagulable state D68.61
- antiphosphatidylinositol R76.0
  - with
    - hemorrhagic disorder D68.312
    - hypercoagulable state D68.61
- antiphosphatidylserine R76.0
  - with
    - hemorrhagic disorder D68.312
    - hypercoagulable state D68.61
- antiphospholipid R76.0
  - with
    - hemorrhagic disorder D68.312
    - hypercoagulable state D68.61

**Anticardiolipin syndrome** D68.61

**Anticoagulant, circulating** (intrinsic) — *see also* Disorder, hemorrhagic D68.318
- drug-induced (extrinsic) — *see also* Disorder, hemorrhagic D68.32
- iatrogenic D68.32

**Antidiuretic hormone syndrome** E22.2

**Antimonial cholera** — *see* Poisoning, antimony

**Antiphospholipid**
- antibody
  - with hemorrhagic disorder D68.312
  - syndrome D68.61

**Antisocial personality** F60.2

**Antithrombinemia** — *see* Circulating anticoagulants

**Antithromboplastinemia** D68.318

**Antithromboplastinogenemia** D68.318

**Antitoxin complication or reaction** — *see* Complications, vaccination

**Antlophobia** F40.228

**Antritis** J32.0
- maxilla J32.0
  - acute J01.00
    - recurrent J01.01
- stomach K29.50
  - with bleeding K29.51

**Antrum, antral** — *see* condition

**Anuria** R34
- calculous (impacted) (recurrent) — *see also* Calculus, urinary N20.9
- following
  - abortion — *see* Abortion by type complicated by, renal failure
  - ectopic or molar pregnancy O08.4
- newborn P96.0
- postprocedural N99.0
- postrenal N13.8
- puerperal O90.49
- traumatic (following crushing) T79.5- ☑

**Anus, anal** — *see* condition

**Anusitis** K62.89

**Anxiety** F41.9
- depression F41.8
- episodic paroxysmal F41.0
- generalized F41.1
- hysteria F41.8
- neurosis F41.1
- panic type F41.0

**Anxiety** — *continued*
- reaction F41.1
- separation, abnormal (of childhood) F93.0
- specified NEC F41.8
- state F41.1

**Aorta, aortic** — *see* condition

**Aortectasia** — *see* Ectasia, aorta
- with aneurysm — *see* Aneurysm, aorta

**Aortitis** (nonsyphilitic) (calcific) I77.6
- arteriosclerotic I70.0
- Doehle-Heller A52.02
- luetic A52.02
- rheumatic — *see* Endocarditis, acute, rheumatic
- specific (syphilitic) A52.02
- syphilitic A52.02
  - congenital A50.54 *[I79.1]*

**Apathetic thyroid storm** — *see* Thyrotoxicosis

**Apathy** R45.3

**Apeirophobia** F40.228

**Apepsia** K30
- psychogenic F45.8

**Aperistalsis, esophagus** K22.0

**Apertognathia** M26.29

**Apert's syndrome** Q87.0

**Aphagia** R13.0
- psychogenic F50.9

**Aphakia** (acquired) (postoperative) H27.0- ☑
- congenital Q12.3

**Aphasia** (amnestic) (global) (nominal) (semantic) (syntactic) R47.01
- acquired, with epilepsy (Landau-Kleffner syndrome) — *see* Epilepsy, specified NEC
- auditory (developmental) F80.2
- developmental (receptive type) F80.2
  - expressive type F80.1
  - Wernicke's F80.2
- following
  - cerebrovascular disease I69.920
    - cerebral infarction I69.320
    - intracerebral hemorrhage I69.120
    - nontraumatic intracranial hemorrhage NEC I69.220
    - specified disease NEC I69.820
    - subarachnoid hemorrhage I69.020
- primary progressive — *see also* Dementia, in, diseases specified elsewhere G31.01 *[F02.80]*
  - with behavioral disturbance — *see also* Dementia, in, diseases specified elsewhere G31.01 *[F02.81-]* ☑
- progressive isolated — *see also* Dementia, in, diseases specified elsewhere G31.01 *[F02.80]*
  - with behavioral disturbance — *see also* Dementia, in, diseases specified elsewhere G31.01 *[F02.81-]* ☑
- sensory F80.2
- syphilis, tertiary A52.19
- Wernicke's (developmental) F80.2

**Aphonia** (organic) R49.1
- hysterical F44.4
- psychogenic F44.4

**Aphthae, aphthous** — *see also* condition
- Bednar's K12.0
- cachectic K14.0
- epizootic B08.8
- fever B08.8
- oral (recurrent) K12.0
- stomatitis (major) (minor) K12.0
- thrush B37.0
- ulcer (oral) (recurrent) K12.0
  - genital organ(s) NEC
    - female N76.6
    - male N50.89
  - larynx J38.7

**Apical** — *see* condition

**Apiphobia** F40.218

**APL** (acquired partial lipodystrophy) E88.11

**Aplasia** — *see also* Agenesis
- abdominal muscle syndrome Q79.4
- alveolar process (acquired) — *see* Anomaly, alveolar
  - congenital Q38.6
- aorta (congenital) Q25.41
- axialis extracorticalis (congenita) E75.29
- bone marrow (myeloid) D61.9
  - congenital D61.01
- brain Q00.0
  - part of Q04.3
- bronchus Q32.4
- cementum K00.4
- cerebellum Q04.3
- cervix (congenital) Q51.5

**Aplasia** — *continued*
- congenital pure red cell D61.Ø1
- corpus callosum QØ4.Ø
- cutis congenita Q84.8
- erythrocyte congenital D61.Ø1
- extracortical axial E75.29
- eye Q11.1
- fovea centralis (congenital) Q14.1
- gallbladder, congenital Q44.Ø
- iris Q13.1
- labyrinth, membranous Q16.5
- limb (congenital) Q73.8
  - lower — *see* Defect, reduction, lower limb
  - upper — *see* Agenesis, arm
- lung, congenital (bilateral) (unilateral) Q33.3
- pancreas Q45.Ø
- parathyroid-thymic D82.1
- Pelizaeus-Merzbacher E75.27
- penis Q55.5
- prostate Q55.4
- red cell (with thymoma) D6Ø.9
  - acquired D6Ø.9
    - due to drugs D6Ø.9
  - adult D6Ø.9
  - chronic D6Ø.Ø
  - congenital D61.Ø1
  - constitutional D61.Ø1
  - due to drugs D6Ø.9
  - hereditary D61.Ø1
  - of infants D61.Ø1
  - primary D61.Ø1
  - pure D61.Ø1
    - due to drugs D6Ø.9
  - specified type NEC D6Ø.8
  - transient D6Ø.1
- round ligament Q52.8
- skin Q84.8
- spermatic cord Q55.4
- spleen Q89.Ø1
- testicle Q55.Ø
- thymic, with immunodeficiency D82.1
- thyroid (congenital) (with myxedema) EØ3.1
- uterus Q51.Ø
- ventral horn cell QØ6.1

**Apnea, apneic** (of) (spells) RØ6.81
- newborn P28.4Ø
  - central P28.41
  - mixed P28.43
  - obstructive P28.42
  - sleep
    - primary P28.3Ø
      - central P28.31
      - mixed P28.33
      - obstructive P28.32
      - specified NEC P28.39
  - specified NEC P28.49
- prematurity P28.49
- sleep G47.3Ø
  - central (primary) G47.31
    - idiopathic G47.31
    - in conditions classified elsewhere G47.37
  - obstructive (adult) (pediatric) G47.33
    - hypopnea G47.33
  - primary central G47.31
  - specified NEC G47.39

**Apneumatosis, newborn** P28.Ø

**Apocrine metaplasia** (breast) — *see* Dysplasia, mammary, specified type NEC

**Apophysitis** (bone) — *see also* Osteochondropathy
- calcaneus M92.6- ☑
- juvenile M92.9

**Apoplectiform convulsions** (cerebral ischemia) I67.82

**Apoplexia, apoplexy, apoplectic**
- adrenal A39.1
- heart (auricle) (ventricle) — *see* Infarct, myocardium
- heat T67.Ø1- ☑
- hemorrhagic (stroke) — *see* Hemorrhage, intracranial
- meninges, hemorrhagic — *see* Hemorrhage, intracranial, subarachnoid
- uremic N18.9 *[I68.8]*

**Appearance**
- bizarre R46.1
- specified NEC R46.89
- very low level of personal hygiene R46.Ø

**Appendage**
- epididymal (organ of Morgagni) Q55.4
- intestine (epiploic) Q43.8
- preauricular Q17.Ø
- testicular (organ of Morgagni) Q55.29

**Appendicitis** (pneumococcal) (retrocecal) K37
- with
  - gangrene K35.891
    - with localized peritonitis K35.31
  - perforation NOS K35.32
  - peritoneal abscess K35.33
  - peritonitis NEC K35.33
    - generalized K35.2Ø9
      - with
        - abscess K35.219
          - with perforation or rupture K35.211
          - following rupture or perforation of appendix NOS K35.211
          - without perforation or rupture K35.21Ø
        - perforation or rupture K35.2Ø1
      - following rupture or perforation of appendix NOS K35.2Ø1
      - without rupture or perforation of appendix K35.2ØØ
    - localized K35.3Ø
      - with
        - gangrene K35.31
        - perforation K35.32
          - and abscess K35.33
    - rupture (with localized peritonitis) K35.32
- acute (catarrhal) (fulminating) (obstructive) (retrocecal) (suppurative) K35.8Ø
  - with
    - gangrene K35.891
    - peritoneal abscess K35.33
    - peritonitis NEC K35.33
      - generalized K35.2Ø9
        - with
          - abscess K35.219
            - with perforation or rupture K35.211
            - following rupture or perforation of appendix NOS K35.211
            - without perforation or rupture K35.21Ø
          - perforation or rupture K35.2Ø1
        - following rupture or perforation of appendix NOS K35.2Ø1
        - without rupture or perforation of appendix K35.2ØØ
      - localized K35.3Ø
        - with
          - gangrene K35.31
          - perforation K35.32
            - and abscess K35.33
  - specified NEC K35.89Ø
    - with gangrene K35.891
      - with localized peritonitis K35.31
- amebic AØ6.89
- chronic (recurrent) K36
- exacerbation — *see* Appendicitis, with, gangrene
- gangrenous — *see* Appendicitis, acute
- healed (obliterative) K36
- interval K36
- neurogenic K36
- obstructive K36
- recurrent K36
- relapsing K36
- ruptured NOS (with localized peritonitis) K35.32
- subacute (adhesive) K36
- subsiding K36
- suppurative — *see* Appendicitis, acute
- tuberculous A18.32

**Appendicopathia oxyurica** B8Ø

**Appendix, appendicular** — *see also* condition
- epididymis Q55.4
- Morgagni
  - female Q5Ø.5
  - male (epididymal) Q55.4
    - testicular Q55.29
- testis Q55.29

**Appetite**
- depraved — *see* Pica
- excessive R63.2
- lack or loss — *see also* Anorexia R63.Ø
  - nonorganic origin F5Ø.89
  - psychogenic F5Ø.89
- perverted (hysterical) — *see* Pica

**Apple peel syndrome** Q41.1

**Apprehension state** F41.1

**Apprehensiveness, abnormal** F41.9

**Approximal wear** KØ3.Ø

**Apraxia** (classic) (ideational) (ideokinetic) (ideomotor) (motor) (verbal) R48.2

**Apraxia** — *continued*
- following
  - cerebrovascular disease I69.99Ø
    - cerebral infarction I69.39Ø
    - intracerebral hemorrhage I69.19Ø
    - nontraumatic intracranial hemorrhage NEC I69.29Ø
    - specified disease NEC I69.89Ø
    - subarachnoid hemorrhage I69.Ø9Ø
- oculomotor, congenital H51.8
- primary progressive, of speech G31.87

**Aptyalism** K11.7

**Apudoma** — *see* Neoplasm, uncertain behavior, by site

**Aqueous misdirection** H4Ø.83- ☑

**Arabicum elephantiasis** — *see* Infestation, filarial

**Arachnitis** — *see* Meningitis

**Arachnodactyly** — *see* Syndrome, Marfan

**Arachnoiditis** (acute) (adhesive) (basal) (brain) (cerebrospinal) — *see* Meningitis

**Arachnophobia** F4Ø.21Ø

**Arboencephalitis, Australian** A83.4

**Arborization block** (heart) I45.5

**ARC** (AIDS-related complex) B2Ø

**Arc-welder's lung** J63.4

**Arch**
- aortic Q25.49
- bovine Q25.49

**Arches** — *see* condition

**Arcuate uterus** Q51.81Ø

**Arcuatus uterus** Q51.81Ø

**Arcus** (cornea) senilis — *see* Degeneration, cornea, senile

**Areflexia** R29.2

**Areola** — *see* condition

**Argentaffinoma** — *see also* Neoplasm, uncertain behavior, by site
- malignant — *see* Neoplasm, malignant, by site
- syndrome E34.Ø9

**Argininemia** E72.21

**Arginosuccinic aciduria** E72.22

**Argyll Robertson phenomenon, pupil or syndrome** (syphilitic) A52.19
- atypical H57.Ø9
- nonsyphilitic H57.Ø9

**Argyria, argyriasis**
- conjunctival H11.13- ☑
- from drug or medicament — *see* Table of Drugs and Chemicals, by substance

**Argyrosis, conjunctival** H11.13- ☑

**Arhinencephaly** QØ4.1

**Ariboflavinosis** E53.Ø

**Arm** — *see* condition

**Arnold-Chiari disease, obstruction or syndrome** (type II) QØ7.ØØ
- with
  - hydrocephalus QØ7.Ø2
    - with spina bifida QØ7.Ø3
  - spina bifida QØ7.Ø1
    - with hydrocephalus QØ7.Ø3
- type III — *see* Encephalocele
- type IV QØ4.8

**Aromatic amino-acid metabolism disorder** E7Ø.9
- specified NEC E7Ø.89

**Arousals, confusional** G47.51

**Arrest, arrested**
- cardiac I46.9
  - complicating
    - abortion — *see* Abortion, by type, complicated by, cardiac arrest
    - anesthesia (general) (local) or other sedation — *see* Table of Drugs and Chemicals, by drug
      - in labor and delivery O74.2
      - in pregnancy O29.11- ☑
      - postpartum, puerperal O89.1
    - delivery (cesarean) (instrumental) O75.4
  - due to
    - cardiac condition I46.2
    - specified condition NEC I46.8
  - intraoperative I97.71- ☑
  - newborn P29.81
  - personal history, successfully resuscitated Z86.74
  - postprocedural I97.12- ☑
    - obstetric procedure O75.4
- cardiorespiratory — *see* Arrest, cardiac
- circulatory — *see* Arrest, cardiac
- deep transverse O64.Ø- ☑
- development or growth
  - bone — *see* Disorder, bone, development or growth
  - child R62.5Ø
  - tracheal rings Q32.1

- **Arrest, arrested** — *continued*
  - epiphyseal
    - complete
      - femur M89.15- ☑
      - humerus M89.12- ☑
      - tibia M89.16- ☑
      - ulna M89.13- ☑
    - forearm M89.13- ☑
      - specified NEC M89.13- ☑
      - ulna — *see* Arrest, epiphyseal, by type, ulna
    - lower leg M89.16- ☑
      - specified NEC M89.168
      - tibia — *see* Arrest, epiphyseal, by type, tibia
    - partial
      - femur M89.15- ☑
      - humerus M89.12- ☑
      - tibia M89.16- ☑
      - ulna M89.13- ☑
    - specified NEC M89.18
  - granulopoiesis — *see* Agranulocytosis
  - growth plate — *see* Arrest, epiphyseal
  - heart — *see* Arrest, cardiac
  - legal, anxiety concerning Z65.3
  - physeal — *see* Arrest, epiphyseal
  - respiratory RØ9.2
    - newborn P28.81
  - sinus I45.5
  - spermatogenesis (complete) — *see* Azoospermia
    - incomplete — *see* Oligospermia
  - transverse (deep) O64.Ø- ☑
- **Arrhenoblastoma**
  - benign
    - specified site — *see* Neoplasm, benign, by site
    - unspecified site
      - female D27.9
      - male D29.2Ø
  - malignant
    - specified site — *see* Neoplasm, malignant, by site
    - unspecified site
      - female C56.9
      - male C62.9Ø
  - specified site — *see* Neoplasm, uncertain behavior, by site
  - unspecified site
    - female D39.1Ø
    - male D4Ø.1Ø
- **Arrhythmia** (auricle) (cardiac) (juvenile) (nodal) (reflex) (supraventricular) (transitory) (ventricle) I49.9
  - block I45.9
  - extrasystolic I49.49
  - newborn
    - bradycardia P29.12
    - occurring before birth PØ3.819
      - before onset of labor PØ3.81Ø
      - during labor PØ3.811
    - tachycardia P29.11
  - psychogenic F45.8
  - sinus I49.89
  - specified NEC I49.89
  - vagal R55
  - ventricular re-entry I47.Ø
- **Arrillaga-Ayerza syndrome** (pulmonary sclerosis with pulmonary hypertension) I27.Ø
- **Arsenical pigmentation** L81.8
  - from drug or medicament — *see* Table of Drugs and Chemicals
- **Arsenism** — *see* Poisoning, arsenic
- **Arterial** — *see* condition
- **Arteriofibrosis** — *see* Arteriosclerosis
- **Arteriolar sclerosis** — *see* Arteriosclerosis
- **Arteriolith** — *see* Arteriosclerosis
- **Arteriolitis** I77.6
  - necrotizing, kidney I77.5
  - renal — *see* Hypertension, kidney
- **Arteriolosclerosis** — *see* Arteriosclerosis
- **Arterionephrosclerosis** — *see* Hypertension, kidney
- **Arteriopathy** I77.9
  - cerebral autosomal dominant, with subcortical infarcts and leukoencephalopathy (CADASIL) I67.85Ø
- **Arteriosclerosis, arteriosclerotic** (diffuse) (obliterans) (of) (senile) (with calcification) I7Ø.9Ø
  - with
    - chronic limb-threatening ischemia — *see* Arteriosclerosis, with critical limb ischemia
    - critical limb ischemia
      - bypass graft I7Ø.329
        - autologous vein graft I7Ø.429
          - leg I7Ø.429

- **Arteriosclerosis, arteriosclerotic** — *continued*
  - with — *continued*
    - critical limb ischemia — *continued*
      - bypass graft — *continued*
        - autologous vein graft — *continued*
          - leg — *continued*
            - with
              - gangrene (and intermittent claudication, rest pain, and ulcer) I7Ø.469
              - rest pain (and intermittent claudication) I7Ø.429
            - bilateral I7Ø.423
              - with
                - gangrene (and intermittent claudication, rest pain, and ulcer) I7Ø.463
                - rest pain (and intermittent claudication) I7Ø.423
            - left I7Ø.422
              - with
                - gangrene (and intermittent claudication, rest pain, and ulcer) I7Ø.462
                - rest pain (and intermittent claudication) I7Ø.422
                - ulceration (and intermittent claudication and rest pain) I7Ø.449
                  - ankle I7Ø.443
                  - calf I7Ø.442
                  - foot site NEC I7Ø.445
                  - heel I7Ø.444
                  - lower leg NEC I7Ø.448
                  - mid foot I7Ø.444
                  - thigh I7Ø.441
            - right I7Ø.421
              - with
                - gangrene (and intermittent claudication, rest pain, and ulcer) I7Ø.461
                - rest pain (and intermittent claudication) I7Ø.421
                - ulceration (and intermittent claudication and rest pain) I7Ø.439
                  - ankle I7Ø.433
                  - calf I7Ø.432
                  - foot site NEC I7Ø.435
                  - heel I7Ø.434
                  - lower leg NEC I7Ø.438
                  - midfoot I7Ø.434
                  - thigh I7Ø.431
        - leg I7Ø.329
          - with
            - gangrene (and intermittent claudication, rest pain, and ulcer) I7Ø.369
            - rest pain (and intermittent claudication) I7Ø.329
          - bilateral I7Ø.323
            - with
              - gangrene (and intermittent claudication, rest pain, and ulcer) I7Ø.363
              - rest pain (and intermittent claudication) I7Ø.323
          - left I7Ø.322
            - with
              - gangrene (and intermittent claudication, rest pain, and ulcer) I7Ø.362
              - rest pain (and intermittent claudication) I7Ø.322
              - ulceration (and intermittent claudication and rest pain) I7Ø.349
                - ankle I7Ø.343
                - calf I7Ø.342
                - foot site NEC I7Ø.345
                - heel I7Ø.344
                - lower leg NEC I7Ø.348
                - midfoot I7Ø.344
                - thigh I7Ø.341
          - right I7Ø.321
            - with
              - gangrene (and intermittent claudication, rest pain, and ulcer) I7Ø.361
              - rest pain (and intermittent claudication) I7Ø.321

- **Arteriosclerosis, arteriosclerotic** — *continued*
  - with — *continued*
    - critical limb ischemia — *continued*
      - bypass graft — *continued*
        - leg — *continued*
          - right — *continued*
            - with — *continued*
              - ulceration (and intermittent claudication and rest pain) I7Ø.339
                - ankle I7Ø.333
                - calf I7Ø.332
                - foot site NEC I7Ø.335
                - heel I7Ø.334
                - lower leg NEC I7Ø.338
                - midfoot I7Ø.334
                - thigh I7Ø.331
        - nonautologous biological graft I7Ø.529
          - leg I7Ø.529
            - with
              - gangrene (and intermittent claudication, rest pain, and ulcer) I7Ø.569
              - rest pain (and intermittent claudication) I7Ø.529
            - bilateral I7Ø.523
              - with
                - gangrene (and intermittent claudication, rest pain, and ulcer) I7Ø.563
                - rest pain (and intermittent claudication) I7Ø.523
            - left I7Ø.522
              - with
                - gangrene (and intermittent claudication, rest pain, and ulcer) I7Ø.562
                - rest pain (and intermittent claudication) I7Ø.522
                - ulceration (and intermittent claudication and rest pain) I7Ø.549
                  - ankle I7Ø.543
                  - calf I7Ø.542
                  - foot site NEC I7Ø.545
                  - heel I7Ø.544
                  - lower leg NEC I7Ø.548
                  - midfoot I7Ø.544
                  - thigh I7Ø.541
            - right I7Ø.521
              - with
                - gangrene (and intermittent claudication, rest pain, and ulcer) I7Ø.561
                - rest pain (and intermittent claudication) I7Ø.521
                - ulceration (and intermittent claudication and rest pain) I7Ø.539
                  - ankle I7Ø.533
                  - calf I7Ø.532
                  - foot site NEC I7Ø.535
                  - heel I7Ø.534
                  - lower leg NEC I7Ø.538
                  - midfoot I7Ø.534
                  - thigh I7Ø.531
        - nonbiological graft I7Ø.629
          - leg I7Ø.629
            - with
              - gangrene (and intermittent claudication, rest pain, and ulcer) I7Ø.669
              - rest pain (and intermittent claudication) I7Ø.629
            - bilateral I7Ø.623
              - with
                - gangrene (and intermittent claudication, rest pain, and ulcer) I7Ø.663
                - rest pain (intermittent claudication) I7Ø.623
            - left I7Ø.622
              - with
                - gangrene (and intermittent claudication, rest pain, and ulcer) I7Ø.662
                - rest pain (and intermittent claudication) I7Ø.622

- **Arteriosclerosis, arteriosclerotic** — *continued*
  - with — *continued*
    - critical limb ischemia — *continued*
      - bypass graft — *continued*
        - nonbiological graft — *continued*
          - leg — *continued*
            - left — *continued*
              - with — *continued*
                - ulceration (and intermittent claudication and rest pain) I7Ø.649
                  - ankle I7Ø.643
                  - calf I7Ø.642
                  - foot site NEC I7Ø.645
                  - heel I7Ø.644
                  - lower leg NEC I7Ø.648
                  - midfoot I7Ø.644
                  - thigh I7Ø.641
            - right I7Ø.621
              - with
                - gangrene (and intermittent claudication, rest pain, and ulcer) I7Ø.661
                - rest pain (and intermittent claudication) I7Ø.621
                - ulceration (and intermittent claudication and rest pain) I7Ø.639
                  - ankle I7Ø.633
                  - calf I7Ø.632
                  - foot site NEC I7Ø.635
                  - heel I7Ø.634
                  - lower leg NEC I7Ø.638
                  - midfoot I7Ø.634
                  - thigh I7Ø.631
        - specified graft NEC I7Ø.729
          - leg I7Ø.729
            - with
              - gangrene (and intermittent claudication, rest pain, and ulcer) I7Ø.769
              - rest pain (and intermittent claudication) I7Ø.729
            - bilateral I7Ø.723
              - with
                - gangrene (and intermittent claudication, rest pain, and ulcer) I7Ø.763
                - rest pain (and intermittent claudication) I7Ø.723
            - left I7Ø.722
              - with
                - gangrene (and intermittent claudication, rest pain, and ulcer) I7Ø.762
                - rest pain (and intermittent claudication) I7Ø.722
                - ulceration (and intermittent claudication and rest pain) I7Ø.749
                  - ankle I7Ø.743
                  - calf I7Ø.742
                  - foot site NEC I7Ø.745
                  - heel I7Ø.744
                  - lower leg NEC I7Ø.748
                  - midfoot I7Ø.744
                  - thigh I7Ø.741
            - right I7Ø.721
              - with
                - gangrene (and intermittent claudication, rest pain, and ulcer) I7Ø.761
                - rest pain (and intermittent claudication) I7Ø.721
                - ulceration (and intermittent claudication and rest pain) I7Ø.739
                  - ankle I7Ø.733
                  - calf I7Ø.732
                  - foot site NEC I7Ø.735
                  - heel I7Ø.734
                  - lower leg NEC I7Ø.738
                  - midfoot I7Ø.734
                  - thigh I7Ø.731
      - leg I7Ø.229
        - with
          - gangrene (and intermittent claudication, rest pain, and ulcer) I7Ø.269

- **Arteriosclerosis, arteriosclerotic** — *continued*
  - with — *continued*
    - critical limb ischemia — *continued*
      - leg — *continued*
        - with — *continued*
          - rest pain (and intermittent claudication) I7Ø.229
        - bilateral I7Ø.223
          - with
            - gangrene (and intermittent claudication, rest pain, and ulcer) I7Ø.263
            - rest pain (and intermittent claudication) I7Ø.223
        - left I7Ø.222
          - with
            - gangrene (and intermittent claudication, rest pain, and ulcer) I7Ø.262
            - rest pain (and intermittent claudication) I7Ø.222
            - ulceration (and intermittent claudication and rest pain) I7Ø.249
              - ankle I7Ø.243
              - calf I7Ø.242
              - foot site NEC I7Ø.245
              - heel I7Ø.244
              - lower leg NEC I7Ø.248
              - midfoot I7Ø.244
              - thigh I7Ø.241
        - right I7Ø.221
          - with
            - gangrene (and intermittent claudication, rest pain, and ulcer) I7Ø.261
            - rest pain (and intermittent claudication) I7Ø.221
            - ulceration (and intermittent claudication and rest pain) I7Ø.239
              - ankle I7Ø.233
              - calf I7Ø.232
              - foot site NEC I7Ø.235
              - heel I7Ø.234
              - lower leg NEC I7Ø.238
              - midfoot I7Ø.234
              - thigh I7Ø.231
  - aorta I7Ø.Ø
  - arteries of extremities — *see* Arteriosclerosis, extremities
    - with
      - chronic limb-threatening ischemia — *see* Arteriosclerosis, with critical limb ischemia
      - critical limb ischemia — *see* Arteriosclerosis, with critical limb ischemia
  - brain I67.2
    - with infarction — *see* Occlusion, artery, brain or cerebral, with infarction
  - bypass graft
    - with
      - chronic limb-threatening ischemia — *see* Arteriosclerosis, with critical limb ischemia
      - critical limb ischemia — *see* Arteriosclerosis, with critical limb ischemia
    - coronary — *see* Arteriosclerosis, coronary, bypass graft
    - extremities — *see* Arteriosclerosis, extremities, bypass graft
  - cardiac — *see* Disease, heart, ischemic, atherosclerotic
  - cardiopathy — *see* Disease, heart, ischemic, atherosclerotic
  - cardiorenal — *see* Hypertension, cardiorenal
  - cardiovascular — *see* Disease, heart, ischemic, atherosclerotic
  - carotid — *see also* Occlusion, artery, carotid I65.2- ☑
  - central nervous system I67.2
    - with infarction — *see* Occlusion, artery, cerebral or precerebral, with infarction
  - cerebral I67.2
    - with infarction — *see* Occlusion, artery, brain or cerebral, with infarction
  - cerebrovascular I67.2
    - with infarction — *see* Occlusion, artery, brain or cerebral, with infarction
  - coronary (artery) I25.1Ø
    - due to
      - calcified coronary lesion (severely) I25.84
      - lipid rich plaque I25.83
    - bypass graft I25.81Ø
      - with
        - angina pectoris I25.7Ø9
          - with documented spasm I25.7Ø1
          - refractory I25.7Ø2
          - specified type NEC I25.7Ø8

- **Arteriosclerosis, arteriosclerotic** — *continued*
  - coronary — *continued*
    - bypass graft — *continued*
      - with — *continued*
        - angina pectoris — *continued*
          - unstable I25.7ØØ
        - ischemic chest pain I25.7Ø9
      - autologous artery I25.81Ø
        - with
          - angina pectoris I25.729
            - with documented spasm I25.721
            - refractory I25.722
            - specified type I25.728
            - unstable I25.72Ø
          - ischemic chest pain I25.729
      - autologous vein I25.81Ø
        - with
          - angina pectoris I25.719
            - with documented spasm I25.711
            - refractory I25.712
            - specified type I25.718
            - unstable I25.71Ø
          - ischemic chest pain I25.719
      - nonautologous biological I25.81Ø
        - with
          - angina pectoris I25.739
            - with documented spasm I25.731
            - refractory I25.732
            - specified type I25.738
            - unstable I25.73Ø
          - ischemic chest pain I25.739
      - specified type NEC I25.81Ø
        - with
          - angina pectoris I25.799
            - with documented spasm I25.791
            - refractory I25.792
            - specified type I25.798
            - unstable I25.79Ø
          - ischemic chest pain I25.799
    - native vessel
      - with
        - angina pectoris I25.119
          - with documented spasm I25.111
          - refractory I25.112
          - specified type NEC I25.118
          - unstable I25.11Ø
        - ischemic chest pain I25.119
    - transplanted heart I25.811
      - bypass graft I25.812
        - with
          - angina pectoris I25.769
            - with documented spasm I25.761
            - refractory I25.762
            - specified type I25.768
            - unstable I25.76Ø
          - ischemic chest pain I25.769
      - native coronary artery I25.811
        - with
          - angina pectoris I25.759
            - with documented spasm I25.751
            - refractory I25.752
            - specified type I25.758
            - unstable I25.75Ø
          - ischemic chest pain I25.759
  - extremities (native arteries) I7Ø.2Ø9
    - with
      - chronic limb-threatening ischemia — *see* Arteriosclerosis, with critical limb ischemia
      - critical limb ischemia — *see* Arteriosclerosis, with critical limb ischemia
    - bypass graft I7Ø.3Ø9
      - with
        - chronic limb-threatening ischemia — *see* Arteriosclerosis, with critical limb ischemia
        - critical limb ischemia — *see* Arteriosclerosis, with critical limb ischemia
      - autologous vein graft I7Ø.4Ø9
        - leg I7Ø.4Ø9
          - with
            - gangrene (and intermittent claudication, rest pain and ulcer) I7Ø.469
            - intermittent claudication I7Ø.419
            - rest pain (and intermittent claudication) I7Ø.429
          - bilateral I7Ø.4Ø3
            - with
              - gangrene (and intermittent claudication, rest pain and ulcer) I7Ø.463

**Artificial** — *continued*
opening status — *continued*
colostomy Z93.3
cystostomy Z93.5Ø
appendico-vesicostomy Z93.52
cutaneous Z93.51
specified NEC Z93.59
enterostomy Z93.4
gastrostomy Z93.1
ileostomy (ileal pouch) (Kock pouch) Z93.2
intestinal tract NEC Z93.4
jejunostomy Z93.4
nephrostomy Z93.6
specified site NEC Z93.8
tracheostomy Z93.Ø
ureterostomy Z93.6
urethrostomy Z93.6
urinary tract NEC Z93.6
vagina Z93.8
vagina status Z93.8
**Arytenoid** — *see* condition
**Asadollahi-Rauch syndrome** Q87.85
**Asbestosis** (occupational) J61
**ASC-H** (atypical squamous cells cannot exclude high grade squamous intraepithelial lesion on cytologic smear)
anus R85.611
cervix R87.611
vagina R87.621
**ASC-US** (atypical squamous cells of undetermined significance on cytologic smear)
anus R85.61Ø
cervix R87.61Ø
vagina R87.62Ø
**Ascariasis** B77.9
with
complications NEC B77.89
intestinal complications B77.Ø
pneumonia, pneumonitis B77.81
**Ascaridosis, ascaridiasis** — *see* Ascariasis
**Ascaris** (infection) (infestation) (lumbricoides) — *see* Ascariasis
**Ascending** — *see* condition
**Aschoff's bodies** — *see* Myocarditis, rheumatic
**Ascites** (abdominal) R18.8
cardiac — *see also* Failure, heart, right I5Ø.81Ø
chylous (nonfilarial) I89.8
filarial — *see* Infestation, filarial
due to
cirrhosis, alcoholic K7Ø.31
hepatitis — *see also* Hepatitis
alcoholic K7Ø.11
chronic active — *see also* Hepatitis, chronic active K73.2
with toxic liver disease K71.51
S. japonicum B65.2
heart — *see also* Failure, heart, right I5Ø.81Ø
malignant R18.Ø
pseudochylous R18.8
syphilitic A52.74
tuberculous A18.31
**Aseptic** — *see* condition
**Asherman's syndrome** N85.6
**Asialia** K11.7
**Asiatic cholera** — *see* Cholera
**Asimultagnosia** (simultanagnosia) R48.3
**Askin's tumor** — *see* Neoplasm, connective tissue, malignant
**Asocial personality** F6Ø.2
**Asomatognosia** R41.4
**Aspartylglucosaminuria** E77.1
**Asperger's disease or syndrome** F84.5
**Aspergilloma** — *see* Aspergillosis
**Aspergillosis** (with pneumonia) B44.9
bronchopulmonary, allergic B44.81
disseminated B44.7
generalized B44.7
pulmonary NEC B44.1
allergic B44.81
invasive B44.Ø
specified NEC B44.89
tonsillar B44.2
**Aspergillus** (flavus) (fumigatus) (infection) (terreus) — *see* Aspergillosis
**Aspermatogenesis** — *see* Azoospermia
**Aspermia** (testis) — *see* Azoospermia
**Asphyxia, asphyxiation** (by) RØ9.Ø1
antenatal P84
birth P84
**Asphyxia, asphyxiation** — *continued*
bunny bag — *see* Asphyxia, due to, mechanical threat to breathing, trapped in bed clothes
crushing S28.Ø- ☑
drowning T75.1- ☑
gas, fumes, or vapor — *see* Table of Drugs and Chemicals
inhalation — *see* Inhalation
intrauterine P84
local I73.ØØ
with gangrene I73.Ø1
mucus — *see also* Foreign body, respiratory tract, causing, asphyxiation
newborn P84
pathological RØ9.Ø1
postnatal P84
mechanical — *see* Asphyxia, due to, mechanical threat to breathing
prenatal P84
reticularis R23.1
strangulation — *see* Asphyxia, due to, mechanical threat to breathing
submersion T75.1- ☑
traumatic T71.9- ☑
due to
crushed chest S28.Ø- ☑
foreign body (in) — *see* Foreign body, respiratory tract, causing asphyxia
low oxygen content of ambient air T71.2Ø- ☑
due to
being trapped in
low oxygen environment T71.29- ☑
in car trunk T71.221- ☑
circumstances undetermined T71.224- ☑
done with intent to harm by
another person T71.223- ☑
self T71.222- ☑
in refrigerator T71.231- ☑
circumstances undetermined T71.234- ☑
done with intent to harm by
another person T71.233- ☑
self T71.232- ☑
cave-in T71.21- ☑
mechanical threat to breathing (accidental) T71.191- ☑
circumstances undetermined T71.194- ☑
done with intent to harm by
another person T71.193- ☑
self T71.192- ☑
hanging T71.161- ☑
circumstances undetermined T71.164- ☑
done with intent to harm by
another person T71.163- ☑
self T71.162- ☑
plastic bag T71.121- ☑
circumstances undetermined T71.124- ☑
done with intent to harm by
another person T71.123- ☑
self T71.122- ☑
smothering
in furniture T71.151- ☑
circumstances undetermined T71.154- ☑
done with intent to harm by
another person T71.153- ☑
self T71.152- ☑
under
another person's body T71.141- ☑
circumstances undetermined T71.144- ☑
done with intent to harm T71.143- ☑
pillow T71.111- ☑
circumstances undetermined T71.114- ☑
done with intent to harm by
another person T71.113- ☑
self T71.112- ☑
trapped in bed clothes T71.131- ☑
circumstances undetermined T71.134- ☑
done with intent to harm by
another person T71.133- ☑
self T71.132- ☑
vomiting, vomitus — *see* Foreign body, respiratory tract, causing asphyxia
**Aspiration**
amniotic (clear) fluid (newborn) P24.1Ø
**Aspiration** — *continued*
amniotic fluid — *continued*
with
pneumonia (pneumonitis) P24.11
respiratory symptoms P24.11
blood
newborn (without respiratory symptoms) P24.2Ø
with
pneumonia (pneumonitis) P24.21
respiratory symptoms P24.21
specified age NEC — *see* Foreign body, respiratory tract
bronchitis J69.Ø
food or foreign body — *see* Foreign body, by site
liquor (amnii) (newborn) P24.1Ø
with
pneumonia (pneumonitis) P24.11
respiratory symptoms P24.11
meconium (newborn) (without respiratory symptoms) P24.ØØ
with
pneumonitis (pneumonitis) P24.Ø1
respiratory symptoms P24.Ø1
milk (newborn) (without respiratory symptoms) P24.3Ø
with
pneumonia (pneumonitis) P24.31
respiratory symptoms P24.31
specified age NEC — *see* Foreign body, respiratory tract
mucus — *see also* Foreign body, by site, causing asphyxia
newborn P24.1Ø
with
pneumonia (pneumonitis) P24.11
respiratory symptoms P24.11
neonatal P24.9
specific NEC (without respiratory symptoms) P24.8Ø
with
pneumonia (pneumonitis) P24.81
respiratory symptoms P24.81
newborn P24.9
specific NEC (without respiratory symptoms) P24.8Ø
with
pneumonia (pneumonitis) P24.81
respiratory symptoms P24.81
pneumonia J69.Ø
pneumonitis J69.Ø
syndrome of newborn — *see* Aspiration, by substance, with pneumonia
vernix caseosa (newborn) P24.8Ø
with
pneumonia (pneumonitis) P24.81
respiratory symptoms P24.81
vomitus — *see also* Foreign body, respiratory tract
newborn (without respiratory symptoms) P24.3Ø
with
pneumonia (pneumonitis) P24.31
respiratory symptoms P24.31
**Asplenia** (congenital) Q89.Ø1
functional D73.Ø
postsurgical Z9Ø.81
**Assam fever** B55.Ø
**Assault, sexual** — *see* Maltreatment
**Assmann's focus NEC** A15.Ø
**Astasia** (-abasia) (hysterical) F44.4
**Asteatosis cutis** L85.3
**Astereognosia, astereognosis** R48.1
**Asterixis** R27.8
in liver disease K71.3
**Asteroid hyalitis** — *see* Deposit, crystalline
**Asthenia, asthenic** R53.1
cardiac — *see also* Failure, heart I5Ø.9
psychogenic F45.8
cardiovascular — *see also* Failure, heart I5Ø.9
psychogenic F45.8
heart — *see also* Failure, heart I5Ø.9
psychogenic F45.8
hysterical F44.4
myocardial — *see also* Failure, heart I5Ø.9
psychogenic F45.8
nervous F48.8
neurocirculatory F45.8
neurotic F48.8
psychogenic F48.8
psychoneurotic F48.8
psychophysiologic F48.8
reaction (psychophysiologic) F48.8
senile R54
**Asthenopia** — *see also* Discomfort, visual
hysterical F44.6

- **Asthenopia** — *continued*
  - psychogenic F44.6
- **Asthenospermia** — *see* Abnormal, specimen, male genital organs
- **Asthma, asthmatic** (bronchial) (catarrh) (spasmodic) J45.9Ø9
  - with
    - chronic obstructive bronchitis J44.89
      - with
        - acute lower respiratory infection J44.Ø
        - exacerbation (acute) J44.1
    - chronic obstructive pulmonary disease J44.89
      - with
        - acute lower respiratory infection J44.Ø
        - exacerbation (acute) J44.1
    - exacerbation (acute) J45.9Ø1
    - hay fever — *see* Asthma, allergic extrinsic
    - rhinitis, allergic — *see* Asthma, allergic extrinsic
    - status asthmaticus J45.9Ø2
  - allergic extrinsic J45.9Ø9
    - with
      - exacerbation (acute) J45.9Ø1
      - status asthmaticus J45.9Ø2
  - atopic — *see* Asthma, allergic extrinsic
  - cardiac — *see* Failure, ventricular, left
  - cardiobronchial I5Ø.1
  - childhood J45.9Ø9
    - with
      - exacerbation (acute) J45.9Ø1
      - status asthmaticus J45.9Ø2
  - chronic obstructive J44.89
    - with
      - acute lower respiratory infection J44.Ø
      - exacerbation (acute) J44.1
  - collier's J6Ø
  - cough variant J45.991
  - detergent J69.8
  - due to
    - detergent J69.8
    - inhalation of fumes J68.3
  - eosinophilic J82.83
  - extrinsic, allergic — *see* Asthma, allergic extrinsic
  - grinder's J62.8
  - hay — *see* Asthma, allergic extrinsic
  - heart I5Ø.1
  - idiosyncratic — *see* Asthma, nonallergic
  - intermittent (mild) J45.2Ø
    - with
      - exacerbation (acute) J45.21
      - status asthmaticus J45.22
  - intrinsic, nonallergic — *see* Asthma, nonallergic
  - Kopp's E32.8
  - late-onset J45.9Ø9
    - with
      - exacerbation (acute) J45.9Ø1
      - status asthmaticus J45.9Ø2
  - mild intermittent J45.2Ø
    - with
      - exacerbation (acute) J45.21
      - status asthmaticus J45.22
  - mild persistent J45.3Ø
    - with
      - exacerbation (acute) J45.31
      - status asthmaticus J45.32
  - Millar's (laryngismus stridulus) J38.5
  - miner's J6Ø
  - mixed J45.9Ø9
    - with
      - exacerbation (acute) J45.9Ø1
      - status asthmaticus J45.9Ø2
  - moderate persistent J45.4Ø
    - with
      - exacerbation (acute) J45.41
      - status asthmaticus J45.42
  - nervous — *see* Asthma, nonallergic
  - nonallergic (intrinsic) J45.9Ø9
    - with
      - exacerbation (acute) J45.9Ø1
      - status asthmaticus J45.9Ø2
  - persistent
    - mild J45.3Ø
      - with
        - exacerbation (acute) J45.31
        - status asthmaticus J45.32
    - moderate J45.4Ø
      - with
        - exacerbation (acute) J45.41
        - status asthmaticus J45.42
    - severe J45.5Ø

- **Asthma, asthmatic** — *continued*
  - persistent — *continued*
    - severe — *continued*
      - with
        - exacerbation (acute) J45.51
        - status asthmaticus J45.52
  - platinum J45.998
  - pneumoconiotic NEC J64
  - potter's J62.8
  - predominantly allergic J45.9Ø9
  - psychogenic F54
  - pulmonary eosinophilic J82.83
  - red cedar J67.8
  - Rostan's I5Ø.1
  - sandblaster's J62.8
  - sequoiosis J67.8
  - severe persistent J45.5Ø
    - with
      - exacerbation (acute) J45.51
      - status asthmaticus J45.52
  - specified NEC J45.998
  - stonemason's J62.8
  - thymic E32.8
  - tuberculous — *see* Tuberculosis, pulmonary
  - Wichmann's (laryngismus stridulus) J38.5
  - wood J67.8
- **Astigmatism** (compound) (congenital) H52.2Ø- ☑
  - irregular H52.21- ☑
  - regular H52.22- ☑
- **Astraphobia** F4Ø.22Ø
- **Astroblastoma**
  - specified site — *see* Neoplasm, malignant, by site
  - unspecified site C71.9
- **Astrocytoma** (cystic)
  - anaplastic
    - specified site — *see* Neoplasm, malignant, by site
    - unspecified site C71.9
  - fibrillary
    - specified site — *see* Neoplasm, malignant, by site
    - unspecified site C71.9
  - fibrous
    - specified site — *see* Neoplasm, malignant, by site
    - unspecified site C71.9
  - gemistocytic
    - specified site — *see* Neoplasm, malignant, by site
    - unspecified site C71.9
  - juvenile
    - specified site — *see* Neoplasm, malignant, by site
    - unspecified site C71.9
  - pilocytic
    - specified site — *see* Neoplasm, malignant, by site
    - unspecified site C71.9
  - piloid
    - specified site — *see* Neoplasm, malignant, by site
    - unspecified site C71.9
  - protoplasmic
    - specified site — *see* Neoplasm, malignant, by site
    - unspecified site C71.9
  - specified site NEC — *see* Neoplasm, malignant, by site
  - subependymal D43.2
    - giant cell
      - specified site — *see* Neoplasm, uncertain behavior, by site
      - unspecified site D43.2
    - specified site — *see* Neoplasm, uncertain behavior, by site
    - unspecified site D43.2
  - unspecified site C71.9
- **Astroglioma**
  - specified site — *see* Neoplasm, malignant, by site
  - unspecified site C71.9
- **Asymbolia** R48.8
- **Asymmetry** — *see also* Distortion
  - between native and reconstructed breast N65.1
  - face Q67.Ø
  - jaw (lower) — *see* Anomaly, dentofacial, jaw-cranial base relationship, asymmetry
- **Asynergia, asynergy** R27.8
  - ventricular I51.89
- **Asystole** (heart) — *see* Arrest, cardiac
- **At risk**
  - for
    - dental caries Z91.849
      - high Z91.843
      - low Z91.841
      - moderate Z91.842
    - falling Z91.81
    - feeling loneliness Z65.8
    - social isolation Z91.89

- **Ataxia, ataxy, ataxic** R27.Ø
  - acute R27.8
  - autosomal recessive Friedreich G11.11
  - brain (hereditary) G11.9
  - cerebellar (hereditary) G11.9
    - with defective DNA repair G11.3
    - alcoholic G31.2
    - early-onset G11.1Ø
      - with
        - essential tremor G11.19
        - myoclonus [Hunt's ataxia] G11.19
        - retained tendon reflexes G11.19
    - in
      - alcoholism G31.2
      - myxedema EØ3.9 *[G13.2]*
      - neoplastic disease — *see also* Neoplasm D49.9 *[G32.81]*
      - specified disease NEC G32.81
    - late-onset (Marie's) G11.2
  - cerebral (hereditary) G11.9
  - congenital nonprogressive G11.Ø
  - family, familial — *see* Ataxia, hereditary
  - following
    - cerebrovascular disease I69.993
      - cerebral infarction I69.393
      - intracerebral hemorrhage I69.193
      - nontraumatic intracranial hemorrhage NEC I69.293
      - specified disease NEC I69.893
      - subarachnoid hemorrhage I69.Ø93
  - Friedreich's (heredofamilial) (cerebellar) (spinal) (with retained reflexes) G11.11
  - gait R26.Ø
    - hysterical F44.4
  - general R27.8
  - gluten M35.9 *[G32.81]*
    - with celiac disease K9Ø.Ø *[G32.81]*
  - hereditary G11.9
    - with neuropathy G6Ø.2
    - cerebellar — *see* Ataxia, cerebellar
    - spastic G11.4
    - specified NEC G11.8
    - spinal (Friedreich's) G11.11
  - heredofamilial — *see* Ataxia, hereditary
  - Hunt's G11.19
  - hysterical F44.4
  - locomotor (progressive) (syphilitic) (partial) (spastic) A52.11
    - diabetic — *see* Diabetes, ataxia
  - Marie's (cerebellar) (heredofamilial) (late- onset) G11.2
  - nonorganic origin F44.4
  - nonprogressive, congenital G11.Ø
  - psychogenic F44.4
  - Roussy-Levy G6Ø.Ø
  - Sanger-Brown's (hereditary) G11.2
  - spastic hereditary G11.4
  - spinal
    - hereditary (Friedreich's) G11.11
    - progressive (syphilitic) A52.11
  - spinocerebellar, X-linked recessive G11.19
  - telangiectasia (Louis-Bar) G11.3
- **Ataxia-telangiectasia** (Louis-Bar) G11.3
- **Atelectasis** (massive) (partial) (pressure) (pulmonary) J98.11
  - newborn P28.1Ø
    - due to resorption P28.11
    - partial P28.19
    - primary P28.Ø
    - secondary P28.19
  - primary (newborn) P28.Ø
  - tuberculous — *see* Tuberculosis, pulmonary
- **Atelocardia** Q24.9
- **Atelomyelia** QØ6.1
- **Atheroembolism**
  - of
    - extremities
      - lower I75.Ø2- ☑
      - upper I75.Ø1- ☑
    - kidney I75.81
    - specified NEC I75.89
- **Atheroma, atheromatous** — *see also* Arteriosclerosis I7Ø.9Ø
  - aorta, aortic I7Ø.Ø
    - valve — *see also* Endocarditis, aortic I35.8
  - aorto-iliac I7Ø.Ø
  - artery — *see* Arteriosclerosis
  - basilar (artery) I67.2
  - carotid (artery) (common) (internal) I67.2
  - cerebral (arteries) I67.2
  - coronary (artery) I25.1Ø
    - with angina pectoris — *see* Arteriosclerosis, coronary (artery),

**Atheroma, atheromatous** — *continued*
- degeneration — *see* Arteriosclerosis
- heart, cardiac — *see* Disease, heart, ischemic, atherosclerotic
- mitral (valve) I34.89
- myocardium, myocardial — *see* Disease, heart, ischemic, atherosclerotic
- pulmonary valve (heart) — *see also* Endocarditis, pulmonary I37.8
- tricuspid (heart) (valve) I36.8
- valve, valvular — *see* Endocarditis
- vertebral (artery) I67.2

**Atheromatosis** — *see* Arteriosclerosis

**Atherosclerosis** — *see also* Arteriosclerosis
- coronary
  - artery I25.1Ø
    - with angina pectoris — *see* Arteriosclerosis, coronary (artery),
    - due to
      - calcified coronary lesion (severely) I25.84
      - lipid rich plaque I25.83
- transplanted heart I25.811
  - bypass graft I25.812
    - with angina pectoris — *see* Arteriosclerosis, coronary (artery),
  - native coronary artery I25.811
    - with angina pectoris — *see* Arteriosclerosis, coronary (artery),

**Athetosis** (acquired) R25.8
- bilateral (congenital) G8Ø.3
- congenital (bilateral) (double) G8Ø.3
- double (congenital) G8Ø.3
- unilateral R25.8

**Athlete's**
- foot B35.3
- heart I51.7

**Athrepsia** E41

**Athyrea** (acquired) — *see also* Hypothyroidism
- congenital EØ3.1

**Atonia, atony, atonic**
- bladder (sphincter) (neurogenic) N31.2
- capillary I78.8
- cecum K59.89
  - psychogenic F45.8
- colon — *see* Atony, intestine
- congenital P94.2
- esophagus K22.89
- intestine K59.89
  - psychogenic F45.8
- stomach K31.89
  - neurotic or psychogenic F45.8
- uterus (during labor) O62.2
  - with hemorrhage (postpartum) O72.1
  - postpartum (with hemorrhage) O72.1
    - without hemorrhage O75.89

**Atopy** — *see* History, allergy

**Atransferrinemia, congenital** E88.Ø9

**Atresia, atretic**
- alimentary organ or tract NEC Q45.8
  - upper Q4Ø.8
- ani, anus, anal (canal) Q42.3
  - with fistula Q42.2
- aorta (ring) Q25.29
- aortic (orifice) (valve) Q23.Ø
  - arch Q25.21
  - congenital with hypoplasia of ascending aorta and defective development of left ventricle (with mitral stenosis) Q23.4
  - in hypoplastic left heart syndrome Q23.4
- aqueduct of Sylvius QØ3.Ø
  - with spina bifida — *see* Spina bifida, with hydrocephalus
- artery NEC Q27.8
  - cerebral Q28.3
  - coronary Q24.5
  - digestive system Q27.8
  - eye Q15.8
  - lower limb Q27.8
  - pulmonary Q25.5
  - specified site NEC Q27.8
  - umbilical Q27.Ø
  - upper limb Q27.8
- auditory canal (external) Q16.1
- bile duct (common) (congenital) (hepatic) Q44.2
  - acquired — *see* Obstruction, bile duct
- bladder (neck) Q64.39
  - obstruction Q64.31
- bronchus Q32.4
- cecum Q42.8

**Atresia, atretic** — *continued*
- cervix (acquired) N88.2
  - congenital Q51.828
  - in pregnancy or childbirth — *see* Anomaly, cervix, in pregnancy or childbirth
    - causing obstructed labor O65.5
- choana Q3Ø.Ø
- colon Q42.9
  - specified NEC Q42.8
- common duct Q44.2
- cricoid cartilage Q31.8
- cystic duct Q44.2
  - acquired K82.8
    - with obstruction K82.Ø
- digestive organs NEC Q45.8
- duodenum Q41.Ø
- ear canal Q16.1
- ejaculatory duct Q55.4
- epiglottis Q31.8
- esophagus Q39.Ø
  - with tracheoesophageal fistula Q39.1
- eustachian tube Q17.8
- fallopian tube (congenital) Q5Ø.6
  - acquired N97.1
- follicular cyst N83.Ø- ☑
- foramen of
  - Luschka QØ3.1
    - with spina bifida — *see* Spina bifida, with hydrocephalus
  - Magendie QØ3.1
    - with spina bifida — *see* Spina bifida, with hydrocephalus
- gallbladder Q44.1
- genital organ
  - external
    - female Q52.79
    - male Q55.8
  - internal
    - female Q52.8
    - male Q55.8
- glottis Q31.8
- gullet Q39.Ø
  - with tracheoesophageal fistula Q39.1
- heart valve NEC Q24.8
  - pulmonary Q22.Ø
  - tricuspid Q22.4
- hymen Q52.3
  - acquired (postinfective) N89.6
- ileum Q41.2
- intestine (small) Q41.9
  - large Q42.9
    - specified NEC Q42.8
- iris, filtration angle Q15.Ø
- jejunum Q41.1
- lacrimal apparatus Q1Ø.4
- larynx Q31.8
- meatus urinarius Q64.33
- mitral valve Q23.2
  - in hypoplastic left heart syndrome Q23.4
- nares (anterior) (posterior) Q3Ø.Ø
- nasopharynx Q34.8
- nose, nostril Q3Ø.Ø
  - acquired J34.89
- organ or site NEC Q89.89
- osseous meatus (ear) Q16.1
- oviduct (congenital) Q5Ø.6
  - acquired N97.1
- parotid duct Q38.4
  - acquired K11.8
- pulmonary (artery) Q25.5
  - valve Q22.Ø
- pulmonic Q22.Ø
- pupil Q13.2
- rectum Q42.1
  - with fistula Q42.Ø
- salivary duct Q38.4
  - acquired K11.8
- sublingual duct Q38.4
  - acquired K11.8
- submandibular duct Q38.4
  - acquired K11.8
- submaxillary duct Q38.4
  - acquired K11.8
- thyroid cartilage Q31.8
- trachea Q32.1
- tricuspid valve Q22.4
- ureter Q62.1Ø
  - pelvic junction Q62.11
  - vesical orifice Q62.12

**Atresia, atretic** — *continued*
- ureteropelvic junction Q62.11
- ureterovesical orifice Q62.12
- urethra (valvular) Q64.39
  - stricture Q64.32
- urinary tract NEC Q64.8
- uterus Q51.818
  - acquired N85.8
- vagina (congenital) Q52.4
  - acquired (postinfectional) (senile) N89.5
- vas deferens Q55.3
- vascular NEC Q27.8
  - cerebral Q28.3
  - digestive system Q27.8
  - lower limb Q27.8
  - specified site NEC Q27.8
  - upper limb Q27.8
- vein NEC Q27.8
  - digestive system Q27.8
  - great Q26.8
  - lower limb Q27.8
  - portal Q26.5
  - pulmonary Q26.4
    - partial Q26.3
    - total Q26.2
  - specified site NEC Q27.8
  - upper limb Q27.8
- vena cava (inferior) (superior) Q26.8
- vesicourethral orifice Q64.31
- vulva Q52.79
  - acquired N9Ø.5

**Atrichia, atrichosis** — *see* Alopecia

**Atrophia** — *see also* Atrophy
- cutis senilis L9Ø.8
  - due to radiation L57.8
- gyrata of choroid and retina H31.23
- senilis R54
  - dermatological L9Ø.8
    - due to radiation (nonionizing) (solar) L57.8
- unguium L6Ø.3
  - congenita Q84.6

**Atrophie blanche** (en plaque) (de Milian) L95.Ø

**Atrophoderma, atrophodermia** (of) L9Ø.9
- diffusum (idiopathic) L9Ø.4
- maculatum L9Ø.8
  - et striatum L9Ø.8
    - due to syphilis A52.79
  - syphilitic A51.39
- neuriticum L9Ø.8
- Pasini and Pierini L9Ø.3
- pigmentosum Q82.1
- reticulatum symmetricum faciei L66.4
- senile L9Ø.8
  - due to radiation (nonionizing) (solar) L57.8
- vermiculata (cheeks) L66.4

**Atrophy, atrophic** (of)
- adrenal (capsule) (gland) E27.49
  - primary (autoimmune) E27.1
- alveolar process or ridge (edentulous) KØ8.2Ø
- anal sphincter (disuse) N81.84
- appendix K38.8
- arteriosclerotic — *see* Arteriosclerosis
- bile duct (common) (hepatic) K83.8
- bladder N32.89
  - neurogenic N31.8
- blanche (en plaque) (of Milian) L95.Ø
- bone (senile) NEC — *see also* Disorder, bone, specified type NEC
  - due to
    - tabes dorsalis (neurogenic) A52.11
- brain (cortex) (progressive) G31.9
  - frontotemporal circumscribed — *see also* Dementia, in, diseases specified elsewhere G31.Ø1 *[FØ2.8Ø]*
    - with behavioral disturbance — *see also* Dementia, in, diseases specified elsewhere G31.Ø1 *[FØ2.81-]* ☑
  - senile NEC G31.1
- breast N64.2
  - obstetric — *see* Disorder, breast, specified type NEC
- buccal cavity K13.79
- cardiac — *see* Degeneration, myocardial
- cartilage (infectional) (joint) — *see* Disorder, cartilage, specified NEC
- cerebellar — *see* Atrophy, brain
- cerebral — *see* Atrophy, brain
- cervix (mucosa) (senile) (uteri) N88.8
  - menopausal N95.8
- Charcot-Marie-Tooth G6Ø.Ø
- choroid (central) (macular) (myopic) (retina) H31.1Ø- ☑

- **Atrophy, atrophic** — *continued*
  - choroid — *continued*
    - diffuse secondary H31.12- ☑
    - gyrate H31.23
    - senile H31.11- ☑
  - ciliary body — *see* Atrophy, iris
  - conjunctiva (senile) H11.89
  - corpus cavernosum N48.89
  - cortical — *see* Atrophy, brain
  - cystic duct K82.8
  - Dejerine-Thomas G23.8
  - disuse NEC — *see* Atrophy, muscle
  - Duchenne-Aran G12.21
  - ear H93.8- ☑
  - edentulous alveolar ridge K08.2Ø
  - endometrium (senile) N85.8
    - cervix N88.8
  - enteric K63.89
  - epididymis N5Ø.89
  - eyeball — *see* Disorder, globe, degenerated condition, atrophy
  - eyelid (senile) — *see* Disorder, eyelid, degenerative
  - facial (skin) L9Ø.9
  - fallopian tube (senile) N83.32- ☑
    - with ovary N83.33- ☑
  - fascioscapulohumeral (Landouzy- Dejerine) G71.Ø2
  - fatty, thymus (gland) E32.8
  - gallbladder K82.8
  - gastric K29.4Ø
    - with bleeding K29.41
  - gastrointestinal K63.89
  - glandular I89.8
  - globe H44.52- ☑
  - gum — *see* Recession, gingival
  - hair L67.8
  - heart (brown) — *see* Degeneration, myocardial
  - hemifacial Q67.4
    - Romberg G51.8
  - infantile E41
    - paralysis, acute — *see* Poliomyelitis, paralytic
  - intestine K63.89
  - iris (essential) (progressive) H21.26- ☑
    - specified NEC H21.29
  - kidney (senile) (terminal) — *see also* Sclerosis, renal N26.1
    - congenital or infantile Q6Ø.5
      - bilateral Q6Ø.4
      - unilateral Q6Ø.3
    - hydronephrotic — *see* Hydronephrosis
  - lacrimal gland (primary) HØ4.14- ☑
    - secondary HØ4.15- ☑
  - Landouzy-Dejerine G71.Ø2
  - laryngitis, infective J37.Ø
  - larynx J38.7
  - Leber's optic (hereditary) H47.22
  - lip K13.Ø
  - liver (yellow) K72.9Ø
    - with coma K72.91
    - acute, subacute K72.ØØ
      - with coma K72.Ø1
    - chronic K72.1Ø
      - with coma K72.11
  - lung (senile) J98.4
  - macular (dermatological) L9Ø.8
    - syphilitic, skin A51.39
      - striated A52.79
  - mandible (edentulous) KØ8.2Ø
    - minimal KØ8.21
    - moderate KØ8.22
    - severe KØ8.23
  - maxilla KØ8.2Ø
    - minimal KØ8.24
    - moderate KØ8.25
    - severe KØ8.26
  - muscle, muscular (diffuse) (general) (idiopathic) (primary) M62.5Ø
    - ankle M62.57- ☑
    - back M62.5A9
      - cervical M62.5AØ
      - lumbosacral M62.5A2
      - thoracic M62.5A1
    - Duchenne-Aran G12.21
    - foot M62.57- ☑
    - forearm M62.53- ☑
    - hand M62.54- ☑
    - infantile spinal G12.Ø
    - lower leg M62.56- ☑
    - multiple sites M62.59
    - myelopathic — *see* Atrophy, muscle, spinal

- **Atrophy, atrophic** — *continued*
  - muscle, muscular — *continued*
    - myotonic G71.11
    - neuritic G58.9
    - neuropathic (peroneal) (progressive) G6Ø.Ø
    - pelvic (disuse) N81.84
    - peroneal G6Ø.Ø
    - progressive (bulbar) G12.21
      - adult G12.1
      - infantile (spinal) G12.Ø
      - spinal G12.25
        - adult G12.1
        - infantile G12.Ø
    - pseudohypertrophic G71.Ø2
    - shoulder region M62.51- ☑
    - specified site NEC M62.58
    - spinal G12.9
      - adult form G12.1
      - Aran-Duchenne G12.21
      - childhood form, type II G12.1
      - distal G12.1
      - hereditary NEC G12.1
      - infantile, type I (Werdnig-Hoffmann) G12.Ø
      - juvenile form, type III (Kugelberg- Welander) G12.1
      - progressive G12.25
      - scapuloperoneal form G12.1
      - specified NEC G12.8
    - syphilitic A52.78
    - thigh M62.55- ☑
    - upper arm M62.52- ☑
  - myocardium — *see* Degeneration, myocardial
  - myometrium (senile) N85.8
    - cervix N88.8
  - myopathic NEC — *see* Atrophy, muscle
  - myotonia G71.11
  - nail L6Ø.3
  - nasopharynx J31.1
  - nerve — *see also* Disorder, nerve
    - abducens — *see* Strabismus, paralytic, sixth nerve
    - accessory G52.8
    - acoustic or auditory H93.3- ☑
    - cranial G52.9
      - eighth (auditory) H93.3- ☑
      - eleventh (accessory) G52.8
      - fifth (trigeminal) G5Ø.8
      - first (olfactory) G52.Ø
      - fourth (trochlear) — *see* Strabismus, paralytic, fourth nerve
      - second (optic) H47.2Ø
      - sixth (abducens) — *see* Strabismus, paralytic, sixth nerve
      - tenth (pneumogastric) (vagus) G52.2
      - third (oculomotor) — *see* Strabismus, paralytic, third nerve
      - twelfth (hypoglossal) G52.3
    - hypoglossal G52.3
    - oculomotor — *see* Strabismus, paralytic, third nerve
    - olfactory G52.Ø
    - optic (papillomacular bundle)
      - syphilitic (late) A52.15
        - congenital A5Ø.44
    - pneumogastric G52.2
    - trigeminal G5Ø.8
    - trochlear — *see* Strabismus, paralytic, fourth nerve
    - vagus (pneumogastric) G52.2
  - neurogenic, bone, tabetic A52.11
  - nutritional E43
    - with marasmus E41
  - old age R54
  - olivopontocerebellar G23.8
  - optic (nerve) H47.2Ø
    - glaucomatous H47.23- ☑
    - hereditary H47.22
    - primary H47.21- ☑
    - specified type NEC H47.29- ☑
    - syphilitic (late) A52.15
      - congenital A5Ø.44
  - orbit HØ5.31- ☑
  - ovary (senile) N83.31- ☑
    - with fallopian tube N83.33- ☑
  - oviduct (senile) — *see* Atrophy, fallopian tube
  - palsy, diffuse (progressive) G12.22
  - pancreas (duct) (senile) K86.89
  - parotid gland K11.Ø
  - pelvic muscle N81.84
  - penis N48.89
  - pharynx J39.2
  - pluriglandular E31.8

- **Atrophy, atrophic** — *continued*
  - pluriglandular — *continued*
    - autoimmune E31.Ø
  - polyarthritis M15.9
  - prostate N42.89
  - pseudohypertrophic (muscle) G71.Ø2
  - renal — *see also* Sclerosis, renal N26.1
  - retina, retinal (postinfectional) H35.89
  - rhinitis J31.Ø
  - salivary gland K11.Ø
  - scar L9Ø.5
  - sclerosis, lobar (of brain) — *see also* Dementia, in, diseases specified elsewhere G31.Ø9 *[FØ2.8Ø]*
    - with behavioral disturbance — *see also* Dementia, in, diseases specified elsewhere G31.Ø9 *[FØ2.81-]* ☑
  - scrotum N5Ø.89
  - seminal vesicle N5Ø.89
  - senile R54
    - due to radiation (nonionizing) (solar) L57.8
  - skin (patches) (spots) L9Ø.9
    - degenerative (senile) L9Ø.8
    - due to radiation (nonionizing) (solar) L57.8
    - senile L9Ø.8
  - spermatic cord N5Ø.89
  - spinal (acute) (cord) G95.89
    - muscular — *see* Atrophy, muscle, spinal
    - paralysis G12.2Ø
      - acute — *see* Poliomyelitis, paralytic
      - meaning progressive muscular atrophy G12.25
  - spine (column) — *see* Spondylopathy, specified NEC
  - spleen (senile) D73.Ø
  - stomach K29.4Ø
    - with bleeding K29.41
  - striate (skin) L9Ø.6
    - syphilitic A52.79
  - subcutaneous L9Ø.9
  - sublingual gland K11.Ø
  - submandibular gland K11.Ø
  - submaxillary gland K11.Ø
  - Sudeck's — *see* Algoneurodystrophy
  - suprarenal (capsule) (gland) E27.49
    - primary E27.1
  - systemic affecting central nervous system
    - in
      - myxedema EØ3.9 *[G13.2]*
      - neoplastic disease — *see also* Neoplasm D49.9 *[G13.1]*
      - specified disease NEC G13.8
  - tarso-orbital fascia, congenital Q1Ø.3
  - testis N5Ø.Ø
  - thenar, partial — *see* Syndrome, carpal tunnel
  - thymus (fatty) E32.8
  - thyroid (gland) (acquired) EØ3.4
    - with cretinism EØ3.1
    - congenital (with myxedema) EØ3.1
  - tongue (senile) K14.8
    - papillae K14.4
  - trachea J39.8
  - tunica vaginalis N5Ø.89
  - turbinate J34.89
  - tympanic membrane (nonflaccid) H73.82- ☑
    - flaccid H73.81- ☑
  - upper respiratory tract J39.8
  - uterus, uterine (senile) N85.8
    - cervix N88.8
    - due to radiation (intended effect) N85.8
      - adverse effect or misadventure N99.89
  - vagina (senile) N95.2
  - vas deferens N5Ø.89
  - vascular I99.8
  - vertebra (senile) — *see* Spondylopathy, specified NEC
  - vulva (senile) N9Ø.5
  - Werdnig-Hoffmann G12.Ø
  - yellow — *see* Failure, hepatic
- **Attack, attacks**
  - with alteration of consciousness (with automatisms) — *see* Epilepsy, localization-related, symptomatic, with complex partial seizures
  - Adams-Stokes I45.9
  - akinetic — *see* Epilepsy, generalized, specified NEC
  - angina — *see* Angina
  - atonic — *see* Epilepsy, generalized, specified NEC
  - benign shuddering G25.83
  - cataleptic — *see* Catalepsy
  - coronary — *see* Infarct, myocardium
  - cyanotic, newborn P28.2
  - drop NEC R55
  - epileptic — *see* Epilepsy

**Attack, attacks** — *continued*
- heart — *see* infarct, myocardium
- hysterical F44.9
- jacksonian — *see* Epilepsy, localization-related, symptomatic, with simple partial seizures
- myocardium, myocardial — *see* Infarct, myocardium
- myoclonic — *see* Epilepsy, generalized, specified NEC
- panic F41.Ø
- psychomotor — *see* Epilepsy, localization-related, symptomatic, with complex partial seizures
- salaam — *see* Epilepsy, spasms
- schizophreniform, brief F23
- shuddering, benign G25.83
- Stokes-Adams I45.9
- syncope R55
- transient ischemic (TIA) G45.9
  - specified NEC G45.8
- unconsciousness R55
  - hysterical F44.89
- vasomotor R55
- vasovagal (paroxysmal) (idiopathic) R55
- without alteration of consciousness — *see* Epilepsy, localization-related, symptomatic, with simple partial seizures

**Attention** (to)
- artificial
  - opening (of) Z43.9
    - digestive tract NEC Z43.4
      - colon Z43.3
      - ilium Z43.2
      - stomach Z43.1
    - specified NEC Z43.8
    - trachea Z43.Ø
    - urinary tract NEC Z43.6
      - cystostomy Z43.5
      - nephrostomy Z43.6
      - ureterostomy Z43.6
      - urethrostomy Z43.6
  - vagina Z43.7
- colostomy Z43.3
- cystostomy Z43.5
- deficit disorder or syndrome F98.8
  - with hyperactivity — *see* Disorder, attention-deficit hyperactivity
- gastrostomy Z43.1
- ileostomy Z43.2
- jejunostomy Z43.4
- nephrostomy Z43.6
- surgical dressings Z48.Ø1
- sutures Z48.Ø2
- tracheostomy Z43.Ø
- ureterostomy Z43.6
- urethrostomy Z43.6

**Attrition**
- gum — *see* Recession, gingival
- tooth, teeth (excessive) (hard tissues) KØ3.Ø

**Atypical, atypism** — *see also* condition
- cells (on cytological smear) (endocervical) (endometrial) (glandular)
- cervical N87.9
- endometrium N85.9
  - hyperplasia N85.ØØ
- parenting situation Z62.9
  - cervix R87.619
  - vagina R87.629

**Auditory** — *see* condition
**Aujeszky's disease** B33.8
**Aurantiasis, cutis** E67.1
**Auricle, auricular** — *see also* condition
- cervical Q18.2

**Auriculotemporal syndrome** G5Ø.8
**Austin Flint murmur** (aortic insufficiency) I35.1
**Australian**
- Q fever A78
- X disease A83.4

**Autism, autistic** (childhood) (infantile) F84.Ø
- atypical F84.9
- spectrum disorder F84.Ø

**Autoantibodies, multiple confirmed islet, with normoglycemia** E1Ø.A1
**Autodigestion** R68.89
**Autoerythrocyte sensitization** (syndrome) D69.2
**Autographism** L5Ø.3
**Autoimmune**
- disease (systemic) M35.9
- inhibitors to clotting factors D68.311
- lymphoproliferative syndrome [ALPS] D89.82
- thyroiditis EØ6.3

**Autoimmunity, confirmed islet, with dysglycemia** E1Ø.A2
**Autointoxication** R68.89
**Automatism** G93.89
- with temporal sclerosis G93.81
- epileptic — *see* Epilepsy, localization-related, symptomatic, with complex partial seizures
- paroxysmal, idiopathic — *see* Epilepsy, localization-related, symptomatic, with complex partial seizures

**Autonomic, autonomous**
- bladder (neurogenic) N31.2
- hysteria seizure F44.5

**Autosensitivity, erythrocyte** D69.2
**Autosensitization, cutaneous** L3Ø.2
**Autosome** — *see* condition by chromosome involved
**Autotopagnosia** R48.1
**Autotoxemia** R68.89
**Autumn** — *see* condition
**Avellis' syndrome** G46.8
**Aversion**
- oral R63.39
  - newborn P92.8
  - nonorganic origin F98.2- ☑
- sexual F52.1

**Aviator's**
- disease or sickness — *see* Effect, adverse, high altitude
- ear T7Ø.Ø- ☑

**Avitaminosis** (multiple) — *see also* Deficiency, vitamin E56.9
- B E53.9
  - with
    - beriberi E51.11
    - pellagra E52
- B2 E53.Ø
- B6 E53.1
- B12 E53.8
- D E55.9
  - with rickets E55.Ø
- G E53.Ø
- K E56.1
- nicotinic acid E52

**AVNRT** (atrioventricular nodal re-entrant tachycardia) I47.19
**AVRT** (atrioventricular nodal re-entrant tachycardia) I47.19
**Avulsion** (traumatic)
- blood vessel — *see* Injury, blood vessel
- bone — *see* Fracture, by site
- cartilage — *see also* Dislocation, by site
  - symphyseal (inner), complicating delivery O71.6
- external site other than limb — *see* Wound, open, by site
- eye SØ5.7- ☑
- head (intracranial)
  - external site NEC SØ8.89- ☑
  - scalp SØ8.Ø- ☑
- internal organ or site — *see* Injury, by site
- joint — *see also* Dislocation, by site
  - capsule — *see* Sprain, by site
- kidney S37.Ø6- ☑
- ligament — *see* Sprain, by site
- limb — *see also* Amputation, traumatic, by site
  - skin and subcutaneous tissue — *see* Wound, open, by site
- muscle — *see* Injury, muscle
- nerve (root) — *see* Injury, nerve
- scalp SØ8.Ø- ☑
- skin and subcutaneous tissue — *see* Wound, open, by site
- spleen S36.Ø32- ☑
- symphyseal cartilage (inner), complicating delivery O71.6
- tendon — *see* Injury, muscle
- tooth SØ3.2- ☑

**Awareness of heart beat** RØØ.2
**Axenfeld's**
- anomaly or syndrome Q15.Ø
- degeneration (calcareous) Q13.4

**Axilla, axillary** — *see also* condition
- breast Q83.1

**Axonotmesis** — *see* Injury, nerve
**Ayerza's disease or syndrome** (pulmonary artery sclerosis with pulmonary hypertension) I27.Ø
**Azoospermia** (organic) N46.Ø1
- due to
  - drug therapy N46.Ø21
  - efferent duct obstruction N46.Ø23
  - infection N46.Ø22
  - radiation N46.Ø24
  - specified cause NEC N46.Ø29
  - systemic disease N46.Ø25

**Azotemia** R79.89
- meaning uremia N19

**Aztec ear** Q17.3
**Azygos**
- continuation inferior vena cava Q26.8
- lobe (lung) Q33.1

# B

**Baastrup's disease** — *see* Kissing spine
**Babesiosis** B6Ø.ØØ
- due to
  - Babesia
    - divergens B6Ø.Ø3
    - duncani B6Ø.Ø2
    - KO-1 B6Ø.Ø9
    - microti B6Ø.Ø1
    - MO-1 B6Ø.Ø3
    - species
      - unspecified B6Ø.ØØ
    - venatorum B6Ø.Ø9
  - specified NEC B6Ø.Ø9

**Babington's disease** (familial hemorrhagic telangiectasia) I78.Ø
**Babinski's syndrome** A52.79
**Baby**
- crying constantly R68.11
- floppy (syndrome) P94.2

**Bacillary** — *see* condition
**Bacilluria** R82.71
**Bacillus** — *see also* Infection, bacillus
- abortus infection A23.1
- anthracis infection A22.9
- coli infection — *see also* Escherichia coli B96.2Ø
- Flexner's AØ3.1
- mallei infection A24.Ø
- Shiga's AØ3.Ø
- suipestifer infection — *see* Infection, salmonella

**Back** — *see* condition
**Backache** (postural) M54.9
- sacroiliac M53.3
- specified NEC M54.89

**Backflow** — *see* Reflux
**Backward reading** (dyslexia) F81.Ø
**Bacteremia** R78.81
- with sepsis — *see* Sepsis

**Bactericholia** — *see* Cholecystitis, acute
**Bacterid, bacteride** (pustular) L4Ø.3
**Bacterium, bacteria, bacterial**
- agent NEC, as cause of disease classified elsewhere B96.89
- in blood — *see* Bacteremia
- in urine — *see* Bacteriuria

**Bacteriuria, bacteruria** (asymptomatic) R82.71
**Bacteroides**
- fragilis, as cause of disease classified elsewhere B96.6

**Bad**
- heart — *see* Disease, heart
- trip
  - due to drug abuse — *see* Abuse, drug, hallucinogen
  - due to drug dependence — *see* Dependence, drug, hallucinogen

**Baelz's disease** (cheilitis glandularis apostematosa) K13.Ø
**Baerensprung's disease** (eczema marginatum) B35.6
**Bagasse disease or pneumonitis** J67.1
**Bagassosis** J67.1
**Baker's cyst** — *see* Cyst, Baker's
**Bakwin-Krida syndrome** (metaphyseal dysplasia) Q78.5
**Balancing side interference** M26.56
**Balanitis** (circinata) (erosiva) (gangrenosa) (phagedenic) (vulgaris) N48.1
- amebic AØ6.82
- candidal B37.42
- due to Haemophilus ducreyi A57
- gonococcal (acute) (chronic) A54.23
- xerotica obliterans N48.Ø

**Balanoposthitis** N47.6
- gonococcal (acute) (chronic) A54.23
- ulcerative (specific) A63.8

**Balanorrhagia** — *see* Balanitis
**Balantidiasis, balantidiosis** AØ7.Ø
**Bald tongue** K14.4
**Baldness** — *see also* Alopecia
- male-pattern — *see* Alopecia, androgenic

**Balkan grippe** A78
**Ball, pulmonary fungal** J4B
**Balloon disease** — *see* Effect, adverse, high altitude
**Balo's disease** (concentric sclerosis) G37.5
**Bamberger-Marie disease** — *see* Osteoarthropathy, hypertrophic, specified type NEC
**Bancroft's filariasis** B74.Ø

**Band**(s)
- adhesive — *see* Adhesions, peritoneum
- anomalous or congenital — *see also* Anomaly, by site
  - heart (atrial) (ventricular) Q24.8
  - intestine Q43.3
  - omentum Q43.3
- cervix N88.1
- constricting, congenital Q79.8
- gallbladder (congenital) Q44.1
- intestinal (adhesive) — *see* Adhesions, peritoneum
- obstructive
  - intestine K56.5Ø
    - complete K56.52
    - incomplete K56.51
    - partial K56.51
  - peritoneum K56.5Ø
    - complete K56.52
    - incomplete K56.51
    - partial K56.51
- periappendiceal, congenital Q43.3
- peritoneal (adhesive) — *see* Adhesions, peritoneum
- uterus N73.6
  - internal N85.6
- vagina N89.5

**Bandemia** D72.825
**Bandl's ring** (contraction), complicating delivery O62.4
**Bangkok hemorrhagic fever** A91
**Bang's disease** (brucella abortus) A23.1
**Bankruptcy** (anxiety concerning) Z59.868
**Bannister's disease** T78.3- ☑
- hereditary D84.1

**Banti's disease or syndrome** (with cirrhosis) (with portal hypertension) K76.6
**Bar, median, prostate** — *see* Enlargement, enlarged, prostate
**Barcoo disease or rot** — *see* Ulcer, skin
**Barlow's disease** E54
**Barodontalgia** T7Ø.29- ☑
**Baron Munchausen syndrome** — *see* Disorder, factitious
**Barosinusitis** T7Ø.1- ☑
**Barotitis** T7Ø.Ø- ☑
**Barotrauma** T7Ø.29- ☑
- odontalgia T7Ø.29- ☑
- otitic T7Ø.Ø- ☑
- sinus T7Ø.1- ☑

**Barraquer** (-Simons) **disease or syndrome** (progressive lipodystrophy) E88.11
**Barre-Guillain disease or syndrome** G61.Ø
**Barre-Lieou syndrome** (posterior cervical sympathetic) M53.Ø
**Barrel chest** M95.4
**Barrett's**
- disease — *see* Barrett's, esophagus
- esophagus K22.7Ø
  - with dysplasia K22.719
    - high grade K22.711
    - low grade K22.71Ø
  - without dysplasia K22.7Ø
- syndrome — *see* Barrett's, esophagus
- ulcer K22.1Ø
  - with bleeding K22.11
  - without bleeding K22.1Ø

**Barsony** (-Polgar) (-Teschendorf) **syndrome** (corkscrew esophagus) K22.4
**Barth syndrome** E78.71
**Bartholinitis** (suppurating) N75.8
- gonococcal (acute) (chronic) (with abscess) A54.1

**Bartonellosis** A44.9
- cutaneous A44.1
- mucocutaneous A44.1
- specified NEC A44.8
- systemic A44.Ø

**Barton's fracture** S52.56- ☑
**Bartter's syndrome** E26.81
**Basal** — *see* condition
**Basan's** (hidrotic) ectodermal dysplasia Q82.4
**Baseball finger** — *see* Dislocation, finger
**Basedow's disease** (exophthalmic goiter) — *see* Hyperthyroidism, with, goiter
**Basic** — *see* condition
**Basilar** — *see* condition
**Bason's** (hidrotic) ectodermal dysplasia Q82.4
**Basopenia** — *see* Agranulocytosis
**Basophilia** D72.824
**Basophilism** (cortico-adrenal) (Cushing's) (pituitary) E24.Ø
**Bassen-Kornzweig disease or syndrome** E78.6
**Bat ear** Q17.5
**Bateman's**
- disease B Ø8.1
- purpura (senile) D69.2

**Bathing cramp** T75.1- ☑
**Bathophobia** F4Ø.248
**Batten** (-Mayou) **disease** E75.4
- retina E75.4 *[H36.89]*

**Batten-Steinert syndrome** G71.11
**Battered** — *see* Maltreatment
**Battey Mycobacterium infection** A31.Ø
**Battle exhaustion** F43.Ø
**Battledore placenta** O43.19- ☑
**Baumgarten-Cruveilhier cirrhosis, disease or syndrome** K74.69
**Bauxite fibrosis** (of lung) J63.1
**Bayle's disease** (general paresis) A52.17
**Bazin's disease** (primary) (tuberculous) A18.4
**Beach ear** — *see* Swimmer's, ear
**Beaded hair** (congenital) Q84.1
**Beal conjunctivitis or syndrome** B3Ø.2
**Beard's disease** (neurasthenia) F48.8
**Beat**(s)
- atrial, premature I49.1
- ectopic I49.49
- elbow — *see* Bursitis, elbow
- escaped, heart I49.49
- hand — *see* Bursitis, hand
- knee — *see* Bursitis, knee
- premature I49.4Ø
  - atrial I49.1
  - auricular I49.1
  - supraventricular I49.1

**Beau's**
- disease or syndrome — *see* Degeneration, myocardial
- lines (transverse furrows on fingernails) L6Ø.4

**Bechterev's syndrome** — *see* Spondylitis, ankylosing
**Becker's**
- cardiomyopathy I42.89
- disease
  - idiopathic mural endomyocardial disease I42.3
  - myotonia congenita, recessive form G71.12
- dystrophy G71.Ø1
- pigmented hairy nevus D22.5

**Beck's syndrome** (anterior spinal artery occlusion) I65.8
**Beckwith-Wiedemann syndrome** Q87.3
**Bed confinement status** Z74.Ø1
**Bed-sharing, infant** Z72.823
**Bed sore** — *see* Ulcer, pressure, by site
**Bedbug bite**(s) — *see* Bite(s), by site, superficial, insect
**Bedclothes, asphyxiation or suffocation by** — *see* Asphyxia, traumatic, due to, mechanical, trapped
**Bednar's**
- aphthae K12.Ø
- tumor — *see* Neoplasm, malignant, by site

**Bedridden** Z74.Ø1
**Bedsore** — *see* Ulcer, pressure, by site
**Bedwetting** — *see* Enuresis
**Bee sting** (with allergic or anaphylactic shock) T63.44- ☑
**Beer drinker's heart** (disease) I42.6
**Begbie's disease** (exophthalmic goiter) — *see* Hyperthyroidism, with, goiter
**Behavior**
- antisocial
  - adult Z72.811
  - child or adolescent Z72.81Ø
- disorder, disturbance — *see* Disorder, conduct
- disruptive — *see* Disorder, conduct
- drug seeking Z76.5
- inexplicable R46.2
- marked evasiveness R46.5
- obsessive-compulsive R46.81
- overactivity R46.3
- poor responsiveness R46.4
- self-damaging (life-style) Z72.89
- sleep-incompatible Z72.821
- slowness R46.4
- specified NEC R46.89
- strange (and inexplicable) R46.2
- suspiciousness R46.5
- type A pattern Z73.1
- undue concern or preoccupation with stressful events R46.6
- verbosity and circumstantial detail obscuring reason for contact R46.7

**Behcet's disease or syndrome** M35.2
**Behr's disease** — *see* Degeneration, macula
**Beigel's disease or morbus** (white piedra) B36.2
**Bejel** A65
**Bekhterev's syndrome** — *see* Spondylitis, ankylosing
**Belching** — *see* Eructation
**Bell's**
- mania F3Ø.8
- palsy, paralysis G51.Ø
  - infant or newborn P11.3
- spasm G51.3- ☑

**Bence Jones albuminuria or proteinuria NEC** R8Ø.3
**Bends** T7Ø.3- ☑
**Benedikt's paralysis or syndrome** G46.3
**Benign** — *see also* condition
- prostatic hyperplasia — *see* Hyperplasia, prostate

**Bennett's fracture** (displaced) S62.21- ☑
**Benson's disease** — *see* Deposit, crystalline
**Bent**
- back (hysterical) F44.4
- nose M95.Ø
  - congenital Q67.4

**Bereavement** (uncomplicated) Z63.4
**Bergeron's disease** (hysterical chorea) F44.4
**Berger's disease** — *see* Nephropathy, IgA
**Beriberi** (dry) E51.11
- heart (disease) E51.12
- polyneuropathy E51.11
- wet E51.12
  - involving circulatory system E51.11

**Berlin's disease or edema** (traumatic) SØ5.8X- ☑
**Berlock** (berloque) **dermatitis** L56.2
**Bernard-Horner syndrome** G9Ø.2
**Bernard-Soulier disease or thrombopathia** D69.19
**Bernhardt** (-Roth) **disease** — *see* Mononeuropathy, lower limb, meralgia paresthetica
**Bernheim's syndrome** — *see* Failure, heart, right
**Bertielliasis** B71.8
**Berylliosis** (lung) J63.2
**Besnier-Boeck** (-Schaumann) **disease** — *see* Sarcoidosis
**Besnier's**
- lupus pernio D86.3
- prurigo L2Ø.Ø

**Bestiality** F65.89
**Best's disease** H35.5Ø
**Beta-mercaptolactate-cysteine disulfiduria** E72.Ø9
**Betalipoproteinemia, broad or floating** E78.2
**Betting and gambling** Z72.6
- pathological (compulsive) F63.Ø

**Bezoar** T18.9- ☑
- intestine T18.3- ☑
- stomach T18.2- ☑

**Bezold's abscess** — *see* Mastoiditis, acute
**BI-RADS** — *see* Breast, Imaging Reporting and Data System
**Bianchi's syndrome** R48.8
**Bicornate or bicornis uterus** Q51.3
- in pregnancy or childbirth O34.ØØ
  - causing obstructed labor O65.5

**Bicuspid aortic valve** (at birth) (congenital) Q23.81
- functional, with stenosis — *see* Stenosis, aortic (valve)

**Biedl-Bardet syndrome** Q87.83
**Bielschowsky** (-Jansky) disease E75.4
**Biermer's** (pernicious) anemia or disease D51.Ø
**Biett's disease** L93.Ø
**Bifid** (congenital)
- apex, heart Q24.8
- clitoris Q52.6
- kidney Q63.8
- nose Q3Ø.2
- patella Q74.1
- scrotum Q55.29
- toe NEC Q74.2
- tongue Q38.3
- ureter Q62.8
- uterus Q51.3
- uvula Q35.7

**Biforis uterus** (suprasimplex) Q51.3
**Bifurcation** (congenital)
- gallbladder Q44.1
- kidney pelvis Q63.8
- renal pelvis Q63.8
- rib Q76.6
- tongue, congenital Q38.3
- trachea Q32.1
- ureter Q62.8
- urethra Q64.74
- vertebra Q76.49

**Big spleen syndrome** D73.1
**Bigeminal pulse** RØØ.8
**Bigeminy, ventricular** I49.82
**Bigorexia** F45.22
**Bilateral** — *see* condition

- **Bile**
  - duct — *see* condition
  - pigments in urine R82.2
- **Bilharziasis** — *see also* Schistosomiasis
  - chyluria B65.Ø
  - cutaneous B65.3
  - galacturia B65.Ø
  - hematochyluria B65.Ø
  - intestinal B65.1
  - lipemia B65.9
  - lipuria B65.Ø
  - oriental B65.2
  - piarhemia B65.9
  - pulmonary NOS B65.9 *[J99]*
    - pneumonia B65.9 *[J17]*
  - tropical hematuria B65.Ø
  - vesical B65.Ø
- **Biliary** — *see* condition
- **Bilirubin metabolism disorder** E8Ø.7
  - specified NEC E8Ø.6
- **Bilirubinemia, familial nonhemolytic** E8Ø.4
- **Bilirubinuria** R82.2
- **Biliuria** R82.2
- **Bilocular stomach** K31.2
- **Binswanger's disease** I67.3
- **Biparta, bipartite**
  - carpal scaphoid Q74.Ø
  - patella Q74.1
  - vagina Q52.1Ø
- **Bird**
  - face Q75.8
  - fancier's disease or lung J67.2
- **Birt-Hogg-Dube syndrome** Q87.89
- **Birth**
  - complications in mother — *see* Delivery, complicated
  - compression during NOS P15.9
  - defect — *see* Anomaly
  - immature (less than 37 completed weeks) — *see* Preterm, newborn
    - extremely (less than 28 completed weeks) — *see* Immaturity, extreme
  - inattention, at or after — *see* Maltreatment, child, neglect
  - injury NOS P15.9
    - basal ganglia P11.1
    - brachial plexus NEC P14.3
    - brain (compression) (pressure) P11.2
    - central nervous system NOS P11.9
    - cerebellum P11.1
    - cerebral hemorrhage P1Ø.1
    - external genitalia P15.5
    - eye P15.3
    - face P15.4
    - fracture
      - bone P13.9
        - specified NEC P13.8
      - clavicle P13.4
      - femur P13.2
      - humerus P13.3
      - long bone, except femur P13.3
      - radius and ulna P13.3
      - skull P13.Ø
      - spine P11.5
      - tibia and fibula P13.3
    - intracranial P11.2
      - laceration or hemorrhage P1Ø.9
        - specified NEC P1Ø.8
    - intraventricular hemorrhage P1Ø.2
    - laceration
      - brain P1Ø.1
      - by scalpel P15.8
      - peripheral nerve P14.9
    - liver P15.Ø
    - meninges
      - brain P11.1
      - spinal cord P11.5
    - nerve
      - brachial plexus P14.3
      - cranial NEC (except facial) P11.4
      - facial P11.3
      - peripheral P14.9
      - phrenic (paralysis) P14.2
    - paralysis
      - facial nerve P11.3
      - spinal P11.5
    - penis P15.5
    - rupture
      - spinal cord P11.5
    - scalp P12.9
    - scalpel wound P15.8
- **Birth** — *continued*
  - injury — *continued*
    - scrotum P15.5
    - skull NEC P13.1
      - fracture P13.Ø
    - specified type NEC P15.8
    - spinal cord P11.5
    - spine P11.5
    - spleen P15.1
    - sternomastoid (hematoma) P15.2
    - subarachnoid hemorrhage P1Ø.3
    - subcutaneous fat necrosis P15.6
    - subdural hemorrhage P1Ø.Ø
    - tentorial tear P1Ø.4
    - testes P15.5
    - vulva P15.5
  - lack of care, at or after — *see* Maltreatment, child, neglect
  - neglect, at or after — *see* Maltreatment, child, neglect
  - palsy or paralysis, newborn, NOS (birth injury) P14.9
  - premature (infant) — *see* Preterm, newborn
  - shock, newborn P96.89
  - trauma — *see* Birth, injury
  - weight
    - low (2499 grams or less) — *see* Low, birthweight
      - extremely (999 grams or less) — *see* Low, birthweight, extreme
    - 4ØØØ grams to 4499 grams PØ8.1
    - 45ØØ grams or more PØ8.Ø
- **Birthmark** Q82.5
- **Bisalbuminemia** E88.Ø9
- **Biskra's button** B55.1
- **Bite**(s) (animal) (human)
  - abdomen, abdominal
    - wall S31.159- ☑
      - with penetration into peritoneal cavity S31.659- ☑
      - epigastric region S31.152- ☑
        - with penetration into peritoneal cavity S31.652- ☑
      - left
        - lower quadrant S31.154- ☑
          - with penetration into peritoneal cavity S31.654- ☑
        - upper quadrant S31.151- ☑
          - with penetration into peritoneal cavity S31.651- ☑
      - periumbilic region S31.155- ☑
        - with penetration into peritoneal cavity S31.655- ☑
      - right
        - lower quadrant S31.153- ☑
          - with penetration into peritoneal cavity S31.653- ☑
        - upper quadrant S31.15Ø- ☑
          - with penetration into peritoneal cavity S31.65Ø- ☑
      - superficial NEC S3Ø.871- ☑
        - insect S3Ø.861- ☑
  - alveolar (process) — *see* Bite, oral cavity
  - amphibian (venomous) — *see* Table of Drugs and Chemicals, by animal or substance, poisoning
  - animal — *see also* Bite, by site
    - venomous — *see* Table of Drugs and Chemicals, by animal or substance, poisoning
  - ankle S91.Ø5- ☑
    - superficial NEC S9Ø.57- ☑
      - insect S9Ø.56- ☑
  - antecubital space — *see* Bite, elbow
  - anus S31.835- ☑
    - superficial NEC S3Ø.877- ☑
      - insect S3Ø.867- ☑
  - arm (upper) S41.15- ☑
    - lower — *see* Bite, forearm
    - superficial NEC S4Ø.87- ☑
      - insect S4Ø.86- ☑
  - arthropod NEC — *see* Table of Drugs and Chemicals, by animal or substance, poisoning
  - auditory canal (external) (meatus) — *see* Bite, ear
  - auricle, ear — *see* Bite, ear
  - axilla — *see* Bite, arm
  - back — *see also* Bite, thorax, back
    - lower S31.Ø5Ø- ☑
      - with penetration into retroperitoneal space S31.Ø51- ☑
      - superficial NEC S3Ø.87Ø- ☑
        - insect S3Ø.86Ø- ☑
  - bedbug — *see* Bite(s), by site, superficial, insect
  - breast S21.Ø5- ☑
- **Bite**(s) — *continued*
  - breast — *continued*
    - superficial NEC S2Ø.17- ☑
      - insect S2Ø.16- ☑
  - brow — *see* Bite, head, specified site NEC
  - buttock S31.8Ø5- ☑
    - left S31.825- ☑
    - right S31.815- ☑
    - superficial NEC S3Ø.87Ø- ☑
      - insect S3Ø.86Ø- ☑
  - calf — *see* Bite, leg
  - canaliculus lacrimalis — *see* Bite, eyelid
  - canthus, eye — *see* Bite, eyelid
  - centipede — *see* Table of Drugs and Chemicals, by animal or substance, poisoning
  - cheek (external) SØ1.45- ☑
    - internal — *see* Bite, oral cavity
    - superficial NEC SØØ.87- ☑
      - insect SØØ.86- ☑
  - chest wall — *see* Bite, thorax
  - chigger B88.Ø9
  - chin — *see* Bite, head, specified site NEC
  - clitoris — *see* Bite, vulva
  - costal region — *see* Bite, thorax
  - digit(s)
    - hand — *see* Bite, finger
    - toe — *see* Bite, toe
  - ear (canal) (external) SØ1.35- ☑
    - superficial NEC SØØ.47- ☑
      - insect SØØ.46- ☑
  - elbow S51.Ø5- ☑
    - superficial NEC S5Ø.37- ☑
      - insect S5Ø.36- ☑
  - epididymis — *see* Bite, testis
  - epigastric region — *see* Bite, abdomen
  - epiglottis — *see* Bite, neck, specified site NEC
  - esophagus, cervical S11.25- ☑
    - superficial NEC S1Ø.17- ☑
      - insect S1Ø.16- ☑
  - eyebrow — *see* Bite, eyelid
  - eyelid SØ1.15- ☑
    - superficial NEC SØØ.27- ☑
      - insect SØØ.26- ☑
  - face NEC — *see* Bite, head, specified site NEC
  - finger(s) S61.259- ☑
    - with
      - damage to nail S61.359- ☑
    - index S61.258- ☑
      - with
        - damage to nail S61.358- ☑
      - left S61.251- ☑
        - with
          - damage to nail S61.351- ☑
      - right S61.25Ø- ☑
        - with
          - damage to nail S61.35Ø- ☑
      - superficial NEC S6Ø.478- ☑
        - insect S6Ø.46- ☑
    - little S61.25- ☑
      - with
        - damage to nail S61.35- ☑
      - superficial NEC S6Ø.47- ☑
        - insect S6Ø.46- ☑
    - middle S61.25- ☑
      - with
        - damage to nail S61.35- ☑
      - superficial NEC S6Ø.47- ☑
        - insect S6Ø.46- ☑
    - ring S61.25- ☑
      - with
        - damage to nail S61.35- ☑
      - superficial NEC S6Ø.47- ☑
        - insect S6Ø.46- ☑
    - superficial NEC S6Ø.479- ☑
      - insect S6Ø.469- ☑
    - thumb — *see* Bite, thumb
  - flank S31.15A- ☑
    - with penetration into peritoneal cavity S31.65A- ☑
    - left S31.157- ☑
      - with penetration into peritoneal cavity S31.657- ☑
    - right S31.156- ☑
      - with penetration into peritoneal cavity S31.656- ☑
    - superficial S3Ø.87A- ☑
      - insect S3Ø.86A- ☑
  - flea — *see* Bite, by site, superficial, insect
  - foot (except toe(s) alone) S91.35- ☑

**Bite**(s) — *continued*
- foot(s alone) — *continued*
  - superficial NEC S9Ø.87- ☑
    - insect S9Ø.86- ☑
  - toe — *see* Bite, toe
- forearm S51.85- ☑
  - elbow only — *see* Bite, elbow
  - superficial NEC S5Ø.87- ☑
    - insect S5Ø.86- ☑
- forehead — *see* Bite, head, specified site NEC
- genital organs, external
  - female S31.552- ☑
    - superficial NEC S3Ø.876- ☑
      - insect S3Ø.866- ☑
    - vagina and vulva — *see* Bite, vulva
  - male S31.551- ☑
    - penis — *see* Bite, penis
    - scrotum — *see* Bite, scrotum
    - superficial NEC S3Ø.875- ☑
      - insect S3Ø.865- ☑
    - testes — *see* Bite, testis
- groin — *see* Bite, abdomen, wall
- gum — *see* Bite, oral cavity
- hand S61.45- ☑
  - finger — *see* Bite, finger
  - superficial NEC S6Ø.57- ☑
    - insect S6Ø.56- ☑
  - thumb — *see* Bite, thumb
- head SØ1.95- ☑
  - cheek — *see* Bite, cheek
  - ear — *see* Bite, ear
  - eyelid — *see* Bite, eyelid
  - lip — *see* Bite, lip
  - nose — *see* Bite, nose
  - oral cavity — *see* Bite, oral cavity
  - scalp — *see* Bite, scalp
  - specified site NEC SØ1.85- ☑
    - superficial NEC SØØ.87- ☑
      - insect SØØ.86- ☑
  - superficial NEC SØØ.97- ☑
    - insect SØØ.96- ☑
  - temporomandibular area — *see* Bite, cheek
- heel — *see* Bite, foot
- hip S71.Ø5- ☑
  - superficial NEC S7Ø.27- ☑
    - insect S7Ø.26- ☑
- hymen S31.45- ☑
- hypochondrium — *see* Bite, abdomen, wall
- hypogastric region — *see* Bite, abdomen, wall
- inguinal region — *see* Bite, abdomen, wall
- insect — *see* Bite, by site, superficial, insect
- instep — *see* Bite, foot
- interscapular region — *see* Bite, thorax, back
- jaw — *see* Bite, head, specified site NEC
- knee S81.Ø5- ☑
  - superficial NEC S8Ø.27- ☑
    - insect S8Ø.26- ☑
- labium (majus) (minus) — *see* Bite, vulva
- lacrimal duct — *see* Bite, eyelid
- larynx S11.Ø15- ☑
  - superficial NEC S1Ø.17- ☑
    - insect S1Ø.16- ☑
- leg (lower) S81.85- ☑
  - ankle — *see* Bite, ankle
  - foot — *see* Bite, foot
  - knee — *see* Bite, knee
  - superficial NEC S8Ø.87- ☑
    - insect S8Ø.86- ☑
  - toe — *see* Bite, toe
  - upper — *see* Bite, thigh
- lip SØ1.551- ☑
  - superficial NEC SØØ.571- ☑
    - insect SØØ.561- ☑
- lizard (venomous) — *see* Table of Drugs and Chemicals, by animal or substance, poisoning
- loin — *see* Bite, abdomen, wall
- lower back — *see* Bite, back, lower
- lumbar region — *see* Bite, back, lower
- malar region — *see* Bite, head, specified site NEC
- mammary — *see* Bite, breast
- marine animals (venomous) — *see* Table of Drugs and Chemicals, by animal or substance, poisoning
- mastoid region — *see* Bite, head, specified site NEC
- mouth — *see* Bite, oral cavity
- nail
  - finger — *see* Bite, finger
  - toe — *see* Bite, toe

**Bite**(s) — *continued*
- nape — *see* Bite, neck, specified site NEC
- nasal (septum) (sinus) — *see* Bite, nose
- nasopharynx — *see* Bite, head, specified site NEC
- neck S11.95- ☑
  - involving
    - cervical esophagus — *see* Bite, esophagus, cervical
    - larynx — *see* Bite, larynx
    - pharynx — *see* Bite, pharynx
    - thyroid gland S11.15- ☑
    - trachea — *see* Bite, trachea
  - specified site NEC S11.85- ☑
    - superficial NEC S1Ø.87- ☑
      - insect S1Ø.86- ☑
  - superficial NEC S1Ø.97- ☑
    - insect S1Ø.96- ☑
  - throat S11.85- ☑
    - superficial NEC S1Ø.17- ☑
      - insect S1Ø.16- ☑
- nose (septum) (sinus) SØ1.25- ☑
  - superficial NEC SØØ.37- ☑
    - insect SØØ.36- ☑
- occipital region — *see* Bite, scalp
- oral cavity SØ1.552- ☑
  - superficial NEC SØØ.572- ☑
    - insect SØØ.562- ☑
- orbital region — *see* Bite, eyelid
- palate — *see* Bite, oral cavity
- palm — *see* Bite, hand
- parietal region — *see* Bite, scalp
- pelvis S31.Ø5Ø- ☑
  - with penetration into retroperitoneal space S31.Ø51- ☑
  - superficial NEC S3Ø.87Ø- ☑
    - insect S3Ø.86Ø- ☑
- penis S31.25- ☑
  - superficial NEC S3Ø.872- ☑
    - insect S3Ø.862- ☑
- perineum
  - female — *see* Bite, vulva
  - male — *see* Bite, pelvis
- periocular area (with or without lacrimal passages) — *see* Bite, eyelid
- phalanges
  - finger — *see* Bite, finger
  - toe — *see* Bite, toe
- pharynx S11.25- ☑
  - superficial NEC S1Ø.17- ☑
    - insect S1Ø.16- ☑
- pinna — *see* Bite, ear
- poisonous — *see* Table of Drugs and Chemicals, by animal or substance, poisoning
- popliteal space — *see* Bite, knee
- prepuce — *see* Bite, penis
- pubic region — *see* Bite, abdomen, wall
- rectovaginal septum — *see* Bite, vulva
- red bug B88.Ø9
- reptile NEC — *see* Table of Drugs and Chemicals, by animal or substance, poisoning
  - snake — *see* Table of Drugs and Chemicals, by animal or substance, poisoning
- sacral region — *see* Bite, back, lower
- sacroiliac region — *see* Bite, back, lower
- salivary gland — *see* Bite, oral cavity
- scalp SØ1.Ø5- ☑
  - superficial NEC SØØ.Ø7- ☑
    - insect SØØ.Ø6- ☑
- scapular region — *see* Bite, shoulder
- scrotum S31.35- ☑
  - superficial NEC S3Ø.873- ☑
    - insect S3Ø.863- ☑
- sea-snake (venomous) — *see* Table of Drugs and Chemicals, by animal or substance, poisoning
- shin — *see* Bite, leg
- shoulder S41.Ø5- ☑
  - superficial NEC S4Ø.27- ☑
    - insect S4Ø.26- ☑
- snake — *see also* Table of Drugs and Chemicals, by animal or substance, poisoning
- spermatic cord — *see* Bite, testis
- spider (venomous) — *see* Table of Drugs and Chemicals, by animal or substance, poisoning
- sternal region — *see* Bite, thorax, front
- submaxillary region — *see* Bite, head, specified site NEC
- submental region — *see* Bite, head, specified site NEC
- subungual
  - finger(s) — *see* Bite, finger

**Bite**(s) — *continued*
- subungual — *continued*
  - toe — *see* Bite, toe
- superficial — *see* Bite, by site, superficial
- supraclavicular fossa S11.85- ☑
- supraorbital — *see* Bite, head, specified site NEC
- temple, temporal region — *see* Bite, head, specified site NEC
- temporomandibular area — *see* Bite, cheek
- testis S31.35- ☑
  - superficial NEC S3Ø.873- ☑
    - insect S3Ø.863- ☑
- thigh S71.15- ☑
  - superficial NEC S7Ø.37- ☑
    - insect S7Ø.36- ☑
- thorax, thoracic (wall) S21.95- ☑
  - back S21.25- ☑
    - with penetration into thoracic cavity S21.45- ☑
  - breast — *see* Bite, breast
  - front S21.15- ☑
    - with penetration into thoracic cavity S21.35- ☑
  - superficial NEC S2Ø.97- ☑
    - back S2Ø.47- ☑
    - front S2Ø.37- ☑
    - insect S2Ø.96- ☑
      - back S2Ø.46- ☑
      - front S2Ø.36- ☑
- throat — *see* Bite, neck, throat
- thumb S61.Ø5- ☑
  - with
    - damage to nail S61.15- ☑
  - superficial NEC S6Ø.37- ☑
    - insect S6Ø.36- ☑
- thyroid S11.15- ☑
  - superficial NEC S1Ø.87- ☑
    - insect S1Ø.86- ☑
- toe(s) S91.15- ☑
  - with
    - damage to nail S91.25- ☑
  - great S91.15- ☑
    - with
      - damage to nail S91.25- ☑
  - lesser S91.15- ☑
    - with
      - damage to nail S91.25- ☑
  - superficial NEC S9Ø.47- ☑
    - great S9Ø.47- ☑
    - insect S9Ø.46- ☑
      - great S9Ø.46- ☑
- tongue SØ1.552- ☑
- trachea S11.Ø25- ☑
  - superficial NEC S1Ø.17- ☑
    - insect S1Ø.16- ☑
- tunica vaginalis — *see* Bite, testis
- tympanum, tympanic membrane — *see* Bite, ear
- umbilical region S31.155- ☑
- uvula — *see* Bite, oral cavity
- vagina — *see* Bite, vulva
- venomous — *see* Table of Drugs and Chemicals, by animal or substance, poisoning
- vocal cords S11.Ø35- ☑
  - superficial NEC S1Ø.17- ☑
    - insect S1Ø.16- ☑
- vulva S31.45- ☑
  - superficial NEC S3Ø.874- ☑
    - insect S3Ø.864- ☑
- wrist S61.55- ☑
  - superficial NEC S6Ø.87- ☑
    - insect S6Ø.86- ☑
  - nonvenomous — *see* Bite, by site
  - nonvenomous — *see* Bite, by site
  - nonvenomous — *see* Bite, by site, superficial, insect

**Biting, cheek or lip** K13.1

**Biventricular failure** (heart) I5Ø.82

**Bjorck** (-Thorson) **syndrome** (malignant carcinoid) E34.Ø9

**Black**
- death A2Ø.9
- eye SØØ.1- ☑
- hairy tongue K14.3
- heel (foot) S9Ø.3- ☑
- lung (disease) J6Ø
- palm (hand) S6Ø.22- ☑

**Blackfan-Diamond anemia or syndrome** (congenital hypoplastic anemia) D61.Ø1

**Blackhead** L7Ø.Ø

**Blackout** R55

**Bladder** — *see* condition
**Blast** (air) (hydraulic) (immersion) (underwater)
  blindness SØ5.8X- ☑
  injury
    abdomen or thorax — *see* Injury, by site
    ear (acoustic nerve trauma) — *see* Injury, nerve, acoustic, specified type NEC
    syndrome NEC T7Ø.8- ☑
**Blastoma** — *see* Neoplasm, malignant, by site
  pulmonary — *see* Neoplasm, lung, malignant
**Blastomycosis, blastomycotic** B4Ø.9
  Brazilian — *see* Paracoccidioidomycosis
  cutaneous B4Ø.3
  disseminated B4Ø.7
  European — *see* Cryptococcosis
  generalized B4Ø.7
  keloidal B48.Ø
  North American B4Ø.9
  primary pulmonary B4Ø.Ø
  pulmonary B4Ø.2
    acute B4Ø.Ø
    chronic B4Ø.1
  skin B4Ø.3
  South American — *see* Paracoccidioidomycosis
  specified NEC B4Ø.89
**Bleb**(s) R23.8
  emphysematous (lung) (solitary) J43.9
  endophthalmitis H59.43
  filtering (vitreous), after glaucoma surgery Z98.83
  inflamed (infected), postprocedural H59.4Ø
    stage 1 H59.41
    stage 2 H59.42
    stage 3 H59.43
  lung (ruptured) J43.9
    congenital — *see* Atelectasis
    newborn P25.8
  subpleural (emphysematous) J43.9
**Blebitis, postprocedural** H59.4Ø
  stage 1 H59.41
  stage 2 H59.42
  stage 3 H59.43
**Bleeder** (familial) (hereditary) — *see* Hemophilia
**Bleeding** — *see also* Hemorrhage
  anal K62.5
  anovulatory N97.Ø
  atonic, following delivery O72.1
  capillary I78.8
    puerperal O72.2
  contact (postcoital) N93.Ø
  due to uterine subinvolution N85.3
  ear — *see* Otorrhagia
  excessive, associated with menopausal onset N92.4
  familial — *see* Defect, coagulation
  following intercourse N93.Ø
  gastrointestinal K92.2
  hemorrhoids — *see* Hemorrhoids
  intermenstrual (regular) N92.3
    irregular N92.1
  intraoperative — *see* Complication, intraoperative, hemorrhage
  irregular N92.6
  menopausal N92.4
  newborn, intraventricular — *see* Newborn, affected by, hemorrhage, intraventricular
  nipple N64.59
  nose RØ4.Ø
  ovulation N92.3
  perimenopausal N92.4
  postclimacteric N95.Ø
  postcoital N93.Ø
  postmenopausal N95.Ø
  postoperative — *see* Complication, postprocedural, hemorrhage
  preclimacteric N92.4
  pre-pubertal vaginal N93.1
  puberty (excessive, with onset of menstrual periods) N92.2
  rectum, rectal K62.5
    newborn P54.2
  tendencies — *see* Defect, coagulation
  throat RØ4.1
  tooth socket (post-extraction) K91.84Ø
  umbilical stump P51.9
  uterus, uterine NEC N93.9
    climacteric N92.4
    dysfunctional or functional N93.8
    menopausal N92.4
    preclimacteric or premenopausal N92.4
    unrelated to menstrual cycle N93.9

**Bleeding** — *continued*
  vagina, vaginal (abnormal) N93.9
    dysfunctional or functional N93.8
    newborn P54.6
    pre-pubertal N93.1
  vicarious N94.89
**Blennorrhagia, blennorrhagic** — *see* Gonorrhea
**Blennorrhea** (acute) (chronic) — *see also* Gonorrhea
  inclusion (neonatal) (newborn) P39.1
  lower genitourinary tract (gonococcal) A54.ØØ
  neonatorum (gonococcal ophthalmia) A54.31
**Blepharelosis** — *see* Entropion
**Blepharitis** (angularis) (ciliaris) (eyelid) (marginal) (nonulcerative) HØ1.ØØ9
  herpes zoster BØ2.39
  left HØ1.ØØ6
    lower HØ1.ØØ5
    upper HØ1.ØØ4
    upper and lower HØ1.ØØB
  right HØ1.ØØ3
    lower HØ1.ØØ2
    upper HØ1.ØØ1
    upper and lower HØ1.ØØA
  squamous HØ1.Ø29
    left HØ1.Ø26
      lower HØ1.Ø25
      upper HØ1.Ø24
      upper and lower HØ1.Ø2B
    right HØ1.Ø23
      lower HØ1.Ø22
      upper HØ1.Ø21
      upper and lower HØ1.Ø2A
  ulcerative HØ1.Ø19
    left HØ1.Ø16
      lower HØ1.Ø15
      upper HØ1.Ø14
      upper and lower HØ1.Ø1B
    right HØ1.Ø13
      lower HØ1.Ø12
      upper HØ1.Ø11
      upper and lower HØ1.Ø1A
**Blepharochalasis** HØ2.3Ø
  congenital Q1Ø.Ø
  left HØ2.36
    lower HØ2.35
    upper HØ2.34
  right HØ2.33
    lower HØ2.32
    upper HØ2.31
**Blepharoclonus** HØ2.59
**Blepharoconjunctivitis** H1Ø.5Ø- ☑
  angular H1Ø.52- ☑
  contact H1Ø.53- ☑
  ligneous H1Ø.51- ☑
**Blepharophimosis** (eyelid) HØ2.529
  congenital Q1Ø.3
  left HØ2.526
    lower HØ2.525
    upper HØ2.524
  right HØ2.523
    lower HØ2.522
    upper HØ2.521
**Blepharoptosis** HØ2.4Ø- ☑
  congenital Q1Ø.Ø
  mechanical HØ2.41- ☑
  myogenic HØ2.42- ☑
  neurogenic HØ2.43- ☑
  paralytic HØ2.43- ☑
**Blepharopyorrhea, gonococcal** A54.39
**Blepharospasm** G24.5
  drug induced G24.Ø1
**Blighted ovum** OØ2.Ø
**Blind** — *see also* Blindness
  bronchus (congenital) Q32.4
  loop syndrome K9Ø.2
    congenital Q43.8
  sac, fallopian tube (congenital) Q5Ø.6
  spot, enlarged — *see* Defect, visual field, localized, scotoma, blind spot area
  tract or tube, congenital NEC — *see* Atresia, by site
**Blindness** (acquired) (congenital) (both eyes) H54.ØX- ☑
  blast SØ5.8X- ☑
  color — *see* Deficiency, color vision
  concussion SØ5.8X- ☑
  cortical H47.619
    left brain H47.612
    right brain H47.611
  day H53.11

**Blindness** — *continued*
  due to injury (current episode) SØ5.9- ☑
    sequelae — *code to* injury with seventh character S
  eclipse (total) — *see* Retinopathy, solar
  emotional (hysterical) F44.6
  face H53.16
  hysterical F44.6
  legal (both eyes) (USA definition) H54.8
  mind R48.8
  night H53.6Ø
    abnormal dark adaptation curve H53.61
    acquired H53.62
    congenital H53.63
    specified type NEC H53.69
    vitamin A deficiency E5Ø.5
  one eye (other eye normal) H54.4Ø
    left (normal vision on right) H54.42- ☑
      low vision on right H54.12- ☑
    low vision, other eye H54.1Ø
    right (normal vision on left) H54.41- ☑
      low vision on left H54.11- ☑
  psychic R48.8
  river B73.Ø1
  snow — *see* Photokeratitis
  sun, solar — *see* Retinopathy, solar
  transient — *see* Disturbance, vision, subjective, loss, transient
  traumatic (current episode) SØ5.9- ☑
  word (developmental) F81.Ø
    acquired R48.Ø
    secondary to organic lesion R48.Ø
**Blister** (nonthermal)
  abdominal wall S3Ø.821- ☑
  alveolar process SØØ.522- ☑
  ankle S9Ø.52- ☑
  antecubital space — *see* Blister, elbow
  anus S3Ø.827- ☑
  arm (upper) S4Ø.82- ☑
  auditory canal — *see* Blister, ear
  auricle — *see* Blister, ear
  axilla — *see* Blister, arm
  back, lower S3Ø.82Ø- ☑
  beetle dermatitis L24.89
  breast S2Ø.12- ☑
  brow SØØ.82- ☑
  calf — *see* Blister, leg
  canthus — *see* Blister, eyelid
  cheek SØØ.82- ☑
    internal SØØ.522- ☑
  chest wall — *see* Blister, thorax
  chin SØØ.82- ☑
  costal region — *see* Blister, thorax
  digit(s)
    foot — *see* Blister, toe
    hand — *see* Blister, finger
  due to burn — *see* Burn, by site, second degree
  ear SØØ.42- ☑
  elbow S5Ø.32- ☑
  epiglottis S1Ø.12- ☑
  esophagus, cervical S1Ø.12- ☑
  eyebrow — *see* Blister, eyelid
  eyelid SØØ.22- ☑
  face SØØ.82- ☑
  fever BØØ.1
  finger(s) S6Ø.429- ☑
    index S6Ø.42- ☑
    little S6Ø.42- ☑
    middle S6Ø.42- ☑
    ring S6Ø.42- ☑
  flank S3Ø.82A- ☑
  foot (except toe(s) alone) S9Ø.82- ☑
    toe — *see* Blister, toe
  forearm S5Ø.82- ☑
    elbow only — *see* Blister, elbow
  forehead SØØ.82- ☑
  fracture — *omit code*
  genital organ
    female S3Ø.826- ☑
    male S3Ø.825- ☑
  gum SØØ.522- ☑
  hand S6Ø.52- ☑
  head SØØ.92- ☑
    ear — *see* Blister, ear
    eyelid — *see* Blister, eyelid
    lip SØØ.521- ☑
    nose SØØ.32- ☑
    oral cavity SØØ.522- ☑

- **Blister** — *continued*
  - head — *continued*
    - scalp S00.02- ☑
    - specified site NEC S00.82- ☑
  - heel — *see* Blister, foot
  - hip S70.22- ☑
  - interscapular region S20.429- ☑
  - jaw S00.82- ☑
  - knee S80.22- ☑
  - larynx S10.12- ☑
  - leg (lower) S80.82- ☑
    - knee — *see* Blister, knee
    - upper — *see* Blister, thigh
  - lip S00.521- ☑
  - malar region S00.82- ☑
  - mammary — *see* Blister, breast
  - mastoid region S00.82- ☑
  - mouth S00.522- ☑
  - multiple, skin, nontraumatic R23.8
  - nail
    - finger — *see* Blister, finger
    - toe — *see* Blister, toe
  - nasal S00.32- ☑
  - neck S10.92- ☑
    - specified site NEC S10.82- ☑
    - throat S10.12- ☑
  - nose S00.32- ☑
  - occipital region S00.02- ☑
  - oral cavity S00.522- ☑
  - orbital region — *see* Blister, eyelid
  - palate S00.522- ☑
  - palm — *see* Blister, hand
  - parietal region S00.02- ☑
  - pelvis S30.820- ☑
  - penis S30.822- ☑
  - periocular area — *see* Blister, eyelid
  - phalanges
    - finger — *see* Blister, finger
    - toe — *see* Blister, toe
  - pharynx S10.12- ☑
  - pinna — *see* Blister, ear
  - popliteal space — *see* Blister, knee
  - scalp S00.02- ☑
  - scapular region — *see* Blister, shoulder
  - scrotum S30.823- ☑
  - shin — *see* Blister, leg
  - shoulder S40.22- ☑
  - sternal region S20.329- ☑
  - submaxillary region S00.82- ☑
  - submental region S00.82- ☑
  - subungual
    - finger(s) — *see* Blister, finger
    - toe(s) — *see* Blister, toe
  - supraclavicular fossa S10.82- ☑
  - supraorbital S00.82- ☑
  - temple S00.82- ☑
  - temporal region S00.82- ☑
  - testis S30.823- ☑
  - thermal — *see* Burn, by site, second degree
  - thigh S70.32- ☑
  - thorax, thoracic (wall) S20.92- ☑
    - back S20.42- ☑
    - front S20.32- ☑
  - throat S10.12- ☑
  - thumb S60.32- ☑
  - toe(s) S90.42- ☑
    - great S90.42- ☑
  - tongue S00.522- ☑
  - trachea S10.12- ☑
  - tympanum, tympanic membrane — *see* Blister, ear
  - upper arm — *see* Blister, arm (upper)
  - uvula S00.522- ☑
  - vagina S30.824- ☑
  - vocal cords S10.12- ☑
  - vulva S30.824- ☑
  - wrist S60.82- ☑
- **Bloating** R14.0
- **Bloch-Sulzberger disease or syndrome** Q82.3
- **Block, blocked**
  - alveolocapillary J84.10
  - arborization (heart) I45.5
  - arrhythmic I45.9
  - atrioventricular (incomplete) (partial) I44.30
    - with atrioventricular dissociation I44.2
    - complete I44.2
      - congenital Q24.6
- **Block, blocked** — *continued*
  - atrioventricular — *continued*
    - congenital Q24.6
    - first degree I44.0
    - second degree (types I and II) I44.1
    - specified NEC I44.39
    - third degree I44.2
    - types I and II I44.1
  - auriculoventricular — *see* Block, atrioventricular
  - bifascicular (cardiac) I45.2
  - bundle-branch (complete) (false) (incomplete) I45.4
    - bilateral I45.2
    - left I44.7
      - with right bundle branch block I45.2
      - hemiblock I44.60
        - anterior I44.4
        - posterior I44.5
      - incomplete I44.7
        - with right bundle branch block I45.2
    - right I45.10
      - with
        - left bundle branch block I45.2
        - left fascicular block I45.2
      - specified NEC I45.19
    - Wilson's type I45.19
  - cardiac I45.9
  - conduction I45.9
    - complete I44.2
  - fascicular (left) I44.60
    - anterior I44.4
    - posterior I44.5
    - right I45.0
    - specified NEC I44.69
  - foramen Magendie (acquired) G91.1
    - congenital Q03.1
      - with spina bifida — *see* Spina bifida, by site, with hydrocephalus
  - heart I45.9
    - bundle branch I45.4
      - bilateral I45.2
    - complete (atrioventricular) I44.2
    - congenital Q24.6
    - first degree (atrioventricular) I44.0
    - second degree (atrioventricular) I44.1
    - specified type NEC I45.5
    - third degree (atrioventricular) I44.2
  - hepatic vein I82.0
  - intraventricular (nonspecific) I45.4
    - bundle branch
      - bilateral I45.2
  - kidney N28.9
    - postcystoscopic or postprocedural N99.0
  - Mobitz (types I and II) I44.1
  - myocardial — *see* Block, heart
  - nodal I45.5
  - organ or site, congenital NEC — *see* Atresia, by site
  - portal (vein) I81
  - second degree (types I and II) I44.1
  - sinoatrial I45.5
  - sinoauricular I45.5
  - third degree I44.2
  - trifascicular I45.3
  - tubal N97.1
  - vein NOS I82.90
  - Wenckebach (types I and II) I44.1
- **Blockage** — *see* Obstruction
- **Blocq's disease** F44.4
- **Blood**
  - constituents, abnormal R78.9
  - disease D75.9
  - donor — *see* Donor, blood
  - dyscrasia D75.9
    - with
      - abortion — *see* Abortion, by type, complicated by, hemorrhage
      - ectopic pregnancy O08.1
      - molar pregnancy O08.1
    - following ectopic or molar pregnancy O08.1
    - newborn P61.9
    - puerperal, postpartum O72.3
  - flukes NEC — *see* Schistosomiasis
  - in
    - feces K92.1
      - occult R19.5
    - urine — *see* Hematuria
  - mole O02.0
  - occult in feces R19.5
  - pressure
    - decreased, due to shock following injury T79.4- ☑
- **Blood** — *continued*
  - pressure — *continued*
    - examination only Z01.30
    - fluctuating I99.8
    - high — *see* Hypertension
      - borderline R03.0
      - incidental reading, without diagnosis of hypertension R03.0
    - low — *see also* Hypotension
      - incidental reading, without diagnosis of hypotension R03.1
  - spitting — *see* Hemoptysis
  - staining cornea — *see* Pigmentation, cornea, stromal
  - transfusion
    - reaction or complication — *see* Complications, transfusion
  - type
    - A (Rh positive) Z67.10
      - Rh negative Z67.11
    - AB (Rh positive) Z67.30
      - Rh negative Z67.31
    - B (Rh positive) Z67.20
      - Rh negative Z67.21
    - O (Rh positive) Z67.40
      - Rh negative Z67.41
    - Rh (positive) Z67.90
      - negative Z67.91
  - vessel rupture — *see* Hemorrhage
  - vomiting — *see* Hematemesis
- **Blood-forming organs, disease** D75.9
- **Bloodgood's disease** — *see* Mastopathy, cystic
- **Bloom** (-Machacek)(-Torre) **syndrome** Q82.8
- **Blount disease or osteochondrosis** M92.51- ☑
- **Blue**
  - baby Q24.9
  - diaper syndrome E72.09
  - dome cyst (breast) — *see* Cyst, breast
  - dot cataract Q12.0
  - nevus D22.9
  - sclera Q13.5
    - with fragility of bone and deafness Q78.0
  - toe syndrome I75.02- ☑
- **Blueness** — *see* Cyanosis
- **Blues, postpartal** O90.6
  - baby O90.6
- **Blurring, visual** H53.8
- **Blushing** (abnormal) (excessive) R23.2
- **BMI** — *see* Body, mass index
- **Boarder, hospital NEC** Z76.4
  - accompanying sick person Z76.3
  - healthy infant or child Z76.2
    - foundling Z76.1
- **Bockhart's impetigo** L01.02
- **Bodechtel-Guttman disease** (subacute sclerosing panencephalitis) A81.1
- **Boder-Sedgwick syndrome** (ataxia-telangiectasia) G11.3
- **Body, bodies**
  - Aschoff's — *see* Myocarditis, rheumatic
  - asteroid, vitreous — *see* Deposit, crystalline
  - cytoid (retina) — *see* Occlusion, artery, retina
  - drusen (degenerative) (macula) (retinal) — *see also* Degeneration, macula, drusen
    - optic disc — *see* Drusen, optic disc
  - foreign — *see* Foreign body
  - loose
    - joint, except knee — *see* Loose, body, joint
      - knee M23.4- ☑
    - sheath, tendon — *see* Disorder, tendon, specified type NEC
  - mass index (BMI)
    - adult
      - 18.4 or less, adult Z68.18
      - 18.5-19.9 Z68.19
      - 20.0-20.9 Z68.20
      - 21.0-21.9 Z68.21
      - 22.0-22.9 Z68.22
      - 23.0-23.9 Z68.23
      - 24.0-24.9 Z68.24
      - 25.0-25.9 Z68.25
      - 26.0-26.9 Z68.26
      - 27.0-27.9 Z68.27
      - 28.0-28.9 Z68.28
      - 29.0-29.9 Z68.29
      - 30.0-30.9 Z68.30
      - 31.0-31.9 Z68.31
      - 32.0-32.9 Z68.32
      - 33.0-33.9 Z68.33
      - 34.0-34.9 Z68.34
      - 35.0-35.9 Z68.35

**Body, bodies** — *continued*
  mass index — *continued*
    adult — *continued*
      36.0-36.9 Z68.36
      37.0-37.9 Z68.37
      38.0-38.9 Z68.38
      39.0-39.9 Z68.39
      40.0-44.9 Z68.41
      45.0-49.9 Z68.42
      50.0-59.9 Z68.43
      60.0-69.9 Z68.44
      70 and over Z68.45
    pediatric
      5th percentile to less than 85th percentile for age Z68.52
      85th percentile to less than 95th percentile for age Z68.53
      95th percentile for age to less than 120% of the 95th percentile for age Z68.54
      120% of the 95th percentile for age to less than 140% of the 95th percentile for age Z68.55
      greater than or equal to 140% of the 95th percentile for age Z68.56
      less than fifth percentile for age Z68.51
  Mooser's A75.2
  rice — *see also* Loose, body, joint
    knee M23.4- ☑
  rocking F98.4
**Boeck's**
  disease or sarcoid — *see* Sarcoidosis
  lupoid (miliary) D86.3
**Boerhaave's syndrome** (spontaneous esophageal rupture) K22.3
**Boggy**
  cervix N88.8
  uterus N85.8
**Boil** — *see also* Furuncle, by site
  Aleppo B55.1
  Baghdad B55.1
  Delhi B55.1
  lacrimal
    gland — *see* Dacryoadenitis
    passages (duct) (sac) — *see* Inflammation, lacrimal, passages, acute
  Natal B55.1
  orbit, orbital — *see* Abscess, orbit
  tropical B55.1
**Bold hives** — *see* Urticaria
**Bombé, iris** — *see* Membrane, pupillary
**Bone** — *see* condition
**Bonnevie-Ullrich syndrome** — *see also* Turner's syndrome Q87.19
**Bonnier's syndrome** H81.8- ☑
**Bonvale dam fever** T73.3- ☑
**Bony block of joint** — *see* Ankylosis
**BOOP** (bronchiolitis obliterans organized pneumonia) J84.89
**Borderline**
  diabetes mellitus R73.03
  hypertension R03.0
  osteopenia M85.8- ☑
  pelvis, with obstruction during labor O65.1
  personality F60.3
**Borna disease** A83.9
**Bornholm disease** B33.0
**Boston exanthem** A88.0
**Botalli, ductus** (patent) (persistent) Q25.0
**Bothriocephalus latus infestation** B70.0
**Botulism** (foodborne intoxication) A05.1
  infant A48.51
  non-foodborne A48.52
  wound A48.52
**Bouba** — *see* Yaws
**Bouchard's nodes** (with arthropathy) M15.2
**Bouffée délirante** F23
**Bouillaud's disease or syndrome** (rheumatic heart disease) I01.9
**Bourneville's disease** Q85.1
**Boutonniere deformity** (finger) — *see* Deformity, finger, boutonniere
**Bouveret** (-Hoffmann) **syndrome** (paroxysmal tachycardia) I47.9
**Bovine heart** — *see* Hypertrophy, cardiac
**Bowel** — *see* condition
**Bowen's**
  dermatosis (precancerous) — *see* Neoplasm, skin, in situ
  disease — *see* Neoplasm, skin, in situ
  epithelioma — *see* Neoplasm, skin, in situ
**Bowen's** — *continued*
  type
    epidermoid carcinoma-in-situ — *see* Neoplasm, skin, in situ
    intraepidermal squamous cell carcinoma — *see* Neoplasm, skin, in situ
**Bowing**
  femur — *see also* Deformity, limb, specified type NEC, thigh
    congenital Q68.3
  fibula — *see also* Deformity, limb, specified type NEC, lower leg
    congenital Q68.4
  forearm — *see* Deformity, limb, specified type NEC, forearm
  leg(s), long bones, congenital Q68.5
  radius — *see* Deformity, limb, specified type NEC, forearm
  tibia — *see also* Deformity, limb, specified type NEC, lower leg
    congenital Q68.4
**Bowleg**(s) (acquired) M21.16- ☑
  congenital Q68.5
  rachitic E64.3
**Boyd's dysentery** A03.2
**Brachial** — *see* condition
**Brachycardia** R00.1
**Brachycephaly, non-deformational** Q75.022
**Bradley's disease** A08.19
**Bradyarrhythmia, cardiac** I49.89
**Bradycardia** (sinoatrial) (sinus) (vagal) R00.1
  neonatal P29.12
  reflex G90.09
  tachycardia syndrome I49.5
**Bradykinesia** R25.8
**Bradypnea** R06.89
**Bradytachycardia** I49.5
**Brailsford's disease or osteochondrosis** — *see* Osteochondrosis, juvenile, radius
**Brain** — *see also* condition
  death G93.82
  syndrome — *see* Syndrome, brain
**Branched-chain amino-acid disorder** E71.2
**Branchial** — *see* condition
  cartilage, congenital Q18.2
**Branchiogenic remnant** (in neck) Q18.0
**Brandt's syndrome** (acrodermatitis enteropathica) E83.2
**Brash** (water) R12
**Bravais-jacksonian epilepsy** — *see* Epilepsy, localization-related, symptomatic, with simple partial seizures
**Braxton Hicks contractions** — *see* False, labor
**Brazilian leishmaniasis** B55.2
**BRBPR** K62.5
**Break, retina** (without detachment) H33.30- ☑
  with retinal detachment — *see* Detachment, retina
  horseshoe tear H33.31- ☑
  multiple H33.33- ☑
  round hole H33.32- ☑
**Breakdown**
  device, graft or implant — *see also* Complications, by site and type, mechanical T85.618- ☑
    arterial graft NEC — *see* Complication, cardiovascular device, mechanical, vascular
    breast (implant) T85.41- ☑
    catheter NEC T85.618- ☑
      cystostomy T83.010- ☑
      dialysis (renal) T82.41- ☑
        intraperitoneal T85.611- ☑
      Hopkins T83.018- ☑
      ileostomy T83.018- ☑
      infusion NEC T82.514- ☑
        cranial T85.610- ☑
        epidural T85.610- ☑
        intrathecal T85.610- ☑
        spinal T85.610- ☑
        subarachnoid T85.610- ☑
        subdural T85.610- ☑
      nephrostomy T83.012- ☑
      urethral indwelling T83.011- ☑
      urinary NEC T83.018- ☑
      urostomy T83.018- ☑
    electronic (electrode) (pulse generator) (stimulator)
      bone T84.310- ☑
      cardiac T82.119- ☑
        electrode T82.110- ☑
        pulse generator T82.111- ☑
        specified type NEC T82.118- ☑
**Breakdown** — *continued*
  device, graft or implant — *see also* Complications, by site and type, mechanical — *continued*
    electronic — *continued*
      nervous system — *see* Complication, prosthetic device, mechanical, electronic nervous system stimulator
      urinary — *see* Complication, genitourinary, device, urinary, mechanical
    fixation, internal (orthopedic) NEC — *see* Complication, fixation device, mechanical
    gastrointestinal — *see* Complications, prosthetic device, mechanical, gastrointestinal device
    genital NEC T83.418- ☑
      intrauterine contraceptive device T83.31- ☑
      penile prosthesis (cylinder) (implanted) (pump) (reservoir) T83.410- ☑
      testicular prosthesis T83.411- ☑
    heart NEC — *see* Complication, cardiovascular device, mechanical
    intrathecal infusion pump T85.615- ☑
    joint prosthesis — *see* Complications, joint prosthesis, internal, mechanical, by site
    nervous system, specified device NEC T85.615- ☑
    ocular NEC — *see* Complications, prosthetic device, mechanical, ocular device
    orthopedic NEC — *see* Complication, orthopedic, device, mechanical
    specified NEC T85.618- ☑
    subcutaneous device pocket
      nervous system prosthetic device, implant, or graft T85.890- ☑
      other internal prosthetic device, implant, or graft T85.898- ☑
    sutures, permanent T85.612- ☑
      used in bone repair — *see* Complications, fixation device, internal (orthopedic), mechanical
    urinary NEC T83.118- ☑
      graft T83.21- ☑
      sphincter, implanted T83.111- ☑
      stent (ileal conduit) (nephroureteral) T83.113- ☑
        ureteral indwelling T83.112- ☑
    vascular NEC — *see* Complication, cardiovascular device, mechanical
    ventricular intracranial shunt T85.01- ☑
  nervous F48.8
  perineum O90.1
  respirator J95.850
    specified NEC J95.859
  ventilator J95.850
    specified NEC J95.859
**Breast** — *see also* condition
  buds E30.1
    in newborn P96.89
  dense R92.3- ☑
  Imaging Reporting and Data System (BI-RADS) : A R92.31- ☑
  Imaging Reporting and Data System (BI-RADS) : B R92.32- ☑
  Imaging Reporting and Data System (BI-RADS) : C R92.33- ☑
  Imaging Reporting and Data System (BI-RADS) : D R92.34- ☑
  Imaging Reporting and Data System (BI-RADS) : 1 R92.31- ☑
  Imaging Reporting and Data System (BI-RADS) : 2 R92.32- ☑
  Imaging Reporting and Data System (BI-RADS) : 3 R92.33- ☑
  nodule — *see also* Lump, breast N63.0
  Imaging Reporting and Data System (BI-RADS) : 4 R92.34- ☑
**Breath**
  foul R19.6
  holder, child R06.89
  holding spell R06.89
  shortness R06.02
**Breathing**
  labored — *see* Hyperventilation
  mouth R06.5
    causing malocclusion M26.59
  periodic R06.3
    high altitude G47.32
**Breathlessness** R06.81
**Breda's disease** — *see* Yaws
**Breech presentation** (mother) O32.1- ☑
  causing obstructed labor O64.1- ☑

- **Breech presentation** — *continued*
  - footling O32.8- ☑
    - causing obstructed labor O64.8- ☑
  - incomplete O32.8- ☑
    - causing obstructed labor O64.8- ☑
- **Breisky's disease** N9Ø.4
- **Brennemann's syndrome** I88.Ø
- **Brenner**
  - tumor (benign) D27.9
    - borderline malignancy D39.1- ☑
    - malignant C56.- ☑
    - proliferating D39.1- ☑
- **Bretonneau's disease or angina** A36.Ø
- **Breus' mole** OØ2.Ø
- **Brevicollis** Q76.49
- **Brickmakers' anemia** B76.9 *[D63.8]*
- **Bridge, myocardial** Q24.5
- **Bright red blood per rectum** (BRBPR) K62.5
- **Bright's disease** — *see also* Nephritis
  - arteriosclerotic — *see* Hypertension, kidney
- **Brill** (-Zinsser) **disease** (recrudescent typhus) A75.1
- **Brill-Symmers' disease** C82.9Ø
- **Brion-Kayser disease** — *see* Fever, paratyphoid
- **Briquet's disorder or syndrome** F45.Ø
- **Brissaud's**
  - infantilism or dwarfism E23.Ø
  - motor-verbal tic F95.2
- **Brittle**
  - bones disease Q78.Ø
  - nails L6Ø.3
    - congenital Q84.6
- **Broad** — *see also* condition
  - beta disease E78.2
  - ligament laceration syndrome N83.8
- **Broad- or floating-betalipoproteinemia** E78.2
- **Brock's syndrome** (atelectasis due to enlarged lymph nodes) J98.19
- **Brocq-Duhring disease** (dermatitis herpetiformis) L13.Ø
- **Brodie's abscess or disease** M86.8X- ☑
- **Broken**
  - arches — *see also* Deformity, limb, flat foot
  - arm (meaning upper limb) — *see* Fracture, arm
  - back — *see* Fracture, vertebra
  - bone — *see* Fracture
  - implant or internal device — *see* Complications, by site and type, mechanical
  - leg (meaning lower limb) — *see* Fracture, leg
  - nose SØ2.2- ☑
  - tooth, teeth — *see* Fracture, tooth
- **Bromhidrosis, bromidrosis** L75.Ø
- **Bromidism, bromism** G92.8
  - due to
    - correct substance properly administered — *see* Table of Drugs and Chemicals, by drug, adverse effect
    - overdose or wrong substance given or taken — *see* Table of Drugs and Chemicals, by drug, poisoning
  - chronic (dependence) F13.2Ø
- **Bromidrosiphobia** F4Ø.298
- **Bronchi, bronchial** — *see* condition
- **Bronchiectasis** (cylindrical) (diffuse) (fusiform) (localized) (saccular) J47.9
  - with
    - acute
      - bronchitis J47.Ø
      - lower respiratory infection J47.Ø
    - exacerbation (acute) J47.1
  - congenital Q33.4
  - tuberculous NEC — *see* Tuberculosis, pulmonary
- **Bronchiolectasis** — *see* Bronchiectasis
- **Bronchiolitis** (acute) (infective) (subacute) J21.9
  - with
    - bronchospasm or obstruction J21.9
    - influenza, flu or grippe — *see* Influenza, with, respiratory manifestations NEC
  - chemical (chronic) J68.4
    - acute J68.Ø
  - chronic (fibrosing) J44.89
    - obliterative J44.81
  - due to
    - external agent — *see* Bronchitis, acute, due to
    - human metapneumovirus J21.1
    - respiratory syncytial virus (RSV) J21.Ø
    - specified organism NEC J21.8
  - fibrosa obliterans J44.81
  - influenzal — *see* Influenza, with, respiratory manifestations NEC
  - obliterans — *see also* Bronchiolitis, obliterative J44.81
- **Bronchiolitis** — *continued*
  - obliterans — *see also* Bronchiolitis, obliterative — *continued*
    - with organizing pneumonia (BOOP) J84.89
    - syndrome J44.81
  - obliterative (chronic) (subacute) — *see also* Bronchiolitis, obliterans J44.81
    - due to chemicals, gases, fumes or vapors (inhalation) — *see also* Disease, respiratory, chronic, due to chemicals, gases, fumes or vapors J44.81
    - due to fumes or vapors — *see also* Disease, respiratory, chronic, due to chemicals, gases, fumes or vapors J44.81
  - respiratory, interstitial lung disease J84.115
- **Bronchitis** (diffuse) (fibrinous) (hypostatic) (infective) (membranous) J4Ø
  - with
    - influenza, flu or grippe — *see* Influenza, with, respiratory manifestations NEC
    - obstruction (airway) (lung) J44.89
    - tracheitis (15 years of age and above) J4Ø
      - acute or subacute J2Ø.9
      - chronic J42
      - under 15 years of age J2Ø.9
  - acute or subacute (with bronchospasm or obstruction) J2Ø.9
    - with
      - bronchiectasis J47.Ø
      - chronic obstructive pulmonary disease J44.Ø
    - chemical (due to gases, fumes or vapors) J68.Ø
    - due to
      - fumes or vapors J68.Ø
      - Haemophilus influenzae J2Ø.1
      - Mycoplasma pneumoniae J2Ø.Ø
      - radiation J7Ø.Ø
      - specified organism NEC J2Ø.8
      - Streptococcus J2Ø.2
      - virus
        - coxsackie J2Ø.3
        - echovirus J2Ø.7
        - parainfluenzae J2Ø.4
        - respiratory syncytial (RSV) J2Ø.5
        - rhinovirus J2Ø.6
    - viral NEC J2Ø.8
  - allergic (acute) J45.9Ø9
    - with
      - exacerbation (acute) J45.9Ø1
      - status asthmaticus J45.9Ø2
  - arachidic T17.528- ☑
  - aspiration (due to food and vomit) J69.Ø
  - asthmatic J45.9- ☑
    - chronic J44.89
      - with
        - acute lower respiratory infection J44.Ø
        - exacerbation (acute) J44.1
  - capillary — *see* Pneumonia, broncho
  - caseous (tuberculous) A15.5
  - Castellani's A69.8
  - catarrhal (15 years of age and above) J4Ø
    - acute — *see* Bronchitis, acute
    - chronic J41.Ø
    - under 15 years of age J2Ø.9
  - chemical (acute) (subacute) J68.Ø
    - chronic J68.4
    - due to fumes or vapors — *see also* Disease, respiratory, chronic, due to chemicals, gases, fumes or vapors J68.4
      - chronic J68.4
  - chronic J42
    - with
      - airways obstruction J44.89
      - tracheitis (chronic) J42
    - asthmatic (obstructive) J44.89
    - catarrhal J41.Ø
    - chemical (due to fumes or vapors) J68.4
    - due to
      - chemicals, gases, fumes or vapors (inhalation) J68.4
      - radiation J7Ø.1
      - tobacco smoking J41.Ø
    - emphysematous J44.89
    - mucopurulent J41.1
    - non-obstructive J41.Ø
    - obliterans — *see* Bronchiolitis, obliterans
    - obstructive J44.89
    - purulent J41.1
    - simple J41.Ø
  - croupous — *see* Bronchitis, acute
  - due to gases, fumes or vapors (chemical) J68.Ø
- **Bronchitis** — *continued*
  - emphysematous (obstructive) J44.89
  - exudative — *see* Bronchitis, acute
  - fetid J41.1
  - grippal — *see* Influenza, with, respiratory manifestations NEC
  - in those under 15 years age — *see* Bronchitis, acute
    - chronic — *see* Bronchitis, chronic
  - influenzal — *see* Influenza, with, respiratory manifestations NEC
  - mixed simple and mucopurulent J41.8
  - moulder's J62.8
  - mucopurulent (chronic) (recurrent) J41.1
    - acute or subacute J2Ø.9
    - simple (mixed) J41.8
  - obliterans (chronic) — *see* Bronchiolitis, obliterans
  - obstructive (chronic) (diffuse) J44.89
  - pituitous J41.1
  - pneumococcal, acute or subacute J2Ø.2
  - pseudomembranous, acute or subacute — *see* Bronchitis, acute
  - purulent (chronic) (recurrent) J41.1
    - acute or subacute — *see* Bronchitis, acute
  - putrid J41.1
  - senile (chronic) J42
  - simple and mucopurulent (mixed) J41.8
  - smokers' J41.Ø
  - spirochetal NEC A69.8
  - subacute — *see* Bronchitis, acute
  - suppurative (chronic) J41.1
    - acute or subacute — *see* Bronchitis, acute
  - tuberculous A15.5
  - under 15 years of age — *see* Bronchitis, acute
    - chronic — *see* Bronchitis, chronic
  - viral NEC, acute or subacute — *see also* Bronchitis, acute J2Ø.8
- **Bronchoalveolitis** J18.Ø
- **Bronchoaspergillosis** B44.1
- **Bronchocele meaning goiter** EØ4.Ø
- **Broncholithiasis** J98.Ø9
  - tuberculous NEC A15.5
- **Bronchomalacia** J98.Ø9
  - congenital Q32.2
- **Bronchomycosis NOS** B49 *[J99]*
  - candidal B37.1
- **Bronchopleuropneumonia** — *see* Pneumonia, broncho
- **Bronchopneumonia** — *see* Pneumonia, broncho
- **Bronchopneumonitis** — *see* Pneumonia, broncho
- **Bronchopulmonary** — *see* condition
- **Bronchopulmonitis** — *see* Pneumonia, broncho
- **Bronchorrhagia** — *see* Hemoptysis
- **Bronchorrhea** J98.Ø9
  - acute J2Ø.9
  - chronic (infective) (purulent) J42
- **Bronchospasm** (acute) J98.Ø1
  - with
    - bronchiolitis, acute J21.9
    - bronchitis, acute (conditions in J2Ø) — *see* Bronchitis, acute
  - due to external agent — *see* condition, respiratory, acute, due to
  - exercise induced J45.99Ø
- **Bronchospirochetosis** A69.8
  - Castellani A69.8
- **Bronchostenosis** J98.Ø9
- **Bronchus** — *see* condition
- **Brontophobia** F4Ø.22Ø
- **Bronze baby syndrome** P83.88
- **Brooke's tumor** — *see* Neoplasm, skin, benign
- **Brown enamel of teeth** (hereditary) KØØ.5
- **Brown-Sequard disease, paralysis or syndrome** G83.81
- **Brown's sheath syndrome** H5Ø.61- ☑
- **Bruce sepsis** A23.Ø
- **Brucellosis** (infection) A23.9
  - abortus A23.1
  - canis A23.3
  - dermatitis A23.9
  - melitensis A23.Ø
  - mixed A23.8
  - sepsis A23.9
    - melitensis A23.Ø
    - specified NEC A23.8
  - suis A23.2
- **Bruck-de Lange disease** Q87.19
- **Bruck's disease** — *see* Deformity, limb
- **BRUE** (brief resolved unexplained event) R68.13
- **Brugsch's syndrome** Q82.8
- **Bruise** (skin surface intact) — *see also* Contusion

- **Bruise** — *continued*
  - with
    - open wound — *see* Wound, open
  - internal organ — *see* Injury, by site
  - newborn P54.5
  - scalp, due to birth injury, newborn P12.3
  - umbilical cord O69.5- ☑
- **Bruit** (arterial) RØ9.89
  - cardiac RØ1.1
- **Brush burn** — *see* Abrasion, by site
- **Bruton's X-linked agammaglobulinemia** D8Ø.Ø
- **Bruxism**
  - psychogenic F45.8
  - sleep related G47.63
- **Bubbly lung syndrome** P27.Ø
- **Bubo** I88.8
  - blennorrhagic (gonococcal) A54.89
  - chancroidal A57
  - climatic A55
  - due to Haemophilus ducreyi A57
  - gonococcal A54.89
  - indolent (nonspecific) I88.8
  - inguinal (nonspecific) I88.8
    - chancroidal A57
    - climatic A55
    - due to H. ducreyi A57
    - infective I88.8
  - scrofulous (tuberculous) A18.2
  - soft chancre A57
  - suppurating — *see* Lymphadenitis, acute
  - syphilitic (primary) A51.Ø
    - congenital A5Ø.Ø7
  - tropical A55
  - virulent (chancroidal) A57
- **Bubonic plague** A2Ø.Ø
- **Bubonocele** — *see* Hernia, inguinal
- **Buccal** — *see* condition
- **Buchanan's disease or osteochondrosis** M91.Ø
- **Buchem's syndrome** (hyperostosis corticalis) M85.2
- **Bucket-handle fracture or tear** (semilunar cartilage) — *see* Tear, meniscus
- **Budd-Chiari syndrome** (hepatic vein thrombosis) I82.Ø
- **Budgerigar fancier's disease or lung** J67.2
- **Buds**
  - breast E3Ø.1
    - in newborn P96.89
- **Buerger's disease** (thromboangiitis obliterans) I73.1
- **Bulbar** — *see* condition
- **Bulbus cordis** (left ventricle) (persistent) Q21.8
- **Bulimia** (nervosa) F5Ø.2- ☑
  - atypical F5Ø.9
  - normal weight F5Ø.9
- **Bulky**
  - stools R19.5
  - uterus N85.2
- **Bulla** (e) R23.8
  - lung (emphysematous) (solitary) J43.9
    - newborn P25.8
- **Bullet wound** — *see also* Puncture
  - fracture — *code as* Fracture, by site
  - internal organ — *see* Injury, by site
- **Bundle**
  - branch block (complete) (false) (incomplete) — *see* Block, bundle-branch
  - of His — *see* condition
- **Bunion** M21.61- ☑
  - tailor's M21.62- ☑
- **Bunionette** M21.62- ☑
- **Buphthalmia, buphthalmos** (congenital) Q15.Ø
- **Burdwan fever** B55.Ø
- **Burger-Grutz disease or syndrome** E78.3
- **Buried**
  - penis (congenital) Q55.64
    - acquired N48.83
  - roots KØ8.3
- **Burke's syndrome** K86.89
- **Burkholderia**
  - cepacia A49.8
  - mallei A24.Ø
  - pseudomallei — *see* Melioidosis
- **Burkitt**
  - cell leukemia C91.Ø- ☑
  - lymphoma (malignant) C83.7- ☑
    - small noncleaved, diffuse C83.7- ☑
    - spleen C83.77
    - undifferentiated C83.7- ☑
  - tumor C83.7- ☑
- **Burkitt** — *continued*
  - type
    - acute lymphoblastic leukemia C91.Ø- ☑
    - undifferentiated C83.7- ☑
- **Burn** (electricity) (flame) (hot gas, liquid or hot object) (radiation) (steam) (thermal) T3Ø.Ø
  - abdomen, abdominal (muscle) (wall) T21.Ø2- ☑
    - first degree T21.12- ☑
    - second degree T21.22- ☑
    - third degree T21.32- ☑
  - above elbow T22.Ø39- ☑
    - first degree T22.139- ☑
    - left T22.Ø32- ☑
      - first degree T22.132- ☑
      - second degree T22.232- ☑
      - third degree T22.332- ☑
    - right T22.Ø31- ☑
      - first degree T22.131- ☑
      - second degree T22.231- ☑
      - third degree T22.331- ☑
    - second degree T22.239- ☑
    - third degree T22.339- ☑
  - acid (caustic) (external) (internal) — *see* Corrosion, by site
  - alimentary tract NEC T28.2- ☑
    - esophagus T28.1- ☑
    - mouth T28.Ø- ☑
    - pharynx T28.Ø- ☑
  - alkaline (caustic) (external) (internal) — *see* Corrosion, by site
  - ankle T25.Ø19- ☑
    - first degree T25.119- ☑
    - left T25.Ø12- ☑
      - first degree T25.112- ☑
      - second degree T25.212- ☑
      - third degree T25.312- ☑
    - multiple with foot — *see* Burn, lower, limb, multiple, ankle and foot
    - right T25.Ø11- ☑
      - first degree T25.111- ☑
      - second degree T25.211- ☑
      - third degree T25.311- ☑
    - second degree T25.219- ☑
    - third degree T25.319- ☑
  - anus — *see* Burn, buttock
  - arm (lower) (upper) — *see* Burn, upper, limb
  - axilla T22.Ø49- ☑
    - first degree T22.149- ☑
    - left T22.Ø42- ☑
      - first degree T22.142- ☑
      - second degree T22.242- ☑
      - third degree T22.342- ☑
    - right T22.Ø41- ☑
      - first degree T22.141- ☑
      - second degree T22.241- ☑
      - third degree T22.341- ☑
    - second degree T22.249- ☑
    - third degree T22.349- ☑
  - back (lower) T21.Ø4- ☑
    - first degree T21.14- ☑
    - second degree T21.24- ☑
    - third degree T21.34- ☑
    - upper T21.Ø3- ☑
      - first degree T21.13- ☑
      - second degree T21.23- ☑
      - third degree T21.33- ☑
  - blisters — *code as* Burn, second degree, by site
  - breast(s) — *see* Burn, chest wall
  - buttock(s) T21.Ø5- ☑
    - first degree T21.15- ☑
    - second degree T21.25- ☑
    - third degree T21.35- ☑
  - calf T24.Ø39- ☑
    - first degree T24.139- ☑
    - left T24.Ø32- ☑
      - first degree T24.132- ☑
      - second degree T24.232- ☑
      - third degree T24.332- ☑
    - right T24.Ø31- ☑
      - first degree T24.131- ☑
      - second degree T24.231- ☑
      - third degree T24.331- ☑
    - second degree T24.239- ☑
    - third degree T24.339- ☑
  - canthus (eye) — *see* Burn, eyelid
- **Burn** — *continued*
  - caustic acid or alkaline — *see* Corrosion, by site
  - cervix T28.3- ☑
  - cheek T2Ø.Ø6- ☑
    - first degree T2Ø.16- ☑
    - second degree T2Ø.26- ☑
    - third degree T2Ø.36- ☑
  - chemical (acids) (alkalines) (caustics) (external) (internal) — *see* Corrosion, by site
  - chest wall T21.Ø1- ☑
    - first degree T21.11- ☑
    - second degree T21.21- ☑
    - third degree T21.31- ☑
  - chin T2Ø.Ø3- ☑
    - first degree T2Ø.13- ☑
    - second degree T2Ø.23- ☑
    - third degree T2Ø.33- ☑
  - colon T28.2- ☑
  - conjunctiva (and cornea) — *see* Burn, cornea
  - cornea (and conjunctiva) T26.1- ☑
    - chemical — *see* Corrosion, cornea
  - corrosion (external) (internal) — *see* Corrosion, by site
  - deep necrosis of underlying tissue — *code as* Burn, third degree, by site
  - dorsum of hand T23.Ø69- ☑
    - first degree T23.169- ☑
    - left T23.Ø62- ☑
      - first degree T23.162- ☑
      - second degree T23.262- ☑
      - third degree T23.362- ☑
    - right T23.Ø61- ☑
      - first degree T23.161- ☑
      - second degree T23.261- ☑
      - third degree T23.361- ☑
    - second degree T23.269- ☑
    - third degree T23.369- ☑
  - due to ingested chemical agent — *see* Corrosion, by site
  - ear (auricle) (external) (canal) T2Ø.Ø1- ☑
    - first degree T2Ø.11- ☑
    - second degree T2Ø.21- ☑
    - third degree T2Ø.31- ☑
  - elbow T22.Ø29- ☑
    - first degree T22.129- ☑
    - left T22.Ø22- ☑
      - first degree T22.122- ☑
      - second degree T22.222- ☑
      - third degree T22.322- ☑
    - right T22.Ø21- ☑
      - first degree T22.121- ☑
      - second degree T22.221- ☑
      - third degree T22.321- ☑
    - second degree T22.229- ☑
    - third degree T22.329- ☑
  - epidermal loss — *code as* Burn, second degree, by site
  - erythema, erythematous — *code as* Burn, first degree, by site
  - esophagus T28.1- ☑
  - extent (percentage of body surface)
    - less than 1Ø percent T31.Ø
    - 1Ø-19 percent T31.1Ø
      - with Ø-9 percent third degree burns T31.1Ø
      - with 1Ø-19 percent third degree burns T31.11
    - 2Ø-29 percent T31.2Ø
      - with Ø-9 percent third degree burns T31.2Ø
      - with 1Ø-19 percent third degree burns T31.21
      - with 2Ø-29 percent third degree burns T31.22
    - 3Ø-39 percent T31.3Ø
      - with Ø-9 percent third degree burns T31.3Ø
      - with 1Ø-19 percent third degree burns T31.31
      - with 2Ø-29 percent third degree burns T31.32
      - with 3Ø-39 percent third degree burns T31.33
    - 4Ø-49 percent T31.4Ø
      - with Ø-9 percent third degree burns T31.4Ø
      - with 1Ø-19 percent third degree burns T31.41
      - with 2Ø-29 percent third degree burns T31.42
      - with 3Ø-39 percent third degree burns T31.43
      - with 4Ø-49 percent third degree burns T31.44
    - 5Ø-59 percent T31.5Ø
      - with Ø-9 percent third degree burns T31.5Ø
      - with 1Ø-19 percent third degree burns T31.51
      - with 2Ø-29 percent third degree burns T31.52
      - with 3Ø-39 percent third degree burns T31.53
      - with 4Ø-49 percent third degree burns T31.54
      - with 5Ø-59 percent third degree burns T31.55
    - 6Ø-69 percent T31.6Ø
      - with Ø-9 percent third degree burns T31.6Ø
      - with 1Ø-19 percent third degree burns T31.61

**Burn** — *continued*
- extent — *continued*
  - 60-69 percent — *continued*
    - with 20-29 percent third degree burns T31.62
    - with 30-39 percent third degree burns T31.63
    - with 40-49 percent third degree burns T31.64
    - with 50-59 percent third degree burns T31.65
    - with 60-69 percent third degree burns T31.66
  - 70-79 percent T31.70
    - with 0-9 percent third degree burns T31.70
    - with 10-19 percent third degree burns T31.71
    - with 20-29 percent third degree burns T31.72
    - with 30-39 percent third degree burns T31.73
    - with 40-49 percent third degree burns T31.74
    - with 50-59 percent third degree burns T31.75
    - with 60-69 percent third degree burns T31.76
    - with 70-79 percent third degree burns T31.77
  - 80-89 percent T31.80
    - with 0-9 percent third degree burns T31.80
    - with 10-19 percent third degree burns T31.81
    - with 20-29 percent third degree burns T31.82
    - with 30-39 percent third degree burns T31.83
    - with 40-49 percent third degree burns T31.84
    - with 50-59 percent third degree burns T31.85
    - with 60-69 percent third degree burns T31.86
    - with 70-79 percent third degree burns T31.87
    - with 80-89 percent third degree burns T31.88
  - 90 percent or more T31.90
    - with 0-9 percent third degree burns T31.90
    - with 10-19 percent third degree burns T31.91
    - with 20-29 percent third degree burns T31.92
    - with 30-39 percent third degree burns T31.93
    - with 40-49 percent third degree burns T31.94
    - with 50-59 percent third degree burns T31.95
    - with 60-69 percent third degree burns T31.96
    - with 70-79 percent third degree burns T31.97
    - with 80-89 percent third degree burns T31.98
    - with 90 percent or more third degree burns T31.99
- extremity — *see* Burn, limb
- eye(s) and adnexa T26.4- ☑
  - with resulting rupture and destruction of eyeball T26.2- ☑
  - conjunctival sac — *see* Burn, cornea
  - cornea — *see* Burn, cornea
  - lid — *see* Burn, eyelid
  - periocular area — *see* Burn, eyelid
  - specified site NEC T26.3- ☑
- eyeball — *see* Burn, eye
- eyelid(s) T26.0- ☑
  - chemical — *see* Corrosion, eyelid
- face — *see* Burn, head
- finger T23.029- ☑
  - first degree T23.129- ☑
  - left T23.022- ☑
    - first degree T23.122- ☑
    - second degree T23.222- ☑
    - third degree T23.322- ☑
  - multiple sites (without thumb) T23.039- ☑
    - with thumb T23.049- ☑
      - first degree T23.149- ☑
      - left T23.042- ☑
        - first degree T23.142- ☑
        - second degree T23.242- ☑
        - third degree T23.342- ☑
      - right T23.041- ☑
        - first degree T23.141- ☑
        - second degree T23.241- ☑
        - third degree T23.341- ☑
      - second degree T23.249- ☑
      - third degree T23.349- ☑
    - first degree T23.139- ☑
    - left T23.032- ☑
      - first degree T23.132- ☑
      - second degree T23.232- ☑
      - third degree T23.332- ☑
    - right T23.031- ☑
      - first degree T23.131- ☑
      - second degree T23.231- ☑
      - third degree T23.331- ☑
    - second degree T23.239- ☑
    - third degree T23.339- ☑
  - right T23.021- ☑
    - first degree T23.121- ☑
    - second degree T23.221- ☑
    - third degree T23.321- ☑
  - second degree T23.229- ☑
  - third degree T23.329- ☑
- flank — *see* Burn, abdominal wall
- foot T25.029- ☑
  - first degree T25.129- ☑
  - left T25.022- ☑
    - first degree T25.122- ☑
    - second degree T25.222- ☑
    - third degree T25.322- ☑
  - multiple with ankle — *see* Burn, lower, limb, multiple, ankle and foot
  - right T25.021- ☑
    - first degree T25.121- ☑
    - second degree T25.221- ☑
    - third degree T25.321- ☑
  - second degree T25.229- ☑
  - third degree T25.329- ☑
- forearm T22.019- ☑
  - first degree T22.119- ☑
  - left T22.012- ☑
    - first degree T22.112- ☑
    - second degree T22.212- ☑
    - third degree T22.312- ☑
  - right T22.011- ☑
    - first degree T22.111- ☑
    - second degree T22.211- ☑
    - third degree T22.311- ☑
  - second degree T22.219- ☑
  - third degree T22.319- ☑
- forehead T20.06- ☑
  - first degree T20.16- ☑
  - second degree T20.26- ☑
  - third degree T20.36- ☑
- fourth degree — *code as* Burn, third degree, by site
- friction — *see* Burn, by site
- from swallowing caustic or corrosive substance NEC — *see* Corrosion, by site
- full thickness skin loss — *code as* Burn, third degree, by site
- gastrointestinal tract NEC T28.2- ☑
  - from swallowing caustic or corrosive substance T28.7- ☑
- genital organs
  - external
    - female T21.07- ☑
      - first degree T21.17- ☑
      - second degree T21.27- ☑
      - third degree T21.37- ☑
    - male T21.06- ☑
      - first degree T21.16- ☑
      - second degree T21.26- ☑
      - third degree T21.36- ☑
  - internal T28.3- ☑
    - from caustic or corrosive substance T28.8- ☑
- groin — *see* Burn, abdominal wall
- hand(s) T23.009- ☑
  - back — *see* Burn, dorsum of hand
  - finger — *see* Burn, finger
  - first degree T23.109- ☑
  - left T23.002- ☑
    - first degree T23.102- ☑
    - second degree T23.202- ☑
    - third degree T23.302- ☑
  - multiple sites with wrist T23.099- ☑
    - first degree T23.199- ☑
    - left T23.092- ☑
      - first degree T23.192- ☑
      - second degree T23.292- ☑
      - third degree T23.392- ☑
    - right T23.091- ☑
      - first degree T23.191- ☑
      - second degree T23.291- ☑
      - third degree T23.391- ☑
    - second degree T23.299- ☑
    - third degree T23.399- ☑
  - palm — *see* Burn, palm
  - right T23.001- ☑
    - first degree T23.101- ☑
    - second degree T23.201- ☑
    - third degree T23.301- ☑
  - second degree T23.209- ☑
  - third degree T23.309- ☑
  - thumb — *see* Burn, thumb
- head (and face) (and neck) T20.00- ☑
  - cheek — *see* Burn, cheek
  - chin — *see* Burn, chin
  - ear — *see* Burn, ear
  - eye(s) only — *see* Burn, eye
  - first degree T20.10- ☑
  - forehead — *see* Burn, forehead
  - lip — *see* Burn, lip
  - multiple sites T20.09- ☑
    - first degree T20.19- ☑
    - second degree T20.29- ☑
    - third degree T20.39- ☑
  - neck — *see* Burn, neck
  - nose — *see* Burn, nose
  - scalp — *see* Burn, scalp
  - second degree T20.20- ☑
  - third degree T20.30- ☑
- hip(s) — *see* Burn, thigh
- inhalation — *see* Burn, respiratory tract
  - caustic or corrosive substance (fumes) — *see* Corrosion, respiratory tract
- internal organ(s) T28.40- ☑
  - alimentary tract T28.2- ☑
    - esophagus T28.1- ☑
  - eardrum T28.41- ☑
  - esophagus T28.1- ☑
  - from caustic or corrosive substance (swallowing) NEC — *see* Corrosion, by site
  - genitourinary T28.3- ☑
  - mouth T28.0- ☑
  - pharynx T28.0- ☑
  - respiratory tract — *see* Burn, respiratory tract
  - specified organ NEC T28.49- ☑
- interscapular region — *see* Burn, back, upper
- intestine (large) (small) T28.2- ☑
- knee T24.029- ☑
  - first degree T24.129- ☑
  - left T24.022- ☑
    - first degree T24.122- ☑
    - second degree T24.222- ☑
    - third degree T24.322- ☑
  - right T24.021- ☑
    - first degree T24.121- ☑
    - second degree T24.221- ☑
    - third degree T24.321- ☑
  - second degree T24.229- ☑
  - third degree T24.329- ☑
- labium (majus) (minus) — *see* Burn, genital organs, external, female
- lacrimal apparatus, duct, gland or sac — *see* Burn, eye, specified site NEC
- larynx T27.0- ☑
  - with lung T27.1- ☑
- leg(s) (lower) (upper) — *see* Burn, lower, limb
- lightning — *see* Burn, by site
- limb(s)
  - lower (except ankle or foot alone) — *see* Burn, lower, limb
  - upper — *see* Burn, upper limb
- lip(s) T20.02- ☑
  - first degree T20.12- ☑
  - second degree T20.22- ☑
  - third degree T20.32- ☑
- lower
  - back — *see* Burn, back
  - limb T24.009- ☑
    - ankle — *see* Burn, ankle
    - calf — *see* Burn, calf
    - first degree T24.109- ☑
    - foot — *see* Burn, foot
    - hip — *see* Burn, thigh
    - knee — *see* Burn, knee
    - left T24.002- ☑
      - first degree T24.102- ☑
      - second degree T24.202- ☑
      - third degree T24.302- ☑
    - multiple sites, except ankle and foot T24.099- ☑
      - ankle and foot T25.099- ☑
        - first degree T25.199- ☑
        - left T25.092- ☑
          - first degree T25.192- ☑
          - second degree T25.292- ☑
          - third degree T25.392- ☑
        - right T25.091- ☑
          - first degree T25.191- ☑
          - second degree T25.291- ☑
          - third degree T25.391- ☑
        - second degree T25.299- ☑

- **Burn** — *continued*
  - upper limb — *continued*
    - forearm — *see* Burn, forearm
    - hand — *see* Burn, hand
    - interscapular region — *see* Burn, back, upper
    - multiple sites T22.Ø99- ☑
      - first degree T22.199- ☑
      - left T22.Ø92- ☑
        - first degree T22.192- ☑
        - second degree T22.292- ☑
        - third degree T22.392- ☑
      - right T22.Ø91- ☑
        - first degree T22.191- ☑
        - second degree T22.291- ☑
        - third degree T22.391- ☑
      - second degree T22.299- ☑
      - third degree T22.399- ☑
    - scapular region — *see* Burn, scapular region
    - second degree T22.2Ø- ☑
    - shoulder — *see* Burn, shoulder
    - third degree T22.3Ø- ☑
    - wrist — *see* Burn, wrist
  - uterus T28.3- ☑
  - vagina T28.3- ☑
  - vulva — *see* Burn, genital organs, external, female
  - wrist T23.Ø79- ☑
    - first degree T23.179- ☑
    - left T23.Ø72- ☑
      - first degree T23.172- ☑
      - second degree T23.272- ☑
      - third degree T23.372- ☑
    - multiple sites with hand T23.Ø99- ☑
      - first degree T23.199- ☑
      - left T23.Ø92- ☑
        - first degree T23.192- ☑
        - second degree T23.292- ☑
        - third degree T23.392- ☑
      - right T23.Ø91- ☑
        - first degree T23.191- ☑
        - second degree T23.291- ☑
        - third degree T23.391- ☑
      - second degree T23.299- ☑
      - third degree T23.399- ☑
    - right T23.Ø71- ☑
      - first degree T23.171- ☑
      - second degree T23.271- ☑
      - third degree T23.371- ☑
    - second degree T23.279- ☑
    - third degree T23.379- ☑
- **Burn-out** (state) Z73.Ø
- **Burnett's syndrome** E83.52
- **Burning**
  - feet syndrome E53.9
  - sensation R2Ø.8
  - tongue K14.6
- **Burns' disease or osteochondrosis** — *see* Osteochondrosis, juvenile, ulna
- **Bursa** — *see* condition
- **Bursitis** M71.9
  - Achilles — *see* Tendinitis, Achilles
  - adhesive — *see* Bursitis, specified NEC
  - ankle — *see* Enthesopathy, ankle and tarsus
  - calcaneal — *see* Enthesopathy, foot, specified type NEC
  - collateral ligament, tibial — *see* Bursitis, tibial collateral
  - due to use, overuse, pressure — *see also* Disorder, soft tissue, due to use, specified type NEC
    - specified NEC — *see* Disorder, soft tissue, due to use, specified NEC
  - Duplay's M75.Ø- ☑
  - elbow NEC M7Ø.3- ☑
    - olecranon M7Ø.2- ☑
  - finger — *see* Disorder, soft tissue, due to use, specified type NEC, hand
  - foot — *see* Enthesopathy, foot, specified type NEC
  - gonococcal A54.49
  - gouty — *see* Gout
  - hand M7Ø.1- ☑
  - hip NEC M7Ø.7- ☑
    - trochanteric M7Ø.6- ☑
  - infective NEC M71.1Ø
    - abscess — *see* Abscess, bursa
    - ankle M71.17- ☑
    - elbow M71.12- ☑
    - foot M71.17- ☑
    - hand M71.14- ☑
    - hip M71.15- ☑
- **Bursitis** — *continued*
  - infective — *continued*
    - knee M71.16- ☑
    - multiple sites M71.19
    - shoulder M71.11- ☑
    - specified site NEC M71.18
    - wrist M71.13- ☑
  - ischial — *see* Bursitis, hip
  - knee NEC M7Ø.5- ☑
    - prepatellar M7Ø.4- ☑
  - occupational NEC — *see also* Disorder, soft tissue, due to, use
  - olecranon — *see* Bursitis, elbow, olecranon
  - pharyngeal J39.1
  - popliteal — *see* Bursitis, knee
  - prepatellar M7Ø.4- ☑
  - radiohumeral M7Ø.3- ☑
  - rheumatoid MØ6.2Ø
    - ankle MØ6.27- ☑
    - elbow MØ6.22- ☑
    - foot joint MØ6.27- ☑
    - hand joint MØ6.24- ☑
    - hip MØ6.25- ☑
    - knee MØ6.26- ☑
    - multiple site MØ6.29
    - shoulder MØ6.21- ☑
    - vertebra MØ6.28
    - wrist MØ6.23- ☑
  - scapulohumeral — *see* Bursitis, shoulder
  - semimembranous muscle (knee) — *see* Bursitis, knee
  - shoulder M75.5- ☑
    - adhesive — *see* Capsulitis, adhesive
  - specified NEC M71.5Ø
    - ankle M71.57- ☑
    - due to use, overuse or pressure — *see* Disorder, soft tissue, due to, use
    - elbow M71.52- ☑
    - foot M71.57- ☑
    - hand M71.54- ☑
    - hip M71.55- ☑
    - knee M71.56- ☑
    - shoulder — *see* Bursitis, shoulder
    - specified site NEC M71.58
    - tibial collateral M76.4- ☑
    - wrist M71.53- ☑
  - subacromial — *see* Bursitis, shoulder
  - subcoracoid — *see* Bursitis, shoulder
  - subdeltoid — *see* Bursitis, shoulder
  - syphilitic A52.78
  - Thornwaldt, Tornwaldt J39.2
  - tibial collateral M76.4- ☑
  - toe — *see* Enthesopathy, foot, specified type NEC
  - trochanteric (area) — *see* Bursitis, hip, trochanteric
  - wrist — *see* Bursitis, hand
- **Bursopathy** M71.9
  - specified type NEC M71.8Ø
    - ankle M71.87- ☑
    - elbow M71.82- ☑
    - foot M71.87- ☑
    - hand M71.84- ☑
    - hip M71.85- ☑
    - knee M71.86- ☑
    - multiple sites M71.89
    - shoulder M71.81- ☑
    - specified site NEC M71.88
    - wrist M71.83- ☑
- **Burst stitches or sutures** (complication of surgery) T81.31- ☑
  - external operation wound T81.31- ☑
  - internal operation wound — *see also* Dehiscence, closure T81.328- ☑
    - abdominal wall muscle or fascia T81.321- ☑
    - specified NEC T81.328- ☑
- **Buruli ulcer** A31.1
- **Bury's disease** L95.1
- **Buschke's**
  - disease — *see* Cryptococcosis by site
  - scleredema — *see* Sclerosis, systemic
- **Busse-Buschke disease** — *see* Cryptococcosis by site
- **Buttock** — *see* condition
- **Button**
  - Biskra B55.1
  - Delhi B55.1
  - oriental B55.1
- **Buttonhole deformity** (finger) — *see* Deformity, finger, boutonniere
- **Bwamba fever** A92.8
- **Byssinosis** J66.Ø
- **Bywaters' syndrome** T79.5- ☑

## C

- **Cachexia** R64
  - cancerous R64
  - cardiac — *see* Disease, heart
  - dehydration E86.Ø
  - due to
    - malnutrition — *see also* Malnutrition, severe E88.A
    - underlying condition E88.A
  - exophthalmic — *see* Hyperthyroidism
  - heart — *see* Disease, heart
  - hypophyseal E23.Ø
  - hypopituitary E23.Ø
  - lead — *see* Poisoning, lead
  - malignant R64
  - marsh — *see* Malaria
  - nervous F48.8
  - old age R54
  - paludal — *see* Malaria
  - pituitary E23.Ø
  - pulmonary R64
  - renal N28.9
  - saturnine — *see* Poisoning, lead
  - senile R54
  - Simmonds' E23.Ø
  - splenica D73.Ø
  - strumipriva EØ3.4
  - tuberculous NEC — *see* Tuberculosis
- **CADASIL** (cerebral autosomal dominant arteriopathy with subcortical infarcts and leukoencephalopathy) I67.85Ø
- **Cafe, au lait spots** L81.3
- **Caffeine-induced**
  - anxiety disorder F15.98Ø
  - sleep disorder F15.982
- **Caffey's syndrome** Q78.8
- **Caisson disease** T7Ø.3- ☑
- **Cake kidney** Q63.1
- **Caked breast** (puerperal, postpartum) O92.79
- **Calabar swelling** B74.3
- **Calcaneal spur** — *see* Spur, bone, calcaneal
- **Calcaneo-apophysitis** M92.6- ☑
- **Calcareous** — *see* condition
- **Calcicosis** J62.8
- **Calciferol** (vitamin D) **deficiency** E55.9
  - with rickets E55.Ø
- **Calcification**
  - adrenal (capsule) (gland) E27.49
    - tuberculous B9Ø.8 *[E35]*
  - aorta I7Ø.Ø
  - arterial
    - generalized, of infancy E83.82Ø
      - with
        - ABCC6 deficiency E83.823
        - ENPP1 deficiency E83.821
        - unspecified genetic causality E83.82Ø
  - artery (annular) — *see* Arteriosclerosis
  - auricle (ear) — *see* Disorder, pinna, specified type NEC
  - basal ganglia G23.8
  - bladder N32.89
    - due to Schistosoma hematobium B65.Ø
  - brain (cortex) — *see* Calcification, cerebral
  - bronchus J98.Ø9
  - bursa M71.4Ø
    - ankle M71.47- ☑
    - elbow M71.42- ☑
    - foot M71.47- ☑
    - hand M71.44- ☑
    - hip M71.45- ☑
    - knee M71.46- ☑
    - multiple sites M71.49
    - shoulder M75.3- ☑
    - specified site NEC M71.48
    - wrist M71.43- ☑
  - cardiac — *see* Degeneration, myocardial
  - cerebral (cortex) G93.89
    - artery I67.2
  - cervix (uteri) N88.8
  - choroid plexus G93.89
  - conjunctiva — *see* Concretion, conjunctiva
  - corpora cavernosa (penis) N48.89
  - cortex (brain) — *see* Calcification, cerebral
  - dental pulp (nodular) KØ4.2
  - dentinal papilla KØØ.4
  - fallopian tube N83.8
  - falx cerebri G96.198

- **Calcification** — *continued*
  - gallbladder K82.8
  - general E83.59
  - heart — *see also* Degeneration, myocardial
    - valve — *see also* Endocarditis
      - mitral — *see* Calcification, mitral
  - idiopathic infantile arterial (IIAC) — *see* Calcification, arterial, generalized, of infancy
  - intervertebral cartilage or disc (postinfective) — *see* Disorder, disc, specified NEC
  - intracranial — *see* Calcification, cerebral
  - joint — *see* Disorder, joint, specified type NEC
  - kidney N28.89
    - tuberculous N29 *[B9Ø.1]*
  - larynx (senile) J38.7
  - lens — *see* Cataract, specified NEC
  - lung (active) (postinfectional) J98.4
    - tuberculous B9Ø.9
  - lymph gland or node (postinfectional) I89.8
    - tuberculous — *see also* Tuberculosis, lymph gland B9Ø.8
  - mammographic R92.1
  - massive (paraplegic) — *see* Myositis, ossificans, in, quadriplegia
  - medial — *see* Arteriosclerosis, extremities
  - meninges (cerebral) (spinal) G96.198
  - metastatic E83.59
  - mitral (valve)
    - annular I34.81
      - nonrheumatic I34.81
      - rheumatic IØ5.8
    - annulus I34.81
      - nonrheumatic I34.81
      - rheumatic IØ5.8
  - Monckeberg's — *see* Arteriosclerosis, extremities
  - muscle M61.9
    - due to burns — *see* Myositis, ossificans, in, burns
    - paralytic — *see* Myositis, ossificans, in, quadriplegia
    - specified type NEC M61.4Ø
      - ankle M61.47- ☑
      - foot M61.47- ☑
      - forearm M61.43- ☑
      - hand M61.44- ☑
      - lower leg M61.46- ☑
      - multiple sites M61.49
      - pelvic region M61.45- ☑
      - shoulder region M61.41- ☑
      - specified site NEC M61.48
      - thigh M61.45- ☑
      - upper arm M61.42- ☑
  - myocardium, myocardial — *see* Degeneration, myocardial
  - ovary N83.8
  - pancreas K86.89
  - penis N48.89
  - periarticular — *see* Disorder, joint, specified type NEC
  - pericardium — *see also* Pericarditis I31.1
  - pineal gland E34.8
  - pleura J94.8
    - postinfectional J94.8
    - tuberculous NEC B9Ø.9
  - pulpal (dental) (nodular) KØ4.2
  - sclera H15.89
  - spleen D73.89
  - subcutaneous L94.2
  - suprarenal (capsule) (gland) E27.49
  - tendon (sheath) — *see also* Tenosynovitis, specified type NEC
    - with bursitis, synovitis or tenosynovitis — *see* Tendinitis, calcific
  - trachea J39.8
  - ureter N28.89
  - uterus N85.8
  - vitreous — *see* Deposit, crystalline
- **Calcified** — *see* Calcification
- **Calcinosis** (interstitial) (tumoral) (universalis) E83.59
  - with Raynaud's phenomenon, esophageal dysfunction, sclerodactyly, telangiectasia (CREST syndrome) M34.1
  - circumscripta (skin) L94.2
  - cutis L94.2
- **Calciphylaxis** — *see also* Calcification, by site E83.59
- **Calcium**
  - deposits — *see* Calcification, by site
  - metabolism disorder E83.5Ø
  - salts or soaps in vitreous — *see* Deposit, crystalline
- **Calciuria** R82.994
- **Calculi** — *see* Calculus
- **Calculosis, intrahepatic** — *see* Calculus, bile duct
- **Calculus, calculi, calculous**
  - ampulla of Vater — *see* Calculus, bile duct
  - anuria (impacted) (recurrent) — *see also* Calculus, urinary N2Ø.9
  - appendix K38.1
  - bile duct (common) (hepatic) K8Ø.5Ø
    - with
      - calculus of gallbladder — *see* Calculus, gallbladder and bile duct
      - cholangitis K8Ø.3Ø
        - with
          - cholecystitis — *see* Calculus, bile duct, with cholecystitis
          - obstruction K8Ø.31
        - acute K8Ø.32
          - with
            - chronic cholangitis K8Ø.36
              - with obstruction K8Ø.37
            - obstruction K8Ø.33
        - chronic K8Ø.34
          - with
            - acute cholangitis K8Ø.36
              - with obstruction K8Ø.37
            - obstruction K8Ø.35
      - cholecystitis (with cholangitis) K8Ø.4Ø
        - with obstruction K8Ø.41
        - acute K8Ø.42
          - with
            - chronic cholecystitis K8Ø.46
              - with obstruction K8Ø.47
            - obstruction K8Ø.43
        - chronic K8Ø.44
          - with
            - acute cholecystitis K8Ø.46
              - with obstruction K8Ø.47
            - obstruction K8Ø.45
  - biliary — *see also* Calculus, gallbladder
    - with bile duct involvement — *see also* Calculus, bile duct
    - specified NEC K8Ø.8Ø
      - with obstruction K8Ø.81
  - bilirubin, multiple — *see* Calculus, gallbladder
  - bladder (encysted) (impacted) (urinary) (diverticulum) N21.Ø
  - bronchus J98.Ø9
  - calyx (kidney) (renal) — *see* Calculus, kidney
  - cholesterol (pure) (solitary) — *see* Calculus, gallbladder
  - common duct (bile) — *see* Calculus, bile duct
  - conjunctiva — *see* Concretion, conjunctiva
  - cystic N21.Ø
    - duct — *see* Calculus, gallbladder
  - dental (subgingival) (supragingival) KØ3.6
  - diverticulum
    - bladder N21.Ø
    - kidney N2Ø.Ø
  - epididymis N5Ø.89
  - gallbladder K8Ø.2Ø
    - with
      - bile duct calculus — *see* Calculus, gallbladder and bile duct
      - cholecystitis K8Ø.1Ø
        - with obstruction K8Ø.11
        - acute K8Ø.ØØ
          - with
            - chronic cholecystitis K8Ø.12
              - with obstruction K8Ø.13
            - obstruction K8Ø.Ø1
        - chronic K8Ø.1Ø
          - with
            - acute cholecystitis K8Ø.12
              - with obstruction K8Ø.13
            - obstruction K8Ø.11
        - specified NEC K8Ø.18
          - with obstruction K8Ø.19
      - obstruction K8Ø.21
  - gallbladder and bile duct K8Ø.7Ø
    - with
      - cholecystitis K8Ø.6Ø
        - with obstruction K8Ø.61
        - acute K8Ø.62
          - with
            - chronic cholecystitis K8Ø.66
              - with obstruction K8Ø.67
            - obstruction K8Ø.63
        - chronic K8Ø.64
          - with
            - acute cholecystitis K8Ø.66
              - with obstruction K8Ø.67
- **Calculus, calculi, calculous** — *continued*
  - gallbladder and bile duct — *continued*
    - with — *continued*
      - cholecystitis — *continued*
        - chronic — *continued*
          - with — *continued*
            - obstruction K8Ø.65
      - obstruction K8Ø.71
  - hepatic (duct) — *see* Calculus, bile duct
  - ileal conduit N21.8
  - intestinal (impaction) (obstruction) K56.49
  - kidney (impacted) (multiple) (pelvis) (recurrent) (staghorn) N2Ø.Ø
    - with calculus, ureter N2Ø.2
      - with hydronephrosis N13.2
        - with infection N13.6
    - congenital Q63.8
      - with hydronephrosis N13.2
        - with infection N13.6
  - lacrimal passages — *see* Dacryolith
  - liver (impacted) — *see* Calculus, bile duct
  - lung J98.4
  - mammographic R92.1
  - nephritic (impacted) (recurrent) — *see* Calculus, kidney
  - nose J34.89
  - pancreas (duct) K86.89
  - parotid duct or gland K11.5
  - pelvis, encysted — *see* Calculus, kidney
  - prostate N42.Ø
  - pulmonary J98.4
  - pyelitis (impacted) (recurrent) N2Ø.Ø
    - with hydronephrosis N13.6
  - pyelonephritis (impacted) (recurrent) — *see* category N2Ø.- ☑
    - with hydronephrosis N13.6
  - renal (impacted) (recurrent) — *see* Calculus, kidney
  - salivary (duct) (gland) K11.5
  - seminal vesicle N5Ø.89
  - staghorn — *see* Calculus, kidney
  - Stensen's duct K11.5
  - stomach K31.89
  - sublingual duct or gland K11.5
    - congenital Q38.4
  - submandibular duct, gland or region K11.5
  - submaxillary duct, gland or region K11.5
  - suburethral N21.8
  - tonsil J35.8
  - tooth, teeth (subgingival) (supragingival) KØ3.6
  - tunica vaginalis N5Ø.89
  - ureter (impacted) (recurrent) N2Ø.1
    - with calculus, kidney N2Ø.2
      - with hydronephrosis N13.2
        - with infection N13.6
    - with hydronephrosis N13.2
      - with infection N13.6
  - ureteropelvic junction N2Ø.1
  - urethra (impacted) N21.1
  - urinary (duct) (impacted) (passage) (tract) N2Ø.9
    - with hydronephrosis N13.2
      - with infection N13.6
    - in (due to)
    - lower N21.9
      - specified NEC N21.8
  - vagina N89.8
  - vesical (impacted) N21.Ø
  - Wharton's duct K11.5
  - xanthine E79.82 *[N22]*
- **Calicectasis** N28.89
- **Caliectasis** N28.89
- **California**
  - disease B38.9
  - encephalitis A83.5
- **Caligo cornea** — *see* Opacity, cornea, central
- **Callositas, callosity** (infected) L84
- **Callus** (infected) L84
  - bone — *see* Osteophyte
    - excessive, following fracture — *code as* Sequelae of fracture
- **CALME** (childhood asymmetric labium majus enlargement) N9Ø.61
- **Calorie deficiency or malnutrition** — *see also* Malnutrition E46
- **Calpainopathy** (primary) G71.Ø32
  - autosomal dominant G71.Ø31
  - autosomal recessive G71.Ø32
- **Calve-Perthes disease** — *see* Legg-Calve-Perthes disease
- **Calve's disease** — *see* Osteochondrosis, juvenile, spine
- **Calvities** — *see* Alopecia, androgenic
- **Cameroon fever** — *see* Malaria

☑ **Additional Character Required — Refer to the Tabular List for Character Selection**

Index

Carcinoma — Carcinoma

- **Carcinoma** — *continued*
  - solid — *continued*
    - microinvasive — *continued*
      - unspecified site C53.9
  - sweat gland — *see* Neoplasm, skin, malignant
  - theca cell C56.- ☑
  - thymic C37
  - unspecified site (primary) C8Ø.1
  - water-clear cell C75.Ø
- **Carcinoma-in-situ** — *see also* Neoplasm, in situ, by site
  - breast NOS DØ5.9- ☑
    - specified type NEC DØ5.8- ☑
  - epidermoid — *see also* Neoplasm, in situ, by site
    - with questionable stromal invasion
      - cervix DØ6.9
      - specified site NEC — *see* Neoplasm, in situ, by site
      - unspecified site DØ6.9
    - Bowen's type — *see* Neoplasm, skin, in situ
  - intraductal
    - breast DØ5.1- ☑
    - specified site NEC — *see* Neoplasm, in situ, by site
    - unspecified site DØ5.1- ☑
  - lobular
    - with
      - infiltrating duct
        - breast (female) C5Ø.91- ☑
          - male C5Ø.92- ☑
        - specified site NEC — *see* Neoplasm, malignant
        - unspecified site (female) C5Ø.91- ☑
          - male C5Ø.92- ☑
      - intraductal
        - breast DØ5.8- ☑
        - specified site NEC — *see* Neoplasm, in situ, by site
        - unspecified site (female) DØ5.8- ☑
    - breast DØ5.Ø- ☑
    - specified site NEC — *see* Neoplasm, in situ, by site
    - unspecified site DØ5.Ø- ☑
  - squamous cell — *see also* Neoplasm, in situ, by site
    - with questionable stromal invasion
      - cervix DØ6.9
      - specified site NEC — *see* Neoplasm, in situ, by site
      - unspecified site DØ6.9
- **Carcinomaphobia** F45.29
- **Carcinomatosis** C8Ø.Ø
  - peritonei C78.6
  - unspecified site (primary) (secondary) C8Ø.Ø
- **Carcinosarcoma** — *see* Neoplasm, malignant, by site
  - embryonal — *see* Neoplasm, malignant, by site
- **Cardia, cardial** — *see* condition
- **Cardiac** — *see also* condition
  - death, sudden — *see* Arrest, cardiac
  - pacemaker
    - in situ Z95.Ø
    - management or adjustment Z45.Ø18
  - tamponade I31.4
- **Cardialgia** — *see* Pain, precordial
- **Cardiectasis** — *see* Hypertrophy, cardiac
- **Cardiochalasia** K21.9
- **Cardiomalacia** I51.5
- **Cardiomegalia glycogenica diffusa** E74.Ø2 *[I43]*
- **Cardiomegaly** — *see also* Hypertrophy, cardiac
  - congenital Q24.8
  - glycogen E74.Ø2 *[I43]*
  - idiopathic I51.7
- **Cardiomyoliposis** I51.5
- **Cardiomyopathy** (familial) (idiopathic) I42.9
  - alcoholic I42.6
  - amyloid E85.4 *[I43]*
    - transthyretin-related (ATTR) familial E85.4 *[I43]*
  - arrhythmogenic I42.81
    - biventricular I42.81
    - ventricular (left) (right) I42.81
  - arteriosclerotic — *see* Disease, heart, ischemic, atherosclerotic
  - beriberi E51.12
  - cobalt-beer I42.6
  - congenital I42.4
  - congestive I42.ØØ
  - constrictive NOS I42.5
  - dilated I42.ØØ
    - familial-genetic I42.Ø1
    - specified (nonfamilial) NEC I42.Ø9
  - due to
    - alcohol I42.6
    - beriberi E51.12
    - cardiac glycogenosis E74.Ø2 *[I43]*
    - drugs I42.7
- **Cardiomyopathy** — *continued*
  - due to — *continued*
    - external agents NEC I42.7
    - Friedreich's ataxia G11.11
    - myotonia atrophica G71.11 *[I43]*
    - progressive muscular dystrophy — *see also* Dystrophy, muscular, by type G71.Ø9 *[I43]*
  - glycogen storage E74.Ø2 *[I43]*
  - hypertensive — *see* Hypertension, heart
  - hypertrophic (nonobstructive) I42.2
    - obstructive I42.1
      - congenital Q24.8
  - in
    - Chagas' disease (chronic) B57.2
      - acute B57.Ø
    - sarcoidosis D86.85
  - ischemic I25.5
  - metabolic E88.9 *[I43]*
    - thyrotoxic EØ5.9Ø *[I43]*
      - with thyroid storm EØ5.91 *[I43]*
  - newborn I42.89
    - congenital I42.4
  - non-ischemic — *see also* by cause I42.89
  - nutritional E63.9 *[I43]*
    - beriberi E51.12
  - obscure of Africa I42.89
  - peripartum O9Ø.3
  - postpartum O9Ø.3
  - restrictive NEC I42.5
  - rheumatic IØ9.Ø
  - secondary I42.9
  - specified NEC I42.89
  - stress induced I51.81
  - takotsubo I51.81
  - thyrotoxic EØ5.9Ø *[I43]*
    - with thyroid storm EØ5.91 *[I43]*
  - toxic NEC I42.7
  - transthyretin-related (ATTR) familial amyloid E85.4
  - tuberculous A18.84
  - viral B33.24
- **Cardionephritis** — *see* Hypertension, cardiorenal
- **Cardionephropathy** — *see* Hypertension, cardiorenal
- **Cardionephrosis** — *see* Hypertension, cardiorenal
- **Cardiopathia nigra** I27.Ø
- **Cardiopathy** — *see also* Disease, heart I51.9
  - idiopathic I42.9
  - mucopolysaccharidosis E76.3 *[I52]*
- **Cardiopericarditis** — *see* Pericarditis
- **Cardiophobia** F45.29
- **Cardiorenal** — *see* condition
- **Cardiorrhexis** — *see* Infarct, myocardium
- **Cardiosclerosis** — *see* Disease, heart, ischemic, atherosclerotic
- **Cardiosis** — *see* Disease, heart
- **Cardiospasm** (esophagus) (reflex) (stomach) K22.Ø
  - congenital Q39.5
    - with megaesophagus Q39.5
- **Cardiostenosis** — *see* Disease, heart
- **Cardiosymphysis** I31.Ø
- **Cardiovascular** — *see* condition
- **Carditis** (acute) (bacterial) (chronic) (subacute) I51.89
  - meningococcal A39.5Ø
  - rheumatic — *see* Disease, heart, rheumatic
  - rheumatoid — *see* Rheumatoid, carditis
  - viral B33.2Ø
- **Care** (of) (for) (following)
  - child (routine) Z76.2
  - comfort Z51.5
  - family member (handicapped) (sick)
    - creating problem for family Z63.6
    - provided away from home for holiday relief Z75.5
    - unavailable, due to
      - absence (person rendering care) (sufferer) Z74.2
      - inability (any reason) of person rendering care Z74.2
  - foundling Z76.1
  - holiday relief Z75.5
  - hospice Z51.5
  - improper — *see* Maltreatment
  - lack of (at or after birth) (infant) — *see* Maltreatment, child, neglect
  - lactating mother Z39.1
  - palliative Z51.5
  - postpartum
    - immediately after delivery Z39.Ø
    - routine follow-up Z39.2
  - respite Z75.5
  - unavailable, due to
    - absence of person rendering care Z74.2
- **Care** — *continued*
  - unavailable, due to — *continued*
    - inability (any reason) of person rendering care Z74.2
  - well-baby Z76.2
- **Caries**
  - bone NEC A18.Ø3
  - dental (dentino enamel junction) (early childhood) (of dentine) (pre-eruptive) (recurrent) (to the pulp) KØ2.9
    - arrested (coronal) (root) KØ2.3
    - chewing surface
      - limited to enamel KØ2.51
      - penetrating into dentin KØ2.52
      - penetrating into pulp KØ2.53
    - coronal surface
      - chewing surface
        - limited to enamel KØ2.51
        - penetrating into dentin KØ2.52
        - penetrating into pulp KØ2.53
      - pit and fissure surface
        - limited to enamel KØ2.51
        - penetrating into dentin KØ2.52
        - penetrating into pulp KØ2.53
      - smooth surface
        - limited to enamel KØ2.61
        - penetrating into dentin KØ2.62
        - penetrating into pulp KØ2.63
    - pit and fissure surface
      - limited to enamel KØ2.51
      - penetrating into dentin KØ2.52
      - penetrating into pulp KØ2.53
    - primary, cervical origin KØ2.52
    - root KØ2.7
    - smooth surface
      - limited to enamel KØ2.61
      - penetrating into dentin KØ2.62
      - penetrating into pulp KØ2.63
  - external meatus — *see* Disorder, ear, external, specified type NEC
  - hip (tuberculous) A18.Ø2
  - initial (tooth)
    - chewing surface KØ2.51
    - pit and fissure surface KØ2.51
    - smooth surface KØ2.61
  - knee (tuberculous) A18.Ø2
  - labyrinth H83.8- ☑
  - limb NEC (tuberculous) A18.Ø3
  - mastoid process (chronic) — *see* Mastoiditis, chronic
    - tuberculous A18.Ø3
  - middle ear H74.8- ☑
  - nose (tuberculous) A18.Ø3
  - orbit (tuberculous) A18.Ø3
  - ossicles, ear — *see* Abnormal, ear ossicles
  - petrous bone — *see* Petrositis
  - root (dental) (tooth) KØ2.7
  - sacrum (tuberculous) A18.Ø1
  - spine, spinal (column) (tuberculous) A18.Ø1
  - syphilitic A52.77
    - congenital (early) A5Ø.Ø2 *[M9Ø.8Ø]*
  - tooth, teeth — *see* Caries, dental
  - tuberculous A18.Ø3
  - vertebra (column) (tuberculous) A18.Ø1
- **Carious teeth** — *see* Caries, dental
- **Carneous mole** OØ2.Ø
- **Carnitine insufficiency** E71.4Ø
- **Carotenemia** (dietary) E67.1
- **Carotenosis** (cutis) (skin) E67.1
- **Carotid body or sinus syndrome** G9Ø.Ø1
- **Carotidynia** G9Ø.Ø1
- **Carpal tunnel syndrome** — *see* Syndrome, carpal tunnel
- **Carpenter's syndrome** Q87.Ø
- **Carpopedal spasm** — *see* Tetany
- **Carr-Barr-Plunkett syndrome** Q97.1
- **Carrier** (suspected) of
  - Acinetobacter baumannii Z22.349
    - carbapenem-resistant Z22.34Ø
    - carbapenem-sensitive Z22.341
  - amebiasis Z22.1
  - bacterial disease NEC Z22.39
    - diphtheria Z22.2
    - intestinal infectious NEC Z22.1
      - typhoid Z22.Ø
    - meningococcal Z22.31
    - sexually transmitted Z22.4
    - specified NEC Z22.39
    - staphylococcal (Methicillin susceptible) Z22.321
      - Methicillin resistant Z22.322
    - streptococcal Z22.338
      - group B Z22.33Ø

- **Carrier** of — *continued*
  - bacterial disease — *continued*
    - streptococcal — *continued*
      - group B — *continued*
        - complicating pregnancy or delivery O99.82- ☑
    - typhoid Z22.0
  - cholera Z22.1
  - diphtheria Z22.2
  - E. coli (Escherichia coli) Z22.35- ☑
  - Enterobacterales Z22.359
    - carbapenem-resistant Z22.350
    - carbapenem-sensitive Z22.358
    - Enterobacterales, specified type NEC Z22.358
    - ESBL-producing Z22.358
    - extended-spectrum beta-lactamase producing Z22.358
  - gastrointestinal pathogens NEC Z22.1
  - genetic Z14.8
    - cystic fibrosis Z14.1
    - hemophilia A (asymptomatic) Z14.01
      - symptomatic Z14.02
  - gestational, pregnant Z33.1
  - gonorrhea Z22.4
  - HAA (hepatitis Australian-antigen) B18.8
  - HB (c)(s)-AG B18.1
  - hepatitis (viral) B18.9
    - Australia-antigen (HAA) B18.8
    - B surface antigen (HBsAg) B18.1
      - with acute delta- (super)infection B17.0
    - C B18.2
    - specified NEC B18.8
  - human T-cell lymphotropic virus type-1 (HTLV-1) infection Z22.6
  - infectious organism Z22.9
    - specified NEC Z22.8
  - K. pneumoniae (Klebsiella pneumoniae) Z22.35- ☑
  - meningococci Z22.31
  - Salmonella typhosa Z22.0
  - serum hepatitis — *see* Carrier, hepatitis
  - staphylococci (Methicillin susceptible) Z22.321
    - Methicillin resistant Z22.322
  - streptococci Z22.338
    - group B Z22.330
      - complicating pregnancy or delivery O99.82- ☑
  - syphilis Z22.4
  - typhoid Z22.0
  - venereal disease NEC Z22.4
- **Carrion's disease** A44.0
- **Carter's relapsing fever** (Asiatic) A68.1
- **Cartilage** — *see* condition
- **Caruncle** (inflamed)
  - conjunctiva (acute) — *see* Conjunctivitis, acute
  - labium (majus) (minus) N90.89
  - lacrimal — *see* Inflammation, lacrimal, passages
  - myrtiform N89.8
  - urethral (benign) N36.2
- **Cascade stomach** K31.2
- **Caseation lymphatic gland** (tuberculous) A18.2
- **Cassidy** (-Scholte) **syndrome** (malignant carcinoid) E34.09
- **Castellani's disease** A69.8
- **Castration, traumatic, male** S38.231- ☑
- **Casts in urine** R82.998
- **Cat**
  - cry syndrome Q93.4
  - ear Q17.3
  - eye syndrome Q92.8
- **Cat-scratch** — *see also* Abrasion
  - disease or fever A28.1
- **Catabolism, senile** R54
- **Catalepsy** (hysterical) F44.2
  - schizophrenic F20.2
- **Cataplexy** (idiopathic) — *see* Narcolepsy
- **Cataract** (cortical) (immature) (incipient) H26.9
  - with
    - neovascularization — *see* Cataract, complicated
  - age-related — *see* Cataract, senile
  - anterior
    - and posterior axial embryonal Q12.0
    - pyramidal Q12.0
  - associated with
    - galactosemia E74.21 *[H28]*
    - myotonic disorders G71.19 *[H28]*
  - blue Q12.0
  - central Q12.0
  - cerulean Q12.0
  - complicated H26.20
    - with
      - neovascularization H26.21- ☑
- **Cataract** — *continued*
  - complicated — *continued*
    - with — *continued*
      - ocular disorder H26.22- ☑
    - glaucomatous flecks H26.23- ☑
  - congenital Q12.0
  - coraliform Q12.0
  - coronary Q12.0
  - crystalline Q12.0
  - diabetic — *see* Diabetes, cataract
  - drug-induced H26.3- ☑
  - due to
    - ocular disorder — *see* Cataract, complicated
    - radiation H26.8
  - electric H26.8
  - extraction status Z98.4- ☑
  - glass-blower's H26.8
  - heat ray H26.8
  - heterochromic — *see* Cataract, complicated
  - hypermature — *see* Cataract, senile, morgagnian type
  - in (due to)
    - chronic iridocyclitis — *see* Cataract, complicated
    - diabetes — *see* Diabetes, cataract
    - endocrine disease E34.9 *[H28]*
    - eye disease — *see* Cataract, complicated
    - hypoparathyroidism E20.9 *[H28]*
    - malnutrition-dehydration E46 *[H28]*
    - metabolic disease E88.9 *[H28]*
    - myotonic disorders G71.19 *[H28]*
    - nutritional disease E63.9 *[H28]*
  - infantile — *see* Cataract, presenile
  - irradiational — *see* Cataract, specified NEC
  - juvenile — *see* Cataract, presenile
  - malnutrition-dehydration E46 *[H28]*
  - morgagnian — *see* Cataract, senile, morgagnian type
  - myotonic G71.19 *[H28]*
  - myxedema E03.9 *[H28]*
  - nuclear
    - embryonal Q12.0
    - sclerosis — *see* Cataract, senile, nuclear
  - presenile H26.00- ☑
    - combined forms H26.06- ☑
    - cortical H26.01- ☑
    - lamellar — *see* Cataract, presenile, cortical
    - nuclear H26.03- ☑
    - specified NEC H26.09
    - subcapsular polar (anterior) H26.04- ☑
      - posterior H26.05- ☑
    - zonular — *see* Cataract, presenile, cortical
  - secondary H26.40
    - Soemmering's ring H26.41- ☑
    - specified NEC H26.49- ☑
    - to eye disease — *see* Cataract, complicated
  - senile H25.9
    - brunescens — *see* Cataract, senile, nuclear
    - combined forms H25.81- ☑
    - coronary — *see* Cataract, senile, incipient
    - cortical H25.01- ☑
    - hypermature — *see* Cataract, senile, morgagnian type
    - incipient (mature) (total) H25.09- ☑
      - cortical — *see* Cataract, senile, cortical
      - subcapsular — *see* Cataract, senile, subcapsular
    - morgagnian type (hypermature) H25.2- ☑
    - nuclear (sclerosis) H25.1- ☑
    - polar subcapsular (anterior) (posterior) — *see* Cataract, senile, incipient
    - punctate — *see* Cataract, senile, incipient
    - specified NEC H25.89
    - subcapsular polar (anterior) H25.03- ☑
      - posterior H25.04- ☑
  - snowflake — *see* Diabetes, cataract
  - specified NEC H26.8
  - toxic — *see* Cataract, drug-induced
  - traumatic H26.10- ☑
    - localized H26.11- ☑
    - partially resolved H26.12- ☑
    - total H26.13- ☑
  - zonular (perinuclear) Q12.0
- **Cataracta** — *see also* Cataract
  - brunescens — *see* Cataract, senile, nuclear
  - centralis pulverulenta Q12.0
  - cerulea Q12.0
  - complicata — *see* Cataract, complicated
  - congenita Q12.0
  - coralliformis Q12.0
  - coronaria Q12.0
  - diabetic — *see* Diabetes, cataract
- **Cataracta** — *continued*
  - membranacea
    - accreta — *see* Cataract, secondary
    - congenita Q12.0
  - nigra — *see* Cataract, senile, nuclear
  - sunflower — *see* Cataract, complicated
- **Catarrh, catarrhal** (acute) (febrile) (infectious) (inflammation) — *see also* condition J00
  - bronchial — *see* Bronchitis
  - chest — *see* Bronchitis
  - chronic J31.0
  - due to congenital syphilis A50.03
  - enteric — *see* Enteritis
  - eustachian H68.009
  - fauces — *see* Pharyngitis
  - gastrointestinal — *see* Enteritis
  - gingivitis K05.00
    - nonplaque induced K05.01
    - plaque induced K05.00
  - hay — *see* Fever, hay
  - intestinal — *see* Enteritis
  - larynx, chronic J37.0
  - liver B15.9
    - with hepatic coma B15.0
  - lung — *see* Bronchitis
  - middle ear, chronic — *see* Otitis, media, nonsuppurative, chronic, serous
  - mouth K12.1
  - nasal (chronic) — *see* Rhinitis
  - nasobronchial J31.1
  - nasopharyngeal (chronic) J31.1
    - acute J00
  - pulmonary — *see* Bronchitis
  - spring (eye) (vernal) — *see* Conjunctivitis, acute, atopic
  - summer (hay) — *see* Fever, hay
  - throat J31.2
  - tubotympanal — *see also* Otitis, media, nonsuppurative
    - chronic — *see* Otitis, media, nonsuppurative, chronic, serous
- **Catatonia** (schizophrenic) F20.2
- **Catatonic**
  - disorder due to known physiologic condition F06.1
  - schizophrenia F20.2
  - stupor R40.1
- **Cauda equina** — *see* condition
- **Cauliflower ear** M95.1- ☑
- **Causalgia** (upper limb) G56.4- ☑
  - lower limb G57.7- ☑
- **Cause**
  - external, general effects T75.89- ☑
- **Caustic burn** — *see* Corrosion, by site
- **Cavare's disease** (familial periodic paralysis) G72.3
- **Cave-in, injury**
  - crushing (severe) — *see* Crush
  - suffocation — *see* Asphyxia, traumatic, due to low oxygen, due to cave-in
- **Cavernitis** (penis) N48.29
- **Cavernositis** N48.29
- **Cavernous** — *see* condition
- **Cavitation of lung** — *see also* Tuberculosis, pulmonary
  - nontuberculous J98.4
- **Cavities, dental** — *see* Caries, dental
- **Cavity**
  - lung — *see* Cavitation of lung
  - optic papilla Q14.2
  - pulmonary — *see* Cavitation of lung
- **Cavovarus foot, congenital** Q66.1- ☑
- **Cavus foot** (congenital) Q66.7- ☑
  - acquired — *see* Deformity, limb, foot, specified NEC
- **Cazenave's disease** L10.2
- **CCCA** (central centrifugal cicatricial alopecia) L66.81
- **CDKL5** (Cyclin-Dependent Kinase-Like 5 Deficiency Disorder) G40.42
- **Cecitis** K52.9
  - with perforation, peritonitis, or rupture K65.8
- **Cecoureterocele** Q62.32
- **Cecum** — *see* condition
- **Celiac**
  - artery compression syndrome I77.4
  - disease (with steatorrhea) K90.0
  - infantilism K90.0
- **Cell**(s), **cellular** — *see also* condition
  - in urine R82.998
- **Cellulitis** (diffuse) (phlegmonous) (septic) (suppurative) L03.90
  - abdominal wall L03.311
  - anaerobic A48.0
  - ankle — *see* Cellulitis, lower limb

**Cellulitis** — *continued*
- anus K61.Ø
- arm — *see* Cellulitis, upper limb
- auricle (ear) — *see* Cellulitis, ear
- axilla LØ3.11- ☑
- back (any part except buttock and flank) LØ3.312
- breast (acute) (nonpuerperal) (subacute) N61.Ø
  - nipple N61.Ø
- broad ligament
  - acute N73.Ø
- buttock LØ3.317
- cervical (meaning neck) LØ3.221
- cervix (uteri) — *see* Cervicitis
- cheek (external) LØ3.211
  - internal K12.2
- chest wall LØ3.313
- chronic LØ3.9Ø
- clostridial A48.Ø
- corpus cavernosum N48.22
- digit
  - finger — *see* Cellulitis, finger
  - toe — *see* Cellulitis, toe
- Douglas' cul-de-sac or pouch
  - acute N73.Ø
- drainage site (following operation) T81.49- ☑
- ear (external) H6Ø.1- ☑
- eosinophilic (granulomatous) L98.3
- erysipelatous — *see* Erysipelas
- external auditory canal — *see* Cellulitis, ear
- eyelid — *see* Abscess, eyelid
- face NEC LØ3.211
- finger (intrathecal) (periosteal) (subcutaneous) (subcuticular) LØ3.Ø1- ☑
- flank LØ3.31A
- foot — *see* Cellulitis, lower limb
- gangrenous — *see* Gangrene
- genital organ NEC
  - female (external) N76.4
  - male N49.9
    - multiple sites N49.8
    - specified NEC N49.8
- gluteal (region) LØ3.317
- gonococcal A54.89
- groin LØ3.314
- hand — *see* Cellulitis, upper limb
- head NEC LØ3.811
  - face (any part, except ear, eye and nose) LØ3.211
- heel — *see* Cellulitis, lower limb
- hip — *see* Cellulitis, lower limb
- jaw (region) LØ3.211
- knee — *see* Cellulitis, lower limb
- labium (majus) (minus) — *see* Vulvitis
- lacrimal passages — *see* Inflammation, lacrimal, passages
- larynx J38.7
- leg — *see* Cellulitis, lower limb
- lip K13.Ø
- lower limb LØ3.11- ☑
  - toe — *see* Cellulitis, toe
- mouth (floor) K12.2
- multiple sites, so stated LØ3.9Ø
- nasopharynx J39.1
- navel LØ3.316
  - newborn P38.9
    - with mild hemorrhage P38.1
    - without hemorrhage P38.9
- neck (region) LØ3.221
- nipple (acute) (nonpuerperal) (subacute) N61.Ø
- nose (septum) (external) J34.Ø
- orbit, orbital HØ5.Ø1- ☑
- palate (soft) K12.2
- pectoral (region) LØ3.313
- pelvis, pelvic (chronic)
  - female — *see also* Disease, pelvis, inflammatory N73.2
    - acute N73.Ø
  - following ectopic or molar pregnancy OØ8.Ø
  - male K65.Ø
- penis N48.22
- perineal, perineum LØ3.315
- periorbital LØ3.213
- perirectal K61.1
- peritonsillar J36
- periurethral N34.Ø
- periuterine — *see also* Disease, pelvis, inflammatory N73.2
  - acute N73.Ø
- pharynx J39.1
- preseptal LØ3.213
- rectum K61.1

**Cellulitis** — *continued*
- retroperitoneal K68.9
- round ligament
  - acute N73.Ø
- scalp (any part) LØ3.811
- scrotum N49.2
- seminal vesicle N49.Ø
- shoulder — *see* Cellulitis, upper limb
- specified site NEC LØ3.818
- submandibular (region) (space) (triangle) K12.2
  - gland K11.3
- submaxillary (region) K12.2
  - gland K11.3
- thigh — *see* Cellulitis, lower limb
- thumb (intrathecal) (periosteal) (subcutaneous) (subcuticular) — *see* Cellulitis, finger
- toe (intrathecal) (periosteal) (subcutaneous) (subcuticular) LØ3.Ø3- ☑
- tonsil J36
- trunk LØ3.319
  - abdominal wall LØ3.311
  - back (any part except buttock and flank) LØ3.312
  - buttock LØ3.317
  - chest wall LØ3.313
  - groin LØ3.314
  - perineal, perineum LØ3.315
  - umbilicus LØ3.316
- tuberculous (primary) A18.4
- umbilicus LØ3.316
- upper limb LØ3.11- ☑
  - axilla — *see* Cellulitis, axilla
  - finger — *see* Cellulitis, finger
  - thumb — *see* Cellulitis, finger
- vaccinal T88.Ø- ☑
- vocal cord J38.3
- vulva — *see* Vulvitis
- wrist — *see* Cellulitis, upper limb

**Cementoblastoma, benign** — *see* Cyst, calcifying odontogenic

**Cementoma** — *see* Cyst, calcifying odontogenic

**Cementoperiostitis** — *see* Periodontitis

**Cementosis** KØ3.4

**Central auditory processing disorder** H93.25

**Central pain syndrome** G89.Ø

**Cephalematocele, cephal** (o)hematocele
- newborn P52.8
  - birth injury P1Ø.8
- traumatic — *see* Hematoma, brain

**Cephalematoma, cephalhematoma** (calcified)
- newborn (birth injury) P12.Ø
- traumatic — *see* Hematoma, brain

**Cephalgia, cephalalgia** — *see also* Headache
- histamine G44.ØØ9
  - intractable G44.ØØ1
  - not intractable G44.ØØ9
- trigeminal autonomic (TAC) NEC G44.Ø99
  - intractable G44.Ø91
  - not intractable G44.Ø99

**Cephalic** — *see* condition

**Cephalitis** — *see* Encephalitis

**Cephalocele** — *see* Encephalocele

**Cephalomenia** N94.89

**Cephalopelvic** — *see* condition

**Cerclage** (with cervical incompetence) in pregnancy — *see* Incompetence, cervix, in pregnancy

**Cerebellitis** — *see* Encephalitis

**Cerebellum, cerebellar** — *see* condition

**Cerebral** — *see* condition

**Cerebritis** — *see* Encephalitis

**Cerebro-hepato-renal syndrome** Q87.89

**Cerebromalacia** — *see* Softening, brain
- sequelae of cerebrovascular disease I69.398

**Cerebroside lipidosis** E75.22

**Cerebrospasticity** (congenital) G8Ø.1

**Cerebrospinal** — *see* condition

**Cerebrum** — *see* condition

**Ceroid-lipofuscinosis, neuronal** E75.4

**Cerumen** (accumulation) (impacted) H61.2- ☑

**Cervical** — *see also* condition
- auricle Q18.2
- dysplasia in pregnancy — *see* Abnormal, cervix, in pregnancy or childbirth
- erosion in pregnancy — *see* Abnormal, cervix, in pregnancy or childbirth
- fibrosis in pregnancy — *see* Abnormal, cervix, in pregnancy or childbirth
- fusion syndrome Q76.1
- rib Q76.5

**Cervical** — *continued*
- shortening (complicating pregnancy) O26.87- ☑

**Cervicalgia** M54.2

**Cervicitis** (acute) (atrophic) (chronic) (nonvenereal) (senile) (subacute) (with ulceration) N72
- with
  - abortion — *see* Abortion, by type complicated by genital tract and pelvic infection
  - ectopic pregnancy OØ8.Ø
  - molar pregnancy OØ8.Ø
- chlamydial A56.Ø9
- gonococcal A54.Ø3
- herpesviral A6Ø.Ø3
- puerperal (postpartum) O86.11
- syphilitic A52.76
- trichomonal A59.Ø9
- tuberculous A18.16

**Cervicocolpitis** (emphysematosa) — *see also* Cervicitis N72

**Cervix** — *see* condition

**Cesarean delivery, previous, affecting management of pregnancy** O34.219
- classical (vertical) scar O34.212
- isthmocele (non-pregnant state) N85.A
  - maternal care for O34.22
- low transverse scar O34.211
- mid-transverse T incision O34.218
- scar
  - defect (non-pregnant state) N85.A
    - maternal care for O34.22
  - specified type NEC O34.218

**Cestan** (-Chenais) **paralysis or syndrome** G46.3

**Cestan-Raymond syndrome** I65.8

**Cestode infestation** B71.9
- specified type NEC B71.8

**Cestodiasis** B71.9

**CGL** (congenital generalized lipodystrophy) E88.12

**Chabert's disease** A22.9

**Chacaleh** E53.8

**Chafing** L3Ø.4

**Chagas'** (-Mazza) disease (chronic) B57.2
- with
  - cardiovascular involvement NEC B57.2
  - digestive system involvement B57.3Ø
    - megacolon B57.32
    - megaesophagus B57.31
    - other specified B57.39
  - megacolon B57.32
  - megaesophagus B57.31
  - myocarditis B57.2
  - nervous system involvement B57.4Ø
    - meningitis B57.41
    - meningoencephalitis B57.42
    - other specified B57.49
  - specified organ involvement NEC B57.5
- acute (with) B57.1
  - cardiovascular NEC B57.Ø
  - myocarditis B57.Ø

**Chagres fever** B5Ø.9

**Chairridden** Z74.Ø9

**Chalasia** (cardiac sphincter) K21.9

**Chalazion** HØØ.19
- left HØØ.16
  - lower HØØ.15
  - upper HØØ.14
- right HØØ.13
  - lower HØØ.12
  - upper HØØ.11

**Chalcosis** — *see also* Disorder, globe, degenerative, chalcosis
- cornea — *see* Deposit, cornea
- crystalline lens — *see* Cataract, complicated
- retina H35.89

**Chalicosis** (pulmonum) J62.8

**Chancre** (any genital site) (hard) (hunterian) (mixed) (primary) (seronegative) (seropositive) (syphilitic) A51.Ø
- congenital A5Ø.Ø7
- conjunctiva NEC A51.2
- ducreyi A57
- Ducrey's A57
- extragenital A51.2
- eyelid A51.2
- lip A51.2
- nipple A51.2
- Nisbet's A57
- of
  - carate A67.Ø
  - pinta A67.Ø
  - yaws A66.Ø
- palate, soft A51.2

**Chancre** — *continued*
- phagedenic A57
- simple A57
- soft A57
  - bubo A57
  - palate A51.2
- urethra A51.Ø
- yaws A66.Ø

**Chancroid** (anus) (genital) (penis) (perineum) (rectum) (urethra) (vulva) A57

**Chandler's disease** (osteochondritis dissecans, hip) — *see* Osteochondritis, dissecans, hip

**Change**(s) (in) (of) — *see also* Removal
- arteriosclerotic — *see* Arteriosclerosis
- bone — *see also* Disorder, bone
  - diabetic — *see* Diabetes, by type, with complication, specified NEC
- bowel habit R19.4
- cardiorenal (vascular) — *see* Hypertension, cardiorenal
- cardiovascular — *see* Disease, cardiovascular
- circulatory I99.9
- cognitive (mild) (organic) R41.89
- color, tooth, teeth
  - during formation KØØ.8
  - posteruptive KØ3.7
- contraceptive device Z3Ø.433
- corneal membrane H18.3Ø
  - Bowman's membrane fold or rupture H18.31- ☑
  - Descemet's membrane
    - fold H18.32- ☑
    - rupture H18.33- ☑
- coronary — *see* Disease, heart, ischemic
- degenerative, spine or vertebra — *see* Spondylosis
- dental pulp, regressive KØ4.2
- dressing (nonsurgical) Z48.ØØ
  - surgical Z48.Ø1
- heart — *see* Disease, heart
- hip joint — *see* Derangement, joint, hip
- hyperplastic larynx J38.7
- hypertrophic
  - nasal sinus J34.89
  - turbinate, nasal J34.3
  - upper respiratory tract J39.8
- indwelling catheter Z46.6
- inflammatory — *see also* Inflammation
  - sacroiliac M46.1
- job, anxiety concerning Z56.1
- joint — *see* Derangement, joint
- life — *see* Menopause
- mental status R41.82
- minimal (glomerular) — *see also* NØØ-NØ7 with fourth character .Ø NØ5.Ø
- myocardium, myocardial — *see* Degeneration, myocardial
- of life — *see* Menopause
- pacemaker Z45.Ø18
  - pulse generator Z45.Ø1Ø
- personality (enduring) F68.8
  - due to (secondary to)
    - general medical condition FØ7.Ø
  - secondary (nonspecific) F6Ø.89
- regressive, dental pulp KØ4.2
- renal — *see* Disease, renal
- retina H35.9
  - myopic — *see also* Myopia, degenerative H44.2- ☑
- sacroiliac joint M53.3
- senile — *see also* condition R54
- sensory R2Ø.8
- skin R23.9
  - acute, due to ultraviolet radiation L56.9
    - specified NEC L56.8
  - chronic, due to nonionizing radiation L57.9
    - specified NEC L57.8
  - cyanosis R23.Ø
  - flushing R23.2
  - pallor R23.1
  - petechiae R23.3
  - specified change NEC R23.8
  - swelling — *see* Mass, localized
  - texture R23.4
- trophic
  - arm — *see* Mononeuropathy, upper limb
  - leg — *see* Mononeuropathy, lower limb
- vascular I99.9
- vasomotor I73.9
- voice R49.9
  - psychogenic F44.4
  - specified NEC R49.8

**Changing sleep-work schedule, affecting sleep** G47.26

**Changuinola fever** A93.1

**Chapping skin** T69.8- ☑

**Charcot-Marie-Tooth disease, paralysis or syndrome** G6Ø.Ø

**Charcot's**
- arthropathy — *see* Arthropathy, neuropathic
- cirrhosis K74.3
- disease (tabetic arthropathy) A52.16
- joint (disease) (tabetic) A52.16
  - diabetic — *see* Diabetes, with, arthropathy
  - syringomyelic G95.Ø
- syndrome (intermittent claudication) I73.9

**CHARGE association** Q89.89

**Charley-horse** (quadriceps) M62.831
- traumatic (quadriceps) S76.11- ☑

**Charlouis' disease** — *see* Yaws

**Cheadle's disease** E54

**Check-up** — *see* Examination

**Checking** (of)
- cardiac pacemaker (battery) (electrode(s)) Z45.Ø18
  - pulse generator Z45.Ø1Ø
- implantable subdermal contraceptive Z3Ø.46
- intrauterine contraceptive device Z3Ø.431
- wound Z48.Ø- ☑
  - due to injury — code to Injury, by site, using appropriate seventh character for subsequent encounter
  - postoperative — *see* Aftercare

**Chediak-Higashi** (-Steinbrinck) **syndrome** (congenital gigantism of peroxidase granules) E7Ø.33Ø

**Cheek** — *see* condition

**Cheese itch** B88.Ø9

**Cheese-washer's lung** J67.8

**Cheese-worker's lung** J67.8

**Cheilitis** (acute) (angular) (catarrhal) (chronic) (exfoliative) (gangrenous) (glandular) (infectional) (suppurative) (ulcerative) (vesicular) K13.Ø
- actinic (due to sun) L56.8
  - other than from sun L59.8
- candidal B37.83

**Cheilodynia** K13.Ø

**Cheiloschisis** — *see* Cleft, lip

**Cheilosis** (angular) K13.Ø
- with pellagra E52
- due to
  - vitamin B2 (riboflavin) deficiency E53.Ø

**Cheiromegaly** M79.89

**Cheiropompholyx** L3Ø.1

**Cheloid** — *see* Keloid

**Chemical burn** — *see* Corrosion, by site

**Chemodectoma** — *see* Paraganglioma, nonchromaffin

**Chemosis, conjunctiva** — *see* Edema, conjunctiva

**Chemotherapy** (session) (for)
- cancer Z51.11
- neoplasm Z51.11

**Cherubism** M27.8

**Chest** — *see* condition

**Cheyne-Stokes breathing** (respiration) RØ6.3

**Chiari's**
- disease or syndrome (hepatic vein thrombosis) I82.Ø
- malformation
  - type I G93.5
  - type II — *see* Spina bifida
- net Q24.8

**Chicago disease** B4Ø.9

**Chickenpox** — *see* Varicella

**Chiclero ulcer or sore** B55.1

**Chigger** (infestation) B88.Ø9

**Chignon** (disease) B36.8
- newborn (from vacuum extraction) (birth injury) P12.1

**Chilaiditi's syndrome** (subphrenic displacement, colon) Q43.3

**Chilblain**(s) (lupus) T69.1- ☑

**Child** — *see also* Problem, child
- custody dispute Z65.3

**Childbirth** — *see* Delivery

**Childhood**
- cerebral X-linked adrenoleukodystrophy E71.52Ø
- period of rapid growth ZØØ.2

**Chill**(s) R68.83
- with fever R5Ø.9
- congestive in malarial regions B54
- without fever R68.83

**Chilomastigiasis** AØ7.8

**Chimera 46,XX/46,XY** Q99.Ø

**Chin** — *see* condition

**Chinese dysentery** AØ3.9

**Chionophobia** F4Ø.228

**Chitral fever** A93.1

**Chlamydia, chlamydial** A74.9
- cervicitis A56.Ø9
- conjunctivitis A74.Ø
- cystitis A56.Ø1
- endometritis A56.11
- epididymitis A56.19
- female
  - pelvic inflammatory disease A56.11
  - pelviperitonitis A56.11
- orchitis A56.19
- peritonitis A74.81
- pharyngitis A56.4
- proctitis A56.3
- psittaci (infection) A7Ø
- salpingitis A56.11
- sexually-transmitted infection NEC A56.8
- specified NEC A74.89
- urethritis A56.Ø1
- vulvovaginitis A56.Ø2

**Chlamydiosis** — *see* Chlamydia

**Chloasma** (skin) (idiopathic) (symptomatic) L81.1
- eyelid HØ2.71- ☑
  - hyperthyroid EØ5.9Ø *[HØ2.71-]* ☑
    - with thyroid storm EØ5.91 *[HØ2.71-]* ☑
  - left HØ2.716
    - lower HØ2.715
    - upper HØ2.714
  - right HØ2.713
    - lower HØ2.712
    - upper HØ2.711

**Chloroma** C92.3- ☑

**Chlorosis** D5Ø.9
- Egyptian B76.9 *[D63.8]*
- miner's B76.9 *[D63.8]*

**Chlorotic anemia** D5Ø.8

**Chocolate cyst** (ovary) N8Ø.1Ø- ☑

**Choked**
- disc or disk — *see* Papilledema
- on food, phlegm, or vomitus NOS — *see* Foreign body, by site
- while vomiting NOS — *see* Foreign body, by site

**Chokes** (resulting from bends) T7Ø.3- ☑

**Choking sensation** RØ9.89

**Cholangiectasis** K83.8

**Cholangiocarcinoma**
- with hepatocellular carcinoma, combined C22.Ø
- liver C22.1
- specified site NEC — *see* Neoplasm, malignant, by site
- unspecified site C22.1

**Cholangiohepatitis** K83.8
- due to fluke infestation B66.1

**Cholangiohepatoma** C22.Ø

**Cholangiolitis** (acute) (chronic) (extrahepatic) (gangrenous) (intrahepatic) K83.Ø9
- paratyphoidal — *see* Fever, paratyphoid
- typhoidal AØ1.Ø9

**Cholangioma** D13.4
- malignant — *see* Cholangiocarcinoma

**Cholangitis** (ascending) (recurrent) (secondary) (stenosing) (suppurative) K83.Ø9
- with calculus, bile duct — *see* Calculus, bile duct, with cholangitis
- chronic nonsuppurative destructive K74.3
- primary K83.Ø9
  - sclerosing K83.Ø1
- sclerosing K83.Ø9

**Cholecystectasia** K82.8

**Cholecystitis** K81.9
- with
  - calculus, stones in
    - bile duct (common) (hepatic) — *see* Calculus, bile duct, with cholecystitis
    - cystic duct — *see* Calculus, gallbladder, with cholecystitis
    - gallbladder — *see* Calculus, gallbladder, with cholecystitis
  - choledocholithiasis — *see* Calculus, bile duct, with cholecystitis
  - cholelithiasis — *see* Calculus, gallbladder, with cholecystitis
  - gangrene of gallbladder K82.A1
  - perforation of gallbladder K82.A2
- acute (emphysematous) (gangrenous) (suppurative) K81.Ø
  - with
    - calculus, stones in
      - cystic duct — *see* Calculus, gallbladder, with cholecystitis, acute



Index

Chancre — Cholecystitis

☑ **Additional Character Required — Refer to the Tabular List for Character Selection**

- **Chromaffinoma** — *see also* Neoplasm, benign, by site
  - malignant — *see* Neoplasm, malignant, by site
- **Chromatopsia** — *see* Deficiency, color vision
- **Chromhidrosis, chromidrosis** L75.1
- **Chromoblastomycosis** — *see* Chromomycosis
- **Chromoconversion** R82.91
- **Chromomycosis** B43.9
  - brain abscess B43.1
  - cerebral B43.1
  - cutaneous B43.0
  - skin B43.0
  - specified NEC B43.8
  - subcutaneous abscess or cyst B43.2
- **Chromophytosis** B36.0
- **Chromosome** — *see* Anomaly, by chromosome involved
  - D (1) — *see* Anomaly, chromosome 13
  - E (3) — *see* Anomaly, chromosome 18
  - G — *see* Anomaly, chromosome 21
- **Chromotrichomycosis** B36.8
- **Chronic** — *see* condition
  - fracture — *see* Fracture, pathological
- **Churg-Strauss syndrome** M30.1
- **Chyle cyst, mesentery** I89.8
- **Chylocele** (nonfilarial) I89.8
  - filarial — *see also* Infestation, filarial B74.9 *[N51]*
  - tunica vaginalis N50.89
    - filarial — *see also* Infestation, filarial B74.9 *[N51]*
- **Chylomicronemia** (fasting) (with hyperprebetalipoproteinemia) E78.3
- **Chylopericardium** I31.39
  - acute I30.9
- **Chylothorax** (nonfilarial) J94.0
  - filarial — *see also* Infestation, filarial B74.9 *[J91.8]*
- **Chylous** — *see* condition
- **Chyluria** (nonfilarial) R82.0
  - due to
    - bilharziasis B65.0
    - Brugia (malayi) B74.1
      - timori B74.2
    - schistosomiasis (bilharziasis) B65.0
    - Wuchereria (bancrofti) B74.0
  - filarial — *see* Infestation, filarial
- **Cicatricial** (deformity) — *see* Cicatrix
- **Cicatrix** (adherent) (contracted) (painful) (vicious) — *see also* Scar L90.5
  - adenoid (and tonsil) J35.8
  - alveolar process M26.79
  - anus K62.89
  - auricle — *see* Disorder, pinna, specified type NEC
  - bile duct (common) (hepatic) K83.8
  - bladder N32.89
  - bone — *see* Disorder, bone, specified type NEC
  - brain G93.89
  - cervix (postoperative) (postpartal) N88.1
  - common duct K83.8
  - cornea H17.9
    - tuberculous A18.59
  - duodenum (bulb), obstructive K31.5
  - esophagus K22.2
  - eyelid — *see* Disorder, eyelid function
  - hypopharynx J39.2
  - lacrimal passages — *see* Obstruction, lacrimal
  - larynx J38.7
  - lung J98.4
  - middle ear H74.8- ☑
  - mouth K13.79
  - muscle M62.89
    - with contracture — *see* Contraction, muscle NEC
  - nasopharynx J39.2
  - palate (soft) K13.79
  - penis N48.89
  - pharynx J39.2
  - prostate N42.89
  - rectum K62.89
  - retina — *see* Scar, chorioretinal
  - semilunar cartilage — *see* Derangement, meniscus
  - seminal vesicle N50.89
  - skin L90.5
    - infected L08.89
    - postinfective L90.5
    - tuberculous B90.8
  - specified site NEC L90.5
  - throat J39.2
  - tongue K14.8
  - tonsil (and adenoid) J35.8
  - trachea J39.8
  - tuberculous NEC B90.9
  - urethra N36.8
  - uterus N85.8
- **Cicatrix** — *continued*
  - vagina N89.8
    - postoperative N99.2
  - vocal cord J38.3
  - wrist, constricting (annular) L90.5
- **CIDP** (chronic inflammatory demyelinating polyneuropathy) G61.81
- **CIN** — *see* Neoplasia, intraepithelial, cervix
- **CINCA** (chronic infantile neurological, cutaneous and articular syndrome) M04.2
- **Cinchonism** — *see* Deafness, ototoxic
  - correct substance properly administered — *see* Table of Drugs and Chemicals, by drug, adverse effect
  - overdose or wrong substance given or taken — *see* Table of Drugs and Chemicals, by drug, poisoning
- **Circle of Willis** — *see* condition
- **Circular** — *see* condition
- **Circulating anticoagulants** — *see also* Disorder, hemorrhagic D68.318
  - due to drugs — *see also* Disorder, hemorrhagic D68.32
  - following childbirth O72.3
- **Circulation**
  - collateral, any site I99.8
  - defective (lower extremity) I99.9
    - congenital Q28.9
  - embryonic Q28.9
  - failure (peripheral) R57.9
    - newborn P29.89
  - fetal, persistent P29.38
  - Fontan related I27.849
    - with
      - Fontan-associated condition, specified NEC I27.848
      - Fontan-associated liver disease [FALD] I27.840
      - Fontan-associated lymphatic dysfunction I27.841
  - heart, incomplete Q28.9
- **Circulatory system** — *see* condition
- **Circulus senilis** (cornea) — *see* Degeneration, cornea, senile
- **Circumcision** (in absence of medical indication) (ritual) (routine) Z41.2
- **Circumscribed** — *see* condition
- **Circumvallate placenta** O43.11- ☑
- **Cirrhosis, cirrhotic** (hepatic) (liver) K74.60
  - alcoholic K70.30
    - with ascites K70.31
  - atrophic — *see* Cirrhosis, liver
  - Baumgarten-Cruveilhier K74.69
  - biliary (cholangiolitic) (cholangitic) (hypertrophic) (obstructive) (pericholangiolitic) K74.5
    - due to
      - Clonorchiasis B66.1
      - flukes B66.3
    - primary K74.3
    - secondary K74.4
  - cardiac (of liver) K76.1
  - Charcot's K74.3
  - cholangiolitic, cholangitic, cholostatic (primary) K74.3
  - congestive K76.1
  - Cruveilhier-Baumgarten K74.69
  - cryptogenic (liver) K74.69
  - due to
    - hepatolenticular degeneration E83.01
    - Wilson's disease E83.01
    - xanthomatosis E78.2
  - fatty K76.0
    - alcoholic K70.0
  - Hanot's (hypertrophic) K74.3
  - hepatic — *see* Cirrhosis, liver
  - hypertrophic K74.3
  - Indian childhood K74.69
  - kidney — *see* Sclerosis, renal
  - Laennec's K70.30
    - with ascites K70.31
    - alcoholic K70.30
      - with ascites K70.31
    - nonalcoholic K74.69
  - liver K74.60
    - alcoholic K70.30
      - with ascites K70.31
      - fatty K70.0
    - congenital P78.81
    - syphilitic A52.74
  - lung (chronic) J84.10
  - macronodular K74.69
    - alcoholic K70.30
      - with ascites K70.31
  - micronodular K74.69
    - alcoholic K70.30
      - with ascites K70.31
  - mixed type K74.69
- **Cirrhosis, cirrhotic** — *continued*
  - monolobular K74.3
  - nephritis — *see* Sclerosis, renal
  - nutritional K74.69
    - alcoholic K70.30
      - with ascites K70.31
  - obstructive — *see* Cirrhosis, biliary
  - ovarian N83.8
  - pancreas (duct) K86.89
  - pigmentary E83.110
  - portal K74.69
    - alcoholic K70.30
      - with ascites K70.31
  - postnecrotic K74.69
    - alcoholic K70.30
      - with ascites K70.31
  - pulmonary J84.10
  - renal — *see* Sclerosis, renal
  - spleen D73.2
  - stasis K76.1
  - Todd's K74.3
  - unilobar K74.3
  - xanthomatous (biliary) K74.5
    - due to xanthomatosis (familial) (metabolic) (primary) E78.2
- **Cistern, subarachnoid** R93.0
- **Citrullinemia** E72.23
- **Citrullinuria** E72.23
- **Civatte's disease or poikiloderma** L57.3
- **CLAD** — *see* Dysfunction, chronic, lung allograft
- **Clam digger's itch** B65.3
- **Clammy skin** R23.1
- **Clap** — *see* Gonorrhea
- **Clarke-Hadfield syndrome** (pancreatic infantilism) K86.89
- **Clark's paralysis** G80.9
- **Clastothrix** L67.8
- **Claude Bernard-Horner syndrome** G90.2
  - traumatic — *see* Injury, nerve, cervical sympathetic
- **Claude's disease or syndrome** G46.3
- **Claudicatio venosa intermittens** I87.8
- **Claudication** (intermittent) I73.9
  - cerebral (artery) G45.9
  - spinal cord (arteriosclerotic) G95.19
    - syphilitic A52.09
  - venous (axillary) I87.8
- **Claustrophobia** F40.240
- **Clavus** (infected) L84
- **Clawfoot** (congenital) Q66.89
  - acquired — *see* Deformity, limb, clawfoot
- **Clawhand** (acquired) — *see also* Deformity, limb, clawhand
  - congenital Q68.1
- **Clawtoe** (congenital) Q66.89
  - acquired — *see* Deformity, toe, specified NEC
- **Clay eating** — *see* Pica
- **Cleansing of artificial opening** — *see* Attention to, artificial, opening
- **Cleft** (congenital) — *see also* Imperfect, closure
  - alveolar process M26.79
  - branchial (persistent) Q18.2
    - cyst Q18.0
      - fistula Q18.0
      - sinus Q18.0
  - cricoid cartilage, posterior Q31.8
  - cyst Q18.0
    - fistula Q18.0
    - sinus Q18.0
  - foot Q72.7- ☑
  - hand Q71.6- ☑
  - lip (unilateral) Q36.9
    - with cleft palate Q37.9
      - hard Q37.1
        - with soft Q37.5
      - soft Q37.3
        - with hard Q37.5
    - bilateral Q36.0
      - with cleft palate Q37.8
        - hard Q37.0
          - with soft Q37.4
        - soft Q37.2
          - with hard Q37.4
    - median Q36.1
  - mitral valve leaflet (at birth) (congenital) Q23.82
  - nose Q30.2
  - palate Q35.9
    - with cleft lip (unilateral) Q37.9
      - bilateral Q37.8
    - hard Q35.1
      - with
        - cleft lip (unilateral) Q37.1

- **Cleft** — *continued*
  - palate — *continued*
    - hard — *continued*
      - with — *continued*
        - cleft lip — *continued*
          - bilateral Q37.Ø
        - soft Q35.5
          - with cleft lip (unilateral) Q37.5
            - bilateral Q37.4
    - medial Q35.5
    - soft Q35.3
      - with
        - cleft lip (unilateral) Q37.3
          - bilateral Q37.2
        - hard Q35.5
          - with cleft lip (unilateral) Q37.5
            - bilateral Q37.4
  - penis Q55.69
  - scrotum Q55.29
  - thyroid cartilage Q31.8
  - uvula Q35.7
- **Cleidocranial dysostosis** Q74.Ø
- **Cleptomania** F63.2
- **Clicking hip** (newborn) R29.4
- **Climacteric** (female) — *see also* Menopause
  - arthritis (any site) NEC — *see* Arthritis, specified form NEC
  - depression (single episode) F32.89
    - recurrent episode F33.8
  - male (symptoms) (syndrome) NEC N5Ø.89
  - melancholia (single episode) F32.89
    - recurrent episode F33.8
  - paranoid state F22
  - polyarthritis NEC — *see* Arthritis, specified form NEC
  - symptoms (female) N95.1
- **Clinical research investigation** (clinical trial) (control subject) (normal comparison) (participant) ZØØ.6
- **Clitoris** — *see* condition
- **Cloaca** (persistent) Q43.7
- **Clonorchiasis, clonorchis infection** (liver) B66.1
- **Clonus** R25.8
- **Closed bite** M26.29
- **Clostridium** (C.) **perfringens, as cause of disease classified elsewhere** B96.7
- **Closure**
  - congenital, nose Q3Ø.Ø
  - cranial sutures, premature Q75.ØØ9
  - defective or imperfect NEC — *see* Imperfect, closure
  - fistula, delayed — *see* Fistula
  - foramen ovale, imperfect Q21.12
  - hymen N89.6
  - interauricular septum, defective Q21.19
  - interventricular septum, defective Q21.Ø
  - lacrimal duct — *see also* Stenosis, lacrimal, duct
    - congenital Q1Ø.5
  - nose (congenital) Q3Ø.Ø
    - acquired M95.Ø
  - of artificial opening — *see* Attention to, artificial, opening
  - vagina N89.5
  - valve — *see* Endocarditis
  - vulva N9Ø.5
- **Clot** (blood) — *see also* Embolism
  - artery (obstruction) (occlusion) — *see* Embolism
  - bladder N32.89
  - brain (intradural or extradural) — *see* Occlusion, artery, cerebral
  - circulation I74.9
  - heart — *see also* Infarct, myocardium
    - not resulting in infarction I51.3
  - vein — *see* Thrombosis
- **Clouded state** R4Ø.1
  - epileptic — *see* Epilepsy, specified NEC
  - paroxysmal — *see* Epilepsy, specified NEC
- **Cloudy antrum, antra** J32.Ø
- **Clouston's** (hidrotic) **ectodermal dysplasia** Q82.4
- **Cloverleaf skull** Q75.Ø51
- **Clubbed nail pachydermoperiostosis** M89.4Ø *[L62]*
- **Clubbing of finger**(s) (nails) R68.3
- **Clubfinger** R68.3
  - congenital Q68.1
- **Clubfoot** (congenital) Q66.89
  - acquired — *see* Deformity, limb, clubfoot
  - equinovarus Q66.Ø- ☑
  - paralytic — *see* Deformity, limb, clubfoot
- **Clubhand** (congenital) (radial) Q71.4- ☑
  - acquired — *see* Deformity, limb, clubhand
- **Clubnail** R68.3
  - congenital Q84.6
- **Clump, kidney** Q63.1
- **Clumsiness, clumsy child syndrome** F82
- **Cluttering** F8Ø.81
- **Clutton's joints** A5Ø.51 *[M12.8Ø]*
- **Coagulation, intravascular** (diffuse) (disseminated) — *see also* Defibrination syndrome
  - complicating abortion — *see* Abortion, by type, complicated by, intravascular coagulation
  - COVID-19 associated — *see also* COVID-19 D65
  - following ectopic or molar pregnancy OØ8.1
- **Coagulopathy** — *see also* Defect, coagulation
  - consumption D65
  - intravascular D65
    - newborn P6Ø
- **Coalition**
  - calcaneo-scaphoid Q66.89
  - tarsal Q66.89
- **Coalminer's**
  - elbow — *see* Bursitis, elbow, olecranon
  - lung or pneumoconiosis J6Ø
- **Coalworker's lung or pneumoconiosis** J6Ø
- **Coarctation**
  - aorta (preductal) (postductal) Q25.1
  - pulmonary artery Q25.71
- **Coated tongue** K14.3
- **Coats' disease** (exudative retinopathy) — *see* Retinopathy, exudative
- **Cocaine-induced**
  - anxiety disorder F14.98Ø
  - bipolar and related disorder F14.94
  - depressive disorder F14.94
  - obsessive-compulsive and related disorder F14.988
  - psychotic disorder F14.959
  - sexual dysfunction F14.981
  - sleep disorder F14.982
- **Cocainism** — *see* Disorder, cocaine use
- **Coccidioidomycosis** B38.9
  - cutaneous B38.3
  - disseminated B38.7
  - generalized B38.7
  - meninges B38.4
  - prostate B38.81
  - pulmonary B38.2
    - acute B38.Ø
    - chronic B38.1
  - skin B38.3
  - specified NEC B38.89
- **Coccidioidosis** — *see* Coccidioidomycosis
- **Coccidiosis** (intestinal) AØ7.3
- **Coccydynia, coccygodynia** M53.3
- **Coccyx** — *see* condition
- **Cochin-China diarrhea** K9Ø.1
- **Cockayne's syndrome** Q87.19
- **Cocked up toe** — *see* Deformity, toe, specified NEC
- **Cock's peculiar tumor** L72.3
- **Codman's tumor** — *see* Neoplasm, bone, benign
- **Coenurosis** B71.8
- **Coffee-worker's lung** J67.8
- **Cogan's syndrome** H16.32- ☑
  - oculomotor apraxia H51.8
- **Coitus, painful** (female) N94.1Ø
  - male N53.12
  - psychogenic F52.6
- **Cold** JØØ
  - with influenza, flu, or grippe — *see* Influenza, with, respiratory manifestations NEC
  - agglutinin disease or hemoglobinuria (chronic) D59.12
  - bronchial — *see* Bronchitis
  - chest — *see* Bronchitis
  - common (head) JØØ
  - effects of T69.9- ☑
    - specified effect NEC T69.8- ☑
  - excessive, effects of T69.9- ☑
    - specified effect NEC T69.8- ☑
  - exhaustion from T69.8- ☑
  - exposure to T69.9- ☑
    - specified effect NEC T69.8- ☑
  - head JØØ
  - injury syndrome (newborn) P8Ø.Ø
  - on lung — *see* Bronchitis
  - rose J3Ø.1
  - sensitivity, auto-immune D59.12
  - symptoms JØØ
  - virus JØØ
- **Coldsore** BØØ.1
- **Colibacillosis** A49.8
  - as the cause of other disease — *see also* Escherichia coli B96.2Ø
  - generalized — *see also* Sepsis, Escherichia coli A41.51
- **Colic** (bilious) (infantile) (intestinal) (recurrent) (spasmodic) R1Ø.83
  - abdomen R1Ø.83
    - psychogenic F45.8
  - appendix, appendicular K38.8
  - bile duct — *see* Calculus, bile duct
  - biliary — *see* Calculus, bile duct
  - common duct — *see* Calculus, bile duct
  - cystic duct — *see* Calculus, gallbladder
  - Devonshire NEC — *see* Poisoning, lead
  - gallbladder — *see* Calculus, gallbladder
  - gallstone — *see* Calculus, gallbladder
    - gallbladder or cystic duct — *see* Calculus, gallbladder
  - hepatic (duct) — *see* Calculus, bile duct
  - hysterical F45.8
  - kidney N23
  - lead NEC — *see* Poisoning, lead
  - mucous K58.9
    - with diarrhea K58.Ø
    - psychogenic F54
  - nephritic N23
  - painter's NEC — *see* Poisoning, lead
  - pancreas K86.89
  - psychogenic F45.8
  - renal N23
  - saturnine NEC — *see* Poisoning, lead
  - ureter N23
  - urethral N36.8
    - due to calculus N21.1
  - uterus NEC N94.89
    - menstrual — *see* Dysmenorrhea
  - worm NOS B83.9
- **Colicystitis** — *see* Cystitis
- **Colitis** (acute) (catarrhal) (chronic) (noninfective) (hemorrhagic) — *see also* Enteritis K52.9
  - allergic K52.29
    - with
      - food protein-induced enterocolitis syndrome K52.21
      - proctocolitis K52.29
  - amebic (acute) — *see also* Amebiasis AØ6.Ø
    - nondysenteric AØ6.2
  - anthrax A22.2
  - bacillary — *see* Infection, Shigella
  - balantidial AØ7.Ø
  - Clostridioides difficile
    - not specified as recurrent AØ4.72
    - recurrent AØ4.71
  - Clostridium difficile
    - not specified as recurrent AØ4.72
    - recurrent AØ4.71
  - coccidial AØ7.3
  - collagenous K52.831
  - cystica superficialis K52.89
  - dietary counseling and surveillance (for) Z71.3
  - dietetic — *see also* Colitis, allergic K52.29
  - drug-induced K52.1
  - due to radiation K52.Ø
  - eosinophilic K52.82
  - food hypersensitivity — *see also* Colitis, allergic K52.29
  - giardial AØ7.1
  - granulomatous — *see* Enteritis, regional, large intestine
  - indeterminate, so stated K52.3
  - infectious — *see* Enteritis, infectious
  - ischemic K55.9
    - acute (subacute) — *see also* Ischemia, intestine, acute K55.Ø39
    - chronic K55.1
    - due to mesenteric artery insufficiency K55.1
    - fulminant (acute) — *see also* Ischemia, intestine, acute K55.Ø39
  - left sided K51.5Ø
    - with
      - abscess K51.514
      - complication K51.519
        - specified NEC K51.518
      - fistula K51.513
      - obstruction K51.512
      - rectal bleeding K51.511
  - lymphocytic K52.832
  - membranous
    - psychogenic F54
  - microscopic K52.839
    - specified NEC K52.838
  - mucous — *see* Syndrome, irritable, bowel
    - psychogenic F54
  - noninfective K52.9
    - specified NEC K52.89
  - polyposa — *see* Polyp, colon, inflammatory

- **Colitis** — *continued*
  - protozoal AØ7.9
  - pseudomembranous
    - not specified as recurrent AØ4.72
    - recurrent AØ4.71
  - pseudomucinous — *see* Syndrome, irritable, bowel
  - regional — *see* Enteritis, regional, large intestine
    - infectious AØ9
  - segmental — *see* Enteritis, regional, large intestine
  - septic — *see* Enteritis, infectious
  - spastic K58.9
    - with diarrhea K58.Ø
    - psychogenic F54
  - staphylococcal AØ4.8
    - foodborne AØ5.Ø
  - subacute ischemic — *see also* Ischemia, intestine, acute K55.Ø39
  - thromboulcerative — *see also* Ischemia, intestine, acute K55.Ø39
  - toxic NEC K52.1
    - due to
      - Clostridioides difficile
        - not specified as recurrent AØ4.72
        - recurrent AØ4.71
      - Clostridium difficile
        - not specified as recurrent AØ4.72
        - recurrent AØ4.71
  - transmural — *see* Enteritis, regional, large intestine
  - trichomonal AØ7.8
  - tuberculous (ulcerative) A18.32
  - ulcerative (chronic) K51.9Ø
    - with
      - complication K51.919
        - abscess K51.914
        - fistula K51.913
        - obstruction K51.912
        - rectal bleeding K51.911
        - specified complication NEC K51.918
    - enterocolitis — *see* Enterocolitis, ulcerative
    - ileocolitis — *see* Ileocolitis, ulcerative
    - mucosal proctocolitis — *see* Proctocolitis, mucosal
    - proctitis — *see* Proctitis, ulcerative
    - pseudopolyposis — *see* Polyp, colon, inflammatory
    - psychogenic F54
    - rectosigmoiditis — *see* Rectosigmoiditis, ulcerative
    - specified type NEC K51.8Ø
      - with
        - complication K51.819
          - abscess K51.814
          - fistula K51.813
          - obstruction K51.812
          - rectal bleeding K51.811
          - specified complication NEC K51.818
- **Collagenosis, collagen disease** (nonvascular) (vascular) M35.9
  - cardiovascular I42.89
  - reactive perforating L87.1
  - specified NEC M35.89
- **Collapse** R55
  - adrenal E27.2
  - cardiorespiratory R57.Ø
  - cardiovascular R57.Ø
    - newborn P29.89
  - circulatory (peripheral) R57.9
    - during or after labor and delivery O75.1
    - following ectopic or molar pregnancy OØ8.3
    - newborn P29.89
  - during or
    - after labor and delivery O75.1
    - resulting from a procedure, not elsewhere classified T81.1Ø- ☑
  - external ear canal — *see* Stenosis, external ear canal
  - general R55
  - heart — *see* Disease, heart
  - heat T67.1- ☑
  - hysterical F44.89
  - labyrinth, membranous (congenital) Q16.5
  - lung (massive) — *see also* Atelectasis J98.19
    - pressure due to anesthesia (general) (local) or other sedation T88.2- ☑
      - during labor and delivery O74.1
      - in pregnancy O29.Ø2- ☑
      - postpartum, puerperal O89.Ø9
  - myocardial — *see* Disease, heart
  - nasal valve J34.829
    - external J34.821Ø
      - dynamic J34.8212
      - static J34.8211
    - internal J34.82ØØ
- **Collapse** — *continued*
  - nasal valve — *continued*
    - internal — *continued*
      - dynamic J34.82Ø2
      - static J34.82Ø1
  - nervous F48.8
  - neurocirculatory F45.8
  - nose M95.Ø
    - lower sidewall or nostril, on inspiration J34.8212
    - upper, middle sidewall, on inspiration J34.82Ø2
  - postoperative T81.1Ø- ☑
  - pulmonary — *see also* Atelectasis J98.19
    - newborn — *see* Atelectasis
  - trachea J39.8
  - tracheobronchial J98.Ø9
  - valvular — *see* Endocarditis
  - vascular (peripheral) R57.9
    - during or after labor and delivery O75.1
    - following ectopic or molar pregnancy OØ8.3
    - newborn P29.89
  - vertebra M48.5Ø- ☑
    - cervical region M48.52- ☑
    - cervicothoracic region M48.53- ☑
    - in (due to)
      - neoplasm (metastasis) M84.58- ☑
      - osteoporosis — *see also* Osteoporosis M8Ø.88- ☑
        - cervical region M8Ø.88- ☑
        - cervicothoracic region M8Ø.88- ☑
        - lumbar region M8Ø.88- ☑
        - lumbosacral region M8Ø.88- ☑
        - multiple sites M8Ø.88- ☑
        - occipito-atlanto-axial region M8Ø.88- ☑
        - sacrococcygeal region M8Ø.88- ☑
        - thoracic region M8Ø.88- ☑
        - thoracolumbar region M8Ø.88- ☑
      - specified disease NEC M48.5Ø- ☑
        - cervical region M48.52- ☑
        - cervicothoracic region M48.53- ☑
        - lumbar region M48.56- ☑
        - lumbosacral region M48.57- ☑
        - occipito-atlanto-axial region M48.51- ☑
        - sacrococcygeal region M48.58- ☑
        - thoracic region M48.54- ☑
        - thoracolumbar region M48.55- ☑
    - lumbar region M48.56- ☑
    - lumbosacral region M48.57- ☑
    - occipito-atlanto-axial region M48.51- ☑
    - sacrococcygeal region M48.58- ☑
    - thoracic region M48.54- ☑
    - thoracolumbar region M48.55- ☑
- **Collateral** — *see also* condition
  - circulation (venous) I87.8
  - dilation, veins I87.8
- **Colles' fracture** S52.53- ☑
- **Collet** (-Sicard) **syndrome** G52.7
- **Collier's asthma or lung** J6Ø
- **Collodion baby** Q8Ø.2
- **Colloid nodule** (of thyroid) (cystic) EØ4.1
- **Coloboma** (iris) Q13.Ø
  - eyelid Q1Ø.3
  - fundus Q14.8
  - lens Q12.2
  - optic disc (congenital) Q14.2
    - acquired H47.31- ☑
- **Coloenteritis** — *see* Enteritis
- **Colon** — *see* condition
- **Colonization**
  - MRSA (Methicillin resistant Staphylococcus aureus) Z22.322
  - MSSA (Methicillin susceptible Staphylococcus aureus) Z22.321
  - status — *see* Carrier (suspected) of
- **Coloptosis** K63.4
- **Color blindness** — *see* Deficiency, color vision
- **Colostomy**
  - attention to Z43.3
  - fitting or adjustment Z46.89
  - malfunctioning K94.Ø3
  - status Z93.3
- **Colpitis** (acute) — *see* Vaginitis
- **Colpocele** N81.5
- **Colpocystitis** — *see* Vaginitis
- **Colpospasm** N94.2
- **Column, spinal, vertebral** — *see* condition
- **Coma** R4Ø.2Ø
  - with
    - motor response (none) R4Ø.231- ☑
- **Coma** — *continued*
  - with — *continued*
    - motor response — *continued*
      - abnormal extensor posturing to pain or noxious stimuli (< 2 years of age) R4Ø.232- ☑
      - abnormal flexure posturing to pain or noxious stimuli (Ø-5 years of age) R4Ø.233- ☑
      - extensor posturing to pain or noxious stimuli (2-5 years of age) R4Ø.232- ☑
      - flexion/decorticate posturing (< 2 years of age) R4Ø.233- ☑
      - localizes pain (2-5 years of age) R4Ø.235- ☑
      - normal or spontaneous movement (< 2 years of age) R4Ø.236- ☑
      - obeys commands (2-5 years of age) R4Ø.236- ☑
      - score of
        - 1 R4Ø.231- ☑
        - 2 R4Ø.232- ☑
        - 3 R4Ø.233- ☑
        - 4 R4Ø.234- ☑
        - 5 R4Ø.235- ☑
        - 6 R4Ø.236- ☑
      - withdraws from pain or noxious stimuli (Ø-5 years of age) R4Ø.234- ☑
      - withdraws to touch (< 2 years of age) R4Ø.235- ☑
    - opening of eyes (never) R4Ø.211- ☑
      - in response to
        - pain R4Ø.212- ☑
        - sound R4Ø.213- ☑
      - score of
        - 1 R4Ø.211- ☑
        - 2 R4Ø.212- ☑
        - 3 R4Ø.213- ☑
        - 4 R4Ø.214- ☑
      - spontaneous R4Ø.214- ☑
    - verbal response (none) R4Ø.221- ☑
      - confused conversation R4Ø.224- ☑
      - cooing or babbling or crying appropriately (<2 years of age) R4Ø.225- ☑
      - inappropriate crying or screaming (< 2 years of age) R4Ø.223- ☑
      - inappropriate words R4Ø.223- ☑
      - inappropriate words (2-5 years of age) R4Ø.224- ☑
      - incomprehensible sounds (2-5 years of age) R4Ø.222- ☑
      - incomprehensible words R4Ø.222- ☑
      - irritable cries (< 2 years of age) R4Ø.224- ☑
      - moans/grunts to pain; restless (< 2 years old) R4Ø.222- ☑
      - oriented R4Ø.225- ☑
      - score of
        - 1 R4Ø.221- ☑
        - 2 R4Ø.222- ☑
        - 3 R4Ø.223- ☑
        - 4 R4Ø.224- ☑
        - 5 R4Ø.225- ☑
      - screaming (2-5 years of age) R4Ø.223- ☑
      - uses appropriate words (2-5 years of age) R4Ø.225- ☑
  - eclamptic — *see* Eclampsia
  - epileptic — *see* Epilepsy
  - Glasgow, scale score — *see* Glasgow coma scale
  - hepatic — *see* Failure, hepatic, by type, with coma
  - hyperglycemic (diabetic) — *see* Diabetes, by type, with hyperosmolarity, with coma
  - hyperosmolar (diabetic) — *see* Diabetes, by type, with hyperosmolarity, with coma
  - hypoglycemic (diabetic) — *see* Diabetes, by type, with hypoglycemia, with coma
    - nondiabetic E15
  - in diabetes — *see* Diabetes, coma
  - insulin-induced — *see* Coma, hypoglycemic
  - ketoacidotic (diabetic) — *see* Diabetes, by type, with ketoacidosis, with coma
  - myxedematous EØ3.5
  - newborn P91.5
  - nontraumatic, due to underlying condition R4Ø.2A
  - persistent vegetative state R4Ø.3
  - secondary R4Ø.2A
  - specified NEC, without documented Glasgow coma scale score, or with partial Glasgow coma scale score reported R4Ø.244- ☑
- **Comatose** — *see* Coma
- **Combat fatigue** F43.Ø
- **Combined** — *see* condition
- **Comedo, comedones** (giant) L7Ø.Ø
- **Comedocarcinoma** — *see also* Neoplasm, breast, malignant

**Comedocarcinoma** — *continued*
- noninfiltrating
  - breast DØ5.8- ☑
  - specified site — *see* Neoplasm, in situ, by site
  - unspecified site DØ5.8- ☑

**Comedomastitis** — *see* Ectasia, mammary duct

**Comminuted fracture** — *code as* Fracture, closed

**Common**
- arterial trunk Q2Ø.Ø
- atrioventricular canal Q21.23
- atrium Q21.19
- cold (head) JØØ
- truncus (arteriosus) Q2Ø.Ø
- variable immunodeficiency — *see* Immunodeficiency, common variable
- ventricle Q2Ø.4

**Commotio, commotion** (current)
- brain — *see* Injury, intracranial, concussion
- cerebri — *see* Injury, intracranial, concussion
- retinae SØ5.8X- ☑
- spinal cord — *see* Injury, spinal cord, by region
- spinalis — *see* Injury, spinal cord, by region

**Communication**
- between
  - base of aorta and pulmonary artery Q21.4
  - left ventricle and right atrium Q2Ø.5
  - pericardial sac and pleural sac Q34.8
  - pulmonary artery and pulmonary vein, congenital Q25.72
- congenital between uterus and digestive or urinary tract Q51.7

**Compartment syndrome** (deep) (posterior) (traumatic) T79.AØ- ☑ (*following* T79.7)
- abdomen T79.A3- ☑ (*following* T79.7)
- lower extremity (hip, buttock, thigh, leg, foot, toes) T79.A2- ☑ (*following* T79.7)
- nontraumatic
  - abdomen M79.A3 (*following* M79.7)
  - lower extremity (hip, buttock, thigh, leg, foot, toes) M79.A2- ☑ (*following* M79.7)
  - specified site NEC M79.A9 (*following* M79.7)
  - upper extremity (shoulder, arm, forearm, wrist, hand, fingers) M79.A1- ☑ (*following* M79.7)
- specified site NEC T79.A9- ☑ (*following* T79.7)
- upper extremity (shoulder, arm, forearm, wrist, hand, fingers) T79.A1- ☑ (*following* T79.7)

**Compensation**
- failure — *see* Disease, heart
- neurosis, psychoneurosis — *see* Disorder, factitious

**Complaint** — *see also* Disease
- bowel, functional K59.9
  - psychogenic F45.8
- intestine, functional K59.9
  - psychogenic F45.8
- kidney — *see* Disease, renal
- miners' J6Ø

**Complete** — *see* condition

**Complex**
- Addison-Schilder E71.528
- cardiorenal — *see* Hypertension, cardiorenal
- Costen's M26.69
- disseminated mycobacterium avium- intracellulare (DMAC) A31.2
- Eisenmenger's (ventricular septal defect) I27.83
- hypersexual F52.8
- jumped process, spine — *see* Dislocation, vertebra
- primary, tuberculous A15.7
- Schilder-Addison E71.528
- subluxation (vertebral) M99.19
  - abdomen M99.19
  - acromioclavicular M99.17
  - cervical region M99.11
  - cervicothoracic M99.11
  - costochondral M99.18
  - costovertebral M99.18
  - head region M99.1Ø
  - hip M99.15
  - lower extremity M99.16
  - lumbar region M99.13
  - lumbosacral M99.13
  - occipitocervical M99.1Ø
  - pelvic region M99.15
  - pubic M99.15
  - rib cage M99.18
  - sacral region M99.14
  - sacrococcygeal M99.14
  - sacroiliac M99.14
  - specified NEC M99.19

**Complex** — *continued*
- subluxation — *continued*
  - sternochondral M99.18
  - sternoclavicular M99.17
  - thoracic region M99.12
  - thoracolumbar M99.12
  - upper extremity M99.17
- Taussig-Bing (transposition, aorta and overriding pulmonary artery) Q2Ø.1

**Complication**(s) (from) (of)
- accidental puncture or laceration during a procedure (of) — *see* Complications, intraoperative (intraprocedural), puncture or laceration
- amputation stump (surgical) (late) NEC T87.9
  - dehiscence T87.81
  - infection or inflammation T87.4Ø
    - lower limb T87.4- ☑
    - upper limb T87.4- ☑
  - necrosis T87.5Ø
    - lower limb T87.5- ☑
    - upper limb T87.5- ☑
  - neuroma T87.3Ø
    - lower limb T87.3- ☑
    - upper limb T87.3- ☑
  - specified type NEC T87.89
- anastomosis (and bypass) — *see also* Complications, prosthetic device or implant
  - intestinal (internal) NEC K91.89
    - involving urinary tract N99.89
  - urinary tract (involving intestinal tract) N99.89
  - vascular — *see* Complications, cardiovascular device or implant
- anesthesia, anesthetic — *see also* Anesthesia, complication T88.59- ☑
  - brain, postpartum, puerperal O89.2
  - cardiac
    - in
      - labor and delivery O74.2
      - pregnancy O29.19- ☑
    - postpartum, puerperal O89.1
  - central nervous system
    - in
      - labor and delivery O74.3
      - pregnancy O29.29- ☑
    - postpartum, puerperal O89.2
  - difficult or failed intubation T88.4- ☑
    - in pregnancy O29.6- ☑
  - failed sedation (conscious) (moderate) during procedure T88.52- ☑
  - general, unintended awareness during procedure T88.53- ☑
  - hyperthermia, malignant T88.3- ☑
  - hypothermia T88.51- ☑
  - intubation failure T88.4- ☑
  - malignant hyperthermia T88.3- ☑
  - pulmonary
    - in
      - labor and delivery O74.1
      - pregnancy NEC O29.Ø9- ☑
    - postpartum, puerperal O89.Ø9
  - shock T88.2- ☑
  - spinal and epidural
    - in
      - labor and delivery NEC O74.6
        - headache O74.5
      - pregnancy NEC O29.5X- ☑
    - postpartum, puerperal NEC O89.5
      - headache O89.4
  - unintended awareness under general anesthesia during procedure T88.53- ☑
- anti-reflux device — *see* Complications, esophageal anti-reflux device
- aortic (bifurcation) graft — *see* Complications, graft, vascular
- aortocoronary (bypass) graft — *see* Complications, coronary artery (bypass) graft
- aortofemoral (bypass) graft — *see* Complications, extremity artery (bypass) graft
- arteriovenous
  - fistula, surgically created T82.9- ☑
    - embolism T82.818- ☑
    - fibrosis T82.828- ☑
    - hemorrhage T82.838- ☑
    - infection or inflammation T82.7- ☑
    - mechanical
      - breakdown T82.51Ø- ☑
      - displacement T82.52Ø- ☑

**Complication**(s) — *continued*
- arteriovenous — *continued*
  - fistula, surgically created — *continued*
    - mechanical — *continued*
      - leakage T82.53Ø- ☑
      - malposition T82.52Ø- ☑
      - obstruction T82.59Ø- ☑
      - perforation T82.59Ø- ☑
      - protrusion T82.59Ø- ☑
    - pain T82.848- ☑
    - specified type NEC T82.898- ☑
    - stenosis T82.858- ☑
    - thrombosis T82.868- ☑
  - shunt, surgically created T82.9- ☑
    - embolism T82.818- ☑
    - fibrosis T82.828- ☑
    - hemorrhage T82.838- ☑
    - infection or inflammation T82.7- ☑
    - mechanical
      - breakdown T82.511- ☑
      - displacement T82.521- ☑
      - leakage T82.531- ☑
      - malposition T82.521- ☑
      - obstruction T82.591- ☑
      - perforation T82.591- ☑
      - protrusion T82.591- ☑
    - pain T82.848- ☑
    - specified type NEC T82.898- ☑
    - stenosis T82.858- ☑
    - thrombosis T82.868- ☑
- arthroplasty — *see* Complications, joint prosthesis
- artificial
  - fertilization or insemination N98.9
    - attempted introduction (of)
      - embryo in embryo transfer N98.3
      - ovum following in vitro fertilization N98.2
    - hyperstimulation of ovaries N98.1
    - infection N98.Ø
    - specified NEC N98.8
  - heart T82.9- ☑
    - embolism T82.817- ☑
    - fibrosis T82.827- ☑
    - hemorrhage T82.837- ☑
    - infection or inflammation T82.7- ☑
    - mechanical
      - breakdown T82.512- ☑
      - displacement T82.522- ☑
      - leakage T82.532- ☑
      - malposition T82.522- ☑
      - obstruction T82.592- ☑
      - perforation T82.592- ☑
      - protrusion T82.592- ☑
    - pain T82.847- ☑
    - specified type NEC T82.897- ☑
    - stenosis T82.857- ☑
    - thrombosis T82.867- ☑
  - opening
    - cecostomy — *see* Complications, colostomy
    - colostomy — *see* Complications, colostomy
    - cystostomy — *see* Complications, cystostomy
    - enterostomy — *see* Complications, enterostomy
    - gastrostomy — *see* Complications, gastrostomy
    - ileostomy — *see* Complications, enterostomy
    - jejunostomy — *see* Complications, enterostomy
    - nephrostomy — *see* Complications, stoma, urinary tract
    - tracheostomy — *see* Complications, tracheostomy
    - ureterostomy — *see* Complications, stoma, urinary tract
    - urethrostomy — *see* Complications, stoma, urinary tract
- balloon implant or device
  - gastrointestinal T85.9- ☑
    - embolism T85.818- ☑
    - fibrosis T85.828- ☑
    - hemorrhage T85.838- ☑
    - infection and inflammation T85.79- ☑
    - pain T85.848- ☑
    - specified type NEC T85.898- ☑
    - stenosis T85.858- ☑
    - thrombosis T85.868- ☑
  - vascular (counterpulsation) T82.9- ☑
    - embolism T82.818- ☑
    - fibrosis T82.828- ☑
    - hemorrhage T82.838- ☑
    - infection or inflammation T82.7- ☑

- **Complication**(s) — *continued*
  - balloon implant or device — *continued*
    - vascular — *continued*
      - mechanical
        - breakdown T82.513- ☑
        - displacement T82.523- ☑
        - leakage T82.533- ☑
        - malposition T82.523- ☑
        - obstruction T82.593- ☑
        - perforation T82.593- ☑
        - protrusion T82.593- ☑
      - pain T82.848- ☑
      - specified type NEC T82.898- ☑
      - stenosis T82.858- ☑
      - thrombosis T82.868- ☑
  - bariatric procedure
    - gastric band procedure K95.09
      - infection K95.01
    - specified procedure NEC K95.89
      - infection K95.81
  - bile duct implant (prosthetic) T85.9- ☑
    - embolism T85.818- ☑
    - fibrosis T85.828- ☑
    - hemorrhage T85.838- ☑
    - infection and inflammation T85.79- ☑
    - mechanical
      - breakdown T85.510- ☑
      - displacement T85.520- ☑
      - malfunction T85.510- ☑
      - malposition T85.520- ☑
      - obstruction T85.590- ☑
      - perforation T85.590- ☑
      - protrusion T85.590- ☑
      - specified NEC T85.590- ☑
    - pain T85.848- ☑
    - specified type NEC T85.898- ☑
    - stenosis T85.858- ☑
    - thrombosis T85.868- ☑
  - bladder device (auxiliary) — *see* Complications, genitourinary, device or implant, urinary system
  - bleeding (postoperative) — *see* Complication, postoperative, hemorrhage
    - intraoperative — *see* Complication, intraoperative, hemorrhage
  - blood vessel graft — *see* Complications, graft, vascular
  - bone
    - device NEC T84.9- ☑
      - embolism T84.81- ☑
      - fibrosis T84.82- ☑
      - hemorrhage T84.83- ☑
      - infection or inflammation T84.7- ☑
      - mechanical
        - breakdown T84.318- ☑
        - displacement T84.328- ☑
        - malposition T84.328- ☑
        - obstruction T84.398- ☑
        - perforation T84.398- ☑
        - protrusion T84.398- ☑
      - pain T84.84- ☑
      - specified type NEC T84.89- ☑
      - stenosis T84.85- ☑
      - thrombosis T84.86- ☑
    - graft — *see* Complications, graft, bone
    - growth stimulator (electrode) — *see* Complications, electronic stimulator device, bone
    - marrow transplant — *see* Complications, transplant, bone, marrow
  - brain neurostimulator (electrode) — *see* Complications, electronic stimulator device, brain
  - breast implant (prosthetic) T85.9- ☑
    - capsular contracture T85.44- ☑
    - embolism T85.818- ☑
    - fibrosis T85.828- ☑
    - hemorrhage T85.838- ☑
    - infection and inflammation T85.79- ☑
    - mechanical
      - breakdown T85.41- ☑
      - displacement T85.42- ☑
      - leakage T85.43- ☑
      - malposition T85.42- ☑
      - obstruction T85.49- ☑
      - perforation T85.49- ☑
      - protrusion T85.49- ☑
      - specified NEC T85.49- ☑
    - pain T85.848- ☑
    - specified type NEC T85.898- ☑

- **Complication**(s) — *continued*
  - breast implant — *continued*
    - stenosis T85.858- ☑
    - thrombosis T85.868- ☑
  - bypass — *see also* Complications, prosthetic device or implant
    - aortocoronary — *see* Complications, coronary artery (bypass) graft
    - arterial — *see also* Complications, graft, vascular
      - extremity — *see* Complications, extremity artery (bypass) graft
  - cardiac — *see also* Disease, heart
    - device, implant or graft T82.9- ☑
      - embolism T82.817- ☑
      - fibrosis T82.827- ☑
      - hemorrhage T82.837- ☑
      - infection or inflammation T82.7- ☑
        - valve prosthesis T82.6- ☑
      - mechanical
        - breakdown T82.519- ☑
          - specified device NEC T82.518- ☑
        - displacement T82.529- ☑
          - specified device NEC T82.528- ☑
        - leakage T82.539- ☑
          - specified device NEC T82.538- ☑
        - malposition T82.529- ☑
          - specified device NEC T82.528- ☑
        - obstruction T82.599- ☑
          - specified device NEC T82.598- ☑
        - perforation T82.599- ☑
          - specified device NEC T82.598- ☑
        - protrusion T82.599- ☑
          - specified device NEC T82.598- ☑
      - pain T82.847- ☑
      - specified type NEC T82.897- ☑
      - stenosis T82.857- ☑
      - thrombosis T82.867- ☑
  - cardiovascular device, graft or implant T82.9- ☑
    - aortic graft — *see* Complications, graft, vascular
    - arteriovenous
      - fistula, artificial — *see* Complication, arteriovenous, fistula, surgically created
      - shunt — *see* Complication, arteriovenous, shunt, surgically created
    - artificial heart — *see* Complication, artificial, heart
    - balloon (counterpulsation) device — *see* Complication, balloon implant, vascular
    - carotid artery graft — *see* Complications, graft, vascular
    - coronary bypass graft — *see* Complication, coronary artery (bypass) graft
    - dialysis catheter (vascular) — *see* Complication, catheter, dialysis
    - electronic T82.9- ☑
      - electrode T82.9- ☑
        - embolism T82.817- ☑
        - fibrosis T82.827- ☑
        - hemorrhage T82.837- ☑
        - infection T82.7- ☑
        - mechanical
          - breakdown T82.110- ☑
          - displacement T82.120- ☑
          - leakage T82.190- ☑
          - obstruction T82.190- ☑
          - perforation T82.190- ☑
          - protrusion T82.190- ☑
          - specified type NEC T82.190- ☑
        - pain T82.847- ☑
        - specified NEC T82.897- ☑
        - stenosis T82.857- ☑
        - thrombosis T82.867- ☑
      - embolism T82.817- ☑
      - fibrosis T82.827- ☑
      - hemorrhage T82.837- ☑
      - infection T82.7- ☑
      - mechanical
        - breakdown T82.119- ☑
        - displacement T82.129- ☑
        - leakage T82.199- ☑
        - obstruction T82.199- ☑
        - perforation T82.199- ☑
        - protrusion T82.199- ☑
        - specified type NEC T82.199- ☑
      - pain T82.847- ☑
      - pulse generator T82.9- ☑
        - embolism T82.817- ☑

- **Complication**(s) — *continued*
  - cardiovascular device, graft or implant — *continued*
    - electronic — *continued*
      - pulse generator — *continued*
        - fibrosis T82.827- ☑
        - hemorrhage T82.837- ☑
        - infection T82.7- ☑
        - mechanical
          - breakdown T82.111- ☑
          - displacement T82.121- ☑
          - leakage T82.191- ☑
          - obstruction T82.191- ☑
          - perforation T82.191- ☑
          - protrusion T82.191- ☑
          - specified type NEC T82.191- ☑
        - pain T82.847- ☑
        - specified NEC T82.897- ☑
        - stenosis T82.857- ☑
        - thrombosis T82.867- ☑
      - specified condition NEC T82.897- ☑
      - specified device NEC T82.9- ☑
        - embolism T82.817- ☑
        - fibrosis T82.827- ☑
        - hemorrhage T82.837- ☑
        - infection T82.7- ☑
        - mechanical
          - breakdown T82.118- ☑
          - displacement T82.128- ☑
          - leakage T82.198- ☑
          - obstruction T82.198- ☑
          - perforation T82.198- ☑
          - protrusion T82.198- ☑
          - specified type NEC T82.198- ☑
        - pain T82.847- ☑
        - specified NEC T82.897- ☑
        - stenosis T82.857- ☑
        - thrombosis T82.867- ☑
      - stenosis T82.857- ☑
      - thrombosis T82.867- ☑
    - extremity artery graft — *see* Complication, extremity artery (bypass) graft
    - femoral artery graft — *see* Complication, extremity artery (bypass) graft
    - heart
      - transplant — *see* Complication, transplant, heart
      - valve — *see* Complication, prosthetic device, heart valve
        - graft — *see* Complication, heart, valve, graft
    - heart-lung transplant — *see* Complication, transplant, heart, with lung
    - infection or inflammation T82.7- ☑
    - umbrella device — *see* Complication, umbrella device, vascular
    - vascular graft (or anastomosis) — *see* Complication, graft, vascular
  - carotid artery (bypass) graft — *see* Complications, graft, vascular
  - catheter (device) NEC — *see also* Complications, prosthetic device or implant
    - cranial infusion
      - infection and inflammation T85.735- ☑
      - mechanical
        - breakdown T85.610- ☑
        - displacement T85.620- ☑
        - leakage T85.630- ☑
        - malfunction T85.690- ☑
        - malposition T85.620- ☑
        - obstruction T85.690- ☑
        - perforation T85.690- ☑
        - protrusion T85.690- ☑
        - specified NEC T85.690- ☑
    - cystostomy T83.9- ☑
      - embolism T83.81- ☑
      - fibrosis T83.82- ☑
      - hemorrhage T83.83- ☑
      - infection and inflammation T83.510- ☑
      - mechanical
        - breakdown T83.010- ☑
        - displacement T83.020- ☑
        - leakage T83.030- ☑
        - malposition T83.020- ☑
        - obstruction T83.090- ☑
        - perforation T83.090- ☑
        - protrusion T83.090- ☑
        - specified NEC T83.090- ☑
      - pain T83.84- ☑

Index — Complication — Complication

- **Complication**(s) — *continued*
  - eye — *continued*
    - implant — *continued*
      - pain T85.848- ☑
      - specified type NEC T85.898- ☑
      - stenosis T85.858- ☑
      - thrombosis T85.868- ☑
    - intraocular lens — *see* Complications, intraocular lens
    - orbital prosthesis — *see* Complications, orbital prosthesis
    - postprocedural H59.- ☑
  - female genital N94.9
    - device, implant or graft NEC — *see* Complications, genitourinary, device or implant, genital tract
  - femoral artery (bypass) graft — *see* Complication, extremity artery (bypass) graft
  - fixation device, internal (orthopedic) T84.9- ☑
    - infection and inflammation T84.6Ø- ☑
      - arm T84.61- ☑
        - humerus T84.61- ☑
        - radius T84.61- ☑
        - ulna T84.61- ☑
      - leg T84.629- ☑
        - femur T84.62- ☑
        - fibula T84.62- ☑
        - tibia T84.62- ☑
      - specified site NEC T84.89- ☑
      - spine T84.63- ☑
    - mechanical
      - breakdown
        - limb T84.119- ☑
          - carpal T84.21Ø- ☑
          - femur T84.11- ☑
          - fibula T84.11- ☑
          - humerus T84.11- ☑
          - metacarpal T84.21Ø- ☑
          - metatarsal T84.213- ☑
          - phalanx
            - foot T84.213- ☑
            - hand T84.21Ø- ☑
          - radius T84.11- ☑
          - tarsal T84.213- ☑
          - tibia T84.11- ☑
          - ulna T84.11- ☑
        - specified bone NEC T84.218- ☑
        - spine T84.216- ☑
      - displacement
        - limb T84.129- ☑
          - carpal T84.22Ø- ☑
          - femur T84.12- ☑
          - fibula T84.12- ☑
          - humerus T84.12- ☑
          - metacarpal T84.22Ø- ☑
          - metatarsal T84.223- ☑
          - phalanx
            - foot T84.223- ☑
            - hand T84.22Ø- ☑
          - radius T84.12- ☑
          - tarsal T84.223- ☑
          - tibia T84.12- ☑
          - ulna T84.12- ☑
        - specified bone NEC T84.228- ☑
        - spine T84.226- ☑
      - malposition — *see* Complications, fixation device, internal, mechanical, displacement
      - obstruction — *see* Complications, fixation device, internal, mechanical, specified type NEC
      - perforation — *see* Complications, fixation device, internal, mechanical, specified type NEC
      - protrusion — *see* Complications, fixation device, internal, mechanical, specified type NEC
      - specified type NEC
        - limb T84.199- ☑
          - carpal T84.29Ø- ☑
          - femur T84.19- ☑
          - fibula T84.19- ☑
          - humerus T84.19- ☑
          - metacarpal T84.29Ø- ☑
          - metatarsal T84.293- ☑
          - phalanx
            - foot T84.293- ☑
            - hand T84.29Ø- ☑
          - radius T84.19- ☑
          - tarsal T84.293- ☑
          - tibia T84.19- ☑
          - ulna T84.19- ☑

- **Complication**(s) — *continued*
  - fixation device, internal — *continued*
    - mechanical — *continued*
      - specified type — *continued*
        - specified bone NEC T84.298- ☑
        - vertebra T84.296- ☑
    - specified type NEC T84.89- ☑
      - embolism T84.81- ☑
      - fibrosis T84.82- ☑
      - hemorrhage T84.83- ☑
      - pain T84.84- ☑
      - specified complication NEC T84.89- ☑
      - stenosis T84.85- ☑
      - thrombosis T84.86- ☑
  - following
    - acute myocardial infarction NEC I23.8
      - aneurysm (false) (of cardiac wall) (of heart wall) (ruptured) I23.3
      - angina I23.7
      - atrial
        - septal defect I23.1
        - thrombosis I23.6
      - cardiac wall rupture I23.3
      - chordae tendineae rupture I23.4
      - defect
        - septal
          - atrial (heart) I23.1
          - ventricular (heart) I23.2
      - hemopericardium I23.Ø
      - papillary muscle rupture I23.5
      - rupture
        - cardiac wall I23.3
          - with hemopericardium I23.Ø
        - chordae tendineae I23.4
        - papillary muscle I23.5
      - specified NEC I23.8
      - thrombosis
        - atrium I23.6
        - auricular appendage I23.6
        - ventricle (heart) I23.6
      - ventricular
        - septal defect I23.2
        - thrombosis I23.6
    - ectopic or molar pregnancy OØ8.9
      - cardiac arrest OØ8.81
      - sepsis OØ8.82
      - specified type NEC OØ8.89
      - urinary tract infection OØ8.83
    - termination of pregnancy — *see* Abortion
  - gastrointestinal K92.9
    - bile duct prosthesis — *see* Complications, bile duct implant
    - esophageal anti-reflux device — *see* Complications, esophageal anti-reflux device
    - postoperative
      - colostomy — *see* Complications, colostomy
      - dumping syndrome K91.1
      - enterostomy — *see* Complications, enterostomy
      - gastrostomy — *see* Complications, gastrostomy
      - malabsorption NEC K91.2
      - obstruction — *see also* Obstruction, intestine, postoperative K91.3Ø
      - postcholecystectomy syndrome K91.5
      - specified NEC K91.89
      - vomiting after GI surgery K91.Ø
    - prosthetic device or implant
      - bile duct prosthesis — *see* Complications, bile duct implant
      - esophageal anti-reflux device — *see* Complications, esophageal anti-reflux device
      - specified type NEC
        - embolism T85.818- ☑
        - fibrosis T85.828- ☑
        - hemorrhage T85.838- ☑
        - mechanical
          - breakdown T85.518- ☑
          - displacement T85.528- ☑
          - malfunction T85.518- ☑
          - malposition T85.528- ☑
          - obstruction T85.598- ☑
          - perforation T85.598- ☑
          - protrusion T85.598- ☑
          - specified NEC T85.598- ☑
        - pain T85.848- ☑
        - specified complication NEC T85.898- ☑
        - stenosis T85.858- ☑
        - thrombosis T85.868- ☑
  - gastrostomy (stoma) K94.2Ø

- **Complication**(s) — *continued*
  - gastrostomy — *continued*
    - hemorrhage K94.21
    - infection K94.22
    - malfunction K94.23
    - mechanical K94.23
    - specified complication NEC K94.29
  - genitourinary
    - device or implant T83.9- ☑
      - genital tract T83.9- ☑
        - infection or inflammation T83.69- ☑
        - intrauterine contraceptive device — *see* Complications, intrauterine, contraceptive device
        - mechanical — *see* Complications, by device, mechanical
        - mesh — *see* Complications, prosthetic device or implant, mesh
        - penile prosthesis — *see* Complications, prosthetic device, penile
        - specified type NEC T83.89- ☑
          - embolism T83.81- ☑
          - fibrosis T83.82- ☑
          - hemorrhage T83.83- ☑
          - pain T83.84- ☑
          - specified complication NEC T83.89- ☑
          - stenosis T83.85- ☑
          - thrombosis T83.86- ☑
        - vaginal mesh — *see* Complications, prosthetic device or implant, mesh
      - urinary system T83.9- ☑
        - cystostomy catheter — *see* Complication, catheter, cystostomy
        - electronic stimulator — *see* Complications, electronic stimulator device, urinary
        - indwelling urethral catheter — *see* Complications, catheter, urethral, indwelling
        - infection or inflammation T83.598- ☑
          - indwelling urethral catheter T83.511- ☑
        - kidney transplant — *see* Complication, transplant, kidney
        - organ graft — *see* Complication, graft, urinary organ
        - specified type NEC T83.89- ☑
          - embolism T83.81- ☑
          - fibrosis T83.82- ☑
          - hemorrhage T83.83- ☑
          - mechanical T83.198- ☑
            - breakdown T83.118- ☑
            - displacement T83.128- ☑
            - malfunction T83.118- ☑
            - malposition T83.128- ☑
            - obstruction T83.198- ☑
            - perforation T83.198- ☑
            - protrusion T83.198- ☑
            - specified NEC T83.198- ☑
        - sphincter implant — *see* Complications, implant, urinary sphincter
        - sphincter, implanted T83.191- ☑
        - stent (ileal conduit) (nephroureteral) T83.193- ☑
          - pain T83.84- ☑
          - specified complication NEC T83.89- ☑
          - stenosis T83.85- ☑
          - thrombosis T83.86- ☑
          - ureteral indwelling T83.192- ☑
    - postprocedural
      - pelvic peritoneal adhesions N99.4
      - renal failure N99.Ø
      - specified NEC N99.89
      - stoma — *see* Complications, stoma, urinary tract
      - urethral stricture — *see* Stricture, urethra, postprocedural
      - vaginal
        - adhesions N99.2
        - vault prolapse N99.3
  - graft (bypass) (patch) — *see also* Complications, prosthetic device or implant
    - aorta — *see* Complications, graft, vascular
    - arterial — *see* Complication, graft, vascular
    - bone T86.839
      - failure T86.831
      - infection T86.832
      - mechanical T84.318- ☑
        - breakdown T84.318- ☑
        - displacement T84.328- ☑
        - protrusion T84.398- ☑

- **Complication**(s) — *continued*
  - intraoperative — *continued*
    - cardiac functional disturbance NEC — *see also* Infarct, myocardium, associated with revascularization procedure
      - during cardiac surgery I97.79Ø
      - during other surgery I97.791
    - hemorrhage (hematoma) (of)
      - circulatory system organ or structure
        - during cardiac bypass I97.411
        - during cardiac catheterization I97.41Ø
        - during other circulatory system procedure I97.418
        - during other procedure I97.42
      - digestive system organ
        - during procedure on digestive system K91.61
        - during procedure on other organ K91.62
      - ear
        - during procedure on ear and mastoid process H95.21
        - during procedure on other organ H95.22
      - endocrine system organ or structure
        - during procedure on endocrine system organ or structure E36.Ø1
        - during procedure on other organ E36.Ø2
      - eye and adnexa
        - during ophthalmic procedure H59.11- ☑
        - during other procedure H59.12- ☑
      - genitourinary organ or structure
        - during procedure on genitourinary organ or structure N99.61
        - during procedure on other organ N99.62
      - mastoid process
        - during procedure on ear and mastoid process H95.21
        - during procedure on other organ H95.22
      - musculoskeletal structure
        - during musculoskeletal surgery M96.81Ø
        - during non-orthopedic surgery M96.811
        - during orthopedic surgery M96.81Ø
      - nervous system
        - during a nervous system procedure G97.31
        - during other procedure G97.32
      - respiratory system
        - during other procedure J95.62
        - during procedure on respiratory system organ or structure J95.61
      - skin and subcutaneous tissue
        - during a dermatologic procedure L76.Ø1
        - during a procedure on other organ L76.Ø2
      - spleen
        - during a procedure on other organ D78.Ø2
        - during a procedure on the spleen D78.Ø1
    - puncture or laceration (accidental) (unintentional) (of)
      - brain
        - during a nervous system procedure G97.48
        - during other procedure G97.49
      - circulatory system organ or structure
        - during circulatory system procedure I97.51
        - during other procedure I97.52
      - digestive system
        - during procedure on digestive system K91.71
        - during procedure on other organ K91.72
      - ear
        - during procedure on ear and mastoid process H95.31
        - during procedure on other organ H95.32
      - endocrine system organ or structure
        - during procedure on endocrine system organ or structure E36.11
        - during procedure on other organ E36.12
      - eye and adnexa
        - during ophthalmic procedure H59.21- ☑
        - during other procedure H59.22- ☑
      - genitourinary organ or structure
        - during procedure on genitourinary organ or structure N99.71
        - during procedure on other organ N99.72
      - mastoid process
        - during procedure on ear and mastoid process H95.31
        - during procedure on other organ H95.32
      - musculoskeletal structure
        - during musculoskeletal surgery M96.82Ø
        - during non-orthopedic surgery M96.821
        - during orthopedic surgery M96.82Ø
      - nervous system
        - during a nervous system procedure G97.48

- **Complication**(s) — *continued*
  - intraoperative — *continued*
    - puncture or laceration — *continued*
      - nervous system — *continued*
        - during other procedure G97.49
      - respiratory system
        - during other procedure J95.72
        - during procedure on respiratory system organ or structure J95.71
      - skin and subcutaneous tissue
        - during a dermatologic procedure L76.11
        - during a procedure on other organ L76.12
      - spleen
        - during a procedure on other organ D78.12
        - during a procedure on the spleen D78.11
    - specified NEC
      - circulatory system I97.88
      - digestive system K91.81
      - ear H95.88
      - endocrine system E36.8
      - eye and adnexa H59.88
      - genitourinary system N99.81
      - mastoid process H95.88
      - musculoskeletal structure M96.89
      - nervous system G97.81
      - respiratory system J95.88
      - skin and subcutaneous tissue L76.81
      - spleen D78.81
  - intraperitoneal catheter (dialysis) (infusion) — *see* Complication(s), catheter, intraperitoneal dialysis
  - intrathecal infusion pump
    - infection and inflammation T85.738- ☑
    - mechanical
      - breakdown T85.615- ☑
      - displacement T85.625- ☑
      - leakage T85.635- ☑
      - malfunction T85.695- ☑
      - malposition T85.625- ☑
      - obstruction T85.695- ☑
      - perforation T85.695- ☑
      - protrusion T85.695- ☑
      - specified NEC T85.695- ☑
  - intrauterine
    - contraceptive device
      - embolism T83.81- ☑
      - fibrosis T83.82- ☑
      - hemorrhage T83.83- ☑
      - infection and inflammation T83.69- ☑
      - mechanical
        - breakdown T83.31- ☑
        - displacement T83.32- ☑
        - malposition T83.32- ☑
        - obstruction T83.39- ☑
        - perforation T83.39- ☑
        - protrusion T83.39- ☑
        - specified NEC T83.39- ☑
      - pain T83.84- ☑
      - specified type NEC T83.89- ☑
      - stenosis T83.85- ☑
      - thrombosis T83.86- ☑
    - procedure (fetal), to newborn P96.5
  - jejunostomy (stoma) — *see* Complications, enterostomy
  - joint prosthesis, internal T84.9- ☑
    - breakage (fracture) T84.Ø1- ☑
    - dislocation T84.Ø2- ☑
    - fracture T84.Ø1- ☑
    - infection or inflammation T84.5Ø- ☑
      - hip T84.5- ☑
      - knee T84.5- ☑
      - specified joint NEC T84.59- ☑
    - instability T84.Ø2- ☑
    - malposition — *see* Complications, joint prosthesis, mechanical, displacement
    - mechanical
      - breakage, broken T84.Ø1- ☑
      - dislocation T84.Ø2- ☑
      - displacement T84.Ø2- ☑
      - fracture T84.Ø1- ☑
      - instability T84.Ø2- ☑
      - leakage — *see* Complications, joint prosthesis, mechanical, specified NEC
      - loosening T84.Ø39- ☑
        - hip T84.Ø3- ☑
        - knee T84.Ø3- ☑
        - specified joint NEC T84.Ø38- ☑
      - obstruction — *see* Complications, joint prosthesis, mechanical, specified NEC

- **Complication**(s) — *continued*
  - joint prosthesis, internal — *continued*
    - mechanical — *continued*
      - osteolysis T84.Ø59- ☑
        - hip T84.Ø5- ☑
        - knee T84.Ø5- ☑
      - perforation — *see* Complications, joint prosthesis, mechanical, specified NEC
        - osteolysis T84.Ø59- ☑
          - other specified joint T84.Ø58- ☑
      - periprosthetic osteolysis, by site T84.Ø5- ☑
      - protrusion — *see* Complications, joint prosthesis, mechanical, specified NEC
      - specified complication NEC T84.Ø99- ☑
        - hip T84.Ø9- ☑
        - knee T84.Ø9- ☑
        - other specified joint T84.Ø98- ☑
      - subluxation T84.Ø2- ☑
      - wear of articular bearing surface T84.Ø69- ☑
        - hip T84.Ø6- ☑
        - knee T84.Ø6- ☑
        - other specified joint T84.Ø68- ☑
    - specified joint NEC T84.89- ☑
      - embolism T84.81- ☑
      - fibrosis T84.82- ☑
      - hemorrhage T84.83- ☑
      - pain T84.84- ☑
      - specified complication NEC T84.89- ☑
      - stenosis T84.85- ☑
      - thrombosis T84.86- ☑
    - subluxation T84.Ø2- ☑
  - kidney transplant — *see* Complications, transplant, kidney
  - labor O75.9
    - specified NEC O75.89
  - liver transplant (immune or nonimmune) — *see* Complications, transplant, liver
  - lumbar puncture G97.1
    - cerebrospinal fluid leak G97.Ø
    - headache or reaction G97.1
  - lung transplant — *see* Complications, transplant, lung
    - and heart — *see* Complications, transplant, lung, with heart
  - male genital N5Ø.9
    - device, implant or graft — *see* Complications, genitourinary, device or implant, genital tract
    - postprocedural or postoperative — *see* Complications, genitourinary, postprocedural
      - specified NEC N99.89
  - mastoid (process) procedure
    - intraoperative H95.88
      - hematoma — *see* Complications, intraoperative, hemorrhage (hematoma) (of), mastoid process
      - hemorrhage — *see* Complications, intraoperative, hemorrhage (hematoma) (of), mastoid process
      - laceration — *see* Complications, intraoperative, puncture or laceration, mastoid process
      - specified NEC H95.88
    - postmastoidectomy — *see* Complications, postmastoidectomy
    - postoperative H95.89
      - external ear canal stenosis H95.81- ☑
      - hematoma — *see* Complications, postprocedural, hematoma (of), mastoid process
      - hemorrhage — *see* Complications, postprocedural, hemorrhage (of), mastoid process
      - postmastoidectomy — *see* Complications, postmastoidectomy
      - seroma — *see* Complications, postprocedural, seroma (of), mastoid process
      - specified NEC H95.89
  - mastoidectomy cavity — *see* Complications, postmastoidectomy
  - mechanical — *see* Complications, by site and type, mechanical
  - medical procedures — *see also* Complication(s), intraoperative T88.9- ☑
  - metabolic E88.9
    - postoperative E89.89
      - specified NEC E89.89
  - molar pregnancy NOS OØ8.9
    - damage to pelvic organs OØ8.6
    - embolism OØ8.2
    - genital infection OØ8.Ø
    - hemorrhage (delayed) (excessive) OØ8.1
    - metabolic disorder OØ8.5

- **Complication**(s) — *continued*
  - molar pregnancy — *continued*
    - renal failure O08.4
    - shock O08.3
    - specified type NEC O08.Ø
    - venous complication NEC O08.7
  - musculoskeletal system — *see also* Complication, intraoperative (intraprocedural), by site
    - device, implant or graft NEC — *see* Complications, orthopedic, device or implant
    - internal fixation (nail) (plate) (rod) — *see* Complications, fixation device, internal
    - joint prosthesis — *see* Complications, joint prosthesis
    - post radiation M96.89
      - kyphosis M96.2
      - scoliosis M96.5
      - specified complication NEC M96.89
    - postoperative (postprocedural) M96.89
      - with osteoporosis — *see* Osteoporosis
      - fracture following insertion of device — *see* Fracture, following insertion of orthopedic implant, joint prosthesis or bone plate
      - joint instability after prosthesis removal M96.89
      - lordosis M96.4
      - postlaminectomy syndrome NEC M96.1
        - kyphosis M96.3
      - pseudarthrosis M96.Ø
      - specified complication NEC M96.89
  - nephrostomy (stoma) — *see* Complications, stoma, urinary tract, external NEC
  - nervous system G98.8
    - central G96.9
    - device, implant or graft — *see also* Complication, prosthetic device or implant, specified NEC
      - electronic stimulator (electrode(s)) — *see* Complications, electronic stimulator device
      - specified NEC
        - infection and inflammation T85.738- ☑
        - mechanical T85.695- ☑
          - breakdown T85.615- ☑
          - displacement T85.625- ☑
          - leakage T85.635- ☑
          - malfunction T85.695- ☑
          - malposition T85.625- ☑
          - obstruction T85.695- ☑
          - perforation T85.695- ☑
          - protrusion T85.695- ☑
          - specified NEC T85.695- ☑
      - ventricular shunt — *see* Complications, ventricular shunt
    - electronic stimulator (electrode(s)) — *see* Complications, electronic stimulator device
    - postprocedural G97.82
      - intracranial hypotension G97.2
      - specified NEC G97.82
      - spinal fluid leak G97.Ø
  - newborn, due to intrauterine (fetal) procedure P96.5
  - nonabsorbable (permanent) sutures — *see* Complication, sutures, permanent
  - obstetric O75.9
    - procedure (instrumental) (manual) (surgical) specified NEC O75.4
    - specified NEC O75.89
    - surgical wound NEC O9Ø.89
      - hematoma O9Ø.2
      - infection O86.ØØ
  - ocular lens implant — *see* Complications, intraocular lens
  - ophthalmologic
    - postprocedural bleb — *see* Blebitis
  - orbital prosthesis T85.9- ☑
    - embolism T85.818- ☑
    - fibrosis T85.828- ☑
    - hemorrhage T85.838- ☑
    - infection and inflammation T85.79- ☑
    - mechanical
      - breakdown T85.31- ☑
      - displacement T85.32- ☑
      - malposition T85.32- ☑
      - obstruction T85.39- ☑
      - perforation T85.39- ☑
      - protrusion T85.39- ☑
      - specified NEC T85.39- ☑
    - pain T85.848- ☑
    - specified type NEC T85.898- ☑
    - stenosis T85.858- ☑
    - thrombosis T85.868- ☑

- **Complication**(s) — *continued*
  - organ or tissue transplant (partial) (total) — *see* Complications, transplant
  - orthopedic — *see also* Disorder, soft tissue
    - device or implant T84.9- ☑
      - bone
        - device or implant — *see* Complication, bone, device NEC
        - graft — *see* Complication, graft, bone
      - breakdown T84.418- ☑
      - displacement T84.428- ☑
      - electronic bone stimulator — *see* Complications, electronic stimulator device, bone
      - embolism T84.81- ☑
      - fibrosis T84.82- ☑
      - fixation device — *see* Complication, fixation device, internal
      - hemorrhage T84.83- ☑
      - infection or inflammation T84.7- ☑
      - joint prosthesis — *see* Complication, joint prosthesis, internal
      - malfunction T84.418- ☑
      - malposition T84.428- ☑
      - mechanical NEC T84.498- ☑
      - muscle graft — *see* Complications, graft, muscle
      - obstruction T84.498- ☑
      - pain T84.84- ☑
      - perforation T84.498- ☑
      - protrusion T84.498- ☑
      - specified complication NEC T84.89- ☑
      - stenosis T84.85- ☑
      - tendon graft — *see* Complications, graft, tendon
      - thrombosis T84.86- ☑
    - fracture (following insertion of device) — *see* Fracture, following insertion of orthopedic implant, joint prosthesis or bone plate
    - postprocedural M96.89
      - fracture — *see* Fracture, following insertion of orthopedic implant, joint prosthesis or bone plate
      - postlaminectomy syndrome NEC M96.1
        - kyphosis M96.3
        - lordosis M96.4
      - postradiation
        - kyphosis M96.2
        - scoliosis M96.5
      - pseudarthrosis post-fusion M96.Ø
      - specified type NEC M96.89
  - pacemaker (cardiac) — *see* Complications, cardiovascular device or implant, electronic
  - pancreas transplant — *see* Complications, transplant, pancreas
  - penile prosthesis (implant) — *see* Complications, prosthetic device, penile
  - perfusion NEC T8Ø.9Ø- ☑
  - perineal repair (obstetrical) NEC O9Ø.89
    - disruption O9Ø.1
    - hematoma O9Ø.2
    - infection (following delivery) O86.Ø9
  - phototherapy T88.9- ☑
    - specified NEC T88.8- ☑
  - postmastoidectomy NEC H95.19- ☑
    - cyst, mucosal H95.13- ☑
    - granulation H95.12- ☑
    - inflammation, chronic H95.11- ☑
    - recurrent cholesteatoma H95.Ø- ☑
  - postoperative — *see* Complications, postprocedural
    - circulatory — *see* Complications, circulatory system
    - ear — *see* Complications, ear
    - endocrine — *see* Complications, endocrine
    - eye — *see* Complications, eye
    - lumbar puncture G97.1
      - cerebrospinal fluid leak G97.Ø
    - nervous system (central) (peripheral) — *see* Complications, nervous system
    - respiratory system — *see* Complications, respiratory system
  - postprocedural — *see also* Complications, surgical procedure
    - cardiac arrest — *see also* Infarct, myocardium, associated with revascularization procedure
      - following cardiac surgery I97.12Ø
      - following other surgery I97.121
    - cardiac functional disturbance NEC — *see also* Infarct, myocardium, associated with revascularization procedure
      - following cardiac surgery I97.19Ø
      - following other surgery I97.191

- **Complication**(s) — *continued*
  - postprocedural — *see also* Complications, surgical procedure — *continued*
    - cardiac insufficiency
      - following cardiac surgery I97.11Ø
      - following other surgery I97.111
    - chorioretinal scars following retinal surgery H59.81- ☑
    - following cataract surgery
      - cataract (lens) fragments H59.Ø2- ☑
      - cystoid macular edema H59.Ø3- ☑
      - specified NEC H59.Ø9- ☑
      - vitreous (touch) syndrome H59.Ø1- ☑
    - heart failure
      - following cardiac surgery I97.13Ø
      - following other surgery I97.131
    - hematoma (of)
      - circulatory system organ or structure
        - following cardiac bypass I97.631
        - following cardiac catheterization I97.63Ø
        - following other circulatory system procedure I97.638
        - following other procedure I97.621
      - digestive system
        - following procedure on digestive system K91.87Ø
        - following procedure on other organ K91.871
      - ear
        - following other procedure H95.52
        - following procedure on ear and mastoid process H95.51
      - endocrine system
        - following endocrine system procedure E89.82Ø
        - following other procedure E89.821
      - eye and adnexa
        - following ophthalmic procedure H59.33- ☑
        - following other procedure H59.34- ☑
      - genitourinary organ or structure
        - following procedure on genitourinary organ or structure N99.84Ø
        - following procedure on other organ N99.841
      - mastoid process
        - following other procedure H95.52
        - following procedure on ear and mastoid process H95.51
      - musculoskeletal structure
        - following musculoskeletal surgery M96.84Ø
        - following non-orthopedic surgery M96.841
        - following orthopedic surgery M96.84Ø
      - nervous system
        - following nervous system procedure G97.61
        - following other procedure G97.62
      - respiratory system
        - following other procedure J95.861
        - following procedure on respiratory system organ or structure J95.86Ø
      - skin and subcutaneous tissue
        - following dermatologic procedure L76.31
        - following procedure on other organ L76.32
      - spleen
        - following procedure on other organ D78.32
        - following procedure on the spleen D78.31
    - hemorrhage (of)
      - circulatory system organ or structure
        - following cardiac bypass I97.611
        - following cardiac catheterization I97.61Ø
        - following other circulatory system procedure I97.618
        - following other procedure I97.62Ø
      - digestive system
        - following procedure on digestive system K91.84Ø
        - following procedure on other organ K91.841
      - ear
        - following other procedure H95.42
        - following procedure on ear and mastoid process H95.41
      - endocrine system
        - following endocrine system procedure E89.81Ø
        - following other procedure E89.811
      - eye and adnexa
        - following ophthalmic procedure H59.31- ☑
        - following other procedure H59.32- ☑
      - genitourinary organ or structure
        - following procedure on genitourinary organ or structure N99.82Ø
        - following procedure on other organ N99.821

- **Complication**(s) — *continued*
  - transfusion — *continued*
    - incompatibility reaction — *continued*
      - ABO — *continued*
        - hemolytic transfusion reaction (HTR) (unspecified time after transfusion) T80.319- ☑
          - acute (AHTR) (less than 24 hours after transfusion) T80.310- ☑
          - delayed (DHTR) (24 hours or more after transfusion) T80.311- ☑
        - specified NEC T80.39- ☑
      - acute (antigen unspecified) T80.910- ☑
      - delayed (antigen unspecified) T80.911- ☑
      - delayed serologic (DSTR) T80.89- ☑
      - non-ABO (minor antigens (Duffy) (K) (Kell) (Kidd) (Lewis) (M) (N) (P) (S)) T80.A0- ☑ (*following* T80.4)
        - delayed serologic (DSTR) T80.A9- ☑ (*following* T80.4)
        - hemolytic transfusion reaction (HTR) (unspecified time after transfusion) T80.A19- ☑ (*following* T80.4)
          - acute (AHTR) (less than 24 hours after transfusion) T80.A10- ☑ (*following* T80.4)
          - delayed (DHTR) (24 hours or more after transfusion) T80.A11- ☑ (*following* T80.4)
        - specified NEC T80.A9- ☑ (*following* T80.4)
      - Rh (antigens (C) (c) (D) (E) (e)) (factor) T80.40- ☑
        - delayed serologic (DSTR) T80.49- ☑
        - hemolytic transfusion reaction (HTR) (unspecified time after transfusion) T80.419- ☑
          - acute (AHTR) (less than 24 hours after transfusion) T80.410- ☑
          - delayed (DHTR) (24 hours or more after transfusion) T80.411- ☑
        - specified NEC T80.49- ☑
    - infection T80.29- ☑
      - acute T80.22- ☑
    - reaction NEC T80.89- ☑
    - sepsis T80.29- ☑
    - shock T80.89- ☑
  - transplant T86.90
    - bone T86.839
      - failure T86.831
      - infection T86.832
      - rejection T86.830
      - specified type NEC T86.838
    - bone marrow T86.00
      - failure T86.02
      - infection T86.03
      - rejection T86.01
      - specified type NEC T86.09
    - cornea T86.849- ☑
      - failure T86.841- ☑
      - infection T86.842- ☑
      - rejection T86.840- ☑
      - specified type NEC T86.848- ☑
    - failure T86.92
    - heart T86.20
      - with lung T86.30
      - cardiac allograft vasculopathy T86.290
        - failure T86.32
        - infection T86.33
        - rejection T86.31
        - specified type NEC T86.39
      - failure T86.22
      - infection T86.23
      - rejection T86.21
      - specified type NEC T86.298
    - infection T86.93
    - intestine T86.859
      - failure T86.851
      - infection T86.852
      - rejection T86.850
      - specified type NEC T86.858
    - kidney T86.10
      - failure T86.12
      - infection T86.13
      - rejection T86.11
      - specified type NEC T86.19
    - liver T86.40
      - failure T86.42
      - infection T86.43
      - rejection T86.41
      - specified type NEC T86.49

- **Complication**(s) — *continued*
  - transplant — *continued*
    - lung T86.819
      - with heart T86.30
        - failure T86.32
        - infection T86.33
        - rejection T86.31
        - specified type NEC T86.39
      - failure T86.811
      - infection T86.812
      - rejection T86.810
      - specified type NEC T86.818
    - malignant neoplasm C80.2
    - pancreas T86.899
      - failure T86.891
      - infection T86.892
      - rejection T86.890
      - specified type NEC T86.898
    - peripheral blood stem cells T86.5
    - post-transplant lymphoproliferative disorder (PTLD) D47.Z1 (*following* D47.4)
    - rejection T86.91
    - skin T86.829
      - failure T86.821
      - infection T86.822
      - rejection T86.820
      - specified type NEC T86.828
    - specified
      - tissue T86.899
        - failure T86.891
        - infection T86.892
        - rejection T86.890
        - specified type NEC T86.898
      - type NEC T86.99
    - stem cell (from peripheral blood) (from umbilical cord) T86.5
    - umbilical cord stem cells T86.5
  - trauma (early) T79.9- ☑
    - specified NEC T79.8- ☑
  - ultrasound therapy NEC T88.9- ☑
  - umbilical cord NEC
    - complicating delivery O69.9- ☑
      - specified NEC O69.89- ☑
  - umbrella device, vascular T82.9- ☑
    - embolism T82.818- ☑
    - fibrosis T82.828- ☑
    - hemorrhage T82.838- ☑
    - infection or inflammation T82.7- ☑
    - mechanical
      - breakdown T82.515- ☑
      - displacement T82.525- ☑
      - leakage T82.535- ☑
      - malposition T82.525- ☑
      - obstruction T82.595- ☑
      - perforation T82.595- ☑
      - protrusion T82.595- ☑
    - pain T82.848- ☑
    - specified type NEC T82.898- ☑
    - stenosis T82.858- ☑
    - thrombosis T82.868- ☑
  - urethral catheter — *see* Complications, catheter, urethral, indwelling
  - vaccination T88.1- ☑
    - anaphylaxis NEC T80.52- ☑
    - arthropathy — *see* Arthropathy, postimmunization
    - cellulitis T88.0- ☑
    - encephalitis or encephalomyelitis G04.02
    - infection (general) (local) NEC T88.0- ☑
    - meningitis G03.8
    - myelitis G04.02
    - protein sickness T80.62- ☑
    - rash T88.1- ☑
    - reaction (allergic) T88.1- ☑
      - serum T80.62- ☑
    - sepsis T88.0- ☑
    - serum intoxication, sickness, rash, or other serum reaction NEC T80.62- ☑
      - anaphylactic shock T80.52- ☑
    - shock (allergic) (anaphylactic) T80.52- ☑
    - vaccinia (generalized) (localized) T88.1- ☑
  - vas deferens device or implant — *see* Complications, genitourinary, device or implant, genital tract
  - vascular I99.9
    - device or implant T82.9- ☑
      - embolism T82.818- ☑
      - fibrosis T82.828- ☑
      - hemorrhage T82.838- ☑

- **Complication**(s) — *continued*
  - vascular — *continued*
    - device or implant — *continued*
      - infection or inflammation T82.7- ☑
      - mechanical
        - breakdown T82.519- ☑
          - specified device NEC T82.518- ☑
        - displacement T82.529- ☑
          - specified device NEC T82.528- ☑
        - leakage T82.539- ☑
          - specified device NEC T82.538- ☑
        - malposition T82.529- ☑
          - specified device NEC T82.528- ☑
        - obstruction T82.599- ☑
          - specified device NEC T82.598- ☑
        - perforation T82.599- ☑
          - specified device NEC T82.598- ☑
        - protrusion T82.599- ☑
          - specified device NEC T82.598- ☑
      - pain T82.848- ☑
      - specified type NEC T82.898- ☑
      - stenosis T82.858- ☑
      - thrombosis T82.868- ☑
    - dialysis catheter — *see* Complication, catheter, dialysis
    - following infusion, therapeutic injection or transfusion T80.1- ☑
    - graft T82.9- ☑
      - embolism T82.818- ☑
      - fibrosis T82.828- ☑
      - hemorrhage T82.838- ☑
      - mechanical
        - breakdown T82.319- ☑
          - aorta (bifurcation) T82.310- ☑
          - carotid artery T82.311- ☑
          - specified vessel NEC T82.318- ☑
        - displacement T82.329- ☑
          - aorta (bifurcation) T82.320- ☑
          - carotid artery T82.321- ☑
          - specified vessel NEC T82.328- ☑
        - leakage T82.339- ☑
          - aorta (bifurcation) T82.330- ☑
          - carotid artery T82.331- ☑
          - femoral artery T82.332- ☑
          - specified vessel NEC T82.338- ☑
        - malposition T82.329- ☑
          - aorta (bifurcation) T82.320- ☑
          - carotid artery T82.321- ☑
          - specified vessel NEC T82.328- ☑
        - obstruction T82.399- ☑
          - aorta (bifurcation) T82.390- ☑
          - carotid artery T82.391- ☑
          - specified vessel NEC T82.398- ☑
        - perforation T82.399- ☑
          - aorta (bifurcation) T82.390- ☑
          - carotid artery T82.391- ☑
          - specified vessel NEC T82.398- ☑
        - protrusion T82.399- ☑
          - aorta (bifurcation) T82.390- ☑
          - carotid artery T82.391- ☑
          - specified vessel NEC T82.398- ☑
      - pain T82.848- ☑
      - specified complication NEC T82.898- ☑
      - stenosis T82.858- ☑
      - thrombosis T82.868- ☑
    - postoperative — *see* Complications, postoperative, circulatory
  - vena cava device (filter) (sieve) (umbrella) — *see* Complications, umbrella device, vascular
  - ventilation therapy NEC T81.81- ☑
  - ventilator
    - mechanical J95.850
      - specified NEC J95.859
  - ventricular (communicating) shunt (device) T85.9- ☑
    - embolism T85.810- ☑
    - fibrosis T85.820- ☑
    - hemorrhage T85.830- ☑
    - infection and inflammation T85.730- ☑
    - mechanical
      - breakdown T85.01- ☑
      - displacement T85.02- ☑
      - leakage T85.03- ☑
      - malposition T85.02- ☑
      - obstruction T85.09- ☑
      - perforation T85.09- ☑
      - protrusion T85.09- ☑

**Complication**(s) — *continued*
- ventricular shunt — *continued*
  - mechanical — *continued*
    - specified NEC T85.09- ☑
  - pain T85.840- ☑
  - specified type NEC T85.890- ☑
  - stenosis T85.850- ☑
  - thrombosis T85.860- ☑
- wire suture, permanent (implanted) — *see* Complications, suture, permanent

**Compressed air disease** T70.3- ☑

**Compression**
- with injury — *code by* Nature of injury
- artery I77.1
  - celiac, syndrome I77.4
- brachial plexus G54.0
- brain (stem) G93.5
  - due to
    - contusion (diffuse) — *see also* Injury, intracranial, diffuse S06.A0- ☑
      - with herniation S06.A1- ☑
      - focal — *see also* Injury, intracranial, focal S06.A0- ☑
        - with herniation S06.A1- ☑
    - injury NEC — *see also* Injury, intracranial, diffuse S06.A0- ☑
  - nontraumatic G93.5
  - traumatic — *see also* Injury, intracranial, diffuse S06.A0- ☑
    - with herniation S06.A1- ☑
- bronchus J98.09
- cauda equina G83.4
- celiac (artery) (axis) I77.4
- cerebral — *see* Compression, brain
- cervical plexus G54.2
- cord
  - spinal — *see* Compression, spinal
  - umbilical — *see* Compression, umbilical cord
- cranial nerve G52.9
  - eighth H93.3- ☑
  - eleventh G52.8
  - fifth G50.8
  - first G52.0
  - fourth — *see* Strabismus, paralytic, fourth nerve
  - ninth G52.1
  - second — *see* Disorder, nerve, optic
  - seventh G51.8
  - sixth — *see* Strabismus, paralytic, sixth nerve
  - tenth G52.2
  - third — *see* Strabismus, paralytic, third nerve
  - twelfth G52.3
- diver's squeeze T70.3- ☑
- during birth (newborn) P15.9
- esophagus K22.2
- eustachian tube — *see* Obstruction, eustachian tube, cartilagenous
- facies Q67.1
- fracture
  - nontraumatic NOS — *see* Collapse, vertebra
  - pathological — *see* Fracture, pathological
  - traumatic — *see* Fracture, traumatic
- heart — *see* Disease, heart
- intestine — *see* Obstruction, intestine
- laryngeal nerve, recurrent G52.2
  - with paralysis of vocal cords and larynx J38.00
    - bilateral J38.02
    - unilateral J38.01
- lumbosacral plexus G54.1
- lung J98.4
- lymphatic vessel I89.0
- medulla — *see* Compression, brain
- nerve — *see also* Disorder, nerve G58.9
  - arm NEC — *see* Mononeuropathy, upper limb
  - axillary G54.0
  - cranial — *see* Compression, cranial nerve
  - leg NEC — *see* Mononeuropathy, lower limb
  - median (in carpal tunnel) — *see* Syndrome, carpal tunnel
  - optic — *see* Disorder, nerve, optic
  - plantar — *see* Lesion, nerve, plantar
  - posterior tibial (in tarsal tunnel) — *see* Syndrome, tarsal tunnel
  - root or plexus NOS (in) G54.9
    - intervertebral disc disorder NEC — *see* Disorder, disc, with, radiculopathy
      - with myelopathy — *see* Disorder, disc, with, myelopathy

**Compression** — *continued*
- nerve — *see also* Disorder, nerve — *continued*
  - root or plexus — *continued*
    - neoplastic disease — *see also* Neoplasm D49.9 *[G55]*
    - spondylosis — *see* Spondylosis, with radiculopathy
  - sciatic (acute) — *see* Lesion, nerve, sciatic
  - sympathetic G90.89
  - traumatic — *see* Injury, nerve
  - ulnar — *see* Lesion, nerve, ulnar
  - upper extremity NEC — *see* Mononeuropathy, upper limb
- spinal (cord) G95.20
  - by displacement of intervertebral disc NEC — *see also* Disorder, disc, with, myelopathy
  - nerve root NOS G54.9
    - due to displacement of intervertebral disc NEC — *see* Disorder, disc, with, radiculopathy
      - with myelopathy — *see* Disorder, disc, with, myelopathy
  - specified NEC G95.29
  - spondylogenic (cervical) (lumbar, lumbosacral) (thoracic) — *see* Spondylosis, with myelopathy NEC
    - anterior — *see* Syndrome, anterior, spinal artery, compression
  - traumatic — *see* Injury, spinal cord, by region
- subcostal nerve (syndrome) — *see* Mononeuropathy, upper limb, specified NEC
- sympathetic nerve NEC G90.89
- syndrome T79.5- ☑
- trachea J39.8
- ulnar nerve (by scar tissue) — *see* Lesion, nerve, ulnar
- umbilical cord
  - complicating delivery O69.2- ☑
    - cord around neck O69.1- ☑
    - prolapse O69.0- ☑
    - specified NEC O69.2- ☑
- ureter N13.5
- vein I87.1
- vena cava (inferior) (superior) I87.1

**Compulsion, compulsive**
- gambling F63.0
- neurosis F42.8
- personality F60.5
- states F42.8
- swearing F42.8
  - in Gilles de la Tourette's syndrome F95.2
- tics and spasms F95.9

**Concato's disease** (pericardial polyserositis) A19.9
- nontubercular I31.1
- pleural — *see* Pleurisy, with effusion

**Concavity chest wall** M95.4

**Concealed penis** Q55.64

**Concern** (normal) **about sick person in family** Z63.6

**Concrescence** (teeth) K00.2

**Concretio cordis** I31.1
- rheumatic I09.2

**Concretion** — *see also* Calculus
- appendicular K38.1
- canaliculus — *see* Dacryolith
- clitoris N90.89
- conjunctiva H11.12- ☑
- eyelid — *see* Disorder, eyelid, specified type NEC
- lacrimal passages — *see* Dacryolith
- prepuce (male) N47.8
- salivary gland (any) K11.5
- seminal vesicle N50.89
- tonsil J35.8

**Concussion** (brain) (cerebral) (current) S06.0X9- ☑
- with
  - loss of consciousness
    - 30 minutes or less S06.0X1- ☑
    - brief S06.0X1- ☑
    - status unknown S06.0XA- ☑
    - unspecified duration S06.0X9- ☑
  - no loss of consciousness S06.0X0- ☑
- blast (air) (hydraulic) (immersion) (underwater)
  - abdomen or thorax — *see* Injury, blast, by site
  - ear with acoustic nerve injury — *see* Injury, nerve, acoustic, specified type NEC
- cauda equina S34.3- ☑
- conus medullaris S34.02- ☑
- ocular S05.8X- ☑
- spinal (cord)
  - cervical S14.0- ☑
  - lumbar S34.01- ☑
  - sacral S34.02- ☑
  - thoracic S24.0- ☑

**Concussion** — *continued*
- syndrome F07.81
- without loss of consciousness S06.0X0- ☑

**Condition** — *see also* Disease
- Fontan-associated, specified NEC I27.848
- post COVID-19 U09.9

**Conditions arising in the perinatal period** — *see* Newborn, affected by

**Conduct disorder** — *see* Disorder, conduct

**Condyloma** A63.0
- acuminatum A63.0
- gonorrheal A54.09
- latum A51.31
- syphilitic A51.31
  - congenital A50.07
- venereal, syphilitic A51.31

**Conflagration** — *see also* Burn
- asphyxia (by inhalation of gases, fumes or vapors) — *see also* Table of Drugs and Chemicals T59.9- ☑

**Conflict** (with) — *see also* Discord
- family Z63.8
- grandparent-child Z62.831
- group home staff-child Z62.833
- kinship-care child Z62.831
- marital Z63.0
  - involving divorce or estrangement Z63.5
- non-parental relative-child Z62.831
- non-parental relative legal guardian-child Z62.831
- non-relative guardian-child Z62.832
- other relative-child Z62.831
- parent-child Z62.820
  - parent-adopted child Z62.821
  - parent-biological child Z62.820
  - parent-foster child Z62.822
  - parent-step child Z62.823
- social role NEC Z73.5

**Confluent** — *see* condition

**Confusion, confused** R41.0
- acute R41.0
  - with dementia F05
- epileptic F05
- mental state (psychogenic) F44.89
- psychogenic F44.89
- reactive (from emotional stress, psychological trauma) F44.89

**Confusional arousals** G47.51

**Congelation** T69.9- ☑

**Congenital** — *see also* condition
- aortic septum Q25.49
- intrinsic factor deficiency D51.0
- malformation — *see* Anomaly

**Congestion, congestive**
- bladder N32.89
- bowel K63.89
- brain G93.89
- breast N64.59
- bronchial J98.09
- catarrhal J31.0
- chest R09.89
- chill, malarial — *see* Malaria
- circulatory NEC I99.8
- duodenum K31.89
- eye — *see* Hyperemia, conjunctiva
- facial, due to birth injury P15.4
- general R68.89
- glottis J37.0
- heart — *see* Failure, heart, congestive
- hepatic K76.1
- hypostatic (lung) — *see* Edema, lung
- intestine K63.89
- kidney N28.89
- labyrinth H83.8- ☑
- larynx J37.0
- liver K76.1
- lung R09.89
  - active or acute — *see* Pneumonia
- malaria, malarial — *see* Malaria
- nasal R09.81
- nose R09.81
- orbit, orbital — *see also* Exophthalmos
  - inflammatory (chronic) — *see* Inflammation, orbit
- ovary N83.8
- pancreas K86.89
- pelvic, female N94.89
- pleural J94.8
- prostate (active) N42.1
- pulmonary — *see* Congestion, lung
- renal N28.89
- retina H35.81

- **Corrosion** — *continued*
  - hand(s) — *continued*
    - thumb — *see* Corrosion, thumb
  - head (and face) (and neck) T2Ø.4Ø- ☑
    - cheek — *see* Corrosion, cheek
    - chin — *see* Corrosion, chin
    - ear — *see* Corrosion, ear
    - eye(s) only — *see* Corrosion, eye
    - first degree T2Ø.5Ø- ☑
    - forehead — *see* Corrosion, forehead
    - lip — *see* Corrosion, lip
    - multiple sites T2Ø.49- ☑
      - first degree T2Ø.59- ☑
      - second degree T2Ø.69- ☑
      - third degree T2Ø.79- ☑
    - neck — *see* Corrosion, neck
    - nose — *see* Corrosion, nose
    - scalp — *see* Corrosion, scalp
    - second degree T2Ø.6Ø- ☑
    - third degree T2Ø.7Ø- ☑
  - hip(s) — *see* Corrosion, lower, limb
  - inhalation — *see* Corrosion, respiratory tract
  - internal organ(s) — *see also* Corrosion, by site T28.9Ø- ☑
    - alimentary tract T28.7- ☑
      - esophagus T28.6- ☑
    - esophagus T28.6- ☑
    - genitourinary T28.8- ☑
    - mouth T28.5- ☑
    - pharynx T28.5- ☑
    - specified organ NEC T28.99- ☑
  - interscapular region — *see* Corrosion, back, upper
  - intestine (large) (small) T28.7- ☑
  - knee T24.429- ☑
    - first degree T24.529- ☑
    - left T24.422- ☑
      - first degree T24.522- ☑
      - second degree T24.622- ☑
      - third degree T24.722- ☑
    - right T24.421- ☑
      - first degree T24.521- ☑
      - second degree T24.621- ☑
      - third degree T24.721- ☑
    - second degree T24.629- ☑
    - third degree T24.729- ☑
  - labium (majus) (minus) — *see* Corrosion, genital organs, external, female
  - lacrimal apparatus, duct, gland or sac — *see* Corrosion, eye, specified site NEC
  - larynx T27.4- ☑
    - with lung T27.5- ☑
  - leg(s) (meaning lower limb(s)) — *see* Corrosion, lower limb
  - limb(s)
    - lower — *see* Corrosion, lower, limb
    - upper — *see* Corrosion, upper limb
  - lip(s) T2Ø.42- ☑
    - first degree T2Ø.52- ☑
    - second degree T2Ø.62- ☑
    - third degree T2Ø.72- ☑
  - lower
    - back — *see* Corrosion, back
    - limb T24.4Ø9- ☑
      - ankle — *see* Corrosion, ankle
      - calf — *see* Corrosion, calf
      - first degree T24.5Ø9- ☑
      - foot — *see* Corrosion, foot
      - knee — *see* Corrosion, knee
      - left T24.4Ø2- ☑
        - first degree T24.5Ø2- ☑
        - second degree T24.6Ø2- ☑
        - third degree T24.7Ø2- ☑
      - multiple sites, except ankle and foot T24.499- ☑
        - ankle and foot T25.499- ☑
          - first degree T25.599- ☑
          - left T25.492- ☑
            - first degree T25.592- ☑
            - second degree T25.692- ☑
            - third degree T25.792- ☑
          - right T25.491- ☑
            - first degree T25.591- ☑
            - second degree T25.691- ☑
            - third degree T25.791- ☑
          - second degree T25.699- ☑
          - third degree T25.799- ☑
        - first degree T24.599- ☑
        - left T24.492- ☑

- **Corrosion** — *continued*
  - lower — *continued*
    - limb — *continued*
      - multiple sites, except ankle and foot — *continued*
        - left — *continued*
          - first degree T24.592- ☑
          - second degree T24.692- ☑
          - third degree T24.792- ☑
        - right T24.491- ☑
          - first degree T24.591- ☑
          - second degree T24.691- ☑
          - third degree T24.791- ☑
        - second degree T24.699- ☑
        - third degree T24.799- ☑
      - right T24.4Ø1- ☑
        - first degree T24.5Ø1- ☑
        - second degree T24.6Ø1- ☑
        - third degree T24.7Ø1- ☑
      - second degree T24.6Ø9- ☑
      - thigh — *see* Corrosion, thigh
      - third degree T24.7Ø9- ☑
  - lung (with larynx and trachea) T27.5- ☑
  - mouth T28.5- ☑
  - neck T2Ø.47- ☑
    - first degree T2Ø.57- ☑
    - second degree T2Ø.67- ☑
    - third degree T2Ø.77- ☑
  - nose (septum) T2Ø.44- ☑
    - first degree T2Ø.54- ☑
    - second degree T2Ø.64- ☑
    - third degree T2Ø.74- ☑
  - ocular adnexa — *see* Corrosion, eye
  - orbit region — *see* Corrosion, eyelid
  - palm T23.459- ☑
    - first degree T23.559- ☑
    - left T23.452- ☑
      - first degree T23.552- ☑
      - second degree T23.652- ☑
      - third degree T23.752- ☑
    - right T23.451- ☑
      - first degree T23.551- ☑
      - second degree T23.651- ☑
      - third degree T23.751- ☑
    - second degree T23.659- ☑
    - third degree T23.759- ☑
  - partial thickness — *code as* Corrosion, unspecified degree, by site
  - pelvis — *see* Corrosion, trunk
  - penis — *see* Corrosion, genital organs, external, male
  - perineum
    - female — *see* Corrosion, genital organs, external, female
    - male — *see* Corrosion, genital organs, external, male
  - periocular area — *see* Corrosion, eyelid
  - pharynx T28.5- ☑
  - rectum T28.7- ☑
  - respiratory tract T27.7- ☑
    - larynx — *see* Corrosion, larynx
    - specified part NEC T27.6- ☑
    - trachea — *see* Corrosion, larynx
  - sac, lacrimal — *see* Corrosion, eye, specified site NEC
  - scalp T2Ø.45- ☑
    - first degree T2Ø.55- ☑
    - second degree T2Ø.65- ☑
    - third degree T2Ø.75- ☑
  - scapular region T22.469- ☑
    - first degree T22.569- ☑
    - left T22.462- ☑
      - first degree T22.562- ☑
      - second degree T22.662- ☑
      - third degree T22.762- ☑
    - right T22.461- ☑
      - first degree T22.561- ☑
      - second degree T22.661- ☑
      - third degree T22.761- ☑
    - second degree T22.669- ☑
    - third degree T22.769- ☑
  - sclera — *see* Corrosion, eye, specified site NEC
  - scrotum — *see* Corrosion, genital organs, external, male
  - shoulder T22.459- ☑
    - first degree T22.559- ☑
    - left T22.452- ☑
      - first degree T22.552- ☑
      - second degree T22.652- ☑
      - third degree T22.752- ☑

- **Corrosion** — *continued*
  - shoulder — *continued*
    - right T22.451- ☑
      - first degree T22.551- ☑
      - second degree T22.651- ☑
      - third degree T22.751- ☑
    - second degree T22.659- ☑
    - third degree T22.759- ☑
  - stomach T28.7- ☑
  - temple — *see* Corrosion, head
  - testis — *see* Corrosion, genital organs, external, male
  - thigh T24.419- ☑
    - first degree T24.519- ☑
    - left T24.412- ☑
      - first degree T24.512- ☑
      - second degree T24.612- ☑
      - third degree T24.712- ☑
    - right T24.411- ☑
      - first degree T24.511- ☑
      - second degree T24.611- ☑
      - third degree T24.711- ☑
    - second degree T24.619- ☑
    - third degree T24.719- ☑
  - thorax (external) — *see* Corrosion, trunk
  - throat (meaning pharynx) T28.5- ☑
  - thumb(s) T23.419- ☑
    - first degree T23.519- ☑
    - left T23.412- ☑
      - first degree T23.512- ☑
      - second degree T23.612- ☑
      - third degree T23.712- ☑
    - multiple sites with fingers T23.449- ☑
      - first degree T23.549- ☑
      - left T23.442- ☑
        - first degree T23.542- ☑
        - second degree T23.642- ☑
        - third degree T23.742- ☑
      - right T23.441- ☑
        - first degree T23.541- ☑
        - second degree T23.641- ☑
        - third degree T23.741- ☑
      - second degree T23.649- ☑
      - third degree T23.749- ☑
    - right T23.411- ☑
      - first degree T23.511- ☑
      - second degree T23.611- ☑
      - third degree T23.711- ☑
    - second degree T23.619- ☑
    - third degree T23.719- ☑
  - toe T25.439- ☑
    - first degree T25.539- ☑
    - left T25.432- ☑
      - first degree T25.532- ☑
      - second degree T25.632- ☑
      - third degree T25.732- ☑
    - right T25.431- ☑
      - first degree T25.531- ☑
      - second degree T25.631- ☑
      - third degree T25.731- ☑
    - second degree T25.639- ☑
    - third degree T25.739- ☑
  - tongue T28.5- ☑
  - tonsil(s) T28.5- ☑
  - total body — *see* Corrosion, multiple body regions
  - trachea T27.4- ☑
    - with lung T27.5- ☑
  - trunk T21.4Ø- ☑
    - abdominal wall — *see* Corrosion, abdominal wall
    - anus — *see* Corrosion, buttock
    - axilla — *see* Corrosion, upper limb
    - back — *see* Corrosion, back
    - breast — *see* Corrosion, chest wall
    - buttock — *see* Corrosion, buttock
    - chest wall — *see* Corrosion, chest wall
    - first degree T21.5Ø- ☑
    - flank — *see* Corrosion, abdominal wall
    - genital
      - female — *see* Corrosion, genital organs, external, female
      - male — *see* Corrosion, genital organs, external, male
    - groin — *see* Corrosion, abdominal wall
    - interscapular region — *see* Corrosion, back, upper
    - labia — *see* Corrosion, genital organs, external, female
    - lower back — *see* Corrosion, back
    - penis — *see* Corrosion, genital organs, external, male

**Corrosion** — *continued*
- trunk — *continued*
  - perineum
    - female — *see* Corrosion, genital organs, external, female
    - male — *see* Corrosion, genital organs, external, male
  - scapular region — *see* Corrosion, upper limb
  - scrotum — *see* Corrosion, genital organs, external, male
  - second degree T21.6Ø- ☑
  - shoulder — *see* Corrosion, upper limb
  - specified site NEC T21.49- ☑
    - first degree T21.59- ☑
    - second degree T21.69- ☑
    - third degree T21.79- ☑
  - testes — *see* Corrosion, genital organs, external, male
  - third degree T21.7Ø- ☑
  - upper back — *see* Corrosion, back, upper
  - vagina T28.8- ☑
  - vulva — *see* Corrosion, genital organs, external, female
- unspecified site with extent of body surface involved specified
  - less than 1Ø percent T32.Ø
  - 1Ø-19 percent (Ø-9 percent third degree) T32.1Ø
    - with 1Ø-19 percent third degree T32.11
  - 2Ø-29 percent (Ø-9 percent third degree) T32.2Ø
    - with
      - 1Ø-19 percent third degree T32.21
      - 2Ø-29 percent third degree T32.22
  - 3Ø-39 percent (Ø-9 percent third degree) T32.3Ø
    - with
      - 1Ø-19 percent third degree T32.31
      - 2Ø-29 percent third degree T32.32
      - 3Ø-39 percent third degree T32.33
  - 4Ø-49 percent (Ø-9 percent third degree) T32.4Ø
    - with
      - 1Ø-19 percent third degree T32.41
      - 2Ø-29 percent third degree T32.42
      - 3Ø-39 percent third degree T32.43
      - 4Ø-49 percent third degree T32.44
  - 5Ø-59 percent (Ø-9 percent third degree) T32.5Ø
    - with
      - 1Ø-19 percent third degree T32.51
      - 2Ø-29 percent third degree T32.52
      - 3Ø-39 percent third degree T32.53
      - 4Ø-49 percent third degree T32.54
      - 5Ø-59 percent third degree T32.55
  - 6Ø-69 percent (Ø-9 percent third degree) T32.6Ø
    - with
      - 1Ø-19 percent third degree T32.61
      - 2Ø-29 percent third degree T32.62
      - 3Ø-39 percent third degree T32.63
      - 4Ø-49 percent third degree T32.64
      - 5Ø-59 percent third degree T32.65
      - 6Ø-69 percent third degree T32.66
  - 7Ø-79 percent (Ø-9 percent third degree) T32.7Ø
    - with
      - 1Ø-19 percent third degree T32.71
      - 2Ø-29 percent third degree T32.72
      - 3Ø-39 percent third degree T32.73
      - 4Ø-49 percent third degree T32.74
      - 5Ø-59 percent third degree T32.75
      - 6Ø-69 percent third degree T32.76
      - 7Ø-79 percent third degree T32.77
  - 8Ø-89 percent (Ø-9 percent third degree) T32.8Ø
    - with
      - 1Ø-19 percent third degree T32.81
      - 2Ø-29 percent third degree T32.82
      - 3Ø-39 percent third degree T32.83
      - 4Ø-49 percent third degree T32.84
      - 5Ø-59 percent third degree T32.85
      - 6Ø-69 percent third degree T32.86
      - 7Ø-79 percent third degree T32.87
      - 8Ø-89 percent third degree T32.88
  - 9Ø percent or more (Ø-9 percent third degree) T32.9Ø
    - with
      - 1Ø-19 percent third degree T32.91
      - 2Ø-29 percent third degree T32.92
      - 3Ø-39 percent third degree T32.93
      - 4Ø-49 percent third degree T32.94
      - 5Ø-59 percent third degree T32.95
      - 6Ø-69 percent third degree T32.96
      - 7Ø-79 percent third degree T32.97
      - 8Ø-89 percent third degree T32.98
      - 9Ø-99 percent third degree T32.99
- upper limb (axilla) (scapular region) T22.4Ø- ☑

**Corrosion** — *continued*
- upper limb — *continued*
  - above elbow — *see* Corrosion, above elbow
  - axilla — *see* Corrosion, axilla
  - elbow — *see* Corrosion, elbow
  - first degree T22.5Ø- ☑
  - forearm — *see* Corrosion, forearm
  - hand — *see* Corrosion, hand
  - interscapular region — *see* Corrosion, back, upper
  - multiple sites T22.499- ☑
    - first degree T22.599- ☑
    - left T22.492- ☑
      - first degree T22.592- ☑
      - second degree T22.692- ☑
      - third degree T22.792- ☑
    - right T22.491- ☑
      - first degree T22.591- ☑
      - second degree T22.691- ☑
      - third degree T22.791- ☑
    - second degree T22.699- ☑
    - third degree T22.799- ☑
  - scapular region — *see* Corrosion, scapular region
  - second degree T22.6Ø- ☑
  - shoulder — *see* Corrosion, shoulder
  - third degree T22.7Ø- ☑
  - wrist — *see* Corrosion, hand
- uterus T28.8- ☑
- vagina T28.8- ☑
- vulva — *see* Corrosion, genital organs, external, female
- wrist T23.479- ☑
  - first degree T23.579- ☑
  - left T23.472- ☑
    - first degree T23.572- ☑
    - second degree T23.672- ☑
    - third degree T23.772- ☑
  - multiple sites with hand T23.499- ☑
    - first degree T23.599- ☑
    - left T23.492- ☑
      - first degree T23.592- ☑
      - second degree T23.692- ☑
      - third degree T23.792- ☑
    - right T23.491- ☑
      - first degree T23.591- ☑
      - second degree T23.691- ☑
      - third degree T23.791- ☑
    - second degree T23.699- ☑
    - third degree T23.799- ☑
  - right T23.471- ☑
    - first degree T23.571- ☑
    - second degree T23.671- ☑
    - third degree T23.771- ☑
  - second degree T23.679- ☑
  - third degree T23.779- ☑

**Corrosive burn** — *see* Corrosion

**Corsican fever** — *see* Malaria

**Cortical** — *see* condition

**Cortico-adrenal** — *see* condition

**Coryza** (acute) JØØ
- with grippe or influenza — *see* Influenza, with, respiratory manifestations NEC
- syphilitic
  - congenital (chronic) A5Ø.Ø5

**Co-sleeping, child-caregiver** Z72.823

**Costen's syndrome or complex** M26.69

**Costiveness** — *see* Constipation

**Costochondritis** M94.Ø

**Cot death** R99

**Cotard's syndrome** F22

**Cotia virus** BØ8.8

**Cotton wool spots** (retinal) H35.81

**Cotugno disease** — *see* Sciatica

**Cough** (affected) (epidemic) (nervous) RØ5.9
- with hemorrhage — *see* Hemoptysis
- acute RØ5.1
- bronchial RØ5.8
  - with grippe or influenza — *see* Influenza, with, respiratory manifestations NEC
- chronic RØ5.3
- functional F45.8
- hysterical F45.8
- laryngeal, spasmodic RØ5.8
- paroxysmal, due to Bordetella pertussis (without pneumonia) A37.ØØ
  - with pneumonia A37.Ø1
- persistent RØ5.3
- psychogenic F45.8
- refractory RØ5.3

**Cough** — *continued*
- smokers' J41.Ø
- specified NEC RØ5.8
- subacute RØ5.2
- syncope RØ5.4
- tea taster's B49
- unexplained RØ5.3

**Counseling** (for) Z71.9
- abuse NEC
  - perpetrator Z69.82
  - victim Z69.81
- alcohol abuser Z71.41
  - family Z71.42
- child abuse
  - nonparental
    - perpetrator Z69.Ø21
    - victim Z69.Ø2Ø
  - parental
    - perpetrator Z69.Ø11
    - victim Z69.Ø1Ø
- consanguinity Z71.89
- contraceptive Z3Ø.Ø9
- dietary Z71.3
- drug abuser Z71.51
  - family member Z71.52
- exercise Z71.82
- family Z71.89
- fertility preservation (prior to cancer therapy) (prior to removal of gonads) Z31.62
- for non-attending third party Z71.Ø
  - related to sexual behavior or orientation Z7Ø.2
- genetic
  - nonprocreative Z71.83
  - procreative NEC Z31.5
- gestational carrier Z31.7
- health (advice) (education) (instruction) — *see* Counseling, medical
  - risk for travel (international) Z71.84
- human immunodeficiency virus (HIV) Z71.7
- immunization safety Z71.85
- impotence Z7Ø.1
- insulin pump use Z46.81
- medical (for) Z71.9
  - boarding school resident Z59.3
  - consanguinity Z71.89
  - feared complaint and no disease found Z71.1
  - human immunodeficiency virus (HIV) Z71.7
  - institutional resident Z59.3
  - on behalf of another Z71.Ø
    - related to sexual behavior or orientation Z7Ø.2
  - person living alone — *see also* Consultation, specified reason NEC Z6Ø.2
  - specified reason NEC Z71.89
- natural family planning
  - procreative Z31.61
  - to avoid pregnancy Z3Ø.Ø2
- pediatric-to-adult transition Z71.87
- perpetrator (of)
  - abuse NEC Z69.82
  - child abuse
    - non-parental Z69.Ø21
    - parental Z69.Ø11
  - rape NEC Z69.82
  - spousal abuse Z69.12
- procreative NEC Z31.69
  - fertility preservation (prior to cancer therapy) (prior to removal of gonads) Z31.62
  - using natural family planning Z31.61
- promiscuity Z7Ø.1
- rape victim Z69.81
- religious Z71.81
- safety for travel (international) Z71.84
- sex, sexual (related to) Z7Ø.9
  - attitude(s) Z7Ø.Ø
  - behavior or orientation Z7Ø.1
  - combined concerns Z7Ø.3
  - non-responsiveness Z7Ø.1
  - on behalf of third party Z7Ø.2
  - specified reason NEC Z7Ø.8
- socioeconomic factors Z71.88
- specified reason NEC Z71.89
- spiritual Z71.81
- spousal abuse (perpetrator) Z69.12
  - victim Z69.11
- substance abuse Z71.89
  - alcohol Z71.41
  - drug Z71.51
  - tobacco Z71.6
- tobacco use Z71.6

- **Counseling** — *continued*
  - travel (international) Z71.84
  - use (of)
    - insulin pump Z46.81
  - vaccine product safety Z71.85
  - victim (of)
    - abuse Z69.81
    - child abuse
      - by parent Z69.Ø1Ø
      - non-parental Z69.Ø2Ø
    - rape NEC Z69.81
- **Coupled rhythm** RØØ.8
- **Couvelaire syndrome or uterus** (complicating delivery) O45.8X- ☑
- **COVID-19** UØ7.1
  - condition post UØ9.9
  - contact (with) Z2Ø.822
  - exposure (to) Z2Ø.822
  - history of (personal) Z86.16
  - long (haul) UØ9.9
  - partially vaccinated (for) Z28.311
  - pneumonia J12.82
  - screening Z11.52
  - sequelae (post acute) UØ9.9
  - unvaccinated (for) Z28.31Ø
- **Cowperitis** — *see* Urethritis
- **Cowper's gland** — *see* condition
- **Cowpox** BØ8.Ø1Ø
  - due to vaccination T88.1- ☑
- **Coxa**
  - magna M91.4- ☑
  - plana M91.2- ☑
  - valga (acquired) — *see also* Deformity, limb, specified type NEC, thigh
    - congenital Q65.81
    - sequelae (late effect) of rickets E64.3
  - vara (acquired) — *see also* Deformity, limb, specified type NEC, thigh
    - congenital Q65.82
    - sequelae (late effect) of rickets E64.3
- **Coxalgia, coxalgic** (nontuberculous) — *see also* Pain, joint, hip
  - tuberculous A18.Ø2
- **Coxitis** — *see* Monoarthritis, hip
- **Coxsackie** (virus) (infection) B34.1
  - as cause of disease classified elsewhere B97.11
  - carditis B33.2Ø
  - central nervous system NEC A88.8
  - endocarditis B33.21
  - enteritis AØ8.39
  - meningitis (aseptic) A87.Ø
  - myocarditis B33.22
  - pericarditis B33.23
  - pharyngitis BØ8.5
  - pleurodynia B33.Ø
  - specific disease NEC B33.8
- **CPVT** (catecholaminergic polymorphic ventricular tachycardia) I47.22
- **Crabs, meaning pubic lice** B85.3
- **Crack baby** PØ4.41
- **Cracked nipple** N64.Ø
  - associated with
    - lactation O92.13
    - pregnancy O92.11- ☑
    - puerperium O92.12
- **Cracked tooth** KØ3.81
- **Cradle cap** L21.Ø
- **Craft neurosis** F48.8
- **Cramp**(s) R25.2
  - abdominal — *see* Pain, abdominal
  - bathing T75.1- ☑
  - colic R1Ø.83
    - psychogenic F45.8
  - due to immersion T75.1- ☑
  - fireman T67.2- ☑
  - heat T67.2- ☑
  - immersion T75.1- ☑
  - intestinal — *see* Pain, abdominal
    - psychogenic F45.8
  - leg, sleep related G47.62
  - limb (lower) (upper) NEC R25.2
    - sleep related G47.62
  - linotypist's F48.8
    - organic G25.89
  - muscle (limb) (general) R25.2
    - due to immersion T75.1- ☑
    - psychogenic F45.8
  - occupational (hand) F48.8
- **Cramp**(s) — *continued*
  - occupational — *continued*
    - organic G25.89
  - salt-depletion E87.1
  - sleep related, leg G47.62
  - stoker's T67.2- ☑
  - swimmer's T75.1- ☑
  - telegrapher's F48.8
    - organic G25.89
  - typist's F48.8
    - organic G25.89
  - uterus N94.89
    - menstrual — *see* Dysmenorrhea
  - writer's F48.8
    - organic G25.89
- **Cranial** — *see* condition
- **Craniocleidodysostosis** Q74.Ø
- **Craniofenestria** (skull) Q75.8
- **Craniolacunia** (skull) Q75.8
- **Craniopagus** Q89.4
- **Craniopathy, metabolic** M85.2
- **Craniopharyngeal** — *see* condition
- **Craniopharyngioma** D44.4
- **Craniorachischisis** (totalis) QØØ.1
- **Cranioschisis** Q75.8
- **Craniostenosis** Q75.ØØ9
- **Craniosynostosis** Q75.ØØ9
  - bilateral Q75.ØØ2
  - coronal Q75.Ø29
    - bilateral Q75.Ø22
    - unilateral Q75.Ø21
  - lambdoid Q75.Ø49
    - bilateral Q75.Ø42
    - unilateral Q75.Ø41
  - metopic Q75.Ø3
  - multi-suture, specified NEC Q75.Ø58
  - sagittal Q75.Ø1
  - single-suture, specified NEC Q75.Ø8
  - unilateral Q75.ØØ1
- **Craniotabes** (cause unknown) M83.8
  - neonatal P96.3
  - rachitic E64.3
  - syphilitic A5Ø.56
- **Cranium** — *see* condition
- **Craw-craw** — *see* Onchocerciasis
- **Creaking joint** — *see* Derangement, joint, specified type NEC
- **Creeping**
  - eruption B76.9
  - palsy or paralysis G12.22
- **Crenated tongue** K14.8
- **Creotoxism** AØ5.9
- **Crepitus**
  - caput Q75.8
  - joint — *see* Derangement, joint, specified type NEC
- **Crescent or conus choroid, congenital** Q14.3
- **CREST syndrome** M34.1
- **Cretin, cretinism** (congenital) (endemic) (nongoitrous) (sporadic) EØØ.9
  - pelvis
    - with disproportion (fetopelvic) O33.Ø
      - causing obstructed labor O65.Ø
  - type
    - hypothyroid EØØ.1
    - mixed EØØ.2
    - myxedematous EØØ.1
    - neurological EØØ.Ø
- **Creutzfeldt-Jakob disease or syndrome** (with dementia) A81.ØØ
  - familial A81.Ø9
  - iatrogenic A81.Ø9
  - specified NEC A81.Ø9
  - sporadic A81.Ø9
  - variant (vCJD) A81.Ø1
- **Cri-du-chat syndrome** Q93.4
- **Crib death** R99
- **Cribriform hymen** Q52.3
- **Crigler-Najjar disease or syndrome** E8Ø.5
- **Crime, victim of** Z65.4
- **Crimean hemorrhagic fever** A98.Ø
- **Criminalism** F6Ø.2
- **Crisis**
  - abdomen R1Ø.Ø
  - acute reaction F43.Ø
  - addisonian E27.2
  - adrenal (cortical) E27.2
  - celiac K9Ø.Ø
  - Dietl's N13.8
  - emotional — *see also* Disorder, adjustment
- **Crisis** — *continued*
  - emotional — *see also* Disorder, adjustment — *continued*
    - acute reaction to stress F43.Ø
    - specific to childhood and adolescence F93.8
  - glaucomatocyclitic — *see* Glaucoma, secondary, inflammation
  - heart — *see* Failure, heart
  - nitritoid I95.2
    - correct substance properly administered — *see* Table of Drugs and Chemicals, by drug, adverse effect
    - overdose or wrong substance given or taken — *see* Table of Drugs and Chemicals, by drug, poisoning
  - oculogyric H51.8
    - psychogenic F45.8
  - Pel's (tabetic) A52.11
  - psychosexual identity F64.2
  - renal N28.Ø
  - sickle-cell — *see also* Disease, sickle-cell, by type, with crisis D57.ØØ
    - with
      - acute chest syndrome D57.Ø1
      - cerebral vascular involvement D57.Ø3
      - complication specified NEC D57.Ø9
      - pain (vaso-occlusive) D57.ØØ
      - splenic sequestration D57.Ø2
  - state (acute reaction) F43.Ø
  - tabetic A52.11
  - thyroid — *see* Thyrotoxicosis with thyroid storm
  - thyrotoxic — *see* Thyrotoxicosis with thyroid storm
- **Crocq's disease** (acrocyanosis) I73.89
- **Crohn's disease** — *see* Enteritis, regional
- **Crooked septum, nasal** J34.2
- **Cross-eye** — *see* Strabismus, convergent concomitant
- **Cross syndrome** E7Ø.328
- **Crossbite** (anterior) (posterior) M26.24
- **Croup, croupous** (catarrhal) (infectious) (inflammatory) (nondiphtheritic) JØ5.Ø
  - bronchial J2Ø.9
  - diphtheritic A36.2
  - false J38.5
  - spasmodic J38.5
    - diphtheritic A36.2
  - stridulous J38.5
    - diphtheritic A36.2
- **Crouzon's disease** Q75.1
- **Crowding, tooth, teeth, fully erupted** M26.31
- **CRST syndrome** M34.1
- **Cruchet's disease** A85.8
- **Cruelty in children** — *see also* Disorder, conduct
- **Crural ulcer** — *see* Ulcer, lower limb
- **Crush, crushed, crushing** T14.8- ☑
  - abdomen S38.1- ☑
  - ankle S97.Ø- ☑
  - arm (upper) (and shoulder) S47.- ☑
  - axilla — *see* Crush, arm
  - back, lower S38.1- ☑
  - buttock S38.1- ☑
  - cheek SØ7.Ø- ☑
  - chest S28.Ø- ☑
  - cranium SØ7.1- ☑
  - ear SØ7.Ø- ☑
  - elbow S57.Ø- ☑
  - extremity
    - lower
      - ankle — *see* Crush, ankle
      - below knee — *see* Crush, leg
      - foot — *see* Crush, foot
      - hip — *see* Crush, hip
      - knee — *see* Crush, knee
      - thigh — *see* Crush, thigh
      - toe — *see* Crush, toe
    - upper
      - below elbow S67.9- ☑
      - elbow — *see* Crush, elbow
      - finger — *see* Crush, finger
      - forearm — *see* Crush, forearm
      - hand — *see* Crush, hand
      - thumb — *see* Crush, thumb
      - upper arm — *see* Crush, arm
      - wrist — *see* Crush, wrist
  - face SØ7.Ø- ☑
  - finger(s) S67.1- ☑
    - with hand (and wrist) — *see* Crush, hand, specified site NEC
    - index S67.19- ☑
    - little S67.19- ☑

**Crush, crushed, crushing** — *continued*
- finger(s) — *continued*
  - middle S67.19- ☑
  - ring S67.19- ☑
  - thumb — *see* Crush, thumb
- foot S97.8- ☑
  - toe — *see* Crush, toe
- forearm S57.8- ☑
- genitalia, external
  - female S38.002- ☑
    - vagina S38.03- ☑
    - vulva S38.03- ☑
  - male S38.001- ☑
    - penis S38.01- ☑
    - scrotum S38.02- ☑
    - testis S38.02- ☑
- hand (except fingers alone) S67.2- ☑
  - with wrist S67.4- ☑
- head S07.9- ☑
  - specified NEC S07.8- ☑
- heel — *see* Crush, foot
- hip S77.0- ☑
  - with thigh S77.2- ☑
- internal organ (abdomen, chest, or pelvis) NEC T14.8- ☑
- knee S87.0- ☑
- labium (majus) (minus) S38.03- ☑
- larynx S17.0- ☑
- leg (lower) S87.8- ☑
  - knee — *see* Crush, knee
- lip S07.0- ☑
- lower
  - back S38.1- ☑
  - leg — *see* Crush, leg
- neck S17.9- ☑
- nerve — *see* Injury, nerve
- nose S07.0- ☑
- pelvis S38.1- ☑
- penis S38.01- ☑
- scalp S07.8- ☑
- scapular region — *see* Crush, arm
- scrotum S38.02- ☑
- severe, unspecified site T14.8- ☑
- shoulder (and upper arm) — *see* Crush, arm
- skull S07.1- ☑
- syndrome (complication of trauma) T79.5- ☑
- testis S38.02- ☑
- thigh S77.1- ☑
  - with hip S77.2- ☑
- throat S17.8- ☑
- thumb S67.0- ☑
  - with hand (and wrist) — *see* Crush, hand, specified site NEC
- toe(s) S97.10- ☑
  - great S97.11- ☑
  - lesser S97.12- ☑
- trachea S17.0- ☑
- vagina S38.03- ☑
- vulva S38.03- ☑
- wrist S67.3- ☑
  - with hand S67.4- ☑

**Crusta lactea** L21.0

**Crusts** R23.4

**Crutch paralysis** — *see* Injury, brachial plexus

**Cruveilhier-Baumgarten cirrhosis, disease or syndrome** K74.69

**Cruveilhier's atrophy or disease** G12.8

**Crying** (constant) (continuous) (excessive)
- child, adolescent, or adult R45.83
- infant (baby) (newborn) R68.11

**Cryofibrinogenemia** D89.2

**Cryoglobulinemia** (essential) (idiopathic) (mixed) (primary) (purpura) (secondary) (vasculitis) D89.1
- with lung involvement D89.1 *[J99]*

**Cryptitis** (anal) (rectal) K62.89

**Cryptococcosis, cryptococcus** (infection) (neoformans) B45.9
- bone B45.3
- cerebral B45.1
- cutaneous B45.2
- disseminated B45.7
- generalized B45.7
- meningitis B45.1
- meningocerebralis B45.1
- osseous B45.3
- pulmonary B45.0
- skin B45.2
- specified NEC B45.8

**Cryptopapillitis** (anus) K62.89

**Cryptophthalmos** Q11.2
- syndrome Q87.0

**Cryptorchid, cryptorchism, cryptorchidism** Q53.9
- bilateral Q53.20
  - abdominal Q53.211
  - perineal Q53.22
- unilateral Q53.10
  - abdominal Q53.111
  - perineal Q53.12

**Cryptosporidiosis** A07.2
- hepatobiliary B88.8
- respiratory B88.8

**Cryptostromosis** J67.6

**Crystalluria** R82.998

**Cubitus**
- congenital Q68.8
- valgus (acquired) M21.02- ☑
  - congenital Q68.8
  - sequelae (late effect) of rickets E64.3
- varus (acquired) M21.12- ☑
  - congenital Q68.8
  - sequelae (late effect) of rickets E64.3

**Cultural deprivation or shock** Z60.3

**Curling esophagus** K22.4

**Curling's ulcer** — *see* Ulcer, peptic, acute

**Curschmann** (-Batten) (-Steinert) **disease or syndrome** G71.11

**Curse, Ondine's** — *see* Apnea, sleep

**Curvature**
- organ or site, congenital NEC — *see* Distortion
- penis (lateral) Q55.61
- Pott's (spinal) A18.01
- radius, idiopathic, progressive (congenital) Q74.0
- spine (acquired) (angular) (idiopathic) (incorrect) (postural) — *see* Dorsopathy, deforming
  - congenital Q67.5
  - due to or associated with
    - Charcot-Marie-Tooth disease — *see also* subcategory M49.8 G60.0
    - osteitis
      - deformans M88.88
      - fibrosa cystica — *see also* subcategory M49.8 E21.0
    - tuberculosis (Pott's curvature) A18.01
  - sequelae (late effect) of rickets E64.3
  - tuberculous A18.01

**Cushingoid due to steroid therapy** E24.2
- correct substance properly administered — *see* Table of Drugs and Chemicals, by drug, adverse effect
- overdose or wrong substance given or taken — *see* Table of Drugs and Chemicals, by drug, poisoning

**Cushing's**
- syndrome or disease E24.9
  - drug-induced E24.2
  - iatrogenic E24.2
  - pituitary-dependent E24.0
  - specified NEC E24.8
- ulcer — *see* Ulcer, peptic, acute

**Cusp, Carabelli** — *omit code*

**Cut** (external) — *see also* Laceration
- muscle — *see* Injury, muscle

**Cutaneous** — *see also* condition
- hemorrhage R23.3
- larva migrans B76.9

**Cutis** — *see also* condition
- hyperelastica Q82.8
  - acquired L57.4
- laxa (hyperelastica) — *see* Dermatolysis
- marmorata R23.8
- osteosis L94.2
- pendula — *see* Dermatolysis
- rhomboidalis nuchae L57.2
- verticis gyrata Q82.8
  - acquired L91.8

**Cyanosis** R23.0
- due to
  - patent foramen botalli Q21.12
  - persistent foramen ovale Q21.12
- enterogenous D74.8
- paroxysmal digital — *see* Raynaud's disease
  - with gangrene I73.01
- retina, retinal H35.89

**Cyanotic heart disease** I24.9
- congenital Q24.9

**Cycle**
- anovulatory N97.0
- menstrual, irregular N92.6

**Cyclencephaly** Q04.9

**Cyclical vomiting, in migraine** — *see also* Vomiting, cyclical G43.A0 (*following* G43.7)
- psychogenic F50.89

**Cyclitis** — *see also* Iridocyclitis H20.9
- chronic — *see* Iridocyclitis, chronic
- Fuchs' heterochromic H20.81- ☑
- granulomatous — *see* Iridocyclitis, chronic
- lens-induced — *see* Iridocyclitis, lens-induced
- posterior H30.2- ☑

**Cycloid personality** F34.0

**Cyclophoria** H50.54

**Cyclopia, cyclops** Q87.0

**Cyclopism** Q87.0

**Cyclosporiasis** A07.4

**Cyclothymia** F34.0

**Cyclothymic personality** F34.0

**Cyclotropia** H50.41- ☑

**Cylindroma** — *see also* Neoplasm, malignant, by site
- eccrine dermal — *see* Neoplasm, skin, benign
- skin — *see* Neoplasm, skin, benign

**Cylindruria** R82.998

**Cynanche**
- diphtheritic A36.2
- tonsillaris J36

**Cynophobia** F40.218

**Cynorexia** R63.2

**Cyphosis** — *see* Kyphosis

**Cyprus fever** — *see* Brucellosis

**Cyst** (colloid) (mucous) (simple) (retention)
- adenoid (infected) J35.8
- adrenal gland E27.8
  - congenital Q89.1
- air, lung J98.4
- allantoic Q64.4
- alveolar process (jaw bone) M27.40
- amnion, amniotic O41.8X- ☑
- aneurysmal M27.49
- anterior
  - chamber (eye) — *see* Cyst, iris
  - nasopalatine K09.1
- antrum J34.1
- anus K62.89
- apical (tooth) (periodontal) K04.8
- appendix K38.8
- arachnoid, brain (acquired) G93.0
  - congenital Q04.6
- arytenoid J38.7
- Baker's M71.2- ☑
  - ruptured M66.0
  - tuberculous A18.02
- Bartholin's gland N75.0
- bile duct (common) (hepatic) K83.5
- bladder (multiple) (trigone) N32.89
- blue dome (breast) — *see* Cyst, breast
- bone (local) NEC M85.60
  - aneurysmal M85.50
    - ankle M85.57- ☑
    - foot M85.57- ☑
    - forearm M85.53- ☑
    - hand M85.54- ☑
    - jaw M27.49
    - lower leg M85.56- ☑
    - multiple site M85.59
    - neck M85.58
    - rib M85.58
    - shoulder M85.51- ☑
    - skull M85.58
    - specified site NEC M85.58
    - thigh M85.55- ☑
    - toe M85.57- ☑
    - upper arm M85.52- ☑
    - vertebra M85.58
  - solitary M85.40
    - ankle M85.47- ☑
    - fibula M85.46- ☑
    - foot M85.47- ☑
    - hand M85.44- ☑
    - humerus M85.42- ☑
    - jaw M27.49
    - neck M85.48
    - pelvis M85.45- ☑
    - radius M85.43- ☑
    - rib M85.48
    - shoulder M85.41- ☑
    - skull M85.48
    - specified site NEC M85.48
    - tibia M85.46- ☑
    - toe M85.47- ☑

- **Cyst** — *continued*
  - bone — *continued*
    - solitary — *continued*
      - ulna M85.43- ☑
      - vertebra M85.48
    - specified type NEC M85.6Ø
      - ankle M85.67- ☑
      - foot M85.67- ☑
      - forearm M85.63- ☑
      - hand M85.64- ☑
      - jaw M27.4Ø
        - developmental (nonodontogenic) KØ9.1
          - odontogenic KØ9.Ø
        - latent M27.Ø
      - lower leg M85.66- ☑
      - multiple site M85.69
      - neck M85.68
      - rib M85.68
      - shoulder M85.61- ☑
      - skull M85.68
      - specified site NEC M85.68
      - thigh M85.65- ☑
      - toe M85.67- ☑
      - upper arm M85.62- ☑
      - vertebra M85.68
  - brain (acquired) G93.Ø
    - congenital QØ4.6
    - hydatid B67.99 *[G94]*
    - third ventricle (colloid), congenital QØ4.6
  - branchial (cleft) Q18.Ø
  - branchiogenic Q18.Ø
  - breast (benign) (blue dome) (pedunculated) (solitary) N6Ø.Ø- ☑
    - involution — *see* Dysplasia, mammary, specified type NEC
    - sebaceous — *see* Dysplasia, mammary, specified type NEC
  - broad ligament (benign) N83.8
  - bronchogenic (mediastinal) (sequestration) J98.4
    - congenital Q33.Ø
  - buccal KØ9.8
  - bulbourethral gland N36.8
  - bursa, bursal NEC M71.3Ø
    - with rupture — *see* Rupture, synovium
    - ankle M71.37- ☑
    - elbow M71.32- ☑
    - foot M71.37- ☑
    - hand M71.34- ☑
    - hip M71.35- ☑
    - multiple sites M71.39
    - pharyngeal J39.2
    - popliteal space — *see* Cyst, Baker's
    - shoulder M71.31- ☑
    - specified site NEC M71.38
    - wrist M71.33- ☑
  - calcifying odontogenic D16.5
    - upper jaw (bone) (maxilla) D16.4
  - canal of Nuck (female) N94.89
    - congenital Q52.4
  - canthus — *see* Cyst, conjunctiva
  - carcinomatous — *see* Neoplasm, malignant, by site
  - cauda equina G95.89
  - cavum septi pellucidi — *see* Cyst, brain
  - celomic (pericardium) Q24.8
  - cerebellopontine (angle) — *see* Cyst, brain
  - cerebellum — *see* Cyst, brain
  - cerebral — *see* Cyst, brain
  - cervical lateral Q18.Ø
  - cervix NEC N88.8
    - embryonic Q51.6
    - nabothian N88.8
  - chiasmal optic NEC — *see* Disorder, optic, chiasm
  - chocolate (ovary) N8Ø.1Ø- ☑
  - choledochus, congenital Q44.4
  - chorion O41.8X- ☑
  - choroid plexus G93.Ø
    - congenital QØ4.6
  - ciliary body — *see* Cyst, iris
  - clitoris N9Ø.7
  - colon K63.89
  - common (bile) duct K83.5
  - congenital NEC Q89.89
    - adrenal gland Q89.1
    - epiglottis Q31.8
    - esophagus Q39.8
    - fallopian tube Q5Ø.4
    - kidney Q61.ØØ
      - more than one (multiple) Q61.Ø2

- **Cyst** — *continued*
  - congenital — *continued*
    - kidney — *continued*
      - more than one — *continued*
        - specified as polycystic Q61.3
          - adult type Q61.2
          - infantile type NEC Q61.19
            - collecting duct dilation Q61.11
      - solitary Q61.Ø1
    - larynx Q31.8
    - liver Q44.6
    - lung Q33.Ø
    - mediastinum Q34.1
    - ovary Q5Ø.1
    - oviduct Q5Ø.4
    - periurethral (tissue) Q64.79
    - prepuce Q55.69
    - salivary gland (any) Q38.4
    - sublingual Q38.6
    - submaxillary gland Q38.6
    - thymus (gland) Q89.2
    - tongue Q38.3
    - ureterovesical orifice Q62.8
    - vulva Q52.79
  - conjunctiva H11.44- ☑
  - cornea H18.89- ☑
  - corpora quadrigemina G93.Ø
  - corpus
    - albicans N83.29- ☑
    - luteum (hemorrhagic) (ruptured) N83.1- ☑
  - Cowper's gland (benign) (infected) N36.8
  - cranial meninges G93.Ø
  - craniobuccal pouch E23.6
  - craniopharyngeal pouch E23.6
  - cystic duct K82.8
  - Cysticercus — *see* Cysticercosis
  - Dandy-Walker QØ3.1
    - with spina bifida — *see* Spina bifida
  - dental (root) KØ4.8
    - developmental KØ9.Ø
    - eruption KØ9.Ø
    - primordial KØ9.Ø
  - dentigerous (mandible) (maxilla) KØ9.Ø
  - dermoid — *see* Neoplasm, benign, by site
    - with malignant transformation C56.- ☑
    - implantation
      - external area or site (skin) NEC L72.Ø
      - iris — *see* Cyst, iris, implantation
      - vagina N89.8
      - vulva N9Ø.7
    - mouth KØ9.8
    - oral soft tissue KØ9.8
    - sacrococcygeal — *see* Cyst, pilonidal
  - developmental KØ9.1
    - odontogenic KØ9.Ø
    - oral region (nonodontogenic) KØ9.1
    - ovary, ovarian Q5Ø.1
  - dura (cerebral) G93.Ø
    - spinal G96.198
  - ear (external) Q18.1
  - echinococcal — *see* Echinococcus
  - embryonic
    - cervix uteri Q51.6
    - fallopian tube Q5Ø.4
    - vagina Q52.4
  - endometrium, endometrial (uterus) N85.8
    - ectopic — *see* Endometriosis
  - enterogenous Q43.8
  - epidermal, epidermoid (inclusion) — *see also* Cyst, skin L72.Ø
    - mouth KØ9.8
    - oral soft tissue KØ9.8
  - epididymis N5Ø.3
  - epiglottis J38.7
  - epiphysis cerebri E34.8
  - epithelial (inclusion) L72.Ø
  - epoophoron Q5Ø.5
  - eruption KØ9.Ø
  - esophagus K22.89
  - ethmoid sinus J34.1
  - external female genital organs NEC N9Ø.7
  - eye NEC H57.89
    - congenital Q15.8
  - eyelid (sebaceous) HØ2.829
    - infected — *see* Hordeolum
    - left HØ2.826
      - lower HØ2.825
      - upper HØ2.824

- **Cyst** — *continued*
  - eyelid — *continued*
    - right HØ2.823
      - lower HØ2.822
      - upper HØ2.821
  - fallopian tube N83.8
    - congenital Q5Ø.4
  - fimbrial (twisted) Q5Ø.4
  - fissural (oral region) KØ9.1
  - follicle (graafian) (hemorrhagic) N83.Ø- ☑
    - nabothian N88.8
  - follicular (atretic) (hemorrhagic) (ovarian) N83.Ø- ☑
    - dentigerous KØ9.Ø
    - odontogenic KØ9.Ø
    - skin L72.9
      - specified NEC L72.8
  - frontal sinus J34.1
  - gallbladder K82.8
  - ganglion — *see* Ganglion
  - Gartner's duct Q52.4
  - gingiva KØ9.Ø
  - gland of Moll — *see* Cyst, eyelid
  - globulomaxillary KØ9.1
  - graafian follicle (hemorrhagic) N83.Ø- ☑
  - granulosal lutein (hemorrhagic) N83.1- ☑
  - hemangiomatous D18.ØØ
    - intra-abdominal D18.Ø3
    - intracranial D18.Ø2
    - skin D18.Ø1
    - specified site NEC D18.Ø9
  - hemorrhagic M27.49
  - hydatid — *see also* Echinococcus B67.9Ø
    - brain B67.99 *[G94]*
    - liver — *see also* Cyst, liver, hydatid B67.8
    - lung NEC B67.99 *[J99]*
    - Morgagni
      - female Q5Ø.5
      - male (epididymal) Q55.4
        - testicular Q55.29
    - specified site NEC B67.99
  - hymen N89.8
    - embryonic Q52.4
  - hypopharynx J39.2
  - hypophysis, hypophyseal (duct) (recurrent) E23.6
    - cerebri E23.6
  - implantation (dermoid)
    - external area or site (skin) NEC L72.Ø
    - iris — *see* Cyst, iris, implantation
    - vagina N89.8
    - vulva N9Ø.7
  - incisive canal KØ9.1
  - inclusion (epidermal) (epithelial) (epidermoid) (squamous) L72.Ø
    - not of skin — *code under* Cyst, by site
  - intestine (large) (small) K63.89
  - intracranial — *see* Cyst, brain
  - intraligamentous — *see also* Disorder, ligament
    - knee — *see* Derangement, knee
  - intrasellar E23.6
  - iris H21.3Ø9
    - exudative H21.31- ☑
    - idiopathic H21.3Ø- ☑
    - implantation H21.32- ☑
    - parasitic H21.33- ☑
    - pars plana (primary) H21.34- ☑
      - exudative H21.35- ☑
  - jaw (bone) M27.4Ø
    - aneurysmal M27.49
    - developmental (odontogenic) KØ9.Ø
    - fissural KØ9.1
    - hemorrhagic M27.49
    - traumatic M27.49
  - joint NEC — *see* Disorder, joint, specified type NEC
  - kidney N28.1
    - acquired N28.1
    - calyceal — *see* Hydronephrosis
    - congenital Q61.ØØ
    - more than one (multiple) Q61.Ø2
      - specified as polycystic Q61.3
        - adult type (autosomal dominant) Q61.2
        - infantile type (autosomal recessive) NEC Q61.19
          - collecting duct dilation Q61.11
    - pyelogenic — *see* Hydronephrosis
    - simple N28.1
    - solitary (single) N28.1
      - acquired N28.1
      - congenital Q61.Ø1
  - labium (majus) (minus) N9Ø.7

# D



Index

d-glycericacidemia — Defect, defective

**Defect, defective** — *continued*
- ventricular septal — *continued*
  - concurrent with acute myocardial infarction — *see* Infarct, myocardium
  - following acute myocardial infarction (current complication) I23.2
  - in tetralogy of Fallot Q21.3
- vision NEC H54.7
- visual field H53.4Ø
  - bilateral
    - heteronymous H53.47
    - homonymous H53.46- ☑
  - generalized contraction H53.48- ☑
  - localized
    - arcuate H53.43- ☑
    - scotoma (central area) H53.41- ☑
      - blind spot area H53.42- ☑
    - sector H53.43- ☑
    - specified type NEC H53.45- ☑
- voice R49.9
  - specified NEC R49.8
- wedge, tooth, teeth (abrasion) KØ3.1

**Deferentitis** N49.1
- gonorrheal (acute) (chronic) A54.23

**Defibrination** (syndrome) D65
- antepartum — *see* Hemorrhage, antepartum, with coagulation defect, disseminated intravascular coagulation
- following ectopic or molar pregnancy OØ8.1
- intrapartum O67.Ø
- newborn P6Ø
- postpartum O72.3

**Deficiency, deficient**
- 3-beta hydroxysteroid dehydrogenase E25.Ø
- 5-alpha reductase (with male pseudohermaphroditism) E29.1
- 11-hydroxylase E25.Ø
- 21-hydroxylase E25.Ø
- ABCC6
  - causing generalized arterial calcification of infancy E83.823
  - pseudoxanthoma elasticum E83.824
- AADC (aromatic L-amino acid decarboxylase) E7Ø.81
- abdominal muscle syndrome Q79.4
- AC globulin (congenital) (hereditary) D68.2
  - acquired D68.4
- accelerator globulin (Ac G) (blood) D68.2
- acid phosphatase E83.39
- acid sphingomyelinase (ASMD) E75.249
  - type
    - A E75.24Ø
    - A/B E75.244
    - B E75.241
- activating factor (blood) D68.2
- ADA2 (adenosine deaminase 2) D81.32
- adenosine deaminase (ADA) D81.3Ø
  - with severe combined immunodeficiency (SCID) D81.31
  - partial (type 1) D81.39
  - specified NEC D81.39
  - type 1 (without SCID) (without severe combined immunodeficiency) D81.39
  - type 2 D81.32
- aldolase (hereditary) E74.19
- alpha-1-antitrypsin E88.Ø1
- amino-acids E72.9
- anemia — *see* Anemia
- aneurin E51.9
- anti-hemophilic
  - factor (A) D66
    - B D67
    - C D68.1
  - globulin (AHG) NEC D66
- antibody with
  - hyperimmunoglobulinemia D8Ø.6
  - near-normal immunoglobins D8Ø.6
- antidiuretic hormone E23.2
- antithrombin (antithrombin III) D68.59
- aromatic L-amino acid decarboxylase (AADC) E7Ø.81
- ascorbic acid E54
- attention (disorder) (syndrome) F98.8
  - with hyperactivity — *see* Disorder, attention-deficit hyperactivity
- autoprothrombin
  - I D68.2
  - II D67
  - C D68.2
- beta-glucuronidase E76.29

**Deficiency, deficient** — *continued*
- biotin E53.8
- biotin-dependent carboxylase D81.819
- biotinidase D81.81Ø
- brancher enzyme (amylopectinosis) E74.Ø3
- C1 esterase inhibitor (C1-INH) D84.1
- calciferol E55.9
  - with
    - adult osteomalacia M83.8
    - rickets — *see* Rickets
- calcium (dietary) E58
- calorie, severe E43
  - with marasmus E41
    - and kwashiorkor E42
- cardiac — *see* Insufficiency, myocardial
- carnitine E71.4Ø
  - due to
    - hemodialysis E71.43
    - inborn errors of metabolism E71.42
    - Valproic acid therapy E71.43
  - iatrogenic E71.43
  - muscle palmityltransferase E71.314
  - primary E71.41
  - secondary E71.448
- carotene E5Ø.9
- CD73 deficiency causing arterial calcification E83.825
- central nervous system G96.89
- ceruloplasmin (Wilson) E83.Ø1
- choline E53.8
- Christmas factor D67
- chromium E61.4
- chronic neurovisceral acid sphingomyelinase E75.244
- chronic visceral acid sphingomyelinase E75.241
- clotting (blood) — *see also* Deficiency, coagulation factor D68.9
- clotting factor NEC (hereditary) — *see also* Deficiency, factor D68.2
- coagulation NOS D68.9
  - with
    - ectopic pregnancy OØ8.1
    - molar pregnancy OØ8.1
  - acquired (any) D68.4
  - antepartum hemorrhage — *see* Hemorrhage, antepartum, with coagulation defect
  - clotting factor NEC — *see also* Deficiency, factor D68.2
  - due to
    - hyperprothrombinemia D68.4
    - liver disease D68.4
    - vitamin K deficiency D68.4
  - newborn, transient P61.6
  - postpartum O72.3
  - specified NEC D68.8
- cognitive FØ9
- color vision H53.5Ø
  - achromatopsia H53.51
  - acquired H53.52
  - deuteranomaly H53.53
  - protanomaly H53.54
  - specified type NEC H53.59
  - tritanomaly H53.55
- combined glucocorticoid and mineralocorticoid E27.49
- contact factor D68.2
- copper (nutritional) E61.Ø
- corticoadrenal E27.4Ø
  - primary E27.1
- craniofacial axis Q75.ØØ9
- cyanocobalamin E53.8
- debrancher enzyme (limit dextrinosis) E74.Ø3
- dehydrogenase
  - long chain/very long chain acyl CoA E71.31Ø
  - medium chain acyl CoA E71.311
  - short chain acyl CoA E71.312
- diet E63.9
- dihydropyrimidine dehydrogenase (DPD) E88.89
- disaccharidase E73.9
- edema — *see* Malnutrition, severe
- endocrine E34.9
- energy-supply — *see* Malnutrition
- ENPP1
  - causing
    - autosomal recessive hypophosphatemic rickets type 2 E83.822
    - generalized arterial calcification of infancy E83.821
- enzymes, circulating NEC E88.Ø9
- ergosterol E55.9
  - with
    - adult osteomalacia M83.8
    - rickets — *see* Rickets
- essential fatty acid (EFA) E63.Ø

**Deficiency, deficient** — *continued*
- eye movements
  - saccadic H55.81
  - smooth pursuit H55.82
- factor — *see also* Deficiency, coagulation
  - Hageman D68.2
  - I (congenital) (hereditary) D68.2
  - II (congenital) (hereditary) D68.2
  - IX (congenital) (functional) (hereditary) (with functional defect) D67
  - multiple (congenital) D68.8
    - acquired D68.4
  - V (congenital) (hereditary) D68.2
  - VII (congenital) (hereditary) D68.2
  - VIII (congenital) (functional) (hereditary) (with functional defect) D66
    - with vascular defect — *see* Disease, von Willebrand
  - X (congenital) (hereditary) D68.2
  - XI (congenital) (hereditary) D68.1
  - XII (congenital) (hereditary) D68.2
  - XIII (congenital) (hereditary) D68.2
- femoral, proximal focal (congenital) — *see* Defect, reduction, lower limb, longitudinal, femur
- fibrin-stabilizing factor (congenital) (hereditary) D68.2
  - acquired D68.4
- fibrinase D68.2
- fibrinogen (congenital) (hereditary) D68.2
  - acquired D65
- folate E53.8
- folic acid E53.8
- foreskin N47.3
- fructokinase E74.11
- fructose-1-phosphate aldolase E74.19
- fructose 1,6-diphosphatase E74.19
- GABA-T (gamma aminobutyric acid transaminase) E72.81
- GABA (gamma aminobutyric acid) transaminase E72.81
- GABA transporter 1 QAØ.Ø131
- galactokinase E74.29
- galactose-1-phosphate uridyl transferase E74.29
- gammaglobulin in blood D8Ø.1
  - hereditary D8Ø.Ø
- glass factor D68.2
- glucocorticoid E27.49
  - mineralocorticoid E27.49
- glucose-6-phosphatase E74.Ø1
- glucose-6-phosphate dehydrogenase
  - anemia D55.Ø
  - without anemia D75.A
- glucose transporter protein type 1 E74.81Ø
- glucuronyl transferase E8Ø.5
- Glut1 E74.81Ø
- glycogen synthetase E74.Ø9
- gonadotropin (isolated) E23.Ø
- growth hormone (idiopathic) (isolated) E23.Ø
- Hageman factor D68.2
- hemoglobin D64.9
- hepatophosphorylase E74.Ø9
- homogentisate 1,2-dioxygenase E7Ø.29
- hormone
  - anterior pituitary (partial) NEC E23.Ø
    - growth E23.Ø
  - growth (isolated) E23.Ø
  - pituitary E23.Ø
  - testicular E29.1
- hypoxanthine- (guanine)-phosphoribosyltransferase (HG- PRT) (total H-PRT) E79.1
- immunity D84.9
  - cell-mediated D84.89
    - with thrombocytopenia and eczema D82.Ø
  - combined D81.9
  - humoral D8Ø.9
  - IgA (secretory) D8Ø.2
  - IgG D8Ø.3
  - IgM D8Ø.4
- immuno — *see* Immunodeficiency
- immunoglobulin, selective
  - A (IgA) D8Ø.2
  - G (IgG) (subclasses) D8Ø.3
  - M (IgM) D8Ø.4
- infantile neurovisceral acid sphingomyelinase E75.24Ø
- inositol (B complex) E53.8
- intrinsic
  - factor (congenital) D51.Ø
  - sphincter N36.42
    - with urethral hypermobility N36.43
- iodine E61.8
  - congenital syndrome — *see* Syndrome, iodine-deficiency, congenital
- iron E61.1

Index

Defect, defective — Deficiency, deficient

Index
Deficit — Deformity

- **Delay, delayed** — *continued*
  - menarche E30.Ø
  - menstruation (cause unknown) N91.Ø
  - milestone R62.Ø
  - passage of meconium (newborn) P76.Ø
  - primary respiration P28.9
  - puberty (constitutional) E30.Ø
  - separation of umbilical cord P96.82
  - sexual maturation, female E30.Ø
  - sleep phase syndrome G47.21
  - union, fracture — *see* Fracture, by site
  - vaccination Z28.9
- **Deletion**(s)
  - autosome Q93.9
    - identified by fluorescence in situ hybridization (FISH) Q93.89
    - identified by in situ hybridization (ISH) Q93.89
  - chromosome
    - with complex rearrangements NEC Q93.7
    - part of NEC Q93.59
    - seen only at prometaphase Q93.89
    - short arm
      - 4 Q93.3
      - 5p Q93.4
      - 22q11.2 Q93.81
    - specified NEC Q93.89
  - long arm chromosome 18 or 21 Q93.89
    - with complex rearrangements NEC Q93.7
  - microdeletions NEC Q93.88
- **Delhi boil or button** B55.1
- **Delinquency** (juvenile) (neurotic) F91.8
  - group Z72.81Ø
- **Delinquent immunization status** Z28.39
  - COVID-19 Z28.31- ☑
- **Delirium, delirious** (acute or subacute) (not alcohol- or drug-induced) R41.Ø
  - with
    - dementia — *see also* Dementia FØ5
  - alcoholic (acute) (tremens) (withdrawal) F1Ø.921
    - with intoxication F1Ø.921
      - in
        - abuse F1Ø.121
        - dependence F1Ø.221
  - due to (secondary to)
    - alcohol
      - intoxication F1Ø.921
        - in
          - abuse F1Ø.121
          - dependence F1Ø.221
      - withdrawal F1Ø.231
    - amphetamine intoxication F15.921
      - in
        - abuse F15.121
        - dependence F15.221
    - anxiolytic
      - intoxication F13.921
        - in
          - abuse F13.121
          - dependence F13.221
      - withdrawal F13.231
    - cannabis intoxication (acute) F12.921
      - in
        - abuse F12.121
        - dependence F12.221
    - cocaine intoxication (acute) F14.921
      - in
        - abuse F14.121
        - dependence F14.221
    - general medical condition FØ5
    - hallucinogen intoxication F16.921
      - in
        - abuse F16.121
        - dependence F16.221
    - hypnotic
      - intoxication F13.921
        - in
          - abuse F13.121
          - dependence F13.221
      - withdrawal F13.231
    - inhalant intoxication (acute) F18.921
      - in
        - abuse F18.121
        - dependence F18.221
    - multiple etiologies FØ5
    - opioid intoxication (acute) F11.921
      - in
        - abuse F11.121
        - dependence F11.221
    - other (or unknown) substance F19.921
- **Delirium, delirious** — *continued*
  - due to — *continued*
    - phencyclidine intoxication (acute) F16.921
      - in
        - abuse F16.121
        - dependence F16.221
    - psychoactive substance NEC intoxication (acute) F19.921
      - in
        - abuse F19.121
        - dependence F19.221
    - sedative
      - intoxication F13.921
        - in
          - abuse F13.121
          - dependence F13.221
      - withdrawal F13.231
    - unknown etiology R41.Ø
  - exhaustion F43.Ø
  - hysterical F44.89
  - postprocedural (postoperative) FØ5
  - puerperal FØ5
  - thyroid — *see* Thyrotoxicosis with thyroid storm
  - traumatic — *see* Injury, intracranial
  - tremens (alcohol-induced) F1Ø.231
    - sedative-induced F13.231
- **Delivery** (childbirth) (labor)
  - arrested active phase O62.1
  - cesarean (for)
    - abnormal
      - pelvis (bony) (deformity) (major) NEC with disproportion (fetopelvic) O33.Ø
        - with obstructed labor O65.Ø
      - presentation or position O32.9- ☑
    - abruptio placentae — *see also* Abruptio placentae O45.9- ☑
    - acromion presentation O32.2- ☑
    - atony, uterus O62.2
    - breech presentation O32.1- ☑
      - incomplete O32.8- ☑
    - brow presentation O32.3- ☑
    - cephalopelvic disproportion O33.9
    - cerclage O34.3- ☑
    - chin presentation O32.3- ☑
    - cicatrix of cervix O34.4- ☑
    - contracted pelvis (general)
      - inlet O33.2
      - outlet O33.3- ☑
    - cord presentation or prolapse O69.Ø- ☑
    - cystocele O34.8- ☑
    - deformity (acquired) (congenital)
      - pelvic organs or tissues NEC O34.8- ☑
      - pelvis (bony) NEC O33.Ø
    - disproportion NOS O33.9
    - eclampsia — *see* Eclampsia
    - face presentation O32.3- ☑
    - failed
      - forceps O66.5
      - induction of labor O61.9
        - instrumental O61.1
        - mechanical O61.1
        - medical O61.Ø
        - specified NEC O61.8
        - surgical O61.1
      - trial of labor NOS O66.4Ø
        - following previous cesarean delivery O66.41
      - vacuum extraction O66.5
      - ventouse O66.5
    - fetal-maternal hemorrhage O43.Ø1- ☑
    - hemorrhage (intrapartum) O67.9
      - with coagulation defect O67.Ø
      - specified cause NEC O67.8
    - high head at term O32.4- ☑
    - hydrocephalic fetus O33.6- ☑
    - incarceration of uterus O34.51- ☑
    - incoordinate uterine action O62.4
    - increased size, fetus O33.5- ☑
    - inertia, uterus O62.2
      - primary O62.Ø
      - secondary O62.1
    - isthmocele O34.22
    - lateroversion, uterus O34.59- ☑
    - mal lie O32.9- ☑
    - malposition
      - fetus O32.9- ☑
      - pelvic organs or tissues NEC O34.8- ☑
      - uterus NEC O34.59- ☑
    - malpresentation NOS O32.9- ☑
- **Delivery** — *continued*
  - cesarean — *continued*
    - oblique presentation O32.2- ☑
    - occurring after 37 completed weeks of gestation but before 39 completed weeks gestation due to (spontaneous) onset of labor O75.82
    - oversize fetus O33.5- ☑
    - pelvic tumor NEC O34.8- ☑
    - placenta previa O44.Ø- ☑
      - complete O44.Ø- ☑
        - with hemorrhage O44.1- ☑
    - placental insufficiency O36.51- ☑
    - planned, occurring after 37 completed weeks of gestation but before 39 completed weeks gestation due to (spontaneous) onset of labor O75.82
    - polyp, cervix O34.4- ☑
      - causing obstructed labor O65.5
    - poor dilatation, cervix O62.Ø
    - pre-eclampsia O14.94
      - mild O14.Ø4
      - moderate O14.Ø4
      - severe O14.14
        - with hemolysis, elevated liver enzymes and low platelet count (HELLP) O14.24
    - previous
      - cesarean delivery O34.219
        - classical (vertical) scar O34.212
        - isthmocele O34.22
        - low transverse scar O34.211
        - mid-transverse T incision O34.218
        - scar
          - defect (isthmocele) O34.22
          - specified type NEC O34.218
      - surgery (to)
        - cervix O34.4- ☑
        - gynecological NEC O34.8- ☑
        - rectum O34.7- ☑
        - uterus O34.29
        - vagina O34.6- ☑
    - prolapse
      - arm or hand O32.2- ☑
      - uterus O34.52- ☑
    - prolonged labor NOS O63.9
    - rectocele O34.8- ☑
    - retroversion
      - uterus O34.53- ☑
    - rigid
      - cervix O34.4- ☑
      - pelvic floor O34.8- ☑
      - perineum O34.7- ☑
      - vagina O34.6- ☑
      - vulva O34.7- ☑
    - sacculation, pregnant uterus O34.59- ☑
    - scar(s)
      - cervix O34.4- ☑
      - cesarean delivery O34.219
        - classical (vertical) O34.212
        - isthmocele O34.22
        - low transverse O34.211
        - mid-transverse T incision O34.218
        - scar
          - defect (isthmocele) O34.22
          - specified type NEC O34.218
      - defect (isthmocele) O34.22
      - transmural uterine O34.29
      - uterus O34.29
    - Shirodkar suture in situ O34.3- ☑
    - shoulder presentation O32.2- ☑
    - stenosis or stricture, cervix O34.4- ☑
    - streptococcus group B (GBS) carrier state O99.824
    - transmural uterine scar O34.29
    - transverse presentation or lie O32.2- ☑
    - tumor, pelvic organs or tissues NEC O34.8- ☑
      - cervix O34.4- ☑
    - umbilical cord presentation or prolapse O69.Ø- ☑
    - without indication O82
  - completely normal case O8Ø
  - complicated O75.9
    - by
      - abnormal, abnormality (of)
        - forces of labor O62.9
          - specified type NEC O62.8
        - glucose O99.814
        - uterine contractions NOS O62.9
      - abruptio placentae — *see also* Abruptio placentae O45.9- ☑
      - abuse

**Delivery** — *continued*
complicated — *continued*
by — *continued*
abuse — *continued*
physical O9A.32 (*following* O99)
psychological O9A.52 (*following* O99)
sexual O9A.42 (*following* O99)
adherent placenta O72.Ø
without hemorrhage O73.Ø
alcohol use O99.314
anemia (pre-existing) O99.Ø2
anesthetic death O74.8
annular detachment of cervix O71.3
atony, uterus O62.2
attempted vacuum extraction and forceps O66.5
Bandl's ring O62.4
bariatric surgery status O99.844
biliary tract disorder O26.62
bleeding — *see* Delivery, complicated by, hemorrhage
blood disorder NEC O99.12
cervical dystocia (hypotonic) O62.2
primary O62.Ø
secondary O62.1
circulatory system disorder O99.42
compression of cord (umbilical) NEC O69.2- ☑
condition NEC O99.892
contraction, contracted ring O62.4
cord (umbilical)
around neck
with compression O69.1- ☑
without compression O69.81- ☑
bruising O69.5- ☑
complication O69.9- ☑
specified NEC O69.89- ☑
compression NEC O69.2- ☑
entanglement O69.2- ☑
without compression O69.82- ☑
hematoma O69.5- ☑
presentation O69.Ø- ☑
prolapse O69.Ø- ☑
short O69.3- ☑
thrombosis (vessels) O69.5- ☑
vascular lesion O69.5- ☑
Couvelaire uterus O45.8X- ☑
damage to (injury to) NEC
perineum O71.82
periurethral tissue O71.82
vulva O71.82
delay following rupture of membranes (spontaneous) — *see* Pregnancy, complicated by, premature rupture of membranes
depressed fetal heart tones O76
diabetes O24.92
gestational O24.429
diet controlled O24.42Ø
insulin controlled O24.424
oral drug controlled (antidiabetic) (hypoglycemic) O24.425
pre-existing O24.32
specified NEC O24.82
type 1 O24.Ø2
type 2 O24.12
diastasis recti (abdominis) O71.89
dilatation
bladder O66.8
cervix incomplete, poor or slow O62.Ø
disease NEC O99.892
disruptio uteri — *see* Delivery, complicated by, rupture, uterus
drug use O99.324
dysfunction, uterus NOS O62.9
hypertonic O62.4
hypotonic O62.2
primary O62.Ø
secondary O62.1
incoordinate O62.4
eclampsia O15.1
embolism (pulmonary) — *see* Embolism, obstetric
endocrine, nutritional or metabolic disease NEC O99.284
failed
attempted vaginal birth after previous cesarean delivery O66.41
induction of labor O61.9
instrumental O61.1
mechanical O61.1
medical O61.Ø

**Delivery** — *continued*
complicated — *continued*
by — *continued*
failed — *continued*
induction of labor — *continued*
specified NEC O61.8
surgical O61.1
trial of labor O66.4Ø
female genital mutilation O65.5
fetal
abnormal acid-base balance O68
acidemia O68
acidosis O68
alkalosis O68
death, early OØ2.1
deformity O66.3
heart rate or rhythm (abnormal) (non-reassuring) O76
hypoxia O77.8
stress O77.9
due to drug administration O77.1
electrocardiographic evidence of O77.8
specified NEC O77.8
ultrasound evidence of O77.8
fever during labor O75.2
gastric banding status O99.844
gastric bypass status O99.844
gastrointestinal disease NEC O99.62
gestational
diabetes O24.429
diet controlled O24.42Ø
insulin (and diet) controlled O24.424
oral drug controlled (antidiabetic) (hypoglycemic) O24.425
edema O12.Ø4
with proteinuria O12.24
proteinuria O12.14
gonorrhea O98.22
hematoma O71.7
ischial spine O71.7
pelvic O71.7
vagina O71.7
vulva or perineum O71.7
hemorrhage (uterine) O67.9
associated with
afibrinogenemia O67.Ø
coagulation defect O67.Ø
hyperfibrinolysis O67.Ø
hypofibrinogenemia O67.Ø
due to
low implantation of placenta O44.5- ☑
low-lying placenta O44.5- ☑
placenta previa O44.1- ☑
marginal O44.3- ☑
partial O44.3- ☑
premature separation of placenta (normally implanted) — *see also* Abruptio placentae O45.9- ☑
retained placenta O72.Ø
uterine leiomyoma O67.8
placenta NEC O67.8
postpartum NEC (atonic) (immediate) O72.1
with retained or trapped placenta O72.Ø
delayed O72.2
secondary O72.2
third stage O72.Ø
hourglass contraction, uterus O62.4
hypertension, hypertensive (pre-existing) — *see* Hypertension, complicated by, childbirth (labor)
hypotension O26.5- ☑
incomplete dilatation (cervix) O62.Ø
incoordinate uterus contractions O62.4
inertia, uterus O62.2
during latent phase of labor O62.Ø
primary O62.Ø
secondary O62.1
infection (maternal) O98.92
carrier state NEC O99.834
gonorrhea O98.22
human immunodeficiency virus (HIV) O98.72
sexually transmitted NEC O98.32
specified NEC O98.82
syphilis O98.12
tuberculosis O98.Ø2
viral hepatitis O98.42
viral NEC O98.52

**Delivery** — *continued*
complicated — *continued*
by — *continued*
injury (to mother) — *see also* Delivery, complicated, by, damage to O71.9
nonobstetric O9A.22 (*following* O99)
caused by abuse — *see* Delivery, complicated by, abuse
intrauterine fetal death, early OØ2.1
inversion, uterus O71.2
laceration (perineal) O7Ø.9
anus (sphincter) O7Ø.4
with third degree laceration — *see also* Delivery, complicated, by, laceration, perineum, third degree O7Ø.2Ø
with mucosa O7Ø.3
without third degree laceration O7Ø.2- ☑
bladder (urinary) O71.5
bowel O71.5
cervix (uteri) O71.3
fourchette O7Ø.Ø
hymen O7Ø.Ø
labia O7Ø.Ø
pelvic
floor O7Ø.1
organ NEC O71.5
perineum, perineal O7Ø.9
first degree O7Ø.Ø
fourth degree O7Ø.3
muscles O7Ø.1
second degree O7Ø.1
skin O7Ø.Ø
slight O7Ø.Ø
third degree O7Ø.2Ø
with
both external anal sphincter (EAS) and internal anal sphincter (IAS) torn (IIIc) O7Ø.23
less than 5Ø% of external anal sphincter (EAS) thickness torn (IIIa) O7Ø.21
more than 5Ø% external anal sphincter (EAS) thickness torn (IIIb) O7Ø.22
IIIa O7Ø.21
IIIb O7Ø.22
IIIc O7Ø.23
peritoneum (pelvic) O71.5
rectovaginal (septum) (without perineal laceration) O71.4
with perineum — *see also* Delivery, complicated, by, laceration, perineum, third degree O7Ø.2Ø
with anal or rectal mucosa O7Ø.3
specified NEC O71.89
sphincter ani — *see* Delivery, complicated, by, laceration, anus (sphincter)
urethra O71.5
uterus O71.81
before labor O71.81
vagina, vaginal (deep) (high) (without perineal laceration) O71.4
with perineum O7Ø.Ø
muscles, with perineum O7Ø.1
vulva O7Ø.Ø
liver disorder O26.62
malignancy O9A.12 (*following* O99)
malnutrition O25.2
malposition, malpresentation
uterus or cervix O65.5
placenta O44.Ø- ☑
with hemorrhage O44.1- ☑
without obstruction — *see also* Delivery, complicated by, obstructed labor O32.9- ☑
breech O32.1- ☑
compound O32.6- ☑
face (brow) (chin) O32.3- ☑
footling O32.8- ☑
high head O32.4- ☑
oblique O32.2- ☑
specified NEC O32.8- ☑
transverse O32.2- ☑
unstable lie O32.Ø- ☑
meconium in amniotic fluid O77.Ø
mental disorder NEC O99.344
metrorrhexis — *see* Delivery, complicated by, rupture, uterus
nervous system disorder O99.354

- **Delivery** — *continued*
  - complicated — *continued*
    - by — *continued*
      - obesity (pre-existing) O99.214
      - obesity surgery status O99.844
      - obstetric trauma O71.9
        - specified NEC O71.89
      - obstructed labor
        - due to
          - breech (complete) (frank) presentation O64.1- ☑
            - incomplete O64.8- ☑
          - brow presentation O64.3- ☑
          - buttock presentation O64.1- ☑
          - chin presentation O64.2- ☑
          - compound presentation O64.5- ☑
          - contracted pelvis O65.1
          - deep transverse arrest O64.Ø- ☑
          - deformed pelvis O65.Ø
          - dystocia (fetal) O66.9
            - due to
              - conjoined twins O66.3
              - fetal
                - abnormality NEC O66.3
                - ascites O66.3
                - hydrops O66.3
                - meningomyelocele O66.3
                - sacral teratoma O66.3
                - tumor O66.3
              - hydrocephalic fetus O66.3
            - shoulder O66.Ø
          - face presentation O64.2- ☑
          - fetopelvic disproportion O65.4
          - footling presentation O64.8- ☑
          - impacted shoulders O66.Ø
          - incomplete rotation of fetal head O64.Ø- ☑
          - large fetus O66.2
          - locked twins O66.1
          - malposition O64.9- ☑
            - specified NEC O64.8- ☑
          - malpresentation O64.9- ☑
            - specified NEC O64.8- ☑
          - multiple fetuses NEC O66.6
          - pelvic
            - abnormality (maternal) O65.9
              - organ O65.5
              - specified NEC O65.8
            - contraction
              - inlet O65.2
              - mid-cavity O65.3
              - outlet O65.3
          - persistent (position)
            - occipitoiliac O64.Ø- ☑
            - occipitoposterior O64.Ø- ☑
            - occipitosacral O64.Ø- ☑
            - occipitotransverse O64.Ø- ☑
          - prolapsed arm O64.4- ☑
          - shoulder presentation O64.4- ☑
        - specified NEC O66.8
      - pathological retraction ring, uterus O62.4
      - penetration, pregnant uterus by instrument O71.1
      - perforation — *see* Delivery, complicated by, laceration
      - placenta, placental
        - ablatio — *see also* Abruptio placentae O45.9- ☑
        - abnormality O43.9- ☑
          - specified NEC O43.89- ☑
        - abruptio — *see also* Abruptio placentae O45.9- ☑
        - accreta O43.21- ☑
        - adherent (with hemorrhage) O72.Ø
          - without hemorrhage O73.Ø
        - detachment (premature) — *see also* Abruptio placentae O45.9- ☑
        - disorder O43.9- ☑
          - specified NEC O43.89- ☑
        - hemorrhage NEC O67.8
        - increta O43.22- ☑
        - low (implantation) (lying) O44.4- ☑
          - with hemorrhage O44.5- ☑
        - malformation O43.1Ø- ☑
        - malposition O44.Ø- ☑
          - without hemorrhage O44.1- ☑
        - percreta O43.23- ☑
        - previa (central) (complete) (lateral) (total) O44.Ø- ☑

- **Delivery** — *continued*
  - complicated — *continued*
    - by — *continued*
      - placenta, placental — *continued*
        - previa — *continued*
          - with hemorrhage O44.1- ☑
          - marginal O44.2- ☑
            - with hemorrhage O44.3- ☑
          - partial O44.2- ☑
            - with hemorrhage O44.3- ☑
        - retained (with hemorrhage) O72.Ø
          - without hemorrhage O73.Ø
        - separation (premature) O45.9- ☑
          - specified NEC O45.8X- ☑
        - vicious insertion O44.1- ☑
      - precipitate labor O62.3
      - premature rupture, membranes — *see also* Pregnancy, complicated by, premature rupture of membranes O42.9Ø
      - prolapse
        - arm or hand O32.2- ☑
        - cord (umbilical) O69.Ø- ☑
        - foot or leg O32.8- ☑
        - uterus O34.52- ☑
      - prolonged labor O63.9
        - first stage O63.Ø
        - second stage O63.1
      - protozoal disease (maternal) O98.62
      - respiratory disease NEC O99.52
      - retained membranes or portions of placenta O72.2
        - without hemorrhage O73.1
      - retarded birth O63.9
      - retention of secundines (with hemorrhage) O72.Ø
        - without hemorrhage O73.Ø
        - partial O72.2
          - without hemorrhage O73.1
      - rupture
        - bladder (urinary) O71.5
        - cervix O71.3
        - pelvic organ NEC O71.5
        - urethra O71.5
        - uterus (during or after labor) O71.1
          - before labor O71.Ø- ☑
      - separation, pubic bone (symphysis pubis) O71.6
      - shock O75.1
      - shoulder presentation O64.4- ☑
      - skin disorder NEC O99.72
      - spasm, cervix O62.4
      - stenosis or stricture, cervix O65.5
      - streptococcus group B (GBS) carrier state O99.824
      - subluxation of symphysis (pubis) O26.72
      - syphilis (maternal) O98.12
      - tear — *see* Delivery, complicated by, laceration
      - tetanic uterus O62.4
      - trauma (obstetrical) — *see also* Delivery, complicated, by, damage to O71.9
        - non-obstetric O9A.22 (*following* O99)
        - periurethral O71.82
        - specified NEC O71.89
      - tuberculosis (maternal) O98.Ø2
      - tumor, pelvic organs or tissues NEC O65.5
      - umbilical cord around neck
        - with compression O69.1- ☑
        - without compression O69.81- ☑
      - uterine inertia O62.2
        - during latent phase of labor O62.Ø
        - primary O62.Ø
        - secondary O62.1
      - vasa previa O69.4- ☑
      - velamentous insertion of cord O43.12- ☑
    - specified complication NEC O75.89
  - delayed NOS O63.9
    - following rupture of membranes
      - artificial O75.5
    - second twin, triplet, etc. O63.2
  - forceps, low following failed vacuum extraction O66.5
  - missed (at or near term) O36.4- ☑
  - normal O8Ø
  - obstructed — *see* Delivery, complicated by, obstructed labor
  - precipitate O62.3
  - preterm — *see also* Pregnancy, complicated by, preterm labor O6Ø.1Ø- ☑
  - spontaneous O8Ø
  - term pregnancy NOS O8Ø
  - uncomplicated O8Ø
  - vaginal, following previous cesarean delivery O34.219
    - classical (vertical) scar O34.212

- **Delivery** — *continued*
  - vaginal, following previous cesarean delivery — *continued*
    - low transverse scar O34.211
    - mid-transverse T incision O34.218
    - scar
      - defect (isthmocele) O34.22
      - specified type NEC O34.218
- **Delusions** (paranoid) — *see* Disorder, delusional
- **Dementia** (degenerative (primary)) (persisting) (unspecified severity) (without behavioral disturbance, psychotic disturbance, mood disturbance, and anxiety) FØ3.9Ø
  - with
    - aberrant motor behavior (exit-seeking) (pacing) (restlessness) (rocking) FØ3.911
    - acute confusional state FØ5
    - agitation FØ3.911
    - anxiety FØ3.94
    - behavioral disturbances (sexual disinhibition) (sleep disturbance) (social disinhibition) FØ3.918
      - specified NEC FØ3.918
    - Lewy bodies — *see also* Dementia, in, diseases specified elsewhere G31.83 *[FØ2.8Ø]*
      - with behavioral disturbance — *see also* Dementia, in, diseases specified elsewhere G31.83 *[FØ2.81-]* ☑
    - mood disturbance (anhedonia) (apathy) (depression) FØ3.93
    - Parkinsonism — *see also* Dementia, in, diseases specified elsewhere G2Ø.C *[FØ2.8Ø]*
      - with behavioral disturbance — *see also* Dementia, in, diseases specified elsewhere G2Ø.C *[FØ2.81-]* ☑
    - Parkinson's disease — *see also* Dementia, in, diseases specified elsewhere G2Ø.A1 *[FØ2.8Ø]*
      - with behavioral disturbance — *see also* Dementia, in, diseases specified elsewhere G2Ø.A1 *[FØ2.81-]* ☑
    - psychotic disturbance (delusional state) (hallucinations) (paranoia) (suspiciousness) FØ3.92
    - verbal or physical behaviors (anger) (aggression) (combativeness) (profanity) (shouting) (threatening) (violence) FØ3.911
  - alcoholic F1Ø.97
    - with dependence F1Ø.27
  - Alzheimer's type — *see* Disease, Alzheimer's
  - arteriosclerotic — *see* Dementia, vascular
  - atypical, Alzheimer's type — *see* Disease, Alzheimer's, specified NEC
  - congenital — *see* Disability, intellectual
  - frontal (lobe) — *see also* Dementia, in, diseases specified elsewhere G31.Ø9 *[FØ2.8Ø]*
    - with behavioral disturbance — *see also* Dementia, in, diseases specified elsewhere G31.Ø9 *[FØ2.81-]* ☑
  - frontotemporal G31.Ø9 *[FØ2.8Ø]*
    - with behavioral disturbance G31.Ø9 *[FØ2.81-]* ☑
    - specified NEC — *see also* Dementia, in, diseases specified elsewhere G31.Ø9 *[FØ2.8Ø]*
      - with behavioral disturbance — *see also* Dementia, in, diseases specified elsewhere G31.Ø9 *[FØ2.81-]* ☑
  - in (due to)
    - alcohol F1Ø.97
      - with dependence F1Ø.27
    - Alzheimer's disease — *see* Disease, Alzheimer's
    - arteriosclerotic brain disease — *see* Dementia, vascular
    - cerebral lipidoses — *see also* Dementia, in, diseases specified elsewhere E75.- ☑ *[FØ2.8Ø]*
      - with behavioral disturbance — *see also* Dementia, in, diseases specified elsewhere E75.- ☑ *[FØ2.81-]* ☑
    - Creutzfeldt-Jakob disease — *see also* Creutzfeldt-Jakob disease or syndrome (with dementia) A81.ØØ
    - diseases specified elsewhere (unspecified severity) (without behavioral disturbance, psychotic disturbance, mood disturbance, and anxiety) FØ2.8Ø
      - with
        - aberrant motor behavior (exit-seeking) (pacing) (restlessness) (rocking) FØ2.811
        - agitation FØ2.811
        - anxiety FØ2.84
        - behavioral disturbances (sexual disinhibition) (sleep disturbance) (social disinhibition) FØ2.818

Index

Delivery — Dementia

- **Dementia** — *continued*
  - in — *continued*
    - diseases specified elsewhere — *continued*
      - with — *continued*
        - behavioral disturbances — *continued*
          - specified NEC FØ2.818
        - mood disturbance (anhedonia) (apathy) (depression) FØ2.83
        - psychotic disturbance (delusional state) (hallucinations) (paranoia) (suspiciousness) FØ2.82
        - verbal or physical behaviors (anger) (aggression) (combativeness) (profanity) (shouting) (threatening) (violence) FØ2.811
      - mild FØ2.AØ
        - with
          - aberrant motor behavior (exit-seeking) (pacing) (restlessness) (rocking) FØ2.A11
          - agitation FØ2.A11
          - anxiety FØ2.A4
          - behavioral disturbances (sexual disinhibition) (sleep disturbance) (social disinhibition) FØ2.A18
            - specified NEC FØ2.A18
          - mood disturbance (anhedonia) (apathy) (depression) FØ2.A3
          - psychotic disturbance (delusional state) (hallucinations) (paranoia) (suspiciousness) FØ2.A2
          - verbal or physical behaviors (anger) (aggression) (combativeness) (profanity) (shouting) (threatening) (violence) FØ2.A11
      - moderate FØ2.BØ
        - with
          - aberrant motor behavior (exit-seeking) (pacing) (restlessness) (rocking) FØ2.B11
          - agitation FØ2.B11
          - anxiety FØ2.B4
          - behavioral disturbances (sexual disinhibition) (sleep disturbance) (social disinhibition) FØ2.B18
            - specified NEC FØ2.B18
          - mood disturbance (anhedonia) (apathy) (depression) FØ2.B3
          - psychotic disturbance (delusional state) (hallucinations) (paranoia) (suspiciousness) FØ2.B2
          - verbal or physical behaviors (anger) (aggression) (combativeness) (profanity) (shouting) (threatening) (violence) FØ2.B11
      - severe FØ2.CØ
        - with
          - aberrant motor behavior (exit-seeking) (pacing) (restlessness) (rocking) FØ2.C11
          - agitation FØ2.C11
          - anxiety FØ2.C4
          - behavioral disturbances (sexual disinhibition) (sleep disturbance) (social disinhibition) FØ2.C18
            - specified NEC FØ2.C18
          - mood disturbance (anhedonia) (apathy) (depression) FØ2.C3
          - psychotic disturbance (delusional state) (hallucinations) (paranoia) (suspiciousness) FØ2.C2
          - verbal or physical behaviors (anger) (aggression) (combativeness) (profanity) (shouting) (threatening) (violence) FØ2.C11
    - epilepsy — *see also* Dementia, in, diseases specified elsewhere G4Ø.- ☑ *[FØ2.8Ø]*
      - with behavioral disturbance — *see also* Dementia, in, diseases specified elsewhere G4Ø.- ☑ *[FØ2.81-]* ☑
    - hepatolenticular degeneration — *see also* Dementia, in, diseases specified elsewhere E83.Ø1 *[FØ2.8Ø]*
      - with behavioral disturbance — *see also* Dementia, in, diseases specified elsewhere E83.Ø1 *[FØ2.81-]* ☑
    - human immunodeficiency virus (HIV) disease — *see also* Dementia, in, diseases specified elsewhere B2Ø *[FØ2.8Ø]*

- **Dementia** — *continued*
  - in — *continued*
    - human immunodeficiency virus disease — *see also* Dementia, in, diseases specified elsewhere — *continued*
      - with behavioral disturbance — *see also* Dementia, in, diseases specified elsewhere B2Ø *[FØ2.81-]* ☑
    - Huntington's disease or chorea — *see also* Dementia, in, diseases specified elsewhere G1Ø *[FØ2.8Ø]*
      - with behavioral disturbance — *see also* Dementia, in, diseases specified elsewhere G1Ø *[FØ2.81-]* ☑
    - hypercalcemia — *see also* Dementia, in, diseases specified elsewhere E83.52 *[FØ2.8Ø]*
      - with behavioral disturbance — *see also* Dementia, in, diseases specified elsewhere E83.52 *[FØ2.81-]* ☑
    - hypothyroidism, acquired — *see also* Dementia, in, diseases specified elsewhere EØ3.9 *[FØ2.8Ø]*
      - with behavioral disturbance — *see also* Dementia, in, diseases specified elsewhere EØ3.9 *[FØ2.81-]* ☑
      - due to iodine deficiency — *see also* Dementia, in, diseases specified elsewhere EØ1.8 *[FØ2.8Ø]*
        - with behavioral disturbance — *see also* Dementia, in, diseases specified elsewhere EØ1.8 *[FØ2.81-]* ☑
    - inhalants F18.97
      - with dependence F18.27
    - multiple
      - etiologies FØ3.- ☑
      - sclerosis — *see also* Dementia, in, diseases specified elsewhere G35.D *[FØ2.8Ø]*
        - with behavioral disturbance — *see also* Dementia, in, diseases specified elsewhere G35.D *[FØ2.81-]* ☑
    - neurosyphilis — *see also* Dementia, in, diseases specified elsewhere A52.17 *[FØ2.8Ø]*
      - with behavioral disturbance — *see also* Dementia, in, diseases specified elsewhere A52.17 *[FØ2.81-]* ☑
      - juvenile — *see also* Dementia, in, diseases specified elsewhere A5Ø.49 *[FØ2.8Ø]*
        - with behavioral disturbance — *see also* Dementia, in, diseases specified elsewhere A5Ø.49 *[FØ2.81-]* ☑
    - niacin deficiency — *see also* Dementia, in, diseases specified elsewhere E52 *[FØ2.8Ø]*
      - with behavioral disturbance — *see also* Dementia, in, diseases specified elsewhere E52 *[FØ2.81-]* ☑
    - paralysis agitans — *see also* Dementia, in, diseases specified elsewhere G2Ø.C *[FØ2.8Ø]*
      - with behavioral disturbance — *see also* Dementia, in, diseases specified elsewhere G2Ø.C *[FØ2.81-]* ☑
    - Parkinson's disease — *see also* Dementia, in, diseases specified elsewhere G2Ø.A1 *[FØ2.8Ø]*
    - pellagra — *see also* Dementia, in, diseases specified elsewhere E52 *[FØ2.8Ø]*
      - with behavioral disturbance — *see also* Dementia, in, diseases specified elsewhere E52 *[FØ2.81-]* ☑
    - Pick's — *see also* Dementia, in, diseases specified elsewhere G31.Ø1 *[FØ2.8Ø]*
      - with behavioral disturbance — *see also* Dementia, in, diseases specified elsewhere G31.Ø1 *[FØ2.81-]* ☑
    - polyarteritis nodosa — *see also* Dementia, in, diseases specified elsewhere M3Ø.Ø *[FØ2.8Ø]*
      - with behavioral disturbance — *see also* Dementia, in, diseases specified elsewhere M3Ø.Ø *[FØ2.81-]* ☑
    - psychoactive drug F19.97
      - with dependence F19.27
      - inhalants F18.97
        - with dependence F18.27
      - sedatives, hypnotics or anxiolytics F13.97
        - with dependence F13.27
    - sedatives, hypnotics or anxiolytics F13.97
      - with dependence F13.27
    - systemic lupus erythematosus — *see also* Dementia, in, diseases specified elsewhere M32.- ☑ *[FØ2.8Ø]*
      - with behavioral disturbance — *see also* Dementia, in, diseases specified elsewhere M32.- ☑ *[FØ2.81-]* ☑

- **Dementia** — *continued*
  - in — *continued*
    - trypanosomiasis
      - African — *see also* Dementia, in, diseases specified elsewhere B56.9 *[FØ2.8Ø]*
        - with behavioral disturbance — *see also* Dementia, in, diseases specified elsewhere B56.9 *[FØ2.81-]* ☑
    - unknown etiology FØ3.- ☑
    - vitamin B12 deficiency — *see also* Dementia, in, diseases specified elsewhere E53.8 *[FØ2.8Ø]*
      - with behavioral disturbance — *see also* Dementia, in, diseases specified elsewhere E53.8 *[FØ2.81-]* ☑
    - volatile solvents F18.97
      - with dependence F18.27
  - infantile, infantilis F84.3
  - Lewy body — *see also* Dementia, in, diseases specified elsewhere G31.83 *[FØ2.8Ø]*
    - with behavioral disturbance — *see also* Dementia, in, diseases specified elsewhere G31.83 *[FØ2.81-]* ☑
  - mild FØ3.AØ
    - with
      - aberrant motor behavior (exit-seeking) (pacing) (restlessness) (rocking) FØ3.A11
      - agitation FØ3.A11
      - anxiety FØ3.A4
      - behavioral disturbances (sexual disinhibition) (sleep disturbance) (social disinhibition) FØ3.A18
        - specified NEC FØ3.A18
      - mood disturbance (anhedonia) (apathy) (depression) FØ3.A3
      - psychotic disturbance (delusional state) (hallucinations) (paranoia) (suspiciousness) FØ3.A2
      - verbal or physical behaviors (anger) (aggression) (combativeness) (profanity) (shouting) (threatening) (violence) FØ3.A11
  - moderate FØ3.BØ
    - with
      - aberrant motor behavior (exit-seeking) (pacing) (restlessness) (rocking) FØ3.B11
      - agitation FØ3.B11
      - anxiety FØ3.B4
      - behavioral disturbances (sexual disinhibition) (sleep disturbance) (social disinhibition) FØ3.B18
        - specified NEC FØ3.B18
      - mood disturbance (anhedonia) (apathy) (depression) FØ3.B3
      - psychotic disturbance (delusional state) (hallucinations) (paranoia) (suspiciousness) FØ3.B2
      - verbal or physical behaviors (anger) (aggression) (combativeness) (profanity) (shouting) (threatening) (violence) FØ3.B11
  - multi-infarct — *see* Dementia, vascular
  - old age (senile) FØ3.- ☑
    - Alzheimer's type — *see* Disease, Alzheimer's, late onset
  - paralytica, paralytic (syphilitic) — *see also* Dementia, in, diseases specified elsewhere A52.17 *[FØ2.8Ø]*
    - with behavioral disturbance — *see also* Dementia, in, diseases specified elsewhere A52.17 *[FØ2.81-]* ☑
    - juvenilis A5Ø.45
  - paretic A52.17
  - praecox — *see* Schizophrenia
  - presenile FØ3.- ☑
    - Alzheimer's type — *see* Disease, Alzheimer's, early onset
  - primary degenerative FØ3.- ☑
  - progressive, syphilitic A52.17
  - senile FØ3.- ☑
    - Alzheimer's type — *see* Disease, Alzheimer's, late onset
    - depressed or paranoid type FØ3.- ☑
  - severe FØ3.CØ
    - with
      - aberrant motor behavior (exit-seeking) (pacing) (restlessness) (rocking) FØ3.C11
      - agitation FØ3.C11
      - anxiety FØ3.C4
      - behavioral disturbances (sexual disinhibition) (sleep disturbance) (social disinhibition) FØ3.C18
        - specified NEC FØ3.C18

☑ **Additional Character Required — Refer to the Tabular List for Character Selection**

- **Dependence** — *continued*
  - drug — *continued*
    - inhalant — *continued*
      - with — *continued*
        - other specified disorder F18.288
        - psychosis F18.259
          - delusions F18.25Ø
          - hallucinations F18.251
        - unspecified disorder F18.29
      - in remission F18.21
    - nicotine F17.2ØØ
      - with disorder F17.2Ø9
        - in remission F17.2Ø1
        - specified disorder NEC F17.2Ø8
        - withdrawal F17.2Ø3
      - chewing tobacco F17.22Ø
        - with disorder F17.229
          - in remission F17.221
          - specified disorder NEC F17.228
          - withdrawal F17.223
      - cigarettes F17.21Ø
        - with disorder F17.219
          - in remission F17.211
          - specified disorder NEC F17.218
          - withdrawal F17.213
      - specified product NEC F17.29Ø
        - with disorder F17.299
          - remission F17.291
          - specified disorder NEC F17.298
          - withdrawal F17.293
    - opioid F11.2Ø
      - with
        - intoxication F11.229
          - with
            - delirium F11.221
            - perceptual disturbance F11.222
          - uncomplicated F11.22Ø
        - mood disorder F11.24
        - opioid-associated amnestic syndrome F11.288
        - other specified disorder F11.288
        - psychosis F11.259
          - delusions F11.25Ø
          - hallucinations F11.251
        - sexual dysfunction F11.281
        - sleep disorder F11.282
        - unspecified disorder F11.29
        - withdrawal F11.23
      - in remission F11.21
    - psychoactive NEC F19.2Ø
      - with
        - amnestic disorder F19.26
        - anxiety disorder F19.28Ø
        - dementia F19.27
        - intoxication F19.229
          - with
            - delirium F19.221
            - perceptual disturbance F19.222
          - uncomplicated F19.22Ø
        - mood disorder F19.24
        - other specified disorder F19.288
        - psychosis F19.259
          - delusions F19.25Ø
          - hallucinations F19.251
        - sexual dysfunction F19.281
        - sleep disorder F19.282
        - unspecified disorder F19.29
        - withdrawal F19.239
          - with
            - delirium F19.231
            - perceptual disturbance F19.232
          - uncomplicated F19.23Ø
      - in remission F19.21
    - sedative, hypnotic or anxiolytic F13.2Ø
      - with
        - amnestic disorder F13.26
        - anxiety disorder F13.28Ø
        - dementia, persisting F13.27
        - intoxication F13.229
          - with delirium F13.221
          - uncomplicated F13.22Ø
        - mood disorder F13.24
        - other specified disorder F13.288
        - psychosis F13.259
          - delusions F13.25Ø
          - hallucinations F13.251
        - sexual dysfunction F13.281
        - sleep disorder F13.282
        - unspecified disorder F13.29
        - withdrawal F13.239

- **Dependence** — *continued*
  - drug — *continued*
    - sedative, hypnotic or anxiolytic — *continued*
      - with — *continued*
        - withdrawal — *continued*
          - with
            - delirium F13.231
            - perceptual disturbance F13.232
          - uncomplicated F13.23Ø
      - in remission F13.21
    - stimulant NEC F15.2Ø
      - with
        - anxiety disorder F15.28Ø
        - intoxication F15.229
          - with
            - delirium F15.221
            - perceptual disturbance F15.222
          - uncomplicated F15.22Ø
        - mood disorder F15.24
        - other specified disorder F15.288
        - psychosis F15.259
          - delusions F15.25Ø
          - hallucinations F15.251
        - sexual dysfunction F15.281
        - sleep disorder F15.282
        - unspecified disorder F15.29
        - withdrawal F15.23
      - in remission F15.21
  - ethyl
    - alcohol (without remission) F1Ø.2Ø
      - with remission F1Ø.21
    - bromide — *see* Dependence, drug, sedative
    - carbamate F19.2Ø
    - chloride F19.2Ø
    - morphine — *see* Dependence, drug, opioid
  - ganja — *see* Dependence, drug, cannabis
  - glue (airplane) (sniffing) — *see* Dependence, drug, inhalant
  - glutethimide — *see* Dependence, drug, sedative
  - hallucinogenics — *see* Dependence, drug, hallucinogen
  - hashish — *see* Dependence, drug, cannabis
  - hemp — *see* Dependence, drug, cannabis
  - heroin (salt) (any) — *see* Dependence, drug, opioid
  - hypnotic NEC — *see* Dependence, drug, sedative
  - Indian hemp — *see* Dependence, drug, cannabis
  - inhalants — *see* Dependence, drug, inhalant
  - khat — *see* Dependence, drug, stimulant NEC
  - laudanum — *see* Dependence, drug, opioid
  - LSD (-25) (derivatives) — *see* Dependence, drug, hallucinogen
  - luminal — *see* Dependence, drug, sedative
  - lysergic acid — *see* Dependence, drug, hallucinogen
  - maconha — *see* Dependence, drug, cannabis
  - marihuana — *see* Dependence, drug, cannabis
  - meprobamate — *see* Dependence, drug, sedative
  - mescaline — *see* Dependence, drug, hallucinogen
  - methadone — *see* Dependence, drug, opioid
  - methamphetamine(s) — *see* Dependence, drug, stimulant NEC
  - methaqualone — *see* Dependence, drug, sedative
  - methyl
    - alcohol (without remission) F1Ø.2Ø
      - with remission F1Ø.21
    - bromide — *see* Dependence, drug, sedative
    - morphine — *see* Dependence, drug, opioid
    - phenidate — *see* Dependence, drug, stimulant NEC
    - sulfonal — *see* Dependence, drug, sedative
  - morphine (sulfate) (sulfite) (type) — *see* Dependence, drug, opioid
  - narcotic (drug) NEC — *see* Dependence, drug, opioid
  - nembutal — *see* Dependence, drug, sedative
  - neraval — *see* Dependence, drug, sedative
  - neravan — *see* Dependence, drug, sedative
  - neurobarb — *see* Dependence, drug, sedative
  - nicotine — *see* Dependence, drug, nicotine
  - nitrous oxide F19.2Ø
  - nonbarbiturate sedatives and tranquilizers with similar effect — *see* Dependence, drug, sedative
  - on
    - artificial heart (fully implantable) (mechanical) Z95.812
    - aspirator Z99.Ø
    - care provider (because of) Z74.9
      - impaired mobility Z74.Ø9
      - need for
        - assistance with personal care Z74.1
        - continuous supervision Z74.3
      - no other household member able to render care Z74.2

- **Dependence** — *continued*
  - on — *continued*
    - care provider — *continued*
      - specified reason NEC Z74.8
    - machine Z99.89
      - enabling NEC Z99.89
      - specified type NEC Z99.89
    - renal dialysis (hemodialysis) (peritoneal) Z99.2
    - respirator Z99.11
    - ventilator Z99.11
    - wheelchair Z99.3
  - opiate — *see* Dependence, drug, opioid
  - opioids — *see* Dependence, drug, opioid
  - opium (alkaloids) (derivatives) (tincture) — *see* Dependence, drug, opioid
  - oxygen (long-term) (supplemental) Z99.81
  - paraldehyde — *see* Dependence, drug, sedative
  - paregoric — *see* Dependence, drug, opioid
  - PCP (phencyclidine) (or related substance) — *see* Dependence, drug, hallucinogen
  - pentobarbital — *see* Dependence, drug, sedative
  - pentobarbitone (sodium) — *see* Dependence, drug, sedative
  - pentothal — *see* Dependence, drug, sedative
  - peyote — *see* Dependence, drug, hallucinogen
  - phencyclidine (PCP) (or related substance) — *see* Dependence, drug, hallucinogen
  - phenmetrazine — *see* Dependence, drug, stimulant NEC
  - phenobarbital — *see* Dependence, drug, sedative
  - polysubstance F19.2Ø
  - psilocibin, psilocin, psilocyn, psilocyline — *see* Dependence, drug, hallucinogen
  - psychostimulant NEC — *see* Dependence, drug, stimulant NEC
  - secobarbital — *see* Dependence, drug, sedative
  - seconal — *see* Dependence, drug, sedative
  - sedative NEC — *see* Dependence, drug, sedative
  - specified drug NEC — *see* Dependence, drug
  - stimulant NEC — *see* Dependence, drug, stimulant NEC
  - substance NEC — *see* Dependence, drug
  - supplemental oxygen Z99.81
  - tobacco — *see* Dependence, drug, nicotine
    - counseling and surveillance Z71.6
  - tranquilizer NEC — *see* Dependence, drug, sedative
  - vitamin B6 E53.1
  - volatile solvents — *see* Dependence, drug, inhalant
- **Dependency**
  - care-provider Z74.9
  - passive F6Ø.7
  - reactions (persistent) F6Ø.7
- **Depersonalization** (in neurotic state) (neurotic) (syndrome) F48.1
- **Depletion**
  - extracellular fluid E86.9
  - plasma E86.1
  - potassium E87.6
    - nephropathy N25.89
  - salt or sodium E87.1
    - causing heat exhaustion or prostration T67.4- ☑
    - nephropathy N28.9
  - volume NOS E86.9
- **Deployment** (current) (military) status Z56.82
  - in theater or in support of military war, peacekeeping and humanitarian operations Z56.82
  - personal history of Z91.82
    - military war, peacekeeping and humanitarian deployment (current or past conflict) Z91.82
  - returned from Z91.82
- **Depolarization, premature** I49.4Ø
  - atrial I49.1
  - junctional I49.2
  - specified NEC I49.49
  - ventricular I49.3
- **Deposit**
  - bone in Boeck's sarcoid D86.89
  - calcareous, calcium — *see* Calcification
  - cholesterol
    - retina H35.89
    - vitreous (body) (humor) — *see* Deposit, crystalline
  - conjunctiva H11.11- ☑
  - cornea H18.ØØ- ☑
    - argentous H18.Ø2- ☑
    - due to metabolic disorder H18.Ø3- ☑
    - Kayser-Fleischer ring H18.Ø4- ☑
    - pigmentation — *see* Pigmentation, cornea
  - crystalline, vitreous (body) (humor) H43.2- ☑
  - hemosiderin in old scars of cornea — *see* Pigmentation, cornea, stromal

Index

Dermatitis — Dermatitis

**Diabetes, diabetic** — *continued*
- type 2 — *continued*
  - with — *continued*
    - ophthalmic complication NEC E11.39
    - oral complication NEC E11.638
    - osteomyelitis E11.69
    - periodontal disease E11.63Ø
    - peripheral angiopathy E11.51
      - with gangrene E11.52
    - polyneuropathy E11.42
    - renal complication NEC E11.29
    - renal tubular degeneration E11.29
    - retinal, hemorrhage E11.39
    - retinopathy E11.319
      - with macular edema E11.311
      - resolved following treatment E11.37- ☑
      - nonproliferative E11.329- ☑
        - with macular edema E11.321- ☑
        - mild E11.329- ☑
          - with macular edema E11.321- ☑
        - moderate E11.339- ☑
          - with macular edema E11.331- ☑
        - severe E11.349- ☑
          - with macular edema E11.341- ☑
      - proliferative E11.359- ☑
        - with
          - combined traction retinal detachment and rhegmatogenous retinal detachment E11.354- ☑
          - macular edema E11.351- ☑
          - stable proliferative diabetic retinopathy E11.355- ☑
          - traction retinal detachment involving the macula E11.352- ☑
          - traction retinal detachment not involving the macula E11.353- ☑
    - skin complication NEC E11.628
    - skin ulcer NEC E11.622
  - without complications in remission E11.A
- uncontrolled
  - meaning
    - hyperglycemia — *see* Diabetes, by type, with, hyperglycemia
    - hypoglycemia — *see* Diabetes, by type, with, hypoglycemia
- without complications in remission E11.A

**Diacyclothrombopathia** D69.19

**Diagnosis deferred** R69

**Dialysis** (intermittent) (treatment)
- noncompliance (with) Z91.158
  - due to financial hardship Z91.151
- renal (hemodialysis) (peritoneal), status Z99.2
- retina, retinal — *see* Detachment, retina, with retinal, dialysis

**Diamond-Blackfan anemia** (congenital hypoplastic) D61.Ø1

**Diamond-Gardener syndrome** (autoerythrocyte sensitization) D69.2

**Diaper rash** L22

**Diaphoresis** (excessive) R61

**Diaphragm** — *see* condition

**Diaphragmalgia** RØ7.1

**Diaphragmatitis, diaphragmitis** J98.6

**Diaphysial aclasis** Q78.6

**Diaphysitis** — *see* Osteomyelitis, specified type NEC

**Diarrhea, diarrheal** (disease) (infantile) (inflammatory) R19.7
- with
  - melena K92.1
- achlorhydric K31.83
- allergic K52.29
  - due to
    - colitis — *see* Colitis, allergic
    - enteritis — *see* Enteritis, allergic
- amebic — *see also* Amebiasis AØ6.Ø
  - with abscess — *see* Abscess, amebic
  - acute AØ6.Ø
  - chronic AØ6.1
  - nondysenteric AØ6.2
- bacillary — *see* Dysentery, bacillary
- balantidial AØ7.Ø
- cachectic NEC K52.89
- Chilomastix AØ7.8
- choleriformis AØØ.1
- chronic (noninfectious) K52.9
- coccidial AØ7.3
- Cochin-China K9Ø.1
  - strongyloidiasis B78.Ø
- Dientamoeba AØ7.8

**Diarrhea, diarrheal** — *continued*
- dietetic — *see also* Diarrhea, allergic K52.29
- drug-induced K52.1
- due to
  - bacteria AØ4.9
    - specified NEC AØ4.8
  - Campylobacter AØ4.5
  - Capillaria philippinensis B81.1
  - Clostridium difficile
    - not specified as recurrent AØ4.72
    - recurrent AØ4.71
  - Clostridium perfringens (C) (F) AØ4.8
  - Cryptosporidium AØ7.2
  - drugs K52.1
  - Escherichia coli AØ4.4
    - enteroaggregative AØ4.4
    - enterohemorrhagic AØ4.3
    - enteroinvasive AØ4.2
    - enteropathogenic AØ4.Ø
    - enterotoxigenic AØ4.1
    - specified NEC AØ4.4
  - food hypersensitivity — *see also* Diarrhea, allergic K52.29
  - Necator americanus B76.1
  - S. japonicum B65.2
  - specified organism NEC AØ8.8
    - bacterial AØ4.8
    - viral AØ8.39
  - Staphylococcus AØ4.8
  - Trichuris trichiuria B79
  - virus — *see* Enteritis, viral
  - Yersinia enterocolitica AØ4.6
- dysenteric AØ9
- endemic AØ9
- epidemic AØ9
- flagellate AØ7.9
- Flexner's (ulcerative) AØ3.1
- functional K59.1
  - following gastrointestinal surgery K91.89
  - psychogenic F45.8
- Giardia lamblia AØ7.1
- giardial AØ7.1
- hill K9Ø.1
- infectious AØ9
- malarial — *see* Malaria
- mite B88.Ø9
- mycotic NEC B49
- neonatal (noninfectious) P78.3
- nervous F45.8
- neurogenic K59.1
- noninfectious K52.9
- postgastrectomy K91.1
- postvagotomy K91.1
- protozoal AØ7.9
  - specified NEC AØ7.8
- psychogenic F45.8
- specified
  - bacterium NEC AØ4.8
  - virus NEC AØ8.39
- strongyloidiasis B78.Ø
- toxic K52.1
- trichomonal AØ7.8
- tropical K9Ø.1
- tuberculous A18.32
- viral — *see* Enteritis, viral

**Diastasis**
- cranial bones M84.88
  - congenital NEC Q75.8
- joint (traumatic) — *see* Dislocation
- muscle M62.ØØ
  - ankle M62.Ø7- ☑
  - congenital Q79.8
  - foot M62.Ø7- ☑
  - forearm M62.Ø3- ☑
  - hand M62.Ø4- ☑
  - lower leg M62.Ø6- ☑
  - pelvic region M62.Ø5- ☑
  - shoulder region M62.Ø1- ☑
  - specified site NEC M62.Ø8
  - thigh M62.Ø5- ☑
  - upper arm M62.Ø2- ☑
- recti (abdomen)
  - complicating delivery O71.89
  - congenital Q79.59

**Diastema, tooth, teeth, fully erupted** M26.32

**Diastematomyelia** QØ6.2

**Diataxia, cerebral** G8Ø.4

**Diathesis**
- allergic — *see* History, allergy
- bleeding (familial) D69.9
- cystine (familial) E72.ØØ
- gouty — *see* Gout
- hemorrhagic (familial) D69.9
  - newborn NEC P53
- spasmophilic R29.Ø

**Diaz's disease or osteochondrosis** (juvenile) (talus) — *see* Osteochondrosis, juvenile, tarsus

**Dibothriocephalus, dibothriocephaliasis** (latus) (infection) (infestation) B7Ø.Ø
- larval B7Ø.1

**Dicephalus, dicephaly** Q89.4

**Dichotomy, teeth** KØØ.2

**Dichromat, dichromatopsia** (congenital) — *see* Deficiency, color vision

**Dichuchwa** A65

**Dicroceliasis** B66.2

**Didelphia, didelphys** — *see* Double uterus

**Didymytis** N45.1
- with orchitis N45.3

**Dietary**
- inadequacy or deficiency E63.9
- surveillance and counseling Z71.3

**Dietl's crisis** N13.8

**Dieulafoy lesion** (hemorrhagic)
- duodenum K31.82
- esophagus K22.89
- intestine (colon) K63.81
- stomach K31.82

**Difficult, difficulty** (in)
- acculturation Z6Ø.3
- feeding R63.3Ø
  - elderly R63.39
  - infant NOS R63.39
  - newborn P92.9
    - breast P92.5
    - specified NEC P92.8
  - nonorganic (infant or child) F98.29
  - specified NEC R63.39
- intubation, in anesthesia T88.4- ☑
- mechanical, gastroduodenal stoma K91.89
  - causing obstruction — *see also* Obstruction, intestine, postoperative K91.3Ø
- micturition
  - need to immediately re-void R39.191
  - position dependent R39.192
  - specified NEC R39.198
- reading (developmental) F81.Ø
  - secondary to emotional disorders F93.9
- spelling (specific) F81.81
  - with reading disorder F81.89
  - due to inadequate teaching Z55.8
- swallowing — *see* Dysphagia
- understanding
  - health related information Z55.6
  - medication instructions Z55.6
- walking R26.2
- work
  - conditions NEC Z56.5
  - schedule Z56.3

**Diffuse** — *see* condition

**Digestive** — *see* condition

**Dihydropyrimidine dehydrogenase disease** (DPD) E88.89

**Diktyoma** — *see* Neoplasm, malignant, by site

**Dilaceration, tooth** KØØ.4

**Dilatation**
- anus K59.89
  - venule — *see* Hemorrhoids
- aorta (focal) (general) — *see* Ectasia, aorta
  - with aneurysm — *see* Aneurysm, aorta
  - congenital Q25.44
- artery — *see* Aneurysm
- bladder (sphincter) N32.89
  - congenital Q64.79
- blood vessel I99.8
- bronchial J47.9
  - with
    - exacerbation (acute) J47.1
    - lower respiratory infection J47.Ø
- calyx N28.89
  - due to obstruction — *see* Hydronephrosis
- capillaries I78.8
- cardiac (acute) (chronic) — *see also* Hypertrophy, cardiac
  - congenital Q24.8
    - valve NEC Q24.8
      - pulmonary Q22.3
  - valve — *see* Endocarditis

**Dilatation** — *continued*
- cavum septi pellucidi QØ6.8
- cervix (uteri) — *see also* Incompetency, cervix
  - incomplete, poor, slow complicating delivery O62.Ø
- colon K59.39
  - congenital Q43.1
  - psychogenic F45.8
  - toxic K59.31
- common duct (acquired) K83.8
  - congenital Q44.5
- cystic duct (acquired) K82.8
  - congenital Q44.5
- duct, mammary — *see* Ectasia, mammary duct
- duodenum K59.89
- esophagus K22.89
  - congenital Q39.5
  - due to achalasia K22.Ø
- eustachian tube, congenital Q17.8
- gallbladder K82.8
- gastric — *see* Dilatation, stomach
- heart (acute) (chronic) — *see also* Hypertrophy, cardiac
  - congenital Q24.8
  - valve — *see* Endocarditis
- ileum K59.89
  - psychogenic F45.8
- jejunum K59.89
  - psychogenic F45.8
- kidney (calyx) (collecting structures) (cystic) (parenchyma) (pelvis) (idiopathic) N28.89
  - due to obstruction — *see* Hydronephrosis
- lacrimal passages or duct — *see* Disorder, lacrimal system, changes
- lymphatic vessel I89.Ø
- mammary duct — *see* Ectasia, mammary duct
- Meckel's diverticulum (congenital) Q43.Ø
  - malignant — *see* Table of Neoplasms, small intestine, malignant
- myocardium (acute) (chronic) — *see* Hypertrophy, cardiac
- organ or site, congenital NEC — *see* Distortion
- pancreatic duct K86.89
- pericardium — *see* Pericarditis
- pharynx J39.2
- prostate N42.89
- pulmonary
  - artery (idiopathic) I28.8
  - valve, congenital Q22.3
- pupil H57.Ø4
- rectum K59.39
- saccule, congenital Q16.5
- salivary gland (duct) K11.8
- sphincter ani K62.89
- stomach K31.89
  - acute K31.Ø
  - psychogenic F45.8
- submaxillary duct K11.8
- trachea, congenital Q32.1
- ureter (idiopathic) N28.82
  - congenital Q62.2
  - due to obstruction N13.4
- urethra (acquired) N36.8
- vasomotor I73.9
- vein I86.8
- ventricular, ventricle (acute) (chronic) — *see also* Hypertrophy, cardiac
  - cerebral, congenital QØ4.8
- venule NEC I86.8
- vesical orifice N32.89

**Dilated, dilation** — *see* Dilatation

**Diminished, diminution**
- hearing (acuity) — *see* Deafness
- sense or sensation (cold) (heat) (tactile) (vibratory) R2Ø.8
- vision NEC H54.7
- vital capacity R94.2

**Diminuta taenia** B71.Ø

**Dimitri-Sturge-Weber disease** Q85.89

**Dimple**
- congenital sacral Q82.6
- parasacral Q82.6
- pilonidal or postanal — *see* Cyst, pilonidal

**Dioctophyme renalis** (infection) (infestation) B83.8

**Dipetalonemiasis** B74.4

**Diphallus** Q55.69

**Diphtheria, diphtheritic** (gangrenous) (hemorrhagic) A36.9
- carrier (suspected) Z22.2
- cutaneous A36.3
- faucial A36.Ø
- infection of wound A36.3
- laryngeal A36.2
- myocarditis A36.81

**Diphtheria, diphtheritic** — *continued*
- nasal, anterior A36.89
- nasopharyngeal A36.1
- neurological complication A36.89
- pharyngeal A36.Ø
- specified site NEC A36.89
- tonsillar A36.Ø

**Diphyllobothriasis** (intestine) B7Ø.Ø
- larval B7Ø.1

**Diplacusis** H93.22- ☑

**Diplegia** (upper limbs) G83.Ø
- congenital (cerebral) G8Ø.8
- facial G51.Ø
- lower limbs G82.2Ø
- spastic G8Ø.1

**Diplococcus, diplococcal** — *see* condition

**Diplopia** H53.2

**Dipsomania** F1Ø.2Ø
- with
  - psychosis — *see* Psychosis, alcoholic
  - remission F1Ø.21

**Dipylidiasis** B71.1

**DIRA** (deficiency of interleukin 1 receptor antagonist) MØ4.8

**Direction, teeth, abnormal, fully erupted** M26.3Ø

**Dirofilariasis** B74.8

**Dirt-eating child** F98.3

**Disability, disabilities**
- heart — *see* Disease, heart
- intellectual F79
  - with
    - autistic features F84.9
    - pathogenic CHAMP1 (genetic) (variant) F78.A9
    - pathogenic HNRNPH2 (genetic) (variant) F78.A9
    - pathogenic SATB2 (genetic) (variant) F78.A9
    - pathogenic SETBP1 (genetic) (variant) F78.A9
    - pathogenic STXBP1 (genetic) (variant) F78.A9
    - pathogenic SYNGAP1 (genetic) (variant) F78.A1
  - autosomal dominant F78.A9
  - autosomal recessive F78.A9
  - genetic related F78.A9
    - with
      - pathogenic CHAMP1 (variant) F78.A9
      - pathogenic HNRNPH2 (variant) F78.A9
      - pathogenic SATB2 (variant) F78.A9
      - pathogenic SETBP1 (variant) F78.A9
      - pathogenic STXBP1 (variant) F78.A9
      - pathogenic SYNGAP1 (variant) F78.A1
    - specified NEC F78.A9
    - SYNGAP1-related F78.A1
  - in
    - autosomal dominant mental retardation F78.A9
    - autosomal recessive mental retardation F78.A9
    - SATB2-associated syndrome F78.A9
    - SETBP1 disorder F78.A9
    - STXBP1 encephalopathy with epilepsy — *see also* Encephalopathy; and — *see also* Epilepsy
    - X-linked mental retardation (syndromic) (Bain type) F78.A9
  - mild (I.Q. 5Ø-69) F7Ø
  - moderate (I.Q. 35-49) F71
  - profound (I.Q. under 2Ø) F73
  - severe (I.Q. 2Ø-34) F72
  - specified level NEC F78.A9
  - SYNGAP1-related F78.A1
  - X-linked (syndromic) (Bain type) F78.A9
- knowledge acquisition F81.9
- learning F81.9
- limiting activities Z73.6
- spelling, specific F81.81

**Disappearance of family member** Z63.4

**Disarticulation** — *see* Amputation
- meaning traumatic amputation — *see* Amputation, traumatic

**Discharge** (from)
- abnormal finding in — *see* Abnormal, specimen
- breast (female) (male) N64.52
- diencephalic autonomic idiopathic — *see* Epilepsy, specified NEC
- ear — *see also* Otorrhea
  - blood — *see* Otorrhagia
- excessive urine R35.89
- nipple N64.52
- penile R36.9
- postnasal RØ9.82
- prison, anxiety concerning Z65.2
- urethral R36.9
  - without blood R36.Ø
  - hematospermia R36.1
- vaginal N89.8

**Discitis, diskitis** M46.4Ø
- cervical region M46.42
- cervicothoracic region M46.43
- lumbar region M46.46
- lumbosacral region M46.47
- multiple sites M46.49
- occipito-atlanto-axial region M46.41
- pyogenic — *see* Infection, intervertebral disc, pyogenic
- sacrococcygeal region M46.48
- thoracic region M46.44
- thoracolumbar region M46.45

**Discoid**
- meniscus (congenital) Q68.6
- semilunar cartilage (congenital) — *see* Derangement, knee, meniscus, specified NEC

**Discoloration**
- nails L6Ø.8
- teeth (posteruptive) KØ3.7
  - during formation KØØ.8

**Discomfort**
- chest RØ7.89
- visual H53.14- ☑

**Discontinuity, ossicles, ear** H74.2- ☑

**Discord** (with)
- boss Z56.4
- classmates Z55.4
- counselor Z64.4
- employer Z56.4
- family Z63.8
- fellow employees Z56.4
- in-laws Z63.1
- landlord Z59.2
- lodgers Z59.2
- neighbors Z59.2
- probation officer Z64.4
- social worker Z64.4
- teachers Z55.4
- workmates Z56.4

**Discordant connection**
- atrioventricular (congenital) Q2Ø.5
- ventriculoarterial Q2Ø.3

**Discrepancy**
- centric occlusion maximum intercuspation M26.55
- leg length (acquired) — *see* Deformity, limb, unequal length
  - congenital — *see* Defect, reduction, lower limb
- uterine size date O26.84- ☑

**Discrimination**
- ethnic Z6Ø.5
- political Z6Ø.5
- racial Z6Ø.5
- religious Z6Ø.5
- sex Z6Ø.5

**Disease, diseased** — *see also* Syndrome
- absorbent system I87.8
- acid-peptic K3Ø
- Acosta's T7Ø.29- ☑
- Adams-Stokes (-Morgagni) (syncope with heart block) I45.9
- Addison's anemia (pernicious) D51.Ø
- adenoids (and tonsils) J35.9
- adrenal (capsule) (cortex) (gland) (medullary) E27.9
  - hyperfunction E27.Ø
  - specified NEC E27.8
- ainhum L94.6
- airway
  - obstructive, chronic J44.9
    - due to
      - cotton dust J66.Ø
      - specific organic dusts NEC J66.8
  - reactive — *see* Asthma
- akamushi (scrub typhus) A75.3
- Albers-Schonberg (marble bones) Q78.2
- Albert's — *see* Tendinitis, Achilles
- Alexander G31.86
- alimentary canal K63.9
- alligator-skin Q8Ø.9
  - acquired L85.Ø
- alpha heavy chain C88.3- ☑
- alpine T7Ø.29- ☑
- altitude T7Ø.2Ø- ☑
- alveolar ridge
  - edentulous KØ6.9
    - specified NEC KØ6.8
- alveoli, teeth KØ8.9
- Alzheimer's — *see also* Dementia, in, diseases specified elsewhere G3Ø.9 *[FØ2.8Ø]*

**Disease, diseased** — *continued*
- high fetal gene or hemoglobin thalassemia D56.9
- Hildenbrand's — *see* Typhus
- hip (joint) M25.9
  - congenital Q65.89
  - suppurative MØØ.9
  - tuberculous A18.Ø2
- His (-Werner) (trench fever) A79.Ø
- Hodgson's — *see also* Aneurysm, aorta, thorax I71.2Ø
  - ruptured — *see also* Aneurysm, aorta, thorax, ruptured I71.1Ø
- Holla — *see* Spherocytosis
- hookworm B76.9
  - specified NEC B76.8
- host-versus-graft D89.813
  - acute D89.81Ø
  - acute on chronic D89.812
  - chronic D89.811
- human immunodeficiency virus (HIV) B2Ø
- Huntington's G1Ø
  - with dementia — *see also* Dementia, in, diseases specified elsewhere G1Ø *[FØ2.8Ø]*
- Hunt's (herpetic geniculate ganglionitis) (neuralgia) BØ2.21
  - dyssynergia cerebellaris myoclonica G11.19
- Hutchinson's (cheiropompholyx) — *see* Hutchinson's disease
- hyaline (diffuse) (generalized)
  - membrane (lung) (newborn) P22.Ø
    - adult J8Ø
- hydatid — *see* Echinococcus
- hydroxyapatite deposition M11.ØØ
  - ankle M11.Ø7- ☑
  - elbow M11.Ø2- ☑
  - foot joint M11.Ø7- ☑
  - hand joint M11.Ø4- ☑
  - hip M11.Ø5- ☑
  - knee M11.Ø6- ☑
  - multiple site M11.Ø9
  - shoulder M11.Ø1- ☑
  - vertebra M11.Ø8
  - wrist M11.Ø3- ☑
- hyperkinetic — *see* Hyperkinesia
- hypertensive — *see* Hypertension
- hypophysis E23.7
- I-cell E77.Ø
- Iceland G93.39
- IgG4-related D89.84
- immune D89.9
- immunoglobulin G4-related D89.84
- immunoproliferative (malignant) C88.9- ☑
  - small intestinal C88.3- ☑
  - specified NEC C88.8- ☑
- inclusion B25.9
  - salivary gland B25.9
- infectious, infective B99.9
  - congenital P37.9
    - specified NEC P37.8
    - viral P35.9
      - specified type NEC P35.8
  - specified NEC B99.8
- inflammatory
  - penis N48.29
    - abscess N48.21
    - cellulitis N48.22
  - prepuce N47.7
    - balanoposthitis N47.6
  - tubo-ovarian — *see* Salpingo-oophoritis
- intervertebral disc — *see also* Disorder, disc
  - with myelopathy — *see* Disorder, disc, with, myelopathy
  - cervical, cervicothoracic — *see* Disorder, disc, cervical
    - with
      - myelopathy — *see* Disorder, disc, cervical, with myelopathy
      - neuritis, radiculitis or radiculopathy — *see* Disorder, disc, cervical, with neuritis
      - specified NEC — *see* Disorder, disc, cervical, specified type NEC
  - lumbar (with)
    - myelopathy M51.Ø6
    - neuritis, radiculitis, radiculopathy or sciatica M51.16
    - specified NEC M51.86
  - lumbosacral (with)
    - neuritis, radiculitis, radiculopathy or sciatica M51.17
    - specified NEC M51.87

**Disease, diseased** — *continued*
- intervertebral disc — *see also* Disorder, disc — *continued*
  - specified NEC — *see* Disorder, disc, specified NEC
  - thoracic (with)
    - myelopathy M51.Ø4
    - neuritis, radiculitis or radiculopathy M51.14
    - specified NEC M51.84
  - thoracolumbar (with)
    - myelopathy M51.Ø5
    - neuritis, radiculitis or radiculopathy M51.15
    - specified NEC M51.85
- intestine K63.9
  - functional K59.9
    - psychogenic F45.8
    - specified NEC K59.89
  - organic K63.9
  - protozoal AØ7.9
  - specified NEC K63.89
- iris H21.9
  - specified NEC H21.89
- iron metabolism or storage E83.1Ø
- island (scrub typhus) A75.3
- itai-itai — *see* Poisoning, cadmium
- Jakob-Creutzfeldt — *see* Creutzfeldt-Jakob disease or syndrome
- jaw M27.9
  - fibrocystic M27.49
  - specified NEC M27.8
- jigger B88.1
- joint — *see also* Disorder, joint
  - Charcot's — *see* Arthropathy, neuropathic (Charcot)
  - degenerative — *see* Osteoarthritis
    - multiple M15.9
    - spine — *see* Spondylosis
  - facet joint — *see also* Spondylosis M47.819
  - hypertrophic — *see* Osteoarthritis
  - sacroiliac M53.3
  - specified NEC — *see* Disorder, joint, specified type NEC
  - spine NEC — *see* Dorsopathy
  - suppurative — *see* Arthritis, pyogenic or pyemic
- Jourdain's (acute gingivitis) KØ5.ØØ
  - nonplaque induced KØ5.Ø1
  - plaque induced KØ5.ØØ
- Kaschin-Beck (endemic polyarthritis) M12.1Ø
  - ankle M12.17- ☑
  - elbow M12.12- ☑
  - foot joint M12.17- ☑
  - hand joint M12.14- ☑
  - hip M12.15- ☑
  - knee M12.16- ☑
  - multiple site M12.19
  - shoulder M12.11- ☑
  - vertebra M12.18
  - wrist M12.13- ☑
- Katayama B65.2
- Kedani (scrub typhus) A75.3
- Keshan E59
- kidney (functional) (pelvis) N28.9
  - chronic N18.9
    - hypertensive — *see* Hypertension, kidney
    - stage 1 N18.1
    - stage 2 (mild) N18.2
    - stage 3 (moderate) N18.3Ø
    - stage 3a N18.31
    - stage 3b N18.32
    - stage 4 (severe) N18.4
    - stage 5 N18.5
  - complicating pregnancy — *see* Pregnancy, complicated by, renal disease
  - cystic (congenital) Q61.9
  - fibrocystic (congenital) Q61.8
  - hypertensive — *see* Hypertension, kidney
  - in (due to)
    - schistosomiasis (bilharziasis) B65.9 *[N29]*
  - multicystic Q61.4
  - polycystic Q61.3
    - adult type Q61.2
    - childhood type NEC Q61.19
      - collecting duct dilatation Q61.11
- Kimmelstiel (-Wilson) (intercapillary polycystic (congenital) glomerulosclerosis) — *see* EØ8-E13 with .21
- Kinnier Wilson's (hepatolenticular degeneration) E83.Ø1
- kissing — *see* Mononucleosis, infectious
- Klebs' — *see also* Glomerulonephritis NØ5.- ☑
- Klippel-Feil (brevicollis) Q76.1

**Disease, diseased** — *continued*
- Kohler-Pellegrini-Stieda (calcification, knee joint) — *see* Bursitis, tibial collateral
- Kok Q89.89
- Konig's (osteochondritis dissecans) — *see* Osteochondritis, dissecans
- Korsakoff's (nonalcoholic) FØ4
  - alcoholic F1Ø.96
    - with dependence F1Ø.26
- Kostmann's (infantile genetic agranulocytosis) D7Ø.Ø
- kuru A81.81
- Kyasanur Forest A98.2
- labyrinth, ear — *see* Disorder, ear, inner
- lacrimal system — *see* Disorder, lacrimal system
- Lafora body — *see also* Epilepsy, progressive, Lafora G4Ø.CØ9
- Lancereaux-Mathieu (leptospiral jaundice) A27.Ø
- Landry's G61.Ø
- Larrey-Weil (leptospiral jaundice) A27.Ø
- larynx J38.7
- Ledderhose M72.2- ☑
- legionnaires' A48.1
  - nonpneumonic A48.2
- Lenegre's I44.2
- lens H27.9
  - specified NEC H27.8
- Lev's (acquired complete heart block) I44.2
- Lewy body (dementia) — *see also* Dementia, in, diseases specified elsewhere G31.83 *[FØ2.8Ø]*
  - with behavioral disturbance — *see also* Dementia, in, diseases specified elsewhere G31.83 *[FØ2.81-]* ☑
- Lichtheim's (subacute combined sclerosis with pernicious anemia) D51.Ø
- Lightwood's (renal tubular acidosis) N25.89
- Lignac's (cystinosis) E72.Ø4
- lip K13.Ø
- lipid-storage E75.6
  - specified NEC E75.5
- Lipschutz's N76.6
- liver (chronic) (organic) K76.9
  - alcoholic (chronic) K7Ø.9
    - acute — *see* Disease, liver, alcoholic, hepatitis
    - cirrhosis K7Ø.3Ø
      - with ascites K7Ø.31
    - failure K7Ø.4Ø
      - with coma K7Ø.41
    - fatty liver K7Ø.Ø
    - fibrosis K7Ø.2
    - hepatitis K7Ø.1Ø
      - with ascites K7Ø.11
    - sclerosis K7Ø.2
  - cystic, congenital Q44.6
  - drug-induced (idiosyncratic) (toxic) (predictable) (unpredictable) — *see* Disease, liver, toxic
  - end stage K72.1- ☑
    - due to hepatitis — *see* Hepatitis
    - with coma K72.11
  - fatty, nonalcoholic (NAFLD) K76.Ø
    - alcoholic K7Ø.Ø
  - fibrocystic (congenital) Q44.6
  - fluke
    - Chinese B66.1
    - oriental B66.1
    - sheep B66.3
  - Fontan-associated (FALD) I27.84Ø
  - gestational alloimmune (GALD) P78.84
  - glycogen storage E74.Ø9 *[K77]*
  - in (due to)
    - schistosomiasis (bilharziasis) B65.9 *[K77]*
  - inflammatory K75.9
    - alcoholic K7Ø.1- ☑
    - specified NEC K75.89
  - intestinal failure-associated (IFALD) K76.83
  - metabolic dysfunction-associated steatotic (MASLD) K76.Ø
  - polycystic (congenital) Q44.6
  - toxic K71.9
    - with
      - cholestasis K71.Ø
      - cirrhosis (liver) K71.7
      - fibrosis (liver) K71.7
      - focal nodular hyperplasia K71.8
      - hepatic granuloma K71.8
      - hepatic necrosis K71.1Ø
        - with coma K71.11
      - hepatitis NEC K71.6
        - acute K71.2

**Disease, diseased** — *continued*
- parodontal K05.6
- Parrot's (syphilitic osteochondritis) A50.02
- Parry's (exophthalmic goiter) — *see* Hyperthyroidism, with, goiter (diffuse)
- Parson's (exophthalmic goiter) — *see* Hyperthyroidism, with, goiter (diffuse)
- Paxton's (white piedra) B36.2
- pearl-worker's — *see* Osteomyelitis, specified type NEC
- Pellegrini-Stieda (calcification, knee joint) — *see* Bursitis, tibial collateral
- pelvis, pelvic K6A.8
  - female NOS N94.9
    - specified NEC N94.89
  - gonococcal (acute) (chronic) A54.24
  - inflammatory (female) N73.9
    - acute N73.0
    - chlamydial A56.11
    - chronic N73.1
    - specified NEC N73.8
    - syphilitic (secondary) A51.42
      - late A52.76
    - tuberculous A18.17
  - male K6A.8
  - organ, female N94.9
  - peritoneum, female NEC N94.89
- penis N48.9
  - inflammatory N48.29
    - abscess N48.21
    - cellulitis N48.22
  - specified NEC N48.89
- periapical tissues NOS K04.90
- periodontal K05.6
  - specified NEC K05.5
- periosteum — *see* Disorder, bone, specified type NEC
- peripheral
  - arterial I73.9
  - autonomic nervous system G90.9
  - nerves — *see* Polyneuropathy
  - vascular NOS I73.9
    - in diabetes mellitus — *see* Diabetes, by type, with peripheral angiopathy
- peritoneum K66.9
  - pelvic, female NEC N94.89
  - specified NEC K66.8
- persistent mucosal (middle ear) H66.20
  - left H66.22
    - with right H66.23
  - right H66.21
    - with left H66.23
- Petit's — *see* Hernia, abdomen, specified site NEC
- pharynx J39.2
  - specified NEC J39.2
- Phocas' — *see* Mastopathy, cystic
- photochromogenic (acid-fast bacilli) (pulmonary) A31.0
  - nonpulmonary A31.9
- Pick's — *see also* Dementia, in, diseases specified elsewhere G31.01 *[F02.80]*
  - with behavioral disturbance — *see also* Dementia, in, diseases specified elsewhere G31.01 *[F02.81-]* ☑
  - brain G31.01 *[F02.80]*
    - with behavioral disturbance — *see also* Dementia, in, diseases specified elsewhere G31.01 *[F02.81-]* ☑
  - of pericardium (pericardial pseudocirrhosis of liver) I31.1
- pigeon fancier's J67.2
- pineal gland E34.8
- pink — *see* Poisoning, mercury
- Pinkus' (lichen nitidus) L44.1
- pinworm B80
- Piry virus A93.8
- pituitary (gland) E23.7
- pituitary-snuff-taker's J67.8
- pleura (cavity) J94.9
  - specified NEC J94.8
- pneumatic drill (hammer) T75.21- ☑
- Pollitzer's (hidradenitis suppurativa) L73.2
- polycystic
  - kidney or renal Q61.3
    - adult type Q61.2
    - childhood type NEC Q61.19
      - collecting duct dilatation Q61.11
  - liver or hepatic Q44.6
  - lung or pulmonary J98.4
    - congenital Q33.0
  - ovary, ovaries E28.2
  - spleen Q89.09

**Disease, diseased** — *continued*
- polyethylene T84.05- ☑
- Pompe's (glycogenosis II) E74.02
- Posadas-Wernicke B38.9
- Potain's (pulmonary edema) — *see* Edema, lung
- prepuce N47.8
  - inflammatory N47.7
    - balanoposthitis N47.6
- Pringle's (tuberous sclerosis) Q85.1
- prion, central nervous system A81.9
  - specified NEC A81.89
- prostate N42.9
  - specified NEC N42.89
- protozoal B64
  - acanthamebiasis — *see* Acanthamebiasis
  - African trypanosomiasis — *see* African trypanosomiasis
  - babesiosis — *see also* Babesiosis B60.00
  - Chagas disease — *see* Chagas disease
  - intestine, intestinal A07.9
  - leishmaniasis — *see* Leishmaniasis
  - malaria — *see* Malaria
  - naegleriasis B60.2
  - pneumocystosis B59
  - specified organism NEC B60.8
  - toxoplasmosis — *see* Toxoplasmosis
- pseudo-Hurler's E77.0
- psychiatric F99
- psychotic — *see* Psychosis
- Puente's (simple glandular cheilitis) K13.0
- puerperal — *see also* Puerperal O90.89
- pulmonary — *see also* Disease, lung
  - artery I28.9
  - chronic obstructive J44.9
    - with
      - acute bronchitis J44.0
      - exacerbation (acute) J44.1
      - lower respiratory infection (acute) J44.0
    - decompensated J44.1
      - with
        - exacerbation (acute) J44.1
  - heart I27.9
    - specified NEC I27.89
  - hypertensive (vascular) — *see also* Hypertension, pulmonary I27.20
    - NEC I27.2- ☑
    - primary (idiopathic) I27.0
  - valve I37.9
    - rheumatic I09.89
- pulp (dental) NOS K04.90
- pulseless M31.4
- Putnam's (subacute combined sclerosis with pernicious anemia) D51.0
- Pyle (-Cohn) (metaphyseal dysplasia) Q78.5
- ragpicker's or ragsorter's A22.1
- Raynaud's — *see* Raynaud's disease
- reactive airway — *see* Asthma
- Reclus' (cystic) — *see* Mastopathy, cystic
- rectum K62.9
  - specified NEC K62.89
- Refsum's (heredopathia atactica polyneuritiformis) G60.1
- renal (functional) (pelvis) — *see also* Disease, kidney N28.9
  - with
    - edema — *see* Nephrosis
    - glomerular lesion — *see* Glomerulonephritis
      - with edema — *see* Nephrosis
    - interstitial nephritis N12
  - acute N28.9
  - chronic — *see also* Disease, kidney, chronic N18.9
  - cystic, congenital Q61.9
  - diabetic — *see* E08-E13 with .22
  - end-stage (failure) N18.6
    - due to hypertension I12.0
  - fibrocystic (congenital) Q61.8
  - hypertensive — *see* Hypertension, kidney
  - lupus M32.14
  - phosphate-losing (tubular) N25.0
  - polycystic (congenital) Q61.3
    - adult type Q61.2
    - childhood type NEC Q61.19
      - collecting duct dilatation Q61.11
  - rapidly progressive N01.9
  - subacute N01.9
- Rendu-Osler-Weber (familial hemorrhagic telangiectasia) I78.0
- renovascular (arteriosclerotic) — *see* Hypertension, kidney
- respiratory (tract) J98.9

**Disease, diseased** — *continued*
- respiratory — *continued*
  - acute or subacute NOS J06.9
    - due to
      - chemicals, gases, fumes or vapors (inhalation) J68.3
      - external agent J70.9
        - specified NEC J70.8
      - radiation J70.0
      - smoke inhalation J70.5
    - noninfectious J39.8
  - chronic NOS J98.9
    - due to
      - chemicals, gases, fumes or vapors J68.4
      - external agent J70.9
        - specified NEC J70.8
      - radiation J70.1
    - newborn P27.9
      - specified NEC P27.8
  - due to
    - chemicals, gases, fumes or vapors J68.9
      - acute or subacute NEC J68.3
      - chronic J68.4
    - external agent J70.9
      - specified NEC J70.8
  - newborn P28.9
    - specified type NEC P28.89
  - upper J39.9
    - acute or subacute J06.9
    - noninfectious NEC J39.8
    - specified NEC J39.8
    - streptococcal J06.9
- retina, retinal H35.9
  - Batten's or Batten-Mayou E75.4 *[H36.89]*
  - specified NEC H35.89
- rheumatoid — *see* Arthritis, rheumatoid
- rickettsial NOS A79.9
  - specified type NEC A79.89
- Riga (-Fede) (cachectic aphthae) K14.0
- Riggs' (compound periodontitis) — *see* Periodontitis
- Ritter's L00
- Rivalta's (cervicofacial actinomycosis) A42.2
- Robles' (onchocerciasis) B73.01
- rod body G71.21
- Roger's (congenital interventricular septal defect) Q21.0
- Rosenthal's (factor XI deficiency) D68.1
- Ross River B33.1
- Rossbach's (hyperchlorhydria) K31.89
  - psychogenic F45.8
- Rotes Querol — *see* Hyperostosis, ankylosing
- Roth (-Bernhardt) — *see* Mononeuropathy, lower limb, meralgia paresthetica
- Runeberg's (progressive pernicious anemia) D51.0
- sacroiliac NEC M53.3
- salivary gland or duct K11.9
  - inclusion B25.9
  - specified NEC K11.8
  - virus B25.9
- sandworm B76.9
- Schimmelbusch's — *see* Mastopathy, cystic
- Schmorl's — *see* Schmorl's disease or nodes
- Schonlein (-Henoch) (purpura rheumatica) D69.0
- Schottmuller's — *see* Fever, paratyphoid
- Schultz's (agranulocytosis) — *see* Agranulocytosis
- Schwalbe-Ziehen-Oppenheim G24.1
- Schwartz-Jampel G71.13
- sclera H15.9
  - specified NEC H15.89
- scrofulous (tuberculous) A18.2
- scrotum N50.9
- sebaceous glands L73.9
- semilunar cartilage, cystic — *see also* Derangement, knee, meniscus, cystic
- seminal vesicle N50.9
- serum NEC — *see also* Reaction, serum T80.69- ☑
- sexually transmitted A64
  - anogenital
    - herpesviral infection — *see* Herpes, anogenital
    - warts A63.0
  - chancroid A57
  - chlamydial infection — *see* Chlamydia
  - gonorrhea — *see* Gonorrhea
  - granuloma inguinale A58
  - specified organism NEC A63.8
  - syphilis — *see* Syphilis
  - trichomoniasis — *see* Trichomoniasis
- Sezary C84.1- ☑
- shimamushi (scrub typhus) A75.3
- shipyard B30.0

- **Disease, diseased** — *continued*
  - vas deferens N50.9
  - vascular I99.9
    - arteriosclerotic — *see* Arteriosclerosis
    - ciliary body NEC — *see* Disorder, iris, vascular
    - hypertensive — *see* Hypertension
    - iris NEC — *see* Disorder, iris, vascular
    - obliterative I77.1
      - peripheral I73.9
    - occlusive I99.8
    - peripheral (occlusive) I73.9
      - in diabetes mellitus — *see* E08-E13 with .51
  - vasomotor I73.9
  - vasospastic I73.9
  - vein I87.9
  - venereal — *see also* Disease, sexually transmitted A64
    - chlamydial NEC A56.8
      - anus A56.3
      - genitourinary NOS A56.2
      - pharynx A56.4
      - rectum A56.3
    - fifth A55
    - sixth A55
    - specified nature or type NEC A63.8
  - vertebra, vertebral — *see also* Spondylopathy
    - disc — *see* Disorder, disc
  - vibration — *see* Vibration, adverse effects
  - viral, virus — *see also* Disease, by type of virus B34.9
    - arbovirus NOS A94
    - arthropod-borne NOS A94
    - congenital P35.9
      - specified NEC P35.8
    - Hanta (with renal manifestations) (Dobrava) (Puumala) (Seoul) A98.5
      - with pulmonary manifestations (Andes) (Bayou) (Bermejo) (Black Creek Canal) (Choclo) (Juquitiba) (Laguna negra) (Lechiguanas) (New York) (Oran) (Sin nombre) B33.4
    - Hantaan (Korean hemorrhagic fever) A98.5
    - human immunodeficiency (HIV) B20
    - Kunjin A83.4
    - nonarthropod-borne NOS B34.9
    - Powassan A84.81
    - Rocio (encephalitis) A83.6
    - Sin nombre (Hantavirus) (cardio)-pulmonary syndrome) B33.4
    - Tahyna B33.8
    - vesicular stomatitis A93.8
  - vitreous H43.9
    - specified NEC H43.89
  - vocal cord J38.3
  - Volkmann's, acquired T79.6- ☑
  - von Eulenburg's (congenital paramyotonia) G71.19
  - von Gierke's (glycogenosis I) E74.01
  - von Graefe's — *see* Strabismus, paralytic, ophthalmoplegia, progressive
  - von Willebrand (-Jurgens) (angiohemophilia) D68.00
    - acquired D68.04
    - platelet-type D68.09
    - pseudo D68.09
    - specified NEC D68.09
    - type 1 D68.01
    - type 1C D68.01
    - type 2 D68.029
      - type 2A D68.020
      - type 2B D68.021
      - type 2M D68.022
      - type 2N D68.023
    - type 3 D68.03
  - Vrolik's (osteogenesis imperfecta) Q78.0
  - vulva (noninflammatory) N90.9
    - inflammatory NEC N76.89
    - specified NEC N90.89
  - Wallgren's (obstruction of splenic vein with collateral circulation) I87.8
  - Wassilieff's (leptospiral jaundice) A27.0
  - wasting NEC E88.A
    - due to
      - malnutrition E43
        - with marasmus E41
      - underlying condition E88.A
      - with marasmus E41
  - Waterhouse-Friderichsen A39.1
  - Wegner's (syphilitic osteochondritis) A50.02
  - Weil's (leptospiral jaundice of lung) A27.0
  - Weir Mitchell's (erythromelalgia) I73.81
  - Werdnig-Hoffmann G12.0
  - Wermer's E31.21
  - Werner-His (trench fever) A79.0

- **Disease, diseased** — *continued*
  - Werner-Schultz (neutropenic splenomegaly) D73.81
  - Wernicke-Posadas B38.9
  - whipworm B79
  - white blood cells D72.9
    - specified NEC D72.89
  - white matter R90.82
  - white-spot, meaning lichen sclerosus et atrophicus L90.0
    - penis N48.0
    - vulva N90.4
  - Wilkie's K55.1
  - Wilkinson-Sneddon (subcorneal pustular dermatosis) L13.1
  - Willis' — *see* Diabetes
  - Wilson's (hepatolenticular degeneration) E83.01
  - woolsorter's A22.1
  - yaba monkey tumor B08.72
  - yaba pox (virus) B08.72
  - Zika virus A92.5
    - congenital P35.4
  - zoonotic, bacterial A28.9
    - specified type NEC A28.8
- **Disfigurement** (due to scar) L90.5
- **Disgerminoma** — *see* Dysgerminoma
- **DISH** (diffuse idiopathic skeletal hyperostosis) — *see* Hyperostosis, ankylosing
- **Disinsertion, retina** — *see* Detachment, retina
- **Dislocatable hip, congenital** Q65.6
- **Dislocation** (articular)
  - with fracture — *see* Fracture
  - acromioclavicular (joint) S43.10- ☑
    - with displacement
      - 100%-200% S43.12- ☑
      - more than 200% S43.13- ☑
    - inferior S43.14- ☑
    - posterior S43.15- ☑
  - ankle S93.0- ☑
  - astragalus — *see* Dislocation, ankle
  - atlantoaxial S13.121- ☑
  - atlantooccipital S13.111- ☑
  - atloidooccipital S13.111- ☑
  - breast bone S23.29- ☑
  - capsule, joint — *code by* site under Dislocation
  - carpal (bone) — *see* Dislocation, wrist
  - carpometacarpal (joint) NEC S63.05- ☑
    - thumb S63.04- ☑
  - cartilage (joint) — *code by* site under Dislocation
  - cervical spine (vertebra) — *see* Dislocation, vertebra, cervical
  - chronic — *see* Dislocation, recurrent
  - clavicle — *see* Dislocation, acromioclavicular joint
  - coccyx S33.2- ☑
  - congenital NEC Q68.8
  - coracoid — *see* Dislocation, shoulder
  - costal cartilage S23.29- ☑
  - costochondral S23.29- ☑
  - cricoarytenoid articulation S13.29- ☑
  - cricothyroid articulation S13.29- ☑
  - dorsal vertebra — *see* Dislocation, vertebra, thoracic
  - ear ossicle — *see* Discontinuity, ossicles, ear
  - elbow S53.10- ☑
    - congenital Q68.8
    - pathological — *see* Dislocation, pathological NEC, elbow
    - radial head alone — *see* Dislocation, radial head
    - recurrent — *see* Dislocation, recurrent, elbow
    - traumatic S53.10- ☑
      - anterior S53.11- ☑
      - lateral S53.14- ☑
      - medial S53.13- ☑
      - posterior S53.12- ☑
      - specified type NEC S53.19- ☑
  - eye, nontraumatic — *see* Luxation, globe
  - eyeball, nontraumatic — *see* Luxation, globe
  - femur
    - distal end — *see* Dislocation, knee
    - proximal end — *see* Dislocation, hip
  - fibula
    - distal end — *see* Dislocation, ankle
    - proximal end — *see* Dislocation, knee
  - finger S63.25- ☑
    - index S63.25- ☑
    - interphalangeal S63.27- ☑
      - distal S63.29- ☑
        - index S63.29- ☑
        - little S63.29- ☑
        - middle S63.29- ☑

- **Dislocation** — *continued*
  - finger — *continued*
    - interphalangeal — *continued*
      - distal — *continued*
        - ring S63.29- ☑
      - index S63.27- ☑
      - little S63.27- ☑
      - middle S63.27- ☑
      - proximal S63.28- ☑
        - index S63.28- ☑
        - little S63.28- ☑
        - middle S63.28- ☑
        - ring S63.28- ☑
      - ring S63.27- ☑
    - little S63.25- ☑
    - metacarpophalangeal S63.26- ☑
      - index S63.26- ☑
      - little S63.26- ☑
      - middle S63.26- ☑
      - ring S63.26- ☑
    - middle S63.25- ☑
    - recurrent — *see* Dislocation, recurrent, finger
    - ring S63.25- ☑
    - thumb — *see* Dislocation, thumb
  - foot S93.30- ☑
    - recurrent — *see* Dislocation, recurrent, foot
    - specified site NEC S93.33- ☑
    - tarsal joint S93.31- ☑
    - tarsometatarsal joint S93.32- ☑
    - toe — *see* Dislocation, toe
  - fracture — *see* Fracture
  - glenohumeral (joint) — *see* Dislocation, shoulder
  - glenoid — *see* Dislocation, shoulder
  - habitual — *see* Dislocation, recurrent
  - hip S73.00- ☑
    - anterior S73.03- ☑
      - obturator S73.02- ☑
    - central S73.04- ☑
    - congenital (total) Q65.2
      - bilateral Q65.1
      - partial Q65.5
        - bilateral Q65.4
        - unilateral Q65.3- ☑
      - unilateral Q65.0- ☑
    - developmental M24.85- ☑
    - pathological — *see* Dislocation, pathological NEC, hip
    - posterior S73.01- ☑
    - recurrent — *see* Dislocation, recurrent, hip
  - humerus, proximal end — *see* Dislocation, shoulder
  - incomplete — *see* Subluxation, by site
  - incus — *see* Discontinuity, ossicles, ear
  - infracoracoid — *see* Dislocation, shoulder
  - innominate (pubic junction) (sacral junction) S33.39- ☑
    - acetabulum — *see* Dislocation, hip
  - interphalangeal (joint(s))
    - finger S63.279- ☑
      - distal S63.29- ☑
        - index S63.29- ☑
        - little S63.29- ☑
        - middle S63.29- ☑
        - ring S63.29- ☑
      - index S63.27- ☑
      - little S63.27- ☑
      - middle S63.27- ☑
      - proximal S63.28- ☑
        - index S63.28- ☑
        - little S63.28- ☑
        - middle S63.28- ☑
        - ring S63.28- ☑
      - ring S63.27- ☑
    - foot or toe — *see* Dislocation, toe
    - thumb S63.12- ☑
  - jaw (cartilage) (meniscus) S03.0- ☑
  - joint prosthesis — *see* Complications, joint prosthesis, mechanical, displacement, by site
  - knee S83.106- ☑
    - cap — *see* Dislocation, patella
    - congenital Q68.2
    - old M23.8X- ☑
    - patella — *see* Dislocation, patella
    - pathological — *see* Dislocation, pathological NEC, knee
    - proximal tibia
      - anteriorly S83.11- ☑
      - laterally S83.14- ☑
      - medially S83.13- ☑

- **Dislocation** — *continued*
  - knee — *continued*
    - proximal tibia — *continued*
      - posteriorly S83.12- ☑
    - recurrent — *see also* Derangement, knee, specified NEC
    - specified type NEC S83.19- ☑
  - lacrimal gland HØ4.16- ☑
  - lens (complete) H27.1Ø
    - anterior H27.12- ☑
    - congenital Q12.1
    - ocular implant — *see* Complications, intraocular lens
    - partial H27.11- ☑
    - posterior H27.13- ☑
    - traumatic SØ5.8X- ☑
  - ligament — *code by* site under Dislocation
  - lumbar (vertebra) — *see* Dislocation, vertebra, lumbar
  - lumbosacral (vertebra) — *see also* Dislocation, vertebra, lumbar
    - congenital Q76.49
  - mandible SØ3.Ø- ☑
  - meniscus (knee) — *see* Tear, meniscus
    - other sites - code by site under Dislocation
  - metacarpal (bone)
    - distal end — *see* Dislocation, finger
    - proximal end S63.Ø6- ☑
  - metacarpophalangeal (joint)
    - finger S63.26- ☑
      - index S63.26- ☑
      - little S63.26- ☑
      - middle S63.26- ☑
      - ring S63.26- ☑
    - thumb S63.11- ☑
  - metatarsal (bone) — *see* Dislocation, foot
  - metatarsophalangeal (joint(s)) — *see* Dislocation, toe
  - midcarpal (joint) S63.Ø3- ☑
  - midtarsal (joint) — *see* Dislocation, foot
  - neck S13.2Ø- ☑
    - specified site NEC S13.29- ☑
    - vertebra — *see* Dislocation, vertebra, cervical
  - nose (septal cartilage) SØ3.1- ☑
  - occipitoatloid S13.111- ☑
  - old — *see* Derangement, joint, specified type NEC
  - ossicles, ear — *see* Discontinuity, ossicles, ear
  - partial — *see* Subluxation, by site
  - patella S83.ØØ6- ☑
    - congenital Q74.1
    - lateral S83.Ø1- ☑
    - recurrent (nontraumatic) M22.Ø- ☑
      - incomplete M22.1- ☑
    - specified type NEC S83.Ø9- ☑
  - pathological NEC M24.3Ø
    - ankle M24.37- ☑
    - elbow M24.32- ☑
    - foot joint M24.37- ☑
    - hand joint M24.34- ☑
    - hip M24.35- ☑
    - knee M24.36- ☑
    - lumbosacral joint — *see* subcategory M53.2- ☑
    - pelvic region — *see* Dislocation, pathological, hip
    - sacroiliac — *see* subcategory M53.2- ☑
    - shoulder M24.31- ☑
    - specified site NEC M24.39
    - wrist M24.33- ☑
  - pelvis NEC S33.3Ø- ☑
    - specified NEC S33.39- ☑
  - phalanx
    - finger or hand — *see* Dislocation, finger
    - foot or toe — *see* Dislocation, toe
  - prosthesis, internal — *see* Complications, prosthetic device, by site, mechanical
  - radial head S53.ØØ6- ☑
    - anterior S53.Ø1- ☑
    - posterior S53.Ø2- ☑
    - specified type NEC S53.Ø9- ☑
  - radiocarpal (joint) S63.Ø2- ☑
  - radiohumeral (joint) — *see* Dislocation, radial head
  - radioulnar (joint)
    - distal S63.Ø1- ☑
    - proximal — *see* Dislocation, elbow
  - radius
    - distal end — *see* Dislocation, wrist
    - proximal end — *see* Dislocation, radial head
  - recurrent M24.4Ø
    - ankle M24.47- ☑
    - elbow M24.42- ☑
    - finger M24.44- ☑
    - foot joint M24.47- ☑
    - hand joint M24.44- ☑
    - hip M24.45- ☑
    - knee M24.46- ☑
      - patella — *see* Dislocation, patella, recurrent
    - patella — *see* Dislocation, patella, recurrent
    - sacroiliac — *see* subcategory M53.2- ☑
    - shoulder M24.41- ☑
    - specified site NEC M24.49
    - toe M24.47- ☑
    - vertebra — *see also* subcategory M43.5- ☑
      - atlantoaxial M43.4
        - with myelopathy M43.3
    - wrist M24.43- ☑
  - rib (cartilage) S23.29- ☑
  - sacrococcygeal S33.2- ☑
  - sacroiliac (joint) (ligament) S33.2- ☑
    - congenital Q74.2
    - recurrent — *see* subcategory M53.2- ☑
  - sacrum S33.2- ☑
  - scaphoid (bone) (hand) (wrist) — *see* Dislocation, wrist
    - foot — *see* Dislocation, foot
  - scapula — *see* Dislocation, shoulder, girdle, scapula
  - semilunar cartilage, knee — *see* Tear, meniscus
  - septal cartilage (nose) SØ3.1- ☑
  - septum (nasal) (old) J34.2
  - sesamoid bone — *code by* site under Dislocation
  - shoulder (blade) (ligament) (joint) (traumatic) S43.ØØ6- ☑
    - acromioclavicular — *see* Dislocation, acromioclavicular
    - chronic — *see* Dislocation, recurrent, shoulder
    - congenital Q68.8
    - girdle S43.3Ø- ☑
      - scapula S43.31- ☑
      - specified site NEC S43.39- ☑
    - humerus S43.ØØ- ☑
      - anterior S43.Ø1- ☑
      - inferior S43.Ø3- ☑
      - posterior S43.Ø2- ☑
    - pathological — *see* Dislocation, pathological NEC, shoulder
    - recurrent — *see* Dislocation, recurrent, shoulder
    - specified type NEC S43.Ø8- ☑
  - spine
    - cervical — *see* Dislocation, vertebra, cervical
    - congenital Q76.49
    - due to birth trauma P11.5
    - lumbar — *see* Dislocation, vertebra, lumbar
    - thoracic — *see* Dislocation, vertebra, thoracic
  - spontaneous — *see* Dislocation, pathological
  - sternoclavicular (joint) S43.2Ø6- ☑
    - anterior S43.21- ☑
    - posterior S43.22- ☑
  - sternum S23.29- ☑
  - subglenoid — *see* Dislocation, shoulder
  - symphysis pubis S33.4- ☑
  - talus — *see* Dislocation, ankle
  - tarsal (bone(s)) (joint(s)) — *see* Dislocation, foot
  - tarsometatarsal (joint(s)) — *see* Dislocation, foot
  - temporomandibular (joint) SØ3.Ø- ☑
  - thigh, proximal end — *see* Dislocation, hip
  - thorax S23.2Ø- ☑
    - specified site NEC S23.29- ☑
    - vertebra — *see* Dislocation, vertebra
  - thumb S63.1Ø- ☑
    - interphalangeal joint — *see* Dislocation, interphalangeal (joint), thumb
    - metacarpophalangeal joint — *see* Dislocation, metacarpophalangeal (joint), thumb
  - thyroid cartilage S13.29- ☑
  - tibia
    - distal end — *see* Dislocation, ankle
    - proximal end — *see* Dislocation, knee
  - tibiofibular (joint)
    - distal — *see* Dislocation, ankle
    - superior — *see* Dislocation, knee
  - toe(s) S93.1Ø6- ☑
    - great S93.1Ø- ☑
      - interphalangeal joint S93.11- ☑
      - metatarsophalangeal joint S93.12- ☑
    - interphalangeal joint S93.119- ☑
    - lesser S93.1Ø6- ☑
      - interphalangeal joint S93.11- ☑
      - metatarsophalangeal joint S93.12- ☑
    - metatarsophalangeal joint S93.12- ☑
  - tooth SØ3.2- ☑
  - trachea S23.29- ☑
  - ulna
    - distal end S63.Ø7- ☑
    - proximal end — *see* Dislocation, elbow
  - ulnohumeral (joint) — *see* Dislocation, elbow
  - vertebra (articular process) (body) (traumatic)
    - cervical S13.1Ø1- ☑
      - atlantoaxial joint S13.121- ☑
      - atlantooccipital joint S13.111- ☑
      - atloidooccipital joint S13.111- ☑
      - joint between
        - CØ and C1 S13.111- ☑
        - C1 and C2 S13.121- ☑
        - C2 and C3 S13.131- ☑
        - C3 and C4 S13.141- ☑
        - C4 and C5 S13.151- ☑
        - C5 and C6 S13.161- ☑
        - C6 and C7 S13.171- ☑
        - C7 and T1 S13.181- ☑
      - occipitoatloid joint S13.111- ☑
    - congenital Q76.49
    - lumbar S33.1Ø1- ☑
      - joint between
        - L1 and L2 S33.111- ☑
        - L2 and L3 S33.121- ☑
        - L3 and L4 S33.131- ☑
        - L4 and L5 S33.141- ☑
    - nontraumatic — *see* Displacement, intervertebral disc
    - partial — *see* Subluxation, by site
    - recurrent NEC — *see* subcategory M43.5- ☑
    - thoracic S23.1Ø1- ☑
      - joint between
        - T1 and T2 S23.111- ☑
        - T2 and T3 S23.121- ☑
        - T3 and T4 S23.123- ☑
        - T4 and T5 S23.131- ☑
        - T5 and T6 S23.133- ☑
        - T6 and T7 S23.141- ☑
        - T7 and T8 S23.143- ☑
        - T8 and T9 S23.151- ☑
        - T1Ø and T11 S23.161- ☑
        - T11 and T12 S23.163- ☑
        - T12 and L1 S23.171- ☑
        - T9 and T1Ø S23.153- ☑
  - wrist (carpal bone) S63.ØØ6- ☑
    - carpometacarpal joint — *see* Dislocation, carpometacarpal (joint)
    - distal radioulnar joint — *see* Dislocation, radioulnar (joint), distal
    - metacarpal bone, proximal — *see* Dislocation, metacarpal (bone), proximal end
    - midcarpal — *see* Dislocation, midcarpal (joint)
    - radiocarpal joint — *see* Dislocation, radiocarpal (joint)
    - recurrent — *see* Dislocation, recurrent, wrist
    - specified site NEC S63.Ø9- ☑
    - ulna — *see* Dislocation, ulna, distal end
  - xiphoid cartilage S23.29- ☑
- **Disorder** (of) — *see also* Disease
  - acantholytic L11.9
    - specified NEC L11.8
  - acute
    - psychotic — *see* Psychosis, acute
    - stress F43.Ø
  - adjustment (grief) F43.2Ø
    - with
      - anxiety F43.22
        - with depressed mood F43.23
      - conduct disturbance F43.24
        - with emotional disturbance F43.25
      - depressed mood F43.21
        - with anxiety F43.23
      - other specified symptom F43.29
  - adrenal (capsule) (gland) (medullary) E27.9
    - specified NEC E27.8
  - adrenogenital — *see also* Adrenogenital syndrome E25.9
    - drug-induced E25.8
    - iatrogenic E25.8
    - idiopathic E25.8
  - adult personality (and behavior) F69
    - specified NEC F68.8
  - affective (mood) — *see* Disorder, mood
  - aggressive, unsocialized F91.1
  - alcohol-related F1Ø.99


☑ **Additional Character Required — Refer to the Tabular List for Character Selection**

- **Disorder** — *continued*
  - alcohol-related — *continued*
    - with
      - amnestic disorder, persisting F1Ø.96
      - anxiety disorder F1Ø.98Ø
      - dementia, persisting F1Ø.97
      - intoxication F1Ø.929
        - with delirium F1Ø.921
        - uncomplicated F1Ø.92Ø
      - mood disorder F1Ø.94
      - other specified F1Ø.988
      - psychotic disorder F1Ø.959
        - with
          - delusions F1Ø.95Ø
          - hallucinations F1Ø.951
      - sexual dysfunction F1Ø.981
      - sleep disorder F1Ø.982
  - alcohol use
    - mild F1Ø.1Ø
      - with
        - alcohol-induced
          - anxiety disorder F1Ø.18Ø
          - bipolar and related disorder F1Ø.14
          - depressive disorder F1Ø.14
          - psychotic disorder F1Ø.159
          - sexual dysfunction F1Ø.181
          - sleep disorder F1Ø.182
        - alcohol intoxication F1Ø.129
          - delirium F1Ø.121
      - in remission (early) (sustained) F1Ø.11
    - moderate or severe F1Ø.2Ø
      - with
        - alcohol-induced
          - anxiety disorder F1Ø.28Ø
          - bipolar and related disorder F1Ø.24
          - depressive disorder F1Ø.24
          - major neurocognitive disorder, amnestic-confabulatory type F1Ø.26
          - major neurocognitive disorder, nonamnestic-confabulatory type F1Ø.27
          - mild neurocognitive disorder F1Ø.288
          - psychotic disorder F1Ø.259
          - sexual dysfunction F1Ø.281
          - sleep disorder F1Ø.282
        - alcohol intoxication F1Ø.229
          - delirium F1Ø.221
      - in remission (early) (sustained) F1Ø.21
  - allergic — *see* Allergy
  - alveolar NEC J84.Ø9
  - amino-acid
    - cystathioninuria E72.19
    - cystinosis E72.Ø4
    - cystinuria E72.Ø1
    - glycinuria E72.Ø9
    - homocystinuria E72.11
    - metabolism — *see* Disturbance, metabolism, amino-acid
      - specified NEC E72.89
    - neonatal, transitory P74.8
    - renal transport NEC E72.Ø9
    - transport NEC E72.Ø9
  - amnesic, amnestic
    - alcohol-induced F1Ø.96
      - with dependence F1Ø.26
    - due to (secondary to) general medical condition FØ4
    - psychoactive NEC-induced F19.96
      - with
        - abuse F19.16
        - dependence F19.26
    - sedative, hypnotic or anxiolytic-induced F13.96
      - with dependence F13.26
  - amphetamine-type substance use
    - mild F15.1Ø
      - in remission (early) (sustained) F15.11
    - moderate F15.2Ø
      - in remission (early) (sustained) F15.21
    - severe F15.2Ø
      - in remission (early) (sustained) F15.21
  - amphetamine (or other stimulant) use
    - mild
      - with
        - amphetamine, cocaine, or other stimulant intoxication
          - with perceptual disturbances F15.122
          - without perceptual disturbances F15.129
        - amphetamine (or other stimulant) -induced
          - anxiety disorder F15.18Ø
          - bipolar and related disorder F15.14
          - depressive disorder F15.14

- **Disorder** — *continued*
  - amphetamine use — *continued*
    - mild — *continued*
      - with — *continued*
        - amphetamine -induced — *continued*
          - obsessive-compulsive and related disorder F15.188
          - psychotic disorder F15.159
          - sexual dysfunction F15.181
        - intoxication delirium F15.121
    - moderate or severe
      - with
        - amphetamine, cocaine, or other stimulant intoxication
          - with perceptual disturbances F15.222
          - without perceptual disturbances F15.229
        - amphetamine (or other stimulant) -induced
          - anxiety disorder F15.28Ø
          - bipolar and related disorder F15.24
          - depressive disorder F15.24
          - obsessive-compulsive and related disorder F15.288
          - psychotic disorder F15.259
          - sexual dysfunction F15.281
        - intoxication delirium F15.221
  - anaerobic glycolysis with anemia D55.29
  - anxiety F41.9
    - due to (secondary to)
      - alcohol F1Ø.98Ø
        - in
          - abuse F1Ø.18Ø
          - dependence F1Ø.28Ø
      - amphetamine F15.98Ø
        - in
          - abuse F15.18Ø
          - dependence F15.28Ø
      - anxiolytic F13.98Ø
        - in
          - abuse F13.18Ø
          - dependence F13.28Ø
      - caffeine F15.98Ø
        - in
          - abuse F15.18Ø
          - dependence F15.28Ø
      - cannabis F12.98Ø
        - in
          - abuse F12.18Ø
          - dependence F12.28Ø
      - cocaine F14.98Ø
        - in
          - abuse F14.18Ø
          - dependence F14.18Ø
      - general medical condition FØ6.4
      - hallucinogen F16.98Ø
        - in
          - abuse F16.18Ø
          - dependence F16.28Ø
      - hypnotic F13.98Ø
        - in
          - abuse F13.18Ø
          - dependence F13.28Ø
      - inhalant F18.98Ø
        - in
          - abuse F18.18Ø
          - dependence F18.28Ø
      - phencyclidine F16.98Ø
        - in
          - abuse F16.18Ø
          - dependence F16.28Ø
      - psychoactive substance NEC F19.98Ø
        - in
          - abuse F19.18Ø
          - dependence F19.28Ø
      - sedative F13.98Ø
        - in
          - abuse F13.18Ø
          - dependence F13.28Ø
      - volatile solvents F18.98Ø
        - in
          - abuse F18.18Ø
          - dependence F18.28Ø
    - generalized F41.1
    - illness F45.21
    - mixed
      - with depression (mild) F41.8
      - specified NEC F41.3
    - organic FØ6.4
    - phobic F4Ø.9
      - of childhood F4Ø.8

- **Disorder** — *continued*
  - anxiety — *continued*
    - specified NEC F41.8
  - aortic valve — *see* Endocarditis, aortic
  - aromatic amino-acid metabolism E7Ø.9
    - specified NEC E7Ø.89
  - arteriole NEC I77.89
  - artery NEC I77.89
  - articulation — *see* Disorder, joint
  - attachment (childhood)
    - disinhibited F94.2
    - reactive F94.1
  - attention-deficit hyperactivity (adolescent) (adult) (child) F9Ø.9
    - combined
      - presentation F9Ø.2
      - type F9Ø.2
    - hyperactive
      - impulsive presentation F9Ø.1
      - type F9Ø.1
    - inattentive
      - presentation F9Ø.Ø
      - type F9Ø.Ø
    - specified type NEC F9Ø.8
  - attention-deficit without hyperactivity (adolescent) (adult) (child) F98.8
  - auditory processing (central) H93.25
  - autism spectrum F84.Ø
  - autistic F84.Ø
  - autoimmune D89.89
  - autonomic nervous system G9Ø.9
    - specified NEC G9Ø.89
  - avoidant
    - child or adolescent F4Ø.1Ø
    - restrictive food intake F5Ø.82
  - balance
    - acid-base E87.8
      - mixed E87.4
    - electrolyte E87.8
    - fluid NEC E87.8
  - behavioral (disruptive) — *see* Disorder, conduct
  - bereavement, persistent complex F43.81
  - beta-amino-acid metabolism E72.89
  - bile acid and cholesterol metabolism E78.7Ø
    - Barth syndrome E78.71
    - other specified E78.79
    - Smith-Lemli-Opitz syndrome E78.72
  - bilirubin excretion E8Ø.6
  - binge eating F5Ø.81- ☑
  - binocular
    - movement H51.9
      - convergence
        - excess H51.12
        - insufficiency H51.11
      - internuclear ophthalmoplegia — *see* Ophthalmoplegia, internuclear
      - palsy of conjugate gaze H51.Ø
      - specified type NEC H51.8
    - vision NEC — *see* Disorder, vision, binocular
  - bipolar (I) (seasonal) (type I) F31.9
    - and related due to a known physiological condition
      - with
        - manic features FØ6.33
        - manic- or hypomanic-like episodes FØ6.33
        - mixed features FØ6.34
    - current (or most recent) episode
      - depressed F31.9
        - with psychotic features F31.5
        - without psychotic features F31.3Ø
          - mild F31.31
          - moderate F31.32
          - severe (without psychotic features) F31.4
            - with psychotic features F31.5
      - hypomanic F31.Ø
      - manic F31.9
        - with psychotic features F31.2
        - without psychotic features F31.1Ø
          - mild F31.11
          - moderate F31.12
          - severe (without psychotic features) F31.13
            - with psychotic features F31.2
      - mixed F31.6Ø
        - mild F31.61
        - moderate F31.62
        - severe (without psychotic features) F31.63
          - with psychotic features F31.64
      - severe depression (without psychotic features) F31.4
        - with psychotic features F31.5

- **Disorder** — *continued*
  - conduct — *continued*
    - hyperkinetic — *see* Disorder, attention-deficit hyperactivity
    - oppositional defiance F91.3
    - socialized F91.2
    - solitary aggressive type F91.1
    - specified NEC F91.8
    - unsocialized (aggressive) F91.1
  - conduction, heart I45.9
  - congenital glycosylation (CDG) E74.89
  - conjunctiva H11.9
    - infection — *see* Conjunctivitis
  - connective tissue, localized L94.9
    - specified NEC L94.8
  - conversion (functional neurological symptom disorder)
    - with
      - abnormal movement F44.4
      - anesthesia or sensory loss F44.6
      - attacks or seizures F44.5
      - mixed symptoms F44.7
      - special sensory symptoms F44.6
      - speech symptoms F44.4
      - swallowing symptoms F44.4
      - weakness or paralysis F44.4
  - convulsive (secondary) — *see* Convulsions
  - cornea H18.9
    - deformity — *see* Deformity, cornea
    - degeneration — *see* Degeneration, cornea
    - deposits — *see* Deposit, cornea
    - due to contact lens H18.82- ☑
      - specified as edema — *see* Edema, cornea
    - edema — *see* Edema, cornea
    - keratitis — *see* Keratitis
    - keratoconjunctivitis — *see* Keratoconjunctivitis
    - membrane change — *see* Change, corneal membrane
    - neovascularization — *see* Neovascularization, cornea
    - scar — *see* Opacity, cornea
    - specified type NEC H18.89- ☑
    - ulcer — *see* Ulcer, cornea
  - corpus cavernosum N48.9
  - cranial nerve — *see* Disorder, nerve, cranial
  - Cyclin-Dependent Kinase-Like 5 Deficiency (CDKL5) G4Ø.42
  - cyclothymic F34.Ø
  - defiant oppositional F91.3
  - delusional (persistent) (systematized) F22
    - induced F24
  - depersonalization F48.1
  - depressive F32.A
    - due to known physiological condition
      - with
        - depressive features FØ6.31
        - major depressive-like episode FØ6.32
        - mixed features FØ6.34
    - major F32.9
      - with psychotic symptoms F32.3
      - in remission (full) F32.5
        - partial F32.4
      - recurrent F33.9
        - with psychotic features F33.3
      - single episode F32.9
        - mild F32.Ø
        - moderate F32.1
        - severe (without psychotic symptoms) F32.2
          - with psychotic symptoms F32.3
    - organic FØ6.31
    - persistent F34.1
    - recurrent F33.9
      - current episode
        - mild F33.Ø
        - moderate F33.1
        - severe (without psychotic symptoms) F33.2
          - with psychotic symptoms F33.3
      - in remission F33.4Ø
        - full F33.42
        - partial F33.41
      - specified NEC F33.8
    - single episode — *see* Episode, depressive
    - specified NEC F32.89
  - developmental F89
    - arithmetical skills F81.2
    - coordination (motor) F82
    - expressive writing F81.81
    - language F8Ø.9
      - expressive F8Ø.1
      - mixed receptive and expressive F8Ø.2
      - receptive type F8Ø.2
      - specified NEC F8Ø.89

- **Disorder** — *continued*
  - developmental — *continued*
    - learning F81.9
      - arithmetical F81.2
      - reading F81.Ø
    - mixed F88
    - motor coordination or function F82
    - pervasive F84.9
      - specified NEC F84.8
    - phonological F8Ø.Ø
    - reading F81.Ø
    - scholastic skills — *see also* Disorder, learning
      - mixed F81.89
    - specified NEC F88
    - speech F8Ø.9
      - articulation F8Ø.Ø
      - specified NEC F8Ø.89
    - written expression F81.81
  - diaphragm J98.6
  - digestive (system) K92.9
    - newborn P78.9
      - specified NEC P78.89
    - postprocedural — *see* Complication, gastrointestinal
    - psychogenic F45.8
  - disc (intervertebral) M51.9
    - with
      - myelopathy
        - cervical region M5Ø.ØØ
        - cervicothoracic region M5Ø.Ø3
        - high cervical region M5Ø.Ø1
        - lumbar region M51.Ø6
        - mid-cervical region M5Ø.Ø2Ø
        - sacrococcygeal region M53.3
        - thoracic region M51.Ø4
        - thoracolumbar region M51.Ø5
      - radiculopathy
        - cervical region M5Ø.1Ø
        - cervicothoracic region M5Ø.13
        - high cervical region M5Ø.11
        - lumbar region M51.16
        - lumbosacral region M51.17
        - mid-cervical region M5Ø.12Ø
        - sacrococcygeal region M53.3
        - thoracic region M51.14
        - thoracolumbar region M51.15
    - cervical M5Ø.9Ø
      - with
        - myelopathy M5Ø.ØØ
          - C2-C3 M5Ø.Ø1
          - C3-C4 M5Ø.Ø1
          - C4-C5 M5Ø.Ø21
          - C5-C6 M5Ø.Ø22
          - C6-C7 M5Ø.Ø23
          - C7-T1 M5Ø.Ø3
          - cervicothoracic region M5Ø.Ø3
          - high cervical region M5Ø.Ø1
          - mid-cervical region M5Ø.Ø2Ø
        - neuritis, radiculitis or radiculopathy M5Ø.1Ø
          - C2-C3 M5Ø.11
          - C3-C4 M5Ø.11
          - C4-C5 M5Ø.121
          - C5-C6 M5Ø.122
          - C6-C7 M5Ø.123
          - C7-T1 M5Ø.13
          - cervicothoracic region M5Ø.13
          - high cervical region M5Ø.11
          - mid-cervical region M5Ø.12Ø
      - C2-C3 M5Ø.91
      - C3-C4 M5Ø.91
      - C4-C5 M5Ø.921
      - C5-C6 M5Ø.922
      - C6-C7 M5Ø.923
      - C7-T1 M5Ø.93
      - cervicothoracic region M5Ø.93
      - degeneration M5Ø.3Ø
        - C2-C3 M5Ø.31
        - C3-C4 M5Ø.31
        - C4-C5 M5Ø.321
        - C5-C6 M5Ø.322
        - C6-C7 M5Ø.323
        - C7-T1 M5Ø.33
        - cervicothoracic region M5Ø.33
        - high cervical region M5Ø.31
        - mid-cervical region M5Ø.32Ø
      - displacement M5Ø.2Ø
        - C2-C3 M5Ø.21
        - C3-C4 M5Ø.21
        - C4-C5 M5Ø.221
        - C5-C6 M5Ø.222

- **Disorder** — *continued*
  - disc — *continued*
    - cervical — *continued*
      - displacement — *continued*
        - C6-C7 M5Ø.223
        - C7-T1 M5Ø.23
        - cervicothoracic region M5Ø.23
        - high cervical region M5Ø.21
        - mid-cervical region M5Ø.22Ø
      - high cervical region M5Ø.91
      - mid-cervical region M5Ø.92Ø
      - specified type NEC M5Ø.8Ø
        - C2-C3 M5Ø.81
        - C3-C4 M5Ø.81
        - C4-C5 M5Ø.821
        - C5-C6 M5Ø.822
        - C6-C7 M5Ø.823
        - C7-T1 M5Ø.83
        - cervicothoracic region M5Ø.83
        - high cervical region M5Ø.81
        - mid-cervical region M5Ø.82Ø
    - specified NEC
      - lumbar region M51.86
      - lumbosacral region M51.87
      - sacrococcygeal region M53.3
      - thoracic region M51.84
      - thoracolumbar region M51.85
  - disinhibited attachment (childhood) F94.2
  - disintegrative, childhood NEC F84.3
  - disruptive F91.9
    - mood dysregulation F34.81
    - specified NEC F91.8
  - disruptive behavior — *see* Disorder, conduct
  - dissocial personality F6Ø.2
  - dissociative F44.9
    - affecting
      - motor function F44.4
        - and sensation F44.7
      - sensation F44.6
        - and motor function F44.7
    - brief reactive F43.Ø
    - due to (secondary to) general medical condition FØ6.8
    - mixed F44.7
    - organic FØ6.8
    - other specified NEC F44.89
  - double heterozygous sickling — *see* Disease, sickle-cell
  - dream anxiety F51.5
  - drug induced hemorrhagic D68.32
  - drug related F19.99
    - abuse — *see* Abuse, drug
    - dependence — *see* Dependence, drug
  - dysmorphic body F45.22
  - dysthymic F34.1
  - ear H93.9- ☑
    - bleeding — *see* Otorrhagia
    - deafness — *see* Deafness
    - degenerative H93.Ø9- ☑
    - discharge — *see* Otorrhea
    - external H61.9- ☑
      - auditory canal stenosis — *see* Stenosis, external ear canal
      - exostosis — *see* Exostosis, external ear canal
      - impacted cerumen — *see* Impaction, cerumen
      - otitis — *see* Otitis, externa
      - perichondritis — *see* Perichondritis, ear
      - pinna — *see* Disorder, pinna
      - specified type NEC H61.89- ☑
    - inner H83.9- ☑
      - vestibular dysfunction — *see* Disorder, vestibular function
    - middle H74.9- ☑
      - adhesive H74.1- ☑
      - ossicle — *see* Abnormal, ear ossicles
      - polyp — *see* Polyp, ear (middle)
      - specified NEC, in diseases classified elsewhere H75.8- ☑
    - postprocedural — *see* Complications, ear, procedure
    - specified NEC, in diseases classified elsewhere H94.8- ☑
  - eating (adult) (psychogenic) F5Ø.9
    - anorexia — *see* Anorexia
    - binge F5Ø.81- ☑
    - bulimia F5Ø.2- ☑
    - child F98.29
      - pica (in remission) F98.3
      - rumination disorder (in remission) F98.21
    - pica F5Ø.89
      - adult (in remission) F5Ø.83

- **Disorder** — *continued*
  - eating — *continued*
    - pica — *continued*
      - childhood (in remission) F98.3
    - rumination — *see also* Rumination R11.10
      - adult (in remission) F50.84
      - infancy or childhood (in remission) F98.21
    - specified NEC F50.89
  - electrolyte (balance) NEC E87.8
    - with
      - abortion — *see* Abortion by type complicated by specified condition NEC
      - ectopic pregnancy O08.5
      - molar pregnancy O08.5
    - acidosis (lactic) (metabolic) E87.20
      - acute E87.21
      - chronic E87.22
      - respiratory E87.29
      - specified NEC E87.29
    - alkalosis (metabolic) (respiratory) E87.3
  - elimination, transepidermal L87.9
    - specified NEC L87.8
  - emotional (persistent) F34.9
    - of childhood F93.9
      - specified NEC F93.8
  - endocrine E34.9
    - postprocedural E89.89
      - specified NEC E89.89
  - erectile (male) (organic) — *see also* Dysfunction, sexual, male, erectile N52.9
    - nonorganic F52.21
  - erythematous — *see* Erythema
  - esophagus K22.9
    - functional K22.4
    - psychogenic F45.8
  - eustachian tube H69.9- ☑
    - infection — *see* Salpingitis, eustachian
    - obstruction — *see* Obstruction, eustachian tube
    - patulous — *see* Patulous, eustachian tube
    - specified NEC H69.8- ☑
  - exhibitionistic F65.2
  - extrapyramidal G25.9
    - in diseases classified elsewhere — *see* category G26
    - specified type NEC G25.89
  - eye H57.9
    - postprocedural — *see* Complication, postprocedural, eye
  - eyelid H02.9
    - cyst — *see* Cyst, eyelid
    - degenerative H02.70
      - chloasma — *see* Chloasma, eyelid
      - madarosis — *see* Madarosis
      - specified type NEC H02.79
      - vitiligo — *see* Vitiligo, eyelid
      - xanthelasma — *see* Xanthelasma
    - dermatochalasis — *see* Dermatochalasis
    - edema — *see* Edema, eyelid
    - elephantiasis — *see* Elephantiasis, eyelid
    - foreign body, retained — *see* Foreign body, retained, eyelid
    - function H02.59
      - abnormal innervation syndrome — *see* Syndrome, abnormal innervation
      - blepharochalasis — *see* Blepharochalasis
      - blepharoclonus — *see* Blepharoclonus
      - blepharophimosis — *see* Blepharophimosis
      - blepharoptosis — *see* Blepharoptosis
      - lagophthalmos — *see* Lagophthalmos
      - lid retraction — *see* Retraction, lid
    - hypertrichosis — *see* Hypertrichosis, eyelid
    - specified type NEC H02.89
    - vascular H02.879
      - left H02.876
        - lower H02.875
        - upper H02.874
      - right H02.873
        - lower H02.872
        - upper H02.871
  - factitious
    - by proxy F68.A
    - imposed on another F68.A
    - imposed on self F68.10
      - with predominantly
        - psychological symptoms F68.11
          - with physical symptoms F68.13
        - physical symptoms F68.12
          - with psychological symptoms F68.13
  - factor, coagulation — *see* Defect, coagulation

- **Disorder** — *continued*
  - fatty acid
    - metabolism E71.30
      - specified NEC E71.39
    - oxidation
      - LCAD E71.310
      - MCAD E71.311
      - SCAD E71.312
      - specified deficiency NEC E71.318
  - feeding (infant or child) — *see also* Disorder, eating R63.30
    - or eating disorder F50.9
    - pediatric
      - acute R63.31
      - chronic R63.32
    - specified NEC F50.9
  - feigned (with obvious motivation) Z76.5
    - without obvious motivation — *see* Disorder, factitious
  - female
    - hypoactive sexual desire F52.0
    - orgasmic F52.31
    - sexual interest/arousal F52.22
  - fetishistic F65.0
  - fibroblastic M72.9
    - specified NEC M72.8
  - fluency
    - adult onset F98.5
    - childhood onset F80.81
    - following
      - cerebral infarction I69.323
      - cerebrovascular disease I69.923
        - specified disease NEC I69.823
      - intracerebral hemorrhage I69.123
      - nontraumatic intracranial hemorrhage NEC I69.223
      - subarachnoid hemorrhage I69.023
    - in conditions classified elsewhere R47.82
  - fluid balance E87.8
  - follicular (skin) L73.9
    - specified NEC L73.8
  - FOXG1-related QA0.0151
  - frotteuristic F65.81
  - fructose metabolism E74.10
    - essential fructosuria E74.11
    - fructokinase deficiency E74.11
    - fructose-1, 6-diphosphatase deficiency E74.19
    - hereditary fructose intolerance E74.12
    - other specified E74.19
  - functional polymorphonuclear neutrophils D71.9
    - specified NEC D71.8
  - gallbladder, biliary tract and pancreas in diseases classified elsewhere K87
  - gambling F63.0
  - gamma aminobutyric acid (GABA) metabolism E72.81
  - gamma-glutamyl cycle E72.89
  - gastric (functional) K31.9
    - motility K30
    - psychogenic F45.8
    - secretion K30
  - gastrointestinal (functional) NOS K92.9
    - newborn P78.9
    - psychogenic F45.8
  - gender-identity or -role F64.9
    - childhood F64.2
    - effect on relationship F66
    - in remission F64.A
    - of adolescence or adulthood F64.0
      - nontranssexual F64.8
    - specified NEC F64.8
    - uncertainty F66
  - gender incongruence F64.9
    - in adolescents and adults F64.0
    - of childhood F64.2
  - genito-pelvic pain penetration F52.6
  - genitourinary system
    - female N94.9
    - male N50.9
    - psychogenic F45.8
  - globe H44.9
    - degenerated condition H44.50
      - absolute glaucoma H44.51- ☑
      - atrophy H44.52- ☑
      - leucocoria H44.53- ☑
    - degenerative H44.30
      - chalcosis H44.31- ☑
      - myopia — *see also* Myopia, degenerative H44.2- ☑
      - siderosis H44.32- ☑
      - specified type NEC H44.39- ☑
    - endophthalmitis — *see* Endophthalmitis

- **Disorder** — *continued*
  - globe — *continued*
    - foreign body, retained — *see* Foreign body, intraocular, old, retained
    - hemophthalmos — *see* Hemophthalmos
    - hypotony H44.40
      - due to
        - ocular fistula H44.42- ☑
        - specified disorder NEC H44.43- ☑
      - flat anterior chamber H44.41- ☑
      - primary H44.44- ☑
    - luxation — *see* Luxation, globe
    - specified type NEC H44.89
  - glomerular (in) N05.9
    - amyloidosis E85.4 *[N08]*
    - cryoglobulinemia D89.1 *[N08]*
    - disseminated intravascular coagulation D65 *[N08]*
    - Fabry's disease E75.21 *[N08]*
    - familial lecithin cholesterol acyltransferase deficiency E78.6 *[N08]*
    - Goodpasture's syndrome M31.0
    - hemolytic-uremic syndrome — *see* Syndrome, hemolytic-uremic
    - Henoch (-Schonlein) purpura D69.0 *[N08]*
    - malariae malaria B52.0
    - microscopic polyangiitis M31.7 *[N08]*
    - multiple myeloma C90.0- ☑ *[N08]*
    - mumps B26.83
    - schistosomiasis B65.9 *[N08]*
    - sepsis NEC A41.- ☑ *[N08]*
      - streptococcal A40.- ☑ *[N08]*
    - sickle-cell disorders D57.- ☑ *[N08]*
    - strongyloidiasis B78.9 *[N08]*
    - subacute bacterial endocarditis I33.0 *[N08]*
    - syphilis A52.75
    - systemic lupus erythematosus M32.14
    - thrombotic thrombocytopenic purpura M31.19 *[N08]*
    - Waldenstrom macroglobulinemia C88.0- ☑ *[N08]*
    - Wegener's granulomatosis M31.31
  - gluconeogenesis E74.4
  - glucosaminoglycan metabolism — *see* Disorder, metabolism, glucosaminoglycan
  - glucose transport E74.819
    - specified NEC E74.818
  - glycine metabolism E72.50
    - d-glycericacidemia E72.59
    - hyperhydroxyprolinemia E72.59
    - hyperoxaluria R82.992
      - dietary E72.540
      - enteric E72.541
      - primary E72.539
        - specified type NEC E72.538
        - type 1 E72.530
        - type 2 E72.538
        - type 3 E72.538
      - secondary E72.549
        - specified type NEC E72.548
    - hyperprolinemia E72.59
    - non-ketotic hyperglycinemia E72.51
    - oxalosis E72.53- ☑
    - oxaluria E72.53- ☑
    - sarcosinemia E72.59
    - trimethylaminuria E72.52
  - glycoprotein metabolism E77.9
    - specified NEC E77.8
  - grief
    - complicated F43.81
    - prolonged F43.81
  - habit (and impulse) F63.9
    - involving sexual behavior NEC F65.9
    - specified NEC F63.89
  - hallucinogen use
    - mild F16.10
      - with
        - hallucinogen-induced
          - anxiety disorder F16.180
          - bipolar and related disorder F16.14
          - depressive disorder F16.14
          - psychotic disorder F16.159
        - hallucinogen intoxication delirium F16.121
        - other hallucinogen intoxication F16.129
      - in remission (early) (sustained) F16.11
    - moderate or severe F16.20
      - with
        - hallucinogen-induced
          - anxiety disorder F16.280
          - bipolar and related disorder F16.24
          - depressive disorder F16.24

- **Disorder** — *continued*
  - hallucinogen use — *continued*
    - moderate or severe — *continued*
      - with — *continued*
        - hallucinogen-induced — *continued*
          - psychotic disorder F16.259
        - hallucinogen intoxication delirium F16.221
        - other hallucinogen intoxication F16.229
      - in remission (early) (sustained) F16.21
  - heart action I49.9
  - hematological D75.9
    - newborn (transient) P61.9
      - specified NEC P61.8
  - hematopoietic organs D75.9
  - hemorrhagic NEC D69.9
    - drug-induced D68.32
    - due to
      - extrinsic circulating anticoagulants D68.32
      - increase in
        - anti-IIa D68.32
        - anti-Xa D68.32
      - intrinsic
        - circulating anticoagulants D68.318
        - increase in
          - anti-VIIIa D68.318
          - anti-IXa D68.318
          - anti-XIa D68.318
          - antithrombin D68.318
    - following childbirth O72.3
  - hemostasis — *see* Defect, coagulation
  - histidine metabolism E7Ø.4Ø
    - histidinemia E7Ø.41
    - other specified E7Ø.49
  - hoarding F42.3
  - hyperkinetic — *see* Disorder, attention-deficit hyperactivity
  - hyperleucine-isoleucinemia E71.19
  - hypervalinemia E71.19
  - hypoactive sexual desire F52.Ø
  - hypochondriacal F45.2Ø
    - body dysmorphic F45.22
    - neurosis F45.21
    - other specified F45.29
  - identity
    - dissociative F44.81
    - illness anxiety F45.21
    - of childhood F93.8
  - immune mechanism (immunity) D89.9
    - specified type NEC D89.89
  - impaired renal tubular function N25.9
    - specified NEC N25.89
  - impulse (control) F63.9
  - inflammatory
    - pelvic, in diseases classified elsewhere — *see* category N74
    - penis N48.29
      - abscess N48.21
      - cellulitis N48.22
  - inhalant use
    - mild F18.1Ø
      - with
        - inhalant-induced
          - anxiety disorder F18.18Ø
          - depressive disorder F18.14
          - major neurocognitive disorder F18.17
          - mild neurocognitive disorder F18.188
          - psychotic disorder F18.159
        - inhalant intoxication F18.129
        - inhalant intoxication delirium F18.121
      - in remission (early) (sustained) F18.11
    - moderate or severe F18.2Ø
      - with
        - inhalant-induced
          - anxiety disorder F18.28Ø
          - depressive disorder F18.24
          - major neurocognitive disorder F18.27
          - mild neurocognitive disorder F18.288
          - psychotic disorder F18.259
        - inhalant intoxication F18.229
        - inhalant intoxication delirium F18.221
      - in remission (early) (sustained) F18.21
  - integument, newborn P83.9
    - specified NEC P83.88
  - intermittent explosive F63.81
  - internal secretion pancreas — *see* Increased, secretion, pancreas, endocrine
  - intestine, intestinal
    - carbohydrate absorption NEC E74.39
      - postoperative K91.2

- **Disorder** — *continued*
  - intestine, intestinal — *continued*
    - functional NEC K59.9
      - postoperative K91.89
    - psychogenic F45.8
    - vascular K55.9
      - chronic K55.1
      - specified NEC K55.8
  - intraoperative (intraprocedural) — *see* Complications, intraoperative
  - involuntary emotional expression (IEED) FØ7.89
  - iris H21.9
    - adhesions — *see* Adhesions, iris
    - atrophy — *see* Atrophy, iris
    - chamber angle recession — *see* Recession, chamber angle
    - cyst — *see* Cyst, iris
    - degeneration — *see* Degeneration, iris
    - in diseases classified elsewhere H22
    - iridodialysis — *see* Iridodialysis
    - iridoschisis — *see* Iridoschisis
    - miotic pupillary cyst — *see* Cyst, pupillary
    - pupillary
      - abnormality — *see* Abnormality, pupillary
      - membrane — *see* Membrane, pupillary
    - specified type NEC H21.89
    - vascular NEC H21.1X- ☑
  - iron metabolism E83.1Ø
    - specified NEC E83.19
  - isovaleric acidemia E71.11Ø
  - jaw, developmental M27.Ø
    - temporomandibular — *see also* Anomaly, dentofacial, temporomandibular joint M26.6Ø- ☑
  - joint M25.9
    - derangement — *see* Derangement, joint
    - effusion — *see* Effusion, joint
    - fistula — *see* Fistula, joint
    - hemarthrosis — *see* Hemarthrosis
    - instability — *see* Instability, joint
    - osteophyte — *see* Osteophyte
    - pain — *see* Pain, joint
    - psychogenic F45.8
    - specified type NEC M25.8Ø
      - ankle M25.87- ☑
      - elbow M25.82- ☑
      - foot joint M25.87- ☑
      - hand joint M25.84- ☑
      - hip M25.85- ☑
      - knee M25.86- ☑
      - shoulder M25.81- ☑
      - wrist M25.83- ☑
    - stiffness — *see* Stiffness, joint
  - ketone metabolism E71.32
  - kidney N28.9
    - functional (tubular) N25.9
    - in
      - schistosomiasis B65.9 *[N29]*
    - tubular function N25.9
      - specified NEC N25.89
  - lacrimal system HØ4.9
    - changes HØ4.69
      - fistula — *see* Fistula, lacrimal
    - gland HØ4.19
      - atrophy — *see* Atrophy, lacrimal gland
      - cyst — *see* Cyst, lacrimal, gland
      - dacryops — *see* Dacryops
      - dislocation — *see* Dislocation, lacrimal gland
      - dry eye syndrome — *see* Syndrome, dry eye
      - infection — *see* Dacryoadenitis
    - granuloma — *see* Granuloma, lacrimal
    - inflammation — *see* Inflammation, lacrimal
    - obstruction — *see* Obstruction, lacrimal
    - specified NEC HØ4.89
  - lactation NEC O92.79
  - language (developmental) F8Ø.9
    - expressive F8Ø.1
    - mixed receptive and expressive F8Ø.2
    - receptive F8Ø.2
  - late luteal phase dysphoric N94.89
  - learning (specific) F81.9
    - acalculia R48.8
    - alexia R48.Ø
    - mathematics F81.2
    - reading F81.Ø
    - specified
      - with impairment in
        - mathematics F81.2
        - reading F81.Ø

- **Disorder** — *continued*
  - learning — *continued*
    - specified — *continued*
      - with impairment in — *continued*
        - written expression F81.81
    - specified NEC F81.89
    - spelling F81.81
    - written expression F81.81
  - lens H27.9
    - aphakia — *see* Aphakia
    - cataract — *see* Cataract
    - dislocation — *see* Dislocation, lens
    - specified type NEC H27.8
  - ligament M24.2Ø
    - ankle M24.27- ☑
    - attachment, spine — *see* Enthesopathy, spinal
    - elbow M24.22- ☑
    - foot joint M24.27- ☑
    - hand joint M24.24- ☑
    - hip M24.25- ☑
    - knee — *see* Derangement, knee, specified NEC
    - shoulder M24.21- ☑
    - specified site NEC M24.29
    - vertebra M24.28
    - wrist M24.23- ☑
  - ligamentous attachments — *see also* Enthesopathy
    - spine — *see* Enthesopathy, spinal
  - lipid
    - metabolism, congenital E78.9
    - storage E75.6
      - specified NEC E75.5
  - lipoprotein
    - deficiency (familial) E78.6
    - metabolism E78.9
      - specified NEC E78.89
  - liver K76.9
    - malarial B54 *[K77]*
  - low back — *see also* Dorsopathy, specified NEC
  - lumbosacral
    - plexus G54.1
    - root (nerve) NEC G54.4
  - lung, interstitial, drug-induced J7Ø.4
    - acute J7Ø.2
    - chronic J7Ø.3
    - dabbing (related) UØ7.Ø
    - e-cigarette (related) UØ7.Ø
    - electronic cigarette (related) UØ7.Ø
    - vaping (associated) (device) (product) (related) (use) UØ7.Ø
  - lymphoproliferative, post-transplant (PTLD) D47.Z1 (*following* D47.4)
  - lysine and hydroxylysine metabolism E72.3
  - major neurocognitive — *see also* Dementia, in (due to) FØ3.- ☑
  - male
    - erectile (organic) — *see also* Dysfunction, sexual, male, erectile N52.9
      - nonorganic F52.21
    - hypoactive sexual desire F52.Ø
    - orgasmic F52.32
  - manic F3Ø.9
    - organic FØ6.33
  - mast cell activation — *see* Activation, mast cell
  - mastoid — *see also* Disorder, ear, middle
    - postprocedural — *see* Complications, ear, procedure
  - meninges, specified type NEC G96.198
  - meniscus — *see* Derangement, knee, meniscus
  - menopausal N95.9
    - specified NEC N95.8
  - menstrual N92.6
    - psychogenic F45.8
    - specified NEC N92.5
  - mental (or behavioral) (nonpsychotic) F99
    - due to (secondary to)
      - amphetamine
        - due to drug abuse — *see* Abuse, drug, stimulant
        - due to drug dependence — *see* Dependence, drug, stimulant
      - brain disease, damage and dysfunction FØ9
      - caffeine use
        - due to drug abuse — *see* Abuse, drug, stimulant
        - due to drug dependence — *see* Dependence, drug, stimulant
      - cannabis use
        - due to drug abuse — *see* Abuse, drug, cannabis

- **Disorder** — *continued*
  - mental — *continued*
    - due to — *continued*
      - cannabis use — *continued*
        - due to drug dependence — *see* Dependence, drug, cannabis
      - general medical condition F09
      - sedative or hypnotic use
        - due to drug abuse — *see* Abuse, drug, sedative
        - due to drug dependence — *see* Dependence, drug, sedative
      - tobacco (nicotine) use — *see* Dependence, drug, nicotine
    - following organic brain damage F07.9
      - frontal lobe syndrome F07.0
      - personality change F07.0
      - postconcussional syndrome F07.81
      - specified NEC F07.89
    - infancy, childhood or adolescence F98.9
    - neurotic — *see* Neurosis
    - organic or symptomatic F09
    - presenile, psychotic F03.- ☑
    - problem NEC
    - psychoneurotic — *see* Neurosis
    - psychotic — *see* Psychosis
    - puerperal F53.0
    - senile, psychotic NEC F03.- ☑
  - metabolic, amino acid, transitory, newborn P74.8
  - metabolism NOS E88.9
    - amino-acid E72.9
      - aromatic E70.9
        - albinism — *see* Albinism
        - histidine E70.40
          - histidinemia E70.41
          - other specified E70.49
        - hyperphenylalaninemia E70.1
          - classical phenylketonuria E70.0
        - other specified E70.89
        - tryptophan E70.5
        - tyrosine E70.20
          - hypertyrosinemia E70.21
          - other specified E70.29
      - branched chain E71.2
        - 3-methylglutaconic aciduria E71.111
        - hyperleucine-isoleucinemia E71.19
        - hypervalinemia E71.19
        - isovaleric acidemia E71.110
        - maple syrup urine disease E71.0
        - methylmalonic acidemia E71.120
        - organic aciduria NEC E71.118
        - other specified E71.19
        - propionate NEC E71.128
        - propionic acidemia E71.121
      - glycine E72.50
        - d-glycericacidemia E72.59
        - hyperhydroxyprolinemia E72.59
        - hyperoxaluria R82.992
          - primary E72.53- ☑
        - hyperprolinemia E72.59
        - non-ketotic hyperglycinemia E72.51
        - other specified E72.59
        - sarcosinemia E72.59
        - trimethylaminuria E72.52
      - hydroxylysine E72.3
      - lysine E72.3
      - ornithine E72.4
      - other specified E72.89
        - beta-amino acid E72.89
        - gamma-glutamyl cycle E72.89
      - straight-chain E72.89
      - sulfur-bearing E72.10
        - homocystinuria E72.11
        - methylenetetrahydrofolate reductase deficiency E72.12
        - other specified E72.19
    - bile acid and cholesterol metabolism E78.70
    - bilirubin E80.7
      - specified NEC E80.6
    - calcium E83.50
      - hypercalcemia E83.52
      - hypocalcemia E83.51
      - other specified E83.59
    - carbohydrate E74.9
      - specified NEC E74.89
    - cholesterol and bile acid metabolism E78.70
    - citrate NEC E74.829
    - congenital E88.9
    - copper E83.00
      - specified type NEC E83.09

- **Disorder** — *continued*
  - metabolism — *continued*
    - copper — *continued*
      - Wilson's disease E83.01
    - cystinuria E72.01
    - fructose E74.10
    - galactose E74.20
    - glucosaminoglycan E76.9
      - mucopolysaccharidosis — *see* Mucopolysaccharidosis
      - specified NEC E76.8
    - glutamine E72.89
    - glycine E72.50
    - glycogen storage (hepatorenal) E74.09
    - glycoprotein E77.9
      - specified NEC E77.8
    - glycosaminoglycan E76.9
      - specified NEC E76.8
    - in labor and delivery O75.89
    - iron E83.10
    - isoleucine E71.19
    - leucine E71.19
    - lipoid E78.9
    - lipoprotein E78.9
      - specified NEC E78.89
    - magnesium E83.40
      - hypermagnesemia E83.41
      - hypomagnesemia E83.42
      - other specified E83.49
    - mineral E83.9
      - specified NEC E83.89
    - mitochondrial E88.40
      - aminoacyl-tRNA synthetase E88.43
      - ARS2-related E88.43
      - MELAS syndrome E88.41
      - MERRF syndrome (myoclonic epilepsy associated with ragged-red fibers) E88.42
      - other specified E88.49
      - tRNA synthetases E88.43
    - ornithine E72.4
    - phosphatases E83.30
    - phosphorus E83.30
      - acid phosphatase deficiency E83.39
      - hypophosphatasia E83.39
      - hypophosphatemia E83.39
        - familial E83.31
      - other specified E83.39
      - pseudovitamin D deficiency E83.32
    - plasma protein NEC E88.09
    - porphyrin — *see* Porphyria
    - postprocedural E89.89
      - specified NEC E89.89
    - purine E79.9
      - specified NEC E79.89
    - pyrimidine E79.9
      - specified NEC E79.89
    - pyruvate E74.4
    - serine E72.89
    - sodium E87.8
    - specified NEC E88.89
    - threonine E72.89
    - valine E71.19
    - zinc E83.2
  - methylmalonic acidemia E71.120
  - micturition NEC — *see also* Difficulty, micturition R39.198
    - feeling of incomplete emptying R39.14
    - hesitancy R39.11
    - poor stream R39.12
    - psychogenic F45.8
    - split stream R39.13
    - straining R39.16
    - urgency R39.15
  - mild neurocognitive G31.84
    - due to known physiological condition (without behavioral disturbance) F06.70
      - with behavioral disturbance F06.71
  - mitochondrial metabolism E88.40
  - mitral (valve) — *see* Endocarditis, mitral
  - mixed
    - anxiety and depressive F41.8
    - of scholastic skills (developmental) F81.89
    - receptive expressive language F80.2
  - mood F39
    - bipolar — *see* Disorder, bipolar
    - depressive — *see* Disorder, depressive
    - due to (secondary to)
      - alcohol F10.94
      - amphetamine F15.94

- **Disorder** — *continued*
  - mood — *continued*
    - due to — *continued*
      - amphetamine — *continued*
        - in
          - abuse F15.14
          - dependence F15.24
      - anxiolytic F13.94
        - in
          - abuse F13.14
          - dependence F13.24
      - cocaine F14.94
        - in
          - abuse F14.14
          - dependence F14.24
      - general medical condition F06.30
      - hallucinogen F16.94
        - in
          - abuse F16.14
          - dependence F16.24
      - hypnotic F13.94
        - in
          - abuse F13.14
          - dependence F13.24
      - inhalant F18.94
        - in
          - abuse F18.14
          - dependence F18.24
      - opioid F11.94
        - in
          - abuse F11.14
          - dependence F11.24
      - phencyclidine (PCP) F16.94
        - in
          - abuse F16.14
          - dependence F16.24
      - physiological condition F06.30
        - with
          - depressive features F06.31
          - major depressive-like episode F06.32
          - manic features F06.33
          - mixed features F06.34
      - psychoactive substance NEC F19.94
        - in
          - abuse F19.14
          - dependence F19.24
      - sedative F13.94
        - in
          - abuse F13.14
          - dependence F13.24
      - volatile solvents F18.94
        - in
          - abuse F18.14
          - dependence F18.24
    - manic episode F30.9
      - with psychotic symptoms F30.2
      - in remission (full) F30.4
        - partial F30.3
      - specified type NEC F30.8
      - without psychotic symptoms F30.10
        - mild F30.11
        - moderate F30.12
        - severe F30.13
    - organic F06.30
      - right hemisphere F07.89
    - persistent F34.9
      - cyclothymia F34.0
      - dysthymia F34.1
      - specified type NEC F34.89
    - recurrent F39
    - right hemisphere organic F07.89
  - movement G25.9
    - drug-induced G25.70
      - akathisia G25.71
      - specified NEC G25.79
    - hysterical F44.4
    - in diseases classified elsewhere — *see* category G26
    - periodic limb G47.61
      - sleep related G47.61
    - sleep related NEC G47.69
    - specified NEC G25.89
    - stereotyped F98.4
    - treatment-induced G25.9
  - multiple personality F44.81
  - muscle M62.9
    - attachment, spine — *see* Enthesopathy, spinal
    - in trichinellosis — *see* Trichinellosis, with muscle disorder
    - psychogenic F45.8

- **Disorder** — *continued*
  - muscle — *continued*
    - specified type NEC M62.89
    - tone, newborn P94.9
      - specified NEC P94.8
  - muscular
    - attachments — *see also* Enthesopathy
      - spine — *see* Enthesopathy, spinal
    - urethra N36.44
  - musculoskeletal system, soft tissue — *see* Disorder, soft tissue
    - postprocedural M96.89
    - psychogenic F45.8
  - myoneural G70.9
    - due to lead G70.1
    - specified NEC G70.89
    - toxic G70.1
  - myotonic NEC G71.19
  - nail, in diseases classified elsewhere L62
  - neck region NEC — *see* Dorsopathy, specified NEC
  - neonatal onset multisystemic inflammatory (NOMID) M04.2
  - nerve G58.9
    - abducent NEC — *see* Strabismus, paralytic, sixth nerve
    - accessory G52.8
    - acoustic — *see* subcategory H93.3- ☑
    - auditory — *see* subcategory H93.3- ☑
    - auriculotemporal G50.8
    - axillary G54.0
    - cerebral — *see* Disorder, nerve, cranial
    - cranial G52.9
      - eighth — *see* subcategory H93.3- ☑
      - eleventh G52.8
      - fifth G50.9
      - first G52.0
      - fourth NEC — *see* Strabismus, paralytic, fourth nerve
      - multiple G52.7
      - ninth G52.1
      - second NEC — *see* Disorder, nerve, optic
      - seventh NEC G51.8
      - sixth NEC — *see* Strabismus, paralytic, sixth nerve
      - specified NEC G52.8
      - tenth G52.2
      - third NEC — *see* Strabismus, paralytic, third nerve
      - twelfth G52.3
    - entrapment — *see* Neuropathy, entrapment
    - facial G51.9
      - specified NEC G51.8
    - femoral — *see* Lesion, nerve, femoral
    - glossopharyngeal NEC G52.1
    - hypoglossal G52.3
    - intercostal G58.0
    - lateral
      - cutaneous of thigh — *see* Mononeuropathy, lower limb, meralgia paresthetica
      - popliteal — *see* Lesion, nerve, popliteal
    - lower limb — *see* Mononeuropathy, lower limb
    - medial popliteal — *see* Lesion, nerve, popliteal, medial
    - median NEC — *see* Lesion, nerve, median
    - multiple G58.7
    - oculomotor NEC — *see* Strabismus, paralytic, third nerve
    - olfactory G52.0
    - optic NEC H47.09- ☑
      - hemorrhage into sheath — *see* Hemorrhage, optic nerve
      - ischemic H47.01- ☑
    - peroneal — *see* Lesion, nerve, popliteal
    - phrenic G58.8
    - plantar — *see* Lesion, nerve, plantar
    - pneumogastric G52.2
    - posterior tibial — *see* Syndrome, tarsal tunnel
    - radial — *see* Lesion, nerve, radial
    - recurrent laryngeal G52.2
    - root G54.9
      - cervical G54.2
      - lumbosacral G54.1
      - specified NEC G54.8
      - thoracic G54.3
    - sciatic NEC — *see* Lesion, nerve, sciatic
    - specified NEC G58.8
      - lower limb — *see* Mononeuropathy, lower limb, specified NEC
      - upper limb — *see* Mononeuropathy, upper limb, specified NEC
    - sympathetic G90.9
    - tibial — *see* Lesion, nerve, popliteal, medial

- **Disorder** — *continued*
  - nerve — *continued*
    - trigeminal G50.9
      - specified NEC G50.8
    - trochlear NEC — *see* Strabismus, paralytic, fourth nerve
    - ulnar — *see* Lesion, nerve, ulnar
    - upper limb — *see* Mononeuropathy, upper limb
    - vagus G52.2
  - nervous system G98.8
    - autonomic (peripheral) G90.9
      - specified NEC G90.89
    - central G96.9
      - specified NEC G96.89
    - parasympathetic G90.9
    - specified NEC G98.8
    - sympathetic G90.9
    - vegetative G90.9
  - neurocognitive R41.9
    - with Lewy bodies — *see also* Dementia, in, diseases specified elsewhere G31.83 *[F02.-]* ☑
    - frontotemporal, specified NEC — *see also* Dementia, in, diseases specified elsewhere G31.09 *[F02.-]* ☑
    - major — *see also* Dementia F03.- ☑
      - due to vascular disease — *see* Dementia, vascular
        - mild — *see* Dementia, vascular, mild
        - moderate — *see* Dementia, vascular, moderate
        - severe — *see* Dementia, vascular, severe
      - in (due to) (other diseases classified elsewhere) — *see also* Dementia, in (due to) F02.80
        - with
          - aggressive behavior — *see also* Dementia, in (due to) F02.81- ☑
          - combative behavior — *see also* Dementia, in (due to) F02.81- ☑
          - violent behavior — *see also* Dementia, in (due to) F02.81- ☑
    - mild (of uncertain or unknown etiology) — *see also* Disorder, mild neurocognitive G31.84
  - neurodevelopmental F89
    - CACNA1A-related QA0.0102
    - DLG4-related synaptopathy QA0.0142
    - FOXG1-related QA0.0151
    - GRIA1-related QA0.011
    - GRIA2-related QA0.011
    - GRIA3-related QA0.011
    - GRIA4-related QA0.011
    - GRIK2-related QA0.011
    - GRIN1-related QA0.011
    - GRIN2A-related QA0.011
    - GRIN2B-related QA0.011
    - GRIN2D-related QA0.011
    - other
      - glutamate receptor, ionotropic, related QA0.011
      - ion channel gene related QA0.0109
      - receptor gene related QA0.012
      - related to other genes associated with transcription and gene expression QA0.0159
      - synapse related gene QA0.0149
      - transporter or solute carrier gene related QA0.0139
    - SCN2A-related QA0.0101
    - SLC6A1-related QA0.0131
    - specified NEC F88
      - related to pathogenic variants in specific genes NEC QA0.8
    - STXBP1-related QA0.0141
    - syntaxin-binding protein 1-related QA0.0141
  - neurohypophysis NEC E23.3
  - neurological NEC R29.818
    - TUBB4A-related G23.3
  - neuromuscular G70.9
    - hereditary NEC G71.9
    - specified NEC G70.89
    - toxic G70.1
  - neurotic F48.9
    - specified NEC F48.8
  - neutrophil, polymorphonuclear D71.9
    - specified NEC D71.8
  - nicotine use — *see* Dependence, drug, nicotine
  - nightmare F51.5
  - non-rapid eye movement sleep arousal
    - sleep terror type F51.4
    - sleepwalking type F51.3
  - nose J34.9
    - specified NEC J34.89
  - obsessive-compulsive F42.9

- **Disorder** — *continued*
  - obsessive-compulsive — *continued*
    - and related disorder due to a known physiological condition F06.8
  - odontogenesis NOS K00.9
  - opioid use
    - with
      - opioid-induced psychotic disorder F11.959
        - with
          - delusions F11.950
          - hallucinations F11.951
    - due to drug abuse — *see* Abuse, drug, opioid
    - due to drug dependence — *see* Dependence, drug, opioid
    - mild F11.10
      - with
        - opioid-induced
          - anxiety disorder F11.188
          - depressive disorder F11.14
          - sexual dysfunction F11.181
        - opioid intoxication
          - with perceptual disturbances F11.122
          - delirium F11.121
          - without perceptual disturbances F11.129
      - in remission (early) (sustained) F11.11
    - moderate or severe F11.20
      - with
        - opioid-induced
          - anxiety disorder F11.288
          - depressive disorder F11.24
          - sexual dysfunction F11.281
        - opioid intoxication
          - with perceptual disturbances F11.222
          - delirium F11.221
          - without perceptual disturbances F11.229
      - in remission (early) (sustained) F11.21
  - oppositional defiant F91.3
  - optic
    - chiasm H47.49
      - due to
        - inflammatory disorder H47.41
        - neoplasm H47.42
        - vascular disorder H47.43
    - disc H47.39- ☑
      - coloboma — *see* Coloboma, optic disc
      - drusen — *see* Drusen, optic disc
      - pseudopapilledema — *see* Pseudopapilledema
    - radiations — *see* Disorder, visual, pathway
    - tracts — *see* Disorder, visual, pathway
  - orbit H05.9
    - cyst — *see* Cyst, orbit
    - deformity — *see* Deformity, orbit
    - edema — *see* Edema, orbit
    - enophthalmos — *see* Enophthalmos
    - exophthalmos — *see* Exophthalmos
    - hemorrhage — *see* Hemorrhage, orbit
    - inflammation — *see* Inflammation, orbit
    - myopathy — *see* Myopathy, extraocular muscles
    - retained foreign body — *see* Foreign body, orbit, old
    - specified type NEC H05.89
  - organic
    - anxiety F06.4
    - catatonic NOS F06.1
    - delusional F06.2
    - dissociative F06.8
    - emotionally labile (asthenic) F06.8
    - mood (affective) F06.30
    - schizophrenia-like F06.2
  - orgasmic (female) F52.31
    - male F52.32
  - ornithine metabolism E72.4
  - overanxious F41.1
    - of childhood F93.8
  - pain
    - with related psychological factors F45.42
    - exclusively related to psychological factors F45.41
    - genito-pelvic penetration disorder F52.6
  - pancreatic internal secretion E16.9
    - specified NEC E16.8
  - panic F41.0
    - with agoraphobia F40.01
  - papulosquamous L44.9
    - in diseases classified elsewhere L45
    - specified NEC L44.8
  - paranoid F22
    - induced F24
    - shared F24
  - paraphilic F65.9
    - specified NEC F65.89

**Displacement, displaced** — *continued*
- brachial plexus (congenital) QØ7.8
- brain stem, caudal (congenital) QØ4.8
- canaliculus (lacrimalis), congenital Q1Ø.6
- cardia through esophageal hiatus (congenital) Q4Ø.1
- cerebellum, caudal (congenital) QØ4.8
- cervix — *see* Malposition, uterus
- colon (congenital) Q43.3
- device, implant or graft — *see also* Complications, by site and type, mechanical T85.628- ☑
  - arterial graft NEC — *see* Complication, cardiovascular device, mechanical, vascular
  - breast (implant) T85.42- ☑
  - catheter NEC T85.628- ☑
    - dialysis (renal) T82.42- ☑
      - intraperitoneal T85.621- ☑
    - infusion NEC T82.524- ☑
      - spinal (epidural) (subdural) T85.62Ø- ☑
    - urinary
      - cystostomy T83.Ø2Ø- ☑
      - Hopkins T83.Ø28- ☑
      - ileostomy T83.Ø28- ☑
      - indwelling T83.Ø21- ☑
      - nephrostomy T83.Ø22- ☑
      - specified NEC T83.Ø28- ☑
      - urostomy T83.Ø28- ☑
  - electronic (electrode) (pulse generator) (stimulator) — *see* Complication, electronic stimulator
  - fixation, internal (orthopedic) NEC — *see* Complication, fixation device, mechanical
  - gastrointestinal — *see* Complications, prosthetic device, mechanical, gastrointestinal device
  - genital NEC T83.428- ☑
    - intrauterine contraceptive device (string) T83.32- ☑
    - penile prosthesis (cylinder) (implanted) (pump) (reservoir) T83.42Ø- ☑
    - testicular prosthesis T83.421- ☑
  - heart NEC — *see* Complication, cardiovascular device, mechanical
  - joint prosthesis — *see* Complications, joint prosthesis, mechanical
  - ocular — *see* Complications, prosthetic device, mechanical, ocular device
  - orthopedic NEC — *see* Complication, orthopedic, device or graft, mechanical
  - specified NEC T85.628- ☑
  - urinary NEC T83.128- ☑
    - graft T83.22- ☑
    - sphincter, implanted T83.121- ☑
    - stent (ileal conduit) (nephroureteral) T83.123- ☑
      - ureteral indwelling T83.122- ☑
  - vascular NEC — *see* Complication, cardiovascular device, mechanical
  - ventricular intracranial shunt T85.Ø2- ☑
- electronic stimulator
  - bone T84.32Ø- ☑
  - cardiac — *see* Complications, cardiac device, electronic
  - nervous system — *see* Complication, prosthetic device, mechanical, electronic nervous system stimulator
  - urinary — *see* Complications, electronic stimulator, urinary
- esophageal mucosa into cardia of stomach, congenital Q39.8
- esophagus (acquired) K22.89
  - congenital Q39.8
- eyeball (acquired) (lateral) (old) — *see* Displacement, globe
  - congenital Q15.8
  - current — *see* Avulsion, eye
- fallopian tube (acquired) N83.4- ☑
  - congenital Q5Ø.6
  - opening (congenital) Q5Ø.6
- gallbladder (congenital) Q44.1
- gastric mucosa (congenital) Q4Ø.2
- globe (acquired) (old) (lateral) HØ5.21- ☑
  - current — *see* Avulsion, eye
- heart (congenital) Q24.8
  - acquired I51.89
- hymen (upward) (congenital) Q52.4
- intervertebral disc NEC
  - with myelopathy — *see* Disorder, disc, with, myelopathy
  - cervical, cervicothoracic (with) M5Ø.2Ø

**Displacement, displaced** — *continued*
- intervertebral disc — *continued*
  - cervical, cervicothoracic — *continued*
    - myelopathy — *see* Disorder, disc, cervical, with myelopathy
    - neuritis, radiculitis or radiculopathy — *see* Disorder, disc, cervical, with neuritis
  - due to trauma — *see* Dislocation, vertebra
  - lumbar region M51.26
    - with
      - myelopathy M51.Ø6
      - neuritis, radiculitis, radiculopathy or sciatica M51.16
  - lumbosacral region M51.27
    - with
      - neuritis, radiculitis, radiculopathy or sciatica M51.17
  - sacrococcygeal region M53.3
  - thoracic region M51.24
    - with
      - myelopathy M51.Ø4
      - neuritis, radiculitis, radiculopathy M51.14
  - thoracolumbar region M51.25
    - with
      - myelopathy M51.Ø5
      - neuritis, radiculitis, radiculopathy M51.15
- intrauterine device (string) T83.32- ☑
- kidney (acquired) N28.83
  - congenital Q63.2
- lachrymal, lacrimal apparatus or duct (congenital) Q1Ø.6
- lens, congenital Q12.1
- macula (congenital) Q14.1
- Meckel's diverticulum Q43.Ø
  - malignant — *see* Table of Neoplasms, small intestine, malignant
- nail (congenital) Q84.6
  - acquired L6Ø.8
- opening of Wharton's duct in mouth Q38.4
- organ or site, congenital NEC — *see* Malposition, congenital
- ovary (acquired) N83.4- ☑
  - congenital Q5Ø.39
  - free in peritoneal cavity (congenital) Q5Ø.39
    - into hernial sac N83.4- ☑
- oviduct (acquired) N83.4- ☑
  - congenital Q5Ø.6
- parathyroid (gland) E21.4
- parotid gland (congenital) Q38.4
- punctum lacrimale (congenital) Q1Ø.6
- sacro-iliac (joint) (congenital) Q74.2
  - current injury S33.2- ☑
  - old — *see* subcategory M53.2- ☑
- salivary gland (any) (congenital) Q38.4
- spleen (congenital) Q89.Ø9
- stomach, congenital Q4Ø.2
- sublingual duct Q38.4
- tongue (downward) (congenital) Q38.3
- tooth, teeth, fully erupted M26.3Ø
  - horizontal M26.33
  - vertical M26.34
- trachea (congenital) Q32.1
- ureter or ureteric opening or orifice (congenital) Q62.62
- uterine opening of oviducts or fallopian tubes Q5Ø.6
- uterus, uterine — *see* Malposition, uterus
- ventricular septum Q21.Ø
  - with rudimentary ventricle Q2Ø.4

**Disproportion**
- between native and reconstructed breast N65.1
- fiber-type G71.2Ø
  - congenital G71.29

**Disruptio uteri** — *see* Rupture, uterus

**Disruption** (of)
- ciliary body NEC H21.89
- closure of
  - abdominal wall muscle or fascia T81.321- ☑
  - cornea T81.31- ☑
  - craniotomy T81.328- ☑
  - fascia (muscular) (superficial) T81.328- ☑
  - gastrointestinal tract anastomosis, repair, or closure T81.32Ø- ☑
  - internal organ or tissue T81.328- ☑
  - laceration (external) (internal) T81.33- ☑
  - ligament T81.328- ☑
  - mucosa T81.31- ☑
  - muscle or muscle flap T81.328- ☑
  - ribs or rib cage T81.328- ☑
  - skin and subcutaneous tissue (full-thickness) (superficial) T81.31- ☑

**Disruption** — *continued*
- closure of — *continued*
  - skull T81.328- ☑
  - sternum (sternotomy) T81.328- ☑
  - tendon T81.328- ☑
  - traumatic laceration (external) (internal) T81.33- ☑
- family Z63.8
  - due to
    - absence of family member due to military deployment Z63.31
    - absence of family member NEC Z63.32
    - alcoholism and drug addiction in family Z63.72
    - bereavement Z63.4
    - death (assumed) or disappearance of family member Z63.4
    - divorce or separation Z63.5
    - drug addiction in family Z63.72
    - return of family member from military deployment (current or past conflict) Z63.71
    - stressful life events NEC Z63.79
- iris NEC H21.89
- ligament(s) — *see also* Sprain
  - knee
    - current injury — *see* Dislocation, knee
    - old (chronic) — *see* Derangement, knee, instability
    - spontaneous NEC — *see* Derangement, knee, disruption ligament
- ossicular chain — *see* Discontinuity, ossicles, ear
- pelvic ring (stable) S32.81Ø- ☑
  - unstable S32.811- ☑
- traumatic injury wound repair T81.33- ☑
- wound T81.3Ø- ☑
  - episiotomy O9Ø.1
  - operation T81.31- ☑
    - cesarean O9Ø.Ø
    - deep T81.329- ☑
    - external operation wound (superficial) T81.31- ☑
    - internal operation wound (deep) T81.329- ☑
      - abdominal wall muscle or fascia T81.321- ☑
      - specified NEC T81.328- ☑
  - perineal (obstetric) O9Ø.1
  - traumatic injury repair T81.33- ☑

**Dissatisfaction with**
- employment Z56.9
- school environment Z55.4

**Dissecting** — *see* condition

**Dissection**
- aorta I71.ØØ
  - abdominal I71.Ø2
  - thoracic I71.Ø19
    - aortic arch I71.Ø11
    - ascending aorta I71.Ø1Ø
    - descending thoracic aorta I71.Ø12
  - thoracoabdominal I71.Ø3
- artery I77.7Ø
  - basilar (trunk) I77.75
  - carotid I77.71
  - cerebral (nonruptured) I67.Ø
    - ruptured — *see* Hemorrhage, intracranial, subarachnoid
  - coronary I25.42
  - extremity
    - lower I77.77
    - upper I77.76
  - iliac I77.72
  - precerebral
    - congenital (nonruptured) Q28.1
    - specified site NEC I77.75
  - renal I77.73
  - specified NEC I77.79
  - vertebral I77.74
- precerebral artery, congenital (nonruptured) Q28.1
- traumatic — *see* Wound, open, by site
- vascular I99.8
- wound — *see* Wound, open

**Disseminated** — *see* condition

**Dissociation**
- auriculoventricular or atrioventricular (AV) (any degree) (isorhythmic) I45.89
  - with heart block I44.2
- interference I45.89

**Dissociative reaction, state** F44.9

**Dissolution, vertebra** — *see* Osteoporosis

**Distension, distention**
- abdomen R14.Ø
- bladder N32.89
- cecum K63.89
- colon K63.89

**Dix-Hallpike neurolabyrinthitis** — *see* Neuronitis, vestibular
**Dizziness** R42
  hysterical F44.89
  psychogenic F45.8
**DMAC** (disseminated mycobacterium avium- intracellulare complex) A31.2
**DNR** (do not resuscitate) Z66
**Doan-Wiseman syndrome** (primary splenic neutropenia) — *see* Agranulocytosis
**Doehle-Heller aortitis** A52.Ø2
**Dog bite** — *see* External Cause of Injuries Index - Bite, bitten by, dog
**Dohle body panmyelopathic syndrome** D72.Ø
**Dolichocephaly** Q67.2
  non-deformational Q75.Ø1
**Dolichocolon** Q43.8
**Dolichostenomelia** — *see* Syndrome, Marfan
**Donohue's syndrome** E34.8
**Donor** (organ or tissue) Z52.9
  blood (whole) Z52.ØØØ
    autologous Z52.Ø1Ø
    specified component (lymphocytes) (platelets) NEC Z52.ØØ8
      autologous Z52.Ø18
      specified donor NEC Z52.Ø98
    specified donor NEC Z52.Ø9Ø
    stem cells Z52.ØØ1
      autologous Z52.Ø11
      specified donor NEC Z52.Ø91
  bone Z52.2Ø
    autologous Z52.21
    marrow Z52.3
    specified type NEC Z52.29
  cornea Z52.5
  egg (Oocyte) Z52.819
    age 35 and over Z52.812
      anonymous recipient Z52.812
      designated recipient Z52.813
    under age 35 Z52.81Ø
      anonymous recipient Z52.81Ø
      designated recipient Z52.811
  kidney Z52.4
  liver Z52.6
  lung Z52.89
  lymphocyte — *see* Donor, blood, specified components NEC
  Oocyte — *see* Donor, egg
  platelets Z52.ØØ8
  potential, examination of ZØØ.5
  semen Z52.89
  skin Z52.1Ø
    autologous Z52.11
    specified type NEC Z52.19
  specified organ or tissue NEC Z52.89
  sperm Z52.89
**Donovanosis** A58
**Dorsalgia** M54.9
  psychogenic F45.41
  specified NEC M54.89
**Dorsopathy** M53.9
  deforming M43.9
    specified NEC — *see* subcategory M43.8- ☑
  specified NEC M53.8Ø
    cervical region M53.82
    cervicothoracic region M53.83
    lumbar region M53.86
    lumbosacral region M53.87
    occipito-atlanto-axial region M53.81
    sacrococcygeal region M53.88
    thoracic region M53.84
    thoracolumbar region M53.85
**Double**
  albumin E88.Ø9
  aortic arch Q25.45
  auditory canal Q17.8
  auricle (heart) Q2Ø.8
  bladder Q64.79
  cervix Q51.82Ø
    with doubling of uterus (and vagina) Q51.1Ø
      with obstruction Q51.11
  inlet ventricle Q2Ø.4
  kidney with double pelvis (renal) Q63.Ø
  meatus urinarius Q64.75
  monster Q89.4
  outlet
    left ventricle Q2Ø.2
    right ventricle Q2Ø.1
  pelvis (renal) with double ureter Q62.5
**Double** — *continued*
  tongue Q38.3
  ureter (one or both sides) Q62.5
    with double pelvis (renal) Q62.5
  urethra Q64.74
  urinary meatus Q64.75
  uterus Q51.28
    with
      doubling of cervix (and vagina) Q51.1Ø
        with obstruction Q51.11
    complete Q51.21
    in pregnancy or childbirth O34.Ø- ☑
      causing obstructed labor O65.5
    partial Q51.22
    specified NEC Q51.28
  vagina Q52.1Ø
    with doubling of uterus (and cervix) Q51.1Ø
      with obstruction Q51.11
  vision H53.2
  vulva Q52.79
**Doubled up** Z59.Ø1
**Douglas' pouch, cul-de-sac** — *see* condition
**Down syndrome** Q9Ø.9
  meiotic nondisjunction Q9Ø.Ø
  mitotic nondisjunction Q9Ø.1
  mosaicism Q9Ø.1
  translocation Q9Ø.2
**DPD** (dihydropyrimidine dehydrogenase deficiency) E88.89
**Dracontiasis** B72
**Dracunculiasis, dracunculosis** B72
**Dream state, hysterical** F44.89
**Drepanocytic anemia** — *see* Disease, sickle-cell
**Dresbach's syndrome** (elliptocytosis) D58.1
**Dreschlera** (hawaiiensis) (infection) B43.8
**Dressler's syndrome** I24.1
**Drift, ulnar** — *see* Deformity, limb, specified type NEC, forearm
**Drinking** (alcohol)
  excessive, to excess NEC (without dependence) F1Ø.1Ø
    habitual (continual) (without remission) F1Ø.2Ø
      with remission F1Ø.21
**Drip, postnasal** (chronic) RØ9.82
  due to
    allergic rhinitis — *see* Rhinitis, allergic
    common cold JØØ
    gastroesophageal reflux — *see* Reflux, gastroesophageal
    nasopharyngitis — *see* Nasopharyngitis
    other known condition — *code to* condition
    sinusitis — *see* Sinusitis
**Droop**
  facial R29.81Ø
    cerebrovascular disease I69.992
      cerebral infarction I69.392
      intracerebral hemorrhage I69.192
      nontraumatic intracranial hemorrhage NEC I69.292
      specified disease NEC I69.892
      subarachnoid hemorrhage I69.Ø92
**Drop** (in)
  attack NEC R55
  finger — *see* Deformity, finger
  foot — *see* Deformity, limb, foot, drop
  hematocrit (precipitous) R71.Ø
  hemoglobin R71.Ø
  toe — *see* Deformity, toe, specified NEC
  wrist — *see* Deformity, limb, wrist drop
**Dropped heart beats** I45.9
**Dropsy, dropsical** — *see also* Hydrops
  abdomen R18.8
  brain — *see* Hydrocephalus
  cardiac, heart — *see* Failure, heart, congestive
  gangrenous — *see* Gangrene
  heart — *see* Failure, heart, congestive
  kidney — *see* Nephrosis
  lung — *see* Edema, lung
  newborn due to isoimmunization P56.Ø
  pericardium — *see* Pericarditis
**Drowned, drowning** (near) T75.1- ☑
**Drowsiness** R4Ø.Ø
**Drug**
  abuse counseling and surveillance Z71.51
  addiction — *see* Dependence
  dependence — *see* Dependence
  habit — *see* Dependence
  harmful use — *see* Abuse, drug
  induced fever R5Ø.2
  overdose — *see* Table of Drugs and Chemicals, by drug, poisoning
**Drug** — *continued*
  poisoning — *see* Table of Drugs and Chemicals, by drug, poisoning
  resistant organism infection — *see also* Resistant, organism, to, drug Z16.3Ø
  therapy
    long term (current) (prophylactic) — *see* Therapy, drug long-term (current) (prophylactic)
    short term — *omit code*
  wrong substance given or taken in error — *see* Table of Drugs and Chemicals, by drug, poisoning
**Drunkenness** (without dependence) F1Ø.129
  acute in alcoholism F1Ø.229
  chronic (without remission) F1Ø.2Ø
    with remission F1Ø.21
  pathological (without dependence) F1Ø.129
    with dependence F1Ø.229
  sleep F51.9
**Drusen**
  macula (degenerative) (retina) — *see* Degeneration, macula, drusen
  optic disc H47.32- ☑
**Dry, dryness** — *see also* condition
  larynx J38.7
  mouth R68.2
    due to dehydration E86.Ø
  nose J34.89
  socket (teeth) M27.3
  throat J39.2
**DSAP** L56.5
**Duane's syndrome** H5Ø.81- ☑
**Dubin-Johnson disease or syndrome** E8Ø.6
**Dubois' disease** (thymus gland) A5Ø.59 *[E35]*
**Dubowitz' syndrome** Q87.19
**Duchenne-Aran muscular atrophy** G12.21
**Duchenne-Griesinger disease** G71.Ø1
**Duchenne's**
  disease or syndrome
    motor neuron disease G12.22
    muscular dystrophy G71.Ø1
  locomotor ataxia (syphilitic) A52.11
  paralysis
    birth injury P14.Ø
    due to or associated with
      motor neuron disease G12.22
      muscular dystrophy G71.Ø1
**Ducreyi chancre** A57
**Ducrey's chancre** A57
**Duct, ductus** — *see* condition
**Duffy phenotype** — *see* Phenotype, Duffy
**Duhring's disease** (dermatitis herpetiformis) L13.Ø
**Dullness, cardiac** (decreased) (increased) RØ1.2
**Dumb ague** — *see* Malaria
**Dumbness** — *see* Aphasia
**Dumdum fever** B55.Ø
**Dumping syndrome** (postgastrectomy) K91.1
**Duodenitis** (nonspecific) (peptic) K29.8Ø
  with bleeding K29.81
  erosive — *see* Ulcer, duodenum
**Duodenocholangitis** — *see* Cholangitis
**Duodenum, duodenal** — *see* condition
**Duplay's bursitis or periarthritis** M75.Ø- ☑
**Duplication, duplex** — *see also* Accessory
  alimentary tract Q45.8
  anus Q43.4
  appendix (and cecum) Q43.4
  biliary duct (any) Q44.5
  bladder Q64.79
  cecum (and appendix) Q43.4
  cervix Q51.82Ø
  chromosome NEC — *see also* Trisomy
    with complex rearrangements NEC Q92.5
    seen only at prometaphase Q92.8
  cystic duct Q44.5
  digestive organs Q45.8
  esophagus Q39.8
  frontonasal process Q75.8
  intestine (large) (small) Q43.4
  kidney Q63.Ø
  liver Q44.79
  pancreas Q45.3
  penis Q55.69
  respiratory organs NEC Q34.8
  salivary duct Q38.4
  spinal cord (incomplete) QØ6.2
  stomach Q4Ø.2
**Dupre's disease** (meningism) R29.1
**Dupuytren's contraction or disease** M72.Ø
**Durand-Nicolas-Favre disease** A55

- **Durotomy** (inadvertent) (incidental) G97.41
- **Duroziez's disease** (congenital mitral stenosis) Q23.2
- **Dutton's relapsing fever** (West African) A68.1
- **Dwarfism** — *see also* Short, stature E34.328
  - achondroplastic Q77.4
  - congenital — *see also* Short, stature E34.328
  - constitutional E34.31
  - hypochondroplastic Q77.4
  - hypophyseal E23.Ø
  - infantile — *see also* Short, stature E34.328
  - Laron-type — *see also* Short, stature E34.321
  - Lorain (-Levi) type E23.Ø
  - metatropic Q77.8
  - nephrotic-glycosuric (with hypophosphatemic rickets) E72.Ø9
  - nutritional E45
  - pancreatic K86.89
  - pituitary E23.Ø
  - renal N25.Ø
  - thanatophoric Q77.1
- **Dyke-Young anemia** (secondary) (symptomatic) D59.19
- **Dysacusis** — *see* Abnormal, auditory perception
- **Dysadrenocortism** E27.9
  - hyperfunction E27.Ø
- **Dysarthria** R47.1
  - following
    - cerebral infarction I69.322
    - cerebrovascular disease I69.922
      - specified disease NEC I69.822
    - intracerebral hemorrhage I69.122
    - nontraumatic intracranial hemorrhage NEC I69.222
    - subarachnoid hemorrhage I69.Ø22
- **Dysautonomia** (familial) G9Ø.1
- **Dysbarism** T7Ø.3- ☑
- **Dysbasia** R26.2
  - angiosclerotica intermittens I73.9
  - hysterical F44.4
  - lordotica (progressiva) G24.1
  - nonorganic origin F44.4
  - psychogenic F44.4
- **Dysbetalipoproteinemia** (familial) E78.2
- **Dyscalculia** R48.8
  - developmental F81.2
- **Dyschezia** K59.ØØ
- **Dyschondroplasia** (with hemangiomata) Q78.4
- **Dyschromia** (skin) L81.9
- **Dyscollagenosis** M35.9
- **Dyscranio-pygo-phalangy** Q87.Ø
- **Dyscrasia**
  - blood (with) D75.9
    - antepartum hemorrhage — *see* Hemorrhage, antepartum, with coagulation defect
    - intrapartum hemorrhage O67.Ø
    - newborn P61.9
      - specified type NEC P61.8
    - puerperal, postpartum O72.3
  - polyglandular, pluriglandular E31.9
- **Dysendocrinism** E34.9
- **Dysentery, dysenteric** (catarrhal) (diarrhea) (epidemic) (hemorrhagic) (infectious) (sporadic) (tropical) AØ9
  - abscess, liver AØ6.4
  - amebic — *see also* Amebiasis AØ6.Ø
    - with abscess — *see* Abscess, amebic
    - acute AØ6.Ø
    - chronic AØ6.1
  - arthritis — *see also* category MØ1 AØ9
    - bacillary — *see also* category MØ1 AØ3.9
  - bacillary AØ3.9
    - arthritis — *see also* category MØ1 AØ3.9
    - Boyd AØ3.2
    - Flexner AØ3.1
    - Schmitz (-Stutzer) AØ3.Ø
    - Shiga (-Kruse) AØ3.Ø
    - Shigella AØ3.9
      - boydii AØ3.2
      - dysenteriae AØ3.Ø
      - flexneri AØ3.1
      - group A AØ3.Ø
      - group B AØ3.1
      - group C AØ3.2
      - group D AØ3.3
      - sonnei AØ3.3
      - specified type NEC AØ3.8
    - Sonne AØ3.3
    - specified type NEC AØ3.8
  - balantidial AØ7.Ø
  - Balantidium coli AØ7.Ø
  - Boyd's AØ3.2
  - candidal B37.82

- **Dysentery, dysenteric** — *continued*
  - Chilomastix AØ7.8
  - Chinese AØ3.9
  - coccidial AØ7.3
  - Dientamoeba (fragilis) AØ7.8
  - Embadomonas AØ7.8
  - Entamoeba, entamebic — *see* Dysentery, amebic
  - Flexner-Boyd AØ3.2
  - Flexner's AØ3.1
  - Giardia lamblia AØ7.1
  - Hiss-Russell AØ3.1
  - Lamblia AØ7.1
  - leishmanial B55.Ø
  - malarial — *see* Malaria
  - metazoal B82.Ø
  - monilial B37.82
  - protozoal AØ7.9
  - Salmonella AØ2.Ø
  - schistosomal B65.1
  - Schmitz (-Stutzer) AØ3.Ø
  - Shiga (-Kruse) AØ3.Ø
  - Shigella NOS — *see* Dysentery, bacillary
  - Sonne AØ3.3
  - strongyloidiasis B78.Ø
  - trichomonal AØ7.8
  - viral — *see also* Enteritis, viral AØ8.4
- **Dysequilibrium** R42
- **Dysesthesia** R2Ø.8
  - hysterical F44.6
- **Dysferlinopathy** G71.Ø33
- **Dysfibrinogenemia** (congenital) D68.2
- **Dysfunction**
  - adrenal E27.9
    - hyperfunction E27.Ø
  - autonomic
    - due to alcohol G31.2
    - somatoform F45.8
  - bladder N31.9
    - neurogenic NOS — *see* Dysfunction, bladder, neuromuscular
    - neuromuscular NOS N31.9
      - atonic (motor) (sensory) N31.2
      - autonomous N31.2
      - flaccid N31.2
      - nonreflex N31.2
      - reflex N31.1
      - specified NEC N31.8
      - uninhibited N31.Ø
  - bleeding, uterus N93.8
  - cerebral G93.89
  - chronic
    - coronary microvascular I25.85
    - lung allograft J4A.9
      - mixed J4A.Ø
      - specified NEC J4A.8
  - colon K59.9
    - psychogenic F45.8
  - colostomy K94.Ø3
  - coronary microvascular I25.85
    - with
      - angina pectoris I2Ø.81
      - myocardial infarction I21.B
    - acute I24.81
    - chronic I25.85
  - cystic duct K82.8
  - cystostomy (stoma) — *see* Complications, cystostomy
  - ejaculatory N53.19
    - anejaculatory orgasm N53.13
    - painful N53.12
    - premature F52.4
    - retarded N53.11
  - endocrine NOS E34.9
  - endometrium N85.8
  - enterostomy K94.13
  - erectile — *see* Dysfunction, sexual, male, erectile
  - feeding, pediatric
    - acute R63.31
    - chronic R63.32
  - gallbladder K82.8
  - gastrostomy (stoma) K94.23
  - gland, glandular NOS E34.9
    - meibomian, of eyelid — *see* Dysfunction, meibomian gland
  - heart I51.89
  - hemoglobin D75.89
  - hepatic K76.89
  - hypophysis E23.7
  - hypothalamic NEC E23.3
  - ileostomy (stoma) K94.13

- **Dysfunction** — *continued*
  - jejunostomy (stoma) K94.13
  - kidney — *see* Disease, renal
  - labyrinthine — *see* subcategory H83.2- ☑
  - left ventricular, following sudden emotional stress I51.81
  - liver K76.89
  - lymphatic
    - Fontan-associated I27.841
  - male — *see* Dysfunction, sexual, male
  - meibomian gland, of eyelid HØ2.889
    - left HØ2.886
      - lower HØ2.885
      - upper HØ2.884
      - upper and lower eyelids HØ2.88B
    - right HØ2.883
      - lower HØ2.882
      - upper HØ2.881
      - upper and lower eyelids HØ2.88A
  - multifidus muscles, lumbar region M62.85
  - orgasmic (female) F52.31
    - male F52.32
  - ovary E28.9
    - specified NEC E28.8
  - papillary muscle I51.89
  - parathyroid E21.4
  - physiological NEC R68.89
    - psychogenic F59
  - pineal gland E34.8
  - pituitary (gland) E23.3
  - platelets D69.19
  - polyglandular E31.9
    - specified NEC E31.8
  - psychophysiologic F59
  - psychosexual F52.9
    - with
      - dyspareunia F52.6
      - premature ejaculation F52.4
      - vaginismus F52.5
  - pylorus K31.9
  - rectum K59.9
    - psychogenic F45.8
  - reflex (sympathetic) — *see* Syndrome, pain, complex regional I
  - segmental — *see* Dysfunction, somatic
  - senile R54
  - sexual (due to) R37
    - alcohol F1Ø.981
      - in
        - abuse F1Ø.181
        - dependence F1Ø.281
    - amphetamine F15.981
      - in
        - abuse F15.181
        - dependence F15.281
    - anxiolytic F13.981
      - in
        - abuse F13.181
        - dependence F13.281
    - cocaine F14.981
      - in
        - abuse F14.181
        - dependence F14.281
    - excessive sexual drive F52.8
    - failure of genital response (male) F52.21
      - female F52.22
    - female N94.9
      - aversion F52.1
      - dyspareunia N94.1Ø
        - psychogenic F52.6
      - frigidity F52.22
      - nymphomania F52.8
      - orgasmic F52.31
      - psychogenic F52.9
        - aversion F52.1
        - dyspareunia F52.6
        - frigidity F52.22
        - nymphomania F52.8
        - orgasmic F52.31
        - vaginismus F52.5
      - vaginismus N94.2
        - psychogenic F52.5
    - hypnotic F13.981
      - in
        - abuse F13.181
        - dependence F13.281
    - inhibited orgasm (female) F52.31
      - male F52.32
    - lack
      - of sexual enjoyment F52.1

- **Dysfunction** — *continued*
  - sexual — *continued*
    - lack — *continued*
      - or loss of sexual desire F52.0
    - male N53.9
      - anejaculatory orgasm N53.13
      - ejaculatory N53.19
        - painful N53.12
        - premature F52.4
        - retarded N53.11
      - erectile N52.9
        - drug induced N52.2
        - due to
          - disease classified elsewhere N52.1
          - drug N52.2
        - postoperative (postprocedural) N52.39
          - following
            - cryotherapy N52.37
            - interstitial seed therapy N52.36
            - prostate ablative therapy N52.37
            - prostatectomy N52.34
              - radical N52.31
            - radiation therapy N52.35
            - radical cystectomy N52.32
            - ultrasound ablative therapy N52.37
            - urethral surgery N52.33
        - psychogenic F52.21
        - specified cause NEC N52.8
        - vasculogenic
          - arterial insufficiency N52.01
            - with corporo-venous occlusive N52.03
          - corporo-venous occlusive N52.02
            - with arterial insufficiency N52.03
      - impotence — *see* Dysfunction, sexual, male, erectile
      - psychogenic F52.9
        - aversion F52.1
        - erectile F52.21
        - orgasmic F52.32
        - premature ejaculation F52.4
        - satyriasis F52.8
        - specified type NEC F52.8
      - specified type NEC N53.8
    - nonorganic F52.9
      - specified NEC F52.8
    - opioid F11.981
      - in
        - abuse F11.181
        - dependence F11.281
    - orgasmic dysfunction (female) F52.31
      - male F52.32
    - premature ejaculation F52.4
    - psychoactive substances NEC F19.981
      - in
        - abuse F19.181
        - dependence F19.281
    - psychogenic F52.9
    - sedative F13.981
      - in
        - abuse F13.181
        - dependence F13.281
    - sexual aversion F52.1
    - vaginismus (nonorganic) (psychogenic) F52.5
  - sinoatrial node I49.5
  - somatic M99.09
    - abdomen M99.09
    - acromioclavicular M99.07
    - cervical region M99.01
    - cervicothoracic M99.01
    - costochondral M99.08
    - costovertebral M99.08
    - head region M99.00
    - hip M99.05
    - lower extremity M99.06
    - lumbar region M99.03
    - lumbosacral M99.03
    - occipitocervical M99.00
    - pelvic region M99.05
    - pubic M99.05
    - rib cage M99.08
    - sacral region M99.04
    - sacrococcygeal M99.04
    - sacroiliac M99.04
    - specified NEC M99.09
    - sternochondral M99.08
    - sternoclavicular M99.07
    - thoracic region M99.02
    - thoracolumbar M99.02
    - upper extremity M99.07
- **Dysfunction** — *continued*
  - somatoform autonomic F45.8
  - stomach K31.89
    - psychogenic F45.8
  - suprarenal E27.9
    - hyperfunction E27.0
  - symbolic R48.9
    - specified type NEC R48.8
  - temporomandibular (joint) M26.69
    - joint-pain syndrome M26.62- ☑
  - testicular (endocrine) E29.9
    - specified NEC E29.8
  - thymus E32.9
  - thyroid E07.9
  - ureterostomy (stoma) — *see* Complications, stoma, urinary tract
  - urethrostomy (stoma) — *see* Complications, stoma, urinary tract
  - uterus, complicating delivery O62.9
    - hypertonic O62.4
    - hypotonic O62.2
      - primary O62.0
      - secondary O62.1
  - ventricular I51.9
    - with congestive heart failure — *see also* Failure, heart I50.9
    - left, reversible, following sudden emotional stress I51.81
- **Dysgenesis**
  - gonadal (due to chromosomal anomaly) Q96.9
    - pure Q99.1
  - renal Q60.5
    - bilateral Q60.4
    - unilateral Q60.3
  - reticular D72.0
  - tidal platelet D69.3
- **Dysgerminoma**
  - specified site — *see* Neoplasm, malignant, by site
  - unspecified site
    - female C56.9
    - male C62.90
- **Dysgeusia** R43.2
- **Dysgraphia** R27.8
- **Dyshidrosis, dysidrosis** L30.1
- **Dyskaryotic cervical smear** R87.619
- **Dyskeratosis** L85.8
  - cervix — *see* Dysplasia, cervix
  - congenital Q82.8
  - uterus NEC N85.8
- **Dyskinesia** G24.9
  - biliary (cystic duct or gallbladder) K82.8
  - drug induced
    - orofacial G24.01
  - esophagus K22.4
  - hysterical F44.4
  - intestinal K59.89
  - nonorganic origin F44.4
  - orofacial (idiopathic) G24.4
    - drug induced G24.01
  - psychogenic F44.4
  - subacute, drug induced G24.01
  - tardive G24.01
    - neuroleptic induced G24.01
  - trachea J39.8
  - tracheobronchial J98.09
- **Dyslalia** (developmental) F80.0
- **Dyslexia** R48.0
  - developmental F81.0
- **Dyslipidemia** E78.5
  - depressed HDL cholesterol E78.6
  - elevated fasting triglycerides E78.1
- **Dysmaturity** — *see also* Light for dates
  - pulmonary (newborn) (Wilson-Mikity) P27.0
- **Dysmenorrhea** (essential) (exfoliative) N94.6
  - congestive (syndrome) N94.6
  - primary N94.4
  - psychogenic F45.8
  - secondary N94.5
- **Dysmetabolic syndrome X** E88.810
- **Dysmetria** R27.8
- **Dysmorphia**
  - muscle F45.22
- **Dysmorphism** (due to)
  - alcohol Q86.0
  - exogenous cause NEC Q86.8
  - hydantoin Q86.1
  - warfarin Q86.2
- **Dysmorphophobia** (nondelusional) F45.22
  - delusional F22
- **Dysnomia** R47.01
- **Dysorexia** R63.0
  - psychogenic F50.89
- **Dysostosis**
  - cleidocranial, cleidocranialis Q74.0
  - craniofacial Q75.1
  - Fairbank's (idiopathic familial generalized osteophytosis) Q78.9
  - mandibulofacial (incomplete) Q75.4
  - multiplex E76.01
  - oculomandibular Q75.5
- **Dyspareunia** (female) N94.10
  - deep N94.12
  - male N53.12
  - nonorganic F52.6
  - psychogenic F52.6
  - secondary N94.19
  - specified NEC N94.19
  - superficial (introital) N94.11
- **Dyspepsia** R10.13
  - atonic K30
  - functional (allergic) (congenital) (gastrointestinal) (occupational) (reflex) K30
  - intestinal K59.89
  - nervous F45.8
  - neurotic F45.8
  - psychogenic F45.8
- **Dysphagia** R13.10
  - cervical R13.19
  - following
    - cerebral infarction I69.391
    - cerebrovascular disease I69.991
      - specified NEC I69.891
    - intracerebral hemorrhage I69.191
    - nontraumatic intracranial hemorrhage NEC I69.291
    - specified disease NEC I69.891
    - subarachnoid hemorrhage I69.091
  - functional (hysterical) F45.8
  - hysterical F45.8
  - nervous (hysterical) F45.8
  - neurogenic R13.19
  - oral phase R13.11
  - oropharyngeal phase R13.12
  - pharyngeal phase R13.13
  - pharyngoesophageal phase R13.14
  - psychogenic F45.8
  - sideropenic D50.1
  - spastica K22.4
  - specified NEC R13.19
- **Dysphagocytosis, congenital** D71.8
- **Dysphasia** R47.02
  - developmental
    - expressive type F80.1
    - receptive type F80.2
  - following
    - cerebrovascular disease I69.921
      - cerebral infarction I69.321
      - intracerebral hemorrhage I69.121
      - nontraumatic intracranial hemorrhage NEC I69.221
      - specified disease NEC I69.821
      - subarachnoid hemorrhage I69.021
- **Dysphonia** R49.0
  - functional F44.4
  - hysterical F44.4
  - psychogenic F44.4
  - spastica J38.3
- **Dysphoria**
  - gender F64.9
    - in
      - adolescence and adulthood F64.0
      - children F64.2
      - remission (desistance) F64.A
    - specified NEC F64.8
  - postpartal O90.6
- **Dyspituitarism** E23.3
- **Dysplasia** — *see also* Anomaly
  - acetabular, congenital Q65.89
  - alveolar capillary, with vein misalignment J84.843
  - anus (histologically confirmed) (mild) (moderate) K62.82
    - severe D01.3
  - arrhythmogenic right ventricular I42.81
  - arterial, fibromuscular I77.3
  - asphyxiating thoracic (congenital) Q77.2
  - brain Q07.9
  - bronchopulmonary, perinatal P27.1
  - cervix (uteri) N87.9
    - mild N87.0
    - moderate N87.1
    - severe D06.9

- **Embolism** — *continued*
  - vein — *continued*
    - brachial I82.62- ☑
      - chronic I82.72- ☑
    - brachiocephalic (innominate) I82.290
      - chronic I82.291
    - calf, muscle I82.46- ☑
      - chronic I82.56- ☑
    - cephalic I82.61- ☑
      - chronic I82.71- ☑
    - chronic I82.91
    - deep (DVT) I82.40- ☑
      - calf I82.4Z- ☑
        - chronic I82.5Z- ☑
      - lower leg I82.4Z- ☑
        - chronic I82.5Z- ☑
      - thigh I82.4Y- ☑
        - chronic I82.5Y- ☑
      - upper leg I82.4Y- ☑
        - chronic I82.5Y-
    - femoral I82.41- ☑
      - chronic I82.51- ☑
    - gastrocnemial I82.46- ☑
      - chronic I82.56- ☑
    - iliac (iliofemoral) I82.42- ☑
      - chronic I82.52- ☑
    - innominate I82.290
      - chronic I82.291
    - internal jugular I82.C1- ☑ (*following* I82.7)
      - chronic I82.C2- ☑ (*following* I82.7)
    - lower extremity
      - deep I82.40- ☑
        - chronic I82.50- ☑
        - specified NEC I82.49- ☑
          - chronic NEC I82.59- ☑
      - distal
        - deep I82.4Z- ☑
      - proximal
        - deep I82.4Y- ☑
          - chronic I82.5Y- ☑
      - superficial I82.81- ☑
    - peroneal I82.45- ☑
      - chronic I82.55- ☑
    - popliteal I82.43- ☑
      - chronic I82.53- ☑
    - radial I82.62- ☑
      - chronic I82.72- ☑
    - renal I82.3
    - saphenous (greater) (lesser) I82.81- ☑
    - soleal I82.46- ☑
      - chronic I82.56- ☑
    - specified NEC I82.890
      - chronic NEC I82.891
    - subclavian I82.B1- ☑ (*following* I82.7)
      - chronic I82.B2- ☑ (*following* I82.7)
    - thoracic NEC I82.290
      - chronic I82.291
    - tibial I82.44- ☑
      - chronic I82.54- ☑
    - ulnar I82.62- ☑
      - chronic I82.72- ☑
    - upper extremity I82.60- ☑
      - chronic I82.70- ☑
      - deep I82.62- ☑
        - chronic I82.72- ☑
      - superficial I82.61- ☑
        - chronic I82.71- ☑
  - vena cava
    - inferior (acute) I82.220
      - chronic I82.221
    - superior (acute) I82.210
      - chronic I82.211
  - venous sinus G08
  - vessels of brain — *see* Occlusion, artery, cerebral
- **Embolus** — *see* Embolism
- **Embryoma** — *see also* Neoplasm, uncertain behavior, by site
  - benign — *see* Neoplasm, benign, by site
  - kidney C64.- ☑
  - liver C22.0
  - malignant — *see also* Neoplasm, malignant, by site
    - kidney C64.- ☑
    - liver C22.0
    - testis C62.9- ☑
      - descended (scrotal) C62.1- ☑
      - undescended C62.0- ☑
- **Embryoma** — *continued*
  - testis C62.9- ☑
    - descended (scrotal) C62.1- ☑
    - undescended C62.0- ☑
- **Embryonic**
  - circulation Q28.9
  - heart Q28.9
  - vas deferens Q55.4
- **Embryopathia NOS** Q89.9
- **Embryotoxon** Q13.4
- **Emesis** — *see* Vomiting
- **Emotional lability** R45.86
- **Emotionality, pathological** F60.3
- **Emotogenic disease** — *see* Disorder, psychogenic
- **Emphysema** (atrophic) (bullous) (chronic) (interlobular) (lung) (obstructive) (pulmonary) (senile) (vesicular) J43.9
  - cellular tissue (traumatic) T79.7- ☑
    - surgical T81.82- ☑
  - centrilobular J43.2
  - compensatory J98.3
  - congenital (interstitial) P25.0
  - conjunctiva H11.89
  - connective tissue (traumatic) T79.7- ☑
    - surgical T81.82- ☑
  - due to chemicals, gases, fumes or vapors — *see also* Disease, respiratory, chronic, due to chemicals, gases, fumes or vapors J43.- ☑
  - eyelid(s) — *see* Disorder, eyelid, specified type NEC
    - surgical T81.82- ☑
    - traumatic T79.7- ☑
  - interstitial J98.2
    - congenital P25.0
    - perinatal period P25.0
  - laminated tissue T79.7- ☑
    - surgical T81.82- ☑
  - mediastinal J98.2
    - newborn P25.2
  - orbit, orbital — *see* Disorder, orbit, specified type NEC
  - panacinar J43.1
  - panlobular J43.1
  - specified NEC J43.8
  - subcutaneous (traumatic) T79.7- ☑
    - nontraumatic J98.2
    - postprocedural T81.82- ☑
    - surgical T81.82- ☑
  - surgical T81.82- ☑
  - thymus (gland) (congenital) E32.8
  - traumatic (subcutaneous) T79.7- ☑
  - unilateral J43.0
- **Empty nest syndrome** Z60.0
- **Empyema** (acute) (chest) (double) (pleura) (supradiaphragmatic) (thorax) J86.9
  - with fistula J86.0
  - accessory sinus (chronic) — *see* Sinusitis
  - antrum (chronic) — *see* Sinusitis, maxillary
  - brain (any part) — *see* Abscess, brain
  - ethmoidal (chronic) (sinus) — *see* Sinusitis, ethmoidal
  - extradural — *see* Abscess, extradural
  - frontal (chronic) (sinus) — *see* Sinusitis, frontal
  - gallbladder K81.0
  - mastoid (process) (acute) — *see* Mastoiditis, acute
  - maxilla, maxillary M27.2
    - sinus (chronic) — *see* Sinusitis, maxillary
  - nasal sinus (chronic) — *see* Sinusitis
  - sinus (accessory) (chronic) (nasal) — *see* Sinusitis
  - sphenoidal (sinus) (chronic) — *see* Sinusitis, sphenoidal
  - subarachnoid — *see* Abscess, extradural
  - subdural — *see* Abscess, subdural
  - tuberculous A15.6
  - ureter — *see* Ureteritis
  - ventricular — *see* Abscess, brain
- **En coup de sabre lesion** L94.1
- **Enamel pearls** K00.2
- **Enameloma** K00.2
- **Enanthema, viral** B09
- **Encephalitis** (chronic) (hemorrhagic) (idiopathic) (nonepidemic) (spurious) (subacute) G04.90
  - acute — *see also* Encephalitis, viral A86
    - disseminated G04.00
      - infectious G04.01
      - noninfectious G04.81
      - postimmunization (postvaccination) G04.02
      - postinfectious G04.01
    - inclusion body A85.8
    - necrotizing hemorrhagic G04.30
      - postimmunization G04.32
      - postinfectious G04.31
- **Encephalitis** — *continued*
  - acute — *see also* Encephalitis, viral — *continued*
    - necrotizing hemorrhagic — *continued*
      - specified NEC G04.39
  - arboviral, arbovirus NEC A85.2
  - arthropod-borne NEC (viral) A85.2
  - Australian A83.4
  - California (virus) A83.5
  - Central European (tick-borne) A84.1
  - Czechoslovakian A84.1
  - Dawson's (inclusion body) A81.1
  - diffuse sclerosing A81.1
  - disseminated, acute G04.00
  - due to
    - cat scratch disease A28.1
    - human immunodeficiency virus (HIV) disease B20 *[G05.3]*
    - malaria — *see* Malaria
    - rickettsiosis — *see* Rickettsiosis
    - smallpox inoculation G04.02
    - typhus — *see* Typhus
  - Eastern equine A83.2
  - endemic (viral) A86
  - epidemic NEC (viral) A86
  - equine (acute) (infectious) (viral) A83.9
    - Eastern A83.2
    - Venezuelan A92.2
    - Western A83.1
  - Far Eastern (tick-borne) A84.0
  - following vaccination or other immunization procedure G04.02
  - herpes zoster B02.0
  - herpesviral B00.4
    - due to herpesvirus 6 B10.01
    - due to herpesvirus 7 B10.09
    - specified NEC B10.09
  - Ilheus (virus) A83.8
  - in (due to)
    - actinomycosis A42.82
    - adenovirus A85.1
    - African trypanosomiasis B56.9 *[G05.3]*
    - Chagas' disease (chronic) B57.42
    - cytomegalovirus B25.8
    - enterovirus A85.0
    - herpes (simplex) virus B00.4
      - due to herpesvirus 6 B10.01
      - due to herpesvirus 7 B10.09
      - specified NEC B10.09
    - infectious disease NEC B99.- ☑ *[G05.3]*
    - influenza — *see* Influenza, with, encephalopathy
    - listeriosis A32.12
    - measles B05.0
    - mumps B26.2
    - naegleriasis B60.2
    - parasitic disease NEC B89 *[G05.3]*
    - poliovirus A80.9 *[G05.3]*
    - rubella B06.01
    - syphilis
      - congenital A50.42
      - late A52.14
    - systemic lupus erythematosus M32.19 *[G05.3]*
    - toxoplasmosis (acquired) B58.2
      - congenital P37.1
    - tuberculosis A17.82
    - zoster B02.0
  - inclusion body A81.1
  - infectious (acute) (virus) NEC A86
  - Japanese (B type) A83.0
  - La Crosse A83.5
  - lead — *see* Poisoning, lead
  - lethargica (acute) (infectious) A85.8
  - louping ill A84.89
  - lupus erythematosus, systemic M32.19 *[G05.3]*
  - lymphatica A87.2
  - Mengo A85.8
  - meningococcal A39.81
  - Murray Valley A83.4
  - otitic NEC H66.40 *[G05.3]*
  - parasitic NOS B71.9
  - periaxial G37.0
  - periaxialis (concentrica) (diffuse) G37.5
  - postchickenpox B01.11
  - postexanthematous NEC B09
  - postimmunization G04.02
  - postinfectious NEC G04.01
  - postmeasles B05.0
  - postvaccinal G04.02
  - postvaricella B01.11
  - postviral NEC A86

- **Encephalitis** — *continued*
  - Powassan A84.81
  - Rasmussen GØ4.81
  - Rio Bravo A85.8
  - Russian
    - autumnal A83.Ø
    - spring-summer (taiga) A84.Ø
  - saturnine — *see* Poisoning, lead
  - specified NEC GØ4.81
  - St. Louis A83.3
  - subacute sclerosing A81.1
  - summer A83.Ø
  - suppurative GØ4.81
  - tick-borne A84.9
  - Torula, torular (cryptococcal) B45.1
  - toxic NEC G92.8
  - trichinosis B75 *[GØ5.3]*
  - type
    - B A83.Ø
    - C A83.3
  - van Bogaert's A81.1
  - Venezuelan equine A92.2
  - Vienna A85.8
  - viral, virus A86
    - arthropod-borne NEC A85.2
      - mosquito-borne A83.9
        - Australian X disease A83.4
        - California virus A83.5
        - Eastern equine A83.2
        - Japanese (B type) A83.Ø
        - Murray Valley A83.4
        - specified NEC A83.8
        - St. Louis A83.3
        - type B A83.Ø
        - type C A83.3
        - Western equine A83.1
      - tick-borne A84.9
        - biundulant A84.1
        - central European A84.1
        - Czechoslovakian A84.1
        - diphasic meningoencephalitis A84.1
        - Far Eastern A84.Ø
        - Russian spring-summer (taiga) A84.Ø
        - specified NEC A84.89
    - specified type NEC A85.8
    - tick-borne, specified NEC A84.89
  - Western equine A83.1
- **Encephalocele** QØ1.9
  - frontal QØ1.Ø
  - nasofrontal QØ1.1
  - occipital QØ1.2
  - specified NEC QØ1.8
- **Encephalocystocele** — *see* Encephalocele
- **Encephaloduroarteriomyosynangiosis** (EDAMS) I67.5
- **Encephalomalacia** (brain) (cerebellar) (cerebral) — *see* Softening, brain
- **Encephalomeningitis** — *see* Meningoencephalitis
- **Encephalomeningocele** — *see* Encephalocele
- **Encephalomeningomyelitis** — *see* Meningoencephalitis
- **Encephalomyelitis** — *see also* Encephalitis GØ4.9Ø
  - acute disseminated GØ4.ØØ
    - infectious GØ4.Ø1
    - noninfectious GØ4.81
    - postimmunization GØ4.Ø2
    - postinfectious GØ4.Ø1
  - acute necrotizing hemorrhagic GØ4.3Ø
    - postimmunization GØ4.32
    - postinfectious GØ4.31
    - specified NEC GØ4.39
  - equine A83.9
    - Eastern A83.2
    - Venezuelan A92.2
    - Western A83.1
  - in diseases classified elsewhere GØ5.3
  - myalgic G93.32
    - chronic fatigue syndrome [ME/CFS] G93.32
  - postchickenpox BØ1.11
  - postinfectious NEC GØ4.Ø1
  - postmeasles BØ5.Ø
  - postvaccinal GØ4.Ø2
  - postvaricella BØ1.11
  - rubella BØ6.Ø1
  - specified NEC GØ4.81
  - Venezuelan equine A92.2
- **Encephalomyelocele** — *see* Encephalocele
- **Encephalomyelomeningitis** — *see* Meningoencephalitis
- **Encephalomyelopathy** G96.9
- **Encephalomyeloradiculitis** (acute) G61.Ø
- **Encephalomyeloradiculoneuritis** (acute) (Guillain-Barre) G61.Ø
- **Encephalomyeloradiculopathy** G96.9
- **Encephalopathia hyperbilirubinemica, newborn** P57.9
  - due to isoimmunization (conditions in P55) P57.Ø
- **Encephalopathy** (acute) G93.4Ø
  - acute necrotizing hemorrhagic GØ4.3Ø
    - postimmunization GØ4.32
    - postinfectious GØ4.31
    - specified NEC GØ4.39
  - alcoholic G31.2
  - anoxic — *see* Damage, brain, anoxic
  - arteriosclerotic I67.2
  - centrolobar progressive (Schilder) G37.Ø
  - congenital QØ7.9
  - degenerative, in specified disease NEC G32.89
  - demyelinating callosal G37.1
  - developmental and epileptic G93.45
  - due to
    - drugs — *see also* Table of Drugs and Chemicals G92.8
  - early infantile epileptic G93.45
  - FOXG1-related QAØ.Ø151
  - hepatic (without coma) K76.82
  - hyperbilirubinemic, newborn P57.9
    - due to isoimmunization (conditions in P55) P57.Ø
  - hypertensive I67.4
  - hypoglycemic E16.2
  - hypoxic — *see* Damage, brain, anoxic
  - hypoxic ischemic P91.6Ø
    - mild P91.61
    - moderate P91.62
    - severe P91.63
  - in (due to) (with)
    - birth injury P11.1
    - hyperinsulinism E16.1 *[G94]*
    - influenza — *see* Influenza, with, encephalopathy
    - lack of vitamin — *see also* Deficiency, vitamin E56.9 *[G32.89]*
    - neoplastic disease — *see also* Neoplasm D49.9 *[G13.1]*
    - serum — *see also* Reaction, serum T8Ø.69- ☑
    - syphilis A52.17
    - trauma (postconcussional) FØ7.81
      - current injury — *see* Injury, intracranial
    - vaccination GØ4.Ø2
  - lead — *see* Poisoning, lead
  - metabolic G93.41
    - drug induced G92.8
    - toxic G92.8
  - myoclonic, early, symptomatic — *see* Epilepsy, generalized, specified NEC
  - necrotizing, subacute (Leigh) G31.82
  - neonatal P91.819
    - in diseases classified elsewhere P91.811
  - pellagrous E52 *[G32.89]*
  - portal-systemic K76.82
  - postcontusional FØ7.81
    - current injury — *see* Injury, intracranial, diffuse
  - posthypoglycemic (coma) E16.1 *[G94]*
  - postradiation G93.89
  - saturnine — *see* Poisoning, lead
  - septic G93.41
  - specified NEC G93.49
  - spongiform, subacute (viral) A81.Ø9
  - toxic G92.9
    - metabolic G92.8
  - traumatic (postconcussional) FØ7.81
    - current injury — *see* Injury, intracranial
  - vitamin B deficiency NEC E53.9 *[G32.89]*
    - vitamin B1 E51.2
  - Wernicke's E51.2
- **Encephalorrhagia** — *see* Hemorrhage, intracranial, intracerebral
- **Encephalosis, posttraumatic** FØ7.81
- **Enchondroma** — *see also* Neoplasm, bone, benign
- **Enchondromatosis** (cartilaginous) (multiple) Q78.4
- **Encopresis** R15.9
  - functional F98.1
  - nonorganic origin F98.1
  - psychogenic F98.1
- **Encounter** (with health service) (for) Z76.89
  - adjustment and management (of)
    - breast implant Z45.81- ☑
    - implanted device NEC Z45.89
    - myringotomy device (stent) (tube) Z45.82
    - neurostimulator (brain) (gastric) (peripheral nerve) (sacral nerve) (spinal cord) (vagus nerve) Z45.42
  - administrative purpose only ZØ2.9
    - examination for
      - adoption ZØ2.82
- **Encounter** — *continued*
  - administrative purpose only — *continued*
    - examination for — *continued*
      - armed forces ZØ2.3
      - child welfare ZØ2.84
      - disability determination ZØ2.71
      - driving license ZØ2.4
      - employment ZØ2.1
      - insurance ZØ2.6
      - medical certificate NEC ZØ2.79
      - paternity testing ZØ2.81
      - residential institution admission ZØ2.2
      - school admission ZØ2.Ø
      - sports ZØ2.5
    - specified reason NEC ZØ2.89
  - aftercare — *see* Aftercare
  - antenatal screening Z36.9
    - cervical length Z36.86
    - chromosomal anomalies Z36.Ø
    - congenital cardiac abnormalities Z36.83
    - Down syndrome Z36.Ø
    - elevated maternal serum alphafetoprotein Z36.1
    - fetal aneuploidy Z36.Ø
    - fetal growth retardation Z36.4
    - fetal lung maturity Z36.84
    - fetal macrosomia Z36.88
    - hydrops fetalis Z36.81
    - intrauterine growth restriction (IUGR) /small-for-dates Z36.4
    - isoimmunization Z36.5
    - large-for-dates Z36.88
    - malformations Z36.3
    - non-visualized anatomy on a previous scan Z36.2
    - nuchal translucency Z36.82
    - Patau syndrome Z36.Ø
    - raised alphafetoprotein level Z36.1
    - risk of pre-term labor Z36.86
    - specified follow-up NEC Z36.2
    - specified genetic defects NEC Z36.8A
    - specified type NEC Z36.89
    - Streptococcus B Z36.85
    - suspected anomaly Z36.3
    - Trisomy 13 Z36.Ø
    - Trisomy 21 Z36.Ø
    - uncertain dates Z36.87
  - assisted reproductive fertility procedure cycle Z31.83
  - blood typing ZØ1.83
    - Rh typing ZØ1.83
  - breast augmentation or reduction Z41.1
  - breast implant exchange (different material) (different size) Z45.81- ☑
  - breast reconstruction following mastectomy Z42.1
  - check-up — *see* Examination
  - chemotherapy for neoplasm Z51.11
  - child welfare screening exam ZØ2.84
  - colonoscopy, screening Z12.11
  - comfort Z51.5
  - counseling — *see* Counseling
  - delivery, full-term, uncomplicated O8Ø
    - cesarean, without indication O82
  - desensitization to allergens Z51.6
  - ear piercing Z41.3
  - examination — *see* Examination
  - expectant parent(s) (adoptive) pre-birth pediatrician visit Z76.81
  - fertility preservation procedure (prior to cancer therapy) (prior to removal of gonads) Z31.84
  - fitting (of) — *see* Fitting (and adjustment) (of)
  - genetic
    - counseling
      - nonprocreative Z71.83
      - procreative Z31.5
    - testing — *see* Test, genetic
  - hearing conservation and treatment ZØ1.12
  - HIV
    - pre-exposure prophylaxis Z29.81
    - PrEP Z29.81
  - hospice Z51.5
  - immunotherapy for neoplasm Z51.12
  - in vitro fertilization cycle Z31.83
  - instruction (in)
    - child care (postpartal) (prenatal) Z32.3
    - childbirth Z32.2
    - natural family planning
      - procreative Z31.61
      - to avoid pregnancy Z3Ø.Ø2
  - insulin pump titration Z46.81

Index

Encephalitis — Encounter

**Endocarditis** — *continued*
- mitral — *continued*
  - specified NEC I05.8
- monilial B37.6
- multiple valves I08.9
  - specified disorders I08.8
- mycotic (acute) (any valve) (subacute) I33.Ø
- pneumococcal (acute) (any valve) (subacute) I33.Ø
- pulmonary (chronic) (heart) (valve) I37.8
  - with rheumatic fever (conditions in IØØ)
    - active — *see* Endocarditis, acute, rheumatic
    - inactive or quiescent (with chorea) IØ9.89
      - with aortic, mitral or tricuspid disease IØ8.8
  - acute or subacute I33.9
    - rheumatic IØ1.1
      - with chorea (acute) (rheumatic) (Sydenham's) IØ2.Ø
  - arteriosclerotic I37.8
  - congenital Q22.2
  - rheumatic (chronic) (inactive) (with chorea) IØ9.89
    - active or acute IØ1.1
      - with chorea (acute) (rheumatic) (Sydenham's) IØ2.Ø
  - syphilitic A52.Ø3
- purulent (acute) (any valve) (subacute) I33.Ø
- Q fever A78 *[I39]*
- rheumatic (chronic) (inactive) (with chorea) IØ9.1
  - active or acute (aortic) (mitral) (pulmonary) (tricuspid) IØ1.1
    - with chorea (acute) (rheumatic) (Sydenham's) IØ2.Ø
- rheumatoid — *see* Rheumatoid, carditis
- septic (acute) (any valve) (subacute) I33.Ø
- streptococcal (acute) (any valve) (subacute) I33.Ø
- subacute — *see* Endocarditis, acute
- suppurative (acute) (any valve) (subacute) I33.Ø
- syphilitic A52.Ø3
- toxic I33.9
- tricuspid (chronic) (heart) (inactive) (rheumatic) (valve) (with chorea) IØ7.9
  - with
    - aortic (valve) disease IØ8.2
      - mitral (valve) disease IØ8.3
    - mitral (valve) disease IØ8.1
      - aortic (valve) disease IØ8.3
    - rheumatic fever (conditions in IØØ)
      - active — *see* Endocarditis, acute, rheumatic
      - inactive or quiescent (with chorea) IØ7.8
  - active or acute IØ1.1
    - with chorea (acute) (rheumatic) (Sydenham's) IØ2.Ø
  - arteriosclerotic I36.8
  - nonrheumatic I36.8
    - acute or subacute I33.9
  - specified cause, except rheumatic I36.8
- tuberculous — *see* Tuberculosis, endocarditis
- typhoid AØ1.Ø2
- ulcerative (acute) (any valve) (subacute) I33.Ø
- vegetative (acute) (any valve) (subacute) I33.Ø
- verrucous (atypical) (nonbacterial) (nonrheumatic) M32.11

**Endocardium, endocardial** — *see also* condition
- cushion defect Q21.2Ø

**Endocervicitis** — *see also* Cervicitis
- due to intrauterine (contraceptive) device T83.69- ☑
- hyperplastic N72

**Endocrine** — *see* condition

**Endocrinopathy, pluriglandular** E31.9

**Endodontic**
- overfill M27.52
- underfill M27.53

**Endodontitis** KØ4.Ø1
- irreversible KØ4.Ø2
- reversible KØ4.Ø1

**Endomastoiditis** — *see* Mastoiditis

**Endometrioma** N8Ø.12- ☑

**Endometriosis** N8Ø.9
- abdomen, abdominal N8Ø.CØ
  - specified site, NEC N8Ø.C9
  - wall N8Ø.C19
    - fascia and muscular layers N8Ø.C11
    - subcutaneous tissue N8Ø.C1Ø
    - unspecified depth N8Ø.C19
- appendix N8Ø.549
  - deep N8Ø.542
  - superficial N8Ø.541
- bladder (unspecified depth) N8Ø.AØ
  - deep N8Ø.A2
  - superficial N8Ø.A1
- bowel N8Ø.5Ø
- broad ligament N8Ø.3C- ☑

**Endometriosis** — *continued*
- cardiothoracic space N8Ø.B6
- cecum N8Ø.539
  - deep N8Ø.532
  - superficial N8Ø.531
- cervix N8Ø.Ø- ☑
- colon N8Ø.559
  - descending N8Ø.559
    - deep N8Ø.552
    - superficial N8Ø.551
  - sigmoid N8Ø.529
    - deep N8Ø.522
    - superficial N8Ø.521
  - transverse N8Ø.559
    - deep N8Ø.552
    - superficial N8Ø.551
- cul-de-sac (Douglas')
  - anterior (unspecified depth) N8Ø.319
    - deep N8Ø.312
    - superficial N8Ø.311
  - posterior (unspecified depth) N8Ø.329
    - deep N8Ø.322
    - superficial N8Ø.321
- deep
  - involving muscular wall of fallopian tube N8Ø.22- ☑
  - retrocervical N8Ø.Ø2
- diaphragm N8Ø.B39
  - deep N8Ø.B32
  - superficial N8Ø.B31
  - unspecified depth N8Ø.B39
- exocervix N8Ø.Ø1
- extra-pelvic abdominal peritoneum N8Ø.C4
- fallopian tube (unspecified depth) N8Ø.2Ø- ☑
  - deep N8Ø.22- ☑
  - superficial N8Ø.21- ☑
- female genital organ NEC N8Ø.8
- gallbladder N8Ø.8
- in scar of skin N8Ø.6
- inguinal canal N8Ø.C3
- internal N8Ø.Ø2
- intestine N8Ø.5Ø
  - small N8Ø.569
    - deep (multifocal) N8Ø.562
    - superficial N8Ø.561
- lung N8Ø.B2
- mediastinal space N8Ø.B5
- myometrium N8Ø.Ø3
- nerve
  - femoral N8Ø.D6
  - obturator N8Ø.D3
  - pelvic N8Ø.DØ
    - splanchnic N8Ø.D1
  - pudendal N8Ø.D5
  - retroperitoneum, NEC N8Ø.D9
  - sacral splanchnic N8Ø.D1
  - sciatic N8Ø.D4
  - specified, NEC N8Ø.D9
- ovary (unspecified depth) N8Ø.1Ø- ☑
  - deep N8Ø.12- ☑
  - superficial N8Ø.11- ☑
- parametrium N8Ø.399
- pelvic
  - brim N8Ø.38- ☑
    - deep N8Ø.37- ☑
    - superficial N8Ø.36- ☑
  - peritoneum N8Ø.3Ø
    - specified sites, NEC N8Ø.399
      - deep N8Ø.392
      - superficial N8Ø.391
  - sidewall N8Ø.35- ☑
    - deep N8Ø.34- ☑
    - superficial N8Ø.33- ☑
- pericardial space N8Ø.B4
- peritoneal (pelvic) N8Ø.3Ø
- pleura N8Ø.B1
- rectovaginal septum N8Ø.4Ø
  - with involvement of vagina N8Ø.42
  - without involvement of vagina N8Ø.41
- rectum N8Ø.519
  - deep (multifocal) N8Ø.512
  - superficial N8Ø.511
- retroperitoneum N8Ø.3Ø
- round ligament N8Ø.3C9
- sacral nerve roots N8Ø.D2
- skin (scar) N8Ø.6
- specified site NEC N8Ø.8
- stromal D39.Ø
- thorax N8Ø.B- ☑

**Endometriosis** — *continued*
- umbilicus N8Ø.C2
- ureter N8Ø.A69
  - deep N8Ø.A5- ☑
  - extrinsic N8Ø.A4- ☑
  - intrinsic N8Ø.A5- ☑
  - superficial N8Ø.A4- ☑
  - unspecified depth N8Ø.A6- ☑
- uterosacral ligament(s) N8Ø.3C- ☑
  - deep N8Ø.3B- ☑
  - superficial N8Ø.3A- ☑
- uterus N8Ø.ØØ
  - deep N8Ø.Ø2
  - internal N8Ø.Ø2
  - superficial N8Ø.Ø1
- vagina N8Ø.42
- vulva N8Ø.8

**Endometritis** (decidual) (nonspecific) (purulent) (senile) (atrophic) (suppurative) N71.9
- with ectopic pregnancy OØ8.Ø
- acute N71.Ø
- blennorrhagic (gonococcal) (acute) (chronic) A54.24
- cervix, cervical (with erosion or ectropion) — *see also* Cervicitis
  - hyperplastic N72
- chlamydial A56.11
- chronic N71.1
- following
  - abortion — *see* Abortion by type complicated by genital infection
  - ectopic or molar pregnancy OØ8.Ø
- gonococcal, gonorrheal (acute) (chronic) A54.24
- hyperplastic — *see also* Hyperplasia, endometrial N85.ØØ
  - cervix N72
- puerperal, postpartum, childbirth O86.12
- subacute N71.Ø
- tuberculous A18.17

**Endometrium** — *see* condition

**Endomyocardiopathy, South African** I42.3

**Endomyocarditis** — *see* Endocarditis

**Endomyofibrosis** I42.3

**Endomyometritis** — *see* Endometritis

**Endopericarditis** — *see* Endocarditis

**Endoperineuritis** — *see* Disorder, nerve

**Endophlebitis** — *see* Phlebitis

**Endophthalmia** — *see* Endophthalmitis, purulent

**Endophthalmitis** (acute) (infective) (metastatic) (subacute) H44.ØØ9
- bleb associated — *see also* Bleb, inflamed (infected), postprocedural H59.4- ☑
- gonorrheal A54.39
- in (due to)
  - cysticercosis B69.1
  - onchocerciasis B73.Ø1
  - toxocariasis B83.Ø
- panuveitis — *see* Panuveitis
- parasitic H44.12- ☑
- purulent H44.ØØ- ☑
  - panophthalmitis — *see* Panophthalmitis
  - vitreous abscess H44.Ø2- ☑
- specified NEC H44.19
- sympathetic — *see* Uveitis, sympathetic

**Endosalpingioma** D28.2

**Endosalpingiosis** N94.89

**Endosteitis** — *see* Osteomyelitis

**Endothelioma, bone** — *see* Neoplasm, bone, malignant

**Endotheliosis** (hemorrhagic infectional) D69.8

**Endotoxemia** — code to condition

**Endotrachelitis** — *see* Cervicitis

**Engelmann** (-Camurati) **syndrome** Q78.3

**English disease** — *see* Rickets

**Engman's disease** L3Ø.3

**Engorgement**
- breast N64.59
  - newborn P83.4
  - puerperal, postpartum O92.79
- lung (passive) — *see* Edema, lung
- pulmonary (passive) — *see* Edema, lung
- stomach K31.89
- venous, retina — *see* Occlusion, retina, vein, engorgement

**Enlargement, enlarged** — *see also* Hypertrophy
- adenoids J35.2
  - with tonsils J35.3
- alveolar ridge KØ8.89
  - congenital — *see* Anomaly, alveolar
- apertures of diaphragm (congenital) Q79.1
- gingival KØ6.1

**Enlargement, enlarged** — *continued*
- heart, cardiac — *see* Hypertrophy, cardiac
- labium majus, childhood asymmetric (CALME) N9Ø.61
- lacrimal gland, chronic HØ4.Ø3- ☑
- liver — *see* Hypertrophy, liver
- lymph gland or node R59.9
  - generalized R59.1
  - localized R59.Ø
- orbit HØ5.34- ☑
- organ or site, congenital NEC — *see* Anomaly, by site
- parathyroid (gland) E21.Ø
- pituitary fossa R93.Ø
- prostate N4Ø.Ø
  - with lower urinary tract symptoms (LUTS) N4Ø.1
    - nodular N4Ø.3
  - nodular N4Ø.2
    - with lower urinary tract symptoms (LUTS) N4Ø.3
  - without lower urinary tract symptoms (LUTS) N4Ø.Ø
    - nodular N4Ø.2
- sella turcica R93.Ø
- spleen — *see* Splenomegaly
- thymus (gland) (congenital) E32.Ø
- thyroid (gland) — *see* Goiter
- tongue K14.8
- tonsils J35.1
  - with adenoids J35.3
- uterus N85.2
- vestibular aqueduct Q16.5

**Enophthalmos** HØ5.4Ø- ☑
- due to
  - orbital tissue atrophy HØ5.41- ☑
  - trauma or surgery HØ5.42- ☑

**Enostosis** M27.8

**Entamebic, entamebiasis** — *see* Amebiasis

**Entanglement**
- umbilical cord(s) O69.82- ☑
  - with compression O69.2- ☑
  - around neck
    - with compression O69.1- ☑
    - without compression O69.81- ☑
  - of twins in monoamniotic sac O69.2- ☑
  - other, with compression O69.2- ☑
  - other, without compression O69.82- ☑
  - without compression O69.82- ☑

**Enteralgia** — *see* Pain, abdominal

**Enteric** — *see* condition

**Enteritis** (acute) (diarrheal) (hemorrhagic) (noninfective) K52.9
- adenovirus AØ8.2
- aertrycke infection AØ2.Ø
- allergic K52.29
  - with
    - eosinophilic gastritis or gastroenteritis K52.81
    - food protein-induced enterocolitis syndrome K52.21
    - food protein-induced enteropathy K52.22
    - FPIES K52.21
- amebic (acute) AØ6.Ø
  - with abscess — *see* Abscess, amebic
  - chronic AØ6.1
    - with abscess — *see* Abscess, amebic
    - nondysenteric AØ6.2
  - nondysenteric AØ6.2
- astrovirus AØ8.32
- bacillary NOS AØ3.9
- bacterial AØ4.9
  - specified NEC AØ4.8
- calicivirus AØ8.31
- candidal B37.82
- Chilomastix AØ7.8
- choleriformis AØØ.1
- chronic (noninfectious) K52.9
  - ulcerative — *see* Colitis, ulcerative
- cicatrizing (chronic) — *see* Enteritis, regional, small intestine
- Clostridioides difficile
  - not specified as recurrent AØ4.72
  - recurrent AØ4.71
- Clostridium
  - botulinum (food poisoning) AØ5.1
  - difficile
    - not specified as recurrent AØ4.72
    - recurrent AØ4.71
- coccidial AØ7.3
- coxsackie virus AØ8.39
- dietetic — *see also* Enteritis, allergic K52.29
- drug-induced K52.1

**Enteritis** — *continued*
- due to
  - astrovirus AØ8.32
  - calicivirus AØ8.31
  - coxsackie virus AØ8.39
  - drugs K52.1
  - echovirus AØ8.39
  - enterovirus NEC AØ8.39
  - food hypersensitivity — *see also* Enteritis, allergic K52.29
  - infectious organism (bacterial) (viral) — *see* Enteritis, infectious
  - torovirus AØ8.39
  - Yersinia enterocolitica AØ4.6
- echovirus AØ8.39
- eltor AØØ.1
- enterovirus NEC AØ8.39
- eosinophilic K52.81
- epidemic (infectious) AØ9
- fulminant — *see also* Ischemia, intestine, acute K55.Ø19
- gangrenous — *see* Enteritis, infectious
- giardial AØ7.1
- infectious NOS AØ9
  - due to
    - adenovirus AØ8.2
    - Aerobacter aerogenes AØ4.8
    - Arizona (bacillus) AØ2.Ø
    - bacteria NOS AØ4.9
      - specified NEC AØ4.8
    - Campylobacter AØ4.5
    - Clostridioides difficile
      - not specified as recurrent AØ4.72
      - recurrent AØ4.71
    - Clostridium difficile
      - not specified as recurrent AØ4.72
      - recurrent AØ4.71
    - Clostridium perfringens AØ4.8
    - Enterobacter aerogenes AØ4.8
    - enterovirus AØ8.39
    - Escherichia coli AØ4.4
      - enteroaggregative AØ4.4
      - enterohemorrhagic AØ4.3
      - enteroinvasive AØ4.2
      - enteropathogenic AØ4.Ø
      - enterotoxigenic AØ4.1
      - specified NEC AØ4.4
    - specified
      - bacteria NEC AØ4.8
      - virus NEC AØ8.39
    - Staphylococcus AØ4.8
    - virus NEC AØ8.4
      - specified type NEC AØ8.39
    - Yersinia enterocolitica AØ4.6
  - specified organism NEC AØ8.8
- influenzal — *see* Influenza, with, digestive manifestations
- ischemic K55.9
  - acute — *see also* Ischemia, intestine, acute K55.Ø19
  - chronic K55.1
- microsporidial AØ7.8
- mucomembranous, myxomembranous — *see* Syndrome, irritable bowel
- mucous — *see* Syndrome, irritable bowel
- necroticans AØ5.2
- necrotizing of newborn — *see* Enterocolitis, necrotizing, in newborn
- neurogenic — *see* Syndrome, irritable bowel
- newborn necrotizing — *see* Enterocolitis, necrotizing, in newborn
- noninfectious K52.9
- norovirus AØ8.11
- parasitic NEC B82.9
- paratyphoid (fever) — *see* Fever, paratyphoid
- protozoal AØ7.9
  - specified NEC AØ7.8
- radiation K52.Ø
- regional (of) K5Ø.9Ø
  - with
    - complication K5Ø.919
      - abscess K5Ø.914
      - fistula K5Ø.913
      - intestinal obstruction K5Ø.912
      - rectal bleeding K5Ø.911
      - specified complication NEC K5Ø.918
  - colon — *see* Enteritis, regional, large intestine
  - duodenum — *see* Enteritis, regional, small intestine
  - ileum — *see* Enteritis, regional, small intestine
  - jejunum — *see* Enteritis, regional, small intestine
  - large bowel — *see* Enteritis, regional, large intestine
  - large intestine (colon) (rectum) K5Ø.1Ø

**Enteritis** — *continued*
- regional — *continued*
  - large intestine — *continued*
    - with
      - complication K5Ø.119
        - abscess K5Ø.114
        - fistula K5Ø.113
        - intestinal obstruction K5Ø.112
        - rectal bleeding K5Ø.111
        - small intestine (duodenum) (ileum) (jejunum) involvement K5Ø.8Ø
          - with
            - complication K5Ø.819
              - abscess K5Ø.814
              - fistula K5Ø.813
              - intestinal obstruction K5Ø.812
              - rectal bleeding K5Ø.811
              - specified complication NEC K5Ø.818
        - specified complication NEC K5Ø.118
  - rectum — *see* Enteritis, regional, large intestine
  - small intestine (duodenum) (ileum) (jejunum) K5Ø.ØØ
    - with
      - complication K5Ø.Ø19
        - abscess K5Ø.Ø14
        - fistula K5Ø.Ø13
        - intestinal obstruction K5Ø.Ø12
        - large intestine (colon) (rectum) involvement K5Ø.8Ø
          - with
            - complication K5Ø.819
              - abscess K5Ø.814
              - fistula K5Ø.813
              - intestinal obstruction K5Ø.812
              - rectal bleeding K5Ø.811
              - specified complication NEC K5Ø.818
        - rectal bleeding K5Ø.Ø11
        - specified complication NEC K5Ø.Ø18
- rotaviral AØ8.Ø
- Salmonella, salmonellosis (arizonae) (cholerae-suis) (enteritidis) (typhimurium) AØ2.Ø
- segmental — *see* Enteritis, regional
- septic AØ9
- Shigella — *see* Infection, Shigella
- small round structured NEC AØ8.19
- spasmodic, spastic — *see* Syndrome, irritable bowel
- staphylococcal AØ4.8
  - due to food AØ5.Ø
- torovirus AØ8.39
- toxic NEC K52.1
  - due to
    - Clostridioides difficile
      - not specified as recurrent AØ4.72
      - recurrent AØ4.71
    - Clostridium difficile
      - not specified as recurrent AØ4.72
      - recurrent AØ4.71
- trichomonal AØ7.8
- tuberculous A18.32
- typhosa AØ1.ØØ
- ulcerative (chronic) — *see* Colitis, ulcerative
- viral AØ8.4
  - adenovirus AØ8.2
  - enterovirus AØ8.39
  - Rotavirus AØ8.Ø
  - small round structured NEC AØ8.19
  - specified NEC AØ8.39
  - virus specified NEC AØ8.39

**Enterobiasis** B8Ø

**Enterobius vermicularis** (infection) (infestation) B8Ø

**Enterocele** — *see also* Hernia, abdomen
- pelvic, pelvis (acquired) (congenital) N81.5
- vagina, vaginal (acquired) (congenital) NEC N81.5

**Enterocolitis** — *see also* Enteritis K52.9
- due to
  - Clostridioides difficile
    - not specified as recurrent AØ4.72
    - recurrent AØ4.71
  - Clostridium difficile
    - not specified as recurrent AØ4.72
    - recurrent AØ4.71
- fulminant ischemic — *see also* Ischemia, intestine, acute K55.Ø59
- granulomatous — *see* Enteritis, regional
- hemorrhagic (acute) — *see also* Ischemia, intestine, acute K55.Ø59
  - chronic K55.1
- infectious NEC AØ9

**Enterocolitis** — *continued*
- ischemic K55.9
- necrotizing K55.3Ø
  - with
    - perforation K55.33
    - pneumatosis K55.32
      - and perforation K55.33
  - due to
    - Clostridioides difficile
      - not specified as recurrent AØ4.72
      - recurrent AØ4.71
    - Clostridium difficile
      - not specified as recurrent AØ4.72
      - recurrent AØ4.71
  - in non-newborn K55.3Ø
    - stage 1 (without pneumatosis, without perforation) K55.31
    - stage 2 (with pneumatosis, without perforation) K55.32
    - stage 3 (with pneumatosis, with perforation) K55.33
  - in newborn P77.9
    - stage 1 (without pneumatosis, without perforation) P77.1
    - stage 2 (with pneumatosis, without perforation) P77.2
    - stage 3 (with pneumatosis, with perforation) P77.3
  - without pneumatosis or perforation K55.31
- noninfectious K52.9
  - newborn — *see* Enterocolitis, necrotizing, in newborn
- pseudomembranous (newborn)
  - not specified as recurrent AØ4.72
  - recurrent AØ4.71
- radiation K52.Ø
  - newborn — *see* Enterocolitis, necrotizing, in newborn
- ulcerative (chronic) — *see* Pancolitis, ulcerative (chronic)

**Enterogastritis** — *see* Enteritis

**Enteropathy** K63.9
- celiac-gluten-sensitive K9Ø.Ø
  - non-celiac K9Ø.41
- food protein-induced K52.22
- hemorrhagic, terminal — *see also* Ischemia, intestine, acute K55.Ø59
- protein-losing K9Ø.49

**Enteroperitonitis** — *see* Peritonitis

**Enteroptosis** K63.4

**Enterorrhagia** K92.2

**Enterospasm** — *see also* Syndrome, irritable, bowel
- psychogenic F45.8

**Enterostenosis** — *see also* Obstruction, intestine, specified NEC K56.699

**Enterostomy**
- complication — *see* Complication, enterostomy
- status Z93.4

**Enterovirus, as cause of disease classified elsewhere** B97.1Ø
- coxsackievirus B97.11
- echovirus B97.12
- other specified B97.19

**Enthesopathy** (peripheral) M77.9
- Achilles tendinitis — *see* Tendinitis, Achilles
- ankle and tarsus M77.5- ☑
  - specified type NEC — *see* Enthesopathy, foot, specified type NEC
- anterior tibial syndrome M76.81- ☑
- calcaneal spur — *see* Spur, bone, calcaneal
- elbow region M77.8
  - lateral epicondylitis — *see* Epicondylitis, lateral
  - medial epicondylitis — *see* Epicondylitis, medial
- foot NEC M77.8
  - metatarsalgia — *see* Metatarsalgia
  - specified type NEC M77.5- ☑
- forearm M77.8
- gluteal tendinitis — *see* Tendinitis, gluteal
- hand M77.8
- hip — *see* Enthesopathy, lower limb, specified type NEC
- iliac crest spur — *see* Spur, bone, iliac crest
- iliotibial band syndrome — *see* Syndrome, iliotibial band
- knee — *see* Enthesopathy, lower limb, lower leg, specified type NEC
- lateral epicondylitis — *see* Epicondylitis, lateral
- lower limb (excluding foot) M76.9
  - Achilles tendinitis — *see* Tendinitis, Achilles
  - ankle and tarsus M77.5- ☑
    - specified type NEC — *see* Enthesopathy, foot, specified type NEC
  - anterior tibial syndrome M76.81- ☑
  - gluteal tendinitis — *see* Tendinitis, gluteal

**Enthesopathy** — *continued*
- lower limb — *continued*
  - iliac crest spur — *see* Spur, bone, iliac crest
  - iliotibial band syndrome — *see* Syndrome, iliotibial band
  - patellar tendinitis — *see* Tendinitis, patellar
  - pelvic region — *see* Enthesopathy, lower limb, specified type NEC
  - peroneal tendinitis — *see* Tendinitis, peroneal
  - posterior tibial syndrome M76.82- ☑
  - psoas tendinitis — *see* Tendinitis, psoas
  - specified type NEC M76.89- ☑
  - tibial collateral bursitis — *see* Bursitis, tibial collateral
- medial epicondylitis — *see* Epicondylitis, medial
- metatarsalgia — *see* Metatarsalgia
- multiple sites M77.8
- patellar tendinitis — *see* Tendinitis, patellar
- pelvis M77.8
- periarthritis of wrist — *see* Periarthritis, wrist
- peroneal tendinitis — *see* Tendinitis, peroneal
- posterior tibial syndrome M76.82- ☑
- psoas tendinitis — *see* Tendinitis, psoas
- shoulder region — *see* Lesion, shoulder
- specified type NEC M77.8
- spinal M46.ØØ
  - cervical region M46.Ø2
  - cervicothoracic region M46.Ø3
  - lumbar region M46.Ø6
  - lumbosacral region M46.Ø7
  - multiple sites M46.Ø9
  - occipito-atlanto-axial region M46.Ø1
  - sacrococcygeal region M46.Ø8
  - thoracic region M46.Ø4
  - thoracolumbar region M46.Ø5
- tibial collateral bursitis — *see* Bursitis, tibial collateral
- upper arm M77.8
- wrist and carpus NEC M77.8
  - calcaneal spur — *see* Spur, bone, calcaneal
  - periarthritis of wrist — *see* Periarthritis, wrist

**Entomophobia** F4Ø.218

**Entomophthoromycosis** B46.8

**Entrance, air into vein** — *see* Embolism, air

**Entrapment**
- muscle
  - eye
    - extraocular H5Ø.68- ☑
    - oblique
      - inferior H5Ø.62- ☑
      - superior H5Ø.66- ☑
    - rectus
      - inferior H5Ø.63- ☑
      - lateral H5Ø.64- ☑
      - medial H5Ø.65- ☑
      - superior H5Ø.67- ☑
- nerve — *see* Neuropathy, entrapment

**Entropion** (eyelid) (paralytic) HØ2.ØØ9
- cicatricial HØ2.Ø19
  - left HØ2.Ø16
    - lower HØ2.Ø15
    - upper HØ2.Ø14
  - right HØ2.Ø13
    - lower HØ2.Ø12
    - upper HØ2.Ø11
- congenital Q1Ø.2
- left HØ2.ØØ6
  - lower HØ2.ØØ5
  - upper HØ2.ØØ4
- mechanical HØ2.Ø29
  - left HØ2.Ø26
    - lower HØ2.Ø25
    - upper HØ2.Ø24
  - right HØ2.Ø23
    - lower HØ2.Ø22
    - upper HØ2.Ø21
- right HØ2.ØØ3
  - lower HØ2.ØØ2
  - upper HØ2.ØØ1
- senile HØ2.Ø39
  - left HØ2.Ø36
    - lower HØ2.Ø35
    - upper HØ2.Ø34
  - right HØ2.Ø33
    - lower HØ2.Ø32
    - upper HØ2.Ø31
- spastic HØ2.Ø49
  - left HØ2.Ø46
    - lower HØ2.Ø45
    - upper HØ2.Ø44

**Entropion** — *continued*
- spastic — *continued*
  - right HØ2.Ø43
    - lower HØ2.Ø42
    - upper HØ2.Ø41

**Enucleated eye** (traumatic, current) SØ5.7- ☑

**Enuresis** R32
- functional F98.Ø
- habit disturbance F98.Ø
- nocturnal N39.44
  - psychogenic F98.Ø
- nonorganic origin F98.Ø
- psychogenic F98.Ø

**Eosinopenia** — *see* Agranulocytosis

**Eosinophilia** (allergic) (idiopathic) (secondary) D72.1Ø
- with
  - angiolymphoid hyperplasia (ALHE) D18.Ø1
- familial D72.19
- hereditary D72.19
- in disease classified elsewhere D72.18
- infiltrative — *see* Eosinophilia, pulmonary
- Loffler's J82.89
- peritoneal — *see* Peritonitis, eosinophilic
- pulmonary NEC J82.89
  - acute J82.82
  - asthmatic J82.83
  - chronic J82.81
- specified NEC D72.19
- tropical (pulmonary) J82.89

**Eosinophilia-myalgia syndrome** M35.89

**Ependymitis** (acute) (cerebral) (chronic) (granular) — *see* Encephalomyelitis

**Ependymoblastoma**
- specified site — *see* Neoplasm, malignant, by site
- unspecified site C71.9

**Ependymoma** (epithelial) (malignant)
- anaplastic
  - specified site — *see* Neoplasm, malignant, by site
  - unspecified site C71.9
- benign
  - specified site — *see* Neoplasm, benign, by site
  - unspecified site D33.2
- myxopapillary D43.2
  - specified site — *see* Neoplasm, uncertain behavior, by site
  - unspecified site D43.2
- papillary D43.2
  - specified site — *see* Neoplasm, uncertain behavior, by site
  - unspecified site D43.2
- specified site — *see* Neoplasm, malignant, by site
- unspecified site C71.9

**Ependymopathy** G93.89

**Ephelis, ephelides** L81.2

**Epiblepharon** (congenital) Q1Ø.3

**Epicanthus, epicanthic fold** (eyelid) (congenital) Q1Ø.3

**Epicondylitis** (elbow)
- lateral M77.1- ☑
- medial M77.Ø- ☑

**Epicystitis** — *see* Cystitis

**Epidemic** — *see* condition

**Epidermidalization, cervix** — *see* Dysplasia, cervix

**Epidermis, epidermal** — *see* condition

**Epidermodysplasia verruciformis** BØ7.8

**Epidermolysis**
- bullosa (congenital) Q81.9
  - acquired L12.3Ø
    - drug-induced L12.31
    - specified cause NEC L12.35
  - dystrophica Q81.2
  - letalis Q81.1
  - simplex Q81.Ø
  - specified NEC Q81.8
- necroticans combustiformis L51.2
  - due to drug — *see* Table of Drugs and Chemicals, by drug

**Epidermophytid** — *see* Dermatophytosis

**Epidermophytosis** (infected) — *see* Dermatophytosis

**Epididymis** — *see* condition

**Epididymitis** (acute) (nonvenereal) (recurrent) (residual) N45.1
- with orchitis N45.3
- blennorrhagic (gonococcal) A54.23
- caseous (tuberculous) A18.15
- chlamydial A56.19
- filarial — *see also* Infestation, filarial B74.9 *[N51]*
- gonococcal A54.23
- syphilitic A52.76
- tuberculous A18.15

**Erythrophagocytosis** D75.89
**Erythrophobia** F4Ø.298
**Erythroplakia, oral epithelium, and tongue** K13.29
**Erythroplasia** (Queyrat) DØ7.4
- specified site — *see* Neoplasm, skin, in situ
- unspecified site DØ7.4

**Escherichia coli** (E. coli), **as cause of disease classified elsewhere** B96.2Ø
- non-O157 Shiga toxin-producing (with known O group) B96.22
- non-Shiga toxin-producing B96.29
- O157 B96.21
- O157 with confirmation of Shiga toxin when H antigen is unknown, or is not H7 B96.21
- O157:H- (nonmotile) with confirmation of Shiga toxin B96.21
- O157:H7 with or without confirmation of Shiga toxin-production B96.21
  - specified NEC B96.22
- Shiga toxin-producing (with unspecified O group) (STEC) B96.23
- specified NEC B96.29

**Esophagismus** K22.4
**Esophagitis** (acute) (alkaline) (chemical) (chronic) (infectional) (necrotic) (peptic) (postoperative) (without bleeding) K2Ø.9Ø
- with bleeding K2Ø.91
- candidal B37.81
- due to gastrointestinal reflux disease (without bleeding) K21.ØØ
  - with bleeding K21.Ø1
- eosinophilic K2Ø.Ø
- reflux K21.ØØ
  - with bleeding K21.Ø1
- specified NEC (without bleeding) K2Ø.8Ø
  - with bleeding K2Ø.81
- tuberculous A18.83
- ulcerative K22.1Ø
  - with bleeding K22.11

**Esophagocele** K22.5
**Esophagomalacia** K22.89
**Esophagospasm** K22.4
**Esophagostenosis** K22.2
**Esophagostomiasis** B81.8
**Esophagotracheal** — *see* condition
**Esophagus** — *see* condition
**Esophoria** H5Ø.51
- convergence, excess H51.12
- divergence, insufficiency H51.8

**Esotropia** — *see* Strabismus, convergent concomitant
**Espundia** B55.2
**Essential** — *see* condition
**Esthesioneuroblastoma** C3Ø.Ø
**Esthesioneurocytoma** C3Ø.Ø
**Esthesioneuroepithelioma** C3Ø.Ø
**Esthiomene** A55
**Estivo-autumnal malaria** (fever) B5Ø.9
**Estrangement** (marital) Z63.5
- parent-child NEC Z62.89Ø

**Estriasis** — *see* Myiasis
**Ethanolism** — *see* Alcoholism
**Etherism** — *see* Dependence, drug, inhalant
**Ethmoid, ethmoidal** — *see* condition
**Ethmoiditis** (chronic) (nonpurulent) (purulent) — *see also* Sinusitis, ethmoidal
- influenzal — *see* Influenza, with, respiratory manifestations NEC
- Woakes' J33.1

**Ethylism** — *see* Alcoholism
**Eulenburg's disease** (congenital paramyotonia) G71.19
**Eumycetoma** B47.Ø
**Eunuchoidism** E29.1
- hypogonadotropic E23.Ø

**European blastomycosis** — *see* Cryptococcosis
**Eustachian** — *see* condition
**EVALI** (e-cigarette, or vaping, product use associated lung injury) UØ7.Ø
**Evaluation** (for) (of)
- development state
  - adolescent ZØØ.3
  - period of
    - delayed growth in childhood ZØØ.7Ø
      - with abnormal findings ZØØ.71
    - rapid growth in childhood ZØØ.2
  - puberty ZØØ.3
- growth and developmental state (period of rapid growth) ZØØ.2
  - delayed growth ZØØ.7Ø
    - with abnormal findings ZØØ.71

**Evaluation** — *continued*
- mental health (status) ZØØ.8
  - requested by authority ZØ4.6
- period of
  - delayed growth in childhood ZØØ.7Ø
    - with abnormal findings ZØØ.71
  - rapid growth in childhood ZØØ.2
- suspected condition — *see* Observation

**Evans syndrome** D69.41
**Event**
- apparent life threatening in newborn and infant (ALTE) R68.13
- brief resolved unexplained event (BRUE) R68.13

**Eventration** — *see also* Hernia, ventral
- colon into chest — *see* Hernia, diaphragm
- diaphragm (congenital) Q79.1

**Eversion**
- bladder N32.89
- cervix (uteri) N86
  - with cervicitis N72
- foot NEC — *see also* Deformity, valgus, ankle
  - congenital Q66.6
- punctum lacrimale (postinfectional) (senile) HØ4.52- ☑
- ureter (meatus) N28.89
- urethra (meatus) N36.8
- uterus N81.4

**Evidence**
- cytologic
  - of malignancy on anal smear R85.614
  - of malignancy on cervical smear R87.614
  - of malignancy on vaginal smear R87.624

**Evisceration**
- birth injury P15.8
- traumatic NEC
  - eye — *see* Enucleated eye

**Evulsion** — *see* Avulsion
**Ewing's sarcoma or tumor** — *see* Neoplasm, bone, malignant
**Examination** (for) (following) (general) (of) (routine) ZØØ.ØØ
- with abnormal findings ZØØ.Ø1
- abuse, physical (alleged), ruled out
  - adult ZØ4.71
  - child ZØ4.72
- adolescent (development state) ZØØ.3
- alleged rape or sexual assault (victim), ruled out
  - adult ZØ4.41
  - child ZØ4.42
- allergy ZØ1.82
- annual (adult) (periodic) (physical) ZØØ.ØØ
  - with abnormal findings ZØØ.Ø1
  - gynecological ZØ1.419
    - with abnormal findings ZØ1.411
- antibody response ZØ1.84
- blood — *see* Examination, laboratory
- blood pressure ZØ1.3Ø
  - with abnormal findings ZØ1.31
- health — *see* Examination, medical
- hearing ZØ1.1Ø
  - with abnormal findings NEC ZØ1.118
  - following failed hearing screening ZØ1.11Ø
  - infant or child (over 28 days old) ZØØ.129
    - with abnormal findings ZØØ.121
- immunity status testing ZØ1.84
- laboratory (as part of a general medical examination) ZØØ.ØØ
  - with abnormal findings ZØØ.Ø1
  - preprocedural ZØ1.812
- lactating mother Z39.1
- medical (adult) (for) (of) ZØØ.ØØ
  - with abnormal findings ZØØ.Ø1
  - administrative purpose only ZØ2.9
    - specified NEC ZØ2.89
  - admission to
    - armed forces ZØ2.3
    - old age home ZØ2.2
    - prison ZØ2.89
    - residential institution ZØ2.2
    - school ZØ2.Ø
      - following illness or medical treatment ZØ2.Ø
    - summer camp ZØ2.89
  - adoption ZØ2.82
  - blood alcohol or drug level ZØ2.83
  - camp (summer) ZØ2.89
  - clinical research, normal subject (control) (participant) ZØØ.6
  - control subject in clinical research (normal comparison) (participant) ZØØ.6
  - donor (potential) ZØØ.5
  - driving license ZØ2.4

**Examination** — *continued*
- medical — *continued*
  - general (adult) ZØØ.ØØ
    - with abnormal findings ZØØ.Ø1
  - immigration ZØ2.89
  - insurance purposes ZØ2.6
  - marriage ZØ2.89
  - medicolegal reasons NEC ZØ4.89
  - naturalization ZØ2.89
  - participation in sport ZØ2.5
  - paternity testing ZØ2.81
  - population survey ZØØ.8
  - pre-employment ZØ2.1
  - pre-operative — *see* Examination, pre-procedural
  - pre-procedural
    - cardiovascular ZØ1.81Ø
    - respiratory ZØ1.811
    - specified NEC ZØ1.818
  - preschool children
    - for admission to school ZØ2.Ø
  - prisoners
    - for entrance into prison ZØ2.89
  - recruitment for armed forces ZØ2.3
  - specified NEC ZØØ.8
  - sport competition ZØ2.5
- medicolegal reason NEC ZØ4.89
  - following
    - forced sexual exploitation ZØ4.81
    - forced labor exploitation ZØ4.82
- newborn — *see* Newborn, examination
- pelvic (annual) (periodic) ZØ1.419
  - with abnormal findings ZØ1.411
- period of rapid growth in childhood ZØØ.2
- periodic (adult) (annual) (routine) ZØØ.ØØ
  - with abnormal findings ZØØ.Ø1
- physical (adult) — *see also* Examination, medical ZØØ.ØØ
  - sports ZØ2.5
- postpartum
  - immediately after delivery Z39.Ø
  - routine follow-up Z39.2
- pre-chemotherapy (antineoplastic) ZØ1.818
- prenatal (normal pregnancy) — *see also* Pregnancy, normal Z34.9- ☑
- pre-procedural (pre-operative)
  - cardiovascular ZØ1.81Ø
  - laboratory ZØ1.812
  - respiratory ZØ1.811
  - specified NEC ZØ1.818
- prior to chemotherapy (antineoplastic) ZØ1.818
- psychiatric NEC ZØØ.8
  - follow-up not needing further care ZØ9
  - requested by authority ZØ4.6
- radiological (as part of a general medical examination) ZØØ.ØØ
  - with abnormal findings ZØØ.Ø1
- repeat cervical smear to confirm findings of recent normal smear following initial abnormal smear ZØ1.42
- skin (hypersensitivity) ZØ1.82
- special — *see also* Examination, by type ZØ1.89
  - specified type NEC ZØ1.89
- specified type or reason NEC ZØ4.89
- teeth ZØ1.2Ø
  - with abnormal findings ZØ1.21
- urine — *see* Examination, laboratory
- vision ZØ1.ØØ
  - with abnormal findings ZØ1.Ø1
  - following failed vision screening ZØ1.Ø2Ø
    - with abnormal findings ZØ1.Ø21
  - infant or child (over 28 days old) ZØØ.129
    - with abnormal findings ZØØ.121
- cancer staging — *see* Neoplasm, malignant, by site
- cervical Papanicolaou smear Z12.4
  - as part of routine gynecological examination ZØ1.419
    - with abnormal findings ZØ1.411
- child (over 28 days old) ZØØ.129
  - with abnormal findings ZØØ.121
  - under 28 days old — *see* Newborn, examination
- clinical research control or normal comparison (control) (participant) ZØØ.6
- contraceptive (drug) maintenance (routine) Z3Ø.8
  - device (intrauterine) Z3Ø.431
- dental ZØ1.2Ø
  - with abnormal findings ZØ1.21
- developmental — *see* Examination, child
- donor (potential) ZØØ.5
- ear ZØ1.1Ø
  - with abnormal findings NEC ZØ1.118
- eye ZØ1.ØØ
  - with abnormal findings ZØ1.Ø1

**Examination** — *continued*
  eye — *continued*
    following failed vision screening Z01.020
      with abnormal findings Z01.021
  follow-up (routine) (following) Z09
    chemotherapy NEC Z09
      malignant neoplasm Z08
    fracture Z09
    malignant neoplasm Z08
    postpartum Z39.2
    psychotherapy Z09
    radiotherapy NEC Z09
      malignant neoplasm Z08
    surgery NEC Z09
      malignant neoplasm Z08
  following
    accident NEC Z04.3
      transport Z04.1
      work Z04.2
    assault, alleged, ruled out
      adult Z04.71
      child Z04.72
    motor vehicle accident Z04.1
    treatment (for) Z09
      combined NEC Z09
        fracture Z09
        malignant neoplasm Z08
      malignant neoplasm Z08
      mental disorder Z09
      specified condition NEC Z09
  forced sexual exploitation Z04.81
  forced labor exploitation Z04.82
  gynecological Z01.419
    with abnormal findings Z01.411
    for contraceptive maintenance Z30.8
**Exanthem, exanthema** — *see also* Rash
  with enteroviral vesicular stomatitis B08.4
  Boston A88.0
  epidemic with meningitis A88.0 *[G02]*
  subitum B08.20
    due to human herpesvirus 6 B08.21
    due to human herpesvirus 7 B08.22
  viral, virus B09
    specified type NEC B08.8
**Excess, excessive, excessively**
  alcohol level in blood R78.0
  androgen (ovarian) E28.1
  attrition, tooth, teeth K03.0
  carotene, carotin (dietary) E67.1
  cold, effects of T69.9- ☑
    specified effect NEC T69.8- ☑
  convergence H51.12
  crying
    in child, adolescent, or adult R45.83
    in infant R68.11
  development, breast N62
  divergence H51.8
  drinking (alcohol) NEC (without dependence) F10.10
    habitual (continual) (without remission) F10.20
  eating R63.2
  estrogen E28.0
  fat — *see also* Obesity
    in heart — *see* Degeneration, myocardial
    localized E65
  foreskin N47.8
  gas R14.0
  glucagon E16.3
  heat — *see* Heat
  intermaxillary vertical dimension of fully erupted teeth M26.37
  interocclusal distance of fully erupted teeth M26.37
  kalium E87.5
  large
    colon K59.39
      congenital Q43.8
    infant P08.0
    organ or site, congenital NEC — *see* Anomaly, by site
  long
    organ or site, congenital NEC — *see* Anomaly, by site
  menstruation (with regular cycle) N92.0
    with irregular cycle N92.1
  napping Z72.821
  natrium E87.0
  number of teeth K00.1
  nutrient (dietary) NEC R63.2
  potassium (K) E87.5
  salivation K11.7
  secretion — *see also* Hypersecretion
    milk O92.6

**Excess, excessive, excessively** — *continued*
  secretion — *see also* Hypersecretion — *continued*
    sputum R09.3
    sweat R61
  sexual drive F52.8
  short
    organ or site, congenital NEC — *see* Anomaly, by site
    umbilical cord in labor or delivery O69.3- ☑
  skin L98.7
    and subcutaneous tissue L98.7
    eyelid (acquired) — *see* Blepharochalasis
      congenital Q10.3
  sodium (Na) E87.0
  spacing of fully erupted teeth M26.32
  sputum R09.3
  sweating R61
  thirst R63.1
    due to deprivation of water T73.1- ☑
  transportation time Z59.82
  tuberosity of jaw M26.07
  vitamin
    A (dietary) E67.0
      administered as drug (prolonged intake) — *see* Table of Drugs and Chemicals, vitamins, adverse effect
      overdose or wrong substance given or taken — *see* Table of Drugs and Chemicals, vitamins, poisoning
    D (dietary) E67.3
      administered as drug (prolonged intake) — *see* Table of Drugs and Chemicals, vitamins, adverse effect
      overdose or wrong substance given or taken — *see* Table of Drugs and Chemicals, vitamins, poisoning
  weight
    gain R63.5
    loss R63.4
**Excitability, abnormal, under minor stress** (personality disorder) F60.3
**Excitation**
  anomalous atrioventricular I45.6
  psychogenic F30.8
  reactive (from emotional stress, psychological trauma) F30.8
**Excitement**
  hypomanic F30.8
  manic F30.9
  mental, reactive (from emotional stress, psychological trauma) F30.8
  state, reactive (from emotional stress, psychological trauma) F30.8
**Excoriation** (traumatic) — *see also* Abrasion
  neurotic L98.1
  skin picking disorder F42.4
**Exfoliation**
  due to erythematous conditions according to extent of body surface involved L49.0
    10-19 percent of body surface L49.1
    20-29 percent of body surface L49.2
    30-39 percent of body surface L49.3
    40-49 percent of body surface L49.4
    50-59 percent of body surface L49.5
    60-69 percent of body surface L49.6
    70-79 percent of body surface L49.7
    80-89 percent of body surface L49.8
    90-99 percent of body surface L49.9
    less than 10 percent of body surface L49.0
  teeth, due to systemic causes K08.0
**Exfoliative** — *see* condition
**Exhaustion, exhaustive** (physical NEC) R53.83
  battle F43.0
  cardiac — *see* Failure, heart
  delirium F43.0
  due to
    cold T69.8- ☑
    excessive exertion T73.3- ☑
    exposure T73.2- ☑
    neurasthenia F48.8
  heart — *see* Failure, heart
  heat — *see also* Heat, exhaustion T67.5- ☑
    due to
      salt depletion T67.4- ☑
      water depletion T67.3- ☑
  maternal, complicating delivery O75.81
  mental F48.8
  myocardium, myocardial — *see* Failure, heart
  nervous F48.8

**Exhaustion, exhaustive** — *continued*
  old age R54
  psychogenic F48.8
  psychosis F43.0
  senile R54
  vital NEC Z73.0
**Exhibitionism** F65.2
**Exocervicitis** — *see* Cervicitis
**Exomphalos** Q79.2
  meaning hernia — *see* Hernia, umbilicus
**Exophoria** H50.52
  convergence, insufficiency H51.11
  divergence, excess H51.8
**Exophthalmos** H05.2- ☑
  congenital Q15.8
  constant NEC H05.24- ☑
  displacement, globe — *see* Displacement, globe
  due to thyrotoxicosis (hyperthyroidism) — *see* Hyperthyroidism, with, goiter (diffuse)
  dysthyroid — *see* Hyperthyroidism, with, goiter (diffuse)
  goiter — *see* Hyperthyroidism, with, goiter (diffuse)
  intermittent NEC H05.25- ☑
  malignant — *see* Hyperthyroidism, with, goiter (diffuse)
  orbital
    edema — *see* Edema, orbit
    hemorrhage — *see* Hemorrhage, orbit
  pulsating NEC H05.26- ☑
  thyrotoxic, thyrotropic — *see* Hyperthyroidism, with, goiter (diffuse)
**Exostosis** — *see also* Disorder, bone
  cartilaginous — *see* Neoplasm, bone, benign
  congenital (multiple) Q78.6
  external ear canal H61.81- ☑
  gonococcal A54.49
  jaw (bone) M27.8
  multiple, congenital Q78.6
  orbit H05.35- ☑
  osteocartilaginous — *see* Neoplasm, bone, benign
  syphilitic A52.77
**Exotropia** — *see* Strabismus, divergent concomitant
**Explanation of**
  investigation finding Z71.2
  medication Z71.89
**Exploitation**
  labor
    confirmed
      adult forced T74.61- ☑
      child forced T74.62- ☑
    suspected
      adult forced T76.61- ☑
      child forced T76.62- ☑
  sexual
    confirmed
      adult forced T74.51- ☑
      child T74.52- ☑
    suspected
      adult forced T76.51- ☑
      child T76.52- ☑
**Exposure** (to) — *see also* Contact, with T75.89- ☑
  acariasis Z20.7
  Agent Orange Z77.33
  AIDS virus Z20.6
  air pollution Z77.110
  algae and algae toxins Z77.121
  algae bloom Z77.121
  anthrax Z20.810
  aromatic amines Z77.020
  aromatic (hazardous) compounds NEC Z77.028
  aromatic dyes NOS Z77.028
  arsenic Z77.010
  asbestos Z77.090
  bacterial disease NEC Z20.818
  benzene Z77.021
  blast overpressure NOS Z77.40
    high-level (HLB) Z77.42
    low-level (LLB) Z77.41
    specified NEC Z77.49
  blue-green algae bloom Z77.121
  body fluids (potentially hazardous) Z77.21
  brown tide Z77.121
  burn pits in war theater Z77.32
  chemicals (chiefly nonmedicinal) (hazardous) NEC Z77.098
  cholera Z20.09
  chromium compounds Z77.018
  cold, effects of T69.9- ☑
    specified effect NEC T69.8- ☑
  communicable disease Z20.9

**Exposure** — *continued*
- communicable disease — *continued*
  - bacterial NEC Z20.818
  - specified NEC Z20.89
  - viral NEC Z20.828
  - Zika virus Z20.821
- coronavirus (disease) (novel) 2019 Z20.822
- COVID-19 Z20.822
- cyanobacteria bloom Z77.121
- disaster Z65.5
- discrimination Z60.5
- dyes Z77.098
- effects of T73.9- ☑
- environmental tobacco smoke (acute) (chronic) Z77.22
- Escherichia coli (E. coli) Z20.01
- exhaustion due to T73.2- ☑
- fiberglass — *see* Table of Drugs and Chemicals, fiberglass
- gadolinium Z77.013
- German measles Z20.4
- gonorrhea Z20.2
- hazardous metals NEC Z77.018
- hazardous substances NEC Z77.29
- hazards in the physical environment NEC Z77.128
- hazards to health NEC Z77.9
- human immunodeficiency virus (HIV) Z20.6
- human T-lymphotropic virus type-1 (HTLV-1) Z20.89
- implanted
  - mesh — *see* Complications, prosthetic device or implant, mesh
  - prosthetic materials NEC — *see* Complications, prosthetic materials NEC
- infestation (parasitic) NEC Z20.7
- intestinal infectious disease NEC Z20.09
  - Escherichia coli (E. coli) Z20.01
- lead Z77.011
- meningococcus Z20.811
- mold (toxic) Z77.120
- nickel dust Z77.018
- noise Z77.122
- occupational
  - air contaminants NEC Z57.39
  - dust Z57.2
  - environmental tobacco smoke Z57.31
  - extreme temperature Z57.6
  - noise Z57.0
  - radiation Z57.1
  - risk factors Z57.9
    - specified NEC Z57.8
  - toxic agents (gases) (liquids) (solids) (vapors) in agriculture Z57.4
  - toxic agents (gases) (liquids) (solids) (vapors) in industry NEC Z57.5
  - vibration Z57.7
- parasitic disease NEC Z20.7
- pediculosis Z20.7
- persecution Z60.5
- pfiesteria piscicida Z77.121
- poliomyelitis Z20.89
- pollution
  - air Z77.110
  - environmental NEC Z77.118
  - soil Z77.112
  - water Z77.111
- polycyclic aromatic hydrocarbons Z77.028
- prenatal (drugs) (toxic chemicals) — *see* Newborn, affected by, noxious substances transmitted via placenta or breast milk
- rabies Z20.3
- radiation, naturally occurring NEC Z77.123
- radon Z77.123
- red tide (Florida) Z77.121
- risk factor, personal, to diethylstilbestrol (DES) (in utero) Z91.B
- rubella Z20.4
- SARS-CoV-2 Z20.822
- second hand tobacco smoke (acute) (chronic) Z77.22
  - in the perinatal period P96.81
- sexually-transmitted disease Z20.2
- smallpox (laboratory) Z20.89
- syphilis Z20.2
- terrorism Z65.4
- torture Z65.4
- tuberculosis Z20.1
- uranium Z77.012
- varicella Z20.820
- venereal disease Z20.2
- viral disease NEC Z20.828
- war Z65.5
  - theater, burn pits in Z77.32

**Exposure** — *continued*
- water pollution Z77.111
- Zika virus Z20.821

**Exsanguination** — *see* Hemorrhage

**Exstrophy**
- abdominal contents Q45.8
- bladder Q64.10
  - cloacal Q64.12
  - specified type NEC Q64.19
  - supravesical fissure Q64.11

**Extensive** — *see* condition

**Extra** — *see also* Accessory
- marker chromosomes (normal individual) Q92.61
  - in abnormal individual Q92.62
- rib Q76.6
  - cervical Q76.5

**Extrasystoles** (supraventricular) I49.49
- atrial I49.1
- auricular I49.1
- junctional I49.2
- ventricular I49.3

**Extrauterine gestation or pregnancy** — *see* Pregnancy, by site

**Extravasation**
- blood R58
- chyle into mesentery I89.8
- pelvicalyceal N13.8
- pyelosinus N13.8
- urine (from ureter) R39.0
- vesicant agent
  - antineoplastic chemotherapy T80.810- ☑
  - other agent NEC T80.818- ☑

**Extremity** — *see* condition, limb

**Extrophy** — *see* Exstrophy

**Extroversion**
- bladder Q64.19
- uterus N81.4
  - complicating delivery O71.2
  - postpartal (old) N81.4

**Extruded tooth** (teeth) M26.34

**Extrusion**
- breast implant (prosthetic) T85.42- ☑
- eye implant (globe) (ball) T85.328- ☑
- intervertebral disc — *see* Displacement, intervertebral disc
- ocular lens implant (prosthetic) — *see* Complications, intraocular lens
- vitreous — *see* Prolapse, vitreous

**Exudate**
- causing irritant dermatitis L24.A9
- pleural — *see* Effusion, pleura
- retina H35.89
- wound fluids causing irritant dermatitis L24.A9

**Exudative** — *see* condition

**Eye, eyeball, eyelid** — *see* condition

**Eyestrain** — *see* Disturbance, vision, subjective

**Eyeworm disease of Africa** B74.3

# F

**Faber's syndrome** (achlorhydric anemia) D50.9

**Fabry (-Anderson) disease** E75.21

**Facet syndrome** M47.89- ☑

**Faciocephalalgia, autonomic** — *see also* Neuropathy, peripheral, autonomic G90.09

**Factor**(s)
- psychic, associated with diseases classified elsewhere F54
- psychological
  - affecting physical conditions F54
  - or behavioral
    - affecting general medical condition F54
    - associated with disorders or diseases classified elsewhere F54

**Fahr disease** (of brain) G23.8

**Fahr Volhard disease** (of kidney) I12.- ☑

**Failure, failed**
- abortion — *see* Abortion, attempted
- aortic (valve) I35.8
  - rheumatic I06.8
- attempted abortion — *see* Abortion, attempted
- biventricular I50.82
  - due to left heart failure I50.814
- bone marrow — *see* Anemia, aplastic
- cardiac — *see* Failure, heart
- cardiorenal (chronic) — *see also* Failure, renal, and Failure, heart I50.9
  - hypertensive I13.2

**Failure, failed** — *continued*
- cardiorespiratory — *see also* Failure, heart R09.2
- cardiovascular (chronic) — *see* Failure, heart
- cerebrovascular I67.9
- cervical dilatation in labor O62.0
- circulation, circulatory (peripheral) R57.9
  - newborn P29.89
- compensation — *see* Disease, heart
- compliance with medical treatment or regimen — *see* Noncompliance
- congestive — *see* Failure, heart, congestive
- dental implant (endosseous) M27.69
  - due to
    - failure of dental prosthesis M27.63
    - lack of attached gingiva M27.62
    - occlusal trauma (poor prosthetic design) M27.62
    - parafunctional habits M27.62
    - periodontal infection (peri-implantitis) M27.62
    - poor oral hygiene M27.62
  - osseointegration M27.61
    - due to
      - complications of systemic disease M27.61
      - poor bone quality M27.61
    - iatrogenic M27.61
  - post-osseointegration
    - biological M27.62
    - due to complications of systemic disease M27.62
    - iatrogenic M27.62
    - mechanical M27.63
  - pre-integration M27.61
  - pre-osseointegration M27.61
  - specified NEC M27.69
- descent of head (at term) of pregnancy (mother) O32.4- ☑
- endosseous dental implant — *see* Failure, dental implant
- engagement of head (term of pregnancy) (mother) O32.4- ☑
- erection (penile) — *see also* Dysfunction, sexual, male, erectile N52.9
  - nonorganic F52.21
- examination(s), anxiety concerning Z55.2
- expansion terminal respiratory units (newborn) (primary) P28.0
- forceps NOS (with subsequent cesarean delivery) O66.5
- gain weight (child over 28 days old) R62.51
  - adult R62.7
  - newborn P92.6
- genital response (male) F52.21
  - female F52.22
- heart (acute) (senile) (sudden) I50.9
  - with
    - acute pulmonary edema — *see* Failure, ventricular, left
    - decompensation I50.9
      - with
        - normal ejection fraction I50.33
        - preserved ejection fraction I50.33
        - reduced ejection fraction I50.23
          - with diastolic dysfunction I50.43
      - combined systolic and diastolic I50.43
      - diastolic I50.33
      - right I50.813
      - systolic I50.23
    - dilatation — *see* Disease, heart
    - hypertension — *see* Hypertension, heart
    - normal ejection fraction — *see* Failure, heart, diastolic
    - preserved ejection fraction — *see* Failure, heart, diastolic
    - reduced ejection fraction — *see* Failure, heart, systolic
  - arteriosclerotic I70.90
  - biventricular I50.82
    - due to left heart failure I50.814
  - combined left-right sided I50.82
    - due to left heart failure I50.814
  - compensated — *see also* Failure, heart, by type as diastolic or systolic, chronic I50.9
  - complicating
    - anesthesia (general) (local) or other sedation
      - in labor and delivery O74.2
      - in pregnancy O29.12- ☑
      - postpartum, puerperal O89.1
    - delivery (cesarean) (instrumental) O75.4
  - congestive I50.9
    - with rheumatic fever (conditions in I00)
      - active I01.8
      - inactive or quiescent (with chorea) I09.81
    - newborn P29.0

- **Failure, failed** — *continued*
  - heart — *continued*
    - congestive — *continued*
      - rheumatic (chronic) (inactive) (with chorea) I09.81
        - active or acute I01.8
          - with chorea I02.0
    - decompensated — *see also* Failure, heart, by type as diastolic or systolic, acute and chronic I50.9
    - degenerative — *see* Degeneration, myocardial
    - diastolic (congestive) (left ventricular) I50.30
      - acute (congestive) I50.31
        - and (on) chronic (congestive) I50.33
      - chronic (congestive) I50.32
        - and (on) acute (congestive) I50.33
      - combined with systolic (congestive) I50.40
        - acute (congestive) I50.41
          - and (on) chronic (congestive) I50.43
        - chronic (congestive) I50.42
          - and (on) acute (congestive) I50.43
    - due to presence of cardiac prosthesis I97.13- ☑
    - end stage — *see also* Failure, heart, by type as diastolic or systolic, chronic I50.84
    - following cardiac surgery I97.130
    - following other surgery I97.131
    - high output NOS I50.83
    - hypertensive — *see* Hypertension, heart
    - left (ventricular) — *see also* Failure, ventricular, left
      - combined diastolic and systolic — *see* Failure, heart, diastolic, combined with systolic
      - diastolic — *see* Failure, heart, diastolic
      - systolic — *see* Failure, heart, systolic
    - low output (syndrome) NOS I50.9
    - newborn P29.0
    - organic — *see* Disease, heart
    - peripartum O90.3
    - postprocedural I97.13- ☑
    - rheumatic (chronic) (inactive) I09.9
    - right (isolated) (ventricular) I50.810
      - acute I50.811
        - and (on) chronic I50.813
      - chronic I50.812
        - and acute I50.813
      - secondary to left heart failure I50.814
    - specified NEC I50.89

*Note: heart failure stages A, B, C, and D are based on the American College of Cardiology and American Heart Association stages of heart failure, which complement and should not be confused with the New York Heart Association Classification of Heart Failure, into Class I, Class II, Class III, and Class IV*

- 
  - 
    - stage A Z91.89
    - stage B — *see also* Failure, heart, by type as diastolic or systolic, if known I50.9
    - stage C — *see also* Failure, heart, by type as diastolic or systolic, if known I50.9
    - stage D — *see also* Failure, heart, by type as diastolic or systolic, chronic I50.84
    - systolic (congestive) (left ventricular) I50.20
      - acute (congestive) I50.21
        - and (on) chronic (congestive) I50.23
      - chronic (congestive) I50.22
        - and (on) acute (congestive) I50.23
      - combined with diastolic (congestive) I50.40
        - acute (congestive) I50.41
          - and (on) chronic (congestive) I50.43
        - chronic (congestive) I50.42
          - and (on) acute (congestive) I50.43
    - thyrotoxic — *see also* Thyrotoxicosis E05.90 *[I43]*
      - with
        - high output — *see also* Thyrotoxicosis I50.83
        - thyroid storm E05.91 *[I43]*
          - high output — *see also* Thyrotoxicosis I50.83
    - valvular — *see* Endocarditis
  - hepatic K72.90
    - with coma K72.91
    - acute or subacute K72.00
      - with coma K72.01
      - due to drugs K71.10
        - with coma K71.11
    - alcoholic (acute) (chronic) (subacute) K70.40
      - with coma K70.41
    - chronic K72.10
      - with coma K72.11
      - due to drugs (acute) (subacute) (chronic) K71.10
        - with coma K71.11
    - due to drugs (acute) (subacute) (chronic) K71.10
      - with coma K71.11

- **Failure, failed** — *continued*
  - hepatic — *continued*
    - end stage K72.10
      - with coma K72.11
    - postprocedural K91.82
  - hepatorenal K76.7
  - induction (of labor) O61.9
    - abortion — *see* Abortion, attempted
    - by
      - oxytocic drugs O61.0
      - prostaglandins O61.0
    - instrumental O61.1
    - mechanical O61.1
    - medical O61.0
    - specified NEC O61.8
    - surgical O61.1
  - intestinal K90.83
  - intubation during anesthesia T88.4- ☑
    - in pregnancy O29.6- ☑
    - labor and delivery O74.7
    - postpartum, puerperal O89.6
  - involution, thymus (gland) E32.0
  - kidney — *see also* Disease, kidney, chronic N19
    - acute — *see also* Failure, renal, acute N17.9
  - lactation (complete) O92.3
    - partial O92.4
  - Leydig's cell, adult E29.1
  - liver — *see* Failure, hepatic
  - menstruation at puberty N91.0
  - mitral I05.8
  - myocardial, myocardium — *see also* Failure, heart I50.9
    - chronic — *see also* Failure, heart, congestive I50.9
    - congestive — *see also* Failure, heart, congestive I50.9
  - newborn screening — *see* Abnormal, neonatal screening
    - neonatal congenital heart disease P09.5
  - orgasm (female) (psychogenic) F52.31
    - male F52.32
  - ovarian (primary) E28.39
    - iatrogenic E89.40
      - asymptomatic E89.40
      - symptomatic E89.41
    - postprocedural (postablative) (postirradiation) (postsurgical) E89.40
      - asymptomatic E89.40
      - symptomatic E89.41
  - ovulation causing infertility N97.0
  - polyglandular, autoimmune E31.0
  - prosthetic joint implant — *see* Complications, joint prosthesis, mechanical, breakdown, by site
  - renal N19
    - with
      - tubular necrosis (acute) N17.0
    - acute N17.9
      - with
        - cortical necrosis N17.1
        - medullary necrosis N17.2
        - tubular necrosis N17.0
      - specified NEC N17.8
    - chronic N18.9
      - hypertensive — *see* Hypertension, kidney
    - congenital P96.0
    - end stage (chronic) N18.6
      - due to hypertension I12.0
    - following
      - abortion — *see* Abortion by type complicated by specified condition NEC
      - crushing T79.5- ☑
      - ectopic or molar pregnancy O08.4
      - labor and delivery (acute) O90.49
    - hypertensive — *see* Hypertension, kidney
    - postprocedural N99.0
  - respiration, respiratory J96.90
    - with
      - hypercapnia J96.92
      - hypercarbia J96.92
      - hypoxia J96.91
    - acute J96.00
      - with
        - hypercapnia J96.02
        - hypercarbia J96.02
        - hypoxia J96.01
    - center G93.89
    - acute and (on) chronic J96.20
      - with
        - hypercapnia J96.22
        - hypercarbia J96.22
        - hypoxia J96.21
    - chronic J96.10

- **Failure, failed** — *continued*
  - respiration, respiratory — *continued*
    - chronic — *continued*
      - with
        - hypercapnia J96.12
        - hypercarbia J96.12
        - hypoxia J96.11
    - newborn P28.5
    - postprocedural (acute) J95.821
      - acute and chronic J95.822
  - rotation
    - cecum Q43.3
    - colon Q43.3
    - intestine Q43.3
    - kidney Q63.2
  - sedation (conscious) (moderate) during procedure T88.52- ☑
    - history of Z92.83
  - segmentation — *see also* Fusion
    - fingers — *see* Syndactylism, complex, fingers
    - vertebra Q76.49
      - with scoliosis Q76.3
  - seminiferous tubule, adult E29.1
  - senile (general) R54
  - sexual arousal (male) F52.21
    - female F52.22
  - testicular endocrine function E29.1
  - to thrive (child over 28 days old) R62.51
    - adult R62.7
    - newborn P92.6
  - transplant T86.92
    - bone T86.831
      - marrow T86.02
    - cornea T86.841- ☑
    - heart T86.22
      - with lung(s) T86.32
    - intestine T86.851
    - kidney T86.12
    - liver T86.42
    - lung(s) T86.811
      - with heart T86.32
    - pancreas T86.891
    - skin (allograft) (autograft) T86.821
    - specified organ or tissue NEC T86.891
    - stem cell (peripheral blood) (umbilical cord) T86.5
  - trial of labor (with subsequent cesarean delivery) O66.40
    - following previous cesarean delivery O66.41
  - tubal ligation N99.89
  - urinary — *see* Disease, kidney, chronic
  - vacuum extraction NOS (with subsequent cesarean delivery) O66.5
  - vasectomy N99.89
  - ventouse NOS (with subsequent cesarean delivery) O66.5
  - ventricular — *see also* Failure, heart I50.9
    - left — *see also* Failure, heart, left I50.1
      - with rheumatic fever (conditions in I00)
        - active I01.8
          - with chorea I02.0
        - inactive or quiescent (with chorea) I09.81
      - rheumatic (chronic) (inactive) (with chorea) I09.81
        - active or acute I01.8
          - with chorea I02.0
    - right — *see* Failure, heart, right
  - vital centers, newborn P91.88
- **Fainting** (fit) R55
- **Fallen arches** — *see* Deformity, limb, flat foot
- **Falling, falls** (repeated) R29.6
  - any organ or part — *see* Prolapse
- **Fallopian**
  - insufflation Z31.41
  - tube — *see* condition
- **Fallot's**
  - pentalogy Q21.8
  - tetrad or tetralogy Q21.3
  - triad or trilogy Q22.3
- **False** — *see also* condition
  - croup J38.5
  - joint — *see* Nonunion, fracture
  - labor (pains) O47.9
    - at or after 37 completed weeks of gestation O47.1
    - before 37 completed weeks of gestation O47.0- ☑
  - passage, urethra (prostatic) N36.5
  - pregnancy F45.8
- **Faltering growth** R62.51
- **Family, familial** — *see also* condition
  - disruption Z63.8
    - involving divorce or separation Z63.5
  - Li-Fraumeni (syndrome) Z15.01
  - planning advice Z30.09

- **Family, familial** — *continued*
  - problem Z63.9
    - specified NEC Z63.8
  - retinoblastoma C69.2- ☑
- **Famine** (effects of) T73.Ø- ☑
  - edema — *see* Malnutrition, severe
- **Fanconi** ('s) **anemia** D61.Ø3
- **Fanconi hypoplastic anemia** D61.Ø3
- **Fanconi panmyelopathy** D61.Ø3
- **Fanconi** (-de Toni)(-Debre) **syndrome** E72.Ø9
  - with cystinosis E72.Ø4
- **Farber's disease or syndrome** E75.29
- **Farcy** A24.Ø
- **Farmer's**
  - lung J67.Ø
  - skin L57.8
- **Farsightedness** — *see* Hypermetropia
- **Fascia** — *see* condition
- **Fasciculation** R25.3
- **Fasciitis** M72.9
  - diffuse (eosinophilic) M35.4
  - infective M72.8
    - necrotizing M72.6
  - necrotizing M72.6
  - nodular M72.4
  - perirenal (with ureteral obstruction) N13.5
    - with infection N13.6
  - plantar (foot) M67.AØ- ☑
  - specified NEC M72.8
  - traumatic (old) M72.8
    - current — *code by* site under Sprain
- **Fascioliasis** B66.3
- **Fasciolopsis, fasciolopsiasis** (intestinal) B66.5
- **Fascioscapulohumeral myopathy** G71.Ø2
- **Fast pulse** RØØ.Ø
- **Fat**
  - embolism — *see* Embolism, fat
  - excessive — *see also* Obesity
    - in heart — *see* Degeneration, myocardial
  - in stool R19.5
  - localized (pad) E65
    - heart — *see* Degeneration, myocardial
    - knee M79.4
    - retropatellar M79.4
  - necrosis
    - breast N64.1
    - mesentery K65.4
    - omentum K65.4
  - pad E65
    - knee M79.4
- **Fatigue** R53.83
  - auditory deafness — *see* Deafness
  - chronic R53.82
  - combat F43.Ø
  - general R53.83
    - psychogenic F48.8
  - heat (transient) T67.6- ☑
  - muscle M62.89
  - myocardium — *see* Failure, heart
  - neoplasm-related R53.Ø
  - nervous, neurosis F48.8
  - operational F48.8
  - psychogenic (general) F48.8
  - senile R54
  - voice R49.8
- **Fatness** — *see* Obesity
- **Fatty** — *see also* condition
  - apron E65
  - degeneration — *see* Degeneration, fatty
  - heart (enlarged) — *see* Degeneration, myocardial
  - liver NEC K76.Ø
    - alcoholic K7Ø.Ø
    - nonalcoholic K76.Ø
  - necrosis — *see* Degeneration, fatty
- **Fauces** — *see* condition
- **Fauchard's disease** (periodontitis) — *see* Periodontitis
- **Faucitis** JØ2.9
- **Favism** (anemia) D55.Ø
- **Favus** — *see* Dermatophytosis
- **Fazio-Londe disease or syndrome** G12.1
- **Fear complex or reaction** F4Ø.9
- **Fear of** — *see* Phobia
- **Feared complaint unfounded** Z71.1
- **Febris, febrile** — *see also* Fever
  - flava — *see also* Fever, yellow A95.9
  - melitensis A23.Ø
  - pestis — *see* Plague
  - recurrens — *see* Fever, relapsing
  - rubra A38.9
- **Fecal**
  - incontinence R15.9
  - smearing R15.1
  - soiling R15.1
  - urgency R15.2
- **Fecalith** (impaction) K56.41
  - appendix K38.1
  - congenital P76.8
- **Fede's disease** K14.Ø
- **Feeble-minded** F7Ø
- **Feeble rapid pulse due to shock following injury** T79.4- ☑
- **Feeding**
  - difficulties R63.3Ø
  - problem (elderly) (infant) R63.39
    - newborn P92.9
      - specified NEC P92.8
    - nonorganic (adult) — *see* Disorder, eating
- **Feeling** (of)
  - foreign body in throat RØ9.A2
- **Feer's disease** — *see* Poisoning, mercury
- **Feet** — *see* condition
- **Feigned illness** Z76.5
- **Feil-Klippel syndrome** (brevicollis) Q76.1
- **Feinmesser's** (hidrotic) **ectodermal dysplasia** Q82.4
- **Felinophobia** F4Ø.218
- **Felon** — *see also* Cellulitis, digit
  - with lymphangitis — *see* Lymphangitis, acute, digit
- **Felty's syndrome** MØ5.ØØ
  - ankle MØ5.Ø7- ☑
  - elbow MØ5.Ø2- ☑
  - foot joint MØ5.Ø7- ☑
  - hand joint MØ5.Ø4- ☑
  - hip MØ5.Ø5- ☑
  - knee MØ5.Ø6- ☑
  - multiple site MØ5.Ø9
  - shoulder MØ5.Ø1- ☑
  - vertebra — *see* Spondylitis, ankylosing
  - wrist MØ5.Ø3- ☑
- **Female genital cutting status** — *see* Female genital mutilation status (FGM)
- **Female genital mutilation status** (FGM) N9Ø.81Ø
  - specified NEC N9Ø.818
  - type I (clitorectomy status) N9Ø.811
  - type II (clitorectomy with excision of labia minora status) N9Ø.812
  - type III (infibulation status) N9Ø.813
  - type IV N9Ø.818
- **Femur, femoral** — *see* condition
- **Fenestration, fenestrated** — *see also* Imperfect, closure
  - aortico-pulmonary Q21.4
  - atrial septum Q21.11
  - cusps, heart valve NEC Q24.8
    - pulmonary Q22.3
  - pulmonic cusps Q22.3
- **Fernell's disease** (aortic aneurysm) I71.9
- **Fertile eunuch syndrome** E23.Ø
- **Fetid**
  - breath R19.6
  - sweat L75.Ø
- **Fetishism** F65.Ø
  - transvestic F65.1
- **Fetus, fetal** — *see also* condition
  - alcohol syndrome (dysmorphic) Q86.Ø
  - compressus O31.Ø- ☑
  - hydantoin syndrome Q86.1
  - lung tissue P28.Ø
  - papyraceous O31.Ø- ☑
- **Fever** (inanition) (of unknown origin) (persistent) (with chills) (with rigor) R5Ø.9
  - abortus A23.1
  - Aden (dengue) A9Ø
  - African tick bite A77.8
  - African tick-borne A68.1
  - American
    - mountain (tick) A93.2
    - spotted A77.Ø
  - aphthous BØ8.8
  - arbovirus, arboviral A94
    - hemorrhagic A94
    - specified NEC A93.8
  - Argentinian hemorrhagic A96.Ø
  - Assam B55.Ø
  - Australian Q A78
  - Bangkok hemorrhagic A91
  - Barmah forest A92.8
  - Bartonella A44.Ø
  - bilious, hemoglobinuric B5Ø.8
- **Fever** — *continued*
  - blackwater B5Ø.8
  - blister BØØ.1
  - Bolivian hemorrhagic A96.1
  - Bonvale dam T73.3- ☑
  - boutonneuse A77.1
  - brain — *see* Encephalitis
  - Brazilian purpuric A48.4
  - breakbone A9Ø
  - Bullis A77.Ø
  - Bunyamwera A92.8
  - Burdwan B55.Ø
  - Bwamba A92.8
  - Cameroon — *see* Malaria
  - Canton A75.9
  - cat-scratch A28.1
  - catarrhal (acute) JØØ
    - chronic J31.Ø
  - Central Asian hemorrhagic A98.Ø
  - cerebral — *see* Encephalitis
  - cerebrospinal meningococcal A39.Ø
  - Chagres B5Ø.9
  - Chandipura A92.8
  - Changuinola A93.1
  - Charcot's (biliary) (hepatic) (intermittent) — *see* Calculus, bile duct
  - Chikungunya (viral) (hemorrhagic) A92.Ø
  - Chitral A93.1
  - Colombo — *see* Fever, paratyphoid
  - Colorado tick (virus) A93.2
  - congestive (remittent) — *see* Malaria
  - Congo virus A98.Ø
  - continued malarial B5Ø.9
  - Corsican — *see* Malaria
  - Crimean-Congo hemorrhagic A98.Ø
  - Cyprus — *see* Brucellosis
  - dandy A9Ø
  - deer fly — *see* Tularemia
  - dengue (virus) A9Ø
    - hemorrhagic A91
    - sandfly A93.1
  - desert B38.Ø
  - drug induced R5Ø.2
  - due to
    - conditions classified elsewhere R5Ø.81
    - heat T67.Ø1- ☑
  - enteric AØ1.ØØ
  - enteroviral exanthematous (Boston exanthem) A88.Ø
  - ephemeral (of unknown origin) R5Ø.9
  - epidemic hemorrhagic A98.5
  - erysipelatous — *see* Erysipelas
  - estivo-autumnal (malarial) B5Ø.9
  - famine A75.Ø
  - five day A79.Ø
  - following delivery O86.4
  - Fort Bragg A27.89
  - gastroenteric AØ1.ØØ
  - gastromalarial — *see* Malaria
  - Gibraltar — *see* Brucellosis
  - glandular — *see* Mononucleosis, infectious
  - Guama (viral) A92.8
  - Haverhill A25.1
  - hay (allergic) J3Ø.1
    - with asthma (bronchial) J45.9Ø9
      - with
        - exacerbation (acute) J45.9Ø1
        - status asthmaticus J45.9Ø2
    - due to
      - allergen other than pollen J3Ø.89
      - pollen, any plant or tree J3Ø.1
  - heat (effects) T67.Ø1- ☑
  - hematuric, bilious B5Ø.8
  - hemoglobinuric (malarial) (bilious) B5Ø.8
  - hemorrhagic (arthropod-borne) NOS A94
    - with renal syndrome A98.5
    - arenaviral A96.9
      - specified NEC A96.8
    - Argentinian A96.Ø
    - Bangkok A91
    - Bolivian A96.1
    - Central Asian A98.Ø
    - Chikungunya A92.Ø
    - Crimean-Congo A98.Ø
    - dengue (virus) A91
    - epidemic A98.5
    - Junin (virus) A96.Ø
    - Korean A98.5
    - Kyasanur forest A98.2
    - Machupo (virus) A96.1

- **Fibrosis, fibrotic** — *continued*
  - seminal vesicle N5Ø.89
  - senile R54
  - skin L9Ø.5
  - spermatic cord N5Ø.89
  - spleen D73.89
    - in schistosomiasis (bilharziasis) B65.9 *[D77]*
  - subepidermal nodular — *see* Neoplasm, skin, benign
  - submucous (oral) (tongue) K13.5
  - testis N44.8
    - chronic, due to syphilis A52.76
  - thymus (gland) E32.8
  - tongue, submucous K13.5
  - tunica vaginalis N5Ø.89
  - uterus (non-neoplastic) N85.8
  - vagina N89.8
  - valve, heart — *see* Endocarditis
  - vas deferens N5Ø.89
  - vein I87.8
- **Fibrositis** (periarticular) M79.7
  - nodular, chronic (Jaccoud's) (rheumatoid) — *see* Arthropathy, postrheumatic, chronic
- **Fibrothorax** J94.1
- **Fibrotic** — *see* Fibrosis
- **Fibrous** — *see* condition
- **Fibroxanthoma** — *see also* Neoplasm, connective tissue, benign
  - atypical — *see* Neoplasm, connective tissue, uncertain behavior
  - malignant — *see* Neoplasm, connective tissue, malignant
- **Fibroxanthosarcoma** — *see* Neoplasm, connective tissue, malignant
- **Fiedler's**
  - disease (icterohemorrhagic leptospirosis) A27.Ø
  - myocarditis (acute) I4Ø.1
- **Fifth disease** BØ8.3
  - venereal A55
- **Filaria, filarial, filariasis** — *see* Infestation, filarial
- **Filatov's disease** — *see* Mononucleosis, infectious
- **File-cutter's disease** — *see* Poisoning, lead
- **Filling defect**
  - biliary tract R93.2
  - bladder R93.41
  - duodenum R93.3
  - gallbladder R93.2
  - gastrointestinal tract R93.3
  - intestine R93.3
  - kidney R93.42- ☑
  - stomach R93.3
  - ureter R93.41
  - urinary organs, specified NEC R93.49
- **Fimbrial cyst** Q5Ø.4
- **Financial problem affecting care NOS** Z59.9
  - bankruptcy Z59.868
  - foreclosure on loan Z59.89
    - home loan Z59.81- ☑
  - insecurity Z59.869
    - paying for utilities (electricity) (heat) (oil) (water bill) Z59.861
  - strain Z59.868
- **Findings, abnormal, inconclusive, without diagnosis** — *see also* Abnormal
  - 17-ketosteroids, elevated R82.5
  - acetonuria R82.4
  - alcohol in blood R78.Ø
  - anisocytosis R71.8
  - antenatal screening of mother O28.9
    - biochemical O28.1
    - chromosomal O28.5
    - cytological O28.2
    - genetic O28.5
    - hematological O28.Ø
    - radiological O28.4
    - specified NEC O28.8
    - ultrasonic O28.3
  - antibody titer, elevated R76.Ø
  - anticardiolipin antibody R76.Ø
  - antiphosphatidylglycerol antibody R76.Ø
  - antiphosphatidylinositol antibody R76.Ø
  - antiphosphatidylserine antibody R76.Ø
  - antiphospholipid antibody R76.Ø
  - bacteriuria R82.71
  - bicarbonate E87.8
  - bile in urine R82.2
  - blood sugar R73.Ø9
    - high R73.9
    - low (transient) E16.2
  - body fluid or substance, specified NEC R88.8
  - casts, urine R82.998

- **Findings, abnormal, inconclusive, without diagnosis** — *continued*
  - catecholamines R82.5
  - cells, urine R82.998
  - chloride E87.8
  - cholesterol E78.9
    - high E78.ØØ
      - with high triglycerides E78.2
  - chyluria R82.Ø
  - cloudy
    - dialysis effluent R88.Ø
    - urine R82.9Ø
  - creatinine clearance R94.4
  - crystals, urine R82.998
  - culture
    - blood R78.81
    - positive — *see* Positive, culture
  - echocardiogram R93.1
  - electrolyte level, urinary R82.998
  - function study NEC R94.8
    - bladder R94.8
    - endocrine NEC R94.7
      - thyroid R94.6
    - kidney R94.4
    - liver R94.5
    - pancreas R94.8
    - placenta R94.8
    - pulmonary R94.2
    - spleen R94.8
  - gallbladder, nonvisualization R93.2
  - glucose (tolerance test) (non-fasting) R73.Ø9
  - glycosuria R81
  - heart
    - shadow R93.1
    - sounds RØ1.2
  - hematinuria R82.3
  - hematocrit drop (precipitous) R71.Ø
  - hemoglobinuria R82.3
  - human papillomavirus (HPV) DNA test positive
    - cervix
      - high risk R87.81Ø
      - low risk R87.82Ø
    - vagina
      - high risk R87.811
      - low risk R87.821
  - in blood (of substance not normally found in blood) R78.9
    - addictive drug NEC R78.4
    - alcohol (excessive level) R78.Ø
    - cocaine R78.2
    - gadolinium level R78.72
    - hallucinogen R78.3
    - heavy metals (abnormal level) R78.79
    - lead R78.71
    - lithium (abnormal level) R78.89
    - opiate drug R78.1
    - psychotropic drug R78.5
    - specified substance NEC R78.89
    - steroid agent R78.6
  - indoleacetic acid, elevated R82.5
  - ketonuria R82.4
  - lactic acid dehydrogenase (LDH) R74.Ø2
  - liver function test — *see also* Elevated, liver function, test R79.89
  - mammogram NEC R92.8
    - calcification (calculus) R92.1
    - inconclusive result R92.2
    - microcalcification R92.Ø
  - mediastinal shift R93.89
  - melanin, urine R82.998
  - myoglobinuria R82.1
  - neonatal screening — *see* Abnormal, neonatal screening
  - newborn screens, state mandated — *see* Abnormal, neonatal screening
  - nonvisualization of gallbladder R93.2
  - odor of urine NOS R82.9Ø
  - Papanicolaou cervix R87.619
    - non-atypical endometrial cells R87.618
  - pneumoencephalogram R93.Ø
  - poikilocytosis R71.8
  - potassium (deficiency) E87.6
    - excess E87.5
  - PPD R76.11
  - radiologic (X-ray) R93.89
    - abdomen R93.5
    - biliary tract R93.2
    - breast R92.8
    - gastrointestinal tract R93.3
    - genitourinary organs R93.89
    - head R93.Ø

- **Findings, abnormal, inconclusive, without diagnosis** — *continued*
  - radiologic — *continued*
    - inconclusive due to excess body fat of patient R93.9
    - intrathoracic organs NEC R93.1
    - musculoskeletal
      - limbs R93.6
      - other than limb R93.7
    - placenta R93.89
    - retroperitoneum R93.5
    - skin R93.89
    - skull R93.Ø
    - subcutaneous tissue R93.89
    - testis R93.81- ☑
  - red blood cell (count) (morphology) (sickling) (volume) R71.8
  - scan NEC R94.8
    - bladder R94.8
    - bone R94.8
    - kidney R94.4
    - liver R93.2
    - lung R94.2
    - pancreas R94.8
    - placental R94.8
    - spleen R94.8
    - thyroid R94.6
  - sedimentation rate, elevated R7Ø.Ø
  - SGOT R74.Ø1
  - SGPT R74.Ø1
  - sodium (deficiency) E87.1
    - excess E87.Ø
  - specified body fluid NEC R88.8
  - stress test R94.39
  - testis R93.81- ☑
  - thyroid (function) (metabolic rate) (scan) (uptake) R94.6
  - transaminase (level) R74.Ø1
  - triglycerides E78.9
    - high E78.1
      - with high cholesterol E78.2
  - tuberculin skin test (without active tuberculosis) R76.11
  - urine R82.9Ø
    - acetone R82.4
    - bacteria R82.71
    - bile R82.2
    - casts or cells R82.998
    - chyle R82.Ø
    - culture positive R82.79
    - glucose R81
    - hemoglobin R82.3
    - ketone R82.4
    - sugar R81
  - vanillylmandelic acid (VMA), elevated R82.5
  - vectorcardiogram (VCG) R94.39
  - ventriculogram R93.Ø
  - white blood cell (count) (differential) (morphology) D72.9
  - xerography R92.8
- **Finger** — *see* condition
- **Fire, Saint Anthony's** — *see* Erysipelas
- **Fire-setting**
  - pathological (compulsive) F63.1
- **Fish hook stomach** K31.89
- **Fishmeal-worker's lung** J67.8
- **Fissure, fissured**
  - anus, anal K6Ø.2
    - acute K6Ø.Ø
    - chronic K6Ø.1
    - congenital Q43.8
  - ear, lobule, congenital Q17.8
  - epiglottis (congenital) Q31.8
  - larynx J38.7
    - congenital Q31.8
  - lip K13.Ø
    - congenital — *see* Cleft, lip
  - nipple N64.Ø
    - associated with
      - lactation O92.13
      - pregnancy O92.11- ☑
      - puerperium O92.12
  - nose Q3Ø.2
  - palate (congenital) — *see* Cleft, palate
  - skin R23.4
  - spine (congenital) — *see also* Spina bifida
    - with hydrocephalus — *see* Spina bifida, by site, with hydrocephalus
  - tongue (acquired) K14.5
    - congenital Q38.3
- **Fistula** (cutaneous) L98.8
  - abdomen (wall) K63.2
    - bladder N32.2

- **Fistula** — *continued*
  - abdomen — *continued*
    - intestine NEC K63.2
    - ureter N28.89
    - uterus N82.5
  - abdominorectal K63.2
  - abdominosigmoidal K63.2
  - abdominothoracic J86.Ø
  - abdominouterine N82.5
    - congenital Q51.7
  - abdominovesical N32.2
  - accessory sinuses — *see* Sinusitis
  - actinomycotic — *see* Actinomycosis
  - alveolar antrum — *see* Sinusitis, maxillary
  - alveolar process KØ4.6
  - anorectal (infectional) K6Ø.5Ø
    - complex K6Ø.529
      - chronic K6Ø.522
      - initial K6Ø.521
      - new K6Ø.521
      - occurring following complete healing K6Ø.523
      - persistent K6Ø.522
      - recurrent K6Ø.523
    - extrasphincteric K6Ø.52- ☑
    - high intersphincteric K6Ø.52- ☑
    - low intersphincteric K6Ø.51- ☑
    - simple K6Ø.519
      - chronic K6Ø.512
      - initial K6Ø.511
      - new K6Ø.511
      - occurring following complete healing K6Ø.513
      - persistent K6Ø.512
      - recurrent K6Ø.513
    - superficial K6Ø.51- ☑
    - suprasphincteric K6Ø.52- ☑
    - transsphincteric K6Ø.52- ☑
  - antrobuccal — *see* Sinusitis, maxillary
  - antrum — *see* Sinusitis, maxillary
  - anus, anal (recurrent) (infectional) K6Ø.3Ø
    - complex K6Ø.329
      - chronic K6Ø.322
      - initial K6Ø.321
      - new K6Ø.321
      - occurring following complete healing K6Ø.323
      - persistent K6Ø.322
      - recurrent K6Ø.323
    - congenital Q43.6
      - with absence, atresia and stenosis Q42.2
    - extrasphincteric K6Ø.32- ☑
    - high intersphincteric K6Ø.32- ☑
    - low intersphincteric K6Ø.31- ☑
    - simple K6Ø.319
      - chronic K6Ø.312
      - initial K6Ø.311
      - new K6Ø.311
      - occurring following complete healing K6Ø.313
      - persistent K6Ø.312
      - recurrent K6Ø.313
    - superficial K6Ø.31- ☑
    - suprasphincteric K6Ø.32- ☑
    - transsphincteric K6Ø.32- ☑
    - tuberculous A18.32
  - aorta-duodenal I77.2
  - appendix, appendicular K38.3
  - arteriovenous (acquired) (nonruptured) I77.Ø
    - brain I67.1
      - congenital Q28.2
        - ruptured — *see* Fistula, arteriovenous, brain, ruptured
      - ruptured I6Ø.8
        - intracerebral I61.8
        - intraparenchymal I61.8
        - intraventricular I61.5
        - subarachnoid I6Ø.8
    - cerebral — *see* Fistula, arteriovenous, brain
    - congenital (peripheral) — *see also* Malformation, arteriovenous
      - brain Q28.2
        - ruptured — *see* Fistula, arteriovenous, brain, ruptured
      - coronary Q24.5
      - pulmonary Q25.72
    - coronary I25.41
      - congenital Q24.5
    - pulmonary I28.Ø
      - congenital Q25.72
    - surgically created (for dialysis) Z99.2

- **Fistula** — *continued*
  - arteriovenous — *continued*
    - surgically created — *continued*
      - complication — *see* Complication, arteriovenous, fistula, surgically created
    - traumatic — *see* Injury, blood vessel
  - artery I77.2
  - aural (mastoid) — *see* Mastoiditis, chronic
  - auricle — *see also* Disorder, pinna, specified type NEC
    - congenital Q18.1
  - Bartholin's gland N82.8
  - bile duct (common) (hepatic) K83.3
    - with calculus, stones — *see also* Calculus, bile duct K83.3
  - biliary (tract) — *see* Fistula, bile duct
  - bladder (sphincter) NEC — *see also* Fistula, vesico- N32.2
    - into seminal vesicle N32.2
  - bone — *see also* Disorder, bone, specified type NEC
    - with osteomyelitis, chronic — *see* Osteomyelitis, chronic, with draining sinus
  - brain G93.89
    - arteriovenous (acquired) — *see also* Fistula, arteriovenous, brain I67.1
      - congenital Q28.2
  - branchial (cleft) Q18.Ø
  - branchiogenous Q18.Ø
  - breast N61.Ø
    - puerperal, postpartum or gestational, due to mastitis (purulent) — *see* Mastitis, obstetric, purulent
  - bronchial J86.Ø
  - bronchocutaneous, bronchomediastinal, bronchopleural, bronchopleuromediastinal (infective) J86.Ø
    - tuberculous NEC A15.5
  - bronchoesophageal J86.Ø
    - congenital Q39.2
      - with atresia of esophagus Q39.1
  - bronchovisceral J86.Ø
  - buccal cavity (infective) K12.2
  - cecosigmoidal K63.2
  - cecum K63.2
  - cerebrospinal (fluid) G96.Ø8
  - cervical, lateral Q18.1
  - cervicoaural Q18.1
  - cervicosigmoidal N82.4
  - cervicovesical N82.1
  - cervix N82.8
  - chest (wall) J86.Ø
  - cholecystenteric — *see* Fistula, gallbladder
  - cholecystocolic — *see* Fistula, gallbladder
  - cholecystocolonic — *see* Fistula, gallbladder
  - cholecystoduodenal — *see* Fistula, gallbladder
  - cholecystogastric — *see* Fistula, gallbladder
  - cholecystointestinal — *see* Fistula, gallbladder
  - choledochoduodenal — *see* Fistula, bile duct
  - cholocolic K82.3
  - coccyx — *see* Sinus, pilonidal
  - colon K63.2
  - colostomy K94.Ø9
  - colovesical N32.1
  - common duct — *see* Fistula, bile duct
  - congenital, site not listed — *see* Anomaly, by site
  - coronary, arteriovenous I25.41
    - congenital Q24.5
  - costal region J86.Ø
  - cul-de-sac, Douglas' N82.8
  - cystic duct — *see also* Fistula, gallbladder
    - congenital Q44.5
  - dental KØ4.6
  - diaphragm J86.Ø
  - duodenum K31.6
  - ear (external) (canal) — *see* Disorder, ear, external, specified type NEC
  - enterocolic K63.2
  - enterocutaneous K63.2
  - enterouterine N82.4
    - congenital Q51.7
  - enterovaginal N82.4
    - congenital Q52.2
    - large intestine N82.3
    - small intestine N82.2
  - enterovesical N32.1
  - epididymis N5Ø.89
    - tuberculous A18.15
  - esophagobronchial J86.Ø
    - congenital Q39.2
      - with atresia of esophagus Q39.1
  - esophagocutaneous K22.89
  - esophagopleural-cutaneous J86.Ø
  - esophagotracheal J86.Ø

- **Fistula** — *continued*
  - esophagotracheal — *continued*
    - congenital Q39.2
      - with atresia of esophagus Q39.1
  - esophagus K22.89
    - congenital Q39.2
      - with atresia of esophagus Q39.1
  - ethmoid — *see* Sinusitis, ethmoidal
  - eyeball (cornea) (sclera) — *see* Disorder, globe, hypotony
  - eyelid HØ1.8- ☑
  - fallopian tube, external N82.5
  - fecal K63.2
    - congenital Q43.6
  - from periapical abscess KØ4.6
  - frontal sinus — *see* Sinusitis, frontal
  - gallbladder K82.3
    - with calculus, cholelithiasis, stones — *see* Calculus, gallbladder
  - gastric K31.6
  - gastrocolic K31.6
    - congenital Q4Ø.2
    - tuberculous A18.32
  - gastroenterocolic K31.6
  - gastroesophageal K31.6
  - gastrojejunal K31.6
  - gastrojejunocolic K31.6
  - genital tract (female) N82.9
    - specified NEC N82.8
    - to intestine NEC N82.4
    - to skin N82.5
  - hepatic artery-portal vein, congenital Q26.6
  - hepatopleural J86.Ø
  - hepatopulmonary J86.Ø
  - ileorectal or ileosigmoidal K63.2
  - ileovaginal N82.2
  - ileovesical N32.1
  - ileum K63.2
  - in ano K6Ø.3Ø
    - tuberculous A18.32
  - inner ear (labyrinth) — *see* subcategory H83.1- ☑
  - intestine NEC K63.2
  - intestinocolonic (abdominal) K63.2
  - intestinoureteral N28.89
  - intestinouterine N82.4
  - intestinovaginal N82.4
    - large intestine N82.3
    - small intestine N82.2
  - intestinovesical N32.1
  - ischiorectal (fossa) K61.39
  - jejunum K63.2
  - joint M25.1Ø
    - ankle M25.17- ☑
    - elbow M25.12- ☑
    - foot joint M25.17- ☑
    - hand joint M25.14- ☑
    - hip M25.15- ☑
    - knee M25.16- ☑
    - shoulder M25.11- ☑
    - specified joint NEC M25.18
    - tuberculous — *see* Tuberculosis, joint
    - vertebrae M25.18
    - wrist M25.13- ☑
  - kidney N28.89
  - labium (majus) (minus) N82.8
  - labyrinth — *see* subcategory H83.1- ☑
  - lacrimal (gland) (sac) HØ4.61- ☑
  - lacrimonasal duct — *see* Fistula, lacrimal
  - laryngotracheal, congenital Q34.8
  - larynx J38.7
  - lip K13.Ø
    - congenital Q38.Ø
  - lumbar, tuberculous A18.Ø1
  - lung J86.Ø
  - lymphatic I89.8
  - mammary (gland) N61.Ø
  - mastoid (process) (region) — *see* Mastoiditis, chronic
  - maxillary J32.Ø
  - medial, face and neck Q18.8
  - mediastinal J86.Ø
  - mediastinobronchial J86.Ø
  - mediastinocutaneous J86.Ø
  - middle ear — *see* subcategory H74.8- ☑
  - mouth K12.2
  - nasal J34.89
    - sinus — *see* Sinusitis
  - nasopharynx J39.2
  - nipple N64.Ø
  - nose J34.89

**Fitting** — *continued*
- wheelchair Z46.89

**Fitzhugh-Curtis syndrome**
- due to
  - Chlamydia trachomatis A74.81
  - Neisseria gonorrhea (gonococcal peritonitis) A54.85

**Fitz's syndrome** (acute hemorrhagic pancreatitis) — *see also* Pancreatitis, acute K85.80

**Fixation**
- joint — *see* Ankylosis
- larynx J38.7
- stapes — *see* Ankylosis, ear ossicles
  - deafness — *see* Deafness, conductive
- uterus (acquired) — *see* Malposition, uterus
- vocal cord J38.3

**Flabby ridge** K06.8

**Flaccid** — *see also* condition
- palate, congenital Q38.5

**Flail**
- chest S22.5- ☑
  - associated with chest compression and cardiopulmonary resuscitation M96.A4
  - newborn (birth injury) P13.8
- joint (paralytic) M25.20
  - ankle M25.27- ☑
  - elbow M25.22- ☑
  - foot joint M25.27- ☑
  - hand joint M25.24- ☑
  - hip M25.25- ☑
  - knee M25.26- ☑
  - shoulder M25.21- ☑
  - specified joint NEC M25.28
  - wrist M25.23- ☑

**Flajani's disease** — *see* Hyperthyroidism, with, goiter (diffuse)

**Flap, liver** K71.3

**Flashbacks** (residual to hallucinogen use) F16.283

**Flat**
- affect R45.89
- chamber (eye) — *see* Disorder, globe, hypotony, flat anterior chamber
- chest, congenital Q67.8
- foot (acquired) (fixed type) (painful) (postural) — *see also* Deformity, limb, flat foot
  - congenital (rigid) (spastic (everted)) Q66.5- ☑
  - rachitic sequelae (late effect) E64.3
- organ or site, congenital NEC — *see* Anomaly, by site
- pelvis M95.5
  - with disproportion (fetopelvic) O33.0
    - causing obstructed labor O65.0
  - congenital Q74.2

**Flatau-Schilder disease** G37.0

**Flatback syndrome** M40.30
- lumbar region M40.36
- lumbosacral region M40.37
- thoracolumbar region M40.35

**Flattening**
- head, femur M89.8X5
- hip — *see* Coxa, plana
- lip (congenital) Q18.8
- nose (congenital) Q67.4
  - acquired M95.0

**Flatulence** R14.3
- psychogenic F45.8

**Flatus** R14.3
- vaginalis N89.8

**Flax-dresser's disease** J66.1

**Flea bite** — *see* Injury, bite, by site, superficial, insect

**Flecks, glaucomatous** (subcapsular) — *see* Cataract, complicated

**Fleischer** (-Kayser) **ring** (cornea) H18.04- ☑

**Fleshy mole** O02.0

**Flexibilitas cerea** — *see* Catalepsy

**Flexion**
- amputation stump (surgical) T87.89
- cervix — *see* Malposition, uterus
- contracture, joint — *see* Contraction, joint
- deformity, joint — *see also* Deformity, limb, flexion M21.20
  - hip, congenital Q65.89
- uterus — *see also* Malposition, uterus
  - lateral — *see* Lateroversion, uterus

**Flexner-Boyd dysentery** A03.2

**Flexner's dysentery** A03.1

**Flexure** — *see* Flexion

**Flint murmur** (aortic insufficiency) I35.1

**Floater, vitreous** — *see* Opacity, vitreous

**Floating**
- cartilage (joint) — *see also* Loose, body, joint
  - knee — *see* Derangement, knee, loose body
- gallbladder, congenital Q44.1
- kidney N28.89
  - congenital Q63.8
- spleen D73.89

**Flooding** N92.0

**Floor** — *see* condition

**Floppy**
- baby syndrome (nonspecific) P94.2
- iris syndrome (intraoperative) (IFIS) H21.81
- nonrheumatic mitral valve syndrome I34.1

**Flu** — *see also* Influenza
- avian — *see also* Influenza, due to, identified novel influenza A virus J09.X2
- bird — *see also* Influenza, due to, identified novel influenza A virus J09.X2
- intestinal NEC A08.4
- swine (viruses that normally cause infections in pigs) — *see also* Influenza, due to, identified novel influenza A virus J09.X2

**Fluctuating blood pressure** I99.8

**Fluid**
- abdomen R18.8
- chest J94.8
- heart — *see* Failure, heart, congestive
- joint — *see* Effusion, joint
- loss (acute) E86.9
- lung — *see* Edema, lung
- overload E87.70
  - specified NEC E87.79
- peritoneal cavity R18.8
- pleural cavity J94.8
- retention R60.9

**Flukes NEC** — *see also* Infestation, fluke
- blood NEC — *see* Schistosomiasis
- liver B66.3

**Fluor** (vaginalis) N89.8
- trichomonal or due to Trichomonas (vaginalis) A59.00

**Fluorosis**
- dental K00.3
- skeletal M85.10
  - ankle M85.17- ☑
  - foot M85.17- ☑
  - forearm M85.13- ☑
  - hand M85.14- ☑
  - lower leg M85.16- ☑
  - multiple site M85.19
  - neck M85.18
  - rib M85.18
  - shoulder M85.11- ☑
  - skull M85.18
  - specified site NEC M85.18
  - thigh M85.15- ☑
  - toe M85.17- ☑
  - upper arm M85.12- ☑
  - vertebra M85.18

**Flush syndrome** E34.09

**Flushing** R23.2
- menopausal N95.1

**Flutter**
- atrial or auricular I48.92
  - atypical I48.4
  - type I I48.3
  - type II I48.4
  - typical I48.3
- heart I49.89
  - atrial or auricular I48.92
    - atypical I48.4
    - type I I48.3
    - type II I48.4
    - typical I48.3
  - ventricular I49.02
- ventricular I49.02

**FNHTR** (febrile nonhemolytic transfusion reaction) R50.84

**Fochier's abscess** — *code by* site under Abscess

**Focus, Assmann's** — *see* Tuberculosis, pulmonary

**Fogo selvagem** L10.3

**Foix-Alajouanine syndrome** G95.19

**Fold, folds** (anomalous) — *see also* Anomaly, by site
- Descemet's membrane — *see* Change, corneal membrane, Descemet's, fold
- epicanthic Q10.3
- heart Q24.8

**Folie a deux** F24

**Follicle**
- cervix (nabothian) (ruptured) N88.8

**Follicle** — *continued*
- graafian, ruptured, with hemorrhage N83.0- ☑
- nabothian N88.8

**Follicular** — *see* condition

**Folliculitis** (superficial) L73.9
- abscedens et suffodiens L66.3
- cyst N83.0- ☑
- decalvans L66.2
- deep — *see* Furuncle, by site
- gonococcal (acute) (chronic) A54.01
- keloid, keloidalis L73.0
- pustular L01.02
- ulerythematosa reticulata L66.4

**Folliculome lipidique**
- specified site — *see* Neoplasm, benign, by site
- unspecified site
  - female D27.9
  - male D29.20

**Følling's disease** E70.0

**Follow-up** — *see* Examination, follow-up

**Fong's syndrome** (hereditary osteo-onychodysplasia) Q87.2

**Food**
- allergy L27.2
- asphyxia (from aspiration or inhalation) — *see* Foreign body, by site
- choked on — *see* Foreign body, by site
- deprivation T73.0- ☑
  - specified kind of food NEC E63.8
- insecurity Z59.41
- intoxication — *see* Poisoning, food
- lack of T73.0- ☑
- poisoning — *see* Poisoning, food
- rejection NEC — *see* Disorder, eating
- strangulation or suffocation — *see* Foreign body, by site
- toxemia — *see* Poisoning, food

**Foot** — *see* condition

**Foramen ovale** (nonclosure) (patent) (persistent) Q21.12

**Forbes' glycogen storage disease** E74.03

**Fordyce-Fox disease** L75.2

**Fordyce's disease** (mouth) Q38.6

**Forearm** — *see* condition

**Foreclosure on loan** Z59.89

**Foreign body**
- with
  - laceration — *see* Laceration, by site, with foreign body
  - puncture wound — *see* Puncture, by site, with foreign body
- accidentally left following a procedure T81.509- ☑
  - aspiration T81.506- ☑
    - resulting in
      - adhesions T81.516- ☑
      - obstruction T81.526- ☑
      - perforation T81.536- ☑
      - specified complication NEC T81.596- ☑
  - cardiac catheterization T81.505- ☑
    - resulting in
      - acute reaction T81.60- ☑
        - aseptic peritonitis T81.61- ☑
        - specified NEC T81.69- ☑
      - adhesions T81.515- ☑
      - obstruction T81.525- ☑
      - perforation T81.535- ☑
      - specified complication NEC T81.595- ☑
  - causing
    - acute reaction T81.60- ☑
      - aseptic peritonitis T81.61- ☑
      - specified complication NEC T81.69- ☑
    - adhesions T81.519- ☑
    - aseptic peritonitis T81.61- ☑
    - obstruction T81.529- ☑
    - perforation T81.539- ☑
    - specified complication NEC T81.599- ☑
  - endoscopy T81.504- ☑
    - resulting in
      - adhesions T81.514- ☑
      - obstruction T81.524- ☑
      - perforation T81.534- ☑
      - specified complication NEC T81.594- ☑
  - immunization T81.503- ☑
    - resulting in
      - adhesions T81.513- ☑
      - obstruction T81.523- ☑
      - perforation T81.533- ☑
      - specified complication NEC T81.593- ☑
  - infusion T81.501- ☑
    - resulting in
      - adhesions T81.511- ☑

**Foreign body** — *continued*
- accidentally left following a procedure — *continued*
  - infusion — *continued*
    - resulting in — *continued*
      - obstruction T81.521- ☑
      - perforation T81.531- ☑
      - specified complication NEC T81.591- ☑
  - injection T81.5Ø3- ☑
    - resulting in
      - adhesions T81.513- ☑
      - obstruction T81.523- ☑
      - perforation T81.533- ☑
      - specified complication NEC T81.593- ☑
  - kidney dialysis T81.5Ø2- ☑
    - resulting in
      - adhesions T81.512- ☑
      - obstruction T81.522- ☑
      - perforation T81.532- ☑
      - specified complication NEC T81.592- ☑
  - packing removal T81.5Ø7- ☑
    - resulting in
      - acute reaction T81.6Ø- ☑
        - aseptic peritonitis T81.61- ☑
        - specified NEC T81.69- ☑
      - adhesions T81.517- ☑
      - obstruction T81.527- ☑
      - perforation T81.537- ☑
      - specified complication NEC T81.597- ☑
  - puncture T81.5Ø6- ☑
    - resulting in
      - adhesions T81.516- ☑
      - obstruction T81.526- ☑
      - perforation T81.536- ☑
      - specified complication NEC T81.596- ☑
  - specified procedure NEC T81.5Ø8- ☑
    - resulting in
      - acute reaction T81.6Ø- ☑
        - aseptic peritonitis T81.61- ☑
        - specified NEC T81.69- ☑
      - adhesions T81.518- ☑
      - obstruction T81.528- ☑
      - perforation T81.538- ☑
      - specified complication NEC T81.598- ☑
  - surgical operation T81.5ØØ- ☑
    - resulting in
      - acute reaction T81.6Ø- ☑
        - aseptic peritonitis T81.61- ☑
        - specified NEC T81.69- ☑
      - adhesions T81.51Ø- ☑
      - obstruction T81.52Ø- ☑
      - perforation T81.53Ø- ☑
      - specified complication NEC T81.59Ø- ☑
  - transfusion T81.5Ø1- ☑
    - resulting in
      - adhesions T81.511- ☑
      - obstruction T81.521- ☑
      - perforation T81.531- ☑
      - specified complication NEC T81.591- ☑
- alimentary tract T18.9- ☑
  - anus T18.5- ☑
  - colon T18.4- ☑
  - esophagus — *see* Foreign body, esophagus
  - mouth T18.Ø- ☑
  - multiple sites T18.8- ☑
  - rectosigmoid (junction) T18.5- ☑
  - rectum T18.5- ☑
  - small intestine T18.3- ☑
  - specified site NEC T18.8- ☑
  - stomach T18.2- ☑
- anterior chamber (eye) SØ5.5- ☑
- auditory canal — *see* Foreign body, entering through orifice, ear
- bronchus T17.5Ø8- ☑
  - causing
    - asphyxiation T17.5ØØ- ☑
      - food (bone) (seed) T17.52Ø- ☑
      - gastric contents (vomitus) T17.51Ø- ☑
      - specified type NEC T17.59Ø- ☑
    - injury NEC T17.5Ø8- ☑
      - food (bone) (seed) T17.528- ☑
      - gastric contents (vomitus) T17.518- ☑
      - specified type NEC T17.598- ☑
- canthus — *see* Foreign body, conjunctival sac
- ciliary body (eye) SØ5.5- ☑
- conjunctival sac T15.1- ☑

**Foreign body** — *continued*
- cornea T15.Ø- ☑
- entering through orifice
  - accessory sinus T17.Ø- ☑
  - alimentary canal T18.9- ☑
    - multiple parts T18.8- ☑
    - specified part NEC T18.8- ☑
  - alveolar process T18.Ø- ☑
  - antrum (Highmore's) T17.Ø- ☑
  - anus T18.5- ☑
  - appendix T18.4- ☑
  - auditory canal — *see* Foreign body, entering through orifice, ear
  - auricle — *see* Foreign body, entering through orifice, ear
  - bladder T19.1- ☑
  - bronchioles — *see* Foreign body, respiratory tract, specified site NEC
  - bronchus (main) — *see* Foreign body, bronchus
  - buccal cavity T18.Ø- ☑
  - canthus (inner) — *see* Foreign body, conjunctival sac
  - cecum T18.4- ☑
  - cervix (canal) (uteri) T19.3- ☑
  - colon T18.4- ☑
  - conjunctival sac — *see* Foreign body, conjunctival sac
  - cornea — *see* Foreign body, cornea
  - digestive organ or tract NOS T18.9- ☑
    - multiple parts T18.8- ☑
    - specified part NEC T18.8- ☑
  - duodenum T18.3- ☑
  - ear (external) T16.- ☑
  - esophagus — *see* Foreign body, esophagus
  - eye (external) NOS T15.9- ☑
    - conjunctival sac — *see* Foreign body, conjunctival sac
    - cornea — *see* Foreign body, cornea
    - specified part NEC T15.8- ☑
  - eyeball — *see also* Foreign body, entering through orifice, eye, specified part NEC
    - with penetrating wound — *see* Puncture, eyeball
  - eyelid — *see also* Foreign body, conjunctival sac
    - with
      - laceration — *see* Laceration, eyelid, with foreign body
      - puncture — *see* Puncture, eyelid, with foreign body
      - superficial injury — *see* Foreign body, superficial, eyelid
  - gastrointestinal tract T18.9- ☑
    - multiple parts T18.8- ☑
    - specified part NEC T18.8- ☑
  - genitourinary tract T19.9- ☑
    - multiple parts T19.8- ☑
    - specified part NEC T19.8- ☑
  - globe — *see* Foreign body, entering through orifice, eyeball
  - gum T18.Ø- ☑
  - Highmore's antrum T17.Ø- ☑
  - hypopharynx — *see* Foreign body, pharynx
  - ileum T18.3- ☑
  - intestine (small) T18.3- ☑
    - large T18.4- ☑
  - lacrimal apparatus (punctum) — *see* Foreign body, entering through orifice, eye, specified part NEC
  - large intestine T18.4- ☑
  - larynx — *see* Foreign body, larynx
  - lung — *see* Foreign body, respiratory tract, specified site NEC
  - maxillary sinus T17.Ø- ☑
  - mouth T18.Ø- ☑
  - nasal sinus T17.Ø- ☑
  - nasopharynx — *see* Foreign body, pharynx
  - nose (passage) T17.1- ☑
  - nostril T17.1- ☑
  - oral cavity T18.Ø- ☑
  - palate T18.Ø- ☑
  - penis T19.4- ☑
  - pharynx — *see* Foreign body, pharynx
  - piriform sinus — *see* Foreign body, pharynx
  - rectosigmoid (junction) T18.5- ☑
  - rectum T18.5- ☑
  - respiratory tract — *see* Foreign body, respiratory tract
  - sinus (accessory) (frontal) (maxillary) (nasal) T17.Ø- ☑
    - piriform — *see* Foreign body, pharynx
  - small intestine T18.3- ☑
  - stomach T18.2- ☑

**Foreign body** — *continued*
- entering through orifice — *continued*
  - suffocation by — *see* Foreign body, by site
  - tear ducts or glands — *see* Foreign body, entering through orifice, eye, specified part NEC
  - throat — *see* Foreign body, pharynx
  - tongue T18.Ø- ☑
  - tonsil, tonsillar (fossa) — *see* Foreign body, pharynx
  - trachea — *see* Foreign body, trachea
  - ureter T19.8- ☑
  - urethra T19.Ø- ☑
  - uterus (any part) T19.3- ☑
  - vagina T19.2- ☑
  - vulva T19.2- ☑
- esophagus T18.1Ø8- ☑
  - causing
    - injury NEC T18.1Ø8- ☑
      - food (bone) (seed) T18.128- ☑
      - gastric contents (vomitus) T18.118- ☑
      - specified type NEC T18.198- ☑
    - tracheal compression T18.1ØØ- ☑
      - food (bone) (seed) T18.12Ø- ☑
      - gastric contents (vomitus) T18.11Ø- ☑
      - specified type NEC T18.19Ø- ☑
- feeling of, in throat RØ9.A2
- fragment — *see* Retained, foreign body fragments (type of)
- genitourinary tract T19.9- ☑
  - bladder T19.1- ☑
  - multiple parts T19.8- ☑
  - penis T19.4- ☑
  - specified site NEC T19.8- ☑
  - urethra T19.Ø- ☑
  - uterus T19.3- ☑
    - IUD Z97.5
  - vagina T19.2- ☑
    - contraceptive device Z97.5
  - vulva T19.2- ☑
- granuloma (old) (soft tissue) — *see also* Granuloma, foreign body
  - skin L92.3
- in
  - laceration — *see* Laceration, by site, with foreign body
  - puncture wound — *see* Puncture, by site, with foreign body
  - soft tissue (residual) M79.5
- inadvertently left in operation wound — *see* Foreign body, accidentally left during a procedure
- ingestion, ingested NOS T18.9- ☑
- inhalation or inspiration — *see* Foreign body, by site
- internal organ, not entering through a natural orifice — code as specific injury with foreign body
- intraocular SØ5.5- ☑
  - old, retained (nonmagnetic) H44.7Ø- ☑
    - anterior chamber H44.71- ☑
    - ciliary body H44.72- ☑
    - iris H44.72- ☑
    - lens H44.73- ☑
    - magnetic H44.6Ø- ☑
      - anterior chamber H44.61- ☑
      - ciliary body H44.62- ☑
      - iris H44.62- ☑
      - lens H44.63- ☑
      - posterior wall H44.64- ☑
      - specified site NEC H44.69- ☑
      - vitreous body H44.65- ☑
    - posterior wall H44.74- ☑
    - specified site NEC H44.79- ☑
    - vitreous body H44.75- ☑
- iris — *see* Foreign body, intraocular
- lacrimal punctum — *see* Foreign body, entering through orifice, eye, specified part NEC
- larynx T17.3Ø8- ☑
  - causing
    - asphyxiation T17.3ØØ- ☑
      - food (bone) (seed) T17.32Ø- ☑
      - gastric contents (vomitus) T17.31Ø- ☑
      - specified type NEC T17.39Ø- ☑
    - injury NEC T17.3Ø8- ☑
      - food (bone) (seed) T17.328- ☑
      - gastric contents (vomitus) T17.318- ☑
      - specified type NEC T17.398- ☑
- lens — *see* Foreign body, intraocular
- ocular muscle SØ5.4- ☑
  - old, retained — *see* Foreign body, orbit, old

**Foreign body** — *continued*
- old or residual
  - soft tissue (residual) M79.5
- operation wound, left accidentally — *see* Foreign body, accidentally left during a procedure
- orbit S05.4- ☑
  - old, retained H05.5- ☑
- pharynx T17.208- ☑
  - causing
    - asphyxiation T17.200- ☑
      - food (bone) (seed) T17.220- ☑
      - gastric contents (vomitus) T17.210- ☑
      - specified type NEC T17.290- ☑
    - injury NEC T17.208- ☑
      - food (bone) (seed) T17.228- ☑
      - gastric contents (vomitus) T17.218- ☑
      - specified type NEC T17.298- ☑
- respiratory tract T17.908- ☑
  - bronchioles — *see* Foreign body, respiratory tract, specified site NEC
  - bronchus — *see* Foreign body, bronchus
  - causing
    - asphyxiation T17.900- ☑
      - food (bone) (seed) T17.920- ☑
      - gastric contents (vomitus) T17.910- ☑
      - specified type NEC T17.990- ☑
    - injury NEC T17.908- ☑
      - food (bone) (seed) T17.928- ☑
      - gastric contents (vomitus) T17.918- ☑
      - specified type NEC T17.998- ☑
  - larynx — *see* Foreign body, larynx
  - lung — *see* Foreign body, respiratory tract, specified site NEC
  - multiple parts — *see* Foreign body, respiratory tract, specified site NEC
  - nasal sinus T17.0- ☑
  - nasopharynx — *see* Foreign body, pharynx
  - nose T17.1- ☑
  - nostril T17.1- ☑
  - pharynx — *see* Foreign body, pharynx
  - specified site NEC T17.808- ☑
    - causing
      - asphyxiation T17.800- ☑
        - food (bone) (seed) T17.820- ☑
        - gastric contents (vomitus) T17.810- ☑
        - specified type NEC T17.890- ☑
      - injury NEC T17.808- ☑
        - food (bone) (seed) T17.828- ☑
        - gastric contents (vomitus) T17.818- ☑
        - specified type NEC T17.898- ☑
  - throat — *see* Foreign body, pharynx
  - trachea — *see* Foreign body, trachea
- retained (old) (nonmagnetic) (in)
  - anterior chamber (eye) — *see* Foreign body, intraocular, old, retained, anterior chamber
    - magnetic — *see* Foreign body, intraocular, old, retained, magnetic, anterior chamber
  - ciliary body — *see* Foreign body, intraocular, old, retained, ciliary body
    - magnetic — *see* Foreign body, intraocular, old, retained, magnetic, ciliary body
  - eyelid H02.819
    - left H02.816
      - lower H02.815
      - upper H02.814
    - right H02.813
      - lower H02.812
      - upper H02.811
  - fragments — *see* Retained, foreign body fragments (type of)
  - globe — *see* Foreign body, intraocular, old, retained
    - magnetic — *see* Foreign body, intraocular, old, retained, magnetic
  - intraocular — *see* Foreign body, intraocular, old, retained
    - magnetic — *see* Foreign body, intraocular, old, retained, magnetic
  - iris — *see* Foreign body, intraocular, old, retained, iris
    - magnetic — *see* Foreign body, intraocular, old, retained, magnetic, iris
  - lens — *see* Foreign body, intraocular, old, retained, lens
    - magnetic — *see* Foreign body, intraocular, old, retained, magnetic, lens
  - muscle — *see* Foreign body, retained, soft tissue
  - orbit — *see* Foreign body, orbit, old

**Foreign body** — *continued*
- retained — *continued*
  - posterior wall of globe — *see* Foreign body, intraocular, old, retained, posterior wall
    - magnetic — *see* Foreign body, intraocular, old, retained, magnetic, posterior wall
  - retrobulbar — *see* Foreign body, orbit, old, retrobulbar
  - soft tissue M79.5
  - vitreous — *see* Foreign body, intraocular, old, retained, vitreous body
    - magnetic — *see* Foreign body, intraocular, old, retained, magnetic, vitreous body
- retina S05.5- ☑
- sensation — *see* Sensation, foreign body
- superficial, without open wound
  - abdomen, abdominal (wall) S30.851- ☑
  - alveolar process S00.552- ☑
  - ankle S90.55- ☑
  - antecubital space — *see* Foreign body, superficial, forearm
  - anus S30.857- ☑
  - arm (upper) S40.85- ☑
  - auditory canal — *see* Foreign body, superficial, ear
  - auricle — *see* Foreign body, superficial, ear
  - axilla — *see* Foreign body, superficial, arm
  - back, lower S30.850- ☑
  - breast S20.15- ☑
  - brow S00.85- ☑
  - buttock S30.850- ☑
  - calf — *see* Foreign body, superficial, leg
  - canthus — *see* Foreign body, superficial, eyelid
  - cheek S00.85- ☑
    - internal S00.552- ☑
  - chest wall — *see* Foreign body, superficial, thorax
  - chin S00.85- ☑
  - clitoris S30.854- ☑
  - costal region — *see* Foreign body, superficial, thorax
  - digit(s)
    - foot — *see* Foreign body, superficial, toe
    - hand — *see* Foreign body, superficial, finger
  - ear S00.45- ☑
  - elbow S50.35- ☑
  - epididymis S30.853- ☑
  - epigastric region S30.851- ☑
  - epiglottis S10.15- ☑
  - esophagus, cervical S10.15- ☑
  - eyebrow — *see* Foreign body, superficial, eyelid
  - eyelid S00.25- ☑
  - face S00.85- ☑
  - finger(s) S60.459- ☑
    - index S60.45- ☑
    - little S60.45- ☑
    - middle S60.45- ☑
    - ring S60.45- ☑
  - flank S30.85A- ☑
  - foot (except toe(s) alone) S90.85- ☑
    - toe — *see* Foreign body, superficial, toe
  - forearm S50.85- ☑
    - elbow only — *see* Foreign body, superficial, elbow
  - forehead S00.85- ☑
  - genital organs, external
    - female S30.856- ☑
    - male S30.855- ☑
  - groin S30.851- ☑
  - gum S00.552- ☑
  - hand S60.55- ☑
  - head S00.95- ☑
    - ear — *see* Foreign body, superficial, ear
    - eyelid — *see* Foreign body, superficial, eyelid
    - lip S00.551- ☑
    - nose S00.35- ☑
    - oral cavity S00.552- ☑
    - scalp S00.05- ☑
    - specified site NEC S00.85- ☑
  - heel — *see* Foreign body, superficial, foot
  - hip S70.25- ☑
  - inguinal region S30.851- ☑
  - interscapular region S20.459- ☑
  - jaw S00.85- ☑
  - knee S80.25- ☑
  - labium (majus) (minus) S30.854- ☑
  - larynx S10.15- ☑
  - leg (lower) S80.85- ☑
    - knee — *see* Foreign body, superficial, knee
    - upper — *see* Foreign body, superficial, thigh

**Foreign body** — *continued*
- superficial, without open wound — *continued*
  - lip S00.551- ☑
  - lower back S30.850- ☑
  - lumbar region S30.850- ☑
  - malar region S00.85- ☑
  - mammary — *see* Foreign body, superficial, breast
  - mastoid region S00.85- ☑
  - mouth S00.552- ☑
  - nail
    - finger — *see* Foreign body, superficial, finger
    - toe — *see* Foreign body, superficial, toe
  - nape S10.85- ☑
  - nasal S00.35- ☑
  - neck S10.95- ☑
    - specified site NEC S10.85- ☑
    - throat S10.15- ☑
  - nose S00.35- ☑
  - occipital region S00.05- ☑
  - oral cavity S00.552- ☑
  - orbital region — *see* Foreign body, superficial, eyelid
  - palate S00.552- ☑
  - palm — *see* Foreign body, superficial, hand
  - parietal region S00.05- ☑
  - pelvis S30.850- ☑
  - penis S30.852- ☑
  - perineum
    - female S30.854- ☑
    - male S30.850- ☑
  - periocular area — *see* Foreign body, superficial, eyelid
  - phalanges
    - finger — *see* Foreign body, superficial, finger
    - toe — *see* Foreign body, superficial, toe
  - pharynx S10.15- ☑
  - pinna — *see* Foreign body, superficial, ear
  - popliteal space — *see* Foreign body, superficial, knee
  - prepuce S30.852- ☑
  - pubic region S30.850- ☑
  - pudendum
    - female S30.856- ☑
    - male S30.855- ☑
  - sacral region S30.850- ☑
  - scalp S00.05- ☑
  - scapular region — *see* Foreign body, superficial, shoulder
  - scrotum S30.853- ☑
  - shin — *see* Foreign body, superficial, leg
  - shoulder S40.25- ☑
  - sternal region S20.359- ☑
  - submaxillary region S00.85- ☑
  - submental region S00.85- ☑
  - subungual
    - finger(s) — *see* Foreign body, superficial, finger
    - toe(s) — *see* Foreign body, superficial, toe
  - supraclavicular fossa S10.85- ☑
  - supraorbital S00.85- ☑
  - temple S00.85- ☑
  - temporal region S00.85- ☑
  - testis S30.853- ☑
  - thigh S70.35- ☑
  - thorax, thoracic (wall) S20.95- ☑
    - back S20.45- ☑
    - front S20.35- ☑
  - throat S10.15- ☑
  - thumb S60.35- ☑
  - toe(s) (lesser) S90.456- ☑
    - great S90.45- ☑
  - tongue S00.552- ☑
  - trachea S10.15- ☑
  - tunica vaginalis S30.853- ☑
  - tympanum, tympanic membrane — *see* Foreign body, superficial, ear
  - uvula S00.552- ☑
  - vagina S30.854- ☑
  - vocal cords S10.15- ☑
  - vulva S30.854- ☑
  - wrist S60.85- ☑
- swallowed T18.9- ☑
- trachea T17.408- ☑
  - causing
    - asphyxiation T17.400- ☑
      - food (bone) (seed) T17.420- ☑
      - gastric contents (vomitus) T17.410- ☑
      - specified type NEC T17.490- ☑
    - injury NEC T17.408- ☑
      - food (bone) (seed) T17.428- ☑

- **Foreign body** — *continued*
  - trachea — *continued*
    - causing — *continued*
      - injury — *continued*
        - gastric contents (vomitus) T17.418- ☑
        - specified type NEC T17.498- ☑
  - type of fragment — *see* Retained, foreign body fragments (type of)
  - vitreous (humor) S05.5- ☑
- **Forestier's disease** (rhizomelic pseudopolyarthritis) M35.3
  - meaning ankylosing hyperostosis — *see* Hyperostosis, ankylosing
- **Formation**
  - hyalin in cornea — *see* Degeneration, cornea
  - sequestrum in bone (due to infection) — *see* Osteomyelitis, chronic
  - valve
    - colon, congenital Q43.8
    - ureter (congenital) Q62.39
- **Formication** R20.2
- **Fort Bragg fever** A27.89
- **Fossa** — *see also* condition
  - pyriform — *see* condition
- **Foster-Kennedy syndrome** H47.14- ☑
- **Fothergill's**
  - disease (trigeminal neuralgia) — *see also* Neuralgia, trigeminal
    - scarlatina anginosa A38.9
- **Foul breath** R19.6
- **Foundling** Z76.1
- **Fournier disease or gangrene** N49.3
  - female N76.82
  - vagina and vulva N76.82
- **Fourth**
  - cranial nerve — *see* condition
  - molar K00.1
- **Foville's** (peduncular) **disease or syndrome** G46.3
- **Fox** (-Fordyce) disease (apocrine miliaria) L75.2
- **FPIES (food protein-induced enterocolitis syndrome)** K52.21
- **FPVT** (familial polymorphic ventricular tachycardia) I47.22
- **Fracture, burst** — *see* Fracture, traumatic, by site
- **Fracture, chronic** — *see* Fracture, pathological, by site
- **Fracture, insufficiency** — *see* Fracture, pathological, by site
- **Fracture, nontraumatic, NEC**
  - atypical
    - femur M84.750- ☑
      - complete
        - oblique M84.759- ☑
          - left side M84.758- ☑
          - right side M84.757- ☑
        - transverse M84.756- ☑
          - left side M84.755- ☑
          - right side M84.754- ☑
      - incomplete M84.753- ☑
        - left side M84.752- ☑
        - right side M84.751- ☑
- **Fracture, pathological** (pathologic) — *see also* Fracture, traumatic M84.40- ☑
  - ankle M84.47- ☑
  - carpus M84.44- ☑
  - clavicle M84.41- ☑
  - compression (not due to trauma) — *see also* Collapse, vertebra M48.50- ☑
  - dental implant M27.63
  - dental restorative material K08.539
    - with loss of material K08.531
    - without loss of material K08.530
  - due to
    - neoplastic disease NEC — *see also* Neoplasm M84.50- ☑
      - ankle M84.57- ☑
      - carpus M84.54- ☑
      - clavicle M84.51- ☑
      - femur M84.55- ☑
      - fibula M84.56- ☑
      - finger M84.54- ☑
      - hip M84.559- ☑
      - humerus M84.52- ☑
      - ilium M84.550- ☑
      - ischium M84.550- ☑
      - metacarpus M84.54- ☑
      - metatarsus M84.57- ☑
      - neck M84.58- ☑
      - pelvis M84.550- ☑
      - radius M84.53- ☑

- **Fracture, pathological** — *continued*
  - due to — *continued*
    - neoplastic disease — *see also* Neoplasm — *continued*
      - rib M84.58- ☑
      - scapula M84.51- ☑
      - skull M84.58- ☑
      - specified site NEC M84.58- ☑
      - tarsus M84.57- ☑
      - tibia M84.56- ☑
      - toe M84.57- ☑
      - ulna M84.53- ☑
      - vertebra M84.58- ☑
    - osteoporosis M80.00- ☑
      - disuse — *see* Osteoporosis, specified type NEC, with pathological fracture
      - drug-induced — *see* Osteoporosis, drug induced, with pathological fracture
      - idiopathic — *see* Osteoporosis, specified type NEC, with pathological fracture
      - postmenopausal — *see* Osteoporosis, postmenopausal, with pathological fracture
      - postoophorectomy — *see* Osteoporosis, postoophorectomy, with pathological fracture
      - postsurgical malabsorption — *see* Osteoporosis, specified type NEC, with pathological fracture
      - specified cause NEC — *see* Osteoporosis, specified type NEC, with pathological fracture
    - specified disease NEC M84.60- ☑
      - ankle M84.67- ☑
      - carpus M84.64- ☑
      - clavicle M84.61- ☑
      - femur M84.65- ☑
      - fibula M84.66- ☑
      - finger M84.64- ☑
      - hip M84.65- ☑
      - humerus M84.62- ☑
      - ilium M84.650- ☑
      - ischium M84.650- ☑
      - metacarpus M84.64- ☑
      - metatarsus M84.67- ☑
      - neck M84.68- ☑
      - radius M84.63- ☑
      - rib M84.68- ☑
      - scapula M84.61- ☑
      - skull M84.68- ☑
      - tarsus M84.67- ☑
      - tibia M84.66- ☑
      - toe M84.67- ☑
      - ulna M84.63- ☑
      - vertebra M84.68- ☑
  - femur M84.45- ☑
  - fibula M84.46- ☑
  - finger M84.44- ☑
  - hip M84.459- ☑
  - humerus M84.42- ☑
  - ilium M84.454- ☑
  - ischium M84.454- ☑
  - joint prosthesis — *see* Complications, joint prosthesis, mechanical, breakdown, by site
    - periprosthetic — *see* Fracture, pathological, periprosthetic
  - metacarpus M84.44- ☑
  - metatarsus M84.47- ☑
  - neck M84.48- ☑
  - pelvis M84.454- ☑
  - periprosthetic M97.9- ☑
    - ankle M97.2- ☑
    - elbow M97.4- ☑
    - finger M97.8- ☑
    - hip M97.0- ☑
    - knee M97.1- ☑
    - other specified joint M97.8- ☑
    - shoulder M97.3- ☑
    - spinal joint M97.8- ☑
    - toe joint M97.8- ☑
    - wrist joint M97.8- ☑
  - radius M84.43- ☑
  - restorative material (dental) K08.539
    - with loss of material K08.531
    - without loss of material K08.530
  - rib M84.48- ☑
  - scapula M84.41- ☑
  - skull M84.48- ☑
  - tarsus M84.47- ☑

- **Fracture, pathological** — *continued*
  - tibia M84.46- ☑
  - toe M84.47- ☑
  - ulna M84.43- ☑
  - vertebra M84.48- ☑
- **Fracture, traumatic** (abduction) (adduction) (separation) — *see also* Fracture, pathological T14.8- ☑
  - acetabulum S32.40- ☑
    - column
      - anterior (displaced) (iliopubic) S32.43- ☑
        - nondisplaced S32.436- ☑
      - posterior (displaced) (ilioischial) S32.443- ☑
        - nondisplaced S32.44- ☑
    - dome (displaced) S32.48- ☑
      - nondisplaced S32.48- ☑
    - specified NEC S32.49- ☑
    - transverse (displaced) S32.45- ☑
      - with associated posterior wall fracture (displaced) S32.46- ☑
        - nondisplaced S32.46- ☑
      - nondisplaced S32.45- ☑
    - wall
      - anterior (displaced) S32.41- ☑
        - nondisplaced S32.41- ☑
      - medial (displaced) S32.47- ☑
        - nondisplaced S32.47- ☑
      - posterior (displaced) S32.42- ☑
        - with associated transverse fracture (displaced) S32.46- ☑
          - nondisplaced S32.46- ☑
        - nondisplaced S32.42- ☑
  - acromion — *see* Fracture, scapula, acromial process
  - ankle S82.899- ☑
    - bimalleolar (displaced) S82.84- ☑
      - nondisplaced S82.84- ☑
    - lateral malleolus only (displaced) S82.6- ☑
      - nondisplaced S82.6- ☑
    - medial malleolus (displaced) S82.5- ☑
      - associated with Maisonneuve's fracture — *see* Fracture, Maisonneuve's
      - nondisplaced S82.5- ☑
    - talus — *see* Fracture, tarsal, talus
    - trimalleolar (displaced) S82.85- ☑
      - nondisplaced S82.85- ☑
  - arm (upper) — *see also* Fracture, humerus, shaft
    - humerus — *see* Fracture, humerus
    - radius — *see* Fracture, radius
    - ulna — *see* Fracture, ulna
  - associated with chest compression and cardiopulmonary resuscitation M96.A9
  - astragalus — *see* Fracture, tarsal, talus
  - atlas — *see* Fracture, neck, cervical vertebra, first
  - axis — *see* Fracture, neck, cervical vertebra, second
  - back — *see* Fracture, vertebra
  - Barton's — *see* Barton's fracture
  - base of skull — *see* Fracture, skull, base
  - basicervical (basal) (femoral) S72.04- ☑
  - Bennett's — *see* Bennett's fracture
  - bimalleolar — *see* Fracture, ankle, bimalleolar
  - blow-out S02.3- ☑
  - bone NEC T14.8- ☑
    - birth injury P13.9
    - following insertion of orthopedic implant, joint prosthesis or bone plate — *see* Fracture, following insertion of orthopedic implant, joint prosthesis or bone plate
    - in (due to) neoplastic disease NEC — *see* Fracture, pathological, due to, neoplastic disease
    - pathological (cause unknown) — *see* Fracture, pathological
  - breast bone — *see* Fracture, sternum
  - bucket handle (semilunar cartilage) — *see* Tear, meniscus
  - buckle — *see* Fracture, by site, torus
  - burst — *see* Fracture, traumatic, by site
  - calcaneus — *see* Fracture, tarsal, calcaneus
  - carpal bone(s) S62.10- ☑
    - capitate (displaced) S62.13- ☑
      - nondisplaced S62.13- ☑
    - cuneiform — *see* Fracture, carpal bone, triquetrum
    - hamate (body) (displaced) S62.143- ☑
      - hook process (displaced) S62.15- ☑
        - nondisplaced S62.15- ☑
      - nondisplaced S62.14- ☑
    - larger multangular — *see* Fracture, carpal bones, trapezium
    - lunate (displaced) S62.12- ☑
      - nondisplaced S62.12- ☑

- **Fracture, traumatic** — *continued*
  - carpal bone(s) — *continued*
    - navicular S62.00- ☑
      - distal pole (displaced) S62.01- ☑
        - nondisplaced S62.01- ☑
      - middle third (displaced) S62.02- ☑
        - nondisplaced S62.02- ☑
      - proximal third (displaced) S62.03- ☑
        - nondisplaced S62.03- ☑
      - volar tuberosity — *see* Fracture, carpal bones, navicular, distal pole
    - os magnum — *see* Fracture, carpal bones, capitate
    - pisiform (displaced) S62.16- ☑
      - nondisplaced S62.16- ☑
    - semilunar — *see* Fracture, carpal bones, lunate
    - smaller multangular — *see* Fracture, carpal bones, trapezoid
    - trapezium (displaced) S62.17- ☑
      - nondisplaced S62.17- ☑
    - trapezoid (displaced) S62.18- ☑
      - nondisplaced S62.18- ☑
    - triquetrum (displaced) S62.11- ☑
      - nondisplaced S62.11- ☑
    - unciform — *see* Fracture, carpal bones, hamate
  - cervical — *see* Fracture, vertebra, cervical
  - clavicle S42.00- ☑
    - acromial end (displaced) S42.03- ☑
      - nondisplaced S42.03- ☑
    - birth injury P13.4
    - lateral end — *see* Fracture, clavicle, acromial end
    - shaft (displaced) S42.02- ☑
      - nondisplaced S42.02- ☑
    - sternal end (anterior) (displaced) S42.01- ☑
      - nondisplaced S42.01- ☑
      - posterior S42.01- ☑
  - coccyx S32.2- ☑
  - collapsed — *see* Collapse, vertebra
  - collar bone — *see* Fracture, clavicle
  - Colles' — *see* Colles' fracture
  - coronoid process — *see* Fracture, ulna, upper end, coronoid process
  - corpus cavernosum penis S39.840- ☑
  - costochondral cartilage S23.41- ☑
  - costochondral, costosternal junction — *see* Fracture, rib
  - cranium — *see* Fracture, skull
  - cricoid cartilage S12.8- ☑
  - cuboid (ankle) — *see* Fracture, tarsal, cuboid
  - cuneiform
    - foot — *see* Fracture, tarsal, cuneiform
    - wrist — *see* Fracture, carpal, triquetrum
  - delayed union — *see* Delay, union, fracture
  - dental restorative material K08.539
    - with loss of material K08.531
    - without loss of material K08.530
  - due to
    - birth injury — *see* Birth, injury, fracture
    - osteoporosis — *see* Osteoporosis, with fracture
  - Dupuytren's — *see* Fracture, ankle, lateral malleolus
  - elbow S42.40- ☑
  - ethmoid (bone) (sinus) — *see* Fracture, skull, base
  - face bone S02.92- ☑
  - fatigue — *see also* Fracture, stress
    - vertebra M48.40- ☑
      - cervical region M48.42- ☑
      - cervicothoracic region M48.43- ☑
      - lumbar region M48.46- ☑
      - lumbosacral region M48.47- ☑
      - occipito-atlanto-axial region M48.41- ☑
      - sacrococcygeal region M48.48- ☑
      - thoracic region M48.44- ☑
      - thoracolumbar region M48.45- ☑
  - femur, femoral S72.9- ☑
    - basicervical (basal) S72.04- ☑
    - birth injury P13.2
    - capital epiphyseal S79.01- ☑
    - condyles, epicondyles — *see* Fracture, femur, lower end
    - distal end — *see* Fracture, femur, lower end
    - epiphysis
      - head — *see* Fracture, femur, upper end, epiphysis
      - lower — *see* Fracture, femur, lower end, epiphysis
      - upper — *see* Fracture, femur, upper end, epiphysis
    - following insertion of implant, prosthesis or plate M96.66- ☑
    - head — *see* Fracture, femur, upper end, head
    - intertrochanteric — *see* Fracture, femur, trochanteric
    - intratrochanteric — *see* Fracture, femur, trochanteric

- **Fracture, traumatic** — *continued*
  - femur, femoral — *continued*
    - lower end S72.40- ☑
      - condyle (displaced) S72.41- ☑
        - lateral (displaced) S72.42- ☑
          - nondisplaced S72.42- ☑
        - medial (displaced) S72.43- ☑
          - nondisplaced S72.43- ☑
        - nondisplaced S72.41- ☑
      - epiphysis (displaced) S72.44- ☑
        - nondisplaced S72.44- ☑
      - physeal S79.10- ☑
        - Salter-Harris
          - Type I S79.11- ☑
          - Type II S79.12- ☑
          - Type III S79.13- ☑
          - Type IV S79.14- ☑
        - specified NEC S79.19- ☑
      - specified NEC S72.49- ☑
      - supracondylar (displaced) S72.45- ☑
        - with intracondylar extension (displaced) S72.46- ☑
          - nondisplaced S72.46- ☑
        - nondisplaced S72.45- ☑
      - torus S72.47- ☑
    - neck — *see* Fracture, femur, upper end, neck
    - pertrochanteric — *see* Fracture, femur, trochanteric
    - shaft (lower third) (middle third) (upper third) S72.30- ☑
      - comminuted (displaced) S72.35- ☑
        - nondisplaced S72.35- ☑
      - oblique (displaced) S72.33- ☑
        - nondisplaced S72.33- ☑
      - segmental (displaced) S72.36- ☑
        - nondisplaced S72.36- ☑
      - specified NEC S72.39- ☑
      - spiral (displaced) S72.34- ☑
        - nondisplaced S72.34- ☑
      - transverse (displaced) S72.32- ☑
        - nondisplaced S72.32- ☑
    - specified site NEC — *see* subcategory S72.8- ☑
    - subcapital (displaced) S72.01- ☑
    - subtrochanteric (region) (section) (displaced) S72.2- ☑
      - nondisplaced S72.2- ☑
    - transcervical — *see* Fracture, femur, midcervical
    - transtrochanteric — *see* Fracture, femur, trochanteric
    - trochanteric S72.10- ☑
      - apophyseal (displaced) S72.13- ☑
        - nondisplaced S72.13- ☑
      - greater trochanter (displaced) S72.11- ☑
        - nondisplaced S72.11- ☑
      - intertrochanteric (displaced) S72.14- ☑
        - nondisplaced S72.14- ☑
      - lesser trochanter (displaced) S72.12- ☑
        - nondisplaced S72.12- ☑
    - upper end S72.00- ☑
      - apophyseal (displaced) S72.13- ☑
        - nondisplaced S72.13- ☑
      - cervicotrochanteric — *see* Fracture, femur, upper end, neck, base
      - epiphysis (displaced) S72.02- ☑
        - nondisplaced S72.02- ☑
      - head S72.05- ☑
        - articular (displaced) S72.06- ☑
          - nondisplaced S72.06- ☑
        - specified NEC S72.09- ☑
      - intertrochanteric (displaced) S72.14- ☑
        - nondisplaced S72.14- ☑
      - intracapsular S72.01- ☑
      - midcervical (displaced) S72.03- ☑
        - nondisplaced S72.03- ☑
      - neck S72.00- ☑
        - base (displaced) S72.04- ☑
          - nondisplaced S72.04- ☑
        - specified NEC S72.09- ☑
      - pertrochanteric — *see* Fracture, femur, upper end, trochanteric
      - physeal S79.00- ☑
        - Salter-Harris type I S79.01- ☑
        - specified NEC S79.09- ☑
      - subcapital (displaced) S72.01- ☑
      - subtrochanteric (displaced) S72.2- ☑
        - nondisplaced S72.2- ☑

- **Fracture, traumatic** — *continued*
  - femur, femoral — *continued*
    - upper end — *continued*
      - transcervical — *see* Fracture, femur, upper end, midcervical
      - trochanteric S72.10- ☑
        - greater (displaced) S72.11- ☑
          - nondisplaced S72.11- ☑
        - lesser (displaced) S72.12- ☑
          - nondisplaced S72.12- ☑
  - fibula (shaft) (styloid) S82.40- ☑
    - comminuted (displaced) S82.45- ☑
      - nondisplaced S82.45- ☑
    - following insertion of implant, prosthesis or plate M96.67- ☑
    - involving ankle or malleolus — *see* Fracture, fibula, lateral malleolus
    - lateral malleolus (displaced) S82.6- ☑
      - nondisplaced S82.6- ☑
    - lower end
      - physeal S89.30- ☑
        - Salter-Harris
          - Type I S89.31- ☑
          - Type II S89.32- ☑
        - specified NEC S89.39- ☑
      - specified NEC S82.83- ☑
      - torus S82.82- ☑
    - oblique (displaced) S82.43- ☑
      - nondisplaced S82.43- ☑
    - segmental (displaced) S82.46- ☑
      - nondisplaced S82.46- ☑
    - specified NEC S82.49- ☑
    - spiral (displaced) S82.44- ☑
      - nondisplaced S82.44- ☑
    - transverse (displaced) S82.42- ☑
      - nondisplaced S82.42- ☑
    - upper end
      - physeal S89.20- ☑
        - Salter-Harris
          - Type I S89.21- ☑
          - Type II S89.22- ☑
        - specified NEC S89.29- ☑
      - specified NEC S82.83- ☑
      - torus S82.81- ☑
  - finger (except thumb) S62.60- ☑
    - distal phalanx (displaced) S62.63- ☑
      - nondisplaced S62.66- ☑
    - index S62.60- ☑
      - distal phalanx (displaced) S62.63- ☑
        - nondisplaced S62.66- ☑
      - middle phalanx (displaced) S62.62- ☑
        - nondisplaced S62.65- ☑
      - proximal phalanx (displaced) S62.61- ☑
        - nondisplaced S62.64- ☑
    - little S62.60- ☑
      - distal phalanx (displaced) S62.63- ☑
        - nondisplaced S62.66- ☑
      - middle phalanx (displaced) S62.62- ☑
        - nondisplaced S62.65- ☑
      - proximal phalanx (displaced) S62.61- ☑
        - nondisplaced S62.64- ☑
    - middle S62.60- ☑
      - distal phalanx (displaced) S62.63- ☑
        - nondisplaced S62.66- ☑
      - middle phalanx (displaced) S62.62- ☑
        - nondisplaced S62.65- ☑
      - proximal phalanx (displaced) S62.61- ☑
        - nondisplaced S62.64- ☑
    - middle phalanx (displaced) S62.62- ☑
      - nondisplaced S62.65- ☑
    - proximal phalanx (displaced) S62.61- ☑
      - nondisplaced S62.64- ☑
    - ring S62.60- ☑
      - distal phalanx (displaced) S62.63- ☑
        - nondisplaced S62.66- ☑
      - middle phalanx (displaced) S62.62- ☑
        - nondisplaced S62.65- ☑
      - proximal phalanx (displaced) S62.61- ☑
        - nondisplaced S62.64- ☑
    - thumb — *see* Fracture, thumb
  - following insertion (intraoperative) (postoperative) of orthopedic implant, joint prosthesis or bone plate M96.69
    - femur M96.66- ☑
    - fibula M96.67- ☑

**Fracture, traumatic** — *continued*
- following insertion of orthopedic implant, joint prosthesis or bone plate — *continued*
  - humerus M96.62- ☑
  - pelvis M96.65
  - radius M96.63- ☑
  - specified bone NEC M96.69
  - tibia M96.67- ☑
  - ulna M96.63- ☑
- foot S92.9Ø- ☑
  - astragalus — *see* Fracture, tarsal, talus
  - calcaneus — *see* Fracture, tarsal, calcaneus
  - cuboid — *see* Fracture, tarsal, cuboid
  - cuneiform — *see* Fracture, tarsal, cuneiform
  - metatarsal — *see* Fracture, metatarsal
  - navicular — *see* Fracture, tarsal, navicular
  - sesamoid S92.81- ☑
  - specified NEC S92.81- ☑
  - talus — *see* Fracture, tarsal, talus
  - tarsal — *see* Fracture, tarsal
  - toe — *see* Fracture, toe
- forearm S52.9- ☑
  - radius — *see* Fracture, radius
  - ulna — *see* Fracture, ulna
- fossa (anterior) (middle) (posterior) SØ2.19- ☑
- fragility — *see* Fracture, pathological, due to osteoporosis
- frontal (bone) (skull) SØ2.Ø- ☑
  - sinus SØ2.19- ☑
- glenoid (cavity) (scapula) — *see* Fracture, scapula, glenoid cavity
- greenstick — *see* Fracture, by site
- hallux — *see* Fracture, toe, great
- hand S62.9- ☑
  - carpal — *see* Fracture, carpal bone
  - finger (except thumb) — *see* Fracture, finger
  - metacarpal — *see* Fracture, metacarpal
  - navicular (scaphoid) (hand) — *see* Fracture, carpal bone, navicular
  - thumb — *see* Fracture, thumb
- healed or old
  - with complications — *code by* Nature of the complication
- heel bone — *see* Fracture, tarsal, calcaneus
- Hill-Sachs S42.29- ☑
- hip — *see* Fracture, femur, neck
- humerus S42.3Ø- ☑
  - anatomical neck — *see* Fracture, humerus, upper end
  - articular process — *see* Fracture, humerus, lower end
  - capitellum — *see* Fracture, humerus, lower end, condyle, lateral
  - distal end — *see* Fracture, humerus, lower end
  - epiphysis
    - lower — *see* Fracture, humerus, lower end, physeal
    - upper — *see* Fracture, humerus, upper end, physeal
  - external condyle — *see* Fracture, humerus, lower end, condyle, lateral
  - following insertion of implant, prosthesis or plate M96.62- ☑
  - great tuberosity — *see* Fracture, humerus, upper end, greater tuberosity
  - intercondylar — *see* Fracture, humerus, lower end
  - internal epicondyle — *see* Fracture, humerus, lower end, epicondyle, medial
  - lesser tuberosity — *see* Fracture, humerus, upper end, lesser tuberosity
  - lower end S42.4Ø- ☑
    - condyle
      - lateral (displaced) S42.45- ☑
        - nondisplaced S42.45- ☑
      - medial (displaced) S42.46- ☑
        - nondisplaced S42.46- ☑
    - epicondyle
      - lateral (displaced) S42.43- ☑
        - nondisplaced S42.43- ☑
      - medial (displaced) S42.44- ☑
        - incarcerated S42.44- ☑
        - nondisplaced S42.44- ☑
    - physeal S49.1Ø- ☑
      - Salter-Harris
        - Type I S49.11- ☑
        - Type II S49.12- ☑
        - Type III S49.13- ☑
        - Type IV S49.14- ☑
      - specified NEC S49.19- ☑
    - specified NEC (displaced) S42.49- ☑
      - nondisplaced S42.49- ☑

**Fracture, traumatic** — *continued*
- humerus — *continued*
  - lower end — *continued*
    - supracondylar (simple) (displaced) S42.41- ☑
      - with intercondylar fracture — *see* Fracture, humerus, lower end
      - comminuted (displaced) S42.42- ☑
        - nondisplaced S42.42- ☑
      - nondisplaced S42.41- ☑
    - torus S42.48- ☑
    - transcondylar (displaced) S42.47- ☑
      - nondisplaced S42.47- ☑
  - proximal end — *see* Fracture, humerus, upper end
  - shaft S42.3Ø- ☑
    - comminuted (displaced) S42.35- ☑
      - nondisplaced S42.35- ☑
    - greenstick S42.31- ☑
    - oblique (displaced) S42.33- ☑
      - nondisplaced S42.33- ☑
    - segmental (displaced) S42.36- ☑
      - nondisplaced S42.36- ☑
    - specified NEC S42.39- ☑
    - spiral (displaced) S42.34- ☑
      - nondisplaced S42.34- ☑
    - transverse (displaced) S42.32- ☑
      - nondisplaced S42.32- ☑
  - supracondylar — *see* Fracture, humerus, lower end
  - surgical neck — *see* Fracture, humerus, upper end, surgical neck
  - trochlea — *see* Fracture, humerus, lower end, condyle, medial
  - tuberosity — *see* Fracture, humerus, upper end
  - upper end S42.2Ø- ☑
    - anatomical neck — *see* Fracture, humerus, upper end, specified NEC
    - articular head — *see* Fracture, humerus, upper end, specified NEC
    - epiphysis — *see* Fracture, humerus, upper end, physeal
    - greater tuberosity (displaced) S42.25- ☑
      - nondisplaced S42.25- ☑
    - lesser tuberosity (displaced) S42.26- ☑
      - nondisplaced S42.26- ☑
    - physeal S49.ØØ- ☑
      - Salter-Harris
        - Type I S49.Ø1- ☑
        - Type II S49.Ø2- ☑
        - Type III S49.Ø3- ☑
        - Type IV S49.Ø4- ☑
      - specified NEC S49.Ø9- ☑
    - specified NEC (displaced) S42.29- ☑
      - nondisplaced S42.29- ☑
    - surgical neck (displaced) S42.21- ☑
      - four-part S42.24- ☑
      - nondisplaced S42.21- ☑
      - three-part S42.23- ☑
      - two-part (displaced) S42.22- ☑
        - nondisplaced S42.22- ☑
    - torus S42.27- ☑
    - transepiphyseal — *see* Fracture, humerus, upper end, physeal
- hyoid bone S12.8- ☑
- ilium S32.3Ø- ☑
  - with disruption of pelvic ring — *see* Disruption, pelvic ring
  - avulsion (displaced) S32.31- ☑
    - nondisplaced S32.31- ☑
  - specified NEC S32.39- ☑
- impaction, impacted — *code as* Fracture, by site
- innominate bone — *see* Fracture, ilium
- instep — *see* Fracture, foot
- ischium S32.6Ø- ☑
  - with disruption of pelvic ring — *see* Disruption, pelvic ring
  - avulsion (displaced) S32.61- ☑
    - nondisplaced S32.61- ☑
  - specified NEC S32.69- ☑
- jaw (bone) (lower) — *see* Fracture, mandible
  - upper — *see* Fracture, maxilla
- joint prosthesis — *see* Complications, joint prosthesis, mechanical, breakdown, by site
  - periprosthetic — *see* Fracture, traumatic, periprosthetic
- knee cap — *see* Fracture, patella
- larynx S12.8- ☑
- late effects — *see* Sequelae, fracture

**Fracture, traumatic** — *continued*
- leg (lower) S82.9- ☑
  - ankle — *see* Fracture, ankle
  - femur — *see* Fracture, femur
  - fibula — *see* Fracture, fibula
  - malleolus — *see* Fracture, ankle
  - patella — *see* Fracture, patella
  - specified site NEC S82.89- ☑
  - tibia — *see* Fracture, tibia
- lumbar spine — *see* Fracture, vertebra, lumbar
- lumbosacral spine S32.9- ☑
- Maisonneuve's (displaced) S82.86- ☑
  - nondisplaced S82.86- ☑
- malar bone — *see also* Fracture, maxilla SØ2.4ØØ- ☑
  - left side SØ2.4ØB- ☑
  - right side SØ2.4ØA- ☑
- malleolus — *see* Fracture, ankle
- malunion — *see* Fracture, by site
- mandible (lower jaw (bone)) SØ2.6Ø9- ☑
  - alveolus SØ2.67- ☑
  - angle (of jaw) SØ2.65- ☑
  - body, unspecified SØ2.6ØØ- ☑
    - left side SØ2.6Ø2- ☑
    - right side SØ2.6Ø1- ☑
  - condylar process SØ2.61- ☑
  - coronoid process SØ2.63- ☑
  - ramus, unspecified SØ2.64- ☑
  - specified site NEC SØ2.69- ☑
  - subcondylar process SØ2.62- ☑
  - symphysis SØ2.66- ☑
- manubrium (sterni) S22.21- ☑
  - dissociation from sternum S22.23- ☑
- march — *see* Fracture, traumatic, stress, by site
- maxilla, maxillary (bone) (sinus) (superior) (upper jaw) SØ2.4Ø1- ☑
  - alveolus SØ2.42- ☑
  - inferior — *see* Fracture, mandible
  - LeFort I SØ2.411- ☑
  - LeFort II SØ2.412- ☑
  - LeFort III SØ2.413- ☑
  - left side SØ2.4ØD- ☑
  - right side SØ2.4ØC- ☑
- metacarpal S62.3Ø9- ☑
  - base (displaced) S62.319- ☑
    - nondisplaced S62.349- ☑
  - fifth S62.3Ø- ☑
    - base (displaced) S62.31- ☑
      - nondisplaced S62.34- ☑
    - neck (displaced) S62.33- ☑
      - nondisplaced S62.36- ☑
    - shaft (displaced) S62.32- ☑
      - nondisplaced S62.35- ☑
    - specified NEC S62.398- ☑
  - first S62.2Ø- ☑
    - base NEC (displaced) S62.23- ☑
      - nondisplaced S62.23- ☑
    - Bennett's — *see* Bennett's fracture
    - neck (displaced) S62.25- ☑
      - nondisplaced S62.25- ☑
    - shaft (displaced) S62.24- ☑
      - nondisplaced S62.24- ☑
    - specified NEC S62.29- ☑
  - fourth S62.3Ø- ☑
    - base (displaced) S62.31- ☑
      - nondisplaced S62.34- ☑
    - neck (displaced) S62.33- ☑
      - nondisplaced S62.36- ☑
    - shaft (displaced) S62.32- ☑
      - nondisplaced S62.35- ☑
    - specified NEC S62.39- ☑
  - neck (displaced) S62.33- ☑
    - nondisplaced S62.36- ☑
  - Rolando's — *see* Rolando's fracture
  - second S62.3Ø- ☑
    - base (displaced) S62.31- ☑
      - nondisplaced S62.34- ☑
    - neck (displaced) S62.33- ☑
      - nondisplaced S62.36- ☑
    - shaft (displaced) S62.32- ☑
      - nondisplaced S62.35- ☑
    - specified NEC S62.39- ☑
  - shaft (displaced) S62.32- ☑
    - nondisplaced S62.35- ☑
  - specified NEC S62.399- ☑
  - third S62.3Ø- ☑

Index

Fracture, traumatic — Fracture, traumatic

**Friction** — *continued*
- precordial RØ1.2
- sounds, chest RØ9.89

**Friderichsen-Waterhouse syndrome or disease** A39.1
**Friedlander's B** (bacillus) **NEC** — *see also* condition A49.8
**Friedreich's**
- ataxia G11.11
- combined systemic disease G11.11
- facial hemihypertrophy Q67.4
- sclerosis (cerebellum) (spinal cord) G11.11

**Frigidity** F52.22
**Frohlich's syndrome** E23.6
**Frontal** — *see also* condition
- lobe syndrome FØ7.Ø

**Frostbite** (superficial) T33.9Ø- ☑
- with
  - partial thickness skin loss — *see* Frostbite (superficial), by site
  - tissue necrosis T34.9Ø- ☑
- abdominal wall T33.3- ☑
  - with tissue necrosis T34.3- ☑
- ankle T33.81- ☑
  - with tissue necrosis T34.81- ☑
- arm T33.4- ☑
  - with tissue necrosis T34.4- ☑
  - finger(s) — *see* Frostbite, finger
  - hand — *see* Frostbite, hand
  - wrist — *see* Frostbite, wrist
- ear T33.Ø1- ☑
  - with tissue necrosis T34.Ø1- ☑
- face T33.Ø9- ☑
  - with tissue necrosis T34.Ø9- ☑
- finger T33.53- ☑
  - with tissue necrosis T34.53- ☑
- foot T33.82- ☑
  - with tissue necrosis T34.82- ☑
- hand T33.52- ☑
  - with tissue necrosis T34.52- ☑
- head T33.Ø9- ☑
  - with tissue necrosis T34.Ø9- ☑
  - ear — *see* Frostbite, ear
  - nose — *see* Frostbite, nose
- hip (and thigh) T33.6- ☑
  - with tissue necrosis T34.6- ☑
- knee T33.7- ☑
  - with tissue necrosis T34.7- ☑
- leg T33.99- ☑
  - with tissue necrosis — *see also* Frostbite, by specific site on leg, if specified T34.99- ☑
  - ankle — *see* Frostbite, ankle
  - foot — *see* Frostbite, foot
  - knee — *see* Frostbite, knee
  - lower T33.7- ☑
    - with tissue necrosis T34.7- ☑
  - thigh — *see* Frostbite, hip
  - toe — *see* Frostbite, toe
- limb
  - lower T33.99- ☑
    - with tissue necrosis T34.99- ☑
  - upper — *see* Frostbite, arm
- neck T33.1- ☑
  - with tissue necrosis T34.1- ☑
- nose T33.Ø2- ☑
  - with tissue necrosis T34.Ø2- ☑
- pelvis T33.3- ☑
  - with tissue necrosis T34.3- ☑
- specified site NEC T33.99- ☑
  - with tissue necrosis T34.99- ☑
- thigh — *see* Frostbite, hip
- thorax T33.2- ☑
  - with tissue necrosis T34.2- ☑
- toes T33.83- ☑
  - with tissue necrosis T34.83- ☑
- trunk T33.99- ☑
  - with tissue necrosis T34.99- ☑
- wrist T33.51- ☑
  - with tissue necrosis T34.51- ☑

**Frotteurism** F65.81
**Frozen** — *see also* Effect, adverse, cold T69.9- ☑
- pelvis (female) N94.89
  - male K66.8
- shoulder — *see* Capsulitis, adhesive

**Fructokinase deficiency** E74.11
**Fructose 1,6 diphosphatase deficiency** E74.19
**Fructosemia** (benign) (essential) E74.12
**Fructosuria** (benign) (essential) E74.11
**Fuchs'**
- black spot (myopic) — *see also* Myopia, degenerative H44.2- ☑
- dystrophy (corneal endothelium) H18.51- ☑
- heterochromic cyclitis — *see* Cyclitis, Fuchs' heterochromic

**Fucosidosis** E77.1
**Fugue** R68.89
- dissociative F44.1
- hysterical (dissociative) F44.1
- postictal in epilepsy — *see* Epilepsy
- reaction to exceptional stress (transient) F43.Ø

**Fulminant, fulminating** — *see* condition
**Functional** — *see also* condition
- bleeding (uterus) N93.8

**Functioning, intellectual, borderline** R41.83
**Fundus** — *see* condition
**Fungemia NOS** B49
- candida B37.7

**Fungus, fungous**
- cerebral G93.89
- disease NOS B49
- infection — *see* Infection, fungus

**Funiculitis** (acute) (chronic) (endemic) N49.1
- gonococcal (acute) (chronic) A54.23
- tuberculous A18.15

**Funnel**
- breast (acquired) M95.4
  - congenital Q67.6
  - sequelae (late effect) of rickets E64.3
- chest (acquired) M95.4
  - congenital Q67.6
  - sequelae (late effect) of rickets E64.3
- pelvis (acquired) M95.5
  - with disproportion (fetopelvic) O33.3- ☑
    - causing obstructed labor O65.3
  - congenital Q74.2

**FUO** (fever of unknown origin) R5Ø.9
**Furfur** L21.Ø
- microsporon B36.Ø

**Furloughed** Z56.89
**Furrier's lung** J67.8
**Furrowed** K14.5
- nail(s) (transverse) L6Ø.4
  - congenital Q84.6
- tongue K14.5
  - congenital Q38.3

**Furuncle** LØ2.92
- abdominal wall LØ2.221
- ankle — *see* Furuncle, lower limb
- antecubital space — *see* Furuncle, upper limb
- anus K61.Ø
- arm — *see* Furuncle, upper limb
- auditory canal, external — *see* Abscess, ear, external
- auricle (ear) — *see* Abscess, ear, external
- axilla (region) LØ2.42- ☑
- back (any part except buttock and flank) LØ2.222
- breast N61.1
- buttock LØ2.32
- cheek (external) LØ2.Ø2
- chest wall LØ2.223
- chin LØ2.Ø2
- corpus cavernosum N48.21
- ear, external — *see* Abscess, ear, external
- external auditory canal — *see* Abscess, ear, external
- eyelid — *see* Abscess, eyelid
- face LØ2.Ø2
- femoral (region) — *see* Furuncle, lower limb
- finger — *see* Furuncle, hand
- flank LØ2.227
- foot LØ2.62- ☑
- forehead LØ2.Ø2
- gluteal (region) LØ2.32
- groin LØ2.224
- hand LØ2.52- ☑
- head LØ2.821
  - face LØ2.Ø2
- hip — *see* Furuncle, lower limb
- kidney — *see* Abscess, kidney
- knee — *see* Furuncle, lower limb
- labium (majus) (minus) N76.4
- lacrimal
  - gland — *see* Dacryoadenitis
  - passages (duct) (sac) — *see* Inflammation, lacrimal, passages, acute
- leg (any part) — *see* Furuncle, lower limb
- lower limb LØ2.42- ☑
- malignant A22.Ø

**Furuncle** — *continued*
- mouth K12.2
- navel LØ2.226
- neck LØ2.12
- nose J34.Ø
- orbit, orbital — *see* Abscess, orbit
- palmar (space) — *see* Furuncle, hand
- partes posteriores LØ2.32
- pectoral region LØ2.223
- penis N48.21
- perineum LØ2.225
- pinna — *see* Abscess, ear, external
- popliteal — *see* Furuncle, lower limb
- prepatellar — *see* Furuncle, lower limb
- scalp LØ2.821
- seminal vesicle N49.Ø
- shoulder — *see* Furuncle, upper limb
- specified site NEC LØ2.828
- submandibular K12.2
- temple (region) LØ2.Ø2
- thumb — *see* Furuncle, hand
- toe — *see* Furuncle, foot
- trunk LØ2.229
  - abdominal wall LØ2.221
  - back LØ2.222
  - chest wall LØ2.223
  - groin LØ2.224
  - perineum LØ2.225
  - umbilicus LØ2.226
- umbilicus LØ2.226
- upper limb LØ2.42- ☑
- vulva N76.4

**Furunculosis** — *see* Furuncle
**Fused** — *see* Fusion, fused
**Fusion, fused** (congenital)
- astragaloscaphoid Q74.2
- atria Q21.19
- auditory canal Q16.1
- auricles, heart Q21.19
- binocular with defective stereopsis H53.32
- bone Q79.8
- cervical spine M43.22
- choanal Q3Ø.Ø
- commissure, mitral valve Q23.2
- cusps, heart valve NEC Q24.8
  - mitral Q23.2
  - pulmonary Q22.1
  - tricuspid Q22.4
- ear ossicles Q16.3
- fingers Q7Ø.Ø- ☑
- hymen Q52.3
- joint (acquired) — *see also* Ankylosis
  - congenital Q74.8
- kidneys (incomplete) Q63.1
- labium (majus) (minus) Q52.5
- larynx and trachea Q34.8
- limb, congenital Q74.8
  - lower Q74.2
  - upper Q74.Ø
- lobes, lung Q33.8
- lumbosacral (acquired) M43.27
  - arthrodesis status Z98.1
  - congenital Q76.49
  - postprocedural status Z98.1
- nares, nose, nasal, nostril(s) Q3Ø.Ø
- organ or site not listed — *see* Anomaly, by site
- ossicles Q79.9
  - auditory Q16.3
- pulmonic cusps Q22.1
- ribs Q76.6
- sacroiliac (joint) (acquired) M43.28
  - arthrodesis status Z98.1
  - congenital Q74.2
  - postprocedural status Z98.1
- spine (acquired) NEC M43.2Ø
  - arthrodesis status Z98.1
  - cervical region M43.22
  - cervicothoracic region M43.23
  - congenital Q76.49
  - lumbar M43.26
  - lumbosacral region M43.27
  - occipito-atlanto-axial region M43.21
  - postoperative status Z98.1
  - sacrococcygeal region M43.28
  - thoracic region M43.24
  - thoracolumbar region M43.25
- sublingual duct with submaxillary duct at opening in mouth Q38.4
- testes Q55.1

# G

- **Gain in weight** (abnormal) (excessive) — *see also* Weight, gain
- **Gaisbock's disease** (polycythemia hypertonica) D75.1
- **Gait abnormality** R26.9
  - ataxic R26.0
  - falling R29.6
  - hysterical (ataxic) (staggering) F44.4
  - paralytic R26.1
  - spastic R26.1
  - specified type NEC R26.89
  - staggering R26.0
  - unsteadiness R26.81
  - walking difficulty NEC R26.2
- **Galactocele** (breast) N64.89
  - puerperal, postpartum O92.79
- **Galactokinase deficiency** E74.29
- **Galactophoritis** N61.0
  - gestational, puerperal, postpartum O91.2- ☑
- **Galactorrhea** O92.6
  - not associated with childbirth N64.3
- **Galactosemia** (classic) (congenital) E74.21
- **Galactosuria** E74.29
- **Galacturia** R82.0
  - schistosomiasis (bilharziasis) B65.0
- **GALD** (gestational alloimmune liver disease) P78.84
- **Galeazzi's fracture** S52.37- ☑
- **Galen's vein** — *see* condition
- **Galeophobia** F40.218
- **Gall duct** — *see* condition
- **Gallbladder** — *see also* condition
  - acute K81.0
- **Gallop rhythm** R00.8
- **Gallstone** (colic) (cystic duct) (gallbladder) (impacted) (multiple) — *see also* Calculus, gallbladder
  - with
    - cholecystitis — *see* Calculus, gallbladder, with cholecystitis
  - bile duct (common) (hepatic) — *see* Calculus, bile duct
  - causing intestinal obstruction K56.3
  - specified NEC K80.80
    - with obstruction K80.81
- **Gambling** Z72.6
  - pathological (compulsive) F63.0
- **Gammopathy** (of undetermined significance [MGUS]) D47.2
  - associated with lymphoplasmacytic dyscrasia D47.2
  - monoclonal D47.2
  - polyclonal D89.0
- **Gamna's disease** (siderotic splenomegaly) D73.1
- **Gamophobia** F40.298
- **Gampsodactylia** (congenital) Q66.7- ☑
- **Gamstorp's disease** (adynamia episodica hereditaria) G72.3
- **Gandy-Nanta disease** (siderotic splenomegaly) D73.1
- **Gang**
  - membership offenses Z72.810
- **Gangliocytoma** D36.10
- **Ganglioglioma** — *see* Neoplasm, uncertain behavior, by site
- **Ganglion** (compound) (diffuse) (joint) (tendon (sheath)) M67.40
  - ankle M67.47- ☑
  - foot M67.47- ☑
  - forearm M67.43- ☑
  - hand M67.44- ☑
  - lower leg M67.46- ☑
  - multiple sites M67.49
  - of yaws (early) (late) A66.6
  - pelvic region M67.45- ☑
  - periosteal — *see* Periostitis
  - shoulder region M67.41- ☑
  - specified site NEC M67.48
  - thigh region M67.45- ☑
  - tuberculous A18.09
  - upper arm M67.42- ☑
  - wrist M67.43- ☑
- **Ganglioneuroblastoma** — *see* Neoplasm, nerve, malignant
- **Ganglioneuroma** D36.10
  - malignant — *see* Neoplasm, nerve, malignant
- **Ganglioneuromatosis** D36.10
- **Ganglionitis**
  - fifth nerve — *see* Neuralgia, trigeminal
  - gasserian (postherpetic) (postzoster) B02.21
  - geniculate G51.1
    - newborn (birth injury) P11.3
    - postherpetic, postzoster B02.21
  - herpes zoster B02.21
- **Ganglionitis** — *continued*
  - postherpetic geniculate B02.21
- **Gangliosidosis** E75.10
  - GM1 E75.19
  - GM2 E75.00
    - other specified E75.09
    - Sandhoff disease E75.01
    - Tay-Sachs disease E75.02
  - GM3 E75.19
  - mucolipidosis IV E75.11
- **Gangosa** A66.5
- **Gangrene, gangrenous** (connective tissue) (dropsical) (dry) (moist) (skin) (ulcer) — *see also* Necrosis I96
  - with diabetes (mellitus) — *see* Diabetes, with, gangrene
  - abdomen (wall) I96
  - alveolar M27.3
  - appendix K35.80
    - with
      - peritonitis, localized — *see also* Appendicitis K35.31
  - arteriosclerotic (general) (senile) — *see* Arteriosclerosis, extremities, with, gangrene
  - auricle I96
  - Bacillus welchii A48.0
  - bladder (infectious) — *see* Cystitis, specified type NEC
  - bowel, cecum, or colon — *see* Gangrene, intestine
  - Clostridium perfringens or welchii A48.0
  - cornea H18.89- ☑
  - corpora cavernosa N48.29
    - noninfective N48.89
  - cutaneous, spreading I96
  - decubital — *see* Ulcer, pressure, by site
  - diabetic (any site) — *see* Diabetes, with, gangrene
  - emphysematous — *see* Gangrene, gas
  - epidemic — *see* Poisoning, food, noxious, plant
  - epididymis (infectional) N45.1
  - erysipelas — *see* Erysipelas
  - extremity (lower) (upper) I96
  - Fournier N49.3
    - female N76.82
    - vagina and vulva N76.82
  - fusospirochetal A69.0
  - gallbladder — *see* Cholecystitis, acute
  - gas (bacillus) A48.0
    - following
      - abortion — *see* Abortion by type complicated by infection
      - ectopic or molar pregnancy O08.0
  - glossitis K14.0
  - hernia — *see* Hernia, by site, with gangrene
  - intestine, intestinal (hemorrhagic) (massive) — *see also* Infarct, intestine K55.069
    - with
      - mesenteric embolism — *see also* Infarct, intestine K55.069
      - obstruction — *see* Obstruction, intestine
  - laryngitis J04.0
  - limb (lower) (upper) I96
  - lung J85.0
    - spirochetal A69.8
  - lymphangitis I89.1
  - Meleney's (synergistic) — *see* Ulcer, skin
  - mesentery — *see also* Infarct, intestine K55.069
    - with
      - embolism — *see also* Infarct, intestine K55.069
      - intestinal obstruction — *see* Obstruction, intestine
  - mouth A69.0
  - ovary — *see* Oophoritis
  - pancreas — *see* Pancreatitis, acute
  - penis N48.29
    - noninfective N48.89
  - perineum I96
  - pharynx — *see also* Pharyngitis
    - Vincent's A69.1
  - presenile I73.1
  - progressive synergistic — *see* Ulcer, skin
  - pulmonary J85.0
  - pulpal (dental) K04.1
  - quinsy J36
  - Raynaud's (symmetric gangrene) I73.01
  - retropharyngeal J39.2
  - scrotum N49.3
    - noninfective N50.89
  - senile (atherosclerotic) — *see* Arteriosclerosis, extremities, with, gangrene
  - spermatic cord N49.1
    - noninfective N50.89
  - spine I96
  - spirochetal NEC A69.8
- **Gangrene, gangrenous** — *continued*
  - spreading cutaneous I96
  - stomatitis A69.0
  - symmetrical I73.01
  - testis (infectional) N45.2
    - noninfective N44.8
  - throat — *see also* Pharyngitis
    - diphtheritic A36.0
    - Vincent's A69.1
  - thyroid (gland) E07.89
  - tooth (pulp) K04.1
  - tuberculous NEC — *see* Tuberculosis
  - tunica vaginalis N49.1
    - noninfective N50.89
  - umbilicus I96
  - uterus — *see* Endometritis
  - uvulitis K12.2
  - vas deferens N49.1
    - noninfective N50.89
  - vulva N76.82
- **Ganister disease** J62.8
- **Ganser's syndrome** (hysterical) F44.89
- **Gardner-Diamond syndrome** (autoerythrocyte sensitization) D69.2
- **Gargoylism** E76.01
- **Garre's disease, osteitis** (sclerosing), osteomyelitis — *see* Osteomyelitis, specified type NEC
- **Garrod's pad, knuckle** M72.1
- **Gartner's duct**
  - cyst Q52.4
  - persistent Q50.6
- **Gas** R14.3
  - asphyxiation, inhalation, poisoning, suffocation NEC — *see* Table of Drugs and Chemicals
  - excessive R14.0
  - gangrene A48.0
    - following
      - abortion — *see* Abortion by type complicated by infection
      - ectopic or molar pregnancy O08.0
  - on stomach R14.0
  - pains R14.1
- **Gastralgia** — *see also* Pain, abdominal
- **Gastrectasis** K31.0
  - psychogenic F45.8
- **Gastric** — *see* condition
- **Gastrinoma**
  - malignant
    - pancreas C25.4
    - specified site NEC — *see* Neoplasm, malignant, by site
    - unspecified site C25.4
  - specified site — *see* Neoplasm, uncertain behavior
  - unspecified site D37.9
- **Gastritis** (simple) K29.70
  - with bleeding K29.71
  - acute (erosive) K29.00
    - with bleeding K29.01
  - alcoholic K29.20
    - with bleeding K29.21
  - allergic K29.60
    - with bleeding K29.61
  - atrophic (chronic) K29.40
    - with bleeding K29.41
  - chronic (antral) (fundal) K29.50
    - with bleeding K29.51
    - atrophic K29.40
      - with bleeding K29.41
    - superficial K29.30
      - with bleeding K29.31
  - dietary counseling and surveillance Z71.3
  - due to diet deficiency E63.9
  - eosinophilic K52.81
  - giant hypertrophic K29.60
    - with bleeding K29.61
  - granulomatous K29.60
    - with bleeding K29.61
  - hypertrophic (mucosa) K29.60
    - with bleeding K29.61
  - nervous F54
  - spastic K29.60
    - with bleeding K29.61
  - specified NEC K29.60
    - with bleeding K29.61
  - superficial chronic K29.30
    - with bleeding K29.31
  - tuberculous A18.83
  - viral NEC A08.4
- **Gastrocarcinoma** — *see* Neoplasm, malignant, stomach

**Gastrocolic** — *see* condition
**Gastrodisciasis, gastrodiscoidiasis** B66.8
**Gastroduodenitis** K29.90
- with bleeding K29.91
- virus, viral A08.4
  - specified type NEC A08.39

**Gastrodynia** — *see* Pain, abdominal
**Gastroenteritis** (acute) (chronic) (noninfectious) — *see also* Enteritis K52.9
- allergic K52.29
  - with
    - eosinophilic gastritis or gastroenteritis K52.81
    - food protein-induced enterocolitis syndrome K52.21
    - food protein-induced enteropathy K52.22
- dietetic — *see also* Gastroenteritis, allergic K52.29
- drug-induced K52.1
- due to
  - Cryptosporidium A07.2
  - drugs K52.1
  - food poisoning — *see* Intoxication, foodborne
  - radiation K52.0
- eosinophilic K52.81
- epidemic (infectious) A09
- food hypersensitivity — *see also* Gastroenteritis, allergic K52.29
- infectious — *see* Enteritis, infectious
- influenzal — *see* Influenza, with gastroenteritis
- noninfectious K52.9
  - specified NEC K52.89
- rotaviral A08.0
- Salmonella A02.0
- toxic K52.1
- viral NEC A08.4
  - acute infectious A08.39
    - type Norwalk A08.11
  - infantile (acute) A08.39
  - Norwalk agent A08.11
  - rotaviral A08.0
  - severe of infants A08.39
  - specified type NEC A08.39

**Gastroenteropathy** — *see also* Gastroenteritis K52.9
- acute, due to Norovirus A08.11
- acute, due to Norwalk agent A08.11
- infectious A09

**Gastroenteroptosis** K63.4
**Gastroesophageal laceration- hemorrhage syndrome** K22.6
**Gastrointestinal** — *see* condition
**Gastrojejunal** — *see* condition
**Gastrojejunitis** — *see also* Enteritis K52.9
**Gastrojejunocolic** — *see* condition
**Gastroliths** K31.89
**Gastromalacia** K31.89
**Gastroparalysis** K31.84
- diabetic — *see* Diabetes, gastroparalysis

**Gastroparesis** K31.84
- diabetic — *see* Diabetes, by type, with gastroparesis

**Gastropathy** K31.9
- congestive portal — *see also* Hypertension, portal K31.89
- erythematous K29.70
- exudative K90.89
- portal hypertensive — *see also* Hypertension, portal K31.89
- specified NEC K31.89

**Gastroptosis** K31.89
**Gastrorrhagia** K92.2
- psychogenic F45.8

**Gastroschisis** (congenital) Q79.3
**Gastrospasm** (neurogenic) (reflex) K31.89
- neurotic F45.8
- psychogenic F45.8

**Gastrostaxis** — *see* Gastritis, with bleeding
**Gastrostenosis** K31.89
**Gastrostomy**
- attention to Z43.1
- status Z93.1

**Gastrosuccorrhea** (continuous) (intermittent) K31.89
- neurotic F45.8
- psychogenic F45.8

**Gatophobia** F40.218
**Gaucher's disease or splenomegaly** (adult) (infantile) E75.22
**Gee** (-Herter)(-Thaysen) **disease** (nontropical sprue) K90.0
**Gelineau's syndrome** G47.419
- with cataplexy G47.411

**Gemination, tooth, teeth** K00.2
**Gemistocytoma**
- specified site — *see* Neoplasm, malignant, by site
- unspecified site C71.9

**General, generalized** — *see* condition
**Genetic**
- carrier (status)
  - cystic fibrosis Z14.1
  - hemophilia A (asymptomatic) Z14.01
    - symptomatic Z14.02
  - specified NEC Z14.8
- susceptibility to disease NEC Z15.89
  - epilepsy Z15.1
  - kidney disease Z15.3
  - malignant neoplasm Z15.09
    - biliary tract Z15.068
    - breast Z15.01
    - colorectal Z15.060
    - digestive system NEC Z15.068
    - endometrium Z15.04
    - fallopian tube(s) Z15.05
    - gastric Z15.068
    - ovary Z15.02
    - pancreas Z15.068
    - prostate Z15.03
    - small bowel Z15.068
    - specified NEC Z15.09
    - urinary tract Z15.07
  - multiple endocrine neoplasia Z15.81
  - neurodevelopmental disorders Z15.1
  - obesity Z15.2

**Genital** — *see* condition
**Genito-anorectal syndrome** A55
**Genitourinary system** — *see* condition
**Genu**
- congenital Q74.1
- extrorsum (acquired) — *see also* Deformity, varus, knee
  - congenital Q74.1
  - sequelae (late effect) of rickets E64.3
- introrsum (acquired) — *see also* Deformity, valgus, knee
  - congenital Q74.1
  - sequelae (late effect) of rickets E64.3
- rachitic (old) E64.3
- recurvatum (acquired) — *see also* Deformity, limb, specified type NEC, lower leg
  - congenital Q68.2
  - sequelae (late effect) of rickets E64.3
- valgum (acquired) (knock-knee) M21.06- ☑
  - congenital Q74.1
  - sequelae (late effect) of rickets E64.3
- varum (acquired) (bowleg) M21.16- ☑
  - congenital Q74.1
  - sequelae (late effect) of rickets E64.3

**Geographic tongue** K14.1
**Geophagia** — *see* Pica
**Geotrichosis** B48.3
- stomatitis B48.3

**Gephyrophobia** F40.242
**Gerbode defect** Q21.0
**GERD** (gastroesophageal reflux disease) — *see also* Disease, gastroesophageal reflux K21.9
**Gerhardt's**
- disease (erythromelalgia) I73.81
- syndrome (vocal cord paralysis) J38.00
  - bilateral J38.02
  - unilateral J38.01

**German measles** — *see also* Rubella
- exposure to Z20.4

**Germinoblastoma** (diffuse) C85.9- ☑
- follicular C82.9- ☑

**Germinoma** — *see* Neoplasm, malignant, by site
**Gerontoxon** — *see* Degeneration, cornea, senile
**Gerstmann-Straussler-Scheinker syndrome** (GSS) A81.82
**Gerstmann's syndrome** R48.8
- developmental F81.2

**Gestation** (period) — *see also* Pregnancy
- ectopic — *see* Pregnancy, by site
- multiple O30.9- ☑
  - greater than quadruplets — *see* Pregnancy, multiple (gestation), specified NEC
  - specified NEC — *see* Pregnancy, multiple (gestation), specified NEC

**Gestational**
- mammary abscess O91.11- ☑
- purulent mastitis O91.11- ☑
- subareolar abscess O91.11- ☑

**Ghon tubercle, primary infection** A15.7
**Ghost**
- teeth K00.4
- vessels (cornea) H16.41- ☑

**Ghoul hand** A66.3
**Gianotti-Crosti disease** L44.4
**Giant**
- cell
  - epulis K06.8
  - peripheral granuloma K06.8
- esophagus, congenital Q39.5
- kidney, congenital Q63.3
- urticaria T78.3- ☑
  - hereditary D84.1

**Giardiasis** A07.1
**Gibert's disease or pityriasis** L42
**Giddiness** R42
- hysterical F44.89
- psychogenic F45.8

**Gierke's disease** (glycogenosis I) E74.01
**Gigantism** (cerebral) (hypophyseal) (pituitary) E22.0
- constitutional E34.4

**Gilbert's disease or syndrome** E80.4
**Gilchrist's disease** B40.9
**Gilford-Hutchinson disease** E34.8
**Gilles de la Tourette's disease or syndrome** (motor-verbal tic) F95.2
**Gingivitis** K05.10
- acute (catarrhal) K05.00
  - necrotizing A69.1
  - nonplaque induced K05.01
  - plaque induced K05.00
- chronic (desquamative) (hyperplastic) (simple marginal) (pregnancy associated) (ulcerative) K05.10
  - nonplaque induced K05.11
  - plaque induced K05.10
- expulsiva — *see* Periodontitis
- necrotizing ulcerative (acute) A69.1
- pellagrous E52
  - acute necrotizing A69.1
- Vincent's A69.1

**Gingivoglossitis** K14.0
**Gingivopericementitis** — *see* Periodontitis
**Gingivosis** — *see* Gingivitis, chronic
**Gingivostomatitis** K05.10
- herpesviral B00.2
- necrotizing ulcerative (acute) A69.1

**Gland, glandular** — *see* condition
**Glanders** A24.0
**Glanzmann** (-Naegeli) **disease or thrombasthenia** D69.11
**Glasgow coma scale**
- total score
  - 3-8 R40.243- ☑
  - 9-12 R40.242- ☑
  - 13-15 R40.241- ☑

**Glass-blower's disease** (cataract) — *see* Cataract, specified NEC
**Glaucoma** H40.9
- with
  - increased episcleral venous pressure H40.81- ☑
  - pseudoexfoliation of lens — *see* Glaucoma, open angle, primary, capsular
- absolute H44.51- ☑
- angle-closure (primary) H40.20- ☑
  - acute (attack) (crisis) H40.21- ☑
  - chronic H40.22- ☑
  - intermittent H40.23- ☑
  - residual stage H40.24- ☑
  - secondary, neovascular H40.84- ☑
- borderline H40.00- ☑
- capsular (with pseudoexfoliation of lens) — *see* Glaucoma, open angle, primary, capsular
- childhood Q15.0
- closed angle — *see* Glaucoma, angle-closure
- congenital Q15.0
- corticosteroid-induced — *see* Glaucoma, secondary, drugs
- hypersecretion H40.82- ☑
- in (due to)
  - amyloidosis E85.4 *[H42]*
  - aniridia Q13.1 *[H42]*
  - concussion of globe — *see* Glaucoma, secondary, trauma
  - dislocation of lens — *see* Glaucoma, secondary
  - disorder of lens NEC — *see* Glaucoma, secondary
  - drugs — *see* Glaucoma, secondary, drugs
  - endocrine disease NOS E34.9 *[H42]*
  - eye
    - inflammation — *see* Glaucoma, secondary, inflammation
    - trauma — *see* Glaucoma, secondary, trauma
  - hypermature cataract — *see* Glaucoma, secondary

**Glaucoma** — *continued*
- in — *continued*
  - iridocyclitis — *see* Glaucoma, secondary, inflammation
  - lens disorder — *see* Glaucoma, secondary
  - Lowe's syndrome E72.Ø3 *[H42]*
  - metabolic disease NOS E88.9 *[H42]*
  - ocular disorders NEC — *see* Glaucoma, secondary
  - onchocerciasis B73.Ø2
  - pupillary block — *see* Glaucoma, secondary
  - retinal vein occlusion — *see* Glaucoma, secondary
  - Rieger anomaly Q13.81 *[H42]*
  - rubeosis of iris — *see* Glaucoma, secondary
  - tumor of globe — *see* Glaucoma, secondary
- infantile Q15.Ø
- low tension — *see* Glaucoma, open angle, primary, low-tension
- malignant H4Ø.83- ☑
- narrow angle — *see* Glaucoma, angle-closure
- neovascular secondary angle closure H4Ø.84- ☑
- newborn Q15.Ø
- noncongestive (chronic) — *see* Glaucoma, open angle
- nonobstructive — *see* Glaucoma, open angle
- obstructive — *see also* Glaucoma, angle-closure
  - due to lens changes — *see* Glaucoma, secondary
- open angle H4Ø.1Ø- ☑
  - primary H4Ø.11- ☑
    - capsular (with pseudoexfoliation of lens) H4Ø.14- ☑
    - low-tension H4Ø.12- ☑
    - pigmentary H4Ø.13- ☑
    - residual stage H4Ø.15- ☑
- phacolytic — *see* Glaucoma, secondary
- pigmentary — *see* Glaucoma, open angle, primary, pigmentary
- postinfectious — *see* Glaucoma, secondary, inflammation
- secondary (to) H4Ø.5- ☑
  - drugs H4Ø.6- ☑
  - inflammation H4Ø.4- ☑
  - trauma H4Ø.3- ☑
- simple (chronic) H4Ø.11- ☑
- simplex H4Ø.11- ☑
- specified type NEC H4Ø.89
- suspect H4Ø.ØØ- ☑
- syphilitic A52.71
- traumatic — *see also* Glaucoma, secondary, trauma
  - newborn (birth injury) P15.3
- tuberculous A18.59

**Glaucomatous flecks** (subcapsular) — *see* Cataract, complicated

**Glazed tongue** K14.4

**Gleet** (gonococcal) A54.Ø1

**Glenard's disease** K63.4

**Glioblastoma** (multiforme)
- with sarcomatous component
  - specified site — *see* Neoplasm, malignant, by site
  - unspecified site C71.9
- giant cell
  - specified site — *see* Neoplasm, malignant, by site
  - unspecified site C71.9
- specified site — *see* Neoplasm, malignant, by site
- unspecified site C71.9

**Glioma** (malignant)
- astrocytic
  - specified site — *see* Neoplasm, malignant, by site
  - unspecified site C71.9
- mixed
  - specified site — *see* Neoplasm, malignant, by site
  - unspecified site C71.9
- nose Q3Ø.8
- specified site NEC — *see* Neoplasm, malignant, by site
- subependymal D43.2
  - specified site — *see* Neoplasm, uncertain behavior, by site
  - unspecified site D43.2
- unspecified site C71.9

**Gliomatosis cerebri** C71.Ø

**Glioneuroma** — *see* Neoplasm, uncertain behavior, by site

**Gliosarcoma**
- specified site — *see* Neoplasm, malignant, by site
- unspecified site C71.9

**Gliosis** (cerebral) G93.89
- spinal G95.89

**Glisson's disease** — *see* Rickets

**Globinuria** R82.3

**Globus** (hystericus) F45.8

**Glomangioma** D18.ØØ
- intra-abdominal D18.Ø3
- intracranial D18.Ø2

**Glomangioma** — *continued*
- skin D18.Ø1
- specified site NEC D18.Ø9

**Glomangiomyoma** D18.ØØ
- intra-abdominal D18.Ø3
- intracranial D18.Ø2
- skin D18.Ø1
- specified site NEC D18.Ø9

**Glomangiosarcoma** — *see* Neoplasm, connective tissue, malignant

**Glomerular**
- disease in syphilis A52.75
- nephritis — *see* Glomerulonephritis

**Glomerulitis** — *see* Glomerulonephritis

**Glomerulonephritis** — *see also* Nephritis NØ5.9
- with
  - C3
    - glomerulonephritis NØ5.A
    - glomerulopathy NØ5.A
      - with dense deposit disease NØ5.6
  - edema — *see* Nephrosis
  - minimal change NØ5.Ø
  - minor glomerular abnormality NØ5.Ø
- acute NØØ.9
- chronic NØ3.9
- crescentic (diffuse) NEC — *see also* NØØ-NØ7 with fourth character .7 NØ5.7
- dense deposit — *see also* NØØ-NØ7 with fourth character .6 NØ5.6
- diffuse
  - crescentic — *see also* NØØ-NØ7 with fourth character .7 NØ5.7
  - endocapillary proliferative — *see also* NØØ-NØ7 with fourth character .4 NØ5.4
  - membranous — *see also* NØØ-NØ7 with fourth character .2 NØ5.2
  - mesangial proliferative — *see also* NØØ-NØ7 with fourth character .3 NØ5.3
  - mesangiocapillary — *see also* NØØ-NØ7 with fourth character .5 NØ5.5
  - sclerosing N18.9
- endocapillary proliferative (diffuse) NEC — *see also* NØØ-NØ7 with fourth character .4 NØ5.4
- extracapillary NEC — *see also* NØØ-NØ7 with fourth character .7 NØ5.7
- focal (and segmental) — *see also* NØØ-NØ7 with fourth character .1 NØ5.1
- hypocomplementemic — *see* Glomerulonephritis, membranoproliferative
- IgA — *see* Nephropathy, IgA
- immune complex (circulating) NEC NØ5.8
- in (due to)
  - amyloidosis E85.4 *[NØ8]*
  - bilharziasis B65.9 *[NØ8]*
  - cryoglobulinemia D89.1 *[NØ8]*
  - defibrination syndrome D65 *[NØ8]*
  - diabetes mellitus — *see* Diabetes, glomerulosclerosis
  - disseminated intravascular coagulation D65 *[NØ8]*
  - Fabry (-Anderson) disease E75.21 *[NØ8]*
  - Goodpasture's syndrome M31.Ø
  - hemolytic-uremic syndrome — *see* Syndrome, hemolytic-uremic
  - Henoch (-Schonlein) purpura D69.Ø *[NØ8]*
  - lecithin cholesterol acyltransferase deficiency E78.6 *[NØ8]*
  - microscopic polyangiitis M31.7 *[NØ8]*
  - multiple myeloma C9Ø.Ø- ☑ *[NØ8]*
  - Plasmodium malariae B52.Ø
  - schistosomiasis B65.9 *[NØ8]*
  - sepsis A41.9 *[NØ8]*
    - streptococcal A4Ø.- ☑ *[NØ8]*
  - sickle-cell disorders D57.- ☑ *[NØ8]*
  - strongyloidiasis B78.9 *[NØ8]*
  - subacute bacterial endocarditis I33.Ø *[NØ8]*
  - syphilis (late) congenital A5Ø.59 *[NØ8]*
  - systemic lupus erythematosus M32.14
  - thrombotic thrombocytopenic purpura M31.19 *[NØ8]*
  - typhoid fever AØ1.Ø9
  - Waldenstrom macroglobulinemia C88.Ø- ☑ *[NØ8]*
  - Wegener's granulomatosis M31.31
- latent or quiescent NØ3.9
- lobular, lobulonodular — *see* Glomerulonephritis, membranoproliferative
- membranoproliferative (diffuse)(type 1 or 3) — *see also* NØØ-NØ7 with fourth character .5 NØ5.5
  - dense deposit (type 2) NEC — *see also* NØØ-NØ7 with fourth character .6 NØ5.6
- membranous (diffuse) NEC — *see also* NØØ-NØ7 with fourth character .2 NØ5.2

**Glomerulonephritis** — *continued*
- mesangial
  - IgA/IgG — *see* Nephropathy, IgA
  - proliferative (diffuse) NEC — *see also* NØØ-NØ7 with fourth character .3 NØ5.3
- mesangiocapillary (diffuse) NEC — *see also* NØØ-NØ7 with fourth character .5 NØ5.5
- necrotic, necrotizing NEC — *see also* NØØ- NØ7 with fourth character .8 NØ5.8
- nodular — *see* Glomerulonephritis, membranoproliferative
- poststreptococcal NEC NØ5.9
  - acute NØØ.9
  - chronic NØ3.9
  - rapidly progressive NØ1.9
- proliferative NEC — *see also* NØØ-NØ7 with fourth character .8 NØ5.8
  - diffuse (lupus) M32.14
- rapidly progressive NØ1.9
- sclerosing, diffuse N18.9
- specified pathology NEC — *see also* NØØ- NØ7 with fourth character .8 NØ5.8
- subacute NØ1.9

**Glomerulopathy** — *see* Glomerulonephritis

**Glomerulosclerosis** — *see also* Sclerosis, renal
- intercapillary (nodular) (with diabetes) — *see* Diabetes, glomerulosclerosis
- intracapillary — *see* Diabetes, glomerulosclerosis

**Glossagra** K14.6

**Glossalgia** K14.6

**Glossitis** (chronic superficial) (gangrenous) (Moeller's) K14.Ø
- areata exfoliativa K14.1
- atrophic K14.4
- benign migratory K14.1
- cortical superficial, sclerotic K14.Ø
- Hunter's D51.Ø
- interstitial, sclerous K14.Ø
- median rhomboid K14.2
- pellagrous E52
- superficial, chronic K14.Ø

**Glossocele** K14.8

**Glossodynia** K14.6
- exfoliativa K14.4

**Glossoncus** K14.8

**Glossopathy** K14.9

**Glossophytia** K14.3

**Glossoplegia** K14.8

**Glossoptosis** K14.8

**Glossopyrosis** K14.6

**Glossotrichia** K14.3

**Glossy skin** L9Ø.8

**Glottis** — *see* condition

**Glottitis** — *see also* Laryngitis JØ4.Ø

**Glucagonoma**
- pancreas
  - benign D13.7
  - malignant C25.4
  - uncertain behavior D37.8
- specified site NEC
  - benign — *see* Neoplasm, benign, by site
  - malignant — *see* Neoplasm, malignant, by site
  - uncertain behavior — *see* Neoplasm, uncertain behavior, by site
- unspecified site
  - benign D13.7
  - malignant C25.4
  - uncertain behavior D37.8

**Glucoglycinuria** E72.51

**Glucose-galactose malabsorption** E74.39

**Glue**
- ear — *see* Otitis, media, nonsuppurative, chronic, mucoid
- sniffing (airplane) — *see* Abuse, drug, inhalant
  - dependence — *see* Dependence, drug, inhalant

**GLUT1 deficiency syndrome 1, infantile onset** E74.81Ø

**GLUT1 deficiency syndrome 2, childhood onset** E74.81Ø

**Glutaric aciduria** E72.3

**Glycinemia** E72.51

**Glycinuria** (renal) (with ketosis) E72.Ø9

**Glycogen**
- infiltration — *see* Disease, glycogen storage
- storage disease — *see* Disease, glycogen storage

**Glycogenosis** (diffuse) (generalized) — *see also* Disease, glycogen storage
- cardiac E74.Ø2 *[I43]*
- diabetic, secondary — *see* Diabetes, glycogenosis, secondary
- pulmonary interstitial J84.842

**Glycopenia** E16.2

**Glycosuria** R81

- **Gumma** (syphilitic) A52.79
  - artery A52.09
    - cerebral A52.04
  - bone A52.77
    - of yaws (late) A66.6
  - brain A52.19
  - cauda equina A52.19
  - central nervous system A52.3
  - ciliary body A52.71
  - congenital A50.59
  - eyelid A52.71
  - heart A52.06
  - intracranial A52.19
  - iris A52.71
  - kidney A52.75
  - larynx A52.73
  - leptomeninges A52.19
  - liver A52.74
  - meninges A52.19
  - myocardium A52.06
  - nasopharynx A52.73
  - neurosyphilitic A52.3
  - nose A52.73
  - orbit A52.71
  - palate (soft) A52.79
  - penis A52.76
  - pericardium A52.06
  - pharynx A52.73
  - pituitary A52.79
  - scrofulous (tuberculous) A18.4
  - skin A52.79
  - specified site NEC A52.79
  - spinal cord A52.19
  - tongue A52.79
  - tonsil A52.73
  - trachea A52.73
  - tuberculous A18.4
  - ulcerative due to yaws A66.4
  - ureter A52.75
  - yaws A66.4
    - bone A66.6
- **Gunn's syndrome** Q07.8
- **Gunshot wound** — *see also* Puncture, open
  - fracture — *code as* Fracture, by site
  - internal organs — *see* Injury, by site
- **Gynandrism** Q56.0
- **Gynandroblastoma**
  - specified site — *see* Neoplasm, uncertain behavior, by site
  - unspecified site
    - female D39.10
    - male D40.10
- **Gynecological examination** (periodic) (routine) Z01.419
  - with abnormal findings Z01.411
- **Gynecomastia** N62
- **Gynephobia** F40.291
- **Gyrate scalp** Q82.8

# H

- **H-ABC** (hypomyelination with atrophy of the basal ganglia and cerebellum) G23.3
- **H** (Hartnup's) **disease** E72.02
- **Haas' disease or osteochondrosis** (juvenile) (head of humerus) — *see* Osteochondrosis, juvenile, humerus
- **Habit, habituation**
  - bad sleep Z72.821
  - chorea F95.8
  - disturbance, child F98.9
  - drug — *see* Dependence, drug
  - irregular sleep Z72.821
  - laxative F55.2
  - spasm — *see* Tic
  - tic — *see* Tic
- **Haemophilus** (H.) **influenzae, as cause of disease classified elsewhere** B96.3
- **Haff disease** — *see* Poisoning, mercury
- **HAFOUS** (Hao-Fountain syndrome) Q87.87
- **Hageman's factor defect, deficiency or disease** D68.2
- **Haglund's disease or osteochondrosis** (juvenile) (os tibiale externum) — *see* Osteochondrosis, juvenile, tarsus
- **Hailey-Hailey disease** Q82.8
- **Hair** — *see also* condition
  - plucking F63.3
    - in stereotyped movement disorder F98.4
  - tourniquet syndrome — *see also* Constriction, external, by site
    - finger S60.44- ☑

- **Hair** — *continued*
  - tourniquet syndrome — *see also* Constriction, external, by site — *continued*
    - penis S30.842- ☑
    - thumb S60.34- ☑
    - toe S90.44- ☑
- **Hair-pulling, pathological** (compulsive) F63.3
- **Hairball in stomach** T18.2- ☑
- **Hairy black tongue** K14.3
- **Half vertebra** Q76.49
- **Halitosis** R19.6
- **Hallerman-Streiff syndrome** Q87.0
- **Hallervorden-Spatz disease** G23.0
- **Hallopeau's acrodermatitis or disease** L40.2
- **Hallucination** R44.3
  - auditory R44.0
  - gustatory R44.2
  - olfactory R44.2
  - specified NEC R44.2
  - tactile R44.2
  - visual R44.1
- **Hallucinosis** (chronic) F28
  - alcoholic (acute) F10.951
    - in
      - abuse F10.151
      - dependence F10.251
  - drug-induced F19.951
    - cannabis F12.951
    - cocaine F14.951
    - hallucinogen F16.151
    - in
      - abuse F19.151
        - cannabis F12.151
        - cocaine F14.151
        - hallucinogen F16.151
        - inhalant F18.151
        - opioid F11.151
        - sedative, anxiolytic or hypnotic F13.151
        - stimulant NEC F15.151
      - dependence F19.251
        - cannabis F12.251
        - cocaine F14.251
        - hallucinogen F16.251
        - inhalant F18.251
        - opioid F11.251
        - sedative, anxiolytic or hypnotic F13.251
        - stimulant NEC F15.251
    - inhalant F18.951
    - opioid F11.951
    - sedative, anxiolytic or hypnotic F13.951
    - stimulant NEC F15.951
  - organic F06.0
- **Hallux**
  - deformity (acquired) NEC M20.5X- ☑
  - limitus M20.5X- ☑
  - malleus (acquired) NEC M20.3- ☑
  - rigidus (acquired) M20.2- ☑
    - congenital Q74.2
    - sequelae (late effect) of rickets E64.3
  - valgus (acquired) M20.1- ☑
    - congenital Q66.6
  - varus (acquired) M20.3- ☑
    - congenital Q66.3- ☑
- **Halo, visual** H53.19
- **Hamartoma, hamartoblastoma** Q85.9
  - epithelial (gingival), odontogenic, central or peripheral — *see* Cyst, calcifying odontogenic
- **Hamartosis** Q85.9
- **Hamman-Rich syndrome** J84.114
- **Hammer toe** (acquired) NEC — *see also* Deformity, toe, hammer toe
  - congenital Q66.89
  - sequelae (late effect) of rickets E64.3
- **Hand** — *see* condition
- **Hand-foot syndrome** L27.1
- **Hand-Schuller-Christian disease or syndrome** C96.5
- **Handicap, handicapped**
  - educational Z55.9
    - specified NEC Z55.8
- **Hanging** (asphyxia) (strangulation) (suffocation) — *see* Asphyxia, traumatic, due to mechanical threat
- **Hangnail** — *see also* Cellulitis, digit
  - with lymphangitis — *see* Lymphangitis, acute, digit
- **Hangover** (alcohol) F10.129
- **Hanhart's syndrome** Q87.0
- **Hanot-Chauffard** (-Troisier) **syndrome** E83.19
- **Hanot's cirrhosis or disease** K74.3
- **Hansen's disease** — *see* Leprosy

- **Hantaan virus disease** (Korean hemorrhagic fever) A98.5
- **Hantavirus disease** (with renal manifestations) (Dobrava) (Puumala) (Seoul) A98.5
  - with pulmonary manifestations (Andes) (Bayou) (Bermejo) (Black Creek Canal) (Choclo) (Juquitiba) (Laguna negra) (Lechiguanas) (New York) (Oran) (Sin nombre) B33.4
- **Happy puppet syndrome** Q93.51
- **Harada's disease or syndrome** H30.81- ☑
- **Hardening**
  - artery — *see* Arteriosclerosis
  - brain G93.89
- **Hardship, material, due to limited financial resources, specified NEC** Z59.87
- **Harelip** (complete) (incomplete) — *see* Cleft, lip
- **Harlequin** (newborn) Q80.4
- **Harley's disease** D59.6
- **Harmful use** (of)
  - alcohol F10.10
  - anxiolytics — *see* Abuse, drug, sedative
  - cannabinoids — *see* Abuse, drug, cannabis
  - cocaine — *see* Abuse, drug, cocaine
  - drug — *see* Abuse, drug
  - hallucinogens — *see* Abuse, drug, hallucinogen
  - hypnotics — *see* Abuse, drug, sedative
  - opioids — *see* Abuse, drug, opioid
  - PCP (phencyclidine) — *see* Abuse, drug, hallucinogen
  - sedatives — *see* Abuse, drug, sedative
  - stimulants NEC — *see* Abuse, drug, stimulant
- **Harris' lines** — *see* Arrest, epiphyseal
- **Hartnup's disease** E72.02
- **Harvester's lung** J67.0
- **Harvesting ovum for in vitro fertilization** Z31.83
- **Hashimoto's disease or thyroiditis** E06.3
- **Hashitoxicosis** (transient) E06.3
- **Hassal-Henle bodies or warts** (cornea) H18.49
- **Haut mal** — *see* Epilepsy, generalized, specified NEC
- **Haverhill fever** A25.1
- **Hay fever** — *see also* Fever, hay J30.1
- **Hayem-Widal syndrome** D59.8
- **Haygarth's nodes** M15.8
- **Haymaker's lung** J67.0
- **Hb** (abnormal)
  - Bart's disease D56.0
  - disease — *see* Disease, hemoglobin
  - trait — *see* Trait
- **Head** — *see* condition
- **Headache** R51.9
  - with
    - orthostatic component NEC R51.0
    - positional component NEC R51.0
  - allergic NEC G44.89
  - associated with sexual activity G44.82
  - cervicogenic G44.86
  - chronic daily R51.9
  - cluster G44.009
    - chronic G44.029
      - intractable G44.021
      - not intractable G44.029
    - episodic G44.019
      - intractable G44.011
      - not intractable G44.019
    - intractable G44.001
    - not intractable G44.009
  - cough (primary) G44.83
  - daily chronic R51.9
  - drug-induced NEC G44.40
    - intractable G44.41
    - not intractable G44.40
  - exertional (primary) G44.84
  - histamine G44.009
    - intractable G44.001
    - not intractable G44.009
  - hypnic G44.81
  - lumbar puncture G97.1
  - medication overuse G44.40
    - intractable G44.41
    - not intractable G44.40
  - menstrual — *see* Migraine, menstrual
  - migraine (type) — *see also* Migraine G43.909
  - nasal septum R51.9
  - neuralgiform, short lasting unilateral, with conjunctival injection and tearing (SUNCT) G44.059
    - intractable G44.051
    - not intractable G44.059
  - new daily persistent (NDPH) G44.52
  - orgasmic G44.82
  - periodic syndromes in adults and children G43.C0 (*following* G43.7)

**Headache** — *continued*
- periodic syndromes in adults and children — *continued*
  - with refractory migraine G43.C1 (*following* G43.7)
  - intractable G43.C1 (*following* G43.7)
  - not intractable G43.CØ (*following* G43.7)
  - without refractory migraine G43.CØ (*following* G43.7)
- postspinal puncture G97.1
- post-traumatic G44.3Ø9
  - acute G44.319
    - intractable G44.311
    - not intractable G44.319
  - chronic G44.329
    - intractable G44.321
    - not intractable G44.329
  - intractable G44.3Ø1
  - not intractable G44.3Ø9
- pre-menstrual — *see* Migraine, menstrual
- preorgasmic G44.82
- primary
  - cough G44.83
  - exertional G44.84
  - stabbing G44.85
  - thunderclap G44.53
- rebound G44.4Ø
  - intractable G44.41
  - not intractable G44.4Ø
- short lasting unilateral neuralgiform, with conjunctival injection and tearing (SUNCT) G44.Ø59
  - intractable G44.Ø51
  - not intractable G44.Ø59
- specified syndrome NEC G44.89
- spinal and epidural anesthesia - induced T88.59- ☑
  - in labor and delivery O74.5
  - in pregnancy O29.4- ☑
  - postpartum, puerperal O89.4
- spinal fluid loss (from puncture) G97.1
- stabbing (primary) G44.85
- tension (-type) G44.2Ø9
  - chronic G44.229
    - intractable G44.221
    - not intractable G44.229
  - episodic G44.219
    - intractable G44.211
    - not intractable G44.219
  - intractable G44.2Ø1
  - not intractable G44.2Ø9
- thunderclap (primary) G44.53
- vascular NEC G44.1

**Healthy**
- infant
  - accompanying sick mother Z76.3
  - receiving care Z76.2
- person accompanying sick person Z76.3

**Hearing examination** ZØ1.1Ø
- with abnormal findings NEC ZØ1.118
- following failed hearing screening ZØ1.11Ø
- for hearing conservation and treatment ZØ1.12
- infant or child (over 28 days old) ZØØ.129
  - with abnormal findings ZØØ.121

**Heart** — *see* condition
- carcinoid — *see* Syndrome, carcinoid, heart

**Heart beat**
- abnormality RØØ.9
  - specified NEC RØØ.8
- awareness RØØ.2
- rapid RØØ.Ø
- slow RØØ.1

**Heartburn** R12
- psychogenic F45.8

**Heartland virus disease** A93.8

**Heat** (effects) T67.9- ☑
- apoplexy T67.Ø1- ☑
- burn — *see also* Burn L55.9
- collapse T67.1- ☑
- cramps T67.2- ☑
- dermatitis or eczema L59.Ø
- edema T67.7- ☑
- erythema — *code by site under* Burn, first degree
- excessive T67.9- ☑
  - specified effect NEC T67.8- ☑
- exhaustion T67.5- ☑
  - anhydrotic T67.3- ☑
  - due to
    - salt (and water) depletion T67.4- ☑
    - water depletion T67.3- ☑
      - with salt depletion T67.4- ☑
- fatigue (transient) T67.6- ☑
- fever T67.Ø1- ☑
- hyperpyrexia T67.Ø1- ☑
- prickly L74.Ø
- prostration — *see* Heat, exhaustion
- pyrexia T67.Ø1- ☑
- rash L74.Ø
- specified effect NEC T67.8- ☑
- stroke T67.Ø1- ☑
  - exertional T67.Ø2- ☑
  - specified NEC T67.Ø9- ☑
- sunburn — *see* Sunburn
- syncope T67.1- ☑

**Heavy-for-dates NEC** (infant) (4ØØØg to 4499g) PØ8.1
- exceptionally (45ØØg or more) PØ8.Ø

**Hebephrenia, hebephrenic** (schizophrenia) F2Ø.1

**Heberden's disease or nodes** (with arthropathy) M15.1

**Hebra's**
- pityriasis L26
- prurigo L28.2

**Heel** — *see* condition

**Heerfordt's disease** D86.89

**HeFH** (heterozygous familial hypercholesterolemia) E78.Ø11

**Hegglin's anomaly or syndrome** D72.Ø

**Heilmeyer-Schoner disease** D45

**Heine-Medin disease** A8Ø.9

**Heinz body anemia, congenital** D58.2

**Heliophobia** F4Ø.228

**Heller's disease or syndrome** F84.3

**HELLP syndrome** (hemolysis, elevated liver enzymes and low platelet count) O14.2- ☑
- complicating
  - childbirth O14.24
  - puerperium O14.25

**Helminthiasis** — *see also* Infestation, helminth
- Ancylostoma B76.Ø
- intestinal B82.Ø
  - mixed types (types classifiable to more than one of the titles B65.Ø-B81.3 and B81.8) B81.4
  - specified type NEC B81.8
- mixed types (intestinal) (types classifiable to more than one of the titles B65.Ø-B81.3 and B81.8) B81.4
- Necator (americanus) B76.1
- specified type NEC B83.8

**Heloma** L84

**Hemangioblastoma** — *see* Neoplasm, connective tissue, uncertain behavior
- malignant — *see* Neoplasm, connective tissue, malignant

**Hemangioendothelioma** — *see also* Neoplasm, uncertain behavior, by site
- benign D18.ØØ
  - intra-abdominal D18.Ø3
  - intracranial D18.Ø2
  - skin D18.Ø1
  - specified site NEC D18.Ø9
- bone (diffuse) — *see* Neoplasm, bone, malignant
- epithelioid — *see also* Neoplasm, uncertain behavior, by site
  - malignant — *see* Neoplasm, malignant, by site
- malignant — *see* Neoplasm, connective tissue, malignant

**Hemangiofibroma** — *see* Neoplasm, benign, by site

**Hemangiolipoma** — *see* Lipoma

**Hemangioma** D18.ØØ
- arteriovenous D18.ØØ
  - intra-abdominal D18.Ø3
  - intracranial D18.Ø2
  - skin D18.Ø1
  - specified site NEC D18.Ø9
- capillary I78.1
  - intra-abdominal D18.Ø3
  - intracranial D18.Ø2
  - skin D18.Ø1
  - specified site NEC D18.Ø9
- cavernous D18.ØØ
  - intra-abdominal D18.Ø3
  - intracranial D18.Ø2
  - skin D18.Ø1
  - specified site NEC D18.Ø9
- epithelioid D18.ØØ
  - intra-abdominal D18.Ø3
  - intracranial D18.Ø2
  - skin D18.Ø1
  - specified site NEC D18.Ø9
- histiocytoid D18.ØØ
  - intra-abdominal D18.Ø3
  - intracranial D18.Ø2
  - skin D18.Ø1
  - specified site NEC D18.Ø9

**Hemangioma** — *continued*
- infantile D18.ØØ
  - intra-abdominal D18.Ø3
  - intracranial D18.Ø2
  - skin D18.Ø1
  - specified site NEC D18.Ø9
- intra-abdominal D18.Ø3
- intracranial D18.Ø2
- intramuscular D18.ØØ
  - intra-abdominal D18.Ø3
  - intracranial D18.Ø2
  - skin D18.Ø1
  - specified site NEC D18.Ø9
- intrathoracic structures D18.Ø9
- juvenile D18.ØØ
- malignant — *see* Neoplasm, connective tissue, malignant
- plexiform D18.ØØ
  - intra-abdominal D18.Ø3
  - intracranial D18.Ø2
  - skin D18.Ø1
  - specified site NEC D18.Ø9
- racemose D18.ØØ
  - intra-abdominal D18.Ø3
  - intracranial D18.Ø2
  - skin D18.Ø1
  - specified site NEC D18.Ø9
- sclerosing — *see* Neoplasm, skin, benign
- simplex D18.ØØ
  - intra-abdominal D18.Ø3
  - intracranial D18.Ø2
  - skin D18.Ø1
  - specified site NEC D18.Ø9
- skin D18.Ø1
- specified site NEC D18.Ø9
- venous D18.ØØ
  - intra-abdominal D18.Ø3
  - intracranial D18.Ø2
  - skin D18.Ø1
  - specified site NEC D18.Ø9
- verrucous keratotic D18.ØØ
  - intra-abdominal D18.Ø3
  - intracranial D18.Ø2
  - skin D18.Ø1
  - specified site NEC D18.Ø9

**Hemangiomatosis** (systemic) I78.8
- involving single site — *see* Hemangioma

**Hemangiopericytoma** — *see also* Neoplasm, connective tissue, uncertain behavior
- benign — *see* Neoplasm, connective tissue, benign
- malignant — *see* Neoplasm, connective tissue, malignant

**Hemangiosarcoma** — *see* Neoplasm, connective tissue, malignant

**Hemarthrosis** (nontraumatic) M25.ØØ
- ankle M25.Ø7- ☑
- elbow M25.Ø2- ☑
- foot joint M25.Ø7- ☑
- hand joint M25.Ø4- ☑
- hip M25.Ø5- ☑
- in hemophilic arthropathy — *see* Arthropathy, hemophilic
- knee M25.Ø6- ☑
- shoulder M25.Ø1- ☑
- specified joint NEC M25.Ø8
- traumatic — *see* Sprain, by site
- vertebrae M25.Ø8
- wrist M25.Ø3- ☑

**Hematemesis** K92.Ø
- with ulcer — *code by site under* Ulcer, with hemorrhage K27.4
- newborn, neonatal P54.Ø
  - due to swallowed maternal blood P78.2

**Hematidrosis** L74.8

**Hematinuria** — *see also* Hemoglobinuria
- malarial B5Ø.8

**Hematobilia** K83.8

**Hematocele**
- female NEC N94.89
  - with ectopic pregnancy OØØ.9Ø
    - with intrauterine pregnancy OØØ.91
  - ovary N83.8
- male N5Ø.1

**Hematochezia** — *see also* Melena K92.1

**Hematochyluria** — *see also* Infestation, filarial
- schistosomiasis (bilharziasis) B65.Ø

**Hematocolpos** (with hematometra or hematosalpinx) N89.7

**Hematocornea** — *see* Pigmentation, cornea, stromal

**Hematogenous** — *see* condition

- **Hematoma** (traumatic) (skin surface intact) — *see also* Contusion
  - with
    - injury of internal organs — *see* Injury, by site
    - open wound — *see* Wound, open
  - amputation stump (surgical) (late) T87.89
  - aorta, dissecting I71.00
    - abdominal I71.02
    - thoracic — *see also* Dissection, aorta, thoracic I71.019
    - thoracoabdominal I71.03
  - aortic intramural — *see* Dissection, aorta
  - arterial (complicating trauma) — *see* Injury, blood vessel, by site
  - auricle — *see* Contusion, ear
    - nontraumatic — *see* Disorder, pinna, hematoma
  - birth injury NEC P15.8
  - brain (traumatic)
    - with
      - cerebral laceration or contusion (diffuse) — *see* Injury, intracranial, diffuse
        - focal — *see* Injury, intracranial, focal
    - cerebellar, traumatic S06.37- ☑
    - intracerebral, traumatic — *see* Injury, intracranial, intracerebral hemorrhage
    - newborn NEC P52.4
      - birth injury P10.0
    - nontraumatic — *see* Hemorrhage, intracranial
    - subarachnoid, arachnoid, traumatic — *see* Injury, intracranial, subarachnoid hemorrhage
    - subdural, traumatic — *see* Injury, intracranial, subdural hemorrhage
  - breast (nontraumatic) N64.89
  - broad ligament (nontraumatic) N83.7
    - traumatic S37.892- ☑
  - cerebellar, traumatic S06.37- ☑
  - cerebral — *see* Hematoma, brain
  - cerebrum S06.36- ☑
    - left S06.35- ☑
    - right S06.34- ☑
  - cesarean delivery wound O90.2
  - complicating delivery (perineal) (pelvic) (vagina) (vulva) O71.7
  - corpus cavernosum (nontraumatic) N48.89
  - epididymis (nontraumatic) N50.1
  - epidural (traumatic) — *see* Injury, intracranial, epidural hemorrhage
    - spinal — *see* Injury, spinal cord, by region
  - episiotomy O90.2
  - face, birth injury P15.4
  - genital organ NEC (nontraumatic)
    - female (nonobstetric) N94.89
      - traumatic S30.202- ☑
    - male N50.1
      - traumatic S30.201- ☑
  - internal organs — *see* Injury, by site
  - intracerebral, traumatic — *see* Injury, intracranial, intracerebral hemorrhage
  - intraoperative — *see* Complications, intraoperative, hemorrhage
  - labia (nontraumatic) (nonobstetric) N90.89
  - liver (subcapsular) (nontraumatic) K76.89
    - birth injury P15.0
  - mediastinum — *see* Injury, intrathoracic
  - mesosalpinx (nontraumatic) N83.7
    - traumatic S37.898- ☑
  - muscle — code by site under Contusion
  - nontraumatic
    - muscle M79.81
    - soft tissue M79.81
  - obstetrical surgical wound O90.2
  - orbit, orbital (nontraumatic) — *see also* Hemorrhage, orbit
    - traumatic — *see* Contusion, orbit
  - pelvis K6A.8
    - female (nontraumatic) (nonobstetric) N94.89
    - male K6A.8
    - obstetric O71.7
    - traumatic — *see* Injury, by site
  - penis (nontraumatic) N48.89
    - birth injury P15.5
  - perianal (nontraumatic) K64.5
  - perineal S30.23- ☑
    - complicating delivery O71.7
  - perirenal — *see* Injury, kidney
  - peritoneal K66.1
  - pinna — *see* Contusion, ear
    - nontraumatic — *see* Disorder, pinna, hematoma
  - placenta O43.89- ☑

**Hematoma** — *continued*

  - postoperative (postprocedural) — *see* Complication, postprocedural, hematoma
  - retroperitoneal (nontraumatic) K68.3
    - traumatic S36.892- ☑
  - scrotum, superficial S30.22- ☑
    - birth injury P15.5
  - seminal vesicle (nontraumatic) N50.1
    - traumatic S37.892- ☑
  - spermatic cord (traumatic) S37.892- ☑
    - nontraumatic N50.1
  - spinal (cord) (meninges) — *see also* Injury, spinal cord, by region
    - newborn (birth injury) P11.5
  - spleen D73.5
    - intraoperative — *see* Complications, intraoperative, hemorrhage, spleen
    - postprocedural (postoperative) — *see* Complications, postprocedural, hemorrhage, spleen
  - sternocleidomastoid, birth injury P15.2
  - sternomastoid, birth injury P15.2
  - subarachnoid (traumatic) — *see* Injury, intracranial, subarachnoid hemorrhage
    - newborn (nontraumatic) P52.5
      - due to birth injury P10.3
    - nontraumatic — *see* Hemorrhage, intracranial, subarachnoid
  - subdural (traumatic) — *see* Injury, intracranial, subdural hemorrhage
    - newborn (localized) P52.8
      - birth injury P10.0
    - nontraumatic — *see* Hemorrhage, intracranial, subdural
  - superficial, newborn P54.5
  - testis (nontraumatic) N50.1
    - birth injury P15.5
  - tunica vaginalis (nontraumatic) N50.1
  - umbilical cord, complicating delivery O69.5- ☑
  - uterine ligament (broad) (nontraumatic) N83.7
    - traumatic S37.892- ☑
  - vagina (ruptured) (nontraumatic) N89.8
    - complicating delivery O71.7
  - vas deferens (nontraumatic) N50.1
    - traumatic S37.892- ☑
  - vitreous — *see* Hemorrhage, vitreous
  - vulva (nontraumatic) (nonobstetric) N90.89
    - complicating delivery O71.7
    - newborn (birth injury) P15.5
- **Hematometra** N85.7
  - with hematocolpos N89.7
- **Hematomyelia** (central) G95.19
  - newborn (birth injury) P11.5
  - traumatic T14.8- ☑
- **Hematomyelitis** G04.90
- **Hematoperitoneum** — *see* Hemoperitoneum
- **Hematophobia** F40.230
- **Hematopneumothorax** — *see* Hemothorax
- **Hematopoiesis, cyclic** D70.4
- **Hematoporphyria** — *see* Porphyria
- **Hematorachis, hematorrhachis** G95.19
  - newborn (birth injury) P11.5
- **Hematosalpinx** N83.6
  - with
    - hematocolpos N89.7
    - hematometra N85.7
      - with hematocolpos N89.7
  - infectional — *see* Salpingitis
- **Hematospermia** R36.1
- **Hematothorax** — *see* Hemothorax
- **Hematuria** R31.9
  - benign (familial) (of childhood) — *see also* Hematuria, idiopathic
    - essential microscopic R31.1
  - due to sulphonamide, sulfonamide — *see* Table of Drugs and Chemicals, by drug
  - endemic — *see also* Schistosomiasis B65.0
  - gross R31.0
  - idiopathic N02.9
    - with glomerular lesion
      - C3
        - glomerulonephritis N02.A
        - glomerulopathy N02.A
          - with dense deposit disease N02.6
      - crescentic (diffuse) glomerulonephritis N02.7
      - dense deposit disease N02.6
      - endocapillary proliferative glomerulonephritis N02.4
      - focal and segmental hyalinosis or sclerosis N02.1

**Hematuria** — *continued*

  - idiopathic — *continued*
    - with glomerular lesion — *continued*
      - membranoproliferative (diffuse) N02.5
      - membranous (diffuse) N02.2
      - mesangial proliferative (diffuse) N02.3
      - mesangiocapillary (diffuse) N02.5
      - minor abnormality N02.0
      - proliferative NEC N02.8
      - specified pathology NEC N02.8
  - intermittent — *see* Hematuria, idiopathic
  - malarial B50.8
  - microscopic NEC (with symptoms) R31.29
    - asymptomatic R31.21
    - benign essential R31.1
  - paroxysmal — *see also* Hematuria, idiopathic
    - nocturnal D59.5
  - persistent — *see* Hematuria, idiopathic
  - recurrent — *see* Hematuria, idiopathic
  - tropical — *see also* Schistosomiasis B65.0
  - tuberculous A18.13
- **Hemeralopia** (day blindness) H53.11
  - vitamin A deficiency E50.5
- **Hemi-akinesia** R41.4
- **Hemi-inattention** R41.4
- **Hemianalgesia** R20.0
- **Hemianencephaly** Q00.0
- **Hemianesthesia** R20.0
- **Hemianopia, hemianopsia** (heteronymous) H53.47
  - homonymous H53.46- ☑
  - syphilitic A52.71
- **Hemiathetosis** R25.8
- **Hemiatrophy** R68.89
  - cerebellar G31.9
  - face, facial, progressive (Romberg) G51.8
  - tongue K14.8
- **Hemiballism** (us) G25.5
- **Hemicardia** Q24.8
- **Hemicephalus, hemicephaly** Q00.0
- **Hemichorea** G25.5
- **Hemicolitis, left** — *see* Colitis, left sided
- **Hemicrania**
  - congenital malformation Q00.0
  - continua G44.51
  - meaning migraine — *see also* Migraine G43.909
  - paroxysmal G44.039
    - chronic G44.049
      - intractable G44.041
      - not intractable G44.049
    - episodic G44.039
      - intractable G44.031
      - not intractable G44.039
    - intractable G44.031
    - not intractable G44.039
- **Hemidystrophy** — *see* Hemiatrophy
- **Hemiectromelia** Q73.8
- **Hemihypalgesia** R20.8
- **Hemihypesthesia** R20.1
- **Hemimegalencephaly** Q04.5
- **Hemimelia** Q73.8
  - lower limb — *see* Defect, reduction, lower limb, specified type NEC
  - upper limb — *see* Defect, reduction, upper limb, specified type NEC
- **Hemiparalysis** — *see* Hemiplegia
- **Hemiparesis** — *see* Hemiplegia
- **Hemiparesthesia** R20.2
- **Hemiparkinsonism** G20.C
- **Hemiplegia** G81.9- ☑
  - alternans facialis G83.89
  - ascending NEC G81.90
    - spinal G95.89
  - congenital (cerebral) G80.8
    - spastic G80.2
  - embolic (current episode) I63.4- ☑
  - flaccid G81.0- ☑
  - following
    - cerebrovascular disease I69.959
      - cerebral infarction I69.35- ☑
      - intracerebral hemorrhage I69.15- ☑
      - nontraumatic intracranial hemorrhage NEC I69.25- ☑
      - specified disease NEC I69.85- ☑
      - stroke NOS I69.35- ☑
      - subarachnoid hemorrhage I69.05- ☑
  - hysterical F44.4
  - newborn NEC P91.88
    - birth injury P11.9

- **Hemiplegia** — *continued*
  - spastic G81.1- ☑
    - congenital G8Ø.2
  - thrombotic (current episode) I63.3- ☑
- **Hemisection, spinal cord** — *see* Injury, spinal cord, by region
- **Hemispasm** (facial) R25.2
- **Hemisporosis** B48.8
- **Hemitremor** R25.1
- **Hemivertebra** Q76.49
  - failure of segmentation with scoliosis Q76.3
  - fusion with scoliosis Q76.3
- **Hemochromatosis** E83.119
  - with refractory anemia D46.1
  - due to repeated red blood cell transfusion E83.111
  - hereditary (primary) E83.11Ø
  - neonatal P78.84
  - primary E83.11Ø
  - specified NEC E83.118
- **Hemoglobin** — *see also* condition
  - abnormal (disease) — *see* Disease, hemoglobin
  - AS genotype D57.3
  - Constant Spring D58.2
  - E-beta thalassemia D56.5
  - fetal, hereditary persistence (HPFH) D56.4
  - H Constant Spring D56.Ø
  - low NOS D64.9
  - S (Hb S), heterozygous D57.3
- **Hemoglobinemia** D59.9
  - due to blood transfusion T8Ø.89- ☑
  - paroxysmal D59.6
    - nocturnal D59.5
- **Hemoglobinopathy** (mixed) D58.2
  - with thalassemia D56.8
  - sickle-cell D57.1
    - with thalassemia D57.4Ø
      - with
        - acute chest syndrome D57.411
        - cerebral vascular involvement D57.413
        - crisis (painful) D57.419
          - with
            - dactylitis D57.414
            - specified complication NEC D57.418
        - pain (vaso-occlusive) D57.419
        - splenic sequestration D57.412
      - without crisis D57.4Ø
- **Hemoglobinuria** R82.3
  - with anemia, hemolytic, acquired (chronic) NEC D59.6
  - cold (paroxysmal) (with Raynaud's syndrome) D59.6
    - agglutinin D59.12
  - due to exertion or hemolysis NEC D59.6
  - intermittent D59.6
  - malarial B5Ø.8
  - march D59.6
  - nocturnal (paroxysmal) D59.5
  - paroxysmal (cold) D59.6
    - nocturnal D59.5
- **Hemolymphangioma** D18.1
- **Hemolysis**
  - intravascular
    - with
      - abortion — *see* Abortion, by type, complicated by, hemorrhage
      - ectopic or molar pregnancy OØ8.1
      - hemorrhage
        - antepartum — *see* Hemorrhage, antepartum, with coagulation defect
        - intrapartum — *see also* Hemorrhage, complicating, delivery O67.Ø
    - postpartum O72.3
  - neonatal (excessive) P58.9
    - specified NEC P58.8
- **Hemolytic** — *see* condition
- **Hemopericardium** I31.2
  - following acute myocardial infarction (current complication) I23.Ø
  - newborn P54.8
  - traumatic — *see* Injury, heart, with hemopericardium
- **Hemoperitoneum** K66.1
  - infectional K65.9
  - traumatic S36.899- ☑
    - with open wound — *see* Wound, open, abdominal, wall, by site if known, with penetration into peritoneal cavity
- **Hemophilia** (classical) (familial) (hereditary) D66
  - A D66
  - acquired D68.311
  - autoimmune D68.311
  - B D67
  - C D68.1
  - calcipriva — *see also* Defect, coagulation D68.4
  - nonfamilial — *see also* Defect, coagulation D68.4
  - secondary D68.311
  - vascular — *see* Disease, von Willebrand
- **Hemophthalmos** H44.81- ☑
- **Hemopneumothorax** — *see also* Hemothorax
  - traumatic S27.2- ☑
- **Hemoptysis** RØ4.2
  - newborn P26.9
  - tuberculous — *see* Tuberculosis, pulmonary
- **Hemorrhage, hemorrhagic** (concealed) R58
  - abdomen R58
  - accidental antepartum — *see* Hemorrhage, antepartum
  - acute idiopathic pulmonary, in infants RØ4.81
  - adenoid J35.8
  - adrenal (capsule) (gland) E27.49
    - medulla E27.8
    - newborn P54.4
  - after delivery — *see* Hemorrhage, postpartum
  - alveolar
    - lung, newborn P26.8
    - process KØ8.89
  - alveolus KØ8.89
  - amputation stump (surgical) T87.89
  - anemia (chronic) D5Ø.Ø
    - acute D62
  - antepartum (with) O46.9Ø
    - with coagulation defect O46.ØØ- ☑
      - afibrinogenemia O46.Ø1- ☑
      - disseminated intravascular coagulation O46.Ø2- ☑
      - hypofibrinogenemia O46.Ø1- ☑
      - specified defect NEC O46.Ø9- ☑
    - before 2Ø weeks gestation O2Ø.9
      - specified type NEC O2Ø.8
      - threatened abortion O2Ø.Ø
    - due to
      - abruptio placenta — *see also* Abruptio placentae O45.9- ☑
      - leiomyoma, uterus — *see* Hemorrhage, antepartum, specified cause NEC
      - placenta previa O44.1- ☑
    - specified cause NEC — *see* subcategory O46.8X- ☑
  - anus (sphincter) K62.5
  - apoplexy (stroke) — *see* Hemorrhage, intracranial, intracerebral
  - arachnoid — *see* Hemorrhage, intracranial, subarachnoid
  - artery R58
    - brain — *see* Hemorrhage, intracranial, intracerebral
  - basilar (ganglion) I61.Ø
  - bladder N32.89
  - bowel K92.2
    - newborn P54.3
  - brain (miliary) (nontraumatic) — *see* Hemorrhage, intracranial, intracerebral
    - due to
      - birth injury P1Ø.1
      - syphilis A52.Ø5
    - epidural or extradural (traumatic) — *see* Injury, intracranial, epidural hemorrhage
    - newborn P52.4
      - birth injury P1Ø.1
    - subarachnoid — *see* Hemorrhage, intracranial, subarachnoid
    - subdural — *see* Hemorrhage, intracranial, subdural
  - brainstem (nontraumatic) I61.3
    - traumatic SØ6.38- ☑
  - breast N64.59
  - bronchial tube — *see* Hemorrhage, lung
  - bronchopulmonary — *see* Hemorrhage, lung
  - bronchus — *see* Hemorrhage, lung
  - bulbar I61.5
  - capillary I78.8
    - primary D69.8
  - cecum K92.2
  - cerebellar, cerebellum (nontraumatic) I61.4
    - newborn P52.6
    - traumatic SØ6.37- ☑
  - cerebral, cerebrum — *see also* Hemorrhage, intracranial, intracerebral
    - lobe I61.1
    - newborn (anoxic) P52.4
      - birth injury P1Ø.1
  - cerebromeningeal I61.8
  - cerebrospinal — *see* Hemorrhage, intracranial, intracerebral
  - cervix (uteri) (stump) NEC N88.8
  - chamber, anterior (eye) — *see* Hyphema
  - childbirth — *see* Hemorrhage, complicating, delivery
  - choroid H31.3Ø- ☑
    - expulsive H31.31- ☑
  - ciliary body — *see* Hyphema
  - cochlea — *see* subcategory H83.8- ☑
  - colon K92.2
  - complicating
    - abortion — *see* Abortion, by type, complicated by, hemorrhage
    - delivery O67.9
      - associated with coagulation defect (afibrinogenemia) (DIC) (hyperfibrinolysis) O67.Ø
      - specified cause NEC O67.8
    - surgical procedure — *see* Hemorrhage, intraoperative
  - conjunctiva H11.3- ☑
    - newborn P54.8
  - cord, newborn (stump) P51.9
  - corpus luteum (ruptured) cyst N83.1- ☑
  - cortical (brain) I61.1
  - cranial — *see* Hemorrhage, intracranial
  - cutaneous R23.3
    - due to autosensitivity, erythrocyte D69.2
    - newborn P54.5
  - delayed
    - following ectopic or molar pregnancy OØ8.1
    - postpartum O72.2
  - diathesis (familial) D69.9
  - disease D69.9
    - newborn P53
    - specified type NEC D69.8
  - due to or associated with
    - afibrinogenemia or other coagulation defect (conditions in categories D65- D69)
      - antepartum — *see* Hemorrhage, antepartum, with coagulation defect
      - intrapartum O67.Ø
    - dental implant M27.61
    - device, implant or graft — *see also* Complications, by site and type, specified NEC T85.838- ☑
      - arterial graft NEC T82.838- ☑
      - breast T85.838- ☑
      - catheter NEC T85.838- ☑
        - dialysis (renal) T82.838- ☑
          - intraperitoneal T85.838- ☑
        - infusion NEC T82.838- ☑
          - spinal (epidural) (subdural) T85.83Ø- ☑
        - urinary (indwelling) T83.83- ☑
      - electronic (electrode) (pulse generator) (stimulator)
        - bone T84.83- ☑
        - cardiac T82.837- ☑
        - nervous system (brain) (peripheral nerve) (spinal) T85.83Ø- ☑
        - urinary T83.83- ☑
      - fixation, internal (orthopedic) NEC T84.83- ☑
      - gastrointestinal (bile duct) (esophagus) T85.838- ☑
      - genital NEC T83.83- ☑
      - heart NEC T82.837- ☑
      - joint prosthesis T84.83- ☑
      - ocular (corneal graft) (orbital implant) NEC T85.838- ☑
      - orthopedic NEC T84.83- ☑
        - bone graft T86.838
      - specified NEC T85.838- ☑
      - urinary NEC T83.83- ☑
      - vascular NEC T82.838- ☑
      - ventricular intracranial shunt T85.83Ø- ☑
  - duodenum, duodenal K92.2
    - ulcer — *see* Ulcer, duodenum, with hemorrhage
  - dura mater — *see* Hemorrhage, intracranial, subdural
  - endotracheal — *see* Hemorrhage, lung
  - epicranial subaponeurotic (massive), birth injury P12.2
  - epidural (traumatic) — *see also* Injury, intracranial, epidural hemorrhage
    - nontraumatic I62.1
  - esophagus K22.89
    - varix I85.Ø1
      - secondary I85.11
  - excessive, following ectopic gestation (subsequent episode) OØ8.1
  - extradural (traumatic) — *see* Injury, intracranial, epidural hemorrhage
    - birth injury P1Ø.8
    - newborn (anoxic) (nontraumatic) P52.8

**Hemorrhage, hemorrhagic** — *continued*
- extradural — *see* Injury, intracranial, epidural hemorrhage — *continued*
  - nontraumatic I62.1
- eye NEC H57.89
  - fundus — *see* Hemorrhage, retina
  - lid — *see* Disorder, eyelid, specified type NEC
- fallopian tube N83.6
- fibrinogenolysis — *see* Fibrinolysis
- fibrinolytic (acquired) — *see* Fibrinolysis
- from
  - ear (nontraumatic) — *see* Otorrhagia
  - tracheostomy stoma J95.Ø1
- fundus, eye — *see* Hemorrhage, retina
- funis — *see* Hemorrhage, umbilicus, cord
- gastric — *see* Hemorrhage, stomach
- gastroenteric K92.2
  - newborn P54.3
- gastrointestinal (tract) K92.2
  - newborn P54.3
- genital organ, male N5Ø.1
- genitourinary (tract) NOS R31.9
- gingiva KØ6.8
- globe (eye) — *see* Hemophthalmos
- graafian follicle cyst (ruptured) N83.Ø- ☑
- gum KØ6.8
- heart I51.89
- hypopharyngeal (throat) RØ4.1
- intermenstrual (regular) N92.3
  - irregular N92.1
- internal (organs) NEC R58
  - capsule I61.Ø
  - ear — *see* subcategory H83.8- ☑
  - newborn P54.8
- intestine K92.2
  - newborn P54.3
- intra-abdominal R58
- intra-alveolar (lung), newborn P26.8
- intracerebral (nontraumatic) — *see* Hemorrhage, intracranial, intracerebral
- intracranial (nontraumatic) I62.9
  - birth injury P1Ø.9
  - epidural, nontraumatic I62.1
  - extradural, nontraumatic I62.1
  - intracerebral (nontraumatic) (in) I61.9
    - brain stem I61.3
    - cerebellum I61.4
    - hemisphere I61.2
      - cortical (superficial) I61.1
      - subcortical (deep) I61.Ø
    - intraoperative
      - during a nervous system procedure G97.31
      - during other procedure G97.32
    - intraventricular I61.5
    - multiple localized I61.6
    - newborn P52.4
      - birth injury P1Ø.1
    - postprocedural
      - following a nervous system procedure G97.51
      - following other procedure G97.52
    - specified NEC I61.8
    - superficial I61.1
    - traumatic — *see* Injury, intracranial, intracerebral hemorrhage, traumatic
  - newborn P52.9
    - specified NEC P52.8
  - subarachnoid (nontraumatic) (from) I6Ø.9
    - intracranial (cerebral) artery I6Ø.7
      - anterior communicating I6Ø.2
      - basilar I6Ø.4
      - carotid siphon and bifurcation I6Ø.Ø- ☑
      - communicating I6Ø.7
        - anterior I6Ø.2
        - posterior I6Ø.3- ☑
      - middle cerebral I6Ø.1- ☑
      - posterior communicating I6Ø.3- ☑
      - specified artery NEC I6Ø.6
      - vertebral I6Ø.5- ☑
    - newborn P52.5
      - birth injury P1Ø.3
    - specified NEC I6Ø.8
    - traumatic SØ6.6X- ☑
  - subdural (nontraumatic) I62.ØØ
    - acute I62.Ø1
    - birth injury P1Ø.Ø
    - chronic I62.Ø3
    - newborn (anoxic) (hypoxic) P52.8
      - birth injury P1Ø.Ø

**Hemorrhage, hemorrhagic** — *continued*
- intracranial — *continued*
  - subdural — *continued*
    - spinal G95.19
    - subacute I62.Ø2
    - traumatic — *see* Injury, intracranial, subdural hemorrhage
  - traumatic — *see* Injury, intracranial, focal brain injury
- intramedullary NEC G95.19
- intraocular — *see* Hemophthalmos
- intraoperative, intraprocedural — *see* Complication, hemorrhage (hematoma), intraoperative (intraprocedural), by site
- intrapartum — *see* Hemorrhage, complicating, delivery
- intrapelvic
  - female N94.89
  - male K66.1
- intraperitoneal K66.1
- intrapontine I61.3
- intraprocedural — *see* Complication, hemorrhage (hematoma), intraoperative (intraprocedural), by site
- intrauterine N85.7
  - complicating delivery — *see also* Hemorrhage, complicating, delivery O67.9
  - postpartum — *see* Hemorrhage, postpartum
- intraventricular I61.5
  - newborn (nontraumatic) — *see also* Newborn, affected by, hemorrhage P52.3
    - due to birth injury P1Ø.2
    - grade
      - 1 P52.Ø
      - 2 P52.1
      - 3 P52.21
      - 4 P52.22
- intravesical N32.89
- iris (postinfectional) (postinflammatory) (toxic) — *see* Hyphema
- joint (nontraumatic) — *see* Hemarthrosis
- kidney N28.89
- knee (joint) (nontraumatic) — *see* Hemarthrosis, knee
- labyrinth — *see* subcategory H83.8- ☑
- lenticular striate artery I61.Ø
- ligature, vessel — *see* Hemorrhage, postoperative
- liver K76.89
- lung RØ4.89
  - newborn P26.9
    - massive P26.1
    - specified NEC P26.8
  - tuberculous — *see* Tuberculosis, pulmonary
- massive umbilical, newborn P51.Ø
- mediastinum — *see* Hemorrhage, lung
- medulla I61.3
- membrane (brain) I6Ø.8
  - spinal cord — *see* Hemorrhage, spinal cord
- meninges, meningeal (brain) (middle) I6Ø.8
  - spinal cord — *see* Hemorrhage, spinal cord
- mesentery K66.1
- metritis — *see* Endometritis
- mouth K13.79
- mucous membrane NEC R58
  - newborn P54.8
- muscle M62.89
- nail (subungual) L6Ø.8
- nasal turbinate RØ4.Ø
  - newborn P54.8
- navel, newborn P51.9
- newborn P54.9
  - specified NEC P54.8
- nipple N64.59
- nose RØ4.Ø
  - newborn P54.8
- omentum K66.1
- optic nerve (sheath) H47.Ø2- ☑
- orbit, orbital HØ5.23- ☑
- ovary NEC N83.8
- oviduct N83.6
- pancreas K86.89
- parathyroid (gland) (spontaneous) E21.4
- parturition — *see* Hemorrhage, complicating, delivery
- penis N48.89
- pericardium, pericarditis I31.2
- peritoneum, peritoneal K66.1
- peritonsillar tissue J35.8
  - due to infection J36
- petechial R23.3
  - due to autosensitivity, erythrocyte D69.2
- pituitary (gland) E23.6
- pleura — *see* Hemorrhage, lung

**Hemorrhage, hemorrhagic** — *continued*
- polioencephalitis, superior E51.2
- polymyositis — *see* Polymyositis
- pons, pontine I61.3
- posterior fossa (nontraumatic) I61.8
  - newborn P52.6
- postmenopausal N95.Ø
- postnasal RØ4.Ø
- postoperative — *see* Complications, postprocedural, hemorrhage, by site
- postpartum NEC (following delivery of placenta) O72.1
  - delayed or secondary O72.2
  - retained placenta O72.Ø
  - third stage O72.Ø
- pregnancy — *see* Hemorrhage, antepartum
- preretinal — *see* Hemorrhage, retina
- prostate N42.1
- puerperal — *see* Hemorrhage, postpartum
  - delayed or secondary O72.2
- pulmonary RØ4.89
  - newborn P26.9
    - massive P26.1
    - specified NEC P26.8
  - tuberculous — *see* Tuberculosis, pulmonary
- purpura (primary) D69.3
- rectum (sphincter) K62.5
  - newborn P54.2
- recurring, following initial hemorrhage at time of injury T79.2- ☑
- renal N28.89
- respiratory passage or tract RØ4.9
  - specified NEC RØ4.89
- retina, retinal (vessels) H35.6- ☑
  - diabetic — *see* Microaneurysm, retinal, diabetic
- retroperitoneal K68.3
- scalp R58
- scrotum N5Ø.1
- secondary (nontraumatic) R58
  - following initial hemorrhage at time of injury T79.2- ☑
- seminal vesicle N5Ø.1
- skin R23.3
  - newborn P54.5
- slipped umbilical ligature P51.8
- spermatic cord N5Ø.1
- spinal (cord) G95.19
  - newborn (birth injury) P11.5
- spleen D73.5
  - intraoperative — *see* Complications, intraoperative, hemorrhage, spleen
  - postprocedural — *see* Complications, postprocedural, hemorrhage, spleen
- stomach K92.2
  - newborn P54.3
  - ulcer — *see* Ulcer, stomach, with hemorrhage
- subarachnoid (nontraumatic) — *see* Hemorrhage, intracranial, subarachnoid
- subconjunctival — *see also* Hemorrhage, conjunctiva
  - birth injury P15.3
- subcortical (brain) I61.Ø
- subcutaneous R23.3
- subdiaphragmatic R58
- subdural (acute) (nontraumatic) — *see* Hemorrhage, intracranial, subdural
- subependymal
  - newborn P52.Ø
    - with intraventricular extension P52.1
      - and intracerebral extension P52.22
- subgaleal P12.2
- subhyaloid — *see* Hemorrhage, retina
- subperiosteal — *see* Disorder, bone, specified type NEC
- subretinal — *see* Hemorrhage, retina
- subtentorial — *see* Hemorrhage, intracranial, subdural
- subungual L6Ø.8
- suprarenal (capsule) (gland) E27.49
  - newborn P54.4
- tentorium (traumatic) NEC — *see* Hemorrhage, brain
  - newborn (birth injury) P1Ø.4
- testis N5Ø.1
- third stage (postpartum) O72.Ø
- thorax — *see* Hemorrhage, lung
- throat RØ4.1
- thymus (gland) E32.8
- thyroid (cyst) (gland) EØ7.89
- tongue K14.8
- tonsil J35.8
- trachea — *see* Hemorrhage, lung
- tracheobronchial RØ4.89
  - newborn P26.Ø

**Herpes, herpesvirus, herpetic** — *continued*
eye (zoster) BØ2.3Ø
simplex BØØ.5Ø
eyelid (zoster) BØ2.39
simplex BØØ.59
facialis BØØ.1
febrilis BØØ.1
geniculate ganglionitis BØ2.21
genital, genitalis A6Ø.ØØ
female A6Ø.Ø9
male A6Ø.Ø2
gestational, gestationis O26.4- ☑
gingivostomatitis BØØ.2
human BØØ.9
1 — *see* Herpes, simplex
2 — *see* Herpes, simplex
3 — *see* Varicella
4 — *see* Mononucleosis, Epstein-Barr (virus)
5 — *see* Disease, cytomegalic inclusion (generalized)
6
encephalitis B1Ø.Ø1
specified NEC B1Ø.81
7
encephalitis B1Ø.Ø9
specified NEC B1Ø.82
8 B1Ø.89
infection NEC B1Ø.89
Kaposi's sarcoma associated B1Ø.89
iridocyclitis (simplex) BØØ.51
zoster BØ2.32
iris (vesicular erythema multiforme) L51.9
iritis (simplex) BØØ.51
Kaposi's sarcoma associated B1Ø.89
keratitis (simplex) (dendritic) (disciform) (interstitial) BØØ.52
zoster (interstitial) BØ2.33
keratoconjunctivitis (simplex) BØØ.52
zoster BØ2.33
labialis BØØ.1
lip BØØ.1
meningitis (simplex) BØØ.3
zoster BØ2.1
ophthalmicus (zoster) NEC BØ2.3Ø
simplex BØØ.5Ø
penis A6Ø.Ø1
perianal skin A6Ø.1
pharyngitis, pharyngotonsillitis BØØ.2
rectum A6Ø.1
scrotum A6Ø.Ø2
sepsis BØØ.7
simplex BØØ.9
complicated NEC BØØ.89
congenital P35.2
conjunctivitis BØØ.53
external ear BØØ.1
eyelid BØØ.59
hepatitis BØØ.81
keratitis (interstitial) BØØ.52
myelitis BØØ.82
specified complication NEC BØØ.89
visceral BØØ.89
stomatitis BØØ.2
tonsurans B35.Ø
visceral BØØ.89
vulva A6Ø.Ø4
whitlow BØØ.89
zoster — *see also* condition BØ2.9
auricularis BØ2.21
complicated NEC BØ2.8
conjunctivitis BØ2.31
disseminated BØ2.7
encephalitis BØ2.Ø
eye (lid) BØ2.39
geniculate ganglionitis BØ2.21
keratitis (interstitial) BØ2.33
meningitis BØ2.1
myelitis BØ2.24
neuritis, neuralgia BØ2.29
ophthalmicus NEC BØ2.3Ø
oticus BØ2.21
polyneuropathy BØ2.23
specified complication NEC BØ2.8
trigeminal neuralgia BØ2.22
**Herpesvirus** (human) — *see* Herpes
**Herpetophobia** F4Ø.218
**Herrick's anemia** — *see* Disease, sickle-cell
**Hers' disease** E74.Ø9
**Herter-Gee syndrome** K9Ø.Ø
**Herxheimer's reaction** R68.89
**Hesitancy**
of micturition R39.11
urinary R39.11
**Hesselbach's hernia** — *see* Hernia, femoral, specified site NEC
**Heterochromia** (congenital) Q13.2
cataract — *see* Cataract, complicated
cyclitis (Fuchs) — *see* Cyclitis, Fuchs' heterochromic
hair L67.1
iritis — *see* Cyclitis, Fuchs' heterochromic
retained metallic foreign body (nonmagnetic) — *see* Foreign body, intraocular, old, retained
magnetic — *see* Foreign body, intraocular, old, retained, magnetic
uveitis — *see* Cyclitis, Fuchs' heterochromic
**Heterophoria** — *see* Strabismus, heterophoria
**Heterophyes, heterophyiasis** (small intestine) B66.8
**Heterotopia, heterotopic** — *see also* Malposition, congenital
cerebralis QØ4.8
**Heterotropia** — *see* Strabismus
**Heubner-Herter disease** K9Ø.Ø
**Hexadactylism** Q69.9
**HGSIL** (cytology finding) (high grade squamous intraepithelial lesion on cytologic smear) (Pap smear finding)
anus R85.613
cervix R87.613
biopsy (histology) finding — *see* Neoplasia, intraepithelial, cervix, grade II or grade III
vagina R87.623
biopsy (histology) finding — *see* Neoplasia, intraepithelial, cervix, grade II or grade III
**Hibernoma** — *see* Lipoma
**Hiccup, hiccough** RØ6.6
epidemic B33.Ø
psychogenic F45.8
**Hidden penis** (congenital) Q55.64
acquired N48.83
**Hidradenitis** (axillaris) (suppurative) L73.2
**Hidradenoma** (nodular) — *see also* Neoplasm, skin, benign
clear cell — *see* Neoplasm, skin, benign
papillary — *see* Neoplasm, skin, benign
**Hidrocystoma** — *see* Neoplasm, skin, benign
**High**
altitude effects T7Ø.2Ø- ☑
anoxia T7Ø.29- ☑
on
ears T7Ø.Ø- ☑
sinuses T7Ø.1- ☑
polycythemia D75.1
arch
foot Q66.7- ☑
palate, congenital Q38.5
arterial tension — *see* Hypertension
basal metabolic rate R94.8
blood pressure — *see also* Hypertension
borderline RØ3.Ø
reading (incidental) (isolated) (nonspecific), without diagnosis of hypertension RØ3.Ø
cholesterol E78.ØØ
with high triglycerides E78.2
diaphragm (congenital) Q79.1
expressed emotional level within family Z63.8
head at term O32.4- ☑
palate, congenital Q38.5
risk
infant NEC Z76.2
sexual behavior (heterosexual) Z72.51
bisexual Z72.53
homosexual Z72.52
scrotal testis, testes
bilateral Q53.23
unilateral Q53.13
temperature (of unknown origin) R5Ø.9
thoracic rib Q76.6
triglycerides E78.1
with high cholesterol E78.2
**Hildenbrand's disease** A75.Ø
**Hilum** — *see* condition
**Hip** — *see* condition
**Hippel's disease** Q85.83
**Hippophobia** F4Ø.218
**Hippus** H57.Ø9
**Hirschsprung's disease or megacolon** Q43.1
**Hirsutism, hirsuties** L68.Ø
**Hirudiniasis**
external B88.3
internal B83.4
**His-Werner disease** A79.Ø
**Hiss-Russell dysentery** AØ3.1
**Histidinemia, histidinuria** E7Ø.41
**Histiocytoma** — *see also* Neoplasm, skin, benign
fibrous — *see also* Neoplasm, skin, benign
atypical — *see* Neoplasm, connective tissue, uncertain behavior
malignant — *see* Neoplasm, connective tissue, malignant
**Histiocytosis** D76.3
acute differentiated progressive C96.Ø
Langerhans' cell NEC C96.6
multifocal X
multisystemic (disseminated) C96.Ø
unisystemic C96.5
pulmonary, adult (adult PLCH) J84.82
unifocal (X) C96.6
lipid, lipoid D76.3
essential E75.29
malignant C96.A (*following* C96.6)
mononuclear phagocytes NEC D76.1
Langerhans' cells C96.6
non-Langerhans cell D76.3
polyostotic sclerosing D76.3
sinus, with massive lymphadenopathy D76.3
syndrome NEC D76.3
X NEC C96.6
acute (progressive) C96.Ø
chronic C96.6
multifocal C96.5
multisystemic C96.Ø
unifocal C96.6
**Histoplasmosis** B39.9
with pneumonia NEC B39.2
African B39.5
American — *see* Histoplasmosis, capsulati
capsulati B39.4
disseminated B39.3
generalized B39.3
pulmonary B39.2
acute B39.Ø
chronic B39.1
Darling's B39.4
duboisii B39.5
lung NEC B39.2
**History**
family (of) — *see also* History, personal (of)
adenomatous polyposis Z83.72
alcohol abuse Z81.1
allergy NEC Z84.89
anemia Z83.2
arthritis Z82.61
asthma Z82.5
blindness Z82.1
cardiac death (sudden) Z82.41
carrier of genetic disease Z84.81
chromosomal anomaly Z82.79
chronic
disabling disease NEC Z82.8
lower respiratory disease Z82.5
colonic polyps Z83.719
adenomatous and serrated Z83.71Ø
hyperplastic Z83.711
inflammatory Z83.718
specified, NEC Z83.718
tubular adenoma Z83.71Ø
tubulovillous adenoma Z83.71Ø
villous adenoma Z83.71Ø
congenital malformations and deformations Z82.79
polycystic kidney Z82.71
consanguinity Z84.3
deafness Z82.2
diabetes mellitus Z83.3
disability NEC Z82.8
disease or disorder (of)
allergic NEC Z84.89
behavioral NEC Z81.8
blood and blood-forming organs Z83.2
cardiovascular NEC Z82.49
chronic disabling NEC Z82.8
digestive Z83.79
ear NEC Z83.52
elevated lipoprotein (a) (Lp(a)) Z83.43Ø
endocrine NEC Z83.49
eye NEC Z83.518
glaucoma Z83.511
familial hypercholesterolemia Z83.42
genitourinary NEC Z84.2
glaucoma Z83.511

- **History** — *continued*
  - family — *see also* History, personal — *continued*
    - disease or disorder — *continued*
      - hematological Z83.2
      - immune mechanism Z83.2
      - infectious NEC Z83.1
      - ischemic heart Z82.49
      - kidney Z84.19
        - APOL1-mediated (AMKD) Z84.11
      - lipoprotein metabolism Z83.438
      - mental NEC Z81.8
      - metabolic Z83.49
      - musculoskeletal NEC Z82.69
      - neurological NEC Z82.0
      - nutritional Z83.49
      - parasitic NEC Z83.1
      - psychiatric NEC Z81.8
      - respiratory NEC Z83.6
      - skin and subcutaneous tissue NEC Z84.0
      - specified NEC Z84.89
    - drug abuse NEC Z81.3
    - elevated lipoprotein (a) (Lp(a)) Z83.430
    - epilepsy Z82.0
    - exposure to diethylstilbestrol (DES) Z84.A
    - familial hypercholesterolemia Z83.42
    - genetic disease carrier Z84.81
    - glaucoma Z83.511
    - hearing loss Z82.2
    - human immunodeficiency virus (HIV) infection Z83.0
    - Huntington's chorea Z82.0
    - hyperlipidemia, familial combined Z83.438
    - intellectual disability Z81.0
    - leukemia Z80.6
    - lipidemia NEC Z83.438
    - malignant neoplasm (of) NOS Z80.9
      - bladder Z80.52
      - breast Z80.3
      - bronchus Z80.1
      - digestive organ Z80.0
      - fallopian tube(s) Z80.44
      - gastrointestinal tract Z80.0
      - genital organ Z80.49
        - fallopian tube(s) Z80.44
        - ovary Z80.41
        - prostate Z80.42
        - specified organ NEC Z80.49
        - testis Z80.43
      - hematopoietic NEC Z80.7
      - intrathoracic organ NEC Z80.2
      - kidney Z80.51
      - lung Z80.1
      - lymphatic NEC Z80.7
      - ovary Z80.41
      - prostate Z80.42
      - respiratory organ NEC Z80.2
      - specified site NEC Z80.8
      - testis Z80.43
      - trachea Z80.1
      - urinary organ or tract Z80.59
        - bladder Z80.52
        - kidney Z80.51
    - mental
      - disorder NEC Z81.8
    - multiple endocrine neoplasia (MEN) syndrome Z83.41
    - osteoporosis Z82.62
    - polycystic kidney Z82.71
    - polyposis, adenomatous Z83.72
    - polyps (colon) — *see also* History, family, colonic polyps Z83.719
    - psychiatric disorder Z81.8
    - psychoactive substance abuse NEC Z81.3
    - respiratory condition NEC Z83.6
      - asthma and other lower respiratory conditions Z82.5
    - self-harmful behavior Z81.8
    - SIDS (sudden infant death syndrome) Z84.82
    - skin condition Z84.0
    - specified condition NEC Z84.89
    - stroke (cerebrovascular) Z82.3
    - substance abuse NEC Z81.4
      - alcohol Z81.1
      - drug NEC Z81.3
      - psychoactive NEC Z81.3
      - tobacco Z81.2
    - sudden
      - cardiac death Z82.41
      - infant death syndrome (SIDS) Z84.82
    - tobacco abuse Z81.2
    - violence, violent behavior Z81.8

- **History** — *continued*
  - family — *see also* History, personal — *continued*
    - visual loss Z82.1
  - personal (of) — *see also* History, family (of)
    - abuse
      - adult Z91.419
        - financial Z91.413
        - forced labor or sexual exploitation Z91.42
        - intimate partner Z91.414
        - physical and sexual Z91.410
        - psychological Z91.411
      - childhood Z62.819
        - financial Z62.814
        - forced labor or sexual exploitation in childhood Z62.813
        - intimate partner Z62.815
        - physical Z62.810
        - psychological Z62.811
        - sexual Z62.810
      - in adolescence — *see* History, personal, abuse, childhood
    - alcohol dependence F10.21
    - allergy (to) Z88.9
      - analgesic agent NEC Z88.6
      - anesthetic Z88.4
      - anti-infective agent NEC Z88.3
      - antibiotic agent NEC Z88.1
      - contrast media Z91.041
      - drugs, medicaments and biological substances Z88.9
        - specified NEC Z88.8
      - food Z91.018
        - additives Z91.02
        - beef Z91.014
        - eggs Z91.0120
          - with
            - reactivity to baked egg Z91.0122
            - tolerance to baked egg Z91.0121
        - lamb Z91.014
        - mammalian meats Z91.014
        - milk products Z91.0110
          - with
            - reactivity to baked milk Z91.0112
            - tolerance to baked milk Z91.0111
        - peanuts Z91.010
        - pork Z91.014
        - red meats Z91.014
        - seafood Z91.013
        - specified food NEC Z91.018
      - insect Z91.038
        - bee Z91.030
      - latex Z91.040
      - medicinal agents Z88.9
        - specified NEC Z88.8
      - narcotic agent NEC Z88.5
      - nonmedicinal agents Z91.048
      - penicillin Z88.0
      - serum Z88.7
      - specified NEC Z91.09
      - sulfonamides Z88.2
      - vaccine Z88.7
    - anaphylactic shock Z87.892
    - anaphylaxis Z87.892
    - behavioral disorders Z86.59
    - benign carcinoid tumor Z86.012
    - benign neoplasm Z86.018
      - brain Z86.011
      - carcinoid Z86.012
      - colonic polyps — *see* History, personal, neoplasm, benign, colon polyp
    - brain injury (traumatic) Z87.820
    - breast implant removal Z98.86
    - calculi, renal Z87.442
    - cancer — *see* History, personal (of), malignant neoplasm (of)
    - CAR-T (Chimeric Antigen Receptor T-cell) therapy Z92.850
    - cardiac arrest (death), successfully resuscitated Z86.74
    - cellular therapy Z92.859
      - specified NEC Z92.858
    - cerebral infarction without residual deficit Z86.73
    - certain (corrected) conditions arising in the perinatal period, specified NEC Z87.68
    - cervical dysplasia Z87.410
    - chemotherapy for neoplastic condition Z92.21
    - childhood abuse — *see* History, personal (of), abuse
    - Chimeric Antigen Receptor T-cell (CAR-T) therapy Z92.850
    - cleft lip (corrected) Z87.730

- **History** — *continued*
  - personal — *see also* History, family — *continued*
    - cleft palate (corrected) Z87.730
    - cloaca, persistent Z87.732
    - cloacal malformations Z87.732
    - Clostridium difficile
      - colitis (fulminant) (nonfulminant) Z86.17
      - difficile infection Z86.17
      - foodborne intoxication Z86.17
    - collapsed vertebra (healed) Z87.311
      - due to osteoporosis Z87.310
    - combat and operational stress reaction Z86.51
    - congenital malformation (corrected) Z87.798
      - circulatory system (corrected) Z87.74
      - diaphragmatic hernia Z87.760
      - digestive system (corrected) NEC Z87.738
      - ear (corrected) Z87.721
      - eye (corrected) Z87.720
      - face and neck (corrected) Z87.790
      - gastroschisis Z87.761
      - genitourinary system (corrected) NEC Z87.718
      - heart (corrected) Z87.74
      - integument (corrected) Z87.768
      - limb(s) (corrected) Z87.768
      - malformations
        - abdominal wall Z87.763
        - diaphragm NEC Z87.760
        - integument Z87.768
        - limbs Z87.768
        - musculoskeletal system Z87.768
        - prune belly Z87.762
      - musculoskeletal system (corrected) Z87.768
      - neck (corrected) Z87.790
      - nervous system (corrected) NEC Z87.728
      - respiratory system (corrected) Z87.75
      - sense organs (corrected) NEC Z87.728
      - specified NEC Z87.798
    - contraception Z92.0
    - coronavirus (disease) (novel) 2019 Z86.16
    - COVID-19 Z86.16
    - deployment (military) Z91.82
    - diabetic foot ulcer Z86.31
    - disease or disorder (of) Z87.898
      - anaphylaxis Z87.892
      - blood and blood-forming organs Z86.2
      - circulatory system Z86.79
        - specified condition NEC Z86.79
      - connective tissue Z87.39
      - digestive system Z87.19
        - colonic polyp — *see* History, personal, neoplasm, benign, colon polyp
        - peptic ulcer disease Z87.11
        - specified condition NEC Z87.19
      - ear Z86.69
      - endocrine Z86.39
        - diabetic foot ulcer Z86.31
        - gestational diabetes Z86.32
        - specified type NEC Z86.39
      - eye Z86.69
      - genital (track) system NEC
        - female Z87.42
        - male Z87.438
      - hematological Z86.2
      - Hodgkin Z85.71
      - immune mechanism Z86.2
      - infectious Z86.19
        - coronavirus (disease) (novel) 2019 Z86.16
        - COVID-19 Z86.16
        - malaria Z86.13
        - Methicillin resistant Staphylococcus aureus (MRSA) Z86.14
        - poliomyelitis Z86.12
        - SARS-CoV-2 Z86.16
        - specified NEC Z86.19
        - tuberculosis Z86.11
      - mental NEC Z86.59
      - metabolic Z86.39
        - diabetic foot ulcer Z86.31
        - gestational diabetes Z86.32
        - specified type NEC Z86.39
      - musculoskeletal NEC Z87.39
      - nervous system Z86.69
      - nutritional Z86.39
      - parasitic Z86.19
      - respiratory system NEC Z87.09
      - sense organs Z86.69
      - skin Z87.2
      - specified site or type NEC Z87.898
      - subcutaneous tissue Z87.2

**History** — *continued*
- personal — *see also* History, family — *continued*
  - disease or disorder — *continued*
    - trophoblastic Z87.59
    - urinary system NEC Z87.448
  - drug dependence — *see* Dependence, drug, by type, in remission
  - drug therapy
    - antineoplastic chemotherapy Z92.21
    - estrogen Z92.23
    - ICI (immune checkpoint inhibitor) drug therapy Z92.26
    - immunosuppression Z92.25
    - inhaled steroids Z92.240
    - monoclonal drug Z92.22
    - specified NEC Z92.29
    - steroid Z92.241
    - systemic steroids Z92.241
  - dysplasia
    - cervical (mild) (moderate) Z87.410
      - severe (grade III) Z86.001
    - prostatic Z87.430
    - vaginal (mild) (moderate) Z87.411
      - severe (grade III) Z86.002
    - vulvar (mild) (moderate) Z87.412
      - severe (grade III) Z86.002
  - embolism (venous) Z86.718
    - pulmonary Z86.711
  - encephalitis Z86.61
  - estrogen therapy Z92.23
  - extracorporeal membrane oxygenation (ECMO) Z92.81
  - failed conscious sedation Z92.83
  - failed moderate sedation Z92.83
  - fall, falling Z91.81
  - forced labor or sexual exploitation Z91.42
    - in childhood Z62.813
  - fracture (healed)
    - fatigue Z87.312
    - fragility Z87.310
    - osteoporosis Z87.310
    - pathological NEC Z87.311
    - stress Z87.312
    - traumatic Z87.81
  - gene therapy Z92.86
  - gestational diabetes Z86.32
  - hepatitis
    - B Z86.19
    - C Z86.19
  - Hodgkin disease Z85.71
  - hyperthermia, malignant Z88.4
  - hypospadias (corrected) Z87.710
  - hysterectomy Z90.710
  - ICI (immune checkpoint inhibitor) drug therapy Z92.26
  - immune checkpoint inhibitor (ICI) therapy Z92.26
  - immunosuppression therapy Z92.25
  - in situ neoplasm
    - breast Z86.000
    - cervix uteri Z86.001
    - digestive organs, specified NEC Z86.004
    - esophagus Z86.003
    - fallopian tube(s) Z86.00A
    - genital organs, specified NEC Z86.002
    - melanoma Z86.006
    - middle ear Z86.005
    - oral cavity Z86.003
    - respiratory system Z86.005
    - skin Z86.007
    - specified NEC Z86.008
    - stomach Z86.003
  - in utero procedure during pregnancy Z98.870
  - in utero procedure while a fetus Z98.871
  - infection NEC Z86.19
    - central nervous system Z86.61
    - Clostridioides (Clostridium) difficile (colitis) (infection) Z86.17
    - coronavirus (disease) (novel) 2019 Z86.16
    - COVID-19 Z86.16
    - latent tuberculosis Z86.15
    - Methicillin resistant Staphylococcus aureus (MRSA) Z86.14
    - SARS-CoV-2 Z86.16
    - urinary (recurrent) (tract) Z87.440
  - injury NEC Z87.828
  - irradiation Z92.3
  - kidney stones Z87.442
  - latent tuberculosis infection Z86.15
  - leukemia Z85.6
  - lymphoma (non-Hodgkin) Z85.72

**History** — *continued*
- personal — *see also* History, family — *continued*
  - malignant melanoma (skin) Z85.820
  - malignant neoplasm (of) Z85.9
    - accessory sinuses Z85.22
    - anus NEC Z85.048
      - carcinoid Z85.040
    - bladder Z85.51
    - bone Z85.830
    - brain Z85.841
    - breast Z85.3
    - bronchus NEC Z85.118
      - carcinoid Z85.110
    - carcinoid — *see* History, personal (of), malignant neoplasm, by site, carcinoid
    - cervix Z85.41
    - colon NEC Z85.038
      - carcinoid Z85.030
    - digestive organ Z85.00
      - specified NEC Z85.09
    - endocrine gland NEC Z85.858
    - epididymis Z85.48
    - esophagus Z85.01
    - eye Z85.840
    - fallopian tube(s) Z85.4A
    - gastrointestinal tract — *see* History, malignant neoplasm, digestive organ
    - genital organ
      - female Z85.40
        - specified NEC Z85.44
      - male Z85.45
        - specified NEC Z85.49
    - hematopoietic NEC Z85.79
    - intrathoracic organ Z85.20
    - kidney NEC Z85.528
      - carcinoid Z85.520
    - large intestine NEC Z85.038
      - carcinoid Z85.030
    - larynx Z85.21
    - liver Z85.05
    - lung NEC Z85.118
      - carcinoid Z85.110
    - mediastinum Z85.29
    - Merkel cell Z85.821
    - middle ear Z85.22
    - nasal cavities Z85.22
    - nervous system NEC Z85.848
    - oral cavity Z85.819
      - specified site NEC Z85.818
    - ovary Z85.43
    - pancreas Z85.07
    - pelvis Z85.53
    - pharynx Z85.819
      - specified site NEC Z85.818
    - pleura Z85.29
    - prostate Z85.46
    - Pseudomembraneous colitis Z86.17
    - rectosigmoid junction NEC Z85.048
      - carcinoid Z85.040
    - rectum NEC Z85.048
      - carcinoid Z85.040
    - respiratory organ Z85.20
    - sinuses, accessory Z85.22
    - skin NEC Z85.828
      - melanoma Z85.820
      - Merkel cell Z85.821
    - small intestine NEC Z85.068
      - carcinoid Z85.060
    - soft tissue Z85.831
    - specified site NEC Z85.89
    - stomach NEC Z85.028
      - carcinoid Z85.020
    - testis Z85.47
    - thymus NEC Z85.238
      - carcinoid Z85.230
    - thyroid Z85.850
    - tongue Z85.810
    - trachea Z85.12
    - urinary organ or tract Z85.50
      - specified NEC Z85.59
    - uterus Z85.42
  - maltreatment Z91.89
  - medical treatment NEC Z92.89
  - melanoma Z85.820
    - in situ Z86.006
    - malignant (skin) Z85.820
  - meningitis Z86.61
  - mental disorder Z86.59
  - Merkel cell carcinoma (skin) Z85.821

**History** — *continued*
- personal — *see also* History, family — *continued*
  - Methicillin resistant Staphylococcus aureus (MRSA) Z86.14
  - military deployment Z91.82
  - military service Z91.85
  - military war, peacekeeping and humanitarian deployment (current or past conflict) Z91.82
  - myocardial infarction (old) I25.2
  - necrotizing enterocolitis of newborn (corrected) Z87.61
  - neglect (in)
    - adult Z91.412
    - childhood Z62.812
  - neoplasia
    - anal intraepithelial, III [AIN III] Z86.004
    - high-grade prostatic intraepithelial, III [HGPIN III] Z86.002
    - vaginal intraepithelial, III [VAIN III] Z86.002
    - vulvar intraepithelial, III [VIN III] Z86.002
  - neoplasm
    - benign Z86.018
      - brain Z86.011
      - colon polyp Z86.0100
        - adenomatous (sessile) Z86.0101
        - hyperplastic Z86.0102
        - serrated (sessile) Z86.0101
        - specified NEC Z86.0109
        - traditional serrated adenoma Z86.0101
        - tubular adenoma Z86.0101
        - tubulovillous adenoma Z86.0101
        - villous adenoma Z86.0101
    - in situ
      - breast Z86.000
      - cervix uteri Z86.001
      - digestive organs, specified NEC Z86.004
      - esophagus Z86.003
      - genital organs, specified NEC Z86.002
      - melanoma Z86.006
      - middle ear Z86.005
      - oral cavity Z86.003
      - respiratory system Z86.005
      - skin Z86.007
      - specified NEC Z86.008
      - stomach Z86.003
    - malignant — *see* History of, malignant neoplasm
    - uncertain behavior Z86.03
  - nephrotic syndrome Z87.441
  - nicotine dependence Z87.891
  - noncompliance with medical treatment or regimen — *see* Noncompliance
  - nutritional deficiency Z86.39
  - obstetric complications Z87.59
    - childbirth Z87.59
    - pregnancy Z87.59
    - pre-term labor Z87.51
    - puerperium Z87.59
  - osteoporosis fractures Z87.310
  - parasuicide (attempt) Z91.51
  - physical trauma NEC Z87.828
    - self-harm or suicide attempt Z91.51
  - pneumonia (recurrent) Z87.01
  - poisoning NEC Z91.89
    - self-harm or suicide attempt Z91.51
  - poor personal hygiene Z91.89
  - preterm labor Z87.51
  - procedure during pregnancy Z98.870
  - procedure while a fetus Z98.871
  - prolonged reversible ischemic neurologic deficit (PRIND) Z86.73
  - prostatic dysplasia Z87.430
  - psychological
    - abuse
      - adult Z91.411
      - child Z62.811
    - trauma, specified NEC Z91.49
  - radiation therapy Z92.3
  - removal
    - implant
      - breast Z98.86
  - renal calculi Z87.442
  - respiratory condition NEC Z87.09
  - retained foreign body fully removed Z87.821
  - risk factors NEC Z91.89
  - SARS-CoV-2 infection Z86.16
  - self-harm
    - nonsuicidal Z91.52
    - suicidal Z91.51
  - self-inflicted injury without suicidal intent Z91.52

- **Hyperemesis** — *continued*
  - gravidarum — *continued*
    - with — *continued*
      - dehydration O21.1
      - electrolyte imbalance O21.1
      - metabolic disturbance O21.1
    - severe (with metabolic disturbance) O21.1
  - projectile R11.12
  - psychogenic F45.8
- **Hyperemia** (acute) (passive) R68.89
  - anal mucosa K62.89
  - bladder N32.89
  - cerebral I67.89
  - conjunctiva H11.43- ☑
  - ear internal, acute — *see* subcategory H83.Ø- ☑
  - enteric K59.89
  - eye — *see* Hyperemia, conjunctiva
  - eyelid (active) (passive) — *see* Disorder, eyelid, specified type NEC
  - intestine K59.89
  - iris — *see* Disorder, iris, vascular
  - kidney N28.89
  - labyrinth — *see* subcategory H83.Ø- ☑
  - liver (active) K76.89
  - lung (passive) — *see* Edema, lung
  - pulmonary (passive) — *see* Edema, lung
  - renal N28.89
  - retina H35.89
  - stomach K31.89
- **Hyperesthesia** (body surface) R2Ø.3
  - larynx (reflex) J38.7
    - hysterical F44.89
  - pharynx (reflex) J39.2
    - hysterical F44.89
- **Hyperestrogenism** (drug-induced) (iatrogenic) E28.Ø
- **Hyperexplexia** Q89.89
- **Hyperfibrinolysis** — *see* Fibrinolysis
- **Hyperfructosemia** E74.19
- **Hyperfunction**
  - adrenal cortex, not associated with Cushing's syndrome E27.Ø
    - medulla E27.5
      - adrenomedullary E27.5
    - virilism E25.9
      - congenital E25.Ø
  - ovarian E28.8
  - pancreas K86.89
  - parathyroid (gland) E21.3
  - pituitary (gland) (anterior) E22.9
    - specified NEC E22.8
  - polyglandular E31.1
  - testicular E29.Ø
- **Hypergammaglobulinemia** D89.2
  - polyclonal D89.Ø
  - Waldenstrom D89.Ø
- **Hypergastrinemia** E16.4
- **Hyperglobulinemia** R77.1
- **Hyperglycemia, hyperglycemic** (transient) R73.9
  - coma — *see* Diabetes, by type, with coma
  - postpancreatectomy E89.1
- **Hyperglyceridemia** (endogenous) (essential) (familial) (hereditary) (pure) E78.1
  - mixed E78.3
- **Hyperglycinemia** (non-ketotic) E72.51
- **Hypergonadism**
  - ovarian E28.8
  - testicular (primary) (infantile) E29.Ø
- **Hyperheparinemia** D68.32
- **Hyperhidrosis, hyperidrosis** R61
  - focal
    - primary L74.519
      - axilla L74.51Ø
      - face L74.511
      - palms L74.512
      - soles L74.513
    - secondary L74.52
  - generalized R61
  - localized
    - primary L74.519
      - axilla L74.51Ø
      - face L74.511
      - palms L74.512
      - soles L74.513
    - secondary L74.52
  - psychogenic F45.8
  - secondary R61
    - focal L74.52
- **Hyperhistidinemia** E7Ø.41
- **Hyperhomocysteinemia** E72.11
- **Hyperhydroxyprolinemia** E72.59
- **Hyperinsulinism** (functional) E16.1
  - with
    - coma (hypoglycemic) E15
    - encephalopathy E16.1 *[G94]*
  - ectopic E16.1
  - therapeutic misadventure (from administration of insulin) — *see* subcategory T38.3- ☑
- **Hyperkalemia** E87.5
- **Hyperkeratosis** — *see also* Keratosis L85.9
  - cervix N88.Ø
  - due to yaws (early) (late) (palmar or plantar) A66.3
  - follicularis Q82.8
    - penetrans (in cutem) L87.Ø
  - palmoplantaris climacterica L85.1
  - pinta A67.1
  - senile (with pruritus) L57.Ø
  - universalis congenita Q8Ø.8
  - vocal cord J38.3
  - vulva N9Ø.4
- **Hyperkinesia, hyperkinetic** (disease) (reaction) (syndrome) (childhood) (adolescence) — *see also* Disorder, attention-deficit hyperactivity
  - heart I51.89
- **Hyperleucine-isoleucinemia** E71.19
- **Hyperlipemia, hyperlipidemia** E78.5
  - combined E78.2
    - familial E78.49
  - group
    - A E78.ØØ
    - B E78.1
    - C E78.2
    - D E78.3
  - mixed E78.2
  - specified NEC E78.49
- **Hyperlipidosis** E75.6
  - hereditary NEC E75.5
- **Hyperlipoproteinemia** E78.5
  - Fredrickson's type
    - I E78.3
    - IIa E78.ØØ
    - IIb E78.2
    - III E78.2
    - IV E78.1
    - V E78.3
  - low-density-lipoprotein-type (LDL) E78.ØØ
  - very-low-density-lipoprotein-type (VLDL) E78.1
- **Hyperlucent lung, unilateral** J43.Ø
- **Hyperlysinemia** E72.3
- **Hypermagnesemia** E83.41
  - neonatal P71.8
- **Hypermenorrhea** N92.Ø
- **Hypermethioninemia** E72.19
- **Hypermetropia** (congenital) H52.Ø- ☑
- **Hypermobility, hypermotility**
  - cecum — *see* Syndrome, irritable bowel
  - coccyx — *see* subcategory M53.2- ☑
  - colon — *see* Syndrome, irritable bowel
    - psychogenic F45.8
  - ileum K58.9
  - intestine — *see also* Syndrome, irritable bowel K58.9
    - psychogenic F45.8
  - meniscus (knee) — *see* Derangement, knee, meniscus
  - scapula — *see* Instability, joint, shoulder
  - stomach K31.89
    - psychogenic F45.8
  - syndrome M35.7
  - urethra N36.41
    - with intrinsic sphincter deficiency N36.43
- **Hypernasality** R49.21
- **Hypernatremia** E87.Ø
- **Hypernephroma** C64.- ☑
- **Hyperopia** — *see* Hypermetropia
- **Hyperorexia nervosa** F5Ø.2- ☑
- **Hyperornithinemia** E72.4
- **Hyperosmia** R43.1
- **Hyperosmolality** — *see also* Diabetes, by type, with hyperosmolarity E87.Ø
- **Hyperostosis** (monomelic) — *see also* Disorder, bone, density and structure, specified NEC
  - ankylosing (spine) M48.1Ø
    - cervical region M48.12
    - cervicothoracic region M48.13
    - lumbar region M48.16
    - lumbosacral region M48.17
    - multiple sites M48.19
    - occipito-atlanto-axial region M48.11
    - sacrococcygeal region M48.18
- **Hyperostosis** — *continued*
  - ankylosing — *continued*
    - thoracic region M48.14
    - thoracolumbar region M48.15
  - cortical (skull) M85.2
    - infantile M89.8X- ☑
  - frontal, internal of skull M85.2
  - interna frontalis M85.2
  - skeletal, diffuse idiopathic — *see* Hyperostosis, ankylosing
  - skull M85.2
    - congenital Q75.8
  - vertebral, ankylosing — *see* Hyperostosis, ankylosing
- **Hyperovarism** E28.8
- **Hyperoxaluria** R82.992
  - primary E72.53- ☑
- **Hyperparathyroidism** E21.3
  - primary E21.Ø
  - secondary (renal) N25.81
    - non-renal E21.1
  - specified NEC E21.2
  - tertiary E21.2
- **Hyperpathia** R2Ø.8
- **Hyperperistalsis** R19.2
  - psychogenic F45.8
- **Hyperpermeability, capillary** I78.8
- **Hyperphagia** R63.2
- **Hyperphenylalaninemia NEC** E7Ø.1
- **Hyperphoria** (alternating) H5Ø.53
- **Hyperphosphatemia** E83.39
- **Hyperpiesis, hyperpiesia** — *see* Hypertension
- **Hyperpigmentation** — *see also* Pigmentation
  - melanin NEC L81.4
  - postinflammatory L81.Ø
- **Hyperpinealism** E34.8
- **Hyperpituitarism** E22.9
- **Hyperplasia, hyperplastic**
  - adenoids J35.2
  - adrenal (capsule) (cortex) (gland) E27.8
    - with
      - sexual precocity (male) E25.9
        - congenital E25.Ø
      - virilism, adrenal E25.9
        - congenital E25.Ø
      - virilization (female) E25.9
        - congenital E25.Ø
    - congenital E25.Ø
      - salt-losing E25.Ø
  - adrenomedullary E27.5
  - angiolymphoid, eosinophilia (ALHE) D18.Ø1
  - appendix (lymphoid) K38.Ø
  - artery, fibromuscular I77.3
  - bone — *see also* Hypertrophy, bone
    - marrow D75.89
  - breast — *see also* Hypertrophy, breast
    - atypical, atypia N6Ø.9- ☑
      - ductal N6Ø.9- ☑
      - lobular N6Ø.9- ☑
  - C-cell, thyroid EØ7.Ø
  - cementation (tooth) (teeth) KØ3.4
  - cervical gland R59.Ø
  - cervix (uteri) (basal cell) (endometrium) (polypoid) — *see also* Dysplasia, cervix
    - congenital Q51.828
  - clitoris, congenital Q52.6
  - denture KØ6.2
  - endocervicitis N72
  - endometrium, endometrial (adenomatous) (cystic) (glandular) (glandular-cystic) (polypoid) N85.ØØ
    - with atypia N85.Ø2
    - benign N85.Ø1
    - cervix — *see* Dysplasia, cervix
    - complex (without atypia) N85.Ø1
    - simple (without atypia) N85.Ø1
  - epithelial L85.9
    - focal, oral, including tongue K13.29
    - nipple N62
    - skin L85.9
    - tongue K13.29
    - vaginal wall N89.3
  - erythroid D75.89
  - fibromuscular of artery (carotid) (renal) I77.3
  - genital
    - female NEC N94.89
    - male N5Ø.89
  - gingiva KØ6.1
  - glandularis cystica uteri (interstitialis) — *see also* Hyperplasia, endometrial N85.ØØ

**Hyperplasia, hyperplastic** — *continued*
- gum KØ6.1
- hymen, congenital Q52.4
- irritative, edentulous (alveolar) KØ6.2
- jaw M26.Ø9
  - alveolar M26.79
  - lower M26.Ø3
    - alveolar M26.72
  - upper M26.Ø1
    - alveolar M26.71
- kidney (congenital) Q63.3
- labia N9Ø.69
  - epithelial N9Ø.3
- liver (congenital) Q44.79
  - nodular, focal K76.89
- lymph gland or node R59.9
- mandible, mandibular M26.Ø3
  - alveolar M26.72
  - unilateral condylar M27.8
- maxilla, maxillary M26.Ø1
  - alveolar M26.71
- myometrium, myometrial N85.2
- neuroendocrine cell, of infancy J84.841
- nose
  - lymphoid J34.89
  - polypoid J33.9
- oral mucosa (irritative) K13.6
- organ or site, congenital NEC — *see* Anomaly, by site
- ovary N83.8
- palate, papillary (irritative) K13.6
- pancreatic islet cells E16.9
  - alpha E16.8
    - with excess
      - gastrin E16.4
      - glucagon E16.3
  - beta E16.1
- parathyroid (gland) E21.Ø
- pharynx (lymphoid) J39.2
- prostate (adenofibromatous) N4Ø.Ø
  - with lower urinary tract symptoms (LUTS) N4Ø.1
    - nodular N4Ø.3
  - nodular N4Ø.2
    - with lower urinary tract symptoms (LUTS) N4Ø.3
  - without lower urinary tract symptoms (LUTS) N4Ø.Ø
    - nodular N4Ø.2
- renal artery I77.89
- reticulo-endothelial (cell) D75.89
- salivary gland (any) K11.1
- Schimmelbusch's — *see* Mastopathy, cystic
- suprarenal capsule (gland) E27.8
- thymus (gland) (persistent) E32.Ø
- thyroid (gland) — *see* Goiter
- tonsils (faucial) (infective) (lingual) (lymphoid) J35.1
  - with adenoids J35.3
- unilateral condylar M27.8
- uterus, uterine N85.2
  - endometrium (glandular) — *see also* Hyperplasia, endometrial N85.ØØ
- vulva N9Ø.69
  - epithelial N9Ø.3

**Hyperpnea** — *see* Hyperventilation

**Hyperpotassemia** E87.5

**Hyperprebetalipoproteinemia** (familial) E78.1

**Hyperprolactinemia** E22.1

**Hyperprolinemia** (type I) (type II) E72.59

**Hyperproteinemia** E88.Ø9

**Hyperprothrombinemia, causing coagulation factor deficiency** D68.4

**Hyperpyrexia** R5Ø.9
- heat (effects) T67.Ø1- ☑
- malignant, due to anesthetic T88.3- ☑
- rheumatic — *see* Fever, rheumatic
- unknown origin R5Ø.9

**Hypersalivation** K11.7

**Hypersecretion**
- ACTH (not associated with Cushing's syndrome) E27.Ø
  - pituitary E24.Ø
- adrenaline E27.5
- adrenomedullary E27.5
- androgen (testicular) E29.Ø
  - ovarian (drug-induced) (iatrogenic) E28.1
- calcitonin EØ7.Ø
- catecholamine E27.5
- corticoadrenal E24.9
- cortisol E24.9
- epinephrine E27.5
- estrogen E28.Ø
- gastric K31.89
  - psychogenic F45.8

**Hypersecretion** — *continued*
- gastrin E16.4
- glucagon E16.3
- hormone(s)
  - ACTH (not associated with Cushing's syndrome) E27.Ø
    - pituitary E24.Ø
  - antidiuretic E22.2
  - growth E22.Ø
  - intestinal NEC E34.1
  - ovarian androgen E28.1
  - pituitary E22.9
  - testicular E29.Ø
  - thyroid stimulating EØ5.8Ø
    - with thyroid storm EØ5.81
- insulin — *see* Hyperinsulinism
- lacrimal glands — *see* Epiphora
- medulloadrenal E27.5
- milk O92.6
- ovarian androgens E28.1
- salivary gland (any) K11.7
- thyrocalcitonin EØ7.Ø
- upper respiratory J39.8

**Hypersegmentation, leukocytic, hereditary** D72.Ø

**Hypersensitive, hypersensitiveness, hypersensitivity** — *see also* Allergy
- carotid sinus G9Ø.Ø1
- colon — *see* Irritable, colon
- drug T88.7- ☑
- gastrointestinal K52.29
  - immediate K52.29
  - psychogenic F45.8
- labyrinth — *see* subcategory H83.2- ☑
- pain R2Ø.8
- pneumonitis — *see* Pneumonitis, allergic
- reaction T78.4Ø- ☑
  - upper respiratory tract NEC J39.3

**Hypersomnia** (organic) G47.1Ø
- due to
  - alcohol
    - abuse F1Ø.182
    - dependence F1Ø.282
    - use F1Ø.982
  - amphetamines
    - abuse F15.182
    - dependence F15.282
    - use F15.982
  - caffeine
    - abuse F15.182
    - dependence F15.282
    - use F15.982
  - cocaine
    - abuse F14.182
    - dependence F14.282
    - use F14.982
  - drug NEC
    - abuse F19.182
    - dependence F19.282
    - use F19.982
  - medical condition G47.14
  - mental disorder F51.13
  - opioid
    - abuse F11.182
    - dependence F11.282
    - use F11.982
  - psychoactive substance NEC
    - abuse F19.182
    - dependence F19.282
    - use F19.982
  - sedative, hypnotic, or anxiolytic
    - abuse F13.182
    - dependence F13.282
    - use F13.982
  - stimulant NEC
    - abuse F15.182
    - dependence F15.282
    - use F15.982
- idiopathic G47.11
  - with long sleep time G47.11
  - without long sleep time G47.12
- menstrual related G47.13
- nonorganic origin F51.11
  - specified NEC F51.19
- not due to a substance or known physiological condition F51.11
  - specified NEC F51.19
- primary F51.11
- recurrent G47.13
- specified NEC G47.19

**Hypersplenia, hypersplenism** D73.1

**Hyperstimulation, ovaries** (associated with induced ovulation) N98.1

**Hypersusceptibility** — *see* Allergy

**Hypertelorism** (ocular) (orbital) Q75.2

**Hypertension, hypertensive** (accelerated) (benign) (essential) (idiopathic) (malignant) (systemic) I1Ø
- with
  - heart failure (congestive) I11.Ø
  - heart involvement (conditions in I5Ø.- or I51.4-I51.7, I51.89, I51.9, due to hypertension) — *see* Hypertension, heart
  - kidney involvement — *see* Hypertension, kidney
- benign, intracranial G93.2
- borderline RØ3.Ø
- cardiorenal (disease) I13.1Ø
  - with heart failure I13.Ø
    - with stage 1 through stage 4 chronic kidney disease I13.Ø
    - with stage 5 or end stage renal disease I13.2
  - without heart failure I13.1Ø
    - with stage 1 through stage 4 chronic kidney disease I13.1Ø
    - with stage 5 or end stage renal disease I13.11
- cardiovascular
  - disease (arteriosclerotic) (sclerotic) — *see* Hypertension, heart
  - renal (disease) — *see* Hypertension, cardiorenal
- chronic venous — *see* Hypertension, venous (chronic)
- complicating
  - childbirth (labor) O16.4
    - pre-existing O1Ø.92
      - with
        - heart disease O1Ø.12
          - with renal disease O1Ø.32
        - pre-eclampsia O11.4
        - renal disease O1Ø.22
          - with heart disease O1Ø.32
      - essential O1Ø.Ø2
    - secondary O1Ø.42
  - pregnancy O16.- ☑
    - with edema — *see also* Pre-eclampsia O14.9- ☑
    - gestational (pregnancy induced) (without proteinuria) O13.- ☑
      - with proteinuria O14.9- ☑
        - mild pre-eclampsia O14.Ø- ☑
        - moderate pre-eclampsia O14.Ø- ☑
        - severe pre-eclampsia O14.1- ☑
          - with hemolysis, elevated liver enzymes and low platelet count (HELLP) O14.2- ☑
    - pre-existing O1Ø.91- ☑
      - with
        - heart disease O1Ø.11- ☑
          - with renal disease O1Ø.31- ☑
        - pre-eclampsia — *see* category O11
        - renal disease O1Ø.21- ☑
          - with heart disease O1Ø.31- ☑
      - essential O1Ø.Ø1- ☑
      - secondary O1Ø.41- ☑
    - transient O13.- ☑
  - puerperium, pre-existing O16.5
    - pre-existing
      - with
        - heart disease O1Ø.13
          - with renal disease O1Ø.33
        - pre-eclampsia O11.5
        - renal disease O1Ø.23
          - with heart disease O1Ø.33
      - essential O1Ø.Ø3
    - pregnancy-induced O13.9
    - secondary O1Ø.43
- crisis I16.9
- due to
  - endocrine disorders I15.2
  - pheochromocytoma — *see also* Pheochromocytoma, by type I15.2
  - renal disorders NEC I15.1
    - arterial I15.Ø
  - renovascular disorders I15.Ø
  - specified disease NEC I15.8
- emergency I16.1
- encephalopathy I67.4
- gestational (without significant proteinuria) (pregnancy-induced) (transient) O13.- ☑
  - with significant proteinuria — *see* Pre-eclampsia
  - complicating
    - delivery O13.4
    - puerperium O13.5

- **Hypertension, hypertensive** — *continued*
  - Goldblatt's I7Ø.1
  - heart (disease) (conditions in I51.4-I51.9 due to hypertension) I11.9
    - with
      - heart failure (congestive) I11.Ø
      - kidney disease (chronic) — *see* Hypertension, cardiorenal
  - intracranial, benign G93.2
  - kidney I12.9
    - with
      - heart disease — *see* Hypertension, cardiorenal
      - stage 1 through stage 4 chronic kidney disease I12.9
      - stage 5 chronic kidney disease (CKD) or end stage renal disease (ESRD) I12.Ø
  - lesser circulation I27.Ø
  - maternal O16.- ☑
  - newborn P29.2
    - pulmonary (persistent) P29.3Ø
  - ocular H4Ø.Ø5- ☑
  - pancreatic duct — *code to* underlying condition
    - with chronic pancreatitis K86.1
  - portal (due to chronic liver disease) (idiopathic) K76.6
    - gastropathy K31.89
    - in (due to) schistosomiasis (bilharziasis) B65.9 *[K77]*
  - postoperative I97.3
  - psychogenic F45.8
  - pulmonary I27.2Ø
    - with
      - cor pulmonale (chronic) I27.29
        - acute I26.Ø9
      - right heart ventricular strain/failure I27.29
        - acute I26.Ø9
      - right to left shunt related to congenital heart disease I27.83
      - unclear multifactorial mechanisms I27.29
    - arterial (associated) (drug-induced) (toxin-induced) I27.21
    - chronic thromboembolic I27.24
    - due to
      - hematologic disorders I27.29
      - kyphoscoliotic heart disease I27.1
      - left heart disease I27.22
      - lung diseases and hypoxia I27.23
      - metabolic disorders I27.29
      - specified systemic disorders I27.29
    - group 1 (associated) (drug-induced) (toxin-induced) I27.21
    - group 2 I27.22
    - group 3 I27.23
    - group 4 I27.24
    - group 5 I27.29
    - of newborn (persistent) P29.3Ø
    - primary (idiopathic) I27.Ø
    - secondary
      - arterial I27.21
      - specified NEC I27.29
  - renal — *see* Hypertension, kidney
  - renovascular I15.Ø
  - resistant (apparent treatment) (treatment) (true) I1A.Ø
  - secondary NEC I15.9
    - due to
      - endocrine disorders I15.2
      - pheochromocytoma — *see also* Pheochromocytoma, by type I15.2
      - renal disorders NEC I15.1
        - arterial I15.Ø
      - renovascular disorders I15.Ø
    - specified NEC I15.8
  - transient RØ3.Ø
    - of pregnancy O13.- ☑
  - urgency I16.Ø
  - venous (chronic)
    - due to
      - deep vein thrombosis — *see* Syndrome, postthrombotic
    - idiopathic I87.3Ø9
      - with
        - inflammation I87.32- ☑
          - with ulcer I87.33- ☑
        - specified complication NEC I87.39- ☑
        - ulcer I87.31- ☑
          - with inflammation I87.33- ☑
      - asymptomatic I87.3Ø- ☑
- **Hypertensive urgency** — *see* Hypertension
- **Hyperthecosis ovary** E28.8
- **Hyperthermia** (of unknown origin) — *see also* Hyperpyrexia
- **Hyperthermia** — *continued*
  - malignant, due to anesthesia T88.3- ☑
  - newborn P81.9
    - environmental P81.Ø
- **Hyperthyroid** (recurrent) — *see* Hyperthyroidism
- **Hyperthyroidism** (latent) (pre-adult) (recurrent) EØ5.9Ø
  - with
    - goiter (diffuse) EØ5.ØØ
      - with thyroid storm EØ5.Ø1
      - nodular (multinodular) EØ5.2Ø
        - with thyroid storm EØ5.21
        - uninodular EØ5.1Ø
          - with thyroid storm EØ5.11
    - storm EØ5.91
  - due to ectopic thyroid tissue EØ5.3Ø
    - with thyroid storm EØ5.31
  - neonatal, transitory P72.1
  - specified NEC EØ5.8Ø
    - with thyroid storm EØ5.81
- **Hypertony, hypertonia, hypertonicity**
  - bladder N31.8
  - congenital P94.1
  - stomach K31.89
    - psychogenic F45.8
  - uterus, uterine (contractions) (complicating delivery) O62.4
- **Hypertrichosis** L68.9
  - congenital Q84.2
  - eyelid HØ2.869
    - left HØ2.866
      - lower HØ2.865
      - upper HØ2.864
    - right HØ2.863
      - lower HØ2.862
      - upper HØ2.861
  - lanuginosa Q84.2
    - acquired L68.1
  - localized L68.2
  - specified NEC L68.8
- **Hypertriglyceridemia, essential** E78.1
- **Hypertrophy, hypertrophic**
  - adenofibromatous, prostate — *see* Enlargement, enlarged, prostate
  - adenoids (infective) J35.2
    - with tonsils J35.3
  - adrenal cortex E27.8
  - alveolar process or ridge — *see* Anomaly, alveolar
  - anal papillae K62.89
  - artery I77.89
    - congenital NEC Q27.8
      - digestive system Q27.8
      - lower limb Q27.8
      - specified site NEC Q27.8
      - upper limb Q27.8
  - auricular — *see* Hypertrophy, cardiac
  - Bartholin's gland N75.8
  - bile duct (common) (hepatic) K83.8
  - bladder (sphincter) (trigone) N32.89
  - bone M89.3Ø
    - carpus M89.34- ☑
    - clavicle M89.31- ☑
    - femur M89.35- ☑
    - fibula M89.36- ☑
    - finger M89.34- ☑
    - humerus M89.32- ☑
    - ilium M89.38
    - ischium M89.38
    - metacarpus M89.34- ☑
    - metatarsus M89.37- ☑
    - multiple sites M89.39
    - neck M89.38
    - pubic ramus [pubis] M89.38
    - radius M89.33- ☑
    - rib M89.38
    - scapula M89.31- ☑
    - skull M89.38
    - tarsus M89.37- ☑
    - tibia M89.36- ☑
    - toe M89.37- ☑
    - ulna M89.33- ☑
    - vertebra M89.38
  - brain G93.89
  - breast N62
    - cystic — *see* Mastopathy, cystic
    - newborn P83.4
    - pubertal, massive N62
    - puerperal, postpartum — *see* Disorder, breast, specified type NEC
- **Hypertrophy, hypertrophic** — *continued*
  - breast — *continued*
    - senile (parenchymatous) N62
  - cardiac (chronic) (idiopathic) I51.7
    - with rheumatic fever (conditions in IØØ)
      - active IØ1.8
      - inactive or quiescent (with chorea) IØ9.89
    - congenital NEC Q24.8
    - fatty — *see* Degeneration, myocardial
    - hypertensive — *see* Hypertension, heart
    - rheumatic (with chorea) IØ9.89
      - active or acute IØ1.8
        - with chorea IØ2.Ø
    - valve — *see* Endocarditis
  - cartilage — *see* Disorder, cartilage, specified type NEC
  - cecum — *see* Megacolon
  - cervix (uteri) N88.8
    - congenital Q51.828
    - elongation N88.4
  - clitoris (cirrhotic) N9Ø.89
    - congenital Q52.6
  - colon — *see also* Megacolon
    - congenital Q43.2
  - conjunctiva, lymphoid H11.89
  - corpora cavernosa N48.89
  - cystic duct K82.8
  - duodenum K31.89
  - endometrium (glandular) — *see also* Hyperplasia, endometrial N85.ØØ
    - cervix N88.8
  - epididymis N5Ø.89
  - esophageal hiatus (congenital) Q79.1
    - with hernia — *see* Hernia, hiatal
  - eyelid — *see* Disorder, eyelid, specified type NEC
  - facet joint — *see also* Spondylosis M47.819
  - fat pad E65
    - knee (infrapatellar) (popliteal) (prepatellar) (retropatellar) M79.4
  - foot (congenital) Q74.2
  - frenulum, frenum (tongue) K14.8
    - lip K13.Ø
  - gallbladder K82.8
  - gastric mucosa K29.6Ø
    - with bleeding K29.61
  - gland, glandular R59.9
    - generalized R59.1
    - localized R59.Ø
  - gum (mucous membrane) KØ6.1
  - heart (idiopathic) — *see also* Hypertrophy, cardiac
    - valve — *see also* Endocarditis I38
  - hemifacial Q67.4
  - hepatic — *see* Hypertrophy, liver
  - hiatus (esophageal) Q79.1
  - hilus gland R59.Ø
  - hymen, congenital Q52.4
  - ileum K63.89
  - intestine NEC K63.89
  - jejunum K63.89
  - kidney (compensatory) N28.81
    - congenital Q63.3
  - labium (majus) (minus) N9Ø.6Ø
  - ligament — *see* Disorder, ligament
  - lingual tonsil (infective) J35.1
    - with adenoids J35.3
  - lip K13.Ø
    - congenital Q18.6
  - liver R16.Ø
    - acute K76.89
    - cirrhotic — *see* Cirrhosis, liver
    - congenital Q44.79
    - fatty — *see* Fatty, liver
  - lymph, lymphatic gland R59.9
    - generalized R59.1
    - localized R59.Ø
    - tuberculous — *see* Tuberculosis, lymph gland
  - mammary gland — *see* Hypertrophy, breast
  - Meckel's diverticulum (congenital) Q43.Ø
    - malignant — *see* Table of Neoplasms, small intestine, malignant
  - median bar — *see* Hyperplasia, prostate
  - meibomian gland — *see* Chalazion
  - meniscus, knee, congenital Q74.1
  - metatarsal head — *see* Hypertrophy, bone, metatarsus
  - metatarsus — *see* Hypertrophy, bone, metatarsus
  - mucous membrane
    - alveolar ridge KØ6.2
    - gum KØ6.1
    - nose (turbinate) J34.3
  - muscle M62.89

- **Hypoparathyroidism** — *continued*
  - idiopathic E2Ø.Ø
  - neonatal, transitory P71.4
  - postprocedural E89.2
  - secondary, in diseases classified elsewhere E2Ø.811
  - specified NEC E2Ø.89
    - due to impaired parathyroid hormone secretion E2Ø.818
- **Hypoperfusion** (in)
  - newborn P96.89
- **Hypopharyngitis** — *see* Laryngopharyngitis
- **Hypophoria** H5Ø.53
- **Hypophosphatemia, hypophosphatasia** (acquired) (congenital) (renal) E83.39
  - familial E83.31
- **Hypophyseal, hypophysis** — *see also* condition
  - dwarfism E23.Ø
  - gigantism E22.Ø
- **Hypopiesis** — *see* Hypotension
- **Hypopinealism** E34.8
- **Hypopituitarism** (juvenile) E23.Ø
  - drug-induced E23.1
  - due to
    - hypophysectomy E89.3
    - radiotherapy E89.3
  - iatrogenic NEC E23.1
  - postirradiation E89.3
  - postpartum O99.285
  - postprocedural E89.3
- **Hypoplasia, hypoplastic**
  - adrenal (gland), congenital Q89.1
  - alimentary tract, congenital Q45.8
    - upper Q4Ø.8
  - anus, anal (canal) Q42.3
    - with fistula Q42.2
  - aorta, aortic Q25.42
    - ascending, in hypoplastic left heart syndrome Q23.4
    - valve Q23.1
      - in hypoplastic left heart syndrome Q23.4
  - areola, congenital Q83.8
  - arm (congenital) — *see* Defect, reduction, upper limb
  - artery (peripheral) Q27.8
    - brain (congenital) Q28.3
    - coronary Q24.5
    - digestive system Q27.8
    - lower limb Q27.8
    - pulmonary Q25.79
      - functional, unilateral J43.Ø
    - retinal (congenital) Q14.1
    - specified site NEC Q27.8
    - umbilical Q27.Ø
    - upper limb Q27.8
  - auditory canal Q17.8
    - causing impairment of hearing Q16.9
  - biliary duct or passage Q44.5
  - bone NOS Q79.9
    - face Q75.8
    - marrow D61.9
      - megakaryocytic D69.49
    - skull — *see* Hypoplasia, skull
  - brain QØ2
    - gyri QØ4.3
    - part of QØ4.3
  - breast (areola) N64.82
  - bronchus Q32.4
  - cardiac Q24.8
  - carpus — *see* Defect, reduction, upper limb, specified type NEC
  - cartilage hair Q78.8
  - cecum Q42.8
  - cementum KØØ.4
  - cephalic QØ2
  - cerebellum QØ4.3
  - cervix (uteri), congenital Q51.821
  - clavicle (congenital) Q74.Ø
  - coccyx Q76.49
  - colon Q42.9
    - specified NEC Q42.8
  - corpus callosum QØ4.Ø
  - cricoid cartilage Q31.2
  - digestive organ(s) or tract NEC Q45.8
    - upper (congenital) Q4Ø.8
  - ear (auricle) (lobe) Q17.2
    - middle Q16.4
  - enamel of teeth (neonatal) (postnatal) (prenatal) KØØ.4
  - endocrine (gland) NEC Q89.2
  - endometrium N85.8
  - epididymis (congenital) Q55.4
  - epiglottis Q31.2

- **Hypoplasia, hypoplastic** — *continued*
  - erythroid, congenital D61.Ø1
  - esophagus (congenital) Q39.8
  - eustachian tube Q17.8
  - eye Q11.2
  - eyelid (congenital) Q1Ø.3
  - face Q18.8
    - bone(s) Q75.8
  - femur (congenital) — *see* Defect, reduction, lower limb, specified type NEC
  - fibula (congenital) — *see* Defect, reduction, lower limb, specified type NEC
  - finger (congenital) — *see* Defect, reduction, upper limb, specified type NEC
  - focal dermal Q82.8
  - foot — *see* Defect, reduction, lower limb, specified type NEC
  - gallbladder Q44.Ø
  - genitalia, genital organ(s)
    - female, congenital Q52.8
      - external Q52.79
      - internal NEC Q52.8
    - in adiposogenital dystrophy E23.6
  - glottis Q31.2
  - hair Q84.2
  - hand (congenital) — *see* Defect, reduction, upper limb, specified type NEC
  - heart Q24.8
  - humerus (congenital) — *see* Defect, reduction, upper limb, specified type NEC
  - intestine (small) Q41.9
    - large Q42.9
      - specified NEC Q42.8
  - jaw M26.Ø9
    - alveolar M26.79
    - lower M26.Ø4
      - alveolar M26.74
    - upper M26.Ø2
      - alveolar M26.73
  - kidney(s) Q6Ø.5
    - bilateral Q6Ø.4
    - unilateral Q6Ø.3
  - labium (majus) (minus), congenital Q52.79
  - larynx Q31.2
  - left heart syndrome Q23.4
  - leg (congenital) — *see* Defect, reduction, lower limb
  - limb Q73.8
    - lower (congenital) — *see* Defect, reduction, lower limb
    - upper (congenital) — *see* Defect, reduction, upper limb
  - liver Q44.79
  - lung (lobe) (not associated with short gestation) Q33.6
    - associated with immaturity, low birth weight, prematurity, or short gestation P28.Ø
  - mammary (areola), congenital Q83.8
  - mandible, mandibular M26.Ø4
    - alveolar M26.74
    - unilateral condylar M27.8
  - maxillary M26.Ø2
    - alveolar M26.73
  - medullary D61.9
  - megakaryocytic D69.49
  - metacarpus — *see* Defect, reduction, upper limb, specified type NEC
  - metatarsus — *see* Defect, reduction, lower limb, specified type NEC
  - muscle Q79.8
  - nail(s) Q84.6
  - nose, nasal Q3Ø.1
  - optic nerve H47.Ø3- ☑
  - osseous meatus (ear) Q17.8
  - ovary, congenital Q5Ø.39
  - pancreas Q45.Ø
  - parathyroid (gland) Q89.2
  - parotid gland Q38.4
  - patella Q74.1
  - pelvis, pelvic girdle Q74.2
  - penis (congenital) Q55.62
  - peripheral vascular system Q27.8
    - digestive system Q27.8
    - lower limb Q27.8
    - specified site NEC Q27.8
    - upper limb Q27.8
  - pituitary (gland) (congenital) Q89.2
  - pulmonary (not associated with short gestation) Q33.6
    - artery, functional J43.Ø
    - associated with short gestation P28.Ø

- **Hypoplasia, hypoplastic** — *continued*
  - radioulnar — *see* Defect, reduction, upper limb, specified type NEC
  - radius — *see* Defect, reduction, upper limb
  - rectum Q42.1
    - with fistula Q42.Ø
  - respiratory system NEC Q34.8
  - rib Q76.6
  - right heart syndrome Q22.6
  - sacrum Q76.49
  - scapula Q74.Ø
  - scrotum Q55.1
  - shoulder girdle Q74.Ø
  - skin Q82.8
  - skull (bone) Q75.8
    - with
      - anencephaly QØØ.Ø
      - encephalocele — *see* Encephalocele
      - hydrocephalus QØ3.9
        - with spina bifida — *see* Spina bifida, by site, with hydrocephalus
      - microcephaly QØ2
  - spinal (cord) (ventral horn cell) QØ6.1
  - spine Q76.49
  - sternum Q76.7
  - tarsus — *see* Defect, reduction, lower limb, specified type NEC
  - testis Q55.1
  - thymic, with immunodeficiency D82.1
  - thymus (gland) Q89.2
    - with immunodeficiency D82.1
  - thyroid (gland) EØ3.1
    - cartilage Q31.2
  - tibiofibular (congenital) — *see* Defect, reduction, lower limb, specified type NEC
  - toe — *see* Defect, reduction, lower limb, specified type NEC
  - tongue Q38.3
  - Turner's KØØ.4
  - ulna (congenital) — *see* Defect, reduction, upper limb
  - umbilical artery Q27.Ø
  - unilateral condylar M27.8
  - ureter Q62.8
  - uterus, congenital Q51.811
  - vagina Q52.4
  - vascular NEC peripheral Q27.8
    - brain Q28.3
    - digestive system Q27.8
    - lower limb Q27.8
    - specified site NEC Q27.8
    - upper limb Q27.8
  - vein(s) (peripheral) Q27.8
    - brain Q28.3
    - digestive system Q27.8
    - great Q26.8
    - lower limb Q27.8
    - specified site NEC Q27.8
    - upper limb Q27.8
  - vena cava (inferior) (superior) Q26.8
  - vertebra Q76.49
  - vulva, congenital Q52.79
  - zonule (ciliary) Q12.8
- **Hypoplasminogenemia** E88.Ø2
- **Hypopnea, obstructive sleep apnea** G47.33
- **Hypopotassemia** E87.6
- **Hypoproconvertinemia, congenital** (hereditary) D68.2
- **Hypoproteinemia** E77.8
- **Hypoprothrombinemia** (congenital) (hereditary) (idiopathic) D68.2
  - acquired D68.4
  - newborn, transient P61.6
- **Hypoptyalism** K11.7
- **Hypopyon** (eye) (anterior chamber) — *see* Iridocyclitis, acute, hypopyon
- **Hypopyrexia** R68.Ø
- **Hyporeflexia** R29.2
- **Hyposecretion**
  - ACTH E23.Ø
  - antidiuretic hormone E23.2
  - ovary E28.39
  - salivary gland (any) K11.7
  - vasopressin E23.2
- **Hyposegmentation, leukocytic, hereditary** D72.Ø
- **Hyposiderinemia** D5Ø.9
- **Hypospadias** Q54.9
  - balanic Q54.Ø
  - coronal Q54.Ø
  - glandular Q54.Ø
  - penile Q54.1

**Hypospadias** — *continued*
- penoscrotal Q54.2
- perineal Q54.3
- specified NEC Q54.8

**Hypospermatogenesis** — *see* Oligospermia
**Hyposplenism** D73.Ø
**Hypostasis pulmonary, passive** — *see* Edema, lung
**Hypostatic** — *see* condition
**Hyposthenuria** N28.89
**Hypotension** (arterial) (constitutional) I95.9
- chronic I95.89
- due to (of) hemodialysis I95.3
- drug-induced I95.2
- iatrogenic I95.89
- idiopathic (permanent) I95.Ø
- intra-dialytic I95.3
- intracranial G96.81Ø
  - following
    - lumbar cerebrospinal fluid shunting G97.83
    - specified procedure NEC G97.84
    - ventricular shunting (ventriculostomy) G97.2
  - specified NEC G96.819
  - spontaneous G96.811
- maternal, syndrome (following labor and delivery) O26.5- ☑
- neurogenic, orthostatic G9Ø.3
- orthostatic (chronic) I95.1
  - due to drugs I95.2
  - neurogenic G9Ø.3
- postoperative I95.81
- postural I95.1
- specified NEC I95.89

**Hypothermia** (accidental) T68.- ☑
- due to anesthesia, anesthetic T88.51- ☑
- low environmental temperature T68.- ☑
- neonatal P8Ø.9
  - environmental (mild) NEC P8Ø.8
  - mild P8Ø.8
  - severe (chronic) (cold injury syndrome) P8Ø.Ø
  - specified NEC P8Ø.8
- not associated with low environmental temperature R68.Ø

**Hypothyroidism** (acquired) EØ3.9
- autoimmune — *see* Thyroiditis, autoimmune
- congenital (without goiter) EØ3.1
  - with goiter (diffuse) EØ3.Ø
- due to
  - exogenous substance NEC EØ3.2
  - iodine-deficiency, acquired EØ1.8
    - subclinical EØ2
  - irradiation therapy E89.Ø
  - medicament NEC EØ3.2
  - P-aminosalicylic acid (PAS) EØ3.2
  - phenylbutazone EØ3.2
  - resorcinol EØ3.2
  - sulfonamide EØ3.2
  - surgery E89.Ø
  - thiourea group drugs EØ3.2
- iatrogenic NEC EØ3.2
- iodine-deficiency (acquired) EØ1.8
  - congenital — *see* Syndrome, iodine- deficiency, congenital
  - subclinical EØ2
- neonatal, transitory P72.2
- postinfectious EØ3.3
- postirradiation E89.Ø
- postprocedural E89.Ø
- postsurgical E89.Ø
- specified NEC EØ3.8
- subclinical, iodine-deficiency related EØ2

**Hypotonia, hypotonicity, hypotony**
- bladder N31.2
- congenital (benign) P94.2
- eye — *see* Disorder, globe, hypotony

**Hypotrichosis** — *see* Alopecia
**Hypotropia** H5Ø.2- ☑
**Hypoventilation** RØ6.89
- congenital central alveolar G47.35
- sleep related
  - idiopathic nonobstructive alveolar G47.34
  - in conditions classified elsewhere G47.36

**Hypovitaminosis** — *see* Deficiency, vitamin
**Hypovolemia** E86.1
- surgical shock T81.19- ☑
- traumatic (shock) T79.4- ☑

**Hypoxemia** RØ9.Ø2
- newborn P84
- sleep related, in conditions classified elsewhere G47.36

**Hypoxia** — *see also* Anoxia RØ9.Ø2
- cerebral, during a procedure NEC G97.81
  - postprocedural NEC G97.82
- intrauterine P84
- myocardial — *see* Insufficiency, coronary
- newborn P84
- sleep-related G47.34

**Hypsarrhythmia** — *see* Epilepsy, generalized, specified NEC
**Hysteralgia, pregnant uterus** O26.89- ☑
**Hysteria, hysterical** (conversion) (dissociative state) F44.9
- anxiety F41.8
- convulsions F44.5
- psychosis, acute F44.9

**Hysteroepilepsy** F44.5

## I

**IBDU** (colonic inflammatory bowel disease unclassified) K52.3
**ICANS** (immune effector cell-associated neurotoxicity syndrome) — *see* Syndrome, immune effector cell-associated neurotoxicity
**Ichthyoparasitism due to Vandellia cirrhosa** B88.8
**Ichthyosis** (congenital) Q8Ø.9
- acquired L85.Ø
- fetalis Q8Ø.4
- hystrix Q8Ø.8
- lamellar Q8Ø.2
- lingual K13.29
- palmaris and plantaris Q82.8
- simplex Q8Ø.Ø
- vera Q8Ø.8
- vulgaris Q8Ø.Ø
- X-linked Q8Ø.1

**Ichthyotoxism** — *see* Poisoning, fish
- bacterial — *see* Intoxication, foodborne

**Icteroanemia, hemolytic** (acquired) D59.9
- congenital — *see* Spherocytosis

**Icterus** — *see also* Jaundice
- conjunctiva R17
- gravis, newborn P55.Ø
- hematogenous (acquired) D59.9
- hemolytic (acquired) D59.9
  - congenital — *see* Spherocytosis
- hemorrhagic (acute) (leptospiral) (spirochetal) A27.Ø
  - newborn P53
- infectious B15.9
  - with hepatic coma B15.Ø
  - leptospiral A27.Ø
  - spirochetal A27.Ø
- neonatorum — *see* Jaundice, newborn
- newborn P59.9
- spirochetal A27.Ø

**Ictus solaris, solis** T67.Ø1- ☑
**Id reaction** (due to bacteria) L3Ø.2
**Ideation**
- homicidal R45.85Ø
- suicidal R45.851

**Identity disorder** (child) F64.9
- gender role F64.2
- psychosexual F64.2

**Idioglossia** F8Ø.Ø
**Idiopathic** — *see* condition
**Idiot, idiocy** (congenital) F73
- amaurotic (Bielschowsky(-Jansky)) (family) (infantile (late)) (juvenile (late)) (Vogt-Spielmeyer) E75.4
- microcephalic QØ2

**IFALD** (intestinal failure-associated liver disease) K76.83
**IgE asthma** J45.9Ø9
**IIAC** (idiopathic infantile arterial calcification) — *see* Calcification, arterial, generalized, of infancy
**Ileitis** (chronic) (noninfectious) — *see also* Enteritis K52.9
- backwash — *see* Pancolitis, ulcerative (chronic)
- infectious AØ9
- regional (ulcerative) — *see* Enteritis, regional, small intestine
- segmental — *see* Enteritis, regional
- terminal (ulcerative) — *see* Enteritis, regional, small intestine

**Ileocolitis** — *see also* Enteritis K52.9
- infectious AØ9
- regional — *see* Enteritis, regional
- ulcerative K51.Ø- ☑

**Ileostomy**
- attention to Z43.2
- malfunctioning K94.13
- status (ileal pouch) (Kock pouch) Z93.2

**Ileostomy** — *continued*
- status — *continued*
  - with complication — *see* Complications, enterostomy

**Ileotyphus** — *see* Typhoid
**Ileum** — *see* condition
**Ileus** (bowel) (colon) (inhibitory) (intestine) K56.7
- adynamic K56.Ø
- due to gallstone (in intestine) K56.3
- duodenal (chronic) K31.5
- gallstone K56.3
- mechanical NEC — *see also* Obstruction, intestine, specified NEC K56.699
- meconium P76.Ø
  - in cystic fibrosis E84.11
  - meaning meconium plug (without cystic fibrosis) P76.Ø
- myxedema K59.89
- neurogenic K56.Ø
  - Hirschsprung's disease or megacolon Q43.1
- newborn
  - due to meconium P76.Ø
    - in cystic fibrosis E84.11
    - meaning meconium plug (without cystic fibrosis) P76.Ø
  - transitory P76.1
- obstructive — *see also* Obstruction, intestine, specified NEC K56.699
- paralytic K56.Ø
- postoperative K91.89

**Iliac** — *see* condition
**Iliotibial band syndrome** M76.3- ☑
**Illiteracy** Z55.Ø
- health Z55.6

**Illness** — *see also* Disease R69
- Gulf war T75.83Ø- ☑
- manic-depressive — *see* Disorder, bipolar

**Imbalance** R26.89
- autonomic G9Ø.89
- constituents of food intake E63.1
- electrolyte E87.8
  - with
    - abortion — *see* Abortion by type, complicated by, electrolyte imbalance
    - molar pregnancy OØ8.5
  - due to hyperemesis gravidarum O21.1
  - following ectopic or molar pregnancy OØ8.5
  - neonatal, transitory NEC P74.49
    - potassium
      - hyperkalemia P74.31
      - hypokalemia P74.32
    - sodium
      - hypernatremia P74.21
      - hyponatremia P74.22
- endocrine E34.9
- eye muscle NOS H5Ø.9
- hormone E34.9
- hysterical F44.4
- labyrinth — *see* subcategory H83.2- ☑
- posture R29.3
- protein-energy — *see* Malnutrition
- sympathetic G9Ø.89

**Imbecile, imbecility** (I.Q. 35-49) F71
**Imbedding, intrauterine device** T83.39- ☑
**Imbibition, cholesterol** (gallbladder) K82.4
**Imbrication, teeth,, fully erupted** M26.3Ø
**Imerslund** (-Gräsbeck) **syndrome** D51.1
**Immature** — *see also* Immaturity
- birth (less than 37 completed weeks) — *see* Preterm, newborn
  - extremely (less than 28 completed weeks) — *see* Immaturity, extreme
- personality F6Ø.89

**Immaturity** (less than 37 completed weeks) — *see also* Preterm, newborn
- extreme of newborn (less than 28 completed weeks of gestation) (less than 196 completed days of gestation) (unspecified weeks of gestation) PØ7.2Ø
  - gestational age
    - 23 completed weeks (23 weeks, Ø days through 23 weeks, 6 days) PØ7.22
    - 24 completed weeks (24 weeks, Ø days through 24 weeks, 6 days) PØ7.23
    - 25 completed weeks (25 weeks, Ø days through 25 weeks, 6 days) PØ7.24
    - 26 completed weeks (26 weeks, Ø days through 26 weeks, 6 days) PØ7.25
    - 27 completed weeks (27 weeks, Ø days through 27 weeks, 6 days) PØ7.26
    - less than 23 completed weeks PØ7.21

- **Immaturity** — *continued*
  - fetus or infant light-for-dates — *see* Light-for-dates
  - lung, newborn P28.Ø
  - organ or site NEC — *see* Hypoplasia
  - pulmonary, newborn P28.Ø
  - reaction F6Ø.89
  - sexual (female) (male), after puberty E3Ø.Ø
- **Immersion** T75.1- ☑
  - foot T69.Ø2- ☑
  - hand T69.Ø1- ☑
- **Immobile, immobility**
  - complete, due to severe physical disability or frailty R53.2
  - intestine K59.89
  - syndrome (paraplegic) M62.3
- **Immune reconstitution** (inflammatory) syndrome [IRIS] D89.3
- **Immunization** — *see also* Vaccination
  - ABO — *see* Incompatibility, ABO
    - in newborn P55.1
  - appropriate for age
    - child (over 28 days old) ZØØ.129
      - with abnormal findings ZØØ.121
  - complication — *see* Complications, vaccination
  - encounter for Z23
  - not done (not carried out) — *see also* Underimmunization status Z28.9
    - because (of)
      - acute illness of patient Z28.Ø1
      - allergy to vaccine (or component) Z28.Ø4
      - caregiver refusal Z28.82
      - chronic illness of patient Z28.Ø2
      - contraindication NEC Z28.Ø9
      - delay in delivery of vaccine Z28.83
      - group pressure Z28.1
      - guardian refusal Z28.82
      - immune compromised state of patient Z28.Ø3
      - lack of availability of vaccine Z28.83
      - manufacturer delay of vaccine Z28.83
      - parent refusal Z28.82
      - patient had disease being vaccinated against Z28.81
      - patient refusal Z28.21
      - patient's belief Z28.1
      - religious beliefs of patient Z28.1
      - specified reason NEC Z28.89
        - of patient Z28.29
      - unavailability of vaccine Z28.83
      - unspecified patient reason Z28.2Ø
  - partial — *see also* Underimmunization status
    - for COVID-19 Z28.311
  - Rh factor
    - affecting management of pregnancy NEC O36.Ø9- ☑
      - anti-D antibody O36.Ø1- ☑
    - from transfusion — *see* Complication(s), transfusion, incompatibility reaction, Rh (factor)
- **Immunocompromised NOS** D84.9
- **Immunocytoma** C83.Ø- ☑
- **Immunodeficiency** D84.9
  - with
    - adenosine-deaminase deficiency — *see also* Deficiency, adenosine deaminase D81.3Ø
    - antibody defects D8Ø.9
      - specified type NEC D8Ø.8
    - hyperimmunoglobulinemia D8Ø.6
    - increased immunoglobulin M (IgM) D8Ø.5
    - major defect D82.9
      - specified type NEC D82.8
    - partial albinism D82.8
    - short-limbed stature D82.2
    - thrombocytopenia and eczema D82.Ø
  - antibody with
    - hyperimmunoglobulinemia D8Ø.6
    - near-normal immunoglobulins D8Ø.6
  - autosomal recessive, Swiss type D8Ø.Ø
  - combined D81.9
    - biotin-dependent carboxylase D81.819
      - biotinidase D81.81Ø
      - holocarboxylase synthetase D81.818
      - specified type NEC D81.818
    - severe (SCID) D81.9
      - with
        - low or normal B-cell numbers D81.2
        - low T- and B-cell numbers D81.1
        - reticular dysgenesis D81.Ø
    - specified type NEC D81.89
  - common variable D83.9

- **Immunodeficiency** — *continued*
  - common variable — *continued*
    - with
      - abnormalities of B-cell numbers and function D83.Ø
      - autoantibodies to B- or T-cells D83.2
      - immunoregulatory T-cell disorders D83.1
    - specified type NEC D83.8
  - due to
    - conditions classified elsewhere D84.81
    - drugs D84.821
    - external causes D84.822
    - medication (current or past) D84.821
  - following hereditary defective response to Epstein-Barr virus (EBV) D82.3
  - selective, immunoglobulin
    - A (IgA) D8Ø.2
    - G (IgG) (subclasses) D8Ø.3
    - M (IgM) D8Ø.4
  - severe combined (SCID) D81.9
    - due to adenosine deaminase deficiency D81.31
  - specified type NEC D84.89
  - X-linked, with increased IgM D8Ø.5
- **Immunodeficient NOS** D84.9
- **Immunosuppressed NOS** D84.9
- **Immunotherapy** (encounter for)
  - antineoplastic Z51.12
- **Impaction, impacted**
  - bowel, colon, rectum — *see also* Impaction, fecal K56.49
    - by gallstone K56.3
  - calculus — *see* Calculus
  - cerumen (ear) (external) H61.2- ☑
  - cuspid — *see* Impaction, tooth
  - dental (same or adjacent tooth) KØ1.1
  - fecal, feces K56.41
  - fracture — *see* Fracture, by site
  - gallbladder — *see* Calculus, gallbladder
  - gallstone(s) — *see* Calculus, gallbladder
    - bile duct (common) (hepatic) — *see* Calculus, bile duct
    - cystic duct — *see* Calculus, gallbladder
    - in intestine, with obstruction (any part) K56.3
  - intestine (calculous) NEC — *see also* Impaction, fecal K56.49
    - gallstone, with ileus K56.3
  - intrauterine device (IUD) T83.39- ☑
  - molar — *see* Impaction, tooth
  - shoulder, causing obstructed labor O66.Ø
  - tooth, teeth KØ1.1
  - turbinate J34.89
- **Impaired, impairment** (function)
  - auditory discrimination — *see* Abnormal, auditory perception
  - cognitive, mild, of uncertain or unknown etiology G31.84
  - dual sensory Z73.82
  - fasting glucose R73.Ø1
  - glucose tolerance (oral) R73.Ø2
  - hearing — *see* Deafness
  - heart — *see* Disease, heart
  - kidney N28.9
    - disorder resulting from N25.9
      - specified NEC N25.89
  - liver K72.9Ø
    - with coma K72.91
  - mastication KØ8.89
  - mild cognitive G31.84
    - of uncertain or unknown etiology G31.84
  - mild neurocognitive
    - due to known physiological condition (without behavioral disturbance) FØ6.7Ø
      - with behavioral disturbance FØ6.71
  - mobility
    - ear ossicles — *see* Ankylosis, ear ossicles
    - requiring care provider Z74.Ø9
  - myocardium, myocardial — *see* Insufficiency, myocardial
  - rectal sphincter R19.8
  - renal (acute) (chronic) N28.9
    - disorder resulting from N25.9
      - specified NEC N25.89
  - vision NEC H54.7
    - both eyes H54.3
- **Impediment, speech** — *see also* Disorder, speech R47.9
  - psychogenic (childhood) F98.8
  - slurring R47.81
  - specified NEC R47.89
- **Impending**
  - coronary syndrome I2Ø.Ø
  - delirium tremens F1Ø.239
  - myocardial infarction I2Ø.Ø

- **Imperception auditory** (acquired) — *see also* Deafness
  - congenital H93.25
- **Imperfect**
  - aeration, lung (newborn) NEC — *see* Atelectasis
  - closure (congenital)
    - alimentary tract NEC Q45.8
      - lower Q43.8
      - upper Q4Ø.8
    - atrioventricular ostium Q21.2Ø
    - atrium (secundum) Q21.11
    - branchial cleft NOS Q18.2
      - cyst Q18.Ø
      - fistula Q18.Ø
      - sinus Q18.Ø
    - choroid Q14.3
    - cricoid cartilage Q31.8
    - cusps, heart valve NEC Q24.8
      - pulmonary Q22.3
    - ductus
      - arteriosus Q25.Ø
      - Botalli Q25.Ø
    - ear drum (causing impairment of hearing) Q16.4
    - esophagus with communication to bronchus or trachea Q39.1
    - eyelid Q1Ø.3
    - foramen
      - botalli Q21.12
      - ovale Q21.12
    - genitalia, genital organ(s) or system
      - female Q52.8
        - external Q52.79
        - internal NEC Q52.8
      - male Q55.8
    - glottis Q31.8
    - interatrial ostium or septum Q21.19
    - interauricular ostium or septum Q21.19
    - interventricular ostium or septum Q21.Ø
    - larynx Q31.8
    - lip — *see* Cleft, lip
    - nasal septum Q3Ø.3
    - nose Q3Ø.2
    - omphalomesenteric duct Q43.Ø
    - optic nerve entry Q14.2
    - organ or site not listed — *see* Anomaly, by site
    - ostium
      - interatrial Q21.19
      - interauricular Q21.19
      - interventricular Q21.Ø
    - palate — *see* Cleft, palate
    - preauricular sinus Q18.1
    - retina Q14.1
    - roof of orbit Q75.8
    - sclera Q13.5
    - septum
      - aorticopulmonary Q21.4
      - atrial (secundum) Q21.19
      - between aorta and pulmonary artery Q21.4
      - heart Q21.9
      - interatrial (secundum) Q21.19
      - interauricular (secundum) Q21.19
      - interventricular Q21.Ø
        - in tetralogy of Fallot Q21.3
      - nasal Q3Ø.3
      - ventricular Q21.Ø
        - with pulmonary stenosis or atresia, dextraposition of aorta, and hypertrophy of right ventricle Q21.3
        - in tetralogy of Fallot Q21.3
    - skull Q75.ØØ9
      - with
        - anencephaly QØØ.Ø
        - encephalocele — *see* Encephalocele
        - hydrocephalus QØ3.9
          - with spina bifida — *see* Spina bifida, by site, with hydrocephalus
        - microcephaly QØ2
    - spine (with meningocele) — *see* Spina bifida
    - trachea Q32.1
    - tympanic membrane (causing impairment of hearing) Q16.4
    - uterus Q51.818
    - vitelline duct Q43.Ø
  - erection — *see* Dysfunction, sexual, male, erectile
  - fusion — *see* Imperfect, closure
  - inflation, lung (newborn) — *see* Atelectasis
  - posture R29.3
  - rotation, intestine Q43.3
  - septum, ventricular Q21.Ø
- **Imperfectly descended testis** — *see* Cryptorchid

- **Incontinence** R32
  - anal sphincter R15.9
  - coital N39.491
  - feces R15.9
    - nonorganic origin F98.1
  - insensible (urinary) N39.42
  - overflow N39.49Ø
  - postural (urinary) N39.492
  - psychogenic F45.8
  - rectal R15.9
  - reflex N39.498
  - stress (female) (male) N39.3
    - and urge N39.46
  - urethral sphincter R32
  - urge N39.41
    - and stress (female) (male) N39.46
  - urine (urinary) R32
    - continuous N39.45
    - due to cognitive impairment, or severe physical disability or immobility R39.81
    - functional R39.81
    - insensible N39.42
    - mixed (stress and urge) N39.46
    - nocturnal N39.44
    - nonorganic origin F98.Ø
    - overflow N39.49Ø
    - post dribbling N39.43
    - postural N39.492
    - reflex N39.498
    - specified NEC N39.498
    - stress (female) (male) N39.3
      - and urge N39.46
    - total N39.498
    - unaware N39.42
    - urge N39.41
      - and stress (female) (male) N39.46
- **Incontinentia pigmenti** Q82.3
- **Incoordinate, incoordination**
  - esophageal-pharyngeal (newborn) — *see* Dysphagia
  - muscular R27.8
  - uterus (action) (contractions) (complicating delivery) O62.4
- **Increase, increased**
  - abnormal, in development R63.8
  - androgens (ovarian) E28.1
  - anticoagulants (antithrombin) (anti-VIIIa) (anti-IXa) (anti-Xa) (anti-XIa) — *see* Circulating anticoagulants
  - cold sense R2Ø.8
  - estrogen E28.Ø
  - function
    - adrenal
      - cortex — *see* Cushing's, syndrome
      - medulla E27.5
    - pituitary (gland) (anterior) (lobe) E22.9
      - posterior E22.2
  - heat sense R2Ø.8
  - intracranial pressure (benign) G93.2
  - permeability, capillaries I78.8
  - pressure, intracranial G93.2
  - secretion
    - gastrin E16.4
    - glucagon E16.3
    - pancreas, endocrine E16.9
      - growth hormone-releasing hormone E16.8
      - pancreatic polypeptide E16.8
      - somatostatin E16.8
      - vasoactive-intestinal polypeptide E16.8
  - sphericity, lens Q12.4
  - splenic activity D73.1
  - venous pressure I87.8
    - portal K76.6
- **Increta placenta** O43.22- ☑
- **Incrustation, cornea, foreign body** (lead)(zinc) — *see* Foreign body, cornea
- **Incyclophoria** H5Ø.54
- **Incyclotropia** — *see* Cyclotropia
- **Indeterminate sex** Q56.4
- **India rubber skin** Q82.8
- **Indigestion** (acid) (bilious) (functional) K3Ø
  - catarrhal K31.89
  - due to decomposed food NOS AØ5.9
  - nervous F45.8
  - psychogenic F45.8
- **Indirect** — *see* condition
- **Induratio penis plastica** N48.6
- **Induration, indurated**
  - brain G93.89
  - breast (fibrous) N64.51
    - puerperal, postpartum O92.29

**Induration, indurated** — *continued*

  - broad ligament N83.8
  - chancre
    - anus A51.1
    - congenital A5Ø.Ø7
    - extragenital NEC A51.2
  - corpora cavernosa (penis) (plastic) N48.6
  - liver (chronic) K76.89
  - lung (black) (chronic) (fibroid) — *see also* Fibrosis, lung J84.1Ø
    - essential brown J84.Ø3
  - penile (plastic) N48.6
  - phlebitic — *see* Phlebitis
  - skin R23.4
- **Inebriety** (without dependence) — *see* Alcohol, intoxication
- **Inefficiency, kidney** N28.9
- **Inelasticity, skin** R23.4
- **Inequality, leg** (length) (acquired) — *see also* Deformity, limb, unequal length
  - congenital — *see* Defect, reduction, lower limb
  - lower leg — *see* Deformity, limb, unequal length
- **Inertia**
  - bladder (neurogenic) N31.2
  - stomach K31.89
    - psychogenic F45.8
  - uterus, uterine during labor O62.2
    - during latent phase of labor O62.Ø
    - primary O62.Ø
    - secondary O62.1
  - vesical (neurogenic) N31.2
- **Infancy, infantile, infantilism** — *see also* condition
  - celiac K9Ø.Ø
  - genitalia, genitals (after puberty) E3Ø.Ø
  - Herter's (nontropical sprue) K9Ø.Ø
  - intestinal K9Ø.Ø
  - Lorain E23.Ø
  - pancreatic K86.89
  - pelvis M95.5
    - with disproportion (fetopelvic) O33.1
      - causing obstructed labor O65.1
  - pituitary E23.Ø
  - renal N25.Ø
  - uterus — *see* Infantile, genitalia
- **Infant**(s) — *see also* Infancy
  - excessive crying R68.11
  - irritable child R68.12
  - lack of care — *see* Neglect
  - liveborn (singleton) Z38.2
    - born in hospital Z38.ØØ
      - by cesarean Z38.Ø1
    - born outside hospital Z38.1
    - multiple NEC Z38.8
      - born in hospital Z38.68
        - by cesarean Z38.69
      - born outside hospital Z38.7
    - quadruplet Z38.8
      - born in hospital Z38.63
        - by cesarean Z38.64
      - born outside hospital Z38.7
    - quintuplet Z38.8
      - born in hospital Z38.65
        - by cesarean Z38.66
      - born outside hospital Z38.7
    - triplet Z38.8
      - born in hospital Z38.61
        - by cesarean Z38.62
      - born outside hospital Z38.7
    - twin Z38.5
      - born in hospital Z38.3Ø
        - by cesarean Z38.31
      - born outside hospital Z38.4
  - of diabetic mother (syndrome of) P7Ø.1
    - gestational diabetes P7Ø.Ø
- **Infantile** — *see also* condition
  - genitalia, genitals E3Ø.Ø
  - os, uterine E3Ø.Ø
  - penis E3Ø.Ø
  - testis E29.1
  - uterus E3Ø.Ø
- **Infantilism** — *see* Infancy
- **Infarct, infarction**
  - adrenal (capsule) (gland) E27.49
  - appendices epiploicae — *see also* Infarct, intestine K55.Ø69
  - bowel — *see also* Infarct, intestine K55.Ø69
  - brain (stem) — *see* Infarct, cerebral
  - breast N64.89
  - brewer's (kidney) N28.Ø
  - cardiac — *see* Infarct, myocardium

**Infarct, infarction** — *continued*

  - cerebellar — *see* Infarct, cerebral
  - cerebral (acute) — *see also* Occlusion, artery cerebral or precerebral, with infarction I63.9
    - aborted I63.9
    - chronic (imaging) (old) (remote) (without sequelae) Z86.73
      - with residual defects — *see* Sequelae, disease, cerebrovascular
    - cortical I63.9
    - due to
      - cerebral venous thrombosis, nonpyogenic I63.6
      - embolism
        - cerebral arteries I63.4- ☑
        - precerebral arteries I63.1- ☑
      - occlusion NEC
        - cerebral arteries I63.5- ☑
        - precerebral arteries I63.2- ☑
        - small artery I63.81
      - stenosis NEC
        - cerebral arteries I63.5- ☑
        - precerebral arteries I63.2- ☑
        - small artery I63.81
      - thrombosis
        - cerebral artery I63.3- ☑
        - precerebral artery I63.Ø- ☑
    - intraoperative
      - during cardiac surgery I97.81Ø
      - during other surgery I97.811
    - neonatal P91.82- ☑
    - perinatal (arterial ischemic) P91.82- ☑
    - postprocedural
      - following cardiac surgery I97.82Ø
      - following other surgery I97.821
    - specified NEC I63.89
  - colon (acute) (agnogenic) (embolic) (hemorrhagic) (nonocclusive) (nonthrombotic) (occlusive) (segmental) (thrombotic) (with gangrene) — *see also* Infarct, intestine K55.Ø49
  - coronary artery — *see* Infarct, myocardium
  - embolic — *see* Embolism
  - fallopian tube N83.8
  - gallbladder K82.8
  - heart — *see* Infarct, myocardium
  - hepatic K76.3
  - hypophysis (anterior lobe) E23.6
  - impending (myocardium) I2Ø.Ø
  - intestine (acute) (agnogenic) (embolic) (hemorrhagic) (nonocclusive) (nonthrombotic) (occlusive) (thrombotic) (with gangrene) K55.Ø69
    - diffuse K55.Ø62
    - focal K55.Ø61
    - large K55.Ø49
      - diffuse K55.Ø42
      - focal K55.Ø41
    - small K55.Ø29
      - diffuse K55.Ø22
      - focal K55.Ø21
  - kidney N28.Ø
  - lacunar I63.81
  - liver K76.3
  - lung (embolic) (thrombotic) — *see* Embolism, pulmonary
  - lymph node I89.8
  - mesentery, mesenteric (embolic) (thrombotic) (with gangrene) — *see also* Infarct, intestine K55.Ø69
  - muscle (ischemic) M62.2Ø
    - ankle M62.27- ☑
    - foot M62.27- ☑
    - forearm M62.23- ☑
    - hand M62.24- ☑
    - lower leg M62.26- ☑
    - pelvic region M62.25- ☑
    - shoulder region M62.21- ☑
    - specified site NEC M62.28
    - thigh M62.25- ☑
    - upper arm M62.22- ☑
  - myocardium, myocardial (acute) (with stated duration of 4 weeks or less) I21.9
    - with
      - coronary microvascular disease I21.B
      - coronary microvascular dysfunction I21.B
      - nonobstructive coronary arteries [MINOCA] with microvascular disease I21.B
    - associated with revascularization procedure I21.A9
    - diagnosed on ECG, but presenting no symptoms I25.2
    - due to
      - demand ischemia I21.A1
      - ischemic imbalance I21.A1

- **Infarct, infarction** — *continued*
  - myocardium, myocardial — *continued*
    - healed or old I25.2
    - intraoperative — *see also* Infarct, myocardium, associated with revascularization procedure
      - during cardiac surgery I97.79Ø
      - during other surgery I97.791
    - non-Q wave I21.4
    - non-ST elevation (NSTEMI) I21.4
      - subsequent I22.2
    - nontransmural I21.4
    - past (diagnosed on ECG or other investigation, but currently presenting no symptoms) I25.2
    - postprocedural — *see also* Infarct, myocardium, associated with revascularization procedure
      - following cardiac surgery — *see also* Infarct, myocardium, type 4 or type 5 I97.19Ø
      - following other surgery I97.191
    - Q wave — *see also* Infarct, myocardium, ST elevation, by site I21.3
    - secondary to
      - demand ischemia I21.A1
      - ischemic imbalance I21.A1
    - ST elevation (STEMI) I21.3
      - anterior (anteroapical) (anterolateral) (anteroseptal) (Q wave) (wall) I21.Ø9
        - subsequent I22.Ø
      - inferior (diaphragmatic) (inferolateral) (inferoposterior) (wall) NEC I21.19
        - subsequent I22.1
      - inferoposterior transmural (Q wave) I21.11
      - involving
        - coronary artery of anterior wall NEC I21.Ø9
        - coronary artery of inferior wall NEC I21.19
        - diagonal coronary artery I21.Ø2
        - left anterior descending coronary artery I21.Ø2
        - left circumflex coronary artery I21.21
        - left main coronary artery I21.Ø1
        - oblique marginal coronary artery I21.21
        - right coronary artery I21.11
      - lateral (apical-lateral) (basal-lateral) (high) I21.29
        - subsequent I22.8
      - posterior (posterobasal) (posterolateral) (posteroseptal) (true) I21.29
        - subsequent I22.8
      - septal I21.29
        - subsequent I22.8
      - specified NEC I21.29
        - subsequent I22.8
      - subsequent I22.9
    - subsequent (recurrent) (reinfarction) I22.9
      - anterior (anteroapical) (anterolateral) (anteroseptal) (wall) I22.Ø
      - diaphragmatic (wall) I22.1
      - inferior (diaphragmatic) (inferolateral) (inferoposterior) (wall) I22.1
      - lateral (apical-lateral) (basal-lateral) (high) I22.8
      - non-ST elevation (NSTEMI) I22.2
      - posterior (posterobasal) (posterolateral) (posteroseptal) (true) I22.8
      - septal I22.8
      - specified NEC I22.8
      - ST elevation I22.9
        - anterior (anteroapical) (anterolateral) (anteroseptal) (wall) I22.Ø
        - inferior (diaphragmatic) (inferolateral) (inferoposterior) (wall) I22.1
        - specified NEC I22.8
      - subendocardial I22.2
      - transmural I22.9
        - anterior (anteroapical) (anterolateral) (anteroseptal) (wall) I22.Ø
        - diaphragmatic (wall) I22.1
        - inferior (diaphragmatic) (inferolateral) (inferoposterior) (wall) I22.1
        - lateral (apical-lateral) (basal-lateral) (high) I22.8
        - posterior (posterobasal) (posterolateral) (posteroseptal) (true) I22.8
        - specified NEC I22.8
      - type 1 — *see also* Infarction, myocardial, subsequent, by site, or by ST elevation or non-ST elevation I22.9
      - type 2 I21.A1
      - type 3 I21.A9
      - type 4 I21.A9
      - type 5 I21.A9
    - syphilitic A52.Ø6
    - transmural — *see also*, Infarct, myocardium, ST elevation, by site I21.3

- **Infarct, infarction** — *continued*
  - myocardium, myocardial — *continued*
    - transmural — *see also*, Infarct, myocardium, ST elevation, by site — *continued*
      - anterior (anteroapical) (anterolateral) (anteroseptal) (Q wave) (wall) NEC I21.Ø9
      - inferior (diaphragmatic) (inferolateral) (inferoposterior) (Q wave) (wall) NEC I21.19
      - inferoposterior (Q wave) I21.11
      - lateral (apical-lateral) (basal-lateral) (high) NEC I21.29
      - posterior (posterobasal) (posterolateral) (posteroseptal) (true) NEC I21.29
      - septal NEC I21.29
      - specified NEC I21.29
    - type 1 — *see also* Infarction, myocardial, by site, or by ST elevation or non-ST elevation I21.9
    - type 2 I21.A1
    - type 3 I21.A9
    - type 4 (a) (b) (c) I21.A9
    - type 5 I21.A9
  - nontransmural I21.4
  - omentum — *see also* Infarct, intestine K55.Ø69
  - ovary N83.8
  - pancreas K86.89
  - papillary muscle — *see* Infarct, myocardium
  - parathyroid gland E21.4
  - pituitary (gland) E23.6
  - placenta O43.81- ☑
  - prostate N42.89
  - pulmonary (artery) (vein) (hemorrhagic) — *see* Embolism, pulmonary
  - renal (embolic) (thrombotic) N28.Ø
  - retina, retinal (artery) — *see* Occlusion, artery, retina
  - spinal (cord) (acute) (embolic) (nonembolic) G95.11
  - spleen D73.5
    - embolic or thrombotic I74.8
  - subendocardial (acute) (nontransmural) I21.4
  - suprarenal (capsule) (gland) E27.49
  - testis N5Ø.1
  - thrombotic — *see also* Thrombosis
    - artery, arterial — *see* Embolism
  - thyroid (gland) EØ7.89
  - ventricle (heart) — *see* Infarct, myocardium
- **Infecting** — *see* condition
- **Infection, infected, infective** (opportunistic) B99.9
  - with
    - drug resistant organism — *see* Resistance (to), drug — *see also* specific organism
    - lymphangitis — *see* Lymphangitis
    - organ dysfunction (acute) R65.2Ø
      - with septic shock R65.21
  - abscess (skin) — *code by* site under Abscess
  - Absidia — *see* Mucormycosis
  - Acanthamoeba — *see* Acanthamebiasis
  - Acanthocheilonema (perstans) (streptocerca) B74.4
  - accessory sinus (chronic) — *see* Sinusitis
  - achorion — *see* Dermatophytosis
  - Acinetobacter baumannii, as cause of disease classified elsewhere B96.83
  - Acremonium falciforme B47.Ø
  - acromioclavicular MØØ.9
  - Actinobacillus (actinomycetem-comitans) A28.8
    - mallei A24.Ø
    - muris A25.1
  - Actinomadura B47.1
  - Actinomyces (israelii) — *see also* Actinomycosis A42.9
  - Actinomycetales — *see* Actinomycosis
  - actinomycotic NOS — *see* Actinomycosis
  - adenoid (and tonsil) JØ3.9Ø
    - chronic J35.Ø2
  - adenovirus NEC
    - as cause of disease classified elsewhere B97.Ø
    - unspecified nature or site B34.Ø
  - aerogenes capsulatus A48.Ø
  - aertrycke — *see* Infection, salmonella
  - alimentary canal NOS — *see* Enteritis, infectious
  - Allescheria boydii B48.2
  - Alternaria B48.8
  - alveolus, alveolar (process) KØ4.7
  - Ameba, amebic (histolytica) — *see* Amebiasis
  - amniotic fluid, sac or cavity O41.1Ø- ☑
    - chorioamnionitis O41.12- ☑
    - placentitis O41.14- ☑
  - amputation stump (surgical) — *see* Complication, amputation stump, infection
  - Ancylostoma (duodenalis) B76.Ø
  - Anisakiasis, Anisakis larvae B81.Ø
  - anthrax — *see* Anthrax

- **Infection, infected, infective** — *continued*
  - antrum (chronic) — *see* Sinusitis, maxillary
  - anus, anal (papillae) (sphincter) K62.89
  - arbovirus (arbor virus) A94
    - specified type NEC A93.8
  - artificial insemination N98.Ø
  - Ascaris lumbricoides — *see* Ascariasis
  - Ascomycetes B47.Ø
  - Aspergillus (flavus) (fumigatus) (terreus) — *see* Aspergillosis
  - atypical
    - acid-fast (bacilli) — *see* Mycobacterium, atypical
    - mycobacteria — *see* Mycobacterium, atypical
    - virus A81.9
      - specified type NEC A81.89
  - auditory meatus (external) — *see* Otitis, externa, infective
  - auricle (ear) — *see* Otitis, externa, infective
  - axillary gland (lymph) LØ4.2
  - Bacillus A49.9
    - abortus A23.1
    - anthracis — *see* Anthrax
    - ducreyi (any location) A57
    - Flexner's AØ3.1
    - Friedlander's NEC A49.8
    - gas (gangrene) A48.Ø
    - mallei A24.Ø
    - melitensis A23.Ø
    - paratyphoid, paratyphosus AØ1.4
      - A AØ1.1
      - B AØ1.2
      - C AØ1.3
    - Shiga (-Kruse) AØ3.Ø
    - suipestifer — *see* Infection, salmonella
    - swimming pool A31.1
    - typhosa AØ1.ØØ
    - welchii — *see* Gangrene, gas
  - bacterial NOS A49.9
    - as cause of disease classified elsewhere B96.89
      - Acinetobacter baumannii B96.83
      - Bacteroides fragilis [B. fragilis] B96.6
      - Clostridium perfringens [C. perfringens] B96.7
      - Cronobacter (sakazakii) A49.8
      - Enterobacter sakazakii B96.89
      - Enterococcus B95.2
      - Escherichia coli [E. coli] — *see also* Escherichia coli B96.2Ø
      - Helicobacter pylori [H.pylori] B96.81
      - Hemophilus influenzae [H. influenzae] B96.3
      - Klebsiella pneumoniae [K. pneumoniae] B96.1
      - Mycoplasma pneumoniae [M. pneumoniae] B96.Ø
      - Proteus (mirabilis) (morganii) B96.4
      - Pseudomonas (aeruginosa) (mallei) (pseudomallei) B96.5
      - Staphylococcus B95.8
        - aureus (methicillin susceptible) (MSSA) B95.61
          - methicillin resistant (MRSA) B95.62
        - specified NEC B95.7
      - Streptococcus B95.5
        - group A B95.Ø
        - group B B95.1
        - pneumoniae B95.3
        - specified NEC B95.4
      - Vibrio vulnificus B96.82
    - specified NEC A48.8
  - Bacterium
    - paratyphosum AØ1.4
      - A AØ1.1
      - B AØ1.2
      - C AØ1.3
    - typhosum AØ1.ØØ
  - Bacteroides NEC A49.8
    - fragilis, as cause of disease classified elsewhere B96.6
  - Balantidium coli AØ7.Ø
  - Bartholin's gland N75.8
  - Basidiobolus B46.8
  - bile duct (common) (hepatic) — *see* Cholangitis
  - bladder — *see* Cystitis
  - Blastomyces, blastomycotic — *see also* Blastomycosis
    - brasiliensis — *see* Paracoccidioidomycosis
    - dermatitidis — *see* Blastomycosis
    - European — *see* Cryptococcosis
    - Loboi B48.Ø
    - North American B4Ø.9
    - South American — *see* Paracoccidioidomycosis
  - bleb, postprocedure — *see* Blebitis
  - bone — *see* Osteomyelitis
  - Bordetella — *see* Whooping cough
  - Borrelia bergdorfi A69.2Ø
  - brain — *see also* Encephalitis GØ4.9Ø

**Infection, infected, infective** — *continued*
- brain — *see also* Encephalitis — *continued*
  - membranes — *see* Meningitis
  - septic G06.0
    - meninges — *see* Meningitis, bacterial
- branchial cyst Q18.0
- breast — *see* Mastitis
- bronchus — *see* Bronchitis
- Brucella A23.9
  - abortus A23.1
  - canis A23.3
  - melitensis A23.0
  - mixed A23.8
  - specified NEC A23.8
  - suis A23.2
- Brugia (malayi) B74.1
  - timori B74.2
- bursa — *see* Bursitis, infective
- buttocks (skin) L08.9
- Campylobacter, intestinal A04.5
  - as cause of disease classified elsewhere B96.81
- Candida (albicans) (tropicalis) — *see* Candidiasis
- candiru B88.8
- Capillaria (intestinal) B81.1
  - hepatica B83.8
  - philippinensis B81.1
- cartilage — *see* Disorder, cartilage, specified type NEC
- cat liver fluke B66.0
- catheter-related bloodstream (CRBSI) T80.211- ☑
- cellulitis — *code by* site under Cellulitis
- central line-associated T80.219- ☑
  - bloodstream (CLABSI) T80.211- ☑
  - specified NEC T80.218- ☑
- Cephalosporium falciforme B47.0
- cerebrospinal — *see* Meningitis
- cervical gland (lymph) L04.0
- cervix — *see* Cervicitis
- cesarean delivery wound (puerperal) O86.00
- cestodes — *see* Infestation, cestodes
- chest J22
- Chilomastix (intestinal) A07.8
- Chlamydia, chlamydial A74.9
  - anus A56.3
  - genitourinary tract A56.2
    - lower A56.00
    - specified NEC A56.19
  - lymphogranuloma A55
  - pharynx A56.4
  - psittaci A70
  - rectum A56.3
  - sexually transmitted NEC A56.8
- cholera — *see* Cholera
- Cladosporium
  - bantianum (brain abscess) B43.1
  - carrionii B43.0
  - castellanii B36.1
  - trichoides (brain abscess) B43.1
  - werneckii B36.1
- Clonorchis (sinensis) (liver) B66.1
- Clostridioides
  - difficile
    - as cause of disease classified elsewhere B96.89
    - foodborne (disease)
      - not specified as recurrent A04.72
      - recurrent A04.71
    - gas gangrene A48.0
    - necrotizing enterocolitis
      - not specified as recurrent A04.72
      - recurrent A04.71
    - sepsis A41.4
- Clostridium NEC
  - bifermentans A48.0
  - botulinum (food poisoning) A05.1
    - infant A48.51
    - wound A48.52
  - difficile
    - as cause of disease classified elsewhere B96.89
    - foodborne (disease)
      - not specified as recurrent A04.72
      - recurrent A04.71
    - gas gangrene A48.0
    - necrotizing enterocolitis
      - not specified as recurrent A04.72
      - recurrent A04.71
    - sepsis A41.4
  - gas-forming NEC A48.0
  - histolyticum A48.0
  - novyi, causing gas gangrene A48.0
  - oedematiens A48.0

**Infection, infected, infective** — *continued*
- Clostridium — *continued*
  - perfringens
    - as cause of disease classified elsewhere B96.7
    - due to food A05.2
    - foodborne (disease) A05.2
    - gas gangrene A48.0
    - sepsis A41.4
  - septicum, causing gas gangrene A48.0
  - sordellii, causing gas gangrene A48.0
  - welchii
    - as cause of disease classified elsewhere B96.7
    - foodborne (disease) A05.2
    - gas gangrene A48.0
    - necrotizing enteritis A05.2
    - sepsis A41.4
- Coccidioides (immitis) — *see* Coccidioidomycosis
- colon — *see* Enteritis, infectious
- colostomy K94.02
- common duct — *see* Cholangitis
- congenital P39.9
  - Candida (albicans) P37.5
  - cytomegalovirus P35.1
  - hepatitis, viral P35.3
  - herpes simplex P35.2
  - infectious or parasitic disease P37.9
    - specified NEC P37.8
  - listeriosis (disseminated) P37.2
  - malaria NEC P37.4
    - falciparum P37.3
  - Plasmodium falciparum P37.3
  - poliomyelitis P35.8
  - rubella P35.0
  - skin P39.4
  - toxoplasmosis (acute) (subacute) (chronic) P37.1
  - tuberculosis P37.0
  - urinary (tract) P39.3
  - vaccinia P35.8
  - virus P35.9
    - specified type NEC P35.8
- Conidiobolus B46.8
- coronavirus-2019 U07.1
- coronavirus NEC B34.2
  - as cause of disease classified elsewhere B97.29
  - severe acute respiratory syndrome (SARS associated) B97.21
- corpus luteum — *see* Salpingo-oophoritis
- Corynebacterium diphtheriae — *see* Diphtheria
- cotia virus B08.8
- COVID-19 — *see also* COVID-19 U07.1
- Coxiella burnetii A78
- coxsackie — *see* Coxsackie
- Cronobacter (sakazakii) A49.8
  - as cause of disease classified elsewhere B96.89
  - generalized A41.59
- Cryptococcus neoformans — *see* Cryptococcosis
- Cryptosporidium A07.2
- Cunninghamella — *see* Mucormycosis
- cyst — *see* Cyst
- cystic duct — *see also* Cholecystitis K81.9
- Cysticercus cellulosae — *see* Cysticercosis
- cytomegalovirus, cytomegaloviral B25.9
  - congenital P35.1
  - maternal, maternal care for (suspected) damage to fetus O35.3- ☑
  - mononucleosis B27.10
    - with
      - complication NEC B27.19
      - meningitis B27.12
      - polyneuropathy B27.11
- delta-agent (acute), in hepatitis B carrier B17.0
- dental (pulpal origin) K04.7
- Deuteromycetes B47.0
- Dicrocoelium dendriticum B66.2
- Dipetalonema (perstans) (streptocerca) B74.4
- diphtherial — *see* Diphtheria
- Diphyllobothrium (adult) (latum) (pacificum) B70.0
  - larval B70.1
- Diplogonoporus (grandis) B71.8
- Dipylidium caninum B67.4
- Dirofilaria B74.8
- Dracunculus medinensis B72
- Drechslera (hawaiiensis) B43.8
- ducreyi Haemophilus (any location) A57
- due to or resulting from
  - artificial insemination N98.0
  - Babesia
    - divergens (-like) strain B60.03
    - duncani (-type) species B60.02

**Infection, infected, infective** — *continued*
- due to or resulting from — *continued*
  - Babesia — *continued*
    - microti B60.01
    - species
      - specified NEC B60.09
  - central venous catheter T80.219- ☑
    - bloodstream T80.211- ☑
    - exit or insertion site T80.212- ☑
    - localized T80.212- ☑
    - port or reservoir T80.212- ☑
    - specified NEC T80.218- ☑
    - tunnel T80.212- ☑
  - device, implant or graft — *see also* Complications, by site and type, infection or inflammation T85.79- ☑
    - arterial graft NEC T82.7- ☑
    - breast (implant) T85.79- ☑
    - catheter NEC T85.79- ☑
      - dialysis (renal) T82.7- ☑
        - central line T80.211- ☑
        - intraperitoneal T85.71- ☑
      - infusion NEC T82.7- ☑
        - cranial T85.735- ☑
        - intrathecal T85.735- ☑
        - spinal (epidural) (subdural) T85.735- ☑
        - subarachnoid T85.735- ☑
      - urinary T83.518- ☑
        - cystostomy T83.510- ☑
        - Hopkins T83.518- ☑
        - ileostomy T83.518- ☑
        - nephrostomy T83.512- ☑
        - specified NEC T83.518- ☑
        - urethral indwelling T83.511- ☑
        - urostomy T83.518- ☑
    - electronic (electrode) (pulse generator) (stimulator)
      - bone T84.7- ☑
      - cardiac T82.7- ☑
      - nervous system T85.738- ☑
        - brain T85.731- ☑
        - cranial nerve T85.732- ☑
        - gastric nerve T85.732- ☑
        - generator pocket T85.734- ☑
        - neurostimulator generator T85.734- ☑
        - peripheral nerve T85.732- ☑
        - sacral nerve T85.732- ☑
        - spinal cord T85.733- ☑
        - vagal nerve T85.732- ☑
      - urinary (indwelling) T83.51- ☑
    - fixation, internal (orthopedic) NEC — *see* Complication, fixation device, infection
    - gastrointestinal (bile duct) (esophagus) T85.79- ☑
      - neurostimulator electrode (lead) T85.732- ☑
    - genital NEC T83.69- ☑
    - heart NEC T82.7- ☑
      - valve (prosthesis) T82.6- ☑
        - graft T82.7- ☑
    - joint prosthesis — *see* Complication, joint prosthesis, infection
    - ocular (corneal graft) (orbital implant) NEC T85.79- ☑
    - orthopedic NEC T84.7- ☑
    - penile (cylinder) (pump) (reservoir) T83.61- ☑
    - specified NEC T85.79- ☑
    - testicular T83.62- ☑
    - urinary NEC T83.598- ☑
      - ileal conduit stent T83.593- ☑
      - implanted neurostimulation T83.590- ☑
      - implanted sphincter T83.591- ☑
      - indwelling ureteral stent T83.592- ☑
      - nephroureteral stent T83.593- ☑
      - specified stent NEC T83.593- ☑
    - vascular NEC T82.7- ☑
    - ventricular intracranial (communicating) shunt T85.730- ☑
  - Hickman catheter T80.219- ☑
    - bloodstream T80.211- ☑
    - localized T80.212- ☑
    - specified NEC T80.218- ☑
  - immunization or vaccination T88.0- ☑
  - infusion, injection or transfusion NEC T80.29- ☑
  - injury NEC — *code by* site under Wound, open
  - peripherally inserted central catheter (PICC) T80.219- ☑
    - bloodstream T80.211- ☑

- **Infection, infected, infective** — *continued*
  - due to or resulting from — *continued*
    - peripherally inserted central catheter — *continued*
      - localized T8Ø.212- ☑
      - specified NEC T8Ø.218- ☑
    - portacath (port-a-cath) T8Ø.219- ☑
      - bloodstream T8Ø.211- ☑
      - localized T8Ø.212- ☑
      - specified NEC T8Ø.218- ☑
    - protozoa of the order Piroplasmida NEC B6Ø.Ø9
    - pulmonary artery catheter — *see* Infection, due to or resulting from, central venous catheter
    - surgery T81.4Ø- ☑
    - Swan Ganz catheter — *see* Infection, due to or resulting from, central venous catheter
    - triple lumen catheter T8Ø.219- ☑
      - bloodstream T8Ø.211- ☑
      - localized T8Ø.212- ☑
      - specified NEC T8Ø.218- ☑
    - umbilical venous catheter T8Ø.219- ☑
      - bloodstream T8Ø.211- ☑
      - localized T8Ø.212- ☑
      - specified NEC T8Ø.218- ☑
  - during labor NEC O75.3
  - ear (middle) — *see also* Otitis media
    - external — *see* Otitis, externa, infective
    - inner — *see* subcategory H83.Ø- ☑
  - Eberthella typhosa AØ1.ØØ
  - Echinococcus — *see* Echinococcus
  - echovirus
    - as cause of disease classified elsewhere B97.12
    - unspecified nature or site B34.1
  - endocardium I33.Ø
  - endocervix — *see* Cervicitis
  - Entamoeba — *see* Amebiasis
  - enteric — *see* Enteritis, infectious
  - Enterobacter sakazakii B96.89
  - Enterobius vermicularis B8Ø
  - enterostomy K94.12
  - enterovirus B34.1
    - as cause of disease classified elsewhere B97.1Ø
      - coxsackievirus B97.11
      - echovirus B97.12
      - specified NEC B97.19
  - Entomophthora B46.8
  - Epidermophyton — *see* Dermatophytosis
  - epididymis — *see* Epididymitis
  - episiotomy (puerperal) O86.Ø9
  - Erysipelothrix (insidiosa) (rhusiopathiae) — *see* Erysipeloid
  - erythema infectiosum BØ8.3
  - Escherichia (E.) coli NEC A49.8
    - as cause of disease classified elsewhere — *see also* Escherichia coli B96.2Ø
    - congenital P39.8
      - sepsis P36.4
    - generalized A41.51
    - intestinal — *see* Enteritis, infectious, due to, Escherichia coli
  - ethmoidal (chronic) (sinus) — *see* Sinusitis, ethmoidal
  - eustachian tube (ear) — *see* Salpingitis, eustachian
  - external auditory canal (meatus) NEC — *see* Otitis, externa, infective
  - eye (purulent) — *see* Endophthalmitis, purulent
  - eyelid — *see* Inflammation, eyelid
  - fallopian tube — *see* Salpingo-oophoritis
  - Fasciola (gigantica) (hepatica) (indica) B66.3
  - Fasciolopsis (buski) B66.5
  - filarial — *see* Infestation, filarial
  - finger (skin) LØ8.9
    - nail LØ3.Ø1- ☑
      - fungus B35.1
  - fish tapeworm B7Ø.Ø
    - larval B7Ø.1
  - flagellate, intestinal AØ7.9
  - fluke — *see* Infestation, fluke
  - focal
    - teeth (pulpal origin) KØ4.7
    - tonsils J35.Ø1
  - Fonsecaea (compactum) (pedrosoi) B43.Ø
  - food — *see* Intoxication, foodborne
  - foot (skin) LØ8.9
    - dermatophytic fungus B35.3
  - Francisella tularensis — *see* Tularemia
  - frontal (sinus) (chronic) — *see* Sinusitis, frontal
  - fungus NOS B49
    - beard B35.Ø

- **Infection, infected, infective** — *continued*
  - fungus — *continued*
    - dermatophytic — *see* Dermatophytosis
    - foot B35.3
    - groin B35.6
    - hand B35.2
    - nail B35.1
    - pathogenic to compromised host only B48.8
    - perianal (area) B35.6
    - scalp B35.Ø
    - skin B36.9
      - foot B35.3
      - hand B35.2
      - toenails B35.1
  - Fusarium B48.8
  - gallbladder — *see* Cholecystitis
  - gas bacillus — *see* Gangrene, gas
  - gastrointestinal — *see* Enteritis, infectious
  - generalized NEC — *see* Sepsis
  - generator pocket, implanted electronic neurostimulator T85.734- ☑
  - genital organ or tract
    - female — *see* Disease, pelvis, inflammatory
    - male N49.9
      - multiple sites N49.8
      - specified NEC N49.8
  - Ghon tubercle, primary A15.7
  - Giardia lamblia AØ7.1
  - gingiva (chronic) KØ5.1Ø
    - acute KØ5.ØØ
      - nonplaque induced KØ5.Ø1
      - plaque induced KØ5.ØØ
    - nonplaque induced KØ5.11
    - plaque induced KØ5.1Ø
  - glanders A24.Ø
  - glenosporopsis B48.Ø
  - Gnathostoma (spinigerum) B83.1
  - Gongylonema B83.8
  - gonococcal — *see* Gonococcus
  - gram-negative bacilli NOS A49.9
  - guinea worm B72
  - gum (chronic) KØ5.1Ø
    - acute KØ5.ØØ
      - nonplaque induced KØ5.Ø1
      - plaque induced KØ5.ØØ
    - nonplaque induced KØ5.11
    - plaque induced KØ5.1Ø
  - Haemophilus — *see* Infection, Hemophilus
  - heart — *see* Carditis
  - Helicobacter pylori AØ4.8
    - as cause of disease classified elsewhere B96.81
  - helminths B83.9
    - intestinal B82.Ø
      - mixed (types classifiable to more than one of the titles B65.Ø-B81.3 and B81.8) B81.4
      - specified type NEC B81.8
    - specified type NEC B83.8
  - Hemophilus
    - aegyptius, systemic A48.4
    - ducreyi (any location) A57
    - generalized A41.3
    - influenzae NEC A49.2
      - as cause of disease classified elsewhere B96.3
  - herpes (simplex) — *see also* Herpes
    - congenital P35.2
    - disseminated BØØ.7
    - zoster BØ2.9
  - herpesvirus, herpesviral — *see* Herpes
  - Heterophyes (heterophyes) B66.8
  - hip (joint) NEC MØØ.9
    - due to internal joint prosthesis
      - left T84.52- ☑
      - right T84.51- ☑
    - skin NEC LØ8.9
  - Histoplasma — *see* Histoplasmosis
    - American B39.4
    - capsulatum B39.4
  - hookworm B76.9
  - human
    - papilloma virus A63.Ø
    - T-cell lymphotropic virus type-1 (HTLV-1) B33.3
  - hydrocele N43.Ø
  - Hymenolepis B71.Ø
  - hypopharynx — *see* Pharyngitis
  - inguinal (lymph) glands LØ4.1
    - due to soft chancre A57
  - intervertebral disc, pyogenic M46.3Ø
    - cervical region M46.32
    - cervicothoracic region M46.33

- **Infection, infected, infective** — *continued*
  - intervertebral disc, pyogenic — *continued*
    - lumbar region M46.36
    - lumbosacral region M46.37
    - multiple sites M46.39
    - occipito-atlanto-axial region M46.31
    - sacrococcygeal region M46.38
    - thoracic region M46.34
    - thoracolumbar region M46.35
  - intestine, intestinal — *see* Enteritis, infectious
    - specified NEC AØ8.8
  - intra-amniotic affecting newborn NEC P39.2
  - intrauterine inflammation O41.12- ☑
  - Isospora belli or hominis AØ7.3
  - Japanese B encephalitis A83.Ø
  - jaw (bone) (lower) (upper) M27.2
  - joint NEC MØØ.9
    - due to internal joint prosthesis T84.5Ø- ☑
  - kidney (cortex) (hematogenous) N15.9
    - with calculus N2Ø.Ø
      - with hydronephrosis N13.6
    - following ectopic gestation OØ8.83
    - pelvis and ureter (cystic) N28.85
    - puerperal (postpartum) O86.21
    - specified NEC N15.8
  - Klebsiella (K.) pneumoniae NEC A49.8
    - as cause of disease classified elsewhere B96.1
  - knee (joint) NEC MØØ.9
    - joint MØØ.9
    - due to internal joint prosthesis
      - left T84.54- ☑
      - right T84.53- ☑
    - skin LØ8.9
  - Koch's — *see* Tuberculosis
  - labia (majora) (minora) (acute) — *see* Vulvitis
  - lacrimal
    - gland — *see* Dacryoadenitis
    - passages (duct) (sac) — *see* Inflammation, lacrimal, passages
  - lancet fluke B66.2
  - larynx NEC J38.7
  - leg (skin) NOS LØ8.9
  - Legionella pneumophila A48.1
    - nonpneumonic A48.2
  - Leishmania — *see also* Leishmaniasis
    - aethiopica B55.1
    - braziliensis B55.2
    - chagasi B55.Ø
    - donovani B55.Ø
    - infantum B55.Ø
    - major B55.1
    - mexicana B55.1
    - tropica B55.1
  - lentivirus, as cause of disease classified elsewhere B97.31
  - Leptosphaeria senegalensis B47.Ø
  - Leptospira interrogans A27.9
    - autumnalis A27.89
    - canicola A27.89
    - hebdomadis A27.89
    - icterohaemorrhagiae A27.Ø
    - pomona A27.89
    - specified type NEC A27.89
  - leptospirochetal NEC — *see* Leptospirosis
  - Listeria monocytogenes — *see also* Listeriosis
    - congenital P37.2
  - Loa loa B74.3
    - with conjunctival infestation B74.3
    - eyelid B74.3
  - Loboa loboi B48.Ø
  - local, skin (staphylococcal) (streptococcal) LØ8.9
    - abscess — *code by* site under Abscess
    - cellulitis — *code by* site under Cellulitis
    - specified NEC LØ8.89
    - ulcer — *see* Ulcer, skin
  - Loefflerella mallei A24.Ø
  - lung — *see also* Pneumonia J18.9
    - atypical Mycobacterium A31.Ø
    - spirochetal A69.8
    - tuberculous — *see* Tuberculosis, pulmonary
    - virus — *see* Pneumonia, viral
  - lymph gland — *see also* Lymphadenitis, acute
    - mesenteric I88.Ø
  - lymphoid tissue, base of tongue or posterior pharynx, NEC (chronic) J35.Ø3
  - Madurella (grisea) (mycetomii) B47.Ø
  - major
    - following ectopic or molar pregnancy OØ8.Ø
    - puerperal, postpartum, childbirth O85
  - Malassezia furfur B36.Ø

- **Infection, infected, infective** — *continued*
  - Salmonella — *continued*
    - localized — *continued*
      - pyelonephritis AØ2.25
      - specified NEC AØ2.29
    - paratyphi AØ1.4
      - A AØ1.1
      - B AØ1.2
      - C AØ1.3
    - schottmuelleri AØ1.2
    - typhi, typhosa — *see* Typhoid
  - Sarcocystis AØ7.8
  - SARS-CoV-2 — *see* Infection, COVID-19
  - scabies B86
  - Schistosoma — *see* Infestation, Schistosoma
  - scrotum (acute) NEC N49.2
  - seminal vesicle — *see* Vesiculitis
  - septic
    - localized, skin — *see* Abscess
  - Serratia NEC A49.8
    - as cause of disease classified elsewhere B96.89
    - generalized A41.53
  - sheep liver fluke B66.3
  - Shigella AØ3.9
    - boydii AØ3.2
    - dysenteriae AØ3.Ø
    - flexneri AØ3.1
    - group
      - A AØ3.Ø
      - B AØ3.1
      - C AØ3.2
      - D AØ3.3
    - Schmitz (-Stutzer) AØ3.Ø
    - schmitzii AØ3.Ø
    - shigae AØ3.Ø
    - sonnei AØ3.3
    - specified NEC AØ3.8
  - shoulder (joint) NEC MØØ.9
    - due to internal joint prosthesis T84.59- ☑
    - skin NEC LØ8.9
  - sinus (accessory) (chronic) (nasal) — *see also* Sinusitis
    - pilonidal — *see* Sinus, pilonidal
    - skin NEC LØ8.89
  - Skene's duct or gland — *see* Urethritis
  - skin (local) (staphylococcal) (streptococcal) LØ8.9
    - abscess — *code by* site under Abscess
    - cellulitis — *code by* site under Cellulitis
    - due to fungus B36.9
      - specified type NEC B36.8
    - mycotic B36.9
      - specified type NEC B36.8
    - newborn P39.4
    - ulcer — *see* Ulcer, skin
  - slow virus A81.9
    - specified NEC A81.89
  - Sparganum (mansoni) (proliferum) (baxteri) B7Ø.1
  - specific — *see also* Syphilis
    - to perinatal period — *see* Infection, congenital
  - specified NEC B99.8
  - spermatic cord NEC N49.1
  - sphenoidal (sinus) — *see* Sinusitis, sphenoidal
  - spinal cord NOS — *see also* Myelitis GØ4.91
    - abscess GØ6.1
    - meninges — *see* Meningitis
    - streptococcal GØ4.89
  - Spirillum A25.Ø
  - spirochetal NOS A69.9
    - lung A69.8
    - specified NEC A69.8
  - Spirometra larvae B7Ø.1
  - spleen D73.89
  - Sporotrichum, Sporothrix (schenckii) — *see* Sporotrichosis
  - staphylococcal, unspecified site
    - as cause of disease classified elsewhere B95.8
      - aureus (methicillin susceptible) (MSSA) B95.61
        - methicillin resistant (MRSA) B95.62
      - specified NEC B95.7
    - aureus (methicillin susceptible) (MSSA) A49.Ø1
      - methicillin resistant (MRSA) A49.Ø2
    - food poisoning AØ5.Ø
    - generalized (purulent) A41.2
    - pneumonia — *see* Pneumonia, staphylococcal
  - Stellantchasmus falcatus B66.8
  - streptobacillus moniliformis A25.1
  - streptococcal NEC A49.1
    - as cause of disease classified elsewhere B95.5
    - B genitourinary complicating
      - childbirth O98.82

- **Infection, infected, infective** — *continued*
  - streptococcal — *continued*
    - B genitourinary complicating — *continued*
      - pregnancy O98.81- ☑
      - puerperium O98.83
    - congenital
      - sepsis P36.1Ø
        - group B P36.Ø
        - specified NEC P36.19
    - generalized (purulent) A4Ø.9
  - Streptomyces B47.1
  - Strongyloides (stercoralis) — *see* Strongyloidiasis
  - stump (amputation) (surgical) — *see* Complication, amputation stump, infection
  - subcutaneous tissue, local LØ8.9
  - suipestifer — *see* Infection, salmonella
  - swimming pool bacillus A31.1
  - Taenia — *see* Infestation, Taenia
  - Taeniarhynchus saginatus B68.1
  - tapeworm — *see* Infestation, tapeworm
  - tendon (sheath) — *see* Tenosynovitis, infective NEC
  - Ternidens diminutus B81.8
  - testis — *see* Orchitis
  - threadworm B8Ø
  - throat — *see* Pharyngitis
  - thyroglossal duct K14.8
  - toe (skin) LØ8.9
    - cellulitis LØ3.Ø3- ☑
      - fungus B35.1
    - nail LØ3.Ø3- ☑
      - fungus B35.1
  - tongue NEC K14.Ø
    - parasitic B37.Ø
  - tonsil (and adenoid) (faucial) (lingual) (pharyngeal) — *see* Tonsillitis
  - tooth, teeth KØ4.7
    - periapical KØ4.7
    - peridental, periodontal KØ5.2Ø
      - generalized — *see* Periodontitis, aggressive, generalized
      - localized — *see* Periodontitis, aggressive, localized
    - pulp KØ4.Ø1
      - irreversible KØ4.Ø2
      - reversible KØ4.Ø1
    - socket M27.3
  - TORCH — *see* Infection, congenital
    - without active infection PØØ.2
  - Torula histolytica — *see* Cryptococcosis
  - Toxocara (canis) (cati) (felis) B83.Ø
  - Toxoplasma gondii — *see* Toxoplasma
  - trachea, chronic J42
  - trematode NEC — *see* Infestation, fluke
  - trench fever A79.Ø
  - Treponema pallidum — *see* Syphilis
  - Trichinella (spiralis) B75
  - Trichomonas A59.9
    - cervix A59.Ø9
    - intestine AØ7.8
    - prostate A59.Ø2
    - specified site NEC A59.8
    - urethra A59.Ø3
    - urogenitalis A59.ØØ
    - vagina A59.Ø1
    - vulva A59.Ø1
  - Trichophyton, trichophytic — *see* Dermatophytosis
  - Trichosporon (beigelii) cutaneum B36.2
  - Trichostrongylus B81.2
  - Trichuris (trichiura) B79
  - Trombicula (irritans) B88.Ø9
  - Trypanosoma
    - brucei
      - gambiense B56.Ø
      - rhodesiense B56.1
    - cruzi — *see* Chagas' disease
  - tubal — *see* Salpingo-oophoritis
  - tuberculous
    - latent (LTBI) Z22.7
    - NEC — *see* Tuberculosis
  - tubo-ovarian — *see* Salpingo-oophoritis
  - tunica vaginalis N49.1
  - tunnel T8Ø.212- ☑
  - tympanic membrane NEC — *see* Myringitis
  - typhoid (abortive) (ambulant) (bacillus) — *see* Typhoid
  - typhus A75.9
    - flea-borne A75.2
    - mite-borne A75.3
    - recrudescent A75.1
    - tick-borne A77.9
      - African A77.1

- **Infection, infected, infective** — *continued*
  - typhus — *continued*
    - tick-borne — *continued*
      - North Asian A77.2
  - umbilicus LØ8.82
  - ureter — *see* Ureteritis
  - urethra — *see* Urethritis
  - urinary (tract) N39.Ø
    - bladder — *see* Cystitis
    - complicating
      - pregnancy O23.4- ☑
        - specified type NEC O23.3- ☑
    - kidney — *see* Infection, kidney
    - newborn P39.3
    - puerperal (postpartum) O86.2Ø
    - tuberculous A18.13
    - urethra — *see* Urethritis
  - uterus, uterine — *see* Endometritis
  - vaccination T88.Ø- ☑
  - vaccinia not from vaccination BØ8.Ø11
  - vagina (acute) — *see* Vaginitis
  - varicella BØ1.9
  - varicose veins — *see* Varix
  - vas deferens NEC N49.1
  - vesical — *see* Cystitis
  - Vibrio
    - cholerae AØØ.Ø
      - El Tor AØØ.1
    - parahaemolyticus (food poisoning) AØ5.3
    - vulnificus
      - as cause of disease classified elsewhere B96.82
      - foodborne intoxication AØ5.5
  - Vincent's (gum) (mouth) (tonsil) A69.1
  - virus, viral NOS B34.9
    - adenovirus
      - as cause of disease classified elsewhere B97.Ø
      - unspecified nature or site B34.Ø
    - arborvirus, arbovirus arthropod-borne A94
    - as cause of disease classified elsewhere B97.89
      - adenovirus B97.Ø
      - coronavirus B97.29
        - SARS-associated B97.21
      - coxsackievirus B97.11
      - echovirus B97.12
      - enterovirus B97.1Ø
        - coxsackievirus B97.11
        - echovirus B97.12
        - specified NEC B97.19
      - human
        - immunodeficiency, type 2 (HIV 2) B97.35
        - metapneumovirus B97.81
        - T-cell lymphotropic,
          - type I (HTLV-I) B97.33
          - type II (HTLV-II) B97.34
      - papillomavirus B97.7
      - parvovirus B97.6
      - reovirus B97.5
      - respiratory syncytial (RSV) — *see* Infection, virus, respiratory syncytial (RSV)
      - retrovirus B97.3Ø
        - human
          - immunodeficiency, type 2 (HIV 2) B97.35
          - T-cell lymphotropic,
            - type I (HTLV-I) B97.33
            - type II (HTLV-II) B97.34
        - lentivirus B97.31
        - oncovirus B97.32
        - specified NEC B97.39
      - specified NEC B97.89
    - central nervous system A89
      - atypical A81.9
        - specified NEC A81.89
      - enterovirus NEC A88.8
        - meningitis A87.Ø
      - slow virus A81.9
        - specified NEC A81.89
      - specified NEC A88.8
    - chest J98.8
    - cotia BØ8.8
    - COVID-19 UØ7.1
    - coxsackie — *see also* Infection, coxsackie B34.1
      - as cause of disease classified elsewhere B97.11
    - ECHO
      - as cause of disease classified elsewhere B97.12
      - unspecified nature or site B34.1
    - encephalitis, tick-borne A84.9
    - enterovirus, as cause of disease classified elsewhere B97.1Ø
      - coxsackievirus B97.11

- **Infection, infected, infective** — *continued*
  - virus, viral — *continued*
    - enterovirus, as cause of disease classified elsewhere — *continued*
      - echovirus B97.12
      - specified NEC B97.19
    - exanthem NOS BØ9
    - human metapneumovirus as cause of disease classified elsewhere B97.81
    - human papilloma as cause of disease classified elsewhere B97.7
    - intestine — *see* Enteritis, viral
    - respiratory syncytial (RSV)
      - as cause of disease classified elsewhere B97.4
      - bronchiolitis J21.Ø
      - bronchitis J2Ø.5
      - bronchopneumonia J12.1
      - otitis media H65.- ☑ *[B97.4]*
      - pneumonia J12.1
      - upper respiratory infection JØ6.9 *[B97.4]*
    - rhinovirus
      - as cause of disease classified elsewhere B97.89
      - unspecified nature or site B34.8
    - slow A81.9
      - specified NEC A81.89
    - specified type NEC B33.8
      - as cause of disease classified elsewhere B97.89
      - unspecified nature or site B34.8
    - unspecified nature or site B34.9
    - West Nile — *see* Virus, West Nile
  - vulva (acute) — *see* Vulvitis
  - West Nile — *see* Virus, West Nile
  - whipworm B79
  - worms B83.9
    - specified type NEC B83.8
  - Wuchereria (bancrofti) B74.Ø
    - malayi B74.1
  - yatapoxvirus BØ8.7Ø
    - specified NEC BØ8.79
  - yeast — *see also* Candidiasis B37.9
  - yellow fever — *see* Fever, yellow
  - Yersinia
    - enterocolitica (intestinal) AØ4.6
    - pestis — *see* Plague
    - pseudotuberculosis A28.2
  - Zeis' gland — *see* Hordeolum
  - Zika virus A92.5
    - congenital P35.4
  - zoonotic bacterial NOS A28.9
  - Zopfia senegalensis B47.Ø
- **Infective, infectious** — *see* condition
- **Infertility**
  - female N97.9
    - age-related N97.8
    - associated with
      - anovulation N97.Ø
      - cervical (mucus) disease or anomaly N88.3
      - congenital anomaly
        - cervix N88.3
        - fallopian tube N97.1
        - uterus N97.2
        - vagina N97.8
      - dysmucorrhea N88.3
      - fallopian tube disease or anomaly N97.1
      - pituitary-hypothalamic origin E23.Ø
      - specified origin NEC N97.8
      - Stein-Leventhal syndrome E28.2
      - uterine disease or anomaly N97.2
      - vaginal disease or anomaly N97.8
    - due to
      - cervical anomaly N88.3
      - fallopian tube anomaly N97.1
      - ovarian failure E28.39
      - Stein-Leventhal syndrome E28.2
      - uterine anomaly N97.2
      - vaginal anomaly N97.8
    - nonimplantation N97.2
    - origin
      - cervical N88.3
      - tubal (block) (occlusion) (stenosis) N97.1
      - uterine N97.2
      - vaginal N97.8
  - male N46.9
    - azoospermia N46.Ø1
      - extratesticular cause N46.Ø29
        - drug therapy N46.Ø21
        - efferent duct obstruction N46.Ø23
        - infection N46.Ø22
        - radiation N46.Ø24
- **Infertility** — *continued*
  - male — *continued*
    - azoospermia — *continued*
      - extratesticular cause — *continued*
        - specified cause NEC N46.Ø29
        - systemic disease N46.Ø25
    - oligospermia N46.11
      - extratesticular cause N46.129
        - drug therapy N46.121
        - efferent duct obstruction N46.123
        - infection N46.122
        - radiation N46.124
        - specified cause NEC N46.129
        - systemic disease N46.125
    - specified type NEC N46.8
- **Infestation** B88.9
  - Acanthocheilonema (perstans) (streptocerca) B74.4
  - Acariasis B88.Ø9
    - demodex folliculorum B88.Ø1
    - sarcoptes scabiei B86
    - trombiculae B88.Ø9
  - Agamofilaria streptocerca B74.4
  - Ancylostoma, ankylostoma (braziliense) (caninum) (ceylanicum) (duodenale) B76.Ø
    - americanum B76.1
    - new world B76.1
  - Anisakis larvae, anisakiasis B81.Ø
  - arthropod NEC B88.2
  - Ascaris lumbricoides — *see* Ascariasis
  - Balantidium coli AØ7.Ø
  - beef tapeworm B68.1
  - Bothriocephalus (latus) B7Ø.Ø
    - larval B7Ø.1
  - broad tapeworm B7Ø.Ø
    - larval B7Ø.1
  - Brugia (malayi) B74.1
    - timori B74.2
  - candiru B88.8
  - Capillaria
    - hepatica B83.8
    - philippinensis B81.1
  - cat liver fluke B66.Ø
  - cestodes B71.9
    - diphyllobothrium — *see* Infestation, diphyllobothrium
    - dipylidiasis B71.1
    - hymenolepiasis B71.Ø
    - specified type NEC B71.8
  - chigger B88.Ø9
  - chigo, chigoe B88.1
  - Clonorchis (sinensis) (liver) B66.1
  - coccidial AØ7.3
  - crab-lice B85.3
  - Cysticercus cellulosae — *see* Cysticercosis
  - Demodex (brevis) (folliculorum) B88.Ø1
  - Dermanyssus gallinae B88.Ø9
  - Dermatobia (hominis) — *see* Myiasis
  - Dibothriocephalus (latus) B7Ø.Ø
    - larval B7Ø.1
  - Dicrocoelium dendriticum B66.2
  - Diphyllobothrium (adult) (latum) (intestinal) (pacificum) B7Ø.Ø
    - larval B7Ø.1
  - Diplogonoporus (grandis) B71.8
  - Dipylidium caninum B67.4
  - Distoma hepaticum B66.3
  - dog tapeworm B67.4
  - Dracunculus medinensis B72
  - dragon worm B72
  - dwarf tapeworm B71.Ø
  - Echinococcus — *see* Echinococcus
  - Echinostomum ilocanum B66.8
  - Entamoeba (histolytica) — *see* Infection, Ameba
  - Enterobius vermicularis B8Ø
  - eyelid
    - in (due to)
      - leishmaniasis B55.1
      - loiasis B74.3
      - onchocerciasis B73.Ø9
      - phthiriasis B85.3
    - parasitic NOS B89
  - eyeworm B74.3
  - Fasciola (gigantica) (hepatica) (indica) B66.3
  - Fasciolopsis (buski) (intestine) B66.5
  - filarial B74.9
    - bancroftian B74.Ø
    - conjunctiva B74.9
    - due to
      - Acanthocheilonema (perstans) (streptocerca) B74.4
      - Brugia (malayi) B74.1
- **Infestation** — *continued*
  - filarial — *continued*
    - due to — *continued*
      - Brugia — *continued*
        - timori B74.2
      - Dracunculus medinensis B72
      - guinea worm B72
      - loa loa B74.3
      - Mansonella (ozzardi) (perstans) (streptocerca) B74.4
      - Onchocerca volvulus B73.ØØ
        - eye B73.ØØ
        - eyelid B73.Ø9
      - Wuchereria (bancrofti) B74.Ø
    - Malayan B74.1
    - ozzardi B74.4
    - specified type NEC B74.8
  - fish tapeworm B7Ø.Ø
    - larval B7Ø.1
  - fluke B66.9
    - blood NOS — *see* Schistosomiasis
    - cat liver B66.Ø
    - intestinal B66.5
    - lancet B66.2
    - liver (sheep) B66.3
      - cat B66.Ø
      - Chinese B66.1
      - due to clonorchiasis B66.1
      - oriental B66.1
    - lung (oriental) B66.4
    - sheep liver B66.3
    - specified type NEC B66.8
  - fly larvae — *see* Myiasis
  - Gasterophilus (intestinalis) — *see* Myiasis
  - Gastrodiscoides hominis B66.8
  - Giardia lamblia AØ7.1
  - Gnathostoma (spinigerum) B83.1
  - Gongylonema B83.8
  - guinea worm B72
  - helminth B83.9
    - angiostrongyliasis B83.2
      - intestinal B81.3
    - gnathostomiasis B83.1
    - hirudiniasis, internal B83.4
    - intestinal B82.Ø
      - angiostrongyliasis B81.3
      - anisakiasis B81.Ø
      - ascariasis — *see* Ascariasis
      - capillariasis B81.1
      - cysticercosis — *see* Cysticercosis
      - diphyllobothriasis — *see* Infestation, diphyllobothriasis
      - dracunculiasis B72
      - echinococcus — *see* Echinococcosis
      - enterobiasis B8Ø
      - filariasis — *see* Infestation, filarial
      - fluke — *see* Infestation, fluke
      - hookworm — *see* Infestation, hookworm
      - mixed (types classifiable to more than one of the titles B65.Ø-B81.3 and B81.8) B81.4
      - onchocerciasis — *see* Onchocerciasis
      - schistosomiasis — *see* Infestation, schistosoma
      - specified
        - cestode NEC — *see* Infestation, cestode
        - type NEC B81.8
      - strongyloidiasis — *see* Strongyloidiasis
      - taenia — *see* Infestation, taenia
      - trichinellosis B75
      - trichostrongyliasis B81.2
      - trichuriasis B79
    - specified type NEC B83.8
    - syngamiasis B83.3
    - visceral larva migrans B83.Ø
  - Heterophyes (heterophyes) B66.8
  - hookworm B76.9
    - ancylostomiasis B76.Ø
    - necatoriasis B76.1
    - specified type NEC B76.8
  - Hymenolepis (diminuta) (nana) B71.Ø
  - intestinal NEC B82.9
  - leeches (aquatic) (land) — *see* Hirudiniasis
  - Leishmania — *see* Leishmaniasis
  - lice, louse — *see* Infestation, Pediculus
  - Linguatula B88.8
  - Liponyssoides sanguineus B88.Ø9
  - Loa loa B74.3
    - conjunctival B74.3
    - eyelid B74.3
  - louse — *see* Infestation, Pediculus

**Infestation** — *continued*
- maggots — *see* Myiasis
- Mansonella (ozzardi) (perstans) (streptocerca) B74.4
- Medina (worm) B72
- Metagonimus (yokogawai) B66.8
- microfilaria streptocerca — *see* Onchocerciasis
  - eye B73.ØØ
  - eyelid B73.Ø9
- mites B88.9
  - Demodex B88.Ø1
  - scabic B86
- Monilia (albicans) — *see* Candidiasis
- mouth B37.Ø
- Necator americanus B76.1
- nematode NEC (intestinal) B82.Ø
  - Ancylostoma B76.Ø
  - conjunctiva NEC B83.9
  - Enterobius vermicularis B8Ø
  - Gnathostoma spinigerum B83.1
  - physaloptera B8Ø
  - specified NEC B81.8
  - trichostrongylus B81.2
  - trichuris (trichuria) B79
- Oesophagostomum (apiostomum) B81.8
- Oestrus ovis — *see also* Myiasis B87.9
- Onchocerca (volvulus) — *see* Onchocerciasis
- Opisthorchis (felineus) (viverrini) B66.Ø
- orbit, parasitic NOS B89
- Oxyuris vermicularis B8Ø
- Paragonimus (westermani) B66.4
- parasite, parasitic B89
  - eyelid B89
  - intestinal NOS B82.9
  - mouth B37.Ø
  - skin B88.9
  - tongue B37.Ø
- Parastrongylus
  - cantonensis B83.2
  - costaricensis B81.3
- Pediculus B85.2
  - body B85.1
  - capitis (humanus) (any site) B85.Ø
  - corporis (humanus) (any site) B85.1
  - head B85.Ø
  - mixed (classifiable to more than one of the titles B85.Ø - B85.3) B85.4
  - pubis (any site) B85.3
- Pentastoma B88.8
- pest Z59.19
- Phthirus (pubis) (any site) B85.3
  - with any infestation classifiable to B85.Ø - B85.2 B85.4
- pinworm B8Ø
- pork tapeworm (adult) B68.Ø
- protozoal NEC B64
  - intestinal AØ7.9
    - specified NEC AØ7.8
  - specified NEC B6Ø.8
- pubic, louse B85.3
- rat tapeworm B71.Ø
- red bug B88.Ø9
- roundworm (large) NEC B82.Ø
  - Ascariasis — *see also* Ascariasis B77.9
- sandflea B88.1
- Sarcoptes scabiei B86
- scabies B86
- Schistosoma B65.9
  - bovis B65.8
  - cercariae B65.3
  - haematobium B65.Ø
  - intercalatum B65.8
  - japonicum B65.2
  - mansoni B65.1
  - mattheei B65.8
  - mekongi B65.8
  - specified type NEC B65.8
  - spindale B65.8
- screw worms — *see* Myiasis
- skin NOS B88.9
- Sparganum (mansoni) (proliferum) (baxteri) B7Ø.1
  - larval B7Ø.1
- specified type NEC B88.8
- Spirometra larvae B7Ø.1
- Stellantchasmus falcatus B66.8
- Strongyloides stercoralis — *see* Strongyloidiasis
- Taenia B68.9
  - diminuta B71.Ø
  - echinococcus — *see* Echinococcus
  - mediocanellata B68.1
  - nana B71.Ø

**Infestation** — *continued*
- Taenia — *continued*
  - saginata B68.1
  - solium (intestinal form) B68.Ø
    - larval form — *see* Cysticercosis
- Taeniarhynchus saginatus B68.1
- tapeworm B71.9
  - beef B68.1
  - broad B7Ø.Ø
    - larval B7Ø.1
  - dog B67.4
  - dwarf B71.Ø
  - fish B7Ø.Ø
    - larval B7Ø.1
  - pork B68.Ø
  - rat B71.Ø
- Ternidens diminutus B81.8
- Tetranychus molestissimus B88.Ø9
- threadworm B8Ø
- tongue B37.Ø
- Toxocara (canis) (cati) (felis) B83.Ø
- trematode(s) NEC — *see* Infestation, fluke
- Trichinella (spiralis) B75
- Trichocephalus B79
- Trichomonas — *see* Trichomoniasis
- Trichostrongylus B81.2
- Trichuris (trichiura) B79
- Trombicula (irritans) B88.Ø9
- Tunga penetrans B88.1
- Uncinaria americana B76.1
- Vandellia cirrhosa B88.8
- whipworm B79
- worms B83.9
  - intestinal B82.Ø
- Wuchereria (bancrofti) B74.Ø

**Infiltrate, infiltration**
- amyloid (generalized) (localized) — *see* Amyloidosis
- calcareous NEC R89.7
  - localized — *see* Degeneration, by site
- calcium salt R89.7
- cardiac
  - fatty — *see* Degeneration, myocardial
  - glycogenic E74.Ø2 *[I43]*
- corneal — *see* Edema, cornea
- eyelid — *see* Inflammation, eyelid
- glycogen, glycogenic — *see* Disease, glycogen storage
- heart, cardiac
  - fatty — *see* Degeneration, myocardial
  - glycogenic E74.Ø2 *[I43]*
- inflammatory in vitreous H43.89
- kidney N28.89
- leukemic — *see* Leukemia
- liver K76.89
  - fatty — *see* Fatty, liver NEC
  - glycogen — *see also* Disease, glycogen storage E74.Ø3 *[K77]*
- lung R91.8
  - eosinophilic — *see* Eosinophilia, pulmonary
- lymphatic — *see also* Leukemia, lymphatic C91.9- ☑
  - gland I88.9
- muscle, fatty M62.89
- myocardium, myocardial
  - fatty — *see* Degeneration, myocardial
  - glycogenic E74.Ø2 *[I43]*
- on chest x-ray R91.8
- pulmonary R91.8
  - with eosinophilia — *see* Eosinophilia, pulmonary
- skin (lymphocytic) L98.6
- thymus (gland) (fatty) E32.8
- urine R39.Ø
- vesicant agent
  - antineoplastic chemotherapy T8Ø.81Ø- ☑
  - other agent NEC T8Ø.818- ☑
- vitreous body H43.89

**Infirmity** R68.89
- senile R54

**Inflammation, inflamed, inflammatory** (with exudation)
- abducent (nerve) — *see* Strabismus, paralytic, sixth nerve
- accessory sinus (chronic) — *see* Sinusitis
- adrenal (gland) E27.8
- alveoli, teeth M27.3
  - scorbutic E54
- anal canal, anus K62.89
- antrum (chronic) — *see* Sinusitis, maxillary
- appendix — *see* Appendicitis
- arachnoid — *see* Meningitis
- areola N61.Ø
  - puerperal, postpartum or gestational — *see* Infection, nipple

**Inflammation, inflamed, inflammatory** — *continued*
- areolar tissue NOS LØ8.9
- artery — *see* Arteritis
- auditory meatus (external) — *see* Otitis, externa
- Bartholin's gland N75.8
- bile duct (common) (hepatic) or passage — *see* Cholangitis
- bladder — *see* Cystitis
- bone — *see* Osteomyelitis
- brain — *see also* Encephalitis
  - membrane — *see* Meningitis
- breast N61.Ø
  - cancer — *see* Table of Neoplasms
  - neoplasm — *see* Table of Neoplasms
  - puerperal, postpartum, gestational — *see* Mastitis, obstetric
- broad ligament — *see* Disease, pelvis, inflammatory
- bronchi — *see* Bronchitis
- catarrhal JØØ
- cecum — *see* Appendicitis
- cerebral — *see also* Encephalitis
  - membrane — *see* Meningitis
- cerebrospinal
  - meningococcal A39.Ø
- cervix (uteri) — *see* Cervicitis
- chest J98.8
- chorioretinal H3Ø.9- ☑
  - cyclitis — *see* Cyclitis
  - disseminated H3Ø.1Ø- ☑
    - generalized H3Ø.13- ☑
    - peripheral H3Ø.12- ☑
    - posterior pole H3Ø.11- ☑
  - epitheliopathy — *see* Epitheliopathy
  - focal H3Ø.ØØ- ☑
    - juxtapapillary H3Ø.Ø1- ☑
    - macular H3Ø.Ø4- ☑
    - paramacular — *see* Inflammation, chorioretinal, focal, macular
    - peripheral H3Ø.Ø3- ☑
    - posterior pole H3Ø.Ø2- ☑
  - specified type NEC H3Ø.89- ☑
- choroid — *see* Inflammation, chorioretinal
- chronic, postmastoidectomy cavity — *see* Complications, postmastoidectomy, inflammation
- colon — *see* Enteritis
- connective tissue (diffuse) NEC — *see* Disorder, soft tissue, specified type NEC
- cornea — *see* Keratitis
- corpora cavernosa N48.29
- cranial nerve — *see* Disorder, nerve, cranial
- Douglas' cul-de-sac or pouch (chronic) N73.Ø
- due to device, implant or graft — *see also* Complications, by site and type, infection or inflammation
  - arterial graft T82.7- ☑
  - breast (implant) T85.79- ☑
  - catheter T85.79- ☑
    - dialysis (renal) T82.7- ☑
      - intraperitoneal T85.71- ☑
    - infusion T82.7- ☑
      - cranial T85.735- ☑
      - intrathecal T85.735- ☑
      - spinal (epidural) (subdural) T85.735- ☑
      - subarachnoid T85.735- ☑
    - urinary T83.518- ☑
      - cystostomy T83.51Ø- ☑
      - Hopkins T83.518- ☑
      - ileostomy T83.518- ☑
      - nephrostomy T83.512- ☑
      - specified NEC T83.518- ☑
      - urethral indwelling T83.511- ☑
      - urostomy T83.518- ☑
  - electronic (electrode) (pulse generator) (stimulator)
    - bone T84.7- ☑
    - cardiac T82.7- ☑
    - nervous system T85.738- ☑
      - brain T85.731- ☑
      - cranial nerve T85.732- ☑
      - gastric nerve T85.732- ☑
      - neurostimulator generator T85.734- ☑
      - peripheral nerve T85.732- ☑
      - sacral nerve T85.732- ☑
      - spinal cord T85.733- ☑
      - vagal nerve T85.732- ☑
    - urinary T83.59Ø- ☑
  - fixation, internal (orthopedic) NEC — *see* Complication, fixation device, infection
  - gastrointestinal (bile duct) (esophagus) T85.79- ☑

**Influenza** — *continued*
- due to — *continued*
  - identified novel influenza A virus — *continued*
    - with — *continued*
      - specified manifestation NEC JØ9.X9
      - upper respiratory symptoms JØ9.X2
  - novel (2ØØ9) H1N1 influenza — *see also* Influenza, due to, identified influenza virus NEC J1Ø.1
  - novel influenza A/H1N1 — *see also* Influenza, due to, identified influenza virus NEC J1Ø.1
  - of other animal origin, not bird or swine — *see also* Influenza, due to, identified novel influenza A virus JØ9.X2
  - swine (viruses that normally cause infections in pigs) — *see also* Influenza, due to, identified novel influenza A virus JØ9.X2

**Influenza-like disease** — *see* Influenza

**Influenzal** — *see* Influenza

**Infraction, Freiberg's** (metatarsal head) — *see* Osteochondrosis, juvenile, metatarsus

**Infraeruption of tooth** (teeth) M26.34

**Infusion complication, misadventure, or reaction** — *see* Complications, infusion

**Ingestion**
- chemical — *see* Table of Drugs and Chemicals, by substance, poisoning
- drug or medicament
  - correct substance properly administered — *see* Table of Drugs and Chemicals, by drug, adverse effect
  - overdose or wrong substance given or taken — *see* Table of Drugs and Chemicals, by drug, poisoning
- foreign body — *see* Foreign body, alimentary tract
- multiple drug — *see* Table of Drugs and Chemicals, multiple
- tularemia A21.3

**Ingrowing**
- hair (beard) L73.1
- nail (finger) (toe) L6Ø.Ø

**Inguinal** — *see also* condition
- testicle Q53.9
  - bilateral Q53.212
  - unilateral Q53.112

**Inhalant-induced**
- anxiety disorder F18.98Ø
- depressive disorder F18.94
- major neurocognitive disorder F18.97
- mild neurocognitive disorder F18.988
- psychotic disorder F18.959

**Inhalation**
- anthrax A22.1
- flame T27.3- ☑
- food or foreign body — *see* Foreign body, by site
- gases, fumes, or vapors T59.9- ☑
  - specified agent NEC — *see* Table of Drugs and Chemicals, by substance T59.89- ☑
- liquid or vomitus — *see* Asphyxia
- meconium (newborn) P24.ØØ
  - with
    - with respiratory symptoms P24.Ø1
    - pneumonia (pneumonitis) P24.Ø1
- mucus — *see* Asphyxia, mucus
- oil or gasoline (causing suffocation) — *see* Foreign body, by site
- smoke T59.81- ☑
  - with respiratory conditions J7Ø.5
    - due to chemicals, gases, fumes and vapors J68.9
- steam — *see also* Burn, respiratory tract T59.9- ☑
- stomach contents or secretions — *see* Foreign body, by site
  - due to anesthesia (general) (local) or other sedation T88.59- ☑
    - in labor and delivery O74.Ø
    - in pregnancy O29.Ø1- ☑
    - postpartum, puerperal O89.Ø1

**Inhibition, orgasm**
- female F52.31
- male F52.32

**Inhibitor, systemic lupus erythematosus** (presence of) D68.62

**Iniencephalus, iniencephaly** QØØ.2

**Injection, traumatic jet** (air) (industrial) (water) (paint or dye) T7Ø.4- ☑

**Injury** — *see also* specified injury type T14.9Ø- ☑
- abdomen, abdominal S39.91- ☑
  - blood vessel — *see* Injury, blood vessel, abdomen
  - cavity — *see* Injury, intra-abdominal
  - contusion S3Ø.11- ☑

**Injury** — *continued*
- abdomen, abdominal — *continued*
  - internal — *see* Injury, intra-abdominal
  - intra-abdominal organ — *see* Injury, intra-abdominal
  - nerve — *see* Injury, nerve, abdomen
  - open — *see* Wound, open, abdomen
  - specified NEC S39.81- ☑
  - superficial — *see* Injury, superficial, abdomen
- Achilles tendon S86.ØØ- ☑
  - laceration S86.Ø2- ☑
  - specified type NEC S86.Ø9- ☑
  - strain S86.Ø1- ☑
- acoustic, resulting in deafness — *see* Injury, nerve, acoustic
- adrenal (gland) S37.819- ☑
  - contusion S37.812- ☑
  - laceration S37.813- ☑
  - specified type NEC S37.818- ☑
- alveolar (process) SØ9.93- ☑
- ankle S99.91- ☑
  - contusion — *see* Contusion, ankle
  - dislocation — *see* Dislocation, ankle
  - fracture — *see* Fracture, ankle
  - nerve — *see* Injury, nerve, ankle
  - open — *see* Wound, open, ankle
  - specified type NEC S99.81- ☑
  - sprain — *see* Sprain, ankle
  - superficial — *see* Injury, superficial, ankle
- anterior chamber, eye — *see* Injury, eye, specified site NEC
- anus — *see* Injury, abdomen
- aorta (thoracic) S25.ØØ- ☑
  - abdominal S35.ØØ- ☑
    - laceration (minor) (superficial) S35.Ø1- ☑
      - major S35.Ø2- ☑
    - specified type NEC S35.Ø9- ☑
  - laceration (minor) (superficial) S25.Ø1- ☑
    - major S25.Ø2- ☑
  - specified type NEC S25.Ø9- ☑
- arm (upper) S49.9- ☑
  - blood vessel — *see* Injury, blood vessel, arm
  - contusion — *see* Contusion, arm, upper
  - fracture — *see* Fracture, humerus
  - lower — *see* Injury, forearm
  - muscle — *see* Injury, muscle, shoulder
  - nerve — *see* Injury, nerve, arm
  - open — *see* Wound, open, arm
  - specified type NEC S49.8- ☑
  - superficial — *see* Injury, superficial, arm
- artery (complicating trauma) — *see also* Injury, blood vessel, by site
  - cerebral or meningeal — *see* Injury, intracranial
- auditory canal (external) (meatus) SØ9.91- ☑
- auricle, auris, ear SØ9.91- ☑
- axilla — *see* Injury, shoulder
- back — *see* Injury, back, lower
- bile duct S36.13- ☑
- birth — *see also* Birth, injury P15.9
- bladder (sphincter) S37.2Ø- ☑
  - at delivery O71.5
  - contusion S37.22- ☑
  - laceration S37.23- ☑
  - obstetrical trauma O71.5
  - specified type NEC S37.29- ☑
- blast (air) (hydraulic) (immersion) (underwater) NEC T14.8- ☑
  - acoustic nerve trauma — *see* Injury, nerve, acoustic
  - bladder — *see* Injury, bladder
  - brain — *see* Concussion
    - primary, specified NEC SØ6.8A- ☑
  - colon — *see* Injury, intestine, large
  - ear (primary) SØ9.31- ☑
    - secondary SØ9.39- ☑
  - generalized T7Ø.8- ☑
  - lung — *see* Injury, intrathoracic, lung
  - multiple body organs T7Ø.8- ☑
  - peritoneum S36.81- ☑
  - rectum S36.61- ☑
  - retroperitoneum S36.898- ☑
  - small intestine S36.419- ☑
    - duodenum S36.41Ø- ☑
    - specified site NEC S36.418- ☑
  - specified
    - intra-abdominal organ NEC S36.898- ☑
    - pelvic organ NEC S37.899- ☑
- blood vessel NEC T14.8- ☑
  - abdomen S35.9- ☑

**Injury** — *continued*
- blood vessel — *continued*
  - abdomen — *continued*
    - aorta — *see* Injury, aorta, abdominal
    - celiac artery — *see* Injury, blood vessel, celiac artery
    - iliac vessel — *see* Injury, blood vessel, iliac
    - laceration S35.91- ☑
    - mesenteric vessel — *see* Injury, mesenteric
    - portal vein — *see* Injury, blood vessel, portal vein
    - renal vessel — *see* Injury, blood vessel, renal
    - specified vessel NEC S35.8X- ☑
    - splenic vessel — *see* Injury, blood vessel, splenic
    - vena cava — *see* Injury, vena cava, inferior
  - ankle — *see* Injury, blood vessel, foot
  - aorta (abdominal) (thoracic) — *see* Injury, aorta
  - arm (upper) NEC S45.9Ø- ☑
    - forearm — *see* Injury, blood vessel, forearm
    - laceration S45.91- ☑
    - specified
      - site NEC S45.8Ø- ☑
        - laceration S45.81- ☑
        - specified type NEC S45.89- ☑
      - type NEC S45.99- ☑
    - superficial vein S45.3Ø- ☑
      - laceration S45.31- ☑
      - specified type NEC S45.39- ☑
  - axillary
    - artery S45.ØØ- ☑
      - laceration S45.Ø1- ☑
      - specified type NEC S45.Ø9- ☑
    - vein S45.2Ø- ☑
      - laceration S45.21- ☑
      - specified type NEC S45.29- ☑
  - azygos vein — *see* Injury, blood vessel, thoracic, specified site NEC
  - brachial
    - artery S45.1Ø- ☑
      - laceration S45.11- ☑
      - specified type NEC S45.19- ☑
    - vein S45.2Ø- ☑
      - laceration S45.219- ☑
      - specified type NEC S45.29- ☑
  - carotid artery (common) (external) (internal, extracranial) S15.ØØ- ☑
    - internal, intracranial SØ6.8- ☑
    - laceration (minor) (superficial) S15.Ø1- ☑
      - major S15.Ø2- ☑
    - specified type NEC S15.Ø9- ☑
  - celiac artery S35.219- ☑
    - branch S35.299- ☑
      - laceration (minor) (superficial) S35.291- ☑
        - major S35.292- ☑
      - specified NEC S35.298- ☑
    - laceration (minor) (superficial) S35.211- ☑
      - major S35.212- ☑
    - specified type NEC S35.218- ☑
  - cerebral — *see* Injury, intracranial
  - deep plantar — *see* Injury, blood vessel, plantar artery
  - digital (hand) — *see* Injury, blood vessel, finger
  - dorsal
    - artery (foot) S95.ØØ- ☑
      - laceration S95.Ø1- ☑
      - specified type NEC S95.Ø9- ☑
    - vein (foot) S95.2Ø- ☑
      - laceration S95.21- ☑
      - specified type NEC S95.29- ☑
  - due to accidental laceration during procedure — *see* Laceration, accidental complicating surgery
  - extremity — *see* Injury, blood vessel, limb
  - femoral
    - artery (common) (superficial) S75.ØØ- ☑
      - laceration (minor) (superficial) S75.Ø1- ☑
        - major S75.Ø2- ☑
      - specified type NEC S75.Ø9- ☑
    - vein (hip level) (thigh level) S75.1Ø- ☑
      - laceration (minor) (superficial) S75.11- ☑
        - major S75.12- ☑
      - specified type NEC S75.19- ☑
  - finger S65.5Ø- ☑
    - index S65.5Ø- ☑
      - laceration S65.51- ☑
      - specified type NEC S65.59- ☑
    - laceration S65.51- ☑
    - little S65.5Ø- ☑
      - laceration S65.51- ☑



Index

Influenza — Injury

- **Injury** — *continued*
  - intrathoracic — *continued*
    - bronchus — *continued*
      - laceration S27.439- ☑
        - bilateral S27.432- ☑
        - unilateral S27.431- ☑
      - specified type NEC S27.499- ☑
        - bilateral S27.492- ☑
        - unilateral S27.491- ☑
      - unilateral S27.4Ø1- ☑
    - diaphragm S27.8Ø9- ☑
      - contusion S27.8Ø2- ☑
      - laceration S27.8Ø3- ☑
      - specified type NEC S27.8Ø8- ☑
    - esophagus (thoracic) S27.819- ☑
      - contusion S27.812- ☑
      - laceration S27.813- ☑
      - specified type NEC S27.818- ☑
    - heart — *see* Injury, heart
    - hemopneumothorax S27.2- ☑
    - hemothorax S27.1- ☑
    - lung S27.3Ø9- ☑
      - aspiration J69.Ø
      - bilateral S27.3Ø2- ☑
      - blast injury (primary) S27.319- ☑
        - bilateral S27.312- ☑
        - secondary — *see* Injury, intrathoracic, lung, specified type NEC
        - unilateral S27.311- ☑
      - contusion S27.329- ☑
        - bilateral S27.322- ☑
        - unilateral S27.321- ☑
      - laceration S27.339- ☑
        - bilateral S27.332- ☑
        - unilateral S27.331- ☑
      - specified type NEC S27.399- ☑
        - bilateral S27.392- ☑
        - unilateral S27.391- ☑
      - unilateral S27.3Ø1- ☑
    - pleura S27.6Ø- ☑
      - laceration S27.63- ☑
      - specified type NEC S27.69- ☑
    - pneumothorax S27.Ø- ☑
    - specified organ NEC S27.899- ☑
      - contusion S27.892- ☑
      - laceration S27.893- ☑
      - specified type NEC S27.898- ☑
    - thoracic duct — *see* Injury, intrathoracic, specified organ NEC
    - thymus gland — *see* Injury, intrathoracic, specified organ NEC
    - trachea, thoracic S27.5Ø- ☑
      - blast (primary) S27.51- ☑
      - contusion S27.52- ☑
      - laceration S27.53- ☑
      - specified type NEC S27.59- ☑
  - iris — *see* Injury, eye, specified site NEC
    - penetrating — *see* Injury, eyeball, penetrating
  - jaw SØ9.93- ☑
  - jejunum — *see* Injury, intestine, small
  - joint NOS T14.8- ☑
    - old or residual — *see* Disorder, joint, specified type NEC
  - kidney S37.ØØ- ☑
    - acute (nontraumatic) N17.9
    - contusion — *see* Contusion, kidney
    - laceration — *see* Laceration, kidney
    - specified NEC S37.Ø9- ☑
  - knee S89.9- ☑
    - contusion — *see* Contusion, knee
    - dislocation — *see* Dislocation, knee
    - meniscus (lateral) (medial) — *see* Sprain, knee, specified site NEC
      - old injury or tear — *see* Derangement, knee, meniscus, due to old injury
    - open — *see* Wound, open, knee
    - specified NEC S89.8- ☑
    - sprain — *see* Sprain, knee
    - superficial — *see* Injury, superficial, knee
  - labium (majus) (minus) S39.94- ☑
  - labyrinth, ear SØ9.3Ø- ☑
  - lacrimal apparatus, duct, gland, or sac — *see* Injury, eye, specified site NEC
  - larynx NEC S19.81- ☑
  - leg (lower) S89.9- ☑
    - blood vessel — *see* Injury, blood vessel, leg

- **Injury** — *continued*
  - leg — *continued*
    - contusion — *see* Contusion, leg
    - fracture — *see* Fracture, leg
    - muscle — *see* Injury, muscle, leg
    - nerve — *see* Injury, nerve, leg
    - open — *see* Wound, open, leg
    - specified NEC S89.8- ☑
    - superficial — *see* Injury, superficial, leg
  - lens, eye — *see* Injury, eye, specified site NEC
    - penetrating — *see* Injury, eyeball, penetrating
  - limb NEC T14.8- ☑
  - lip SØ9.93- ☑
  - liver S36.119- ☑
    - contusion S36.112- ☑
    - laceration S36.113- ☑
      - major (stellate) S36.116- ☑
      - minor S36.114- ☑
      - moderate S36.115- ☑
    - specified NEC S36.118- ☑
  - lower back S39.92- ☑
    - specified NEC S39.82- ☑
  - lumbar, lumbosacral (region) S39.92- ☑
    - plexus — *see* Injury, lumbosacral plexus
  - lumbosacral plexus S34.4- ☑
  - lung — *see also* Injury, intrathoracic, lung
    - aspiration J69.Ø
    - dabbing (related) UØ7.Ø
    - electronic cigarette (related) UØ7.Ø
    - EVALI [e-cigarette, or vaping, product use associated] UØ7.Ø
    - transfusion-related (TRALI) J95.84
    - vaping (associated) (device) (product) (use) UØ7.Ø
  - lymphatic thoracic duct — *see* Injury, intrathoracic, specified organ NEC
  - malar region SØ9.93- ☑
  - mastoid region SØ9.9Ø- ☑
  - maxilla SØ9.93- ☑
  - mediastinum — *see* Injury, intrathoracic, specified organ NEC
  - membrane, brain — *see* Injury, intracranial
  - meningeal artery — *see* Injury, intracranial, subdural hemorrhage
  - meninges (cerebral) — *see* Injury, intracranial
  - mesenteric
    - artery
      - branch S35.299- ☑
        - laceration (minor) (superficial) S35.291- ☑
          - major S35.292- ☑
        - specified NEC S35.298- ☑
      - inferior S35.239- ☑
        - laceration (minor) (superficial) S35.231- ☑
          - major S35.232- ☑
        - specified NEC S35.238- ☑
      - superior S35.229- ☑
        - laceration (minor) (superficial) S35.221- ☑
          - major S35.222- ☑
        - specified NEC S35.228- ☑
    - plexus (inferior) (superior) — *see* Injury, nerve, lumbosacral, sympathetic
    - vein
      - inferior S35.349- ☑
        - laceration S35.341- ☑
        - specified NEC S35.348- ☑
      - superior S35.339- ☑
        - laceration S35.331- ☑
        - specified NEC S35.338- ☑
  - mesentery — *see* Injury, intra-abdominal, specified site NEC
  - mesosalpinx — *see* Injury, pelvic organ, specified site NEC
  - middle ear SØ9.3Ø- ☑
  - midthoracic region NOS S29.9- ☑
  - mouth SØ9.93- ☑
  - multiple NOS TØ7.- ☑
  - muscle (and fascia) (and tendon)
    - abdomen S39.ØØ1- ☑
      - laceration S39.Ø21- ☑
      - specified type NEC S39.Ø91- ☑
      - strain S39.Ø11- ☑
    - abductor
      - thumb, forearm level — *see* Injury, muscle, thumb, abductor
    - adductor
      - thigh S76.2Ø- ☑
        - laceration S76.22- ☑
        - specified type NEC S76.29- ☑

- **Injury** — *continued*
  - muscle — *continued*
    - adductor — *continued*
      - thigh — *continued*
        - strain S76.21- ☑
    - ankle — *see* Injury, muscle, foot
    - anterior muscle group, at leg level (lower) S86.2Ø- ☑
      - laceration S86.22- ☑
      - specified type NEC S86.29- ☑
      - strain S86.21- ☑
    - arm (upper) — *see* Injury, muscle, shoulder
    - biceps (parts NEC) S46.2Ø- ☑
      - laceration S46.22- ☑
      - long head S46.1Ø- ☑
        - laceration S46.12- ☑
        - specified type NEC S46.19- ☑
        - strain S46.11- ☑
      - specified type NEC S46.29- ☑
      - strain S46.21- ☑
    - extensor
      - finger(s) (other than thumb) — *see* Injury, muscle, finger by site, extensor
      - forearm level, specified NEC — *see* Injury, muscle, forearm, extensor
      - thumb — *see* Injury, muscle, thumb, extensor
      - toe (large) (ankle level) (foot level) — *see* Injury, muscle, toe, extensor
    - finger
      - extensor (forearm level) S56.4Ø- ☑
        - hand level S66.3Ø9- ☑
          - laceration S66.329- ☑
          - specified type NEC S66.399- ☑
          - strain S66.319- ☑
        - laceration S56.429- ☑
        - specified type NEC S56.499- ☑
        - strain S56.419- ☑
      - flexor (forearm level) S56.1Ø- ☑
        - hand level S66.1Ø9- ☑
          - laceration S66.129- ☑
          - specified type NEC S66.199- ☑
          - strain S66.119- ☑
        - laceration S56.129- ☑
        - specified type NEC S56.199- ☑
        - strain S56.119- ☑
      - index
        - extensor (forearm level)
          - hand level S66.3Ø8- ☑
            - laceration S66.32- ☑
            - specified type NEC S66.39- ☑
            - strain S66.31- ☑
          - specified type NEC S56.492- ☑
        - flexor (forearm level)
          - hand level S66.1Ø8- ☑
            - laceration S66.12- ☑
            - specified type NEC S66.19- ☑
            - strain S66.11- ☑
          - specified type NEC S56.19- ☑
          - strain S56.11- ☑
        - intrinsic S66.5Ø- ☑
          - laceration S66.52- ☑
          - specified type NEC S66.59- ☑
          - strain S66.51- ☑
      - intrinsic S66.5Ø9- ☑
        - laceration S66.529- ☑
        - specified type NEC S66.599- ☑
        - strain S66.519- ☑
      - little
        - extensor (forearm level)
          - hand level S66.3Ø- ☑
            - laceration S66.32- ☑
            - specified type NEC S66.39- ☑
            - strain S66.31- ☑
          - laceration S56.42- ☑
          - specified type NEC S56.49- ☑
          - strain S56.41- ☑
        - flexor (forearm level)
          - hand level S66.1Ø- ☑
            - laceration S66.12- ☑
            - specified type NEC S66.19- ☑
            - strain S66.11- ☑
          - laceration S56.12- ☑
          - specified type NEC S56.19- ☑
          - strain S56.11- ☑
        - intrinsic S66.5Ø- ☑
          - laceration S66.52- ☑
          - specified type NEC S66.59- ☑

- **Injury** — *continued*
  - nerve — *continued*
    - ulnar (forearm level) S54.Ø- ☑
      - arm (upper) (level) S44.Ø- ☑
      - hand (level) S64.Ø- ☑
      - wrist (level) — *see* Injury, nerve, ulnar, hand
    - vagus SØ4.89- ☑
      - specified type NEC SØ4.89- ☑
    - wrist (level) — *see* Injury, nerve, hand
  - ninth cranial nerve (glossopharyngeal) — *see* Injury, nerve, glossopharyngeal
  - nose (septum) SØ9.92- ☑
  - obstetrical O71.9
    - specified NEC O71.89
  - occipital (region) (scalp) SØ9.9Ø- ☑
    - lobe — *see* Injury, intracranial
  - optic chiasm SØ4.Ø2- ☑
  - optic radiation SØ4.Ø3- ☑
  - optic tract and pathways SØ4.Ø3- ☑
  - orbit, orbital (region) — *see* Injury, eye
    - penetrating (with foreign body) — *see* Injury, eye, orbit, penetrating
    - specified NEC — *see* Injury, eye, specified site NEC
  - ovary, ovarian S37.4Ø9- ☑
    - bilateral S37.4Ø2- ☑
      - contusion S37.422- ☑
      - laceration S37.432- ☑
      - specified type NEC S37.492- ☑
    - blood vessel — *see* Injury, blood vessel, ovarian
    - contusion S37.429- ☑
      - bilateral S37.422- ☑
      - unilateral S37.421- ☑
    - laceration S37.439- ☑
      - bilateral S37.432- ☑
      - unilateral S37.431- ☑
    - specified type NEC S37.499- ☑
      - bilateral S37.492- ☑
      - unilateral S37.491- ☑
    - unilateral S37.4Ø1- ☑
      - contusion S37.421- ☑
      - laceration S37.431- ☑
      - specified type NEC S37.491- ☑
  - palate (hard) (soft) SØ9.93- ☑
  - pancreas S36.2Ø9- ☑
    - body S36.2Ø1- ☑
      - contusion S36.221- ☑
      - laceration S36.231- ☑
        - major S36.261- ☑
        - minor S36.241- ☑
        - moderate S36.251- ☑
      - specified type NEC S36.291- ☑
    - contusion S36.229- ☑
    - head S36.2ØØ- ☑
      - contusion S36.22Ø- ☑
      - laceration S36.23Ø- ☑
        - major S36.26Ø- ☑
        - minor S36.24Ø- ☑
        - moderate S36.25Ø- ☑
      - specified type NEC S36.29Ø- ☑
    - laceration S36.239- ☑
      - major S36.269- ☑
      - minor S36.249- ☑
      - moderate S36.259- ☑
    - specified type NEC S36.299- ☑
    - tail S36.2Ø2- ☑
      - contusion S36.222- ☑
      - laceration S36.232- ☑
        - major S36.262- ☑
        - minor S36.242- ☑
        - moderate S36.252- ☑
      - specified type NEC S36.292- ☑
  - parietal (region) (scalp) SØ9.9Ø- ☑
    - lobe — *see* Injury, intracranial
  - patellar ligament (tendon) S76.1Ø- ☑
    - laceration S76.12- ☑
    - specified NEC S76.19- ☑
    - strain S76.11- ☑
  - pelvis, pelvic (floor) S39.93- ☑
    - complicating delivery O7Ø.1
    - joint or ligament, complicating delivery O71.6
    - organ S37.9Ø- ☑
      - with ectopic or molar pregnancy OØ8.6
      - complication of abortion — *see* Abortion
      - contusion S37.92- ☑
      - following ectopic or molar pregnancy OØ8.6
      - laceration S37.93- ☑

- **Injury** — *continued*
  - pelvis, pelvic — *continued*
    - organ — *continued*
      - obstetrical trauma NEC O71.5
      - specified
        - site NEC S37.899- ☑
          - contusion S37.892- ☑
          - laceration S37.893- ☑
          - specified type NEC S37.898- ☑
        - type NEC S37.99- ☑
    - specified NEC S39.83- ☑
  - penis S39.94- ☑
  - perineum S39.94- ☑
  - peritoneum S36.81- ☑
    - laceration S36.893- ☑
  - periurethral tissue — *see* Injury, urethra
    - complicating delivery O71.82
  - phalanges
    - foot — *see* Injury, foot
    - hand — *see* Injury, hand
  - pharynx NEC S19.85- ☑
  - pleura — *see* Injury, intrathoracic, pleura
  - plexus
    - brachial — *see* Injury, brachial plexus
    - cardiac — *see* Injury, nerve, thorax, sympathetic
    - celiac, coeliac — *see* Injury, nerve, lumbosacral, sympathetic
    - esophageal — *see* Injury, nerve, thorax, sympathetic
    - hypogastric — *see* Injury, nerve, lumbosacral, sympathetic
    - lumbar, lumbosacral — *see* Injury, lumbosacral plexus
    - mesenteric — *see* Injury, nerve, lumbosacral, sympathetic
    - pulmonary — *see* Injury, nerve, thorax, sympathetic
  - postcardiac surgery (syndrome) I97.Ø
  - prepuce S39.94- ☑
  - pressure
    - injury — *see* Ulcer, pressure, by site
  - prostate S37.829- ☑
    - contusion S37.822- ☑
    - laceration S37.823- ☑
    - specified type NEC S37.828- ☑
  - pubic region S39.94- ☑
  - pudendum S39.94- ☑
  - pulmonary plexus — *see* Injury, nerve, thorax, sympathetic
  - rectovaginal septum NEC S39.83- ☑
  - rectum — *see* Injury, intestine, large, rectum
  - retina — *see* Injury, eye, specified site NEC
    - penetrating — *see* Injury, eyeball, penetrating
  - retroperitoneal — *see* Injury, intra-abdominal, specified site NEC
  - rotator cuff (muscle(s)) (tendon(s)) S46.ØØ- ☑
    - laceration S46.Ø2- ☑
    - specified type NEC S46.Ø9- ☑
    - strain S46.Ø1- ☑
  - round ligament — *see* Injury, pelvic organ, specified site NEC
  - sacral plexus — *see* Injury, lumbosacral plexus
  - salivary duct or gland SØ9.93- ☑
  - scalp SØ9.9Ø- ☑
    - newborn (birth injury) P12.9
      - due to monitoring (electrode) (sampling incision) P12.4
      - specified NEC P12.89
        - caput succedaneum P12.81
  - scapular region — *see* Injury, shoulder
  - sclera — *see* Injury, eye, specified site NEC
    - penetrating — *see* Injury, eyeball, penetrating
  - scrotum S39.94- ☑
  - second cranial nerve (optic) — *see* Injury, nerve, optic
  - self-inflicted, without suicidal intent R45.88
  - seminal vesicle — *see* Injury, pelvic organ, specified site NEC
  - seventh cranial nerve (facial) — *see* Injury, nerve, facial
  - shoulder S49.9- ☑
    - blood vessel — *see* Injury, blood vessel, arm
    - contusion — *see* Contusion, shoulder
    - dislocation — *see* Dislocation, shoulder
    - fracture — *see* Fracture, shoulder
    - muscle — *see* Injury, muscle, shoulder
    - nerve — *see* Injury, nerve, shoulder
    - open — *see* Wound, open, shoulder
    - specified type NEC S49.8- ☑
    - sprain — *see* Sprain, shoulder girdle
    - superficial — *see* Injury, superficial, shoulder

- **Injury** — *continued*
  - sinus
    - cavernous — *see* Injury, intracranial
    - nasal SØ9.92- ☑
  - sixth cranial nerve (abducent) — *see* Injury, nerve, abducens
  - skeleton, birth injury P13.9
    - specified part NEC P13.8
  - skin NEC T14.8- ☑
    - surface intact — *see* Injury, superficial
  - skull NEC SØ9.9Ø- ☑
  - specified NEC T14.8- ☑
  - spermatic cord (pelvic region) S37.898- ☑
    - scrotal region S39.848- ☑
  - spinal (cord)
    - cervical (neck) S14.1Ø9- ☑
      - anterior cord syndrome S14.139- ☑
        - C1 level S14.131- ☑
        - C2 level S14.132- ☑
        - C3 level S14.133- ☑
        - C4 level S14.134- ☑
        - C5 level S14.135- ☑
        - C6 level S14.136- ☑
        - C7 level S14.137- ☑
        - C8 level S14.138- ☑
      - Brown-Sequard syndrome S14.149- ☑
        - C1 level S14.141- ☑
        - C2 level S14.142- ☑
        - C3 level S14.143- ☑
        - C4 level S14.144- ☑
        - C5 level S14.145- ☑
        - C6 level S14.146- ☑
        - C7 level S14.147- ☑
        - C8 level S14.148- ☑
      - C1 level S14.1Ø1- ☑
      - C2 level S14.1Ø2- ☑
      - C3 level S14.1Ø3- ☑
      - C4 level S14.1Ø4- ☑
      - C5 level S14.1Ø5- ☑
      - C6 level S14.1Ø6- ☑
      - C7 level S14.1Ø7- ☑
      - C8 level S14.1Ø8- ☑
      - central cord syndrome S14.129- ☑
        - C1 level S14.121- ☑
        - C2 level S14.122- ☑
        - C3 level S14.123- ☑
        - C4 level S14.124- ☑
        - C5 level S14.125- ☑
        - C6 level S14.126- ☑
        - C7 level S14.127- ☑
        - C8 level S14.128- ☑
      - complete lesion S14.119- ☑
        - C1 level S14.111- ☑
        - C2 level S14.112- ☑
        - C3 level S14.113- ☑
        - C4 level S14.114- ☑
        - C5 level S14.115- ☑
        - C6 level S14.116- ☑
        - C7 level S14.117- ☑
        - C8 level S14.118- ☑
      - concussion S14.Ø- ☑
      - edema S14.Ø- ☑
      - incomplete lesion specified NEC S14.159- ☑
        - C1 level S14.151- ☑
        - C2 level S14.152- ☑
        - C3 level S14.153- ☑
        - C4 level S14.154- ☑
        - C5 level S14.155- ☑
        - C6 level S14.156- ☑
        - C7 level S14.157- ☑
        - C8 level S14.158- ☑
      - posterior cord syndrome S14.159- ☑
        - C1 level S14.151- ☑
        - C2 level S14.152- ☑
        - C3 level S14.153- ☑
        - C4 level S14.154- ☑
        - C5 level S14.155- ☑
        - C6 level S14.156- ☑
        - C7 level S14.157- ☑
        - C8 level S14.158- ☑
    - dorsal — *see* Injury, spinal, thoracic
    - lumbar S34.1Ø9- ☑
      - complete lesion S34.119- ☑
        - L1 level S34.111- ☑
        - L2 level S34.112- ☑

- **Injury** — *continued*
  - urinary organ — *continued*
    - specified
      - site NEC S37.899- ☑
        - contusion S37.892- ☑
        - laceration S37.893- ☑
        - specified type NEC S37.898- ☑
      - type NEC S37.99- ☑
  - uterus, uterine S37.6Ø- ☑
    - with ectopic or molar pregnancy OØ8.6
    - blood vessel — *see* Injury, blood vessel, iliac
    - contusion S37.62- ☑
    - laceration S37.63- ☑
      - cervix at delivery O71.3
    - rupture associated with obstetrics — *see* Rupture, uterus
    - specified type NEC S37.69- ☑
  - uvula SØ9.93- ☑
  - vagina S39.93- ☑
    - abrasion S3Ø.814- ☑
    - bite S31.45- ☑
      - insect S3Ø.864- ☑
      - superficial NEC S3Ø.874- ☑
    - contusion S3Ø.23- ☑
    - crush S38.Ø3- ☑
    - during delivery — *see* Laceration, vagina, during delivery
    - external constriction S3Ø.844- ☑
    - insect bite S3Ø.864- ☑
    - laceration S31.41- ☑
      - with foreign body S31.42- ☑
    - open wound S31.4Ø- ☑
    - puncture S31.43- ☑
      - with foreign body S31.44- ☑
    - superficial S3Ø.95- ☑
      - foreign body S3Ø.854- ☑
  - vas deferens — *see* Injury, pelvic organ, specified site NEC
  - vascular NEC T14.8- ☑
  - vein — *see* Injury, blood vessel
  - vena cava (superior) S25.2Ø- ☑
    - inferior S35.1Ø- ☑
      - laceration (minor) (superficial) S35.11- ☑
        - major S35.12- ☑
      - specified type NEC S35.19- ☑
    - laceration (minor) (superficial) S25.21- ☑
      - major S25.22- ☑
    - specified type NEC S25.29- ☑
  - vesical (sphincter) — *see* Injury, bladder
  - visual cortex SØ4.Ø4- ☑
  - vitreous (humor) SØ5.9Ø- ☑
    - specified NEC SØ5.8X- ☑
  - vocal cord NEC S19.83- ☑
  - vulva S39.94- ☑
    - abrasion S3Ø.814- ☑
    - bite S31.45- ☑
      - insect S3Ø.864- ☑
      - superficial NEC S3Ø.874- ☑
    - contusion S3Ø.23- ☑
    - crush S38.Ø3- ☑
    - during delivery — *see* Laceration, perineum, female, during delivery
    - external constriction S3Ø.844- ☑
    - insect bite S3Ø.864- ☑
    - laceration S31.41- ☑
      - with foreign body S31.42- ☑
    - open wound S31.4Ø- ☑
    - puncture S31.43- ☑
      - with foreign body S31.44- ☑
    - superficial S3Ø.95- ☑
      - foreign body S3Ø.854- ☑
  - whiplash (cervical spine) S13.4- ☑
  - wrist S69.9- ☑
    - blood vessel — *see* Injury, blood vessel, hand
    - contusion — *see* Contusion, wrist
    - dislocation — *see* Dislocation, wrist
    - fracture — *see* Fracture, wrist
    - muscle — *see* Injury, muscle, hand
    - nerve — *see* Injury, nerve, hand
    - open — *see* Wound, open, wrist
    - specified NEC S69.8- ☑
    - sprain — *see* Sprain, wrist
    - superficial — *see* Injury, superficial, wrist
- **Inoculation** — *see also* Vaccination
  - complication or reaction — *see* Complications, vaccination
- **Insanity, insane** — *see also* Psychosis
  - adolescent — *see* Schizophrenia
  - confusional F28
    - acute or subacute FØ5
  - delusional F22
  - senile FØ3.- ☑
- **Insect**
  - bite — *see* Bite, by site, superficial, insect
  - venomous, poisoning NEC (by) — *see* Venom, arthropod
- **Insecurity**
  - financial Z59.869
  - food Z59.41
  - transportation Z59.82
- **Insensitivity**
  - adrenocorticotropin hormone (ACTH) E27.49
  - androgen E34.5Ø
    - complete E34.51
    - partial E34.52
- **Insertion**
  - cord (umbilical) lateral or velamentous O43.12- ☑
  - intrauterine contraceptive device (encounter for) — *see* Intrauterine contraceptive device
- **Insolation** (sunstroke) T67.Ø1- ☑
- **Insomnia** (organic) G47.ØØ
  - adjustment F51.Ø2
  - adjustment disorder F51.Ø2
  - behavioral, of childhood Z73.819
    - combined type Z73.812
    - limit setting type Z73.811
    - sleep-onset association type Z73.81Ø
  - childhood Z73.819
  - chronic F51.Ø4
    - somatized tension F51.Ø4
  - conditioned F51.Ø4
  - due to
    - alcohol
      - abuse F1Ø.182
      - dependence F1Ø.282
      - use F1Ø.982
    - amphetamines
      - abuse F15.182
      - dependence F15.282
      - use F15.982
    - anxiety disorder F51.Ø5
    - caffeine
      - abuse F15.182
      - dependence F15.282
      - use F15.982
    - cocaine
      - abuse F14.182
      - dependence F14.282
      - use F14.982
    - depression F51.Ø5
    - drug NEC
      - abuse F19.182
      - dependence F19.282
      - use F19.982
    - medical condition G47.Ø1
    - mental disorder NEC F51.Ø5
    - opioid
      - abuse F11.182
      - dependence F11.282
      - use F11.982
    - psychoactive substance NEC
      - abuse F19.182
      - dependence F19.182
      - use F19.982
    - sedative, hypnotic, or anxiolytic
      - abuse F13.182
      - dependence F13.282
      - use F13.982
    - stimulant NEC
      - abuse F15.182
      - dependence F15.282
      - use F15.982
  - fatal familial (FFI) A81.83
  - idiopathic F51.Ø1
  - learned F51.3
  - nonorganic origin F51.Ø1
  - not due to a substance or known physiological condition F51.Ø1
    - specified NEC F51.Ø9
  - paradoxical F51.Ø3
  - primary F51.Ø1
  - psychiatric F51.Ø5
  - psychophysiologic F51.Ø4
  - related to psychopathology F51.Ø5
  - short-term F51.Ø2
  - specified NEC G47.Ø9
- **Insomnia** — *continued*
  - stress-related F51.Ø2
  - transient F51.Ø2
  - without objective findings F51.Ø2
- **Inspiration**
  - food or foreign body — *see* Foreign body, by site
  - mucus — *see* Asphyxia, mucus
- **Inspissated bile syndrome** (newborn) P59.1
- **Instability**
  - emotional (excessive) F6Ø.3
  - housing
    - housed Z59.819
      - with risk of homelessness Z59.811
      - homelessness in past 12 months Z59.812
  - joint (post-traumatic) M25.3Ø
    - ankle M25.37- ☑
    - due to old ligament injury — *see* Disorder, ligament
    - elbow M25.32- ☑
    - flail — *see* Flail, joint
    - foot M25.37- ☑
    - hand M25.34- ☑
    - hip M25.35- ☑
    - knee M25.36- ☑
    - lumbosacral — *see* subcategory M53.2- ☑
    - prosthesis — *see* Complications, joint prosthesis, mechanical, displacement, by site
    - sacroiliac — *see* subcategory M53.2- ☑
    - secondary to
      - old ligament injury — *see* Disorder, ligament
      - removal of joint prosthesis M96.89
    - shoulder (region) M25.31- ☑
    - specified site NEC M25.39
    - spine — *see* subcategory M53.2- ☑
    - wrist M25.33- ☑
  - knee (chronic) M23.5- ☑
  - lumbosacral — *see* subcategory M53.2- ☑
  - nervous F48.8
  - personality (emotional) F6Ø.3
  - spine — *see* Instability, joint, spine
  - vasomotor R55
- **Institutional syndrome** (childhood) F94.2
- **Institutionalization, affecting child** Z62.22
  - disinhibited attachment F94.2
- **Insufficiency, insufficient**
  - accommodation, old age H52.4
  - adrenal (gland) E27.4Ø
    - primary E27.1
  - adrenocortical E27.4Ø
    - drug-induced E27.3
    - iatrogenic E27.3
    - primary E27.1
  - anatomic crown height KØ8.89
  - anterior (occlusal) guidance M26.54
  - anus K62.89
  - aortic (valve) I35.1
    - with
      - mitral (valve) disease IØ8.Ø
        - with tricuspid (valve) disease IØ8.3
      - stenosis I35.2
      - tricuspid (valve) disease IØ8.2
        - with mitral (valve) disease IØ8.3
    - congenital Q23.1
    - rheumatic IØ6.1
      - with
        - mitral (valve) disease IØ8.Ø
          - with tricuspid (valve) disease IØ8.3
        - stenosis IØ6.2
          - with mitral (valve) disease IØ8.Ø
            - with tricuspid (valve) disease IØ8.3
        - tricuspid (valve) disease IØ8.2
          - with mitral (valve) disease IØ8.3
    - specified cause NEC I35.1
    - syphilitic A52.Ø3
  - arterial I77.1
    - basilar G45.Ø
    - carotid (hemispheric) G45.1
    - cerebral I67.81
    - coronary (acute or subacute) I24.89
    - mesenteric K55.1
    - peripheral I73.9
    - precerebral (multiple) (bilateral) G45.2
    - vertebral G45.Ø
  - arteriovenous I99.8
  - biliary K83.8
  - cardiac — *see also* Insufficiency, myocardial
    - due to presence of (cardiac) prosthesis I97.11- ☑
    - postprocedural I97.11- ☑
  - cardiorenal, hypertensive I13.2

- **Insufficiency, insufficient** — *continued*
  - cardiovascular — *see* Disease, cardiovascular
  - cerebrovascular (acute) I67.81
    - with transient focal neurological signs and symptoms G45.8
  - circulatory NEC I99.8
    - newborn P29.89
  - clinical crown length KØ8.89
  - convergence H51.11
  - coronary (acute or subacute) I24.89
    - chronic or with a stated duration of over 4 weeks I25.89
  - corticoadrenal E27.4Ø
    - primary E27.1
  - dietary E63.9
  - divergence H51.8
  - food T73.Ø- ☑
  - gastroesophageal K22.89
  - gonadal
    - ovary E28.39
    - testis E29.1
  - health insurance coverage Z59.71
  - heart — *see also* Insufficiency, myocardial
    - newborn P29.Ø
    - valve — *see* Endocarditis
  - hepatic — *see* Failure, hepatic
  - idiopathic autonomic G9Ø.Ø9
  - interocclusal distance of fully erupted teeth (ridge) M26.36
  - kidney N28.9
    - acute N28.9
    - chronic N18.9
  - lacrimal (secretion) HØ4.12- ☑
    - passages — *see* Stenosis, lacrimal
  - liver — *see* Failure, hepatic
  - lung — *see* Insufficiency, pulmonary
  - mental (congenital) — *see* Disability, intellectual
  - mesenteric K55.1
  - mitral (valve) I34.Ø
    - with
      - aortic valve disease IØ8.Ø
        - with tricuspid (valve) disease IØ8.3
      - obstruction or stenosis IØ5.2
        - with aortic valve disease IØ8.Ø
      - tricuspid (valve) disease IØ8.1
        - with aortic (valve) disease IØ8.3
    - congenital Q23.3
    - rheumatic IØ5.1
      - with
        - aortic valve disease IØ8.Ø
          - with tricuspid (valve) disease IØ8.3
        - obstruction or stenosis IØ5.2
          - with aortic valve disease IØ8.Ø
            - with tricuspid (valve) disease IØ8.3
        - tricuspid (valve) disease IØ8.1
          - with aortic (valve) disease IØ8.3
      - active or acute IØ1.1
        - with chorea, rheumatic (Sydenham's) IØ2.Ø
    - specified cause, except rheumatic I34.Ø
  - muscle — *see also* Disease, muscle
    - heart — *see* Insufficiency, myocardial
    - ocular NEC H5Ø.9
  - myocardial, myocardium (with arteriosclerosis) — *see also* Failure, heart I5Ø.9
    - with
      - rheumatic fever (conditions in IØØ) IØ9.Ø
        - active, acute or subacute IØ1.2
          - with chorea IØ2.Ø
        - inactive or quiescent (with chorea) IØ9.Ø
    - congenital Q24.8
    - hypertensive — *see* Hypertension, heart
    - newborn P29.Ø
    - rheumatic IØ9.Ø
      - active, acute, or subacute IØ1.2
    - syphilitic A52.Ø6
  - nourishment — *see also* Nutrition deficient T73.Ø- ☑
  - pancreatic K86.89
    - exocrine K86.81
  - parathyroid (gland) E2Ø.9
  - peripheral vascular (arterial) I73.9
  - pituitary E23.Ø
  - placental (mother) O36.51- ☑
  - platelets D69.6
  - prenatal care affecting management of pregnancy OØ9.3- ☑
  - progressive pluriglandular E31.Ø
  - pulmonary J98.4
    - acute, following surgery (nonthoracic) J95.2

- **Insufficiency, insufficient** — *continued*
  - pulmonary — *continued*
    - acute, following surgery — *continued*
      - thoracic J95.1
    - chronic, following surgery J95.3
    - following
      - shock J98.4
      - trauma J98.4
    - newborn P28.89
    - valve I37.1
      - with stenosis I37.2
      - congenital Q22.2
      - rheumatic IØ9.89
        - with aortic, mitral or tricuspid (valve) disease IØ8.8
  - pyloric K31.89
  - renal (acute) N28.9
    - chronic N18.9
  - respiratory RØ6.89
    - newborn P28.5
  - rotation — *see* Malrotation
  - sleep syndrome F51.12
  - social insurance Z59.71
  - suprarenal E27.4Ø
    - primary E27.1
  - tarso-orbital fascia, congenital Q1Ø.3
  - testis E29.1
  - thyroid (gland) (acquired) EØ3.9
    - congenital EØ3.1
  - tricuspid (valve) (rheumatic) IØ7.1
    - with
      - aortic (valve) disease IØ8.2
        - with mitral (valve) disease IØ8.3
      - mitral (valve) disease IØ8.1
        - with aortic (valve) disease IØ8.3
      - obstruction or stenosis IØ7.2
        - with aortic (valve) disease IØ8.2
          - with mitral (valve) disease IØ8.3
    - congenital Q22.8
    - nonrheumatic I36.1
      - with stenosis I36.2
  - urethral sphincter R32
  - valve, valvular (heart) I38
    - aortic — *see* Insufficiency, aortic (valve)
    - congenital Q24.8
    - mitral — *see* Insufficiency, mitral (valve)
    - pulmonary — *see* Insufficiency, pulmonary, valve
    - tricuspid — *see* Insufficiency, tricuspid (valve)
  - vascular I99.8
    - intestine K55.9
      - acute — *see also* Ischemia, intestine, acute K55.Ø59
    - mesenteric K55.1
    - peripheral I73.9
    - renal — *see* Hypertension, kidney
  - velopharyngeal
    - acquired K13.79
    - congenital Q38.8
  - venous (chronic) (peripheral) I87.2
  - ventricular — *see* Insufficiency, myocardial
  - welfare support Z59.72
- **Insufflation, fallopian** Z31.41
- **Insular** — *see* condition
- **Insulinoma**
  - pancreas
    - benign D13.7
    - malignant C25.4
    - uncertain behavior D37.8
  - specified site
    - benign — *see* Neoplasm, by site, benign
    - malignant — *see* Neoplasm, by site, malignant
    - uncertain behavior — *see* Neoplasm, by site, uncertain behavior
  - unspecified site
    - benign D13.7
    - malignant C25.4
    - uncertain behavior D37.8
- **Insuloma** — *see* Insulinoma
- **Interference**
  - balancing side M26.56
  - non-working side M26.56
- **Intermenstrual** — *see* condition
- **Intermittent** — *see* condition
- **Internal** — *see* condition
- **Interrogation**
  - cardiac defibrillator (automatic) (implantable) Z45.Ø2
  - cardiac pacemaker Z45.Ø18
  - cardiac (event) (loop) recorder Z45.Ø9
  - infusion pump (implanted) (intrathecal) Z45.1
  - neurostimulator Z46.2

- **Interruption**
  - aortic arch Q25.21
  - bundle of His I44.3Ø
  - phase-shift, sleep cycle — *see* Disorder, sleep, circadian rhythm
  - sleep phase-shift, or 24 hour sleep-wake cycle — *see* Disorder, sleep, circadian rhythm
- **Interstitial** — *see* condition
- **Intertrigo** L3Ø.4
  - labialis K13.Ø
- **Intervertebral disc** — *see* condition
- **Intestine, intestinal** — *see* condition
- **Intolerance**
  - carbohydrate K9Ø.49
  - disaccharide, hereditary E73.Ø
  - fat NEC K9Ø.49
    - pancreatic K9Ø.3
  - food K9Ø.49
    - dietary counseling and surveillance Z71.3
  - fructose E74.1Ø
    - hereditary E74.12
  - glucose (-galactose) E74.39
  - gluten K9Ø.41
  - lactose E73.9
    - specified NEC E73.8
  - lysine E72.3
  - milk NEC K9Ø.49
    - lactose E73.9
  - orthostatic, chronic G9Ø.A
  - protein K9Ø.49
  - starch NEC K9Ø.49
  - sucrose (-isomaltose) E74.31
- **Intoxicated NEC** (without dependence) — *see* Alcohol, intoxication
- **Intoxication**
  - acid — *see also* Acidosis E87.29
  - alcoholic (acute) (without dependence) — *see* Alcohol, intoxication
  - alimentary canal K52.1
  - amphetamine (without dependence) — *see also* Abuse, drug, stimulant, with intoxication
    - with dependence — *see* Dependence, drug, stimulant, with intoxication
    - stimulant NEC F15.1Ø
      - with
        - anxiety disorder F15.18Ø
        - intoxication F15.129
          - with
            - delirium F15.121
            - perceptual disturbance F15.122
  - anxiolytic (acute) (without dependence) — *see* Abuse, drug, sedative, with intoxication
    - with dependence — *see* Dependence, drug, sedative, with intoxication
  - caffeine F15.929
    - with dependence — *see* Dependence, drug, stimulant, with intoxication
  - cannabinoids (acute) (without dependence) — *see* Use, cannabis, with intoxication
    - with
      - abuse — *see* Abuse, drug, cannabis, with intoxication
      - dependence — *see* Dependence, drug, cannabis, with intoxication
  - chemical — *see* Table of Drugs and Chemicals
    - via placenta or breast milk — *see* - Absorption, chemical, through placenta
  - cocaine (acute) (without dependence) — *see* Abuse, drug, cocaine, with intoxication
    - with dependence — *see* Dependence, drug, cocaine, with intoxication
  - drug
    - acute (without dependence) — *see* Abuse, drug, by type with intoxication
      - with dependence — *see* Dependence, drug, by type with intoxication
    - addictive
      - via placenta or breast milk — *see* Absorption, drug, addictive, through placenta
    - newborn P93.8
      - gray baby syndrome P93.Ø
    - overdose or wrong substance given or taken — *see* Table of Drugs and Chemicals, by drug, poisoning
  - enteric K52.1
  - foodborne AØ5.9
    - bacterial AØ5.9
    - classical (Clostridium botulinum) AØ5.1

- **Intoxication** — *continued*
  - foodborne — *continued*
    - due to
      - Bacillus cereus A05.4
      - bacterium A05.9
        - specified NEC A05.8
      - Clostridium
        - botulinum A05.1
        - perfringens A05.2
        - welchii A05.2
      - Salmonella A02.9
        - with
          - (gastro)enteritis A02.0
          - localized infection(s) A02.20
            - arthritis A02.23
            - meningitis A02.21
            - osteomyelitis A02.24
            - pneumonia A02.22
            - pyelonephritis A02.25
            - specified NEC A02.29
          - sepsis A02.1
          - specified manifestation NEC A02.8
      - Staphylococcus A05.0
      - Vibrio
        - parahaemolyticus A05.3
        - vulnificus A05.5
    - enterotoxin, staphylococcal A05.0
    - noxious — *see* Poisoning, food, noxious
  - gastrointestinal K52.1
  - hallucinogenic (without dependence) — *see* Abuse, drug, hallucinogen, with intoxication
    - with dependence — *see* Dependence, drug, hallucinogen, with intoxication
  - hepatocerebral K76.82
  - hypnotic (acute) (without dependence) — *see* Abuse, drug, sedative, with intoxication
    - with dependence — *see* Dependence, drug, sedative, with intoxication
  - inhalant (acute) (without dependence) — *see* Abuse, drug, inhalant, with intoxication
    - with dependence — *see* Dependence, drug, inhalant, with intoxication
  - meaning
    - inebriation — *see* category F10.- ☑
    - poisoning — *see* Table of Drugs and Chemicals
  - methyl alcohol (acute) (without dependence) — *see* Alcohol, intoxication
  - opioid (acute) (without dependence) — *see* Abuse, drug, opioid, with intoxication
    - with dependence — *see* Dependence, drug, opioid, with intoxication
  - pathologic NEC (without dependence) — *see* Alcohol, intoxication
  - phencyclidine (without dependence) — *see* Abuse, drug, hallucinogen, with intoxication
    - with dependence — *see* Dependence, drug, hallucinogen, with intoxication
  - potassium (K) E87.5
  - psychoactive substance NEC (without dependence) — *see* Abuse, drug, psychoactive NEC, with intoxication
    - with dependence — *see* Dependence, drug, psychoactive NEC, with intoxication
  - sedative (acute) (without dependence) — *see* Abuse, drug, sedative, with intoxication
    - with dependence — *see* Dependence, drug, sedative, with intoxication
  - serum — *see also* Reaction, serum T80.69- ☑
  - uremic — *see* Uremia
  - volatile solvents (acute) (without dependence) — *see* Abuse, drug, inhalant, with intoxication
    - with dependence — *see* Dependence, drug, inhalant, with intoxication
  - water E87.79
- **Intraabdominal testis, testes**
  - bilateral Q53.211
  - unilateral Q53.111
- **Intracranial** — *see* condition
- **Intrahepatic gallbladder** Q44.1
- **Intraligamentous** — *see* condition
- **Intrathoracic** — *see also* condition
  - kidney Q63.2
- **Intrauterine contraceptive device**
  - checking Z30.431
  - in situ Z97.5
  - insertion Z30.430
    - immediately following removal Z30.433
  - management Z30.431
  - reinsertion Z30.433
- **Intrauterine contraceptive device** — *continued*
  - removal Z30.432
  - replacement Z30.433
  - retention in pregnancy O26.3- ☑
- **Intraventricular** — *see* condition
- **Intrinsic deformity** — *see* Deformity
- **Intubation, difficult or failed** T88.4- ☑
- **Intumescence, lens** (eye) (cataract) — *see* Cataract
- **Intussusception** (bowel) (colon) (enteric) (ileocecal) (ileocolic) (intestine) ( rectum) K56.1
  - appendix K38.8
  - congenital Q43.8
  - ureter (with obstruction) N13.5
- **Invagination** (bowel, colon, intestine or rectum) K56.1
- **Inversion**
  - albumin-globulin (A-G) ratio E88.09
  - bladder N32.89
  - cecum — *see* Intussusception
  - cervix N88.8
  - chromosome in normal individual Q95.1
  - circadian rhythm — *see* Disorder, sleep, circadian rhythm
  - nipple N64.59
    - congenital Q83.8
    - gestational — *see* Retraction, nipple
    - puerperal, postpartum — *see* Retraction, nipple
  - nyctohemeral rhythm — *see* Disorder, sleep, circadian rhythm
  - optic papilla Q14.2
  - organ or site, congenital NEC — *see* Anomaly, by site
  - sleep rhythm — *see* Disorder, sleep, circadian rhythm
  - testis (congenital) Q55.29
  - uterus (chronic) (postinfectional) (postpartal, old) N85.5
    - postpartum O71.2
  - vagina (posthysterectomy) N99.3
  - ventricular Q20.5
- **Investigation** — *see also* Examination Z04.9
  - clinical research subject (control) (normal comparison) (participant) Z00.6
- **Involuntary movement, abnormal** R25.9
- **Involution, involutional** — *see also* condition
  - breast, cystic — *see* Dysplasia, mammary, specified type NEC
  - depression (single episode) F32.89
    - recurrent episode F33.9
  - melancholia (single episode) F32.89
    - recurrent episode F33.8
  - ovary, senile — *see* Atrophy, ovary
  - thymus failure E32.8
- **I.Q.**
  - 20-34 F72
  - 35-49 F71
  - 50-69 F70
  - under 20 F73
- **IRDS** (type I) P22.0
  - type II P22.1
- **Irideremia** Q13.1
- **Iridis rubeosis** — *see* Disorder, iris, vascular
- **Iridochoroiditis** (panuveitis) — *see* Panuveitis
- **Iridocyclitis** H20.9
  - acute H20.0- ☑
    - hypopyon H20.05- ☑
    - primary H20.01- ☑
    - recurrent H20.02- ☑
    - secondary (noninfectious) H20.04- ☑
      - infectious H20.03- ☑
  - chronic H20.1- ☑
  - due to allergy — *see* Iridocyclitis, acute, secondary
  - endogenous — *see* Iridocyclitis, acute, primary
  - Fuchs' — *see* Cyclitis, Fuchs' heterochromic
  - gonococcal A54.32
  - granulomatous — *see* Iridocyclitis, chronic
  - herpes, herpetic (simplex) B00.51
    - zoster B02.32
  - hypopyon — *see* Iridocyclitis, acute, hypopyon
  - in (due to)
    - ankylosing spondylitis M45.9
    - gonococcal infection A54.32
    - herpes (simplex) virus B00.51
      - zoster B02.32
    - infectious disease NOS B99.- ☑
    - parasitic disease NOS B89 *[H22]*
    - sarcoidosis D86.83
    - syphilis A51.43
    - tuberculosis A18.54
    - zoster B02.32
  - lens-induced H20.2- ☑
  - nongranulomatous — *see* Iridocyclitis, acute
  - recurrent — *see* Iridocyclitis, acute, recurrent
- **Iridocyclitis** — *continued*
  - rheumatic — *see* Iridocyclitis, chronic
  - subacute — *see* Iridocyclitis, acute
  - sympathetic — *see* Uveitis, sympathetic
  - syphilitic (secondary) A51.43
  - tuberculous (chronic) A18.54
  - Vogt-Koyanagi H20.82- ☑
- **Iridocyclochoroiditis** (panuveitis) — *see* Panuveitis
- **Iridodialysis** H21.53- ☑
- **Iridodonesis** H21.89
- **Iridoplegia** (complete) (partial) (reflex) H57.09
- **Iridoschisis** H21.25- ☑
- **Iris** — *see also* condition
  - bombé — *see* Membrane, pupillary
- **Iritis** — *see also* Iridocyclitis
  - chronic — *see* Iridocyclitis, chronic
  - diabetic — *see* E08-E13 with .39
  - due to
    - herpes simplex B00.51
    - leprosy A30.9 *[H22]*
  - gonococcal A54.32
  - gouty — *see also* Gout, by type M10.9 *[H22]*
  - granulomatous — *see* Iridocyclitis, chronic
  - lens induced — *see* Iridocyclitis, lens-induced
  - papulosa (syphilitic) A52.71
  - rheumatic — *see* Iridocyclitis, chronic
  - syphilitic (secondary) A51.43
    - congenital (early) A50.01
    - late A52.71
  - tuberculous A18.54
- **Iron** — *see* condition
- **Iron-miner's lung** J63.4
- **Irradiated enamel** (tooth, teeth) K03.89
- **Irradiation effects, adverse** T66.- ☑
- **Irreducible, irreducibility** — *see* condition
- **Irregular, irregularity**
  - action, heart I49.9
  - alveolar process K08.89
  - bleeding N92.6
  - breathing R06.89
  - contour of cornea (acquired) — *see* Deformity, cornea
    - congenital Q13.4
  - contour, reconstructed breast N65.0
  - dentin (in pulp) K04.3
  - eye movements H55.89
    - deficient
      - saccadic H55.81
      - smooth H55.82
    - nystagmus — *see* Nystagmus
  - labor O62.2
  - menstruation (cause unknown) N92.6
  - periods N92.6
  - prostate N42.9
  - pupil — *see* Abnormality, pupillary
  - reconstructed breast N65.0
  - respiratory R06.89
  - septum (nasal) J34.2
  - shape, organ or site, congenital NEC — *see* Distortion
  - sleep-wake pattern (rhythm) G47.23
- **Irritable, irritability** R45.4
  - bladder N32.89
  - bowel (syndrome) K58.9
    - with
      - constipation K58.1
      - diarrhea K58.0
    - mixed K58.2
    - psychogenic F45.8
    - specified NEC K58.8
  - bronchial — *see* Bronchitis
  - cerebral, in newborn P91.3
  - colon — *see also* Irritable, bowel K58.9
    - with diarrhea K58.0
    - psychogenic F45.8
  - duodenum K59.89
  - heart (psychogenic) F45.8
  - hip — *see* Derangement, joint, specified type NEC, hip
  - ileum K59.89
  - infant R68.12
  - jejunum K59.89
  - rectum K59.89
  - stomach K31.89
    - psychogenic F45.8
  - sympathetic G90.89
  - urethra N36.8
  - without diarrhea K58.9
- **Irritation**
  - anus K62.89
  - axillary nerve G54.0
  - bladder N32.89

- **Irritation** — *continued*
  - brachial plexus G54.Ø
  - bronchial — *see* Bronchitis
  - cervical plexus G54.2
  - cervix — *see* Cervicitis
  - choroid, sympathetic — *see* Endophthalmitis
  - cranial nerve — *see* Disorder, nerve, cranial
  - gastric K31.89
    - psychogenic F45.8
  - globe, sympathetic — *see* Uveitis, sympathetic
  - labyrinth — *see* subcategory H83.2- ☑
  - lumbosacral plexus G54.1
  - meninges (traumatic) — *see* Injury, intracranial
    - nontraumatic — *see* Meningismus
  - nerve — *see* Disorder, nerve
  - nervous R45.Ø
  - penis N48.89
  - perineum NEC L29.3
  - peripheral autonomic nervous system G9Ø.89
  - peritoneum — *see* Peritonitis
  - pharynx J39.2
  - plantar nerve — *see* Lesion, nerve, plantar
  - spinal (cord) (traumatic) — *see also* Injury, spinal cord, by region
    - nerve G58.9
      - root NEC — *see* Radiculopathy
    - nontraumatic — *see* Myelopathy
  - stomach K31.89
    - psychogenic F45.8
  - sympathetic nerve NEC G9Ø.89
  - ulnar nerve — *see* Lesion, nerve, ulnar
  - vagina N89.8
- **Ischemia, ischemic** I99.8
  - bowel (transient)
    - acute — *see also* Ischemia, intestine, acute K55.Ø59
    - chronic K55.1
    - due to mesenteric artery insufficiency K55.1
  - brain — *see* Ischemia, cerebral
  - cardiac — *see* Disease, heart, ischemic
  - cardiomyopathy I25.5
  - cerebral (chronic) (generalized) I67.82
    - arteriosclerotic I67.2
    - intermittent G45.9
    - newborn P91.Ø
    - recurrent focal G45.8
    - transient G45.9
  - colon chronic (due to mesenteric artery insufficiency) K55.1
  - coronary — *see* Disease, heart, ischemic
  - demand (coronary) — *see also* Angina I24.89
    - with myocardial infarction I21.A1
    - resulting in myocardial infarction I21.A1
  - heart (chronic or with a stated duration of over 4 weeks) I25.9
    - acute or with a stated duration of 4 weeks or less I24.9
    - subacute I24.9
  - infarction, muscle — *see* Infarct, muscle
  - intestine (large) (small) (transient) K55.9
    - acute K55.Ø59
      - diffuse K55.Ø52
      - focal K55.Ø51
      - large K55.Ø39
        - diffuse K55.Ø32
        - focal K55.Ø31
      - small K55.Ø19
        - diffuse K55.Ø12
        - focal K55.Ø11
    - chronic K55.1
    - due to mesenteric artery insufficiency K55.1
  - kidney N28.Ø
  - limb, critical — *see* Arteriosclerosis, with critical limb ischemia
  - limb-threatening, chronic — *see* Arteriosclerosis, with critical limb ischemia
  - mesenteric, acute — *see also* Ischemia, intestine, acute K55.Ø59
  - muscle, traumatic T79.6- ☑
  - myocardium, myocardial (chronic or with a stated duration of over 4 weeks) I25.9
    - acute, without myocardial infarction I51.3
    - silent (asymptomatic) I25.6
    - transient of newborn P29.4
  - nipple, intraoperative and postprocedural N99.86Ø
  - renal N28.Ø
  - retina, retinal — *see* Occlusion, artery, retina
  - small bowel
    - acute K55.Ø19
      - diffuse K55.Ø12
      - focal K55.Ø11
- **Ischemia, ischemic** — *continued*
  - small bowel — *continued*
    - chronic K55.1
    - due to mesenteric artery insufficiency K55.1
  - spinal cord G95.11
  - subendocardial — *see* Insufficiency, coronary
  - supply (coronary) — *see also* Angina I25.9
    - due to vasospasm I2Ø.1
- **Ischial spine** — *see* condition
- **Ischialgia** — *see* Sciatica
- **Ischiopagus** Q89.4
- **Ischium, ischial** — *see* condition
- **Ischuria** R34
- **Iselin's disease or osteochondrosis** — *see* Osteochondrosis, juvenile, metatarsus
- **Islands of**
  - parotid tissue in
    - lymph nodes Q38.6
    - neck structures Q38.6
  - submaxillary glands in
    - fascia Q38.6
    - lymph nodes Q38.6
    - neck muscles Q38.6
- **Islet cell tumor, pancreas** D13.7
- **Isoimmunization NEC** — *see also* Incompatibility
  - affecting management of pregnancy (ABO) (with hydrops fetalis) O36.11- ☑
    - anti-A sensitization O36.11- ☑
    - anti-B sensitization O36.19- ☑
    - anti-C sensitization O36.Ø9- ☑
    - anti-c sensitization O36.Ø9- ☑
    - anti-E sensitization O36.Ø9- ☑
    - anti-e sensitization O36.Ø9- ☑
    - Rh NEC O36.Ø9- ☑
      - anti-D antibody O36.Ø1- ☑
    - specified NEC O36.19- ☑
  - newborn P55.9
    - with
      - hydrops fetalis P56.Ø
      - kernicterus P57.Ø
    - ABO (blood groups) P55.1
    - Rhesus (Rh) factor P55.Ø
    - specified type NEC P55.8
- **Isolation, isolated**
  - dwelling Z59.89
  - family Z63.79
  - social Z6Ø.4
- **Isoleucinosis** E71.19
- **Isomerism atrial appendages** (with asplenia or polysplenia) Q2Ø.6
- **Isosporiasis, isosporosis** AØ7.3
- **Isovaleric acidemia** E71.11Ø
- **Issue of**
  - medical certificate ZØ2.79
    - for disability determination ZØ2.71
  - repeat prescription (appliance) (glasses) (medicinal substance, medicament, medicine) Z76.Ø
    - contraception — *see* Contraception
- **IST** (inappropriate sinus tachycardia, so stated) I47.11
- **Itch, itching** — *see also* Pruritus
  - baker's L23.6
  - barber's B35.Ø
  - bricklayer's L24.5
  - cheese B88.Ø9
  - clam digger's B65.3
  - coolie B76.9
  - copra B88.Ø9
  - dew B76.9
  - dhobi B35.6
  - filarial — *see* Infestation, filarial
  - grain B88.Ø9
  - grocer's B88.Ø9
  - ground B76.9
  - harvest B88.Ø9
  - jock B35.6
  - Malabar B35.5
    - beard B35.Ø
    - foot B35.3
    - scalp B35.Ø
  - meaning scabies B86
  - Norwegian B86
  - perianal L29.Ø
  - poultrymen's B88.Ø9
  - sarcoptic B86
  - scabies B86
  - scrub B88.Ø9
  - straw B88.Ø9
  - swimmer's B65.3
- **Itch, itching** — *continued*
  - water B76.9
  - winter L29.89
- **Ivemark's syndrome** (asplenia with congenital heart disease) Q89.Ø1
- **Ivory bones** Q78.2
- **Ixodiasis NEC** B88.8

# J

- **Jaccoud's syndrome** — *see* Arthropathy, postrheumatic, chronic
- **Jackson's**
  - membrane Q43.3
  - paralysis or syndrome G83.89
  - veil Q43.3
- **Jacquet's dermatitis** (diaper dermatitis) L22
- **Jadassohn-Pellizari's disease or anetoderma** L9Ø.2
- **Jadassohn's**
  - blue nevus — *see* Nevus
  - intraepidermal epithelioma — *see* Neoplasm, skin, benign
- **Jaffe-Lichtenstein** (-Uehlinger) **syndrome** — *see* Dysplasia, fibrous, bone NEC
- **Jakob-Creutzfeldt disease or syndrome** — *see* Creutzfeldt-Jakob disease or syndrome
- **Jaksch-Luzet disease** D64.89
- **Jamaican**
  - neuropathy G92.8
  - paraplegic tropical ataxic-spastic syndrome G92.8
- **Janet's disease** F48.8
- **Janiceps** Q89.4
- **Jansky-Bielschowsky amaurotic idiocy** E75.4
- **Japanese**
  - B-type encephalitis A83.Ø
  - river fever A75.3
- **Jaundice** (yellow) R17
  - acholuric (familial) (splenomegalic) — *see also* Spherocytosis
    - acquired D59.8
  - breast-milk (inhibitor) P59.3
  - catarrhal (acute) B15.9
    - with hepatic coma B15.Ø
  - cholestatic (benign) R17
  - due to or associated with
    - delayed conjugation P59.8
      - associated with (due to) preterm delivery P59.Ø
    - preterm delivery P59.Ø
  - epidemic (catarrhal) B15.9
    - with hepatic coma B15.Ø
    - leptospiral A27.Ø
    - spirochetal A27.Ø
  - familial nonhemolytic (congenital) (Gilbert) E8Ø.4
    - Crigler-Najjar E8Ø.5
  - febrile (acute) B15.9
    - with hepatic coma B15.Ø
    - leptospiral A27.Ø
    - spirochetal A27.Ø
  - hematogenous D59.9
  - hemolytic (acquired) D59.9
    - congenital — *see* Spherocytosis
  - hemorrhagic (acute) (leptospiral) (spirochetal) A27.Ø
  - infectious (acute) (subacute) B15.9
    - with hepatic coma B15.Ø
    - leptospiral A27.Ø
    - spirochetal A27.Ø
  - leptospiral (hemorrhagic) A27.Ø
  - malignant (without coma) K72.9Ø
    - with coma K72.91
  - neonatal — *see* Jaundice, newborn
  - newborn P59.9
    - due to or associated with
      - ABO
        - antibodies P55.1
        - incompatibility, maternal/fetal P55.1
        - isoimmunization P55.1
      - absence or deficiency of enzyme system for bilirubin conjugation (congenital) P59.8
      - bleeding P58.1
      - breast milk inhibitors to conjugation P59.3
        - associated with preterm delivery P59.Ø
      - bruising P58.Ø
      - Crigler-Najjar syndrome E8Ø.5
      - delayed conjugation P59.8
        - associated with preterm delivery P59.Ø
      - drugs or toxins
        - given to newborn P58.42
        - transmitted from mother P58.41
      - excessive hemolysis P58.9

**Jaundice** — *continued*
  newborn — *continued*
    due to or associated with — *continued*
      excessive hemolysis — *continued*
        due to
          bleeding P58.1
          bruising P58.Ø
          drugs or toxins
            given to newborn P58.42
            transmitted from mother P58.41
          infection P58.2
          polycythemia P58.3
          swallowed maternal blood P58.5
        specified type NEC P58.8
      galactosemia E74.21
      Gilbert syndrome E8Ø.4
      hemolytic disease P55.9
        ABO isoimmunization P55.1
        Rh isoimmunization P55.Ø
        specified NEC P55.8
      hepatocellular damage P59.2Ø
        specified NEC P59.29
      hereditary hemolytic anemia P58.8
      hypothyroidism, congenital EØ3.1
      incompatibility, maternal/fetal NOS P55.9
      infection P58.2
      inspissated bile syndrome P59.1
      isoimmunization NOS P55.9
      mucoviscidosis E84.9
      polycythemia P58.3
      preterm delivery P59.Ø
      Rh
        antibodies P55.Ø
        incompatibility, maternal/fetal P55.Ø
        isoimmunization P55.Ø
      specified cause NEC P59.8
      swallowed maternal blood P58.5
    spherocytosis (congenital) D58.Ø
  nonhemolytic congenital familial (Gilbert) E8Ø.4
  nuclear, newborn — *see also* Kernicterus of newborn P57.9
  obstructive — *see also* Obstruction, bile duct K83.1
  post-immunization — *see* Hepatitis, viral, type, B
  post-transfusion — *see* Hepatitis, viral, type, B
  regurgitation — *see also* Obstruction, bile duct K83.1
  serum (homologous) (prophylactic) (therapeutic) — *see* Hepatitis, viral, type, B
  spirochetal (hemorrhagic) A27.Ø
  symptomatic R17
    newborn P59.9
**Jaw** — *see* condition
**Jaw-winking phenomenon or syndrome** QØ7.8
**Jealousy**
  alcoholic F1Ø.988
  childhood F93.8
  sibling F93.8
**Jejunitis** — *see* Enteritis
**Jejunostomy status** Z93.4
**Jejunum, jejunal** — *see* condition
**Jensen's disease** — *see* Inflammation, chorioretinal, focal, juxtapapillary
**Jerks, myoclonic** G25.3
**Jervell-Lange-Nielsen syndrome** I45.81
**Jeune's disease** Q77.2
**Jigger disease** B88.1
**Job's syndrome** (chronic granulomatous disease) D71.8
**Joint** — *see also* condition
  mice — *see* Loose, body, joint
    knee M23.4- ☑
**Jordan's anomaly or syndrome** D72.Ø
**Joseph-Diamond-Blackfan anemia** (congenital hypoplastic) D61.Ø1
**Jungle yellow fever** A95.Ø
**Jüngling's disease** — *see* Sarcoidosis
**Juvenile** — *see* condition

# K

**Kahler's disease** C9Ø.Ø- ☑
**Kakke** E51.11
**Kala-azar** B55.Ø
**Kallmann's syndrome** E23.Ø
**Kanner's syndrome** (autism) — *see* Psychosis, childhood
**Kaposi's**
  dermatosis (xeroderma pigmentosum) Q82.1
  lichen ruber L44.Ø
    acuminatus L44.Ø
**Kaposi's** — *continued*
  sarcoma
    colon C46.4
    connective tissue C46.1
    gastrointestinal organ C46.4
    lung C46.5- ☑
    lymph node (multiple) C46.3
    palate (hard) (soft) C46.2
    rectum C46.4
    skin (multiple sites) C46.Ø
    specified site NEC C46.7
    stomach C46.4
    unspecified site C46.9
  varicelliform eruption BØØ.Ø
    vaccinia T88.1- ☑
**Kartagener's syndrome or triad** (sinusitis, bronchiectasis, situs inversus) Q89.3
**Karyotype**
  with abnormality except iso (Xq) Q96.2
  45,X Q96.Ø
  46,X
    iso (Xq) Q96.1
  46,XX Q98.3
    with streak gonads Q5Ø.32
    hermaphrodite (true) Q99.1
    male Q98.3
  46,XY
    with streak gonads Q56.1
    female Q97.3
    hermaphrodite (true) Q99.1
  47,XXX Q97.Ø
  47,XXY Q98.Ø
  47,XYY Q98.5
**Kaschin-Beck disease** — *see* Disease, Kaschin-Beck
**Katayama's disease or fever** B65.2
**Kawasaki's syndrome** M3Ø.3
**Kayser-Fleischer ring** (cornea) (pseudosclerosis) H18.Ø4- ☑
**Kaznelson's syndrome** (congenital hypoplastic anemia) D61.Ø1
**Kearns-Sayre syndrome** H49.81- ☑
**Kedani fever** A75.3
**Kelis** L91.Ø
**Kelly** (-Patterson) **syndrome** (sideropenic dysphagia) D5Ø.1
**Keloid, cheloid** L91.Ø
  acne L73.Ø
  Addison's L94.Ø
  cornea — *see* Opacity, cornea
  Hawkin's L91.Ø
  scar L91.Ø
**Keloma** L91.Ø
**Kenya fever** A77.1
**Keratectasia** — *see also* Ectasia, cornea
  congenital Q13.4
**Keratinization of alveolar ridge mucosa**
  excessive K13.23
  minimal K13.22
**Keratinized residual ridge mucosa**
  excessive K13.23
  minimal K13.22
**Keratitis** (nodular) (nonulcerative) (simple) (zonular) H16.9
  with ulceration (central) (marginal) (perforated) (ring) — *see* Ulcer, cornea
  actinic — *see* Photokeratitis
  arborescens (herpes simplex) BØØ.52
  areolar H16.11- ☑
  bullosa H16.8
  deep H16.3Ø9
    specified type NEC H16.399
  dendritic (a) (herpes simplex) BØØ.52
  disciform (is) (herpes simplex) BØØ.52
    varicella BØ1.81
  filamentary H16.12- ☑
  gonococcal (congenital or prenatal) A54.33
  herpes, herpetic (simplex) BØØ.52
    zoster BØ2.33
  in (due to)
    acanthamebiasis B6Ø.13
    adenovirus B3Ø.Ø
    exanthema — *see also* Exanthem BØ9
    herpes (simplex) virus BØØ.52
    measles BØ5.81
    syphilis A5Ø.31
    tuberculosis A18.52
    zoster BØ2.33
  interstitial (nonsyphilitic) H16.3Ø- ☑
    diffuse H16.32- ☑
    herpes, herpetic (simplex) BØØ.52
      zoster BØ2.33
**Keratitis** — *continued*
  interstitial — *continued*
    sclerosing H16.33- ☑
    specified type NEC H16.39- ☑
    syphilitic (congenital) (late) A5Ø.31
    tuberculous A18.52
  macular H16.11- ☑
  nummular H16.11- ☑
  oyster shuckers' H16.8
  parenchymatous — *see* Keratitis, interstitial
  petrificans H16.8
  postmeasles BØ5.81
  punctata
    leprosa A3Ø.9 *[H16.14-]* ☑
    syphilitic (profunda) A5Ø.31
  punctate H16.14- ☑
  purulent H16.8
  rosacea L71.8
  sclerosing H16.33- ☑
  specified type NEC H16.8
  stellate H16.11- ☑
  striate H16.11- ☑
  superficial H16.1Ø- ☑
    with conjunctivitis — *see* Keratoconjunctivitis
    due to light — *see* Photokeratitis
  suppurative H16.8
  syphilitic (congenital) (prenatal) A5Ø.31
  trachomatous A71.1
    sequelae B94.Ø
  tuberculous A18.52
  vesicular H16.8
  xerotic — *see also* Keratomalacia H16.8
    vitamin A deficiency E5Ø.4
**Kerato-uveitis** — *see* Iridocyclitis
**Keratoacanthoma** L85.8
**Keratocele** — *see* Descemetocele
**Keratoconjunctivitis** H16.2Ø- ☑
  Acanthamoeba B6Ø.13
  adenoviral B3Ø.Ø
  epidemic B3Ø.Ø
  exposure H16.21- ☑
  herpes, herpetic (simplex) BØØ.52
    zoster BØ2.33
  in exanthema — *see also* Exanthem BØ9
  infectious B3Ø.Ø
  lagophthalmic — *see* Keratoconjunctivitis, specified type NEC
  neurotrophic H16.23- ☑
  phlyctenular H16.25- ☑
  postmeasles BØ5.81
  shipyard B3Ø.Ø
  sicca (Sjogren's) M35.Ø- ☑
    not Sjogren's H16.22- ☑
  specified type NEC H16.29- ☑
  tuberculous (phlyctenular) A18.52
  vernal H16.26- ☑
**Keratoconus** H18.6Ø- ☑
  congenital Q13.4
  stable H18.61- ☑
  unstable H18.62- ☑
**Keratocyst** (dental) (odontogenic) — *see* Cyst, calcifying odontogenic
**Keratoderma, keratodermia** (congenital) (palmaris et plantaris) (symmetrical) Q82.8
  acquired L85.1
    in diseases classified elsewhere L86
  climactericum L85.1
  gonococcal A54.89
  gonorrheal A54.89
  punctata L85.2
  Reiter's — *see* Reiter's disease
**Keratodermatocele** — *see* Descemetocele
**Keratoglobus** H18.79- ☑
  congenital Q15.8
    with glaucoma Q15.Ø
**Keratohemia** — *see* Pigmentation, cornea, stromal
**Keratoiritis** — *see also* Iridocyclitis
  syphilitic A5Ø.39
  tuberculous A18.54
**Keratoma** L57.Ø
  palmaris and plantaris hereditarium Q82.8
  senile L57.Ø
**Keratomalacia** H18.44- ☑
  vitamin A deficiency E5Ø.4
**Keratomegaly** Q13.4
**Keratomycosis** B49
  nigrans, nigricans (palmaris) B36.1
**Keratopathy** H18.9

**Laceration** — *continued*
- submental region — *see* Laceration, head, specified site NEC
- subungual
  - finger(s) — *see* Laceration, finger, with damage to nail
  - toe(s) — *see* Laceration, toe, with damage to nail
- suprarenal gland — *see* Laceration, adrenal gland
- temple, temporal region — *see* Laceration, head, specified site NEC
- temporomandibular area — *see* Laceration, cheek
- tendon — *see* Injury, muscle, by site, laceration
  - Achilles S86.Ø2- ☑
- tentorium cerebelli — *see* Injury, intracranial, diffuse
- testis S31.31- ☑
  - with foreign body S31.32- ☑
- thigh S71.11- ☑
  - with foreign body S71.12- ☑
- thorax, thoracic (wall) S21.91- ☑
  - with foreign body S21.92- ☑
    - back S21.22- ☑
      - with penetration into thoracic cavity S21.42- ☑
    - front S21.12- ☑
      - with penetration into thoracic cavity S21.32- ☑
  - back S21.21- ☑
    - with
      - foreign body S21.22- ☑
        - with penetration into thoracic cavity S21.42- ☑
      - penetration into thoracic cavity S21.41- ☑
  - breast — *see* Laceration, breast
  - front S21.11- ☑
    - with
      - foreign body S21.12- ☑
        - with penetration into thoracic cavity S21.32- ☑
      - penetration into thoracic cavity S21.31- ☑
- thumb S61.Ø19- ☑
  - with
    - damage to nail S61.119- ☑
      - with
        - foreign body S61.129- ☑
    - foreign body S61.Ø29- ☑
  - left S61.Ø12- ☑
    - with
      - damage to nail S61.112- ☑
        - with
          - foreign body S61.122- ☑
      - foreign body S61.Ø22- ☑
  - right S61.Ø11- ☑
    - with
      - damage to nail S61.111- ☑
        - with
          - foreign body S61.121- ☑
      - foreign body S61.Ø21- ☑
- thyroid gland S11.11- ☑
  - with foreign body S11.12- ☑
- toe(s) S91.119- ☑
  - with
    - damage to nail S91.219- ☑
      - with
        - foreign body S91.229- ☑
    - foreign body S91.129- ☑
  - great S91.113- ☑
    - with
      - damage to nail S91.213- ☑
        - with
          - foreign body S91.223- ☑
      - foreign body S91.123- ☑
    - left S91.112- ☑
      - with
        - damage to nail S91.212- ☑
          - with
            - foreign body S91.222- ☑
        - foreign body S91.122- ☑
    - right S91.111- ☑
      - with
        - damage to nail S91.211- ☑
          - with
            - foreign body S91.221- ☑
        - foreign body S91.121- ☑
  - lesser S91.116- ☑
    - with
      - damage to nail S91.216- ☑
        - with
          - foreign body S91.226- ☑

**Laceration** — *continued*
- toe(s) — *continued*
  - lesser — *continued*
    - with — *continued*
      - foreign body S91.126- ☑
    - left S91.115- ☑
      - with
        - damage to nail S91.215- ☑
          - with
            - foreign body S91.225- ☑
        - foreign body S91.125- ☑
    - right S91.114- ☑
      - with
        - damage to nail S91.214- ☑
          - with
            - foreign body S91.224- ☑
        - foreign body S91.124- ☑
- tongue — *see* Laceration, oral cavity
- trachea S11.Ø21- ☑
  - with foreign body S11.Ø22- ☑
- tunica vaginalis — *see* Laceration, testis
- tympanum, tympanic membrane — *see* Laceration, ear, drum
- umbilical region S31.115- ☑
  - with foreign body S31.125- ☑
- ureter S37.13- ☑
- urethra S37.33- ☑
  - with or following ectopic or molar pregnancy OØ8.6
  - obstetrical trauma O71.5
- urinary organ NEC S37.893- ☑
- uterus S37.63- ☑
  - with ectopic or molar pregnancy OØ8.6
  - following ectopic or molar pregnancy OØ8.6
  - nonpuerperal, nontraumatic N85.8
  - obstetrical trauma NEC O71.81
  - old (postpartal) N85.8
- uvula — *see* Laceration, oral cavity
- vagina S31.41- ☑
  - with
    - ectopic or molar pregnancy OØ8.6
    - foreign body S31.42- ☑
  - during delivery O71.4
    - with perineal laceration — *see* Laceration, perineum, female, during delivery
  - following ectopic or molar pregnancy OØ8.6
  - nonpuerperal, nontraumatic N89.8
  - old (postpartal) N89.8
- vas deferens S37.893- ☑
- vesical — *see* Laceration, bladder
- vocal cords S11.Ø31- ☑
  - with foreign body S11.Ø32- ☑
- vulva S31.41- ☑
  - with
    - ectopic or molar pregnancy OØ8.6
    - foreign body S31.42- ☑
  - complicating delivery O7Ø.Ø
  - following ectopic or molar pregnancy OØ8.6
  - nonpuerperal, nontraumatic N9Ø.89
  - old (postpartal) N9Ø.89
- wrist S61.519- ☑
  - with
    - foreign body S61.529- ☑
  - left S61.512- ☑
    - with
      - foreign body S61.522- ☑
  - right S61.511- ☑
    - with
      - foreign body S61.521- ☑

**Lack of**
- achievement in school Z55.3
- adequate
  - food Z59.48
  - intermaxillary vertical dimension of fully erupted teeth M26.36
  - sleep Z72.82Ø
- air conditioning Z59.11
- appetite — *see* Anorexia R63.Ø
- awareness R41.9
- basic services in physical environment Z58.81
- care
  - in home Z74.2
  - of infant (at or after birth) T76.Ø2- ☑
    - confirmed T74.Ø2- ☑
- cognitive functions R41.9
- coordination R27.9
  - ataxia R27.Ø
  - specified type NEC R27.8

**Lack of** — *continued*
- development (physiological) R62.5Ø
  - failure to thrive (child over 28 days old) R62.51
    - adult R62.7
    - newborn P92.6
  - short stature R62.52
  - specified type NEC R62.59
- electricity services Z59.12
- emotional support Z6Ø.8
- energy R53.83
- financial resources Z59.6
- food Z59.48
- gas services Z59.12
- growth R62.52
- heating Z59.11
- housing (permanent) (temporary) Z59.ØØ
  - adequate Z59.1Ø
- learning experiences in childhood Z62.898
- leisure time (affecting life-style) Z73.2
- material resources due to limited financial resources, specified NEC Z59.87
- memory — *see also* Amnesia
  - mild, following organic brain damage FØ6.8
- oil services Z59.12
- ovulation N97.Ø
- parental supervision or control of child Z62.Ø
- person able to render necessary care Z74.2
- physical exercise Z72.3
- play experience in childhood Z62.898
- posterior occlusal support M26.57
- relaxation (affecting life-style) Z73.2
- safe drinking water Z58.6
- sexual
  - desire F52.Ø
  - enjoyment F52.1
- shelter Z59.Ø2
- sleep (adequate) Z72.82Ø
- supervision of child by parent Z62.Ø
- support, posterior occlusal M26.57
- transportation Z59.82
- water T73.1- ☑
  - safe drinking Z58.6
  - services Z59.12

**Lacrimal** — *see* condition

**Lacrimation, abnormal** — *see* Epiphora

**Lacrimonasal duct** — *see* condition

**Lactate, elevated** — *see* Acidosis, lactic

**Lactation, lactating** (breast) (puerperal, postpartum)
- associated
  - cracked nipple O92.13
  - retracted nipple O92.Ø3
- defective O92.4
- disorder NEC O92.79
- excessive O92.6
- failed (complete) O92.3
  - partial O92.4
- mastitis NEC — *see* Mastitis, obstetric
- mother (care and/or examination) Z39.1
- nonpuerperal N64.3

**Lacticemia, excessive** — *see also* Acidosis E87.2Ø

**Lacunar skull** Q75.8

**LAD** (leukocyte adhesion deficiency) (LAD-I) (LAD-II) (LAD-III) D71.1

**Laennec's cirrhosis** K7Ø.3Ø
- with ascites K7Ø.31
- nonalcoholic K74.69

**Lafora disease** — *see also* Epilepsy, progressive, Lafora G4Ø.CØ9

**Lag, lid** (nervous) — *see* Retraction, lid

**Lagophthalmos** (eyelid) (nervous) HØ2.2Ø9
- bilateral, upper and lower eyelids HØ2.2ØC
- cicatricial HØ2.219
  - bilateral, upper and lower eyelids HØ2.21C
  - left HØ2.216
    - lower HØ2.215
    - upper HØ2.214
    - upper and lower eyelids HØ2.21B
  - right HØ2.213
    - lower HØ2.212
    - upper HØ2.211
    - upper and lower eyelids HØ2.21A
- keratoconjunctivitis — *see* Keratoconjunctivitis
- left HØ2.2Ø6
  - lower HØ2.2Ø5
  - upper HØ2.2Ø4
  - upper and lower eyelids HØ2.2ØB
- mechanical HØ2.229
  - bilateral, upper and lower eyelids HØ2.22C
  - left HØ2.226

- **Lagophthalmos** — *continued*
  - mechanical — *continued*
    - left — *continued*
      - lower HØ2.225
      - upper HØ2.224
      - upper and lower eyelids HØ2.22B
    - right HØ2.223
      - lower HØ2.222
      - upper HØ2.221
      - upper and lower eyelids HØ2.22A
  - paralytic HØ2.239
    - bilateral, upper and lower eyelids HØ2.23C
    - left HØ2.236
      - lower HØ2.235
      - upper HØ2.234
      - upper and lower eyelids HØ2.23B
    - right HØ2.233
      - lower HØ2.232
      - upper HØ2.231
      - upper and lower eyelids HØ2.23A
  - right HØ2.2Ø3
    - lower HØ2.2Ø2
    - upper HØ2.2Ø1
    - upper and lower eyelids HØ2.2ØA
- **Laki-Lorand factor deficiency** — *see* Defect, coagulation, specified type NEC
- **Lalling** F8Ø.Ø
- **Lambert-Eaton syndrome** — *see* Syndrome, Lambert-Eaton
- **Lambliasis, lambliosis** AØ7.1
- **Landau-Kleffner syndrome** — *see* Epilepsy, specified NEC
- **Landouzy-Dejerine dystrophy or facioscapulohumeral atrophy** G71.Ø2
- **Landouzy's disease** (icterohemorrhagic leptospirosis) A27.Ø
- **Landry-Guillain-Barre, syndrome or paralysis** G61.Ø
- **Landry's disease or paralysis** G61.Ø
- **Lane's**
  - band Q43.3
  - kink — *see* Obstruction, intestine
  - syndrome K9Ø.2
- **Langdon Down syndrome** — *see* Trisomy, 21
- **Lapsed immunization schedule status** Z28.39
- **Large**
  - baby (regardless of gestational age) (4ØØØg to 4499g) PØ8.1
  - ear, congenital Q17.1
  - physiological cup Q14.2
  - stature R68.89
- **Large-for-dates NEC** (infant) (4ØØØg to 4499g) PØ8.1
  - affecting management of pregnancy O36.6- ☑
  - exceptionally (45ØØg or more) PØ8.Ø
- **Larsen-Johansson disease or osteochondrosis** — *see* Osteochondrosis, juvenile, patella
- **Larsen's syndrome** (flattened facies and multiple congenital dislocations) Q74.8
- **Larva migrans**
  - cutaneous B76.9
    - Ancylostoma B76.Ø
  - visceral B83.Ø
- **Laryngeal** — *see* condition
- **Laryngismus** (stridulus) J38.5
  - congenital P28.89
  - diphtheritic A36.2
- **Laryngitis** (acute) (edematous) (fibrinous) (infective) (infiltrative) (malignant) (membranous) (phlegmonous) (pneumococcal) (pseudomembranous) (septic) (subglottic) (suppurative) (ulcerative) JØ4.Ø
  - with
    - influenza, flu, or grippe — *see* Influenza, with, laryngitis
    - tracheitis (acute) — *see* Laryngotracheitis
  - atrophic J37.Ø
  - catarrhal J37.Ø
  - chronic J37.Ø
    - with tracheitis (chronic) J37.1
  - diphtheritic A36.2
  - due to external agent — *see* Inflammation, respiratory, upper, due to
  - H. influenzae JØ4.Ø
  - Hemophilus influenzae JØ4.Ø
  - hypertrophic J37.Ø
  - influenzal — *see* Influenza, with, respiratory manifestations NEC
  - obstructive JØ5.Ø
  - sicca J37.Ø
  - spasmodic JØ5.Ø
    - acute JØ4.Ø
  - streptococcal JØ4.Ø
  - stridulous JØ5.Ø
- **Laryngitis** — *continued*
  - syphilitic (late) A52.73
    - congenital A5Ø.59 *[J99]*
      - early A5Ø.Ø3 *[J99]*
  - tuberculous A15.5
  - Vincent's A69.1
- **Laryngocele** (congenital) (ventricular) Q31.3
- **Laryngofissure** J38.7
  - congenital Q31.8
- **Laryngomalacia** (congenital) Q31.5
- **Laryngopharyngitis** (acute) JØ6.Ø
  - chronic J37.Ø
  - due to external agent — *see* Inflammation, respiratory, upper, due to
- **Laryngoplegia** J38.ØØ
  - bilateral J38.Ø2
  - unilateral J38.Ø1
- **Laryngoptosis** J38.7
- **Laryngospasm** J38.5
- **Laryngostenosis** J38.6
- **Laryngotracheitis** (acute) (Infectional) (infective) (viral) JØ4.2
  - atrophic J37.1
  - catarrhal J37.1
  - chronic J37.1
  - diphtheritic A36.2
  - due to external agent — *see* Inflammation, respiratory, upper, due to
  - Hemophilus influenzae JØ4.2
  - hypertrophic J37.1
  - influenzal — *see* Influenza, with, respiratory manifestations NEC
  - pachydermic J38.7
  - sicca J37.1
  - spasmodic J38.5
    - acute JØ5.Ø
  - streptococcal JØ4.2
  - stridulous J38.5
  - syphilitic (late) A52.73
    - congenital A5Ø.59 *[J99]*
      - early A5Ø.Ø3 *[J99]*
  - tuberculous A15.5
  - Vincent's A69.1
- **Laryngotracheobronchitis** — *see* Bronchitis
- **Larynx, laryngeal** — *see* condition
- **Lassa fever** A96.2
- **Lassitude** — *see* Weakness
- **Late**
  - talker R62.Ø
  - walker R62.Ø
- **Late effect**(s) — *see* Sequelae
- **Latent** — *see* condition
- **Laterocession** — *see* Lateroversion
- **Lateroflexion** — *see* Lateroversion
- **Lateroversion**
  - cervix — *see* Lateroversion, uterus
  - uterus, uterine (cervix) (postinfectional) (postpartal, old) N85.4
    - congenital Q51.818
    - in pregnancy or childbirth O34.59- ☑
- **Lathyrism** — *see* Poisoning, food, noxious, plant
- **Launois-Bensaude adenolipomatosis** E88.89
- **Launois' syndrome** (pituitary gigantism) E22.Ø
- **Laurence-Moon syndrome** Q87.84
- **Lax, laxity** — *see also* Relaxation
  - ligament (ous) — *see also* Disorder, ligament
    - familial M35.7
    - knee — *see* Derangement, knee
  - skin (acquired) L57.4
    - congenital Q82.8
- **Laxative habit** F55.2
- **Lazy leukocyte syndrome** D7Ø.8
- **LBSL** (leukoencephalopathy with brainstem - spinal cord involvement - lactate elevation) E88.43
- **Lead miner's lung** J63.6
- **Leak, leakage**
  - air NEC J93.82
    - postprocedural J95.812
  - amniotic fluid — *see* Rupture, membranes, premature
  - blood (microscopic), fetal, into maternal circulation affecting management of pregnancy — *see* Pregnancy, complicated by
  - cerebrospinal fluid G96.ØØ
    - cranial
      - postoperative G96.Ø8
      - specified NEC G96.Ø8
      - spontaneous G96.Ø1
      - traumatic G96.Ø8
    - from spinal (lumbar) puncture G97.Ø
- **Leak, leakage** — *continued*
  - cerebrospinal fluid — *continued*
    - spinal
      - postoperative G96.Ø9
      - post-traumatic G96.Ø9
      - specified NEC G96.Ø9
      - spontaneous G96.Ø2
    - spontaneous
      - from
        - skull base G96.Ø1
        - spine G96.Ø2
  - CSF — *see* Leak, cerebrospinal fluid
  - device, implant or graft — *see also* Complications, by site and type, mechanical
    - arterial graft NEC — *see* Complication, vascular, graft, mechanical, leakage T82.838- ☑
    - breast (implant) T85.43- ☑
    - catheter NEC T85.638- ☑
      - dialysis (renal) T82.43- ☑
        - intraperitoneal T85.631- ☑
      - infusion NEC T82.534- ☑
        - spinal (epidural) (subdural) T85.63Ø- ☑
      - urinary T83.Ø38- ☑
        - cystostomy T83.Ø3Ø- ☑
        - Hopkins T83.Ø38- ☑
        - ileostomy T83.Ø38- ☑
        - indwelling T83.Ø31- ☑
        - nephrostomy T83.Ø32- ☑
        - specified T83.Ø38- ☑
        - urostomy T83.Ø38- ☑
    - gastrointestinal — *see* Complications, prosthetic device, mechanical, gastrointestinal device
    - genital NEC T83.498- ☑
      - penile prosthesis (cylinder) (implanted) (pump) (reservoir) T83.49Ø- ☑
      - testicular prosthesis T83.491- ☑
    - heart NEC — *see* Complication, cardiovascular device, mechanical
    - joint prosthesis — *see* Complications, joint prosthesis, mechanical, specified NEC, by site
    - ocular NEC — *see* Complications, prosthetic device, mechanical, ocular device
    - orthopedic NEC — *see* Complication, orthopedic, device, mechanical
    - persistent air J93.82
    - specified NEC T85.638- ☑
    - urinary NEC — *see also* Complication, genitourinary, device, urinary, mechanical
      - graft T83.23- ☑
    - vascular NEC — *see* Complication, cardiovascular device, mechanical
    - ventricular intracranial shunt T85.Ø3- ☑
  - urine — *see* Incontinence
- **Leaky heart** — *see* Endocarditis
- **Learning defect** (specific) F81.9
- **Leather bottle stomach** C16.9
- **Leber's**
  - congenital amaurosis H35.5Ø
  - optic atrophy (hereditary) H47.22
- **Lederer's anemia** D59.19
- **Leeches** (external) — *see* Hirudiniasis
- **Leg** — *see* condition
- Legg (-Calve)-**Perthes disease, syndrome or osteochondrosis** M91.1- ☑
- **Legionellosis** A48.1
  - nonpneumonic A48.2
- **Legionnaires'**
  - disease A48.1
    - nonpneumonic A48.2
  - pneumonia A48.1
- **Leigh's disease** G31.82
- **Leiner's disease** L21.1
- **Leiofibromyoma** — *see* Leiomyoma
- **Leiomyoblastoma** — *see* Neoplasm, connective tissue, benign
- **Leiomyofibroma** — *see also* Neoplasm, connective tissue benign
  - uterus (cervix) (corpus) D25.9
- **Leiomyoma** — *see also* Neoplasm, connective tissue, benign
  - bizarre — *see* Neoplasm, connective tissue, benign
  - cellular — *see* Neoplasm, connective tissue, benign
  - epithelioid — *see* Neoplasm, connective tissue, benign
  - uterus (cervix) (corpus) D25.9
    - intramural D25.1
    - submucous D25.Ø
    - subserosal D25.2
  - vascular — *see* Neoplasm, connective tissue, benign

**Littre's**
- gland — *see* condition
- hernia — *see* Hernia, abdomen

**Littritis** — *see* Urethritis
**Livedo** (annularis) (racemosa) (reticularis) R23.1
**Liver** — *see* condition
**Lives in a homeless encampment** Z59.Ø2
**Living alone** (problems with) Z6Ø.2
- with handicapped person Z74.2

**Living in a shelter** (motel) (scattered site housing) (temporary or transitional living situation) Z59.Ø1
**Lloyd's syndrome** — *see* Adenomatosis, endocrine
**Loa loa** (loiasis) B74.3
**Lobar** — *see* condition
**Lobomycosis** B48.Ø
**Lobo's disease** B48.Ø
**Lobotomy syndrome** FØ7.Ø
**Lobstein** (-Ekman) **disease or syndrome** Q78.Ø
**Lobster-claw hand** Q71.6- ☑
**Lobulation** (congenital) — *see also* Anomaly, by site
- kidney, Q63.1
- liver, abnormal Q44.79
- spleen Q89.Ø9

**Lobule, lobular** — *see* condition
**Local, localized** — *see* condition
**Locked-in state** G83.5
**Locked twins causing obstructed labor** O66.1
**Locking**
- joint — *see* Derangement, joint, specified type NEC
  - knee — *see* Derangement, knee

**Lockjaw** — *see* Tetanus
**Loffler's**
- endocarditis I42.3
- eosinophilia J82.89
- pneumonia J82.89
- syndrome (eosinophilic pneumonitis) J82.89

**Loiasis** (with conjunctival infestation) (eyelid) B74.3
**Lone Star fever** A77.Ø
**Loneliness** R45.89
**Long**
- COVID (-19) — *see also* COVID-19 UØ9.9
- labor O63.9
  - first stage O63.Ø
  - second stage O63.1
- QT syndrome I45.81

**Long-term** (current) (prophylactic) **drug therapy** (use of)
- 5-fluorouracil Z79.631
- 6-mercaptopurine Z79.631
- adalimumab Z79.62Ø
- agents affecting estrogen receptors and estrogen levels NEC Z79.818
- alkylating agent Z79.63Ø
- anastrozole (Arimidex) Z79.811
- anti-inflammatory, non-steroidal (NSAID) Z79.1
- antibiotics Z79.2
  - short-term use — *omit code*
- anticoagulants Z79.Ø1
- antidiabetic drugs, injectable, non-insulin Z79.85
- antimetabolite agent Z79.631
- antiplatelet Z79.Ø2
- antithrombotics Z79.Ø2
- antitumor antibiotic Z79.632
- apremilast Z79.61
- aromatase inhibitors Z79.811
- aspirin Z79.82
- azathioprine Z79.624
- birth control pill or patch Z79.3
- bisphosphonates Z79.83
- bleomycin Z79.632
- calcineurin inhibitor Z79.621
- chlorambucil Z79.63Ø
- cisplatin Z79.63Ø
- contraceptive, oral Z79.3
- cyclophosphamide Z79.63Ø
- cyclosporine Z79.621
- cytarabine Z79.631
- doxorubicin Z79.632
- drug, specified NEC Z79.899
- estrogen receptor downregulators Z79.818
- etanercept Z79.62Ø
- etoposide Z79.634
- Evista Z79.81Ø
- exemestane (Aromasin) Z79.811
- Fareston Z79.81Ø
- fulvestrant (Faslodex) Z79.818
- gonadotropin-releasing hormone (GnRH) agonist Z79.818
- goserelin acetate (Zoladex) Z79.818
- hormone replacement Z79.89Ø
- hydroxyurea Z79.64

**Long-term** (current) (prophylactic) **drug therapy** — *continued*
- immunomodulators, unspecified Z79.6Ø
  - specified NEC Z79.69
- immunomodulatory imide drug Z79.61
- immunosuppressants, unspecified Z79.6Ø
  - specified NEC Z79.69
- immunosuppressive biologic Z79.62Ø
- infliximab Z79.62Ø
- inhibitors of nucleotide synthesis Z79.624
- insulin Z79.4
- irinotecan Z79.634
- Janus kinase inhibitor Z79.622
- lenalidomide Z79.61
- letrozole (Femara) Z79.811
- leuprolide acetate (leuprorelin) (Lupron) Z79.818
- mammalian target of rapamycin (mTOR) inhibitor Z79.623
- megestrol acetate (Megace) Z79.818
- methadone for pain management Z79.891
- mitomycin C Z79.632
- mitotic inhibitor Z79.633
- monoclonal antibodies Z79.62Ø
- mycophenolate Z79.624
- myelosuppressive agent Z79.64
- Nolvadex Z79.81Ø
- non-insulin antidiabetic drug, injectable Z79.85
- non-steroidal anti-inflammatories (NSAID) Z79.1
- opiate analgesic Z79.891
- oral
  - antidiabetic Z79.84
  - contraceptive Z79.3
  - hypoglycemic Z79.84
- paclitaxel Z79.633
- plant alkaloids Z79.633
- pomalidomide Z79.61
- purine synthesis (IMDH) inhibitors Z79.624
- raloxifene (Evista) Z79.81Ø
- selective estrogen receptor modulators (SERMs) Z79.81Ø
- sirolimus Z79.623
- steroids
  - inhaled Z79.51
  - systemic Z79.52
- tacrolimus Z79.621
- tamoxifen (Nolvadex) Z79.81Ø
- tofacitinib Z79.622
- topoisomerase inhibitor Z79.634
- topotecan Z79.634
- toremifene (Fareston) Z79.81Ø
- vinblastine Z79.633
- vincristine Z79.633

**Longitudinal stripes or grooves, nails** L6Ø.8
- congenital Q84.6

**Loop**
- intestine — *see* Volvulus
- vascular on papilla (optic) Q14.2

**Loose** — *see also* condition
- body
  - joint M24.ØØ
    - ankle M24.Ø7- ☑
    - elbow M24.Ø2- ☑
    - hand M24.Ø4- ☑
    - hip M24.Ø5- ☑
    - knee M23.4- ☑
    - shoulder (region) M24.Ø1- ☑
    - specified site NEC M24.Ø8
    - temporomandibular M24.Ø8
    - toe M24.Ø7- ☑
    - vertebra M24.Ø8
    - wrist M24.Ø3- ☑
  - knee M23.4- ☑
  - sheath, tendon — *see* Disorder, tendon, specified type NEC
- cartilage — *see* Loose, body, joint
- skin and subcutaneous tissue (following bariatric surgery weight loss) (following dietary weight loss) L98.7
- tooth, teeth KØ8.89

**Loosening**
- aseptic
  - joint prosthesis — *see* Complications, joint prosthesis, mechanical, loosening, by site
- epiphysis — *see* Osteochondropathy
- mechanical
  - joint prosthesis — *see* Complications, joint prosthesis, mechanical, loosening, by site

**Looser-Milkman** (-Debray) **syndrome** M83.8
**Lop ear** (deformity) Q17.3
**Lorain** (-Levi) **short stature syndrome** E23.Ø

**Lordosis** M4Ø.5Ø
- acquired — *see* Lordosis, specified type NEC
- congenital Q76.429
  - lumbar region Q76.426
  - lumbosacral region Q76.427
  - sacral region Q76.428
  - sacrococcygeal region Q76.428
  - thoracolumbar region Q76.425
- lumbar region M4Ø.56
- lumbosacral region M4Ø.57
- postsurgical M96.4
- postural — *see* Lordosis, specified type NEC
- rachitic (late effect) (sequelae) E64.3
- sequelae of rickets E64.3
- specified type NEC M4Ø.4Ø
  - lumbar region M4Ø.46
  - lumbosacral region M4Ø.47
  - thoracolumbar region M4Ø.45
- thoracolumbar region M4Ø.55
- tuberculous A18.Ø1

**Loss** (of)
- appetite — *see also* Anorexia R63.Ø
  - hysterical F5Ø.89
  - nonorganic origin F5Ø.89
  - psychogenic F5Ø.89
- blood — *see* Hemorrhage
- bone —*see* Loss, substance of, bone
- consciousness, transient R55
  - traumatic — *see* Injury, intracranial
- control, sphincter, rectum R15.9
  - nonorganic origin F98.1
- elasticity, skin R23.4
- family (member) in childhood Z62.898
- fluid (acute) E86.9
- function of labyrinth — *see* subcategory H83.2- ☑
- hair, nonscarring — *see* Alopecia
- hearing — *see also* Deafness
  - central NOS H9Ø.5
  - conductive H9Ø.2
    - bilateral H9Ø.Ø
    - unilateral
      - with
        - restricted hearing on the contralateral side H9Ø.A1- ☑
        - unrestricted hearing on the contralateral side H9Ø.1- ☑
  - mixed conductive and sensorineural hearing loss H9Ø.8
    - bilateral H9Ø.6
    - unilateral
      - with
        - restricted hearing on the contralateral side H9Ø.A3- ☑
        - unrestricted hearing on the contralateral side H9Ø.7- ☑
  - neural NOS H9Ø.5
  - perceptive NOS H9Ø.5
  - sensorineural NOS H9Ø.5
    - bilateral H9Ø.3
    - unilateral
      - with
        - restricted hearing on the contralateral side H9Ø.A2- ☑
        - unrestricted hearing on the contralateral side H9Ø.4- ☑
  - sensory NOS H9Ø.5
- height R29.89Ø
- limb or member, traumatic, current — *see* Amputation, traumatic
- love relationship in childhood Z62.898
- memory — *see also* Amnesia
  - mild, following organic brain damage FØ6.8
- mind — *see* Psychosis
- occlusal vertical dimension of fully erupted teeth M26.37
- organ or part — *see* Absence, by site, acquired
- ossicles, ear (partial) H74.32- ☑
- parent in childhood Z63.4
- pregnancy, recurrent N96
  - care in current pregnancy O26.2- ☑
  - without current pregnancy N96
- recurrent pregnancy — *see* Loss, pregnancy, recurrent
- self-esteem, in childhood Z62.898
- sense of
  - smell — *see* Disturbance, sensation, smell
  - taste — *see* Disturbance, sensation, taste
  - touch R2Ø.8
- sensory R44.9
  - dissociative F44.6

**Loss** — *continued*
- sexual desire F52.Ø
- sight (acquired) (complete) (congenital) — *see* Blindness
- substance of
  - bone — *see* Disorder, bone, density and structure, specified NEC
    - horizontal alveolar KØ6.3
  - cartilage — *see* Disorder, cartilage, specified type NEC
    - auricle (ear) — *see* Disorder, pinna, specified type NEC
  - vitreous (humor) H15.89
- tooth, teeth — *see* Absence, teeth, acquired
- vision, visual H54.7
  - both eyes H54.3
  - one eye H54.6Ø
    - left (normal vision on right) H54.62
    - right (normal vision on left) H54.61
  - specified as blindness — *see* Blindness
  - subjective
    - sudden H53.13- ☑
    - transient H53.12- ☑
- vitreous — *see* Prolapse, vitreous
- voice — *see* Aphonia
- weight (abnormal) (cause unknown) R63.4

**Louis-Bar syndrome** (ataxia-telangiectasia) G11.3
**Louping ill** (encephalitis) A84.89
**Louse, lousiness** — *see* Lice
**Low**
- achiever, school Z55.3
- back syndrome M54.5Ø
- basal metabolic rate R94.8
- birthweight (2499 grams or less) PØ7.1Ø
  - with weight of
    - 1ØØØ-1249 grams PØ7.14
    - 125Ø-1499 grams PØ7.15
    - 15ØØ-1749 grams PØ7.16
    - 175Ø-1999 grams PØ7.17
    - 2ØØØ-2499 grams PØ7.18
  - extreme (999 grams or less) PØ7.ØØ
    - with weight of
      - 499 grams or less PØ7.Ø1
      - 5ØØ-749 grams PØ7.Ø2
      - 75Ø-999 grams PØ7.Ø3
  - for gestational age — *see* Light for dates
- blood pressure — *see also* Hypotension
  - reading (incidental) (isolated) (nonspecific) RØ3.1
- cardiac reserve — *see* Disease, heart
- function — *see also* Hypofunction
  - kidney N28.9
- hematocrit D64.9
- hemoglobin D64.9
- income Z59.6
- level of literacy Z55.Ø
- lying
  - kidney N28.89
  - organ or site, congenital — *see* Malposition, congenital
- output syndrome (cardiac) — *see* Failure, heart
- platelets (blood) — *see* Thrombocytopenia
- reserve, kidney N28.89
- salt syndrome E87.1
- self esteem R45.81
- set ears Q17.4
- vision H54.2X- ☑
  - one eye (other eye normal) H54.5Ø
    - left (normal vision on right)
      - category 1 H54.52A1
      - category 2 H54.52A2
    - other eye blind — *see* Blindness
    - right (normal vision on left)
      - category 1 H54.511A
      - category 2 H54.512A
- von Willebrand factor R79.1

**Low-density-lipoprotein-type** (LDL) **hyperlipoproteinemia** E78.ØØ
**Lowe's syndrome** E72.Ø3
**Lown-Ganong-Levine syndrome** I45.6
**LSD reaction** (acute) (without dependence) F16.9Ø
- with dependence F16.2Ø

**LTBI** (latent tuberculosis infection) Z22.7
**LTBL** (leukoencephalopathy with thalamus - brainstem involvement - high lactate) E88.43
**Ludwig's angina or disease** K12.2
**Lues** (venerea), **luetic** — *see* Syphilis
**Luetscher's syndrome** (dehydration) E86.Ø
**Lumbago, lumbalgia** M54.5Ø
- with sciatica M54.4- ☑
  - due to intervertebral disc disorder M51.17
- due to displacement, intervertebral disc M51.27

**Lumbago, lumbalgia** — *continued*
- due to displacement, intervertebral disc — *continued*
  - with sciatica M51.17

**Lumbar** — *see* condition
**Lumbarization, vertebra, congenital** Q76.49
**Lumbermen's itch** B88.Ø9
**Lump** — *see also* Mass
- breast N63.Ø
  - axillary tail
    - left N63.32
    - right N63.31
  - left
    - lower inner quadrant N63.24
    - lower outer quadrant N63.23
    - overlapping quadrants N63.25
    - unspecified quadrant N63.2Ø
    - upper inner quadrant N63.22
    - upper outer quadrant N63.21
  - right
    - lower inner quadrant N63.14
    - lower outer quadrant N63.13
    - overlapping quadrants N63.15
    - unspecified quadrant N63.1Ø
    - upper inner quadrant N63.12
    - upper outer quadrant N63.11
  - subareolar
    - left N63.42
    - right N63.41

**Lunacy** — *see* Psychosis
**Lung** — *see* condition
**Lupoid** (miliary) **of Boeck** D86.3
**Lupus**
- anticoagulant D68.62
  - with
    - hemorrhagic disorder D68.312
    - hypercoagulable state D68.62
  - finding without diagnosis R76.Ø
- discoid (local) L93.Ø
- erythematosus (discoid) (local) L93.Ø
  - disseminated — *see* Lupus, erythematosus, systemic
  - eyelid HØ1.129
    - left HØ1.126
      - lower HØ1.125
      - upper HØ1.124
    - right HØ1.123
      - lower HØ1.122
      - upper HØ1.121
  - profundus L93.2
  - specified NEC L93.2
  - subacute cutaneous L93.1
  - systemic M32.9
    - with organ or system involvement M32.1Ø
      - endocarditis M32.11
      - lung M32.13
      - pericarditis M32.12
      - renal (glomerular) M32.14
        - tubulo-interstitial M32.15
      - specified organ or system NEC M32.19
    - drug-induced M32.Ø
    - inhibitor (presence of) D68.62
      - with
        - hemorrhagic disorder D68.312
        - hypercoagulable state D68.62
      - finding without diagnosis R76.Ø
    - specified NEC M32.8
- exedens A18.4
- hydralazine M32.Ø
  - correct substance properly administered — *see* Table of Drugs and Chemicals, by drug, adverse effect
  - overdose or wrong substance given or taken — *see* Table of Drugs and Chemicals, by drug, poisoning
- nephritis (chronic) M32.14
- nontuberculous, not disseminated L93.Ø
- panniculitis L93.2
- pernio (Besnier) D86.3
- systemic — *see* Lupus, erythematosus, systemic
- tuberculous A18.4
  - eyelid A18.4
- vulgaris A18.4
  - eyelid A18.4

**Luteinoma** D27.- ☑
**Lutembacher's disease or syndrome** (atrial septal defect with mitral stenosis) Q21.19
**Luteoma** D27.- ☑
**Lutz** (-Splendore-de Almeida) **disease** — *see* Paracoccidioidomycosis
**Luxation** — *see also* Dislocation

**Luxation** — *continued*
- eyeball (nontraumatic) — *see* Luxation, globe
  - birth injury P15.3
- globe, nontraumatic H44.82- ☑
- lacrimal gland — *see* Dislocation, lacrimal gland
- lens (old) (partial) (spontaneous)
  - congenital Q12.1
    - syphilitic A5Ø.39

**Lycanthropy** F22
**Lyell's syndrome** L51.2
- due to drug L51.2
  - correct substance properly administered — *see* Table of Drugs and Chemicals, by drug, adverse effect
  - overdose or wrong substance given or taken — *see* Table of Drugs and Chemicals, by drug, poisoning

**Lyme disease** A69.2Ø
**Lymph**
- gland or node — *see* condition
- scrotum — *see* Infestation, filarial

**Lymphadenitis** I88.9
- with ectopic or molar pregnancy OØ8.Ø
- acute LØ4.9
  - axilla LØ4.2
  - face LØ4.Ø
  - flank LØ3.32A
  - head LØ4.Ø
  - hip LØ4.3
  - limb
    - lower LØ4.3
    - upper LØ4.2
  - neck LØ4.Ø
  - shoulder LØ4.2
  - specified site NEC LØ4.8
  - trunk LØ4.1
- anthracosis (occupational) J6Ø
- any site, except mesenteric I88.9
  - chronic I88.1
  - subacute I88.1
- breast
  - gestational — *see* Mastitis, obstetric
  - puerperal, postpartum (nonpurulent) O91.22
- chancroidal (congenital) A57
- chronic I88.1
  - mesenteric I88.Ø
- due to
  - Brugia (malayi) B74.1
    - timori B74.2
  - chlamydial lymphogranuloma A55
  - diphtheria (toxin) A36.89
  - lymphogranuloma venereum A55
  - Wuchereria bancrofti B74.Ø
- following ectopic or molar pregnancy OØ8.Ø
- gonorrheal A54.89
- infective — *see* Lymphadenitis, acute
- mesenteric (acute) (chronic) (nonspecific) (subacute) I88.Ø
  - due to Salmonella typhi AØ1.Ø9
  - tuberculous A18.39
- mycobacterial A31.8
- purulent — *see* Lymphadenitis, acute
- pyogenic — *see* Lymphadenitis, acute
- regional, nonbacterial I88.8
- septic — *see* Lymphadenitis, acute
- subacute, unspecified site I88.1
- suppurative — *see* Lymphadenitis, acute
- syphilitic (early) (secondary) A51.49
  - late A52.79
- tuberculous — *see* Tuberculosis, lymph gland
- venereal (chlamydial) A55

**Lymphadenoid goiter** EØ6.3
**Lymphadenopathy** (generalized) R59.1
- angioimmunoblastic, with dysproteinemia (AILD) C86.5- ☑
- due to toxoplasmosis (acquired) B58.89
  - congenital (acute) (subacute) (chronic) P37.1
- localized R59.Ø
- syphilitic (early) (secondary) A51.49

**Lymphadenosis** R59.1
**Lymphangiectasis** I89.Ø
- conjunctiva H11.89
- postinfectional I89.Ø
- scrotum I89.Ø

**Lymphangiectatic elephantiasis, nonfilarial** I89.Ø
**Lymphangioendothelioma** D18.1
- malignant — *see* Neoplasm, connective tissue, malignant

**Lymphangioleiomyomatosis** J84.81
**Lymphangioma** D18.1
- capillary D18.1

**Lymphangioma** — *continued*
  cavernous D18.1
  cystic D18.1
  malignant — *see* Neoplasm, connective tissue, malignant
**Lymphangiomyoma** D18.1
**Lymphangiomyomatosis** J84.81
**Lymphangiosarcoma** — *see* Neoplasm, connective tissue, malignant
**Lymphangitis** I89.1
  with
    abscess — *code by* site under Abscess
    cellulitis — *code by* site under Cellulitis
    ectopic or molar pregnancy O08.Ø
  acute LØ3.91
    abdominal wall LØ3.321
    ankle — *see* Lymphangitis, acute, lower limb
    arm — *see* Lymphangitis, acute, upper limb
    auricle (ear) — *see* Lymphangitis, acute, ear
    axilla LØ3.12- ☑
    back (any part except buttock and flank) LØ3.322
    buttock LØ3.327
    cervical (meaning neck) LØ3.222
    cheek (external) LØ3.212
    chest wall LØ3.323
    digit
      finger — *see* Lymphangitis, acute, finger
      toe — *see* Lymphangitis, acute, toe
    ear (external) H6Ø.1- ☑
    external auditory canal — *see* Lymphangitis, acute, ear
    eyelid — *see* Abscess, eyelid
    face NEC LØ3.212
    finger (intrathecal) (periosteal) (subcutaneous) (subcuticular) LØ3.Ø2- ☑
    flank LØ3.32A
    foot — *see* Lymphangitis, acute, lower limb
    gluteal (region) LØ3.327
    groin LØ3.324
    hand — *see* Lymphangitis, acute, upper limb
    head NEC LØ3.891
      face (any part, except ear, eye and nose) LØ3.212
    heel — *see* Lymphangitis, acute, lower limb
    hip — *see* Lymphangitis, acute, lower limb
    jaw (region) LØ3.212
    knee — *see* Lymphangitis, acute, lower limb
    leg — *see* Lymphangitis, acute, lower limb
    lower limb LØ3.12- ☑
      toe — *see* Lymphangitis, acute, toe
    navel LØ3.326
    neck (region) LØ3.222
    orbit, orbital — *see* Cellulitis, orbit
    pectoral (region) LØ3.323
    perineal, perineum LØ3.325
    scalp (any part) LØ3.891
    shoulder — *see* Lymphangitis, acute, upper limb
    specified site NEC LØ3.898
    thigh — *see* Lymphangitis, acute, lower limb
    thumb (intrathecal) (periosteal) (subcutaneous) (subcuticular) — *see* Lymphangitis, acute, finger
    toe (intrathecal) (periosteal) (subcutaneous) (subcuticular) LØ3.Ø4- ☑
    trunk LØ3.329
      abdominal wall LØ3.321
      back (any part except buttock and flank) LØ3.322
      buttock LØ3.327
      chest wall LØ3.323
      groin LØ3.324
      perineal, perineum LØ3.325
      umbilicus LØ3.326
    umbilicus LØ3.326
    upper limb LØ3.12- ☑
      axilla — *see* Lymphangitis, acute, axilla
      finger — *see* Lymphangitis, acute, finger
      thumb — *see* Lymphangitis, acute, finger
    wrist — *see* Lymphangitis, acute, upper limb
  breast
    gestational — *see* Mastitis, obstetric
  chancroidal A57
  chronic (any site) I89.1
  due to
    Brugia (malayi) B74.1
      timori B74.2
    Wuchereria bancrofti B74.Ø
  following ectopic or molar pregnancy O08.89
  penis
    acute N48.29
    gonococcal (acute) (chronic) A54.Ø9

**Lymphangitis** — *continued*
  puerperal, postpartum, childbirth O86.89
  strumous, tuberculous A18.2
  subacute (any site) I89.1
  tuberculous — *see* Tuberculosis, lymph gland
**Lymphatic** (vessel) — *see* condition
**Lymphatism** E32.8
**Lymphectasia** I89.Ø
**Lymphedema** (acquired) — *see also* Elephantiasis
  congenital Q82.Ø
  hereditary (chronic) (idiopathic) Q82.Ø
  postmastectomy I97.2
  praecox I89.Ø
  secondary I89.Ø
  surgical NEC I97.89
    postmastectomy (syndrome) I97.2
**Lymphoblastic** — *see* condition
**Lymphoblastoma** (diffuse) — *see* Lymphoma, lymphoblastic (diffuse)
  giant follicular — *see* Lymphoma, lymphoblastic (diffuse)
  macrofollicular — *see* Lymphoma, lymphoblastic (diffuse)
**Lymphocele** I89.8
**Lymphocytic**
  chorioencephalitis (acute) (serous) A87.2
  choriomeningitis (acute) (serous) A87.2
  meningoencephalitis A87.2
**Lymphocytoma, benign cutis** L98.8
**Lymphocytopenia** D72.81Ø
**Lymphocytosis** (symptomatic) D72.82Ø
  infectious (acute) B33.8
**Lymphoepithelioma** — *see* Neoplasm, malignant, by site
**Lymphogranuloma** (malignant) — *see also* Lymphoma, Hodgkin
  chlamydial A55
  inguinale A55
  venereum (any site) (chlamydial) (with stricture of rectum) A55
**Lymphogranulomatosis** (malignant) — *see also* Lymphoma, Hodgkin
  benign (Boeck's sarcoid) (Schaumann's) D86.1
**Lymphohistiocytosis, hemophagocytic** (familial) D76.1
**Lymphoid** — *see* condition
**Lymphoma** (of) (malignant) C85.9Ø
  adult T-cell (HTLV-1-associated) (acute variant) (chronic variant) (lymphomatoid variant) (smouldering variant) C91.5- ☑
  anaplastic large cell
    ALK-negative C84.7- ☑
    ALK-positive C84.6- ☑
    breast implant associated (BIA-ALCL) C84.7A
    CD3Ø-positive C84.6- ☑
    primary cutaneous C86.6- ☑
  angioimmunoblastic T-cell C86.5- ☑
  B-cell C85.1- ☑
  B-precursor C83.5- ☑
  BALT C88.4- ☑
  blastic NK-cell C86.4- ☑
  blastic plasmacytoid dendritic cell neoplasm (BPDCN) C86.4- ☑
  brain, primary — *see* Lymphoma, primary central nervous system
  bronchial-associated lymphoid tissue [BALT-lymphoma] C88.4- ☑
  Burkitt (atypical) C83.7- ☑
  Burkitt-like C83.7- ☑
  central nervous system, primary — *see* Lymphoma, primary central nervous system
  centrocytic C83.1- ☑
  cutaneous follicle center C82.6- ☑
  cutaneous T-cell C84.A- ☑ (*following* C84.7)
  diffuse follicle center C82.5- ☑
  diffuse large cell C83.3- ☑
    anaplastic C83.3- ☑
    B-cell C83.3- ☑
    CD3Ø-positive C83.3- ☑
    centroblastic C83.3- ☑
    extranodal and solid organ sites NEC C83.398
    immunoblastic C83.3- ☑
    plasmablastic C83.3- ☑
    primary central nervous system (brain) (meninges) (PCNSL) (spinal cord) C83.39Ø
    subtype not specified C83.3- ☑
    T-cell rich C83.3- ☑
  enteropathy-type (associated) (intestinal) T-cell C86.2- ☑
  extranodal marginal zone B-cell lymphoma of mucosa-associated lymphoid tissue [MALT-lymphoma] C88.4- ☑

**Lymphoma** — *continued*
  extranodal NK/T-cell, nasal type C86.Ø- ☑
  follicular C82.9- ☑
    grade
      I C82.Ø- ☑
      II C82.1- ☑
      III C82.2- ☑
      IIIa C82.3- ☑
      IIIb C82.4- ☑
    specified NEC C82.8- ☑
  hepatosplenic T-cell (alpha-beta) (gamma-delta) C86.1- ☑
  histiocytic C85.9- ☑
    true C96.A (*following* C96.6)
  Hodgkin C81.9- ☑
    lymphocyte depleted (classical) C81.3- ☑
    lymphocyte-rich (classical) C81.4- ☑
    mixed cellularity (classical) C81.2- ☑
    nodular
      lymphocyte predominant C81.Ø- ☑
      sclerosis (classical) C81.1- ☑
    nodular sclerosis (classical) C81.1- ☑
    specified NEC (classical) C81.7- ☑
  intravascular large B-cell C83.8- ☑
  Lennert's C84.4- ☑
  lymphoblastic (diffuse) C83.5- ☑
  lymphoblastic B-cell C83.5- ☑
  lymphoblastic T-cell C83.5- ☑
  lymphoepithelioid C84.4- ☑
  lymphoplasmacytic C83.Ø- ☑
    with IgM-production C88.Ø- ☑
  MALT C88.4- ☑
  mantle cell C83.1- ☑
  mature T-cell NEC C84.4- ☑
  mature T/NK-cell C84.9- ☑
    specified NEC C84.Z- ☑ (*following* C84.7)
  mediastinal (thymic) large B-cell C85.2- ☑
  Mediterranean C88.3- ☑
  meninges, primary — *see* Lymphoma, primary central nervous system
  mucosa-associated lymphoid tissue [MALT-lymphoma] C88.4- ☑
  NK/T cell C84.9- ☑
  nodal marginal zone C83.Ø- ☑
  non-follicular (diffuse) C83.9- ☑
    specified NEC C83.8- ☑
  non-Hodgkin — *see also* Lymphoma, by type C85.9- ☑
    specified NEC C85.8- ☑
  non-leukemic variant of B-CLL C83.Ø- ☑
  peripheral T-cell NEC C84.4- ☑
  primary central nervous system (brain) (meninges) (PCNSL) (spinal cord) C83.39Ø
    Burkitt C83.79
    diffuse large B-cell C83.39Ø
    lymphoblastic C83.59
    peripheral T-cell C84.49
  primary cutaneous
    anaplastic large cell C86.6- ☑
    CD3Ø-positive large T-cell C86.6- ☑
  primary effusion B-cell C83.8- ☑
  SALT C88.4- ☑
  skin-associated lymphoid tissue [SALT-lymphoma] C88.4- ☑
  small cell B-cell C83.Ø- ☑
  spinal cord, primary — *see* Lymphoma, primary central nervous system
  splenic marginal zone C83.Ø- ☑
  subcutaneous panniculitis-like T-cell C86.3- ☑
  T-precursor C83.5- ☑
  true histiocytic C96.A (*following* C96.6)
**Lymphomatosis** — *see* Lymphoma
**Lymphopathia venereum, veneris** A55
**Lymphopenia** D72.81Ø
**Lymphoplasmacytic leukemia** — *see* Leukemia, chronic lymphocytic, B-cell type
**Lymphoproliferation, X-linked disease** D82.3
**Lymphoreticulosis, benign** (of inoculation) A28.1
**Lymphorrhea** I89.8
**Lymphosarcoma** (diffuse) — *see also* Lymphoma C85.9- ☑
**Lymphostasis** I89.8
**Lypemania** — *see* Melancholia
**Lysine and hydroxylysine metabolism disorder** E72.3
**Lyssa** — *see* Rabies

# M

- **Malformation** — *continued*
  - arteriovenous, aneurysmatic — *continued*
    - peripheral — *continued*
      - renal vessel Q27.34
      - upper limb Q27.31
    - precerebral vessels (nonruptured) Q28.Ø
  - auricle
    - ear (congenital) Q17.3
      - acquired H61.119
        - left H61.112
          - with right H61.113
        - right H61.111
          - with left H61.113
  - bile duct Q44.5
  - bladder Q64.79
    - aplasia Q64.5
    - diverticulum Q64.6
    - exstrophy — *see* Exstrophy, bladder
    - neck obstruction Q64.31
  - bone Q79.9
    - face Q75.9
      - specified type NEC Q75.8
    - skull Q75.9
      - specified type NEC Q75.8
  - brain (multiple) QØ4.9
    - arteriovenous Q28.2
    - specified type NEC QØ4.8
  - branchial cleft Q18.2
  - breast Q83.9
    - specified type NEC Q83.8
  - broad ligament Q5Ø.6
  - bronchus Q32.4
  - bursa Q79.9
  - cardiac
    - chambers Q2Ø.9
      - specified type NEC Q2Ø.8
    - septum Q21.9
      - specified type NEC Q21.8
  - cerebral QØ4.9
    - vessels Q28.3
  - cervix uteri Q51.9
    - specified type NEC Q51.828
  - Chiari
    - Type I G93.5
    - Type II QØ7.Ø1
  - choroid (congenital) Q14.3
    - plexus QØ7.8
  - circulatory system Q28.9
  - cochlea Q16.5
  - cornea Q13.4
  - coronary vessels Q24.5
  - corpus callosum (congenital) QØ4.Ø
  - diaphragm Q79.1
  - digestive system NEC, specified type NEC Q45.8
  - dura QØ7.9
    - brain QØ4.9
    - spinal QØ6.9
  - ear Q17.9
    - causing impairment of hearing Q16.9
    - external Q17.9
      - accessory auricle Q17.Ø
      - causing impairment of hearing Q16.9
        - absence of
          - auditory canal Q16.1
          - auricle Q16.Ø
      - macrotia Q17.1
      - microtia Q17.2
      - misplacement Q17.4
      - misshapen NEC Q17.3
      - prominence Q17.5
      - specified type NEC Q17.8
    - inner Q16.5
    - middle Q16.4
      - absence of eustachian tube Q16.2
      - ossicles (fusion) Q16.3
    - ossicles Q16.3
    - specified type NEC Q17.8
  - epididymis Q55.4
  - esophagus Q39.9
    - specified type NEC Q39.8
  - eye Q15.9
    - lid Q1Ø.3
    - specified NEC Q15.8
  - fallopian tube Q5Ø.6
  - genital organ — *see* Anomaly, genitalia
  - great
    - artery Q25.9
      - aorta — *see* Malformation, aorta

- **Malformation** — *continued*
  - great — *continued*
    - artery — *continued*
      - pulmonary artery — *see* Malformation, pulmonary, artery
      - specified type NEC Q25.8
    - vein Q26.9
      - anomalous
        - portal venous connection Q26.5
        - pulmonary venous connection Q26.4
          - partial Q26.3
          - total Q26.2
      - persistent left superior vena cava Q26.1
      - portal vein-hepatic artery fistula Q26.6
      - specified type NEC Q26.8
      - vena cava stenosis, congenital Q26.Ø
  - gum Q38.6
  - hair Q84.2
  - heart Q24.9
    - specified type NEC Q24.8
  - integument Q84.9
    - specified type NEC Q84.8
  - internal ear Q16.5
  - intestine Q43.9
    - specified type NEC Q43.8
  - iris Q13.2
  - joint Q74.9
    - ankle Q74.2
    - lumbosacral Q76.49
    - sacroiliac Q74.2
    - specified type NEC Q74.8
  - kidney Q63.9
    - accessory Q63.Ø
    - giant Q63.3
    - horseshoe Q63.1
    - hydronephrosis Q62.Ø
    - malposition Q63.2
    - specified type NEC Q63.8
  - lacrimal apparatus Q1Ø.6
  - lingual Q38.3
  - lip Q38.Ø
  - liver Q44.7Ø
  - lung Q33.9
  - meninges or membrane (congenital) QØ7.9
    - cerebral QØ4.8
    - spinal (cord) QØ6.9
  - middle ear Q16.4
    - ossicles Q16.3
  - mitral valve Q23.9
    - specified NEC Q23.88
  - Mondini's (congenital) (malformation, cochlea) Q16.5
  - mouth (congenital) Q38.6
  - multiple types NEC Q89.7
  - musculoskeletal system Q79.9
  - myocardium Q24.8
  - nail Q84.6
  - nervous system (central) QØ7.9
  - nose Q3Ø.9
    - specified type NEC Q3Ø.8
  - optic disc Q14.2
  - orbit Q1Ø.7
  - ovary Q5Ø.39
  - palate Q38.5
  - parathyroid gland Q89.2
  - pelvic organs or tissues NEC
    - in pregnancy or childbirth O34.8- ☑
      - causing obstructed labor O65.5
  - penis Q55.69
    - aplasia Q55.5
    - curvature (lateral) Q55.61
    - hypoplasia Q55.62
  - pericardium Q24.8
  - peripheral vascular system Q27.9
    - specified type NEC Q27.8
  - pharynx Q38.8
  - precerebral vessels Q28.1
  - prostate Q55.4
  - pulmonary
    - arteriovenous Q25.72
    - artery Q25.9
      - atresia Q25.5
      - specified type NEC Q25.79
      - stenosis Q25.6
    - valve Q22.3
  - renal artery Q27.2
  - respiratory system Q34.9
  - retina Q14.1
  - scrotum — *see* Malformation, testis and scrotum
  - seminal vesicles Q55.4

- **Malformation** — *continued*
  - sense organs NEC QØ7.9
  - skin Q82.9
  - specified NEC Q89.89
  - spinal
    - cord QØ6.9
    - nerve root QØ7.8
  - spine Q76.49
    - kyphosis — *see* Kyphosis, congenital
    - lordosis — *see* Lordosis, congenital
  - spleen Q89.Ø9
  - stomach Q4Ø.3
    - specified type NEC Q4Ø.2
  - teeth, tooth KØØ.9
  - tendon Q79.9
  - testis and scrotum Q55.2Ø
    - aplasia Q55.Ø
    - hypoplasia Q55.1
    - polyorchism Q55.21
    - retractile testis Q55.22
    - scrotal transposition Q55.23
    - specified NEC Q55.29
  - thorax, bony Q76.9
  - throat Q38.8
  - thyroid gland Q89.2
  - tongue (congenital) Q38.3
    - hypertrophy Q38.2
    - tie Q38.1
  - trachea Q32.1
  - tricuspid valve Q22.9
    - specified type NEC Q22.8
  - umbilical cord NEC (complicating delivery) O69.89- ☑
  - umbilicus Q89.9
  - ureter Q62.8
    - agenesis Q62.4
    - duplication Q62.5
    - malposition — *see* Malposition, congenital, ureter
    - obstructive defect — *see* Defect, obstructive, ureter
    - vesico-uretero-renal reflux Q62.7
  - urethra Q64.79
    - aplasia Q64.5
    - duplication Q64.74
    - posterior valves Q64.2
    - prolapse Q64.71
    - stricture Q64.32
  - urinary system Q64.9
  - uterus Q51.9
    - specified type NEC Q51.818
  - vagina Q52.4
  - vas deferens Q55.4
    - atresia Q55.3
  - vascular system, peripheral Q27.9
  - venous — *see* Anomaly, vein(s)
  - vulva Q52.7Ø
- **Malfunction** — *see also* Dysfunction
  - cardiac electronic device T82.119- ☑
    - electrode T82.11Ø- ☑
    - pulse generator T82.111- ☑
    - specified type NEC T82.118- ☑
  - catheter device NEC T85.618- ☑
    - cystostomy T83.Ø1Ø- ☑
    - dialysis (renal) (vascular) T82.41- ☑
      - intraperitoneal T85.611- ☑
    - infusion NEC T82.514- ☑
      - cranial — *see also* Complication(s), catheter, cranial infusion, mechanical T85.69Ø- ☑
      - epidural — *see also* Complication(s), catheter, cranial infusion, mechanical T85.69Ø- ☑
      - intrathecal — *see also* Complication(s), catheter, cranial infusion, mechanical T85.69Ø- ☑
      - spinal — *see also* Complication(s), catheter, cranial infusion, mechanical T85.69Ø- ☑
      - subarachnoid — *see also* Complication(s), catheter, cranial infusion, mechanical T85.69Ø- ☑
      - subdural — *see also* Complication(s), catheter, cranial infusion, mechanical T85.69Ø- ☑
    - urinary — *see also* Breakdown, device, catheter T83.Ø18- ☑
  - colostomy K94.Ø3
    - valve K94.Ø3
  - cystostomy (stoma) N99.512
    - catheter T83.Ø1Ø- ☑
  - enteric stoma K94.13
  - enterostomy K94.13
  - esophagostomy K94.33
  - gastroenteric K31.89
  - gastrostomy K94.23
  - ileostomy K94.13

- **Malposition** — *continued*
  - uterus — *continued*
    - anteflexion or anteversion N85.4
      - congenital Q51.818
    - flexion N85.4
      - lateral — *see* Lateroversion, uterus
    - inversion N85.5
    - lateral (flexion) (version) — *see* Lateroversion, uterus
      - in pregnancy or childbirth — *see* subcategory O34.5- ☑
    - retroflexion or retroversion — *see* Retroversion, uterus
- **Malposture** R29.3
- **Malrotation**
  - cecum Q43.3
  - colon Q43.3
  - intestine Q43.3
  - kidney Q63.2
- **Malta fever** — *see* Brucellosis
- **Maltreatment**
  - adult
    - abandonment
      - confirmed T74.Ø1- ☑
      - suspected T76.Ø1- ☑
    - bullying
      - confirmed T74.31- ☑
      - suspected T76.31- ☑
    - confirmed T74.91- ☑
    - financial
      - confirmed T74.A1- ☑
      - suspected T76.A1- ☑
    - history of Z91.419
    - intimidation (through social media)
      - confirmed T74.31- ☑
      - suspected T76.31- ☑
    - neglect
      - confirmed T74.Ø1- ☑
      - suspected T76.Ø1- ☑
    - physical abuse
      - confirmed T74.11- ☑
      - suspected T76.11- ☑
    - psychological abuse
      - confirmed T74.31- ☑
      - history of Z91.411
      - suspected T76.31- ☑
    - sexual abuse
      - confirmed T74.21- ☑
      - suspected T76.21- ☑
    - suspected T76.91- ☑
    - threatened abuse (harm) (physical violence) (sexual abuse)
      - confirmed T74.31- ☑
      - suspected T76.31- ☑
  - child
    - abandonment
      - confirmed T74.Ø2- ☑
      - suspected T76.Ø2- ☑
    - bullying
      - confirmed T74.32- ☑
      - suspected T76.32- ☑
    - confirmed T74.92- ☑
    - financial
      - confirmed T74.A2- ☑
      - suspected T76.A2- ☑
    - history of — *see* History, personal (of), abuse
    - intimidation (through social media)
      - confirmed T74.32- ☑
      - suspected T76.32- ☑
    - neglect
      - confirmed T74.Ø2- ☑
      - history of — *see* History, personal (of), abuse
      - suspected T76.Ø2- ☑
    - physical abuse
      - confirmed T74.12- ☑
      - history of — *see* History, personal (of), abuse
      - suspected T76.12- ☑
    - psychological abuse
      - confirmed T74.32- ☑
      - history of — *see* History, personal (of), abuse
      - suspected T76.32- ☑
    - sexual abuse
      - confirmed T74.22- ☑
      - history of — *see* History, personal (of), abuse
      - suspected T76.22- ☑
    - suspected T76.92- ☑
    - threatened abuse (harm) (physical violence) (sexual abuse)
      - confirmed T74.32- ☑

- **Maltreatment** — *continued*
  - child — *continued*
    - threatened abuse — *continued*
      - suspected T76.32- ☑
  - personal history of Z91.89
- **Maltworker's lung** J67.4
- **Malunion, fracture** — *see* Fracture, by site
- **Mammillitis** N61.Ø
  - puerperal, postpartum O91.Ø2
- **Mammitis** — *see* Mastitis
- **Mammogram** (examination) Z12.39
  - routine Z12.31
- **Mammoplasia** N62
- **Management** (of)
  - bone conduction hearing device (implanted) Z45.32Ø
  - cardiac pacemaker NEC Z45.Ø18
  - cerebrospinal fluid drainage device Z45.41
  - cochlear device (implanted) Z45.321
  - contraceptive Z3Ø.9
    - specified NEC Z3Ø.8
  - implanted device Z45.9
    - specified NEC Z45.89
  - infusion pump Z45.1
  - procreative Z31.9
    - male factor infertility in female Z31.81
    - specified NEC Z31.89
  - prosthesis (external) — *see also* Fitting Z44.9
    - implanted Z45.9
      - specified NEC Z45.89
  - renal dialysis catheter Z49.Ø1
  - vascular access device Z45.2
- **Mangled** — *see* specified injury by site
- **Mania** (monopolar) — *see also* Disorder, mood, manic episode
  - with psychotic symptoms F3Ø.2
  - without psychotic symptoms F3Ø.1Ø
    - mild F3Ø.11
    - moderate F3Ø.12
    - severe F3Ø.13
  - Bell's F3Ø.8
  - chronic (recurrent) F31.89
  - hysterical F44.89
  - puerperal F3Ø.8
  - recurrent F31.89
- **Manic depression** F31.9
- **Manic-depressive insanity, psychosis, or syndrome** — *see* Disorder, bipolar
- **Mannosidosis** E77.1
- **Mansonelliasis, mansonellosis** B74.4
- **Manson's**
  - disease B65.1
  - schistosomiasis B65.1
- **Manual** — *see* condition
- **Maple-bark-stripper's lung** (disease) J67.6
- **Maple-syrup-urine disease** E71.Ø
- **Marable's syndrome** (celiac artery compression) I77.4
- **Marasmus** E41
  - due to malnutrition E41
  - intestinal E41
  - nutritional E41
  - senile R54
  - tuberculous NEC — *see* Tuberculosis
- **Marble**
  - bones Q78.2
  - skin R23.8
- **Marburg virus disease** A98.3
- **March**
  - fracture — *see* Fracture, traumatic, stress, by site
  - hemoglobinuria D59.6
- **Marchesani** (-Weill) **syndrome** Q87.Ø
- **Marchiafava-Micheli syndrome** D59.5
- **Marchiafava** (-Bignami) **syndrome or disease** G37.1
- **Marcus Gunn's syndrome** QØ7.8
- **Marfan syndrome** — *see* Syndrome, Marfan
- **Marie-Bamberger disease** — *see* Osteoarthropathy, hypertrophic, specified NEC
- **Marie-Charcot-Tooth neuropathic muscular atrophy** G6Ø.Ø
- **Marie-Strumpell arthritis, disease or spondylitis** — *see* Spondylitis, ankylosing
- **Marie's**
  - cerebellar ataxia (late-onset) G11.2
  - disease or syndrome (acromegaly) E22.Ø
- **Marion's disease** (bladder neck obstruction) N32.Ø
- **Marital conflict** Z63.Ø
- **Mark**
  - port wine Q82.5
  - raspberry Q82.5
  - strawberry Q82.5

- **Mark** — *continued*
  - stretch L9Ø.6
  - tattoo L81.8
- **Marker heterochromatin** — *see* Extra, marker chromosomes
- **Maroteaux-Lamy syndrome** (mild) (severe) E76.29
- **Marrow** (bone)
  - arrest D61.9
  - poor function D75.89
- **Marseilles fever** A77.1
- **Marsh fever** — *see* Malaria
- **Marshall's** (hidrotic) **ectodermal dysplasia** Q82.4
- **Marsh's disease** (exophthalmic goiter) EØ5.ØØ
  - with storm EØ5.Ø1
- **Masculinization** (female) **with adrenal hyperplasia** E25.9
  - congenital E25.Ø
- **Masculinovoblastoma** D27.- ☑
- **Masochism** (sexual) F65.51
- **Mason's lung** J62.8
- **Mass**
  - abdominal R19.ØØ
    - epigastric R19.Ø6
    - generalized R19.Ø7
    - left lower quadrant R19.Ø4
    - left upper quadrant R19.Ø2
    - periumbilic R19.Ø5
    - right lower quadrant R19.Ø3
    - right upper quadrant R19.Ø1
    - specified site NEC R19.Ø9
  - breast — *see also* Lump, breast N63.Ø
  - chest R22.2
  - cystic — *see* Cyst
  - ear H93.8- ☑
  - head R22.Ø
  - intra-abdominal (diffuse) (generalized) — *see* Mass, abdominal
  - kidney N28.89
  - liver R16.Ø
  - localized (skin) R22.9
    - chest R22.2
    - head R22.Ø
    - limb
      - lower R22.4- ☑
      - upper R22.3- ☑
    - neck R22.1
    - trunk R22.2
  - lung R91.8
  - malignant — *see* Neoplasm, malignant, by site
  - neck R22.1
  - pelvic (diffuse) (generalized) — *see* Mass, abdominal
  - specified organ NEC — *see* Disease, by site
  - splenic R16.1
  - substernal thyroid — *see* Goiter
  - superficial (localized) R22.9
  - umbilical (diffuse) (generalized) R19.Ø9
- **Massive** — *see* condition
- **Mast cell**
  - disease, systemic tissue D47.Ø2
  - leukemia C94.3- ☑
  - neoplasm
    - malignant C96.2Ø
      - specified type NEC C96.29
    - of uncertain behavior NEC D47.Ø9
  - sarcoma C96.22
  - tumor D47.Ø9
- **Mastalgia** N64.4
- **Masters-Allen syndrome** N83.8
- **Mastitis** (acute) (diffuse) (nonpuerperal) (subacute) N61.Ø
  - with abscess N61.1
  - chronic (cystic) — *see* Mastopathy, cystic
  - cystic (Schimmelbusch's type) — *see* Mastopathy, cysti
  - fibrocystic — *see* Mastopathy, cystic
  - granulomatous N61.2- ☑
  - infective N61.Ø
    - newborn P39.Ø
  - interstitial, gestational or puerperal — *see* Mastitis, obstetric
  - neonatal (noninfective) P83.4
    - infective P39.Ø
  - obstetric (interstitial) (nonpurulent)
    - associated with
      - lactation O91.23
      - pregnancy O91.21- ☑
      - puerperium O91.22
    - purulent
      - associated with
        - lactation O91.13
        - pregnancy O91.11- ☑

**Mastitis** — *continued*
obstetric — *continued*
purulent — *continued*
associated with — *continued*
puerperium O91.12
periductal — *see* Ectasia, mammary duct
phlegmonous — *see* Mastopathy, cystic
plasma cell — *see* Ectasia, mammary duct
without abscess N61.Ø
**Mastocytoma** (extracutaneous) D47.Ø9
malignant C96.29
solitary D47.Ø1
**Mastocytosis** D47.Ø9
aggressive systemic C96.21
cutaneous (diffuse) (maculopapular) D47.Ø1
congenital Q82.2
of neonatal onset Q82.2
of newborn onset Q82.2
indolent systemic D47.Ø2
isolated bone marrow D47.Ø2
malignant C96.29
systemic (indolent) (smoldering)
with an associated hematological non-mast cell lineage disease (SM-AHNMD) D47.Ø2
**Mastodynia** N64.4
**Mastoid** — *see* condition
**Mastoidalgia** — *see* subcategory H92.Ø- ☑
**Mastoiditis** (coalescent) (hemorrhagic) (suppurative) H7Ø.9- ☑
acute, subacute H7Ø.ØØ- ☑
complicated NEC H7Ø.Ø9- ☑
subperiosteal H7Ø.Ø1- ☑
chronic (necrotic) (recurrent) H7Ø.1- ☑
in (due to)
infectious disease NEC B99.- ☑ *[H75.Ø-]* ☑
parasitic disease NEC B89 *[H75.Ø-]* ☑
tuberculosis A18.Ø3
petrositis — *see* Petrositis
postauricular fistula — *see* Fistula, postauricular
specified NEC H7Ø.89- ☑
tuberculous A18.Ø3
**Mastopathy, mastopathia** N64.9
chronica cystica — *see* Mastopathy, cystic
cystic (chronic) (diffuse) N6Ø.1- ☑
with epithelial proliferation N6Ø.3- ☑
diffuse cystic — *see* Mastopathy, cystic
estrogenic, oestrogenica, oestrogenic N64.89
ovarian origin N64.89
**Mastoplasia, mastoplastia** N62
**Masturbation** (excessive) F98.8
**Maternal care** (for) — *see* Pregnancy (complicated by) (management affected by)
**Matheiu's disease** (leptospiral jaundice) A27.Ø
**Mauclaire's disease or osteochondrosis** — *see* Osteochondrosis, juvenile, hand, metacarpal
**Maxcy's disease** A75.2
**Maxilla, maxillary** — *see* condition
**May** (-Hegglin) **anomaly or syndrome** D72.Ø
**McArdle** (-Schmid)(-Pearson) **disease** (glycogen storage) E74.Ø4
**McCune-Albright syndrome** Q78.1
**McQuarrie's syndrome** (idiopathic familial hypoglycemia) E16.2
**ME/CFS** (myalgic encephalomyelitis/chronic fatigue syndrome) G93.32
**Meadow's syndrome** Q86.1
**Measles** (black) (hemorrhagic) (suppressed) BØ5.9
with
complications NEC BØ5.89
encephalitis BØ5.Ø
intestinal complications BØ5.4
keratitis (keratoconjunctivitis) BØ5.81
meningitis BØ5.1
otitis media BØ5.3
pneumonia BØ5.2
French — *see* Rubella
German — *see* Rubella
Liberty — *see* Rubella
**Meat-wrappers' asthma** J68.9
**Meatitis, urethral** — *see* Urethritis
**Meatus, meatal** — *see* condition
**Meckel-Gruber syndrome** Q61.9
**Meckel's diverticulitis, diverticulum** (displaced) (hypertrophic) Q43.Ø
malignant — *see* Table of Neoplasms, small intestine, malignant
**Meconium**
ileus, newborn P76.Ø

**Meconium** — *continued*
ileus, newborn — *continued*
in cystic fibrosis E84.11
meaning meconium plug (without cystic fibrosis) P76.Ø
obstruction, newborn P76.Ø
due to fecaliths P76.Ø
in mucoviscidosis E84.11
peritonitis P78.Ø
plug syndrome (newborn) NEC P76.Ø
**MED13L** (mediator complex subunit 13L) **syndrome** Q87.85
**Median** — *see also* condition
arcuate ligament syndrome I77.4
bar (prostate) (vesical orifice) — *see* Hyperplasia, prostate
rhomboid glossitis K14.2
**Mediastinal shift** R93.89
**Mediastinitis** (acute) (chronic) J98.51
syphilitic A52.73
tuberculous A15.8
**Mediastinopericarditis** — *see also* Pericarditis
acute I3Ø.9
adhesive I31.Ø
chronic I31.8
rheumatic IØ9.2
**Mediastinum, mediastinal** — *see* condition
**Mediator complex subunit 13L** (MED13L) **syndrome** Q87.85
**Medicine poisoning** — *see* Table of Drugs and Chemicals, by drug, poisoning
**Mediterranean**
fever — *see* Brucellosis
familial MØ4.1
tick A77.1
kala-azar B55.Ø
leishmaniasis B55.Ø
tick fever A77.1
**Medulla** — *see* condition
**Medullary cystic kidney** Q61.5
**Medullated fibers**
optic (nerve) Q14.8
retina Q14.1
**Medulloblastoma**
desmoplastic C71.6
specified site — *see* Neoplasm, malignant, by site
unspecified site C71.6
**Medulloepithelioma** — *see also* Neoplasm, malignant, by site
teratoid — *see* Neoplasm, malignant, by site
**Medullomyoblastoma**
specified site — *see* Neoplasm, malignant, by site
unspecified site C71.6
**Meekeren-Ehlers-Danlos syndrome** — *see also* Syndrome, Ehlers-Danlos Q79.69
**Megacolon** (acquired) (functional) (not Hirschsprung's disease) (in) K59.39
Chagas' disease B57.32
congenital, congenitum (aganglionic) Q43.1
Hirschsprung's (disease) Q43.1
toxic NEC K59.31
due to
Clostridioides difficile
not specified as recurrent AØ4.72
recurrent AØ4.71
Clostridium difficile
not specified as recurrent AØ4.72
recurrent AØ4.71
**Megaesophagus** (functional) K22.Ø
congenital Q39.5
in (due to) Chagas' disease B57.31
**Megalencephaly** QØ4.5
**Megalerythema** (epidemic) BØ8.3
**Megaloappendix** Q43.8
**Megalocephalus, megalocephaly NEC** Q75.3
**Megalocornea** Q15.8
with glaucoma Q15.Ø
**Megalocytic anemia** D53.1
**Megalodactylia** (fingers) (thumbs) (congenital) Q74.Ø
toes Q74.2
**Megaloduodenum** Q43.8
**Megaloesophagus** (functional) K22.Ø
congenital Q39.5
**Megalogastria** (acquired) K31.89
congenital Q4Ø.2
**Megalophthalmos** Q11.3
**Megalopsia** H53.15
**Megalosplenia** — *see* Splenomegaly
**Megaloureter** N28.82
congenital Q62.2
**Megarectum** K62.89

**Megasigmoid** K59.39
congenital Q43.2
**Megaureter** N28.82
congenital Q62.2
**Megavitamin-B6 syndrome** E67.2
**Megrim** — *see* Migraine
**Meibomian**
cyst, infected — *see* Hordeolum
gland — *see* condition
sty, stye — *see* Hordeolum
**Meibomitis** — *see* Hordeolum
**Meige-Milroy disease** (chronic hereditary edema) Q82.Ø
**Meige's syndrome** Q82.Ø
**Melalgia, nutritional** E53.8
**Melancholia** F32.A
climacteric (single episode) F32.89
recurrent episode F33.8
hypochondriac F45.29
intermittent (single episode) F32.89
recurrent episode F33.8
involutional (single episode) F32.89
recurrent episode F33.8
menopausal (single episode) F32.89
recurrent episode F33.8
puerperal F32.89
reactive (emotional stress or trauma) F32.3
recurrent F33.9
senile FØ3.- ☑
stuporous (single episode) F32.89
recurrent episode F33.8
**Melanemia** R79.89
**Melanoameloblastoma** — *see* Neoplasm, bone, benign
**Melanoblastoma** — *see* Melanoma
**Melanocarcinoma** — *see* Melanoma
**Melanocytoma, eyeball** D31.9- ☑
**Melanocytosis, neurocutaneous** Q82.8
**Melanoderma, melanodermia** L81.4
**Melanodontia, infantile** KØ3.89
**Melanodontoclasia** KØ3.89
**Melanoepithelioma** — *see* Melanoma
**Melanoma** (malignant) C43.9
acral lentiginous, malignant — *see* Melanoma, skin, by site
amelanotic — *see* Melanoma, skin, by site
balloon cell — *see* Melanoma, skin, by site
benign — *see* Nevus
desmoplastic, malignant — *see* Melanoma, skin, by site
epithelioid cell — *see* Melanoma, skin, by site
with spindle cell, mixed — *see* Melanoma, skin, by site
in
giant pigmented nevus — *see* Melanoma, skin, by site
Hutchinson's melanotic freckle — *see* Melanoma, skin, by site
junctional nevus — *see* Melanoma, skin, by site
precancerous melanosis — *see* Melanoma, skin, by site
in situ DØ3.9
abdominal wall DØ3.59
ala nasi DØ3.39
ankle DØ3.7- ☑
anus, anal (margin) (skin) DØ3.51
arm DØ3.6- ☑
auditory canal DØ3.2- ☑
auricle (ear) DØ3.2- ☑
auricular canal (external) DØ3.2- ☑
axilla, axillary fold DØ3.59
back DØ3.59
breast DØ3.52
brow DØ3.39
buttock DØ3.59
canthus (eye) DØ3.1- ☑
cheek (external) DØ3.39
chest wall DØ3.59
chin DØ3.39
choroid DØ3.8
conjunctiva DØ3.8
ear (external) DØ3.2- ☑
external meatus (ear) DØ3.2- ☑
eye DØ3.8
eyebrow DØ3.39
eyelid (lower) (upper) DØ3.1- ☑
face DØ3.3Ø
specified NEC DØ3.39
female genital organ (external) NEC DØ3.8
finger DØ3.6- ☑
flank DØ3.59

**Melanoma** — *continued*
  in situ — *continued*
    foot D03.7- ☑
    forearm D03.6- ☑
    forehead D03.39
    foreskin D03.8
    gluteal region D03.59
    groin D03.59
    hand D03.6- ☑
    heel D03.7- ☑
    helix D03.2- ☑
    hip D03.7- ☑
    interscapular region D03.59
    iris D03.8
    jaw D03.39
    knee D03.7- ☑
    labium (majus) (minus) D03.8
    lacrimal gland D03.8
    leg D03.7- ☑
    lip (lower) (upper) D03.0
    lower limb NEC D03.7- ☑
    male genital organ (external) NEC D03.8
    nail D03.9
      finger D03.6- ☑
      toe D03.7- ☑
    neck D03.4
    nose (external) D03.39
    orbit D03.8
    penis D03.8
    perianal skin D03.51
    perineum D03.51
    pinna D03.2- ☑
    popliteal fossa or space D03.7- ☑
    prepuce D03.8
    pudendum D03.8
    retina D03.8
    retrobulbar D03.8
    scalp D03.4
    scrotum D03.8
    shoulder D03.6- ☑
    specified site NEC D03.8
    submammary fold D03.52
    temple D03.39
    thigh D03.7- ☑
    toe D03.7- ☑
    trunk NEC D03.59
    umbilicus D03.59
    upper limb NEC D03.6- ☑
    vulva D03.8
  juvenile — *see* Nevus
  malignant, of soft parts except skin — *see* Neoplasm, connective tissue, malignant
  metastatic
    breast C79.81
    genital organ C79.82
    specified site NEC C79.89
  neurotropic, malignant — *see* Melanoma, skin, by site
  nodular — *see* Melanoma, skin, by site
  regressing, malignant — *see* Melanoma, skin, by site
  skin C43.9
    abdominal wall C43.59
    ala nasi C43.31
    ankle C43.7- ☑
    anus, anal (skin) C43.51
    arm C43.6- ☑
    auditory canal (external) C43.2- ☑
    auricle (ear) C43.2- ☑
    auricular canal (external) C43.2- ☑
    axilla, axillary fold C43.59
    back C43.59
    breast (female) (male) C43.52
    brow C43.39
    buttock C43.59
    canthus (eye) C43.1- ☑
    cheek (external) C43.39
    chest wall C43.59
    chin C43.39
    ear (external) C43.2- ☑
    elbow C43.6- ☑
    external meatus (ear) C43.2- ☑
    eyebrow C43.39
    eyelid (lower) (upper) C43.1- ☑
    face C43.30
      specified NEC C43.39
    female genital organ (external) NEC C51.9
    finger C43.6- ☑
    flank C43.59

**Melanoma** — *continued*
  skin — *continued*
    foot C43.7- ☑
    forearm C43.6- ☑
    forehead C43.39
    foreskin C60.0
    glabella C43.39
    gluteal region C43.59
    groin C43.59
    hand C43.6- ☑
    heel C43.7- ☑
    helix C43.2- ☑
    hip C43.7- ☑
    interscapular region C43.59
    jaw (external) C43.39
    knee C43.7- ☑
    labium C51.9
      majus C51.0
      minus C51.1
    leg C43.7- ☑
    lip (lower) (upper) C43.0
    lower limb NEC C43.7- ☑
    male genital organ (external) NEC C63.9
    nail
      finger C43.6- ☑
      toe C43.7- ☑
    nasolabial groove C43.39
    nates C43.59
    neck C43.4
    nose (external) C43.31
    overlapping site C43.8
    palpebra C43.1- ☑
    penis C60.9
    perianal skin C43.51
    perineum C43.51
    pinna C43.2- ☑
    popliteal fossa or space C43.7- ☑
    prepuce C60.0
    pudendum C51.9
    scalp C43.4
    scrotum C63.2
    shoulder C43.6- ☑
    skin NEC C43.9
    submammary fold C43.52
    temple C43.39
    thigh C43.7- ☑
    toe C43.7- ☑
    trunk NEC C43.59
    umbilicus C43.59
    upper limb NEC C43.6- ☑
    vulva C51.9
      overlapping sites C51.8
  spindle cell
    with epithelioid, mixed — *see* Melanoma, skin, by site
    type A C69.4- ☑
    type B C69.4- ☑
  superficial spreading — *see* Melanoma, skin, by site
**Melanosarcoma** — *see also* Melanoma
  epithelioid cell — *see* Melanoma
**Melanosis** L81.4
  addisonian E27.1
    tuberculous A18.7
  adrenal E27.1
  colon K63.89
  conjunctiva — *see* Pigmentation, conjunctiva
    congenital Q13.89
  cornea (presenile) (senile) — *see also* Pigmentation, cornea
    congenital Q13.4
  eye NEC H57.89
    congenital Q15.8
  lenticularis progressiva Q82.1
  liver K76.89
  precancerous — *see also* Melanoma, in situ
    malignant melanoma in — *see* Melanoma
  Riehl's L81.4
  sclera H15.89
    congenital Q13.89
  suprarenal E27.1
  tar L81.4
  toxic L81.4
**Melanuria** R82.998
**MELAS syndrome** E88.41
**Melasma** L81.1
  adrenal (gland) E27.1
  suprarenal (gland) E27.1
**Melena** K92.1

**Melena** — *continued*
  with ulcer — *code by* site under Ulcer, with hemorrhage K27.4
  due to swallowed maternal blood P78.2
  newborn, neonatal P54.1
    due to swallowed maternal blood P78.2
**Meleney's**
  gangrene (cutaneous) — *see* Ulcer, skin
  ulcer (chronic undermining) — *see* Ulcer, skin
**Melioidosis** A24.9
  acute A24.1
  chronic A24.2
  fulminating A24.1
  pneumonia A24.1
  pulmonary (chronic) A24.2
    acute A24.1
    subacute A24.2
  sepsis A24.1
  specified NEC A24.3
  subacute A24.2
**Melitensis, febris** A23.0
**Melkersson** (-Rosenthal) **syndrome** G51.2
**Mellitus, diabetes** — *see* Diabetes
**Melorheostosis** (bone) — *see* Disorder, bone, density and structure, specified NEC
**Meloschisis** Q18.4
**Melotia** Q17.4
**Membrana**
  capsularis lentis posterior Q13.89
  epipapillaris Q14.2
**Membranacea placenta** O43.19- ☑
**Membranaceous uterus** N85.8
**Membrane**(s), membranous — *see also* condition
  cyclitic — *see* Membrane, pupillary
  folds, congenital — *see* Web
  Jackson's Q43.3
  over face of newborn P28.9
  premature rupture — *see* Rupture, membranes, premature
  pupillary H21.4- ☑
    persistent Q13.89
  retained (with hemorrhage) (complicating delivery) O72.2
    without hemorrhage O73.1
  secondary cataract — *see* Cataract, secondary
  unruptured (causing asphyxia) — *see* Asphyxia, newborn
  vitreous — *see* Opacity, vitreous, membranes and strands
**Membranitis** — *see* Chorioamnionitis
**Memory disturbance, lack or loss** — *see also* Amnesia
  mild, following organic brain damage F06.8
**Menadione deficiency** E56.1
**Menarche**
  delayed E30.0
  precocious E30.1
**Mendacity, pathologic** F60.2
**Mendelson's syndrome** (due to anesthesia) J95.4
  in labor and delivery O74.0
  in pregnancy O29.01- ☑
  obstetric O74.0
  postpartum, puerperal O89.01
**Menetrier's disease or syndrome** K29.60
  with bleeding K29.61
**Meniere's disease, syndrome or vertigo** H81.0- ☑
**Meninges, meningeal** — *see* condition
**Meningioma** — *see also* Neoplasm, meninges, benign
  angioblastic — *see* Neoplasm, meninges, benign
  angiomatous — *see* Neoplasm, meninges, benign
  atypical — *see* Neoplasm, meninges, uncertain behavior
  endotheliomatous — *see* Neoplasm, meninges, benign
  fibroblastic — *see* Neoplasm, meninges, benign
  fibrous — *see* Neoplasm, meninges, benign
  hemangioblastic — *see* Neoplasm, meninges, benign
  hemangiopericytic — *see* Neoplasm, meninges, benign
  malignant — *see* Neoplasm, meninges, malignant
  meningiothelial — *see* Neoplasm, meninges, benign
  meningotheliomatous — *see* Neoplasm, meninges, benign
  mixed — *see* Neoplasm, meninges, benign
  multiple — *see* Neoplasm, meninges, uncertain behavior
  papillary — *see* Neoplasm, meninges, uncertain behavior
  psammomatous — *see* Neoplasm, meninges, benign
  syncytial — *see* Neoplasm, meninges, benign
  transitional — *see* Neoplasm, meninges, benign
**Meningiomatosis** (diffuse) — *see* Neoplasm, meninges, uncertain behavior
**Meningism** — *see* Meningismus
**Meningismus** (infectional) (pneumococcal) R29.1
  due to serum or vaccine R29.1
  influenzal — *see* Influenza, with, manifestations NEC

**Menstruation** — *continued*
- latent N92.5
- membranous N92.5
- painful — *see also* Dysmenorrhea N94.6
  - primary N94.4
  - psychogenic F45.8
  - secondary N94.5
- passage of clots N92.Ø
- precocious E3Ø.1
- protracted N92.5
- rare — *see* Oligomenorrhea
- retained N94.89
- retrograde N92.5
- scanty — *see* Oligomenorrhea
- suppression N94.89
- vicarious (nasal) N94.89

**Mental** — *see also* condition
- deficiency — *see* Disability, intellectual
- deterioration — *see* Psychosis
- disorder — *see* Disorder, mental
- exhaustion F48.8
- insufficiency (congenital) — *see* Disability, intellectual
- observation without need for further medical care ZØ3.89
- retardation — *see* Disability, intellectual
- subnormality — *see* Disability, intellectual
- upset — *see* Disorder, mental

**Meralgia paresthetica** G57.1- ☑

**Mercurial** — *see* condition

**Mercurialism** — *see* subcategory T56.1- ☑

**Merkel cell tumor** — *see* Carcinoma, Merkel cell

**Merocele** — *see* Hernia, femoral

**Meromelia**
- lower limb — *see* Defect, reduction, lower limb
  - intercalary
    - femur — *see* Defect, reduction, lower limb, specified type NEC
      - tibiofibular (complete) (incomplete) — *see* Defect, reduction, lower limb
- upper limb — *see* Defect, reduction, upper limb
  - intercalary, humeral, radioulnar — *see* Agenesis, arm, with hand present

**MERRF syndrome** (myoclonic epilepsy associated with ragged-red fiber) E88.42

**Merzbacher-Pelizaeus disease** E75.27

**Mesaortitis** — *see* Aortitis

**Mesarteritis** — *see* Arteritis

**Mesencephalitis** — *see* Encephalitis

**Mesenchymoma** — *see also* Neoplasm, connective tissue, uncertain behavior
- benign — *see* Neoplasm, connective tissue, benign
- malignant — *see* Neoplasm, connective tissue, malignant

**Mesenteritis**
- retractile K65.4
- sclerosing K65.4

**Mesentery, mesenteric** — *see* condition

**Mesio-occlusion** M26.213

**Mesiodens, mesiodentes** KØØ.1

**Mesocolon** — *see* condition

**Mesonephroma** (malignant) — *see* Neoplasm, malignant, by site
- benign — *see* Neoplasm, benign, by site

**Mesophlebitis** — *see* Phlebitis

**Mesostromal dysgenesia** Q13.89

**Mesothelioma** (malignant) C45.9
- benign
  - mesentery D19.1
  - mesocolon D19.1
  - omentum D19.1
  - peritoneum D19.1
  - pleura D19.Ø
  - specified site NEC D19.7
  - unspecified site D19.9
- biphasic C45.9
  - benign
    - mesentery D19.1
    - mesocolon D19.1
    - omentum D19.1
    - peritoneum D19.1
    - pleura D19.Ø
    - specified site NEC D19.7
    - unspecified site D19.9
- cystic D48.4
- epithelioid C45.9
  - benign
    - mesentery D19.1
    - mesocolon D19.1
    - omentum D19.1
    - peritoneum D19.1
    - pleura D19.Ø

**Mesothelioma** — *continued*
- epithelioid — *continued*
  - benign — *continued*
    - specified site NEC D19.7
    - unspecified site D19.9
- fibrous C45.9
  - benign
    - mesentery D19.1
    - mesocolon D19.1
    - omentum D19.1
    - peritoneum D19.1
    - pleura D19.Ø
    - specified site NEC D19.7
    - unspecified site D19.9
- site classification
  - liver C45.7
  - lung C45.7
  - mediastinum C45.7
  - mesentery C45.1
  - mesocolon C45.1
  - omentum C45.1
  - pericardium C45.2
  - peritoneum C45.1
  - pleura C45.Ø
    - parietal C45.Ø
  - retroperitoneum C45.7
  - specified site NEC C45.7
  - unspecified C45.9

**Metabolic syndrome** E88.81Ø

**Metagonimiasis** B66.8

**Metagonimus infestation** (intestine) B66.8

**Metal**
- pigmentation L81.8
- polisher's disease J62.8

**Metamorphopsia** H53.15

**Metaplasia**
- apocrine (breast) — *see* Dysplasia, mammary, specified type NEC
- cervix (squamous) — *see* Dysplasia, cervix
- endometrium (squamous) (uterus) N85.8
- esophagus K22.7- ☑
- gastric intestinal K31.AØ
  - with dysplasia K31.A29
    - high grade K31.A22
    - low grade K31.A21
  - indefinite for dysplasia K31.AØ
  - without dysplasia K31.A19
    - involving
      - antrum K31.A11
      - body (corpus) K31.A12
      - cardia K31.A14
      - fundus K31.A13
      - multiple sites K31.A15
- kidney (pelvis) (squamous) N28.89
- myelogenous D73.1
- myeloid (agnogenic) (megakaryocytic) D73.1
- spleen D73.1
- squamous cell, bladder N32.89

**Metastasis, metastatic**
- abscess — *see* Abscess
- calcification E83.59
- cancer
  - from specified site — *see* Neoplasm, malignant, by site
  - to specified site — *see* Neoplasm, secondary, by site
- deposits (in) — *see* Neoplasm, secondary, by site
- disease — *see also* Neoplasm, secondary, by site C79.9
- spread (to) — *see* Neoplasm, secondary, by site

**Metastrongyliasis** B83.8

**Metatarsalgia** M77.4- ☑
- anterior G57.6- ☑
- Morton's G57.6- ☑

**Metatarsus, metatarsal** — *see also* condition
- adductus, congenital Q66.22- ☑
- valgus (abductus), congenital Q66.6
- varus (congenital) Q66.22- ☑
  - primus Q66.21- ☑

**Methadone use** — *see* Use, opioid

**Methemoglobinemia** D74.9
- acquired (with sulfhemoglobinemia) D74.8
- congenital D74.Ø
- enzymatic (congenital) D74.Ø
- Hb M disease D74.Ø
- hereditary D74.Ø
- toxic D74.8

**Methemoglobinuria** — *see* Hemoglobinuria

**Methioninemia** E72.19

**Methylmalonic acidemia** E71.12Ø

**Metritis** (catarrhal) (hemorrhagic) (septic) (suppurative) — *see also* Endometritis
- cervical — *see* Cervicitis

**Metropathia hemorrhagica** N93.8

**Metroperitonitis** — *see* Peritonitis, pelvic, female

**Metrorrhagia** N92.1
- climacteric N92.4
- menopausal N92.4
- perimenopausal N92.4
- postpartum NEC (atonic) (following delivery of placenta) O72.1
  - delayed or secondary O72.2
- preclimacteric or premenopausal N92.4
- psychogenic F45.8

**Metrorrhexis** — *see* Rupture, uterus

**Metrosalpingitis** N7Ø.91

**Metrostaxis** N93.8

**Metrovaginitis** — *see* Endometritis

**Meyer-Schwickerath and Weyers syndrome** Q87.Ø

**Meynert's amentia** (nonalcoholic) FØ4
- alcoholic F1Ø.96
  - with dependence F1Ø.26

**Mibelli's disease** (porokeratosis) Q82.8

**Mice, joint** — *see* Loose, body, joint
- knee M23.4- ☑

**Micrencephalon, micrencephaly** QØ2

**Microalbuminuria** R8Ø.9

**Microaneurysm, retinal** — *see also* Disorder, retina, microaneurysms
- diabetic — *see* EØ8-E13 with .31

**Microangiopathy** (peripheral) I73.9
- thrombotic M31.1Ø
  - hematopoietic stem cell transplantation-associated [HSCT-TMA] M31.11

**Microcalcifications, breast** R92.Ø

**Microcephalus, microcephalic, microcephaly** QØ2
- due to toxoplasmosis (congenital) P37.1

**Microcheilia** Q18.7

**Microcolon** (congenital) Q43.8

**Microcornea** (congenital) Q13.4

**Microcytic** — *see* condition

**Microdeletions NEC** Q93.88

**Microdontia** KØØ.2

**Microdrepanocytosis** D57.4Ø
- with
  - acute chest syndrome D57.411
  - cerebral vascular involvement D57.413
  - crisis (painful) D57.419
    - with specified complication NEC D57.418
  - pain (vaso-occlusive) D57.419
  - splenic sequestration D57.412

**Microembolism**
- atherothrombotic — *see* Atheroembolism
- retinal — *see* Occlusion, artery, retina

**Microencephalon** QØ2

**Microfilaria streptocerca infestation** — *see* Onchocerciasis

**Microgastria** (congenital) Q4Ø.2

**Microgenia** M26.Ø6

**Microgenitalia, congenital**
- female Q52.8
- male Q55.8

**Microglioma** — *see* Lymphoma, non-Hodgkin, specified NEC

**Microglossia** (congenital) Q38.3

**Micrognathia, micrognathism** (congenital) (mandibular) (maxillary) M26.Ø9

**Microgyria** (congenital) QØ4.3

**Microinfarct of heart** — *see* Insufficiency, coronary

**Microlentia** (congenital) Q12.8

**Microlithiasis, alveolar, pulmonary** J84.Ø2

**Micromastia** N64.82

**Micromyelia** (congenital) QØ6.8

**Micropenis** Q55.62

**Microphakia** (congenital) Q12.8

**Microphthalmos, microphthalmia** (congenital) Q11.2
- due to toxoplasmosis P37.1

**Micropsia** H53.15

**Microscopic polyangiitis** (polyarteritis) M31.7

**Microsporidiosis** B6Ø.8
- intestinal AØ7.8

**Microsporon furfur infestation** B36.Ø

**Microsporosis** — *see also* Dermatophytosis
- nigra B36.1

**Microstomia** (congenital) Q18.5

**Microtia** (congenital) (external ear) Q17.2

**Microtropia** H5Ø.4Ø

**Microvillus inclusion disease** (MVD) (MVID) Q43.8

**Mosaicism, mosaic** (autosomal) (chromosomal)
- 45,X/46,XX Q96.3
- 45,X/other cell lines NEC with abnormal sex chromosome Q96.4
- sex chromosome
  - female Q97.8
  - lines with various numbers of X chromosomes Q97.2
  - male Q98.7
- XY Q96.3

**Moschowitz' disease** M31.19
**Mother yaw** A66.Ø
**Motion sickness** (from travel, any vehicle) (from roundabouts or swings) T75.3- ☑
**Mottled, mottling, teeth** (enamel) (endemic) (nonendemic) KØØ.3
**Mounier-Kuhn syndrome** Q32.4
- with bronchiectasis J47.9
  - exacerbation (acute) J47.1
  - lower respiratory infection J47.Ø
- acquired J98.Ø9
  - with bronchiectasis J47.9
    - with
      - exacerbation (acute) J47.1
      - lower respiratory infection J47.Ø

**Mountain**
- sickness T7Ø.29- ☑
  - with polycythemia , acquired (acute) D75.1
- tick fever A93.2

**Mouse, joint** — *see* Loose, body, joint
- knee M23.4- ☑

**Mouth** — *see* condition
**Movable**
- coccyx — *see* subcategory M53.2- ☑
- kidney N28.89
  - congenital Q63.8
- spleen D73.89

**Movements, dystonic** R25.8
**Moyamoya disease** I67.5
**Mpox** BØ4
**MRSA** (Methicillin resistant Staphylococcus aureus)
- infection A49.Ø2
  - as the cause of diseases classified elsewhere B95.62
- sepsis A41.Ø2

**MSD** (multiple sulfatase deficiency) E75.26
**MSSA** (Methicillin susceptible Staphylococcus aureus)
- infection A49.Ø1
  - as the cause of diseases classified elsewhere B95.61
- sepsis A41.Ø1

**Mucha-Habermann disease** L41.Ø
**Mucinosis** (cutaneous) (focal) (papular) (skin) L98.5
- oral K13.79

**Mucocele**
- appendix K38.8
- buccal cavity K13.79
- gallbladder K82.1
- lacrimal sac, chronic HØ4.43- ☑
- nasal sinus J34.1
- nose J34.1
- salivary gland (any) K11.6
- sinus (accessory) (nasal) J34.1
- turbinate (bone) (middle) (nasal) J34.1
- uterus N85.8

**Mucolipidosis**
- I E77.1
- II, III E77.Ø
- IV E75.11

**Mucopolysaccharidosis** E76.3
- beta-gluduronidase deficiency E76.29
- cardiopathy E76.3 *[I52]*
- Hunter's syndrome E76.1
- Hurler-Scheie syndrome E76.Ø2
- Hurler's syndrome E76.Ø1
- Maroteaux-Lamy syndrome E76.29
- Morquio syndrome E76.219
  - A E76.21Ø
  - B E76.211
  - classic E76.21Ø
- Sanfilippo syndrome E76.22
- Scheie's syndrome E76.Ø3
- specified NEC E76.29
- type
  - I
    - Hurler-Scheie syndrome E76.Ø2
    - Hurler's syndrome E76.Ø1
    - Scheie's syndrome E76.Ø3
  - II E76.1
  - III E76.22
  - IV E76.219

**Mucopolysaccharidosis** — *continued*
- type — *continued*
  - IVA E76.21Ø
  - IVB E76.211
  - VI E76.29
  - VII E76.29

**Mucormycosis** B46.5
- cutaneous B46.3
- disseminated B46.4
- gastrointestinal B46.2
- generalized B46.4
- pulmonary B46.Ø
- rhinocerebral B46.1
- skin B46.3
- subcutaneous B46.3

**Mucositis** (ulcerative) K12.3Ø
- due to drugs NEC K12.32
- gastrointestinal K92.81
- mouth (oral) (oropharyngeal) K12.3Ø
  - due to antineoplastic therapy K12.31
  - due to drugs NEC K12.32
  - due to radiation K12.33
  - specified NEC K12.39
  - viral K12.39
- nasal J34.81
- oral cavity — *see* Mucositis, mouth
- oral soft tissues — *see* Mucositis, mouth
- vagina and vulva N76.81

**Mucositis necroticans agranulocytica** — *see* Agranulocytosis
**Mucous** — *see also* condition
- patches (syphilitic) A51.39
  - congenital A5Ø.Ø7

**Mucoviscidosis** E84.9
- with meconium obstruction E84.11

**Mucus**
- asphyxia or suffocation — *see* Asphyxia, mucus
- in stool R19.5
- plug — *see* Asphyxia, mucus

**Muguet** B37.Ø
**Mulberry molars** (congenital syphilis) A5Ø.52
**Mullerian mixed tumor**
- specified site — *see* Neoplasm, malignant, by site
- unspecified site C54.9

**Multicystic kidney** (development) Q61.4
**Multiparity** (grand) Z64.1
- affecting management of pregnancy, labor and delivery (supervision only) OØ9.4- ☑
- requiring contraceptive management — *see* Contraception

**Multipartita placenta** O43.19- ☑
**Multiple, multiplex** — *see also* condition
- digits (congenital) Q69.9
- endocrine neoplasia — *see* Neoplasia, endocrine, multiple (MEN)
- personality F44.81

**Multisystem inflammatory syndrome** (in adult) (in children) M35.81
**Mumps** B26.9
- arthritis B26.85
- complication NEC B26.89
- encephalitis B26.2
- hepatitis B26.81
- meningitis (aseptic) B26.1
- meningoencephalitis B26.2
- myocarditis B26.82
- oophoritis B26.89
- orchitis B26.Ø
- pancreatitis B26.3
- polyneuropathy B26.84

**Mumu** — *see also* Infestation, filarial B74.9 *[N51]*
**Munchhausen's syndrome** — *see* Disorder, factitious
**Munchmeyer's syndrome** — *see* Myositis, ossificans, progressiva
**Mural** — *see* condition
**Murmur** (cardiac) (heart) (organic) RØ1.1
- abdominal R19.15
- aortic (valve) — *see* Endocarditis, aortic
- benign RØ1.Ø
- diastolic — *see* Endocarditis
- Flint I35.1
- functional RØ1.Ø
- Graham Steell I37.1
- innocent RØ1.Ø
- mitral (valve) — *see* Insufficiency, mitral
- nonorganic RØ1.Ø
- presystolic, mitral — *see* Insufficiency, mitral
- pulmonic (valve) I37.8
- systolic RØ1.1

**Murmur** — *continued*
- tricuspid (valve) IØ7.9
- valvular — *see* Endocarditis

**Murri's disease** (intermittent hemoglobinuria) D59.6
**Muscle, muscular** — *see also* condition
- carnitine (palmityltransferase) deficiency E71.314

**Musculoneuralgia** — *see* Neuralgia
**Mushroom-workers' (pickers') disease or lung** J67.5
**Mushrooming hip** — *see* Derangement, joint, specified NEC, hip
**Mutation**(s)
- factor V Leiden D68.51
- prothrombin gene D68.52
- surfactant, of lung J84.83

**Mutism** — *see also* Aphasia
- deaf (acquired) (congenital) NEC H91.3
- elective (adjustment reaction) (childhood) F94.Ø
- hysterical F44.4
- selective (childhood) F94.Ø

**MVD** (microvillus inclusion disease) Q43.8
**MVID** (microvillus inclusion disease) Q43.8
**Myalgia** M79.1Ø
- auxiliary muscles, head and neck M79.12
- epidemic (cervical) B33.Ø
- mastication muscle M79.11
- site specified NEC M79.18
- traumatic NEC T14.8- ☑

**Myasthenia** G7Ø.9
- congenital G7Ø.2
- cordis — *see* Failure, heart
- developmental G7Ø.2
- gravis G7Ø.ØØ
  - with exacerbation (acute) G7Ø.Ø1
  - in crisis G7Ø.Ø1
  - neonatal, transient P94.Ø
  - pseudoparalytica G7Ø.ØØ
    - with exacerbation (acute) G7Ø.Ø1
    - in crisis G7Ø.Ø1
- stomach, psychogenic F45.8
- syndrome
  - in
    - diabetes mellitus — *see* EØ8-E13 with .44
    - neoplastic disease — *see also* Neoplasm D49.9 *[G73.3]*
    - pernicious anemia D51.Ø *[G73.3]*
    - thyrotoxicosis EØ5.9Ø *[G73.3]*
      - with thyroid storm EØ5.91 *[G73.3]*

**Myasthenic** M62.81
**Mycelium infection** B49
**Mycetismus** — *see* Poisoning, food, noxious, mushroom
**Mycetoma** B47.9
- actinomycotic B47.1
- bone (mycotic) B47.9 *[M9Ø.8Ø]*
- eumycotic B47.Ø
- foot B47.9
  - actinomycotic B47.1
  - mycotic B47.Ø
- madurae NEC B47.9
  - mycotic B47.Ø
- maduromycotic B47.Ø
- mycotic B47.Ø
- nocardial B47.1
- pulmonary J4B

**Mycobacteriosis** — *see* Mycobacterium
**Mycobacterium, mycobacterial** (infection) A31.9
- anonymous A31.9
- atypical A31.9
  - cutaneous A31.1
  - pulmonary A31.Ø
    - tuberculous — *see* Tuberculosis, pulmonary
  - specified site NEC A31.8
- avium (intracellulare complex) A31.Ø
- balnei A31.1
- Battey A31.Ø
- chelonei A31.8
- cutaneous A31.1
- extrapulmonary systemic A31.8
- fortuitum A31.8
- intracellulare (Battey bacillus) A31.Ø
- kakaferifu A31.8
- kansasii (yellow bacillus) A31.Ø
- kasongo A31.8
- leprae — *see also* Leprosy A3Ø.9
- luciflavum A31.1
- marinum (M. balnei) A31.1
- nonspecific — *see* Mycobacterium, atypical
- pulmonary (atypical) A31.Ø
  - tuberculous — *see* Tuberculosis, pulmonary
- scrofulaceum A31.8

- **Myoclonus, myoclonic, myoclonia** — *continued*
  - pharyngeal G25.3
- **Myocytolysis** I51.5
- **Myodiastasis** — *see* Diastasis, muscle
- **Myoendocarditis** — *see* Endocarditis
- **Myoepithelioma** — *see* Neoplasm, benign, by site
- **Myofasciitis** (acute) — *see* Myositis
- **Myofibroma** — *see also* Neoplasm, connective tissue, benign
  - uterus (cervix) (corpus) — *see* Leiomyoma
- **Myofibromatosis** D48.19
  - infantile Q89.89
- **Myofibrosis** M62.89
  - heart — *see* Myocarditis
  - scapulohumeral — *see* Lesion, shoulder, specified NEC
- **Myofibrositis** M79.7
  - scapulohumeral — *see* Lesion, shoulder, specified NEC
- **Myoglobulinuria, myoglobinuria** (primary) R82.1
- **Myokymia, facial** G51.4
- **Myolipoma** — *see* Lipoma
- **Myoma** — *see also* Neoplasm, connective tissue, benign
  - malignant — *see* Neoplasm, connective tissue, malignant
  - prostate D29.1
  - uterus (cervix) (corpus) — *see* Leiomyoma
- **Myomalacia** M62.89
- **Myometritis** — *see* Endometritis
- **Myometrium** — *see* condition
- **Myonecrosis, clostridial** A48.Ø
- **Myopathy** G72.9
  - acute
    - necrotizing G72.81
    - quadriplegic G72.81
  - alcoholic G72.1
  - benign congenital G71.2Ø
  - central core G71.29
  - centronuclear G71.228
    - autosomal (dominant) (recessive) G71.228
    - other specified NEC G71.228
  - congenital (benign) G71.2Ø
  - critical illness G72.81
  - distal G71.Ø9
  - drug-induced G72.Ø
  - endocrine NEC E34.9 *[G73.7]*
  - extraocular muscles HØ5.82- ☑
  - facioscapulohumeral G71.Ø2
  - hereditary G71.9
    - specified NEC G71.8
  - hyaline body G71.29
  - immune NEC G72.49
  - in (due to)
    - Addison's disease E27.1 *[G73.7]*
    - alcohol G72.1
    - amyloidosis E85.Ø *[G73.7]*
    - cretinism EØØ.9 *[G73.7]*
    - Cushing's syndrome E24.9 *[G73.7]*
    - drugs G72.Ø
    - endocrine disease NEC E34.9 *[G73.7]*
    - giant cell arteritis M31.6 *[G73.7]*
    - glycogen storage disease E74.ØØ *[G73.7]*
    - hyperadrenocorticism E24.9 *[G73.7]*
    - hyperparathyroidism NEC E21.3 *[G73.7]*
    - hypoparathyroidism E2Ø.9 *[G73.7]*
    - hypopituitarism E23.Ø *[G73.7]*
    - hypothyroidism EØ3.9 *[G73.7]*
    - infectious disease NEC B99.- ☑ *[G73.7]*
    - lipid storage disease E75.6 *[G73.7]*
    - metabolic disease NEC E88.9 *[G73.7]*
    - myxedema EØ3.9 *[G73.7]*
    - parasitic disease NEC B89 *[G73.7]*
    - polyarteritis nodosa M3Ø.Ø *[G73.7]*
    - rheumatoid arthritis — *see* Rheumatoid, myopathy
    - sarcoidosis D86.87
    - scleroderma M34.82
    - sicca syndrome M35.Ø3
    - Sjogren's syndrome M35.Ø3
    - systemic lupus erythematosus M32.19
    - thyrotoxicosis (hyperthyroidism) EØ5.9Ø *[G73.7]*
      - with thyroid storm EØ5.91 *[G73.7]*
    - toxic agent NEC G72.2
  - inflammatory NEC G72.49
  - intensive care (ICU) G72.81
  - limb-girdle — *see* Dystrophy, muscular, limb-girdle
  - mitochondrial NEC G71.3
  - Miyoshi, type 3 G71.Ø35
  - myosin storage G71.29
  - myotonic, proximal (PROMM) G71.11
  - myotubular (centronuclear) G71.22Ø
    - X-linked G71.22Ø
  - nemaline G71.21
- **Myopathy** — *continued*
  - ocular G71.Ø9
  - oculopharyngeal G71.Ø9
  - of critical illness G72.81
  - primary G71.9
    - specified NEC G71.8
  - progressive NEC G72.89
  - proximal myotonic (PROMM) G71.11
  - rod (body) G71.21
  - scapulohumeral G71.Ø2
  - specified NEC G72.89
  - toxic G72.2
- **Myopericarditis** — *see also* Pericarditis
  - chronic rheumatic IØ9.2
- **Myopia** (axial) (congenital) H52.1- ☑
  - degenerative (malignant) H44.2Ø
    - with
      - choroidal neovascularization H44.2A- ☑
      - foveoschisis H44.2D- ☑
      - macular hole H44.2B- ☑
      - retinal detachment H44.2C- ☑
      - specified maculopathy NEC H44.2E- ☑
    - bilateral H44.23
    - left eye H44.22
    - right eye H44.21
  - malignant — *see also* Myopia, degenerative H44.2- ☑
  - pernicious — *see also* Myopia, degenerative H44.2- ☑
  - progressive high (degenerative) — *see also* Myopia, degenerative H44.2- ☑
- **Myosarcoma** — *see* Neoplasm, connective tissue, malignant
- **Myosis** (pupil) H57.Ø3
  - stromal (endolymphatic) D39.Ø
- **Myositis** M6Ø.9
  - clostridial A48.Ø
  - due to posture — *see* Myositis, specified type NEC
  - epidemic B33.Ø
  - fibrosa or fibrous (chronic), Volkmann's T79.6- ☑
  - foreign body granuloma — *see* Granuloma, foreign body
  - in (due to)
    - bilharziasis B65.9 *[M63.8-]* ☑
    - cysticercosis B69.81
    - leprosy A3Ø.9 *[M63.8-]* ☑
    - mycosis B49 *[M63.8-]* ☑
    - sarcoidosis D86.87
    - schistosomiasis B65.9 *[M63.8-]* ☑
    - syphilis
      - late A52.78
      - secondary A51.49
    - toxoplasmosis (acquired) B58.82
    - trichinellosis B75 *[M63.8-]* ☑
    - tuberculosis A18.Ø9
  - inclusion body [IBM] G72.41
  - infective M6Ø.ØØ9
    - arm M6Ø.ØØ2
      - left M6Ø.ØØ1
      - right M6Ø.ØØØ
    - leg M6Ø.ØØ5
      - left M6Ø.ØØ4
      - right M6Ø.ØØ3
    - lower limb M6Ø.ØØ5
      - ankle M6Ø.Ø7- ☑
      - foot M6Ø.Ø7- ☑
      - lower leg M6Ø.Ø6- ☑
      - thigh M6Ø.Ø5- ☑
      - toe M6Ø.Ø7- ☑
    - multiple sites M6Ø.Ø9
    - specified site NEC M6Ø.Ø8
    - upper limb M6Ø.ØØ2
      - finger M6Ø.Ø4- ☑
      - forearm M6Ø.Ø3- ☑
      - hand M6Ø.Ø4- ☑
      - shoulder region M6Ø.Ø1- ☑
      - upper arm M6Ø.Ø2- ☑
  - interstitial M6Ø.1Ø
    - ankle M6Ø.17- ☑
    - foot M6Ø.17- ☑
    - forearm M6Ø.13- ☑
    - hand M6Ø.14- ☑
    - lower leg M6Ø.16- ☑
    - multiple sites M6Ø.19
    - shoulder region M6Ø.11- ☑
    - specified site NEC M6Ø.18
    - thigh M6Ø.15- ☑
    - upper arm M6Ø.12- ☑
  - mycotic B49 *[M63.8-]* ☑
  - orbital, chronic HØ5.12- ☑
- **Myositis** — *continued*
  - ossificans or ossifying (circumscripta) — *see also* Ossification, muscle, specified NEC
    - in (due to)
      - burns M61.3Ø
        - ankle M61.37- ☑
        - foot M61.37- ☑
        - forearm M61.33- ☑
        - hand M61.34- ☑
        - lower leg M61.36- ☑
        - multiple sites M61.39
        - pelvic region M61.35- ☑
        - shoulder region M61.31- ☑
        - specified site NEC M61.38
        - thigh M61.35- ☑
        - upper arm M61.32- ☑
      - quadriplegia or paraplegia M61.2Ø
        - ankle M61.27- ☑
        - foot M61.27- ☑
        - forearm M61.23- ☑
        - hand M61.24- ☑
        - lower leg M61.26- ☑
        - multiple sites M61.29
        - pelvic region M61.25- ☑
        - shoulder region M61.21- ☑
        - specified site NEC M61.28
        - thigh M61.25- ☑
        - upper arm M61.22- ☑
    - progressiva M61.1Ø
      - ankle M61.17- ☑
      - finger M61.14- ☑
      - foot M61.17- ☑
      - forearm M61.13- ☑
      - hand M61.14- ☑
      - lower leg M61.16- ☑
      - multiple sites M61.19
      - pelvic region M61.15- ☑
      - shoulder region M61.11- ☑
      - specified site NEC M61.18
      - thigh M61.15- ☑
      - toe M61.17- ☑
      - upper arm M61.12- ☑
    - traumatica M61.ØØ
      - ankle M61.Ø7- ☑
      - foot M61.Ø7- ☑
      - forearm M61.Ø3- ☑
      - hand M61.Ø4- ☑
      - lower leg M61.Ø6- ☑
      - multiple sites M61.Ø9
      - pelvic region M61.Ø5- ☑
      - shoulder region M61.Ø1- ☑
      - specified site NEC M61.Ø8
      - thigh M61.Ø5- ☑
      - upper arm M61.Ø2- ☑
  - purulent — *see* Myositis, infective
  - specified type NEC M6Ø.8Ø
    - ankle M6Ø.87- ☑
    - foot M6Ø.87- ☑
    - forearm M6Ø.83- ☑
    - hand M6Ø.84- ☑
    - lower leg M6Ø.86- ☑
    - multiple sites M6Ø.89
    - pelvic region M6Ø.85- ☑
    - shoulder region M6Ø.81- ☑
    - specified site NEC M6Ø.88
    - thigh M6Ø.85- ☑
    - upper arm M6Ø.82- ☑
  - suppurative — *see* Myositis, infective
  - traumatic (old) — *see* Myositis, specified type NEC
- **Myospasia impulsiva** F95.2
- **Myotonia** (acquisita) (intermittens) M62.89
  - atrophica G71.11
  - chondrodystrophic G71.13
  - congenita (acetazolamide responsive) (dominant) (recessive) G71.12
  - drug-induced G71.14
  - dystrophica G71.11
  - fluctuans G71.19
  - levior G71.12
  - permanens G71.19
  - symptomatic G71.19
- **Myotonic pupil** — *see* Anomaly, pupil, function, tonic pupil
- **Myriapodiasis** B88.2
- **Myringitis** H73.2- ☑
  - with otitis media — *see* Otitis, media
  - acute H73.ØØ- ☑

Index

Myoclonus, myoclonic, myoclonia — Myringitis

# N

- **Nephropathy** — *continued*
  - hereditary — *continued*
    - with
      - APOL1-mediated kidney disease (AMKD) NØ7.B
      - C3
        - glomerulonephritis NØ7.A
        - glomerulopathy NØ7.A
          - with dense deposit disease NØ7.6
      - dense deposit disease NØ7.6
      - diffuse
        - crescentic glomerulonephritis NØ7.7
        - endocapillary proliferative glomerulonephritis NØ7.4
        - membranous glomerulonephritis NØ7.2
        - mesangial proliferative glomerulonephritis NØ7.3
        - mesangiocapillary glomerulonephritis NØ7.5
      - focal and segmental glomerular lesions NØ7.1
      - minor glomerular abnormality NØ7.Ø
      - specified morphological changes NEC NØ7.8
  - hypercalcemic N25.89
  - hypertensive — *see* Hypertension, kidney
  - hypokalemic (vacuolar) N25.89
  - IgA NØ2.B- ☑
    - with
      - focal and segmental hyalinosis or sclerosis NØ2.B2
      - glomerular lesion NØ2.B1
        - focal and segmental NØ2.B2
      - glomerulonephritis
        - membranoproliferative (diffuse) NØ2.B3
        - membranous (diffuse) NØ2.B4
        - mesangial proliferative (diffuse) NØ2.B5
        - mesangiocapillary (diffuse) NØ2.B6
    - proliferative NEC NØ2.B9
    - specified pathology NEC NØ2.B9
  - lead N14.3
  - membranoproliferative (diffuse) NØ2.5
  - membranous (diffuse) NØ6.2Ø
    - with
      - nephrotic syndrome NØ4.2Ø
        - primary NØ4.21
        - secondary NØ4.22
    - idiopathic, with nephrotic syndrome NØ4.21
    - primary NØ6.21
      - with nephrotic syndrome NØ4.21
    - secondary NØ6.22
      - with nephrotic syndrome NØ4.22
  - mesangial (IgA/IgG) — *see* Nephropathy, IgA
    - proliferative (diffuse) NØ2.3
  - mesangiocapillary (diffuse) NØ2.5
  - obstructive N13.8
  - phenacetin N17.2
  - phosphate-losing N25.Ø
  - potassium depletion N25.89
  - pregnancy-related O26.83- ☑
  - proliferative NEC — *see also* NØØ-NØ7 with fourth character .8 NØ5.8
  - protein-losing N25.89
  - saturnine N14.3
  - sickle-cell D57.- ☑ *[NØ8]*
  - toxic NEC N14.4
    - due to
      - drugs N14.2
        - analgesic N14.Ø
        - specified NEC N14.19
      - heavy metals N14.3
  - vasomotor N17.Ø
  - water-losing N25.89
- **Nephroptosis** N28.83
- **Nephropyosis** — *see* Abscess, kidney
- **Nephrorrhagia** N28.89
- **Nephrosclerosis** (arteriolar) (arteriosclerotic) (chronic) (hyaline) — *see also* Hypertension, kidney
  - hyperplastic — *see* Hypertension, kidney
  - senile N26.9
- **Nephrosis, nephrotic** (Epstein's) (syndrome) (congenital) NØ4.9
  - with
    - foot process disease NØ4.9
    - glomerular lesion NØ4.1
      - hypocomplementemic NØ4.5
  - acute NØ4.9
  - anoxic — *see* Nephrosis, tubular
  - chemical — *see* Nephrosis, tubular
  - cholemic K76.7
  - diabetic — *see* EØ8-E13 with .21
  - Finnish type (congenital) Q89.89
  - hemoglobin N1Ø
  - hemoglobinuric — *see* Nephrosis, tubular
- **Nephrosis, nephrotic** — *continued*
  - in
    - amyloidosis E85.4 *[NØ8]*
    - diabetes mellitus — *see* EØ8-E13 with .21
    - epidemic hemorrhagic fever A98.5
    - malaria (malariae) B52.Ø
  - ischemic — *see* Nephrosis, tubular
  - lipoid NØ4.9
  - lower nephron — *see* Nephrosis, tubular
  - malarial (malariae) B52.Ø
  - minimal change NØ4.Ø
  - myoglobin N1Ø
  - necrotizing — *see* Nephrosis, tubular
  - osmotic (sucrose) N25.89
  - radiation NØ4.9
  - syphilitic (late) A52.75
  - toxic — *see* Nephrosis, tubular
  - tubular (acute) N17.Ø
    - postprocedural N99.Ø
    - radiation NØ4.9
- **Nephrosonephritis, hemorrhagic** (endemic) A98.5
- **Nephrostomy**
  - attention to Z43.6
  - status Z93.6
- **Nerve** — *see also* condition
  - injury — *see* Injury, nerve, by body site
- **Nerves** R45.Ø
- **Nervous** — *see also* condition R45.Ø
  - heart F45.8
  - stomach F45.8
  - tension R45.Ø
- **Nervousness** R45.Ø
- **Nesidioblastoma**
  - pancreas D13.7
  - specified site NEC — *see* Neoplasm, benign, by site
  - unspecified site D13.7
- **Nettleship's syndrome** — *see* Urticaria pigmentosa
- **Neumann's disease or syndrome** L1Ø.1
- **Neuralgia, neuralgic** (acute) M79.2
  - accessory (nerve) G52.8
  - acoustic (nerve) — *see* subcategory H93.3- ☑
  - auditory (nerve) — *see* subcategory H93.3- ☑
  - ciliary G44.ØØ9
    - intractable G44.ØØ1
    - not intractable G44.ØØ9
  - cranial
    - nerve — *see also* Disorder, nerve, cranial
      - fifth or trigeminal — *see* Neuralgia, trigeminal
    - postherpetic, postzoster BØ2.29
  - ear — *see* subcategory H92.Ø- ☑
  - facialis vera G51.1
  - Fothergill's — *see* Neuralgia, trigeminal
  - glossopharyngeal (nerve) G52.1
  - Horton's G44.Ø99
    - intractable G44.Ø91
    - not intractable G44.Ø99
  - Hunt's BØ2.21
  - hypoglossal (nerve) G52.3
  - infraorbital — *see* Neuralgia, trigeminal
  - malarial — *see* Malaria
  - migrainous G44.ØØ9
    - intractable G44.ØØ1
    - not intractable G44.ØØ9
  - Morton's G57.6- ☑
  - nerve, cranial — *see* Disorder, nerve, cranial
  - nose G52.Ø
  - occipital M54.81
  - olfactory G52.Ø
  - penis N48.9
  - perineum R1Ø.2Ø
    - bilateral R1Ø.23
    - left R1Ø.22
    - right R1Ø.21
  - postherpetic NEC BØ2.29
    - trigeminal BØ2.22
  - pubic region R1Ø.2Ø
    - bilateral R1Ø.23
    - left R1Ø.22
    - right R1Ø.21
  - scrotum R1Ø.2Ø
  - Sluder's G44.89
  - specified nerve NEC G58.8
  - spermatic cord R1Ø.2Ø
  - sphenopalatine (ganglion) G9Ø.Ø9
  - trifacial — *see* Neuralgia, trigeminal
  - trigeminal G5Ø.Ø
    - postherpetic, postzoster BØ2.22
  - vagus (nerve) G52.2
  - writer's F48.8
- **Neuralgia, neuralgic** — *continued*
  - writer's — *continued*
    - organic G25.89
- **Neurapraxia** — *see* Injury, nerve
- **Neurasthenia** F48.8
  - cardiac F45.8
  - gastric F45.8
  - heart F45.8
- **Neurilemmoma** — *see also* Neoplasm, nerve, benign
  - acoustic (nerve) D33.3
  - malignant — *see also* Neoplasm, nerve, malignant
    - acoustic (nerve) C72.4- ☑
- **Neurilemmosarcoma** — *see* Neoplasm, nerve, malignant
- **Neurinoma** — *see* Neoplasm, nerve, benign
- **Neurinomatosis** — *see* Neoplasm, nerve, uncertain behavior
- **Neuritis** (rheumatoid) M79.2
  - abducens (nerve) — *see* Strabismus, paralytic, sixth nerve
  - accessory (nerve) G52.8
  - acoustic (nerve) — *see also* subcategory H93.3- ☑
    - in (due to)
      - infectious disease NEC B99.- ☑ *[H94.Ø-]* ☑
      - parasitic disease NEC B89 *[H94.Ø-]* ☑
    - syphilitic A52.15
  - alcoholic G62.1
    - with psychosis — *see* Psychosis, alcoholic
  - amyloid, any site E85.4 *[G63]*
  - auditory (nerve) — *see* subcategory H93.3- ☑
  - brachial — *see* Radiculopathy
    - due to displacement, intervertebral disc — *see* Disorder, disc, cervical, with neuritis
  - cranial nerve
    - due to Lyme disease A69.22
    - eighth or acoustic or auditory — *see* subcategory H93.3- ☑
    - eleventh or accessory G52.8
    - fifth or trigeminal G5Ø.- ☑
    - first or olfactory G52.Ø
    - fourth or trochlear — *see* Strabismus, paralytic, fourth nerve
    - second or optic — *see* Neuritis, optic
    - seventh or facial G51.8
      - newborn (birth injury) P11.3
    - sixth or abducent — *see* Strabismus, paralytic, sixth nerve
    - tenth or vagus G52.2
    - third or oculomotor — *see* Strabismus, paralytic, third nerve
    - twelfth or hypoglossal G52.3
  - Dejerine-Sottas G6Ø.Ø
  - diabetic (mononeuropathy) — *see* EØ8-E13 with .41
    - polyneuropathy — *see* EØ8-E13 with .42
  - due to
    - beriberi E51.11
    - displacement, prolapse or rupture, intervertebral disc — *see* Disorder, disc, with, radiculopathy
    - herniation, nucleus pulposus M51.9 *[G55]*
  - endemic E51.11
  - facial G51.8
    - newborn (birth injury) P11.3
  - general — *see* Polyneuropathy
  - geniculate ganglion G51.1
    - due to herpes (zoster) BØ2.21
  - gouty — *see also* Gout, by type M1Ø.9 *[G63]*
  - hypoglossal (nerve) G52.3
  - ilioinguinal (nerve) G57.9- ☑
  - infectious (multiple) NEC G61.Ø
  - interstitial hypertrophic progressive G6Ø.Ø
  - lumbar M54.16
  - lumbosacral M54.17
  - multiple — *see also* Polyneuropathy
    - endemic E51.11
    - infective, acute G61.Ø
  - multiplex endemica E51.11
  - nerve root — *see* Radiculopathy
  - oculomotor (nerve) — *see* Strabismus, paralytic, third nerve
  - olfactory nerve G52.Ø
  - optic (nerve) (hereditary) (sympathetic) H46.9
    - with demyelination G36.Ø
    - in myelitis G36.Ø
    - nutritional H46.2
    - papillitis — *see* Papillitis, optic
    - retrobulbar H46.1- ☑
    - specified type NEC H46.8
    - toxic H46.3
  - peripheral (nerve) G62.9
    - multiple — *see* Polyneuropathy

**Neurosis, neurotic** — *continued*
- rumination F45.8
- sexual F65.9
- situational F48.8
- social F4Ø.1Ø
  - generalized F4Ø.11
- specified type NEC F48.8
- state F48.9
  - with depersonalization episode F48.1
- stomach F45.8
- traumatic F43.1Ø
  - acute F43.11
  - chronic F43.12
- vasomotor F45.8
- visceral F45.8
- war F48.8

**Neurospongioblastosis diffusa** Q85.1

**Neurosyphilis** (arrested) (early) (gumma) (late) (latent) (recurrent) (relapse) A52.3
- with ataxia (cerebellar) (locomotor) (spastic) (spinal) A52.19
- aneurysm (cerebral) A52.Ø5
- arachnoid (adhesive) A52.13
- arteritis (any artery) (cerebral) A52.Ø4
- asymptomatic A52.2
- congenital A5Ø.4Ø
- dura (mater) A52.13
- general paresis A52.17
- hemorrhagic A52.Ø5
- juvenile (asymptomatic) (meningeal) A5Ø.4Ø
- leptomeninges (aseptic) A52.13
- meningeal, meninges (adhesive) A52.13
- meningitis A52.13
- meningovascular (diffuse) A52.13
- optic atrophy A52.15
- parenchymatous (degenerative) A52.19
- paresis, paretic A52.17
  - juvenile A5Ø.45
- remission in (sustained) A52.3
- serological (without symptoms) A52.2
- specified nature or site NEC A52.19
- tabes, tabetic (dorsalis) A52.11
  - juvenile A5Ø.45
- taboparesis (taboparetic) A52.17
  - juvenile A5Ø.45
- thrombosis (cerebral) A52.Ø5
- vascular (cerebral) NEC A52.Ø5

**Neurothekeoma** — *see* Neoplasm, nerve, benign

**Neurotic** — *see* Neurosis

**Neurotoxemia** — *see* Toxemia

**Neutroclusion** M26.211

**Neutropenia, neutropenic** (chronic) (genetic) (idiopathic) (immune) (infantile) (malignant) (pernicious) (splenic) D7Ø.9
- benign ethnic — *see* Phenotype, Duffy, null
- congenital (primary) D7Ø.Ø
- cyclic D7Ø.4
- cytoreductive cancer chemotherapy sequela D7Ø.1
- drug-induced D7Ø.2
  - due to cytoreductive cancer chemotherapy D7Ø.1
- due to infection D7Ø.3
- fever D7Ø.9
- neonatal, transitory (isoimmune) (maternal transfer) P61.5
- periodic D7Ø.4
- secondary (cyclic) (periodic) (splenic) D7Ø.4
  - drug-induced D7Ø.2
    - due to cytoreductive cancer chemotherapy D7Ø.1
- specified NEC D7Ø.8
- toxic D7Ø.8

**Neutrophilia, hereditary giant** D72.Ø

**Nevocarcinoma** — *see* Melanoma

**Nevus** D22.9
- achromic — *see* Neoplasm, skin, benign
- amelanotic — *see* Neoplasm, skin, benign
- angiomatous D18.ØØ
  - intra-abdominal D18.Ø3
  - intracranial D18.Ø2
  - skin D18.Ø1
  - specified site NEC D18.Ø9
- araneus I78.1
- balloon cell — *see* Neoplasm, skin, benign
- bathing trunk D48.5
- blue — *see* Neoplasm, skin, benign
  - cellular — *see* Neoplasm, skin, benign
  - giant — *see* Neoplasm, skin, benign
  - Jadassohn's — *see* Neoplasm, skin, benign
  - malignant — *see* Melanoma
- capillary D18.ØØ

**Nevus** — *continued*
- capillary — *continued*
  - intra-abdominal D18.Ø3
  - intracranial D18.Ø2
  - skin D18.Ø1
  - specified site NEC D18.Ø9
- cavernous D18.ØØ
  - intra-abdominal D18.Ø3
  - intracranial D18.Ø2
  - skin D18.Ø1
  - specified site NEC D18.Ø9
- cellular — *see* Neoplasm, skin, benign
  - blue — *see* Neoplasm, skin, benign
- choroid D31.3- ☑
- comedonicus Q82.5
- conjunctiva D31.Ø- ☑
- dermal — *see* Neoplasm, skin, benign
  - with epidermal nevus — *see* Neoplasm, skin, benign
- dysplastic — *see* Neoplasm, skin, benign
- eye D31.9- ☑
- flammeus Q82.5
- hemangiomatous D18.ØØ
  - intra-abdominal D18.Ø3
  - intracranial D18.Ø2
  - skin D18.Ø1
  - specified site NEC D18.Ø9
- iris D31.4- ☑
- lacrimal gland D31.5- ☑
- lymphatic D18.1
- magnocellular
  - specified site — *see* Neoplasm, benign, by site
  - unspecified site D31.4Ø
- malignant — *see* Melanoma
- meaning hemangioma D18.ØØ
  - intra-abdominal D18.Ø3
  - intracranial D18.Ø2
  - skin D18.Ø1
  - specified site NEC D18.Ø9
- mouth (mucosa) D1Ø.3Ø
  - specified site NEC D1Ø.39
  - white sponge Q38.6
- multiplex Q85.1
- non-neoplastic I78.1
- oral mucosa D1Ø.3Ø
  - specified site NEC D1Ø.39
  - white sponge Q38.6
- orbit D31.6- ☑
- pigmented
  - giant — *see also* Neoplasm, skin, uncertain behavior D48.5
    - malignant melanoma in — *see* Melanoma
- portwine Q82.5
- retina D31.2- ☑
- retrobulbar D31.6- ☑
- sanguineous Q82.5
- senile I78.1
- skin D22.9
  - abdominal wall D22.5
  - ala nasi D22.39
  - ankle D22.7- ☑
  - anus, anal D22.5
  - arm D22.6- ☑
  - auditory canal (external) D22.2- ☑
  - auricle (ear) D22.2- ☑
  - auricular canal (external) D22.2- ☑
  - axilla, axillary fold D22.5
  - back D22.5
  - breast D22.5
  - brow D22.39
  - buttock D22.5
  - canthus (eye) D22.1- ☑
  - cheek (external) D22.39
  - chest wall D22.5
  - chin D22.39
  - ear (external) D22.2- ☑
  - external meatus (ear) D22.2- ☑
  - eyebrow D22.39
  - eyelid (lower) (upper) D22.1- ☑
  - face D22.3Ø
    - specified NEC D22.39
  - female genital organ (external) NEC D28.Ø
  - finger D22.6- ☑
  - flank D22.5
  - foot D22.7- ☑
  - forearm D22.6- ☑
  - forehead D22.39
  - foreskin D29.Ø

**Nevus** — *continued*
- skin — *continued*
  - genital organ (external) NEC
    - female D28.Ø
    - male D29.9
  - gluteal region D22.5
  - groin D22.5
  - hand D22.6- ☑
  - heel D22.7- ☑
  - helix D22.2- ☑
  - hip D22.7- ☑
  - interscapular region D22.5
  - jaw D22.39
  - knee D22.7- ☑
  - labium (majus) (minus) D28.Ø
  - leg D22.7- ☑
  - lip (lower) (upper) D22.Ø
  - lower limb D22.7- ☑
  - male genital organ (external) D29.9
  - nail D22.9
    - finger D22.6- ☑
    - toe D22.7- ☑
  - nasolabial groove D22.39
  - nates D22.5
  - neck D22.4
  - nose (external) D22.39
  - palpebra D22.1- ☑
  - penis D29.Ø
  - perianal skin D22.5
  - perineum D22.5
  - pinna D22.2- ☑
  - popliteal fossa or space D22.7- ☑
  - prepuce D29.Ø
  - pudendum D28.Ø
  - scalp D22.4
  - scrotum D29.4
  - shoulder D22.6- ☑
  - submammary fold D22.5
  - temple D22.39
  - thigh D22.7- ☑
  - toe D22.7- ☑
  - trunk NEC D22.5
  - umbilicus D22.5
  - upper limb D22.6- ☑
  - vulva D28.Ø
- specified site NEC — *see* Neoplasm, by site, benign
- spider I78.1
- stellar I78.1
- strawberry Q82.5
- Sutton's benign D22.9
- unius lateris Q82.5
- Unna's Q82.5
- vascular Q82.5
- verrucous Q82.5

**Newborn** (infant) (liveborn) (singleton) Z38.2
- abstinence syndrome P96.1
- acne L7Ø.4
- affected by
  - abnormalities of membranes PØ2.9
    - specified NEC PØ2.8
  - abruptio placenta PØ2.1
  - amino-acid metabolic disorder, transitory P74.8
  - amniocentesis (while in utero) PØØ.6
  - amnionitis PØ2.78
  - apparent life threatening event (ALTE) R68.13
  - bleeding (into)
    - cerebral cortex P52.22
    - germinal matrix P52.Ø
    - ventricles P52.1
  - breech delivery PØ3.Ø
  - cardiac arrest P29.81
  - cardiomyopathy I42.89
    - congenital I42.4
  - cerebral ischemia P91.Ø
  - Cesarean delivery PØ3.4
  - chemotherapy agents PØ4.11
  - chorioamnionitis PØ2.78
  - cocaine (crack) PØ4.41
  - complications of labor and delivery PØ3.9
    - specified NEC PØ3.89
  - compression of umbilical cord NEC PØ2.5
  - contracted pelvis PØ3.1
  - cyanosis P28.2
  - delivery PØ3.9
    - Cesarean PØ3.4
    - forceps PØ3.2
    - vacuum extractor PØ3.3
  - drugs of addiction PØ4.4Ø

**Nocardiosis, nocardiasis** — *continued*
- cutaneous A43.1
- lung A43.Ø
- pneumonia A43.Ø
- pulmonary A43.Ø
- specified site NEC A43.8

**Nocturia** R35.1
- psychogenic F45.8

**Nocturnal** — *see* condition

**Nodal rhythm** I49.89

**Node**(s) — *see also* Nodule
- Bouchard's (with arthropathy) M15.2
- Haygarth's M15.8
- Heberden's (with arthropathy) M15.1
- larynx J38.7
- lymph — *see* condition
- milker's BØ8.Ø3
- Osler's I33.Ø
- Schmorl's — *see* Schmorl's disease
- singer's J38.2
- teacher's J38.2
- tuberculous — *see* Tuberculosis, lymph gland
- vocal cord J38.2

**Nodule(s), nodular**
- actinomycotic — *see* Actinomycosis
- breast NEC — *see also* Lump, breast N63.Ø
- colloid (cystic), thyroid EØ4.1
- cutaneous — *see* Swelling, localized
- endometrial (stromal) D26.1
- Haygarth's M15.8
- inflammatory — *see* Inflammation
- juxta-articular
  - syphilitic A52.77
  - yaws A66.7
- larynx J38.7
- lung, solitary (subsegmental branch of the bronchial tree) R91.1
  - multiple R91.8
- milker's BØ8.Ø3
- prostate N4Ø.2
  - with lower urinary tract symptoms (LUTS) N4Ø.3
  - without lower urinary tract symptoms (LUTS) N4Ø.2
- pulmonary, solitary (subsegmental branch of the bronchial tree) R91.1
- retrocardiac RØ9.89
- rheumatoid MØ6.3Ø
  - ankle MØ6.37- ☑
  - elbow MØ6.32- ☑
  - foot joint MØ6.37- ☑
  - hand joint MØ6.34- ☑
  - hip MØ6.35- ☑
  - knee MØ6.36- ☑
  - multiple site MØ6.39
  - shoulder MØ6.31- ☑
  - vertebra MØ6.38
  - wrist MØ6.33- ☑
- scrotum (inflammatory) N49.2
- singer's J38.2
- solitary, lung (subsegmental branch of the bronchial tree) R91.1
  - multiple R91.8
- subcutaneous — *see* Swelling, localized
- teacher's J38.2
- thyroid (cold) (gland) (nontoxic) EØ4.1
  - with thyrotoxicosis EØ5.2Ø
    - with thyroid storm EØ5.21
  - toxic or with hyperthyroidism EØ5.2Ø
    - with thyroid storm EØ5.21
- vocal cord J38.2

**Noma** (gangrenous) (hospital) (infective) A69.Ø
- auricle I96
- mouth A69.Ø
- pudendi N76.89
- vulvae N76.89

**Nomad, nomadism** Z59.ØØ

**NOMID** (neonatal onset multisystemic inflammatory disorder) MØ4.2

**Non-accidental trauma** — *see* Abuse, physical

**Non-Hodgkin lymphoma NEC** — *see* Lymphoma, non-Hodgkin

**Non-ketotic hyperglycinemia** E72.51

**Non-palpable testicle**(s)
- bilateral R39.84
- unilateral R39.83

**Non-working side interference** M26.56

**Nonadherence to medical treatment, specified NEC** Z91.199

**Nonadherence to medical treatment, specified** — *continued*
- due to
  - financial hardship Z91.19Ø
  - specified reason NEC Z91.198

**Nonautoimmune hemolytic anemia** D59.4
- drug-induced D59.2

**Nonclosure** — *see also* Imperfect, closure
- ductus arteriosus (Botallo's) Q25.Ø
- foramen
  - botalli Q21.12
  - ovale Q21.12

**Noncompliance** Z91.199
- with
  - dialysis Z91.158
    - due to financial hardship Z91.151
  - dietary regimen Z91.119
    - due to
      - financial hardship Z91.11Ø
      - specified reason NEC Z91.118
  - medical treatment, specified NEC Z91.199
    - due to
      - financial hardship Z91.19Ø
      - specified reason NEC Z91.198
  - medication regimen NEC Z91.148
    - due to financial hardship Z91.141
    - underdosing — *see also* Table of Drugs and Chemicals, categories T36-T5Ø, with final character 6 Z91.148
      - intentional NEC Z91.128
        - by caregiver
          - due to
            - financial hardship Z91.A2Ø
            - specified reason NEC Z91.A28
        - due to financial hardship of patient Z91.12Ø
      - unintentional NEC Z91.138
        - by caregiver Z91.A3
        - due to patient's age related debility Z91.13Ø
  - renal dialysis Z91.158
    - due to financial hardship Z91.151
- caregiver
  - with patient's
    - dietary regimen
      - due to
        - financial hardship Z91.A1Ø
        - specified reason NEC Z91.A18
    - medical treatment and regimen
      - due to financial hardship Z91.A91
      - specified reason NEC Z91.A98
    - medication regimen
      - due to financial hardship Z91.A41
      - specified reason NEC Z91.A48
    - renal dialysis
      - due to financial hardship Z91.A51
      - specified reason NEC Z91.A58

**Nondescent** (congenital) — *see also* Malposition, congenital
- cecum Q43.3
- colon Q43.3
- testicle Q53.9
  - bilateral Q53.2Ø
    - abdominal Q53.211
    - perineal Q53.22
  - unilateral Q53.1Ø
    - abdominal Q53.111
    - perineal Q53.12

**Nondevelopment**
- brain QØ2
  - part of QØ4.3
- heart Q24.8
- organ or site, congenital NEC — *see* Hypoplasia

**Nonengagement**
- head NEC O32.4- ☑
  - in labor, causing obstructed labor O64.8- ☑

**Nonexanthematous tick fever** A93.2

**Nonexpansion, lung** (newborn) P28.Ø

**Nonfunctioning**
- cystic duct — *see also* Disease, gallbladder K82.8
- gallbladder — *see also* Disease, gallbladder K82.8
- kidney N28.9
- labyrinth — *see* subcategory H83.2- ☑

**Nonimplantation, ovum** N97.2

**Noninsufflation, fallopian tube** N97.1

**Nonne-Milroy syndrome** Q82.Ø

**Nonovulation** N97.Ø

**Nonpatent fallopian tube** N97.1

**Nonpneumatization, lung NEC** P28.Ø

**Nonrotation** — *see* Malrotation

**Nonsecretion, urine** — *see* Anuria

**Nonunion**
- fracture — *see* Fracture, by site
- joint, following fusion or arthrodesis M96.Ø
- organ or site, congenital NEC — *see* Imperfect, closure
- symphysis pubis, congenital Q74.2

**Nonvisualization, gallbladder** R93.2

**Nonvital, nonvitalized tooth** KØ4.99

**Noonan's syndrome** Q87.19

**Normocytic anemia** (infectional) due to blood loss (chronic) D5Ø.Ø
- acute D62

**Norrie's disease** (congenital) Q15.8

**North American blastomycosis** B4Ø.9

**Norwegian itch** B86

**Nose, nasal** — *see* condition

**Nose-picking** F98.8

**Nosebleed** RØ4.Ø

**Nosomania** F45.21

**Nosophobia** F45.22

**Nostalgia** F43.2Ø

**Notch of iris** Q13.2

**Notching nose, congenital** (tip) Q3Ø.2

**Nothnagel's**
- syndrome — *see* Strabismus, paralytic, third nerve
- vasomotor acroparesthesia I73.89

**Novy's relapsing fever** A68.9
- louse-borne A68.Ø
- tick-borne A68.1

**Noxious**
- foodstuffs, poisoning by — *see* Poisoning, food, noxious, plant
- substances transmitted through placenta or breast milk PØ4.9

**Nucleus pulposus** — *see* condition

**Numbness** R2Ø.Ø

**Nuns' knee** — *see* Bursitis, prepatellar

**Nursemaid's elbow** S53.Ø3- ☑

**Nutcracker esophagus** K22.4

**Nutmeg liver** K76.1

**Nutrient element deficiency** E61.9
- specified NEC E61.8

**Nutrition deficient or insufficient** — *see also* Malnutrition E63.9
- due to
  - insufficient food T73.Ø- ☑
  - lack of
    - care (child) T76.Ø2- ☑
      - adult T76.Ø1- ☑
    - food T73.Ø- ☑
  - specific element deficiency — *see* Nutrient element deficiency, or by element
- sequelae — *see* Sequelae, nutritional deficiency
- specified NEC E63.8

**Nutritional stunting** E45

**Nyctalopia** (night blindness) — *see* Blindness, night

**Nycturia** R35.1
- psychogenic F45.8

**Nymphomania** F52.8

**Nystagmus** H55.ØØ
- benign paroxysmal — *see* Vertigo, benign paroxysmal
- central positional H81.4
- congenital H55.Ø1
- dissociated H55.Ø4
- latent H55.Ø2
- miners' H55.Ø9
- positional
  - benign paroxysmal H81.4
  - central H81.4
- specified form NEC H55.Ø9
- visual deprivation H55.Ø3

# O

**Obermeyer's relapsing fever** (European) A68.Ø

**Obesity** E66.9
- with alveolar hypoventilation E66.2
- adrenal E27.8
- class
  - 1 E66.811
  - 2 E66.812
  - 3 E66.813
- complicating
  - childbirth O99.214
  - pregnancy O99.21- ☑
  - puerperium O99.215
- constitutional E66.89
- dietary counseling and surveillance Z71.3

- **Obstruction, obstructed, obstructive** — *continued*
  - foramen of Monro — *continued*
    - with spina bifida — *see* Spina bifida, by site, with hydrocephalus
  - foreign body — *see* Foreign body
  - gallbladder K82.Ø
    - with calculus, stones K8Ø.21
    - congenital Q44.1
  - gastric outlet K31.1
  - gastrointestinal — *see* Obstruction, intestine
  - hepatic K76.89
    - duct (noncalculous) K83.1
  - ileum — *see* Obstruction, intestine
  - iliofemoral (artery) I74.5
  - intestine K56.6Ø9
    - with
      - adhesions (intestinal) (peritoneal) K56.5Ø
        - complete K56.52
        - incomplete K56.51
        - partial K56.51
    - adynamic K56.Ø
    - by gallstone K56.3
    - complete K56.6Ø1
    - congenital (small) Q41.9
      - large Q42.9
        - specified part NEC Q42.8
    - incomplete K56.6ØØ
    - neurogenic K56.Ø
      - Hirschsprung's disease or megacolon Q43.1
    - newborn P76.9
      - due to
        - fecaliths P76.8
        - inspissated milk P76.2
        - meconium (plug) P76.Ø
          - in mucoviscidosis E84.11
      - specified NEC P76.8
    - partial K56.6ØØ
    - postoperative K91.3Ø
      - complete K91.32
      - incomplete K91.31
      - partial K91.31
    - reflex K56.Ø
    - specified NEC K56.699
      - complete K56.691
      - incomplete K56.69Ø
      - partial K56.69Ø
    - volvulus K56.2
  - intracardiac ball valve prosthesis T82.Ø9- ☑
  - jejunum — *see* Obstruction, intestine
  - joint prosthesis — *see* Complications, joint prosthesis, mechanical, specified NEC, by site
  - kidney (calices) — *see also* Hydronephrosis N28.89
  - labor — *see* Delivery
  - lacrimal (passages) (duct)
    - by
      - dacryolith — *see* Dacryolith
      - stenosis — *see* Stenosis, lacrimal
    - congenital Q1Ø.5
    - neonatal HØ4.53- ☑
  - lacrimonasal duct — *see* Obstruction, lacrimal
  - lacteal, with steatorrhea K9Ø.2
  - laryngitis — *see* Laryngitis
  - larynx NEC J38.6
    - congenital Q31.8
  - lung J98.4
    - disease, chronic J44.9
  - lymphatic I89.Ø
  - meconium (plug)
    - newborn P76.Ø
      - due to fecaliths P76.Ø
      - in mucoviscidosis E84.11
  - mitral — *see* Stenosis, mitral
  - nasal J34.89
  - nasolacrimal duct — *see also* Obstruction, lacrimal
    - congenital Q1Ø.5
  - nasopharynx J39.2
  - nose J34.89
  - organ or site, congenital NEC — *see* Atresia, by site
  - pancreatic duct K86.89
  - parotid duct or gland K11.8
  - pelviureteral junction N13.5
    - with hydronephrosis N13.Ø
    - congenital Q62.39
  - pharynx J39.2
  - portal (circulation) (vein) I81
  - prostate — *see also* Hyperplasia, prostate
    - valve (urinary) N32.Ø
  - pulmonary valve (heart) I37.Ø
  - pyelonephritis (chronic) N11.1
- **Obstruction, obstructed, obstructive** — *continued*
  - pylorus
    - adult K31.1
    - congenital Q4Ø.Ø
  - rectosigmoid — *see* Obstruction, intestine
  - rectum K62.4
  - renal — *see also* Hydronephrosis N28.89
    - outflow N13.8
    - pelvis, congenital Q62.39
  - respiratory J98.8
    - chronic J44.9
  - retinal (vessels) H34.9
  - salivary duct (any) K11.8
    - with calculus K11.5
  - sigmoid — *see* Obstruction, intestine
  - sinus (accessory) (nasal) J34.89
  - Stensen's duct K11.8
  - stomach NEC K31.89
    - acute K31.Ø
    - congenital Q4Ø.2
    - due to pylorospasm K31.3
  - submandibular duct K11.8
  - submaxillary gland K11.8
    - with calculus K11.5
  - thoracic duct I89.Ø
  - thrombotic — *see* Thrombosis
  - trachea J39.8
  - tracheostomy airway J95.Ø3
  - tricuspid (valve) — *see* Stenosis, tricuspid
  - upper respiratory, congenital Q34.8
  - ureter (functional) (pelvic junction) NEC N13.5
    - with
      - hydronephrosis N13.1
        - with infection N13.6
        - congenital Q62.39
      - pyelonephritis (chronic) N11.1
    - congenital Q62.39
    - due to calculus — *see* Calculus, ureter
  - urethra NEC N36.8
    - congenital Q64.39
  - urinary (moderate) N13.9
    - due to hyperplasia (hypertrophy) of prostate — *see* Hyperplasia, prostate
    - organ or tract (lower) N13.9
    - prostatic valve N32.Ø
    - specified NEC N13.8
  - uropathy N13.9
  - uterus N85.8
  - vagina N89.5
  - valvular — *see* Endocarditis
  - vein, venous I87.1
    - caval (inferior) (superior) I87.1
    - thrombotic — *see* Thrombosis
  - vena cava (inferior) (superior) I87.1
  - vesical NEC N32.Ø
  - vesicourethral orifice N32.Ø
    - congenital Q64.31
  - vessel NEC I99.8
    - stent — *see* Restenosis, stent
- **Obturator** — *see* condition
- **Occlusal wear, teeth** KØ3.Ø
- **Occlusio pupillae** — *see* Membrane, pupillary
- **Occlusion, occluded**
  - anus K62.4
    - congenital Q42.3
      - with fistula Q42.2
  - aortoiliac (chronic) I74.Ø9
  - aqueduct of Sylvius G91.1
    - congenital QØ3.Ø
      - with spina bifida — *see* Spina bifida, by site, with hydrocephalus
  - artery — *see also* Atherosclerosis, artery I7Ø.9- ☑
    - auditory, internal I65.8
    - basilar I65.1
      - with
        - infarction I63.22
          - due to
            - embolism I63.12
            - thrombosis I63.Ø2
    - brain or cerebral I66.9
      - with infarction (due to) I63.5- ☑
        - embolism I63.4- ☑
        - thrombosis I63.3- ☑
    - carotid I65.2- ☑
      - with
        - infarction I63.23- ☑
          - due to
            - embolism I63.13- ☑
- **Occlusion, occluded** — *continued*
  - artery — *see also* Atherosclerosis, artery — *continued*
    - carotid — *continued*
      - with — *continued*
        - infarction — *continued*
          - due to — *continued*
            - thrombosis I63.Ø3- ☑
    - cerebellar (anterior inferior) (posterior inferior) (superior) I66.3
      - with infarction I63.54- ☑
        - due to
          - embolism I63.44- ☑
          - thrombosis I63.34- ☑
    - cerebral I66.9
      - with infarction I63.5Ø
        - due to
          - embolism I63.4Ø
            - specified NEC I63.49
          - thrombosis I63.3Ø
            - specified NEC I63.39
      - anterior I66.1- ☑
        - with infarction I63.52- ☑
          - due to
            - embolism I63.42- ☑
            - thrombosis I63.32- ☑
      - middle I66.Ø- ☑
        - with infarction I63.51- ☑
          - due to
            - embolism I63.41- ☑
            - thrombosis I63.31- ☑
      - posterior I66.2- ☑
        - with infarction I63.53- ☑
          - due to
            - embolism I63.43- ☑
            - thrombosis I63.33- ☑
      - specified NEC I66.8
        - with infarction I63.59
          - due to
            - embolism I63.4- ☑
            - thrombosis I63.3- ☑
    - choroidal (anterior) — *see* Occlusion, artery, precerebral, specified NEC
    - communicating posterior — *see* Occlusion, artery, precerebral, specified NEC
    - complete
      - coronary I25.82
      - extremities I7Ø.92
    - coronary (acute) (thrombotic) (without myocardial infarction) I24.Ø
      - with myocardial infarction — *see* Infarction, myocardium
      - chronic total I25.82
      - complete I25.82
      - healed or old I25.2
      - total (chronic) I25.82
    - hypophyseal — *see* Occlusion, artery, precerebral, specified NEC
    - iliac I74.5
    - lower extremities due to stenosis or stricture I77.1
    - mesenteric (embolic) (thrombotic) — *see also* Infarct, intestine K55.Ø69
    - perforating — *see* Occlusion, artery, cerebral, specified NEC
    - peripheral I77.9
      - thrombotic or embolic I74.4
    - pontine — *see* Occlusion, artery, precerebral, specified NEC
    - precerebral I65.9
      - with infarction I63.2Ø
        - specified NEC I63.29
        - due to
          - embolism I63.1Ø
            - specified NEC I63.19
          - thrombosis I63.ØØ
            - specified NEC I63.Ø9
      - basilar — *see* Occlusion, artery, basilar
      - carotid — *see* Occlusion, artery, carotid
      - puerperal O88.23
      - specified NEC I65.8
        - with infarction I63.29
          - due to
            - embolism I63.19
            - thrombosis I63.Ø9
      - vertebral — *see* Occlusion, artery, vertebral
    - renal N28.Ø
    - retinal
      - branch H34.23- ☑
      - central H34.1- ☑

Index

Obstruction, obstructed, obstructive — Occlusion, occluded

- **Opacity, opacities** — *continued*
  - enamel (teeth) (fluoride) (nonfluoride) KØØ.3
  - lens — *see* Cataract
  - snowball — *see* Deposit, crystalline
  - vitreous (humor) NEC H43.39- ☑
    - congenital Q14.Ø
    - membranes and strands H43.31- ☑
- **Opalescent dentin** (hereditary) KØØ.5
- **Open, opening**
  - abnormal, organ or site, congenital — *see* Imperfect, closure
  - angle with
    - borderline
      - findings
        - high risk H4Ø.Ø2- ☑
        - low risk H4Ø.Ø1- ☑
      - intraocular pressure H4Ø.ØØ- ☑
    - cupping of discs H4Ø.Ø1- ☑
    - glaucoma (primary) — *see* Glaucoma, open angle
  - bite
    - anterior M26.22Ø
    - posterior M26.221
  - false — *see* Imperfect, closure
  - margin on tooth restoration KØ8.51
  - restoration margins of tooth KØ8.51
  - wound — *see* Wound, open
- **Operational fatigue** F48.8
- **Operative** — *see* condition
- **Operculitis** — *see* Periodontitis
- **Operculum** — *see* Break, retina
- **Ophiasis** L63.2
- **Ophthalmia** — *see also* Conjunctivitis H1Ø.9
  - actinic rays — *see* Photokeratitis
  - allergic (acute) — *see* Conjunctivitis, acute, atopic
  - blennorrhagic (gonococcal) (neonatorum) A54.31
  - diphtheritic A36.86
  - Egyptian A71.1
  - electrica — *see* Photokeratitis
  - gonococcal (neonatorum) A54.31
  - metastatic — *see* Endophthalmitis, purulent
  - migraine — *see* Migraine, ophthalmoplegic
  - neonatorum, newborn P39.1
    - gonococcal A54.31
  - nodosa H16.24- ☑
  - purulent — *see* Conjunctivitis, acute, mucopurulent
  - spring — *see* Conjunctivitis, acute, atopic
  - sympathetic — *see* Uveitis, sympathetic
- **Ophthalmitis** — *see* Ophthalmia
- **Ophthalmocele** (congenital) Q15.8
- **Ophthalmoneuromyelitis** G36.Ø
- **Ophthalmopathy, Graves'** HØ5.83- ☑
- **Ophthalmoplegia** — *see also* Strabismus, paralytic
  - anterior internuclear — *see* Ophthalmoplegia, internuclear
  - ataxia-areflexia G61.Ø
  - diabetic — *see* EØ8-E13 with .39
  - exophthalmic EØ5.ØØ
    - with thyroid storm EØ5.Ø1
  - external H49.88- ☑
    - progressive H49.4- ☑
      - with pigmentary retinopathy — *see* Kearns-Sayre syndrome
    - total H49.3- ☑
  - internal (complete) (total) H52.51- ☑
  - internuclear H51.2- ☑
  - migraine — *see* Migraine, ophthalmoplegic
  - Parinaud's H49.88- ☑
  - progressive external — *see* Ophthalmoplegia, external, progressive
  - supranuclear, progressive G23.1
  - total (external) — *see* Ophthalmoplegia, external, total
- **Opioid**(s)
  - abuse — *see* Abuse, drug, opioids
  - dependence — *see* Dependence, drug, opioids
  - induced, without use disorder
    - anxiety disorder F11.288
    - delirium F11.921
    - depressive disorder F11.24
    - sexual dysfunction F11.281
    - sleep disorder F11.982
- **Opisthognathism** M26.Ø9
- **Opisthorchiasis** (felineus) (viverrini) B66.Ø
- **Opitz' disease** D73.2
- **Opiumism** — *see* Dependence, drug, opioid
- **Oppenheim-Urbach disease** (necrobiosis lipoidica diabeticorum) — *see* EØ8-E13 with .62Ø
- **Oppenheim's disease** G7Ø.2
- **Opportunistic salpingectomy** Z4Ø.82
- **Optic nerve** — *see* condition
- **Orbit** — *see* condition
- **Orbitopathy** (Graves') (thyroid) HØ5.83- ☑
- **Orchioblastoma** C62.9- ☑
- **Orchitis** (gangrenous) (nonspecific) (septic) (suppurative) N45.2
  - blennorrhagic (gonococcal) (acute) (chronic) A54.23
  - chlamydial A56.19
  - filarial — *see also* Infestation, filarial B74.9 *[N51]*
  - gonococcal (acute) (chronic) A54.23
  - mumps B26.Ø
  - syphilitic A52.76
  - tuberculous A18.15
- **Orf** (virus disease) BØ8.Ø2
- **Organic** — *see also* condition
  - brain syndrome FØ9
  - heart — *see* Disease, heart
  - mental disorder FØ9
  - psychosis FØ9
- **Orgasm**
  - anejaculatory N53.13
- **Oriental**
  - bilharziasis B65.2
  - schistosomiasis B65.2
- **Orifice** — *see* condition
- **Origin of both great vessels from right ventricle** Q2Ø.1
- **Ormond's disease** (with ureteral obstruction) N13.5
  - with infection N13.6
- **Ornithine metabolism disorder** E72.4
- **Ornithinemia** (Type I) (Type II) E72.4
- **Ornithosis** A7Ø
- **Orotaciduria, oroticaciduria** (congenital) (hereditary) (pyrimidine deficiency) E79.89
  - anemia D53.Ø
- **Orthodontics**
  - adjustment Z46.4
  - fitting Z46.4
- **Orthopnea** RØ6.Ø1
- **Orthopoxvirus** BØ8.Ø9
- **Os, uterus** — *see* condition
- **Osgood-Schlatter disease or osteochondrosis** M92.52- ☑
- **Osler** (-Weber)-**Rendu disease** I78.Ø
- **Osler's nodes** I33.Ø
- **Osmidrosis** L75.Ø
- **Osseous** — *see* condition
- **Ossification**
  - artery — *see* Arteriosclerosis
  - auricle (ear) — *see* Disorder, pinna, specified type NEC
  - bronchial J98.Ø9
  - cardiac — *see* Degeneration, myocardial
  - cartilage (senile) — *see* Disorder, cartilage, specified type NEC
  - coronary (artery) — *see* Disease, heart, ischemic, atherosclerotic
  - diaphragm J98.6
  - ear, middle — *see* Otosclerosis
  - falx cerebri G96.198
  - fontanel, premature Q75.ØØ9
  - heart — *see also* Degeneration, myocardial
    - valve — *see* Endocarditis
  - larynx J38.7
  - ligament — *see* Disorder, tendon, specified type NEC
    - posterior longitudinal — *see* Spondylopathy, specified NEC
  - meninges (cerebral) (spinal) G96.198
  - multiple, eccentric centers — *see* Disorder, bone, development or growth
  - muscle — *see also* Calcification, muscle
    - due to burns — *see* Myositis, ossificans, in, burns
    - paralytic — *see* Myositis, ossificans, in, quadriplegia
    - progressive — *see* Myositis, ossificans, progressiva
    - specified NEC M61.5Ø
      - ankle M61.57- ☑
      - foot M61.57- ☑
      - forearm M61.53- ☑
      - hand M61.54- ☑
      - lower leg M61.56- ☑
      - multiple sites M61.59
      - pelvic region M61.55- ☑
      - shoulder region M61.51- ☑
      - specified site NEC M61.58
      - thigh M61.55- ☑
      - upper arm M61.52- ☑
    - traumatic — *see* Myositis, ossificans, traumatica
  - myocardium, myocardial — *see* Degeneration, myocardial
  - penis N48.89
  - periarticular — *see* Disorder, joint, specified type NEC
- **Ossification** — *continued*
  - pinna — *see* Disorder, pinna, specified type NEC
  - rider's bone — *see* Ossification, muscle, specified NEC
  - sclera H15.89
  - subperiosteal, post-traumatic M89.8X- ☑
  - tendon — *see* Disorder, tendon, specified type NEC
  - trachea J39.8
  - tympanic membrane — *see* Disorder, tympanic membrane, specified NEC
  - vitreous (humor) — *see* Deposit, crystalline
- **Osteitis** — *see also* Osteomyelitis
  - alveolar M27.3
  - condensans M85.3Ø
    - ankle M85.37- ☑
    - foot M85.37- ☑
    - forearm M85.33- ☑
    - hand M85.34- ☑
    - lower leg M85.36- ☑
    - multiple site M85.39
    - neck M85.38
    - rib M85.38
    - shoulder M85.31- ☑
    - skull M85.38
    - specified site NEC M85.38
    - thigh M85.35- ☑
    - toe M85.37- ☑
    - upper arm M85.32- ☑
    - vertebra M85.38
  - deformans — *see also* Paget's disease, bone M88.9
    - in (due to)
      - malignant neoplasm of bone — *see also* Neoplasm, malignant, by site C41.9 *[M9Ø.6Ø]*
      - neoplastic disease — *see also* Neoplasm, by type and site D49.9 *[M9Ø.6Ø]*
        - carpus D49.2 *[M9Ø.64-]* ☑
        - clavicle D49.2 *[M9Ø.61-]* ☑
        - femur D49.2 *[M9Ø.65-]* ☑
        - fibula D49.2 *[M9Ø.66-]* ☑
        - finger D49.2 *[M9Ø.64-]* ☑
        - humerus D49.2 *[M9Ø.62-]* ☑
        - ilium D49.2 *[M9Ø.68]*
        - ischium D49.2 *[M9Ø.68]*
        - metacarpus D49.2 *[M9Ø.64-]* ☑
        - metatarsus D49.2 *[M9Ø.67-]* ☑
        - multiple sites D49.89 *[M9Ø.69]*
        - neck D49.2 *[M9Ø.68]*
        - pubic ramus [pubis] D49.2 *[M9Ø.68]*
        - radius D49.2 *[M9Ø.63-]* ☑
        - rib D49.2 *[M9Ø.68]*
        - scapula D49.2 *[M9Ø.61-]* ☑
        - skull D49.2 *[M9Ø.68]*
        - tarsus D49.2 *[M9Ø.67-]* ☑
        - tibia D49.2 *[M9Ø.66-]* ☑
        - toe D49.2 *[M9Ø.67-]* ☑
        - ulna D49.2 *[M9Ø.63-]* ☑
        - vertebra D49.2 *[M9Ø.68]*
    - skull M88.Ø
    - specified NEC — *see* Paget's disease, bone, by site
    - vertebra M88.1
  - due to yaws A66.6
  - fibrosa NEC — *see* Cyst, bone, by site
    - circumscripta — *see* Dysplasia, fibrous, bone NEC
    - cystica (generalisata) E21.Ø
    - disseminata Q78.1
    - osteoplastica E21.Ø
  - fragilitans Q78.Ø
  - Garr's (sclerosing) — *see* Osteomyelitis, specified type NEC
  - jaw (acute) (chronic) (lower) (suppurative) (upper) M27.2
  - parathyroid E21.Ø
  - petrous bone (acute) (chronic) — *see* Petrositis
  - sclerotic, nonsuppurative — *see* Osteomyelitis, specified type NEC
  - tuberculosa A18.Ø9
    - cystica D86.89
    - multiplex cystoides D86.89
- **Osteo-onycho-arthro-dysplasia** Q87.2
- **Osteo-onychodysplasia, hereditary** Q87.2
- **Osteoarthritis** M19.9Ø
  - ankle M19.Ø7- ☑
    - post-traumatic M19.17- ☑
    - primary M19.Ø7- ☑
    - secondary M19.27- ☑
  - elbow M19.Ø2- ☑
    - post-traumatic M19.12- ☑
    - primary M19.Ø2- ☑
    - secondary M19.22- ☑

- **Osteoarthritis** — *continued*
  - foot joint M19.Ø7- ☑
    - post-traumatic M19.17- ☑
    - primary M19.Ø7- ☑
    - secondary M19.27- ☑
  - generalized (multiple joints) M15.9
    - erosive M15.4
    - primary M15.Ø
    - specified NEC M15.8
  - hand joint M19.Ø4- ☑
    - first carpometacarpal joint M18.9
      - post-traumatic — *see* Osteoarthritis, post-traumatic NEC, hand joint, first carpometacarpal joint
      - primary — *see* Osteoarthritis, primary, hand joint, first carpometacarpal joint
      - secondary — *see* Osteoarthritis, secondary, hand joint, first carpometacarpal joint
    - post-traumatic M19.14- ☑
    - primary M19.Ø4- ☑
    - secondary M19.24- ☑
  - hip M16.9
    - bilateral M16.Ø
      - due to hip dysplasia M16.2
      - post-traumatic M16.4
      - secondary M16.6
    - due to hip dysplasia (unilateral) M16.3- ☑
      - bilateral M16.2
    - post-traumatic — *see* Osteoarthritis, post-traumatic, hip
    - primary M16.1- ☑
    - secondary — *see* Osteoarthritis, secondary, hip
    - unilateral M16.1- ☑
      - due to hip dysplasia M16.3- ☑
      - post-traumatic M16.5- ☑
      - primary M16.1- ☑
      - secondary NEC M16.7
  - interphalangeal
    - distal (Heberden) M15.1
    - proximal (Bouchard) M15.2
  - knee M17.9
    - bilateral M17.Ø
      - post-traumatic M17.2
      - secondary M17.4
    - post-traumatic — *see* Osteoarthritis, post-traumatic, knee
    - primary M17.1- ☑
      - bilateral M17.Ø
    - secondary — *see* Osteoarthritis, secondary, knee
    - unilateral M17.1- ☑
      - post-traumatic M17.3- ☑
      - primary M17.1- ☑
      - secondary NEC M17.5
  - post-traumatic NEC M19.92
    - ankle M19.17- ☑
    - elbow M19.12- ☑
    - foot joint M19.17- ☑
    - hand joint M19.14- ☑
      - first carpometacarpal joint M18.3- ☑
        - bilateral M18.2
    - hip M16.5- ☑
      - bilateral M16.4
    - knee M17.3- ☑
      - bilateral M17.2
    - shoulder M19.11- ☑
    - specified site NEC M19.19
    - wrist M19.13- ☑
  - primary M19.91
    - ankle M19.Ø7- ☑
    - elbow M19.Ø2- ☑
    - foot joint M19.Ø7- ☑
    - hand joint M19.Ø4- ☑
      - first carpometacarpal joint M18.1- ☑
        - bilateral M18.Ø
    - hip M16.1- ☑
      - bilateral M16.Ø
    - knee M17.1- ☑
      - bilateral M17.Ø
    - multiple sites M15.9
    - shoulder M19.Ø1- ☑
    - specified site NEC M19.Ø9
    - spine — *see* Spondylosis
    - wrist M19.Ø3- ☑
  - secondary M19.93
    - ankle M19.27- ☑
    - elbow M19.22- ☑
    - foot joint M19.27- ☑

- **Osteoarthritis** — *continued*
  - secondary — *continued*
    - hand joint M19.24- ☑
      - first carpometacarpal joint M18.5- ☑
        - bilateral M18.4
    - hip M16.7
      - bilateral M16.6
    - knee M17.5
      - bilateral M17.4
    - multiple M15.3
    - shoulder M19.21- ☑
    - specified site NEC M19.29
    - spine — *see* Spondylosis
    - wrist M19.23- ☑
  - shoulder M19.Ø1- ☑
    - post-traumatic M19.11- ☑
    - primary M19.Ø1- ☑
    - secondary M19.21- ☑
  - specified site NEC M19.Ø9
  - spine — *see* Spondylosis
  - wrist M19.Ø3- ☑
    - first carpometacarpal joint — *see* Osteoarthritis, hand joint, first carpometacarpal joint
    - post-traumatic M19.13- ☑
    - primary M19.Ø3- ☑
    - secondary M19.23- ☑
- **Osteoarthropathy** (hypertrophic) M19.9Ø
  - ankle — *see* Osteoarthritis, primary, ankle
  - elbow — *see* Osteoarthritis, primary, elbow
  - foot joint — *see* Osteoarthritis, primary, foot
  - hand joint — *see* Osteoarthritis, primary, hand joint
  - knee joint — *see* Osteoarthritis, primary, knee
  - multiple site — *see* Osteoarthritis, primary, multiple joint
  - pulmonary — *see also* Osteoarthropathy, specified type NEC
    - hypertrophic — *see* Osteoarthropathy, hypertrophic, specified type NEC
  - secondary — *see* Osteoarthropathy, specified type NEC
  - secondary hypertrophic — *see* Osteoarthropathy, specified type NEC
  - shoulder — *see* Osteoarthritis, primary, shoulder
  - specified joint NEC — *see* Osteoarthritis, primary, specified joint NEC
  - specified type NEC M89.4Ø
    - carpus M89.44- ☑
    - clavicle M89.41- ☑
    - femur M89.45- ☑
    - fibula M89.46- ☑
    - finger M89.44- ☑
    - humerus M89.42- ☑
    - ilium M89.48
    - ischium M89.48
    - metacarpus M89.44- ☑
    - metatarsus M89.47- ☑
    - multiple sites M89.49
    - neck M89.48
    - pubic ramus [pubis] M89.48
    - radius M89.43- ☑
    - rib M89.48
    - scapula M89.41- ☑
    - skull M89.48
    - tarsus M89.47- ☑
    - tibia M89.46- ☑
    - toe M89.47- ☑
    - ulna M89.43- ☑
    - vertebra M89.48
  - spine — *see* Spondylosis
  - wrist — *see* Osteoarthritis, primary, wrist
- **Osteoarthrosis** (degenerative) (hypertrophic) (joint) — *see also* Osteoarthritis
  - deformans alkaptonurica E7Ø.29 *[M36.8]*
  - erosive M15.4
  - generalized M15.9
    - primary M15.Ø
  - polyarticular M15.9
  - spine — *see* Spondylosis
- **Osteoblastoma** — *see* Neoplasm, bone, benign
  - aggressive — *see* Neoplasm, bone, uncertain behavior
- **Osteochondritis** — *see also* Osteochondropathy, by site
  - Brailsford's — *see* Osteochondrosis, juvenile, radius
  - dissecans M93.2Ø
    - ankle M93.27- ☑
    - elbow M93.22- ☑
    - foot M93.27- ☑
    - hand M93.24- ☑
    - hip M93.25- ☑
    - knee M93.26- ☑

- **Osteochondritis** — *continued*
  - dissecans — *continued*
    - multiple sites M93.29
    - shoulder joint M93.21- ☑
    - specified site NEC M93.28
    - wrist M93.23- ☑
  - juvenile M92.9
    - patellar — *see* Osteochondrosis, juvenile, patella
  - syphilitic (congenital) (early) A5Ø.Ø2 *[M9Ø.8Ø]*
    - ankle A5Ø.Ø2 *[M9Ø.87-]* ☑
    - elbow A5Ø.Ø2 *[M9Ø.82-]* ☑
    - foot A5Ø.Ø2 *[M9Ø.87-]* ☑
    - forearm A5Ø.Ø2 *[M9Ø.83-]* ☑
    - hand A5Ø.Ø2 *[M9Ø.84-]* ☑
    - hip A5Ø.Ø2 *[M9Ø.85-]* ☑
    - knee A5Ø.Ø2 *[M9Ø.86-]* ☑
    - multiple sites A5Ø.Ø2 *[M9Ø.89]*
    - shoulder joint A5Ø.Ø2 *[M9Ø.81-]* ☑
    - specified site NEC A5Ø.Ø2 *[M9Ø.88]*
- **Osteochondroarthrosis deformans endemica** — *see* Disease, Kaschin-Beck
- **Osteochondrodysplasia** Q78.9
  - with defects of growth of tubular bones and spine Q77.9
    - specified NEC Q77.8
  - specified NEC Q78.8
- **Osteochondrodystrophy** E78.9
- **Osteochondrolysis** — *see* Osteochondritis, dissecans
- **Osteochondroma** — *see* Neoplasm, bone, benign
- **Osteochondromatosis** D16.9
  - syndrome Q78.4
- **Osteochondromyxosarcoma** — *see* Neoplasm, bone, malignant
- **Osteochondropathy** M93.9Ø
  - ankle M93.97- ☑
  - elbow M93.92- ☑
  - foot M93.97- ☑
  - hand M93.94- ☑
  - hip M93.95- ☑
  - Kienbock's disease of adults M93.1
  - knee M93.96- ☑
  - multiple joints M93.99
  - osteochondritis dissecans — *see* Osteochondritis, dissecans
  - osteochondrosis — *see* Osteochondrosis
  - shoulder region M93.91- ☑
  - slipped upper femoral epiphysis — *see* Slipped, epiphysis, upper femoral
  - specified joint NEC M93.98
  - specified type NEC M93.8Ø
    - ankle M93.87- ☑
    - elbow M93.82- ☑
    - foot M93.87- ☑
    - hand M93.84- ☑
    - hip M93.85- ☑
    - knee M93.86- ☑
    - multiple joints M93.89
    - shoulder region M93.81- ☑
    - specified joint NEC M93.88
    - wrist M93.83- ☑
  - syphilitic, congenital
    - early A5Ø.Ø2 *[M9Ø.8Ø]*
    - late A5Ø.56 *[M9Ø.8Ø]*
  - wrist M93.93- ☑
- **Osteochondrosarcoma** — *see* Neoplasm, bone, malignant
- **Osteochondrosis** — *see also* Osteochondropathy, by site
  - acetabulum (juvenile) M91.Ø
  - adult — *see* Osteochondropathy, specified type NEC, by site
  - astragalus (juvenile) — *see* Osteochondrosis, juvenile, tarsus
  - Blount M92.51- ☑
  - Buchanan's M91.Ø
  - Burns' — *see* Osteochondrosis, juvenile, ulna
  - calcaneus (juvenile) — *see* Osteochondrosis, juvenile, tarsus
  - capitular epiphysis (femur) (juvenile) — *see* Legg-Calve-Perthes disease
  - carpal (juvenile) (lunate) (scaphoid) — *see* Osteochondrosis, juvenile, hand, carpal lunate
    - adult M93.1
  - coxae juvenilis — *see* Legg-Calve-Perthes disease
  - deformans juvenilis, coxae — *see* Legg-Calve-Perthes disease
  - Diaz's — *see* Osteochondrosis, juvenile, tarsus
  - dissecans (knee) (shoulder) — *see* Osteochondritis, dissecans

- **Osteonecrosis** — *continued*
  - secondary — *continued*
    - due to — *continued*
      - trauma — *continued*
        - fibula M87.26- ☑
        - finger M87.24- ☑
        - humerus M87.22- ☑
        - ilium M87.25Ø
        - ischium M87.25Ø
        - metacarpus M87.24- ☑
        - metatarsus M87.27- ☑
        - multiple sites M87.29
        - neck M87.28
        - pubic ramus [pubis] M87.25Ø
        - radius M87.23- ☑
        - rib M87.28
        - scapula M87.21- ☑
        - skull M87.28
        - tarsus M87.27- ☑
        - tibia M87.26- ☑
        - toe M87.27- ☑
        - ulna M87.23- ☑
        - vertebra M87.28
    - femur M87.35- ☑
    - fibula M87.36- ☑
    - finger M87.34- ☑
    - humerus M87.32- ☑
    - ilium M87.35Ø
    - in
      - caisson disease T7Ø.3- ☑ *[M9Ø.5Ø]*
        - carpus T7Ø.3- ☑ *[M9Ø.54-]* ☑
        - clavicle T7Ø.3- ☑ *[M9Ø.51-]* ☑
        - femur T7Ø.3- ☑ *[M9Ø.55-]* ☑
        - fibula T7Ø.3- ☑ *[M9Ø.56-]* ☑
        - finger T7Ø.3- ☑ *[M9Ø.54-]* ☑
        - humerus T7Ø.3- ☑ *[M9Ø.52-]* ☑
        - ilium T7Ø.3- ☑ *[M9Ø.58]*
        - ischium T7Ø.3- ☑ *[M9Ø.58]*
        - metacarpus T7Ø.3- ☑ *[M9Ø.54-]* ☑
        - metatarsus T7Ø.3- ☑ *[M9Ø.57-]* ☑
        - multiple sites T7Ø.3- ☑ *[M9Ø.59]*
        - neck T7Ø.3- ☑ *[M9Ø.58]*
        - pubic ramus [pubis] T7Ø.3- ☑ *[M9Ø.58]*
        - radius T7Ø.3- ☑ *[M9Ø.53-]* ☑
        - rib T7Ø.3- ☑ *[M9Ø.58]*
        - scapula T7Ø.3- ☑ *[M9Ø.51-]* ☑
        - skull T7Ø.3- ☑ *[M9Ø.58]*
        - tarsus T7Ø.3- ☑ *[M9Ø.57-]* ☑
        - tibia T7Ø.3- ☑ *[M9Ø.56-]* ☑
        - toe T7Ø.3- ☑ *[M9Ø.57-]* ☑
        - ulna T7Ø.3- ☑ *[M9Ø.53-]* ☑
        - vertebra T7Ø.3- ☑ *[M9Ø.58]*
    - ischium M87.35Ø
    - metacarpus M87.34- ☑
    - metatarsus M87.37- ☑
    - multiple site M87.39
    - neck M87.38
    - pubic ramus [pubis] M87.35Ø
    - radius M87.33- ☑
    - rib M87.38
    - scapula M87.319
    - skull M87.38
    - tarsus M87.379
    - tibia M87.366
    - toe M87.379
    - ulna M87.33- ☑
    - vertebra M87.38
  - specified type NEC M87.8Ø
    - carpus M87.83- ☑
    - clavicle M87.81- ☑
    - femur M87.85- ☑
    - fibula M87.86- ☑
    - finger M87.84- ☑
    - humerus M87.82- ☑
    - ilium M87.85Ø
    - ischium M87.85Ø
    - metacarpus M87.84- ☑
    - metatarsus M87.87- ☑
    - multiple sites M87.89
    - neck M87.88
    - pubic ramus [pubis] M87.85Ø
    - radius M87.83- ☑
    - rib M87.88
    - scapula M87.81- ☑
    - skull M87.88
    - tarsus M87.87- ☑

- **Osteonecrosis** — *continued*
  - specified type — *continued*
    - tibia M87.86- ☑
    - toe M87.87- ☑
    - ulna M87.83- ☑
    - vertebra M87.88
- **Osteopathia condensans disseminata** Q78.8
- **Osteopathy** — *see also* Osteomyelitis, Osteonecrosis, Osteoporosis
  - after poliomyelitis M89.6Ø
    - carpus M89.64- ☑
    - clavicle M89.61- ☑
    - femur M89.65- ☑
    - fibula M89.66- ☑
    - finger M89.64- ☑
    - humerus M89.62- ☑
    - ilium M89.68
    - ischium M89.68
    - metacarpus M89.64- ☑
    - metatarsus M89.67- ☑
    - multiple sites M89.69
    - neck M89.68
    - pubic ramus [pubis] M89.68
    - radius M89.63- ☑
    - rib M89.68
    - scapula M89.61- ☑
    - skull M89.68
    - tarsus M89.67- ☑
    - tibia M89.66- ☑
    - toe M89.67- ☑
    - ulna M89.63- ☑
    - vertebra M89.68
  - in (due to)
    - renal osteodystrophy N25.Ø
    - specified diseases classified elsewhere — *see* subcategory M9Ø.8- ☑
- **Osteopenia** M85.8- ☑
  - borderline M85.8- ☑
- **Osteoperiostitis** — *see* Osteomyelitis, specified type NEC
- **Osteopetrosis** (familial) Q78.2
- **Osteophyte** M25.7Ø
  - ankle M25.77- ☑
  - elbow M25.72- ☑
  - foot joint M25.77- ☑
  - hand joint M25.74- ☑
  - hip M25.75- ☑
  - knee M25.76- ☑
  - shoulder M25.71- ☑
  - spine M25.78
  - vertebrae M25.78
  - wrist M25.73- ☑
- **Osteopoikilosis** Q78.8
- **Osteoporosis** (female) (male) M81.Ø
  - with current pathological fracture M8Ø.ØØ- ☑
  - age-related M81.Ø
    - with current pathologic fracture M8Ø.ØØ- ☑
      - carpus M8Ø.Ø4- ☑
      - clavicle M8Ø.Ø1- ☑
      - femur M8Ø.Ø5- ☑
      - fibula M8Ø.Ø6- ☑
      - finger M8Ø.Ø4- ☑
      - hip M8Ø.Ø5- ☑
      - humerus M8Ø.Ø2- ☑
      - ilium M8Ø.ØB- ☑
      - ischium M8Ø.ØB- ☑
      - metacarpus M8Ø.Ø4- ☑
      - metatarsus M8Ø.Ø7- ☑
      - pelvis M8Ø.ØB- ☑
      - pubic ramus [pubis] M8Ø.ØB- ☑
      - radius M8Ø.Ø3- ☑
      - rib(s) M8Ø.ØA- ☑
      - scapula M8Ø.Ø1- ☑
      - site specified NEC M8Ø.ØA- ☑
      - tarsus M8Ø.Ø7- ☑
      - tibia M8Ø.Ø6- ☑
      - toe M8Ø.Ø7- ☑
      - ulna M8Ø.Ø3- ☑
      - vertebra M8Ø.Ø8- ☑
  - disuse M81.8
    - with current pathological fracture M8Ø.8Ø- ☑
      - carpus M8Ø.84- ☑
      - clavicle M8Ø.81- ☑
      - femur M8Ø.85- ☑
      - fibula M8Ø.86- ☑
      - finger M8Ø.84- ☑
      - hip M8Ø.85- ☑

- **Osteoporosis** — *continued*
  - disuse — *continued*
    - with current pathological fracture — *continued*
      - humerus M8Ø.82- ☑
      - ilium M8Ø.8B- ☑
      - ischium M8Ø.8B- ☑
      - metacarpus M8Ø.84- ☑
      - metatarsus M8Ø.87- ☑
      - pelvis M8Ø.8B- ☑
      - pubic ramus [pubis] M8Ø.8B- ☑
      - radius M8Ø.83- ☑
      - scapula M8Ø.81- ☑
      - site specified NEC M8Ø.8A- ☑
      - tarsus M8Ø.87- ☑
      - tibia M8Ø.86- ☑
      - toe M8Ø.87- ☑
      - ulna M8Ø.83- ☑
      - vertebra M8Ø.88- ☑
  - drug-induced — *see* Osteoporosis, specified type NEC
  - idiopathic — *see* Osteoporosis, specified type NEC
  - involutional — *see* Osteoporosis, age-related
  - Lequesne M81.6
  - localized M81.6
  - postmenopausal M81.Ø
    - with pathological fracture M8Ø.ØØ- ☑
      - carpus M8Ø.Ø4- ☑
      - clavicle M8Ø.Ø1- ☑
      - femur M8Ø.Ø5- ☑
      - fibula M8Ø.Ø6- ☑
      - finger M8Ø.Ø4- ☑
      - hip M8Ø.Ø5- ☑
      - humerus M8Ø.Ø2- ☑
      - ilium M8Ø.ØA- ☑
      - ischium M8Ø.ØA- ☑
      - metacarpus M8Ø.Ø4- ☑
      - metatarsus M8Ø.Ø7- ☑
      - pelvis M8Ø.ØB- ☑
      - pubic ramus [pubis] M8Ø.8B- ☑
      - radius M8Ø.Ø3- ☑
      - scapula M8Ø.Ø1- ☑
      - site specified NEC M8Ø.ØA- ☑
      - tarsus M8Ø.Ø7- ☑
      - tibia M8Ø.Ø6- ☑
      - toe M8Ø.Ø7- ☑
      - ulna M8Ø.Ø3- ☑
      - vertebra M8Ø.Ø8- ☑
  - postoophorectomy — *see* Osteoporosis, specified type NEC
  - postsurgical malabsorption — *see* Osteoporosis, specified type NEC
  - post-traumatic — *see* Osteoporosis, specified type NEC
  - senile — *see* Osteoporosis, age-related
  - specified type NEC M81.8
    - with pathological fracture M8Ø.8Ø- ☑
      - carpus M8Ø.84- ☑
      - clavicle M8Ø.81- ☑
      - femur M8Ø.85- ☑
      - fibula M8Ø.86- ☑
      - finger M8Ø.84- ☑
      - hip M8Ø.85- ☑
      - humerus M8Ø.82- ☑
      - ilium M8Ø.8B- ☑
      - ischium M8Ø.8B- ☑
      - metacarpus M8Ø.84- ☑
      - metatarsus M8Ø.87- ☑
      - pelvis M8Ø.8B- ☑
      - pubic ramus [pubis] M8Ø.8B- ☑
      - radius M8Ø.83- ☑
      - scapula M8Ø.81- ☑
      - site specified NEC M8Ø.8A- ☑
      - tarsus M8Ø.87- ☑
      - tibia M8Ø.86- ☑
      - toe M8Ø.87- ☑
      - ulna M8Ø.83- ☑
      - vertebra M8Ø.88- ☑
- **Osteopsathyrosis** (idiopathica) Q78.Ø
- **Osteoradionecrosis, jaw** (acute) (chronic) (lower) (suppurative) (upper) M27.2
- **Osteosarcoma** (any form) — *see* Neoplasm, bone, malignant
- **Osteosclerosis** Q78.2
  - acquired M85.8- ☑
  - congenita Q77.4
  - fragilitas (generalisata) Q78.2
  - myelofibrosis D75.81
- **Osteosclerotic anemia** D64.89

**Overjet** (excessive horizontal) M26.23
**Overlaid, overlying** (suffocation) — *see* Asphyxia, traumatic, due to mechanical threat
**Overlap, excessive horizontal** (teeth) M26.23
**Overlapping toe** (acquired) — *see also* Deformity, toe, specified NEC
- congenital (fifth toe) Q66.89

**Overload**
- circulatory, due to transfusion (blood) (blood components) (TACO) E87.71
- fluid E87.70
  - due to transfusion (blood) (blood components) E87.71
  - specified NEC E87.79
- iron, due to repeated red blood cell transfusions E83.111
- potassium (K) E87.5
- sodium (Na) E87.0

**Overnutrition** — *see* Hyperalimentation
**Overproduction** — *see also* Hypersecretion
- ACTH E27.0
- catecholamine E27.5
- growth hormone E22.0

**Overprotection, child by parent** Z62.1
**Overriding**
- aorta Q25.49
- finger (acquired) — *see* Deformity, finger
  - congenital Q68.1
- toe (acquired) — *see also* Deformity, toe, specified NEC
  - congenital Q66.89

**Overstrained** R53.83
- heart — *see* Hypertrophy, cardiac

**Overuse, muscle NEC** M70.8- ☑
**Overweight** E66.3
**Overworked** R53.83
**Oviduct** — *see* condition
**Ovotestis** Q56.0
**Ovulation** (cycle)
- failure or lack of N97.0
- pain N94.0

**Ovum** — *see* condition
**Owren's disease or syndrome** (parahemophilia) D68.2
**Ox heart** — *see* Hypertrophy, cardiac
**Oxalosis** E72.53- ☑
**Oxaluria** E72.53- ☑
**Oxycephaly, oxycephalic** Q75.009
- syphilitic, congenital A50.02

**Oxyuriasis** B80
**Oxyuris vermicularis** (infestation) B80
**Ozena** J31.0

# P

**Pachyderma, pachydermia** L85.9
- larynx (verrucosa) J38.7

**Pachydermatocele** (congenital) Q82.8
**Pachydermoperiostosis** — *see also* Osteoarthropathy, hypertrophic, specified type NEC
- clubbed nail M89.40 *[L62]*

**Pachygyria** Q04.3
**Pachymeningitis** (adhesive) (basal) (brain) (cervical) (chronic) (circumscribed) (external) (fibrous) (hemorrhagic) (hypertrophic) (internal) (purulent) (spinal) (suppurative) — *see* Meningitis
**Pachyonychia** (congenital) Q84.5
**Pacinian tumor** — *see* Neoplasm, skin, benign
**Pad, knuckle or Garrod's** M72.1
**Paget-Schroetter syndrome** I82.890
**Paget's disease**
- with infiltrating duct carcinoma — *see* Neoplasm, breast, malignant
- bone M88.9
  - carpus M88.84- ☑
  - clavicle M88.81- ☑
  - femur M88.85- ☑
  - fibula M88.86- ☑
  - finger M88.84- ☑
  - humerus M88.82- ☑
  - ilium M88.88
  - in neoplastic disease — *see* Osteitis, deformans, in neoplastic disease
  - ischium M88.88
  - metacarpus M88.84- ☑
  - metatarsus M88.87- ☑
  - multiple sites M88.89
  - neck M88.88
  - pubic ramus [pubis] M88.88
  - radius M88.83- ☑
  - rib M88.88
  - scapula M88.81- ☑

**Paget's disease** — *continued*
- bone — *continued*
  - skull M88.0
  - specified NEC M88.88
  - tarsus M88.87- ☑
  - tibia M88.86- ☑
  - toe M88.87- ☑
  - ulna M88.83- ☑
  - vertebra M88.1
- breast (female) C50.01- ☑
  - male C50.02- ☑
- extramammary — *see also* Neoplasm, skin, malignant
  - anus C21.0
    - margin C44.590
    - skin C44.590
- intraductal carcinoma — *see* Neoplasm, breast, malignant
- malignant — *see* Neoplasm, skin, malignant
  - breast (female) C50.01- ☑
    - male C50.02- ☑
  - unspecified site (female) C50.01- ☑
    - male C50.02- ☑
- mammary — *see* Paget's disease, breast
- nipple — *see* Paget's disease, breast
- osteitis deformans — *see* Paget's disease, bone

**Pain**(s) — *see also* Painful R52
- abdominal R10.9
  - colic R10.83
  - generalized R10.84
    - with acute abdomen R10.0
  - lower R10.30
    - left quadrant R10.32
    - pelvic or perineal R10.20
      - bilateral R10.23
      - left R10.22
      - right R10.21
    - periumbilical R10.33
    - right quadrant R10.31
  - multiple sites R10.85
  - rebound — *see* Tenderness, abdominal, rebound
  - severe with abdominal rigidity R10.0
  - tenderness — *see* Tenderness, abdominal
  - upper R10.10
    - epigastric R10.13
    - left quadrant R10.12
    - right quadrant R10.11
- acute R52
  - due to trauma G89.11
  - neoplasm related G89.3
  - postprocedural NEC G89.18
  - post-thoracotomy G89.12
  - specified by site — *code to* Pain, by site
- adnexa (uteri) R10.20
- anginoid — *see* Pain, precordial
- anus K62.89
- arm — *see* Pain, limb, upper
- axillary (axilla) M79.62- ☑
- back (postural) M54.9
- bladder R39.89
  - associated with micturition — *see* Micturition, painful
  - chronic R39.82
- bone — *see* Disorder, bone, specified type NEC
- breast N64.4
- broad ligament R10.20
- cancer associated (acute) (chronic) G89.3
- cecum — *see* Pain, abdominal
- cervicobrachial M53.1
- chest (central) R07.9
  - anterior wall R07.89
  - atypical R07.89
  - ischemic I20.9
  - musculoskeletal R07.89
  - non-cardiac R07.89
  - on breathing R07.1
  - pleurodynia R07.81
  - precordial R07.2
  - wall (anterior) R07.89
- chronic G89.29
  - associated with significant psychosocial dysfunction G89.4
  - due to trauma G89.21
  - neoplasm related G89.3
  - postoperative NEC G89.28
  - postprocedural NEC G89.28
  - post-thoracotomy G89.22
  - specified NEC G89.29
- coccyx M53.3
- colon — *see* Pain, abdominal

**Pain(s)** — *continued*
- coronary — *see* Angina
- costochondral R07.1
- diaphragm R07.1
- due to cancer G89.3
- due to device, implant or graft — *see also* Complications, by site and type, specified NEC T85.848- ☑
  - arterial graft NEC T82.848- ☑
  - breast (implant) T85.848- ☑
  - catheter NEC T85.848- ☑
    - dialysis (renal) T82.848- ☑
      - intraperitoneal T85.848- ☑
    - infusion NEC T82.848- ☑
      - spinal (epidural) (subdural) T85.840- ☑
    - urinary (indwelling) T83.84- ☑
  - electronic (electrode) (pulse generator) (stimulator)
    - bone T85.840- ☑
    - cardiac T82.847- ☑
    - nervous system (brain) (peripheral nerve) (spinal) T85.84- ☑
    - urinary T83.84- ☑
  - fixation, internal (orthopedic) NEC T84.84- ☑
  - gastrointestinal (bile duct) (esophagus) T85.848- ☑
  - genital NEC T83.84- ☑
  - heart NEC T82.847- ☑
  - infusion NEC T85.848- ☑
  - joint prosthesis T84.84- ☑
  - ocular (corneal graft) (orbital implant) NEC T85.848- ☑
  - orthopedic NEC T84.84- ☑
  - specified NEC T85.848- ☑
  - urinary NEC T83.84- ☑
  - vascular NEC T82.848- ☑
  - ventricular intracranial shunt T85.840- ☑
- due to malignancy (primary) (secondary) G89.3
- ear — *see* subcategory H92.0- ☑
- epigastric, epigastrium R10.13
- eye — *see* Pain, ocular
- face, facial R51.9
  - atypical G50.1
- female genital organs NEC N94.89
- finger — *see* Pain, limb, upper
- flank R10.A0
  - bilateral R10.A3
  - left R10.A2
  - right R10.A1
- foot — *see* Pain, limb, lower
- gallbladder K82.9
- gas (intestinal) R14.1
- gastric — *see* Pain, abdominal
- generalized NOS R52
- genital organ
  - female N94.89
  - male N50.89
- groin — *see* Pain, abdominal, lower
- hand — *see* Pain, limb, upper
- head — *see* Headache
- heart — *see* Pain, precordial
- infra-orbital — *see* Neuralgia, trigeminal
- intercostal R07.82
- intermenstrual N94.0
- jaw R68.84
- joint M25.50
  - ankle M25.57- ☑
  - elbow M25.52- ☑
  - finger M25.54- ☑
  - foot M25.57- ☑
  - hand M25.54- ☑
  - hip M25.55- ☑
  - knee M25.56- ☑
  - shoulder M25.51- ☑
  - specified site NEC M25.59
  - toe M25.57- ☑
  - wrist M25.53- ☑
- kidney N23
- laryngeal R07.0
- leg — *see* Pain, limb, lower
- limb M79.609
  - lower M79.60- ☑
    - foot M79.67- ☑
    - lower leg M79.66- ☑
    - thigh M79.65- ☑
    - toe M79.67- ☑
  - upper M79.60- ☑
    - axilla M79.62- ☑
    - finger M79.64- ☑
    - forearm M79.63- ☑

**Pain(s)** — *continued*
- limb — *continued*
  - upper — *continued*
    - hand M79.64- ☑
    - upper arm M79.62- ☑
- loin M54.5Ø
- low back M54.5Ø
  - specified NEC M54.59
  - vertebral end plate M54.51
  - vertebrogenic M54.51
- lumbar region M54.5Ø
  - vertebral end plate M54.51
  - vertebrogenic M54.51
- mandibular R68.84
- mastoid — *see* subcategory H92.Ø- ☑
- maxilla R68.84
- menstrual — *see also* Dysmenorrhea N94.6
- metacarpophalangeal (joint) — *see* Pain, joint, hand
- metatarsophalangeal (joint) — *see* Pain, joint, foot
- mouth K13.79
- muscle — *see* Myalgia
- musculoskeletal — *see also* Pain, by site M79.18
- myofascial M79.18
- nasal J34.89
- nasopharynx J39.2
- neck NEC M54.2
- nerve NEC — *see* Neuralgia
- neuromuscular — *see* Neuralgia
- nose J34.89
- ocular H57.1- ☑
- ophthalmic — *see* Pain, ocular
- orbital region — *see* Pain, ocular
- ovary N94.89
- over heart — *see* Pain, precordial
- ovulation N94.Ø
- pelvic (female) R1Ø.2Ø
  - bilateral R1Ø.23
  - left R1Ø.22
  - right R1Ø.21
- penis N48.89
- pericardial — *see* Pain, precordial
- perineal, perineum R1Ø.2Ø
  - bilateral R1Ø.23
  - left R1Ø.22
  - right R1Ø.21
- pharynx J39.2
- pleura, pleural, pleuritic RØ7.81
- postoperative NOS G89.18
- postprocedural NOS G89.18
- post-thoracotomy G89.12
- precordial (region) RØ7.2
- premenstrual N94.3
- psychogenic (persistent) (any site) F45.41
- radicular (spinal) — *see* Radiculopathy
- rectum K62.89
- respiration RØ7.1
- retrosternal RØ7.2
- rheumatoid, muscular — *see* Myalgia
- rib RØ7.89
- root (spinal) — *see* Radiculopathy
- round ligament (stretch) R1Ø.2Ø
- sacroiliac M53.3
- sciatic — *see* Sciatica
- scrotum N5Ø.82
- seminal vesicle N5Ø.89
- shoulder M25.51- ☑
- spermatic cord N5Ø.89
- spinal root — *see* Radiculopathy
- spine M54.9
  - cervical M54.2
  - low back M54.5Ø
    - with sciatica M54.4- ☑
  - thoracic M54.6
- stomach — *see* Pain, abdominal
- substernal RØ7.2
- suprapubic R1Ø.24
- temporomandibular (joint) M26.62- ☑
- testis N5Ø.81- ☑
- thoracic spine M54.6
  - with radicular and visceral pain M54.14
- throat RØ7.Ø
- tibia — *see* Pain, limb, lower
- toe — *see* Pain, limb, lower
- tongue K14.6
- tooth KØ8.89
- trigeminal — *see* Neuralgia, trigeminal
- tumor associated G89.3
- ureter N23

**Pain(s)** — *continued*
- urinary (organ) (system) N23
- uterus NEC N94.89
- vagina R1Ø.2Ø
- vertebral end plate — *see* Pain, vertebrogenic
- vertebrogenic M54.89
  - low back M54.51
  - lumbar M54.51
  - syndrome M54.89
- vesical R39.89
  - associated with micturition — *see* Micturition, painful
- vulva R1Ø.2Ø

**Painful** — *see also* Pain
- coitus
  - female N94.1Ø
  - male N53.12
  - psychogenic F52.6
- ejaculation (semen) N53.12
  - psychogenic F52.6
- erection — *see* Priapism
- feet syndrome E53.8
- joint replacement (hip) (knee) T84.84- ☑
- menstruation — *see* Dysmenorrhea
  - psychogenic F45.8
- micturition — *see* Micturition, painful
- respiration RØ7.1
- scar NEC L9Ø.5
- wire sutures T81.89- ☑

**Painter's colic** — *see* subcategory T56.Ø- ☑

**Palate** — *see* condition

**Palatoplegia** K13.79

**Palatoschisis** — *see* Cleft, palate

**Palilalia** R48.8

**Palliative care** Z51.5

**Pallor** R23.1
- optic disc, temporal — *see* Atrophy, optic

**Palmar** — *see also* condition
- fascia — *see* condition

**Palpable**
- cecum K63.89
- kidney N28.89
- ovary N83.8
- prostate N42.9
- spleen — *see* Splenomegaly

**Palpitations** (heart) RØØ.2
- psychogenic F45.8

**Palsy** — *see also* Paralysis G83.9
- atrophic diffuse (progressive) G12.22
- Bell's — *see also* Palsy, facial
  - newborn P11.3
- brachial plexus NEC G54.Ø
  - newborn (birth injury) P14.3
- brain — *see* Palsy, cerebral
- bulbar (progressive) (chronic) G12.22
  - of childhood (Fazio-Londe) G12.1
  - pseudo NEC G12.29
  - supranuclear (progressive) G23.1
- cerebral (congenital) G8Ø.9
  - ataxic G8Ø.4
  - athetoid G8Ø.3
  - choreathetoid G8Ø.3
  - diplegic G8Ø.8
    - spastic G8Ø.1
  - dyskinetic G8Ø.3
    - athetoid G8Ø.3
    - choreathetoid G8Ø.3
    - distonic G8Ø.3
  - dystonic G8Ø.3
  - hemiplegic G8Ø.8
    - spastic G8Ø.2
  - mixed G8Ø.8
  - monoplegic G8Ø.8
    - spastic G8Ø.1
  - paraplegic G8Ø.8
    - spastic G8Ø.1
  - quadriplegic G8Ø.8
    - spastic G8Ø.Ø
  - spastic G8Ø.1
    - diplegic G8Ø.1
    - hemiplegic G8Ø.2
    - monoplegic G8Ø.1
    - quadriplegic G8Ø.Ø
    - specified NEC G8Ø.1
    - tetraplegic G8Ø.Ø
  - specified NEC G8Ø.8
  - syphilitic A52.12
    - congenital A5Ø.49
  - tetraplegic G8Ø.8
    - spastic G8Ø.Ø

**Palsy** — *continued*
- cranial nerve — *see also* Disorder, nerve, cranial
  - multiple G52.7
    - in
      - infectious disease B99.- ☑ *[G53]*
      - neoplastic disease — *see also* Neoplasm D49.9 *[G53]*
      - parasitic disease B89 *[G53]*
      - sarcoidosis D86.82
- creeping G12.22
- diver's T7Ø.3- ☑
- Erb's P14.Ø
- facial G51.Ø
  - newborn (birth injury) P11.3
- glossopharyngeal G52.1
- Klumpke (-Dejerine) P14.1
- lead — *see* subcategory T56.Ø- ☑
- median nerve (tardy) G56.1- ☑
- nerve G58.9
  - specified NEC G58.8
- peroneal nerve (acute) (tardy) G57.3- ☑
- progressive supranuclear G23.1
- pseudobulbar NEC G12.29
- radial nerve (acute) G56.3- ☑
- seventh nerve — *see also* Palsy, facial
  - newborn P11.3
- shaking — *see* Parkinsonism
- spastic (cerebral) (spinal) G8Ø.1
- ulnar nerve (tardy) G56.2- ☑
- wasting G12.29

**Paludism** — *see* Malaria

**Panangiitis** M3Ø.Ø

**Panaris, panaritium** — *see also* Cellulitis, digit
- with lymphangitis — *see* Lymphangitis, acute, digit

**Panarteritis nodosa** M3Ø.Ø
- brain or cerebral I67.7

**Pancake heart** R93.1
- with cor pulmonale (chronic) I27.81

**Pancarditis** (acute) (chronic) I51.89
- rheumatic IØ9.89
  - active or acute IØ1.8

**Pancoast's syndrome or tumor** C34.1- ☑

**Pancolitis** — *see also* Colitis
- ulcerative (chronic) K51.ØØ
  - with
    - abscess K51.Ø14
    - complication K51.Ø19
    - fistula K51.Ø13
    - obstruction K51.Ø12
    - rectal bleeding K51.Ø11
    - specified complication NEC K51.Ø18

**Pancreas, pancreatic** — *see* condition

**Pancreatitis** (annular) (apoplectic) (calcareous) (edematous) (hemorrhagic) (malignant) (subacute) (suppurative) K85.9Ø
- with necrosis (uninfected) K85.91
  - infected K85.92
- acute (without necrosis or infection) K85.9Ø
  - with necrosis (uninfected) K85.91
    - infected K85.92
  - alcohol induced (without necrosis or infection) K85.2Ø
    - with necrosis (uninfected) K85.21
      - infected K85.22
  - biliary (without necrosis or infection) K85.1Ø
    - with necrosis (uninfected) K85.11
      - infected K85.12
  - drug induced (without necrosis or infection) K85.3Ø
    - with necrosis (uninfected) K85.31
      - infected K85.32
  - gallstone (without necrosis or infection) K85.1Ø
    - with necrosis (uninfected) K85.11
      - infected K85.12
  - idiopathic (without necrosis or infection) K85.ØØ
    - with necrosis (uninfected) K85.Ø1
      - infected K85.Ø2
  - specified NEC (without necrosis or infection) K85.8Ø
    - with necrosis (uninfected) K85.81
      - infected K85.82
- chronic (infectious) K86.1
  - alcohol-induced K86.Ø
  - recurrent K86.1
  - relapsing K86.1
- cystic (chronic) K86.1
- cytomegaloviral B25.2
- fibrous (chronic) K86.1
- gallstone (without necrosis or infection) K85.1Ø
  - with necrosis (uninfected) K85.11
    - infected K85.12

- **Paralysis, paralytic** — *continued*
  - throat — *continued*
    - diphtheritic A36.Ø
    - muscle J39.2
  - thrombotic (current episode) I63.3- ☑
  - thumb G56.9- ☑
  - tick — *see* Toxicity, venom, arthropod, specified NEC
  - Todd's (postepileptic transitory paralysis) G83.84
  - toe G57.6- ☑
  - tongue K14.8
  - transient R29.5
    - arm or leg NEC R29.818
    - traumatic NEC — *see* Injury, nerve
  - trapezius G52.8
  - traumatic, transient NEC — *see* Injury, nerve
  - trembling — *see* Parkinsonism
  - triceps brachii G56.9- ☑
  - trigeminal nerve G5Ø.9
  - trochlear (nerve) — *see* Strabismus, paralytic, fourth nerve
  - ulnar nerve G56.2- ☑
  - upper limb — *see* Monoplegia, upper limb
  - uremic N18.9 *[G99.8]*
  - uveoparotitic D86.89
  - uvula K13.79
    - postdiphtheritic A36.Ø
  - vagus nerve G52.2
  - vasomotor NEC G9Ø.89
  - velum palati K13.79
  - vesical — *see* Paralysis, bladder
  - vestibular nerve (except Vertigo) H93.3- ☑
  - vocal cords J38.ØØ
    - bilateral J38.Ø2
    - unilateral J38.Ø1
  - Volkmann's (complicating trauma) T79.6- ☑
  - wasting G12.29
  - Weber's G46.3
  - wrist G56.9- ☑
- **Paramedial urethrovesical orifice** Q64.79
- **Paramenia** N92.6
- **Parametritis** — *see also* Disease, pelvis, inflammatory N73.2
  - acute N73.Ø
  - complicating abortion — *see* Abortion, by type, complicated by, parametritis
- **Parametrium, parametric** — *see* condition
- **Paramnesia** — *see* Amnesia
- **Paramolar** KØØ.1
- **Paramyloidosis** E85.89
- **Paramyoclonus multiplex** G25.3
- **Paramyotonia** (congenita) G71.19
- **Parangi** — *see* Yaws
- **Paranoia** (querulans) F22
  - senile FØ3.- ☑
- **Paranoid**
  - dementia (senile) FØ3.- ☑
    - praecox — *see* Schizophrenia
  - personality F6Ø.Ø
  - psychosis (climacteric) (involutional) (menopausal) F22
    - psychogenic (acute) F23
    - senile FØ3.- ☑
  - reaction (acute) F23
    - chronic F22
  - schizophrenia F2Ø.Ø
  - state (climacteric) (involutional) (menopausal) (simple) F22
    - senile FØ3.- ☑
  - tendencies F6Ø.Ø
  - traits F6Ø.Ø
  - trends F6Ø.Ø
  - type, psychopathic personality F6Ø.Ø
- **Paraparesis** — *see* Paraplegia
- **Paraphasia** R47.Ø2
- **Paraphilia** F65.9
- **Paraphimosis** (congenital) N47.2
  - chancroidal A57
- **Paraphrenia, paraphrenic** (late) F22
  - schizophrenia F2Ø.Ø
- **Paraplegia** (lower) G82.2Ø
  - ataxic — *see* Degeneration, combined, spinal cord
  - complete G82.21
  - congenital (cerebral) G8Ø.8
    - spastic G8Ø.1
  - familial spastic G11.4
  - functional (hysterical) F44.4
  - hereditary, spastic G11.4
  - hysterical F44.4
  - incomplete G82.22
  - Pott's A18.Ø1
- **Paraplegia** — *continued*
  - psychogenic F44.4
  - spastic
    - Erb's spinal, syphilitic A52.17
    - hereditary G11.4
    - tropical GØ4.1
  - syphilitic (spastic) A52.17
  - traumatic
    - current injury — code to injury with seventh character A
      - sequela of previous injury — code to injury with seventh character S
  - tropical spastic GØ4.1
- **Parapoxvirus** BØ8.6Ø
  - specified NEC BØ8.69
- **Paraproteinemia** D89.2
  - benign (familial) D89.2
  - monoclonal D47.2
  - secondary to malignant disease D47.2
- **Parapsoriasis** L41.9
  - en plaques L41.4
  - guttata L41.1
  - large plaque L41.4
  - retiform, retiformis L41.5
  - small plaque L41.3
  - specified NEC L41.8
  - varioliformis (acuta) L41.Ø
- **Parasitic** — *see also* condition
  - disease NEC B89
  - stomatitis B37.Ø
  - sycosis (beard) (scalp) B35.Ø
  - twin Q89.4
- **Parasitism** B89
  - intestinal B82.9
  - skin B88.9
  - specified — *see* Infestation
- **Parasitophobia** F4Ø.218
- **Parasomnia** G47.5Ø
  - due to
    - alcohol
      - abuse F1Ø.182
      - dependence F1Ø.282
      - use F1Ø.982
    - amphetamines
      - abuse F15.182
      - dependence F15.282
      - use F15.982
    - caffeine
      - abuse F15.182
      - dependence F15.282
      - use F15.982
    - cocaine
      - abuse F14.182
      - dependence F14.282
      - use F14.982
    - drug NEC
      - abuse F19.182
      - dependence F19.282
      - use F19.982
    - opioid
      - abuse F11.182
      - dependence F11.282
      - use F11.982
    - psychoactive substance NEC
      - abuse F19.182
      - dependence F19.282
      - use F19.982
    - sedative, hypnotic, or anxiolytic
      - abuse F13.182
      - dependence F13.282
      - use F13.982
    - stimulant NEC
      - abuse F15.182
      - dependence F15.282
      - use F15.982
  - in conditions classified elsewhere G47.54
  - nonorganic origin F51.8
  - organic G47.5Ø
  - specified NEC G47.59
- **Paraspadias** Q54.9
- **Paraspasmus facialis** G51.8
- **Parasuicide** (attempt)
  - history of (personal) Z91.51
    - in family Z81.8
- **Parathyroid gland** — *see* condition
- **Parathyroid tetany** E2Ø.9
- **Paratrachoma** A74.Ø
- **Paratyphilitis** — *see* Appendicitis
- **Paratyphoid** (fever) — *see* Fever, paratyphoid
- **Paratyphus** — *see* Fever, paratyphoid
- **Paraurethral duct** Q64.79
- **Paraurethritis** — *see also* Urethritis
  - gonococcal (acute) (chronic) (with abscess) A54.1
- **Paravaccinia NEC** BØ8.Ø4
- **Paravaginitis** — *see* Vaginitis
- **Parencephalitis** — *see also* Encephalitis
  - sequelae GØ9
- **Parent-child conflict** — *see* Conflict, parent-child
  - estrangement NEC Z62.89Ø
- **Paresis** — *see also* Paralysis
  - accommodation — *see* Paresis, of accommodation
  - Bernhardt's G57.1- ☑
  - bladder (sphincter) — *see also* Paralysis, bladder
    - tabetic A52.17
  - bowel, colon or intestine K56.Ø
  - extrinsic muscle, eye H49.9
  - general (progressive) (syphilitic) A52.17
    - juvenile A5Ø.45
  - heart — *see* Failure, heart
  - insane (syphilitic) A52.17
  - juvenile (general) A5Ø.45
  - of accommodation H52.52- ☑
  - peripheral progressive (idiopathic) G6Ø.3
  - pseudohypertrophic — *see also* Dystrophy, muscular, by type, if applicable G71.Ø9
  - senile G83.9
  - syphilitic (general) A52.17
    - congenital A5Ø.45
  - vesical NEC N31.2
- **Paresthesia** — *see also* Disturbance, sensation, skin R2Ø.2
  - Bernhardt G57.1- ☑
- **Paretic** — *see* condition
- **Parinaud's**
  - conjunctivitis H1Ø.89
  - oculoglandular syndrome H1Ø.89
  - ophthalmoplegia H49.88- ☑
- **Parkinsonism** (idiopathic) (primary) G2Ø.C
  - with neurogenic orthostatic hypotension (symptomatic) G9Ø.3
  - arteriosclerotic G21.4
  - dementia — *see also* Dementia, in, diseases specified elsewhere G2Ø.C *[FØ2.8Ø]*
    - with behavioral disturbance — *see also* Dementia, in, diseases specified elsewhere G2Ø.C *[FØ2.81-]* ☑
  - due to
    - drugs NEC G21.19
      - neuroleptic G21.11
    - Parkinson's disease — *see* Disease, Parkinson's
  - medication-induced NEC G21.19
  - neuroleptic induced G21.11
  - postencephalitic G21.3
  - secondary G21.9
    - due to
      - arteriosclerosis G21.4
      - drugs NEC G21.19
        - neuroleptic G21.11
      - encephalitis G21.3
      - external agents NEC G21.2
      - syphilis A52.19
    - specified NEC G21.8
  - syphilitic A52.19
  - treatment-induced NEC G21.19
  - vascular G21.4
- **Parkinson's disease** — *see* Disease, Parkinson's
- **Parkinson's syndrome or tremor** — *see* Parkinsonism
- **Parodontitis** — *see* Periodontitis
- **Parodontosis** KØ5.4
- **Paronychia** — *see also* Cellulitis, digit
  - with lymphangitis — *see* Lymphangitis, acute, digit
  - candidal (chronic) B37.2
  - tuberculous (primary) A18.4
- **Parorexia** (psychogenic) F5Ø.89
- **Parosmia** R43.1
  - psychogenic F45.8
- **Parotid gland** — *see* condition
- **Parotitis, parotiditis** (allergic) (nonspecific toxic) (purulent) (septic) (suppurative) — *see also* Sialoadenitis
  - epidemic — *see* Mumps
  - infectious — *see* Mumps
  - postoperative K91.89
  - surgical K91.89
- **Parrot fever** A7Ø
- **Parrot's disease** (early congenital syphilitic pseudoparalysis) A5Ø.Ø2
- **Parry-Romberg syndrome** G51.8
- **Parry's disease or syndrome** EØ5.ØØ
  - with thyroid storm EØ5.Ø1

- **Pars planitis** — *see* Cyclitis
- **Parsonage** (-Aldren)-**Turner syndrome** G54.5
- **Parson's disease** (exophthalmic goiter) EØ5.ØØ
  - with thyroid storm EØ5.Ø1
- **Particolored infant** Q82.8
- **Parturition** — *see* Delivery
- **Parulis** KØ4.7
  - with sinus KØ4.6
- **Parvovirus, as cause of disease classified elsewhere** B97.6
- **Pasini and Pierini's atrophoderma** L9Ø.3
- **Passage**
  - false, urethra N36.5
  - meconium (newborn) during delivery PØ3.82
  - of sounds or bougies — *see* Attention to, artificial, opening
- **Passive** — *see* condition
  - smoking Z77.22
- **Past due on rent or mortgage** Z59.81- ☑
- **Pasteurella septica** A28.Ø
- **Pasteurellosis** — *see* Infection, Pasteurella
- **PAT** (paroxysmal atrial tachycardia) I47.19
- **Patau's syndrome** — *see* Trisomy, 13
- **Patches**
  - mucous (syphilitic) A51.39
    - congenital A5Ø.Ø7
  - smokers' (mouth) K13.24
- **Patellar** — *see* condition
- **Patent** — *see also* Imperfect, closure
  - canal of Nuck Q52.4
  - cervix N88.3
  - ductus arteriosus or Botallo's Q25.Ø
  - foramen
    - botalli Q21.12
    - ovale Q21.12
  - interauricular septum Q21.19
  - interventricular septum Q21.Ø
  - omphalomesenteric duct Q43.Ø
  - os (uteri) — *see* Patent, cervix
  - ostium secundum (type II) Q21.11
  - urachus Q64.4
  - vitelline duct Q43.Ø
- **Paterson** (-Brown) (-Kelly) **syndrome or web** D5Ø.1
- **Pathologic, pathological** — *see also* condition
  - asphyxia RØ9.Ø1
  - fire-setting F63.1
  - gambling F63.Ø
  - ovum OØ2.Ø
  - resorption, tooth KØ3.3
  - stealing F63.2
- **Pathology** (of) — *see* Disease
  - periradicular, associated with previous endodontic treatment NEC M27.59
- **Pattern, sleep-wake, irregular** G47.23
- **Patulous** — *see also* Imperfect, closure (congenital)
  - alimentary tract Q45.8
    - lower Q43.8
    - upper Q4Ø.8
  - eustachian tube H69.Ø- ☑
- **Pause, sinoatrial** I49.5
- **Paxton's disease** B36.2
- **Pearl(s)**
  - enamel KØØ.2
  - Epstein's KØ9.8
- **Pearl-worker's disease** — *see* Osteomyelitis, specified type NEC
- **Pectenosis** K62.4
- **Pectoral** — *see* condition
- **Pectus**
  - carinatum (congenital) Q67.7
    - acquired M95.4
    - rachitic sequelae (late effect) E64.3
  - excavatum (congenital) Q67.6
    - acquired M95.4
    - rachitic sequelae (late effect) E64.3
  - recurvatum (congenital) Q67.6
- **Pedatrophia** E41
- **Pederosis** F65.4
- **Pediatric inflammatory multisystem syndrome** M35.81
- **Pediculosis** (infestation) B85.2
  - capitis (head-louse) (any site) B85.Ø
  - corporis (body-louse) (any site) B85.1
  - eyelid B85.Ø
  - mixed (classifiable to more than one of the titles B85.Ø-B85.3) B85.4
  - pubis (pubic louse) (any site) B85.3
  - vestimenti B85.1
  - vulvae B85.3
- **Pediculus** (infestation) — *see* Pediculosis
- **Pedophilia** F65.4
- **Peg-shaped teeth** KØØ.2
- **Pelade** — *see* Alopecia, areata
- **Pelger-Huet anomaly or syndrome** D72.Ø
- **Peliosis** (rheumatica) D69.Ø
  - hepatis K76.4
    - with toxic liver disease K71.8
- **Pelizaeus-Merzbacher disease** E75.27
- **Pellagra** (alcoholic) E52
  - with
    - polyneuropathy E52 *[G63]*
- **Pellagra-cerebellar-ataxia-renal aminoaciduria syndrome** E72.Ø2
- **Pellegrini** (-Stieda) **disease or syndrome** — *see* Bursitis, tibial collateral
- **Pellizzi's syndrome** E34.8
- **Pel's crisis** A52.11
- **Pelvic** — *see also* condition
  - examination (periodic) (routine) ZØ1.419
    - with abnormal findings ZØ1.411
  - kidney, congenital Q63.2
- **Pelviolithiasis** — *see* Calculus, kidney
- **Pelviperitonitis** — *see also* Peritonitis, pelvic
  - gonococcal A54.24
  - puerperal O85
- **Pelvis** — *see* condition or type
- **Pemphigoid** L12.9
  - benign, mucous membrane L12.1
  - bullous L12.Ø
  - cicatricial L12.1
  - juvenile L12.2
  - ocular L12.1
  - specified NEC L12.8
- **Pemphigus** L1Ø.9
  - benign familial (chronic) Q82.8
  - Brazilian L1Ø.3
  - circinatus L13.Ø
  - conjunctiva L12.1
  - drug-induced L1Ø.5
  - erythematosus L1Ø.4
  - foliaceous L1Ø.2
  - gangrenous — *see* Gangrene
  - neonatorum LØ1.Ø3
  - ocular L12.1
  - paraneoplastic L1Ø.81
  - specified NEC L1Ø.89
  - syphilitic (congenital) A5Ø.Ø6
  - vegetans L1Ø.1
  - vulgaris L1Ø.Ø
  - wildfire L1Ø.3
- **Pendred's syndrome** EØ7.1
- **Pendulous**
  - abdomen, in pregnancy — *see* Pregnancy, complicated by, abnormal, pelvic organs or tissues NEC
  - breast N64.89
- **Penetrating wound** — *see also* Puncture
  - with internal injury — *see* Injury, by site
  - eyeball — *see* Puncture, eyeball
  - orbit (with or without foreign body) — *see* Puncture, orbit
  - uterus by instrument with or following ectopic or molar pregnancy OØ8.6
- **Penicillosis** B48.4
- **Penis** — *see* condition
- **Penitis** N48.29
- **Pentalogy of Fallot** Q21.8
- **Pentasomy X syndrome** Q97.1
- **Pentosuria** (essential) E74.89
- **Percreta placenta** - O43.23- ☑
- **Peregrinating patient** — *see* Disorder, factitious
- **Perforation, perforated** (nontraumatic) (of)
  - accidental during procedure (blood vessel) (nerve) (organ) — *see* Complication, accidental puncture or laceration
  - antrum — *see* Sinusitis, maxillary
  - appendix K35.32
    - with localized peritonitis K35.32
  - atrial septum, multiple Q21.19
  - attic, ear — *see* Perforation, tympanum, attic
  - bile duct (common) (hepatic) K83.2
    - cystic K82.2
  - bladder (urinary)
    - with or following ectopic or molar pregnancy OØ8.6
    - obstetrical trauma O71.5
    - traumatic S37.29- ☑
      - at delivery O71.5
  - bowel K63.1
    - with or following ectopic or molar pregnancy OØ8.6
    - newborn P78.Ø

**Perforation, perforated** — *continued*

  - bowel — *continued*
    - obstetrical trauma O71.5
    - traumatic — *see* Laceration, intestine
  - broad ligament N83.8
    - with or following ectopic or molar pregnancy OØ8.6
    - obstetrical trauma O71.6
  - by
    - device, implant or graft — *see also* Complications, by site and type, mechanical T85.628- ☑
      - arterial graft NEC — *see* Complication, cardiovascular device, mechanical, vascular
      - breast (implant) T85.49- ☑
      - catheter NEC T85.698- ☑
        - cystostomy T83.Ø9Ø- ☑
        - dialysis (renal) T82.49- ☑
          - intraperitoneal T85.691- ☑
        - infusion NEC T82.594- ☑
          - spinal (epidural) (subdural) T85.69Ø- ☑
        - urinary — *see also* Complications, catheter, urinary T83.Ø98- ☑
      - electronic (electrode) (pulse generator) (stimulator)
        - bone T84.39Ø- ☑
        - cardiac T82.199- ☑
          - electrode T82.19Ø- ☑
          - pulse generator T82.191- ☑
          - specified type NEC T82.198- ☑
        - nervous system — *see* Complication, prosthetic device, mechanical, electronic nervous system stimulator
        - urinary — *see* Complication, genitourinary, device, urinary, mechanical
      - fixation, internal (orthopedic) NEC — *see* Complication, fixation device, mechanical
      - gastrointestinal — *see* Complications, prosthetic device, mechanical, gastrointestinal device
      - genital NEC T83.498- ☑
        - intrauterine contraceptive device T83.39- ☑
        - penile prosthesis T83.49Ø- ☑
      - heart NEC — *see* Complication, cardiovascular device, mechanical
      - joint prosthesis — *see* Complications, joint prosthesis, mechanical, specified NEC, by site
      - ocular NEC — *see* Complications, prosthetic device, mechanical, ocular device
      - orthopedic NEC — *see* Complication, orthopedic, device, mechanical
      - specified NEC T85.628- ☑
      - urinary NEC — *see also* Complication, genitourinary, device, urinary, mechanical
        - graft T83.29- ☑
      - vascular NEC — *see* Complication, cardiovascular device, mechanical
      - ventricular intracranial shunt T85.Ø9- ☑
    - foreign body left accidentally in operative wound T81.539- ☑
    - instrument (any) during a procedure, accidental — *see* Puncture, accidental complicating surgery
  - cecum K35.32
    - with localized peritonitis K35.32
  - cervix (uteri) N88.8
    - with or following ectopic or molar pregnancy OØ8.6
    - obstetrical trauma O71.3
  - colon K63.1
    - newborn P78.Ø
    - obstetrical trauma O71.5
    - traumatic — *see* Laceration, intestine, large
  - common duct (bile) K83.2
  - cornea (due to ulceration) — *see* Ulcer, cornea, perforated
  - cystic duct K82.2
  - diverticulum (intestine) K57.8Ø
    - with bleeding K57.81
    - large intestine K57.2Ø
      - with
        - bleeding K57.21
        - small intestine K57.4Ø
          - with bleeding K57.41
    - small intestine K57.ØØ
      - with
        - bleeding K57.Ø1
        - large intestine K57.4Ø
          - with bleeding K57.41
  - ear drum — *see* Perforation, tympanum
  - esophagus K22.3
  - ethmoidal sinus — *see* Sinusitis, ethmoidal
  - frontal sinus — *see* Sinusitis, frontal



Index

Pars planitis — Perforation, perforated

**Perforation, perforated** — *continued*
- gallbladder K82.2
- heart valve — *see* Endocarditis
- ileum K63.1
  - newborn P78.Ø
  - obstetrical trauma O71.5
  - traumatic — *see* Laceration, intestine, small
- instrumental, surgical (accidental) (blood vessel) (nerve) (organ) — *see* Puncture, accidental complicating surgery
- intestine NEC K63.1
  - with ectopic or molar pregnancy OØ8.6
  - newborn P78.Ø
  - obstetrical trauma O71.5
  - traumatic — *see* Laceration, intestine
  - ulcerative NEC K63.1
    - newborn P78.Ø
- jejunum, jejunal K63.1
  - obstetrical trauma O71.5
  - traumatic — *see* Laceration, intestine, small
  - ulcer — *see* Ulcer, gastrojejunal, with perforation
- joint prosthesis — *see* Complications, joint prosthesis, mechanical, specified NEC, by site
- mastoid (antrum) (cell) — *see* Disorder, mastoid, specified NEC
- maxillary sinus — *see* Sinusitis, maxillary
- membrana tympani — *see* Perforation, tympanum
- nasal
  - septum J34.89
    - congenital Q3Ø.3
    - syphilitic A52.73
  - sinus J34.89
    - congenital Q3Ø.8
    - due to sinusitis — *see* Sinusitis
- palate — *see also* Cleft, palate Q35.9
  - syphilitic A52.79
- palatine vault — *see also* Cleft, palate, hard Q35.1
  - syphilitic A52.79
    - congenital A5Ø.59
- pars flaccida (ear drum) — *see* Perforation, tympanum, attic
- pelvic
  - floor S31.Ø3Ø- ☑
    - with
      - ectopic or molar pregnancy OØ8.6
      - penetration into retroperitoneal space S31.Ø31- ☑
      - retained foreign body S31.Ø4Ø- ☑
        - with penetration into retroperitoneal space S31.Ø41- ☑
    - following ectopic or molar pregnancy OØ8.6
    - obstetrical trauma O7Ø.1
  - organ S37.99- ☑
    - adrenal gland S37.818- ☑
    - bladder — *see* Perforation, bladder
    - fallopian tube S37.599- ☑
      - bilateral S37.592- ☑
      - unilateral S37.591- ☑
    - kidney S37.Ø9- ☑
    - obstetrical trauma O71.5
    - ovary S37.499- ☑
      - bilateral S37.492- ☑
      - unilateral S37.491- ☑
    - prostate S37.828- ☑
    - specified organ NEC S37.898- ☑
    - ureter — *see* Perforation, ureter
    - urethra — *see* Perforation, urethra
    - uterus — *see* Perforation, uterus
- perineum — *see* Laceration, perineum
- pharynx J39.2
- rectum K63.1
  - newborn P78.Ø
  - obstetrical trauma O71.5
  - traumatic S36.63- ☑
- root canal space due to endodontic treatment M27.51
- sigmoid K63.1
  - newborn P78.Ø
  - obstetrical trauma O71.5
  - traumatic S36.533- ☑
- sinus (accessory) (chronic) (nasal) J34.89
- sphenoidal sinus — *see* Sinusitis, sphenoidal
- surgical (accidental) (by instrument) (blood vessel) (nerve) (organ) — *see* Puncture, accidental complicating surgery
- traumatic
  - external — *see* Puncture
  - eye — *see* Puncture, eyeball
  - internal organ — *see* Injury, by site

**Perforation, perforated** — *continued*
- tympanum, tympanic (membrane) (persistent post-traumatic) (postinflammatory) H72.9- ☑
  - attic H72.1- ☑
    - multiple — *see* Perforation, tympanum, multiple
    - total — *see* Perforation, tympanum, total
  - central H72.Ø- ☑
    - multiple — *see* Perforation, tympanum, multiple
    - total — *see* Perforation, tympanum, total
  - marginal NEC — *see* subcategory H72.2- ☑
  - multiple H72.81- ☑
  - pars flaccida — *see* Perforation, tympanum, attic
  - total H72.82- ☑
  - traumatic, current episode SØ9.2- ☑
- typhoid, gastrointestinal — *see* Typhoid
- ulcer — *see* Ulcer, by site, with perforation
- ureter N28.89
  - traumatic S37.19- ☑
- urethra N36.8
  - with ectopic or molar pregnancy OØ8.6
  - following ectopic or molar pregnancy OØ8.6
  - obstetrical trauma O71.5
  - traumatic S37.39- ☑
    - at delivery O71.5
- uterus
  - with ectopic or molar pregnancy OØ8.6
  - by intrauterine contraceptive device T83.39- ☑
  - following ectopic or molar pregnancy OØ8.6
  - obstetrical trauma O71.1
  - traumatic S37.69- ☑
    - obstetric O71.1
- uvula K13.79
  - syphilitic A52.79
- vagina O71.4
  - obstetrical trauma O71.4
  - other trauma — *see* Puncture, vagina

**Periadenitis mucosa necrotica recurrens** K12.Ø

**Periappendicitis** (acute) — *see* Appendicitis

**Periarteritis nodosa** (disseminated) (infectious) (necrotizing) M3Ø.Ø

**Periarthritis** (joint) — *see also* Enthesopathy
- Duplay's M75.Ø- ☑
- gonococcal A54.42
- humeroscapularis — *see* Capsulitis, adhesive
- scapulohumeral — *see* Capsulitis, adhesive
- shoulder — *see* Capsulitis, adhesive
- wrist M77.2- ☑

**Periarthrosis** (angioneural) — *see* Enthesopathy

**Pericapsulitis, adhesive** (shoulder) — *see* Capsulitis, adhesive

**Pericarditis** (with decompensation) (with effusion) I31.9
- with rheumatic fever (conditions in IØØ)
  - active — *see* Pericarditis, rheumatic
  - inactive or quiescent IØ9.2
- acute (hemorrhagic) (nonrheumatic) (Sicca) I3Ø.9
  - with chorea (acute) (rheumatic) (Sydenham's) IØ2.Ø
  - benign I3Ø.8
  - nonspecific I3Ø.Ø
  - rheumatic IØ1.Ø
    - with chorea (acute) (Sydenham's) IØ2.Ø
- adhesive or adherent (chronic) (external) (internal) I31.Ø
  - acute — *see* Pericarditis, acute
  - rheumatic IØ9.2
- bacterial (acute) (subacute) (with serous or seropurulent effusion) I3Ø.1
- calcareous I31.1
- cholesterol (chronic) I31.8
  - acute I3Ø.9
- chronic (nonrheumatic) I31.9
  - rheumatic IØ9.2
- constrictive (chronic) I31.1
- coxsackie B33.23
- fibrinocaseous (tuberculous) A18.84
- fibrinopurulent I3Ø.1
- fibrinous I3Ø.8
- fibrous I31.Ø
- gonococcal A54.83
- idiopathic I3Ø.Ø
- in systemic lupus erythematosus M32.12
- infective I3Ø.1
- meningococcal A39.53
- neoplastic (chronic) I31.8
  - acute I3Ø.9
- obliterans, obliterating I31.Ø
- plastic I31.Ø
- pneumococcal I3Ø.1
- postinfarction I24.1
- purulent I3Ø.1

**Pericarditis** — *continued*
- rheumatic (active) (acute) (with effusion) (with pneumonia) IØ1.Ø
  - with chorea (acute) (rheumatic) (Sydenham's) IØ2.Ø
  - chronic or inactive (with chorea) IØ9.2
- rheumatoid — *see* Rheumatoid, carditis
- septic I3Ø.1
- serofibrinous I3Ø.8
- staphylococcal I3Ø.1
- streptococcal I3Ø.1
- suppurative I3Ø.1
- syphilitic A52.Ø6
- tuberculous A18.84
- uremic N18.9 *[I32]*
- viral I3Ø.1

**Pericardium, pericardial** — *see* condition

**Pericellulitis** — *see* Cellulitis

**Pericementitis** (chronic) (suppurative) — *see also* Periodontitis
- acute KØ5.2Ø
  - generalized — *see* Periodontitis, aggressive, generalized
  - localized — *see* Periodontitis, aggressive, localized

**Perichondritis**
- auricle — *see* Perichondritis, ear
- bronchus J98.Ø9
- ear (external) H61.ØØ- ☑
  - acute H61.Ø1- ☑
  - chronic H61.Ø2- ☑
- external auditory canal — *see* Perichondritis, ear
- larynx J38.7
  - syphilitic A52.73
  - typhoid AØ1.Ø9
- nose J34.89
- pinna — *see* Perichondritis, ear
- trachea J39.8

**Periclasia** KØ5.4

**Pericoronitis** — *see* Periodontitis

**Pericystitis** N3Ø.9Ø
- with hematuria N3Ø.91

**Peridiverticulitis** (intestine) K57.92
- cecum — *see* Diverticulitis, intestine, large
- colon — *see* Diverticulitis, intestine, large
- duodenum — *see* Diverticulitis, intestine, small
- intestine — *see* Diverticulitis, intestine
- jejunum — *see* Diverticulitis, intestine, small
- rectosigmoid — *see* Diverticulitis, intestine, large
- rectum — *see* Diverticulitis, intestine, large
- sigmoid — *see* Diverticulitis, intestine, large

**Periendocarditis** — *see* Endocarditis

**Periepididymitis** N45.1

**Perifolliculitis** LØ1.Ø2
- abscedens, caput, scalp L66.3
- capitis, abscedens (et suffodiens) L66.3
- superficial pustular LØ1.Ø2

**Perihepatitis** K65.8

**Perilabyrinthitis** (acute) — *see* subcategory H83.Ø- ☑

**Perimeningitis** — *see* Meningitis

**Perimetritis** — *see* Endometritis

**Perimetrosalpingitis** — *see* Salpingo-oophoritis

**Perineocele** N81.81

**Perinephric, perinephritic** — *see* condition

**Perinephritis** — *see also* Infection, kidney
- purulent — *see* Abscess, kidney

**Perineum, perineal** — *see* condition

**Perineuritis NEC** — *see* Neuralgia

**Periodic** — *see* condition

**Periodontitis** (chronic) (complex) (compound) (local) (simplex) KØ5.3Ø
- acute KØ5.2Ø
  - generalized KØ5.229
    - moderate KØ5.222
    - severe KØ5.223
    - slight KØ5.221
  - localized KØ5.219
    - moderate KØ5.212
    - severe KØ5.213
    - slight KØ5.211
- aggressive KØ5.2Ø
  - generalized KØ5.229
    - moderate KØ5.222
    - severe KØ5.223
    - slight KØ5.221
  - localized KØ5.219
    - moderate KØ5.212
    - severe KØ5.213
    - slight KØ5.211
- apical KØ4.5
  - acute (pulpal origin) KØ4.4

Index

Perforation, perforated — Periodontitis

- **Periodontitis** — *continued*
  - generalized KØ5.329
    - moderate KØ5.322
    - severe KØ5.323
    - slight KØ5.321
  - localized KØ5.319
    - moderate KØ5.312
    - severe KØ5.313
    - slight KØ5.311
- **Periodontoclasia** KØ5.4
- **Periodontosis** (juvenile) KØ5.4
- **Periods** — *see also* Menstruation
  - heavy N92.Ø
  - irregular N92.6
  - shortened intervals (irregular) N92.1
- **Perionychia** — *see also* Cellulitis, digit
  - with lymphangitis — *see* Lymphangitis, acute, digit
- **Perioophoritis** — *see* Salpingo-oophoritis
- **Periorchitis** N45.2
- **Periosteum, periosteal** — *see* condition
- **Periostitis** (albuminosa) (circumscribed) (diffuse) (infective) (monomelic) — *see also* Osteomyelitis
  - alveolar M27.3
  - alveolodental M27.3
  - dental M27.3
  - gonorrheal A54.43
  - jaw (lower) (upper) M27.2
  - orbit HØ5.Ø3- ☑
  - syphilitic A52.77
    - congenital (early) A5Ø.Ø2 *[M9Ø.8Ø]*
    - secondary A51.46
  - tuberculous — *see* Tuberculosis, bone
  - yaws (hypertrophic) (early) (late) A66.6 *[M9Ø.8Ø]*
- **Periostosis** (hyperplastic) — *see also* Disorder, bone, specified type NEC
  - with osteomyelitis — *see* Osteomyelitis, specified type NEC
- **Peripartum**
  - cardiomyopathy O9Ø.3
- **Periphlebitis** — *see* Phlebitis
- **Periproctitis** K62.89
- **Periprostatitis** — *see* Prostatitis
- **Perirectal** — *see* condition
- **Perirenal** — *see* condition
- **Perisalpingitis** — *see* Salpingo-oophoritis
- **Perisplenitis** (infectional) D73.89
- **Peristalsis, visible or reversed** R19.2
- **Peritendinitis** — *see* Enthesopathy
- **Peritoneum, peritoneal** — *see* condition
- **Peritonitis** (adhesive) (bacterial) (fibrinous) (hemorrhagic) (idiopathic) (localized) (perforative) (primary) (with adhesions) (with effusion) K65.9
  - with or following
    - abscess K65.1
    - appendicitis
      - with perforation or rupture K35.32
      - generalized — *see also* Appendicitis K35.2Ø9
      - localized — *see also* Appendicitis K35.3Ø
    - diverticular disease (intestine) K57.8Ø
      - with bleeding K57.81
      - ectopic or molar pregnancy OØ8.Ø
      - large intestine K57.2Ø
        - with
          - bleeding K57.21
          - small intestine K57.4Ø
            - with bleeding K57.41
      - small intestine K57.ØØ
        - with
          - bleeding K57.Ø1
          - large intestine K57.4Ø
            - with bleeding K57.41
  - acute (generalized) K65.Ø
  - aseptic T81.61- ☑
  - bile, biliary K65.3
  - chemical T81.61- ☑
  - chlamydial A74.81
  - chronic proliferative K65.8
  - complicating abortion — *see* Abortion, by type, complicated by, pelvic peritonitis
  - congenital P78.1
  - diaphragmatic K65.Ø
  - diffuse K65.Ø
  - diphtheritic A36.89
  - disseminated K65.Ø
  - due to
    - bile K65.3
    - foreign
      - body or object accidentally left during a procedure (instrument) (sponge) (swab) T81.599- ☑

- **Peritonitis** — *continued*
  - due to — *continued*
    - foreign — *continued*
      - substance accidentally left during a procedure (chemical) (powder) (talc) T81.61- ☑
    - talc T81.61- ☑
    - urine K65.8
  - eosinophilic K65.8
    - acute K65.Ø
  - fibrocaseous (tuberculous) A18.31
  - fibropurulent K65.Ø
  - following ectopic or molar pregnancy OØ8.Ø
  - general (ized) K65.Ø
  - gonococcal A54.85
  - meconium (newborn) P78.Ø
  - neonatal P78.1
    - meconium P78.Ø
  - pancreatic K65.Ø
  - paroxysmal, familial E85.Ø
    - benign E85.Ø
  - pelvic — *see also, if applicable,* Abscess, abdominopelvic)
    - female N73.5
      - acute N73.3
      - chronic N73.4
        - with adhesions N73.6
    - male K65.Ø
  - periodic, familial E85.Ø
  - proliferative, chronic K65.8
  - puerperal, postpartum, childbirth O85
  - purulent K65.Ø
  - septic K65.Ø
  - specified NEC K65.8
  - spontaneous bacterial K65.2
  - subdiaphragmatic K65.Ø
  - subphrenic K65.Ø
  - suppurative K65.Ø
  - syphilitic A52.74
    - congenital (early) A5Ø.Ø8 *[K67]*
  - talc T81.61- ☑
  - tuberculous A18.31
  - urine K65.8
- **Peritonsillar** — *see* condition
- **Peritonsillitis** J36
- **Perityphlitis** — *see also* Cecitis K37
- **Periureteritis** N28.89
- **Periurethral** — *see* condition
- **Periurethritis** (gangrenous) — *see* Urethritis
- **Periuterine** — *see* condition
- **Perivaginitis** — *see* Vaginitis
- **Perivasculitis, retinal** H35.Ø6- ☑
- **Perivasitis** (chronic) N49.1
- **Perivesiculitis** (seminal) — *see* Vesiculitis
- **Perlèche NEC** K13.Ø
  - due to
    - candidiasis B37.83
    - moniliasis B37.83
    - riboflavin deficiency E53.Ø
    - vitamin B2 (riboflavin) deficiency E53.Ø
- **Pernicious** — *see* condition
- **Pernio, perniosis** T69.1- ☑
- **Perpetrator** (of abuse) — *see* Index to External Causes of Injury, Perpetrator
- **Persecution**
  - delusion F22
  - social Z6Ø.5
- **Perseveration** (tonic) R48.8
- **Persistence, persistent** (congenital)
  - anal membrane Q42.3
    - with fistula Q42.2
  - arteria stapedia Q16.3
  - atrioventricular canal Q21.2Ø
  - branchial cleft NOS Q18.2
    - cyst Q18.Ø
    - fistula Q18.Ø
    - sinus Q18.Ø
  - bulbus cordis in left ventricle Q21.8
  - canal of Cloquet Q14.Ø
  - capsule (opaque) Q12.8
  - cilioretinal artery or vein Q14.8
  - cloaca Q43.7
  - communication — *see* Fistula, congenital
  - convolutions
    - aortic arch Q25.46
    - fallopian tube Q5Ø.6
    - oviduct Q5Ø.6
    - uterine tube Q5Ø.6
  - double aortic arch Q25.45
  - ductus arteriosus (Botalli) Q25.Ø

- **Persistence, persistent** — *continued*
  - fetal
    - circulation P29.38
    - form of cervix (uteri) Q51.828
    - hemoglobin, hereditary (HPFH) D56.4
  - foramen
    - Botalli Q21.12
    - ovale Q21.12
  - Gartner's duct Q52.4
  - hemoglobin, fetal (hereditary) (HPFH) D56.4
  - hyaloid
    - artery (generally incomplete) Q14.Ø
    - system Q14.8
  - hymen, in pregnancy or childbirth — *see* Pregnancy, complicated by, abnormal, vulva
  - lanugo Q84.2
  - left
    - posterior cardinal vein Q26.8
    - root with right arch of aorta Q25.49
    - superior vena cava Q26.1
  - Meckel's diverticulum Q43.Ø
    - malignant — *see* Table of Neoplasms, small intestine malignant
  - mucosal disease (middle ear) — *see* Otitis, media, suppurative, chronic, tubotympanic
  - nail(s), anomalous Q84.6
  - omphalomesenteric duct Q43.Ø
  - organ or site not listed — *see* Anomaly, by site
  - ostium
    - atrioventriculare commune Q21.23
    - primum Q21.2Ø
    - secundum Q21.11
  - ovarian rests in fallopian tube Q5Ø.6
  - pancreatic tissue in intestinal tract Q43.8
  - primary (deciduous)
    - teeth KØØ.6
    - vitreous hyperplasia Q14.Ø
  - pupillary membrane Q13.89
  - rhesus (Rh) titer — *see* Complication(s), transfusion, incompatibility reaction, Rh (factor)
  - right aortic arch Q25.47
  - sinus
    - urogenitalis
      - female Q52.8
      - male Q55.8
    - venosus with imperfect incorporation in right auricle Q26.8
  - thymus (gland) (hyperplasia) E32.Ø
  - thyroglossal duct Q89.2
  - thyrolingual duct Q89.2
  - truncus arteriosus or communis Q2Ø.Ø
  - tunica vasculosa lentis Q12.2
  - umbilical sinus Q64.4
  - urachus Q64.4
  - vitelline duct Q43.Ø
- **Person** (with)
  - admitted for clinical research, as a control subject (normal comparison) (participant) ZØØ.6
  - awaiting admission to adequate facility elsewhere Z75.1
  - concern (normal) about sick person in family Z63.6
  - consulting on behalf of another Z71.Ø
  - feigning illness Z76.5
  - living (in)
    - alone Z6Ø.2
    - boarding school Z59.3
    - residential institution Z59.3
    - without
      - adequate housing Z59.1Ø
        - air conditioning Z59.11
        - environmental temperature Z59.11
        - heating Z59.11
        - space Z59.19
      - housing (permanent) (temporary) Z59.ØØ
      - person able to render necessary care Z74.2
      - shelter Z59.Ø2
  - on waiting list Z75.1
  - sick or handicapped in family Z63.6
- **Personality** (disorder) F6Ø.9
  - accentuation of traits (type A pattern) Z73.1
  - affective F34.Ø
  - aggressive F6Ø.3
  - amoral F6Ø.2
  - anacastic, anankastic F6Ø.5
  - antisocial F6Ø.2
  - anxious F6Ø.6
  - asocial F6Ø.2
  - asthenic F6Ø.7
  - avoidant F6Ø.6
  - borderline F6Ø.3

**ersonality** — *continued*
- change due to organic condition (enduring) F07.Ø
- compulsive F6Ø.5
- cycloid F34.Ø
- cyclothymic F34.Ø
- dependent F6Ø.7
- depressive F34.1
- dissocial F6Ø.2
- dual F44.81
- eccentric F6Ø.89
- emotionally unstable F6Ø.3
- expansive paranoid F6Ø.Ø
- explosive F6Ø.3
- fanatic F6Ø.Ø
- haltlose type F6Ø.89
- histrionic F6Ø.4
- hyperthymic F34.Ø
- hypothymic F34.1
- hysterical F6Ø.4
- immature F6Ø.89
- inadequate F6Ø.7
- labile (emotional) F6Ø.3
- mixed (nonspecific) F6Ø.89
- morally defective F6Ø.2
- multiple F44.81
- narcissistic F6Ø.81
- obsessional F6Ø.5
- obsessive (-compulsive) F6Ø.5
- organic FØ7.Ø
- overconscientious F6Ø.5
- paranoid F6Ø.Ø
- passive (-dependent) F6Ø.7
- passive-aggressive F6Ø.89
- pathologic F6Ø.9
- pattern defect or disturbance F6Ø.9
- pseudopsychopathic (organic) FØ7.Ø
- pseudoretarded (organic) FØ7.Ø
- psychoinfantile F6Ø.4
- psychoneurotic NEC F6Ø.89
- psychopathic F6Ø.2
- querulant F6Ø.Ø
- sadistic F6Ø.89
- schizoid F6Ø.1
- self-defeating F6Ø.89
- sensitive paranoid F6Ø.Ø
- sociopathic (amoral) (antisocial) (asocial) (dissocial) F6Ø.2
- specified NEC F6Ø.89
- type A Z73.1
- unstable (emotional) F6Ø.3

**erthes' disease** — *see* Legg-Calve-Perthes disease

**ertussis** — *see also* Whooping cough A37.9Ø

**erversion, perverted**
- appetite F5Ø.89
  - psychogenic F5Ø.89
- function
  - pituitary gland E23.2
    - posterior lobe E22.2
- sense of smell and taste R43.8
  - psychogenic F45.8
- sexual — *see* Deviation, sexual

**ervious, congenital** — *see also* Imperfect, closure
- ductus arteriosus Q25.Ø

**es** (congenital) — *see also* Talipes
- acquired — *see also* Deformity, limb, foot, specified NEC
  - planus — *see* Deformity, limb, flat foot
- adductus Q66.89
- cavus Q66.7- ☑
- deformity NEC, acquired — *see* Deformity, limb, foot, specified NEC
- planus (acquired) (any degree) — *see also* Deformity, limb, flat foot
  - rachitic sequelae (late effect) E64.3
- valgus Q66.6

**est, pestis** — *see* Plague

**etechia, petechiae** R23.3
- newborn P54.5

**etechial typhus** A75.9

**eter's anomaly** Q13.4

**etit mal seizure** — *see* Epilepsy, childhood, absence

**etit's hernia** — *see* Hernia, abdomen, specified site NEC

**etrellidosis** B48.2

**etrositis** H7Ø.2Ø- ☑
- acute H7Ø.21- ☑
- chronic H7Ø.22- ☑

**eutz-Jeghers disease or syndrome** Q85.89

**eyronie's disease** N48.6

**FAPA** (periodic fever, aphthous stomatitis, pharyngitis, and adenopathy syndrome) MØ4.8

**feiffer's disease** — *see* Mononucleosis, infectious

**Phagedena** (dry) (moist) (sloughing) — *see also* Gangrene
- geometric L88
- penis N48.29
- tropical — *see* Ulcer, skin
- vulva N76.6

**Phagedenic** — *see* condition

**Phakoma** H35.89

**Phakomatosis** — *see also* specific eponymous syndromes Q85.9
- Bourneville's Q85.1
- specified NEC Q85.89

**Phantom limb syndrome** (without pain) G54.7
- with pain G54.6

**Pharyngeal pouch syndrome** D82.1

**Pharyngitis** (acute) (catarrhal) (gangrenous) (infective) (malignant) (membranous) (phlegmonous) (pseudomembranous) (simple) (subacute) (suppurative) (ulcerative) JØ2.9
- with influenza, flu, or grippe — *see* Influenza, with, pharyngitis
- aphthous BØ8.5
- atrophic J31.2
- chlamydial A56.4
- chronic (atrophic) (granular) (hypertrophic) J31.2
- coxsackievirus BØ8.5
- diphtheritic A36.Ø
- enteroviral vesicular BØ8.5
- follicular (chronic) J31.2
- fusospirochetal A69.1
- gonococcal A54.5
- granular (chronic) J31.2
- herpesviral BØØ.2
- hypertrophic J31.2
- infectional, chronic J31.2
- influenzal — *see* Influenza, with, respiratory manifestations NEC
- lymphonodular, acute (enteroviral) BØ8.8
- pneumococcal JØ2.8
- purulent JØ2.9
- putrid JØ2.9
- septic JØ2.Ø
- sicca J31.2
- specified organism NEC JØ2.8
- staphylococcal JØ2.8
- streptococcal JØ2.Ø
- syphilitic, congenital (early) A5Ø.Ø3
- tuberculous A15.8
- vesicular, enteroviral BØ8.5
- viral NEC JØ2.8

**Pharyngoconjunctivitis, viral** B3Ø.2

**Pharyngolaryngitis** (acute) JØ6.Ø
- chronic J37.Ø

**Pharyngoplegia** J39.2

**Pharyngotonsillitis, herpesviral** BØØ.2

**Pharyngotracheitis, chronic** J42

**Pharynx, pharyngeal** — *see* condition

**Phelan-McDermid syndrome** Q93.52

**Phencyclidine-induced**
- anxiety disorder F16.98Ø
- bipolar and related disorder F16.94
- depressive disorder F16.94
- psychotic disorder F16.959

**Phenomenon**
- Arthus' — *see* Arthus' phenomenon
- jaw-winking QØ7.8
- lupus erythematosus (LE) cell M32.9
- Raynaud's (secondary) I73.ØØ
  - with gangrene I73.Ø1
- vasomotor R55
- vasospastic I73.9
- vasovagal R55
- Wenckebach's I44.1

**Phenotype**
- Duffy
  - a positive Z67.A2
  - a and b positive Z67.A4
  - b positive Z67.A3
  - Fy (a+b-) Z67.A2
  - Fy (a-b-) Z67.A1
  - Fy (a-b+) Z67.A3
  - Fy (a+b+) Z67.A4
  - null Z67.A1

**Phenylketonuria** E7Ø.1
- classical E7Ø.Ø
- maternal E7Ø.1

**Pheochromoblastoma**
- specified site — *see* Neoplasm, malignant, by site
- unspecified site C74.1Ø

**Pheochromocytoma**
- malignant
  - specified site — *see* Neoplasm, malignant, by site
  - unspecified site C74.1Ø
- specified site — *see* Neoplasm, benign, by site
- unspecified site D35.ØØ

**Pheohyphomycosis** — *see* Chromomycosis

**Pheomycosis** — *see* Chromomycosis

**Phimosis** (congenital) (due to infection) N47.1
- chancroidal A57

**Phlebectasia** — *see also* Varix
- congenital Q27.4

**Phlebitis** (infective) (pyemic) (septic) (suppurative) I8Ø.9
- antepartum — *see* Thrombophlebitis, antepartum
- blue — *see* Phlebitis, leg, deep
- breast, superficial I8Ø.8
- calf muscular vein (NOS) I8Ø.25- ☑
- cavernous (venous) sinus — *see* Phlebitis, intracranial (venous) sinus
- cerebral (venous) sinus — *see* Phlebitis, intracranial (venous) sinus
- chest wall, superficial I8Ø.8
- cranial (venous) sinus — *see* Phlebitis, intracranial (venous) sinus
- deep (vessels) — *see* Phlebitis, leg, deep
- due to implanted device — *see* Complications, by site and type, specified NEC
- during or resulting from a procedure T81.72- ☑
- femoral vein (superficial) I8Ø.1- ☑
- femoropopliteal vein I8Ø.Ø- ☑
- gastrocnemial vein I8Ø.25- ☑
- gestational — *see* Phlebopathy, gestational
- hepatic veins I8Ø.8
- iliac vein (common) (external) (internal) I8Ø.21- ☑
- iliofemoral — *see* Phlebitis, femoral vein
- intracranial (venous) sinus (any) GØ8
  - nonpyogenic I67.6
- intraspinal venous sinuses and veins GØ8
  - nonpyogenic G95.19
- lateral (venous) sinus — *see* Phlebitis, intracranial (venous) sinus
- leg I8Ø.3
  - antepartum — *see* Thrombophlebitis, antepartum
  - deep (vessels) NEC I8Ø.2Ø- ☑
    - iliac I8Ø.21- ☑
    - popliteal vein I8Ø.22- ☑
    - specified vessel NEC I8Ø.29- ☑
    - tibial vein (anterior) (posterior) I8Ø.23- ☑
  - femoral vein (superficial) I8Ø.1- ☑
  - superficial (vessels) I8Ø.Ø- ☑
- longitudinal sinus — *see* Phlebitis, intracranial (venous) sinus
- lower limb — *see* Phlebitis, leg
- migrans, migrating (superficial) I82.1
- pelvic
  - with ectopic or molar pregnancy OØ8.Ø
  - following ectopic or molar pregnancy OØ8.Ø
  - puerperal, postpartum O87.1
- peroneal vein I8Ø.24- ☑
- popliteal vein — *see* Phlebitis, leg, deep, popliteal
- portal (vein) K75.1
- postoperative T81.72- ☑
- pregnancy — *see* Thrombophlebitis, antepartum
- puerperal, postpartum, childbirth O87.Ø
  - deep O87.1
  - pelvic O87.1
  - superficial O87.Ø
- retina — *see* Vasculitis, retina
- saphenous (accessory) (great) (long) (small) — *see* Phlebitis, leg, superficial
- sinus (meninges) — *see* Phlebitis, intracranial (venous) sinus
- soleal vein I8Ø.25- ☑
- specified site NEC I8Ø.8
- syphilitic A52.Ø9
- tibial vein — *see* Phlebitis, leg, deep, tibial
- ulcerative I8Ø.9
  - leg — *see* Phlebitis, leg
- umbilicus I8Ø.8
- uterus (septic) — *see* Endometritis
- varicose (leg) (lower limb) — *see* Varix, leg, with, inflammation

**Phlebofibrosis** I87.8

**Phleboliths** I87.8

**Phlebopathy,**
- gestational O22.9- ☑
- puerperal O87.9

**Phlebosclerosis** I87.8

Index

**Phlebothrombosis** — *see also* Thrombosis
antepartum — *see* Thrombophlebitis, antepartum
pregnancy — *see* Thrombophlebitis, antepartum
puerperal — *see* Thrombophlebitis, puerperal
**Phlebotomus fever** A93.1
**Phlegmasia**
alba dolens O87.1
nonpuerperal — *see* Phlebitis, femoral vein
cerulea dolens — *see* Phlebitis, leg, deep
**Phlegmon** — *see* Abscess
**Phlegmonous** — *see* condition
**Phlyctenulosis** (allergic) (keratoconjunctivitis) (nontuberculous) — *see also* Keratoconjunctivitis
cornea — *see* Keratoconjunctivitis
tuberculous A18.52
**Phobia, phobic** F4Ø.9
animal F4Ø.218
spiders F4Ø.21Ø
examination F4Ø.298
reaction F4Ø.9
simple F4Ø.298
social F4Ø.1Ø
generalized F4Ø.11
specific (isolated) F4Ø.298
animal F4Ø.218
spiders F4Ø.21Ø
blood F4Ø.23Ø
injection F4Ø.231
injury F4Ø.233
men F4Ø.29Ø
natural environment F4Ø.228
thunderstorms F4Ø.22Ø
situational F4Ø.248
bridges F4Ø.242
closed in spaces F4Ø.24Ø
flying F4Ø.243
heights F4Ø.241
specified focus NEC F4Ø.298
transfusion F4Ø.231
women F4Ø.291
specified NEC F4Ø.8
medical care NEC F4Ø.232
state F4Ø.9
**Phocas' disease** — *see* Mastopathy, cystic
**Phocomelia** Q73.1
lower limb — *see* Agenesis, leg, with foot present
upper limb — *see* Agenesis, arm, with hand present
**Phoria** H5Ø.5Ø
**Phosphate-losing tubular disorder** N25.Ø
**Phosphatemia** E83.39
**Phosphaturia** E83.39
**Photodermatitis** (sun) L56.8
chronic L57.8
due to drug L56.8
light other than sun L59.8
**Photokeratitis** H16.13- ☑
**Photophobia** H53.14- ☑
**Photophthalmia** — *see* Photokeratitis
**Photopsia** H53.19
**Photoretinitis** — *see* Retinopathy, solar
**Photosensitivity, photosensitization** (sun) skin L56.8
light other than sun L59.8
**Phrenitis** — *see* Encephalitis
**Phrynoderma** (vitamin A deficiency) E5Ø.8
**Phthiriasis** (pubis) B85.3
with any infestation classifiable to B85.Ø-B85.2 B85.4
**Phthirus infestation** — *see* Phthiriasis
**Phthisis** — *see also* Tuberculosis
bulbi (infectional) — *see* Disorder, globe, degenerated condition, atrophy
eyeball (due to infection) — *see* Disorder, globe, degenerated condition, atrophy
**PHTS** Q85.81
**Phycomycosis** — *see* Zygomycosis
**Physalopteriasis** B81.8
**Physical restraint status** Z78.1
**Phytobezoar** T18.9- ☑
intestine T18.3- ☑
stomach T18.2- ☑
**Pian** — *see* Yaws
**Pianoma** A66.1
**Pica** F5Ø.89
in adults (in remission) F5Ø.83
infant or child (in remission) F98.3
**Pick-Niemann disease** — *see* Niemann-Pick disease or syndrome
**Picking, nose** F98.8
**Pick's**
cerebral atrophy — *see also* Dementia, in, diseases specified elsewhere G31.Ø1 *[FØ2.8Ø]*
with behavioral disturbance — *see also* Dementia, in, diseases specified elsewhere G31.Ø1 *[FØ2.81-]* ☑
disease or syndrome (brain) — *see also* Dementia, in, diseases specified elsewhere G31.Ø1 *[FØ2.8Ø]*
with behavioral disturbance — *see also* Dementia, in, diseases specified elsewhere G31.Ø1 *[FØ2.81-]* ☑
brain — *see also* Dementia, in, diseases specified elsewhere G31.Ø1 *[FØ2.8Ø]*
with behavioral disturbance — *see also* Dementia, in, diseases specified elsewhere G31.Ø1 *[FØ2.81-]* ☑
pericardium (pericardial pseudocirrhosis of liver) I31.1
syndrome
brain — *see also* Dementia, in, diseases specified elsewhere G31.Ø1 *[FØ2.8Ø]*
with behavioral disturbance — *see also* Dementia, in, diseases specified elsewhere G31.Ø1 *[FØ2.81-]* ☑
of heart (pericardial pseudocirrhosis of liver) I31.1
**Pickwickian syndrome** E66.2
**Piebaldism** E7Ø.39
**Piedra** (beard) (scalp) B36.8
black B36.3
white B36.2
**Pierre Robin deformity or syndrome** Q87.Ø
**Pierson's disease or osteochondrosis** M91.Ø
**Pig-bel** AØ5.2
**Pigeon**
breast or chest (acquired) M95.4
congenital Q67.7
rachitic sequelae (late effect) E64.3
breeder's disease or lung J67.2
fancier's disease or lung J67.2
toe — *see* Deformity, toe, specified NEC
**Pigmentation** (abnormal) (anomaly) L81.9
conjunctiva H11.13- ☑
cornea (anterior) H18.Ø1- ☑
posterior H18.Ø5- ☑
stromal H18.Ø6- ☑
diminished melanin formation NEC L81.6
iron L81.8
lids, congenital Q82.8
limbus corneae — *see* Pigmentation, cornea
metals L81.8
optic papilla, congenital Q14.2
retina, congenital (grouped) (nevoid) Q14.1
scrotum, congenital Q82.8
tattoo L81.8
**Piles** — *see also* Hemorrhoids K64.9
**Pili**
annulati or torti (congenital) Q84.1
incarnati L73.1
**Pilomatrixoma** — *see* Neoplasm, skin, benign
malignant — *see* Neoplasm, skin, malignant
**Pilonidal** — *see* condition
**Pimple** R23.8
**PIMS** M35.81
**PIN** — *see* Neoplasia, intraepithelial, prostate
**Pinched nerve** — *see* Neuropathy, entrapment
**Pindborg tumor** — *see* Cyst, calcifying odontogenic
**Pineal body or gland** — *see* condition
**Pinealoblastoma** C75.3
**Pinealoma** D44.5
malignant C75.3
**Pineoblastoma** C75.3
**Pineocytoma** D44.5
**Pinguecula** H11.15- ☑
**Pingueculitis** H1Ø.81- ☑
**Pinhole meatus** — *see also* Stricture, urethra N35.919
**Pink**
disease — *see* subcategory T56.1- ☑
eye — *see* Conjunctivitis, acute, mucopurulent
**Pinkus' disease** (lichen nitidus) L44.1
**Pinpoint**
meatus — *see* Stricture, urethra
os (uteri) — *see* Stricture, cervix
**Pins and needles** R2Ø.2
**Pinta** A67.9
cardiovascular lesions A67.2
chancre (primary) A67.Ø
erythematous plaques A67.1
hyperchromic lesions A67.1
hyperkeratosis A67.1
**Pinta** — *continued*
lesions A67.9
cardiovascular A67.2
hyperchromic A67.1
intermediate A67.1
late A67.2
mixed A67.3
primary A67.Ø
skin (achromic) (cicatricial) (dyschromic) A67.2
hyperchromic A67.1
mixed (achromic and hyperchromic) A67.3
papule (primary) A67.Ø
skin lesions (achromic) (cicatricial) (dyschromic) A67.2
hyperchromic A67.1
mixed (achromic and hyperchromic) A67.3
vitiligo A67.2
**Pintids** A67.1
**Pinworm** (disease) (infection) (infestation) B8Ø
**Piroplasmosis** — *see also* Babesiosis B6Ø.ØØ
specified NEC B6Ø.Ø9
**Pistol wound** — *see* Gunshot wound
**Pitchers' elbow** — *see* Derangement, joint, specified typ
NEC, elbow
**Pithecoid pelvis** Q74.2
with disproportion (fetopelvic) O33.Ø
causing obstructed labor O65.Ø
**Pithiatism** F48.8
**Pitted** — *see* Pitting
**Pitting** — *see also* Edema R6Ø.9
lip R6Ø.Ø
nail L6Ø.8
teeth KØØ.4
**Pituitary gland** — *see* condition
**Pituitary-snuff-taker's disease** J67.8
**Pityriasis** (capitis) L21.Ø
alba L3Ø.5
circinata (et maculata) L42
furfuracea L21.Ø
Hebra's L26
lichenoides L41.Ø
chronica L41.1
et varioliformis (acuta) L41.Ø
maculata (et circinata) L3Ø.5
nigra B36.1
pilaris, Hebra's L44.Ø
rosea L42
rotunda L44.8
rubra (Hebra) pilaris L44.Ø
simplex L3Ø.5
specified type NEC L3Ø.5
streptogenes L3Ø.5
versicolor (scrotal) B36.Ø
**Placenta, placental** — *see* Pregnancy, complicated by (car
of) (management affected by), specified condition
**Placentitis** O41.14- ☑
**Plagiocephaly** Q67.3
non-deformational
anterior Q75.Ø21
posterior Q75.Ø4- ☑
**Plague** A2Ø.9
abortive A2Ø.8
ambulatory A2Ø.8
asymptomatic A2Ø.8
bubonic A2Ø.Ø
cellulocutaneous A2Ø.1
cutaneobubonic A2Ø.1
lymphatic gland A2Ø.Ø
meningitis A2Ø.3
pharyngeal A2Ø.8
pneumonic (primary) (secondary) A2Ø.2
pulmonary, pulmonic A2Ø.2
septicemic A2Ø.7
tonsillar A2Ø.8
septicemic A2Ø.7
**Planning, family**
contraception Z3Ø.9
procreation Z31.69
**Plaque(s)**
artery, arterial — *see* Arteriosclerosis
calcareous — *see* Calcification
coronary, lipid rich I25.83
epicardial I31.8
erythematous, of pinta A67.1
Hollenhorst's — *see* Occlusion, artery, retina
lipid rich, coronary I25.83
pleural (without asbestos) J92.9
with asbestos J92.Ø
tongue K13.29
**Plasmacytoma** C9Ø.3- ☑

Phlebothrombosis — Plasmacytoma

- **Plasmacytoma** — *continued*
  - extramedullary C90.2- ☑
  - medullary C90.0- ☑
  - solitary C90.3- ☑
- **Plasmacytopenia** D72.818
- **Plasmacytosis** D72.822
- **Plaster ulcer** — *see* Ulcer, pressure, by site
- **Plateau iris syndrome** (post-iridectomy) (postprocedural) (without glaucoma) H21.82
  - with glaucoma H40.22- ☑
- **Platybasia** Q75.8
- **Platyonychia** (congenital) Q84.6
  - acquired L60.8
- **Platypelloid pelvis** M95.5
  - with disproportion (fetopelvic) O33.0
    - causing obstructed labor O65.0
  - congenital Q74.2
- **Platyspondylisis** Q76.49
- **Plaut** (-Vincent) **disease** — *see also* Vincent's A69.1
- **Plethora** R23.2
  - newborn P61.1
- **Pleura, pleural** — *see* condition
- **Pleuralgia** R07.81
- **Pleurisy** (acute) (adhesive) (chronic) (costal) (diaphragmatic) (double) (dry) (fibrinous) (fibrous) (interlobar) (latent) (plastic) (primary) (residual) (sicca) (sterile) (subacute) (unresolved) R09.1
  - with
    - adherent pleura J86.0
    - effusion J90
      - chylous, chyliform J94.0
      - tuberculous (non primary) A15.6
        - primary (progressive) A15.7
    - tuberculosis — *see* Pleurisy, tuberculous (non primary)
  - encysted — *see* Pleurisy, with effusion
  - exudative — *see* Pleurisy, with effusion
  - fibrinopurulent, fibropurulent — *see* Pyothorax
  - hemorrhagic — *see* Hemothorax
  - pneumococcal J90
  - purulent — *see* Pyothorax
  - septic — *see* Pyothorax
  - serofibrinous — *see* Pleurisy, with effusion
  - seropurulent — *see* Pyothorax
  - serous — *see* Pleurisy, with effusion
  - staphylococcal J86.9
  - streptococcal J90
  - suppurative — *see* Pyothorax
  - traumatic (post) (current) — *see* Injury, intrathoracic, pleura
  - tuberculous (with effusion) (non primary) A15.6
    - primary (progressive) A15.7
- **Pleuritis sicca** — *see* Pleurisy
- **Pleuro-pneumonia-like-organism** (PPLO), as cause of disease classified elsewhere B96.0
- **Pleurobronchopneumonia** — *see* Pneumonia, broncho-
- **Pleurodynia** R07.81
  - epidemic B33.0
  - viral B33.0
- **Pleuropericarditis** — *see also* Pericarditis
  - acute I30.9
- **Pleuropneumonia** (acute) (bilateral) (double) (septic) — *see also* Pneumonia J18.8
  - chronic — *see* Fibrosis, lung
- **Pleurorrhea** — *see* Pleurisy, with effusion
- **Plexitis, brachial** G54.0
- **Plica**
  - polonica B85.0
  - syndrome, knee M67.5- ☑
  - tonsil J35.8
- **Plicated tongue** K14.5
- **Plug**
  - bronchus NEC J98.09
  - meconium (newborn) NEC syndrome P76.0
  - mucus — *see* Asphyxia, mucus
- **Plumbism** — *see* subcategory T56.0- ☑
- **Plummer-Vinson syndrome** D50.1
- **Plummer's disease** E05.20
  - with thyroid storm E05.21
- **Pluricarential syndrome of infancy** E40
- **Plus** (and minus) **hand** (intrinsic) — *see* Deformity, limb, specified type NEC, forearm
- **PMEI** (polymorphic epilepsy in infancy) G40.83- ☑
- **Pneumathemia** — *see* Air, embolism
- **Pneumatic hammer** (drill) syndrome T75.21- ☑
- **Pneumatocele** (lung) J98.4
  - intracranial G93.89
  - tension J98.8
- **Pneumatosis**
  - cystoides intestinalis K63.89
  - intestinalis K63.89
  - peritonei K66.8
- **Pneumaturia** R39.89
- **Pneumoblastoma** — *see* Neoplasm, lung, malignant
- **Pneumocephalus** G93.89
- **Pneumococcemia** A40.3
- **Pneumococcus, pneumococcal** — *see* condition
- **Pneumoconiosis** (due to) (inhalation of) J64
  - with tuberculosis (any type in A15) J65
  - aluminum J63.0
  - asbestos J61
  - bagasse, bagassosis J67.1
  - bauxite J63.1
  - beryllium J63.2
  - coal miners' (simple) J60
  - coalworkers' (simple) J60
  - collier's J60
  - cotton dust J66.0
  - diatomite (diatomaceous earth) J62.8
  - dust
    - inorganic NEC J63.6
    - lime J62.8
    - marble J62.8
    - organic NEC J66.8
  - fumes or vapors (from silo) J68.9
  - graphite J63.3
  - grinder's J62.8
  - kaolin J62.8
  - mica J62.8
  - millstone maker's J62.8
  - mineral fibers NEC J61
  - miner's J60
  - moldy hay J67.0
  - potter's J62.8
  - rheumatoid — *see* Rheumatoid, lung
  - sandblaster's J62.8
  - silica, silicate NEC J62.8
    - with carbon J60
  - stonemason's J62.8
  - talc (dust) J62.0
- **Pneumocystis carinii pneumonia** B59
- **Pneumocystis jirovecii** (pneumonia) B59
- **Pneumocystosis** (with pneumonia) B59
- **Pneumohemopericardium** I31.2
- **Pneumohemothorax** J94.2
  - traumatic S27.2- ☑
- **Pneumohydropericardium** — *see* Pericarditis
- **Pneumohydrothorax** — *see* Hydrothorax
- **Pneumomediastinum** J98.2
  - congenital or perinatal P25.2
- **Pneumomycosis** B49 *[J99]*
- **Pneumonia** (acute) (double) (migratory) (purulent) (septic) (unresolved) J18.9
  - with
    - influenza — *see* Influenza, with, pneumonia
    - lung abscess J85.1
      - due to specified organism — *see* Pneumonia, in (due to)
  - 2019 (novel) coronavirus J12.82
  - adenoviral J12.0
  - adynamic J18.2
  - alba A50.04
  - allergic — *see also* Pneumonitis, hypersensitivity J82.89
  - alveolar — *see* Pneumonia, lobar
  - anaerobes J15.8
  - anthrax A22.1
  - apex, apical — *see* Pneumonia, lobar
  - Ascaris B77.81
  - aspiration J69.0
    - due to
      - aspiration of microorganisms
        - bacterial J15.9
        - viral J12.9
      - food (regurgitated) J69.0
      - gastric secretions J69.0
      - milk (regurgitated) J69.0
      - oils, essences J69.1
      - solids, liquids NEC J69.8
      - vomitus J69.0
    - newborn P24.81
      - amniotic fluid (clear) P24.11
      - blood P24.21
      - food (regurgitated) P24.31
      - liquor (amnii) P24.11
      - meconium P24.01
      - milk P24.31
      - mucus P24.11
- **Pneumonia** — *continued*
  - aspiration — *continued*
    - newborn — *continued*
      - specified NEC P24.81
      - stomach contents P24.31
    - postprocedural J95.4
  - atypical NEC J18.9
  - bacillus J15.9
    - specified NEC J15.8
  - bacterial J15.9
    - specified NEC J15.8
  - Bacteroides (fragilis) (oralis) (melaninogenicus) J15.8
  - basal, basic, basilar — *see* Pneumonia, by type
  - bronchiolitis obliterans organized (BOOP) J84.89
  - broncho-, bronchial (confluent) (croupous) (diffuse) (disseminated) (hemorrhagic) (involving lobes) (lobar) (terminal) J18.0
    - allergic — *see also* Pneumonitis, hypersensitivity J82.89
    - aspiration — *see* Pneumonia, aspiration
    - bacterial J15.9
      - specified NEC J15.8
    - chronic — *see* Fibrosis, lung
    - diplococcal J13
    - Eaton's agent J15.7
    - Escherichia coli (E. coli) J15.5
    - Friedlander's bacillus J15.0
    - Hemophilus influenzae J14
    - hypostatic J18.2
    - inhalation — *see also* Pneumonia, aspiration
      - due to fumes or vapors (chemical) J68.0
      - of oils or essences J69.1
    - Klebsiella (pneumoniae) J15.0
    - lipid, lipoid J69.1
      - endogenous J84.89
    - Mycoplasma (pneumoniae) J15.7
    - pleuro-pneumonia-like-organisms (PPLO) J15.7
    - pneumococcal J13
    - Proteus J15.69
    - Pseudomonas J15.1
    - Serratia marcescens J15.69
    - specified organism NEC J16.8
    - staphylococcal — *see* Pneumonia, staphylococcal
    - streptococcal NEC J15.4
      - group B J15.3
      - pneumoniae J13
    - viral, virus — *see* Pneumonia, viral
  - Butyrivibrio (fibriosolvens) J15.8
  - Candida B37.1
  - caseous — *see* Tuberculosis, pulmonary
  - catarrhal — *see* Pneumonia, broncho
  - chlamydial J16.0
    - congenital P23.1
  - cholesterol J84.89
  - cirrhotic (chronic) — *see* Fibrosis, lung
  - Clostridium (haemolyticum) (novyi) J15.8
  - confluent — *see* Pneumonia, broncho
  - congenital (infective) P23.9
    - due to
      - bacterium NEC P23.6
      - Chlamydia P23.1
      - Escherichia coli P23.4
      - Haemophilus influenzae P23.6
      - infective organism NEC P23.8
      - Klebsiella pneumoniae P23.6
      - Mycoplasma P23.6
      - Pseudomonas P23.5
      - Staphylococcus P23.2
      - Streptococcus (except group B) P23.6
        - group B P23.3
      - viral agent P23.0
    - specified NEC P23.8
  - coronavirus (novel) (disease) 2019 J12.82
  - COVID-19 J12.82
  - croupous — *see* Pneumonia, lobar
  - cryptogenic organizing J84.116
  - cytomegalic inclusion B25.0
  - cytomegaloviral B25.0
  - deglutition — *see* Pneumonia, aspiration
  - desquamative interstitial J84.117
  - diffuse — *see* Pneumonia, broncho
  - diplococcal, diplococcus (broncho-) (lobar) J13
  - disseminated (focal) — *see* Pneumonia, broncho
  - Eaton's agent J15.7
  - embolic, embolism — *see* Embolism, pulmonary
  - Enterobacter J15.69
  - eosinophilic J82.81
    - acute J82.82
    - chronic J82.81

- **Pneumonia** — *continued*
  - Escherichia coli (E. coli) J15.5
  - Eubacterium J15.8
  - fibrinous — *see* Pneumonia, lobar
  - fibroid, fibrous (chronic) — *see* Fibrosis, lung
  - Friedlander's bacillus J15.Ø
  - Fusobacterium (nucleatum) J15.8
  - gangrenous J85.Ø
  - giant cell (measles) BØ5.2
  - gonococcal A54.84
  - gram-negative bacteria NEC J15.69
    - anaerobic J15.8
  - Hemophilus influenzae (broncho) (lobar) J14
  - human metapneumovirus J12.3
  - hypostatic (broncho) (lobar) J18.2
  - in (due to)
    - Acinetobacter baumannii J15.61
    - actinomycosis A42.Ø
    - adenovirus J12.Ø
    - anthrax A22.1
    - ascariasis B77.81
    - aspergillosis B44.9
    - Bacillus anthracis A22.1
    - Bacterium anitratum J15.69
    - candidiasis B37.1
    - chickenpox BØ1.2
    - Chlamydia J16.Ø
      - neonatal P23.1
    - coccidioidomycosis B38.2
      - acute B38.Ø
      - chronic B38.1
    - cytomegalovirus disease B25.Ø
    - Diplococcus (pneumoniae) J13
    - Eaton's agent J15.7
    - Enterobacter J15.69
    - Escherichia coli (E. coli) J15.5
    - Friedlander's bacillus J15.Ø
    - fumes and vapors (chemical) (inhalation) J68.Ø
    - gonorrhea A54.84
    - Hemophilus influenzae (H. influenzae) J14
    - Herellea J15.69
    - histoplasmosis B39.2
      - acute B39.Ø
      - chronic B39.1
    - human metapneumovirus J12.3
    - Klebsiella (pneumoniae) J15.Ø
    - measles BØ5.2
    - Mycoplasma (pneumoniae) J15.7
    - nocardiosis, nocardiasis A43.Ø
    - ornithosis A7Ø
    - parainfluenza virus J12.2
    - pleuro-pneumonia-like-organism (PPLO) J15.7
    - pneumococcus J13
    - pneumocystosis (Pneumocystis carinii) (Pneumocystis jirovecii) B59
    - Proteus J15.69
    - Pseudomonas NEC J15.1
      - pseudomallei A24.1
    - psittacosis A7Ø
    - Q fever A78
    - respiratory syncytial virus (RSV) J12.1
    - rheumatic fever IØØ *[J17]*
    - rubella BØ6.81
    - Salmonella (infection) AØ2.22
      - typhi AØ1.Ø3
    - schistosomiasis B65.9 *[J17]*
    - Serratia marcescens J15.69
    - specified
      - bacterium NEC J15.8
      - organism NEC J16.8
    - spirochetal NEC A69.8
    - Staphylococcus J15.2Ø
      - aureus (methicillin susceptible) (MSSA) J15.211
        - methicillin resistant (MRSA) J15.212
      - specified NEC J15.29
    - Streptococcus J15.4
      - group B J15.3
      - pneumoniae J13
      - specified NEC J15.4
    - toxoplasmosis B58.3
    - tularemia A21.2
    - typhoid (fever) AØ1.Ø3
    - varicella BØ1.2
    - virus — *see* Pneumonia, viral
    - whooping cough A37.91
      - due to
        - Bordetella parapertussis A37.11
        - Bordetella pertussis A37.Ø1
        - specified NEC A37.81

- **Pneumonia** — *continued*
  - in — *continued*
    - Yersinia pestis A2Ø.2
  - inhalation of food or vomit — *see* Pneumonia, aspiration
  - interstitial J84.9
    - chronic J84.111
    - desquamative J84.117
    - due to
      - collagen vascular disease J84.178
      - known underlying cause J84.178
    - idiopathic NOS J84.111
    - in disease classified elsewhere J84.178
    - lymphocytic (due to collagen vascular disease) (in diseases classified elsewhere) J84.178
    - lymphoid J84.2
    - non-specific J84.89
      - due to
        - collagen vascular disease J84.178
        - known underlying cause J84.178
      - idiopathic J84.113
      - in diseases classified elsewhere J84.178
    - plasma cell B59
    - pseudomonas J15.1
    - usual J84.112
      - due to collagen vascular disease J84.178
      - idiopathic J84.112
      - in diseases classified elsewhere J84.178
  - Klebsiella (pneumoniae) J15.Ø
  - lipid, lipoid (exogenous) J69.1
    - endogenous J84.89
  - lobar (disseminated) (double) (interstitial) J18.1
    - bacterial J15.9
      - specified NEC J15.8
    - chronic — *see* Fibrosis, lung
    - Escherichia coli (E. coli) J15.5
    - Friedlander's bacillus J15.Ø
    - Hemophilus influenzae J14
    - hypostatic J18.2
    - Klebsiella (pneumoniae) J15.Ø
    - pneumococcal J13
    - Proteus J15.69
    - Pseudomonas J15.1
    - specified organism NEC J16.8
    - staphylococcal — *see* Pneumonia, staphylococcal
    - streptococcal NEC J15.4
    - Streptococcus pneumoniae J13
    - viral, virus — *see* Pneumonia, viral
  - lobular — *see* Pneumonia, broncho
  - Loffler's J82.89
  - lymphoid interstitial J84.2
  - massive — *see* Pneumonia, lobar
  - meconium P24.Ø1
  - MRSA (methicillin resistant Staphylococcus aureus) J15.212
  - MSSA (methicillin susceptible Staphylococcus aureus) J15.211
  - multilobar — *see* Pneumonia, by type
  - Mycoplasma (pneumoniae) J15.7
  - necrotic J85.Ø
  - neonatal P23.9
    - aspiration — *see* Aspiration, by substance, with pneumonia
  - nitrogen dioxide J68.Ø
  - organizing J84.89
    - due to
      - collagen vascular disease J84.178
      - known underlying cause J84.178
    - in diseases classified elsewhere J84.178
  - orthostatic J18.2
  - parainfluenza virus J12.2
  - parenchymatous — *see* Fibrosis, lung
  - passive J18.2
  - patchy — *see* Pneumonia, broncho
  - Peptococcus J15.8
  - Peptostreptococcus J15.8
  - plasma cell (of infants) B59
  - pleuro-pneumonia-like organism (PPLO) J15.7
  - pleurolobar — *see* Pneumonia, lobar
  - pneumococcal (broncho) (lobar) J13
  - Pneumocystis (carinii) (jirovecii) B59
  - postinfectional NEC B99.- ☑ *[J17]*
  - postmeasles BØ5.2
  - Proteus J15.69
  - Pseudomonas J15.1
  - psittacosis A7Ø
  - radiation J7Ø.Ø
  - respiratory syncytial virus (RSV) J12.1
  - resulting from a procedure J95.89
  - rheumatic IØØ *[J17]*

- **Pneumonia** — *continued*
  - Salmonella (arizonae) (cholerae-suis) (enteritidis) (typhimurium) AØ2.22
    - typhi AØ1.Ø3
    - typhoid fever AØ1.Ø3
  - SARS-associated coronavirus J12.81
  - SARS-CoV-2 J12.82
  - segmented, segmental — *see* Pneumonia, broncho-
  - Serratia marcescens J15.69
  - specified NEC J18.8
    - bacterium NEC J15.8
    - organism NEC J16.8
    - virus NEC J12.89
  - spirochetal NEC A69.8
  - staphylococcal (broncho) (lobar) J15.2Ø
    - aureus (methicillin susceptible) (MSSA) J15.211
      - methicillin resistant (MRSA) J15.212
    - specified NEC J15.29
  - static, stasis J18.2
  - streptococcal NEC (broncho) (lobar) J15.4
    - group
      - A J15.4
      - B J15.3
      - specified NEC J15.4
  - Streptococcus pneumoniae J13
  - syphilitic, congenital (early) A5Ø.Ø4
  - traumatic (complication) (early) (secondary) T79.8- ☑
  - tuberculous (any) — *see* Tuberculosis, pulmonary
  - tularemic A21.2
  - varicella BØ1.2
  - Veillonella J15.8
  - ventilator associated J95.851
  - viral, virus (broncho) (interstitial) (lobar) J12.9
    - adenoviral J12.Ø
    - congenital P23.Ø
    - human metapneumovirus J12.3
    - parainfluenza J12.2
    - respiratory syncytial (RSV) J12.1
    - SARS-associated coronavirus J12.81
    - specified NEC J12.89
  - white (congenital) A5Ø.Ø4
- **Pneumonic** — *see* condition
- **Pneumonitis** (acute) (primary) — *see also* Pneumonia J98.4
  - air-conditioner J67.7
  - allergic (due to) J67.9
    - organic dust NEC J67.8
    - red cedar dust J67.8
    - sequoiosis J67.8
    - wood dust J67.8
  - aspiration J69.Ø
    - due to
      - anesthesia J95.4
        - during
          - labor and delivery O74.Ø
          - pregnancy O29.Ø1- ☑
          - puerperium O89.Ø1
      - fumes or gases J68.Ø
    - obstetric O74.Ø
  - chemical (due to gases, fumes or vapors) (inhalation) J68.Ø
    - due to anesthesia J95.4
  - chemotherapy J7Ø.4
    - acute J7Ø.2
    - chronic J7Ø.3
  - cholesterol J84.89
  - chronic — *see* Fibrosis, lung
  - congenital rubella P35.Ø
  - crack (cocaine) J68.Ø
  - due to
    - beryllium J68.Ø
    - cadmium J68.Ø
    - crack (cocaine) J68.Ø
    - detergent J69.8
    - fluorocarbon-polymer J68.Ø
    - food, vomit (aspiration) J69.Ø
    - fumes or vapors J68.Ø
    - gases, fumes or vapors (inhalation) J68.Ø
    - inhalation
      - blood J69.8
      - essences J69.1
      - food (regurgitated), milk, vomit J69.Ø
      - oils, essences J69.1
      - saliva J69.Ø
      - solids, liquids NEC J69.8
    - manganese J68.Ø
    - nitrogen dioxide J68.Ø
    - oils, essences J69.1
    - solids, liquids NEC J69.8
    - toxoplasmosis (acquired) B58.3

- **Polycythemia** — *continued*
  - emotional D75.1
  - erythropoietin D75.1
  - familial (benign) D75.Ø
  - Gaisbock's (hypertonica) D75.1
  - high altitude D75.1
  - hypertonica D75.1
  - hypoxemic D75.1
  - neonatorum P61.1
  - nephrogenous D75.1
  - relative D75.1
  - secondary D75.1
  - spurious D75.1
  - stress D75.1
  - vera D45
- **Polycytosis cryptogenica** D75.1
- **Polydactylism, polydactyly** Q69.9
  - fingers Q69.Ø
  - thumb Q69.1
  - toes Q69.2
- **Polydipsia** R63.1
- **Polydystrophy, pseudo-Hurler** E77.Ø
- **Polyembryoma** — *see* Neoplasm, malignant, by site
- **Polyglandular**
  - deficiency E31.Ø
  - dyscrasia E31.9
  - dysfunction E31.9
  - syndrome E31.8
- **Polyhydramnios** O4Ø.- ☑
- **Polymastia** Q83.1
- **Polymenorrhea** N92.Ø
- **Polymyalgia** M35.3
  - arteritica, giant cell M31.5
  - rheumatica M35.3
    - with giant cell arteritis M31.5
- **Polymyositis** (acute) (chronic) (hemorrhagic) M33.2Ø
  - with
    - myopathy M33.22
    - respiratory involvement M33.21
    - skin involvement — *see* Dermatopolymyositis
    - specified organ involvement NEC M33.29
  - ossificans (generalisata) (progressiva) — *see* Myositis, ossificans, progressiva
- **Polyneuritis, polyneuritic** — *see also* Polyneuropathy
  - acute (post-)infective G61.Ø
  - alcoholic G62.1
  - cranialis G52.7
  - demyelinating, chronic inflammatory (CIDP) G61.81
  - diabetic — *see* Diabetes, polyneuropathy
  - diphtheritic A36.83
  - due to lack of vitamin NEC E56.9 *[G63]*
  - endemic E51.11
  - erythredema — *see* subcategory T56.1- ☑
  - febrile, acute G61.Ø
  - hereditary ataxic G6Ø.1
  - idiopathic, acute G61.Ø
  - infective (acute) G61.Ø
  - inflammatory, chronic demyelinating (CIDP) G61.81
  - nutritional E63.9 *[G63]*
  - postinfective (acute) G61.Ø
  - specified NEC G62.89
- **Polyneuropathy** (peripheral) G62.9
  - alcoholic G62.1
  - amyloid (Portuguese) E85.1 *[G63]*
    - transthyretin-related (ATTR) familial E85.1 *[G63]*
  - arsenical G62.2
  - critical illness G62.81
  - demyelinating, chronic inflammatory (CIDP) G61.81
  - diabetic — *see* Diabetes, polyneuropathy
  - drug-induced G62.Ø
  - hereditary G6Ø.9
    - specified NEC G6Ø.8
  - idiopathic G6Ø.9
    - progressive G6Ø.3
  - in (due to)
    - alcohol G62.1
      - sequelae G65.2
    - amyloidosis, familial (Portuguese) E85.1 *[G63]*
    - antitetanus serum G61.1
    - arsenic G62.2
      - sequelae G65.2
    - avitaminosis NEC E56.9 *[G63]*
    - beriberi E51.11
    - collagen vascular disease NEC M35.9 *[G63]*
    - deficiency (of)
      - B (-complex) vitamins E53.9 *[G63]*
      - vitamin B6 E53.1 *[G63]*
    - diabetes — *see* Diabetes, polyneuropathy
    - diphtheria A36.83

- **Polyneuropathy** — *continued*
  - in — *continued*
    - drug or medicament G62.Ø
      - correct substance properly administered — *see* Table of Drugs and Chemicals, by drug, adverse effect
      - overdose or wrong substance given or taken — *see* Table of Drugs and Chemicals, by drug, poisoning
    - endocrine disease NEC E34.9 *[G63]*
    - herpes zoster BØ2.23
    - hypoglycemia E16.2 *[G63]*
    - infectious
      - disease NEC B99.- ☑ *[G63]*
      - mononucleosis B27.91
    - lack of vitamin NEC E56.9 *[G63]*
    - lead G62.2
      - sequelae G65.2
    - leprosy A3Ø.9 *[G63]*
    - Lyme disease A69.22
    - metabolic disease NEC E88.9 *[G63]*
    - microscopic polyangiitis M31.7 *[G63]*
    - mumps B26.84
    - neoplastic disease — *see also* Neoplasm D49.9 *[G63]*
    - nutritional deficiency NEC E63.9 *[G63]*
    - organophosphate compounds G62.2
      - sequelae G65.2
    - parasitic disease NEC B89 *[G63]*
    - pellagra E52 *[G63]*
    - polyarteritis nodosa M3Ø.Ø
    - porphyria E8Ø.2Ø *[G63]*
    - radiation G62.82
    - rheumatoid arthritis — *see* Rheumatoid, polyneuropathy
    - sarcoidosis D86.89
    - serum G61.1
    - syphilis (late) A52.15
      - congenital A5Ø.43
    - systemic
      - connective tissue disorder M35.9 *[G63]*
      - lupus erythematosus M32.19
    - toxic agent NEC G62.2
      - sequelae G65.2
    - transthyretin-related (ATTR) familial amyloid E85.1
    - triorthocresyl phosphate G62.2
      - sequelae G65.2
    - tuberculosis A17.89
    - uremia N18.9 *[G63]*
    - vitamin B12 deficiency E53.8 *[G63]*
      - with anemia (pernicious) D51.Ø *[G63]*
        - due to dietary deficiency D51.3 *[G63]*
    - zoster BØ2.23
  - inflammatory G61.9
    - chronic demyelinating (CIDP) G61.81
    - sequelae G65.1
    - specified NEC G61.89
  - lead G62.2
    - sequelae G65.2
  - nutritional NEC E63.9 *[G63]*
  - postherpetic (zoster) BØ2.23
  - progressive G6Ø.3
  - radiation-induced G62.82
  - sensory (hereditary) (idiopathic) G6Ø.8
  - specified NEC G62.89
  - syphilitic (late) A52.15
    - congenital A5Ø.43
- **Polyopia** H53.8
- **Polyorchism, polyorchidism** Q55.21
- **Polyosteoarthritis** — *see also* Osteoarthritis, generalized M15.9
  - post-traumatic M15.3
  - specified NEC M15.8
- **Polyostotic fibrous dysplasia** Q78.1
- **Polyotia** Q17.Ø
- **Polyp, polypus**
  - accessory sinus J33.8
  - adenocarcinoma in — *see* Neoplasm, malignant, by site
  - adenocarcinoma in situ in — *see* Neoplasm, in situ, by site
  - adenoid tissue J33.Ø
  - adenomatous — *see also* Neoplasm, benign, by site
    - adenocarcinoma in — *see* Neoplasm, malignant, by site
    - adenocarcinoma in situ in — *see* Neoplasm, in situ, by site
    - carcinoma in — *see* Neoplasm, malignant, by site
    - carcinoma in situ in — *see* Neoplasm, in situ, by site
    - multiple — *see* Neoplasm, benign

- **Polyp, polypus** — *continued*
  - adenomatous — *see also* Neoplasm, benign, by site — *continued*
    - multiple — *see* Neoplasm, benign — *continued*
      - adenocarcinoma in — *see* Neoplasm, malignant, by site
      - adenocarcinoma in situ in — *see* Neoplasm, in situ, by site
  - antrum J33.8
  - anus, anal (canal) K62.Ø
  - Bartholin's gland N84.3
  - bladder D41.4
  - carcinoma in — *see* Neoplasm, malignant, by site
  - carcinoma in situ in — *see* Neoplasm, in situ, by site
  - cecum K63.5
    - adenomatous D12.6
  - cervix (uteri) N84.1
    - in pregnancy or childbirth — *see* Pregnancy, complicated by, abnormal, cervix
    - mucous N84.1
    - nonneoplastic N84.1
  - choanal J33.Ø
  - cholesterol K82.4
  - clitoris N84.3
  - colon K63.5
    - adenomatous D12.6
      - ascending D12.2
      - cecum D12.Ø
      - descending D12.4
      - sigmoid D12.5
      - transverse D12.3
    - ascending K63.5
    - cecum K63.5
    - descending K63.5
    - hyperplastic, (any site) K63.5
    - inflammatory K51.4Ø
      - with
        - abscess K51.414
        - complication K51.419
          - specified NEC K51.418
        - fistula K51.413
        - intestinal obstruction K51.412
        - rectal bleeding K51.411
    - sigmoid K63.5
    - transverse K63.5
  - corpus uteri N84.Ø
  - dental KØ4.Ø1
    - irreversible KØ4.Ø2
    - reversible KØ4.Ø1
  - duodenum K31.7
  - ear (middle) H74.4- ☑
  - endometrium N84.Ø
  - esophageal K22.81
  - esophagogastric junction K22.82
  - ethmoidal (sinus) J33.8
  - fallopian tube N84.8
  - female genital tract N84.9
    - specified NEC N84.8
  - frontal (sinus) J33.8
  - gallbladder K82.4
  - gingiva, gum KØ6.8
  - labia, labium (majus) (minus) N84.3
  - larynx (mucous) J38.1
    - adenomatous D14.1
  - malignant — *see* Neoplasm, malignant, by site
  - maxillary (sinus) J33.8
  - middle ear — *see* Polyp, ear (middle)
  - myometrium N84.Ø
  - nares
    - anterior J33.9
    - posterior J33.Ø
  - nasal (mucous) J33.9
    - cavity J33.Ø
    - septum J33.Ø
  - nasopharyngeal J33.Ø
  - nose (mucous) J33.9
  - oviduct N84.8
  - pharynx J39.2
  - placenta O9Ø.89
  - prostate — *see* Enlargement, enlarged, prostate
  - pudenda, pudendum N84.3
  - pulpal (dental) KØ4.Ø1
    - irreversible KØ4.Ø2
    - reversible KØ4.Ø1
  - rectum (nonadenomatous) K62.1
    - adenomatous — *see* Polyp, adenomatous
  - septum (nasal) J33.Ø
  - sinus (accessory) (ethmoidal) (frontal) (maxillary) (sphenoidal) J33.8

**Polyp, polypus** — *continued*
- sphenoidal (sinus) J33.8
- stomach K31.7
  - adenomatous D13.1
- tube, fallopian N84.8
- turbinate, mucous membrane J33.8
- umbilical, newborn P83.6
- ureter N28.89
- urethra N36.2
- uterus (body) (corpus) (mucous) N84.Ø
  - cervix N84.1
  - in pregnancy or childbirth — *see* Pregnancy, complicated by, tumor, uterus
- vagina N84.2
- vocal cord (mucous) J38.1
- vulva N84.3

**Polyphagia** R63.2

**Polyploidy** Q92.7

**Polypoid** — *see* condition

**Polyposis** — *see also* Polyp
- adenomatous D13.91
- coli D12.6
  - adenocarcinoma in C18.9
  - adenocarcinoma in situ in — *see* Neoplasm, in situ, by site
  - carcinoma in C18.9
- colon D12.6
- familial D12.6
  - adenocarcinoma in situ in — *see* Neoplasm, in situ, by site
  - adenomatous D13.91
- intestinal D12.6
  - adenomatous D13.91
- malignant lymphomatous C83.1- ☑
- multiple, adenomatous — *see also* Neoplasm, benign D36.9

**Polyradiculitis** — *see* Polyneuropathy

**Polyradiculoneuropathy** (acute) (postinfective) (segmentally demyelinating) G61.Ø

**Polyserositis**
- due to pericarditis I31.1
- pericardial I31.1
- periodic, familial E85.Ø
- tuberculous A19.9
  - acute A19.1
  - chronic A19.8

**Polysplenia syndrome** Q89.Ø9

**Polysyndactyly** — *see also* Syndactylism, syndactyly Q7Ø.4

**Polytrichia** L68.3

**Polyunguia** Q84.6

**Polyuria** R35.89
- nocturnal R35.81
- psychogenic F45.8
- specified NEC R35.89

**Pompe's disease** (glycogen storage) E74.Ø2

**Pompholyx** L3Ø.1

**Poncet's disease** (tuberculous rheumatism) A18.Ø9

**Pond fracture** — *see* Fracture, skull

**Ponos** B55.Ø

**Pons, pontine** — *see* condition

**Poor**
- aesthetic of existing restoration of tooth KØ8.56
- contractions, labor O62.2
- gingival margin to tooth restoration KØ8.51
- housing weatherization Z59.19
- personal hygiene R46.Ø
- prenatal care, affecting management of pregnancy — *see* Pregnancy, complicated by, insufficient, prenatal care
- sucking reflex (newborn) R29.2
- urinary stream R39.12
- vision NEC H54.7

**Poradenitis, nostras inguinalis or venerea** A55

**Porencephaly** (congenital) (developmental) (true) QØ4.6
- acquired G93.Ø
- nondevelopmental G93.Ø
- traumatic (post) FØ7.89

**Porocephaliasis** B88.8

**Porokeratosis** Q82.8

**Poroma, eccrine** — *see* Neoplasm, skin, benign

**Porphyria** (South African) E8Ø.2Ø
- acquired E8Ø.2Ø
- acute intermittent (hepatic) (Swedish) E8Ø.21
- cutanea tarda (hereditary) (symptomatic) E8Ø.1
- due to drugs E8Ø.2Ø
  - correct substance properly administered — *see* Table of Drugs and Chemicals, by drug, adverse effect

**Porphyria** — *continued*
- due to drugs — *continued*
  - overdose or wrong substance given or taken — *see* Table of Drugs and Chemicals, by drug, poisoning
- erythropoietic (congenital) (hereditary) E8Ø.Ø
- hepatocutaneous type E8Ø.1
- secondary E8Ø.2Ø
- toxic NEC E8Ø.2Ø
- variegata E8Ø.2Ø

**Porphyrinuria** — *see* Porphyria

**Porphyruria** — *see* Porphyria

**Port wine nevus, mark, or stain** Q82.5

**Portal** — *see* condition

**Posadas-Wernicke disease** B38.9

**Positive**
- culture (nonspecific)
  - blood R78.81
  - bronchial washings R84.5
  - cerebrospinal fluid R83.5
  - cervix uteri R87.5
  - nasal secretions R84.5
  - nipple discharge R89.5
  - nose R84.5
    - staphylococcus (Methicillin susceptible) Z22.321
      - Methicillin resistant Z22.322
  - peritoneal fluid R85.5
  - pleural fluid R84.5
  - prostatic secretions R86.5
  - saliva R85.5
  - seminal fluid R86.5
  - sputum R84.5
  - synovial fluid R89.5
  - throat scrapings R84.5
  - urine R82.79
  - vagina R87.5
  - vulva R87.5
  - wound secretions R89.5
- PPD (skin test) R76.11
- serology for syphilis A53.Ø
  - false R76.89
  - with signs or symptoms — *code as* Syphilis, by site and stage
- skin test, tuberculin (without active tuberculosis) R76.11
- test, human immunodeficiency virus (HIV) R75
- VDRL A53.Ø
  - with signs or symptoms — *code by* site and stage under Syphilis A53.9
- Wassermann reaction A53.Ø

**Post COVID-19 condition, unspecified** UØ9.9

**Postcardiotomy syndrome** I97.Ø

**Postcaval ureter** Q62.62

**Postcholecystectomy syndrome** K91.5

**Postclimacteric bleeding** N95.Ø

**Postcommissurotomy syndrome** I97.Ø

**Postconcussional syndrome** FØ7.81

**Postcontusional syndrome** FØ7.81

**Postcricoid region** — *see* condition

**Post-dates** (4Ø-42 weeks) (pregnancy) (mother) O48.Ø
- more than 42 weeks gestation O48.1

**Postencephalitic syndrome** FØ7.89

**Posterior** — *see* condition

**Posterolateral sclerosis** (spinal cord) — *see* Degeneration, combined

**Postexanthematous** — *see* condition

**Postfebrile** — *see* condition

**Postgastrectomy dumping syndrome** K91.1

**Posthemiplegic chorea** — *see* Monoplegia

**Posthemorrhagic anemia** (chronic) D5Ø.Ø
- acute D62
- newborn P61.3

**Postherpetic neuralgia** (zoster) BØ2.29
- trigeminal BØ2.22

**Posthitis** N47.7

**Postimmunization complication or reaction** — *see* Complications, vaccination

**Postinfectious** — *see* condition

**Postlaminectomy syndrome NEC** M96.1

**Postleukotomy syndrome** FØ7.Ø

**Postmastectomy lymphedema** (syndrome) I97.2

**Postmaturity, postmature** (over 42 weeks)
- maternal (over 42 weeks gestation) O48.1
- newborn PØ8.22

**Postmeasles complication NEC** — *see also* condition BØ5.89

**Postmenopausal**
- endometrium (atrophic) N95.8
  - suppurative — *see also* Endometritis N71.9
- osteoporosis — *see* Osteoporosis, postmenopausal

**Postnasal drip** RØ9.82
- due to
  - allergic rhinitis — *see* Rhinitis, allergic
  - common cold JØØ
  - gastroesophageal reflux — *see* Reflux, gastroesophageal
  - nasopharyngitis — *see* Nasopharyngitis
  - other known condition — *code to* condition
  - sinusitis — *see* Sinusitis

**Postnatal** — *see* condition

**Postoperative** (postprocedural) — *see also* Complication, postoperative
- pneumothorax, therapeutic Z98.3
- state NEC Z98.89Ø
- visit — *see* Aftercare
- wound check — *see* Aftercare

**Postpancreatectomy hyperglycemia** E89.1

**Postpartum** — *see* Puerperal

**Postphlebitic syndrome** — *see* Syndrome, postthrombotic

**Postpolio** (myelitic) **syndrome** G14

**Postpoliomyelitic** — *see also* condition
- osteopathy — *see* Osteopathy, after poliomyelitis

**Postprocedural** — *see also* Postoperative
- hypoinsulinemia E89.1

**Postschizophrenic depression** F32.89

**Postsurgery status** — *see also* Status (post)
- pneumothorax, therapeutic Z98.3

**Post-term** (4Ø-42 weeks) (pregnancy) (mother) O48.Ø
- infant PØ8.21
- more than 42 weeks gestation (mother) O48.1

**Post-traumatic brain syndrome, nonpsychotic** FØ7.81

**Post-typhoid abscess** AØ1.Ø9

**Postures, hysterical** F44.2

**Postvaccinal reaction or complication** — *see* Complications, vaccination

**Postvalvulotomy syndrome** I97.Ø

**Potain's**
- disease (pulmonary edema) — *see* Edema, lung
- syndrome (gastrectasis with dyspepsia) K31.Ø

**POTS** (postural orthostatic tachycardia syndrome) G9Ø.A

**Potter's**
- asthma J62.8
- facies Q6Ø.6
- lung J62.8
- syndrome (with renal agenesis) Q6Ø.6

**Pott's**
- curvature (spinal) A18.Ø1
- disease or paraplegia A18.Ø1
- spinal curvature A18.Ø1
- tumor, puffy M86.8X8- ☑

**Pouch**
- bronchus Q32.4
- Douglas' — *see* condition
- esophagus, esophageal, congenital Q39.6
  - acquired K22.5
- gastric K31.4
- Hartmann's K82.8
- pharynx, pharyngeal (congenital) Q38.7

**Pouchitis** K91.85Ø

**Poultrymen's itch** B88.Ø9

**Poverty NEC** Z59.6
- extreme Z59.5

**Poxvirus NEC** BØ8.8

**Prader-Willi-like syndrome** Q87.19

**Prader-Willi syndrome** Q87.11

**Preauricular appendage or tag** Q17.Ø

**Prebetalipoproteinemia** (acquired) (essential) (familial) (hereditary) (primary) (secondary) E78.1
- with chylomicronemia E78.3

**Precipitate labor or delivery** O62.3

**Preclimacteric bleeding** (menorrhagia) N92.4

**Precocious**
- adrenarche E3Ø.1
- menarche E3Ø.1
- menstruation E3Ø.1
- pubarche E3Ø.1
- puberty E3Ø.1
  - central E22.8
- sexual development NEC E3Ø.1
- thelarche E3Ø.8

**Precocity, sexual** (constitutional) (cryptogenic) (female) (idiopathic) (male) E3Ø.1
- with adrenal hyperplasia E25.9
  - congenital E25.Ø

**Precordial pain** RØ7.2

**Predeciduous teeth** KØØ.2

**Prediabetes, prediabetic** R73.Ø3

- **Prediabetes, prediabetic** — *continued*
  - complicating
    - pregnancy — *see* Pregnancy, complicated by, diseases of, specified type or system NEC
    - puerperium O99.893
- **Predislocation status of hip at birth** Q65.6
- **Pre-eclampsia** O14.9- ☑
  - with pre-existing hypertension — *see* Hypertension, complicating pregnancy, pre-existing, with, pre-eclampsia
  - complicating
    - childbirth O14.94
    - puerperium O14.95
  - mild O14.Ø- ☑
    - complicating
      - childbirth O14.Ø4
      - puerperium O14.Ø5
  - moderate O14.Ø- ☑
    - complicating
      - childbirth O14.Ø4
      - puerperium O14.Ø5
  - severe O14.1- ☑
    - with hemolysis, elevated liver enzymes and low platelet count (HELLP) O14.2- ☑
      - complicating
        - childbirth O14.24
        - puerperium O14.25
    - complicating
      - childbirth O14.14
      - puerperium O14.15
- **Pre-eruptive color change, teeth, tooth** KØØ.8
- **Pre-excitation atrioventricular conduction** I45.6
- **Preglaucoma** H4Ø.ØØ- ☑
- **Pregnancy** (single) (uterine) — *see also* Delivery and Puerperal Z33.1

> *Note: The Tabular must be reviewed for assignment of appropriate seventh character for multiple gestation codes in Chapter 15*

> *Note: The Tabular must be reviewed for assignment of the appropriate character indicating the trimester of the pregnancy*

  - abdominal (ectopic) OØØ.ØØ
    - with intrauterine pregnancy OØØ.Ø1
    - with viable fetus O36.7- ☑
  - ampullar OØØ.1Ø- ☑
    - with intrauterine pregnancy OØØ.11- ☑
  - biochemical OØ2.81
  - broad ligament OØØ.8Ø
    - with intrauterine pregnancy OØØ.81
  - cervical OØØ.41
    - with intrauterine pregnancy OØØ.42
  - chemical OØ2.81
  - complicated by (care of) (management affected by)
    - abnormal, abnormality
      - cervix O34.4- ☑
        - causing obstructed labor O65.5
      - cord (umbilical) O69.9- ☑
      - fetal heart rate or rhythm O36.83- ☑
      - findings on antenatal screening of mother O28.9
        - biochemical O28.1
        - chromosomal O28.5
        - cytological O28.2
        - genetic O28.5
        - hematological O28.Ø
        - radiological O28.4
        - specified NEC O28.8
        - ultrasonic O28.3
      - glucose (tolerance) NEC O99.81Ø
      - pelvic organs O34.9- ☑
        - specified NEC O34.8- ☑
          - causing obstructed labor O65.5
      - pelvis (bony) (major) NEC O33.Ø
      - perineum O34.7- ☑
      - position
        - placenta O44.Ø- ☑
          - with hemorrhage O44.1- ☑
        - uterus O34.59- ☑
      - uterus O34.59- ☑
        - causing obstructed labor O65.5
        - congenital O34.Ø- ☑
      - vagina O34.6- ☑
        - causing obstructed labor O65.5
      - vulva O34.7- ☑
        - causing obstructed labor O65.5
    - abruptio placentae — *see* Abruptio placentae

- **Pregnancy** — *continued*
  - complicated by — *continued*
    - abscess or cellulitis
      - bladder O23.1- ☑
      - breast O91.11- ☑
      - genital organ or tract O23.9- ☑
    - abuse
      - physical O9A.31- ☑ *(following O99)*
      - psychological O9A.51- ☑ *(following O99)*
      - sexual O9A.41- ☑ *(following O99)*
    - adverse effect anesthesia O29.9- ☑
      - aspiration pneumonitis O29.Ø1- ☑
      - cardiac arrest O29.11- ☑
      - cardiac complication NEC O29.19- ☑
      - cardiac failure O29.12- ☑
      - central nervous system complication NEC O29.29- ☑
      - cerebral anoxia O29.21- ☑
      - failed or difficult intubation O29.6- ☑
      - inhalation of stomach contents or secretions NOS O29.Ø1- ☑
      - local, toxic reaction O29.3X- ☑
      - Mendelson's syndrome O29.Ø1- ☑
      - pressure collapse of lung O29.Ø2- ☑
      - pulmonary complications NEC O29.Ø9- ☑
      - specified NEC O29.8X- ☑
      - spinal and epidural type NEC O29.5X- ☑
        - induced headache O29.4- ☑
    - albuminuria — *see also* Proteinuria, gestational O12.1- ☑
    - alcohol use O99.31- ☑
    - amnionitis O41.12- ☑
    - anaphylactoid syndrome of pregnancy O88.Ø1- ☑
    - anemia (conditions in D5Ø-D64) (pre-existing) O99.Ø1- ☑
      - complicating childbirth O99.Ø2
      - complicating the puerperium O99.Ø3
    - antepartum hemorrhage O46.9- ☑
      - with coagulation defect — *see* Hemorrhage, antepartum, with coagulation defect
      - specified NEC O46.8X- ☑
    - appendicitis O99.61- ☑
    - atrophy (yellow) (acute) liver (subacute) O26.61- ☑
    - bariatric surgery status O99.84- ☑
    - bicornis or bicornuate uterus O34.Ø- ☑
    - biliary tract problems O26.61- ☑
    - breech presentation O32.1- ☑
    - cardiovascular diseases (conditions in IØØ-IØ9, I2Ø-I52, I7Ø-I99) O99.41- ☑
    - cerebrovascular disorders (conditions in I6Ø-I69) O99.41- ☑
    - cervical shortening O26.87- ☑
    - cervicitis O23.51- ☑
    - cesarean scar defect (isthmocele) O34.22
    - chloasma (gravidarum) O26.89- ☑
    - cholecystitis O99.61- ☑
    - cholestasis (intrahepatic) O26.61- ☑
    - chorioamnionitis O41.12- ☑
    - circulatory system disorder (conditions in IØØ-IØ9, I2Ø-I99, O99.41-)
    - compound presentation O32.6- ☑
    - conjoined twins O3Ø.Ø2- ☑
    - connective system disorders (conditions in MØØ-M99) O99.891
    - contracted pelvis (general) O33.1
      - inlet O33.2
      - outlet O33.3- ☑
    - convulsions (eclamptic) (uremic) — *see also* Eclampsia O15.9
    - cracked nipple O92.11- ☑
    - cystitis O23.1- ☑
    - cystocele O34.8- ☑
    - death of fetus (near term) O36.4- ☑
      - early pregnancy OØ2.1
      - of one fetus or more in multiple gestation O31.2- ☑
    - deciduitis O41.14- ☑
    - decreased fetal movement O36.81- ☑
    - dental problems O99.61- ☑
    - diabetes (mellitus) O24.91- ☑
      - gestational (pregnancy induced) — *see* Diabetes, gestational
      - pre-existing O24.31- ☑
        - specified NEC O24.81- ☑
        - type 1 O24.Ø1- ☑
        - type 2 O24.11- ☑

- **Pregnancy** — *continued*
  - complicated by — *continued*
    - digestive system disorders (conditions in KØØ-K93) O99.61- ☑
    - diseases of — *see* Pregnancy, complicated by, specified body system disease
      - biliary tract O26.61- ☑
      - blood NEC (conditions in D65-D77) O99.11- ☑
      - liver O26.61- ☑
      - specified NEC O99.891
    - disorders of — *see* Pregnancy, complicated by, specified body system disorder
      - amniotic fluid and membranes O41.9- ☑
        - specified NEC O41.8X- ☑
      - biliary tract O26.61- ☑
      - ear and mastoid process (conditions in H6Ø-H95) O99.891
      - eye and adnexa (conditions in HØØ-H59) O99.891
      - liver O26.61- ☑
      - skin (conditions in LØØ-L99) O99.71- ☑
      - specified NEC O99.891
    - displacement, uterus NEC O34.59- ☑
      - causing obstructed labor O65.5
    - disproportion (due to) O33.9
      - fetal (ascites) (hydrops) (meningomyelocele) (sacral teratoma) (tumor) deformities NEC O33.7- ☑
      - generally contracted pelvis O33.1
      - hydrocephalic fetus O33.6- ☑
      - inlet contraction of pelvis O33.2
      - mixed maternal and fetal origin O33.4- ☑
      - specified NEC O33.8
    - double uterus O34.Ø- ☑
      - causing obstructed labor O65.5
    - drug use (conditions in F11-F19) O99.32- ☑
    - eclampsia, eclamptic (coma) (convulsions) (delirium) (nephritis) (uremia) — *see also* Eclampsia O15.- ☑
    - ectopic pregnancy — *see* Pregnancy, ectopic
    - edema O12.Ø- ☑
      - with
        - gestational hypertension, mild — *see also* Pre-eclampsia O14.Ø- ☑
        - proteinuria O12.2- ☑
    - effusion, amniotic fluid — *see* Pregnancy, complicated by, premature rupture of membranes
    - elderly
      - multigravida OØ9.52- ☑
      - primigravida OØ9.51- ☑
    - embolism — *see also* Embolism, obstetric, pregnancy O88.- ☑
    - endocrine diseases NEC O99.28- ☑
    - endometritis O86.12
    - excessive weight gain O26.Ø- ☑
    - exhaustion O26.81- ☑
      - during labor and delivery O75.81
    - face presentation O32.3- ☑
    - failed induction of labor O61.9
      - instrumental O61.1
      - mechanical O61.1
      - medical O61.Ø
      - specified NEC O61.8
      - surgical O61.1
    - failed or difficult intubation for anesthesia O29.6- ☑
    - false labor (pains) O47.9
      - at or after 37 completed weeks of pregnancy O47.1
      - before 37 completed weeks of pregnancy O47.Ø- ☑
    - fatigue O26.81- ☑
      - during labor and delivery O75.81
    - fatty metamorphosis of liver O26.61- ☑
    - female genital mutilation O34.8- ☑ *[N9Ø.81-]* ☑
    - fetal (maternal care for)
      - abnormality or damage O35.9- ☑
        - acid-base balance O68
        - specified type NEC O35.8- ☑
      - acidemia O68
      - acidosis O68
      - agenesis of corpus callosum O35.Ø1- ☑
      - alkalosis O68
      - anemia and thrombocytopenia O36.82- ☑
      - anencephaly O35.Ø2- ☑
      - bradycardia O36.83- ☑
      - cardiac anomalies O35.B- ☑
      - central nervous system malformation or damage O35.ØØ- ☑
        - specified type NEC O35.Ø9- ☑

**Pregnancy** — *continued*
- ectopic — *continued*
  - ovarian — *continued*
    - with intrauterine pregnancy OØØ.21- ☑
  - specified site NEC OØØ.8Ø
    - with intrauterine pregnancy OØØ.81
  - tubal (ruptured) OØØ.1Ø- ☑
    - with intrauterine pregnancy OØØ.11- ☑
- examination (normal) Z34.9- ☑
  - first Z34.Ø- ☑
  - high-risk — *see* Pregnancy, supervision of, high-risk
  - specified Z34.8- ☑
- extrauterine — *see* Pregnancy, ectopic
- fallopian OØØ.1Ø- ☑
  - with intrauterine pregnancy OØØ.11- ☑
- false F45.8
- gestational carrier Z33.3
- heptachorionic, hepta-amniotic (septuplets) O3Ø.83- ☑
- hexachorionic, hexa-amniotic (sextuplets) O3Ø.83- ☑
- hidden OØ9.3- ☑
- high-risk — *see* Pregnancy, supervision of, high-risk
- incidental finding Z33.1
- interstitial OØØ.12- ☑
  - with intrauterine pregnancy OØØ.13- ☑
- intraligamentous OØØ.8Ø
  - with intrauterine pregnancy OØØ.81
- intramural OØØ.8Ø
  - with intrauterine pregnancy OØØ.81
- intraperitoneal OØØ.ØØ
  - with intrauterine pregnancy OØØ.Ø1
- isthmian OØØ.1Ø- ☑
  - with intrauterine pregnancy OØØ.11- ☑
- mesometric (mural) OØØ.8Ø
  - with intrauterine pregnancy OØØ.81
- molar NEC OØ2.Ø
  - complicated (by) OØ8.9
    - afibrinogenemia OØ8.1
    - cardiac arrest OØ8.81
    - chemical damage of pelvic organ(s) OØ8.6
    - circulatory collapse OØ8.3
    - defibrination syndrome OØ8.1
    - electrolyte imbalance OØ8.5
    - embolism (amniotic fluid) (blood clot) (pulmonary) (septic) OØ8.2
    - endometritis OØ8.Ø
    - genital tract and pelvic infection OØ8.Ø
    - hemorrhage (delayed) (excessive) OØ8.1
    - infection
      - genital tract or pelvic OØ8.Ø
      - kidney OØ8.83
      - urinary tract OØ8.83
    - intravascular coagulation OØ8.1
    - laceration of pelvic organ(s) OØ8.6
    - metabolic disorder OØ8.5
    - oliguria OØ8.4
    - oophoritis OØ8.Ø
    - parametritis OØ8.Ø
    - pelvic peritonitis OØ8.Ø
    - perforation of pelvic organ(s) OØ8.6
    - renal failure or shutdown OØ8.4
    - salpingitis or salpingo-oophoritis OØ8.Ø
    - sepsis OØ8.82
    - shock OØ8.3
      - septic OØ8.82
    - specified condition NEC OØ8.89
    - tubular necrosis (renal) OØ8.4
    - uremia OØ8.4
    - urinary infection OØ8.83
    - venous complication NEC OØ8.7
      - embolism OØ8.2
  - hydatidiform — *see also* Mole, hydatidiform OØ1.9
- multiple (gestation) O3Ø.9- ☑
  - greater than quadruplets — *see* Pregnancy, multiple (gestation), specified NEC
  - specified NEC O3Ø.8Ø- ☑
    - with
      - two or more monoamniotic fetuses O3Ø.82- ☑
      - two or more monochorionic fetuses O3Ø.81- ☑
    - number of chorions and amnions are both equal to the number of fetuses O3Ø.83- ☑
    - two or more monoamniotic fetuses O3Ø.82- ☑
    - two or more monochorionic fetuses O3Ø.81- ☑
    - unable to determine number of placenta and number of amniotic sacs O3Ø.89- ☑
    - unspecified number of placenta and unspecified number of amniotic sacs O3Ø.8Ø- ☑
- mural OØØ.8Ø
  - with intrauterine pregnancy OØØ.81

**Pregnancy** — *continued*
- normal (supervision of) Z34.9- ☑
  - first Z34.Ø- ☑
  - high-risk — *see* Pregnancy, supervision of, high-risk
  - specified Z34.8- ☑
- ovarian OØØ.2Ø- ☑
  - with intrauterine pregnancy OØØ.21- ☑
- pentachorionic, penta-amniotic (quintuplets) O3Ø.83- ☑
- postmature (4Ø to 42 weeks) O48.Ø
  - more than 42 weeks gestation O48.1
- post-term (4Ø to 42 weeks) O48.Ø
- prenatal care only Z34.9- ☑
  - first Z34.Ø- ☑
  - high-risk — *see* Pregnancy, supervision of, high-risk
  - specified Z34.8- ☑
- prolonged (more than 42 weeks gestation) O48.1
- quadruplet O3Ø.2Ø- ☑
  - with
    - two or more monoamniotic fetuses O3Ø.22- ☑
    - two or more monochorionic fetuses O3Ø.21- ☑
  - quadrachorionic/quadra-amniotic O3Ø.23- ☑
  - two or more monoamniotic fetuses O3Ø.22- ☑
  - two or more monochorionic fetuses O3Ø.21- ☑
  - unable to determine number of placenta and number of amniotic sacs O3Ø.29- ☑
  - unspecified number of placenta and unspecified number of amniotic sacs O3Ø.2Ø- ☑
- quintuplet — *see* Pregnancy, multiple (gestation), specified NEC
- sextuplet — *see* Pregnancy, multiple (gestation), specified NEC
- supervision of
  - concealed pregnancy OØ9.3- ☑
  - elderly mother
    - multigravida OØ9.52- ☑
    - primigravida OØ9.51- ☑
  - hidden pregnancy OØ9.3- ☑
  - high-risk OØ9.9- ☑
    - due to (history of)
      - ectopic pregnancy OØ9.1- ☑
      - elderly — *see* Pregnancy, supervision, elderly mother
      - grand multiparity OØ9.4- ☑
      - in utero procedure during previous pregnancy OØ9.82- ☑
      - in vitro fertilization OØ9.81- ☑
      - infertility OØ9.Ø- ☑
      - insufficient prenatal care OØ9.3- ☑
      - molar pregnancy OØ9.A- ☑
      - multiple previous pregnancies OØ9.4- ☑
      - older mother — *see* Pregnancy, supervision of, elderly mother
      - poor reproductive or obstetric history NEC OØ9.29- ☑
      - pre-term labor OØ9.21- ☑
      - previous
        - neonatal death OØ9.29- ☑
      - social problems OØ9.7- ☑
      - specified NEC OØ9.89- ☑
      - very young mother — *see* Pregnancy, supervision, young mother
    - resulting from in vitro fertilization OØ9.81- ☑
  - normal Z34.9- ☑
    - first Z34.Ø- ☑
    - specified NEC Z34.8- ☑
  - young mother
    - multigravida OØ9.62- ☑
    - primigravida OØ9.61- ☑
- triplet O3Ø.1Ø- ☑
  - with
    - two or more monoamniotic fetuses O3Ø.12- ☑
    - two or more monochorionic fetuses O3Ø.11- ☑
  - trichorionic/triamniotic O3Ø.13- ☑
  - two or more monoamniotic fetuses O3Ø.12- ☑
  - two or more monochorionic fetuses O3Ø.11- ☑
  - unable to determine number of placenta and number of amniotic sacs O3Ø.19- ☑
  - unspecified number of placenta and unspecified number of amniotic sacs O3Ø.1Ø- ☑
- tubal (with abortion) (with rupture) OØØ.1Ø- ☑
  - with intrauterine pregnancy OØØ.11- ☑
- twin O3Ø.ØØ- ☑
  - conjoined O3Ø.Ø2- ☑
  - dichorionic/diamniotic (two placenta, two amniotic sacs) O3Ø.Ø4- ☑

**Pregnancy** — *continued*
- twin — *continued*
  - monochorionic/diamniotic (one placenta, two amniotic sacs) O3Ø.Ø3- ☑
  - monochorionic/monoamniotic (one placenta, one amniotic sac) O3Ø.Ø1- ☑
  - unable to determine number of placenta and number of amniotic sacs O3Ø.Ø9- ☑
  - unspecified number of placenta and unspecified number of amniotic sacs O3Ø.ØØ- ☑
- unwanted Z64.Ø
- weeks of gestation
  - 8 weeks Z3A.Ø8 (*following* Z36)
  - 9 weeks Z3A.Ø9 (*following* Z36)
  - 1Ø weeks Z3A.1Ø (*following* Z36)
  - 11 weeks Z3A.11 (*following* Z36)
  - 12 weeks Z3A.12 (*following* Z36)
  - 13 weeks Z3A.13 (*following* Z36)
  - 14 weeks Z3A.14 (*following* Z36)
  - 15 weeks Z3A.15 (*following* Z36)
  - 16 weeks Z3A.16 (*following* Z36)
  - 17 weeks Z3A.17 (*following* Z36)
  - 18 weeks Z3A.18 (*following* Z36)
  - 19 weeks Z3A.19 (*following* Z36)
  - 2Ø weeks Z3A.2Ø (*following* Z36)
  - 21 weeks Z3A.21 (*following* Z36)
  - 22 weeks Z3A.22 (*following* Z36)
  - 23 weeks Z3A.23 (*following* Z36)
  - 24 weeks Z3A.24 (*following* Z36)
  - 25 weeks Z3A.25 (*following* Z36)
  - 26 weeks Z3A.26 (*following* Z36)
  - 27 weeks Z3A.27 (*following* Z36)
  - 28 weeks Z3A.28 (*following* Z36)
  - 29 weeks Z3A.29 (*following* Z36)
  - 3Ø weeks Z3A.3Ø (*following* Z36)
  - 31 weeks Z3A.31 (*following* Z36)
  - 32 weeks Z3A.32 (*following* Z36)
  - 33 weeks Z3A.33 (*following* Z36)
  - 34 weeks Z3A.34 (*following* Z36)
  - 35 weeks Z3A.35 (*following* Z36)
  - 36 weeks Z3A.36 (*following* Z36)
  - 37 weeks Z3A.37 (*following* Z36)
  - 38 weeks Z3A.38 (*following* Z36)
  - 39 weeks Z3A.39 (*following* Z36)
  - 4Ø weeks Z3A.4Ø (*following* Z36)
  - 41 weeks Z3A.41 (*following* Z36)
  - 42 weeks Z3A.42 (*following* Z36)
  - greater than 42 weeks Z3A.49 (*following* Z36)
  - less than 8 weeks Z3A.Ø1 (*following* Z36)
  - not specified Z3A.ØØ (*following* Z36)

**Preiser's disease** — *see* Osteonecrosis, secondary, due to, trauma, metacarpus

**Pre-kwashiorkor** — *see* Malnutrition, severe

**Preleukemia** (syndrome) D46.9

**Preluxation, hip, congenital** Q65.6

**Premature** — *see also* condition
- adrenarche E27.Ø
- aging E34.8
- beats I49.4Ø
  - atrial I49.1
  - auricular I49.1
  - supraventricular I49.1
- birth NEC — *see* Preterm, newborn
- closure, foramen ovale Q21.8
- contraction
  - atrial I49.1
  - atrioventricular I49.2
  - auricular I49.1
  - auriculoventricular I49.49
  - heart (extrasystole) I49.49
  - junctional I49.2
  - ventricular I49.3
- delivery — *see also* Pregnancy, complicated by, preterm labor O6Ø.1Ø- ☑
- ejaculation F52.4
- infant NEC — *see* Preterm, newborn
  - light-for-dates — *see* Light for dates
- labor — *see* Pregnancy, complicated by, preterm labor
- lungs P28.Ø
- menopause E28.319
  - asymptomatic E28.319
  - symptomatic E28.31Ø
- newborn
  - extreme (less than 28 completed weeks) — *see* Immaturity, extreme
  - less than 37 completed weeks — *see* Preterm, newborn
- puberty E3Ø.1

**Premature** — *continued*
- rupture membranes or amnion — *see* Pregnancy, complicated by, premature rupture of membranes
- senility E34.8
- thelarche E3Ø.8
- ventricular systole I49.3

**Prematurity NEC** (less than 37 completed weeks) — *see* Preterm, newborn
- extreme (less than 28 completed weeks) — *see* Immaturity, extreme

**Premenstrual**
- dysphoric disorder (PMDD) F32.81
- tension (syndrome) N94.3

**Premolarization, cuspids** KØØ.2

**Prenatal**
- care, normal pregnancy — *see* Pregnancy, normal
- screening of mother — *see also* Encounter, antenatal screening Z36.9
- teeth KØØ.6

**Preparatory care for subsequent treatment NEC**
- for dialysis Z49.Ø1
  - peritoneal Z49.Ø2

**Prepartum** — *see* condition

**Preponderance, left or right ventricular** I51.7

**Prepuce** — *see* condition

**PRES** (posterior reversible encephalopathy syndrome) I67.83

**Presbycardia** R54

**Presbycusis, presbyacusia** H91.1- ☑

**Presbyesophagus** K22.89

**Presbyophrenia** FØ3.- ☑

**Presbyopia** H52.4

**Prescription of contraceptives** (initial) Z3Ø.Ø19
- barrier Z3Ø.Ø18
- diaphragm Z3Ø.Ø18
- emergency (postcoital) Z3Ø.Ø12
- implantable subdermal Z3Ø.Ø17
- injectable Z3Ø.Ø13
- intrauterine contraceptive device Z3Ø.Ø14
- pills Z3Ø.Ø11
- postcoital (emergency) Z3Ø.Ø12
- repeat Z3Ø.4Ø
  - barrier Z3Ø.49
  - diaphragm Z3Ø.49
  - implantable subdermal Z3Ø.46
  - injectable Z3Ø.42
  - pills Z3Ø.41
  - specified type NEC Z3Ø.49
  - transdermal patch hormonal Z3Ø.45
  - vaginal ring hormonal Z3Ø.44
- specified type NEC Z3Ø.Ø18
  - transdermal patch hormonal Z3Ø.Ø16
  - vaginal ring hormonal Z3Ø.Ø15

**Presence** (of)
- ankle-joint implant (functional) (prosthesis) Z96.66- ☑
- aortocoronary (bypass) graft Z95.1
- arterial-venous shunt (dialysis) Z99.2
- artificial
  - eye (globe) Z97.Ø
  - heart (fully implantable) (mechanical) Z95.812
    - valve Z95.2
  - larynx Z96.3
  - lens (intraocular) Z96.1
  - limb (complete) (partial) Z97.1- ☑
    - arm Z97.1- ☑
      - bilateral Z97.15
    - leg Z97.1- ☑
      - bilateral Z97.16
- audiological implant (functional) Z96.29
- bladder implant (functional) Z96.Ø
- bone
  - conduction hearing device Z96.29
  - implant (functional) NEC Z96.7
  - joint (prosthesis) — *see* Presence, joint implant
- cardiac
  - defibrillator (functional) (with synchronous cardiac pacemaker) Z95.81Ø
  - implant or graft Z95.9
    - specified type NEC Z95.818
  - pacemaker Z95.Ø
  - resynchronization therapy
    - defibrillator Z95.81Ø
    - pacemaker Z95.Ø
- cardioverter-defibrillator (ICD) Z95.81Ø
- cerebrospinal fluid drainage device Z98.2
- cochlear implant (functional) Z96.21
- contact lens (es) Z97.3
- coronary artery graft or prosthesis Z95.5

**Presence** — *continued*
- CRT-D (cardiac resynchronization therapy defibrillator) Z95.81Ø
- CRT-P (cardiac resynchronization therapy pacemaker) Z95.Ø
- CSF shunt Z98.2
- dental prosthesis device Z97.2
- dentures Z97.2
- device (external) NEC Z97.8
  - cardiac NEC Z95.818
  - heart assist Z95.811
  - implanted (functional) Z96.9
    - specified NEC Z96.89
  - prosthetic Z97.8
- ear implant Z96.2Ø
  - cochlear implant Z96.21
  - myringotomy tube Z96.22
  - specified type NEC Z96.29
- elbow-joint implant (functional) (prosthesis) Z96.62- ☑
- endocrine implant (functional) NEC Z96.49
- eustachian tube stent or device (functional) Z96.29
- external hearing-aid or device Z97.4
- finger-joint implant (functional) (prosthetic) Z96.69- ☑
- functional implant Z96.9
  - specified NEC Z96.89
- graft
  - cardiac NEC Z95.818
  - vascular NEC Z95.828
- hearing-aid or device (external) Z97.4
  - implant (bone) (cochlear) (functional) Z96.21
- heart assist device Z95.811
- heart valve implant (functional) Z95.2
  - prosthetic Z95.2
  - specified type NEC Z95.4
  - xenogenic Z95.3
- hip-joint implant (functional) (prosthesis) Z96.64- ☑
- ICD (cardioverter-defibrillator) Z95.81Ø
- implanted device (artificial) (functional) (prosthetic) Z96.9
  - automatic cardiac defibrillator (with synchronous cardiac pacemaker) Z95.81Ø
  - cardiac pacemaker Z95.Ø
  - cochlear Z96.21
  - dental Z96.5
  - heart Z95.812
  - heart valve Z95.2
    - prosthetic Z95.2
    - specified NEC Z95.4
    - xenogenic Z95.3
  - insulin pump Z96.41
  - intraocular lens Z96.1
  - joint Z96.6Ø
    - ankle Z96.66- ☑
    - elbow Z96.62- ☑
    - finger Z96.69- ☑
    - hip Z96.64- ☑
    - knee Z96.65- ☑
    - shoulder Z96.61- ☑
    - specified NEC Z96.698
    - wrist Z96.63- ☑
  - larynx Z96.3
  - myringotomy tube Z96.22
  - otological Z96.2Ø
    - cochlear Z96.21
    - eustachian stent Z96.29
    - myringotomy Z96.22
    - specified NEC Z96.29
    - stapes Z96.29
  - skin Z96.81
  - skull plate Z96.7
  - specified NEC Z96.89
  - urogenital Z96.Ø
- insulin pump (functional) Z96.41
- intestinal bypass or anastomosis Z98.Ø
- intraocular lens (functional) Z96.1
- intrauterine contraceptive device (IUD) Z97.5
- intravascular implant (functional) (prosthetic) NEC Z95.9
  - coronary artery Z95.5
  - defibrillator (with synchronous cardiac pacemaker) Z95.81Ø
  - peripheral vessel (with angioplasty) Z95.82Ø
- joint implant (prosthetic) (any) Z96.6Ø
  - ankle — *see* Presence, ankle joint implant
  - elbow — *see* Presence, elbow joint implant
  - finger — *see* Presence, finger joint implant
  - hip — *see* Presence, hip joint implant
  - knee — *see* Presence, knee joint implant
  - shoulder — *see* Presence, shoulder joint implant
  - specified joint NEC Z96.698

**Presence** — *continued*
- joint implant — *continued*
  - wrist — *see* Presence, wrist joint implant
- knee-joint implant (functional) (prosthesis) Z96.65- ☑
- laryngeal implant (functional) Z96.3
- mandibular implant (dental) Z96.5
- myringotomy tube(s) Z96.22
- neurostimulator (brain) (gastric) (peripheral nerve) (sacra nerve) (spinal cord) (vagus nerve) Z96.82
- orthopedic-joint implant (prosthetic) (any) — *see* Presence, joint implant
- otological implant (functional) Z96.29
- shoulder-joint implant (functional) (prosthesis) Z96.61- ☑
- skull-plate implant Z96.7
- spectacles Z97.3
- stapes implant (functional) Z96.29
- systemic lupus erythematosus [SLE] inhibitor D68.62
- tendon implant (functional) (graft) Z96.7
- tooth root(s) implant Z96.5
- ureteral stent Z96.Ø
- urethral stent Z96.Ø
- urogenital implant (functional) Z96.Ø
- vascular implant or device Z95.9
  - access port device Z95.828
  - specified type NEC Z95.828
- wrist-joint implant (functional) (prosthesis) Z96.63- ☑

**Presenile** — *see also* condition
- dementia FØ3.- ☑
- premature aging E34.8

**Presentation, fetal** — *see* Delivery, complicated by, malpo sition

**Prespondylolisthesis** (congenital) Q76.2

**Pressure**
- area, skin — *see* Ulcer, pressure, by site
- brachial plexus G54.Ø
- brain G93.5
  - injury at birth NEC P11.1
- cerebral — *see* Pressure, brain
- chest RØ7.89
- cone, tentorial G93.5
- hyposystolic — *see also* Hypotension
  - incidental reading, without diagnosis of hypotensio RØ3.1
- increased
  - intracranial benign G93.2
    - injury at birth P11.Ø
  - intraocular H4Ø.Ø5- ☑
- injury — *see* Ulcer, pressure, by site
- lumbosacral plexus G54.1
- mediastinum J98.59
- necrosis (chronic) — *see* Ulcer, pressure, by site
- parental, inappropriate (excessive) Z62.6
- sore (chronic) — *see* Ulcer, pressure, by site
- spinal cord G95.2Ø
- ulcer (chronic) — *see* Ulcer, pressure, by site
- venous, increased I87.8

**Pre-syncope** R55

**Preterm**
- delivery — *see also* Pregnancy, complicated by, preterr labor O6Ø.1Ø- ☑
- labor — *see* Pregnancy, complicated by, preterm labo
- newborn (infant) PØ7.3Ø
  - gestational age
    - 28 completed weeks (28 weeks, Ø days through 28 weeks, 6 days) PØ7.31
    - 29 completed weeks (29 weeks, Ø days through 29 weeks, 6 days) PØ7.32
    - 3Ø completed weeks (3Ø weeks, Ø days through 3Ø weeks, 6 days) PØ7.33
    - 31 completed weeks (31 weeks, Ø days through 31 weeks, 6 days) PØ7.34
    - 32 completed weeks (32 weeks, Ø days through 32 weeks, 6 days) PØ7.35
    - 33 completed weeks (33 weeks, Ø days through 33 weeks, 6 days) PØ7.36
    - 34 completed weeks (34 weeks, Ø days through 34 weeks, 6 days) PØ7.37
    - 35 completed weeks (35 weeks, Ø days through 35 weeks, 6 days) PØ7.38
    - 36 completed weeks (36 weeks, Ø days through 36 weeks, 6 days) PØ7.39

**Previa**
- placenta (total) (without hemorrhage) O44.Ø- ☑
  - with hemorrhage O44.1- ☑
  - complete O44.Ø- ☑
    - with hemorrhage O44.1- ☑

**Previa** — *continued*
  placenta — *continued*
    low — *see also* Delivery, complicated, by, placenta, low O44.4- ☑
      with hemorrhage O44.5- ☑
    marginal O44.2- ☑
      with hemorrhage O44.3- ☑
    partial O44.2- ☑
      with hemorrhage O44.3- ☑
  vasa O69.4- ☑
**Priapism** N48.3Ø
  due to
    disease classified elsewhere N48.32
    drug N48.33
    sickle-cell disease — *see* Disease, sickle-cell, by type, with priapism
    specified cause NEC N48.39
    trauma N48.31
**Prickling sensation** (skin) R2Ø.2
**Prickly heat** L74.Ø
**Primary** — *see* condition
**Primigravida**
  elderly, affecting management of pregnancy, labor and delivery (supervision only) — *see* Pregnancy, complicated by, elderly, primigravida
  older, affecting management of pregnancy, labor and delivery (supervision only) — *see* Pregnancy, complicated by, elderly, primigravida
  very young, affecting management of pregnancy, labor and delivery (supervision only) — *see* Pregnancy, complicated by, young mother, primigravida
**Primipara**
  elderly, affecting management of pregnancy, labor and delivery (supervision only) — *see* Pregnancy, complicated by, elderly, primigravida
  older, affecting management of pregnancy, labor and delivery (supervision only) — *see* Pregnancy, complicated by, elderly, primigravida
  very young, affecting management of pregnancy, labor and delivery (supervision only) — *see* Pregnancy, complicated by, young mother, primigravida
**Primus varus** Q66.21- ☑
**PRIND** (Prolonged reversible ischemic neurologic deficit) I63.9
**Pringle's disease** (tuberous sclerosis) Q85.1
**Prinzmetal angina** I2Ø.1
**Prizefighter ear** — *see* Cauliflower ear
**Problem** (with) (related to)
  academic Z55.8
  acculturation Z6Ø.3
  adjustment (to)
    change of job Z56.1
    life-cycle transition Z6Ø.Ø
    pension Z6Ø.Ø
    retirement Z6Ø.Ø
  adopted child Z62.821
  alcoholism in family Z63.72
  atypical parenting situation Z62.9
  bankruptcy Z59.89
  behavioral (adult) F69
    drug seeking Z76.5
  birth of sibling affecting child Z62.898
  care (of)
    provider dependency Z74.9
      specified NEC Z74.8
    sick or handicapped person in family or household Z63.6
  child
    abuse (affecting the child) — *see* Maltreatment, child
    custody or support proceedings Z65.3
    in
      care of non-parental family member Z62.23
      custody of
        grandparent Z62.23
        non-parental relative Z62.23
        non-relative guardian Z62.24
      foster care Z62.21
      kinship care Z62.23
      welfare
        custody Z62.21
        guardianship Z62.21
    leaving living situation without permission Z62.892
    living in
      group home Z62.22
      orphanage Z62.22
  child-rearing Z62.9
    specified NEC Z62.898
  communication (developmental) F8Ø.9

**Problem** — *continued*
  completing medical forms Z55.6
  conflict or discord (with)
    boss Z56.4
    classmates Z55.4
    counselor Z64.4
    employer Z56.4
    family Z63.9
      specified NEC Z63.8
    probation officer Z64.4
    social worker Z64.4
    teachers Z55.4
    workmates Z56.4
  conviction in legal proceedings Z65.Ø
    with imprisonment Z65.1
  counselor Z64.4
  creditors Z59.89
  digestive K92.9
  drug addict in family Z63.72
  ear — *see* Disorder, ear
  economic Z59.9
    affecting care Z59.9
    specified NEC Z59.89
    strain Z59.868
  education Z55.9
    specified NEC Z55.8
  employment Z56.9
    change of job Z56.1
    discord Z56.4
    environment Z56.5
    sexual harassment Z56.81
    specified NEC Z56.89
    stress NEC Z56.6
    stressful schedule Z56.3
    threat of job loss Z56.2
    unemployment Z56.Ø
  enuresis, child F98.Ø
  eye H57.9
  failed examinations (school) Z55.2
  falling Z91.81
  family — *see also* Disruption, family Z63.9
    specified NEC Z63.8
  feeding (elderly) (infant) NOS R63.39
    newborn P92.9
      breast P92.5
      overfeeding P92.4
      slow P92.2
      specified NEC P92.8
      underfeeding P92.3
    nonorganic F5Ø.89
  finance Z59.9
    specified NEC Z59.89
  foreclosure on loan Z59.89
  foster child Z62.822
  frightening experience(s) in childhood Z62.898
  genital NEC
    female N94.9
    male N5Ø.9
  health care Z75.9
    specified NEC Z75.8
  health literacy Z55.6
  hearing — *see* Deafness
  homelessness Z59.ØØ
  housing Z59.9
    inadequate Z59.1Ø
    isolated Z59.89
    specified NEC Z59.89
  identity (of childhood) F93.8
  illegitimate pregnancy (unwanted) Z64.Ø
  illiteracy Z55.Ø
  impaired mobility Z74.Ø9
  imprisonment or incarceration Z65.1
  in-law Z63.1
  inadequate teaching affecting education Z55.8
  inappropriate (excessive) parental pressure Z62.6
  influencing health status NEC Z78.9
  institutionalization, affecting child Z62.22
  intrafamilial communication Z63.8
  jealousy, child F93.8
  landlord Z59.2
  language (developmental) F8Ø.9
  learning (developmental) F81.9
  legal Z65.3
    conviction without imprisonment Z65.Ø
    imprisonment Z65.1
    release from prison Z65.2
  life-management Z73.9
    specified NEC Z73.89
  life-style Z72.9

**Problem** — *continued*
  life-style — *continued*
    gambling Z72.6
    high-risk sexual behavior (heterosexual) Z72.51
      bisexual Z72.53
      homosexual Z72.52
    inappropriate eating habits Z72.4
    self-damaging behavior NEC Z72.89
    specified NEC Z72.89
    tobacco use Z72.Ø
  literacy Z55.9
    low level Z55.Ø
    specified NEC Z55.8
  living alone Z6Ø.2
  lodgers Z59.2
  loss of love relationship in childhood Z62.898
  marital Z63.Ø
    involving
      divorce Z63.5
      estrangement Z63.5
      gender identity F66
  mastication KØ8.89
  medical
    care, within family Z63.6
    facilities Z75.9
      specified NEC Z75.8
  mental F48.9
  money Z59.868
  multiparity Z64.1
  negative life events in childhood Z62.9
    altered pattern of family relationships Z62.898
    frightening experience Z62.898
    loss of
      love relationship Z62.898
      self-esteem Z62.898
    physical abuse (alleged) — *see* Maltreatment, child
    removal from home Z62.29
    specified event NEC Z62.898
  neighbor Z59.2
  neurological NEC R29.818
  new step-parent affecting child Z62.823
  none (feared complaint unfounded) Z71.1
  occupational NEC Z56.89
  parent-child — *see* Conflict, parent-child
  personal hygiene Z91.89
  personality F69
  phase-of-life transition, adjustment Z6Ø.Ø
  presence of sick or disabled person in family or household Z63.79
    needing care Z63.6
  primary support group (family) Z63.9
    specified NEC Z63.8
  probation officer Z64.4
  psychiatric F99
  psychosexual (development) F66
  psychosocial Z65.9
    religious or spiritual Z65.8
    specified NEC Z65.8
  related to physical environment, specified NEC Z58.89
  relationship Z63.9
    childhood F93.8
  release from prison Z65.2
    religious or spiritual Z65.8
  removal from home affecting child Z62.29
  seeking and accepting known hazardous and harmful
    behavioral or psychological interventions Z65.8
    chemical, nutritional or physical interventions Z65.8
  sexual function (nonorganic) F52.9
  sight H54.7
  sleep disorder, child F51.9
  smell — *see* Disturbance, sensation, smell
  social
    environment Z6Ø.9
      specified NEC Z6Ø.8
    exclusion and rejection Z6Ø.4
    worker Z64.4
  speech R47.9
    developmental F8Ø.9
    specified NEC R47.89
  swallowing — *see* Dysphagia
  taste — *see* Disturbance, sensation, taste
  tic, child F95.Ø
  underachievement in school Z55.3
  unemployment Z56.Ø
    threatened Z56.2
  unwanted pregnancy Z64.Ø
  upbringing Z62.9
    specified NEC Z62.898
  urinary N39.9

- **Problem** — *continued*
  - voice production R47.89
  - work schedule (stressful) Z56.3
- **Procedure** (surgical)
  - converted
    - arthroscopic to open Z53.33
    - laparoscopic to open Z53.31
    - specified procedure NEC to open Z53.39
    - thoracoscopic to open Z53.32
  - for purpose other than remedying health state Z41.9
    - specified NEC Z41.8
  - not done Z53.9
    - because of
      - administrative reasons Z53.8
      - contraindication Z53.Ø9
        - smoking Z53.Ø1
      - patient's decision Z53.2Ø
        - for reasons of belief or group pressure Z53.1
        - left against medical advice (AMA) Z53.29
        - left without being seen Z53.21
        - specified reason NEC Z53.29
      - specified reason NEC Z53.8
- **Procidentia** (uteri) N81.3
- **Proctalgia** K62.89
  - fugax K59.4
  - spasmodic K59.4
- **Proctitis** K62.89
  - amebic (acute) AØ6.Ø
  - chlamydial A56.3
  - gonococcal A54.6
  - granulomatous — *see* Enteritis, regional, large intestine
  - herpetic A6Ø.1
  - radiation K62.7
  - tuberculous A18.32
  - ulcerative (chronic) K51.2Ø
    - with
      - complication K51.219
        - abscess K51.214
        - fistula K51.213
        - obstruction K51.212
        - rectal bleeding K51.211
        - specified NEC K51.218
- **Proctocele**
  - female (without uterine prolapse) N81.6
    - with uterine prolapse N81.2
      - complete N81.3
  - male K62.3
- **Proctocolitis**
  - allergic K52.29
  - food-induced eosinophilic K52.29
  - food protein-induced K52.29
  - milk protein-induced K52.29
  - mucosal — *see* Rectosigmoiditis, ulcerative
- **Proctoptosis** K62.3
- **Proctorrhagia** K62.5
- **Proctosigmoiditis** K63.89
  - ulcerative (chronic) — *see* Rectosigmoiditis, ulcerative
- **Proctospasm** K59.4
  - psychogenic F45.8
- **Profichet's disease** — *see* Disorder, soft tissue, specified type NEC
- **Progeria** E34.8
- **Prognathism** (mandibular) (maxillary) M26.19
- **Progonoma** (melanotic) — *see* Neoplasm, benign, by site
- **Progressive** — *see* condition
- **Prolactinoma**
  - specified site — *see* Neoplasm, benign, by site
  - unspecified site D35.2
- **Prolapse, prolapsed**
  - anus, anal (canal) (sphincter) K62.2
  - arm or hand O32.2- ☑
    - causing obstructed labor O64.4- ☑
  - bladder (mucosa) (sphincter) (acquired)
    - congenital Q79.4
    - female — *see* Cystocele
    - male N32.89
  - breast implant (prosthetic) T85.49- ☑
  - cecostomy K94.Ø9
  - cecum K63.4
  - cervix, cervical (hypertrophied) N81.2
    - anterior lip, obstructing labor O65.5
    - congenital Q51.828
    - postpartal, old N81.2
    - stump N81.85
  - ciliary body (traumatic) — *see* Laceration, eye(ball), with prolapse or loss of interocular tissue
  - colon (pedunculated) K63.4
  - colostomy K94.Ø9
- **Prolapse, prolapsed** — *continued*
  - disc (intervertebral) — *see* Displacement, intervertebral disc
  - eye implant (orbital) T85.398- ☑
    - lens (ocular) — *see* Complications, intraocular lens
  - fallopian tube N83.4- ☑
  - gastric (mucosa) K31.89
  - genital, female N81.9
    - specified NEC N81.89
  - globe, nontraumatic — *see* Luxation, globe
  - ileostomy bud K94.19
  - intervertebral disc — *see* Displacement, intervertebral disc
  - intestine (small) K63.4
  - iris (traumatic) — *see* Laceration, eye(ball), with prolapse or loss of interocular tissue
    - nontraumatic H21.89
  - kidney N28.83
    - congenital Q63.2
  - laryngeal muscles or ventricle J38.7
  - liver K76.89
  - meatus urinarius N36.8
  - mitral (valve) I34.1
  - ocular lens implant — *see* Complications, intraocular lens
  - organ or site, congenital NEC — *see* Malposition, congenital
  - ovary N83.4- ☑
  - pelvic floor, female N81.89
  - perineum, female N81.89
  - rectum (mucosa) (sphincter) K62.3
    - due to trichuris trichuria B79
  - spleen D73.89
  - stomach K31.89
  - umbilical cord
    - complicating delivery O69.Ø- ☑
  - urachus, congenital Q64.4
  - ureter N28.89
    - with obstruction N13.5
      - with infection N13.6
  - ureterovesical orifice N28.89
  - urethra (acquired) (infected) (mucosa) N36.8
    - congenital Q64.71
  - urinary meatus N36.8
    - congenital Q64.72
  - uterovaginal N81.4
    - complete N81.3
    - incomplete N81.2
  - uterus (with prolapse of vagina) N81.4
    - complete N81.3
    - congenital Q51.818
    - first degree N81.2
    - in pregnancy or childbirth — *see* Pregnancy, complicated by, abnormal, uterus
    - incomplete N81.2
    - postpartal (old) N81.4
    - second degree N81.2
    - third degree N81.3
  - uveal (traumatic) — *see* Laceration, eye(ball), with prolapse or loss of interocular tissue
  - vagina (anterior) (wall) — *see* Cystocele
    - with prolapse of uterus N81.4
      - complete N81.3
      - incomplete N81.2
    - posterior wall N81.6
    - posthysterectomy N99.3
  - vitreous (humor) H43.Ø- ☑
    - in wound — *see* Laceration, eye(ball), with prolapse or loss of interocular tissue
  - womb — *see* Prolapse, uterus
- **Prolapsus, female** N81.9
  - specified NEC N81.89
- **Proliferation(s)**
  - primary cutaneous CD3Ø-positive large T-cell C86.6- ☑
  - prostate, atypical small acinar N42.32
- **Proliferative** — *see* condition
- **Prolonged, prolongation** (of)
  - bleeding (time) (idiopathic) R79.1
  - coagulation (time) R79.1
  - gestation (over 42 completed weeks)
    - mother O48.1
    - newborn PØ8.22
  - interval I44.Ø
  - labor O63.9
    - first stage O63.Ø
    - second stage O63.1
  - partial thromboplastin time (PTT) R79.1
  - pregnancy (more than 42 weeks gestation) O48.1
- **Prolonged, prolongation** — *continued*
  - prothrombin time R79.1
  - QT interval R94.31
  - uterine contractions in labor O62.4
- **Prominence, prominent**
  - auricle (congenital) (ear) Q17.5
  - ischial spine or sacral promontory with disproportion (fetopelvic) O33.Ø
    - causing obstructed labor O65.Ø
  - nose (congenital) acquired M95.Ø
- **Promiscuity** — *see* High, risk, sexual behavior
- **Pronation**
  - ankle — *see* Deformity, limb, foot, specified NEC
  - foot — *see also* Deformity, limb, foot, specified NEC
    - congenital Q74.2
- **Prophylactic**
  - administration of
    - antibiotics, long-term Z79.2
      - short-term use — *omit code*
    - drug — *see also* Long-term (current) drug therapy (use of) Z79.899
  - medication Z79.899
  - organ removal (for neoplasia management) **Z4Ø.ØØ**
    - breast Z4Ø.Ø1
    - fallopian tube(s) Z4Ø.Ø3
      - with ovary(s) Z4Ø.Ø2
    - ovary(s) Z4Ø.Ø2
    - specified site NEC Z4Ø.Ø9
  - surgery Z4Ø.9
    - for risk factors related to malignant neoplasm — *see* Prophylactic, organ removal
    - specified NEC Z4Ø.89
  - vaccination Z23
- **Propionic acidemia** E71.121
- **Proptosis** (ocular) — *see also* Exophthalmos
  - thyroid — *see* Hyperthyroidism, with goiter
- **Prosecution, anxiety concerning** Z65.3
- **Prosopagnosia** R48.3
- **Prostadynia** N42.81
- **Prostate, prostatic** — *see* condition
- **Prostatism** — *see* Hyperplasia, prostate
- **Prostatitis** (congestive) (suppurative) (with cystitis) N41.9
  - acute N41.Ø
  - cavitary N41.8
  - chronic N41.1
  - diverticular N41.8
  - due to Trichomonas (vaginalis) A59.Ø2
  - fibrous N41.1
  - gonococcal (acute) (chronic) A54.22
  - granulomatous N41.4
  - hypertrophic N41.1
  - subacute N41.1
  - trichomonal A59.Ø2
  - tuberculous A18.14
- **Prostatocystitis** N41.3
- **Prostatorrhea** N42.89
- **Prostatosis** N42.82
- **Prostration** R53.83
  - heat — *see also* Heat, exhaustion
    - anhydrotic T67.3- ☑
    - due to
      - salt (and water) depletion T67.4- ☑
      - water depletion T67.3- ☑
  - nervous F48.8
  - senile R54
- **Protanomaly** (anomalous trichromat) H53.54
- **Protanopia** (complete) (incomplete) H53.54
- **Protection** (against) (from) — *see* Prophylactic
- **Protein**
  - deficiency NEC — *see* Malnutrition
  - malnutrition — *see* Malnutrition
  - sickness — *see also* Reaction, serum T8Ø.69- ☑
- **Proteinemia** R77.9
- **Proteinosis**
  - alveolar (pulmonary) J84.Ø1
  - lipid or lipoid (of Urbach) E78.89
- **Proteinuria** R8Ø.9
  - Bence Jones R8Ø.3
  - complicating pregnancy — *see* Proteinuria, gestational
  - gestational
    - complicating
      - childbirth O12.14
      - pregnancy O12.1- ☑
        - with edema O12.2- ☑
      - puerperium O12.15
  - idiopathic R8Ø.Ø
  - isolated R8Ø.Ø
    - with glomerular lesion NØ6.9

**Proteinuria** — *continued*
- isolated — *continued*
  - with glomerular lesion — *continued*
    - C3
      - glomerulonephritis NØ6.A
      - glomerulopathy NØ6.A
        - with dense deposit disease NØ6.6
    - dense deposit disease NØ6.6
    - diffuse
      - crescentic glomerulonephritis NØ6.7
      - endocapillary proliferative glomerulonephritis NØ6.4
      - mesangiocapillary glomerulonephritis NØ6.5
    - focal and segmental hyalinosis or sclerosis NØ6.1
    - membranous (diffuse) — *see also* Nephropathy, membranous NØ6.2Ø
      - with diffuse membranous glomerulonephritis NØ6.29
    - mesangial proliferative (diffuse) NØ6.3
    - minimal change NØ6.Ø
    - specified pathology NEC NØ6.8
- orthostatic R8Ø.2
  - with glomerular lesion — *see* Proteinuria, isolated, with glomerular lesion
- persistent R8Ø.1
  - with glomerular lesion — *see* Proteinuria, isolated, with glomerular lesion
- postural R8Ø.2
  - with glomerular lesion — *see* Proteinuria, isolated, with glomerular lesion
- pre-eclamptic — *see* Pre-eclampsia
- puerperal O12.15
- specified type NEC R8Ø.8

**Proteolysis, pathologic** D65

**Proteus** (mirabilis) (morganii), **as cause of disease classified elsewhere** B96.4

**Prothrombin gene mutation** D68.52

**Protoporphyria, erythropoietic** E8Ø.Ø

**Protozoal** — *see also* condition
- disease B64
  - specified NEC B6Ø.8

**Protrusion, protrusio**
- acetabuli M24.7
- acetabulum (into pelvis) M24.7
- device, implant or graft — *see also* Complications, by site and type, mechanical T85.698- ☑
  - arterial graft NEC — *see* Complication, vascular, mechanical, protrusion
  - breast (implant) T85.49- ☑
  - catheter NEC T85.698- ☑
    - cystostomy T83.Ø9Ø- ☑
    - dialysis (renal) T82.49- ☑
      - intraperitoneal T85.691- ☑
    - infusion NEC T82.594- ☑
      - spinal (epidural) (subdural) T85.69Ø- ☑
    - urinary — *see also* Complications, catheter, urinary T83.Ø98- ☑
  - electronic (electrode) (pulse generator) (stimulator)
    - bone T84.39Ø- ☑
    - nervous system — *see* Complication, prosthetic device, mechanical, electronic nervous system stimulator
  - fixation, internal (orthopedic) NEC — *see* Complication, fixation device, mechanical
  - gastrointestinal — *see* Complications, prosthetic device, mechanical, gastrointestinal device
  - genital NEC T83.498- ☑
    - intrauterine contraceptive device T83.39- ☑
    - penile prosthesis (cylinder) (implanted) (pump) (reservoir) T83.49Ø- ☑
    - testicular prosthesis T83.491- ☑
  - heart NEC — *see* Complication, cardiovascular device, mechanical
  - joint prosthesis — *see* Complications, joint prosthesis, mechanical, specified NEC, by site
  - ocular NEC — *see* Complications, prosthetic device, mechanical, ocular device
  - orthopedic NEC — *see* Complication, orthopedic, device, mechanical
  - specified NEC T85.628- ☑
  - urinary NEC — *see also* Complication, genitourinary, device, urinary, mechanical
    - graft T83.29- ☑
  - vascular NEC — *see* Complication, cardiovascular device, mechanical
  - ventricular intracranial shunt T85.Ø9- ☑
- intervertebral disc — *see* Displacement, intervertebral disc

**Protrusion, protrusio** — *continued*
- joint prosthesis — *see* Complications, joint prosthesis, mechanical, specified NEC, by site
- nucleus pulposus — *see* Displacement, intervertebral disc

**Prune belly** (syndrome) Q79.4

**Prurigo** (ferox) (gravis) (Hebrae) (Hebra's) (mitis) (simplex) L28.2
- Besnier's L2Ø.Ø
- estivalis L56.4
- nodularis L28.1
- psychogenic F45.8

**Pruritus, pruritic** (essential) L29.9
- ani, anus L29.Ø
  - psychogenic F45.8
- anogenital L29.3
  - psychogenic F45.8
- cholestatic L29.81
- due to onchocerca volvulus B73.1
- gravidarum — *see* Pregnancy, complicated by, specified pregnancy-related condition NEC
- hiemalis L29.89
- neurogenic (any site) F45.8
- perianal L29.Ø
- psychogenic (any site) F45.8
- scroti, scrotum L29.1
  - psychogenic F45.8
- senile, senilis L29.89
- specified NEC L29.89
  - psychogenic F45.8
- Trichomonas A59.9
- vulva, vulvae L29.2
  - psychogenic F45.8

**Pseudarthrosis, pseudoarthrosis** (bone) — *see* Nonunion, fracture
- clavicle, congenital Q74.Ø
- joint, following fusion or arthrodesis M96.Ø

**Pseudo-Cushing's syndrome, alcohol-induced** E24.4

**Pseudo-Hurler's polydystrophy** E77.Ø

**Pseudo-obstruction intestine** (acute) (chronic) (idiopathic) (intermittent secondary) (primary) K59.89
- colonic K59.81

**Pseudoaneurysm** — *see* Aneurysm

**Pseudoangina** (pectoris) — *see* Angina

**Pseudoangioma** I81

**Pseudoarteriosus** Q28.8

**Pseudoarthrosis** — *see* Pseudarthrosis

**Pseudobulbar affect** (PBA) F48.2

**Pseudochromhidrosis** L67.8

**Pseudocirrhosis, liver, pericardial** I31.1

**Pseudocowpox** BØ8.Ø3

**Pseudocoxalgia** M91.3- ☑

**Pseudocroup** J38.5

**Pseudocyesis** F45.8

**Pseudocyst**
- lung J98.4
- pancreas K86.3
- retina — *see* Cyst, retina

**Pseudoelephantiasis neuroarthritica** Q82.Ø

**Pseudoexfoliation, capsule** (lens) — *see* Cataract, specified NEC

**Pseudofolliculitis barbae** L73.1

**Pseudoglioma** H44.89

**Pseudohemophilia** (Bernuth's) (hereditary) (type B) — *see* Disease, von Willebrand
- Type A D69.8
- vascular D69.8

**Pseudohermaphroditism** Q56.3
- adrenal E25.8
- female — *see also* Disorder, adrenogenital Q56.2
  - with adrenocortical disorder E25.8
  - without adrenocortical disorder Q56.2
  - adrenal (congenital) E25.Ø
- male — *see also* Disorder, adrenogenital Q56.1
  - with
    - 5-alpha-reductase deficiency E29.1
    - adrenocortical disorder E25.8
    - androgen resistance E34.51
    - cleft scrotum Q56.1
    - feminizing testis E34.51
  - without gonadal disorder Q56.1
  - adrenal E25.8

**Pseudohydrocephalus** G93.2

**Pseudohypertrophic muscular dystrophy** (Erb's) G71.Ø2

**Pseudohypertrophy, muscle** — *see also* Dystrophy, muscular, by type, if applicable G71.Ø9

**Pseudohypoparathyroidism** E2Ø.1

**Pseudoinsomnia** F51.Ø3

**Pseudoleukemia, infantile** D64.89

**Pseudomembranous** — *see* condition

**Pseudomeningocele** (cerebral) (infective) (post-traumatic) G96.198
- postprocedural (spinal) G97.82

**Pseudomenses** (newborn) P54.6

**Pseudomenstruation** (newborn) P54.6

**Pseudomonas**
- aeruginosa, as cause of disease classified elsewhere B96.5
- mallei infection A24.Ø
  - as cause of disease classified elsewhere B96.5
- pseudomallei, as cause of disease classified elsewhere B96.5

**Pseudomyotonia** G71.19

**Pseudomyxoma peritonei** C78.6

**Pseudoneuritis, optic** (nerve) (disc) (papilla), **congenital** Q14.2

**Pseudopapilledema** H47.33- ☑
- congenital Q14.2

**Pseudoparalysis**
- arm or leg R29.818
- atonic, congenital P94.2

**Pseudopelade** L66.Ø

**Pseudophakia** Z96.1

**Pseudopolyarthritis, rhizomelic** M35.3

**Pseudopolycythemia** D75.1

**Pseudopseudohypoparathyroidism** E2Ø.1

**Pseudopterygium** H11.81- ☑

**Pseudoptosis** (eyelid) — *see* Blepharochalasis

**Pseudopuberty, precocious**
- female heterosexual E25.8
- male isosexual E25.8

**Pseudorickets** (renal) N25.Ø

**Pseudorubella** BØ8.2Ø

**Pseudosclerema, newborn** P83.88

**Pseudosclerosis** (brain)
- Jakob's — *see* Creutzfeldt-Jakob disease or syndrome
- of Westphal (Strumpell) E83.Ø1
- spastic — *see* Creutzfeldt-Jakob disease or syndrome

**Pseudotetanus** — *see* Convulsions

**Pseudotetany** R29.Ø
- hysterical F44.5

**Pseudotruncus arteriosus** Q25.49

**Pseudotuberculosis** A28.2
- enterocolitis AØ4.8
- pasteurella (infection) A28.Ø

**Pseudotumor** G93.2
- cerebri G93.2
- orbital HØ5.11- ☑

**Pseudoxanthoma elasticum** Q82.8

**Psilosis** (sprue) (tropical) K9Ø.1
- nontropical K9Ø.Ø

**Psittacosis** A7Ø

**Psoitis** M6Ø.88

**Psoriasis** L4Ø.9
- arthropathic L4Ø.5Ø
  - arthritis mutilans L4Ø.52
  - distal interphalangeal L4Ø.51
  - juvenile L4Ø.54
  - other specified L4Ø.59
  - spondylitis L4Ø.53
- buccal K13.29
- flexural L4Ø.8
- guttate L4Ø.4
- mouth K13.29
- nummular L4Ø.Ø
- plaque L4Ø.Ø
- psychogenic F54
- pustular (generalized) L4Ø.1
  - palmaris et plantaris L4Ø.3
- specified NEC L4Ø.8
- vulgaris L4Ø.Ø

**Psychasthenia** F48.8

**Psychiatric disorder or problem** F99

**Psychogenic** — *see also* condition
- factors associated with physical conditions F54

**Psychological and behavioral factors affecting medical condition** F59

**Psychoneurosis, psychoneurotic** — *see also* Neurosis
- anxiety (state) F41.1
- depersonalization F48.1
- hypochondriacal F45.21
- hysteria F44.9
- neurasthenic F48.8
- personality NEC F6Ø.89

**Psychopathy, psychopathic**
- affectionless F94.2
- autistic F84.5
- constitution, post-traumatic FØ7.81
- personality — *see* Disorder, personality

- **Puerperal, puerperium** — *continued*
  - venous O87.9
  - vulvitis O86.19
  - vulvovaginitis O86.13
  - white leg O87.1
- **Puerperium** — *see* Puerperal
- **Pulmolithiasis** J98.4
- **Pulmonary** — *see* condition
- **Pulpitis** (acute) (anachoretic) (chronic) (hyperplastic) (putrescent) (suppurative) (ulcerative) K04.01
  - irreversible K04.02
  - reversible K04.01
- **Pulpless tooth** K04.99
- **Pulse**
  - alternating R00.8
  - bigeminal R00.8
  - fast R00.0
  - feeble, rapid due to shock following injury T79.4- ☑
  - rapid R00.0
  - weak R09.89
- **Pulsus alternans or trigeminus** R00.8
- **Punch drunk** F07.81
- **Punctum lacrimale occlusion** — *see* Obstruction, lacrimal
- **Puncture**
  - abdomen, abdominal
    - wall S31.139- ☑
      - with
        - foreign body S31.149- ☑
        - penetration into peritoneal cavity S31.639- ☑
          - with foreign body S31.649- ☑
      - epigastric region S31.132- ☑
        - with
          - foreign body S31.142- ☑
          - penetration into peritoneal cavity S31.632- ☑
            - with foreign body S31.642- ☑
      - left
        - lower quadrant S31.134- ☑
          - with
            - foreign body S31.144- ☑
            - penetration into peritoneal cavity S31.634- ☑
              - with foreign body S31.644- ☑
        - upper quadrant S31.131- ☑
          - with
            - foreign body S31.141- ☑
            - penetration into peritoneal cavity S31.631- ☑
              - with foreign body S31.641- ☑
      - periumbilic region S31.135- ☑
        - with
          - foreign body S31.145- ☑
          - penetration into peritoneal cavity S31.635- ☑
            - with foreign body S31.645- ☑
      - right
        - lower quadrant S31.133- ☑
          - with
            - foreign body S31.143- ☑
            - penetration into peritoneal cavity S31.633- ☑
              - with foreign body S31.643- ☑
        - upper quadrant S31.130- ☑
          - with
            - foreign body S31.140- ☑
            - penetration into peritoneal cavity S31.630- ☑
              - with foreign body S31.640- ☑
  - accidental, complicating surgery — *see* Complication, accidental puncture or laceration
  - alveolar (process) — *see* Puncture, oral cavity
  - ankle S91.039- ☑
    - with
      - foreign body S91.049- ☑
    - left S91.032- ☑
      - with
        - foreign body S91.042- ☑
    - right S91.031- ☑
      - with
        - foreign body S91.041- ☑
  - anus S31.833- ☑
    - with foreign body S31.834- ☑
  - arm (upper) S41.139- ☑
    - with foreign body S41.149- ☑
    - left S41.132- ☑
      - with foreign body S41.142- ☑
    - lower — *see* Puncture, forearm

- **Puncture** — *continued*
  - arm — *continued*
    - right S41.131- ☑
      - with foreign body S41.141- ☑
  - auditory canal (external) (meatus) — *see* Puncture, ear
  - auricle, ear — *see* Puncture, ear
  - axilla — *see* Puncture, arm
  - back — *see also* Puncture, thorax, back
    - lower S31.030- ☑
      - with
        - foreign body S31.040- ☑
          - with penetration into retroperitoneal space S31.041- ☑
        - penetration into retroperitoneal space S31.031- ☑
  - bladder (traumatic) S37.29- ☑
    - nontraumatic N32.89
  - breast S21.039- ☑
    - with foreign body S21.049- ☑
    - left S21.032- ☑
      - with foreign body S21.042- ☑
    - right S21.031- ☑
      - with foreign body S21.041- ☑
  - buttock S31.803- ☑
    - with foreign body S31.804- ☑
    - left S31.823- ☑
      - with foreign body S31.824- ☑
    - right S31.813- ☑
      - with foreign body S31.814- ☑
  - by
    - device, implant or graft — *see* Complications, by site and type, mechanical
    - foreign body left accidentally in operative wound T81.539- ☑
    - instrument (any) during a procedure, accidental — *see* Puncture, accidental complicating surgery
  - calf — *see* Puncture, leg
  - canaliculus lacrimalis — *see* Puncture, eyelid
  - canthus, eye — *see* Puncture, eyelid
  - cervical esophagus S11.23- ☑
    - with foreign body S11.24- ☑
  - cheek (external) S01.439- ☑
    - with foreign body S01.449- ☑
    - internal — *see* Puncture, oral cavity
    - left S01.432- ☑
      - with foreign body S01.442- ☑
    - right S01.431- ☑
      - with foreign body S01.441- ☑
  - chest wall — *see* Puncture, thorax
  - chin — *see* Puncture, head, specified site NEC
  - clitoris — *see* Puncture, vulva
  - costal region — *see* Puncture, thorax
  - digit(s)
    - foot — *see* Puncture, toe
    - hand — *see* Puncture, finger
  - ear (canal) (external) S01.339- ☑
    - with foreign body S01.349- ☑
    - drum S09.2- ☑
    - left S01.332- ☑
      - with foreign body S01.342- ☑
    - right S01.331- ☑
      - with foreign body S01.341- ☑
  - elbow S51.039- ☑
    - with
      - foreign body S51.049- ☑
    - left S51.032- ☑
      - with
        - foreign body S51.042- ☑
    - right S51.031- ☑
      - with
        - foreign body S51.041- ☑
  - epididymis — *see* Puncture, testis
  - epigastric region — *see* Puncture, abdomen, wall, epigastric
  - epiglottis S11.83- ☑
    - with foreign body S11.84- ☑
  - esophagus
    - cervical S11.23- ☑
      - with foreign body S11.24- ☑
    - thoracic S27.818- ☑
  - eyeball S05.6- ☑
    - with foreign body S05.5- ☑
  - eyebrow — *see* Puncture, eyelid
  - eyelid S01.13- ☑
    - with foreign body S01.14- ☑
    - left S01.132- ☑

- **Puncture** — *continued*
  - eyelid — *continued*
    - left — *continued*
      - with foreign body S01.142- ☑
    - right S01.131- ☑
      - with foreign body S01.141- ☑
  - face NEC — *see* Puncture, head, specified site NEC
  - finger(s) S61.239- ☑
    - with
      - damage to nail S61.339- ☑
        - with
          - foreign body S61.349- ☑
      - foreign body S61.249- ☑
    - index S61.238- ☑
      - with
        - damage to nail S61.338- ☑
          - with
            - foreign body S61.348- ☑
        - foreign body S61.248- ☑
      - left S61.231- ☑
        - with
          - damage to nail S61.331- ☑
            - with
              - foreign body S61.341- ☑
          - foreign body S61.241- ☑
      - right S61.230- ☑
        - with
          - damage to nail S61.330- ☑
            - with
              - foreign body S61.340- ☑
          - foreign body S61.240- ☑
    - little S61.238- ☑
      - with
        - damage to nail S61.338- ☑
          - with
            - foreign body S61.348- ☑
        - foreign body S61.248- ☑
      - left S61.237- ☑
        - with
          - damage to nail S61.337- ☑
            - with
              - foreign body S61.347- ☑
          - foreign body S61.247- ☑
      - right S61.236- ☑
        - with
          - damage to nail S61.336- ☑
            - with
              - foreign body S61.346- ☑
          - foreign body S61.246- ☑
    - middle S61.238- ☑
      - with
        - damage to nail S61.338- ☑
          - with
            - foreign body S61.348- ☑
        - foreign body S61.248- ☑
      - left S61.233- ☑
        - with
          - damage to nail S61.333- ☑
            - with
              - foreign body S61.343- ☑
          - foreign body S61.243- ☑
      - right S61.232- ☑
        - with
          - damage to nail S61.332- ☑
            - with
              - foreign body S61.342- ☑
          - foreign body S61.242- ☑
    - ring S61.238- ☑
      - with
        - damage to nail S61.338- ☑
          - with
            - foreign body S61.348- ☑
        - foreign body S61.248- ☑
      - left S61.235- ☑
        - with
          - damage to nail S61.335- ☑
            - with
              - foreign body S61.345- ☑
          - foreign body S61.245- ☑
      - right S61.234- ☑
        - with
          - damage to nail S61.334- ☑
            - with
              - foreign body S61.344- ☑
          - foreign body S61.244- ☑
  - flank S31.13A- ☑

- **Puncture** — *continued*
  - flank — *continued*
    - with
      - foreign body S31.14A- ☑
      - penetration into peritoneal cavity S31.63A- ☑
        - with foreign body S31.64A- ☑
    - left S31.137- ☑
      - with
        - foreign body S31.147- ☑
        - penetration into peritoneal cavity S31.637- ☑
          - with foreign body S31.647- ☑
    - right S31.136- ☑
      - with
        - foreign body S31.146- ☑
        - penetration into peritoneal cavity S31.636- ☑
          - with foreign body S31.646- ☑
  - foot (except toe(s) alone) S91.339- ☑
    - with foreign body S91.349- ☑
    - left S91.332- ☑
      - with foreign body S91.342- ☑
    - right S91.331- ☑
      - with foreign body S91.341- ☑
    - toe — *see* Puncture, toe
  - forearm S51.839- ☑
    - with
      - foreign body S51.849- ☑
    - elbow only — *see* Puncture, elbow
    - left S51.832- ☑
      - with
        - foreign body S51.842- ☑
    - right S51.831- ☑
      - with
        - foreign body S51.841- ☑
  - forehead — *see* Puncture, head, specified site NEC
  - genital organs, external
    - female S31.532- ☑
      - with foreign body S31.542- ☑
      - vagina — *see* Puncture, vagina
      - vulva — *see* Puncture, vulva
    - male S31.531- ☑
      - with foreign body S31.541- ☑
      - penis — *see* Puncture, penis
      - scrotum — *see* Puncture, scrotum
      - testis — *see* Puncture, testis
  - groin — *see* Puncture, abdomen, wall
  - gum — *see* Puncture, oral cavity
  - hand S61.439- ☑
    - with
      - foreign body S61.449- ☑
    - finger — *see* Puncture, finger
    - left S61.432- ☑
      - with
        - foreign body S61.442- ☑
    - right S61.431- ☑
      - with
        - foreign body S61.441- ☑
    - thumb — *see* Puncture, thumb
  - head SØ1.93- ☑
    - with foreign body SØ1.94- ☑
    - cheek — *see* Puncture, cheek
    - ear — *see* Puncture, ear
    - eyelid — *see* Puncture, eyelid
    - lip — *see* Puncture, oral cavity
    - nose — *see* Puncture, nose
    - oral cavity — *see* Puncture, oral cavity
    - scalp SØ1.Ø3- ☑
      - with foreign body SØ1.Ø4- ☑
    - specified site NEC SØ1.83- ☑
      - with foreign body SØ1.84- ☑
    - temporomandibular area — *see* Puncture, cheek
  - heart S26.99- ☑
    - with hemopericardium S26.Ø9- ☑
    - without hemopericardium S26.19- ☑
  - heel — *see* Puncture, foot
  - hip S71.Ø39- ☑
    - with foreign body S71.Ø49- ☑
    - left S71.Ø32- ☑
      - with foreign body S71.Ø42- ☑
    - right S71.Ø31- ☑
      - with foreign body S71.Ø41- ☑
  - hymen — *see* Puncture, vagina
  - hypochondrium — *see* Puncture, abdomen, wall
  - hypogastric region — *see* Puncture, abdomen, wall
  - inguinal region — *see* Puncture, abdomen, wall
  - instep — *see* Puncture, foot
  - internal organs — *see* Injury, by site

- **Puncture** — *continued*
  - interscapular region — *see* Puncture, thorax, back
  - intestine
    - large
      - colon S36.599- ☑
        - ascending S36.59Ø- ☑
        - descending S36.592- ☑
        - sigmoid S36.593- ☑
        - specified site NEC S36.598- ☑
        - transverse S36.591- ☑
      - rectum S36.69- ☑
    - small S36.499- ☑
      - duodenum S36.49Ø- ☑
      - specified site NEC S36.498- ☑
  - intra-abdominal organ S36.99- ☑
    - gallbladder S36.128- ☑
    - intestine — *see* Puncture, intestine
    - liver S36.118- ☑
    - pancreas — *see* Puncture, pancreas
    - peritoneum S36.81- ☑
    - specified site NEC S36.898- ☑
    - spleen S36.Ø9- ☑
    - stomach S36.39- ☑
  - jaw — *see* Puncture, head, specified site NEC
  - knee S81.Ø39- ☑
    - with foreign body S81.Ø49- ☑
    - left S81.Ø32- ☑
      - with foreign body S81.Ø42- ☑
    - right S81.Ø31- ☑
      - with foreign body S81.Ø41- ☑
  - labium (majus) (minus) — *see* Puncture, vulva
  - lacrimal duct — *see* Puncture, eyelid
  - larynx S11.Ø13- ☑
    - with foreign body S11.Ø14- ☑
  - leg (lower) S81.839- ☑
    - with foreign body S81.849- ☑
    - foot — *see* Puncture, foot
    - knee — *see* Puncture, knee
    - left S81.832- ☑
      - with foreign body S81.842- ☑
    - right S81.831- ☑
      - with foreign body S81.841- ☑
    - upper — *see* Puncture, thigh
  - lip SØ1.531- ☑
    - with foreign body SØ1.541- ☑
  - loin — *see* Puncture, abdomen, wall
  - lower back — *see* Puncture, back, lower
  - lumbar region — *see* Puncture, back, lower
  - malar region — *see* Puncture, head, specified site NEC
  - mammary — *see* Puncture, breast
  - mastoid region — *see* Puncture, head, specified site NEC
  - mouth — *see* Puncture, oral cavity
  - nail
    - finger — *see* Puncture, finger, with damage to nail
    - toe — *see* Puncture, toe, with damage to nail
  - nasal (septum) (sinus) — *see* Puncture, nose
  - nasopharynx — *see* Puncture, head, specified site NEC
  - neck S11.93- ☑
    - with foreign body S11.94- ☑
    - involving
      - cervical esophagus — *see* Puncture, cervical esophagus
      - larynx — *see* Puncture, larynx
      - pharynx — *see* Puncture, pharynx
      - thyroid gland — *see* Puncture, thyroid gland
      - trachea — *see* Puncture, trachea
    - specified site NEC S11.83- ☑
      - with foreign body S11.84- ☑
  - nose (septum) (sinus) SØ1.23- ☑
    - with foreign body SØ1.24- ☑
  - ocular — *see* Puncture, eyeball
  - oral cavity SØ1.532- ☑
    - with foreign body SØ1.542- ☑
  - orbit SØ5.4- ☑
  - palate — *see* Puncture, oral cavity
  - palm — *see* Puncture, hand
  - pancreas S36.299- ☑
    - body S36.291- ☑
    - head S36.29Ø- ☑
    - tail S36.292- ☑
  - pelvis — *see* Puncture, back, lower
  - penis S31.23- ☑
    - with foreign body S31.24- ☑
  - perineum
    - female S31.43- ☑
      - with foreign body S31.44- ☑

- **Puncture** — *continued*
  - perineum — *continued*
    - male S31.139- ☑
      - with foreign body S31.149- ☑
  - periocular area (with or without lacrimal passages) — *see* Puncture, eyelid
  - phalanges
    - finger — *see* Puncture, finger
    - toe — *see* Puncture, toe
  - pharynx S11.23- ☑
    - with foreign body S11.24- ☑
  - pinna — *see* Puncture, ear
  - popliteal space — *see* Puncture, knee
  - prepuce — *see* Puncture, penis
  - pubic region S31.139- ☑
    - with foreign body S31.149- ☑
  - pudendum — *see* Puncture, genital organs, external
  - rectovaginal septum — *see* Puncture, vagina
  - sacral region — *see* Puncture, back, lower
  - sacroiliac region — *see* Puncture, back, lower
  - salivary gland — *see* Puncture, oral cavity
  - scalp SØ1.Ø3- ☑
    - with foreign body SØ1.Ø4- ☑
  - scapular region — *see* Puncture, shoulder
  - scrotum S31.33- ☑
    - with foreign body S31.34- ☑
  - shin — *see* Puncture, leg
  - shoulder S41.Ø39- ☑
    - with foreign body S41.Ø49- ☑
    - left S41.Ø32- ☑
      - with foreign body S41.Ø42- ☑
    - right S41.Ø31- ☑
      - with foreign body S41.Ø41- ☑
  - spermatic cord — *see* Puncture, testis
  - sternal region — *see* Puncture, thorax, front
  - submaxillary region — *see* Puncture, head, specified site NEC
  - submental region — *see* Puncture, head, specified site NEC
  - subungual
    - finger(s) — *see* Puncture, finger, with damage to nail
    - toe — *see* Puncture, toe, with damage to nail
  - supraclavicular fossa — *see* Puncture, neck, specified site NEC
  - temple, temporal region — *see* Puncture, head, specified site NEC
  - temporomandibular area — *see* Puncture, cheek
  - testis S31.33- ☑
    - with foreign body S31.34- ☑
  - thigh S71.139- ☑
    - with foreign body S71.149- ☑
    - left S71.132- ☑
      - with foreign body S71.142- ☑
    - right S71.131- ☑
      - with foreign body S71.141- ☑
  - thorax, thoracic (wall) S21.93- ☑
    - with foreign body S21.94- ☑
    - back S21.23- ☑
      - with
        - foreign body S21.24- ☑
          - with penetration S21.44- ☑
        - penetration S21.43- ☑
    - breast — *see* Puncture, breast
    - front S21.13- ☑
      - with
        - foreign body S21.14- ☑
          - with penetration S21.34- ☑
        - penetration S21.33- ☑
  - throat — *see* Puncture, neck
  - thumb S61.Ø39- ☑
    - with
      - damage to nail S61.139- ☑
        - with
          - foreign body S61.149- ☑
      - foreign body S61.Ø49- ☑
    - left S61.Ø32- ☑
      - with
        - damage to nail S61.132- ☑
          - with
            - foreign body S61.142- ☑
        - foreign body S61.Ø42- ☑
    - right S61.Ø31- ☑
      - with
        - damage to nail S61.131- ☑
          - with
            - foreign body S61.141- ☑
        - foreign body S61.Ø41- ☑

- **Puncture** — *continued*
  - thyroid gland S11.13- ☑
    - with foreign body S11.14- ☑
  - toe(s) S91.139- ☑
    - with
      - damage to nail S91.239- ☑
        - with
          - foreign body S91.249- ☑
      - foreign body S91.149- ☑
    - great S91.133- ☑
      - with
        - damage to nail S91.233- ☑
          - with
            - foreign body S91.243- ☑
        - foreign body S91.143- ☑
      - left S91.132- ☑
        - with
          - damage to nail S91.232- ☑
            - with
              - foreign body S91.242- ☑
          - foreign body S91.142- ☑
      - right S91.131- ☑
        - with
          - damage to nail S91.231- ☑
            - with
              - foreign body S91.241- ☑
          - foreign body S91.141- ☑
    - lesser S91.136- ☑
      - with
        - damage to nail S91.236- ☑
          - with
            - foreign body S91.246- ☑
        - foreign body S91.146- ☑
      - left S91.135- ☑
        - with
          - damage to nail S91.235- ☑
            - with
              - foreign body S91.245- ☑
          - foreign body S91.145- ☑
      - right S91.134- ☑
        - with
          - damage to nail S91.234- ☑
            - with
              - foreign body S91.244- ☑
          - foreign body S91.144- ☑
  - tongue — *see* Puncture, oral cavity
  - trachea S11.Ø23- ☑
    - with foreign body S11.Ø24- ☑
  - tunica vaginalis — *see* Puncture, testis
  - tympanum, tympanic membrane SØ9.2- ☑
  - umbilical region S31.135- ☑
    - with foreign body S31.145- ☑
  - uvula — *see* Puncture, oral cavity
  - vagina S31.43- ☑
    - with foreign body S31.44- ☑
  - vocal cords S11.Ø33- ☑
    - with foreign body S11.Ø34- ☑
  - vulva S31.43- ☑
    - with foreign body S31.44- ☑
  - wrist S61.539- ☑
    - with
      - foreign body S61.549- ☑
    - left S61.532- ☑
      - with
        - foreign body S61.542- ☑
    - right S61.531- ☑
      - with
        - foreign body S61.541- ☑
- **PUO** (pyrexia of unknown origin) R5Ø.9
- **Pupillary membrane** (persistent) Q13.89
- **Pupillotonia** — *see* Anomaly, pupil, function, tonic pupil
- **Purpura** D69.2
  - abdominal D69.Ø
  - allergic D69.Ø
  - anaphylactoid D69.Ø
  - annularis telangiectodes L81.7
  - arthritic D69.Ø
  - autoerythrocyte sensitization D69.2
  - autoimmune D69.Ø
  - bacterial D69.Ø
  - Bateman's (senile) D69.2
  - capillary fragility (hereditary) (idiopathic) D69.8
  - cryoglobulinemic D89.1
  - Devil's pinches D69.2
  - fibrinolytic — *see* Fibrinolysis
  - fulminans, fulminous D65
  - gangrenous D65
- **Purpura** — *continued*
  - hemorrhagic, hemorrhagica D69.3
    - not due to thrombocytopenia D69.Ø
  - Henoch (-Schonlein) (allergic) D69.Ø
  - hypergammaglobulinemic (benign) (Waldenstrom) D89.Ø
  - idiopathic (thrombocytopenic) D69.3
    - nonthrombocytopenic D69.Ø
  - immune thrombocytopenic D69.3
  - infectious D69.Ø
  - malignant D69.Ø
  - neonatorum P54.5
  - nervosa D69.Ø
  - newborn P54.5
  - nonthrombocytopenic D69.2
    - hemorrhagic D69.Ø
    - idiopathic D69.Ø
  - nonthrombopenic D69.2
  - peliosis rheumatica D69.Ø
  - posttransfusion (post-transfusion) (from (fresh) whole blood or blood products) D69.51
  - primary D69.49
  - red cell membrane sensitivity D69.2
  - rheumatica D69.Ø
  - Schonlein (-Henoch) (allergic) D69.Ø
  - scorbutic E54 *[D77]*
  - senile D69.2
  - simplex D69.2
  - symptomatica D69.Ø
  - telangiectasia annularis L81.7
  - thrombocytopenic D69.49
    - congenital D69.42
    - hemorrhagic D69.3
    - hereditary D69.42
    - idiopathic D69.3
    - immune D69.3
    - neonatal, transitory P61.Ø
    - thrombotic M31.19
  - thrombohemolytic — *see* Fibrinolysis
  - thrombolytic — *see* Fibrinolysis
  - thrombopenic D69.49
  - thrombotic, thrombocytopenic M31.19
  - toxic D69.Ø
  - vascular D69.Ø
  - visceral symptoms D69.Ø
- **Purpuric spots** R23.3
- **Purulent** — *see* condition
- **Pus**
  - in
    - stool R19.5
    - urine N39.Ø
  - tube (rupture) — *see* Salpingo-oophoritis
- **Pustular rash** LØ8.Ø
- **Pustule** (nonmalignant) LØ8.9
  - malignant A22.Ø
- **Pustulosis palmaris et plantaris** L4Ø.3
- **Putnam** (-Dana) **disease or syndrome** — *see* Degeneration, combined
- **Putrescent pulp** (dental) KØ4.1
- **Pyarthritis, pyarthrosis** — *see* Arthritis, pyogenic or pyemic
  - tuberculous — *see* Tuberculosis, joint
- **Pyelectasis** — *see* Hydronephrosis
- **Pyelitis** (congenital) (uremic) — *see also* Pyelonephritis
  - with
    - calculus — *see* category N2Ø.- ☑
      - with hydronephrosis N13.6
    - contracted kidney N11.9
  - acute N1Ø
  - chronic N11.9
    - with calculus — *see* category N2Ø.- ☑
      - with hydronephrosis N13.6
  - cystica N28.84
  - puerperal (postpartum) O86.21
  - tuberculous A18.11
- **Pyelocystitis** — *see* Pyelonephritis
- **Pyelonephritis** — *see also* Nephritis, tubulo-interstitial
  - with
    - calculus — *see* category N2Ø.- ☑
      - with hydronephrosis N13.6
    - contracted kidney N11.9
  - acute N1Ø
  - calculous — *see* category N2Ø.- ☑
    - with hydronephrosis N13.6
  - chronic N11.9
    - with calculus — *see* category N2Ø.- ☑
      - with hydronephrosis N13.6
    - associated with ureteral obstruction or stricture N11.1
    - nonobstructive N11.8
      - with reflux (vesicoureteral) N11.Ø
- **Pyelonephritis** — *continued*
  - chronic — *continued*
    - obstructive N11.1
    - specified NEC N11.8
  - in (due to)
    - brucellosis A23.9 *[N16]*
    - cryoglobulinemia (mixed) D89.1 *[N16]*
    - cystinosis E72.Ø4
    - diphtheria A36.84
    - glycogen storage disease E74.Ø9 *[N16]*
    - leukemia NEC C95.9- ☑ *[N16]*
    - lymphoma NEC C85.9Ø *[N16]*
    - multiple myeloma C9Ø.Ø- ☑ *[N16]*
    - obstruction N11.1
    - Salmonella infection AØ2.25
    - sarcoidosis D86.84
    - sepsis A41.9 *[N16]*
    - Sjogren's disease M35.Ø4
    - toxoplasmosis B58.83
    - transplant rejection T86.91 *[N16]*
    - Wilson's disease E83.Ø1 *[N16]*
  - nonobstructive N12
    - with reflux (vesicoureteral) N11.Ø
    - chronic N11.8
  - syphilitic A52.75
- **Pyelonephrosis** (obstructive) N11.1
  - chronic N11.9
- **Pyelophlebitis** I8Ø.8
- **Pyeloureteritis cystica** N28.85
- **Pyemia, pyemic** (fever) (infection) (purulent) — *see also* Sepsis
  - joint — *see* Arthritis, pyogenic or pyemic
  - liver K75.1
  - pneumococcal A4Ø.3
  - portal K75.1
  - postvaccinal T88.Ø- ☑
  - puerperal, postpartum, childbirth O85
  - specified organism NEC A41.89
  - tuberculous — *see* Tuberculosis, miliary
- **Pygopagus** Q89.4
- **Pyknoepilepsy** (idiopathic) — *see* Pyknolepsy
- **Pyknolepsy** G4Ø.AØ9 (*following* G4Ø.3)
  - intractable G4Ø.A19 (*following* G4Ø.3)
    - with status epilepticus G4Ø.A11 (*following* G4Ø.3)
    - without status epilepticus G4Ø.A19 (*following* G4Ø.3)
  - not intractable G4Ø.AØ9 (*following* G4Ø.3)
    - with status epilepticus G4Ø.AØ1 (*following* G4Ø.3)
    - without status epilepticus G4Ø.AØ9 (*following* G4Ø.3)
- **Pylephlebitis** K75.1
- **Pyle's syndrome** Q78.5
- **Pylethrombophlebitis** K75.1
- **Pylethrombosis** K75.1
- **Pyloritis** K29.9Ø
  - with bleeding K29.91
- **Pylorospasm** (reflex) **NEC** K31.3
  - congenital Q4Ø.Ø
  - neurotic F45.8
  - newborn Q4Ø.Ø
  - psychogenic F45.8
- **Pylorus, pyloric** — *see* condition
- **Pyo-oophoritis** — *see* Salpingo-oophoritis
- **Pyo-ovarium** — *see* Salpingo-oophoritis
- **Pyoarthrosis** — *see* Arthritis, pyogenic or pyemic
- **Pyocele**
  - mastoid — *see* Mastoiditis, acute
  - sinus (accessory) — *see* Sinusitis
  - turbinate (bone) J32.9
  - urethra — *see also* Urethritis N34.Ø
- **Pyocolpos** — *see* Vaginitis
- **Pyocystitis** N3Ø.8Ø
  - with hematuria N3Ø.81
- **Pyoderma, pyodermia** LØ8.Ø
  - gangrenosum L88
  - newborn P39.4
  - phagedenic L88
  - vegetans LØ8.81
- **Pyodermatitis** LØ8.Ø
  - vegetans LØ8.81
- **Pyogenic** — *see* condition
- **Pyohydronephrosis** N13.6
- **Pyometra, pyometrium, pyometritis** — *see* Endometritis
- **Pyomyositis** (tropical) — *see* Myositis, infective
- **Pyonephritis** N12
- **Pyonephrosis** N13.6
  - tuberculous A18.11
- **Pyopericarditis, pyopericardium** I3Ø.1
- **Pyophlebitis** — *see* Phlebitis
- **Pyopneumopericardium** I3Ø.1
- **Pyopneumothorax** (infective) J86.9

- **Pyopneumothorax** — *continued*
  - with fistula J86.Ø
  - tuberculous NEC A15.6
- **Pyosalpinx, pyosalpingitis** — *see also* Salpingo-oophoritis
- **Pyothorax** J86.9
  - with fistula J86.Ø
  - tuberculous NEC A15.6
- **Pyoureter** N28.89
  - tuberculous A18.11
- **Pyramidopallidonigral syndrome** G2Ø.C
- **Pyrexia** (of unknown origin) R5Ø.9
  - atmospheric T67.Ø1- ☑
  - during labor NEC O75.2
  - heat T67.Ø1- ☑
  - newborn P81.9
    - environmentally-induced P81.Ø
  - persistent R5Ø.9
  - puerperal O86.4
- **Pyroglobulinemia NEC** E88.Ø9
- **Pyromania** F63.1
- **Pyrosis** R12
- **Pyuria** (bacterial) (sterile) R82.81

# Q

- **Q fever** A78
  - with pneumonia A78
- **Quadricuspid aortic valve** Q23.88
- **Quadrilateral fever** A78
- **Quadriparesis** — *see* Quadriplegia
  - meaning muscle weakness M62.81
- **Quadriplegia** G82.5Ø
  - complete
    - C1-C4 level G82.51
    - C5-C7 level G82.53
  - congenital (cerebral) (spinal) G8Ø.8
    - spastic G8Ø.Ø
  - embolic (current episode) I63.4- ☑
  - functional R53.2
  - incomplete
    - C1-C4 level G82.52
    - C5-C7 level G82.54
  - thrombotic (current episode) I63.3- ☑
  - traumatic — *code to* injury with seventh character S
    - current episode — *see* Injury, spinal (cord), cervical
- **Quadruplet, pregnancy** — *see* Pregnancy, quadruplet
- **Quarrelsomeness** F6Ø.3
- **Queensland fever** A77.3
- **Quervain's disease** M65.4
  - thyroid EØ6.1
- **Queyrat's erythroplasia** DØ7.4
  - penis DØ7.4
  - specified site — *see* Neoplasm, skin, in situ
  - unspecified site DØ7.4
- **Quincke's disease or edema** T78.3- ☑
  - hereditary D84.1
- **Quinsy** (gangrenous) J36
- **Quintan fever** A79.Ø
- **Quintuplet, pregnancy** — *see* Pregnancy, quintuplet

# R

- **Rabbit fever** — *see* Tularemia
- **Rabies** A82.9
  - contact Z2Ø.3
  - exposure to Z2Ø.3
  - inoculation reaction — *see* Complications, vaccination
  - sylvatic A82.Ø
  - urban A82.1
- **Rachischisis** — *see* Spina bifida
- **Rachitic** — *see also* condition
  - deformities of spine (late effect) (sequelae) E64.3
  - pelvis (late effect) (sequelae) E64.3
    - with disproportion (fetopelvic) O33.Ø
      - causing obstructed labor O65.Ø
- **Rachitis, rachitism** (acute) (tarda) — *see also* Rickets
  - renalis N25.Ø
  - sequelae E64.3
- **Radial nerve** — *see* condition
- **Radiation**
  - burn — *see* Burn
  - effects NOS T66.- ☑
  - sickness NOS T66.- ☑
  - therapy, encounter for Z51.Ø
- **Radiculitis** (pressure) (vertebrogenic) — *see* Radiculopathy
- **Radiculomyelitis** — *see also* Encephalitis
  - toxic, due to
    - Clostridium tetani A35
- **Radiculomyelitis** — *continued*
  - toxic, due to — *continued*
    - Corynebacterium diphtheriae A36.82
- **Radiculopathy** M54.1Ø
  - cervical region M54.12
  - cervicothoracic region M54.13
  - due to
    - disc disorder
      - C3 M5Ø.11
      - C4 M5Ø.11
      - C5 M5Ø.121
      - C6 M5Ø.122
      - C7 M5Ø.123
    - displacement of intervertebral disc — *see* Disorder, disc, with, radiculopathy
  - leg M54.1- ☑
  - lumbar region M54.16
  - lumbosacral region M54.17
  - occipito-atlanto-axial region M54.11
  - postherpetic BØ2.29
  - sacrococcygeal region M54.18
  - syphilitic A52.11
  - thoracic region (with visceral pain) M54.14
  - thoracolumbar region M54.15
- **Radiodermal burns** (acute, chronic, or occupational) — *see* Burn
- **Radiodermatitis** L58.9
  - acute L58.Ø
  - chronic L58.1
- **Radiotherapy session** Z51.Ø
- **RAEB** (refractory anemia with excess blasts) D46.2- ☑
- **Rage, meaning rabies** — *see* Rabies
- **Ragpicker's disease** A22.1
- **Ragsorter's disease** A22.1
- **Raillietiniasis** B71.8
- **Railroad neurosis** F48.8
- **Railway spine** F48.8
- **Raised** — *see also* Elevated
  - antibody titer R76.Ø
- **Rake teeth, tooth** M26.39
- **Rales** RØ9.89
- **Ramifying renal pelvis** Q63.8
- **Ramsay-Hunt disease or syndrome** — *see also* Hunt's, disease BØ2.21
  - meaning dyssynergia cerebellaris myoclonica G11.19
- **Ranula** K11.6
  - congenital Q38.4
- **Rape**
  - adult
    - confirmed T74.21- ☑
    - suspected T76.21- ☑
  - alleged, observation or examination, ruled out
    - adult ZØ4.41
    - child ZØ4.42
  - child
    - confirmed T74.22- ☑
    - suspected T76.22- ☑
- **Rapid**
  - feeble pulse, due to shock, following injury T79.4- ☑
  - heart (beat) RØØ.Ø
    - psychogenic F45.8
  - second stage (delivery) O62.3
  - time-zone change syndrome G47.25
- **Rarefaction, bone** — *see* Disorder, bone, density and structure, specified NEC
- **Rash** (toxic) R21
  - canker A38.9
  - diaper L22
  - drug (internal use) L27.Ø
    - contact — *see also* Dermatitis, due to, drugs, external L25.1
  - following immunization T88.1- ☑
  - food — *see* Dermatitis, due to, food
  - heat L74.Ø
  - napkin (psoriasiform) L22
  - nettle — *see* Urticaria
  - pustular LØ8.Ø
  - rose R21
    - epidemic BØ6.9
  - scarlet A38.9
  - serum — *see also* Reaction, serum T8Ø.69- ☑
  - wandering tongue K14.1
- **Rasmussen aneurysm** — *see* Tuberculosis, pulmonary
- **Rasmussen encephalitis** GØ4.81
- **Rat-bite fever** A25.9
  - due to Streptobacillus moniliformis A25.1
  - spirochetal (morsus muris) A25.Ø
- **Rathke's pouch tumor** D44.3
- **Raymond** (-Cestan) **syndrome** I65.8
- **Raynaud's disease, phenomenon or syndrome** (secondary) I73.ØØ
  - with gangrene (symmetric) I73.Ø1
- **RDS** (newborn) (type I) P22.Ø
  - type II P22.1
- **Reaction** — *see also* Disorder
  - adaptation — *see* Disorder, adjustment
  - adjustment (anxiety) (conduct disorder) (depressiveness) (distress) — *see* Disorder, adjustment
    - with
      - mutism, elective (child) (adolescent) F94.Ø
  - adverse
    - food (any) (ingested) NEC T78.19- ☑
      - anaphylactic — *see* Shock, anaphylactic, due to food
  - affective — *see* Disorder, mood
  - allergic — *see* Allergy
  - anaphylactic — *see* Shock, anaphylactic
  - anaphylactoid — *see* Shock, anaphylactic
  - anesthesia — *see* Anesthesia, complication
  - antitoxin (prophylactic) (therapeutic) — *see* Complications, vaccination
  - anxiety F41.1
  - Arthus — *see* Arthus' phenomenon
  - asthenic F48.8
  - combat and operational stress F43.Ø
  - compulsive F42.8
  - conversion F44.9
  - crisis, acute F43.Ø
  - deoxyribonuclease (DNA) (DNase) hypersensitivity D69.2
  - depressive (single episode) F32.9
    - affective (single episode) F31.4
      - recurrent episode F33.9
    - neurotic F34.1
    - psychoneurotic F34.1
    - psychotic F32.3
    - recurrent — *see* Disorder, depressive, recurrent
  - dissociative F44.9
  - drug NEC T88.7- ☑
    - addictive — *see* Dependence, drug
      - transmitted via placenta or breast milk — *see* Absorption, drug, addictive, through placenta
    - allergic — *see* Allergy, drug
    - lichenoid L43.2
    - newborn P93.8
      - gray baby syndrome P93.Ø
    - overdose or poisoning (by accident) — *see* Table of Drugs and Chemicals, by drug, poisoning
    - photoallergic L56.1
    - phototoxic L56.Ø
    - withdrawal — *see* Dependence, by drug, with, withdrawal
      - infant of dependent mother P96.1
      - newborn P96.1
    - wrong substance given or taken (by accident) — *see* Table of Drugs and Chemicals, by drug, poisoning
  - fear F4Ø.9
    - child (abnormal) F93.8
  - febrile nonhemolytic transfusion (FNHTR) R5Ø.84
  - fluid loss, cerebrospinal G97.1
  - foreign
    - body NEC — *see* Granuloma, foreign body
      - in operative wound (inadvertently left) — *see* Foreign body, accidentally left during a procedure
    - substance accidentally left during a procedure (chemical) (powder) (talc) T81.6Ø- ☑
      - aseptic peritonitis T81.61- ☑
      - body or object (instrument) (sponge) (swab) — *see* Foreign body, accidentally left during a procedure
      - specified reaction NEC T81.69- ☑
  - grief — *see* Disorder, adjustment
  - Herxheimer's R68.89
  - hyperkinetic — *see* Hyperkinesia
  - hypochondriacal F45.2Ø
  - hypoglycemic, due to insulin E16.Ø
    - with coma (diabetic) — *see* Diabetes, coma
      - nondiabetic E15
    - therapeutic misadventure — *see* subcategory T38.3- ☑
  - hypomanic F3Ø.8
  - hysterical F44.9
  - immunization — *see* Complications, vaccination

Index Pyopneumothorax — Reaction

- **Rejection**
  - food, psychogenic F5Ø.89
  - transplant T86.91
    - bone T86.83Ø
      - marrow T86.Ø1
    - cornea T86.84Ø- ☑
    - heart T86.21
      - with lung(s) T86.31
    - intestine T86.85Ø
    - kidney T86.11
    - liver T86.41
    - lung(s) T86.81Ø
      - with heart T86.31
    - organ (immune or nonimmune cause) T86.91
    - pancreas T86.89Ø
    - skin (allograft) (autograft) T86.82Ø
    - specified NEC T86.89Ø
    - stem cell (peripheral blood) (umbilical cord) T86.5
- **Relapsing fever** A68.9
  - Carter's (Asiatic) A68.1
  - Dutton's (West African) A68.1
  - Koch's A68.9
  - louse-borne (epidemic) A68.Ø
  - Novy's (American) A68.1
  - Obermeyer's (European) A68.Ø
  - Spirillum A68.9
  - tick-borne (endemic) A68.1
- **Relationship**
  - occlusal
    - open anterior M26.22Ø
    - open posterior M26.221
- **Relaxation**
  - anus (sphincter) K62.89
    - psychogenic F45.8
  - arch (foot) — *see also* Deformity, limb, flat foot
  - back ligaments — *see* Instability, joint, spine
  - bladder (sphincter) N31.2
  - cardioesophageal K21.9
  - cervix — *see* Incompetency, cervix
  - diaphragm J98.6
  - joint (capsule) (ligament) (paralytic) — *see* Flail, joint
    - congenital NEC Q74.8
  - lumbosacral (joint) — *see* subcategory M53.2- ☑
  - pelvic floor N81.89
  - perineum N81.89
  - posture R29.3
  - rectum (sphincter) K62.89
  - sacroiliac (joint) — *see* subcategory M53.2- ☑
  - scrotum N5Ø.89
  - urethra (sphincter) N36.44
  - vesical N31.2
- **Release from prison, anxiety concerning** Z65.2
- **Remains**
  - canal of Cloquet Q14.Ø
  - capsule (opaque) Q14.8
- **Remittent fever** (malarial) B54
- **Remnant**
  - canal of Cloquet Q14.Ø
  - capsule (opaque) Q14.8
  - cervix, cervical stump (acquired) (postoperative) N88.8
  - cystic duct, postcholecystectomy K91.5
  - fingernail L6Ø.8
    - congenital Q84.6
  - meniscus, knee — *see* Derangement, knee, meniscus, specified NEC
  - thyroglossal duct Q89.2
  - tonsil J35.8
    - infected (chronic) J35.Ø1
  - urachus Q64.4
- **Removal** (from) (of)
  - artificial
    - arm Z44.ØØ- ☑
      - complete Z44.Ø1- ☑
      - partial Z44.Ø2- ☑
    - eye Z44.2- ☑
    - leg Z44.1Ø- ☑
      - complete Z44.11- ☑
      - partial Z44.12- ☑
  - breast implant Z45.81- ☑
  - cardiac pulse generator (battery) (end-of-life) Z45.Ø1Ø
  - catheter (urinary) (indwelling) Z46.6
    - from artificial opening — *see* Attention to, artificial, opening
    - non-vascular Z46.82
    - vascular NEC Z45.2
  - device Z46.9
    - contraceptive Z3Ø.432
      - implantable subdermal Z3Ø.46

- **Removal** — *continued*
  - device — *continued*
    - implanted NEC Z45.89
    - specified NEC Z46.89
  - drains Z48.Ø3
  - dressing (nonsurgical) Z48.ØØ
    - surgical Z48.Ø1
  - external
    - fixation device — *code to* fracture with seventh character D
    - prosthesis, prosthetic device Z44.9
      - breast Z44.3- ☑
      - specified NEC Z44.8
  - home in childhood (to foster home or institution) Z62.29
  - ileostomy Z43.2
  - insulin pump Z46.81
  - myringotomy device (stent) (tube) Z45.82
  - nervous system device NEC Z46.2
    - brain neuropacemaker Z46.2
    - visual substitution device Z46.2
      - implanted Z45.31
  - non-vascular catheter Z46.82
  - organ, prophylactic (for neoplasia management) — *see* Prophylactic, organ removal
  - orthodontic device Z46.4
  - staples Z48.Ø2
  - stent
    - ureteral Z46.6
  - suture Z48.Ø2
  - urinary device Z46.6
  - vascular access device or catheter Z45.2
- **Ren**
  - arcuatus Q63.1
  - mobile, mobilis N28.89
    - congenital Q63.8
  - unguliformis Q63.1
- **Renal** — *see* condition
- **Rendu-Osler-Weber disease or syndrome** I78.Ø
- **Reninoma** D41.Ø- ☑
- **Renon-Delille syndrome** E23.3
- **Reovirus, as cause of disease classified elsewhere** B97.5
- **Repeated falls NEC** R29.6
- **Replaced chromosome by dicentric ring** Q93.2
- **Replacement by artificial or mechanical device or prosthesis of**
  - bladder Z96.Ø
  - blood vessel NEC Z95.828
  - bone NEC Z96.7
  - cochlea Z96.21
  - coronary artery Z95.5
  - eustachian tube Z96.29
  - eye globe Z97.Ø
  - heart Z95.812
    - valve Z95.2
      - prosthetic Z95.2
      - specified NEC Z95.4
      - xenogenic Z95.3
  - intestine Z96.89
  - joint Z96.6Ø
    - hip — *see* Presence, hip joint implant
    - knee — *see* Presence, knee joint implant
    - specified site NEC Z96.698
  - larynx Z96.3
  - lens Z96.1
  - limb(s) — *see* Presence, artificial, limb
  - mandible NEC (for tooth root implant(s)) Z96.5
  - organ NEC Z96.89
  - peripheral vessel NEC Z95.828
  - stapes Z96.29
  - teeth Z97.2
  - tendon Z96.7
  - tissue NEC Z96.89
  - tooth root(s) Z96.5
  - vessel NEC Z95.828
    - coronary (artery) Z95.5
- **Request for expert evidence** ZØ4.89
- **Reserve, decreased or low**
  - cardiac — *see* Disease, heart
  - kidney N28.89
- **Residing**
  - in place not meant for human habitation (abandoned building) (car) (park) (sidewalk) Z59.Ø2
  - on the street Z59.Ø2
- **Residual** — *see also* condition
  - ovary syndrome N99.83
  - state, schizophrenic F2Ø.5
  - urine R39.198
- **Resistance, resistant** (to)
  - activated protein C D68.51

- **Resistance, resistant** — *continued*
  - insulin E88.819
    - complicating pregnancy O26.89- ☑
    - specified type NEC E88.818
  - organism(s)
    - to
      - drug Z16.3Ø
        - aminoglycosides Z16.29
        - amoxicillin Z16.11
        - ampicillin Z16.11
        - antibiotic(s) Z16.2Ø
          - multiple Z16.24
          - specified NEC Z16.29
        - antifungal Z16.32
        - antimicrobial (single) Z16.3Ø
          - multiple Z16.35
          - specified NEC Z16.39
        - antimycobacterial (single) Z16.341
          - multiple Z16.342
        - antiparasitic Z16.31
        - antiviral Z16.33
        - beta lactam antibiotics Z16.1Ø
          - specified NEC Z16.19
        - carbapenem Z16.13
        - cephalosporins Z16.19
        - extended beta lactamase (ESBL) Z16.12
        - fluoroquinolones Z16.23
        - macrolides Z16.29
        - methicillin — *see* MRSA
        - multiple drugs (MDRO)
          - antibiotics Z16.24
          - antimicrobial Z16.35
          - antimycobacterials Z16.342
        - penicillins Z16.11
        - quinine (and related compounds) Z16.31
        - quinolones Z16.23
        - sulfonamides Z16.29
        - tetracyclines Z16.29
        - tuberculostatics (single) Z16.341
          - multiple Z16.342
        - vancomycin Z16.21
          - related antibiotics Z16.22
  - thyroid hormone EØ7.89
- **Resorption**
  - dental (roots) KØ3.3
    - alveoli M26.79
  - teeth (external) (internal) (pathological) (roots) KØ3.3
- **Respiration**
  - Cheyne-Stokes RØ6.3
  - decreased due to shock, following injury T79.4- ☑
  - disorder of, psychogenic F45.8
  - insufficient, or poor RØ6.89
    - newborn P28.5
  - painful RØ7.1
  - sighing, psychogenic F45.8
- **Respiratory** — *see also* condition
  - distress syndrome (newborn) (type I) P22.Ø
    - type II P22.1
  - syncytial virus, as cause of disease classified elsewhere — *see also* Virus, respiratory syncytial (RSV) B97.4
- **Respite care** Z75.5
- **Response** (drug)
  - photoallergic L56.1
  - phototoxic L56.Ø
- **Restenosis**
  - stent
    - vascular
      - end stent
        - adjacent to stent — *see* Arteriosclerosis
        - within the stent
          - coronary T82.855- ☑
          - peripheral T82.856- ☑
      - in stent
        - coronary vessel T82.855- ☑
        - peripheral vessel T82.856- ☑
- **Restless legs** (syndrome) G25.81
- **Restlessness** R45.1
- **Restoration** (of)
  - dental
    - aesthetically inadequate or displeasing KØ8.56
    - defective KØ8.5Ø
      - specified NEC KØ8.59
    - failure of marginal integrity KØ8.51
    - failure of periodontal anatomical integrity KØ8.54
  - organ continuity from previous sterilization (tuboplasty) (vasoplasty) Z31.Ø
    - aftercare Z31.42

**Retroperineal** — *see* condition
**Retroperitoneal** — *see* condition
**Retroperitonitis** K68.9
**Retropharyngeal** — *see* condition
**Retroplacental** — *see* condition
**Retroposition** — *see* Retroversion
**Retroprosthetic membrane** T85.398- ☑
**Retrosternal thyroid** (congenital) Q89.2
**Retroversion, retroverted**
- cervix — *see* Retroversion, uterus
- female NEC — *see* Retroversion, uterus
- iris H21.89
- testis (congenital) Q55.29
- uterus (acquired) (acute) (any degree) (asymptomatic) (cervix) (postinfectional) (postpartal, old) N85.4
  - congenital Q51.818
  - in pregnancy O34.53- ☑

**Retrovirus, as cause of disease classified elsewhere** B97.30
- human
  - immunodeficiency, type 2 (HIV 2) B97.35
  - T-cell lymphotropic
    - type I (HTLV-I) B97.33
    - type II (HTLV-II) B97.34
- lentivirus B97.31
- oncovirus B97.32
- specified NEC B97.39

**Retrusion, premaxilla** (developmental) M26.09
**Rett's disease or syndrome** F84.2
**Reverse peristalsis** R19.2
**Reye's syndrome** G93.7
**Rh** (factor)
- hemolytic disease (newborn) P55.0
- incompatibility, immunization or sensitization
  - affecting management of pregnancy NEC O36.09- ☑
    - anti-D antibody O36.01- ☑
  - newborn P55.0
  - transfusion reaction — *see* Complication(s), transfusion, incompatibility reaction, Rh (factor)
- negative mother affecting newborn P55.0
- titer elevated — *see* Complication(s), transfusion, incompatibility reaction, Rh (factor)
- transfusion reaction — *see* Complication(s), transfusion, incompatibility reaction, Rh (factor)

**Rhabdomyolysis** (idiopathic) NEC M62.82
- traumatic T79.6- ☑

**Rhabdomyoma** — *see also* Neoplasm, connective tissue, benign
- adult — *see* Neoplasm, connective tissue, benign
- fetal — *see* Neoplasm, connective tissue, benign
- glycogenic — *see* Neoplasm, connective tissue, benign

**Rhabdomyosarcoma** (any type) — *see* Neoplasm, connective tissue, malignant
**Rhabdosarcoma** — *see* Rhabdomyosarcoma
**Rhesus** (factor) **incompatibility** — *see* Rh, incompatibility
**Rheumatic** (acute) (subacute)
- adherent pericardium I09.2
- chronic I09.89
- coronary arteritis I01.8
- degeneration, myocardium I09.0
- fever (acute) — *see* Fever, rheumatic
- heart — *see* Disease, heart, rheumatic
- myocardial degeneration — *see* Degeneration, myocardium
- myocarditis (chronic) (inactive) (with chorea) I09.0
  - active or acute I01.2
  - with chorea (acute) (rheumatic) (Sydenham's) I02.0
- pancarditis, acute I01.8
  - with chorea (acute (rheumatic) Sydenham's) I02.0
- pericarditis (active) (acute) (with effusion) (with pneumonia) I01.0
  - with chorea (acute) (rheumatic) (Sydenham's) I02.0
  - chronic or inactive I09.2
- pneumonia I00 *[J17]*
- torticollis M43.6
- typhoid fever A01.09

**Rheumatism** (articular) (neuralgic) (nonarticular) M79.0
- gout — *see* Arthritis, rheumatoid
- intercostal, meaning Tietze's disease M94.0
- palindromic (any site) M12.30
  - ankle M12.37- ☑
  - elbow M12.32- ☑
  - foot joint M12.37- ☑
  - hand joint M12.34- ☑
  - hip M12.35- ☑
  - knee M12.36- ☑
  - multiple site M12.39
  - shoulder M12.31- ☑

**Rheumatism** — *continued*
- palindromic — *continued*
  - specified joint NEC M12.38
  - vertebrae M12.38
  - wrist M12.33- ☑
- sciatic M54.4- ☑

**Rheumatoid** — *see also* condition
- arthritis — *see also* Arthritis, rheumatoid
  - with involvement of organs NEC M05.60
    - ankle M05.67- ☑
    - elbow M05.62- ☑
    - foot joint M05.67- ☑
    - hand joint M05.64- ☑
    - hip M05.65- ☑
    - knee M05.66- ☑
    - multiple site M05.69
    - shoulder M05.61- ☑
    - vertebra — *see* Spondylitis, ankylosing
    - wrist M05.63- ☑
  - seronegative — *see* Arthritis, rheumatoid, seronegative
  - seropositive — *see* Arthritis, rheumatoid, seropositive
- carditis M05.30
  - ankle M05.37- ☑
  - elbow M05.32- ☑
  - foot joint M05.37- ☑
  - hand joint M05.34- ☑
  - hip M05.35- ☑
  - knee M05.36- ☑
  - multiple site M05.39
  - shoulder M05.31- ☑
  - vertebra — *see* Spondylitis, ankylosing
  - wrist M05.33- ☑
- endocarditis — *see* Rheumatoid, carditis
- lung (disease) M05.10
  - ankle M05.17- ☑
  - elbow M05.12- ☑
  - foot joint M05.17- ☑
  - hand joint M05.14- ☑
  - hip M05.15- ☑
  - knee M05.16- ☑
  - multiple site M05.19
  - shoulder M05.11- ☑
  - vertebra — *see* Spondylitis, ankylosing
  - wrist M05.13- ☑
- myocarditis — *see* Rheumatoid, carditis
- myopathy M05.40
  - ankle M05.47- ☑
  - elbow M05.42- ☑
  - foot joint M05.47- ☑
  - hand joint M05.44- ☑
  - hip M05.45- ☑
  - knee M05.46- ☑
  - multiple site M05.49
  - shoulder M05.41- ☑
  - vertebra — *see* Spondylitis, ankylosing
  - wrist M05.43- ☑
- pericarditis — *see* Rheumatoid, carditis
- polyarthritis — *see* Arthritis, rheumatoid
- polyneuropathy M05.50
  - ankle M05.57- ☑
  - elbow M05.52- ☑
  - foot joint M05.57- ☑
  - hand joint M05.54- ☑
  - hip M05.55- ☑
  - knee M05.56- ☑
  - multiple site M05.59
  - shoulder M05.51- ☑
  - vertebra — *see* Spondylitis, ankylosing
  - wrist M05.53- ☑
- vasculitis M05.20
  - ankle M05.27- ☑
  - elbow M05.22- ☑
  - foot joint M05.27- ☑
  - hand joint M05.24- ☑
  - hip M05.25- ☑
  - knee M05.26- ☑
  - multiple site M05.29
  - shoulder M05.21- ☑
  - vertebra — *see* Spondylitis, ankylosing
  - wrist M05.23- ☑

**Rhinitis** (atrophic) (catarrhal) (chronic) (croupous) (fibrinous) (granulomatous) (hyperplastic) (hypertrophic) (membranous) (obstructive) (purulent) (suppurative) (ulcerative) J31.0

**Rhinitis** — *continued*
- with
  - sore throat — *see* Nasopharyngitis
- acute J00
- allergic J30.9
  - with asthma J45.909
    - with
      - exacerbation (acute) J45.901
      - status asthmaticus J45.902
  - due to
    - food J30.5
    - pollen J30.1
  - nonseasonal J30.89
  - perennial J30.89
  - seasonal NEC J30.2
  - specified NEC J30.89
- infective J00
- pneumococcal J00
- syphilitic A52.73
  - congenital A50.05 *[J99]*
- tuberculous A15.8
- vasomotor J30.0

**Rhinoantritis** (chronic) — *see* Sinusitis, maxillary
**Rhinodacryolith** — *see* Dacryolith
**Rhinolith** (nasal sinus) J34.89
**Rhinomegaly** J34.89
**Rhinopharyngitis** (acute) (subacute) — *see also* Nasopharyngitis
- chronic J31.1
- destructive ulcerating A66.5
- mutilans A66.5

**Rhinophyma** L71.1
**Rhinorrhea** J34.89
- cerebrospinal (fluid) G96.01
  - postoperative G96.08
  - specified NEC G96.08
  - spontaneous G96.01
  - traumatic G96.08
- paroxysmal — *see* Rhinitis, allergic
- spasmodic — *see* Rhinitis, allergic

**Rhinosalpingitis** — *see* Salpingitis, eustachian
**Rhinoscleroma** A48.8
**Rhinosinusitis** — *see* Sinusitis
**Rhinosporidiosis** B48.1
**Rhinovirus infection NEC** B34.8
**Rhizomelic chondrodysplasia punctata** E71.540
**Rhythm**
- atrioventricular nodal I49.89
- disorder I49.9
  - coronary sinus I49.89
  - ectopic I49.89
  - nodal I49.89
- escape I49.9
- heart, abnormal I49.9
- idioventricular I44.2
- nodal I49.89
- sleep, inversion G47.2- ☑
  - nonorganic origin — *see* Disorder, sleep, circadian rhythm, psychogenic

**Rhytidosis facialis** L98.8
**Rib** — *see also* condition
- cervical Q76.5

**Riboflavin deficiency** E53.0
**Rice bodies** — *see also* Loose, body, joint
- knee M23.4- ☑

**Richter syndrome** — *see* Leukemia, chronic lymphocytic, B-cell type
**Richter's hernia** — *see* Hernia, abdomen, with obstruction
**Ricinism** — *see* Poisoning, food, noxious, plant
**Rickets** (active) (acute) (adolescent) (chest wall) (congenital) (current) (infantile) (intestinal) E55.0
- adult — *see* Osteomalacia
- celiac K90.0
- hypophosphatemic with nephrotic-glycosuric dwarfism E72.09
- inactive E64.3
- kidney N25.0
- renal N25.0
- sequelae, any E64.3
- vitamin-D-resistant E83.31 *[M90.80]*

**Rickettsia 364D/R. philipii** (Pacific Coast tick fever) A77.8
**Rickettsial disease** A79.9
- specified type NEC A79.89

**Rickettsialpox** (Rickettsia akari) A79.1
**Rickettsiosis** A79.9
- due to
  - Ehrlichia sennetsu A79.81
  - Neorickettsia sennetsu A79.81
  - Rickettsia akari (rickettsialpox) A79.1

**Rickettsiosis** — *continued*
specified type NEC A79.89
tick-borne A77.9
vesicular A79.1
**Rider's bone** — *see* Ossification, muscle, specified NEC
**Ridge, alveolus** — *see also* condition
flabby K06.8
**Ridged ear, congenital** Q17.3
**Riedel's**
lobe, liver Q44.79
struma, thyroiditis or disease E06.5
**Rieger anomaly or syndrome** Q13.81
**Riehl's melanosis** L81.4
**Rietti-Greppi-Micheli anemia** D56.9
**Rieux's hernia** — *see* Hernia, abdomen, specified site NEC
**Riga** (-Fede) **disease** K14.0
**Riggs' disease** — *see* Periodontitis
**Right aortic arch** Q25.47
**Right middle lobe syndrome** J98.11
**Rigid, rigidity** — *see also* condition
abdominal R19.30
with severe abdominal pain R10.0
epigastric R19.36
generalized R19.37
left lower quadrant R19.34
left upper quadrant R19.32
periumbilic R19.35
right lower quadrant R19.33
right upper quadrant R19.31
articular, multiple, congenital Q68.8
cervix (uteri) in pregnancy — *see* Pregnancy, complicated by, abnormal, cervix
hymen (acquired) (congenital) N89.6
nuchal R29.1
pelvic floor in pregnancy — *see* Pregnancy, complicated by, abnormal, pelvic organs or tissues NEC
perineum or vulva in pregnancy — *see* Pregnancy, complicated by, abnormal, vulva
spine — *see* Dorsopathy, specified NEC
vagina in pregnancy — *see* Pregnancy, complicated by, abnormal, vagina
**Rigors** R68.89
with fever R50.9
**Riley-Day syndrome** G90.1
**RIND** (reversible ischemic neurologic deficit) I63.9
**Ring(s)**
aorta (vascular) Q25.45
Bandl's O62.4
contraction, complicating delivery O62.4
esophageal, lower (muscular) K22.2
Fleischer's (cornea) H18.04- ☑
hymenal, tight (acquired) (congenital) N89.6
Kayser-Fleischer (cornea) H18.04- ☑
retraction, uterus, pathological O62.4
Schatzki's (esophagus) (lower) K22.2
congenital Q39.3
Soemmerring's — *see* Cataract, secondary
vascular (congenital) Q25.8
aorta Q25.45
**Ringed hair** (congenital) Q84.1
**Ringworm** B35.9
beard B35.0
black dot B35.0
body B35.4
Burmese B35.5
corporeal B35.4
foot B35.3
groin B35.6
hand B35.2
honeycomb B35.0
nails B35.1
perianal (area) B35.6
scalp B35.0
specified NEC B35.8
Tokelau B35.5
**Rise, venous pressure** I87.8
**Rising, PSA following treatment for malignant neoplasm of prostate** R97.21
**Risk**
for
dental caries Z91.849
high Z91.843
low Z91.841
moderate Z91.842
homelessness, imminent Z59.811
suffocation (smothering) under another while sleeping Z72.823
suicidal
meaning personal history of attempted suicide Z91.51

**Risk** — *continued*
suicidal — *continued*
meaning suicidal ideation — *see* Ideation, suicidal
**Ritter's disease** L00
**Rivalry, sibling** Z62.891
**Rivalta's disease** A42.2
**River blindness** B73.01
**Robert's pelvis** Q74.2
with disproportion (fetopelvic) O33.0
causing obstructed labor O65.0
**Robin** (-Pierre) **syndrome** Q87.0
**Robinow-Silverman-Smith syndrome** Q87.19
**Robinson's** (hidrotic) **ectodermal dysplasia or syndrome** Q82.4
**Robles' disease** B73.01
**Rocky Mountain** (spotted) **fever** A77.0
**Roetheln** — *see* Rubella
**Roger's disease** Q21.0
**Rokitansky-Aschoff sinuses** (gallbladder) K82.8
**Rolando's fracture** (displaced) S62.22- ☑
nondisplaced S62.22- ☑
**Romano-Ward** (prolonged QT interval) **syndrome** I45.81
**Romberg's disease or syndrome** G51.8
**Roof, mouth** — *see* condition
**Rosacea** L71.9
acne L71.9
keratitis L71.8
specified NEC L71.8
**Rosary, rachitic** E55.0
**Rose**
cold J30.1
fever J30.1
rash R21
epidemic B06.9
**Rosenbach's erysipeloid** A26.0
**Rosenthal's disease or syndrome** D68.1
**Roseola** B09
infantum B08.20
due to human herpesvirus 6 B08.21
due to human herpesvirus 7 B08.22
**Ross River disease or fever** B33.1
**Rossbach's disease** K31.89
psychogenic F45.8
**Rostan's asthma** (cardiac) — *see* Failure, ventricular, left
**Rotation**
anomalous, incomplete or insufficient, intestine Q43.3
cecum (congenital) Q43.3
colon (congenital) Q43.3
spine, incomplete or insufficient — *see* Dorsopathy, deforming, specified NEC
tooth, teeth, fully erupted M26.35
vertebra, incomplete or insufficient — *see* Dorsopathy, deforming, specified NEC
**Rotes Querol disease or syndrome** — *see* Hyperostosis, ankylosing
**Roth** (-Bernhardt) **disease or syndrome** — *see* Meralgia paraesthetica
**Rothmund** (-Thomson) **syndrome** Q82.8
**Rotor's disease or syndrome** E80.6
**Round**
back (with wedging of vertebrae) — *see* Kyphosis
sequelae (late effect) of rickets E64.3
worms (large) (infestation) NEC B82.0
Ascariasis — *see also* Ascariasis B77.9
**Roussy-Levy syndrome** G60.0
**Rubella** (German measles) B06.9
complication NEC B06.09
neurological B06.00
congenital P35.0
contact Z20.4
exposure to Z20.4
maternal
care for (suspected) damage to fetus O35.3- ☑
manifest rubella in infant P35.0
suspected damage to fetus affecting management of pregnancy O35.3- ☑
specified complications NEC B06.89
**Rubeola** (meaning measles) — *see* Measles
meaning rubella — *see* Rubella
**Rubeosis, iris** — *see* Disorder, iris, vascular
**Rubinstein-Taybi syndrome** Q87.2
**Rudimentary** (congenital) — *see also* Agenesis
arm — *see* Defect, reduction, upper limb
bone Q79.9
cervix uteri Q51.828
eye Q11.2
lobule of ear Q17.3
patella Q74.1
respiratory organs in thoracopagus Q89.4

**Rudimentary** — *continued*
tracheal bronchus Q32.4
uterus Q51.818
in male Q56.1
vagina Q52.0
**Ruled out condition** — *see* Observation, suspected
**Rumination** R11.10
with nausea R11.2
disorder of infancy or childhood (in remission) F98.21
in adults (in remission) F50.84
neurotic F42.8
newborn P92.1
obsessional F42.8
psychogenic F42.8
**Runaway** [from current living environment] Z62.892
**Runeberg's disease** D51.0
**Running out of money** Z59.868
**Runny nose** R09.89
**Rupia** (syphilitic) A51.39
congenital A50.06
tertiary A52.79
**Rupture, ruptured**
abscess (spontaneous) — *code by* site under Abscess
aneurysm — *see* Aneurysm
anus (sphincter) — *see* Laceration, anus
aorta, aortic I71.8
abdominal I71.30
infrarenal I71.33
juxtarenal I71.32
pararenal I71.31
arch I71.12
ascending I71.11
descending I71.8
abdominal I71.30
thoracic I71.13
syphilitic A52.01
thoracoabdominal I71.50
paravisceral I71.52
supraceliac I71.51
thorax, thoracic I71.10
transverse I71.12
traumatic — *see* Injury, aorta, laceration, major
valve or cusp — *see also* Endocarditis, aortic I35.8
appendix (with peritonitis) — *see also* Appendicitis K35.32
with localized peritonitis — *see also* Appendicitis K35.32
arteriovenous fistula, brain — *see* Fistula, arteriovenous, brain, ruptured
artery I77.2
brain — *see* Hemorrhage, intracranial, intracerebral
coronary — *see* Infarct, myocardium
heart — *see* Infarct, myocardium
pulmonary I28.8
traumatic (complication) — *see* Injury, blood vessel
bile duct (common) (hepatic) K83.2
cystic K82.2
bladder (sphincter) (nontraumatic) (spontaneous) N32.89
following ectopic or molar pregnancy O08.6
obstetrical trauma O71.5
traumatic S37.29- ☑
blood vessel — *see also* Hemorrhage
brain — *see* Hemorrhage, intracranial, intracerebral
heart — *see* Infarct, myocardium
traumatic (complication) — *see* Injury, blood vessel, laceration, major, by site
bone — *see* Fracture
bowel (nontraumatic) K63.1
brain
aneurysm (congenital) — *see also* Hemorrhage, intracranial, subarachnoid
syphilitic A52.05
hemorrhagic — *see* Hemorrhage, intracranial, intracerebral
capillaries I78.8
cardiac (auricle) (ventricle) (wall) I23.3
with hemopericardium I23.0
infectional I40.9
traumatic — *see* Injury, heart
cartilage (articular) (current) — *see also* Sprain
knee S83.3- ☑
semilunar — *see* Tear, meniscus
cecum (with peritonitis) K65.0
with peritoneal abscess K35.33
traumatic S36.598- ☑
celiac artery, traumatic — *see* Injury, blood vessel, celiac artery, laceration, major
cerebral aneurysm (congenital) — *see* Hemorrhage, intracranial, subarachnoid

Index
Rupture, ruptured — Rupture, ruptured

- **Rupture, ruptured** — *continued*
  - traumatic — *continued*
    - ligament — *see also* Sprain — *continued*
      - finger — *continued*
        - index S63.40- ☑
        - little S63.40- ☑
        - middle S63.40- ☑
        - palmar S63.42- ☑
          - index S63.42- ☑
          - little S63.42- ☑
          - middle S63.42- ☑
          - ring S63.42- ☑
        - ring S63.40- ☑
        - specified site NEC S63.499- ☑
          - index S63.49- ☑
          - little S63.49- ☑
          - middle S63.49- ☑
          - ring S63.49- ☑
        - volar plate S63.43- ☑
          - index S63.43- ☑
          - little S63.43- ☑
          - middle S63.43- ☑
          - ring S63.43- ☑
      - foot — *see* Sprain, foot
      - radial collateral S53.2- ☑
      - radiocarpal — *see* Rupture, traumatic, ligament, wrist, radiocarpal
      - ulnar collateral S53.3- ☑
      - ulnocarpal — *see* Rupture, traumatic, ligament, wrist, ulnocarpal
      - wrist S63.30- ☑
        - collateral S63.31- ☑
        - radiocarpal S63.32- ☑
        - specified site NEC S63.39- ☑
        - ulnocarpal (palmar) S63.33- ☑
    - liver S36.116- ☑
    - membrana tympani — *see* Rupture, ear drum, traumatic
    - muscle or tendon — *see* Strain
    - myocardium — *see* Injury, heart
    - pancreas S36.299- ☑
    - rectum S36.69- ☑
    - sigmoid S36.593- ☑
    - spleen S36.09- ☑
    - stomach S36.39- ☑
    - symphysis pubis S33.4- ☑
    - tympanum, tympanic (membrane) — *see* Rupture, ear drum, traumatic
    - ureter S37.19- ☑
    - uterus S37.69- ☑
    - vagina — *see* Injury, vagina
    - vena cava — *see* Injury, vena cava, laceration, major
  - tricuspid (heart) (valve) I07.8
  - tube, tubal (nonobstetric) (nontraumatic) N83.8
    - abscess — *see* Salpingitis
    - due to pregnancy O00.10- ☑
      - with intrauterine pregnancy O00.11- ☑
  - tympanum, tympanic (membrane) (nontraumatic) — *see also* Perforation, tympanic membrane H72.9- ☑
    - traumatic — *see* Rupture, ear drum, traumatic
  - umbilical cord, complicating delivery O69.89- ☑
  - ureter (traumatic) S37.19- ☑
    - nontraumatic N28.89
  - urethra (nontraumatic) N36.8
    - with ectopic or molar pregnancy O08.6
    - following ectopic or molar pregnancy O08.6
    - obstetrical trauma O71.5
    - traumatic S37.39- ☑
  - uterosacral ligament (nonobstetric) (nontraumatic) N83.8
  - uterus (traumatic) S37.69- ☑
    - before labor O71.0- ☑
    - during or after labor O71.1
    - nonpuerperal, nontraumatic N85.8
    - pregnant (during labor) O71.1
      - before labor O71.0- ☑
  - vagina — *see* Injury, vagina
  - valve, valvular (heart) — *see* Endocarditis
  - varicose vein — *see* Varix
  - varix — *see* Varix
  - vena cava R58
    - traumatic — *see* Injury, vena cava, laceration, major
  - vesical (urinary) N32.89
  - vessel (blood) R58
    - pulmonary I28.8
    - traumatic — *see* Injury, blood vessel
  - viscus R19.8

- **Rupture, ruptured** — *continued*
  - vulva complicating delivery O70.0
- **Russell-Silver syndrome** Q87.19
- **Russian spring-summer type encephalitis** A84.0
- **Rust's disease** (tuberculous cervical spondylitis) A18.01
- **Ruvalcaba-Myhre-Smith syndrome** E71.440
- **Rytand-Lipsitch syndrome** I44.2

# S

- **Saber, sabre shin or tibia** (syphilitic) A50.56 *[M90.86-]* ☑
- **Sac lacrimal** — *see* condition
- **Saccharomyces infection** B37.9
- **Saccharopinuria** E72.3
- **Saccular** — *see* condition
- **Sacculation**
  - aorta (nonsyphilitic) — *see* Aneurysm, aorta
  - bladder N32.3
  - intralaryngeal (congenital) (ventricular) Q31.3
  - larynx (congenital) (ventricular) Q31.3
  - organ or site, congenital — *see* Distortion
  - pregnant uterus — *see* Pregnancy, complicated by, abnormal, uterus
  - ureter N28.89
  - urethra N36.1
  - vesical N32.3
- **Sachs' amaurotic familial idiocy or disease** E75.02
- **Sachs-Tay disease** E75.02
- **Sacks-Libman disease** M32.11
- **Sacralgia** M53.3
- **Sacralization** Q76.49
- **Sacrodynia** M53.3
- **Sacroiliac joint** — *see* condition
- **Sacroiliitis NEC** M46.1
- **Sacrum** — *see* condition
- **Saddle**
  - back — *see* Lordosis
  - embolus
    - abdominal aorta I74.01
    - pulmonary artery I26.92
      - with acute cor pulmonale I26.02
  - injury — *code to* condition
  - nose M95.0
    - due to syphilis A50.57
- **Sadism** (sexual) F65.52
- **Sadness, postpartal** O90.6
- **Sadomasochism** F65.50
- **Saemisch's ulcer** (cornea) — *see* Ulcer, cornea, central
- **Sagging**
  - skin and subcutaneous tissue (following bariatric surgery weight loss) (following dietary weight loss) L98.7
- **Sahib disease** B55.0
- **Sailors' skin** L57.8
- **Saint**
  - Anthony's fire — *see* Erysipelas
  - triad — *see* Hernia, diaphragm
  - Vitus' dance — *see* Chorea, Sydenham's
- **Salaam**
  - attack(s) — *see* Epilepsy, spasms
  - tic R25.8
- **Salicylism**
  - abuse F55.8
  - overdose or wrong substance given — *see* Table of Drugs and Chemicals, by drug, poisoning
- **Salivary duct or gland** — *see* condition
- **Salivation, excessive** K11.7
- **Salmonella** — *see* Infection, Salmonella
- **Salmonellosis** A02.0
- **Salpingitis** (catarrhal) (fallopian tube) (nodular) (pseudofollicular) (purulent) (septic) N70.91
  - with oophoritis N70.93
  - acute N70.01
    - with oophoritis N70.03
  - chlamydial A56.11
  - chronic N70.11
    - with oophoritis N70.13
  - complicating abortion — *see* Abortion, by type, complicated by, salpingitis
  - ear — *see* Salpingitis, eustachian
  - eustachian (tube) H68.00- ☑
    - acute H68.01- ☑
    - chronic H68.02- ☑
  - follicularis N70.11
    - with oophoritis N70.13
  - gonococcal (acute) (chronic) A54.24
  - interstitial, chronic N70.11
    - with oophoritis N70.13
  - isthmica nodosa N70.11

- **Salpingitis** — *continued*
  - isthmica nodosa — *continued*
    - with oophoritis N70.13
  - specific (gonococcal) (acute) (chronic) A54.24
  - tuberculous (acute) (chronic) A18.17
  - venereal (gonococcal) (acute) (chronic) A54.24
- **Salpingo-oophoritis** (catarrhal) (purulent) (ruptured) (septic) (suppurative) N70.93
  - acute N70.03
    - with ectopic or molar pregnancy O08.0
    - following ectopic or molar pregnancy O08.0
    - gonococcal A54.24
  - chronic N70.13
  - following ectopic or molar pregnancy O08.0
  - gonococcal (acute) (chronic) A54.24
  - puerperal O86.19
  - specific (gonococcal) (acute) (chronic) A54.24
  - subacute N70.03
  - tuberculous (acute) (chronic) A18.17
  - venereal (gonococcal) (acute) (chronic) A54.24
- **Salpingo-ovaritis** — *see* Salpingo-oophoritis
- **Salpingocele** N83.4- ☑
- **Salpingoperitonitis** — *see* Salpingo-oophoritis
- **Salzmann's nodular dystrophy** — *see* Degeneration, cornea, nodular
- **Sampson's cyst or tumor** N80.10- ☑
- **San Joaquin** (Valley) **fever** B38.0
- **Sandblaster's asthma, lung or pneumoconiosis** J62.8
- **Sander's disease** (paranoia) F22
- **Sandfly fever** A93.1
- **Sandhoff's disease** E75.01
- **Sanfilippo** (Type B) (Type C) (Type D) **syndrome** E76.22
- **Sanger-Brown ataxia** G11.2
- **Sao Paulo fever or typhus** A77.0
- **Saponification, mesenteric** K65.8
- **Sarcocele** (benign)
  - syphilitic A52.76
    - congenital A50.59
- **Sarcocystosis** A07.8
- **Sarcoepiplocele** — *see* Hernia
- **Sarcoepiplomphalocele** Q79.2
- **Sarcoglycanopathy** G71.0340
  - alpha G71.0341
  - beta G71.0342
  - delta G71.0349
  - gamma G71.0349
- **Sarcoid** — *see also* Sarcoidosis
  - arthropathy D86.86
  - Boeck's D86.9
  - Darier-Roussy D86.3
  - iridocyclitis D86.83
  - meningitis D86.81
  - myocarditis D86.85
  - myositis D86.87
  - pyelonephritis D86.84
  - Spiegler-Fendt L08.89
- **Sarcoidosis** D86.9
  - with
    - cranial nerve palsies D86.82
    - hepatic granuloma D86.89
    - polyarthritis D86.86
    - tubulo-interstitial nephropathy D86.84
  - combined sites NEC D86.89
  - lung D86.0
    - and lymph nodes D86.2
  - lymph nodes D86.1
    - and lung D86.2
  - meninges D86.81
  - skin D86.3
  - specified type NEC D86.89
- **Sarcoma** (of) — *see also* Neoplasm, connective tissue, malignant
  - alveolar soft part — *see* Neoplasm, connective tissue, malignant
  - ameloblastic C41.1
    - upper jaw (bone) C41.0
  - botryoid — *see* Neoplasm, connective tissue, malignant
  - botryoides — *see* Neoplasm, connective tissue, malignant
  - cerebellar C71.6
    - circumscribed (arachnoidal) C71.6
  - circumscribed (arachnoidal) cerebellar C71.6
  - clear cell — *see also* Neoplasm, connective tissue, malignant
    - kidney C64.- ☑
  - dendritic cells (accessory cells) C96.4
  - embryonal — *see* Neoplasm, connective tissue, malignant
  - endometrial (stromal) C54.1
    - isthmus C54.0

- **Sarcoma** — *continued*
  - epithelioid (cell) — *see* Neoplasm, connective tissue, malignant
  - Ewing's — *see* Neoplasm, bone, malignant
  - follicular dendritic cell C96.4
  - germinoblastic (diffuse) — *see* Lymphoma, diffuse large cell
    - follicular — *see* Lymphoma, follicular, specified NEC
  - giant cell (except of bone) — *see also* Neoplasm, connective tissue, malignant
    - bone — *see* Neoplasm, bone, malignant
  - glomoid — *see* Neoplasm, connective tissue, malignant
  - granulocytic C92.3- ☑
  - hemangioendothelial — *see* Neoplasm, connective tissue, malignant
  - hemorrhagic, multiple — *see* Sarcoma, Kaposi's
  - histiocytic C96.A (*following* C96.6)
  - Hodgkin — *see* Lymphoma, Hodgkin
  - immunoblastic (diffuse) — *see* Lymphoma, diffuse large cell
  - interdigitating dendritic cell C96.4
  - Kaposi's
    - colon C46.4
    - connective tissue C46.1
    - gastrointestinal organ C46.4
    - lung C46.5- ☑
    - lymph node(s) C46.3
    - palate (hard) (soft) C46.2
    - rectum C46.4
    - skin C46.0
    - specified site NEC C46.7
    - stomach C46.4
    - unspecified site C46.9
  - Kupffer cell C22.3
  - Langerhans cell C96.4
  - leptomeningeal — *see* Neoplasm, meninges, malignant
  - liver NEC C22.4
  - lymphangioendothelial — *see* Neoplasm, connective tissue, malignant
  - lymphoblastic — *see* Lymphoma, lymphoblastic (diffuse)
  - lymphocytic — *see* Lymphoma, small cell B-cell
  - mast cell C96.22
  - melanotic — *see* Melanoma
  - meningeal — *see* Neoplasm, meninges, malignant
  - meningothelial — *see* Neoplasm, meninges, malignant
  - mesenchymal — *see also* Neoplasm, connective tissue, malignant
    - mixed — *see* Neoplasm, connective tissue, malignant
  - mesothelial — *see* Mesothelioma
  - monstrocellular
    - specified site — *see* Neoplasm, malignant, by site
    - unspecified site C71.9
  - myeloid C92.3- ☑
  - neurogenic — *see* Neoplasm, nerve, malignant
  - odontogenic C41.1
    - upper jaw (bone) C41.0
  - osteoblastic — *see* Neoplasm, bone, malignant
  - osteogenic — *see also* Neoplasm, bone, malignant
    - juxtacortical — *see* Neoplasm, bone, malignant
    - periosteal — *see* Neoplasm, bone, malignant
  - periosteal — *see also* Neoplasm, bone, malignant
    - osteogenic — *see* Neoplasm, bone, malignant
  - pleomorphic cell — *see* Neoplasm, connective tissue, malignant
  - reticulum cell (diffuse) — *see* Lymphoma, diffuse large cell
    - nodular — *see* Lymphoma, follicular
    - pleomorphic cell type — *see* Lymphoma, diffuse large cell
  - rhabdoid — *see* Neoplasm, malignant, by site
  - round cell — *see* Neoplasm, connective tissue, malignant
  - small cell — *see* Neoplasm, connective tissue, malignant
  - soft tissue — *see* Neoplasm, connective tissue, malignant
  - spindle cell — *see* Neoplasm, connective tissue, malignant
  - stromal (endometrial) C54.1
    - isthmus C54.0
  - synovial — *see also* Neoplasm, connective tissue, malignant
    - biphasic — *see* Neoplasm, connective tissue, malignant
    - epithelioid cell — *see* Neoplasm, connective tissue, malignant
    - spindle cell — *see* Neoplasm, connective tissue, malignant
- **Sarcomatosis**
  - meningeal — *see* Neoplasm, meninges, malignant
  - specified site NEC — *see* Neoplasm, connective tissue, malignant
- **Sarcomatosis** — *continued*
  - unspecified site C80.1
- **Sarcopenia** (age-related) M62.84
- **Sarcosinemia** E72.59
- **Sarcosporidiosis** (intestinal) A07.8
- **SARS-CoV-2** — *see also* COVID-19
  - sequelae (post acute) U09.9
- **Satiety, early** R68.81
- **Saturnine** — *see* condition
- **Saturnism**
  - overdose or wrong substance given or taken — *see* Table of Drugs and Chemicals, by drug, poisoning
- **Satyriasis** F52.8
- **Sauriasis** — *see* Ichthyosis
- **SBE** (subacute bacterial endocarditis) I33.0
- **Scabies** (any site) B86
- **Scabs** R23.4
- **Scaglietti-Dagnini syndrome** E22.0
- **Scald** — *see* Burn
- **Scalenus anticus** (anterior) **syndrome** G54.0
- **Scales** R23.4
- **Scaling, skin** R23.4
- **Scalp** — *see* condition
- **Scapegoating affecting child** Z62.3
- **Scaphocephaly, non-deformational** Q75.01
- **Scapulalgia** M89.8X1
- **Scapulohumeral myopathy** G71.02
- **Scar, scarring** — *see also* Cicatrix L90.5
  - adherent L90.5
  - atrophic L90.5
  - cervix
    - in pregnancy or childbirth — *see* Pregnancy, complicated by, abnormal cervix
  - cheloid L91.0
  - chorioretinal H31.00- ☑
    - posterior pole macula H31.01- ☑
    - postsurgical H59.81- ☑
    - solar retinopathy H31.02- ☑
    - specified type NEC H31.09- ☑
  - choroid — *see* Scar, chorioretinal
  - conjunctiva H11.24- ☑
  - cornea H17.9
    - xerophthalmic — *see also* Opacity, cornea
      - vitamin A deficiency E50.6
  - defect (isthmocele) O34.22
  - duodenum, obstructive K31.5
  - hypertrophic L91.0
  - keloid L91.0
  - labia N90.89
  - lung (base) J98.4
  - macula — *see* Scar, chorioretinal, posterior pole
  - muscle M62.89
  - myocardium, myocardial I25.2
  - painful L90.5
  - posterior pole (eye) — *see* Scar, chorioretinal, posterior pole
  - retina — *see* Scar, chorioretinal
  - trachea J39.8
  - transmural uterine, in pregnancy O34.29
  - uterus N85.8
    - in pregnancy O34.29
  - vagina N89.8
    - postoperative N99.2
  - vulva N90.89
- **Scarabiasis** B88.2
- **Scarlatina** (anginosa) (maligna) A38.9
  - myocarditis (acute) A38.1
    - old — *see* Myocarditis
  - otitis media A38.0
  - ulcerosa A38.8
- **Scarlet fever** (albuminuria) (angina) A38.9
- **Schamberg's disease** (progressive pigmentary dermatosis) L81.7
- **Schatzki's ring** (acquired) (esophagus) (lower) K22.2
  - congenital Q39.3
- **Schaufenster krankheit** I20.89
- **Schaumann's**
  - benign lymphogranulomatosis D86.1
  - disease or syndrome — *see* Sarcoidosis
- **Scheie's syndrome** E76.03
- **Schenck's disease** B42.1
- **Scheuermann's disease or osteochondrosis** — *see* Osteochondrosis, juvenile, spine
- **Schilder** (-Flatau) **disease** G37.0
- **Schilling-type monocytic leukemia** C93.0- ☑
- **Schimmelbusch's disease, cystic mastitis, or hyperplasia** — *see* Mastopathy, cystic
- **Schistosoma infestation** — *see* Infestation, Schistosoma
- **Schistosomiasis** B65.9
  - with muscle disorder B65.9 *[M63.80]*
    - ankle B65.9 *[M63.87-]* ☑
    - foot B65.9 *[M63.87-]* ☑
    - forearm B65.9 *[M63.83-]* ☑
    - hand B65.9 *[M63.84-]* ☑
    - lower leg B65.9 *[M63.86-]* ☑
    - multiple sites B65.9 *[M63.89]*
    - pelvic region B65.9 *[M63.85-]* ☑
    - shoulder region B65.9 *[M63.81-]* ☑
    - specified site NEC B65.9 *[M63.88]*
    - thigh B65.9 *[M63.85-]* ☑
    - upper arm B65.9 *[M63.82-]* ☑
  - Asiatic B65.2
  - bladder B65.0
  - chestermani B65.8
  - colon B65.1
  - cutaneous B65.3
  - due to
    - S. haematobium B65.0
    - S. japonicum B65.2
    - S. mansoni B65.1
    - S. mattheii B65.8
  - Eastern B65.2
  - genitourinary tract B65.0
  - intestinal B65.1
  - lung NEC B65.9 *[J99]*
    - pneumonia B65.9 *[J17]*
  - Manson's (intestinal) B65.1
  - oriental B65.2
  - pulmonary NEC B65.9 *[J99]*
    - pneumonia B65.9
  - Schistosoma
    - haematobium B65.0
    - japonicum B65.2
    - mansoni B65.1
  - specified type NEC B65.8
  - urinary B65.0
  - vesical B65.0
- **Schizencephaly** Q04.6
- **Schizoaffective psychosis** F25.9
- **Schizodontia** K00.2
- **Schizoid personality** F60.1
- **Schizophrenia, schizophrenic** F20.9
  - acute (brief) (undifferentiated) F23
  - atypical (form) F20.3
  - borderline F21
  - catalepsy F20.2
  - catatonic (type) (excited) (withdrawn) F20.2
  - cenesthopathic, cenesthesiopathic F20.89
  - childhood type F20.9
  - chronic undifferentiated F20.9
  - cyclic F25.0
  - disorganized (type) F20.1
  - flexibilitas cerea F20.2
  - hebephrenic (type) F20.1
  - incipient F21
  - latent F21
  - negative type F20.5
  - paranoid (type) F20.0
  - paraphrenic F20.0
  - post-psychotic depression F32.89
  - prepsychotic F21
  - prodromal F21
  - pseudoneurotic F21
  - pseudopsychopathic F21
  - reaction F23
  - residual (state) (type) F20.5
  - restzustand F20.5
  - schizoaffective (type) — *see* Psychosis, schizoaffective
  - simple (type) F20.89
  - simplex F20.89
  - specified type NEC F20.89
  - spectrum and other psychotic disorder F29
    - specified NEC F28
  - stupor F20.2
  - syndrome of childhood F84.5
  - undifferentiated (type) F20.3
    - chronic F20.9
- **Schizothymia** (persistent) F60.1
- **Schlatter-Osgood disease or osteochondrosis** M92.52- ☑
- **Schlatter's tibia** — *see* Osteochondrosis, juvenile, tibia
- **Schmidt's syndrome** (polyglandular, autoimmune) E31.0
- **Schmincke's carcinoma or tumor** — *see* Neoplasm, nasopharynx, malignant
- **Schmitz** (-Stutzer) **dysentery** A03.0
- **Schmorl's disease or nodes**
  - lumbar region M51.46

**Screening** — *continued*
  parasitic infestation Z11.9
    specified NEC Z11.8
  phenylketonuria Z13.228
  plague Z11.2
  poisoning (chemical) (heavy metal) Z13.88
  poliomyelitis Z11.59
  postnatal, chromosomal abnormalities Z13.89
  prenatal, of mother — *see also* Encounter, antenatal screening Z36.9
  protozoal disease Z11.6
    intestinal Z11.Ø
  pulmonary tuberculosis Z11.1
  radiation exposure Z13.88
  respiratory condition Z13.83
  respiratory tuberculosis Z11.1
  rheumatoid arthritis Z13.828
  rubella Z11.59
  SARS-CoV-2 Z11.52
  schistosomiasis Z11.6
  sexually-transmitted disease NEC Z11.3
    human immunodeficiency virus (HIV) Z11.4
  sickle-cell disease or trait Z13.Ø
  skin condition Z13.89
  sleeping sickness Z11.6
  special Z13.9
    specified NEC Z13.89
  syphilis Z11.3
  tetanus Z11.2
  trachoma Z11.8
  traumatic brain injury Z13.85Ø
  trypanosomiasis Z11.6
  tuberculosis, respiratory Z11.1
    active Z11.1
    latent Z11.7
  venereal disease Z11.3
  viral encephalitis (mosquito- or tick-borne) Z11.59
  whooping cough Z11.2
  worms, intestinal Z11.6
  yaws Z11.8
  yellow fever Z11.59
**Scrofula, scrofulosis** (tuberculosis of cervical lymph glands) A18.2
**Scrofulide** (primary) (tuberculous) A18.4
**Scrofuloderma, scrofulodermia** (any site) (primary) A18.4
**Scrofulosus lichen** (primary) (tuberculous) A18.4
**Scrofulous** — *see* condition
**Scrotal tongue** K14.5
**Scrotum** — *see* condition
**Scurvy, scorbutic** E54
  anemia D53.2
  gum E54
  infantile E54
  rickets E55.Ø *[M9Ø.8Ø]*
**Sealpox** BØ8.62
**Seasickness** T75.3- ☑
**Seatworm** (infection) (infestation) B8Ø
**Sebaceous** — *see also* condition
  cyst — *see* Cyst, sebaceous
**Seborrhea, seborrheic** L21.9
  capillitii R23.8
  capitis L21.Ø
  dermatitis L21.9
    infantile L21.1
  eczema L21.9
    infantile L21.1
  sicca L21.Ø
**Seckel's syndrome** Q87.19
**Seclusion, pupil** — *see* Membrane, pupillary
**Second hand tobacco smoke exposure** (acute) (chronic) Z77.22
  in the perinatal period P96.81
**Secondary**
  dentin (in pulp) KØ4.3
  neoplasm, secondaries — *see* Table of Neoplasms, secondary
**Secretion**
  antidiuretic hormone, inappropriate E22.2
  catecholamine, by pheochromocytoma — *see also* Pheochromocytoma, by type E27.5
  hormone
    antidiuretic, inappropriate (syndrome) E22.2
    by
      carcinoid tumor — *see also* Tumor, carcinoid E34.Ø9
      pheochromocytoma — *see also* Pheochromocytoma, by type E27.5
    ectopic NEC E34.2

**Secretion** — *continued*
  urinary
    excessive R35.89
    suppression R34
**Section**
  nerve, traumatic — *see* Injury, nerve
**Sedative, hypnotic, or anxiolytic-induced**
  anxiety disorder F13.98Ø
  bipolar and related disorder F13.94
  delirium F13.921
  depressive disorder F13.94
  major neurocognitive disorder F13.97
  mild neurocognitive disorder F13.988
  psychotic disorder F13.959
  sexual dysfunction F13.981
  sleep disorder F13.982
**Segmentation, incomplete** (congenital) — *see also* Fusion
  bone NEC Q78.8
  lumbosacral (joint) (vertebra) Q76.49
**SEID** (systemic exertion intolerance disease) G93.32
**Seitelberger's syndrome** (infantile neuraxonal dystrophy) G31.89
**Seizure(s)** — *see also* Convulsions R56.9
  absence G4Ø.A- ☑ (*following* G4Ø.3)
  akinetic — *see* Epilepsy, generalized, specified NEC
  atonic — *see* Epilepsy, generalized, specified NEC
  autonomic (hysterical) F44.5
  convulsive — *see* Convulsions
  cortical (focal) (motor) — *see* Epilepsy, localization-related, symptomatic, with simple partial seizures
  disorder — *see also* Epilepsy G4Ø.9Ø9
  due to stroke — *see* Sequelae (of), disease, cerebrovascular, by type, specified NEC
  epileptic — *see* Epilepsy
  febrile (simple) R56.ØØ
    with status epilepticus G4Ø.9Ø1
    complex (atypical) (complicated) R56.Ø1
      with status epilepticus G4Ø.9Ø1
  grand mal G4Ø.4Ø9
    intractable G4Ø.419
      with status epilepticus G4Ø.411
      without status epilepticus G4Ø.419
    not intractable G4Ø.4Ø9
      with status epilepticus G4Ø.4Ø1
      without status epilepticus G4Ø.4Ø9
  heart — *see* Disease, heart
  hysterical F44.5
  intractable G4Ø.919
    with status epilepticus G4Ø.911
  Jacksonian (focal) (motor type) (sensory type) — *see* Epilepsy, localization-related, symptomatic, with simple partial seizures
  newborn P9Ø
  nonspecific epileptic
    atonic — *see* Epilepsy, generalized, specified NEC
    clonic — *see* Epilepsy, generalized, specified NEC
    myoclonic — *see* Epilepsy, generalized, specified NEC
    tonic — *see* Epilepsy, generalized, specified NEC
    tonic-clonic — *see* Epilepsy, generalized, specified NEC
  partial, developing into secondarily generalized seizures
    complex — *see* Epilepsy, localization-related, symptomatic, with complex partial seizures
    simple — *see* Epilepsy, localization-related, symptomatic, with simple partial seizures
  petit mal G4Ø.A- ☑ (*following* G4Ø.3)
    intractable G4Ø.A1- ☑ (*following* G4Ø.3)
      with status epilepticus G4Ø.A11 (*following* G4Ø.3)
      without status epilepticus G4Ø.A19 (*following* G4Ø.3)
    not intractable G4Ø.AØ- ☑ (*following* G4Ø.3)
      with status epilepticus G4Ø.AØ1 (*following* G4Ø.3)
      without status epilepticus G4Ø.AØ9 (*following* G4Ø.3)
  post traumatic R56.1
  recurrent G4Ø.9Ø9
  specified NEC G4Ø.89
  uncinate — *see* Epilepsy, localization-related, symptomatic, with complex partial seizures
**Selenium deficiency, dietary** E59
**Self-damaging behavior** (life-style) Z72.89
**Self-harm** (attempted)
  history (personal)
    in family Z81.8
    nonsuicidal Z91.52
    suicidal Z91.51
  nonsuicidal R45.88
**Self-injury, nonsuicidal** R45.88
  personal history Z91.52

**Self-mutilation** (attempted)
  history (personal)
    in family Z81.8
    nonsuicidal Z91.52
    suicidal Z91.51
  nonsuicidal R45.88
**Self-poisoning**
  history (personal) Z91.51
    in family Z81.8
  observation following (alleged) attempt ZØ3.6
**Semicoma** R4Ø.1
**Seminal vesiculitis** N49.Ø
**Seminoma** C62.9- ☑
  specified site — *see* Neoplasm, malignant, by site
**Senear-Usher disease or syndrome** L1Ø.4
**Senectus** R54
**Senescence** (without mention of psychosis) R54
**Senile, senility** — *see also* condition R41.81
  with
    acute confusional state FØ5
    mental changes NOS FØ3.- ☑
    psychosis NEC — *see* Psychosis, senile
  asthenia R54
  cervix (atrophic) N88.8
  debility R54
  endometrium (atrophic) N85.8
  fallopian tube (atrophic) — *see* Atrophy, fallopian tube
  heart (failure) R54
  ovary (atrophic) — *see* Atrophy, ovary
  premature E34.8
  vagina, vaginitis (atrophic) N95.2
  wart L82.1
**Sensation**
  burning (skin) R2Ø.8
    tongue K14.6
  foreign body RØ9.AØ
    eye H57.8A- ☑
    globus RØ9.A2
    nose RØ9.A1
    specified site NEC RØ9.A9
    throat RØ9.A2
  loss of R2Ø.8
  prickling (skin) R2Ø.2
  tingling (skin) R2Ø.2
**Sense loss**
  smell — *see* Disturbance, sensation, smell
  taste — *see* Disturbance, sensation, taste
  touch R2Ø.8
**Sensibility disturbance** (cortical) (deep) (vibratory) R2Ø.9
**Sensitive, sensitivity** — *see also* Allergy
  carotid sinus G9Ø.Ø1
  child (excessive) F93.8
  cold, autoimmune D59.12
  dentin KØ3.89
  gluten (non-celiac) K9Ø.41
  latex Z91.Ø4Ø
  methemoglobin D74.8
  tuberculin, without clinical or radiological symptoms R76.11
  visual
    glare H53.71
    impaired contrast H53.72
**Sensitiver Beziehungswahn** F22
**Sensitization, auto-erythrocytic** D69.2
**Separation**
  anxiety, abnormal (of childhood) F93.Ø
  apophysis, traumatic — *code as* Fracture, by site
  choroid — *see* Detachment, choroid
  epiphysis, epiphyseal
    nontraumatic — *see also* Osteochondropathy, specified type NEC
      upper femoral — *see* Slipped, epiphysis, upper femoral
    traumatic — *code as* Fracture, by site
  fracture — *see* Fracture
  infundibulum cardiac from right ventricle by a partition Q24.3
  joint (traumatic) (current) — *code by* site under Dislocation
  muscle (nontraumatic) — *see* Diastasis, muscle
  pubic bone, obstetrical trauma O71.6
  retina, retinal — *see* Detachment, retina
  symphysis pubis, obstetrical trauma O71.6
  tracheal ring, incomplete, congenital Q32.1
**Sepsis** (generalized) (unspecified organism) A41.9
  with
    ectopic or molar pregnancy OØ8.82
    organ dysfunction (acute) (multiple) R65.2Ø
      with septic shock R65.21

**Sepsis** — *continued*
- Acinetobacter baumannii A41.54
- actinomycotic A42.7
- adrenal hemorrhage syndrome (meningococcal) A39.1
- anaerobic A41.4
- Bacillus anthracis A22.7
- Brucella — *see also* Brucellosis A23.9
- candidal B37.7
- Cronobacter A41.59
- cryptogenic A41.9
- due to device, implant or graft T85.79- ☑
  - arterial graft NEC T82.7- ☑
  - breast (implant) T85.79- ☑
  - catheter NEC T85.79- ☑
    - dialysis (renal) T82.7- ☑
      - intraperitoneal T85.71- ☑
    - infusion NEC T82.7- ☑
      - spinal (cranial) (epidural) (intrathecal) (spinal) (subarachnoid) (subdural) T85.735- ☑
    - urethral indwelling T83.511- ☑
    - urinary T83.518- ☑
  - electronic (electrode) (pulse generator) (stimulator)
    - bone T84.7- ☑
    - cardiac T82.7- ☑
    - nervous system T85.738- ☑
      - brain T85.731- ☑
      - neurostimulator generator T85.734- ☑
      - peripheral nerve T85.732- ☑
      - spinal cord T85.733- ☑
    - urinary T83.590- ☑
  - fixation, internal (orthopedic) — *see* Complication, fixation device, infection
  - gastrointestinal (bile duct) (esophagus) T85.79- ☑
    - neurostimulator electrode (lead) T85.732- ☑
  - genital T83.69- ☑
  - heart NEC T82.7- ☑
    - valve (prosthesis) T82.6- ☑
      - graft T82.7- ☑
  - joint prosthesis — *see* Complication, joint prosthesis, infection
  - ocular (corneal graft) (orbital implant) T85.79- ☑
  - orthopedic NEC T84.7- ☑
    - fixation device, internal — *see* Complication, fixation device, infection
  - specified NEC T85.79- ☑
  - vascular T82.7- ☑
  - ventricular intracranial (communicating) shunt T85.730- ☑
- during labor O75.3
- Enterococcus A41.81
- Erysipelothrix (rhusiopathiae) (erysipeloid) A26.7
- Escherichia coli (E. coli) A41.51
- extraintestinal yersiniosis A28.2
- following
  - abortion (subsequent episode) O08.0
    - current episode — *see* Abortion
  - ectopic or molar pregnancy O08.82
  - immunization T88.0- ☑
  - infusion, therapeutic injection or transfusion NEC T80.29- ☑
  - obstetrical procedure O86.04
- gangrenous A41.9
- gonococcal A54.86
- Gram-negative (organism) A41.50
  - anaerobic A41.4
- Haemophilus influenzae A41.3
- herpesviral B00.7
- intra-abdominal K65.1
- intraocular — *see* Endophthalmitis, purulent
- Listeria monocytogenes A32.7
- localized — *code to* specific localized infection
  - in operation wound T81.49- ☑
  - skin — *see* Abscess
- malleus A24.0
- melioidosis A24.1
- meningeal — *see* Meningitis
- meningococcal A39.4
  - acute A39.2
  - chronic A39.3
- MRSA (Methicillin resistant Staphylococcus aureus) A41.02
- MSSA (Methicillin susceptible Staphylococcus aureus) A41.01
- newborn P36.9
  - due to
    - anaerobes NEC P36.5
    - Escherichia coli P36.4
    - Staphylococcus P36.30
      - aureus P36.2
      - specified NEC P36.39
    - Streptococcus P36.10
      - group B P36.0
      - specified NEC P36.19
  - specified NEC P36.8
- other gram-negative A41.59
- Pasteurella multocida A28.0
- pelvic, puerperal, postpartum, childbirth O85
- pneumococcal A40.3
- postprocedural T81.44- ☑
- Pseudomonas (pseudomonas aeruginosa) A41.52
- puerperal, postpartum, childbirth (pelvic) O85
- Salmonella (arizonae) (cholerae-suis) (enteritidis) (typhimurium) A02.1
- Serratia A41.53
- severe R65.20
  - with septic shock R65.21
- Shigella — *see also* Dysentery, bacillary A03.9
- skin, localized — *see* Abscess
- specified organism NEC A41.89
- Staphylococcus, staphylococcal A41.2
  - aureus (methicillin susceptible) (MSSA) A41.01
    - methicillin resistant (MRSA) A41.02
  - coagulase-negative A41.1
  - specified NEC A41.1
- Streptococcus, streptococcal A40.9
  - agalactiae A40.1
  - group
    - A A40.0
    - B A40.1
    - D A41.81
  - neonatal P36.10
    - group B P36.0
    - specified NEC P36.19
  - pneumoniae A40.3
  - pyogenes A40.0
  - specified NEC A40.8
- tracheostomy stoma J95.02
- tularemic A21.7
- umbilical, umbilical cord (newborn) — *see* Sepsis, newborn
- Yersinia pestis A20.7

**Septate** — *see* Septum

**Septic** — *see* condition
- arm — *see* Cellulitis, upper limb
  - with lymphangitis — *see* Lymphangitis, acute, upper limb
- embolus — *see* Embolism
- finger — *see* Cellulitis, digit
  - with lymphangitis — *see* Lymphangitis, acute, digit
- foot — *see* Cellulitis, lower limb
  - with lymphangitis — *see* Lymphangitis, acute, lower limb
- gallbladder (acute) K81.0
- hand — *see* Cellulitis, upper limb
  - with lymphangitis — *see* Lymphangitis, acute, upper limb
- joint — *see* Arthritis, pyogenic or pyemic
- leg — *see* Cellulitis, lower limb
  - with lymphangitis — *see* Lymphangitis, acute, lower limb
- nail — *see also* Cellulitis, digit
  - with lymphangitis — *see* Lymphangitis, acute, digit
- sore — *see also* Abscess
  - throat J02.0
    - streptococcal J02.0
- spleen (acute) D73.89
- teeth, tooth (pulpal origin) K04.4
- throat — *see* Pharyngitis
- thrombus — *see* Thrombosis
- toe — *see* Cellulitis, digit
  - with lymphangitis — *see* Lymphangitis, acute, digit
- tonsils, chronic J35.01
  - with adenoiditis J35.03
- uterus — *see* Endometritis

**Septicemia** A41.9
- meaning sepsis — *see* Sepsis

**Septum, septate** (congenital) — *see also* Anomaly, by site
- anal Q42.3
  - with fistula Q42.2
- aqueduct of Sylvius Q03.0
  - with spina bifida — *see* Spina bifida, by site, with hydrocephalus
- uterus Q51.28
  - complete Q51.21
  - partial Q51.22
  - specified NEC Q51.28
- vagina Q52.10
  - in pregnancy — *see* Pregnancy, complicated by, abnormal vagina
    - causing obstructed labor O65.5
  - longitudinal Q52.129
    - microperforate
      - left side Q52.124
      - right side Q52.123
    - nonobstruction Q52.120
    - obstructing Q52.129
      - left side Q52.122
      - right side Q52.121
  - transverse Q52.11

**Sequelae** (of) — *see also* condition
- abscess, intracranial or intraspinal (conditions in G06) G09
- amputation — *code to* injury with seventh character S
- burn and corrosion — *code to* injury with seventh character S
- calcium deficiency E64.8
- cerebrovascular disease — *see* Sequelae, disease, cerebrovascular
- childbirth O94
- contusion — *code to* injury with seventh character S
- corrosion — *see* Sequelae, burn and corrosion
- COVID-19 (post acute) U09.9
- crushing injury — *code to* injury with seventh character S
- disease
  - cerebrovascular I69.90
    - alteration of sensation I69.998
    - aphasia I69.920
    - apraxia I69.990
    - ataxia I69.993
    - cognitive deficits I69.91- ☑
    - disturbance of vision I69.998
    - dysarthria I69.922
    - dysphagia I69.991
    - dysphasia I69.921
    - facial droop I69.992
    - facial weakness I69.992
    - fluency disorder I69.923
    - hemiplegia I69.95- ☑
    - hemorrhage
      - intracerebral — *see* Sequelae, hemorrhage, intracerebral
      - intracranial, nontraumatic NEC — *see* Sequelae, hemorrhage, intracranial, nontraumatic
      - subarachnoid — *see* Sequelae, hemorrhage, subarachnoid
    - language deficit I69.928
    - monoplegia
      - lower limb I69.94- ☑
      - upper limb I69.93- ☑
    - paralytic syndrome I69.96- ☑
    - specified effect NEC I69.998
    - specified type NEC I69.80
      - alteration of sensation I69.898
      - aphasia I69.820
      - apraxia I69.890
      - ataxia I69.893
      - cognitive deficits I69.81- ☑
      - disturbance of vision I69.898
      - dysarthria I69.822
      - dysphagia I69.891
      - dysphasia I69.821
      - facial droop I69.892
      - facial weakness I69.892
      - fluency disorder I69.823
      - hemiplegia I69.85- ☑
      - language deficit I69.828
      - monoplegia
        - lower limb I69.84- ☑
        - upper limb I69.83- ☑
      - paralytic syndrome I69.86- ☑
      - specified effect NEC I69.898
    - speech deficit I69.928
      - speech deficit I69.828
    - stroke NOS — *see* Sequelae, stroke NOS
- dislocation — *code to* injury with seventh character S
- encephalitis or encephalomyelitis (conditions in G04) G09
  - in infectious disease NEC B94.8

- **Sequelae** — *continued*
  - encephalitis or encephalomyelitis — *continued*
    - viral B94.1
  - external cause — *code to* injury with seventh character S
  - foreign body entering natural orifice — *code to* injury with seventh character S
  - fracture — *code to* injury with seventh character S
  - frostbite — *code to* injury with seventh character S
  - Hansen's disease B92
  - hemorrhage
    - intracerebral I69.1Ø
      - alteration of sensation I69.198
      - aphasia I69.12Ø
      - apraxia I69.19Ø
      - ataxia I69.193
      - cognitive deficits I69.11- ☑
      - disturbance of vision I69.198
      - dysarthria I69.122
      - dysphagia I69.191
      - dysphasia I69.121
      - facial droop I69.192
      - facial weakness I69.192
      - fluency disorder I69.123
      - hemiplegia I69.15- ☑
      - language deficit NEC I69.128
      - monoplegia
        - lower limb I69.14- ☑
        - upper limb I69.13- ☑
      - paralytic syndrome I69.16- ☑
      - specified effect NEC I69.198
      - speech deficit NEC I69.128
    - intracranial, nontraumatic NEC I69.2Ø
      - alteration of sensation I69.298
      - aphasia I69.22Ø
      - apraxia I69.29Ø
      - ataxia I69.293
      - cognitive deficits I69.21- ☑
      - disturbance of vision I69.298
      - dysarthria I69.222
      - dysphagia I69.291
      - dysphasia I69.221
      - facial droop I69.292
      - facial weakness I69.292
      - fluency disorder I69.223
      - hemiplegia I69.25- ☑
      - language deficit NEC I69.228
      - monoplegia
        - lower limb I69.24- ☑
        - upper limb I69.23- ☑
      - paralytic syndrome I69.26- ☑
      - specified effect NEC I69.298
      - speech deficit NEC I69.228
    - subarachnoid I69.ØØ
      - alteration of sensation I69.Ø98
      - aphasia I69.Ø2Ø
      - apraxia I69.Ø9Ø
      - ataxia I69.Ø93
      - cognitive deficits — *see* subcategory I69.Ø1- ☑
      - disturbance of vision I69.Ø98
      - dysarthria I69.Ø22
      - dysphagia I69.Ø91
      - dysphasia I69.Ø21
      - facial droop I69.Ø92
      - facial weakness I69.Ø92
      - fluency disorder I69.Ø23
      - hemiplegia I69.Ø5- ☑
      - language deficit NEC I69.Ø28
      - monoplegia
        - lower limb I69.Ø4- ☑
        - upper limb I69.Ø3- ☑
      - paralytic syndrome I69.Ø6- ☑
      - specified effect NEC I69.Ø98
      - speech deficit NEC I69.Ø28
  - hepatitis, viral B94.2
  - hyperalimentation E68
  - infarction
    - cerebral I69.3Ø
      - alteration of sensation I69.398
      - aphasia I69.32Ø
      - apraxia I69.39Ø
      - ataxia I69.393
      - cognitive deficits I69.31- ☑
      - disturbance of vision I69.398
      - dysarthria I69.322
      - dysphagia I69.391
      - dysphasia I69.321
      - facial droop I69.392

- **Sequelae** — *continued*
  - infarction — *continued*
    - cerebral — *continued*
      - facial weakness I69.392
      - fluency disorder I69.323
      - hemiplegia I69.35- ☑
      - language deficit NEC I69.328
      - monoplegia
        - lower limb I69.34- ☑
        - upper limb I69.33- ☑
      - paralytic syndrome I69.36- ☑
      - specified effect NEC I69.398
      - speech deficit NEC I69.328
  - infection, pyogenic, intracranial or intraspinal GØ9
  - infectious disease B94.9
    - specified NEC B94.8
  - injury — *code to* injury with seventh character S
  - leprosy B92
  - meningitis
    - bacterial (conditions in GØØ) GØ9
    - other or unspecified cause (conditions in GØ3) GØ9
  - muscle (and tendon) injury — *code to* injury with seventh character S
  - myelitis — *see* Sequelae, encephalitis
  - niacin deficiency E64.8
  - nutritional deficiency E64.9
    - specified NEC E64.8
  - obstetrical condition O94
  - parasitic disease B94.9
  - phlebitis or thrombophlebitis of intracranial or intraspinal venous sinuses and veins (conditions in GØ8) GØ9
  - poisoning — *code to* poisoning with seventh character S
    - nonmedicinal substance — *see* Sequelae, toxic effect, nonmedicinal substance
  - poliomyelitis (acute) B91
  - pregnancy O94
  - protein-energy malnutrition E64.Ø
  - puerperium O94
  - rickets E64.3
  - SARS-CoV-2 (post acute) UØ9.9
  - selenium deficiency E64.8
  - sprain and strain — *code to* injury with seventh character S
  - stroke NOS I69.3Ø
    - alteration in sensation I69.398
    - aphasia I69.32Ø
    - apraxia I69.39Ø
    - ataxia I69.393
    - cognitive deficits I69.31- ☑
    - disturbance of vision I69.398
    - dysarthria I69.322
    - dysphagia I69.391
    - dysphasia I69.321
    - facial droop I69.392
    - facial weakness I69.392
    - hemiplegia I69.35- ☑
    - language deficit NEC I69.328
    - monoplegia
      - lower limb I69.34- ☑
      - upper limb I69.33- ☑
    - paralytic syndrome I69.36- ☑
    - specified effect NEC I69.398
    - speech deficit NEC I69.328
  - tendon and muscle injury — *code to* injury with seventh character S
  - thiamine deficiency E64.8
  - trachoma B94.Ø
  - tuberculosis B9Ø.9
    - bones and joints B9Ø.2
    - central nervous system B9Ø.Ø
    - genitourinary B9Ø.1
    - pulmonary (respiratory) B9Ø.9
    - specified organs NEC B9Ø.8
  - viral
    - encephalitis B94.1
    - hepatitis B94.2
  - vitamin deficiency NEC E64.8
    - A E64.1
    - B E64.8
    - C E64.2
  - wound, open — *code to* injury with seventh character S
- **Sequestration** — *see also* Sequestrum
  - disc — *see* Displacement, intervertebral disc
  - lung, congenital Q33.2
- **Sequestrum**
  - bone — *see* Osteomyelitis, chronic
  - dental M27.2

- **Sequestrum** — *continued*
  - jaw bone M27.2
  - orbit — *see* Osteomyelitis, orbit
  - sinus (accessory) (nasal) — *see* Sinusitis
- **Sequoiosis lung or pneumonitis** J67.8
- **Serology for syphilis**
  - doubtful
    - with signs or symptoms — *code by* site and stage under Syphilis
    - follow-up of latent syphilis — *see* Syphilis, latent
  - negative, with signs or symptoms — *code by* site and stage under Syphilis
  - positive A53.Ø
    - with signs or symptoms — *code by* site and stage under Syphilis
  - reactivated A53.Ø
- **Seroma** — *see also* Hematoma
  - postprocedural — *see* Complication, postprocedural, seroma
  - traumatic, secondary and recurrent T79.2- ☑
- **Seropurulent** — *see* condition
- **Serositis, multiple** K65.8
  - pericardial I31.1
  - peritoneal K65.8
- **Serous** — *see* condition
- **Sertoli cell**
  - adenoma
    - specified site — *see* Neoplasm, benign, by site
    - unspecified site
      - female D27.9
      - male D29.2Ø
  - carcinoma
    - specified site — *see* Neoplasm, malignant, by site
    - unspecified site (male) C62.9- ☑
      - female C56.9
  - tumor
    - with lipid storage
      - specified site — *see* Neoplasm, benign, by site
      - unspecified site
        - female D27.9
        - male D29.2Ø
    - specified site — *see* Neoplasm, benign, by site
    - unspecified site
      - female D27.9
      - male D29.2Ø
- **Sertoli-Leydig cell tumor** — *see* Neoplasm, benign, by site
  - specified site — *see* Neoplasm, benign, by site
  - unspecified site
    - female D27.9
    - male D29.2Ø
- **Serum**
  - allergy, allergic reaction — *see also* Reaction, serum T8Ø.69- ☑
    - shock — *see also* Shock, anaphylactic T8Ø.59- ☑
  - arthritis — *see also* Reaction, serum T8Ø.69- ☑
  - complication or reaction NEC — *see also* Reaction, serum T8Ø.69- ☑
  - disease NEC — *see also* Reaction, serum T8Ø.69- ☑
  - hepatitis — *see also* Hepatitis, viral, type B
    - carrier (suspected) of B18.1
  - intoxication — *see also* Reaction, serum T8Ø.69- ☑
  - neuritis — *see also* Reaction, serum T8Ø.69- ☑
  - neuropathy G61.1
  - poisoning NEC — *see also* Reaction, serum T8Ø.69- ☑
  - rash NEC — *see also* Reaction, serum T8Ø.69- ☑
  - reaction NEC — *see also* Reaction, serum T8Ø.69- ☑
  - sickness NEC — *see also* Reaction, serum T8Ø.69- ☑
  - urticaria — *see also* Reaction, serum T8Ø.69- ☑
- **Sesamoiditis** M25.8- ☑
- **Severe sepsis** R65.2Ø
  - with septic shock R65.21
- **Sever's disease or osteochondrosis** — *see* Osteochondrosis, juvenile, tarsus
- **Sex**
  - chromosome mosaics Q97.8
    - lines with various numbers of X chromosomes Q97.2
  - education Z7Ø.8
  - reassignment surgery status Z87.89Ø- ☑
- **Sextuplet pregnancy** — *see* Pregnancy, sextuplet
- **Sexual**
  - function, disorder of (psychogenic) F52.9
  - immaturity (female) (male) E3Ø.Ø
  - impotence (psychogenic) organic origin NEC — *see* Dysfunction, sexual, male
  - precocity (constitutional) (cryptogenic) (female) (idiopathic) (male) E3Ø.1
- **Sexuality, pathologic** — *see* Deviation, sexual
- **Sezary disease** C84.1- ☑

- **Shy-Drager syndrome** G9Ø.3
- **Sialadenitis, sialadenosis** (any gland) (chronic) (periodic) (suppurative) — *see* Sialoadenitis
- **Sialectasia** K11.8
- **Sialidosis** E77.1
- **Sialitis, silitis** (any gland) (chronic) (suppurative) — *see* Sialoadenitis
- **Sialoadenitis** (any gland) (periodic) (suppurative) K11.2Ø
  - acute K11.21
    - recurrent K11.22
  - chronic K11.23
- **Sialoadenopathy** K11.9
- **Sialoangitis** — *see* Sialoadenitis
- **Sialodochitis** (fibrinosa) — *see* Sialoadenitis
- **Sialodocholithiasis** K11.5
- **Sialolithiasis** K11.5
- **Sialometaplasia, necrotizing** K11.8
- **Sialorrhea** — *see also* Ptyalism
  - periodic — *see* Sialoadenitis
- **Sialosis** K11.7
- **Siamese twin** Q89.4
- **Sibling rivalry** Z62.891
- **Sicard's syndrome** G52.7
- **Sicca syndrome** — *see* Syndrome, Sjogren
- **Sick** R69
  - or handicapped person in family Z63.79
    - needing care at home Z63.6
  - sinus (syndrome) I49.5
- **Sick-euthyroid syndrome** EØ7.81
- **Sickle-cell**
  - anemia — *see* Disease, sickle-cell
  - beta plus — *see* Disease, sickle-cell, thalassemia, beta plus
  - beta zero — *see* Disease, sickle-cell, thalassemia, beta zero
  - trait D57.3
- **Sicklemia** — *see also* Disease, sickle-cell
  - trait D57.3
- **Sickness**
  - air (travel) T75.3- ☑
  - airplane T75.3- ☑
  - alpine T7Ø.29- ☑
  - altitude T7Ø.2Ø- ☑
  - Andes T7Ø.29- ☑
  - aviator's T7Ø.29- ☑
  - balloon T7Ø.29- ☑
  - car T75.3- ☑
  - compressed air T7Ø.3- ☑
  - decompression T7Ø.3- ☑
  - green D5Ø.8
  - milk — *see* Poisoning, food, noxious
  - motion T75.3- ☑
  - mountain T7Ø.29- ☑
    - acute D75.1
  - protein — *see also* Reaction, serum T8Ø.69- ☑
  - radiation T66.- ☑
  - roundabout (motion) T75.3- ☑
  - sea T75.3- ☑
  - serum NEC — *see also* Reaction, serum T8Ø.69- ☑
  - sleeping (African) B56.9
    - by Trypanosoma B56.9
      - brucei
        - gambiense B56.Ø
        - rhodesiense B56.1
    - East African B56.1
    - Gambian B56.Ø
    - Rhodesian B56.1
    - West African B56.Ø
  - swing (motion) T75.3- ☑
  - train (railway) (travel) T75.3- ☑
  - travel (any vehicle) T75.3- ☑
- **Sideropenia** — *see* Anemia, iron deficiency
- **Siderosilicosis** J62.8
- **Siderosis** (lung) J63.4
  - brain G93.89
  - eye (globe) — *see* Disorder, globe, degenerative, siderosis
- **Siemens' syndrome** (ectodermal dysplasia) Q82.8
- **Sighing** RØ6.89
  - psychogenic F45.8
- **Sigmoid** — *see also* condition
  - flexure — *see* condition
  - kidney Q63.1
- **Sigmoiditis** — *see also* Enteritis K52.9
  - infectious AØ9
  - noninfectious K52.9
- **Silfverskold's syndrome** Q78.9
- **Silicosiderosis** J62.8
- **Silicosis, silicotic** (simple) (complicated) J62.8
  - with tuberculosis J65
- **Silicotuberculosis** J65
- **Silo-fillers' disease** J68.8
  - bronchitis J68.Ø
  - pneumonitis J68.Ø
  - pulmonary edema J68.1
- **Silver's syndrome** Q87.19
- **Simian malaria** B53.1
- **Simmonds' cachexia or disease** E23.Ø
- **Simons' disease or syndrome** (progressive lipodystrophy) E88.11
- **Simple, simplex** — *see* condition
- **Simulation, conscious** (of illness) Z76.5
- **Simultanagnosia** (asimultagnosia) R48.3
- **Sin Nombre virus disease** (Hantavirus) (cardio)-pulmonary syndrome B33.4
- **Sinding-Larsen disease or osteochondrosis** — *see* Osteochondrosis, juvenile, patella
- **Singapore hemorrhagic fever** A91
- **Singer's node or nodule** J38.2
- **Single**
  - atrium Q21.2Ø
  - coronary artery Q24.5
  - umbilical artery Q27.Ø
  - ventricle Q2Ø.4
- **Singultus** RØ6.6
  - epidemicus B33.Ø
- **Sinus** — *see also* Fistula
  - abdominal K63.89
  - arrest I45.5
  - arrhythmia I49.89
  - bradycardia RØØ.1
  - branchial cleft (internal) (external) Q18.Ø
  - coccygeal — *see* Sinus, pilonidal
  - dental KØ4.6
  - dermal (congenital) QØ6.8
    - with abscess QØ6.8
    - coccygeal, pilonidal — *see* Sinus, coccygeal
  - infected, skin NEC LØ8.89
  - marginal, ruptured or bleeding — *see* Hemorrhage, antepartum, specified cause NEC
  - medial, face and neck Q18.8
  - pause I45.5
  - pericranii QØ1.9
  - pilonidal (infected) (rectum) LØ5.92
    - with abscess LØ5.Ø2
  - preauricular Q18.1
  - rectovaginal N82.3
  - Rokitansky-Aschoff (gallbladder) K82.8
  - sacrococcygeal (dermoid) (infected) — *see* Sinus, pilonidal
  - tachycardia RØØ.Ø
    - paroxysmal I47.19
  - tarsi syndrome M25.57- ☑
  - testis N5Ø.89
  - tract (postinfective) — *see* Fistula
  - urachus Q64.4
- **Sinusitis** (accessory) (chronic) (hyperplastic) (nasal) (nonpurulent) (purulent) J32.9
  - acute JØ1.9Ø
    - ethmoidal JØ1.2Ø
      - recurrent JØ1.21
    - frontal JØ1.1Ø
      - recurrent JØ1.11
    - involving more than one sinus, other than pansinusitis JØ1.8Ø
      - recurrent JØ1.81
    - maxillary JØ1.ØØ
      - recurrent JØ1.Ø1
    - pansinusitis JØ1.4Ø
      - recurrent JØ1.41
    - recurrent JØ1.91
    - specified NEC JØ1.8Ø
      - recurrent JØ1.81
    - sphenoidal JØ1.3Ø
      - recurrent JØ1.31
  - allergic — *see* Rhinitis, allergic
  - due to high altitude T7Ø.1- ☑
  - ethmoidal J32.2
    - acute JØ1.2Ø
      - recurrent JØ1.21
  - frontal J32.1
    - acute JØ1.1Ø
      - recurrent JØ1.11
  - influenzal — *see* Influenza, with, respiratory manifestations NEC
  - involving more than one sinus but not pansinusitis J32.8
    - acute JØ1.8Ø

**Sinusitis** — *continued*
  - involving more than one sinus but not pansinusitis — *continued*
    - acute — *continued*
      - recurrent JØ1.81
  - maxillary J32.Ø
    - acute JØ1.ØØ
      - recurrent JØ1.Ø1
  - odontogenic NOS J34.839
    - ethmoid sinus J34.831
    - frontal sinus J34.832
    - maxillary sinus J34.83Ø
    - sphenoid sinus J34.833
  - sphenoidal J32.3
    - acute JØ1.3Ø
      - recurrent JØ1.31
  - tuberculous, any sinus A15.8
- **Sinusitis-bronchiectasis-situs inversus** (syndrome) (triad) Q89.3
- **Sipple's syndrome** E31.22
- **Sirenomelia** (syndrome) Q87.2
- **Siriasis** T67.Ø1- ☑
- **Sirkari's disease** B55.Ø
- **Siti** A65
- **Situation, psychiatric** F99
- **Situational**
  - disturbance (transient) — *see* Disorder, adjustment
    - acute F43.Ø
  - maladjustment — *see* Disorder, adjustment
  - reaction — *see* Disorder, adjustment
    - acute F43.Ø
- **Situs inversus or transversus** (abdominalis) (thoracis) Q89.3
- **Sixth disease** BØ8.2Ø
  - due to human herpesvirus 6 BØ8.21
  - due to human herpesvirus 7 BØ8.22
- **Sjogren-Larsson syndrome** Q87.19
- **Sjogren's syndrome or disease** — *see* Syndrome, Sjogren
- **Skeletal** — *see* condition
- **Skene's gland** — *see* condition
- **Skenitis** — *see* Urethritis
- **Skerljevo** A65
- **Skevas-Zerfus disease** — *see* Toxicity, venom, marine animal, sea anemone
- **Skin** — *see also* condition
  - clammy R23.1
  - donor — *see* Donor, skin
  - dry L85.3
  - hidebound M35.9
- **Slate-dressers' or slate-miners' lung** J62.8
- **Sleep**
  - apnea — *see* Apnea, sleep
  - deprivation Z72.82Ø
  - disorder or disturbance G47.9
    - child F51.9
    - nonorganic origin F51.9
    - specified NEC G47.8
  - disturbance G47.9
    - nonorganic origin F51.9
  - drunkenness F51.9
  - rhythm inversion G47.2- ☑
  - terrors F51.4
  - walking F51.3
    - hysterical F44.89
- **Sleep hygiene**
  - abuse Z72.821
  - inadequate Z72.821
  - poor Z72.821
- **Sleep-wake schedule disorder** G47.2Ø
- **Sleeping sickness** — *see* Sickness, sleeping
- **Sleeplessness** — *see* Insomnia
  - menopausal N95.1
- **Slim disease** (in HIV infection) B2Ø
- **Slipped, slipping**
  - epiphysis (traumatic) — *see also* Osteochondropathy, specified type NEC
    - capital femoral (traumatic) [SCFE]
      - acute (on chronic) S79.Ø1- ☑
      - nontraumatic M93.ØØ- ☑
    - current traumatic — *code as* Fracture, by site
    - upper femoral (nontraumatic) [SUFE] M93.ØØ- ☑
      - acute M93.Ø1- ☑
        - on chronic M93.Ø3- ☑
      - chronic M93.Ø2- ☑
  - intervertebral disc — *see* Displacement, intervertebral disc
  - ligature, umbilical P51.8
  - patella — *see* Disorder, patella, derangement NEC

**Slipped, slipping** — *continued*
  rib M89.8X8
  sacroiliac joint — *see* subcategory M53.2- ☑
  tendon — *see* Disorder, tendon
  ulnar nerve, nontraumatic — *see* Lesion, nerve, ulnar
  vertebra NEC — *see* Spondylolisthesis
**Slocumb's syndrome** E27.Ø
**Sloughing** (multiple) (phagedena) (skin) — *see also* Gangrene
  abscess — *see* Abscess
  appendix K38.8
  fascia — *see* Disorder, soft tissue, specified type NEC
  scrotum N5Ø.89
  tendon — *see* Disorder, tendon
  transplanted organ — *see* Rejection, transplant
  ulcer — *see* Ulcer, skin
**Slow**
  feeding, newborn P92.2
  flow syndrome, coronary I2Ø.89
  heart (beat) RØØ.1
**Slowing, urinary stream** R39.198
**Sluder's neuralgia** (syndrome) G44.89
**Slurred, slurring speech** R47.81
**Small** (ness)
  for gestational age — *see* Small for dates
  introitus, vagina N89.6
  kidney (unknown cause) N27.9
    bilateral N27.1
    unilateral N27.Ø
  ovary (congenital) Q5Ø.39
  pelvis
    with disproportion (fetopelvic) O33.1
      causing obstructed labor O65.1
  uterus N85.8
  white kidney NØ3.9
**Small-and-light-for-dates** — *see* Small for dates
**Small-for-dates** (infant) PØ5.1Ø
  with weight of
    499 grams or less PØ5.11
    5ØØ-749 grams PØ5.12
    75Ø-999 grams PØ5.13
    1ØØØ-1249 grams PØ5.14
    125Ø-1499 grams PØ5.15
    15ØØ-1749 grams PØ5.16
    175Ø-1999 grams PØ5.17
    2ØØØ-2499 grams PØ5.18
    25ØØ grams and over PØ5.19
  specified NEC PØ5.19
**Smallpox** BØ3
**Smearing, fecal** R15.1
**SMEI** (severe myoclonic epilepsy in infancy) G4Ø.83- ☑
**Smith-Lemli-Opitz syndrome** E78.72
**Smith's fracture** S52.54- ☑
**Smoker** — *see* Dependence, drug, nicotine
**Smoker's**
  bronchitis J41.Ø
  cough J41.Ø
  palate K13.24
  throat J31.2
  tongue K13.24
**Smoking**
  passive Z77.22
**Smothering spells** RØ6.81
**Snaggle teeth, tooth** M26.39
**Snapping**
  finger — *see* Trigger finger
  hip — *see* Derangement, joint, specified type NEC, hip
    involving the iliotibial band M76.3- ☑
  knee — *see* Derangement, knee
    involving the iliotibial band M76.3- ☑
**Sneddon-Wilkinson disease or syndrome** (sub-corneal pustular dermatosis) L13.1
**Sneezing** (intractable) RØ6.7
**Sniffing**
  cocaine
    abuse — *see* Abuse, drug, cocaine
    dependence — *see* Dependence, drug, cocaine
  gasoline
    abuse — *see* Abuse, drug, inhalant
    dependence — *see* Dependence, drug, inhalant
  glue (airplane)
    abuse — *see* Abuse, drug, inhalant
    drug dependence — *see* Dependence, drug, inhalant
**Sniffles**
  newborn P28.89
**Snoring** RØ6.83
**Snow blindness** — *see* Photokeratitis
**Snuffles** (non-syphilitic) RØ6.5
**Snuffles** — *continued*
  newborn P28.89
  syphilitic (infant) A5Ø.Ø5 *[J99]*
**Social**
  exclusion Z6Ø.4
    due to discrimination or persecution (perceived) Z6Ø.5
  migrant Z59.ØØ
    acculturation difficulty Z6Ø.3
  rejection Z6Ø.4
    due to discrimination or persecution Z6Ø.5
  role conflict NEC Z73.5
  skills inadequacy NEC Z73.4
  transplantation Z6Ø.3
**Sodoku** A25.Ø
**Soemmerring's ring** — *see* Cataract, secondary
**Soft** — *see also* condition
  nails L6Ø.3
**Softening**
  bone — *see* Osteomalacia
  brain (necrotic) (progressive) G93.89
    congenital QØ4.8
    embolic I63.4- ☑
    hemorrhagic — *see* Hemorrhage, intracranial, intracerebral
    occlusive I63.5- ☑
    thrombotic I63.3- ☑
  cartilage M94.2- ☑
    patella M22.4- ☑
  cerebellar — *see* Softening, brain
  cerebral — *see* Softening, brain
  cerebrospinal — *see* Softening, brain
  myocardial, heart — *see* Degeneration, myocardial
  spinal cord G95.89
  stomach K31.89
**Soldier's**
  heart F45.8
  patches I31.Ø
**Solitary**
  cyst, kidney N28.1
  kidney, congenital Q6Ø.Ø
**Solvent abuse** — *see* Abuse, drug, inhalant
  dependence — *see* Dependence, drug, inhalant
**Somatization reaction, somatic reaction** — *see* Disorder, somatoform
**Somnambulism** F51.3
  hysterical F44.89
**Somnolence** R4Ø.Ø
  nonorganic origin F51.11
**Sonne dysentery** AØ3.3
**Soor** B37.Ø
**Sore**
  bed — *see* Ulcer, pressure, by site
  chiclero B55.1
  Delhi B55.1
  desert — *see* Ulcer, skin
  eye H57.1- ☑
  Lahore B55.1
  mouth K13.79
    canker K12.Ø
  muscle M79.1Ø
  Naga — *see* Ulcer, skin
  of skin — *see* Ulcer, skin
  oriental B55.1
  pressure — *see* Ulcer, pressure, by site
  skin L98.9
  soft A57
  throat (acute) — *see also* Pharyngitis
    with influenza, flu, or grippe — *see* Influenza, with, respiratory manifestations NEC
    chronic J31.2
    coxsackie (virus) BØ8.5
    diphtheritic A36.Ø
    herpesviral BØØ.2
    influenzal — *see* Influenza, with, respiratory manifestations NEC
    septic JØ2.Ø
    streptococcal (ulcerative) JØ2.Ø
    viral NEC JØ2.8
      coxsackie BØ8.5
  tropical — *see* Ulcer, skin
  veldt — *see* Ulcer, skin
**Soto's syndrome** (cerebral gigantism) Q87.3
**South African cardiomyopathy syndrome** I42.89
**Southeast Asian hemorrhagic fever** A91
**Spacing**
  abnormal, tooth, teeth, fully erupted M26.3Ø
  excessive, tooth, fully erupted M26.32
**Spade-like hand** (congenital) Q68.1
**Spading nail** L6Ø.8
  congenital Q84.6
**Spanish collar** N47.1
**Sparganosis** B7Ø.1
**Spasm**(s), **spastic, spasticity** — *see also* condition R25.2
  accommodation — *see* Spasm, of accommodation
  ampulla of Vater K83.4
  anus, ani (sphincter) (reflex) K59.4
    psychogenic F45.8
  artery I73.9
    cerebral G45.9
  Bell's G51.3- ☑
  bladder (sphincter, external or internal) N32.89
    psychogenic F45.8
  bronchus, bronchiole J98.Ø1
  cardia K22.Ø
  cardiac I2Ø.1
  carpopedal — *see* Tetany
  cerebral (arteries) (vascular) G45.9
  cervix, complicating delivery O62.4
  ciliary body (of accommodation) — *see* Spasm, of accommodation
  colon — *see also* Irritable, bowel K58.9
    with diarrhea K58.Ø
    psychogenic F45.8
  common duct K83.8
  compulsive — *see* Tic
  conjugate H51.8
  coronary (artery) I2Ø.1
  diaphragm (reflex) RØ6.6
    epidemic B33.Ø
    psychogenic F45.8
  duodenum K59.89
  epidemic diaphragmatic (transient) B33.Ø
  esophagus (diffuse) K22.4
    psychogenic F45.8
  facial G51.3- ☑
  fallopian tube N83.8
  gastrointestinal (tract) K31.89
    psychogenic F45.8
  glottis J38.5
    hysterical F44.4
    psychogenic F45.8
      conversion reaction F44.4
    reflex through recurrent laryngeal nerve J38.5
  habit — *see* Tic
  heart I2Ø.1
  hemifacial (clonic) G51.3- ☑
  hourglass — *see* Contraction, hourglass
  hysterical F44.4
  infantile — *see* Epilepsy, spasms
  inferior oblique, eye H51.8
  intestinal — *see also* Syndrome, irritable bowel K58.9
    psychogenic F45.8
  larynx, laryngeal J38.5
    hysterical F44.4
    psychogenic F45.8
      conversion reaction F44.4
  levator palpebrae superioris — *see* Disorder, eyelid function
  muscle NEC M62.838
    back M62.83Ø
  nerve, trigeminal G5Ø.Ø
  nervous F45.8
  nodding F98.4
  occupational F48.8
  oculogyric H51.8
    psychogenic F45.8
  of accommodation H52.53- ☑
  ophthalmic artery — *see* Occlusion, artery, retina
  perineal, female N94.89
  peroneo-extensor — *see also* Deformity, limb, flat foot
  pharynx (reflex) J39.2
    hysterical F45.8
    psychogenic F45.8
  psychogenic F45.8
  pylorus NEC K31.3
    adult hypertrophic K31.89
    congenital Q4Ø.Ø
    psychogenic F45.8
  rectum (sphincter) K59.4
    psychogenic F45.8
  retinal (artery) — *see* Occlusion, artery, retina
  sigmoid — *see also* Syndrome, irritable bowel K58.9
    psychogenic F45.8
  sphincter of Oddi K83.4
  stomach K31.89
    neurotic F45.8
  throat J39.2

Index

Slipped, slipping — Spasm

**Spasm(s), spastic, spasticity** — *continued*
- throat — *continued*
  - hysterical F45.8
  - psychogenic F45.8
- tic F95.9
  - chronic F95.1
  - transient of childhood F95.Ø
- tongue K14.8
- torsion (progressive) G24.1
- trigeminal nerve — *see* Neuralgia, trigeminal
- ureter N13.5
- urethra (sphincter) N35.919
- uterus N85.8
  - complicating labor O62.4
- vagina N94.2
  - psychogenic F52.5
- vascular I73.9
- vasomotor I73.9
- vein NEC I87.8
- viscera — *see* Pain, abdominal

**Spasmodic** — *see* condition
**Spasmophilia** — *see* Tetany
**Spasmus nutans** F98.4
**Spastic, spasticity** — *see also* Spasm
- child (cerebral) (congenital) (paralysis) G8Ø.1

**Speaker's throat** R49.8
**Specific, specified** — *see* condition
**Speech**
- defect, disorder, disturbance, impediment — *see* Disorder, speech R47.9
  - psychogenic, in childhood and adolescence F98.8
  - slurring R47.81
  - specified NEC R47.89

**Spells, transient oxygen desaturation of newborn** — *see also* Apnea, newborn P28.4Ø
- during sleep — *see also* Apnea, newborn, sleep, primary P28.3Ø

**Spencer's disease** AØ8.19
**Spens' syndrome** (syncope with heart block) I45.9
**Sperm counts** (fertility testing) Z31.41
- postvasectomy Z3Ø.8
  - reversal Z31.42

**Spermatic cord** — *see* condition
**Spermatocele** N43.4Ø
- congenital Q55.4
- multiple N43.42
- single N43.41

**Spermatocystitis** N49.Ø
**Spermatocytoma** C62.9- ☑
- specified site — *see* Neoplasm, malignant, by site

**Spermatorrhea** N5Ø.89
**Sphacelus** — *see* Gangrene
**Sphenoidal** — *see* condition
**Sphenoiditis** (chronic) — *see* Sinusitis, sphenoidal
**Sphenopalatine ganglion neuralgia** G9Ø.Ø9
**Sphericity, increased, lens** (congenital) Q12.4
**Spherocytosis** (congenital) (familial) (hereditary) D58.Ø
- hemoglobin disease D58.Ø
- sickle-cell (disease) D57.8- ☑

**Spherophakia** Q12.4
**Sphincter** — *see* condition
**Sphincteritis, sphincter of Oddi** — *see* Cholangitis
**Sphingolipidosis** E75.3
- specified NEC E75.29

**Sphingomyelinosis** E75.3
**Spicule tooth** KØØ.2
**Spider**
- bite — *see* Toxicity, venom, spider
  - nonvenomous — *see* Bite, by site, superficial, insect
- fingers — *see* Syndrome, Marfan
- nevus I78.1
- toes — *see* Syndrome, Marfan
- vascular I78.1

**Spiegler-Fendt**
- benign lymphocytoma L98.8
- sarcoid LØ8.89

**Spielmeyer-Vogt disease** E75.4
**Spina bifida** (aperta) QØ5.9
- with hydrocephalus NEC QØ5.4
- cervical QØ5.5
  - with hydrocephalus QØ5.Ø
- dorsal QØ5.6
  - with hydrocephalus QØ5.1
- lumbar QØ5.7
  - with hydrocephalus QØ5.2
- lumbosacral QØ5.7
  - with hydrocephalus QØ5.2
- occulta Q76.Ø
- sacral QØ5.8

**Spina bifida** — *continued*
- sacral — *continued*
  - with hydrocephalus QØ5.3
- thoracic QØ5.6
  - with hydrocephalus QØ5.1
- thoracolumbar QØ5.6
  - with hydrocephalus QØ5.1

**Spindle, Krukenberg's** — *see* Pigmentation, cornea, posterior
**Spine, spinal** — *see* condition
**Spiradenoma** (eccrine) — *see* Neoplasm, skin, benign
**Spirillosis** A25.Ø
**Spirillum**
- minus A25.Ø
- obermeieri infection A68.Ø

**Spirochetal** — *see* condition
**Spirochetosis** A69.9
- arthritic, arthritica A69.9
- bronchopulmonary A69.8
- icterohemorrhagic A27.Ø
- lung A69.8

**Spirometrosis** B7Ø.1
**Spitting blood** — *see* Hemoptysis
**Splanchnoptosis** K63.4
**Spleen, splenic** — *see* condition
**Splenectasis** — *see* Splenomegaly
**Splenitis** (interstitial) (malignant) (nonspecific) D73.89
- malarial — *see also* Malaria B54 *[D77]*
- tuberculous A18.85

**Splenocele** D73.89
**Splenomegaly, splenomegalia** (Bengal) (cryptogenic) (idiopathic) (tropical) R16.1
- with hepatomegaly R16.2
- cirrhotic D73.2
- congenital Q89.Ø9
- congestive, chronic D73.2
- Egyptian B65.1
- Gaucher's E75.22
- malarial — *see also* Malaria B54 *[D77]*
- neutropenic D73.81
- Niemann-Pick — *see* Niemann-Pick disease or syndrome
- siderotic D73.2
- syphilitic A52.79
  - congenital (early) A5Ø.Ø8 *[D77]*

**Splenopathy** D73.9
**Splenoptosis** D73.89
**Splenosis** D73.89
**Splinter** — *see* Foreign body, superficial, by site
**Split, splitting**
- foot Q72.7- ☑
- hand Q71.6- ☑
- heart sounds RØ1.2
- lip, congenital — *see* Cleft, lip
- nails L6Ø.3
- urinary stream R39.13

**Spondylarthrosis** — *see* Spondylosis
**Spondylitis** (chronic) — *see also* Spondylopathy, inflammatory
- ankylopoietica — *see* Spondylitis, ankylosing
- ankylosing (chronic) M45.9
  - with lung involvement M45.9 *[J99]*
  - cervical region M45.2
  - cervicothoracic region M45.3
  - juvenile MØ8.1
  - lumbar region M45.6
  - lumbosacral region M45.7
  - multiple sites M45.Ø
  - occipito-atlanto-axial region M45.1
  - sacrococcygeal region M45.8
  - thoracic region M45.4
  - thoracolumbar region M45.5
- atrophic (ligamentous) — *see* Spondylitis, ankylosing
- deformans (chronic) — *see* Spondylosis
- gonococcal A54.41
- gouty — *see also* Gout, by type, vertebrae M1Ø.Ø8
- in (due to)
  - brucellosis A23.9 *[M49.8Ø]*
    - cervical region A23.9 *[M49.82]*
    - cervicothoracic region A23.9 *[M49.83]*
    - lumbar region A23.9 *[M49.86]*
    - lumbosacral region A23.9 *[M49.87]*
    - multiple sites A23.9 *[M49.89]*
    - occipito-atlanto-axial region A23.9 *[M49.81]*
    - sacrococcygeal region A23.9 *[M49.88]*
    - thoracic region A23.9 *[M49.84]*
    - thoracolumbar region A23.9 *[M49.85]*
  - enterobacteria — *see also* subcategory M49.8 AØ4.9
  - tuberculosis A18.Ø1
- infectious NEC — *see* Spondylopathy, infective

**Spondylitis** — *continued*
- juvenile ankylosing (chronic) MØ8.1
- Kummell's — *see* Spondylopathy, traumatic
- Marie-Strumpell — *see* Spondylitis, ankylosing
- muscularis — *see* Spondylopathy, specified NEC
- psoriatic L4Ø.53
- rheumatoid — *see* Spondylitis, ankylosing
- rhizomelica — *see* Spondylitis, ankylosing
- sacroiliac NEC M46.1
- senescent, senile — *see* Spondylosis
- traumatic (chronic) or post-traumatic — *see* Spondylopathy, traumatic
- tuberculous A18.Ø1
- typhosa AØ1.Ø5

**Spondyloarthritis**
- axial — *see also* Spondylitis, ankylosing
  - non-radiographic M45.AØ
    - cervical M45.A2
    - cervicothoracic M45.A3
    - lumbar M45.A6
    - lumbosacral M45.A7
    - multiple sites M45.AB
    - occipito-atlanto-axial region M45.A1
    - sacral and sacrococcygeal M45.A8
    - thoracic M45.A4
    - thoracolumbar M45.A5

**Spondylolisthesis** (acquired) (degenerative) M43.1Ø
- with disproportion (fetopelvic) O33.Ø
  - causing obstructed labor O65.Ø
- cervical region M43.12
- cervicothoracic region M43.13
- congenital Q76.2
- lumbar region M43.16
- lumbosacral region M43.17
- multiple sites M43.19
- occipito-atlanto-axial region M43.11
- sacrococcygeal region M43.18
- thoracic region M43.14
- thoracolumbar region M43.15
- traumatic (old) M43.1Ø
  - acute
    - fifth cervical (displaced) S12.43Ø- ☑
      - nondisplaced S12.431- ☑
      - specified type NEC (displaced) S12.45Ø- ☑
        - nondisplaced S12.451- ☑
      - type III S12.44- ☑
    - fourth cervical (displaced) S12.33Ø- ☑
      - nondisplaced S12.331- ☑
      - specified type NEC (displaced) S12.35Ø- ☑
        - nondisplaced S12.351- ☑
      - type III S12.34- ☑
    - second cervical (displaced) S12.13Ø- ☑
      - nondisplaced S12.131- ☑
      - specified type NEC (displaced) S12.15Ø- ☑
        - nondisplaced S12.151- ☑
      - type III S12.14- ☑
    - seventh cervical (displaced) S12.63Ø- ☑
      - nondisplaced S12.631- ☑
      - specified type NEC (displaced) S12.65Ø- ☑
        - nondisplaced S12.651- ☑
      - type III S12.64- ☑
    - sixth cervical (displaced) S12.53Ø- ☑
      - nondisplaced S12.531- ☑
      - specified type NEC (displaced) S12.55Ø- ☑
        - nondisplaced S12.551- ☑
      - type III S12.54- ☑
    - third cervical (displaced) S12.23Ø- ☑
      - nondisplaced S12.231- ☑
      - specified type NEC (displaced) S12.25Ø- ☑
        - nondisplaced S12.251- ☑
      - type III S12.24- ☑

**Spondylolysis** (acquired) M43.ØØ
- cervical region M43.Ø2
- cervicothoracic region M43.Ø3
- congenital Q76.2
- lumbar region M43.Ø6
- lumbosacral region M43.Ø7
  - with disproportion (fetopelvic) O33.Ø
    - causing obstructed labor O65.8
- multiple sites M43.Ø9
- occipito-atlanto-axial region M43.Ø1
- sacrococcygeal region M43.Ø8
- thoracic region M43.Ø4
- thoracolumbar region M43.Ø5

**Spondylopathy** M48.9
- infective NEC M46.5Ø
  - cervical region M46.52

**Spondylopathy** — *continued*
- infective — *continued*
  - cervicothoracic region M46.53
  - lumbar region M46.56
  - lumbosacral region M46.57
  - multiple sites M46.59
  - occipito-atlanto-axial region M46.51
  - sacrococcygeal region M46.58
  - thoracic region M46.54
  - thoracolumbar region M46.55
- inflammatory M46.90
  - cervical region M46.92
  - cervicothoracic region M46.93
  - lumbar region M46.96
  - lumbosacral region M46.97
  - multiple sites M46.99
  - occipito-atlanto-axial region M46.91
  - sacrococcygeal region M46.98
  - specified type NEC M46.80
    - cervical region M46.82
    - cervicothoracic region M46.83
    - lumbar region M46.86
    - lumbosacral region M46.87
    - multiple sites M46.89
    - occipito-atlanto-axial region M46.81
    - sacrococcygeal region M46.88
    - thoracic region M46.84
    - thoracolumbar region M46.85
  - thoracic region M46.94
  - thoracolumbar region M46.95
- neuropathic, in
  - syringomyelia and syringobulbia G95.0
  - tabes dorsalis A52.11
- specified NEC — *see* subcategory M48.8- ☑
- traumatic M48.30
  - cervical region M48.32
  - cervicothoracic region M48.33
  - lumbar region M48.36
  - lumbosacral region M48.37
  - occipito-atlanto-axial region M48.31
  - sacrococcygeal region M48.38
  - thoracic region M48.34
  - thoracolumbar region M48.35

**Spondylosis** M47.9
- with
  - disproportion (fetopelvic) O33.0
    - causing obstructed labor O65.0
  - myelopathy NEC M47.10
    - cervical region M47.12
    - cervicothoracic region M47.13
    - lumbar region M47.16
    - occipito-atlanto-axial region M47.11
    - thoracic region M47.14
    - thoracolumbar region M47.15
  - radiculopathy M47.20
    - cervical region M47.22
    - cervicothoracic region M47.23
    - lumbar region M47.26
    - lumbosacral region M47.27
    - occipito-atlanto-axial region M47.21
    - sacrococcygeal region M47.28
    - thoracic region M47.24
    - thoracolumbar region M47.25
- specified NEC M47.899
  - cervical region M47.892
  - cervicothoracic region M47.893
  - facet joint M47.819
  - lumbar region M47.896
  - lumbosacral region M47.897
  - occipito-atlanto-axial region M47.891
  - sacrococcygeal region M47.898
  - thoracic region M47.894
  - thoracolumbar region M47.895
- traumatic — *see* Spondylopathy, traumatic
- without myelopathy or radiculopathy M47.819
  - cervical region M47.812
  - cervicothoracic region M47.813
  - lumbar region M47.816
  - lumbosacral region M47.817
  - occipito-atlanto-axial region M47.811
  - sacrococcygeal region M47.818
  - thoracic region M47.814
  - thoracolumbar region M47.815

**Sponge**
- inadvertently left in operation wound — *see* Foreign body, accidentally left during a procedure
- kidney (medullary) Q61.5

**Sponge-diver's disease** — *see* Toxicity, venom, marine animal, sea anemone

**Spongioblastoma** (any type) — *see* Neoplasm, malignant, by site
- specified site — *see* Neoplasm, malignant, by site
- unspecified site C71.9

**Spongioneuroblastoma** — *see* Neoplasm, malignant, by site

**Spontaneous** — *see also* condition
- fracture (cause unknown) — *see* Fracture, pathological

**Spoon nail** L60.3
- congenital Q84.6

**Sporadic** — *see* condition

**Sporothrix schenckii infection** — *see* Sporotrichosis

**Sporotrichosis** B42.9
- arthritis B42.82
- disseminated B42.7
- generalized B42.7
- lymphocutaneous (fixed) (progressive) B42.1
- pulmonary B42.0
- specified NEC B42.89

**Spots, spotting** (in) (of)
- Bitot's — *see also* Pigmentation, conjunctiva
  - in the young child E50.1
  - vitamin A deficiency E50.1
- cafe, au lait L81.3
- Cayenne pepper I78.1
- cotton wool, retina — *see* Occlusion, artery, retina
- de Morgan's (senile angiomas) D18.- ☑
- Fuchs' black (myopic) — *see also* Myopia, degenerative H44.2- ☑
- intermenstrual (regular) N92.0
  - irregular N92.1
- Koplik's B05.9
- liver L81.4
- pregnancy O26.85- ☑
- purpuric R23.3
- ruby I78.1

**Spotted fever** — *see* Fever, spotted A77.9

**Sprain** (joint) (ligament)
- acromioclavicular joint or ligament S43.5- ☑
- ankle S93.40- ☑
  - calcaneofibular ligament S93.41- ☑
  - deltoid ligament S93.42- ☑
  - internal collateral ligament — *see* Sprain, ankle, specified ligament NEC
  - specified ligament NEC S93.49- ☑
  - talofibular ligament — *see* Sprain, ankle, specified ligament NEC
  - tibiofibular ligament S93.43- ☑
- anterior longitudinal, cervical S13.4- ☑
- atlas, atlanto-axial, atlanto-occipital S13.4- ☑
- breast bone — *see* Sprain, sternum
- calcaneofibular — *see* Sprain, ankle
- carpal — *see* Sprain, wrist
- carpometacarpal — *see* Sprain, hand, specified site NEC
- cartilage
  - costal S23.41- ☑
  - semilunar (knee) — *see* Sprain, knee, specified site NEC
    - with current tear — *see* Tear, meniscus
  - thyroid region S13.5- ☑
  - xiphoid — *see* Sprain, sternum
- cervical, cervicodorsal, cervicothoracic S13.4- ☑
- chondrosternal S23.421- ☑
- coracoclavicular S43.8- ☑
- coracohumeral S43.41- ☑
- coronary, knee — *see* Sprain, knee, specified site NEC
- costal cartilage S23.41- ☑
- cricoarytenoid articulation or ligament S13.5- ☑
- cricothyroid articulation S13.5- ☑
- cruciate, knee — *see* Sprain, knee, cruciate
- deltoid, ankle — *see* Sprain, ankle
- dorsal (spine) S23.3- ☑
- elbow S53.40- ☑
  - radial collateral ligament S53.43- ☑
  - radiohumeral S53.41- ☑
  - rupture
    - radial collateral ligament — *see* Rupture, traumatic, ligament, radial collateral
    - ulnar collateral ligament — *see* Rupture, traumatic, ligament, ulnar collateral
  - specified type NEC S53.49- ☑
  - ulnar collateral ligament S53.44- ☑
  - ulnohumeral S53.42- ☑
- femur, head — *see* Sprain, hip
- fibular collateral, knee — *see* Sprain, knee, collateral
- fibulocalcaneal — *see* Sprain, ankle
- finger(s) S63.61- ☑

**Sprain** — *continued*
- finger(s) — *continued*
  - index S63.61- ☑
  - interphalangeal (joint) S63.63- ☑
    - index S63.63- ☑
    - little S63.63- ☑
    - middle S63.63- ☑
    - ring S63.63- ☑
  - little S63.61- ☑
  - metacarpophalangeal (joint) S63.65- ☑
  - middle S63.61- ☑
  - ring S63.61- ☑
  - specified site NEC S63.69- ☑
    - index S63.69- ☑
    - little S63.69- ☑
    - middle S63.69- ☑
    - ring S63.69- ☑
- foot S93.60- ☑
  - specified ligament NEC S93.69- ☑
  - tarsal ligament S93.61- ☑
  - tarsometatarsal ligament S93.62- ☑
  - toe — *see* Sprain, toe
- hand S63.9- ☑
  - finger — *see* Sprain, finger
  - specified site NEC — *see* subcategory S63.8- ☑
  - thumb — *see* Sprain, thumb
- head S03.9- ☑
- hip S73.10- ☑
  - iliofemoral ligament S73.11- ☑
  - ischiocapsular (ligament) S73.12- ☑
  - specified NEC S73.19- ☑
- iliofemoral — *see* Sprain, hip
- innominate
  - acetabulum — *see* Sprain, hip
  - sacral junction S33.6- ☑
- internal
  - collateral, ankle — *see* Sprain, ankle
  - semilunar cartilage — *see* Sprain, knee, specified site NEC
- interphalangeal
  - finger — *see* Sprain, finger, interphalangeal (joint)
  - toe — *see* Sprain, toe, interphalangeal joint
- ischiocapsular — *see* Sprain, hip
- ischiofemoral — *see* Sprain, hip
- jaw (articular disc) (cartilage) (meniscus) S03.4- ☑
  - old M26.69
- knee S83.9- ☑
  - collateral ligament S83.40- ☑
    - lateral (fibular) S83.42- ☑
    - medial (tibial) S83.41- ☑
  - cruciate ligament S83.50- ☑
    - anterior S83.51- ☑
    - posterior S83.52- ☑
  - lateral (fibular) collateral ligament S83.42- ☑
  - medial (tibial) collateral ligament S83.41- ☑
  - patellar ligament S76.11- ☑
  - specified site NEC S83.8X- ☑
  - superior tibiofibular joint (ligament) S83.6- ☑
- lateral collateral, knee — *see* Sprain, knee, collateral
- lumbar (spine) S33.5- ☑
- lumbosacral S33.9- ☑
- mandible (articular disc) S03.4- ☑
  - old M26.69
- medial collateral, knee — *see* Sprain, knee, collateral
- meniscus
  - jaw S03.4- ☑
    - old M26.69
  - knee — *see* Sprain, knee, specified site NEC
    - with current tear — *see* Tear, meniscus
      - old — *see* Derangement, knee, meniscus, due to old tear
  - mandible S03.4- ☑
    - old M26.69
- metacarpal (distal) (proximal) — *see* Sprain, hand, specified site NEC
- metacarpophalangeal — *see* Sprain, finger, metacarpophalangeal (joint)
- metatarsophalangeal — *see* Sprain, toe, metatarsophalangeal joint
- midcarpal — *see* Sprain, hand, specified site NEC
- midtarsal — *see* Sprain, foot, specified site NEC
- neck S13.9- ☑
  - anterior longitudinal cervical ligament S13.4- ☑
  - atlanto-axial joint S13.4- ☑
  - atlanto-occipital joint S13.4- ☑
  - cervical spine S13.4- ☑

- **Sprain** — *continued*
  - neck — *continued*
    - cricoarytenoid ligament S13.5- ☑
    - cricothyroid ligament S13.5- ☑
    - specified site NEC S13.8- ☑
    - thyroid region (cartilage) S13.5- ☑
  - nose SØ3.8- ☑
  - orbicular, hip — *see* Sprain, hip
  - patella — *see* Sprain, knee, specified site NEC
  - patellar ligament S76.11- ☑
  - pelvis NEC S33.8- ☑
  - phalanx
    - finger — *see* Sprain, finger
    - toe — *see* Sprain, toe
  - pubofemoral — *see* Sprain, hip
  - radiocarpal — *see* Sprain, wrist
  - radiohumeral — *see* Sprain, elbow
  - radius, collateral — *see* Rupture, traumatic, ligament, radial collateral
  - rib (cage) S23.41- ☑
  - rotator cuff (capsule) S43.42- ☑
  - sacroiliac (region)
    - chronic or old — *see* subcategory M53.2- ☑
    - joint S33.6- ☑
  - scaphoid (hand) — *see* Sprain, hand, specified site NEC
  - scapula (r) — *see* Sprain, shoulder girdle, specified site NEC
  - semilunar cartilage (knee) — *see* Sprain, knee, specified site NEC
    - with current tear — *see* Tear, meniscus
      - old — *see* Derangement, knee, meniscus, due to old tear
  - shoulder joint S43.4Ø- ☑
    - acromioclavicular joint (ligament) — *see* Sprain, acromioclavicular joint
    - blade — *see* Sprain, shoulder, girdle, specified site NEC
    - coracoclavicular joint (ligament) — *see* Sprain, coracoclavicular joint
    - coracohumeral ligament — *see* Sprain, coracohumeral joint
    - girdle S43.9- ☑
      - specified site NEC S43.8- ☑
    - rotator cuff — *see* Sprain, rotator cuff
    - specified site NEC S43.49- ☑
    - sternoclavicular joint (ligament) — *see* Sprain, sternoclavicular joint
  - spine
    - cervical S13.4- ☑
    - lumbar S33.5- ☑
    - thoracic S23.3- ☑
  - sternoclavicular joint S43.6- ☑
  - sternum S23.429- ☑
    - chondrosternal joint S23.421- ☑
    - specified site NEC S23.428- ☑
    - sternoclavicular (joint) (ligament) S43.6- ☑
  - symphysis
    - jaw SØ3.4- ☑
      - old M26.69
    - mandibular SØ3.4- ☑
      - old M26.69
  - talofibular — *see* Sprain, ankle
  - tarsal — *see* Sprain, foot, specified site NEC
  - tarsometatarsal — *see* Sprain, foot, specified site NEC
  - temporomandibular SØ3.4- ☑
    - old M26.69
  - thorax S23.9- ☑
    - ribs S23.41- ☑
    - specified site NEC S23.8- ☑
    - spine S23.3- ☑
    - sternum — *see* Sprain, sternum
  - thumb S63.6Ø- ☑
    - interphalangeal (joint) S63.62- ☑
    - metacarpophalangeal (joint) S63.64- ☑
    - specified site NEC S63.68- ☑
  - thyroid cartilage or region S13.5- ☑
  - tibia (proximal end) — *see* Sprain, knee, specified site NEC
  - tibial collateral, knee — *see* Sprain, knee, collateral
  - tibiofibular
    - distal — *see* Sprain, ankle
    - superior — *see* Sprain, knee, specified site NEC
  - toe(s) S93.5Ø- ☑
    - great S93.5Ø- ☑
    - interphalangeal joint S93.51- ☑
      - great S93.51- ☑
      - lesser S93.51- ☑

- **Sprain** — *continued*
  - toe(s) — *continued*
    - lesser S93.5Ø- ☑
    - metatarsophalangeal joint S93.52- ☑
      - great S93.52- ☑
      - lesser S93.52- ☑
  - ulna, collateral — *see* Rupture, traumatic, ligament, ulnar collateral
  - ulnohumeral — *see* Sprain, elbow
  - wrist S63.5Ø- ☑
    - carpal S63.51- ☑
    - radiocarpal S63.52- ☑
    - specified site NEC S63.59- ☑
  - xiphoid cartilage — *see* Sprain, sternum
- **Sprengel's deformity** (congenital) Q74.3
- **Sprue** (tropical) K9Ø.1
  - celiac K9Ø.Ø
  - idiopathic K9Ø.49
  - meaning thrush B37.Ø
  - nontropical K9Ø.Ø
- **Spur, bone** — *see also* Enthesopathy
  - calcaneal M77.3- ☑
  - iliac crest M76.2- ☑
  - nose (septum) J34.89
- **Spurway's syndrome** Q78.Ø
- **Sputum**
  - abnormal (amount) (color) (odor) (purulent) RØ9.3
  - blood-stained RØ4.2
  - excessive (cause unknown) RØ9.3
- **Squamous** — *see also* condition
  - epithelium in
    - cervical canal (congenital) Q51.828
    - uterine mucosa (congenital) Q51.818
- **Squashed nose** M95.Ø
  - congenital Q67.4
- **Squeeze, diver's** T7Ø.3- ☑
- **Squint** — *see also* Strabismus
  - accommodative — *see* Strabismus, convergent concomitant
- **SSADHD** (succinic semialdehyde dehydrogenase deficiency) E72.81
- **St. Hubert's disease** A82.9
- **Stab** — *see also* Laceration
  - internal organs — *see* Injury, by site
- **Stafne's cyst or cavity** M27.Ø
- **Staggering gait** R26.Ø
  - hysterical F44.4
- **Staghorn calculus** — *see* Calculus, kidney
- **Stahli's line** (cornea) (pigment) — *see* Pigmentation, cornea, anterior
- **Stain, staining**
  - meconium (newborn) P96.83
  - port wine Q82.5
  - tooth, teeth (hard tissues) (extrinsic) KØ3.6
    - due to
      - accretions KØ3.6
      - deposits (betel) (black) (green) (materia alba) (orange) (soft) (tobacco) KØ3.6
      - metals (copper) (silver) KØ3.7
      - nicotine KØ3.6
      - pulpal bleeding KØ3.7
      - tobacco KØ3.6
    - intrinsic KØØ.8
- **Stammering** — *see also* Disorder, fluency F8Ø.81
- **Standstill**
  - auricular I45.5
  - cardiac — *see* Arrest, cardiac
  - sinoatrial I45.5
  - ventricular — *see* Arrest, cardiac
- **Stannosis** J63.5
- **Stanton's disease** — *see* Melioidosis
- **Staphylitis** (acute) (catarrhal) (chronic) (gangrenous) (membranous) (suppurative) (ulcerative) K12.2
- **Staphylococcal scalded skin syndrome** LØØ
- **Staphylococcemia** A41.2
- **Staphylococcus, staphylococcal** — *see also* condition
  - as cause of disease classified elsewhere B95.8
    - aureus (methicillin susceptible) (MSSA) B95.61
      - methicillin resistant (MRSA) B95.62
  - specified NEC, as cause of disease classified elsewhere B95.7
- **Staphyloma** (sclera)
  - cornea H18.72- ☑
  - equatorial H15.81- ☑
  - localized (anterior) H15.82- ☑
  - posticum H15.83- ☑
  - ring H15.85- ☑
- **Stargardt's disease** — *see* Dystrophy, retina

- **Starvation** (inanition) (due to lack of food) T73.Ø- ☑
  - edema — *see* Malnutrition, severe
- **Stasis**
  - bile (noncalculous) K83.1
  - bronchus J98.Ø9
    - with infection — *see* Bronchitis
  - cardiac — *see* Failure, heart, congestive
  - cecum K59.89
  - colon K59.89
  - dermatitis I87.2
    - with
      - varicose ulcer — *see* Varix, leg, with ulcer, with inflammation
      - varicose veins — *see* Varix, leg, with, inflammation
    - due to postthrombotic syndrome — *see* Syndrome, postthrombotic
  - duodenal K31.5
  - eczema — *see* Varix, leg, with, inflammation
  - edema — *see* Hypertension, venous (chronic), idiopathic
  - foot T69.Ø2- ☑
  - ileocecal coil K59.89
  - ileum K59.89
  - intestinal K59.89
  - jejunum K59.89
  - kidney N19
  - liver (cirrhotic) K76.1
  - lymphatic I89.8
  - pneumonia J18.2
  - pulmonary — *see* Edema, lung
  - rectal K59.89
  - renal N19
    - tubular N17.Ø
  - ulcer — *see* Varix, leg, with, ulcer
    - without varicose veins — *see also* Ulcer, by site I87.2
  - urine — *see* Retention, urine
  - venous I87.8
- **State** (of)
  - affective and paranoid, mixed, organic psychotic FØ6.8
  - agitated R45.1
    - acute reaction to stress F43.Ø
  - anxiety (neurotic) F41.1
  - apprehension F41.1
  - burn-out Z73.Ø
  - climacteric, female Z78.Ø
    - symptomatic N95.1
  - compulsive F42.8
    - mixed with obsessional thoughts F42.2
  - confusional (psychogenic) F44.89
    - acute — *see also* Delirium
      - with
        - arteriosclerotic dementia — *see also* Dementia vascular FØ1.5Ø
          - with behavioral disturbance — *see* Dementia, vascular
        - senility or dementia FØ5
      - alcoholic F1Ø.231
    - epileptic FØ5
    - reactive (from emotional stress, psychological trauma) F44.89
    - subacute — *see* Delirium
  - convulsive — *see* Convulsions
  - crisis F43.Ø
  - depressive F32.A
    - neurotic F34.1
  - dissociative F44.9
  - emotional shock (stress) R45.7
  - hypercoagulation — *see* Hypercoagulable
  - locked-in G83.5
  - menopausal Z78.Ø
    - symptomatic N95.1
  - neurotic F48.9
    - with depersonalization F48.1
  - obsessional F42.8
  - oneiroid (schizophrenia-like) F23
  - organic
    - hallucinatory (nonalcoholic) FØ6.Ø
    - paranoid (-hallucinatory) FØ6.2
  - panic F41.Ø
  - paranoid F22
    - climacteric F22
    - involutional F22
    - menopausal F22
    - organic FØ6.2
    - senile FØ3.- ☑
    - simple F22
  - persistent vegetative R4Ø.3
  - phobic F4Ø.9
  - postleukotomy FØ7.Ø

**Stone(s)** — *see also* Calculus
  bladder (diverticulum) N21.Ø
  cystine E72.Ø9
  heart syndrome I5Ø.1
  kidney N2Ø.Ø
  prostate N42.Ø
  pulpal (dental) KØ4.2
  renal N2Ø.Ø
  salivary gland or duct (any) K11.5
  urethra (impacted) N21.1
  urinary (duct) (impacted) (passage) N2Ø.9
    bladder (diverticulum) N21.Ø
    lower tract N21.9
    specified NEC N21.8
  xanthine E79.82 *[N22]*
**Stonecutter's lung** J62.8
**Stonemason's asthma, disease, lung or pneumoconiosis** J62.8
**Stoppage**
  heart — *see* Arrest, cardiac
  urine — *see* Retention, urine
**Storm, thyroid** — *see* Thyrotoxicosis
**Strabismus** (congenital) (nonparalytic) H5Ø.9
  concomitant H5Ø.4Ø
    convergent — *see* Strabismus, convergent concomitant
    divergent — *see* Strabismus, divergent concomitant
  convergent concomitant H5Ø.ØØ
    accommodative component H5Ø.43
    alternating H5Ø.Ø5
      with
        A pattern H5Ø.Ø6
        specified nonconcomitances NEC H5Ø.Ø8
        V pattern H5Ø.Ø7
    monocular H5Ø.Ø1- ☑
      with
        A pattern H5Ø.Ø2- ☑
        specified nonconcomitances NEC H5Ø.Ø4- ☑
        V pattern H5Ø.Ø3- ☑
      intermittent H5Ø.31- ☑
        alternating H5Ø.32
  cyclotropia H5Ø.41- ☑
  divergent concomitant H5Ø.1Ø
    alternating H5Ø.15
      with
        A pattern H5Ø.16
        specified noncomitances NEC H5Ø.18
        V pattern H5Ø.17
    monocular H5Ø.11- ☑
      with
        A pattern H5Ø.12- ☑
        specified noncomitances NEC H5Ø.14- ☑
        V pattern H5Ø.13- ☑
      intermittent H5Ø.33- ☑
        alternating H5Ø.34
  Duane's syndrome H5Ø.81- ☑
  due to adhesions, scars H5Ø.69
  heterophoria H5Ø.5Ø
    alternating H5Ø.55
    cyclophoria H5Ø.54
    esophoria H5Ø.51
    exophoria H5Ø.52
    vertical H5Ø.53
  heterotropia H5Ø.4Ø
    intermittent H5Ø.3Ø
  hypertropia H5Ø.2- ☑
  hypotropia — *see* Hypertropia
  latent H5Ø.5Ø
  mechanical H5Ø.6Ø
    Brown's sheath syndrome H5Ø.61- ☑
    specified type NEC H5Ø.69
  monofixation syndrome H5Ø.42
  paralytic H49.9
    abducens nerve H49.2- ☑
    fourth nerve H49.1- ☑
    Kearns-Sayre syndrome H49.81- ☑
    ophthalmoplegia (external)
      progressive H49.4- ☑
        with pigmentary retinopathy H49.81- ☑
      total H49.3- ☑
    sixth nerve H49.2- ☑
    specified type NEC H49.88- ☑
    third nerve H49.Ø- ☑
    trochlear nerve H49.1- ☑
  specified type NEC H5Ø.89
  vertical H5Ø.2- ☑
**Strain**
  back S39.Ø12- ☑
**Strain** — *continued*
  cervical S16.1- ☑
  eye NEC — *see* Disturbance, vision, subjective
  heart — *see* Disease, heart
  low back S39.Ø12- ☑
  mental NOS Z73.3
    work-related Z56.6
  muscle (tendon) — *see* Injury, muscle, by site, strain
  neck S16.1- ☑
  physical NOS Z73.3
    work-related Z56.6
  postural — *see also* Disorder, soft tissue, due to use
  psychological NEC Z73.3
  tendon — *see* Injury, muscle, by site, strain
**Straining, on urination** R39.16
**Strand, vitreous** — *see* Opacity, vitreous, membranes and strands
**Strangulation, strangulated** — *see also* Asphyxia, traumatic
  appendix K38.8
  bladder-neck N32.Ø
  bowel or colon K56.2
  food or foreign body — *see* Foreign body, by site
  hemorrhoids — *see* Hemorrhoids, with complication
  hernia — *see also* Hernia, by site, with obstruction
    with gangrene — *see* Hernia, by site, with gangrene
  intestine (large) (small) K56.2
    with hernia — *see also* Hernia, by site, with obstruction
      with gangrene — *see* Hernia, by site, with gangrene
  mesentery K56.2
  mucus — *see* Asphyxia, mucus
  omentum K56.2
  organ or site, congenital NEC — *see* Atresia, by site
  ovary — *see* Torsion, ovary
  penis N48.89
    foreign body T19.4- ☑
  rupture — *see* Hernia, by site, with obstruction
  stomach due to hernia — *see also* Hernia, by site, with obstruction
    with gangrene — *see* Hernia, by site, with gangrene
  vesicourethral orifice N32.Ø
**Strangury** R3Ø.Ø
**Straw itch** B88.Ø9
**Strawberry**
  gallbladder K82.4
  mark Q82.5
  tongue (red) (white) K14.3
**Streak**(s)
  macula, angioid H35.33
  ovarian Q5Ø.32
**Strephosymbolia** F81.Ø
  secondary to organic lesion R48.8
**Streptobacillary fever** A25.1
**Streptobacillosis** A25.1
**Streptobacillus moniliformis** A25.1
**Streptococcus, streptococcal** — *see also* condition
  as cause of disease classified elsewhere B95.5
  group
    A, as cause of disease classified elsewhere B95.Ø
    B, as cause of disease classified elsewhere B95.1
    D, as cause of disease classified elsewhere B95.2
  pneumoniae, as cause of disease classified elsewhere B95.3
  specified NEC, as cause of disease classified elsewhere B95.4
**Streptomycosis** B47.1
**Streptotrichosis** A48.8
**Stress** F43.9
  family — *see* Disruption, family
  fetal P84
    complicating pregnancy O77.9
      due to drug administration O77.1
  mental NEC Z73.3
    work-related Z56.6
  physical NEC Z73.3
    work-related Z56.6
  polycythemia D75.1
  reaction — *see also* Reaction, stress F43.9
  work schedule Z56.3
  workplace Z56.6
**Stretching, nerve** — *see* Injury, nerve
**Striae albicantes, atrophicae or distensae** (cutis) L9Ø.6
**Stricture** — *see also* Stenosis
  ampulla of Vater K83.1
  anus (sphincter) K62.4
    congenital Q42.3
      with fistula Q42.2
**Stricture** — *continued*
  anus — *continued*
    infantile Q42.3
      with fistula Q42.2
  aorta (ascending) (congenital) Q25.1
    arteriosclerotic I7Ø.Ø
    calcified I7Ø.Ø
    supravalvular, congenital Q25.3
  aortic (valve) — *see* Stenosis, aortic
  aqueduct of Sylvius (congenital) QØ3.Ø
    with spina bifida — *see* Spina bifida, by site, with hydrocephalus
    acquired G91.1
  artery I77.1
    basilar — *see* Occlusion, artery, basilar
    carotid — *see* Occlusion, artery, carotid
    celiac (compression) I77.4
      arteriosclerotic I7Ø.8
      atherosclerosis I7Ø.8
    congenital (peripheral) Q27.8
      cerebral Q28.3
      coronary Q24.5
      digestive system Q27.8
      lower limb Q27.8
      retinal Q14.1
      specified site NEC Q27.8
      umbilical Q27.Ø
      upper limb Q27.8
    coronary — *see* Disease, heart, ischemic, atherosclerotic
      congenital Q24.5
    precerebral — *see* Occlusion, artery, precerebral
    pulmonary (congenital) Q25.6
      acquired I28.8
    renal I7Ø.1
    vertebral — *see* Occlusion, artery, vertebral
  auditory canal (external) (congenital)
    acquired — *see* Stenosis, external ear canal
  bile duct (common) (hepatic) K83.1
    congenital Q44.3
    postoperative K91.89
  bladder N32.89
    neck N32.Ø
  bowel — *see* Obstruction, intestine
  brain G93.89
  bronchus J98.Ø9
    congenital Q32.3
    syphilitic A52.72
  cardia (stomach) K22.2
    congenital Q39.3
  cardiac — *see also* Disease, heart
    orifice (stomach) K22.2
  cecum — *see* Obstruction, intestine
  cervix, cervical (canal) N88.2
    congenital Q51.828
    in pregnancy — *see* Pregnancy, complicated by, abnormal cervix
      causing obstructed labor O65.5
  colon — *see also* Obstruction, intestine
    congenital Q42.9
      specified NEC Q42.8
  colostomy K94.Ø3
  common (bile) duct K83.1
  coronary (artery) — *see* Disease, heart, ischemic, atherosclerotic
  cystic duct — *see* Obstruction, gallbladder
  digestive organs NEC, congenital Q45.8
  duodenum K31.5
    congenital Q41.Ø
  ear canal (external) (congenital) Q16.1
    acquired — *see* Stricture, auditory canal, acquired
  ejaculatory duct N5Ø.89
  enterostomy K94.13
  esophagus K22.2
    congenital Q39.3
    syphilitic A52.79
      congenital A5Ø.59 *[K23]*
  eustachian tube — *see also* Obstruction, eustachian tube
    congenital Q17.8
  fallopian tube N97.1
    gonococcal A54.24
    tuberculous A18.17
  gallbladder — *see* Obstruction, gallbladder
  glottis J38.6
  heart — *see also* Disease, heart
    valve — *see also* Endocarditis I38
      aortic Q23.Ø
      mitral Q23.2
      pulmonary Q22.1

- **Struma** — *continued*
  - nodosa — *continued*
    - toxic or with hyperthyroidism — *continued*
      - uninodular EØ5.1Ø
        - with thyroid storm EØ5.11
    - toxicosa EØ5.2Ø
      - with thyroid storm EØ5.21
      - multinodular EØ5.2Ø
        - with thyroid storm EØ5.21
      - uninodular EØ5.1Ø
        - with thyroid storm EØ5.11
    - uninodular EØ4.1
  - ovarii D27.- ☑
  - Riedel's EØ6.5
- **Strumipriva cachexia** EØ3.4
- **Strumpell-Marie spine** — *see* Spondylitis, ankylosing
- **Strumpell-Westphal pseudosclerosis** E83.Ø1
- **Stuart deficiency disease** (factor X) D68.2
- **Stuart-Prower factor deficiency** (factor X) D68.2
- **Student's elbow** — *see* Bursitis, elbow, olecranon
- **Stump** — *see* Amputation
- **Stunned myocardium, neurogenic** I5A
- **Stunting, nutritional** E45
- **Stupor** (catatonic) R4Ø.1
  - depressive (single episode) F32.89
    - recurrent episode F33.8
  - dissociative F44.2
  - manic F3Ø.2
  - manic-depressive F31.89
  - psychogenic (anergic) F44.2
  - reaction to exceptional stress (transient) F43.Ø
- **Sturge** (-Weber) (-Dimitri) (-Kalischer) **disease or syndrome** Q85.89
- **Stuttering** F8Ø.81
  - adult onset F98.5
  - childhood onset F8Ø.81
  - following cerebrovascular disease — *see* Disorder, fluency. following cerebrovascular disease
  - in conditions classified elsewhere R47.82
- **Sty, stye** (external) (internal) (meibomian) (zeisian) — *see* Hordeolum
- **Subacidity, gastric** K31.89
  - psychogenic F45.8
- **Subacute** — *see* condition
- **Subarachnoid** — *see* condition
- **Subcortical** — *see* condition
- **Subcostal syndrome, nerve compression** — *see* Mononeuropathy, upper limb, specified site NEC
- **Subcutaneous, subcuticular** — *see* condition
- **Subdural** — *see* condition
- **Subendocardium** — *see* condition
- **Subependymoma**
  - specified site — *see* Neoplasm, uncertain behavior, by site
  - unspecified site D43.2
- **Suberosis** J67.3
- **Subglossitis** — *see* Glossitis
- **Subhemophilia** D66
- **Subinvolution**
  - breast (postlactational) (postpuerperal) N64.89
  - puerperal O9Ø.89
  - uterus (chronic) (nonpuerperal) N85.3
    - puerperal O9Ø.89
- **Sublingual** — *see* condition
- **Sublinguitis** — *see* Sialoadenitis
- **Subluxatable hip** Q65.6
- **Subluxation** — *see also* Dislocation
  - acromioclavicular S43.11- ☑
  - ankle S93.Ø- ☑
  - atlantoaxial, recurrent M43.4
    - with myelopathy M43.3
  - carpometacarpal (joint) NEC S63.Ø5- ☑
    - thumb S63.Ø4- ☑
  - complex, vertebral — *see* Complex, subluxation
  - congenital — *see also* Malposition, congenital
    - hip — *see* Dislocation, hip, congenital, partial
    - joint (excluding hip)
      - lower limb Q68.8
      - shoulder Q68.8
      - upper limb Q68.8
  - elbow (traumatic) S53.1Ø- ☑
    - anterior S53.11- ☑
    - lateral S53.14- ☑
    - medial S53.13- ☑
    - posterior S53.12- ☑
    - specified type NEC S53.19- ☑
  - finger S63.2Ø- ☑
    - index S63.2Ø- ☑

- **Subluxation** — *continued*
  - finger — *continued*
    - interphalangeal S63.22- ☑
      - distal S63.24- ☑
        - index S63.24- ☑
        - little S63.24- ☑
        - middle S63.24- ☑
        - ring S63.24- ☑
      - index S63.22- ☑
      - little S63.22- ☑
      - middle S63.22- ☑
      - proximal S63.23- ☑
        - index S63.23- ☑
        - little S63.23- ☑
        - middle S63.23- ☑
        - ring S63.23- ☑
      - ring S63.22- ☑
    - little S63.2Ø- ☑
    - metacarpophalangeal S63.21- ☑
      - index S63.21- ☑
      - little S63.21- ☑
      - middle S63.21- ☑
      - ring S63.21- ☑
    - middle S63.2Ø- ☑
    - ring S63.2Ø- ☑
  - foot S93.3Ø- ☑
    - specified site NEC S93.33- ☑
    - tarsal joint S93.31- ☑
    - tarsometatarsal joint S93.32- ☑
    - toe — *see* Subluxation, toe
  - hip S73.ØØ- ☑
    - anterior S73.Ø3- ☑
      - obturator S73.Ø2- ☑
    - central S73.Ø4- ☑
    - posterior S73.Ø1- ☑
  - interphalangeal (joint)
    - finger S63.22- ☑
      - distal joint S63.24- ☑
        - index S63.24- ☑
        - little S63.24- ☑
        - middle S63.24- ☑
        - ring S63.24- ☑
      - index S63.22- ☑
      - little S63.22- ☑
      - middle S63.22- ☑
      - proximal joint S63.23- ☑
        - index S63.23- ☑
        - little S63.23- ☑
        - middle S63.23- ☑
        - ring S63.23- ☑
      - ring S63.22- ☑
    - thumb S63.12- ☑
    - toe S93.13- ☑
      - great S93.13- ☑
      - lesser S93.13- ☑
  - joint prosthesis — *see* Complications, joint prosthesis, mechanical, displacement, by site
  - knee S83.1Ø- ☑
    - cap — *see* Subluxation, patella
    - patella — *see* Subluxation, patella
    - proximal tibia
      - anteriorly S83.11- ☑
      - laterally S83.14- ☑
      - medially S83.13- ☑
      - posteriorly S83.12- ☑
    - specified type NEC S83.19- ☑
  - lens — *see* Dislocation, lens, partial
  - ligament, traumatic — *see* Sprain, by site
  - metacarpal (bone)
    - proximal end S63.Ø6- ☑
  - metacarpophalangeal (joint)
    - finger S63.21- ☑
      - index S63.21- ☑
      - little S63.21- ☑
      - middle S63.21- ☑
      - ring S63.21- ☑
    - thumb S63.11- ☑
  - metatarsophalangeal joint S93.14- ☑
    - great toe S93.14- ☑
    - lesser toe S93.14- ☑
  - midcarpal (joint) S63.Ø3- ☑
  - patella S83.ØØ- ☑
    - lateral S83.Ø1- ☑
    - recurrent (nontraumatic) — *see* Dislocation, patella, recurrent, incomplete

- **Subluxation** — *continued*
  - patella — *continued*
    - specified type NEC S83.Ø9- ☑
  - pathological — *see* Dislocation, pathological
  - radial head S53.ØØ- ☑
    - anterior S53.Ø1- ☑
    - nursemaid's elbow S53.Ø3- ☑
    - posterior S53.Ø2- ☑
    - specified type NEC S53.Ø9- ☑
  - radiocarpal (joint) S63.Ø2- ☑
  - radioulnar (joint)
    - distal S63.Ø1- ☑
    - proximal — *see* Subluxation, elbow
  - shoulder
    - congenital Q68.8
    - girdle S43.3Ø- ☑
      - scapula S43.31- ☑
      - specified site NEC S43.39- ☑
    - traumatic S43.ØØ- ☑
      - anterior S43.Ø1- ☑
      - inferior S43.Ø3- ☑
      - posterior S43.Ø2- ☑
      - specified type NEC S43.Ø8- ☑
  - sternoclavicular (joint) S43.2Ø- ☑
    - anterior S43.21- ☑
    - posterior S43.22- ☑
  - symphysis (pubis) — *see also* Dislocation, symphysis pubis
  - thumb S63.1Ø3- ☑
    - interphalangeal joint — *see* Subluxation, interphalangeal (joint), thumb
    - metacarpophalangeal joint — *see* Subluxation, metacarpophalangeal (joint), thumb
  - toe(s) S93.1Ø- ☑
    - great S93.1Ø- ☑
      - interphalangeal joint S93.13- ☑
      - metatarsophalangeal joint S93.14- ☑
    - interphalangeal joint S93.13- ☑
    - lesser S93.1Ø- ☑
      - interphalangeal joint S93.13- ☑
      - metatarsophalangeal joint S93.14- ☑
    - metatarsophalangeal joint S93.149- ☑
  - ulna
    - distal end S63.Ø7- ☑
    - proximal end — *see* Subluxation, elbow
  - ulnohumeral joint — *see* Subluxation, elbow
  - vertebral
    - recurrent NEC — *see* subcategory M43.5- ☑
    - traumatic
      - cervical S13.1ØØ- ☑
        - atlantoaxial joint S13.12Ø- ☑
        - atlantooccipital joint S13.11Ø- ☑
        - atloidooccipital joint S13.11Ø- ☑
        - joint between
          - CØ and C1 S13.11Ø- ☑
          - C1 and C2 S13.12Ø- ☑
          - C2 and C3 S13.13Ø- ☑
          - C3 and C4 S13.14Ø- ☑
          - C4 and C5 S13.15Ø- ☑
          - C5 and C6 S13.16Ø- ☑
          - C6 and C7 S13.17Ø- ☑
          - C7 and T1 S13.18Ø- ☑
        - occipitoatloid joint S13.11Ø- ☑
      - lumbar S33.1ØØ- ☑
        - joint between
          - L1 and L2 S33.11Ø- ☑
          - L2 and L3 S33.12Ø- ☑
          - L3 and L4 S33.13Ø- ☑
          - L4 and L5 S33.14Ø- ☑
      - thoracic S23.1ØØ- ☑
        - joint between
          - T1 and T2 S23.11Ø- ☑
          - T2 and T3 S23.12Ø- ☑
          - T3 and T4 S23.122- ☑
          - T4 and T5 S23.13Ø- ☑
          - T5 and T6 S23.132- ☑
          - T6 and T7 S23.14Ø- ☑
          - T7 and T8 S23.142- ☑
          - T8 and T9 S23.15Ø- ☑
          - T1Ø and T11 S23.16Ø- ☑
          - T11 and T12 S23.162- ☑
          - T12 and L1 S23.17Ø- ☑
          - T9 and T1Ø S23.152- ☑
  - wrist (carpal bone) S63.ØØ- ☑
    - carpometacarpal joint — *see* Subluxation, carpometacarpal (joint)

☑ **Additional Character Required — Refer to the Tabular List for Character Selection**

**Syndrome** — *continued*
- Hoppe-Goldflam G7Ø.ØØ
  - with exacerbation (acute) G7Ø.Ø1
  - in crisis G7Ø.Ø1
- Horner's G9Ø.2
- hungry bone E83.81
- hunterian glossitis D51.Ø
- Hunt's (herpetic geniculate ganglionitis) (neuralgia) BØ2.21
  - dyssynergia cerebellaris myoclonica G11.19
- Hutchinson's triad A5Ø.53
- hyperabduction G54.Ø
- hyperammonemia-hyperornithinemia-homocitrullinemia E72.4
- hypereosinophilic (HES) D72.119
  - idiopathic (IHES) D72.11Ø
  - lymphocytic variant (LHES) D72.111
  - myeloid D72.118
  - specified NEC D72.118
- hyperimmunoglobulin D MØ4.1
- hyperimmunoglobulin E (IgE) D82.4
- hyperkalemic E87.5
- hyperkinetic — *see* Hyperkinesia
- hypermobility M35.7
- hypernatremia E87.Ø
- hyperosmolarity — *see also* Diabetes, by type, with hyperosmolarity E87.Ø
- hyperperfusion G97.82
- hypersplenic D73.1
- hypertransfusion, newborn P61.1
- hyperventilation F45.8
- hyperviscosity (of serum)
  - polycythemic D75.1
  - sclerothymic D58.8
- hypoglycemic (familial) (neonatal) E16.2
- hypokalemic E87.6
- hyponatremic E87.1
- hypopituitarism E23.Ø
- hypoplastic left-heart Q23.4
- hypopotassemia E87.6
- hyposmolality E87.1
- hypotension, maternal O26.5- ☑
- hypothenar hammer I73.89
- hypoventilation, obesity (OHS) E66.2
- ICF (intravascular coagulation-fibrinolysis) D65
- idiopathic
  - cardiorespiratory distress, newborn P22.Ø
  - nephrotic (infantile) NØ4.9
- iliotibial band M76.3- ☑
- immobility, immobilization (paraplegic) M62.3
- immune effector cell-associated neurotoxicity (ICANS) G92.ØØ
  - grade
    - 1 G92.Ø1
    - 2 G92.Ø2
    - 3 G92.Ø3
    - 4 G92.Ø4
    - 5 G92.Ø5
    - unspecified G92.ØØ
- immune reconstitution D89.3
- immune reconstitution inflammatory [IRIS] D89.3
- immunity deficiency, combined D81.9
- immunodeficiency
  - acquired — *see* Human, immunodeficiency virus (HIV) disease
  - combined D81.9
- impending coronary I2Ø.Ø
- impingement, shoulder M75.4- ☑
- inappropriate secretion of antidiuretic hormone E22.2
- infant
  - gestational diabetes P7Ø.Ø
  - of diabetic mother P7Ø.1
- infantilism (pituitary) E23.Ø
- inferior vena cava I87.1
- inherited neoplasm predisposition syndrome of multiple systems, specified NEC QA1.798
- inspissated bile (newborn) P59.1
- institutional (childhood) F94.2
- insufficient sleep F51.12
- insulin resistance
  - type A E88.811
  - type B E88.818
- intermediate coronary (artery) I2Ø.Ø
- interspinous ligament — *see* Spondylopathy, specified NEC
- intestinal
  - carcinoid E34.Ø9
  - knot K56.2
- intravascular coagulation-fibrinolysis (ICF) D65

**Syndrome** — *continued*
- iodine-deficiency, congenital EØØ.9
  - type
    - mixed EØØ.2
    - myxedematous EØØ.1
    - neurological EØØ.Ø
- IRDS (idiopathic respiratory distress, newborn) P22.Ø
- irritable
  - bowel K58.9
    - with
      - constipation K58.1
      - diarrhea K58.Ø
    - mixed K58.2
    - psychogenic F45.8
    - specified NEC K58.8
  - heart (psychogenic) F45.8
  - weakness F48.8
- ischemic
  - bowel (transient) K55.9
    - chronic K55.1
    - due to mesenteric artery insufficiency K55.1
  - steal T82.898- ☑
- IVC (intravascular coagulopathy) D65
- Ivemark's Q89.Ø1
- Jaccoud's — *see* Arthropathy, postrheumatic, chronic
- Jackson's G83.89
- Jakob-Creutzfeldt — *see* Creutzfeldt-Jakob disease or syndrome
- jaw-winking QØ7.8
- Jervell-Lange-Nielsen I45.81
- jet lag G47.25
- Job's D71.8
- Joseph-Diamond-Blackfan D61.Ø1
- jugular foramen G52.7
- Kabuki (type 1, due to KMT2D mutation) (type 2, due to KDM6A mutation) Q89.81
- Kanner's (autism) F84.Ø
- Kartagener's Q89.3
- Kelly's D5Ø.1
- Kimmelstiel-Wilson — *see* Diabetes, specified type, with Kimmelstiel-Wilson disease
- Kleefstra Q87.86
- Klein (e)-Levine G47.13
- Klippel-Feil (brevicollis) Q76.1
- Kohler-Pellegrini-Stieda — *see* Bursitis, tibial collateral
- Konig's K59.89
- Korsakoff (-Wernicke) (nonalcoholic) FØ4
  - alcoholic F1Ø.9- ☑
    - with dependence F1Ø.2- ☑
- Kostmann's D7Ø.Ø
- Krabbe's congenital muscle hypoplasia Q79.8
- labyrinthine — *see* subcategory H83.2- ☑
- lacunar NEC G46.7
- Lambert-Eaton G7Ø.8Ø
  - in
    - neoplastic disease G73.1
    - specified disease NEC G7Ø.81
- Landau-Kleffner — *see* Epilepsy, specified NEC
- Larsen's Q74.8
- Lassueur Graham-Little Piccardi L66.19
- lateral
  - cutaneous nerve of thigh G57.1- ☑
  - medullary G46.4
- Launois' E22.Ø
- Laurence-Moon Q87.84
- Lawrence E88.12
- lazy
  - leukocyte D7Ø.8
  - posture M62.3
- Lemierre I8Ø.8
- Lennox-Gastaut G4Ø.812
  - intractable G4Ø.814
    - with status epilepticus G4Ø.813
    - without status epilepticus G4Ø.814
  - not intractable G4Ø.812
    - with status epilepticus G4Ø.811
    - without status epilepticus G4Ø.812
- lenticular, progressive E83.Ø1
- Leopold-Levi's EØ5.9Ø
- Lev's I44.2
- Li-Fraumeni QA1.792
- Lichtheim's D51.Ø
- Lightwood's N25.89
- Lignac (de Toni) (-Fanconi) (-Debre) E72.Ø9
  - with cystinosis E72.Ø4
- Likoff's I2Ø.89
- limbic epilepsy personality FØ7.Ø
- liver-kidney K76.7

**Syndrome** — *continued*
- lobotomy FØ7.Ø
- Loeys-Dietz Q87.A
- Loffler's J82.89
- long arm 18 or 21 deletion Q93.89
- long QT I45.81
- Louis-Barre G11.3
- low
  - atmospheric pressure T7Ø.29- ☑
  - back M54.5Ø
  - output (cardiac) I5Ø.9
- lower radicular, newborn (birth injury) P14.8
- Luetscher's (dehydration) E86.Ø
- Lupus anticoagulant D68.62
- Lutembacher's Q21.19
- Lynch (due to EPCAM) (due to MLH1) (due to MSH2) (due to MSH6) (due to PMS2) QA1.71
- macrophage activation D76.1
  - due to infection D76.2
- magnesium-deficiency R29.Ø
- Majeed MØ4.8
- Mal de Debarquement R42
- malabsorption K9Ø.9
  - postsurgical K91.2
- malformation, congenital, due to
  - alcohol Q86.Ø
  - exogenous cause NEC Q86.8
  - hydantoin Q86.1
  - warfarin Q86.2
- malignant
  - carcinoid E34.ØØ
  - neuroleptic G21.Ø
- Mallory-Weiss K22.6
- mandibulofacial dysostosis Q75.4
- manic-depressive — *see* Disorder, bipolar
- maple-syrup-urine E71.Ø
- Marable's I77.4
- Marfan Q87.4Ø
  - with
    - cardiovascular manifestations Q87.418
      - aortic dilation Q87.41Ø
    - ocular manifestations Q87.42
    - skeletal manifestations Q87.43
- Marie's (acromegaly) E22.Ø
- mast cell activation — *see* Activation, mast cell
- maternal hypotension — *see* Syndrome, hypotension, maternal
- May (-Hegglin) D72.Ø
- McArdle (-Schmidt) (-Pearson) E74.Ø4
- McQuarrie's E16.2
- meconium plug (newborn) P76.Ø
- MED13L (mediator complex subunit 13L) Q87.85
- median arcuate ligament I77.4
- mediator complex subunit 13L (MED13L) Q87.85
- Meekeren-Ehlers-Danlos Q79.6- ☑
- megavitamin-B6 E67.2
- Meige G24.4
- MELAS E88.41
- Mendelson's O74.Ø
- MERRF (myoclonic epilepsy associated with ragged-red fibers) E88.42
- mesenteric
  - artery (superior) K55.1
  - vascular insufficiency K55.1
- metabolic E88.81Ø
- metastatic carcinoid E34.ØØ
- micrognathia-glossoptosis Q87.Ø
- midbrain NEC G93.89
- middle lobe (lung) J98.19
- middle radicular G54.Ø
- migraine — *see also* Migraine G43.9Ø9
- Mikulicz' K11.8
- milk-alkali E83.52
- Millard-Gubler G46.3
- Miller-Dieker Q93.88
- Miller-Fisher G61.Ø
- Minkowski-Chauffard D58.Ø
- Mirizzi's K83.1
- MNGIE (Mitochondrial Neurogastrointestinal Encephalopathy) E88.49
- Mobius, ophthalmoplegic migraine — *see* Migraine, ophthalmoplegic
- monofixation H5Ø.42
- Morel-Moore M85.2
- Morel-Morgagni M85.2
- Morgagni (-Morel) (-Stewart) M85.2
- Morgagni-Adams-Stokes I45.9
- Mounier-Kuhn Q32.4
  - with bronchiectasis J47.9

**Syndrome** — *continued*
- Mounier-Kuhn — *continued*
  - with bronchiectasis — *continued*
    - with
      - exacerbation (acute) J47.1
      - lower respiratory infection J47.Ø
  - acquired J98.Ø9
    - with bronchiectasis J47.9
      - with
        - exacerbation (acute) J47.1
        - lower respiratory infection J47.Ø
- Muckle-Wells MØ4.2
- mucocutaneous lymph node (acute febrile) (MCLS) M3Ø.3
- multiple endocrine neoplasia (MEN) — *see* Neoplasia, endocrine, multiple (MEN)
- multiple operations — *see* Disorder, factitious
- multisystem inflammatory (in adults) (in children) M35.81
- myasthenic G7Ø.9
  - in
    - diabetes mellitus — *see* Diabetes, amyotrophy
    - endocrine disease NEC E34.9 *[G73.3]*
    - neoplastic disease — *see also* Neoplasm D49.9 *[G73.3]*
    - thyrotoxicosis (hyperthyroidism) EØ5.9Ø *[G73.3]*
      - with thyroid storm EØ5.91 *[G73.3]*
- myelodysplastic D46.9
  - with
    - 5q deletion D46.C (*following* D46.2)
    - isolated del (5q) chromosomal abnormality D46.C (*following* D46.2)
    - multilineage dysplasia D46.A (*following* D46.2)
      - with ringed sideroblasts D46.B (*following* D46.2)
    - pancytopenia (acquired) D61.818
  - lesions, low grade D46.2Ø
  - specified NEC D46.Z (*following* D46.4)
- myeloid hypereosinophilic D72.118
- myelopathic pain G89.Ø
- myeloproliferative (chronic) D47.1
- myofascial pain M79.18
- Naffziger's G54.Ø
- nail patella Q87.2
- NARP (Neuropathy, Ataxia and Retinitis pigmentosa) E88.49
- neonatal abstinence P96.1
- nephritic — *see also* Nephritis
  - with edema — *see* Nephrosis
  - acute NØØ.9
  - chronic NØ3.9
  - rapidly progressive NØ1.9
- nephrotic (congenital) — *see also* Nephrosis NØ4.9
  - with
    - C3
      - glomerulonephritis NØ4.A
      - glomerulopathy NØ4.A
        - with dense deposit disease NØ4.6
    - dense deposit disease NØ4.6
    - diffuse
      - crescentic glomerulonephritis NØ4.7
      - endocapillary proliferative glomerulonephritis NØ4.4
      - membranous glomerulonephritis NØ4.2Ø
      - mesangial proliferative glomerulonephritis NØ4.3
      - mesangiocapillary glomerulonephritis NØ4.5
    - focal and segmental glomerular lesions NØ4.1
    - minor glomerular abnormality NØ4.Ø
    - specified morphological changes NEC NØ4.8
  - diabetic — *see* Diabetes, nephrosis
  - specified type NEC with diffuse membranous glomerulonephritis NØ4.29
- neurologic neglect R41.4
- Nezelof's D81.4
- Niikawa-Kuroki Q89.81
- Nonne-Milroy-Meige Q82.Ø
- Nothnagel's vasomotor acroparesthesia I73.89
- obesity hypoventilation (OHS) E66.2
- obliterans
  - bronchiolitis — *see also* Bronchiolitis, obliterative J44.81
- oculomotor H51.9
- Ogilvie K59.81
- Oliver-McFarlane Q87.89
- ophthalmoplegia-cerebellar ataxia — *see* Strabismus, paralytic, third nerve
- oral allergy T78.19- ☑
- oral-facial-digital Q87.Ø
- organic
  - affective FØ6.3Ø
  - amnesic (not alcohol- or drug-induced) FØ4

**Syndrome** — *continued*
- organic — *continued*
  - brain FØ9
  - depressive FØ6.31
  - hallucinosis FØ6.Ø
  - personality FØ7.Ø
- Ormond's N13.5
- oro-facial-digital Q87.Ø
- os trigonum Q68.8
- Osler-Weber-Rendu I78.Ø
- osteoporosis-osteomalacia M83.8
- Osterreicher-Turner Q87.2
- oto-palatal-digital Q87.Ø
- otolith — *see* subcategory H81.8- ☑
- outlet (thoracic) — *see also* Syndrome, thoracic outlet G54.Ø
- ovary
  - polycystic E28.2
  - resistant E28.39
  - sclerocystic E28.2
- Owren's D68.2
- Paget-Schroetter I82.89Ø
- pain — *see also* Pain
  - complex regional I G9Ø.5Ø
    - lower limb G9Ø.52- ☑
    - specified site NEC G9Ø.59
    - upper limb G9Ø.51- ☑
  - complex regional II — *see* Causalgia
- painful
  - bruising D69.2
  - feet E53.8
  - prostate N42.81
- paralysis agitans — *see* Parkinsonism
- paralytic G83.9
  - specified NEC G83.89
- Parinaud's H51.Ø
- parkinsonian — *see* Parkinsonism
- Parkinson's — *see* Parkinsonism
- paroxysmal facial pain G5Ø.Ø
- Parry's EØ5.ØØ
  - with thyroid storm EØ5.Ø1
- Parsonage (-Aldren)-Turner G54.5
- patella clunk M25.86- ☑
- Paterson (-Brown) (-Kelly) D5Ø.1
- pectoral girdle I77.89
- pectoralis minor I77.89
- pediatric acute-onset neuropsychiatric (PANS) D89.89
- pediatric autoimmune neuropsychiatric disorders associated with streptococcal infections (PANDAS) D89.89
- pediatric inflammatory multisystem M35.81
- Pelger-Huet D72.Ø
- pellagra-cerebellar ataxia-renal aminoaciduria E72.Ø2
- pellagroid E52
- Pellegrini-Stieda — *see* Bursitis, tibial collateral
- pelvic congestion-fibrosis, female N94.89
- penta X Q97.1
- peptic ulcer — *see* Ulcer, peptic
- perabduction I77.89
- periodic fever MØ4.1
- periodic fever, aphthous stomatitis, pharyngitis, and adenopathy [PFAPA] MØ4.8
- periodic headache, in adults and children — *see* Headache, periodic syndromes in adults and children
- periurethral fibrosis N13.5
- Peutz-Jeghers Q85.89
- phantom limb (without pain) G54.7
  - with pain G54.6
- pharyngeal pouch D82.1
- Phelan-McDermid Q93.52
- Pick's — *see* Disease, Pick's
- Pickwickian E66.2
- PIE (pulmonary infiltration with eosinophilia) — *see also* Eosinophilia, pulmonary J82.89
- pigmentary pallidal degeneration (progressive) G23.Ø
- pineal E34.8
- pituitary E22.Ø
- placental transfusion — *see* Pregnancy, complicated by, placental transfusion syndromes
- plantar fascia M72.2- ☑
- plateau iris (post-iridectomy) (postprocedural) H21.82
- Plummer-Vinson D5Ø.1
- pluricarential of infancy E4Ø
- plurideficiency E4Ø
- pluriglandular (compensatory) E31.8
  - autoimmune E31.Ø
- pneumatic hammer T75.21- ☑

**Syndrome** — *continued*
- polyangiitis overlap M3Ø.8
- polycarential of infancy E4Ø
- polyglandular E31.8
  - autoimmune E31.Ø
- polysplenia Q89.Ø9
- pontine NEC G93.89
- popliteal
  - artery entrapment I77.89
  - web Q87.89
- post chemoembolization — *code to* associated conditions
- post endometrial ablation N99.85
- postbacterial fatigue G93.39
- postcardiac injury
  - postcardiotomy I97.Ø
  - postmyocardial infarction I24.1
- postcardiotomy I97.Ø
- postcholecystectomy K91.5
- postcommissurotomy I97.Ø
- postconcussional FØ7.81
- postcontusional FØ7.81
- post-COVID (-19) UØ9.9
- postencephalitic FØ7.89
- posterior
  - cervical sympathetic M53.Ø
  - cord G83.83
  - fossa compression G93.5
  - reversible encephalopathy (PRES) I67.83
- postgastrectomy (dumping) K91.1
- postgastric surgery K91.1
- postinfarction I24.1
- postinfectious fatigue G93.39
- postlaminectomy NEC M96.1
- postleukotomy FØ7.Ø
- postmastectomy lymphedema I97.2
- postmyocardial infarction I24.1
- postoperative NEC T81.9- ☑
  - blind loop K9Ø.2
- postpartum panhypopituitary (Sheehan) E23.Ø
- postpolio (myelitic) G14
- post-polypectomy coagulation K91.89
- postthrombotic I87.ØØ9
  - with
    - inflammation I87.Ø2- ☑
      - with ulcer I87.Ø3- ☑
    - specified complication NEC I87.Ø9- ☑
    - ulcer I87.Ø1- ☑
      - with inflammation I87.Ø3- ☑
  - asymptomatic I87.ØØ- ☑
- postural
  - orthostatic tachycardia [POTS] G9Ø.A
  - tachycardia G9Ø.A
- postvagotomy K91.1
- postvalvulotomy I97.Ø
- postviral NEC G93.31
  - fatigue G93.31
- Potain's K31.Ø
- potassium intoxication E87.5
- Prader-Willi Q87.11
- Prader-Willi-like Q87.19
- precerebral artery (multiple) (bilateral) G45.2
- preinfarction I2Ø.Ø
- preleukemic D46.9
- premature senility E34.8
- premenstrual dysphoric F32.81
- premenstrual tension N94.3
- Prinzmetal-Massumi RØ7.1
- prune belly Q79.4
- pseudo -Turner's Q87.19
- pseudocarpal tunnel (sublimis) — *see* Syndrome, carpal tunnel
- pseudoparalytica G7Ø.ØØ
  - with exacerbation (acute) G7Ø.Ø1
  - in crisis G7Ø.Ø1
- psycho-organic (nonpsychotic severity) FØ7.9
  - acute or subacute FØ5
  - depressive type FØ6.31
  - hallucinatory type FØ6.Ø
  - nonpsychotic severity FØ7.Ø
  - specified NEC FØ7.89
- PTEN (hamartoma) tumor Q85.81
- pulmonary
  - arteriosclerosis I27.Ø
  - dysmaturity (Wilson-Mikity) P27.Ø
  - hypoperfusion (idiopathic) P22.Ø
  - renal (hemorrhagic) (Goodpasture's) M31.Ø
- pure
  - motor lacunar G46.5

- **Syndrome** — *continued*
  - usher — *continued*
    - type 4 Q99.818
  - vacuoles, E1 ubiquitin-activating enzyme, X-linked, autoinflammatory, somatic (VEXAS) MØ4.3
  - vago-hypoglossal G52.7
  - van Buchem's M85.2
  - van der Hoeve's Q78.Ø
  - vanishing twin of one fetus or more O31.4- ☑
  - vascular NEC in cerebrovascular disease G46.8
  - vasoconstriction, reversible cerebrovascular I67.841
  - vasomotor I73.9
  - vasospastic (traumatic) T75.22- ☑
  - vasovagal R55
  - VATER Q87.2
  - velo-cardio-facial Q93.81
  - vena cava (inferior) (superior) (obstruction) I87.1
  - vertebral
    - artery G45.Ø
      - compression — *see* Syndrome, anterior, spinal artery, compression
    - steal G45.Ø
  - vertebro-basilar artery G45.Ø
  - vertebrogenic (pain) — *see also* Pain, vertebrogenic M54.89
  - vertiginous — *see* Disorder, vestibular function
  - VEXAS (vacuoles, E1 ubiquitin-activating enzyme, X-linked, autoinflammatory, somatic) MØ4.3
  - Vinson-Plummer D5Ø.1
  - virus B34.9
  - visceral larva migrans B83.Ø
  - visual disorientation H53.8
  - vitamin B6 deficiency E53.1
  - vitreal corneal H59.Ø1- ☑
  - vitreous (touch) H59.Ø1- ☑
  - Vogt-Koyanagi H2Ø.82- ☑
  - Volkmann's T79.6- ☑
  - von Hippel-Lindau Q85.83
  - von Schroetter's I82.89Ø
  - von Willebrand (-Jurgen) — *see* Disease, von Willebrand
    - acquired — *see also* Disease, von Willebrand D68.Ø4
  - Waldenstrom-Kjellberg D5Ø.1
  - Wallenberg's G46.3
  - wasting (syndrome) due to underlying condition E88.A
  - water retention E87.79
  - Waterhouse (-Friderichsen) A39.1
  - Weber-Gubler G46.3
  - Weber-Leyden G46.3
  - Weber's G46.3
  - Wegener's M31.3Ø
    - with
      - kidney involvement M31.31
      - lung involvement M31.3Ø
        - with kidney involvement M31.31
  - Weingarten's (tropical eosinophilia) J82.89
  - Weiss-Baker G9Ø.Ø9
  - Werdnig-Hoffman G12.Ø
  - Wermer's E31.21
  - Werner's E34.8
  - Wernicke-Korsakoff (nonalcoholic) FØ4
    - alcoholic F1Ø.9- ☑
      - with dependence F1Ø.2- ☑
  - Westphal-Strumpell E83.Ø1
  - West's — *see* Epilepsy, spasms
  - wet
    - feet (maceration) (tropical) T69.Ø2- ☑
    - lung, newborn P22.1
  - whiplash S13.4- ☑
  - whistling face Q87.Ø
  - Wilkie's K55.1
  - Wilkinson-Sneddon L13.1
  - Willebrand (-Jurgens) — *see* Disease, von Willebrand
  - Williams Q93.82
  - Wilson's (hepatolenticular degeneration) E83.Ø1
  - Wiskott-Aldrich D82.Ø
  - withdrawal — *see* Withdrawal, state
    - drug
      - infant of dependent mother P96.1
      - therapeutic use, newborn P96.2
  - Woakes' (ethmoiditis) J33.1
  - Wright's (hyperabduction) G54.Ø
  - X I2Ø.9
  - XXXX Q97.1
  - XXXXX Q97.1
  - XXXXY Q98.1
  - XXY Q98.Ø
  - Yao MØ4.8
  - yellow nail L6Ø.5
- **Syndrome** — *continued*
  - Zahorsky's BØ8.5
  - Zellweger-like syndrome E71.541
  - Zellweger syndrome E71.51Ø
- **Synechia** (anterior) (iris) (posterior) (pupil) — *see also* Adhesions, iris
  - intra-uterine (traumatic) N85.6
- **Synesthesia** R2Ø.8
- **Syngamiasis, syngamosis** B83.3
- **Synodontia** KØØ.2
- **Synorchidism, synorchism** Q55.1
- **Synostosis** (congenital) Q78.8
  - astragalo-scaphoid Q74.2
  - radioulnar Q74.Ø
- **Synovial sarcoma** — *see* Neoplasm, connective tissue, malignant
- **Synovioma** (malignant) — *see also* Neoplasm, connective tissue, malignant
  - benign — *see* Neoplasm, connective tissue, benign
- **Synoviosarcoma** — *see* Neoplasm, connective tissue, malignant
- **Synovitis** — *see also* Tenosynovitis M65.9Ø
  - ankle and foot M65.97- ☑
  - arm, upper M65.92- ☑
  - crepitant
    - hand M7Ø.Ø4- ☑
    - wrist M7Ø.Ø3- ☑
  - forearm M65.93- ☑
  - gonococcal A54.49
  - gouty — *see* Gout
  - hand M65.94- ☑
  - in (due to)
    - crystals M65.8- ☑
    - gonorrhea A54.49
    - syphilis (late) A52.78
    - use, overuse, pressure — *see* Disorder, soft tissue, due to use
  - infective NEC — *see* Tenosynovitis, infective NEC
  - leg, lower M65.96- ☑
  - multiple sites, unspecified type M65.39
  - shoulder M65.91- ☑
  - specified NEC — *see* Tenosynovitis, specified type NEC
  - specified site, unspecified type M65.38
  - syphilitic A52.78
    - congenital (early) A5Ø.Ø2
  - thigh M65.95- ☑
  - toxic — *see* Synovitis, transient
  - transient M67.3- ☑
    - ankle M67.37- ☑
    - elbow M67.32- ☑
    - foot joint M67.37- ☑
    - hand joint M67.34- ☑
    - hip M67.35- ☑
    - knee M67.36- ☑
    - multiple site M67.39
    - pelvic region M67.35- ☑
    - shoulder M67.31- ☑
    - specified joint NEC M67.38
    - wrist M67.33- ☑
  - traumatic, current — *see* Sprain
  - tuberculous — *see* Tuberculosis, synovitis
  - villonodular (pigmented) M12.2- ☑
    - ankle M12.27- ☑
    - elbow M12.22- ☑
    - foot joint M12.27- ☑
    - hand joint M12.24- ☑
    - hip M12.25- ☑
    - knee M12.26- ☑
    - multiple site M12.29
    - pelvic region M12.25- ☑
    - shoulder M12.21- ☑
    - specified joint NEC M12.28
    - vertebrae M12.28
    - wrist M12.23- ☑
- **Syphilid** A51.39
  - congenital A5Ø.Ø6
  - newborn A5Ø.Ø6
  - tubercular (late) A52.79
- **Syphilis, syphilitic** (acquired) A53.9
  - abdomen (late) A52.79
  - acoustic nerve A52.15
  - adenopathy (secondary) A51.49
  - adrenal (gland) (with cortical hypofunction) A52.79
  - age under 2 years NOS — *see also* Syphilis, congenital, early
    - acquired A51.9
  - alopecia (secondary) A51.32
- **Syphilis, syphilitic** — *continued*
  - anemia (late) A52.79 *[D63.8]*
  - aneurysm (aorta) (ruptured) A52.Ø1
    - central nervous system A52.Ø5
    - congenital A5Ø.54 *[I79.Ø]*
  - anus (late) A52.74
    - primary A51.1
    - secondary A51.39
  - aorta (arch) (abdominal) (thoracic) A52.Ø2
    - aneurysm A52.Ø1
  - aortic (insufficiency) (regurgitation) (stenosis) A52.Ø3
    - aneurysm A52.Ø1
  - arachnoid (adhesive) (cerebral) (spinal) A52.13
  - asymptomatic — *see* Syphilis, latent
  - ataxia (locomotor) A52.11
  - atrophoderma maculatum A51.39
  - auricular fibrillation A52.Ø6
  - bladder (late) A52.76
  - bone A52.77
    - secondary A51.46
  - brain A52.17
  - breast (late) A52.79
  - bronchus (late) A52.72
  - bubo (primary) A51.Ø
  - bulbar palsy A52.19
  - bursa (late) A52.78
  - cardiac decompensation A52.Ø6
  - cardiovascular A52.ØØ
  - central nervous system (late) (recurrent) (relapse) (tertiary) A52.3
    - with
      - ataxia A52.11
      - general paralysis A52.17
        - juvenile A5Ø.45
      - paresis (general) A52.17
        - juvenile A5Ø.45
      - tabes (dorsalis) A52.11
        - juvenile A5Ø.45
      - taboparesis A52.17
        - juvenile A5Ø.45
    - aneurysm A52.Ø5
    - congenital A5Ø.4Ø
    - juvenile A5Ø.4Ø
    - remission in (sustained) A52.3
    - serology doubtful, negative, or positive A52.3
    - specified nature or site NEC A52.19
    - vascular A52.Ø5
  - cerebral A52.17
    - meningovascular A52.13
    - nerves (multiple palsies) A52.15
    - sclerosis A52.17
    - thrombosis A52.Ø5
  - cerebrospinal (tabetic type) A52.12
  - cerebrovascular A52.Ø5
  - cervix (late) A52.76
  - chancre (multiple) A51.Ø
    - extragenital A51.2
    - Rollet's A51.Ø
  - Charcot's joint A52.16
  - chorioretinitis A51.43
    - congenital A5Ø.Ø1
    - late A52.71
    - prenatal A5Ø.Ø1
  - choroiditis — *see* Syphilitic chorioretinitis
  - choroidoretinitis — *see* Syphilitic chorioretinitis
  - ciliary body (secondary) A51.43
    - late A52.71
  - colon (late) A52.74
  - combined spinal sclerosis A52.11
  - condyloma (latum) A51.31
  - congenital A5Ø.9
    - with
      - paresis (general) A5Ø.45
      - tabes (dorsalis) A5Ø.45
      - taboparesis A5Ø.45
    - chorioretinitis, choroiditis A5Ø.Ø1 *[H32]*
    - early, or less than 2 years after birth NEC A5Ø.2
      - with manifestations — *see* Syphilis, congenital, early, symptomatic
      - latent (without manifestations) A5Ø.1
        - negative spinal fluid test A5Ø.1
        - serology positive A5Ø.1
      - symptomatic A5Ø.Ø9
        - cutaneous A5Ø.Ø6
        - mucocutaneous A5Ø.Ø7
        - oculopathy A5Ø.Ø1
        - osteochondropathy A5Ø.Ø2
        - pharyngitis A5Ø.Ø3
        - pneumonia A5Ø.Ø4

# T

- **T-shaped incisors** KØØ.2
- **Tabacism, tabacosis, tabagism** — *see also* Poisoning, tobacco
  - meaning dependence (without remission) — *see* Dependence, drug, nicotine
- **Tabardillo** A75.9
  - flea-borne A75.2
  - louse-borne A75.Ø
- **Tabes, tabetic** A52.1Ø
  - with
    - central nervous system syphilis A52.1Ø
    - Charcot's joint A52.16
    - cord bladder A52.19
    - crisis, viscera (any) A52.19
    - paralysis, general A52.17
    - paresis (general) A52.17
    - perforating ulcer (foot) A52.19
  - arthropathy (Charcot) A52.16
  - bladder A52.19
  - bone A52.11
  - cerebrospinal A52.12
  - congenital A5Ø.45
  - conjugal A52.1Ø
  - dorsalis A52.11
    - juvenile A5Ø.49
  - juvenile A5Ø.49
  - latent A52.19
  - mesenterica A18.39
  - paralysis, insane, general A52.17
  - spasmodic A52.17
  - syphilis (cerebrospinal) A52.12
- **Taboparalysis** A52.17
- **Taboparesis** (remission) A52.17
  - juvenile A5Ø.45
- **TAC** (trigeminal autonomic cephalgia) **NEC** G44.Ø99
  - intractable G44.Ø91
  - not intractable G44.Ø99
- **Tache noir** S6Ø.22- ☑
- **Tachyalimentation** K91.2
- **Tachyarrhythmia, tachyrhythmia** — *see* Tachycardia
- **Tachycardia** RØØ.Ø
  - atrial (paroxysmal) I47.19
  - auricular I47.19
  - AV nodal re-entry (re-entrant) I47.19
  - junctional (paroxysmal) I47.19
  - newborn P29.11
  - nodal (paroxysmal) I47.19
  - non-paroxysmal AV nodal I45.89
  - paroxysmal (sustained) (nonsustained) I47.9
    - with sinus bradycardia I49.5
    - atrial (PAT) I47.19
    - atrioventricular (AV) (re-entrant) I47.19
      - psychogenic F54
    - junctional I47.19
      - ectopic I47.19
    - nodal I47.19
    - psychogenic (atrial) (supraventricular) (ventricular) F54
    - supraventricular (sustained) I47.1Ø
      - psychogenic F54
    - ventricular I47.2Ø
      - catecholaminergic polymorphic (CPVT) I47.22
      - familial polymorphic (FPVT) I47.22
      - psychogenic F54
      - specified type NEC I47.29
  - psychogenic F45.8
  - sick sinus I49.5
  - sinoauricular NOS RØØ.Ø
    - paroxysmal I47.19
  - sinus [sinusal] NOS RØØ.Ø
    - inappropriate, so stated (IST) I47.11
    - paroxysmal I47.19
  - supraventricular I47.1Ø
  - ventricular (paroxysmal) (sustained) I47.2Ø
    - psychogenic F54
    - specified NEC I47.29
- **Tachygastria** K31.89
- **Tachypnea** RØ6.82
  - hysterical F45.8
  - newborn (idiopathic) (transitory) P22.1
  - psychogenic F45.8
  - transitory, of newborn P22.1
- **TACO** (transfusion associated circulatory overload) E87.71
- **TAD** (transfusion-associated dyspnea) J95.87
- **Taenia** (infection) (infestation) B68.9
  - diminuta B71.Ø
- **Taenia** — *continued*
  - echinococcal infestation B67.9Ø
  - mediocanellata B68.1
  - nana B71.Ø
  - saginata B68.1
  - solium (intestinal form) B68.Ø
    - larval form — *see* Cysticercosis
- **Taeniasis** (intestine) — *see* Taenia
- **Tag** (hypertrophied skin) (infected) L91.8
  - adenoid J35.8
  - anus K64.4
  - hemorrhoidal K64.4
  - hymen N89.8
  - perineal N9Ø.89
  - preauricular Q17.Ø
  - sentinel K64.4
  - skin L91.8
    - accessory (congenital) Q82.8
    - anus K64.4
    - congenital Q82.8
    - preauricular Q17.Ø
  - tonsil J35.8
  - urethra, urethral N36.8
  - vulva N9Ø.89
- **Tahyna fever** B33.8
- **Takahara's disease** E8Ø.3
- **Takayasu's disease or syndrome** M31.4
- **Talaromycosis** B48.4
- **Talcosis** (pulmonary) J62.Ø
- **Talipes** (congenital) Q66.89
  - acquired, planus — *see* Deformity, limb, flat foot
  - asymmetric Q66.89
  - calcaneovalgus Q66.4- ☑
  - calcaneovarus Q66.1- ☑
  - calcaneus Q66.89
  - cavus Q66.7- ☑
  - equinovalgus Q66.6
  - equinovarus Q66.Ø- ☑
  - equinus Q66.89
  - percavus Q66.7- ☑
  - planovalgus Q66.6
  - planus (acquired) (any degree) — *see also* Deformity, limb, flat foot
    - congenital Q66.5- ☑
    - due to rickets (sequelae) E64.3
  - valgus Q66.6
  - varus Q66.3- ☑
- **Tall stature, constitutional** E34.4
- **Talma's disease** M62.89
- **Talon noir** S9Ø.3- ☑
  - hand S6Ø.22- ☑
  - heel S9Ø.3- ☑
  - toe S9Ø.1- ☑
- **Tamponade, heart** I31.4
- **Tanapox** (virus disease) BØ8.71
- **Tangier disease** E78.6
- **Tantrum, child problem** F91.8
- **Tapeworm** (infection) (infestation) — *see* Infestation, tapeworm
- **Tapia's syndrome** G52.7
- **TAR** (thrombocytopenia with absent radius) **syndrome** Q87.2
- **Tarral-Besnier disease** L44.Ø
- **Tarsal tunnel syndrome** — *see* Syndrome, tarsal tunnel
- **Tarsalgia** — *see* Pain, limb, lower
- **Tarsitis** (eyelid) HØ1.8- ☑
  - syphilitic A52.71
  - tuberculous A18.4
- **Tartar** (teeth) (dental calculus) KØ3.6
- **Tattoo** (mark) L81.8
- **Tauri's disease** E74.Ø9
- **Taurodontism** KØØ.2
- **Taussig-Bing syndrome** Q2Ø.1
- **Tay-Sachs amaurotic familial idiocy or disease** E75.Ø2
- **Taybi's syndrome** Q87.2
- **TBI** (traumatic brain injury) SØ6.9- ☑
- **Teacher's node or nodule** J38.2
- **Tear-stone** — *see* Dacryolith
- **Tear, torn** (traumatic) — *see also* Laceration
  - with abortion — *see* Abortion
  - annular fibrosis M51.35
  - anus, anal (sphincter) S31.831- ☑
    - complicating delivery
      - with third degree perineal laceration — *see also* Delivery, complicated, by, laceration, perineum, third degree O7Ø.2Ø
        - with mucosa O7Ø.3
      - without third degree perineal laceration O7Ø.4
- **Tear, torn** — *continued*
  - anus, anal — *continued*
    - nontraumatic (healed) (old) K62.81
  - articular cartilage, old — *see* Derangement, joint, articular cartilage, by site
  - bladder
    - with ectopic or molar pregnancy OØ8.6
    - following ectopic or molar pregnancy OØ8.6
    - obstetrical O71.5
    - traumatic — *see* Injury, bladder
  - bowel
    - with ectopic or molar pregnancy OØ8.6
    - following ectopic or molar pregnancy OØ8.6
    - obstetrical trauma O71.5
  - broad ligament
    - with ectopic or molar pregnancy OØ8.6
    - following ectopic or molar pregnancy OØ8.6
    - obstetrical trauma O71.6
  - bucket handle (knee) (meniscus) — *see* Tear, meniscus
  - capsule, joint — *see* Sprain
  - cartilage — *see also* Sprain
    - articular, old — *see* Derangement, joint, articular cartilage, by site
  - cervix
    - with ectopic or molar pregnancy OØ8.6
    - following ectopic or molar pregnancy OØ8.6
    - obstetrical trauma (current) O71.3
    - old N88.1
    - traumatic — *see* Injury, uterus
  - dural G97.41
    - nontraumatic G96.11
  - internal organ — *see* Injury, by site
  - knee cartilage
    - articular (current) S83.3- ☑
    - old — *see* Derangement, knee, meniscus, due to old tear
  - ligament — *see* Sprain
  - meniscus (knee) (current injury) S83.2Ø9- ☑
    - bucket-handle S83.2Ø- ☑
    - lateral
      - bucket-handle S83.25- ☑
      - complex S83.27- ☑
      - peripheral S83.26- ☑
      - specified type NEC S83.28- ☑
    - medial
      - bucket-handle S83.21- ☑
      - complex S83.23- ☑
      - peripheral S83.22- ☑
      - specified type NEC S83.24- ☑
    - old — *see* Derangement, knee, meniscus, due to old tear
    - site other than knee — *code as* Sprain
    - specified type NEC S83.2Ø- ☑
  - muscle — *see* Strain
  - pelvic
    - floor, complicating delivery O7Ø.1
    - organ NEC, obstetrical trauma O71.5
      - with ectopic or molar pregnancy OØ8.6
      - following ectopic or molar pregnancy OØ8.6
  - perineal, secondary O9Ø.1
  - periurethral tissue, obstetrical trauma O71.82
    - with ectopic or molar pregnancy OØ8.6
    - following ectopic or molar pregnancy OØ8.6
  - rectovaginal septum — *see* Laceration, vagina
  - retina, retinal (without detachment) (horseshoe) — *see also* Break, retina, horseshoe
    - with detachment — *see* Detachment, retina, with retinal, break
  - rotator cuff (nontraumatic) M75.1Ø- ☑
    - complete M75.12- ☑
    - incomplete M75.11- ☑
    - traumatic S46.Ø1- ☑
      - capsule S43.42- ☑
  - semilunar cartilage, knee — *see* Tear, meniscus
  - supraspinatus (complete) (incomplete) (nontraumatic) — *see also* Tear, rotator cuff M75.1Ø- ☑
  - tendon — *see* Strain
  - tentorial, at birth P1Ø.4
  - umbilical cord
    - complicating delivery O69.89- ☑
  - urethra
    - with ectopic or molar pregnancy OØ8.6
    - following ectopic or molar pregnancy OØ8.6
    - obstetrical trauma O71.5
  - uterus — *see* Injury, uterus
  - vagina — *see* Laceration, vagina
  - vessel, from catheter — *see* Puncture, accidental complicating surgery

- **Tear, torn** — *continued*
  - vulva, complicating delivery O7Ø.Ø
- **Teeth** — *see also* condition
  - grinding
    - psychogenic F45.8
    - sleep related G47.63
- **Teething** (syndrome) KØØ.7
- **Telangiectasia, telangiectasis** (verrucous) I78.1
  - ataxic (cerebellar) (Louis-Bar) G11.3
  - familial I78.Ø
  - hemorrhagic, hereditary (congenital) (senile) I78.Ø
  - hereditary, hemorrhagic (congenital) (senile) I78.Ø
  - juxtafoveal H35.Ø7- ☑
  - macular H35.Ø7- ☑
  - macularis eruptiva perstans D47.Ø1
  - parafoveal H35.Ø7- ☑
  - retinal (idiopathic) (juxtafoveal) (macular) (parafoveal) H35.Ø7- ☑
  - spider I78.1
- **Telephone scatologia** F65.89
- **Telescoped bowel or intestine** K56.1
  - congenital Q43.8
- **Temperature**
  - body, high (of unknown origin) R5Ø.9
  - cold, trauma from T69.9- ☑
    - newborn P8Ø.Ø
    - specified effect NEC T69.8- ☑
- **Temple** — *see* condition
- **Temporal** — *see* condition
- **Temporomandibular joint pain-dysfunction syndrome** M26.62- ☑
- **Temporosphenoidal** — *see* condition
- **Tendency**
  - bleeding — *see* Defect, coagulation
  - suicide
    - meaning personal history of attempted suicide Z91.51
    - meaning suicidal ideation — *see* Ideation, suicidal
  - to fall R29.6
- **Tenderness, abdominal** R1Ø.819
  - costovertebral (angle) R39.859
    - bilateral R39.853
    - left R39.852
    - right R39.851
  - epigastric R1Ø.816
  - flank R1Ø.8A9
    - left R1Ø.8A2
    - right R1Ø.8A1
  - generalized R1Ø.817
  - left lower quadrant R1Ø.814
  - left upper quadrant R1Ø.812
  - periumbilic R1Ø.815
  - rebound R1Ø.829
    - epigastric R1Ø.826
    - generalized R1Ø.827
    - left lower quadrant R1Ø.824
    - left upper quadrant R1Ø.822
    - periumbilic R1Ø.825
    - right lower quadrant R1Ø.823
    - right upper quadrant R1Ø.821
  - right lower quadrant R1Ø.813
  - right upper quadrant R1Ø.811
  - suprapubic R1Ø.8A3
- **Tendinitis, tendonitis** — *see also* Enthesopathy
  - Achilles M76.6- ☑
  - adhesive — *see* Tenosynovitis, specified type NEC
    - shoulder — *see* Capsulitis, adhesive
  - bicipital M75.2- ☑
  - calcific M65.2- ☑
    - ankle M65.27- ☑
    - foot M65.27- ☑
    - forearm M65.23- ☑
    - hand M65.24- ☑
    - lower leg M65.26- ☑
    - multiple sites M65.29
    - pelvic region M65.25- ☑
    - shoulder M75.3- ☑
    - specified site NEC M65.28
    - thigh M65.25- ☑
    - upper arm M65.22- ☑
  - due to use, overuse, pressure — *see also* Disorder, soft tissue, due to use
    - specified NEC — *see* Disorder, soft tissue, due to use, specified NEC
  - gluteal M76.Ø- ☑
  - patellar M76.5- ☑
  - peroneal M76.7- ☑
  - psoas M76.1- ☑
  - tibial (posterior) M76.82- ☑
- **Tendinitis, tendonitis** — *continued*
  - tibial — *continued*
    - anterior M76.81- ☑
  - trochanteric — *see* Bursitis, hip, trochanteric
- **Tendon** — *see* condition
- **Tendosynovitis** — *see* Tenosynovitis
- **Tenesmus** (rectal) R19.8
  - vesical R3Ø.1
- **Tennis elbow** — *see* Epicondylitis, lateral
- **Tenonitis** — *see also* Tenosynovitis
  - eye (capsule) HØ5.Ø4- ☑
- **Tenontosynovitis** — *see* Tenosynovitis
- **Tenontothecitis** — *see* Tenosynovitis
- **Tenophyte** — *see* Disorder, synovium, specified type NEC
- **Tenosynovitis** — *see also* Synovitis M65.9Ø
  - adhesive — *see* Tenosynovitis, specified type NEC
    - shoulder — *see* Capsulitis, adhesive
  - bicipital (calcifying) — *see* Tendinitis, bicipital
  - gonococcal A54.49
  - in (due to)
    - crystals M65.8- ☑
    - gonorrhea A54.49
    - syphilis (late) A52.78
    - use, overuse, pressure — *see also* Disorder, soft tissue, due to use
      - specified NEC — *see* Disorder, soft tissue, due to use, specified NEC
  - infective NEC M65.1- ☑
    - ankle M65.17- ☑
    - foot M65.17- ☑
    - forearm M65.13- ☑
    - hand M65.14- ☑
    - lower leg M65.16- ☑
    - multiple sites M65.19
    - pelvic region M65.15- ☑
    - shoulder region M65.11- ☑
    - specified site NEC M65.18
    - thigh M65.15- ☑
    - upper arm M65.12- ☑
  - radial styloid M65.4
  - shoulder region M65.81- ☑
    - adhesive — *see* Capsulitis, adhesive
  - specified type NEC M65.88
    - ankle M65.87- ☑
    - foot M65.87- ☑
    - forearm M65.83- ☑
    - hand M65.84- ☑
    - lower leg M65.86- ☑
    - multiple sites M65.89
    - pelvic region M65.85- ☑
    - shoulder region M65.81- ☑
    - specified site NEC M65.88
    - thigh M65.85- ☑
    - upper arm M65.82- ☑
  - tuberculous — *see* Tuberculosis, tenosynovitis
- **Tenovaginitis** — *see* Tenosynovitis
- **Tension**
  - arterial, high — *see also* Hypertension
    - without diagnosis of hypertension RØ3.Ø
  - headache G44.2Ø9
    - intractable G44.2Ø1
    - not intractable G44.2Ø9
  - nervous R45.Ø
  - pneumothorax J93.Ø
  - premenstrual N94.3
  - state (mental) F48.9
- **Tentorium** — *see* condition
- **Teratencephalus** Q89.89
- **Teratism** Q89.7
- **Teratoblastoma** (malignant) — *see* Neoplasm, malignant, by site
- **Teratocarcinoma** — *see also* Neoplasm, malignant, by site
  - liver C22.7
- **Teratoma** (solid) — *see also* Neoplasm, uncertain behavior, by site
  - with embryonal carcinoma, mixed — *see* Neoplasm, malignant, by site
  - with malignant transformation — *see* Neoplasm, malignant, by site
  - adult (cystic) — *see* Neoplasm, benign, by site
  - benign — *see* Neoplasm, benign, by site
  - combined with choriocarcinoma — *see* Neoplasm, malignant, by site
  - cystic (adult) — *see* Neoplasm, benign, by site
  - differentiated — *see* Neoplasm, benign, by site
  - embryonal — *see also* Neoplasm, malignant, by site
    - liver C22.7
  - immature — *see* Neoplasm, malignant, by site
- **Teratoma** — *continued*
  - liver C22.7
    - adult, benign, cystic, differentiated type or mature D13.4
  - malignant — *see also* Neoplasm, malignant, by site
    - anaplastic — *see* Neoplasm, malignant, by site
    - intermediate — *see* Neoplasm, malignant, by site
      - specified site — *see* Neoplasm, malignant, by site
      - unspecified site C62.9Ø
    - undifferentiated — *see* Neoplasm, malignant, by site
  - mature — *see* Neoplasm, uncertain behavior, by site
    - malignant — *see* Neoplasm, by site, malignant, by site
  - ovary D27.- ☑
    - embryonal, immature or malignant C56.- ☑
  - solid — *see* Neoplasm, uncertain behavior, by site
  - testis C62.9- ☑
    - adult, benign, cystic, differentiated type or mature D29.2- ☑
    - scrotal C62.1- ☑
    - undescended C62.Ø- ☑
- **Termination**
  - anomalous — *see also* Malposition, congenital
    - right pulmonary vein Q26.3
  - pregnancy, elective Z33.2
- **Ternidens diminutus infestation** B81.8
- **Ternidensiasis** B81.8
- **Terror(s) night** (child) F51.4
- **Terrorism, victim of** Z65.4
- **Terry's syndrome** — *see also* Myopia, degenerative H44.2- ☑
- **Tertiary** — *see* condition
- **Test, tests, testing** (for)
  - adequacy (for dialysis)
    - hemodialysis Z49.31
    - peritoneal Z49.32
  - blood-alcohol ZØ2.83
    - positive — *see* Findings, abnormal, in blood
  - blood-drug ZØ2.83
    - positive — *see* Findings, abnormal, in blood
  - blood pressure ZØ1.3Ø
    - abnormal reading — *see* Blood, pressure
  - blood typing ZØ1.83
    - Rh typing ZØ1.83
  - cardiac pulse generator (battery) Z45.Ø1Ø
  - fertility Z31.41
  - genetic
    - disease carrier status for procreative management
      - female Z31.43Ø
      - male Z31.44Ø
    - male partner of patient with recurrent pregnancy loss Z31.441
    - procreative management NEC
      - female Z31.438
      - male Z31.448
  - hearing ZØ1.1Ø
    - with abnormal findings NEC ZØ1.118
    - infant or child (over 28 days old) ZØØ.129
      - with abnormal findings ZØØ.121
  - HIV (human immunodeficiency virus)
    - nonconclusive (in infants) R75
    - positive Z21
    - seropositive Z21
  - immunity status ZØ1.84
  - intelligence NEC ZØ1.89
  - laboratory (as part of a general medical examination) ZØØ.ØØ
    - with abnormal finding ZØØ.Ø1
    - for medicolegal reason NEC ZØ4.89
  - male partner of patient with recurrent pregnancy loss Z31.441
  - Mantoux (for tuberculosis) Z11.1
    - abnormal result R76.11
  - pregnancy, positive first pregnancy — *see* Pregnancy, normal, first
  - procreative Z31.49
    - fertility Z31.41
  - skin, diagnostic
    - allergy ZØ1.82
      - special screening examination — *see* Screening, by name of disease
    - Mantoux Z11.1
    - tuberculin Z11.1
  - specified NEC ZØ1.89
  - tuberculin Z11.1
    - abnormal result R76.11
  - vision ZØ1.ØØ
    - with abnormal findings ZØ1.Ø1

**Test, tests, testing** — *continued*
- vision — *continued*
  - following failed vision screening Z01.020
    - with abnormal findings Z01.021
  - infant or child (over 28 days old) Z00.129
    - with abnormal findings Z00.121
- Wassermann Z11.3
  - positive — *see* Serology for syphilis, positive

**Testicle, testicular, testis** — *see also* condition
- feminization syndrome — *see also* Syndrome, androgen insensitivity E34.51
- migrans Q55.29

**Tetanus, tetanic** (cephalic) (convulsions) A35
- with
  - abortion A34
  - ectopic or molar pregnancy O08.0
- following ectopic or molar pregnancy O08.0
- inoculation reaction (due to serum) — *see* Complications, vaccination
- neonatorum A33
- obstetrical A34
- puerperal, postpartum, childbirth A34

**Tetany** (due to) R29.0
- alkalosis E87.3
- associated with rickets E55.0
- convulsions R29.0
  - hysterical F44.5
- functional (hysterical) F44.5
- hyperkinetic R29.0
  - hysterical F44.5
- hyperpnea R06.4
  - hysterical F44.5
  - psychogenic F45.8
- hyperventilation — *see also* Hyperventilation R06.4
  - hysterical F44.5
- neonatal (without calcium or magnesium deficiency) P71.3
- parathyroid (gland) E20.9
- parathyroprival E89.2
- post- (para)thyroidectomy E89.2
- postoperative E89.2
- pseudotetany R29.0
- psychogenic (conversion reaction) F44.5

**Tetralogy of Fallot** Q21.3

**Tetraplegia** (chronic) — *see also* Quadriplegia G82.50

**Thailand hemorrhagic fever** A91

**Thalassanemia** — *see* Thalassemia

**Thalassemia** (anemia) (disease) D56.9
- with other hemoglobinopathy D56.8
- alpha (major) (severe) (triple gene defect) D56.0
  - minor D56.3
  - silent carrier D56.3
  - trait D56.3
- beta (severe) D56.1
  - homozygous D56.1
  - major D56.1
  - minor D56.3
  - trait D56.3
- delta-beta (homozygous) D56.2
  - minor D56.3
  - trait D56.3
- dominant D56.8
- hemoglobin
  - C D56.8
  - E-beta D56.5
- intermedia D56.1
- major D56.1
- minor D56.3
- mixed D56.8
- sickle-cell — *see* Disease, sickle-cell, thalassemia
- specified type NEC D56.8
- trait D56.3
- variants D56.8

**Thanatophoric dwarfism or short stature** Q77.1

**Thaysen-Gee disease** (nontropical sprue) K90.0

**Thaysen's disease** K90.0

**Thecoma** D27.- ☑
- luteinized D27.- ☑
- malignant C56.- ☑

**Thelarche, premature** E30.8

**Thelaziasis** B83.8

**Thelitis** N61.0
- puerperal, postpartum or gestational — *see* Infection, nipple

**Therapeutic** — *see* condition

**Therapy**
- drug, long-term (current) (prophylactic)
  - agents affecting estrogen receptors and estrogen levels NEC Z79.818

**Therapy** — *continued*
- drug, long-term — *continued*
  - anastrozole (Arimidex) Z79.811
  - anti-inflammatory Z79.1
  - antibiotics Z79.2
    - short-term use — *omit code*
  - anticoagulants Z79.01
  - antiplatelet Z79.02
  - antithrombotics Z79.02
  - aromatase inhibitors Z79.811
  - aspirin Z79.82
  - birth control pill or patch Z79.3
  - bisphosphonates Z79.83
  - contraceptive, oral Z79.3
  - drug, specified NEC Z79.899
  - estrogen receptor downregulators Z79.818
  - Evista Z79.810
  - exemestane (Aromasin) Z79.811
  - Fareston Z79.810
  - fulvestrant (Faslodex) Z79.818
  - gonadotropin-releasing hormone (GnRH) agonist Z79.818
  - goserelin acetate (Zoladex) Z79.818
  - hormone replacement Z79.890
  - insulin Z79.4
  - letrozole (Femara) Z79.811
  - leuprolide acetate (leuprorelin) (Lupron) Z79.818
  - megestrol acetate (Megace) Z79.818
  - methadone
    - for pain management Z79.891
    - maintenance therapy F11.20
  - Nolvadex Z79.810
  - opiate analgesic Z79.891
  - oral antidiabetic Z79.84
  - oral contraceptive Z79.3
  - oral hypoglycemic Z79.84
  - raloxifene (Evista) Z79.810
  - selective estrogen receptor modulators (SERMs) Z79.810
  - short term — *omit code*
  - steroids
    - inhaled Z79.51
    - systemic Z79.52
  - tamoxifen (Nolvadex) Z79.810
  - toremifene (Fareston) Z79.810

**Thermic** — *see* condition

**Thermography** (abnormal) — *see also* Abnormal, diagnostic imaging R93.89
- breast R92.8

**Thermoplegia** T67.01- ☑

**Thesaurismosis, glycogen** — *see* Disease, glycogen storage

**Thiamin deficiency** E51.9
- specified NEC E51.8

**Thiaminic deficiency with beriberi** E51.11

**Thibierge-Weissenbach syndrome** — *see* Sclerosis, systemic

**Thickening**
- bone — *see* Hypertrophy, bone
- breast N64.59
- endometrium R93.89
- epidermal L85.9
  - specified NEC L85.8
- hymen N89.6
- larynx J38.7
- nail L60.2
  - congenital Q84.5
- periosteal — *see* Hypertrophy, bone
- pleura J92.9
  - with asbestos J92.0
- skin R23.4
- subepiglottic J38.7
- tongue K14.8
- valve, heart — *see* Endocarditis

**Thigh** — *see* condition

**Thinning vertebra** — *see* Spondylopathy, specified NEC

**Thirst, excessive** R63.1
- due to deprivation of water T73.1- ☑

**Thomsen disease** G71.12

**Thoracic** — *see also* condition
- kidney Q63.2
- outlet syndrome — *see also* Syndrome, thoracic outlet G54.0

**Thoracogastroschisis** (congenital) Q79.8

**Thoracopagus** Q89.4

**Thorax** — *see* condition

**Thorn's syndrome** N28.89

**Thorson-Bjorck syndrome** E34.09

**Threadworm** (infection) (infestation) B80

**Threatened**
- abortion O20.0
  - with subsequent abortion O03.9
- abuse (harm)
  - adult — *see* Maltreatment, adult, threatened abuse
  - child — *see* Maltreatment, child, threatened abuse
- job loss, anxiety concerning Z56.2
- labor (without delivery) O47.9
  - at or after 37 completed weeks of gestation O47.1
  - before 37 completed weeks of gestation O47.0- ☑
- loss of job, anxiety concerning Z56.2
- miscarriage O20.0
- unemployment, anxiety concerning Z56.2

**Three-day fever** A93.1

**Threshers' lung** J67.0

**Thrix annulata** (congenital) Q84.1

**Throat** — *see* condition

**Thrombasthenia** (Glanzmann) (hemorrhagic) (hereditary) D69.11

**Thromboangiitis** I73.1
- obliterans (general) I73.1
  - cerebral I67.89
  - vessels
    - brain I67.89
    - spinal cord I67.89

**Thromboarteritis** — *see* Arteritis

**Thromboasthenia** (Glanzmann) (hemorrhagic) (hereditary) D69.11

**Thrombocytasthenia** (Glanzmann) D69.11

**Thrombocythemia** (hemorrhagic) *see also* Thrombocytosis D75.839
- essential D47.3
- idiopathic D47.3
- primary D47.3

**Thrombocytopathy** (dystrophic) (granulopenic) D69.19

**Thrombocytopenia, thrombocytopenic** D69.6
- with absent radius (TAR) Q87.2
- congenital D69.42
- dilutional D69.59
- due to
  - (massive) blood transfusion D69.59
  - drugs D69.59
  - extracorporeal circulation of blood D69.59
  - platelet alloimmunization D69.59
- essential D69.3
- heparin-associated D75.821
- heparin induced (HIT) D75.829
  - delayed-onset D75.828
  - immune-mediated D75.822
  - non-immune D75.821
  - persisting D75.828
  - syndrome
    - autoimmune D75.828
    - specified NEC D75.828
    - spontaneous (without heparin exposure) D75.84
  - type 1 D75.821
  - type 2 D75.822
- hereditary D69.42
- idiopathic D69.3
- neonatal, transitory P61.0
  - due to
    - exchange transfusion P61.0
    - idiopathic maternal thrombocytopenia P61.0
    - isoimmunization P61.0
- primary NEC D69.49
  - idiopathic D69.3
- puerperal, postpartum O72.3
- secondary D69.59
- transient neonatal P61.0
- vaccine-induced thrombotic D75.84

**Thrombocytosis** D75.839
- essential D47.3
- idiopathic D47.3
- primary D47.3
- reactive D75.838
- secondary D75.838
- specified NEC D75.838

**Thromboembolism** — *see* Embolism

**Thrombopathy** (Bernard-Soulier) D69.19
- constitutional — *see* Disease, von Willebrand
- Willebrand-Jurgens — *see* Disease, von Willebrand

**Thrombopenia** — *see* Thrombocytopenia

**Thrombophilia** D68.59
- primary NEC D68.59
- secondary NEC D68.69
- specified NEC D68.69

**Thrombophlebitis** I80.9
- antepartum O22.2- ☑
  - deep O22.3- ☑

**Thrombophlebitis** — *continued*
- antepartum — *continued*
  - superficial O22.2- ☑
- calf muscular vein (NOS) I8Ø.25- ☑
- cavernous (venous) sinus GØ8
  - complicating pregnancy O22.5- ☑
  - nonpyogenic I67.6
- cerebral (sinus) (vein) GØ8
  - nonpyogenic I67.6
  - sequelae GØ9
- due to implanted device — *see* Complications, by site and type, specified NEC
- during or resulting from a procedure NEC T81.72- ☑
- femoral vein (superficial) I8Ø.1- ☑
- femoropopliteal vein I8Ø.Ø- ☑
- gastrocnemial vein I8Ø.25- ☑
- hepatic (vein) I8Ø.8
- idiopathic, recurrent I82.1
- iliac vein (common) (external) (internal) I8Ø.21- ☑
- iliofemoral I8Ø.1- ☑
- intracranial venous sinus (any) GØ8
  - nonpyogenic I67.6
  - sequelae GØ9
- intraspinal venous sinuses and veins GØ8
  - nonpyogenic G95.19
- lateral (venous) sinus GØ8
  - nonpyogenic I67.6
- leg — *see* Phlebitis, leg
- longitudinal (venous) sinus GØ8
  - nonpyogenic I67.6
- lower extremity — *see* Phlebitis, leg
  - deep — *see also* Phlebitis, leg, deep I8Ø.29- ☑
- migrans, migrating I82.1
- pelvic
  - with ectopic or molar pregnancy OØ8.Ø
  - following ectopic or molar pregnancy OØ8.Ø
  - puerperal O87.1
- peroneal vein I8Ø.24- ☑
- popliteal vein — *see* Phlebitis, leg, deep, popliteal
- portal (vein) K75.1
- postoperative T81.72- ☑
- pregnancy — *see* Thrombophlebitis, antepartum
- puerperal, postpartum, childbirth O87.Ø
  - deep O87.1
  - pelvic O87.1
  - septic O86.81
  - superficial O87.Ø
- saphenous (greater) (lesser) I8Ø.Ø- ☑
- sinus (intracranial) GØ8
  - nonpyogenic I67.6
- soleal vein I8Ø.25- ☑
- specified site NEC I8Ø.8
- tibial vein (anterior) (posterior) I8Ø.23- ☑

**Thrombosis, thrombotic** (bland) (multiple) (progressive) (silent) (vessel) I82.9Ø
- anal K64.5
- antepartum — *see* Thrombophlebitis, antepartum
- aorta, aortic I74.1Ø
  - abdominal I74.Ø9
    - saddle I74.Ø1
  - bifurcation I74.Ø9
  - saddle I74.Ø1
  - specified site NEC I74.19
  - terminal I74.Ø9
  - thoracic I74.11
  - valve — *see* Endocarditis, aortic
- apoplexy I63.3- ☑
- artery, arteries (postinfectional) I74.9
  - auditory, internal — *see* Occlusion, artery, precerebral, specified NEC
  - basilar — *see* Occlusion, artery, basilar
  - carotid (common) (internal) — *see* Occlusion, artery, carotid
  - cerebellar (anterior inferior) (posterior inferior) (superior) — *see* Occlusion, artery, cerebellar
  - cerebral — *see* Occlusion, artery, cerebral
  - choroidal (anterior) — *see* Occlusion, artery, precerebral, specified NEC
  - communicating, posterior — *see* Occlusion, artery, precerebral, specified NEC
  - coronary — *see also* Infarct, myocardium
    - not resulting in infarction I24.Ø
  - hepatic I74.8
  - hypophyseal — *see* Occlusion, artery, precerebral, specified NEC
  - iliac I74.5
  - limb I74.4
    - lower I74.3

**Thrombosis, thrombotic** — *continued*
- artery, arteries — *continued*
  - limb — *continued*
    - upper I74.2
  - meningeal, anterior or posterior — *see* Occlusion, artery, cerebral, specified NEC
  - mesenteric (with gangrene) — *see also* Infarct, intestine K55.Ø69
  - ophthalmic — *see* Occlusion, artery, retina
  - pontine — *see* Occlusion, artery, precerebral, specified NEC
  - precerebral — *see* Occlusion, artery, precerebral
  - pulmonary (iatrogenic) — *see* Embolism, pulmonary
  - renal N28.Ø
  - retinal — *see* Occlusion, artery, retina
  - spinal, anterior or posterior G95.11
  - traumatic NEC T14.8- ☑
  - vertebral — *see* Occlusion, artery, vertebral
- atrium, auricular — *see also* Infarct, myocardium
  - following acute myocardial infarction (current complication) I23.6
  - not resulting in infarction I51.3
  - old I51.3
- basilar (artery) — *see* Occlusion, artery, basilar
- brain (artery) (stem) — *see also* Occlusion, artery, cerebral
  - due to syphilis A52.Ø5
  - puerperal O99.43
  - sinus — *see* Thrombosis, intracranial, venous sinus
- capillary I78.8
- cardiac — *see also* Infarct, myocardium
  - not resulting in infarction I51.3
  - old I51.3
  - valve — *see* Endocarditis
- carotid (artery) (common) (internal) — *see* Occlusion, artery, carotid
- cavernous (venous) sinus — *see* Thrombosis, intracranial, venous sinus
- cerebellar artery (anterior inferior) (posterior inferior) (superior) I66.3
- cerebral (artery) — *see* Occlusion, artery, cerebral
- cerebrovenous sinus — *see also* Thrombosis, intracranial, venous sinus
  - puerperium O87.3
- chronic I82.91
- coronary (artery) (vein) — *see also* Infarct, myocardium
  - not resulting in infarction I24.Ø
- corpus cavernosum N48.89
- cortical I66.9
- deep — *see* Embolism, vein, lower extremity
- due to device, implant or graft — *see also* Complications, by site and type, specified NEC T85.868- ☑
  - arterial graft NEC T82.868- ☑
  - breast (implant) T85.868- ☑
  - catheter NEC T85.868- ☑
    - dialysis (renal) T82.868- ☑
      - intraperitoneal T85.868- ☑
    - infusion NEC T82.868- ☑
      - spinal (epidural) (subdural) T85.86Ø- ☑
    - urinary (indwelling) T83.86- ☑
  - electronic (electrode) (pulse generator) (stimulator)
    - bone T84.86- ☑
    - cardiac T82.867- ☑
    - nervous system (brain) (peripheral nerve) (spinal) T85.86Ø- ☑
    - urinary T83.86- ☑
  - fixation, internal (orthopedic) NEC T84.86- ☑
  - gastrointestinal (bile duct) (esophagus) T85.868- ☑
  - genital NEC T83.86- ☑
  - heart T82.867- ☑
  - joint prosthesis T84.86- ☑
  - ocular (corneal graft) (orbital implant) NEC T85.868- ☑
  - orthopedic NEC T84.86- ☑
  - specified NEC T85.868- ☑
  - urinary NEC T83.86- ☑
  - vascular NEC T82.868- ☑
  - ventricular intracranial shunt T85.86Ø- ☑
- during the puerperium — *see* Thrombosis, puerperal
- endocardial — *see also* Infarct, myocardium
  - not resulting in infarction I51.3
- eye — *see* Occlusion, retina
- genital organ
  - female NEC N94.89
    - pregnancy — *see* Thrombophlebitis, antepartum
  - male N5Ø.1
- gestational — *see* Phlebopathy, gestational
- heart (chamber) — *see also* Infarct, myocardium
  - not resulting in infarction I51.3

**Thrombosis, thrombotic** — *continued*
- heart — *see also* Infarct, myocardium — *continued*
  - old I51.3
- hepatic (vein) I82.Ø
  - artery I74.8
- history (of) Z86.718
- intestine (with gangrene) — *see also* Infarct, intestine K55.Ø69
- intracardiac NEC (apical) (atrial) (auricular) (ventricular) (old) I51.3
- intracranial (arterial) I66.9
  - venous sinus (any) I67.6
    - nonpyogenic I67.6
    - nonpyogenic origin I67.6
    - puerperium O87.3
- intramural — *see also* Infarct, myocardium
  - not resulting in infarction I51.3
  - old I51.3
- intraspinal venous sinuses and veins GØ8
  - nonpyogenic G95.19
- kidney (artery) N28.Ø
- lateral (venous) sinus — *see* Thrombosis, intracranial, venous sinus
- leg — *see* Thrombosis, vein, lower extremity
  - arterial I74.3
- liver (venous) I82.Ø
  - artery I74.8
  - portal vein I81
- longitudinal (venous) sinus — *see* Thrombosis, intracranial, venous sinus
- lower limb — *see* Thrombosis, vein, lower extremity
- lung (iatrogenic) (postoperative) — *see* Embolism, pulmonary
- meninges (brain) (arterial) I66.8
- mesenteric (artery) (with gangrene) — *see also* Infarct, intestine K55.Ø69
  - vein (inferior) (superior) K55.Ø- ☑
- mitral I34.89
- mural — *see also* Infarct, myocardium
  - due to syphilis A52.Ø6
  - not resulting in infarction I51.3
  - old I51.3
- omentum (with gangrene) — *see also* Infarct, intestine K55.Ø69
- ophthalmic — *see* Occlusion, retina
- pampiniform plexus (male) N5Ø.1
- parietal — *see also* Infarct, myocardium
  - not resulting in infarction I24.Ø
- penis, superficial vein N48.81
- perianal venous K64.5
- peripheral arteries I74.4
  - upper I74.2
- personal history (of) Z86.718
- portal I81
  - due to syphilis A52.Ø9
- precerebral artery — *see* Occlusion, artery, precerebral
- puerperal, postpartum O87.Ø
  - brain (artery) O99.43
    - venous (sinus) O87.3
  - cardiac O99.43
  - cerebral (artery) O99.43
    - venous (sinus) O87.3
  - superficial O87.Ø
- pulmonary (artery) (iatrogenic) (postoperative) (vein) — *see* Embolism, pulmonary
- renal (artery) N28.Ø
  - vein I82.3
- resulting from presence of device, implant or graft — *see* Complications, by site and type, specified NEC
- retina, retinal — *see* Occlusion, retina
- scrotum N5Ø.1
- seminal vesicle N5Ø.1
- sigmoid (venous) sinus — *see* Thrombosis, intracranial venous sinus
- sinus, intracranial (any) — *see* Thrombosis, intracranial venous sinus
- specified site NEC I82.89Ø
  - chronic I82.891
- spermatic cord N5Ø.1
- spinal cord (arterial) G95.11
  - due to syphilis A52.Ø9
  - pyogenic origin GØ6.1
- spleen, splenic D73.5
  - artery I74.8
- testis N5Ø.1
- traumatic NEC T14.8- ☑
- tricuspid IØ7.8
- tumor — *see* Neoplasm, unspecified behavior, by site
- tunica vaginalis N5Ø.1

**Thrombosis, thrombotic** — *continued*
- umbilical cord (vessels), complicating delivery O69.5- ☑
- vas deferens N50.1
- vein (acute) I82.90
  - antecubital I82.61- ☑
    - chronic I82.71- ☑
  - axillary I82.A1- ☑ *(following* I82.7)
    - chronic I82.A2- ☑ *(following* I82.7)
  - basilic I82.61- ☑
    - chronic I82.71- ☑
  - brachial I82.62- ☑
    - chronic I82.72- ☑
  - brachiocephalic (innominate) I82.290
    - chronic I82.291
  - calf muscular I82.46- ☑
    - chronic I82.56- ☑
  - cephalic I82.61- ☑
    - chronic I82.71- ☑
  - cerebral, nonpyogenic I67.6
  - chronic I82.91
  - deep (DVT) I82.40- ☑
    - calf I82.4Z- ☑
      - chronic I82.5Z- ☑
    - lower leg I82.4Z- ☑
      - chronic I82.5Z- ☑
    - thigh I82.4Y- ☑
      - chronic I82.5Y- ☑
    - upper leg I82.4Y- ☑
      - chronic I82.5Y- ☑
  - femoral I82.41- ☑
    - chronic I82.51- ☑
  - iliac (iliofemoral) I82.42- ☑
    - chronic I82.52- ☑
  - innominate I82.290
    - chronic I82.291
  - internal jugular I82.C1- ☑ *(following* I82.7)
    - chronic I82.C2- ☑ *(following* I82.7)
  - lower extremity
    - deep I82.40- ☑
      - chronic I82.50- ☑
      - specified NEC I82.49- ☑
        - chronic NEC I82.59- ☑
    - distal
      - deep I82.4Z- ☑
    - proximal
      - deep I82.4Y- ☑
        - chronic I82.5Y- ☑
    - superficial I82.81- ☑
  - perianal K64.5
  - peroneal I82.45- ☑
    - chronic I82.55- ☑
  - popliteal I82.43- ☑
    - chronic I82.53- ☑
  - radial I82.62- ☑
    - chronic I82.72- ☑
  - renal I82.3
  - saphenous (greater) (lesser) I82.81- ☑
  - specified NEC I82.890
    - chronic NEC I82.891
  - subclavian I82.B1- ☑ *(following* I82.7)
    - chronic I82.B2- ☑ *(following* I82.7)
  - thoracic NEC I82.290
    - chronic I82.291
  - tibial I82.44- ☑
    - chronic I82.54- ☑
  - ulnar I82.62- ☑
    - chronic I82.72- ☑
  - upper extremity I82.60- ☑
    - chronic I82.70- ☑
    - deep I82.62- ☑
      - chronic I82.72- ☑
    - superficial I82.61- ☑
      - chronic I82.71- ☑
- vena cava
  - inferior I82.220
    - chronic I82.221
  - superior I82.210
    - chronic I82.211
- venous, perianal K64.5
- ventricle — *see also* Infarct, myocardium
  - following acute myocardial infarction (current complication) I23.6
  - not resulting in infarction I24.0
  - old I51.3

**Thrombus** — *see* Thrombosis

**Thrush** — *see also* Candidiasis
- newborn P37.5
- oral B37.0
- vaginal (acute) B37.31
  - chronic (recurrent) B37.32

**Thumb** — *see also* condition
- sucking (child problem) F98.8

**Thymitis** E32.8

**Thymoma** — *see also* Neoplasm, thymus, by type
- malignant C37
- metaplastic C37
- microscopic D15.0
- sclerosing C37
- type A C37
- type AB C37
- type B1 C37
- type B2 C37
- type B3 C37

**Thymus, thymic** (gland) — *see* condition

**Thyrocele** — *see* Goiter

**Thyroglossal** — *see also* condition
- cyst Q89.2
- duct, persistent Q89.2

**Thyroid** (gland) (body) — *see also* condition
- hormone resistance E07.89
- lingual Q89.2
- nodule (cystic) (nontoxic) (single) E04.1

**Thyroiditis** E06.9
- acute (nonsuppurative) (pyogenic) (suppurative) E06.0
- autoimmune E06.3
- chronic (nonspecific) (sclerosing) E06.5
  - with thyrotoxicosis, transient E06.2
  - fibrous E06.5
  - lymphadenoid E06.3
  - lymphocytic E06.3
  - lymphoid E06.3
- de Quervain's E06.1
- drug-induced E06.4
- fibrous (chronic) E06.5
- giant-cell (follicular) E06.1
- granulomatous (de Quervain) (subacute) E06.1
- Hashimoto's (struma lymphomatosa) E06.3
- iatrogenic E06.4
- ligneous E06.5
- lymphocytic (chronic) E06.3
- lymphoid E06.3
- lymphomatous E06.3
- nonsuppurative E06.1
- postpartum, puerperal O90.5
- pseudotuberculous E06.1
- pyogenic E06.0
- radiation E06.4
- Riedel's E06.5
- subacute (granulomatous) E06.1
- suppurative E06.0
- tuberculous A18.81
- viral E06.1
- woody E06.5

**Thyrolingual duct, persistent** Q89.2

**Thyromegaly** E01.0

**Thyrotoxic**
- crisis — *see* Thyrotoxicosis
- heart disease or failure — *see also* Thyrotoxicosis E05.90 *[I43]*
  - with thyroid storm E05.91 *[I43]*
- storm — *see* Thyrotoxicosis

**Thyrotoxicosis** (recurrent) E05.90
- with
  - goiter (diffuse) E05.00
    - with thyroid storm E05.01
    - adenomatous uninodular E05.10
      - with thyroid storm E05.11
    - multinodular E05.20
      - with thyroid storm E05.21
    - nodular E05.20
      - with thyroid storm E05.21
    - uninodular E05.10
      - with thyroid storm E05.11
  - infiltrative
    - dermopathy E05.00
      - with thyroid storm E05.01
    - ophthalmopathy E05.00
      - with thyroid storm E05.01
  - single thyroid nodule E05.10
    - with thyroid storm E05.11
  - thyroid storm E05.91
- due to
  - ectopic thyroid nodule or tissue E05.30
    - with thyroid storm E05.31
  - ingestion of (excessive) thyroid material E05.40
    - with thyroid storm E05.41
  - overproduction of thyroid-stimulating hormone E05.80
    - with thyroid storm E05.81
  - specified cause NEC E05.80
    - with thyroid storm E05.81
- factitia E05.40
  - with thyroid storm E05.41
- heart — *see also* Failure, heart, high-output E05.90 *[I43]*
  - with thyroid storm — *see also* Failure, heart, high-output E05.91 *[I43]*
  - failure — *see also* Failure, heart, high-output E05.90 *[I43]*
- neonatal (transient) P72.1
- transient with chronic thyroiditis E06.2

**Tibia vara** M92.51- ☑

**Tic** (disorder) F95.9
- breathing F95.8
- child problem F95.0
- compulsive F95.1
- de la Tourette F95.2
- degenerative (generalized) (localized) G25.69
  - facial G25.69
- disorder
  - chronic
    - motor F95.1
    - vocal F95.1
  - combined vocal and multiple motor F95.2
  - transient F95.0
- douloureux G50.0
  - atypical G50.1
  - postherpetic, postzoster B02.22
- drug-induced G25.61
- eyelid F95.8
- habit F95.9
  - chronic F95.1
  - transient of childhood F95.0
- lid, transient of childhood F95.0
- motor-verbal F95.2
- occupational F48.8
- orbicularis F95.8
  - transient of childhood F95.0
- organic origin G25.69
- postchoreic G25.69
- provisional F95.0
- psychogenic, compulsive F95.1
- salaam R25.8
- spasm (motor or vocal) F95.9
  - chronic F95.1
  - transient of childhood F95.0
- specified NEC F95.8

**Tick-borne** — *see* condition

**Tietze's disease or syndrome** M94.0

**Tight, tightness**
- anus K62.89
- chest R07.89
- fascia (lata) M62.89
- foreskin (congenital) N47.1
- hymen, hymenal ring N89.6
- introitus (acquired) (congenital) N89.6
- rectal sphincter K62.89
- tendon — *see* Short, tendon
- urethral sphincter N35.919

**Tilting vertebra** — *see* Dorsopathy, deforming, specified NEC

**Timidity, child** F93.8

**Tin-miner's lung** J63.5

**Tinea** (intersecta) (tarsi) B35.9
- amiantacea L44.8
- asbestina B35.0
- barbae B35.0
- beard B35.0
- black dot B35.0
- blanca B36.2
- capitis B35.0
- corporis B35.4
- cruris B35.6
- flava B36.0
- foot B35.3
- furfuracea B36.0
- imbricata (Tokelau) B35.5
- kerion B35.0
- manuum B35.2
- microsporic — *see* Dermatophytosis
- nigra B36.1
- nodosa — *see* Piedra

- **Tinea** — *continued*
  - pedis B35.3
  - scalp B35.Ø
  - specified NEC B35.8
  - sycosis B35.Ø
  - tonsurans B35.Ø
  - trichophytic — *see* Dermatophytosis
  - unguium B35.1
  - versicolor B36.Ø
- **Tingling sensation** (skin) R2Ø.2
- **Tinnitus NOS** H93.1- ☑
  - audible H93.1- ☑
  - aurium H93.1- ☑
  - pulsatile H93.A- ☑
  - subjective H93.1- ☑
- **Tipped tooth** (teeth) M26.33
- **Tipping**
  - pelvis M95.5
    - with disproportion (fetopelvic) O33.Ø
      - causing obstructed labor O65.Ø
  - tooth (teeth), fully erupted M26.33
- **Tiredness** R53.83
- **Tissue** — *see* condition
- **Tobacco** (nicotine)
  - abuse — *see* Tobacco, use
  - dependence — *see* Dependence, drug, nicotine
  - harmful use Z72.Ø
  - heart — *see* Tobacco, toxic effect
  - maternal use, affecting newborn PØ4.2
  - toxic effect — *see* Table of Drugs and Chemicals, by substance, poisoning
    - chewing tobacco — *see* Table of Drugs and Chemicals, by substance, poisoning
    - cigarettes — *see* Table of Drugs and Chemicals, by substance, poisoning
  - use Z72.Ø
    - complicating
      - childbirth O99.334
      - pregnancy O99.33- ☑
      - puerperium O99.335
    - counseling and surveillance Z71.6
    - history Z87.891
  - withdrawal state — *see also* Dependence, drug, nicotine F17.2Ø3
- **Tocopherol deficiency** E56.Ø
- **Todd's**
  - cirrhosis K74.3
  - paralysis (postepileptic) (transitory) G83.84
- **Toe** — *see* condition
- **Toilet, artificial opening** — *see* Attention to, artificial, opening
- **Tokelau** (ringworm) B35.5
- **Tollwut** — *see* Rabies
- **Tommaselli's disease** R31.9
  - correct substance properly administered — *see* Table of Drugs and Chemicals, by drug, adverse effect
  - overdose or wrong substance given or taken — *see* Table of Drugs and Chemicals, by drug, poisoning
- **Tongue** — *see also* condition
  - tie Q38.1
- **Toni-Fanconi syndrome** (cystinosis) E72.Ø9
  - with cystinosis E72.Ø4
- **Tonic pupil** — *see* Anomaly, pupil, function, tonic pupil
- **Tonsil** — *see* condition
- **Tonsillitis** (acute) (catarrhal) (croupous) (follicular) (gangrenous) (infective) (lacunar) (lingual) (malignant) (membranous) (parenchymatous) (phlegmonous) (pseudomembranous) (purulent) (septic) (subacute) (suppurative) (toxic) (ulcerative) (vesicular) (viral) JØ3.9Ø
  - chronic J35.Ø1
    - with adenoiditis J35.Ø3
  - diphtheritic A36.Ø
  - hypertrophic J35.Ø1
    - with adenoiditis J35.Ø3
  - recurrent JØ3.91
  - specified organism NEC JØ3.8Ø
    - recurrent JØ3.81
  - staphylococcal JØ3.8Ø
    - recurrent JØ3.81
  - streptococcal JØ3.ØØ
    - recurrent JØ3.Ø1
  - tuberculous A15.8
  - Vincent's A69.1
- **Tooth, teeth** — *see* condition
- **Toothache** KØ8.89
- **Topagnosis** R2Ø.8
- **Tophi** — *see* Gout, chronic
- **TORCH infection** — *see* Infection, congenital
  - without active infection PØØ.2
- **Torn** — *see* Tear
- **Tornwaldt's cyst or disease** J39.2
- **Torsades de pointes** I47.21
- **Torsion**
  - accessory tube — *see* Torsion, fallopian tube
  - adnexa (female) — *see* Torsion, fallopian tube
  - aorta, acquired I77.1
  - appendix epididymis N44.Ø4
  - appendix testis N44.Ø3
  - bile duct (common) (hepatic) K83.8
    - congenital Q44.5
  - bowel, colon or intestine K56.2
  - cervix — *see* Malposition, uterus
  - cystic duct K82.8
  - dystonia — *see* Dystonia, torsion
  - epididymis (appendix) N44.Ø4
  - fallopian tube N83.52- ☑
    - with ovary N83.53
  - gallbladder K82.8
    - congenital Q44.1
  - hydatid of Morgagni
    - female N83.52- ☑
    - male N44.Ø3
  - kidney (pedicle) (leading to infarction) N28.Ø
  - Meckel's diverticulum (congenital) Q43.Ø
    - malignant — *see* Table of Neoplasms, small intestine, malignant
  - mesentery K56.2
  - omentum K56.2
  - organ or site, congenital NEC — *see* Anomaly, by site
  - ovary (pedicle) N83.51- ☑
    - with fallopian tube N83.53
    - congenital Q5Ø.2
  - oviduct — *see* Torsion, fallopian tube
  - penis (acquired) N48.82
    - congenital Q55.63
  - spasm — *see* Dystonia, torsion
  - spermatic cord N44.Ø2
    - extravaginal N44.Ø1
    - intravaginal N44.Ø2
  - spleen D73.5
  - testis, testicle N44.ØØ
    - appendix N44.Ø3
  - tibia — *see* Deformity, limb, specified type NEC, lower leg
  - uterus — *see* Malposition, uterus
- **Torticollis** (intermittent) (spastic) M43.6
  - congenital (sternomastoid) Q68.Ø
  - due to birth injury P15.8
  - hysterical F44.4
  - ocular R29.891
  - psychogenic F45.8
    - conversion reaction F44.4
  - rheumatic M43.6
  - rheumatoid MØ6.88
  - spasmodic G24.3
  - traumatic, current S13.4- ☑
- **Tortipelvis** G24.1
- **Tortuous**
  - aortic arch Q25.46
  - artery I77.1
  - organ or site, congenital NEC — *see* Distortion
  - retinal vessel, congenital Q14.1
  - ureter N13.8
  - urethra N36.8
  - vein — *see* Varix
- **Torture, victim of** Z65.4
- **Torula, torular** (histolytica) (infection) — *see* Cryptococcosis
- **Torulosis** — *see* Cryptococcosis
- **Torus** (mandibularis) (palatinus) M27.Ø
  - fracture — *see* Fracture, by site, torus
- **Touraine's syndrome** Q79.8
- **Tourette's syndrome** F95.2
- **Tourniquet syndrome** — *see* Constriction, external, by site
- **Tower skull** Q75.Ø58
  - with exophthalmos Q87.Ø
- **Toxemia** R68.89
  - bacterial — *see* Sepsis
  - burn — *see* Burn
  - eclamptic (with pre-existing hypertension) — *see* Eclampsia
  - erysipelatous — *see* Erysipelas
  - fatigue R68.89
  - food — *see* Poisoning, food
  - gastrointestinal K52.1
  - intestinal K52.1
  - kidney — *see* Uremia
- **Toxemia** — *continued*
  - malarial — *see* Malaria
  - myocardial — *see* Myocarditis, toxic
  - of pregnancy — *see* Pre-eclampsia
  - pre-eclamptic — *see* Pre-eclampsia
  - small intestine K52.1
  - staphylococcal, due to food AØ5.Ø
  - stasis R68.89
  - uremic — *see* Uremia
  - urinary — *see* Uremia
- **Toxemica cerebropathia psychica** (nonalcoholic) FØ4
  - alcoholic — *see* Alcohol, amnestic disorder
- **Toxic** (poisoning) — *see also* condition T65.91- ☑
  - effect — *see* Table of Drugs and Chemicals, by substance, poisoning
  - shock syndrome A48.3
  - thyroid (gland) — *see* Thyrotoxicosis
- **Toxicemia** — *see* Toxemia
- **Toxicity** — *see* Table of Drugs and Chemicals, by substance, poisoning
  - fava bean D55.Ø
  - food, noxious — *see* Poisoning, food
  - from drug or nonmedicinal substance — *see* Table of Drugs and Chemicals, by drug
- **Toxicosis** — *see also* Toxemia
  - capillary, hemorrhagic D69.Ø
- **Toxinfection, gastrointestinal** K52.1
- **Toxocariasis** B83.Ø
- **Toxoplasma, toxoplasmosis** (acquired) B58.9
  - with
    - hepatitis B58.1
    - meningoencephalitis B58.2
    - ocular involvement B58.ØØ
    - other organ involvement B58.89
    - pneumonia, pneumonitis B58.3
  - congenital (acute) (subacute) (chronic) P37.1
  - maternal, manifest toxoplasmosis in infant (acute) (subacute) (chronic) P37.1
- **tPA** (rtPA) **administration in a different facility within the last 24 hours prior to admission to current facility** Z92.82
- **Trabeculation, bladder** N32.89
- **Trachea** — *see* condition
- **Tracheitis** (catarrhal) (infantile) (membranous) (plastic) (septal) (suppurative) (viral) JØ4.1Ø
  - with
    - bronchitis (15 years of age and above) J4Ø
      - acute or subacute — *see* Bronchitis, acute
      - chronic J42
      - tuberculous NEC A15.5
      - under 15 years of age J2Ø.9
    - laryngitis (acute) JØ4.2
      - chronic J37.1
      - tuberculous NEC A15.5
  - acute JØ4.1Ø
    - with obstruction JØ4.11
  - chronic J42
    - with
      - bronchitis (chronic) J42
      - laryngitis (chronic) J37.1
  - diphtheritic (membranous) A36.89
  - due to external agent — *see* Inflammation, respiratory, upper, due to
  - syphilitic A52.73
  - tuberculous A15.5
- **Trachelitis** (nonvenereal) — *see* Cervicitis
- **Tracheobronchial** — *see* condition
- **Tracheobronchitis** (15 years of age and above) — *see also* Bronchitis
  - due to
    - Bordetella bronchiseptica A37.8Ø
      - with pneumonia A37.81
    - Francisella tularensis A21.8
- **Tracheobronchomegaly** Q32.4
  - with bronchiectasis J47.9
    - with
      - exacerbation (acute) J47.1
      - lower respiratory infection J47.Ø
  - acquired J98.Ø9
    - with bronchiectasis J47.9
      - with
        - exacerbation (acute) J47.1
        - lower respiratory infection J47.Ø
- **Tracheobronchopneumonitis** — *see* Pneumonia, broncho
- **Tracheocele** (external) (internal) J39.8
  - congenital Q32.1
- **Tracheomalacia** J39.8
  - congenital Q32.Ø
- **Tracheopharyngitis** (acute) JØ6.9





☑ **Additional Character Required — Refer to the Tabular List for Character Selection**

**Tracheopharyngitis** — *continued*
- chronic J42
- due to external agent — *see* Inflammation, respiratory, upper, due to

**Tracheostenosis** J39.8

**Tracheostomy**
- complication — *see* Complication, tracheostomy
- status Z93.Ø
  - attention to Z43.Ø
  - malfunctioning J95.Ø3

**Trachoma, trachomatous** A71.9
- active (stage) A71.1
- contraction of conjunctiva A71.1
- dubium A71.Ø
- healed or sequelae B94.Ø
- initial (stage) A71.Ø
- pannus A71.1
- Türck's J37.Ø

**Traction, vitreomacular** H43.82- ☑

**Train sickness** T75.3- ☑

**Trait**(s)
- Hb-S D57.3
- hemoglobin
  - abnormal NEC D58.2
    - with thalassemia D56.3
  - C — *see* Disease, hemoglobin C
  - S (Hb-S) D57.3
- Lepore D56.3
- personality, accentuated Z73.1
- sickle-cell D57.3
  - with elliptocytosis or spherocytosis D57.3
- type A personality Z73.1

**Tramp** Z59.ØØ

**Trance** R41.89
- hysterical F44.89

**Transaminasemia** R74.Ø1

**Transection**
- abdomen (partial) S38.3- ☑
- aorta (incomplete) — *see also* Injury, aorta
  - complete — *see* Injury, aorta, laceration, major
- carotid artery (incomplete) — *see also* Injury, blood vessel, carotid, laceration
  - complete — *see* Injury, blood vessel, carotid, laceration, major
- celiac artery (incomplete) S35.211- ☑
  - branch (incomplete) S35.291- ☑
    - complete S35.292- ☑
  - complete S35.212- ☑
- innominate
  - artery (incomplete) — *see also* Injury, blood vessel, thoracic, innominate, artery, laceration
    - complete — *see* Injury, blood vessel, thoracic, innominate, artery, laceration, major
  - vein (incomplete) — *see also* Injury, blood vessel, thoracic, innominate, vein, laceration
    - complete — *see* Injury, blood vessel, thoracic, innominate, vein, laceration, major
- jugular vein (external) (incomplete) — *see also* Injury, blood vessel, jugular vein, laceration
  - complete — *see* Injury, blood vessel, jugular vein, laceration, major
  - internal (incomplete) — *see also* Injury, blood vessel, jugular vein, internal, laceration
    - complete — *see* Injury, blood vessel, jugular vein, internal, laceration, major
- mesenteric artery (incomplete) — *see also* Injury, mesenteric, artery, laceration
  - complete — *see* Injury, mesenteric artery, laceration, major
- pulmonary vessel (incomplete) — *see also* Injury, blood vessel, thoracic, pulmonary, laceration
  - complete — *see* Injury, blood vessel, thoracic, pulmonary, laceration, major
- subclavian — *see* Transection, innominate
- vena cava (incomplete) — *see also* Injury, vena cava
  - complete — *see* Injury, vena cava, laceration, major
- vertebral artery (incomplete) — *see also* Injury, blood vessel, vertebral, laceration
  - complete — *see* Injury, blood vessel, vertebral, laceration, major

**Transfusion**
- associated (red blood cell) hemochromatosis E83.111
- blood
  - ABO incompatible — *see* Complication(s), transfusion, incompatibility reaction, ABO
  - minor blood group (Duffy) (E) (K) (Kell) (Kidd) (Lewis) (M) (N) (P) (S) T8Ø.89- ☑

**Transfusion** — *continued*
- blood — *continued*
  - reaction or complication — *see* Complications, transfusion
- fetomaternal (mother) — *see* Pregnancy, complicated by, placenta, transfusion syndrome
- maternofetal (mother) — *see* Pregnancy, complicated by, placenta, transfusion syndrome
- placental (syndrome) (mother) — *see* Pregnancy, complicated by, placenta, transfusion syndrome
- reaction (adverse) — *see* Complications, transfusion
- related acute lung injury (TRALI) J95.84
- twin-to-twin — *see* Pregnancy, complicated by, placenta, transfusion syndrome, fetus to fetus

**Transgender** F64.Ø

**Transient** (meaning homeless) — *see also* condition Z59.ØØ

**Translocation**
- balanced autosomal Q95.9
  - in normal individual Q95.Ø
- chromosomes NEC Q99.8- ☑
  - balanced and insertion in normal individual Q95.Ø
- Down syndrome Q9Ø.2
- trisomy
  - 13 Q91.6
  - 18 Q91.2
  - 21 Q9Ø.2

**Translucency, iris** — *see* Degeneration, iris

**Transmission of chemical substances through the placenta** — *see* Absorption, chemical, through placenta

**Transparency, lung, unilateral** J43.Ø

**Transplant** (ed) (status) Z94.9
- awaiting organ Z76.82
- bone Z94.6
  - marrow Z94.81
- candidate Z76.82
- complication — *see* Complication, transplant
- cornea Z94.7
- heart Z94.1
  - and lung(s) Z94.3
  - valve Z95.2
    - prosthetic Z95.2
    - specified NEC Z95.4
    - xenogenic Z95.3
- intestine Z94.82
- kidney Z94.Ø
- liver Z94.4
- lung(s) Z94.2
  - and heart Z94.3
- organ (failure) (infection) (rejection) Z94.9
  - removal status Z98.85
- pancreas Z94.83
- skin Z94.5
- social Z6Ø.3
- specified organ or tissue NEC Z94.89
- stem cells Z94.84
- tissue Z94.9

**Transplants, ovarian, endometrial** N8Ø.1Ø- ☑

**Transposed** — *see* Transposition

**Transposition** (congenital) — *see also* Malposition, congenital
- abdominal viscera Q89.3
- aorta (dextra) Q2Ø.3
- appendix Q43.8
- colon Q43.8
- corrected Q2Ø.5
- great vessels (complete) (partial) Q2Ø.3
- heart Q24.Ø
  - with complete transposition of viscera Q89.3
- intestine (large) (small) Q43.8
- reversed jejunal (for bypass) (status) Z98.Ø
- scrotum Q55.23
- stomach Q4Ø.2
  - with general transposition of viscera Q89.3
- tooth, teeth, fully erupted M26.3Ø
- vessels, great (complete) (partial) Q2Ø.3
- viscera (abdominal) (thoracic) Q89.3

**Transsexualism** F64.Ø

**Transverse** — *see also* condition
- arrest (deep), in labor O64.Ø- ☑
- lie (mother) O32.2- ☑
  - causing obstructed labor O64.8- ☑

**Transvestism, transvestitism** (dual-role) F64.1
- fetishistic F65.1

**Trapped placenta** (with hemorrhage) O72.Ø
- without hemorrhage O73.Ø

**TRAPS** (tumor necrosis factor receptor associated periodic syndrome) MØ4.1

**Trauma, traumatism** — *see also* Injury

**Trauma, traumatism** — *continued*
- acoustic — *see* subcategory H83.3- ☑
- birth — *see* Birth, injury
- complicating ectopic or molar pregnancy OØ8.6
- during delivery O71.9
- following ectopic or molar pregnancy OØ8.6
- non-accidental — *see* Abuse, physical
- obstetric O71.9
  - specified NEC O71.89
- occusal
  - primary KØ8.81
  - secondary KØ8.82

**Traumatic** — *see also* condition
- brain injury SØ6.9- ☑

**Treacher Collins syndrome** Q75.4

**Treitz's hernia** — *see* Hernia, abdomen, specified site NEC

**Trematode infestation** — *see* Infestation, fluke

**Trematodiasis** — *see* Infestation, fluke

**Trembling paralysis** — *see* Parkinsonism

**Tremor(s)** R25.1
- drug induced G25.1
- essential (benign) G25.Ø
- familial G25.Ø
- hereditary G25.Ø
- hysterical F44.4
- intention G25.2
- medication induced postural G25.1
- mercurial — *see* subcategory T56.1- ☑
- Parkinson's — *see* Parkinsonism
- psychogenic (conversion reaction) F44.4
- senilis R54
- specified type NEC G25.2

**Trench**
- fever A79.Ø
- foot — *see* Immersion, foot
- mouth A69.1

**Treponema pallidum infection** — *see* Syphilis

**Treponematosis**
- due to
  - T. pallidum — *see* Syphilis
  - T. pertenue — *see* Yaws

**Triad**
- Hutchinson's (congenital syphilis) A5Ø.53
- Kartagener's Q89.3
- Saint's — *see* Hernia, diaphragm

**Trichiasis** (eyelid) HØ2.Ø59
- with entropion — *see* Entropion
- left HØ2.Ø56
  - lower HØ2.Ø55
  - upper HØ2.Ø54
- right HØ2.Ø53
  - lower HØ2.Ø52
  - upper HØ2.Ø51

**Trichinella spiralis** (infection) (infestation) B75

**Trichinellosis, trichiniasis, trichinelliasis, trichinosis** B75
- with muscle disorder B75 *[M63.8Ø]*
  - ankle B75 *[M63.87-]* ☑
  - foot B75 *[M63.87-]* ☑
  - forearm B75 *[M63.83-]* ☑
  - hand B75 *[M63.84-]* ☑
  - lower leg B75 *[M63.86-]* ☑
  - multiple sites B75 *[M63.89]*
  - pelvic region B75 *[M63.85-]* ☑
  - shoulder region B75 *[M63.81-]* ☑
  - specified site NEC B75 *[M63.88]*
  - thigh B75 *[M63.85-]* ☑
  - upper arm B75 *[M63.82-]* ☑

**Trichobezoar** T18.9- ☑
- intestine T18.3- ☑
- stomach T18.2- ☑

**Trichocephaliasis, trichocephalosis** B79

**Trichocephalus infestation** B79

**Trichoclasis** L67.8

**Trichoepithelioma** — *see also* Neoplasm, skin, benign
- malignant — *see* Neoplasm, skin, malignant

**Trichofolliculoma** — *see* Neoplasm, skin, benign

**Tricholemmoma** — *see* Neoplasm, skin, benign

**Trichomoniasis** A59.9
- bladder A59.Ø3
- cervix A59.Ø9
- intestinal AØ7.8
- prostate A59.Ø2
- seminal vesicles A59.Ø9
- specified site NEC A59.8
- urethra A59.Ø3
- urogenitalis A59.ØØ
- vagina A59.Ø1
- vulva A59.Ø1

**Trichomycosis**
  axillaris A48.8
  nodosa, nodularis B36.8
**Trichonodosis** L67.8
**Trichophytid, trichophyton infection** — *see* Dermatophytosis
**Trichophytobezoar** T18.9- ☑
  intestine T18.3- ☑
  stomach T18.2- ☑
**Trichophytosis** — *see* Dermatophytosis
**Trichoptilosis** L67.8
**Trichorrhexis** (nodosa) (invaginata) L67.Ø
**Trichosis axillaris** A48.8
**Trichosporosis nodosa** B36.2
**Trichostasis spinulosa** (congenital) Q84.1
**Trichostrongyliasis, trichostrongylosis** (small intestine) B81.2
**Trichostrongylus infection** B81.2
**Trichotillomania** F63.3
**Trichromat, trichromatopsia, anomalous** (congenital) H53.55
**Trichuriasis** B79
**Trichuris trichiura** (infection) (infestation) (any site) B79
**Tricuspid** (valve) — *see* condition
**Trifid** — *see also* Accessory
  kidney (pelvis) Q63.8
  tongue Q38.3
**Trigeminal neuralgia** — *see* Neuralgia, trigeminal
**Trigeminy** RØØ.8
**Trigger finger** (acquired) M65.3Ø
  congenital Q74.Ø
  index finger M65.32- ☑
  little finger M65.35- ☑
  middle finger M65.33- ☑
  ring finger M65.34- ☑
  thumb M65.31- ☑
**Trigonitis** (bladder) (chronic) (pseudomembranous) N3Ø.3Ø
  with hematuria N3Ø.31
**Trigonocephaly** Q75.Ø3
**Trilocular heart** — *see* Cor triloculare
**Trimethylaminuria** E72.52
**Tripartite placenta** O43.19- ☑
**Triphalangeal thumb** Q74.Ø
**Triple** — *see also* Accessory
  kidneys Q63.Ø
  negative breast cancer (TNBC) Z17.421
  uteri Q51.818
  X, female Q97.Ø
**Triple I** O41.12- ☑
**Triplegia** G83.89
  congenital G8Ø.8
**Triplet** (newborn) — *see also* Newborn, triplet
  complicating pregnancy — *see* Pregnancy, triplet
**Triplication** — *see* Accessory
**Triploidy** Q92.7
**Trismus** R25.2
  neonatorum A33
  newborn A33
**Trisomy** (syndrome) Q92.9
  13 (partial) Q91.7
    meiotic nondisjunction Q91.4
    mitotic nondisjunction Q91.5
    mosaicism Q91.5
    translocation Q91.6
  18 (partial) Q91.3
    meiotic nondisjunction Q91.Ø
    mitotic nondisjunction Q91.1
    mosaicism Q91.1
    translocation Q91.2
  2Ø Q92.8
  21 (partial) Q9Ø.9
    meiotic nondisjunction Q9Ø.Ø
    mitotic nondisjunction Q9Ø.1
    mosaicism Q9Ø.1
    translocation Q9Ø.2
  22 Q92.8
  autosomes Q92.9
  chromosome specified NEC Q92.8
    partial Q92.2
      due to unbalanced translocation Q92.5
    specified NEC Q92.8
    whole (nonsex chromosome)
      meiotic nondisjunction Q92.Ø
      mitotic nondisjunction Q92.1
      mosaicism Q92.1
  due to
    dicentrics — *see* Extra, marker chromosomes
    extra rings — *see* Extra, marker chromosomes

**Trisomy** — *continued*
  due to — *continued*
    isochromosomes — *see* Extra, marker chromosomes
  specified NEC Q92.8
  whole chromosome Q92.9
    meiotic nondisjunction Q92.Ø
    mitotic nondisjunction Q92.1
    mosaicism Q92.1
    partial Q92.9
    specified NEC Q92.8
**Tritanomaly, tritanopia** H53.55
**Trombiculosis, trombiculiasis, trombidiosis** B88.Ø9
**Trophedema** (congenital) (hereditary) Q82.Ø
**Trophoblastic disease** — *see also* Mole, hydatidiform OØ1.9
**Tropholymphedema** Q82.Ø
**Trophoneurosis NEC** G96.89
  disseminated M34.9
**Tropical** — *see* condition
**Trouble** — *see also* Disease
  heart — *see* Disease, heart
  kidney — *see* Disease, renal
  nervous R45.Ø
  sinus — *see* Sinusitis
**Trousseau's syndrome** (thrombophlebitis migrans) I82.1
**Truancy, childhood**
  from school Z72.81Ø
**Truncus**
  arteriosus (persistent) Q2Ø.Ø
  communis Q2Ø.Ø
**Trunk** — *see* condition
**Trypanosomiasis**
  African B56.9
    by Trypanosoma brucei
      gambiense B56.Ø
      rhodesiense B56.1
  American — *see* Chagas' disease
  Brazilian — *see* Chagas' disease
  by Trypanosoma
    brucei gambiense B56.Ø
    brucei rhodesiense B56.1
    cruzi — *see* Chagas' disease
  gambiensis, Gambian B56.Ø
  rhodesiensis, Rhodesian B56.1
  South American — *see* Chagas' disease
  where
    African trypanosomiasis is prevalent B56.9
    Chagas' disease is prevalent B57.2
**Tryptasemia, hereditary alpha** D89.44
**Tsutsugamushi** (disease) (fever) A75.3
**Tube, tubal, tubular** — *see* condition
**Tubercle** — *see also* Tuberculosis
  brain, solitary A17.81
  Darwin's Q17.8
  Ghon, primary infection A15.7
**Tuberculid, tuberculide** (indurating, subcutaneous) (lichenoid) (miliary) (papulonecrotic) (primary) (skin) A18.4
**Tuberculoma** — *see also* Tuberculosis
  brain A17.81
  meninges (cerebral) (spinal) A17.1
  spinal cord A17.81
**Tuberculosis, tubercular, tuberculous** (calcification) (calcified) (caseous) (chromogenic acid-fast bacilli) (degeneration) (fibrocaseous) (fistula) (interstitial) (isolated circumscribed lesions) (necrosis) (parenchymatous) (ulcerative) A15.9
  with pneumoconiosis (any condition in J6Ø-J64) J65
  abdomen (lymph gland) A18.39
  abscess (respiratory) A15.9
    bone A18.Ø3
      hip A18.Ø2
      knee A18.Ø2
      sacrum A18.Ø1
      specified site NEC A18.Ø3
      spinal A18.Ø1
      vertebra A18.Ø1
    brain A17.81
    breast A18.89
    Cowper's gland A18.15
    dura (mater) (cerebral) (spinal) A17.81
    epidural (cerebral) (spinal) A17.81
    female pelvis A18.17
    frontal sinus A15.8
    genital organs NEC A18.1Ø
    genitourinary A18.1Ø
    gland (lymphatic) — *see* Tuberculosis, lymph gland
    hip A18.Ø2
    intestine A18.32
    ischiorectal A18.32

**Tuberculosis, tubercular, tuberculous** — *continued*
  abscess — *continued*
    joint NEC A18.Ø2
      hip A18.Ø2
      knee A18.Ø2
      specified NEC A18.Ø2
      vertebral A18.Ø1
    kidney A18.11
    knee A18.Ø2
    latent Z22.7
    lumbar (spine) A18.Ø1
    lung — *see* Tuberculosis, pulmonary
    meninges (cerebral) (spinal) A17.Ø
    muscle A18.Ø9
    perianal (fistula) A18.32
    perinephritic A18.11
    perirectal A18.32
    rectum A18.32
    retropharyngeal A15.8
    sacrum A18.Ø1
    scrofulous A18.2
    scrotum A18.15
    skin (primary) A18.4
    spinal cord A17.81
    spine or vertebra (column) A18.Ø1
    subdiaphragmatic A18.31
    testis A18.15
    urinary A18.13
    uterus A18.17
  accessory sinus — *see* Tuberculosis, sinus
  Addison's disease A18.7
  adenitis — *see* Tuberculosis, lymph gland
  adenoids A15.8
  adenopathy — *see* Tuberculosis, lymph gland
  adherent pericardium A18.84
  adnexa (uteri) A18.17
  adrenal (capsule) (gland) A18.7
  alimentary canal A18.32
  anemia A18.89
  ankle (joint) (bone) A18.Ø2
  anus A18.32
  apex, apical — *see* Tuberculosis, pulmonary
  appendicitis, appendix A18.32
  arachnoid A17.Ø
  artery, arteritis A18.89
    cerebral A18.89
  arthritis (chronic) (synovial) A18.Ø2
    spine or vertebra (column) A18.Ø1
  articular — *see* Tuberculosis, joint
  ascites A18.31
  asthma — *see* Tuberculosis, pulmonary
  axilla, axillary (gland) A18.2
  bladder A18.12
  bone A18.Ø3
    hip A18.Ø2
    knee A18.Ø2
    limb NEC A18.Ø3
    sacrum A18.Ø1
    spine or vertebral column A18.Ø1
  bowel (miliary) A18.32
  brain A17.81
  breast A18.89
  broad ligament A18.17
  bronchi, bronchial, bronchus A15.5
    ectasia, ectasis (bronchiectasis) — *see* Tuberculosis, pulmonary
    fistula A15.5
      primary (progressive) A15.7
    gland or node A15.4
      primary (progressive) A15.7
    lymph gland or node A15.4
      primary (progressive) A15.7
  bronchiectasis — *see* Tuberculosis, pulmonary
  bronchitis A15.5
  bronchopleural A15.6
  bronchopneumonia, bronchopneumonic — *see* Tuberculosis, pulmonary
  bronchorrhagia A15.5
  bronchotracheal A15.5
  bronze disease A18.7
  buccal cavity A18.83
  bulbourethral gland A18.15
  bursa A18.Ø9
  cachexia A15.9
  cardiomyopathy A18.84
  caries — *see* Tuberculosis, bone
  cartilage A18.Ø2
    intervertebral A18.Ø1
  catarrhal — *see* Tuberculosis, respiratory

- **Tuberculosis, tubercular, tuberculous** — *continued*
  - retina, retinitis A18.53
  - retroperitoneal (lymph gland or node) A18.39
  - rheumatism NEC A18.Ø9
  - rhinitis A15.8
  - sacroiliac (joint) A18.Ø1
  - sacrum A18.Ø1
  - salivary gland A18.83
  - salpingitis (acute) (chronic) A18.17
  - sandblaster's J65
  - sclera A18.51
  - scoliosis A18.Ø1
  - scrofulous A18.2
  - scrotum A18.15
  - seminal tract or vesicle A18.15
  - senile A15.9
  - septic — *see* Tuberculosis, miliary
  - shoulder (joint) A18.Ø2
    - blade A18.Ø3
  - sigmoid A18.32
  - sinus (any nasal) A15.8
    - bone A18.Ø3
    - epididymis A18.15
  - skeletal NEC A18.Ø3
  - skin (any site) (primary) A18.4
  - small intestine A18.32
  - soft palate A18.83
  - spermatic cord A18.15
  - spine, spinal (column) A18.Ø1
    - cord A17.81
    - medulla A17.81
    - membrane A17.Ø
    - meninges A17.Ø
  - spleen, splenitis A18.85
  - spondylitis A18.Ø1
  - sternoclavicular joint A18.Ø2
  - stomach A18.83
  - stonemason's J65
  - subcutaneous tissue (cellular) (primary) A18.4
  - subcutis (primary) A18.4
  - subdeltoid bursa A18.83
  - submaxillary (region) A18.83
  - supraclavicular gland A18.2
  - suprarenal (capsule) (gland) A18.7
  - swelling, joint — *see also* category MØ1 — *see also* Tuberculosis, joint A18.Ø2
  - symphysis pubis A18.Ø2
  - synovitis A18.Ø9
    - articular A18.Ø2
    - spine or vertebra A18.Ø1
  - systemic — *see* Tuberculosis, miliary
  - tarsitis A18.4
  - tendon (sheath) — *see* Tuberculosis, tenosynovitis
  - tenosynovitis A18.Ø9
    - spine or vertebra A18.Ø1
  - testis A18.15
  - throat A15.8
  - thymus gland A18.82
  - thyroid gland A18.81
  - tongue A18.83
  - tonsil, tonsillitis A15.8
  - trachea, tracheal A15.5
    - lymph gland or node A15.4
      - primary (progressive) A15.7
  - tracheobronchial A15.5
    - lymph gland or node A15.4
      - primary (progressive) A15.7
  - tubal (acute) (chronic) A18.17
  - tunica vaginalis A18.15
  - ulcer (skin) (primary) A18.4
    - bowel or intestine A18.32
    - specified NEC — *see* Tuberculosis, by site
  - unspecified site A15.9
  - ureter A18.11
  - urethra, urethral (gland) A18.13
  - urinary organ or tract A18.13
  - uterus A18.17
  - uveal tract A18.54
  - uvula A18.83
  - vagina A18.18
  - vas deferens A18.15
  - verruca, verrucosa (cutis) (primary) A18.4
  - vertebra (column) A18.Ø1
  - vesiculitis A18.15
  - vulva A18.18
  - wrist (joint) A18.Ø2
- **Tuberculum**
  - Carabelli — *see* Excludes Note at KØØ.2
  - occlusal — *see* Excludes Note at KØØ.2
- **Tuberculum** — *continued*
  - paramolare KØØ.2
- **Tuberosity, entire maxillary** M26.Ø7
- **Tuberous sclerosis** (brain) Q85.1
- **Tubo-ovarian** — *see* condition
- **Tuboplasty, after previous sterilization** Z31.Ø
  - aftercare Z31.42
- **Tubotympanitis, catarrhal** (chronic) — *see* Otitis, media, nonsuppurative, chronic, serous
- **Tularemia** A21.9
  - with
    - conjunctivitis A21.1
    - pneumonia A21.2
  - abdominal A21.3
  - bronchopneumonic A21.2
  - conjunctivitis A21.1
  - cryptogenic A21.3
  - enteric A21.3
  - gastrointestinal A21.3
  - generalized A21.7
  - ingestion A21.3
  - intestinal A21.3
  - oculoglandular A21.1
  - ophthalmic A21.1
  - pneumonia (any), pneumonic A21.2
  - pulmonary A21.2
  - sepsis A21.7
  - specified NEC A21.8
  - typhoidal A21.7
  - ulceroglandular A21.Ø
- **Tularensis conjunctivitis** A21.1
- **Tumefaction** — *see also* Swelling
  - liver — *see* Hypertrophy, liver
- **Tumor** — *see also* Neoplasm, unspecified behavior, by site
  - acinar cell — *see* Neoplasm, uncertain behavior, by site
  - acinic cell — *see* Neoplasm, uncertain behavior, by site
  - adenocarcinoid — *see* Neoplasm, malignant, by site
  - adenomatoid — *see also* Neoplasm, benign, by site
    - odontogenic — *see* Cyst, calcifying odontogenic
  - adnexal (skin) — *see* Neoplasm, skin, benign, by site
  - adrenal
    - cortical (benign) D35.Ø- ☑
      - malignant C74.Ø- ☑
    - rest — *see* Neoplasm, benign, by site
  - alpha-cell
    - malignant
      - pancreas C25.4
      - specified site NEC — *see* Neoplasm, malignant, by site
      - unspecified site C25.4
    - pancreas D13.7
    - specified site NEC — *see* Neoplasm, benign, by site
    - unspecified site D13.7
  - aneurysmal — *see* Aneurysm
  - aortic body D44.7
    - malignant C75.5
  - Askin's — *see* Neoplasm, connective tissue, malignant
  - basal cell — *see also* Neoplasm, skin, uncertain behavior D48.5
  - Bednar — *see* Neoplasm, skin, malignant
  - benign (unclassified) — *see* Neoplasm, benign, by site
  - beta-cell
    - malignant
      - pancreas C25.4
      - specified site NEC — *see* Neoplasm, malignant, by site
      - unspecified site C25.4
    - pancreas D13.7
    - specified site NEC — *see* Neoplasm, benign, by site
    - unspecified site D13.7
  - Brenner D27.9
    - borderline malignancy D39.1- ☑
    - malignant C56.- ☑
    - proliferating D39.1- ☑
  - bronchial alveolar, intravascular D38.1
  - Brooke's — *see* Neoplasm, skin, benign
  - brown fat — *see* Lipoma
  - Burkitt — *see* Lymphoma, Burkitt
  - calcifying epithelial odontogenic — *see* Cyst, calcifying odontogenic
  - carcinoid D3A.ØØ (*following* D36)
    - benign D3A.ØØ (*following* D36)
      - appendix D3A.Ø2Ø (*following* D36)
      - ascending colon D3A.Ø22 (*following* D36)
      - bronchus (lung) D3A.Ø9Ø (*following* D36)
      - cecum D3A.Ø21 (*following* D36)
      - colon D3A.Ø29 (*following* D36)
      - descending colon D3A.Ø24 (*following* D36)
- **Tumor** — *continued*
  - carcinoid — *continued*
    - benign — *continued*
      - duodenum D3A.Ø1Ø (*following* D36)
      - foregut NOS D3A.Ø94 (*following* D36)
      - hindgut NOS D3A.Ø96 (*following* D36)
      - ileum D3A.Ø12 (*following* D36)
      - jejunum D3A.Ø11 (*following* D36)
      - kidney D3A.Ø93 (*following* D36)
      - large intestine D3A.Ø29 (*following* D36)
      - lung (bronchus) D3A.Ø9Ø (*following* D36)
      - midgut NOS D3A.Ø95 (*following* D36)
      - rectum D3A.Ø26 (*following* D36)
      - sigmoid colon D3A.Ø25 (*following* D36)
      - small intestine D3A.Ø19 (*following* D36)
      - specified NEC D3A.Ø98 (*following* D36)
      - stomach D3A.Ø92 (*following* D36)
      - thymus D3A.Ø91 (*following* D36)
      - transverse colon D3A.Ø23 (*following* D36)
    - malignant C7A.ØØ (*following* C75)
      - appendix C7A.Ø2Ø (*following* C75)
      - ascending colon C7A.Ø22 (*following* C75)
      - bronchus (lung) C7A.Ø9Ø (*following* C75)
      - cecum C7A.Ø21 (*following* C75)
      - colon C7A.Ø29 (*following* C75)
      - descending colon C7A.Ø24 (*following* C75)
      - duodenum C7A.Ø1Ø (*following* C75)
      - foregut NOS C7A.Ø94 (*following* C75)
      - hindgut NOS C7A.Ø96 (*following* C75)
      - ileum C7A.Ø12 (*following* C75)
      - jejunum C7A.Ø11 (*following* C75)
      - kidney C7A.Ø93 (*following* C75)
      - large intestine C7A.Ø29 (*following* C75)
      - lung (bronchus) C7A.Ø9Ø (*following* C75)
      - midgut NOS C7A.Ø95 (*following* C75)
      - rectum C7A.Ø26 (*following* C75)
      - sigmoid colon C7A.Ø25 (*following* C75)
      - small intestine C7A.Ø19 (*following* C75)
      - specified NEC C7A.Ø98 (*following* C75)
      - stomach C7A.Ø92 (*following* C75)
      - thymus C7A.Ø91 (*following* C75)
      - transverse colon C7A.Ø23 (*following* C75)
    - mesentery metastasis C7B.Ø4 (*following* C75)
    - secondary C7B.ØØ (*following* C75)
      - bone C7B.Ø3 (*following* C75)
      - distant lymph nodes C7B.Ø1 (*following* C75)
      - liver C7B.Ø2 (*following* C75)
      - peritoneum C7B.Ø4 (*following* C75)
      - specified NEC C7B.Ø9 (*following* C75)
  - carotid body D44.6
    - malignant C75.4
  - cells — *see also* Neoplasm, unspecified behavior, by sit
    - benign — *see* Neoplasm, benign, by site
    - malignant — *see* Neoplasm, malignant, by site
    - uncertain whether benign or malignant — *see* Neoplasm, uncertain behavior, by site
  - cervix, in pregnancy or childbirth — *see* Pregnancy, complicated by, tumor, cervix
  - chondromatous giant cell — *see* Neoplasm, bone, benig
  - chromaffin — *see also* Neoplasm, benign, by site
    - malignant — *see* Neoplasm, malignant, by site
  - Cock's peculiar L72.3
  - Codman's — *see* Neoplasm, bone, benign
  - dentigerous, mixed — *see* Cyst, calcifying odontogeni
  - dermoid — *see* Neoplasm, benign, by site
    - with malignant transformation C56.- ☑
  - desmoid (extra-abdominal) — *see also* Neoplasm, connective tissue, uncertain behavior
    - abdominal — *see* Neoplasm, connective tissue, uncertain behavior
  - embolus — *see* Neoplasm, secondary, by site
  - embryonal (mixed) — *see also* Neoplasm, uncertain behavior, by site
    - liver C22.7
  - endodermal sinus
    - specified site — *see* Neoplasm, malignant, by site
    - unspecified site
      - female C56.- ☑
      - male C62.9Ø
  - epithelial
    - benign — *see* Neoplasm, benign, by site
    - malignant — *see* Neoplasm, malignant, by site
  - Ewing's — *see* Neoplasm, bone, malignant, by site
  - fatty — *see* Lipoma
  - fibroid — *see* Leiomyoma
  - G cell
    - malignant
      - pancreas C25.4

# U

**Ulcer, ulcerated, ulcerating, ulceration, ulcerative** — *continued*
- due to — *continued*
  - trophic disturbance (any region) — *see* Ulcer, skin
  - X-ray L58.1
- duodenum, duodenal (eroded) (peptic) K26.9
  - with
    - hemorrhage K26.4
      - and perforation K26.6
    - perforation K26.5
  - acute K26.3
    - with
      - hemorrhage K26.Ø
        - and perforation K26.2
      - perforation K26.1
  - chronic (erosive) K26.7
    - with
      - hemorrhage K26.4
        - and perforation K26.6
      - perforation K26.5
- dysenteric AØ9
- elusive — *see* Cystitis, interstitial
- endocarditis (acute) (chronic) (subacute) I28.8
- epiglottis J38.7
- esophagus (peptic) K22.1Ø
  - with bleeding K22.11
  - due to
    - aspirin K22.1Ø
      - with bleeding K22.11
    - gastrointestinal reflux disease (without bleeding) K21.ØØ
      - with bleeding K21.Ø1
    - ingestion of chemical or medicament K22.1Ø
      - with bleeding K22.11
  - fungal K22.1Ø
    - with bleeding K22.11
  - infective K22.1Ø
    - with bleeding K22.11
  - varicose — *see* Varix, esophagus
- eyelid (region) HØ1.8- ☑
- face L98.469
  - with
    - bone involvement without evidence of necrosis L98.466
    - bone necrosis L98.464
    - exposed fat layer L98.462
    - muscle involvement without evidence of necrosis L98.465
    - muscle necrosis L98.463
    - skin breakdown only L98.461
    - specified severity NEC L98.468
- fauces J39.2
- Fenwick (-Hunner) (solitary) — *see* Cystitis, interstitial
- fistulous — *see* Ulcer, skin
- foot (indolent) (trophic) — *see* Ulcer, lower limb
- forearm L98.A299
  - with
    - bone involvement without evidence of necrosis L98.A296
    - bone necrosis L98.A294
    - exposed fat layer L98.A292
    - muscle involvement without evidence of necrosis L98.A295
    - muscle necrosis L98.A293
    - skin breakdown only L98.A291
    - specified severity NEC L98.A298
  - left L98.A229
    - with
      - bone involvement without evidence of necrosis L98.A226
      - bone necrosis L98.A224
      - exposed fat layer L98.A222
      - muscle involvement without evidence of necrosis L98.A225
      - muscle necrosis L98.A223
      - skin breakdown only L98.A221
      - specified severity NEC L98.A228
  - right L98.A219
    - with
      - bone involvement without evidence of necrosis L98.A216
      - bone necrosis L98.A214
      - exposed fat layer L98.A212
      - muscle involvement without evidence of necrosis L98.A215
      - muscle necrosis L98.A213
      - skin breakdown only L98.A211
      - specified severity NEC L98.A218
- frambesial, initial A66.Ø

**Ulcer, ulcerated, ulcerating, ulceration, ulcerative** — *continued*
- frenum (tongue) K14.Ø
- gallbladder or duct K82.8
- gangrenous — *see* Gangrene
- gastric — *see* Ulcer, stomach
- gastrocolic — *see* Ulcer, gastrojejunal
- gastroduodenal — *see* Ulcer, peptic
- gastroesophageal — *see* Ulcer, stomach
- gastrointestinal — *see* Ulcer, gastrojejunal
- gastrojejunal (peptic) K28.9
  - with
    - hemorrhage K28.4
      - and perforation K28.6
    - perforation K28.5
  - acute K28.3
    - with
      - hemorrhage K28.Ø
        - and perforation K28.2
      - perforation K28.1
  - chronic K28.7
    - with
      - hemorrhage K28.4
        - and perforation K28.6
      - perforation K28.5
- gastrojejunocolic — *see* Ulcer, gastrojejunal
- gingiva KØ6.8
- gingivitis KØ5.1Ø
  - nonplaque induced KØ5.11
  - plaque induced KØ5.1Ø
- glottis J38.7
- granuloma of pudenda A58
- groin L98.479
  - with
    - bone involvement without evidence of necrosis L98.476
    - bone necrosis L98.474
    - exposed fat layer L98.472
    - muscle involvement without evidence of necrosis L98.475
    - muscle necrosis L98.473
    - skin breakdown only L98.471
    - specified severity NEC L98.478
- gum KØ6.8
- gumma, due to yaws A66.4
- hand L98.A399
  - with
    - bone involvement without evidence of necrosis L98.A396
    - bone necrosis L98.A394
    - exposed fat layer L98.A392
    - muscle involvement without evidence of necrosis L98.A395
    - muscle necrosis L98.A393
    - skin breakdown only L98.A391
    - specified severity NEC L98.A398
  - left L98.A329
    - with
      - bone involvement without evidence of necrosis L98.A326
      - bone necrosis L98.A324
      - exposed fat layer L98.A322
      - muscle involvement without evidence of necrosis L98.A325
      - muscle necrosis L98.A323
      - skin breakdown only L98.A321
      - specified severity NEC L98.A328
  - right L98.A319
    - with
      - bone involvement without evidence of necrosis L98.A316
      - bone necrosis L98.A314
      - exposed fat layer L98.A312
      - muscle involvement without evidence of necrosis L98.A315
      - muscle necrosis L98.A313
      - skin breakdown only L98.A311
      - specified severity NEC L98.A318
- heel — *see* Ulcer, lower limb
- hemorrhoid — *see also* Hemorrhoids, by degree K64.8
- Hunner's — *see* Cystitis, interstitial
- hypopharynx J39.2
- hypopyon (chronic) (subacute) — *see* Ulcer, cornea, with hypopyon
- hypostaticum — *see* Ulcer, varicose
- ileum — *see* Ulcer, intestine
- intestine, intestinal K63.3
  - with perforation K63.1
  - amebic AØ6.1

**Ulcer, ulcerated, ulcerating, ulceration, ulcerative** — *continued*
- intestine, intestinal — *continued*
  - duodenal — *see* Ulcer, duodenum
  - granulocytopenic (with hemorrhage) — *see* Neutropenia
  - marginal — *see* Ulcer, gastrojejunal
  - perforating K63.1
    - newborn P78.Ø
  - primary, small intestine K63.3
  - rectum K62.6
  - stercoraceous, stercoral K63.3
  - tuberculous A18.32
  - typhoid (fever) — *see* Typhoid
  - varicose I86.8
- jejunum, jejunal — *see* Ulcer, gastrojejunal
- keratitis — *see* Ulcer, cornea
- knee — *see* Ulcer, lower limb
- labium (majus) (minus) N76.6
- laryngitis — *see* Laryngitis
- larynx (aphthous) (contact) J38.7
  - diphtheritic A36.2
- leg — *see* Ulcer, lower limb
- lip K13.Ø
- Lipschütz's N76.6
- lower limb (atrophic) (chronic) (neurogenic) (perforating) (pyogenic) (trophic) (tropical) L97.9Ø9
  - with
    - bone involvement without evidence of necrosis L97.9Ø6
    - bone necrosis L97.9Ø4
    - exposed fat layer L97.9Ø2
    - muscle involvement without evidence of necrosis L97.9Ø5
    - muscle necrosis L97.9Ø3
    - skin breakdown only L97.9Ø1
    - specified severity NEC L97.9Ø8
  - ankle L97.3Ø9
    - with
      - bone involvement without evidence of necrosis L97.3Ø6
      - bone necrosis L97.3Ø4
      - exposed fat layer L97.3Ø2
      - muscle involvement without evidence of necrosis L97.3Ø5
      - muscle necrosis L97.3Ø3
      - skin breakdown only L97.3Ø1
      - specified severity NEC L97.3Ø8
    - left L97.329
      - with
        - bone involvement without evidence of necrosis L97.326
        - bone necrosis L97.324
        - exposed fat layer L97.322
        - muscle involvement without evidence of necrosis L97.325
        - muscle necrosis L97.323
        - skin breakdown only L97.321
        - specified severity NEC L97.328
    - right L97.319
      - with
        - bone involvement without evidence of necrosis L97.316
        - bone necrosis L97.314
        - exposed fat layer L97.312
        - muscle involvement without evidence of necrosis L97.315
        - muscle necrosis L97.313
        - skin breakdown only L97.311
        - specified severity NEC L97.318
  - calf L97.2Ø9
    - with
      - bone involvement without evidence of necrosis L97.2Ø6
      - bone necrosis L97.2Ø4
      - exposed fat layer L97.2Ø2
      - muscle involvement without evidence of necrosis L97.2Ø5
      - muscle necrosis L97.2Ø3
      - skin breakdown only L97.2Ø1
      - specified severity NEC L97.2Ø8
    - left L97.229
      - with
        - bone involvement without evidence of necrosis L97.226
        - bone necrosis L97.224
        - exposed fat layer L97.222
        - muscle involvement without evidence of necrosis L97.225

Ulcer, ulcerated, ulcerating, ulceration, ulcerative — *continued*
  lower limb — *continued*
    toe — *continued*
      left — *continued*
        with
          bone involvement without evidence of necrosis L97.526
          bone necrosis L97.524
          exposed fat layer L97.522
          muscle involvement without evidence of necrosis L97.525
          muscle necrosis L97.523
          skin breakdown only L97.521
          specified severity NEC L97.528
      right L97.519
        with
          bone involvement without evidence of necrosis L97.516
          bone necrosis L97.514
          exposed fat layer L97.512
          muscle involvement without evidence of necrosis L97.515
          muscle necrosis L97.513
          skin breakdown only L97.511
          specified severity NEC L97.518
    varicose — *see* Varix, leg, with, ulcer
  luetic — *see* Ulcer, syphilitic
  lung J98.4
    tuberculous — *see* Tuberculosis, pulmonary
  malignant — *see* Neoplasm, malignant, by site
  marginal NEC — *see* Ulcer, gastrojejunal
  meatus (urinarius) N34.2
  Meckel's diverticulum Q43.Ø
    malignant — *see* Table of Neoplasms, small intestine, malignant
  Meleney's (chronic undermining) — *see* Ulcer, skin
  Mooren's (cornea) — *see* Ulcer, cornea, Mooren's
  mycobacterial (skin) A31.1
  nasopharynx J39.2
  neck L98.459
    with
      bone involvement without evidence of necrosis L98.456
      bone necrosis L98.454
      exposed fat layer L98.452
      muscle involvement without evidence of necrosis L98.455
      muscle necrosis L98.453
      skin breakdown only L98.451
      specified severity NEC L98.458
    uterus N86
  neurogenic NEC — *see* Ulcer, skin
  nose, nasal (passage) (infective) (septum) J34.Ø
    skin — *see* Ulcer, skin
    spirochetal A69.8
    varicose (bleeding) I86.8
  oral mucosa (traumatic) K12.1
  palate (soft) K12.1
  penis (chronic) N48.5
  peptic (site unspecified) K27.9
    with
      hemorrhage K27.4
        and perforation K27.6
      perforation K27.5
    acute K27.3
      with
        hemorrhage K27.Ø
          and perforation K27.2
        perforation K27.1
    chronic K27.7
      with
        hemorrhage K27.4
          and perforation K27.6
        perforation K27.5
    esophagus K22.1Ø
      with bleeding K22.11
    newborn P78.82
  perforating K27.5
    skin — *see* Ulcer, skin
  peritonsillar J35.8
  phagedenic (tropical) — *see* Ulcer, skin
  pharynx J39.2
  phlebitis — *see* Phlebitis
  plaster — *see* Ulcer, pressure, by site
  popliteal space — *see* Ulcer, lower limb
  postpyloric — *see* Ulcer, duodenum
  prepuce N47.7
  prepyloric — *see* Ulcer, stomach

Ulcer, ulcerated, ulcerating, ulceration, ulcerative — *continued*
  pressure (pressure area) L89.9- ☑
    ankle L89.5- ☑
    back L89.1- ☑
    buttock L89.3- ☑
    coccyx L89.15- ☑
    contiguous site of back, buttock, hip L89.4- ☑
    elbow L89.Ø- ☑
    face L89.81- ☑
    head L89.81- ☑
    heel L89.6- ☑
    hip L89.2- ☑
    sacral region (tailbone) L89.15- ☑
    specified site NEC L89.89- ☑
    stage 1 (healing) (pre-ulcer skin changes limited to persistent focal edema)
      ankle L89.5- ☑
      back L89.1- ☑
      buttock L89.3- ☑
      coccyx L89.15- ☑
      contiguous site of back, buttock, hip L89.4- ☑
      elbow L89.Ø- ☑
      face L89.81- ☑
      head L89.81- ☑
      heel L89.6- ☑
      hip L89.2- ☑
      sacral region (tailbone) L89.15- ☑
      specified site NEC L89.89- ☑
    stage 2 (healing) (abrasion, blister, partial thickness skin loss involving epidermis and/or dermis)
      ankle L89.5- ☑
      back L89.1- ☑
      buttock L89.3- ☑
      coccyx L89.15- ☑
      contiguous site of back, buttock, hip L89.4- ☑
      elbow L89.Ø- ☑
      face L89.81- ☑
      head L89.81- ☑
      heel L89.6- ☑
      hip L89.2- ☑
      sacral region (tailbone) L89.15- ☑
      specified site NEC L89.89- ☑
    stage 3 (healing) (full thickness skin loss involving damage or necrosis of subcutaneous tissue)
      ankle L89.5- ☑
      back L89.1- ☑
      buttock L89.3- ☑
      coccyx L89.15- ☑
      contiguous site of back, buttock, hip L89.4- ☑
      elbow L89.Ø- ☑
      face L89.81- ☑
      head L89.81- ☑
      heel L89.6- ☑
      hip L89.2- ☑
      sacral region (tailbone) L89.15- ☑
      specified site NEC L89.89- ☑
    stage 4 (healing) (necrosis of soft tissues through to underlying muscle, tendon, or bone)
      ankle L89.5- ☑
      back L89.1- ☑
      buttock L89.3- ☑
      coccyx L89.15- ☑
      contiguous site of back, buttock, hip L89.4- ☑
      elbow L89.Ø- ☑
      face L89.81- ☑
      head L89.81- ☑
      heel L89.6- ☑
      hip L89.2- ☑
      sacral region (tailbone) L89.15- ☑
      specified site NEC L89.89- ☑
    unspecified stage
      ankle L89.5- ☑
      back L89.1- ☑
      buttock L89.3- ☑
      coccyx L89.15- ☑
      contiguous site of back, buttock, hip L89.4- ☑
      elbow L89.Ø- ☑
      face L89.81- ☑
      head L89.81- ☑
      heel L89.6- ☑
      hip L89.2- ☑
      sacral region (tailbone) L89.15- ☑
      specified site NEC L89.89- ☑

Ulcer, ulcerated, ulcerating, ulceration, ulcerative — *continued*
  pressure — *continued*
    unstageable
      ankle L89.5- ☑
      back L89.1- ☑
      buttock L89.3- ☑
      coccyx L89.15- ☑
      contiguous site of back, buttock, hip L89.4- ☑
      elbow L89.Ø- ☑
      face L89.81- ☑
      head L89.81- ☑
      heel L89.6- ☑
      hip L89.2- ☑
      sacral region (tailbone) L89.15- ☑
      specified site NEC L89.89- ☑
  primary of intestine K63.3
    with perforation K63.1
  prostate N41.9
  pyloric — *see* Ulcer, stomach
  rectosigmoid K63.3
    with perforation K63.1
  rectum (sphincter) (solitary) K62.6
    stercoraceous, stercoral K62.6
  retina — *see* Inflammation, chorioretinal
  rodent — *see also* Neoplasm, skin, malignant
  sclera — *see* Scleritis
  scrofulous (tuberculous) A18.2
  scrotum N5Ø.89
    tuberculous A18.15
    varicose I86.1
  seminal vesicle N5Ø.89
  sigmoid — *see* Ulcer, intestine
  skin (atrophic) (chronic) (neurogenic) (non-healing) (perforating) (pyogenic) (trophic) (tropical) L98.499
    with gangrene — *see* Gangrene
    amebic AØ6.7
    back — *see* Ulcer, back
    buttock — *see* Ulcer, buttock
    decubitus — *see* Ulcer, pressure
    lower limb — *see* Ulcer, lower limb
    mycobacterial A31.1
    specified site NEC L98.499
      with
        bone involvement without evidence of necrosis L98.496
        bone necrosis L98.494
        exposed fat layer L98.492
        muscle involvement without evidence of necrosis L98.495
        muscle necrosis L98.493
        skin breakdown only L98.491
        specified severity NEC L98.498
    tuberculous (primary) A18.4
    upper limb — *see* Ulcer, upper limb
    varicose — *see* Ulcer, varicose
  sloughing — *see* Ulcer, skin
  solitary, anus or rectum (sphincter) K62.6
  sore throat JØ2.9
    streptococcal JØ2.Ø
  spermatic cord N5Ø.89
  spine (tuberculous) A18.Ø1
  stasis (venous) — *see* Varix, leg, with, ulcer
    without varicose veins — *see also* Ulcer, by site I87.2
  stercoraceous, stercoral K63.3
    with perforation K63.1
    anus or rectum K62.6
  stoma, stomal — *see* Ulcer, gastrojejunal
  stomach (eroded) (peptic) (round) K25.9
    with
      hemorrhage K25.4
        and perforation K25.6
      perforation K25.5
    acute K25.3
      with
        hemorrhage K25.Ø
          and perforation K25.2
        perforation K25.1
    chronic K25.7
      with
        hemorrhage K25.4
          and perforation K25.6
        perforation K25.5
  stomal — *see* Ulcer, gastrojejunal
  stomatitis K12.1
  stress — *see* Ulcer, peptic
  strumous (tuberculous) A18.2
  submucosal, bladder — *see* Cystitis, interstitial

- **Urea**
  - blood, high — *see* Uremia
  - cycle metabolism disorder — *see* Disorder, urea cycle metabolism
- **Uremia, uremic** N19
  - with
    - ectopic or molar pregnancy O08.4
    - polyneuropathy N18.9 *[G63]*
  - chronic NOS — *see also* Disease, kidney, chronic N18.9
    - due to hypertension — *see* Hypertensive, kidney
  - complicating
    - ectopic or molar pregnancy O08.4
  - congenital P96.Ø
  - extrarenal R39.2
  - following ectopic or molar pregnancy O08.4
  - newborn P96.Ø
  - prerenal R39.2
- **Ureter, ureteral** — *see* condition
- **Ureteralgia** N23
- **Ureterectasis** — *see* Hydroureter
- **Ureteritis** N28.89
  - cystica N28.86
  - due to calculus N2Ø.1
    - with calculus, kidney N2Ø.2
      - with hydronephrosis N13.2
  - gonococcal (acute) (chronic) A54.21
  - nonspecific N28.89
- **Ureterocele** N28.89
  - congenital (orthotopic) Q62.31
    - ectopic Q62.32
- **Ureterolith, ureterolithiasis** — *see* Calculus, ureter
- **Ureterostomy**
  - attention to Z43.6
  - status Z93.6
- **Urethra, urethral** — *see* condition
- **Urethralgia** R39.89
- **Urethritis** (anterior) (posterior) N34.2
  - calculous N21.1
  - candidal B37.41
  - chlamydial A56.Ø1
  - diplococcal (gonococcal) A54.Ø1
    - with abscess (accessory gland) (periurethral) A54.1
  - gonococcal A54.Ø1
    - with abscess (accessory gland) (periurethral) A54.1
  - nongonococcal N34.1
    - Reiter's — *see* Reiter's disease
  - nonspecific N34.1
  - nonvenereal N34.1
  - postmenopausal N34.2
  - puerperal O86.22
  - Reiter's — *see* Reiter's disease
  - specified NEC N34.2
  - trichomonal or due to Trichomonas (vaginalis) A59.Ø3
- **Urethrocele** N81.Ø
  - with
    - cystocele — *see* Cystocele
    - prolapse of uterus — *see* Prolapse, uterus
- **Urethrolithiasis** (with colic or infection) N21.1
- **Urethrorectal** — *see* condition
- **Urethrorrhagia** N36.8
- **Urethrorrhea** R36.9
- **Urethrostomy**
  - attention to Z43.6
  - status Z93.6
- **Urethrotrigonitis** — *see* Trigonitis
- **Urethrovaginal** — *see* condition
- **Urgency**
  - fecal R15.2
  - hypertensive — *see* Hypertension
  - urinary R39.15
- **Urhidrosis, uridrosis** L74.8
- **Uric acid in blood** (increased) E79.Ø
- **Uricacidemia** (asymptomatic) E79.Ø
- **Uricemia** (asymptomatic) E79.Ø
- **Uricosuria** R82.998
- **Urinary** — *see* condition
- **Urination**
  - frequent R35.Ø
  - painful R3Ø.9
- **Urine**
  - blood in — *see* Hematuria
  - discharge, excessive R35.89
  - enuresis, nonorganic origin F98.Ø
  - extravasation R39.Ø
  - frequency R35.Ø
  - incontinence R32
    - nonorganic origin F98.Ø
  - intermittent stream R39.198
  - pus in N39.Ø
- **Urine** — *continued*
  - retention or stasis R33.9
    - organic R33.8
      - drug-induced R33.Ø
    - psychogenic F45.8
  - secretion
    - deficient R34
    - excessive R35.89
    - frequency R35.Ø
  - stream
    - intermittent R39.198
    - slowing R39.198
    - splitting R39.13
    - weak R39.12
- **Urinemia** — *see* Uremia
- **Urinoma, urethra** N36.8
- **Uroarthritis, infectious** (Reiter's) — *see* Reiter's disease
- **Urodialysis** R34
- **Urolithiasis** — *see* Calculus, urinary
- **Uronephrosis** — *see* Hydronephrosis
- **Uropathy** N39.9
  - obstructive N13.9
    - specified NEC N13.8
  - reflux N13.9
    - specified NEC N13.8
  - vesicoureteral reflux-associated — *see* Reflux, vesicoureteral
- **Urosepsis** — *code to* condition
- **Urticaria** L5Ø.9
  - with angioneurotic edema T78.3- ☑
    - hereditary D84.1
  - allergic L5Ø.Ø
  - cholinergic L5Ø.5
  - chronic L5Ø.8
  - cold, familial L5Ø.2
  - contact L5Ø.6
  - dermatographic L5Ø.3
  - due to
    - cold or heat L5Ø.2
    - drugs L5Ø.Ø
    - food L5Ø.Ø
    - inhalants L5Ø.Ø
    - plants L5Ø.6
    - serum — *see also* Reaction, serum T8Ø.69- ☑
  - factitial L5Ø.3
  - familial cold MØ4.2
  - giant T78.3- ☑
    - hereditary D84.1
  - gigantea T78.3- ☑
  - idiopathic L5Ø.1
  - larynx T78.3- ☑
    - hereditary D84.1
  - neonatorum P83.88
  - nonallergic L5Ø.1
  - papulosa (Hebra) L28.2
  - pigmentosa D47.Ø1
    - congenital Q82.2
    - of neonatal onset Q82.2
    - of newborn onset Q82.2
  - recurrent periodic L5Ø.8
  - serum — *see also* Reaction, serum T8Ø.69- ☑
  - solar L56.3
  - specified type NEC L5Ø.8
  - thermal (cold) (heat) L5Ø.2
  - vibratory L5Ø.4
  - xanthelasmoidea — *see* Urticaria pigmentosa
- **Use** (of)
  - alcohol — *see also* Alcohol, alcoholic, by disorder F1Ø.9Ø
    - with
      - anxiety disorder F1Ø.98Ø
      - intoxication F1Ø.929
      - sleep disorder F1Ø.982
      - withdrawal F1Ø.939
        - with
          - perceptual disturbance F1Ø.932
        - delirium F1Ø.931
        - uncomplicated F1Ø.93Ø
    - harmful — *see* Abuse, alcohol
    - in remission F1Ø.91
  - amphetamines — *see* Use, stimulant NEC
  - caffeine — *see* Use, stimulant NEC
  - cannabis F12.9Ø
    - with
      - anxiety disorder F12.98Ø
      - intoxication F12.929
        - with
          - delirium F12.921
          - perceptual disturbance F12.922
- **Use** — *continued*
  - cannabis — *continued*
    - with — *continued*
      - intoxication — *continued*
        - uncomplicated F12.92Ø
      - other specified disorder F12.988
      - psychosis F12.959
        - delusions F12.95Ø
        - hallucinations F12.951
      - unspecified disorder F12.99
      - withdrawal F12.93
    - in remission F12.91
  - cocaine F14.9Ø
    - with
      - anxiety disorder F14.98Ø
      - intoxication F14.929
        - with
          - delirium F14.921
          - perceptual disturbance F14.922
        - uncomplicated F14.92Ø
      - other specified disorder F14.988
      - psychosis F14.959
        - delusions F14.95Ø
        - hallucinations F14.951
      - sexual dysfunction F14.981
      - sleep disorder F14.982
      - unspecified disorder F14.99
      - withdrawal F14.93
    - harmful — *see* Abuse, drug, cocaine
    - in remission F14.91
  - drug(s) NEC F19.9Ø
    - with sleep disorder F19.982
    - harmful — *see* Abuse, drug, by type
  - hallucinogen NEC F16.9Ø
    - with
      - anxiety disorder F16.98Ø
      - intoxication F16.929
        - with
          - delirium F16.921
        - uncomplicated F16.92Ø
      - mood disorder F16.94
      - other specified disorder F16.988
      - perception disorder (flashbacks) F16.983
      - psychosis F16.959
        - delusions F16.95Ø
        - hallucinations F16.951
      - unspecified disorder F16.99
    - harmful — *see* Abuse, drug, hallucinogen NEC
    - in remission F16.91
  - inhalants F18.9Ø
    - with
      - anxiety disorder F18.98Ø
      - intoxication F18.929
        - with delirium F18.921
        - uncomplicated F18.92Ø
      - mood disorder F18.94
      - other specified disorder F18.988
      - persisting dementia F18.97
      - psychosis F18.959
        - delusions F18.95Ø
        - hallucinations F18.951
      - unspecified disorder F18.99
    - harmful — *see* Abuse, drug, inhalant
    - in remission F18.91
  - methadone — *see* Use, opioid
  - nonprescribed drugs F19.9Ø
    - harmful — *see* Abuse, non-psychoactive substance
  - opioid F11.9Ø
    - with
      - disorder F11.99
        - mood F11.94
        - sleep F11.982
        - specified type NEC F11.988
      - intoxication F11.929
        - with
          - delirium F11.921
          - perceptual disturbance F11.922
        - uncomplicated F11.92Ø
      - opioid-associated amnestic syndrome F11.288
      - withdrawal F11.93
    - harmful — *see* Abuse, drug, opioid
    - in remission F11.91
  - patent medicines F19.9Ø
    - harmful — *see* Abuse, non-psychoactive substance
  - psychoactive drug NEC F19.9Ø
    - with
      - anxiety disorder F19.98Ø
      - intoxication F19.929

☑ **Additional Character Required — Refer to the Tabular List for Character Selection**

- **Use** — *continued*
  - psychoactive drug — *continued*
    - with — *continued*
      - intoxication — *continued*
        - with
          - delirium F19.921
          - perceptual disturbance F19.922
        - uncomplicated F19.92Ø
      - mood disorder F19.94
      - other specified disorder F19.988
      - persisting
        - amnestic disorder F19.96
        - dementia F19.97
      - psychosis F19.959
        - delusions F19.95Ø
        - hallucinations F19.951
      - sexual dysfunction F19.981
      - sleep disorder F19.982
      - unspecified disorder F19.99
      - withdrawal F19.939
        - with
          - delirium F19.931
          - perceptual disturbance F19.932
        - uncomplicated F19.93Ø
    - harmful — *see* Abuse, drug NEC, psychoactive NEC
    - in remission F19.91
  - sedative, hypnotic, or anxiolytic F13.9Ø
    - with
      - anxiety disorder F13.98Ø
      - intoxication F13.929
        - with
          - delirium F13.921
        - uncomplicated F13.92Ø
      - other specified disorder F13.988
      - persisting
        - amnestic disorder F13.96
        - dementia F13.97
      - psychosis F13.959
        - delusions F13.95Ø
        - hallucinations F13.951
      - sexual dysfunction F13.981
      - sleep disorder F13.982
      - unspecified disorder F13.99
    - harmful — *see* Abuse, drug, sedative, hypnotic, or anxiolytic
    - in remission F13.91
  - stimulant NEC F15.9Ø
    - with
      - anxiety disorder F15.98Ø
      - intoxication F15.929
        - with
          - delirium F15.921
          - perceptual disturbance F15.922
        - uncomplicated F15.92Ø
      - mood disorder F15.94
      - other specified disorder F15.988
      - psychosis F15.959
        - delusions F15.95Ø
        - hallucinations F15.951
      - sexual dysfunction F15.981
      - sleep disorder F15.982
      - unspecified disorder F15.99
      - withdrawal F15.93
    - harmful — *see* Abuse, drug, stimulant NEC
    - in remission F15.91
  - tobacco Z72.Ø
    - with dependence — *see* Dependence, drug, nicotine
  - volatile solvents — *see also* Use, inhalant F18.9Ø
    - harmful — *see* Abuse, drug, inhalant
- **Usher-Senear disease or syndrome** L1Ø.4
- **Uta** B55.1
- **Uteromegaly** N85.2
- **Uterovaginal** — *see* condition
- **Uterovesical** — *see* condition
- **Uveal** — *see* condition
- **Uveitis** (anterior) — *see also* Iridocyclitis
  - acute — *see* Iridocyclitis, acute
  - chronic — *see* Iridocyclitis, chronic
  - due to toxoplasmosis (acquired) B58.Ø9
    - congenital P37.1
  - granulomatous — *see* Iridocyclitis, chronic
  - heterochromic — *see* Cyclitis, Fuchs' heterochromic
  - lens-induced — *see* Iridocyclitis, lens-induced
  - posterior — *see* Chorioretinitis
  - sympathetic H44.13- ☑
  - syphilitic (secondary) A51.43
    - congenital (early) A5Ø.Ø1
    - late A52.71
  - tuberculous A18.54
- **Uveoencephalitis** — *see* Inflammation, chorioretinal
- **Uveokeratitis** — *see* Iridocyclitis
- **Uveoparotitis** D86.89
- **Uvula** — *see* condition
- **Uvulitis** (acute) (catarrhal) (chronic) (membranous) (suppurative) (ulcerative) K12.2

# V

- **Vaccination** (prophylactic)
  - complication or reaction — *see* Complications, vaccination
  - delayed Z28.9
  - encounter for Z23
  - not done — *see* Immunization, not done
  - partial — *see also* Underimmunization status
    - for COVID-19 Z28.311
- **Vaccinia** (generalized) (localized) T88.1- ☑
  - congenital P35.8
  - without vaccination BØ8.Ø11
- **Vacuum, in sinus** (accessory) (nasal) J34.89
- **Vagabond, vagabondage** Z59.ØØ
- **Vagabond's disease** B85.1
- **Vagina, vaginal** — *see* condition
- **Vaginalitis** (tunica) (testis) N49.1
- **Vaginismus** (reflex) N94.2
  - functional F52.5
  - nonorganic F52.5
  - psychogenic F52.5
  - secondary N94.2
- **Vaginitis** (acute) (circumscribed) (diffuse) (emphysematous) (nonvenereal) (ulcerative) N76.Ø
  - with ectopic or molar pregnancy OØ8.Ø
  - amebic AØ6.82
  - atrophic, postmenopausal N95.2
  - bacterial N76.Ø
  - blennorrhagic (gonococcal) A54.Ø2
  - candidal (acute) B37.31
    - chronic (recurrent) B37.32
  - chlamydial A56.Ø2
  - chronic N76.1
  - due to Trichomonas (vaginalis) A59.Ø1
  - following ectopic or molar pregnancy OØ8.Ø
  - gonococcal A54.Ø2
    - with abscess (accessory gland) (periurethral) A54.1
  - granuloma A58
  - in (due to)
    - candidiasis (acute) B37.31
      - chronic (recurrent) B37.32
    - herpesviral (herpes simplex) infection A6Ø.Ø4
    - pinworm infection B8Ø *[N77.1]*
  - monilial (acute) B37.31
    - chronic (recurrent) B37.32
  - mycotic (candidal) (acute) B37.31
    - chronic (recurrent) B37.32
  - postmenopausal atrophic N95.2
  - puerperal (postpartum) O86.13
  - senile (atrophic) N95.2
  - subacute or chronic N76.1
  - syphilitic (early) A51.Ø
    - late A52.76
  - trichomonal A59.Ø1
  - tuberculous A18.18
- **Vaginosis** — *see* Vaginitis
- **Vagotonia** G52.2
- **Vagrancy** Z59.ØØ
- **VAIN** — *see* Neoplasia, intraepithelial, vagina
- **Vallecula** — *see* condition
- **Valley fever** B38.Ø
- **Valsuani's disease** O99.Ø3
- **Valve, valvular** (formation) — *see also* condition
  - cerebral ventricle (communicating) in situ Z98.2
  - cervix, internal os Q51.828
  - congenital NEC — *see* Atresia, by site
  - ureter (pelvic junction) (vesical orifice) Q62.39
  - urethra (congenital) (posterior) Q64.2
- **Valvulitis** (chronic) — *see* Endocarditis
- **Valvulopathy** — *see* Endocarditis
- **Van Bogaert-Scherer-Epstein disease or syndrome** E75.5
- **Van Bogaert's leukoencephalopathy** (sclerosing) (subacute) A81.1
- **Van Buchem's syndrome** M85.2
- **Van Creveld-von Gierke disease** E74.Ø1
- **Van der Hoeve** (-de Kleyn) **syndrome** Q78.Ø
- **Van der Woude's syndrome** Q38.Ø
- **Van Neck's disease or osteochondrosis** M91.Ø
- **Vanishing lung** J44.89
- **Vapor asphyxia or suffocation** T59.9- ☑
- **Vapor asphyxia or suffocation** — *continued*
  - specified agent — *see* Table of Drugs and Chemicals
- **Variance, lethal ball, prosthetic heart valve** T82.Ø9- ☑
- **Variants, thalassemic** D56.8
- **Variations in hair color** L67.1
- **Varicella** BØ1.9
  - with
    - complications NEC BØ1.89
    - encephalitis BØ1.11
    - encephalomyelitis BØ1.11
    - meningitis BØ1.Ø
    - myelitis BØ1.12
    - pneumonia BØ1.2
  - congenital P35.8
- **Varices** — *see* Varix
- **Varicocele** (scrotum) (thrombosed) I86.1
  - ovary I86.2
  - perineum I86.3
  - spermatic cord (ulcerated) I86.1
- **Varicose**
  - aneurysm (ruptured) I77.Ø
  - dermatitis — *see* Varix, leg, with, inflammation
  - eczema — *see* Varix, leg, with, inflammation
  - phlebitis — *see* Varix, with, inflammation
  - tumor — *see* Varix
  - ulcer (lower limb, any part) — *see also* Varix, leg, with, ulcer
    - anus — *see also* Hemorrhoids K64.8
    - esophagus — *see* Varix, esophagus
    - inflamed or infected — *see* Varix, leg, with ulcer, with inflammation
    - nasal septum I86.8
    - perineum I86.3
    - scrotum I86.1
    - specified site NEC I86.8
  - vein — *see* Varix
  - vessel — *see* Varix, leg
- **Varicosis, varicosities, varicosity** — *see* Varix
- **Variola** (major) (minor) BØ3
- **Varioloid** BØ3
- **Varix** (lower limb) I83.9Ø
  - with
    - bleeding I83.899
    - edema I83.899
    - inflammation I83.1Ø
      - with ulcer (venous) I83.2Ø9
    - pain I83.819
    - rupture I83.899
    - specified complication NEC I83.899
    - stasis dermatitis I83.1Ø
      - with ulcer (venous) I83.2Ø9
    - swelling I83.899
    - ulcer I83.ØØ9
      - with inflammation I83.2Ø9
  - aneurysmal I77.Ø
  - asymptomatic I83.9- ☑
  - bladder I86.2
  - broad ligament I86.2
  - complicating
    - childbirth (lower extremity) O87.4
      - anus or rectum O87.2
      - genital (vagina, vulva or perineum) O87.8
    - pregnancy (lower extremity) O22.Ø- ☑
      - anus or rectum O22.4- ☑
      - genital (vagina, vulva or perineum) O22.1- ☑
    - puerperium (lower extremity) O87.4
      - anus or rectum O87.2
      - genital (vagina, vulva, perineum) O87.8
  - congenital (any site) Q27.8
  - esophagus (idiopathic) (primary) (ulcerated) I85.ØØ
    - bleeding I85.Ø1
    - congenital Q27.8
    - in (due to)
      - alcoholic liver disease I85.1Ø
        - bleeding I85.11
      - cirrhosis of liver I85.1Ø
        - bleeding I85.11
      - portal hypertension I85.1Ø
        - bleeding I85.11
      - schistosomiasis I85.1Ø
        - bleeding I85.11
      - toxic liver disease I85.1Ø
        - bleeding I85.11
    - secondary I85.1Ø
      - bleeding I85.11
  - gastric I86.4
  - inflamed or infected I83.1Ø
    - ulcerated I83.2Ø9

**Vestige, vestigial** — *continued*
- structures in vitreous Q14.Ø

**Vibration**
- adverse effects T75.2Ø- ☑
  - pneumatic hammer syndrome T75.21- ☑
  - specified effect NEC T75.29- ☑
  - vasospastic syndrome T75.22- ☑
  - vertigo from infrasound T75.23- ☑
- exposure (occupational) Z57.7
- vertigo T75.23- ☑

**Vibriosis** A28.9
**Victim** (of)
- crime Z65.4
- disaster Z65.5
- terrorism Z65.4
- torture Z65.4
- war Z65.5

**Vidal's disease** L28.Ø
**Villaret's syndrome** G52.7
**Villous** — *see* condition
**VIN** — *see* Neoplasia, intraepithelial, vulva
**Vincent's infection** (angina) (gingivitis) A69.1
- stomatitis NEC A69.1

**Vinson-Plummer syndrome** D5Ø.1
**Violence, physical** R45.6
**Viosterol deficiency** — *see* Deficiency, calciferol
**Vipoma** — *see* Neoplasm, malignant, by site
**Viremia** B34.9
**Virilism** (adrenal) E25.9
- congenital E25.Ø

**Virilization** (female) (suprarenal) E25.9
- congenital E25.Ø
- isosexual E28.2

**Virulent bubo** A57
**Virus, viral** — *see also* condition
- as cause of disease classified elsewhere B97.89
  - respiratory syncytial virus (RSV) — *see* Virus, respiratory syncytial (RSV)
- cytomegalovirus B25.9
- human immunodeficiency (HIV) — *see* Human, immunodeficiency virus (HIV) disease
- infection — *see* Infection, virus
- respiratory syncytial (RSV)
  - as cause of disease classified elsewhere B97.4
  - bronchiolitis J21.Ø
  - bronchitis J2Ø.5
  - bronchopneumonia J12.1
  - otitis media H65.- ☑ *[B97.4]*
  - pneumonia J12.1
  - upper respiratory infection JØ6.9 *[B97.4]*
- specified NEC B34.8
- swine influenza (viruses that normally cause infections in pigs) — *see also* Influenza, due to, identified novel influenza A virus JØ9.X2
- West Nile (fever) A92.3Ø
  - with
    - complications NEC A92.39
    - cranial nerve disorders A92.32
    - encephalitis A92.31
    - encephalomyelitis A92.31
    - neurologic manifestation NEC A92.32
    - optic neuritis A92.32
    - polyradiculitis A92.32

**Viscera, visceral** — *see* condition
**Visceroptosis** K63.4
**Visible peristalsis** R19.2
**Vision, visual**
- binocular, suppression H53.34
- blurred, blurring H53.8
  - hysterical F44.6
- defect, defective NEC H54.7
- disorientation (syndrome) H53.8
- disturbance H53.9
  - hysterical F44.6
- double H53.2
- examination ZØ1.ØØ
  - with abnormal findings ZØ1.Ø1
  - following failed vision screening ZØ1.Ø2Ø
    - with abnormal findings ZØ1.Ø21
- field, limitation (defect) — *see* Defect, visual field
- hallucinations R44.1
- halos H53.19
- loss — *see* Loss, vision
  - sudden — *see* Disturbance, vision, subjective, loss, sudden
- low (both eyes) — *see* Low, vision
- perception, simultaneous without fusion H53.33

**Vitality, lack or want of** R53.83

**Vitality, lack or want of** — *continued*
- newborn P96.89

**Vitamin deficiency** — *see* Deficiency, vitamin
**Vitelline duct, persistent** Q43.Ø
**Vitiligo** L8Ø
- eyelid HØ2.739
  - left HØ2.736
    - lower HØ2.735
    - upper HØ2.734
  - right HØ2.733
    - lower HØ2.732
    - upper HØ2.731
- pinta A67.2
- vulva N9Ø.89

**Vitreal corneal syndrome** H59.Ø1- ☑
**Vitreoretinopathy, proliferative** — *see also* Retinopathy, proliferative
- with retinal detachment — *see* Detachment, retina, traction

**Vitreous** — *see also* condition
- touch syndrome — *see* Complication, postprocedural, following cataract surgery

**Vocal cord** — *see* condition
**Vogt-Koyanagi syndrome** H2Ø.82- ☑
**Vogt-Spielmeyer amaurotic idiocy or disease** E75.4
**Vogt's disease or syndrome** G8Ø.3
**Voice**
- change R49.9
  - specified NEC R49.8
- loss — *see* Aphonia

**Volhynian fever** A79.Ø
**Volkmann's ischemic contracture or paralysis** (complicating trauma) T79.6- ☑
**Volvulus** (bowel) (colon) (intestine) K56.2
- with perforation K56.2
- congenital Q43.8
- duodenum K31.5
- fallopian tube — *see* Torsion, fallopian tube
- oviduct — *see* Torsion, fallopian tube
- stomach (due to absence of gastrocolic ligament) K31.89

**Vomiting** R11.1Ø
- with nausea R11.2
- asphyxia — *see* Foreign body, by site, causing asphyxia, gastric contents
- bilious (cause unknown) R11.14
  - following gastro-intestinal surgery K91.Ø
  - in newborn P92.Ø1
- blood — *see* Hematemesis
- causing asphyxia, choking, or suffocation — *see* Foreign body, by site
- cyclical, in migraine G43.AØ (*following* G43.7)
  - with refractory migraine G43.A1 (*following* G43.7)
  - intractable G43.A1 (*following* G43.7)
  - not intractable G43.AØ (*following* G43.7)
  - psychogenic F5Ø.89
  - without refractory migraine G43.AØ (*following* G43.7)
- cyclical syndrome NOS (unrelated to migraine) R11.15
- fecal matter R11.13
- following gastrointestinal surgery K91.Ø
  - psychogenic F5Ø.89
- functional K31.89
- hysterical F5Ø.89
- nervous F5Ø.89
- neurotic F5Ø.89
- newborn NEC P92.Ø9
  - bilious P92.Ø1
- periodic R11.1Ø
  - psychogenic F5Ø.89
- persistent R11.15
- projectile R11.12
- psychogenic F5Ø.89
- uremic — *see* Uremia
- without nausea R11.11

**Vomito negro** — *see* Fever, yellow
**Von Bezold's abscess** — *see* Mastoiditis, acute
**Von Economo-Cruchet disease** A85.8
**Von Eulenburg's disease** G71.19
**Von Gierke's disease** E74.Ø1
**Von Hippel** (-Lindau) **disease or syndrome** Q85.83
**Von Jaksch's anemia or disease** D64.89
**Von Recklinghausen**
- disease (neurofibromatosis) Q85.Ø1
  - bones E21.Ø

**Von Schroetter's syndrome** I82.89Ø
**Von Willebrand** (-Jurgens) (-Minot) **disease or syndrome** — *see* Disease, von Willebrand
**Von Zumbusch's disease** L4Ø.1
**Voyeurism** F65.3
**Vrolik's disease** Q78.Ø

**Vulva** — *see* condition
**Vulvismus** N94.2
**Vulvitis** (acute) (allergic) (atrophic) (hypertrophic) (intertriginous) (senile) N76.2
- with ectopic or molar pregnancy OØ8.Ø
- adhesive, congenital Q52.79
- blennorrhagic (gonococcal) A54.Ø2
- candidal (acute) B37.31
  - chronic (recurrent) B37.32
- chlamydial A56.Ø2
- due to Haemophilus ducreyi A57
- following ectopic or molar pregnancy OØ8.Ø
- gonococcal A54.Ø2
  - with abscess (accessory gland) (periurethral) A54.1
- herpesviral A6Ø.Ø4
- leukoplakic N9Ø.4
- monilial (acute) B37.31
  - chronic (recurrent) B37.32
- puerperal (postpartum) O86.19
- subacute or chronic N76.3
- syphilitic (early) A51.Ø
  - late A52.76
- trichomonal A59.Ø1
- tuberculous A18.18

**Vulvodynia** N94.819
- specified NEC N94.818

**Vulvorectal** — *see* condition
**Vulvovaginitis** (acute) — *see* Vaginitis

# W

**Waiting list, person on** Z75.1
- for organ transplant Z76.82
- undergoing social agency investigation Z75.2

**Waldenstrom**
- hypergammaglobulinemia D89.Ø
- syndrome or macroglobulinemia C88.Ø- ☑

**Waldenstrom-Kjellberg syndrome** D5Ø.1
**Walking**
- difficulty R26.2
  - psychogenic F44.4
- sleep F51.3
  - hysterical F44.89

**Wall, abdominal** — *see* condition
**Wallenberg's disease or syndrome** G46.3
**Wallgren's disease** I87.8
**Wandering**
- gallbladder, congenital Q44.1
- in diseases classified elsewhere Z91.83
- kidney, congenital Q63.8
- organ or site, congenital NEC — *see* Malposition, congenital, by site
- pacemaker (heart) I49.89
- spleen D73.89

**War neurosis** F48.8
**Wart** (due to HPV) (filiform) (infectious) (viral) BØ7.9
- anogenital region (venereal) A63.Ø
- common BØ7.8
- external genital organs (venereal) A63.Ø
- flat BØ7.8
- Hassal-Henle's (of cornea) H18.49
- Peruvian A44.1
- plantar BØ7.Ø
- prosector (tuberculous) A18.4
- seborrheic L82.1
  - inflamed L82.Ø
- senile (seborrheic) L82.1
  - inflamed L82.Ø
- tuberculous A18.4
- venereal A63.Ø

**Warthin's tumor** — *see* Neoplasm, salivary gland or duct, benign
**Wassilieff's disease** A27.Ø
**Wasting**
- disease (syndrome) E88.A
  - due to
    - malnutrition E43
      - with marasmus E41
    - underlying condition E88.A
- extreme (due to malnutrition) E43
  - with marasmus E41
- muscle NEC — *see* Atrophy, muscle

**Water**
- clefts (senile cataract) — *see* Cataract, senile, incipient
- deprivation of T73.1- ☑
- intoxication E87.79
- itch B76.9
- lack of T73.1- ☑



 ☑ **Additional Character Required — Refer to the Tabular List for Character Selection**

**Water** — *continued*
  lack of — *continued*
    safe drinking Z58.6
  loading E87.70
  on
    brain — *see* Hydrocephalus
    chest J94.8
  poisoning E87.79
**Water-losing nephritis** N25.89
**Waterbrash** R12
**Waterhouse** (-Friderichsen) **syndrome or disease** (meningococcal) A39.1
**Watermelon stomach** K31.819
  with hemorrhage K31.811
  without hemorrhage K31.819
**Watsoniasis** B66.8
**Wax in ear** — *see* Impaction, cerumen
**Weak, weakening, weakness** (generalized) R53.1
  arches (acquired) — *see also* Deformity, limb, flat foot
  bladder (sphincter) R32
  facial R29.810
    following
      cerebrovascular disease I69.992
        cerebral infarction I69.392
        intracerebral hemorrhage I69.192
        nontraumatic intracranial hemorrhage NEC I69.292
        specified disease NEC I69.892
        stroke I69.392
        subarachnoid hemorrhage I69.092
  foot (double) — *see also* Weak, arches
  heart, cardiac — *see* Failure, heart
  mind F70
  muscle M62.81
  myocardium — *see* Failure, heart
  newborn P96.89
  pelvic fundus N81.89
  pubocervical tissue N81.82
  rectovaginal tissue N81.83
  senile R54
  urinary stream R39.12
  valvular — *see* Endocarditis
**Wear, worn** (with normal or routine use)
  articular bearing surface of internal joint prosthesis — *see* Complications, joint prosthesis, mechanical, wear of articular bearing surfaces, by site
  device, implant or graft — *see* Complications, by site, mechanical complication
  tooth, teeth (approximal) (hard tissues) (interproximal) (occlusal) K03.0
**Weather, weathered**
  effects of
    cold T69.9- ☑
      specified effect NEC T69.8- ☑
    hot — *see* Heat
  skin L57.8
**Weaver's syndrome** Q87.3
**Web, webbed** (congenital)
  duodenal Q43.8
  esophagus Q39.4
  fingers Q70.1- ☑
  larynx (glottic) (subglottic) Q31.0
  neck (pterygium colli) Q18.3
  Paterson-Kelly D50.1
  popliteal syndrome Q87.89
  toes Q70.3- ☑
**Weber-Christian disease** M35.6
**Weber-Cockayne syndrome** (epidermolysis bullosa) Q81.8
**Weber-Gubler syndrome** G46.3
**Weber-Leyden syndrome** G46.3
**Weber-Osler syndrome** I78.0
**Weber's paralysis or syndrome** G46.3
**Wedge-shaped or wedging vertebra** — *see* Collapse, vertebra NEC
**Wegener's granulomatosis or syndrome** M31.30
  with
    kidney involvement M31.31
    lung involvement M31.30
      with kidney involvement M31.31
**Wegner's disease** A50.02
**Weight**
  1000-2499 grams at birth (low) — *see* Low, birthweight
  999 grams or less at birth (extremely low) — *see* Low, birthweight, extreme
  and length below 10th percentile for gestational age P05.1- ☑
  below but length above 10th percentile for gestational age P05.0- ☑

**Weight** — *continued*
  gain (abnormal) (excessive) R63.5
    in pregnancy — *see* Pregnancy, complicated by, excessive weight gain
      low — *see* Pregnancy, complicated by, insufficient, weight gain
  loss (abnormal) (cause unknown) R63.4
**Weightlessness** (effect of) T75.82- ☑
**Weil (l)-Marchesani syndrome** Q87.19
**Weil's disease** A27.0
**Weingarten's syndrome** J82.89
**Weir Mitchell's disease** I73.81
**Weiss-Baker syndrome** G90.09
**Wells' disease** L98.3
**Wen** — *see* Cyst, sebaceous
**Wenckebach's block or phenomenon** I44.1
**Werdnig-Hoffmann syndrome** (muscular atrophy) G12.0
**Werlhof's disease** D69.3
**Wermer's disease or syndrome** E31.21
**Werner-His disease** A79.0
**Werner's disease or syndrome** E34.8
**Wernicke-Korsakoff's syndrome or psychosis** (alcoholic) F10.9- ☑
  with dependence F10.2- ☑
  drug-induced
    due to drug abuse — *see* Abuse, drug, by type, with amnestic disorder
    due to drug dependence — *see* Dependence, drug, by type, with amnestic disorder
  nonalcoholic F04
**Wernicke-Posadas disease** B38.9
**Wernicke's**
  developmental aphasia F80.2
  disease or syndrome E51.2
  encephalopathy E51.2
  polioencephalitis, superior E51.2
**West African fever** B50.8
**Westphal-Strumpell syndrome** E83.01
**West's syndrome** — *see* Epilepsy, spasms
**Wet**
  feet, tropical (maceration) (syndrome) — *see* Immersion, foot
  lung (syndrome), newborn P22.1
**Wharton's duct** — *see* condition
**Wheal** — *see* Urticaria
**Wheezing** R06.2
**Whiplash injury** S13.4- ☑
**Whipple's disease** — *see also* subcategory M14.8- K90.81
**Whipworm** (disease) (infection) (infestation) B79
**Whistling face** Q87.0
**White** — *see also* condition
  kidney, small N03.9
  leg, puerperal, postpartum, childbirth O87.1
  mouth B37.0
  patches of mouth K13.29
  spot lesions, teeth
    chewing surface K02.51
    pit and fissure surface K02.51
    smooth surface K02.61
**Whitehead** L70.0
**Whitlow** — *see also* Cellulitis, digit
  with lymphangitis — *see* Lymphangitis, acute, digit
  herpesviral B00.89
**Whitmore's disease or fever** — *see* Melioidosis
**Whooping cough** A37.90
  with pneumonia A37.91
    due to Bordetella
      bronchiseptica A37.81
      parapertussis A37.11
      pertussis A37.01
    specified organism NEC A37.81
  due to
    Bordetella
      bronchiseptica A37.80
        with pneumonia A37.81
      parapertussis A37.10
        with pneumonia A37.11
      pertussis A37.00
        with pneumonia A37.01
      specified NEC A37.80
        with pneumonia A37.81
**Wichman's asthma** J38.5
**Wide cranial sutures, newborn** P96.3
**Widening aorta** — *see* Ectasia, aorta
  with aneurysm — *see* Aneurysm, aorta
**Wilkie's disease or syndrome** K55.1
**Wilkinson-Sneddon disease or syndrome** L13.1
**Willebrand** (-Jurgens) **thrombopathy** — *see* Disease, von Willebrand

**Williams syndrome** Q93.82
**Willige-Hunt disease or syndrome** G23.1
**Wilms' tumor** C64.- ☑
**Wilson-Mikity syndrome** P27.0
**Wilson's**
  disease or syndrome E83.01
  hepatolenticular degeneration E83.01
  lichen ruber L43.9
**Window** — *see also* Imperfect, closure
  aorticopulmonary Q21.4
**Winter** — *see* condition
**Wiskott-Aldrich syndrome** D82.0
**Withdrawal state** — *see also* Dependence, drug by type, with withdrawal
  alcohol
    with perceptual disturbances F10.232
      due to alcohol abuse F10.132
      due to alcohol use F10.932
    abuse — *see* Abuse, alcohol, with, withdrawal
    dependence — *see* Dependence, alcohol, with, withdrawal
    use — *see* Use, alcohol, with, withdrawal
    without perceptual disturbances F10.239
      due to alcohol abuse F10.139
      due to alcohol use F10.939
  caffeine F15.93
  cannabis F12.23
  newborn
    correct therapeutic substance properly administered P96.2
    infant of dependent mother P96.1
  therapeutic substance, neonatal P96.2
**Witts' anemia** D50.8
**Witzelsucht** F07.0
**Woakes' ethmoiditis or syndrome** J33.1
**Wolff-Hirschorn syndrome** Q93.3
**Wolff-Parkinson-White syndrome** I45.6
**Wolhynian fever** A79.0
**Wolman's disease** E75.5
**Wood lung or pneumonitis** J67.8
**Woolly, wooly hair** (congenital) (nevus) Q84.1
**Woolsorter's disease** A22.1
**Word**
  blindness (congenital) (developmental) F81.0
  deafness (congenital) (developmental) H93.25
**Worm(s)** (infection) (infestation) — *see also* Infestation, helminth
  guinea B72
  in intestine NEC B82.0
**Worm-eaten soles** A66.3
**Worn out** — *see* Exhaustion
  cardiac
    defibrillator (with synchronous cardiac pacemaker) Z45.02
    pacemaker
      battery Z45.010
      lead Z45.018
  device, implant or graft — *see* Complications, by site, mechanical
**Worried well** Z71.1
**Worries** R45.82
**Wound check** Z48.0- ☑
  due to injury — *code to* Injury, by site, using appropriate seventh character for subsequent encounter
  postoperative — *see* Aftercare
**Wound, open** T14.8- ☑
  abdomen, abdominal
    wall S31.109- ☑
      with penetration into peritoneal cavity S31.609- ☑
      bite — *see* Bite, abdomen, wall
      epigastric region S31.102- ☑
        with penetration into peritoneal cavity S31.602- ☑
        bite — *see* Bite, abdomen, wall, epigastric region
        laceration — *see* Laceration, abdomen, wall, epigastric region
        puncture — *see* Puncture, abdomen, wall, epigastric region
      laceration — *see* Laceration, abdomen, wall
      left
        lower quadrant S31.104- ☑
          with penetration into peritoneal cavity S31.604- ☑
          bite — *see* Bite, abdomen, wall, left, lower quadrant
          laceration — *see* Laceration, abdomen, wall, left, lower quadrant

- **Wound, open** — *continued*
  - abdomen, abdominal — *continued*
    - wall — *continued*
      - left — *continued*
        - lower quadrant — *continued*
          - puncture — *see* Puncture, abdomen, wall, left, lower quadrant
        - upper quadrant S31.1Ø1- ☑
          - with penetration into peritoneal cavity S31.6Ø1- ☑
          - bite — *see* Bite, abdomen, wall, left, upper quadrant
          - laceration — *see* Laceration, abdomen, wall, left, upper quadrant
          - puncture — *see* Puncture, abdomen, wall, left, upper quadrant
      - periumbilic region S31.1Ø5- ☑
        - with penetration into peritoneal cavity S31.6Ø5- ☑
        - bite — *see* Bite, abdomen, wall, periumbilic region
        - laceration — *see* Laceration, abdomen, wall, periumbilic region
        - puncture — *see* Puncture, abdomen, wall, periumbilic region
      - puncture — *see* Puncture, abdomen, wall
      - right
        - lower quadrant S31.1Ø3- ☑
          - with penetration into peritoneal cavity S31.6Ø3- ☑
          - bite — *see* Bite, abdomen, wall, right, lower quadrant
          - laceration — *see* Laceration, abdomen, wall, right, lower quadrant
          - puncture — *see* Puncture, abdomen, wall, right, lower quadrant
        - upper quadrant S31.1ØØ- ☑
          - with penetration into peritoneal cavity S31.6ØØ- ☑
          - bite — *see* Bite, abdomen, wall, right, upper quadrant
          - laceration — *see* Laceration, abdomen, wall, right, upper quadrant
          - puncture — *see* Puncture, abdomen, wall, right, upper quadrant
  - alveolar (process) — *see* Wound, open, oral cavity
  - ankle S91.ØØ- ☑
    - bite — *see* Bite, ankle
    - laceration — *see* Laceration, ankle
    - puncture — *see* Puncture, ankle
  - antecubital space — *see* Wound, open, elbow
  - anterior chamber, eye — *see* Wound, open, ocular
  - anus S31.839- ☑
    - bite S31.835- ☑
    - laceration — *see* Laceration, anus
    - puncture — *see* Puncture, anus
  - arm (upper) S41.1Ø- ☑
    - with amputation — *see* Amputation, traumatic, arm
    - bite — *see* Bite, arm
    - forearm — *see* Wound, open, forearm
    - laceration — *see* Laceration, arm
    - puncture — *see* Puncture, arm
  - auditory canal (external) (meatus) — *see* Wound, open, ear
  - auricle, ear — *see* Wound, open, ear
  - axilla — *see* Wound, open, arm
  - back — *see also* Wound, open, thorax, back
    - lower S31.ØØØ- ☑
      - with penetration into retroperitoneal space S31.ØØ1- ☑
      - bite — *see* Bite, back, lower
      - laceration — *see* Laceration, back, lower
      - puncture — *see* Puncture, back, lower
  - bite — *see* Bite
  - blood vessel — *see* Injury, blood vessel
  - breast S21.ØØ- ☑
    - with amputation — *see* Amputation, traumatic, breast
    - bite — *see* Bite, breast
    - laceration — *see* Laceration, breast
    - puncture — *see* Puncture, breast
  - buttock S31.8Ø9- ☑
    - bite — *see* Bite, buttock
    - laceration — *see* Laceration, buttock
    - left S31.829- ☑
    - puncture — *see* Puncture, buttock
    - right S31.819- ☑
  - calf — *see* Wound, open, leg
  - canaliculus lacrimalis — *see* Wound, open, eyelid

- **Wound, open** — *continued*
  - canthus, eye — *see* Wound, open, eyelid
  - cervical esophagus S11.2Ø- ☑
    - bite S11.25- ☑
    - laceration — *see* Laceration, esophagus, traumatic, cervical
    - puncture — *see* Puncture, cervical esophagus
  - cheek (external) SØ1.4Ø- ☑
    - bite — *see* Bite, cheek
    - internal — *see* Wound, open, oral cavity
    - laceration — *see* Laceration, cheek
    - puncture — *see* Puncture, cheek
  - chest wall — *see* Wound, open, thorax
  - chin — *see* Wound, open, head, specified site NEC
  - choroid — *see* Wound, open, ocular
  - ciliary body (eye) — *see* Wound, open, ocular
  - clitoris S31.4Ø- ☑
    - with amputation — *see* Amputation, traumatic, clitoris
    - bite S31.45- ☑
    - laceration — *see* Laceration, vulva
    - puncture — *see* Puncture, vulva
  - conjunctiva — *see* Wound, open, ocular
  - cornea — *see* Wound, open, ocular
  - costal region — *see* Wound, open, thorax
  - Descemet's membrane — *see* Wound, open, ocular
  - digit(s)
    - foot — *see* Wound, open, toe
    - hand — *see* Wound, open, finger
  - ear (canal) (external) SØ1.3Ø- ☑
    - with amputation — *see* Amputation, traumatic, ear
    - bite — *see* Bite, ear
    - drum SØ9.2- ☑
    - laceration — *see* Laceration, ear
    - puncture — *see* Puncture, ear
  - elbow S51.ØØ- ☑
    - bite — *see* Bite, elbow
    - laceration — *see* Laceration, elbow
    - puncture — *see* Puncture, elbow
  - epididymis — *see* Wound, open, testis
  - epigastric region S31.1Ø2- ☑
    - with penetration into peritoneal cavity S31.6Ø2- ☑
    - bite — *see* Bite, abdomen, wall, epigastric region
    - laceration — *see* Laceration, abdomen, wall, epigastric region
    - puncture — *see* Puncture, abdomen, wall, epigastric region
  - epiglottis — *see* Wound, open, neck, specified site NEC
  - esophagus (thoracic) S27.819- ☑
    - cervical — *see* Wound, open, cervical esophagus
    - laceration S27.813- ☑
    - specified type NEC S27.818- ☑
  - eye — *see* Wound, open, ocular
  - eyeball — *see* Wound, open, ocular
  - eyebrow — *see* Wound, open, eyelid
  - eyelid SØ1.1Ø- ☑
    - bite — *see* Bite, eyelid
    - laceration — *see* Laceration, eyelid
    - puncture — *see* Puncture, eyelid
  - face NEC — *see* Wound, open, head, specified site NEC
  - finger(s) S61.2Ø9- ☑
    - with
      - amputation — *see* Amputation, traumatic, finger
      - damage to nail S61.3Ø9- ☑
    - bite — *see* Bite, finger
    - index S61.2Ø8- ☑
      - with
        - damage to nail S61.3Ø8- ☑
      - left S61.2Ø1- ☑
        - with
          - damage to nail S61.3Ø1- ☑
      - right S61.2ØØ- ☑
        - with
          - damage to nail S61.3ØØ- ☑
    - laceration — *see* Laceration, finger
    - little S61.2Ø8- ☑
      - with
        - damage to nail S61.3Ø8- ☑
      - left S61.2Ø7- ☑
        - with damage to nail S61.3Ø7- ☑
      - right S61.2Ø6- ☑
        - with damage to nail S61.3Ø6- ☑
    - middle S61.2Ø8- ☑
      - with
        - damage to nail S61.3Ø8- ☑
      - left S61.2Ø3- ☑
        - with damage to nail S61.3Ø3- ☑
      - right S61.2Ø2- ☑

- **Wound, open** — *continued*
  - finger(s) — *continued*
    - middle — *continued*
      - right — *continued*
        - with damage to nail S61.3Ø2- ☑
    - puncture — *see* Puncture, finger
    - ring S61.2Ø8- ☑
      - with
        - damage to nail S61.3Ø8- ☑
      - left S61.2Ø5- ☑
        - with damage to nail S61.3Ø5- ☑
      - right S61.2Ø4- ☑
        - with damage to nail S61.3Ø4- ☑
  - flank S31.1ØA- ☑
    - with penetration into peritoneal cavity S31.6ØA- ☑
    - left S31.1Ø7- ☑
      - with penetration into peritoneal cavity S31.6Ø7- ☑
    - right S31.1Ø6- ☑
      - with penetration into peritoneal cavity S31.6Ø6- ☑
  - foot (except toe(s) alone) S91.3Ø- ☑
    - with amputation — *see* Amputation, traumatic, foot
    - bite — *see* Bite, foot
    - laceration — *see* Laceration, foot
    - puncture — *see* Puncture, foot
    - toe — *see* Wound, open, toe
  - forearm S51.8Ø- ☑
    - with
      - amputation — *see* Amputation, traumatic, forearm
    - bite — *see* Bite, forearm
    - elbow only — *see* Wound, open, elbow
    - laceration — *see* Laceration, forearm
    - puncture — *see* Puncture, forearm
  - forehead — *see* Wound, open, head, specified site NEC
  - genital organs, external
    - with amputation — *see* Amputation, traumatic, genital organs
    - bite — *see* Bite, genital organ
    - female S31.5Ø2- ☑
      - vagina S31.4Ø- ☑
      - vulva S31.4Ø- ☑
    - laceration — *see* Laceration, genital organ
    - male S31.5Ø1- ☑
      - penis S31.2Ø- ☑
      - scrotum S31.3Ø- ☑
      - testes S31.3Ø- ☑
    - puncture — *see* Puncture, genital organ
  - globe (eye) — *see* Wound, open, ocular
  - groin — *see* Wound, open, abdomen, wall
  - gum — *see* Wound, open, oral cavity
  - hand S61.4Ø- ☑
    - with
      - amputation — *see* Amputation, traumatic, hand
    - bite — *see* Bite, hand
    - finger(s) — *see* Wound, open, finger
    - laceration — *see* Laceration, hand
    - puncture — *see* Puncture, hand
    - thumb — *see* Wound, open, thumb
  - head SØ1.9Ø- ☑
    - bite — *see* Bite, head
    - cheek — *see* Wound, open, cheek
    - ear — *see* Wound, open, ear
    - eyelid — *see* Wound, open, eyelid
    - laceration — *see* Laceration, head
    - lip — *see* Wound, open, lip
    - nose SØ1.2Ø- ☑
    - oral cavity — *see* Wound, open, oral cavity
    - puncture — *see* Puncture, head
    - scalp — *see* Wound, open, scalp
    - specified site NEC SØ1.8Ø- ☑
    - temporomandibular area — *see* Wound, open, cheek
  - heel — *see* Wound, open, foot
  - hip S71.ØØ- ☑
    - with amputation — *see* Amputation, traumatic, hip
    - bite — *see* Bite, hip
    - laceration — *see* Laceration, hip
    - puncture — *see* Puncture, hip
  - hymen S31.4Ø- ☑
    - bite — *see* Bite, vulva
    - laceration — *see* Laceration, vagina
    - puncture — *see* Puncture, vagina
  - hypochondrium S31.1Ø9- ☑
    - bite — *see* Bite, hypochondrium
    - laceration — *see* Laceration, hypochondrium
    - puncture — *see* Puncture, hypochondrium
  - hypogastric region S31.1Ø9- ☑
    - bite — *see* Bite, hypogastric region
    - laceration — *see* Laceration, hypogastric region

- **Wound, open** — *continued*
  - toe(s) — *continued*
    - lesser — *continued*
      - right — *continued*
        - with
          - damage to nail S91.204- ☑
    - puncture — *see* Puncture, toe
  - tongue — *see* Wound, open, oral cavity
  - trachea (cervical region) — *see* Wound, open, neck, trachea
  - tunica vaginalis — *see* Wound, open, testis
  - tympanum, tympanic membrane S09.2- ☑
    - laceration — *see* Laceration, ear, drum
    - puncture — *see* Puncture, tympanum
  - umbilical region — *see* Wound, open, abdomen, wall, periumbilic region
  - uvula — *see* Wound, open, oral cavity
  - vagina S31.40- ☑
    - bite S31.45- ☑
    - laceration — *see* Laceration, vagina
    - puncture — *see* Puncture, vagina
  - vitreous (humor) — *see* Wound, open, ocular
  - vocal cord S11.039- ☑
    - bite — *see* Bite, vocal cord
    - laceration S11.031- ☑
      - with foreign body S11.032- ☑
    - puncture S11.033- ☑
      - with foreign body S11.034- ☑
  - vulva S31.40- ☑
    - with amputation — *see* Amputation, traumatic, vulva
    - bite S31.45- ☑
    - laceration — *see* Laceration, vulva
    - puncture — *see* Puncture, vulva
  - wrist S61.50- ☑
    - bite — *see* Bite, wrist
    - laceration — *see* Laceration, wrist
    - puncture — *see* Puncture, wrist
- **Wound, superficial** — *see* Injury — *see also* specified injury type
- **Wright's syndrome** G54.0
- **Wrist** — *see* condition
- **Wrong drug** (by accident) (given in error) — *see* Table of Drugs and Chemicals, by drug, poisoning
- **Wry neck** — *see* Torticollis
- **Wuchereria** (bancrofti) **infestation** B74.0
- **Wuchereriasis** B74.0
- **Wuchernde Struma Langhans** C73

## X

- **X-ray** (of)
  - abnormal findings — *see* Abnormal, diagnostic imaging
  - breast (mammogram) (routine) Z12.31
  - chest
    - routine (as part of a general medical examination) Z00.00
      - with abnormal findings Z00.01
  - routine (as part of a general medical examination) Z00.00
    - with abnormal findings Z00.01
- **Xanthelasma** (eyelid) (palpebrarum) H02.60
  - left H02.66
    - lower H02.65
    - upper H02.64
  - right H02.63
    - lower H02.62
    - upper H02.61
- **Xanthelasmatosis** (essential) E78.2
- **Xanthinuria, hereditary** E79.82
- **Xanthoastrocytoma**
  - specified site — *see* Neoplasm, malignant, by site
  - unspecified site C71.9
- **Xanthofibroma** — *see* Neoplasm, connective tissue, benign
- **Xanthogranuloma** D76.3
- **Xanthoma(s), xanthomatosis** (primary) (familial) (hereditary) E78.2
  - with
    - hyperlipoproteinemia
      - Type I E78.3
      - Type III E78.2
      - Type IV E78.1
      - Type V E78.3
  - bone (generalisata) C96.5
  - cerebrotendinous E75.5
  - cutaneotendinous E75.5
  - disseminatum (skin) E78.2
  - eruptive E78.2
  - hypercholesterinemic E78.00
  - hypercholesterolemic E78.00
  - hyperlipidemic E78.5
  - joint E75.5
  - multiple (skin) E78.2
  - tendon (sheath) E75.5
  - tuberosum E78.2
  - tuberous E78.2
  - tubo-eruptive E78.2
  - verrucous, oral mucosa K13.4
- **Xanthosis** R23.8
- **Xenophobia** F40.10
- **Xeroderma** — *see also* Ichthyosis
  - acquired L85.0
    - eyelid H01.149
      - left H01.146
        - lower H01.145
        - upper H01.144
      - right H01.143
        - lower H01.142
        - upper H01.141
  - pigmentosum Q82.1
  - vitamin A deficiency E50.8
- **Xerophthalmia** (vitamin A deficiency) E50.7
  - unrelated to vitamin A deficiency — *see* Keratoconjunctivitis
- **Xerosis**
  - conjunctiva H11.14- ☑
    - with Bitot's spots — *see also* Pigmentation, conjunctiva
      - vitamin A deficiency E50.1
    - vitamin A deficiency E50.0
  - cornea H18.89- ☑
    - with ulceration — *see* Ulcer, cornea
      - vitamin A deficiency E50.3
    - vitamin A deficiency E50.2
  - cutis (dry skin) L85.3
  - skin L85.3
- **Xerostomia** K11.7
- **Xiphopagus** Q89.4
- **XO syndrome** Q96.9
- **XXXXY syndrome** Q98.1
- **XXY syndrome** Q98.0

## Y

- **Yaba pox** (virus disease) B08.72
- **Yatapoxvirus** B08.70
  - specified NEC B08.79
- **Yawning** R06.89
  - psychogenic F45.8
- **Yaws** A66.9
  - bone lesions A66.6
  - butter A66.1
  - chancre A66.0
  - cutaneous, less than five years after infection A66.2
  - early (cutaneous) (macular) (maculopapular) (micropapular) (papular) A66.2
    - frambeside A66.2
    - skin lesions NEC A66.2
  - eyelid A66.2
  - ganglion A66.6
  - gangosis, gangosa A66.5
  - gumma, gummata A66.4
    - bone A66.6
  - gummatous
    - frambeside A66.4
    - osteitis A66.6
    - periostitis A66.6
  - hydrarthrosis — *see also* subcategory M14.8- A66.6
  - hyperkeratosis (early) (late) A66.3
  - initial lesions A66.0
  - joint lesions — *see also* subcategory M14.8- A66.6
  - juxta-articular nodules A66.7
  - late nodular (ulcerated) A66.4
  - latent (without clinical manifestations) (with positive serology) A66.8
  - mother A66.0
  - mucosal A66.7
  - multiple papillomata A66.1
  - nodular, late (ulcerated) A66.4
  - osteitis A66.6
  - papilloma, plantar or palmar A66.1
  - periostitis (hypertrophic) A66.6
  - specified NEC A66.7
  - ulcers A66.4
  - wet crab A66.1
- **Yeast infection** — *see also* Candidiasis B37.9
- **Yellow**
  - atrophy (liver) — *see* Failure, hepatic
  - fever — *see* Fever, yellow
  - jack — *see* Fever, yellow
  - jaundice — *see* Jaundice
  - nail syndrome L60.5
- **Yersiniosis** — *see also* Infection, Yersinia
  - extraintestinal A28.2
  - intestinal A04.6

## Z

- **Zahorsky's syndrome** (herpangina) B08.5
- **Zellweger's syndrome** E71.510
- **Zenker's diverticulum** (esophagus) K22.5
- **Ziehen-Oppenheim disease** G24.1
- **Zieve's syndrome** K70.0
- **Zika NOS** A92.5
  - congenital P35.4
- **Zinc**
  - deficiency, dietary E60
  - metabolism disorder E83.2
- **Zollinger-Ellison syndrome** E16.4
- **Zona** — *see* Herpes, zoster
- **Zoophobia** F40.218
- **Zoster** (herpes) — *see* Herpes, zoster
- **Zygomycosis** B46.9
  - specified NEC B46.8
- **Zymotic** — *see* condition

| | Malignant Primary | Malignant Secondary | Ca in situ | Benign | Uncertain Behavior | Unspecified Behavior |
|---|---|---|---|---|---|---|
| **Neoplasm, neoplastic** | C80.1 | C79.9 | D09.9 | D36.9 | D48.9 | D49.9 |
| abdomen, abdominal | C76.2 | C79.8-☑ | D09.8 | D36.7 | D48.7 | D49.89 |
| cavity | C76.2 | C79.8-☑ | D09.8 | D36.7 | D48.7 | D49.89 |
| organ | C76.2 | C79.8-☑ | D09.8 | D36.7 | D48.7 | D49.89 |
| viscera | C76.2 | C79.8-☑ | D09.8 | D36.7 | D48.7 | D49.89 |
| wall — *see also* Neoplasm, abdomen, wall, skin | C44.509 | C79.2 | D04.5 | D23.5 | D48.5 | D49.2 |
| connective tissue | C49.4 | C79.8-☑ | — | D21.4 | D48.1-☑ | D49.2 |
| skin | C44.509 | — | — | — | — | — |
| basal cell carcinoma | C44.519 | — | — | — | — | — |
| specified type NEC | C44.599 | — | — | — | — | — |
| squamous cell carcinoma | C44.529 | — | — | — | — | — |
| abdominopelvic | C76.8 | C79.8-☑ | — | D36.7 | D48.7 | D49.89 |
| accessory sinus — *see* Neoplasm, sinus | | | | | | |
| acoustic nerve | C72.4-☑ | C79.49 | — | D33.3 | D43.3 | D49.7 |
| adenoid (pharynx) (tissue) | C11.1 | C79.89 | D00.08 | D10.6 | D37.05 | D49.0 |
| adipose tissue — *see also* Neoplasm, connective tissue | C49.4 | C79.89 | — | D21.9 | D48.1-☑ | D49.2 |
| adnexa (uterine) | C57.4 | C79.89 | D07.39 | D28.7 | D39.8 | D49.59 |
| adrenal | C74.9-☑ | C79.7-☑ | D09.3 | D35.0-☑ | D44.1-☑ | D49.7 |
| capsule | C74.9-☑ | C79.7-☑ | D09.3 | D35.0-☑ | D44.1-☑ | D49.7 |
| cortex | C74.0-☑ | C79.7-☑ | D09.3 | D35.0-☑ | D44.1-☑ | D49.7 |
| gland | C74.9-☑ | C79.7-☑ | D09.3 | D35.0-☑ | D44.1-☑ | D49.7 |
| medulla | C74.1-☑ | C79.7-☑ | D09.3 | D35.0-☑ | D44.1-☑ | D49.7 |
| ala nasi (external) — *see also* Neoplasm, skin, nose | C44.301 | C79.2 | D04.39 | D23.39 | D48.5 | D49.2 |
| alimentary canal or tract NEC | C26.9 | C78.80 | D01.9 | D13.99 | D37.9 | D49.0 |
| alveolar | C03.9 | C79.89 | D00.03 | D10.39 | D37.09 | D49.0 |
| mucosa | C03.9 | C79.89 | D00.03 | D10.39 | D37.09 | D49.0 |
| lower | C03.1 | C79.89 | D00.03 | D10.39 | D37.09 | D49.0 |
| upper | C03.0 | C79.89 | D00.03 | D10.39 | D37.09 | D49.0 |
| ridge or process | C41.1 | C79.51 | — | D16.5 | D48.0 | D49.2 |
| carcinoma | C03.9 | C79.8-☑ | — | — | — | — |
| lower | C03.1 | C79.8-☑ | — | — | — | — |
| upper | C03.0 | C79.8-☑ | — | — | — | — |
| lower | C41.1 | C79.51 | — | D16.5 | D48.0 | D49.2 |
| mucosa | C03.9 | C79.89 | D00.03 | D10.39 | D37.09 | D49.0 |
| lower | C03.1 | C79.89 | D00.03 | D10.39 | D37.09 | D49.0 |
| upper | C03.0 | C79.89 | D00.03 | D10.39 | D37.09 | D49.0 |
| upper | C41.0 | C79.51 | — | D16.4 | D48.0 | D49.2 |
| sulcus | C06.1 | C79.89 | D00.02 | D10.39 | D37.09 | D49.0 |
| alveolus | C03.9 | C79.89 | D00.03 | D10.39 | D37.09 | D49.0 |
| lower | C03.1 | C79.89 | D00.03 | D10.39 | D37.09 | D49.0 |
| upper | C03.0 | C79.89 | D00.03 | D10.39 | D37.09 | D49.0 |
| ampulla of Vater | C24.1 | C78.89 | D01.5 | D13.5 | D37.6 | D49.0 |
| ankle NEC | C76.5-☑ | C79.89 | D04.7-☑ | D36.7 | D48.7 | D49.89 |
| anorectum, anorectal (junction) | C21.8 | C78.5 | D01.3 | D12.9 | D37.8 | D49.0 |
| antecubital fossa or space | C76.4-☑ | C79.89 | D04.6-☑ | D36.7 | D48.7 | D49.89 |
| antrum (Highmore) (maxillary) | C31.0 | C78.39 | D02.3 | D14.0 | D38.5 | D49.1 |
| pyloric | C16.3 | C78.89 | D00.2 | D13.1 | D37.1 | D49.0 |
| tympanicum | C30.1 | C78.39 | D02.3 | D14.0 | D38.5 | D49.1 |
| anus, anal | C21.0 | C78.5 | D01.3 | D12.9 | D37.8 | D49.0 |
| canal | C21.1 | C78.5 | D01.3 | D12.9 | D37.8 | D49.0 |
| cloacogenic zone | C21.2 | C78.5 | D01.3 | D12.9 | D37.8 | D49.0 |
| margin — *see also* Neoplasm, anus, skin | C44.500 | C79.2 | D04.5 | D23.5 | D48.5 | D49.2 |
| overlapping lesion with rectosigmoid junction or rectum | C21.8 | — | — | — | — | — |
| skin | C44.500 | C79.2 | D04.5 | D23.5 | D48.5 | D49.2 |
| **Neoplasm, neoplastic** *— continued* | | | | | | |
| anus, anal *— continued* | | | | | | |
| skin *— continued* | | | | | | |
| basal cell carcinoma | C44.510 | — | — | — | — | — |
| specified type NEC | C44.590 | — | — | — | — | — |
| squamous cell carcinoma | C44.520 | — | — | — | — | — |
| sphincter | C21.1 | C78.5 | D01.3 | D12.9 | D37.8 | D49.0 |
| aorta (thoracic) | C49.3 | C79.89 | — | D21.3 | D48.1-☑ | D49.2 |
| abdominal | C49.4 | C79.89 | — | D21.4 | D48.1-☑ | D49.2 |
| aortic body | C75.5 | C79.89 | — | D35.6 | D44.7 | D49.7 |
| aponeurosis | C49.9 | C79.89 | — | D21.9 | D48.1-☑ | D49.2 |
| palmar | C49.1-☑ | C79.89 | — | D21.1-☑ | D48.1-☑ | D49.2 |
| plantar | C49.2-☑ | C79.89 | — | D21.2-☑ | D48.1-☑ | D49.2 |
| appendix | C18.1 | C78.5 | D01.0 | D12.1 | D37.3 | D49.0 |
| arachnoid | C70.9 | C79.49 | — | D32.9 | D42.9 | D49.7 |
| cerebral | C70.0 | C79.32 | — | D32.0 | D42.0 | D49.7 |
| spinal | C70.1 | C79.49 | — | D32.1 | D42.1 | D49.7 |
| areola | C50.0-☑ | C79.81 | D05.-☑ | D24.-☑ | D48.6-☑ | D49.3 |
| arm NEC | C76.4-☑ | C79.89 | D04.6-☑ | D36.7 | D48.7 | D49.89 |
| artery — *see* Neoplasm, connective tissue | | | | | | |
| aryepiglottic fold | C13.1 | C79.89 | D00.08 | D10.7 | D37.05 | D49.0 |
| hypopharyngeal aspect | C13.1 | C79.89 | D00.08 | D10.7 | D37.05 | D49.0 |
| laryngeal aspect | C32.1 | C78.31 | D02.0 | D14.1 | D38.0 | D49.1 |
| marginal zone | C13.1 | C79.89 | D00.08 | D10.7 | D37.05 | D49.0 |
| arytenoid (cartilage) | C32.3 | C78.31 | D02.0 | D14.1 | D38.0 | D49.1 |
| fold — *see* Neoplasm, aryepiglottic | | | | | | |
| associated with transplanted organ | C80.2 | — | — | — | — | — |
| atlas | C41.2 | C79.51 | — | D16.6 | D48.0 | D49.2 |
| atrium, cardiac | C38.0 | C79.89 | — | D15.1 | D48.7 | D49.89 |
| auditory | | | | | | |
| canal (external) (skin) | C44.20-☑ | C79.2 | D04.2-☑ | D23.2-☑ | D48.5 | D49.2 |
| internal | C30.1 | C78.39 | D02.3 | D14.0 | D38.5 | D49.1 |
| nerve | C72.4-☑ | C79.49 | — | D33.3 | D43.3 | D49.7 |
| tube | C30.1 | C78.39 | D02.3 | D14.0 | D38.5 | D49.1 |
| opening | C11.2 | C79.89 | D00.08 | D10.6 | D37.05 | D49.0 |
| auricle, ear — *see also* Neoplasm, skin, ear | C44.20-☑ | C79.2 | D04.2-☑ | D23.2-☑ | D48.5 | D49.2 |
| auricular canal (external) — *see also* Neoplasm, skin, ear | C44.20-☑ | C79.2 | D04.2-☑ | D23.2-☑ | D48.5 | D49.2 |
| internal | C30.1 | C78.39 | D02.3 | D14.0 | D38.5 | D49.2 |
| autonomic nerve or nervous system NEC (see Neoplasm, nerve, peripheral) | | | | | | |
| axilla, axillary | C76.1 | C79.89 | D09.8 | D36.7 | D48.7 | D49.89 |
| fold — *see also* Neoplasm, skin, trunk | C44.509 | C79.2 | D04.5 | D23.5 | D48.5 | D49.2 |
| back NEC | C76.8 | C79.89 | D04.5 | D36.7 | D48.7 | D49.89 |
| Bartholin's gland | C51.0 | C79.82 | D07.1 | D28.0 | D39.8 | D49.59 |
| basal ganglia | C71.0 | C79.31 | — | D33.0 | D43.0 | D49.6 |
| basis pedunculi | C71.7 | C79.31 | — | D33.1 | D43.1 | D49.6 |
| bile or biliary (tract) | C24.9 | C78.89 | D01.5 | D13.5 | D37.6 | D49.0 |
| canaliculi (biliferi) (intrahepatic) | C22.1 | C78.7 | D01.5 | D13.4 | D37.6 | D49.0 |
| canals, interlobular | C22.1 | C78.89 | D01.5 | D13.4 | D37.6 | D49.0 |
| duct or passage (common) (cystic) (extrahepatic) | C24.0 | C78.89 | D01.5 | D13.5 | D37.6 | D49.0 |
| interlobular | C22.1 | C78.89 | D01.5 | D13.4 | D37.6 | D49.0 |
| intrahepatic | C22.1 | C78.7 | D01.5 | D13.4 | D37.6 | D49.0 |
| and extrahepatic | C24.8 | C78.89 | D01.5 | D13.5 | D37.6 | D49.0 |
| bladder (urinary) | C67.9 | C79.11 | D09.0 | D30.3 | D41.4 | D49.4 |
| dome | C67.1 | C79.11 | D09.0 | D30.3 | D41.4 | D49.4 |
| neck | C67.5 | C79.11 | D09.0 | D30.3 | D41.4 | D49.4 |
| orifice | C67.9 | C79.11 | D09.0 | D30.3 | D41.4 | D49.4 |

| | Malignant Primary | Malignant Secondary | Ca in situ | Benign | Uncertain Behavior | Unspecified Behavior |
|---|---|---|---|---|---|---|
| **Neoplasm, neoplastic** — *continued* | | | | | | |
| bladder — *continued* | | | | | | |
| orifice — *continued* | | | | | | |
| ureteric | C67.6 | C79.11 | DØ9.Ø | D3Ø.3 | D41.4 | D49.4 |
| urethral | C67.5 | C79.11 | DØ9.Ø | D3Ø.3 | D41.4 | D49.4 |
| overlapping lesion | C67.8 | — | — | — | — | — |
| sphincter | C67.8 | C79.11 | DØ9.Ø | D3Ø.3 | D41.4 | D49.4 |
| trigone | C67.Ø | C79.11 | DØ9.Ø | D3Ø.3 | D41.4 | D49.4 |
| urachus | C67.7 | C79.11 | DØ9.Ø | D3Ø.3 | D41.4 | D49.4 |
| wall | C67.9 | C79.11 | DØ9.Ø | D3Ø.3 | D41.4 | D49.4 |
| anterior | C67.3 | C79.11 | DØ9.Ø | D3Ø.3 | D41.4 | D49.4 |
| lateral | C67.2 | C79.11 | DØ9.Ø | D3Ø.3 | D41.4 | D49.4 |
| posterior | C67.4 | C79.11 | DØ9.Ø | D3Ø.3 | D41.4 | D49.4 |
| blood vessel — *see* Neoplasm, connective tissue | | | | | | |
| bone (periosteum) | C41.9 | C79.51 | — | D16.9 | D48.Ø | D49.2 |
| acetabulum | | | | | | |
| ankle | C4Ø.3-☑ | C79.51 | — | D16.3-☑ | — | — |
| arm NEC | C4Ø.Ø-☑ | C79.51 | — | D16.Ø-☑ | — | — |
| astragalus | C4Ø.3-☑ | C79.51 | — | D16.3-☑ | — | — |
| atlas | C41.2 | C79.51 | — | D16.6 | D48.Ø | D49.2 |
| axis | C41.2 | C79.51 | — | D16.6 | D48.Ø | D49.2 |
| back NEC | C41.2 | C79.51 | — | D16.6 | D48.Ø | D49.2 |
| calcaneus | C4Ø.3-☑ | C79.51 | — | D16.3-☑ | — | — |
| calvarium | C41.Ø | C79.51 | — | D16.4 | D48.Ø | D49.2 |
| carpus (any) | C4Ø.1-☑ | C79.51 | — | D16.1-☑ | — | — |
| cartilage NEC | C41.9 | C79.51 | — | D16.9 | D48.Ø | D49.2 |
| clavicle | C41.3 | C79.51 | — | D16.7 | D48.Ø | D49.2 |
| clivus | C41.Ø | C79.51 | — | D16.4 | D48.Ø | D49.2 |
| coccygeal vertebra | C41.4 | C79.51 | — | D16.8 | D48.Ø | D49.2 |
| coccyx | C41.4 | C79.51 | — | D16.8 | D48.Ø | D49.2 |
| costal cartilage | C41.3 | C79.51 | — | D16.7 | D48.Ø | D49.2 |
| costovertebral joint | C41.3 | C79.51 | — | D16.7 | D48.Ø | D49.2 |
| cranial | C41.Ø | C79.51 | — | D16.4 | D48.Ø | D49.2 |
| cuboid | C4Ø.3-☑ | C79.51 | — | D16.3-☑ | — | — |
| cuneiform | C41.9 | C79.51 | — | D16.9 | D48.Ø | D49.2 |
| elbow | C4Ø.Ø-☑ | C79.51 | — | D16.Ø-☑ | — | — |
| ethmoid (labyrinth) | C41.Ø | C79.51 | — | D16.4 | D48.Ø | D49.2 |
| face | C41.Ø | C79.51 | — | D16.4 | D48.Ø | D49.2 |
| femur (any part) | C4Ø.2-☑ | C79.51 | — | D16.2-☑ | — | — |
| fibula (any part) | C4Ø.2-☑ | C79.51 | — | D16.2-☑ | — | — |
| finger (any) | C4Ø.1-☑ | C79.51 | — | D16.1-☑ | — | — |
| foot | C4Ø.3-☑ | C79.51 | — | D16.3-☑ | — | — |
| forearm | C4Ø.Ø-☑ | C79.51 | — | D16.Ø-☑ | — | — |
| frontal | C41.Ø | C79.51 | — | D16.4 | D48.Ø | D49.2 |
| hand | C4Ø.1-☑ | C79.51 | — | D16.1-☑ | — | — |
| heel | C4Ø.3-☑ | C79.51 | — | D16.3-☑ | — | — |
| hip | C41.4 | C79.51 | — | D16.8 | D48.Ø | D49.2 |
| humerus (any part) | C4Ø.Ø-☑ | C79.51 | — | D16.Ø-☑ | — | — |
| hyoid | C41.Ø | C79.51 | — | D16.4 | D48.Ø | D49.2 |
| ilium | C41.4 | C79.51 | — | D16.8 | D48.Ø | D49.2 |
| innominate | C41.4 | C79.51 | — | D16.8 | D48.Ø | D49.2 |
| intervertebral cartilage or disc | C41.2 | C79.51 | — | D16.6 | D48.Ø | D49.2 |
| ischium | C41.4 | C79.51 | — | D16.8 | D48.Ø | D49.2 |
| jaw (lower) | C41.1 | C79.51 | — | D16.5 | D48.Ø | D49.2 |
| knee | C4Ø.2-☑ | C79.51 | — | D16.2-☑ | — | — |
| leg NEC | C4Ø.2-☑ | C79.51 | — | D16.2-☑ | — | — |
| limb NEC | C4Ø.9-☑ | C79.51 | — | D16.9 | — | — |
| lower (long bones) | C4Ø.2-☑ | C79.51 | — | D16.2-☑ | — | — |
| short bones | C4Ø.3-☑ | C79.51 | — | D16.3-☑ | — | — |
| upper (long bones) | C4Ø.Ø-☑ | C79.51 | — | D16.Ø-☑ | — | — |
| short bones | C4Ø.1-☑ | C79.51 | — | D16.1-☑ | — | — |
| malar | C41.Ø | C79.51 | — | D16.4 | D48.Ø | D49.2 |
| mandible | C41.1 | C79.51 | — | D16.5 | D48.Ø | D49.2 |
| marrow NEC (any bone) | C96.9 | C79.52 | — | — | D47.9 | D49.89 |
| mastoid | C41.Ø | C79.51 | — | D16.4 | D48.Ø | D49.2 |
| maxilla, maxillary (superior) | C41.Ø | C79.51 | — | D16.4 | D48.Ø | D49.2 |
| inferior | C41.1 | C79.51 | — | D16.5 | D48.Ø | D49.2 |

| | Malignant Primary | Malignant Secondary | Ca in situ | Benign | Uncertain Behavior | Unspecified Behavior |
|---|---|---|---|---|---|---|
| **Neoplasm, neoplastic** — *continued* | | | | | | |
| bone — *continued* | | | | | | |
| metacarpus (any) | C4Ø.1-☑ | C79.51 | — | D16.1-☑ | — | — |
| metatarsus (any) | C4Ø.3-☑ | C79.51 | — | D16.3-☑ | — | — |
| navicular | | | | | | |
| ankle | C4Ø.3-☑ | C79.51 | — | — | — | — |
| hand | C4Ø.1-☑ | C79.51 | — | — | — | — |
| nose, nasal | C41.Ø | C79.51 | — | D16.4 | D48.Ø | D49.2 |
| occipital | C41.Ø | C79.51 | — | D16.4 | D48.Ø | D49.2 |
| orbit | C41.Ø | C79.51 | — | D16.4 | D48.Ø | D49.2 |
| overlapping sites | C4Ø.8-☑ | — | — | — | — | — |
| parietal | C41.Ø | C79.51 | — | D16.4 | D48.Ø | D49.2 |
| patella | C4Ø.2-☑ | C79.51 | — | — | — | — |
| pelvic | C41.4 | C79.51 | — | D16.8 | D48.Ø | D49.2 |
| phalanges | | | | | | |
| foot | C4Ø.3-☑ | C79.51 | — | — | — | — |
| hand | C4Ø.1-☑ | C79.51 | — | — | — | — |
| pubic | C41.4 | C79.51 | — | D16.8 | D48.Ø | D49.2 |
| radius (any part) | C4Ø.Ø-☑ | C79.51 | — | D16.Ø-☑ | — | — |
| rib | C41.3 | C79.51 | — | D16.7 | D48.Ø | D49.2 |
| sacral vertebra | C41.4 | C79.51 | — | D16.8 | D48.Ø | D49.2 |
| sacrum | C41.4 | C79.51 | — | D16.8 | D48.Ø | D49.2 |
| scaphoid | | | | | | |
| of ankle | C4Ø.3-☑ | C79.51 | — | — | — | — |
| of hand | C4Ø.1-☑ | C79.51 | — | — | — | — |
| scapula (any part) | C4Ø.Ø-☑ | C79.51 | — | D16.Ø-☑ | — | — |
| sella turcica | C41.Ø | C79.51 | — | D16.4 | D48.Ø | D49.2 |
| shoulder | C4Ø.Ø-☑ | C79.51 | — | D16.Ø-☑ | — | — |
| skull | C41.Ø | C79.51 | — | D16.4 | D48.Ø | D49.2 |
| sphenoid | C41.Ø | C79.51 | — | D16.4 | D48.Ø | D49.2 |
| spine, spinal (column) | C41.2 | C79.51 | — | D16.6 | D48.Ø | D49.2 |
| coccyx | C41.4 | C79.51 | — | D16.8 | D48.Ø | D49.2 |
| sacrum | C41.4 | C79.51 | — | D16.8 | D48.Ø | D49.2 |
| sternum | C41.3 | C79.51 | — | D16.7 | D48.Ø | D49.2 |
| tarsus (any) | C4Ø.3-☑ | C79.51 | — | — | — | — |
| temporal | C41.Ø | C79.51 | — | D16.4 | D48.Ø | D49.2 |
| thumb | C4Ø.1-☑ | C79.51 | — | — | — | — |
| tibia (any part) | C4Ø.2-☑ | C79.51 | — | — | — | — |
| toe (any) | C4Ø.3-☑ | C79.51 | — | — | — | — |
| trapezium | C4Ø.1-☑ | C79.51 | — | — | — | — |
| trapezoid | C4Ø.1-☑ | C79.51 | — | — | — | — |
| turbinate | C41.Ø | C79.51 | — | D16.4 | D48.Ø | D49.2 |
| ulna (any part) | C4Ø.Ø-☑ | C79.51 | — | D16.Ø-☑ | — | — |
| unciform | C4Ø.1-☑ | C79.51 | — | — | — | — |
| vertebra (column) | C41.2 | C79.51 | — | D16.6 | D48.Ø | D49.2 |
| coccyx | C41.4 | C79.51 | — | D16.8 | D48.Ø | D49.2 |
| sacrum | C41.4 | C79.51 | — | D16.8 | D48.Ø | D49.2 |
| vomer | C41.Ø | C79.51 | — | D16.4 | D48.Ø | D49.2 |
| wrist | C4Ø.1-☑ | C79.51 | — | — | — | — |
| xiphoid process | C41.3 | C79.51 | — | D16.7 | D48.Ø | D49.2 |
| zygomatic | C41.Ø | C79.51 | — | D16.4 | D48.Ø | D49.2 |
| book-leaf (mouth) — *ventral surface of tongue and floor of mouth* | CØ6.89 | C79.89 | DØØ.ØØ | D1Ø.39 | D37.Ø9 | D49.Ø |
| bowel — *see* Neoplasm, intestine | | | | | | |
| brachial plexus | C47.1-☑ | C79.89 | — | D36.12 | D48.2 | D49.2 |
| brain NEC | C71.9 | C79.31 | — | D33.2 | D43.2 | D49.6 |
| basal ganglia | C71.Ø | C79.31 | — | D33.Ø | D43.Ø | D49.6 |
| cerebellopontine angle | C71.6 | C79.31 | — | D33.1 | D43.1 | D49.6 |
| cerebellum NOS | C71.6 | C79.31 | — | D33.1 | D43.1 | D49.6 |
| cerebrum | C71.Ø | C79.31 | — | D33.Ø | D43.Ø | D49.6 |
| choroid plexus | C71.7 | C79.31 | — | D33.1 | D43.1 | D49.6 |
| corpus callosum | C71.8 | C79.31 | — | D33.2 | D43.2 | D49.6 |
| corpus striatum | C71.Ø | C79.31 | — | D33.Ø | D43.Ø | D49.6 |
| cortex (cerebral) | C71.Ø | C79.31 | — | D33.Ø | D43.Ø | D49.6 |
| frontal lobe | C71.1 | C79.31 | — | D33.Ø | D43.Ø | D49.6 |
| globus pallidus | C71.Ø | C79.31 | — | D33.Ø | D43.Ø | D49.6 |
| hippocampus | C71.2 | C79.31 | — | D33.Ø | D43.Ø | D49.6 |
| hypothalamus | C71.Ø | C79.31 | — | D33.Ø | D43.Ø | D49.6 |
| internal capsule | C71.Ø | C79.31 | — | D33.Ø | D43.Ø | D49.6 |

| | Malignant Primary | Malignant Secondary | Ca in situ | Benign | Uncertain Behavior | Unspecified Behavior |
|---|---|---|---|---|---|---|
| **Neoplasm, neoplastic** *— continued* | | | | | | |
| brain *— continued* | | | | | | |
| medulla oblongata | C71.7 | C79.31 | — | D33.1 | D43.1 | D49.6 |
| meninges | C7Ø.Ø | C79.32 | — | D32.Ø | D42.Ø | D49.7 |
| midbrain | C71.7 | C79.31 | — | D33.1 | D43.1 | D49.6 |
| occipital lobe | C71.4 | C79.31 | — | D33.Ø | D43.Ø | D49.6 |
| overlapping lesion | C71.8 | C79.31 | — | — | — | — |
| parietal lobe | C71.3 | C79.31 | — | D33.Ø | D43.Ø | D49.6 |
| peduncle | C71.7 | C79.31 | — | D33.1 | D43.1 | D49.6 |
| pons | C71.7 | C79.31 | — | D33.1 | D43.1 | D49.6 |
| stem | C71.7 | C79.31 | — | D33.1 | D43.1 | D49.6 |
| tapetum | C71.8 | C79.31 | — | D33.2 | D43.2 | D49.6 |
| temporal lobe | C71.2 | C79.31 | — | D33.Ø | D43.Ø | D49.6 |
| thalamus | C71.Ø | C79.31 | — | D33.Ø | D43.Ø | D49.6 |
| uncus | C71.2 | C79.31 | — | D33.Ø | D43.Ø | D49.6 |
| ventricle (floor) | C71.5 | C79.31 | — | D33.Ø | D43.Ø | D49.6 |
| fourth | C71.7 | C79.31 | — | D33.1 | D43.1 | D49.6 |
| branchial (cleft) (cyst) (vestiges) | C1Ø.4 | C79.89 | DØØ.Ø8 | D1Ø.5 | D37.Ø5 | D49.Ø |
| breast (connective tissue) (glandular tissue) (soft parts) | C5Ø.9-☑ | C79.81 | DØ5.-☑ | D24.-☑ | D48.6-☑ | D49.3 |
| areola | C5Ø.Ø-☑ | C79.81 | DØ5.-☑ | D24.-☑ | D48.6-☑ | D49.3 |
| axillary tail | C5Ø.6-☑ | C79.81 | DØ5.-☑ | D24.-☑ | D48.6-☑ | D49.3 |
| central portion | C5Ø.1-☑ | C79.81 | DØ5.-☑ | D24.-☑ | D48.6-☑ | D49.3 |
| inflammatory | C5Ø.A-☑ | — | — | — | — | — |
| inner | C5Ø.8-☑ | C79.81 | DØ5.-☑ | D24.-☑ | D48.6-☑ | D49.3 |
| lower | C5Ø.8-☑ | C79.81 | DØ5.-☑ | D24.-☑ | D48.6-☑ | D49.3 |
| lower-inner quadrant | C5Ø.3-☑ | C79.81 | DØ5.-☑ | D24.-☑ | D48.6-☑ | D49.3 |
| lower-outer quadrant | C5Ø.5-☑ | C79.81 | DØ5.-☑ | D24.-☑ | D48.6-☑ | D49.3 |
| mastectomy site (skin) *— see also* Neoplasm, breast, skin | C44.5Ø1 | C79.2 | — | — | — | — |
| specified as breast tissue | C5Ø.8-☑ | C79.81 | — | — | — | — |
| midline | C5Ø.8-☑ | C79.81 | DØ5.-☑ | D24.-☑ | D48.6-☑ | D49.3 |
| nipple | C5Ø.Ø-☑ | C79.81 | DØ5.-☑ | D24.-☑ | D48.6-☑ | D49.3 |
| outer | C5Ø.8-☑ | C79.81 | DØ5.-☑ | D24.-☑ | D48.6-☑ | D49.3 |
| overlapping lesion | C5Ø.8-☑ | — | — | — | — | — |
| skin | C44.5Ø1 | C79.2 | DØ4.5 | D23.5 | D48.5 | D49.2 |
| basal cell carcinoma | C44.511 | — | — | — | — | — |
| specified type NEC | C44.591 | — | — | — | — | — |
| squamous cell carcinoma | C44.521 | — | — | — | — | — |
| tail (axillary) | C5Ø.6-☑ | C79.81 | DØ5.-☑ | D24.-☑ | D48.6-☑ | D49.3 |
| upper | C5Ø.8-☑ | C79.81 | DØ5.-☑ | D24.-☑ | D48.6-☑ | D49.3 |
| upper-inner quadrant | C5Ø.2-☑ | C79.81 | DØ5.-☑ | D24.-☑ | D48.6-☑ | D49.3 |
| upper-outer quadrant | C5Ø.4-☑ | C79.81 | DØ5.-☑ | D24.-☑ | D48.6-☑ | D49.3 |
| broad ligament | C57.1-☑ | C79.82 | DØ7.39 | D28.2 | D39.8 | D49.59 |
| bronchiogenic, bronchogenic (lung) | C34.9-☑ | C78.Ø-☑ | DØ2.2-☑ | D14.3-☑ | D38.1 | D49.1 |
| bronchiole | C34.9-☑ | C78.Ø-☑ | DØ2.2-☑ | D14.3-☑ | D38.1 | D49.1 |
| bronchus | C34.9-☑ | C78.Ø-☑ | DØ2.2-☑ | D14.3-☑ | D38.1 | D49.1 |
| carina | C34.Ø-☑ | C78.Ø-☑ | DØ2.2-☑ | D14.3-☑ | D38.1 | D49.1 |
| lower lobe of lung | C34.3-☑ | C78.Ø-☑ | DØ2.2-☑ | D14.3-☑ | D38.1 | D49.1 |
| main | C34.Ø-☑ | C78.Ø-☑ | DØ2.2-☑ | D14.3-☑ | D38.1 | D49.1 |
| middle lobe of lung | C34.2 | C78.Ø-☑ | DØ2.21 | D14.31 | D38.1 | D49.1 |
| overlapping lesion | C34.8-☑ | — | — | — | — | — |
| upper lobe of lung | C34.1-☑ | C78.Ø-☑ | DØ2.2-☑ | D14.3-☑ | D38.1 | D49.1 |
| brow | C44.3Ø9 | C79.2 | DØ4.39 | D23.39 | D48.5 | D49.2 |
| basal cell carcinoma | C44.319 | — | — | — | — | — |
| specified type NEC | C44.399 | — | — | — | — | — |

| | Malignant Primary | Malignant Secondary | Ca in situ | Benign | Uncertain Behavior | Unspecified Behavior |
|---|---|---|---|---|---|---|
| **Neoplasm, neoplastic** *— continued* | | | | | | |
| brow *— continued* | | | | | | |
| squamous cell carcinoma | C44.329 | — | — | — | — | — |
| buccal (cavity) | CØ6.9 | C79.89 | DØØ.ØØ | D1Ø.39 | D37.Ø9 | D49.Ø |
| commissure | CØ6.Ø | C79.89 | DØØ.Ø2 | D1Ø.39 | D37.Ø9 | D49.Ø |
| groove (lower) (upper) | CØ6.1 | C79.89 | DØØ.Ø2 | D1Ø.39 | D37.Ø9 | D49.Ø |
| mucosa | CØ6.Ø | C79.89 | DØØ.Ø2 | D1Ø.39 | D37.Ø9 | D49.Ø |
| sulcus (lower) (upper) | CØ6.1 | C79.89 | DØØ.Ø2 | D1Ø.39 | D37.Ø9 | D49.Ø |
| bulbourethral gland | C68.Ø | C79.19 | DØ9.19 | D3Ø.4 | D41.3 | D49.59 |
| bursa *— see* Neoplasm, connective tissue | | | | | | |
| buttock NEC | C76.3 | C79.89 | DØ4.5 | D36.7 | D48.7 | D49.89 |
| calf | C76.5-☑ | C79.89 | DØ4.7-☑ | D36.7 | D48.7 | D49.89 |
| calvarium | C41.Ø | C79.51 | — | D16.4 | D48.Ø | D49.2 |
| calyx, renal | C65.-☑ | C79.Ø-☑ | DØ9.19 | D3Ø.1-☑ | D41.1-☑ | D49.51-☑ |
| canal | | | | | | |
| anal | C21.1 | C78.5 | DØ1.3 | D12.9 | D37.8 | D49.Ø |
| auditory (external) *— see also* Neoplasm, skin, ear | C44.2Ø-☑ | C79.2 | DØ4.2-☑ | D23.2-☑ | D48.5 | D49.2 |
| auricular (external) *— see also* Neoplasm, skin, ear | C44.2Ø-☑ | C79.2 | DØ4.2-☑ | D23.2-☑ | D48.5 | D49.2 |
| canaliculi, biliary (biliferi) (intrahepatic) | C22.1 | C78.7 | DØ1.5 | D13.4 | D37.6 | D49.Ø |
| canthus (eye) (inner) (outer) | C44.1Ø-☑ | C79.2 | DØ4.1-☑ | D23.1-☑ | D48.5 | D49.2 |
| basal cell carcinoma | C44.11-☑ | — | — | — | — | — |
| sebaceous cell | C44.13-☑ | — | — | — | — | — |
| specified type NEC | C44.19-☑ | — | — | — | — | — |
| squamous cell carcinoma | C44.12-☑ | — | — | — | — | — |
| capillary *— see* Neoplasm, connective tissue | | | | | | |
| caput coli | C18.Ø | C78.5 | DØ1.Ø | D12.Ø | D37.4 | D49.Ø |
| carcinoid *— see* Tumor, carcinoid | | | | | | |
| cardia (gastric) | C16.Ø | C78.89 | DØØ.2 | D13.1 | D37.1 | D49.Ø |
| cardiac orifice (stomach) | C16.Ø | C78.89 | DØØ.2 | D13.1 | D37.1 | D49.Ø |
| cardio-esophageal junction | C16.Ø | C78.89 | DØØ.2 | D13.1 | D37.1 | D49.Ø |
| cardio-esophagus | C16.Ø | C78.89 | DØØ.2 | D13.1 | D37.1 | D49.Ø |
| carina (bronchus) | C34.Ø-☑ | C78.Ø-☑ | DØ2.2-☑ | D14.3-☑ | D38.1 | D49.1 |
| carotid (artery) | C49.Ø | C79.89 | — | D21.Ø | D48.1-☑ | D49.2 |
| body | C75.4 | C79.89 | — | D35.5 | D44.6 | D49.7 |
| carpus (any bone) | C4Ø.1-☑ | C79.51 | — | D16.1-☑ | — | — |
| cartilage (articular) (joint) NEC *— see also* Neoplasm, bone | C41.9 | C79.51 | — | D16.9 | D48.Ø | D49.2 |
| arytenoid | C32.3 | C78.31 | DØ2.Ø | D14.1 | D38.Ø | D49.1 |
| auricular | C49.Ø | C79.89 | — | D21.Ø | D48.1-☑ | D49.2 |
| bronchi | C34.Ø-☑ | C78.39 | — | D14.3-☑ | D38.1 | D49.1 |
| costal | C41.3 | C79.51 | — | D16.7 | D48.Ø | D49.2 |
| cricoid | C32.3 | C78.31 | DØ2.Ø | D14.1 | D38.Ø | D49.1 |
| cuneiform | C32.3 | C78.31 | DØ2.Ø | D14.1 | D38.Ø | D49.1 |
| ear (external) | C49.Ø | C79.89 | — | D21.Ø | D48.1-☑ | D49.2 |
| ensiform | C41.3 | C79.51 | — | D16.7 | D48.Ø | D49.2 |
| epiglottis | C32.1 | C78.31 | DØ2.Ø | D14.1 | D38.Ø | D49.1 |
| anterior surface | C1Ø.1 | C79.89 | DØØ.Ø8 | D1Ø.5 | D37.Ø5 | D49.Ø |
| eyelid | C49.Ø | C79.89 | — | D21.Ø | D48.1-☑ | D49.2 |
| intervertebral | C41.2 | C79.51 | — | D16.6 | D48.Ø | D49.2 |
| larynx, laryngeal | C32.3 | C78.31 | DØ2.Ø | D14.1 | D38.Ø | D49.1 |
| nose, nasal | C3Ø.Ø | C78.39 | DØ2.3 | D14.Ø | D38.5 | D49.1 |
| pinna | C49.Ø | C79.89 | — | D21.Ø | D48.1-☑ | D49.2 |
| rib | C41.3 | C79.51 | — | D16.7 | D48.Ø | D49.2 |
| semilunar (knee) | C4Ø.2-☑ | C79.51 | — | D16.2-☑ | D48.Ø | D49.2 |
| thyroid | C32.3 | C78.39 | DØ2.Ø | D14.1 | D38.Ø | D49.1 |
| trachea | C33 | C78.39 | DØ2.1 | D14.2 | D38.1 | D49.1 |

| | Malignant Primary | Malignant Secondary | Ca in situ | Benign | Uncertain Behavior | Unspecified Behavior |
|---|---|---|---|---|---|---|
| **Neoplasm, neoplastic** — *continued* | | | | | | |
| cauda equina | C72.1 | C79.49 | — | D33.4 | D43.4 | D49.7 |
| cavity | | | | | | |
| buccal | CØ6.9 | C79.89 | DØØ.ØØ | D1Ø.3Ø | D37.Ø9 | D49.Ø |
| nasal | C3Ø.Ø | C78.39 | DØ2.3 | D14.Ø | D38.5 | D49.1 |
| oral | CØ6.9 | C79.89 | DØØ.ØØ | D1Ø.3Ø | D37.Ø9 | D49.Ø |
| peritoneal | C48.2 | C78.6 | — | D2Ø.1 | D48.4 | D49.Ø |
| tympanic | C3Ø.1 | C78.39 | DØ2.3 | D14.Ø | D38.5 | D49.1 |
| cecum | C18.Ø | C78.5 | DØ1.Ø | D12.Ø | D37.4 | D49.Ø |
| central nervous system | C72.9 | C79.4Ø | — | — | — | — |
| cerebellopontine (angle) | C71.6 | C79.31 | — | D33.1 | D43.1 | D49.6 |
| cerebellum, cerebellar | C71.6 | C79.31 | — | D33.1 | D43.1 | D49.6 |
| cerebrum, cerebral (cortex) (hemisphere) (white matter) | C71.Ø | C79.31 | — | D33.Ø | D43.Ø | D49.6 |
| meninges | C7Ø.Ø | C79.32 | — | D32.Ø | D42.Ø | D49.7 |
| peduncle | C71.7 | C79.31 | — | D33.1 | D43.1 | D49.6 |
| ventricle | C71.5 | C79.31 | — | D33.Ø | D43.Ø | D49.6 |
| fourth | C71.7 | C79.31 | — | D33.1 | D43.1 | D49.6 |
| cervical region | C76.Ø | C79.89 | DØ9.8 | D36.7 | D48.7 | D49.89 |
| cervix (cervical) (uteri) (uterus) | C53.9 | C79.82 | DØ6.9 | D26.Ø | D39.Ø | D49.59 |
| canal | C53.Ø | C79.82 | DØ6.Ø | D26.Ø | D39.Ø | D49.59 |
| endocervix (canal) (gland) | C53.Ø | C79.82 | DØ6.Ø | D26.Ø | D39.Ø | D49.59 |
| exocervix | C53.1 | C79.82 | DØ6.1 | D26.Ø | D39.Ø | D49.59 |
| external os | C53.1 | C79.82 | DØ6.1 | D26.Ø | D39.Ø | D49.59 |
| internal os | C53.Ø | C79.82 | DØ6.Ø | D26.Ø | D39.Ø | D49.59 |
| nabothian gland | C53.Ø | C79.82 | DØ6.Ø | D26.Ø | D39.Ø | D49.59 |
| overlapping lesion | C53.8 | — | — | — | — | — |
| squamocolumnar junction | C53.8 | C79.82 | DØ6.7 | D26.Ø | D39.Ø | D49.59 |
| stump | C53.8 | C79.82 | DØ6.7 | D26.Ø | D39.Ø | D49.59 |
| cheek | C76.Ø | C79.89 | DØ9.8 | D36.7 | D48.7 | D49.89 |
| external | C44.3Ø9 | C79.2 | DØ4.39 | D23.39 | D48.5 | D49.2 |
| basal cell carcinoma | C44.319 | — | — | — | — | — |
| specified type NEC | C44.399 | — | — | — | — | — |
| squamous cell carcinoma | C44.329 | — | — | — | — | — |
| inner aspect | CØ6.Ø | C79.89 | DØØ.Ø2 | D1Ø.39 | D37.Ø9 | D49.Ø |
| internal | CØ6.Ø | C79.89 | DØØ.Ø2 | D1Ø.39 | D37.Ø9 | D49.Ø |
| mucosa | CØ6.Ø | C79.89 | DØØ.Ø2 | D1Ø.39 | D37.Ø9 | D49.Ø |
| chest (wall) NEC | C76.1 | C79.89 | DØ9.8 | D36.7 | D48.7 | D49.89 |
| chiasma opticum | C72.3-☑ | C79.49 | — | D33.3 | D43.3 | D49.7 |
| chin | C44.3Ø9 | C79.2 | DØ4.39 | D23.39 | D48.5 | D49.2 |
| basal cell carcinoma | C44.319 | — | — | — | — | — |
| specified type NEC | C44.399 | — | — | — | — | — |
| squamous cell carcinoma | C44.329 | — | — | — | — | — |
| choana | C11.3 | C79.89 | DØØ.Ø8 | D1Ø.6 | D37.Ø5 | D49.Ø |
| cholangiole | C22.1 | C78.89 | DØ1.5 | D13.4 | D37.6 | D49.Ø |
| choledochal duct | C24.Ø | C78.89 | DØ1.5 | D13.5 | D37.6 | D49.Ø |
| choroid | C69.3-☑ | C79.49 | DØ9.2-☑ | D31.3-☑ | D48.7 | D49.81 |
| plexus | C71.5 | C79.31 | — | D33.Ø | D43.Ø | D49.6 |
| ciliary body | C69.4-☑ | C79.49 | DØ9.2-☑ | D31.4-☑ | D48.7 | D49.89 |
| clavicle | C41.3 | C79.51 | — | D16.7 | D48.Ø | D49.2 |
| clitoris | C51.2 | C79.82 | DØ7.1 | D28.Ø | D39.8 | D49.59 |
| clivus | C41.Ø | C79.51 | — | D16.4 | D48.Ø | D49.2 |
| cloacogenic zone | C21.2 | C78.5 | DØ1.3 | D12.9 | D37.8 | D49.Ø |
| coccygeal | | | | | | |
| body or glomus | C49.5 | C79.89 | — | D21.5 | D48.1-☑ | D49.2 |
| vertebra | C41.4 | C79.51 | — | D16.8 | D48.Ø | D49.2 |
| coccyx | C41.4 | C79.51 | — | D16.8 | D48.Ø | D49.2 |
| colon — *see also* Neoplasm, intestine, large | C18.9 | C78.5 | — | — | — | — |
| with rectum | C19 | C78.5 | DØ1.1 | D12.7 | D37.5 | D49.Ø |
| column, spinal — *see* Neoplasm, spine | | | | | | |
| columnella — *see also* Neoplasm, skin, face | C44.39Ø | C79.2 | DØ4.39 | D23.39 | D48.5 | D49.2 |

| | Malignant Primary | Malignant Secondary | Ca in situ | Benign | Uncertain Behavior | Unspecified Behavior |
|---|---|---|---|---|---|---|
| **Neoplasm, neoplastic** — *continued* | | | | | | |
| commissure | | | | | | |
| labial, lip | CØØ.6 | C79.89 | DØØ.Ø1 | D1Ø.39 | D37.Ø1 | D49.Ø |
| laryngeal | C32.Ø | C78.31 | DØ2.Ø | D14.1 | D38.Ø | D49.1 |
| common (bile) duct | C24.Ø | C78.89 | DØ1.5 | D13.5 | D37.6 | D49.Ø |
| concha — *see also* Neoplasm, skin, ear | C44.2Ø-☑ | C79.2 | DØ4.2-☑ | D23.2-☑ | D48.5 | D49.2 |
| nose | C3Ø.Ø | C78.39 | DØ2.3 | D14.Ø | D38.5 | D49.1 |
| conjunctiva | C69.Ø-☑ | C79.49 | DØ9.2-☑ | D31.Ø-☑ | D48.7 | D49.89 |
| connective tissue NEC | C49.9 | C79.89 | — | D21.9 | D48.1-☑ | D49.2 |

Note: For neoplasms of connective tissue (blood vessel, bursa, fascia, ligament, muscle, peripheral nerves, sympathetic and parasympathetic nerves and ganglia, synovia, tendon, etc.) or of morphological types that indicate connective tissue, code according to the list under "Neoplasm, connective tissue". For sites that do not appear in this list, code to neoplasm of that site; e.g., fibrosarcoma, pancreas (C25.9)

Note: Morphological types that indicate connective tissue appear in their proper place in the alphabetic index with the instruction "see Neoplasm, connective tissue ...."

| | Malignant Primary | Malignant Secondary | Ca in situ | Benign | Uncertain Behavior | Unspecified Behavior |
|---|---|---|---|---|---|---|
| abdomen | C49.4 | C79.89 | — | D21.4 | D48.1-☑ | D49.2 |
| abdominal wall | C49.4 | C79.89 | — | D21.4 | D48.1-☑ | D49.2 |
| ankle | C49.2-☑ | C79.89 | — | D21.2-☑ | D48.1-☑ | D49.2 |
| antecubital fossa or space | C49.1-☑ | C79.89 | — | D21.1-☑ | D48.1-☑ | D49.2 |
| arm | C49.1-☑ | C79.89 | — | D21.1-☑ | D48.1-☑ | D49.2 |
| auricle (ear) | C49.Ø | C79.89 | — | D21.Ø | D48.1-☑ | D49.2 |
| axilla | C49.3 | C79.89 | — | D21.3 | D48.1-☑ | D49.2 |
| back | C49.6 | C79.89 | — | D21.6 | D48.1-☑ | D49.2 |
| breast — *see* Neoplasm, breast | | | | | | |
| buttock | C49.5 | C79.89 | — | D21.5 | D48.1-☑ | D49.2 |
| calf | C49.2-☑ | C79.89 | — | D21.2-☑ | D48.1-☑ | D49.2 |
| cervical region | C49.Ø | C79.89 | — | D21.Ø | D48.1-☑ | D49.2 |
| cheek | C49.Ø | C79.89 | — | D21.Ø | D48.1-☑ | D49.2 |
| chest (wall) | C49.3 | C79.89 | — | D21.3 | D48.1-☑ | D49.2 |
| chin | C49.Ø | C79.89 | — | D21.Ø | D48.1-☑ | D49.2 |
| diaphragm | C49.3 | C79.89 | — | D21.3 | D48.1-☑ | D49.2 |
| ear (external) | C49.Ø | C79.89 | — | D21.Ø | D48.1-☑ | D49.2 |
| elbow | C49.1-☑ | C79.89 | — | D21.1-☑ | D48.1-☑ | D49.2 |
| extrarectal | C49.5 | C79.89 | — | D21.5 | D48.1-☑ | D49.2 |
| extremity | C49.9 | C79.89 | — | D21.9 | D48.1-☑ | D49.2 |
| lower | C49.2-☑ | C79.89 | — | D21.2-☑ | D48.1-☑ | D49.2 |
| upper | C49.1-☑ | C79.89 | — | D21.1-☑ | D48.1-☑ | D49.2 |
| eyelid | C49.Ø | C79.89 | — | D21.Ø | D48.1-☑ | D49.2 |
| face | C49.Ø | C79.89 | — | D21.Ø | D48.1-☑ | D49.2 |
| finger | C49.1-☑ | C79.89 | — | D21.1-☑ | D48.1-☑ | D49.2 |
| flank | C49.6 | C79.89 | — | D21.6 | D48.1-☑ | D49.2 |
| foot | C49.2-☑ | C79.89 | — | D21.2-☑ | D48.1-☑ | D49.2 |
| forearm | C49.1-☑ | C79.89 | — | D21.1-☑ | D48.1-☑ | D49.2 |
| forehead | C49.Ø | C79.89 | — | D21.Ø | D48.1-☑ | D49.2 |
| gastric | C49.4 | C79.89 | — | D21.4 | D48.1-☑ | D49.2 |
| gastrointestinal | C49.4 | C79.89 | — | D21.4 | D48.1-☑ | D49.2 |
| gluteal region | C49.5 | C79.89 | — | D21.5 | D48.1-☑ | D49.2 |
| great vessels NEC | C49.3 | C79.89 | — | D21.3 | D48.1-☑ | D49.2 |
| groin | C49.5 | C79.89 | — | D21.5 | D48.1-☑ | D49.2 |
| hand | C49.1-☑ | C79.89 | — | D21.1-☑ | D48.1-☑ | D49.2 |
| head | C49.Ø | C79.89 | — | D21.Ø | D48.1-☑ | D49.2 |
| heel | C49.2-☑ | C79.89 | — | D21.2-☑ | D48.1-☑ | D49.2 |
| hip | C49.2-☑ | C79.89 | — | D21.2-☑ | D48.1-☑ | D49.2 |
| hypochondrium | C49.4 | C79.89 | — | D21.4 | D48.1-☑ | D49.2 |
| iliopsoas muscle | C49.5 | C79.89 | — | D21.5 | D48.1-☑ | D49.2 |
| infraclavicular region | C49.3 | C79.89 | — | D21.3 | D48.1-☑ | D49.2 |
| inguinal (canal) (region) | C49.5 | C79.89 | — | D21.5 | D48.1-☑ | D49.2 |
| intestinal | C49.4 | C79.89 | — | D21.4 | D48.1-☑ | D49.2 |
| intrathoracic | C49.3 | C79.89 | — | D21.3 | D48.1-☑ | D49.2 |
| ischiorectal fossa | C49.5 | C79.89 | — | D21.5 | D48.1-☑ | D49.2 |
| jaw | CØ3.9 | C79.89 | DØØ.Ø3 | D1Ø.39 | D48.1-☑ | D49.Ø |
| knee | C49.2-☑ | C79.89 | — | D21.2-☑ | D48.1-☑ | D49.2 |

| | Malignant Primary | Malignant Secondary | Ca in situ | Benign | Uncertain Behavior | Unspecified Behavior |
|---|---|---|---|---|---|---|
| **Neoplasm, neoplastic** — *continued* | | | | | | |
| connective tissue — *continued* | | | | | | |
| leg | C49.2-☑ | C79.89 | — | D21.2-☑ | D48.1-☑ | D49.2 |
| limb NEC | C49.9 | C79.89 | — | D21.9 | D48.1-☑ | D49.2 |
| lower | C49.2-☑ | C79.89 | — | D21.2-☑ | D48.1-☑ | D49.2 |
| upper | C49.1-☑ | C79.89 | — | D21.1-☑ | D48.1-☑ | D49.2 |
| nates | C49.5 | C79.89 | — | D21.5 | D48.1-☑ | D49.2 |
| neck | C49.0 | C79.89 | — | D21.0 | D48.1-☑ | D49.2 |
| orbit | C69.6-☑ | C79.49 | D09.2-☑ | D31.6-☑ | D48.1-☑ | D49.89 |
| overlapping lesion | C49.8 | — | — | — | — | — |
| para-urethral | C49.5 | C79.89 | — | D21.5 | D48.1-☑ | D49.2 |
| pararectal | C49.5 | C79.89 | — | D21.5 | D48.1-☑ | D49.2 |
| paravaginal | C49.5 | C79.89 | — | D21.5 | D48.1-☑ | D49.2 |
| pelvis (floor) | C49.5 | C79.89 | — | D21.5 | D48.1-☑ | D49.2 |
| pelvo-abdominal | C49.8 | C79.89 | — | D21.6 | D48.1-☑ | D49.2 |
| perineum | C49.5 | C79.89 | — | D21.5 | D48.1-☑ | D49.2 |
| perirectal (tissue) | C49.5 | C79.89 | — | D21.5 | D48.1-☑ | D49.2 |
| periurethral (tissue) | C49.5 | C79.89 | — | D21.5 | D48.1-☑ | D49.2 |
| popliteal fossa or space | C49.2-☑ | C79.89 | — | D21.2-☑ | D48.1-☑ | D49.2 |
| presacral | C49.5 | C79.89 | — | D21.5 | D48.1-☑ | D49.2 |
| psoas muscle | C49.4 | C79.89 | — | D21.4 | D48.1-☑ | D49.2 |
| pterygoid fossa | C49.0 | C79.89 | — | D21.0 | D48.1-☑ | D49.2 |
| rectovaginal septum or wall | C49.5 | C79.89 | — | D21.5 | D48.1-☑ | D49.2 |
| rectovesical | C49.5 | C79.89 | — | D21.5 | D48.1-☑ | D49.2 |
| retroperitoneum | C48.0 | C78.6 | — | D20.0 | D48.3 | D49.0 |
| sacrococcygeal region | C49.5 | C79.89 | — | D21.5 | D48.1-☑ | D49.2 |
| scalp | C49.0 | C79.89 | — | D21.0 | D48.1-☑ | D49.2 |
| scapular region | C49.3 | C79.89 | — | D21.3 | D48.1-☑ | D49.2 |
| shoulder | C49.1-☑ | C79.89 | — | D21.1-☑ | D48.1-☑ | D49.2 |
| skin (dermis) NEC — *see also* Neoplasm, skin, by site | C44.90 | C79.2 | D04.9 | D23.9 | D48.5 | D49.2 |
| stomach | C49.4 | C79.89 | — | D21.4 | D48.1-☑ | D49.2 |
| submental | C49.0 | C79.89 | — | D21.0 | D48.1-☑ | D49.2 |
| supraclavicular region | C49.0 | C79.89 | — | D21.0 | D48.1-☑ | D49.2 |
| temple | C49.0 | C79.89 | — | D21.0 | D48.1-☑ | D49.2 |
| temporal region | C49.0 | C79.89 | — | D21.0 | D48.1-☑ | D49.2 |
| thigh | C49.2-☑ | C79.89 | — | D21.2-☑ | D48.1-☑ | D49.2 |
| thoracic (duct) (wall) | C49.3 | C79.89 | — | D21.3 | D48.1-☑ | D49.2 |
| thorax | C49.3 | C79.89 | — | D21.3 | D48.1-☑ | D49.2 |
| thumb | C49.1-☑ | C79.89 | — | D21.1-☑ | D48.1-☑ | D49.2 |
| toe | C49.2-☑ | C79.89 | — | D21.2-☑ | D48.1-☑ | D49.2 |
| trunk | C49.6 | C79.89 | — | D21.6 | D48.1-☑ | D49.2 |
| umbilicus | C49.4 | C79.89 | — | D21.4 | D48.1-☑ | D49.2 |
| vesicorectal | C49.5 | C79.89 | — | D21.5 | D48.1-☑ | D49.2 |
| wrist | C49.1-☑ | C79.89 | — | D21.1-☑ | D48.1-☑ | D49.2 |
| conus medullaris | C72.0 | C79.49 | — | D33.4 | D43.4 | D49.7 |
| cord (true) (vocal) | C32.0 | C78.31 | D02.0 | D14.1 | D38.0 | D49.1 |
| false | C32.1 | C78.31 | D02.0 | D14.1 | D38.0 | D49.1 |
| spermatic | C63.1-☑ | C79.82 | D07.69 | D29.8 | D40.8 | D49.59 |
| spinal (cervical) (lumbar) (thoracic) | C72.0 | C79.49 | — | D33.4 | D43.4 | D49.7 |
| cornea (limbus) | C69.1-☑ | C79.49 | D09.2-☑ | D31.1-☑ | D48.7 | D49.89 |
| corpus | | | | | | |
| albicans | C56.-☑ | C79.6-☑ | D07.39 | D27.-☑ | D39.1-☑ | D49.59 |
| callosum, brain | C71.0 | C79.31 | — | D33.2 | D43.2 | D49.6 |
| cavernosum | C60.2 | C79.82 | D07.4 | D29.0 | D40.8 | D49.59 |
| gastric | C16.2 | C78.89 | D00.2 | D13.1 | D37.1 | D49.0 |
| overlapping sites | C54.8 | — | — | — | — | — |
| penis | C60.2 | C79.82 | D07.4 | D29.0 | D40.8 | D49.59 |
| striatum, cerebrum | C71.0 | C79.31 | — | D33.0 | D43.0 | D49.6 |
| uteri | C54.9 | C79.82 | D07.0 | D26.1 | D39.0 | D49.59 |
| isthmus | C54.0 | C79.82 | D07.0 | D26.1 | D39.0 | D49.59 |
| cortex | | | | | | |
| adrenal | C74.0-☑ | C79.7-☑ | D09.3 | D35.0-☑ | D44.1-☑ | D49.7 |
| cerebral | C71.0 | C79.31 | — | D33.0 | D43.0 | D49.6 |
| **Neoplasm, neoplastic** — *continued* | | | | | | |
| costal cartilage | C41.3 | C79.51 | — | D16.7 | D48.0 | D49.2 |
| costovertebral joint | C41.3 | C79.51 | — | D16.7 | D48.0 | D49.2 |
| Cowper's gland | C68.0 | C79.19 | D09.19 | D30.4 | D41.3 | D49.59 |
| cranial (fossa, any) | C71.9 | C79.31 | — | D33.2 | D43.2 | D49.6 |
| meninges | C70.0 | C79.32 | — | D32.0 | D42.0 | D49.7 |
| nerve | C72.50 | C79.49 | — | D33.3 | D43.3 | D49.7 |
| specified NEC | C72.59 | C79.49 | — | D33.3 | D43.3 | D49.7 |
| craniobuccal pouch | C75.2 | C79.89 | D09.3 | D35.2 | D44.3 | D49.7 |
| craniopharyngeal (duct) (pouch) | C75.2 | C79.89 | D09.3 | D35.3 | D44.4 | D49.7 |
| cricoid | C13.0 | C79.89 | D00.08 | D10.7 | D37.05 | D49.0 |
| cartilage | C32.3 | C78.31 | D02.0 | D14.1 | D38.0 | D49.1 |
| cricopharynx | C13.0 | C79.89 | D00.08 | D10.7 | D37.05 | D49.0 |
| crypt of Morgagni | C21.8 | C78.5 | D01.3 | D12.9 | D37.8 | D49.0 |
| crystalline lens | C69.4-☑ | C79.49 | D09.2-☑ | D31.4-☑ | D48.7 | D49.89 |
| cul-de-sac (Douglas') | C48.1 | C78.6 | — | D20.1 | D48.4 | D49.0 |
| cuneiform cartilage | C32.3 | C78.31 | D02.0 | D14.1 | D38.0 | D49.1 |
| cutaneous — *see* Neoplasm, skin | | | | | | |
| cutis — *see* Neoplasm, skin | | | | | | |
| cystic (bile) duct (common) | C24.0 | C78.89 | D01.5 | D13.5 | D37.6 | D49.0 |
| dermis — *see* Neoplasm, skin | | | | | | |
| diaphragm | C49.3 | C79.89 | — | D21.3 | D48.1-☑ | D49.2 |
| digestive organs, system, tube, or tract NEC | C26.9 | C78.89 | D01.9 | D13.99 | D37.9 | D49.0 |
| disc, intervertebral | C41.2 | C79.51 | — | D16.6 | D48.0 | D49.2 |
| disease, generalized | C80.0 | — | — | — | — | — |
| disseminated | C80.0 | — | — | — | — | — |
| Douglas' cul-de-sac or pouch | C48.1 | C78.6 | — | D20.1 | D48.4 | D49.0 |
| duodenojejunal junction | C17.8 | C78.4 | D01.49 | D13.39 | D37.2 | D49.0 |
| duodenum | C17.0 | C78.4 | D01.49 | D13.2 | D37.2 | D49.0 |
| dura (cranial) (mater) | C70.9 | C79.49 | — | D32.9 | D42.9 | D49.7 |
| cerebral | C70.0 | C79.32 | — | D32.0 | D42.0 | D49.7 |
| spinal | C70.1 | C79.49 | — | D32.1 | D42.1 | D49.7 |
| ear (external) — *see also* Neoplasm, skin, ear | C44.20-☑ | C79.2 | D04.2-☑ | D23.2-☑ | D48.5 | D49.2 |
| auricle or auris — *see also* Neoplasm, skin, ear | C44.20-☑ | C79.2 | D04.2-☑ | D23.2-☑ | D48.5 | D49.2 |
| canal, external — *see also* Neoplasm, skin, ear | C44.20-☑ | C79.2 | D04.2-☑ | D23.2-☑ | D48.5 | D49.2 |
| cartilage | C49.0 | C79.89 | — | D21.0 | D48.1-☑ | D49.2 |
| external meatus — *see also* Neoplasm, skin, ear | C44.20-☑ | C79.2 | D04.2-☑ | D23.2-☑ | D48.5 | D49.2 |
| inner | C30.1 | C78.39 | D02.3 | D14.0 | D38.5 | D49.1 |
| lobule — *see also* Neoplasm, skin, ear | C44.20-☑ | C79.2 | D04.2-☑ | D23.2-☑ | D48.5 | D49.2 |
| middle | C30.1 | C78.39 | D02.3 | D14.0 | D38.5 | D49.1 |
| overlapping lesion with accessory sinuses | C31.8 | — | — | — | — | — |
| skin | C44.20-☑ | C79.2 | D04.2-☑ | D23.2-☑ | D48.5 | D49.2 |
| basal cell carcinoma | C44.21-☑ | — | — | — | — | — |
| specified type NEC | C44.29-☑ | — | — | — | — | — |
| squamous cell carcinoma | C44.22-☑ | — | — | — | — | — |
| earlobe | C44.20-☑ | C79.2 | D04.2-☑ | D23.2-☑ | D48.5 | D49.2 |
| basal cell carcinoma | C44.21-☑ | — | — | — | — | — |
| specified type NEC | C44.29-☑ | — | — | — | — | — |

| | Malignant Primary | Malignant Secondary | Ca in situ | Benign | Uncertain Behavior | Unspecified Behavior |
|---|---|---|---|---|---|---|
| **Neoplasm, neoplastic** *— continued* | | | | | | |
| earlobe *— continued* | | | | | | |
| squamous cell carcinoma | C44.22-☑ | — | — | — | — | — |
| ejaculatory duct | C63.7 | C79.82 | D07.69 | D29.8 | D40.8 | D49.59 |
| elbow NEC | C76.4-☑ | C79.89 | D04.6-☑ | D36.7 | D48.7 | D49.89 |
| endocardium | C38.0 | C79.89 | — | D15.1 | D48.7 | D49.89 |
| endocervix (canal) (gland) | C53.0 | C79.82 | D06.0 | D26.0 | D39.0 | D49.59 |
| endocrine gland NEC | C75.9 | C79.89 | D09.3 | D35.9 | D44.9 | D49.7 |
| pluriglandular | C75.8 | C79.89 | D09.3 | D35.7 | D44.9 | D49.7 |
| endometrium (gland) (stroma) | C54.1 | C79.82 | D07.0 | D26.1 | D39.0 | D49.59 |
| ensiform cartilage | C41.3 | C79.51 | — | D16.7 | D48.0 | D49.2 |
| enteric *— see* Neoplasm, intestine | | | | | | |
| ependyma (brain) | C71.5 | C79.31 | — | D33.0 | D43.0 | D49.6 |
| fourth ventricle | C71.7 | C79.31 | — | D33.1 | D43.1 | D49.6 |
| epicardium | C38.0 | C79.89 | — | D15.1 | D48.7 | D49.89 |
| epididymis | C63.0-☑ | C79.82 | D07.69 | D29.3-☑ | D40.8 | D49.59 |
| epidural | C72.9 | C79.49 | — | D33.9 | D43.9 | D49.7 |
| epiglottis | C32.1 | C78.31 | D02.0 | D14.1 | D38.0 | D49.1 |
| anterior aspect or surface | C10.1 | C79.89 | D00.08 | D10.5 | D37.05 | D49.0 |
| cartilage | C32.3 | C78.31 | D02.0 | D14.1 | D38.0 | D49.1 |
| free border (margin) | C10.1 | C79.89 | D00.08 | D10.5 | D37.05 | D49.0 |
| junctional region | C10.8 | C79.89 | D00.08 | D10.5 | D37.05 | D49.0 |
| posterior (laryngeal) surface | C32.1 | C78.31 | D02.0 | D14.1 | D38.0 | D49.1 |
| suprahyoid portion | C32.1 | C78.31 | D02.0 | D14.1 | D38.0 | D49.1 |
| esophagogastric junction | C16.0 | C78.89 | D00.2 | D13.1 | D37.1 | D49.0 |
| esophagus | C15.9 | C78.89 | D00.1 | D13.0 | D37.8 | D49.0 |
| abdominal | C15.5 | C78.89 | D00.1 | D13.0 | D37.8 | D49.0 |
| cervical | C15.3 | C78.89 | D00.1 | D13.0 | D37.8 | D49.0 |
| distal (third) | C15.5 | C78.89 | D00.1 | D13.0 | D37.8 | D49.0 |
| lower (third) | C15.5 | C78.89 | D00.1 | D13.0 | D37.8 | D49.0 |
| middle (third) | C15.4 | C78.89 | D00.1 | D13.0 | D37.8 | D49.0 |
| overlapping lesion | C15.8 | — | — | — | — | — |
| proximal (third) | C15.3 | C78.89 | D00.1 | D13.0 | D37.8 | D49.0 |
| thoracic | C15.4 | C78.89 | D00.1 | D13.0 | D37.8 | D49.0 |
| upper (third) | C15.3 | C78.89 | D00.1 | D13.0 | D37.8 | D49.0 |
| ethmoid (sinus) | C31.1 | C78.39 | D02.3 | D14.0 | D38.5 | D49.1 |
| bone or labyrinth | C41.0 | C79.51 | — | D16.4 | D48.0 | D49.2 |
| eustachian tube | C30.1 | C78.39 | D02.3 | D14.0 | D38.5 | D49.1 |
| exocervix | C53.1 | C79.82 | D06.1 | D26.0 | D39.0 | D49.59 |
| external | | | | | | |
| meatus (ear) *— see also* Neoplasm, skin, ear | C44.20-☑ | C79.2 | D04.2-☑ | D23.2-☑ | D48.5 | D49.2 |
| os, cervix uteri | C53.1 | C79.82 | D06.1 | D26.0 | D39.0 | D49.59 |
| extradural | C72.9 | C79.49 | — | D33.9 | D43.9 | D49.7 |
| extrahepatic (bile) duct | C24.0 | C78.89 | D01.5 | D13.5 | D37.6 | D49.0 |
| overlapping lesion with gallbladder | C24.8 | — | — | — | — | — |
| extraocular muscle | C69.6-☑ | C79.49 | D09.2-☑ | D31.6-☑ | D48.7 | D49.89 |
| extrarectal | C76.3 | C79.89 | D09.8 | D36.7 | D48.7 | D49.89 |
| extremity | C76.8 | C79.89 | D04.8 | D36.7 | D48.7 | D49.89 |
| lower | C76.5-☑ | C79.89 | D04.7-☑ | D36.7 | D48.7 | D49.89 |
| upper | C76.4-☑ | C79.89 | D04.6-☑ | D36.7 | D48.7 | D49.89 |
| eye NEC | C69.9-☑ | C79.49 | D09.2-☑ | D31.9-☑ | D48.7 | D49.89 |
| overlapping sites | C69.8-☑ | — | — | — | — | — |
| eyeball | C69.9-☑ | C79.49 | D09.2-☑ | D31.9-☑ | D48.7 | D49.89 |
| eyebrow | C44.309 | C79.2 | D04.39 | D23.39 | D48.5 | D49.2 |
| basal cell carcinoma | C44.319 | — | — | — | — | — |
| specified type NEC | C44.399 | — | — | — | — | — |
| squamous cell carcinoma | C44.329 | — | — | — | — | — |

| | Malignant Primary | Malignant Secondary | Ca in situ | Benign | Uncertain Behavior | Unspecified Behavior |
|---|---|---|---|---|---|---|
| **Neoplasm, neoplastic** *— continued* | | | | | | |
| eyelid (lower) (skin) (upper) | C44.10-☑ | — | — | — | — | — |
| basal cell carcinoma | C44.11-☑ | — | — | — | — | — |
| cartilage | C49.0 | C79.89 | — | D21.0 | D48.1-☑ | D49.2 |
| sebaceous cell | C44.13-☑ | — | — | — | — | — |
| specified type NEC | C44.19-☑ | — | — | — | — | — |
| squamous cell carcinoma | C44.12-☑ | — | — | — | — | — |
| face NEC | C76.0 | C79.89 | D04.39 | D36.7 | D48.7 | D49.89 |
| fallopian tube (accessory) | C57.0-☑ | C79.82 | D07.39 | D28.2 | D39.8 | D49.59 |
| falx (cerebella) (cerebri) | C70.0 | C79.32 | — | D32.0 | D42.0 | D49.7 |
| fascia *— see also* Neoplasm, connective tissue | | | | | | |
| palmar | C49.1-☑ | C79.89 | — | D21.1-☑ | D48.1-☑ | D49.2 |
| plantar | C49.2-☑ | C79.89 | — | D21.2-☑ | D48.1-☑ | D49.2 |
| fatty tissue *— see* Neoplasm, connective tissue | | | | | | |
| fauces, faucial NEC | C10.9 | C79.89 | D00.08 | D10.5 | D37.05 | D49.0 |
| pillars | C09.1 | C79.89 | D00.08 | D10.5 | D37.05 | D49.0 |
| tonsil | C09.9 | C79.89 | D00.08 | D10.4 | D37.05 | D49.0 |
| femur (any part) | C40.2-☑ | C79.51 | — | D16.2-☑ | — | — |
| fetal membrane | C58 | C79.82 | D07.0 | D26.7 | D39.2 | D49.59 |
| fibrous tissue *— see* Neoplasm, connective tissue | | | | | | |
| fibula (any part) | C40.2-☑ | C79.51 | — | D16.2-☑ | — | — |
| filum terminale | C72.0 | C79.49 | — | D33.4 | D43.4 | D49.7 |
| finger NEC | C76.4-☑ | C79.89 | D04.6-☑ | D36.7 | D48.7 | D49.89 |
| flank NEC | C76.8 | C79.89 | D04.5 | D36.7 | D48.7 | D49.89 |
| follicle, nabothian | C53.0 | C79.82 | D06.0 | D26.0 | D39.0 | D49.59 |
| foot NEC | C76.5-☑ | C79.89 | D04.7-☑ | D36.7 | D48.7 | D49.89 |
| forearm NEC | C76.4-☑ | C79.89 | D04.6-☑ | D36.7 | D48.7 | D49.89 |
| forehead (skin) | C44.309 | C79.2 | D04.39 | D23.39 | D48.5 | D49.2 |
| basal cell carcinoma | C44.319 | — | — | — | — | — |
| specified type NEC | C44.399 | — | — | — | — | — |
| squamous cell carcinoma | C44.329 | — | — | — | — | — |
| foreskin | C60.0 | C79.82 | D07.4 | D29.0 | D40.8 | D49.59 |
| fornix | | | | | | |
| pharyngeal | C11.3 | C79.89 | D00.08 | D10.6 | D37.05 | D49.0 |
| vagina | C52 | C79.82 | D07.2 | D28.1 | D39.8 | D49.59 |
| fossa (of) | | | | | | |
| anterior (cranial) | C71.9 | C79.31 | — | D33.2 | D43.2 | D49.6 |
| cranial | C71.9 | C79.31 | — | D33.2 | D43.2 | D49.6 |
| ischiorectal | C76.3 | C79.89 | D09.8 | D36.7 | D48.7 | D49.89 |
| middle (cranial) | C71.9 | C79.31 | — | D33.2 | D43.2 | D49.6 |
| piriform | C12 | C79.89 | D00.08 | D10.7 | D37.05 | D49.0 |
| pituitary | C75.1 | C79.89 | D09.3 | D35.2 | D44.3 | D49.7 |
| posterior (cranial) | C71.9 | C79.31 | — | D33.2 | D43.2 | D49.6 |
| pterygoid | C49.0 | C79.89 | — | D21.0 | D48.1-☑ | D49.2 |
| pyriform | C12 | C79.89 | D00.08 | D10.7 | D37.05 | D49.0 |
| Rosenmuller | C11.2 | C79.89 | D00.08 | D10.6 | D37.05 | D49.0 |
| tonsillar | C09.0 | C79.89 | D00.08 | D10.5 | D37.05 | D49.0 |
| fourchette | C51.9 | C79.82 | D07.1 | D28.0 | D39.8 | D49.59 |
| frenulum | | | | | | |
| labii *— see* Neoplasm, lip, internal | | | | | | |
| linguae | C02.2 | C79.89 | D00.07 | D10.1 | D37.02 | D49.0 |
| frontal | | | | | | |
| bone | C41.0 | C79.51 | — | D16.4 | D48.0 | D49.2 |
| lobe, brain | C71.1 | C79.31 | — | D33.0 | D43.0 | D49.6 |
| pole | C71.1 | C79.31 | — | D33.0 | D43.0 | D49.6 |
| sinus | C31.2 | C78.39 | D02.3 | D14.0 | D38.5 | D49.1 |
| fundus | | | | | | |
| stomach | C16.1 | C78.89 | D00.2 | D13.1 | D37.1 | D49.0 |
| uterus | C54.3 | C79.82 | D07.0 | D26.1 | D39.0 | D49.59 |
| gall duct (extrahepatic) | C24.0 | C78.89 | D01.5 | D13.5 | D37.6 | D49.0 |
| intrahepatic | C22.1 | C78.7 | D01.5 | D13.4 | D37.6 | D49.0 |
| gallbladder | C23 | C78.89 | D01.5 | D13.5 | D37.6 | D49.0 |

| | Malignant Primary | Malignant Secondary | Ca in situ | Benign | Uncertain Behavior | Unspecified Behavior |
|---|---|---|---|---|---|---|
| **Neoplasm, neoplastic** — *continued* | | | | | | |
| gallbladder — *continued* | | | | | | |
| overlapping lesion with extrahepatic bile ducts | C24.8 | — | — | — | — | — |
| ganglia — *see also* Neoplasm, nerve, peripheral | C47.9 | C79.89 | — | D36.1Ø | D48.2 | D49.2 |
| basal | C71.Ø | C79.31 | — | D33.Ø | D43.Ø | D49.6 |
| cranial nerve | C72.5Ø | C79.49 | — | D33.3 | D43.3 | D49.7 |
| Gartner's duct | C52 | C79.82 | DØ7.2 | D28.1 | D39.8 | D49.59 |
| gastric — *see* Neoplasm, stomach | | | | | | |
| gastrocolic | C26.9 | C78.89 | DØ1.9 | D13.99 | D37.9 | D49.Ø |
| gastroesophageal junction | C16.Ø | C78.89 | DØØ.2 | D13.1 | D37.1 | D49.Ø |
| gastrointestinal (tract) NEC | C26.9 | C78.89 | DØ1.9 | D13.99 | D37.9 | D49.Ø |
| generalized | C8Ø.Ø | — | — | — | — | — |
| genital organ or tract | | | | | | |
| female NEC | C57.9 | C79.82 | DØ7.3Ø | D28.9 | D39.9 | D49.59 |
| overlapping lesion | C57.8 | — | — | — | — | — |
| specified site NEC | C57.7 | C79.82 | DØ7.39 | D28.7 | D39.8 | D49.59 |
| male NEC | C63.9 | C79.82 | DØ7.6Ø | D29.9 | D4Ø.9 | D49.59 |
| overlapping lesion | C63.8 | — | — | — | — | — |
| specified site NEC | C63.7 | C79.82 | DØ7.69 | D29.8 | D4Ø.8 | D49.59 |
| genitourinary tract | | | | | | |
| female | C57.9 | C79.82 | DØ7.3Ø | D28.9 | D39.9 | D49.59 |
| male | C63.9 | C79.82 | DØ7.6Ø | D29.9 | D4Ø.9 | D49.59 |
| gingiva (alveolar) (marginal) | CØ3.9 | C79.89 | DØØ.Ø3 | D1Ø.39 | D37.Ø9 | D49.Ø |
| lower | CØ3.1 | C79.89 | DØØ.Ø3 | D1Ø.39 | D37.Ø9 | D49.Ø |
| mandibular | CØ3.1 | C79.89 | DØØ.Ø3 | D1Ø.39 | D37.Ø9 | D49.Ø |
| maxillary | CØ3.Ø | C79.89 | DØØ.Ø3 | D1Ø.39 | D37.Ø9 | D49.Ø |
| upper | CØ3.Ø | C79.89 | DØØ.Ø3 | D1Ø.39 | D37.Ø9 | D49.Ø |
| gland, glandular (lymphatic) (system) — *see also* Neoplasm, lymph gland | | | | | | |
| endocrine NEC | C75.9 | C79.89 | DØ9.3 | D35.9 | D44.9 | D49.7 |
| salivary — *see* Neoplasm, salivary gland | | | | | | |
| glans penis | C6Ø.1 | C79.82 | DØ7.4 | D29.Ø | D4Ø.8 | D49.59 |
| globus pallidus | C71.Ø | C79.31 | — | D33.Ø | D43.Ø | D49.6 |
| glomus | | | | | | |
| coccygeal | C49.5 | C79.89 | — | D21.5 | D48.1-☑ | D49.2 |
| jugularis | C75.5 | C79.89 | — | D35.6 | D44.7 | D49.7 |
| glosso-epiglottic fold(s) | C1Ø.1 | C79.89 | DØØ.Ø8 | D1Ø.5 | D37.Ø5 | D49.Ø |
| glossopalatine fold | CØ9.1 | C79.89 | DØØ.Ø8 | D1Ø.5 | D37.Ø5 | D49.Ø |
| glossopharyngeal sulcus | CØ9.Ø | C79.89 | DØØ.Ø8 | D1Ø.5 | D37.Ø5 | D49.Ø |
| glottis | C32.Ø | C78.31 | DØ2.Ø | D14.1 | D38.Ø | D49.1 |
| gluteal region | C76.3 | C79.89 | DØ4.5 | D36.7 | D48.7 | D49.89 |
| great vessels NEC | C49.3 | C79.89 | — | D21.3 | D48.1-☑ | D49.2 |
| groin NEC | C76.3 | C79.89 | DØ4.5 | D36.7 | D48.7 | D49.89 |
| gum | CØ3.9 | C79.89 | DØØ.Ø3 | D1Ø.39 | D37.Ø9 | D49.Ø |
| lower | CØ3.1 | C79.89 | DØØ.Ø3 | D1Ø.39 | D37.Ø9 | D49.Ø |
| upper | CØ3.Ø | C79.89 | DØØ.Ø3 | D1Ø.39 | D37.Ø9 | D49.Ø |
| hand NEC | C76.4-☑ | C79.89 | DØ4.6-☑ | D36.7 | D48.7 | D49.89 |
| head NEC | C76.Ø | C79.89 | DØ4.4 | D36.7 | D48.7 | D49.89 |
| heart | C38.Ø | C79.89 | — | D15.1 | D48.7 | D49.89 |
| heel NEC | C76.5-☑ | C79.89 | DØ4.7-☑ | D36.7 | D48.7 | D49.89 |
| helix — *see also* Neoplasm, skin, ear | C44.2Ø-☑ | C79.2 | DØ4.2-☑ | D23.2-☑ | D48.5 | D49.2 |
| hematopoietic, hemopoietic tissue NEC | C96.9 | — | — | — | — | — |
| specified NEC | C96.Z | — | — | — | — | — |
| hemisphere, cerebral | C71.Ø | C79.31 | — | D33.Ø | D43.Ø | D49.6 |
| **Neoplasm, neoplastic** — *continued* | | | | | | |
| hemorrhoidal zone | C21.1 | C78.5 | DØ1.3 | D12.9 | D37.8 | D49.Ø |
| hepatic — *see also* Index to disease, by histology | C22.9 | C78.7 | DØ1.5 | D13.4 | D37.6 | D49.Ø |
| duct (bile) | C24.Ø | C78.89 | DØ1.5 | D13.5 | D37.6 | D49.Ø |
| flexure (colon) | C18.3 | C78.5 | DØ1.Ø | D12.3 | D37.4 | D49.Ø |
| primary | C22.8 | C78.7 | DØ1.5 | D13.4 | D37.6 | D49.Ø |
| hepatobiliary | C24.9 | C78.89 | DØ1.5 | D13.5 | D37.6 | D49.Ø |
| hepatoblastoma | C22.2 | C78.7 | DØ1.5 | D13.4 | D37.6 | D49.Ø |
| hepatoma | C22.Ø | C78.7 | DØ1.5 | D13.4 | D37.6 | D49.Ø |
| hilus of lung | C34.Ø-☑ | C78.Ø-☑ | DØ2.2-☑ | D14.3-☑ | D38.1 | D49.1 |
| hip NEC | C76.5-☑ | C79.89 | DØ4.7-☑ | D36.7 | D48.7 | D49.89 |
| hippocampus, brain | C71.2 | C79.31 | — | D33.Ø | D43.Ø | D49.6 |
| humerus (any part) | C4Ø.Ø-☑ | C79.51 | — | D16.Ø-☑ | — | — |
| hymen | C52 | C79.82 | DØ7.2 | D28.1 | D39.8 | D49.59 |
| hypopharynx, hypopharyngeal NEC | C13.9 | C79.89 | DØØ.Ø8 | D1Ø.7 | D37.Ø5 | D49.Ø |
| overlapping lesion | C13.8 | — | — | — | — | — |
| postcricoid region | C13.Ø | C79.89 | DØØ.Ø8 | D1Ø.7 | D37.Ø5 | D49.Ø |
| posterior wall | C13.2 | C79.89 | DØØ.Ø8 | D1Ø.7 | D37.Ø5 | D49.Ø |
| pyriform fossa (sinus) | C12 | C79.89 | DØØ.Ø8 | D1Ø.7 | D37.Ø5 | D49.Ø |
| hypophysis | C75.1 | C79.89 | DØ9.3 | D35.2 | D44.3 | D49.7 |
| hypothalamus | C71.Ø | C79.31 | — | D33.Ø | D43.Ø | D49.6 |
| ileocecum, ileocecal (coil) (junction) (valve) | C18.Ø | C78.5 | DØ1.Ø | D12.Ø | D37.4 | D49.Ø |
| ileum | C17.2 | C78.4 | DØ1.49 | D13.39 | D37.2 | D49.Ø |
| ilium | C41.4 | C79.51 | — | D16.8 | D48.Ø | D49.2 |
| immunoproliferative NEC | C88.9-☑ | — | — | — | — | — |
| infraclavicular (region) | C76.1 | C79.89 | DØ4.5 | D36.7 | D48.7 | D49.89 |
| inguinal (region) | C76.3 | C79.89 | DØ4.5 | D36.7 | D48.7 | D49.89 |
| insula | C71.Ø | C79.31 | — | D33.Ø | D43.Ø | D49.6 |
| insular tissue (pancreas) | C25.4 | C78.89 | DØ1.7 | D13.7 | D37.8 | D49.Ø |
| brain | C71.Ø | C79.31 | — | D33.Ø | D43.Ø | D49.6 |
| interarytenoid fold | C13.1 | C79.89 | DØØ.Ø8 | D1Ø.7 | D37.Ø5 | D49.Ø |
| hypopharyngeal aspect | C13.1 | C79.89 | DØØ.Ø8 | D1Ø.7 | D37.Ø5 | D49.Ø |
| laryngeal aspect | C32.1 | C78.31 | DØ2.Ø | D14.1 | D38.Ø | D49.1 |
| marginal zone | C13.1 | C79.89 | DØØ.Ø8 | D1Ø.7 | D37.Ø5 | D49.Ø |
| interdental papillae | CØ3.9 | C79.89 | DØØ.Ø3 | D1Ø.39 | D37.Ø9 | D49.Ø |
| lower | CØ3.1 | C79.89 | DØØ.Ø3 | D1Ø.39 | D37.Ø9 | D49.Ø |
| upper | CØ3.Ø | C79.89 | DØØ.Ø3 | D1Ø.39 | D37.Ø9 | D49.Ø |
| internal | | | | | | |
| capsule | C71.Ø | C79.31 | — | D33.Ø | D43.Ø | D49.6 |
| os (cervix) | C53.Ø | C79.82 | DØ6.Ø | D26.Ø | D39.Ø | D49.59 |
| intervertebral cartilage or disc | C41.2 | C79.51 | — | D16.6 | D48.Ø | D49.2 |
| intestine, intestinal | C26.Ø | C78.8Ø | DØ1.4Ø | D13.99 | D37.8 | D49.Ø |
| large | C18.9 | C78.5 | DØ1.Ø | D12.6 | D37.4 | D49.Ø |
| appendix | C18.1 | C78.5 | DØ1.Ø | D12.1 | D37.3 | D49.Ø |
| caput coli | C18.Ø | C78.5 | DØ1.Ø | D12.Ø | D37.4 | D49.Ø |
| cecum | C18.Ø | C78.5 | DØ1.Ø | D12.Ø | D37.4 | D49.Ø |
| colon | C18.9 | C78.5 | DØ1.Ø | D12.6 | D37.4 | D49.Ø |
| and rectum | C19 | C78.5 | DØ1.1 | D12.7 | D37.5 | D49.Ø |
| ascending | C18.2 | C78.5 | DØ1.Ø | D12.2 | D37.4 | D49.Ø |
| caput | C18.Ø | C78.5 | DØ1.Ø | D12.Ø | D37.4 | D49.Ø |
| descending | C18.6 | C78.5 | DØ1.Ø | D12.4 | D37.4 | D49.Ø |
| distal | C18.6 | C78.5 | DØ1.Ø | D12.4 | D37.4 | D49.Ø |
| left | C18.6 | C78.5 | DØ1.Ø | D12.4 | D37.4 | D49.Ø |
| overlapping lesion | C18.8 | — | — | — | — | — |
| pelvic | C18.7 | C78.5 | DØ1.Ø | D12.5 | D37.4 | D49.Ø |
| right | C18.2 | C78.5 | DØ1.Ø | D12.2 | D37.4 | D49.Ø |
| sigmoid (flexure) | C18.7 | C78.5 | DØ1.Ø | D12.5 | D37.4 | D49.Ø |
| transverse | C18.4 | C78.5 | DØ1.Ø | D12.3 | D37.4 | D49.Ø |
| hepatic flexure | C18.3 | C78.5 | DØ1.Ø | D12.3 | D37.4 | D49.Ø |

| | Malignant Primary | Malignant Secondary | Ca in situ | Benign | Uncertain Behavior | Unspecified Behavior |
|---|---|---|---|---|---|---|
| **Neoplasm, neoplastic** — *continued* | | | | | | |
| intestine, intestinal — *continued* | | | | | | |
| large — *continued* | | | | | | |
| ileocecum, ileocecal (coil) (valve) | C18.0 | C78.5 | D01.0 | D12.0 | D37.4 | D49.0 |
| overlapping lesion | C18.8 | — | — | — | — | — |
| sigmoid flexure (lower) (upper) | C18.7 | C78.5 | D01.0 | D12.5 | D37.4 | D49.0 |
| splenic flexure | C18.5 | C78.5 | D01.0 | D12.3 | D37.4 | D49.0 |
| small | C17.9 | C78.4 | D01.40 | D13.30 | D37.2 | D49.0 |
| duodenum | C17.0 | C78.4 | D01.49 | D13.2 | D37.2 | D49.0 |
| ileum | C17.2 | C78.4 | D01.49 | D13.39 | D37.2 | D49.0 |
| jejunum | C17.1 | C78.4 | D01.49 | D13.39 | D37.2 | D49.0 |
| overlapping lesion | C17.8 | — | — | — | — | — |
| tract NEC | C26.0 | C78.89 | D01.40 | D13.99 | D37.8 | D49.0 |
| intra-abdominal | C76.2 | C79.89 | D09.8 | D36.7 | D48.7 | D49.89 |
| intracranial NEC | C71.9 | C79.31 | — | D33.2 | D43.2 | D49.6 |
| intrahepatic (bile) duct | C22.1 | C78.7 | D01.5 | D13.4 | D37.6 | D49.0 |
| intraocular | C69.9-☑ | C79.49 | D09.2-☑ | D31.9-☑ | D48.7 | D49.89 |
| intraorbital | C69.6-☑ | C79.49 | D09.2-☑ | D31.6-☑ | D48.7 | D49.89 |
| intrasellar | C75.1 | C79.89 | D09.3 | D35.2 | D44.3 | D49.7 |
| intrathoracic (cavity) (organs) | C76.1 | C79.89 | D09.8 | D15.9 | D48.7 | D49.89 |
| specified NEC | C76.1 | C79.89 | D09.8 | D15.7 | — | — |
| iris | C69.4-☑ | C79.49 | D09.2-☑ | D31.4-☑ | D48.7 | D49.89 |
| ischiorectal (fossa) | C76.3 | C79.89 | D09.8 | D36.7 | D48.7 | D49.89 |
| ischium | C41.4 | C79.51 | — | D16.8 | D48.0 | D49.2 |
| island of Reil | C71.0 | C79.31 | — | D33.0 | D43.0 | D49.6 |
| islands or islets of Langerhans | C25.4 | C78.89 | D01.7 | D13.7 | D37.8 | D49.0 |
| isthmus uteri | C54.0 | C79.82 | D07.0 | D26.1 | D39.0 | D49.59 |
| jaw | C76.0 | C79.89 | D09.8 | D36.7 | D48.7 | D49.89 |
| bone | C41.1 | C79.51 | — | D16.5 | D48.0 | D49.2 |
| lower | C41.1 | C79.51 | — | D16.5 | — | — |
| upper | C41.0 | C79.51 | — | D16.4 | — | — |
| carcinoma (any type) (lower) (upper) | C76.0 | C79.89 | — | — | — | — |
| skin — *see also* Neoplasm, skin, face | C44.309 | C79.2 | D04.39 | D23.39 | D48.5 | D49.2 |
| soft tissues | C03.9 | C79.89 | D00.03 | D10.39 | D37.09 | D49.0 |
| lower | C03.1 | C79.89 | D00.03 | D10.39 | D37.09 | D49.0 |
| upper | C03.0 | C79.89 | D00.03 | D10.39 | D37.09 | D49.0 |
| jejunum | C17.1 | C78.4 | D01.49 | D13.39 | D37.2 | D49.0 |
| joint NEC — *see also* Neoplasm, bone | C41.9 | C79.51 | — | D16.9 | D48.0 | D49.2 |
| acromioclavicular | C40.0-☑ | C79.51 | — | D16.0-☑ | — | — |
| bursa or synovial membrane — *see* Neoplasm, connective tissue | | | | | | |
| costovertebral | C41.3 | C79.51 | — | D16.7 | D48.0 | D49.2 |
| sternocostal | C41.3 | C79.51 | — | D16.7 | D48.0 | D49.2 |
| temporomandibular | C41.1 | C79.51 | — | D16.5 | D48.0 | D49.2 |
| junction | | | | | | |
| anorectal | C21.8 | C78.5 | D01.3 | D12.9 | D37.8 | D49.0 |
| cardioesophageal | C16.0 | C78.89 | D00.2 | D13.1 | D37.1 | D49.0 |
| esophagogastric | C16.0 | C78.89 | D00.2 | D13.1 | D37.1 | D49.0 |
| gastroesophageal | C16.0 | C78.89 | D00.2 | D13.1 | D37.1 | D49.0 |
| hard and soft palate | C05.9 | C79.89 | D00.00 | D10.39 | D37.09 | D49.0 |
| ileocecal | C18.0 | C78.5 | D01.0 | D12.0 | D37.4 | D49.0 |
| pelvirectal | C19 | C78.5 | D01.1 | D12.7 | D37.5 | D49.0 |
| pelviureteric | C65.-☑ | C79.0-☑ | D09.19 | D30.1-☑ | D41.1-☑ | D49.59 |
| rectosigmoid | C19 | C78.5 | D01.1 | D12.7 | D37.5 | D49.0 |
| squamocolumnar, of cervix | C53.8 | C79.82 | D06.7 | D26.0 | D39.0 | D49.59 |
| Kaposi's sarcoma — *see* Kaposi's, sarcoma | | | | | | |
| kidney (parenchymal) | C64.-☑ | C79.0-☑ | D09.19 | D30.0-☑ | D41.0-☑ | D49.51-☑ |
| calyx | C65.-☑ | C79.0-☑ | D09.19 | D30.1-☑ | D41.1-☑ | D49.51-☑ |
| hilus | C65.-☑ | C79.0-☑ | D09.19 | D30.1-☑ | D41.1-☑ | D49.51-☑ |
| **Neoplasm, neoplastic** — *continued* | | | | | | |
| kidney — *continued* | | | | | | |
| pelvis | C65.-☑ | C79.0-☑ | D09.19 | D30.1-☑ | D41.1-☑ | D49.51-☑ |
| knee NEC | C76.5-☑ | C79.89 | D04.7-☑ | D36.7 | D48.7 | D49.89 |
| labia (skin) | C51.9 | C79.82 | D07.1 | D28.0 | D39.8 | D49.59 |
| majora | C51.0 | C79.82 | D07.1 | D28.0 | D39.8 | D49.59 |
| minora | C51.1 | C79.82 | D07.1 | D28.0 | D39.8 | D49.59 |
| labial — *see also* Neoplasm, lip | C00.9 | C79.89 | D00.01 | D10.0 | D37.01 | D49.0 |
| sulcus (lower) (upper) | C06.1 | C79.89 | D00.02 | D10.39 | D37.09 | D49.0 |
| labium (skin) | C51.9 | C79.82 | D07.1 | D28.0 | D39.8 | D49.59 |
| majus | C51.0 | C79.82 | D07.1 | D28.0 | D39.8 | D49.59 |
| minus | C51.1 | C79.82 | D07.1 | D28.0 | D39.8 | D49.59 |
| lacrimal | | | | | | |
| canaliculi | C69.5-☑ | C79.49 | D09.2-☑ | D31.5-☑ | D48.7 | D49.89 |
| duct (nasal) | C69.5-☑ | C79.49 | D09.2-☑ | D31.5-☑ | D48.7 | D49.89 |
| gland | C69.5-☑ | C79.49 | D09.2-☑ | D31.5-☑ | D48.7 | D49.89 |
| punctum | C69.5-☑ | C79.49 | D09.2-☑ | D31.5-☑ | D48.7 | D49.89 |
| sac | C69.5-☑ | C79.49 | D09.2-☑ | D31.5-☑ | D48.7 | D49.89 |
| Langerhans, islands or islets | C25.4 | C78.89 | D01.7 | D13.7 | D37.8 | D49.0 |
| laryngopharynx | C13.9 | C79.89 | D00.08 | D10.7 | D37.05 | D49.0 |
| larynx, laryngeal NEC | C32.9 | C78.31 | D02.0 | D14.1 | D38.0 | D49.1 |
| aryepiglottic fold | C32.1 | C78.31 | D02.0 | D14.1 | D38.0 | D49.1 |
| cartilage (arytenoid) (cricoid) (cuneiform) (thyroid) | C32.3 | C78.31 | D02.0 | D14.1 | D38.0 | D49.1 |
| commissure (anterior) (posterior) | C32.0 | C78.31 | D02.0 | D14.1 | D38.0 | D49.1 |
| extrinsic NEC | C32.1 | C78.31 | D02.0 | D14.1 | D38.0 | D49.1 |
| meaning hypopharynx | C13.9 | C79.89 | D00.08 | D10.7 | D37.05 | D49.0 |
| interarytenoid fold | C32.1 | C78.31 | D02.0 | D14.1 | D38.0 | D49.1 |
| intrinsic | C32.0 | C78.31 | D02.0 | D14.1 | D38.0 | D49.1 |
| overlapping lesion | C32.8 | — | — | — | — | — |
| ventricular band | C32.1 | C78.31 | D02.0 | D14.1 | D38.0 | D49.1 |
| leg NEC | C76.5-☑ | C79.89 | D04.7-☑ | D36.7 | D48.7 | D49.89 |
| lens, crystalline | C69.4-☑ | C79.49 | D09.2-☑ | D31.4-☑ | D48.7 | D49.89 |
| lid (lower) (upper) | C44.10-☑ | C79.2 | D04.1-☑ | D23.1-☑ | D48.5 | D49.2 |
| basal cell carcinoma | C44.11-☑ | — | — | — | — | — |
| sebaceous cell | C44.13-☑ | — | — | — | — | — |
| specified type NEC | C44.19-☑ | — | — | — | — | — |
| squamous cell carcinoma | C44.12-☑ | — | — | — | — | — |
| ligament — *see also* Neoplasm, connective tissue | | | | | | |
| broad | C57.1-☑ | C79.82 | D07.39 | D28.2 | D39.8 | D49.59 |
| Mackenrodt's | C57.7 | C79.82 | D07.39 | D28.7 | D39.8 | D49.59 |
| non-uterine — *see* Neoplasm, connective tissue | | | | | | |
| round | C57.2-☑ | C79.82 | — | D28.2 | D39.8 | D49.59 |
| sacro-uterine | C57.3 | C79.82 | — | D28.2 | D39.8 | D49.59 |
| uterine | C57.3 | C79.82 | — | D28.2 | D39.8 | D49.59 |
| utero-ovarian | C57.7 | C79.82 | D07.39 | D28.2 | D39.8 | D49.59 |
| uterosacral | C57.3 | C79.82 | — | D28.2 | D39.8 | D49.59 |
| limb | C76.8 | C79.89 | D04.8 | D36.7 | D48.7 | D49.89 |
| lower | C76.5-☑ | C79.89 | D04.7-☑ | D36.7 | D48.7 | D49.89 |
| upper | C76.4-☑ | C79.89 | D04.6-☑ | D36.7 | D48.7 | D49.89 |
| limbus of cornea | C69.1-☑ | C79.49 | D09.2-☑ | D31.1-☑ | D48.7 | D49.89 |
| lingual NEC — *see also* Neoplasm, tongue | C02.9 | C79.89 | D00.07 | D10.1 | D37.02 | D49.0 |
| lingula, lung | C34.1-☑ | C78.0-☑ | D02.2-☑ | D14.3-☑ | D38.1 | D49.1 |
| lip | C00.9 | C79.89 | D00.01 | D10.0 | D37.01 | D49.0 |
| buccal aspect — *see* Neoplasm, lip, internal | | | | | | |
| commissure | C00.6 | C79.89 | D00.01 | D10.0 | D37.01 | D49.0 |
| external | C00.2 | C79.89 | D00.01 | D10.0 | D37.01 | D49.0 |
| lower | C00.1 | C79.89 | D00.01 | D10.0 | D37.01 | D49.0 |

| | Malignant Primary | Malignant Secondary | Ca in situ | Benign | Uncertain Behavior | Unspecified Behavior |
|---|---|---|---|---|---|---|
| **Neoplasm, neoplastic** — *continued* | | | | | | |
| lip — *continued* | | | | | | |
| external — *continued* | | | | | | |
| upper | CØØ.Ø | C79.89 | DØØ.Ø1 | D1Ø.Ø | D37.Ø1 | D49.Ø |
| frenulum — *see* Neoplasm, lip, internal | | | | | | |
| inner aspect — *see* Neoplasm, lip, internal | | | | | | |
| internal | CØØ.5 | C79.89 | DØØ.Ø1 | D1Ø.Ø | D37.Ø1 | D49.Ø |
| lower | CØØ.4 | C79.89 | DØØ.Ø1 | D1Ø.Ø | D37.Ø1 | D49.Ø |
| upper | CØØ.3 | C79.89 | DØØ.Ø1 | D1Ø.Ø | D37.Ø1 | D49.Ø |
| lipstick area | CØØ.2 | C79.89 | DØØ.Ø1 | D1Ø.Ø | D37.Ø1 | D49.Ø |
| lower | CØØ.1 | C79.89 | DØØ.Ø1 | D1Ø.Ø | D37.Ø1 | D49.Ø |
| upper | CØØ.Ø | C79.89 | DØØ.Ø1 | D1Ø.Ø | D37.Ø1 | D49.Ø |
| lower | CØØ.1 | C79.89 | DØØ.Ø1 | D1Ø.Ø | D37.Ø1 | D49.Ø |
| internal | CØØ.4 | C79.89 | DØØ.Ø1 | D1Ø.Ø | D37.Ø1 | D49.Ø |
| mucosa — *see* Neoplasm, lip, internal | | | | | | |
| oral aspect — *see* Neoplasm, lip, internal | | | | | | |
| overlapping lesion | CØØ.8 | — | — | — | — | — |
| with oral cavity or pharynx | C14.8 | C79.89 | — | — | — | — |
| skin (commissure) (lower) (upper) | C44.ØØ | C79.2 | DØ4.Ø | D23.Ø | D48.5 | D49.2 |
| basal cell carcinoma | C44.Ø1 | — | — | — | — | — |
| specified type NEC | C44.Ø9 | — | — | — | — | — |
| squamous cell carcinoma | C44.Ø2 | — | — | — | — | — |
| upper | CØØ.Ø | C79.89 | DØØ.Ø1 | D1Ø.Ø | D37.Ø1 | D49.Ø |
| internal | CØØ.3 | C79.89 | DØØ.Ø1 | D1Ø.Ø | D37.Ø1 | D49.Ø |
| vermilion border | CØØ.2 | C79.89 | DØØ.Ø1 | D1Ø.Ø | D37.Ø1 | D49.Ø |
| lower | CØØ.1 | C79.89 | DØØ.Ø1 | D1Ø.Ø | D37.Ø1 | D49.Ø |
| upper | CØØ.Ø | C79.89 | DØØ.Ø1 | D1Ø.Ø | D37.Ø1 | D49.Ø |
| lipomatous — *see* Lipoma, by site | | | | | | |
| liver — *see also* Index to disease, by histology | C22.9 | C78.7 | DØ1.5 | D13.4 | D37.6 | D49.Ø |
| primary | C22.8 | C78.7 | DØ1.5 | D13.4 | D37.6 | D49.Ø |
| lumbosacral plexus | C47.5 | C79.89 | — | D36.16 | D48.2 | D49.2 |
| lung | C34.9-☑ | C78.Ø-☑ | DØ2.2-☑ | D14.3-☑ | D38.1 | D49.1 |
| azygos lobe | C34.1-☑ | C78.Ø-☑ | DØ2.2-☑ | D14.3-☑ | D38.1 | D49.1 |
| carina | C34.Ø-☑ | C78.Ø-☑ | DØ2.2-☑ | D14.3-☑ | D38.1 | D49.1 |
| hilus | C34.Ø-☑ | C78.Ø-☑ | DØ2.2-☑ | D14.3-☑ | D38.1 | D49.1 |
| lingula | C34.1-☑ | C78.Ø-☑ | DØ2.2-☑ | D14.3-☑ | D38.1 | D49.1 |
| lobe NEC | C34.9-☑ | C78.Ø-☑ | DØ2.2-☑ | D14.3-☑ | D38.1 | D49.1 |
| lower lobe | C34.3-☑ | C78.Ø-☑ | DØ2.2-☑ | D14.3-☑ | D38.1 | D49.1 |
| main bronchus | C34.Ø-☑ | C78.Ø-☑ | DØ2.2-☑ | D14.3-☑ | D38.1 | D49.1 |
| mesothelioma — *see* Mesothelioma | | | | | | |
| middle lobe | C34.2 | C78.Ø-☑ | DØ2.21 | D14.31 | D38.1 | D49.1 |
| overlapping lesion | C34.8-☑ | — | — | — | — | — |
| upper lobe | C34.1-☑ | C78.Ø-☑ | DØ2.2-☑ | D14.3-☑ | D38.1 | D49.1 |
| lymph, lymphatic channel NEC | C49.9 | C79.89 | — | D21.9 | D48.1-☑ | D49.2 |
| gland (secondary) | — | C77.9 | — | D36.Ø | D48.7 | D49.89 |
| abdominal | — | C77.2 | — | D36.Ø | D48.7 | D49.89 |
| aortic | — | C77.2 | — | D36.Ø | D48.7 | D49.89 |
| arm | — | C77.3 | — | D36.Ø | D48.7 | D49.89 |
| auricular (anterior) (posterior) | — | C77.Ø | — | D36.Ø | D48.7 | D49.89 |
| axilla, axillary | — | C77.3 | — | D36.Ø | D48.7 | D49.89 |
| brachial | — | C77.3 | — | D36.Ø | D48.7 | D49.89 |
| bronchial | — | C77.1 | — | D36.Ø | D48.7 | D49.89 |
| bronchopulmonary | — | C77.1 | — | D36.Ø | D48.7 | D49.89 |
| celiac | — | C77.2 | — | D36.Ø | D48.7 | D49.89 |
| cervical | — | C77.Ø | — | D36.Ø | D48.7 | D49.89 |
| cervicofacial | — | C77.Ø | — | D36.Ø | D48.7 | D49.89 |
| **Neoplasm, neoplastic** — *continued* | | | | | | |
| lymph, lymphatic channel — *continued* | | | | | | |
| gland — *continued* | | | | | | |
| Cloquet | — | C77.4 | — | D36.Ø | D48.7 | D49.89 |
| colic | — | C77.2 | — | D36.Ø | D48.7 | D49.89 |
| common duct | — | C77.2 | — | D36.Ø | D48.7 | D49.89 |
| cubital | — | C77.3 | — | D36.Ø | D48.7 | D49.89 |
| diaphragmatic | — | C77.1 | — | D36.Ø | D48.7 | D49.89 |
| epigastric, inferior | — | C77.1 | — | D36.Ø | D48.7 | D49.89 |
| epitrochlear | — | C77.3 | — | D36.Ø | D48.7 | D49.89 |
| esophageal | — | C77.1 | — | D36.Ø | D48.7 | D49.89 |
| face | — | C77.Ø | — | D36.Ø | D48.7 | D49.89 |
| femoral | — | C77.4 | — | D36.Ø | D48.7 | D49.89 |
| gastric | — | C77.2 | — | D36.Ø | D48.7 | D49.89 |
| groin | — | C77.4 | — | D36.Ø | D48.7 | D49.89 |
| head | — | C77.Ø | — | D36.Ø | D48.7 | D49.89 |
| hepatic | — | C77.2 | — | D36.Ø | D48.7 | D49.89 |
| hilar (pulmonary) | — | C77.1 | — | D36.Ø | D48.7 | D49.89 |
| splenic | — | C77.2 | — | D36.Ø | D48.7 | D49.89 |
| hypogastric | — | C77.5 | — | D36.Ø | D48.7 | D49.89 |
| ileocolic | — | C77.2 | — | D36.Ø | D48.7 | D49.89 |
| iliac | — | C77.5 | — | D36.Ø | D48.7 | D49.89 |
| infraclavicular | — | C77.3 | — | D36.Ø | D48.7 | D49.89 |
| inguina, inguinal | — | C77.4 | — | D36.Ø | D48.7 | D49.89 |
| innominate | — | C77.1 | — | D36.Ø | D48.7 | D49.89 |
| intercostal | — | C77.1 | — | D36.Ø | D48.7 | D49.89 |
| intestinal | — | C77.2 | — | D36.Ø | D48.7 | D49.89 |
| intrabdominal | — | C77.2 | — | D36.Ø | D48.7 | D49.89 |
| intrapelvic | — | C77.5 | — | D36.Ø | D48.7 | D49.89 |
| intrathoracic | — | C77.1 | — | D36.Ø | D48.7 | D49.89 |
| jugular | — | C77.Ø | — | D36.Ø | D48.7 | D49.89 |
| leg | — | C77.4 | — | D36.Ø | D48.7 | D49.89 |
| limb | | | | | | |
| lower | — | C77.4 | — | D36.Ø | D48.7 | D49.89 |
| upper | — | C77.3 | — | D36.Ø | D48.7 | D49.89 |
| lower limb | — | C77.4 | — | D36.Ø | D48.7 | D49.89 |
| lumbar | — | C77.2 | — | D36.Ø | D48.7 | D49.89 |
| mandibular | — | C77.Ø | — | D36.Ø | D48.7 | D49.89 |
| mediastinal | — | C77.1 | — | D36.Ø | D48.7 | D49.89 |
| mesenteric (inferior) (superior) | — | C77.2 | — | D36.Ø | D48.7 | D49.89 |
| midcolic | — | C77.2 | — | D36.Ø | D48.7 | D49.89 |
| multiple sites in categories C77.0 - C77.5 | — | C77.8 | — | D36.Ø | D48.7 | D49.89 |
| neck | — | C77.Ø | — | D36.Ø | D48.7 | D49.89 |
| obturator | — | C77.5 | — | D36.Ø | D48.7 | D49.89 |
| occipital | — | C77.Ø | — | D36.Ø | D48.7 | D49.89 |
| pancreatic | — | C77.2 | — | D36.Ø | D48.7 | D49.89 |
| para-aortic | — | C77.2 | — | D36.Ø | D48.7 | D49.89 |
| paracervical | — | C77.5 | — | D36.Ø | D48.7 | D49.89 |
| parametrial | — | C77.5 | — | D36.Ø | D48.7 | D49.89 |
| parasternal | — | C77.1 | — | D36.Ø | D48.7 | D49.89 |
| parotid | — | C77.Ø | — | D36.Ø | D48.7 | D49.89 |
| pectoral | — | C77.3 | — | D36.Ø | D48.7 | D49.89 |
| pelvic | — | C77.5 | — | D36.Ø | D48.7 | D49.89 |
| peri-aortic | — | C77.2 | — | D36.Ø | D48.7 | D49.89 |
| peripancreatic | — | C77.2 | — | D36.Ø | D48.7 | D49.89 |
| popliteal | — | C77.4 | — | D36.Ø | D48.7 | D49.89 |
| porta hepatis | — | C77.2 | — | D36.Ø | D48.7 | D49.89 |
| portal | — | C77.2 | — | D36.Ø | D48.7 | D49.89 |
| preauricular | — | C77.Ø | — | D36.Ø | D48.7 | D49.89 |
| prelaryngeal | — | C77.Ø | — | D36.Ø | D48.7 | D49.89 |
| presymphysial | — | C77.5 | — | D36.Ø | D48.7 | D49.89 |
| pretracheal | — | C77.Ø | — | D36.Ø | D48.7 | D49.89 |
| primary (any site) NEC | C96.9 | — | — | — | — | — |
| pulmonary (hiler) | — | C77.1 | — | D36.Ø | D48.7 | D49.89 |
| pyloric | — | C77.2 | — | D36.Ø | D48.7 | D49.89 |
| retroperitoneal | — | C77.2 | — | D36.Ø | D48.7 | D49.89 |
| retropharyngeal | — | C77.Ø | — | D36.Ø | D48.7 | D49.89 |
| Rosenmuller's | — | C77.4 | — | D36.Ø | D48.7 | D49.89 |
| sacral | — | C77.5 | — | D36.Ø | D48.7 | D49.89 |
| scalene | — | C77.Ø | — | D36.Ø | D48.7 | D49.89 |
| site NEC | — | C77.9 | — | D36.Ø | D48.7 | D49.89 |

| | Malignant Primary | Malignant Secondary | Ca in situ | Benign | Uncertain Behavior | Unspecified Behavior |
|---|---|---|---|---|---|---|
| **Neoplasm, neoplastic** — *continued* | | | | | | |
| lymph, lymphatic channel — *continued* | | | | | | |
| . gland — *continued* | | | | | | |
| . . splenic (hilar) | — | C77.2 | — | D36.Ø | D48.7 | D49.89 |
| . . subclavicular | — | C77.3 | — | D36.Ø | D48.7 | D49.89 |
| . . subinguinal | — | C77.4 | — | D36.Ø | D48.7 | D49.89 |
| . . sublingual | — | C77.Ø | — | D36.Ø | D48.7 | D49.89 |
| . . submandibular | — | C77.Ø | — | D36.Ø | D48.7 | D49.89 |
| . . submaxillary | — | C77.Ø | — | D36.Ø | D48.7 | D49.89 |
| . . submental | — | C77.Ø | — | D36.Ø | D48.7 | D49.89 |
| . . subscapular | — | C77.3 | — | D36.Ø | D48.7 | D49.89 |
| . . supraclavicular | — | C77.Ø | — | D36.Ø | D48.7 | D49.89 |
| . . thoracic | — | C77.1 | — | D36.Ø | D48.7 | D49.89 |
| . . tibial | — | C77.4 | — | D36.Ø | D48.7 | D49.89 |
| . . tracheal | — | C77.1 | — | D36.Ø | D48.7 | D49.89 |
| . . tracheobronchial | — | C77.1 | — | D36.Ø | D48.7 | D49.89 |
| . . upper limb | — | C77.3 | — | D36.Ø | D48.7 | D49.89 |
| . . Virchow's | — | C77.Ø | — | D36.Ø | D48.7 | D49.89 |
| . node — *see also* Neoplasm, lymph gland | | | | | | |
| . . primary NEC | C96.9 | — | — | — | — | — |
| . vessel — *see also* Neoplasm, connective tissue | C49.9 | C79.89 | — | D21.9 | D48.1-☑ | D49.2 |
| Mackenrodt's ligament | C57.7 | C79.82 | DØ7.39 | D28.7 | D39.8 | D49.59 |
| malar | C41.Ø | C79.51 | — | D16.4 | D48.Ø | D49.2 |
| . region — *see* Neoplasm, cheek | | | | | | |
| mammary gland — *see* Neoplasm, breast | | | | | | |
| mandible | C41.1 | C79.51 | — | D16.5 | D48.Ø | D49.2 |
| . alveolar | | | | | | |
| . . mucosa (carcinoma) | CØ3.1 | C79.89 | DØØ.Ø3 | D1Ø.39 | D37.Ø9 | D49.Ø |
| . . ridge or process | C41.1 | C79.51 | — | D16.5 | D48.Ø | D49.2 |
| marrow (bone) NEC | C96.9 | C79.52 | — | — | D47.9 | D49.89 |
| mastectomy site (skin) — *see also* Neoplasm, breast, skin | C44.5Ø1 | C79.2 | — | — | — | — |
| . specified as breast tissue | C5Ø.8-☑ | C79.81 | — | — | — | — |
| mastoid (air cells) (antrum) (cavity) | C3Ø.1 | C78.39 | DØ2.3 | D14.Ø | D38.5 | D49.1 |
| . bone or process | C41.Ø | C79.51 | — | D16.4 | D48.Ø | D49.2 |
| maxilla, maxillary (superior) | C41.Ø | C79.51 | — | D16.4 | D48.Ø | D49.2 |
| . alveolar | | | | | | |
| . . mucosa | CØ3.Ø | C79.89 | DØØ.Ø3 | D1Ø.39 | D37.Ø9 | D49.Ø |
| . . ridge or process (carcinoma) | C41.Ø | C79.51 | — | D16.4 | D48.Ø | D49.2 |
| . antrum | C31.Ø | C78.39 | DØ2.3 | D14.Ø | D38.5 | D49.1 |
| . carcinoma | CØ3.Ø | C79.51 | — | — | — | — |
| . inferior — *see* Neoplasm, mandible | | | | | | |
| . sinus | C31.Ø | C78.39 | DØ2.3 | D14.Ø | D38.5 | D49.1 |
| meatus external (ear) — *see also* Neoplasm, skin, ear | C44.2Ø-☑ | C79.2 | DØ4.2-☑ | D23.2-☑ | D48.5 | D49.2 |
| Meckel diverticulum, malignant | C17.3 | C78.4 | DØ1.49 | D13.39 | D37.2 | D49.Ø |
| mediastinum, mediastinal | C38.3 | C78.1 | — | D15.2 | D38.3 | D49.89 |
| . anterior | C38.1 | C78.1 | — | D15.2 | D38.3 | D49.89 |
| . posterior | C38.2 | C78.1 | — | D15.2 | D38.3 | D49.89 |
| medulla | | | | | | |
| . adrenal | C74.1-☑ | C79.7-☑ | DØ9.3 | D35.Ø-☑ | D44.1-☑ | D49.7 |
| . oblongata | C71.7 | C79.31 | — | D33.1 | D43.1 | D49.6 |
| meibomian gland | C44.1Ø-☑ | C79.2 | DØ4.1-☑ | D23.1-☑ | D48.5 | D49.2 |
| . basal cell carcinoma | C44.11-☑ | — | — | — | — | — |
| . sebaceous cell | C44.13-☑ | — | — | — | — | — |
| **Neoplasm, neoplastic** — *continued* | | | | | | |
| meibomian gland — *continued* | | | | | | |
| . specified type NEC | C44.19-☑ | — | — | — | — | — |
| . squamous cell carcinoma | C44.12-☑ | — | — | — | — | — |
| melanoma — *see* Melanoma | | | | | | |
| meninges | C7Ø.9 | C79.49 | — | D32.9 | D42.9 | D49.7 |
| . brain | C7Ø.Ø | C79.32 | — | D32.Ø | D42.Ø | D49.7 |
| . cerebral | C7Ø.Ø | C79.32 | — | D32.Ø | D42.Ø | D49.7 |
| . cranial | C7Ø.Ø | C79.32 | — | D32.Ø | D42.Ø | D49.7 |
| . intracranial | C7Ø.Ø | C79.32 | — | D32.Ø | D42.Ø | D49.7 |
| . spinal (cord) | C7Ø.1 | C79.49 | — | D32.1 | D42.1 | D49.7 |
| meniscus, knee joint (lateral) (medial) | C4Ø.2-☑ | C79.51 | — | D16.2-☑ | D48.Ø | D49.2 |
| Merkel cell — *see* Carcinoma, Merkel cell | | | | | | |
| mesentery, mesenteric | C48.1 | C78.6 | — | D2Ø.1 | D48.4 | D49.Ø |
| mesoappendix | C48.1 | C78.6 | — | D2Ø.1 | D48.4 | D49.Ø |
| mesocolon | C48.1 | C78.6 | — | D2Ø.1 | D48.4 | D49.Ø |
| mesopharynx — *see* Neoplasm, oropharynx | | | | | | |
| mesosalpinx | C57.1-☑ | C79.82 | DØ7.39 | D28.2 | D39.8 | D49.59 |
| mesothelial tissue — *see* Mesothelioma | | | | | | |
| mesothelioma — *see* Mesothelioma | | | | | | |
| mesovarium | C57.1-☑ | C79.82 | DØ7.39 | D28.2 | D39.8 | D49.59 |
| metacarpus (any bone) | C4Ø.1-☑ | C79.51 | — | D16.1-☑ | — | — |
| metastatic NEC — *see also* Neoplasm, by site, secondary | — | C79.9 | — | — | — | — |
| metatarsus (any bone) | C4Ø.3-☑ | C79.51 | — | D16.3-☑ | — | — |
| midbrain | C71.7 | C79.31 | — | D33.1 | D43.1 | D49.6 |
| milk duct — *see* Neoplasm, breast | | | | | | |
| mons | | | | | | |
| . pubis | C51.9 | C79.82 | DØ7.1 | D28.Ø | D39.8 | D49.59 |
| . veneris | C51.9 | C79.82 | DØ7.1 | D28.Ø | D39.8 | D49.59 |
| motor tract | C72.9 | C79.49 | — | D33.9 | D43.9 | D49.7 |
| . brain | C71.9 | C79.31 | — | D33.2 | D43.2 | D49.6 |
| . cauda equina | C72.1 | C79.49 | — | D33.4 | D43.4 | D49.7 |
| . spinal | C72.Ø | C79.49 | — | D33.4 | D43.4 | D49.7 |
| mouth | CØ6.9 | C79.89 | DØØ.ØØ | D1Ø.3Ø | D37.Ø9 | D49.Ø |
| . book-leaf | CØ6.89 | C79.89 | — | — | — | — |
| . floor | CØ4.9 | C79.89 | DØØ.Ø6 | D1Ø.2 | D37.Ø9 | D49.Ø |
| . . anterior portion | CØ4.Ø | C79.89 | DØØ.Ø6 | D1Ø.2 | D37.Ø9 | D49.Ø |
| . . lateral portion | CØ4.1 | C79.89 | DØØ.Ø6 | D1Ø.2 | D37.Ø9 | D49.Ø |
| . . overlapping lesion | CØ4.8 | — | — | — | — | — |
| . overlapping NEC | CØ6.8Ø | — | — | — | — | — |
| . roof | CØ5.9 | C79.89 | DØØ.ØØ | D1Ø.39 | D37.Ø9 | D49.Ø |
| . specified part NEC | CØ6.89 | C79.89 | DØØ.ØØ | D1Ø.39 | D37.Ø9 | D49.Ø |
| . vestibule | CØ6.1 | C79.89 | DØØ.ØØ | D1Ø.39 | D37.Ø9 | D49.Ø |
| mucosa | | | | | | |
| . alveolar (ridge or process) | CØ3.9 | C79.89 | DØØ.Ø3 | D1Ø.39 | D37.Ø9 | D49.Ø |
| . . lower | CØ3.1 | C79.89 | DØØ.Ø3 | D1Ø.39 | D37.Ø9 | D49.Ø |
| . . upper | CØ3.Ø | C79.89 | DØØ.Ø3 | D1Ø.39 | D37.Ø9 | D49.Ø |
| . buccal | CØ6.Ø | C79.89 | DØØ.Ø2 | D1Ø.39 | D37.Ø9 | D49.Ø |
| . cheek | CØ6.Ø | C79.89 | DØØ.Ø2 | D1Ø.39 | D37.Ø9 | D49.Ø |
| . lip — *see* Neoplasm, lip, internal | | | | | | |
| . nasal | C3Ø.Ø | C78.39 | DØ2.3 | D14.Ø | D38.5 | D49.1 |
| . oral | CØ6.Ø | C79.89 | DØØ.Ø2 | D1Ø.39 | D37.Ø9 | D49.Ø |
| Mullerian duct | | | | | | |
| . female | C57.7 | C79.82 | DØ7.39 | D28.7 | D39.8 | D49.59 |
| . male | C63.7 | C79.82 | DØ7.69 | D29.8 | D4Ø.8 | D49.59 |
| muscle — *see also* Neoplasm, connective tissue | | | | | | |

| | Malignant Primary | Malignant Secondary | Ca in situ | Benign | Uncertain Behavior | Unspecified Behavior |
|---|---|---|---|---|---|---|
| **Neoplasm, neoplastic** *— continued* | | | | | | |
| muscle *— see also* Neoplasm, connective tissue *— continued* | | | | | | |
| extraocular | C69.6-☑ | C79.49 | D09.2-☑ | D31.6-☑ | D48.7 | D49.89 |
| myocardium | C38.0 | C79.89 | — | D15.1 | D48.7 | D49.89 |
| myometrium | C54.2 | C79.82 | D07.0 | D26.1 | D39.0 | D49.59 |
| myopericardium | C38.0 | C79.89 | — | D15.1 | D48.7 | D49.89 |
| nabothian gland (follicle) | C53.0 | C79.82 | D06.0 | D26.0 | D39.0 | D49.59 |
| nail *— see also* Neoplasm, skin, limb | C44.90 | C79.2 | D04.9 | D23.9 | D48.5 | D49.2 |
| finger *— see also* Neoplasm, skin, limb, upper | C44.60-☑ | C79.2 | D04.6-☑ | D23.6-☑ | D48.5 | D49.2 |
| toe *— see also* Neoplasm, skin, limb, lower | C44.70-☑ | C79.2 | D04.7-☑ | D23.7-☑ | D48.5 | D49.2 |
| nares, naris (anterior) (posterior) | C30.0 | C78.39 | D02.3 | D14.0 | D38.5 | D49.1 |
| nasal *— see* Neoplasm, nose | | | | | | |
| nasolabial groove *— see also* Neoplasm, skin, face | C44.309 | C79.2 | D04.39 | D23.39 | D48.5 | D49.2 |
| nasolacrimal duct | C69.5-☑ | C79.49 | D09.2-☑ | D31.5-☑ | D48.7 | D49.89 |
| nasopharynx, nasopharyngeal | C11.9 | C79.89 | D00.08 | D10.6 | D37.05 | D49.0 |
| floor | C11.3 | C79.89 | D00.08 | D10.6 | D37.05 | D49.0 |
| overlapping lesion | C11.8 | — | — | — | — | — |
| roof | C11.0 | C79.89 | D00.08 | D10.6 | D37.05 | D49.0 |
| wall | C11.9 | C79.89 | D00.08 | D10.6 | D37.05 | D49.0 |
| anterior | C11.3 | C79.89 | D00.08 | D10.6 | D37.05 | D49.0 |
| lateral | C11.2 | C79.89 | D00.08 | D10.6 | D37.05 | D49.0 |
| posterior | C11.1 | C79.89 | D00.08 | D10.6 | D37.05 | D49.0 |
| superior | C11.0 | C79.89 | D00.08 | D10.6 | D37.05 | D49.0 |
| nates *— see also* Neoplasm, skin, trunk | C44.509 | C79.2 | D04.5 | D23.5 | D48.5 | D49.2 |
| neck NEC | C76.0 | C79.89 | D09.8 | D36.7 | D48.7 | D49.89 |
| skin | C44.40 | — | — | — | — | — |
| basal cell carcinoma | C44.41 | — | — | — | — | — |
| specified type NEC | C44.49 | — | — | — | — | — |
| squamous cell carcinoma | C44.42 | — | — | — | — | — |
| nerve (ganglion) | C47.9 | C79.89 | — | D36.10 | D48.2 | D49.2 |
| abducens | C72.59 | C79.49 | — | D33.3 | D43.3 | D49.7 |
| accessory (spinal) | C72.59 | C79.49 | — | D33.3 | D43.3 | D49.7 |
| acoustic | C72.4-☑ | C79.49 | — | D33.3 | D43.3 | D49.7 |
| auditory | C72.4-☑ | C79.49 | — | D33.3 | D43.3 | D49.7 |
| autonomic NEC *— see also* Neoplasm, nerve, peripheral | C47.9 | C79.89 | — | D36.10 | D48.2 | D49.2 |
| brachial | C47.1-☑ | C79.89 | — | D36.12 | D48.2 | D49.2 |
| cranial | C72.50 | C79.49 | — | D33.3 | D43.3 | D49.7 |
| specified NEC | C72.59 | C79.49 | — | D33.3 | D43.3 | D49.7 |
| facial | C72.59 | C79.49 | — | D33.3 | D43.3 | D49.7 |
| femoral | C47.2-☑ | C79.89 | — | D36.13 | D48.2 | D49.2 |
| ganglion NEC *— see also* Neoplasm, nerve, peripheral | C47.9 | C79.89 | — | D36.10 | D48.2 | D49.2 |
| glossopharyngeal | C72.59 | C79.49 | — | D33.3 | D43.3 | D49.7 |
| hypoglossal | C72.59 | C79.49 | — | D33.3 | D43.3 | D49.7 |
| intercostal | C47.3 | C79.89 | — | D36.14 | D48.2 | D49.2 |
| lumbar | C47.6 | C79.89 | — | D36.17 | D48.2 | D49.2 |
| median | C47.1-☑ | C79.89 | — | D36.12 | D48.2 | D49.2 |
| obturator | C47.2-☑ | C79.89 | — | D36.13 | D48.2 | D49.2 |
| oculomotor | C72.59 | C79.49 | — | D33.3 | D43.3 | D49.7 |
| olfactory | C47.2-☑ | C79.49 | — | D33.3 | D43.3 | D49.7 |
| optic | C72.3-☑ | C79.49 | — | D33.3 | D43.3 | D49.7 |
| parasympathetic NEC | C47.9 | C79.89 | — | D36.10 | D48.2 | D49.2 |
| peripheral NEC | C47.9 | C79.89 | — | D36.10 | D48.2 | D49.2 |
| abdomen | C47.4 | C79.89 | — | D36.15 | D48.2 | D49.2 |

| | Malignant Primary | Malignant Secondary | Ca in situ | Benign | Uncertain Behavior | Unspecified Behavior |
|---|---|---|---|---|---|---|
| **Neoplasm, neoplastic** *— continued* | | | | | | |
| nerve *— continued* | | | | | | |
| peripheral *— continued* | | | | | | |
| abdominal wall | C47.4 | C79.89 | — | D36.15 | D48.2 | D49.2 |
| ankle | C47.2-☑ | C79.89 | — | D36.13 | D48.2 | D49.2 |
| antecubital fossa or space | C47.1-☑ | C79.89 | — | D36.12 | D48.2 | D49.2 |
| arm | C47.1-☑ | C79.89 | — | D36.12 | D48.2 | D49.2 |
| auricle (ear) | C47.0 | C79.89 | — | D36.11 | D48.2 | D49.2 |
| axilla | C47.3 | C79.89 | — | D36.12 | D48.2 | D49.2 |
| back | C47.6 | C79.89 | — | D36.17 | D48.2 | D49.2 |
| buttock | C47.5 | C79.89 | — | D36.16 | D48.2 | D49.2 |
| calf | C47.2-☑ | C79.89 | — | D36.13 | D48.2 | D49.2 |
| cervical region | C47.0 | C79.89 | — | D36.11 | D48.2 | D49.2 |
| cheek | C47.0 | C79.89 | — | D36.11 | D48.2 | D49.2 |
| chest (wall) | C47.3 | C79.89 | — | D36.14 | D48.2 | D49.2 |
| chin | C47.0 | C79.89 | — | D36.11 | D48.2 | D49.2 |
| ear (external) | C47.0 | C79.89 | — | D36.11 | D48.2 | D49.2 |
| elbow | C47.1-☑ | C79.89 | — | D36.12 | D48.2 | D49.2 |
| extrarectal | C47.5 | C79.89 | — | D36.16 | D48.2 | D49.2 |
| extremity | C47.9 | C79.89 | — | D36.10 | D48.2 | D49.2 |
| lower | C47.2-☑ | C79.89 | — | D36.13 | D48.2 | D49.2 |
| upper | C47.1-☑ | C79.89 | — | D36.12 | D48.2 | D49.2 |
| eyelid | C47.0 | C79.89 | — | D36.11 | D48.2 | D49.2 |
| face | C47.0 | C79.89 | — | D36.11 | D48.2 | D49.2 |
| finger | C47.1-☑ | C79.89 | — | D36.12 | D48.2 | D49.2 |
| flank | C47.6 | C79.89 | — | D36.17 | D48.2 | D49.2 |
| foot | C47.2-☑ | C79.89 | — | D36.13 | D48.2 | D49.2 |
| forearm | C47.1-☑ | C79.89 | — | D36.12 | D48.2 | D49.2 |
| forehead | C47.0 | C79.89 | — | D36.11 | D48.2 | D49.2 |
| gluteal region | C47.5 | C79.89 | — | D36.16 | D48.2 | D49.2 |
| groin | C47.5 | C79.89 | — | D36.16 | D48.2 | D49.2 |
| hand | C47.1-☑ | C79.89 | — | D36.12 | D48.2 | D49.2 |
| head | C47.0 | C79.89 | — | D36.11 | D48.2 | D49.2 |
| heel | C47.2-☑ | C79.89 | — | D36.13 | D48.2 | D49.2 |
| hip | C47.2-☑ | C79.89 | — | D36.13 | D48.2 | D49.2 |
| infraclavicular region | C47.3 | C79.89 | — | D36.14 | D48.2 | D49.2 |
| inguinal (canal) (region) | C47.5 | C79.89 | — | D36.16 | D48.2 | D49.2 |
| intrathoracic | C47.3 | C79.89 | — | D36.14 | D48.2 | D49.2 |
| ischiorectal fossa | C47.5 | C79.89 | — | D36.16 | D48.2 | D49.2 |
| knee | C47.2-☑ | C79.89 | — | D36.13 | D48.2 | D49.2 |
| leg | C47.2-☑ | C79.89 | — | D36.13 | D48.2 | D49.2 |
| limb NEC | C47.9 | C79.89 | — | D36.10 | D48.2 | D49.2 |
| lower | C47.2-☑ | C79.89 | — | D36.13 | D48.2 | D49.2 |
| upper | C47.1-☑ | C79.89 | — | D36.12 | D48.2 | D49.2 |
| nates | C47.5 | C79.89 | — | D36.16 | D48.2 | D49.2 |
| neck | C47.0 | C79.89 | — | D36.11 | D48.2 | D49.2 |
| orbit | C69.6-☑ | C79.49 | — | D31.6-☑ | D48.7 | D49.2 |
| pararectal | C47.5 | C79.89 | — | D36.16 | D48.2 | D49.2 |
| paraurethral | C47.5 | C79.89 | — | D36.16 | D48.2 | D49.2 |
| paravaginal | C47.5 | C79.89 | — | D36.16 | D48.2 | D49.2 |
| pelvis (floor) | C47.5 | C79.89 | — | D36.16 | D48.2 | D49.2 |
| pelvoabdominal | C47.8 | C79.89 | — | D36.17 | D48.2 | D49.2 |
| perineum | C47.5 | C79.89 | — | D36.16 | D48.2 | D49.2 |
| perirectal (tissue) | C47.5 | C79.89 | — | D36.16 | D48.2 | D49.2 |
| periurethral (tissue) | C47.5 | C79.89 | — | D36.16 | D48.2 | D49.2 |
| popliteal fossa or space | C47.2-☑ | C79.89 | — | D36.13 | D48.2 | D49.2 |
| presacral | C47.5 | C79.89 | — | D36.16 | D48.2 | D49.2 |
| pterygoid fossa | C47.0 | C79.89 | — | D36.11 | D48.2 | D49.2 |
| rectovaginal septum or wall | C47.5 | C79.89 | — | D36.16 | D48.2 | D49.2 |
| rectovesical | C47.5 | C79.89 | — | D36.16 | D48.2 | D49.2 |
| sacrococcygeal region | C47.5 | C79.89 | — | D36.16 | D48.2 | D49.2 |
| scalp | C47.0 | C79.89 | — | D36.11 | D48.2 | D49.2 |
| scapular region | C47.3 | C79.89 | — | D36.14 | D48.2 | D49.2 |
| shoulder | C47.1-☑ | C79.89 | — | D36.12 | D48.2 | D49.2 |
| submental | C47.0 | C79.89 | — | D36.11 | D48.2 | D49.2 |
| supraclavicular region | C47.0 | C79.89 | — | D36.11 | D48.2 | D49.2 |

| | Malignant Primary | Malignant Secondary | Ca in situ | Benign | Uncertain Behavior | Unspecified Behavior |
|---|---|---|---|---|---|---|
| **Neoplasm, neoplastic** — *continued* | | | | | | |
| nerve — *continued* | | | | | | |
| peripheral — *continued* | | | | | | |
| temple | C47.0 | C79.89 | — | D36.11 | D48.2 | D49.2 |
| temporal region | C47.0 | C79.89 | — | D36.11 | D48.2 | D49.2 |
| thigh | C47.2-☑ | C79.89 | — | D36.13 | D48.2 | D49.2 |
| thoracic (duct) (wall) | C47.3 | C79.89 | — | D36.14 | D48.2 | D49.2 |
| thorax | C47.3 | C79.89 | — | D36.14 | D48.2 | D49.2 |
| thumb | C47.1-☑ | C79.89 | — | D36.12 | D48.2 | D49.2 |
| toe | C47.2-☑ | C79.89 | — | D36.13 | D48.2 | D49.2 |
| trunk | C47.6 | C79.89 | — | D36.17 | D48.2 | D49.2 |
| umbilicus | C47.4 | C79.89 | — | D36.15 | D48.2 | D49.2 |
| vesicorectal | C47.5 | C79.89 | — | D36.16 | D48.2 | D49.2 |
| wrist | C47.1-☑ | C79.89 | — | D36.12 | D48.2 | D49.2 |
| radial | C47.1-☑ | C79.89 | — | D36.12 | D48.2 | D49.2 |
| sacral | C47.5 | C79.89 | — | D36.16 | D48.2 | D49.2 |
| sciatic | C47.2-☑ | C79.89 | — | D36.13 | D48.2 | D49.2 |
| spinal NEC | C47.9 | C79.89 | — | D36.10 | D48.2 | D49.2 |
| accessory | C72.59 | C79.49 | — | D33.3 | D43.3 | D49.7 |
| sympathetic NEC — *see also* Neoplasm, nerve, peripheral | C47.9 | C79.89 | — | D36.10 | D48.2 | D49.2 |
| trigeminal | C72.59 | C79.49 | — | D33.3 | D43.3 | D49.7 |
| trochlear | C72.59 | C79.49 | — | D33.3 | D43.3 | D49.7 |
| ulnar | C47.1-☑ | C79.89 | — | D36.12 | D48.2 | D49.2 |
| vagus | C72.59 | C79.49 | — | D33.3 | D43.3 | D49.7 |
| nervous system (central) | C72.9 | C79.40 | — | D33.9 | D43.9 | D49.7 |
| autonomic — *see* Neoplasm, nerve, peripheral | | | | | | |
| parasympathetic — *see* Neoplasm, nerve, peripheral | | | | | | |
| specified site NEC | — | C79.49 | — | D33.7 | D43.8 | — |
| sympathetic — *see* Neoplasm, nerve, peripheral | | | | | | |
| nevus — *see* Nevus | | | | | | |
| nipple | C50.0-☑ | C79.81 | D05.-☑ | D24.-☑ | — | — |
| nose, nasal | C76.0 | C79.89 | D09.8 | D36.7 | D48.7 | D49.89 |
| ala (external) (nasi) — *see also* Neoplasm, nose, skin | C44.301 | C79.2 | D04.39 | D23.39 | D48.5 | D49.2 |
| bone | C41.0 | C79.51 | — | D16.4 | D48.0 | D49.2 |
| cartilage | C30.0 | C78.39 | D02.3 | D14.0 | D38.5 | D49.1 |
| cavity | C30.0 | C78.39 | D02.3 | D14.0 | D38.5 | D49.1 |
| choana | C11.3 | C79.89 | D00.08 | D10.6 | D37.05 | D49.0 |
| external (skin) — *see also* Neoplasm, nose, skin | C44.301 | C79.2 | D04.39 | D23.39 | D48.5 | D49.2 |
| fossa | C30.0 | C78.39 | D02.3 | D14.0 | D38.5 | D49.1 |
| internal | C30.0 | C78.39 | D02.3 | D14.0 | D38.5 | D49.1 |
| mucosa | C30.0 | C78.39 | D02.3 | D14.0 | D38.5 | D49.1 |
| septum | C30.0 | C78.39 | D02.3 | D14.0 | D38.5 | D49.1 |
| posterior margin | C11.3 | C79.89 | D00.08 | D10.6 | D37.05 | D49.0 |
| sinus — *see* Neoplasm, sinus | | | | | | |
| skin | C44.301 | C79.2 | D04.39 | D23.39 | D48.5 | D49.2 |
| basal cell carcinoma | C44.311 | — | — | — | — | — |
| specified type NEC | C44.391 | — | — | — | — | — |
| squamous cell carcinoma | C44.321 | — | — | — | — | — |
| turbinate (mucosa) | C30.0 | C78.39 | D02.3 | D14.0 | D38.5 | D49.1 |
| bone | C41.0 | C79.51 | — | D16.4 | D48.0 | D49.2 |
| vestibule | C30.0 | C78.39 | D02.3 | D14.0 | D38.5 | D49.1 |
| nostril | C30.0 | C78.39 | D02.3 | D14.0 | D38.5 | D49.1 |
| nucleus pulposus | C41.2 | C79.51 | — | D16.6 | D48.0 | D49.2 |
| occipital | | | | | | |
| bone | C41.0 | C79.51 | — | D16.4 | D48.0 | D49.2 |
| lobe or pole, brain | C71.4 | C79.31 | — | D33.0 | D43.0 | D49.6 |
| **Neoplasm, neoplastic** — *continued* | | | | | | |
| odontogenic — *see* Neoplasm, jaw, bone | | | | | | |
| olfactory nerve or bulb | C72.2-☑ | C79.49 | — | D33.3 | D43.3 | D49.7 |
| olive (brain) | C71.7 | C79.31 | — | D33.1 | D43.1 | D49.6 |
| omentum | C48.1 | C78.6 | — | D20.1 | D48.4 | D49.0 |
| operculum (brain) | C71.0 | C79.31 | — | D33.0 | D43.0 | D49.6 |
| optic nerve, chiasm, or tract | C72.3-☑ | C79.49 | — | D33.3 | D43.3 | D49.7 |
| oral (cavity) | C06.9 | C79.83 | D00.00 | D10.30 | D37.09 | D49.0 |
| ill-defined | C14.8 | C79.83 | D00.00 | D10.30 | D37.09 | D49.0 |
| mucosa | C06.0 | C79.83 | D00.02 | D10.39 | D37.09 | D49.0 |
| orbit | C69.6-☑ | C79.49 | D09.2-☑ | D31.6-☑ | D48.7 | D49.89 |
| autonomic nerve | C69.6-☑ | C79.49 | — | D31.6-☑ | D48.7 | D49.2 |
| bone | C41.0 | C79.51 | — | D16.4 | D48.0 | D49.2 |
| eye | C69.6-☑ | C79.49 | D09.2-☑ | D31.6-☑ | D48.7 | D49.89 |
| peripheral nerves | C69.6-☑ | C79.49 | — | D31.6-☑ | D48.7 | D49.2 |
| soft parts | C69.6-☑ | C79.49 | D09.2-☑ | D31.6-☑ | D48.7 | D49.89 |
| organ of Zuckerkandl | C75.5 | C79.89 | — | D35.6 | D44.7 | D49.7 |
| oropharynx | C10.9 | C79.89 | D00.08 | D10.5 | D37.05 | D49.0 |
| branchial cleft (vestige) | C10.4 | C79.89 | D00.08 | D10.5 | D37.05 | D49.0 |
| junctional region | C10.8 | C79.89 | D00.08 | D10.5 | D37.05 | D49.0 |
| lateral wall | C10.2 | C79.89 | D00.08 | D10.5 | D37.05 | D49.0 |
| overlapping lesion | C10.8 | — | — | — | — | — |
| pillars or fauces | C09.1 | C79.89 | D00.08 | D10.5 | D37.05 | D49.0 |
| posterior wall | C10.3 | C79.89 | D00.08 | D10.5 | D37.05 | D49.0 |
| vallecula | C10.0 | C79.89 | D00.08 | D10.5 | D37.05 | D49.0 |
| os | | | | | | |
| external | C53.1 | C79.82 | D06.1 | D26.0 | D39.0 | D49.59 |
| internal | C53.0 | C79.82 | D06.0 | D26.0 | D39.0 | D49.59 |
| ovary | C56.-☑ | C79.6-☑ | D07.39 | D27.-☑ | D39.1-☑ | D49.59 |
| oviduct | C57.0-☑ | C79.82 | D07.39 | D28.2 | D39.8 | D49.59 |
| palate | C05.9 | C79.89 | D00.00 | D10.39 | D37.09 | D49.0 |
| hard | C05.0 | C79.89 | D00.05 | D10.39 | D37.09 | D49.0 |
| junction of hard and soft palate | C05.9 | C79.89 | D00.00 | D10.39 | D37.09 | D49.0 |
| overlapping lesions | C05.8 | — | — | — | — | — |
| soft | C05.1 | C79.89 | D00.04 | D10.39 | D37.09 | D49.0 |
| nasopharyngeal surface | C11.3 | C79.89 | D00.08 | D10.6 | D37.05 | D49.0 |
| posterior surface | C11.3 | C79.89 | D00.08 | D10.6 | D37.05 | D49.0 |
| superior surface | C11.3 | C79.89 | D00.08 | D10.6 | D37.05 | D49.0 |
| palatoglossal arch | C09.1 | C79.89 | D00.00 | D10.5 | D37.09 | D49.0 |
| palatopharyngeal arch | C09.1 | C79.89 | D00.00 | D10.5 | D37.09 | D49.0 |
| pallium | C71.0 | C79.31 | — | D33.0 | D43.0 | D49.6 |
| palpebra | C44.10-☑ | C79.2 | D04.1-☑ | D23.1-☑ | D48.5 | D49.2 |
| basal cell carcinoma | C44.11-☑ | — | — | — | — | — |
| sebaceous cell | C44.13-☑ | — | — | — | — | — |
| specified type NEC | C44.19-☑ | — | — | — | — | — |
| squamous cell carcinoma | C44.12-☑ | — | — | — | — | — |
| pancreas | C25.9 | C78.89 | D01.7 | D13.6 | D37.8 | D49.0 |
| body | C25.1 | C78.89 | D01.7 | D13.6 | D37.8 | D49.0 |
| duct (of Santorini) (of Wirsung) | C25.3 | C78.89 | D01.7 | D13.6 | D37.8 | D49.0 |
| ectopic tissue | C25.7 | C78.89 | — | D13.6 | D37.8 | D49.0 |
| head | C25.0 | C78.89 | D01.7 | D13.6 | D37.8 | D49.0 |
| islet cells | C25.4 | C78.89 | D01.7 | D13.7 | D37.8 | D49.0 |
| neck | C25.7 | C78.89 | D01.7 | D13.6 | D37.8 | D49.0 |
| overlapping lesion | C25.8 | — | — | — | — | — |
| tail | C25.2 | C78.89 | D01.7 | D13.6 | D37.8 | D49.0 |
| para-aortic body | C75.5 | C79.89 | — | D35.6 | D44.7 | D49.7 |
| paraganglion NEC | C75.5 | C79.89 | — | D35.6 | D44.7 | D49.7 |
| parametrium | C57.3 | C79.82 | — | D28.2 | D39.8 | D49.59 |
| paranephric | C48.0 | C78.6 | — | D20.0 | D48.3 | D49.0 |
| pararectal | C76.3 | C79.89 | — | D36.7 | D48.7 | D49.89 |



☑ **Additional Character Required — Refer to the Tabular List for Character Selection**

| | Malignant Primary | Malignant Secondary | Ca in situ | Benign | Uncertain Behavior | Unspecified Behavior |
|---|---|---|---|---|---|---|
| **Neoplasm, neoplastic** — *continued* | | | | | | |
| parasagittal (region) | C76.0 | C79.89 | D09.8 | D36.7 | D48.7 | D49.89 |
| parasellar | C72.9 | C79.49 | — | D33.9 | D43.8 | D49.7 |
| parathyroid (gland) | C75.0 | C79.89 | D09.3 | D35.1 | D44.2 | D49.7 |
| paraurethral | C76.3 | C79.89 | — | D36.7 | D48.7 | D49.89 |
| gland | C68.1 | C79.19 | D09.19 | D30.8 | D41.8 | D49.59 |
| paravaginal | C76.3 | C79.89 | — | D36.7 | D48.7 | D49.89 |
| parenchyma, kidney | C64.-☑ | C79.0-☑ | D09.19 | D30.0-☑ | D41.0-☑ | D49.51-☑ |
| parietal | | | | | | |
| bone | C41.0 | C79.51 | — | D16.4 | D48.0 | D49.2 |
| lobe, brain | C71.3 | C79.31 | — | D33.0 | D43.0 | D49.6 |
| paroophoron | C57.1-☑ | C79.82 | D07.39 | D28.2 | D39.8 | D49.59 |
| parotid (duct) (gland) | C07 | C79.89 | D00.00 | D11.0 | D37.030 | D49.0 |
| parovarium | C57.1-☑ | C79.82 | D07.39 | D28.2 | D39.8 | D49.59 |
| patella | C40.2-☑ | C79.51 | — | — | — | — |
| peduncle, cerebral | C71.7 | C79.31 | — | D33.1 | D43.1 | D49.6 |
| pelvirectal junction | C19 | C78.5 | D01.1 | D12.7 | D37.5 | D49.0 |
| pelvis, pelvic | C76.3 | C79.89 | D09.8 | D36.7 | D48.7 | D49.89 |
| bone | C41.4 | C79.51 | — | D16.8 | D48.0 | D49.2 |
| floor | C76.3 | C79.89 | D09.8 | D36.7 | D48.7 | D49.89 |
| renal | C65.-☑ | C79.0-☑ | D09.19 | D30.1-☑ | D41.1-☑ | D49.51-☑ |
| viscera | C76.3 | C79.89 | D09.8 | D36.7 | D48.7 | D49.89 |
| wall | C76.3 | C79.89 | D09.8 | D36.7 | D48.7 | D49.89 |
| pelvo-abdominal | C76.8 | C79.89 | D09.8 | D36.7 | D48.7 | D49.89 |
| penis | C60.9 | C79.82 | D07.4 | D29.0 | D40.8 | D49.59 |
| body | C60.2 | C79.82 | D07.4 | D29.0 | D40.8 | D49.59 |
| corpus (cavernosum) | C60.2 | C79.82 | D07.4 | D29.0 | D40.8 | D49.59 |
| glans | C60.1 | C79.82 | D07.4 | D29.0 | D40.8 | D49.59 |
| overlapping sites | C60.8 | — | — | — | — | — |
| skin NEC | C60.9 | C79.82 | D07.4 | D29.0 | D40.8 | D49.59 |
| periadrenal (tissue) | C48.0 | C78.6 | — | D20.0 | D48.3 | D49.0 |
| perianal (skin) — *see also* Neoplasm, anus, skin | C44.500 | C79.2 | D04.5 | D23.5 | D48.5 | D49.2 |
| pericardium | C38.0 | C79.89 | — | D15.1 | D48.7 | D49.89 |
| perinephric | C48.0 | C78.6 | — | D20.0 | D48.3 | D49.0 |
| perineum | C76.3 | C79.89 | D09.8 | D36.7 | D48.7 | D49.89 |
| periodontal tissue NEC | C03.9 | C79.89 | D00.03 | D10.39 | D37.09 | D49.0 |
| periosteum — *see* Neoplasm, bone | | | | | | |
| peripancreatic | C48.0 | C78.6 | — | D20.0 | D48.3 | D49.0 |
| peripheral nerve NEC | C47.9 | C79.89 | — | D36.10 | D48.2 | D49.2 |
| perirectal (tissue) | C76.3 | C79.89 | — | D36.7 | D48.7 | D49.89 |
| perirenal (tissue) | C48.0 | C78.6 | — | D20.0 | D48.3 | D49.0 |
| peritoneum, peritoneal (cavity) | C48.2 | C78.6 | — | D20.1 | D48.4 | D49.0 |
| benign mesothelial tissue — *see* Mesothelioma, benign | | | | | | |
| overlapping lesion | C48.8 | — | — | — | — | — |
| with digestive organs | C26.9 | — | — | — | — | — |
| parietal | C48.1 | C78.6 | — | D20.1 | D48.4 | D49.0 |
| pelvic | C48.1 | C78.6 | — | D20.1 | D48.4 | D49.0 |
| specified part NEC | C48.1 | C78.6 | — | D20.1 | D48.4 | D49.0 |
| peritonsillar (tissue) | C76.0 | C79.89 | D09.8 | D36.7 | D48.7 | D49.89 |
| periurethral tissue | C76.3 | C79.89 | — | D36.7 | D48.7 | D49.89 |
| phalanges | | | | | | |
| foot | C40.3-☑ | C79.51 | — | D16.3-☑ | — | — |
| hand | C40.1-☑ | C79.51 | — | D16.1-☑ | — | — |
| pharynx, pharyngeal | C14.0 | C78.32 | D00.08 | D10.9 | D37.05 | D49.0 |
| bursa | C11.1 | C79.89 | D00.08 | D10.6 | D37.05 | D49.0 |
| fornix | C11.3 | C79.89 | D00.08 | D10.6 | D37.05 | D49.0 |
| recess | C11.2 | C79.89 | D00.08 | D10.6 | D37.05 | D49.0 |
| region | C14.0 | C79.89 | D00.08 | D10.9 | D37.05 | D49.0 |
| tonsil | C11.1 | C79.89 | D00.08 | D10.6 | D37.05 | D49.0 |
| **Neoplasm, neoplastic** — *continued* | | | | | | |
| pharynx, pharyngeal — *continued* | | | | | | |
| wall (lateral) (posterior) | C14.0 | C79.89 | D00.08 | D10.9 | D37.05 | D49.0 |
| pia mater | C70.9 | C79.40 | — | D32.9 | D42.9 | D49.7 |
| cerebral | C70.0 | C79.32 | — | D32.0 | D42.0 | D49.7 |
| cranial | C70.0 | C79.32 | — | D32.0 | D42.0 | D49.7 |
| spinal | C70.1 | C79.49 | — | D32.1 | D42.1 | D49.7 |
| pillars of fauces | C09.1 | C79.89 | D00.08 | D10.5 | D37.05 | D49.0 |
| pineal (body) (gland) | C75.3 | C79.89 | D09.3 | D35.4 | D44.5 | D49.7 |
| pinna (ear) NEC — *see also* Neoplasm, skin, ear | C44.20-☑ | C79.2 | D04.2-☑ | D23.2-☑ | D48.5 | D49.2 |
| piriform fossa or sinus | C12 | C79.89 | D00.08 | D10.7 | D37.05 | D49.0 |
| pituitary (body) (fossa) (gland) (lobe) | C75.1 | C79.89 | D09.3 | D35.2 | D44.3 | D49.7 |
| placenta | C58 | C79.82 | D07.0 | D26.7 | D39.2 | D49.59 |
| pleura, pleural (cavity) | C38.4 | C78.2 | — | D19.0 | D38.2 | D49.1 |
| overlapping lesion with heart or mediastinum | C38.8 | — | — | — | — | — |
| parietal | C38.4 | C78.2 | — | D19.0 | D38.2 | D49.1 |
| visceral | C38.4 | C78.2 | — | D19.0 | D38.2 | D49.1 |
| plexus | | | | | | |
| brachial | C47.1-☑ | C79.89 | — | D36.12 | D48.2 | D49.2 |
| cervical | C47.0 | C79.89 | — | D36.11 | D48.2 | D49.2 |
| choroid | C71.5 | C79.31 | — | D33.0 | D43.0 | D49.6 |
| lumbosacral | C47.5 | C79.89 | — | D36.16 | D48.2 | D49.2 |
| sacral | C47.5 | C79.89 | — | D36.16 | D48.2 | D49.2 |
| pluriendocrine | C75.8 | C79.89 | D09.3 | D35.7 | D44.9 | D49.7 |
| pole | | | | | | |
| frontal | C71.1 | C79.31 | — | D33.0 | D43.0 | D49.6 |
| occipital | C71.4 | C79.31 | — | D33.0 | D43.0 | D49.6 |
| pons (varolii) | C71.7 | C79.31 | — | D33.1 | D43.1 | D49.6 |
| popliteal fossa or space | C76.5-☑ | C79.89 | D04.7-☑ | D36.7 | D48.7 | D49.89 |
| postcricoid (region) | C13.0 | C79.89 | D00.08 | D10.7 | D37.05 | D49.0 |
| posterior fossa (cranial) | C71.9 | C79.31 | — | D33.2 | D43.2 | D49.6 |
| postnasal space | C11.9 | C79.89 | D00.08 | D10.6 | D37.05 | D49.0 |
| prepuce | C60.0 | C79.82 | D07.4 | D29.0 | D40.8 | D49.59 |
| prepylorus | C16.4 | C78.89 | D00.2 | D13.1 | D37.1 | D49.0 |
| presacral (region) | C76.3 | C79.89 | — | D36.7 | D48.7 | D49.89 |
| prostate (gland) | C61 | C79.82 | D07.5 | D29.1 | D40.0 | D49.59 |
| utricle | C68.0 | C79.19 | D09.19 | D30.4 | D41.3 | D49.59 |
| pterygoid fossa | C49.0 | C79.89 | — | D21.0 | D48.1-☑ | D49.2 |
| pubic bone | C41.4 | C79.51 | — | D16.8 | D48.0 | D49.2 |
| pudenda, pudendum (female) | C51.9 | C79.82 | D07.1 | D28.0 | D39.8 | D49.59 |
| pulmonary — *see also* Neoplasm, lung | C34.9-☑ | C78.0-☑ | D02.2-☑ | D14.3-☑ | D38.1 | D49.1 |
| putamen | C71.0 | C79.31 | — | D33.0 | D43.0 | D49.6 |
| pyloric | | | | | | |
| antrum | C16.3 | C78.89 | D00.2 | D13.1 | D37.1 | D49.0 |
| canal | C16.4 | C78.89 | D00.2 | D13.1 | D37.1 | D49.0 |
| pylorus | C16.4 | C78.89 | D00.2 | D13.1 | D37.1 | D49.0 |
| pyramid (brain) | C71.7 | C79.31 | — | D33.1 | D43.1 | D49.6 |
| pyriform fossa or sinus | C12 | C79.89 | D00.08 | D10.7 | D37.05 | D49.0 |
| radius (any part) | C40.0-☑ | C79.51 | — | D16.0-☑ | — | — |
| Rathke's pouch | C75.1 | C79.89 | D09.3 | D35.2 | D44.3 | D49.7 |
| rectosigmoid (junction) | C19 | C78.5 | D01.1 | D12.7 | D37.5 | D49.0 |
| overlapping lesion with anus or rectum | C21.8 | — | — | — | — | — |
| rectouterine pouch | C48.1 | C78.6 | — | D20.1 | D48.4 | D49.0 |
| rectovaginal septum or wall | C76.3 | C79.89 | D09.8 | D36.7 | D48.7 | D49.89 |
| rectovesical septum | C76.3 | C79.89 | D09.8 | D36.7 | D48.7 | D49.89 |
| rectum (ampulla) | C20 | C78.5 | D01.2 | D12.8 | D37.5 | D49.0 |
| and colon | C19 | C78.5 | D01.1 | D12.7 | D37.5 | D49.0 |
| overlapping lesion with anus or | C21.8 | — | — | — | — | — |

| | Malignant Primary | Malignant Secondary | Ca in situ | Benign | Uncertain Behavior | Unspecified Behavior |
|---|---|---|---|---|---|---|
| **Neoplasm, neoplastic** — *continued* | | | | | | |
| rectum — *continued* | | | | | | |
| overlapping lesion | | | | | | |
| with anus or rectosigmoid junction — *continued* | | | | | | |
| rectosigmoid junction | | | | | | |
| renal | C64.-☑ | C79.0-☑ | D09.19 | D30.0-☑ | D41.0-☑ | D49.51-☑ |
| calyx | C65.-☑ | C79.0-☑ | D09.19 | D30.1-☑ | D41.1-☑ | D49.51-☑ |
| hilus | C65.-☑ | C79.0-☑ | D09.19 | D30.1-☑ | D41.1-☑ | D49.51-☑ |
| parenchyma | C64.-☑ | C79.0-☑ | D09.19 | D30.0-☑ | D41.0-☑ | D49.51-☑ |
| pelvis | C65.-☑ | C79.0-☑ | D09.19 | D30.1-☑ | D41.1-☑ | D49.51-☑ |
| respiratory | | | | | | |
| organs or system NEC | C39.9 | C78.30 | D02.4 | D14.4 | D38.6 | D49.1 |
| tract NEC | C39.9 | C78.30 | D02.4 | D14.4 | D38.5 | D49.1 |
| upper | C39.0 | C78.30 | D02.4 | D14.4 | D38.5 | D49.1 |
| retina | C69.2-☑ | C79.49 | D09.2-☑ | D31.2-☑ | D48.7 | D49.81 |
| retro-orbital | C76.0 | C79.89 | D09.8 | D36.7 | D48.7 | D49.89 |
| retrobulbar | C69.6-☑ | C79.49 | — | D31.6-☑ | D48.7 | D49.89 |
| retrocecal | C48.0 | C78.6 | — | D20.0 | D48.3 | D49.0 |
| retromolar (area) (triangle) (trigone) | C06.2 | C79.89 | D00.00 | D10.39 | D37.09 | D49.0 |
| retroperitoneal (space) (tissue) | C48.0 | C78.6 | — | D20.0 | D48.3 | D49.0 |
| retroperitoneum | C48.0 | C78.6 | — | D20.0 | D48.3 | D49.0 |
| retropharyngeal | C14.0 | C79.89 | D00.08 | D10.9 | D37.05 | D49.0 |
| retrovesical (septum) | C76.3 | C79.89 | D09.8 | D36.7 | D48.7 | D49.89 |
| rhinencephalon | C71.0 | C79.31 | — | D33.0 | D43.0 | D49.6 |
| rib | C41.3 | C79.51 | — | D16.7 | D48.0 | D49.2 |
| Rosenmuller's fossa | C11.2 | C79.89 | D00.08 | D10.6 | D37.05 | D49.0 |
| round ligament | C57.2-☑ | C79.82 | — | D28.2 | D39.8 | D49.59 |
| sacrococcyx, sacrococcygeal | C41.4 | C79.51 | — | D16.8 | D48.0 | D49.2 |
| region | C76.3 | C79.89 | D09.8 | D36.7 | D48.7 | D49.89 |
| sacrouterine ligament | C57.3 | C79.82 | — | D28.2 | D39.8 | D49.59 |
| sacrum, sacral (vertebra) | C41.4 | C79.51 | — | D16.8 | D48.0 | D49.2 |
| salivary gland or duct (major) | C08.9 | C79.89 | D00.00 | D11.9 | D37.039 | D49.0 |
| minor NEC | C06.9 | C79.89 | D00.00 | D10.39 | D37.04 | D49.0 |
| overlapping lesion | C08.9 | — | — | — | — | — |
| parotid | C07 | C79.89 | D00.00 | D11.0 | D37.030 | D49.0 |
| pluriglandular | C08.9 | C79.89 | D00.00 | D11.9 | D37.039 | D49.0 |
| sublingual | C08.1 | C79.89 | D00.00 | D11.7 | D37.031 | D49.0 |
| submandibular | C08.0 | C79.89 | D00.00 | D11.7 | D37.032 | D49.0 |
| submaxillary | C08.0 | C79.89 | D00.00 | D11.7 | D37.032 | D49.0 |
| salpinx (uterine) | C57.0-☑ | C79.82 | D07.39 | D28.2 | D39.8 | D49.59 |
| Santorini's duct | C25.3 | C78.89 | D01.7 | D13.6 | D37.8 | D49.0 |
| scalp | C44.40 | C79.2 | D04.4 | D23.4 | D48.5 | D49.2 |
| basal cell carcinoma | C44.41 | — | — | — | — | — |
| specified type NEC | C44.49 | — | — | — | — | — |
| squamous cell carcinoma | C44.42 | — | — | — | — | — |
| scapula (any part) | C40.0-☑ | C79.51 | — | D16.0-☑ | — | — |
| scapular region | C76.1 | C79.89 | D09.8 | D36.7 | D48.7 | D49.89 |
| scar NEC — *see also* Neoplasm, skin, by site | C44.90 | C79.2 | D04.9 | D23.9 | D48.5 | D49.2 |
| sciatic nerve | C47.2-☑ | C79.89 | — | D36.13 | D48.2 | D49.2 |
| sclera | C69.4-☑ | C79.49 | D09.2-☑ | D31.4-☑ | D48.7 | D49.89 |
| scrotum (skin) | C63.2 | C79.82 | D07.61 | D29.4 | D40.8 | D49.59 |
| sebaceous gland — *see* Neoplasm, skin | | | | | | |
| sella turcica | C75.1 | C79.89 | D09.3 | D35.2 | D44.3 | D49.7 |
| bone | C41.0 | C79.51 | — | D16.4 | D48.0 | D49.2 |
| semilunar cartilage (knee) | C40.2-☑ | C79.51 | — | D16.2-☑ | D48.0 | D49.2 |
| seminal vesicle | C63.7 | C79.82 | D07.69 | D29.8 | D40.8 | D49.59 |
| septum | | | | | | |
| nasal | C30.0 | C78.39 | D02.3 | D14.0 | D38.5 | D49.1 |
| posterior margin | C11.3 | C79.89 | D00.08 | D10.6 | D37.05 | D49.0 |
| **Neoplasm, neoplastic** — *continued* | | | | | | |
| septum — *continued* | | | | | | |
| rectovaginal | C76.3 | C79.89 | D09.8 | D36.7 | D48.7 | D49.89 |
| rectovesical | C76.3 | C79.89 | D09.8 | D36.7 | D48.7 | D49.89 |
| urethrovaginal | C57.9 | C79.82 | D07.30 | D28.9 | D39.9 | D49.59 |
| vesicovaginal | C57.9 | C79.82 | D07.30 | D28.9 | D39.9 | D49.59 |
| shoulder NEC | C76.4-☑ | C79.89 | D04.6-☑ | D36.7 | D48.7 | D49.89 |
| sigmoid flexure (lower) (upper) | C18.7 | C78.5 | D01.0 | D12.5 | D37.4 | D49.0 |
| sinus (accessory) | C31.9 | C78.39 | D02.3 | D14.0 | D38.5 | D49.1 |
| bone (any) | C41.0 | C79.51 | — | D16.4 | D48.0 | D49.2 |
| ethmoidal | C31.1 | C78.39 | D02.3 | D14.0 | D38.5 | D49.1 |
| frontal | C31.2 | C78.39 | D02.3 | D14.0 | D38.5 | D49.1 |
| maxillary | C31.0 | C78.39 | D02.3 | D14.0 | D38.5 | D49.1 |
| nasal, paranasal NEC | C31.9 | C78.39 | D02.3 | D14.0 | D38.5 | D49.1 |
| overlapping lesion | C31.8 | — | — | — | — | — |
| pyriform | C12 | C79.89 | D00.08 | D10.7 | D37.05 | D49.0 |
| sphenoid | C31.3 | C78.39 | D02.3 | D14.0 | D38.5 | D49.1 |
| skeleton, skeletal NEC | C41.9 | C79.51 | — | D16.9 | D48.0 | D49.2 |
| Skene's gland | C68.1 | C79.19 | D09.19 | D30.8 | D41.8 | D49.59 |
| skin NOS | C44.90 | C79.2 | D04.9 | D23.9 | D48.5 | D49.2 |
| abdominal wall | C44.509 | C79.2 | D04.5 | D23.5 | D48.5 | D49.2 |
| basal cell carcinoma | C44.519 | — | — | — | — | — |
| specified type NEC | C44.599 | — | — | — | — | — |
| squamous cell carcinoma | C44.529 | — | — | — | — | — |
| ala nasi — *see also* Neoplasm, nose, skin | C44.301 | C79.2 | D04.39 | D23.39 | D48.5 | D49.2 |
| ankle — *see also* Neoplasm, skin, limb, lower | C44.70-☑ | C79.2 | D04.7-☑ | D23.7-☑ | D48.5 | D49.2 |
| antecubital space — *see also* Neoplasm, skin, limb, upper | C44.60-☑ | C79.2 | D04.6-☑ | D23.6-☑ | D48.5 | D49.2 |
| anus | C44.500 | C79.2 | D04.5 | D23.5 | D48.5 | D49.2 |
| basal cell carcinoma | C44.510 | — | — | — | — | — |
| specified type NEC | C44.590 | — | — | — | — | — |
| squamous cell carcinoma | C44.520 | — | — | — | — | — |
| arm — *see also* Neoplasm, skin, limb, upper | C44.60-☑ | C79.2 | D04.6-☑ | D23.6-☑ | D48.5 | D49.2 |
| auditory canal (external) — *see also* Neoplasm, skin, ear | C44.20-☑ | C79.2 | D04.2-☑ | D23.2-☑ | D48.5 | D49.2 |
| auricle (ear) — *see also* Neoplasm, skin, ear | C44.20-☑ | C79.2 | D04.2-☑ | D23.2-☑ | D48.5 | D49.2 |
| auricular canal (external) — *see also* Neoplasm, skin, ear | C44.20-☑ | C79.2 | D04.2-☑ | D23.2-☑ | D48.5 | D49.2 |
| axilla, axillary fold — *see also* Neoplasm, skin, trunk | C44.509 | C79.2 | D04.5 | D23.5 | D48.5 | D49.2 |
| back — *see also* Neoplasm, skin, trunk | C44.509 | C79.2 | D04.5 | D23.5 | D48.5 | D49.2 |
| basal cell carcinoma | C44.91 | — | — | — | — | — |
| breast | C44.501 | C79.2 | D04.5 | D23.5 | D48.5 | D49.2 |
| basal cell carcinoma | C44.511 | — | — | — | — | — |
| specified type NEC | C44.591 | — | — | — | — | — |
| squamous cell carcinoma | C44.521 | — | — | — | — | — |
| brow — *see also* Neoplasm, skin, face | C44.309 | C79.2 | D04.39 | D23.39 | D48.5 | D49.2 |

| | Malignant Primary | Malignant Secondary | Ca in situ | Benign | Uncertain Behavior | Unspecified Behavior |
|---|---|---|---|---|---|---|
| **Neoplasm, neoplastic** *— continued* | | | | | | |
| skin *— continued* | | | | | | |
| buttock *— see also* Neoplasm, skin, trunk | C44.5Ø9 | C79.2 | DØ4.5 | D23.5 | D48.5 | D49.2 |
| calf *— see also* Neoplasm, skin, limb, lower | C44.7Ø-☑ | C79.2 | DØ4.7-☑ | D23.7-☑ | D48.5 | D49.2 |
| canthus (eye) (inner) (outer) | C44.1Ø-☑ | C79.2 | DØ4.1-☑ | D23.1-☑ | D48.5 | D49.2 |
| basal cell carcinoma | C44.11-☑ | — | — | — | — | — |
| sebaceous cell | C44.13-☑ | — | — | — | — | — |
| specified type NEC | C44.19-☑ | — | — | — | — | — |
| squamous cell carcinoma | C44.12-☑ | — | — | — | — | — |
| cervical region *— see also* Neoplasm, skin, neck | C44.4Ø | C79.2 | DØ4.4 | D23.4 | D48.5 | D49.2 |
| cheek (external) *— see also* Neoplasm, skin, face | C44.3Ø9 | C79.2 | DØ4.39 | D23.39 | D48.5 | D49.2 |
| chest (wall) *— see also* Neoplasm, skin, trunk | C44.5Ø9 | C79.2 | DØ4.5 | D23.5 | D48.5 | D49.2 |
| chin *— see also* Neoplasm, skin, face | C44.3Ø9 | C79.2 | DØ4.39 | D23.39 | D48.5 | D49.2 |
| clavicular area *— see also* Neoplasm, skin, trunk | C44.5Ø9 | C79.2 | DØ4.5 | D23.5 | D48.5 | D49.2 |
| clitoris | C51.2 | C79.82 | DØ7.1 | D28.Ø | D39.8 | D49.59 |
| columnella *— see also* Neoplasm, skin, face | C44.3Ø9 | C79.2 | DØ4.39 | D23.39 | D48.5 | D49.2 |
| concha *— see also* Neoplasm, skin, ear | C44.2Ø-☑ | C79.2 | DØ4.2-☑ | D23.2-☑ | D48.5 | D49.2 |
| ear (external) | C44.2Ø-☑ | C79.2 | DØ4.2-☑ | D23.2-☑ | D48.5 | D49.2 |
| basal cell carcinoma | C44.21-☑ | — | — | — | — | — |
| specified type NEC | C44.29-☑ | — | — | — | — | — |
| squamous cell carcinoma | C44.22-☑ | — | — | — | — | — |
| elbow *— see also* Neoplasm, skin, limb, upper | C44.6Ø-☑ | C79.2 | DØ4.6-☑ | D23.6-☑ | D48.5 | D49.2 |
| eyebrow *— see also* Neoplasm, skin, face | C44.3Ø9 | C79.2 | DØ4.39 | D23.39 | D48.5 | D49.2 |
| eyelid | C44.1Ø-☑ | C79.2 | DØ4.1-☑ | D23.1-☑ | D48.5 | D49.2 |
| basal cell carcinoma | C44.11-☑ | — | — | — | — | — |
| sebaceous cell | C44.13-☑ | — | — | — | — | — |
| specified type NEC | C44.19-☑ | — | — | — | — | — |
| squamous cell carcinoma | C44.12-☑ | — | — | — | — | — |
| face NOS | C44.3ØØ | C79.2 | DØ4.3Ø | D23.3Ø | D48.5 | D49.2 |
| basal cell carcinoma | C44.31Ø | — | — | — | — | — |
| specified type NEC | C44.39Ø | — | — | — | — | — |
| squamous cell carcinoma | C44.32Ø | — | — | — | — | — |
| female genital organs (external) | C51.9 | C79.82 | DØ7.1 | D28.Ø | D39.8 | D49.59 |
| clitoris | C51.2 | C79.82 | DØ7.1 | D28.Ø | D39.8 | D49.59 |
| labium NEC | C51.9 | C79.82 | DØ7.1 | D28.Ø | D39.8 | D49.59 |
| majus | C51.Ø | C79.82 | DØ7.1 | D28.Ø | D39.8 | D49.59 |
| minus | C51.1 | C79.82 | DØ7.1 | D28.Ø | D39.8 | D49.59 |
| pudendum | C51.9 | C79.82 | DØ7.1 | D28.Ø | D39.8 | D49.59 |
| vulva | C51.9 | C79.82 | DØ7.1 | D28.Ø | D39.8 | D49.59 |
| finger *— see also* Neoplasm, skin, limb, upper | C44.6Ø-☑ | C79.2 | DØ4.6-☑ | D23.6-☑ | D48.5 | D49.2 |
| flank *— see also* Neoplasm, skin, trunk | C44.5Ø9 | C79.2 | DØ4.5 | D23.5 | D48.5 | D49.2 |
| **Neoplasm, neoplastic** *— continued* | | | | | | |
| skin *— continued* | | | | | | |
| foot *— see also* Neoplasm, skin, limb, lower | C44.7Ø-☑ | C79.2 | DØ4.7-☑ | D23.7-☑ | D48.5 | D49.2 |
| forearm *— see also* Neoplasm, skin, limb, upper | C44.6Ø-☑ | C79.2 | DØ4.6-☑ | D23.6-☑ | D48.5 | D49.2 |
| forehead *— see also* Neoplasm, skin, face | C44.3Ø9 | C79.2 | DØ4.39 | D23.39 | D48.5 | D49.2 |
| glabella *— see also* Neoplasm, skin, face | C44.3Ø9 | C79.2 | DØ4.39 | D23.39 | D48.5 | D49.2 |
| gluteal region *— see also* Neoplasm, skin, trunk | C44.5Ø9 | C79.2 | DØ4.5 | D23.5 | D48.5 | D49.2 |
| groin *— see also* Neoplasm, skin, trunk | C44.5Ø9 | C79.2 | DØ4.5 | D23.5 | D48.5 | D49.2 |
| hand *— see also* Neoplasm, skin, limb, upper | C44.6Ø-☑ | C79.2 | DØ4.6-☑ | D23.6-☑ | D48.5 | D49.2 |
| head NEC *— see also* Neoplasm, skin, scalp | C44.4Ø | C79.2 | DØ4.4 | D23.4 | D48.5 | D49.2 |
| heel *— see also* Neoplasm, skin, limb, lower | C44.7Ø-☑ | C79.2 | DØ4.7-☑ | D23.7-☑ | D48.5 | D49.2 |
| helix *— see also* Neoplasm, skin, ear | C44.2Ø-☑ | C79.2 | DØ4.2-☑ | D23.2-☑ | D48.5 | D49.2 |
| hip *— see also* Neoplasm, skin, limb, lower | C44.7Ø-☑ | C79.2 | DØ4.7-☑ | D23.7-☑ | D48.5 | D49.2 |
| infraclavicular region *— see also* Neoplasm, skin, trunk | C44.5Ø9 | C79.2 | DØ4.5 | D23.5 | D48.5 | D49.2 |
| inguinal region *— see also* Neoplasm, skin, trunk | C44.5Ø9 | C79.2 | DØ4.5 | D23.5 | D48.5 | D49.2 |
| jaw *— see also* Neoplasm, skin, face | C44.3Ø9 | C79.2 | DØ4.39 | D23.39 | D48.5 | D49.2 |
| Kaposi's sarcoma *— see* Kaposi's, sarcoma, skin | | | | | | |
| knee *— see also* Neoplasm, skin, limb, lower | C44.7Ø-☑ | C79.2 | DØ4.7-☑ | D23.7-☑ | D48.5 | D49.2 |
| labia | | | | | | |
| majora | C51.Ø | C79.82 | DØ7.1 | D28.Ø | D39.8 | D49.59 |
| minora | C51.1 | C79.82 | DØ7.1 | D28.Ø | D39.8 | D49.59 |
| leg *— see also* Neoplasm, skin, limb, lower | C44.7Ø-☑ | C79.2 | DØ4.7-☑ | D23.7-☑ | D48.5 | D49.2 |
| lid (lower) (upper) | C44.1Ø-☑ | C79.2 | DØ4.1-☑ | D23.1-☑ | D48.5 | D49.2 |
| basal cell carcinoma | C44.11-☑ | — | — | — | — | — |
| sebaceous cell | C44.13-☑ | — | — | — | — | — |
| specified type NEC | C44.19-☑ | — | — | — | — | — |
| squamous cell carcinoma | C44.12-☑ | — | — | — | — | — |
| limb NEC | C44.9Ø | C79.2 | DØ4.9 | D23.9 | D48.5 | D49.2 |
| basal cell carcinoma | C44.91 | — | — | — | — | — |
| lower | C44.7Ø-☑ | C79.2 | DØ4.7-☑ | D23.7-☑ | D48.5 | D49.2 |
| basal cell carcinoma | C44.71-☑ | — | — | — | — | — |
| specified type NEC | C44.79-☑ | — | — | — | — | — |
| squamous cell carcinoma | C44.72-☑ | — | — | — | — | — |
| upper | C44.6Ø-☑ | C79.2 | DØ4.6-☑ | D23.6-☑ | D48.5 | D49.2 |
| basal cell carcinoma | C44.61-☑ | — | — | — | — | — |
| specified type NEC | C44.69-☑ | — | — | — | — | — |

| | Malignant Primary | Malignant Secondary | Ca in situ | Benign | Uncertain Behavior | Unspecified Behavior |
|---|---|---|---|---|---|---|
| **Neoplasm, neoplastic** — *continued* | | | | | | |
| skin — *continued* | | | | | | |
| limb — *continued* | | | | | | |
| upper — *continued* | | | | | | |
| squamous cell carcinoma | C44.62-☑ | — | — | — | — | — |
| lip (lower) (upper) | C44.ØØ | C79.2 | DØ4.Ø | D23.Ø | D48.5 | D49.2 |
| basal cell carcinoma | C44.Ø1 | — | — | — | — | — |
| specified type NEC | C44.Ø9 | — | — | — | — | — |
| squamous cell carcinoma | C44.Ø2 | — | — | — | — | — |
| male genital organs | C63.9 | C79.82 | DØ7.6Ø | D29.9 | D4Ø.8 | D49.59 |
| penis | C6Ø.9 | C79.82 | DØ7.4 | D29.Ø | D4Ø.8 | D49.59 |
| prepuce | C6Ø.Ø | C79.82 | DØ7.4 | D29.Ø | D4Ø.8 | D49.59 |
| scrotum | C63.2 | C79.82 | DØ7.61 | D29.4 | D4Ø.8 | D49.59 |
| mastectomy site (skin) — *see also* Neoplasm, skin, breast | C44.5Ø1 | C79.2 | — | — | — | — |
| specified as breast tissue | C5Ø.8-☑ | C79.81 | — | — | — | — |
| meatus, acoustic (external) — *see also* Neoplasm, skin, ear | C44.2Ø-☑ | C79.2 | DØ4.2-☑ | D23.2-☑ | D48.5 | D49.2 |
| melanotic — *see* Melanoma | | | | | | |
| Merkel cell — *see* Carcinoma, Merkel cell | | | | | | |
| nates — *see also* Neoplasm, skin, trunk | C44.5Ø9 | C79.2 | DØ4.5 | D23.5 | D48.5 | D49.2 |
| neck | C44.4Ø | C79.2 | DØ4.4 | D23.4 | D48.5 | D49.2 |
| basal cell carcinoma | C44.41 | — | — | — | — | — |
| specified type NEC | C44.49 | — | — | — | — | — |
| squamous cell carcinoma | C44.42 | — | — | — | — | — |
| nevus — *see* Nevus, skin | | | | | | |
| nose (external) — *see also* Neoplasm, nose, skin | C44.3Ø1 | C79.2 | DØ4.39 | D23.39 | D48.5 | D49.2 |
| overlapping lesion | C44.8Ø | — | — | — | — | — |
| basal cell carcinoma | C44.81 | — | — | — | — | — |
| specified type NEC | C44.89 | — | — | — | — | — |
| squamous cell carcinoma | C44.82 | — | — | — | — | — |
| palm — *see also* Neoplasm, skin, limb, upper | C44.6Ø-☑ | C79.2 | DØ4.6-☑ | D23.6-☑ | D48.5 | D49.2 |
| palpebra | C44.1Ø-☑ | C79.2 | DØ4.1-☑ | D23.1-☑ | D48.5 | D49.2 |
| basal cell carcinoma | C44.11-☑ | — | — | — | — | — |
| sebaceous cell | C44.13-☑ | — | — | — | — | — |
| specified type NEC | C44.19-☑ | — | — | — | — | — |
| squamous cell carcinoma | C44.12-☑ | — | — | — | — | — |
| penis NEC | C6Ø.9 | C79.82 | DØ7.4 | D29.Ø | D4Ø.8 | D49.59 |
| perianal — *see also* Neoplasm, skin, anus | C44.5ØØ | C79.2 | DØ4.5 | D23.5 | D48.5 | D49.2 |
| perineum — *see also* Neoplasm, skin, anus | C44.5ØØ | C79.2 | DØ4.5 | D23.5 | D48.5 | D49.2 |
| pinna — *see also* Neoplasm, skin, ear | C44.2Ø-☑ | C79.2 | DØ4.2-☑ | D23.2-☑ | D48.5 | D49.2 |
| plantar — *see also* Neoplasm, skin, limb, lower | C44.7Ø-☑ | C79.2 | DØ4.7-☑ | D23.7-☑ | D48.5 | D49.2 |
| popliteal fossa or space — *see also* | C44.7Ø-☑ | C79.2 | DØ4.7-☑ | D23.7-☑ | D48.5 | D49.2 |
| **Neoplasm, neoplastic** — *continued* | | | | | | |
| skin — *continued* | | | | | | |
| popliteal fossa or space — *see also* Neoplasm, skin, limb, lower — *continued* | | | | | | |
| Neoplasm, skin, limb, lower | | | | | | |
| prepuce | C6Ø.Ø | C79.82 | DØ7.4 | D29.Ø | D4Ø.8 | D49.59 |
| pubes — *see also* Neoplasm, skin, trunk | C44.5Ø9 | C79.2 | DØ4.5 | D23.5 | D48.5 | D49.2 |
| sacrococcygeal region — *see also* Neoplasm, skin, trunk | C44.5Ø9 | C79.2 | DØ4.5 | D23.5 | D48.5 | D49.2 |
| scalp | C44.4Ø | C79.2 | DØ4.4 | D23.4 | D48.5 | D49.2 |
| basal cell carcinoma | C44.41 | — | — | — | — | — |
| specified type NEC | C44.49 | — | — | — | — | — |
| squamous cell carcinoma | C44.42 | — | — | — | — | — |
| scapular region — *see also* Neoplasm, skin, trunk | C44.5Ø9 | C79.2 | DØ4.5 | D23.5 | D48.5 | D49.2 |
| scrotum | C63.2 | C79.82 | DØ7.61 | D29.4 | D4Ø.8 | D49.59 |
| shoulder — *see also* Neoplasm, skin, limb, upper | C44.6Ø-☑ | C79.2 | DØ4.6-☑ | D23.6-☑ | D48.5 | D49.2 |
| sole (foot) — *see also* Neoplasm, skin, limb, lower | C44.7Ø-☑ | C79.2 | DØ4.7-☑ | D23.7-☑ | D48.5 | D49.2 |
| specified sites NEC | C44.8Ø | C79.2 | DØ4.8 | D23.9 | D48.5 | D49.2 |
| basal cell carcinoma | C44.81 | — | — | — | — | — |
| specified type NEC | C44.89 | — | — | — | — | — |
| squamous cell carcinoma | C44.82 | — | — | — | — | — |
| specified type NEC | C44.99 | — | — | — | — | — |
| squamous cell carcinoma | C44.92 | — | — | — | — | — |
| submammary fold — *see also* Neoplasm, skin, trunk | C44.5Ø9 | C79.2 | DØ4.5 | D23.5 | D48.5 | D49.2 |
| supraclavicular region — *see also* Neoplasm, skin, neck | C44.4Ø | C79.2 | DØ4.4 | D23.4 | D48.5 | D49.2 |
| temple — *see also* Neoplasm, skin, face | C44.3Ø9 | C79.2 | DØ4.39 | D23.39 | D48.5 | D49.2 |
| thigh — *see also* Neoplasm, skin, limb, lower | C44.7Ø-☑ | C79.2 | DØ4.7-☑ | D23.7-☑ | D48.5 | D49.2 |
| thoracic wall — *see also* Neoplasm, skin, trunk | C44.5Ø9 | C79.2 | DØ4.5 | D23.5 | D48.5 | D49.2 |
| thumb — *see also* Neoplasm, skin, limb, upper | C44.6Ø-☑ | C79.2 | DØ4.6-☑ | D23.6-☑ | D48.5 | D49.2 |
| toe — *see also* Neoplasm, skin, limb, lower | C44.7Ø-☑ | C79.2 | DØ4.7-☑ | D23.7-☑ | D48.5 | D49.2 |
| tragus — *see also* Neoplasm, skin, ear | C44.2Ø-☑ | C79.2 | DØ4.2-☑ | D23.2-☑ | D48.5 | D49.2 |
| trunk | C44.5Ø9 | C79.2 | DØ4.5 | D23.5 | D48.5 | D49.2 |
| basal cell carcinoma | C44.519 | — | — | — | — | — |
| specified type NEC | C44.599 | — | — | — | — | — |
| squamous cell carcinoma | C44.529 | — | — | — | — | — |
| umbilicus — *see also* Neoplasm, skin, trunk | C44.5Ø9 | C79.2 | DØ4.5 | D23.5 | D48.5 | D49.2 |

| | Malignant Primary | Malignant Secondary | Ca in situ | Benign | Uncertain Behavior | Unspecified Behavior |
|---|---|---|---|---|---|---|
| **Neoplasm, neoplastic** — *continued* | | | | | | |
| skin — *continued* | | | | | | |
| vulva | C51.9 | C79.82 | D07.1 | D28.0 | D39.8 | D49.59 |
| overlapping lesion | C51.8 | — | — | — | — | — |
| wrist — *see also* Neoplasm, skin, limb, upper | C44.60-☑ | C79.2 | D04.6-☑ | D23.6-☑ | D48.5 | D49.2 |
| skull | C41.0 | C79.51 | — | D16.4 | D48.0 | D49.2 |
| soft parts or tissues — *see* Neoplasm, connective tissue | | | | | | |
| specified site NEC | C76.8 | C79.89 | D09.8 | D36.7 | D48.7 | D49.89 |
| spermatic cord | C63.1-☑ | C79.82 | D07.69 | D29.8 | D40.8 | D49.59 |
| sphenoid | C31.3 | C78.39 | D02.3 | D14.0 | D38.5 | D49.1 |
| bone | C41.0 | C79.51 | — | D16.4 | D48.0 | D49.2 |
| sinus | C31.3 | C78.39 | D02.3 | D14.0 | D38.5 | D49.1 |
| sphincter | | | | | | |
| anal | C21.1 | C78.5 | D01.3 | D12.9 | D37.8 | D49.0 |
| of Oddi | C24.0 | C78.89 | D01.5 | D13.5 | D37.6 | D49.0 |
| spine, spinal (column) | C41.2 | C79.51 | — | D16.6 | D48.0 | D49.2 |
| bulb | C71.7 | C79.31 | — | D33.1 | D43.1 | D49.6 |
| coccyx | C41.4 | C79.51 | — | D16.8 | D48.0 | D49.2 |
| cord (cervical) (lumbar) (sacral) (thoracic) | C72.0 | C79.49 | — | D33.4 | D43.4 | D49.7 |
| dura mater | C70.1 | C79.49 | — | D32.1 | D42.1 | D49.7 |
| lumbosacral | C41.2 | C79.51 | — | D16.6 | D48.0 | D49.2 |
| marrow NEC | C96.9 | C79.52 | — | — | D47.9 | D49.89 |
| membrane | C70.1 | C79.49 | — | D32.1 | D42.1 | D49.7 |
| meninges | C70.1 | C79.49 | — | D32.1 | D42.1 | D49.7 |
| nerve (root) | C47.9 | C79.89 | — | D36.10 | D48.2 | D49.2 |
| pia mater | C70.1 | C79.49 | — | D32.1 | D42.1 | D49.7 |
| root | C47.9 | C79.89 | — | D36.10 | D48.2 | D49.2 |
| sacrum | C41.4 | C79.51 | — | D16.8 | D48.0 | D49.2 |
| spleen, splenic NEC | C26.1 | C78.89 | D01.7 | D13.99 | D37.8 | D49.0 |
| flexure (colon) | C18.5 | C78.5 | D01.0 | D12.3 | D37.4 | D49.0 |
| stem, brain | C71.7 | C79.31 | — | D33.1 | D43.1 | D49.6 |
| Stensen's duct | C07 | C79.89 | D00.00 | D11.0 | D37.030 | D49.0 |
| sternum | C41.3 | C79.51 | — | D16.7 | D48.0 | D49.2 |
| stomach | C16.9 | C78.89 | D00.2 | D13.1 | D37.1 | D49.0 |
| antrum (pyloric) | C16.3 | C78.89 | D00.2 | D13.1 | D37.1 | D49.0 |
| body | C16.2 | C78.89 | D00.2 | D13.1 | D37.1 | D49.0 |
| cardia | C16.0 | C78.89 | D00.2 | D13.1 | D37.1 | D49.0 |
| cardiac orifice | C16.0 | C78.89 | D00.2 | D13.1 | D37.1 | D49.0 |
| corpus | C16.2 | C78.89 | D00.2 | D13.1 | D37.1 | D49.0 |
| fundus | C16.1 | C78.89 | D00.2 | D13.1 | D37.1 | D49.0 |
| greater curvature NEC | C16.6 | C78.89 | D00.2 | D13.1 | D37.1 | D49.0 |
| lesser curvature NEC | C16.5 | C78.89 | D00.2 | D13.1 | D37.1 | D49.0 |
| overlapping lesion | C16.8 | — | — | — | — | — |
| prepylorus | C16.4 | C78.89 | D00.2 | D13.1 | D37.1 | D49.0 |
| pylorus | C16.4 | C78.89 | D00.2 | D13.1 | D37.1 | D49.0 |
| wall NEC | C16.9 | C78.89 | D00.2 | D13.1 | D37.1 | D49.0 |
| anterior NEC | C16.8 | C78.89 | D00.2 | D13.1 | D37.1 | D49.0 |
| posterior NEC | C16.8 | C78.89 | D00.2 | D13.1 | D37.1 | D49.0 |
| stroma, endometrial | C54.1 | C79.82 | D07.0 | D26.1 | D39.0 | D49.59 |
| stump, cervical | C53.8 | C79.82 | D06.7 | D26.0 | D39.0 | D49.59 |
| subcutaneous (nodule) (tissue) NEC — *see* Neoplasm, connective tissue | | | | | | |
| subdural | C70.9 | C79.32 | — | D32.9 | D42.9 | D49.7 |
| subglottis, subglottic | C32.2 | C78.31 | D02.0 | D14.1 | D38.0 | D49.1 |
| sublingual | C04.9 | C79.89 | D00.06 | D10.2 | D37.09 | D49.0 |
| gland or duct | C08.1 | C79.89 | D00.00 | D11.7 | D37.031 | D49.0 |
| submandibular gland | C08.0 | C79.89 | D00.00 | D11.7 | D37.032 | D49.0 |
| submaxillary gland or duct | C08.0 | C79.89 | D00.00 | D11.7 | D37.032 | D49.0 |
| submental | C76.0 | C79.89 | D09.8 | D36.7 | D48.7 | D49.89 |
| subpleural | C34.9-☑ | C78.0-☑ | D02.2-☑ | D14.3-☑ | D38.1 | D49.1 |
| substernal | C38.1 | C78.1 | — | D15.2 | D38.3 | D49.89 |
| sudoriferous, sudoriparous gland, site unspecified | C44.90 | C79.2 | D04.9 | D23.9 | D48.5 | D49.2 |
| **Neoplasm, neoplastic** — *continued* | | | | | | |
| sudoriferous, sudoriparous gland, site unspecified — *continued* | | | | | | |
| specified site — *see* Neoplasm, skin | | | | | | |
| supraclavicular region | C76.0 | C79.89 | D09.8 | D36.7 | D48.7 | D49.89 |
| supraglottis | C32.1 | C78.31 | D02.0 | D14.1 | D38.0 | D49.1 |
| suprarenal | C74.9-☑ | C79.7-☑ | D09.3 | D35.0-☑ | D44.1-☑ | D49.7 |
| capsule | C74.9-☑ | C79.7-☑ | D09.3 | D35.0-☑ | D44.1-☑ | D49.7 |
| cortex | C74.0-☑ | C79.7-☑ | D09.3 | D35.0-☑ | D44.1-☑ | D49.7 |
| gland | C74.9-☑ | C79.7-☑ | D09.3 | D35.0-☑ | D44.1-☑ | D49.7 |
| medulla | C74.1-☑ | C79.7-☑ | D09.3 | D35.0-☑ | D44.1-☑ | D49.7 |
| suprasellar (region) | C71.9 | C79.31 | — | D33.2 | D43.2 | D49.6 |
| supratentorial (brain) NEC | C71.0 | C79.31 | — | D33.0 | D43.0 | D49.6 |
| sweat gland (apocrine) (eccrine), site unspecified | C44.90 | C79.2 | D04.9 | D23.9 | D48.5 | D49.2 |
| specified site — *see* Neoplasm, skin | | | | | | |
| sympathetic nerve or nervous system NEC | C47.9 | C79.89 | — | D36.10 | D48.2 | D49.2 |
| symphysis pubis | C41.4 | C79.51 | — | D16.8 | D48.0 | D49.2 |
| synovial membrane — *see* Neoplasm, connective tissue | | | | | | |
| tapetum, brain | C71.8 | C79.31 | — | D33.2 | D43.2 | D49.6 |
| tarsus (any bone) | C40.3-☑ | C79.51 | — | D16.3-☑ | — | — |
| temple (skin) — *see also* Neoplasm, skin, face | C44.309 | C79.2 | D04.39 | D23.39 | D48.5 | D49.2 |
| temporal | | | | | | |
| bone | C41.0 | C79.51 | — | D16.4 | D48.0 | D49.2 |
| lobe or pole | C71.2 | C79.31 | — | D33.0 | D43.0 | D49.6 |
| region | C76.0 | C79.89 | D09.8 | D36.7 | D48.7 | D49.89 |
| skin — *see also* Neoplasm, skin, face | C44.309 | C79.2 | D04.39 | D23.39 | D48.5 | D49.2 |
| tendon (sheath) — *see* Neoplasm, connective tissue | | | | | | |
| tentorium (cerebelli) | C70.0 | C79.32 | — | D32.0 | D42.0 | D49.7 |
| testis, testes | C62.9-☑ | C79.82 | D07.69 | D29.2-☑ | D40.1-☑ | D49.59 |
| descended | C62.1-☑ | C79.82 | D07.69 | D29.2-☑ | D40.1-☑ | D49.59 |
| ectopic | C62.0-☑ | C79.82 | D07.69 | D29.2-☑ | D40.1-☑ | D49.59 |
| retained | C62.0-☑ | C79.82 | D07.69 | D29.2-☑ | D40.1-☑ | D49.59 |
| scrotal | C62.1-☑ | C79.82 | D07.69 | D29.2-☑ | D40.1-☑ | D49.59 |
| undescended | C62.0-☑ | C79.82 | D07.69 | D29.2-☑ | D40.1-☑ | D49.59 |
| unspecified whether descended or undescended | C62.9-☑ | C79.82 | D07.69 | D29.2-☑ | D40.1-☑ | D49.59 |
| thalamus | C71.0 | C79.31 | — | D33.0 | D43.0 | D49.6 |
| thigh NEC | C76.5-☑ | C79.89 | D04.7-☑ | D36.7 | D48.7 | D49.89 |
| thorax, thoracic (cavity) (organs NEC) | C76.1 | C79.89 | D09.8 | D36.7 | D48.7 | D49.89 |
| duct | C49.3 | C79.89 | — | D21.3 | D48.1-☑ | D49.2 |
| wall NEC | C76.1 | C79.89 | D09.8 | D36.7 | D48.7 | D49.89 |
| throat | C14.0 | C79.89 | D00.08 | D10.9 | D37.05 | D49.0 |
| thumb NEC | C76.4-☑ | C79.89 | D04.6-☑ | D36.7 | D48.7 | D49.89 |
| thymus (gland) | C37 | C79.89 | D09.3 | D15.0 | D38.4 | D49.89 |
| thyroglossal duct | C73 | C79.89 | D09.3 | D34 | D44.0 | D49.7 |
| thyroid (gland) | C73 | C79.89 | D09.3 | D34 | D44.0 | D49.7 |
| cartilage | C32.3 | C78.39 | D02.0 | D14.1 | D38.0 | D49.1 |
| tibia (any part) | C40.2-☑ | C79.51 | — | D16.2-☑ | — | — |
| toe NEC | C76.5-☑ | C79.89 | D04.7-☑ | D36.7 | D48.7 | D49.89 |
| tongue | C02.9 | C79.89 | D00.07 | D10.1 | D37.02 | D49.0 |
| anterior (two-thirds) NEC | C02.3 | C79.89 | D00.07 | D10.1 | D37.02 | D49.0 |
| dorsal surface | C02.0 | C79.89 | D00.07 | D10.1 | D37.02 | D49.0 |
| ventral surface | C02.2 | C79.89 | D00.07 | D10.1 | D37.02 | D49.0 |
| base (dorsal surface) | C01 | C79.89 | D00.07 | D10.1 | D37.02 | D49.0 |
| border (lateral) | C02.1 | C79.89 | D00.07 | D10.1 | D37.02 | D49.0 |

☑ **Additional Character Required — Refer to the Tabular List for Character Selection**

| | Malignant Primary | Malignant Secondary | Ca in situ | Benign | Uncertain Behavior | Unspecified Behavior |
|---|---|---|---|---|---|---|
| **Neoplasm, neoplastic** *— continued* | | | | | | |
| tongue *— continued* | | | | | | |
| dorsal surface NEC | C02.0 | C79.89 | D00.07 | D10.1 | D37.02 | D49.0 |
| fixed part NEC | C01 | C79.89 | D00.07 | D10.1 | D37.02 | D49.0 |
| foramen cecum | C02.0 | C79.89 | D00.07 | D10.1 | D37.02 | D49.0 |
| frenulum linguae | C02.2 | C79.89 | D00.07 | D10.1 | D37.02 | D49.0 |
| junctional zone | C02.8 | C79.89 | D00.07 | D10.1 | D37.02 | D49.0 |
| margin (lateral) | C02.1 | C79.89 | D00.07 | D10.1 | D37.02 | D49.0 |
| midline NEC | C02.0 | C79.89 | D00.07 | D10.1 | D37.02 | D49.0 |
| mobile part NEC | C02.3 | C79.89 | D00.07 | D10.1 | D37.02 | D49.0 |
| overlapping lesion | C02.8 | — | — | — | — | — |
| posterior (third) | C01 | C79.89 | D00.07 | D10.1 | D37.02 | D49.0 |
| root | C01 | C79.89 | D00.07 | D10.1 | D37.02 | D49.0 |
| surface (dorsal) | C02.0 | C79.89 | D00.07 | D10.1 | D37.02 | D49.0 |
| base | C01 | C79.89 | D00.07 | D10.1 | D37.02 | D49.0 |
| ventral | C02.2 | C79.89 | D00.07 | D10.1 | D37.02 | D49.0 |
| tip | C02.1 | C79.89 | D00.07 | D10.1 | D37.02 | D49.0 |
| tonsil | C02.4 | C79.89 | D00.07 | D10.1 | D37.02 | D49.0 |
| tonsil | C09.9 | C79.89 | D00.08 | D10.4 | D37.05 | D49.0 |
| fauces, faucial | C09.9 | C79.89 | D00.08 | D10.4 | D37.05 | D49.0 |
| lingual | C02.4 | C79.89 | D00.07 | D10.1 | D37.02 | D49.0 |
| overlapping sites | C09.8 | — | — | — | — | — |
| palatine | C09.9 | C79.89 | D00.08 | D10.4 | D37.05 | D49.0 |
| pharyngeal | C11.1 | C79.89 | D00.08 | D10.6 | D37.05 | D49.0 |
| pillar (anterior) (posterior) | C09.1 | C79.89 | D00.08 | D10.5 | D37.05 | D49.0 |
| tonsillar fossa | C09.0 | C79.89 | D00.08 | D10.5 | D37.05 | D49.0 |
| tooth socket NEC | C03.9 | C79.89 | D00.03 | D10.39 | D37.09 | D49.0 |
| trachea (cartilage) (mucosa) | C33 | C78.39 | D02.1 | D14.2 | D38.1 | D49.1 |
| overlapping lesion with bronchus or lung | C34.8-☑ | — | — | — | — | — |
| tracheobronchial | C34.8-☑ | C78.39 | D02.1 | D14.2 | D38.1 | D49.1 |
| overlapping lesion with lung | C34.8-☑ | — | — | — | — | — |
| tragus *— see also* Neoplasm, skin, ear | C44.20-☑ | C79.2 | D04.2-☑ | D23.2-☑ | D48.5 | D49.2 |
| trunk NEC | C76.8 | C79.89 | D04.5 | D36.7 | D48.7 | D49.89 |
| tubo-ovarian | C57.8 | C79.82 | D07.39 | D28.7 | D39.8 | D49.59 |
| tunica vaginalis | C63.7 | C79.82 | D07.69 | D29.8 | D40.8 | D49.59 |
| turbinate (bone) | C41.0 | C79.51 | — | D16.4 | D48.0 | D49.2 |
| nasal | C30.0 | C78.39 | D02.3 | D14.0 | D38.5 | D49.1 |
| tympanic cavity | C30.1 | C78.39 | D02.3 | D14.0 | D38.5 | D49.1 |
| ulna (any part) | C40.0-☑ | C79.51 | — | D16.0-☑ | — | — |
| umbilicus, umbilical *— see also* Neoplasm, skin, trunk | C44.509 | C79.2 | D04.5 | D23.5 | D48.5 | D49.2 |
| uncus, brain | C71.2 | C79.31 | — | D33.0 | D43.0 | D49.6 |
| unknown site or unspecified | C80.1 | C79.9 | D09.9 | D36.9 | D48.9 | D49.9 |
| urachus | C67.7 | C79.11 | D09.0 | D30.3 | D41.4 | D49.4 |
| ureter-bladder (junction) | C67.6 | C79.11 | D09.0 | D30.3 | D41.4 | D49.4 |
| ureter, ureteral | C66.-☑ | C79.19 | D09.19 | D30.2-☑ | D41.2-☑ | D49.59 |
| orifice (bladder) | C67.6 | C79.11 | D09.0 | D30.3 | D41.4 | D49.4 |
| urethra, urethral (gland) | C68.0 | C79.19 | D09.19 | D30.4 | D41.3 | D49.59 |
| orifice, internal | C67.5 | C79.11 | D09.0 | D30.3 | D41.4 | D49.4 |
| urethrovaginal (septum) | C57.9 | C79.82 | D07.30 | D28.9 | D39.8 | D49.59 |
| urinary organ or system | C68.9 | C79.10 | D09.10 | D30.9 | D41.9 | D49.59 |
| bladder *— see* Neoplasm, bladder | | | | | | |
| overlapping lesion | C68.8 | — | — | — | — | — |
| specified sites NEC | C68.8 | C79.19 | D09.19 | D30.8 | D41.8 | D49.59 |
| utero-ovarian | C57.8 | C79.82 | D07.39 | D28.7 | D39.8 | D49.59 |
| ligament | C57.1-☑ | C79.82 | D07.39 | D28.2 | D39.8 | D49.59 |
| uterosacral ligament | C57.3 | C79.82 | — | D28.2 | D39.8 | D49.59 |
| uterus, uteri, uterine | C55 | C79.82 | D07.0 | D26.9 | D39.0 | D49.59 |
| adnexa NEC | C57.4 | C79.82 | D07.39 | D28.7 | D39.8 | D49.59 |
| **Neoplasm, neoplastic** *— continued* | | | | | | |
| uterus, uteri, uterine *— continued* | | | | | | |
| body | C54.9 | C79.82 | D07.0 | D26.1 | D39.0 | D49.59 |
| cervix | C53.9 | C79.82 | D06.9 | D26.0 | D39.0 | D49.59 |
| cornu | C54.9 | C79.82 | D07.0 | D26.1 | D39.0 | D49.59 |
| corpus | C54.9 | C79.82 | D07.0 | D26.1 | D39.0 | D49.59 |
| endocervix (canal) (gland) | C53.0 | C79.82 | D06.0 | D26.0 | D39.0 | D49.59 |
| endometrium | C54.1 | C79.82 | D07.0 | D26.1 | D39.0 | D49.59 |
| exocervix | C53.1 | C79.82 | D06.1 | D26.0 | D39.0 | D49.59 |
| external os | C53.1 | C79.82 | D06.1 | D26.0 | D39.0 | D49.59 |
| fundus | C54.3 | C79.82 | D07.0 | D26.1 | D39.0 | D49.59 |
| internal os | C53.0 | C79.82 | D06.0 | D26.0 | D39.0 | D49.59 |
| isthmus | C54.0 | C79.82 | D07.0 | D26.1 | D39.0 | D49.59 |
| ligament | C57.3 | C79.82 | — | D28.2 | D39.8 | D49.59 |
| broad | C57.1-☑ | C79.82 | D07.39 | D28.2 | D39.8 | D49.59 |
| round | C57.2-☑ | C79.82 | — | D28.2 | D39.8 | D49.59 |
| lower segment | C54.0 | C79.82 | D07.0 | D26.1 | D39.0 | D49.59 |
| myometrium | C54.2 | C79.82 | D07.0 | D26.1 | D39.0 | D49.59 |
| overlapping sites | C54.8 | — | — | — | — | — |
| squamocolumnar junction | C53.8 | C79.82 | D06.7 | D26.0 | D39.0 | D49.59 |
| tube | C57.0-☑ | C79.82 | D07.39 | D28.2 | D39.8 | D49.59 |
| utricle, prostatic | C68.0 | C79.19 | D09.19 | D30.4 | D41.3 | D49.59 |
| uveal tract | C69.4-☑ | C79.49 | D09.2-☑ | D31.4-☑ | D48.7 | D49.89 |
| uvula | C05.2 | C79.89 | D00.04 | D10.39 | D37.09 | D49.0 |
| vagina, vaginal (fornix) (vault) (wall) | C52 | C79.82 | D07.2 | D28.1 | D39.8 | D49.59 |
| vaginovesical | C57.9 | C79.82 | D07.30 | D28.9 | D39.9 | D49.59 |
| septum | C57.9 | C79.82 | D07.30 | D28.9 | D39.9 | D49.59 |
| vallecula (epiglottis) | C10.0 | C79.89 | D00.08 | D10.5 | D37.05 | D49.0 |
| vas deferens | C63.1-☑ | C79.82 | D07.69 | D29.8 | D40.8 | D49.59 |
| vascular *— see* Neoplasm, connective tissue | | | | | | |
| Vater's ampulla | C24.1 | C78.89 | D01.5 | D13.5 | D37.6 | D49.0 |
| vein, venous *— see* Neoplasm, connective tissue | | | | | | |
| vena cava (abdominal) (inferior) | C49.4 | C79.89 | — | D21.4 | D48.1-☑ | D49.2 |
| superior | C49.3 | C79.89 | — | D21.3 | D48.1-☑ | D49.2 |
| ventricle (cerebral) (floor) (lateral) (third) | C71.5 | C79.31 | — | D33.0 | D43.0 | D49.6 |
| cardiac (left) (right) | C38.0 | C79.89 | — | D15.1 | D48.7 | D49.89 |
| fourth | C71.7 | C79.31 | — | D33.1 | D43.1 | D49.6 |
| ventricular band of larynx | C32.1 | C78.31 | D02.0 | D14.1 | D38.0 | D49.1 |
| ventriculus *— see* Neoplasm, stomach | | | | | | |
| vermillion border *— see* Neoplasm, lip | | | | | | |
| vermis, cerebellum | C71.6 | C79.31 | — | D33.1 | D43.1 | D49.6 |
| vertebra (column) | C41.2 | C79.51 | — | D16.6 | D48.0 | D49.2 |
| coccyx | C41.4 | C79.51 | — | D16.8 | D48.0 | D49.2 |
| marrow NEC | C96.9 | C79.52 | — | — | D47.9 | D49.89 |
| sacrum | C41.4 | C79.51 | — | D16.8 | D48.0 | D49.2 |
| vesical *— see* Neoplasm, bladder | | | | | | |
| vesicle, seminal | C63.7 | C79.82 | D07.69 | D29.8 | D40.8 | D49.59 |
| vesicocervical tissue | C57.9 | C79.82 | D07.30 | D28.9 | D39.9 | D49.59 |
| vesicorectal | C76.3 | C79.82 | D09.8 | D36.7 | D48.7 | D49.89 |
| vesicovaginal | C57.9 | C79.82 | D07.30 | D28.9 | D39.9 | D49.59 |
| septum | C57.9 | C79.82 | D07.30 | D28.9 | D39.8 | D49.59 |
| vessel (blood) *— see* Neoplasm, connective tissue | | | | | | |
| vestibular gland, greater | C51.0 | C79.82 | D07.1 | D28.0 | D39.8 | D49.59 |
| vestibule | | | | | | |
| mouth | C06.1 | C79.89 | D00.00 | D10.39 | D37.09 | D49.0 |
| nose | C30.0 | C78.39 | D02.3 | D14.0 | D38.5 | D49.1 |
| Virchow's gland | C77.0 | C77.0 | — | D36.0 | D48.7 | D49.89 |
| viscera NEC | C76.8 | C79.89 | D09.8 | D36.7 | D48.7 | D49.89 |





☑ **Additional Character Required — Refer to the Tabular List for Character Selection**

| | Malignant Primary | Malignant Secondary | Ca in situ | Benign | Uncertain Behavior | Unspecified Behavior |
|---|---|---|---|---|---|---|
| **Neoplasm, neoplastic** — *continued* | | | | | | |
| vocal cords (true) | C32.Ø | C78.31 | DØ2.Ø | D14.1 | D38.Ø | D49.1 |
| false | C32.1 | C78.31 | DØ2.Ø | D14.1 | D38.Ø | D49.1 |
| vomer | C41.Ø | C79.51 | — | D16.4 | D48.Ø | D49.2 |
| vulva | C51.9 | C79.82 | DØ7.1 | D28.Ø | D39.8 | D49.59 |
| vulvovaginal gland | C51.Ø | C79.82 | DØ7.1 | D28.Ø | D39.8 | D49.59 |
| Waldeyer's ring | C14.2 | C79.89 | DØØ.Ø8 | D1Ø.9 | D37.Ø5 | D49.Ø |
| Wharton's duct | CØ8.Ø | C79.89 | DØØ.ØØ | D11.7 | D37.Ø32 | D49.Ø |
| white matter (central) (cerebral) | C71.Ø | C79.31 | — | D33.Ø | D43.Ø | D49.6 |
| windpipe | C33 | C78.39 | DØ2.1 | D14.2 | D38.1 | D49.1 |
| Wirsung's duct | C25.3 | C78.89 | DØ1.7 | D13.6 | D37.8 | D49.Ø |
| wolffian (body) (duct) | | | | | | |
| female | C57.7 | C79.82 | DØ7.39 | D28.7 | D39.8 | D49.59 |
| male | C63.7 | C79.82 | DØ7.69 | D29.8 | D4Ø.8 | D49.59 |
| womb — *see* Neoplasm, uterus | | | | | | |
| wrist NEC | C76.4-☑ | C79.89 | DØ4.6-☑ | D36.7 | D48.7 | D49.89 |
| xiphoid process | C41.3 | C79.51 | — | D16.7 | D48.Ø | D49.2 |
| Zuckerkandl organ | C75.5 | C79.89 | — | D35.6 | D44.7 | D49.7 |

**Note:** The list below gives the code number for neoplasms by anatomical site. For each site there are six possible code numbers according to whether the neoplasm in question is malignant, benign, in situ, of uncertain behavior, or of unspecified nature. The description of the neoplasm will often indicate which of the six columns is appropriate; e.g., malignant melanoma of skin, benign fibroadenoma of breast, carcinoma in situ of cervix uteri. Where such descriptors are not present, the remainder of the Index should be consulted where guidance is given to the appropriate column for each morphological (histological) variety listed; e.g., Mesonephroma – see Neoplasm, malignant; Embryoma — see also Neoplasm, uncertain behavior; Disease, Bowen's – see Neoplasm, skin, in situ. However, the guidance in the Index can be overridden if one of the descriptors mentioned above is present; e.g., malignant adenoma of colon is coded to C18.9 and not to D12.6 as the adjective "malignant" overrides the Index entry "Adenoma — *see also* Neoplasm, benign, by site." Codes listed with a dash -, following the code have a required additional character for laterality. The tabular list must be reviewed for the complete code.

| Substance | Poisoning, Accidental (unintentional) | Poisoning, Intentional Self-harm | Poisoning, Assault | Poisoning, Undetermined | Adverse Effect | Under-dosing |
|---|---|---|---|---|---|---|
| **1-Propanol** | T51.3X1 | T51.3X2 | T51.3X3 | T51.3X4 | — | — |
| **14-hydroxydihydro-morphinone** | T40.2X1 | T40.2X2 | T40.2X3 | T40.2X4 | T40.2X5 | T40.2X6 |
| **2-Deoxy-5-fluorouridine** | T45.1X1 | T45.1X2 | T45.1X3 | T45.1X4 | T45.1X5 | T45.1X6 |
| **2-Ethoxyethanol** | T52.3X1 | T52.3X2 | T52.3X3 | T52.3X4 | — | — |
| **2-Methoxyethanol** | T52.3X1 | T52.3X2 | T52.3X3 | T52.3X4 | — | — |
| **2-Propanol** | T51.2X1 | T51.2X2 | T51.2X3 | T51.2X4 | — | — |
| **2,3,7,8-Tetrachlorodibenzo-p-dioxin** | T53.7X1 | T53.7X2 | T53.7X3 | T53.7X4 | — | — |
| **2,4-D** (dichlorophen-oxyacetic acid) | T60.3X1 | T60.3X2 | T60.3X3 | T60.3X4 | — | — |
| **2,4-Toluene diisocyanate** | T65.0X1 | T65.0X2 | T65.0X3 | T65.0X4 | — | — |
| **2,4,5-T** (trichloro-phenoxyacetic acid) | T60.1X1 | T60.1X2 | T60.1X3 | T60.1X4 | — | — |
| **2,4,5-Trichlorophen-oxyacetic acid** | T60.3X1 | T60.3X2 | T60.3X3 | T60.3X4 | — | — |
| **3,4-methylenedioxymeth-amphetamine** | T43.641 | T43.642 | T43.643 | T43.644 | — | — |
| **4-Aminobutyric acid** | T43.8X1 | T43.8X2 | T43.8X3 | T43.8X4 | T43.8X5 | T43.8X6 |
| **4-Aminophenol derivatives** | T39.1X1 | T39.1X2 | T39.1X3 | T39.1X4 | T39.1X5 | T39.1X6 |
| **5-Deoxy-5-fluorouridine** | T45.1X1 | T45.1X2 | T45.1X3 | T45.1X4 | T45.1X5 | T45.1X6 |
| **5-Methoxypsoralen** (5-MOP) | T50.991 | T50.992 | T50.993 | T50.994 | T50.995 | T50.996 |
| **8-Aminoquinoline drugs** | T37.2X1 | T37.2X2 | T37.2X3 | T37.2X4 | T37.2X5 | T37.2X6 |
| **8-Methoxypsoralen** (8-MOP) | T50.991 | T50.992 | T50.993 | T50.994 | T50.995 | T50.996 |
| **9-hydoxyrisperidone*** | T43.591 | T43.592 | T43.593 | T43.594 | T43.595 | T43.596 |
| **ABOB** | T37.5X1 | T37.5X2 | T37.5X3 | T37.5X4 | T37.5X5 | T37.5X6 |
| **Abrine** | T62.2X1 | T62.2X2 | T62.2X3 | T62.2X4 | — | — |
| **Abrus** (seed) | T62.2X1 | T62.2X2 | T62.2X3 | T62.2X4 | — | — |
| **Absinthe** | T51.0X1 | T51.0X2 | T51.0X3 | T51.0X4 | — | — |
| beverage | T51.0X1 | T51.0X2 | T51.0X3 | T51.0X4 | — | — |
| **Acaricide** | T60.8X1 | T60.8X2 | T60.8X3 | T60.8X4 | — | — |
| **Acebutolol** | T44.7X1 | T44.7X2 | T44.7X3 | T44.7X4 | T44.7X5 | T44.7X6 |
| **Acecarbromal** | T42.6X1 | T42.6X2 | T42.6X3 | T42.6X4 | T42.6X5 | T42.6X6 |
| **Aceclidine** | T44.1X1 | T44.1X2 | T44.1X3 | T44.1X4 | T44.1X5 | T44.1X6 |
| **Acedapsone** | T37.0X1 | T37.0X2 | T37.0X3 | T37.0X4 | T37.0X5 | T37.0X6 |
| **Acefylline piperazine** | T48.6X1 | T48.6X2 | T48.6X3 | T48.6X4 | T48.6X5 | T48.6X6 |
| **Acemorphan** | T40.2X1 | T40.2X2 | T40.2X3 | T40.2X4 | T40.2X5 | T40.2X6 |
| **Acenocoumarin** | T45.511 | T45.512 | T45.513 | T45.514 | T45.515 | T45.516 |
| **Acenocoumarol** | T45.511 | T45.512 | T45.513 | T45.514 | T45.515 | T45.516 |
| **Aceon*** | T46.4X1 | T46.4X2 | T46.4X3 | T46.4X4 | T46.4X5 | T46.4X6 |
| **Acepifylline** | T48.6X1 | T48.6X2 | T48.6X3 | T48.6X4 | T48.6X5 | T48.6X6 |
| **Acepromazine** | T43.3X1 | T43.3X2 | T43.3X3 | T43.3X4 | T43.3X5 | T43.3X6 |
| **Acesulfamethoxypyridazine** | T37.0X1 | T37.0X2 | T37.0X3 | T37.0X4 | T37.0X5 | T37.0X6 |
| **Acetal** | T52.891 | T52.892 | T52.893 | T52.894 | — | — |
| **Acetaldehyde** (vapor) | T52.891 | T52.892 | T52.893 | T52.894 | — | — |
| liquid | T65.891 | T65.892 | T65.893 | T65.894 | — | — |
| **Acetaminophen** | T39.1X1 | T39.1X2 | T39.1X3 | T39.1X4 | T39.1X5 | T39.1X6 |
| **Acetaminosalol** | T39.1X1 | T39.1X2 | T39.1X3 | T39.1X4 | T39.1X5 | T39.1X6 |
| **Acetanilide** | T39.1X1 | T39.1X2 | T39.1X3 | T39.1X4 | T39.1X5 | T39.1X6 |
| **Acetarsol** | T37.3X1 | T37.3X2 | T37.3X3 | T37.3X4 | T37.3X5 | T37.3X6 |
| **Acetazolamide** | T50.2X1 | T50.2X2 | T50.2X3 | T50.2X4 | T50.2X5 | T50.2X6 |
| **Acetiamine** | T45.2X1 | T45.2X2 | T45.2X3 | T45.2X4 | T45.2X5 | T45.2X6 |
| **Acetic** | | | | | | |
| acid | T54.2X1 | T54.2X2 | T54.2X3 | T54.2X4 | — | — |
| with sodium acetate (ointment) | T49.3X1 | T49.3X2 | T49.3X3 | T49.3X4 | T49.3X5 | T49.3X6 |
| ester (solvent)(vapor) | T52.891 | T52.892 | T52.893 | T52.894 | — | — |
| irrigating solution | T50.3X1 | T50.3X2 | T50.3X3 | T50.3X4 | T50.3X5 | T50.3X6 |
| medicinal (lotion) | T49.2X1 | T49.2X2 | T49.2X3 | T49.2X4 | T49.2X5 | T49.2X6 |
| anhydride | T65.891 | T65.892 | T65.893 | T65.894 | — | — |
| ether (vapor) | T52.891 | T52.892 | T52.893 | T52.894 | — | — |
| **Acetohexamide** | T38.3X1 | T38.3X2 | T38.3X3 | T38.3X4 | T38.3X5 | T38.3X6 |
| **Acetohydroxamic acid** | T50.991 | T50.992 | T50.993 | T50.994 | T50.995 | T50.996 |
| **Acetomenaphthone** | T45.7X1 | T45.7X2 | T45.7X3 | T45.7X4 | T45.7X5 | T45.7X6 |
| **Acetomorphine** | T40.1X1 | T40.1X2 | T40.1X3 | T40.1X4 | — | — |
| **Acetone** (oils) | T52.4X1 | T52.4X2 | T52.4X3 | T52.4X4 | — | — |
| chlorinated | T52.4X1 | T52.4X2 | T52.4X3 | T52.4X4 | — | — |
| vapor | T52.4X1 | T52.4X2 | T52.4X3 | T52.4X4 | — | — |
| **Acetonitrile** | T52.891 | T52.892 | T52.893 | T52.894 | — | — |
| **Acetophenazine** | T43.3X1 | T43.3X2 | T43.3X3 | T43.3X4 | T43.3X5 | T43.3X6 |
| **Acetophenetedin** | T39.1X1 | T39.1X2 | T39.1X3 | T39.1X4 | T39.1X5 | T39.1X6 |
| **Acetophenone** | T52.4X1 | T52.4X2 | T52.4X3 | T52.4X4 | — | — |
| **Acetorphine** | T40.2X1 | T40.2X2 | T40.2X3 | T40.2X4 | — | — |
| **Acetosulfone** (sodium) | T37.1X1 | T37.1X2 | T37.1X3 | T37.1X4 | T37.1X5 | T37.1X6 |
| **Acetrizoate** (sodium) | T50.8X1 | T50.8X2 | T50.8X3 | T50.8X4 | T50.8X5 | T50.8X6 |
| **Acetrizoic acid** | T50.8X1 | T50.8X2 | T50.8X3 | T50.8X4 | T50.8X5 | T50.8X6 |
| **Acetyl** | | | | | | |
| bromide | T53.6X1 | T53.6X2 | T53.6X3 | T53.6X4 | — | — |
| chloride | T53.6X1 | T53.6X2 | T53.6X3 | T53.6X4 | — | — |
| **Acetylcarbromal** | T42.6X1 | T42.6X2 | T42.6X3 | T42.6X4 | T42.6X5 | T42.6X6 |
| **Acetylcholine** | | | | | | |

| Substance | Poisoning, Accidental (unintentional) | Poisoning, Intentional Self-harm | Poisoning, Assault | Poisoning, Undetermined | Adverse Effect | Under-dosing |
|---|---|---|---|---|---|---|
| **Acetylcholine** — *continued* | | | | | | |
| chloride | T44.1X1 | T44.1X2 | T44.1X3 | T44.1X4 | T44.1X5 | T44.1X6 |
| derivative | T44.1X1 | T44.1X2 | T44.1X3 | T44.1X4 | T44.1X5 | T44.1X6 |
| **Acetylcysteine** | T48.4X1 | T48.4X2 | T48.4X3 | T48.4X4 | T48.4X5 | T48.4X6 |
| **Acetyldigitoxin** | T46.0X1 | T46.0X2 | T46.0X3 | T46.0X4 | T46.0X5 | T46.0X6 |
| **Acetyldigoxin** | T46.0X1 | T46.0X2 | T46.0X3 | T46.0X4 | T46.0X5 | T46.0X6 |
| **Acetyldihydrocodeine** | T40.2X1 | T40.2X2 | T40.2X3 | T40.2X4 | — | — |
| **Acetyldihydrocodeinone** | T40.2X1 | T40.2X2 | T40.2X3 | T40.2X4 | — | — |
| **Acetylene** (gas) | T59.891 | T59.892 | T59.893 | T59.894 | — | — |
| dichloride | T53.6X1 | T53.6X2 | T53.6X3 | T53.6X4 | — | — |
| incomplete combustion of | T58.11 | T58.12 | T58.13 | T58.14 | — | — |
| industrial | T59.891 | T59.892 | T59.893 | T59.894 | — | — |
| tetrachloride | T53.6X1 | T53.6X2 | T53.6X3 | T53.6X4 | — | — |
| vapor | T53.6X1 | T53.6X2 | T53.6X3 | T53.6X4 | — | — |
| **Acetylpheneturide** | T42.6X1 | T42.6X2 | T42.6X3 | T42.6X4 | T42.6X5 | T42.6X6 |
| **Acetylphenylhydrazine** | T39.8X1 | T39.8X2 | T39.8X3 | T39.8X4 | T39.8X5 | T39.8X6 |
| **Acetylsalicylic acid** (salts) | T39.011 | T39.012 | T39.013 | T39.014 | T39.015 | T39.016 |
| enteric coated | T39.011 | T39.012 | T39.013 | T39.014 | T39.015 | T39.016 |
| **Acetylsulfamethoxypyridazine** | T37.0X1 | T37.0X2 | T37.0X3 | T37.0X4 | T37.0X5 | T37.0X6 |
| **Achromycin** | T36.4X1 | T36.4X2 | T36.4X3 | T36.4X4 | T36.4X5 | T36.4X6 |
| ophthalmic preparation | T49.5X1 | T49.5X2 | T49.5X3 | T49.5X4 | T49.5X5 | T49.5X6 |
| topical NEC | T49.0X1 | T49.0X2 | T49.0X3 | T49.0X4 | T49.0X5 | T49.0X6 |
| **Aciclovir** | T37.5X1 | T37.5X2 | T37.5X3 | T37.5X4 | T37.5X5 | T37.5X6 |
| **Acid** (corrosive) **NEC** | T54.2X1 | T54.2X2 | T54.2X3 | T54.2X4 | — | — |
| **Acidifying agent NEC** | T50.901 | T50.902 | T50.903 | T50.904 | T50.905 | T50.906 |
| **AcipHex*** | T47.1X1 | T47.1X2 | T47.1X3 | T47.1X4 | T47.1X5 | T47.1X6 |
| **Acipimox** | T46.6X1 | T46.6X2 | T46.6X3 | T46.6X4 | T46.6X5 | T46.6X6 |
| **Acitretin** | T50.991 | T50.992 | T50.993 | T50.994 | T50.995 | T50.996 |
| **Aclarubicin** | T45.1X1 | T45.1X2 | T45.1X3 | T45.1X4 | T45.1X5 | T45.1X6 |
| **Aclatonium napadisilate** | T48.1X1 | T48.1X2 | T48.1X3 | T48.1X4 | T48.1X5 | T48.1X6 |
| **Aconite** (wild) | T46.991 | T46.992 | T46.993 | T46.994 | T46.995 | T46.996 |
| **Aconitine** | T46.991 | T46.992 | T46.993 | T46.994 | T46.995 | T46.996 |
| **Aconitum ferox** | T46.991 | T46.992 | T46.993 | T46.994 | T46.995 | T46.996 |
| **Acridine** | T65.6X1 | T65.6X2 | T65.6X3 | T65.6X4 | — | — |
| vapor | T59.891 | T59.892 | T59.893 | T59.894 | — | — |
| **Acriflavine** | T37.91 | T37.92 | T37.93 | T37.94 | T37.95 | T37.96 |
| **Acriflavinium chloride** | T49.0X1 | T49.0X2 | T49.0X3 | T49.0X4 | T49.0X5 | T49.0X6 |
| **Acrinol** | T49.0X1 | T49.0X2 | T49.0X3 | T49.0X4 | T49.0X5 | T49.0X6 |
| **Acrisorcin** | T49.0X1 | T49.0X2 | T49.0X3 | T49.0X4 | T49.0X5 | T49.0X6 |
| **Acrivastine** | T45.0X1 | T45.0X2 | T45.0X3 | T45.0X4 | T45.0X5 | T45.0X6 |
| **Acrolein** (gas) | T59.891 | T59.892 | T59.893 | T59.894 | — | — |
| liquid | T54.1X1 | T54.1X2 | T54.1X3 | T54.1X4 | — | — |
| **Acrylamide** | T65.891 | T65.892 | T65.893 | T65.894 | — | — |
| **Acrylic resin** | T49.3X1 | T49.3X2 | T49.3X3 | T49.3X4 | T49.3X5 | T49.3X6 |
| **Acrylonitrile** | T65.891 | T65.892 | T65.893 | T65.894 | — | — |
| **Actaea spicata** | T62.2X1 | T62.2X2 | T62.2X3 | T62.2X4 | — | — |
| berry | T62.1X1 | T62.1X2 | T62.1X3 | T62.1X4 | — | — |
| **Acterol** | T37.3X1 | T37.3X2 | T37.3X3 | T37.3X4 | T37.3X5 | T37.3X6 |
| **ACTH** | T38.811 | T38.812 | T38.813 | T38.814 | T38.815 | T38.816 |
| **Acticlate*** | T36.4X1 | T36.4X2 | T36.4X3 | T36.4X4 | T36.4X5 | T36.4X6 |
| **Actinomycin C** | T45.1X1 | T45.1X2 | T45.1X3 | T45.1X4 | T45.1X5 | T45.1X6 |
| **Actinomycin D** | T45.1X1 | T45.1X2 | T45.1X3 | T45.1X4 | T45.1X5 | T45.1X6 |
| **Activated charcoal** — *see also* Charcoal, medicinal | T47.6X1 | T47.6X2 | T47.6X3 | T47.6X4 | T47.6X5 | T47.6X6 |
| **Activella*** | T38.5X1 | T38.5X2 | T38.5X3 | T38.5X4 | T38.5X5 | T38.5X6 |
| **Acyclovir** | T37.5X1 | T37.5X2 | T37.5X3 | T37.5X4 | T37.5X5 | T37.5X6 |
| **Adenine** | T45.2X1 | T45.2X2 | T45.2X3 | T45.2X4 | T45.2X5 | T45.2X6 |
| arabinoside | T37.5X1 | T37.5X2 | T37.5X3 | T37.5X4 | T37.5X5 | T37.5X6 |
| **Adenosine** (phosphate) | T46.2X1 | T46.2X2 | T46.2X3 | T46.2X4 | T46.2X5 | T46.2X6 |
| **ADH** | T38.891 | T38.892 | T38.893 | T38.894 | T38.895 | T38.896 |
| **Adhesive NEC** | T65.891 | T65.892 | T65.893 | T65.894 | — | — |
| **Adicillin** | T36.0X1 | T36.0X2 | T36.0X3 | T36.0X4 | T36.0X5 | T36.0X6 |
| **Adiphenine** | T44.3X1 | T44.3X2 | T44.3X3 | T44.3X4 | T44.3X5 | T44.3X6 |
| **Adipiodone** | T50.8X1 | T50.8X2 | T50.8X3 | T50.8X4 | T50.8X5 | T50.8X6 |
| **Adjunct, pharmaceutical** | T50.901 | T50.902 | T50.903 | T50.904 | T50.905 | T50.906 |
| **Adrenal** (extract, cortex or medulla) (glucocorticoids) (hormones) (mineralocorticoids) | T38.0X1 | T38.0X2 | T38.0X3 | T38.0X4 | T38.0X5 | T38.0X6 |
| ENT agent | T49.6X1 | T49.6X2 | T49.6X3 | T49.6X4 | T49.6X5 | T49.6X6 |
| ophthalmic preparation | T49.5X1 | T49.5X2 | T49.5X3 | T49.5X4 | T49.5X5 | T49.5X6 |
| topical NEC | T49.0X1 | T49.0X2 | T49.0X3 | T49.0X4 | T49.0X5 | T49.0X6 |
| **Adrenalin** — *see* Adrenaline | | | | | | |
| **Adrenaline** | T44.5X1 | T44.5X2 | T44.5X3 | T44.5X4 | T44.5X5 | T44.5X6 |
| **Adrenergic NEC** | T44.901 | T44.902 | T44.903 | T44.904 | T44.905 | T44.906 |
| blocking agent NEC | T44.8X1 | T44.8X2 | T44.8X3 | T44.8X4 | T44.8X5 | T44.8X6 |
| beta, heart | T44.7X1 | T44.7X2 | T44.7X3 | T44.7X4 | T44.7X5 | T44.7X6 |
| specified NEC | T44.991 | T44.992 | T44.993 | T44.994 | T44.995 | T44.996 |
| **Adrenochrome** | | | | | | |
| (mono) semicarbazone | T46.991 | T46.992 | T46.993 | T46.994 | T46.995 | T46.996 |
| derivative | T46.991 | T46.992 | T46.993 | T46.994 | T46.995 | T46.996 |
| **Adrenocorticotrophic hormone** | T38.811 | T38.812 | T38.813 | T38.814 | T38.815 | T38.816 |





☑ **Additional Character May Be Required — Refer to the Tabular List for Character Selection**

***Optum Value-Added**

| Substance | Poisoning, Accidental (unintentional) | Poisoning, Intentional Self-harm | Poisoning, Assault | Poisoning, Undetermined | Adverse Effect | Under-dosing |
|---|---|---|---|---|---|---|
| **Adrenocorticotrophin** | T38.811 | T38.812 | T38.813 | T38.814 | T38.815 | T38.816 |
| **Adriamycin** | T45.1X1 | T45.1X2 | T45.1X3 | T45.1X4 | T45.1X5 | T45.1X6 |
| **Adrucil*** | T45.1X1 | T45.1X2 | T45.1X3 | T45.1X4 | T45.1X5 | T45.1X6 |
| **Aerosol spray NEC** | T65.91 | T65.92 | T65.93 | T65.94 | — | — |
| **Aerosporin** | T36.8X1 | T36.8X2 | T36.8X3 | T36.8X4 | T36.8X5 | T36.8X6 |
| ENT agent | T49.6X1 | T49.6X2 | T49.6X3 | T49.6X4 | T49.6X5 | T49.6X6 |
| ophthalmic preparation | T49.5X1 | T49.5X2 | T49.5X3 | T49.5X4 | T49.5X5 | T49.5X6 |
| topical NEC | T49.0X1 | T49.0X2 | T49.0X3 | T49.0X4 | T49.0X5 | T49.0X6 |
| **Aethusa cynapium** | T62.2X1 | T62.2X2 | T62.2X3 | T62.2X4 | — | — |
| **Afghanistan black** | T40.711 | T40.712 | T40.713 | T40.714 | T40.715 | T40.716 |
| **Aflatoxin** | T64.01 | T64.02 | T64.03 | T64.04 | — | — |
| **Afloqualone** | T42.8X1 | T42.8X2 | T42.8X3 | T42.8X4 | T42.8X5 | T42.8X6 |
| **African boxwood** | T62.2X1 | T62.2X2 | T62.2X3 | T62.2X4 | — | — |
| **Agar** | T47.4X1 | T47.4X2 | T47.4X3 | T47.4X4 | T47.4X5 | T47.4X6 |
| **Agonist** | | | | | | |
| predominantly | | | | | | |
| alpha-adrenoreceptor | T44.4X1 | T44.4X2 | T44.4X3 | T44.4X4 | T44.4X5 | T44.4X6 |
| beta-adrenoreceptor | T44.5X1 | T44.5X2 | T44.5X3 | T44.5X4 | T44.5X5 | T44.5X6 |
| **Agricultural agent NEC** | T65.91 | T65.92 | T65.93 | T65.94 | — | — |
| **Agrypnal** | T42.3X1 | T42.3X2 | T42.3X3 | T42.3X4 | T42.3X5 | T42.3X6 |
| **AHLG** | T50.Z11 | T50.Z12 | T50.Z13 | T50.Z14 | T50.Z15 | T50.Z16 |
| **Air contaminant**(s), **source/type NOS** | T65.91 | T65.92 | T65.93 | T65.94 | — | — |
| **Ajmaline** | T46.2X1 | T46.2X2 | T46.2X3 | T46.2X4 | T46.2X5 | T46.2X6 |
| **Akee** | T62.1X1 | T62.1X2 | T62.1X3 | T62.1X4 | — | — |
| **Akne-Mycin*** | T49.0X1 | T49.0X2 | T49.0X3 | T49.0X4 | T49.0X5 | T49.0X6 |
| **Akrinol** | T49.0X1 | T49.0X2 | T49.0X3 | T49.0X4 | T49.0X5 | T49.0X6 |
| **Akritoin** | T37.8X1 | T37.8X2 | T37.8X3 | T37.8X4 | T37.8X5 | T37.8X6 |
| **Alacepril** | T46.4X1 | T46.4X2 | T46.4X3 | T46.4X4 | T46.4X5 | T46.4X6 |
| **Alantolactone** | T37.4X1 | T37.4X2 | T37.4X3 | T37.4X4 | T37.4X5 | T37.4X6 |
| **Albamycin** | T36.8X1 | T36.8X2 | T36.8X3 | T36.8X4 | T36.8X5 | T36.8X6 |
| **Albendazole** | T37.4X1 | T37.4X2 | T37.4X3 | T37.4X4 | T37.4X5 | T37.4X6 |
| **Albigutide*** | T38.3X1 | T38.3X2 | T38.3X3 | T38.3X4 | T38.3X5 | T38.3X6 |
| **Albumin** | | | | | | |
| bovine | T45.8X1 | T45.8X2 | T45.8X3 | T45.8X4 | T45.8X5 | T45.8X6 |
| human serum | T45.8X1 | T45.8X2 | T45.8X3 | T45.8X4 | T45.8X5 | T45.8X6 |
| salt-poor | T45.8X1 | T45.8X2 | T45.8X3 | T45.8X4 | T45.8X5 | T45.8X6 |
| normal human serum | T45.8X1 | T45.8X2 | T45.8X3 | T45.8X4 | T45.8X5 | T45.8X6 |
| **Albuterol** | T48.6X1 | T48.6X2 | T48.6X3 | T48.6X4 | T48.6X5 | T48.6X6 |
| **Albutoin** | T42.0X1 | T42.0X2 | T42.0X3 | T42.0X4 | T42.0X5 | T42.0X6 |
| **Alclometasone** | T49.0X1 | T49.0X2 | T49.0X3 | T49.0X4 | T49.0X5 | T49.0X6 |
| **Alcohol** | T51.91 | T51.92 | T51.93 | T51.94 | — | — |
| absolute | T51.0X1 | T51.0X2 | T51.0X3 | T51.0X4 | — | — |
| beverage | T51.0X1 | T51.0X2 | T51.0X3 | T51.0X4 | — | — |
| allyl | T51.8X1 | T51.8X2 | T51.8X3 | T51.8X4 | — | — |
| amyl | T51.3X1 | T51.3X2 | T51.3X3 | T51.3X4 | — | — |
| antifreeze | T51.1X1 | T51.1X2 | T51.1X3 | T51.1X4 | — | — |
| beverage | T51.0X1 | T51.0X2 | T51.0X3 | T51.0X4 | — | — |
| butyl | T51.3X1 | T51.3X2 | T51.3X3 | T51.3X4 | — | — |
| dehydrated | T51.0X1 | T51.0X2 | T51.0X3 | T51.0X4 | — | — |
| beverage | T51.0X1 | T51.0X2 | T51.0X3 | T51.0X4 | — | — |
| denatured | T51.0X1 | T51.0X2 | T51.0X3 | T51.0X4 | — | — |
| deterrent NEC | T50.6X1 | T50.6X2 | T50.6X3 | T50.6X4 | T50.6X5 | T50.6X6 |
| diagnostic (gastric function) | T50.8X1 | T50.8X2 | T50.8X3 | T50.8X4 | T50.8X5 | T50.8X6 |
| ethyl | T51.0X1 | T51.0X2 | T51.0X3 | T51.0X4 | — | — |
| beverage | T51.0X1 | T51.0X2 | T51.0X3 | T51.0X4 | — | — |
| grain | T51.0X1 | T51.0X2 | T51.0X3 | T51.0X4 | — | — |
| beverage | T51.0X1 | T51.0X2 | T51.0X3 | T51.0X4 | — | — |
| industrial | T51.0X1 | T51.0X2 | T51.0X3 | T51.0X4 | — | — |
| isopropyl | T51.2X1 | T51.2X2 | T51.2X3 | T51.2X4 | — | — |
| methyl | T51.1X1 | T51.1X2 | T51.1X3 | T51.1X4 | — | — |
| preparation for consumption | T51.0X1 | T51.0X2 | T51.0X3 | T51.0X4 | — | — |
| propyl | T51.3X1 | T51.3X2 | T51.3X3 | T51.3X4 | — | — |
| secondary | T51.2X1 | T51.2X2 | T51.2X3 | T51.2X4 | — | — |
| radiator | T51.1X1 | T51.1X2 | T51.1X3 | T51.1X4 | — | — |
| rubbing | T51.2X1 | T51.2X2 | T51.2X3 | T51.2X4 | — | — |
| specified type NEC | T51.8X1 | T51.8X2 | T51.8X3 | T51.8X4 | — | — |
| surgical | T51.0X1 | T51.0X2 | T51.0X3 | T51.0X4 | — | — |
| vapor (from any type of Alcohol) | T59.891 | T59.892 | T59.893 | T59.894 | — | — |
| wood | T51.1X1 | T51.1X2 | T51.1X3 | T51.1X4 | — | — |
| **Alcuronium** (chloride) | T48.1X1 | T48.1X2 | T48.1X3 | T48.1X4 | T48.1X5 | T48.1X6 |
| **Aldactone** | T50.0X1 | T50.0X2 | T50.0X3 | T50.0X4 | T50.0X5 | T50.0X6 |
| **Aldesulfone sodium** | T37.1X1 | T37.1X2 | T37.1X3 | T37.1X4 | T37.1X5 | T37.1X6 |
| **Aldicarb** | T60.0X1 | T60.0X2 | T60.0X3 | T60.0X4 | — | — |
| **Aldomet** | T46.5X1 | T46.5X2 | T46.5X3 | T46.5X4 | T46.5X5 | T46.5X6 |
| **Aldosterone** | T50.0X1 | T50.0X2 | T50.0X3 | T50.0X4 | T50.0X5 | T50.0X6 |
| **Aldrin** (dust) | T60.1X1 | T60.1X2 | T60.1X3 | T60.1X4 | — | — |
| **Aleve** — *see* Naproxen | | | | | | |
| **Alexitol sodium** | T47.1X1 | T47.1X2 | T47.1X3 | T47.1X4 | T47.1X5 | T47.1X6 |
| **Alfacalcidol** | T45.2X1 | T45.2X2 | T45.2X3 | T45.2X4 | T45.2X5 | T45.2X6 |
| **Alfadolone** | T41.1X1 | T41.1X2 | T41.1X3 | T41.1X4 | T41.1X5 | T41.1X6 |
| **Alfaxalone** | T41.1X1 | T41.1X2 | T41.1X3 | T41.1X4 | T41.1X5 | T41.1X6 |
| **Alfentanil** | T40.411 | T40.412 | T40.413 | T40.414 | T40.415 | T40.416 |
| **Alfuzosin** (hydrochloride) | T44.8X1 | T44.8X2 | T44.8X3 | T44.8X4 | T44.8X5 | T44.8X6 |
| **Algae** (harmful) (toxin) | T65.821 | T65.822 | T65.823 | T65.824 | — | — |
| **Algeldrate** | T47.1X1 | T47.1X2 | T47.1X3 | T47.1X4 | T47.1X5 | T47.1X6 |
| **Algin** | T47.8X1 | T47.8X2 | T47.8X3 | T47.8X4 | T47.8X5 | T47.8X6 |
| **Alglucerase** | T45.3X1 | T45.3X2 | T45.3X3 | T45.3X4 | T45.3X5 | T45.3X6 |
| **Alidase** | T45.3X1 | T45.3X2 | T45.3X3 | T45.3X4 | T45.3X5 | T45.3X6 |
| **Alimemazine** | T43.3X1 | T43.3X2 | T43.3X3 | T43.3X4 | T43.3X5 | T43.3X6 |
| **Aliphatic thiocyanates** | T65.0X1 | T65.0X2 | T65.0X3 | T65.0X4 | — | — |
| **Alitretinoin*** | T49.0X1 | T49.0X2 | T49.0X3 | T49.0X4 | T49.0X5 | T49.0X6 |
| **Alizapride** | T45.0X1 | T45.0X2 | T45.0X3 | T45.0X4 | T45.0X5 | T45.0X6 |
| **Alka-seltzer** | T39.011 | T39.012 | T39.013 | T39.014 | T39.015 | T39.016 |
| **Alkali** (caustic) | T54.3X1 | T54.3X2 | T54.3X3 | T54.3X4 | — | — |
| **Alkaline antiseptic solution** (aromatic) | T49.6X1 | T49.6X2 | T49.6X3 | T49.6X4 | T49.6X5 | T49.6X6 |
| **Alkalinizing agents** (medicinal) | T50.901 | T50.902 | T50.903 | T50.904 | T50.905 | T50.906 |
| **Alkalizing agent NEC** | T50.901 | T50.902 | T50.903 | T50.904 | T50.905 | T50.906 |
| **Alkavervir** | T46.5X1 | T46.5X2 | T46.5X3 | T46.5X4 | T46.5X5 | T46.5X6 |
| **Alkenes** | T52.811 | T52.812 | T52.813 | T52.814 | — | — |
| **Alkeran*** | T45.1X1 | T45.1X2 | T45.1X3 | T45.1X4 | T45.1X5 | T45.1X6 |
| **Alkonium** (bromide) | T49.0X1 | T49.0X2 | T49.0X3 | T49.0X4 | T49.0X5 | T49.0X6 |
| **Alkylating drug NEC** | T45.1X1 | T45.1X2 | T45.1X3 | T45.1X4 | T45.1X5 | T45.1X6 |
| antimyeloproliferative | T45.1X1 | T45.1X2 | T45.1X3 | T45.1X4 | T45.1X5 | T45.1X6 |
| lymphatic | T45.1X1 | T45.1X2 | T45.1X3 | T45.1X4 | T45.1X5 | T45.1X6 |
| **Alkylisocyanate** | T65.0X1 | T65.0X2 | T65.0X3 | T65.0X4 | — | — |
| **Allantoin** | T49.4X1 | T49.4X2 | T49.4X3 | T49.4X4 | T49.4X5 | T49.4X6 |
| **Allegron** | T43.011 | T43.012 | T43.013 | T43.014 | T43.015 | T43.016 |
| **Allethrin** | T49.0X1 | T49.0X2 | T49.0X3 | T49.0X4 | T49.0X5 | T49.0X6 |
| **Allobarbital** | T42.3X1 | T42.3X2 | T42.3X3 | T42.3X4 | T42.3X5 | T42.3X6 |
| **Allopurinol** | T50.4X1 | T50.4X2 | T50.4X3 | T50.4X4 | T50.4X5 | T50.4X6 |
| **Allyl** | | | | | | |
| alcohol | T51.8X1 | T51.8X2 | T51.8X3 | T51.8X4 | — | — |
| disulfide | T46.6X1 | T46.6X2 | T46.6X3 | T46.6X4 | T46.6X5 | T46.6X6 |
| **Allylestrenol** | T38.5X1 | T38.5X2 | T38.5X3 | T38.5X4 | T38.5X5 | T38.5X6 |
| **Allylisopropylacetylurea** | T42.6X1 | T42.6X2 | T42.6X3 | T42.6X4 | T42.6X5 | T42.6X6 |
| **Allylisopropylmalonylurea** | T42.3X1 | T42.3X2 | T42.3X3 | T42.3X4 | T42.3X5 | T42.3X6 |
| **Allylthiourea** | T49.3X1 | T49.3X2 | T49.3X3 | T49.3X4 | T49.3X5 | T49.3X6 |
| **Allyltribromide** | T42.6X1 | T42.6X2 | T42.6X3 | T42.6X4 | T42.6X5 | T42.6X6 |
| **Allypropymal** | T42.3X1 | T42.3X2 | T42.3X3 | T42.3X4 | T42.3X5 | T42.3X6 |
| **Almagate** | T47.1X1 | T47.1X2 | T47.1X3 | T47.1X4 | T47.1X5 | T47.1X6 |
| **Almasilate** | T47.1X1 | T47.1X2 | T47.1X3 | T47.1X4 | T47.1X5 | T47.1X6 |
| **Almitrine** | T50.7X1 | T50.7X2 | T50.7X3 | T50.7X4 | T50.7X5 | T50.7X6 |
| **Aloes** | T47.2X1 | T47.2X2 | T47.2X3 | T47.2X4 | T47.2X5 | T47.2X6 |
| **Aloglutamol** | T47.1X1 | T47.1X2 | T47.1X3 | T47.1X4 | T47.1X5 | T47.1X6 |
| **Aloin** | T47.2X1 | T47.2X2 | T47.2X3 | T47.2X4 | T47.2X5 | T47.2X6 |
| **Aloxidone** | T42.2X1 | T42.2X2 | T42.2X3 | T42.2X4 | T42.2X5 | T42.2X6 |
| **Alpha** | | | | | | |
| acetyldigoxin | T46.0X1 | T46.0X2 | T46.0X3 | T46.0X4 | T46.0X5 | T46.0X6 |
| adrenergic blocking drug | T44.6X1 | T44.6X2 | T44.6X3 | T44.6X4 | T44.6X5 | T44.6X6 |
| amylase | T45.3X1 | T45.3X2 | T45.3X3 | T45.3X4 | T45.3X5 | T45.3X6 |
| tocoferol (acetate) | T45.2X1 | T45.2X2 | T45.2X3 | T45.2X4 | T45.2X5 | T45.2X6 |
| tocopherol | T45.2X1 | T45.2X2 | T45.2X3 | T45.2X4 | T45.2X5 | T45.2X6 |
| **Alphadolone** | T41.1X1 | T41.1X2 | T41.1X3 | T41.1X4 | T41.1X5 | T41.1X6 |
| **Alphaprodine** | T40.491 | T40.492 | T40.493 | T40.494 | T40.495 | T40.496 |
| **Alphaxalone** | T41.1X1 | T41.1X2 | T41.1X3 | T41.1X4 | T41.1X5 | T41.1X6 |
| **Alprazolam** | T42.4X1 | T42.4X2 | T42.4X3 | T42.4X4 | T42.4X5 | T42.4X6 |
| **Alprenolol** | T44.7X1 | T44.7X2 | T44.7X3 | T44.7X4 | T44.7X5 | T44.7X6 |
| **Alprostadil** | T46.7X1 | T46.7X2 | T46.7X3 | T46.7X4 | T46.7X5 | T46.7X6 |
| **Alsactide** | T38.811 | T38.812 | T38.813 | T38.814 | T38.815 | T38.816 |
| **Alseroxylon** | T46.5X1 | T46.5X2 | T46.5X3 | T46.5X4 | T46.5X5 | T46.5X6 |
| **Alteplase** | T45.611 | T45.612 | T45.613 | T45.614 | T45.615 | T45.616 |
| **Altizide** | T50.2X1 | T50.2X2 | T50.2X3 | T50.2X4 | T50.2X5 | T50.2X6 |
| **Altoprev*** | T46.6X1 | T46.6X2 | T46.6X3 | T46.6X4 | T46.6X5 | T46.6X6 |
| **Altretamine** | T45.1X1 | T45.1X2 | T45.1X3 | T45.1X4 | T45.1X5 | T45.1X6 |
| **Alum** (medicinal) | T49.4X1 | T49.4X2 | T49.4X3 | T49.4X4 | T49.4X5 | T49.4X6 |
| nonmedicinal (ammonium) (potassium) | T56.891 | T56.892 | T56.893 | T56.894 | — | — |
| **Aluminium, aluminum** | | | | | | |
| acetate | T49.2X1 | T49.2X2 | T49.2X3 | T49.2X4 | T49.2X5 | T49.2X6 |
| solution | T49.0X1 | T49.0X2 | T49.0X3 | T49.0X4 | T49.0X5 | T49.0X6 |
| aspirin | T39.011 | T39.012 | T39.013 | T39.014 | T39.015 | T39.016 |
| bis (acetylsalicylate) | T39.011 | T39.012 | T39.013 | T39.014 | T39.015 | T39.016 |
| carbonate (gel, basic) | T47.1X1 | T47.1X2 | T47.1X3 | T47.1X4 | T47.1X5 | T47.1X6 |
| chlorhydroxide-complex | T47.1X1 | T47.1X2 | T47.1X3 | T47.1X4 | T47.1X5 | T47.1X6 |
| chloride | T49.2X1 | T49.2X2 | T49.2X3 | T49.2X4 | T49.2X5 | T49.2X6 |
| clofibrate | T46.6X1 | T46.6X2 | T46.6X3 | T46.6X4 | T46.6X5 | T46.6X6 |
| diacetate | T49.2X1 | T49.2X2 | T49.2X3 | T49.2X4 | T49.2X5 | T49.2X6 |
| glycinate | T47.1X1 | T47.1X2 | T47.1X3 | T47.1X4 | T47.1X5 | T47.1X6 |
| hydroxide (gel) | T47.1X1 | T47.1X2 | T47.1X3 | T47.1X4 | T47.1X5 | T47.1X6 |

| Substance | Poisoning, Accidental (unintentional) | Poisoning, Intentional Self-harm | Poisoning, Assault | Poisoning, Undetermined | Adverse Effect | Under-dosing |
|---|---|---|---|---|---|---|
| **Aluminium, aluminum** — *continued* | | | | | | |
| hydroxide-magnesium carb. gel | T47.1X1 | T47.1X2 | T47.1X3 | T47.1X4 | T47.1X5 | T47.1X6 |
| magnesium silicate | T47.1X1 | T47.1X2 | T47.1X3 | T47.1X4 | T47.1X5 | T47.1X6 |
| nicotinate | T46.7X1 | T46.7X2 | T46.7X3 | T46.7X4 | T46.7X5 | T46.7X6 |
| ointment (surgical) (topical) | T49.3X1 | T49.3X2 | T49.3X3 | T49.3X4 | T49.3X5 | T49.3X6 |
| phosphate | T47.1X1 | T47.1X2 | T47.1X3 | T47.1X4 | T47.1X5 | T47.1X6 |
| salicylate | T39.Ø91 | T39.Ø92 | T39.Ø93 | T39.Ø94 | T39.Ø95 | T39.Ø96 |
| silicate | T47.1X1 | T47.1X2 | T47.1X3 | T47.1X4 | T47.1X5 | T47.1X6 |
| sodium silicate | T47.1X1 | T47.1X2 | T47.1X3 | T47.1X4 | T47.1X5 | T47.1X6 |
| subacetate | T49.2X1 | T49.2X2 | T49.2X3 | T49.2X4 | T49.2X5 | T49.2X6 |
| sulfate | T49.ØX1 | T49.ØX2 | T49.ØX3 | T49.ØX4 | T49.ØX5 | T49.ØX6 |
| tannate | T47.6X1 | T47.6X2 | T47.6X3 | T47.6X4 | T47.6X5 | T47.6X6 |
| topical NEC | T49.3X1 | T49.3X2 | T49.3X3 | T49.3X4 | T49.3X5 | T49.3X6 |
| **Alurate** | T42.3X1 | T42.3X2 | T42.3X3 | T42.3X4 | T42.3X5 | T42.3X6 |
| **Alverine** | T44.3X1 | T44.3X2 | T44.3X3 | T44.3X4 | T44.3X5 | T44.3X6 |
| **Alvodine** | T4Ø.2X1 | T4Ø.2X2 | T4Ø.2X3 | T4Ø.2X4 | T4Ø.2X5 | T4Ø.2X6 |
| **Amanita phalloides** | T62.ØX1 | T62.ØX2 | T62.ØX3 | T62.ØX4 | — | — |
| **Amanitine** | T62.ØX1 | T62.ØX2 | T62.ØX3 | T62.ØX4 | — | — |
| **Amantadine** | T42.8X1 | T42.8X2 | T42.8X3 | T42.8X4 | T42.8X5 | T42.8X6 |
| **Ambazone** | T49.6X1 | T49.6X2 | T49.6X3 | T49.6X4 | T49.6X5 | T49.6X6 |
| **Ambenonium** (chloride) | T44.ØX1 | T44.ØX2 | T44.ØX3 | T44.ØX4 | T44.ØX5 | T44.ØX6 |
| **Ambien*** | T42.6X1 | T42.6X2 | T42.6X3 | T42.6X4 | T42.6X5 | T42.6X6 |
| **Ambroxol** | T48.4X1 | T48.4X2 | T48.4X3 | T48.4X4 | T48.4X5 | T48.4X6 |
| **Ambuphylline** | T48.6X1 | T48.6X2 | T48.6X3 | T48.6X4 | T48.6X5 | T48.6X6 |
| **Ambutonium bromide** | T44.3X1 | T44.3X2 | T44.3X3 | T44.3X4 | T44.3X5 | T44.3X6 |
| **Amcinonide** | T49.ØX1 | T49.ØX2 | T49.ØX3 | T49.ØX4 | T49.ØX5 | T49.ØX6 |
| **Amdinocilline** | T36.ØX1 | T36.ØX2 | T36.ØX3 | T36.ØX4 | T36.ØX5 | T36.ØX6 |
| **Americaine*** | T41.3X1 | T41.3X2 | T41.3X3 | T41.3X4 | T41.3X5 | T41.3X6 |
| **Ametazole** | T5Ø.8X1 | T5Ø.8X2 | T5Ø.8X3 | T5Ø.8X4 | T5Ø.8X5 | T5Ø.8X6 |
| **Amethocaine** | T41.3X1 | T41.3X2 | T41.3X3 | T41.3X4 | T41.3X5 | T41.3X6 |
| regional | T41.3X1 | T41.3X2 | T41.3X3 | T41.3X4 | T41.3X5 | T41.3X6 |
| spinal | T41.3X1 | T41.3X2 | T41.3X3 | T41.3X4 | T41.3X5 | T41.3X6 |
| **Amethopterin** | T45.1X1 | T45.1X2 | T45.1X3 | T45.1X4 | T45.1X5 | T45.1X6 |
| **Amezinium metilsulfate** | T44.991 | T44.992 | T44.993 | T44.994 | T44.995 | T44.996 |
| **Amfebutamone** | T43.291 | T43.292 | T43.293 | T43.294 | T43.295 | T43.296 |
| **Amfepramone** | T5Ø.5X1 | T5Ø.5X2 | T5Ø.5X3 | T5Ø.5X4 | T5Ø.5X5 | T5Ø.5X6 |
| **Amfetamine** | T43.621 | T43.622 | T43.623 | T43.624 | T43.625 | T43.626 |
| **Amfetaminil** | T43.621 | T43.622 | T43.623 | T43.624 | T43.625 | T43.626 |
| **Amfomycin** | T36.8X1 | T36.8X2 | T36.8X3 | T36.8X4 | T36.8X5 | T36.8X6 |
| **Amidefrine mesilate** | T48.5X1 | T48.5X2 | T48.5X3 | T48.5X4 | T48.5X5 | T48.5X6 |
| **Amidone** | T4Ø.3X1 | T4Ø.3X2 | T4Ø.3X3 | T4Ø.3X4 | T4Ø.3X5 | T4Ø.3X6 |
| **Amidopyrine** | T39.2X1 | T39.2X2 | T39.2X3 | T39.2X4 | T39.2X5 | T39.2X6 |
| **Amidotrizoate** | T5Ø.8X1 | T5Ø.8X2 | T5Ø.8X3 | T5Ø.8X4 | T5Ø.8X5 | T5Ø.8X6 |
| **Amiflamine** | T43.1X1 | T43.1X2 | T43.1X3 | T43.1X4 | T43.1X5 | T43.1X6 |
| **Amikacin** | T36.5X1 | T36.5X2 | T36.5X3 | T36.5X4 | T36.5X5 | T36.5X6 |
| **Amikhelline** | T46.3X1 | T46.3X2 | T46.3X3 | T46.3X4 | T46.3X5 | T46.3X6 |
| **Amiloride** | T5Ø.2X1 | T5Ø.2X2 | T5Ø.2X3 | T5Ø.2X4 | T5Ø.2X5 | T5Ø.2X6 |
| **Aminacrine** | T49.ØX1 | T49.ØX2 | T49.ØX3 | T49.ØX4 | T49.ØX5 | T49.ØX6 |
| **Amineptine** | T43.Ø11 | T43.Ø12 | T43.Ø13 | T43.Ø14 | T43.Ø15 | T43.Ø16 |
| **Aminitrozole** | T37.3X1 | T37.3X2 | T37.3X3 | T37.3X4 | T37.3X5 | T37.3X6 |
| **Amino acids** | T5Ø.3X1 | T5Ø.3X2 | T5Ø.3X3 | T5Ø.3X4 | T5Ø.3X5 | T5Ø.3X6 |
| **Aminoacetic acid** (derivatives) | T5Ø.3X1 | T5Ø.3X2 | T5Ø.3X3 | T5Ø.3X4 | T5Ø.3X5 | T5Ø.3X6 |
| **Aminoacridine** | T49.ØX1 | T49.ØX2 | T49.ØX3 | T49.ØX4 | T49.ØX5 | T49.ØX6 |
| **Aminobenzoic acid** (-p) | T49.3X1 | T49.3X2 | T49.3X3 | T49.3X4 | T49.3X5 | T49.3X6 |
| **Aminocaproic acid** | T45.621 | T45.622 | T45.623 | T45.624 | T45.625 | T45.626 |
| **Aminoethylisothiourium** | T45.8X1 | T45.8X2 | T45.8X3 | T45.8X4 | T45.8X5 | T45.8X6 |
| **Aminofenazone** | T39.2X1 | T39.2X2 | T39.2X3 | T39.2X4 | T39.2X5 | T39.2X6 |
| **Aminoglutethimide** | T45.1X1 | T45.1X2 | T45.1X3 | T45.1X4 | T45.1X5 | T45.1X6 |
| **Aminoglycosides*** | T36.5X1 | T36.5X2 | T36.5X3 | T36.5X4 | T36.5X5 | T36.5X6 |
| **Aminohippuric acid** | T5Ø.8X1 | T5Ø.8X2 | T5Ø.8X3 | T5Ø.8X4 | T5Ø.8X5 | T5Ø.8X6 |
| **Aminomethylbenzoic acid** | T45.691 | T45.692 | T45.693 | T45.694 | T45.695 | T45.696 |
| **Aminometradine** | T5Ø.2X1 | T5Ø.2X2 | T5Ø.2X3 | T5Ø.2X4 | T5Ø.2X5 | T5Ø.2X6 |
| **Aminopentamide** | T44.3X1 | T44.3X2 | T44.3X3 | T44.3X4 | T44.3X5 | T44.3X6 |
| **Aminophenazone** | T39.2X1 | T39.2X2 | T39.2X3 | T39.2X4 | T39.2X5 | T39.2X6 |
| **Aminophenol** | T54.ØX1 | T54.ØX2 | T54.ØX3 | T54.ØX4 | — | — |
| **Aminophenylpyridone** | T43.591 | T43.592 | T43.593 | T43.594 | T43.595 | T43.596 |
| **Aminophylline** | T48.6X1 | T48.6X2 | T48.6X3 | T48.6X4 | T48.6X5 | T48.6X6 |
| **Aminopterin sodium** | T45.1X1 | T45.1X2 | T45.1X3 | T45.1X4 | T45.1X5 | T45.1X6 |
| **Aminopyrine** | T39.2X1 | T39.2X2 | T39.2X3 | T39.2X4 | T39.2X5 | T39.2X6 |
| **Aminorex** | T5Ø.5X1 | T5Ø.5X2 | T5Ø.5X3 | T5Ø.5X4 | T5Ø.5X5 | T5Ø.5X6 |
| **Aminosalicylic acid** | T37.1X1 | T37.1X2 | T37.1X3 | T37.1X4 | T37.1X5 | T37.1X6 |
| **Aminosalylum** | T37.1X1 | T37.1X2 | T37.1X3 | T37.1X4 | T37.1X5 | T37.1X6 |
| **Amiodarone** | T46.2X1 | T46.2X2 | T46.2X3 | T46.2X4 | T46.2X5 | T46.2X6 |
| **Amiphenazole** | T5Ø.7X1 | T5Ø.7X2 | T5Ø.7X3 | T5Ø.7X4 | T5Ø.7X5 | T5Ø.7X6 |
| **Amiquinsin** | T46.5X1 | T46.5X2 | T46.5X3 | T46.5X4 | T46.5X5 | T46.5X6 |
| **Amisometradine** | T5Ø.2X1 | T5Ø.2X2 | T5Ø.2X3 | T5Ø.2X4 | T5Ø.2X5 | T5Ø.2X6 |
| **Amisulpride** | T43.591 | T43.592 | T43.593 | T43.594 | T43.595 | T43.596 |
| **Amitriptyline** | T43.Ø11 | T43.Ø12 | T43.Ø13 | T43.Ø14 | T43.Ø15 | T43.Ø16 |
| **Amitriptylinoxide** | T43.Ø11 | T43.Ø12 | T43.Ø13 | T43.Ø14 | T43.Ø15 | T43.Ø16 |

| Substance | Poisoning, Accidental (unintentional) | Poisoning, Intentional Self-harm | Poisoning, Assault | Poisoning, Undetermined | Adverse Effect | Under-dosing |
|---|---|---|---|---|---|---|
| **Amlexanox** | T48.6X1 | T48.6X2 | T48.6X3 | T48.6X4 | T48.6X5 | T48.6X |
| **Amlodipine*** | T46.1X1 | T46.1X2 | T46.1X3 | T46.1X4 | T46.1X5 | T46.1X |
| **Ammonia** (fumes) (gas) (vapor) | T59.891 | T59.892 | T59.893 | T59.894 | — | — |
| aromatic spirit | T48.991 | T48.992 | T48.993 | T48.994 | T48.995 | T48.99 |
| liquid (household) | T54.3X1 | T54.3X2 | T54.3X3 | T54.3X4 | — | — |
| **Ammoniated mercury** | T49.ØX1 | T49.ØX2 | T49.ØX3 | T49.ØX4 | T49.ØX5 | T49.ØX |
| **Ammonium** | | | | | | |
| acid tartrate | T49.5X1 | T49.5X2 | T49.5X3 | T49.5X4 | T49.5X5 | T49.5X |
| bromide | T42.6X1 | T42.6X2 | T42.6X3 | T42.6X4 | T42.6X5 | T42.6X |
| carbonate | T54.3X1 | T54.3X2 | T54.3X3 | T54.3X4 | — | — |
| chloride | T5Ø.991 | T5Ø.992 | T5Ø.993 | T5Ø.994 | T5Ø.995 | T5Ø.99 |
| expectorant | T48.4X1 | T48.4X2 | T48.4X3 | T48.4X4 | T48.4X5 | T48.4X |
| compounds (household) NEC | T54.3X1 | T54.3X2 | T54.3X3 | T54.3X4 | — | — |
| fumes (any usage) | T59.891 | T59.892 | T59.893 | T59.894 | — | — |
| industrial | T54.3X1 | T54.3X2 | T54.3X3 | T54.3X4 | — | — |
| ichthyosulronate | T49.4X1 | T49.4X2 | T49.4X3 | T49.4X4 | T49.4X5 | T49.4X |
| mandelate | T37.91 | T37.92 | T37.93 | T37.94 | T37.95 | T37.9 |
| sulfamate | T6Ø.3X1 | T6Ø.3X2 | T6Ø.3X3 | T6Ø.3X4 | — | — |
| sulfonate resin | T47.8X1 | T47.8X2 | T47.8X3 | T47.8X4 | T47.8X5 | T47.8X |
| **Amobarbital** (sodium) | T42.3X1 | T42.3X2 | T42.3X3 | T42.3X4 | T42.3X5 | T42.3X |
| **Amodiaquine** | T37.2X1 | T37.2X2 | T37.2X3 | T37.2X4 | T37.2X5 | T37.2X |
| **Amopyroquin** (e) | T37.2X1 | T37.2X2 | T37.2X3 | T37.2X4 | T37.2X5 | T37.2X |
| **Amoxapine** | T43.Ø11 | T43.Ø12 | T43.Ø13 | T43.Ø14 | T43.Ø15 | T43.Ø1 |
| **Amoxicillin** | T36.ØX1 | T36.ØX2 | T36.ØX3 | T36.ØX4 | T36.ØX5 | T36.ØX |
| **Amperozide** | T43.591 | T43.592 | T43.593 | T43.594 | T43.595 | T43.59 |
| **Amphenidone** | T43.591 | T43.592 | T43.593 | T43.594 | T43.595 | T43.59 |
| **Amphetamine NEC** | T43.621 | T43.622 | T43.623 | T43.624 | T43.625 | T43.62 |
| **Amphogel*** | T47.1X1 | T47.1X2 | T47.1X3 | T47.1X4 | T47.1X5 | T47.1X |
| **Amphomycin** | T36.8X1 | T36.8X2 | T36.8X3 | T36.8X4 | T36.8X5 | T36.8X |
| **Amphotalide** | T37.4X1 | T37.4X2 | T37.4X3 | T37.4X4 | T37.4X5 | T37.4X |
| **Amphotericin B** | T36.7X1 | T36.7X2 | T36.7X3 | T36.7X4 | T36.7X5 | T36.7X |
| topical | T49.ØX1 | T49.ØX2 | T49.ØX3 | T49.ØX4 | T49.ØX5 | T49.ØX |
| **Ampicillin** | T36.ØX1 | T36.ØX2 | T36.ØX3 | T36.ØX4 | T36.ØX5 | T36.ØX |
| **Amprotropine** | T44.3X1 | T44.3X2 | T44.3X3 | T44.3X4 | T44.3X5 | T44.3X |
| **Amsacrine** | T45.1X1 | T45.1X2 | T45.1X3 | T45.1X4 | T45.1X5 | T45.1X |
| **Amygdaline** | T62.2X1 | T62.2X2 | T62.2X3 | T62.2X4 | — | — |
| **Amyl** | | | | | | |
| acetate | T52.891 | T52.892 | T52.893 | T52.894 | — | — |
| vapor | T59.891 | T59.892 | T59.893 | T59.894 | — | — |
| alcohol | T51.3X1 | T51.3X2 | T51.3X3 | T51.3X4 | — | — |
| chloride | T53.6X1 | T53.6X2 | T53.6X3 | T53.6X4 | — | — |
| formate | T52.891 | T52.892 | T52.893 | T52.894 | — | — |
| nitrite | T46.3X1 | T46.3X2 | T46.3X3 | T46.3X4 | T46.3X5 | T46.3X |
| propionate | T65.891 | T65.892 | T65.893 | T65.894 | — | — |
| **Amylase** | T47.5X1 | T47.5X2 | T47.5X3 | T47.5X4 | T47.5X5 | T47.5X |
| **Amyleine, regional** | T41.3X1 | T41.3X2 | T41.3X3 | T41.3X4 | T41.3X5 | T41.3X |
| **Amylene** | | | | | | |
| dichloride | T53.6X1 | T53.6X2 | T53.6X3 | T53.6X4 | — | — |
| hydrate | T51.3X1 | T51.3X2 | T51.3X3 | T51.3X4 | — | — |
| **Amylmetacresol** | T49.6X1 | T49.6X2 | T49.6X3 | T49.6X4 | T49.6X5 | T49.6X |
| **Amylobarbitone** | T42.3X1 | T42.3X2 | T42.3X3 | T42.3X4 | T42.3X5 | T42.3X |
| **Amylocaine, regional** | T41.3X1 | T41.3X2 | T41.3X3 | T41.3X4 | T41.3X5 | T41.3X |
| infiltration (subcutaneous) | T41.3X1 | T41.3X2 | T41.3X3 | T41.3X4 | T41.3X5 | T41.3X |
| nerve block (peripheral) (plexus) | T41.3X1 | T41.3X2 | T41.3X3 | T41.3X4 | T41.3X5 | T41.3X |
| spinal | T41.3X1 | T41.3X2 | T41.3X3 | T41.3X4 | T41.3X5 | T41.3X |
| topical (surface) | T41.3X1 | T41.3X2 | T41.3X3 | T41.3X4 | T41.3X5 | T41.3X |
| **Amylopectin** | T47.6X1 | T47.6X2 | T47.6X3 | T47.6X4 | T47.6X5 | T47.6X |
| **Amytal** (sodium) | T42.3X1 | T42.3X2 | T42.3X3 | T42.3X4 | T42.3X5 | T42.3X |
| **Anabolic steroid** | T38.7X1 | T38.7X2 | T38.7X3 | T38.7X4 | T38.7X5 | T38.7X |
| **Anacaine*** | T41.3X1 | T41.3X2 | T41.3X3 | T41.3X4 | T41.3X5 | T41.3X |
| **Analeptic NEC** | T5Ø.7X1 | T5Ø.7X2 | T5Ø.7X3 | T5Ø.7X4 | T5Ø.7X5 | T5Ø.7X |
| **Analgesic** | T39.91 | T39.92 | T39.93 | T39.94 | T39.95 | T39.9 |
| anti-inflammatory NEC | T39.91 | T39.92 | T39.93 | T39.94 | T39.95 | T39.9 |
| propionic acid derivative | T39.311 | T39.312 | T39.313 | T39.314 | T39.315 | T39.31 |
| antirheumatic NEC | T39.4X1 | T39.4X2 | T39.4X3 | T39.4X4 | T39.4X5 | T39.4X |
| aromatic NEC | T39.1X1 | T39.1X2 | T39.1X3 | T39.1X4 | T39.1X5 | T39.1X |
| narcotic NEC | T4Ø.6Ø1 | T4Ø.6Ø2 | T4Ø.6Ø3 | T4Ø.6Ø4 | T4Ø.6Ø5 | T4Ø.6Ø |
| combination | T4Ø.6Ø1 | T4Ø.6Ø2 | T4Ø.6Ø3 | T4Ø.6Ø4 | T4Ø.6Ø5 | T4Ø.6Ø |
| obstetric | T4Ø.6Ø1 | T4Ø.6Ø2 | T4Ø.6Ø3 | T4Ø.6Ø4 | T4Ø.6Ø5 | T4Ø.6Ø |
| non-narcotic NEC | T39.91 | T39.92 | T39.93 | T39.94 | T39.95 | T39.9 |
| combination | T39.91 | T39.92 | T39.93 | T39.94 | T39.95 | T39.9 |
| pyrazole | T39.2X1 | T39.2X2 | T39.2X3 | T39.2X4 | T39.2X5 | T39.2X |
| specified NEC | T39.8X1 | T39.8X2 | T39.8X3 | T39.8X4 | T39.8X5 | T39.8X |
| **Analgin** | T39.2X1 | T39.2X2 | T39.2X3 | T39.2X4 | T39.2X5 | T39.2X |
| **Anamirta cocculus** | T62.1X1 | T62.1X2 | T62.1X3 | T62.1X4 | — | — |
| **Ancillin** | T36.ØX1 | T36.ØX2 | T36.ØX3 | T36.ØX4 | T36.ØX5 | T36.ØX |
| **Ancrod** | T45.691 | T45.692 | T45.693 | T45.694 | T45.695 | T45.69 |
| **Androgen** | T38.7X1 | T38.7X2 | T38.7X3 | T38.7X4 | T38.7X5 | T38.7X |
| **Androgen-estrogen mixture** | T38.7X1 | T38.7X2 | T38.7X3 | T38.7X4 | T38.7X5 | T38.7X |





☑ **Additional Character May Be Required — Refer to the Tabular List for Character Selection**

***Optum Value-Add**

| Substance | Poisoning, Accidental (unintentional) | Poisoning, Intentional Self-harm | Poisoning, Assault | Poisoning, Undetermined | Adverse Effect | Under-dosing |
|---|---|---|---|---|---|---|
| **Androstalone** | T38.7X1 | T38.7X2 | T38.7X3 | T38.7X4 | T38.7X5 | T38.7X6 |
| **Androstanolone** | T38.7X1 | T38.7X2 | T38.7X3 | T38.7X4 | T38.7X5 | T38.7X6 |
| **Androsterone** | T38.7X1 | T38.7X2 | T38.7X3 | T38.7X4 | T38.7X5 | T38.7X6 |
| **Anemone pulsatilla** | T62.2X1 | T62.2X2 | T62.2X3 | T62.2X4 | — | — |
| **Anesthesia** | | | | | | |
| caudal | T41.3X1 | T41.3X2 | T41.3X3 | T41.3X4 | T41.3X5 | T41.3X6 |
| endotracheal | T41.ØX1 | T41.ØX2 | T41.ØX3 | T41.ØX4 | T41.ØX5 | T41.ØX6 |
| epidural | T41.3X1 | T41.3X2 | T41.3X3 | T41.3X4 | T41.3X5 | T41.3X6 |
| inhalation | T41.ØX1 | T41.ØX2 | T41.ØX3 | T41.ØX4 | T41.ØX5 | T41.ØX6 |
| local | T41.3X1 | T41.3X2 | T41.3X3 | T41.3X4 | T41.3X5 | T41.3X6 |
| mucosal | T41.3X1 | T41.3X2 | T41.3X3 | T41.3X4 | T41.3X5 | T41.3X6 |
| muscle relaxation | T48.1X1 | T48.1X2 | T48.1X3 | T48.1X4 | T48.1X5 | T48.1X6 |
| nerve blocking | T41.3X1 | T41.3X2 | T41.3X3 | T41.3X4 | T41.3X5 | T41.3X6 |
| plexus blocking | T41.3X1 | T41.3X2 | T41.3X3 | T41.3X4 | T41.3X5 | T41.3X6 |
| potentiated | T41.2Ø1 | T41.2Ø2 | T41.2Ø3 | T41.2Ø4 | T41.2Ø5 | T41.2Ø6 |
| rectal | T41.2Ø1 | T41.2Ø2 | T41.2Ø3 | T41.2Ø4 | T41.2Ø5 | T41.2Ø6 |
| general | T41.2Ø1 | T41.2Ø2 | T41.2Ø3 | T41.2Ø4 | T41.2Ø5 | T41.2Ø6 |
| local | T41.3X1 | T41.3X2 | T41.3X3 | T41.3X4 | T41.3X5 | T41.3X6 |
| regional | T41.3X1 | T41.3X2 | T41.3X3 | T41.3X4 | T41.3X5 | T41.3X6 |
| surface | T41.3X1 | T41.3X2 | T41.3X3 | T41.3X4 | T41.3X5 | T41.3X6 |
| **Anesthetic NEC** — *see also* Anesthesia | T41.41 | T41.42 | T41.43 | T41.44 | T41.45 | T41.46 |
| gaseous NEC | T41.ØX1 | T41.ØX2 | T41.ØX3 | T41.ØX4 | T41.ØX5 | T41.ØX6 |
| general NEC | T41.2Ø1 | T41.2Ø2 | T41.2Ø3 | T41.2Ø4 | T41.2Ø5 | T41.2Ø6 |
| halogenated hydrocarbon derivatives NEC | T41.ØX1 | T41.ØX2 | T41.ØX3 | T41.ØX4 | T41.ØX5 | T41.ØX6 |
| infiltration NEC | T41.3X1 | T41.3X2 | T41.3X3 | T41.3X4 | T41.3X5 | T41.3X6 |
| intravenous NEC | T41.1X1 | T41.1X2 | T41.1X3 | T41.1X4 | T41.1X5 | T41.1X6 |
| local NEC | T41.3X1 | T41.3X2 | T41.3X3 | T41.3X4 | T41.3X5 | T41.3X6 |
| rectal | T41.2Ø1 | T41.2Ø2 | T41.2Ø3 | T41.2Ø4 | T41.2Ø5 | T41.2Ø6 |
| general | T41.2Ø1 | T41.2Ø2 | T41.2Ø3 | T41.2Ø4 | T41.2Ø5 | T41.2Ø6 |
| local | T41.3X1 | T41.3X2 | T41.3X3 | T41.3X4 | T41.3X5 | T41.3X6 |
| regional NEC | T41.3X1 | T41.3X2 | T41.3X3 | T41.3X4 | T41.3X5 | T41.3X6 |
| spinal NEC | T41.3X1 | T41.3X2 | T41.3X3 | T41.3X4 | T41.3X5 | T41.3X6 |
| thiobarbiturate | T41.1X1 | T41.1X2 | T41.1X3 | T41.1X4 | T41.1X5 | T41.1X6 |
| topical | T41.3X1 | T41.3X2 | T41.3X3 | T41.3X4 | T41.3X5 | T41.3X6 |
| with muscle relaxant | T41.2Ø1 | T41.2Ø2 | T41.2Ø3 | T41.2Ø4 | T41.2Ø5 | T41.2Ø6 |
| general | T41.2Ø1 | T41.2Ø2 | T41.2Ø3 | T41.2Ø4 | T41.2Ø5 | T41.2Ø6 |
| local | T41.3X1 | T41.3X2 | T41.3X3 | T41.3X4 | T41.3X5 | T41.3X6 |
| **Aneurine** | T45.2X1 | T45.2X2 | T45.2X3 | T45.2X4 | T45.2X5 | T45.2X6 |
| **Angeliq*** | T38.5X1 | T38.5X2 | T38.5X3 | T38.5X4 | T38.5X5 | T38.5X6 |
| **Angio-Conray** | T5Ø.8X1 | T5Ø.8X2 | T5Ø.8X3 | T5Ø.8X4 | T5Ø.8X5 | T5Ø.8X6 |
| **Angiotensin** | T44.5X1 | T44.5X2 | T44.5X3 | T44.5X4 | T44.5X5 | T44.5X6 |
| **Angiotensinamide** | T44.991 | T44.992 | T44.993 | T44.994 | T44.995 | T44.996 |
| **Anhydrohydroxy-progesterone** | T38.5X1 | T38.5X2 | T38.5X3 | T38.5X4 | T38.5X5 | T38.5X6 |
| **Anhydron** | T5Ø.2X1 | T5Ø.2X2 | T5Ø.2X3 | T5Ø.2X4 | T5Ø.2X5 | T5Ø.2X6 |
| **Anileridine** | T4Ø.491 | T4Ø.492 | T4Ø.493 | T4Ø.494 | T4Ø.495 | T4Ø.496 |
| **Aniline** (dye) (liquid) | T65.3X1 | T65.3X2 | T65.3X3 | T65.3X4 | — | — |
| analgesic | T39.1X1 | T39.1X2 | T39.1X3 | T39.1X4 | T39.1X5 | T39.1X6 |
| derivatives, therapeutic NEC | T39.1X1 | T39.1X2 | T39.1X3 | T39.1X4 | T39.1X5 | T39.1X6 |
| vapor | T65.3X1 | T65.3X2 | T65.3X3 | T65.3X4 | — | — |
| **Aniscoropine** | T44.3X1 | T44.3X2 | T44.3X3 | T44.3X4 | T44.3X5 | T44.3X6 |
| **Anise oil** | T47.5X1 | T47.5X2 | T47.5X3 | T47.5X4 | T47.5X5 | T47.5X6 |
| **Anisidine** | T65.3X1 | T65.3X2 | T65.3X3 | T65.3X4 | — | — |
| **Anisindione** | T45.511 | T45.512 | T45.513 | T45.514 | T45.515 | T45.516 |
| **Anisotropine methyl-bromide** | T44.3X1 | T44.3X2 | T44.3X3 | T44.3X4 | T44.3X5 | T44.3X6 |
| **Anistreplase** | T45.611 | T45.612 | T45.613 | T45.614 | T45.615 | T45.616 |
| **Anorexiant** (central) | T5Ø.5X1 | T5Ø.5X2 | T5Ø.5X3 | T5Ø.5X4 | T5Ø.5X5 | T5Ø.5X6 |
| **Anorexic agents** | T5Ø.5X1 | T5Ø.5X2 | T5Ø.5X3 | T5Ø.5X4 | T5Ø.5X5 | T5Ø.5X6 |
| **Ansaid*** | T39.311 | T39.312 | T39.313 | T39.314 | T39.315 | T39.316 |
| **Ansamycin** | T36.6X1 | T36.6X2 | T36.6X3 | T36.6X4 | T36.6X5 | T36.6X6 |
| **Ant** (bite) (sting) | T63.421 | T63.422 | T63.423 | T63.424 | — | — |
| **Ant poison** — *see* Insecticide | | | | | | |
| **Antabuse** | T5Ø.6X1 | T5Ø.6X2 | T5Ø.6X3 | T5Ø.6X4 | T5Ø.6X5 | T5Ø.6X6 |
| **Antacid NEC** | T47.1X1 | T47.1X2 | T47.1X3 | T47.1X4 | T47.1X5 | T47.1X6 |
| **Antagonist** | | | | | | |
| Aldosterone | T5Ø.ØX1 | T5Ø.ØX2 | T5Ø.ØX3 | T5Ø.ØX4 | T5Ø.ØX5 | T5Ø.ØX6 |
| alpha-adrenoreceptor | T44.6X1 | T44.6X2 | T44.6X3 | T44.6X4 | T44.6X5 | T44.6X6 |
| anticoagulant | T45.7X1 | T45.7X2 | T45.7X3 | T45.7X4 | T45.7X5 | T45.7X6 |
| beta-adrenoreceptor | T44.7X1 | T44.7X2 | T44.7X3 | T44.7X4 | T44.7X5 | T44.7X6 |
| extrapyramidal NEC | T44.3X1 | T44.3X2 | T44.3X3 | T44.3X4 | T44.3X5 | T44.3X6 |
| folic acid | T45.1X1 | T45.1X2 | T45.1X3 | T45.1X4 | T45.1X5 | T45.1X6 |
| H2 receptor | T47.ØX1 | T47.ØX2 | T47.ØX3 | T47.ØX4 | T47.ØX5 | T47.ØX6 |
| heavy metal | T45.8X1 | T45.8X2 | T45.8X3 | T45.8X4 | T45.8X5 | T45.8X6 |
| narcotic analgesic | T5Ø.7X1 | T5Ø.7X2 | T5Ø.7X3 | T5Ø.7X4 | T5Ø.7X5 | T5Ø.7X6 |
| opiate | T5Ø.7X1 | T5Ø.7X2 | T5Ø.7X3 | T5Ø.7X4 | T5Ø.7X5 | T5Ø.7X6 |
| pyrimidine | T45.1X1 | T45.1X2 | T45.1X3 | T45.1X4 | T45.1X5 | T45.1X6 |
| serotonin | T46.5X1 | T46.5X2 | T46.5X3 | T46.5X4 | T46.5X5 | T46.5X6 |
| **Antazolin** (e) | T45.ØX1 | T45.ØX2 | T45.ØX3 | T45.ØX4 | T45.ØX5 | T45.ØX6 |
| **Anterior pituitary hormone NEC** | T38.811 | T38.812 | T38.813 | T38.814 | T38.815 | T38.816 |

| Substance | Poisoning, Accidental (unintentional) | Poisoning, Intentional Self-harm | Poisoning, Assault | Poisoning, Undetermined | Adverse Effect | Under-dosing |
|---|---|---|---|---|---|---|
| **Anthelmintic NEC** | T37.4X1 | T37.4X2 | T37.4X3 | T37.4X4 | T37.4X5 | T37.4X6 |
| **Anthiolimine** | T37.4X1 | T37.4X2 | T37.4X3 | T37.4X4 | T37.4X5 | T37.4X6 |
| **Anthralin** | T49.4X1 | T49.4X2 | T49.4X3 | T49.4X4 | T49.4X5 | T49.4X6 |
| **Anthramycin** | T45.1X1 | T45.1X2 | T45.1X3 | T45.1X4 | T45.1X5 | T45.1X6 |
| **Anti-anemic** (drug) (preparation) | T45.8X1 | T45.8X2 | T45.8X3 | T45.8X4 | T45.8X5 | T45.8X6 |
| **Anti-common-cold drug NEC** | T48.5X1 | T48.5X2 | T48.5X3 | T48.5X4 | T48.5X5 | T48.5X6 |
| **Anti-D immunoglobulin** (human) | T5Ø.Z11 | T5Ø.Z12 | T5Ø.Z13 | T5Ø.Z14 | T5Ø.Z15 | T5Ø.Z16 |
| **Anti-gastric-secretion drug NEC** | T47.1X1 | T47.1X2 | T47.1X3 | T47.1X4 | T47.1X5 | T47.1X6 |
| **Anti-human lymphocytic globulin** | T5Ø.Z11 | T5Ø.Z12 | T5Ø.Z13 | T5Ø.Z14 | T5Ø.Z15 | T5Ø.Z16 |
| **Anti-infective NEC** | T37.91 | T37.92 | T37.93 | T37.94 | T37.95 | T37.96 |
| anthelmintic | T37.4X1 | T37.4X2 | T37.4X3 | T37.4X4 | T37.4X5 | T37.4X6 |
| antibiotics | T36.91 | T36.92 | T36.93 | T36.94 | T36.95 | T36.96 |
| specified NEC | T36.8X1 | T36.8X2 | T36.8X3 | T36.8X4 | T36.8X5 | T36.8X6 |
| antimalarial | T37.2X1 | T37.2X2 | T37.2X3 | T37.2X4 | T37.2X5 | T37.2X6 |
| antimycobacterial NEC | T37.1X1 | T37.1X2 | T37.1X3 | T37.1X4 | T37.1X5 | T37.1X6 |
| antibiotics | T36.5X1 | T36.5X2 | T36.5X3 | T36.5X4 | T36.5X5 | T36.5X6 |
| antiprotozoal NEC | T37.3X1 | T37.3X2 | T37.3X3 | T37.3X4 | T37.3X5 | T37.3X6 |
| blood | T37.2X1 | T37.2X2 | T37.2X3 | T37.2X4 | T37.2X5 | T37.2X6 |
| antiviral | T37.5X1 | T37.5X2 | T37.5X3 | T37.5X4 | T37.5X5 | T37.5X6 |
| arsenical | T37.8X1 | T37.8X2 | T37.8X3 | T37.8X4 | T37.8X5 | T37.8X6 |
| bismuth, local | T49.ØX1 | T49.ØX2 | T49.ØX3 | T49.ØX4 | T49.ØX5 | T49.ØX6 |
| ENT | T49.6X1 | T49.6X2 | T49.6X3 | T49.6X4 | T49.6X5 | T49.6X6 |
| eye NEC | T49.5X1 | T49.5X2 | T49.5X3 | T49.5X4 | T49.5X5 | T49.5X6 |
| heavy metals NEC | T37.8X1 | T37.8X2 | T37.8X3 | T37.8X4 | T37.8X5 | T37.8X6 |
| local NEC | T49.ØX1 | T49.ØX2 | T49.ØX3 | T49.ØX4 | T49.ØX5 | T49.ØX6 |
| specified NEC | T49.ØX1 | T49.ØX2 | T49.ØX3 | T49.ØX4 | T49.ØX5 | T49.ØX6 |
| mixed | T37.91 | T37.92 | T37.93 | T37.94 | T37.95 | T37.96 |
| ophthalmic preparation | T49.5X1 | T49.5X2 | T49.5X3 | T49.5X4 | T49.5X5 | T49.5X6 |
| topical NEC | T49.ØX1 | T49.ØX2 | T49.ØX3 | T49.ØX4 | T49.ØX5 | T49.ØX6 |
| **Anti-inflammatory drug NEC** | T39.391 | T39.392 | T39.393 | T39.394 | T39.395 | T39.396 |
| local | T49.ØX1 | T49.ØX2 | T49.ØX3 | T49.ØX4 | T49.ØX5 | T49.ØX6 |
| nonsteroidal NEC | T39.391 | T39.392 | T39.393 | T39.394 | T39.395 | T39.396 |
| propionic acid derivative | T39.311 | T39.312 | T39.313 | T39.314 | T39.315 | T39.316 |
| specified NEC | T39.391 | T39.392 | T39.393 | T39.394 | T39.395 | T39.396 |
| **Antiadrenergic NEC** | T44.8X1 | T44.8X2 | T44.8X3 | T44.8X4 | T44.8X5 | T44.8X6 |
| **Antiallergic NEC** | T45.ØX1 | T45.ØX2 | T45.ØX3 | T45.ØX4 | T45.ØX5 | T45.ØX6 |
| **Antiandrogen NEC** | T38.6X1 | T38.6X2 | T38.6X3 | T38.6X4 | T38.6X5 | T38.6X6 |
| **Antianxiety drug NEC** | T43.5Ø1 | T43.5Ø2 | T43.5Ø3 | T43.5Ø4 | T43.5Ø5 | T43.5Ø6 |
| **Antiaris toxicaria** | T65.891 | T65.892 | T65.893 | T65.894 | — | — |
| **Antiarteriosclerotic drug** | T46.6X1 | T46.6X2 | T46.6X3 | T46.6X4 | T46.6X5 | T46.6X6 |
| **Antiasthmatic drug NEC** | T48.6X1 | T48.6X2 | T48.6X3 | T48.6X4 | T48.6X5 | T48.6X6 |
| **Antibiotic NEC** | T36.91 | T36.92 | T36.93 | T36.94 | T36.95 | T36.96 |
| aminoglycoside | T36.5X1 | T36.5X2 | T36.5X3 | T36.5X4 | T36.5X5 | T36.5X6 |
| anticancer | T45.1X1 | T45.1X2 | T45.1X3 | T45.1X4 | T45.1X5 | T45.1X6 |
| antifungal | T36.7X1 | T36.7X2 | T36.7X3 | T36.7X4 | T36.7X5 | T36.7X6 |
| antimycobacterial | T36.5X1 | T36.5X2 | T36.5X3 | T36.5X4 | T36.5X5 | T36.5X6 |
| antineoplastic | T45.1X1 | T45.1X2 | T45.1X3 | T45.1X4 | T45.1X5 | T45.1X6 |
| b-lactam NEC | T36.1X1 | T36.1X2 | T36.1X3 | T36.1X4 | T36.1X5 | T36.1X6 |
| cephalosporin (group) | T36.1X1 | T36.1X2 | T36.1X3 | T36.1X4 | T36.1X5 | T36.1X6 |
| chloramphenicol (group) | T36.2X1 | T36.2X2 | T36.2X3 | T36.2X4 | T36.2X5 | T36.2X6 |
| ENT | T49.6X1 | T49.6X2 | T49.6X3 | T49.6X4 | T49.6X5 | T49.6X6 |
| eye | T49.5X1 | T49.5X2 | T49.5X3 | T49.5X4 | T49.5X5 | T49.5X6 |
| fungicidal (local) | T49.ØX1 | T49.ØX2 | T49.ØX3 | T49.ØX4 | T49.ØX5 | T49.ØX6 |
| intestinal | T36.8X1 | T36.8X2 | T36.8X3 | T36.8X4 | T36.8X5 | T36.8X6 |
| local | T49.ØX1 | T49.ØX2 | T49.ØX3 | T49.ØX4 | T49.ØX5 | T49.ØX6 |
| macrolides | T36.3X1 | T36.3X2 | T36.3X3 | T36.3X4 | T36.3X5 | T36.3X6 |
| polypeptide | T36.8X1 | T36.8X2 | T36.8X3 | T36.8X4 | T36.8X5 | T36.8X6 |
| specified NEC | T36.8X1 | T36.8X2 | T36.8X3 | T36.8X4 | T36.8X5 | T36.8X6 |
| tetracycline (group) | T36.4X1 | T36.4X2 | T36.4X3 | T36.4X4 | T36.4X5 | T36.4X6 |
| throat | T49.6X1 | T49.6X2 | T49.6X3 | T49.6X4 | T49.6X5 | T49.6X6 |
| **Antibiotic Otic Suspension (Solution)*** | T49.6X1 | T49.6X2 | T49.6X3 | T49.6X4 | T49.6X5 | T49.6X6 |
| **Anticancer agents NEC** | T45.1X1 | T45.1X2 | T45.1X3 | T45.1X4 | T45.1X5 | T45.1X6 |
| **Anticholesterolemic drug NEC** | T46.6X1 | T46.6X2 | T46.6X3 | T46.6X4 | T46.6X5 | T46.6X6 |
| **Anticholinergic NEC** | T44.3X1 | T44.3X2 | T44.3X3 | T44.3X4 | T44.3X5 | T44.3X6 |
| **Anticholinesterase** | T44.ØX1 | T44.ØX2 | T44.ØX3 | T44.ØX4 | T44.ØX5 | T44.ØX6 |
| organophosphorus | T44.ØX1 | T44.ØX2 | T44.ØX3 | T44.ØX4 | T44.ØX5 | T44.ØX6 |
| insecticide | T6Ø.ØX1 | T6Ø.ØX2 | T6Ø.ØX3 | T6Ø.ØX4 | — | — |
| nerve gas | T59.891 | T59.892 | T59.893 | T59.894 | — | — |
| reversible | T44.ØX1 | T44.ØX2 | T44.ØX3 | T44.ØX4 | T44.ØX5 | T44.ØX6 |
| ophthalmological | T49.5X1 | T49.5X2 | T49.5X3 | T49.5X4 | T49.5X5 | T49.5X6 |
| **Anticoagulant NEC** | T45.511 | T45.512 | T45.513 | T45.514 | T45.515 | T45.516 |
| Antagonist | T45.7X1 | T45.7X2 | T45.7X3 | T45.7X4 | T45.7X5 | T45.7X6 |
| **Anticonvulsant** | T42.71 | T42.72 | T42.73 | T42.74 | T42.75 | T42.76 |
| barbiturate | T42.3X1 | T42.3X2 | T42.3X3 | T42.3X4 | T42.3X5 | T42.3X6 |

| Substance | Poisoning, Accidental (unintentional) | Poisoning, Intentional Self-harm | Poisoning, Assault | Poisoning, Undetermined | Adverse Effect | Under-dosing |
|---|---|---|---|---|---|---|
| **Anticonvulsant** — *continued* | | | | | | |
| combination (with barbiturate) | T42.3X1 | T42.3X2 | T42.3X3 | T42.3X4 | T42.3X5 | T42.3X6 |
| hydantoin | T42.ØX1 | T42.ØX2 | T42.ØX3 | T42.ØX4 | T42.ØX5 | T42.ØX6 |
| hypnotic NEC | T42.6X1 | T42.6X2 | T42.6X3 | T42.6X4 | T42.6X5 | T42.6X6 |
| oxazolidinedione | T42.2X1 | T42.2X2 | T42.2X3 | T42.2X4 | T42.2X5 | T42.2X6 |
| pyrimidinedione | T42.6X1 | T42.6X2 | T42.6X3 | T42.6X4 | T42.6X5 | T42.6X6 |
| specified NEC | T42.6X1 | T42.6X2 | T42.6X3 | T42.6X4 | T42.6X5 | T42.6X6 |
| succinimide | T42.2X1 | T42.2X2 | T42.2X3 | T42.2X4 | T42.2X5 | T42.2X6 |
| **Antidepressant** | T43.2Ø1 | T43.2Ø2 | T43.2Ø3 | T43.2Ø4 | T43.2Ø5 | T43.2Ø6 |
| monoamine oxidase inhibitor | T43.1X1 | T43.1X2 | T43.1X3 | T43.1X4 | T43.1X5 | T43.1X6 |
| selective serotonin norepinephrine reuptake inhibitor | T43.211 | T43.212 | T43.213 | T43.214 | T43.215 | T43.216 |
| selective serotonin reuptake inhibitor | T43.221 | T43.222 | T43.223 | T43.224 | T43.225 | T43.226 |
| specified NEC | T43.291 | T43.292 | T43.293 | T43.294 | T43.295 | T43.296 |
| tetracyclic | T43.Ø21 | T43.Ø22 | T43.Ø23 | T43.Ø24 | T43.Ø25 | T43.Ø26 |
| triazolopyridine | T43.211 | T43.212 | T43.213 | T43.214 | T43.215 | T43.216 |
| tricyclic | T43.Ø11 | T43.Ø12 | T43.Ø13 | T43.Ø14 | T43.Ø15 | T43.Ø16 |
| **Antidiabetic NEC** | T38.3X1 | T38.3X2 | T38.3X3 | T38.3X4 | T38.3X5 | T38.3X6 |
| biguanide | T38.3X1 | T38.3X2 | T38.3X3 | T38.3X4 | T38.3X5 | T38.3X6 |
| and sulfonyl combined | T38.3X1 | T38.3X2 | T38.3X3 | T38.3X4 | T38.3X5 | T38.3X6 |
| combined | T38.3X1 | T38.3X2 | T38.3X3 | T38.3X4 | T38.3X5 | T38.3X6 |
| sulfonylurea | T38.3X1 | T38.3X2 | T38.3X3 | T38.3X4 | T38.3X5 | T38.3X6 |
| **Antidiarrheal drug NEC** | T47.6X1 | T47.6X2 | T47.6X3 | T47.6X4 | T47.6X5 | T47.6X6 |
| absorbent | T47.6X1 | T47.6X2 | T47.6X3 | T47.6X4 | T47.6X5 | T47.6X6 |
| **Antidiphtheria serum** | T5Ø.Z11 | T5Ø.Z12 | T5Ø.Z13 | T5Ø.Z14 | T5Ø.Z15 | T5Ø.Z16 |
| **Antidiuretic hormone** | T38.891 | T38.892 | T38.893 | T38.894 | T38.895 | T38.896 |
| **Antidote NEC** | T5Ø.6X1 | T5Ø.6X2 | T5Ø.6X3 | T5Ø.6X4 | T5Ø.6X5 | T5Ø.6X6 |
| heavy metal | T45.8X1 | T45.8X2 | T45.8X3 | T45.8X4 | T45.8X5 | T45.8X6 |
| **Antidysrhythmic NEC** | T46.2X1 | T46.2X2 | T46.2X3 | T46.2X4 | T46.2X5 | T46.2X6 |
| **Antiemetic drug** | T45.ØX1 | T45.ØX2 | T45.ØX3 | T45.ØX4 | T45.ØX5 | T45.ØX6 |
| **Antiepilepsy agent** | T42.71 | T42.72 | T42.73 | T42.74 | T42.75 | T42.76 |
| combination | T42.5X1 | T42.5X2 | T42.5X3 | T42.5X4 | T42.5X5 | T42.5X6 |
| mixed | T42.5X1 | T42.5X2 | T42.5X3 | T42.5X4 | T42.5X5 | T42.5X6 |
| specified, NEC | T42.6X1 | T42.6X2 | T42.6X3 | T42.6X4 | T42.6X5 | T42.6X6 |
| **Antiestrogen NEC** | T38.6X1 | T38.6X2 | T38.6X3 | T38.6X4 | T38.6X5 | T38.6X6 |
| **Antifertility pill** | T38.4X1 | T38.4X2 | T38.4X3 | T38.4X4 | T38.4X5 | T38.4X6 |
| **Antifibrinolytic drug** | T45.621 | T45.622 | T45.623 | T45.624 | T45.625 | T45.626 |
| **Antifilarial drug** | T37.4X1 | T37.4X2 | T37.4X3 | T37.4X4 | T37.4X5 | T37.4X6 |
| **Antiflatulent** | T47.5X1 | T47.5X2 | T47.5X3 | T47.5X4 | T47.5X5 | T47.5X6 |
| **Antifreeze** | T65.91 | T65.92 | T65.93 | T65.94 | — | — |
| alcohol | T51.1X1 | T51.1X2 | T51.1X3 | T51.1X4 | — | — |
| ethylene glycol | T51.8X1 | T51.8X2 | T51.8X3 | T51.8X4 | — | — |
| **Antifungal** | | | | | | |
| anti-infective NEC | T37.91 | T37.92 | T37.93 | T37.94 | T37.95 | T37.96 |
| antibiotic (systemic) | T36.7X1 | T36.7X2 | T36.7X3 | T36.7X4 | T36.7X5 | T36.7X6 |
| disinfectant, local | T49.ØX1 | T49.ØX2 | T49.ØX3 | T49.ØX4 | T49.ØX5 | T49.ØX6 |
| nonmedicinal (spray) | T6Ø.3X1 | T6Ø.3X2 | T6Ø.3X3 | T6Ø.3X4 | — | — |
| topical | T49.ØX1 | T49.ØX2 | T49.ØX3 | T49.ØX4 | T49.ØX5 | T49.ØX6 |
| **Antigonadotrophin NEC** | T38.6X1 | T38.6X2 | T38.6X3 | T38.6X4 | T38.6X5 | T38.6X6 |
| **Antihallucinogen** | T43.5Ø1 | T43.5Ø2 | T43.5Ø3 | T43.5Ø4 | T43.5Ø5 | T43.5Ø6 |
| **Antihelmintics** | T37.4X1 | T37.4X2 | T37.4X3 | T37.4X4 | T37.4X5 | T37.4X6 |
| **Antihemophilic** | | | | | | |
| factor | T45.8X1 | T45.8X2 | T45.8X3 | T45.8X4 | T45.8X5 | T45.8X6 |
| fraction | T45.8X1 | T45.8X2 | T45.8X3 | T45.8X4 | T45.8X5 | T45.8X6 |
| globulin concentrate | T45.7X1 | T45.7X2 | T45.7X3 | T45.7X4 | T45.7X5 | T45.7X6 |
| human plasma | T45.8X1 | T45.8X2 | T45.8X3 | T45.8X4 | T45.8X5 | T45.8X6 |
| plasma, dried | T45.7X1 | T45.7X2 | T45.7X3 | T45.7X4 | T45.7X5 | T45.7X6 |
| **Antihemorrhoidal preparation** | T49.2X1 | T49.2X2 | T49.2X3 | T49.2X4 | T49.2X5 | T49.2X6 |
| **Antiheparin drug** | T45.7X1 | T45.7X2 | T45.7X3 | T45.7X4 | T45.7X5 | T45.7X6 |
| **Antihistamine** | T45.ØX1 | T45.ØX2 | T45.ØX3 | T45.ØX4 | T45.ØX5 | T45.ØX6 |
| **Antihookworm drug** | T37.4X1 | T37.4X2 | T37.4X3 | T37.4X4 | T37.4X5 | T37.4X6 |
| **Antihyperlipidemic drug** | T46.6X1 | T46.6X2 | T46.6X3 | T46.6X4 | T46.6X5 | T46.6X6 |
| **Antihypertensive drug NEC** | T46.5X1 | T46.5X2 | T46.5X3 | T46.5X4 | T46.5X5 | T46.5X6 |
| **Antikaluretic** | T5Ø.3X1 | T5Ø.3X2 | T5Ø.3X3 | T5Ø.3X4 | T5Ø.3X5 | T5Ø.3X6 |
| **Antiknock** (tetraethyl lead) | T56.ØX1 | T56.ØX2 | T56.ØX3 | T56.ØX4 | — | — |
| **Antilipemic drug NEC** | T46.6X1 | T46.6X2 | T46.6X3 | T46.6X4 | T46.6X5 | T46.6X6 |
| **Antilysin*** | T45.621 | T45.622 | T45.623 | T45.624 | T45.625 | T45.626 |
| **Antimalarial** | T37.2X1 | T37.2X2 | T37.2X3 | T37.2X4 | T37.2X5 | T37.2X6 |
| prophylactic NEC | T37.2X1 | T37.2X2 | T37.2X3 | T37.2X4 | T37.2X5 | T37.2X6 |
| pyrimidine derivative | T37.2X1 | T37.2X2 | T37.2X3 | T37.2X4 | T37.2X5 | T37.2X6 |
| **Antimetabolite** | T45.1X1 | T45.1X2 | T45.1X3 | T45.1X4 | T45.1X5 | T45.1X6 |
| **Antimitotic agent** | T45.1X1 | T45.1X2 | T45.1X3 | T45.1X4 | T45.1X5 | T45.1X6 |
| **Antimony** (compounds) (vapor) **NEC** | T56.891 | T56.892 | T56.893 | T56.894 | — | — |
| anti-infectives | T37.8X1 | T37.8X2 | T37.8X3 | T37.8X4 | T37.8X5 | T37.8X6 |
| dimercaptosuccinate | T37.3X1 | T37.3X2 | T37.3X3 | T37.3X4 | T37.3X5 | T37.3X6 |
| hydride | T56.891 | T56.892 | T56.893 | T56.894 | — | — |
| **Antimony** (compounds) (vapor) **NEC** — *continued* | | | | | | |
| pesticide (vapor) | T6Ø.8X1 | T6Ø.8X2 | T6Ø.8X3 | T6Ø.8X4 | — | — |
| potassium (sodium) tartrate | T37.8X1 | T37.8X2 | T37.8X3 | T37.8X4 | T37.8X5 | T37.8X6 |
| sodium dimercaptosuccinate | T37.3X1 | T37.3X2 | T37.3X3 | T37.3X4 | T37.3X5 | T37.3X6 |
| tartrated | T37.8X1 | T37.8X2 | T37.8X3 | T37.8X4 | T37.8X5 | T37.8X6 |
| **Antimuscarinic NEC** | T44.3X1 | T44.3X2 | T44.3X3 | T44.3X4 | T44.3X5 | T44.3X6 |
| **Antimycobacterial drug NEC** | T37.1X1 | T37.1X2 | T37.1X3 | T37.1X4 | T37.1X5 | T37.1X6 |
| antibiotics | T36.5X1 | T36.5X2 | T36.5X3 | T36.5X4 | T36.5X5 | T36.5X6 |
| combination | T37.1X1 | T37.1X2 | T37.1X3 | T37.1X4 | T37.1X5 | T37.1X6 |
| **Antinausea drug** | T45.ØX1 | T45.ØX2 | T45.ØX3 | T45.ØX4 | T45.ØX5 | T45.ØX6 |
| **Antinematode drug** | T37.4X1 | T37.4X2 | T37.4X3 | T37.4X4 | T37.4X5 | T37.4X6 |
| **Antineoplastic NEC** | T45.1X1 | T45.1X2 | T45.1X3 | T45.1X4 | T45.1X5 | T45.1X6 |
| alkaloidal | T45.1X1 | T45.1X2 | T45.1X3 | T45.1X4 | T45.1X5 | T45.1X6 |
| antibiotics | T45.1X1 | T45.1X2 | T45.1X3 | T45.1X4 | T45.1X5 | T45.1X6 |
| combination | T45.1X1 | T45.1X2 | T45.1X3 | T45.1X4 | T45.1X5 | T45.1X6 |
| estrogen | T38.5X1 | T38.5X2 | T38.5X3 | T38.5X4 | T38.5X5 | T38.5X6 |
| steroid | T38.7X1 | T38.7X2 | T38.7X3 | T38.7X4 | T38.7X5 | T38.7X6 |
| **Antiparasitic drug** (systemic) | T37.91 | T37.92 | T37.93 | T37.94 | T37.95 | T37.96 |
| local | T49.ØX1 | T49.ØX2 | T49.ØX3 | T49.ØX4 | T49.ØX5 | T49.ØX6 |
| specified NEC | T37.8X1 | T37.8X2 | T37.8X3 | T37.8X4 | T37.8X5 | T37.8X6 |
| **Antiparkinsonism drug NEC** | T42.8X1 | T42.8X2 | T42.8X3 | T42.8X4 | T42.8X5 | T42.8X6 |
| **Antiperspirant NEC** | T49.2X1 | T49.2X2 | T49.2X3 | T49.2X4 | T49.2X5 | T49.2X6 |
| **Antiphlogistic NEC** | T39.4X1 | T39.4X2 | T39.4X3 | T39.4X4 | T39.4X5 | T39.4X6 |
| **Antiplatyhelmintic drug** | T37.4X1 | T37.4X2 | T37.4X3 | T37.4X4 | T37.4X5 | T37.4X6 |
| **Antiprotozoal drug NEC** | T37.3X1 | T37.3X2 | T37.3X3 | T37.3X4 | T37.3X5 | T37.3X6 |
| blood | T37.2X1 | T37.2X2 | T37.2X3 | T37.2X4 | T37.2X5 | T37.2X6 |
| local | T49.ØX1 | T49.ØX2 | T49.ØX3 | T49.ØX4 | T49.ØX5 | T49.ØX6 |
| **Antipruritic drug NEC** | T49.1X1 | T49.1X2 | T49.1X3 | T49.1X4 | T49.1X5 | T49.1X6 |
| **Antipsychotic drug** | T43.5Ø1 | T43.5Ø2 | T43.5Ø3 | T43.5Ø4 | T43.5Ø5 | T43.5Ø6 |
| specified NEC | T43.591 | T43.592 | T43.593 | T43.594 | T43.595 | T43.596 |
| **Antipyretic** | T39.91 | T39.92 | T39.93 | T39.94 | T39.95 | T39.96 |
| specified NEC | T39.8X1 | T39.8X2 | T39.8X3 | T39.8X4 | T39.8X5 | T39.8X6 |
| **Antipyrine** | T39.2X1 | T39.2X2 | T39.2X3 | T39.2X4 | T39.2X5 | T39.2X6 |
| **Antirabies hyperimmune serum** | T5Ø.Z11 | T5Ø.Z12 | T5Ø.Z13 | T5Ø.Z14 | T5Ø.Z15 | T5Ø.Z16 |
| **Antirheumatic NEC** | T39.4X1 | T39.4X2 | T39.4X3 | T39.4X4 | T39.4X5 | T39.4X6 |
| **Antirigidity drug NEC** | T42.8X1 | T42.8X2 | T42.8X3 | T42.8X4 | T42.8X5 | T42.8X6 |
| **Antischistosomal drug** | T37.4X1 | T37.4X2 | T37.4X3 | T37.4X4 | T37.4X5 | T37.4X6 |
| **Antiscorpion sera** | T5Ø.Z11 | T5Ø.Z12 | T5Ø.Z13 | T5Ø.Z14 | T5Ø.Z15 | T5Ø.Z16 |
| **Antiseborrheics** | T49.4X1 | T49.4X2 | T49.4X3 | T49.4X4 | T49.4X5 | T49.4X6 |
| **Antiseptics** (external) (medicinal) | T49.ØX1 | T49.ØX2 | T49.ØX3 | T49.ØX4 | T49.ØX5 | T49.ØX6 |
| **Antistine** | T45.ØX1 | T45.ØX2 | T45.ØX3 | T45.ØX4 | T45.ØX5 | T45.ØX6 |
| **Antitapeworm drug** | T37.4X1 | T37.4X2 | T37.4X3 | T37.4X4 | T37.4X5 | T37.4X6 |
| **Antitetanus immunoglobulin** | T5Ø.Z11 | T5Ø.Z12 | T5Ø.Z13 | T5Ø.Z14 | T5Ø.Z15 | T5Ø.Z16 |
| **Antithrombin III*** | T45.511 | T45.512 | T45.513 | T45.514 | T45.515 | T45.516 |
| **Antithrombotic** | T45.521 | T45.522 | T45.523 | T45.524 | T45.525 | T45.526 |
| **Antithyroid drug NEC** | T38.2X1 | T38.2X2 | T38.2X3 | T38.2X4 | T38.2X5 | T38.2X6 |
| **Antitoxin** | T5Ø.Z11 | T5Ø.Z12 | T5Ø.Z13 | T5Ø.Z14 | T5Ø.Z15 | T5Ø.Z16 |
| diphtheria | T5Ø.Z11 | T5Ø.Z12 | T5Ø.Z13 | T5Ø.Z14 | T5Ø.Z15 | T5Ø.Z16 |
| gas gangrene | T5Ø.Z11 | T5Ø.Z12 | T5Ø.Z13 | T5Ø.Z14 | T5Ø.Z15 | T5Ø.Z16 |
| tetanus | T5Ø.Z11 | T5Ø.Z12 | T5Ø.Z13 | T5Ø.Z14 | T5Ø.Z15 | T5Ø.Z16 |
| **Antitrichomonal drug** | T37.3X1 | T37.3X2 | T37.3X3 | T37.3X4 | T37.3X5 | T37.3X6 |
| **Antituberculars** | T37.1X1 | T37.1X2 | T37.1X3 | T37.1X4 | T37.1X5 | T37.1X6 |
| antibiotics | T36.5X1 | T36.5X2 | T36.5X3 | T36.5X4 | T36.5X5 | T36.5X6 |
| **Antitussive NEC** | T48.3X1 | T48.3X2 | T48.3X3 | T48.3X4 | T48.3X5 | T48.3X6 |
| codeine mixture | T4Ø.2X1 | T4Ø.2X2 | T4Ø.2X3 | T4Ø.2X4 | T4Ø.2X5 | T4Ø.2X6 |
| opiate | T4Ø.2X1 | T4Ø.2X2 | T4Ø.2X3 | T4Ø.2X4 | T4Ø.2X5 | T4Ø.2X6 |
| **Antivaricose drug** | T46.8X1 | T46.8X2 | T46.8X3 | T46.8X4 | T46.8X5 | T46.8X6 |
| **Antivenin, antivenom** (sera) | T5Ø.Z11 | T5Ø.Z12 | T5Ø.Z13 | T5Ø.Z14 | T5Ø.Z15 | T5Ø.Z16 |
| crotaline | T5Ø.Z11 | T5Ø.Z12 | T5Ø.Z13 | T5Ø.Z14 | T5Ø.Z15 | T5Ø.Z16 |
| spider bite | T5Ø.Z11 | T5Ø.Z12 | T5Ø.Z13 | T5Ø.Z14 | T5Ø.Z15 | T5Ø.Z16 |
| **Antivert*** | T45.ØX1 | T45.ØX2 | T45.ØX3 | T45.ØX4 | T45.ØX5 | T45.ØX6 |
| **Antivertigo drug** | T45.ØX1 | T45.ØX2 | T45.ØX3 | T45.ØX4 | T45.ØX5 | T45.ØX6 |
| **Antiviral drug NEC** | T37.5X1 | T37.5X2 | T37.5X3 | T37.5X4 | T37.5X5 | T37.5X6 |
| eye | T49.5X1 | T49.5X2 | T49.5X3 | T49.5X4 | T49.5X5 | T49.5X6 |
| **Antiwhipworm drug** | T37.4X1 | T37.4X2 | T37.4X3 | T37.4X4 | T37.4X5 | T37.4X6 |
| **Antrol** — *see also* by specific chemical substance | T6Ø.91 | T6Ø.92 | T6Ø.93 | T6Ø.94 | — | — |
| fungicide | T6Ø.91 | T6Ø.92 | T6Ø.93 | T6Ø.94 | — | — |
| **ANTU** (alpha naphthylthiourea) | T6Ø.4X1 | T6Ø.4X2 | T6Ø.4X3 | T6Ø.4X4 | — | — |
| **Apalcillin** | T36.ØX1 | T36.ØX2 | T36.ØX3 | T36.ØX4 | T36.ØX5 | T36.ØX6 |
| **APC** | T48.5X1 | T48.5X2 | T48.5X3 | T48.5X4 | T48.5X5 | T48.5X6 |
| **Aplonidine** | T44.4X1 | T44.4X2 | T44.4X3 | T44.4X4 | T44.4X5 | T44.4X6 |





☑ **Additional Character May Be Required — Refer to the Tabular List for Character Selection**

***Optum Value-Add**

| Substance | Poisoning, Accidental (unintentional) | Poisoning, Intentional Self-harm | Poisoning, Assault | Poisoning, Undetermined | Adverse Effect | Under-dosing |
|---|---|---|---|---|---|---|
| **Apomorphine** | T47.7X1 | T47.7X2 | T47.7X3 | T47.7X4 | T47.7X5 | T47.7X6 |
| **Appetite depressants, central** | T5Ø.5X1 | T5Ø.5X2 | T5Ø.5X3 | T5Ø.5X4 | T5Ø.5X5 | T5Ø.5X6 |
| **Apraclonidine** (hydrochloride) | T44.4X1 | T44.4X2 | T44.4X3 | T44.4X4 | T44.4X5 | T44.4X6 |
| **Apresoline** | T46.5X1 | T46.5X2 | T46.5X3 | T46.5X4 | T46.5X5 | T46.5X6 |
| **Apri*** | T38.4X1 | T38.4X2 | T38.4X3 | T38.4X4 | T38.4X5 | T38.4X6 |
| **Aprindine** | T46.2X1 | T46.2X2 | T46.2X3 | T46.2X4 | T46.2X5 | T46.2X6 |
| **Aprobarbital** | T42.3X1 | T42.3X2 | T42.3X3 | T42.3X4 | T42.3X5 | T42.3X6 |
| **Apronalide** | T42.6X1 | T42.6X2 | T42.6X3 | T42.6X4 | T42.6X5 | T42.6X6 |
| **Aprotinin** | T45.621 | T45.622 | T45.623 | T45.624 | T45.625 | T45.626 |
| **Aptocaine** | T41.3X1 | T41.3X2 | T41.3X3 | T41.3X4 | T41.3X5 | T41.3X6 |
| **Aqua fortis** | T54.2X1 | T54.2X2 | T54.2X3 | T54.2X4 | — | — |
| **Ara-A** | T37.5X1 | T37.5X2 | T37.5X3 | T37.5X4 | T37.5X5 | T37.5X6 |
| **Ara-C** | T45.1X1 | T45.1X2 | T45.1X3 | T45.1X4 | T45.1X5 | T45.1X6 |
| **Arachis oil** | T49.3X1 | T49.3X2 | T49.3X3 | T49.3X4 | T49.3X5 | T49.3X6 |
| cathartic | T47.4X1 | T47.4X2 | T47.4X3 | T47.4X4 | T47.4X5 | T47.4X6 |
| **Aralen** | T37.2X1 | T37.2X2 | T37.2X3 | T37.2X4 | T37.2X5 | T37.2X6 |
| **Arecoline** | T44.1X1 | T44.1X2 | T44.1X3 | T44.1X4 | T44.1X5 | T44.1X6 |
| **Arginine** | T5Ø.991 | T5Ø.992 | T5Ø.993 | T5Ø.994 | T5Ø.995 | T5Ø.996 |
| glutamate | T5Ø.991 | T5Ø.992 | T5Ø.993 | T5Ø.994 | T5Ø.995 | T5Ø.996 |
| **Argyrol** | T49.ØX1 | T49.ØX2 | T49.ØX3 | T49.ØX4 | T49.ØX5 | T49.ØX6 |
| ENT agent | T49.6X1 | T49.6X2 | T49.6X3 | T49.6X4 | T49.6X5 | T49.6X6 |
| ophthalmic preparation | T49.5X1 | T49.5X2 | T49.5X3 | T49.5X4 | T49.5X5 | T49.5X6 |
| **Aristocort** | T38.ØX1 | T38.ØX2 | T38.ØX3 | T38.ØX4 | T38.ØX5 | T38.ØX6 |
| ENT agent | T49.6X1 | T49.6X2 | T49.6X3 | T49.6X4 | T49.6X5 | T49.6X6 |
| ophthalmic preparation | T49.5X1 | T49.5X2 | T49.5X3 | T49.5X4 | T49.5X5 | T49.5X6 |
| topical NEC | T49.ØX1 | T49.ØX2 | T49.ØX3 | T49.ØX4 | T49.ØX5 | T49.ØX6 |
| **Armour*** | T38.1X1 | T38.1X2 | T38.1X3 | T38.1X4 | T38.1X5 | T38.1X6 |
| **Aromatics, corrosive** | T54.1X1 | T54.1X2 | T54.1X3 | T54.1X4 | — | — |
| disinfectants | T54.1X1 | T54.1X2 | T54.1X3 | T54.1X4 | — | — |
| **Arsenate of lead** | T57.ØX1 | T57.ØX2 | T57.ØX3 | T57.ØX4 | — | — |
| herbicide | T57.ØX1 | T57.ØX2 | T57.ØX3 | T57.ØX4 | — | — |
| **Arsenic, arsenicals** (compounds) (dust) (vapor) **NEC** | T57.ØX1 | T57.ØX2 | T57.ØX3 | T57.ØX4 | — | — |
| anti-infectives | T37.8X1 | T37.8X2 | T37.8X3 | T37.8X4 | T37.8X5 | T37.8X6 |
| pesticide (dust) (fumes) | T57.ØX1 | T57.ØX2 | T57.ØX3 | T57.ØX4 | — | — |
| **Arsine** (gas) | T57.ØX1 | T57.ØX2 | T57.ØX3 | T57.ØX4 | — | — |
| **Arsobal*** | T37.3X1 | T37.3X2 | T37.3X3 | T37.3X4 | T37.3X5 | T37.3X6 |
| **Arsphenamine** (silver) | T37.8X1 | T37.8X2 | T37.8X3 | T37.8X4 | T37.8X5 | T37.8X6 |
| **Arsthinol** | T37.3X1 | T37.3X2 | T37.3X3 | T37.3X4 | T37.3X5 | T37.3X6 |
| **Artane** | T44.3X1 | T44.3X2 | T44.3X3 | T44.3X4 | T44.3X5 | T44.3X6 |
| **Arthropod** (venomous) **NEC** | T63.481 | T63.482 | T63.483 | T63.484 | — | — |
| **Articaine** | T41.3X1 | T41.3X2 | T41.3X3 | T41.3X4 | T41.3X5 | T41.3X6 |
| **Asbestos** | T57.8X1 | T57.8X2 | T57.8X3 | T57.8X4 | — | — |
| **Ascaridole** | T37.4X1 | T37.4X2 | T37.4X3 | T37.4X4 | T37.4X5 | T37.4X6 |
| **Ascorbic acid** | T45.2X1 | T45.2X2 | T45.2X3 | T45.2X4 | T45.2X5 | T45.2X6 |
| **Asiaticoside** | T49.ØX1 | T49.ØX2 | T49.ØX3 | T49.ØX4 | T49.ØX5 | T49.ØX6 |
| **Asparaginase** | T45.1X1 | T45.1X2 | T45.1X3 | T45.1X4 | T45.1X5 | T45.1X6 |
| **Aspidium** (oleoresin) | T37.4X1 | T37.4X2 | T37.4X3 | T37.4X4 | T37.4X5 | T37.4X6 |
| **Aspirin** (aluminum) (soluble) | T39.Ø11 | T39.Ø12 | T39.Ø13 | T39.Ø14 | T39.Ø15 | T39.Ø16 |
| **Aspoxicillin** | T36.ØX1 | T36.ØX2 | T36.ØX3 | T36.ØX4 | T36.ØX5 | T36.ØX6 |
| **Astemizole** | T45.ØX1 | T45.ØX2 | T45.ØX3 | T45.ØX4 | T45.ØX5 | T45.ØX6 |
| **Astringent** (local) | T49.2X1 | T49.2X2 | T49.2X3 | T49.2X4 | T49.2X5 | T49.2X6 |
| specified NEC | T49.2X1 | T49.2X2 | T49.2X3 | T49.2X4 | T49.2X5 | T49.2X6 |
| **Astromicin** | T36.5X1 | T36.5X2 | T36.5X3 | T36.5X4 | T36.5X5 | T36.5X6 |
| **Ataractic drug NEC** | T43.5Ø1 | T43.5Ø2 | T43.5Ø3 | T43.5Ø4 | T43.5Ø5 | T43.5Ø6 |
| **Atenolol** | T44.7X1 | T44.7X2 | T44.7X3 | T44.7X4 | T44.7X5 | T44.7X6 |
| **Atonia drug, intestinal** | T47.4X1 | T47.4X2 | T47.4X3 | T47.4X4 | T47.4X5 | T47.4X6 |
| **Atophan** | T5Ø.4X1 | T5Ø.4X2 | T5Ø.4X3 | T5Ø.4X4 | T5Ø.4X5 | T5Ø.4X6 |
| **Atorvastatin*** | T46.6X1 | T46.6X2 | T46.6X3 | T46.6X4 | T46.6X5 | T46.6X6 |
| **Atracurium besilate** | T48.1X1 | T48.1X2 | T48.1X3 | T48.1X4 | T48.1X5 | T48.1X6 |
| **Atropine** | T44.3X1 | T44.3X2 | T44.3X3 | T44.3X4 | T44.3X5 | T44.3X6 |
| derivative | T44.3X1 | T44.3X2 | T44.3X3 | T44.3X4 | T44.3X5 | T44.3X6 |
| methonitrate | T44.3X1 | T44.3X2 | T44.3X3 | T44.3X4 | T44.3X5 | T44.3X6 |
| **Atrovent*** | T48.6X1 | T48.6X2 | T48.6X3 | T48.6X4 | T48.6X5 | T48.6X6 |
| **Attapulgite** | T47.6X1 | T47.6X2 | T47.6X3 | T47.6X4 | T47.6X5 | T47.6X6 |
| **Augmentin (ES-600) (XR)*** | T36.ØX1 | T36.ØX2 | T36.ØX3 | T36.ØX4 | T36.ØX5 | T36.ØX6 |
| **Auramine** | T65.891 | T65.892 | T65.893 | T65.894 | — | — |
| dye | T65.6X1 | T65.6X2 | T65.6X3 | T65.6X4 | — | — |
| fungicide | T6Ø.3X1 | T6Ø.3X2 | T6Ø.3X3 | T6Ø.3X4 | — | — |
| **Auranofin** | T39.4X1 | T39.4X2 | T39.4X3 | T39.4X4 | T39.4X5 | T39.4X6 |
| **Aurantiin** | T46.991 | T46.992 | T46.993 | T46.994 | T46.995 | T46.996 |
| **Aureomycin** | T36.4X1 | T36.4X2 | T36.4X3 | T36.4X4 | T36.4X5 | T36.4X6 |
| ophthalmic preparation | T49.5X1 | T49.5X2 | T49.5X3 | T49.5X4 | T49.5X5 | T49.5X6 |
| topical NEC | T49.ØX1 | T49.ØX2 | T49.ØX3 | T49.ØX4 | T49.ØX5 | T49.ØX6 |
| **Aurothioglucose** | T39.4X1 | T39.4X2 | T39.4X3 | T39.4X4 | T39.4X5 | T39.4X6 |
| **Aurothioglycanide** | T39.4X1 | T39.4X2 | T39.4X3 | T39.4X4 | T39.4X5 | T39.4X6 |
| **Aurothiomalate sodium** | T39.4X1 | T39.4X2 | T39.4X3 | T39.4X4 | T39.4X5 | T39.4X6 |
| **Aurotioprol** | T39.4X1 | T39.4X2 | T39.4X3 | T39.4X4 | T39.4X5 | T39.4X6 |
| **Automobile fuel** | T52.ØX1 | T52.ØX2 | T52.ØX3 | T52.ØX4 | — | — |
| **Autonomic nervous system agent NEC** | T44.9Ø1 | T44.9Ø2 | T44.9Ø3 | T44.9Ø4 | T44.9Ø5 | T44.9Ø6 |
| **Avelox*** | T36.8X1 | T36.8X2 | T36.8X3 | T36.8X4 | T36.8X5 | T36.8X6 |
| **Avlosulfon** | T37.1X1 | T37.1X2 | T37.1X3 | T37.1X4 | T37.1X5 | T37.1X6 |
| **Avomine** | T42.6X1 | T42.6X2 | T42.6X3 | T42.6X4 | T42.6X5 | T42.6X6 |
| **Axerophthol** | T45.2X1 | T45.2X2 | T45.2X3 | T45.2X4 | T45.2X5 | T45.2X6 |
| **Azacitidine** | T45.1X1 | T45.1X2 | T45.1X3 | T45.1X4 | T45.1X5 | T45.1X6 |
| **Azacyclonol** | T43.591 | T43.592 | T43.593 | T43.594 | T43.595 | T43.596 |
| **Azadirachta** | T6Ø.2X1 | T6Ø.2X2 | T6Ø.2X3 | T6Ø.2X4 | — | — |
| **Azanidazole** | T37.3X1 | T37.3X2 | T37.3X3 | T37.3X4 | T37.3X5 | T37.3X6 |
| **Azapetine** | T46.7X1 | T46.7X2 | T46.7X3 | T46.7X4 | T46.7X5 | T46.7X6 |
| **Azapropazone** | T39.2X1 | T39.2X2 | T39.2X3 | T39.2X4 | T39.2X5 | T39.2X6 |
| **Azaribine** | T45.1X1 | T45.1X2 | T45.1X3 | T45.1X4 | T45.1X5 | T45.1X6 |
| **Azaserine** | T45.1X1 | T45.1X2 | T45.1X3 | T45.1X4 | T45.1X5 | T45.1X6 |
| **Azatadine** | T45.ØX1 | T45.ØX2 | T45.ØX3 | T45.ØX4 | T45.ØX5 | T45.ØX6 |
| **Azatepa** | T45.1X1 | T45.1X2 | T45.1X3 | T45.1X4 | T45.1X5 | T45.1X6 |
| **Azathioprine** | T45.1X1 | T45.1X2 | T45.1X3 | T45.1X4 | T45.1X5 | T45.1X6 |
| **Azelaic acid** | T49.ØX1 | T49.ØX2 | T49.ØX3 | T49.ØX4 | T49.ØX5 | T49.ØX6 |
| **Azelastine** | T45.ØX1 | T45.ØX2 | T45.ØX3 | T45.ØX4 | T45.ØX5 | T45.ØX6 |
| **Azidocillin** | T36.ØX1 | T36.ØX2 | T36.ØX3 | T36.ØX4 | T36.ØX5 | T36.ØX6 |
| **Azidothymidine** | T37.5X1 | T37.5X2 | T37.5X3 | T37.5X4 | T37.5X5 | T37.5X6 |
| **Azinphos** (ethyl) (methyl) | T6Ø.ØX1 | T6Ø.ØX2 | T6Ø.ØX3 | T6Ø.ØX4 | — | — |
| **Aziridine** (chelating) | T54.1X1 | T54.1X2 | T54.1X3 | T54.1X4 | — | — |
| **Azithromycin** | T36.3X1 | T36.3X2 | T36.3X3 | T36.3X4 | T36.3X5 | T36.3X6 |
| **Azlocillin** | T36.ØX1 | T36.ØX2 | T36.ØX3 | T36.ØX4 | T36.ØX5 | T36.ØX6 |
| **Azo-Standard*** | T49.ØX1 | T49.ØX2 | T49.ØX3 | T49.ØX4 | T49.ØX5 | T49.ØX6 |
| **Azobenzene smoke** | T65.3X1 | T65.3X2 | T65.3X3 | T65.3X4 | — | — |
| acaricide | T6Ø.8X1 | T6Ø.8X2 | T6Ø.8X3 | T6Ø.8X4 | — | — |
| **Azosulfamide** | T37.ØX1 | T37.ØX2 | T37.ØX3 | T37.ØX4 | T37.ØX5 | T37.ØX6 |
| **AZT** | T37.5X1 | T37.5X2 | T37.5X3 | T37.5X4 | T37.5X5 | T37.5X6 |
| **Aztreonam** | T36.1X1 | T36.1X2 | T36.1X3 | T36.1X4 | T36.1X5 | T36.1X6 |
| **Azulfidine** | T37.ØX1 | T37.ØX2 | T37.ØX3 | T37.ØX4 | T37.ØX5 | T37.ØX6 |
| **Azuresin** | T5Ø.8X1 | T5Ø.8X2 | T5Ø.8X3 | T5Ø.8X4 | T5Ø.8X5 | T5Ø.8X6 |
| **b-acetyldigoxin** | T46.ØX1 | T46.ØX2 | T46.ØX3 | T46.ØX4 | T46.ØX5 | T46.ØX6 |
| **b-benzalbutyramide** | T46.6X1 | T46.6X2 | T46.6X3 | T46.6X4 | T46.6X5 | T46.6X6 |
| **b-eucaine** | T49.1X1 | T49.1X2 | T49.1X3 | T49.1X4 | T49.1X5 | T49.1X6 |
| **b-Galactosidase** | T47.5X1 | T47.5X2 | T47.5X3 | T47.5X4 | T47.5X5 | T47.5X6 |
| **b-sitosterol**(s) | T46.6X1 | T46.6X2 | T46.6X3 | T46.6X4 | T46.6X5 | T46.6X6 |
| **Bacampicillin** | T36.ØX1 | T36.ØX2 | T36.ØX3 | T36.ØX4 | T36.ØX5 | T36.ØX6 |
| **Bacillus** | | | | | | |
| lactobacillus | T47.8X1 | T47.8X2 | T47.8X3 | T47.8X4 | T47.8X5 | T47.8X6 |
| subtilis | T47.6X1 | T47.6X2 | T47.6X3 | T47.6X4 | T47.6X5 | T47.6X6 |
| **Bacimycin** | T49.ØX1 | T49.ØX2 | T49.ØX3 | T49.ØX4 | T49.ØX5 | T49.ØX6 |
| ophthalmic preparation | T49.5X1 | T49.5X2 | T49.5X3 | T49.5X4 | T49.5X5 | T49.5X6 |
| **Bacitracin zinc** | T49.ØX1 | T49.ØX2 | T49.ØX3 | T49.ØX4 | T49.ØX5 | T49.ØX6 |
| ENT agent | T49.6X1 | T49.6X2 | T49.6X3 | T49.6X4 | T49.6X5 | T49.6X6 |
| ophthalmic preparation | T49.5X1 | T49.5X2 | T49.5X3 | T49.5X4 | T49.5X5 | T49.5X6 |
| topical NEC | T49.ØX1 | T49.ØX2 | T49.ØX3 | T49.ØX4 | T49.ØX5 | T49.ØX6 |
| with neomycin | T49.ØX1 | T49.ØX2 | T49.ØX3 | T49.ØX4 | T49.ØX5 | T49.ØX6 |
| **Baclofen** | T42.8X1 | T42.8X2 | T42.8X3 | T42.8X4 | T42.8X5 | T42.8X6 |
| **Bactrim*** | T36.8X1 | T36.8X2 | T36.8X3 | T36.8X4 | T36.8X5 | T36.8X6 |
| **Baking soda** | T5Ø.991 | T5Ø.992 | T5Ø.993 | T5Ø.994 | T5Ø.995 | T5Ø.996 |
| **BAL** | T45.8X1 | T45.8X2 | T45.8X3 | T45.8X4 | T45.8X5 | T45.8X6 |
| **Bambuterol** | T48.6X1 | T48.6X2 | T48.6X3 | T48.6X4 | T48.6X5 | T48.6X6 |
| **Bamethan** (sulfate) | T46.7X1 | T46.7X2 | T46.7X3 | T46.7X4 | T46.7X5 | T46.7X6 |
| **Bamifylline** | T48.6X1 | T48.6X2 | T48.6X3 | T48.6X4 | T48.6X5 | T48.6X6 |
| **Bamipine** | T45.ØX1 | T45.ØX2 | T45.ØX3 | T45.ØX4 | T45.ØX5 | T45.ØX6 |
| **Baneberry** — *see* Actaea spicata | | | | | | |
| **Banewort** — *see* Belladonna | | | | | | |
| **Barbenyl** | T42.3X1 | T42.3X2 | T42.3X3 | T42.3X4 | T42.3X5 | T42.3X6 |
| **Barbexaclone** | T42.6X1 | T42.6X2 | T42.6X3 | T42.6X4 | T42.6X5 | T42.6X6 |
| **Barbital** | T42.3X1 | T42.3X2 | T42.3X3 | T42.3X4 | T42.3X5 | T42.3X6 |
| sodium | T42.3X1 | T42.3X2 | T42.3X3 | T42.3X4 | T42.3X5 | T42.3X6 |
| **Barbitone** | T42.3X1 | T42.3X2 | T42.3X3 | T42.3X4 | T42.3X5 | T42.3X6 |
| **Barbiturate NEC** | T42.3X1 | T42.3X2 | T42.3X3 | T42.3X4 | T42.3X5 | T42.3X6 |
| anesthetic (intravenous) | T41.1X1 | T41.1X2 | T41.1X3 | T41.1X4 | T41.1X5 | T41.1X6 |
| with tranquilizer | T42.3X1 | T42.3X2 | T42.3X3 | T42.3X4 | T42.3X5 | T42.3X6 |
| **Barium** (carbonate) (chloride) (sulfite) | T57.8X1 | T57.8X2 | T57.8X3 | T57.8X4 | — | — |
| diagnostic agent | T5Ø.8X1 | T5Ø.8X2 | T5Ø.8X3 | T5Ø.8X4 | T5Ø.8X5 | T5Ø.8X6 |
| pesticide | T6Ø.4X1 | T6Ø.4X2 | T6Ø.4X3 | T6Ø.4X4 | — | — |
| rodenticide | T6Ø.4X1 | T6Ø.4X2 | T6Ø.4X3 | T6Ø.4X4 | — | — |
| sulfate (medicinal) | T5Ø.8X1 | T5Ø.8X2 | T5Ø.8X3 | T5Ø.8X4 | T5Ø.8X5 | T5Ø.8X6 |
| **Barrier cream** | T49.3X1 | T49.3X2 | T49.3X3 | T49.3X4 | T49.3X5 | T49.3X6 |
| **Basic fuchsin** | T49.ØX1 | T49.ØX2 | T49.ØX3 | T49.ØX4 | T49.ØX5 | T49.ØX6 |
| **Basiliximab*** | T45.1X1 | T45.1X2 | T45.1X3 | T45.1X4 | T45.1X5 | T45.1X6 |
| **Battery acid or fluid** | T54.2X1 | T54.2X2 | T54.2X3 | T54.2X4 | — | — |
| **Bay rum** | T51.8X1 | T51.8X2 | T51.8X3 | T51.8X4 | — | — |
| **BCG** (vaccine) | T5Ø.A91 | T5Ø.A92 | T5Ø.A93 | T5Ø.A94 | T5Ø.A95 | T5Ø.A96 |
| **BCNU** | T45.1X1 | T45.1X2 | T45.1X3 | T45.1X4 | T45.1X5 | T45.1X6 |
| **Bearsfoot** | T62.2X1 | T62.2X2 | T62.2X3 | T62.2X4 | — | — |
| **Beclamide** | T42.6X1 | T42.6X2 | T42.6X3 | T42.6X4 | T42.6X5 | T42.6X6 |
| **Beclomethasone** | T44.5X1 | T44.5X2 | T44.5X3 | T44.5X4 | T44.5X5 | T44.5X6 |

*Optum Value-Add

☑ Additional Character May Be Required — Refer to the Tabular List for Character Selection

| Substance | Poisoning, Accidental (unintentional) | Poisoning, Intentional Self-harm | Poisoning, Assault | Poisoning, Undetermined | Adverse Effect | Under-dosing |
|---|---|---|---|---|---|---|
| **Bee** (sting) (venom) | T63.441 | T63.442 | T63.443 | T63.444 | — | — |
| **Befunolol** | T49.5X1 | T49.5X2 | T49.5X3 | T49.5X4 | T49.5X5 | T49.5X6 |
| **Bekanamycin** | T36.5X1 | T36.5X2 | T36.5X3 | T36.5X4 | T36.5X5 | T36.5X6 |
| **Belladonna** — *see also* Nightshade | | | | | | |
| alkaloids | T44.3X1 | T44.3X2 | T44.3X3 | T44.3X4 | T44.3X5 | T44.3X6 |
| extract | T44.3X1 | T44.3X2 | T44.3X3 | T44.3X4 | T44.3X5 | T44.3X6 |
| herb | T44.3X1 | T44.3X2 | T44.3X3 | T44.3X4 | T44.3X5 | T44.3X6 |
| **Belviq*** | T5Ø.5X1 | T5Ø.5X2 | T5Ø.5X3 | T5Ø.5X4 | T5Ø.5X5 | T5Ø.5X6 |
| **Bemegride** | T5Ø.7X1 | T5Ø.7X2 | T5Ø.7X3 | T5Ø.7X4 | T5Ø.7X5 | T5Ø.7X6 |
| **Benactyzine** | T44.3X1 | T44.3X2 | T44.3X3 | T44.3X4 | T44.3X5 | T44.3X6 |
| **Benadryl** | T45.ØX1 | T45.ØX2 | T45.ØX3 | T45.ØX4 | T45.ØX5 | T45.ØX6 |
| **Benaprizine** | T44.3X1 | T44.3X2 | T44.3X3 | T44.3X4 | T44.3X5 | T44.3X6 |
| **Benazepril** | T46.4X1 | T46.4X2 | T46.4X3 | T46.4X4 | T46.4X5 | T46.4X6 |
| **Bencyclane** | T46.7X1 | T46.7X2 | T46.7X3 | T46.7X4 | T46.7X5 | T46.7X6 |
| **Bendazol** | T46.3X1 | T46.3X2 | T46.3X3 | T46.3X4 | T46.3X5 | T46.3X6 |
| **Bendrofluazide** | T5Ø.2X1 | T5Ø.2X2 | T5Ø.2X3 | T5Ø.2X4 | T5Ø.2X5 | T5Ø.2X6 |
| **Bendroflumethiazide** | T5Ø.2X1 | T5Ø.2X2 | T5Ø.2X3 | T5Ø.2X4 | T5Ø.2X5 | T5Ø.2X6 |
| **Benemid** | T5Ø.4X1 | T5Ø.4X2 | T5Ø.4X3 | T5Ø.4X4 | T5Ø.4X5 | T5Ø.4X6 |
| **Benethamine penicillin** | T36.ØX1 | T36.ØX2 | T36.ØX3 | T36.ØX4 | T36.ØX5 | T36.ØX6 |
| **Benexate** | T47.1X1 | T47.1X2 | T47.1X3 | T47.1X4 | T47.1X5 | T47.1X6 |
| **Benfluorex** | T46.6X1 | T46.6X2 | T46.6X3 | T46.6X4 | T46.6X5 | T46.6X6 |
| **Benfotiamine** | T45.2X1 | T45.2X2 | T45.2X3 | T45.2X4 | T45.2X5 | T45.2X6 |
| **Benisone** | T49.ØX1 | T49.ØX2 | T49.ØX3 | T49.ØX4 | T49.ØX5 | T49.ØX6 |
| **Benomyl** | T6Ø.ØX1 | T6Ø.ØX2 | T6Ø.ØX3 | T6Ø.ØX4 | — | — |
| **Benoquin** | T49.8X1 | T49.8X2 | T49.8X3 | T49.8X4 | T49.8X5 | T49.8X6 |
| **Benoxinate** | T41.3X1 | T41.3X2 | T41.3X3 | T41.3X4 | T41.3X5 | T41.3X6 |
| **Benperidol** | T43.4X1 | T43.4X2 | T43.4X3 | T43.4X4 | T43.4X5 | T43.4X6 |
| **Benproperine** | T48.3X1 | T48.3X2 | T48.3X3 | T48.3X4 | T48.3X5 | T48.3X6 |
| **Benserazide** | T42.8X1 | T42.8X2 | T42.8X3 | T42.8X4 | T42.8X5 | T42.8X6 |
| **Bentazepam** | T42.4X1 | T42.4X2 | T42.4X3 | T42.4X4 | T42.4X5 | T42.4X6 |
| **Bentiromide** | T5Ø.8X1 | T5Ø.8X2 | T5Ø.8X3 | T5Ø.8X4 | T5Ø.8X5 | T5Ø.8X6 |
| **Bentonite** | T49.3X1 | T49.3X2 | T49.3X3 | T49.3X4 | T49.3X5 | T49.3X6 |
| **Benzalbutyramide** | T46.6X1 | T46.6X2 | T46.6X3 | T46.6X4 | T46.6X5 | T46.6X6 |
| **Benzalkonium** (chloride) | T49.ØX1 | T49.ØX2 | T49.ØX3 | T49.ØX4 | T49.ØX5 | T49.ØX6 |
| ophthalmic preparation | T49.5X1 | T49.5X2 | T49.5X3 | T49.5X4 | T49.5X5 | T49.5X6 |
| **Benzamidosalicylate** (calcium) | T37.1X1 | T37.1X2 | T37.1X3 | T37.1X4 | T37.1X5 | T37.1X6 |
| **Benzamine** | T41.3X1 | T41.3X2 | T41.3X3 | T41.3X4 | T41.3X5 | T41.3X6 |
| lactate | T49.1X1 | T49.1X2 | T49.1X3 | T49.1X4 | T49.1X5 | T49.1X6 |
| **Benzamphetamine** | T5Ø.5X1 | T5Ø.5X2 | T5Ø.5X3 | T5Ø.5X4 | T5Ø.5X5 | T5Ø.5X6 |
| **Benzapril hydrochloride** | T46.5X1 | T46.5X2 | T46.5X3 | T46.5X4 | T46.5X5 | T46.5X6 |
| **Benzathine benzylpenicillin** | T36.ØX1 | T36.ØX2 | T36.ØX3 | T36.ØX4 | T36.ØX5 | T36.ØX6 |
| **Benzathine penicillin** | T36.ØX1 | T36.ØX2 | T36.ØX3 | T36.ØX4 | T36.ØX5 | T36.ØX6 |
| **Benzatropine** | T42.8X1 | T42.8X2 | T42.8X3 | T42.8X4 | T42.8X5 | T42.8X6 |
| **Benzbromarone** | T5Ø.4X1 | T5Ø.4X2 | T5Ø.4X3 | T5Ø.4X4 | T5Ø.4X5 | T5Ø.4X6 |
| **Benzcarbimine** | T45.1X1 | T45.1X2 | T45.1X3 | T45.1X4 | T45.1X5 | T45.1X6 |
| **Benzedrex** | T44.991 | T44.992 | T44.993 | T44.994 | T44.995 | T44.996 |
| **Benzedrine** (amphetamine) | T43.621 | T43.622 | T43.623 | T43.624 | T43.625 | T43.626 |
| **Benzenamine** | T65.3X1 | T65.3X2 | T65.3X3 | T65.3X4 | — | — |
| **Benzene** | T52.1X1 | T52.1X2 | T52.1X3 | T52.1X4 | — | — |
| homologues (acetyl) (dimethyl) (methyl) (solvent) | T52.2X1 | T52.2X2 | T52.2X3 | T52.2X4 | — | — |
| **Benzethonium** (chloride) | T49.ØX1 | T49.ØX2 | T49.ØX3 | T49.ØX4 | T49.ØX5 | T49.ØX6 |
| **Benzfetamine** | T5Ø.5X1 | T5Ø.5X2 | T5Ø.5X3 | T5Ø.5X4 | T5Ø.5X5 | T5Ø.5X6 |
| **Benzhexol** | T44.3X1 | T44.3X2 | T44.3X3 | T44.3X4 | T44.3X5 | T44.3X6 |
| **Benzhydramine** (chloride) | T45.ØX1 | T45.ØX2 | T45.ØX3 | T45.ØX4 | T45.ØX5 | T45.ØX6 |
| **Benzidine** | T65.891 | T65.892 | T65.893 | T65.894 | — | — |
| **Benzilonium bromide** | T44.3X1 | T44.3X2 | T44.3X3 | T44.3X4 | T44.3X5 | T44.3X6 |
| **Benzimidazole** | T6Ø.3X1 | T6Ø.3X2 | T6Ø.3X3 | T6Ø.3X4 | — | — |
| **Benzin** (e) — *see* Ligroin | | | | | | |
| **Benziodarone** | T46.3X1 | T46.3X2 | T46.3X3 | T46.3X4 | T46.3X5 | T46.3X6 |
| **Benznidazole** | T37.3X1 | T37.3X2 | T37.3X3 | T37.3X4 | T37.3X5 | T37.3X6 |
| **Benzocaine** | T41.3X1 | T41.3X2 | T41.3X3 | T41.3X4 | T41.3X5 | T41.3X6 |
| **Benzocol*** | T41.3X1 | T41.3X2 | T41.3X3 | T41.3X4 | T41.3X5 | T41.3X6 |
| **Benzodiapin** | T42.4X1 | T42.4X2 | T42.4X3 | T42.4X4 | T42.4X5 | T42.4X6 |
| **Benzodiazepine NEC** | T42.4X1 | T42.4X2 | T42.4X3 | T42.4X4 | T42.4X5 | T42.4X6 |
| **Benzoic acid** | T49.ØX1 | T49.ØX2 | T49.ØX3 | T49.ØX4 | T49.ØX5 | T49.ØX6 |
| with salicylic acid | T49.ØX1 | T49.ØX2 | T49.ØX3 | T49.ØX4 | T49.ØX5 | T49.ØX6 |
| **Benzoin** (tincture) | T48.5X1 | T48.5X2 | T48.5X3 | T48.5X4 | T48.5X5 | T48.5X6 |
| **Benzol** (benzene) | T52.1X1 | T52.1X2 | T52.1X3 | T52.1X4 | — | — |
| vapor | T52.ØX1 | T52.ØX2 | T52.ØX3 | T52.ØX4 | — | — |
| **Benzomorphan** | T4Ø.2X1 | T4Ø.2X2 | T4Ø.2X3 | T4Ø.2X4 | T4Ø.2X5 | T4Ø.2X6 |
| **Benzonatate** | T48.3X1 | T48.3X2 | T48.3X3 | T48.3X4 | T48.3X5 | T48.3X6 |
| **Benzophenones** | T49.3X1 | T49.3X2 | T49.3X3 | T49.3X4 | T49.3X5 | T49.3X6 |
| **Benzopyrone** | T46.991 | T46.992 | T46.993 | T46.994 | T46.995 | T46.996 |
| **Benzothiadiazides** | T5Ø.2X1 | T5Ø.2X2 | T5Ø.2X3 | T5Ø.2X4 | T5Ø.2X5 | T5Ø.2X6 |
| **Benzoxonium chloride** | T49.ØX1 | T49.ØX2 | T49.ØX3 | T49.ØX4 | T49.ØX5 | T49.ØX6 |
| **Benzoyl peroxide** | T49.ØX1 | T49.ØX2 | T49.ØX3 | T49.ØX4 | T49.ØX5 | T49.ØX6 |
| **Benzoylpas calcium** | T37.1X1 | T37.1X2 | T37.1X3 | T37.1X4 | T37.1X5 | T37.1X6 |
| **Benzperidin** | T43.591 | T43.592 | T43.593 | T43.594 | T43.595 | T43.596 |
| **Benzperidol** | T43.591 | T43.592 | T43.593 | T43.594 | T43.595 | T43.596 |

| Substance | Poisoning, Accidental (unintentional) | Poisoning, Intentional Self-harm | Poisoning, Assault | Poisoning, Undetermined | Adverse Effect | Under-dosing |
|---|---|---|---|---|---|---|
| **Benzphetamine** | T5Ø.5X1 | T5Ø.5X2 | T5Ø.5X3 | T5Ø.5X4 | T5Ø.5X5 | T5Ø.5X6 |
| **Benzpyrinium bromide** | T44.1X1 | T44.1X2 | T44.1X3 | T44.1X4 | T44.1X5 | T44.1X6 |
| **Benzquinamide** | T45.ØX1 | T45.ØX2 | T45.ØX3 | T45.ØX4 | T45.ØX5 | T45.ØX6 |
| **Benzthiazide** | T5Ø.2X1 | T5Ø.2X2 | T5Ø.2X3 | T5Ø.2X4 | T5Ø.2X5 | T5Ø.2X6 |
| **Benztropine** | | | | | | |
| anticholinergic | T44.3X1 | T44.3X2 | T44.3X3 | T44.3X4 | T44.3X5 | T44.3X6 |
| antiparkinson | T42.8X1 | T42.8X2 | T42.8X3 | T42.8X4 | T42.8X5 | T42.8X6 |
| **Benzydamine** | T49.ØX1 | T49.ØX2 | T49.ØX3 | T49.ØX4 | T49.ØX5 | T49.ØX6 |
| **Benzyl** | | | | | | |
| acetate | T52.891 | T52.892 | T52.893 | T52.894 | — | — |
| alcohol | T49.ØX1 | T49.ØX2 | T49.ØX3 | T49.ØX4 | T49.ØX5 | T49.ØX6 |
| benzoate | T49.ØX1 | T49.ØX2 | T49.ØX3 | T49.ØX4 | T49.ØX5 | T49.ØX6 |
| Benzoic acid | T49.ØX1 | T49.ØX2 | T49.ØX3 | T49.ØX4 | T49.ØX5 | T49.ØX6 |
| hydroquinone* | T49.4X1 | T49.4X2 | T49.4X3 | T49.4X4 | T49.4X5 | T49.4X6 |
| morphine | T4Ø.2X1 | T4Ø.2X2 | T4Ø.2X3 | T4Ø.2X4 | — | — |
| nicotinate | T46.6X1 | T46.6X2 | T46.6X3 | T46.6X4 | T46.6X5 | T46.6X6 |
| penicillin | T36.ØX1 | T36.ØX2 | T36.ØX3 | T36.ØX4 | T36.ØX5 | T36.ØX6 |
| **Benzylhydrochlorothiazide** | T5Ø.2X1 | T5Ø.2X2 | T5Ø.2X3 | T5Ø.2X4 | T5Ø.2X5 | T5Ø.2X6 |
| **Benzylpenicillin** | T36.ØX1 | T36.ØX2 | T36.ØX3 | T36.ØX4 | T36.ØX5 | T36.ØX6 |
| **Benzylthiouracil** | T38.2X1 | T38.2X2 | T38.2X3 | T38.2X4 | T38.2X5 | T38.2X6 |
| **Bephenium hydroxynaphthoate** | T37.4X1 | T37.4X2 | T37.4X3 | T37.4X4 | T37.4X5 | T37.4X6 |
| **Bepridil** | T46.1X1 | T46.1X2 | T46.1X3 | T46.1X4 | T46.1X5 | T46.1X6 |
| **Bergamot oil** | T65.891 | T65.892 | T65.893 | T65.894 | — | — |
| **Bergapten** | T5Ø.991 | T5Ø.992 | T5Ø.993 | T5Ø.994 | T5Ø.995 | T5Ø.996 |
| **Berries, poisonous** | T62.1X1 | T62.1X2 | T62.1X3 | T62.1X4 | — | — |
| **Beryllium** (compounds) | T56.7X1 | T56.7X2 | T56.7X3 | T56.7X4 | — | — |
| **beta adrenergic blocking agent, heart** | T44.7X1 | T44.7X2 | T44.7X3 | T44.7X4 | T44.7X5 | T44.7X6 |
| **Beta-Chlor** | T42.6X1 | T42.6X2 | T42.6X3 | T42.6X4 | T42.6X5 | T42.6X6 |
| **Betacarotene** | T45.2X1 | T45.2X2 | T45.2X3 | T45.2X4 | T45.2X5 | T45.2X6 |
| **Betahistine** | T46.7X1 | T46.7X2 | T46.7X3 | T46.7X4 | T46.7X5 | T46.7X6 |
| **Betaine** | T47.5X1 | T47.5X2 | T47.5X3 | T47.5X4 | T47.5X5 | T47.5X6 |
| **Betamethasone** | T49.ØX1 | T49.ØX2 | T49.ØX3 | T49.ØX4 | T49.ØX5 | T49.ØX6 |
| topical | T49.ØX1 | T49.ØX2 | T49.ØX3 | T49.ØX4 | T49.ØX5 | T49.ØX6 |
| **Betamicin** | T36.8X1 | T36.8X2 | T36.8X3 | T36.8X4 | T36.8X5 | T36.8X6 |
| **Betanidine** | T46.5X1 | T46.5X2 | T46.5X3 | T46.5X4 | T46.5X5 | T46.5X6 |
| **Betaxolol** | T44.7X1 | T44.7X2 | T44.7X3 | T44.7X4 | T44.7X5 | T44.7X6 |
| **Betazole** | T5Ø.8X1 | T5Ø.8X2 | T5Ø.8X3 | T5Ø.8X4 | T5Ø.8X5 | T5Ø.8X6 |
| **Bethanechol** | T44.1X1 | T44.1X2 | T44.1X3 | T44.1X4 | T44.1X5 | T44.1X6 |
| chloride | T44.1X1 | T44.1X2 | T44.1X3 | T44.1X4 | T44.1X5 | T44.1X6 |
| **Bethanidine** | T46.5X1 | T46.5X2 | T46.5X3 | T46.5X4 | T46.5X5 | T46.5X6 |
| **Betoxycaine** | T41.3X1 | T41.3X2 | T41.3X3 | T41.3X4 | T41.3X5 | T41.3X6 |
| **Betula oil** | T49.3X1 | T49.3X2 | T49.3X3 | T49.3X4 | T49.3X5 | T49.3X6 |
| **Bevantolol** | T44.7X1 | T44.7X2 | T44.7X3 | T44.7X4 | T44.7X5 | T44.7X6 |
| **Bevonium metilsulfate** | T44.3X1 | T44.3X2 | T44.3X3 | T44.3X4 | T44.3X5 | T44.3X6 |
| **Bezafibrate** | T46.6X1 | T46.6X2 | T46.6X3 | T46.6X4 | T46.6X5 | T46.6X6 |
| **Bezitramide** | T4Ø.491 | T4Ø.492 | T4Ø.493 | T4Ø.494 | T4Ø.495 | T4Ø.496 |
| **BHA** | T5Ø.991 | T5Ø.992 | T5Ø.993 | T5Ø.994 | T5Ø.995 | T5Ø.996 |
| **Bhang+C394** | T4Ø.711 | T4Ø.712 | T4Ø.713 | T4Ø.714 | T4Ø.715 | T4Ø.716 |
| **BHC** (medicinal) | T49.ØX1 | T49.ØX2 | T49.ØX3 | T49.ØX4 | T49.ØX5 | T49.ØX6 |
| nonmedicinal (vapor) | T53.6X1 | T53.6X2 | T53.6X3 | T53.6X4 | — | — |
| **Bialamicol** | T37.3X1 | T37.3X2 | T37.3X3 | T37.3X4 | T37.3X5 | T37.3X6 |
| **Bibenzonium bromide** | T48.3X1 | T48.3X2 | T48.3X3 | T48.3X4 | T48.3X5 | T48.3X6 |
| **Bibrocathol** | T49.5X1 | T49.5X2 | T49.5X3 | T49.5X4 | T49.5X5 | T49.5X6 |
| **Bichloride of mercury** — *see* Mercury, chloride | | | | | | |
| **Bichromates** (calcium) (potassium)(sodium) (crystals) | T57.8X1 | T57.8X2 | T57.8X3 | T57.8X4 | — | — |
| fumes | T56.2X1 | T56.2X2 | T56.2X3 | T56.2X4 | — | — |
| **Biclotymol** | T49.6X1 | T49.6X2 | T49.6X3 | T49.6X4 | T49.6X5 | T49.6X6 |
| **BiCNU*** | T45.1X1 | T45.1X2 | T45.1X3 | T45.1X4 | T45.1X5 | T45.1X6 |
| **Bicucculine** | T5Ø.7X1 | T5Ø.7X2 | T5Ø.7X3 | T5Ø.7X4 | T5Ø.7X5 | T5Ø.7X6 |
| **Bifemelane** | T43.291 | T43.292 | T43.293 | T43.294 | T43.295 | T43.296 |
| **Biguanide derivatives, oral** | T38.3X1 | T38.3X2 | T38.3X3 | T38.3X4 | T38.3X5 | T38.3X6 |
| **Bile salts** | T47.5X1 | T47.5X2 | T47.5X3 | T47.5X4 | T47.5X5 | T47.5X6 |
| **Biligrafin** | T5Ø.8X1 | T5Ø.8X2 | T5Ø.8X3 | T5Ø.8X4 | T5Ø.8X5 | T5Ø.8X6 |
| **Bilopaque** | T5Ø.8X1 | T5Ø.8X2 | T5Ø.8X3 | T5Ø.8X4 | T5Ø.8X5 | T5Ø.8X6 |
| **Binifibrate** | T46.6X1 | T46.6X2 | T46.6X3 | T46.6X4 | T46.6X5 | T46.6X6 |
| **Binitrobenzol** | T65.3X1 | T65.3X2 | T65.3X3 | T65.3X4 | — | — |
| **Bioflavonoid**(s) | T46.991 | T46.992 | T46.993 | T46.994 | T46.995 | T46.996 |
| **Biological substance NEC** | T5Ø.9Ø1 | T5Ø.9Ø2 | T5Ø.9Ø3 | T5Ø.9Ø4 | T5Ø.9Ø5 | T5Ø.9Ø6 |
| **Biotin** | T45.2X1 | T45.2X2 | T45.2X3 | T45.2X4 | T45.2X5 | T45.2X6 |
| **Biperiden** | T44.3X1 | T44.3X2 | T44.3X3 | T44.3X4 | T44.3X5 | T44.3X6 |
| **Bisacodyl** | T47.2X1 | T47.2X2 | T47.2X3 | T47.2X4 | T47.2X5 | T47.2X6 |
| **Bisbentiamine** | T45.2X1 | T45.2X2 | T45.2X3 | T45.2X4 | T45.2X5 | T45.2X6 |
| **Bisbutiamine** | T45.2X1 | T45.2X2 | T45.2X3 | T45.2X4 | T45.2X5 | T45.2X6 |
| **Bisdequalinium** (salts) (diacetate) | T49.6X1 | T49.6X2 | T49.6X3 | T49.6X4 | T49.6X5 | T49.6X6 |
| **Bishydroxycoumarin** | T45.511 | T45.512 | T45.513 | T45.514 | T45.515 | T45.516 |
| **Bismarsen** | T37.8X1 | T37.8X2 | T37.8X3 | T37.8X4 | T37.8X5 | T37.8X6 |

| Substance | Poisoning, Accidental (unintentional) | Poisoning, Intentional Self-harm | Poisoning, Assault | Poisoning, Undetermined | Adverse Effect | Under-dosing |
|---|---|---|---|---|---|---|
| **Bismuth salts** | T47.6X1 | T47.6X2 | T47.6X3 | T47.6X4 | T47.6X5 | T47.6X6 |
| aluminate | T47.1X1 | T47.1X2 | T47.1X3 | T47.1X4 | T47.1X5 | T47.1X6 |
| anti-infectives | T37.8X1 | T37.8X2 | T37.8X3 | T37.8X4 | T37.8X5 | T37.8X6 |
| formic iodide | T49.ØX1 | T49.ØX2 | T49.ØX3 | T49.ØX4 | T49.ØX5 | T49.ØX6 |
| glycolylarsenate | T49.ØX1 | T49.ØX2 | T49.ØX3 | T49.ØX4 | T49.ØX5 | T49.ØX6 |
| nonmedicinal (compounds) NEC | T65.91 | T65.92 | T65.93 | T65.94 | — | — |
| subcarbonate | T47.6X1 | T47.6X2 | T47.6X3 | T47.6X4 | T47.6X5 | T47.6X6 |
| subsalicylate | T37.8X1 | T37.8X2 | T37.8X3 | T37.8X4 | T37.8X5 | T37.8X6 |
| sulfarsphenamine | T37.8X1 | T37.8X2 | T37.8X3 | T37.8X4 | T37.8X5 | T37.8X6 |
| **Bisoprolol** | T44.7X1 | T44.7X2 | T44.7X3 | T44.7X4 | T44.7X5 | T44.7X6 |
| **Bisoxatin** | T47.2X1 | T47.2X2 | T47.2X3 | T47.2X4 | T47.2X5 | T47.2X6 |
| **Bisulepin** (hydrochloride) | T45.ØX1 | T45.ØX2 | T45.ØX3 | T45.ØX4 | T45.ØX5 | T45.ØX6 |
| **Bithionol** | T37.8X1 | T37.8X2 | T37.8X3 | T37.8X4 | T37.8X5 | T37.8X6 |
| anthelmintic | T37.4X1 | T37.4X2 | T37.4X3 | T37.4X4 | T37.4X5 | T37.4X6 |
| **Bitolterol** | T48.6X1 | T48.6X2 | T48.6X3 | T48.6X4 | T48.6X5 | T48.6X6 |
| **Bitoscanate** | T37.4X1 | T37.4X2 | T37.4X3 | T37.4X4 | T37.4X5 | T37.4X6 |
| **Bitter almond oil** | T62.8X1 | T62.8X2 | T62.8X3 | T62.8X4 | — | — |
| **Bittersweet** | T62.2X1 | T62.2X2 | T62.2X3 | T62.2X4 | — | — |
| **Bivalirudin*** | T45.511 | T45.512 | T45.513 | T45.514 | T45.515 | T45.516 |
| **Black** | | | | | | |
| flag | T6Ø.91 | T6Ø.92 | T6Ø.93 | T6Ø.94 | — | — |
| henbane | T62.2X1 | T62.2X2 | T62.2X3 | T62.2X4 | — | — |
| leaf (40) | T6Ø.91 | T6Ø.92 | T6Ø.93 | T6Ø.94 | — | — |
| widow spider (bite) | T63.311 | T63.312 | T63.313 | T63.314 | — | — |
| antivenin | T5Ø.Z11 | T5Ø.Z12 | T5Ø.Z13 | T5Ø.Z14 | T5Ø.Z15 | T5Ø.Z16 |
| **Blast furnace gas** (carbon monoxide from) | T58.8X1 | T58.8X2 | T58.8X3 | T58.8X4 | — | — |
| **Bleach** | T54.91 | T54.92 | T54.93 | T54.94 | — | — |
| **Bleaching agent** (medicinal) | T49.4X1 | T49.4X2 | T49.4X3 | T49.4X4 | T49.4X5 | T49.4X6 |
| **Bleomycin** | T45.1X1 | T45.1X2 | T45.1X3 | T45.1X4 | T45.1X5 | T45.1X6 |
| **Blockain** | T41.3X1 | T41.3X2 | T41.3X3 | T41.3X4 | T41.3X5 | T41.3X6 |
| infiltration (subcutaneous) | T41.3X1 | T41.3X2 | T41.3X3 | T41.3X4 | T41.3X5 | T41.3X6 |
| nerve block (peripheral) (plexus) | T41.3X1 | T41.3X2 | T41.3X3 | T41.3X4 | T41.3X5 | T41.3X6 |
| topical (surface) | T41.3X1 | T41.3X2 | T41.3X3 | T41.3X4 | T41.3X5 | T41.3X6 |
| **Blockers, calcium channel** | T46.1X1 | T46.1X2 | T46.1X3 | T46.1X4 | T46.1X5 | T46.1X6 |
| **Blood** (derivatives) (natural) (plasma) (whole) | T45.8X1 | T45.8X2 | T45.8X3 | T45.8X4 | T45.8X5 | T45.8X6 |
| dried | T45.8X1 | T45.8X2 | T45.8X3 | T45.8X4 | T45.8X5 | T45.8X6 |
| drug affecting NEC | T45.91 | T45.92 | T45.93 | T45.94 | T45.95 | T45.96 |
| expander NEC | T45.8X1 | T45.8X2 | T45.8X3 | T45.8X4 | T45.8X5 | T45.8X6 |
| fraction NEC | T45.8X1 | T45.8X2 | T45.8X3 | T45.8X4 | T45.8X5 | T45.8X6 |
| substitute (macromolecular) | T45.8X1 | T45.8X2 | T45.8X3 | T45.8X4 | T45.8X5 | T45.8X6 |
| **Blue velvet** | T4Ø.2X1 | T4Ø.2X2 | T4Ø.2X3 | T4Ø.2X4 | — | — |
| **Bone meal** | T62.8X1 | T62.8X2 | T62.8X3 | T62.8X4 | — | — |
| **Bonine** | T45.ØX1 | T45.ØX2 | T45.ØX3 | T45.ØX4 | T45.ØX5 | T45.ØX6 |
| **Bontril*** | T5Ø.5X1 | T5Ø.5X2 | T5Ø.5X3 | T5Ø.5X4 | T5Ø.5X5 | T5Ø.5X6 |
| **Bopindolol** | T44.7X1 | T44.7X2 | T44.7X3 | T44.7X4 | T44.7X5 | T44.7X6 |
| **Boracic acid** | T49.ØX1 | T49.ØX2 | T49.ØX3 | T49.ØX4 | T49.ØX5 | T49.ØX6 |
| ENT agent | T49.6X1 | T49.6X2 | T49.6X3 | T49.6X4 | T49.6X5 | T49.6X6 |
| ophthalmic preparation | T49.5X1 | T49.5X2 | T49.5X3 | T49.5X4 | T49.5X5 | T49.5X6 |
| **Borane complex** | T57.8X1 | T57.8X2 | T57.8X3 | T57.8X4 | — | — |
| **Borate**(s) | T57.8X1 | T57.8X2 | T57.8X3 | T57.8X4 | — | — |
| buffer | T5Ø.991 | T5Ø.992 | T5Ø.993 | T5Ø.994 | T5Ø.995 | T5Ø.996 |
| cleanser | T54.91 | T54.92 | T54.93 | T54.94 | — | — |
| sodium | T57.8X1 | T57.8X2 | T57.8X3 | T57.8X4 | — | — |
| **Borax** (cleanser) | T54.91 | T54.92 | T54.93 | T54.94 | — | — |
| **Bordeaux mixture** | T6Ø.3X1 | T6Ø.3X2 | T6Ø.3X3 | T6Ø.3X4 | — | — |
| **Boric acid** | T49.ØX1 | T49.ØX2 | T49.ØX3 | T49.ØX4 | T49.ØX5 | T49.ØX6 |
| ENT agent | T49.6X1 | T49.6X2 | T49.6X3 | T49.6X4 | T49.6X5 | T49.6X6 |
| ophthalmic preparation | T49.5X1 | T49.5X2 | T49.5X3 | T49.5X4 | T49.5X5 | T49.5X6 |
| **Bornaprine** | T44.3X1 | T44.3X2 | T44.3X3 | T44.3X4 | T44.3X5 | T44.3X6 |
| **Boron** | T57.8X1 | T57.8X2 | T57.8X3 | T57.8X4 | — | — |
| hydride NEC | T57.8X1 | T57.8X2 | T57.8X3 | T57.8X4 | — | — |
| fumes or gas | T57.8X1 | T57.8X2 | T57.8X3 | T57.8X4 | — | — |
| trifluoride | T59.891 | T59.892 | T59.893 | T59.894 | — | — |
| **Botox** | T48.291 | T48.292 | T48.293 | T48.294 | T48.295 | T48.296 |
| **Botulinus anti-toxin** (type A, B) | T5Ø.Z11 | T5Ø.Z12 | T5Ø.Z13 | T5Ø.Z14 | T5Ø.Z15 | T5Ø.Z16 |
| **Brake fluid vapor** | T59.891 | T59.892 | T59.893 | T59.894 | — | — |
| **Brallobarbital** | T42.3X1 | T42.3X2 | T42.3X3 | T42.3X4 | T42.3X5 | T42.3X6 |
| **Bran** (wheat) | T47.4X1 | T47.4X2 | T47.4X3 | T47.4X4 | T47.4X5 | T47.4X6 |
| **Brass** (fumes) | T56.891 | T56.892 | T56.893 | T56.894 | — | — |
| **Brasso** | T52.ØX1 | T52.ØX2 | T52.ØX3 | T52.ØX4 | — | — |
| **Bretylium tosilate** | T46.2X1 | T46.2X2 | T46.2X3 | T46.2X4 | T46.2X5 | T46.2X6 |
| **Brevital** (sodium) | T41.1X1 | T41.1X2 | T41.1X3 | T41.1X4 | T41.1X5 | T41.1X6 |
| **Brinase** | T45.3X1 | T45.3X2 | T45.3X3 | T45.3X4 | T45.3X5 | T45.3X6 |
| **British antilewisite** | T45.8X1 | T45.8X2 | T45.8X3 | T45.8X4 | T45.8X5 | T45.8X6 |
| **Brodalumab*** | T5Ø.991 | T5Ø.992 | T5Ø.993 | T5Ø.994 | T5Ø.995 | T5Ø.996 |
| **Brodifacoum** | T6Ø.4X1 | T6Ø.4X2 | T6Ø.4X3 | T6Ø.4X4 | — | — |

| Substance | Poisoning, Accidental (unintentional) | Poisoning, Intentional Self-harm | Poisoning, Assault | Poisoning, Undetermined | Adverse Effect | Under-dosing |
|---|---|---|---|---|---|---|
| **Bromal** (hydrate) | T42.6X1 | T42.6X2 | T42.6X3 | T42.6X4 | T42.6X5 | T42.6X6 |
| **Bromazepam** | T42.4X1 | T42.4X2 | T42.4X3 | T42.4X4 | T42.4X5 | T42.4X6 |
| **Bromazine** | T45.ØX1 | T45.ØX2 | T45.ØX3 | T45.ØX4 | T45.ØX5 | T45.ØX6 |
| **Brombenzylcyanide** | T59.3X1 | T59.3X2 | T59.3X3 | T59.3X4 | — | — |
| **Bromelains** | T45.3X1 | T45.3X2 | T45.3X3 | T45.3X4 | T45.3X5 | T45.3X6 |
| **Bromethalin** | T6Ø.4X1 | T6Ø.4X2 | T6Ø.4X3 | T6Ø.4X4 | — | — |
| **Bromhexine** | T48.4X1 | T48.4X2 | T48.4X3 | T48.4X4 | T48.4X5 | T48.4X6 |
| **Bromide salts** | T42.6X1 | T42.6X2 | T42.6X3 | T42.6X4 | T42.6X5 | T42.6X6 |
| **Bromindione** | T45.511 | T45.512 | T45.513 | T45.514 | T45.515 | T45.516 |
| **Bromine** | | | | | | |
| compounds (medicinal) | T42.6X1 | T42.6X2 | T42.6X3 | T42.6X4 | T42.6X5 | T42.6X6 |
| sedative | T42.6X1 | T42.6X2 | T42.6X3 | T42.6X4 | T42.6X5 | T42.6X6 |
| vapor | T59.891 | T59.892 | T59.893 | T59.894 | — | — |
| **Bromisoval** | T42.6X1 | T42.6X2 | T42.6X3 | T42.6X4 | T42.6X5 | T42.6X6 |
| **Bromisovalum** | T42.6X1 | T42.6X2 | T42.6X3 | T42.6X4 | T42.6X5 | T42.6X6 |
| **Bromo-seltzer** | T39.1X1 | T39.1X2 | T39.1X3 | T39.1X4 | T39.1X5 | T39.1X6 |
| **Bromobenzylcyanide** | T59.3X1 | T59.3X2 | T59.3X3 | T59.3X4 | — | — |
| **Bromochlorosalicylanilide** | T49.ØX1 | T49.ØX2 | T49.ØX3 | T49.ØX4 | T49.ØX5 | T49.ØX6 |
| **Bromocriptine** | T42.8X1 | T42.8X2 | T42.8X3 | T42.8X4 | T42.8X5 | T42.8X6 |
| **Bromodiphenhydramine** | T45.ØX1 | T45.ØX2 | T45.ØX3 | T45.ØX4 | T45.ØX5 | T45.ØX6 |
| **Bromoform** | T42.6X1 | T42.6X2 | T42.6X3 | T42.6X4 | T42.6X5 | T42.6X6 |
| **Bromophenol blue reagent** | T5Ø.991 | T5Ø.992 | T5Ø.993 | T5Ø.994 | T5Ø.995 | T5Ø.996 |
| **Bromopride** | T47.8X1 | T47.8X2 | T47.8X3 | T47.8X4 | T47.8X5 | T47.8X6 |
| **Bromosalicylchloranitide** | T49.ØX1 | T49.ØX2 | T49.ØX3 | T49.ØX4 | T49.ØX5 | T49.ØX6 |
| **Bromosalicylhydroxamic acid** | T37.1X1 | T37.1X2 | T37.1X3 | T37.1X4 | T37.1X5 | T37.1X6 |
| **Bromoxynil** | T6Ø.3X1 | T6Ø.3X2 | T6Ø.3X3 | T6Ø.3X4 | — | — |
| **Bromperidol** | T43.4X1 | T43.4X2 | T43.4X3 | T43.4X4 | T43.4X5 | T43.4X6 |
| **Brompheniramine** | T45.ØX1 | T45.ØX2 | T45.ØX3 | T45.ØX4 | T45.ØX5 | T45.ØX6 |
| **Bromsulfophthalein** | T5Ø.8X1 | T5Ø.8X2 | T5Ø.8X3 | T5Ø.8X4 | T5Ø.8X5 | T5Ø.8X6 |
| **Bromural** | T42.6X1 | T42.6X2 | T42.6X3 | T42.6X4 | T42.6X5 | T42.6X6 |
| **Bromvaletone** | T42.6X1 | T42.6X2 | T42.6X3 | T42.6X4 | T42.6X5 | T42.6X6 |
| **Bronchodilator NEC** | T48.6X1 | T48.6X2 | T48.6X3 | T48.6X4 | T48.6X5 | T48.6X6 |
| **Brotizolam** | T42.4X1 | T42.4X2 | T42.4X3 | T42.4X4 | T42.4X5 | T42.4X6 |
| **Brovincamine** | T46.7X1 | T46.7X2 | T46.7X3 | T46.7X4 | T46.7X5 | T46.7X6 |
| **Brown recluse spider** (bite) (venom) | T63.331 | T63.332 | T63.333 | T63.334 | — | — |
| **Brown spider** (bite) (venom) | T63.391 | T63.392 | T63.393 | T63.394 | — | — |
| **Broxaterol** | T48.6X1 | T48.6X2 | T48.6X3 | T48.6X4 | T48.6X5 | T48.6X6 |
| **Broxuridine** | T45.1X1 | T45.1X2 | T45.1X3 | T45.1X4 | T45.1X5 | T45.1X6 |
| **Broxyquinoline** | T37.8X1 | T37.8X2 | T37.8X3 | T37.8X4 | T37.8X5 | T37.8X6 |
| **Bruceine** | T48.291 | T48.292 | T48.293 | T48.294 | T48.295 | T48.296 |
| **Brucia** | T62.2X1 | T62.2X2 | T62.2X3 | T62.2X4 | — | — |
| **Brucine** | T65.1X1 | T65.1X2 | T65.1X3 | T65.1X4 | — | — |
| **Brunswick green** — *see* Copper | | | | | | |
| **Bruten** — *see* Ibuprofen | | | | | | |
| **Bryonia** | T47.2X1 | T47.2X2 | T47.2X3 | T47.2X4 | T47.2X5 | T47.2X6 |
| **Buclizine** | T45.ØX1 | T45.ØX2 | T45.ØX3 | T45.ØX4 | T45.ØX5 | T45.ØX6 |
| **Buclosamide** | T49.ØX1 | T49.ØX2 | T49.ØX3 | T49.ØX4 | T49.ØX5 | T49.ØX6 |
| **Budesonide** | T44.5X1 | T44.5X2 | T44.5X3 | T44.5X4 | T44.5X5 | T44.5X6 |
| **Budralazine** | T46.5X1 | T46.5X2 | T46.5X3 | T46.5X4 | T46.5X5 | T46.5X6 |
| **Bufferin** | T39.Ø11 | T39.Ø12 | T39.Ø13 | T39.Ø14 | T39.Ø15 | T39.Ø16 |
| **Buflomedil** | T46.7X1 | T46.7X2 | T46.7X3 | T46.7X4 | T46.7X5 | T46.7X6 |
| **Buformin** | T38.3X1 | T38.3X2 | T38.3X3 | T38.3X4 | T38.3X5 | T38.3X6 |
| **Bufotenine** | T4Ø.991 | T4Ø.992 | T4Ø.993 | T4Ø.994 | — | — |
| **Bufrolin** | T48.6X1 | T48.6X2 | T48.6X3 | T48.6X4 | T48.6X5 | T48.6X6 |
| **Bufylline** | T48.6X1 | T48.6X2 | T48.6X3 | T48.6X4 | T48.6X5 | T48.6X6 |
| **Bulgaricum IB*** | T47.6X1 | T47.6X2 | T47.6X3 | T47.6X4 | T47.6X5 | T47.6X6 |
| **Bulk filler** | T5Ø.5X1 | T5Ø.5X2 | T5Ø.5X3 | T5Ø.5X4 | T5Ø.5X5 | T5Ø.5X6 |
| cathartic | T47.4X1 | T47.4X2 | T47.4X3 | T47.4X4 | T47.4X5 | T47.4X6 |
| **Bumetanide** | T5Ø.1X1 | T5Ø.1X2 | T5Ø.1X3 | T5Ø.1X4 | T5Ø.1X5 | T5Ø.1X6 |
| **Bunaftine** | T46.2X1 | T46.2X2 | T46.2X3 | T46.2X4 | T46.2X5 | T46.2X6 |
| **Bunamiodyl** | T5Ø.8X1 | T5Ø.8X2 | T5Ø.8X3 | T5Ø.8X4 | T5Ø.8X5 | T5Ø.8X6 |
| **Bunazosin** | T44.6X1 | T44.6X2 | T44.6X3 | T44.6X4 | T44.6X5 | T44.6X6 |
| **Bunitrolol** | T44.7X1 | T44.7X2 | T44.7X3 | T44.7X4 | T44.7X5 | T44.7X6 |
| **Buphenine** | T46.7X1 | T46.7X2 | T46.7X3 | T46.7X4 | T46.7X5 | T46.7X6 |
| **Bupivacaine** | T41.3X1 | T41.3X2 | T41.3X3 | T41.3X4 | T41.3X5 | T41.3X6 |
| infiltration (subcutaneous) | T41.3X1 | T41.3X2 | T41.3X3 | T41.3X4 | T41.3X5 | T41.3X6 |
| nerve block (peripheral) (plexus) | T41.3X1 | T41.3X2 | T41.3X3 | T41.3X4 | T41.3X5 | T41.3X6 |
| spinal | T41.3X1 | T41.3X2 | T41.3X3 | T41.3X4 | T41.3X5 | T41.3X6 |
| **Bupranolol** | T44.7X1 | T44.7X2 | T44.7X3 | T44.7X4 | T44.7X5 | T44.7X6 |
| **Buprenorphine** | T4Ø.491 | T4Ø.492 | T4Ø.493 | T4Ø.494 | T4Ø.495 | T4Ø.496 |
| **Bupropion** | T43.291 | T43.292 | T43.293 | T43.294 | T43.295 | T43.296 |
| **Burimamide** | T47.1X1 | T47.1X2 | T47.1X3 | T47.1X4 | T47.1X5 | T47.1X6 |
| **Buserelin** | T38.891 | T38.892 | T38.893 | T38.894 | T38.895 | T38.896 |
| **Buspirone** | T43.591 | T43.592 | T43.593 | T43.594 | T43.595 | T43.596 |
| **Busulfan, busulphan** | T45.1X1 | T45.1X2 | T45.1X3 | T45.1X4 | T45.1X5 | T45.1X6 |
| **Busulfex*** | T45.1X1 | T45.1X2 | T45.1X3 | T45.1X4 | T45.1X5 | T45.1X6 |
| **Butabarbital** (sodium) | T42.3X1 | T42.3X2 | T42.3X3 | T42.3X4 | T42.3X5 | T42.3X6 |
| **Butabarbitone** | T42.3X1 | T42.3X2 | T42.3X3 | T42.3X4 | T42.3X5 | T42.3X6 |

| Substance | Poisoning, Accidental (unintentional) | Poisoning, Intentional Self-harm | Poisoning, Assault | Poisoning, Undetermined | Adverse Effect | Under-dosing |
|---|---|---|---|---|---|---|
| **Butabarpal** | T42.3X1 | T42.3X2 | T42.3X3 | T42.3X4 | T42.3X5 | T42.3X6 |
| **Butacaine** | T41.3X1 | T41.3X2 | T41.3X3 | T41.3X4 | T41.3X5 | T41.3X6 |
| **Butalamine** | T46.7X1 | T46.7X2 | T46.7X3 | T46.7X4 | T46.7X5 | T46.7X6 |
| **Butalbital** | T42.3X1 | T42.3X2 | T42.3X3 | T42.3X4 | T42.3X5 | T42.3X6 |
| **Butallylonal** | T42.3X1 | T42.3X2 | T42.3X3 | T42.3X4 | T42.3X5 | T42.3X6 |
| **Butamben** | T41.3X1 | T41.3X2 | T41.3X3 | T41.3X4 | T41.3X5 | T41.3X6 |
| **Butamirate** | T48.3X1 | T48.3X2 | T48.3X3 | T48.3X4 | T48.3X5 | T48.3X6 |
| **Butane** (distributed in mobile container) | T59.891 | T59.892 | T59.893 | T59.894 | — | — |
| distributed through pipes | T59.891 | T59.892 | T59.893 | T59.894 | — | — |
| incomplete combustion | T58.11 | T58.12 | T58.13 | T58.14 | — | — |
| **Butanilicaine** | T41.3X1 | T41.3X2 | T41.3X3 | T41.3X4 | T41.3X5 | T41.3X6 |
| **Butanol** | T51.3X1 | T51.3X2 | T51.3X3 | T51.3X4 | — | — |
| **Butanone, 2-butanone** | T52.4X1 | T52.4X2 | T52.4X3 | T52.4X4 | — | — |
| **Butantrone** | T49.4X1 | T49.4X2 | T49.4X3 | T49.4X4 | T49.4X5 | T49.4X6 |
| **Butaperazine** | T43.3X1 | T43.3X2 | T43.3X3 | T43.3X4 | T43.3X5 | T43.3X6 |
| **Butazolidin** | T39.2X1 | T39.2X2 | T39.2X3 | T39.2X4 | T39.2X5 | T39.2X6 |
| **Butetamate** | T48.6X1 | T48.6X2 | T48.6X3 | T48.6X4 | T48.6X5 | T48.6X6 |
| **Butethal** | T42.3X1 | T42.3X2 | T42.3X3 | T42.3X4 | T42.3X5 | T42.3X6 |
| **Butethamate** | T44.3X1 | T44.3X2 | T44.3X3 | T44.3X4 | T44.3X5 | T44.3X6 |
| **Buthalitone** (sodium) | T41.1X1 | T41.1X2 | T41.1X3 | T41.1X4 | T41.1X5 | T41.1X6 |
| **Butisol** (sodium) | T42.3X1 | T42.3X2 | T42.3X3 | T42.3X4 | T42.3X5 | T42.3X6 |
| **Butizide** | T5Ø.2X1 | T5Ø.2X2 | T5Ø.2X3 | T5Ø.2X4 | T5Ø.2X5 | T5Ø.2X6 |
| **Butobarbital** | T42.3X1 | T42.3X2 | T42.3X3 | T42.3X4 | T42.3X5 | T42.3X6 |
| sodium | T42.3X1 | T42.3X2 | T42.3X3 | T42.3X4 | T42.3X5 | T42.3X6 |
| **Butobarbitone** | T42.3X1 | T42.3X2 | T42.3X3 | T42.3X4 | T42.3X5 | T42.3X6 |
| **Butoconazole** (nitrate) | T49.ØX1 | T49.ØX2 | T49.ØX3 | T49.ØX4 | T49.ØX5 | T49.ØX6 |
| **Butorphanol** | T4Ø.491 | T4Ø.492 | T4Ø.493 | T4Ø.494 | T4Ø.495 | T4Ø.496 |
| **Butriptyline** | T43.Ø11 | T43.Ø12 | T43.Ø13 | T43.Ø14 | T43.Ø15 | T43.Ø16 |
| **Butropium bromide** | T44.3X1 | T44.3X2 | T44.3X3 | T44.3X4 | T44.3X5 | T44.3X6 |
| **Butter of antimony** — *see* Antimony | | | | | | |
| **Buttercups** | T62.2X1 | T62.2X2 | T62.2X3 | T62.2X4 | — | — |
| **Butyl** | | | | | | |
| acetate (secondary) | T52.891 | T52.892 | T52.893 | T52.894 | — | — |
| alcohol | T51.3X1 | T51.3X2 | T51.3X3 | T51.3X4 | — | — |
| aminobenzoate | T41.3X1 | T41.3X2 | T41.3X3 | T41.3X4 | T41.3X5 | T41.3X6 |
| butyrate | T52.891 | T52.892 | T52.893 | T52.894 | — | — |
| carbinol | T51.3X1 | T51.3X2 | T51.3X3 | T51.3X4 | — | — |
| carbitol | T52.3X1 | T52.3X2 | T52.3X3 | T52.3X4 | — | — |
| cellosolve | T52.3X1 | T52.3X2 | T52.3X3 | T52.3X4 | — | — |
| chloral (hydrate) | T42.6X1 | T42.6X2 | T42.6X3 | T42.6X4 | T42.6X5 | T42.6X6 |
| formate | T52.891 | T52.892 | T52.893 | T52.894 | — | — |
| lactate | T52.891 | T52.892 | T52.893 | T52.894 | — | — |
| propionate | T52.891 | T52.892 | T52.893 | T52.894 | — | — |
| scopolamine bromide | T44.3X1 | T44.3X2 | T44.3X3 | T44.3X4 | T44.3X5 | T44.3X6 |
| thiobarbital sodium | T41.1X1 | T41.1X2 | T41.1X3 | T41.1X4 | T41.1X5 | T41.1X6 |
| **Butylated hydroxyanisole** | T5Ø.991 | T5Ø.992 | T5Ø.993 | T5Ø.994 | T5Ø.995 | T5Ø.996 |
| **Butylchloral hydrate** | T42.6X1 | T42.6X2 | T42.6X3 | T42.6X4 | T42.6X5 | T42.6X6 |
| **Butyltoluene** | T52.2X1 | T52.2X2 | T52.2X3 | T52.2X4 | — | — |
| **Butyn** | T41.3X1 | T41.3X2 | T41.3X3 | T41.3X4 | T41.3X5 | T41.3X6 |
| **Butyrophenone** (-based tranquilizers) | T43.4X1 | T43.4X2 | T43.4X3 | T43.4X4 | T43.4X5 | T43.4X6 |
| **Cabazitaxel*** | T45.1X1 | T45.1X2 | T45.1X3 | T45.1X4 | T45.1X5 | T45.1X6 |
| **Cabergoline** | T42.8X1 | T42.8X2 | T42.8X3 | T42.8X4 | T42.8X5 | T42.8X6 |
| **Cacodyl, cacodylic acid** | T57.ØX1 | T57.ØX2 | T57.ØX3 | T57.ØX4 | — | — |
| **Cactinomycin** | T45.1X1 | T45.1X2 | T45.1X3 | T45.1X4 | T45.1X5 | T45.1X6 |
| **Cade oil** | T49.4X1 | T49.4X2 | T49.4X3 | T49.4X4 | T49.4X5 | T49.4X6 |
| **Cadexomer iodine** | T49.ØX1 | T49.ØX2 | T49.ØX3 | T49.ØX4 | T49.ØX5 | T49.ØX6 |
| **Cadmium** (chloride) (fumes) (oxide) | T56.3X1 | T56.3X2 | T56.3X3 | T56.3X4 | — | — |
| sulfide (medicinal) NEC | T49.4X1 | T49.4X2 | T49.4X3 | T49.4X4 | T49.4X5 | T49.4X6 |
| **Cadralazine** | T46.5X1 | T46.5X2 | T46.5X3 | T46.5X4 | T46.5X5 | T46.5X6 |
| **Caffeine** | T43.611 | T43.612 | T43.613 | T43.614 | T43.615 | T43.616 |
| **Calabar bean** | T62.2X1 | T62.2X2 | T62.2X3 | T62.2X4 | — | — |
| **Caladium seguinum** | T62.2X1 | T62.2X2 | T62.2X3 | T62.2X4 | — | — |
| **Calamine** (lotion) | T49.3X1 | T49.3X2 | T49.3X3 | T49.3X4 | T49.3X5 | T49.3X6 |
| **Calcifediol** | T45.2X1 | T45.2X2 | T45.2X3 | T45.2X4 | T45.2X5 | T45.2X6 |
| **Calciferol** | T45.2X1 | T45.2X2 | T45.2X3 | T45.2X4 | T45.2X5 | T45.2X6 |
| **Calcijex*** | T45.2X1 | T45.2X2 | T45.2X3 | T45.2X4 | T45.2X5 | T45.2X6 |
| **Calcitonin** | T5Ø.991 | T5Ø.992 | T5Ø.993 | T5Ø.994 | T5Ø.995 | T5Ø.996 |
| **Calcitriol** | T45.2X1 | T45.2X2 | T45.2X3 | T45.2X4 | T45.2X5 | T45.2X6 |
| **Calcium** | T5Ø.3X1 | T5Ø.3X2 | T5Ø.3X3 | T5Ø.3X4 | T5Ø.3X5 | T5Ø.3X6 |
| actylsalicylate | T39.Ø11 | T39.Ø12 | T39.Ø13 | T39.Ø14 | T39.Ø15 | T39.Ø16 |
| benzamidosalicylate | T37.1X1 | T37.1X2 | T37.1X3 | T37.1X4 | T37.1X5 | T37.1X6 |
| bromide | T42.6X1 | T42.6X2 | T42.6X3 | T42.6X4 | T42.6X5 | T42.6X6 |
| bromolactobionate | T42.6X1 | T42.6X2 | T42.6X3 | T42.6X4 | T42.6X5 | T42.6X6 |
| carbaspirin | T39.Ø11 | T39.Ø12 | T39.Ø13 | T39.Ø14 | T39.Ø15 | T39.Ø16 |
| carbimide | T5Ø.6X1 | T5Ø.6X2 | T5Ø.6X3 | T5Ø.6X4 | T5Ø.6X5 | T5Ø.6X6 |
| carbonate | T47.1X1 | T47.1X2 | T47.1X3 | T47.1X4 | T47.1X5 | T47.1X6 |
| chloride | T5Ø.991 | T5Ø.992 | T5Ø.993 | T5Ø.994 | T5Ø.995 | T5Ø.996 |
| anhydrous | T5Ø.991 | T5Ø.992 | T5Ø.993 | T5Ø.994 | T5Ø.995 | T5Ø.996 |
| cyanide | T57.8X1 | T57.8X2 | T57.8X3 | T57.8X4 | — | — |
| **Calcium** — *continued* | | | | | | |
| dioctyl sulfosuccinate | T47.4X1 | T47.4X2 | T47.4X3 | T47.4X4 | T47.4X5 | T47.4X6 |
| disodium edathamil | T45.8X1 | T45.8X2 | T45.8X3 | T45.8X4 | T45.8X5 | T45.8X6 |
| disodium edetate | T45.8X1 | T45.8X2 | T45.8X3 | T45.8X4 | T45.8X5 | T45.8X6 |
| dobesilate | T46.991 | T46.992 | T46.993 | T46.994 | T46.995 | T46.996 |
| EDTA | T45.8X1 | T45.8X2 | T45.8X3 | T45.8X4 | T45.8X5 | T45.8X6 |
| ferrous citrate | T45.4X1 | T45.4X2 | T45.4X3 | T45.4X4 | T45.4X5 | T45.4X6 |
| folinate | T45.8X1 | T45.8X2 | T45.8X3 | T45.8X4 | T45.8X5 | T45.8X6 |
| glubionate | T5Ø.3X1 | T5Ø.3X2 | T5Ø.3X3 | T5Ø.3X4 | T5Ø.3X5 | T5Ø.3X6 |
| gluconate | T5Ø.3X1 | T5Ø.3X2 | T5Ø.3X3 | T5Ø.3X4 | T5Ø.3X5 | T5Ø.3X6 |
| gluconogalactogluconate | T5Ø.3X1 | T5Ø.3X2 | T5Ø.3X3 | T5Ø.3X4 | T5Ø.3X5 | T5Ø.3X6 |
| hydrate, hydroxide | T54.3X1 | T54.3X2 | T54.3X3 | T54.3X4 | — | — |
| hypochlorite | T54.3X1 | T54.3X2 | T54.3X3 | T54.3X4 | — | — |
| iodide | T48.4X1 | T48.4X2 | T48.4X3 | T48.4X4 | T48.4X5 | T48.4X6 |
| ipodate | T5Ø.8X1 | T5Ø.8X2 | T5Ø.8X3 | T5Ø.8X4 | T5Ø.8X5 | T5Ø.8X6 |
| lactate | T5Ø.3X1 | T5Ø.3X2 | T5Ø.3X3 | T5Ø.3X4 | T5Ø.3X5 | T5Ø.3X6 |
| leucovorin | T45.8X1 | T45.8X2 | T45.8X3 | T45.8X4 | T45.8X5 | T45.8X6 |
| mandelate | T37.91 | T37.92 | T37.93 | T37.94 | T37.95 | T37.96 |
| oxide | T54.3X1 | T54.3X2 | T54.3X3 | T54.3X4 | — | — |
| pantothenate | T45.2X1 | T45.2X2 | T45.2X3 | T45.2X4 | T45.2X5 | T45.2X6 |
| phosphate | T5Ø.3X1 | T5Ø.3X2 | T5Ø.3X3 | T5Ø.3X4 | T5Ø.3X5 | T5Ø.3X6 |
| salicylate | T39.Ø91 | T39.Ø92 | T39.Ø93 | T39.Ø94 | T39.Ø95 | T39.Ø96 |
| salts | T5Ø.3X1 | T5Ø.3X2 | T5Ø.3X3 | T5Ø.3X4 | T5Ø.3X5 | T5Ø.3X6 |
| **Calculus-dissolving drug** | T5Ø.991 | T5Ø.992 | T5Ø.993 | T5Ø.994 | T5Ø.995 | T5Ø.996 |
| **Calomel** | T49.ØX1 | T49.ØX2 | T49.ØX3 | T49.ØX4 | T49.ØX5 | T49.ØX6 |
| **Caloric agent** | T5Ø.3X1 | T5Ø.3X2 | T5Ø.3X3 | T5Ø.3X4 | T5Ø.3X5 | T5Ø.3X6 |
| **Calusterone** | T38.7X1 | T38.7X2 | T38.7X3 | T38.7X4 | T38.7X5 | T38.7X6 |
| **Camazepam** | T42.4X1 | T42.4X2 | T42.4X3 | T42.4X4 | T42.4X5 | T42.4X6 |
| **Camomile** | T49.ØX1 | T49.ØX2 | T49.ØX3 | T49.ØX4 | T49.ØX5 | T49.ØX6 |
| **Camoquin** | T37.2X1 | T37.2X2 | T37.2X3 | T37.2X4 | T37.2X5 | T37.2X6 |
| **Camphor** | | | | | | |
| insecticide | T6Ø.2X1 | T6Ø.2X2 | T6Ø.2X3 | T6Ø.2X4 | — | — |
| medicinal | T49.8X1 | T49.8X2 | T49.8X3 | T49.8X4 | T49.8X5 | T49.8X6 |
| **Camylofin** | T44.3X1 | T44.3X2 | T44.3X3 | T44.3X4 | T44.3X5 | T44.3X6 |
| **Cancer chemotherapy drug regimen** | T45.1X1 | T45.1X2 | T45.1X3 | T45.1X4 | T45.1X5 | T45.1X6 |
| **Candeptin** | T49.ØX1 | T49.ØX2 | T49.ØX3 | T49.ØX4 | T49.ØX5 | T49.ØX6 |
| **Candicidin** | T49.ØX1 | T49.ØX2 | T49.ØX3 | T49.ØX4 | T49.ØX5 | T49.ØX6 |
| **Cankaid*** | T49.6X1 | T49.6X2 | T49.6X3 | T49.6X4 | T49.6X5 | T49.6X6 |
| **Cannabinoids, synthetic** | T4Ø.721 | T4Ø.722 | T4Ø.723 | T4Ø.724 | T4Ø.725 | T4Ø.726 |
| **Cannabinol** | T4Ø.711 | T4Ø.712 | T4Ø.713 | T4Ø.714 | T4Ø.715 | T4Ø.716 |
| **Cannabis** (derivatives) | T4Ø.711 | T4Ø.712 | T4Ø.713 | T4Ø.714 | T4Ø.715 | T4Ø.716 |
| **Canned heat** | T51.1X1 | T51.1X2 | T51.1X3 | T51.1X4 | — | — |
| **Canrenoic acid** | T5Ø.ØX1 | T5Ø.ØX2 | T5Ø.ØX3 | T5Ø.ØX4 | T5Ø.ØX5 | T5Ø.ØX6 |
| **Canrenone** | T5Ø.ØX1 | T5Ø.ØX2 | T5Ø.ØX3 | T5Ø.ØX4 | T5Ø.ØX5 | T5Ø.ØX6 |
| **Cantharides, cantharidin, cantharis** | T49.8X1 | T49.8X2 | T49.8X3 | T49.8X4 | T49.8X5 | T49.8X6 |
| **Canthaxanthin** | T5Ø.991 | T5Ø.992 | T5Ø.993 | T5Ø.994 | T5Ø.995 | T5Ø.996 |
| **Capillary-active drug NEC** | T46.9Ø1 | T46.9Ø2 | T46.9Ø3 | T46.9Ø4 | T46.9Ø5 | T46.9Ø6 |
| **Capreomycin** | T36.8X1 | T36.8X2 | T36.8X3 | T36.8X4 | T36.8X5 | T36.8X6 |
| **Capresla*** | T45.1X1 | T45.1X2 | T45.1X3 | T45.1X4 | T45.1X5 | T45.1X6 |
| **Capsicum** | T49.4X1 | T49.4X2 | T49.4X3 | T49.4X4 | T49.4X5 | T49.4X6 |
| **Captafol** | T6Ø.3X1 | T6Ø.3X2 | T6Ø.3X3 | T6Ø.3X4 | — | — |
| **Captan** | T6Ø.3X1 | T6Ø.3X2 | T6Ø.3X3 | T6Ø.3X4 | — | — |
| **Captodiame, captodiamine** | T43.591 | T43.592 | T43.593 | T43.594 | T43.595 | T43.596 |
| **Captopril** | T46.4X1 | T46.4X2 | T46.4X3 | T46.4X4 | T46.4X5 | T46.4X6 |
| **Caramiphen** | T44.3X1 | T44.3X2 | T44.3X3 | T44.3X4 | T44.3X5 | T44.3X6 |
| **Carazolol** | T44.7X1 | T44.7X2 | T44.7X3 | T44.7X4 | T44.7X5 | T44.7X6 |
| **Carbachol** | T44.1X1 | T44.1X2 | T44.1X3 | T44.1X4 | T44.1X5 | T44.1X6 |
| **Carbacrylamine** (resin) | T5Ø.3X1 | T5Ø.3X2 | T5Ø.3X3 | T5Ø.3X4 | T5Ø.3X5 | T5Ø.3X6 |
| **Carbamate** (insecticide) | T6Ø.ØX1 | T6Ø.ØX2 | T6Ø.ØX3 | T6Ø.ØX4 | — | — |
| **Carbamate** (sedative) | T42.6X1 | T42.6X2 | T42.6X3 | T42.6X4 | T42.6X5 | T42.6X6 |
| herbicide | T6Ø.ØX1 | T6Ø.ØX2 | T6Ø.ØX3 | T6Ø.ØX4 | — | — |
| insecticide | T6Ø.ØX1 | T6Ø.ØX2 | T6Ø.ØX3 | T6Ø.ØX4 | — | — |
| **Carbamazepine** | T42.1X1 | T42.1X2 | T42.1X3 | T42.1X4 | T42.1X5 | T42.1X6 |
| **Carbamide** | T47.3X1 | T47.3X2 | T47.3X3 | T47.3X4 | T47.3X5 | T47.3X6 |
| peroxide | T49.ØX1 | T49.ØX2 | T49.ØX3 | T49.ØX4 | T49.ØX5 | T49.ØX6 |
| topical | T49.8X1 | T49.8X2 | T49.8X3 | T49.8X4 | T49.8X5 | T49.8X6 |
| **Carbamylcholine chloride** | T44.1X1 | T44.1X2 | T44.1X3 | T44.1X4 | T44.1X5 | T44.1X6 |
| **Carbaril** | T6Ø.ØX1 | T6Ø.ØX2 | T6Ø.ØX3 | T6Ø.ØX4 | — | — |
| **Carbarsone** | T37.3X1 | T37.3X2 | T37.3X3 | T37.3X4 | T37.3X5 | T37.3X6 |
| **Carbaryl** | T6Ø.ØX1 | T6Ø.ØX2 | T6Ø.ØX3 | T6Ø.ØX4 | — | — |
| **Carbaspirin** | T39.Ø11 | T39.Ø12 | T39.Ø13 | T39.Ø14 | T39.Ø15 | T39.Ø16 |
| **Carbastat*** | T49.5X1 | T49.5X2 | T49.5X3 | T49.5X4 | T49.5X5 | T49.5X6 |
| **Carbazochrome** (salicylate) (sodium sulfonate) | T49.4X1 | T49.4X2 | T49.4X3 | T49.4X4 | T49.4X5 | T49.4X6 |
| **Carbenicillin** | T36.ØX1 | T36.ØX2 | T36.ØX3 | T36.ØX4 | T36.ØX5 | T36.ØX6 |
| **Carbenoxolone** | T47.1X1 | T47.1X2 | T47.1X3 | T47.1X4 | T47.1X5 | T47.1X6 |
| **Carbetapentane** | T48.3X1 | T48.3X2 | T48.3X3 | T48.3X4 | T48.3X5 | T48.3X6 |
| **Carbethyl salicylate** | T39.Ø91 | T39.Ø92 | T39.Ø93 | T39.Ø94 | T39.Ø95 | T39.Ø96 |
| **Carbidopa** (with levodopa) | T42.8X1 | T42.8X2 | T42.8X3 | T42.8X4 | T42.8X5 | T42.8X6 |
| **Carbimazole** | T38.2X1 | T38.2X2 | T38.2X3 | T38.2X4 | T38.2X5 | T38.2X6 |

| Substance | Poisoning, Accidental (unintentional) | Poisoning, Intentional Self-harm | Poisoning, Assault | Poisoning, Undetermined | Adverse Effect | Under-dosing |
|---|---|---|---|---|---|---|
| **Carbinol** | T51.1X1 | T51.1X2 | T51.1X3 | T51.1X4 | — | — |
| **Carbinoxamine** | T45.ØX1 | T45.ØX2 | T45.ØX3 | T45.ØX4 | T45.ØX5 | T45.ØX6 |
| **Carbiphene** | T39.8X1 | T39.8X2 | T39.8X3 | T39.8X4 | T39.8X5 | T39.8X6 |
| **Carbitol** | T52.3X1 | T52.3X2 | T52.3X3 | T52.3X4 | — | — |
| **Carbo medicinalis** | T47.6X1 | T47.6X2 | T47.6X3 | T47.6X4 | T47.6X5 | T47.6X6 |
| **Carbocaine** | T41.3X1 | T41.3X2 | T41.3X3 | T41.3X4 | T41.3X5 | T41.3X6 |
| infiltration (subcutaneous) | T41.3X1 | T41.3X2 | T41.3X3 | T41.3X4 | T41.3X5 | T41.3X6 |
| nerve block (peripheral) (plexus) | T41.3X1 | T41.3X2 | T41.3X3 | T41.3X4 | T41.3X5 | T41.3X6 |
| topical (surface) | T41.3X1 | T41.3X2 | T41.3X3 | T41.3X4 | T41.3X5 | T41.3X6 |
| **Carbocisteine** | T48.4X1 | T48.4X2 | T48.4X3 | T48.4X4 | T48.4X5 | T48.4X6 |
| **Carbocromen** | T46.3X1 | T46.3X2 | T46.3X3 | T46.3X4 | T46.3X5 | T46.3X6 |
| **Carbol fuchsin** | T49.ØX1 | T49.ØX2 | T49.ØX3 | T49.ØX4 | T49.ØX5 | T49.ØX6 |
| **Carbolic acid** — *see also* Phenol | T54.ØX1 | T54.ØX2 | T54.ØX3 | T54.ØX4 | — | — |
| **Carbolonium** (bromide) | T48.1X1 | T48.1X2 | T48.1X3 | T48.1X4 | T48.1X5 | T48.1X6 |
| **Carbomycin** | T36.8X1 | T36.8X2 | T36.8X3 | T36.8X4 | T36.8X5 | T36.8X6 |
| **Carbon** | | | | | | |
| bisulfide (liquid) | T65.4X1 | T65.4X2 | T65.4X3 | T65.4X4 | — | — |
| vapor | T65.4X1 | T65.4X2 | T65.4X3 | T65.4X4 | — | — |
| dioxide (gas) | T59.7X1 | T59.7X2 | T59.7X3 | T59.7X4 | — | — |
| medicinal | T41.5X1 | T41.5X2 | T41.5X3 | T41.5X4 | T41.5X5 | T41.5X6 |
| nonmedicinal | T59.7X1 | T59.7X2 | T59.7X3 | T59.7X4 | — | — |
| snow | T49.4X1 | T49.4X2 | T49.4X3 | T49.4X4 | T49.4X5 | T49.4X6 |
| disulfide (liquid) | T65.4X1 | T65.4X2 | T65.4X3 | T65.4X4 | — | — |
| vapor | T65.4X1 | T65.4X2 | T65.4X3 | T65.4X4 | — | — |
| monoxide (from incomplete combustion) | T58.91 | T58.92 | T58.93 | T58.94 | — | — |
| blast furnace gas | T58.8X1 | T58.8X2 | T58.8X3 | T58.8X4 | — | — |
| butane (distributed in mobile container) | T58.11 | T58.12 | T58.13 | T58.14 | — | — |
| distributed through pipes | T58.11 | T58.12 | T58.13 | T58.14 | — | — |
| charcoal fumes | T58.2X1 | T58.2X2 | T58.2X3 | T58.2X4 | — | — |
| coal | T58.2X1 | T58.2X2 | T58.2X3 | T58.2X4 | — | — |
| coke (in domestic stoves, fireplaces) | T58.2X1 | T58.2X2 | T58.2X3 | T58.2X4 | — | — |
| exhaust gas (motor) not in transit | T58.Ø1 | T58.Ø2 | T58.Ø3 | T58.Ø4 | — | — |
| combustion engine, any not in watercraft | T58.Ø1 | T58.Ø2 | T58.Ø3 | T58.Ø4 | — | — |
| farm tractor, not in transit | T58.Ø1 | T58.Ø2 | T58.Ø3 | T58.Ø4 | — | — |
| gas engine | T58.Ø1 | T58.Ø2 | T58.Ø3 | T58.Ø4 | — | — |
| motor pump | T58.Ø1 | T58.Ø2 | T58.Ø3 | T58.Ø4 | — | — |
| motor vehicle, not in transit | T58.Ø1 | T58.Ø2 | T58.Ø3 | T58.Ø4 | — | — |
| fuel (in domestic use) | T58.2X1 | T58.2X2 | T58.2X3 | T58.2X4 | — | — |
| gas (piped) | T58.11 | T58.12 | T58.13 | T58.14 | — | — |
| in mobile container | T58.11 | T58.12 | T58.13 | T58.14 | — | — |
| piped (natural) | T58.11 | T58.12 | T58.13 | T58.14 | — | — |
| utility | T58.11 | T58.12 | T58.13 | T58.14 | — | — |
| in mobile container | T58.11 | T58.12 | T58.13 | T58.14 | — | — |
| gas (piped) | T58.11 | T58.12 | T58.13 | T58.14 | — | — |
| illuminating gas | T58.11 | T58.12 | T58.13 | T58.14 | — | — |
| industrial fuels or gases, any | T58.8X1 | T58.8X2 | T58.8X3 | T58.8X4 | — | — |
| kerosene (in domestic stoves, fireplaces) | T58.2X1 | T58.2X2 | T58.2X3 | T58.2X4 | — | — |
| kiln gas or vapor | T58.8X1 | T58.8X2 | T58.8X3 | T58.8X4 | — | — |
| motor exhaust gas, not in transit | T58.Ø1 | T58.Ø2 | T58.Ø3 | T58.Ø4 | — | — |
| piped gas (manufactured) (natural) | T58.11 | T58.12 | T58.13 | T58.14 | — | — |
| producer gas | T58.8X1 | T58.8X2 | T58.8X3 | T58.8X4 | — | — |
| propane (distributed in mobile container) | T58.11 | T58.12 | T58.13 | T58.14 | — | — |
| distributed through pipes | T58.11 | T58.12 | T58.13 | T58.14 | — | — |
| solid (in domestic stoves, fireplaces) | T58.2X1 | T58.2X2 | T58.2X3 | T58.2X4 | — | — |
| specified source NEC | T58.8X1 | T58.8X2 | T58.8X3 | T58.8X4 | — | — |
| stove gas | T58.11 | T58.12 | T58.13 | T58.14 | — | — |
| piped | T58.11 | T58.12 | T58.13 | T58.14 | — | — |
| utility gas | T58.11 | T58.12 | T58.13 | T58.14 | — | — |
| piped | T58.11 | T58.12 | T58.13 | T58.14 | — | — |
| water gas | T58.11 | T58.12 | T58.13 | T58.14 | — | — |
| wood (in domestic stoves, fireplaces) | T58.2X1 | T58.2X2 | T58.2X3 | T58.2X4 | — | — |
| tetrachloride (vapor) NEC | T53.ØX1 | T53.ØX2 | T53.ØX3 | T53.ØX4 | — | — |
| liquid (cleansing agent) NEC | T53.ØX1 | T53.ØX2 | T53.ØX3 | T53.ØX4 | — | — |
| solvent | T53.ØX1 | T53.ØX2 | T53.ØX3 | T53.ØX4 | — | — |
| **Carbonic acid gas** | T59.7X1 | T59.7X2 | T59.7X3 | T59.7X4 | — | — |
| anhydrase inhibitor NEC | T5Ø.2X1 | T5Ø.2X2 | T5Ø.2X3 | T5Ø.2X4 | T5Ø.2X5 | T5Ø.2X6 |
| **Carbophenothion** | T6Ø.ØX1 | T6Ø.ØX2 | T6Ø.ØX3 | T6Ø.ØX4 | — | — |
| **Carboplatin** | T45.1X1 | T45.1X2 | T45.1X3 | T45.1X4 | T45.1X5 | T45.1X6 |
| **Carboprost** | T48.ØX1 | T48.ØX2 | T48.ØX3 | T48.ØX4 | T48.ØX5 | T48.ØX6 |
| **Carboquone** | T45.1X1 | T45.1X2 | T45.1X3 | T45.1X4 | T45.1X5 | T45.1X6 |
| **Carbowax** | T49.3X1 | T49.3X2 | T49.3X3 | T49.3X4 | T49.3X5 | T49.3X6 |
| **Carboxymethylcellulose** | T47.4X1 | T47.4X2 | T47.4X3 | T47.4X4 | T47.4X5 | T47.4X6 |
| **Carbrital** | T42.3X1 | T42.3X2 | T42.3X3 | T42.3X4 | T42.3X5 | T42.3X6 |
| **Carbromal** | T42.6X1 | T42.6X2 | T42.6X3 | T42.6X4 | T42.6X5 | T42.6X6 |
| **Carbutamide** | T38.3X1 | T38.3X2 | T38.3X3 | T38.3X4 | T38.3X5 | T38.3X6 |
| **Carbuterol** | T48.6X1 | T48.6X2 | T48.6X3 | T48.6X4 | T48.6X5 | T48.6X6 |
| **Cardiac** | | | | | | |
| depressants | T46.2X1 | T46.2X2 | T46.2X3 | T46.2X4 | T46.2X5 | T46.2X6 |
| rhythm regulator | T46.2X1 | T46.2X2 | T46.2X3 | T46.2X4 | T46.2X5 | T46.2X6 |
| specified NEC | T46.2X1 | T46.2X2 | T46.2X3 | T46.2X4 | T46.2X5 | T46.2X6 |
| **Cardiografin** | T5Ø.8X1 | T5Ø.8X2 | T5Ø.8X3 | T5Ø.8X4 | T5Ø.8X5 | T5Ø.8X6 |
| **Cardiogreen** | T5Ø.8X1 | T5Ø.8X2 | T5Ø.8X3 | T5Ø.8X4 | T5Ø.8X5 | T5Ø.8X6 |
| **Cardiotonic** (glycoside) **NEC** | T46.ØX1 | T46.ØX2 | T46.ØX3 | T46.ØX4 | T46.ØX5 | T46.ØX6 |
| **Cardiovascular drug NEC** | T46.9Ø1 | T46.9Ø2 | T46.9Ø3 | T46.9Ø4 | T46.9Ø5 | T46.9Ø6 |
| **Cardizem*** | T46.1X1 | T46.1X2 | T46.1X3 | T46.1X4 | T46.1X5 | T46.1X6 |
| **Cardrase** | T5Ø.2X1 | T5Ø.2X2 | T5Ø.2X3 | T5Ø.2X4 | T5Ø.2X5 | T5Ø.2X6 |
| **Carfecillin** | T36.ØX1 | T36.ØX2 | T36.ØX3 | T36.ØX4 | T36.ØX5 | T36.ØX6 |
| **Carfenazine** | T43.3X1 | T43.3X2 | T43.3X3 | T43.3X4 | T43.3X5 | T43.3X6 |
| **Carfusin** | T49.ØX1 | T49.ØX2 | T49.ØX3 | T49.ØX4 | T49.ØX5 | T49.ØX6 |
| **Carindacillin** | T36.ØX1 | T36.ØX2 | T36.ØX3 | T36.ØX4 | T36.ØX5 | T36.ØX6 |
| **Carisoprodol** | T42.8X1 | T42.8X2 | T42.8X3 | T42.8X4 | T42.8X5 | T42.8X6 |
| **Carmellose** | T47.4X1 | T47.4X2 | T47.4X3 | T47.4X4 | T47.4X5 | T47.4X6 |
| **Carminative** | T47.5X1 | T47.5X2 | T47.5X3 | T47.5X4 | T47.5X5 | T47.5X6 |
| **Carmofur** | T45.1X1 | T45.1X2 | T45.1X3 | T45.1X4 | T45.1X5 | T45.1X6 |
| **Carmustine** | T45.1X1 | T45.1X2 | T45.1X3 | T45.1X4 | T45.1X5 | T45.1X6 |
| **Carotene** | T45.2X1 | T45.2X2 | T45.2X3 | T45.2X4 | T45.2X5 | T45.2X6 |
| **Carphenazine** | T43.3X1 | T43.3X2 | T43.3X3 | T43.3X4 | T43.3X5 | T43.3X6 |
| **Carpipramine** | T42.4X1 | T42.4X2 | T42.4X3 | T42.4X4 | T42.4X5 | T42.4X6 |
| **Carprofen** | T39.311 | T39.312 | T39.313 | T39.314 | T39.315 | T39.316 |
| **Carpronium chloride** | T44.3X1 | T44.3X2 | T44.3X3 | T44.3X4 | T44.3X5 | T44.3X6 |
| **Carrageenan** | T47.8X1 | T47.8X2 | T47.8X3 | T47.8X4 | T47.8X5 | T47.8X6 |
| **Carteolol** | T44.7X1 | T44.7X2 | T44.7X3 | T44.7X4 | T44.7X5 | T44.7X6 |
| **Carter's Little Pills** | T47.2X1 | T47.2X2 | T47.2X3 | T47.2X4 | T47.2X5 | T47.2X6 |
| **Cartia*** | T46.1X1 | T46.1X2 | T46.1X3 | T46.1X4 | T46.1X5 | T46.1X6 |
| **Cascara** (sagrada) | T47.2X1 | T47.2X2 | T47.2X3 | T47.2X4 | T47.2X5 | T47.2X6 |
| **Cassava** | T62.2X1 | T62.2X2 | T62.2X3 | T62.2X4 | — | — |
| **Castellani's paint** | T49.ØX1 | T49.ØX2 | T49.ØX3 | T49.ØX4 | T49.ØX5 | T49.ØX6 |
| **Castor** | | | | | | |
| bean | T62.2X1 | T62.2X2 | T62.2X3 | T62.2X4 | — | — |
| oil | T47.2X1 | T47.2X2 | T47.2X3 | T47.2X4 | T47.2X5 | T47.2X6 |
| **Catalase** | T45.3X1 | T45.3X2 | T45.3X3 | T45.3X4 | T45.3X5 | T45.3X6 |
| **Caterpillar** (sting) | T63.431 | T63.432 | T63.433 | T63.434 | — | — |
| **Catha** (edulis) (tea) | T43.691 | T43.692 | T43.693 | T43.694 | — | — |
| **Cathartic NEC** | T47.4X1 | T47.4X2 | T47.4X3 | T47.4X4 | T47.4X5 | T47.4X6 |
| anthacene derivative | T47.2X1 | T47.2X2 | T47.2X3 | T47.2X4 | T47.2X5 | T47.2X6 |
| bulk | T47.4X1 | T47.4X2 | T47.4X3 | T47.4X4 | T47.4X5 | T47.4X6 |
| contact | T47.2X1 | T47.2X2 | T47.2X3 | T47.2X4 | T47.2X5 | T47.2X6 |
| emollient NEC | T47.4X1 | T47.4X2 | T47.4X3 | T47.4X4 | T47.4X5 | T47.4X6 |
| irritant NEC | T47.2X1 | T47.2X2 | T47.2X3 | T47.2X4 | T47.2X5 | T47.2X6 |
| mucilage | T47.4X1 | T47.4X2 | T47.4X3 | T47.4X4 | T47.4X5 | T47.4X6 |
| saline | T47.3X1 | T47.3X2 | T47.3X3 | T47.3X4 | T47.3X5 | T47.3X6 |
| vegetable | T47.2X1 | T47.2X2 | T47.2X3 | T47.2X4 | T47.2X5 | T47.2X6 |
| **Cathine** | T5Ø.5X1 | T5Ø.5X2 | T5Ø.5X3 | T5Ø.5X4 | T5Ø.5X5 | T5Ø.5X6 |
| **Cathomycin** | T36.8X1 | T36.8X2 | T36.8X3 | T36.8X4 | T36.8X5 | T36.8X6 |
| **Cation exchange resin** | T5Ø.3X1 | T5Ø.3X2 | T5Ø.3X3 | T5Ø.3X4 | T5Ø.3X5 | T5Ø.3X6 |
| **Caustic**(s) **NEC** | T54.91 | T54.92 | T54.93 | T54.94 | — | — |
| alkali | T54.3X1 | T54.3X2 | T54.3X3 | T54.3X4 | — | — |
| hydroxide | T54.3X1 | T54.3X2 | T54.3X3 | T54.3X4 | — | — |
| potash | T54.3X1 | T54.3X2 | T54.3X3 | T54.3X4 | — | — |
| soda | T54.3X1 | T54.3X2 | T54.3X3 | T54.3X4 | — | — |
| specified NEC | T54.91 | T54.92 | T54.93 | T54.94 | — | — |
| **Ceepryn** | T49.ØX1 | T49.ØX2 | T49.ØX3 | T49.ØX4 | T49.ØX5 | T49.ØX6 |
| ENT agent | T49.6X1 | T49.6X2 | T49.6X3 | T49.6X4 | T49.6X5 | T49.6X6 |
| lozenges | T49.6X1 | T49.6X2 | T49.6X3 | T49.6X4 | T49.6X5 | T49.6X6 |
| **Cefacetrile** | T36.1X1 | T36.1X2 | T36.1X3 | T36.1X4 | T36.1X5 | T36.1X6 |
| **Cefaclor** | T36.1X1 | T36.1X2 | T36.1X3 | T36.1X4 | T36.1X5 | T36.1X6 |
| **Cefadroxil** | T36.1X1 | T36.1X2 | T36.1X3 | T36.1X4 | T36.1X5 | T36.1X6 |
| **Cefalexin** | T36.1X1 | T36.1X2 | T36.1X3 | T36.1X4 | T36.1X5 | T36.1X6 |
| **Cefaloglycin** | T36.1X1 | T36.1X2 | T36.1X3 | T36.1X4 | T36.1X5 | T36.1X6 |
| **Cefaloridine** | T36.1X1 | T36.1X2 | T36.1X3 | T36.1X4 | T36.1X5 | T36.1X6 |
| **Cefalosporins** | T36.1X1 | T36.1X2 | T36.1X3 | T36.1X4 | T36.1X5 | T36.1X6 |
| **Cefalotin** | T36.1X1 | T36.1X2 | T36.1X3 | T36.1X4 | T36.1X5 | T36.1X6 |
| **Cefamandole** | T36.1X1 | T36.1X2 | T36.1X3 | T36.1X4 | T36.1X5 | T36.1X6 |
| **Cefamycin antibiotic** | T36.1X1 | T36.1X2 | T36.1X3 | T36.1X4 | T36.1X5 | T36.1X6 |
| **Cefapirin** | T36.1X1 | T36.1X2 | T36.1X3 | T36.1X4 | T36.1X5 | T36.1X6 |
| **Cefatrizine** | T36.1X1 | T36.1X2 | T36.1X3 | T36.1X4 | T36.1X5 | T36.1X6 |
| **Cefazedone** | T36.1X1 | T36.1X2 | T36.1X3 | T36.1X4 | T36.1X5 | T36.1X6 |

| Substance | Poisoning, Accidental (unintentional) | Poisoning, Intentional Self-harm | Poisoning, Assault | Poisoning, Undetermined | Adverse Effect | Under-dosing |
|---|---|---|---|---|---|---|
| **Cefazolin** | T36.1X1 | T36.1X2 | T36.1X3 | T36.1X4 | T36.1X5 | T36.1X6 |
| **Cefbuperazone** | T36.1X1 | T36.1X2 | T36.1X3 | T36.1X4 | T36.1X5 | T36.1X6 |
| **Cefetamet** | T36.1X1 | T36.1X2 | T36.1X3 | T36.1X4 | T36.1X5 | T36.1X6 |
| **Cefixime** | T36.1X1 | T36.1X2 | T36.1X3 | T36.1X4 | T36.1X5 | T36.1X6 |
| **Cefmenoxime** | T36.1X1 | T36.1X2 | T36.1X3 | T36.1X4 | T36.1X5 | T36.1X6 |
| **Cefmetazole** | T36.1X1 | T36.1X2 | T36.1X3 | T36.1X4 | T36.1X5 | T36.1X6 |
| **Cefminox** | T36.1X1 | T36.1X2 | T36.1X3 | T36.1X4 | T36.1X5 | T36.1X6 |
| **Cefonicid** | T36.1X1 | T36.1X2 | T36.1X3 | T36.1X4 | T36.1X5 | T36.1X6 |
| **Cefoperazone** | T36.1X1 | T36.1X2 | T36.1X3 | T36.1X4 | T36.1X5 | T36.1X6 |
| **Ceforanide** | T36.1X1 | T36.1X2 | T36.1X3 | T36.1X4 | T36.1X5 | T36.1X6 |
| **Cefotaxime** | T36.1X1 | T36.1X2 | T36.1X3 | T36.1X4 | T36.1X5 | T36.1X6 |
| **Cefotetan** | T36.1X1 | T36.1X2 | T36.1X3 | T36.1X4 | T36.1X5 | T36.1X6 |
| **Cefotiam** | T36.1X1 | T36.1X2 | T36.1X3 | T36.1X4 | T36.1X5 | T36.1X6 |
| **Cefoxitin** | T36.1X1 | T36.1X2 | T36.1X3 | T36.1X4 | T36.1X5 | T36.1X6 |
| **Cefpimizole** | T36.1X1 | T36.1X2 | T36.1X3 | T36.1X4 | T36.1X5 | T36.1X6 |
| **Cefpiramide** | T36.1X1 | T36.1X2 | T36.1X3 | T36.1X4 | T36.1X5 | T36.1X6 |
| **Cefradine** | T36.1X1 | T36.1X2 | T36.1X3 | T36.1X4 | T36.1X5 | T36.1X6 |
| **Cefroxadine** | T36.1X1 | T36.1X2 | T36.1X3 | T36.1X4 | T36.1X5 | T36.1X6 |
| **Cefsulodin** | T36.1X1 | T36.1X2 | T36.1X3 | T36.1X4 | T36.1X5 | T36.1X6 |
| **Ceftazidime** | T36.1X1 | T36.1X2 | T36.1X3 | T36.1X4 | T36.1X5 | T36.1X6 |
| **Cefteram** | T36.1X1 | T36.1X2 | T36.1X3 | T36.1X4 | T36.1X5 | T36.1X6 |
| **Ceftezole** | T36.1X1 | T36.1X2 | T36.1X3 | T36.1X4 | T36.1X5 | T36.1X6 |
| **Ceftin*** | T36.1X1 | T36.1X2 | T36.1X3 | T36.1X4 | T36.1X5 | T36.1X6 |
| **Ceftizoxime** | T36.1X1 | T36.1X2 | T36.1X3 | T36.1X4 | T36.1X5 | T36.1X6 |
| **Ceftriaxone** | T36.1X1 | T36.1X2 | T36.1X3 | T36.1X4 | T36.1X5 | T36.1X6 |
| **Cefuroxime** | T36.1X1 | T36.1X2 | T36.1X3 | T36.1X4 | T36.1X5 | T36.1X6 |
| **Cefuzonam** | T36.1X1 | T36.1X2 | T36.1X3 | T36.1X4 | T36.1X5 | T36.1X6 |
| **Celestone** | T38.ØX1 | T38.ØX2 | T38.ØX3 | T38.ØX4 | T38.ØX5 | T38.ØX6 |
| topical | T49.ØX1 | T49.ØX2 | T49.ØX3 | T49.ØX4 | T49.ØX5 | T49.ØX6 |
| **Celexa*** | T43.221 | T43.222 | T43.223 | T43.224 | T43.225 | T43.226 |
| **Celiprolol** | T44.7X1 | T44.7X2 | T44.7X3 | T44.7X4 | T44.7X5 | T44.7X6 |
| **Cell stimulants and proliferants** | T49.8X1 | T49.8X2 | T49.8X3 | T49.8X4 | T49.8X5 | T49.8X6 |
| **Cellosolve** | T52.91 | T52.92 | T52.93 | T52.94 | — | — |
| **Cellulose** | | | | | | |
| cathartic | T47.4X1 | T47.4X2 | T47.4X3 | T47.4X4 | T47.4X5 | T47.4X6 |
| hydroxyethyl | T47.4X1 | T47.4X2 | T47.4X3 | T47.4X4 | T47.4X5 | T47.4X6 |
| nitrates (topical) | T49.3X1 | T49.3X2 | T49.3X3 | T49.3X4 | T49.3X5 | T49.3X6 |
| oxidized | T49.4X1 | T49.4X2 | T49.4X3 | T49.4X4 | T49.4X5 | T49.4X6 |
| **Centipede** (bite) | T63.411 | T63.412 | T63.413 | T63.414 | — | — |
| **Central nervous system** | | | | | | |
| depressants | T42.71 | T42.72 | T42.73 | T42.74 | T42.75 | T42.76 |
| anesthetic (general) NEC | T41.2Ø1 | T41.2Ø2 | T41.2Ø3 | T41.2Ø4 | T41.2Ø5 | T41.2Ø6 |
| gases NEC | T41.ØX1 | T41.ØX2 | T41.ØX3 | T41.ØX4 | T41.ØX5 | T41.ØX6 |
| intravenous | T41.1X1 | T41.1X2 | T41.1X3 | T41.1X4 | T41.1X5 | T41.1X6 |
| barbiturates | T42.3X1 | T42.3X2 | T42.3X3 | T42.3X4 | T42.3X5 | T42.3X6 |
| benzodiazepines | T42.4X1 | T42.4X2 | T42.4X3 | T42.4X4 | T42.4X5 | T42.4X6 |
| bromides | T42.6X1 | T42.6X2 | T42.6X3 | T42.6X4 | T42.6X5 | T42.6X6 |
| cannabis sativa | T4Ø.711 | T4Ø.712 | T4Ø.713 | T4Ø.714 | T4Ø.715 | T4Ø.716 |
| chloral hydrate | T42.6X1 | T42.6X2 | T42.6X3 | T42.6X4 | T42.6X5 | T42.6X6 |
| ethanol | T51.ØX1 | T51.ØX2 | T51.ØX3 | T51.ØX4 | — | — |
| hallucinogenics | T4Ø.9Ø1 | T4Ø.9Ø2 | T4Ø.9Ø3 | T4Ø.9Ø4 | T4Ø.9Ø5 | T4Ø.9Ø6 |
| hypnotics | T42.71 | T42.72 | T42.73 | T42.74 | T42.75 | T42.76 |
| specified NEC | T42.6X1 | T42.6X2 | T42.6X3 | T42.6X4 | T42.6X5 | T42.6X6 |
| muscle relaxants | T42.8X1 | T42.8X2 | T42.8X3 | T42.8X4 | T42.8X5 | T42.8X6 |
| paraldehyde | T42.6X1 | T42.6X2 | T42.6X3 | T42.6X4 | T42.6X5 | T42.6X6 |
| sedatives; sedative-hypnotics | T42.71 | T42.72 | T42.73 | T42.74 | T42.75 | T42.76 |
| mixed NEC | T42.6X1 | T42.6X2 | T42.6X3 | T42.6X4 | T42.6X5 | T42.6X6 |
| specified NEC | T42.6X1 | T42.6X2 | T42.6X3 | T42.6X4 | T42.6X5 | T42.6X6 |
| muscle-tone depressants | T42.8X1 | T42.8X2 | T42.8X3 | T42.8X4 | T42.8X5 | T42.8X6 |
| stimulants | T43.6Ø1 | T43.6Ø2 | T43.6Ø3 | T43.6Ø4 | T43.6Ø5 | T43.6Ø6 |
| amphetamines | T43.621 | T43.622 | T43.623 | T43.624 | T43.625 | T43.626 |
| analeptics | T5Ø.7X1 | T5Ø.7X2 | T5Ø.7X3 | T5Ø.7X4 | T5Ø.7X5 | T5Ø.7X6 |
| antidepressants | T43.2Ø1 | T43.2Ø2 | T43.2Ø3 | T43.2Ø4 | T43.2Ø5 | T43.2Ø6 |
| opiate antagonists | T5Ø.7X1 | T5Ø.7X2 | T5Ø.7X3 | T5Ø.7X4 | T5Ø.7X5 | T5Ø.7X6 |
| specified NEC | T43.691 | T43.692 | T43.693 | T43.694 | T43.695 | T43.696 |
| **Cepacol*** | T41.3X1 | T41.3X2 | T41.3X3 | T41.3X4 | T41.3X5 | T41.3X6 |
| **Cephalexin** | T36.1X1 | T36.1X2 | T36.1X3 | T36.1X4 | T36.1X5 | T36.1X6 |
| **Cephaloglycin** | T36.1X1 | T36.1X2 | T36.1X3 | T36.1X4 | T36.1X5 | T36.1X6 |
| **Cephaloridine** | T36.1X1 | T36.1X2 | T36.1X3 | T36.1X4 | T36.1X5 | T36.1X6 |
| **Cephalosporins** | T36.1X1 | T36.1X2 | T36.1X3 | T36.1X4 | T36.1X5 | T36.1X6 |
| N (adicillin) | T36.ØX1 | T36.ØX2 | T36.ØX3 | T36.ØX4 | T36.ØX5 | T36.ØX6 |
| **Cephalothin** | T36.1X1 | T36.1X2 | T36.1X3 | T36.1X4 | T36.1X5 | T36.1X6 |
| **Cephalotin** | T36.1X1 | T36.1X2 | T36.1X3 | T36.1X4 | T36.1X5 | T36.1X6 |
| **Cephradine** | T36.1X1 | T36.1X2 | T36.1X3 | T36.1X4 | T36.1X5 | T36.1X6 |
| **Cerbera** (odallam) | T62.2X1 | T62.2X2 | T62.2X3 | T62.2X4 | — | — |
| **Cerberin** | T46.ØX1 | T46.ØX2 | T46.ØX3 | T46.ØX4 | T46.ØX5 | T46.ØX6 |
| **Cerebral stimulants** | T43.6Ø1 | T43.6Ø2 | T43.6Ø3 | T43.6Ø4 | T43.6Ø5 | T43.6Ø6 |
| psychotherapeutic | T43.6Ø1 | T43.6Ø2 | T43.6Ø3 | T43.6Ø4 | T43.6Ø5 | T43.6Ø6 |
| specified NEC | T43.691 | T43.692 | T43.693 | T43.694 | T43.695 | T43.696 |
| **Cerium oxalate** | T45.ØX1 | T45.ØX2 | T45.ØX3 | T45.ØX4 | T45.ØX5 | T45.ØX6 |
| **Cerous oxalate** | T45.ØX1 | T45.ØX2 | T45.ØX3 | T45.ØX4 | T45.ØX5 | T45.ØX6 |

| Substance | Poisoning, Accidental (unintentional) | Poisoning, Intentional Self-harm | Poisoning, Assault | Poisoning, Undetermined | Adverse Effect | Under-dosing |
|---|---|---|---|---|---|---|
| **Ceruletide** | T5Ø.8X1 | T5Ø.8X2 | T5Ø.8X3 | T5Ø.8X4 | T5Ø.8X5 | T5Ø.8X6 |
| **Cetacort*** | T49.ØX1 | T49.ØX2 | T49.ØX3 | T49.ØX4 | T49.ØX5 | T49.ØX6 |
| **Cetalkonium** (chloride) | T49.ØX1 | T49.ØX2 | T49.ØX3 | T49.ØX4 | T49.ØX5 | T49.ØX6 |
| **Cethexonium chloride** | T49.ØX1 | T49.ØX2 | T49.ØX3 | T49.ØX4 | T49.ØX5 | T49.ØX6 |
| **Cetiedil** | T46.7X1 | T46.7X2 | T46.7X3 | T46.7X4 | T46.7X5 | T46.7X6 |
| **Cetirizine** | T45.ØX1 | T45.ØX2 | T45.ØX3 | T45.ØX4 | T45.ØX5 | T45.ØX6 |
| **Cetomacrogol** | T5Ø.991 | T5Ø.992 | T5Ø.993 | T5Ø.994 | T5Ø.995 | T5Ø.996 |
| **Cetotiamine** | T45.2X1 | T45.2X2 | T45.2X3 | T45.2X4 | T45.2X5 | T45.2X6 |
| **Cetoxime** | T45.ØX1 | T45.ØX2 | T45.ØX3 | T45.ØX4 | T45.ØX5 | T45.ØX6 |
| **Cetraxate** | T47.1X1 | T47.1X2 | T47.1X3 | T47.1X4 | T47.1X5 | T47.1X6 |
| **Cetrimide** | T49.ØX1 | T49.ØX2 | T49.ØX3 | T49.ØX4 | T49.ØX5 | T49.ØX6 |
| **Cetrimonium** (bromide) | T49.ØX1 | T49.ØX2 | T49.ØX3 | T49.ØX4 | T49.ØX5 | T49.ØX6 |
| **Cetylpyridinium chloride** | T49.ØX1 | T49.ØX2 | T49.ØX3 | T49.ØX4 | T49.ØX5 | T49.ØX6 |
| ENT agent | T49.6X1 | T49.6X2 | T49.6X3 | T49.6X4 | T49.6X5 | T49.6X6 |
| lozenges | T49.6X1 | T49.6X2 | T49.6X3 | T49.6X4 | T49.6X5 | T49.6X6 |
| **Cevadilla** — *see* Sabadilla | | | | | | |
| **Cevitamic acid** | T45.2X1 | T45.2X2 | T45.2X3 | T45.2X4 | T45.2X5 | T45.2X6 |
| **Chalk, precipitated** | T47.1X1 | T47.1X2 | T47.1X3 | T47.1X4 | T47.1X5 | T47.1X6 |
| **Chamomile** | T49.ØX1 | T49.ØX2 | T49.ØX3 | T49.ØX4 | T49.ØX5 | T49.ØX6 |
| **Ch'an su** | T46.ØX1 | T46.ØX2 | T46.ØX3 | T46.ØX4 | T46.ØX5 | T46.ØX6 |
| **Charcoal** | T47.6X1 | T47.6X2 | T47.6X3 | T47.6X4 | T47.6X5 | T47.6X6 |
| activated — *see also* Charcoal, medicinal | T47.6X1 | T47.6X2 | T47.6X3 | T47.6X4 | T47.6X5 | T47.6X6 |
| fumes (Carbon monoxide) | T58.2X1 | T58.2X2 | T58.2X3 | T58.2X4 | — | — |
| industrial | T58.8X1 | T58.8X2 | T58.8X3 | T58.8X4 | — | — |
| medicinal (activated) | T47.6X1 | T47.6X2 | T47.6X3 | T47.6X4 | T47.6X5 | T47.6X6 |
| antidiarrheal | T47.6X1 | T47.6X2 | T47.6X3 | T47.6X4 | T47.6X5 | T47.6X6 |
| poison control | T47.8X1 | T47.8X2 | T47.8X3 | T47.8X4 | T47.8X5 | T47.8X6 |
| specified use other than for diarrhea | T47.8X1 | T47.8X2 | T47.8X3 | T47.8X4 | T47.8X5 | T47.8X6 |
| topical | T49.8X1 | T49.8X2 | T49.8X3 | T49.8X4 | T49.8X5 | T49.8X6 |
| **Chaulmosulfone** | T37.1X1 | T37.1X2 | T37.1X3 | T37.1X4 | T37.1X5 | T37.1X6 |
| **Chelating agent NEC** | T5Ø.6X1 | T5Ø.6X2 | T5Ø.6X3 | T5Ø.6X4 | T5Ø.6X5 | T5Ø.6X6 |
| **Chelidonium majus** | T62.2X1 | T62.2X2 | T62.2X3 | T62.2X4 | — | — |
| **Chemical substance NEC** | T65.91 | T65.92 | T65.93 | T65.94 | — | — |
| **Chenodeoxycholic acid** | T47.5X1 | T47.5X2 | T47.5X3 | T47.5X4 | T47.5X5 | T47.5X6 |
| **Chenodiol** | T47.5X1 | T47.5X2 | T47.5X3 | T47.5X4 | T47.5X5 | T47.5X6 |
| **Chenopodium** | T37.4X1 | T37.4X2 | T37.4X3 | T37.4X4 | T37.4X5 | T37.4X6 |
| **Cherry laurel** | T62.2X1 | T62.2X2 | T62.2X3 | T62.2X4 | — | — |
| **Chiggertox*** | T41.3X1 | T41.3X2 | T41.3X3 | T41.3X4 | T41.3X5 | T41.3X6 |
| **Chinidin** (e) | T46.2X1 | T46.2X2 | T46.2X3 | T46.2X4 | T46.2X5 | T46.2X6 |
| **Chiniofon** | T37.8X1 | T37.8X2 | T37.8X3 | T37.8X4 | T37.8X5 | T37.8X6 |
| **Chlophedianol** | T48.3X1 | T48.3X2 | T48.3X3 | T48.3X4 | T48.3X5 | T48.3X6 |
| **Chlor-Trimeton** | T45.ØX1 | T45.ØX2 | T45.ØX3 | T45.ØX4 | T45.ØX5 | T45.ØX6 |
| **Chloral** | T42.6X1 | T42.6X2 | T42.6X3 | T42.6X4 | T42.6X5 | T42.6X6 |
| derivative | T42.6X1 | T42.6X2 | T42.6X3 | T42.6X4 | T42.6X5 | T42.6X6 |
| hydrate | T42.6X1 | T42.6X2 | T42.6X3 | T42.6X4 | T42.6X5 | T42.6X6 |
| **Chloralamide** | T42.6X1 | T42.6X2 | T42.6X3 | T42.6X4 | T42.6X5 | T42.6X6 |
| **Chloralodol** | T42.6X1 | T42.6X2 | T42.6X3 | T42.6X4 | T42.6X5 | T42.6X6 |
| **Chloralose** | T6Ø.4X1 | T6Ø.4X2 | T6Ø.4X3 | T6Ø.4X4 | — | — |
| **Chlorambucil** | T45.1X1 | T45.1X2 | T45.1X3 | T45.1X4 | T45.1X5 | T45.1X6 |
| **Chloramine** | T57.8X1 | T57.8X2 | T57.8X3 | T57.8X4 | — | — |
| T | T49.ØX1 | T49.ØX2 | T49.ØX3 | T49.ØX4 | T49.ØX5 | T49.ØX6 |
| topical | T49.ØX1 | T49.ØX2 | T49.ØX3 | T49.ØX4 | T49.ØX5 | T49.ØX6 |
| **Chloramphenicol** | T36.2X1 | T36.2X2 | T36.2X3 | T36.2X4 | T36.2X5 | T36.2X6 |
| ENT agent | T49.6X1 | T49.6X2 | T49.6X3 | T49.6X4 | T49.6X5 | T49.6X6 |
| ophthalmic preparation | T49.5X1 | T49.5X2 | T49.5X3 | T49.5X4 | T49.5X5 | T49.5X6 |
| topical NEC | T49.ØX1 | T49.ØX2 | T49.ØX3 | T49.ØX4 | T49.ØX5 | T49.ØX6 |
| **Chlorate** (potassium) (sodium) **NEC** | T6Ø.3X1 | T6Ø.3X2 | T6Ø.3X3 | T6Ø.3X4 | — | — |
| herbicide | T6Ø.3X1 | T6Ø.3X2 | T6Ø.3X3 | T6Ø.3X4 | — | — |
| **Chlorazanil** | T5Ø.2X1 | T5Ø.2X2 | T5Ø.2X3 | T5Ø.2X4 | T5Ø.2X5 | T5Ø.2X6 |
| **Chlorbenzene, chlorbenzol** | T53.7X1 | T53.7X2 | T53.7X3 | T53.7X4 | — | — |
| **Chlorbenzoxamine** | T44.3X1 | T44.3X2 | T44.3X3 | T44.3X4 | T44.3X5 | T44.3X6 |
| **Chlorbutol** | T42.6X1 | T42.6X2 | T42.6X3 | T42.6X4 | T42.6X5 | T42.6X6 |
| **Chlorcyclizine** | T45.ØX1 | T45.ØX2 | T45.ØX3 | T45.ØX4 | T45.ØX5 | T45.ØX6 |
| **Chlordan** (e) (dust) | T6Ø.1X1 | T6Ø.1X2 | T6Ø.1X3 | T6Ø.1X4 | — | — |
| **Chlordantoin** | T49.ØX1 | T49.ØX2 | T49.ØX3 | T49.ØX4 | T49.ØX5 | T49.ØX6 |
| **Chlordiazepoxide** | T42.4X1 | T42.4X2 | T42.4X3 | T42.4X4 | T42.4X5 | T42.4X6 |
| **Chlordiethyl benzamide** | T49.3X1 | T49.3X2 | T49.3X3 | T49.3X4 | T49.3X5 | T49.3X6 |
| **Chloresium** | T49.8X1 | T49.8X2 | T49.8X3 | T49.8X4 | T49.8X5 | T49.8X6 |
| **Chlorethiazol** | T42.6X1 | T42.6X2 | T42.6X3 | T42.6X4 | T42.6X5 | T42.6X6 |
| **Chlorethyl** — *see* Ethyl, chloride | | | | | | |
| **Chloretone** | T42.6X1 | T42.6X2 | T42.6X3 | T42.6X4 | T42.6X5 | T42.6X6 |
| **Chlorex** | T53.6X1 | T53.6X2 | T53.6X3 | T53.6X4 | — | — |
| insecticide | T6Ø.1X1 | T6Ø.1X2 | T6Ø.1X3 | T6Ø.1X4 | — | — |
| **Chlorfenvinphos** | T6Ø.ØX1 | T6Ø.ØX2 | T6Ø.ØX3 | T6Ø.ØX4 | — | — |
| **Chlorhexadol** | T42.6X1 | T42.6X2 | T42.6X3 | T42.6X4 | T42.6X5 | T42.6X6 |
| **Chlorhexamide** | T45.1X1 | T45.1X2 | T45.1X3 | T45.1X4 | T45.1X5 | T45.1X6 |
| **Chlorhexidine** | T49.ØX1 | T49.ØX2 | T49.ØX3 | T49.ØX4 | T49.ØX5 | T49.ØX6 |
| **Chlorhexidine Gluconate Oral Rinse*** | T49.6X1 | T49.6X2 | T49.6X3 | T49.6X4 | T49.6X5 | T49.6X6 |

| Substance | Poisoning, Accidental (unintentional) | Poisoning, Intentional Self-harm | Poisoning, Assault | Poisoning, Undetermined | Adverse Effect | Under-dosing |
|---|---|---|---|---|---|---|
| **Chlorhydroxyquinolin** | T49.ØX1 | T49.ØX2 | T49.ØX3 | T49.ØX4 | T49.ØX5 | T49.ØX6 |
| **Chloride of lime** (bleach) | T54.3X1 | T54.3X2 | T54.3X3 | T54.3X4 | — | — |
| **Chlorimipramine** | T43.Ø11 | T43.Ø12 | T43.Ø13 | T43.Ø14 | T43.Ø15 | T43.Ø16 |
| **Chlorinated** | | | | | | |
| camphene | T53.6X1 | T53.6X2 | T53.6X3 | T53.6X4 | — | — |
| diphenyl | T53.7X1 | T53.7X2 | T53.7X3 | T53.7X4 | — | — |
| hydrocarbons NEC | T53.91 | T53.92 | T53.93 | T53.94 | — | — |
| solvents | T53.91 | T53.92 | T53.93 | T53.94 | — | — |
| lime (bleach) | T54.3X1 | T54.3X2 | T54.3X3 | T54.3X4 | — | — |
| and boric acid solution | T49.ØX1 | T49.ØX2 | T49.ØX3 | T49.ØX4 | T49.ØX5 | T49.ØX6 |
| naphthalene (insecticide) | T6Ø.1X1 | T6Ø.1X2 | T6Ø.1X3 | T6Ø.1X4 | — | — |
| industrial (non-pesticide) | T53.7X1 | T53.7X2 | T53.7X3 | T53.7X4 | — | — |
| pesticide NEC | T6Ø.8X1 | T6Ø.8X2 | T6Ø.8X3 | T6Ø.8X4 | — | — |
| soda — *see also* sodium hypochlorite | | | | | | |
| solution | T49.ØX1 | T49.ØX2 | T49.ØX3 | T49.ØX4 | T49.ØX5 | T49.ØX6 |
| **Chlorine** (fumes) (gas) | T59.4X1 | T59.4X2 | T59.4X3 | T59.4X4 | — | — |
| bleach | T54.3X1 | T54.3X2 | T54.3X3 | T54.3X4 | — | — |
| compound gas NEC | T59.4X1 | T59.4X2 | T59.4X3 | T59.4X4 | — | — |
| disinfectant | T59.4X1 | T59.4X2 | T59.4X3 | T59.4X4 | — | — |
| releasing agents NEC | T59.4X1 | T59.4X2 | T59.4X3 | T59.4X4 | — | — |
| **Chlorisondamine chloride** | T46.991 | T46.992 | T46.993 | T46.994 | T46.995 | T46.996 |
| **Chlormadinone** | T38.5X1 | T38.5X2 | T38.5X3 | T38.5X4 | T38.5X5 | T38.5X6 |
| **Chlormephos** | T6Ø.ØX1 | T6Ø.ØX2 | T6Ø.ØX3 | T6Ø.ØX4 | — | — |
| **Chlormerodrin** | T5Ø.2X1 | T5Ø.2X2 | T5Ø.2X3 | T5Ø.2X4 | T5Ø.2X5 | T5Ø.2X6 |
| **Chlormethiazole** | T42.6X1 | T42.6X2 | T42.6X3 | T42.6X4 | T42.6X5 | T42.6X6 |
| **Chlormethine** | T45.1X1 | T45.1X2 | T45.1X3 | T45.1X4 | T45.1X5 | T45.1X6 |
| **Chlormethylenecycline** | T36.4X1 | T36.4X2 | T36.4X3 | T36.4X4 | T36.4X5 | T36.4X6 |
| **Chlormezanone** | T42.6X1 | T42.6X2 | T42.6X3 | T42.6X4 | T42.6X5 | T42.6X6 |
| **Chloroacetic acid** | T6Ø.3X1 | T6Ø.3X2 | T6Ø.3X3 | T6Ø.3X4 | — | — |
| **Chloroacetone** | T59.3X1 | T59.3X2 | T59.3X3 | T59.3X4 | — | — |
| **Chloroacetophenone** | T59.3X1 | T59.3X2 | T59.3X3 | T59.3X4 | — | — |
| **Chloroaniline** | T53.7X1 | T53.7X2 | T53.7X3 | T53.7X4 | — | — |
| **Chlorobenzene, chlorobenzol** | T53.7X1 | T53.7X2 | T53.7X3 | T53.7X4 | — | — |
| **Chlorobromomethane** (fire extinguisher) | T53.6X1 | T53.6X2 | T53.6X3 | T53.6X4 | — | — |
| **Chlorobutanol** | T49.ØX1 | T49.ØX2 | T49.ØX3 | T49.ØX4 | T49.ØX5 | T49.ØX6 |
| **Chlorocresol** | T49.ØX1 | T49.ØX2 | T49.ØX3 | T49.ØX4 | T49.ØX5 | T49.ØX6 |
| **Chlorodehydromethyltestosterone** | T38.7X1 | T38.7X2 | T38.7X3 | T38.7X4 | T38.7X5 | T38.7X6 |
| **Chlorodeoxyadenosine*** | T45.1X1 | T45.1X2 | T45.1X3 | T45.1X4 | T45.1X5 | T45.1X6 |
| **Chlorodinitrobenzene** | T53.7X1 | T53.7X2 | T53.7X3 | T53.7X4 | — | — |
| dust or vapor | T53.7X1 | T53.7X2 | T53.7X3 | T53.7X4 | — | — |
| **Chlorodiphenyl** | T53.7X1 | T53.7X2 | T53.7X3 | T53.7X4 | — | — |
| **Chloroethane** — *see* Ethyl, chloride | | | | | | |
| **Chloroethylene** | T53.6X1 | T53.6X2 | T53.6X3 | T53.6X4 | — | — |
| **Chlorofluorocarbons** | T53.5X1 | T53.5X2 | T53.5X3 | T53.5X4 | — | — |
| **Chloroform** (fumes) (vapor) | T53.1X1 | T53.1X2 | T53.1X3 | T53.1X4 | — | — |
| anesthetic | T41.ØX1 | T41.ØX2 | T41.ØX3 | T41.ØX4 | T41.ØX5 | T41.ØX6 |
| solvent | T53.1X1 | T53.1X2 | T53.1X3 | T53.1X4 | — | — |
| water, concentrated | T41.ØX1 | T41.ØX2 | T41.ØX3 | T41.ØX4 | T41.ØX5 | T41.ØX6 |
| **Chloroguanide** | T37.2X1 | T37.2X2 | T37.2X3 | T37.2X4 | T37.2X5 | T37.2X6 |
| **Chloromycetin** | T36.2X1 | T36.2X2 | T36.2X3 | T36.2X4 | T36.2X5 | T36.2X6 |
| ENT agent | T49.6X1 | T49.6X2 | T49.6X3 | T49.6X4 | T49.6X5 | T49.6X6 |
| ophthalmic preparation | T49.5X1 | T49.5X2 | T49.5X3 | T49.5X4 | T49.5X5 | T49.5X6 |
| otic solution | T49.6X1 | T49.6X2 | T49.6X3 | T49.6X4 | T49.6X5 | T49.6X6 |
| topical NEC | T49.ØX1 | T49.ØX2 | T49.ØX3 | T49.ØX4 | T49.ØX5 | T49.ØX6 |
| **Chloronitrobenzene** | T53.7X1 | T53.7X2 | T53.7X3 | T53.7X4 | — | — |
| dust or vapor | T53.7X1 | T53.7X2 | T53.7X3 | T53.7X4 | — | — |
| **Chlorophacinone** | T6Ø.4X1 | T6Ø.4X2 | T6Ø.4X3 | T6Ø.4X4 | — | — |
| **Chlorophenol** | T53.7X1 | T53.7X2 | T53.7X3 | T53.7X4 | — | — |
| **Chlorophenothane** | T6Ø.1X1 | T6Ø.1X2 | T6Ø.1X3 | T6Ø.1X4 | — | — |
| **Chlorophyll** | T5Ø.991 | T5Ø.992 | T5Ø.993 | T5Ø.994 | T5Ø.995 | T5Ø.996 |
| **Chloropicrin** (fumes) | T53.6X1 | T53.6X2 | T53.6X3 | T53.6X4 | — | — |
| fumigant | T6Ø.8X1 | T6Ø.8X2 | T6Ø.8X3 | T6Ø.8X4 | — | — |
| fungicide | T6Ø.3X1 | T6Ø.3X2 | T6Ø.3X3 | T6Ø.3X4 | — | — |
| pesticide | T6Ø.8X1 | T6Ø.8X2 | T6Ø.8X3 | T6Ø.8X4 | — | — |
| **Chloroprocaine** | T41.3X1 | T41.3X2 | T41.3X3 | T41.3X4 | T41.3X5 | T41.3X6 |
| infiltration (subcutaneous) | T41.3X1 | T41.3X2 | T41.3X3 | T41.3X4 | T41.3X5 | T41.3X6 |
| nerve block (peripheral) (plexus) | T41.3X1 | T41.3X2 | T41.3X3 | T41.3X4 | T41.3X5 | T41.3X6 |
| spinal | T41.3X1 | T41.3X2 | T41.3X3 | T41.3X4 | T41.3X5 | T41.3X6 |
| **Chloroptic** | T49.5X1 | T49.5X2 | T49.5X3 | T49.5X4 | T49.5X5 | T49.5X6 |
| **Chloropurine** | T45.1X1 | T45.1X2 | T45.1X3 | T45.1X4 | T45.1X5 | T45.1X6 |
| **Chloropyramine** | T45.ØX1 | T45.ØX2 | T45.ØX3 | T45.ØX4 | T45.ØX5 | T45.ØX6 |
| **Chloropyrifos** | T6Ø.ØX1 | T6Ø.ØX2 | T6Ø.ØX3 | T6Ø.ØX4 | — | — |
| **Chloropyrilene** | T45.ØX1 | T45.ØX2 | T45.ØX3 | T45.ØX4 | T45.ØX5 | T45.ØX6 |
| **Chloroquine** | T37.2X1 | T37.2X2 | T37.2X3 | T37.2X4 | T37.2X5 | T37.2X6 |
| **Chlorostat*** | T49.ØX1 | T49.ØX2 | T49.ØX3 | T49.ØX4 | T49.ØX5 | T49.ØX6 |
| **Chlorothalonil** | T6Ø.3X1 | T6Ø.3X2 | T6Ø.3X3 | T6Ø.3X4 | — | — |

| Substance | Poisoning, Accidental (unintentional) | Poisoning, Intentional Self-harm | Poisoning, Assault | Poisoning, Undetermined | Adverse Effect | Under-dosing |
|---|---|---|---|---|---|---|
| **Chlorothen** | T45.ØX1 | T45.ØX2 | T45.ØX3 | T45.ØX4 | T45.ØX5 | T45.ØX6 |
| **Chlorothiazide** | T5Ø.2X1 | T5Ø.2X2 | T5Ø.2X3 | T5Ø.2X4 | T5Ø.2X5 | T5Ø.2X6 |
| **Chlorothymol** | T49.4X1 | T49.4X2 | T49.4X3 | T49.4X4 | T49.4X5 | T49.4X6 |
| **Chlorotrianisene** | T38.5X1 | T38.5X2 | T38.5X3 | T38.5X4 | T38.5X5 | T38.5X6 |
| **Chlorovinyldichloroarsine, not in war** | T57.ØX1 | T57.ØX2 | T57.ØX3 | T57.ØX4 | — | — |
| **Chloroxine** | T49.4X1 | T49.4X2 | T49.4X3 | T49.4X4 | T49.4X5 | T49.4X6 |
| **Chloroxylenol** | T49.ØX1 | T49.ØX2 | T49.ØX3 | T49.ØX4 | T49.ØX5 | T49.ØX6 |
| **Chlorphenamine** | T45.ØX1 | T45.ØX2 | T45.ØX3 | T45.ØX4 | T45.ØX5 | T45.ØX6 |
| **Chlorphenesin** | T42.8X1 | T42.8X2 | T42.8X3 | T42.8X4 | T42.8X5 | T42.8X6 |
| topical (antifungal) | T49.ØX1 | T49.ØX2 | T49.ØX3 | T49.ØX4 | T49.ØX5 | T49.ØX6 |
| **Chlorpheniramine** | T45.ØX1 | T45.ØX2 | T45.ØX3 | T45.ØX4 | T45.ØX5 | T45.ØX6 |
| **Chlorphenoxamine** | T45.ØX1 | T45.ØX2 | T45.ØX3 | T45.ØX4 | T45.ØX5 | T45.ØX6 |
| **Chlorphentermine** | T5Ø.5X1 | T5Ø.5X2 | T5Ø.5X3 | T5Ø.5X4 | T5Ø.5X5 | T5Ø.5X6 |
| **Chlorprocaine** — *see* Chloroprocaine | | | | | | |
| **Chlorproguanil** | T37.2X1 | T37.2X2 | T37.2X3 | T37.2X4 | T37.2X5 | T37.2X6 |
| **Chlorpromazine** | T43.3X1 | T43.3X2 | T43.3X3 | T43.3X4 | T43.3X5 | T43.3X6 |
| **Chlorpropamide** | T38.3X1 | T38.3X2 | T38.3X3 | T38.3X4 | T38.3X5 | T38.3X6 |
| **Chlorprothixene** | T43.4X1 | T43.4X2 | T43.4X3 | T43.4X4 | T43.4X5 | T43.4X6 |
| **Chlorquinaldol** | T49.ØX1 | T49.ØX2 | T49.ØX3 | T49.ØX4 | T49.ØX5 | T49.ØX6 |
| **Chlorquinol** | T49.ØX1 | T49.ØX2 | T49.ØX3 | T49.ØX4 | T49.ØX5 | T49.ØX6 |
| **Chlortalidone** | T5Ø.2X1 | T5Ø.2X2 | T5Ø.2X3 | T5Ø.2X4 | T5Ø.2X5 | T5Ø.2X6 |
| **Chlortetracycline** | T36.4X1 | T36.4X2 | T36.4X3 | T36.4X4 | T36.4X5 | T36.4X6 |
| **Chlorthalidone** | T5Ø.2X1 | T5Ø.2X2 | T5Ø.2X3 | T5Ø.2X4 | T5Ø.2X5 | T5Ø.2X6 |
| **Chlorthion** | T6Ø.ØX1 | T6Ø.ØX2 | T6Ø.ØX3 | T6Ø.ØX4 | — | — |
| **Chlorthiophos** | T6Ø.ØX1 | T6Ø.ØX2 | T6Ø.ØX3 | T6Ø.ØX4 | — | — |
| **Chlortrianisene** | T38.5X1 | T38.5X2 | T38.5X3 | T38.5X4 | T38.5X5 | T38.5X6 |
| **Chlorzoxazone** | T42.8X1 | T42.8X2 | T42.8X3 | T42.8X4 | T42.8X5 | T42.8X6 |
| **Choke damp** | T59.7X1 | T59.7X2 | T59.7X3 | T59.7X4 | — | — |
| **Cholagogues** | T47.5X1 | T47.5X2 | T47.5X3 | T47.5X4 | T47.5X5 | T47.5X6 |
| **Cholebrine** | T5Ø.8X1 | T5Ø.8X2 | T5Ø.8X3 | T5Ø.8X4 | T5Ø.8X5 | T5Ø.8X6 |
| **Cholecalciferol** | T45.2X1 | T45.2X2 | T45.2X3 | T45.2X4 | T45.2X5 | T45.2X6 |
| **Cholecystokinin** | T5Ø.8X1 | T5Ø.8X2 | T5Ø.8X3 | T5Ø.8X4 | T5Ø.8X5 | T5Ø.8X6 |
| **Cholera vaccine** | T5Ø.A91 | T5Ø.A92 | T5Ø.A93 | T5Ø.A94 | T5Ø.A95 | T5Ø.A96 |
| **Choleretic** | T47.5X1 | T47.5X2 | T47.5X3 | T47.5X4 | T47.5X5 | T47.5X6 |
| **Cholesterol-lowering agents** | T46.6X1 | T46.6X2 | T46.6X3 | T46.6X4 | T46.6X5 | T46.6X6 |
| **Cholestyramine** (resin) | T46.6X1 | T46.6X2 | T46.6X3 | T46.6X4 | T46.6X5 | T46.6X6 |
| **Cholic acid** | T47.5X1 | T47.5X2 | T47.5X3 | T47.5X4 | T47.5X5 | T47.5X6 |
| **Choline** | T48.6X1 | T48.6X2 | T48.6X3 | T48.6X4 | T48.6X5 | T48.6X6 |
| chloride | T5Ø.991 | T5Ø.992 | T5Ø.993 | T5Ø.994 | T5Ø.995 | T5Ø.996 |
| dihydrogen citrate | T5Ø.991 | T5Ø.992 | T5Ø.993 | T5Ø.994 | T5Ø.995 | T5Ø.996 |
| salicylate | T39.Ø91 | T39.Ø92 | T39.Ø93 | T39.Ø94 | T39.Ø95 | T39.Ø96 |
| theophyllinate | T48.6X1 | T48.6X2 | T48.6X3 | T48.6X4 | T48.6X5 | T48.6X6 |
| **Cholinergic** (drug) **NEC** | T44.1X1 | T44.1X2 | T44.1X3 | T44.1X4 | T44.1X5 | T44.1X6 |
| muscle tone enhancer | T44.1X1 | T44.1X2 | T44.1X3 | T44.1X4 | T44.1X5 | T44.1X6 |
| organophosphorus | T44.ØX1 | T44.ØX2 | T44.ØX3 | T44.ØX4 | T44.ØX5 | T44.ØX6 |
| insecticide | T6Ø.ØX1 | T6Ø.ØX2 | T6Ø.ØX3 | T6Ø.ØX4 | — | — |
| nerve gas | T59.891 | T59.892 | T59.893 | T59.894 | — | — |
| trimethyl ammonium propanediol | T44.1X1 | T44.1X2 | T44.1X3 | T44.1X4 | T44.1X5 | T44.1X6 |
| **Cholinesterase reactivator** | T5Ø.6X1 | T5Ø.6X2 | T5Ø.6X3 | T5Ø.6X4 | T5Ø.6X5 | T5Ø.6X6 |
| **Cholografin** | T5Ø.8X1 | T5Ø.8X2 | T5Ø.8X3 | T5Ø.8X4 | T5Ø.8X5 | T5Ø.8X6 |
| **Chorionic gonadotropin** | T38.891 | T38.892 | T38.893 | T38.894 | T38.895 | T38.896 |
| **Chromate** | T56.2X1 | T56.2X2 | T56.2X3 | T56.2X4 | — | — |
| dust or mist | T56.2X1 | T56.2X2 | T56.2X3 | T56.2X4 | — | — |
| lead — *see also* lead | T56.ØX1 | T56.ØX2 | T56.ØX3 | T56.ØX4 | — | — |
| paint | T56.ØX1 | T56.ØX2 | T56.ØX3 | T56.ØX4 | — | — |
| **Chromelin*** | T49.3X1 | T49.3X2 | T49.3X3 | T49.3X4 | T49.3X5 | T49.3X6 |
| **Chromic** | | | | | | |
| acid | T56.2X1 | T56.2X2 | T56.2X3 | T56.2X4 | — | — |
| dust or mist | T56.2X1 | T56.2X2 | T56.2X3 | T56.2X4 | — | — |
| phosphate 32P | T45.1X1 | T45.1X2 | T45.1X3 | T45.1X4 | T45.1X5 | T45.1X6 |
| **Chromium** | T56.2X1 | T56.2X2 | T56.2X3 | T56.2X4 | — | — |
| compounds — *see* Chromate | | | | | | |
| sesquioxide | T5Ø.8X1 | T5Ø.8X2 | T5Ø.8X3 | T5Ø.8X4 | T5Ø.8X5 | T5Ø.8X6 |
| **Chromomycin A3** | T45.1X1 | T45.1X2 | T45.1X3 | T45.1X4 | T45.1X5 | T45.1X6 |
| **Chromonar** | T46.3X1 | T46.3X2 | T46.3X3 | T46.3X4 | T46.3X5 | T46.3X6 |
| **Chromyl chloride** | T56.2X1 | T56.2X2 | T56.2X3 | T56.2X4 | — | — |
| **Chrysarobin** | T49.4X1 | T49.4X2 | T49.4X3 | T49.4X4 | T49.4X5 | T49.4X6 |
| **Chrysazin** | T47.2X1 | T47.2X2 | T47.2X3 | T47.2X4 | T47.2X5 | T47.2X6 |
| **Chymar** | T45.3X1 | T45.3X2 | T45.3X3 | T45.3X4 | T45.3X5 | T45.3X6 |
| ophthalmic preparation | T49.5X1 | T49.5X2 | T49.5X3 | T49.5X4 | T49.5X5 | T49.5X6 |
| **Chymopapain** | T45.3X1 | T45.3X2 | T45.3X3 | T45.3X4 | T45.3X5 | T45.3X6 |
| **Chymotrypsin** | T45.3X1 | T45.3X2 | T45.3X3 | T45.3X4 | T45.3X5 | T45.3X6 |
| ophthalmic preparation | T49.5X1 | T49.5X2 | T49.5X3 | T49.5X4 | T49.5X5 | T49.5X6 |
| **Cialis*** | T46.7X1 | T46.7X2 | T46.7X3 | T46.7X4 | T46.7X5 | T46.7X6 |
| **Cianidanol** | T5Ø.991 | T5Ø.992 | T5Ø.993 | T5Ø.994 | T5Ø.995 | T5Ø.996 |
| **Cianopramine** | T43.Ø11 | T43.Ø12 | T43.Ø13 | T43.Ø14 | T43.Ø15 | T43.Ø16 |
| **Cibenzoline** | T46.2X1 | T46.2X2 | T46.2X3 | T46.2X4 | T46.2X5 | T46.2X6 |
| **Ciclacillin** | T36.ØX1 | T36.ØX2 | T36.ØX3 | T36.ØX4 | T36.ØX5 | T36.ØX6 |

| Substance | Poisoning, Accidental (unintentional) | Poisoning, Intentional Self-harm | Poisoning, Assault | Poisoning, Undetermined | Adverse Effect | Under-dosing |
|---|---|---|---|---|---|---|
| **Ciclobarbital** — *see* Hexobarbital | | | | | | |
| **Ciclonicate** | T46.7X1 | T46.7X2 | T46.7X3 | T46.7X4 | T46.7X5 | T46.7X6 |
| **Ciclopirox** (olamine) | T49.ØX1 | T49.ØX2 | T49.ØX3 | T49.ØX4 | T49.ØX5 | T49.ØX6 |
| **Ciclosporin** | T45.1X1 | T45.1X2 | T45.1X3 | T45.1X4 | T45.1X5 | T45.1X6 |
| **Cicuta maculata or virosa** | T62.2X1 | T62.2X2 | T62.2X3 | T62.2X4 | — | — |
| **Cicutoxin** | T62.2X1 | T62.2X2 | T62.2X3 | T62.2X4 | — | — |
| **Cigarette lighter fluid** | T52.ØX1 | T52.ØX2 | T52.ØX3 | T52.ØX4 | — | — |
| **Cigarettes** (tobacco) | T65.221 | T65.222 | T65.223 | T65.224 | — | — |
| **Ciguatoxin** | T61.Ø1 | T61.Ø2 | T61.Ø3 | T61.Ø4 | — | — |
| **Cilazapril** | T46.4X1 | T46.4X2 | T46.4X3 | T46.4X4 | T46.4X5 | T46.4X6 |
| **Cimetidine** | T47.ØX1 | T47.ØX2 | T47.ØX3 | T47.ØX4 | T47.ØX5 | T47.ØX6 |
| **Cimetropium bromide** | T44.3X1 | T44.3X2 | T44.3X3 | T44.3X4 | T44.3X5 | T44.3X6 |
| **Cinchocaine** | T41.3X1 | T41.3X2 | T41.3X3 | T41.3X4 | T41.3X5 | T41.3X6 |
| topical (surface) | T41.3X1 | T41.3X2 | T41.3X3 | T41.3X4 | T41.3X5 | T41.3X6 |
| **Cinchona** | T37.2X1 | T37.2X2 | T37.2X3 | T37.2X4 | T37.2X5 | T37.2X6 |
| **Cinchonine alkaloids** | T37.2X1 | T37.2X2 | T37.2X3 | T37.2X4 | T37.2X5 | T37.2X6 |
| **Cinchophen** | T5Ø.4X1 | T5Ø.4X2 | T5Ø.4X3 | T5Ø.4X4 | T5Ø.4X5 | T5Ø.4X6 |
| **Cinepazide** | T46.7X1 | T46.7X2 | T46.7X3 | T46.7X4 | T46.7X5 | T46.7X6 |
| **Cinnamedrine** | T48.5X1 | T48.5X2 | T48.5X3 | T48.5X4 | T48.5X5 | T48.5X6 |
| **Cinnarizine** | T45.ØX1 | T45.ØX2 | T45.ØX3 | T45.ØX4 | T45.ØX5 | T45.ØX6 |
| **Cinoxacin** | T37.8X1 | T37.8X2 | T37.8X3 | T37.8X4 | T37.8X5 | T37.8X6 |
| **Ciprofibrate** | T46.6X1 | T46.6X2 | T46.6X3 | T46.6X4 | T46.6X5 | T46.6X6 |
| **Ciprofloxacin** | T36.8X1 | T36.8X2 | T36.8X3 | T36.8X4 | T36.8X5 | T36.8X6 |
| **Cisapride** | T47.8X1 | T47.8X2 | T47.8X3 | T47.8X4 | T47.8X5 | T47.8X6 |
| **Cisplatin** | T45.1X1 | T45.1X2 | T45.1X3 | T45.1X4 | T45.1X5 | T45.1X6 |
| **Citalopram** | T43.221 | T43.222 | T43.223 | T43.224 | T43.225 | T43.226 |
| **Citanest** | T41.3X1 | T41.3X2 | T41.3X3 | T41.3X4 | T41.3X5 | T41.3X6 |
| infiltration (subcutaneous) | T41.3X1 | T41.3X2 | T41.3X3 | T41.3X4 | T41.3X5 | T41.3X6 |
| nerve block (peripheral) (plexus) | T41.3X1 | T41.3X2 | T41.3X3 | T41.3X4 | T41.3X5 | T41.3X6 |
| **Citracel*** | T5Ø.3X1 | T5Ø.3X2 | T5Ø.3X3 | T5Ø.3X4 | T5Ø.3X5 | T5Ø.3X6 |
| **Citric acid** | T47.5X1 | T47.5X2 | T47.5X3 | T47.5X4 | T47.5X5 | T47.5X6 |
| **Citrovorum** (factor) | T45.8X1 | T45.8X2 | T45.8X3 | T45.8X4 | T45.8X5 | T45.8X6 |
| **Claviceps purpurea** | T62.2X1 | T62.2X2 | T62.2X3 | T62.2X4 | — | — |
| **Clavulanic acid** | T36.1X1 | T36.1X2 | T36.1X3 | T36.1X4 | T36.1X5 | T36.1X6 |
| **Cleaner, cleansing agent, type not specified** | T65.891 | T65.892 | T65.893 | T65.894 | — | — |
| of paint or varnish | T52.91 | T52.92 | T52.93 | T52.94 | — | — |
| specified type NEC | T65.891 | T65.892 | T65.893 | T65.894 | — | — |
| **Clebopride** | T47.8X1 | T47.8X2 | T47.8X3 | T47.8X4 | T47.8X5 | T47.8X6 |
| **Clefamide** | T37.3X1 | T37.3X2 | T37.3X3 | T37.3X4 | T37.3X5 | T37.3X6 |
| **Clemastine** | T45.ØX1 | T45.ØX2 | T45.ØX3 | T45.ØX4 | T45.ØX5 | T45.ØX6 |
| **Clematis vitalba** | T62.2X1 | T62.2X2 | T62.2X3 | T62.2X4 | — | — |
| **Clemizole** | T45.ØX1 | T45.ØX2 | T45.ØX3 | T45.ØX4 | T45.ØX5 | T45.ØX6 |
| penicillin | T36.ØX1 | T36.ØX2 | T36.ØX3 | T36.ØX4 | T36.ØX5 | T36.ØX6 |
| **Clenbuterol** | T48.6X1 | T48.6X2 | T48.6X3 | T48.6X4 | T48.6X5 | T48.6X6 |
| **Clidinium bromide** | T44.3X1 | T44.3X2 | T44.3X3 | T44.3X4 | T44.3X5 | T44.3X6 |
| **Climara*** | T38.5X1 | T38.5X2 | T38.5X3 | T38.5X4 | T38.5X5 | T38.5X6 |
| **Clinda-Derm*** | T49.ØX1 | T49.ØX2 | T49.ØX3 | T49.ØX4 | T49.ØX5 | T49.ØX6 |
| **Clindamycin** | T36.8X1 | T36.8X2 | T36.8X3 | T36.8X4 | T36.8X5 | T36.8X6 |
| **Clinofibrate** | T46.6X1 | T46.6X2 | T46.6X3 | T46.6X4 | T46.6X5 | T46.6X6 |
| **Clioquinol** | T37.8X1 | T37.8X2 | T37.8X3 | T37.8X4 | T37.8X5 | T37.8X6 |
| **Cliradon** | T4Ø.2X1 | T4Ø.2X2 | T4Ø.2X3 | T4Ø.2X4 | — | — |
| **Clobazam** | T42.4X1 | T42.4X2 | T42.4X3 | T42.4X4 | T42.4X5 | T42.4X6 |
| **Clobenzorex** | T5Ø.5X1 | T5Ø.5X2 | T5Ø.5X3 | T5Ø.5X4 | T5Ø.5X5 | T5Ø.5X6 |
| **Clobetasol** | T49.ØX1 | T49.ØX2 | T49.ØX3 | T49.ØX4 | T49.ØX5 | T49.ØX6 |
| **Clobetasone** | T49.ØX1 | T49.ØX2 | T49.ØX3 | T49.ØX4 | T49.ØX5 | T49.ØX6 |
| **Clobutinol** | T48.3X1 | T48.3X2 | T48.3X3 | T48.3X4 | T48.3X5 | T48.3X6 |
| **Clocortolone** | T38.ØX1 | T38.ØX2 | T38.ØX3 | T38.ØX4 | T38.ØX5 | T38.ØX6 |
| **Clodantoin** | T49.ØX1 | T49.ØX2 | T49.ØX3 | T49.ØX4 | T49.ØX5 | T49.ØX6 |
| **Clodronic acid** | T5Ø.991 | T5Ø.992 | T5Ø.993 | T5Ø.994 | T5Ø.995 | T5Ø.996 |
| **Clofazimine** | T37.1X1 | T37.1X2 | T37.1X3 | T37.1X4 | T37.1X5 | T37.1X6 |
| **Clofedanol** | T48.3X1 | T48.3X2 | T48.3X3 | T48.3X4 | T48.3X5 | T48.3X6 |
| **Clofenamide** | T5Ø.2X1 | T5Ø.2X2 | T5Ø.2X3 | T5Ø.2X4 | T5Ø.2X5 | T5Ø.2X6 |
| **Clofenotane** | T49.ØX1 | T49.ØX2 | T49.ØX3 | T49.ØX4 | T49.ØX5 | T49.ØX6 |
| **Clofezone** | T39.2X1 | T39.2X2 | T39.2X3 | T39.2X4 | T39.2X5 | T39.2X6 |
| **Clofibrate** | T46.6X1 | T46.6X2 | T46.6X3 | T46.6X4 | T46.6X5 | T46.6X6 |
| **Clofibride** | T46.6X1 | T46.6X2 | T46.6X3 | T46.6X4 | T46.6X5 | T46.6X6 |
| **Cloforex** | T5Ø.5X1 | T5Ø.5X2 | T5Ø.5X3 | T5Ø.5X4 | T5Ø.5X5 | T5Ø.5X6 |
| **Clomethiazole** | T42.6X1 | T42.6X2 | T42.6X3 | T42.6X4 | T42.6X5 | T42.6X6 |
| **Clometocillin** | T36.ØX1 | T36.ØX2 | T36.ØX3 | T36.ØX4 | T36.ØX5 | T36.ØX6 |
| **Clomifene** | T38.5X1 | T38.5X2 | T38.5X3 | T38.5X4 | T38.5X5 | T38.5X6 |
| **Clomiphene** | T38.5X1 | T38.5X2 | T38.5X3 | T38.5X4 | T38.5X5 | T38.5X6 |
| **Clomipramine** | T43.Ø11 | T43.Ø12 | T43.Ø13 | T43.Ø14 | T43.Ø15 | T43.Ø16 |
| **Clomocycline** | T36.4X1 | T36.4X2 | T36.4X3 | T36.4X4 | T36.4X5 | T36.4X6 |
| **Clonazepam** | T42.4X1 | T42.4X2 | T42.4X3 | T42.4X4 | T42.4X5 | T42.4X6 |
| **Clonidine** | T46.5X1 | T46.5X2 | T46.5X3 | T46.5X4 | T46.5X5 | T46.5X6 |
| **Clonixin** | T39.8X1 | T39.8X2 | T39.8X3 | T39.8X4 | T39.8X5 | T39.8X6 |
| **Clopamide** | T5Ø.2X1 | T5Ø.2X2 | T5Ø.2X3 | T5Ø.2X4 | T5Ø.2X5 | T5Ø.2X6 |
| **Clopenthixol** | T43.4X1 | T43.4X2 | T43.4X3 | T43.4X4 | T43.4X5 | T43.4X6 |
| **Cloperastine** | T48.3X1 | T48.3X2 | T48.3X3 | T48.3X4 | T48.3X5 | T48.3X6 |
| **Clophedianol** | T48.3X1 | T48.3X2 | T48.3X3 | T48.3X4 | T48.3X5 | T48.3X6 |

| Substance | Poisoning, Accidental (unintentional) | Poisoning, Intentional Self-harm | Poisoning, Assault | Poisoning, Undetermined | Adverse Effect | Under-dosing |
|---|---|---|---|---|---|---|
| **Cloponone** | T36.2X1 | T36.2X2 | T36.2X3 | T36.2X4 | T36.2X5 | T36.2X |
| **Cloprednol** | T38.ØX1 | T38.ØX2 | T38.ØX3 | T38.ØX4 | T38.ØX5 | T38.ØX |
| **Cloral betaine** | T42.6X1 | T42.6X2 | T42.6X3 | T42.6X4 | T42.6X5 | T42.6X |
| **Cloramfenicol** | T36.2X1 | T36.2X2 | T36.2X3 | T36.2X4 | T36.2X5 | T36.2X |
| **Clorazepate** (dipotassium) | T42.4X1 | T42.4X2 | T42.4X3 | T42.4X4 | T42.4X5 | T42.4X |
| **Clorexolone** | T5Ø.2X1 | T5Ø.2X2 | T5Ø.2X3 | T5Ø.2X4 | T5Ø.2X5 | T5Ø.2X |
| **Clorfenamine** | T45.ØX1 | T45.ØX2 | T45.ØX3 | T45.ØX4 | T45.ØX5 | T45.ØX |
| **Clorgiline** | T43.1X1 | T43.1X2 | T43.1X3 | T43.1X4 | T43.1X5 | T43.1X |
| **Clorotepine** | T44.3X1 | T44.3X2 | T44.3X3 | T44.3X4 | T44.3X5 | T44.3X |
| **Clorox** (bleach) | T54.91 | T54.92 | T54.93 | T54.94 | — | — |
| **Clorprenaline** | T48.6X1 | T48.6X2 | T48.6X3 | T48.6X4 | T48.6X5 | T48.6X |
| **Clortermine** | T5Ø.5X1 | T5Ø.5X2 | T5Ø.5X3 | T5Ø.5X4 | T5Ø.5X5 | T5Ø.5X |
| **Clotiapine** | T43.591 | T43.592 | T43.593 | T43.594 | T43.595 | T43.59 |
| **Clotiazepam** | T42.4X1 | T42.4X2 | T42.4X3 | T42.4X4 | T42.4X5 | T42.4X |
| **Clotibric acid** | T46.6X1 | T46.6X2 | T46.6X3 | T46.6X4 | T46.6X5 | T46.6X |
| **Clotrimazole** | T49.ØX1 | T49.ØX2 | T49.ØX3 | T49.ØX4 | T49.ØX5 | T49.ØX |
| **Cloxacillin** | T36.ØX1 | T36.ØX2 | T36.ØX3 | T36.ØX4 | T36.ØX5 | T36.ØX |
| **Cloxazolam** | T42.4X1 | T42.4X2 | T42.4X3 | T42.4X4 | T42.4X5 | T42.4X |
| **Cloxiquine** | T49.ØX1 | T49.ØX2 | T49.ØX3 | T49.ØX4 | T49.ØX5 | T49.ØX |
| **Clozapine** | T42.4X1 | T42.4X2 | T42.4X3 | T42.4X4 | T42.4X5 | T42.4X |
| **Coagulant NEC** | T45.7X1 | T45.7X2 | T45.7X3 | T45.7X4 | T45.7X5 | T45.7X |
| **Coal** (carbon monoxide from) — *see also* Carbon, monoxide, coal | T58.2X1 | T58.2X2 | T58.2X3 | T58.2X4 | — | — |
| oil — *see* Kerosene | | | | | | |
| tar | T49.1X1 | T49.1X2 | T49.1X3 | T49.1X4 | T49.1X5 | T49.1X |
| fumes | T59.891 | T59.892 | T59.893 | T59.894 | — | — |
| medicinal (ointment) | T49.4X1 | T49.4X2 | T49.4X3 | T49.4X4 | T49.4X5 | T49.4X |
| analgesics NEC | T39.2X1 | T39.2X2 | T39.2X3 | T39.2X4 | T39.2X5 | T39.2X |
| naphtha (solvent) | T52.ØX1 | T52.ØX2 | T52.ØX3 | T52.ØX4 | — | — |
| **Coartem*** | T37.2X1 | T37.2X2 | T37.2X3 | T37.2X4 | T37.2X5 | T37.2X |
| **Cobalamine** | T45.2X1 | T45.2X2 | T45.2X3 | T45.2X4 | T45.2X5 | T45.2X |
| **Cobalt** (nonmedicinal) (fumes) (industrial) | T56.891 | T56.892 | T56.893 | T56.894 | — | — |
| medicinal (trace) (chloride) | T45.8X1 | T45.8X2 | T45.8X3 | T45.8X4 | T45.8X5 | T45.8X |
| **Cobra** (venom) | T63.Ø41 | T63.Ø42 | T63.Ø43 | T63.Ø44 | — | — |
| **Coca** (leaf) | T4Ø.5X1 | T4Ø.5X2 | T4Ø.5X3 | T4Ø.5X4 | T4Ø.5X5 | T4Ø.5X |
| **Cocaine** | T4Ø.5X1 | T4Ø.5X2 | T4Ø.5X3 | T4Ø.5X4 | T4Ø.5X5 | T4Ø.5X |
| topical anesthetic | T41.3X1 | T41.3X2 | T41.3X3 | T41.3X4 | T41.3X5 | T41.3X |
| **Cocarboxylase** | T45.3X1 | T45.3X2 | T45.3X3 | T45.3X4 | T45.3X5 | T45.3X |
| **Coccidioidin** | T5Ø.8X1 | T5Ø.8X2 | T5Ø.8X3 | T5Ø.8X4 | T5Ø.8X5 | T5Ø.8X |
| **Cocculus indicus** | T62.1X1 | T62.1X2 | T62.1X3 | T62.1X4 | — | — |
| **Cochineal** | T65.6X1 | T65.6X2 | T65.6X3 | T65.6X4 | — | — |
| medicinal products | T5Ø.991 | T5Ø.992 | T5Ø.993 | T5Ø.994 | T5Ø.995 | T5Ø.99 |
| **Cod-liver oil** | T45.2X1 | T45.2X2 | T45.2X3 | T45.2X4 | T45.2X5 | T45.2X |
| **Codeine** | T4Ø.2X1 | T4Ø.2X2 | T4Ø.2X3 | T4Ø.2X4 | T4Ø.2X5 | T4Ø.2X |
| **Coenzyme A** | T5Ø.991 | T5Ø.992 | T5Ø.993 | T5Ø.994 | T5Ø.995 | T5Ø.99 |
| **Coffee** | T62.8X1 | T62.8X2 | T62.8X3 | T62.8X4 | — | — |
| **Cogalactoisomerase** | T5Ø.991 | T5Ø.992 | T5Ø.993 | T5Ø.994 | T5Ø.995 | T5Ø.99 |
| **Cogentin** | T44.3X1 | T44.3X2 | T44.3X3 | T44.3X4 | T44.3X5 | T44.3X |
| **Coke fumes or gas** (carbon monoxide) | T58.2X1 | T58.2X2 | T58.2X3 | T58.2X4 | — | — |
| industrial use | T58.8X1 | T58.8X2 | T58.8X3 | T58.8X4 | — | — |
| **Colace** | T47.4X1 | T47.4X2 | T47.4X3 | T47.4X4 | T47.4X5 | T47.4X |
| **Colaspase** | T45.1X1 | T45.1X2 | T45.1X3 | T45.1X4 | T45.1X5 | T45.1X |
| **Colazal*** | T47.8X1 | T47.8X2 | T47.8X3 | T47.8X4 | T47.8X5 | T47.8X |
| **Colchicine** | T5Ø.4X1 | T5Ø.4X2 | T5Ø.4X3 | T5Ø.4X4 | T5Ø.4X5 | T5Ø.4X |
| **Colchicum** | T62.2X1 | T62.2X2 | T62.2X3 | T62.2X4 | — | — |
| **Cold cream** | T49.3X1 | T49.3X2 | T49.3X3 | T49.3X4 | T49.3X5 | T49.3X |
| **Colecalciferol** | T45.2X1 | T45.2X2 | T45.2X3 | T45.2X4 | T45.2X5 | T45.2X |
| **Colestipol** | T46.6X1 | T46.6X2 | T46.6X3 | T46.6X4 | T46.6X5 | T46.6X |
| **Colestyramine** | T46.6X1 | T46.6X2 | T46.6X3 | T46.6X4 | T46.6X5 | T46.6X |
| **Colimycin** | T36.8X1 | T36.8X2 | T36.8X3 | T36.8X4 | T36.8X5 | T36.8X |
| **Colistimethate** | T36.8X1 | T36.8X2 | T36.8X3 | T36.8X4 | T36.8X5 | T36.8X |
| **Colistin** | T36.8X1 | T36.8X2 | T36.8X3 | T36.8X4 | T36.8X5 | T36.8X |
| sulfate (eye preparation) | T49.5X1 | T49.5X2 | T49.5X3 | T49.5X4 | T49.5X5 | T49.5X |
| **Collagen** | T5Ø.991 | T5Ø.992 | T5Ø.993 | T5Ø.994 | T5Ø.995 | T5Ø.99 |
| **Collagenase** | T49.4X1 | T49.4X2 | T49.4X3 | T49.4X4 | T49.4X5 | T49.4X |
| **Collodion** | T49.3X1 | T49.3X2 | T49.3X3 | T49.3X4 | T49.3X5 | T49.3X |
| **Colocynth** | T47.2X1 | T47.2X2 | T47.2X3 | T47.2X4 | T47.2X5 | T47.2X |
| **Colophony adhesive** | T49.3X1 | T49.3X2 | T49.3X3 | T49.3X4 | T49.3X5 | T49.3X |
| **Colorant** — *see also* Dye | T5Ø.991 | T5Ø.992 | T5Ø.993 | T5Ø.994 | T5Ø.995 | T5Ø.99 |
| **Coloring matter** — *see* Dye(s) | | | | | | |
| **Combustion gas** (after combustion) — *see* Carbon, monoxide | | | | | | |
| prior to combustion | T59.891 | T59.892 | T59.893 | T59.894 | — | — |
| **Cometriq*** | T45.1X1 | T45.1X2 | T45.1X3 | T45.1X4 | T45.1X5 | T45.1X |
| **Compazine** | T43.3X1 | T43.3X2 | T43.3X3 | T43.3X4 | T43.3X5 | T43.3X |
| **Compound** | | | | | | |
| 1080 (sodium fluoroacetate) | T6Ø.4X1 | T6Ø.4X2 | T6Ø.4X3 | T6Ø.4X4 | — | — |
| 269 (endrin) | T6Ø.1X1 | T6Ø.1X2 | T6Ø.1X3 | T6Ø.1X4 | — | — |

| Substance | Poisoning, Accidental (unintentional) | Poisoning, Intentional Self-harm | Poisoning, Assault | Poisoning, Undetermined | Adverse Effect | Under-dosing |
|---|---|---|---|---|---|---|
| **Compound** — *continued* | | | | | | |
| 3422 (parathion) | T6Ø.ØX1 | T6Ø.ØX2 | T6Ø.ØX3 | T6Ø.ØX4 | — | — |
| 3911 (phorate) | T6Ø.ØX1 | T6Ø.ØX2 | T6Ø.ØX3 | T6Ø.ØX4 | — | — |
| 3956 (toxaphene) | T6Ø.1X1 | T6Ø.1X2 | T6Ø.1X3 | T6Ø.1X4 | — | — |
| 4049 (malathion) | T6Ø.ØX1 | T6Ø.ØX2 | T6Ø.ØX3 | T6Ø.ØX4 | — | — |
| 4069 (malathion) | T6Ø.ØX1 | T6Ø.ØX2 | T6Ø.ØX3 | T6Ø.ØX4 | — | — |
| 4124 (dicapthon) | T6Ø.ØX1 | T6Ø.ØX2 | T6Ø.ØX3 | T6Ø.ØX4 | — | — |
| 42 (warfarin) | T6Ø.4X1 | T6Ø.4X2 | T6Ø.4X3 | T6Ø.4X4 | — | — |
| 497 (dieldrin) | T6Ø.1X1 | T6Ø.1X2 | T6Ø.1X3 | T6Ø.1X4 | — | — |
| E (cortisone) | T38.ØX1 | T38.ØX2 | T38.ØX3 | T38.ØX4 | T38.ØX5 | T38.ØX6 |
| F (hydrocortisone) | T38.ØX1 | T38.ØX2 | T38.ØX3 | T38.ØX4 | T38.ØX5 | T38.ØX6 |
| **Comvax*** | T5Ø.A21 | T5Ø.A22 | T5Ø.A23 | T5Ø.A24 | T5Ø.A25 | T5Ø.A26 |
| **Congener, anabolic** | T38.7X1 | T38.7X2 | T38.7X3 | T38.7X4 | T38.7X5 | T38.7X6 |
| **Congo red** | T5Ø.8X1 | T5Ø.8X2 | T5Ø.8X3 | T5Ø.8X4 | T5Ø.8X5 | T5Ø.8X6 |
| **Coniine, conine** | T62.2X1 | T62.2X2 | T62.2X3 | T62.2X4 | — | — |
| **Conium** (maculatum) | T62.2X1 | T62.2X2 | T62.2X3 | T62.2X4 | — | — |
| **Conjugated estrogenic substances** | T38.5X1 | T38.5X2 | T38.5X3 | T38.5X4 | T38.5X5 | T38.5X6 |
| **Contac** | T48.5X1 | T48.5X2 | T48.5X3 | T48.5X4 | T48.5X5 | T48.5X6 |
| **Contact lens solution** | T49.5X1 | T49.5X2 | T49.5X3 | T49.5X4 | T49.5X5 | T49.5X6 |
| **Contraceptive** (oral) | T38.4X1 | T38.4X2 | T38.4X3 | T38.4X4 | T38.4X5 | T38.4X6 |
| vaginal | T49.8X1 | T49.8X2 | T49.8X3 | T49.8X4 | T49.8X5 | T49.8X6 |
| **Contrast medium, radiography** | T5Ø.8X1 | T5Ø.8X2 | T5Ø.8X3 | T5Ø.8X4 | T5Ø.8X5 | T5Ø.8X6 |
| **Convallaria glycosides** | T46.ØX1 | T46.ØX2 | T46.ØX3 | T46.ØX4 | T46.ØX5 | T46.ØX6 |
| **Convallaria majalis** | T62.2X1 | T62.2X2 | T62.2X3 | T62.2X4 | — | — |
| berry | T62.1X1 | T62.1X2 | T62.1X3 | T62.1X4 | — | — |
| **Copper** (dust) (fumes) (nonmedicinal) **NEC** | T56.4X1 | T56.4X2 | T56.4X3 | T56.4X4 | — | — |
| arsenate, arsenite | T57.ØX1 | T57.ØX2 | T57.ØX3 | T57.ØX4 | — | — |
| insecticide | T6Ø.2X1 | T6Ø.2X2 | T6Ø.2X3 | T6Ø.2X4 | — | — |
| emetic | T47.7X1 | T47.7X2 | T47.7X3 | T47.7X4 | T47.7X5 | T47.7X6 |
| fungicide | T6Ø.3X1 | T6Ø.3X2 | T6Ø.3X3 | T6Ø.3X4 | — | — |
| gluconate | T49.ØX1 | T49.ØX2 | T49.ØX3 | T49.ØX4 | T49.ØX5 | T49.ØX6 |
| insecticide | T6Ø.2X1 | T6Ø.2X2 | T6Ø.2X3 | T6Ø.2X4 | — | — |
| medicinal (trace) | T45.8X1 | T45.8X2 | T45.8X3 | T45.8X4 | T45.8X5 | T45.8X6 |
| oleate | T49.ØX1 | T49.ØX2 | T49.ØX3 | T49.ØX4 | T49.ØX5 | T49.ØX6 |
| sulfate | T56.4X1 | T56.4X2 | T56.4X3 | T56.4X4 | — | — |
| cupric | T56.4X1 | T56.4X2 | T56.4X3 | T56.4X4 | — | — |
| fungicide | T6Ø.3X1 | T6Ø.3X2 | T6Ø.3X3 | T6Ø.3X4 | — | — |
| medicinal | | | | | | |
| ear | T49.6X1 | T49.6X2 | T49.6X3 | T49.6X4 | T49.6X5 | T49.6X6 |
| emetic | T47.7X1 | T47.7X2 | T47.7X3 | T47.7X4 | T47.7X5 | T47.7X6 |
| eye | T49.5X1 | T49.5X2 | T49.5X3 | T49.5X4 | T49.5X5 | T49.5X6 |
| cuprous | T56.4X1 | T56.4X2 | T56.4X3 | T56.4X4 | — | — |
| fungicide | T6Ø.3X1 | T6Ø.3X2 | T6Ø.3X3 | T6Ø.3X4 | — | — |
| medicinal | | | | | | |
| ear | T49.6X1 | T49.6X2 | T49.6X3 | T49.6X4 | T49.6X5 | T49.6X6 |
| emetic | T47.7X1 | T47.7X2 | T47.7X3 | T47.7X4 | T47.7X5 | T47.7X6 |
| eye | T49.5X1 | T49.5X2 | T49.5X3 | T49.5X4 | T49.5X5 | T49.5X6 |
| **Copperhead snake** (bite) (venom) | T63.Ø61 | T63.Ø62 | T63.Ø63 | T63.Ø64 | — | — |
| **Coral** (sting) | T63.691 | T63.692 | T63.693 | T63.694 | — | — |
| snake (bite) (venom) | T63.Ø21 | T63.Ø22 | T63.Ø23 | T63.Ø24 | — | — |
| **Corbadrine** | T49.6X1 | T49.6X2 | T49.6X3 | T49.6X4 | T49.6X5 | T49.6X6 |
| **Cordite** | T65.891 | T65.892 | T65.893 | T65.894 | — | — |
| vapor | T59.891 | T59.892 | T59.893 | T59.894 | — | — |
| **Cordran** | T49.ØX1 | T49.ØX2 | T49.ØX3 | T49.ØX4 | T49.ØX5 | T49.ØX6 |
| **Coreg*** | T44.7X1 | T44.7X2 | T44.7X3 | T44.7X4 | T44.7X5 | T44.7X6 |
| **Cormax*** | T49.ØX1 | T49.ØX2 | T49.ØX3 | T49.ØX4 | T49.ØX5 | T49.ØX6 |
| **Corn cures** | T49.4X1 | T49.4X2 | T49.4X3 | T49.4X4 | T49.4X5 | T49.4X6 |
| **Corn starch** | T49.3X1 | T49.3X2 | T49.3X3 | T49.3X4 | T49.3X5 | T49.3X6 |
| **Cornhusker's lotion** | T49.3X1 | T49.3X2 | T49.3X3 | T49.3X4 | T49.3X5 | T49.3X6 |
| **Coronary vasodilator NEC** | T46.3X1 | T46.3X2 | T46.3X3 | T46.3X4 | T46.3X5 | T46.3X6 |
| **Corrosive NEC** | T54.91 | T54.92 | T54.93 | T54.94 | — | — |
| acid NEC | T54.2X1 | T54.2X2 | T54.2X3 | T54.2X4 | — | — |
| aromatics | T54.1X1 | T54.1X2 | T54.1X3 | T54.1X4 | — | — |
| disinfectant | T54.1X1 | T54.1X2 | T54.1X3 | T54.1X4 | — | — |
| fumes NEC | T54.91 | T54.92 | T54.93 | T54.94 | — | — |
| specified NEC | T54.91 | T54.92 | T54.93 | T54.94 | — | — |
| sublimate | T56.1X1 | T56.1X2 | T56.1X3 | T56.1X4 | — | — |
| **Cort-Dome** | T38.ØX1 | T38.ØX2 | T38.ØX3 | T38.ØX4 | T38.ØX5 | T38.ØX6 |
| ENT agent | T49.6X1 | T49.6X2 | T49.6X3 | T49.6X4 | T49.6X5 | T49.6X6 |
| ophthalmic preparation | T49.5X1 | T49.5X2 | T49.5X3 | T49.5X4 | T49.5X5 | T49.5X6 |
| topical NEC | T49.ØX1 | T49.ØX2 | T49.ØX3 | T49.ØX4 | T49.ØX5 | T49.ØX6 |
| **Cortate** | T38.ØX1 | T38.ØX2 | T38.ØX3 | T38.ØX4 | T38.ØX5 | T38.ØX6 |
| **Cortef** | T38.ØX1 | T38.ØX2 | T38.ØX3 | T38.ØX4 | T38.ØX5 | T38.ØX6 |
| ENT agent | T49.6X1 | T49.6X2 | T49.6X3 | T49.6X4 | T49.6X5 | T49.6X6 |
| ophthalmic preparation | T49.5X1 | T49.5X2 | T49.5X3 | T49.5X4 | T49.5X5 | T49.5X6 |
| topical NEC | T49.ØX1 | T49.ØX2 | T49.ØX3 | T49.ØX4 | T49.ØX5 | T49.ØX6 |
| **Corticosteroid** | T38.ØX1 | T38.ØX2 | T38.ØX3 | T38.ØX4 | T38.ØX5 | T38.ØX6 |
| ENT agent | T49.6X1 | T49.6X2 | T49.6X3 | T49.6X4 | T49.6X5 | T49.6X6 |
| mineral | T5Ø.ØX1 | T5Ø.ØX2 | T5Ø.ØX3 | T5Ø.ØX4 | T5Ø.ØX5 | T5Ø.ØX6 |

| Substance | Poisoning, Accidental (unintentional) | Poisoning, Intentional Self-harm | Poisoning, Assault | Poisoning, Undetermined | Adverse Effect | Under-dosing |
|---|---|---|---|---|---|---|
| **Corticosteroid** — *continued* | | | | | | |
| ophthalmic | T49.5X1 | T49.5X2 | T49.5X3 | T49.5X4 | T49.5X5 | T49.5X6 |
| topical NEC | T49.ØX1 | T49.ØX2 | T49.ØX3 | T49.ØX4 | T49.ØX5 | T49.ØX6 |
| **Corticotropin** | T38.811 | T38.812 | T38.813 | T38.814 | T38.815 | T38.816 |
| **Cortisol** | T49.ØX1 | T49.ØX2 | T49.ØX3 | T49.ØX4 | T49.ØX5 | T49.ØX6 |
| ENT agent | T49.6X1 | T49.6X2 | T49.6X3 | T49.6X4 | T49.6X5 | T49.6X6 |
| ophthalmic preparation | T49.5X1 | T49.5X2 | T49.5X3 | T49.5X4 | T49.5X5 | T49.5X6 |
| topical NEC | T49.ØX1 | T49.ØX2 | T49.ØX3 | T49.ØX4 | T49.ØX5 | T49.ØX6 |
| **Cortisone** (acetate) | T38.ØX1 | T38.ØX2 | T38.ØX3 | T38.ØX4 | T38.ØX5 | T38.ØX6 |
| ENT agent | T49.6X1 | T49.6X2 | T49.6X3 | T49.6X4 | T49.6X5 | T49.6X6 |
| ophthalmic preparation | T49.5X1 | T49.5X2 | T49.5X3 | T49.5X4 | T49.5X5 | T49.5X6 |
| topical NEC | T49.ØX1 | T49.ØX2 | T49.ØX3 | T49.ØX4 | T49.ØX5 | T49.ØX6 |
| **Cortisporin*** | T49.ØX1 | T49.ØX2 | T49.ØX3 | T49.ØX4 | T49.ØX5 | T49.ØX6 |
| **Cortivazol** | T38.ØX1 | T38.ØX2 | T38.ØX3 | T38.ØX4 | T38.ØX5 | T38.ØX6 |
| **Cortogen** | T38.ØX1 | T38.ØX2 | T38.ØX3 | T38.ØX4 | T38.ØX5 | T38.ØX6 |
| ENT agent | T49.6X1 | T49.6X2 | T49.6X3 | T49.6X4 | T49.6X5 | T49.6X6 |
| ophthalmic preparation | T49.5X1 | T49.5X2 | T49.5X3 | T49.5X4 | T49.5X5 | T49.5X6 |
| **Cortone** | T38.ØX1 | T38.ØX2 | T38.ØX3 | T38.ØX4 | T38.ØX5 | T38.ØX6 |
| ENT agent | T49.6X1 | T49.6X2 | T49.6X3 | T49.6X4 | T49.6X5 | T49.6X6 |
| ophthalmic preparation | T49.5X1 | T49.5X2 | T49.5X3 | T49.5X4 | T49.5X5 | T49.5X6 |
| **Cortril** | T38.ØX1 | T38.ØX2 | T38.ØX3 | T38.ØX4 | T38.ØX5 | T38.ØX6 |
| ENT agent | T49.6X1 | T49.6X2 | T49.6X3 | T49.6X4 | T49.6X5 | T49.6X6 |
| ophthalmic preparation | T49.5X1 | T49.5X2 | T49.5X3 | T49.5X4 | T49.5X5 | T49.5X6 |
| topical NEC | T49.ØX1 | T49.ØX2 | T49.ØX3 | T49.ØX4 | T49.ØX5 | T49.ØX6 |
| **Corynebacterium parvum** | T45.1X1 | T45.1X2 | T45.1X3 | T45.1X4 | T45.1X5 | T45.1X6 |
| **Cosmetic preparation** | T49.8X1 | T49.8X2 | T49.8X3 | T49.8X4 | T49.8X5 | T49.8X6 |
| **Cosmetics** | T49.8X1 | T49.8X2 | T49.8X3 | T49.8X4 | T49.8X5 | T49.8X6 |
| **Cosyntropin** | T38.811 | T38.812 | T38.813 | T38.814 | T38.815 | T38.816 |
| **Cotarnine** | T45.7X1 | T45.7X2 | T45.7X3 | T45.7X4 | T45.7X5 | T45.7X6 |
| **Co-trimoxazole** | T36.8X1 | T36.8X2 | T36.8X3 | T36.8X4 | T36.8X5 | T36.8X6 |
| **Cottonseed oil** | T49.3X1 | T49.3X2 | T49.3X3 | T49.3X4 | T49.3X5 | T49.3X6 |
| **Cough mixture** (syrup) | T48.4X1 | T48.4X2 | T48.4X3 | T48.4X4 | T48.4X5 | T48.4X6 |
| containing opiates | T4Ø.2X1 | T4Ø.2X2 | T4Ø.2X3 | T4Ø.2X4 | T4Ø.2X5 | T4Ø.2X6 |
| expectorants | T48.4X1 | T48.4X2 | T48.4X3 | T48.4X4 | T48.4X5 | T48.4X6 |
| **Coumadin** | T45.511 | T45.512 | T45.513 | T45.514 | T45.515 | T45.516 |
| rodenticide | T6Ø.4X1 | T6Ø.4X2 | T6Ø.4X3 | T6Ø.4X4 | — | — |
| **Coumaphos** | T6Ø.ØX1 | T6Ø.ØX2 | T6Ø.ØX3 | T6Ø.ØX4 | — | — |
| **Coumarin** | T45.511 | T45.512 | T45.513 | T45.514 | T45.515 | T45.516 |
| **Coumetarol** | T45.511 | T45.512 | T45.513 | T45.514 | T45.515 | T45.516 |
| **Cowbane** | T62.2X1 | T62.2X2 | T62.2X3 | T62.2X4 | — | — |
| **Cozaar*** | T46.5X1 | T46.5X2 | T46.5X3 | T46.5X4 | T46.5X5 | T46.5X6 |
| **Cozyme** | T45.2X1 | T45.2X2 | T45.2X3 | T45.2X4 | T45.2X5 | T45.2X6 |
| **Crack** | T4Ø.5X1 | T4Ø.5X2 | T4Ø.5X3 | T4Ø.5X4 | — | — |
| **Crataegus extract** | T46.ØX1 | T46.ØX2 | T46.ØX3 | T46.ØX4 | T46.ØX5 | T46.ØX6 |
| **Creolin** | T54.1X1 | T54.1X2 | T54.1X3 | T54.1X4 | — | — |
| disinfectant | T54.1X1 | T54.1X2 | T54.1X3 | T54.1X4 | — | — |
| **Creosol** (compound) | T49.ØX1 | T49.ØX2 | T49.ØX3 | T49.ØX4 | T49.ØX5 | T49.ØX6 |
| **Creosote** (coal tar) (beechwood) | T49.ØX1 | T49.ØX2 | T49.ØX3 | T49.ØX4 | T49.ØX5 | T49.ØX6 |
| medicinal (expectorant) | T48.4X1 | T48.4X2 | T48.4X3 | T48.4X4 | T48.4X5 | T48.4X6 |
| syrup | T48.4X1 | T48.4X2 | T48.4X3 | T48.4X4 | T48.4X5 | T48.4X6 |
| **Cresol**(s) | T49.ØX1 | T49.ØX2 | T49.ØX3 | T49.ØX4 | T49.ØX5 | T49.ØX6 |
| and soap solution | T49.ØX1 | T49.ØX2 | T49.ØX3 | T49.ØX4 | T49.ØX5 | T49.ØX6 |
| **Crestor*** | T46.6X1 | T46.6X2 | T46.6X3 | T46.6X4 | T46.6X5 | T46.6X6 |
| **Cresyl acetate** | T49.ØX1 | T49.ØX2 | T49.ØX3 | T49.ØX4 | T49.ØX5 | T49.ØX6 |
| **Cresylic acid** | T49.ØX1 | T49.ØX2 | T49.ØX3 | T49.ØX4 | T49.ØX5 | T49.ØX6 |
| **Crimidine** | T6Ø.4X1 | T6Ø.4X2 | T6Ø.4X3 | T6Ø.4X4 | — | — |
| **Croconazole** | T37.8X1 | T37.8X2 | T37.8X3 | T37.8X4 | T37.8X5 | T37.8X6 |
| **Cromoglicic acid** | T48.6X1 | T48.6X2 | T48.6X3 | T48.6X4 | T48.6X5 | T48.6X6 |
| **Cromolyn** | T48.6X1 | T48.6X2 | T48.6X3 | T48.6X4 | T48.6X5 | T48.6X6 |
| **Cromonar** | T46.3X1 | T46.3X2 | T46.3X3 | T46.3X4 | T46.3X5 | T46.3X6 |
| **Cropropamide** | T39.8X1 | T39.8X2 | T39.8X3 | T39.8X4 | T39.8X5 | T39.8X6 |
| with crotethamide | T5Ø.7X1 | T5Ø.7X2 | T5Ø.7X3 | T5Ø.7X4 | T5Ø.7X5 | T5Ø.7X6 |
| **Crotamiton** | T49.ØX1 | T49.ØX2 | T49.ØX3 | T49.ØX4 | T49.ØX5 | T49.ØX6 |
| **Crotethamide** | T39.8X1 | T39.8X2 | T39.8X3 | T39.8X4 | T39.8X5 | T39.8X6 |
| with cropropamide | T5Ø.7X1 | T5Ø.7X2 | T5Ø.7X3 | T5Ø.7X4 | T5Ø.7X5 | T5Ø.7X6 |
| **Croton** (oil) | T47.2X1 | T47.2X2 | T47.2X3 | T47.2X4 | T47.2X5 | T47.2X6 |
| chloral | T42.6X1 | T42.6X2 | T42.6X3 | T42.6X4 | T42.6X5 | T42.6X6 |
| **Crude oil** | T52.ØX1 | T52.ØX2 | T52.ØX3 | T52.ØX4 | — | — |
| **Cryogenine** | T39.8X1 | T39.8X2 | T39.8X3 | T39.8X4 | T39.8X5 | T39.8X6 |
| **Cryolite** (vapor) | T6Ø.1X1 | T6Ø.1X2 | T6Ø.1X3 | T6Ø.1X4 | — | — |
| insecticide | T6Ø.1X1 | T6Ø.1X2 | T6Ø.1X3 | T6Ø.1X4 | — | — |
| **Cryptenamine** (tannates) | T46.5X1 | T46.5X2 | T46.5X3 | T46.5X4 | T46.5X5 | T46.5X6 |
| **Crystal violet** | T49.ØX1 | T49.ØX2 | T49.ØX3 | T49.ØX4 | T49.ØX5 | T49.ØX6 |
| **Cuckoopint** | T62.2X1 | T62.2X2 | T62.2X3 | T62.2X4 | — | — |
| **Cumetharol** | T45.511 | T45.512 | T45.513 | T45.514 | T45.515 | T45.516 |
| **Cupric** | | | | | | |
| acetate | T6Ø.3X1 | T6Ø.3X2 | T6Ø.3X3 | T6Ø.3X4 | — | — |
| acetoarsenite | T57.ØX1 | T57.ØX2 | T57.ØX3 | T57.ØX4 | — | — |
| arsenate | T57.ØX1 | T57.ØX2 | T57.ØX3 | T57.ØX4 | — | — |
| gluconate | T49.ØX1 | T49.ØX2 | T49.ØX3 | T49.ØX4 | T49.ØX5 | T49.ØX6 |
| oleate | T49.ØX1 | T49.ØX2 | T49.ØX3 | T49.ØX4 | T49.ØX5 | T49.ØX6 |
| sulfate | T56.4X1 | T56.4X2 | T56.4X3 | T56.4X4 | — | — |

| Substance | Poisoning, Accidental (unintentional) | Poisoning, Intentional Self-harm | Poisoning, Assault | Poisoning, Undetermined | Adverse Effect | Under-dosing |
|---|---|---|---|---|---|---|
| **Cuprimine*** | T5Ø.6X1 | T5Ø.6X2 | T5Ø.6X3 | T5Ø.6X4 | T5Ø.6X5 | T5Ø.6X6 |
| **Cuprous sulfate** — *see also* Copper, sulfate | T56.4X1 | T56.4X2 | T56.4X3 | T56.4X4 | — | — |
| **Curare, curarine** | T48.1X1 | T48.1X2 | T48.1X3 | T48.1X4 | T48.1X5 | T48.1X6 |
| **Cyamemazine** | T43.3X1 | T43.3X2 | T43.3X3 | T43.3X4 | T43.3X5 | T43.3X6 |
| **Cyamopsis tetragonoloba** | T46.6X1 | T46.6X2 | T46.6X3 | T46.6X4 | T46.6X5 | T46.6X6 |
| **Cyanacetyl hydrazide** | T37.1X1 | T37.1X2 | T37.1X3 | T37.1X4 | T37.1X5 | T37.1X6 |
| **Cyanic acid** (gas) | T59.891 | T59.892 | T59.893 | T59.894 | — | — |
| **Cyanide**(s) (compounds) (potassium) (sodium) **NEC** | T65.ØX1 | T65.ØX2 | T65.ØX3 | T65.ØX4 | — | — |
| dust or gas (inhalation) NEC | T57.3X1 | T57.3X2 | T57.3X3 | T57.3X4 | — | — |
| fumigant | T65.ØX1 | T65.ØX2 | T65.ØX3 | T65.ØX4 | — | — |
| hydrogen | T57.3X1 | T57.3X2 | T57.3X3 | T57.3X4 | — | — |
| mercuric — *see* Mercury | | | | | | |
| pesticide (dust) (fumes) | T65.ØX1 | T65.ØX2 | T65.ØX3 | T65.ØX4 | — | — |
| **Cyanoacrylate adhesive** | T49.3X1 | T49.3X2 | T49.3X3 | T49.3X4 | T49.3X5 | T49.3X6 |
| **Cyanocobalamin** | T45.8X1 | T45.8X2 | T45.8X3 | T45.8X4 | T45.8X5 | T45.8X6 |
| **Cyanogen** (chloride) (gas) **NEC** | T59.891 | T59.892 | T59.893 | T59.894 | — | — |
| **Cyclacillin** | T36.ØX1 | T36.ØX2 | T36.ØX3 | T36.ØX4 | T36.ØX5 | T36.ØX6 |
| **Cyclaine** | T41.3X1 | T41.3X2 | T41.3X3 | T41.3X4 | T41.3X5 | T41.3X6 |
| **Cyclamate** | T5Ø.991 | T5Ø.992 | T5Ø.993 | T5Ø.994 | T5Ø.995 | T5Ø.996 |
| **Cyclamen europaeum** | T62.2X1 | T62.2X2 | T62.2X3 | T62.2X4 | — | — |
| **Cyclandelate** | T46.7X1 | T46.7X2 | T46.7X3 | T46.7X4 | T46.7X5 | T46.7X6 |
| **Cyclazocine** | T5Ø.7X1 | T5Ø.7X2 | T5Ø.7X3 | T5Ø.7X4 | T5Ø.7X5 | T5Ø.7X6 |
| **Cyclizine** | T45.ØX1 | T45.ØX2 | T45.ØX3 | T45.ØX4 | T45.ØX5 | T45.ØX6 |
| **Cycloalkanes** | T52.821 | T52.822 | T52.823 | T52.824 | — | — |
| **Cyclobarbital** | T42.3X1 | T42.3X2 | T42.3X3 | T42.3X4 | T42.3X5 | T42.3X6 |
| **Cyclobarbitone** | T42.3X1 | T42.3X2 | T42.3X3 | T42.3X4 | T42.3X5 | T42.3X6 |
| **Cyclobenzaprine** | T48.1X1 | T48.1X2 | T48.1X3 | T48.1X4 | T48.1X5 | T48.1X6 |
| **Cyclodrine** | T44.3X1 | T44.3X2 | T44.3X3 | T44.3X4 | T44.3X5 | T44.3X6 |
| **Cycloguanil embonate** | T37.2X1 | T37.2X2 | T37.2X3 | T37.2X4 | T37.2X5 | T37.2X6 |
| **Cyclohexane** | T52.821 | T52.822 | T52.823 | T52.824 | — | — |
| **Cyclohexanol** | T51.8X1 | T51.8X2 | T51.8X3 | T51.8X4 | — | — |
| **Cyclohexanone** | T52.4X1 | T52.4X2 | T52.4X3 | T52.4X4 | — | — |
| **Cycloheximide** | T6Ø.3X1 | T6Ø.3X2 | T6Ø.3X3 | T6Ø.3X4 | — | — |
| **Cyclohexyl acetate** | T52.891 | T52.892 | T52.893 | T52.894 | — | — |
| **Cycloleucin** | T45.1X1 | T45.1X2 | T45.1X3 | T45.1X4 | T45.1X5 | T45.1X6 |
| **Cyclomethycaine** | T41.3X1 | T41.3X2 | T41.3X3 | T41.3X4 | T41.3X5 | T41.3X6 |
| **Cycloparaffins** | T52.821 | T52.822 | T52.823 | T52.824 | — | — |
| **Cyclopentamine** | T44.4X1 | T44.4X2 | T44.4X3 | T44.4X4 | T44.4X5 | T44.4X6 |
| **Cyclopenthiazide** | T5Ø.2X1 | T5Ø.2X2 | T5Ø.2X3 | T5Ø.2X4 | T5Ø.2X5 | T5Ø.2X6 |
| **Cyclopentolate** | T44.3X1 | T44.3X2 | T44.3X3 | T44.3X4 | T44.3X5 | T44.3X6 |
| **Cyclophosphamide** | T45.1X1 | T45.1X2 | T45.1X3 | T45.1X4 | T45.1X5 | T45.1X6 |
| **Cycloplegic drug** | T49.5X1 | T49.5X2 | T49.5X3 | T49.5X4 | T49.5X5 | T49.5X6 |
| **Cyclopropane** | T41.291 | T41.292 | T41.293 | T41.294 | T41.295 | T41.296 |
| **Cyclopyrabital** | T39.8X1 | T39.8X2 | T39.8X3 | T39.8X4 | T39.8X5 | T39.8X6 |
| **Cycloserine** | T37.1X1 | T37.1X2 | T37.1X3 | T37.1X4 | T37.1X5 | T37.1X6 |
| **Cyclosporin** | T45.1X1 | T45.1X2 | T45.1X3 | T45.1X4 | T45.1X5 | T45.1X6 |
| **Cyclothiazide** | T5Ø.2X1 | T5Ø.2X2 | T5Ø.2X3 | T5Ø.2X4 | T5Ø.2X5 | T5Ø.2X6 |
| **Cycrimine** | T44.3X1 | T44.3X2 | T44.3X3 | T44.3X4 | T44.3X5 | T44.3X6 |
| **Cyhalothrin** | T6Ø.1X1 | T6Ø.1X2 | T6Ø.1X3 | T6Ø.1X4 | — | — |
| **Cymarin** | T46.ØX1 | T46.ØX2 | T46.ØX3 | T46.ØX4 | T46.ØX5 | T46.ØX6 |
| **Cymbalta*** | T43.221 | T43.222 | T43.223 | T43.224 | T43.225 | T43.226 |
| **Cypermethrin** | T6Ø.1X1 | T6Ø.1X2 | T6Ø.1X3 | T6Ø.1X4 | — | — |
| **Cyphenothrin** | T6Ø.2X1 | T6Ø.2X2 | T6Ø.2X3 | T6Ø.2X4 | — | — |
| **Cyproheptadine** | T45.ØX1 | T45.ØX2 | T45.ØX3 | T45.ØX4 | T45.ØX5 | T45.ØX6 |
| **Cyproterone** | T38.6X1 | T38.6X2 | T38.6X3 | T38.6X4 | T38.6X5 | T38.6X6 |
| **Cystaran*** | T49.5X1 | T49.5X2 | T49.5X3 | T49.5X4 | T49.5X5 | T49.5X6 |
| **Cysteamine** | T5Ø.6X1 | T5Ø.6X2 | T5Ø.6X3 | T5Ø.6X4 | T5Ø.6X5 | T5Ø.6X6 |
| **Cytarabine** | T45.1X1 | T45.1X2 | T45.1X3 | T45.1X4 | T45.1X5 | T45.1X6 |
| **Cytisus** | | | | | | |
| laburnum | T62.2X1 | T62.2X2 | T62.2X3 | T62.2X4 | — | — |
| scoparius | T62.2X1 | T62.2X2 | T62.2X3 | T62.2X4 | — | — |
| **Cytochrome C** | T47.5X1 | T47.5X2 | T47.5X3 | T47.5X4 | T47.5X5 | T47.5X6 |
| **Cytomel** | T38.1X1 | T38.1X2 | T38.1X3 | T38.1X4 | T38.1X5 | T38.1X6 |
| **Cytosine arabinoside** | T45.1X1 | T45.1X2 | T45.1X3 | T45.1X4 | T45.1X5 | T45.1X6 |
| **Cytoxan** | T45.1X1 | T45.1X2 | T45.1X3 | T45.1X4 | T45.1X5 | T45.1X6 |
| **Cytozyme** | T45.7X1 | T45.7X2 | T45.7X3 | T45.7X4 | T45.7X5 | T45.7X6 |
| **D-Con** | T6Ø.91 | T6Ø.92 | T6Ø.93 | T6Ø.94 | — | — |
| insecticide | T6Ø.2X1 | T6Ø.2X2 | T6Ø.2X3 | T6Ø.2X4 | — | — |
| rodenticide | T6Ø.4X1 | T6Ø.4X2 | T6Ø.4X3 | T6Ø.4X4 | — | — |
| **D-lysergic acid diethylamide** | T4Ø.8X1 | T4Ø.8X2 | T4Ø.8X3 | T4Ø.8X4 | — | — |
| **Dabigatran*** | T45.511 | T45.512 | T45.513 | T45.514 | T45.515 | T45.516 |
| **Dacarbazine** | T45.1X1 | T45.1X2 | T45.1X3 | T45.1X4 | T45.1X5 | T45.1X6 |
| **Dactinomycin** | T45.1X1 | T45.1X2 | T45.1X3 | T45.1X4 | T45.1X5 | T45.1X6 |
| **DADPS** | T37.1X1 | T37.1X2 | T37.1X3 | T37.1X4 | T37.1X5 | T37.1X6 |
| **Dakin's solution** | T49.ØX1 | T49.ØX2 | T49.ØX3 | T49.ØX4 | T49.ØX5 | T49.ØX6 |
| **Dalapon** (sodium) | T6Ø.3X1 | T6Ø.3X2 | T6Ø.3X3 | T6Ø.3X4 | — | — |
| **Dalmane** | T42.4X1 | T42.4X2 | T42.4X3 | T42.4X4 | T42.4X5 | T42.4X6 |

| Substance | Poisoning, Accidental (unintentional) | Poisoning, Intentional Self-harm | Poisoning, Assault | Poisoning, Undetermined | Adverse Effect | Under-dosing |
|---|---|---|---|---|---|---|
| **Danazol** | T38.6X1 | T38.6X2 | T38.6X3 | T38.6X4 | T38.6X5 | T38.6X6 |
| **Danilone** | T45.511 | T45.512 | T45.513 | T45.514 | T45.515 | T45.516 |
| **Danthron** | T47.2X1 | T47.2X2 | T47.2X3 | T47.2X4 | T47.2X5 | T47.2X6 |
| **Dantrolene** | T42.8X1 | T42.8X2 | T42.8X3 | T42.8X4 | T42.8X5 | T42.8X6 |
| **Dantron** | T47.2X1 | T47.2X2 | T47.2X3 | T47.2X4 | T47.2X5 | T47.2X6 |
| **Daphne** (gnidium) (mezereum) | T62.2X1 | T62.2X2 | T62.2X3 | T62.2X4 | — | — |
| berry | T62.1X1 | T62.1X2 | T62.1X3 | T62.1X4 | — | — |
| **Dapsone** | T37.1X1 | T37.1X2 | T37.1X3 | T37.1X4 | T37.1X5 | T37.1X6 |
| **Daraprim** | T37.2X1 | T37.2X2 | T37.2X3 | T37.2X4 | T37.2X5 | T37.2X6 |
| **Darnel** | T62.2X1 | T62.2X2 | T62.2X3 | T62.2X4 | — | — |
| **Darvon** | T39.8X1 | T39.8X2 | T39.8X3 | T39.8X4 | T39.8X5 | T39.8X6 |
| **Daunomycin** | T45.1X1 | T45.1X2 | T45.1X3 | T45.1X4 | T45.1X5 | T45.1X6 |
| **Daunorubicin** | T45.1X1 | T45.1X2 | T45.1X3 | T45.1X4 | T45.1X5 | T45.1X6 |
| **DBI** | T38.3X1 | T38.3X2 | T38.3X3 | T38.3X4 | T38.3X5 | T38.3X6 |
| **DDAVP** | T38.891 | T38.892 | T38.893 | T38.894 | T38.895 | T38.896 |
| **DDE** (bis(chlorophenyl)-dichloroethylene) | T6Ø.2X1 | T6Ø.2X2 | T6Ø.2X3 | T6Ø.2X4 | — | — |
| **DDS** | T37.1X1 | T37.1X2 | T37.1X3 | T37.1X4 | T37.1X5 | T37.1X6 |
| **DDT** (dust) | T6Ø.1X1 | T6Ø.1X2 | T6Ø.1X3 | T6Ø.1X4 | — | — |
| **Deadly nightshade** — *see also* Belladonna | T62.2X1 | T62.2X2 | T62.2X3 | T62.2X4 | — | — |
| berry | T62.1X1 | T62.1X2 | T62.1X3 | T62.1X4 | — | — |
| **Deamino-D-arginine vasopressin** | T38.891 | T38.892 | T38.893 | T38.894 | T38.895 | T38.896 |
| **Deanol** (aceglumate) | T5Ø.991 | T5Ø.992 | T5Ø.993 | T5Ø.994 | T5Ø.995 | T5Ø.996 |
| **Debrisoquine** | T46.5X1 | T46.5X2 | T46.5X3 | T46.5X4 | T46.5X5 | T46.5X6 |
| **Decaborane** | T57.8X1 | T57.8X2 | T57.8X3 | T57.8X4 | — | — |
| fumes | T59.891 | T59.892 | T59.893 | T59.894 | — | — |
| **Decadron** | T38.ØX1 | T38.ØX2 | T38.ØX3 | T38.ØX4 | T38.ØX5 | T38.ØX6 |
| ENT agent | T49.6X1 | T49.6X2 | T49.6X3 | T49.6X4 | T49.6X5 | T49.6X6 |
| ophthalmic preparation | T49.5X1 | T49.5X2 | T49.5X3 | T49.5X4 | T49.5X5 | T49.5X6 |
| topical NEC | T49.ØX1 | T49.ØX2 | T49.ØX3 | T49.ØX4 | T49.ØX5 | T49.ØX6 |
| **Decahydronaphthalene** | T52.891 | T52.892 | T52.893 | T52.894 | — | — |
| **Decalin** | T52.891 | T52.892 | T52.893 | T52.894 | — | — |
| **Decamethonium** (bromide) | T48.1X1 | T48.1X2 | T48.1X3 | T48.1X4 | T48.1X5 | T48.1X6 |
| **Decholin** | T47.5X1 | T47.5X2 | T47.5X3 | T47.5X4 | T47.5X5 | T47.5X6 |
| **Declomycin** | T36.4X1 | T36.4X2 | T36.4X3 | T36.4X4 | T36.4X5 | T36.4X6 |
| **Decongestant, nasal** (mucosa) | T48.5X1 | T48.5X2 | T48.5X3 | T48.5X4 | T48.5X5 | T48.5X6 |
| combination | T48.5X1 | T48.5X2 | T48.5X3 | T48.5X4 | T48.5X5 | T48.5X6 |
| **Deet** | T6Ø.8X1 | T6Ø.8X2 | T6Ø.8X3 | T6Ø.8X4 | — | — |
| **Deferoxamine** | T45.8X1 | T45.8X2 | T45.8X3 | T45.8X4 | T45.8X5 | T45.8X6 |
| **Deflazacort** | T38.ØX1 | T38.ØX2 | T38.ØX3 | T38.ØX4 | T38.ØX5 | T38.ØX6 |
| **Deglycyrrhizinized extract of licorice** | T48.4X1 | T48.4X2 | T48.4X3 | T48.4X4 | T48.4X5 | T48.4X6 |
| **Dehydrocholic acid** | T47.5X1 | T47.5X2 | T47.5X3 | T47.5X4 | T47.5X5 | T47.5X6 |
| **Dehydroemetine** | T37.3X1 | T37.3X2 | T37.3X3 | T37.3X4 | T37.3X5 | T37.3X6 |
| **Dekalin** | T52.891 | T52.892 | T52.893 | T52.894 | — | — |
| **Delafloxacin*** | T36.8X1 | T36.8X2 | T36.8X3 | T36.8X4 | T36.8X5 | T36.8X6 |
| **Delalutin** | T38.5X1 | T38.5X2 | T38.5X3 | T38.5X4 | T38.5X5 | T38.5X6 |
| **Delorazepam** | T42.4X1 | T42.4X2 | T42.4X3 | T42.4X4 | T42.4X5 | T42.4X6 |
| **Delphinium** | T62.2X1 | T62.2X2 | T62.2X3 | T62.2X4 | — | — |
| **Deltacortisone*** | T38.ØX1 | T38.ØX2 | T38.ØX3 | T38.ØX4 | T38.ØX5 | T38.ØX6 |
| **Deltamethrin** | T6Ø.1X1 | T6Ø.1X2 | T6Ø.1X3 | T6Ø.1X4 | — | — |
| **Deltasone** | T38.ØX1 | T38.ØX2 | T38.ØX3 | T38.ØX4 | T38.ØX5 | T38.ØX6 |
| **Deltra** | T38.ØX1 | T38.ØX2 | T38.ØX3 | T38.ØX4 | T38.ØX5 | T38.ØX6 |
| **Delvinal** | T42.3X1 | T42.3X2 | T42.3X3 | T42.3X4 | T42.3X5 | T42.3X6 |
| **Demecarium** (bromide) | T49.5X1 | T49.5X2 | T49.5X3 | T49.5X4 | T49.5X5 | T49.5X6 |
| **Demeclocycline** | T36.4X1 | T36.4X2 | T36.4X3 | T36.4X4 | T36.4X5 | T36.4X6 |
| **Demecolcine** | T45.1X1 | T45.1X2 | T45.1X3 | T45.1X4 | T45.1X5 | T45.1X6 |
| **Demegestone** | T38.5X1 | T38.5X2 | T38.5X3 | T38.5X4 | T38.5X5 | T38.5X6 |
| **Demelanizing agents** | T49.8X1 | T49.8X2 | T49.8X3 | T49.8X4 | T49.8X5 | T49.8X6 |
| **Demephion -O and -S** | T6Ø.ØX1 | T6Ø.ØX2 | T6Ø.ØX3 | T6Ø.ØX4 | — | — |
| **Demerol** | T4Ø.2X1 | T4Ø.2X2 | T4Ø.2X3 | T4Ø.2X4 | T4Ø.2X5 | T4Ø.2X6 |
| **Demethylchlortetracycline** | T36.4X1 | T36.4X2 | T36.4X3 | T36.4X4 | T36.4X5 | T36.4X6 |
| **Demethyltetracycline** | T36.4X1 | T36.4X2 | T36.4X3 | T36.4X4 | T36.4X5 | T36.4X6 |
| **Demeton -O and -S** | T6Ø.ØX1 | T6Ø.ØX2 | T6Ø.ØX3 | T6Ø.ØX4 | — | — |
| **Demulcent** (external) | T49.3X1 | T49.3X2 | T49.3X3 | T49.3X4 | T49.3X5 | T49.3X6 |
| specified NEC | T49.3X1 | T49.3X2 | T49.3X3 | T49.3X4 | T49.3X5 | T49.3X6 |
| **Demulen** | T38.4X1 | T38.4X2 | T38.4X3 | T38.4X4 | T38.4X5 | T38.4X6 |
| **Denatured alcohol** | T51.ØX1 | T51.ØX2 | T51.ØX3 | T51.ØX4 | — | — |
| **Dendrid** | T49.5X1 | T49.5X2 | T49.5X3 | T49.5X4 | T49.5X5 | T49.5X6 |
| **Dental drug, topical application NEC** | T49.7X1 | T49.7X2 | T49.7X3 | T49.7X4 | T49.7X5 | T49.7X6 |
| **Dentifrice** | T49.7X1 | T49.7X2 | T49.7X3 | T49.7X4 | T49.7X5 | T49.7X6 |
| **Deodorant spray** (feminine hygiene) | T49.8X1 | T49.8X2 | T49.8X3 | T49.8X4 | T49.8X5 | T49.8X6 |
| **Deoxycortone** | T5Ø.ØX1 | T5Ø.ØX2 | T5Ø.ØX3 | T5Ø.ØX4 | T5Ø.ØX5 | T5Ø.ØX6 |
| **Deoxyribonuclease** (pancreatic) | T45.3X1 | T45.3X2 | T45.3X3 | T45.3X4 | T45.3X5 | T45.3X6 |
| **Depilatory** | T49.4X1 | T49.4X2 | T49.4X3 | T49.4X4 | T49.4X5 | T49.4X6 |
| **Deprenalin** | T42.8X1 | T42.8X2 | T42.8X3 | T42.8X4 | T42.8X5 | T42.8X6 |

| Substance | Poisoning, Accidental (unintentional) | Poisoning, Intentional Self-harm | Poisoning, Assault | Poisoning, Undetermined | Adverse Effect | Under-dosing |
|---|---|---|---|---|---|---|
| **Deprenyl** | T42.8X1 | T42.8X2 | T42.8X3 | T42.8X4 | T42.8X5 | T42.8X6 |
| **Depressant** | | | | | | |
| appetite (central) | T50.5X1 | T50.5X2 | T50.5X3 | T50.5X4 | T50.5X5 | T50.5X6 |
| cardiac | T46.2X1 | T46.2X2 | T46.2X3 | T46.2X4 | T46.2X5 | T46.2X6 |
| central nervous system (anesthetic) — *see also* Central nervous system, depressants | T42.71 | T42.72 | T42.73 | T42.74 | T42.75 | T42.76 |
| general anesthetic | T41.201 | T41.202 | T41.203 | T41.204 | T41.205 | T41.206 |
| muscle tone | T42.8X1 | T42.8X2 | T42.8X3 | T42.8X4 | T42.8X5 | T42.8X6 |
| muscle tone, central | T42.8X1 | T42.8X2 | T42.8X3 | T42.8X4 | T42.8X5 | T42.8X6 |
| psychotherapeutic | T43.501 | T43.502 | T43.503 | T43.504 | T43.505 | T43.506 |
| **Depressant, appetite** | T50.5X1 | T50.5X2 | T50.5X3 | T50.5X4 | T50.5X5 | T50.5X6 |
| **Deptropine** | T45.0X1 | T45.0X2 | T45.0X3 | T45.0X4 | T45.0X5 | T45.0X6 |
| **Dequalinium** (chloride) | T49.0X1 | T49.0X2 | T49.0X3 | T49.0X4 | T49.0X5 | T49.0X6 |
| **Derris root** | T60.2X1 | T60.2X2 | T60.2X3 | T60.2X4 | — | — |
| **Deserpidine** | T46.5X1 | T46.5X2 | T46.5X3 | T46.5X4 | T46.5X5 | T46.5X6 |
| **Desferrioxamine** | T45.8X1 | T45.8X2 | T45.8X3 | T45.8X4 | T45.8X5 | T45.8X6 |
| **Desipramine** | T43.011 | T43.012 | T43.013 | T43.014 | T43.015 | T43.016 |
| **Deslanoside** | T46.0X1 | T46.0X2 | T46.0X3 | T46.0X4 | T46.0X5 | T46.0X6 |
| **Desloughing agent** | T49.4X1 | T49.4X2 | T49.4X3 | T49.4X4 | T49.4X5 | T49.4X6 |
| **Desmethylimipramine** | T43.011 | T43.012 | T43.013 | T43.014 | T43.015 | T43.016 |
| **Desmopressin** | T38.891 | T38.892 | T38.893 | T38.894 | T38.895 | T38.896 |
| **Desocodeine** | T40.2X1 | T40.2X2 | T40.2X3 | T40.2X4 | T40.2X5 | T40.2X6 |
| **Desogestrel** | T38.5X1 | T38.5X2 | T38.5X3 | T38.5X4 | T38.5X5 | T38.5X6 |
| **Desomorphine** | T40.2X1 | T40.2X2 | T40.2X3 | T40.2X4 | — | — |
| **Desonide** | T49.0X1 | T49.0X2 | T49.0X3 | T49.0X4 | T49.0X5 | T49.0X6 |
| **Desoximetasone** | T49.0X1 | T49.0X2 | T49.0X3 | T49.0X4 | T49.0X5 | T49.0X6 |
| **Desoxycorticosteroid** | T50.0X1 | T50.0X2 | T50.0X3 | T50.0X4 | T50.0X5 | T50.0X6 |
| **Desoxycortone** | T50.0X1 | T50.0X2 | T50.0X3 | T50.0X4 | T50.0X5 | T50.0X6 |
| **Desoxyephedrine** | T43.651 | T43.652 | T43.653 | T43.654 | T43.655 | T43.656 |
| **Dessicated thyroid*** | T38.1X1 | T38.1X2 | T38.1X3 | T38.1X4 | T38.1X5 | T38.1X6 |
| **Detaxtran** | T46.6X1 | T46.6X2 | T46.6X3 | T46.6X4 | T46.6X5 | T46.6X6 |
| **Detergent** | T49.2X1 | T49.2X2 | T49.2X3 | T49.2X4 | T49.2X5 | T49.2X6 |
| external medication | T49.2X1 | T49.2X2 | T49.2X3 | T49.2X4 | T49.2X5 | T49.2X6 |
| local | T49.2X1 | T49.2X2 | T49.2X3 | T49.2X4 | T49.2X5 | T49.2X6 |
| medicinal | T49.2X1 | T49.2X2 | T49.2X3 | T49.2X4 | T49.2X5 | T49.2X6 |
| nonmedicinal | T55.1X1 | T55.1X2 | T55.1X3 | T55.1X4 | — | — |
| specified NEC | T55.1X1 | T55.1X2 | T55.1X3 | T55.1X4 | — | — |
| **Deterrent, alcohol** | T50.6X1 | T50.6X2 | T50.6X3 | T50.6X4 | T50.6X5 | T50.6X6 |
| **Detoxifying agent** | T50.6X1 | T50.6X2 | T50.6X3 | T50.6X4 | T50.6X5 | T50.6X6 |
| **Detrothyronine** | T38.1X1 | T38.1X2 | T38.1X3 | T38.1X4 | T38.1X5 | T38.1X6 |
| **Dettol** (external medication) | T49.0X1 | T49.0X2 | T49.0X3 | T49.0X4 | T49.0X5 | T49.0X6 |
| **Dexamethasone** | T38.0X1 | T38.0X2 | T38.0X3 | T38.0X4 | T38.0X5 | T38.0X6 |
| ENT agent | T49.6X1 | T49.6X2 | T49.6X3 | T49.6X4 | T49.6X5 | T49.6X6 |
| ophthalmic preparation | T49.5X1 | T49.5X2 | T49.5X3 | T49.5X4 | T49.5X5 | T49.5X6 |
| topical NEC | T49.0X1 | T49.0X2 | T49.0X3 | T49.0X4 | T49.0X5 | T49.0X6 |
| **Dexamfetamine** | T43.621 | T43.622 | T43.623 | T43.624 | T43.625 | T43.626 |
| **Dexamphetamine** | T43.621 | T43.622 | T43.623 | T43.624 | T43.625 | T43.626 |
| **Dexbrompheniramine** | T45.0X1 | T45.0X2 | T45.0X3 | T45.0X4 | T45.0X5 | T45.0X6 |
| **Dexchlorpheniramine** | T45.0X1 | T45.0X2 | T45.0X3 | T45.0X4 | T45.0X5 | T45.0X6 |
| **Dexedrine** | T43.621 | T43.622 | T43.623 | T43.624 | T43.625 | T43.626 |
| **Dexetimide** | T44.3X1 | T44.3X2 | T44.3X3 | T44.3X4 | T44.3X5 | T44.3X6 |
| **Dexfenfluramine** | T50.5X1 | T50.5X2 | T50.5X3 | T50.5X4 | T50.5X5 | T50.5X6 |
| **Dexpanthenol** | T45.2X1 | T45.2X2 | T45.2X3 | T45.2X4 | T45.2X5 | T45.2X6 |
| **Dextran** (40) (70) (150) | T45.8X1 | T45.8X2 | T45.8X3 | T45.8X4 | T45.8X5 | T45.8X6 |
| **Dextriferron** | T45.4X1 | T45.4X2 | T45.4X3 | T45.4X4 | T45.4X5 | T45.4X6 |
| **Dextro calcium pantothenate** | T45.2X1 | T45.2X2 | T45.2X3 | T45.2X4 | T45.2X5 | T45.2X6 |
| **Dextro pantothenyl alcohol** | T45.2X1 | T45.2X2 | T45.2X3 | T45.2X4 | T45.2X5 | T45.2X6 |
| **Dextroamphetamine** | T43.621 | T43.622 | T43.623 | T43.624 | T43.625 | T43.626 |
| **Dextromethorphan** | T48.3X1 | T48.3X2 | T48.3X3 | T48.3X4 | T48.3X5 | T48.3X6 |
| **Dextromoramide** | T40.491 | T40.492 | T40.493 | T40.494 | — | — |
| topical | T49.8X1 | T49.8X2 | T49.8X3 | T49.8X4 | T49.8X5 | T49.8X6 |
| **Dextropropoxyphene** | T40.491 | T40.492 | T40.493 | T40.494 | T40.495 | T40.496 |
| **Dextrorphan** | T40.2X1 | T40.2X2 | T40.2X3 | T40.2X4 | T40.2X5 | T40.2X6 |
| **Dextrose** | T50.3X1 | T50.3X2 | T50.3X3 | T50.3X4 | T50.3X5 | T50.3X6 |
| concentrated solution, intravenous | T46.8X1 | T46.8X2 | T46.8X3 | T46.8X4 | T46.8X5 | T46.8X6 |
| **Dextrothyroxin** | T38.1X1 | T38.1X2 | T38.1X3 | T38.1X4 | T38.1X5 | T38.1X6 |
| **Dextrothyroxine sodium** | T38.1X1 | T38.1X2 | T38.1X3 | T38.1X4 | T38.1X5 | T38.1X6 |
| **DFP** | T44.0X1 | T44.0X2 | T44.0X3 | T44.0X4 | T44.0X5 | T44.0X6 |
| **DHE** | T37.3X1 | T37.3X2 | T37.3X3 | T37.3X4 | T37.3X5 | T37.3X6 |
| 45 | T46.5X1 | T46.5X2 | T46.5X3 | T46.5X4 | T46.5X5 | T46.5X6 |
| **DiaBeta*** | T38.3X1 | T38.3X2 | T38.3X3 | T38.3X4 | T38.3X5 | T38.3X6 |
| **Diabinese** | T38.3X1 | T38.3X2 | T38.3X3 | T38.3X4 | T38.3X5 | T38.3X6 |
| **Diacetone alcohol** | T52.4X1 | T52.4X2 | T52.4X3 | T52.4X4 | — | — |
| **Diacetyl monoxime** | T50.991 | T50.992 | T50.993 | T50.994 | — | — |
| **Diacetylmorphine** | T40.1X1 | T40.1X2 | T40.1X3 | T40.1X4 | — | — |
| **Diachylon plaster** | T49.4X1 | T49.4X2 | T49.4X3 | T49.4X4 | T49.4X5 | T49.4X6 |
| **Diaethylstilboestrolum** | T38.5X1 | T38.5X2 | T38.5X3 | T38.5X4 | T38.5X5 | T38.5X6 |
| **Diagnostic agent NEC** | T50.8X1 | T50.8X2 | T50.8X3 | T50.8X4 | T50.8X5 | T50.8X6 |

| Substance | Poisoning, Accidental (unintentional) | Poisoning, Intentional Self-harm | Poisoning, Assault | Poisoning, Undetermined | Adverse Effect | Under-dosing |
|---|---|---|---|---|---|---|
| **Dial** (soap) | T49.2X1 | T49.2X2 | T49.2X3 | T49.2X4 | T49.2X5 | T49.2X6 |
| sedative | T42.3X1 | T42.3X2 | T42.3X3 | T42.3X4 | T42.3X5 | T42.3X6 |
| **Dialkyl carbonate** | T52.91 | T52.92 | T52.93 | T52.94 | — | — |
| **Diallylbarbituric acid** | T42.3X1 | T42.3X2 | T42.3X3 | T42.3X4 | T42.3X5 | T42.3X6 |
| **Diallymal** | T42.3X1 | T42.3X2 | T42.3X3 | T42.3X4 | T42.3X5 | T42.3X6 |
| **Dialysis solution** (intraperitoneal) | T50.3X1 | T50.3X2 | T50.3X3 | T50.3X4 | T50.3X5 | T50.3X6 |
| **Diaminodiphenylsulfone** | T37.1X1 | T37.1X2 | T37.1X3 | T37.1X4 | T37.1X5 | T37.1X6 |
| **Diamorphine** | T40.1X1 | T40.1X2 | T40.1X3 | T40.1X4 | — | — |
| **Diamox** | T50.2X1 | T50.2X2 | T50.2X3 | T50.2X4 | T50.2X5 | T50.2X6 |
| **Diamthazole** | T49.0X1 | T49.0X2 | T49.0X3 | T49.0X4 | T49.0X5 | T49.0X6 |
| **Dianthone** | T47.2X1 | T47.2X2 | T47.2X3 | T47.2X4 | T47.2X5 | T47.2X6 |
| **Diaphenylsulfone** | T37.0X1 | T37.0X2 | T37.0X3 | T37.0X4 | T37.0X5 | T37.0X6 |
| **Diasone** (sodium) | T37.1X1 | T37.1X2 | T37.1X3 | T37.1X4 | T37.1X5 | T37.1X6 |
| **Diastase** | T47.5X1 | T47.5X2 | T47.5X3 | T47.5X4 | T47.5X5 | T47.5X6 |
| **Diastat*** | T42.4X1 | T42.4X2 | T42.4X3 | T42.4X4 | T42.4X5 | T42.4X6 |
| **Diatrizoate** | T50.8X1 | T50.8X2 | T50.8X3 | T50.8X4 | T50.8X5 | T50.8X6 |
| **Diazepam** | T42.4X1 | T42.4X2 | T42.4X3 | T42.4X4 | T42.4X5 | T42.4X6 |
| **Diazinon** | T60.0X1 | T60.0X2 | T60.0X3 | T60.0X4 | — | — |
| **Diazomethane** (gas) | T59.891 | T59.892 | T59.893 | T59.894 | — | — |
| **Diazoxide** | T46.5X1 | T46.5X2 | T46.5X3 | T46.5X4 | T46.5X5 | T46.5X6 |
| **Dibekacin** | T36.5X1 | T36.5X2 | T36.5X3 | T36.5X4 | T36.5X5 | T36.5X6 |
| **Dibenamine** | T44.6X1 | T44.6X2 | T44.6X3 | T44.6X4 | T44.6X5 | T44.6X6 |
| **Dibenzepin** | T43.011 | T43.012 | T43.013 | T43.014 | T43.015 | T43.016 |
| **Dibenzheptropine** | T45.0X1 | T45.0X2 | T45.0X3 | T45.0X4 | T45.0X5 | T45.0X6 |
| **Dibenzyline** | T44.6X1 | T44.6X2 | T44.6X3 | T44.6X4 | T44.6X5 | T44.6X6 |
| **Diborane** (gas) | T59.891 | T59.892 | T59.893 | T59.894 | — | — |
| **Dibromochloropropane** | T60.8X1 | T60.8X2 | T60.8X3 | T60.8X4 | — | — |
| **Dibromodulcitol** | T45.1X1 | T45.1X2 | T45.1X3 | T45.1X4 | T45.1X5 | T45.1X6 |
| **Dibromoethane** | T53.6X1 | T53.6X2 | T53.6X3 | T53.6X4 | — | — |
| **Dibromomannitol** | T45.1X1 | T45.1X2 | T45.1X3 | T45.1X4 | T45.1X5 | T45.1X6 |
| **Dibromopropamidine isethionate** | T49.0X1 | T49.0X2 | T49.0X3 | T49.0X4 | T49.0X5 | T49.0X6 |
| **Dibrompropamidine** | T49.0X1 | T49.0X2 | T49.0X3 | T49.0X4 | T49.0X5 | T49.0X6 |
| **Dibucaine** | T41.3X1 | T41.3X2 | T41.3X3 | T41.3X4 | T41.3X5 | T41.3X6 |
| topical (surface) | T41.3X1 | T41.3X2 | T41.3X3 | T41.3X4 | T41.3X5 | T41.3X6 |
| **Dibunate sodium** | T48.3X1 | T48.3X2 | T48.3X3 | T48.3X4 | T48.3X5 | T48.3X6 |
| **Dibutoline sulfate** | T44.3X1 | T44.3X2 | T44.3X3 | T44.3X4 | T44.3X5 | T44.3X6 |
| **Dicamba** | T60.3X1 | T60.3X2 | T60.3X3 | T60.3X4 | — | — |
| **Dicapthon** | T60.0X1 | T60.0X2 | T60.0X3 | T60.0X4 | — | — |
| **Dichlobenil** | T60.3X1 | T60.3X2 | T60.3X3 | T60.3X4 | — | — |
| **Dichlone** | T60.3X1 | T60.3X2 | T60.3X3 | T60.3X4 | — | — |
| **Dichloralphenozone** | T42.6X1 | T42.6X2 | T42.6X3 | T42.6X4 | T42.6X5 | T42.6X6 |
| **Dichlorbenzidine** | T65.3X1 | T65.3X2 | T65.3X3 | T65.3X4 | — | — |
| **Dichlorhydrin** | T52.891 | T52.892 | T52.893 | T52.894 | — | — |
| **Dichlorhydroxyquinoline** | T37.8X1 | T37.8X2 | T37.8X3 | T37.8X4 | T37.8X5 | T37.8X6 |
| **Dichlorobenzene** | T53.7X1 | T53.7X2 | T53.7X3 | T53.7X4 | — | — |
| **Dichlorobenzyl alcohol** | T49.6X1 | T49.6X2 | T49.6X3 | T49.6X4 | T49.6X5 | T49.6X6 |
| **Dichlorodifluoromethane** | T53.5X1 | T53.5X2 | T53.5X3 | T53.5X4 | — | — |
| **Dichloroethane** | T52.891 | T52.892 | T52.893 | T52.894 | — | — |
| **Dichloroethyl sulfide, not in war** | T59.891 | T59.892 | T59.893 | T59.894 | — | — |
| **Dichloroethylene** | T53.6X1 | T53.6X2 | T53.6X3 | T53.6X4 | — | — |
| **Dichloroformoxine, not in war** | T59.891 | T59.892 | T59.893 | T59.894 | — | — |
| **Dichlorohydrin, alpha-dichlorohydrin** | T52.891 | T52.892 | T52.893 | T52.894 | — | — |
| **Dichloromethane** (solvent) | T53.4X1 | T53.4X2 | T53.4X3 | T53.4X4 | — | — |
| vapor | T53.4X1 | T53.4X2 | T53.4X3 | T53.4X4 | — | — |
| **Dichloronaphthoquinone** | T60.3X1 | T60.3X2 | T60.3X3 | T60.3X4 | — | — |
| **Dichlorophen** | T37.4X1 | T37.4X2 | T37.4X3 | T37.4X4 | T37.4X5 | T37.4X6 |
| **Dichloropropene** | T60.3X1 | T60.3X2 | T60.3X3 | T60.3X4 | — | — |
| **Dichloropropionic acid** | T60.3X1 | T60.3X2 | T60.3X3 | T60.3X4 | — | — |
| **Dichlorphenamide** | T50.2X1 | T50.2X2 | T50.2X3 | T50.2X4 | T50.2X5 | T50.2X6 |
| **Dichlorvos** | T60.0X1 | T60.0X2 | T60.0X3 | T60.0X4 | — | — |
| **Dichysterol*** | T45.2X1 | T45.2X2 | T45.2X3 | T45.2X4 | T45.2X5 | T45.2X6 |
| **Diclofenac** | T39.391 | T39.392 | T39.393 | T39.394 | T39.395 | T39.396 |
| **Diclofenamide** | T50.2X1 | T50.2X2 | T50.2X3 | T50.2X4 | T50.2X5 | T50.2X6 |
| **Diclofensine** | T43.291 | T43.292 | T43.293 | T43.294 | T43.295 | T43.296 |
| **Diclonixine** | T39.8X1 | T39.8X2 | T39.8X3 | T39.8X4 | T39.8X5 | T39.8X6 |
| **Dicloxacillin** | T36.0X1 | T36.0X2 | T36.0X3 | T36.0X4 | T36.0X5 | T36.0X6 |
| **Dicophane** | T49.0X1 | T49.0X2 | T49.0X3 | T49.0X4 | T49.0X5 | T49.0X6 |
| **Dicoumarol, dicoumarin, dicumarol** | T45.511 | T45.512 | T45.513 | T45.514 | T45.515 | T45.516 |
| **Dicrotophos** | T60.0X1 | T60.0X2 | T60.0X3 | T60.0X4 | — | — |
| **Dicyanogen** (gas) | T65.0X1 | T65.0X2 | T65.0X3 | T65.0X4 | — | — |
| **Dicyclomine** | T44.3X1 | T44.3X2 | T44.3X3 | T44.3X4 | T44.3X5 | T44.3X6 |
| **Dicycloverine** | T44.3X1 | T44.3X2 | T44.3X3 | T44.3X4 | T44.3X5 | T44.3X6 |
| **Didanosine*** | T37.5X1 | T37.5X2 | T37.5X3 | T37.5X4 | T37.5X5 | T37.5X6 |
| **Dideoxycytidine** | T37.5X1 | T37.5X2 | T37.5X3 | T37.5X4 | T37.5X5 | T37.5X6 |
| **Dideoxyinosine** | T37.5X1 | T37.5X2 | T37.5X3 | T37.5X4 | T37.5X5 | T37.5X6 |
| **Dieldrin** (vapor) | T60.1X1 | T60.1X2 | T60.1X3 | T60.1X4 | — | — |
| **Diemal** | T42.3X1 | T42.3X2 | T42.3X3 | T42.3X4 | T42.3X5 | T42.3X6 |

| Substance | Poisoning, Accidental (unintentional) | Poisoning, Intentional Self-harm | Poisoning, Assault | Poisoning, Undetermined | Adverse Effect | Under-dosing |
|---|---|---|---|---|---|---|
| **Dienestrol** | T38.5X1 | T38.5X2 | T38.5X3 | T38.5X4 | T38.5X5 | T38.5X6 |
| **Dienoestrol** | T38.5X1 | T38.5X2 | T38.5X3 | T38.5X4 | T38.5X5 | T38.5X6 |
| **Dietetic drug NEC** | T5Ø.9Ø1 | T5Ø.9Ø2 | T5Ø.9Ø3 | T5Ø.9Ø4 | T5Ø.9Ø5 | T5Ø.9Ø6 |
| **Diethazine** | T42.8X1 | T42.8X2 | T42.8X3 | T42.8X4 | T42.8X5 | T42.8X6 |
| **Diethyl** | | | | | | |
| barbituric acid | T42.3X1 | T42.3X2 | T42.3X3 | T42.3X4 | T42.3X5 | T42.3X6 |
| carbamazine | T37.4X1 | T37.4X2 | T37.4X3 | T37.4X4 | T37.4X5 | T37.4X6 |
| carbinol | T51.3X1 | T51.3X2 | T51.3X3 | T51.3X4 | — | — |
| carbonate | T52.891 | T52.892 | T52.893 | T52.894 | — | — |
| ether (vapor) — *see also* ether | T41.ØX1 | T41.ØX2 | T41.ØX3 | T41.ØX4 | T41.ØX5 | T41.ØX6 |
| oxide | T52.891 | T52.892 | T52.893 | T52.894 | — | — |
| propion | T5Ø.5X1 | T5Ø.5X2 | T5Ø.5X3 | T5Ø.5X4 | T5Ø.5X5 | T5Ø.5X6 |
| stilbestrol | T38.5X1 | T38.5X2 | T38.5X3 | T38.5X4 | T38.5X5 | T38.5X6 |
| toluamide (nonmedicinal) | T6Ø.8X1 | T6Ø.8X2 | T6Ø.8X3 | T6Ø.8X4 | — | — |
| medicinal | T49.3X1 | T49.3X2 | T49.3X3 | T49.3X4 | T49.3X5 | T49.3X6 |
| **Diethylcarbamazine** | T37.4X1 | T37.4X2 | T37.4X3 | T37.4X4 | T37.4X5 | T37.4X6 |
| **Diethylene** | | | | | | |
| dioxide | T52.891 | T52.892 | T52.893 | T52.894 | — | — |
| glycol (monoacetate) (monobutyl ether) (monoethyl ether) | T52.3X1 | T52.3X2 | T52.3X3 | T52.3X4 | — | — |
| **Diethylhexylphthalate** | T65.891 | T65.892 | T65.893 | T65.894 | — | — |
| **Diethylpropion** | T5Ø.5X1 | T5Ø.5X2 | T5Ø.5X3 | T5Ø.5X4 | T5Ø.5X5 | T5Ø.5X6 |
| **Diethylstilbestrol** | T38.5X1 | T38.5X2 | T38.5X3 | T38.5X4 | T38.5X5 | T38.5X6 |
| **Diethylstilboestrol** | T38.5X1 | T38.5X2 | T38.5X3 | T38.5X4 | T38.5X5 | T38.5X6 |
| **Diethylsulfone-diethylmethane** | T42.6X1 | T42.6X2 | T42.6X3 | T42.6X4 | T42.6X5 | T42.6X6 |
| **Diethyltoluamide** | T49.ØX1 | T49.ØX2 | T49.ØX3 | T49.ØX4 | T49.ØX5 | T49.ØX6 |
| **Diethyltryptamine** (DET) | T4Ø.991 | T4Ø.992 | T4Ø.993 | T4Ø.994 | — | — |
| **Difebarbamate** | T42.3X1 | T42.3X2 | T42.3X3 | T42.3X4 | T42.3X5 | T42.3X6 |
| **Difencloxazine** | T4Ø.2X1 | T4Ø.2X2 | T4Ø.2X3 | T4Ø.2X4 | T4Ø.2X5 | T4Ø.2X6 |
| **Difenidol** | T45.ØX1 | T45.ØX2 | T45.ØX3 | T45.ØX4 | T45.ØX5 | T45.ØX6 |
| **Difenoxin** | T47.6X1 | T47.6X2 | T47.6X3 | T47.6X4 | T47.6X5 | T47.6X6 |
| **Difetarsone** | T37.3X1 | T37.3X2 | T37.3X3 | T37.3X4 | T37.3X5 | T37.3X6 |
| **Diffusin** | T45.3X1 | T45.3X2 | T45.3X3 | T45.3X4 | T45.3X5 | T45.3X6 |
| **Diflorasone** | T49.ØX1 | T49.ØX2 | T49.ØX3 | T49.ØX4 | T49.ØX5 | T49.ØX6 |
| **Diflos** | T44.ØX1 | T44.ØX2 | T44.ØX3 | T44.ØX4 | T44.ØX5 | T44.ØX6 |
| **Diflubenzuron** | T6Ø.1X1 | T6Ø.1X2 | T6Ø.1X3 | T6Ø.1X4 | — | — |
| **Diflucan*** | T37.8X1 | T37.8X2 | T37.8X3 | T37.8X4 | T37.8X5 | T37.8X6 |
| **Diflucortolone** | T49.ØX1 | T49.ØX2 | T49.ØX3 | T49.ØX4 | T49.ØX5 | T49.ØX6 |
| **Diflunisal** | T39.Ø91 | T39.Ø92 | T39.Ø93 | T39.Ø94 | T39.Ø95 | T39.Ø96 |
| **Difluoromethyldopa** | T42.8X1 | T42.8X2 | T42.8X3 | T42.8X4 | T42.8X5 | T42.8X6 |
| **Difluorophate** | T44.ØX1 | T44.ØX2 | T44.ØX3 | T44.ØX4 | T44.ØX5 | T44.ØX6 |
| **Digestant NEC** | T47.5X1 | T47.5X2 | T47.5X3 | T47.5X4 | T47.5X5 | T47.5X6 |
| **Digitalin** (e) | T46.ØX1 | T46.ØX2 | T46.ØX3 | T46.ØX4 | T46.ØX5 | T46.ØX6 |
| **Digitalis** (leaf)(glycoside) | T46.ØX1 | T46.ØX2 | T46.ØX3 | T46.ØX4 | T46.ØX5 | T46.ØX6 |
| lanata | T46.ØX1 | T46.ØX2 | T46.ØX3 | T46.ØX4 | T46.ØX5 | T46.ØX6 |
| purpurea | T46.ØX1 | T46.ØX2 | T46.ØX3 | T46.ØX4 | T46.ØX5 | T46.ØX6 |
| **Digitoxin** | T46.ØX1 | T46.ØX2 | T46.ØX3 | T46.ØX4 | T46.ØX5 | T46.ØX6 |
| **Digitoxose** | T46.ØX1 | T46.ØX2 | T46.ØX3 | T46.ØX4 | T46.ØX5 | T46.ØX6 |
| **Digoxin** | T46.ØX1 | T46.ØX2 | T46.ØX3 | T46.ØX4 | T46.ØX5 | T46.ØX6 |
| **Digoxine** | T46.ØX1 | T46.ØX2 | T46.ØX3 | T46.ØX4 | T46.ØX5 | T46.ØX6 |
| **Dihydralazine** | T46.5X1 | T46.5X2 | T46.5X3 | T46.5X4 | T46.5X5 | T46.5X6 |
| **Dihydrazine** | T46.5X1 | T46.5X2 | T46.5X3 | T46.5X4 | T46.5X5 | T46.5X6 |
| **Dihydrocodeine** | T4Ø.2X1 | T4Ø.2X2 | T4Ø.2X3 | T4Ø.2X4 | T4Ø.2X5 | T4Ø.2X6 |
| **Dihydrocodeinone** | T4Ø.2X1 | T4Ø.2X2 | T4Ø.2X3 | T4Ø.2X4 | T4Ø.2X5 | T4Ø.2X6 |
| **Dihydroergocornine** | T46.7X1 | T46.7X2 | T46.7X3 | T46.7X4 | T46.7X5 | T46.7X6 |
| **Dihydroergocristine** (mesilate) | T46.7X1 | T46.7X2 | T46.7X3 | T46.7X4 | T46.7X5 | T46.7X6 |
| **Dihydroergokryptine** | T46.7X1 | T46.7X2 | T46.7X3 | T46.7X4 | T46.7X5 | T46.7X6 |
| **Dihydroergotamine** | T46.5X1 | T46.5X2 | T46.5X3 | T46.5X4 | T46.5X5 | T46.5X6 |
| **Dihydroergotoxine** | T46.7X1 | T46.7X2 | T46.7X3 | T46.7X4 | T46.7X5 | T46.7X6 |
| mesilate | T46.7X1 | T46.7X2 | T46.7X3 | T46.7X4 | T46.7X5 | T46.7X6 |
| **Dihydrohydroxycodeinone** | T4Ø.2X1 | T4Ø.2X2 | T4Ø.2X3 | T4Ø.2X4 | T4Ø.2X5 | T4Ø.2X6 |
| **Dihydrohydroxymorphinone** | T4Ø.2X1 | T4Ø.2X2 | T4Ø.2X3 | T4Ø.2X4 | T4Ø.2X5 | T4Ø.2X6 |
| **Dihydroisocodeine** | T4Ø.2X1 | T4Ø.2X2 | T4Ø.2X3 | T4Ø.2X4 | T4Ø.2X5 | T4Ø.2X6 |
| **Dihydromorphine** | T4Ø.2X1 | T4Ø.2X2 | T4Ø.2X3 | T4Ø.2X4 | — | — |
| **Dihydromorphinone** | T4Ø.2X1 | T4Ø.2X2 | T4Ø.2X3 | T4Ø.2X4 | T4Ø.2X5 | T4Ø.2X6 |
| **Dihydrostreptomycin** | T36.5X1 | T36.5X2 | T36.5X3 | T36.5X4 | T36.5X5 | T36.5X6 |
| **Dihydrotachysterol** | T45.2X1 | T45.2X2 | T45.2X3 | T45.2X4 | T45.2X5 | T45.2X6 |
| **Dihydroxyacetone*** | T49.3X1 | T49.3X2 | T49.3X3 | T49.3X4 | T49.3X5 | T49.3X6 |
| **Dihydroxyaluminum aminoacetate** | T47.1X1 | T47.1X2 | T47.1X3 | T47.1X4 | T47.1X5 | T47.1X6 |
| **Dihydroxyaluminum sodium carbonate** | T47.1X1 | T47.1X2 | T47.1X3 | T47.1X4 | T47.1X5 | T47.1X6 |
| **Dihydroxyanthraquinone** | T47.2X1 | T47.2X2 | T47.2X3 | T47.2X4 | T47.2X5 | T47.2X6 |
| **Dihydroxycodeinone** | T4Ø.2X1 | T4Ø.2X2 | T4Ø.2X3 | T4Ø.2X4 | T4Ø.2X5 | T4Ø.2X6 |
| **Dihydroxypropyl theophylline** | T5Ø.2X1 | T5Ø.2X2 | T5Ø.2X3 | T5Ø.2X4 | T5Ø.2X5 | T5Ø.2X6 |
| **Diiodohydroxyquin** | T37.8X1 | T37.8X2 | T37.8X3 | T37.8X4 | T37.8X5 | T37.8X6 |
| topical | T49.ØX1 | T49.ØX2 | T49.ØX3 | T49.ØX4 | T49.ØX5 | T49.ØX6 |
| **Diiodohydroxyquinoline** | T37.8X1 | T37.8X2 | T37.8X3 | T37.8X4 | T37.8X5 | T37.8X6 |

| Substance | Poisoning, Accidental (unintentional) | Poisoning, Intentional Self-harm | Poisoning, Assault | Poisoning, Undetermined | Adverse Effect | Under-dosing |
|---|---|---|---|---|---|---|
| **Diiodotyrosine** | T38.2X1 | T38.2X2 | T38.2X3 | T38.2X4 | T38.2X5 | T38.2X |
| **Diisopromine** | T44.3X1 | T44.3X2 | T44.3X3 | T44.3X4 | T44.3X5 | T44.3X |
| **Diisopropylamine** | T46.3X1 | T46.3X2 | T46.3X3 | T46.3X4 | T46.3X5 | T46.3X |
| **Diisopropylfluorophosphonate** | T44.ØX1 | T44.ØX2 | T44.ØX3 | T44.ØX4 | T44.ØX5 | T44.ØX |
| **Dilantin** | T42.ØX1 | T42.ØX2 | T42.ØX3 | T42.ØX4 | T42.ØX5 | T42.ØX |
| **Dilatrate*** | T46.3X1 | T46.3X2 | T46.3X3 | T46.3X4 | T46.3X5 | T46.3X |
| **Dilaudid** | T4Ø.2X1 | T4Ø.2X2 | T4Ø.2X3 | T4Ø.2X4 | T4Ø.2X5 | T4Ø.2X |
| **Dilazep** | T46.3X1 | T46.3X2 | T46.3X3 | T46.3X4 | T46.3X5 | T46.3X |
| **Dill** | T47.5X1 | T47.5X2 | T47.5X3 | T47.5X4 | T47.5X5 | T47.5X |
| **Diloxanide** | T37.3X1 | T37.3X2 | T37.3X3 | T37.3X4 | T37.3X5 | T37.3X |
| **Diltiazem** | T46.1X1 | T46.1X2 | T46.1X3 | T46.1X4 | T46.1X5 | T46.1X |
| **Dimazole** | T49.ØX1 | T49.ØX2 | T49.ØX3 | T49.ØX4 | T49.ØX5 | T49.ØX |
| **Dimefline** | T5Ø.7X1 | T5Ø.7X2 | T5Ø.7X3 | T5Ø.7X4 | T5Ø.7X5 | T5Ø.7X |
| **Dimefox** | T6Ø.ØX1 | T6Ø.ØX2 | T6Ø.ØX3 | T6Ø.ØX4 | — | — |
| **Dimemorfan** | T48.3X1 | T48.3X2 | T48.3X3 | T48.3X4 | T48.3X5 | T48.3X |
| **Dimenhydrinate** | T45.ØX1 | T45.ØX2 | T45.ØX3 | T45.ØX4 | T45.ØX5 | T45.ØX |
| **Dimercaprol** (British anti-lewisite) | T45.8X1 | T45.8X2 | T45.8X3 | T45.8X4 | T45.8X5 | T45.8X |
| **Dimercaptopropanol** | T45.8X1 | T45.8X2 | T45.8X3 | T45.8X4 | T45.8X5 | T45.8X |
| **Dimestrol** | T38.5X1 | T38.5X2 | T38.5X3 | T38.5X4 | T38.5X5 | T38.5X |
| **Dimetane** | T45.ØX1 | T45.ØX2 | T45.ØX3 | T45.ØX4 | T45.ØX5 | T45.ØX |
| **Dimethicone** | T47.1X1 | T47.1X2 | T47.1X3 | T47.1X4 | T47.1X5 | T47.1X |
| **Dimethindene** | T45.ØX1 | T45.ØX2 | T45.ØX3 | T45.ØX4 | T45.ØX5 | T45.ØX |
| **Dimethisoquin** | T49.1X1 | T49.1X2 | T49.1X3 | T49.1X4 | T49.1X5 | T49.1X |
| **Dimethisterone** | T38.5X1 | T38.5X2 | T38.5X3 | T38.5X4 | T38.5X5 | T38.5X |
| **Dimethoate** | T6Ø.ØX1 | T6Ø.ØX2 | T6Ø.ØX3 | T6Ø.ØX4 | — | — |
| **Dimethocaine** | T41.3X1 | T41.3X2 | T41.3X3 | T41.3X4 | T41.3X5 | T41.3X |
| **Dimethoxanate** | T48.3X1 | T48.3X2 | T48.3X3 | T48.3X4 | T48.3X5 | T48.3X |
| **Dimethyl** | | | | | | |
| arsine, arsinic acid | T57.ØX1 | T57.ØX2 | T57.ØX3 | T57.ØX4 | — | — |
| carbinol | T51.2X1 | T51.2X2 | T51.2X3 | T51.2X4 | — | — |
| carbonate | T52.891 | T52.892 | T52.893 | T52.894 | — | — |
| diguanide | T38.3X1 | T38.3X2 | T38.3X3 | T38.3X4 | T38.3X5 | T38.3X6 |
| ketone | T52.4X1 | T52.4X2 | T52.4X3 | T52.4X4 | — | — |
| vapor | T52.4X1 | T52.4X2 | T52.4X3 | T52.4X4 | — | — |
| meperidine | T4Ø.2X1 | T4Ø.2X2 | T4Ø.2X3 | T4Ø.2X4 | T4Ø.2X5 | T4Ø.2X6 |
| parathion | T6Ø.ØX1 | T6Ø.ØX2 | T6Ø.ØX3 | T6Ø.ØX4 | — | — |
| phthlate | T49.3X1 | T49.3X2 | T49.3X3 | T49.3X4 | T49.3X5 | T49.3X6 |
| polysiloxane | T47.8X1 | T47.8X2 | T47.8X3 | T47.8X4 | T47.8X5 | T47.8X6 |
| sulfate (fumes) | T59.891 | T59.892 | T59.893 | T59.894 | — | — |
| liquid | T65.891 | T65.892 | T65.893 | T65.894 | — | — |
| sulfoxide (nonmedicinal) | T52.891 | T52.892 | T52.893 | T52.894 | — | — |
| medicinal | T49.4X1 | T49.4X2 | T49.4X3 | T49.4X4 | T49.4X5 | T49.4X6 |
| tryptamine | T4Ø.991 | T4Ø.992 | T4Ø.993 | T4Ø.994 | — | — |
| tubocurarine | T48.1X1 | T48.1X2 | T48.1X3 | T48.1X4 | T48.1X5 | T48.1X6 |
| **Dimethylamine sulfate** | T49.4X1 | T49.4X2 | T49.4X3 | T49.4X4 | T49.4X5 | T49.4X6 |
| **Dimethylcysteine*** | T5Ø.6X1 | T5Ø.6X2 | T5Ø.6X3 | T5Ø.6X4 | T5Ø.6X5 | T5Ø.6X6 |
| **Dimethylformamide** | T52.891 | T52.892 | T52.893 | T52.894 | — | — |
| **Dimethyltubocurarinium chloride** | T48.1X1 | T48.1X2 | T48.1X3 | T48.1X4 | T48.1X5 | T48.1X6 |
| **Dimeticone** | T47.1X1 | T47.1X2 | T47.1X3 | T47.1X4 | T47.1X5 | T47.1X6 |
| **Dimetilan** | T6Ø.ØX1 | T6Ø.ØX2 | T6Ø.ØX3 | T6Ø.ØX4 | — | — |
| **Dimetindene** | T45.ØX1 | T45.ØX2 | T45.ØX3 | T45.ØX4 | T45.ØX5 | T45.ØX6 |
| **Dimetotiazine** | T43.3X1 | T43.3X2 | T43.3X3 | T43.3X4 | T43.3X5 | T43.3X6 |
| **Dimorpholamine** | T5Ø.7X1 | T5Ø.7X2 | T5Ø.7X3 | T5Ø.7X4 | T5Ø.7X5 | T5Ø.7X6 |
| **Dimoxyline** | T46.3X1 | T46.3X2 | T46.3X3 | T46.3X4 | T46.3X5 | T46.3X6 |
| **Dinitro** (-ortho-)cresol (pesticide) (spray) | T65.3X1 | T65.3X2 | T65.3X3 | T65.3X4 | — | — |
| **Dinitrobenzene** | T65.3X1 | T65.3X2 | T65.3X3 | T65.3X4 | — | — |
| vapor | T59.891 | T59.892 | T59.893 | T59.894 | — | — |
| **Dinitrobenzol** | T65.3X1 | T65.3X2 | T65.3X3 | T65.3X4 | — | — |
| vapor | T59.891 | T59.892 | T59.893 | T59.894 | — | — |
| **Dinitrobutylphenol** | T65.3X1 | T65.3X2 | T65.3X3 | T65.3X4 | — | — |
| **Dinitrocyclohexylphenol** | T65.3X1 | T65.3X2 | T65.3X3 | T65.3X4 | — | — |
| **Dinitrophenol** | T65.3X1 | T65.3X2 | T65.3X3 | T65.3X4 | — | — |
| **Dinoprost** | T48.ØX1 | T48.ØX2 | T48.ØX3 | T48.ØX4 | T48.ØX5 | T48.ØX6 |
| **Dinoprostone** | T48.ØX1 | T48.ØX2 | T48.ØX3 | T48.ØX4 | T48.ØX5 | T48.ØX6 |
| **Dinoseb** | T6Ø.3X1 | T6Ø.3X2 | T6Ø.3X3 | T6Ø.3X4 | — | — |
| **Dioctyl sulfosuccinate** (calcium) (sodium) | T47.4X1 | T47.4X2 | T47.4X3 | T47.4X4 | T47.4X5 | T47.4X6 |
| **Diodone** | T5Ø.8X1 | T5Ø.8X2 | T5Ø.8X3 | T5Ø.8X4 | T5Ø.8X5 | T5Ø.8X6 |
| **Diodoquin** | T37.8X1 | T37.8X2 | T37.8X3 | T37.8X4 | T37.8X5 | T37.8X6 |
| **Dionin** | T4Ø.2X1 | T4Ø.2X2 | T4Ø.2X3 | T4Ø.2X4 | T4Ø.2X5 | T4Ø.2X6 |
| **Diosmin** | T46.991 | T46.992 | T46.993 | T46.994 | T46.995 | T46.996 |
| **Diovan*** | T46.5X1 | T46.5X2 | T46.5X3 | T46.5X4 | T46.5X5 | T46.5X6 |
| **Dioxane** | T52.891 | T52.892 | T52.893 | T52.894 | — | — |
| **Dioxathion** | T6Ø.ØX1 | T6Ø.ØX2 | T6Ø.ØX3 | T6Ø.ØX4 | — | — |
| **Dioxin** | T53.7X1 | T53.7X2 | T53.7X3 | T53.7X4 | — | — |
| **Dioxopromethazine** | T43.3X1 | T43.3X2 | T43.3X3 | T43.3X4 | T43.3X5 | T43.3X6 |
| **Dioxyline** | T46.3X1 | T46.3X2 | T46.3X3 | T46.3X4 | T46.3X5 | T46.3X6 |
| **Dipentene** | T52.891 | T52.892 | T52.893 | T52.894 | — | — |
| **Diperodon** | T41.3X1 | T41.3X2 | T41.3X3 | T41.3X4 | T41.3X5 | T41.3X6 |
| **Diphacinone** | T6Ø.4X1 | T6Ø.4X2 | T6Ø.4X3 | T6Ø.4X4 | — | — |



☑ Additional Character May Be Required — Refer to the Tabular List for Character Selection

*Optum Value-Add

| Substance | Poisoning, Accidental (unintentional) | Poisoning, Intentional Self-harm | Poisoning, Assault | Poisoning, Undetermined | Adverse Effect | Under-dosing |
|---|---|---|---|---|---|---|
| **Diphemanil** | T44.3X1 | T44.3X2 | T44.3X3 | T44.3X4 | T44.3X5 | T44.3X6 |
| metilsulfate | T44.3X1 | T44.3X2 | T44.3X3 | T44.3X4 | T44.3X5 | T44.3X6 |
| **Diphenadione** | T45.511 | T45.512 | T45.513 | T45.514 | T45.515 | T45.516 |
| rodenticide | T6Ø.4X1 | T6Ø.4X2 | T6Ø.4X3 | T6Ø.4X4 | — | — |
| **Diphenhydramine** | T45.ØX1 | T45.ØX2 | T45.ØX3 | T45.ØX4 | T45.ØX5 | T45.ØX6 |
| **Diphenidol** | T45.ØX1 | T45.ØX2 | T45.ØX3 | T45.ØX4 | T45.ØX5 | T45.ØX6 |
| **Diphenoxylate** | T47.6X1 | T47.6X2 | T47.6X3 | T47.6X4 | T47.6X5 | T47.6X6 |
| **Diphenylamine** | T65.3X1 | T65.3X2 | T65.3X3 | T65.3X4 | — | — |
| **Diphenylbutazone** | T39.2X1 | T39.2X2 | T39.2X3 | T39.2X4 | T39.2X5 | T39.2X6 |
| **Diphenylchloroarsine, not in war** | T57.ØX1 | T57.ØX2 | T57.ØX3 | T57.ØX4 | — | — |
| **Diphenylhydantoin** | T42.ØX1 | T42.ØX2 | T42.ØX3 | T42.ØX4 | T42.ØX5 | T42.ØX6 |
| **Diphenylmethane dye** | T52.1X1 | T52.1X2 | T52.1X3 | T52.1X4 | — | — |
| **Diphenylpyraline** | T45.ØX1 | T45.ØX2 | T45.ØX3 | T45.ØX4 | T45.ØX5 | T45.ØX6 |
| **Diphtheria** | | | | | | |
| antitoxin | T5Ø.Z11 | T5Ø.Z12 | T5Ø.Z13 | T5Ø.Z14 | T5Ø.Z15 | T5Ø.Z16 |
| toxoid | T5Ø.A91 | T5Ø.A92 | T5Ø.A93 | T5Ø.A94 | T5Ø.A95 | T5Ø.A96 |
| with tetanus toxoid | T5Ø.A21 | T5Ø.A22 | T5Ø.A23 | T5Ø.A24 | T5Ø.A25 | T5Ø.A26 |
| with pertussis component | T5Ø.A11 | T5Ø.A12 | T5Ø.A13 | T5Ø.A14 | T5Ø.A15 | T5Ø.A16 |
| vaccine | T5Ø.A91 | T5Ø.A92 | T5Ø.A93 | T5Ø.A94 | T5Ø.A95 | T5Ø.A96 |
| combination | | | | | | |
| including pertussis | T5Ø.A11 | T5Ø.A12 | T5Ø.A13 | T5Ø.A14 | T5Ø.A15 | T5Ø.A16 |
| without pertussis | T5Ø.A21 | T5Ø.A22 | T5Ø.A23 | T5Ø.A24 | T5Ø.A25 | T5Ø.A26 |
| **Diphylline** | T5Ø.2X1 | T5Ø.2X2 | T5Ø.2X3 | T5Ø.2X4 | T5Ø.2X5 | T5Ø.2X6 |
| **Dipipanone** | T4Ø.491 | T4Ø.492 | T4Ø.493 | T4Ø.494 | — | — |
| **Dipivefrine** | T49.5X1 | T49.5X2 | T49.5X3 | T49.5X4 | T49.5X5 | T49.5X6 |
| **Diplovax** | T5Ø.B91 | T5Ø.B92 | T5Ø.B93 | T5Ø.B94 | T5Ø.B95 | T5Ø.B96 |
| **Diprophylline** | T5Ø.2X1 | T5Ø.2X2 | T5Ø.2X3 | T5Ø.2X4 | T5Ø.2X5 | T5Ø.2X6 |
| **Dipropyline** | T48.291 | T48.292 | T48.293 | T48.294 | T48.295 | T48.296 |
| **Dipyridamole** | T46.3X1 | T46.3X2 | T46.3X3 | T46.3X4 | T46.3X5 | T46.3X6 |
| **Dipyrone** | T39.2X1 | T39.2X2 | T39.2X3 | T39.2X4 | T39.2X5 | T39.2X6 |
| **Diquat** (dibromide) | T6Ø.3X1 | T6Ø.3X2 | T6Ø.3X3 | T6Ø.3X4 | — | — |
| **Disinfectant** | T65.891 | T65.892 | T65.893 | T65.894 | — | — |
| alkaline | T54.3X1 | T54.3X2 | T54.3X3 | T54.3X4 | — | — |
| aromatic | T54.1X1 | T54.1X2 | T54.1X3 | T54.1X4 | — | — |
| intestinal | T37.8X1 | T37.8X2 | T37.8X3 | T37.8X4 | T37.8X5 | T37.8X6 |
| **Disipal** | T42.8X1 | T42.8X2 | T42.8X3 | T42.8X4 | T42.8X5 | T42.8X6 |
| **Disodium edetate** | T5Ø.6X1 | T5Ø.6X2 | T5Ø.6X3 | T5Ø.6X4 | T5Ø.6X5 | T5Ø.6X6 |
| **Disoprofol** | T41.291 | T41.292 | T41.293 | T41.294 | T41.295 | T41.296 |
| **Disopyramide*** | T46.2X1 | T46.2X2 | T46.2X3 | T46.2X4 | T46.2X5 | T46.2X6 |
| **Distigmine** (bromide) | T44.ØX1 | T44.ØX2 | T44.ØX3 | T44.ØX4 | T44.ØX5 | T44.ØX6 |
| **Disulfamide** | T5Ø.2X1 | T5Ø.2X2 | T5Ø.2X3 | T5Ø.2X4 | T5Ø.2X5 | T5Ø.2X6 |
| **Disulfanilamide** | T37.ØX1 | T37.ØX2 | T37.ØX3 | T37.ØX4 | T37.ØX5 | T37.ØX6 |
| **Disulfiram** | T5Ø.6X1 | T5Ø.6X2 | T5Ø.6X3 | T5Ø.6X4 | T5Ø.6X5 | T5Ø.6X6 |
| **Disulfoton** | T6Ø.ØX1 | T6Ø.ØX2 | T6Ø.ØX3 | T6Ø.ØX4 | — | — |
| **Dithiazanine iodide** | T37.4X1 | T37.4X2 | T37.4X3 | T37.4X4 | T37.4X5 | T37.4X6 |
| **Dithiocarbamate** | T6Ø.ØX1 | T6Ø.ØX2 | T6Ø.ØX3 | T6Ø.ØX4 | — | — |
| **Dithranol** | T49.4X1 | T49.4X2 | T49.4X3 | T49.4X4 | T49.4X5 | T49.4X6 |
| **Diucardin** | T5Ø.2X1 | T5Ø.2X2 | T5Ø.2X3 | T5Ø.2X4 | T5Ø.2X5 | T5Ø.2X6 |
| **Diupres** | T5Ø.2X1 | T5Ø.2X2 | T5Ø.2X3 | T5Ø.2X4 | T5Ø.2X5 | T5Ø.2X6 |
| **Diuretic NEC** | T5Ø.2X1 | T5Ø.2X2 | T5Ø.2X3 | T5Ø.2X4 | T5Ø.2X5 | T5Ø.2X6 |
| benzothiadiazine | T5Ø.2X1 | T5Ø.2X2 | T5Ø.2X3 | T5Ø.2X4 | T5Ø.2X5 | T5Ø.2X6 |
| carbonic acid anhydrase inhibitors | T5Ø.2X1 | T5Ø.2X2 | T5Ø.2X3 | T5Ø.2X4 | T5Ø.2X5 | T5Ø.2X6 |
| furfuryl NEC | T5Ø.2X1 | T5Ø.2X2 | T5Ø.2X3 | T5Ø.2X4 | T5Ø.2X5 | T5Ø.2X6 |
| loop (high-ceiling) | T5Ø.1X1 | T5Ø.1X2 | T5Ø.1X3 | T5Ø.1X4 | T5Ø.1X5 | T5Ø.1X6 |
| mercurial NEC | T5Ø.2X1 | T5Ø.2X2 | T5Ø.2X3 | T5Ø.2X4 | T5Ø.2X5 | T5Ø.2X6 |
| osmotic | T5Ø.2X1 | T5Ø.2X2 | T5Ø.2X3 | T5Ø.2X4 | T5Ø.2X5 | T5Ø.2X6 |
| purine NEC | T5Ø.2X1 | T5Ø.2X2 | T5Ø.2X3 | T5Ø.2X4 | T5Ø.2X5 | T5Ø.2X6 |
| saluretic NEC | T5Ø.2X1 | T5Ø.2X2 | T5Ø.2X3 | T5Ø.2X4 | T5Ø.2X5 | T5Ø.2X6 |
| sulfonamide | T5Ø.2X1 | T5Ø.2X2 | T5Ø.2X3 | T5Ø.2X4 | T5Ø.2X5 | T5Ø.2X6 |
| thiazide NEC | T5Ø.2X1 | T5Ø.2X2 | T5Ø.2X3 | T5Ø.2X4 | T5Ø.2X5 | T5Ø.2X6 |
| xanthine | T5Ø.2X1 | T5Ø.2X2 | T5Ø.2X3 | T5Ø.2X4 | T5Ø.2X5 | T5Ø.2X6 |
| **Diurgin** | T5Ø.2X1 | T5Ø.2X2 | T5Ø.2X3 | T5Ø.2X4 | T5Ø.2X5 | T5Ø.2X6 |
| **Diuril** | T5Ø.2X1 | T5Ø.2X2 | T5Ø.2X3 | T5Ø.2X4 | T5Ø.2X5 | T5Ø.2X6 |
| **Diuron** | T6Ø.3X1 | T6Ø.3X2 | T6Ø.3X3 | T6Ø.3X4 | — | — |
| **Divalproex** | T42.6X1 | T42.6X2 | T42.6X3 | T42.6X4 | T42.6X5 | T42.6X6 |
| **Divinyl ether** | T41.ØX1 | T41.ØX2 | T41.ØX3 | T41.ØX4 | T41.ØX5 | T41.ØX6 |
| **Dixanthogen** | T49.ØX1 | T49.ØX2 | T49.ØX3 | T49.ØX4 | T49.ØX5 | T49.ØX6 |
| **Dixyrazine** | T43.3X1 | T43.3X2 | T43.3X3 | T43.3X4 | T43.3X5 | T43.3X6 |
| **DMCT** | T36.4X1 | T36.4X2 | T36.4X3 | T36.4X4 | T36.4X5 | T36.4X6 |
| **DMSO** — *see* Dimethyl, sulfoxide | | | | | | |
| **DNBP** | T6Ø.3X1 | T6Ø.3X2 | T6Ø.3X3 | T6Ø.3X4 | — | — |
| **DNOC** | T65.3X1 | T65.3X2 | T65.3X3 | T65.3X4 | — | — |
| **Dobutamine** | T44.5X1 | T44.5X2 | T44.5X3 | T44.5X4 | T44.5X5 | T44.5X6 |
| **DOCA** | T38.ØX1 | T38.ØX2 | T38.ØX3 | T38.ØX4 | T38.ØX5 | T38.ØX6 |
| **Docusate sodium** | T47.4X1 | T47.4X2 | T47.4X3 | T47.4X4 | T47.4X5 | T47.4X6 |
| **Dodicin** | T49.ØX1 | T49.ØX2 | T49.ØX3 | T49.ØX4 | T49.ØX5 | T49.ØX6 |
| **Dofamium chloride** | T49.ØX1 | T49.ØX2 | T49.ØX3 | T49.ØX4 | T49.ØX5 | T49.ØX6 |
| **Dolophine** | T4Ø.3X1 | T4Ø.3X2 | T4Ø.3X3 | T4Ø.3X4 | T4Ø.3X5 | T4Ø.3X6 |
| **Doloxene** | T39.8X1 | T39.8X2 | T39.8X3 | T39.8X4 | T39.8X5 | T39.8X6 |

| Substance | Poisoning, Accidental (unintentional) | Poisoning, Intentional Self-harm | Poisoning, Assault | Poisoning, Undetermined | Adverse Effect | Under-dosing |
|---|---|---|---|---|---|---|
| **Domestic gas** (after combustion) — *see* Gas, utility | | | | | | |
| prior to combustion | T59.891 | T59.892 | T59.893 | T59.894 | — | — |
| **Domiodol** | T48.4X1 | T48.4X2 | T48.4X3 | T48.4X4 | T48.4X5 | T48.4X6 |
| **Domiphen** (bromide) | T49.ØX1 | T49.ØX2 | T49.ØX3 | T49.ØX4 | T49.ØX5 | T49.ØX6 |
| **Domperidone** | T45.ØX1 | T45.ØX2 | T45.ØX3 | T45.ØX4 | T45.ØX5 | T45.ØX6 |
| **Donepezil*** | T44.ØX1 | T44.ØX2 | T44.ØX3 | T44.ØX4 | T44.ØX5 | T44.ØX6 |
| **Dopa** | T42.8X1 | T42.8X2 | T42.8X3 | T42.8X4 | T42.8X5 | T42.8X6 |
| **Dopamine** | T44.991 | T44.992 | T44.993 | T44.994 | T44.995 | T44.996 |
| **Doriden** | T42.6X1 | T42.6X2 | T42.6X3 | T42.6X4 | T42.6X5 | T42.6X6 |
| **Dormiral** | T42.3X1 | T42.3X2 | T42.3X3 | T42.3X4 | T42.3X5 | T42.3X6 |
| **Dormison** | T42.6X1 | T42.6X2 | T42.6X3 | T42.6X4 | T42.6X5 | T42.6X6 |
| **Dornase** | T48.4X1 | T48.4X2 | T48.4X3 | T48.4X4 | T48.4X5 | T48.4X6 |
| **Dorsacaine** | T41.3X1 | T41.3X2 | T41.3X3 | T41.3X4 | T41.3X5 | T41.3X6 |
| **Dosulepin** | T43.Ø11 | T43.Ø12 | T43.Ø13 | T43.Ø14 | T43.Ø15 | T43.Ø16 |
| **Dothiepin** | T43.Ø11 | T43.Ø12 | T43.Ø13 | T43.Ø14 | T43.Ø15 | T43.Ø16 |
| **Doxantrazole** | T48.6X1 | T48.6X2 | T48.6X3 | T48.6X4 | T48.6X5 | T48.6X6 |
| **Doxapram** | T5Ø.7X1 | T5Ø.7X2 | T5Ø.7X3 | T5Ø.7X4 | T5Ø.7X5 | T5Ø.7X6 |
| **Doxazosin** | T44.6X1 | T44.6X2 | T44.6X3 | T44.6X4 | T44.6X5 | T44.6X6 |
| **Doxepin** | T43.Ø11 | T43.Ø12 | T43.Ø13 | T43.Ø14 | T43.Ø15 | T43.Ø16 |
| **Doxifluridine** | T45.1X1 | T45.1X2 | T45.1X3 | T45.1X4 | T45.1X5 | T45.1X6 |
| **Doxil*** | T45.1X1 | T45.1X2 | T45.1X3 | T45.1X4 | T45.1X5 | T45.1X6 |
| **Doxorubicin** | T45.1X1 | T45.1X2 | T45.1X3 | T45.1X4 | T45.1X5 | T45.1X6 |
| **Doxycycline** | T36.4X1 | T36.4X2 | T36.4X3 | T36.4X4 | T36.4X5 | T36.4X6 |
| **Doxylamine** | T45.ØX1 | T45.ØX2 | T45.ØX3 | T45.ØX4 | T45.ØX5 | T45.ØX6 |
| **Dramamine** | T45.ØX1 | T45.ØX2 | T45.ØX3 | T45.ØX4 | T45.ØX5 | T45.ØX6 |
| **Drano** (drain cleaner) | T54.3X1 | T54.3X2 | T54.3X3 | T54.3X4 | — | — |
| **Dressing, live pulp** | T49.7X1 | T49.7X2 | T49.7X3 | T49.7X4 | T49.7X5 | T49.7X6 |
| **Drocode** | T4Ø.2X1 | T4Ø.2X2 | T4Ø.2X3 | T4Ø.2X4 | T4Ø.2X5 | T4Ø.2X6 |
| **Dromoran** | T4Ø.2X1 | T4Ø.2X2 | T4Ø.2X3 | T4Ø.2X4 | T4Ø.2X5 | T4Ø.2X6 |
| **Dromostanolone** | T38.7X1 | T38.7X2 | T38.7X3 | T38.7X4 | T38.7X5 | T38.7X6 |
| **Dronabinol** | T4Ø.711 | T4Ø.712 | T4Ø.713 | T4Ø.714 | T4Ø.715 | T4Ø.716 |
| **Droperidol** | T43.591 | T43.592 | T43.593 | T43.594 | T43.595 | T43.596 |
| **Dropropizine** | T48.3X1 | T48.3X2 | T48.3X3 | T48.3X4 | T48.3X5 | T48.3X6 |
| **Drostanolone** | T38.7X1 | T38.7X2 | T38.7X3 | T38.7X4 | T38.7X5 | T38.7X6 |
| **Drotaverine** | T44.3X1 | T44.3X2 | T44.3X3 | T44.3X4 | T44.3X5 | T44.3X6 |
| **Drotrecogin alfa** | T45.511 | T45.512 | T45.513 | T45.514 | T45.515 | T45.516 |
| **Drug NEC** | T5Ø.9Ø1 | T5Ø.9Ø2 | T5Ø.9Ø3 | T5Ø.9Ø4 | T5Ø.9Ø5 | T5Ø.9Ø6 |
| specified NEC | T5Ø.991 | T5Ø.992 | T5Ø.993 | T5Ø.994 | T5Ø.995 | T5Ø.996 |
| **DTIC** | T45.1X1 | T45.1X2 | T45.1X3 | T45.1X4 | T45.1X5 | T45.1X6 |
| **Duboisine** | T44.3X1 | T44.3X2 | T44.3X3 | T44.3X4 | T44.3X5 | T44.3X6 |
| **Dulcolax** | T47.2X1 | T47.2X2 | T47.2X3 | T47.2X4 | T47.2X5 | T47.2X6 |
| **Duponol** (C) (EP) | T49.2X1 | T49.2X2 | T49.2X3 | T49.2X4 | T49.2X5 | T49.2X6 |
| **Durabolin** | T38.7X1 | T38.7X2 | T38.7X3 | T38.7X4 | T38.7X5 | T38.7X6 |
| **Durezol*** | T49.5X1 | T49.5X2 | T49.5X3 | T49.5X4 | T49.5X5 | T49.5X6 |
| **Dyclone** | T41.3X1 | T41.3X2 | T41.3X3 | T41.3X4 | T41.3X5 | T41.3X6 |
| **Dyclonine** | T41.3X1 | T41.3X2 | T41.3X3 | T41.3X4 | T41.3X5 | T41.3X6 |
| **Dydrogesterone** | T38.5X1 | T38.5X2 | T38.5X3 | T38.5X4 | T38.5X5 | T38.5X6 |
| **Dye NEC** | T65.6X1 | T65.6X2 | T65.6X3 | T65.6X4 | — | — |
| antiseptic | T49.ØX1 | T49.ØX2 | T49.ØX3 | T49.ØX4 | T49.ØX5 | T49.ØX6 |
| diagnostic agents | T5Ø.8X1 | T5Ø.8X2 | T5Ø.8X3 | T5Ø.8X4 | T5Ø.8X5 | T5Ø.8X6 |
| pharmaceutical NEC | T5Ø.9Ø1 | T5Ø.9Ø2 | T5Ø.9Ø3 | T5Ø.9Ø4 | T5Ø.9Ø5 | T5Ø.9Ø6 |
| **Dyflos** | T44.ØX1 | T44.ØX2 | T44.ØX3 | T44.ØX4 | T44.ØX5 | T44.ØX6 |
| **Dymelor** | T38.3X1 | T38.3X2 | T38.3X3 | T38.3X4 | T38.3X5 | T38.3X6 |
| **Dynamite** | T65.3X1 | T65.3X2 | T65.3X3 | T65.3X4 | — | — |
| fumes | T59.891 | T59.892 | T59.893 | T59.894 | — | — |
| **Dyphylline** | T44.3X1 | T44.3X2 | T44.3X3 | T44.3X4 | T44.3X5 | T44.3X6 |
| **Ear drug NEC** | T49.6X1 | T49.6X2 | T49.6X3 | T49.6X4 | T49.6X5 | T49.6X6 |
| **Ear preparations** | T49.6X1 | T49.6X2 | T49.6X3 | T49.6X4 | T49.6X5 | T49.6X6 |
| **Echothiophate, echothiopate, ecothiopate** | T49.5X1 | T49.5X2 | T49.5X3 | T49.5X4 | T49.5X5 | T49.5X6 |
| **Econazole** | T49.ØX1 | T49.ØX2 | T49.ØX3 | T49.ØX4 | T49.ØX5 | T49.ØX6 |
| **Ecothiopate iodide** | T49.5X1 | T49.5X2 | T49.5X3 | T49.5X4 | T49.5X5 | T49.5X6 |
| **Ecstasy** | T43.641 | T43.642 | T43.643 | T43.644 | — | — |
| **Ectylurea** | T42.6X1 | T42.6X2 | T42.6X3 | T42.6X4 | T42.6X5 | T42.6X6 |
| **Edathamil disodium** | T45.8X1 | T45.8X2 | T45.8X3 | T45.8X4 | T45.8X5 | T45.8X6 |
| **Edecrin** | T5Ø.1X1 | T5Ø.1X2 | T5Ø.1X3 | T5Ø.1X4 | T5Ø.1X5 | T5Ø.1X6 |
| **Edetate, disodium** (calcium) | T45.8X1 | T45.8X2 | T45.8X3 | T45.8X4 | T45.8X5 | T45.8X6 |
| **Edoxudine** | T49.5X1 | T49.5X2 | T49.5X3 | T49.5X4 | T49.5X5 | T49.5X6 |
| **Edrophonium** | T44.ØX1 | T44.ØX2 | T44.ØX3 | T44.ØX4 | T44.ØX5 | T44.ØX6 |
| chloride | T44.ØX1 | T44.ØX2 | T44.ØX3 | T44.ØX4 | T44.ØX5 | T44.ØX6 |
| **EDTA** | T5Ø.6X1 | T5Ø.6X2 | T5Ø.6X3 | T5Ø.6X4 | T5Ø.6X5 | T5Ø.6X6 |
| **Effexor*** | T43.221 | T43.222 | T43.223 | T43.224 | T43.225 | T43.226 |
| **Eflornithine** | T37.2X1 | T37.2X2 | T37.2X3 | T37.2X4 | T37.2X5 | T37.2X6 |
| **Efloxate** | T46.3X1 | T46.3X2 | T46.3X3 | T46.3X4 | T46.3X5 | T46.3X6 |
| **Elase** | T49.8X1 | T49.8X2 | T49.8X3 | T49.8X4 | T49.8X5 | T49.8X6 |
| **Elastase** | T47.5X1 | T47.5X2 | T47.5X3 | T47.5X4 | T47.5X5 | T47.5X6 |
| **Elaterium** | T47.2X1 | T47.2X2 | T47.2X3 | T47.2X4 | T47.2X5 | T47.2X6 |
| **Elcatonin** | T5Ø.991 | T5Ø.992 | T5Ø.993 | T5Ø.994 | T5Ø.995 | T5Ø.996 |
| **Elder** | T62.2X1 | T62.2X2 | T62.2X3 | T62.2X4 | — | — |
| berry, (unripe) | T62.1X1 | T62.1X2 | T62.1X3 | T62.1X4 | — | — |
| **Electrolyte balance drug** | T5Ø.3X1 | T5Ø.3X2 | T5Ø.3X3 | T5Ø.3X4 | T5Ø.3X5 | T5Ø.3X6 |

| Substance | Poisoning, Accidental (unintentional) | Poisoning, Intentional Self-harm | Poisoning, Assault | Poisoning, Undetermined | Adverse Effect | Under-dosing |
|---|---|---|---|---|---|---|
| **Electrolytes NEC** | T50.3X1 | T50.3X2 | T50.3X3 | T50.3X4 | T50.3X5 | T50.3X6 |
| **Electrolytic agent NEC** | T50.3X1 | T50.3X2 | T50.3X3 | T50.3X4 | T50.3X5 | T50.3X6 |
| **Elemental diet** | T50.901 | T50.902 | T50.903 | T50.904 | T50.905 | T50.906 |
| **Elliptinium acetate** | T45.1X1 | T45.1X2 | T45.1X3 | T45.1X4 | T45.1X5 | T45.1X6 |
| **Elocon*** | T49.ØX1 | T49.ØX2 | T49.ØX3 | T49.ØX4 | T49.ØX5 | T49.ØX6 |
| **Embramine** | T45.ØX1 | T45.ØX2 | T45.ØX3 | T45.ØX4 | T45.ØX5 | T45.ØX6 |
| **Emepronium** (salts) | T44.3X1 | T44.3X2 | T44.3X3 | T44.3X4 | T44.3X5 | T44.3X6 |
| bromide | T44.3X1 | T44.3X2 | T44.3X3 | T44.3X4 | T44.3X5 | T44.3X6 |
| **Emetic NEC** | T47.7X1 | T47.7X2 | T47.7X3 | T47.7X4 | T47.7X5 | T47.7X6 |
| **Emetine** | T37.3X1 | T37.3X2 | T37.3X3 | T37.3X4 | T37.3X5 | T37.3X6 |
| **Emollient NEC** | T49.3X1 | T49.3X2 | T49.3X3 | T49.3X4 | T49.3X5 | T49.3X6 |
| **Emorfazone** | T39.8X1 | T39.8X2 | T39.8X3 | T39.8X4 | T39.8X5 | T39.8X6 |
| **Emylcamate** | T43.591 | T43.592 | T43.593 | T43.594 | T43.595 | T43.596 |
| **Enalapril** | T46.4X1 | T46.4X2 | T46.4X3 | T46.4X4 | T46.4X5 | T46.4X6 |
| **Enalaprilat** | T46.4X1 | T46.4X2 | T46.4X3 | T46.4X4 | T46.4X5 | T46.4X6 |
| **Enbrel*** | T39.4X1 | T39.4X2 | T39.4X3 | T39.4X4 | T39.4X5 | T39.4X6 |
| **Encainide** | T46.2X1 | T46.2X2 | T46.2X3 | T46.2X4 | T46.2X5 | T46.2X6 |
| **Endocaine** | T41.3X1 | T41.3X2 | T41.3X3 | T41.3X4 | T41.3X5 | T41.3X6 |
| **Endosulfan** | T6Ø.2X1 | T6Ø.2X2 | T6Ø.2X3 | T6Ø.2X4 | — | — |
| **Endothall** | T6Ø.3X1 | T6Ø.3X2 | T6Ø.3X3 | T6Ø.3X4 | — | — |
| **Endralazine** | T46.5X1 | T46.5X2 | T46.5X3 | T46.5X4 | T46.5X5 | T46.5X6 |
| **Endrin** | T6Ø.1X1 | T6Ø.1X2 | T6Ø.1X3 | T6Ø.1X4 | — | — |
| **Enflurane** | T41.ØX1 | T41.ØX2 | T41.ØX3 | T41.ØX4 | T41.ØX5 | T41.ØX6 |
| **Enfuvirtide*** | T37.5X1 | T37.5X2 | T37.5X3 | T37.5X4 | T37.5X5 | T37.5X6 |
| **Enhexymal** | T42.3X1 | T42.3X2 | T42.3X3 | T42.3X4 | T42.3X5 | T42.3X6 |
| **Enocitabine** | T45.1X1 | T45.1X2 | T45.1X3 | T45.1X4 | T45.1X5 | T45.1X6 |
| **Enovid** | T38.4X1 | T38.4X2 | T38.4X3 | T38.4X4 | T38.4X5 | T38.4X6 |
| **Enoxacin** | T36.8X1 | T36.8X2 | T36.8X3 | T36.8X4 | T36.8X5 | T36.8X6 |
| **Enoxaparin** (sodium) | T45.511 | T45.512 | T45.513 | T45.514 | T45.515 | T45.516 |
| **Enpiprazole** | T43.591 | T43.592 | T43.593 | T43.594 | T43.595 | T43.596 |
| **Enprofylline** | T48.6X1 | T48.6X2 | T48.6X3 | T48.6X4 | T48.6X5 | T48.6X6 |
| **Enprostil** | T47.1X1 | T47.1X2 | T47.1X3 | T47.1X4 | T47.1X5 | T47.1X6 |
| **ENT preparations** (anti-infectives) | T49.6X1 | T49.6X2 | T49.6X3 | T49.6X4 | T49.6X5 | T49.6X6 |
| **Enterogastrone** | T38.891 | T38.892 | T38.893 | T38.894 | T38.895 | T38.896 |
| **Enviomycin** | T36.8X1 | T36.8X2 | T36.8X3 | T36.8X4 | T36.8X5 | T36.8X6 |
| **Enzodase** | T45.3X1 | T45.3X2 | T45.3X3 | T45.3X4 | T45.3X5 | T45.3X6 |
| **Enzyme NEC** | T45.3X1 | T45.3X2 | T45.3X3 | T45.3X4 | T45.3X5 | T45.3X6 |
| depolymerizing | T49.8X1 | T49.8X2 | T49.8X3 | T49.8X4 | T49.8X5 | T49.8X6 |
| fibrolytic | T45.3X1 | T45.3X2 | T45.3X3 | T45.3X4 | T45.3X5 | T45.3X6 |
| gastric | T47.5X1 | T47.5X2 | T47.5X3 | T47.5X4 | T47.5X5 | T47.5X6 |
| intestinal | T47.5X1 | T47.5X2 | T47.5X3 | T47.5X4 | T47.5X5 | T47.5X6 |
| local action | T49.4X1 | T49.4X2 | T49.4X3 | T49.4X4 | T49.4X5 | T49.4X6 |
| proteolytic | T49.4X1 | T49.4X2 | T49.4X3 | T49.4X4 | T49.4X5 | T49.4X6 |
| thrombolytic | T45.3X1 | T45.3X2 | T45.3X3 | T45.3X4 | T45.3X5 | T45.3X6 |
| **EPAB** | T41.3X1 | T41.3X2 | T41.3X3 | T41.3X4 | T41.3X5 | T41.3X6 |
| **Epanutin** | T42.ØX1 | T42.ØX2 | T42.ØX3 | T42.ØX4 | T42.ØX5 | T42.ØX6 |
| **Ephedra** | T44.991 | T44.992 | T44.993 | T44.994 | T44.995 | T44.996 |
| **Ephedrine** | T44.991 | T44.992 | T44.993 | T44.994 | T44.995 | T44.996 |
| **Epichlorhydrin, epichlorohydrin** | T52.891 | T52.892 | T52.893 | T52.894 | — | — |
| **Epicillin** | T36.ØX1 | T36.ØX2 | T36.ØX3 | T36.ØX4 | T36.ØX5 | T36.ØX6 |
| **Epiestriol** | T38.5X1 | T38.5X2 | T38.5X3 | T38.5X4 | T38.5X5 | T38.5X6 |
| **Epilim** — *see* Sodium, valproate | | | | | | |
| **Epimestrol** | T38.5X1 | T38.5X2 | T38.5X3 | T38.5X4 | T38.5X5 | T38.5X6 |
| **Epinephrine** | T44.5X1 | T44.5X2 | T44.5X3 | T44.5X4 | T44.5X5 | T44.5X6 |
| **EpiPen*** | T44.5X1 | T44.5X2 | T44.5X3 | T44.5X4 | T44.5X5 | T44.5X6 |
| **Epirubicin** | T45.1X1 | T45.1X2 | T45.1X3 | T45.1X4 | T45.1X5 | T45.1X6 |
| **Epitiostanol** | T38.7X1 | T38.7X2 | T38.7X3 | T38.7X4 | T38.7X5 | T38.7X6 |
| **Epitizide** | T5Ø.2X1 | T5Ø.2X2 | T5Ø.2X3 | T5Ø.2X4 | T5Ø.2X5 | T5Ø.2X6 |
| **EPN** | T6Ø.ØX1 | T6Ø.ØX2 | T6Ø.ØX3 | T6Ø.ØX4 | — | — |
| **EPO** | T45.8X1 | T45.8X2 | T45.8X3 | T45.8X4 | T45.8X5 | T45.8X6 |
| **Epoetin alpha** | T45.8X1 | T45.8X2 | T45.8X3 | T45.8X4 | T45.8X5 | T45.8X6 |
| **Epomediol** | T5Ø.991 | T5Ø.992 | T5Ø.993 | T5Ø.994 | T5Ø.995 | T5Ø.996 |
| **Epoprostenol** | T45.521 | T45.522 | T45.523 | T45.524 | T45.525 | T45.526 |
| **Epoxy resin** | T65.891 | T65.892 | T65.893 | T65.894 | — | — |
| **Eprazinone** | T48.4X1 | T48.4X2 | T48.4X3 | T48.4X4 | T48.4X5 | T48.4X6 |
| **Epsilon aminocaproic acid** | T45.621 | T45.622 | T45.623 | T45.624 | T45.625 | T45.626 |
| **Epsom salt** | T47.3X1 | T47.3X2 | T47.3X3 | T47.3X4 | T47.3X5 | T47.3X6 |
| **Eptazocine** | T4Ø.491 | T4Ø.492 | T4Ø.493 | T4Ø.494 | T4Ø.495 | T4Ø.496 |
| **Equanil** | T43.591 | T43.592 | T43.593 | T43.594 | T43.595 | T43.596 |
| **Equisetum** | T62.2X1 | T62.2X2 | T62.2X3 | T62.2X4 | — | — |
| diuretic | T5Ø.2X1 | T5Ø.2X2 | T5Ø.2X3 | T5Ø.2X4 | T5Ø.2X5 | T5Ø.2X6 |
| **Ergobasine** | T48.ØX1 | T48.ØX2 | T48.ØX3 | T48.ØX4 | T48.ØX5 | T48.ØX6 |
| **Ergocalciferol** | T45.2X1 | T45.2X2 | T45.2X3 | T45.2X4 | T45.2X5 | T45.2X6 |
| **Ergoloid mesylates** | T46.7X1 | T46.7X2 | T46.7X3 | T46.7X4 | T46.7X5 | T46.7X6 |
| **Ergometrine** | T48.ØX1 | T48.ØX2 | T48.ØX3 | T48.ØX4 | T48.ØX5 | T48.ØX6 |
| **Ergonovine** | T48.ØX1 | T48.ØX2 | T48.ØX3 | T48.ØX4 | T48.ØX5 | T48.ØX6 |
| **Ergot NEC** | T64.81 | T64.82 | T64.83 | T64.84 | — | — |
| derivative | T48.ØX1 | T48.ØX2 | T48.ØX3 | T48.ØX4 | T48.ØX5 | T48.ØX6 |
| medicinal (alkaloids) | T48.ØX1 | T48.ØX2 | T48.ØX3 | T48.ØX4 | T48.ØX5 | T48.ØX6 |
| prepared | T48.ØX1 | T48.ØX2 | T48.ØX3 | T48.ØX4 | T48.ØX5 | T48.ØX6 |
| **Ergotamine** | T46.5X1 | T46.5X2 | T46.5X3 | T46.5X4 | T46.5X5 | T46.5X6 |

| Substance | Poisoning, Accidental (unintentional) | Poisoning, Intentional Self-harm | Poisoning, Assault | Poisoning, Undetermined | Adverse Effect | Under-dosing |
|---|---|---|---|---|---|---|
| **Ergotocine** | T48.ØX1 | T48.ØX2 | T48.ØX3 | T48.ØX4 | T48.ØX5 | T48.ØX6 |
| **Ergotrate** | T48.ØX1 | T48.ØX2 | T48.ØX3 | T48.ØX4 | T48.ØX5 | T48.ØX6 |
| **Eritrityl tetranitrate** | T46.3X1 | T46.3X2 | T46.3X3 | T46.3X4 | T46.3X5 | T46.3X6 |
| **Erythrityl tetranitrate** | T46.3X1 | T46.3X2 | T46.3X3 | T46.3X4 | T46.3X5 | T46.3X6 |
| **Erythrol tetranitrate** | T46.3X1 | T46.3X2 | T46.3X3 | T46.3X4 | T46.3X5 | T46.3X6 |
| **Erythromycin** (salts) | T36.3X1 | T36.3X2 | T36.3X3 | T36.3X4 | T36.3X5 | T36.3X6 |
| ophthalmic preparation | T49.5X1 | T49.5X2 | T49.5X3 | T49.5X4 | T49.5X5 | T49.5X6 |
| topical NEC | T49.ØX1 | T49.ØX2 | T49.ØX3 | T49.ØX4 | T49.ØX5 | T49.ØX6 |
| **Erythropoietin** | T45.8X1 | T45.8X2 | T45.8X3 | T45.8X4 | T45.8X5 | T45.8X6 |
| human | T45.8X1 | T45.8X2 | T45.8X3 | T45.8X4 | T45.8X5 | T45.8X6 |
| **Esbriet*** | T48.991 | T48.992 | T48.993 | T48.994 | T48.995 | T48.996 |
| **Escin** | T46.991 | T46.992 | T46.993 | T46.994 | T46.995 | T46.996 |
| **Escitalopram*** | T43.221 | T43.222 | T43.223 | T43.224 | T43.225 | T43.226 |
| **Esculin** | T45.2X1 | T45.2X2 | T45.2X3 | T45.2X4 | T45.2X5 | T45.2X6 |
| **Esculoside** | T45.2X1 | T45.2X2 | T45.2X3 | T45.2X4 | T45.2X5 | T45.2X6 |
| **ESDT** (ether-soluble tar distillate) | T49.1X1 | T49.1X2 | T49.1X3 | T49.1X4 | T49.1X5 | T49.1X6 |
| **Eserine** | T49.5X1 | T49.5X2 | T49.5X3 | T49.5X4 | T49.5X5 | T49.5X6 |
| **Esflurbiprofen** | T39.311 | T39.312 | T39.313 | T39.314 | T39.315 | T39.316 |
| **Eskabarb** | T42.3X1 | T42.3X2 | T42.3X3 | T42.3X4 | T42.3X5 | T42.3X6 |
| **Eskalith** | T43.8X1 | T43.8X2 | T43.8X3 | T43.8X4 | T43.8X5 | T43.8X6 |
| **Esmolol** | T44.7X1 | T44.7X2 | T44.7X3 | T44.7X4 | T44.7X5 | T44.7X6 |
| **Estanozolol** | T38.7X1 | T38.7X2 | T38.7X3 | T38.7X4 | T38.7X5 | T38.7X6 |
| **Estazolam** | T42.4X1 | T42.4X2 | T42.4X3 | T42.4X4 | T42.4X5 | T42.4X6 |
| **Estradiol** | T38.5X1 | T38.5X2 | T38.5X3 | T38.5X4 | T38.5X5 | T38.5X6 |
| benzoate | T38.5X1 | T38.5X2 | T38.5X3 | T38.5X4 | T38.5X5 | T38.5X6 |
| with testosterone | T38.7X1 | T38.7X2 | T38.7X3 | T38.7X4 | T38.7X5 | T38.7X6 |
| **Estramustine** | T45.1X1 | T45.1X2 | T45.1X3 | T45.1X4 | T45.1X5 | T45.1X6 |
| **Estriol** | T38.5X1 | T38.5X2 | T38.5X3 | T38.5X4 | T38.5X5 | T38.5X6 |
| **Estrogen** | T38.5X1 | T38.5X2 | T38.5X3 | T38.5X4 | T38.5X5 | T38.5X6 |
| conjugated | T38.5X1 | T38.5X2 | T38.5X3 | T38.5X4 | T38.5X5 | T38.5X6 |
| with progesterone | T38.5X1 | T38.5X2 | T38.5X3 | T38.5X4 | T38.5X5 | T38.5X6 |
| **Estrone** | T38.5X1 | T38.5X2 | T38.5X3 | T38.5X4 | T38.5X5 | T38.5X6 |
| **Estropipate** | T38.5X1 | T38.5X2 | T38.5X3 | T38.5X4 | T38.5X5 | T38.5X6 |
| **Etacrynate sodium** | T5Ø.1X1 | T5Ø.1X2 | T5Ø.1X3 | T5Ø.1X4 | T5Ø.1X5 | T5Ø.1X6 |
| **Etacrynic acid** | T5Ø.1X1 | T5Ø.1X2 | T5Ø.1X3 | T5Ø.1X4 | T5Ø.1X5 | T5Ø.1X6 |
| **Etafedrine** | T48.6X1 | T48.6X2 | T48.6X3 | T48.6X4 | T48.6X5 | T48.6X6 |
| **Etafenone** | T46.3X1 | T46.3X2 | T46.3X3 | T46.3X4 | T46.3X5 | T46.3X6 |
| **Etambutol** | T37.1X1 | T37.1X2 | T37.1X3 | T37.1X4 | T37.1X5 | T37.1X6 |
| **Etamiphyllin** | T48.6X1 | T48.6X2 | T48.6X3 | T48.6X4 | T48.6X5 | T48.6X6 |
| **Etamivan** | T5Ø.7X1 | T5Ø.7X2 | T5Ø.7X3 | T5Ø.7X4 | T5Ø.7X5 | T5Ø.7X6 |
| **Etamsylate** | T45.7X1 | T45.7X2 | T45.7X3 | T45.7X4 | T45.7X5 | T45.7X6 |
| **Etebenecid** | T5Ø.4X1 | T5Ø.4X2 | T5Ø.4X3 | T5Ø.4X4 | T5Ø.4X5 | T5Ø.4X6 |
| **Ethacridine** | T49.ØX1 | T49.ØX2 | T49.ØX3 | T49.ØX4 | T49.ØX5 | T49.ØX6 |
| **Ethacrynate*** | T5Ø.1X1 | T5Ø.1X2 | T5Ø.1X3 | T5Ø.1X4 | T5Ø.1X5 | T5Ø.1X6 |
| **Ethacrynic acid** | T5Ø.1X1 | T5Ø.1X2 | T5Ø.1X3 | T5Ø.1X4 | T5Ø.1X5 | T5Ø.1X6 |
| **Ethadione** | T42.2X1 | T42.2X2 | T42.2X3 | T42.2X4 | T42.2X5 | T42.2X6 |
| **Ethambutol** | T37.1X1 | T37.1X2 | T37.1X3 | T37.1X4 | T37.1X5 | T37.1X6 |
| **Ethamide** | T5Ø.2X1 | T5Ø.2X2 | T5Ø.2X3 | T5Ø.2X4 | T5Ø.2X5 | T5Ø.2X6 |
| **Ethamivan** | T5Ø.7X1 | T5Ø.7X2 | T5Ø.7X3 | T5Ø.7X4 | T5Ø.7X5 | T5Ø.7X6 |
| **Ethamsylate** | T45.7X1 | T45.7X2 | T45.7X3 | T45.7X4 | T45.7X5 | T45.7X6 |
| **Ethanol** | T51.ØX1 | T51.ØX2 | T51.ØX3 | T51.ØX4 | — | — |
| beverage | T51.ØX1 | T51.ØX2 | T51.ØX3 | T51.ØX4 | — | — |
| **Ethanolamine oleate** | T46.8X1 | T46.8X2 | T46.8X3 | T46.8X4 | T46.8X5 | T46.8X6 |
| **Ethaverine** | T44.3X1 | T44.3X2 | T44.3X3 | T44.3X4 | T44.3X5 | T44.3X6 |
| **Ethchlorvynol** | T42.6X1 | T42.6X2 | T42.6X3 | T42.6X4 | T42.6X5 | T42.6X6 |
| **Ethebenecid** | T5Ø.4X1 | T5Ø.4X2 | T5Ø.4X3 | T5Ø.4X4 | T5Ø.4X5 | T5Ø.4X6 |
| **Ether** (vapor) | T41.ØX1 | T41.ØX2 | T41.ØX3 | T41.ØX4 | T41.ØX5 | T41.ØX6 |
| anesthetic | T41.ØX1 | T41.ØX2 | T41.ØX3 | T41.ØX4 | T41.ØX5 | T41.ØX6 |
| divinyl | T41.ØX1 | T41.ØX2 | T41.ØX3 | T41.ØX4 | T41.ØX5 | T41.ØX6 |
| ethyl (medicinal) | T41.ØX1 | T41.ØX2 | T41.ØX3 | T41.ØX4 | T41.ØX5 | T41.ØX6 |
| nonmedicinal | T52.891 | T52.892 | T52.893 | T52.894 | — | — |
| petroleum — *see* Ligroin | | | | | | |
| solvent | T52.891 | T52.892 | T52.893 | T52.894 | — | — |
| **Ethiazide** | T5Ø.2X1 | T5Ø.2X2 | T5Ø.2X3 | T5Ø.2X4 | T5Ø.2X5 | T5Ø.2X6 |
| **Ethidium chloride** (vapor) | T59.891 | T59.892 | T59.893 | T59.894 | — | — |
| **Ethinamate** | T42.6X1 | T42.6X2 | T42.6X3 | T42.6X4 | T42.6X5 | T42.6X6 |
| **Ethinylestradiol, ethinyloestradiol** | T38.5X1 | T38.5X2 | T38.5X3 | T38.5X4 | T38.5X5 | T38.5X6 |
| with | | | | | | |
| levonorgestrel | T38.4X1 | T38.4X2 | T38.4X3 | T38.4X4 | T38.4X5 | T38.4X6 |
| norethisterone | T38.4X1 | T38.4X2 | T38.4X3 | T38.4X4 | T38.4X5 | T38.4X6 |
| **Ethiodized oil** (131 I) | T5Ø.8X1 | T5Ø.8X2 | T5Ø.8X3 | T5Ø.8X4 | T5Ø.8X5 | T5Ø.8X6 |
| **Ethiofos*** | T5Ø.991 | T5Ø.992 | T5Ø.993 | T5Ø.994 | T5Ø.995 | T5Ø.996 |
| **Ethion** | T6Ø.ØX1 | T6Ø.ØX2 | T6Ø.ØX3 | T6Ø.ØX4 | — | — |
| **Ethionamide** | T37.1X1 | T37.1X2 | T37.1X3 | T37.1X4 | T37.1X5 | T37.1X6 |
| **Ethioniamide** | T37.1X1 | T37.1X2 | T37.1X3 | T37.1X4 | T37.1X5 | T37.1X6 |
| **Ethisterone** | T38.5X1 | T38.5X2 | T38.5X3 | T38.5X4 | T38.5X5 | T38.5X6 |
| **Ethobral** | T42.3X1 | T42.3X2 | T42.3X3 | T42.3X4 | T42.3X5 | T42.3X6 |
| **Ethocaine** (infiltration) (topical) | T41.3X1 | T41.3X2 | T41.3X3 | T41.3X4 | T41.3X5 | T41.3X6 |
| nerve block (peripheral) (plexus) | T41.3X1 | T41.3X2 | T41.3X3 | T41.3X4 | T41.3X5 | T41.3X6 |

| Substance | Poisoning, Accidental (unintentional) | Poisoning, Intentional Self-harm | Poisoning, Assault | Poisoning, Undetermined | Adverse Effect | Under-dosing |
|---|---|---|---|---|---|---|
| **Ethocaine** — *continued* | | | | | | |
| spinal | T41.3X1 | T41.3X2 | T41.3X3 | T41.3X4 | T41.3X5 | T41.3X6 |
| **Ethoheptazine** | T4Ø.491 | T4Ø.492 | T4Ø.493 | T4Ø.494 | T4Ø.495 | T4Ø.496 |
| **Ethopropazine** | T44.3X1 | T44.3X2 | T44.3X3 | T44.3X4 | T44.3X5 | T44.3X6 |
| **Ethosuximide** | T42.2X1 | T42.2X2 | T42.2X3 | T42.2X4 | T42.2X5 | T42.2X6 |
| **Ethotoin** | T42.ØX1 | T42.ØX2 | T42.ØX3 | T42.ØX4 | T42.ØX5 | T42.ØX6 |
| **Ethoxazene** | T37.91 | T37.92 | T37.93 | T37.94 | T37.95 | T37.96 |
| **Ethoxazorutoside** | T46.991 | T46.992 | T46.993 | T46.994 | T46.995 | T46.996 |
| **Ethoxzolamide** | T5Ø.2X1 | T5Ø.2X2 | T5Ø.2X3 | T5Ø.2X4 | T5Ø.2X5 | T5Ø.2X6 |
| **Ethyl** | | | | | | |
| acetate | T52.891 | T52.892 | T52.893 | T52.894 | — | — |
| alcohol | T51.ØX1 | T51.ØX2 | T51.ØX3 | T51.ØX4 | — | — |
| beverage | T51.ØX1 | T51.ØX2 | T51.ØX3 | T51.ØX4 | — | — |
| aldehyde (vapor) | T59.891 | T59.892 | T59.893 | T59.894 | — | — |
| liquid | T52.891 | T52.892 | T52.893 | T52.894 | — | — |
| aminobenzoate | T41.3X1 | T41.3X2 | T41.3X3 | T41.3X4 | T41.3X5 | T41.3X6 |
| aminophenothiazine | T43.3X1 | T43.3X2 | T43.3X3 | T43.3X4 | T43.3X5 | T43.3X6 |
| benzoate | T52.891 | T52.892 | T52.893 | T52.894 | — | — |
| biscoumacetate | T45.511 | T45.512 | T45.513 | T45.514 | T45.515 | T45.516 |
| bromide (anesthetic) | T41.ØX1 | T41.ØX2 | T41.ØX3 | T41.ØX4 | T41.ØX5 | T41.ØX6 |
| carbamate | T45.1X1 | T45.1X2 | T45.1X3 | T45.1X4 | T45.1X5 | T45.1X6 |
| carbinol | T51.3X1 | T51.3X2 | T51.3X3 | T51.3X4 | — | — |
| carbonate | T52.891 | T52.892 | T52.893 | T52.894 | — | — |
| chaulmoograte | T37.1X1 | T37.1X2 | T37.1X3 | T37.1X4 | T37.1X5 | T37.1X6 |
| chloride (anesthetic) | T41.ØX1 | T41.ØX2 | T41.ØX3 | T41.ØX4 | T41.ØX5 | T41.ØX6 |
| anesthetic (local) | T41.3X1 | T41.3X2 | T41.3X3 | T41.3X4 | T41.3X5 | T41.3X6 |
| inhaled | T41.ØX1 | T41.ØX2 | T41.ØX3 | T41.ØX4 | T41.ØX5 | T41.ØX6 |
| local | T49.4X1 | T49.4X2 | T49.4X3 | T49.4X4 | T49.4X5 | T49.4X6 |
| solvent | T53.6X1 | T53.6X2 | T53.6X3 | T53.6X4 | — | — |
| dibunate | T48.3X1 | T48.3X2 | T48.3X3 | T48.3X4 | T48.3X5 | T48.3X6 |
| dichloroarsine (vapor) | T57.ØX1 | T57.ØX2 | T57.ØX3 | T57.ØX4 | — | — |
| estranol | T38.7X1 | T38.7X2 | T38.7X3 | T38.7X4 | T38.7X5 | T38.7X6 |
| ether — *see also* ether | T52.891 | T52.892 | T52.893 | T52.894 | — | — |
| formate NEC (solvent) | T52.ØX1 | T52.ØX2 | T52.ØX3 | T52.ØX4 | — | — |
| fumarate | T49.4X1 | T49.4X2 | T49.4X3 | T49.4X4 | T49.4X5 | T49.4X6 |
| hydroxyisobutyrate NEC (solvent) | T52.891 | T52.892 | T52.893 | T52.894 | — | — |
| iodoacetate | T59.3X1 | T59.3X2 | T59.3X3 | T59.3X4 | — | — |
| lactate NEC (solvent) | T52.891 | T52.892 | T52.893 | T52.894 | — | — |
| loflazepate | T42.4X1 | T42.4X2 | T42.4X3 | T42.4X4 | T42.4X5 | T42.4X6 |
| mercuric chloride | T56.1X1 | T56.1X2 | T56.1X3 | T56.1X4 | — | — |
| methylcarbinol | T51.8X1 | T51.8X2 | T51.8X3 | T51.8X4 | — | — |
| morphine | T4Ø.2X1 | T4Ø.2X2 | T4Ø.2X3 | T4Ø.2X4 | T4Ø.2X5 | T4Ø.2X6 |
| noradrenaline | T48.6X1 | T48.6X2 | T48.6X3 | T48.6X4 | T48.6X5 | T48.6X6 |
| oxybutyrate NEC (solvent) | T52.891 | T52.892 | T52.893 | T52.894 | — | — |
| **Ethylene** (gas) | T59.891 | T59.892 | T59.893 | T59.894 | — | — |
| anesthetic (general) | T41.ØX1 | T41.ØX2 | T41.ØX3 | T41.ØX4 | T41.ØX5 | T41.ØX6 |
| chlorohydrin | T52.891 | T52.892 | T52.893 | T52.894 | — | — |
| vapor | T53.6X1 | T53.6X2 | T53.6X3 | T53.6X4 | — | — |
| dichloride | T52.891 | T52.892 | T52.893 | T52.894 | — | — |
| vapor | T53.6X1 | T53.6X2 | T53.6X3 | T53.6X4 | — | — |
| dinitrate | T52.3X1 | T52.3X2 | T52.3X3 | T52.3X4 | — | — |
| glycol(s) | T52.891 | T52.892 | T52.893 | T52.894 | — | — |
| dinitrate | T52.3X1 | T52.3X2 | T52.3X3 | T52.3X4 | — | — |
| monobutyl ether | T52.3X1 | T52.3X2 | T52.3X3 | T52.3X4 | — | — |
| imine | T54.1X1 | T54.1X2 | T54.1X3 | T54.1X4 | — | — |
| oxide (fumigant) (nonmedicinal) | T59.891 | T59.892 | T59.893 | T59.894 | — | — |
| medicinal | T49.ØX1 | T49.ØX2 | T49.ØX3 | T49.ØX4 | T49.ØX5 | T49.ØX6 |
| **Ethylenediamine** | T48.6X1 | T48.6X2 | T48.6X3 | T48.6X4 | T48.6X5 | T48.6X6 |
| **theophylline** | | | | | | |
| **Ethylenediaminetetra-acetic acid** | T5Ø.6X1 | T5Ø.6X2 | T5Ø.6X3 | T5Ø.6X4 | T5Ø.6X5 | T5Ø.6X6 |
| **Ethylenedinitrilotetra-acetate** | T5Ø.6X1 | T5Ø.6X2 | T5Ø.6X3 | T5Ø.6X4 | T5Ø.6X5 | T5Ø.6X6 |
| **Ethylestrenol** | T38.7X1 | T38.7X2 | T38.7X3 | T38.7X4 | T38.7X5 | T38.7X6 |
| **Ethylhydroxycellulose** | T47.4X1 | T47.4X2 | T47.4X3 | T47.4X4 | T47.4X5 | T47.4X6 |
| **Ethylidene** | | | | | | |
| chloride NEC | T53.6X1 | T53.6X2 | T53.6X3 | T53.6X4 | — | — |
| diacetate | T6Ø.3X1 | T6Ø.3X2 | T6Ø.3X3 | T6Ø.3X4 | — | — |
| dicoumarin | T45.511 | T45.512 | T45.513 | T45.514 | T45.515 | T45.516 |
| dicoumarol | T45.511 | T45.512 | T45.513 | T45.514 | T45.515 | T45.516 |
| diethyl ether | T52.ØX1 | T52.ØX2 | T52.ØX3 | T52.ØX4 | — | — |
| **Ethylmorphine** | T4Ø.2X1 | T4Ø.2X2 | T4Ø.2X3 | T4Ø.2X4 | T4Ø.2X5 | T4Ø.2X6 |
| **Ethylnorepinephrine** | T48.6X1 | T48.6X2 | T48.6X3 | T48.6X4 | T48.6X5 | T48.6X6 |
| **Ethylparachlorophen-oxyisobutyrate** | T46.6X1 | T46.6X2 | T46.6X3 | T46.6X4 | T46.6X5 | T46.6X6 |
| **Ethynodiol** | T38.4X1 | T38.4X2 | T38.4X3 | T38.4X4 | T38.4X5 | T38.4X6 |
| with mestranol diacetate | T38.4X1 | T38.4X2 | T38.4X3 | T38.4X4 | T38.4X5 | T38.4X6 |
| **Ethyol*** | T5Ø.991 | T5Ø.992 | T5Ø.993 | T5Ø.994 | T5Ø.995 | T5Ø.996 |
| **Etidocaine** | T41.3X1 | T41.3X2 | T41.3X3 | T41.3X4 | T41.3X5 | T41.3X6 |
| infiltration (subcutaneous) | T41.3X1 | T41.3X2 | T41.3X3 | T41.3X4 | T41.3X5 | T41.3X6 |
| nerve (peripheral) (plexus) | T41.3X1 | T41.3X2 | T41.3X3 | T41.3X4 | T41.3X5 | T41.3X6 |
| **Etidronate** | T5Ø.991 | T5Ø.992 | T5Ø.993 | T5Ø.994 | T5Ø.995 | T5Ø.996 |

| Substance | Poisoning, Accidental (unintentional) | Poisoning, Intentional Self-harm | Poisoning, Assault | Poisoning, Undetermined | Adverse Effect | Under-dosing |
|---|---|---|---|---|---|---|
| **Etidronic acid** (disodium salt) | T5Ø.991 | T5Ø.992 | T5Ø.993 | T5Ø.994 | T5Ø.995 | T5Ø.996 |
| **Etifoxine** | T42.6X1 | T42.6X2 | T42.6X3 | T42.6X4 | T42.6X5 | T42.6X6 |
| **Etilefrine** | T44.4X1 | T44.4X2 | T44.4X3 | T44.4X4 | T44.4X5 | T44.4X6 |
| **Etilfen** | T42.3X1 | T42.3X2 | T42.3X3 | T42.3X4 | T42.3X5 | T42.3X6 |
| **Etinodiol** | T38.4X1 | T38.4X2 | T38.4X3 | T38.4X4 | T38.4X5 | T38.4X6 |
| **Etiroxate** | T46.6X1 | T46.6X2 | T46.6X3 | T46.6X4 | T46.6X5 | T46.6X6 |
| **Etizolam** | T42.4X1 | T42.4X2 | T42.4X3 | T42.4X4 | T42.4X5 | T42.4X6 |
| **Etodolac** | T39.391 | T39.392 | T39.393 | T39.394 | T39.395 | T39.396 |
| **Etofamide** | T37.3X1 | T37.3X2 | T37.3X3 | T37.3X4 | T37.3X5 | T37.3X6 |
| **Etofibrate** | T46.6X1 | T46.6X2 | T46.6X3 | T46.6X4 | T46.6X5 | T46.6X6 |
| **Etofylline** | T46.7X1 | T46.7X2 | T46.7X3 | T46.7X4 | T46.7X5 | T46.7X6 |
| clofibrate | T46.6X1 | T46.6X2 | T46.6X3 | T46.6X4 | T46.6X5 | T46.6X6 |
| **Etoglucid** | T45.1X1 | T45.1X2 | T45.1X3 | T45.1X4 | T45.1X5 | T45.1X6 |
| **Etomidate** | T41.1X1 | T41.1X2 | T41.1X3 | T41.1X4 | T41.1X5 | T41.1X6 |
| **Etomide** | T39.8X1 | T39.8X2 | T39.8X3 | T39.8X4 | T39.8X5 | T39.8X6 |
| **Etomidoline** | T44.3X1 | T44.3X2 | T44.3X3 | T44.3X4 | T44.3X5 | T44.3X6 |
| **Etoposide** | T45.1X1 | T45.1X2 | T45.1X3 | T45.1X4 | T45.1X5 | T45.1X6 |
| **Etorphine** | T4Ø.2X1 | T4Ø.2X2 | T4Ø.2X3 | T4Ø.2X4 | T4Ø.2X5 | T4Ø.2X6 |
| **Etoval** | T42.3X1 | T42.3X2 | T42.3X3 | T42.3X4 | T42.3X5 | T42.3X6 |
| **Etozolin** | T5Ø.1X1 | T5Ø.1X2 | T5Ø.1X3 | T5Ø.1X4 | T5Ø.1X5 | T5Ø.1X6 |
| **Etravirine*** | T37.5X1 | T37.5X2 | T37.5X3 | T37.5X4 | T37.5X5 | T37.5X6 |
| **Etretinate** | T5Ø.991 | T5Ø.992 | T5Ø.993 | T5Ø.994 | T5Ø.995 | T5Ø.996 |
| **Etryptamine** | T43.691 | T43.692 | T43.693 | T43.694 | T43.695 | T43.696 |
| **Etybenzatropine** | T44.3X1 | T44.3X2 | T44.3X3 | T44.3X4 | T44.3X5 | T44.3X6 |
| **Etynodiol** | T38.4X1 | T38.4X2 | T38.4X3 | T38.4X4 | T38.4X5 | T38.4X6 |
| **Eucaine** | T41.3X1 | T41.3X2 | T41.3X3 | T41.3X4 | T41.3X5 | T41.3X6 |
| **Eucalyptus oil** | T49.7X1 | T49.7X2 | T49.7X3 | T49.7X4 | T49.7X5 | T49.7X6 |
| **Eucatropine** | T49.5X1 | T49.5X2 | T49.5X3 | T49.5X4 | T49.5X5 | T49.5X6 |
| **Eucodal** | T4Ø.2X1 | T4Ø.2X2 | T4Ø.2X3 | T4Ø.2X4 | T4Ø.2X5 | T4Ø.2X6 |
| **Euneryl** | T42.3X1 | T42.3X2 | T42.3X3 | T42.3X4 | T42.3X5 | T42.3X6 |
| **Euphthalmine** | T44.3X1 | T44.3X2 | T44.3X3 | T44.3X4 | T44.3X5 | T44.3X6 |
| **Eurax** | T49.ØX1 | T49.ØX2 | T49.ØX3 | T49.ØX4 | T49.ØX5 | T49.ØX6 |
| **Euresol** | T49.4X1 | T49.4X2 | T49.4X3 | T49.4X4 | T49.4X5 | T49.4X6 |
| **Euthroid** | T38.1X1 | T38.1X2 | T38.1X3 | T38.1X4 | T38.1X5 | T38.1X6 |
| **Evans blue** | T5Ø.8X1 | T5Ø.8X2 | T5Ø.8X3 | T5Ø.8X4 | T5Ø.8X5 | T5Ø.8X6 |
| **Evipal** | T42.3X1 | T42.3X2 | T42.3X3 | T42.3X4 | T42.3X5 | T42.3X6 |
| sodium | T41.1X1 | T41.1X2 | T41.1X3 | T41.1X4 | T41.1X5 | T41.1X6 |
| **Evipan** | T42.3X1 | T42.3X2 | T42.3X3 | T42.3X4 | T42.3X5 | T42.3X6 |
| sodium | T41.1X1 | T41.1X2 | T41.1X3 | T41.1X4 | T41.1X5 | T41.1X6 |
| **Ex-Lax** (phenolphthalein) | T47.2X1 | T47.2X2 | T47.2X3 | T47.2X4 | T47.2X5 | T47.2X6 |
| **Exalamide** | T49.ØX1 | T49.ØX2 | T49.ØX3 | T49.ØX4 | T49.ØX5 | T49.ØX6 |
| **Exalgin** | T39.1X1 | T39.1X2 | T39.1X3 | T39.1X4 | T39.1X5 | T39.1X6 |
| **Excipients, pharmaceutical** | T5Ø.9Ø1 | T5Ø.9Ø2 | T5Ø.9Ø3 | T5Ø.9Ø4 | T5Ø.9Ø5 | T5Ø.9Ø6 |
| **Exhaust gas** (engine) (motor vehicle) | T58.Ø1 | T58.Ø2 | T58.Ø3 | T58.Ø4 | — | — |
| **Expectorant NEC** | T48.4X1 | T48.4X2 | T48.4X3 | T48.4X4 | T48.4X5 | T48.4X6 |
| **Extended insulin zinc suspension** | T38.3X1 | T38.3X2 | T38.3X3 | T38.3X4 | T38.3X5 | T38.3X6 |
| **External medications** (skin) (mucous membrane) | T49.91 | T49.92 | T49.93 | T49.94 | T49.95 | T49.96 |
| dental agent | T49.7X1 | T49.7X2 | T49.7X3 | T49.7X4 | T49.7X5 | T49.7X6 |
| ENT agent | T49.6X1 | T49.6X2 | T49.6X3 | T49.6X4 | T49.6X5 | T49.6X6 |
| ophthalmic preparation | T49.5X1 | T49.5X2 | T49.5X3 | T49.5X4 | T49.5X5 | T49.5X6 |
| specified NEC | T49.8X1 | T49.8X2 | T49.8X3 | T49.8X4 | T49.8X5 | T49.8X6 |
| **Extina*** | T49.ØX1 | T49.ØX2 | T49.ØX3 | T49.ØX4 | T49.ØX5 | T49.ØX6 |
| **Extrapyramidal antagonist NEC** | T44.3X1 | T44.3X2 | T44.3X3 | T44.3X4 | T44.3X5 | T44.3X6 |
| **Eye agents** (anti-infective) | T49.5X1 | T49.5X2 | T49.5X3 | T49.5X4 | T49.5X5 | T49.5X6 |
| **Eye drug NEC** | T49.5X1 | T49.5X2 | T49.5X3 | T49.5X4 | T49.5X5 | T49.5X6 |
| **FAC** (fluorouracil + doxorubicin + cyclophosphamide) | T45.1X1 | T45.1X2 | T45.1X3 | T45.1X4 | T45.1X5 | T45.1X6 |
| **Factor** | | | | | | |
| I (fibrinogen) | T45.8X1 | T45.8X2 | T45.8X3 | T45.8X4 | T45.8X5 | T45.8X6 |
| III (thromboplastin) | T45.8X1 | T45.8X2 | T45.8X3 | T45.8X4 | T45.8X5 | T45.8X6 |
| IX complex | T45.7X1 | T45.7X2 | T45.7X3 | T45.7X4 | T45.7X5 | T45.7X6 |
| human | T45.8X1 | T45.8X2 | T45.8X3 | T45.8X4 | T45.8X5 | T45.8X6 |
| VIII (antihemophilic Factor) (concentrate) | T45.8X1 | T45.8X2 | T45.8X3 | T45.8X4 | T45.8X5 | T45.8X6 |
| **Famotidine** | T47.ØX1 | T47.ØX2 | T47.ØX3 | T47.ØX4 | T47.ØX5 | T47.ØX6 |
| **Fat suspension, intravenous** | T5Ø.991 | T5Ø.992 | T5Ø.993 | T5Ø.994 | T5Ø.995 | T5Ø.996 |
| **Fazadinium bromide** | T48.1X1 | T48.1X2 | T48.1X3 | T48.1X4 | T48.1X5 | T48.1X6 |
| **Febarbamate** | T42.3X1 | T42.3X2 | T42.3X3 | T42.3X4 | T42.3X5 | T42.3X6 |
| **Fecal softener** | T47.4X1 | T47.4X2 | T47.4X3 | T47.4X4 | T47.4X5 | T47.4X6 |
| **Fedrilate** | T48.3X1 | T48.3X2 | T48.3X3 | T48.3X4 | T48.3X5 | T48.3X6 |
| **Felodipine** | T46.1X1 | T46.1X2 | T46.1X3 | T46.1X4 | T46.1X5 | T46.1X6 |
| **Felypressin** | T38.891 | T38.892 | T38.893 | T38.894 | T38.895 | T38.896 |
| **Femizol*** | T49.ØX1 | T49.ØX2 | T49.ØX3 | T49.ØX4 | T49.ØX5 | T49.ØX6 |
| **Femoxetine** | T43.221 | T43.222 | T43.223 | T43.224 | T43.225 | T43.226 |
| **Fenalcomine** | T46.3X1 | T46.3X2 | T46.3X3 | T46.3X4 | T46.3X5 | T46.3X6 |
| **Fenamisal** | T37.1X1 | T37.1X2 | T37.1X3 | T37.1X4 | T37.1X5 | T37.1X6 |

| Substance | Poisoning, Accidental (unintentional) | Poisoning, Intentional Self-harm | Poisoning, Assault | Poisoning, Undetermined | Adverse Effect | Under-dosing |
|---|---|---|---|---|---|---|
| **Fenazone** | T39.2X1 | T39.2X2 | T39.2X3 | T39.2X4 | T39.2X5 | T39.2X6 |
| **Fenbendazole** | T37.4X1 | T37.4X2 | T37.4X3 | T37.4X4 | T37.4X5 | T37.4X6 |
| **Fenbutrazate** | T5Ø.5X1 | T5Ø.5X2 | T5Ø.5X3 | T5Ø.5X4 | T5Ø.5X5 | T5Ø.5X6 |
| **Fencamfamine** | T43.691 | T43.692 | T43.693 | T43.694 | T43.695 | T43.696 |
| **Fendiline** | T46.1X1 | T46.1X2 | T46.1X3 | T46.1X4 | T46.1X5 | T46.1X6 |
| **Fenetylline** | T43.691 | T43.692 | T43.693 | T43.694 | T43.695 | T43.696 |
| **Fenflumizole** | T39.391 | T39.392 | T39.393 | T39.394 | T39.395 | T39.396 |
| **Fenfluramine** | T5Ø.5X1 | T5Ø.5X2 | T5Ø.5X3 | T5Ø.5X4 | T5Ø.5X5 | T5Ø.5X6 |
| **Fenobarbital** | T42.3X1 | T42.3X2 | T42.3X3 | T42.3X4 | T42.3X5 | T42.3X6 |
| **Fenofibrate** | T46.6X1 | T46.6X2 | T46.6X3 | T46.6X4 | T46.6X5 | T46.6X6 |
| **Fenoprofen** | T39.311 | T39.312 | T39.313 | T39.314 | T39.315 | T39.316 |
| **Fenoterol** | T48.6X1 | T48.6X2 | T48.6X3 | T48.6X4 | T48.6X5 | T48.6X6 |
| **Fenoverine** | T44.3X1 | T44.3X2 | T44.3X3 | T44.3X4 | T44.3X5 | T44.3X6 |
| **Fenoxazoline** | T48.5X1 | T48.5X2 | T48.5X3 | T48.5X4 | T48.5X5 | T48.5X6 |
| **Fenproporex** | T5Ø.5X1 | T5Ø.5X2 | T5Ø.5X3 | T5Ø.5X4 | T5Ø.5X5 | T5Ø.5X6 |
| **Fenquizone** | T5Ø.2X1 | T5Ø.2X2 | T5Ø.2X3 | T5Ø.2X4 | T5Ø.2X5 | T5Ø.2X6 |
| **Fentanyl (analogs)** | T4Ø.411 | T4Ø.412 | T4Ø.413 | T4Ø.414 | T4Ø.415 | T4Ø.416 |
| **Fentazin** | T43.3X1 | T43.3X2 | T43.3X3 | T43.3X4 | T43.3X5 | T43.3X6 |
| **Fenthion** | T6Ø.ØX1 | T6Ø.ØX2 | T6Ø.ØX3 | T6Ø.ØX4 | — | — |
| **Fenticlor** | T49.ØX1 | T49.ØX2 | T49.ØX3 | T49.ØX4 | T49.ØX5 | T49.ØX6 |
| **Fenylbutazone** | T39.2X1 | T39.2X2 | T39.2X3 | T39.2X4 | T39.2X5 | T39.2X6 |
| **Feprazone** | T39.2X1 | T39.2X2 | T39.2X3 | T39.2X4 | T39.2X5 | T39.2X6 |
| **Fer de lance** (bite) (venom) | T63.Ø61 | T63.Ø62 | T63.Ø63 | T63.Ø64 | — | — |
| **Ferrex*** | T45.4X1 | T45.4X2 | T45.4X3 | T45.4X4 | T45.4X5 | T45.4X6 |
| **Ferric** — *see also* Iron | | | | | | |
| chloride | T45.4X1 | T45.4X2 | T45.4X3 | T45.4X4 | T45.4X5 | T45.4X6 |
| citrate | T45.4X1 | T45.4X2 | T45.4X3 | T45.4X4 | T45.4X5 | T45.4X6 |
| hydroxide | | | | | | |
| colloidal | T45.4X1 | T45.4X2 | T45.4X3 | T45.4X4 | T45.4X5 | T45.4X6 |
| polymaltose | T45.4X1 | T45.4X2 | T45.4X3 | T45.4X4 | T45.4X5 | T45.4X6 |
| pyrophosphate | T45.4X1 | T45.4X2 | T45.4X3 | T45.4X4 | T45.4X5 | T45.4X6 |
| **Ferritin** | T45.4X1 | T45.4X2 | T45.4X3 | T45.4X4 | T45.4X5 | T45.4X6 |
| **Ferrocholinate** | T45.4X1 | T45.4X2 | T45.4X3 | T45.4X4 | T45.4X5 | T45.4X6 |
| **Ferrodextrane** | T45.4X1 | T45.4X2 | T45.4X3 | T45.4X4 | T45.4X5 | T45.4X6 |
| **Ferropolimaler** | T45.4X1 | T45.4X2 | T45.4X3 | T45.4X4 | T45.4X5 | T45.4X6 |
| **Ferrous** — *see also* Iron | | | | | | |
| phosphate | T45.4X1 | T45.4X2 | T45.4X3 | T45.4X4 | T45.4X5 | T45.4X6 |
| salt | T45.4X1 | T45.4X2 | T45.4X3 | T45.4X4 | T45.4X5 | T45.4X6 |
| with folic acid | T45.4X1 | T45.4X2 | T45.4X3 | T45.4X4 | T45.4X5 | T45.4X6 |
| **Ferrous fumerate, gluconate, lactate, salt NEC, sulfate** (medicinal) | T45.4X1 | T45.4X2 | T45.4X3 | T45.4X4 | T45.4X5 | T45.4X6 |
| **Ferrovanadium** (fumes) | T59.891 | T59.892 | T59.893 | T59.894 | — | — |
| **Ferrum** — *see* Iron | | | | | | |
| **Fertilizers NEC** | T65.891 | T65.892 | T65.893 | T65.894 | — | — |
| with herbicide mixture | T6Ø.3X1 | T6Ø.3X2 | T6Ø.3X3 | T6Ø.3X4 | — | — |
| **Fetoxilate** | T47.6X1 | T47.6X2 | T47.6X3 | T47.6X4 | T47.6X5 | T47.6X6 |
| **Fiber, dietary** | T47.4X1 | T47.4X2 | T47.4X3 | T47.4X4 | T47.4X5 | T47.4X6 |
| **Fiberglass** | T65.831 | T65.832 | T65.833 | T65.834 | — | — |
| **Fibrinogen** (human) | T45.8X1 | T45.8X2 | T45.8X3 | T45.8X4 | T45.8X5 | T45.8X6 |
| **Fibrinolysin** (human) | T45.691 | T45.692 | T45.693 | T45.694 | T45.695 | T45.696 |
| **Fibrinolysis** | | | | | | |
| affecting drug | T45.6Ø1 | T45.6Ø2 | T45.6Ø3 | T45.6Ø4 | T45.6Ø5 | T45.6Ø6 |
| inhibitor NEC | T45.621 | T45.622 | T45.623 | T45.624 | T45.625 | T45.626 |
| **Fibrinolytic drug** | T45.611 | T45.612 | T45.613 | T45.614 | T45.615 | T45.616 |
| **Filix mas** | T37.4X1 | T37.4X2 | T37.4X3 | T37.4X4 | T37.4X5 | T37.4X6 |
| **Filtering cream** | T49.3X1 | T49.3X2 | T49.3X3 | T49.3X4 | T49.3X5 | T49.3X6 |
| **Finacea*** | T49.ØX1 | T49.ØX2 | T49.ØX3 | T49.ØX4 | T49.ØX5 | T49.ØX6 |
| **Fiorinal** | T39.Ø11 | T39.Ø12 | T39.Ø13 | T39.Ø14 | T39.Ø15 | T39.Ø16 |
| **Firedamp** | T59.891 | T59.892 | T59.893 | T59.894 | — | — |
| **Fish, noxious, nonbacterial** | T61.91 | T61.92 | T61.93 | T61.94 | — | — |
| ciguatera | T61.Ø1 | T61.Ø2 | T61.Ø3 | T61.Ø4 | — | — |
| scombroid | T61.11 | T61.12 | T61.13 | T61.14 | — | — |
| shell | T61.781 | T61.782 | T61.783 | T61.784 | — | — |
| specified NEC | T61.771 | T61.772 | T61.773 | T61.774 | — | — |
| **Flagyl** | T37.3X1 | T37.3X2 | T37.3X3 | T37.3X4 | T37.3X5 | T37.3X6 |
| **Flavine adenine dinucleotide** | T45.2X1 | T45.2X2 | T45.2X3 | T45.2X4 | T45.2X5 | T45.2X6 |
| **Flavodic acid** | T46.991 | T46.992 | T46.993 | T46.994 | T46.995 | T46.996 |
| **Flavoxate** | T44.3X1 | T44.3X2 | T44.3X3 | T44.3X4 | T44.3X5 | T44.3X6 |
| **Flaxedil** | T48.1X1 | T48.1X2 | T48.1X3 | T48.1X4 | T48.1X5 | T48.1X6 |
| **Flaxseed** (medicinal) | T49.3X1 | T49.3X2 | T49.3X3 | T49.3X4 | T49.3X5 | T49.3X6 |
| **Flecainide** | T46.2X1 | T46.2X2 | T46.2X3 | T46.2X4 | T46.2X5 | T46.2X6 |
| **Fleroxacin** | T36.8X1 | T36.8X2 | T36.8X3 | T36.8X4 | T36.8X5 | T36.8X6 |
| **Floctafenine** | T39.8X1 | T39.8X2 | T39.8X3 | T39.8X4 | T39.8X5 | T39.8X6 |
| **Flomax** | T44.6X1 | T44.6X2 | T44.6X3 | T44.6X4 | T44.6X5 | T44.6X6 |
| **Flomoxef** | T36.1X1 | T36.1X2 | T36.1X3 | T36.1X4 | T36.1X5 | T36.1X6 |
| **Flonase*** | T49.6X1 | T49.6X2 | T49.6X3 | T49.6X4 | T49.6X5 | T49.6X6 |
| **Flopropione** | T44.3X1 | T44.3X2 | T44.3X3 | T44.3X4 | T44.3X5 | T44.3X6 |
| **FLORAjen*** | T47.6X1 | T47.6X2 | T47.6X3 | T47.6X4 | T47.6X5 | T47.6X6 |
| **Florantyrone** | T47.5X1 | T47.5X2 | T47.5X3 | T47.5X4 | T47.5X5 | T47.5X6 |
| **Floraquin** | T37.8X1 | T37.8X2 | T37.8X3 | T37.8X4 | T37.8X5 | T37.8X6 |

| Substance | Poisoning, Accidental (unintentional) | Poisoning, Intentional Self-harm | Poisoning, Assault | Poisoning, Undetermined | Adverse Effect | Under-dosing |
|---|---|---|---|---|---|---|
| **Florinef** | T38.ØX1 | T38.ØX2 | T38.ØX3 | T38.ØX4 | T38.ØX5 | T38.ØX |
| ENT agent | T49.6X1 | T49.6X2 | T49.6X3 | T49.6X4 | T49.6X5 | T49.6X |
| ophthalmic preparation | T49.5X1 | T49.5X2 | T49.5X3 | T49.5X4 | T49.5X5 | T49.5X |
| topical NEC | T49.ØX1 | T49.ØX2 | T49.ØX3 | T49.ØX4 | T49.ØX5 | T49.ØX |
| **Flovent*** | T38.ØX1 | T38.ØX2 | T38.ØX3 | T38.ØX4 | T38.ØX5 | T38.ØX |
| **Flowers of sulfur** | T49.4X1 | T49.4X2 | T49.4X3 | T49.4X4 | T49.4X5 | T49.4X |
| **Floxuridine** | T45.1X1 | T45.1X2 | T45.1X3 | T45.1X4 | T45.1X5 | T45.1X |
| **Fluanisone** | T43.4X1 | T43.4X2 | T43.4X3 | T43.4X4 | T43.4X5 | T43.4X |
| **Flubendazole** | T37.4X1 | T37.4X2 | T37.4X3 | T37.4X4 | T37.4X5 | T37.4X |
| **Fluclorolone acetonide** | T49.ØX1 | T49.ØX2 | T49.ØX3 | T49.ØX4 | T49.ØX5 | T49.ØX |
| **Flucloxacillin** | T36.ØX1 | T36.ØX2 | T36.ØX3 | T36.ØX4 | T36.ØX5 | T36.ØX |
| **Fluconazole** | T37.8X1 | T37.8X2 | T37.8X3 | T37.8X4 | T37.8X5 | T37.8X |
| **Flucytosine** | T37.8X1 | T37.8X2 | T37.8X3 | T37.8X4 | T37.8X5 | T37.8X |
| **Fludeoxyglucose** (18F) | T5Ø.8X1 | T5Ø.8X2 | T5Ø.8X3 | T5Ø.8X4 | T5Ø.8X5 | T5Ø.8X |
| **Fludiazepam** | T42.4X1 | T42.4X2 | T42.4X3 | T42.4X4 | T42.4X5 | T42.4X |
| **Fludrocortisone** | T5Ø.ØX1 | T5Ø.ØX2 | T5Ø.ØX3 | T5Ø.ØX4 | T5Ø.ØX5 | T5Ø.ØX |
| ENT agent | T49.6X1 | T49.6X2 | T49.6X3 | T49.6X4 | T49.6X5 | T49.6X |
| ophthalmic preparation | T49.5X1 | T49.5X2 | T49.5X3 | T49.5X4 | T49.5X5 | T49.5X |
| topical NEC | T49.ØX1 | T49.ØX2 | T49.ØX3 | T49.ØX4 | T49.ØX5 | T49.ØX |
| **Fludroxycortide** | T49.ØX1 | T49.ØX2 | T49.ØX3 | T49.ØX4 | T49.ØX5 | T49.ØX |
| **Flufenamic acid** | T39.391 | T39.392 | T39.393 | T39.394 | T39.395 | T39.39 |
| **Fluindione** | T45.511 | T45.512 | T45.513 | T45.514 | T45.515 | T45.51 |
| **Flumequine** | T37.8X1 | T37.8X2 | T37.8X3 | T37.8X4 | T37.8X5 | T37.8X |
| **Flumethasone** | T49.ØX1 | T49.ØX2 | T49.ØX3 | T49.ØX4 | T49.ØX5 | T49.ØX |
| **Flumethiazide** | T5Ø.2X1 | T5Ø.2X2 | T5Ø.2X3 | T5Ø.2X4 | T5Ø.2X5 | T5Ø.2X |
| **Flumicin** | T37.5X1 | T37.5X2 | T37.5X3 | T37.5X4 | T37.5X5 | T37.5X |
| **Flunarizine** | T46.7X1 | T46.7X2 | T46.7X3 | T46.7X4 | T46.7X5 | T46.7X |
| **Flunidazole** | T37.8X1 | T37.8X2 | T37.8X3 | T37.8X4 | T37.8X5 | T37.8X |
| **Flunisolide** | T48.6X1 | T48.6X2 | T48.6X3 | T48.6X4 | T48.6X5 | T48.6X |
| **Flunitrazepam** | T42.4X1 | T42.4X2 | T42.4X3 | T42.4X4 | T42.4X5 | T42.4X |
| **Fluocinolone** (acetonide) | T49.ØX1 | T49.ØX2 | T49.ØX3 | T49.ØX4 | T49.ØX5 | T49.ØX |
| **Fluocinonide** | T49.ØX1 | T49.ØX2 | T49.ØX3 | T49.ØX4 | T49.ØX5 | T49.ØX |
| **Fluocortin** (butyl) | T49.ØX1 | T49.ØX2 | T49.ØX3 | T49.ØX4 | T49.ØX5 | T49.ØX |
| **Fluocortolone** | T49.ØX1 | T49.ØX2 | T49.ØX3 | T49.ØX4 | T49.ØX5 | T49.ØX |
| **Fluohydrocortisone** | T38.ØX1 | T38.ØX2 | T38.ØX3 | T38.ØX4 | T38.ØX5 | T38.ØX |
| ENT agent | T49.6X1 | T49.6X2 | T49.6X3 | T49.6X4 | T49.6X5 | T49.6X |
| ophthalmic preparation | T49.5X1 | T49.5X2 | T49.5X3 | T49.5X4 | T49.5X5 | T49.5X |
| topical NEC | T49.ØX1 | T49.ØX2 | T49.ØX3 | T49.ØX4 | T49.ØX5 | T49.ØX |
| **Fluonid** | T49.ØX1 | T49.ØX2 | T49.ØX3 | T49.ØX4 | T49.ØX5 | T49.ØX |
| **Fluopromazine** | T43.3X1 | T43.3X2 | T43.3X3 | T43.3X4 | T43.3X5 | T43.3X |
| **Fluoracetate** | T6Ø.8X1 | T6Ø.8X2 | T6Ø.8X3 | T6Ø.8X4 | — | — |
| **Fluorescein** | T5Ø.8X1 | T5Ø.8X2 | T5Ø.8X3 | T5Ø.8X4 | T5Ø.8X5 | T5Ø.8X |
| **Fluorhydrocortisone** | T5Ø.ØX1 | T5Ø.ØX2 | T5Ø.ØX3 | T5Ø.ØX4 | T5Ø.ØX5 | T5Ø.ØX |
| **Fluoride** (nonmedicinal) (pesticide) (sodium) **NEC** | T6Ø.8X1 | T6Ø.8X2 | T6Ø.8X3 | T6Ø.8X4 | — | — |
| hydrogen — *see* Hydrofluoric acid | | | | | | |
| medicinal NEC | T5Ø.991 | T5Ø.992 | T5Ø.993 | T5Ø.994 | T5Ø.995 | T5Ø.99 |
| dental use | T49.7X1 | T49.7X2 | T49.7X3 | T49.7X4 | T49.7X5 | T49.7X |
| not pesticide NEC | T54.91 | T54.92 | T54.93 | T54.94 | — | — |
| stannous | T49.7X1 | T49.7X2 | T49.7X3 | T49.7X4 | T49.7X5 | T49.7X |
| **Fluorigard*** | T47.7X1 | T47.7X2 | T47.7X3 | T47.7X4 | T47.7X5 | T47.7X |
| **Fluorinated corticosteroids** | T38.ØX1 | T38.ØX2 | T38.ØX3 | T38.ØX4 | T38.ØX5 | T38.ØX |
| **Fluorine** (gas) | T59.5X1 | T59.5X2 | T59.5X3 | T59.5X4 | — | — |
| salt — *see* Fluoride(s) | | | | | | |
| **Fluoristan** | T49.7X1 | T49.7X2 | T49.7X3 | T49.7X4 | T49.7X5 | T49.7X |
| **Fluormetholone** | T49.ØX1 | T49.ØX2 | T49.ØX3 | T49.ØX4 | T49.ØX5 | T49.ØX |
| **Fluoroacetate** | T6Ø.8X1 | T6Ø.8X2 | T6Ø.8X3 | T6Ø.8X4 | — | — |
| **Fluorocarbon monomer** | T53.6X1 | T53.6X2 | T53.6X3 | T53.6X4 | — | — |
| **Fluorocytosine** | T37.8X1 | T37.8X2 | T37.8X3 | T37.8X4 | T37.8X5 | T37.8X |
| **Fluorodeoxyuridine** | T45.1X1 | T45.1X2 | T45.1X3 | T45.1X4 | T45.1X5 | T45.1X |
| **Fluorometholone** | T49.ØX1 | T49.ØX2 | T49.ØX3 | T49.ØX4 | T49.ØX5 | T49.ØX |
| ophthalmic preparation | T49.5X1 | T49.5X2 | T49.5X3 | T49.5X4 | T49.5X5 | T49.5X |
| **Fluorophosphate insecticide** | T6Ø.ØX1 | T6Ø.ØX2 | T6Ø.ØX3 | T6Ø.ØX4 | — | — |
| **Fluoroquinolone antibiotics** | T36.AX1 | T36.AX2 | T36.AX3 | T36.AX4 | T36.AX5 | T36.AX |
| **Fluorosol** | T46.3X1 | T46.3X2 | T46.3X3 | T46.3X4 | T46.3X5 | T46.3X |
| **Fluorouracil** | T45.1X1 | T45.1X2 | T45.1X3 | T45.1X4 | T45.1X5 | T45.1X |
| **Fluorphenylalanine** | T49.5X1 | T49.5X2 | T49.5X3 | T49.5X4 | T49.5X5 | T49.5X |
| **Fluothane** | T41.ØX1 | T41.ØX2 | T41.ØX3 | T41.ØX4 | T41.ØX5 | T41.ØX |
| **Fluoxetine** | T43.221 | T43.222 | T43.223 | T43.224 | T43.225 | T43.22 |
| **Fluoxymesterone** | T38.7X1 | T38.7X2 | T38.7X3 | T38.7X4 | T38.7X5 | T38.7X |
| **Flupenthixol** | T43.4X1 | T43.4X2 | T43.4X3 | T43.4X4 | T43.4X5 | T43.4X |
| **Flupentixol** | T43.4X1 | T43.4X2 | T43.4X3 | T43.4X4 | T43.4X5 | T43.4X |
| **Fluphenazine** | T43.3X1 | T43.3X2 | T43.3X3 | T43.3X4 | T43.3X5 | T43.3X |
| **Fluprednidene** | T49.ØX1 | T49.ØX2 | T49.ØX3 | T49.ØX4 | T49.ØX5 | T49.ØX |
| **Fluprednisolone** | T38.ØX1 | T38.ØX2 | T38.ØX3 | T38.ØX4 | T38.ØX5 | T38.ØX |
| **Fluradoline** | T39.8X1 | T39.8X2 | T39.8X3 | T39.8X4 | T39.8X5 | T39.8X |
| **Flurandrenolide** | T49.ØX1 | T49.ØX2 | T49.ØX3 | T49.ØX4 | T49.ØX5 | T49.ØX |
| **Flurandrenolone** | T49.ØX1 | T49.ØX2 | T49.ØX3 | T49.ØX4 | T49.ØX5 | T49.ØX |
| **Flurazepam** | T42.4X1 | T42.4X2 | T42.4X3 | T42.4X4 | T42.4X5 | T42.4X |

| Substance | Poisoning, Accidental (unintentional) | Poisoning, Intentional Self-harm | Poisoning, Assault | Poisoning, Undetermined | Adverse Effect | Under-dosing |
|---|---|---|---|---|---|---|
| **Flurbiprofen** | T39.311 | T39.312 | T39.313 | T39.314 | T39.315 | T39.316 |
| **Flurobate** | T49.ØX1 | T49.ØX2 | T49.ØX3 | T49.ØX4 | T49.ØX5 | T49.ØX6 |
| **Fluroxene** | T41.ØX1 | T41.ØX2 | T41.ØX3 | T41.ØX4 | T41.ØX5 | T41.ØX6 |
| **Fluspirilene** | T43.591 | T43.592 | T43.593 | T43.594 | T43.595 | T43.596 |
| **Flutamide** | T38.6X1 | T38.6X2 | T38.6X3 | T38.6X4 | T38.6X5 | T38.6X6 |
| **Flutazolam** | T38.ØX1 | T38.ØX2 | T38.ØX3 | T38.ØX4 | T38.ØX5 | T38.ØX6 |
| **Fluticasone propionate** | T38.ØX1 | T38.ØX2 | T38.ØX3 | T38.ØX4 | T38.ØX5 | T38.ØX6 |
| **Flutoprazepam** | T42.4X1 | T42.4X2 | T42.4X3 | T42.4X4 | T42.4X5 | T42.4X6 |
| **Flutropium bromide** | T48.6X1 | T48.6X2 | T48.6X3 | T48.6X4 | T48.6X5 | T48.6X6 |
| **Fluvoxamine** | T43.221 | T43.222 | T43.223 | T43.224 | T43.225 | T43.226 |
| **Folacin** | T45.8X1 | T45.8X2 | T45.8X3 | T45.8X4 | T45.8X5 | T45.8X6 |
| **Folic acid** | T45.8X1 | T45.8X2 | T45.8X3 | T45.8X4 | T45.8X5 | T45.8X6 |
| antagonist | T45.1X1 | T45.1X2 | T45.1X3 | T45.1X4 | T45.1X5 | T45.1X6 |
| with ferrous salt | T45.2X1 | T45.2X2 | T45.2X3 | T45.2X4 | T45.2X5 | T45.2X6 |
| **Folinic acid** | T45.8X1 | T45.8X2 | T45.8X3 | T45.8X4 | T45.8X5 | T45.8X6 |
| **Folium stramoniae** | T48.6X1 | T48.6X2 | T48.6X3 | T48.6X4 | T48.6X5 | T48.6X6 |
| **Follicle-stimulating hormone, human** | T38.811 | T38.812 | T38.813 | T38.814 | T38.815 | T38.816 |
| **Folpet** | T6Ø.3X1 | T6Ø.3X2 | T6Ø.3X3 | T6Ø.3X4 | — | — |
| **Fomepizole*** | T5Ø.6X1 | T5Ø.6X2 | T5Ø.6X3 | T5Ø.6X4 | T5Ø.6X5 | T5Ø.6X6 |
| **Fominoben** | T48.3X1 | T48.3X2 | T48.3X3 | T48.3X4 | T48.3X5 | T48.3X6 |
| **Food, foodstuffs, noxious, nonbacterial, NEC** | T62.91 | T62.92 | T62.93 | T62.94 | — | — |
| berries | T62.1X1 | T62.1X2 | T62.1X3 | T62.1X4 | — | — |
| fish — *see also* Fish | T61.91 | T61.92 | T61.93 | T61.94 | — | — |
| mushrooms | T62.ØX1 | T62.ØX2 | T62.ØX3 | T62.ØX4 | — | — |
| plants | T62.2X1 | T62.2X2 | T62.2X3 | T62.2X4 | — | — |
| seafood | T61.91 | T61.92 | T61.93 | T61.94 | — | — |
| specified NEC | T61.8X1 | T61.8X2 | T61.8X3 | T61.8X4 | — | — |
| seeds | T62.2X1 | T62.2X2 | T62.2X3 | T62.2X4 | — | — |
| shellfish | T61.781 | T61.782 | T61.783 | T61.784 | — | — |
| specified NEC | T62.8X1 | T62.8X2 | T62.8X3 | T62.8X4 | — | — |
| **Fool's parsley** | T62.2X1 | T62.2X2 | T62.2X3 | T62.2X4 | — | — |
| **Formaldehyde** (solution), gas or vapor | T59.2X1 | T59.2X2 | T59.2X3 | T59.2X4 | — | — |
| fungicide | T6Ø.3X1 | T6Ø.3X2 | T6Ø.3X3 | T6Ø.3X4 | — | — |
| **Formalin** | T59.2X1 | T59.2X2 | T59.2X3 | T59.2X4 | — | — |
| fungicide | T6Ø.3X1 | T6Ø.3X2 | T6Ø.3X3 | T6Ø.3X4 | — | — |
| vapor | T59.2X1 | T59.2X2 | T59.2X3 | T59.2X4 | — | — |
| **Formic acid** | T54.2X1 | T54.2X2 | T54.2X3 | T54.2X4 | — | — |
| vapor | T59.891 | T59.892 | T59.893 | T59.894 | — | — |
| **Formoterol*** | T48.6X1 | T48.6X2 | T48.6X3 | T48.6X4 | T48.6X5 | T48.6X6 |
| **Fortaz*** | T36.1X1 | T36.1X2 | T36.1X3 | T36.1X4 | T36.1X5 | T36.1X6 |
| **Foscarnet sodium** | T37.5X1 | T37.5X2 | T37.5X3 | T37.5X4 | T37.5X5 | T37.5X6 |
| **Fosfestrol** | T38.5X1 | T38.5X2 | T38.5X3 | T38.5X4 | T38.5X5 | T38.5X6 |
| **Fosfomycin** | T36.8X1 | T36.8X2 | T36.8X3 | T36.8X4 | T36.8X5 | T36.8X6 |
| **Fosfonet sodium** | T37.5X1 | T37.5X2 | T37.5X3 | T37.5X4 | T37.5X5 | T37.5X6 |
| **Fosinopril** | T46.4X1 | T46.4X2 | T46.4X3 | T46.4X4 | T46.4X5 | T46.4X6 |
| sodium | T46.4X1 | T46.4X2 | T46.4X3 | T46.4X4 | T46.4X5 | T46.4X6 |
| **Fowler's solution** | T57.ØX1 | T57.ØX2 | T57.ØX3 | T57.ØX4 | — | — |
| **Foxglove** | T62.2X1 | T62.2X2 | T62.2X3 | T62.2X4 | — | — |
| **Framycetin** | T36.5X1 | T36.5X2 | T36.5X3 | T36.5X4 | T36.5X5 | T36.5X6 |
| **Frangula** | T47.2X1 | T47.2X2 | T47.2X3 | T47.2X4 | T47.2X5 | T47.2X6 |
| extract | T47.2X1 | T47.2X2 | T47.2X3 | T47.2X4 | T47.2X5 | T47.2X6 |
| **Frei antigen** | T5Ø.8X1 | T5Ø.8X2 | T5Ø.8X3 | T5Ø.8X4 | T5Ø.8X5 | T5Ø.8X6 |
| **Freon** | T53.5X1 | T53.5X2 | T53.5X3 | T53.5X4 | — | — |
| **Fructose** | T5Ø.3X1 | T5Ø.3X2 | T5Ø.3X3 | T5Ø.3X4 | T5Ø.3X5 | T5Ø.3X6 |
| **Frusemide** | T5Ø.1X1 | T5Ø.1X2 | T5Ø.1X3 | T5Ø.1X4 | T5Ø.1X5 | T5Ø.1X6 |
| **FSH** | T38.811 | T38.812 | T38.813 | T38.814 | T38.815 | T38.816 |
| **Ftorafur** | T45.1X1 | T45.1X2 | T45.1X3 | T45.1X4 | T45.1X5 | T45.1X6 |
| **Fuel** | | | | | | |
| automobile | T52.ØX1 | T52.ØX2 | T52.ØX3 | T52.ØX4 | — | — |
| exhaust gas, not in transit | T58.Ø1 | T58.Ø2 | T58.Ø3 | T58.Ø4 | — | — |
| vapor NEC | T52.ØX1 | T52.ØX2 | T52.ØX3 | T52.ØX4 | — | — |
| gas (domestic use) — *see also* Carbon, monoxide, fuel, utility | T59.891 | T59.892 | T59.893 | T59.894 | — | — |
| utility | T59.891 | T59.892 | T59.893 | T59.894 | — | — |
| in mobile container | T59.891 | T59.892 | T59.893 | T59.894 | — | — |
| incomplete combustion of — *see* Carbon, monoxide, fuel, utility | | | | | | |
| piped (natural) | T59.891 | T59.892 | T59.893 | T59.894 | — | — |
| industrial, incomplete combustion | T58.8X1 | T58.8X2 | T58.8X3 | T58.8X4 | — | — |
| **Fugillin** | T36.8X1 | T36.8X2 | T36.8X3 | T36.8X4 | T36.8X5 | T36.8X6 |
| **Fulminate of mercury** | T56.1X1 | T56.1X2 | T56.1X3 | T56.1X4 | — | — |
| **Fulvicin** | T36.7X1 | T36.7X2 | T36.7X3 | T36.7X4 | T36.7X5 | T36.7X6 |
| **Fumadil** | T36.8X1 | T36.8X2 | T36.8X3 | T36.8X4 | T36.8X5 | T36.8X6 |
| **Fumagillin** | T36.8X1 | T36.8X2 | T36.8X3 | T36.8X4 | T36.8X5 | T36.8X6 |
| **Fumaric acid** | T49.4X1 | T49.4X2 | T49.4X3 | T49.4X4 | T49.4X5 | T49.4X6 |
| **Fumes** (from) | T59.91 | T59.92 | T59.93 | T59.94 | — | — |
| **Fumes** — *continued* | | | | | | |
| carbon monoxide — *see* Carbon, monoxide | | | | | | |
| charcoal (domestic use) — *see* Charcoal, fumes | | | | | | |
| chloroform — *see* Chloroform | | | | | | |
| coke (in domestic stoves, fireplaces) — *see* Coke fumes | | | | | | |
| corrosive NEC | T54.91 | T54.92 | T54.93 | T54.94 | — | — |
| ether — *see* ether | | | | | | |
| freons | T53.5X1 | T53.5X2 | T53.5X3 | T53.5X4 | — | — |
| hydrocarbons | T59.891 | T59.892 | T59.893 | T59.894 | — | — |
| petroleum (liquefied) | T59.891 | T59.892 | T59.893 | T59.894 | — | — |
| distributed through pipes (pure or mixed with air) | T59.891 | T59.892 | T59.893 | T59.894 | — | — |
| lead — *see* lead | | | | | | |
| metal — *see* Metals, or the specified metal | | | | | | |
| nitrogen dioxide | T59.ØX1 | T59.ØX2 | T59.ØX3 | T59.ØX4 | — | — |
| pesticides — *see* Pesticide | | | | | | |
| petroleum (liquefied) | T59.891 | T59.892 | T59.893 | T59.894 | — | — |
| distributed through pipes (pure or mixed with air) | T59.891 | T59.892 | T59.893 | T59.894 | — | — |
| polyester | T59.891 | T59.892 | T59.893 | T59.894 | — | — |
| specified source NEC — *see also* substance specified | T59.891 | T59.892 | T59.893 | T59.894 | — | — |
| sulfur dioxide | T59.1X1 | T59.1X2 | T59.1X3 | T59.1X4 | — | — |
| **Fumigant NEC** | T6Ø.91 | T6Ø.92 | T6Ø.93 | T6Ø.94 | — | — |
| **Fungi, noxious, used as food** | T62.ØX1 | T62.ØX2 | T62.ØX3 | T62.ØX4 | — | — |
| **Fungicide NEC** (nonmedicinal) | T6Ø.3X1 | T6Ø.3X2 | T6Ø.3X3 | T6Ø.3X4 | — | — |
| **Fungizone** | T36.7X1 | T36.7X2 | T36.7X3 | T36.7X4 | T36.7X5 | T36.7X6 |
| topical | T49.ØX1 | T49.ØX2 | T49.ØX3 | T49.ØX4 | T49.ØX5 | T49.ØX6 |
| **Fungoid*** | T49.ØX1 | T49.ØX2 | T49.ØX3 | T49.ØX4 | T49.ØX5 | T49.ØX6 |
| **Furacin** | T49.ØX1 | T49.ØX2 | T49.ØX3 | T49.ØX4 | T49.ØX5 | T49.ØX6 |
| **Furadantin** | T37.91 | T37.92 | T37.93 | T37.94 | T37.95 | T37.96 |
| **Furazolidone** | T37.8X1 | T37.8X2 | T37.8X3 | T37.8X4 | T37.8X5 | T37.8X6 |
| **Furazolium chloride** | T49.ØX1 | T49.ØX2 | T49.ØX3 | T49.ØX4 | T49.ØX5 | T49.ØX6 |
| **Furfural** | T52.891 | T52.892 | T52.893 | T52.894 | — | — |
| **Furnace** (coal burning) (domestic), gas from | T58.2X1 | T58.2X2 | T58.2X3 | T58.2X4 | — | — |
| industrial | T58.8X1 | T58.8X2 | T58.8X3 | T58.8X4 | — | — |
| **Furniture polish** | T65.891 | T65.892 | T65.893 | T65.894 | — | — |
| **Furosemide** | T5Ø.1X1 | T5Ø.1X2 | T5Ø.1X3 | T5Ø.1X4 | T5Ø.1X5 | T5Ø.1X6 |
| **Furoxone** | T37.91 | T37.92 | T37.93 | T37.94 | T37.95 | T37.96 |
| **Fursultiamine** | T45.2X1 | T45.2X2 | T45.2X3 | T45.2X4 | T45.2X5 | T45.2X6 |
| **Fusafungine** | T36.8X1 | T36.8X2 | T36.8X3 | T36.8X4 | T36.8X5 | T36.8X6 |
| **Fusel oil** (any) (amyl) (butyl) (propyl), vapor | T51.3X1 | T51.3X2 | T51.3X3 | T51.3X4 | — | — |
| **Fusidate** (ethanolamine) (sodium) | T36.8X1 | T36.8X2 | T36.8X3 | T36.8X4 | T36.8X5 | T36.8X6 |
| **Fusidic acid** | T36.8X1 | T36.8X2 | T36.8X3 | T36.8X4 | T36.8X5 | T36.8X6 |
| **Fytic acid, nonasodium** | T5Ø.6X1 | T5Ø.6X2 | T5Ø.6X3 | T5Ø.6X4 | T5Ø.6X5 | T5Ø.6X6 |
| **GABA** | T43.8X1 | T43.8X2 | T43.8X3 | T43.8X4 | T43.8X5 | T43.8X6 |
| **Gabapentin*** | T42.6X1 | T42.6X2 | T42.6X3 | T42.6X4 | T42.6X5 | T42.6X6 |
| **Gabitril*** | T42.6X1 | T42.6X2 | T42.6X3 | T42.6X4 | T42.6X5 | T42.6X6 |
| **Gadolinium** | T56.821 | T56.822 | T56.823 | T56.824 | — | — |
| **Gadopentetic acid** | T5Ø.8X1 | T5Ø.8X2 | T5Ø.8X3 | T5Ø.8X4 | T5Ø.8X5 | T5Ø.8X6 |
| **Galactose** | T5Ø.3X1 | T5Ø.3X2 | T5Ø.3X3 | T5Ø.3X4 | T5Ø.3X5 | T5Ø.3X6 |
| **Galantamine** | T44.ØX1 | T44.ØX2 | T44.ØX3 | T44.ØX4 | T44.ØX5 | T44.ØX6 |
| **Gallamine** (triethiodide) | T48.1X1 | T48.1X2 | T48.1X3 | T48.1X4 | T48.1X5 | T48.1X6 |
| **Gallium citrate** | T5Ø.991 | T5Ø.992 | T5Ø.993 | T5Ø.994 | T5Ø.995 | T5Ø.996 |
| **Gallopamil** | T46.1X1 | T46.1X2 | T46.1X3 | T46.1X4 | T46.1X5 | T46.1X6 |
| **Gamboge** | T47.2X1 | T47.2X2 | T47.2X3 | T47.2X4 | T47.2X5 | T47.2X6 |
| **Gamimune** | T5Ø.Z11 | T5Ø.Z12 | T5Ø.Z13 | T5Ø.Z14 | T5Ø.Z15 | T5Ø.Z16 |
| **Gamma-aminobutyric acid** | T43.8X1 | T43.8X2 | T43.8X3 | T43.8X4 | T43.8X5 | T43.8X6 |
| **Gamma-benzene hexachloride** (medicinal) | T49.ØX1 | T49.ØX2 | T49.ØX3 | T49.ØX4 | T49.ØX5 | T49.ØX6 |
| nonmedicinal, vapor | T53.6X1 | T53.6X2 | T53.6X3 | T53.6X4 | — | — |
| **Gamma-BHC** (medicinal) — *see also* Gamma-benzene hexachloride | T49.ØX1 | T49.ØX2 | T49.ØX3 | T49.ØX4 | T49.ØX5 | T49.ØX6 |
| **Gamma globulin** | T5Ø.Z11 | T5Ø.Z12 | T5Ø.Z13 | T5Ø.Z14 | T5Ø.Z15 | T5Ø.Z16 |
| **Gamulin** | T5Ø.Z11 | T5Ø.Z12 | T5Ø.Z13 | T5Ø.Z14 | T5Ø.Z15 | T5Ø.Z16 |
| **Ganciclovir** (sodium) | T37.5X1 | T37.5X2 | T37.5X3 | T37.5X4 | T37.5X5 | T37.5X6 |
| **Ganglionic blocking drug NEC** | T44.2X1 | T44.2X2 | T44.2X3 | T44.2X4 | T44.2X5 | T44.2X6 |
| specified NEC | T44.2X1 | T44.2X2 | T44.2X3 | T44.2X4 | T44.2X5 | T44.2X6 |
| **Ganja** | T4Ø.711 | T4Ø.712 | T4Ø.713 | T4Ø.714 | T4Ø.715 | T4Ø.716 |

| Substance | Poisoning, Accidental (unintentional) | Poisoning, Intentional Self-harm | Poisoning, Assault | Poisoning, Undetermined | Adverse Effect | Under-dosing |
|---|---|---|---|---|---|---|
| **Garamycin** | T36.5X1 | T36.5X2 | T36.5X3 | T36.5X4 | T36.5X5 | T36.5X6 |
| ophthalmic preparation | T49.5X1 | T49.5X2 | T49.5X3 | T49.5X4 | T49.5X5 | T49.5X6 |
| topical NEC | T49.ØX1 | T49.ØX2 | T49.ØX3 | T49.ØX4 | T49.ØX5 | T49.ØX6 |
| **Gardenal** | T42.3X1 | T42.3X2 | T42.3X3 | T42.3X4 | T42.3X5 | T42.3X6 |
| **Gardepanyl** | T42.3X1 | T42.3X2 | T42.3X3 | T42.3X4 | T42.3X5 | T42.3X6 |
| **Gas NEC** | T59.91 | T59.92 | T59.93 | T59.94 | — | — |
| acetylene | T59.891 | T59.892 | T59.893 | T59.894 | — | — |
| incomplete combustion of | T58.11 | T58.12 | T58.13 | T58.14 | — | — |
| air contaminants, source or type not specified | T59.91 | T59.92 | T59.93 | T59.94 | — | — |
| anesthetic | T41.ØX1 | T41.ØX2 | T41.ØX3 | T41.ØX4 | T41.ØX5 | T41.ØX6 |
| blast furnace | T58.8X1 | T58.8X2 | T58.8X3 | T58.8X4 | — | — |
| butane — *see* butane | | | | | | |
| carbon monoxide — *see* Carbon, monoxide | | | | | | |
| chlorine | T59.4X1 | T59.4X2 | T59.4X3 | T59.4X4 | — | — |
| coal | T58.2X1 | T58.2X2 | T58.2X3 | T58.2X4 | — | — |
| cyanide | T57.3X1 | T57.3X2 | T57.3X3 | T57.3X4 | — | — |
| dicyanogen | T65.ØX1 | T65.ØX2 | T65.ØX3 | T65.ØX4 | — | — |
| domestic — *see* Domestic gas | | | | | | |
| exhaust | T58.Ø1 | T58.Ø2 | T58.Ø3 | T58.Ø4 | — | — |
| from utility (for cooking, heating, or lighting) (after combustion) — *see* Carbon, monoxide, fuel, utility | | | | | | |
| prior to combustion | T59.891 | T59.892 | T59.893 | T59.894 | — | — |
| from wood- or coal-burning stove or fireplace | T58.2X1 | T58.2X2 | T58.2X3 | T58.2X4 | — | — |
| fuel (domestic use) (after combustion) — *see also* Carbon, monoxide, fuel | | | | | | |
| industrial use | T58.8X1 | T58.8X2 | T58.8X3 | T58.8X4 | — | — |
| prior to combustion | T59.891 | T59.892 | T59.893 | T59.894 | — | — |
| utility | T59.891 | T59.892 | T59.893 | T59.894 | — | — |
| in mobile container | T59.891 | T59.892 | T59.893 | T59.894 | — | — |
| incomplete combustion of — *see* Carbon, monoxide, fuel, utility | | | | | | |
| piped (natural) | T59.891 | T59.892 | T59.893 | T59.894 | — | — |
| garage | T58.Ø1 | T58.Ø2 | T58.Ø3 | T58.Ø4 | — | — |
| hydrocarbon NEC | T59.891 | T59.892 | T59.893 | T59.894 | — | — |
| incomplete combustion of — *see* Carbon, monoxide, fuel, utility | | | | | | |
| liquefied — *see* butane | | | | | | |
| piped | T59.891 | T59.892 | T59.893 | T59.894 | — | — |
| hydrocyanic acid | T65.ØX1 | T65.ØX2 | T65.ØX3 | T65.ØX4 | — | — |
| illuminating (after combustion) | T58.11 | T58.12 | T58.13 | T58.14 | — | — |
| prior to combustion | T59.891 | T59.892 | T59.893 | T59.894 | — | — |
| incomplete combustion, any — *see* Carbon, monoxide | | | | | | |
| kiln | T58.8X1 | T58.8X2 | T58.8X3 | T58.8X4 | — | — |
| lacrimogenic | T59.3X1 | T59.3X2 | T59.3X3 | T59.3X4 | — | — |
| liquefied petroleum — *see* butane | | | | | | |
| marsh | T59.891 | T59.892 | T59.893 | T59.894 | — | — |
| motor exhaust, not in transit | T58.Ø1 | T58.Ø2 | T58.Ø3 | T58.Ø4 | — | — |
| mustard, not in war | T59.891 | T59.892 | T59.893 | T59.894 | — | — |
| natural | T59.891 | T59.892 | T59.893 | T59.894 | — | — |
| nerve, not in war | T59.91 | T59.92 | T59.93 | T59.94 | — | — |
| oil | T52.ØX1 | T52.ØX2 | T52.ØX3 | T52.ØX4 | — | — |
| petroleum (liquefied) (distributed in mobile containers) | T59.891 | T59.892 | T59.893 | T59.894 | — | — |
| piped (pure or mixed with air) | T59.891 | T59.892 | T59.893 | T59.894 | — | — |
| piped (manufactured) (natural) NEC | T59.891 | T59.892 | T59.893 | T59.894 | — | — |
| producer | T58.8X1 | T58.8X2 | T58.8X3 | T58.8X4 | — | — |
| propane — *see* propane | | | | | | |
| refrigerant (chlorofluoro-carbon) | T53.5X1 | T53.5X2 | T53.5X3 | T53.5X4 | — | — |
| not chlorofluoro-carbon | T59.891 | T59.892 | T59.893 | T59.894 | — | — |
| sewer | T59.91 | T59.92 | T59.93 | T59.94 | — | — |
| specified source NEC | T59.91 | T59.92 | T59.93 | T59.94 | — | — |
| stove (after combustion) | T58.11 | T58.12 | T58.13 | T58.14 | — | — |
| prior to combustion | T59.891 | T59.892 | T59.893 | T59.894 | — | — |
| tear | T59.3X1 | T59.3X2 | T59.3X3 | T59.3X4 | — | — |
| therapeutic | T41.5X1 | T41.5X2 | T41.5X3 | T41.5X4 | T41.5X5 | T41.5X6 |

| Substance | Poisoning, Accidental (unintentional) | Poisoning, Intentional Self-harm | Poisoning, Assault | Poisoning, Undetermined | Adverse Effect | Under-dosing |
|---|---|---|---|---|---|---|
| **Gas** — *continued* | | | | | | |
| utility (for cooking, heating, or lighting) (piped) NEC | T59.891 | T59.892 | T59.893 | T59.894 | — | — |
| in mobile container | T59.891 | T59.892 | T59.893 | T59.894 | — | — |
| incomplete combustion of — *see* Carbon, monoxide, fuel, utility | | | | | | |
| piped (natural) | T59.891 | T59.892 | T59.893 | T59.894 | — | — |
| water | T58.11 | T58.12 | T58.13 | T58.14 | — | — |
| incomplete combustion of — *see* Carbon, monoxide, fuel, utility | | | | | | |
| **Gaseous substance** — *see* Gas | | | | | | |
| **Gasoline** | T52.ØX1 | T52.ØX2 | T52.ØX3 | T52.ØX4 | — | — |
| vapor | T52.ØX1 | T52.ØX2 | T52.ØX3 | T52.ØX4 | — | — |
| **Gastric enzymes** | T47.5X1 | T47.5X2 | T47.5X3 | T47.5X4 | T47.5X5 | T47.5X6 |
| **Gastrografin** | T5Ø.8X1 | T5Ø.8X2 | T5Ø.8X3 | T5Ø.8X4 | T5Ø.8X5 | T5Ø.8X6 |
| **Gastrointestinal drug** | T47.91 | T47.92 | T47.93 | T47.94 | T47.95 | T47.96 |
| biological | T47.8X1 | T47.8X2 | T47.8X3 | T47.8X4 | T47.8X5 | T47.8X6 |
| specified NEC | T47.8X1 | T47.8X2 | T47.8X3 | T47.8X4 | T47.8X5 | T47.8X6 |
| **Gaultheria procumbens** | T62.2X1 | T62.2X2 | T62.2X3 | T62.2X4 | — | — |
| **Gaviscon*** | T47.1X1 | T47.1X2 | T47.1X3 | T47.1X4 | T47.1X5 | T47.1X6 |
| **Gefarnate** | T44.3X1 | T44.3X2 | T44.3X3 | T44.3X4 | T44.3X5 | T44.3X6 |
| **Gelatin** (intravenous) | T45.8X1 | T45.8X2 | T45.8X3 | T45.8X4 | T45.8X5 | T45.8X6 |
| absorbable (sponge) | T45.7X1 | T45.7X2 | T45.7X3 | T45.7X4 | T45.7X5 | T45.7X6 |
| **Gelfilm** | T49.8X1 | T49.8X2 | T49.8X3 | T49.8X4 | T49.8X5 | T49.8X6 |
| **Gelfoam** | T45.7X1 | T45.7X2 | T45.7X3 | T45.7X4 | T45.7X5 | T45.7X6 |
| **Gelsemine** | T5Ø.991 | T5Ø.992 | T5Ø.993 | T5Ø.994 | T5Ø.995 | T5Ø.996 |
| **Gelsemium** (sempervirens) | T62.2X1 | T62.2X2 | T62.2X3 | T62.2X4 | — | — |
| **Gemeprost** | T48.ØX1 | T48.ØX2 | T48.ØX3 | T48.ØX4 | T48.ØX5 | T48.ØX6 |
| **Gemfibrozil** | T46.6X1 | T46.6X2 | T46.6X3 | T46.6X4 | T46.6X5 | T46.6X6 |
| **Gemonil** | T42.3X1 | T42.3X2 | T42.3X3 | T42.3X4 | T42.3X5 | T42.3X6 |
| **Gentamicin** | T36.5X1 | T36.5X2 | T36.5X3 | T36.5X4 | T36.5X5 | T36.5X6 |
| ophthalmic preparation | T49.5X1 | T49.5X2 | T49.5X3 | T49.5X4 | T49.5X5 | T49.5X6 |
| topical NEC | T49.ØX1 | T49.ØX2 | T49.ØX3 | T49.ØX4 | T49.ØX5 | T49.ØX6 |
| **Gentasol*** | T49.5X1 | T49.5X2 | T49.5X3 | T49.5X4 | T49.5X5 | T49.5X6 |
| **Gentian** | T47.5X1 | T47.5X2 | T47.5X3 | T47.5X4 | T47.5X5 | T47.5X6 |
| violet | T49.ØX1 | T49.ØX2 | T49.ØX3 | T49.ØX4 | T49.ØX5 | T49.ØX6 |
| **Gepefrine** | T44.4X1 | T44.4X2 | T44.4X3 | T44.4X4 | T44.4X5 | T44.4X6 |
| **Gestonorone caproate** | T38.5X1 | T38.5X2 | T38.5X3 | T38.5X4 | T38.5X5 | T38.5X6 |
| **Gexane** | T49.ØX1 | T49.ØX2 | T49.ØX3 | T49.ØX4 | T49.ØX5 | T49.ØX6 |
| **Gila monster** (venom) | T63.111 | T63.112 | T63.113 | T63.114 | — | — |
| **Ginger** | T47.5X1 | T47.5X2 | T47.5X3 | T47.5X4 | T47.5X5 | T47.5X6 |
| Jamaica — *see* Jamaica, ginger | | | | | | |
| **Gitalin** | T46.ØX1 | T46.ØX2 | T46.ØX3 | T46.ØX4 | T46.ØX5 | T46.ØX6 |
| amorphous | T46.ØX1 | T46.ØX2 | T46.ØX3 | T46.ØX4 | T46.ØX5 | T46.ØX6 |
| **Gitaloxin** | T46.ØX1 | T46.ØX2 | T46.ØX3 | T46.ØX4 | T46.ØX5 | T46.ØX6 |
| **Gitoxin** | T46.ØX1 | T46.ØX2 | T46.ØX3 | T46.ØX4 | T46.ØX5 | T46.ØX6 |
| **Glafenine** | T39.8X1 | T39.8X2 | T39.8X3 | T39.8X4 | T39.8X5 | T39.8X6 |
| **Glandular extract** (medicinal) **NEC** | T5Ø.Z91 | T5Ø.Z92 | T5Ø.Z93 | T5Ø.Z94 | T5Ø.Z95 | T5Ø.Z96 |
| **Glaucarubin** | T37.3X1 | T37.3X2 | T37.3X3 | T37.3X4 | T37.3X5 | T37.3X6 |
| **Glibenclamide** | T38.3X1 | T38.3X2 | T38.3X3 | T38.3X4 | T38.3X5 | T38.3X6 |
| **Glibornuride** | T38.3X1 | T38.3X2 | T38.3X3 | T38.3X4 | T38.3X5 | T38.3X6 |
| **Gliclazide** | T38.3X1 | T38.3X2 | T38.3X3 | T38.3X4 | T38.3X5 | T38.3X6 |
| **Glimidine** | T38.3X1 | T38.3X2 | T38.3X3 | T38.3X4 | T38.3X5 | T38.3X6 |
| **Glipizide** | T38.3X1 | T38.3X2 | T38.3X3 | T38.3X4 | T38.3X5 | T38.3X6 |
| **Gliquidone** | T38.3X1 | T38.3X2 | T38.3X3 | T38.3X4 | T38.3X5 | T38.3X6 |
| **Glisolamide** | T38.3X1 | T38.3X2 | T38.3X3 | T38.3X4 | T38.3X5 | T38.3X6 |
| **Glisoxepide** | T38.3X1 | T38.3X2 | T38.3X3 | T38.3X4 | T38.3X5 | T38.3X6 |
| **Globin zinc insulin** | T38.3X1 | T38.3X2 | T38.3X3 | T38.3X4 | T38.3X5 | T38.3X6 |
| **Globulin** | | | | | | |
| antilymphocytic | T5Ø.Z11 | T5Ø.Z12 | T5Ø.Z13 | T5Ø.Z14 | T5Ø.Z15 | T5Ø.Z16 |
| antirhesus | T5Ø.Z11 | T5Ø.Z12 | T5Ø.Z13 | T5Ø.Z14 | T5Ø.Z15 | T5Ø.Z16 |
| antivenin | T5Ø.Z11 | T5Ø.Z12 | T5Ø.Z13 | T5Ø.Z14 | T5Ø.Z15 | T5Ø.Z16 |
| antiviral | T5Ø.Z11 | T5Ø.Z12 | T5Ø.Z13 | T5Ø.Z14 | T5Ø.Z15 | T5Ø.Z16 |
| **Glucagon** | T38.3X1 | T38.3X2 | T38.3X3 | T38.3X4 | T38.3X5 | T38.3X6 |
| **Glucocorticoids** | T38.ØX1 | T38.ØX2 | T38.ØX3 | T38.ØX4 | T38.ØX5 | T38.ØX6 |
| **Glucocorticosteroid** | T38.ØX1 | T38.ØX2 | T38.ØX3 | T38.ØX4 | T38.ØX5 | T38.ØX6 |
| **Gluconic acid** | T5Ø.991 | T5Ø.992 | T5Ø.993 | T5Ø.994 | T5Ø.995 | T5Ø.996 |
| **Glucosamine sulfate** | T39.4X1 | T39.4X2 | T39.4X3 | T39.4X4 | T39.4X5 | T39.4X6 |
| **Glucose** | T5Ø.3X1 | T5Ø.3X2 | T5Ø.3X3 | T5Ø.3X4 | T5Ø.3X5 | T5Ø.3X6 |
| with sodium chloride | T5Ø.3X1 | T5Ø.3X2 | T5Ø.3X3 | T5Ø.3X4 | T5Ø.3X5 | T5Ø.3X6 |
| **Glucosulfone sodium** | T37.1X1 | T37.1X2 | T37.1X3 | T37.1X4 | T37.1X5 | T37.1X6 |
| **Glucotrol*** | T38.3X1 | T38.3X2 | T38.3X3 | T38.3X4 | T38.3X5 | T38.3X6 |
| **Glucurolactone** | T47.8X1 | T47.8X2 | T47.8X3 | T47.8X4 | T47.8X5 | T47.8X6 |
| **Glue NEC** | T52.891 | T52.892 | T52.893 | T52.894 | — | — |
| **Glutamic acid** | T47.5X1 | T47.5X2 | T47.5X3 | T47.5X4 | T47.5X5 | T47.5X6 |
| **Glutaral** (medicinal) | T49.ØX1 | T49.ØX2 | T49.ØX3 | T49.ØX4 | T49.ØX5 | T49.ØX6 |
| nonmedicinal | T65.891 | T65.892 | T65.893 | T65.894 | — | — |
| **Glutaraldehyde** (nonmedicinal) | T65.891 | T65.892 | T65.893 | T65.894 | — | — |
| medicinal | T49.ØX1 | T49.ØX2 | T49.ØX3 | T49.ØX4 | T49.ØX5 | T49.ØX6 |





☑ **Additional Character May Be Required — Refer to the Tabular List for Character Selection**

***Optum Value-Add**

| Substance | Poisoning, Accidental (unintentional) | Poisoning, Intentional Self-harm | Poisoning, Assault | Poisoning, Undetermined | Adverse Effect | Under-dosing |
|---|---|---|---|---|---|---|
| **Glutathione** | T5Ø.6X1 | T5Ø.6X2 | T5Ø.6X3 | T5Ø.6X4 | T5Ø.6X5 | T5Ø.6X6 |
| **Glutethimide** | T42.6X1 | T42.6X2 | T42.6X3 | T42.6X4 | T42.6X5 | T42.6X6 |
| **Glyburide** | T38.3X1 | T38.3X2 | T38.3X3 | T38.3X4 | T38.3X5 | T38.3X6 |
| **Glycerin** | T47.4X1 | T47.4X2 | T47.4X3 | T47.4X4 | T47.4X5 | T47.4X6 |
| **Glycerol** | T47.4X1 | T47.4X2 | T47.4X3 | T47.4X4 | T47.4X5 | T47.4X6 |
| borax | T49.6X1 | T49.6X2 | T49.6X3 | T49.6X4 | T49.6X5 | T49.6X6 |
| intravenous | T5Ø.3X1 | T5Ø.3X2 | T5Ø.3X3 | T5Ø.3X4 | T5Ø.3X5 | T5Ø.3X6 |
| iodinated | T48.4X1 | T48.4X2 | T48.4X3 | T48.4X4 | T48.4X5 | T48.4X6 |
| **Glycerophosphate** | T5Ø.991 | T5Ø.992 | T5Ø.993 | T5Ø.994 | T5Ø.995 | T5Ø.996 |
| **Glyceryl** | | | | | | |
| guaiacolate | T48.4X1 | T48.4X2 | T48.4X3 | T48.4X4 | T48.4X5 | T48.4X6 |
| nitrate | T46.3X1 | T46.3X2 | T46.3X3 | T46.3X4 | T46.3X5 | T46.3X6 |
| triacetate (topical) | T49.ØX1 | T49.ØX2 | T49.ØX3 | T49.ØX4 | T49.ØX5 | T49.ØX6 |
| trinitrate | T46.3X1 | T46.3X2 | T46.3X3 | T46.3X4 | T46.3X5 | T46.3X6 |
| **Glycine** | T5Ø.3X1 | T5Ø.3X2 | T5Ø.3X3 | T5Ø.3X4 | T5Ø.3X5 | T5Ø.3X6 |
| **Glyclopyramide** | T38.3X1 | T38.3X2 | T38.3X3 | T38.3X4 | T38.3X5 | T38.3X6 |
| **Glycobiarsol** | T37.3X1 | T37.3X2 | T37.3X3 | T37.3X4 | T37.3X5 | T37.3X6 |
| **Glycols** (ether) | T52.3X1 | T52.3X2 | T52.3X3 | T52.3X4 | — | — |
| **Glyconiazide** | T37.1X1 | T37.1X2 | T37.1X3 | T37.1X4 | T37.1X5 | T37.1X6 |
| **Glycopyrrolate** | T44.3X1 | T44.3X2 | T44.3X3 | T44.3X4 | T44.3X5 | T44.3X6 |
| **Glycopyrronium** | T44.3X1 | T44.3X2 | T44.3X3 | T44.3X4 | T44.3X5 | T44.3X6 |
| bromide | T44.3X1 | T44.3X2 | T44.3X3 | T44.3X4 | T44.3X5 | T44.3X6 |
| **Glycoside, cardiac** (stimulant) | T46.ØX1 | T46.ØX2 | T46.ØX3 | T46.ØX4 | T46.ØX5 | T46.ØX6 |
| **Glycyclamide** | T38.3X1 | T38.3X2 | T38.3X3 | T38.3X4 | T38.3X5 | T38.3X6 |
| **Glycyrrhiza extract** | T48.4X1 | T48.4X2 | T48.4X3 | T48.4X4 | T48.4X5 | T48.4X6 |
| **Glycyrrhizic acid** | T48.4X1 | T48.4X2 | T48.4X3 | T48.4X4 | T48.4X5 | T48.4X6 |
| **Glycyrrhizinate potassium** | T48.4X1 | T48.4X2 | T48.4X3 | T48.4X4 | T48.4X5 | T48.4X6 |
| **Glymidine sodium** | T38.3X1 | T38.3X2 | T38.3X3 | T38.3X4 | T38.3X5 | T38.3X6 |
| **Glyphosate** | T6Ø.3X1 | T6Ø.3X2 | T6Ø.3X3 | T6Ø.3X4 | — | — |
| **Glyphylline** | T48.6X1 | T48.6X2 | T48.6X3 | T48.6X4 | T48.6X5 | T48.6X6 |
| **Gold** | | | | | | |
| colloidal (I98Au) | T45.1X1 | T45.1X2 | T45.1X3 | T45.1X4 | T45.1X5 | T45.1X6 |
| salts | T39.4X1 | T39.4X2 | T39.4X3 | T39.4X4 | T39.4X5 | T39.4X6 |
| **Golden sulfide of antimony** | T56.891 | T56.892 | T56.893 | T56.894 | — | — |
| **Goldylocks** | T62.2X1 | T62.2X2 | T62.2X3 | T62.2X4 | — | — |
| **Gonadal tissue extract** | T38.9Ø1 | T38.9Ø2 | T38.9Ø3 | T38.9Ø4 | T38.9Ø5 | T38.9Ø6 |
| female | T38.5X1 | T38.5X2 | T38.5X3 | T38.5X4 | T38.5X5 | T38.5X6 |
| male | T38.7X1 | T38.7X2 | T38.7X3 | T38.7X4 | T38.7X5 | T38.7X6 |
| **Gonadorelin** | T38.891 | T38.892 | T38.893 | T38.894 | T38.895 | T38.896 |
| **Gonadotropin** | T38.891 | T38.892 | T38.893 | T38.894 | T38.895 | T38.896 |
| chorionic | T38.891 | T38.892 | T38.893 | T38.894 | T38.895 | T38.896 |
| pituitary | T38.811 | T38.812 | T38.813 | T38.814 | T38.815 | T38.816 |
| **Goserelin** | T45.1X1 | T45.1X2 | T45.1X3 | T45.1X4 | T45.1X5 | T45.1X6 |
| **Grain alcohol** | T51.ØX1 | T51.ØX2 | T51.ØX3 | T51.ØX4 | — | — |
| **Gralise*** | T42.6X1 | T42.6X2 | T42.6X3 | T42.6X4 | T42.6X5 | T42.6X6 |
| **Gramicidin** | T49.ØX1 | T49.ØX2 | T49.ØX3 | T49.ØX4 | T49.ØX5 | T49.ØX6 |
| **Granisetron** | T45.ØX1 | T45.ØX2 | T45.ØX3 | T45.ØX4 | T45.ØX5 | T45.ØX6 |
| **Gratiola officinalis** | T62.2X1 | T62.2X2 | T62.2X3 | T62.2X4 | — | — |
| **Grease** | T65.891 | T65.892 | T65.893 | T65.894 | — | — |
| **Green hellebore** | T62.2X1 | T62.2X2 | T62.2X3 | T62.2X4 | — | — |
| **Green soap** | T49.2X1 | T49.2X2 | T49.2X3 | T49.2X4 | T49.2X5 | T49.2X6 |
| **Grifulvin** | T36.7X1 | T36.7X2 | T36.7X3 | T36.7X4 | T36.7X5 | T36.7X6 |
| **Griseofulvin** | T36.7X1 | T36.7X2 | T36.7X3 | T36.7X4 | T36.7X5 | T36.7X6 |
| **Growth hormone** | T38.811 | T38.812 | T38.813 | T38.814 | T38.815 | T38.816 |
| **Guaiac reagent** | T5Ø.991 | T5Ø.992 | T5Ø.993 | T5Ø.994 | T5Ø.995 | T5Ø.996 |
| **Guaiacol derivatives** | T48.4X1 | T48.4X2 | T48.4X3 | T48.4X4 | T48.4X5 | T48.4X6 |
| **Guaifenesin** | T48.4X1 | T48.4X2 | T48.4X3 | T48.4X4 | T48.4X5 | T48.4X6 |
| **Guaimesal** | T48.4X1 | T48.4X2 | T48.4X3 | T48.4X4 | T48.4X5 | T48.4X6 |
| **Guaiphenesin** | T48.4X1 | T48.4X2 | T48.4X3 | T48.4X4 | T48.4X5 | T48.4X6 |
| **Guaituss*** | T48.4X1 | T48.4X2 | T48.4X3 | T48.4X4 | T48.4X5 | T48.4X6 |
| **Guamecycline** | T36.4X1 | T36.4X2 | T36.4X3 | T36.4X4 | T36.4X5 | T36.4X6 |
| **Guanabenz** | T46.5X1 | T46.5X2 | T46.5X3 | T46.5X4 | T46.5X5 | T46.5X6 |
| **Guanacline** | T46.5X1 | T46.5X2 | T46.5X3 | T46.5X4 | T46.5X5 | T46.5X6 |
| **Guanadrel** | T46.5X1 | T46.5X2 | T46.5X3 | T46.5X4 | T46.5X5 | T46.5X6 |
| **Guanatol** | T37.2X1 | T37.2X2 | T37.2X3 | T37.2X4 | T37.2X5 | T37.2X6 |
| **Guanethidine** | T46.5X1 | T46.5X2 | T46.5X3 | T46.5X4 | T46.5X5 | T46.5X6 |
| **Guanfacine** | T46.5X1 | T46.5X2 | T46.5X3 | T46.5X4 | T46.5X5 | T46.5X6 |
| **Guano** | T65.891 | T65.892 | T65.893 | T65.894 | — | — |
| **Guanochlor** | T46.5X1 | T46.5X2 | T46.5X3 | T46.5X4 | T46.5X5 | T46.5X6 |
| **Guanoclor** | T46.5X1 | T46.5X2 | T46.5X3 | T46.5X4 | T46.5X5 | T46.5X6 |
| **Guanoctine** | T46.5X1 | T46.5X2 | T46.5X3 | T46.5X4 | T46.5X5 | T46.5X6 |
| **Guanoxabenz** | T46.5X1 | T46.5X2 | T46.5X3 | T46.5X4 | T46.5X5 | T46.5X6 |
| **Guanoxan** | T46.5X1 | T46.5X2 | T46.5X3 | T46.5X4 | T46.5X5 | T46.5X6 |
| **Guar gum** (medicinal) | T46.6X1 | T46.6X2 | T46.6X3 | T46.6X4 | T46.6X5 | T46.6X6 |
| **Hachimycin** | T36.7X1 | T36.7X2 | T36.7X3 | T36.7X4 | T36.7X5 | T36.7X6 |
| **Hair** | | | | | | |
| dye | T49.4X1 | T49.4X2 | T49.4X3 | T49.4X4 | T49.4X5 | T49.4X6 |
| preparation NEC | T49.4X1 | T49.4X2 | T49.4X3 | T49.4X4 | T49.4X5 | T49.4X6 |
| **Halazepam** | T42.4X1 | T42.4X2 | T42.4X3 | T42.4X4 | T42.4X5 | T42.4X6 |
| **Halcinolone** | T49.ØX1 | T49.ØX2 | T49.ØX3 | T49.ØX4 | T49.ØX5 | T49.ØX6 |
| **Halcinonide** | T49.ØX1 | T49.ØX2 | T49.ØX3 | T49.ØX4 | T49.ØX5 | T49.ØX6 |

| Substance | Poisoning, Accidental (unintentional) | Poisoning, Intentional Self-harm | Poisoning, Assault | Poisoning, Undetermined | Adverse Effect | Under-dosing |
|---|---|---|---|---|---|---|
| **Halethazole** | T49.ØX1 | T49.ØX2 | T49.ØX3 | T49.ØX4 | T49.ØX5 | T49.ØX6 |
| **Hallucinogen NOS** | T4Ø.9Ø1 | T4Ø.9Ø2 | T4Ø.9Ø3 | T4Ø.9Ø4 | T4Ø.9Ø5 | T4Ø.9Ø6 |
| specified NEC | T4Ø.991 | T4Ø.992 | T4Ø.993 | T4Ø.994 | T4Ø.995 | T4Ø.996 |
| **Halofantrine** | T37.2X1 | T37.2X2 | T37.2X3 | T37.2X4 | T37.2X5 | T37.2X6 |
| **Halofenate** | T46.6X1 | T46.6X2 | T46.6X3 | T46.6X4 | T46.6X5 | T46.6X6 |
| **Halometasone** | T49.ØX1 | T49.ØX2 | T49.ØX3 | T49.ØX4 | T49.ØX5 | T49.ØX6 |
| **Haloperidol** | T43.4X1 | T43.4X2 | T43.4X3 | T43.4X4 | T43.4X5 | T43.4X6 |
| **Haloprogin** | T49.ØX1 | T49.ØX2 | T49.ØX3 | T49.ØX4 | T49.ØX5 | T49.ØX6 |
| **Halotex** | T49.ØX1 | T49.ØX2 | T49.ØX3 | T49.ØX4 | T49.ØX5 | T49.ØX6 |
| **Halothane** | T41.ØX1 | T41.ØX2 | T41.ØX3 | T41.ØX4 | T41.ØX5 | T41.ØX6 |
| **Haloxazolam** | T42.4X1 | T42.4X2 | T42.4X3 | T42.4X4 | T42.4X5 | T42.4X6 |
| **Halquinols** | T49.ØX1 | T49.ØX2 | T49.ØX3 | T49.ØX4 | T49.ØX5 | T49.ØX6 |
| **Hamamelis** | T49.2X1 | T49.2X2 | T49.2X3 | T49.2X4 | T49.2X5 | T49.2X6 |
| **Haptendextran** | T45.8X1 | T45.8X2 | T45.8X3 | T45.8X4 | T45.8X5 | T45.8X6 |
| **Harmonyl** | T46.5X1 | T46.5X2 | T46.5X3 | T46.5X4 | T46.5X5 | T46.5X6 |
| **Hartmann's solution** | T5Ø.3X1 | T5Ø.3X2 | T5Ø.3X3 | T5Ø.3X4 | T5Ø.3X5 | T5Ø.3X6 |
| **Hashish** | T4Ø.711 | T4Ø.712 | T4Ø.713 | T4Ø.714 | T4Ø.715 | T4Ø.716 |
| **Havrix*** | T5Ø.B91 | T5Ø.B92 | T5Ø.B93 | T5Ø.B94 | T5Ø.B95 | T5Ø.B96 |
| **Hawaiian Woodrose seeds** | T4Ø.991 | T4Ø.992 | T4Ø.993 | T4Ø.994 | — | — |
| **HCB** | T6Ø.3X1 | T6Ø.3X2 | T6Ø.3X3 | T6Ø.3X4 | — | — |
| **HCH** | T53.6X1 | T53.6X2 | T53.6X3 | T53.6X4 | — | — |
| medicinal | T49.ØX1 | T49.ØX2 | T49.ØX3 | T49.ØX4 | T49.ØX5 | T49.ØX6 |
| **HCN** | T57.3X1 | T57.3X2 | T57.3X3 | T57.3X4 | — | — |
| **Headache cures, drugs, powders NEC** | T5Ø.9Ø1 | T5Ø.9Ø2 | T5Ø.9Ø3 | T5Ø.9Ø4 | T5Ø.9Ø5 | T5Ø.9Ø6 |
| **Heavenly Blue** (morning glory) | T4Ø.991 | T4Ø.992 | T4Ø.993 | T4Ø.994 | — | — |
| **Heavy metal antidote** | T45.8X1 | T45.8X2 | T45.8X3 | T45.8X4 | T45.8X5 | T45.8X6 |
| **Hedaquinium** | T49.ØX1 | T49.ØX2 | T49.ØX3 | T49.ØX4 | T49.ØX5 | T49.ØX6 |
| **Hedge hyssop** | T62.2X1 | T62.2X2 | T62.2X3 | T62.2X4 | — | — |
| **Heet** | T49.8X1 | T49.8X2 | T49.8X3 | T49.8X4 | T49.8X5 | T49.8X6 |
| **Helenin** | T37.4X1 | T37.4X2 | T37.4X3 | T37.4X4 | T37.4X5 | T37.4X6 |
| **Helium** (nonmedicinal) **NEC** | T59.891 | T59.892 | T59.893 | T59.894 | — | — |
| medicinal | T48.991 | T48.992 | T48.993 | T48.994 | T48.995 | T48.996 |
| **Hellebore** (black) (green) (white) | T62.2X1 | T62.2X2 | T62.2X3 | T62.2X4 | — | — |
| **Hematin** | T45.8X1 | T45.8X2 | T45.8X3 | T45.8X4 | T45.8X5 | T45.8X6 |
| **Hematinic preparation** | T45.8X1 | T45.8X2 | T45.8X3 | T45.8X4 | T45.8X5 | T45.8X6 |
| **Hematological agent** | T45.91 | T45.92 | T45.93 | T45.94 | T45.95 | T45.96 |
| specified NEC | T45.8X1 | T45.8X2 | T45.8X3 | T45.8X4 | T45.8X5 | T45.8X6 |
| **Hemlock** | T62.2X1 | T62.2X2 | T62.2X3 | T62.2X4 | — | — |
| **Hemostatic** | T45.621 | T45.622 | T45.623 | T45.624 | T45.625 | T45.626 |
| drug, systemic | T45.621 | T45.622 | T45.623 | T45.624 | T45.625 | T45.626 |
| **Hemostyptic** | T49.4X1 | T49.4X2 | T49.4X3 | T49.4X4 | T49.4X5 | T49.4X6 |
| **Henbane** | T62.2X1 | T62.2X2 | T62.2X3 | T62.2X4 | — | — |
| **Heparin** (sodium) | T45.511 | T45.512 | T45.513 | T45.514 | T45.515 | T45.516 |
| action reverser | T45.7X1 | T45.7X2 | T45.7X3 | T45.7X4 | T45.7X5 | T45.7X6 |
| **Heparin-fraction** | T45.511 | T45.512 | T45.513 | T45.514 | T45.515 | T45.516 |
| **Heparinoid** (systemic) | T45.511 | T45.512 | T45.513 | T45.514 | T45.515 | T45.516 |
| **Hepatic secretion stimulant** | T47.8X1 | T47.8X2 | T47.8X3 | T47.8X4 | T47.8X5 | T47.8X6 |
| **Hepatitis A vaccine*** | T5Ø.B91 | T5Ø.B92 | T5Ø.B93 | T5Ø.B94 | T5Ø.B95 | T5Ø.B96 |
| **Hepatitis B** | | | | | | |
| immune globulin | T5Ø.Z11 | T5Ø.Z12 | T5Ø.Z13 | T5Ø.Z14 | T5Ø.Z15 | T5Ø.Z16 |
| vaccine | T5Ø.B91 | T5Ø.B92 | T5Ø.B93 | T5Ø.B94 | T5Ø.B95 | T5Ø.B96 |
| **Hepronicate** | T46.7X1 | T46.7X2 | T46.7X3 | T46.7X4 | T46.7X5 | T46.7X6 |
| **Heptabarb** | T42.3X1 | T42.3X2 | T42.3X3 | T42.3X4 | T42.3X5 | T42.3X6 |
| **Heptabarbital** | T42.3X1 | T42.3X2 | T42.3X3 | T42.3X4 | T42.3X5 | T42.3X6 |
| **Heptabarbitone** | T42.3X1 | T42.3X2 | T42.3X3 | T42.3X4 | T42.3X5 | T42.3X6 |
| **Heptachlor** | T6Ø.1X1 | T6Ø.1X2 | T6Ø.1X3 | T6Ø.1X4 | — | — |
| **Heptalgin** | T4Ø.2X1 | T4Ø.2X2 | T4Ø.2X3 | T4Ø.2X4 | T4Ø.2X5 | T4Ø.2X6 |
| **Heptaminol** | T46.3X1 | T46.3X2 | T46.3X3 | T46.3X4 | T46.3X5 | T46.3X6 |
| **Herbicide NEC** | T6Ø.3X1 | T6Ø.3X2 | T6Ø.3X3 | T6Ø.3X4 | — | — |
| **Heroin** | T4Ø.1X1 | T4Ø.1X2 | T4Ø.1X3 | T4Ø.1X4 | — | — |
| **Herplex** | T49.5X1 | T49.5X2 | T49.5X3 | T49.5X4 | T49.5X5 | T49.5X6 |
| **HES** | T45.8X1 | T45.8X2 | T45.8X3 | T45.8X4 | T45.8X5 | T45.8X6 |
| **Hesperidin** | T46.991 | T46.992 | T46.993 | T46.994 | T46.995 | T46.996 |
| **Hetacillin** | T36.ØX1 | T36.ØX2 | T36.ØX3 | T36.ØX4 | T36.ØX5 | T36.ØX6 |
| **Hetastarch** | T45.8X1 | T45.8X2 | T45.8X3 | T45.8X4 | T45.8X5 | T45.8X6 |
| **HETP** | T6Ø.ØX1 | T6Ø.ØX2 | T6Ø.ØX3 | T6Ø.ØX4 | — | — |
| **Hexa-germ** | T49.2X1 | T49.2X2 | T49.2X3 | T49.2X4 | T49.2X5 | T49.2X6 |
| **Hexachlorobenzene** (vapor) | T6Ø.3X1 | T6Ø.3X2 | T6Ø.3X3 | T6Ø.3X4 | — | — |
| **Hexachlorocyclohexane** | T53.6X1 | T53.6X2 | T53.6X3 | T53.6X4 | — | — |
| **Hexachlorophene** | T49.ØX1 | T49.ØX2 | T49.ØX3 | T49.ØX4 | T49.ØX5 | T49.ØX6 |
| **Hexadiline** | T46.3X1 | T46.3X2 | T46.3X3 | T46.3X4 | T46.3X5 | T46.3X6 |
| **Hexadimethrine** (bromide) | T45.7X1 | T45.7X2 | T45.7X3 | T45.7X4 | T45.7X5 | T45.7X6 |
| **Hexadylamine** | T46.3X1 | T46.3X2 | T46.3X3 | T46.3X4 | T46.3X5 | T46.3X6 |
| **Hexaethyl tetraphosphate** | T6Ø.ØX1 | T6Ø.ØX2 | T6Ø.ØX3 | T6Ø.ØX4 | — | — |
| **Hexafluorenium bromide** | T48.1X1 | T48.1X2 | T48.1X3 | T48.1X4 | T48.1X5 | T48.1X6 |
| **Hexafluronium** (bromide) | T48.1X1 | T48.1X2 | T48.1X3 | T48.1X4 | T48.1X5 | T48.1X6 |
| **Hexahydrobenzol** | T52.891 | T52.892 | T52.893 | T52.894 | — | — |
| **Hexahydrocresol**(s) | T51.8X1 | T51.8X2 | T51.8X3 | T51.8X4 | — | — |

| Substance | Poisoning, Accidental (unintentional) | Poisoning, Intentional Self-harm | Poisoning, Assault | Poisoning, Undetermined | Adverse Effect | Under-dosing |
|---|---|---|---|---|---|---|
| **Hexahydrocresol**(s) — *continued* | | | | | | |
| arsenide | T57.ØX1 | T57.ØX2 | T57.ØX3 | T57.ØX4 | — | — |
| arseniurated | T57.ØX1 | T57.ØX2 | T57.ØX3 | T57.ØX4 | — | — |
| cyanide | T57.3X1 | T57.3X2 | T57.3X3 | T57.3X4 | — | — |
| gas | T59.891 | T59.892 | T59.893 | T59.894 | — | — |
| Fluoride (liquid) | T57.8X1 | T57.8X2 | T57.8X3 | T57.8X4 | — | — |
| vapor | T59.891 | T59.892 | T59.893 | T59.894 | — | — |
| phophorated | T6Ø.ØX1 | T6Ø.ØX2 | T6Ø.ØX3 | T6Ø.ØX4 | — | — |
| sulfate | T57.8X1 | T57.8X2 | T57.8X3 | T57.8X4 | — | — |
| sulfide (gas) | T59.6X1 | T59.6X2 | T59.6X3 | T59.6X4 | — | — |
| arseniurated | T57.ØX1 | T57.ØX2 | T57.ØX3 | T57.ØX4 | — | — |
| sulfurated | T57.8X1 | T57.8X2 | T57.8X3 | T57.8X4 | — | — |
| **Hexahydrophenol** | T51.8X1 | T51.8X2 | T51.8X3 | T51.8X4 | — | — |
| **Hexalen** | T51.8X1 | T51.8X2 | T51.8X3 | T51.8X4 | — | — |
| **Hexamethonium bromide** | T44.2X1 | T44.2X2 | T44.2X3 | T44.2X4 | T44.2X5 | T44.2X6 |
| **Hexamethylene** | T52.821 | T52.822 | T52.823 | T52.824 | — | — |
| diisocyanate | T59.821 | T59.822 | T59.823 | T59.824 | — | — |
| **Hexamethylmelamine** | T45.1X1 | T45.1X2 | T45.1X3 | T45.1X4 | T45.1X5 | T45.1X6 |
| **Hexamidine** | T49.ØX1 | T49.ØX2 | T49.ØX3 | T49.ØX4 | T49.ØX5 | T49.ØX6 |
| **Hexamine** (mandelate) | T37.8X1 | T37.8X2 | T37.8X3 | T37.8X4 | T37.8X5 | T37.8X6 |
| **Hexanone, 2-hexanone** | T52.4X1 | T52.4X2 | T52.4X3 | T52.4X4 | — | — |
| **Hexanuorenium** | T48.1X1 | T48.1X2 | T48.1X3 | T48.1X4 | T48.1X5 | T48.1X6 |
| **Hexapropymate** | T42.6X1 | T42.6X2 | T42.6X3 | T42.6X4 | T42.6X5 | T42.6X6 |
| **Hexasonium iodide** | T44.3X1 | T44.3X2 | T44.3X3 | T44.3X4 | T44.3X5 | T44.3X6 |
| **Hexcarbacholine bromide** | T48.1X1 | T48.1X2 | T48.1X3 | T48.1X4 | T48.1X5 | T48.1X6 |
| **Hexemal** | T42.3X1 | T42.3X2 | T42.3X3 | T42.3X4 | T42.3X5 | T42.3X6 |
| **Hexestrol** | T38.5X1 | T38.5X2 | T38.5X3 | T38.5X4 | T38.5X5 | T38.5X6 |
| **Hexethal** (sodium) | T42.3X1 | T42.3X2 | T42.3X3 | T42.3X4 | T42.3X5 | T42.3X6 |
| **Hexetidine** | T37.8X1 | T37.8X2 | T37.8X3 | T37.8X4 | T37.8X5 | T37.8X6 |
| **Hexobarbital** | T42.3X1 | T42.3X2 | T42.3X3 | T42.3X4 | T42.3X5 | T42.3X6 |
| rectal | T41.291 | T41.292 | T41.293 | T41.294 | T41.295 | T41.296 |
| sodium | T41.1X1 | T41.1X2 | T41.1X3 | T41.1X4 | T41.1X5 | T41.1X6 |
| **Hexobendine** | T46.3X1 | T46.3X2 | T46.3X3 | T46.3X4 | T46.3X5 | T46.3X6 |
| **Hexocyclium** | T44.3X1 | T44.3X2 | T44.3X3 | T44.3X4 | T44.3X5 | T44.3X6 |
| metilsulfate | T44.3X1 | T44.3X2 | T44.3X3 | T44.3X4 | T44.3X5 | T44.3X6 |
| **Hexoestrol** | T38.5X1 | T38.5X2 | T38.5X3 | T38.5X4 | T38.5X5 | T38.5X6 |
| **Hexone** | T52.4X1 | T52.4X2 | T52.4X3 | T52.4X4 | — | — |
| **Hexoprenaline** | T48.6X1 | T48.6X2 | T48.6X3 | T48.6X4 | T48.6X5 | T48.6X6 |
| **Hexylcaine** | T41.3X1 | T41.3X2 | T41.3X3 | T41.3X4 | T41.3X5 | T41.3X6 |
| **Hexylresorcinol** | T52.2X1 | T52.2X2 | T52.2X3 | T52.2X4 | — | — |
| **HGH** (human growth hormone) | T38.811 | T38.812 | T38.813 | T38.814 | T38.815 | T38.816 |
| **Hibistat*** | T49.ØX1 | T49.ØX2 | T49.ØX3 | T49.ØX4 | T49.ØX5 | T49.ØX6 |
| **Hinkle's pills** | T47.2X1 | T47.2X2 | T47.2X3 | T47.2X4 | T47.2X5 | T47.2X6 |
| **Histalog** | T5Ø.8X1 | T5Ø.8X2 | T5Ø.8X3 | T5Ø.8X4 | T5Ø.8X5 | T5Ø.8X6 |
| **Histamine** (phosphate) | T5Ø.8X1 | T5Ø.8X2 | T5Ø.8X3 | T5Ø.8X4 | T5Ø.8X5 | T5Ø.8X6 |
| **Histolyn*** | T5Ø.8X1 | T5Ø.8X2 | T5Ø.8X3 | T5Ø.8X4 | T5Ø.8X5 | T5Ø.8X6 |
| **Histoplasmin** | T5Ø.8X1 | T5Ø.8X2 | T5Ø.8X3 | T5Ø.8X4 | T5Ø.8X5 | T5Ø.8X6 |
| **Holly berries** | T62.2X1 | T62.2X2 | T62.2X3 | T62.2X4 | — | — |
| **Homatropine** | T44.3X1 | T44.3X2 | T44.3X3 | T44.3X4 | T44.3X5 | T44.3X6 |
| methylbromide | T44.3X1 | T44.3X2 | T44.3X3 | T44.3X4 | T44.3X5 | T44.3X6 |
| **Homo-tet** | T5Ø.Z11 | T5Ø.Z12 | T5Ø.Z13 | T5Ø.Z14 | T5Ø.Z15 | T5Ø.Z16 |
| **Homochlorcyclizine** | T45.ØX1 | T45.ØX2 | T45.ØX3 | T45.ØX4 | T45.ØX5 | T45.ØX6 |
| **Homosalate** | T49.3X1 | T49.3X2 | T49.3X3 | T49.3X4 | T49.3X5 | T49.3X6 |
| **Hormone** | T38.8Ø1 | T38.8Ø2 | T38.8Ø3 | T38.8Ø4 | T38.8Ø5 | T38.8Ø6 |
| adrenal cortical steroids | T38.ØX1 | T38.ØX2 | T38.ØX3 | T38.ØX4 | T38.ØX5 | T38.ØX6 |
| androgenic | T38.7X1 | T38.7X2 | T38.7X3 | T38.7X4 | T38.7X5 | T38.7X6 |
| anterior pituitary NEC | T38.811 | T38.812 | T38.813 | T38.814 | T38.815 | T38.816 |
| antidiabetic agents | T38.3X1 | T38.3X2 | T38.3X3 | T38.3X4 | T38.3X5 | T38.3X6 |
| antidiuretic | T38.891 | T38.892 | T38.893 | T38.894 | T38.895 | T38.896 |
| cancer therapy | T45.1X1 | T45.1X2 | T45.1X3 | T45.1X4 | T45.1X5 | T45.1X6 |
| follicle stimulating | T38.811 | T38.812 | T38.813 | T38.814 | T38.815 | T38.816 |
| gonadotropic | T38.891 | T38.892 | T38.893 | T38.894 | T38.895 | T38.896 |
| pituitary | T38.811 | T38.812 | T38.813 | T38.814 | T38.815 | T38.816 |
| growth | T38.811 | T38.812 | T38.813 | T38.814 | T38.815 | T38.816 |
| luteinizing | T38.811 | T38.812 | T38.813 | T38.814 | T38.815 | T38.816 |
| ovarian | T38.5X1 | T38.5X2 | T38.5X3 | T38.5X4 | T38.5X5 | T38.5X6 |
| oxytocic | T48.ØX1 | T48.ØX2 | T48.ØX3 | T48.ØX4 | T48.ØX5 | T48.ØX6 |
| parathyroid (derivatives) | T5Ø.991 | T5Ø.992 | T5Ø.993 | T5Ø.994 | T5Ø.995 | T5Ø.996 |
| pituitary (posterior) NEC | T38.891 | T38.892 | T38.893 | T38.894 | T38.895 | T38.896 |
| anterior | T38.811 | T38.812 | T38.813 | T38.814 | T38.815 | T38.816 |
| specified, NEC | T38.891 | T38.892 | T38.893 | T38.894 | T38.895 | T38.896 |
| thyroid | T38.1X1 | T38.1X2 | T38.1X3 | T38.1X4 | T38.1X5 | T38.1X6 |
| **Hornet** (sting) | T63.451 | T63.452 | T63.453 | T63.454 | — | — |
| **Horse anti-human lymphocytic serum** | T5Ø.Z11 | T5Ø.Z12 | T5Ø.Z13 | T5Ø.Z14 | T5Ø.Z15 | T5Ø.Z16 |
| **Horticulture agent NEC** | T65.91 | T65.92 | T65.93 | T65.94 | — | — |
| with pesticide | T6Ø.91 | T6Ø.92 | T6Ø.93 | T6Ø.94 | — | — |
| **Human** | | | | | | |
| albumin | T45.8X1 | T45.8X2 | T45.8X3 | T45.8X4 | T45.8X5 | T45.8X6 |
| growth hormone (HGH) | T38.811 | T38.812 | T38.813 | T38.814 | T38.815 | T38.816 |
| immune serum | T5Ø.Z11 | T5Ø.Z12 | T5Ø.Z13 | T5Ø.Z14 | T5Ø.Z15 | T5Ø.Z16 |

| Substance | Poisoning, Accidental (unintentional) | Poisoning, Intentional Self-harm | Poisoning, Assault | Poisoning, Undetermined | Adverse Effect | Under-dosing |
|---|---|---|---|---|---|---|
| **Hyaluronidase** | T45.3X1 | T45.3X2 | T45.3X3 | T45.3X4 | T45.3X5 | T45.3X |
| **Hyazyme** | T45.3X1 | T45.3X2 | T45.3X3 | T45.3X4 | T45.3X5 | T45.3X |
| **Hycodan** | T4Ø.2X1 | T4Ø.2X2 | T4Ø.2X3 | T4Ø.2X4 | T4Ø.2X5 | T4Ø.2X |
| **Hydantoin derivative NEC** | T42.ØX1 | T42.ØX2 | T42.ØX3 | T42.ØX4 | T42.ØX5 | T42.ØX |
| **Hydeltra** | T38.ØX1 | T38.ØX2 | T38.ØX3 | T38.ØX4 | T38.ØX5 | T38.ØX |
| **Hydergine** | T44.6X1 | T44.6X2 | T44.6X3 | T44.6X4 | T44.6X5 | T44.6X |
| **Hydrabamine penicillin** | T36.ØX1 | T36.ØX2 | T36.ØX3 | T36.ØX4 | T36.ØX5 | T36.ØX |
| **Hydralazine** | T46.5X1 | T46.5X2 | T46.5X3 | T46.5X4 | T46.5X5 | T46.5X |
| **Hydrargaphen** | T49.ØX1 | T49.ØX2 | T49.ØX3 | T49.ØX4 | T49.ØX5 | T49.ØX |
| **Hydrargyri aminochloridum** | T49.ØX1 | T49.ØX2 | T49.ØX3 | T49.ØX4 | T49.ØX5 | T49.ØX |
| **Hydrastine** | T48.291 | T48.292 | T48.293 | T48.294 | T48.295 | T48.29 |
| **Hydrazine** | T54.1X1 | T54.1X2 | T54.1X3 | T54.1X4 | — | — |
| monoamine oxidase inhibitors | T43.1X1 | T43.1X2 | T43.1X3 | T43.1X4 | T43.1X5 | T43.1X |
| **Hydrazoic acid, azides** | T54.2X1 | T54.2X2 | T54.2X3 | T54.2X4 | — | — |
| **Hydriodic acid** | T48.4X1 | T48.4X2 | T48.4X3 | T48.4X4 | T48.4X5 | T48.4X |
| **Hydrisalic*** | T49.4X1 | T49.4X2 | T49.4X3 | T49.4X4 | T49.4X5 | T49.4X |
| **Hydro-ride*** | T5Ø.2X1 | T5Ø.2X2 | T5Ø.2X3 | T5Ø.2X4 | T5Ø.2X5 | T5Ø.2X |
| **Hydrocarbon gas** | T59.891 | T59.892 | T59.893 | T59.894 | — | — |
| incomplete combustion of — *see* Carbon, monoxide, fuel, utility | | | | | | |
| liquefied (mobile container) | T59.891 | T59.892 | T59.893 | T59.894 | — | — |
| piped (natural) | T59.891 | T59.892 | T59.893 | T59.894 | — | — |
| **Hydrochloric acid** (liquid) | T54.2X1 | T54.2X2 | T54.2X3 | T54.2X4 | — | — |
| medicinal (digestant) | T47.5X1 | T47.5X2 | T47.5X3 | T47.5X4 | T47.5X5 | T47.5X |
| vapor | T59.891 | T59.892 | T59.893 | T59.894 | — | — |
| **Hydrochlorothiazide** | T5Ø.2X1 | T5Ø.2X2 | T5Ø.2X3 | T5Ø.2X4 | T5Ø.2X5 | T5Ø.2X |
| **Hydrocodone** | T4Ø.2X1 | T4Ø.2X2 | T4Ø.2X3 | T4Ø.2X4 | T4Ø.2X5 | T4Ø.2X |
| **Hydrocortisone** (derivatives) | T38.ØX1 | T38.ØX2 | T38.ØX3 | T38.ØX4 | T38.ØX5 | T38.ØX |
| aceponate | T49.ØX1 | T49.ØX2 | T49.ØX3 | T49.ØX4 | T49.ØX5 | T49.ØX |
| ENT agent | T49.6X1 | T49.6X2 | T49.6X3 | T49.6X4 | T49.6X5 | T49.6X |
| ophthalmic preparation | T49.5X1 | T49.5X2 | T49.5X3 | T49.5X4 | T49.5X5 | T49.5X |
| topical NEC | T49.ØX1 | T49.ØX2 | T49.ØX3 | T49.ØX4 | T49.ØX5 | T49.ØX |
| **Hydrocortone** | T38.ØX1 | T38.ØX2 | T38.ØX3 | T38.ØX4 | T38.ØX5 | T38.ØX |
| ENT agent | T49.6X1 | T49.6X2 | T49.6X3 | T49.6X4 | T49.6X5 | T49.6X |
| ophthalmic preparation | T49.5X1 | T49.5X2 | T49.5X3 | T49.5X4 | T49.5X5 | T49.5X |
| topical NEC | T49.ØX1 | T49.ØX2 | T49.ØX3 | T49.ØX4 | T49.ØX5 | T49.ØX |
| **Hydrocyanic acid** (liquid) | T57.3X1 | T57.3X2 | T57.3X3 | T57.3X4 | — | — |
| gas | T65.ØX1 | T65.ØX2 | T65.ØX3 | T65.ØX4 | — | — |
| **Hydroflumethiazide** | T5Ø.2X1 | T5Ø.2X2 | T5Ø.2X3 | T5Ø.2X4 | T5Ø.2X5 | T5Ø.2X |
| **Hydrofluoric acid** (liquid) | T54.2X1 | T54.2X2 | T54.2X3 | T54.2X4 | — | — |
| vapor | T59.891 | T59.892 | T59.893 | T59.894 | — | — |
| **Hydrogen** | T59.891 | T59.892 | T59.893 | T59.894 | — | — |
| arsenide | T57.ØX1 | T57.ØX2 | T57.ØX3 | T57.ØX4 | — | — |
| arseniureted | T57.ØX1 | T57.ØX2 | T57.ØX3 | T57.ØX4 | — | — |
| chloride | T57.8X1 | T57.8X2 | T57.8X3 | T57.8X4 | — | — |
| cyanide (salts) | T57.3X1 | T57.3X2 | T57.3X3 | T57.3X4 | — | — |
| gas | T57.3X1 | T57.3X2 | T57.3X3 | T57.3X4 | — | — |
| Fluoride | T59.5X1 | T59.5X2 | T59.5X3 | T59.5X4 | — | — |
| vapor | T59.5X1 | T59.5X2 | T59.5X3 | T59.5X4 | — | — |
| peroxide | T49.ØX1 | T49.ØX2 | T49.ØX3 | T49.ØX4 | T49.ØX5 | T49.ØX |
| phosphureted | T57.1X1 | T57.1X2 | T57.1X3 | T57.1X4 | — | — |
| sulfide | T59.6X1 | T59.6X2 | T59.6X3 | T59.6X4 | — | — |
| arseniureted | T57.ØX1 | T57.ØX2 | T57.ØX3 | T57.ØX4 | — | — |
| sulfureted | T59.6X1 | T59.6X2 | T59.6X3 | T59.6X4 | — | — |
| **Hydromethylpyridine** | T46.7X1 | T46.7X2 | T46.7X3 | T46.7X4 | T46.7X5 | T46.7X |
| **Hydromorphinol** | T4Ø.2X1 | T4Ø.2X2 | T4Ø.2X3 | T4Ø.2X4 | — | — |
| **Hydromorphinone** | T4Ø.2X1 | T4Ø.2X2 | T4Ø.2X3 | T4Ø.2X4 | T4Ø.2X5 | T4Ø.2X |
| **Hydromorphone** | T4Ø.2X1 | T4Ø.2X2 | T4Ø.2X3 | T4Ø.2X4 | T4Ø.2X5 | T4Ø.2X |
| **Hydromox** | T5Ø.2X1 | T5Ø.2X2 | T5Ø.2X3 | T5Ø.2X4 | T5Ø.2X5 | T5Ø.2X |
| **Hydrophilic lotion** | T49.3X1 | T49.3X2 | T49.3X3 | T49.3X4 | T49.3X5 | T49.3X |
| **Hydroquinidine** | T46.2X1 | T46.2X2 | T46.2X3 | T46.2X4 | T46.2X5 | T46.2X |
| **Hydroquinone** | T52.2X1 | T52.2X2 | T52.2X3 | T52.2X4 | — | — |
| vapor | T59.891 | T59.892 | T59.893 | T59.894 | — | — |
| **Hydrosulfuric acid** (gas) | T59.6X1 | T59.6X2 | T59.6X3 | T59.6X4 | — | — |
| **Hydrotalcite** | T47.1X1 | T47.1X2 | T47.1X3 | T47.1X4 | T47.1X5 | T47.1X |
| **Hydrous wool fat** | T49.3X1 | T49.3X2 | T49.3X3 | T49.3X4 | T49.3X5 | T49.3X |
| **Hydroxide, caustic** | T54.3X1 | T54.3X2 | T54.3X3 | T54.3X4 | — | — |
| **Hydroxocobalamin** | T45.8X1 | T45.8X2 | T45.8X3 | T45.8X4 | T45.8X5 | T45.8X |
| **Hydroxyamphetamine** | T49.5X1 | T49.5X2 | T49.5X3 | T49.5X4 | T49.5X5 | T49.5X |
| **Hydroxycarbamide** | T45.1X1 | T45.1X2 | T45.1X3 | T45.1X4 | T45.1X5 | T45.1X |
| **Hydroxychloroquine** | T37.8X1 | T37.8X2 | T37.8X3 | T37.8X4 | T37.8X5 | T37.8X |
| **Hydroxydaunorubicin*** | T45.1X1 | T45.1X2 | T45.1X3 | T45.1X4 | T45.1X5 | T45.1X |
| **Hydroxydihydrocodeinone** | T4Ø.2X1 | T4Ø.2X2 | T4Ø.2X3 | T4Ø.2X4 | T4Ø.2X5 | T4Ø.2X |
| **Hydroxyestrone** | T38.5X1 | T38.5X2 | T38.5X3 | T38.5X4 | T38.5X5 | T38.5X |
| **Hydroxyethyl starch** | T45.8X1 | T45.8X2 | T45.8X3 | T45.8X4 | T45.8X5 | T45.8X |
| **Hydroxymethylpentanone** | T52.4X1 | T52.4X2 | T52.4X3 | T52.4X4 | — | — |
| **Hydroxyphenamate** | T43.591 | T43.592 | T43.593 | T43.594 | T43.595 | T43.59 |
| **Hydroxyphenylbutazone** | T39.2X1 | T39.2X2 | T39.2X3 | T39.2X4 | T39.2X5 | T39.2X |

| Substance | Poisoning, Accidental (unintentional) | Poisoning, Intentional Self-harm | Poisoning, Assault | Poisoning, Undetermined | Adverse Effect | Under-dosing |
|---|---|---|---|---|---|---|
| **Hydroxyprogesterone** | T38.5X1 | T38.5X2 | T38.5X3 | T38.5X4 | T38.5X5 | T38.5X6 |
| caproate | T38.5X1 | T38.5X2 | T38.5X3 | T38.5X4 | T38.5X5 | T38.5X6 |
| **Hydroxyquinoline** (derivatives) **NEC** | T37.8X1 | T37.8X2 | T37.8X3 | T37.8X4 | T37.8X5 | T37.8X6 |
| **Hydroxystilbamidine** | T37.3X1 | T37.3X2 | T37.3X3 | T37.3X4 | T37.3X5 | T37.3X6 |
| **Hydroxytoluene** (nonmedicinal) | T54.ØX1 | T54.ØX2 | T54.ØX3 | T54.ØX4 | — | — |
| medicinal | T49.ØX1 | T49.ØX2 | T49.ØX3 | T49.ØX4 | T49.ØX5 | T49.ØX6 |
| **Hydroxyurea** | T45.1X1 | T45.1X2 | T45.1X3 | T45.1X4 | T45.1X5 | T45.1X6 |
| **Hydroxyzine** | T43.591 | T43.592 | T43.593 | T43.594 | T43.595 | T43.596 |
| antiallergic | T45.ØX1 | T45.ØX2 | T45.ØX3 | T45.ØX4 | T45.ØX5 | T45.ØX6 |
| **Hyoscine** | T44.3X1 | T44.3X2 | T44.3X3 | T44.3X4 | T44.3X5 | T44.3X6 |
| **Hyoscyamine** | T44.3X1 | T44.3X2 | T44.3X3 | T44.3X4 | T44.3X5 | T44.3X6 |
| **Hyoscyamus** | T44.3X1 | T44.3X2 | T44.3X3 | T44.3X4 | T44.3X5 | T44.3X6 |
| dry extract | T44.3X1 | T44.3X2 | T44.3X3 | T44.3X4 | T44.3X5 | T44.3X6 |
| **Hypaque** | T5Ø.8X1 | T5Ø.8X2 | T5Ø.8X3 | T5Ø.8X4 | T5Ø.8X5 | T5Ø.8X6 |
| **HyperRAB*** | T5Ø.Z11 | T5Ø.Z12 | T5Ø.Z13 | T5Ø.Z14 | T5Ø.Z15 | T5Ø.Z16 |
| **Hypertussis** | T5Ø.Z11 | T5Ø.Z12 | T5Ø.Z13 | T5Ø.Z14 | T5Ø.Z15 | T5Ø.Z16 |
| **Hypnotic** | T42.71 | T42.72 | T42.73 | T42.74 | T42.75 | T42.76 |
| anticonvulsant | T42.71 | T42.72 | T42.73 | T42.74 | T42.75 | T42.76 |
| specified NEC | T42.6X1 | T42.6X2 | T42.6X3 | T42.6X4 | T42.6X5 | T42.6X6 |
| **Hypochlorite** | T49.ØX1 | T49.ØX2 | T49.ØX3 | T49.ØX4 | T49.ØX5 | T49.ØX6 |
| **Hypophysis, posterior** | T38.891 | T38.892 | T38.893 | T38.894 | T38.895 | T38.896 |
| **Hypotensive NEC** | T46.5X1 | T46.5X2 | T46.5X3 | T46.5X4 | T46.5X5 | T46.5X6 |
| **Hypromellose** | T49.5X1 | T49.5X2 | T49.5X3 | T49.5X4 | T49.5X5 | T49.5X6 |
| **I-thyroxine sodium** | T38.1X1 | T38.1X2 | T38.1X3 | T38.1X4 | T38.1X5 | T38.1X6 |
| **Ibacitabine** | T37.5X1 | T37.5X2 | T37.5X3 | T37.5X4 | T37.5X5 | T37.5X6 |
| **Ibopamine** | T44.991 | T44.992 | T44.993 | T44.994 | T44.995 | T44.996 |
| **Ibufenac** | T39.311 | T39.312 | T39.313 | T39.314 | T39.315 | T39.316 |
| **Ibuprofen** | T39.311 | T39.312 | T39.313 | T39.314 | T39.315 | T39.316 |
| **Ibuproxam** | T39.311 | T39.312 | T39.313 | T39.314 | T39.315 | T39.316 |
| **Ibuterol** | T48.6X1 | T48.6X2 | T48.6X3 | T48.6X4 | T48.6X5 | T48.6X6 |
| **Ichthammol** | T49.ØX1 | T49.ØX2 | T49.ØX3 | T49.ØX4 | T49.ØX5 | T49.ØX6 |
| **Ichthyol** | T49.4X1 | T49.4X2 | T49.4X3 | T49.4X4 | T49.4X5 | T49.4X6 |
| **Idarubicin** | T45.1X1 | T45.1X2 | T45.1X3 | T45.1X4 | T45.1X5 | T45.1X6 |
| **Idrocilamide** | T42.8X1 | T42.8X2 | T42.8X3 | T42.8X4 | T42.8X5 | T42.8X6 |
| **Ifenprodil** | T46.7X1 | T46.7X2 | T46.7X3 | T46.7X4 | T46.7X5 | T46.7X6 |
| **Ifosfamide** | T45.1X1 | T45.1X2 | T45.1X3 | T45.1X4 | T45.1X5 | T45.1X6 |
| **Iletin** | T38.3X1 | T38.3X2 | T38.3X3 | T38.3X4 | T38.3X5 | T38.3X6 |
| **Ilex** | T62.2X1 | T62.2X2 | T62.2X3 | T62.2X4 | — | — |
| **Illuminating gas** (after combustion) | T58.11 | T58.12 | T58.13 | T58.14 | — | — |
| prior to combustion | T59.891 | T59.892 | T59.893 | T59.894 | — | — |
| **Ilopan** | T45.2X1 | T45.2X2 | T45.2X3 | T45.2X4 | T45.2X5 | T45.2X6 |
| **Iloprost** | T46.7X1 | T46.7X2 | T46.7X3 | T46.7X4 | T46.7X5 | T46.7X6 |
| **Ilotycin** | T36.3X1 | T36.3X2 | T36.3X3 | T36.3X4 | T36.3X5 | T36.3X6 |
| ophthalmic preparation | T49.5X1 | T49.5X2 | T49.5X3 | T49.5X4 | T49.5X5 | T49.5X6 |
| topical NEC | T49.ØX1 | T49.ØX2 | T49.ØX3 | T49.ØX4 | T49.ØX5 | T49.ØX6 |
| **Imdur*** | T46.3X1 | T46.3X2 | T46.3X3 | T46.3X4 | T46.3X5 | T46.3X6 |
| **Imidazole-4-carboxamide** | T45.1X1 | T45.1X2 | T45.1X3 | T45.1X4 | T45.1X5 | T45.1X6 |
| **Iminostilbene** | T42.1X1 | T42.1X2 | T42.1X3 | T42.1X4 | T42.1X5 | T42.1X6 |
| **Imipenem** | T36.ØX1 | T36.ØX2 | T36.ØX3 | T36.ØX4 | T36.ØX5 | T36.ØX6 |
| **Imipramine** | T43.Ø11 | T43.Ø12 | T43.Ø13 | T43.Ø14 | T43.Ø15 | T43.Ø16 |
| **Immu-G** | T5Ø.Z11 | T5Ø.Z12 | T5Ø.Z13 | T5Ø.Z14 | T5Ø.Z15 | T5Ø.Z16 |
| **Immu-tetanus** | T5Ø.Z11 | T5Ø.Z12 | T5Ø.Z13 | T5Ø.Z14 | T5Ø.Z15 | T5Ø.Z16 |
| **Immuglobin** | T5Ø.Z11 | T5Ø.Z12 | T5Ø.Z13 | T5Ø.Z14 | T5Ø.Z15 | T5Ø.Z16 |
| **Immune** | | | | | | |
| checkpoint inhibitors | T45.AX1 | T45.AX2 | T45.AX3 | T45.AX4 | T45.AX5 | T45.AX6 |
| globulin | T5Ø.Z11 | T5Ø.Z12 | T5Ø.Z13 | T5Ø.Z14 | T5Ø.Z15 | T5Ø.Z16 |
| serum globulin | T5Ø.Z11 | T5Ø.Z12 | T5Ø.Z13 | T5Ø.Z14 | T5Ø.Z15 | T5Ø.Z16 |
| **Immunoglobin human** (intravenous) (normal) | T5Ø.Z11 | T5Ø.Z12 | T5Ø.Z13 | T5Ø.Z14 | T5Ø.Z15 | T5Ø.Z16 |
| unmodified | T5Ø.Z11 | T5Ø.Z12 | T5Ø.Z13 | T5Ø.Z14 | T5Ø.Z15 | T5Ø.Z16 |
| **Immunostimulant drug** | T45.AX1 | T45.AX2 | T45.AX3 | T45.AX4 | T45.AX5 | T45.AX6 |
| **Immunosuppressive drug** | T45.1X1 | T45.1X2 | T45.1X3 | T45.1X4 | T45.1X5 | T45.1X6 |
| **Indalpine** | T43.221 | T43.222 | T43.223 | T43.224 | T43.225 | T43.226 |
| **Indanazoline** | T48.5X1 | T48.5X2 | T48.5X3 | T48.5X4 | T48.5X5 | T48.5X6 |
| **Indandione** (derivatives) | T45.511 | T45.512 | T45.513 | T45.514 | T45.515 | T45.516 |
| **Indapamide** | T46.5X1 | T46.5X2 | T46.5X3 | T46.5X4 | T46.5X5 | T46.5X6 |
| **Indendione** (derivatives) | T45.511 | T45.512 | T45.513 | T45.514 | T45.515 | T45.516 |
| **Indenolol** | T44.7X1 | T44.7X2 | T44.7X3 | T44.7X4 | T44.7X5 | T44.7X6 |
| **Inderal** | T44.7X1 | T44.7X2 | T44.7X3 | T44.7X4 | T44.7X5 | T44.7X6 |
| **Indian** | | | | | | |
| hemp | T4Ø.711 | T4Ø.712 | T4Ø.713 | T4Ø.714 | T4Ø.715 | T4Ø.716 |
| tobacco | T62.2X1 | T62.2X2 | T62.2X3 | T62.2X4 | — | — |
| **Indigo carmine** | T5Ø.8X1 | T5Ø.8X2 | T5Ø.8X3 | T5Ø.8X4 | T5Ø.8X5 | T5Ø.8X6 |
| **Indobufen** | T45.521 | T45.522 | T45.523 | T45.524 | T45.525 | T45.526 |
| **Indocin** | T39.2X1 | T39.2X2 | T39.2X3 | T39.2X4 | T39.2X5 | T39.2X6 |
| **Indocyanine green** | T5Ø.8X1 | T5Ø.8X2 | T5Ø.8X3 | T5Ø.8X4 | T5Ø.8X5 | T5Ø.8X6 |
| **Indometacin** | T39.391 | T39.392 | T39.393 | T39.394 | T39.395 | T39.396 |
| **Indomethacin** | T39.391 | T39.392 | T39.393 | T39.394 | T39.395 | T39.396 |
| farnesil | T39.4X1 | T39.4X2 | T39.4X3 | T39.4X4 | T39.4X5 | T39.4X6 |
| **Indoramin** | T44.6X1 | T44.6X2 | T44.6X3 | T44.6X4 | T44.6X5 | T44.6X6 |

| Substance | Poisoning, Accidental (unintentional) | Poisoning, Intentional Self-harm | Poisoning, Assault | Poisoning, Undetermined | Adverse Effect | Under-dosing |
|---|---|---|---|---|---|---|
| **Industrial** | | | | | | |
| alcohol | T51.ØX1 | T51.ØX2 | T51.ØX3 | T51.ØX4 | — | — |
| fumes | T59.891 | T59.892 | T59.893 | T59.894 | — | — |
| solvents (fumes) (vapors) | T52.91 | T52.92 | T52.93 | T52.94 | — | — |
| **Inflectra*** | T39.4X1 | T39.4X2 | T39.4X3 | T39.4X4 | T39.4X5 | T39.4X6 |
| **Influenza vaccine** | T5Ø.B91 | T5Ø.B92 | T5Ø.B93 | T5Ø.B94 | T5Ø.B95 | T5Ø.B96 |
| **Ingested substance NEC** | T65.91 | T65.92 | T65.93 | T65.94 | — | — |
| **INH** | T37.1X1 | T37.1X2 | T37.1X3 | T37.1X4 | T37.1X5 | T37.1X6 |
| **Inhalation, gas** (noxious) — *see* Gas | | | | | | |
| **Inhibitor** | | | | | | |
| angiotensin-converting enzyme | T46.4X1 | T46.4X2 | T46.4X3 | T46.4X4 | T46.4X5 | T46.4X6 |
| carbonic anhydrase | T5Ø.2X1 | T5Ø.2X2 | T5Ø.2X3 | T5Ø.2X4 | T5Ø.2X5 | T5Ø.2X6 |
| fibrinolysis | T45.621 | T45.622 | T45.623 | T45.624 | T45.625 | T45.626 |
| monoamine oxidase NEC | T43.1X1 | T43.1X2 | T43.1X3 | T43.1X4 | T43.1X5 | T43.1X6 |
| hydrazine | T43.1X1 | T43.1X2 | T43.1X3 | T43.1X4 | T43.1X5 | T43.1X6 |
| postsynaptic | T43.8X1 | T43.8X2 | T43.8X3 | T43.8X4 | T43.8X5 | T43.8X6 |
| prothrombin synthesis | T45.511 | T45.512 | T45.513 | T45.514 | T45.515 | T45.516 |
| **Ink** | T65.891 | T65.892 | T65.893 | T65.894 | — | — |
| **Innopran*** | T44.7X1 | T44.7X2 | T44.7X3 | T44.7X4 | T44.7X5 | T44.7X6 |
| **Inorganic substance NEC** | T57.91 | T57.92 | T57.93 | T57.94 | — | — |
| **Inosine pranobex** | T37.5X1 | T37.5X2 | T37.5X3 | T37.5X4 | T37.5X5 | T37.5X6 |
| **Inositol** | T5Ø.991 | T5Ø.992 | T5Ø.993 | T5Ø.994 | T5Ø.995 | T5Ø.996 |
| nicotinate | T46.7X1 | T46.7X2 | T46.7X3 | T46.7X4 | T46.7X5 | T46.7X6 |
| **Inproquone** | T45.1X1 | T45.1X2 | T45.1X3 | T45.1X4 | T45.1X5 | T45.1X6 |
| **Insect** (sting), venomous | T63.481 | T63.482 | T63.483 | T63.484 | — | — |
| ant | T63.421 | T63.422 | T63.423 | T63.424 | — | — |
| bee | T63.441 | T63.442 | T63.443 | T63.444 | — | — |
| caterpillar | T63.431 | T63.432 | T63.433 | T63.434 | — | — |
| hornet | T63.451 | T63.452 | T63.453 | T63.454 | — | — |
| wasp | T63.461 | T63.462 | T63.463 | T63.464 | — | — |
| **Insecticide NEC** | T6Ø.91 | T6Ø.92 | T6Ø.93 | T6Ø.94 | — | — |
| carbamate | T6Ø.ØX1 | T6Ø.ØX2 | T6Ø.ØX3 | T6Ø.ØX4 | — | — |
| chlorinated | T6Ø.1X1 | T6Ø.1X2 | T6Ø.1X3 | T6Ø.1X4 | — | — |
| mixed | T6Ø.91 | T6Ø.92 | T6Ø.93 | T6Ø.94 | — | — |
| organochlorine | T6Ø.1X1 | T6Ø.1X2 | T6Ø.1X3 | T6Ø.1X4 | — | — |
| organophosphorus | T6Ø.ØX1 | T6Ø.ØX2 | T6Ø.ØX3 | T6Ø.ØX4 | — | — |
| **Insular tissue extract** | T38.3X1 | T38.3X2 | T38.3X3 | T38.3X4 | T38.3X5 | T38.3X6 |
| **Insulin** (amorphous) (globin) (isophane) (Lente) (NPH) (Semilente) (Ultralente) | T38.3X1 | T38.3X2 | T38.3X3 | T38.3X4 | T38.3X5 | T38.3X6 |
| defalan | T38.3X1 | T38.3X2 | T38.3X3 | T38.3X4 | T38.3X5 | T38.3X6 |
| human | T38.3X1 | T38.3X2 | T38.3X3 | T38.3X4 | T38.3X5 | T38.3X6 |
| injection, soluble | T38.3X1 | T38.3X2 | T38.3X3 | T38.3X4 | T38.3X5 | T38.3X6 |
| biphasic | T38.3X1 | T38.3X2 | T38.3X3 | T38.3X4 | T38.3X5 | T38.3X6 |
| intermediate acting | T38.3X1 | T38.3X2 | T38.3X3 | T38.3X4 | T38.3X5 | T38.3X6 |
| protamine zinc | T38.3X1 | T38.3X2 | T38.3X3 | T38.3X4 | T38.3X5 | T38.3X6 |
| slow acting | T38.3X1 | T38.3X2 | T38.3X3 | T38.3X4 | T38.3X5 | T38.3X6 |
| zinc | | | | | | |
| protamine injection | T38.3X1 | T38.3X2 | T38.3X3 | T38.3X4 | T38.3X5 | T38.3X6 |
| suspension (amorphous) (crystalline) | T38.3X1 | T38.3X2 | T38.3X3 | T38.3X4 | T38.3X5 | T38.3X6 |
| **Interferon** (alpha) (beta) (gamma) | T37.5X1 | T37.5X2 | T37.5X3 | T37.5X4 | T37.5X5 | T37.5X6 |
| **Intestinal motility control drug** | T47.6X1 | T47.6X2 | T47.6X3 | T47.6X4 | T47.6X5 | T47.6X6 |
| biological | T47.8X1 | T47.8X2 | T47.8X3 | T47.8X4 | T47.8X5 | T47.8X6 |
| **Intranarcon** | T41.1X1 | T41.1X2 | T41.1X3 | T41.1X4 | T41.1X5 | T41.1X6 |
| **Intravenous** | | | | | | |
| amino acids | T5Ø.991 | T5Ø.992 | T5Ø.993 | T5Ø.994 | T5Ø.995 | T5Ø.996 |
| fat suspension | T5Ø.991 | T5Ø.992 | T5Ø.993 | T5Ø.994 | T5Ø.995 | T5Ø.996 |
| **Inulin** | T5Ø.8X1 | T5Ø.8X2 | T5Ø.8X3 | T5Ø.8X4 | T5Ø.8X5 | T5Ø.8X6 |
| **Invanz*** | T36.1X1 | T36.1X2 | T36.1X3 | T36.1X4 | T36.1X5 | T36.1X6 |
| **Invert sugar** | T5Ø.3X1 | T5Ø.3X2 | T5Ø.3X3 | T5Ø.3X4 | T5Ø.3X5 | T5Ø.3X6 |
| **Inza** — *see* Naproxen | | | | | | |
| **Iobenzamic acid** | T5Ø.8X1 | T5Ø.8X2 | T5Ø.8X3 | T5Ø.8X4 | T5Ø.8X5 | T5Ø.8X6 |
| **Iocarmic acid** | T5Ø.8X1 | T5Ø.8X2 | T5Ø.8X3 | T5Ø.8X4 | T5Ø.8X5 | T5Ø.8X6 |
| **Iocetamic acid** | T5Ø.8X1 | T5Ø.8X2 | T5Ø.8X3 | T5Ø.8X4 | T5Ø.8X5 | T5Ø.8X6 |
| **Iodamide** | T5Ø.8X1 | T5Ø.8X2 | T5Ø.8X3 | T5Ø.8X4 | T5Ø.8X5 | T5Ø.8X6 |
| **Iodide NEC** — *see also* Iodine | T49.ØX1 | T49.ØX2 | T49.ØX3 | T49.ØX4 | T49.ØX5 | T49.ØX6 |
| mercury (ointment) | T49.ØX1 | T49.ØX2 | T49.ØX3 | T49.ØX4 | T49.ØX5 | T49.ØX6 |
| methylate | T49.ØX1 | T49.ØX2 | T49.ØX3 | T49.ØX4 | T49.ØX5 | T49.ØX6 |
| potassium (expectorant) NEC | T48.4X1 | T48.4X2 | T48.4X3 | T48.4X4 | T48.4X5 | T48.4X6 |
| **Iodinated** | | | | | | |
| contrast medium | T5Ø.8X1 | T5Ø.8X2 | T5Ø.8X3 | T5Ø.8X4 | T5Ø.8X5 | T5Ø.8X6 |
| glycerol | T48.4X1 | T48.4X2 | T48.4X3 | T48.4X4 | T48.4X5 | T48.4X6 |
| human serum albumin (131I) | T5Ø.8X1 | T5Ø.8X2 | T5Ø.8X3 | T5Ø.8X4 | T5Ø.8X5 | T5Ø.8X6 |
| **Iodine** (antiseptic, external) (tincture) **NEC** | T49.ØX1 | T49.ØX2 | T49.ØX3 | T49.ØX4 | T49.ØX5 | T49.ØX6 |

| Substance | Poisoning, Accidental (unintentional) | Poisoning, Intentional Self-harm | Poisoning, Assault | Poisoning, Undetermined | Adverse Effect | Under-dosing |
|---|---|---|---|---|---|---|
| **Iodine** (antiseptic, external) (tincture) **NEC** — *continued* | | | | | | |
| 125 — *see also* Radiation sickness, and exposure to radioactive isotopes | T5Ø.8X1 | T5Ø.8X2 | T5Ø.8X3 | T5Ø.8X4 | T5Ø.8X5 | T5Ø.8X6 |
| therapeutic | T5Ø.991 | T5Ø.992 | T5Ø.993 | T5Ø.994 | T5Ø.995 | T5Ø.996 |
| 131 — *see also* Radiation sickness, and exposure to radioactive isotopes | T5Ø.8X1 | T5Ø.8X2 | T5Ø.8X3 | T5Ø.8X4 | T5Ø.8X5 | T5Ø.8X6 |
| therapeutic | T38.2X1 | T38.2X2 | T38.2X3 | T38.2X4 | T38.2X5 | T38.2X6 |
| diagnostic | T5Ø.8X1 | T5Ø.8X2 | T5Ø.8X3 | T5Ø.8X4 | T5Ø.8X5 | T5Ø.8X6 |
| for thyroid conditions (antithyroid) | T38.2X1 | T38.2X2 | T38.2X3 | T38.2X4 | T38.2X5 | T38.2X6 |
| solution | T49.ØX1 | T49.ØX2 | T49.ØX3 | T49.ØX4 | T49.ØX5 | T49.ØX6 |
| vapor | T59.891 | T59.892 | T59.893 | T59.894 | — | — |
| **Iodipamide** | T5Ø.8X1 | T5Ø.8X2 | T5Ø.8X3 | T5Ø.8X4 | T5Ø.8X5 | T5Ø.8X6 |
| **Iodized** (poppy seed) oil | T5Ø.8X1 | T5Ø.8X2 | T5Ø.8X3 | T5Ø.8X4 | T5Ø.8X5 | T5Ø.8X6 |
| **Iodobismitol** | T37.8X1 | T37.8X2 | T37.8X3 | T37.8X4 | T37.8X5 | T37.8X6 |
| **Iodochlorhydroxyquin** | T37.8X1 | T37.8X2 | T37.8X3 | T37.8X4 | T37.8X5 | T37.8X6 |
| topical | T49.ØX1 | T49.ØX2 | T49.ØX3 | T49.ØX4 | T49.ØX5 | T49.ØX6 |
| **Iodochlorhydroxyquinoline** | T37.8X1 | T37.8X2 | T37.8X3 | T37.8X4 | T37.8X5 | T37.8X6 |
| **Iodocholesterol** (131I) | T5Ø.8X1 | T5Ø.8X2 | T5Ø.8X3 | T5Ø.8X4 | T5Ø.8X5 | T5Ø.8X6 |
| **Iodoform** | T49.ØX1 | T49.ØX2 | T49.ØX3 | T49.ØX4 | T49.ØX5 | T49.ØX6 |
| **Iodohippuric acid** | T5Ø.8X1 | T5Ø.8X2 | T5Ø.8X3 | T5Ø.8X4 | T5Ø.8X5 | T5Ø.8X6 |
| **Iodopanoic acid** | T5Ø.8X1 | T5Ø.8X2 | T5Ø.8X3 | T5Ø.8X4 | T5Ø.8X5 | T5Ø.8X6 |
| **Iodophthalein** (sodium) | T5Ø.8X1 | T5Ø.8X2 | T5Ø.8X3 | T5Ø.8X4 | T5Ø.8X5 | T5Ø.8X6 |
| **Iodopyracet** | T5Ø.8X1 | T5Ø.8X2 | T5Ø.8X3 | T5Ø.8X4 | T5Ø.8X5 | T5Ø.8X6 |
| **Iodoquinol** | T37.8X1 | T37.8X2 | T37.8X3 | T37.8X4 | T37.8X5 | T37.8X6 |
| **Iodoxamic acid** | T5Ø.8X1 | T5Ø.8X2 | T5Ø.8X3 | T5Ø.8X4 | T5Ø.8X5 | T5Ø.8X6 |
| **Iofendylate** | T5Ø.8X1 | T5Ø.8X2 | T5Ø.8X3 | T5Ø.8X4 | T5Ø.8X5 | T5Ø.8X6 |
| **Ioglycamic acid** | T5Ø.8X1 | T5Ø.8X2 | T5Ø.8X3 | T5Ø.8X4 | T5Ø.8X5 | T5Ø.8X6 |
| **Iohexol** | T5Ø.8X1 | T5Ø.8X2 | T5Ø.8X3 | T5Ø.8X4 | T5Ø.8X5 | T5Ø.8X6 |
| **Ion exchange resin** | | | | | | |
| anion | T47.8X1 | T47.8X2 | T47.8X3 | T47.8X4 | T47.8X5 | T47.8X6 |
| cation | T5Ø.3X1 | T5Ø.3X2 | T5Ø.3X3 | T5Ø.3X4 | T5Ø.3X5 | T5Ø.3X6 |
| cholestyramine | T46.6X1 | T46.6X2 | T46.6X3 | T46.6X4 | T46.6X5 | T46.6X6 |
| intestinal | T47.8X1 | T47.8X2 | T47.8X3 | T47.8X4 | T47.8X5 | T47.8X6 |
| **Iopamidol** | T5Ø.8X1 | T5Ø.8X2 | T5Ø.8X3 | T5Ø.8X4 | T5Ø.8X5 | T5Ø.8X6 |
| **Iopanoic acid** | T5Ø.8X1 | T5Ø.8X2 | T5Ø.8X3 | T5Ø.8X4 | T5Ø.8X5 | T5Ø.8X6 |
| **Iophenoic acid** | T5Ø.8X1 | T5Ø.8X2 | T5Ø.8X3 | T5Ø.8X4 | T5Ø.8X5 | T5Ø.8X6 |
| **Iopodate, sodium** | T5Ø.8X1 | T5Ø.8X2 | T5Ø.8X3 | T5Ø.8X4 | T5Ø.8X5 | T5Ø.8X6 |
| **Iopodic acid** | T5Ø.8X1 | T5Ø.8X2 | T5Ø.8X3 | T5Ø.8X4 | T5Ø.8X5 | T5Ø.8X6 |
| **Iopromide** | T5Ø.8X1 | T5Ø.8X2 | T5Ø.8X3 | T5Ø.8X4 | T5Ø.8X5 | T5Ø.8X6 |
| **Iopydol** | T5Ø.8X1 | T5Ø.8X2 | T5Ø.8X3 | T5Ø.8X4 | T5Ø.8X5 | T5Ø.8X6 |
| **Iotalamic acid** | T5Ø.8X1 | T5Ø.8X2 | T5Ø.8X3 | T5Ø.8X4 | T5Ø.8X5 | T5Ø.8X6 |
| **Iothalamate** | T5Ø.8X1 | T5Ø.8X2 | T5Ø.8X3 | T5Ø.8X4 | T5Ø.8X5 | T5Ø.8X6 |
| **Iothiouracil** | T38.2X1 | T38.2X2 | T38.2X3 | T38.2X4 | T38.2X5 | T38.2X6 |
| **Iotrol** | T5Ø.8X1 | T5Ø.8X2 | T5Ø.8X3 | T5Ø.8X4 | T5Ø.8X5 | T5Ø.8X6 |
| **Iotrolan** | T5Ø.8X1 | T5Ø.8X2 | T5Ø.8X3 | T5Ø.8X4 | T5Ø.8X5 | T5Ø.8X6 |
| **Iotroxate** | T5Ø.8X1 | T5Ø.8X2 | T5Ø.8X3 | T5Ø.8X4 | T5Ø.8X5 | T5Ø.8X6 |
| **Iotroxic acid** | T5Ø.8X1 | T5Ø.8X2 | T5Ø.8X3 | T5Ø.8X4 | T5Ø.8X5 | T5Ø.8X6 |
| **Ioversol** | T5Ø.8X1 | T5Ø.8X2 | T5Ø.8X3 | T5Ø.8X4 | T5Ø.8X5 | T5Ø.8X6 |
| **Ioxaglate** | T5Ø.8X1 | T5Ø.8X2 | T5Ø.8X3 | T5Ø.8X4 | T5Ø.8X5 | T5Ø.8X6 |
| **Ioxaglic acid** | T5Ø.8X1 | T5Ø.8X2 | T5Ø.8X3 | T5Ø.8X4 | T5Ø.8X5 | T5Ø.8X6 |
| **Ioxitalamic acid** | T5Ø.8X1 | T5Ø.8X2 | T5Ø.8X3 | T5Ø.8X4 | T5Ø.8X5 | T5Ø.8X6 |
| **Ipecac** | T47.7X1 | T47.7X2 | T47.7X3 | T47.7X4 | T47.7X5 | T47.7X6 |
| **Ipecacuanha** | T48.4X1 | T48.4X2 | T48.4X3 | T48.4X4 | T48.4X5 | T48.4X6 |
| **Ipodate, calcium** | T5Ø.8X1 | T5Ø.8X2 | T5Ø.8X3 | T5Ø.8X4 | T5Ø.8X5 | T5Ø.8X6 |
| **IPOL*** | T5Ø.B91 | T5Ø.B92 | T5Ø.B93 | T5Ø.B94 | T5Ø.B95 | T5Ø.B96 |
| **Ipral** | T42.3X1 | T42.3X2 | T42.3X3 | T42.3X4 | T42.3X5 | T42.3X6 |
| **Ipratropium** (bromide) | T48.6X1 | T48.6X2 | T48.6X3 | T48.6X4 | T48.6X5 | T48.6X6 |
| **Ipriflavone** | T46.3X1 | T46.3X2 | T46.3X3 | T46.3X4 | T46.3X5 | T46.3X6 |
| **Iprindole** | T43.Ø11 | T43.Ø12 | T43.Ø13 | T43.Ø14 | T43.Ø15 | T43.Ø16 |
| **Iproclozide** | T43.1X1 | T43.1X2 | T43.1X3 | T43.1X4 | T43.1X5 | T43.1X6 |
| **Iprofenin** | T5Ø.8X1 | T5Ø.8X2 | T5Ø.8X3 | T5Ø.8X4 | T5Ø.8X5 | T5Ø.8X6 |
| **Iproheptine** | T49.2X1 | T49.2X2 | T49.2X3 | T49.2X4 | T49.2X5 | T49.2X6 |
| **Iproniazid** | T43.1X1 | T43.1X2 | T43.1X3 | T43.1X4 | T43.1X5 | T43.1X6 |
| **Iproplatin** | T45.1X1 | T45.1X2 | T45.1X3 | T45.1X4 | T45.1X5 | T45.1X6 |
| **Iproveratril** | T46.1X1 | T46.1X2 | T46.1X3 | T46.1X4 | T46.1X5 | T46.1X6 |
| **Irinotecan*** | T45.1X1 | T45.1X2 | T45.1X3 | T45.1X4 | T45.1X5 | T45.1X6 |
| **Iron** (compounds) (medicinal) **NEC** | T45.4X1 | T45.4X2 | T45.4X3 | T45.4X4 | T45.4X5 | T45.4X6 |
| ammonium | T45.4X1 | T45.4X2 | T45.4X3 | T45.4X4 | T45.4X5 | T45.4X6 |
| dextran injection | T45.4X1 | T45.4X2 | T45.4X3 | T45.4X4 | T45.4X5 | T45.4X6 |
| nonmedicinal | T56.891 | T56.892 | T56.893 | T56.894 | — | — |
| salts | T45.4X1 | T45.4X2 | T45.4X3 | T45.4X4 | T45.4X5 | T45.4X6 |
| sorbitex | T45.4X1 | T45.4X2 | T45.4X3 | T45.4X4 | T45.4X5 | T45.4X6 |
| sorbitol citric acid complex | T45.4X1 | T45.4X2 | T45.4X3 | T45.4X4 | T45.4X5 | T45.4X6 |
| **Irrigating fluid** (vaginal) | T49.8X1 | T49.8X2 | T49.8X3 | T49.8X4 | T49.8X5 | T49.8X6 |
| eye | T49.5X1 | T49.5X2 | T49.5X3 | T49.5X4 | T49.5X5 | T49.5X6 |
| **Isepamicin** | T36.5X1 | T36.5X2 | T36.5X3 | T36.5X4 | T36.5X5 | T36.5X6 |
| **Isoaminile** (citrate) | T48.3X1 | T48.3X2 | T48.3X3 | T48.3X4 | T48.3X5 | T48.3X6 |
| **Isoamyl nitrite** | T46.3X1 | T46.3X2 | T46.3X3 | T46.3X4 | T46.3X5 | T46.3X6 |

| Substance | Poisoning, Accidental (unintentional) | Poisoning, Intentional Self-harm | Poisoning, Assault | Poisoning, Undetermined | Adverse Effect | Under-dosing |
|---|---|---|---|---|---|---|
| **Isobenzan** | T6Ø.1X1 | T6Ø.1X2 | T6Ø.1X3 | T6Ø.1X4 | — | — |
| **Isobutyl acetate** | T52.891 | T52.892 | T52.893 | T52.894 | — | — |
| **Isocarboxazid** | T43.1X1 | T43.1X2 | T43.1X3 | T43.1X4 | T43.1X5 | T43.1X6 |
| **Isoconazole** | T49.ØX1 | T49.ØX2 | T49.ØX3 | T49.ØX4 | T49.ØX5 | T49.ØX6 |
| **Isocyanate** | T65.ØX1 | T65.ØX2 | T65.ØX3 | T65.ØX4 | — | — |
| **Isoephedrine** | T44.991 | T44.992 | T44.993 | T44.994 | T44.995 | T44.996 |
| **Isoetarine** | T48.6X1 | T48.6X2 | T48.6X3 | T48.6X4 | T48.6X5 | T48.6X6 |
| **Isoethadione** | T42.2X1 | T42.2X2 | T42.2X3 | T42.2X4 | T42.2X5 | T42.2X6 |
| **Isoetharine** | T44.5X1 | T44.5X2 | T44.5X3 | T44.5X4 | T44.5X5 | T44.5X6 |
| **Isoflurane** | T41.ØX1 | T41.ØX2 | T41.ØX3 | T41.ØX4 | T41.ØX5 | T41.ØX6 |
| **Isoflurophate** | T44.ØX1 | T44.ØX2 | T44.ØX3 | T44.ØX4 | T44.ØX5 | T44.ØX6 |
| **Isomaltose, ferric complex** | T45.4X1 | T45.4X2 | T45.4X3 | T45.4X4 | T45.4X5 | T45.4X6 |
| **Isometheptene** | T44.3X1 | T44.3X2 | T44.3X3 | T44.3X4 | T44.3X5 | T44.3X6 |
| **Isoniazid** | T37.1X1 | T37.1X2 | T37.1X3 | T37.1X4 | T37.1X5 | T37.1X6 |
| with | | | | | | |
| rifampicin | T36.6X1 | T36.6X2 | T36.6X3 | T36.6X4 | T36.6X5 | T36.6X6 |
| thioacetazone | T37.1X1 | T37.1X2 | T37.1X3 | T37.1X4 | T37.1X5 | T37.1X6 |
| **Isonicotinic acid hydrazide** | T37.1X1 | T37.1X2 | T37.1X3 | T37.1X4 | T37.1X5 | T37.1X6 |
| **Isonipecaine** | T4Ø.491 | T4Ø.492 | T4Ø.493 | T4Ø.494 | T4Ø.495 | T4Ø.496 |
| **Isopentaquine** | T37.2X1 | T37.2X2 | T37.2X3 | T37.2X4 | T37.2X5 | T37.2X6 |
| **Isophane insulin** | T38.3X1 | T38.3X2 | T38.3X3 | T38.3X4 | T38.3X5 | T38.3X6 |
| **Isophorone** | T65.891 | T65.892 | T65.893 | T65.894 | — | — |
| **Isophosphamide** | T45.1X1 | T45.1X2 | T45.1X3 | T45.1X4 | T45.1X5 | T45.1X6 |
| **Isopregnenone** | T38.5X1 | T38.5X2 | T38.5X3 | T38.5X4 | T38.5X5 | T38.5X6 |
| **Isoprenaline** | T48.6X1 | T48.6X2 | T48.6X3 | T48.6X4 | T48.6X5 | T48.6X6 |
| **Isopromethazine** | T43.3X1 | T43.3X2 | T43.3X3 | T43.3X4 | T43.3X5 | T43.3X6 |
| **Isopropamide** | T44.3X1 | T44.3X2 | T44.3X3 | T44.3X4 | T44.3X5 | T44.3X6 |
| iodide | T44.3X1 | T44.3X2 | T44.3X3 | T44.3X4 | T44.3X5 | T44.3X6 |
| **Isopropanol** | T51.2X1 | T51.2X2 | T51.2X3 | T51.2X4 | — | — |
| **Isopropyl** | | | | | | |
| acetate | T52.891 | T52.892 | T52.893 | T52.894 | — | — |
| alcohol | T51.2X1 | T51.2X2 | T51.2X3 | T51.2X4 | — | — |
| medicinal | T49.4X1 | T49.4X2 | T49.4X3 | T49.4X4 | T49.4X5 | T49.4X6 |
| ether | T52.891 | T52.892 | T52.893 | T52.894 | — | — |
| **Isopropylaminophenazone** | T39.2X1 | T39.2X2 | T39.2X3 | T39.2X4 | T39.2X5 | T39.2X6 |
| **Isoproterenol** | T48.6X1 | T48.6X2 | T48.6X3 | T48.6X4 | T48.6X5 | T48.6X6 |
| **Isosorbide dinitrate** | T46.3X1 | T46.3X2 | T46.3X3 | T46.3X4 | T46.3X5 | T46.3X6 |
| **Isothipendyl** | T45.ØX1 | T45.ØX2 | T45.ØX3 | T45.ØX4 | T45.ØX5 | T45.ØX6 |
| **Isotretinoin** | T5Ø.991 | T5Ø.992 | T5Ø.993 | T5Ø.994 | T5Ø.995 | T5Ø.996 |
| **Isoxazolyl penicillin** | T36.ØX1 | T36.ØX2 | T36.ØX3 | T36.ØX4 | T36.ØX5 | T36.ØX6 |
| **Isoxicam** | T39.391 | T39.392 | T39.393 | T39.394 | T39.395 | T39.396 |
| **Isoxsuprine** | T46.7X1 | T46.7X2 | T46.7X3 | T46.7X4 | T46.7X5 | T46.7X6 |
| **Ispagula** | T47.4X1 | T47.4X2 | T47.4X3 | T47.4X4 | T47.4X5 | T47.4X6 |
| husk | T47.4X1 | T47.4X2 | T47.4X3 | T47.4X4 | T47.4X5 | T47.4X6 |
| **Isradipine** | T46.1X1 | T46.1X2 | T46.1X3 | T46.1X4 | T46.1X5 | T46.1X6 |
| **Itraconazole** | T37.8X1 | T37.8X2 | T37.8X3 | T37.8X4 | T37.8X5 | T37.8X6 |
| **Itramin tosilate** | T46.3X1 | T46.3X2 | T46.3X3 | T46.3X4 | T46.3X5 | T46.3X6 |
| **Ivarest*** | T41.3X1 | T41.3X2 | T41.3X3 | T41.3X4 | T41.3X5 | T41.3X6 |
| **Ivermectin** | T37.4X1 | T37.4X2 | T37.4X3 | T37.4X4 | T37.4X5 | T37.4X6 |
| **Izoniazid** | T37.1X1 | T37.1X2 | T37.1X3 | T37.1X4 | T37.1X5 | T37.1X6 |
| with thioacetazone | T37.1X1 | T37.1X2 | T37.1X3 | T37.1X4 | T37.1X5 | T37.1X6 |
| **Jalap** | T47.2X1 | T47.2X2 | T47.2X3 | T47.2X4 | T47.2X5 | T47.2X6 |
| **Jamaica** | | | | | | |
| dogwood (bark) | T39.8X1 | T39.8X2 | T39.8X3 | T39.8X4 | T39.8X5 | T39.8X6 |
| ginger | T65.891 | T65.892 | T65.893 | T65.894 | — | — |
| root | T62.2X1 | T62.2X2 | T62.2X3 | T62.2X4 | — | — |
| **Jantoven*** | T45.511 | T45.512 | T45.513 | T45.514 | T45.515 | T45.516 |
| **Jatropha** | T62.2X1 | T62.2X2 | T62.2X3 | T62.2X4 | — | — |
| curcas | T62.2X1 | T62.2X2 | T62.2X3 | T62.2X4 | — | — |
| **Jectofer** | T45.4X1 | T45.4X2 | T45.4X3 | T45.4X4 | T45.4X5 | T45.4X6 |
| **Jellyfish** (sting) | T63.621 | T63.622 | T63.623 | T63.624 | — | — |
| **Jequirity** (bean) | T62.2X1 | T62.2X2 | T62.2X3 | T62.2X4 | — | — |
| **Jimson weed** (stramonium) | T62.2X1 | T62.2X2 | T62.2X3 | T62.2X4 | — | — |
| seeds | T62.2X1 | T62.2X2 | T62.2X3 | T62.2X4 | — | — |
| **Josamycin** | T36.3X1 | T36.3X2 | T36.3X3 | T36.3X4 | T36.3X5 | T36.3X6 |
| **Juniper tar** | T49.1X1 | T49.1X2 | T49.1X3 | T49.1X4 | T49.1X5 | T49.1X6 |
| **Kaletra*** | T37.5X1 | T37.5X2 | T37.5X3 | T37.5X4 | T37.5X5 | T37.5X6 |
| **Kallidinogenase** | T46.7X1 | T46.7X2 | T46.7X3 | T46.7X4 | T46.7X5 | T46.7X6 |
| **Kallikrein** | T46.7X1 | T46.7X2 | T46.7X3 | T46.7X4 | T46.7X5 | T46.7X6 |
| **Kanamycin** | T36.5X1 | T36.5X2 | T36.5X3 | T36.5X4 | T36.5X5 | T36.5X6 |
| **Kantrex** | T36.5X1 | T36.5X2 | T36.5X3 | T36.5X4 | T36.5X5 | T36.5X6 |
| **Kaolin** | T47.6X1 | T47.6X2 | T47.6X3 | T47.6X4 | T47.6X5 | T47.6X6 |
| light | T47.6X1 | T47.6X2 | T47.6X3 | T47.6X4 | T47.6X5 | T47.6X6 |
| **Karaya** (gum) | T47.4X1 | T47.4X2 | T47.4X3 | T47.4X4 | T47.4X5 | T47.4X6 |
| **Kebuzone** | T39.2X1 | T39.2X2 | T39.2X3 | T39.2X4 | T39.2X5 | T39.2X6 |
| **Keflex*** | T36.1X1 | T36.1X2 | T36.1X3 | T36.1X4 | T36.1X5 | T36.1X6 |
| **Kelevan** | T6Ø.1X1 | T6Ø.1X2 | T6Ø.1X3 | T6Ø.1X4 | — | — |
| **Kemithal** | T41.1X1 | T41.1X2 | T41.1X3 | T41.1X4 | T41.1X5 | T41.1X6 |
| **Kenacort** | T38.ØX1 | T38.ØX2 | T38.ØX3 | T38.ØX4 | T38.ØX5 | T38.ØX6 |
| **Keratolytic drug NEC** | T49.4X1 | T49.4X2 | T49.4X3 | T49.4X4 | T49.4X5 | T49.4X6 |
| anthracene | T49.4X1 | T49.4X2 | T49.4X3 | T49.4X4 | T49.4X5 | T49.4X6 |
| **Keratoplastic NEC** | T49.4X1 | T49.4X2 | T49.4X3 | T49.4X4 | T49.4X5 | T49.4X6 |

| Substance | Poisoning, Accidental (unintentional) | Poisoning, Intentional Self-harm | Poisoning, Assault | Poisoning, Undetermined | Adverse Effect | Under-dosing |
|---|---|---|---|---|---|---|
| **Kerosene, kerosine** (fuel) (solvent) **NEC** | T52.ØX1 | T52.ØX2 | T52.ØX3 | T52.ØX4 | — | — |
| insecticide | T52.ØX1 | T52.ØX2 | T52.ØX3 | T52.ØX4 | — | — |
| vapor | T52.ØX1 | T52.ØX2 | T52.ØX3 | T52.ØX4 | — | — |
| **Ketamine** | T41.291 | T41.292 | T41.293 | T41.294 | T41.295 | T41.296 |
| **Ketazolam** | T42.4X1 | T42.4X2 | T42.4X3 | T42.4X4 | T42.4X5 | T42.4X6 |
| **Ketazon** | T39.2X1 | T39.2X2 | T39.2X3 | T39.2X4 | T39.2X5 | T39.2X6 |
| **Ketobemidone** | T4Ø.491 | T4Ø.492 | T4Ø.493 | T4Ø.494 | — | — |
| **Ketoconazole** | T49.ØX1 | T49.ØX2 | T49.ØX3 | T49.ØX4 | T49.ØX5 | T49.ØX6 |
| **Ketols** | T52.4X1 | T52.4X2 | T52.4X3 | T52.4X4 | — | — |
| **Ketone oils** | T52.4X1 | T52.4X2 | T52.4X3 | T52.4X4 | — | — |
| **Ketoprofen** | T39.311 | T39.312 | T39.313 | T39.314 | T39.315 | T39.316 |
| **Ketorolac** | T39.8X1 | T39.8X2 | T39.8X3 | T39.8X4 | T39.8X5 | T39.8X6 |
| **Ketotifen** | T45.ØX1 | T45.ØX2 | T45.ØX3 | T45.ØX4 | T45.ØX5 | T45.ØX6 |
| **Keytruda*** | T45.1X1 | T45.1X2 | T45.1X3 | T45.1X4 | T45.1X5 | T45.1X6 |
| **Khat** | T43.691 | T43.692 | T43.693 | T43.694 | — | — |
| **Khellin** | T46.3X1 | T46.3X2 | T46.3X3 | T46.3X4 | T46.3X5 | T46.3X6 |
| **Khelloside** | T46.3X1 | T46.3X2 | T46.3X3 | T46.3X4 | T46.3X5 | T46.3X6 |
| **Kiln gas or vapor** (carbon monoxide) | T58.8X1 | T58.8X2 | T58.8X3 | T58.8X4 | — | — |
| **Kineret*** | T39.4X1 | T39.4X2 | T39.4X3 | T39.4X4 | T39.4X5 | T39.4X6 |
| **Kitasamycin** | T36.3X1 | T36.3X2 | T36.3X3 | T36.3X4 | T36.3X5 | T36.3X6 |
| **Klonopin*** | T42.4X1 | T42.4X2 | T42.4X3 | T42.4X4 | T42.4X5 | T42.4X6 |
| **Komgiblyze*** | T38.3X1 | T38.3X2 | T38.3X3 | T38.3X4 | T38.3X5 | T38.3X6 |
| **Konsyl** | T47.4X1 | T47.4X2 | T47.4X3 | T47.4X4 | T47.4X5 | T47.4X6 |
| **Kosam seed** | T62.2X1 | T62.2X2 | T62.2X3 | T62.2X4 | — | — |
| **Krait** (venom) | T63.Ø91 | T63.Ø92 | T63.Ø93 | T63.Ø94 | — | — |
| **Kwell** (insecticide) | T6Ø.1X1 | T6Ø.1X2 | T6Ø.1X3 | T6Ø.1X4 | — | — |
| anti-infective (topical) | T49.ØX1 | T49.ØX2 | T49.ØX3 | T49.ØX4 | T49.ØX5 | T49.ØX6 |
| **L-dopa** | T42.8X1 | T42.8X2 | T42.8X3 | T42.8X4 | T42.8X5 | T42.8X6 |
| **L-Tryptophan** — *see* amino acid | | | | | | |
| **Labetalol** | T44.8X1 | T44.8X2 | T44.8X3 | T44.8X4 | T44.8X5 | T44.8X6 |
| **Laburnum** (seeds) | T62.2X1 | T62.2X2 | T62.2X3 | T62.2X4 | — | — |
| leaves | T62.2X1 | T62.2X2 | T62.2X3 | T62.2X4 | — | — |
| **Lachesine** | T49.5X1 | T49.5X2 | T49.5X3 | T49.5X4 | T49.5X5 | T49.5X6 |
| **Lacidipine** | T46.5X1 | T46.5X2 | T46.5X3 | T46.5X4 | T46.5X5 | T46.5X6 |
| **Lacquer** | T65.6X1 | T65.6X2 | T65.6X3 | T65.6X4 | — | — |
| **Lacrimogenic gas** | T59.3X1 | T59.3X2 | T59.3X3 | T59.3X4 | — | — |
| **Lactated potassic saline** | T5Ø.3X1 | T5Ø.3X2 | T5Ø.3X3 | T5Ø.3X4 | T5Ø.3X5 | T5Ø.3X6 |
| **Lactic acid** | T49.8X1 | T49.8X2 | T49.8X3 | T49.8X4 | T49.8X5 | T49.8X6 |
| **Lactobacillus** | | | | | | |
| acidophilus | T47.6X1 | T47.6X2 | T47.6X3 | T47.6X4 | T47.6X5 | T47.6X6 |
| compound | T47.6X1 | T47.6X2 | T47.6X3 | T47.6X4 | T47.6X5 | T47.6X6 |
| bifidus, lyophilized | T47.6X1 | T47.6X2 | T47.6X3 | T47.6X4 | T47.6X5 | T47.6X6 |
| bulgaricus | T47.6X1 | T47.6X2 | T47.6X3 | T47.6X4 | T47.6X5 | T47.6X6 |
| sporogenes | T47.6X1 | T47.6X2 | T47.6X3 | T47.6X4 | T47.6X5 | T47.6X6 |
| **Lactoflavin** | T45.2X1 | T45.2X2 | T45.2X3 | T45.2X4 | T45.2X5 | T45.2X6 |
| **Lactose** (as excipient) | T5Ø.9Ø1 | T5Ø.9Ø2 | T5Ø.9Ø3 | T5Ø.9Ø4 | T5Ø.9Ø5 | T5Ø.9Ø6 |
| **Lactuca** (virosa) (extract) | T42.6X1 | T42.6X2 | T42.6X3 | T42.6X4 | T42.6X5 | T42.6X6 |
| **Lactucarium** | T42.6X1 | T42.6X2 | T42.6X3 | T42.6X4 | T42.6X5 | T42.6X6 |
| **Lactulose** | T47.3X1 | T47.3X2 | T47.3X3 | T47.3X4 | T47.3X5 | T47.3X6 |
| **Laevo** — *see* Levo- | | | | | | |
| **Lanatosides** | T46.ØX1 | T46.ØX2 | T46.ØX3 | T46.ØX4 | T46.ØX5 | T46.ØX6 |
| **Lanolin** | T49.3X1 | T49.3X2 | T49.3X3 | T49.3X4 | T49.3X5 | T49.3X6 |
| **Lanoxin*** | T46.ØX1 | T46.ØX2 | T46.ØX3 | T46.ØX4 | T46.ØX5 | T46.ØX6 |
| **Largactil** | T43.3X1 | T43.3X2 | T43.3X3 | T43.3X4 | T43.3X5 | T43.3X6 |
| **Larkspur** | T62.2X1 | T62.2X2 | T62.2X3 | T62.2X4 | — | — |
| **Laroxyl** | T43.Ø11 | T43.Ø12 | T43.Ø13 | T43.Ø14 | T43.Ø15 | T43.Ø16 |
| **Lasix** | T5Ø.1X1 | T5Ø.1X2 | T5Ø.1X3 | T5Ø.1X4 | T5Ø.1X5 | T5Ø.1X6 |
| **Lassar's paste** | T49.4X1 | T49.4X2 | T49.4X3 | T49.4X4 | T49.4X5 | T49.4X6 |
| **Latamoxef** | T36.1X1 | T36.1X2 | T36.1X3 | T36.1X4 | T36.1X5 | T36.1X6 |
| **Latex** | T65.811 | T65.812 | T65.813 | T65.814 | — | — |
| **Lathyrus** (seed) | T62.2X1 | T62.2X2 | T62.2X3 | T62.2X4 | — | — |
| **Laudanum** | T4Ø.ØX1 | T4Ø.ØX2 | T4Ø.ØX3 | T4Ø.ØX4 | T4Ø.ØX5 | T4Ø.ØX6 |
| **Laudexium** | T48.1X1 | T48.1X2 | T48.1X3 | T48.1X4 | T48.1X5 | T48.1X6 |
| **Laughing gas** | T41.ØX1 | T41.ØX2 | T41.ØX3 | T41.ØX4 | T41.ØX5 | T41.ØX6 |
| **Laurel, black or cherry** | T62.2X1 | T62.2X2 | T62.2X3 | T62.2X4 | — | — |
| **Laurolinium** | T49.ØX1 | T49.ØX2 | T49.ØX3 | T49.ØX4 | T49.ØX5 | T49.ØX6 |
| **Lauryl sulfoacetate** | T49.2X1 | T49.2X2 | T49.2X3 | T49.2X4 | T49.2X5 | T49.2X6 |
| **Laxative NEC** | T47.4X1 | T47.4X2 | T47.4X3 | T47.4X4 | T47.4X5 | T47.4X6 |
| osmotic | T47.3X1 | T47.3X2 | T47.3X3 | T47.3X4 | T47.3X5 | T47.3X6 |
| saline | T47.3X1 | T47.3X2 | T47.3X3 | T47.3X4 | T47.3X5 | T47.3X6 |
| stimulant | T47.2X1 | T47.2X2 | T47.2X3 | T47.2X4 | T47.2X5 | T47.2X6 |
| **Lead** (dust) (fumes) (vapor) **NEC** | T56.ØX1 | T56.ØX2 | T56.ØX3 | T56.ØX4 | — | — |
| acetate | T49.2X1 | T49.2X2 | T49.2X3 | T49.2X4 | T49.2X5 | T49.2X6 |
| alkyl (fuel additive) | T56.ØX1 | T56.ØX2 | T56.ØX3 | T56.ØX4 | — | — |
| anti-infectives | T37.8X1 | T37.8X2 | T37.8X3 | T37.8X4 | T37.8X5 | T37.8X6 |
| antiknock compound (tetraethyl) | T56.ØX1 | T56.ØX2 | T56.ØX3 | T56.ØX4 | — | — |
| arsenate, arsenite (dust)(herbicide) (insecticide) (vapor) | T57.ØX1 | T57.ØX2 | T57.ØX3 | T57.ØX4 | — | — |
| **Lead** (dust) (fumes) (vapor) **NEC** — *continued* | | | | | | |
| carbonate | T56.ØX1 | T56.ØX2 | T56.ØX3 | T56.ØX4 | — | — |
| paint | T56.ØX1 | T56.ØX2 | T56.ØX3 | T56.ØX4 | — | — |
| chromate | T56.ØX1 | T56.ØX2 | T56.ØX3 | T56.ØX4 | — | — |
| paint | T56.ØX1 | T56.ØX2 | T56.ØX3 | T56.ØX4 | — | — |
| dioxide | T56.ØX1 | T56.ØX2 | T56.ØX3 | T56.ØX4 | — | — |
| inorganic | T56.ØX1 | T56.ØX2 | T56.ØX3 | T56.ØX4 | — | — |
| iodide | T56.ØX1 | T56.ØX2 | T56.ØX3 | T56.ØX4 | — | — |
| pigment (paint) | T56.ØX1 | T56.ØX2 | T56.ØX3 | T56.ØX4 | — | — |
| monoxide (dust) | T56.ØX1 | T56.ØX2 | T56.ØX3 | T56.ØX4 | — | — |
| paint | T56.ØX1 | T56.ØX2 | T56.ØX3 | T56.ØX4 | — | — |
| organic | T56.ØX1 | T56.ØX2 | T56.ØX3 | T56.ØX4 | — | — |
| oxide | T56.ØX1 | T56.ØX2 | T56.ØX3 | T56.ØX4 | — | — |
| paint | T56.ØX1 | T56.ØX2 | T56.ØX3 | T56.ØX4 | — | — |
| paint | T56.ØX1 | T56.ØX2 | T56.ØX3 | T56.ØX4 | — | — |
| salts | T56.ØX1 | T56.ØX2 | T56.ØX3 | T56.ØX4 | — | — |
| specified compound NEC | T56.ØX1 | T56.ØX2 | T56.ØX3 | T56.ØX4 | — | — |
| tetra-ethyl | T56.ØX1 | T56.ØX2 | T56.ØX3 | T56.ØX4 | — | — |
| **Lebanese red** | T4Ø.711 | T4Ø.712 | T4Ø.713 | T4Ø.714 | T4Ø.715 | T4Ø.716 |
| **Lefetamine** | T39.8X1 | T39.8X2 | T39.8X3 | T39.8X4 | T39.8X5 | T39.8X6 |
| **Lenperone** | T43.4X1 | T43.4X2 | T43.4X3 | T43.4X4 | T43.4X5 | T43.4X6 |
| **Lente Iletin** (insulin) | T38.3X1 | T38.3X2 | T38.3X3 | T38.3X4 | T38.3X5 | T38.3X6 |
| **Leptazol** | T5Ø.7X1 | T5Ø.7X2 | T5Ø.7X3 | T5Ø.7X4 | T5Ø.7X5 | T5Ø.7X6 |
| **Leptophos** | T6Ø.ØX1 | T6Ø.ØX2 | T6Ø.ØX3 | T6Ø.ØX4 | — | — |
| **Leritine** | T4Ø.2X1 | T4Ø.2X2 | T4Ø.2X3 | T4Ø.2X4 | T4Ø.2X5 | T4Ø.2X6 |
| **Lescol*** | T46.6X1 | T46.6X2 | T46.6X3 | T46.6X4 | T46.6X5 | T46.6X6 |
| **Letosteine** | T48.4X1 | T48.4X2 | T48.4X3 | T48.4X4 | T48.4X5 | T48.4X6 |
| **Letter** | T38.1X1 | T38.1X2 | T38.1X3 | T38.1X4 | T38.1X5 | T38.1X6 |
| **Lettuce opium** | T42.6X1 | T42.6X2 | T42.6X3 | T42.6X4 | T42.6X5 | T42.6X6 |
| **Leucinocaine** | T41.3X1 | T41.3X2 | T41.3X3 | T41.3X4 | T41.3X5 | T41.3X6 |
| **Leucocianidol** | T46.991 | T46.992 | T46.993 | T46.994 | T46.995 | T46.996 |
| **Leucovorin** (factor) | T45.8X1 | T45.8X2 | T45.8X3 | T45.8X4 | T45.8X5 | T45.8X6 |
| **Leukeran** | T45.1X1 | T45.1X2 | T45.1X3 | T45.1X4 | T45.1X5 | T45.1X6 |
| **Leuprolide** | T38.891 | T38.892 | T38.893 | T38.894 | T38.895 | T38.896 |
| **Levalbuterol** | T48.6X1 | T48.6X2 | T48.6X3 | T48.6X4 | T48.6X5 | T48.6X6 |
| **Levallorphan** | T5Ø.7X1 | T5Ø.7X2 | T5Ø.7X3 | T5Ø.7X4 | T5Ø.7X5 | T5Ø.7X6 |
| **Levamisole** | T37.4X1 | T37.4X2 | T37.4X3 | T37.4X4 | T37.4X5 | T37.4X6 |
| **Levanil** | T42.6X1 | T42.6X2 | T42.6X3 | T42.6X4 | T42.6X5 | T42.6X6 |
| **Levarterenol** | T44.4X1 | T44.4X2 | T44.4X3 | T44.4X4 | T44.4X5 | T44.4X6 |
| **Levdropropizine** | T48.3X1 | T48.3X2 | T48.3X3 | T48.3X4 | T48.3X5 | T48.3X6 |
| **Levo-dromoran** | T4Ø.2X1 | T4Ø.2X2 | T4Ø.2X3 | T4Ø.2X4 | T4Ø.2X5 | T4Ø.2X6 |
| **Levo-isomethadone** | T4Ø.3X1 | T4Ø.3X2 | T4Ø.3X3 | T4Ø.3X4 | T4Ø.3X5 | T4Ø.3X6 |
| **Levobunolol** | T49.5X1 | T49.5X2 | T49.5X3 | T49.5X4 | T49.5X5 | T49.5X6 |
| **Levocabastine** (hydrochloride) | T45.ØX1 | T45.ØX2 | T45.ØX3 | T45.ØX4 | T45.ØX5 | T45.ØX6 |
| **Levocarnitine** | T5Ø.991 | T5Ø.992 | T5Ø.993 | T5Ø.994 | T5Ø.995 | T5Ø.996 |
| **Levodopa** | T42.8X1 | T42.8X2 | T42.8X3 | T42.8X4 | T42.8X5 | T42.8X6 |
| with carbidopa | T42.8X1 | T42.8X2 | T42.8X3 | T42.8X4 | T42.8X5 | T42.8X6 |
| **Levoglutamide** | T5Ø.991 | T5Ø.992 | T5Ø.993 | T5Ø.994 | T5Ø.995 | T5Ø.996 |
| **Levoid** | T38.1X1 | T38.1X2 | T38.1X3 | T38.1X4 | T38.1X5 | T38.1X6 |
| **Levomepromazine** | T43.3X1 | T43.3X2 | T43.3X3 | T43.3X4 | T43.3X5 | T43.3X6 |
| **Levonordefrin** | T49.6X1 | T49.6X2 | T49.6X3 | T49.6X4 | T49.6X5 | T49.6X6 |
| **Levonorgestrel** | T38.4X1 | T38.4X2 | T38.4X3 | T38.4X4 | T38.4X5 | T38.4X6 |
| with ethinylestradiol | T38.5X1 | T38.5X2 | T38.5X3 | T38.5X4 | T38.5X5 | T38.5X6 |
| **Levopromazine** | T43.3X1 | T43.3X2 | T43.3X3 | T43.3X4 | T43.3X5 | T43.3X6 |
| **Levoprome** | T42.6X1 | T42.6X2 | T42.6X3 | T42.6X4 | T42.6X5 | T42.6X6 |
| **Levopropoxyphene** | T4Ø.491 | T4Ø.492 | T4Ø.493 | T4Ø.494 | T4Ø.495 | T4Ø.496 |
| **Levopropylhexedrine** | T5Ø.5X1 | T5Ø.5X2 | T5Ø.5X3 | T5Ø.5X4 | T5Ø.5X5 | T5Ø.5X6 |
| **Levoproxyphylline** | T48.6X1 | T48.6X2 | T48.6X3 | T48.6X4 | T48.6X5 | T48.6X6 |
| **Levorphanol** | T4Ø.491 | T4Ø.492 | T4Ø.493 | T4Ø.494 | T4Ø.495 | T4Ø.496 |
| **Levothroid*** | T38.1X1 | T38.1X2 | T38.1X3 | T38.1X4 | T38.1X5 | T38.1X6 |
| **Levothyroxine** | T38.1X1 | T38.1X2 | T38.1X3 | T38.1X4 | T38.1X5 | T38.1X6 |
| sodium | T38.1X1 | T38.1X2 | T38.1X3 | T38.1X4 | T38.1X5 | T38.1X6 |
| **Levoxyl*** | T38.1X1 | T38.1X2 | T38.1X3 | T38.1X4 | T38.1X5 | T38.1X6 |
| **Levsin** | T44.3X1 | T44.3X2 | T44.3X3 | T44.3X4 | T44.3X5 | T44.3X6 |
| **Levulose** | T5Ø.3X1 | T5Ø.3X2 | T5Ø.3X3 | T5Ø.3X4 | T5Ø.3X5 | T5Ø.3X6 |
| **Lewisite** (gas), not in war | T57.ØX1 | T57.ØX2 | T57.ØX3 | T57.ØX4 | — | — |
| **Lexapro*** | T43.221 | T43.222 | T43.223 | T43.224 | T43.225 | T43.226 |
| **Librium** | T42.4X1 | T42.4X2 | T42.4X3 | T42.4X4 | T42.4X5 | T42.4X6 |
| **Lidex** | T49.ØX1 | T49.ØX2 | T49.ØX3 | T49.ØX4 | T49.ØX5 | T49.ØX6 |
| **Lidocaine** | T41.3X1 | T41.3X2 | T41.3X3 | T41.3X4 | T41.3X5 | T41.3X6 |
| regional | T41.3X1 | T41.3X2 | T41.3X3 | T41.3X4 | T41.3X5 | T41.3X6 |
| spinal | T41.3X1 | T41.3X2 | T41.3X3 | T41.3X4 | T41.3X5 | T41.3X6 |
| **Lidofenin** | T5Ø.8X1 | T5Ø.8X2 | T5Ø.8X3 | T5Ø.8X4 | T5Ø.8X5 | T5Ø.8X6 |
| **Lidoflazine** | T46.1X1 | T46.1X2 | T46.1X3 | T46.1X4 | T46.1X5 | T46.1X6 |
| **Lighter fluid** | T52.ØX1 | T52.ØX2 | T52.ØX3 | T52.ØX4 | — | — |
| **Lignin hemicellulose** | T47.6X1 | T47.6X2 | T47.6X3 | T47.6X4 | T47.6X5 | T47.6X6 |
| **Lignocaine** | T41.3X1 | T41.3X2 | T41.3X3 | T41.3X4 | T41.3X5 | T41.3X6 |
| regional | T41.3X1 | T41.3X2 | T41.3X3 | T41.3X4 | T41.3X5 | T41.3X6 |
| spinal | T41.3X1 | T41.3X2 | T41.3X3 | T41.3X4 | T41.3X5 | T41.3X6 |
| **Ligroin** (e) (solvent) | T52.ØX1 | T52.ØX2 | T52.ØX3 | T52.ØX4 | — | — |
| vapor | T59.891 | T59.892 | T59.893 | T59.894 | — | — |

| Substance | Poisoning, Accidental (unintentional) | Poisoning, Intentional Self-harm | Poisoning, Assault | Poisoning, Undetermined | Adverse Effect | Under-dosing |
|---|---|---|---|---|---|---|
| **Ligustrum vulgare** | T62.2X1 | T62.2X2 | T62.2X3 | T62.2X4 | — | — |
| **Lily of the valley** | T62.2X1 | T62.2X2 | T62.2X3 | T62.2X4 | — | — |
| **Lime** (chloride) | T54.3X1 | T54.3X2 | T54.3X3 | T54.3X4 | — | — |
| **Limonene** | T52.891 | T52.892 | T52.893 | T52.894 | — | — |
| **Lincomycin** | T36.8X1 | T36.8X2 | T36.8X3 | T36.8X4 | T36.8X5 | T36.8X6 |
| **Lindane** (insecticide) (nonmedicinal) (vapor) | T53.6X1 | T53.6X2 | T53.6X3 | T53.6X4 | — | — |
| medicinal | T49.ØX1 | T49.ØX2 | T49.ØX3 | T49.ØX4 | T49.ØX5 | T49.ØX6 |
| **Liniments NEC** | T49.91 | T49.92 | T49.93 | T49.94 | T49.95 | T49.96 |
| **Linoleic acid** | T46.6X1 | T46.6X2 | T46.6X3 | T46.6X4 | T46.6X5 | T46.6X6 |
| **Linolenic acid** | T46.6X1 | T46.6X2 | T46.6X3 | T46.6X4 | T46.6X5 | T46.6X6 |
| **Linseed** | T47.4X1 | T47.4X2 | T47.4X3 | T47.4X4 | T47.4X5 | T47.4X6 |
| **Liothyronine** | T38.1X1 | T38.1X2 | T38.1X3 | T38.1X4 | T38.1X5 | T38.1X6 |
| **Liotrix** | T38.1X1 | T38.1X2 | T38.1X3 | T38.1X4 | T38.1X5 | T38.1X6 |
| **Lipancreatin** | T47.5X1 | T47.5X2 | T47.5X3 | T47.5X4 | T47.5X5 | T47.5X6 |
| **Lipitor*** | T46.6X1 | T46.6X2 | T46.6X3 | T46.6X4 | T46.6X5 | T46.6X6 |
| **Lipo-alprostadil** | T46.7X1 | T46.7X2 | T46.7X3 | T46.7X4 | T46.7X5 | T46.7X6 |
| **Lipo-Lutin** | T38.5X1 | T38.5X2 | T38.5X3 | T38.5X4 | T38.5X5 | T38.5X6 |
| **Lipotropic drug NEC** | T5Ø.9Ø1 | T5Ø.9Ø2 | T5Ø.9Ø3 | T5Ø.9Ø4 | T5Ø.9Ø5 | T5Ø.9Ø6 |
| **Liquefied petroleum gases** | T59.891 | T59.892 | T59.893 | T59.894 | — | — |
| piped (pure or mixed with air) | T59.891 | T59.892 | T59.893 | T59.894 | — | — |
| **Liquid** | | | | | | |
| paraffin | T47.4X1 | T47.4X2 | T47.4X3 | T47.4X4 | T47.4X5 | T47.4X6 |
| petrolatum | T47.4X1 | T47.4X2 | T47.4X3 | T47.4X4 | T47.4X5 | T47.4X6 |
| topical | T49.3X1 | T49.3X2 | T49.3X3 | T49.3X4 | T49.3X5 | T49.3X6 |
| specified NEC | T65.891 | T65.892 | T65.893 | T65.894 | — | — |
| substance | T65.91 | T65.92 | T65.93 | T65.94 | — | — |
| **Liquor creosolis compositus** | T65.891 | T65.892 | T65.893 | T65.894 | — | — |
| **Liquorice** | T48.4X1 | T48.4X2 | T48.4X3 | T48.4X4 | T48.4X5 | T48.4X6 |
| extract | T47.8X1 | T47.8X2 | T47.8X3 | T47.8X4 | T47.8X5 | T47.8X6 |
| **Liraglutide*** | T38.3X1 | T38.3X2 | T38.3X3 | T38.3X4 | T38.3X5 | T38.3X6 |
| **Lisinopril** | T46.4X1 | T46.4X2 | T46.4X3 | T46.4X4 | T46.4X5 | T46.4X6 |
| **Lisuride** | T42.8X1 | T42.8X2 | T42.8X3 | T42.8X4 | T42.8X5 | T42.8X6 |
| **Lithane** | T43.8X1 | T43.8X2 | T43.8X3 | T43.8X4 | T43.8X5 | T43.8X6 |
| **Lithium** | T56.891 | T56.892 | T56.893 | T56.894 | — | — |
| gluconate | T43.591 | T43.592 | T43.593 | T43.594 | T43.595 | T43.596 |
| salts (carbonate) | T43.591 | T43.592 | T43.593 | T43.594 | T43.595 | T43.596 |
| **Lithonate** | T43.8X1 | T43.8X2 | T43.8X3 | T43.8X4 | T43.8X5 | T43.8X6 |
| **Liver** | | | | | | |
| extract | T45.8X1 | T45.8X2 | T45.8X3 | T45.8X4 | T45.8X5 | T45.8X6 |
| for parenteral use | T45.8X1 | T45.8X2 | T45.8X3 | T45.8X4 | T45.8X5 | T45.8X6 |
| fraction 1 | T45.8X1 | T45.8X2 | T45.8X3 | T45.8X4 | T45.8X5 | T45.8X6 |
| hydrolysate | T45.8X1 | T45.8X2 | T45.8X3 | T45.8X4 | T45.8X5 | T45.8X6 |
| **Lizard** (bite) (venom) | T63.121 | T63.122 | T63.123 | T63.124 | — | — |
| **LMD** | T45.8X1 | T45.8X2 | T45.8X3 | T45.8X4 | T45.8X5 | T45.8X6 |
| **Lobelia** | T62.2X1 | T62.2X2 | T62.2X3 | T62.2X4 | — | — |
| **Lobeline** | T5Ø.7X1 | T5Ø.7X2 | T5Ø.7X3 | T5Ø.7X4 | T5Ø.7X5 | T5Ø.7X6 |
| **Local action drug NEC** | T49.8X1 | T49.8X2 | T49.8X3 | T49.8X4 | T49.8X5 | T49.8X6 |
| **Locorten** | T49.ØX1 | T49.ØX2 | T49.ØX3 | T49.ØX4 | T49.ØX5 | T49.ØX6 |
| **Lofepramine** | T43.Ø11 | T43.Ø12 | T43.Ø13 | T43.Ø14 | T43.Ø15 | T43.Ø16 |
| **Lolium temulentum** | T62.2X1 | T62.2X2 | T62.2X3 | T62.2X4 | — | — |
| **Lomotil** | T47.6X1 | T47.6X2 | T47.6X3 | T47.6X4 | T47.6X5 | T47.6X6 |
| **Lomustine** | T45.1X1 | T45.1X2 | T45.1X3 | T45.1X4 | T45.1X5 | T45.1X6 |
| **Lonidamine** | T45.1X1 | T45.1X2 | T45.1X3 | T45.1X4 | T45.1X5 | T45.1X6 |
| **LoOvral*** | T38.4X1 | T38.4X2 | T38.4X3 | T38.4X4 | T38.4X5 | T38.4X6 |
| **Loperamide** | T47.6X1 | T47.6X2 | T47.6X3 | T47.6X4 | T47.6X5 | T47.6X6 |
| **Loprazolam** | T42.4X1 | T42.4X2 | T42.4X3 | T42.4X4 | T42.4X5 | T42.4X6 |
| **Lopressor*** | T44.7X1 | T44.7X2 | T44.7X3 | T44.7X4 | T44.7X5 | T44.7X6 |
| **Lorajmine** | T46.2X1 | T46.2X2 | T46.2X3 | T46.2X4 | T46.2X5 | T46.2X6 |
| **Loratidine** | T45.ØX1 | T45.ØX2 | T45.ØX3 | T45.ØX4 | T45.ØX5 | T45.ØX6 |
| **Lorazepam** | T42.4X1 | T42.4X2 | T42.4X3 | T42.4X4 | T42.4X5 | T42.4X6 |
| **Lorcainide** | T46.2X1 | T46.2X2 | T46.2X3 | T46.2X4 | T46.2X5 | T46.2X6 |
| **Lormetazepam** | T42.4X1 | T42.4X2 | T42.4X3 | T42.4X4 | T42.4X5 | T42.4X6 |
| **Losartan*** | T46.5X1 | T46.5X2 | T46.5X3 | T46.5X4 | T46.5X5 | T46.5X6 |
| **Lotions NEC** | T49.91 | T49.92 | T49.93 | T49.94 | T49.95 | T49.96 |
| **Lotrimin*** | T49.ØX1 | T49.ØX2 | T49.ØX3 | T49.ØX4 | T49.ØX5 | T49.ØX6 |
| **Lotusate** | T42.3X1 | T42.3X2 | T42.3X3 | T42.3X4 | T42.3X5 | T42.3X6 |
| **Lovastatin** | T46.6X1 | T46.6X2 | T46.6X3 | T46.6X4 | T46.6X5 | T46.6X6 |
| **Lowila** | T49.2X1 | T49.2X2 | T49.2X3 | T49.2X4 | T49.2X5 | T49.2X6 |
| **Loxapine** | T43.591 | T43.592 | T43.593 | T43.594 | T43.595 | T43.596 |
| **Lozenges** (throat) | T49.6X1 | T49.6X2 | T49.6X3 | T49.6X4 | T49.6X5 | T49.6X6 |
| **LSD** | T4Ø.8X1 | T4Ø.8X2 | T4Ø.8X3 | T4Ø.8X4 | — | — |
| **Lubricant, eye** | T49.5X1 | T49.5X2 | T49.5X3 | T49.5X4 | T49.5X5 | T49.5X6 |
| **Lubricating oil NEC** | T52.ØX1 | T52.ØX2 | T52.ØX3 | T52.ØX4 | — | — |
| **Lucanthone** | T37.4X1 | T37.4X2 | T37.4X3 | T37.4X4 | T37.4X5 | T37.4X6 |
| **Luminal** | T42.3X1 | T42.3X2 | T42.3X3 | T42.3X4 | T42.3X5 | T42.3X6 |
| **Lung irritant** (gas) **NEC** | T59.91 | T59.92 | T59.93 | T59.94 | — | — |
| **Luteinizing hormone** | T38.811 | T38.812 | T38.813 | T38.814 | T38.815 | T38.816 |
| **Lutocylol** | T38.5X1 | T38.5X2 | T38.5X3 | T38.5X4 | T38.5X5 | T38.5X6 |
| **Lutromone** | T38.5X1 | T38.5X2 | T38.5X3 | T38.5X4 | T38.5X5 | T38.5X6 |
| **Lututrin** | T48.291 | T48.292 | T48.293 | T48.294 | T48.295 | T48.296 |

| Substance | Poisoning, Accidental (unintentional) | Poisoning, Intentional Self-harm | Poisoning, Assault | Poisoning, Undetermined | Adverse Effect | Under-dosing |
|---|---|---|---|---|---|---|
| **Luveris*** | T38.891 | T38.892 | T38.893 | T38.894 | T38.895 | T38.89 |
| **Lye** (concentrated) | T54.3X1 | T54.3X2 | T54.3X3 | T54.3X4 | — | — |
| **Lygranum** (skin test) | T5Ø.8X1 | T5Ø.8X2 | T5Ø.8X3 | T5Ø.8X4 | T5Ø.8X5 | T5Ø.8X |
| **Lymecycline** | T36.4X1 | T36.4X2 | T36.4X3 | T36.4X4 | T36.4X5 | T36.4X |
| **Lymphogranuloma venereum antigen** | T5Ø.8X1 | T5Ø.8X2 | T5Ø.8X3 | T5Ø.8X4 | T5Ø.8X5 | T5Ø.8X |
| **Lynestrenol** | T38.4X1 | T38.4X2 | T38.4X3 | T38.4X4 | T38.4X5 | T38.4X |
| **Lyovac Sodium Edecrin** | T5Ø.1X1 | T5Ø.1X2 | T5Ø.1X3 | T5Ø.1X4 | T5Ø.1X5 | T5Ø.1X |
| **Lypressin** | T38.891 | T38.892 | T38.893 | T38.894 | T38.895 | T38.89 |
| **Lysergic acid diethylamide** | T4Ø.8X1 | T4Ø.8X2 | T4Ø.8X3 | T4Ø.8X4 | — | — |
| **Lysergide** | T4Ø.8X1 | T4Ø.8X2 | T4Ø.8X3 | T4Ø.8X4 | — | — |
| **Lysine vasopressin** | T38.891 | T38.892 | T38.893 | T38.894 | T38.895 | T38.89 |
| **Lysol** | T54.1X1 | T54.1X2 | T54.1X3 | T54.1X4 | — | — |
| **Lysozyme** | T49.ØX1 | T49.ØX2 | T49.ØX3 | T49.ØX4 | T49.ØX5 | T49.ØX |
| **Lytta** (vitatta) | T49.8X1 | T49.8X2 | T49.8X3 | T49.8X4 | T49.8X5 | T49.8X |
| **M-AMSA** | T45.1X1 | T45.1X2 | T45.1X3 | T45.1X4 | T45.1X5 | T45.1X |
| **M-vac** | T45.1X1 | T45.1X2 | T45.1X3 | T45.1X4 | T45.1X5 | T45.1X |
| **Mace** | T59.3X1 | T59.3X2 | T59.3X3 | T59.3X4 | — | — |
| **Macrogol** | T5Ø.991 | T5Ø.992 | T5Ø.993 | T5Ø.994 | T5Ø.995 | T5Ø.99 |
| **Macrolide** | | | | | | |
| anabolic drug | T38.7X1 | T38.7X2 | T38.7X3 | T38.7X4 | T38.7X5 | T38.7X |
| antibiotic | T36.3X1 | T36.3X2 | T36.3X3 | T36.3X4 | T36.3X5 | T36.3X |
| **Mafenide** | T49.ØX1 | T49.ØX2 | T49.ØX3 | T49.ØX4 | T49.ØX5 | T49.ØX |
| **Magaldrate** | T47.1X1 | T47.1X2 | T47.1X3 | T47.1X4 | T47.1X5 | T47.1X |
| **Magic mushroom** | T4Ø.991 | T4Ø.992 | T4Ø.993 | T4Ø.994 | — | — |
| **Magnamycin** | T36.8X1 | T36.8X2 | T36.8X3 | T36.8X4 | T36.8X5 | T36.8X |
| **Magnesia magma** | T47.1X1 | T47.1X2 | T47.1X3 | T47.1X4 | T47.1X5 | T47.1X |
| **Magnesium NEC** | T56.891 | T56.892 | T56.893 | T56.894 | — | — |
| carbonate | T47.1X1 | T47.1X2 | T47.1X3 | T47.1X4 | T47.1X5 | T47.1X |
| citrate | T47.4X1 | T47.4X2 | T47.4X3 | T47.4X4 | T47.4X5 | T47.4X |
| hydroxide | T47.1X1 | T47.1X2 | T47.1X3 | T47.1X4 | T47.1X5 | T47.1X |
| oxide | T47.1X1 | T47.1X2 | T47.1X3 | T47.1X4 | T47.1X5 | T47.1X |
| peroxide | T49.ØX1 | T49.ØX2 | T49.ØX3 | T49.ØX4 | T49.ØX5 | T49.ØX |
| salicylate | T39.Ø91 | T39.Ø92 | T39.Ø93 | T39.Ø94 | T39.Ø95 | T39.Ø9 |
| silicofluoride | T5Ø.3X1 | T5Ø.3X2 | T5Ø.3X3 | T5Ø.3X4 | T5Ø.3X5 | T5Ø.3X |
| sulfate | T47.4X1 | T47.4X2 | T47.4X3 | T47.4X4 | T47.4X5 | T47.4X |
| thiosulfate | T45.ØX1 | T45.ØX2 | T45.ØX3 | T45.ØX4 | T45.ØX5 | T45.ØX |
| trisilicate | T47.1X1 | T47.1X2 | T47.1X3 | T47.1X4 | T47.1X5 | T47.1X |
| **Malathion** (medicinal) | T49.ØX1 | T49.ØX2 | T49.ØX3 | T49.ØX4 | T49.ØX5 | T49.ØX |
| insecticide | T6Ø.ØX1 | T6Ø.ØX2 | T6Ø.ØX3 | T6Ø.ØX4 | — | — |
| **Male fern extract** | T37.4X1 | T37.4X2 | T37.4X3 | T37.4X4 | T37.4X5 | T37.4X |
| **Mandelic acid** | T37.8X1 | T37.8X2 | T37.8X3 | T37.8X4 | T37.8X5 | T37.8X |
| **Manganese** (dioxide) (salts) | T57.2X1 | T57.2X2 | T57.2X3 | T57.2X4 | — | — |
| medicinal | T5Ø.991 | T5Ø.992 | T5Ø.993 | T5Ø.994 | T5Ø.995 | T5Ø.99 |
| **Mannitol** | T47.3X1 | T47.3X2 | T47.3X3 | T47.3X4 | T47.3X5 | T47.3X |
| hexanitrate | T46.3X1 | T46.3X2 | T46.3X3 | T46.3X4 | T46.3X5 | T46.3X |
| **Mannomustine** | T45.1X1 | T45.1X2 | T45.1X3 | T45.1X4 | T45.1X5 | T45.1X |
| **MAO inhibitors** | T43.1X1 | T43.1X2 | T43.1X3 | T43.1X4 | T43.1X5 | T43.1X |
| **Mapharsen** | T37.8X1 | T37.8X2 | T37.8X3 | T37.8X4 | T37.8X5 | T37.8X |
| **Maphenide** | T49.ØX1 | T49.ØX2 | T49.ØX3 | T49.ØX4 | T49.ØX5 | T49.ØX |
| **Maprotiline** | T43.Ø21 | T43.Ø22 | T43.Ø23 | T43.Ø24 | T43.Ø25 | T43.Ø2 |
| **Marcaine** | T41.3X1 | T41.3X2 | T41.3X3 | T41.3X4 | T41.3X5 | T41.3X |
| infiltration (subcutaneous) | T41.3X1 | T41.3X2 | T41.3X3 | T41.3X4 | T41.3X5 | T41.3X |
| nerve block (peripheral) (plexus) | T41.3X1 | T41.3X2 | T41.3X3 | T41.3X4 | T41.3X5 | T41.3X |
| **Marezine** | T45.ØX1 | T45.ØX2 | T45.ØX3 | T45.ØX4 | T45.ØX5 | T45.ØX |
| **Marihuana** | T4Ø.711 | T4Ø.712 | T4Ø.713 | T4Ø.714 | T4Ø.715 | T4Ø.71 |
| **Marijuana** | T4Ø.711 | T4Ø.712 | T4Ø.713 | T4Ø.714 | T4Ø.715 | T4Ø.71 |
| **Marine** (sting) | T63.691 | T63.692 | T63.693 | T63.694 | — | — |
| animals (sting) | T63.691 | T63.692 | T63.693 | T63.694 | — | — |
| plants (sting) | T63.711 | T63.712 | T63.713 | T63.714 | — | — |
| **Marplan** | T43.1X1 | T43.1X2 | T43.1X3 | T43.1X4 | T43.1X5 | T43.1X |
| **Marsh gas** | T59.891 | T59.892 | T59.893 | T59.894 | — | — |
| **Marsilid** | T43.1X1 | T43.1X2 | T43.1X3 | T43.1X4 | T43.1X5 | T43.1X |
| **Massengill*** | T49.ØX1 | T49.ØX2 | T49.ØX3 | T49.ØX4 | T49.ØX5 | T49.ØX |
| **Matulane** | T45.1X1 | T45.1X2 | T45.1X3 | T45.1X4 | T45.1X5 | T45.1X |
| **Mazindol** | T5Ø.5X1 | T5Ø.5X2 | T5Ø.5X3 | T5Ø.5X4 | T5Ø.5X5 | T5Ø.5X |
| **MCPA** | T6Ø.3X1 | T6Ø.3X2 | T6Ø.3X3 | T6Ø.3X4 | — | — |
| **MDMA** | T43.641 | T43.642 | T43.643 | T43.644 | — | — |
| **Meadow saffron** | T62.2X1 | T62.2X2 | T62.2X3 | T62.2X4 | — | — |
| **Measles virus vaccine** (attenuated) | T5Ø.B91 | T5Ø.B92 | T5Ø.B93 | T5Ø.B94 | T5Ø.B95 | T5Ø.B9 |
| **Meat, noxious** | T62.8X1 | T62.8X2 | T62.8X3 | T62.8X4 | — | — |
| **Meballymal** | T42.3X1 | T42.3X2 | T42.3X3 | T42.3X4 | T42.3X5 | T42.3X |
| **Mebanazine** | T43.1X1 | T43.1X2 | T43.1X3 | T43.1X4 | T43.1X5 | T43.1X |
| **Mebaral** | T42.3X1 | T42.3X2 | T42.3X3 | T42.3X4 | T42.3X5 | T42.3X |
| **Mebendazole** | T37.4X1 | T37.4X2 | T37.4X3 | T37.4X4 | T37.4X5 | T37.4X |
| **Mebeverine** | T44.3X1 | T44.3X2 | T44.3X3 | T44.3X4 | T44.3X5 | T44.3X |
| **Mebhydrolin** | T45.ØX1 | T45.ØX2 | T45.ØX3 | T45.ØX4 | T45.ØX5 | T45.ØX |
| **Mebumal** | T42.3X1 | T42.3X2 | T42.3X3 | T42.3X4 | T42.3X5 | T42.3X |
| **Mebutamate** | T43.591 | T43.592 | T43.593 | T43.594 | T43.595 | T43.59 |
| **Mecamylamine** | T44.2X1 | T44.2X2 | T44.2X3 | T44.2X4 | T44.2X5 | T44.2X |
| **Mechlorethamine** | T45.1X1 | T45.1X2 | T45.1X3 | T45.1X4 | T45.1X5 | T45.1X |

| Substance | Poisoning, Accidental (unintentional) | Poisoning, Intentional Self-harm | Poisoning, Assault | Poisoning, Undetermined | Adverse Effect | Under-dosing |
|---|---|---|---|---|---|---|
| **Mecillinam** | T36.ØX1 | T36.ØX2 | T36.ØX3 | T36.ØX4 | T36.ØX5 | T36.ØX6 |
| **Meclizine** (hydrochloride) | T45.ØX1 | T45.ØX2 | T45.ØX3 | T45.ØX4 | T45.ØX5 | T45.ØX6 |
| **Meclocycline** | T36.4X1 | T36.4X2 | T36.4X3 | T36.4X4 | T36.4X5 | T36.4X6 |
| **Meclofenamate** | T39.391 | T39.392 | T39.393 | T39.394 | T39.395 | T39.396 |
| **Meclofenamic acid** | T39.391 | T39.392 | T39.393 | T39.394 | T39.395 | T39.396 |
| **Meclofenoxate** | T43.691 | T43.692 | T43.693 | T43.694 | T43.695 | T43.696 |
| **Meclozine** | T45.ØX1 | T45.ØX2 | T45.ØX3 | T45.ØX4 | T45.ØX5 | T45.ØX6 |
| **Mecobalamin** | T45.8X1 | T45.8X2 | T45.8X3 | T45.8X4 | T45.8X5 | T45.8X6 |
| **Mecoprop** | T6Ø.3X1 | T6Ø.3X2 | T6Ø.3X3 | T6Ø.3X4 | — | — |
| **Mecrilate** | T49.3X1 | T49.3X2 | T49.3X3 | T49.3X4 | T49.3X5 | T49.3X6 |
| **Mecysteine** | T48.4X1 | T48.4X2 | T48.4X3 | T48.4X4 | T48.4X5 | T48.4X6 |
| **Medazepam** | T42.4X1 | T42.4X2 | T42.4X3 | T42.4X4 | T42.4X5 | T42.4X6 |
| **Medetomidine** | T65.851 | T65.852 | T65.853 | T65.854 | — | — |
| **Medicament NEC** | T5Ø.9Ø1 | T5Ø.9Ø2 | T5Ø.9Ø3 | T5Ø.9Ø4 | T5Ø.9Ø5 | T5Ø.9Ø6 |
| **Medinal** | T42.3X1 | T42.3X2 | T42.3X3 | T42.3X4 | T42.3X5 | T42.3X6 |
| **Medomin** | T42.3X1 | T42.3X2 | T42.3X3 | T42.3X4 | T42.3X5 | T42.3X6 |
| **Medrogestone** | T38.5X1 | T38.5X2 | T38.5X3 | T38.5X4 | T38.5X5 | T38.5X6 |
| **Medrol*** | T38.ØX1 | T38.ØX2 | T38.ØX3 | T38.ØX4 | T38.ØX5 | T38.ØX6 |
| **Medroxalol** | T44.8X1 | T44.8X2 | T44.8X3 | T44.8X4 | T44.8X5 | T44.8X6 |
| **Medroxyprogesterone acetate** (depot) | T38.5X1 | T38.5X2 | T38.5X3 | T38.5X4 | T38.5X5 | T38.5X6 |
| **Medrysone** | T49.ØX1 | T49.ØX2 | T49.ØX3 | T49.ØX4 | T49.ØX5 | T49.ØX6 |
| **Mefenamic acid** | T39.391 | T39.392 | T39.393 | T39.394 | T39.395 | T39.396 |
| **Mefenorex** | T5Ø.5X1 | T5Ø.5X2 | T5Ø.5X3 | T5Ø.5X4 | T5Ø.5X5 | T5Ø.5X6 |
| **Mefloquine** | T37.2X1 | T37.2X2 | T37.2X3 | T37.2X4 | T37.2X5 | T37.2X6 |
| **Mefoxin*** | T36.1X1 | T36.1X2 | T36.1X3 | T36.1X4 | T36.1X5 | T36.1X6 |
| **Mefruside** | T5Ø.2X1 | T5Ø.2X2 | T5Ø.2X3 | T5Ø.2X4 | T5Ø.2X5 | T5Ø.2X6 |
| **Megahallucinogen** | T4Ø.9Ø1 | T4Ø.9Ø2 | T4Ø.9Ø3 | T4Ø.9Ø4 | T4Ø.9Ø5 | T4Ø.9Ø6 |
| **Megestrol** | T38.5X1 | T38.5X2 | T38.5X3 | T38.5X4 | T38.5X5 | T38.5X6 |
| **Meglumine** | | | | | | |
| antimoniate | T37.8X1 | T37.8X2 | T37.8X3 | T37.8X4 | T37.8X5 | T37.8X6 |
| diatrizoate | T5Ø.8X1 | T5Ø.8X2 | T5Ø.8X3 | T5Ø.8X4 | T5Ø.8X5 | T5Ø.8X6 |
| iodipamide | T5Ø.8X1 | T5Ø.8X2 | T5Ø.8X3 | T5Ø.8X4 | T5Ø.8X5 | T5Ø.8X6 |
| iotroxate | T5Ø.8X1 | T5Ø.8X2 | T5Ø.8X3 | T5Ø.8X4 | T5Ø.8X5 | T5Ø.8X6 |
| **MEK** (methyl ethyl ketone) | T52.4X1 | T52.4X2 | T52.4X3 | T52.4X4 | — | — |
| **Meladinin** | T49.3X1 | T49.3X2 | T49.3X3 | T49.3X4 | T49.3X5 | T49.3X6 |
| **Meladrazine** | T44.3X1 | T44.3X2 | T44.3X3 | T44.3X4 | T44.3X5 | T44.3X6 |
| **Melaleuca alternifolia oil** | T49.ØX1 | T49.ØX2 | T49.ØX3 | T49.ØX4 | T49.ØX5 | T49.ØX6 |
| **Melanizing agents** | T49.3X1 | T49.3X2 | T49.3X3 | T49.3X4 | T49.3X5 | T49.3X6 |
| **Melanocyte-stimulating hormone** | T38.891 | T38.892 | T38.893 | T38.894 | T38.895 | T38.896 |
| **Melarsonyl potassium** | T37.3X1 | T37.3X2 | T37.3X3 | T37.3X4 | T37.3X5 | T37.3X6 |
| **Melarsoprol** | T37.3X1 | T37.3X2 | T37.3X3 | T37.3X4 | T37.3X5 | T37.3X6 |
| **Melia azedarach** | T62.2X1 | T62.2X2 | T62.2X3 | T62.2X4 | — | — |
| **Melitracen** | T43.Ø11 | T43.Ø12 | T43.Ø13 | T43.Ø14 | T43.Ø15 | T43.Ø16 |
| **Mellaril** | T43.3X1 | T43.3X2 | T43.3X3 | T43.3X4 | T43.3X5 | T43.3X6 |
| **Meloxicam*** | T39.391 | T39.392 | T39.393 | T39.394 | T39.395 | T39.396 |
| **Meloxine** | T49.3X1 | T49.3X2 | T49.3X3 | T49.3X4 | T49.3X5 | T49.3X6 |
| **Melperone** | T43.4X1 | T43.4X2 | T43.4X3 | T43.4X4 | T43.4X5 | T43.4X6 |
| **Melphalan** | T45.1X1 | T45.1X2 | T45.1X3 | T45.1X4 | T45.1X5 | T45.1X6 |
| **Memantine** | T43.8X1 | T43.8X2 | T43.8X3 | T43.8X4 | T43.8X5 | T43.8X6 |
| **Menadiol** | T45.7X1 | T45.7X2 | T45.7X3 | T45.7X4 | T45.7X5 | T45.7X6 |
| sodium sulfate | T45.7X1 | T45.7X2 | T45.7X3 | T45.7X4 | T45.7X5 | T45.7X6 |
| **Menadione** | T45.7X1 | T45.7X2 | T45.7X3 | T45.7X4 | T45.7X5 | T45.7X6 |
| sodium bisulfite | T45.7X1 | T45.7X2 | T45.7X3 | T45.7X4 | T45.7X5 | T45.7X6 |
| **Menaphthone** | T45.7X1 | T45.7X2 | T45.7X3 | T45.7X4 | T45.7X5 | T45.7X6 |
| **Menaquinone** | T45.7X1 | T45.7X2 | T45.7X3 | T45.7X4 | T45.7X5 | T45.7X6 |
| **Menatetrenone** | T45.7X1 | T45.7X2 | T45.7X3 | T45.7X4 | T45.7X5 | T45.7X6 |
| **Meningococcal vaccine** | T5Ø.A91 | T5Ø.A92 | T5Ø.A93 | T5Ø.A94 | T5Ø.A95 | T5Ø.A96 |
| **Menningovax** (-AC) (-C) | T5Ø.A91 | T5Ø.A92 | T5Ø.A93 | T5Ø.A94 | T5Ø.A95 | T5Ø.A96 |
| **Menotropins** | T38.811 | T38.812 | T38.813 | T38.814 | T38.815 | T38.816 |
| **Menthol** | T48.5X1 | T48.5X2 | T48.5X3 | T48.5X4 | T48.5X5 | T48.5X6 |
| **Mepacrine** | T37.2X1 | T37.2X2 | T37.2X3 | T37.2X4 | T37.2X5 | T37.2X6 |
| **Meparfynol** | T42.6X1 | T42.6X2 | T42.6X3 | T42.6X4 | T42.6X5 | T42.6X6 |
| **Mepartricin** | T36.7X1 | T36.7X2 | T36.7X3 | T36.7X4 | T36.7X5 | T36.7X6 |
| **Mepazine** | T43.3X1 | T43.3X2 | T43.3X3 | T43.3X4 | T43.3X5 | T43.3X6 |
| **Mepenzolate** | T44.3X1 | T44.3X2 | T44.3X3 | T44.3X4 | T44.3X5 | T44.3X6 |
| bromide | T44.3X1 | T44.3X2 | T44.3X3 | T44.3X4 | T44.3X5 | T44.3X6 |
| **Meperidine** | T4Ø.491 | T4Ø.492 | T4Ø.493 | T4Ø.494 | T4Ø.495 | T4Ø.496 |
| **Mephebarbital** | T42.3X1 | T42.3X2 | T42.3X3 | T42.3X4 | T42.3X5 | T42.3X6 |
| **Mephenamin** (e) | T42.8X1 | T42.8X2 | T42.8X3 | T42.8X4 | T42.8X5 | T42.8X6 |
| **Mephenesin** | T42.8X1 | T42.8X2 | T42.8X3 | T42.8X4 | T42.8X5 | T42.8X6 |
| **Mephenhydramine** | T45.ØX1 | T45.ØX2 | T45.ØX3 | T45.ØX4 | T45.ØX5 | T45.ØX6 |
| **Mephenoxalone** | T42.8X1 | T42.8X2 | T42.8X3 | T42.8X4 | T42.8X5 | T42.8X6 |
| **Mephentermine** | T44.991 | T44.992 | T44.993 | T44.994 | T44.995 | T44.996 |
| **Mephenytoin** | T42.ØX1 | T42.ØX2 | T42.ØX3 | T42.ØX4 | T42.ØX5 | T42.ØX6 |
| with phenobarbital | T42.3X1 | T42.3X2 | T42.3X3 | T42.3X4 | T42.3X5 | T42.3X6 |
| **Mephobarbital** | T42.3X1 | T42.3X2 | T42.3X3 | T42.3X4 | T42.3X5 | T42.3X6 |
| **Mephosfolan** | T6Ø.ØX1 | T6Ø.ØX2 | T6Ø.ØX3 | T6Ø.ØX4 | — | — |
| **Mepindolol** | T44.7X1 | T44.7X2 | T44.7X3 | T44.7X4 | T44.7X5 | T44.7X6 |
| **Mepiperphenidol** | T44.3X1 | T44.3X2 | T44.3X3 | T44.3X4 | T44.3X5 | T44.3X6 |
| **Mepitiostane** | T38.7X1 | T38.7X2 | T38.7X3 | T38.7X4 | T38.7X5 | T38.7X6 |
| **Mepivacaine** | T41.3X1 | T41.3X2 | T41.3X3 | T41.3X4 | T41.3X5 | T41.3X6 |

| Substance | Poisoning, Accidental (unintentional) | Poisoning, Intentional Self-harm | Poisoning, Assault | Poisoning, Undetermined | Adverse Effect | Under-dosing |
|---|---|---|---|---|---|---|
| **Mepivacaine** — *continued* | | | | | | |
| epidural | T41.3X1 | T41.3X2 | T41.3X3 | T41.3X4 | T41.3X5 | T41.3X6 |
| **Meprednisone** | T38.ØX1 | T38.ØX2 | T38.ØX3 | T38.ØX4 | T38.ØX5 | T38.ØX6 |
| **Meprobam** | T43.591 | T43.592 | T43.593 | T43.594 | T43.595 | T43.596 |
| **Meprobamate** | T43.591 | T43.592 | T43.593 | T43.594 | T43.595 | T43.596 |
| **Meproscillarin** | T46.ØX1 | T46.ØX2 | T46.ØX3 | T46.ØX4 | T46.ØX5 | T46.ØX6 |
| **Meprylcaine** | T41.3X1 | T41.3X2 | T41.3X3 | T41.3X4 | T41.3X5 | T41.3X6 |
| **Meptazinol** | T39.8X1 | T39.8X2 | T39.8X3 | T39.8X4 | T39.8X5 | T39.8X6 |
| **Mepyramine** | T45.ØX1 | T45.ØX2 | T45.ØX3 | T45.ØX4 | T45.ØX5 | T45.ØX6 |
| **Mequinol*** | T49.8X1 | T49.8X2 | T49.8X3 | T49.8X4 | T49.8X5 | T49.8X6 |
| **Mequitazine** | T43.3X1 | T43.3X2 | T43.3X3 | T43.3X4 | T43.3X5 | T43.3X6 |
| **Meralluride** | T5Ø.2X1 | T5Ø.2X2 | T5Ø.2X3 | T5Ø.2X4 | T5Ø.2X5 | T5Ø.2X6 |
| **Merbaphen** | T5Ø.2X1 | T5Ø.2X2 | T5Ø.2X3 | T5Ø.2X4 | T5Ø.2X5 | T5Ø.2X6 |
| **Merbromin** | T49.ØX1 | T49.ØX2 | T49.ØX3 | T49.ØX4 | T49.ØX5 | T49.ØX6 |
| **Mercaptobenzothiazole salts** | T49.ØX1 | T49.ØX2 | T49.ØX3 | T49.ØX4 | T49.ØX5 | T49.ØX6 |
| **Mercaptomerin** | T5Ø.2X1 | T5Ø.2X2 | T5Ø.2X3 | T5Ø.2X4 | T5Ø.2X5 | T5Ø.2X6 |
| **Mercaptopurine** | T45.1X1 | T45.1X2 | T45.1X3 | T45.1X4 | T45.1X5 | T45.1X6 |
| **Mercumatilin** | T5Ø.2X1 | T5Ø.2X2 | T5Ø.2X3 | T5Ø.2X4 | T5Ø.2X5 | T5Ø.2X6 |
| **Mercuramide** | T5Ø.2X1 | T5Ø.2X2 | T5Ø.2X3 | T5Ø.2X4 | T5Ø.2X5 | T5Ø.2X6 |
| **Mercurochrome** | T49.ØX1 | T49.ØX2 | T49.ØX3 | T49.ØX4 | T49.ØX5 | T49.ØX6 |
| **Mercurophylline** | T5Ø.2X1 | T5Ø.2X2 | T5Ø.2X3 | T5Ø.2X4 | T5Ø.2X5 | T5Ø.2X6 |
| **Mercury, mercurial, mercuric, mercurous** (compounds) (cyanide) (fumes) (nonmedicinal) (vapor) **NEC** | T56.1X1 | T56.1X2 | T56.1X3 | T56.1X4 | — | — |
| ammoniated | T49.ØX1 | T49.ØX2 | T49.ØX3 | T49.ØX4 | T49.ØX5 | T49.ØX6 |
| anti-infective | | | | | | |
| local | T49.ØX1 | T49.ØX2 | T49.ØX3 | T49.ØX4 | T49.ØX5 | T49.ØX6 |
| systemic | T37.8X1 | T37.8X2 | T37.8X3 | T37.8X4 | T37.8X5 | T37.8X6 |
| topical | T49.ØX1 | T49.ØX2 | T49.ØX3 | T49.ØX4 | T49.ØX5 | T49.ØX6 |
| chloride (ammoniated) | T49.ØX1 | T49.ØX2 | T49.ØX3 | T49.ØX4 | T49.ØX5 | T49.ØX6 |
| fungicide | T56.1X1 | T56.1X2 | T56.1X3 | T56.1X4 | — | — |
| diuretic NEC | T5Ø.2X1 | T5Ø.2X2 | T5Ø.2X3 | T5Ø.2X4 | T5Ø.2X5 | T5Ø.2X6 |
| fungicide | T56.1X1 | T56.1X2 | T56.1X3 | T56.1X4 | — | — |
| organic (fungicide) | T56.1X1 | T56.1X2 | T56.1X3 | T56.1X4 | — | — |
| oxide, yellow | T49.ØX1 | T49.ØX2 | T49.ØX3 | T49.ØX4 | T49.ØX5 | T49.ØX6 |
| **Mersalyl** | T5Ø.2X1 | T5Ø.2X2 | T5Ø.2X3 | T5Ø.2X4 | T5Ø.2X5 | T5Ø.2X6 |
| **Merthiolate** | T49.ØX1 | T49.ØX2 | T49.ØX3 | T49.ØX4 | T49.ØX5 | T49.ØX6 |
| ophthalmic preparation | T49.5X1 | T49.5X2 | T49.5X3 | T49.5X4 | T49.5X5 | T49.5X6 |
| **Meruvax** | T5Ø.B91 | T5Ø.B92 | T5Ø.B93 | T5Ø.B94 | T5Ø.B95 | T5Ø.B96 |
| **Mesalazine** | T47.8X1 | T47.8X2 | T47.8X3 | T47.8X4 | T47.8X5 | T47.8X6 |
| **Mescal buttons** | T4Ø.991 | T4Ø.992 | T4Ø.993 | T4Ø.994 | — | — |
| **Mescaline** | T4Ø.991 | T4Ø.992 | T4Ø.993 | T4Ø.994 | — | — |
| **Mesna** | T48.4X1 | T48.4X2 | T48.4X3 | T48.4X4 | T48.4X5 | T48.4X6 |
| **Mesoglycan** | T46.6X1 | T46.6X2 | T46.6X3 | T46.6X4 | T46.6X5 | T46.6X6 |
| **Mesoridazine** | T43.3X1 | T43.3X2 | T43.3X3 | T43.3X4 | T43.3X5 | T43.3X6 |
| **Mestanolone** | T38.7X1 | T38.7X2 | T38.7X3 | T38.7X4 | T38.7X5 | T38.7X6 |
| **Mesterolone** | T38.7X1 | T38.7X2 | T38.7X3 | T38.7X4 | T38.7X5 | T38.7X6 |
| **Mestranol** | T38.5X1 | T38.5X2 | T38.5X3 | T38.5X4 | T38.5X5 | T38.5X6 |
| **Mesulergine** | T42.8X1 | T42.8X2 | T42.8X3 | T42.8X4 | T42.8X5 | T42.8X6 |
| **Mesulfen** | T49.ØX1 | T49.ØX2 | T49.ØX3 | T49.ØX4 | T49.ØX5 | T49.ØX6 |
| **Mesuximide** | T42.2X1 | T42.2X2 | T42.2X3 | T42.2X4 | T42.2X5 | T42.2X6 |
| **Metabutethamine** | T41.3X1 | T41.3X2 | T41.3X3 | T41.3X4 | T41.3X5 | T41.3X6 |
| **Metactesylacetate** | T49.ØX1 | T49.ØX2 | T49.ØX3 | T49.ØX4 | T49.ØX5 | T49.ØX6 |
| **Metacycline** | T36.4X1 | T36.4X2 | T36.4X3 | T36.4X4 | T36.4X5 | T36.4X6 |
| **Metaldehyde** (snail killer) **NEC** | T6Ø.8X1 | T6Ø.8X2 | T6Ø.8X3 | T6Ø.8X4 | — | — |
| **Metals** (heavy) (nonmedicinal) | T56.91 | T56.92 | T56.93 | T56.94 | — | — |
| dust, fumes, or vapor NEC | T56.91 | T56.92 | T56.93 | T56.94 | — | — |
| gadolinium | T56.821 | T56.822 | T56.823 | T56.824 | — | — |
| light NEC | T56.91 | T56.92 | T56.93 | T56.94 | — | — |
| dust, fumes, or vapor NEC | T56.91 | T56.92 | T56.93 | T56.94 | — | — |
| specified NEC | T56.891 | T56.892 | T56.893 | T56.894 | — | — |
| thallium | T56.811 | T56.812 | T56.813 | T56.814 | — | — |
| **Metamfetamine** | T43.651 | T43.652 | T43.653 | T43.654 | T43.655 | T43.656 |
| **Metamizole sodium** | T39.2X1 | T39.2X2 | T39.2X3 | T39.2X4 | T39.2X5 | T39.2X6 |
| **Metampicillin** | T36.ØX1 | T36.ØX2 | T36.ØX3 | T36.ØX4 | T36.ØX5 | T36.ØX6 |
| **Metamucil** | T47.4X1 | T47.4X2 | T47.4X3 | T47.4X4 | T47.4X5 | T47.4X6 |
| **Metandienone** | T38.7X1 | T38.7X2 | T38.7X3 | T38.7X4 | T38.7X5 | T38.7X6 |
| **Metandrostenolone** | T38.7X1 | T38.7X2 | T38.7X3 | T38.7X4 | T38.7X5 | T38.7X6 |
| **Metaphen** | T49.ØX1 | T49.ØX2 | T49.ØX3 | T49.ØX4 | T49.ØX5 | T49.ØX6 |
| **Metaphos** | T6Ø.ØX1 | T6Ø.ØX2 | T6Ø.ØX3 | T6Ø.ØX4 | — | — |
| **Metapramine** | T43.Ø11 | T43.Ø12 | T43.Ø13 | T43.Ø14 | T43.Ø15 | T43.Ø16 |
| **Metaproterenol** | T48.291 | T48.292 | T48.293 | T48.294 | T48.295 | T48.296 |
| **Metaraminol** | T44.4X1 | T44.4X2 | T44.4X3 | T44.4X4 | T44.4X5 | T44.4X6 |
| **Metaxalone** | T42.8X1 | T42.8X2 | T42.8X3 | T42.8X4 | T42.8X5 | T42.8X6 |
| **Meted*** | T49.4X1 | T49.4X2 | T49.4X3 | T49.4X4 | T49.4X5 | T49.4X6 |
| **Metenolone** | T38.7X1 | T38.7X2 | T38.7X3 | T38.7X4 | T38.7X5 | T38.7X6 |
| **Metergoline** | T42.8X1 | T42.8X2 | T42.8X3 | T42.8X4 | T42.8X5 | T42.8X6 |



*Optum Value-Add

| Substance | Poisoning, Accidental (unintentional) | Poisoning, Intentional Self-harm | Poisoning, Assault | Poisoning, Undetermined | Adverse Effect | Under-dosing |
|---|---|---|---|---|---|---|
| **Metescufylline** | T46.991 | T46.992 | T46.993 | T46.994 | T46.995 | T46.996 |
| **Metetoin** | T42.0X1 | T42.0X2 | T42.0X3 | T42.0X4 | T42.0X5 | T42.0X6 |
| **Metformin** | T38.3X1 | T38.3X2 | T38.3X3 | T38.3X4 | T38.3X5 | T38.3X6 |
| **Methacholine** | T44.1X1 | T44.1X2 | T44.1X3 | T44.1X4 | T44.1X5 | T44.1X6 |
| **Methacycline** | T36.4X1 | T36.4X2 | T36.4X3 | T36.4X4 | T36.4X5 | T36.4X6 |
| **Methadone** | T40.3X1 | T40.3X2 | T40.3X3 | T40.3X4 | T40.3X5 | T40.3X6 |
| **Methadose*** | T40.3X1 | T40.3X2 | T40.3X3 | T40.3X4 | T40.3X5 | T40.3X6 |
| **Methallenestril** | T38.5X1 | T38.5X2 | T38.5X3 | T38.5X4 | T38.5X5 | T38.5X6 |
| **Methallenoestril** | T38.5X1 | T38.5X2 | T38.5X3 | T38.5X4 | T38.5X5 | T38.5X6 |
| **Methamphetamine** | T43.651 | T43.652 | T43.653 | T43.654 | T43.655 | T43.656 |
| **Methampyrone** | T39.2X1 | T39.2X2 | T39.2X3 | T39.2X4 | T39.2X5 | T39.2X6 |
| **Methandienone** | T38.7X1 | T38.7X2 | T38.7X3 | T38.7X4 | T38.7X5 | T38.7X6 |
| **Methandriol** | T38.7X1 | T38.7X2 | T38.7X3 | T38.7X4 | T38.7X5 | T38.7X6 |
| **Methandrostenolone** | T38.7X1 | T38.7X2 | T38.7X3 | T38.7X4 | T38.7X5 | T38.7X6 |
| **Methane** | T59.891 | T59.892 | T59.893 | T59.894 | — | — |
| **Methanethiol** | T59.891 | T59.892 | T59.893 | T59.894 | — | — |
| **Methaniazide** | T37.1X1 | T37.1X2 | T37.1X3 | T37.1X4 | T37.1X5 | T37.1X6 |
| **Methanol** (vapor) | T51.1X1 | T51.1X2 | T51.1X3 | T51.1X4 | — | — |
| **Methantheline** | T44.3X1 | T44.3X2 | T44.3X3 | T44.3X4 | T44.3X5 | T44.3X6 |
| **Methanthelinium bromide** | T44.3X1 | T44.3X2 | T44.3X3 | T44.3X4 | T44.3X5 | T44.3X6 |
| **Methaphenilene** | T45.0X1 | T45.0X2 | T45.0X3 | T45.0X4 | T45.0X5 | T45.0X6 |
| **Methapyrilene** | T45.0X1 | T45.0X2 | T45.0X3 | T45.0X4 | T45.0X5 | T45.0X6 |
| **Methaqualone** (compound) | T42.6X1 | T42.6X2 | T42.6X3 | T42.6X4 | T42.6X5 | T42.6X6 |
| **Metharbital** | T42.3X1 | T42.3X2 | T42.3X3 | T42.3X4 | T42.3X5 | T42.3X6 |
| **Methazolamide** | T50.2X1 | T50.2X2 | T50.2X3 | T50.2X4 | T50.2X5 | T50.2X6 |
| **Methdilazine** | T43.3X1 | T43.3X2 | T43.3X3 | T43.3X4 | T43.3X5 | T43.3X6 |
| **Methedrine** | T43.651 | T43.652 | T43.653 | T43.654 | T43.655 | T43.656 |
| **Methenamine** (mandelate) | T37.8X1 | T37.8X2 | T37.8X3 | T37.8X4 | T37.8X5 | T37.8X6 |
| **Methenolone** | T38.7X1 | T38.7X2 | T38.7X3 | T38.7X4 | T38.7X5 | T38.7X6 |
| **Methergine** | T48.0X1 | T48.0X2 | T48.0X3 | T48.0X4 | T48.0X5 | T48.0X6 |
| **Methetoin** | T42.0X1 | T42.0X2 | T42.0X3 | T42.0X4 | T42.0X5 | T42.0X6 |
| **Methiacil** | T38.2X1 | T38.2X2 | T38.2X3 | T38.2X4 | T38.2X5 | T38.2X6 |
| **Methicillin** | T36.0X1 | T36.0X2 | T36.0X3 | T36.0X4 | T36.0X5 | T36.0X6 |
| **Methimazole** | T38.2X1 | T38.2X2 | T38.2X3 | T38.2X4 | T38.2X5 | T38.2X6 |
| **Methiodal sodium** | T50.8X1 | T50.8X2 | T50.8X3 | T50.8X4 | T50.8X5 | T50.8X6 |
| **Methionine** | T50.991 | T50.992 | T50.993 | T50.994 | T50.995 | T50.996 |
| **Methisazone** | T37.5X1 | T37.5X2 | T37.5X3 | T37.5X4 | T37.5X5 | T37.5X6 |
| **Methisoprinol** | T37.5X1 | T37.5X2 | T37.5X3 | T37.5X4 | T37.5X5 | T37.5X6 |
| **Methitural** | T42.3X1 | T42.3X2 | T42.3X3 | T42.3X4 | T42.3X5 | T42.3X6 |
| **Methixene** | T44.3X1 | T44.3X2 | T44.3X3 | T44.3X4 | T44.3X5 | T44.3X6 |
| **Methobarbital, methobarbitone** | T42.3X1 | T42.3X2 | T42.3X3 | T42.3X4 | T42.3X5 | T42.3X6 |
| **Methocarbamol** | T42.8X1 | T42.8X2 | T42.8X3 | T42.8X4 | T42.8X5 | T42.8X6 |
| skeletal muscle relaxant | T48.1X1 | T48.1X2 | T48.1X3 | T48.1X4 | T48.1X5 | T48.1X6 |
| **Methohexital** | T41.1X1 | T41.1X2 | T41.1X3 | T41.1X4 | T41.1X5 | T41.1X6 |
| **Methohexitone** | T41.1X1 | T41.1X2 | T41.1X3 | T41.1X4 | T41.1X5 | T41.1X6 |
| **Methoin** | T42.0X1 | T42.0X2 | T42.0X3 | T42.0X4 | T42.0X5 | T42.0X6 |
| **Methopholine** | T39.8X1 | T39.8X2 | T39.8X3 | T39.8X4 | T39.8X5 | T39.8X6 |
| **Methopromazine** | T43.3X1 | T43.3X2 | T43.3X3 | T43.3X4 | T43.3X5 | T43.3X6 |
| **Methorate** | T48.3X1 | T48.3X2 | T48.3X3 | T48.3X4 | T48.3X5 | T48.3X6 |
| **Methoserpidine** | T46.5X1 | T46.5X2 | T46.5X3 | T46.5X4 | T46.5X5 | T46.5X6 |
| **Methotrexate** | T45.1X1 | T45.1X2 | T45.1X3 | T45.1X4 | T45.1X5 | T45.1X6 |
| **Methotrimeprazine** | T43.3X1 | T43.3X2 | T43.3X3 | T43.3X4 | T43.3X5 | T43.3X6 |
| **Methoxa-Dome** | T49.3X1 | T49.3X2 | T49.3X3 | T49.3X4 | T49.3X5 | T49.3X6 |
| **Methoxamine** | T44.4X1 | T44.4X2 | T44.4X3 | T44.4X4 | T44.4X5 | T44.4X6 |
| **Methoxsalen** | T50.991 | T50.992 | T50.993 | T50.994 | T50.995 | T50.996 |
| **Methoxy-DDT** | T53.7X1 | T53.7X2 | T53.7X3 | T53.7X4 | — | — |
| **Methoxyaniline** | T65.3X1 | T65.3X2 | T65.3X3 | T65.3X4 | — | — |
| **Methoxybenzyl penicillin** | T36.0X1 | T36.0X2 | T36.0X3 | T36.0X4 | T36.0X5 | T36.0X6 |
| **Methoxychlor** | T53.7X1 | T53.7X2 | T53.7X3 | T53.7X4 | — | — |
| **Methoxyflurane** | T41.0X1 | T41.0X2 | T41.0X3 | T41.0X4 | T41.0X5 | T41.0X6 |
| **Methoxyphenamine** | T48.6X1 | T48.6X2 | T48.6X3 | T48.6X4 | T48.6X5 | T48.6X6 |
| **Methoxypromazine** | T43.3X1 | T43.3X2 | T43.3X3 | T43.3X4 | T43.3X5 | T43.3X6 |
| **Methscopolamine bromide** | T44.3X1 | T44.3X2 | T44.3X3 | T44.3X4 | T44.3X5 | T44.3X6 |
| **Methsuximide** | T42.2X1 | T42.2X2 | T42.2X3 | T42.2X4 | T42.2X5 | T42.2X6 |
| **Methyclothiazide** | T50.2X1 | T50.2X2 | T50.2X3 | T50.2X4 | T50.2X5 | T50.2X6 |
| **Methyl** | | | | | | |
| acetate | T52.4X1 | T52.4X2 | T52.4X3 | T52.4X4 | — | — |
| acetone | T52.4X1 | T52.4X2 | T52.4X3 | T52.4X4 | — | — |
| acrylate | T65.891 | T65.892 | T65.893 | T65.894 | — | — |
| alcohol | T51.1X1 | T51.1X2 | T51.1X3 | T51.1X4 | — | — |
| aminophenol | T65.3X1 | T65.3X2 | T65.3X3 | T65.3X4 | — | — |
| amphetamine | T43.651 | T43.652 | T43.653 | T43.654 | T43.655 | T43.656 |
| androstanolone | T38.7X1 | T38.7X2 | T38.7X3 | T38.7X4 | T38.7X5 | T38.7X6 |
| atropine | T44.3X1 | T44.3X2 | T44.3X3 | T44.3X4 | T44.3X5 | T44.3X6 |
| benzene | T52.2X1 | T52.2X2 | T52.2X3 | T52.2X4 | — | — |
| benzoate | T52.891 | T52.892 | T52.893 | T52.894 | — | — |
| benzol | T52.2X1 | T52.2X2 | T52.2X3 | T52.2X4 | — | — |
| bromide (gas) | T59.891 | T59.892 | T59.893 | T59.894 | — | — |
| fumigant | T60.8X1 | T60.8X2 | T60.8X3 | T60.8X4 | — | — |
| butanol | T51.3X1 | T51.3X2 | T51.3X3 | T51.3X4 | — | — |
| carbinol | T51.1X1 | T51.1X2 | T51.1X3 | T51.1X4 | — | — |

| Substance | Poisoning, Accidental (unintentional) | Poisoning, Intentional Self-harm | Poisoning, Assault | Poisoning, Undetermined | Adverse Effect | Under-dosing |
|---|---|---|---|---|---|---|
| **Methyl** — *continued* | | | | | | |
| carbonate | T52.891 | T52.892 | T52.893 | T52.894 | — | — |
| CCNU | T45.1X1 | T45.1X2 | T45.1X3 | T45.1X4 | T45.1X5 | T45.1X |
| cellosolve | T52.91 | T52.92 | T52.93 | T52.94 | — | — |
| cellulose | T47.4X1 | T47.4X2 | T47.4X3 | T47.4X4 | T47.4X5 | T47.4X |
| chloride (gas) | T59.891 | T59.892 | T59.893 | T59.894 | — | — |
| chloroformate | T59.3X1 | T59.3X2 | T59.3X3 | T59.3X4 | — | — |
| cyclohexane | T52.821 | T52.822 | T52.823 | T52.824 | — | — |
| cyclohexanol | T51.8X1 | T51.8X2 | T51.8X3 | T51.8X4 | — | — |
| cyclohexanone | T52.891 | T52.892 | T52.893 | T52.894 | — | — |
| cyclohexyl acetate | T52.891 | T52.892 | T52.893 | T52.894 | — | — |
| demeton | T60.0X1 | T60.0X2 | T60.0X3 | T60.0X4 | — | — |
| dihydromorphinone | T40.2X1 | T40.2X2 | T40.2X3 | T40.2X4 | T40.2X5 | T40.2X |
| ergometrine | T48.0X1 | T48.0X2 | T48.0X3 | T48.0X4 | T48.0X5 | T48.0X |
| ergonovine | T48.0X1 | T48.0X2 | T48.0X3 | T48.0X4 | T48.0X5 | T48.0X |
| ethyl ketone | T52.4X1 | T52.4X2 | T52.4X3 | T52.4X4 | — | — |
| glucamine antimonate | T37.8X1 | T37.8X2 | T37.8X3 | T37.8X4 | T37.8X5 | T37.8X |
| hydrazine | T65.891 | T65.892 | T65.893 | T65.894 | — | — |
| iodide | T65.891 | T65.892 | T65.893 | T65.894 | — | — |
| isobutyl ketone | T52.4X1 | T52.4X2 | T52.4X3 | T52.4X4 | — | — |
| isothiocyanate | T60.3X1 | T60.3X2 | T60.3X3 | T60.3X4 | — | — |
| mercaptan | T59.891 | T59.892 | T59.893 | T59.894 | — | — |
| morphine NEC | T40.2X1 | T40.2X2 | T40.2X3 | T40.2X4 | T40.2X5 | T40.2X |
| nicotinate | T49.4X1 | T49.4X2 | T49.4X3 | T49.4X4 | T49.4X5 | T49.4X |
| paraben | T49.0X1 | T49.0X2 | T49.0X3 | T49.0X4 | T49.0X5 | T49.0X |
| parafynol | T42.6X1 | T42.6X2 | T42.6X3 | T42.6X4 | T42.6X5 | T42.6X |
| parathion | T60.0X1 | T60.0X2 | T60.0X3 | T60.0X4 | — | — |
| peridol | T43.4X1 | T43.4X2 | T43.4X3 | T43.4X4 | T43.4X5 | T43.4X |
| phenidate | T43.631 | T43.632 | T43.633 | T43.634 | T43.635 | T43.63 |
| prednisolone | T38.0X1 | T38.0X2 | T38.0X3 | T38.0X4 | T38.0X5 | T38.0X |
| ENT agent | T49.6X1 | T49.6X2 | T49.6X3 | T49.6X4 | T49.6X5 | T49.6X |
| ophthalmic preparation | T49.5X1 | T49.5X2 | T49.5X3 | T49.5X4 | T49.5X5 | T49.5X |
| topical NEC | T49.0X1 | T49.0X2 | T49.0X3 | T49.0X4 | T49.0X5 | T49.0X |
| propylcarbinol | T51.3X1 | T51.3X2 | T51.3X3 | T51.3X4 | — | — |
| rosaniline NEC | T49.0X1 | T49.0X2 | T49.0X3 | T49.0X4 | T49.0X5 | T49.0X |
| salicylate | T49.2X1 | T49.2X2 | T49.2X3 | T49.2X4 | T49.2X5 | T49.2X |
| sulfate (fumes) | T59.891 | T59.892 | T59.893 | T59.894 | — | — |
| liquid | T52.891 | T52.892 | T52.893 | T52.894 | — | — |
| sulfonal | T42.6X1 | T42.6X2 | T42.6X3 | T42.6X4 | T42.6X5 | T42.6X |
| testosterone | T38.7X1 | T38.7X2 | T38.7X3 | T38.7X4 | T38.7X5 | T38.7X |
| thiouracil | T38.2X1 | T38.2X2 | T38.2X3 | T38.2X4 | T38.2X5 | T38.2X |
| **Methylacetoxyprogesterone*** | T38.5X1 | T38.5X2 | T38.5X3 | T38.5X4 | T38.5X5 | T38.5X |
| **Methylamphetamine** | T43.651 | T43.652 | T43.653 | T43.654 | T43.655 | T43.65 |
| **Methylated spirit** | T51.1X1 | T51.1X2 | T51.1X3 | T51.1X4 | — | — |
| **Methylatropine nitrate** | T44.3X1 | T44.3X2 | T44.3X3 | T44.3X4 | T44.3X5 | T44.3X |
| **Methylbenactyzium bromide** | T44.3X1 | T44.3X2 | T44.3X3 | T44.3X4 | T44.3X5 | T44.3X |
| **Methylbenzethonium chloride** | T49.0X1 | T49.0X2 | T49.0X3 | T49.0X4 | T49.0X5 | T49.0X |
| **Methylcellulose** | T47.4X1 | T47.4X2 | T47.4X3 | T47.4X4 | T47.4X5 | T47.4X |
| laxative | T47.4X1 | T47.4X2 | T47.4X3 | T47.4X4 | T47.4X5 | T47.4X |
| **Methylchlorophenoxyacetic acid** | T60.3X1 | T60.3X2 | T60.3X3 | T60.3X4 | — | — |
| **Methyldopa** | T46.5X1 | T46.5X2 | T46.5X3 | T46.5X4 | T46.5X5 | T46.5X |
| **Methyldopate** | T46.5X1 | T46.5X2 | T46.5X3 | T46.5X4 | T46.5X5 | T46.5X |
| **Methylene** | | | | | | |
| blue | T50.6X1 | T50.6X2 | T50.6X3 | T50.6X4 | T50.6X5 | T50.6X |
| chloride or dichloride (solvent) NEC | T53.4X1 | T53.4X2 | T53.4X3 | T53.4X4 | — | — |
| **Methylenedioxyamphetamine** | T43.621 | T43.622 | T43.623 | T43.624 | T43.625 | T43.62 |
| **Methylenedioxymeth-amphetamine** | T43.641 | T43.642 | T43.643 | T43.644 | — | — |
| **Methylergometrine** | T48.0X1 | T48.0X2 | T48.0X3 | T48.0X4 | T48.0X5 | T48.0X |
| **Methylergonovine** | T48.0X1 | T48.0X2 | T48.0X3 | T48.0X4 | T48.0X5 | T48.0X |
| **Methylestrenolone** | T38.5X1 | T38.5X2 | T38.5X3 | T38.5X4 | T38.5X5 | T38.5X |
| **Methylethyl cellulose** | T50.991 | T50.992 | T50.993 | T50.994 | T50.995 | T50.99 |
| **Methylhexabital** | T42.3X1 | T42.3X2 | T42.3X3 | T42.3X4 | T42.3X5 | T42.3X |
| **Methylmorphine** | T40.2X1 | T40.2X2 | T40.2X3 | T40.2X4 | T40.2X5 | T40.2X |
| **Methylparaben** (ophthalmic) | T49.5X1 | T49.5X2 | T49.5X3 | T49.5X4 | T49.5X5 | T49.5X |
| **Methylparafynol** | T42.6X1 | T42.6X2 | T42.6X3 | T42.6X4 | T42.6X5 | T42.6X |
| **Methylpentynol, methylpenthynol** | T42.6X1 | T42.6X2 | T42.6X3 | T42.6X4 | T42.6X5 | T42.6X |
| **Methylphenidate** | T43.631 | T43.632 | T43.633 | T43.634 | T43.635 | T43.63 |
| **Methylphenobarbital** | T42.3X1 | T42.3X2 | T42.3X3 | T42.3X4 | T42.3X5 | T42.3X |
| **Methylpolysiloxane** | T47.1X1 | T47.1X2 | T47.1X3 | T47.1X4 | T47.1X5 | T47.1X |
| **Methylprednisolone** — *see* Methyl, prednisolone | | | | | | |
| **Methylrosaniline** | T49.0X1 | T49.0X2 | T49.0X3 | T49.0X4 | T49.0X5 | T49.0X |
| **Methylrosanilinium chloride** | T49.0X1 | T49.0X2 | T49.0X3 | T49.0X4 | T49.0X5 | T49.0X |
| **Methyltestosterone** | T38.7X1 | T38.7X2 | T38.7X3 | T38.7X4 | T38.7X5 | T38.7X |
| **Methylthionine chloride** | T50.6X1 | T50.6X2 | T50.6X3 | T50.6X4 | T50.6X5 | T50.6X |





☑ Additional Character May Be Required — Refer to the Tabular List for Character Selection

*Optum Value-Add

| Substance | Poisoning, Accidental (unintentional) | Poisoning, Intentional Self-harm | Poisoning, Assault | Poisoning, Undetermined | Adverse Effect | Under-dosing |
|---|---|---|---|---|---|---|
| **Methylthioninium chloride** | T5Ø.6X1 | T5Ø.6X2 | T5Ø.6X3 | T5Ø.6X4 | T5Ø.6X5 | T5Ø.6X6 |
| **Methylthiouracil** | T38.2X1 | T38.2X2 | T38.2X3 | T38.2X4 | T38.2X5 | T38.2X6 |
| **Methyprylon** | T42.6X1 | T42.6X2 | T42.6X3 | T42.6X4 | T42.6X5 | T42.6X6 |
| **Methysergide** | T46.5X1 | T46.5X2 | T46.5X3 | T46.5X4 | T46.5X5 | T46.5X6 |
| **Metiamide** | T47.1X1 | T47.1X2 | T47.1X3 | T47.1X4 | T47.1X5 | T47.1X6 |
| **Meticillin** | T36.ØX1 | T36.ØX2 | T36.ØX3 | T36.ØX4 | T36.ØX5 | T36.ØX6 |
| **Meticrane** | T5Ø.2X1 | T5Ø.2X2 | T5Ø.2X3 | T5Ø.2X4 | T5Ø.2X5 | T5Ø.2X6 |
| **Metildigoxin** | T46.ØX1 | T46.ØX2 | T46.ØX3 | T46.ØX4 | T46.ØX5 | T46.ØX6 |
| **Metipranolol** | T49.5X1 | T49.5X2 | T49.5X3 | T49.5X4 | T49.5X5 | T49.5X6 |
| **Metirosine** | T46.5X1 | T46.5X2 | T46.5X3 | T46.5X4 | T46.5X5 | T46.5X6 |
| **Metisazone** | T37.5X1 | T37.5X2 | T37.5X3 | T37.5X4 | T37.5X5 | T37.5X6 |
| **Metixene** | T44.3X1 | T44.3X2 | T44.3X3 | T44.3X4 | T44.3X5 | T44.3X6 |
| **Metizoline** | T48.5X1 | T48.5X2 | T48.5X3 | T48.5X4 | T48.5X5 | T48.5X6 |
| **Metoclopramide** | T45.ØX1 | T45.ØX2 | T45.ØX3 | T45.ØX4 | T45.ØX5 | T45.ØX6 |
| **Metofenazate** | T43.3X1 | T43.3X2 | T43.3X3 | T43.3X4 | T43.3X5 | T43.3X6 |
| **Metofoline** | T39.8X1 | T39.8X2 | T39.8X3 | T39.8X4 | T39.8X5 | T39.8X6 |
| **Metolazone** | T5Ø.2X1 | T5Ø.2X2 | T5Ø.2X3 | T5Ø.2X4 | T5Ø.2X5 | T5Ø.2X6 |
| **Metopon** | T4Ø.2X1 | T4Ø.2X2 | T4Ø.2X3 | T4Ø.2X4 | T4Ø.2X5 | T4Ø.2X6 |
| **Metoprine** | T45.1X1 | T45.1X2 | T45.1X3 | T45.1X4 | T45.1X5 | T45.1X6 |
| **Metoprolol** | T44.7X1 | T44.7X2 | T44.7X3 | T44.7X4 | T44.7X5 | T44.7X6 |
| **Metrifonate** | T6Ø.ØX1 | T6Ø.ØX2 | T6Ø.ØX3 | T6Ø.ØX4 | — | — |
| **Metrizamide** | T5Ø.8X1 | T5Ø.8X2 | T5Ø.8X3 | T5Ø.8X4 | T5Ø.8X5 | T5Ø.8X6 |
| **Metrizoic acid** | T5Ø.8X1 | T5Ø.8X2 | T5Ø.8X3 | T5Ø.8X4 | T5Ø.8X5 | T5Ø.8X6 |
| **MetroGel*** | T49.ØX1 | T49.ØX2 | T49.ØX3 | T49.ØX4 | T49.ØX5 | T49.ØX6 |
| **Metronidazole** | T37.8X1 | T37.8X2 | T37.8X3 | T37.8X4 | T37.8X5 | T37.8X6 |
| **Metycaine** | T41.3X1 | T41.3X2 | T41.3X3 | T41.3X4 | T41.3X5 | T41.3X6 |
| infiltration (subcutaneous) | T41.3X1 | T41.3X2 | T41.3X3 | T41.3X4 | T41.3X5 | T41.3X6 |
| nerve block (peripheral) (plexus) | T41.3X1 | T41.3X2 | T41.3X3 | T41.3X4 | T41.3X5 | T41.3X6 |
| topical (surface) | T41.3X1 | T41.3X2 | T41.3X3 | T41.3X4 | T41.3X5 | T41.3X6 |
| **Metyrapone** | T5Ø.8X1 | T5Ø.8X2 | T5Ø.8X3 | T5Ø.8X4 | T5Ø.8X5 | T5Ø.8X6 |
| **Mevacor*** | T46.6X1 | T46.6X2 | T46.6X3 | T46.6X4 | T46.6X5 | T46.6X6 |
| **Mevinphos** | T6Ø.ØX1 | T6Ø.ØX2 | T6Ø.ØX3 | T6Ø.ØX4 | — | — |
| **Mexazolam** | T42.4X1 | T42.4X2 | T42.4X3 | T42.4X4 | T42.4X5 | T42.4X6 |
| **Mexenone** | T49.3X1 | T49.3X2 | T49.3X3 | T49.3X4 | T49.3X5 | T49.3X6 |
| **Mexiletine** | T46.2X1 | T46.2X2 | T46.2X3 | T46.2X4 | T46.2X5 | T46.2X6 |
| **Mezereon** | T62.2X1 | T62.2X2 | T62.2X3 | T62.2X4 | — | — |
| berries | T62.1X1 | T62.1X2 | T62.1X3 | T62.1X4 | — | — |
| **Mezlocillin** | T36.ØX1 | T36.ØX2 | T36.ØX3 | T36.ØX4 | T36.ØX5 | T36.ØX6 |
| **Mianserin** | T43.Ø21 | T43.Ø22 | T43.Ø23 | T43.Ø24 | T43.Ø25 | T43.Ø26 |
| **Micatin** | T49.ØX1 | T49.ØX2 | T49.ØX3 | T49.ØX4 | T49.ØX5 | T49.ØX6 |
| **Miconazole** | T49.ØX1 | T49.ØX2 | T49.ØX3 | T49.ØX4 | T49.ØX5 | T49.ØX6 |
| **Micronomicin** | T36.5X1 | T36.5X2 | T36.5X3 | T36.5X4 | T36.5X5 | T36.5X6 |
| **Microzide*** | T5Ø.2X1 | T5Ø.2X2 | T5Ø.2X3 | T5Ø.2X4 | T5Ø.2X5 | T5Ø.2X6 |
| **Midazolam** | T42.4X1 | T42.4X2 | T42.4X3 | T42.4X4 | T42.4X5 | T42.4X6 |
| **Midecamycin** | T36.3X1 | T36.3X2 | T36.3X3 | T36.3X4 | T36.3X5 | T36.3X6 |
| **Mifepristone** | T38.6X1 | T38.6X2 | T38.6X3 | T38.6X4 | T38.6X5 | T38.6X6 |
| **Milk of magnesia** | T47.1X1 | T47.1X2 | T47.1X3 | T47.1X4 | T47.1X5 | T47.1X6 |
| **Millipede** (tropical) (venomous) | T63.411 | T63.412 | T63.413 | T63.414 | — | — |
| **Miltown** | T43.591 | T43.592 | T43.593 | T43.594 | T43.595 | T43.596 |
| **Milverine** | T44.3X1 | T44.3X2 | T44.3X3 | T44.3X4 | T44.3X5 | T44.3X6 |
| **Minaprine** | T43.291 | T43.292 | T43.293 | T43.294 | T43.295 | T43.296 |
| **Minaxolone** | T41.291 | T41.292 | T41.293 | T41.294 | T41.295 | T41.296 |
| **Mineral** | | | | | | |
| acids | T54.2X1 | T54.2X2 | T54.2X3 | T54.2X4 | — | — |
| oil (laxative)(medicinal) | T47.4X1 | T47.4X2 | T47.4X3 | T47.4X4 | T47.4X5 | T47.4X6 |
| emulsion | T47.2X1 | T47.2X2 | T47.2X3 | T47.2X4 | T47.2X5 | T47.2X6 |
| nonmedicinal | T52.ØX1 | T52.ØX2 | T52.ØX3 | T52.ØX4 | — | — |
| topical | T49.3X1 | T49.3X2 | T49.3X3 | T49.3X4 | T49.3X5 | T49.3X6 |
| salt NEC | T5Ø.3X1 | T5Ø.3X2 | T5Ø.3X3 | T5Ø.3X4 | T5Ø.3X5 | T5Ø.3X6 |
| spirits | T52.ØX1 | T52.ØX2 | T52.ØX3 | T52.ØX4 | — | — |
| **Mineralocorticosteroid** | T5Ø.ØX1 | T5Ø.ØX2 | T5Ø.ØX3 | T5Ø.ØX4 | T5Ø.ØX5 | T5Ø.ØX6 |
| **Minocycline** | T36.4X1 | T36.4X2 | T36.4X3 | T36.4X4 | T36.4X5 | T36.4X6 |
| **Minoxidil** | T46.7X1 | T46.7X2 | T46.7X3 | T46.7X4 | T46.7X5 | T46.7X6 |
| **Miokamycin** | T36.3X1 | T36.3X2 | T36.3X3 | T36.3X4 | T36.3X5 | T36.3X6 |
| **Miotic drug** | T49.5X1 | T49.5X2 | T49.5X3 | T49.5X4 | T49.5X5 | T49.5X6 |
| **Mipafox** | T6Ø.ØX1 | T6Ø.ØX2 | T6Ø.ØX3 | T6Ø.ØX4 | — | — |
| **Mipomerson*** | T46.6X1 | T46.6X2 | T46.6X3 | T46.6X4 | T46.6X5 | T46.6X6 |
| **Mirex** | T6Ø.1X1 | T6Ø.1X2 | T6Ø.1X3 | T6Ø.1X4 | — | — |
| **Mirtazapine** | T43.Ø21 | T43.Ø22 | T43.Ø23 | T43.Ø24 | T43.Ø25 | T43.Ø26 |
| **Misonidazole** | T37.3X1 | T37.3X2 | T37.3X3 | T37.3X4 | T37.3X5 | T37.3X6 |
| **Misoprostol** | T47.1X1 | T47.1X2 | T47.1X3 | T47.1X4 | T47.1X5 | T47.1X6 |
| **Mithramycin** | T45.1X1 | T45.1X2 | T45.1X3 | T45.1X4 | T45.1X5 | T45.1X6 |
| **Mitobronitol** | T45.1X1 | T45.1X2 | T45.1X3 | T45.1X4 | T45.1X5 | T45.1X6 |
| **Mitoguazone** | T45.1X1 | T45.1X2 | T45.1X3 | T45.1X4 | T45.1X5 | T45.1X6 |
| **Mitolactol** | T45.1X1 | T45.1X2 | T45.1X3 | T45.1X4 | T45.1X5 | T45.1X6 |
| **Mitomycin** | T45.1X1 | T45.1X2 | T45.1X3 | T45.1X4 | T45.1X5 | T45.1X6 |
| **Mitopodozide** | T45.1X1 | T45.1X2 | T45.1X3 | T45.1X4 | T45.1X5 | T45.1X6 |
| **Mitotane** | T45.1X1 | T45.1X2 | T45.1X3 | T45.1X4 | T45.1X5 | T45.1X6 |
| **Mitoxantrone** | T45.1X1 | T45.1X2 | T45.1X3 | T45.1X4 | T45.1X5 | T45.1X6 |
| **Mivacurium chloride** | T48.1X1 | T48.1X2 | T48.1X3 | T48.1X4 | T48.1X5 | T48.1X6 |
| **Miyari bacteria** | T47.6X1 | T47.6X2 | T47.6X3 | T47.6X4 | T47.6X5 | T47.6X6 |
| **Mobic*** | T39.391 | T39.392 | T39.393 | T39.394 | T39.395 | T39.396 |
| **Moclobemide** | T43.1X1 | T43.1X2 | T43.1X3 | T43.1X4 | T43.1X5 | T43.1X6 |
| **Moderil** | T46.5X1 | T46.5X2 | T46.5X3 | T46.5X4 | T46.5X5 | T46.5X6 |
| **Mofebutazone** | T39.2X1 | T39.2X2 | T39.2X3 | T39.2X4 | T39.2X5 | T39.2X6 |
| **Mogadon** — *see* Nitrazepam | | | | | | |
| **Molindone** | T43.591 | T43.592 | T43.593 | T43.594 | T43.595 | T43.596 |
| **Molsidomine** | T46.3X1 | T46.3X2 | T46.3X3 | T46.3X4 | T46.3X5 | T46.3X6 |
| **Mometasone** | T49.ØX1 | T49.ØX2 | T49.ØX3 | T49.ØX4 | T49.ØX5 | T49.ØX6 |
| **Monistat** | T49.ØX1 | T49.ØX2 | T49.ØX3 | T49.ØX4 | T49.ØX5 | T49.ØX6 |
| **Monkshood** | T62.2X1 | T62.2X2 | T62.2X3 | T62.2X4 | — | — |
| **Monoamine oxidase inhibitor NEC** | T43.1X1 | T43.1X2 | T43.1X3 | T43.1X4 | T43.1X5 | T43.1X6 |
| hydrazine | T43.1X1 | T43.1X2 | T43.1X3 | T43.1X4 | T43.1X5 | T43.1X6 |
| **Monobenzone** | T49.4X1 | T49.4X2 | T49.4X3 | T49.4X4 | T49.4X5 | T49.4X6 |
| **Monochloroacetic acid** | T6Ø.3X1 | T6Ø.3X2 | T6Ø.3X3 | T6Ø.3X4 | — | — |
| **Monochlorobenzene** | T53.7X1 | T53.7X2 | T53.7X3 | T53.7X4 | — | — |
| **Monoethanolamine** | T46.8X1 | T46.8X2 | T46.8X3 | T46.8X4 | T46.8X5 | T46.8X6 |
| oleate | T46.8X1 | T46.8X2 | T46.8X3 | T46.8X4 | T46.8X5 | T46.8X6 |
| **Monooctanoin** | T5Ø.991 | T5Ø.992 | T5Ø.993 | T5Ø.994 | T5Ø.995 | T5Ø.996 |
| **Monophenylbutazone** | T39.2X1 | T39.2X2 | T39.2X3 | T39.2X4 | T39.2X5 | T39.2X6 |
| **Monopril*** | T46.4X1 | T46.4X2 | T46.4X3 | T46.4X4 | T46.4X5 | T46.4X6 |
| **Monosodium glutamate** | T65.891 | T65.892 | T65.893 | T65.894 | — | — |
| **Monosulfiram** | T49.ØX1 | T49.ØX2 | T49.ØX3 | T49.ØX4 | T49.ØX5 | T49.ØX6 |
| **Monoxide, carbon** — *see* Carbon, monoxide | | | | | | |
| **Monoxidine hydrochloride** | T46.1X1 | T46.1X2 | T46.1X3 | T46.1X4 | T46.1X5 | T46.1X6 |
| **Montelukast*** | T48.6X1 | T48.6X2 | T48.6X3 | T48.6X4 | T48.6X5 | T48.6X6 |
| **Monuron** | T6Ø.3X1 | T6Ø.3X2 | T6Ø.3X3 | T6Ø.3X4 | — | — |
| **Moperone** | T43.4X1 | T43.4X2 | T43.4X3 | T43.4X4 | T43.4X5 | T43.4X6 |
| **Mopidamol** | T45.1X1 | T45.1X2 | T45.1X3 | T45.1X4 | T45.1X5 | T45.1X6 |
| **MOPP** (mechlorethamine + vincristine + prednisone + procarbazine) | T45.1X1 | T45.1X2 | T45.1X3 | T45.1X4 | T45.1X5 | T45.1X6 |
| **Morfin** | T4Ø.2X1 | T4Ø.2X2 | T4Ø.2X3 | T4Ø.2X4 | T4Ø.2X5 | T4Ø.2X6 |
| **Morinamide** | T37.1X1 | T37.1X2 | T37.1X3 | T37.1X4 | T37.1X5 | T37.1X6 |
| **Morning glory seeds** | T4Ø.991 | T4Ø.992 | T4Ø.993 | T4Ø.994 | — | — |
| **Moroxydine** | T37.5X1 | T37.5X2 | T37.5X3 | T37.5X4 | T37.5X5 | T37.5X6 |
| **Morphazinamide** | T37.1X1 | T37.1X2 | T37.1X3 | T37.1X4 | T37.1X5 | T37.1X6 |
| **Morphine** | T4Ø.2X1 | T4Ø.2X2 | T4Ø.2X3 | T4Ø.2X4 | T4Ø.2X5 | T4Ø.2X6 |
| antagonist | T5Ø.7X1 | T5Ø.7X2 | T5Ø.7X3 | T5Ø.7X4 | T5Ø.7X5 | T5Ø.7X6 |
| **Morpholinylethylmorphine** | T4Ø.2X1 | T4Ø.2X2 | T4Ø.2X3 | T4Ø.2X4 | — | — |
| **Morsuximide** | T42.2X1 | T42.2X2 | T42.2X3 | T42.2X4 | T42.2X5 | T42.2X6 |
| **Mosapramine** | T43.591 | T43.592 | T43.593 | T43.594 | T43.595 | T43.596 |
| **Moth balls** — *see also* Pesticide | T6Ø.2X1 | T6Ø.2X2 | T6Ø.2X3 | T6Ø.2X4 | — | — |
| naphthalene | T6Ø.2X1 | T6Ø.2X2 | T6Ø.2X3 | T6Ø.2X4 | — | — |
| paradichlorobenzene | T6Ø.1X1 | T6Ø.1X2 | T6Ø.1X3 | T6Ø.1X4 | — | — |
| **Motor exhaust gas** | T58.Ø1 | T58.Ø2 | T58.Ø3 | T58.Ø4 | — | — |
| **Motrin*** | T39.311 | T39.312 | T39.313 | T39.314 | T39.315 | T39.316 |
| **Mouthwash** (antiseptic) (zinc chloride) | T49.6X1 | T49.6X2 | T49.6X3 | T49.6X4 | T49.6X5 | T49.6X6 |
| **Moxastine** | T45.ØX1 | T45.ØX2 | T45.ØX3 | T45.ØX4 | T45.ØX5 | T45.ØX6 |
| **Moxaverine** | T44.3X1 | T44.3X2 | T44.3X3 | T44.3X4 | T44.3X5 | T44.3X6 |
| **Moxisylyte** | T46.7X1 | T46.7X2 | T46.7X3 | T46.7X4 | T46.7X5 | T46.7X6 |
| **Mucilage, plant** | T47.4X1 | T47.4X2 | T47.4X3 | T47.4X4 | T47.4X5 | T47.4X6 |
| **Mucolytic drug** | T48.4X1 | T48.4X2 | T48.4X3 | T48.4X4 | T48.4X5 | T48.4X6 |
| **Mucomyst** | T48.4X1 | T48.4X2 | T48.4X3 | T48.4X4 | T48.4X5 | T48.4X6 |
| **Mucous membrane agents** (external) | T49.91 | T49.92 | T49.93 | T49.94 | T49.95 | T49.96 |
| specified NEC | T49.8X1 | T49.8X2 | T49.8X3 | T49.8X4 | T49.8X5 | T49.8X6 |
| **Multaq*** | T46.2X1 | T46.2X2 | T46.2X3 | T46.2X4 | T46.2X5 | T46.2X6 |
| **Multiple unspecified drugs, medicaments and biological substances** | T5Ø.911 | T5Ø.912 | T5Ø.913 | T5Ø.914 | T5Ø.915 | T5Ø.916 |
| **Mumps** | | | | | | |
| immune globulin (human) | T5Ø.Z11 | T5Ø.Z12 | T5Ø.Z13 | T5Ø.Z14 | T5Ø.Z15 | T5Ø.Z16 |
| skin test antigen | T5Ø.8X1 | T5Ø.8X2 | T5Ø.8X3 | T5Ø.8X4 | T5Ø.8X5 | T5Ø.8X6 |
| vaccine | T5Ø.B91 | T5Ø.B92 | T5Ø.B93 | T5Ø.B94 | T5Ø.B95 | T5Ø.B96 |
| **Mumpsvax** | T5Ø.B91 | T5Ø.B92 | T5Ø.B93 | T5Ø.B94 | T5Ø.B95 | T5Ø.B96 |
| **Mupirocin** | T49.ØX1 | T49.ØX2 | T49.ØX3 | T49.ØX4 | T49.ØX5 | T49.ØX6 |
| **Muriatic acid** — *see* Hydrochloric acid | | | | | | |
| **Muromonab-CD3** | T45.1X1 | T45.1X2 | T45.1X3 | T45.1X4 | T45.1X5 | T45.1X6 |
| **Muscle-action drug NEC** | T48.2Ø1 | T48.2Ø2 | T48.2Ø3 | T48.2Ø4 | T48.2Ø5 | T48.2Ø6 |
| **Muscle affecting agents NEC** | T48.2Ø1 | T48.2Ø2 | T48.2Ø3 | T48.2Ø4 | T48.2Ø5 | T48.2Ø6 |
| oxytocic | T48.ØX1 | T48.ØX2 | T48.ØX3 | T48.ØX4 | T48.ØX5 | T48.ØX6 |
| relaxants | T48.2Ø1 | T48.2Ø2 | T48.2Ø3 | T48.2Ø4 | T48.2Ø5 | T48.2Ø6 |
| central nervous system | T42.8X1 | T42.8X2 | T42.8X3 | T42.8X4 | T42.8X5 | T42.8X6 |
| skeletal | T48.1X1 | T48.1X2 | T48.1X3 | T48.1X4 | T48.1X5 | T48.1X6 |
| smooth | T44.3X1 | T44.3X2 | T44.3X3 | T44.3X4 | T44.3X5 | T44.3X6 |

| Substance | Poisoning, Accidental (unintentional) | Poisoning, Intentional Self-harm | Poisoning, Assault | Poisoning, Undetermined | Adverse Effect | Under-dosing |
|---|---|---|---|---|---|---|
| **Muscle relaxant** — *see* Relaxant, muscle | | | | | | |
| **Muscle-tone depressant, central NEC** | T42.8X1 | T42.8X2 | T42.8X3 | T42.8X4 | T42.8X5 | T42.8X6 |
| specified NEC | T42.8X1 | T42.8X2 | T42.8X3 | T42.8X4 | T42.8X5 | T42.8X6 |
| **Mushroom, noxious** | T62.ØX1 | T62.ØX2 | T62.ØX3 | T62.ØX4 | — | — |
| **Mussel, noxious** | T61.781 | T61.782 | T61.783 | T61.784 | — | — |
| **Mustard** (emetic) | T47.7X1 | T47.7X2 | T47.7X3 | T47.7X4 | T47.7X5 | T47.7X6 |
| black | T47.7X1 | T47.7X2 | T47.7X3 | T47.7X4 | T47.7X5 | T47.7X6 |
| gas, not in war | T59.91 | T59.92 | T59.93 | T59.94 | — | — |
| nitrogen | T45.1X1 | T45.1X2 | T45.1X3 | T45.1X4 | T45.1X5 | T45.1X6 |
| **Mustine** | T45.1X1 | T45.1X2 | T45.1X3 | T45.1X4 | T45.1X5 | T45.1X6 |
| **Mycifradin** | T36.5X1 | T36.5X2 | T36.5X3 | T36.5X4 | T36.5X5 | T36.5X6 |
| topical | T49.ØX1 | T49.ØX2 | T49.ØX3 | T49.ØX4 | T49.ØX5 | T49.ØX6 |
| **Mycitracin** | T36.8X1 | T36.8X2 | T36.8X3 | T36.8X4 | T36.8X5 | T36.8X6 |
| ophthalmic preparation | T49.5X1 | T49.5X2 | T49.5X3 | T49.5X4 | T49.5X5 | T49.5X6 |
| **Mycostatin** | T36.7X1 | T36.7X2 | T36.7X3 | T36.7X4 | T36.7X5 | T36.7X6 |
| topical | T49.ØX1 | T49.ØX2 | T49.ØX3 | T49.ØX4 | T49.ØX5 | T49.ØX6 |
| **Mycotoxins** | T64.81 | T64.82 | T64.83 | T64.84 | — | — |
| aflatoxin | T64.Ø1 | T64.Ø2 | T64.Ø3 | T64.Ø4 | — | — |
| specified NEC | T64.81 | T64.82 | T64.83 | T64.84 | — | — |
| **Mydriacyl** | T44.3X1 | T44.3X2 | T44.3X3 | T44.3X4 | T44.3X5 | T44.3X6 |
| **Mydriatic drug** | T49.5X1 | T49.5X2 | T49.5X3 | T49.5X4 | T49.5X5 | T49.5X6 |
| **Myelobromal** | T45.1X1 | T45.1X2 | T45.1X3 | T45.1X4 | T45.1X5 | T45.1X6 |
| **Myleran** | T45.1X1 | T45.1X2 | T45.1X3 | T45.1X4 | T45.1X5 | T45.1X6 |
| **Myochrysin** (e) | T39.2X1 | T39.2X2 | T39.2X3 | T39.2X4 | T39.2X5 | T39.2X6 |
| **Myoneural blocking agents** | T48.1X1 | T48.1X2 | T48.1X3 | T48.1X4 | T48.1X5 | T48.1X6 |
| **Myrac*** | T36.4X1 | T36.4X2 | T36.4X3 | T36.4X4 | T36.4X5 | T36.4X6 |
| **Myralact** | T49.ØX1 | T49.ØX2 | T49.ØX3 | T49.ØX4 | T49.ØX5 | T49.ØX6 |
| **Myristica fragrans** | T62.2X1 | T62.2X2 | T62.2X3 | T62.2X4 | — | — |
| **Myristicin** | T65.891 | T65.892 | T65.893 | T65.894 | — | — |
| **Mysoline** | T42.3X1 | T42.3X2 | T42.3X3 | T42.3X4 | T42.3X5 | T42.3X6 |
| **Nabilone** | T40.711 | T40.712 | T40.713 | T40.714 | T40.715 | T40.716 |
| **Nabumetone** | T39.391 | T39.392 | T39.393 | T39.394 | T39.395 | T39.396 |
| **Nadolol** | T44.7X1 | T44.7X2 | T44.7X3 | T44.7X4 | T44.7X5 | T44.7X6 |
| **Nafcillin** | T36.ØX1 | T36.ØX2 | T36.ØX3 | T36.ØX4 | T36.ØX5 | T36.ØX6 |
| **Nafoxidine** | T38.6X1 | T38.6X2 | T38.6X3 | T38.6X4 | T38.6X5 | T38.6X6 |
| **Naftazone** | T46.991 | T46.992 | T46.993 | T46.994 | T46.995 | T46.996 |
| **Naftidrofuryl** (oxalate) | T46.7X1 | T46.7X2 | T46.7X3 | T46.7X4 | T46.7X5 | T46.7X6 |
| **Naftifine** | T49.ØX1 | T49.ØX2 | T49.ØX3 | T49.ØX4 | T49.ØX5 | T49.ØX6 |
| **Nail polish remover** | T52.91 | T52.92 | T52.93 | T52.94 | — | — |
| **Nalbuphine** | T40.491 | T40.492 | T40.493 | T40.494 | T40.495 | T40.496 |
| **Naled** | T60.ØX1 | T60.ØX2 | T60.ØX3 | T60.ØX4 | — | — |
| **Nalidixic acid** | T37.8X1 | T37.8X2 | T37.8X3 | T37.8X4 | T37.8X5 | T37.8X6 |
| **Nalorphine** | T50.7X1 | T50.7X2 | T50.7X3 | T50.7X4 | T50.7X5 | T50.7X6 |
| **Naloxone** | T50.7X1 | T50.7X2 | T50.7X3 | T50.7X4 | T50.7X5 | T50.7X6 |
| **Naltrexone** | T50.7X1 | T50.7X2 | T50.7X3 | T50.7X4 | T50.7X5 | T50.7X6 |
| **Namenda** | T43.8X1 | T43.8X2 | T43.8X3 | T43.8X4 | T43.8X5 | T43.8X6 |
| **Nandrolone** | T38.7X1 | T38.7X2 | T38.7X3 | T38.7X4 | T38.7X5 | T38.7X6 |
| **Naphazoline** | T48.5X1 | T48.5X2 | T48.5X3 | T48.5X4 | T48.5X5 | T48.5X6 |
| **Naphtha** (painters') (petroleum) | T52.ØX1 | T52.ØX2 | T52.ØX3 | T52.ØX4 | — | — |
| solvent | T52.ØX1 | T52.ØX2 | T52.ØX3 | T52.ØX4 | — | — |
| vapor | T52.ØX1 | T52.ØX2 | T52.ØX3 | T52.ØX4 | — | — |
| **Naphthalene** (non-chlorinated) | T60.2X1 | T60.2X2 | T60.2X3 | T60.2X4 | — | — |
| chlorinated | T60.1X1 | T60.1X2 | T60.1X3 | T60.1X4 | — | — |
| vapor | T60.1X1 | T60.1X2 | T60.1X3 | T60.1X4 | — | — |
| insecticide or moth repellent | T60.2X1 | T60.2X2 | T60.2X3 | T60.2X4 | — | — |
| chlorinated | T60.1X1 | T60.1X2 | T60.1X3 | T60.1X4 | — | — |
| vapor | T60.2X1 | T60.2X2 | T60.2X3 | T60.2X4 | — | — |
| chlorinated | T60.1X1 | T60.1X2 | T60.1X3 | T60.1X4 | — | — |
| **Naphthenes** | T52.821 | T52.822 | T52.823 | T52.824 | — | — |
| **Naphthol** | T65.891 | T65.892 | T65.893 | T65.894 | — | — |
| **Naphthylamine** | T65.891 | T65.892 | T65.893 | T65.894 | — | — |
| **Naphthylthiourea** (ANTU) | T60.4X1 | T60.4X2 | T60.4X3 | T60.4X4 | — | — |
| **Naprosyn** — *see* Naproxen | | | | | | |
| **Naproxen** | T39.311 | T39.312 | T39.313 | T39.314 | T39.315 | T39.316 |
| **Narcotic** (drug) | T40.6Ø1 | T40.6Ø2 | T40.6Ø3 | T40.6Ø4 | T40.6Ø5 | T40.6Ø6 |
| analgesic NEC | T40.6Ø1 | T40.6Ø2 | T40.6Ø3 | T40.6Ø4 | T40.6Ø5 | T40.6Ø6 |
| antagonist | T50.7X1 | T50.7X2 | T50.7X3 | T50.7X4 | T50.7X5 | T50.7X6 |
| specified NEC | T40.691 | T40.692 | T40.693 | T40.694 | T40.695 | T40.696 |
| synthetic | T40.491 | T40.492 | T40.493 | T40.494 | T40.495 | T40.496 |
| **Narcotine** | T48.3X1 | T48.3X2 | T48.3X3 | T48.3X4 | T48.3X5 | T48.3X6 |
| **Nardil** | T43.1X1 | T43.1X2 | T43.1X3 | T43.1X4 | T43.1X5 | T43.1X6 |
| **Nasacort*** | T49.5X1 | T49.5X2 | T49.5X3 | T49.5X4 | T49.5X5 | T49.5X6 |
| **Nasal drug NEC** | T49.6X1 | T49.6X2 | T49.6X3 | T49.6X4 | T49.6X5 | T49.6X6 |
| **Natamycin** | T49.ØX1 | T49.ØX2 | T49.ØX3 | T49.ØX4 | T49.ØX5 | T49.ØX6 |
| **Natrium cyanide** — *see* Cyanide(s) | | | | | | |
| **Natural** | | | | | | |
| **Natural** — *continued* | | | | | | |
| blood (product) | T45.8X1 | T45.8X2 | T45.8X3 | T45.8X4 | T45.8X5 | T45.8X6 |
| gas (piped) | T59.891 | T59.892 | T59.893 | T59.894 | — | — |
| incomplete combustion | T58.11 | T58.12 | T58.13 | T58.14 | — | — |
| **Nealbarbital** | T42.3X1 | T42.3X2 | T42.3X3 | T42.3X4 | T42.3X5 | T42.3X6 |
| **Nectadon** | T48.3X1 | T48.3X2 | T48.3X3 | T48.3X4 | T48.3X5 | T48.3X6 |
| **Nedocromil** | T48.6X1 | T48.6X2 | T48.6X3 | T48.6X4 | T48.6X5 | T48.6X6 |
| **Nefopam** | T39.8X1 | T39.8X2 | T39.8X3 | T39.8X4 | T39.8X5 | T39.8X6 |
| **Nematocyst** (sting) | T63.691 | T63.692 | T63.693 | T63.694 | — | — |
| **Nembutal** | T42.3X1 | T42.3X2 | T42.3X3 | T42.3X4 | T42.3X5 | T42.3X6 |
| **Nemonapride** | T43.591 | T43.592 | T43.593 | T43.594 | T43.595 | T43.596 |
| **Neoarsphenamine** | T37.8X1 | T37.8X2 | T37.8X3 | T37.8X4 | T37.8X5 | T37.8X6 |
| **Neocinchophen** | T50.4X1 | T50.4X2 | T50.4X3 | T50.4X4 | T50.4X5 | T50.4X6 |
| **Neomycin** (derivatives) | T36.5X1 | T36.5X2 | T36.5X3 | T36.5X4 | T36.5X5 | T36.5X6 |
| ENT agent | T49.6X1 | T49.6X2 | T49.6X3 | T49.6X4 | T49.6X5 | T49.6X6 |
| ophthalmic preparation | T49.5X1 | T49.5X2 | T49.5X3 | T49.5X4 | T49.5X5 | T49.5X6 |
| topical NEC | T49.ØX1 | T49.ØX2 | T49.ØX3 | T49.ØX4 | T49.ØX5 | T49.ØX6 |
| with | | | | | | |
| bacitracin | T49.ØX1 | T49.ØX2 | T49.ØX3 | T49.ØX4 | T49.ØX5 | T49.ØX6 |
| neostigmine | T44.ØX1 | T44.ØX2 | T44.ØX3 | T44.ØX4 | T44.ØX5 | T44.ØX6 |
| **Neonal** | T42.3X1 | T42.3X2 | T42.3X3 | T42.3X4 | T42.3X5 | T42.3X6 |
| **Neopham*** | T50.3X1 | T50.3X2 | T50.3X3 | T50.3X4 | T50.3X5 | T50.3X6 |
| **Neoprontosil** | T37.ØX1 | T37.ØX2 | T37.ØX3 | T37.ØX4 | T37.ØX5 | T37.ØX6 |
| **Neosalvarsan** | T37.8X1 | T37.8X2 | T37.8X3 | T37.8X4 | T37.8X5 | T37.8X6 |
| **Neosilversalvarsan** | T37.8X1 | T37.8X2 | T37.8X3 | T37.8X4 | T37.8X5 | T37.8X6 |
| **Neosporin** | T36.8X1 | T36.8X2 | T36.8X3 | T36.8X4 | T36.8X5 | T36.8X6 |
| ENT agent | T49.6X1 | T49.6X2 | T49.6X3 | T49.6X4 | T49.6X5 | T49.6X6 |
| ophthalmic preparation | T49.5X1 | T49.5X2 | T49.5X3 | T49.5X4 | T49.5X5 | T49.5X6 |
| topical NEC | T49.ØX1 | T49.ØX2 | T49.ØX3 | T49.ØX4 | T49.ØX5 | T49.ØX6 |
| **Neostigmine bromide** | T44.ØX1 | T44.ØX2 | T44.ØX3 | T44.ØX4 | T44.ØX5 | T44.ØX6 |
| **Neraval** | T42.3X1 | T42.3X2 | T42.3X3 | T42.3X4 | T42.3X5 | T42.3X6 |
| **Neravan** | T42.3X1 | T42.3X2 | T42.3X3 | T42.3X4 | T42.3X5 | T42.3X6 |
| **Nerium oleander** | T62.2X1 | T62.2X2 | T62.2X3 | T62.2X4 | — | — |
| **Nerlynx*** | T45.1X1 | T45.1X2 | T45.1X3 | T45.1X4 | T45.1X5 | T45.1X6 |
| **Nerve gas, not in war** | T59.91 | T59.92 | T59.93 | T59.94 | — | — |
| **Nesacaine** | T41.3X1 | T41.3X2 | T41.3X3 | T41.3X4 | T41.3X5 | T41.3X6 |
| infiltration (subcutaneous) | T41.3X1 | T41.3X2 | T41.3X3 | T41.3X4 | T41.3X5 | T41.3X6 |
| nerve block (peripheral) (plexus) | T41.3X1 | T41.3X2 | T41.3X3 | T41.3X4 | T41.3X5 | T41.3X6 |
| **Netilmicin** | T36.5X1 | T36.5X2 | T36.5X3 | T36.5X4 | T36.5X5 | T36.5X6 |
| **Neurobarb** | T42.3X1 | T42.3X2 | T42.3X3 | T42.3X4 | T42.3X5 | T42.3X6 |
| **Neuroleptic drug NEC** | T43.5Ø1 | T43.5Ø2 | T43.5Ø3 | T43.5Ø4 | T43.5Ø5 | T43.5Ø6 |
| **Neuromuscular blocking drug** | T48.1X1 | T48.1X2 | T48.1X3 | T48.1X4 | T48.1X5 | T48.1X6 |
| **Neurontin*** | T42.6X1 | T42.6X2 | T42.6X3 | T42.6X4 | T42.6X5 | T42.6X6 |
| **Neutral insulin injection** | T38.3X1 | T38.3X2 | T38.3X3 | T38.3X4 | T38.3X5 | T38.3X6 |
| **Neutral spirits** | T51.ØX1 | T51.ØX2 | T51.ØX3 | T51.ØX4 | — | — |
| beverage | T51.ØX1 | T51.ØX2 | T51.ØX3 | T51.ØX4 | — | — |
| **Niacin** | T46.7X1 | T46.7X2 | T46.7X3 | T46.7X4 | T46.7X5 | T46.7X6 |
| **Niacinamide** | T45.2X1 | T45.2X2 | T45.2X3 | T45.2X4 | T45.2X5 | T45.2X6 |
| **Nialamide** | T43.1X1 | T43.1X2 | T43.1X3 | T43.1X4 | T43.1X5 | T43.1X6 |
| **Niaprazine** | T42.6X1 | T42.6X2 | T42.6X3 | T42.6X4 | T42.6X5 | T42.6X6 |
| **Nicametate** | T46.7X1 | T46.7X2 | T46.7X3 | T46.7X4 | T46.7X5 | T46.7X6 |
| **Nicardipine** | T46.1X1 | T46.1X2 | T46.1X3 | T46.1X4 | T46.1X5 | T46.1X6 |
| **Nicergoline** | T46.7X1 | T46.7X2 | T46.7X3 | T46.7X4 | T46.7X5 | T46.7X6 |
| **Nickel** (carbonyl) (tetra-carbonyl) (fumes) (vapor) | T56.891 | T56.892 | T56.893 | T56.894 | — | — |
| **Nickelocene** | T56.891 | T56.892 | T56.893 | T56.894 | — | — |
| **Niclosamide** | T37.4X1 | T37.4X2 | T37.4X3 | T37.4X4 | T37.4X5 | T37.4X6 |
| **Nicofuranose** | T46.7X1 | T46.7X2 | T46.7X3 | T46.7X4 | T46.7X5 | T46.7X6 |
| **Nicomorphine** | T40.2X1 | T40.2X2 | T40.2X3 | T40.2X4 | — | — |
| **Nicorandil** | T46.3X1 | T46.3X2 | T46.3X3 | T46.3X4 | T46.3X5 | T46.3X6 |
| **Nicotiana** (plant) | T62.2X1 | T62.2X2 | T62.2X3 | T62.2X4 | — | — |
| **Nicotinamide** | T45.2X1 | T45.2X2 | T45.2X3 | T45.2X4 | T45.2X5 | T45.2X6 |
| **Nicotine** (insecticide) (spray) (sulfate) **NEC** | T60.2X1 | T60.2X2 | T60.2X3 | T60.2X4 | — | — |
| from tobacco | T65.291 | T65.292 | T65.293 | T65.294 | — | — |
| cigarettes | T65.221 | T65.222 | T65.223 | T65.224 | — | — |
| not insecticide | T65.291 | T65.292 | T65.293 | T65.294 | — | — |
| **Nicotinic acid** | T46.7X1 | T46.7X2 | T46.7X3 | T46.7X4 | T46.7X5 | T46.7X6 |
| **Nicotinyl alcohol** | T46.7X1 | T46.7X2 | T46.7X3 | T46.7X4 | T46.7X5 | T46.7X6 |
| **Nicoumalone** | T45.511 | T45.512 | T45.513 | T45.514 | T45.515 | T45.516 |
| **Nifedipine** | T46.1X1 | T46.1X2 | T46.1X3 | T46.1X4 | T46.1X5 | T46.1X6 |
| **Nifenazone** | T39.2X1 | T39.2X2 | T39.2X3 | T39.2X4 | T39.2X5 | T39.2X6 |
| **Nifuraldezone** | T37.91 | T37.92 | T37.93 | T37.94 | T37.95 | T37.96 |
| **Nifuratel** | T37.8X1 | T37.8X2 | T37.8X3 | T37.8X4 | T37.8X5 | T37.8X6 |
| **Nifurtimox** | T37.3X1 | T37.3X2 | T37.3X3 | T37.3X4 | T37.3X5 | T37.3X6 |
| **Nifurtoinol** | T37.8X1 | T37.8X2 | T37.8X3 | T37.8X4 | T37.8X5 | T37.8X6 |
| **Nightshade, deadly** (solanum) — *see also* Belladonna | T62.2X1 | T62.2X2 | T62.2X3 | T62.2X4 | — | — |
| berry | T62.1X1 | T62.1X2 | T62.1X3 | T62.1X4 | — | — |
| **Nikethamide** | T50.7X1 | T50.7X2 | T50.7X3 | T50.7X4 | T50.7X5 | T50.7X6 |
| **Nilstat** | T36.7X1 | T36.7X2 | T36.7X3 | T36.7X4 | T36.7X5 | T36.7X6 |

| Substance | Poisoning, Accidental (unintentional) | Poisoning, Intentional Self-harm | Poisoning, Assault | Poisoning, Undetermined | Adverse Effect | Under-dosing |
|---|---|---|---|---|---|---|
| **Nilstat** — *continued* | | | | | | |
| topical | T49.ØX1 | T49.ØX2 | T49.ØX3 | T49.ØX4 | T49.ØX5 | T49.ØX6 |
| **Nilutamide** | T38.6X1 | T38.6X2 | T38.6X3 | T38.6X4 | T38.6X5 | T38.6X6 |
| **Nimesulide** | T39.391 | T39.392 | T39.393 | T39.394 | T39.395 | T39.396 |
| **Nimetazepam** | T42.4X1 | T42.4X2 | T42.4X3 | T42.4X4 | T42.4X5 | T42.4X6 |
| **Nimodipine** | T46.1X1 | T46.1X2 | T46.1X3 | T46.1X4 | T46.1X5 | T46.1X6 |
| **Nimorazole** | T37.3X1 | T37.3X2 | T37.3X3 | T37.3X4 | T37.3X5 | T37.3X6 |
| **Nimustine** | T45.1X1 | T45.1X2 | T45.1X3 | T45.1X4 | T45.1X5 | T45.1X6 |
| **Nipent*** | T45.1X1 | T45.1X2 | T45.1X3 | T45.1X4 | T45.1X5 | T45.1X6 |
| **Niridazole** | T37.4X1 | T37.4X2 | T37.4X3 | T37.4X4 | T37.4X5 | T37.4X6 |
| **Nisentil** | T4Ø.2X1 | T4Ø.2X2 | T4Ø.2X3 | T4Ø.2X4 | T4Ø.2X5 | T4Ø.2X6 |
| **Nisoldipine** | T46.1X1 | T46.1X2 | T46.1X3 | T46.1X4 | T46.1X5 | T46.1X6 |
| **Nitramine** | T65.3X1 | T65.3X2 | T65.3X3 | T65.3X4 | — | — |
| **Nitrate, organic** | T46.3X1 | T46.3X2 | T46.3X3 | T46.3X4 | T46.3X5 | T46.3X6 |
| **Nitrazepam** | T42.4X1 | T42.4X2 | T42.4X3 | T42.4X4 | T42.4X5 | T42.4X6 |
| **Nitrefazole** | T5Ø.6X1 | T5Ø.6X2 | T5Ø.6X3 | T5Ø.6X4 | T5Ø.6X5 | T5Ø.6X6 |
| **Nitrendipine** | T46.1X1 | T46.1X2 | T46.1X3 | T46.1X4 | T46.1X5 | T46.1X6 |
| **Nitric** | | | | | | |
| acid (liquid) | T54.2X1 | T54.2X2 | T54.2X3 | T54.2X4 | — | — |
| vapor | T59.891 | T59.892 | T59.893 | T59.894 | — | — |
| oxide (gas) | T59.ØX1 | T59.ØX2 | T59.ØX3 | T59.ØX4 | — | — |
| **Nitrimidazine** | T37.3X1 | T37.3X2 | T37.3X3 | T37.3X4 | T37.3X5 | T37.3X6 |
| **Nitrite, amyl** (medicinal) (vapor) | T46.3X1 | T46.3X2 | T46.3X3 | T46.3X4 | T46.3X5 | T46.3X6 |
| **Nitroaniline** | T65.3X1 | T65.3X2 | T65.3X3 | T65.3X4 | — | — |
| vapor | T59.891 | T59.892 | T59.893 | T59.894 | — | — |
| **Nitrobenzene, nitrobenzol** | T65.3X1 | T65.3X2 | T65.3X3 | T65.3X4 | — | — |
| vapor | T65.3X1 | T65.3X2 | T65.3X3 | T65.3X4 | — | — |
| **Nitrocellulose** | T65.891 | T65.892 | T65.893 | T65.894 | — | — |
| lacquer | T65.891 | T65.892 | T65.893 | T65.894 | — | — |
| **Nitrodiphenyl** | T65.3X1 | T65.3X2 | T65.3X3 | T65.3X4 | — | — |
| **Nitrofural** | T49.ØX1 | T49.ØX2 | T49.ØX3 | T49.ØX4 | T49.ØX5 | T49.ØX6 |
| **Nitrofurantoin** | T37.8X1 | T37.8X2 | T37.8X3 | T37.8X4 | T37.8X5 | T37.8X6 |
| **Nitrofurazone** | T49.ØX1 | T49.ØX2 | T49.ØX3 | T49.ØX4 | T49.ØX5 | T49.ØX6 |
| **Nitrogen** | T59.ØX1 | T59.ØX2 | T59.ØX3 | T59.ØX4 | — | — |
| mustard | T45.1X1 | T45.1X2 | T45.1X3 | T45.1X4 | T45.1X5 | T45.1X6 |
| **Nitroglycerin, nitroglycerol** (medicinal) | T46.3X1 | T46.3X2 | T46.3X3 | T46.3X4 | T46.3X5 | T46.3X6 |
| nonmedicinal | T65.5X1 | T65.5X2 | T65.5X3 | T65.5X4 | — | — |
| fumes | T65.5X1 | T65.5X2 | T65.5X3 | T65.5X4 | — | — |
| **Nitroglycol** | T52.3X1 | T52.3X2 | T52.3X3 | T52.3X4 | — | — |
| **Nitrohydrochloric acid** | T54.2X1 | T54.2X2 | T54.2X3 | T54.2X4 | — | — |
| **Nitromersol** | T49.ØX1 | T49.ØX2 | T49.ØX3 | T49.ØX4 | T49.ØX5 | T49.ØX6 |
| **Nitronaphthalene** | T65.891 | T65.892 | T65.893 | T65.894 | — | — |
| **Nitrophenol** | T54.ØX1 | T54.ØX2 | T54.ØX3 | T54.ØX4 | — | — |
| **Nitropropane** | T52.891 | T52.892 | T52.893 | T52.894 | — | — |
| **Nitroprusside** | T46.5X1 | T46.5X2 | T46.5X3 | T46.5X4 | T46.5X5 | T46.5X6 |
| **Nitrosodimethylamine** | T65.3X1 | T65.3X2 | T65.3X3 | T65.3X4 | — | — |
| **Nitrothiazol** | T37.4X1 | T37.4X2 | T37.4X3 | T37.4X4 | T37.4X5 | T37.4X6 |
| **Nitrotoluene, nitrotoluol** | T65.3X1 | T65.3X2 | T65.3X3 | T65.3X4 | — | — |
| vapor | T65.3X1 | T65.3X2 | T65.3X3 | T65.3X4 | — | — |
| **Nitrous** | | | | | | |
| acid (liquid) | T54.2X1 | T54.2X2 | T54.2X3 | T54.2X4 | — | — |
| fumes | T59.891 | T59.892 | T59.893 | T59.894 | — | — |
| ether spirit | T46.3X1 | T46.3X2 | T46.3X3 | T46.3X4 | T46.3X5 | T46.3X6 |
| oxide | T41.ØX1 | T41.ØX2 | T41.ØX3 | T41.ØX4 | T41.ØX5 | T41.ØX6 |
| **Nitroxoline** | T37.8X1 | T37.8X2 | T37.8X3 | T37.8X4 | T37.8X5 | T37.8X6 |
| **Nitrozone** | T49.ØX1 | T49.ØX2 | T49.ØX3 | T49.ØX4 | T49.ØX5 | T49.ØX6 |
| **Nizatidine** | T47.ØX1 | T47.ØX2 | T47.ØX3 | T47.ØX4 | T47.ØX5 | T47.ØX6 |
| **Nizofenone** | T43.8X1 | T43.8X2 | T43.8X3 | T43.8X4 | T43.8X5 | T43.8X6 |
| **No Doz*** | T43.611 | T43.612 | T43.613 | T43.614 | T43.615 | T43.616 |
| **Noctec** | T42.6X1 | T42.6X2 | T42.6X3 | T42.6X4 | T42.6X5 | T42.6X6 |
| **Noludar** | T42.6X1 | T42.6X2 | T42.6X3 | T42.6X4 | T42.6X5 | T42.6X6 |
| **Nomegestrol** | T38.5X1 | T38.5X2 | T38.5X3 | T38.5X4 | T38.5X5 | T38.5X6 |
| **Nomifensine** | T43.291 | T43.292 | T43.293 | T43.294 | T43.295 | T43.296 |
| **Nonoxinol** | T49.8X1 | T49.8X2 | T49.8X3 | T49.8X4 | T49.8X5 | T49.8X6 |
| **Nonylphenoxy** (polyethoxyethanol) | T49.8X1 | T49.8X2 | T49.8X3 | T49.8X4 | T49.8X5 | T49.8X6 |
| **Noptil** | T42.3X1 | T42.3X2 | T42.3X3 | T42.3X4 | T42.3X5 | T42.3X6 |
| **Noradrenaline** | T44.4X1 | T44.4X2 | T44.4X3 | T44.4X4 | T44.4X5 | T44.4X6 |
| **Noramidopyrine** | T39.2X1 | T39.2X2 | T39.2X3 | T39.2X4 | T39.2X5 | T39.2X6 |
| methanesulfonate sodium | T39.2X1 | T39.2X2 | T39.2X3 | T39.2X4 | T39.2X5 | T39.2X6 |
| **Norbormide** | T6Ø.4X1 | T6Ø.4X2 | T6Ø.4X3 | T6Ø.4X4 | — | — |
| **Nordazepam** | T42.4X1 | T42.4X2 | T42.4X3 | T42.4X4 | T42.4X5 | T42.4X6 |
| **Norepinephrine** | T44.4X1 | T44.4X2 | T44.4X3 | T44.4X4 | T44.4X5 | T44.4X6 |
| **Norethandrolone** | T38.7X1 | T38.7X2 | T38.7X3 | T38.7X4 | T38.7X5 | T38.7X6 |
| **Norethindrone** | T38.4X1 | T38.4X2 | T38.4X3 | T38.4X4 | T38.4X5 | T38.4X6 |
| **Norethisterone** (acetate) (enantate) | T38.4X1 | T38.4X2 | T38.4X3 | T38.4X4 | T38.4X5 | T38.4X6 |
| with ethinylestradiol | T38.5X1 | T38.5X2 | T38.5X3 | T38.5X4 | T38.5X5 | T38.5X6 |
| **Noretynodrel** | T38.5X1 | T38.5X2 | T38.5X3 | T38.5X4 | T38.5X5 | T38.5X6 |
| **Norfenefrine** | T44.4X1 | T44.4X2 | T44.4X3 | T44.4X4 | T44.4X5 | T44.4X6 |
| **Norfloxacin** | T36.8X1 | T36.8X2 | T36.8X3 | T36.8X4 | T36.8X5 | T36.8X6 |

| Substance | Poisoning, Accidental (unintentional) | Poisoning, Intentional Self-harm | Poisoning, Assault | Poisoning, Undetermined | Adverse Effect | Under-dosing |
|---|---|---|---|---|---|---|
| **Norgestrel** | T38.4X1 | T38.4X2 | T38.4X3 | T38.4X4 | T38.4X5 | T38.4X6 |
| **Norgestrienone** | T38.4X1 | T38.4X2 | T38.4X3 | T38.4X4 | T38.4X5 | T38.4X6 |
| **Norlestrin** | T38.4X1 | T38.4X2 | T38.4X3 | T38.4X4 | T38.4X5 | T38.4X6 |
| **Norlutin** | T38.4X1 | T38.4X2 | T38.4X3 | T38.4X4 | T38.4X5 | T38.4X6 |
| **Normal serum albumin** (human), salt-poor | T45.8X1 | T45.8X2 | T45.8X3 | T45.8X4 | T45.8X5 | T45.8X6 |
| **Normethandrone** | T38.5X1 | T38.5X2 | T38.5X3 | T38.5X4 | T38.5X5 | T38.5X6 |
| **Normison** — *see* Benzodiazepines | | | | | | |
| **Normorphine** | T4Ø.2X1 | T4Ø.2X2 | T4Ø.2X3 | T4Ø.2X4 | — | — |
| **Norpseudoephedrine** | T5Ø.5X1 | T5Ø.5X2 | T5Ø.5X3 | T5Ø.5X4 | T5Ø.5X5 | T5Ø.5X6 |
| **Nortestosterone** (furanpropionate) | T38.7X1 | T38.7X2 | T38.7X3 | T38.7X4 | T38.7X5 | T38.7X6 |
| **Nortriptyline** | T43.Ø11 | T43.Ø12 | T43.Ø13 | T43.Ø14 | T43.Ø15 | T43.Ø16 |
| **Norvasc*** | T46.1X1 | T46.1X2 | T46.1X3 | T46.1X4 | T46.1X5 | T46.1X6 |
| **Noscapine** | T48.3X1 | T48.3X2 | T48.3X3 | T48.3X4 | T48.3X5 | T48.3X6 |
| **Nose preparations** | T49.6X1 | T49.6X2 | T49.6X3 | T49.6X4 | T49.6X5 | T49.6X6 |
| **Novobiocin** | T36.5X1 | T36.5X2 | T36.5X3 | T36.5X4 | T36.5X5 | T36.5X6 |
| **Novocain** (infiltration) (topical) | T41.3X1 | T41.3X2 | T41.3X3 | T41.3X4 | T41.3X5 | T41.3X6 |
| nerve block (peripheral) (plexus) | T41.3X1 | T41.3X2 | T41.3X3 | T41.3X4 | T41.3X5 | T41.3X6 |
| spinal | T41.3X1 | T41.3X2 | T41.3X3 | T41.3X4 | T41.3X5 | T41.3X6 |
| **Noxious foodstuff** | T62.91 | T62.92 | T62.93 | T62.94 | — | — |
| specified NEC | T62.8X1 | T62.8X2 | T62.8X3 | T62.8X4 | — | — |
| **Noxiptiline** | T43.Ø11 | T43.Ø12 | T43.Ø13 | T43.Ø14 | T43.Ø15 | T43.Ø16 |
| **Noxytiolin** | T49.ØX1 | T49.ØX2 | T49.ØX3 | T49.ØX4 | T49.ØX5 | T49.ØX6 |
| **NPH Iletin** (insulin) | T38.3X1 | T38.3X2 | T38.3X3 | T38.3X4 | T38.3X5 | T38.3X6 |
| **Numorphan** | T4Ø.2X1 | T4Ø.2X2 | T4Ø.2X3 | T4Ø.2X4 | T4Ø.2X5 | T4Ø.2X6 |
| **Nunol** | T42.3X1 | T42.3X2 | T42.3X3 | T42.3X4 | T42.3X5 | T42.3X6 |
| **Nupercaine** (spinal anesthetic) | T41.3X1 | T41.3X2 | T41.3X3 | T41.3X4 | T41.3X5 | T41.3X6 |
| topical (surface) | T41.3X1 | T41.3X2 | T41.3X3 | T41.3X4 | T41.3X5 | T41.3X6 |
| **Nutmeg oil** (liniment) | T49.3X1 | T49.3X2 | T49.3X3 | T49.3X4 | T49.3X5 | T49.3X6 |
| **Nutrilipid*** | T5Ø.991 | T5Ø.992 | T5Ø.993 | T5Ø.994 | T5Ø.995 | T5Ø.996 |
| **Nutritional supplement** | T5Ø.9Ø1 | T5Ø.9Ø2 | T5Ø.9Ø3 | T5Ø.9Ø4 | T5Ø.9Ø5 | T5Ø.9Ø6 |
| **Nux vomica** | T65.1X1 | T65.1X2 | T65.1X3 | T65.1X4 | — | — |
| **Nydrazid** | T37.1X1 | T37.1X2 | T37.1X3 | T37.1X4 | T37.1X5 | T37.1X6 |
| **Nylidrin** | T46.7X1 | T46.7X2 | T46.7X3 | T46.7X4 | T46.7X5 | T46.7X6 |
| **Nystatin** | T36.7X1 | T36.7X2 | T36.7X3 | T36.7X4 | T36.7X5 | T36.7X6 |
| topical | T49.ØX1 | T49.ØX2 | T49.ØX3 | T49.ØX4 | T49.ØX5 | T49.ØX6 |
| **Nytol** | T45.ØX1 | T45.ØX2 | T45.ØX3 | T45.ØX4 | T45.ØX5 | T45.ØX6 |
| **Obidoxime chloride** | T5Ø.6X1 | T5Ø.6X2 | T5Ø.6X3 | T5Ø.6X4 | T5Ø.6X5 | T5Ø.6X6 |
| **Octafonium** (chloride) | T49.3X1 | T49.3X2 | T49.3X3 | T49.3X4 | T49.3X5 | T49.3X6 |
| **Octamethyl pyrophosphoramide** | T6Ø.ØX1 | T6Ø.ØX2 | T6Ø.ØX3 | T6Ø.ØX4 | — | — |
| **Octanoin** | T5Ø.991 | T5Ø.992 | T5Ø.993 | T5Ø.994 | T5Ø.995 | T5Ø.996 |
| **Octatropine methylbromide** | T44.3X1 | T44.3X2 | T44.3X3 | T44.3X4 | T44.3X5 | T44.3X6 |
| **Octotiamine** | T45.2X1 | T45.2X2 | T45.2X3 | T45.2X4 | T45.2X5 | T45.2X6 |
| **Octoxinol** (9) | T49.8X1 | T49.8X2 | T49.8X3 | T49.8X4 | T49.8X5 | T49.8X6 |
| **Octreotide** | T38.991 | T38.992 | T38.993 | T38.994 | T38.995 | T38.996 |
| **Octyl nitrite** | T46.3X1 | T46.3X2 | T46.3X3 | T46.3X4 | T46.3X5 | T46.3X6 |
| **Oestradiol** | T38.5X1 | T38.5X2 | T38.5X3 | T38.5X4 | T38.5X5 | T38.5X6 |
| **Oestriol** | T38.5X1 | T38.5X2 | T38.5X3 | T38.5X4 | T38.5X5 | T38.5X6 |
| **Oestrogen** | T38.5X1 | T38.5X2 | T38.5X3 | T38.5X4 | T38.5X5 | T38.5X6 |
| **Oestrone** | T38.5X1 | T38.5X2 | T38.5X3 | T38.5X4 | T38.5X5 | T38.5X6 |
| **Ofloxacin** | T36.8X1 | T36.8X2 | T36.8X3 | T36.8X4 | T36.8X5 | T36.8X6 |
| **Oil** (of) | T65.891 | T65.892 | T65.893 | T65.894 | — | — |
| bitter almond | T62.8X1 | T62.8X2 | T62.8X3 | T62.8X4 | — | — |
| cloves | T49.7X1 | T49.7X2 | T49.7X3 | T49.7X4 | T49.7X5 | T49.7X6 |
| colors | T65.6X1 | T65.6X2 | T65.6X3 | T65.6X4 | — | — |
| fumes | T59.891 | T59.892 | T59.893 | T59.894 | — | — |
| lubricating | T52.ØX1 | T52.ØX2 | T52.ØX3 | T52.ØX4 | — | — |
| Niobe | T52.891 | T52.892 | T52.893 | T52.894 | — | — |
| vitriol (liquid) | T54.2X1 | T54.2X2 | T54.2X3 | T54.2X4 | — | — |
| fumes | T54.2X1 | T54.2X2 | T54.2X3 | T54.2X4 | — | — |
| wintergreen (bitter) NEC | T49.3X1 | T49.3X2 | T49.3X3 | T49.3X4 | T49.3X5 | T49.3X6 |
| **Oily preparation** (for skin) | T49.3X1 | T49.3X2 | T49.3X3 | T49.3X4 | T49.3X5 | T49.3X6 |
| **Ointment NEC** | T49.3X1 | T49.3X2 | T49.3X3 | T49.3X4 | T49.3X5 | T49.3X6 |
| **Olanzapine** | T43.591 | T43.592 | T43.593 | T43.594 | T43.595 | T43.596 |
| **Oleander** | T62.2X1 | T62.2X2 | T62.2X3 | T62.2X4 | — | — |
| **Oleandomycin** | T36.3X1 | T36.3X2 | T36.3X3 | T36.3X4 | T36.3X5 | T36.3X6 |
| **Oleandrin** | T46.ØX1 | T46.ØX2 | T46.ØX3 | T46.ØX4 | T46.ØX5 | T46.ØX6 |
| **Oleic acid** | T46.6X1 | T46.6X2 | T46.6X3 | T46.6X4 | T46.6X5 | T46.6X6 |
| **Oleovitamin A** | T45.2X1 | T45.2X2 | T45.2X3 | T45.2X4 | T45.2X5 | T45.2X6 |
| **Oleum ricini** | T47.2X1 | T47.2X2 | T47.2X3 | T47.2X4 | T47.2X5 | T47.2X6 |
| **Olive oil** (medicinal) **NEC** | T47.4X1 | T47.4X2 | T47.4X3 | T47.4X4 | T47.4X5 | T47.4X6 |
| **Olivomycin** | T45.1X1 | T45.1X2 | T45.1X3 | T45.1X4 | T45.1X5 | T45.1X6 |
| **Olodaterol*** | T48.6X1 | T48.6X2 | T48.6X3 | T48.6X4 | T48.6X5 | T48.6X6 |
| **Olsalazine** | T47.8X1 | T47.8X2 | T47.8X3 | T47.8X4 | T47.8X5 | T47.8X6 |
| **Omeprazole** | T47.1X1 | T47.1X2 | T47.1X3 | T47.1X4 | T47.1X5 | T47.1X6 |
| **OMPA** | T6Ø.ØX1 | T6Ø.ØX2 | T6Ø.ØX3 | T6Ø.ØX4 | — | — |

| Substance | Poisoning, Accidental (unintentional) | Poisoning, Intentional Self-harm | Poisoning, Assault | Poisoning, Undetermined | Adverse Effect | Under-dosing |
|---|---|---|---|---|---|---|
| **Oncovin** | T45.1X1 | T45.1X2 | T45.1X3 | T45.1X4 | T45.1X5 | T45.1X6 |
| **Ondansetron** | T45.ØX1 | T45.ØX2 | T45.ØX3 | T45.ØX4 | T45.ØX5 | T45.ØX6 |
| **Ophthaine** | T41.3X1 | T41.3X2 | T41.3X3 | T41.3X4 | T41.3X5 | T41.3X6 |
| **Ophthetic** | T41.3X1 | T41.3X2 | T41.3X3 | T41.3X4 | T41.3X5 | T41.3X6 |
| **Opiate NEC** | T4Ø.6Ø1 | T4Ø.6Ø2 | T4Ø.6Ø3 | T4Ø.6Ø4 | T4Ø.6Ø5 | T4Ø.6Ø6 |
| antagonists | T5Ø.7X1 | T5Ø.7X2 | T5Ø.7X3 | T5Ø.7X4 | T5Ø.7X5 | T5Ø.7X6 |
| **Opioid NEC** | T4Ø.2X1 | T4Ø.2X2 | T4Ø.2X3 | T4Ø.2X4 | T4Ø.2X5 | T4Ø.2X6 |
| **Opipramol** | T43.Ø11 | T43.Ø12 | T43.Ø13 | T43.Ø14 | T43.Ø15 | T43.Ø16 |
| **Opium alkaloids** (total) | T4Ø.ØX1 | T4Ø.ØX2 | T4Ø.ØX3 | T4Ø.ØX4 | T4Ø.ØX5 | T4Ø.ØX6 |
| standardized powdered | T4Ø.ØX1 | T4Ø.ØX2 | T4Ø.ØX3 | T4Ø.ØX4 | T4Ø.ØX5 | T4Ø.ØX6 |
| tincture (camphorated) | T4Ø.ØX1 | T4Ø.ØX2 | T4Ø.ØX3 | T4Ø.ØX4 | T4Ø.ØX5 | T4Ø.ØX6 |
| **Optivar*** | T49.5X1 | T49.5X2 | T49.5X3 | T49.5X4 | T49.5X5 | T49.5X6 |
| **Oracon** | T38.4X1 | T38.4X2 | T38.4X3 | T38.4X4 | T38.4X5 | T38.4X6 |
| **Oragrafin** | T5Ø.8X1 | T5Ø.8X2 | T5Ø.8X3 | T5Ø.8X4 | T5Ø.8X5 | T5Ø.8X6 |
| **Oral contraceptives** | T38.4X1 | T38.4X2 | T38.4X3 | T38.4X4 | T38.4X5 | T38.4X6 |
| **Oral rehydration salts** | T5Ø.3X1 | T5Ø.3X2 | T5Ø.3X3 | T5Ø.3X4 | T5Ø.3X5 | T5Ø.3X6 |
| **Orazamide** | T5Ø.991 | T5Ø.992 | T5Ø.993 | T5Ø.994 | T5Ø.995 | T5Ø.996 |
| **Orciprenaline** | T48.291 | T48.292 | T48.293 | T48.294 | T48.295 | T48.296 |
| **Organidin** | T48.4X1 | T48.4X2 | T48.4X3 | T48.4X4 | T48.4X5 | T48.4X6 |
| **Organonitrate NEC** | T46.3X1 | T46.3X2 | T46.3X3 | T46.3X4 | T46.3X5 | T46.3X6 |
| **Organophosphates** | T6Ø.ØX1 | T6Ø.ØX2 | T6Ø.ØX3 | T6Ø.ØX4 | — | — |
| **Orimune** | T5Ø.B91 | T5Ø.B92 | T5Ø.B93 | T5Ø.B94 | T5Ø.B95 | T5Ø.B96 |
| **Orinase** | T38.3X1 | T38.3X2 | T38.3X3 | T38.3X4 | T38.3X5 | T38.3X6 |
| **Ormeloxifene** | T38.6X1 | T38.6X2 | T38.6X3 | T38.6X4 | T38.6X5 | T38.6X6 |
| **Ornidazole** | T37.3X1 | T37.3X2 | T37.3X3 | T37.3X4 | T37.3X5 | T37.3X6 |
| **Ornithine aspartate** | T5Ø.991 | T5Ø.992 | T5Ø.993 | T5Ø.994 | T5Ø.995 | T5Ø.996 |
| **Ornoprostil** | T47.1X1 | T47.1X2 | T47.1X3 | T47.1X4 | T47.1X5 | T47.1X6 |
| **Orphenadrine** (hydrochloride) | T42.8X1 | T42.8X2 | T42.8X3 | T42.8X4 | T42.8X5 | T42.8X6 |
| **Ortal** (sodium) | T42.3X1 | T42.3X2 | T42.3X3 | T42.3X4 | T42.3X5 | T42.3X6 |
| **Ortho-Novum** | T38.4X1 | T38.4X2 | T38.4X3 | T38.4X4 | T38.4X5 | T38.4X6 |
| **Orthoboric acid** | T49.ØX1 | T49.ØX2 | T49.ØX3 | T49.ØX4 | T49.ØX5 | T49.ØX6 |
| ENT agent | T49.6X1 | T49.6X2 | T49.6X3 | T49.6X4 | T49.6X5 | T49.6X6 |
| ophthalmic preparation | T49.5X1 | T49.5X2 | T49.5X3 | T49.5X4 | T49.5X5 | T49.5X6 |
| **Orthocaine** | T41.3X1 | T41.3X2 | T41.3X3 | T41.3X4 | T41.3X5 | T41.3X6 |
| **Orthodichlorobenzene** | T53.7X1 | T53.7X2 | T53.7X3 | T53.7X4 | — | — |
| **Orthotolidine** (reagent) | T54.2X1 | T54.2X2 | T54.2X3 | T54.2X4 | — | — |
| **Osmic acid** (liquid) | T54.2X1 | T54.2X2 | T54.2X3 | T54.2X4 | — | — |
| fumes | T54.2X1 | T54.2X2 | T54.2X3 | T54.2X4 | — | — |
| **Osmotic diuretics** | T5Ø.2X1 | T5Ø.2X2 | T5Ø.2X3 | T5Ø.2X4 | T5Ø.2X5 | T5Ø.2X6 |
| **Otilonium bromide** | T44.3X1 | T44.3X2 | T44.3X3 | T44.3X4 | T44.3X5 | T44.3X6 |
| **Otorhinolaryngological drug NEC** | T49.6X1 | T49.6X2 | T49.6X3 | T49.6X4 | T49.6X5 | T49.6X6 |
| **Ouabain** (e) | T46.ØX1 | T46.ØX2 | T46.ØX3 | T46.ØX4 | T46.ØX5 | T46.ØX6 |
| **Ovarian** | | | | | | |
| hormone | T38.5X1 | T38.5X2 | T38.5X3 | T38.5X4 | T38.5X5 | T38.5X6 |
| stimulant | T38.5X1 | T38.5X2 | T38.5X3 | T38.5X4 | T38.5X5 | T38.5X6 |
| **Ovide*** | T49.ØX1 | T49.ØX2 | T49.ØX3 | T49.ØX4 | T49.ØX5 | T49.ØX6 |
| **Ovral** | T38.4X1 | T38.4X2 | T38.4X3 | T38.4X4 | T38.4X5 | T38.4X6 |
| **Ovulen** | T38.4X1 | T38.4X2 | T38.4X3 | T38.4X4 | T38.4X5 | T38.4X6 |
| **Ox bile extract** | T47.5X1 | T47.5X2 | T47.5X3 | T47.5X4 | T47.5X5 | T47.5X6 |
| **Oxacillin** | T36.ØX1 | T36.ØX2 | T36.ØX3 | T36.ØX4 | T36.ØX5 | T36.ØX6 |
| **Oxalic acid** | T54.2X1 | T54.2X2 | T54.2X3 | T54.2X4 | — | — |
| ammonium salt | T5Ø.991 | T5Ø.992 | T5Ø.993 | T5Ø.994 | T5Ø.995 | T5Ø.996 |
| **Oxamniquine** | T37.4X1 | T37.4X2 | T37.4X3 | T37.4X4 | T37.4X5 | T37.4X6 |
| **Oxanamide** | T43.591 | T43.592 | T43.593 | T43.594 | T43.595 | T43.596 |
| **Oxandrolone** | T38.7X1 | T38.7X2 | T38.7X3 | T38.7X4 | T38.7X5 | T38.7X6 |
| **Oxantel** | T37.4X1 | T37.4X2 | T37.4X3 | T37.4X4 | T37.4X5 | T37.4X6 |
| **Oxapium iodide** | T44.3X1 | T44.3X2 | T44.3X3 | T44.3X4 | T44.3X5 | T44.3X6 |
| **Oxaprotiline** | T43.Ø21 | T43.Ø22 | T43.Ø23 | T43.Ø24 | T43.Ø25 | T43.Ø26 |
| **Oxaprozin** | T39.311 | T39.312 | T39.313 | T39.314 | T39.315 | T39.316 |
| **Oxatomide** | T45.ØX1 | T45.ØX2 | T45.ØX3 | T45.ØX4 | T45.ØX5 | T45.ØX6 |
| **Oxazepam** | T42.4X1 | T42.4X2 | T42.4X3 | T42.4X4 | T42.4X5 | T42.4X6 |
| **Oxazimedrine** | T5Ø.5X1 | T5Ø.5X2 | T5Ø.5X3 | T5Ø.5X4 | T5Ø.5X5 | T5Ø.5X6 |
| **Oxazolam** | T42.4X1 | T42.4X2 | T42.4X3 | T42.4X4 | T42.4X5 | T42.4X6 |
| **Oxazolidine derivatives** | T42.2X1 | T42.2X2 | T42.2X3 | T42.2X4 | T42.2X5 | T42.2X6 |
| **Oxazolidinedione** (derivative) | T42.2X1 | T42.2X2 | T42.2X3 | T42.2X4 | T42.2X5 | T42.2X6 |
| **Oxcarbazepine** | T42.1X1 | T42.1X2 | T42.1X3 | T42.1X4 | T42.1X5 | T42.1X6 |
| **Oxedrine** | T44.4X1 | T44.4X2 | T44.4X3 | T44.4X4 | T44.4X5 | T44.4X6 |
| **Oxeladin** (citrate) | T48.3X1 | T48.3X2 | T48.3X3 | T48.3X4 | T48.3X5 | T48.3X6 |
| **Oxendolone** | T38.5X1 | T38.5X2 | T38.5X3 | T38.5X4 | T38.5X5 | T38.5X6 |
| **Oxetacaine** | T41.3X1 | T41.3X2 | T41.3X3 | T41.3X4 | T41.3X5 | T41.3X6 |
| **Oxethazine** | T41.3X1 | T41.3X2 | T41.3X3 | T41.3X4 | T41.3X5 | T41.3X6 |
| **Oxetorone** | T39.8X1 | T39.8X2 | T39.8X3 | T39.8X4 | T39.8X5 | T39.8X6 |
| **Oxiconazole** | T49.ØX1 | T49.ØX2 | T49.ØX3 | T49.ØX4 | T49.ØX5 | T49.ØX6 |
| **Oxidizing agent NEC** | T54.91 | T54.92 | T54.93 | T54.94 | — | — |
| **Oxipurinol** | T5Ø.4X1 | T5Ø.4X2 | T5Ø.4X3 | T5Ø.4X4 | T5Ø.4X5 | T5Ø.4X6 |
| **Oxitriptan** | T43.291 | T43.292 | T43.293 | T43.294 | T43.295 | T43.296 |
| **Oxitropium bromide** | T48.6X1 | T48.6X2 | T48.6X3 | T48.6X4 | T48.6X5 | T48.6X6 |
| **Oxodipine** | T46.1X1 | T46.1X2 | T46.1X3 | T46.1X4 | T46.1X5 | T46.1X6 |
| **Oxolamine** | T48.3X1 | T48.3X2 | T48.3X3 | T48.3X4 | T48.3X5 | T48.3X6 |
| **Oxolinic acid** | T37.8X1 | T37.8X2 | T37.8X3 | T37.8X4 | T37.8X5 | T37.8X6 |

| Substance | Poisoning, Accidental (unintentional) | Poisoning, Intentional Self-harm | Poisoning, Assault | Poisoning, Undetermined | Adverse Effect | Under-dosing |
|---|---|---|---|---|---|---|
| **Oxomemazine** | T43.3X1 | T43.3X2 | T43.3X3 | T43.3X4 | T43.3X5 | T43.3X6 |
| **Oxophenarsine** | T37.3X1 | T37.3X2 | T37.3X3 | T37.3X4 | T37.3X5 | T37.3X6 |
| **Oxprenolol** | T44.7X1 | T44.7X2 | T44.7X3 | T44.7X4 | T44.7X5 | T44.7X6 |
| **Oxsoralen** | T49.3X1 | T49.3X2 | T49.3X3 | T49.3X4 | T49.3X5 | T49.3X6 |
| **Oxtriphylline** | T48.6X1 | T48.6X2 | T48.6X3 | T48.6X4 | T48.6X5 | T48.6X6 |
| **Oxybate sodium** | T41.291 | T41.292 | T41.293 | T41.294 | T41.295 | T41.296 |
| **Oxybuprocaine** | T41.3X1 | T41.3X2 | T41.3X3 | T41.3X4 | T41.3X5 | T41.3X6 |
| **Oxybutynin** | T44.3X1 | T44.3X2 | T44.3X3 | T44.3X4 | T44.3X5 | T44.3X6 |
| **Oxychlorosene** | T49.ØX1 | T49.ØX2 | T49.ØX3 | T49.ØX4 | T49.ØX5 | T49.ØX6 |
| **Oxycodone** | T4Ø.2X1 | T4Ø.2X2 | T4Ø.2X3 | T4Ø.2X4 | T4Ø.2X5 | T4Ø.2X6 |
| **OxyContin*** | T4Ø.2X1 | T4Ø.2X2 | T4Ø.2X3 | T4Ø.2X4 | T4Ø.2X5 | T4Ø.2X6 |
| **Oxyfedrine** | T46.3X1 | T46.3X2 | T46.3X3 | T46.3X4 | T46.3X5 | T46.3X6 |
| **Oxygen** | T41.5X1 | T41.5X2 | T41.5X3 | T41.5X4 | T41.5X5 | T41.5X6 |
| **Oxylone** | T49.ØX1 | T49.ØX2 | T49.ØX3 | T49.ØX4 | T49.ØX5 | T49.ØX6 |
| ophthalmic preparation | T49.5X1 | T49.5X2 | T49.5X3 | T49.5X4 | T49.5X5 | T49.5X6 |
| **Oxymesterone** | T38.7X1 | T38.7X2 | T38.7X3 | T38.7X4 | T38.7X5 | T38.7X6 |
| **Oxymetazoline** | T48.5X1 | T48.5X2 | T48.5X3 | T48.5X4 | T48.5X5 | T48.5X6 |
| **Oxymetholone** | T38.7X1 | T38.7X2 | T38.7X3 | T38.7X4 | T38.7X5 | T38.7X6 |
| **Oxymorphone** | T4Ø.2X1 | T4Ø.2X2 | T4Ø.2X3 | T4Ø.2X4 | T4Ø.2X5 | T4Ø.2X6 |
| **Oxypertine** | T43.591 | T43.592 | T43.593 | T43.594 | T43.595 | T43.596 |
| **Oxyphenbutazone** | T39.2X1 | T39.2X2 | T39.2X3 | T39.2X4 | T39.2X5 | T39.2X6 |
| **Oxyphencyclimine** | T44.3X1 | T44.3X2 | T44.3X3 | T44.3X4 | T44.3X5 | T44.3X6 |
| **Oxyphenisatine** | T47.2X1 | T47.2X2 | T47.2X3 | T47.2X4 | T47.2X5 | T47.2X6 |
| **Oxyphenonium bromide** | T44.3X1 | T44.3X2 | T44.3X3 | T44.3X4 | T44.3X5 | T44.3X6 |
| **Oxypolygelatin** | T45.8X1 | T45.8X2 | T45.8X3 | T45.8X4 | T45.8X5 | T45.8X6 |
| **Oxyquinoline** (derivatives) | T37.8X1 | T37.8X2 | T37.8X3 | T37.8X4 | T37.8X5 | T37.8X6 |
| **Oxytetracycline** | T36.4X1 | T36.4X2 | T36.4X3 | T36.4X4 | T36.4X5 | T36.4X6 |
| **Oxytocic drug NEC** | T48.ØX1 | T48.ØX2 | T48.ØX3 | T48.ØX4 | T48.ØX5 | T48.ØX6 |
| **Oxytocin** (synthetic) | T48.ØX1 | T48.ØX2 | T48.ØX3 | T48.ØX4 | T48.ØX5 | T48.ØX6 |
| **Oxytrol*** | T44.3X1 | T44.3X2 | T44.3X3 | T44.3X4 | T44.3X5 | T44.3X6 |
| **Ozone** | T59.891 | T59.892 | T59.893 | T59.894 | — | — |
| **P-Acetamidophenol** | T39.1X1 | T39.1X2 | T39.1X3 | T39.1X4 | T39.1X5 | T39.1X6 |
| **PABA** | T49.3X1 | T49.3X2 | T49.3X3 | T49.3X4 | T49.3X5 | T49.3X6 |
| **Packed red cells** | T45.8X1 | T45.8X2 | T45.8X3 | T45.8X4 | T45.8X5 | T45.8X6 |
| **Padimate** | T49.3X1 | T49.3X2 | T49.3X3 | T49.3X4 | T49.3X5 | T49.3X6 |
| **Paint NEC** | T65.6X1 | T65.6X2 | T65.6X3 | T65.6X4 | — | — |
| cleaner | T52.91 | T52.92 | T52.93 | T52.94 | — | — |
| fumes NEC | T59.891 | T59.892 | T59.893 | T59.894 | — | — |
| lead (fumes) | T56.ØX1 | T56.ØX2 | T56.ØX3 | T56.ØX4 | — | — |
| solvent NEC | T52.891 | T52.892 | T52.893 | T52.894 | — | — |
| stripper | T52.891 | T52.892 | T52.893 | T52.894 | — | — |
| **Palfium** | T4Ø.2X1 | T4Ø.2X2 | T4Ø.2X3 | T4Ø.2X4 | — | — |
| **Palm kernel oil** | T5Ø.991 | T5Ø.992 | T5Ø.993 | T5Ø.994 | T5Ø.995 | T5Ø.996 |
| **Paludrine** | T37.2X1 | T37.2X2 | T37.2X3 | T37.2X4 | T37.2X5 | T37.2X6 |
| **PAM** (pralidoxime) | T5Ø.6X1 | T5Ø.6X2 | T5Ø.6X3 | T5Ø.6X4 | T5Ø.6X5 | T5Ø.6X6 |
| **Pamaquine** (naphthoute) | T37.2X1 | T37.2X2 | T37.2X3 | T37.2X4 | T37.2X5 | T37.2X6 |
| **Panadol** | T39.1X1 | T39.1X2 | T39.1X3 | T39.1X4 | T39.1X5 | T39.1X6 |
| **Pancreatic** | | | | | | |
| digestive secretion stimulant | T47.8X1 | T47.8X2 | T47.8X3 | T47.8X4 | T47.8X5 | T47.8X6 |
| dornase | T45.3X1 | T45.3X2 | T45.3X3 | T45.3X4 | T45.3X5 | T45.3X6 |
| **Pancreatin** | T47.5X1 | T47.5X2 | T47.5X3 | T47.5X4 | T47.5X5 | T47.5X6 |
| **Pancrelipase** | T47.5X1 | T47.5X2 | T47.5X3 | T47.5X4 | T47.5X5 | T47.5X6 |
| **Pancuronium** (bromide) | T48.1X1 | T48.1X2 | T48.1X3 | T48.1X4 | T48.1X5 | T48.1X6 |
| **Pangamic acid** | T45.2X1 | T45.2X2 | T45.2X3 | T45.2X4 | T45.2X5 | T45.2X6 |
| **Panthenol** | T45.2X1 | T45.2X2 | T45.2X3 | T45.2X4 | T45.2X5 | T45.2X6 |
| topical | T49.8X1 | T49.8X2 | T49.8X3 | T49.8X4 | T49.8X5 | T49.8X6 |
| **Pantopon** | T4Ø.ØX1 | T4Ø.ØX2 | T4Ø.ØX3 | T4Ø.ØX4 | T4Ø.ØX5 | T4Ø.ØX6 |
| **Pantoprazole*** | T47.1X1 | T47.1X2 | T47.1X3 | T47.1X4 | T47.1X5 | T47.1X6 |
| **Pantothenic acid** | T45.2X1 | T45.2X2 | T45.2X3 | T45.2X4 | T45.2X5 | T45.2X6 |
| **Panwarfin** | T45.511 | T45.512 | T45.513 | T45.514 | T45.515 | T45.516 |
| **Papain** | T47.5X1 | T47.5X2 | T47.5X3 | T47.5X4 | T47.5X5 | T47.5X6 |
| digestant | T47.5X1 | T47.5X2 | T47.5X3 | T47.5X4 | T47.5X5 | T47.5X6 |
| **Papaveretum** | T4Ø.ØX1 | T4Ø.ØX2 | T4Ø.ØX3 | T4Ø.ØX4 | T4Ø.ØX5 | T4Ø.ØX6 |
| **Papaverine** | T44.3X1 | T44.3X2 | T44.3X3 | T44.3X4 | T44.3X5 | T44.3X6 |
| **Para-acetamidophenol** | T39.1X1 | T39.1X2 | T39.1X3 | T39.1X4 | T39.1X5 | T39.1X6 |
| **Para-aminobenzoic acid** | T49.3X1 | T49.3X2 | T49.3X3 | T49.3X4 | T49.3X5 | T49.3X6 |
| **Para-aminophenol derivatives** | T39.1X1 | T39.1X2 | T39.1X3 | T39.1X4 | T39.1X5 | T39.1X6 |
| **Para-aminosalicylic acid** | T37.1X1 | T37.1X2 | T37.1X3 | T37.1X4 | T37.1X5 | T37.1X6 |
| **Paracetaldehyde** | T42.6X1 | T42.6X2 | T42.6X3 | T42.6X4 | T42.6X5 | T42.6X6 |
| **Paracetamol** | T39.1X1 | T39.1X2 | T39.1X3 | T39.1X4 | T39.1X5 | T39.1X6 |
| **Parachlorophenol** (camphorated) | T49.ØX1 | T49.ØX2 | T49.ØX3 | T49.ØX4 | T49.ØX5 | T49.ØX6 |
| **Paracodin** | T4Ø.2X1 | T4Ø.2X2 | T4Ø.2X3 | T4Ø.2X4 | T4Ø.2X5 | T4Ø.2X6 |
| **Paradione** | T42.2X1 | T42.2X2 | T42.2X3 | T42.2X4 | T42.2X5 | T42.2X6 |
| **Paraffin**(s) (wax) | T52.ØX1 | T52.ØX2 | T52.ØX3 | T52.ØX4 | — | — |
| liquid (medicinal) | T47.4X1 | T47.4X2 | T47.4X3 | T47.4X4 | T47.4X5 | T47.4X6 |
| nonmedicinal | T52.ØX1 | T52.ØX2 | T52.ØX3 | T52.ØX4 | — | — |
| **Paraformaldehyde** | T6Ø.3X1 | T6Ø.3X2 | T6Ø.3X3 | T6Ø.3X4 | — | — |
| **Paraldehyde** | T42.6X1 | T42.6X2 | T42.6X3 | T42.6X4 | T42.6X5 | T42.6X6 |
| **Paramethadione** | T42.2X1 | T42.2X2 | T42.2X3 | T42.2X4 | T42.2X5 | T42.2X6 |
| **Paramethasone** | T38.ØX1 | T38.ØX2 | T38.ØX3 | T38.ØX4 | T38.ØX5 | T38.ØX6 |

| Substance | Poisoning, Accidental (unintentional) | Poisoning, Intentional Self-harm | Poisoning, Assault | Poisoning, Undetermined | Adverse Effect | Under-dosing |
|---|---|---|---|---|---|---|
| **Paramethasone** — *continued* | | | | | | |
| acetate | T49.ØX1 | T49.ØX2 | T49.ØX3 | T49.ØX4 | T49.ØX5 | T49.ØX6 |
| **Paraoxon** | T6Ø.ØX1 | T6Ø.ØX2 | T6Ø.ØX3 | T6Ø.ØX4 | — | — |
| **Paraquat** | T6Ø.3X1 | T6Ø.3X2 | T6Ø.3X3 | T6Ø.3X4 | — | — |
| **Parasympatholytic NEC** | T44.3X1 | T44.3X2 | T44.3X3 | T44.3X4 | T44.3X5 | T44.3X6 |
| **Parasympathomimetic drug NEC** | T44.1X1 | T44.1X2 | T44.1X3 | T44.1X4 | T44.1X5 | T44.1X6 |
| **Parathion** | T6Ø.ØX1 | T6Ø.ØX2 | T6Ø.ØX3 | T6Ø.ØX4 | — | — |
| **Parathormone** | T5Ø.991 | T5Ø.992 | T5Ø.993 | T5Ø.994 | T5Ø.995 | T5Ø.996 |
| **Parathyroid extract** | T5Ø.991 | T5Ø.992 | T5Ø.993 | T5Ø.994 | T5Ø.995 | T5Ø.996 |
| **Paratyphoid vaccine** | T5Ø.A91 | T5Ø.A92 | T5Ø.A93 | T5Ø.A94 | T5Ø.A95 | T5Ø.A96 |
| **Paredrine** | T44.4X1 | T44.4X2 | T44.4X3 | T44.4X4 | T44.4X5 | T44.4X6 |
| **Paregoric** | T4Ø.ØX1 | T4Ø.ØX2 | T4Ø.ØX3 | T4Ø.ØX4 | T4Ø.ØX5 | T4Ø.ØX6 |
| **Pargyline** | T46.5X1 | T46.5X2 | T46.5X3 | T46.5X4 | T46.5X5 | T46.5X6 |
| **Paris green** | T57.ØX1 | T57.ØX2 | T57.ØX3 | T57.ØX4 | — | — |
| insecticide | T57.ØX1 | T57.ØX2 | T57.ØX3 | T57.ØX4 | — | — |
| **Parnate** | T43.1X1 | T43.1X2 | T43.1X3 | T43.1X4 | T43.1X5 | T43.1X6 |
| **Paromomycin** | T36.5X1 | T36.5X2 | T36.5X3 | T36.5X4 | T36.5X5 | T36.5X6 |
| **Paroxypropione** | T45.1X1 | T45.1X2 | T45.1X3 | T45.1X4 | T45.1X5 | T45.1X6 |
| **Parsabiv*** | T5Ø.991 | T5Ø.992 | T5Ø.993 | T5Ø.994 | T5Ø.995 | T5Ø.996 |
| **Parzone** | T4Ø.2X1 | T4Ø.2X2 | T4Ø.2X3 | T4Ø.2X4 | T4Ø.2X5 | T4Ø.2X6 |
| **PAS** | T37.1X1 | T37.1X2 | T37.1X3 | T37.1X4 | T37.1X5 | T37.1X6 |
| **Pasiniazid** | T37.1X1 | T37.1X2 | T37.1X3 | T37.1X4 | T37.1X5 | T37.1X6 |
| **PBB** (polybrominated biphenyls) | T65.891 | T65.892 | T65.893 | T65.894 | — | — |
| **PCB** | T65.891 | T65.892 | T65.893 | T65.894 | — | — |
| **PCP** | | | | | | |
| meaning pentachlorophenol | T6Ø.1X1 | T6Ø.1X2 | T6Ø.1X3 | T6Ø.1X4 | — | — |
| fungicide | T6Ø.3X1 | T6Ø.3X2 | T6Ø.3X3 | T6Ø.3X4 | — | — |
| herbicide | T6Ø.3X1 | T6Ø.3X2 | T6Ø.3X3 | T6Ø.3X4 | — | — |
| insecticide | T6Ø.1X1 | T6Ø.1X2 | T6Ø.1X3 | T6Ø.1X4 | — | — |
| meaning phencyclidine | T4Ø.991 | T4Ø.992 | T4Ø.993 | T4Ø.994 | — | — |
| **Peach kernel oil** (emulsion) | T47.4X1 | T47.4X2 | T47.4X3 | T47.4X4 | T47.4X5 | T47.4X6 |
| **Peanut oil** (emulsion) **NEC** | T47.4X1 | T47.4X2 | T47.4X3 | T47.4X4 | T47.4X5 | T47.4X6 |
| topical | T49.3X1 | T49.3X2 | T49.3X3 | T49.3X4 | T49.3X5 | T49.3X6 |
| **Pearly Gates** (morning glory seeds) | T4Ø.991 | T4Ø.992 | T4Ø.993 | T4Ø.994 | — | — |
| **Pecazine** | T43.3X1 | T43.3X2 | T43.3X3 | T43.3X4 | T43.3X5 | T43.3X6 |
| **Pectin** | T47.6X1 | T47.6X2 | T47.6X3 | T47.6X4 | T47.6X5 | T47.6X6 |
| **Pediaflor*** | T49.7X1 | T49.7X2 | T49.7X3 | T49.7X4 | T49.7X5 | T49.7X6 |
| **Pefloxacin** | T37.8X1 | T37.8X2 | T37.8X3 | T37.8X4 | T37.8X5 | T37.8X6 |
| **Pegademase, bovine** | T5Ø.Z91 | T5Ø.Z92 | T5Ø.Z93 | T5Ø.Z94 | T5Ø.Z95 | T5Ø.Z96 |
| **Pelletierine tannate** | T37.4X1 | T37.4X2 | T37.4X3 | T37.4X4 | T37.4X5 | T37.4X6 |
| **Pemirolast** (potassium) | T48.6X1 | T48.6X2 | T48.6X3 | T48.6X4 | T48.6X5 | T48.6X6 |
| **Pemoline** | T5Ø.7X1 | T5Ø.7X2 | T5Ø.7X3 | T5Ø.7X4 | T5Ø.7X5 | T5Ø.7X6 |
| **Pempidine** | T44.2X1 | T44.2X2 | T44.2X3 | T44.2X4 | T44.2X5 | T44.2X6 |
| **Penamecillin** | T36.ØX1 | T36.ØX2 | T36.ØX3 | T36.ØX4 | T36.ØX5 | T36.ØX6 |
| **Penbutolol** | T44.7X1 | T44.7X2 | T44.7X3 | T44.7X4 | T44.7X5 | T44.7X6 |
| **Penethamate** | T36.ØX1 | T36.ØX2 | T36.ØX3 | T36.ØX4 | T36.ØX5 | T36.ØX6 |
| **Penfluridol** | T43.591 | T43.592 | T43.593 | T43.594 | T43.595 | T43.596 |
| **Penflutizide** | T5Ø.2X1 | T5Ø.2X2 | T5Ø.2X3 | T5Ø.2X4 | T5Ø.2X5 | T5Ø.2X6 |
| **Pengitoxin** | T46.ØX1 | T46.ØX2 | T46.ØX3 | T46.ØX4 | T46.ØX5 | T46.ØX6 |
| **Penicillamine** | T5Ø.6X1 | T5Ø.6X2 | T5Ø.6X3 | T5Ø.6X4 | T5Ø.6X5 | T5Ø.6X6 |
| **Penicillin** (any) | T36.ØX1 | T36.ØX2 | T36.ØX3 | T36.ØX4 | T36.ØX5 | T36.ØX6 |
| **Penicillinase** | T45.3X1 | T45.3X2 | T45.3X3 | T45.3X4 | T45.3X5 | T45.3X6 |
| **Penicilloyl polylysine** | T5Ø.8X1 | T5Ø.8X2 | T5Ø.8X3 | T5Ø.8X4 | T5Ø.8X5 | T5Ø.8X6 |
| **Penimepicycline** | T36.4X1 | T36.4X2 | T36.4X3 | T36.4X4 | T36.4X5 | T36.4X6 |
| **Pentacel*** | T5Ø.A11 | T5Ø.A12 | T5Ø.A13 | T5Ø.A14 | T5Ø.A15 | T5Ø.A16 |
| **Pentachloroethane** | T53.6X1 | T53.6X2 | T53.6X3 | T53.6X4 | — | — |
| **Pentachloronaphthalene** | T53.7X1 | T53.7X2 | T53.7X3 | T53.7X4 | — | — |
| **Pentachlorophenol** (pesticide) | T6Ø.1X1 | T6Ø.1X2 | T6Ø.1X3 | T6Ø.1X4 | — | — |
| fungicide | T6Ø.3X1 | T6Ø.3X2 | T6Ø.3X3 | T6Ø.3X4 | — | — |
| herbicide | T6Ø.3X1 | T6Ø.3X2 | T6Ø.3X3 | T6Ø.3X4 | — | — |
| insecticide | T6Ø.1X1 | T6Ø.1X2 | T6Ø.1X3 | T6Ø.1X4 | — | — |
| **Pentaerythritol** | T46.3X1 | T46.3X2 | T46.3X3 | T46.3X4 | T46.3X5 | T46.3X6 |
| chloral | T42.6X1 | T42.6X2 | T42.6X3 | T42.6X4 | T42.6X5 | T42.6X6 |
| tetranitrate NEC | T46.3X1 | T46.3X2 | T46.3X3 | T46.3X4 | T46.3X5 | T46.3X6 |
| **Pentaerythrityl tetranitrate** | T46.3X1 | T46.3X2 | T46.3X3 | T46.3X4 | T46.3X5 | T46.3X6 |
| **Pentagastrin** | T5Ø.8X1 | T5Ø.8X2 | T5Ø.8X3 | T5Ø.8X4 | T5Ø.8X5 | T5Ø.8X6 |
| **Pentalin** | T53.6X1 | T53.6X2 | T53.6X3 | T53.6X4 | — | — |
| **Pentamethonium bromide** | T44.2X1 | T44.2X2 | T44.2X3 | T44.2X4 | T44.2X5 | T44.2X6 |
| **Pentamidine** | T37.3X1 | T37.3X2 | T37.3X3 | T37.3X4 | T37.3X5 | T37.3X6 |
| **Pentanol** | T51.3X1 | T51.3X2 | T51.3X3 | T51.3X4 | — | — |
| **Pentapyrrolinium** (bitartrate) | T44.2X1 | T44.2X2 | T44.2X3 | T44.2X4 | T44.2X5 | T44.2X6 |
| **Pentaquine** | T37.2X1 | T37.2X2 | T37.2X3 | T37.2X4 | T37.2X5 | T37.2X6 |
| **Pentazocine** | T4Ø.491 | T4Ø.492 | T4Ø.493 | T4Ø.494 | T4Ø.495 | T4Ø.496 |
| **Pentetrazole** | T5Ø.7X1 | T5Ø.7X2 | T5Ø.7X3 | T5Ø.7X4 | T5Ø.7X5 | T5Ø.7X6 |
| **Penthienate bromide** | T44.3X1 | T44.3X2 | T44.3X3 | T44.3X4 | T44.3X5 | T44.3X6 |
| **Pentifylline** | T46.7X1 | T46.7X2 | T46.7X3 | T46.7X4 | T46.7X5 | T46.7X6 |

| Substance | Poisoning, Accidental (unintentional) | Poisoning, Intentional Self-harm | Poisoning, Assault | Poisoning, Undetermined | Adverse Effect | Under-dosing |
|---|---|---|---|---|---|---|
| **Pentobarbital** | T42.3X1 | T42.3X2 | T42.3X3 | T42.3X4 | T42.3X5 | T42.3X6 |
| sodium | T42.3X1 | T42.3X2 | T42.3X3 | T42.3X4 | T42.3X5 | T42.3X6 |
| **Pentobarbitone** | T42.3X1 | T42.3X2 | T42.3X3 | T42.3X4 | T42.3X5 | T42.3X6 |
| **Pentolonium tartrate** | T44.2X1 | T44.2X2 | T44.2X3 | T44.2X4 | T44.2X5 | T44.2X6 |
| **Pentosan polysulfate** (sodium) | T39.8X1 | T39.8X2 | T39.8X3 | T39.8X4 | T39.8X5 | T39.8X6 |
| **Pentostatin** | T45.1X1 | T45.1X2 | T45.1X3 | T45.1X4 | T45.1X5 | T45.1X6 |
| **Pentothal** | T41.1X1 | T41.1X2 | T41.1X3 | T41.1X4 | T41.1X5 | T41.1X6 |
| **Pentoxifylline** | T46.7X1 | T46.7X2 | T46.7X3 | T46.7X4 | T46.7X5 | T46.7X6 |
| **Pentoxyverine** | T48.3X1 | T48.3X2 | T48.3X3 | T48.3X4 | T48.3X5 | T48.3X6 |
| **Pentrinat** | T46.3X1 | T46.3X2 | T46.3X3 | T46.3X4 | T46.3X5 | T46.3X6 |
| **Pentylenetetrazole** | T5Ø.7X1 | T5Ø.7X2 | T5Ø.7X3 | T5Ø.7X4 | T5Ø.7X5 | T5Ø.7X6 |
| **Pentylsalicylamide** | T37.1X1 | T37.1X2 | T37.1X3 | T37.1X4 | T37.1X5 | T37.1X6 |
| **Pentymal** | T42.3X1 | T42.3X2 | T42.3X3 | T42.3X4 | T42.3X5 | T42.3X6 |
| **Pepcid*** | T47.ØX1 | T47.ØX2 | T47.ØX3 | T47.ØX4 | T47.ØX5 | T47.ØX6 |
| **Peplomycin** | T45.1X1 | T45.1X2 | T45.1X3 | T45.1X4 | T45.1X5 | T45.1X6 |
| **Peppermint** (oil) | T47.5X1 | T47.5X2 | T47.5X3 | T47.5X4 | T47.5X5 | T47.5X6 |
| **Pepsin** | T47.5X1 | T47.5X2 | T47.5X3 | T47.5X4 | T47.5X5 | T47.5X6 |
| digestant | T47.5X1 | T47.5X2 | T47.5X3 | T47.5X4 | T47.5X5 | T47.5X6 |
| **Pepstatin** | T47.1X1 | T47.1X2 | T47.1X3 | T47.1X4 | T47.1X5 | T47.1X6 |
| **Peptavlon** | T5Ø.8X1 | T5Ø.8X2 | T5Ø.8X3 | T5Ø.8X4 | T5Ø.8X5 | T5Ø.8X6 |
| **Perazine** | T43.3X1 | T43.3X2 | T43.3X3 | T43.3X4 | T43.3X5 | T43.3X6 |
| **Percaine** (spinal) | T41.3X1 | T41.3X2 | T41.3X3 | T41.3X4 | T41.3X5 | T41.3X6 |
| topical (surface) | T41.3X1 | T41.3X2 | T41.3X3 | T41.3X4 | T41.3X5 | T41.3X6 |
| **Perchloroethylene** | T53.3X1 | T53.3X2 | T53.3X3 | T53.3X4 | — | — |
| medicinal | T37.4X1 | T37.4X2 | T37.4X3 | T37.4X4 | T37.4X5 | T37.4X6 |
| vapor | T53.3X1 | T53.3X2 | T53.3X3 | T53.3X4 | — | — |
| **Percodan** | T4Ø.2X1 | T4Ø.2X2 | T4Ø.2X3 | T4Ø.2X4 | T4Ø.2X5 | T4Ø.2X6 |
| **Percogesic** — *see also* acetaminophen | T45.ØX1 | T45.ØX2 | T45.ØX3 | T45.ØX4 | T45.ØX5 | T45.ØX6 |
| **Percorten** | T38.ØX1 | T38.ØX2 | T38.ØX3 | T38.ØX4 | T38.ØX5 | T38.ØX6 |
| **Pergolide** | T42.8X1 | T42.8X2 | T42.8X3 | T42.8X4 | T42.8X5 | T42.8X6 |
| **Pergonal** | T38.811 | T38.812 | T38.813 | T38.814 | T38.815 | T38.816 |
| **Perhexilene** | T46.3X1 | T46.3X2 | T46.3X3 | T46.3X4 | T46.3X5 | T46.3X6 |
| **Perhexiline** (maleate) | T46.3X1 | T46.3X2 | T46.3X3 | T46.3X4 | T46.3X5 | T46.3X6 |
| **Periactin** | T45.ØX1 | T45.ØX2 | T45.ØX3 | T45.ØX4 | T45.ØX5 | T45.ØX6 |
| **Periciazine** | T43.3X1 | T43.3X2 | T43.3X3 | T43.3X4 | T43.3X5 | T43.3X6 |
| **Periclor** | T42.6X1 | T42.6X2 | T42.6X3 | T42.6X4 | T42.6X5 | T42.6X6 |
| **Perindopril** | T46.4X1 | T46.4X2 | T46.4X3 | T46.4X4 | T46.4X5 | T46.4X6 |
| **Perisoxal** | T39.8X1 | T39.8X2 | T39.8X3 | T39.8X4 | T39.8X5 | T39.8X6 |
| **Peritoneal dialysis solution** | T5Ø.3X1 | T5Ø.3X2 | T5Ø.3X3 | T5Ø.3X4 | T5Ø.3X5 | T5Ø.3X6 |
| **Peritrate** | T46.3X1 | T46.3X2 | T46.3X3 | T46.3X4 | T46.3X5 | T46.3X6 |
| **Perlapine** | T42.4X1 | T42.4X2 | T42.4X3 | T42.4X4 | T42.4X5 | T42.4X6 |
| **Permanganate** | T65.891 | T65.892 | T65.893 | T65.894 | — | — |
| **Permapen*** | T36.ØX1 | T36.ØX2 | T36.ØX3 | T36.ØX4 | T36.ØX5 | T36.ØX6 |
| **Permethrin** | T6Ø.1X1 | T6Ø.1X2 | T6Ø.1X3 | T6Ø.1X4 | — | — |
| **Pernocton** | T42.3X1 | T42.3X2 | T42.3X3 | T42.3X4 | T42.3X5 | T42.3X6 |
| **Pernoston** | T42.3X1 | T42.3X2 | T42.3X3 | T42.3X4 | T42.3X5 | T42.3X6 |
| **Peronine** | T4Ø.2X1 | T4Ø.2X2 | T4Ø.2X3 | T4Ø.2X4 | — | — |
| **Perphenazine** | T43.3X1 | T43.3X2 | T43.3X3 | T43.3X4 | T43.3X5 | T43.3X6 |
| **Pertofrane** | T43.Ø11 | T43.Ø12 | T43.Ø13 | T43.Ø14 | T43.Ø15 | T43.Ø16 |
| **Pertussis** | | | | | | |
| immune serum (human) | T5Ø.Z11 | T5Ø.Z12 | T5Ø.Z13 | T5Ø.Z14 | T5Ø.Z15 | T5Ø.Z16 |
| vaccine (with diphtheria toxoid) (with tetanus toxoid) | T5Ø.A11 | T5Ø.A12 | T5Ø.A13 | T5Ø.A14 | T5Ø.A15 | T5Ø.A16 |
| **Peruvian balsam** | T49.ØX1 | T49.ØX2 | T49.ØX3 | T49.ØX4 | T49.ØX5 | T49.ØX6 |
| **Peruvoside** | T46.ØX1 | T46.ØX2 | T46.ØX3 | T46.ØX4 | T46.ØX5 | T46.ØX6 |
| **Pesticide** (dust) (fumes) (vapor) **NEC** | T6Ø.91 | T6Ø.92 | T6Ø.93 | T6Ø.94 | — | — |
| arsenic | T57.ØX1 | T57.ØX2 | T57.ØX3 | T57.ØX4 | — | — |
| chlorinated | T6Ø.1X1 | T6Ø.1X2 | T6Ø.1X3 | T6Ø.1X4 | — | — |
| cyanide | T65.ØX1 | T65.ØX2 | T65.ØX3 | T65.ØX4 | — | — |
| kerosene | T52.ØX1 | T52.ØX2 | T52.ØX3 | T52.ØX4 | — | — |
| mixture (of compounds) | T6Ø.91 | T6Ø.92 | T6Ø.93 | T6Ø.94 | — | — |
| naphthalene | T6Ø.2X1 | T6Ø.2X2 | T6Ø.2X3 | T6Ø.2X4 | — | — |
| organochlorine (compounds) | T6Ø.1X1 | T6Ø.1X2 | T6Ø.1X3 | T6Ø.1X4 | — | — |
| petroleum (distillate) (products) NEC | T6Ø.8X1 | T6Ø.8X2 | T6Ø.8X3 | T6Ø.8X4 | — | — |
| specified ingredient NEC | T6Ø.8X1 | T6Ø.8X2 | T6Ø.8X3 | T6Ø.8X4 | — | — |
| strychnine | T65.1X1 | T65.1X2 | T65.1X3 | T65.1X4 | — | — |
| thallium | T6Ø.4X1 | T6Ø.4X2 | T6Ø.4X3 | T6Ø.4X4 | — | — |
| **Pethidine** | T4Ø.491 | T4Ø.492 | T4Ø.493 | T4Ø.494 | T4Ø.495 | T4Ø.496 |
| **Petrichloral** | T42.6X1 | T42.6X2 | T42.6X3 | T42.6X4 | T42.6X5 | T42.6X6 |
| **Petrol** | T52.ØX1 | T52.ØX2 | T52.ØX3 | T52.ØX4 | — | — |
| vapor | T52.ØX1 | T52.ØX2 | T52.ØX3 | T52.ØX4 | — | — |
| **Petrolatum** | T49.3X1 | T49.3X2 | T49.3X3 | T49.3X4 | T49.3X5 | T49.3X6 |
| hydrophilic | T49.3X1 | T49.3X2 | T49.3X3 | T49.3X4 | T49.3X5 | T49.3X6 |
| liquid | T47.4X1 | T47.4X2 | T47.4X3 | T47.4X4 | T47.4X5 | T47.4X6 |
| topical | T49.3X1 | T49.3X2 | T49.3X3 | T49.3X4 | T49.3X5 | T49.3X6 |
| nonmedicinal | T52.ØX1 | T52.ØX2 | T52.ØX3 | T52.ØX4 | — | — |
| red veterinary | T49.3X1 | T49.3X2 | T49.3X3 | T49.3X4 | T49.3X5 | T49.3X6 |

| Substance | Poisoning, Accidental (unintentional) | Poisoning, Intentional Self-harm | Poisoning, Assault | Poisoning, Undetermined | Adverse Effect | Under-dosing |
|---|---|---|---|---|---|---|
| **Petrolatum** — *continued* | | | | | | |
| white | T49.3X1 | T49.3X2 | T49.3X3 | T49.3X4 | T49.3X5 | T49.3X6 |
| **Petroleum** (products) **NEC** | T52.ØX1 | T52.ØX2 | T52.ØX3 | T52.ØX4 | — | — |
| benzine(s) — *see* Ligroin | | | | | | |
| ether — *see* Ligroin | | | | | | |
| jelly — *see* Petrolatum | | | | | | |
| naphtha — *see* Ligroin | | | | | | |
| pesticide | T6Ø.8X1 | T6Ø.8X2 | T6Ø.8X3 | T6Ø.8X4 | — | — |
| solids | T52.ØX1 | T52.ØX2 | T52.ØX3 | T52.ØX4 | — | — |
| solvents | T52.ØX1 | T52.ØX2 | T52.ØX3 | T52.ØX4 | — | — |
| vapor | T52.ØX1 | T52.ØX2 | T52.ØX3 | T52.ØX4 | — | — |
| **Peyote** | T4Ø.991 | T4Ø.992 | T4Ø.993 | T4Ø.994 | — | — |
| **Phanodorm, phanodorn** | T42.3X1 | T42.3X2 | T42.3X3 | T42.3X4 | T42.3X5 | T42.3X6 |
| **Phanquinone** | T37.3X1 | T37.3X2 | T37.3X3 | T37.3X4 | T37.3X5 | T37.3X6 |
| **Phanquone** | T37.3X1 | T37.3X2 | T37.3X3 | T37.3X4 | T37.3X5 | T37.3X6 |
| **Pharmaceutical** | | | | | | |
| adjunct NEC | T5Ø.9Ø1 | T5Ø.9Ø2 | T5Ø.9Ø3 | T5Ø.9Ø4 | T5Ø.9Ø5 | T5Ø.9Ø6 |
| excipient NEC | T5Ø.9Ø1 | T5Ø.9Ø2 | T5Ø.9Ø3 | T5Ø.9Ø4 | T5Ø.9Ø5 | T5Ø.9Ø6 |
| sweetener | T5Ø.9Ø1 | T5Ø.9Ø2 | T5Ø.9Ø3 | T5Ø.9Ø4 | T5Ø.9Ø5 | T5Ø.9Ø6 |
| viscous agent | T5Ø.9Ø1 | T5Ø.9Ø2 | T5Ø.9Ø3 | T5Ø.9Ø4 | T5Ø.9Ø5 | T5Ø.9Ø6 |
| **Phazyme*** | T47.1X1 | T47.1X2 | T47.1X3 | T47.1X4 | T47.1X5 | T47.1X6 |
| **Phemitone** | T42.3X1 | T42.3X2 | T42.3X3 | T42.3X4 | T42.3X5 | T42.3X6 |
| **Phenacaine** | T41.3X1 | T41.3X2 | T41.3X3 | T41.3X4 | T41.3X5 | T41.3X6 |
| **Phenacemide** | T42.6X1 | T42.6X2 | T42.6X3 | T42.6X4 | T42.6X5 | T42.6X6 |
| **Phenacetin** | T39.1X1 | T39.1X2 | T39.1X3 | T39.1X4 | T39.1X5 | T39.1X6 |
| **Phenadoxone** | T4Ø.2X1 | T4Ø.2X2 | T4Ø.2X3 | T4Ø.2X4 | — | — |
| **Phenaglycodol** | T43.591 | T43.592 | T43.593 | T43.594 | T43.595 | T43.596 |
| **Phenantoin** | T42.ØX1 | T42.ØX2 | T42.ØX3 | T42.ØX4 | T42.ØX5 | T42.ØX6 |
| **Phenaphthazine reagent** | T5Ø.991 | T5Ø.992 | T5Ø.993 | T5Ø.994 | T5Ø.995 | T5Ø.996 |
| **Phenazocine** | T4Ø.491 | T4Ø.492 | T4Ø.493 | T4Ø.494 | T4Ø.495 | T4Ø.496 |
| **Phenazone** | T39.2X1 | T39.2X2 | T39.2X3 | T39.2X4 | T39.2X5 | T39.2X6 |
| **Phenazopyridine** | T39.8X1 | T39.8X2 | T39.8X3 | T39.8X4 | T39.8X5 | T39.8X6 |
| **Phenbenicillin** | T36.ØX1 | T36.ØX2 | T36.ØX3 | T36.ØX4 | T36.ØX5 | T36.ØX6 |
| **Phenbutrazate** | T5Ø.5X1 | T5Ø.5X2 | T5Ø.5X3 | T5Ø.5X4 | T5Ø.5X5 | T5Ø.5X6 |
| **Phencyclidine** | T4Ø.991 | T4Ø.992 | T4Ø.993 | T4Ø.994 | T4Ø.995 | T4Ø.996 |
| **Phendimetrazine** | T5Ø.5X1 | T5Ø.5X2 | T5Ø.5X3 | T5Ø.5X4 | T5Ø.5X5 | T5Ø.5X6 |
| **Phenelzine** | T43.1X1 | T43.1X2 | T43.1X3 | T43.1X4 | T43.1X5 | T43.1X6 |
| **Phenemal** | T42.3X1 | T42.3X2 | T42.3X3 | T42.3X4 | T42.3X5 | T42.3X6 |
| **Phenergan** | T42.6X1 | T42.6X2 | T42.6X3 | T42.6X4 | T42.6X5 | T42.6X6 |
| **Pheneticillin** | T36.ØX1 | T36.ØX2 | T36.ØX3 | T36.ØX4 | T36.ØX5 | T36.ØX6 |
| **Pheneturide** | T42.6X1 | T42.6X2 | T42.6X3 | T42.6X4 | T42.6X5 | T42.6X6 |
| **Phenformin** | T38.3X1 | T38.3X2 | T38.3X3 | T38.3X4 | T38.3X5 | T38.3X6 |
| **Phenglutarimide** | T44.3X1 | T44.3X2 | T44.3X3 | T44.3X4 | T44.3X5 | T44.3X6 |
| **Phenicarbazide** | T39.8X1 | T39.8X2 | T39.8X3 | T39.8X4 | T39.8X5 | T39.8X6 |
| **Phenindamine** | T45.ØX1 | T45.ØX2 | T45.ØX3 | T45.ØX4 | T45.ØX5 | T45.ØX6 |
| **Phenindione** | T45.511 | T45.512 | T45.513 | T45.514 | T45.515 | T45.516 |
| **Pheniprazine** | T43.1X1 | T43.1X2 | T43.1X3 | T43.1X4 | T43.1X5 | T43.1X6 |
| **Pheniramine** | T45.ØX1 | T45.ØX2 | T45.ØX3 | T45.ØX4 | T45.ØX5 | T45.ØX6 |
| **Phenisatin** | T47.2X1 | T47.2X2 | T47.2X3 | T47.2X4 | T47.2X5 | T47.2X6 |
| **Phenmetrazine** | T5Ø.5X1 | T5Ø.5X2 | T5Ø.5X3 | T5Ø.5X4 | T5Ø.5X5 | T5Ø.5X6 |
| **Phenobal** | T42.3X1 | T42.3X2 | T42.3X3 | T42.3X4 | T42.3X5 | T42.3X6 |
| **Phenobarbital** | T42.3X1 | T42.3X2 | T42.3X3 | T42.3X4 | T42.3X5 | T42.3X6 |
| sodium | T42.3X1 | T42.3X2 | T42.3X3 | T42.3X4 | T42.3X5 | T42.3X6 |
| with | | | | | | |
| mephenytoin | T42.3X1 | T42.3X2 | T42.3X3 | T42.3X4 | T42.3X5 | T42.3X6 |
| phenytoin | T42.3X1 | T42.3X2 | T42.3X3 | T42.3X4 | T42.3X5 | T42.3X6 |
| **Phenobarbitone** | T42.3X1 | T42.3X2 | T42.3X3 | T42.3X4 | T42.3X5 | T42.3X6 |
| **Phenobutiodil** | T5Ø.8X1 | T5Ø.8X2 | T5Ø.8X3 | T5Ø.8X4 | T5Ø.8X5 | T5Ø.8X6 |
| **Phenoctide** | T49.ØX1 | T49.ØX2 | T49.ØX3 | T49.ØX4 | T49.ØX5 | T49.ØX6 |
| **Phenol** | T49.ØX1 | T49.ØX2 | T49.ØX3 | T49.ØX4 | T49.ØX5 | T49.ØX6 |
| disinfectant | T54.ØX1 | T54.ØX2 | T54.ØX3 | T54.ØX4 | — | — |
| in oil injection | T46.8X1 | T46.8X2 | T46.8X3 | T46.8X4 | T46.8X5 | T46.8X6 |
| medicinal | T49.1X1 | T49.1X2 | T49.1X3 | T49.1X4 | T49.1X5 | T49.1X6 |
| nonmedicinal NEC | T54.ØX1 | T54.ØX2 | T54.ØX3 | T54.ØX4 | — | — |
| pesticide | T6Ø.8X1 | T6Ø.8X2 | T6Ø.8X3 | T6Ø.8X4 | — | — |
| red | T5Ø.8X1 | T5Ø.8X2 | T5Ø.8X3 | T5Ø.8X4 | T5Ø.8X5 | T5Ø.8X6 |
| **Phenolic preparation** | T49.1X1 | T49.1X2 | T49.1X3 | T49.1X4 | T49.1X5 | T49.1X6 |
| **Phenolphthalein** | T47.2X1 | T47.2X2 | T47.2X3 | T47.2X4 | T47.2X5 | T47.2X6 |
| **Phenolsulfonphthalein** | T5Ø.8X1 | T5Ø.8X2 | T5Ø.8X3 | T5Ø.8X4 | T5Ø.8X5 | T5Ø.8X6 |
| **Phenomorphan** | T4Ø.2X1 | T4Ø.2X2 | T4Ø.2X3 | T4Ø.2X4 | — | — |
| **Phenonyl** | T42.3X1 | T42.3X2 | T42.3X3 | T42.3X4 | T42.3X5 | T42.3X6 |
| **Phenoperidine** | T4Ø.491 | T4Ø.492 | T4Ø.493 | T4Ø.494 | — | — |
| **Phenopyrazone** | T46.991 | T46.992 | T46.993 | T46.994 | T46.995 | T46.996 |
| **Phenoquin** | T5Ø.4X1 | T5Ø.4X2 | T5Ø.4X3 | T5Ø.4X4 | T5Ø.4X5 | T5Ø.4X6 |
| **Phenothiazine** (psychotropic) **NEC** | T43.3X1 | T43.3X2 | T43.3X3 | T43.3X4 | T43.3X5 | T43.3X6 |
| insecticide | T6Ø.2X1 | T6Ø.2X2 | T6Ø.2X3 | T6Ø.2X4 | — | — |
| **Phenothrin** | T49.ØX1 | T49.ØX2 | T49.ØX3 | T49.ØX4 | T49.ØX5 | T49.ØX6 |
| **Phenoxybenzamine** | T46.7X1 | T46.7X2 | T46.7X3 | T46.7X4 | T46.7X5 | T46.7X6 |
| **Phenoxyethanol** | T49.ØX1 | T49.ØX2 | T49.ØX3 | T49.ØX4 | T49.ØX5 | T49.ØX6 |
| **Phenoxymethyl penicillin** | T36.ØX1 | T36.ØX2 | T36.ØX3 | T36.ØX4 | T36.ØX5 | T36.ØX6 |
| **Phenprobamate** | T42.8X1 | T42.8X2 | T42.8X3 | T42.8X4 | T42.8X5 | T42.8X6 |
| **Phenprocoumon** | T45.511 | T45.512 | T45.513 | T45.514 | T45.515 | T45.516 |
| **Phensuximide** | T42.2X1 | T42.2X2 | T42.2X3 | T42.2X4 | T42.2X5 | T42.2X |
| **Phentermine** | T5Ø.5X1 | T5Ø.5X2 | T5Ø.5X3 | T5Ø.5X4 | T5Ø.5X5 | T5Ø.5X |
| **Phenthicillin** | T36.ØX1 | T36.ØX2 | T36.ØX3 | T36.ØX4 | T36.ØX5 | T36.ØX |
| **Phentolamine** | T46.7X1 | T46.7X2 | T46.7X3 | T46.7X4 | T46.7X5 | T46.7X |
| **Phenyl** | | | | | | |
| butazone | T39.2X1 | T39.2X2 | T39.2X3 | T39.2X4 | T39.2X5 | T39.2X |
| enediamine | T65.3X1 | T65.3X2 | T65.3X3 | T65.3X4 | — | — |
| hydrazine | T65.3X1 | T65.3X2 | T65.3X3 | T65.3X4 | — | — |
| antineoplastic | T45.1X1 | T45.1X2 | T45.1X3 | T45.1X4 | T45.1X5 | T45.1X |
| mercuric compounds — *see* Mercury | | | | | | |
| salicylate | T49.3X1 | T49.3X2 | T49.3X3 | T49.3X4 | T49.3X5 | T49.3X |
| **Phenylalanine mustard** | T45.1X1 | T45.1X2 | T45.1X3 | T45.1X4 | T45.1X5 | T45.1X |
| **Phenylbutazone** | T39.2X1 | T39.2X2 | T39.2X3 | T39.2X4 | T39.2X5 | T39.2X |
| **Phenylenediamine** | T65.3X1 | T65.3X2 | T65.3X3 | T65.3X4 | — | — |
| **Phenylephrine** | T44.4X1 | T44.4X2 | T44.4X3 | T44.4X4 | T44.4X5 | T44.4X |
| **Phenylethylbiguanide** | T38.3X1 | T38.3X2 | T38.3X3 | T38.3X4 | T38.3X5 | T38.3X |
| **Phenylmercuric** | | | | | | |
| acetate | T49.ØX1 | T49.ØX2 | T49.ØX3 | T49.ØX4 | T49.ØX5 | T49.ØX |
| borate | T49.ØX1 | T49.ØX2 | T49.ØX3 | T49.ØX4 | T49.ØX5 | T49.ØX |
| nitrate | T49.ØX1 | T49.ØX2 | T49.ØX3 | T49.ØX4 | T49.ØX5 | T49.ØX |
| **Phenylmethylbarbitone** | T42.3X1 | T42.3X2 | T42.3X3 | T42.3X4 | T42.3X5 | T42.3X |
| **Phenylpropanol** | T47.5X1 | T47.5X2 | T47.5X3 | T47.5X4 | T47.5X5 | T47.5X |
| **Phenylpropanolamine** | T44.991 | T44.992 | T44.993 | T44.994 | T44.995 | T44.99 |
| **Phenylsulfthion** | T6Ø.ØX1 | T6Ø.ØX2 | T6Ø.ØX3 | T6Ø.ØX4 | — | — |
| **Phenyltoloxamine** | T45.ØX1 | T45.ØX2 | T45.ØX3 | T45.ØX4 | T45.ØX5 | T45.ØX |
| **Phenyramidol, phenyramidon** | T39.8X1 | T39.8X2 | T39.8X3 | T39.8X4 | T39.8X5 | T39.8X |
| **Phenytek*** | T42.ØX1 | T42.ØX2 | T42.ØX3 | T42.ØX4 | T42.ØX5 | T42.ØX |
| **Phenytoin** | T42.ØX1 | T42.ØX2 | T42.ØX3 | T42.ØX4 | T42.ØX5 | T42.ØX |
| with Phenobarbital | T42.3X1 | T42.3X2 | T42.3X3 | T42.3X4 | T42.3X5 | T42.3X |
| **pHisoHex** | T49.2X1 | T49.2X2 | T49.2X3 | T49.2X4 | T49.2X5 | T49.2X |
| **Pholcodine** | T48.3X1 | T48.3X2 | T48.3X3 | T48.3X4 | T48.3X5 | T48.3X |
| **Pholedrine** | T46.991 | T46.992 | T46.993 | T46.994 | T46.995 | T46.99 |
| **Phorate** | T6Ø.ØX1 | T6Ø.ØX2 | T6Ø.ØX3 | T6Ø.ØX4 | — | — |
| **Phosdrin** | T6Ø.ØX1 | T6Ø.ØX2 | T6Ø.ØX3 | T6Ø.ØX4 | — | — |
| **Phosfolan** | T6Ø.ØX1 | T6Ø.ØX2 | T6Ø.ØX3 | T6Ø.ØX4 | — | — |
| **Phosgene** (gas) | T59.891 | T59.892 | T59.893 | T59.894 | — | — |
| **Phosphamidon** | T6Ø.ØX1 | T6Ø.ØX2 | T6Ø.ØX3 | T6Ø.ØX4 | — | — |
| **Phosphate** | T65.891 | T65.892 | T65.893 | T65.894 | — | — |
| laxative | T47.4X1 | T47.4X2 | T47.4X3 | T47.4X4 | T47.4X5 | T47.4X |
| organic | T6Ø.ØX1 | T6Ø.ØX2 | T6Ø.ØX3 | T6Ø.ØX4 | — | — |
| solvent | T52.91 | T52.92 | T52.93 | T52.94 | — | — |
| tricresyl | T65.891 | T65.892 | T65.893 | T65.894 | — | — |
| **Phosphine** | T57.1X1 | T57.1X2 | T57.1X3 | T57.1X4 | — | — |
| fumigant | T57.1X1 | T57.1X2 | T57.1X3 | T57.1X4 | — | — |
| **Phospholine** | T49.5X1 | T49.5X2 | T49.5X3 | T49.5X4 | T49.5X5 | T49.5X |
| **Phosphoric acid** | T54.2X1 | T54.2X2 | T54.2X3 | T54.2X4 | — | — |
| **Phosphorus** (compound) **NEC** | T57.1X1 | T57.1X2 | T57.1X3 | T57.1X4 | — | — |
| pesticide | T6Ø.ØX1 | T6Ø.ØX2 | T6Ø.ØX3 | T6Ø.ØX4 | — | — |
| **Photrexa*** | T49.5X1 | T49.5X2 | T49.5X3 | T49.5X4 | T49.5X5 | T49.5X |
| **Phthalates** | T65.891 | T65.892 | T65.893 | T65.894 | — | — |
| **Phthalic anhydride** | T65.891 | T65.892 | T65.893 | T65.894 | — | — |
| **Phthalimidoglutarimide** | T42.6X1 | T42.6X2 | T42.6X3 | T42.6X4 | T42.6X5 | T42.6X |
| **Phthalylsulfathiazole** | T37.ØX1 | T37.ØX2 | T37.ØX3 | T37.ØX4 | T37.ØX5 | T37.ØX |
| **Phylloquinone** | T45.7X1 | T45.7X2 | T45.7X3 | T45.7X4 | T45.7X5 | T45.7X |
| **Physeptone** | T4Ø.3X1 | T4Ø.3X2 | T4Ø.3X3 | T4Ø.3X4 | T4Ø.3X5 | T4Ø.3X |
| **Physostigma venenosum** | T62.2X1 | T62.2X2 | T62.2X3 | T62.2X4 | — | — |
| **Physostigmine** | T49.5X1 | T49.5X2 | T49.5X3 | T49.5X4 | T49.5X5 | T49.5X |
| **Phytolacca decandra** | T62.2X1 | T62.2X2 | T62.2X3 | T62.2X4 | — | — |
| berries | T62.1X1 | T62.1X2 | T62.1X3 | T62.1X4 | — | — |
| **Phytomenadione** | T45.7X1 | T45.7X2 | T45.7X3 | T45.7X4 | T45.7X5 | T45.7X |
| **Phytonadione** | T45.7X1 | T45.7X2 | T45.7X3 | T45.7X4 | T45.7X5 | T45.7X |
| **Picoperine** | T48.3X1 | T48.3X2 | T48.3X3 | T48.3X4 | T48.3X5 | T48.3X |
| **Picosulfate** (sodium) | T47.2X1 | T47.2X2 | T47.2X3 | T47.2X4 | T47.2X5 | T47.2X |
| **Picric** (acid) | T54.2X1 | T54.2X2 | T54.2X3 | T54.2X4 | — | — |
| **Picrotoxin** | T5Ø.7X1 | T5Ø.7X2 | T5Ø.7X3 | T5Ø.7X4 | T5Ø.7X5 | T5Ø.7X |
| **Piketoprofen** | T49.ØX1 | T49.ØX2 | T49.ØX3 | T49.ØX4 | T49.ØX5 | T49.ØX |
| **Pilocarpine** | T44.1X1 | T44.1X2 | T44.1X3 | T44.1X4 | T44.1X5 | T44.1X |
| **Pilocarpus** (jaborandi) extract | T44.1X1 | T44.1X2 | T44.1X3 | T44.1X4 | T44.1X5 | T44.1X |
| **Pilsicainide** (hydrochloride) | T46.2X1 | T46.2X2 | T46.2X3 | T46.2X4 | T46.2X5 | T46.2X |
| **Pimaricin** | T36.7X1 | T36.7X2 | T36.7X3 | T36.7X4 | T36.7X5 | T36.7X |
| **Pimeclone** | T5Ø.7X1 | T5Ø.7X2 | T5Ø.7X3 | T5Ø.7X4 | T5Ø.7X5 | T5Ø.7X |
| **Pimelic ketone** | T52.891 | T52.892 | T52.893 | T52.894 | — | — |
| **Pimethixene** | T45.ØX1 | T45.ØX2 | T45.ØX3 | T45.ØX4 | T45.ØX5 | T45.ØX |
| **Piminodine** | T4Ø.2X1 | T4Ø.2X2 | T4Ø.2X3 | T4Ø.2X4 | T4Ø.2X5 | T4Ø.2X |
| **Pimozide** | T43.591 | T43.592 | T43.593 | T43.594 | T43.595 | T43.59 |
| **Pinacidil** | T46.5X1 | T46.5X2 | T46.5X3 | T46.5X4 | T46.5X5 | T46.5X |
| **Pinaverium bromide** | T44.3X1 | T44.3X2 | T44.3X3 | T44.3X4 | T44.3X5 | T44.3X |
| **Pinazepam** | T42.4X1 | T42.4X2 | T42.4X3 | T42.4X4 | T42.4X5 | T42.4X |
| **Pindolol** | T44.7X1 | T44.7X2 | T44.7X3 | T44.7X4 | T44.7X5 | T44.7X |

| Substance | Poisoning, Accidental (unintentional) | Poisoning, Intentional Self-harm | Poisoning, Assault | Poisoning, Undetermined | Adverse Effect | Under-dosing |
|---|---|---|---|---|---|---|
| **Pindone** | T6Ø.4X1 | T6Ø.4X2 | T6Ø.4X3 | T6Ø.4X4 | — | — |
| **Pine oil** (disinfectant) | T65.891 | T65.892 | T65.893 | T65.894 | — | — |
| **Pinkroot** | T37.4X1 | T37.4X2 | T37.4X3 | T37.4X4 | T37.4X5 | T37.4X6 |
| **Pipadone** | T4Ø.2X1 | T4Ø.2X2 | T4Ø.2X3 | T4Ø.2X4 | — | — |
| **Pipamazine** | T45.ØX1 | T45.ØX2 | T45.ØX3 | T45.ØX4 | T45.ØX5 | T45.ØX6 |
| **Pipamperone** | T43.4X1 | T43.4X2 | T43.4X3 | T43.4X4 | T43.4X5 | T43.4X6 |
| **Pipazetate** | T48.3X1 | T48.3X2 | T48.3X3 | T48.3X4 | T48.3X5 | T48.3X6 |
| **Pipemidic acid** | T37.8X1 | T37.8X2 | T37.8X3 | T37.8X4 | T37.8X5 | T37.8X6 |
| **Pipenzolate bromide** | T44.3X1 | T44.3X2 | T44.3X3 | T44.3X4 | T44.3X5 | T44.3X6 |
| **Piper cubeba** | T62.2X1 | T62.2X2 | T62.2X3 | T62.2X4 | — | — |
| **Piperacetazine** | T43.3X1 | T43.3X2 | T43.3X3 | T43.3X4 | T43.3X5 | T43.3X6 |
| **Piperacillin** | T36.ØX1 | T36.ØX2 | T36.ØX3 | T36.ØX4 | T36.ØX5 | T36.ØX6 |
| **Piperazine** | T37.4X1 | T37.4X2 | T37.4X3 | T37.4X4 | T37.4X5 | T37.4X6 |
| estrone sulfate | T38.5X1 | T38.5X2 | T38.5X3 | T38.5X4 | T38.5X5 | T38.5X6 |
| **Piperidione** | T48.3X1 | T48.3X2 | T48.3X3 | T48.3X4 | T48.3X5 | T48.3X6 |
| **Piperidolate** | T44.3X1 | T44.3X2 | T44.3X3 | T44.3X4 | T44.3X5 | T44.3X6 |
| **Piperocaine** | T41.3X1 | T41.3X2 | T41.3X3 | T41.3X4 | T41.3X5 | T41.3X6 |
| infiltration (subcutaneous) | T41.3X1 | T41.3X2 | T41.3X3 | T41.3X4 | T41.3X5 | T41.3X6 |
| nerve block (peripheral) (plexus) | T41.3X1 | T41.3X2 | T41.3X3 | T41.3X4 | T41.3X5 | T41.3X6 |
| topical (surface) | T41.3X1 | T41.3X2 | T41.3X3 | T41.3X4 | T41.3X5 | T41.3X6 |
| **Piperonyl butoxide** | T6Ø.8X1 | T6Ø.8X2 | T6Ø.8X3 | T6Ø.8X4 | — | — |
| **Pipethanate** | T44.3X1 | T44.3X2 | T44.3X3 | T44.3X4 | T44.3X5 | T44.3X6 |
| **Pipobroman** | T45.1X1 | T45.1X2 | T45.1X3 | T45.1X4 | T45.1X5 | T45.1X6 |
| **Pipotiazine** | T43.3X1 | T43.3X2 | T43.3X3 | T43.3X4 | T43.3X5 | T43.3X6 |
| **Pipoxizine** | T45.ØX1 | T45.ØX2 | T45.ØX3 | T45.ØX4 | T45.ØX5 | T45.ØX6 |
| **Pipradrol** | T43.691 | T43.692 | T43.693 | T43.694 | T43.695 | T43.696 |
| **Piprinhydrinate** | T45.ØX1 | T45.ØX2 | T45.ØX3 | T45.ØX4 | T45.ØX5 | T45.ØX6 |
| **Pirarubicin** | T45.1X1 | T45.1X2 | T45.1X3 | T45.1X4 | T45.1X5 | T45.1X6 |
| **Pirazinamide** | T37.1X1 | T37.1X2 | T37.1X3 | T37.1X4 | T37.1X5 | T37.1X6 |
| **Pirbuterol** | T48.6X1 | T48.6X2 | T48.6X3 | T48.6X4 | T48.6X5 | T48.6X6 |
| **Pirenzepine** | T47.1X1 | T47.1X2 | T47.1X3 | T47.1X4 | T47.1X5 | T47.1X6 |
| **Piretanide** | T5Ø.1X1 | T5Ø.1X2 | T5Ø.1X3 | T5Ø.1X4 | T5Ø.1X5 | T5Ø.1X6 |
| **Pirfenidone*** | T48.991 | T48.992 | T48.993 | T48.994 | T48.995 | T48.996 |
| **Piribedil** | T42.8X1 | T42.8X2 | T42.8X3 | T42.8X4 | T42.8X5 | T42.8X6 |
| **Piridoxilate** | T46.3X1 | T46.3X2 | T46.3X3 | T46.3X4 | T46.3X5 | T46.3X6 |
| **Piritramide** | T4Ø.491 | T4Ø.492 | T4Ø.493 | T4Ø.494 | — | — |
| **Piromidic acid** | T37.8X1 | T37.8X2 | T37.8X3 | T37.8X4 | T37.8X5 | T37.8X6 |
| **Piroxicam** | T39.391 | T39.392 | T39.393 | T39.394 | T39.395 | T39.396 |
| beta-cyclodextrin complex | T39.8X1 | T39.8X2 | T39.8X3 | T39.8X4 | T39.8X5 | T39.8X6 |
| **Pirozadil** | T46.6X1 | T46.6X2 | T46.6X3 | T46.6X4 | T46.6X5 | T46.6X6 |
| **Piscidia** (bark) (erythrina) | T39.8X1 | T39.8X2 | T39.8X3 | T39.8X4 | T39.8X5 | T39.8X6 |
| **Pitch** | T65.891 | T65.892 | T65.893 | T65.894 | — | — |
| **Pitkin's solution** | T41.3X1 | T41.3X2 | T41.3X3 | T41.3X4 | T41.3X5 | T41.3X6 |
| **Pitocin** | T48.ØX1 | T48.ØX2 | T48.ØX3 | T48.ØX4 | T48.ØX5 | T48.ØX6 |
| **Pitressin** (tannate) | T38.891 | T38.892 | T38.893 | T38.894 | T38.895 | T38.896 |
| **Pituitary extracts** (posterior) | T38.891 | T38.892 | T38.893 | T38.894 | T38.895 | T38.896 |
| anterior | T38.811 | T38.812 | T38.813 | T38.814 | T38.815 | T38.816 |
| **Pituitrin** | T38.891 | T38.892 | T38.893 | T38.894 | T38.895 | T38.896 |
| **Pivampicillin** | T36.ØX1 | T36.ØX2 | T36.ØX3 | T36.ØX4 | T36.ØX5 | T36.ØX6 |
| **Pivmecillinam** | T36.ØX1 | T36.ØX2 | T36.ØX3 | T36.ØX4 | T36.ØX5 | T36.ØX6 |
| **Placental hormone** | T38.891 | T38.892 | T38.893 | T38.894 | T38.895 | T38.896 |
| **Placidyl** | T42.6X1 | T42.6X2 | T42.6X3 | T42.6X4 | T42.6X5 | T42.6X6 |
| **Plague vaccine** | T5Ø.A91 | T5Ø.A92 | T5Ø.A93 | T5Ø.A94 | T5Ø.A95 | T5Ø.A96 |
| **Plant** | | | | | | |
| food or fertilizer NEC | T65.891 | T65.892 | T65.893 | T65.894 | — | — |
| containing herbicide | T6Ø.3X1 | T6Ø.3X2 | T6Ø.3X3 | T6Ø.3X4 | — | — |
| noxious, used as food | T62.2X1 | T62.2X2 | T62.2X3 | T62.2X4 | — | — |
| berries | T62.1X1 | T62.1X2 | T62.1X3 | T62.1X4 | — | — |
| seeds | T62.2X1 | T62.2X2 | T62.2X3 | T62.2X4 | — | — |
| specified type NEC | T62.2X1 | T62.2X2 | T62.2X3 | T62.2X4 | — | — |
| **Plasma** | T45.8X1 | T45.8X2 | T45.8X3 | T45.8X4 | T45.8X5 | T45.8X6 |
| expander NEC | T45.8X1 | T45.8X2 | T45.8X3 | T45.8X4 | T45.8X5 | T45.8X6 |
| protein fraction (human) | T45.8X1 | T45.8X2 | T45.8X3 | T45.8X4 | T45.8X5 | T45.8X6 |
| **Plasmanate** | T45.8X1 | T45.8X2 | T45.8X3 | T45.8X4 | T45.8X5 | T45.8X6 |
| **Plasminogen** (tissue) activator | T45.611 | T45.612 | T45.613 | T45.614 | T45.615 | T45.616 |
| **Plaster dressing** | T49.3X1 | T49.3X2 | T49.3X3 | T49.3X4 | T49.3X5 | T49.3X6 |
| **Plastic dressing** | T49.3X1 | T49.3X2 | T49.3X3 | T49.3X4 | T49.3X5 | T49.3X6 |
| **Plavix*** | T45.521 | T45.522 | T45.523 | T45.524 | T45.525 | T45.526 |
| **Plegicil** | T43.3X1 | T43.3X2 | T43.3X3 | T43.3X4 | T43.3X5 | T43.3X6 |
| **Plicamycin** | T45.1X1 | T45.1X2 | T45.1X3 | T45.1X4 | T45.1X5 | T45.1X6 |
| **Podophyllotoxin** | T49.8X1 | T49.8X2 | T49.8X3 | T49.8X4 | T49.8X5 | T49.8X6 |
| **Podophyllum** (resin) | T49.4X1 | T49.4X2 | T49.4X3 | T49.4X4 | T49.4X5 | T49.4X6 |
| **Poison NEC** | T65.91 | T65.92 | T65.93 | T65.94 | — | — |
| **Poisonous berries** | T62.1X1 | T62.1X2 | T62.1X3 | T62.1X4 | — | — |
| **Pokeweed** (any part) | T62.2X1 | T62.2X2 | T62.2X3 | T62.2X4 | — | — |
| **Poldine metilsulfate** | T44.3X1 | T44.3X2 | T44.3X3 | T44.3X4 | T44.3X5 | T44.3X6 |
| **Polidexide** (sulfate) | T46.6X1 | T46.6X2 | T46.6X3 | T46.6X4 | T46.6X5 | T46.6X6 |
| **Polidocanol** | T46.8X1 | T46.8X2 | T46.8X3 | T46.8X4 | T46.8X5 | T46.8X6 |
| **Poliomyelitis vaccine** | T5Ø.B91 | T5Ø.B92 | T5Ø.B93 | T5Ø.B94 | T5Ø.B95 | T5Ø.B96 |

| Substance | Poisoning, Accidental (unintentional) | Poisoning, Intentional Self-harm | Poisoning, Assault | Poisoning, Undetermined | Adverse Effect | Under-dosing |
|---|---|---|---|---|---|---|
| **Polish** (car) (floor) (furniture) (metal) (porcelain) (silver) | T65.891 | T65.892 | T65.893 | T65.894 | — | — |
| abrasive | T65.891 | T65.892 | T65.893 | T65.894 | — | — |
| porcelain | T65.891 | T65.892 | T65.893 | T65.894 | — | — |
| **Poloxalkol** | T47.4X1 | T47.4X2 | T47.4X3 | T47.4X4 | T47.4X5 | T47.4X6 |
| **Poloxamer** | T47.4X1 | T47.4X2 | T47.4X3 | T47.4X4 | T47.4X5 | T47.4X6 |
| **Poly-Pred*** | T49.5X1 | T49.5X2 | T49.5X3 | T49.5X4 | T49.5X5 | T49.5X6 |
| **Polyaminostyrene resins** | T5Ø.3X1 | T5Ø.3X2 | T5Ø.3X3 | T5Ø.3X4 | T5Ø.3X5 | T5Ø.3X6 |
| **Polycarbophil** | T47.4X1 | T47.4X2 | T47.4X3 | T47.4X4 | T47.4X5 | T47.4X6 |
| **Polychlorinated biphenyl** | T65.891 | T65.892 | T65.893 | T65.894 | — | — |
| **Polycycline** | T36.4X1 | T36.4X2 | T36.4X3 | T36.4X4 | T36.4X5 | T36.4X6 |
| **Polyester fumes** | T59.891 | T59.892 | T59.893 | T59.894 | — | — |
| **Polyester resin hardener** | T52.91 | T52.92 | T52.93 | T52.94 | — | — |
| fumes | T59.891 | T59.892 | T59.893 | T59.894 | — | — |
| **Polyestradiol phosphate** | T38.5X1 | T38.5X2 | T38.5X3 | T38.5X4 | T38.5X5 | T38.5X6 |
| **Polyethanolamine alkyl sulfate** | T49.2X1 | T49.2X2 | T49.2X3 | T49.2X4 | T49.2X5 | T49.2X6 |
| **Polyethylene adhesive** | T49.3X1 | T49.3X2 | T49.3X3 | T49.3X4 | T49.3X5 | T49.3X6 |
| **Polyferose** | T45.4X1 | T45.4X2 | T45.4X3 | T45.4X4 | T45.4X5 | T45.4X6 |
| **Polygeline** | T45.8X1 | T45.8X2 | T45.8X3 | T45.8X4 | T45.8X5 | T45.8X6 |
| **Polymyxin** | T36.8X1 | T36.8X2 | T36.8X3 | T36.8X4 | T36.8X5 | T36.8X6 |
| B | T36.8X1 | T36.8X2 | T36.8X3 | T36.8X4 | T36.8X5 | T36.8X6 |
| ENT agent | T49.6X1 | T49.6X2 | T49.6X3 | T49.6X4 | T49.6X5 | T49.6X6 |
| ophthalmic preparation | T49.5X1 | T49.5X2 | T49.5X3 | T49.5X4 | T49.5X5 | T49.5X6 |
| topical NEC | T49.ØX1 | T49.ØX2 | T49.ØX3 | T49.ØX4 | T49.ØX5 | T49.ØX6 |
| E sulfate (eye preparation) | T49.5X1 | T49.5X2 | T49.5X3 | T49.5X4 | T49.5X5 | T49.5X6 |
| **Polynoxylin** | T49.ØX1 | T49.ØX2 | T49.ØX3 | T49.ØX4 | T49.ØX5 | T49.ØX6 |
| **Polyoestradiol phosphate** | T38.5X1 | T38.5X2 | T38.5X3 | T38.5X4 | T38.5X5 | T38.5X6 |
| **Polyoxymethyleneurea** | T49.ØX1 | T49.ØX2 | T49.ØX3 | T49.ØX4 | T49.ØX5 | T49.ØX6 |
| **Polysilane** | T47.8X1 | T47.8X2 | T47.8X3 | T47.8X4 | T47.8X5 | T47.8X6 |
| **Polytetrafluoroethylene** (inhaled) | T59.891 | T59.892 | T59.893 | T59.894 | — | — |
| **Polythiazide** | T5Ø.2X1 | T5Ø.2X2 | T5Ø.2X3 | T5Ø.2X4 | T5Ø.2X5 | T5Ø.2X6 |
| **Polyvidone** | T45.8X1 | T45.8X2 | T45.8X3 | T45.8X4 | T45.8X5 | T45.8X6 |
| **Polyvinylpyrrolidone** | T45.8X1 | T45.8X2 | T45.8X3 | T45.8X4 | T45.8X5 | T45.8X6 |
| **Pontocaine** (hydrochloride) (infiltration) (topical) | T41.3X1 | T41.3X2 | T41.3X3 | T41.3X4 | T41.3X5 | T41.3X6 |
| nerve block (peripheral) (plexus) | T41.3X1 | T41.3X2 | T41.3X3 | T41.3X4 | T41.3X5 | T41.3X6 |
| spinal | T41.3X1 | T41.3X2 | T41.3X3 | T41.3X4 | T41.3X5 | T41.3X6 |
| **Porfiromycin** | T45.1X1 | T45.1X2 | T45.1X3 | T45.1X4 | T45.1X5 | T45.1X6 |
| **Portactant alfa*** | T48.991 | T48.992 | T48.993 | T48.994 | T48.995 | T48.996 |
| **Posterior pituitary hormone NEC** | T38.891 | T38.892 | T38.893 | T38.894 | T38.895 | T38.896 |
| **Pot** | T4Ø.711 | T4Ø.712 | T4Ø.713 | T4Ø.714 | T4Ø.715 | T4Ø.716 |
| **Potash** (caustic) | T54.3X1 | T54.3X2 | T54.3X3 | T54.3X4 | — | — |
| **Potassic saline injection** (lactated) | T5Ø.3X1 | T5Ø.3X2 | T5Ø.3X3 | T5Ø.3X4 | T5Ø.3X5 | T5Ø.3X6 |
| **Potassium** (salts) **NEC** | T5Ø.3X1 | T5Ø.3X2 | T5Ø.3X3 | T5Ø.3X4 | T5Ø.3X5 | T5Ø.3X6 |
| aminobenzoate | T45.8X1 | T45.8X2 | T45.8X3 | T45.8X4 | T45.8X5 | T45.8X6 |
| aminosalicylate | T37.1X1 | T37.1X2 | T37.1X3 | T37.1X4 | T37.1X5 | T37.1X6 |
| antimony 'tartrate' | T37.8X1 | T37.8X2 | T37.8X3 | T37.8X4 | T37.8X5 | T37.8X6 |
| arsenite (solution) | T57.ØX1 | T57.ØX2 | T57.ØX3 | T57.ØX4 | — | — |
| bichromate | T56.2X1 | T56.2X2 | T56.2X3 | T56.2X4 | — | — |
| bisulfate | T47.3X1 | T47.3X2 | T47.3X3 | T47.3X4 | T47.3X5 | T47.3X6 |
| bromide | T42.6X1 | T42.6X2 | T42.6X3 | T42.6X4 | T42.6X5 | T42.6X6 |
| canrenoate | T5Ø.ØX1 | T5Ø.ØX2 | T5Ø.ØX3 | T5Ø.ØX4 | T5Ø.ØX5 | T5Ø.ØX6 |
| carbonate | T54.3X1 | T54.3X2 | T54.3X3 | T54.3X4 | — | — |
| chlorate NEC | T65.891 | T65.892 | T65.893 | T65.894 | — | — |
| chloride | T5Ø.3X1 | T5Ø.3X2 | T5Ø.3X3 | T5Ø.3X4 | T5Ø.3X5 | T5Ø.3X6 |
| citrate | T5Ø.991 | T5Ø.992 | T5Ø.993 | T5Ø.994 | T5Ø.995 | T5Ø.996 |
| cyanide | T65.ØX1 | T65.ØX2 | T65.ØX3 | T65.ØX4 | — | — |
| ferric hexacyanoferrate (medicinal) | T5Ø.6X1 | T5Ø.6X2 | T5Ø.6X3 | T5Ø.6X4 | T5Ø.6X5 | T5Ø.6X6 |
| nonmedicinal | T65.891 | T65.892 | T65.893 | T65.894 | — | — |
| Fluoride | T57.8X1 | T57.8X2 | T57.8X3 | T57.8X4 | — | — |
| glucaldrate | T47.1X1 | T47.1X2 | T47.1X3 | T47.1X4 | T47.1X5 | T47.1X6 |
| hydroxide | T54.3X1 | T54.3X2 | T54.3X3 | T54.3X4 | — | — |
| iodate | T49.ØX1 | T49.ØX2 | T49.ØX3 | T49.ØX4 | T49.ØX5 | T49.ØX6 |
| iodide | T48.4X1 | T48.4X2 | T48.4X3 | T48.4X4 | T48.4X5 | T48.4X6 |
| nitrate | T57.8X1 | T57.8X2 | T57.8X3 | T57.8X4 | — | — |
| oxalate | T65.891 | T65.892 | T65.893 | T65.894 | — | — |
| perchlorate (nonmedicinal) NEC | T65.891 | T65.892 | T65.893 | T65.894 | — | — |
| antithyroid | T38.2X1 | T38.2X2 | T38.2X3 | T38.2X4 | T38.2X5 | T38.2X6 |
| medicinal | T38.2X1 | T38.2X2 | T38.2X3 | T38.2X4 | T38.2X5 | T38.2X6 |
| Permanganate (nonmedicinal) | T65.891 | T65.892 | T65.893 | T65.894 | — | — |
| medicinal | T49.ØX1 | T49.ØX2 | T49.ØX3 | T49.ØX4 | T49.ØX5 | T49.ØX6 |
| sulfate | T47.2X1 | T47.2X2 | T47.2X3 | T47.2X4 | T47.2X5 | T47.2X6 |
| **Potassium-removing resin** | T5Ø.3X1 | T5Ø.3X2 | T5Ø.3X3 | T5Ø.3X4 | T5Ø.3X5 | T5Ø.3X6 |
| **Potassium-retaining drug** | T5Ø.3X1 | T5Ø.3X2 | T5Ø.3X3 | T5Ø.3X4 | T5Ø.3X5 | T5Ø.3X6 |

| Substance | Poisoning, Accidental (unintentional) | Poisoning, Intentional Self-harm | Poisoning, Assault | Poisoning, Undetermined | Adverse Effect | Under-dosing |
|---|---|---|---|---|---|---|
| **Povidone** | T45.8X1 | T45.8X2 | T45.8X3 | T45.8X4 | T45.8X5 | T45.8X6 |
| iodine | T49.ØX1 | T49.ØX2 | T49.ØX3 | T49.ØX4 | T49.ØX5 | T49.ØX6 |
| **Practolol** | T44.7X1 | T44.7X2 | T44.7X3 | T44.7X4 | T44.7X5 | T44.7X6 |
| **Prajmalium bitartrate** | T46.2X1 | T46.2X2 | T46.2X3 | T46.2X4 | T46.2X5 | T46.2X6 |
| **Pralidoxime** (iodide) | T5Ø.6X1 | T5Ø.6X2 | T5Ø.6X3 | T5Ø.6X4 | T5Ø.6X5 | T5Ø.6X6 |
| chloride | T5Ø.6X1 | T5Ø.6X2 | T5Ø.6X3 | T5Ø.6X4 | T5Ø.6X5 | T5Ø.6X6 |
| **Pramiverine** | T44.3X1 | T44.3X2 | T44.3X3 | T44.3X4 | T44.3X5 | T44.3X6 |
| **Pramlintide*** | T38.3X1 | T38.3X2 | T38.3X3 | T38.3X4 | T38.3X5 | T38.3X6 |
| **Pramocaine** | T49.1X1 | T49.1X2 | T49.1X3 | T49.1X4 | T49.1X5 | T49.1X6 |
| **Pramoxine** | T49.1X1 | T49.1X2 | T49.1X3 | T49.1X4 | T49.1X5 | T49.1X6 |
| **Prasterone** | T38.7X1 | T38.7X2 | T38.7X3 | T38.7X4 | T38.7X5 | T38.7X6 |
| **Pravachol*** | T46.6X1 | T46.6X2 | T46.6X3 | T46.6X4 | T46.6X5 | T46.6X6 |
| **Pravastatin** | T46.6X1 | T46.6X2 | T46.6X3 | T46.6X4 | T46.6X5 | T46.6X6 |
| **Prazepam** | T42.4X1 | T42.4X2 | T42.4X3 | T42.4X4 | T42.4X5 | T42.4X6 |
| **Praziquantel** | T37.4X1 | T37.4X2 | T37.4X3 | T37.4X4 | T37.4X5 | T37.4X6 |
| **Prazitone** | T43.291 | T43.292 | T43.293 | T43.294 | T43.295 | T43.296 |
| **Prazosin** | T44.6X1 | T44.6X2 | T44.6X3 | T44.6X4 | T44.6X5 | T44.6X6 |
| **Prednicarbate** | T49.ØX1 | T49.ØX2 | T49.ØX3 | T49.ØX4 | T49.ØX5 | T49.ØX6 |
| **Prednimustine** | T45.1X1 | T45.1X2 | T45.1X3 | T45.1X4 | T45.1X5 | T45.1X6 |
| **Prednisolone** | T38.ØX1 | T38.ØX2 | T38.ØX3 | T38.ØX4 | T38.ØX5 | T38.ØX6 |
| ENT agent | T49.6X1 | T49.6X2 | T49.6X3 | T49.6X4 | T49.6X5 | T49.6X6 |
| ophthalmic preparation | T49.5X1 | T49.5X2 | T49.5X3 | T49.5X4 | T49.5X5 | T49.5X6 |
| steaglate | T49.ØX1 | T49.ØX2 | T49.ØX3 | T49.ØX4 | T49.ØX5 | T49.ØX6 |
| topical NEC | T49.ØX1 | T49.ØX2 | T49.ØX3 | T49.ØX4 | T49.ØX5 | T49.ØX6 |
| **Prednisone** | T38.ØX1 | T38.ØX2 | T38.ØX3 | T38.ØX4 | T38.ØX5 | T38.ØX6 |
| **Prednylidene** | T38.ØX1 | T38.ØX2 | T38.ØX3 | T38.ØX4 | T38.ØX5 | T38.ØX6 |
| **Pregnandiol** | T38.5X1 | T38.5X2 | T38.5X3 | T38.5X4 | T38.5X5 | T38.5X6 |
| **Pregneninolone** | T38.5X1 | T38.5X2 | T38.5X3 | T38.5X4 | T38.5X5 | T38.5X6 |
| **Preludin** | T43.691 | T43.692 | T43.693 | T43.694 | T43.695 | T43.696 |
| **Premarin** | T38.5X1 | T38.5X2 | T38.5X3 | T38.5X4 | T38.5X5 | T38.5X6 |
| **Premedication anesthetic** | T41.2Ø1 | T41.2Ø2 | T41.2Ø3 | T41.2Ø4 | T41.2Ø5 | T41.2Ø6 |
| **Prenalterol** | T44.5X1 | T44.5X2 | T44.5X3 | T44.5X4 | T44.5X5 | T44.5X6 |
| **Prenoxdiazine** | T48.3X1 | T48.3X2 | T48.3X3 | T48.3X4 | T48.3X5 | T48.3X6 |
| **Prenylamine** | T46.3X1 | T46.3X2 | T46.3X3 | T46.3X4 | T46.3X5 | T46.3X6 |
| **Preparation H** | T49.8X1 | T49.8X2 | T49.8X3 | T49.8X4 | T49.8X5 | T49.8X6 |
| **Preparation, local** | T49.4X1 | T49.4X2 | T49.4X3 | T49.4X4 | T49.4X5 | T49.4X6 |
| **Preservative** (nonmedicinal) | T65.891 | T65.892 | T65.893 | T65.894 | — | — |
| medicinal | T5Ø.9Ø1 | T5Ø.9Ø2 | T5Ø.9Ø3 | T5Ø.9Ø4 | T5Ø.9Ø5 | T5Ø.9Ø6 |
| wood | T6Ø.91 | T6Ø.92 | T6Ø.93 | T6Ø.94 | — | — |
| **Prethcamide** | T5Ø.7X1 | T5Ø.7X2 | T5Ø.7X3 | T5Ø.7X4 | T5Ø.7X5 | T5Ø.7X6 |
| **Prevacid*** | T47.1X1 | T47.1X2 | T47.1X3 | T47.1X4 | T47.1X5 | T47.1X6 |
| **Pride of China** | T62.2X1 | T62.2X2 | T62.2X3 | T62.2X4 | — | — |
| **Pridinol** | T44.3X1 | T44.3X2 | T44.3X3 | T44.3X4 | T44.3X5 | T44.3X6 |
| **Prifinium bromide** | T44.3X1 | T44.3X2 | T44.3X3 | T44.3X4 | T44.3X5 | T44.3X6 |
| **Prilocaine** | T41.3X1 | T41.3X2 | T41.3X3 | T41.3X4 | T41.3X5 | T41.3X6 |
| infiltration (subcutaneous) | T41.3X1 | T41.3X2 | T41.3X3 | T41.3X4 | T41.3X5 | T41.3X6 |
| nerve block (peripheral) (plexus) | T41.3X1 | T41.3X2 | T41.3X3 | T41.3X4 | T41.3X5 | T41.3X6 |
| regional | T41.3X1 | T41.3X2 | T41.3X3 | T41.3X4 | T41.3X5 | T41.3X6 |
| **Prilosec*** | T47.1X1 | T47.1X2 | T47.1X3 | T47.1X4 | T47.1X5 | T47.1X6 |
| **Primaquine** | T37.2X1 | T37.2X2 | T37.2X3 | T37.2X4 | T37.2X5 | T37.2X6 |
| **Primidone** | T42.6X1 | T42.6X2 | T42.6X3 | T42.6X4 | T42.6X5 | T42.6X6 |
| **Primula** (veris) | T62.2X1 | T62.2X2 | T62.2X3 | T62.2X4 | — | — |
| **Prinadol** | T4Ø.2X1 | T4Ø.2X2 | T4Ø.2X3 | T4Ø.2X4 | T4Ø.2X5 | T4Ø.2X6 |
| **Prinivil*** | T46.4X1 | T46.4X2 | T46.4X3 | T46.4X4 | T46.4X5 | T46.4X6 |
| **Priscol, Priscoline** | T44.6X1 | T44.6X2 | T44.6X3 | T44.6X4 | T44.6X5 | T44.6X6 |
| **Pristinamycin** | T36.3X1 | T36.3X2 | T36.3X3 | T36.3X4 | T36.3X5 | T36.3X6 |
| **Pristiq*** | T43.211 | T43.212 | T43.213 | T43.214 | T43.215 | T43.216 |
| **Privet** | T62.2X1 | T62.2X2 | T62.2X3 | T62.2X4 | — | — |
| berries | T62.1X1 | T62.1X2 | T62.1X3 | T62.1X4 | — | — |
| **Privine** | T44.4X1 | T44.4X2 | T44.4X3 | T44.4X4 | T44.4X5 | T44.4X6 |
| **Pro-Banthine** | T44.3X1 | T44.3X2 | T44.3X3 | T44.3X4 | T44.3X5 | T44.3X6 |
| **Probarbital** | T42.3X1 | T42.3X2 | T42.3X3 | T42.3X4 | T42.3X5 | T42.3X6 |
| **Probenecid** | T5Ø.4X1 | T5Ø.4X2 | T5Ø.4X3 | T5Ø.4X4 | T5Ø.4X5 | T5Ø.4X6 |
| **Probucol** | T46.6X1 | T46.6X2 | T46.6X3 | T46.6X4 | T46.6X5 | T46.6X6 |
| **Procainamide** | T46.2X1 | T46.2X2 | T46.2X3 | T46.2X4 | T46.2X5 | T46.2X6 |
| **Procaine** | T41.3X1 | T41.3X2 | T41.3X3 | T41.3X4 | T41.3X5 | T41.3X6 |
| benzylpenicillin | T36.ØX1 | T36.ØX2 | T36.ØX3 | T36.ØX4 | T36.ØX5 | T36.ØX6 |
| nerve block (periphreal) (plexus) | T41.3X1 | T41.3X2 | T41.3X3 | T41.3X4 | T41.3X5 | T41.3X6 |
| penicillin G | T36.ØX1 | T36.ØX2 | T36.ØX3 | T36.ØX4 | T36.ØX5 | T36.ØX6 |
| regional | T41.3X1 | T41.3X2 | T41.3X3 | T41.3X4 | T41.3X5 | T41.3X6 |
| spinal | T41.3X1 | T41.3X2 | T41.3X3 | T41.3X4 | T41.3X5 | T41.3X6 |
| **Procalmidol** | T43.591 | T43.592 | T43.593 | T43.594 | T43.595 | T43.596 |
| **Procarbazine** | T45.1X1 | T45.1X2 | T45.1X3 | T45.1X4 | T45.1X5 | T45.1X6 |
| **Procaterol** | T44.5X1 | T44.5X2 | T44.5X3 | T44.5X4 | T44.5X5 | T44.5X6 |
| **Prochlorperazine** | T43.3X1 | T43.3X2 | T43.3X3 | T43.3X4 | T43.3X5 | T43.3X6 |
| **Procyclidine** | T44.3X1 | T44.3X2 | T44.3X3 | T44.3X4 | T44.3X5 | T44.3X6 |
| **Producer gas** | T58.8X1 | T58.8X2 | T58.8X3 | T58.8X4 | — | — |
| **Profadol** | T4Ø.491 | T4Ø.492 | T4Ø.493 | T4Ø.494 | T4Ø.495 | T4Ø.496 |
| **Profenamine** | T44.3X1 | T44.3X2 | T44.3X3 | T44.3X4 | T44.3X5 | T44.3X6 |
| **Profenil** | T44.3X1 | T44.3X2 | T44.3X3 | T44.3X4 | T44.3X5 | T44.3X6 |
| **Proflavine** | T49.ØX1 | T49.ØX2 | T49.ØX3 | T49.ØX4 | T49.ØX5 | T49.ØX |
| **Progabide** | T42.6X1 | T42.6X2 | T42.6X3 | T42.6X4 | T42.6X5 | T42.6X |
| **Progesterone** | T38.5X1 | T38.5X2 | T38.5X3 | T38.5X4 | T38.5X5 | T38.5X |
| **Progestin** | T38.5X1 | T38.5X2 | T38.5X3 | T38.5X4 | T38.5X5 | T38.5X |
| oral contraceptive | T38.4X1 | T38.4X2 | T38.4X3 | T38.4X4 | T38.4X5 | T38.4X |
| **Progestogen NEC** | T38.5X1 | T38.5X2 | T38.5X3 | T38.5X4 | T38.5X5 | T38.5X |
| **Progestone** | T38.5X1 | T38.5X2 | T38.5X3 | T38.5X4 | T38.5X5 | T38.5X |
| **Proglumide** | T47.1X1 | T47.1X2 | T47.1X3 | T47.1X4 | T47.1X5 | T47.1X |
| **Prograf*** | T45.1X1 | T45.1X2 | T45.1X3 | T45.1X4 | T45.1X5 | T45.1X |
| **Proguanil** | T37.2X1 | T37.2X2 | T37.2X3 | T37.2X4 | T37.2X5 | T37.2X |
| **Prolactin** | T38.811 | T38.812 | T38.813 | T38.814 | T38.815 | T38.81 |
| **Prolintane** | T43.691 | T43.692 | T43.693 | T43.694 | T43.695 | T43.69 |
| **Proloid** | T38.1X1 | T38.1X2 | T38.1X3 | T38.1X4 | T38.1X5 | T38.1X |
| **Proluton** | T38.5X1 | T38.5X2 | T38.5X3 | T38.5X4 | T38.5X5 | T38.5X |
| **Promacetin** | T37.1X1 | T37.1X2 | T37.1X3 | T37.1X4 | T37.1X5 | T37.1X |
| **Promazine** | T43.3X1 | T43.3X2 | T43.3X3 | T43.3X4 | T43.3X5 | T43.3X |
| **Promedol** | T4Ø.2X1 | T4Ø.2X2 | T4Ø.2X3 | T4Ø.2X4 | — | — |
| **Promegestone** | T38.5X1 | T38.5X2 | T38.5X3 | T38.5X4 | T38.5X5 | T38.5X |
| **Promethazine** (teoclate) | T43.3X1 | T43.3X2 | T43.3X3 | T43.3X4 | T43.3X5 | T43.3X |
| **Promin** | T37.1X1 | T37.1X2 | T37.1X3 | T37.1X4 | T37.1X5 | T37.1X |
| **Pronase** | T45.3X1 | T45.3X2 | T45.3X3 | T45.3X4 | T45.3X5 | T45.3X |
| **Pronestyl** (hydrochloride) | T46.2X1 | T46.2X2 | T46.2X3 | T46.2X4 | T46.2X5 | T46.2X |
| **Pronetalol** | T44.7X1 | T44.7X2 | T44.7X3 | T44.7X4 | T44.7X5 | T44.7X |
| **Prontosil** | T37.ØX1 | T37.ØX2 | T37.ØX3 | T37.ØX4 | T37.ØX5 | T37.ØX |
| **Propachlor** | T6Ø.3X1 | T6Ø.3X2 | T6Ø.3X3 | T6Ø.3X4 | — | — |
| **Propafenone** | T46.2X1 | T46.2X2 | T46.2X3 | T46.2X4 | T46.2X5 | T46.2X |
| **Propallylonal** | T42.3X1 | T42.3X2 | T42.3X3 | T42.3X4 | T42.3X5 | T42.3X |
| **Propamidine** | T49.ØX1 | T49.ØX2 | T49.ØX3 | T49.ØX4 | T49.ØX5 | T49.ØX |
| **Propane** (distributed in mobile container) | T59.891 | T59.892 | T59.893 | T59.894 | — | — |
| distributed through pipes | T59.891 | T59.892 | T59.893 | T59.894 | — | — |
| incomplete combustion | T58.11 | T58.12 | T58.13 | T58.14 | — | — |
| **Propanidid** | T41.291 | T41.292 | T41.293 | T41.294 | T41.295 | T41.29 |
| **Propanil** | T6Ø.3X1 | T6Ø.3X2 | T6Ø.3X3 | T6Ø.3X4 | — | — |
| **Propantheline** | T44.3X1 | T44.3X2 | T44.3X3 | T44.3X4 | T44.3X5 | T44.3X |
| bromide | T44.3X1 | T44.3X2 | T44.3X3 | T44.3X4 | T44.3X5 | T44.3X |
| **Proparacaine** | T41.3X1 | T41.3X2 | T41.3X3 | T41.3X4 | T41.3X5 | T41.3X |
| **Propatylnitrate** | T46.3X1 | T46.3X2 | T46.3X3 | T46.3X4 | T46.3X5 | T46.3X |
| **Propicillin** | T36.ØX1 | T36.ØX2 | T36.ØX3 | T36.ØX4 | T36.ØX5 | T36.ØX |
| **Propine*** | T49.5X1 | T49.5X2 | T49.5X3 | T49.5X4 | T49.5X5 | T49.5X |
| **Propiolactone** | T49.ØX1 | T49.ØX2 | T49.ØX3 | T49.ØX4 | T49.ØX5 | T49.ØX |
| **Propiomazine** | T45.ØX1 | T45.ØX2 | T45.ØX3 | T45.ØX4 | T45.ØX5 | T45.ØX |
| **Propion gel** | T49.ØX1 | T49.ØX2 | T49.ØX3 | T49.ØX4 | T49.ØX5 | T49.ØX |
| **Propionaldehyde (medicinal)** | T42.6X1 | T42.6X2 | T42.6X3 | T42.6X4 | T42.6X5 | T42.6X |
| **Propionate** (calcium) (sodium) | T49.ØX1 | T49.ØX2 | T49.ØX3 | T49.ØX4 | T49.ØX5 | T49.ØX |
| **Propitocaine** | T41.3X1 | T41.3X2 | T41.3X3 | T41.3X4 | T41.3X5 | T41.3X |
| infiltration (subcutaneous) | T41.3X1 | T41.3X2 | T41.3X3 | T41.3X4 | T41.3X5 | T41.3X |
| nerve block (peripheral) (plexus) | T41.3X1 | T41.3X2 | T41.3X3 | T41.3X4 | T41.3X5 | T41.3X |
| **Propofol** | T41.291 | T41.292 | T41.293 | T41.294 | T41.295 | T41.29 |
| **Propoxur** | T6Ø.ØX1 | T6Ø.ØX2 | T6Ø.ØX3 | T6Ø.ØX4 | — | — |
| **Propoxycaine** | T41.3X1 | T41.3X2 | T41.3X3 | T41.3X4 | T41.3X5 | T41.3X |
| infiltration (subcutaneous) | T41.3X1 | T41.3X2 | T41.3X3 | T41.3X4 | T41.3X5 | T41.3X |
| nerve block (peripheral) (plexus) | T41.3X1 | T41.3X2 | T41.3X3 | T41.3X4 | T41.3X5 | T41.3X |
| topical (surface) | T41.3X1 | T41.3X2 | T41.3X3 | T41.3X4 | T41.3X5 | T41.3X |
| **Propoxyphene** | T4Ø.491 | T4Ø.492 | T4Ø.493 | T4Ø.494 | T4Ø.495 | T4Ø.49 |
| **Propranolol** | T44.7X1 | T44.7X2 | T44.7X3 | T44.7X4 | T44.7X5 | T44.7X |
| **Propyl** | | | | | | |
| alcohol | T51.3X1 | T51.3X2 | T51.3X3 | T51.3X4 | — | — |
| carbinol | T51.3X1 | T51.3X2 | T51.3X3 | T51.3X4 | — | — |
| hexadrine | T44.4X1 | T44.4X2 | T44.4X3 | T44.4X4 | T44.4X5 | T44.4X |
| iodone | T5Ø.8X1 | T5Ø.8X2 | T5Ø.8X3 | T5Ø.8X4 | T5Ø.8X5 | T5Ø.8X |
| thiouracil | T38.2X1 | T38.2X2 | T38.2X3 | T38.2X4 | T38.2X5 | T38.2X |
| **Propylaminophenothiazine** | T43.3X1 | T43.3X2 | T43.3X3 | T43.3X4 | T43.3X5 | T43.3X |
| **Propylene** | T59.891 | T59.892 | T59.893 | T59.894 | — | — |
| **Propylhexedrine** | T48.5X1 | T48.5X2 | T48.5X3 | T48.5X4 | T48.5X5 | T48.5X |
| **Propyliodone** | T5Ø.8X1 | T5Ø.8X2 | T5Ø.8X3 | T5Ø.8X4 | T5Ø.8X5 | T5Ø.8X |
| **Propylparaben** (ophthalmic) | T49.5X1 | T49.5X2 | T49.5X3 | T49.5X4 | T49.5X5 | T49.5X |
| **Propylthiouracil** | T38.2X1 | T38.2X2 | T38.2X3 | T38.2X4 | T38.2X5 | T38.2X |
| **Propyphenazone** | T39.2X1 | T39.2X2 | T39.2X3 | T39.2X4 | T39.2X5 | T39.2X |
| **Proquazone** | T39.391 | T39.392 | T39.393 | T39.394 | T39.395 | T39.39 |
| **Proscar*** | T38.6X1 | T38.6X2 | T38.6X3 | T38.6X4 | T38.6X5 | T38.6X |
| **Proscillaridin** | T46.ØX1 | T46.ØX2 | T46.ØX3 | T46.ØX4 | T46.ØX5 | T46.ØX |
| **Prostacyclin** | T45.521 | T45.522 | T45.523 | T45.524 | T45.525 | T45.52 |
| **Prostaglandin** (I2) | T45.521 | T45.522 | T45.523 | T45.524 | T45.525 | T45.52 |
| E1 | T46.7X1 | T46.7X2 | T46.7X3 | T46.7X4 | T46.7X5 | T46.7X |
| E2 | T48.ØX1 | T48.ØX2 | T48.ØX3 | T48.ØX4 | T48.ØX5 | T48.ØX |
| F2 alpha | T48.ØX1 | T48.ØX2 | T48.ØX3 | T48.ØX4 | T48.ØX5 | T48.ØX |
| **Prostigmin** | T44.ØX1 | T44.ØX2 | T44.ØX3 | T44.ØX4 | T44.ØX5 | T44.ØX |



☑ Additional Character May Be Required — Refer to the Tabular List for Character Selection

*Optum Value-Add

| Substance | Poisoning, Accidental (unintentional) | Poisoning, Intentional Self-harm | Poisoning, Assault | Poisoning, Undetermined | Adverse Effect | Under-dosing |
|---|---|---|---|---|---|---|
| **Prosultiamine** | T45.2X1 | T45.2X2 | T45.2X3 | T45.2X4 | T45.2X5 | T45.2X6 |
| **Protamine sulfate** | T45.7X1 | T45.7X2 | T45.7X3 | T45.7X4 | T45.7X5 | T45.7X6 |
| zinc insulin | T38.3X1 | T38.3X2 | T38.3X3 | T38.3X4 | T38.3X5 | T38.3X6 |
| **Protease** | T47.5X1 | T47.5X2 | T47.5X3 | T47.5X4 | T47.5X5 | T47.5X6 |
| **Protectant, skin NEC** | T49.3X1 | T49.3X2 | T49.3X3 | T49.3X4 | T49.3X5 | T49.3X6 |
| **Protein hydrolysate** | T5Ø.991 | T5Ø.992 | T5Ø.993 | T5Ø.994 | T5Ø.995 | T5Ø.996 |
| **Prothiaden** — *see* Dothiepin hydrochloride | | | | | | |
| **Prothionamide** | T37.1X1 | T37.1X2 | T37.1X3 | T37.1X4 | T37.1X5 | T37.1X6 |
| **Prothipendyl** | T43.591 | T43.592 | T43.593 | T43.594 | T43.595 | T43.596 |
| **Prothoate** | T6Ø.ØX1 | T6Ø.ØX2 | T6Ø.ØX3 | T6Ø.ØX4 | — | — |
| **Prothrombin** | | | | | | |
| activator | T45.7X1 | T45.7X2 | T45.7X3 | T45.7X4 | T45.7X5 | T45.7X6 |
| synthesis inhibitor | T45.511 | T45.512 | T45.513 | T45.514 | T45.515 | T45.516 |
| **Protionamide** | T37.1X1 | T37.1X2 | T37.1X3 | T37.1X4 | T37.1X5 | T37.1X6 |
| **Protirelin** | T38.891 | T38.892 | T38.893 | T38.894 | T38.895 | T38.896 |
| **Protokylol** | T48.6X1 | T48.6X2 | T48.6X3 | T48.6X4 | T48.6X5 | T48.6X6 |
| **Protonix*** | T47.1X1 | T47.1X2 | T47.1X3 | T47.1X4 | T47.1X5 | T47.1X6 |
| **Protopam** | T5Ø.6X1 | T5Ø.6X2 | T5Ø.6X3 | T5Ø.6X4 | T5Ø.6X5 | T5Ø.6X6 |
| **Protoveratrine**(s) (A) (B) | T46.5X1 | T46.5X2 | T46.5X3 | T46.5X4 | T46.5X5 | T46.5X6 |
| **Protriptyline** | T43.Ø11 | T43.Ø12 | T43.Ø13 | T43.Ø14 | T43.Ø15 | T43.Ø16 |
| **Proventil*** | T48.6X1 | T48.6X2 | T48.6X3 | T48.6X4 | T48.6X5 | T48.6X6 |
| **Provera** | T38.5X1 | T38.5X2 | T38.5X3 | T38.5X4 | T38.5X5 | T38.5X6 |
| **Provitamin A** | T45.2X1 | T45.2X2 | T45.2X3 | T45.2X4 | T45.2X5 | T45.2X6 |
| **Proxibarbal** | T42.3X1 | T42.3X2 | T42.3X3 | T42.3X4 | T42.3X5 | T42.3X6 |
| **Proxymetacaine** | T41.3X1 | T41.3X2 | T41.3X3 | T41.3X4 | T41.3X5 | T41.3X6 |
| **Proxyphylline** | T48.6X1 | T48.6X2 | T48.6X3 | T48.6X4 | T48.6X5 | T48.6X6 |
| **Prozac** — *see* Fluoxetine hydrochloride | | | | | | |
| **Prunus** | | | | | | |
| laurocerasus | T62.2X1 | T62.2X2 | T62.2X3 | T62.2X4 | — | — |
| virginiana | T62.2X1 | T62.2X2 | T62.2X3 | T62.2X4 | — | — |
| **Prussian blue** | | | | | | |
| commercial | T65.891 | T65.892 | T65.893 | T65.894 | — | — |
| therapeutic | T5Ø.6X1 | T5Ø.6X2 | T5Ø.6X3 | T5Ø.6X4 | T5Ø.6X5 | T5Ø.6X6 |
| **Prussic acid** | T65.ØX1 | T65.ØX2 | T65.ØX3 | T65.ØX4 | — | — |
| vapor | T57.3X1 | T57.3X2 | T57.3X3 | T57.3X4 | — | — |
| **Pseudoephedrine** | T44.991 | T44.992 | T44.993 | T44.994 | T44.995 | T44.996 |
| **Psilocin** | T4Ø.991 | T4Ø.992 | T4Ø.993 | T4Ø.994 | — | — |
| **Psilocybin** | T4Ø.991 | T4Ø.992 | T4Ø.993 | T4Ø.994 | — | — |
| **Psilocybine** | T4Ø.991 | T4Ø.992 | T4Ø.993 | T4Ø.994 | — | — |
| **Psoralene** (nonmedicinal) | T65.891 | T65.892 | T65.893 | T65.894 | — | — |
| **Psoralens** (medicinal) | T5Ø.991 | T5Ø.992 | T5Ø.993 | T5Ø.994 | T5Ø.995 | T5Ø.996 |
| **PSP** (phenolsulfonphthalein) | T5Ø.8X1 | T5Ø.8X2 | T5Ø.8X3 | T5Ø.8X4 | T5Ø.8X5 | T5Ø.8X6 |
| **Psychodysleptic drug NOS** | T4Ø.9Ø1 | T4Ø.9Ø2 | T4Ø.9Ø3 | T4Ø.9Ø4 | T4Ø.9Ø5 | T4Ø.9Ø6 |
| specified NEC | T4Ø.991 | T4Ø.992 | T4Ø.993 | T4Ø.994 | T4Ø.995 | T4Ø.996 |
| **Psychostimulant** | T43.6Ø1 | T43.6Ø2 | T43.6Ø3 | T43.6Ø4 | T43.6Ø5 | T43.6Ø6 |
| amphetamine | T43.621 | T43.622 | T43.623 | T43.624 | T43.625 | T43.626 |
| caffeine | T43.611 | T43.612 | T43.613 | T43.614 | T43.615 | T43.616 |
| methylphenidate | T43.631 | T43.632 | T43.633 | T43.634 | T43.635 | T43.636 |
| specified NEC | T43.691 | T43.692 | T43.693 | T43.694 | T43.695 | T43.696 |
| **Psychotherapeutic drug NEC** | T43.91 | T43.92 | T43.93 | T43.94 | T43.95 | T43.96 |
| antidepressants — *see also* Antidepressant | T43.2Ø1 | T43.2Ø2 | T43.2Ø3 | T43.2Ø4 | T43.2Ø5 | T43.2Ø6 |
| specified NEC | T43.8X1 | T43.8X2 | T43.8X3 | T43.8X4 | T43.8X5 | T43.8X6 |
| tranquilizers NEC | T43.5Ø1 | T43.5Ø2 | T43.5Ø3 | T43.5Ø4 | T43.5Ø5 | T43.5Ø6 |
| **Psychotomimetic agents** | T4Ø.9Ø1 | T4Ø.9Ø2 | T4Ø.9Ø3 | T4Ø.9Ø4 | T4Ø.9Ø5 | T4Ø.9Ø6 |
| **Psychotropic drug NEC** | T43.91 | T43.92 | T43.93 | T43.94 | T43.95 | T43.96 |
| specified NEC | T43.8X1 | T43.8X2 | T43.8X3 | T43.8X4 | T43.8X5 | T43.8X6 |
| **Psyllium hydrophilic mucilloid** | T47.4X1 | T47.4X2 | T47.4X3 | T47.4X4 | T47.4X5 | T47.4X6 |
| **Pteroylglutamic acid** | T45.8X1 | T45.8X2 | T45.8X3 | T45.8X4 | T45.8X5 | T45.8X6 |
| **Pteroyltriglutamate** | T45.1X1 | T45.1X2 | T45.1X3 | T45.1X4 | T45.1X5 | T45.1X6 |
| **PTFE** — *see* Polytetrafluoroethylene | | | | | | |
| **Pulmicort*** | T44.5X1 | T44.5X2 | T44.5X3 | T44.5X4 | T44.5X5 | T44.5X6 |
| **Pulp** | | | | | | |
| devitalizing paste | T49.7X1 | T49.7X2 | T49.7X3 | T49.7X4 | T49.7X5 | T49.7X6 |
| dressing | T49.7X1 | T49.7X2 | T49.7X3 | T49.7X4 | T49.7X5 | T49.7X6 |
| **Pulsatilla** | T62.2X1 | T62.2X2 | T62.2X3 | T62.2X4 | — | — |
| **Pumpkin seed extract** | T37.4X1 | T37.4X2 | T37.4X3 | T37.4X4 | T37.4X5 | T37.4X6 |
| **Purex** (bleach) | T54.91 | T54.92 | T54.93 | T54.94 | — | — |
| **Purgative NEC** — *see also* Cathartic | T47.4X1 | T47.4X2 | T47.4X3 | T47.4X4 | T47.4X5 | T47.4X6 |
| **Purine analogue** (antineoplastic) | T45.1X1 | T45.1X2 | T45.1X3 | T45.1X4 | T45.1X5 | T45.1X6 |
| **Purine diuretics** | T5Ø.2X1 | T5Ø.2X2 | T5Ø.2X3 | T5Ø.2X4 | T5Ø.2X5 | T5Ø.2X6 |
| **Purinethol** | T45.1X1 | T45.1X2 | T45.1X3 | T45.1X4 | T45.1X5 | T45.1X6 |
| **PVP** | T45.8X1 | T45.8X2 | T45.8X3 | T45.8X4 | T45.8X5 | T45.8X6 |
| **Pyrabital** | T39.8X1 | T39.8X2 | T39.8X3 | T39.8X4 | T39.8X5 | T39.8X6 |
| **Pyramidon** | T39.2X1 | T39.2X2 | T39.2X3 | T39.2X4 | T39.2X5 | T39.2X6 |

| Substance | Poisoning, Accidental (unintentional) | Poisoning, Intentional Self-harm | Poisoning, Assault | Poisoning, Undetermined | Adverse Effect | Under-dosing |
|---|---|---|---|---|---|---|
| **Pyrantel** | T37.4X1 | T37.4X2 | T37.4X3 | T37.4X4 | T37.4X5 | T37.4X6 |
| **Pyrathiazine** | T45.ØX1 | T45.ØX2 | T45.ØX3 | T45.ØX4 | T45.ØX5 | T45.ØX6 |
| **Pyrazinamide** | T37.1X1 | T37.1X2 | T37.1X3 | T37.1X4 | T37.1X5 | T37.1X6 |
| **Pyrazinoic acid** (amide) | T37.1X1 | T37.1X2 | T37.1X3 | T37.1X4 | T37.1X5 | T37.1X6 |
| **Pyrazole** (derivatives) | T39.2X1 | T39.2X2 | T39.2X3 | T39.2X4 | T39.2X5 | T39.2X6 |
| **Pyrazolone analgesic NEC** | T39.2X1 | T39.2X2 | T39.2X3 | T39.2X4 | T39.2X5 | T39.2X6 |
| **Pyrethrin, pyrethrum** (nonmedicinal) | T6Ø.2X1 | T6Ø.2X2 | T6Ø.2X3 | T6Ø.2X4 | — | — |
| **Pyrethrum extract** | T49.ØX1 | T49.ØX2 | T49.ØX3 | T49.ØX4 | T49.ØX5 | T49.ØX6 |
| **Pyribenzamine** | T45.ØX1 | T45.ØX2 | T45.ØX3 | T45.ØX4 | T45.ØX5 | T45.ØX6 |
| **Pyridine** | T52.891 | T52.892 | T52.893 | T52.894 | — | — |
| aldoxime methiodide | T5Ø.6X1 | T5Ø.6X2 | T5Ø.6X3 | T5Ø.6X4 | T5Ø.6X5 | T5Ø.6X6 |
| aldoxime methyl chloride | T5Ø.6X1 | T5Ø.6X2 | T5Ø.6X3 | T5Ø.6X4 | T5Ø.6X5 | T5Ø.6X6 |
| vapor | T59.891 | T59.892 | T59.893 | T59.894 | — | — |
| **Pyridium** | T39.8X1 | T39.8X2 | T39.8X3 | T39.8X4 | T39.8X5 | T39.8X6 |
| **Pyridostigmine bromide** | T44.ØX1 | T44.ØX2 | T44.ØX3 | T44.ØX4 | T44.ØX5 | T44.ØX6 |
| **Pyridoxal phosphate** | T45.2X1 | T45.2X2 | T45.2X3 | T45.2X4 | T45.2X5 | T45.2X6 |
| **Pyridoxine** | T45.2X1 | T45.2X2 | T45.2X3 | T45.2X4 | T45.2X5 | T45.2X6 |
| **Pyrilamine** | T45.ØX1 | T45.ØX2 | T45.ØX3 | T45.ØX4 | T45.ØX5 | T45.ØX6 |
| **Pyrimethamine** | T37.2X1 | T37.2X2 | T37.2X3 | T37.2X4 | T37.2X5 | T37.2X6 |
| with sulfadoxine | T37.2X1 | T37.2X2 | T37.2X3 | T37.2X4 | T37.2X5 | T37.2X6 |
| **Pyrimidine antagonist** | T45.1X1 | T45.1X2 | T45.1X3 | T45.1X4 | T45.1X5 | T45.1X6 |
| **Pyriminil** | T6Ø.4X1 | T6Ø.4X2 | T6Ø.4X3 | T6Ø.4X4 | — | — |
| **Pyrithione zinc** | T49.4X1 | T49.4X2 | T49.4X3 | T49.4X4 | T49.4X5 | T49.4X6 |
| **Pyrithyldione** | T42.6X1 | T42.6X2 | T42.6X3 | T42.6X4 | T42.6X5 | T42.6X6 |
| **Pyrogallic acid** | T49.ØX1 | T49.ØX2 | T49.ØX3 | T49.ØX4 | T49.ØX5 | T49.ØX6 |
| **Pyrogallol** | T49.ØX1 | T49.ØX2 | T49.ØX3 | T49.ØX4 | T49.ØX5 | T49.ØX6 |
| **Pyroxylin** | T49.3X1 | T49.3X2 | T49.3X3 | T49.3X4 | T49.3X5 | T49.3X6 |
| **Pyrrobutamine** | T45.ØX1 | T45.ØX2 | T45.ØX3 | T45.ØX4 | T45.ØX5 | T45.ØX6 |
| **Pyrrolizidine alkaloids** | T62.8X1 | T62.8X2 | T62.8X3 | T62.8X4 | — | — |
| **Pyrvinium chloride** | T37.4X1 | T37.4X2 | T37.4X3 | T37.4X4 | T37.4X5 | T37.4X6 |
| **PZI** | T38.3X1 | T38.3X2 | T38.3X3 | T38.3X4 | T38.3X5 | T38.3X6 |
| **Qbrelis*** | T46.4X1 | T46.4X2 | T46.4X3 | T46.4X4 | T46.4X5 | T46.4X6 |
| **Quaalude** | T42.6X1 | T42.6X2 | T42.6X3 | T42.6X4 | T42.6X5 | T42.6X6 |
| **Quarternary ammonium** | | | | | | |
| anti-infective | T49.ØX1 | T49.ØX2 | T49.ØX3 | T49.ØX4 | T49.ØX5 | T49.ØX6 |
| ganglion blocking | T44.2X1 | T44.2X2 | T44.2X3 | T44.2X4 | T44.2X5 | T44.2X6 |
| parasympatholytic | T44.3X1 | T44.3X2 | T44.3X3 | T44.3X4 | T44.3X5 | T44.3X6 |
| **Quazepam** | T42.4X1 | T42.4X2 | T42.4X3 | T42.4X4 | T42.4X5 | T42.4X6 |
| **Quicklime** | T54.3X1 | T54.3X2 | T54.3X3 | T54.3X4 | — | — |
| **Quilbron-T*** | T48.6X1 | T48.6X2 | T48.6X3 | T48.6X4 | T48.6X5 | T48.6X6 |
| **Quillaja extract** | T48.4X1 | T48.4X2 | T48.4X3 | T48.4X4 | T48.4X5 | T48.4X6 |
| **Quinacrine** | T37.2X1 | T37.2X2 | T37.2X3 | T37.2X4 | T37.2X5 | T37.2X6 |
| **Quinaglute** | T46.2X1 | T46.2X2 | T46.2X3 | T46.2X4 | T46.2X5 | T46.2X6 |
| **Quinalbarbital** | T42.3X1 | T42.3X2 | T42.3X3 | T42.3X4 | T42.3X5 | T42.3X6 |
| **Quinalbarbitone sodium** | T42.3X1 | T42.3X2 | T42.3X3 | T42.3X4 | T42.3X5 | T42.3X6 |
| **Quinalphos** | T6Ø.ØX1 | T6Ø.ØX2 | T6Ø.ØX3 | T6Ø.ØX4 | — | — |
| **Quinapril** | T46.4X1 | T46.4X2 | T46.4X3 | T46.4X4 | T46.4X5 | T46.4X6 |
| **Quinestradiol** | T38.5X1 | T38.5X2 | T38.5X3 | T38.5X4 | T38.5X5 | T38.5X6 |
| **Quinestradol** | T38.5X1 | T38.5X2 | T38.5X3 | T38.5X4 | T38.5X5 | T38.5X6 |
| **Quinestrol** | T38.5X1 | T38.5X2 | T38.5X3 | T38.5X4 | T38.5X5 | T38.5X6 |
| **Quinethazone** | T5Ø.2X1 | T5Ø.2X2 | T5Ø.2X3 | T5Ø.2X4 | T5Ø.2X5 | T5Ø.2X6 |
| **Quingestanol** | T38.4X1 | T38.4X2 | T38.4X3 | T38.4X4 | T38.4X5 | T38.4X6 |
| **Quinidine** | T46.2X1 | T46.2X2 | T46.2X3 | T46.2X4 | T46.2X5 | T46.2X6 |
| **Quinine** | T37.2X1 | T37.2X2 | T37.2X3 | T37.2X4 | T37.2X5 | T37.2X6 |
| **Quiniobine** | T37.8X1 | T37.8X2 | T37.8X3 | T37.8X4 | T37.8X5 | T37.8X6 |
| **Quinisocaine** | T49.1X1 | T49.1X2 | T49.1X3 | T49.1X4 | T49.1X5 | T49.1X6 |
| **Quinocide** | T37.2X1 | T37.2X2 | T37.2X3 | T37.2X4 | T37.2X5 | T37.2X6 |
| **Quinoline** (derivatives) **NEC** | T37.8X1 | T37.8X2 | T37.8X3 | T37.8X4 | T37.8X5 | T37.8X6 |
| **Quinupramine** | T43.Ø11 | T43.Ø12 | T43.Ø13 | T43.Ø14 | T43.Ø15 | T43.Ø16 |
| **Quixin*** | T49.5X1 | T49.5X2 | T49.5X3 | T49.5X4 | T49.5X5 | T49.5X6 |
| **Quotane** | T41.3X1 | T41.3X2 | T41.3X3 | T41.3X4 | T41.3X5 | T41.3X6 |
| **Rabies** | | | | | | |
| immune globulin (human) | T5Ø.Z11 | T5Ø.Z12 | T5Ø.Z13 | T5Ø.Z14 | T5Ø.Z15 | T5Ø.Z16 |
| vaccine | T5Ø.B91 | T5Ø.B92 | T5Ø.B93 | T5Ø.B94 | T5Ø.B95 | T5Ø.B96 |
| **Racemoramide** | T4Ø.2X1 | T4Ø.2X2 | T4Ø.2X3 | T4Ø.2X4 | — | — |
| **Racemorphan** | T4Ø.2X1 | T4Ø.2X2 | T4Ø.2X3 | T4Ø.2X4 | T4Ø.2X5 | T4Ø.2X6 |
| **Racepinefrin** | T44.5X1 | T44.5X2 | T44.5X3 | T44.5X4 | T44.5X5 | T44.5X6 |
| **Raclopride** | T43.591 | T43.592 | T43.593 | T43.594 | T43.595 | T43.596 |
| **Radiator alcohol** | T51.1X1 | T51.1X2 | T51.1X3 | T51.1X4 | — | — |
| **Radio-opaque** (drugs) (materials) | T5Ø.8X1 | T5Ø.8X2 | T5Ø.8X3 | T5Ø.8X4 | T5Ø.8X5 | T5Ø.8X6 |
| **Radioactive drug NEC** | T5Ø.8X1 | T5Ø.8X2 | T5Ø.8X3 | T5Ø.8X4 | T5Ø.8X5 | T5Ø.8X6 |
| **Ramifenazone** | T39.2X1 | T39.2X2 | T39.2X3 | T39.2X4 | T39.2X5 | T39.2X6 |
| **Ramipril** | T46.4X1 | T46.4X2 | T46.4X3 | T46.4X4 | T46.4X5 | T46.4X6 |
| **Ranitidine** | T47.ØX1 | T47.ØX2 | T47.ØX3 | T47.ØX4 | T47.ØX5 | T47.ØX6 |
| **Ranunculus** | T62.2X1 | T62.2X2 | T62.2X3 | T62.2X4 | — | — |
| **Rat poison NEC** | T6Ø.4X1 | T6Ø.4X2 | T6Ø.4X3 | T6Ø.4X4 | — | — |
| **Rattlesnake** (venom) | T63.Ø11 | T63.Ø12 | T63.Ø13 | T63.Ø14 | — | — |
| **Raubasine** | T46.7X1 | T46.7X2 | T46.7X3 | T46.7X4 | T46.7X5 | T46.7X6 |
| **Raudixin** | T46.5X1 | T46.5X2 | T46.5X3 | T46.5X4 | T46.5X5 | T46.5X6 |
| **Rautensin** | T46.5X1 | T46.5X2 | T46.5X3 | T46.5X4 | T46.5X5 | T46.5X6 |
| **Rautina** | T46.5X1 | T46.5X2 | T46.5X3 | T46.5X4 | T46.5X5 | T46.5X6 |

| Substance | Poisoning, Accidental (unintentional) | Poisoning, Intentional Self-harm | Poisoning, Assault | Poisoning, Undetermined | Adverse Effect | Under-dosing |
|---|---|---|---|---|---|---|
| **Rautotal** | T46.5X1 | T46.5X2 | T46.5X3 | T46.5X4 | T46.5X5 | T46.5X6 |
| **Rauwiloid** | T46.5X1 | T46.5X2 | T46.5X3 | T46.5X4 | T46.5X5 | T46.5X6 |
| **Rauwoldin** | T46.5X1 | T46.5X2 | T46.5X3 | T46.5X4 | T46.5X5 | T46.5X6 |
| **Rauwolfia** (alkaloids) | T46.5X1 | T46.5X2 | T46.5X3 | T46.5X4 | T46.5X5 | T46.5X6 |
| **Razadyne*** | T44.ØX1 | T44.ØX2 | T44.ØX3 | T44.ØX4 | T44.ØX5 | T44.ØX6 |
| **Razoxane** | T45.1X1 | T45.1X2 | T45.1X3 | T45.1X4 | T45.1X5 | T45.1X6 |
| **Realgar** | T57.ØX1 | T57.ØX2 | T57.ØX3 | T57.ØX4 | — | — |
| **Recombinant** (R) — *see* specific protein | | | | | | |
| **Red blood cells, packed** | T45.8X1 | T45.8X2 | T45.8X3 | T45.8X4 | T45.8X5 | T45.8X6 |
| **Red squill** (scilliroside) | T6Ø.4X1 | T6Ø.4X2 | T6Ø.4X3 | T6Ø.4X4 | — | — |
| **Reducing agent, industrial NEC** | T65.891 | T65.892 | T65.893 | T65.894 | — | — |
| **Refrigerant gas** (chlorofluorocarbon) | T53.5X1 | T53.5X2 | T53.5X3 | T53.5X4 | — | — |
| not chlorofluorocarbon | T59.891 | T59.892 | T59.893 | T59.894 | — | — |
| **Regroton** | T5Ø.2X1 | T5Ø.2X2 | T5Ø.2X3 | T5Ø.2X4 | T5Ø.2X5 | T5Ø.2X6 |
| **Rehydration salts** (oral) | T5Ø.3X1 | T5Ø.3X2 | T5Ø.3X3 | T5Ø.3X4 | T5Ø.3X5 | T5Ø.3X6 |
| **Rela** | T42.8X1 | T42.8X2 | T42.8X3 | T42.8X4 | T42.8X5 | T42.8X6 |
| **Relaxant, muscle** | | | | | | |
| anesthetic | T48.1X1 | T48.1X2 | T48.1X3 | T48.1X4 | T48.1X5 | T48.1X6 |
| central nervous system | T42.8X1 | T42.8X2 | T42.8X3 | T42.8X4 | T42.8X5 | T42.8X6 |
| skeletal NEC | T48.1X1 | T48.1X2 | T48.1X3 | T48.1X4 | T48.1X5 | T48.1X6 |
| smooth NEC | T44.3X1 | T44.3X2 | T44.3X3 | T44.3X4 | T44.3X5 | T44.3X6 |
| **Remoxipride** | T43.591 | T43.592 | T43.593 | T43.594 | T43.595 | T43.596 |
| **Renese** | T5Ø.2X1 | T5Ø.2X2 | T5Ø.2X3 | T5Ø.2X4 | T5Ø.2X5 | T5Ø.2X6 |
| **Renografin** | T5Ø.8X1 | T5Ø.8X2 | T5Ø.8X3 | T5Ø.8X4 | T5Ø.8X5 | T5Ø.8X6 |
| **Replacement solution** | T5Ø.3X1 | T5Ø.3X2 | T5Ø.3X3 | T5Ø.3X4 | T5Ø.3X5 | T5Ø.3X6 |
| **Reproterol** | T48.6X1 | T48.6X2 | T48.6X3 | T48.6X4 | T48.6X5 | T48.6X6 |
| **Rescinnamine** | T46.5X1 | T46.5X2 | T46.5X3 | T46.5X4 | T46.5X5 | T46.5X6 |
| **Reserpin** (e) | T46.5X1 | T46.5X2 | T46.5X3 | T46.5X4 | T46.5X5 | T46.5X6 |
| **Resorcin, resorcinol** (nonmedicinal) | T65.891 | T65.892 | T65.893 | T65.894 | — | — |
| medicinal | T49.4X1 | T49.4X2 | T49.4X3 | T49.4X4 | T49.4X5 | T49.4X6 |
| **Respaire** | T48.4X1 | T48.4X2 | T48.4X3 | T48.4X4 | T48.4X5 | T48.4X6 |
| **Respiratory drug NEC** | T48.9Ø1 | T48.9Ø2 | T48.9Ø3 | T48.9Ø4 | T48.9Ø5 | T48.9Ø6 |
| anti-common-cold NEC | T48.5X1 | T48.5X2 | T48.5X3 | T48.5X4 | T48.5X5 | T48.5X6 |
| antiasthmatic NEC | T48.6X1 | T48.6X2 | T48.6X3 | T48.6X4 | T48.6X5 | T48.6X6 |
| expectorant NEC | T48.4X1 | T48.4X2 | T48.4X3 | T48.4X4 | T48.4X5 | T48.4X6 |
| stimulant | T48.9Ø1 | T48.9Ø2 | T48.9Ø3 | T48.9Ø4 | T48.9Ø5 | T48.9Ø6 |
| **Restoril*** | T42.4X1 | T42.4X2 | T42.4X3 | T42.4X4 | T42.4X5 | T42.4X6 |
| **Retinoic acid** | T49.ØX1 | T49.ØX2 | T49.ØX3 | T49.ØX4 | T49.ØX5 | T49.ØX6 |
| **Retinol** | T45.2X1 | T45.2X2 | T45.2X3 | T45.2X4 | T45.2X5 | T45.2X6 |
| **Revatio*** | T46.7X1 | T46.7X2 | T46.7X3 | T46.7X4 | T46.7X5 | T46.7X6 |
| **Rh (D) immune globulin** (human) | T5Ø.Z11 | T5Ø.Z12 | T5Ø.Z13 | T5Ø.Z14 | T5Ø.Z15 | T5Ø.Z16 |
| **Rhodine** | T39.Ø11 | T39.Ø12 | T39.Ø13 | T39.Ø14 | T39.Ø15 | T39.Ø16 |
| **RhoGAM** | T5Ø.Z11 | T5Ø.Z12 | T5Ø.Z13 | T5Ø.Z14 | T5Ø.Z15 | T5Ø.Z16 |
| **Rhubarb** | | | | | | |
| dry extract | T47.2X1 | T47.2X2 | T47.2X3 | T47.2X4 | T47.2X5 | T47.2X6 |
| tincture, compound | T47.2X1 | T47.2X2 | T47.2X3 | T47.2X4 | T47.2X5 | T47.2X6 |
| **Ribavirin** | T37.5X1 | T37.5X2 | T37.5X3 | T37.5X4 | T37.5X5 | T37.5X6 |
| **Riboflavin** | T45.2X1 | T45.2X2 | T45.2X3 | T45.2X4 | T45.2X5 | T45.2X6 |
| **Ribostamycin** | T36.5X1 | T36.5X2 | T36.5X3 | T36.5X4 | T36.5X5 | T36.5X6 |
| **Ricin** | T62.2X1 | T62.2X2 | T62.2X3 | T62.2X4 | — | — |
| **Ricinus communis** | T62.2X1 | T62.2X2 | T62.2X3 | T62.2X4 | — | — |
| **Rickettsial vaccine NEC** | T5Ø.A91 | T5Ø.A92 | T5Ø.A93 | T5Ø.A94 | T5Ø.A95 | T5Ø.A96 |
| **Rifabutin** | T36.6X1 | T36.6X2 | T36.6X3 | T36.6X4 | T36.6X5 | T36.6X6 |
| **Rifamide** | T36.6X1 | T36.6X2 | T36.6X3 | T36.6X4 | T36.6X5 | T36.6X6 |
| **Rifampicin** | T36.6X1 | T36.6X2 | T36.6X3 | T36.6X4 | T36.6X5 | T36.6X6 |
| with isoniazid | T37.1X1 | T37.1X2 | T37.1X3 | T37.1X4 | T37.1X5 | T37.1X6 |
| **Rifampin** | T36.6X1 | T36.6X2 | T36.6X3 | T36.6X4 | T36.6X5 | T36.6X6 |
| **Rifamycin** | T36.6X1 | T36.6X2 | T36.6X3 | T36.6X4 | T36.6X5 | T36.6X6 |
| **Rifaximin** | T36.6X1 | T36.6X2 | T36.6X3 | T36.6X4 | T36.6X5 | T36.6X6 |
| **Rimantadine** | T37.5X1 | T37.5X2 | T37.5X3 | T37.5X4 | T37.5X5 | T37.5X6 |
| **Rimazolium metilsulfate** | T39.8X1 | T39.8X2 | T39.8X3 | T39.8X4 | T39.8X5 | T39.8X6 |
| **Rimifon** | T37.1X1 | T37.1X2 | T37.1X3 | T37.1X4 | T37.1X5 | T37.1X6 |
| **Rimiterol** | T48.6X1 | T48.6X2 | T48.6X3 | T48.6X4 | T48.6X5 | T48.6X6 |
| **Ringer** (lactate) **solution** | T5Ø.3X1 | T5Ø.3X2 | T5Ø.3X3 | T5Ø.3X4 | T5Ø.3X5 | T5Ø.3X6 |
| **Riomet*** | T38.3X1 | T38.3X2 | T38.3X3 | T38.3X4 | T38.3X5 | T38.3X6 |
| **Risperdal*** | T43.591 | T43.592 | T43.593 | T43.594 | T43.595 | T43.596 |
| **Ristocetin** | T36.8X1 | T36.8X2 | T36.8X3 | T36.8X4 | T36.8X5 | T36.8X6 |
| **Ritalin** | T43.631 | T43.632 | T43.633 | T43.634 | T43.635 | T43.636 |
| **Ritodrine** | T44.5X1 | T44.5X2 | T44.5X3 | T44.5X4 | T44.5X5 | T44.5X6 |
| **Roach killer** — *see* Insecticide | | | | | | |
| **Robaxin*** | T48.1X1 | T48.1X2 | T48.1X3 | T48.1X4 | T48.1X5 | T48.1X6 |
| **Robitussin*** | T48.3X1 | T48.3X2 | T48.3X3 | T48.3X4 | T48.3X5 | T48.3X6 |
| **Rociverine** | T44.3X1 | T44.3X2 | T44.3X3 | T44.3X4 | T44.3X5 | T44.3X6 |
| **Rocky Mountain spotted fever vaccine** | T5Ø.A91 | T5Ø.A92 | T5Ø.A93 | T5Ø.A94 | T5Ø.A95 | T5Ø.A96 |
| **Rodenticide NEC** | T6Ø.4X1 | T6Ø.4X2 | T6Ø.4X3 | T6Ø.4X4 | — | — |
| **Rohypnol** | T42.4X1 | T42.4X2 | T42.4X3 | T42.4X4 | T42.4X5 | T42.4X6 |
| **Rokitamycin** | T36.3X1 | T36.3X2 | T36.3X3 | T36.3X4 | T36.3X5 | T36.3X6 |

| Substance | Poisoning, Accidental (unintentional) | Poisoning, Intentional Self-harm | Poisoning, Assault | Poisoning, Undetermined | Adverse Effect | Under-dosing |
|---|---|---|---|---|---|---|
| **Rolaids** | T47.1X1 | T47.1X2 | T47.1X3 | T47.1X4 | T47.1X5 | T47.1X |
| **Rolitetracycline** | T36.4X1 | T36.4X2 | T36.4X3 | T36.4X4 | T36.4X5 | T36.4X |
| **Romilar** | T48.3X1 | T48.3X2 | T48.3X3 | T48.3X4 | T48.3X5 | T48.3X |
| **Ronifibrate** | T46.6X1 | T46.6X2 | T46.6X3 | T46.6X4 | T46.6X5 | T46.6X |
| **Rosaprostol** | T47.1X1 | T47.1X2 | T47.1X3 | T47.1X4 | T47.1X5 | T47.1X |
| **Rose bengal sodium** (131I) | T5Ø.8X1 | T5Ø.8X2 | T5Ø.8X3 | T5Ø.8X4 | T5Ø.8X5 | T5Ø.8X |
| **Rose water ointment** | T49.3X1 | T49.3X2 | T49.3X3 | T49.3X4 | T49.3X5 | T49.3X |
| **Rosoxacin** | T37.8X1 | T37.8X2 | T37.8X3 | T37.8X4 | T37.8X5 | T37.8X |
| **Rotenone** | T6Ø.2X1 | T6Ø.2X2 | T6Ø.2X3 | T6Ø.2X4 | — | — |
| **Rotoxamine** | T45.ØX1 | T45.ØX2 | T45.ØX3 | T45.ØX4 | T45.ØX5 | T45.ØX |
| **Rough-on-rats** | T6Ø.4X1 | T6Ø.4X2 | T6Ø.4X3 | T6Ø.4X4 | — | — |
| **Roxatidine** | T47.ØX1 | T47.ØX2 | T47.ØX3 | T47.ØX4 | T47.ØX5 | T47.ØX |
| **Roxithromycin** | T36.3X1 | T36.3X2 | T36.3X3 | T36.3X4 | T36.3X5 | T36.3X |
| **Rt-PA** | T45.611 | T45.612 | T45.613 | T45.614 | T45.615 | T45.61 |
| **Rubbing alcohol** | T51.2X1 | T51.2X2 | T51.2X3 | T51.2X4 | — | — |
| **Rubefacient** | T49.4X1 | T49.4X2 | T49.4X3 | T49.4X4 | T49.4X5 | T49.4X |
| **Rubella vaccine** | T5Ø.B91 | T5Ø.B92 | T5Ø.B93 | T5Ø.B94 | T5Ø.B95 | T5Ø.B9 |
| **Rubeola vaccine** | T5Ø.B91 | T5Ø.B92 | T5Ø.B93 | T5Ø.B94 | T5Ø.B95 | T5Ø.B9 |
| **Rubidium chloride Rb82** | T5Ø.8X1 | T5Ø.8X2 | T5Ø.8X3 | T5Ø.8X4 | T5Ø.8X5 | T5Ø.8X |
| **Rubidomycin** | T45.1X1 | T45.1X2 | T45.1X3 | T45.1X4 | T45.1X5 | T45.1X |
| **Rue** | T62.2X1 | T62.2X2 | T62.2X3 | T62.2X4 | — | — |
| **Rufocromomycin** | T45.1X1 | T45.1X2 | T45.1X3 | T45.1X4 | T45.1X5 | T45.1X |
| **Russel's viper venin** | T45.7X1 | T45.7X2 | T45.7X3 | T45.7X4 | T45.7X5 | T45.7X |
| **Ruta** (graveolens) | T62.2X1 | T62.2X2 | T62.2X3 | T62.2X4 | — | — |
| **Rutinum** | T46.991 | T46.992 | T46.993 | T46.994 | T46.995 | T46.99 |
| **Rutoside** | T46.991 | T46.992 | T46.993 | T46.994 | T46.995 | T46.99 |
| **S-Carboxymethylcysteine** | T48.4X1 | T48.4X2 | T48.4X3 | T48.4X4 | T48.4X5 | T48.4X |
| **Sabadilla** (plant) | T62.2X1 | T62.2X2 | T62.2X3 | T62.2X4 | — | — |
| pesticide | T6Ø.2X1 | T6Ø.2X2 | T6Ø.2X3 | T6Ø.2X4 | — | — |
| **Sabril*** | T42.6X1 | T42.6X2 | T42.6X3 | T42.6X4 | T42.6X5 | T42.6X |
| **Saccharated iron oxide** | T45.8X1 | T45.8X2 | T45.8X3 | T45.8X4 | T45.8X5 | T45.8X |
| **Saccharin** | T5Ø.9Ø1 | T5Ø.9Ø2 | T5Ø.9Ø3 | T5Ø.9Ø4 | T5Ø.9Ø5 | T5Ø.9Ø |
| **Saccharomyces boulardii** | T47.6X1 | T47.6X2 | T47.6X3 | T47.6X4 | T47.6X5 | T47.6X |
| **Safflower oil** | T46.6X1 | T46.6X2 | T46.6X3 | T46.6X4 | T46.6X5 | T46.6X |
| **Safrazine** | T43.1X1 | T43.1X2 | T43.1X3 | T43.1X4 | T43.1X5 | T43.1X |
| **Salazosulfapyridine** | T37.ØX1 | T37.ØX2 | T37.ØX3 | T37.ØX4 | T37.ØX5 | T37.ØX |
| **Salbutamol** | T48.6X1 | T48.6X2 | T48.6X3 | T48.6X4 | T48.6X5 | T48.6X |
| **Salicylamide** | T39.Ø91 | T39.Ø92 | T39.Ø93 | T39.Ø94 | T39.Ø95 | T39.Ø9 |
| **Salicylate NEC** | T39.Ø91 | T39.Ø92 | T39.Ø93 | T39.Ø94 | T39.Ø95 | T39.Ø9 |
| methyl | T49.3X1 | T49.3X2 | T49.3X3 | T49.3X4 | T49.3X5 | T49.3X |
| theobromine calcium | T5Ø.2X1 | T5Ø.2X2 | T5Ø.2X3 | T5Ø.2X4 | T5Ø.2X5 | T5Ø.2X |
| **Salicylazosulfapyridine** | T37.ØX1 | T37.ØX2 | T37.ØX3 | T37.ØX4 | T37.ØX5 | T37.ØX |
| **Salicylhydroxamic acid** | T49.ØX1 | T49.ØX2 | T49.ØX3 | T49.ØX4 | T49.ØX5 | T49.ØX |
| **Salicylic acid** | T49.4X1 | T49.4X2 | T49.4X3 | T49.4X4 | T49.4X5 | T49.4X |
| congeners | T39.Ø91 | T39.Ø92 | T39.Ø93 | T39.Ø94 | T39.Ø95 | T39.Ø9 |
| derivative | T39.Ø91 | T39.Ø92 | T39.Ø93 | T39.Ø94 | T39.Ø95 | T39.Ø9 |
| salts | T39.Ø91 | T39.Ø92 | T39.Ø93 | T39.Ø94 | T39.Ø95 | T39.Ø9 |
| with benzoic acid | T49.4X1 | T49.4X2 | T49.4X3 | T49.4X4 | T49.4X5 | T49.4X |
| **Salinazid** | T37.1X1 | T37.1X2 | T37.1X3 | T37.1X4 | T37.1X5 | T37.1X |
| **Salmeterol** | T48.6X1 | T48.6X2 | T48.6X3 | T48.6X4 | T48.6X5 | T48.6X |
| **Salol** | T49.3X1 | T49.3X2 | T49.3X3 | T49.3X4 | T49.3X5 | T49.3X |
| **Salsalate** | T39.Ø91 | T39.Ø92 | T39.Ø93 | T39.Ø94 | T39.Ø95 | T39.Ø9 |
| **Salt-replacing drug** | T5Ø.9Ø1 | T5Ø.9Ø2 | T5Ø.9Ø3 | T5Ø.9Ø4 | T5Ø.9Ø5 | T5Ø.9Ø |
| **Salt-retaining mineralocorticoid** | T5Ø.ØX1 | T5Ø.ØX2 | T5Ø.ØX3 | T5Ø.ØX4 | T5Ø.ØX5 | T5Ø.ØX |
| **Salt substitute** | T5Ø.9Ø1 | T5Ø.9Ø2 | T5Ø.9Ø3 | T5Ø.9Ø4 | T5Ø.9Ø5 | T5Ø.9Ø |
| **Saluretic NEC** | T5Ø.2X1 | T5Ø.2X2 | T5Ø.2X3 | T5Ø.2X4 | T5Ø.2X5 | T5Ø.2X |
| **Saluron** | T5Ø.2X1 | T5Ø.2X2 | T5Ø.2X3 | T5Ø.2X4 | T5Ø.2X5 | T5Ø.2X |
| **Salvarsan 606** (neosilver) (silver) | T37.8X1 | T37.8X2 | T37.8X3 | T37.8X4 | T37.8X5 | T37.8X |
| **Sambucus canadensis** | T62.2X1 | T62.2X2 | T62.2X3 | T62.2X4 | — | — |
| berry | T62.1X1 | T62.1X2 | T62.1X3 | T62.1X4 | — | — |
| **Sandril** | T46.5X1 | T46.5X2 | T46.5X3 | T46.5X4 | T46.5X5 | T46.5X |
| **Sanguinaria canadensis** | T62.2X1 | T62.2X2 | T62.2X3 | T62.2X4 | — | — |
| **Saniflush** (cleaner) | T54.2X1 | T54.2X2 | T54.2X3 | T54.2X4 | — | — |
| **Santonin** | T37.4X1 | T37.4X2 | T37.4X3 | T37.4X4 | T37.4X5 | T37.4X |
| **Santyl** | T49.8X1 | T49.8X2 | T49.8X3 | T49.8X4 | T49.8X5 | T49.8X |
| **Saralasin** | T46.5X1 | T46.5X2 | T46.5X3 | T46.5X4 | T46.5X5 | T46.5X |
| **Sarcolysin** | T45.1X1 | T45.1X2 | T45.1X3 | T45.1X4 | T45.1X5 | T45.1X |
| **Sarilumab*** | T39.4X1 | T39.4X2 | T39.4X3 | T39.4X4 | T39.4X5 | T39.4X |
| **Sarkomycin** | T45.1X1 | T45.1X2 | T45.1X3 | T45.1X4 | T45.1X5 | T45.1X |
| **Saroten** | T43.Ø11 | T43.Ø12 | T43.Ø13 | T43.Ø14 | T43.Ø15 | T43.Ø1 |
| **Saturnine** — *see* Lead | | | | | | |
| **Savin** (oil) | T49.4X1 | T49.4X2 | T49.4X3 | T49.4X4 | T49.4X5 | T49.4X |
| **Scammony** | T47.2X1 | T47.2X2 | T47.2X3 | T47.2X4 | T47.2X5 | T47.2X |
| **Scarlet red** | T49.8X1 | T49.8X2 | T49.8X3 | T49.8X4 | T49.8X5 | T49.8X |
| **Scheele's green** | T57.ØX1 | T57.ØX2 | T57.ØX3 | T57.ØX4 | — | — |
| insecticide | T57.ØX1 | T57.ØX2 | T57.ØX3 | T57.ØX4 | — | — |
| **Schizontozide** (blood) (tissue) | T37.2X1 | T37.2X2 | T37.2X3 | T37.2X4 | T37.2X5 | T37.2X |
| **Schradan** | T6Ø.ØX1 | T6Ø.ØX2 | T6Ø.ØX3 | T6Ø.ØX4 | — | — |
| **Schweinfurth green** | T57.ØX1 | T57.ØX2 | T57.ØX3 | T57.ØX4 | — | — |
| insecticide | T57.ØX1 | T57.ØX2 | T57.ØX3 | T57.ØX4 | — | — |

| Substance | Poisoning, Accidental (unintentional) | Poisoning, Intentional Self-harm | Poisoning, Assault | Poisoning, Undetermined | Adverse Effect | Under-dosing |
|---|---|---|---|---|---|---|
| **Scilla, rat poison** | T60.4X1 | T60.4X2 | T60.4X3 | T60.4X4 | — | — |
| **Scillaren** | T60.4X1 | T60.4X2 | T60.4X3 | T60.4X4 | — | — |
| **Sclerosing agent** | T46.8X1 | T46.8X2 | T46.8X3 | T46.8X4 | T46.8X5 | T46.8X6 |
| **Scombrotoxin** | T61.11 | T61.12 | T61.13 | T61.14 | — | — |
| **Scopolamine** | T44.3X1 | T44.3X2 | T44.3X3 | T44.3X4 | T44.3X5 | T44.3X6 |
| **Scopolia extract** | T44.3X1 | T44.3X2 | T44.3X3 | T44.3X4 | T44.3X5 | T44.3X6 |
| **Scouring powder** | T65.891 | T65.892 | T65.893 | T65.894 | — | — |
| **Sea** | | | | | | |
| anemone (sting) | T63.631 | T63.632 | T63.633 | T63.634 | — | — |
| cucumber (sting) | T63.691 | T63.692 | T63.693 | T63.694 | — | — |
| snake (bite) (venom) | T63.091 | T63.092 | T63.093 | T63.094 | — | — |
| urchin spine (puncture) | T63.691 | T63.692 | T63.693 | T63.694 | — | — |
| **Seafood** | T61.91 | T61.92 | T61.93 | T61.94 | — | — |
| specified NEC | T61.8X1 | T61.8X2 | T61.8X3 | T61.8X4 | — | — |
| **Secbutabarbital** | T42.3X1 | T42.3X2 | T42.3X3 | T42.3X4 | T42.3X5 | T42.3X6 |
| **Secbutabarbitone** | T42.3X1 | T42.3X2 | T42.3X3 | T42.3X4 | T42.3X5 | T42.3X6 |
| **Secnidazole** | T37.3X1 | T37.3X2 | T37.3X3 | T37.3X4 | T37.3X5 | T37.3X6 |
| **Secobarbital** | T42.3X1 | T42.3X2 | T42.3X3 | T42.3X4 | T42.3X5 | T42.3X6 |
| **Seconal** | T42.3X1 | T42.3X2 | T42.3X3 | T42.3X4 | T42.3X5 | T42.3X6 |
| **Secretin** | T50.8X1 | T50.8X2 | T50.8X3 | T50.8X4 | T50.8X5 | T50.8X6 |
| **Sectral*** | T44.7X1 | T44.7X2 | T44.7X3 | T44.7X4 | T44.7X5 | T44.7X6 |
| **Sedative NEC** | T42.71 | T42.72 | T42.73 | T42.74 | T42.75 | T42.76 |
| mixed NEC | T42.6X1 | T42.6X2 | T42.6X3 | T42.6X4 | T42.6X5 | T42.6X6 |
| **Sedormid** | T42.6X1 | T42.6X2 | T42.6X3 | T42.6X4 | T42.6X5 | T42.6X6 |
| **Seed disinfectant or dressing** | T60.8X1 | T60.8X2 | T60.8X3 | T60.8X4 | — | — |
| **Seeds** (poisonous) | T62.2X1 | T62.2X2 | T62.2X3 | T62.2X4 | — | — |
| **Selegiline** | T42.8X1 | T42.8X2 | T42.8X3 | T42.8X4 | T42.8X5 | T42.8X6 |
| **Selenium NEC** | T56.891 | T56.892 | T56.893 | T56.894 | — | — |
| disulfide or sulfide | T49.4X1 | T49.4X2 | T49.4X3 | T49.4X4 | T49.4X5 | T49.4X6 |
| fumes | T59.891 | T59.892 | T59.893 | T59.894 | — | — |
| sulfide | T49.4X1 | T49.4X2 | T49.4X3 | T49.4X4 | T49.4X5 | T49.4X6 |
| **Selenomethionine** (75Se) | T50.8X1 | T50.8X2 | T50.8X3 | T50.8X4 | T50.8X5 | T50.8X6 |
| **Selsun** | T49.4X1 | T49.4X2 | T49.4X3 | T49.4X4 | T49.4X5 | T49.4X6 |
| **Semustine** | T45.1X1 | T45.1X2 | T45.1X3 | T45.1X4 | T45.1X5 | T45.1X6 |
| **Senega syrup** | T48.4X1 | T48.4X2 | T48.4X3 | T48.4X4 | T48.4X5 | T48.4X6 |
| **Senna** | T47.2X1 | T47.2X2 | T47.2X3 | T47.2X4 | T47.2X5 | T47.2X6 |
| **Sennoside A+B** | T47.2X1 | T47.2X2 | T47.2X3 | T47.2X4 | T47.2X5 | T47.2X6 |
| **Septisol** | T49.2X1 | T49.2X2 | T49.2X3 | T49.2X4 | T49.2X5 | T49.2X6 |
| **Seractide** | T38.811 | T38.812 | T38.813 | T38.814 | T38.815 | T38.816 |
| **Serax** | T42.4X1 | T42.4X2 | T42.4X3 | T42.4X4 | T42.4X5 | T42.4X6 |
| **Serenesil** | T42.6X1 | T42.6X2 | T42.6X3 | T42.6X4 | T42.6X5 | T42.6X6 |
| **Serenium** (hydrochloride) | T37.91 | T37.92 | T37.93 | T37.94 | T37.95 | T37.96 |
| **Serepax** — *see* Oxazepam | | | | | | |
| **Serevent*** | T48.6X1 | T48.6X2 | T48.6X3 | T48.6X4 | T48.6X5 | T48.6X6 |
| **Sermorelin** | T38.891 | T38.892 | T38.893 | T38.894 | T38.895 | T38.896 |
| **Sernyl** | T41.1X1 | T41.1X2 | T41.1X3 | T41.1X4 | T41.1X5 | T41.1X6 |
| **Serotonin** | T50.991 | T50.992 | T50.993 | T50.994 | T50.995 | T50.996 |
| **Serpasil** | T46.5X1 | T46.5X2 | T46.5X3 | T46.5X4 | T46.5X5 | T46.5X6 |
| **Serrapeptase** | T45.3X1 | T45.3X2 | T45.3X3 | T45.3X4 | T45.3X5 | T45.3X6 |
| **Sertraline*** | T43.221 | T43.222 | T43.223 | T43.224 | T43.225 | T43.226 |
| **Serum** | | | | | | |
| anti-Rh | T50.Z11 | T50.Z12 | T50.Z13 | T50.Z14 | T50.Z15 | T50.Z16 |
| anti-snake-bite | T50.Z11 | T50.Z12 | T50.Z13 | T50.Z14 | T50.Z15 | T50.Z16 |
| antibotulinus | T50.Z11 | T50.Z12 | T50.Z13 | T50.Z14 | T50.Z15 | T50.Z16 |
| anticytotoxic | T50.Z11 | T50.Z12 | T50.Z13 | T50.Z14 | T50.Z15 | T50.Z16 |
| antidiphtheria | T50.Z11 | T50.Z12 | T50.Z13 | T50.Z14 | T50.Z15 | T50.Z16 |
| antimeningococcus | T50.Z11 | T50.Z12 | T50.Z13 | T50.Z14 | T50.Z15 | T50.Z16 |
| antitetanic | T50.Z11 | T50.Z12 | T50.Z13 | T50.Z14 | T50.Z15 | T50.Z16 |
| antitoxic | T50.Z11 | T50.Z12 | T50.Z13 | T50.Z14 | T50.Z15 | T50.Z16 |
| complement (inhibitor) | T45.8X1 | T45.8X2 | T45.8X3 | T45.8X4 | T45.8X5 | T45.8X6 |
| convalescent | T50.Z11 | T50.Z12 | T50.Z13 | T50.Z14 | T50.Z15 | T50.Z16 |
| hemolytic complement | T45.8X1 | T45.8X2 | T45.8X3 | T45.8X4 | T45.8X5 | T45.8X6 |
| immune (human) | T50.Z11 | T50.Z12 | T50.Z13 | T50.Z14 | T50.Z15 | T50.Z16 |
| protective NEC | T50.Z11 | T50.Z12 | T50.Z13 | T50.Z14 | T50.Z15 | T50.Z16 |
| **Setastine** | T45.0X1 | T45.0X2 | T45.0X3 | T45.0X4 | T45.0X5 | T45.0X6 |
| **Setoperone** | T43.591 | T43.592 | T43.593 | T43.594 | T43.595 | T43.596 |
| **Sewer gas** | T59.91 | T59.92 | T59.93 | T59.94 | — | — |
| **Shampoo** | T55.0X1 | T55.0X2 | T55.0X3 | T55.0X4 | — | — |
| **Shellfish, noxious, nonbacterial** | T61.781 | T61.782 | T61.783 | T61.784 | — | — |
| **Sildenafil** | T46.7X1 | T46.7X2 | T46.7X3 | T46.7X4 | T46.7X5 | T46.7X6 |
| **Silibinin** | T50.991 | T50.992 | T50.993 | T50.994 | T50.995 | T50.996 |
| **Silicone NEC** | T65.891 | T65.892 | T65.893 | T65.894 | — | — |
| medicinal | T49.3X1 | T49.3X2 | T49.3X3 | T49.3X4 | T49.3X5 | T49.3X6 |
| **Silvadene** | T49.0X1 | T49.0X2 | T49.0X3 | T49.0X4 | T49.0X5 | T49.0X6 |
| **Silver** | T49.0X1 | T49.0X2 | T49.0X3 | T49.0X4 | T49.0X5 | T49.0X6 |
| anti-infectives | T49.0X1 | T49.0X2 | T49.0X3 | T49.0X4 | T49.0X5 | T49.0X6 |
| arsphenamine | T37.8X1 | T37.8X2 | T37.8X3 | T37.8X4 | T37.8X5 | T37.8X6 |
| colloidal | T49.0X1 | T49.0X2 | T49.0X3 | T49.0X4 | T49.0X5 | T49.0X6 |
| nitrate | T49.0X1 | T49.0X2 | T49.0X3 | T49.0X4 | T49.0X5 | T49.0X6 |
| ophthalmic preparation | T49.5X1 | T49.5X2 | T49.5X3 | T49.5X4 | T49.5X5 | T49.5X6 |
| toughened (keratolytic) | T49.4X1 | T49.4X2 | T49.4X3 | T49.4X4 | T49.4X5 | T49.4X6 |

| Substance | Poisoning, Accidental (unintentional) | Poisoning, Intentional Self-harm | Poisoning, Assault | Poisoning, Undetermined | Adverse Effect | Under-dosing |
|---|---|---|---|---|---|---|
| **Silver** — *continued* | | | | | | |
| nonmedicinal (dust) | T56.891 | T56.892 | T56.893 | T56.894 | — | — |
| protein | T49.5X1 | T49.5X2 | T49.5X3 | T49.5X4 | T49.5X5 | T49.5X6 |
| salvarsan | T37.8X1 | T37.8X2 | T37.8X3 | T37.8X4 | T37.8X5 | T37.8X6 |
| sulfadiazine | T49.4X1 | T49.4X2 | T49.4X3 | T49.4X4 | T49.4X5 | T49.4X6 |
| **Silymarin** | T50.991 | T50.992 | T50.993 | T50.994 | T50.995 | T50.996 |
| **Simaldrate** | T47.1X1 | T47.1X2 | T47.1X3 | T47.1X4 | T47.1X5 | T47.1X6 |
| **Simazine** | T60.3X1 | T60.3X2 | T60.3X3 | T60.3X4 | — | — |
| **Simethicone** | T47.1X1 | T47.1X2 | T47.1X3 | T47.1X4 | T47.1X5 | T47.1X6 |
| **Simfibrate** | T46.6X1 | T46.6X2 | T46.6X3 | T46.6X4 | T46.6X5 | T46.6X6 |
| **Simvastatin** | T46.6X1 | T46.6X2 | T46.6X3 | T46.6X4 | T46.6X5 | T46.6X6 |
| **Sincalide** | T50.8X1 | T50.8X2 | T50.8X3 | T50.8X4 | T50.8X5 | T50.8X6 |
| **Sinequan** | T43.011 | T43.012 | T43.013 | T43.014 | T43.015 | T43.016 |
| **Singoserp** | T46.5X1 | T46.5X2 | T46.5X3 | T46.5X4 | T46.5X5 | T46.5X6 |
| **Singulair*** | T48.6X1 | T48.6X2 | T48.6X3 | T48.6X4 | T48.6X5 | T48.6X6 |
| **Sintrom** | T45.511 | T45.512 | T45.513 | T45.514 | T45.515 | T45.516 |
| **Sisomicin** | T36.5X1 | T36.5X2 | T36.5X3 | T36.5X4 | T36.5X5 | T36.5X6 |
| **Sitosterols** | T46.6X1 | T46.6X2 | T46.6X3 | T46.6X4 | T46.6X5 | T46.6X6 |
| **Skeletal muscle relaxants** | T48.1X1 | T48.1X2 | T48.1X3 | T48.1X4 | T48.1X5 | T48.1X6 |
| **Skin** | | | | | | |
| agents (external) | T49.91 | T49.92 | T49.93 | T49.94 | T49.95 | T49.96 |
| specified NEC | T49.8X1 | T49.8X2 | T49.8X3 | T49.8X4 | T49.8X5 | T49.8X6 |
| test antigen | T50.8X1 | T50.8X2 | T50.8X3 | T50.8X4 | T50.8X5 | T50.8X6 |
| **Sleep-eze** | T45.0X1 | T45.0X2 | T45.0X3 | T45.0X4 | T45.0X5 | T45.0X6 |
| **Sleeping draught, pill** | T42.71 | T42.72 | T42.73 | T42.74 | T42.75 | T42.76 |
| **Smallpox vaccine** | T50.B11 | T50.B12 | T50.B13 | T50.B14 | T50.B15 | T50.B16 |
| **Smelter fumes NEC** | T56.91 | T56.92 | T56.93 | T56.94 | — | — |
| **Smog** | T59.1X1 | T59.1X2 | T59.1X3 | T59.1X4 | — | — |
| **Smoke NEC** | T59.811 | T59.812 | T59.813 | T59.814 | — | — |
| **Smooth muscle relaxant** | T44.3X1 | T44.3X2 | T44.3X3 | T44.3X4 | T44.3X5 | T44.3X6 |
| **Snail killer NEC** | T60.8X1 | T60.8X2 | T60.8X3 | T60.8X4 | — | — |
| **Snake venom or bite** | T63.001 | T63.002 | T63.003 | T63.004 | — | — |
| hemocoagulase | T45.7X1 | T45.7X2 | T45.7X3 | T45.7X4 | T45.7X5 | T45.7X6 |
| **Snuff** | T65.211 | T65.212 | T65.213 | T65.214 | — | — |
| **Soap** (powder) (product) | T55.0X1 | T55.0X2 | T55.0X3 | T55.0X4 | — | — |
| enema | T47.4X1 | T47.4X2 | T47.4X3 | T47.4X4 | T47.4X5 | T47.4X6 |
| medicinal, soft | T49.2X1 | T49.2X2 | T49.2X3 | T49.2X4 | T49.2X5 | T49.2X6 |
| superfatted | T49.2X1 | T49.2X2 | T49.2X3 | T49.2X4 | T49.2X5 | T49.2X6 |
| **Sobrerol** | T48.4X1 | T48.4X2 | T48.4X3 | T48.4X4 | T48.4X5 | T48.4X6 |
| **Soda** (caustic) | T54.3X1 | T54.3X2 | T54.3X3 | T54.3X4 | — | — |
| bicarb | T47.1X1 | T47.1X2 | T47.1X3 | T47.1X4 | T47.1X5 | T47.1X6 |
| chlorinated — *see* Sodium, hypochlorite | | | | | | |
| **Sodium** | | | | | | |
| (L)-triiodothyronine | T38.1X1 | T38.1X2 | T38.1X3 | T38.1X4 | T38.1X5 | T38.1X6 |
| acetosulfone | T37.1X1 | T37.1X2 | T37.1X3 | T37.1X4 | T37.1X5 | T37.1X6 |
| acetrizoate | T50.8X1 | T50.8X2 | T50.8X3 | T50.8X4 | T50.8X5 | T50.8X6 |
| acid phosphate | T50.3X1 | T50.3X2 | T50.3X3 | T50.3X4 | T50.3X5 | T50.3X6 |
| alginate | T47.8X1 | T47.8X2 | T47.8X3 | T47.8X4 | T47.8X5 | T47.8X6 |
| amidotrizoate | T50.8X1 | T50.8X2 | T50.8X3 | T50.8X4 | T50.8X5 | T50.8X6 |
| aminohippurate* | T50.8X1 | T50.8X2 | T50.8X3 | T50.8X4 | T50.8X5 | T50.8X6 |
| aminopterin | T45.1X1 | T45.1X2 | T45.1X3 | T45.1X4 | T45.1X5 | T45.1X6 |
| amylosulfate | T47.8X1 | T47.8X2 | T47.8X3 | T47.8X4 | T47.8X5 | T47.8X6 |
| amytal | T42.3X1 | T42.3X2 | T42.3X3 | T42.3X4 | T42.3X5 | T42.3X6 |
| antimony gluconate | T37.3X1 | T37.3X2 | T37.3X3 | T37.3X4 | T37.3X5 | T37.3X6 |
| arsenate | T57.0X1 | T57.0X2 | T57.0X3 | T57.0X4 | — | — |
| aurothiomalate | T39.4X1 | T39.4X2 | T39.4X3 | T39.4X4 | T39.4X5 | T39.4X6 |
| aurothiosulfate | T39.4X1 | T39.4X2 | T39.4X3 | T39.4X4 | T39.4X5 | T39.4X6 |
| barbiturate | T42.3X1 | T42.3X2 | T42.3X3 | T42.3X4 | T42.3X5 | T42.3X6 |
| basic phosphate | T47.4X1 | T47.4X2 | T47.4X3 | T47.4X4 | T47.4X5 | T47.4X6 |
| bicarbonate | T47.1X1 | T47.1X2 | T47.1X3 | T47.1X4 | T47.1X5 | T47.1X6 |
| bichromate | T57.8X1 | T57.8X2 | T57.8X3 | T57.8X4 | — | — |
| biphosphate | T50.3X1 | T50.3X2 | T50.3X3 | T50.3X4 | T50.3X5 | T50.3X6 |
| bisulfate | T65.891 | T65.892 | T65.893 | T65.894 | — | — |
| borate | | | | | | |
| cleanser | T57.8X1 | T57.8X2 | T57.8X3 | T57.8X4 | — | — |
| eye | T49.5X1 | T49.5X2 | T49.5X3 | T49.5X4 | T49.5X5 | T49.5X6 |
| therapeutic | T49.8X1 | T49.8X2 | T49.8X3 | T49.8X4 | T49.8X5 | T49.8X6 |
| bromide | T42.6X1 | T42.6X2 | T42.6X3 | T42.6X4 | T42.6X5 | T42.6X6 |
| cacodylate (nonmedicinal) NEC | T50.8X1 | T50.8X2 | T50.8X3 | T50.8X4 | T50.8X5 | T50.8X6 |
| anti-infective | T37.8X1 | T37.8X2 | T37.8X3 | T37.8X4 | T37.8X5 | T37.8X6 |
| herbicide | T60.3X1 | T60.3X2 | T60.3X3 | T60.3X4 | — | — |
| calcium edetate | T45.8X1 | T45.8X2 | T45.8X3 | T45.8X4 | T45.8X5 | T45.8X6 |
| carbonate NEC | T54.3X1 | T54.3X2 | T54.3X3 | T54.3X4 | — | — |
| chlorate NEC | T65.891 | T65.892 | T65.893 | T65.894 | — | — |
| herbicide | T54.91 | T54.92 | T54.93 | T54.94 | — | — |
| chloride | T50.3X1 | T50.3X2 | T50.3X3 | T50.3X4 | T50.3X5 | T50.3X6 |
| with glucose | T50.3X1 | T50.3X2 | T50.3X3 | T50.3X4 | T50.3X5 | T50.3X6 |
| chromate | T65.891 | T65.892 | T65.893 | T65.894 | — | — |
| citrate | T50.991 | T50.992 | T50.993 | T50.994 | T50.995 | T50.996 |
| cromoglicate | T48.6X1 | T48.6X2 | T48.6X3 | T48.6X4 | T48.6X5 | T48.6X6 |
| cyanide | T65.0X1 | T65.0X2 | T65.0X3 | T65.0X4 | — | — |

| Substance | Poisoning, Accidental (unintentional) | Poisoning, Intentional Self-harm | Poisoning, Assault | Poisoning, Undetermined | Adverse Effect | Under-dosing |
|---|---|---|---|---|---|---|
| **Sodium** — *continued* | | | | | | |
| cyclamate | T5Ø.3X1 | T5Ø.3X2 | T5Ø.3X3 | T5Ø.3X4 | T5Ø.3X5 | T5Ø.3X6 |
| dehydrocholate | T45.8X1 | T45.8X2 | T45.8X3 | T45.8X4 | T45.8X5 | T45.8X6 |
| diatrizoate | T5Ø.8X1 | T5Ø.8X2 | T5Ø.8X3 | T5Ø.8X4 | T5Ø.8X5 | T5Ø.8X6 |
| dibunate | T48.4X1 | T48.4X2 | T48.4X3 | T48.4X4 | T48.4X5 | T48.4X6 |
| dioctyl sulfosuccinate | T47.4X1 | T47.4X2 | T47.4X3 | T47.4X4 | T47.4X5 | T47.4X6 |
| dipantoyl ferrate | T45.8X1 | T45.8X2 | T45.8X3 | T45.8X4 | T45.8X5 | T45.8X6 |
| edetate | T45.8X1 | T45.8X2 | T45.8X3 | T45.8X4 | T45.8X5 | T45.8X6 |
| ethacrynate | T5Ø.1X1 | T5Ø.1X2 | T5Ø.1X3 | T5Ø.1X4 | T5Ø.1X5 | T5Ø.1X6 |
| etidronate* | T5Ø.991 | T5Ø.992 | T5Ø.993 | T5Ø.994 | T5Ø.995 | T5Ø.996 |
| feredetate | T45.8X1 | T45.8X2 | T45.8X3 | T45.8X4 | T45.8X5 | T45.8X6 |
| Fluoride — *see* Fluoride | | | | | | |
| fluoroacetate (dust) (pesticide) | T6Ø.4X1 | T6Ø.4X2 | T6Ø.4X3 | T6Ø.4X4 | — | — |
| free salt | T5Ø.3X1 | T5Ø.3X2 | T5Ø.3X3 | T5Ø.3X4 | T5Ø.3X5 | T5Ø.3X6 |
| fusidate | T36.8X1 | T36.8X2 | T36.8X3 | T36.8X4 | T36.8X5 | T36.8X6 |
| glucaldrate | T47.1X1 | T47.1X2 | T47.1X3 | T47.1X4 | T47.1X5 | T47.1X6 |
| glucosulfone | T37.1X1 | T37.1X2 | T37.1X3 | T37.1X4 | T37.1X5 | T37.1X6 |
| glutamate | T45.8X1 | T45.8X2 | T45.8X3 | T45.8X4 | T45.8X5 | T45.8X6 |
| hydrogen carbonate | T5Ø.3X1 | T5Ø.3X2 | T5Ø.3X3 | T5Ø.3X4 | T5Ø.3X5 | T5Ø.3X6 |
| hydroxide | T54.3X1 | T54.3X2 | T54.3X3 | T54.3X4 | — | — |
| hypochlorite (bleach) NEC | T54.3X1 | T54.3X2 | T54.3X3 | T54.3X4 | — | — |
| disinfectant | T54.3X1 | T54.3X2 | T54.3X3 | T54.3X4 | — | — |
| medicinal (anti-infective) (external) | T49.ØX1 | T49.ØX2 | T49.ØX3 | T49.ØX4 | T49.ØX5 | T49.ØX6 |
| vapor | T54.3X1 | T54.3X2 | T54.3X3 | T54.3X4 | — | — |
| hyposulfite | T49.ØX1 | T49.ØX2 | T49.ØX3 | T49.ØX4 | T49.ØX5 | T49.ØX6 |
| indigotin disulfonate | T5Ø.8X1 | T5Ø.8X2 | T5Ø.8X3 | T5Ø.8X4 | T5Ø.8X5 | T5Ø.8X6 |
| iodide | T5Ø.991 | T5Ø.992 | T5Ø.993 | T5Ø.994 | T5Ø.995 | T5Ø.996 |
| I-131 | T5Ø.8X1 | T5Ø.8X2 | T5Ø.8X3 | T5Ø.8X4 | T5Ø.8X5 | T5Ø.8X6 |
| therapeutic | T38.2X1 | T38.2X2 | T38.2X3 | T38.2X4 | T38.2X5 | T38.2X6 |
| iodohippurate (131I) | T5Ø.8X1 | T5Ø.8X2 | T5Ø.8X3 | T5Ø.8X4 | T5Ø.8X5 | T5Ø.8X6 |
| iopodate | T5Ø.8X1 | T5Ø.8X2 | T5Ø.8X3 | T5Ø.8X4 | T5Ø.8X5 | T5Ø.8X6 |
| iothalamate | T5Ø.8X1 | T5Ø.8X2 | T5Ø.8X3 | T5Ø.8X4 | T5Ø.8X5 | T5Ø.8X6 |
| iron edetate | T45.4X1 | T45.4X2 | T45.4X3 | T45.4X4 | T45.4X5 | T45.4X6 |
| L-triiodothyronine | T38.1X1 | T38.1X2 | T38.1X3 | T38.1X4 | T38.1X5 | T38.1X6 |
| lactate (compound solution) | T45.8X1 | T45.8X2 | T45.8X3 | T45.8X4 | T45.8X5 | T45.8X6 |
| lauryl (sulfate) | T49.2X1 | T49.2X2 | T49.2X3 | T49.2X4 | T49.2X5 | T49.2X6 |
| magnesium citrate | T5Ø.991 | T5Ø.992 | T5Ø.993 | T5Ø.994 | T5Ø.995 | T5Ø.996 |
| mersalate | T5Ø.2X1 | T5Ø.2X2 | T5Ø.2X3 | T5Ø.2X4 | T5Ø.2X5 | T5Ø.2X6 |
| metasilicate | T65.891 | T65.892 | T65.893 | T65.894 | — | — |
| metrizoate | T5Ø.8X1 | T5Ø.8X2 | T5Ø.8X3 | T5Ø.8X4 | T5Ø.8X5 | T5Ø.8X6 |
| monofluoroacetate (pesticide) | T6Ø.1X1 | T6Ø.1X2 | T6Ø.1X3 | T6Ø.1X4 | — | — |
| morrhuate | T46.8X1 | T46.8X2 | T46.8X3 | T46.8X4 | T46.8X5 | T46.8X6 |
| nafcillin | T36.ØX1 | T36.ØX2 | T36.ØX3 | T36.ØX4 | T36.ØX5 | T36.ØX6 |
| nitrate (oxidizing agent) | T65.891 | T65.892 | T65.893 | T65.894 | — | — |
| nitrite | T5Ø.6X1 | T5Ø.6X2 | T5Ø.6X3 | T5Ø.6X4 | T5Ø.6X5 | T5Ø.6X6 |
| nitroferricyanide | T46.5X1 | T46.5X2 | T46.5X3 | T46.5X4 | T46.5X5 | T46.5X6 |
| nitroprusside | T46.5X1 | T46.5X2 | T46.5X3 | T46.5X4 | T46.5X5 | T46.5X6 |
| oxalate | T65.891 | T65.892 | T65.893 | T65.894 | — | — |
| oxide/peroxide | T65.891 | T65.892 | T65.893 | T65.894 | — | — |
| oxybate | T41.291 | T41.292 | T41.293 | T41.294 | T41.295 | T41.296 |
| para-aminohippurate | T5Ø.8X1 | T5Ø.8X2 | T5Ø.8X3 | T5Ø.8X4 | T5Ø.8X5 | T5Ø.8X6 |
| perborate (nonmedicinal) NEC | T65.891 | T65.892 | T65.893 | T65.894 | — | — |
| medicinal | T49.ØX1 | T49.ØX2 | T49.ØX3 | T49.ØX4 | T49.ØX5 | T49.ØX6 |
| soap | T55.ØX1 | T55.ØX2 | T55.ØX3 | T55.ØX4 | — | — |
| percarbonate — *see* Sodium, perborate | | | | | | |
| pertechnetate Tc99m | T5Ø.8X1 | T5Ø.8X2 | T5Ø.8X3 | T5Ø.8X4 | T5Ø.8X5 | T5Ø.8X6 |
| phosphate | | | | | | |
| cellulose | T45.8X1 | T45.8X2 | T45.8X3 | T45.8X4 | T45.8X5 | T45.8X6 |
| dibasic | T47.2X1 | T47.2X2 | T47.2X3 | T47.2X4 | T47.2X5 | T47.2X6 |
| monobasic | T47.2X1 | T47.2X2 | T47.2X3 | T47.2X4 | T47.2X5 | T47.2X6 |
| phytate | T5Ø.6X1 | T5Ø.6X2 | T5Ø.6X3 | T5Ø.6X4 | T5Ø.6X5 | T5Ø.6X6 |
| picosulfate | T47.2X1 | T47.2X2 | T47.2X3 | T47.2X4 | T47.2X5 | T47.2X6 |
| polyhydroxyaluminium monocarbonate | T47.1X1 | T47.1X2 | T47.1X3 | T47.1X4 | T47.1X5 | T47.1X6 |
| polystyrene sulfonate | T5Ø.3X1 | T5Ø.3X2 | T5Ø.3X3 | T5Ø.3X4 | T5Ø.3X5 | T5Ø.3X6 |
| propionate | T49.ØX1 | T49.ØX2 | T49.ØX3 | T49.ØX4 | T49.ØX5 | T49.ØX6 |
| propyl hydroxybenzoate | T5Ø.991 | T5Ø.992 | T5Ø.993 | T5Ø.994 | T5Ø.995 | T5Ø.996 |
| psylliate | T46.8X1 | T46.8X2 | T46.8X3 | T46.8X4 | T46.8X5 | T46.8X6 |
| removing resins | T5Ø.3X1 | T5Ø.3X2 | T5Ø.3X3 | T5Ø.3X4 | T5Ø.3X5 | T5Ø.3X6 |
| salicylate | T39.Ø91 | T39.Ø92 | T39.Ø93 | T39.Ø94 | T39.Ø95 | T39.Ø96 |
| salt NEC | T5Ø.3X1 | T5Ø.3X2 | T5Ø.3X3 | T5Ø.3X4 | T5Ø.3X5 | T5Ø.3X6 |
| selenate | T6Ø.2X1 | T6Ø.2X2 | T6Ø.2X3 | T6Ø.2X4 | — | — |
| stibogluconate | T37.3X1 | T37.3X2 | T37.3X3 | T37.3X4 | T37.3X5 | T37.3X6 |
| sulfate | T47.4X1 | T47.4X2 | T47.4X3 | T47.4X4 | T47.4X5 | T47.4X6 |
| sulfoxone | T37.1X1 | T37.1X2 | T37.1X3 | T37.1X4 | T37.1X5 | T37.1X6 |
| tetradecyl sulfate | T46.8X1 | T46.8X2 | T46.8X3 | T46.8X4 | T46.8X5 | T46.8X6 |
| thiopental | T41.1X1 | T41.1X2 | T41.1X3 | T41.1X4 | T41.1X5 | T41.1X6 |

| Substance | Poisoning, Accidental (unintentional) | Poisoning, Intentional Self-harm | Poisoning, Assault | Poisoning, Undetermined | Adverse Effect | Under-dosing |
|---|---|---|---|---|---|---|
| **Sodium** — *continued* | | | | | | |
| thiosalicylate | T39.Ø91 | T39.Ø92 | T39.Ø93 | T39.Ø94 | T39.Ø95 | T39.Ø9 |
| thiosulfate | T5Ø.6X1 | T5Ø.6X2 | T5Ø.6X3 | T5Ø.6X4 | T5Ø.6X5 | T5Ø.6X |
| tolbutamide | T38.3X1 | T38.3X2 | T38.3X3 | T38.3X4 | T38.3X5 | T38.3X |
| tyropanoate | T5Ø.8X1 | T5Ø.8X2 | T5Ø.8X3 | T5Ø.8X4 | T5Ø.8X5 | T5Ø.8X |
| valproate | T42.6X1 | T42.6X2 | T42.6X3 | T42.6X4 | T42.6X5 | T42.6X |
| versenate | T5Ø.6X1 | T5Ø.6X2 | T5Ø.6X3 | T5Ø.6X4 | T5Ø.6X5 | T5Ø.6X |
| **Sodium-free salt** | T5Ø.9Ø1 | T5Ø.9Ø2 | T5Ø.9Ø3 | T5Ø.9Ø4 | T5Ø.9Ø5 | T5Ø.9Ø |
| **Sodium-removing resin** | T5Ø.3X1 | T5Ø.3X2 | T5Ø.3X3 | T5Ø.3X4 | T5Ø.3X5 | T5Ø.3X |
| **Soft soap** | T55.ØX1 | T55.ØX2 | T55.ØX3 | T55.ØX4 | — | — |
| **Solanine** | T62.2X1 | T62.2X2 | T62.2X3 | T62.2X4 | — | — |
| berries | T62.1X1 | T62.1X2 | T62.1X3 | T62.1X4 | — | — |
| **Solanum dulcamara** | T62.2X1 | T62.2X2 | T62.2X3 | T62.2X4 | — | — |
| berries | T62.1X1 | T62.1X2 | T62.1X3 | T62.1X4 | — | — |
| **Solapsone** | T37.1X1 | T37.1X2 | T37.1X3 | T37.1X4 | T37.1X5 | T37.1X |
| **Solaquin*** | T49.8X1 | T49.8X2 | T49.8X3 | T49.8X4 | T49.8X5 | T49.8X |
| **Solar lotion** | T49.3X1 | T49.3X2 | T49.3X3 | T49.3X4 | T49.3X5 | T49.3X |
| **Solasulfone** | T37.1X1 | T37.1X2 | T37.1X3 | T37.1X4 | T37.1X5 | T37.1X |
| **Soldering fluid** | T65.891 | T65.892 | T65.893 | T65.894 | — | — |
| **Solid substance** | T65.91 | T65.92 | T65.93 | T65.94 | — | — |
| specified NEC | T65.891 | T65.892 | T65.893 | T65.894 | — | — |
| **Solvent, industrial NEC** | T52.91 | T52.92 | T52.93 | T52.94 | — | — |
| naphtha | T52.ØX1 | T52.ØX2 | T52.ØX3 | T52.ØX4 | — | — |
| petroleum | T52.ØX1 | T52.ØX2 | T52.ØX3 | T52.ØX4 | — | — |
| specified NEC | T52.891 | T52.892 | T52.893 | T52.894 | — | — |
| **Soma** | T42.8X1 | T42.8X2 | T42.8X3 | T42.8X4 | T42.8X5 | T42.8X |
| **Somatorelin** | T38.891 | T38.892 | T38.893 | T38.894 | T38.895 | T38.89 |
| **Somatostatin** | T38.991 | T38.992 | T38.993 | T38.994 | T38.995 | T38.99 |
| **Somatotropin** | T38.811 | T38.812 | T38.813 | T38.814 | T38.815 | T38.81 |
| **Somatrem** | T38.811 | T38.812 | T38.813 | T38.814 | T38.815 | T38.81 |
| **Somatropin** | T38.811 | T38.812 | T38.813 | T38.814 | T38.815 | T38.81 |
| **Sominex** | T45.ØX1 | T45.ØX2 | T45.ØX3 | T45.ØX4 | T45.ØX5 | T45.ØX |
| **Somnos** | T42.6X1 | T42.6X2 | T42.6X3 | T42.6X4 | T42.6X5 | T42.6X |
| **Somonal** | T42.3X1 | T42.3X2 | T42.3X3 | T42.3X4 | T42.3X5 | T42.3X |
| **Soneryl** | T42.3X1 | T42.3X2 | T42.3X3 | T42.3X4 | T42.3X5 | T42.3X |
| **Soothing syrup** | T5Ø.9Ø1 | T5Ø.9Ø2 | T5Ø.9Ø3 | T5Ø.9Ø4 | T5Ø.9Ø5 | T5Ø.9Ø |
| **Sopor** | T42.6X1 | T42.6X2 | T42.6X3 | T42.6X4 | T42.6X5 | T42.6X |
| **Soporific** | T42.71 | T42.72 | T42.73 | T42.74 | T42.75 | T42.7 |
| **Soporific drug** | T42.71 | T42.72 | T42.73 | T42.74 | T42.75 | T42.7 |
| specified type NEC | T42.6X1 | T42.6X2 | T42.6X3 | T42.6X4 | T42.6X5 | T42.6X |
| **Sorbide nitrate** | T46.3X1 | T46.3X2 | T46.3X3 | T46.3X4 | T46.3X5 | T46.3X |
| **Sorbitol** | T47.4X1 | T47.4X2 | T47.4X3 | T47.4X4 | T47.4X5 | T47.4X |
| **Sotalol** | T44.7X1 | T44.7X2 | T44.7X3 | T44.7X4 | T44.7X5 | T44.7X |
| **Sotradecol** | T46.8X1 | T46.8X2 | T46.8X3 | T46.8X4 | T46.8X5 | T46.8X |
| **Soysterol** | T46.6X1 | T46.6X2 | T46.6X3 | T46.6X4 | T46.6X5 | T46.6X |
| **Spacoline** | T44.3X1 | T44.3X2 | T44.3X3 | T44.3X4 | T44.3X5 | T44.3X |
| **Spanish fly** | T49.8X1 | T49.8X2 | T49.8X3 | T49.8X4 | T49.8X5 | T49.8X |
| **Sparine** | T43.3X1 | T43.3X2 | T43.3X3 | T43.3X4 | T43.3X5 | T43.3X |
| **Sparteine** | T48.ØX1 | T48.ØX2 | T48.ØX3 | T48.ØX4 | T48.ØX5 | T48.ØX |
| **Spasmolytic** | | | | | | |
| anticholinergics | T44.3X1 | T44.3X2 | T44.3X3 | T44.3X4 | T44.3X5 | T44.3X |
| autonomic | T44.3X1 | T44.3X2 | T44.3X3 | T44.3X4 | T44.3X5 | T44.3X |
| bronchial NEC | T48.6X1 | T48.6X2 | T48.6X3 | T48.6X4 | T48.6X5 | T48.6X |
| quaternary ammonium | T44.3X1 | T44.3X2 | T44.3X3 | T44.3X4 | T44.3X5 | T44.3X |
| skeletal muscle NEC | T48.1X1 | T48.1X2 | T48.1X3 | T48.1X4 | T48.1X5 | T48.1X |
| **Spectinomycin** | T36.5X1 | T36.5X2 | T36.5X3 | T36.5X4 | T36.5X5 | T36.5X |
| **Spectracef*** | T36.1X1 | T36.1X2 | T36.1X3 | T36.1X4 | T36.1X5 | T36.1X |
| **Speed** | T43.651 | T43.652 | T43.653 | T43.654 | T43.655 | T43.65 |
| **Spermicide** | T49.8X1 | T49.8X2 | T49.8X3 | T49.8X4 | T49.8X5 | T49.8X |
| **Spider** (bite) (venom) | T63.391 | T63.392 | T63.393 | T63.394 | — | — |
| antivenin | T5Ø.Z11 | T5Ø.Z12 | T5Ø.Z13 | T5Ø.Z14 | T5Ø.Z15 | T5Ø.Z1 |
| **Spigelia** (root) | T37.4X1 | T37.4X2 | T37.4X3 | T37.4X4 | T37.4X5 | T37.4X |
| **Spindle inactivator** | T5Ø.4X1 | T5Ø.4X2 | T5Ø.4X3 | T5Ø.4X4 | T5Ø.4X5 | T5Ø.4X |
| **Spiperone** | T43.4X1 | T43.4X2 | T43.4X3 | T43.4X4 | T43.4X5 | T43.4X |
| **Spiramycin** | T36.3X1 | T36.3X2 | T36.3X3 | T36.3X4 | T36.3X5 | T36.3X |
| **Spirapril** | T46.4X1 | T46.4X2 | T46.4X3 | T46.4X4 | T46.4X5 | T46.4X |
| **Spirilene** | T43.591 | T43.592 | T43.593 | T43.594 | T43.595 | T43.59 |
| **Spirit**(s) (neutral) **NEC** | T51.ØX1 | T51.ØX2 | T51.ØX3 | T51.ØX4 | — | — |
| beverage | T51.ØX1 | T51.ØX2 | T51.ØX3 | T51.ØX4 | — | — |
| industrial | T51.ØX1 | T51.ØX2 | T51.ØX3 | T51.ØX4 | — | — |
| mineral | T52.ØX1 | T52.ØX2 | T52.ØX3 | T52.ØX4 | — | — |
| of salt — *see* Hydrochloric acid | | | | | | |
| surgical | T51.ØX1 | T51.ØX2 | T51.ØX3 | T51.ØX4 | — | — |
| **Spiriva*** | T44.3X1 | T44.3X2 | T44.3X3 | T44.3X4 | T44.3X5 | T44.3X |
| **Spironolactone** | T5Ø.ØX1 | T5Ø.ØX2 | T5Ø.ØX3 | T5Ø.ØX4 | T5Ø.ØX5 | T5Ø.ØX |
| **Spiroperidol** | T43.4X1 | T43.4X2 | T43.4X3 | T43.4X4 | T43.4X5 | T43.4X |
| **Sponge, absorbable** (gelatin) | T45.7X1 | T45.7X2 | T45.7X3 | T45.7X4 | T45.7X5 | T45.7X |
| **Sporostacin** | T49.ØX1 | T49.ØX2 | T49.ØX3 | T49.ØX4 | T49.ØX5 | T49.ØX |
| **Spray** (aerosol) | T65.91 | T65.92 | T65.93 | T65.94 | — | — |
| cosmetic | T65.891 | T65.892 | T65.893 | T65.894 | — | — |
| medicinal NEC | T5Ø.9Ø1 | T5Ø.9Ø2 | T5Ø.9Ø3 | T5Ø.9Ø4 | T5Ø.9Ø5 | T5Ø.9Ø |
| pesticides — *see* Pesticide | | | | | | |

| Substance | Poisoning, Accidental (unintentional) | Poisoning, Intentional Self-harm | Poisoning, Assault | Poisoning, Undetermined | Adverse Effect | Under-dosing |
|---|---|---|---|---|---|---|
| **Spray** — *continued* | | | | | | |
| specified content — *see* specific substance | | | | | | |
| **Spurge flax** | T62.2X1 | T62.2X2 | T62.2X3 | T62.2X4 | — | — |
| **Spurges** | T62.2X1 | T62.2X2 | T62.2X3 | T62.2X4 | — | — |
| **Sputum viscosity-lowering drug** | T48.4X1 | T48.4X2 | T48.4X3 | T48.4X4 | T48.4X5 | T48.4X6 |
| **Squill** | T46.ØX1 | T46.ØX2 | T46.ØX3 | T46.ØX4 | T46.ØX5 | T46.ØX6 |
| rat poison | T6Ø.4X1 | T6Ø.4X2 | T6Ø.4X3 | T6Ø.4X4 | — | — |
| **Squirting cucumber** (cathartic) | T47.2X1 | T47.2X2 | T47.2X3 | T47.2X4 | T47.2X5 | T47.2X6 |
| **Stains** | T65.6X1 | T65.6X2 | T65.6X3 | T65.6X4 | — | — |
| **Stannous fluoride** | T49.7X1 | T49.7X2 | T49.7X3 | T49.7X4 | T49.7X5 | T49.7X6 |
| **Stanolone** | T38.7X1 | T38.7X2 | T38.7X3 | T38.7X4 | T38.7X5 | T38.7X6 |
| **Stanozolol** | T38.7X1 | T38.7X2 | T38.7X3 | T38.7X4 | T38.7X5 | T38.7X6 |
| **Staphisagria or stavesacre** (pediculicide) | T49.ØX1 | T49.ØX2 | T49.ØX3 | T49.ØX4 | T49.ØX5 | T49.ØX6 |
| **Starch** | T5Ø.9Ø1 | T5Ø.9Ø2 | T5Ø.9Ø3 | T5Ø.9Ø4 | T5Ø.9Ø5 | T5Ø.9Ø6 |
| **Stavzor*** | T42.6X1 | T42.6X2 | T42.6X3 | T42.6X4 | T42.6X5 | T42.6X6 |
| **Stelazine** | T43.3X1 | T43.3X2 | T43.3X3 | T43.3X4 | T43.3X5 | T43.3X6 |
| **Stemetil** | T43.3X1 | T43.3X2 | T43.3X3 | T43.3X4 | T43.3X5 | T43.3X6 |
| **Stepronin** | T48.4X1 | T48.4X2 | T48.4X3 | T48.4X4 | T48.4X5 | T48.4X6 |
| **Sterculia** | T47.4X1 | T47.4X2 | T47.4X3 | T47.4X4 | T47.4X5 | T47.4X6 |
| **Sternutator gas** | T59.891 | T59.892 | T59.893 | T59.894 | — | — |
| **Steroid** | T38.ØX1 | T38.ØX2 | T38.ØX3 | T38.ØX4 | T38.ØX5 | T38.ØX6 |
| anabolic | T38.7X1 | T38.7X2 | T38.7X3 | T38.7X4 | T38.7X5 | T38.7X6 |
| androgenic | T38.7X1 | T38.7X2 | T38.7X3 | T38.7X4 | T38.7X5 | T38.7X6 |
| antineoplastic, hormone | T38.7X1 | T38.7X2 | T38.7X3 | T38.7X4 | T38.7X5 | T38.7X6 |
| estrogen | T38.5X1 | T38.5X2 | T38.5X3 | T38.5X4 | T38.5X5 | T38.5X6 |
| ENT agent | T49.6X1 | T49.6X2 | T49.6X3 | T49.6X4 | T49.6X5 | T49.6X6 |
| ophthalmic preparation | T49.5X1 | T49.5X2 | T49.5X3 | T49.5X4 | T49.5X5 | T49.5X6 |
| topical NEC | T49.ØX1 | T49.ØX2 | T49.ØX3 | T49.ØX4 | T49.ØX5 | T49.ØX6 |
| **Stibine** | T56.891 | T56.892 | T56.893 | T56.894 | — | — |
| **Stibogluconate** | T37.3X1 | T37.3X2 | T37.3X3 | T37.3X4 | T37.3X5 | T37.3X6 |
| **Stibophen** | T37.4X1 | T37.4X2 | T37.4X3 | T37.4X4 | T37.4X5 | T37.4X6 |
| **Stilbamidine** (isetionate) | T37.3X1 | T37.3X2 | T37.3X3 | T37.3X4 | T37.3X5 | T37.3X6 |
| **Stilbestrol** | T38.5X1 | T38.5X2 | T38.5X3 | T38.5X4 | T38.5X5 | T38.5X6 |
| **Stilboestrol** | T38.5X1 | T38.5X2 | T38.5X3 | T38.5X4 | T38.5X5 | T38.5X6 |
| **Stimulant** | | | | | | |
| central nervous system — *see also* Psychostimulant | T43.6Ø1 | T43.6Ø2 | T43.6Ø3 | T43.6Ø4 | T43.6Ø5 | T43.6Ø6 |
| analeptics | T5Ø.7X1 | T5Ø.7X2 | T5Ø.7X3 | T5Ø.7X4 | T5Ø.7X5 | T5Ø.7X6 |
| opiate antagonist | T5Ø.7X1 | T5Ø.7X2 | T5Ø.7X3 | T5Ø.7X4 | T5Ø.7X5 | T5Ø.7X6 |
| psychotherapeutic NEC — *see also* Psychotherapeutic drug | T43.6Ø1 | T43.6Ø2 | T43.6Ø3 | T43.6Ø4 | T43.6Ø5 | T43.6Ø6 |
| specified NEC | T43.691 | T43.692 | T43.693 | T43.694 | T43.695 | T43.696 |
| respiratory | T48.9Ø1 | T48.9Ø2 | T48.9Ø3 | T48.9Ø4 | T48.9Ø5 | T48.9Ø6 |
| **Stone-dissolving drug** | T5Ø.9Ø1 | T5Ø.9Ø2 | T5Ø.9Ø3 | T5Ø.9Ø4 | T5Ø.9Ø5 | T5Ø.9Ø6 |
| **Storage battery** (cells) (acid) | T54.2X1 | T54.2X2 | T54.2X3 | T54.2X4 | — | — |
| **Stovaine** | T41.3X1 | T41.3X2 | T41.3X3 | T41.3X4 | T41.3X5 | T41.3X6 |
| infiltration (subcutaneous) | T41.3X1 | T41.3X2 | T41.3X3 | T41.3X4 | T41.3X5 | T41.3X6 |
| nerve block (peripheral) (plexus) | T41.3X1 | T41.3X2 | T41.3X3 | T41.3X4 | T41.3X5 | T41.3X6 |
| spinal | T41.3X1 | T41.3X2 | T41.3X3 | T41.3X4 | T41.3X5 | T41.3X6 |
| topical (surface) | T41.3X1 | T41.3X2 | T41.3X3 | T41.3X4 | T41.3X5 | T41.3X6 |
| **Stovarsal** | T37.8X1 | T37.8X2 | T37.8X3 | T37.8X4 | T37.8X5 | T37.8X6 |
| **Stove gas** — *see* Gas, stove | | | | | | |
| **Stoxil** | T49.5X1 | T49.5X2 | T49.5X3 | T49.5X4 | T49.5X5 | T49.5X6 |
| **Stramonium** | T48.6X1 | T48.6X2 | T48.6X3 | T48.6X4 | T48.6X5 | T48.6X6 |
| natural state | T62.2X1 | T62.2X2 | T62.2X3 | T62.2X4 | — | — |
| **Streptodornase** | T45.3X1 | T45.3X2 | T45.3X3 | T45.3X4 | T45.3X5 | T45.3X6 |
| **Streptoduocin** | T36.5X1 | T36.5X2 | T36.5X3 | T36.5X4 | T36.5X5 | T36.5X6 |
| **Streptokinase** | T45.611 | T45.612 | T45.613 | T45.614 | T45.615 | T45.616 |
| **Streptomycin** (derivative) | T36.5X1 | T36.5X2 | T36.5X3 | T36.5X4 | T36.5X5 | T36.5X6 |
| **Streptonivicin** | T36.5X1 | T36.5X2 | T36.5X3 | T36.5X4 | T36.5X5 | T36.5X6 |
| **Streptovarycin** | T36.5X1 | T36.5X2 | T36.5X3 | T36.5X4 | T36.5X5 | T36.5X6 |
| **Streptozocin** | T45.1X1 | T45.1X2 | T45.1X3 | T45.1X4 | T45.1X5 | T45.1X6 |
| **Streptozotocin** | T45.1X1 | T45.1X2 | T45.1X3 | T45.1X4 | T45.1X5 | T45.1X6 |
| **Stripper** (paint) (solvent) | T52.891 | T52.892 | T52.893 | T52.894 | — | — |
| **Strobane** | T6Ø.1X1 | T6Ø.1X2 | T6Ø.1X3 | T6Ø.1X4 | — | — |
| **Strofantina** | T46.ØX1 | T46.ØX2 | T46.ØX3 | T46.ØX4 | T46.ØX5 | T46.ØX6 |
| **Stromectol*** | T37.4X1 | T37.4X2 | T37.4X3 | T37.4X4 | T37.4X5 | T37.4X6 |
| **Strophanthin** (g) (k) | T46.ØX1 | T46.ØX2 | T46.ØX3 | T46.ØX4 | T46.ØX5 | T46.ØX6 |
| **Strophanthus** | T46.ØX1 | T46.ØX2 | T46.ØX3 | T46.ØX4 | T46.ØX5 | T46.ØX6 |
| **Strophantin** | T46.ØX1 | T46.ØX2 | T46.ØX3 | T46.ØX4 | T46.ØX5 | T46.ØX6 |
| **Strophantin-g** | T46.ØX1 | T46.ØX2 | T46.ØX3 | T46.ØX4 | T46.ØX5 | T46.ØX6 |
| **Strychnine** (nonmedicinal) (pesticide) (salts) | T65.1X1 | T65.1X2 | T65.1X3 | T65.1X4 | — | — |
| medicinal | T48.291 | T48.292 | T48.293 | T48.294 | T48.295 | T48.296 |
| **Strychnos** (ignatii) — *see* Strychnine | | | | | | |

| Substance | Poisoning, Accidental (unintentional) | Poisoning, Intentional Self-harm | Poisoning, Assault | Poisoning, Undetermined | Adverse Effect | Under-dosing |
|---|---|---|---|---|---|---|
| **Styramate** | T42.8X1 | T42.8X2 | T42.8X3 | T42.8X4 | T42.8X5 | T42.8X6 |
| **Styrene** | T65.891 | T65.892 | T65.893 | T65.894 | — | — |
| **Succinimide, antiepileptic or anticonvulsant** | T42.2X1 | T42.2X2 | T42.2X3 | T42.2X4 | T42.2X5 | T42.2X6 |
| mercuric — *see* Mercury | | | | | | |
| **Succinylcholine** | T48.1X1 | T48.1X2 | T48.1X3 | T48.1X4 | T48.1X5 | T48.1X6 |
| **Succinylsulfathiazole** | T37.ØX1 | T37.ØX2 | T37.ØX3 | T37.ØX4 | T37.ØX5 | T37.ØX6 |
| **Sucralfate** | T47.1X1 | T47.1X2 | T47.1X3 | T47.1X4 | T47.1X5 | T47.1X6 |
| **Sucrose** | T5Ø.3X1 | T5Ø.3X2 | T5Ø.3X3 | T5Ø.3X4 | T5Ø.3X5 | T5Ø.3X6 |
| **Sufentanil** | T4Ø.411 | T4Ø.412 | T4Ø.413 | T4Ø.414 | T4Ø.415 | T4Ø.416 |
| **Sulbactam** | T36.ØX1 | T36.ØX2 | T36.ØX3 | T36.ØX4 | T36.ØX5 | T36.ØX6 |
| **Sulbenicillin** | T36.ØX1 | T36.ØX2 | T36.ØX3 | T36.ØX4 | T36.ØX5 | T36.ØX6 |
| **Sulbentine** | T49.ØX1 | T49.ØX2 | T49.ØX3 | T49.ØX4 | T49.ØX5 | T49.ØX6 |
| **Sulconazole*** | T49.ØX1 | T49.ØX2 | T49.ØX3 | T49.ØX4 | T49.ØX5 | T49.ØX6 |
| **Sulfacetamide** | T49.ØX1 | T49.ØX2 | T49.ØX3 | T49.ØX4 | T49.ØX5 | T49.ØX6 |
| ophthalmic preparation | T49.5X1 | T49.5X2 | T49.5X3 | T49.5X4 | T49.5X5 | T49.5X6 |
| **Sulfachlorpyridazine** | T37.ØX1 | T37.ØX2 | T37.ØX3 | T37.ØX4 | T37.ØX5 | T37.ØX6 |
| **Sulfacitine** | T37.ØX1 | T37.ØX2 | T37.ØX3 | T37.ØX4 | T37.ØX5 | T37.ØX6 |
| **Sulfadiasulfone sodium** | T37.ØX1 | T37.ØX2 | T37.ØX3 | T37.ØX4 | T37.ØX5 | T37.ØX6 |
| **Sulfadiazine** | T37.ØX1 | T37.ØX2 | T37.ØX3 | T37.ØX4 | T37.ØX5 | T37.ØX6 |
| silver (topical) | T49.ØX1 | T49.ØX2 | T49.ØX3 | T49.ØX4 | T49.ØX5 | T49.ØX6 |
| **Sulfadimethoxine** | T37.ØX1 | T37.ØX2 | T37.ØX3 | T37.ØX4 | T37.ØX5 | T37.ØX6 |
| **Sulfadimidine** | T37.ØX1 | T37.ØX2 | T37.ØX3 | T37.ØX4 | T37.ØX5 | T37.ØX6 |
| **Sulfadoxine** | T37.ØX1 | T37.ØX2 | T37.ØX3 | T37.ØX4 | T37.ØX5 | T37.ØX6 |
| with pyrimethamine | T37.2X1 | T37.2X2 | T37.2X3 | T37.2X4 | T37.2X5 | T37.2X6 |
| **Sulfaethidole** | T37.ØX1 | T37.ØX2 | T37.ØX3 | T37.ØX4 | T37.ØX5 | T37.ØX6 |
| **Sulfafurazole** | T37.ØX1 | T37.ØX2 | T37.ØX3 | T37.ØX4 | T37.ØX5 | T37.ØX6 |
| **Sulfaguanidine** | T37.ØX1 | T37.ØX2 | T37.ØX3 | T37.ØX4 | T37.ØX5 | T37.ØX6 |
| **Sulfalene** | T37.ØX1 | T37.ØX2 | T37.ØX3 | T37.ØX4 | T37.ØX5 | T37.ØX6 |
| **Sulfaloxate** | T37.ØX1 | T37.ØX2 | T37.ØX3 | T37.ØX4 | T37.ØX5 | T37.ØX6 |
| **Sulfaloxic acid** | T37.ØX1 | T37.ØX2 | T37.ØX3 | T37.ØX4 | T37.ØX5 | T37.ØX6 |
| **Sulfamazone** | T39.2X1 | T39.2X2 | T39.2X3 | T39.2X4 | T39.2X5 | T39.2X6 |
| **Sulfamerazine** | T37.ØX1 | T37.ØX2 | T37.ØX3 | T37.ØX4 | T37.ØX5 | T37.ØX6 |
| **Sulfameter** | T37.ØX1 | T37.ØX2 | T37.ØX3 | T37.ØX4 | T37.ØX5 | T37.ØX6 |
| **Sulfamethazine** | T37.ØX1 | T37.ØX2 | T37.ØX3 | T37.ØX4 | T37.ØX5 | T37.ØX6 |
| **Sulfamethizole** | T37.ØX1 | T37.ØX2 | T37.ØX3 | T37.ØX4 | T37.ØX5 | T37.ØX6 |
| **Sulfamethoxazole** | T37.ØX1 | T37.ØX2 | T37.ØX3 | T37.ØX4 | T37.ØX5 | T37.ØX6 |
| with trimethoprim | T36.8X1 | T36.8X2 | T36.8X3 | T36.8X4 | T36.8X5 | T36.8X6 |
| **Sulfamethoxydiazine** | T37.ØX1 | T37.ØX2 | T37.ØX3 | T37.ØX4 | T37.ØX5 | T37.ØX6 |
| **Sulfamethoxypyridazine** | T37.ØX1 | T37.ØX2 | T37.ØX3 | T37.ØX4 | T37.ØX5 | T37.ØX6 |
| **Sulfamethylthiazole** | T37.ØX1 | T37.ØX2 | T37.ØX3 | T37.ØX4 | T37.ØX5 | T37.ØX6 |
| **Sulfametoxydiazine** | T37.ØX1 | T37.ØX2 | T37.ØX3 | T37.ØX4 | T37.ØX5 | T37.ØX6 |
| **Sulfamidopyrine** | T39.2X1 | T39.2X2 | T39.2X3 | T39.2X4 | T39.2X5 | T39.2X6 |
| **Sulfamonomethoxine** | T37.ØX1 | T37.ØX2 | T37.ØX3 | T37.ØX4 | T37.ØX5 | T37.ØX6 |
| **Sulfamoxole** | T37.ØX1 | T37.ØX2 | T37.ØX3 | T37.ØX4 | T37.ØX5 | T37.ØX6 |
| **Sulfamylon** | T49.ØX1 | T49.ØX2 | T49.ØX3 | T49.ØX4 | T49.ØX5 | T49.ØX6 |
| **Sulfan blue** (diagnostic dye) | T5Ø.8X1 | T5Ø.8X2 | T5Ø.8X3 | T5Ø.8X4 | T5Ø.8X5 | T5Ø.8X6 |
| **Sulfanilamide** | T37.ØX1 | T37.ØX2 | T37.ØX3 | T37.ØX4 | T37.ØX5 | T37.ØX6 |
| **Sulfanilylguanidine** | T37.ØX1 | T37.ØX2 | T37.ØX3 | T37.ØX4 | T37.ØX5 | T37.ØX6 |
| **Sulfaperin** | T37.ØX1 | T37.ØX2 | T37.ØX3 | T37.ØX4 | T37.ØX5 | T37.ØX6 |
| **Sulfaphenazole** | T37.ØX1 | T37.ØX2 | T37.ØX3 | T37.ØX4 | T37.ØX5 | T37.ØX6 |
| **Sulfaphenylthiazole** | T37.ØX1 | T37.ØX2 | T37.ØX3 | T37.ØX4 | T37.ØX5 | T37.ØX6 |
| **Sulfaproxyline** | T37.ØX1 | T37.ØX2 | T37.ØX3 | T37.ØX4 | T37.ØX5 | T37.ØX6 |
| **Sulfapyridine** | T37.ØX1 | T37.ØX2 | T37.ØX3 | T37.ØX4 | T37.ØX5 | T37.ØX6 |
| **Sulfapyrimidine** | T37.ØX1 | T37.ØX2 | T37.ØX3 | T37.ØX4 | T37.ØX5 | T37.ØX6 |
| **Sulfarsphenamine** | T37.8X1 | T37.8X2 | T37.8X3 | T37.8X4 | T37.8X5 | T37.8X6 |
| **Sulfasalazine** | T37.ØX1 | T37.ØX2 | T37.ØX3 | T37.ØX4 | T37.ØX5 | T37.ØX6 |
| **Sulfasuxidine** | T37.ØX1 | T37.ØX2 | T37.ØX3 | T37.ØX4 | T37.ØX5 | T37.ØX6 |
| **Sulfasymazine** | T37.ØX1 | T37.ØX2 | T37.ØX3 | T37.ØX4 | T37.ØX5 | T37.ØX6 |
| **Sulfated amylopectin** | T47.8X1 | T47.8X2 | T47.8X3 | T47.8X4 | T47.8X5 | T47.8X6 |
| **Sulfathiazole** | T37.ØX1 | T37.ØX2 | T37.ØX3 | T37.ØX4 | T37.ØX5 | T37.ØX6 |
| **Sulfatostearate** | T49.2X1 | T49.2X2 | T49.2X3 | T49.2X4 | T49.2X5 | T49.2X6 |
| **Sulfatrim*** | T36.8X1 | T36.8X2 | T36.8X3 | T36.8X4 | T36.8X5 | T36.8X6 |
| **Sulfinpyrazone** | T5Ø.4X1 | T5Ø.4X2 | T5Ø.4X3 | T5Ø.4X4 | T5Ø.4X5 | T5Ø.4X6 |
| **Sulfiram** | T49.ØX1 | T49.ØX2 | T49.ØX3 | T49.ØX4 | T49.ØX5 | T49.ØX6 |
| **Sulfisomidine** | T37.ØX1 | T37.ØX2 | T37.ØX3 | T37.ØX4 | T37.ØX5 | T37.ØX6 |
| **Sulfisoxazole** | T37.ØX1 | T37.ØX2 | T37.ØX3 | T37.ØX4 | T37.ØX5 | T37.ØX6 |
| ophthalmic preparation | T49.5X1 | T49.5X2 | T49.5X3 | T49.5X4 | T49.5X5 | T49.5X6 |
| **Sulfobromophthalein** (sodium) | T5Ø.8X1 | T5Ø.8X2 | T5Ø.8X3 | T5Ø.8X4 | T5Ø.8X5 | T5Ø.8X6 |
| **Sulfobromphthalein** | T5Ø.8X1 | T5Ø.8X2 | T5Ø.8X3 | T5Ø.8X4 | T5Ø.8X5 | T5Ø.8X6 |
| **Sulfogaiacol** | T48.4X1 | T48.4X2 | T48.4X3 | T48.4X4 | T48.4X5 | T48.4X6 |
| **Sulfomyxin** | T36.8X1 | T36.8X2 | T36.8X3 | T36.8X4 | T36.8X5 | T36.8X6 |
| **Sulfonal** | T42.6X1 | T42.6X2 | T42.6X3 | T42.6X4 | T42.6X5 | T42.6X6 |
| **Sulfonamide NEC** | T37.ØX1 | T37.ØX2 | T37.ØX3 | T37.ØX4 | T37.ØX5 | T37.ØX6 |
| eye | T49.5X1 | T49.5X2 | T49.5X3 | T49.5X4 | T49.5X5 | T49.5X6 |
| **Sulfonazide** | T37.1X1 | T37.1X2 | T37.1X3 | T37.1X4 | T37.1X5 | T37.1X6 |
| **Sulfones** | T37.1X1 | T37.1X2 | T37.1X3 | T37.1X4 | T37.1X5 | T37.1X6 |
| **Sulfonethylmethane** | T42.6X1 | T42.6X2 | T42.6X3 | T42.6X4 | T42.6X5 | T42.6X6 |
| **Sulfonmethane** | T42.6X1 | T42.6X2 | T42.6X3 | T42.6X4 | T42.6X5 | T42.6X6 |
| **Sulfonphthal, sulfonphthol** | T5Ø.8X1 | T5Ø.8X2 | T5Ø.8X3 | T5Ø.8X4 | T5Ø.8X5 | T5Ø.8X6 |

| Substance | Poisoning, Accidental (unintentional) | Poisoning, Intentional Self-harm | Poisoning, Assault | Poisoning, Undetermined | Adverse Effect | Under-dosing |
|---|---|---|---|---|---|---|
| **Sulfonylurea derivatives, oral** | T38.3X1 | T38.3X2 | T38.3X3 | T38.3X4 | T38.3X5 | T38.3X6 |
| **Sulforidazine** | T43.3X1 | T43.3X2 | T43.3X3 | T43.3X4 | T43.3X5 | T43.3X6 |
| **Sulfoxone** | T37.1X1 | T37.1X2 | T37.1X3 | T37.1X4 | T37.1X5 | T37.1X6 |
| **Sulfur, sulfurated, sulfuric, sulfurous, sulfuryl** (compounds NEC) (medicinal) | T49.4X1 | T49.4X2 | T49.4X3 | T49.4X4 | T49.4X5 | T49.4X6 |
| acid | T54.2X1 | T54.2X2 | T54.2X3 | T54.2X4 | — | — |
| dioxide (gas) | T59.1X1 | T59.1X2 | T59.1X3 | T59.1X4 | — | — |
| ether — *see* Ether(s) | | | | | | |
| hydrogen | T59.6X1 | T59.6X2 | T59.6X3 | T59.6X4 | — | — |
| medicinal (keratolytic) (ointment) NEC | T49.4X1 | T49.4X2 | T49.4X3 | T49.4X4 | T49.4X5 | T49.4X6 |
| ointment | T49.ØX1 | T49.ØX2 | T49.ØX3 | T49.ØX4 | T49.ØX5 | T49.ØX6 |
| pesticide (vapor) | T6Ø.91 | T6Ø.92 | T6Ø.93 | T6Ø.94 | — | — |
| vapor NEC | T59.891 | T59.892 | T59.893 | T59.894 | — | — |
| **Sulfuric acid** | T54.2X1 | T54.2X2 | T54.2X3 | T54.2X4 | — | — |
| **Sulglicotide** | T47.1X1 | T47.1X2 | T47.1X3 | T47.1X4 | T47.1X5 | T47.1X6 |
| **Sulindac** | T39.391 | T39.392 | T39.393 | T39.394 | T39.395 | T39.396 |
| **Sulisatin** | T47.2X1 | T47.2X2 | T47.2X3 | T47.2X4 | T47.2X5 | T47.2X6 |
| **Sulisobenzone** | T49.3X1 | T49.3X2 | T49.3X3 | T49.3X4 | T49.3X5 | T49.3X6 |
| **Sulkowitch's reagent** | T5Ø.8X1 | T5Ø.8X2 | T5Ø.8X3 | T5Ø.8X4 | T5Ø.8X5 | T5Ø.8X6 |
| **Sulmetozine** | T44.3X1 | T44.3X2 | T44.3X3 | T44.3X4 | T44.3X5 | T44.3X6 |
| **Suloctidil** | T46.7X1 | T46.7X2 | T46.7X3 | T46.7X4 | T46.7X5 | T46.7X6 |
| **Sulph-** — *see also* Sulf- | | | | | | |
| **Sulphadiazine** | T37.ØX1 | T37.ØX2 | T37.ØX3 | T37.ØX4 | T37.ØX5 | T37.ØX6 |
| **Sulphadimethoxine** | T37.ØX1 | T37.ØX2 | T37.ØX3 | T37.ØX4 | T37.ØX5 | T37.ØX6 |
| **Sulphadimidine** | T37.ØX1 | T37.ØX2 | T37.ØX3 | T37.ØX4 | T37.ØX5 | T37.ØX6 |
| **Sulphadione** | T37.1X1 | T37.1X2 | T37.1X3 | T37.1X4 | T37.1X5 | T37.1X6 |
| **Sulphafurazole** | T37.ØX1 | T37.ØX2 | T37.ØX3 | T37.ØX4 | T37.ØX5 | T37.ØX6 |
| **Sulphamethizole** | T37.ØX1 | T37.ØX2 | T37.ØX3 | T37.ØX4 | T37.ØX5 | T37.ØX6 |
| **Sulphamethoxazole** | T37.ØX1 | T37.ØX2 | T37.ØX3 | T37.ØX4 | T37.ØX5 | T37.ØX6 |
| **Sulphan blue** | T5Ø.8X1 | T5Ø.8X2 | T5Ø.8X3 | T5Ø.8X4 | T5Ø.8X5 | T5Ø.8X6 |
| **Sulphaphenazole** | T37.ØX1 | T37.ØX2 | T37.ØX3 | T37.ØX4 | T37.ØX5 | T37.ØX6 |
| **Sulphapyridine** | T37.ØX1 | T37.ØX2 | T37.ØX3 | T37.ØX4 | T37.ØX5 | T37.ØX6 |
| **Sulphasalazine** | T37.ØX1 | T37.ØX2 | T37.ØX3 | T37.ØX4 | T37.ØX5 | T37.ØX6 |
| **Sulphinpyrazone** | T5Ø.4X1 | T5Ø.4X2 | T5Ø.4X3 | T5Ø.4X4 | T5Ø.4X5 | T5Ø.4X6 |
| **Sulpiride** | T43.591 | T43.592 | T43.593 | T43.594 | T43.595 | T43.596 |
| **Sulprostone** | T48.ØX1 | T48.ØX2 | T48.ØX3 | T48.ØX4 | T48.ØX5 | T48.ØX6 |
| **Sulpyrine** | T39.2X1 | T39.2X2 | T39.2X3 | T39.2X4 | T39.2X5 | T39.2X6 |
| **Sultamicillin** | T36.ØX1 | T36.ØX2 | T36.ØX3 | T36.ØX4 | T36.ØX5 | T36.ØX6 |
| **Sulthiame** | T42.6X1 | T42.6X2 | T42.6X3 | T42.6X4 | T42.6X5 | T42.6X6 |
| **Sultiame** | T42.6X1 | T42.6X2 | T42.6X3 | T42.6X4 | T42.6X5 | T42.6X6 |
| **Sultopride** | T43.591 | T43.592 | T43.593 | T43.594 | T43.595 | T43.596 |
| **Sumatriptan** | T39.8X1 | T39.8X2 | T39.8X3 | T39.8X4 | T39.8X5 | T39.8X6 |
| **Sumavel*** | T39.8X1 | T39.8X2 | T39.8X3 | T39.8X4 | T39.8X5 | T39.8X6 |
| **Sunflower seed oil** | T46.6X1 | T46.6X2 | T46.6X3 | T46.6X4 | T46.6X5 | T46.6X6 |
| **Superinone** | T48.4X1 | T48.4X2 | T48.4X3 | T48.4X4 | T48.4X5 | T48.4X6 |
| **Suprofen** | T39.311 | T39.312 | T39.313 | T39.314 | T39.315 | T39.316 |
| **Suramin** (sodium) | T37.4X1 | T37.4X2 | T37.4X3 | T37.4X4 | T37.4X5 | T37.4X6 |
| **Surfacaine** | T41.3X1 | T41.3X2 | T41.3X3 | T41.3X4 | T41.3X5 | T41.3X6 |
| **Surital** | T41.1X1 | T41.1X2 | T41.1X3 | T41.1X4 | T41.1X5 | T41.1X6 |
| **Sutilains** | T45.3X1 | T45.3X2 | T45.3X3 | T45.3X4 | T45.3X5 | T45.3X6 |
| **Suxamethonium** (chloride) | T48.1X1 | T48.1X2 | T48.1X3 | T48.1X4 | T48.1X5 | T48.1X6 |
| **Suxethonium** (chloride) | T48.1X1 | T48.1X2 | T48.1X3 | T48.1X4 | T48.1X5 | T48.1X6 |
| **Suxibuzone** | T39.2X1 | T39.2X2 | T39.2X3 | T39.2X4 | T39.2X5 | T39.2X6 |
| **Sweet niter spirit** | T46.3X1 | T46.3X2 | T46.3X3 | T46.3X4 | T46.3X5 | T46.3X6 |
| **Sweet oil** (birch) | T49.3X1 | T49.3X2 | T49.3X3 | T49.3X4 | T49.3X5 | T49.3X6 |
| **Sweetener** | T5Ø.9Ø1 | T5Ø.9Ø2 | T5Ø.9Ø3 | T5Ø.9Ø4 | T5Ø.9Ø5 | T5Ø.9Ø6 |
| **Sylvant*** | T45.1X1 | T45.1X2 | T45.1X3 | T45.1X4 | T45.1X5 | T45.1X6 |
| **Sym-dichloroethyl ether** | T53.6X1 | T53.6X2 | T53.6X3 | T53.6X4 | — | — |
| **Sympatholytic NEC** | T44.8X1 | T44.8X2 | T44.8X3 | T44.8X4 | T44.8X5 | T44.8X6 |
| haloalkylamine | T44.8X1 | T44.8X2 | T44.8X3 | T44.8X4 | T44.8X5 | T44.8X6 |
| **Sympathomimetic NEC** | T44.9Ø1 | T44.9Ø2 | T44.9Ø3 | T44.9Ø4 | T44.9Ø5 | T44.9Ø6 |
| anti-common-cold | T48.5X1 | T48.5X2 | T48.5X3 | T48.5X4 | T48.5X5 | T48.5X6 |
| bronchodilator | T48.6X1 | T48.6X2 | T48.6X3 | T48.6X4 | T48.6X5 | T48.6X6 |
| specified NEC | T44.991 | T44.992 | T44.993 | T44.994 | T44.995 | T44.996 |
| **Synagis** | T5Ø.B91 | T5Ø.B92 | T5Ø.B93 | T5Ø.B94 | T5Ø.B95 | T5Ø.B96 |
| **Synalar** | T49.ØX1 | T49.ØX2 | T49.ØX3 | T49.ØX4 | T49.ØX5 | T49.ØX6 |
| **Synthetic cannabinoids** | T4Ø.721 | T4Ø.722 | T4Ø.723 | T4Ø.724 | T4Ø.725 | T4Ø.726 |
| **Synthroid** | T38.1X1 | T38.1X2 | T38.1X3 | T38.1X4 | T38.1X5 | T38.1X6 |
| **Syntocinon** | T48.ØX1 | T48.ØX2 | T48.ØX3 | T48.ØX4 | T48.ØX5 | T48.ØX6 |
| **Syrosingopine** | T46.5X1 | T46.5X2 | T46.5X3 | T46.5X4 | T46.5X5 | T46.5X6 |
| **Systemic drug** | T45.91 | T45.92 | T45.93 | T45.94 | T45.95 | T45.96 |
| specified NEC | T45.8X1 | T45.8X2 | T45.8X3 | T45.8X4 | T45.8X5 | T45.8X6 |
| **Tablets** — *see also* specified substance | T5Ø.9Ø1 | T5Ø.9Ø2 | T5Ø.9Ø3 | T5Ø.9Ø4 | T5Ø.9Ø5 | T5Ø.9Ø6 |
| **Tace** | T38.5X1 | T38.5X2 | T38.5X3 | T38.5X4 | T38.5X5 | T38.5X6 |
| **Tacrine** | T44.ØX1 | T44.ØX2 | T44.ØX3 | T44.ØX4 | T44.ØX5 | T44.ØX6 |
| **Tadalafil** | T46.7X1 | T46.7X2 | T46.7X3 | T46.7X4 | T46.7X5 | T46.7X6 |
| **Talampicillin** | T36.ØX1 | T36.ØX2 | T36.ØX3 | T36.ØX4 | T36.ØX5 | T36.ØX6 |
| **Talbutal** | T42.3X1 | T42.3X2 | T42.3X3 | T42.3X4 | T42.3X5 | T42.3X6 |
| **Talc powder** | T49.3X1 | T49.3X2 | T49.3X3 | T49.3X4 | T49.3X5 | T49.3X6 |
| **Talcum** | T49.3X1 | T49.3X2 | T49.3X3 | T49.3X4 | T49.3X5 | T49.3X6 |
| **Taleranol** | T38.6X1 | T38.6X2 | T38.6X3 | T38.6X4 | T38.6X5 | T38.6X6 |
| **Taltz*** | T39.391 | T39.392 | T39.393 | T39.394 | T39.395 | T39.396 |
| **Tamoxifen** | T38.6X1 | T38.6X2 | T38.6X3 | T38.6X4 | T38.6X5 | T38.6X6 |
| **Tamsulosin** | T44.6X1 | T44.6X2 | T44.6X3 | T44.6X4 | T44.6X5 | T44.6X6 |
| **Tandearil, tanderil** | T39.2X1 | T39.2X2 | T39.2X3 | T39.2X4 | T39.2X5 | T39.2X6 |
| **Tannic acid** | T49.2X1 | T49.2X2 | T49.2X3 | T49.2X4 | T49.2X5 | T49.2X6 |
| medicinal (astringent) | T49.2X1 | T49.2X2 | T49.2X3 | T49.2X4 | T49.2X5 | T49.2X6 |
| **Tannin** — *see* Tannic acid | | | | | | |
| **Tansy** | T62.2X1 | T62.2X2 | T62.2X3 | T62.2X4 | — | — |
| **TAO** | T36.3X1 | T36.3X2 | T36.3X3 | T36.3X4 | T36.3X5 | T36.3X6 |
| **Tapazole** | T38.2X1 | T38.2X2 | T38.2X3 | T38.2X4 | T38.2X5 | T38.2X6 |
| **Tar NEC** | T52.ØX1 | T52.ØX2 | T52.ØX3 | T52.ØX4 | — | — |
| camphor | T6Ø.1X1 | T6Ø.1X2 | T6Ø.1X3 | T6Ø.1X4 | — | — |
| distillate | T49.1X1 | T49.1X2 | T49.1X3 | T49.1X4 | T49.1X5 | T49.1X6 |
| fumes | T59.891 | T59.892 | T59.893 | T59.894 | — | — |
| medicinal | T49.1X1 | T49.1X2 | T49.1X3 | T49.1X4 | T49.1X5 | T49.1X6 |
| ointment | T49.1X1 | T49.1X2 | T49.1X3 | T49.1X4 | T49.1X5 | T49.1X6 |
| **Taractan** | T43.591 | T43.592 | T43.593 | T43.594 | T43.595 | T43.596 |
| **Tarantula** (venomous) | T63.321 | T63.322 | T63.323 | T63.324 | — | — |
| **Tartar emetic** | T37.8X1 | T37.8X2 | T37.8X3 | T37.8X4 | T37.8X5 | T37.8X6 |
| **Tartaric acid** | T65.891 | T65.892 | T65.893 | T65.894 | — | — |
| **Tartrate, laxative** | T47.4X1 | T47.4X2 | T47.4X3 | T47.4X4 | T47.4X5 | T47.4X6 |
| **Tartrated antimony** (anti-infective) | T37.8X1 | T37.8X2 | T37.8X3 | T37.8X4 | T37.8X5 | T37.8X6 |
| **Tauromustine** | T45.1X1 | T45.1X2 | T45.1X3 | T45.1X4 | T45.1X5 | T45.1X6 |
| **TCA** — *see* Trichloroacetic acid | | | | | | |
| **TCDD** | T53.7X1 | T53.7X2 | T53.7X3 | T53.7X4 | — | — |
| **TDI** (vapor) | T65.ØX1 | T65.ØX2 | T65.ØX3 | T65.ØX4 | — | — |
| **Tear** | | | | | | |
| gas | T59.3X1 | T59.3X2 | T59.3X3 | T59.3X4 | — | — |
| solution | T49.5X1 | T49.5X2 | T49.5X3 | T49.5X4 | T49.5X5 | T49.5X6 |
| **Tecentriq*** | T45.1X1 | T45.1X2 | T45.1X3 | T45.1X4 | T45.1X5 | T45.1X6 |
| **Teclothiazide** | T5Ø.2X1 | T5Ø.2X2 | T5Ø.2X3 | T5Ø.2X4 | T5Ø.2X5 | T5Ø.2X6 |
| **Teclozan** | T37.3X1 | T37.3X2 | T37.3X3 | T37.3X4 | T37.3X5 | T37.3X6 |
| **Tegafur** | T45.1X1 | T45.1X2 | T45.1X3 | T45.1X4 | T45.1X5 | T45.1X6 |
| **Tegretol** | T42.1X1 | T42.1X2 | T42.1X3 | T42.1X4 | T42.1X5 | T42.1X6 |
| **Teicoplanin** | T36.8X1 | T36.8X2 | T36.8X3 | T36.8X4 | T36.8X5 | T36.8X6 |
| **Telepaque** | T5Ø.8X1 | T5Ø.8X2 | T5Ø.8X3 | T5Ø.8X4 | T5Ø.8X5 | T5Ø.8X6 |
| **Tellurium** | T56.891 | T56.892 | T56.893 | T56.894 | — | — |
| fumes | T56.891 | T56.892 | T56.893 | T56.894 | — | — |
| **TEM** | T45.1X1 | T45.1X2 | T45.1X3 | T45.1X4 | T45.1X5 | T45.1X6 |
| **Temazepam** | T42.4X1 | T42.4X2 | T42.4X3 | T42.4X4 | T42.4X5 | T42.4X6 |
| **Temocillin** | T36.ØX1 | T36.ØX2 | T36.ØX3 | T36.ØX4 | T36.ØX5 | T36.ØX6 |
| **Tenamfetamine** | T43.621 | T43.622 | T43.623 | T43.624 | T43.625 | T43.626 |
| **Tenecteplase*** | T45.611 | T45.612 | T45.613 | T45.614 | T45.615 | T45.616 |
| **Teniposide** | T45.1X1 | T45.1X2 | T45.1X3 | T45.1X4 | T45.1X5 | T45.1X6 |
| **Tenitramine** | T46.3X1 | T46.3X2 | T46.3X3 | T46.3X4 | T46.3X5 | T46.3X6 |
| **Tenoglicin** | T48.4X1 | T48.4X2 | T48.4X3 | T48.4X4 | T48.4X5 | T48.4X6 |
| **Tenonitrozole** | T37.3X1 | T37.3X2 | T37.3X3 | T37.3X4 | T37.3X5 | T37.3X6 |
| **Tenormin*** | T44.7X1 | T44.7X2 | T44.7X3 | T44.7X4 | T44.7X5 | T44.7X6 |
| **Tenoxicam** | T39.391 | T39.392 | T39.393 | T39.394 | T39.395 | T39.396 |
| **TEPA** | T45.1X1 | T45.1X2 | T45.1X3 | T45.1X4 | T45.1X5 | T45.1X6 |
| **TEPP** | T6Ø.ØX1 | T6Ø.ØX2 | T6Ø.ØX3 | T6Ø.ØX4 | — | — |
| **Teprotide** | T46.5X1 | T46.5X2 | T46.5X3 | T46.5X4 | T46.5X5 | T46.5X6 |
| **Terazosin** | T44.6X1 | T44.6X2 | T44.6X3 | T44.6X4 | T44.6X5 | T44.6X6 |
| **Terbufos** | T6Ø.ØX1 | T6Ø.ØX2 | T6Ø.ØX3 | T6Ø.ØX4 | — | — |
| **Terbutaline** | T48.6X1 | T48.6X2 | T48.6X3 | T48.6X4 | T48.6X5 | T48.6X6 |
| **Terconazole** | T49.ØX1 | T49.ØX2 | T49.ØX3 | T49.ØX4 | T49.ØX5 | T49.ØX6 |
| **Terfenadine** | T45.ØX1 | T45.ØX2 | T45.ØX3 | T45.ØX4 | T45.ØX5 | T45.ØX6 |
| **Teriparatide** (acetate) | T5Ø.991 | T5Ø.992 | T5Ø.993 | T5Ø.994 | T5Ø.995 | T5Ø.996 |
| **Terizidone** | T37.1X1 | T37.1X2 | T37.1X3 | T37.1X4 | T37.1X5 | T37.1X6 |
| **Terlipressin** | T38.891 | T38.892 | T38.893 | T38.894 | T38.895 | T38.896 |
| **Terodiline** | T46.3X1 | T46.3X2 | T46.3X3 | T46.3X4 | T46.3X5 | T46.3X6 |
| **Teroxalene** | T37.4X1 | T37.4X2 | T37.4X3 | T37.4X4 | T37.4X5 | T37.4X6 |
| **Terpin** (cis) **hydrate** | T48.4X1 | T48.4X2 | T48.4X3 | T48.4X4 | T48.4X5 | T48.4X6 |
| **Terramycin** | T36.4X1 | T36.4X2 | T36.4X3 | T36.4X4 | T36.4X5 | T36.4X6 |
| **Tertatolol** | T44.7X1 | T44.7X2 | T44.7X3 | T44.7X4 | T44.7X5 | T44.7X6 |
| **Tessalon** | T48.3X1 | T48.3X2 | T48.3X3 | T48.3X4 | T48.3X5 | T48.3X6 |
| **Testolactone** | T38.7X1 | T38.7X2 | T38.7X3 | T38.7X4 | T38.7X5 | T38.7X6 |
| **Testosterone** | T38.7X1 | T38.7X2 | T38.7X3 | T38.7X4 | T38.7X5 | T38.7X6 |
| **Tetanus toxoid or vaccine** | T5Ø.A91 | T5Ø.A92 | T5Ø.A93 | T5Ø.A94 | T5Ø.A95 | T5Ø.A96 |
| antitoxin | T5Ø.Z11 | T5Ø.Z12 | T5Ø.Z13 | T5Ø.Z14 | T5Ø.Z15 | T5Ø.Z16 |
| immune globulin (human) | T5Ø.Z11 | T5Ø.Z12 | T5Ø.Z13 | T5Ø.Z14 | T5Ø.Z15 | T5Ø.Z16 |
| toxoid | T5Ø.A91 | T5Ø.A92 | T5Ø.A93 | T5Ø.A94 | T5Ø.A95 | T5Ø.A96 |
| with diphtheria toxoid | T5Ø.A21 | T5Ø.A22 | T5Ø.A23 | T5Ø.A24 | T5Ø.A25 | T5Ø.A26 |
| with pertussis | T5Ø.A11 | T5Ø.A12 | T5Ø.A13 | T5Ø.A14 | T5Ø.A15 | T5Ø.A16 |
| **Tetrabenazine** | T43.591 | T43.592 | T43.593 | T43.594 | T43.595 | T43.596 |
| **Tetracaine** | T41.3X1 | T41.3X2 | T41.3X3 | T41.3X4 | T41.3X5 | T41.3X6 |
| nerve block (peripheral) (plexus) | T41.3X1 | T41.3X2 | T41.3X3 | T41.3X4 | T41.3X5 | T41.3X6 |
| regional | T41.3X1 | T41.3X2 | T41.3X3 | T41.3X4 | T41.3X5 | T41.3X6 |



☑ **Additional Character May Be Required — Refer to the Tabular List for Character Selection**

***Optum Value-Add**

| Substance | Poisoning, Accidental (unintentional) | Poisoning, Intentional Self-harm | Poisoning, Assault | Poisoning, Undetermined | Adverse Effect | Under-dosing |
|---|---|---|---|---|---|---|
| **Tetracaine** — *continued* | | | | | | |
| spinal | T41.3X1 | T41.3X2 | T41.3X3 | T41.3X4 | T41.3X5 | T41.3X6 |
| **Tetrachlorethylene** — *see* Tetrachloroethylene | | | | | | |
| **Tetrachlormethiazide** | T5Ø.2X1 | T5Ø.2X2 | T5Ø.2X3 | T5Ø.2X4 | T5Ø.2X5 | T5Ø.2X6 |
| **Tetrachloroethane** | T53.6X1 | T53.6X2 | T53.6X3 | T53.6X4 | — | — |
| vapor | T53.6X1 | T53.6X2 | T53.6X3 | T53.6X4 | — | — |
| paint or varnish | T53.6X1 | T53.6X2 | T53.6X3 | T53.6X4 | — | — |
| **Tetrachloroethylene** (liquid) | T53.3X1 | T53.3X2 | T53.3X3 | T53.3X4 | — | — |
| medicinal | T37.4X1 | T37.4X2 | T37.4X3 | T37.4X4 | T37.4X5 | T37.4X6 |
| vapor | T53.3X1 | T53.3X2 | T53.3X3 | T53.3X4 | — | — |
| **Tetrachloromethane** — *see* Carbon tetrachloride | | | | | | |
| **Tetracosactide** | T38.811 | T38.812 | T38.813 | T38.814 | T38.815 | T38.816 |
| **Tetracosactrin** | T38.811 | T38.812 | T38.813 | T38.814 | T38.815 | T38.816 |
| **Tetracycline** | T36.4X1 | T36.4X2 | T36.4X3 | T36.4X4 | T36.4X5 | T36.4X6 |
| ophthalmic preparation | T49.5X1 | T49.5X2 | T49.5X3 | T49.5X4 | T49.5X5 | T49.5X6 |
| topical NEC | T49.ØX1 | T49.ØX2 | T49.ØX3 | T49.ØX4 | T49.ØX5 | T49.ØX6 |
| **Tetradifon** | T6Ø.8X1 | T6Ø.8X2 | T6Ø.8X3 | T6Ø.8X4 | — | — |
| **Tetradotoxin** | T61.771 | T61.772 | T61.773 | T61.774 | — | — |
| **Tetraethyl** | | | | | | |
| lead | T56.ØX1 | T56.ØX2 | T56.ØX3 | T56.ØX4 | — | — |
| pyrophosphate | T6Ø.ØX1 | T6Ø.ØX2 | T6Ø.ØX3 | T6Ø.ØX4 | — | — |
| **Tetraethylammonium chloride** | T44.2X1 | T44.2X2 | T44.2X3 | T44.2X4 | T44.2X5 | T44.2X6 |
| **Tetraethylthiuram disulfide** | T5Ø.6X1 | T5Ø.6X2 | T5Ø.6X3 | T5Ø.6X4 | T5Ø.6X5 | T5Ø.6X6 |
| **Tetrahydroaminoacridine** | T44.ØX1 | T44.ØX2 | T44.ØX3 | T44.ØX4 | T44.ØX5 | T44.ØX6 |
| **Tetrahydrocannabinol** | T4Ø.711 | T4Ø.712 | T4Ø.713 | T4Ø.714 | T4Ø.715 | T4Ø.716 |
| **Tetrahydrofuran** | T52.891 | T52.892 | T52.893 | T52.894 | — | — |
| **Tetrahydrolipstatin*** | T47.8X1 | T47.8X2 | T47.8X3 | T47.8X4 | T47.8X5 | T47.8X6 |
| **Tetrahydronaphthalene** | T52.891 | T52.892 | T52.893 | T52.894 | — | — |
| **Tetrahydrozoline** | T49.5X1 | T49.5X2 | T49.5X3 | T49.5X4 | T49.5X5 | T49.5X6 |
| **Tetralin** | T52.891 | T52.892 | T52.893 | T52.894 | — | — |
| **Tetramethrin** | T6Ø.2X1 | T6Ø.2X2 | T6Ø.2X3 | T6Ø.2X4 | — | — |
| **Tetramethylthiuram** (disulfide) **NEC** | T6Ø.3X1 | T6Ø.3X2 | T6Ø.3X3 | T6Ø.3X4 | — | — |
| medicinal | T49.ØX1 | T49.ØX2 | T49.ØX3 | T49.ØX4 | T49.ØX5 | T49.ØX6 |
| **Tetramisole** | T37.4X1 | T37.4X2 | T37.4X3 | T37.4X4 | T37.4X5 | T37.4X6 |
| **Tetranicotinoyl fructose** | T46.7X1 | T46.7X2 | T46.7X3 | T46.7X4 | T46.7X5 | T46.7X6 |
| **Tetrazepam** | T42.4X1 | T42.4X2 | T42.4X3 | T42.4X4 | T42.4X5 | T42.4X6 |
| **Tetronal** | T42.6X1 | T42.6X2 | T42.6X3 | T42.6X4 | T42.6X5 | T42.6X6 |
| **Tetryl** | T65.3X1 | T65.3X2 | T65.3X3 | T65.3X4 | — | — |
| **Tetrylammonium chloride** | T44.2X1 | T44.2X2 | T44.2X3 | T44.2X4 | T44.2X5 | T44.2X6 |
| **Tetryzoline** | T49.5X1 | T49.5X2 | T49.5X3 | T49.5X4 | T49.5X5 | T49.5X6 |
| **Thalidomide** | T45.1X1 | T45.1X2 | T45.1X3 | T45.1X4 | T45.1X5 | T45.1X6 |
| **Thallium** (compounds) (dust) **NEC** | T56.811 | T56.812 | T56.813 | T56.814 | — | — |
| pesticide | T6Ø.4X1 | T6Ø.4X2 | T6Ø.4X3 | T6Ø.4X4 | — | — |
| **THC** | T4Ø.711 | T4Ø.712 | T4Ø.713 | T4Ø.714 | T4Ø.715 | T4Ø.716 |
| **Thebacon** | T48.3X1 | T48.3X2 | T48.3X3 | T48.3X4 | T48.3X5 | T48.3X6 |
| **Thebaine** | T4Ø.2X1 | T4Ø.2X2 | T4Ø.2X3 | T4Ø.2X4 | T4Ø.2X5 | T4Ø.2X6 |
| **Thenoic acid** | T49.6X1 | T49.6X2 | T49.6X3 | T49.6X4 | T49.6X5 | T49.6X6 |
| **Thenyldiamine** | T45.ØX1 | T45.ØX2 | T45.ØX3 | T45.ØX4 | T45.ØX5 | T45.ØX6 |
| **Theobromine** (calcium salicylate) | T48.6X1 | T48.6X2 | T48.6X3 | T48.6X4 | T48.6X5 | T48.6X6 |
| sodium salicylate | T48.6X1 | T48.6X2 | T48.6X3 | T48.6X4 | T48.6X5 | T48.6X6 |
| **Theolair*** | T48.6X1 | T48.6X2 | T48.6X3 | T48.6X4 | T48.6X5 | T48.6X6 |
| **Theophyllamine** | T48.6X1 | T48.6X2 | T48.6X3 | T48.6X4 | T48.6X5 | T48.6X6 |
| **Theophylline** | T48.6X1 | T48.6X2 | T48.6X3 | T48.6X4 | T48.6X5 | T48.6X6 |
| aminobenzoic acid | T48.6X1 | T48.6X2 | T48.6X3 | T48.6X4 | T48.6X5 | T48.6X6 |
| ethylenediamine | T48.6X1 | T48.6X2 | T48.6X3 | T48.6X4 | T48.6X5 | T48.6X6 |
| piperazine p-amino-benzoate | T48.6X1 | T48.6X2 | T48.6X3 | T48.6X4 | T48.6X5 | T48.6X6 |
| **Therevac*** | T47.4X1 | T47.4X2 | T47.4X3 | T47.4X4 | T47.4X5 | T47.4X6 |
| **Thiabendazole** | T37.4X1 | T37.4X2 | T37.4X3 | T37.4X4 | T37.4X5 | T37.4X6 |
| **Thialbarbital** | T41.1X1 | T41.1X2 | T41.1X3 | T41.1X4 | T41.1X5 | T41.1X6 |
| **Thiamazole** | T38.2X1 | T38.2X2 | T38.2X3 | T38.2X4 | T38.2X5 | T38.2X6 |
| **Thiambutosine** | T37.1X1 | T37.1X2 | T37.1X3 | T37.1X4 | T37.1X5 | T37.1X6 |
| **Thiamine** | T45.2X1 | T45.2X2 | T45.2X3 | T45.2X4 | T45.2X5 | T45.2X6 |
| **Thiamphenicol** | T36.2X1 | T36.2X2 | T36.2X3 | T36.2X4 | T36.2X5 | T36.2X6 |
| **Thiamylal** | T41.1X1 | T41.1X2 | T41.1X3 | T41.1X4 | T41.1X5 | T41.1X6 |
| sodium | T41.1X1 | T41.1X2 | T41.1X3 | T41.1X4 | T41.1X5 | T41.1X6 |
| **Thiazesim** | T43.291 | T43.292 | T43.293 | T43.294 | T43.295 | T43.296 |
| **Thiazides** (diuretics) | T5Ø.2X1 | T5Ø.2X2 | T5Ø.2X3 | T5Ø.2X4 | T5Ø.2X5 | T5Ø.2X6 |
| **Thiazinamium metilsulfate** | T43.3X1 | T43.3X2 | T43.3X3 | T43.3X4 | T43.3X5 | T43.3X6 |
| **Thiethylperazine** | T43.3X1 | T43.3X2 | T43.3X3 | T43.3X4 | T43.3X5 | T43.3X6 |
| **Thimerosal** | T49.ØX1 | T49.ØX2 | T49.ØX3 | T49.ØX4 | T49.ØX5 | T49.ØX6 |
| ophthalmic preparation | T49.5X1 | T49.5X2 | T49.5X3 | T49.5X4 | T49.5X5 | T49.5X6 |
| **Thioacetazone** | T37.1X1 | T37.1X2 | T37.1X3 | T37.1X4 | T37.1X5 | T37.1X6 |
| with isoniazid | T37.1X1 | T37.1X2 | T37.1X3 | T37.1X4 | T37.1X5 | T37.1X6 |

| Substance | Poisoning, Accidental (unintentional) | Poisoning, Intentional Self-harm | Poisoning, Assault | Poisoning, Undetermined | Adverse Effect | Under-dosing |
|---|---|---|---|---|---|---|
| **Thiobarbital sodium** | T41.1X1 | T41.1X2 | T41.1X3 | T41.1X4 | T41.1X5 | T41.1X6 |
| **Thiobarbiturate anesthetic** | T41.1X1 | T41.1X2 | T41.1X3 | T41.1X4 | T41.1X5 | T41.1X6 |
| **Thiobismol** | T37.8X1 | T37.8X2 | T37.8X3 | T37.8X4 | T37.8X5 | T37.8X6 |
| **Thiobutabarbital sodium** | T41.1X1 | T41.1X2 | T41.1X3 | T41.1X4 | T41.1X5 | T41.1X6 |
| **Thiocarbamate** (insecticide) | T6Ø.ØX1 | T6Ø.ØX2 | T6Ø.ØX3 | T6Ø.ØX4 | — | — |
| **Thiocarbamide** | T38.2X1 | T38.2X2 | T38.2X3 | T38.2X4 | T38.2X5 | T38.2X6 |
| **Thiocarbarsone** | T37.8X1 | T37.8X2 | T37.8X3 | T37.8X4 | T37.8X5 | T37.8X6 |
| **Thiocarlide** | T37.1X1 | T37.1X2 | T37.1X3 | T37.1X4 | T37.1X5 | T37.1X6 |
| **Thioctamide** | T5Ø.991 | T5Ø.992 | T5Ø.993 | T5Ø.994 | T5Ø.995 | T5Ø.996 |
| **Thioctic acid** | T5Ø.991 | T5Ø.992 | T5Ø.993 | T5Ø.994 | T5Ø.995 | T5Ø.996 |
| **Thiofos** | T6Ø.ØX1 | T6Ø.ØX2 | T6Ø.ØX3 | T6Ø.ØX4 | — | — |
| **Thioglycolate** | T49.4X1 | T49.4X2 | T49.4X3 | T49.4X4 | T49.4X5 | T49.4X6 |
| **Thioglycolic acid** | T65.891 | T65.892 | T65.893 | T65.894 | — | — |
| **Thioguanine** | T45.1X1 | T45.1X2 | T45.1X3 | T45.1X4 | T45.1X5 | T45.1X6 |
| **Thiomercaptomerin** | T5Ø.2X1 | T5Ø.2X2 | T5Ø.2X3 | T5Ø.2X4 | T5Ø.2X5 | T5Ø.2X6 |
| **Thiomerin** | T5Ø.2X1 | T5Ø.2X2 | T5Ø.2X3 | T5Ø.2X4 | T5Ø.2X5 | T5Ø.2X6 |
| **Thiomersal** | T49.ØX1 | T49.ØX2 | T49.ØX3 | T49.ØX4 | T49.ØX5 | T49.ØX6 |
| **Thionazin** | T6Ø.ØX1 | T6Ø.ØX2 | T6Ø.ØX3 | T6Ø.ØX4 | — | — |
| **Thiopental** (sodium) | T41.1X1 | T41.1X2 | T41.1X3 | T41.1X4 | T41.1X5 | T41.1X6 |
| **Thiopentone** (sodium) | T41.1X1 | T41.1X2 | T41.1X3 | T41.1X4 | T41.1X5 | T41.1X6 |
| **Thiopropazate** | T43.3X1 | T43.3X2 | T43.3X3 | T43.3X4 | T43.3X5 | T43.3X6 |
| **Thioproperazine** | T43.3X1 | T43.3X2 | T43.3X3 | T43.3X4 | T43.3X5 | T43.3X6 |
| **Thioridazine** | T43.3X1 | T43.3X2 | T43.3X3 | T43.3X4 | T43.3X5 | T43.3X6 |
| **Thiosinamine** | T49.3X1 | T49.3X2 | T49.3X3 | T49.3X4 | T49.3X5 | T49.3X6 |
| **Thiotepa** | T45.1X1 | T45.1X2 | T45.1X3 | T45.1X4 | T45.1X5 | T45.1X6 |
| **Thiothixene** | T43.4X1 | T43.4X2 | T43.4X3 | T43.4X4 | T43.4X5 | T43.4X6 |
| **Thiouracil** (benzyl) (methyl) (propyl) | T38.2X1 | T38.2X2 | T38.2X3 | T38.2X4 | T38.2X5 | T38.2X6 |
| **Thiourea** | T38.2X1 | T38.2X2 | T38.2X3 | T38.2X4 | T38.2X5 | T38.2X6 |
| **Thiphenamil** | T44.3X1 | T44.3X2 | T44.3X3 | T44.3X4 | T44.3X5 | T44.3X6 |
| **Thiram** | T6Ø.3X1 | T6Ø.3X2 | T6Ø.3X3 | T6Ø.3X4 | — | — |
| medicinal | T49.2X1 | T49.2X2 | T49.2X3 | T49.2X4 | T49.2X5 | T49.2X6 |
| **Thonzylamine** (systemic) | T45.ØX1 | T45.ØX2 | T45.ØX3 | T45.ØX4 | T45.ØX5 | T45.ØX6 |
| mucosal decongestant | T48.5X1 | T48.5X2 | T48.5X3 | T48.5X4 | T48.5X5 | T48.5X6 |
| **Thorazine** | T43.3X1 | T43.3X2 | T43.3X3 | T43.3X4 | T43.3X5 | T43.3X6 |
| **Thorium dioxide suspension** | T5Ø.8X1 | T5Ø.8X2 | T5Ø.8X3 | T5Ø.8X4 | T5Ø.8X5 | T5Ø.8X6 |
| **Thornapple** | T62.2X1 | T62.2X2 | T62.2X3 | T62.2X4 | — | — |
| **Throat drug NEC** | T49.6X1 | T49.6X2 | T49.6X3 | T49.6X4 | T49.6X5 | T49.6X6 |
| **Thrombate 111*** | T45.511 | T45.512 | T45.513 | T45.514 | T45.515 | T45.516 |
| **Thrombin** | T45.7X1 | T45.7X2 | T45.7X3 | T45.7X4 | T45.7X5 | T45.7X6 |
| **Thrombolysin** | T45.611 | T45.612 | T45.613 | T45.614 | T45.615 | T45.616 |
| **Thromboplastin** | T45.7X1 | T45.7X2 | T45.7X3 | T45.7X4 | T45.7X5 | T45.7X6 |
| **Thurfyl nicotinate** | T46.7X1 | T46.7X2 | T46.7X3 | T46.7X4 | T46.7X5 | T46.7X6 |
| **Thymol** | T49.ØX1 | T49.ØX2 | T49.ØX3 | T49.ØX4 | T49.ØX5 | T49.ØX6 |
| **Thymopentin** | T37.5X1 | T37.5X2 | T37.5X3 | T37.5X4 | T37.5X5 | T37.5X6 |
| **Thymoxamine** | T46.7X1 | T46.7X2 | T46.7X3 | T46.7X4 | T46.7X5 | T46.7X6 |
| **Thymus extract** | T38.891 | T38.892 | T38.893 | T38.894 | T38.895 | T38.896 |
| **Thyreotrophic hormone** | T38.811 | T38.812 | T38.813 | T38.814 | T38.815 | T38.816 |
| **Thyroglobulin** | T38.1X1 | T38.1X2 | T38.1X3 | T38.1X4 | T38.1X5 | T38.1X6 |
| **Thyroid** (hormone) | T38.1X1 | T38.1X2 | T38.1X3 | T38.1X4 | T38.1X5 | T38.1X6 |
| **Thyrolar** | T38.1X1 | T38.1X2 | T38.1X3 | T38.1X4 | T38.1X5 | T38.1X6 |
| **Thyrotrophin** | T38.811 | T38.812 | T38.813 | T38.814 | T38.815 | T38.816 |
| **Thyrotropic hormone** | T38.811 | T38.812 | T38.813 | T38.814 | T38.815 | T38.816 |
| **Thyroxine** | T38.1X1 | T38.1X2 | T38.1X3 | T38.1X4 | T38.1X5 | T38.1X6 |
| **Tiabendazole** | T37.4X1 | T37.4X2 | T37.4X3 | T37.4X4 | T37.4X5 | T37.4X6 |
| **Tiamizide** | T5Ø.2X1 | T5Ø.2X2 | T5Ø.2X3 | T5Ø.2X4 | T5Ø.2X5 | T5Ø.2X6 |
| **Tianeptine** | T43.291 | T43.292 | T43.293 | T43.294 | T43.295 | T43.296 |
| **Tiapamil** | T46.1X1 | T46.1X2 | T46.1X3 | T46.1X4 | T46.1X5 | T46.1X6 |
| **Tiapride** | T43.591 | T43.592 | T43.593 | T43.594 | T43.595 | T43.596 |
| **Tiaprofenic acid** | T39.311 | T39.312 | T39.313 | T39.314 | T39.315 | T39.316 |
| **Tiaramide** | T39.8X1 | T39.8X2 | T39.8X3 | T39.8X4 | T39.8X5 | T39.8X6 |
| **Ticagrelor*** | T45.521 | T45.522 | T45.523 | T45.524 | T45.525 | T45.526 |
| **Ticarcillin** | T36.ØX1 | T36.ØX2 | T36.ØX3 | T36.ØX4 | T36.ØX5 | T36.ØX6 |
| **Ticlatone** | T49.ØX1 | T49.ØX2 | T49.ØX3 | T49.ØX4 | T49.ØX5 | T49.ØX6 |
| **Ticlopidine** | T45.521 | T45.522 | T45.523 | T45.524 | T45.525 | T45.526 |
| **Ticrynafen** | T5Ø.1X1 | T5Ø.1X2 | T5Ø.1X3 | T5Ø.1X4 | T5Ø.1X5 | T5Ø.1X6 |
| **Tidiacic** | T5Ø.991 | T5Ø.992 | T5Ø.993 | T5Ø.994 | T5Ø.995 | T5Ø.996 |
| **Tiemonium** | T44.3X1 | T44.3X2 | T44.3X3 | T44.3X4 | T44.3X5 | T44.3X6 |
| iodide | T44.3X1 | T44.3X2 | T44.3X3 | T44.3X4 | T44.3X5 | T44.3X6 |
| **Tienilic acid** | T5Ø.1X1 | T5Ø.1X2 | T5Ø.1X3 | T5Ø.1X4 | T5Ø.1X5 | T5Ø.1X6 |
| **Tifenamil** | T44.3X1 | T44.3X2 | T44.3X3 | T44.3X4 | T44.3X5 | T44.3X6 |
| **Tigan** | T45.ØX1 | T45.ØX2 | T45.ØX3 | T45.ØX4 | T45.ØX5 | T45.ØX6 |
| **Tigloidine** | T44.3X1 | T44.3X2 | T44.3X3 | T44.3X4 | T44.3X5 | T44.3X6 |
| **Tilactase** | T47.5X1 | T47.5X2 | T47.5X3 | T47.5X4 | T47.5X5 | T47.5X6 |
| **Tiletamine** | T41.291 | T41.292 | T41.293 | T41.294 | T41.295 | T41.296 |
| **Tilidine** | T4Ø.491 | T4Ø.492 | T4Ø.493 | T4Ø.494 | — | — |
| **Timepidium bromide** | T44.3X1 | T44.3X2 | T44.3X3 | T44.3X4 | T44.3X5 | T44.3X6 |
| **Timiperone** | T43.4X1 | T43.4X2 | T43.4X3 | T43.4X4 | T43.4X5 | T43.4X6 |
| **Timolol** | T44.7X1 | T44.7X2 | T44.7X3 | T44.7X4 | T44.7X5 | T44.7X6 |

| Substance | Poisoning, Accidental (unintentional) | Poisoning, Intentional Self-harm | Poisoning, Assault | Poisoning, Undetermined | Adverse Effect | Under-dosing |
|---|---|---|---|---|---|---|
| **Tin** (chloride) (dust) (oxide) | T56.6X1 | T56.6X2 | T56.6X3 | T56.6X4 | — | — |
| **NEC** | | | | | | |
| anti-infectives | T37.8X1 | T37.8X2 | T37.8X3 | T37.8X4 | T37.8X5 | T37.8X6 |
| **Tincture, iodine** — *see* Iodine | | | | | | |
| **Tindal** | T43.3X1 | T43.3X2 | T43.3X3 | T43.3X4 | T43.3X5 | T43.3X6 |
| **Tinidazole** | T37.3X1 | T37.3X2 | T37.3X3 | T37.3X4 | T37.3X5 | T37.3X6 |
| **Tinoridine** | T39.8X1 | T39.8X2 | T39.8X3 | T39.8X4 | T39.8X5 | T39.8X6 |
| **Tiocarlide** | T37.1X1 | T37.1X2 | T37.1X3 | T37.1X4 | T37.1X5 | T37.1X6 |
| **Tioclomarol** | T45.511 | T45.512 | T45.513 | T45.514 | T45.515 | T45.516 |
| **Tioconazole** | T49.ØX1 | T49.ØX2 | T49.ØX3 | T49.ØX4 | T49.ØX5 | T49.ØX6 |
| **Tioguanine** | T45.1X1 | T45.1X2 | T45.1X3 | T45.1X4 | T45.1X5 | T45.1X6 |
| **Tiopronin** | T5Ø.991 | T5Ø.992 | T5Ø.993 | T5Ø.994 | T5Ø.995 | T5Ø.996 |
| **Tiotixene** | T43.4X1 | T43.4X2 | T43.4X3 | T43.4X4 | T43.4X5 | T43.4X6 |
| **Tioxolone** | T49.4X1 | T49.4X2 | T49.4X3 | T49.4X4 | T49.4X5 | T49.4X6 |
| **Tipepidine** | T48.3X1 | T48.3X2 | T48.3X3 | T48.3X4 | T48.3X5 | T48.3X6 |
| **Tiquizium bromide** | T44.3X1 | T44.3X2 | T44.3X3 | T44.3X4 | T44.3X5 | T44.3X6 |
| **Tiratricol** | T38.1X1 | T38.1X2 | T38.1X3 | T38.1X4 | T38.1X5 | T38.1X6 |
| **Tisopurine** | T5Ø.4X1 | T5Ø.4X2 | T5Ø.4X3 | T5Ø.4X4 | T5Ø.4X5 | T5Ø.4X6 |
| **Titanium** (compounds) (vapor) | T56.891 | T56.892 | T56.893 | T56.894 | — | — |
| dioxide | T49.3X1 | T49.3X2 | T49.3X3 | T49.3X4 | T49.3X5 | T49.3X6 |
| ointment | T49.3X1 | T49.3X2 | T49.3X3 | T49.3X4 | T49.3X5 | T49.3X6 |
| oxide | T49.3X1 | T49.3X2 | T49.3X3 | T49.3X4 | T49.3X5 | T49.3X6 |
| tetrachloride | T56.891 | T56.892 | T56.893 | T56.894 | — | — |
| **Titanocene** | T56.891 | T56.892 | T56.893 | T56.894 | — | — |
| **Titroid** | T38.1X1 | T38.1X2 | T38.1X3 | T38.1X4 | T38.1X5 | T38.1X6 |
| **Tizanidine** | T42.8X1 | T42.8X2 | T42.8X3 | T42.8X4 | T42.8X5 | T42.8X6 |
| **TMTD** | T6Ø.3X1 | T6Ø.3X2 | T6Ø.3X3 | T6Ø.3X4 | — | — |
| **TNT** (fumes) | T65.3X1 | T65.3X2 | T65.3X3 | T65.3X4 | — | — |
| **Toadstool** | T62.ØX1 | T62.ØX2 | T62.ØX3 | T62.ØX4 | — | — |
| **Tobacco NEC** | T65.291 | T65.292 | T65.293 | T65.294 | — | — |
| cigarettes | T65.221 | T65.222 | T65.223 | T65.224 | — | — |
| Indian | T62.2X1 | T62.2X2 | T62.2X3 | T62.2X4 | — | — |
| smoke, second-hand | T65.221 | T65.222 | T65.223 | T65.224 | — | — |
| **Tobraflex*** | T49.5X1 | T49.5X2 | T49.5X3 | T49.5X4 | T49.5X5 | T49.5X6 |
| **Tobramycin** | T36.5X1 | T36.5X2 | T36.5X3 | T36.5X4 | T36.5X5 | T36.5X6 |
| **Tocainide** | T46.2X1 | T46.2X2 | T46.2X3 | T46.2X4 | T46.2X5 | T46.2X6 |
| **Tocoferol** | T45.2X1 | T45.2X2 | T45.2X3 | T45.2X4 | T45.2X5 | T45.2X6 |
| **Tocopherol** | T45.2X1 | T45.2X2 | T45.2X3 | T45.2X4 | T45.2X5 | T45.2X6 |
| acetate | T45.2X1 | T45.2X2 | T45.2X3 | T45.2X4 | T45.2X5 | T45.2X6 |
| **Tocosamine** | T48.ØX1 | T48.ØX2 | T48.ØX3 | T48.ØX4 | T48.ØX5 | T48.ØX6 |
| **Todralazine** | T46.5X1 | T46.5X2 | T46.5X3 | T46.5X4 | T46.5X5 | T46.5X6 |
| **Tofisopam** | T42.4X1 | T42.4X2 | T42.4X3 | T42.4X4 | T42.4X5 | T42.4X6 |
| **Tofranil** | T43.Ø11 | T43.Ø12 | T43.Ø13 | T43.Ø14 | T43.Ø15 | T43.Ø16 |
| **Toilet deodorizer** | T65.891 | T65.892 | T65.893 | T65.894 | — | — |
| **Tolamolol** | T44.7X1 | T44.7X2 | T44.7X3 | T44.7X4 | T44.7X5 | T44.7X6 |
| **Tolazamide** | T38.3X1 | T38.3X2 | T38.3X3 | T38.3X4 | T38.3X5 | T38.3X6 |
| **Tolazoline** | T46.7X1 | T46.7X2 | T46.7X3 | T46.7X4 | T46.7X5 | T46.7X6 |
| **Tolbutamide** (sodium) | T38.3X1 | T38.3X2 | T38.3X3 | T38.3X4 | T38.3X5 | T38.3X6 |
| **Tolciclate** | T49.ØX1 | T49.ØX2 | T49.ØX3 | T49.ØX4 | T49.ØX5 | T49.ØX6 |
| **Tolmetin** | T39.391 | T39.392 | T39.393 | T39.394 | T39.395 | T39.396 |
| **Tolnaftate** | T49.ØX1 | T49.ØX2 | T49.ØX3 | T49.ØX4 | T49.ØX5 | T49.ØX6 |
| **Tolonidine** | T46.5X1 | T46.5X2 | T46.5X3 | T46.5X4 | T46.5X5 | T46.5X6 |
| **Toloxatone** | T42.6X1 | T42.6X2 | T42.6X3 | T42.6X4 | T42.6X5 | T42.6X6 |
| **Tolperisone** | T44.3X1 | T44.3X2 | T44.3X3 | T44.3X4 | T44.3X5 | T44.3X6 |
| **Tolserol** | T42.8X1 | T42.8X2 | T42.8X3 | T42.8X4 | T42.8X5 | T42.8X6 |
| **Toluene** (liquid) | T52.2X1 | T52.2X2 | T52.2X3 | T52.2X4 | — | — |
| diisocyanate | T65.ØX1 | T65.ØX2 | T65.ØX3 | T65.ØX4 | — | — |
| **Toluidine** | T65.891 | T65.892 | T65.893 | T65.894 | — | — |
| vapor | T59.891 | T59.892 | T59.893 | T59.894 | — | — |
| **Toluol** (liquid) | T52.2X1 | T52.2X2 | T52.2X3 | T52.2X4 | — | — |
| vapor | T52.2X1 | T52.2X2 | T52.2X3 | T52.2X4 | — | — |
| **Toluylenediamine** | T65.3X1 | T65.3X2 | T65.3X3 | T65.3X4 | — | — |
| **Tolylene-2,4-diisocyanate** | T65.ØX1 | T65.ØX2 | T65.ØX3 | T65.ØX4 | — | — |
| **Tonic NEC** | T5Ø.9Ø1 | T5Ø.9Ø2 | T5Ø.9Ø3 | T5Ø.9Ø4 | T5Ø.9Ø5 | T5Ø.9Ø6 |
| **Topical action drug NEC** | T49.91 | T49.92 | T49.93 | T49.94 | T49.95 | T49.96 |
| ear, nose or throat | T49.6X1 | T49.6X2 | T49.6X3 | T49.6X4 | T49.6X5 | T49.6X6 |
| eye | T49.5X1 | T49.5X2 | T49.5X3 | T49.5X4 | T49.5X5 | T49.5X6 |
| skin | T49.91 | T49.92 | T49.93 | T49.94 | T49.95 | T49.96 |
| specified NEC | T49.8X1 | T49.8X2 | T49.8X3 | T49.8X4 | T49.8X5 | T49.8X6 |
| **Toprol*** | T44.7X1 | T44.7X2 | T44.7X3 | T44.7X4 | T44.7X5 | T44.7X6 |
| **Toquizine** | T44.3X1 | T44.3X2 | T44.3X3 | T44.3X4 | T44.3X5 | T44.3X6 |
| **Toremifene** | T38.6X1 | T38.6X2 | T38.6X3 | T38.6X4 | T38.6X5 | T38.6X6 |
| **Tosylchloramide sodium** | T49.8X1 | T49.8X2 | T49.8X3 | T49.8X4 | T49.8X5 | T49.8X6 |
| **Toxaphene** (dust) (spray) | T6Ø.1X1 | T6Ø.1X2 | T6Ø.1X3 | T6Ø.1X4 | — | — |
| **Toxin, diphtheria** (Schick Test) | T5Ø.8X1 | T5Ø.8X2 | T5Ø.8X3 | T5Ø.8X4 | T5Ø.8X5 | T5Ø.8X6 |
| **Toxoid** | | | | | | |
| combined | T5Ø.A21 | T5Ø.A22 | T5Ø.A23 | T5Ø.A24 | T5Ø.A25 | T5Ø.A26 |
| diphtheria | T5Ø.A91 | T5Ø.A92 | T5Ø.A93 | T5Ø.A94 | T5Ø.A95 | T5Ø.A96 |
| tetanus | T5Ø.A91 | T5Ø.A92 | T5Ø.A93 | T5Ø.A94 | T5Ø.A95 | T5Ø.A96 |
| **Trace element NEC** | T45.8X1 | T45.8X2 | T45.8X3 | T45.8X4 | T45.8X5 | T45.8X6 |
| **Tractor fuel NEC** | T52.ØX1 | T52.ØX2 | T52.ØX3 | T52.ØX4 | — | — |

| Substance | Poisoning, Accidental (unintentional) | Poisoning, Intentional Self-harm | Poisoning, Assault | Poisoning, Undetermined | Adverse Effect | Under-dosing |
|---|---|---|---|---|---|---|
| **Tragacanth** | T5Ø.991 | T5Ø.992 | T5Ø.993 | T5Ø.994 | T5Ø.995 | T5Ø.99 |
| **Tramadol** | T4Ø.421 | T4Ø.422 | T4Ø.423 | T4Ø.424 | T4Ø.425 | T4Ø.42 |
| **Tramazoline** | T48.5X1 | T48.5X2 | T48.5X3 | T48.5X4 | T48.5X5 | T48.5X |
| **Tranexamic acid** | T45.621 | T45.622 | T45.623 | T45.624 | T45.625 | T45.62 |
| **Tranilast** | T45.ØX1 | T45.ØX2 | T45.ØX3 | T45.ØX4 | T45.ØX5 | T45.ØX |
| **Tranquilizer NEC** | T43.5Ø1 | T43.5Ø2 | T43.5Ø3 | T43.5Ø4 | T43.5Ø5 | T43.5Ø |
| with hypnotic or sedative | T42.6X1 | T42.6X2 | T42.6X3 | T42.6X4 | T42.6X5 | T42.6X |
| benzodiazepine NEC | T42.4X1 | T42.4X2 | T42.4X3 | T42.4X4 | T42.4X5 | T42.4X |
| butyrophenone NEC | T43.4X1 | T43.4X2 | T43.4X3 | T43.4X4 | T43.4X5 | T43.4X |
| carbamate | T43.591 | T43.592 | T43.593 | T43.594 | T43.595 | T43.59 |
| dimethylamine | T43.3X1 | T43.3X2 | T43.3X3 | T43.3X4 | T43.3X5 | T43.3X |
| ethylamine | T43.3X1 | T43.3X2 | T43.3X3 | T43.3X4 | T43.3X5 | T43.3X |
| hydroxyzine | T43.591 | T43.592 | T43.593 | T43.594 | T43.595 | T43.59 |
| major NEC | T43.5Ø1 | T43.5Ø2 | T43.5Ø3 | T43.5Ø4 | T43.5Ø5 | T43.5Ø |
| penothiazine NEC | T43.3X1 | T43.3X2 | T43.3X3 | T43.3X4 | T43.3X5 | T43.3X |
| phenothiazine-based | T43.3X1 | T43.3X2 | T43.3X3 | T43.3X4 | T43.3X5 | T43.3X |
| piperazine NEC | T43.3X1 | T43.3X2 | T43.3X3 | T43.3X4 | T43.3X5 | T43.3X |
| piperidine | T43.3X1 | T43.3X2 | T43.3X3 | T43.3X4 | T43.3X5 | T43.3X |
| propylamine | T43.3X1 | T43.3X2 | T43.3X3 | T43.3X4 | T43.3X5 | T43.3X |
| specified NEC | T43.591 | T43.592 | T43.593 | T43.594 | T43.595 | T43.59 |
| thioxanthene NEC | T43.591 | T43.592 | T43.593 | T43.594 | T43.595 | T43.59 |
| **Tranxene** | T42.4X1 | T42.4X2 | T42.4X3 | T42.4X4 | T42.4X5 | T42.4X |
| **Tranylcypromine** | T43.1X1 | T43.1X2 | T43.1X3 | T43.1X4 | T43.1X5 | T43.1X |
| **Trapidil** | T46.3X1 | T46.3X2 | T46.3X3 | T46.3X4 | T46.3X5 | T46.3X |
| **Trasentine** | T44.3X1 | T44.3X2 | T44.3X3 | T44.3X4 | T44.3X5 | T44.3X |
| **Travert** | T5Ø.3X1 | T5Ø.3X2 | T5Ø.3X3 | T5Ø.3X4 | T5Ø.3X5 | T5Ø.3X |
| **Trazodone** | T43.211 | T43.212 | T43.213 | T43.214 | T43.215 | T43.21 |
| **Treanda*** | T45.1X1 | T45.1X2 | T45.1X3 | T45.1X4 | T45.1X5 | T45.1X |
| **Trecator** | T37.1X1 | T37.1X2 | T37.1X3 | T37.1X4 | T37.1X5 | T37.1X |
| **Treosulfan** | T45.1X1 | T45.1X2 | T45.1X3 | T45.1X4 | T45.1X5 | T45.1X |
| **Tretamine** | T45.1X1 | T45.1X2 | T45.1X3 | T45.1X4 | T45.1X5 | T45.1X |
| **Tretinoin** | T49.ØX1 | T49.ØX2 | T49.ØX3 | T49.ØX4 | T49.ØX5 | T49.ØX |
| **Tretoquinol** | T48.6X1 | T48.6X2 | T48.6X3 | T48.6X4 | T48.6X5 | T48.6X |
| **Triacetin** | T49.ØX1 | T49.ØX2 | T49.ØX3 | T49.ØX4 | T49.ØX5 | T49.ØX |
| **Triacetoxyanthracene** | T49.4X1 | T49.4X2 | T49.4X3 | T49.4X4 | T49.4X5 | T49.4X |
| **Triacetyloleandomycin** | T36.3X1 | T36.3X2 | T36.3X3 | T36.3X4 | T36.3X5 | T36.3X |
| **Triamcinolone** | T38.ØX1 | T38.ØX2 | T38.ØX3 | T38.ØX4 | T38.ØX5 | T38.ØX |
| ENT agent | T49.6X1 | T49.6X2 | T49.6X3 | T49.6X4 | T49.6X5 | T49.6X |
| hexacetonide | T49.ØX1 | T49.ØX2 | T49.ØX3 | T49.ØX4 | T49.ØX5 | T49.ØX |
| ophthalmic preparation | T49.5X1 | T49.5X2 | T49.5X3 | T49.5X4 | T49.5X5 | T49.5X |
| topical NEC | T49.ØX1 | T49.ØX2 | T49.ØX3 | T49.ØX4 | T49.ØX5 | T49.ØX |
| **Triampyzine** | T44.3X1 | T44.3X2 | T44.3X3 | T44.3X4 | T44.3X5 | T44.3X |
| **Triamterene** | T5Ø.2X1 | T5Ø.2X2 | T5Ø.2X3 | T5Ø.2X4 | T5Ø.2X5 | T5Ø.2X |
| **Triazine** (herbicide) | T6Ø.3X1 | T6Ø.3X2 | T6Ø.3X3 | T6Ø.3X4 | — | — |
| **Triaziquone** | T45.1X1 | T45.1X2 | T45.1X3 | T45.1X4 | T45.1X5 | T45.1X |
| **Triazolam** | T42.4X1 | T42.4X2 | T42.4X3 | T42.4X4 | T42.4X5 | T42.4X |
| **Triazole** (herbicide) | T6Ø.3X1 | T6Ø.3X2 | T6Ø.3X3 | T6Ø.3X4 | — | — |
| **Tribavirin*** | T37.5X1 | T37.5X2 | T37.5X3 | T37.5X4 | T37.5X5 | T37.5X |
| **Tribenoside** | T46.991 | T46.992 | T46.993 | T46.994 | T46.995 | T46.99 |
| **Tribromacetaldehyde** | T42.6X1 | T42.6X2 | T42.6X3 | T42.6X4 | T42.6X5 | T42.6X |
| **Tribromoethanol, rectal** | T41.291 | T41.292 | T41.293 | T41.294 | T41.295 | T41.29 |
| **Tribromomethane** | T42.6X1 | T42.6X2 | T42.6X3 | T42.6X4 | T42.6X5 | T42.6X |
| **Trichlorethane** | T53.2X1 | T53.2X2 | T53.2X3 | T53.2X4 | — | — |
| **Trichlorethylene** | T53.2X1 | T53.2X2 | T53.2X3 | T53.2X4 | — | — |
| **Trichlorfon** | T6Ø.ØX1 | T6Ø.ØX2 | T6Ø.ØX3 | T6Ø.ØX4 | — | — |
| **Trichlormethiazide** | T5Ø.2X1 | T5Ø.2X2 | T5Ø.2X3 | T5Ø.2X4 | T5Ø.2X5 | T5Ø.2X |
| **Trichlormethine** | T45.1X1 | T45.1X2 | T45.1X3 | T45.1X4 | T45.1X5 | T45.1X |
| **Trichloroacetic acid, Trichloracetic acid** | T54.2X1 | T54.2X2 | T54.2X3 | T54.2X4 | — | — |
| medicinal | T49.4X1 | T49.4X2 | T49.4X3 | T49.4X4 | T49.4X5 | T49.4X |
| **Trichloroethane** | T53.2X1 | T53.2X2 | T53.2X3 | T53.2X4 | — | — |
| **Trichloroethanol** | T42.6X1 | T42.6X2 | T42.6X3 | T42.6X4 | T42.6X5 | T42.6X |
| **Trichloroethyl phosphate** | T42.6X1 | T42.6X2 | T42.6X3 | T42.6X4 | T42.6X5 | T42.6X |
| **Trichloroethylene** (liquid) (vapor) | T53.2X1 | T53.2X2 | T53.2X3 | T53.2X4 | — | — |
| anesthetic (gas) | T41.ØX1 | T41.ØX2 | T41.ØX3 | T41.ØX4 | T41.ØX5 | T41.ØX |
| vapor NEC | T53.2X1 | T53.2X2 | T53.2X3 | T53.2X4 | — | — |
| **Trichlorofluoromethane NEC** | T53.5X1 | T53.5X2 | T53.5X3 | T53.5X4 | — | — |
| **Trichloronate** | T6Ø.ØX1 | T6Ø.ØX2 | T6Ø.ØX3 | T6Ø.ØX4 | — | — |
| **Trichloropropane** | T53.6X1 | T53.6X2 | T53.6X3 | T53.6X4 | — | — |
| **Trichlorotriethylamine** | T45.1X1 | T45.1X2 | T45.1X3 | T45.1X4 | T45.1X5 | T45.1X |
| **Trichomonacides NEC** | T37.3X1 | T37.3X2 | T37.3X3 | T37.3X4 | T37.3X5 | T37.3X |
| **Trichomycin** | T36.7X1 | T36.7X2 | T36.7X3 | T36.7X4 | T36.7X5 | T36.7X |
| **Triclobisonium chloride** | T49.ØX1 | T49.ØX2 | T49.ØX3 | T49.ØX4 | T49.ØX5 | T49.ØX |
| **Triclocarban** | T49.ØX1 | T49.ØX2 | T49.ØX3 | T49.ØX4 | T49.ØX5 | T49.ØX |
| **Triclofos** | T42.6X1 | T42.6X2 | T42.6X3 | T42.6X4 | T42.6X5 | T42.6X |
| **Triclosan** | T49.ØX1 | T49.ØX2 | T49.ØX3 | T49.ØX4 | T49.ØX5 | T49.ØX |
| **Tricosal*** | T39.Ø91 | T39.Ø92 | T39.Ø93 | T39.Ø94 | T39.Ø95 | T39.Ø9 |
| **Tricresyl phosphate** | T65.891 | T65.892 | T65.893 | T65.894 | — | — |
| solvent | T52.91 | T52.92 | T52.93 | T52.94 | — | — |
| **Tricyclamol chloride** | T44.3X1 | T44.3X2 | T44.3X3 | T44.3X4 | T44.3X5 | T44.3X |
| **Tridesilon** | T49.ØX1 | T49.ØX2 | T49.ØX3 | T49.ØX4 | T49.ØX5 | T49.ØX |

| Substance | Poisoning, Accidental (unintentional) | Poisoning, Intentional Self-harm | Poisoning, Assault | Poisoning, Undetermined | Adverse Effect | Under-dosing |
|---|---|---|---|---|---|---|
| **Tridihexethyl iodide** | T44.3X1 | T44.3X2 | T44.3X3 | T44.3X4 | T44.3X5 | T44.3X6 |
| **Tridione** | T42.2X1 | T42.2X2 | T42.2X3 | T42.2X4 | T42.2X5 | T42.2X6 |
| **Trientine** | T45.8X1 | T45.8X2 | T45.8X3 | T45.8X4 | T45.8X5 | T45.8X6 |
| **Triethanolamine NEC** | T54.3X1 | T54.3X2 | T54.3X3 | T54.3X4 | — | — |
| detergent | T54.3X1 | T54.3X2 | T54.3X3 | T54.3X4 | — | — |
| trinitrate (biphosphate) | T46.3X1 | T46.3X2 | T46.3X3 | T46.3X4 | T46.3X5 | T46.3X6 |
| **Triethanomelamine** | T45.1X1 | T45.1X2 | T45.1X3 | T45.1X4 | T45.1X5 | T45.1X6 |
| **Triethylenemelamine** | T45.1X1 | T45.1X2 | T45.1X3 | T45.1X4 | T45.1X5 | T45.1X6 |
| **Triethylenephosphoramide** | T45.1X1 | T45.1X2 | T45.1X3 | T45.1X4 | T45.1X5 | T45.1X6 |
| **Triethylenethiophosphoramide** | T45.1X1 | T45.1X2 | T45.1X3 | T45.1X4 | T45.1X5 | T45.1X6 |
| **Trifluoperazine** | T43.3X1 | T43.3X2 | T43.3X3 | T43.3X4 | T43.3X5 | T43.3X6 |
| **Trifluoroethyl vinyl ether** | T41.ØX1 | T41.ØX2 | T41.ØX3 | T41.ØX4 | T41.ØX5 | T41.ØX6 |
| **Trifluperidol** | T43.4X1 | T43.4X2 | T43.4X3 | T43.4X4 | T43.4X5 | T43.4X6 |
| **Triflupromazine** | T43.3X1 | T43.3X2 | T43.3X3 | T43.3X4 | T43.3X5 | T43.3X6 |
| **Trifluridine** | T37.5X1 | T37.5X2 | T37.5X3 | T37.5X4 | T37.5X5 | T37.5X6 |
| **Triflusal** | T45.521 | T45.522 | T45.523 | T45.524 | T45.525 | T45.526 |
| **Trihexyphenidyl** | T44.3X1 | T44.3X2 | T44.3X3 | T44.3X4 | T44.3X5 | T44.3X6 |
| **Triiodothyronine** | T38.1X1 | T38.1X2 | T38.1X3 | T38.1X4 | T38.1X5 | T38.1X6 |
| **Trilene** | T41.ØX1 | T41.ØX2 | T41.ØX3 | T41.ØX4 | T41.ØX5 | T41.ØX6 |
| **Trilostane** | T38.991 | T38.992 | T38.993 | T38.994 | T38.995 | T38.996 |
| **Trimebutine** | T44.3X1 | T44.3X2 | T44.3X3 | T44.3X4 | T44.3X5 | T44.3X6 |
| **Trimecaine** | T41.3X1 | T41.3X2 | T41.3X3 | T41.3X4 | T41.3X5 | T41.3X6 |
| **Trimeprazine** (tartrate) | T44.3X1 | T44.3X2 | T44.3X3 | T44.3X4 | T44.3X5 | T44.3X6 |
| **Trimetaphan camsilate** | T44.2X1 | T44.2X2 | T44.2X3 | T44.2X4 | T44.2X5 | T44.2X6 |
| **Trimetazidine** | T46.7X1 | T46.7X2 | T46.7X3 | T46.7X4 | T46.7X5 | T46.7X6 |
| **Trimethadione** | T42.2X1 | T42.2X2 | T42.2X3 | T42.2X4 | T42.2X5 | T42.2X6 |
| **Trimethaphan** | T44.2X1 | T44.2X2 | T44.2X3 | T44.2X4 | T44.2X5 | T44.2X6 |
| **Trimethidinium** | T44.2X1 | T44.2X2 | T44.2X3 | T44.2X4 | T44.2X5 | T44.2X6 |
| **Trimethobenzamide** | T45.ØX1 | T45.ØX2 | T45.ØX3 | T45.ØX4 | T45.ØX5 | T45.ØX6 |
| **Trimethoprim** | T37.8X1 | T37.8X2 | T37.8X3 | T37.8X4 | T37.8X5 | T37.8X6 |
| with sulfamethoxazole | T36.8X1 | T36.8X2 | T36.8X3 | T36.8X4 | T36.8X5 | T36.8X6 |
| **Trimethylcarbinol** | T51.3X1 | T51.3X2 | T51.3X3 | T51.3X4 | — | — |
| **Trimethylpsoralen** | T49.3X1 | T49.3X2 | T49.3X3 | T49.3X4 | T49.3X5 | T49.3X6 |
| **Trimeton** | T45.ØX1 | T45.ØX2 | T45.ØX3 | T45.ØX4 | T45.ØX5 | T45.ØX6 |
| **Trimetrexate** | T45.1X1 | T45.1X2 | T45.1X3 | T45.1X4 | T45.1X5 | T45.1X6 |
| **Trimipramine** | T43.Ø11 | T43.Ø12 | T43.Ø13 | T43.Ø14 | T43.Ø15 | T43.Ø16 |
| **Trimox*** | T36.ØX1 | T36.ØX2 | T36.ØX3 | T36.ØX4 | T36.ØX5 | T36.ØX6 |
| **Trimustine** | T45.1X1 | T45.1X2 | T45.1X3 | T45.1X4 | T45.1X5 | T45.1X6 |
| **Trinitrine** | T46.3X1 | T46.3X2 | T46.3X3 | T46.3X4 | T46.3X5 | T46.3X6 |
| **Trinitrobenzol** | T65.3X1 | T65.3X2 | T65.3X3 | T65.3X4 | — | — |
| **Trinitrophenol** | T65.3X1 | T65.3X2 | T65.3X3 | T65.3X4 | — | — |
| **Trinitrotoluene** (fumes) | T65.3X1 | T65.3X2 | T65.3X3 | T65.3X4 | — | — |
| **Trional** | T42.6X1 | T42.6X2 | T42.6X3 | T42.6X4 | T42.6X5 | T42.6X6 |
| **Triorthocresyl phosphate** | T65.891 | T65.892 | T65.893 | T65.894 | — | — |
| **Trioxide of arsenic** | T57.ØX1 | T57.ØX2 | T57.ØX3 | T57.ØX4 | — | — |
| **Trioxysalen** | T49.4X1 | T49.4X2 | T49.4X3 | T49.4X4 | T49.4X5 | T49.4X6 |
| **Tripamide** | T5Ø.2X1 | T5Ø.2X2 | T5Ø.2X3 | T5Ø.2X4 | T5Ø.2X5 | T5Ø.2X6 |
| **Triparanol** | T46.6X1 | T46.6X2 | T46.6X3 | T46.6X4 | T46.6X5 | T46.6X6 |
| **Tripelennamine** | T45.ØX1 | T45.ØX2 | T45.ØX3 | T45.ØX4 | T45.ØX5 | T45.ØX6 |
| **Triperiden** | T44.3X1 | T44.3X2 | T44.3X3 | T44.3X4 | T44.3X5 | T44.3X6 |
| **Triperidol** | T43.4X1 | T43.4X2 | T43.4X3 | T43.4X4 | T43.4X5 | T43.4X6 |
| **Triphenylphosphate** | T65.891 | T65.892 | T65.893 | T65.894 | — | — |
| **Triple** | | | | | | |
| bromides | T42.6X1 | T42.6X2 | T42.6X3 | T42.6X4 | T42.6X5 | T42.6X6 |
| carbonate | T47.1X1 | T47.1X2 | T47.1X3 | T47.1X4 | T47.1X5 | T47.1X6 |
| vaccine | | | | | | |
| DPT | T5Ø.A11 | T5Ø.A12 | T5Ø.A13 | T5Ø.A14 | T5Ø.A15 | T5Ø.A16 |
| including pertussis | T5Ø.A11 | T5Ø.A12 | T5Ø.A13 | T5Ø.A14 | T5Ø.A15 | T5Ø.A16 |
| MMR | T5Ø.B91 | T5Ø.B92 | T5Ø.B93 | T5Ø.B94 | T5Ø.B95 | T5Ø.B96 |
| **Triprolidine** | T45.ØX1 | T45.ØX2 | T45.ØX3 | T45.ØX4 | T45.ØX5 | T45.ØX6 |
| **Trisodium hydrogen edetate** | T5Ø.6X1 | T5Ø.6X2 | T5Ø.6X3 | T5Ø.6X4 | T5Ø.6X5 | T5Ø.6X6 |
| **Trisoralen** | T49.3X1 | T49.3X2 | T49.3X3 | T49.3X4 | T49.3X5 | T49.3X6 |
| **Trisulfapyrimidines** | T37.ØX1 | T37.ØX2 | T37.ØX3 | T37.ØX4 | T37.ØX5 | T37.ØX6 |
| **Trithiozine** | T44.3X1 | T44.3X2 | T44.3X3 | T44.3X4 | T44.3X5 | T44.3X6 |
| **Tritiozine** | T44.3X1 | T44.3X2 | T44.3X3 | T44.3X4 | T44.3X5 | T44.3X6 |
| **Tritoqualine** | T45.ØX1 | T45.ØX2 | T45.ØX3 | T45.ØX4 | T45.ØX5 | T45.ØX6 |
| **Trizivir*** | T37.5X1 | T37.5X2 | T37.5X3 | T37.5X4 | T37.5X5 | T37.5X6 |
| **Trofosfamide** | T45.1X1 | T45.1X2 | T45.1X3 | T45.1X4 | T45.1X5 | T45.1X6 |
| **Troleandomycin** | T36.3X1 | T36.3X2 | T36.3X3 | T36.3X4 | T36.3X5 | T36.3X6 |
| **Trolnitrate** (phosphate) | T46.3X1 | T46.3X2 | T46.3X3 | T46.3X4 | T46.3X5 | T46.3X6 |
| **Tromantadine** | T37.5X1 | T37.5X2 | T37.5X3 | T37.5X4 | T37.5X5 | T37.5X6 |
| **Trometamol** | T5Ø.2X1 | T5Ø.2X2 | T5Ø.2X3 | T5Ø.2X4 | T5Ø.2X5 | T5Ø.2X6 |
| **Tromethamine** | T5Ø.2X1 | T5Ø.2X2 | T5Ø.2X3 | T5Ø.2X4 | T5Ø.2X5 | T5Ø.2X6 |
| **Tronothane** | T41.3X1 | T41.3X2 | T41.3X3 | T41.3X4 | T41.3X5 | T41.3X6 |
| **Tropacine** | T44.3X1 | T44.3X2 | T44.3X3 | T44.3X4 | T44.3X5 | T44.3X6 |
| **Tropatepine** | T44.3X1 | T44.3X2 | T44.3X3 | T44.3X4 | T44.3X5 | T44.3X6 |
| **Tropicamide** | T44.3X1 | T44.3X2 | T44.3X3 | T44.3X4 | T44.3X5 | T44.3X6 |
| **Trospium chloride** | T44.3X1 | T44.3X2 | T44.3X3 | T44.3X4 | T44.3X5 | T44.3X6 |
| **Troxerutin** | T46.991 | T46.992 | T46.993 | T46.994 | T46.995 | T46.996 |
| **Troxidone** | T42.2X1 | T42.2X2 | T42.2X3 | T42.2X4 | T42.2X5 | T42.2X6 |
| **Tryparsamide** | T37.3X1 | T37.3X2 | T37.3X3 | T37.3X4 | T37.3X5 | T37.3X6 |

| Substance | Poisoning, Accidental (unintentional) | Poisoning, Intentional Self-harm | Poisoning, Assault | Poisoning, Undetermined | Adverse Effect | Under-dosing |
|---|---|---|---|---|---|---|
| **Trypsin** | T45.3X1 | T45.3X2 | T45.3X3 | T45.3X4 | T45.3X5 | T45.3X6 |
| **Tryptizol** | T43.Ø11 | T43.Ø12 | T43.Ø13 | T43.Ø14 | T43.Ø15 | T43.Ø16 |
| **TSH** | T38.811 | T38.812 | T38.813 | T38.814 | T38.815 | T38.816 |
| **Tuaminoheptane** | T48.5X1 | T48.5X2 | T48.5X3 | T48.5X4 | T48.5X5 | T48.5X6 |
| **Tuberculin, purified protein derivative** (PPD) | T5Ø.8X1 | T5Ø.8X2 | T5Ø.8X3 | T5Ø.8X4 | T5Ø.8X5 | T5Ø.8X6 |
| **Tubocurare** | T48.1X1 | T48.1X2 | T48.1X3 | T48.1X4 | T48.1X5 | T48.1X6 |
| **Tubocurarine** (chloride) | T48.1X1 | T48.1X2 | T48.1X3 | T48.1X4 | T48.1X5 | T48.1X6 |
| **Tulobuterol** | T48.6X1 | T48.6X2 | T48.6X3 | T48.6X4 | T48.6X5 | T48.6X6 |
| **Turpentine** (spirits of) | T52.811 | T52.812 | T52.813 | T52.814 | — | — |
| vapor | T52.811 | T52.812 | T52.813 | T52.814 | — | — |
| **Twinrix*** | T5Ø.B91 | T5Ø.B92 | T5Ø.B93 | T5Ø.B94 | T5Ø.B95 | T5Ø.B96 |
| **Tybamate** | T43.591 | T43.592 | T43.593 | T43.594 | T43.595 | T43.596 |
| **Tygacil*** | T36.4X1 | T36.4X2 | T36.4X3 | T36.4X4 | T36.4X5 | T36.4X6 |
| **Tyloxapol** | T48.4X1 | T48.4X2 | T48.4X3 | T48.4X4 | T48.4X5 | T48.4X6 |
| **Tymazoline** | T48.5X1 | T48.5X2 | T48.5X3 | T48.5X4 | T48.5X5 | T48.5X6 |
| **Tymlos*** | T5Ø.991 | T5Ø.992 | T5Ø.993 | T5Ø.994 | T5Ø.995 | T5Ø.996 |
| **Typhoid-paratyphoid vaccine** | T5Ø.A91 | T5Ø.A92 | T5Ø.A93 | T5Ø.A94 | T5Ø.A95 | T5Ø.A96 |
| **Typhus vaccine** | T5Ø.A91 | T5Ø.A92 | T5Ø.A93 | T5Ø.A94 | T5Ø.A95 | T5Ø.A96 |
| **Tyropanoate** | T5Ø.8X1 | T5Ø.8X2 | T5Ø.8X3 | T5Ø.8X4 | T5Ø.8X5 | T5Ø.8X6 |
| **Tyrothricin** | T49.6X1 | T49.6X2 | T49.6X3 | T49.6X4 | T49.6X5 | T49.6X6 |
| ENT agent | T49.6X1 | T49.6X2 | T49.6X3 | T49.6X4 | T49.6X5 | T49.6X6 |
| ophthalmic preparation | T49.5X1 | T49.5X2 | T49.5X3 | T49.5X4 | T49.5X5 | T49.5X6 |
| **Ufenamate** | T39.391 | T39.392 | T39.393 | T39.394 | T39.395 | T39.396 |
| **Ultraviolet light protectant** | T49.3X1 | T49.3X2 | T49.3X3 | T49.3X4 | T49.3X5 | T49.3X6 |
| **Unasyn*** | T36.ØX1 | T36.ØX2 | T36.ØX3 | T36.ØX4 | T36.ØX5 | T36.ØX6 |
| **Undecenoic acid** | T49.ØX1 | T49.ØX2 | T49.ØX3 | T49.ØX4 | T49.ØX5 | T49.ØX6 |
| **Undecoylium** | T49.ØX1 | T49.ØX2 | T49.ØX3 | T49.ØX4 | T49.ØX5 | T49.ØX6 |
| **Undecylenic acid** (derivatives) | T49.ØX1 | T49.ØX2 | T49.ØX3 | T49.ØX4 | T49.ØX5 | T49.ØX6 |
| **Unithroid*** | T38.1X1 | T38.1X2 | T38.1X3 | T38.1X4 | T38.1X5 | T38.1X6 |
| **Unna's boot** | T49.3X1 | T49.3X2 | T49.3X3 | T49.3X4 | T49.3X5 | T49.3X6 |
| **Unsaturated fatty acid** | T46.6X1 | T46.6X2 | T46.6X3 | T46.6X4 | T46.6X5 | T46.6X6 |
| **Uracil mustard** | T45.1X1 | T45.1X2 | T45.1X3 | T45.1X4 | T45.1X5 | T45.1X6 |
| **Uramustine** | T45.1X1 | T45.1X2 | T45.1X3 | T45.1X4 | T45.1X5 | T45.1X6 |
| **Urapidil** | T46.5X1 | T46.5X2 | T46.5X3 | T46.5X4 | T46.5X5 | T46.5X6 |
| **Urari** | T48.1X1 | T48.1X2 | T48.1X3 | T48.1X4 | T48.1X5 | T48.1X6 |
| **Urate oxidase** | T5Ø.4X1 | T5Ø.4X2 | T5Ø.4X3 | T5Ø.4X4 | T5Ø.4X5 | T5Ø.4X6 |
| **Urea** | T47.3X1 | T47.3X2 | T47.3X3 | T47.3X4 | T47.3X5 | T47.3X6 |
| peroxide | T49.ØX1 | T49.ØX2 | T49.ØX3 | T49.ØX4 | T49.ØX5 | T49.ØX6 |
| stibamine | T37.4X1 | T37.4X2 | T37.4X3 | T37.4X4 | T37.4X5 | T37.4X6 |
| topical | T49.8X1 | T49.8X2 | T49.8X3 | T49.8X4 | T49.8X5 | T49.8X6 |
| **Ureaphil*** | T48.ØX1 | T48.ØX2 | T48.ØX3 | T48.ØX4 | T48.ØX5 | T48.ØX6 |
| **Urethane** | T45.1X1 | T45.1X2 | T45.1X3 | T45.1X4 | T45.1X5 | T45.1X6 |
| **Urginea** (maritima) (scilla) — *see* Squill | | | | | | |
| **Uric acid metabolism drug NEC** | T5Ø.4X1 | T5Ø.4X2 | T5Ø.4X3 | T5Ø.4X4 | T5Ø.4X5 | T5Ø.4X6 |
| **Uricosuric agent** | T5Ø.4X1 | T5Ø.4X2 | T5Ø.4X3 | T5Ø.4X4 | T5Ø.4X5 | T5Ø.4X6 |
| **Urinary anti-infective** | T37.8X1 | T37.8X2 | T37.8X3 | T37.8X4 | T37.8X5 | T37.8X6 |
| **Urofollitropin** | T38.811 | T38.812 | T38.813 | T38.814 | T38.815 | T38.816 |
| **Urokinase** | T45.611 | T45.612 | T45.613 | T45.614 | T45.615 | T45.616 |
| **Urokon** | T5Ø.8X1 | T5Ø.8X2 | T5Ø.8X3 | T5Ø.8X4 | T5Ø.8X5 | T5Ø.8X6 |
| **Ursodeoxycholic acid** | T5Ø.991 | T5Ø.992 | T5Ø.993 | T5Ø.994 | T5Ø.995 | T5Ø.996 |
| **Ursodiol** | T5Ø.991 | T5Ø.992 | T5Ø.993 | T5Ø.994 | T5Ø.995 | T5Ø.996 |
| **Urtica** | T62.2X1 | T62.2X2 | T62.2X3 | T62.2X4 | — | — |
| **Utility gas** — *see* Gas, utility | | | | | | |
| **Vaccine NEC** | T5Ø.Z91 | T5Ø.Z92 | T5Ø.Z93 | T5Ø.Z94 | T5Ø.Z95 | T5Ø.Z96 |
| antineoplastic | T5Ø.Z91 | T5Ø.Z92 | T5Ø.Z93 | T5Ø.Z94 | T5Ø.Z95 | T5Ø.Z96 |
| bacterial NEC | T5Ø.A91 | T5Ø.A92 | T5Ø.A93 | T5Ø.A94 | T5Ø.A95 | T5Ø.A96 |
| mixed NEC | T5Ø.A21 | T5Ø.A22 | T5Ø.A23 | T5Ø.A24 | T5Ø.A25 | T5Ø.A26 |
| with | | | | | | |
| other bacterial component | T5Ø.A21 | T5Ø.A22 | T5Ø.A23 | T5Ø.A24 | T5Ø.A25 | T5Ø.A26 |
| pertussis component | T5Ø.A11 | T5Ø.A12 | T5Ø.A13 | T5Ø.A14 | T5Ø.A15 | T5Ø.A16 |
| viral-rickettsial component | T5Ø.A21 | T5Ø.A22 | T5Ø.A23 | T5Ø.A24 | T5Ø.A25 | T5Ø.A26 |
| BCG | T5Ø.A91 | T5Ø.A92 | T5Ø.A93 | T5Ø.A94 | T5Ø.A95 | T5Ø.A96 |
| cholera | T5Ø.A91 | T5Ø.A92 | T5Ø.A93 | T5Ø.A94 | T5Ø.A95 | T5Ø.A96 |
| diphtheria | T5Ø.A91 | T5Ø.A92 | T5Ø.A93 | T5Ø.A94 | T5Ø.A95 | T5Ø.A96 |
| with tetanus | T5Ø.A21 | T5Ø.A22 | T5Ø.A23 | T5Ø.A24 | T5Ø.A25 | T5Ø.A26 |
| and pertussis | T5Ø.A11 | T5Ø.A12 | T5Ø.A13 | T5Ø.A14 | T5Ø.A15 | T5Ø.A16 |
| influenza | T5Ø.B91 | T5Ø.B92 | T5Ø.B93 | T5Ø.B94 | T5Ø.B95 | T5Ø.B96 |
| measles | T5Ø.B91 | T5Ø.B92 | T5Ø.B93 | T5Ø.B94 | T5Ø.B95 | T5Ø.B96 |
| with mumps and rubella | T5Ø.B91 | T5Ø.B92 | T5Ø.B93 | T5Ø.B94 | T5Ø.B95 | T5Ø.B96 |
| meningococcal | T5Ø.A91 | T5Ø.A92 | T5Ø.A93 | T5Ø.A94 | T5Ø.A95 | T5Ø.A96 |
| mumps | T5Ø.B91 | T5Ø.B92 | T5Ø.B93 | T5Ø.B94 | T5Ø.B95 | T5Ø.B96 |
| paratyphoid | T5Ø.A91 | T5Ø.A92 | T5Ø.A93 | T5Ø.A94 | T5Ø.A95 | T5Ø.A96 |
| pertussis | T5Ø.A11 | T5Ø.A12 | T5Ø.A13 | T5Ø.A14 | T5Ø.A15 | T5Ø.A16 |
| with diphtheria | T5Ø.A11 | T5Ø.A12 | T5Ø.A13 | T5Ø.A14 | T5Ø.A15 | T5Ø.A16 |
| and tetanus | T5Ø.A11 | T5Ø.A12 | T5Ø.A13 | T5Ø.A14 | T5Ø.A15 | T5Ø.A16 |

| Substance | Poisoning, Accidental (unintentional) | Poisoning, Intentional Self-harm | Poisoning, Assault | Poisoning, Undetermined | Adverse Effect | Under-dosing |
|---|---|---|---|---|---|---|
| **Vaccine** — *continued* | | | | | | |
| pertussis — *continued* | | | | | | |
| with other component | T5Ø.A11 | T5Ø.A12 | T5Ø.A13 | T5Ø.A14 | T5Ø.A15 | T5Ø.A16 |
| plague | T5Ø.A91 | T5Ø.A92 | T5Ø.A93 | T5Ø.A94 | T5Ø.A95 | T5Ø.A96 |
| poliomyelitis | T5Ø.B91 | T5Ø.B92 | T5Ø.B93 | T5Ø.B94 | T5Ø.B95 | T5Ø.B96 |
| poliovirus | T5Ø.B91 | T5Ø.B92 | T5Ø.B93 | T5Ø.B94 | T5Ø.B95 | T5Ø.B96 |
| rabies | T5Ø.B91 | T5Ø.B92 | T5Ø.B93 | T5Ø.B94 | T5Ø.B95 | T5Ø.B96 |
| respiratory syncytial virus | T5Ø.B91 | T5Ø.B92 | T5Ø.B93 | T5Ø.B94 | T5Ø.B95 | T5Ø.B96 |
| rickettsial NEC | T5Ø.A91 | T5Ø.A92 | T5Ø.A93 | T5Ø.A94 | T5Ø.A95 | T5Ø.A96 |
| with | | | | | | |
| bacterial component | T5Ø.A21 | T5Ø.A22 | T5Ø.A23 | T5Ø.A24 | T5Ø.A25 | T5Ø.A26 |
| Rocky Mountain spotted fever | T5Ø.A91 | T5Ø.A92 | T5Ø.A93 | T5Ø.A94 | T5Ø.A95 | T5Ø.A96 |
| rubella | T5Ø.B91 | T5Ø.B92 | T5Ø.B93 | T5Ø.B94 | T5Ø.B95 | T5Ø.B96 |
| sabin oral | T5Ø.B91 | T5Ø.B92 | T5Ø.B93 | T5Ø.B94 | T5Ø.B95 | T5Ø.B96 |
| smallpox | T5Ø.B11 | T5Ø.B12 | T5Ø.B13 | T5Ø.B14 | T5Ø.B15 | T5Ø.B16 |
| TAB | T5Ø.A91 | T5Ø.A92 | T5Ø.A93 | T5Ø.A94 | T5Ø.A95 | T5Ø.A96 |
| tetanus | T5Ø.A91 | T5Ø.A92 | T5Ø.A93 | T5Ø.A94 | T5Ø.A95 | T5Ø.A96 |
| typhoid | T5Ø.A91 | T5Ø.A92 | T5Ø.A93 | T5Ø.A94 | T5Ø.A95 | T5Ø.A96 |
| typhus | T5Ø.A91 | T5Ø.A92 | T5Ø.A93 | T5Ø.A94 | T5Ø.A95 | T5Ø.A96 |
| viral NEC | T5Ø.B91 | T5Ø.B92 | T5Ø.B93 | T5Ø.B94 | T5Ø.B95 | T5Ø.B96 |
| yellow fever | T5Ø.B91 | T5Ø.B92 | T5Ø.B93 | T5Ø.B94 | T5Ø.B95 | T5Ø.B96 |
| **Vaccinia immune globulin** | T5Ø.Z11 | T5Ø.Z12 | T5Ø.Z13 | T5Ø.Z14 | T5Ø.Z15 | T5Ø.Z16 |
| **Vaginal contraceptives** | T49.8X1 | T49.8X2 | T49.8X3 | T49.8X4 | T49.8X5 | T49.8X6 |
| **Valacyclovir*** | T37.5X1 | T37.5X2 | T37.5X3 | T37.5X4 | T37.5X5 | T37.5X6 |
| **Valerian** | | | | | | |
| root | T42.6X1 | T42.6X2 | T42.6X3 | T42.6X4 | T42.6X5 | T42.6X6 |
| tincture | T42.6X1 | T42.6X2 | T42.6X3 | T42.6X4 | T42.6X5 | T42.6X6 |
| **Valethamate bromide** | T44.3X1 | T44.3X2 | T44.3X3 | T44.3X4 | T44.3X5 | T44.3X6 |
| **Valisone** | T49.ØX1 | T49.ØX2 | T49.ØX3 | T49.ØX4 | T49.ØX5 | T49.ØX6 |
| **Valium** | T42.4X1 | T42.4X2 | T42.4X3 | T42.4X4 | T42.4X5 | T42.4X6 |
| **Valmid** | T42.6X1 | T42.6X2 | T42.6X3 | T42.6X4 | T42.6X5 | T42.6X6 |
| **Valnoctamide** | T42.6X1 | T42.6X2 | T42.6X3 | T42.6X4 | T42.6X5 | T42.6X6 |
| **Valproate** (sodium) | T42.6X1 | T42.6X2 | T42.6X3 | T42.6X4 | T42.6X5 | T42.6X6 |
| **Valproic acid** | T42.6X1 | T42.6X2 | T42.6X3 | T42.6X4 | T42.6X5 | T42.6X6 |
| **Valpromide** | T42.6X1 | T42.6X2 | T42.6X3 | T42.6X4 | T42.6X5 | T42.6X6 |
| **Vanadium** | T56.891 | T56.892 | T56.893 | T56.894 | — | — |
| **Vancomycin** | T36.8X1 | T36.8X2 | T36.8X3 | T36.8X4 | T36.8X5 | T36.8X6 |
| **Vandazole*** | T49.ØX1 | T49.ØX2 | T49.ØX3 | T49.ØX4 | T49.ØX5 | T49.ØX6 |
| **Vapor** — *see also* Gas | T59.91 | T59.92 | T59.93 | T59.94 | — | — |
| kiln (carbon monoxide) | T58.8X1 | T58.8X2 | T58.8X3 | T58.8X4 | — | — |
| lead — *see* lead | | | | | | |
| specified source NEC | T59.891 | T59.892 | T59.893 | T59.894 | — | — |
| **Vardenafil** | T46.7X1 | T46.7X2 | T46.7X3 | T46.7X4 | T46.7X5 | T46.7X6 |
| **Varicose reduction drug** | T46.8X1 | T46.8X2 | T46.8X3 | T46.8X4 | T46.8X5 | T46.8X6 |
| **Varnish** | T65.4X1 | T65.4X2 | T65.4X3 | T65.4X4 | — | — |
| cleaner | T52.91 | T52.92 | T52.93 | T52.94 | — | — |
| **Vaseline** | T49.3X1 | T49.3X2 | T49.3X3 | T49.3X4 | T49.3X5 | T49.3X6 |
| **Vasodilan** | T46.7X1 | T46.7X2 | T46.7X3 | T46.7X4 | T46.7X5 | T46.7X6 |
| **Vasodilator** | | | | | | |
| coronary NEC | T46.3X1 | T46.3X2 | T46.3X3 | T46.3X4 | T46.3X5 | T46.3X6 |
| peripheral NEC | T46.7X1 | T46.7X2 | T46.7X3 | T46.7X4 | T46.7X5 | T46.7X6 |
| **Vasopressin** | T38.891 | T38.892 | T38.893 | T38.894 | T38.895 | T38.896 |
| **Vasopressor drugs** | T38.891 | T38.892 | T38.893 | T38.894 | T38.895 | T38.896 |
| **Vecuronium bromide** | T48.1X1 | T48.1X2 | T48.1X3 | T48.1X4 | T48.1X5 | T48.1X6 |
| **Vegetable extract, astringent** | T49.2X1 | T49.2X2 | T49.2X3 | T49.2X4 | T49.2X5 | T49.2X6 |
| **Venlafaxine** | T43.211 | T43.212 | T43.213 | T43.214 | T43.215 | T43.216 |
| **Venom, venomous** (bite) (sting) | T63.91 | T63.92 | T63.93 | T63.94 | — | — |
| amphibian NEC | T63.831 | T63.832 | T63.833 | T63.834 | — | — |
| animal NEC | T63.891 | T63.892 | T63.893 | T63.894 | — | — |
| ant | T63.421 | T63.422 | T63.423 | T63.424 | — | — |
| arthropod NEC | T63.481 | T63.482 | T63.483 | T63.484 | — | — |
| bee | T63.441 | T63.442 | T63.443 | T63.444 | — | — |
| centipede | T63.411 | T63.412 | T63.413 | T63.414 | — | — |
| fish | T63.591 | T63.592 | T63.593 | T63.594 | — | — |
| frog | T63.811 | T63.812 | T63.813 | T63.814 | — | — |
| hornet | T63.451 | T63.452 | T63.453 | T63.454 | — | — |
| insect NEC | T63.481 | T63.482 | T63.483 | T63.484 | — | — |
| lizard | T63.121 | T63.122 | T63.123 | T63.124 | — | — |
| marine | | | | | | |
| animals | T63.691 | T63.692 | T63.693 | T63.694 | — | — |
| bluebottle | T63.611 | T63.612 | T63.613 | T63.614 | — | — |
| jellyfish NEC | T63.621 | T63.622 | T63.623 | T63.624 | — | — |
| Portuguese Man-o-war | T63.611 | T63.612 | T63.613 | T63.614 | — | — |
| sea anemone | T63.631 | T63.632 | T63.633 | T63.634 | — | — |
| specified NEC | T63.691 | T63.692 | T63.693 | T63.694 | — | — |
| fish | T63.591 | T63.592 | T63.593 | T63.594 | — | — |
| plants | T63.711 | T63.712 | T63.713 | T63.714 | — | — |
| sting ray | T63.511 | T63.512 | T63.513 | T63.514 | — | — |
| millipede (tropical) | T63.411 | T63.412 | T63.413 | T63.414 | — | — |
| plant NEC | T63.791 | T63.792 | T63.793 | T63.794 | — | — |

| Substance | Poisoning, Accidental (unintentional) | Poisoning, Intentional Self-harm | Poisoning, Assault | Poisoning, Undetermined | Adverse Effect | Under-dosing |
|---|---|---|---|---|---|---|
| **Venom, venomous** — *continued* | | | | | | |
| plant — *continued* | | | | | | |
| marine | T63.711 | T63.712 | T63.713 | T63.714 | — | — |
| reptile | T63.191 | T63.192 | T63.193 | T63.194 | — | — |
| gila monster | T63.111 | T63.112 | T63.113 | T63.114 | — | — |
| lizard NEC | T63.121 | T63.122 | T63.123 | T63.124 | — | — |
| scorpion | T63.2X1 | T63.2X2 | T63.2X3 | T63.2X4 | — | — |
| snake | T63.ØØ1 | T63.ØØ2 | T63.ØØ3 | T63.ØØ4 | — | — |
| African NEC | T63.Ø81 | T63.Ø82 | T63.Ø83 | T63.Ø84 | — | — |
| American (North) (South) NEC | T63.Ø61 | T63.Ø62 | T63.Ø63 | T63.Ø64 | — | — |
| Asian | T63.Ø81 | T63.Ø82 | T63.Ø83 | T63.Ø84 | — | — |
| Australian | T63.Ø71 | T63.Ø72 | T63.Ø73 | T63.Ø74 | — | — |
| cobra | T63.Ø41 | T63.Ø42 | T63.Ø43 | T63.Ø44 | — | — |
| coral snake | T63.Ø21 | T63.Ø22 | T63.Ø23 | T63.Ø24 | — | — |
| rattlesnake | T63.Ø11 | T63.Ø12 | T63.Ø13 | T63.Ø14 | — | — |
| specified NEC | T63.Ø91 | T63.Ø92 | T63.Ø93 | T63.Ø94 | — | — |
| taipan | T63.Ø31 | T63.Ø32 | T63.Ø33 | T63.Ø34 | — | — |
| specified NEC | T63.891 | T63.892 | T63.893 | T63.894 | — | — |
| spider | T63.3Ø1 | T63.3Ø2 | T63.3Ø3 | T63.3Ø4 | — | — |
| black widow | T63.311 | T63.312 | T63.313 | T63.314 | — | — |
| brown recluse | T63.331 | T63.332 | T63.333 | T63.334 | — | — |
| specified NEC | T63.391 | T63.392 | T63.393 | T63.394 | — | — |
| tarantula | T63.321 | T63.322 | T63.323 | T63.324 | — | — |
| sting ray | T63.511 | T63.512 | T63.513 | T63.514 | — | — |
| toad | T63.821 | T63.822 | T63.823 | T63.824 | — | — |
| wasp | T63.461 | T63.462 | T63.463 | T63.464 | — | — |
| **Venous sclerosing drug NEC** | T46.8X1 | T46.8X2 | T46.8X3 | T46.8X4 | T46.8X5 | T46.8X |
| **Ventavis*** | T46.7X1 | T46.7X2 | T46.7X3 | T46.7X4 | T46.7X5 | T46.7X |
| **Ventolin** — *see* Albuterol | | | | | | |
| **Veramon** | T42.3X1 | T42.3X2 | T42.3X3 | T42.3X4 | T42.3X5 | T42.3X |
| **Verapamil** | T46.1X1 | T46.1X2 | T46.1X3 | T46.1X4 | T46.1X5 | T46.1X |
| **Veratrine** | T46.5X1 | T46.5X2 | T46.5X3 | T46.5X4 | T46.5X5 | T46.5X |
| **Veratrum** | | | | | | |
| album | T62.2X1 | T62.2X2 | T62.2X3 | T62.2X4 | — | — |
| alkaloids | T46.5X1 | T46.5X2 | T46.5X3 | T46.5X4 | T46.5X5 | T46.5X |
| viride | T62.2X1 | T62.2X2 | T62.2X3 | T62.2X4 | — | — |
| **Verdigris** | T6Ø.3X1 | T6Ø.3X2 | T6Ø.3X3 | T6Ø.3X4 | — | — |
| **Veronal** | T42.3X1 | T42.3X2 | T42.3X3 | T42.3X4 | T42.3X5 | T42.3X |
| **Veroxil** | T37.4X1 | T37.4X2 | T37.4X3 | T37.4X4 | T37.4X5 | T37.4X |
| **Versenate** | T5Ø.6X1 | T5Ø.6X2 | T5Ø.6X3 | T5Ø.6X4 | T5Ø.6X5 | T5Ø.6X |
| **Versidyne** | T39.8X1 | T39.8X2 | T39.8X3 | T39.8X4 | T39.8X5 | T39.8X |
| **Vetrabutine** | T48.ØX1 | T48.ØX2 | T48.ØX3 | T48.ØX4 | T48.ØX5 | T48.ØX |
| **Vexol*** | T49.5X1 | T49.5X2 | T49.5X3 | T49.5X4 | T49.5X5 | T49.5X |
| **Viagra*** | T46.7X1 | T46.7X2 | T46.7X3 | T46.7X4 | T46.7X5 | T46.7X |
| **Vibramycin*** | T36.4X1 | T36.4X2 | T36.4X3 | T36.4X4 | T36.4X5 | T36.4X |
| **Victrelis*** | T37.5X1 | T37.5X2 | T37.5X3 | T37.5X4 | T37.5X5 | T37.5X |
| **Vidarabine** | T37.5X1 | T37.5X2 | T37.5X3 | T37.5X4 | T37.5X5 | T37.5X |
| **Vienna** | | | | | | |
| green | T57.ØX1 | T57.ØX2 | T57.ØX3 | T57.ØX4 | — | — |
| insecticide | T6Ø.2X1 | T6Ø.2X2 | T6Ø.2X3 | T6Ø.2X4 | — | — |
| red | T57.ØX1 | T57.ØX2 | T57.ØX3 | T57.ØX4 | — | — |
| pharmaceutical dye | T5Ø.991 | T5Ø.992 | T5Ø.993 | T5Ø.994 | T5Ø.995 | T5Ø.99 |
| **Vigabatrin** | T42.6X1 | T42.6X2 | T42.6X3 | T42.6X4 | T42.6X5 | T42.6X |
| **Viloxazine** | T43.291 | T43.292 | T43.293 | T43.294 | T43.295 | T43.29 |
| **Viminol** | T39.8X1 | T39.8X2 | T39.8X3 | T39.8X4 | T39.8X5 | T39.8X |
| **Vinbarbital, vinbarbitone** | T42.3X1 | T42.3X2 | T42.3X3 | T42.3X4 | T42.3X5 | T42.3X |
| **Vinblastine** | T45.1X1 | T45.1X2 | T45.1X3 | T45.1X4 | T45.1X5 | T45.1X |
| **Vinburnine** | T46.7X1 | T46.7X2 | T46.7X3 | T46.7X4 | T46.7X5 | T46.7X |
| **Vincamine** | T45.1X1 | T45.1X2 | T45.1X3 | T45.1X4 | T45.1X5 | T45.1X |
| **Vincristine** | T45.1X1 | T45.1X2 | T45.1X3 | T45.1X4 | T45.1X5 | T45.1X |
| **Vindesine** | T45.1X1 | T45.1X2 | T45.1X3 | T45.1X4 | T45.1X5 | T45.1X |
| **Vinesthene, vinethene** | T41.ØX1 | T41.ØX2 | T41.ØX3 | T41.ØX4 | T41.ØX5 | T41.ØX |
| **Vinorelbine tartrate** | T45.1X1 | T45.1X2 | T45.1X3 | T45.1X4 | T45.1X5 | T45.1X |
| **Vinpocetine** | T46.7X1 | T46.7X2 | T46.7X3 | T46.7X4 | T46.7X5 | T46.7X |
| **Vinyl** | | | | | | |
| acetate | T65.891 | T65.892 | T65.893 | T65.894 | — | — |
| bital | T42.3X1 | T42.3X2 | T42.3X3 | T42.3X4 | T42.3X5 | T42.3X |
| bromide | T65.891 | T65.892 | T65.893 | T65.894 | — | — |
| chloride | T59.891 | T59.892 | T59.893 | T59.894 | — | — |
| ether | T41.ØX1 | T41.ØX2 | T41.ØX3 | T41.ØX4 | T41.ØX5 | T41.ØX |
| **Vinylbital** | T42.3X1 | T42.3X2 | T42.3X3 | T42.3X4 | T42.3X5 | T42.3X |
| **Vinylidene chloride** | T65.891 | T65.892 | T65.893 | T65.894 | — | — |
| **Vioform** | T37.8X1 | T37.8X2 | T37.8X3 | T37.8X4 | T37.8X5 | T37.8X |
| topical | T49.ØX1 | T49.ØX2 | T49.ØX3 | T49.ØX4 | T49.ØX5 | T49.ØX |
| **Viokase*** | T47.5X1 | T47.5X2 | T47.5X3 | T47.5X4 | T47.5X5 | T47.5X |
| **Viomycin** | T36.8X1 | T36.8X2 | T36.8X3 | T36.8X4 | T36.8X5 | T36.8X |
| **Viosterol** | T45.2X1 | T45.2X2 | T45.2X3 | T45.2X4 | T45.2X5 | T45.2X |
| **Viper** (venom) | T63.Ø91 | T63.Ø92 | T63.Ø93 | T63.Ø94 | — | — |
| **Viprynium** | T37.4X1 | T37.4X2 | T37.4X3 | T37.4X4 | T37.4X5 | T37.4X |
| **Viquidil** | T46.7X1 | T46.7X2 | T46.7X3 | T46.7X4 | T46.7X5 | T46.7X |
| **Viral vaccine NEC** | T5Ø.B91 | T5Ø.B92 | T5Ø.B93 | T5Ø.B94 | T5Ø.B95 | T5Ø.B |

| Substance | Poisoning, Accidental (unintentional) | Poisoning, Intentional Self-harm | Poisoning, Assault | Poisoning, Undetermined | Adverse Effect | Under-dosing |
|---|---|---|---|---|---|---|
| **Virginiamycin** | T36.8X1 | T36.8X2 | T36.8X3 | T36.8X4 | T36.8X5 | T36.8X6 |
| **Virugon** | T37.5X1 | T37.5X2 | T37.5X3 | T37.5X4 | T37.5X5 | T37.5X6 |
| **Viscous agent** | T5Ø.9Ø1 | T5Ø.9Ø2 | T5Ø.9Ø3 | T5Ø.9Ø4 | T5Ø.9Ø5 | T5Ø.9Ø6 |
| **Visine** | T49.5X1 | T49.5X2 | T49.5X3 | T49.5X4 | T49.5X5 | T49.5X6 |
| **Visnadine** | T46.3X1 | T46.3X2 | T46.3X3 | T46.3X4 | T46.3X5 | T46.3X6 |
| **Vitamin NEC** | T45.2X1 | T45.2X2 | T45.2X3 | T45.2X4 | T45.2X5 | T45.2X6 |
| A | T45.2X1 | T45.2X2 | T45.2X3 | T45.2X4 | T45.2X5 | T45.2X6 |
| B NEC | T45.2X1 | T45.2X2 | T45.2X3 | T45.2X4 | T45.2X5 | T45.2X6 |
| nicotinic acid | T46.7X1 | T46.7X2 | T46.7X3 | T46.7X4 | T46.7X5 | T46.7X6 |
| B1 | T45.2X1 | T45.2X2 | T45.2X3 | T45.2X4 | T45.2X5 | T45.2X6 |
| B12 | T45.2X1 | T45.2X2 | T45.2X3 | T45.2X4 | T45.2X5 | T45.2X6 |
| B15 | T45.2X1 | T45.2X2 | T45.2X3 | T45.2X4 | T45.2X5 | T45.2X6 |
| B2 | T45.2X1 | T45.2X2 | T45.2X3 | T45.2X4 | T45.2X5 | T45.2X6 |
| B6 | T45.2X1 | T45.2X2 | T45.2X3 | T45.2X4 | T45.2X5 | T45.2X6 |
| C | T45.2X1 | T45.2X2 | T45.2X3 | T45.2X4 | T45.2X5 | T45.2X6 |
| D | T45.2X1 | T45.2X2 | T45.2X3 | T45.2X4 | T45.2X5 | T45.2X6 |
| D2 | T45.2X1 | T45.2X2 | T45.2X3 | T45.2X4 | T45.2X5 | T45.2X6 |
| D3 | T45.2X1 | T45.2X2 | T45.2X3 | T45.2X4 | T45.2X5 | T45.2X6 |
| E | T45.2X1 | T45.2X2 | T45.2X3 | T45.2X4 | T45.2X5 | T45.2X6 |
| E acetate | T45.2X1 | T45.2X2 | T45.2X3 | T45.2X4 | T45.2X5 | T45.2X6 |
| hematopoietic | T45.8X1 | T45.8X2 | T45.8X3 | T45.8X4 | T45.8X5 | T45.8X6 |
| K NEC | T45.7X1 | T45.7X2 | T45.7X3 | T45.7X4 | T45.7X5 | T45.7X6 |
| K1 | T45.7X1 | T45.7X2 | T45.7X3 | T45.7X4 | T45.7X5 | T45.7X6 |
| K2 | T45.7X1 | T45.7X2 | T45.7X3 | T45.7X4 | T45.7X5 | T45.7X6 |
| PP | T45.2X1 | T45.2X2 | T45.2X3 | T45.2X4 | T45.2X5 | T45.2X6 |
| ulceroprotectant | T47.1X1 | T47.1X2 | T47.1X3 | T47.1X4 | T47.1X5 | T47.1X6 |
| **Vleminckx's solution** | T49.4X1 | T49.4X2 | T49.4X3 | T49.4X4 | T49.4X5 | T49.4X6 |
| **Voltaren** — *see* Diclofenac sodium | | | | | | |
| **Voraxaze*** | T5Ø.6X1 | T5Ø.6X2 | T5Ø.6X3 | T5Ø.6X4 | T5Ø.6X5 | T5Ø.6X6 |
| **Warfarin** | T45.511 | T45.512 | T45.513 | T45.514 | T45.515 | T45.516 |
| rodenticide | T6Ø.4X1 | T6Ø.4X2 | T6Ø.4X3 | T6Ø.4X4 | — | — |
| sodium | T45.511 | T45.512 | T45.513 | T45.514 | T45.515 | T45.516 |
| **Wasp** (sting) | T63.461 | T63.462 | T63.463 | T63.464 | — | — |
| **Water** | | | | | | |
| balance drug | T5Ø.3X1 | T5Ø.3X2 | T5Ø.3X3 | T5Ø.3X4 | T5Ø.3X5 | T5Ø.3X6 |
| distilled | T5Ø.3X1 | T5Ø.3X2 | T5Ø.3X3 | T5Ø.3X4 | T5Ø.3X5 | T5Ø.3X6 |
| gas — *see* Gas, water | | | | | | |
| incomplete combustion of — *see* Carbon, monoxide, fuel, utility | | | | | | |
| hemlock | T62.2X1 | T62.2X2 | T62.2X3 | T62.2X4 | — | — |
| moccasin (venom) | T63.Ø61 | T63.Ø62 | T63.Ø63 | T63.Ø64 | — | — |
| purified | T5Ø.3X1 | T5Ø.3X2 | T5Ø.3X3 | T5Ø.3X4 | T5Ø.3X5 | T5Ø.3X6 |
| **Wax** (paraffin) (petroleum) | T52.ØX1 | T52.ØX2 | T52.ØX3 | T52.ØX4 | — | — |
| automobile | T65.891 | T65.892 | T65.893 | T65.894 | — | — |
| floor | T52.ØX1 | T52.ØX2 | T52.ØX3 | T52.ØX4 | — | — |
| **Weed killers NEC** | T6Ø.3X1 | T6Ø.3X2 | T6Ø.3X3 | T6Ø.3X4 | — | — |
| **Wellbutrin*** | T43.291 | T43.292 | T43.293 | T43.294 | T43.295 | T43.296 |
| **Welldorm** | T42.6X1 | T42.6X2 | T42.6X3 | T42.6X4 | T42.6X5 | T42.6X6 |
| **Westcort*** | T49.ØX1 | T49.ØX2 | T49.ØX3 | T49.ØX4 | T49.ØX5 | T49.ØX6 |
| **White** | | | | | | |
| arsenic | T57.ØX1 | T57.ØX2 | T57.ØX3 | T57.ØX4 | — | — |
| hellebore | T62.2X1 | T62.2X2 | T62.2X3 | T62.2X4 | — | — |
| lotion (keratolytic) | T49.4X1 | T49.4X2 | T49.4X3 | T49.4X4 | T49.4X5 | T49.4X6 |
| spirit | T52.ØX1 | T52.ØX2 | T52.ØX3 | T52.ØX4 | — | — |
| **Whitewash** | T65.891 | T65.892 | T65.893 | T65.894 | — | — |
| **Whole blood** (human) | T45.8X1 | T45.8X2 | T45.8X3 | T45.8X4 | T45.8X5 | T45.8X6 |
| **Wild** | | | | | | |
| black cherry | T62.2X1 | T62.2X2 | T62.2X3 | T62.2X4 | — | — |
| poisonous plants NEC | T62.2X1 | T62.2X2 | T62.2X3 | T62.2X4 | — | — |
| **Window cleaning fluid** | T65.891 | T65.892 | T65.893 | T65.894 | — | — |
| **Wintergreen** (oil) | T49.3X1 | T49.3X2 | T49.3X3 | T49.3X4 | T49.3X5 | T49.3X6 |
| **Wisterine** | T62.2X1 | T62.2X2 | T62.2X3 | T62.2X4 | — | — |
| **Witch hazel** | T49.2X1 | T49.2X2 | T49.2X3 | T49.2X4 | T49.2X5 | T49.2X6 |
| **Wood alcohol or spirit** | T51.1X1 | T51.1X2 | T51.1X3 | T51.1X4 | — | — |
| **Wool fat** (hydrous) | T49.3X1 | T49.3X2 | T49.3X3 | T49.3X4 | T49.3X5 | T49.3X6 |
| **Woorali** | T48.1X1 | T48.1X2 | T48.1X3 | T48.1X4 | T48.1X5 | T48.1X6 |
| **Wormseed, American** | T37.4X1 | T37.4X2 | T37.4X3 | T37.4X4 | T37.4X5 | T37.4X6 |
| **Xamoterol** | T44.5X1 | T44.5X2 | T44.5X3 | T44.5X4 | T44.5X5 | T44.5X6 |
| **Xanax*** | T42.4X1 | T42.4X2 | T42.4X3 | T42.4X4 | T42.4X5 | T42.4X6 |
| **Xanthine diuretics** | T5Ø.2X1 | T5Ø.2X2 | T5Ø.2X3 | T5Ø.2X4 | T5Ø.2X5 | T5Ø.2X6 |
| **Xanthinol nicotinate** | T46.7X1 | T46.7X2 | T46.7X3 | T46.7X4 | T46.7X5 | T46.7X6 |
| **Xanthotoxin** | T49.3X1 | T49.3X2 | T49.3X3 | T49.3X4 | T49.3X5 | T49.3X6 |
| **Xantinol nicotinate** | T46.7X1 | T46.7X2 | T46.7X3 | T46.7X4 | T46.7X5 | T46.7X6 |
| **Xantocillin** | T36.ØX1 | T36.ØX2 | T36.ØX3 | T36.ØX4 | T36.ØX5 | T36.ØX6 |
| **Xenon** (127Xe) (133Xe) | T5Ø.8X1 | T5Ø.8X2 | T5Ø.8X3 | T5Ø.8X4 | T5Ø.8X5 | T5Ø.8X6 |
| **Xenysalate** | T49.4X1 | T49.4X2 | T49.4X3 | T49.4X4 | T49.4X5 | T49.4X6 |
| **Xibornol** | T37.8X1 | T37.8X2 | T37.8X3 | T37.8X4 | T37.8X5 | T37.8X6 |
| **Xigris** | T45.511 | T45.512 | T45.513 | T45.514 | T45.515 | T45.516 |
| **Xipamide** | T5Ø.2X1 | T5Ø.2X2 | T5Ø.2X3 | T5Ø.2X4 | T5Ø.2X5 | T5Ø.2X6 |
| **Xylazine** | T65.841 | T65.842 | T65.843 | T65.844 | — | — |
| **Xylene** (vapor) | T52.2X1 | T52.2X2 | T52.2X3 | T52.2X4 | — | — |

| Substance | Poisoning, Accidental (unintentional) | Poisoning, Intentional Self-harm | Poisoning, Assault | Poisoning, Undetermined | Adverse Effect | Under-dosing |
|---|---|---|---|---|---|---|
| **Xylocaine** (infiltration) (topical) | T41.3X1 | T41.3X2 | T41.3X3 | T41.3X4 | T41.3X5 | T41.3X6 |
| nerve block (peripheral) (plexus) | T41.3X1 | T41.3X2 | T41.3X3 | T41.3X4 | T41.3X5 | T41.3X6 |
| spinal | T41.3X1 | T41.3X2 | T41.3X3 | T41.3X4 | T41.3X5 | T41.3X6 |
| **Xylol** (vapor) | T52.2X1 | T52.2X2 | T52.2X3 | T52.2X4 | — | — |
| **Xylometazoline** | T48.5X1 | T48.5X2 | T48.5X3 | T48.5X4 | T48.5X5 | T48.5X6 |
| **Xylose*** | T5Ø.8X1 | T5Ø.8X2 | T5Ø.8X3 | T5Ø.8X4 | T5Ø.8X5 | T5Ø.8X6 |
| **Yaz*** | T38.4X1 | T38.4X2 | T38.4X3 | T38.4X4 | T38.4X5 | T38.4X6 |
| **Yeast** | T45.2X1 | T45.2X2 | T45.2X3 | T45.2X4 | T45.2X5 | T45.2X6 |
| dried | T45.2X1 | T45.2X2 | T45.2X3 | T45.2X4 | T45.2X5 | T45.2X6 |
| **Yellow** | | | | | | |
| fever vaccine | T5Ø.B91 | T5Ø.B92 | T5Ø.B93 | T5Ø.B94 | T5Ø.B95 | T5Ø.B96 |
| jasmine | T62.2X1 | T62.2X2 | T62.2X3 | T62.2X4 | — | — |
| phenolphthalein | T47.2X1 | T47.2X2 | T47.2X3 | T47.2X4 | T47.2X5 | T47.2X6 |
| **Yervoy*** | T45.1X1 | T45.1X2 | T45.1X3 | T45.1X4 | T45.1X5 | T45.1X6 |
| **Yew** | T62.2X1 | T62.2X2 | T62.2X3 | T62.2X4 | — | — |
| **Yohimbic acid** | T4Ø.991 | T4Ø.992 | T4Ø.993 | T4Ø.994 | T4Ø.995 | T4Ø.996 |
| **Zactane** | T39.8X1 | T39.8X2 | T39.8X3 | T39.8X4 | T39.8X5 | T39.8X6 |
| **Zalcitabine** | T37.5X1 | T37.5X2 | T37.5X3 | T37.5X4 | T37.5X5 | T37.5X6 |
| **Zanaflex*** | T48.1X1 | T48.1X2 | T48.1X3 | T48.1X4 | T48.1X5 | T48.1X6 |
| **Zaroxolyn** | T5Ø.2X1 | T5Ø.2X2 | T5Ø.2X3 | T5Ø.2X4 | T5Ø.2X5 | T5Ø.2X6 |
| **Zephiran** (topical) | T49.ØX1 | T49.ØX2 | T49.ØX3 | T49.ØX4 | T49.ØX5 | T49.ØX6 |
| ophthalmic preparation | T49.5X1 | T49.5X2 | T49.5X3 | T49.5X4 | T49.5X5 | T49.5X6 |
| **Zeranol** | T38.7X1 | T38.7X2 | T38.7X3 | T38.7X4 | T38.7X5 | T38.7X6 |
| **Zerone** | T51.1X1 | T51.1X2 | T51.1X3 | T51.1X4 | — | — |
| **Zestril*** | T46.4X1 | T46.4X2 | T46.4X3 | T46.4X4 | T46.4X5 | T46.4X6 |
| **Zidovudine** | T37.5X1 | T37.5X2 | T37.5X3 | T37.5X4 | T37.5X5 | T37.5X6 |
| **Zilactin*** | T41.3X1 | T41.3X2 | T41.3X3 | T41.3X4 | T41.3X5 | T41.3X6 |
| **Zimeldine** | T43.221 | T43.222 | T43.223 | T43.224 | T43.225 | T43.226 |
| **Zinc** (compounds) (fumes) (vapor) NEC | T56.5X1 | T56.5X2 | T56.5X3 | T56.5X4 | — | — |
| anti-infectives | T49.ØX1 | T49.ØX2 | T49.ØX3 | T49.ØX4 | T49.ØX5 | T49.ØX6 |
| antivaricose | T46.8X1 | T46.8X2 | T46.8X3 | T46.8X4 | T46.8X5 | T46.8X6 |
| bacitracin | T49.ØX1 | T49.ØX2 | T49.ØX3 | T49.ØX4 | T49.ØX5 | T49.ØX6 |
| chloride (mouthwash) | T49.6X1 | T49.6X2 | T49.6X3 | T49.6X4 | T49.6X5 | T49.6X6 |
| chromate | T56.5X1 | T56.5X2 | T56.5X3 | T56.5X4 | — | — |
| gelatin | T49.3X1 | T49.3X2 | T49.3X3 | T49.3X4 | T49.3X5 | T49.3X6 |
| oxide | T49.3X1 | T49.3X2 | T49.3X3 | T49.3X4 | T49.3X5 | T49.3X6 |
| plaster | T49.3X1 | T49.3X2 | T49.3X3 | T49.3X4 | T49.3X5 | T49.3X6 |
| peroxide | T49.ØX1 | T49.ØX2 | T49.ØX3 | T49.ØX4 | T49.ØX5 | T49.ØX6 |
| pesticides | T56.5X1 | T56.5X2 | T56.5X3 | T56.5X4 | — | — |
| phosphide | T6Ø.4X1 | T6Ø.4X2 | T6Ø.4X3 | T6Ø.4X4 | — | — |
| pyrithionate | T49.4X1 | T49.4X2 | T49.4X3 | T49.4X4 | T49.4X5 | T49.4X6 |
| stearate | T49.3X1 | T49.3X2 | T49.3X3 | T49.3X4 | T49.3X5 | T49.3X6 |
| sulfate | T49.5X1 | T49.5X2 | T49.5X3 | T49.5X4 | T49.5X5 | T49.5X6 |
| ENT agent | T49.6X1 | T49.6X2 | T49.6X3 | T49.6X4 | T49.6X5 | T49.6X6 |
| ophthalmic solution | T49.5X1 | T49.5X2 | T49.5X3 | T49.5X4 | T49.5X5 | T49.5X6 |
| topical NEC | T49.ØX1 | T49.ØX2 | T49.ØX3 | T49.ØX4 | T49.ØX5 | T49.ØX6 |
| undecylenate | T49.ØX1 | T49.ØX2 | T49.ØX3 | T49.ØX4 | T49.ØX5 | T49.ØX6 |
| **Zineb** | T6Ø.ØX1 | T6Ø.ØX2 | T6Ø.ØX3 | T6Ø.ØX4 | — | — |
| **Zinostatin** | T45.1X1 | T45.1X2 | T45.1X3 | T45.1X4 | T45.1X5 | T45.1X6 |
| **Zipeprol** | T48.3X1 | T48.3X2 | T48.3X3 | T48.3X4 | T48.3X5 | T48.3X6 |
| **Zithromax*** | T36.3X1 | T36.3X2 | T36.3X3 | T36.3X4 | T36.3X5 | T36.3X6 |
| **Zocor*** | T46.6X1 | T46.6X2 | T46.6X3 | T46.6X4 | T46.6X5 | T46.6X6 |
| **Zofenopril** | T46.4X1 | T46.4X2 | T46.4X3 | T46.4X4 | T46.4X5 | T46.4X6 |
| **Zoloft*** | T43.221 | T43.222 | T43.223 | T43.224 | T43.225 | T43.226 |
| **Zolpidem** | T42.6X1 | T42.6X2 | T42.6X3 | T42.6X4 | T42.6X5 | T42.6X6 |
| **Zolpimist*** | T42.6X1 | T42.6X2 | T42.6X3 | T42.6X4 | T42.6X5 | T42.6X6 |
| **Zomepirac** | T39.391 | T39.392 | T39.393 | T39.394 | T39.395 | T39.396 |
| **Zopiclone** | T42.6X1 | T42.6X2 | T42.6X3 | T42.6X4 | T42.6X5 | T42.6X6 |
| **Zorubicin** | T45.1X1 | T45.1X2 | T45.1X3 | T45.1X4 | T45.1X5 | T45.1X6 |
| **Zotepine** | T43.591 | T43.592 | T43.593 | T43.594 | T43.595 | T43.596 |
| **Zovant** | T45.511 | T45.512 | T45.513 | T45.514 | T45.515 | T45.516 |
| **Zoxazolamine** | T42.8X1 | T42.8X2 | T42.8X3 | T42.8X4 | T42.8X5 | T42.8X6 |
| **Zuclopenthixol** | T43.4X1 | T43.4X2 | T43.4X3 | T43.4X4 | T43.4X5 | T43.4X6 |
| **Zyban*** | T43.291 | T43.292 | T43.293 | T43.294 | T43.295 | T43.296 |
| **Zyflo*** | T48.6X1 | T48.6X2 | T48.6X3 | T48.6X4 | T48.6X5 | T48.6X6 |
| **Zygadenus** (venenosus) | T62.2X1 | T62.2X2 | T62.2X3 | T62.2X4 | — | — |
| **Zyprexa** | T43.591 | T43.592 | T43.593 | T43.594 | T43.595 | T43.596 |
| **Zyzal*** | T45.ØX1 | T45.ØX2 | T45.ØX3 | T45.ØX4 | T45.ØX5 | T45.ØX6 |

# A

External Causes Index

Accident — Accident

- **Accident** — *continued*
  - transport — *continued*
    - bus occupant — *continued*
      - hanger-on — *continued*
        - collision — *continued*
          - three wheeled motor vehicle (traffic) V72.7- ☑
            - nontraffic V72.2- ☑
          - truck (traffic) V74.7- ☑
            - nontraffic V74.2- ☑
          - two wheeled motor vehicle (traffic) V72.7- ☑
            - nontraffic V72.2- ☑
          - van (traffic) V73.7- ☑
            - nontraffic V73.2- ☑
        - noncollision accident (traffic) V78.7- ☑
          - nontraffic V78.2- ☑
      - noncollision accident (traffic) V78.9- ☑
        - nontraffic V78.3- ☑
        - while boarding or alighting V78.4- ☑
      - nontraffic V79.3- ☑
      - passenger
        - collision (with)
          - animal (traffic) V70.6- ☑
            - being ridden (traffic) V76.6- ☑
              - nontraffic V76.1- ☑
            - nontraffic V70.1- ☑
          - animal-drawn vehicle (traffic) V76.6- ☑
            - nontraffic V76.1- ☑
          - bus (traffic) V74.6- ☑
            - nontraffic V74.1- ☑
          - car (traffic) V73.6- ☑
            - nontraffic V73.1- ☑
          - motor vehicle NOS (traffic) V79.50- ☑
            - nontraffic V79.10- ☑
            - specified type NEC (traffic) V79.59- ☑
              - nontraffic V79.19- ☑
          - pedal cycle (traffic) V71.6- ☑
            - nontraffic V71.1- ☑
          - pickup truck (traffic) V73.6- ☑
            - nontraffic V73.1- ☑
          - railway vehicle (traffic) V75.6- ☑
            - nontraffic V75.1- ☑
          - specified vehicle NEC (traffic) V76.6- ☑
            - nontraffic V76.1- ☑
          - stationary object (traffic) V77.6- ☑
            - nontraffic V77.1- ☑
          - streetcar (traffic) V76.6- ☑
            - nontraffic V76.1- ☑
          - three wheeled motor vehicle (traffic) V72.6- ☑
            - nontraffic V72.1- ☑
          - truck (traffic) V74.6- ☑
            - nontraffic V74.1- ☑
          - two wheeled motor vehicle (traffic) V72.6- ☑
            - nontraffic V72.1- ☑
          - van (traffic) V73.6- ☑
            - nontraffic V73.1- ☑
        - noncollision accident (traffic) V78.6- ☑
          - nontraffic V78.1- ☑
      - specified type NEC V79.88- ☑
        - military vehicle V79.81- ☑
    - cable car, not on rails V98.0- ☑
      - on rails — *see* Accident, transport, streetcar occupant
    - car occupant V49.9- ☑
      - ambulance occupant — *see* Accident, transport, ambulance occupant
      - collision (with)
        - animal (traffic) V40.9- ☑
          - being ridden (traffic) V46.9- ☑
            - nontraffic V46.3- ☑
            - while boarding or alighting V46.4- ☑
          - nontraffic V40.3- ☑
          - while boarding or alighting V40.4- ☑
        - animal-drawn vehicle (traffic) V46.9- ☑
          - nontraffic V46.3- ☑
          - while boarding or alighting V46.4- ☑
        - bus (traffic) V44.9- ☑
          - nontraffic V44.3- ☑
          - while boarding or alighting V44.4- ☑
        - car (traffic) V43.92- ☑
          - nontraffic V43.32- ☑
          - while boarding or alighting V43.42- ☑

- **Accident** — *continued*
  - transport — *continued*
    - car occupant — *continued*
      - collision — *continued*
        - motor vehicle NOS (traffic) V49.60- ☑
          - nontraffic V49.20- ☑
          - specified type NEC (traffic) V49.69- ☑
            - nontraffic V49.29- ☑
        - pedal cycle (traffic) V41.9- ☑
          - nontraffic V41.3- ☑
          - while boarding or alighting V41.4- ☑
        - pickup truck (traffic) V43.93- ☑
          - nontraffic V43.33- ☑
          - while boarding or alighting V43.43- ☑
        - railway vehicle (traffic) V45.9- ☑
          - nontraffic V45.3- ☑
          - while boarding or alighting V45.4- ☑
        - specified vehicle NEC (traffic) V46.9- ☑
          - nontraffic V46.3- ☑
          - while boarding or alighting V46.4- ☑
        - sport utility vehicle (traffic) V43.91- ☑
          - nontraffic V43.31- ☑
          - while boarding or alighting V43.41- ☑
        - stationary object (traffic) V47.9- ☑
          - nontraffic V47.3- ☑
          - while boarding or alighting V47.4- ☑
        - streetcar (traffic) V46.9- ☑
          - nontraffic V46.3- ☑
          - while boarding or alighting V46.4- ☑
        - three wheeled motor vehicle (traffic) V42.9- ☑
          - nontraffic V42.3- ☑
          - while boarding or alighting V42.4- ☑
        - truck (traffic) V44.9- ☑
          - nontraffic V44.3- ☑
          - while boarding or alighting V44.4- ☑
        - two wheeled motor vehicle (traffic) V42.9- ☑
          - nontraffic V42.3- ☑
          - while boarding or alighting V42.4- ☑
        - van (traffic) V43.94- ☑
          - nontraffic V43.34- ☑
          - while boarding or alighting V43.44- ☑
      - driver
        - collision (with)
          - animal (traffic) V40.5- ☑
            - being ridden (traffic) V46.5- ☑
              - nontraffic V46.0- ☑
            - nontraffic V40.0- ☑
          - animal-drawn vehicle (traffic) V46.5- ☑
            - nontraffic V46.0- ☑
          - bus (traffic) V44.5- ☑
            - nontraffic V44.0- ☑
          - car (traffic) V43.52- ☑
            - nontraffic V43.02- ☑
          - motor vehicle NOS (traffic) V49.40- ☑
            - nontraffic V49.00- ☑
            - specified type NEC (traffic) V49.49- ☑
              - nontraffic V49.09- ☑
          - pedal cycle (traffic) V41.5- ☑
            - nontraffic V41.0- ☑
          - pickup truck (traffic) V43.53- ☑
            - nontraffic V43.03- ☑
          - railway vehicle (traffic) V45.5- ☑
            - nontraffic V45.0- ☑
          - specified vehicle NEC (traffic) V46.5- ☑
            - nontraffic V46.0- ☑
          - sport utility vehicle (traffic) V43.51- ☑
            - nontraffic V43.01- ☑
          - stationary object (traffic) V47.5- ☑
            - nontraffic V47.0- ☑
          - streetcar (traffic) V46.5- ☑
            - nontraffic V46.0- ☑
          - three wheeled motor vehicle (traffic) V42.5- ☑
            - nontraffic V42.0- ☑
          - truck (traffic) V44.5- ☑
            - nontraffic V44.0- ☑
          - two wheeled motor vehicle (traffic) V42.5- ☑
            - nontraffic V42.0- ☑
          - van (traffic) V43.54- ☑
            - nontraffic V43.04- ☑
        - noncollision accident (traffic) V48.5- ☑
          - nontraffic V48.0- ☑

- **Accident** — *continued*
  - transport — *continued*
    - car occupant — *continued*
      - hanger-on
        - collision (with)
          - animal (traffic) V40.7- ☑
            - being ridden (traffic) V46.7- ☑
              - nontraffic V46.2- ☑
            - nontraffic V40.2- ☑
          - animal-drawn vehicle (traffic) V46.7- ☑
            - nontraffic V46.2- ☑
          - bus (traffic) V44.7- ☑
            - nontraffic V44.2- ☑
          - car (traffic) V43.72- ☑
            - nontraffic V43.22- ☑
          - pedal cycle (traffic) V41.7- ☑
            - nontraffic V41.2- ☑
          - pickup truck (traffic) V43.73- ☑
            - nontraffic V43.23- ☑
          - railway vehicle (traffic) V45.7- ☑
            - nontraffic V45.2- ☑
          - specified vehicle NEC (traffic) V46.7- ☑
            - nontraffic V46.2- ☑
          - sport utility vehicle (traffic) V43.71- ☑
            - nontraffic V43.21- ☑
          - stationary object (traffic) V47.7- ☑
            - nontraffic V47.2- ☑
          - streetcar (traffic) V46.7- ☑
            - nontraffic V46.2- ☑
          - three wheeled motor vehicle (traffic) V42.7- ☑
            - nontraffic V42.2- ☑
          - truck (traffic) V44.7- ☑
            - nontraffic V44.2- ☑
          - two wheeled motor vehicle (traffic) V42.7- ☑
            - nontraffic V42.2- ☑
          - van (traffic) V43.74- ☑
            - nontraffic V43.24- ☑
        - noncollision accident (traffic) V48.7- ☑
          - nontraffic V48.2- ☑
      - noncollision accident (traffic) V48.9- ☑
        - nontraffic V48.3- ☑
        - while boarding or alighting V48.4- ☑
      - nontraffic V49.3- ☑
      - passenger
        - collision (with)
          - animal (traffic) V40.6- ☑
            - being ridden (traffic) V46.6- ☑
              - nontraffic V46.1- ☑
            - nontraffic V40.1- ☑
          - animal-drawn vehicle (traffic) V46.6- ☑
            - nontraffic V46.1- ☑
          - bus (traffic) V44.6- ☑
            - nontraffic V44.1- ☑
          - car (traffic) V43.62- ☑
            - nontraffic V43.12- ☑
          - motor vehicle NOS (traffic) V49.50- ☑
            - nontraffic V49.10- ☑
            - specified type NEC (traffic) V49.59- ☑
              - nontraffic V49.19- ☑
          - pedal cycle (traffic) V41.6- ☑
            - nontraffic V41.1- ☑
          - pickup truck (traffic) V43.63- ☑
            - nontraffic V43.13- ☑
          - railway vehicle (traffic) V45.6- ☑
            - nontraffic V45.1- ☑
          - specified vehicle NEC (traffic) V46.6- ☑
            - nontraffic V46.1- ☑
          - sport utility vehicle (traffic) V43.61- ☑
            - nontraffic V43.11- ☑
          - stationary object (traffic) V47.6- ☑
            - nontraffic V47.1- ☑
          - streetcar (traffic) V46.6- ☑
            - nontraffic V46.1- ☑
          - three wheeled motor vehicle (traffic) V42.6- ☑
            - nontraffic V42.1- ☑
          - truck (traffic) V44.6- ☑
            - nontraffic V44.1- ☑
          - two wheeled motor vehicle (traffic) V42.6- ☑
            - nontraffic V42.1- ☑
          - van (traffic) V43.64- ☑
            - nontraffic V43.14- ☑

- **Accident** — *continued*
  - transport — *continued*
    - motorcycle — *continued*
      - collision — *continued*
        - motor vehicle — *continued*
          - nontraffic V29.208- ☑
          - specified type NEC (traffic) V29.698- ☑
            - nontraffic V29.298- ☑
        - pedal cycle (traffic) V21.99- ☑
          - nontraffic V21.29- ☑
          - while boarding or alighting V21.39- ☑
        - pickup truck (traffic) V23.99- ☑
          - nontraffic V23.29- ☑
          - while boarding or alighting V23.39- ☑
        - railway vehicle (traffic) V25.99- ☑
          - nontraffic V25.29- ☑
          - while boarding or alighting V25.39- ☑
        - specified vehicle NEC (traffic) V26.99- ☑
          - nontraffic V26.29- ☑
          - while boarding or alighting V26.39- ☑
        - stationary object (traffic) V27.99- ☑
          - nontraffic V27.29- ☑
          - while boarding or alighting V27.39- ☑
        - streetcar (traffic) V26.99- ☑
          - nontraffic V26.29- ☑
          - while boarding or alighting V26.39- ☑
        - three wheeled motor vehicle (traffic) V22.99- ☑
          - nontraffic V22.29- ☑
          - while boarding or alighting V22.39- ☑
        - truck (traffic) V24.99- ☑
          - nontraffic V24.29- ☑
          - while boarding or alighting V24.39- ☑
        - two wheeled motor vehicle (traffic) V22.99- ☑
          - nontraffic V22.29- ☑
          - while boarding or alighting V22.39- ☑
        - van (traffic) V23.99- ☑
          - nontraffic V23.29- ☑
          - while boarding or alighting V23.39- ☑
      - driver
        - collision (with)
          - animal (traffic) V20.49- ☑
            - being ridden (traffic) V26.49- ☑
              - nontraffic V26.09- ☑
            - nontraffic V20.09- ☑
          - animal-drawn vehicle (traffic) V26.49- ☑
            - nontraffic V26.09- ☑
          - bus (traffic) V24.49- ☑
            - nontraffic V24.09- ☑
          - car (traffic) V23.49- ☑
            - nontraffic V23.09- ☑
          - motor vehicle NOS (traffic) V29.408- ☑
            - nontraffic V29.008- ☑
            - specified type NEC (traffic) V29.498- ☑
              - nontraffic V29.098- ☑
          - pedal cycle (traffic) V21.49- ☑
            - nontraffic V21.09- ☑
          - pedestrian
            - nontraffic V20.09- ☑
            - traffic V20.49- ☑
          - pickup truck (traffic) V23.49- ☑
            - nontraffic V23.09- ☑
          - railway vehicle (traffic) V25.49- ☑
            - nontraffic V25.09- ☑
          - specified vehicle NEC (traffic) V26.49- ☑
            - nontraffic V26.09- ☑
          - stationary object (traffic) V27.49- ☑
            - nontraffic V27.09- ☑
          - streetcar (traffic) V26.49- ☑
            - nontraffic V26.09- ☑
          - three wheeled motor vehicle (traffic) V22.49- ☑
            - nontraffic V22.09- ☑
          - truck (traffic) V24.49- ☑
            - nontraffic V24.09- ☑
          - two wheeled motor vehicle (traffic) V22.49- ☑
            - nontraffic V22.09- ☑
          - van (traffic) V23.49- ☑
            - nontraffic V23.09- ☑
        - noncollision accident (traffic) V28.49- ☑
          - nontraffic V28.09- ☑
      - noncollision accident (traffic) V28.99- ☑
        - nontraffic V28.29- ☑
        - while boarding or alighting V28.39- ☑
      - nontraffic V29.39- ☑

- **Accident** — *continued*
  - transport — *continued*
    - motorcycle — *continued*
      - passenger
        - collision (with)
          - animal (traffic) V20.59- ☑
            - being ridden (traffic) V26.59- ☑
              - nontraffic V26.19- ☑
            - nontraffic V20.19- ☑
          - animal-drawn vehicle (traffic) V26.59- ☑
            - nontraffic V26.19- ☑
          - bus (traffic) V24.59- ☑
            - nontraffic V24.19- ☑
          - car (traffic) V23.59- ☑
            - nontraffic V23.19- ☑
          - motor vehicle NOS (traffic) V29.508- ☑
            - nontraffic V29.108- ☑
            - specified type NEC (traffic) V29.598- ☑
              - nontraffic V29.198- ☑
          - pedal cycle (traffic) V21.59- ☑
            - nontraffic V21.19- ☑
          - pedestrian
            - nontraffic V20.19- ☑
            - traffic V20.59- ☑
          - pickup truck (traffic) V23.59- ☑
            - nontraffic V23.19- ☑
          - railway vehicle (traffic) V25.59- ☑
            - nontraffic V25.19- ☑
          - specified vehicle NEC (traffic) V26.59- ☑
            - nontraffic V26.19- ☑
          - stationary object (traffic) V27.59- ☑
            - nontraffic V27.19- ☑
          - streetcar (traffic) V26.59- ☑
            - nontraffic V26.19- ☑
          - three wheeled motor vehicle (traffic) V22.59- ☑
            - nontraffic V22.19- ☑
          - truck (traffic) V24.59- ☑
            - nontraffic V24.19- ☑
          - two wheeled motor vehicle (traffic) V22.59- ☑
            - nontraffic V22.19- ☑
          - van (traffic) V23.59- ☑
            - nontraffic V23.19- ☑
        - noncollision accident (traffic) V28.59- ☑
          - nontraffic V28.19- ☑
      - specified type NEC V29.888- ☑
        - military vehicle V29.818- ☑
    - occupant (of)
      - aircraft (powered) V95.9- ☑
        - fixed wing
          - commercial — *see* Accident, transport, aircraft, occupant, powered, fixed wing, commercial
          - private — *see* Accident, transport, aircraft, occupant, powered, fixed wing, private
        - nonpowered V96.9- ☑
        - specified NEC V95.8- ☑
      - airport battery-powered vehicle — *see* Accident, transport, industrial vehicle occupant
      - all-terrain vehicle (ATV) — *see* Accident, transport, all-terrain vehicle occupant
      - animal-drawn vehicle — *see* Accident, transport, animal-drawn vehicle occupant
      - automobile — *see* Accident, transport, car occupant
      - balloon V96.00- ☑
      - battery-powered vehicle — *see* Accident, transport, industrial vehicle occupant
      - bicycle — *see* Accident, transport, pedal cyclist
        - motorized — *see* Accident, transport, motorcycle rider
      - boat NEC — *see* Accident, watercraft
      - bulldozer — *see* Accident, transport, construction vehicle occupant
      - bus — *see* Accident, transport, bus occupant
      - cable car (on rails) — *see also* Accident, transport, streetcar occupant
        - not on rails V98.0- ☑
      - car — *see also* Accident, transport, car occupant
        - cable (on rails) — *see also* Accident, transport, streetcar occupant
          - not on rails V98.0- ☑
      - coach — *see* Accident, transport, bus occupant
      - coal-car — *see* Accident, transport, industrial vehicle occupant

- **Accident** — *continued*
  - transport — *continued*
    - occupant — *continued*
      - digger — *see* Accident, transport, construction vehicle occupant
      - dump truck — *see* Accident, transport, construction vehicle occupant
      - earth-leveler — *see* Accident, transport, construction vehicle occupant
      - farm machinery (self-propelled) — *see* Accident, transport, agricultural vehicle occupant
      - forklift — *see* Accident, transport, industrial vehicle occupant
      - glider (unpowered) V96.20- ☑
        - hang V96.10- ☑
        - powered (microlight) (ultralight) — *see* Accident, transport, aircraft, occupant, powered, glider
      - glider (unpowered) NEC V96.20- ☑
      - hang-glider V96.10- ☑
      - harvester — *see* Accident, transport, agricultural vehicle occupant
      - heavy (transport) vehicle — *see* Accident, transport, truck occupant
      - helicopter — *see* Accident, transport, aircraft, occupant, helicopter
      - ice-yacht V98.2- ☑
      - kite (carrying person) V96.8- ☑
      - land-yacht V98.1- ☑
      - logging car — *see* Accident, transport, industrial vehicle occupant
      - mechanical shovel — *see* Accident, transport, construction vehicle occupant
      - microlight — *see* Accident, transport, aircraft, occupant, powered, glider
      - minibus — *see* Accident, transport, pickup truck occupant
      - minivan — *see* Accident, transport, pickup truck occupant
      - moped — *see* Accident, transport, motorcycle
      - motor scooter — *see* Accident, transport, motorcycle
      - motorcycle (with sidecar) — *see* Accident, transport, motorcycle
      - off-road motor-vehicle — *see also* Accident, transport, all-terrain vehicle occupant V86.99- ☑
      - pedal cycle — *see also* Accident, transport, pedal cyclist
      - pick-up (truck) — *see* Accident, transport, pickup truck occupant
      - railway (train) (vehicle) (subterranean) (elevated) — *see* Accident, transport, railway vehicle occupant
      - rickshaw — *see* Accident, transport, pedal cycle
        - motorized — *see* Accident, transport, three-wheeled motor vehicle
        - pedal driven — *see* Accident, transport, pedal cyclist
      - road-roller — *see* Accident, transport, construction vehicle occupant
      - ship NOS V94.9- ☑
      - ski-lift (chair) (gondola) V98.3- ☑
      - snowmobile — *see* Accident, transport, snowmobile occupant
      - spacecraft, spaceship — *see* Accident, transport, aircraft, occupant, spacecraft
      - sport utility vehicle — *see* Accident, transport, pickup truck occupant
      - streetcar (interurban) (operating on public street or highway) — *see* Accident, transport, streetcar occupant
      - SUV — *see* Accident, transport, pickup truck occupant
      - teleferique V98.0- ☑
      - three-wheeled vehicle (motorized) — *see also* Accident, transport, three-wheeled motor vehicle occupant
        - nonmotorized — *see* Accident, transport, pedal cycle
      - tractor (farm) (and trailer) — *see* Accident, transport, agricultural vehicle occupant
      - train — *see* Accident, transport, railway vehicle occupant
      - tram — *see* Accident, transport, streetcar occupant
        - in mine or quarry — *see* Accident, transport, industrial vehicle occupant
      - tricycle — *see* Accident, transport, pedal cycle

- **Accident** — *continued*
  - transport — *continued*
    - occupant — *continued*
      - tricycle — *see* Accident, transport, pedal cycle — *continued*
        - motorized — *see* Accident, transport, three-wheeled motor vehicle
      - trolley — *see* Accident, transport, streetcar occupant
        - in mine or quarry — *see* Accident, transport, industrial vehicle occupant
      - tub, in mine or quarry — *see* Accident, transport, industrial vehicle occupant
      - ultralight — *see* Accident, transport, aircraft, occupant, powered, glider
      - van — *see* Accident, transport, van occupant
      - vehicle NEC V89.9- ☑
        - heavy transport — *see* Accident, transport, truck occupant
        - motor (traffic) NEC V89.2- ☑
          - nontraffic NEC V89.0- ☑
      - watercraft NOS V94.9- ☑
        - causing drowning — *see* Drowning, resulting from accident to boat
    - off-road motor-vehicle — *see also* Accident, transport, all-terrain vehicle occupant V86.99- ☑
    - parachutist V97.29- ☑
      - after accident to aircraft — *see* Accident, transport, aircraft
      - entangled in object V97.21- ☑
      - injured on landing V97.22- ☑
    - pedal cyclist V19.9- ☑
      - collision (with)
        - animal (traffic) V10.9- ☑
          - being ridden (traffic) V16.9- ☑
            - nontraffic V16.2- ☑
            - while boarding or alighting V16.3- ☑
          - nontraffic V10.2- ☑
          - while boarding or alighting V10.3- ☑
        - animal-drawn vehicle (traffic) V16.9- ☑
          - nontraffic V16.2- ☑
          - while boarding or alighting V16.3- ☑
        - bus (traffic) V14.9- ☑
          - nontraffic V14.2- ☑
          - while boarding or alighting V14.3- ☑
        - car (traffic) V13.9- ☑
          - nontraffic V13.2- ☑
          - while boarding or alighting V13.3- ☑
        - motor vehicle NOS (traffic) V19.60- ☑
          - nontraffic V19.20- ☑
          - specified type NEC (traffic) V19.69- ☑
            - nontraffic V19.29- ☑
        - pedal cycle (traffic) V11.9- ☑
          - nontraffic V11.2- ☑
          - while boarding or alighting V11.3- ☑
        - pickup truck (traffic) V13.9- ☑
          - nontraffic V13.2- ☑
          - while boarding or alighting V13.3- ☑
        - railway vehicle (traffic) V15.9- ☑
          - nontraffic V15.2- ☑
          - while boarding or alighting V15.3- ☑
        - specified vehicle NEC (traffic) V16.9- ☑
          - nontraffic V16.2- ☑
          - while boarding or alighting V16.3- ☑
        - stationary object (traffic) V17.9- ☑
          - nontraffic V17.2- ☑
          - while boarding or alighting V17.3- ☑
        - streetcar (traffic) V16.9- ☑
          - nontraffic V16.2- ☑
          - while boarding or alighting V16.3- ☑
        - three wheeled motor vehicle (traffic) V12.9- ☑
          - nontraffic V12.2- ☑
          - while boarding or alighting V12.3- ☑
        - truck (traffic) V14.9- ☑
          - nontraffic V14.2- ☑
          - while boarding or alighting V14.3- ☑
        - two wheeled motor vehicle (traffic) V12.9- ☑
          - nontraffic V12.2- ☑
          - while boarding or alighting V12.3- ☑
        - van (traffic) V13.9- ☑
          - nontraffic V13.2- ☑
          - while boarding or alighting V13.3- ☑
      - driver
        - collision (with)
          - animal (traffic) V10.4- ☑
            - being ridden (traffic) V16.4- ☑

- **Accident** — *continued*
  - transport — *continued*
    - pedal cyclist — *continued*
      - driver — *continued*
        - collision — *continued*
          - animal — *continued*
            - being ridden — *continued*
              - nontraffic V16.0- ☑
            - nontraffic V10.0- ☑
          - animal-drawn vehicle (traffic) V16.4- ☑
            - nontraffic V16.0- ☑
          - bus (traffic) V14.4- ☑
            - nontraffic V14.0- ☑
          - car (traffic) V13.4- ☑
            - nontraffic V13.0- ☑
          - motor vehicle NOS (traffic) V19.40- ☑
            - nontraffic V19.00- ☑
            - specified type NEC (traffic) V19.49- ☑
              - nontraffic V19.09- ☑
          - pedal cycle (traffic) V11.4- ☑
            - nontraffic V11.0- ☑
          - pickup truck (traffic) V13.4- ☑
            - nontraffic V13.0- ☑
          - railway vehicle (traffic) V15.4- ☑
            - nontraffic V15.0- ☑
          - specified vehicle NEC (traffic) V16.4- ☑
            - nontraffic V16.0- ☑
          - stationary object (traffic) V17.4- ☑
            - nontraffic V17.0- ☑
          - streetcar (traffic) V16.4- ☑
            - nontraffic V16.0- ☑
          - three wheeled motor vehicle (traffic) V12.4- ☑
            - nontraffic V12.0- ☑
          - truck (traffic) V14.4- ☑
            - nontraffic V14.0- ☑
          - two wheeled motor vehicle (traffic) V12.4- ☑
            - nontraffic V12.0- ☑
          - van (traffic) V13.4- ☑
            - nontraffic V13.0- ☑
        - noncollision accident (traffic) V18.4- ☑
          - nontraffic V18.0- ☑
      - noncollision accident (traffic) V18.9- ☑
        - nontraffic V18.2- ☑
        - while boarding or alighting V18.3- ☑
      - nontraffic V19.3- ☑
      - passenger
        - collision (with)
          - animal (traffic) V10.5- ☑
            - being ridden (traffic) V16.5- ☑
              - nontraffic V16.1- ☑
            - nontraffic V10.1- ☑
          - animal-drawn vehicle (traffic) V16.5- ☑
            - nontraffic V16.1- ☑
          - bus (traffic) V14.5- ☑
            - nontraffic V14.1- ☑
          - car (traffic) V13.5- ☑
            - nontraffic V13.1- ☑
          - motor vehicle NOS (traffic) V19.50- ☑
            - nontraffic V19.10- ☑
            - specified type NEC (traffic) V19.59- ☑
              - nontraffic V19.19- ☑
          - pedal cycle (traffic) V11.5- ☑
            - nontraffic V11.1- ☑
          - pickup truck (traffic) V13.5- ☑
            - nontraffic V13.1- ☑
          - railway vehicle (traffic) V15.5- ☑
            - nontraffic V15.1- ☑
          - specified vehicle NEC (traffic) V16.5- ☑
            - nontraffic V16.1- ☑
          - stationary object (traffic) V17.5- ☑
            - nontraffic V17.1- ☑
          - streetcar (traffic) V16.5- ☑
            - nontraffic V16.1- ☑
          - three wheeled motor vehicle (traffic) V12.5- ☑
            - nontraffic V12.1- ☑
          - truck (traffic) V14.5- ☑
            - nontraffic V14.1- ☑
          - two wheeled motor vehicle (traffic) V12.5- ☑
            - nontraffic V12.1- ☑
          - van (traffic) V13.5- ☑
            - nontraffic V13.1- ☑

- **Accident** — *continued*
  - transport — *continued*
    - pedal cyclist — *continued*
      - passenger — *continued*
        - noncollision accident (traffic) V18.5- ☑
          - nontraffic V18.1- ☑
      - specified type NEC V19.88- ☑
        - military vehicle V19.81- ☑
    - pedestrian
      - conveyance (occupant) V09.9- ☑
        - baby stroller V00.828- ☑
          - collision (with) V09.9- ☑
            - animal being ridden or animal drawn vehicle V06.99- ☑
              - nontraffic V06.09- ☑
              - traffic V06.19- ☑
            - bus or heavy transport V04.99- ☑
              - nontraffic V04.09- ☑
              - traffic V04.19- ☑
            - car V03.99- ☑
              - nontraffic V03.09- ☑
              - traffic V03.19- ☑
            - pedal cycle V01.99- ☑
              - nontraffic V01.09- ☑
              - traffic V01.19- ☑
            - pick-up truck or van V03.99- ☑
              - nontraffic V03.09- ☑
              - traffic V03.19- ☑
            - railway (train) (vehicle) V05.99- ☑
              - nontraffic V05.09- ☑
              - traffic V05.19- ☑
            - stationary object V00.822- ☑
            - streetcar V06.99- ☑
              - nontraffic V06.09- ☑
              - traffic V06.19- ☑
            - two- or three-wheeled motor vehicle V02.99- ☑
              - nontraffic V02.09- ☑
              - traffic V02.19- ☑
            - vehicle V09.9- ☑
              - animal-drawn V06.99- ☑
                - nontraffic V06.09- ☑
                - traffic V06.19- ☑
              - motor
                - nontraffic V09.00- ☑
                - traffic V09.20- ☑
          - fall V00.821- ☑
          - nontraffic V09.1- ☑
            - involving motor vehicle NEC V09.00- ☑
          - traffic V09.3- ☑
            - involving motor vehicle NEC V09.20- ☑
        - flat-bottomed NEC V00.388- ☑
          - collision (with) V09.9- ☑
            - animal being ridden or animal drawn vehicle V06.99- ☑
              - nontraffic V06.09- ☑
              - traffic V06.19- ☑
            - bus or heavy transport V04.99- ☑
              - nontraffic V04.09- ☑
              - traffic V04.19- ☑
            - car V03.99- ☑
              - nontraffic V03.09- ☑
              - traffic V03.19- ☑
            - pedal cycle V01.99- ☑
              - nontraffic V01.09- ☑
              - traffic V01.19- ☑
            - pick-up truck or van V03.99- ☑
              - nontraffic V03.09- ☑
              - traffic V03.19- ☑
            - railway (train) (vehicle) V05.99- ☑
              - nontraffic V05.09- ☑
              - traffic V05.19- ☑
            - stationary object V00.382- ☑
            - streetcar V06.99- ☑
              - nontraffic V06.09- ☑
              - traffic V06.19- ☑
            - two- or three-wheeled motor vehicle V02.99- ☑
              - nontraffic V02.09- ☑
              - traffic V02.19- ☑
            - vehicle V09.9- ☑
              - animal-drawn V06.99- ☑
                - nontraffic V06.09- ☑
                - traffic V06.19- ☑

- **Accident** — *continued*
  - transport — *continued*
    - person — *continued*
      - collision — *continued*
        - car (with)
          - bus (traffic) V87.3- ☑
            - nontraffic V88.3- ☑
          - heavy transport vehicle (traffic) V87.4- ☑
            - nontraffic V88.4- ☑
          - nontraffic V88.5- ☑
          - pick-up truck or van (traffic) V87.2- ☑
            - nontraffic V88.2- ☑
          - train or railway vehicle (traffic) V87.6- ☑
            - nontraffic V88.6- ☑
          - two-or three-wheeled motor vehicle (traffic) V87.Ø- ☑
            - nontraffic V88.Ø- ☑
        - motor vehicle (traffic) NEC V87.7- ☑
          - nontraffic V88.7- ☑
        - two-or three-wheeled vehicle (with) (traffic)
          - motor vehicle NEC V87.1- ☑
            - nontraffic V88.1- ☑
      - nonmotor vehicle (collision) (noncollision) (traffic) V87.9- ☑
        - nontraffic V88.9- ☑
    - pickup truck occupant V59.9- ☑
      - collision (with)
        - animal (traffic) V5Ø.9- ☑
          - being ridden (traffic) V56.9- ☑
            - nontraffic V56.3- ☑
            - while boarding or alighting V56.4- ☑
          - nontraffic V5Ø.3- ☑
          - while boarding or alighting V5Ø.4- ☑
        - animal-drawn vehicle (traffic) V56.9- ☑
          - nontraffic V56.3- ☑
          - while boarding or alighting V56.4- ☑
        - bus (traffic) V54.9- ☑
          - nontraffic V54.3- ☑
          - while boarding or alighting V54.4- ☑
        - car (traffic) V53.9- ☑
          - nontraffic V53.3- ☑
          - while boarding or alighting V53.4- ☑
        - motor vehicle NOS (traffic) V59.6Ø- ☑
          - nontraffic V59.2Ø- ☑
          - specified type NEC (traffic) V59.69- ☑
            - nontraffic V59.29- ☑
        - pedal cycle (traffic) V51.9- ☑
          - nontraffic V51.3- ☑
          - while boarding or alighting V51.4- ☑
        - pickup truck (traffic) V53.9- ☑
          - nontraffic V53.3- ☑
          - while boarding or alighting V53.4- ☑
        - railway vehicle (traffic) V55.9- ☑
          - nontraffic V55.3- ☑
          - while boarding or alighting V55.4- ☑
        - specified vehicle NEC (traffic) V56.9- ☑
          - nontraffic V56.3- ☑
          - while boarding or alighting V56.4- ☑
        - stationary object (traffic) V57.9- ☑
          - nontraffic V57.3- ☑
          - while boarding or alighting V57.4- ☑
        - streetcar (traffic) V56.9- ☑
          - nontraffic V56.3- ☑
          - while boarding or alighting V56.4- ☑
        - three wheeled motor vehicle (traffic) V52.9- ☑
          - nontraffic V52.3- ☑
          - while boarding or alighting V52.4- ☑
        - truck (traffic) V54.9- ☑
          - nontraffic V54.3- ☑
          - while boarding or alighting V54.4- ☑
        - two wheeled motor vehicle (traffic) V52.9- ☑
          - nontraffic V52.3- ☑
          - while boarding or alighting V52.4- ☑
        - van (traffic) V53.9- ☑
          - nontraffic V53.3- ☑
          - while boarding or alighting V53.4- ☑
      - driver
        - collision (with)
          - animal (traffic) V5Ø.5- ☑
            - being ridden (traffic) V56.5- ☑
              - nontraffic V56.Ø- ☑
            - nontraffic V5Ø.Ø- ☑
          - animal-drawn vehicle (traffic) V56.5- ☑
            - nontraffic V56.Ø- ☑
          - bus (traffic) V54.5- ☑

- **Accident** — *continued*
  - transport — *continued*
    - pickup truck occupant — *continued*
      - driver — *continued*
        - collision — *continued*
          - bus — *continued*
            - nontraffic V54.Ø- ☑
          - car (traffic) V53.5- ☑
            - nontraffic V53.Ø- ☑
          - motor vehicle NOS (traffic) V59.4Ø- ☑
            - nontraffic V59.ØØ- ☑
            - specified type NEC (traffic) V59.49- ☑
              - nontraffic V59.Ø9- ☑
          - pedal cycle (traffic) V51.5- ☑
            - nontraffic V51.Ø- ☑
          - pickup truck (traffic) V53.5- ☑
            - nontraffic V53.Ø- ☑
          - railway vehicle (traffic) V55.5- ☑
            - nontraffic V55.Ø- ☑
          - specified vehicle NEC (traffic) V56.5- ☑
            - nontraffic V56.Ø- ☑
          - stationary object (traffic) V57.5- ☑
            - nontraffic V57.Ø- ☑
          - streetcar (traffic) V56.5- ☑
            - nontraffic V56.Ø- ☑
          - three wheeled motor vehicle (traffic) V52.5- ☑
            - nontraffic V52.Ø- ☑
          - truck (traffic) V54.5- ☑
            - nontraffic V54.Ø- ☑
          - two wheeled motor vehicle (traffic) V52.5- ☑
            - nontraffic V52.Ø- ☑
          - van (traffic) V53.5- ☑
            - nontraffic V53.Ø- ☑
        - noncollision accident (traffic) V58.5- ☑
          - nontraffic V58.Ø- ☑
      - hanger-on
        - collision (with)
          - animal (traffic) V5Ø.7- ☑
            - being ridden (traffic) V56.7- ☑
              - nontraffic V56.2- ☑
            - nontraffic V5Ø.2- ☑
          - animal-drawn vehicle (traffic) V56.7- ☑
            - nontraffic V56.2- ☑
          - bus (traffic) V54.7- ☑
            - nontraffic V54.2- ☑
          - car (traffic) V53.7- ☑
            - nontraffic V53.2- ☑
          - pedal cycle (traffic) V51.7- ☑
            - nontraffic V51.2- ☑
          - pickup truck (traffic) V53.7- ☑
            - nontraffic V53.2- ☑
          - railway vehicle (traffic) V55.7- ☑
            - nontraffic V55.2- ☑
          - specified vehicle NEC (traffic) V56.7- ☑
            - nontraffic V56.2- ☑
          - stationary object (traffic) V57.7- ☑
            - nontraffic V57.2- ☑
          - streetcar (traffic) V56.7- ☑
            - nontraffic V56.2- ☑
          - three wheeled motor vehicle (traffic) V52.7- ☑
            - nontraffic V52.2- ☑
          - truck (traffic) V54.7- ☑
            - nontraffic V54.2- ☑
          - two wheeled motor vehicle (traffic) V52.7- ☑
            - nontraffic V52.2- ☑
          - van (traffic) V53.7- ☑
            - nontraffic V53.2- ☑
        - noncollision accident (traffic) V58.7- ☑
          - nontraffic V58.2- ☑
      - noncollision accident (traffic) V58.9- ☑
        - nontraffic V58.3- ☑
        - while boarding or alighting V58.4- ☑
      - nontraffic V59.3- ☑
      - passenger
        - collision (with)
          - animal (traffic) V5Ø.6- ☑
            - being ridden (traffic) V56.6- ☑
              - nontraffic V56.1- ☑
            - nontraffic V5Ø.1- ☑
          - animal-drawn vehicle (traffic) V56.6- ☑
            - nontraffic V56.1- ☑

- **Accident** — *continued*
  - transport — *continued*
    - pickup truck occupant — *continued*
      - passenger — *continued*
        - collision — *continued*
          - bus (traffic) V54.6- ☑
            - nontraffic V54.1- ☑
          - car (traffic) V53.6- ☑
            - nontraffic V53.1- ☑
          - motor vehicle NOS (traffic) V59.5Ø- ☑
            - nontraffic V59.1Ø- ☑
            - specified type NEC (traffic) V59.59- ☑
              - nontraffic V59.19- ☑
          - pedal cycle (traffic) V51.6- ☑
            - nontraffic V51.1- ☑
          - pickup truck (traffic) V53.6- ☑
            - nontraffic V53.1- ☑
          - railway vehicle (traffic) V55.6- ☑
            - nontraffic V55.1- ☑
          - specified vehicle NEC (traffic) V56.6- ☑
            - nontraffic V56.1- ☑
          - stationary object (traffic) V57.6- ☑
            - nontraffic V57.1- ☑
          - streetcar (traffic) V56.6- ☑
            - nontraffic V56.1- ☑
          - three wheeled motor vehicle (traffic) V52.6- ☑
            - nontraffic V52.1- ☑
          - truck (traffic) V54.6- ☑
            - nontraffic V54.1- ☑
          - two wheeled motor vehicle (traffic) V52.6- ☑
            - nontraffic V52.1- ☑
          - van (traffic) V53.6- ☑
            - nontraffic V53.1- ☑
        - noncollision accident (traffic) V58.6- ☑
          - nontraffic V58.1- ☑
      - specified type NEC V59.88- ☑
        - military vehicle V59.81- ☑
    - quarry truck — *see* Accident, transport, industrial vehicle occupant
    - race car — *see* Accident, transport, motor vehicle NEC occupant
    - railway vehicle occupant V81.9- ☑
      - collision (with) V81.3- ☑
        - motor vehicle (non-military) (traffic) V81.1- ☑
          - military V81.83- ☑
          - nontraffic V81.Ø- ☑
        - rolling stock V81.2- ☑
        - specified object NEC V81.3- ☑
      - during derailment V81.7- ☑
        - with antecedent collision — *see* Accident, transport, railway vehicle occupant, collision
      - explosion V81.81- ☑
      - fall (in railway vehicle) V81.5- ☑
        - during derailment V81.7- ☑
          - with antecedent collision — *see* Accident, transport, railway vehicle occupant, collision
        - from railway vehicle V81.6- ☑
          - during derailment V81.7- ☑
            - with antecedent collision — *see* Accident, transport, railway vehicle occupant, collision
        - while boarding or alighting V81.4- ☑
      - fire V81.81- ☑
      - object falling onto train V81.82- ☑
      - specified type NEC V81.89- ☑
      - while boarding or alighting V81.4- ☑
    - Segway VØØ.848- ☑
    - ski lift V98.3- ☑
    - snowmobile occupant (nontraffic) V86.92- ☑
      - driver V86.52- ☑
      - hanger-on V86.72- ☑
      - passenger V86.62- ☑
      - traffic V86.32- ☑
        - driver V86.Ø2- ☑
        - hanger-on V86.22- ☑
        - passenger V86.12- ☑
      - while boarding or alighting V86.42- ☑
    - specified NEC V98.8- ☑
    - sport utility vehicle occupant — *see also* Accident, transport, pickup truck occupant
    - streetcar occupant V82.9- ☑
      - collision (with) V82.3- ☑

- **Accident** — *continued*
  - transport — *continued*
    - streetcar occupant — *continued*
      - collision — *continued*
        - motor vehicle (traffic) V82.1- ☑
          - nontraffic V82.Ø- ☑
        - rolling stock V82.2- ☑
      - during derailment V82.7- ☑
        - with antecedent collision — *see* Accident, transport, streetcar occupant, collision
      - fall (in streetcar) V82.5- ☑
        - during derailment V82.7- ☑
          - with antecedent collision — *see* Accident, transport, streetcar occupant, collision
        - from streetcar V82.6- ☑
          - during derailment V82.7- ☑
            - with antecedent collision — *see* Accident, transport, streetcar occupant, collision
          - while boarding or alighting V82.4- ☑
        - while boarding or alighting V82.4- ☑
      - specified type NEC V82.8- ☑
      - while boarding or alighting V82.4- ☑
    - three-wheeled motor vehicle occupant V39.9- ☑
      - collision (with)
        - animal (traffic) V3Ø.9- ☑
          - being ridden (traffic) V36.9- ☑
            - nontraffic V36.3- ☑
            - while boarding or alighting V36.4- ☑
          - nontraffic V3Ø.3- ☑
          - while boarding or alighting V3Ø.4- ☑
        - animal-drawn vehicle (traffic) V36.9- ☑
          - nontraffic V36.3- ☑
          - while boarding or alighting V36.4- ☑
        - bus (traffic) V34.9- ☑
          - nontraffic V34.3- ☑
          - while boarding or alighting V34.4- ☑
        - car (traffic) V33.9- ☑
          - nontraffic V33.3- ☑
          - while boarding or alighting V33.4- ☑
        - motor vehicle NOS (traffic) V39.6Ø- ☑
          - nontraffic V39.2Ø- ☑
          - specified type NEC (traffic) V39.69- ☑
            - nontraffic V39.29- ☑
        - pedal cycle (traffic) V31.9- ☑
          - nontraffic V31.3- ☑
          - while boarding or alighting V31.4- ☑
        - pickup truck (traffic) V33.9- ☑
          - nontraffic V33.3- ☑
          - while boarding or alighting V33.4- ☑
        - railway vehicle (traffic) V35.9- ☑
          - nontraffic V35.3- ☑
          - while boarding or alighting V35.4- ☑
        - specified vehicle NEC (traffic) V36.9- ☑
          - nontraffic V36.3- ☑
          - while boarding or alighting V36.4- ☑
        - stationary object (traffic) V37.9- ☑
          - nontraffic V37.3- ☑
          - while boarding or alighting V37.4- ☑
        - streetcar (traffic) V36.9- ☑
          - nontraffic V36.3- ☑
          - while boarding or alighting V36.4- ☑
        - three wheeled motor vehicle (traffic) V32.9- ☑
          - nontraffic V32.3- ☑
          - while boarding or alighting V32.4- ☑
        - truck (traffic) V34.9- ☑
          - nontraffic V34.3- ☑
          - while boarding or alighting V34.4- ☑
        - two wheeled motor vehicle (traffic) V32.9- ☑
          - nontraffic V32.3- ☑
          - while boarding or alighting V32.4- ☑
        - van (traffic) V33.9- ☑
          - nontraffic V33.3- ☑
          - while boarding or alighting V33.4- ☑
      - driver
        - collision (with)
          - animal (traffic) V3Ø.5- ☑
            - being ridden (traffic) V36.5- ☑
              - nontraffic V36.Ø- ☑
            - nontraffic V3Ø.Ø- ☑
          - animal-drawn vehicle (traffic) V36.5- ☑
            - nontraffic V36.Ø- ☑
          - bus (traffic) V34.5- ☑
            - nontraffic V34.Ø- ☑

- **Accident** — *continued*
  - transport — *continued*
    - three-wheeled motor vehicle occupant — *continued*
      - driver — *continued*
        - collision — *continued*
          - car (traffic) V33.5- ☑
            - nontraffic V33.Ø- ☑
          - motor vehicle NOS (traffic) V39.4Ø- ☑
            - nontraffic V39.ØØ- ☑
            - specified type NEC (traffic) V39.49- ☑
              - nontraffic V39.Ø9- ☑
          - pedal cycle (traffic) V31.5- ☑
            - nontraffic V31.Ø- ☑
          - pickup truck (traffic) V33.5- ☑
            - nontraffic V33.Ø- ☑
          - railway vehicle (traffic) V35.5- ☑
            - nontraffic V35.Ø- ☑
          - specified vehicle NEC (traffic) V36.5- ☑
            - nontraffic V36.Ø- ☑
          - stationary object (traffic) V37.5- ☑
            - nontraffic V37.Ø- ☑
          - streetcar (traffic) V36.5- ☑
            - nontraffic V36.Ø- ☑
          - three wheeled motor vehicle (traffic) V32.5- ☑
            - nontraffic V32.Ø- ☑
          - truck (traffic) V34.5- ☑
            - nontraffic V34.Ø- ☑
          - two wheeled motor vehicle (traffic) V32.5- ☑
            - nontraffic V32.Ø- ☑
          - van (traffic) V33.5- ☑
            - nontraffic V33.Ø- ☑
        - noncollision accident (traffic) V38.5- ☑
          - nontraffic V38.Ø- ☑
      - hanger-on
        - collision (with)
          - animal (traffic) V3Ø.7- ☑
            - being ridden (traffic) V36.7- ☑
              - nontraffic V36.2- ☑
            - nontraffic V3Ø.2- ☑
          - animal-drawn vehicle (traffic) V36.7- ☑
            - nontraffic V36.2- ☑
          - bus (traffic) V34.7- ☑
            - nontraffic V34.2- ☑
          - car (traffic) V33.7- ☑
            - nontraffic V33.2- ☑
          - pedal cycle (traffic) V31.7- ☑
            - nontraffic V31.2- ☑
          - pickup truck (traffic) V33.7- ☑
            - nontraffic V33.2- ☑
          - railway vehicle (traffic) V35.7- ☑
            - nontraffic V35.2- ☑
          - specified vehicle NEC (traffic) V36.7- ☑
            - nontraffic V36.2- ☑
          - stationary object (traffic) V37.7- ☑
            - nontraffic V37.2- ☑
          - streetcar (traffic) V36.7- ☑
            - nontraffic V36.2- ☑
          - three wheeled motor vehicle (traffic) V32.7- ☑
            - nontraffic V32.2- ☑
          - truck (traffic) V34.7- ☑
            - nontraffic V34.2- ☑
          - two wheeled motor vehicle (traffic) V32.7- ☑
            - nontraffic V32.2- ☑
          - van (traffic) V33.7- ☑
            - nontraffic V33.2- ☑
        - noncollision accident (traffic) V38.7- ☑
          - nontraffic V38.2- ☑
      - noncollision accident (traffic) V38.9- ☑
        - nontraffic V38.3- ☑
        - while boarding or alighting V38.4- ☑
      - nontraffic V39.3- ☑
      - passenger
        - collision (with)
          - animal (traffic) V3Ø.6- ☑
            - being ridden (traffic) V36.6- ☑
              - nontraffic V36.1- ☑
            - nontraffic V3Ø.1- ☑
          - animal-drawn vehicle (traffic) V36.6- ☑
            - nontraffic V36.1- ☑
          - bus (traffic) V34.6- ☑

- **Accident** — *continued*
  - transport — *continued*
    - three-wheeled motor vehicle occupant — *continued*
      - passenger — *continued*
        - collision — *continued*
          - bus — *continued*
            - nontraffic V34.1- ☑
          - car (traffic) V33.6- ☑
            - nontraffic V33.1- ☑
          - motor vehicle NOS (traffic) V39.5Ø- ☑
            - nontraffic V39.1Ø- ☑
            - specified type NEC (traffic) V39.59- ☑
              - nontraffic V39.19- ☑
          - pedal cycle (traffic) V31.6- ☑
            - nontraffic V31.1- ☑
          - pickup truck (traffic) V33.6- ☑
            - nontraffic V33.1- ☑
          - railway vehicle (traffic) V35.6- ☑
            - nontraffic V35.1- ☑
          - specified vehicle NEC (traffic) V36.6- ☑
            - nontraffic V36.1- ☑
          - stationary object (traffic) V37.6- ☑
            - nontraffic V37.1- ☑
          - streetcar (traffic) V36.6- ☑
            - nontraffic V36.1- ☑
          - three wheeled motor vehicle (traffic) V32.6- ☑
            - nontraffic V32.1- ☑
          - truck (traffic) V34.6- ☑
            - nontraffic V34.1- ☑
          - two wheeled motor vehicle (traffic) V32.6- ☑
            - nontraffic V32.1- ☑
          - van (traffic) V33.6- ☑
            - nontraffic V33.1- ☑
        - noncollision accident (traffic) V38.6- ☑
          - nontraffic V38.1- ☑
      - specified type NEC V39.89- ☑
        - military vehicle V39.81- ☑
    - tractor (farm) (and trailer) — *see* Accident, transport, agricultural vehicle occupant
    - tram — *see* Accident, transport, streetcar
      - in mine or quarry — *see* Accident, transport, industrial vehicle occupant
    - trolley — *see* Accident, transport, streetcar
      - in mine or quarry — *see* Accident, transport, industrial vehicle occupant
    - truck (heavy) occupant V69.9- ☑
      - collision (with)
        - animal (traffic) V6Ø.9- ☑
          - being ridden (traffic) V66.9- ☑
            - nontraffic V66.3- ☑
            - while boarding or alighting V66.4- ☑
          - nontraffic V6Ø.3- ☑
          - while boarding or alighting V6Ø.4- ☑
        - animal-drawn vehicle (traffic) V66.9- ☑
          - nontraffic V66.3- ☑
          - while boarding or alighting V66.4- ☑
        - bus (traffic) V64.9- ☑
          - nontraffic V64.3- ☑
          - while boarding or alighting V64.4- ☑
        - car (traffic) V63.9- ☑
          - nontraffic V63.3- ☑
          - while boarding or alighting V63.4- ☑
        - motor vehicle NOS (traffic) V69.6Ø- ☑
          - nontraffic V69.2Ø- ☑
          - specified type NEC (traffic) V69.69- ☑
            - nontraffic V69.29- ☑
        - pedal cycle (traffic) V61.9- ☑
          - nontraffic V61.3- ☑
          - while boarding or alighting V61.4- ☑
        - pickup truck (traffic) V63.9- ☑
          - nontraffic V63.3- ☑
          - while boarding or alighting V63.4- ☑
        - railway vehicle (traffic) V65.9- ☑
          - nontraffic V65.3- ☑
          - while boarding or alighting V65.4- ☑
        - specified vehicle NEC (traffic) V66.9- ☑
          - nontraffic V66.3- ☑
          - while boarding or alighting V66.4- ☑
        - stationary object (traffic) V67.9- ☑
          - nontraffic V67.3- ☑
          - while boarding or alighting V67.4- ☑
        - streetcar (traffic) V66.9- ☑
          - nontraffic V66.3- ☑

- **Accident** — *continued*
  - transport — *continued*
    - van occupant — *continued*
      - hanger-on — *continued*
        - collision — *continued*
          - bus (traffic) V54.7- ☑
            - nontraffic V54.2- ☑
          - car (traffic) V53.7- ☑
            - nontraffic V53.2- ☑
          - pedal cycle (traffic) V51.7- ☑
            - nontraffic V51.2- ☑
          - pickup truck (traffic) V53.7- ☑
            - nontraffic V53.2- ☑
          - railway vehicle (traffic) V55.7- ☑
            - nontraffic V55.2- ☑
          - specified vehicle NEC (traffic) V56.7- ☑
            - nontraffic V56.2- ☑
          - stationary object (traffic) V57.7- ☑
            - nontraffic V57.2- ☑
          - streetcar (traffic) V56.7- ☑
            - nontraffic V56.2- ☑
          - three wheeled motor vehicle (traffic) V52.7- ☑
            - nontraffic V52.2- ☑
          - truck (traffic) V54.7- ☑
            - nontraffic V54.2- ☑
          - two wheeled motor vehicle (traffic) V52.7- ☑
            - nontraffic V52.2- ☑
          - van (traffic) V53.7- ☑
            - nontraffic V53.2- ☑
        - noncollision accident (traffic) V58.7- ☑
          - nontraffic V58.2- ☑
      - noncollision accident (traffic) V58.9- ☑
        - nontraffic V58.3- ☑
        - while boarding or alighting V58.4- ☑
      - nontraffic V59.3- ☑
      - passenger
        - collision (with)
          - animal (traffic) V5Ø.6- ☑
            - being ridden (traffic) V56.6- ☑
              - nontraffic V56.1- ☑
            - nontraffic V5Ø.1- ☑
          - animal-drawn vehicle (traffic) V56.6- ☑
            - nontraffic V56.1- ☑
          - bus (traffic) V54.6- ☑
            - nontraffic V54.1- ☑
          - car (traffic) V53.6- ☑
            - nontraffic V53.1- ☑
          - motor vehicle NOS (traffic) V59.5Ø- ☑
            - nontraffic V59.1Ø- ☑
            - specified type NEC (traffic) V59.59- ☑
              - nontraffic V59.19- ☑
          - pedal cycle (traffic) V51.6- ☑
            - nontraffic V51.1- ☑
          - pickup truck (traffic) V53.6- ☑
            - nontraffic V53.1- ☑
          - railway vehicle (traffic) V55.6- ☑
            - nontraffic V55.1- ☑
          - specified vehicle NEC (traffic) V56.6- ☑
            - nontraffic V56.1- ☑
          - stationary object (traffic) V57.6- ☑
            - nontraffic V57.1- ☑
          - streetcar (traffic) V56.6- ☑
            - nontraffic V56.1- ☑
          - three wheeled motor vehicle (traffic) V52.6- ☑
            - nontraffic V52.1- ☑
          - truck (traffic) V54.6- ☑
            - nontraffic V54.1- ☑
          - two wheeled motor vehicle (traffic) V52.6- ☑
            - nontraffic V52.1- ☑
          - van (traffic) V53.6- ☑
            - nontraffic V53.1- ☑
        - noncollision accident (traffic) V58.6- ☑
          - nontraffic V58.1- ☑
      - specified type NEC V59.88- ☑
        - military vehicle V59.81- ☑
    - watercraft occupant — *see* Accident, watercraft
  - vehicle NEC V89.9- ☑
    - animal-drawn NEC — *see* Accident, transport, animal-drawn vehicle occupant

- **Accident** — *continued*
  - vehicle — *continued*
    - special
      - agricultural — *see* Accident, transport, agricultural vehicle occupant
      - construction — *see* Accident, transport, construction vehicle occupant
      - industrial — *see* Accident, transport, industrial vehicle occupant
    - three-wheeled NEC (motorized) — *see* Accident, transport, three-wheeled motor vehicle occupant
  - watercraft V94.9- ☑
    - causing
      - drowning — *see* Drowning, due to, accident to, watercraft
      - injury NEC V91.89- ☑
        - crushed between craft and object V91.19- ☑
          - powered craft V91.13- ☑
            - ferry boat V91.11- ☑
            - fishing boat V91.12- ☑
            - jetskis V91.13- ☑
            - liner V91.11- ☑
            - merchant ship V91.1Ø- ☑
            - passenger ship V91.11- ☑
          - unpowered craft V91.18- ☑
            - canoe V91.15- ☑
            - inflatable V91.16- ☑
            - kayak V91.15- ☑
            - sailboat V91.14- ☑
            - surf-board V91.18- ☑
            - windsurfer V91.18- ☑
        - fall on board V91.29- ☑
          - powered craft V91.23- ☑
            - ferry boat V91.21- ☑
            - fishing boat V91.22- ☑
            - jetskis V91.23- ☑
            - liner V91.21- ☑
            - merchant ship V91.2Ø- ☑
            - passenger ship V91.21- ☑
          - unpowered craft
            - canoe V91.25- ☑
            - inflatable V91.26- ☑
            - kayak V91.25- ☑
            - sailboat V91.24- ☑
        - fire on board causing burn V91.Ø9- ☑
          - powered craft V91.Ø3- ☑
            - ferry boat V91.Ø1- ☑
            - fishing boat V91.Ø2- ☑
            - jetskis V91.Ø3- ☑
            - liner V91.Ø1- ☑
            - merchant ship V91.ØØ- ☑
            - passenger ship V91.Ø1- ☑
          - unpowered craft V91.Ø8- ☑
            - canoe V91.Ø5- ☑
            - inflatable V91.Ø6- ☑
            - kayak V91.Ø5- ☑
            - sailboat V91.Ø4- ☑
            - surf-board V91.Ø8- ☑
            - water skis V91.Ø7- ☑
            - windsurfer V91.Ø8- ☑
        - hit by falling object V91.39- ☑
          - powered craft V91.33- ☑
            - ferry boat V91.31- ☑
            - fishing boat V91.32- ☑
            - jetskis V91.33- ☑
            - liner V91.31- ☑
            - merchant ship V91.3Ø- ☑
            - passenger ship V91.31- ☑
          - unpowered craft V91.38- ☑
            - canoe V91.35- ☑
            - inflatable V91.36- ☑
            - kayak V91.35- ☑
            - sailboat V91.34- ☑
            - surf-board V91.38- ☑
            - water skis V91.37- ☑
            - windsurfer V91.38- ☑
        - specified type NEC V91.89- ☑
          - powered craft V91.83- ☑
            - ferry boat V91.81- ☑
            - fishing boat V91.82- ☑
            - jetskis V91.83- ☑
            - liner V91.81- ☑
            - merchant ship V91.8Ø- ☑
            - passenger ship V91.81- ☑

- **Accident** — *continued*
  - watercraft — *continued*
    - causing — *continued*
      - injury — *continued*
        - specified type — *continued*
          - unpowered craft V91.88- ☑
            - canoe V91.85- ☑
            - inflatable V91.86- ☑
            - kayak V91.85- ☑
            - sailboat V91.84- ☑
            - surf-board V91.88- ☑
            - water skis V91.87- ☑
            - windsurfer V91.88- ☑
    - due to, caused by cataclysm — *see* Forces of nature, by type
    - military NEC V94.818- ☑
      - civilian in water injured by V94.811- ☑
      - with civilian watercraft V94.81Ø- ☑
    - nonpowered, struck by
      - nonpowered vessel V94.21- ☑
      - powered vessel V94.22- ☑
    - specified type NEC V94.89- ☑
    - striking swimmer
      - powered V94.11- ☑
      - unpowered V94.12- ☑
- **Acid throwing** (assault) YØ8.89- ☑
- **Activity** (involving) (of victim at time of event) Y93.9
  - aerobic and step exercise (class) Y93.A3 (*following* Y93.7)
  - alpine skiing Y93.23
  - animal care NEC Y93.K9 (*following* Y93.7)
  - arts and handcrafts NEC Y93.D9 (*following* Y93.7)
  - athletics NEC Y93.79
  - athletics played as a team or group NEC Y93.69
  - athletics played individually NEC Y93.59
  - badminton Y93.73
  - baking Y93.G3 (*following* Y93.7)
  - ballet Y93.41
  - barbells Y93.B3 (*following* Y93.7)
  - BASE (Building, Antenna, Span, Earth) jumping Y93.33
  - baseball Y93.64
  - basketball Y93.67
  - bathing (personal) Y93.E1 (*following* Y93.7)
  - beach volleyball Y93.68
  - bike riding Y93.55
  - blackout game Y93.85
  - boogie boarding Y93.18
  - bowling Y93.54
  - boxing Y93.71
  - brass instrument playing Y93.J4 (*following* Y93.7)
  - building construction Y93.H3 (*following* Y93.7)
  - bungee jumping Y93.34
  - calisthenics Y93.A2 (*following* Y93.7)
  - canoeing (in calm and turbulent water) Y93.16
  - capture the flag Y93.6A
  - cardiorespiratory exercise NEC Y93.A9 (*following* Y93.7)
  - caregiving (providing) NEC Y93.F9 (*following* Y93.7)
    - bathing Y93.F1 (*following* Y93.7)
    - lifting Y93.F2 (*following* Y93.7)
  - cellular
    - communication device Y93.C2 (*following* Y93.7)
    - telephone Y93.C2 (*following* Y93.7)
  - challenge course Y93.A5 (*following* Y93.7)
  - cheerleading Y93.45
  - choking game Y93.85
  - circuit training Y93.A4 (*following* Y93.7)
  - cleaning
    - floor Y93.E5 (*following* Y93.7)
  - climbing NEC Y93.39
    - mountain Y93.31
    - rock Y93.31
    - wall Y93.31
  - clothing care and maintenance NEC Y93.E9 (*following* Y93.7)
  - combatives Y93.75
  - computer
    - keyboarding Y93.C1 (*following* Y93.7)
    - technology NEC Y93.C9 (*following* Y93.7)
  - confidence course Y93.A5 (*following* Y93.7)
  - construction (building) Y93.H3 (*following* Y93.7)
  - cooking and baking Y93.G3 (*following* Y93.7)
  - cool down exercises Y93.A2 (*following* Y93.7)
  - cricket Y93.69
  - crocheting Y93.D1 (*following* Y93.7)
  - cross country skiing Y93.24
  - dancing (all types) Y93.41
  - digging
    - dirt Y93.H1 (*following* Y93.7)
  - dirt digging Y93.H1 (*following* Y93.7)

- **Air** — *continued*
  - pressure — *continued*
    - high, prolonged W94.Ø- ☑
    - low, prolonged W94.12- ☑
      - due to residence or long visit at high altitude W94.11- ☑
- **Alpine sickness** W94.11- ☑
- **Altitude sickness** W94.11- ☑
- **Anaphylactic shock, anaphylaxis** — *see* Table of Drugs and Chemicals
- **Andes disease** W94.11- ☑
- **Arachnidism, arachnoidism** X58.- ☑
- **Arson** (with intent to injure or kill) X97.- ☑
- **Asphyxia, asphyxiation**
  - by
    - food (bone) (seed) — *see* categories T17 and T18.- ☑
    - gas — *see also* Table of Drugs and Chemicals
      - legal
        - execution — *see* Legal, intervention, gas
        - intervention — *see* Legal, intervention, gas
  - from
    - fire — *see also* Exposure, fire
      - in war operations — *see* War operations, fire
    - ignition — *see* Ignition
    - vomitus T17.81Ø- ☑
  - in war operations — *see* War operations, restriction of airway
- **Aspiration**
  - food (any type) (into respiratory tract) (with asphyxia, obstruction respiratory tract, suffocation) — *see* categories T17 and T18.- ☑
  - foreign body — *see* Foreign body, aspiration
  - vomitus (with asphyxia, obstruction respiratory tract, suffocation) — *see* Index to Diseases and Injuries, Foreign body, respiratory tract
- **Assassination** (attempt) — *see* Assault
- **Assault** (homicidal) (by) (in) YØ9
  - arson X97.- ☑
  - bite (of human being) YØ4.1- ☑
  - bodily force YØ4.8- ☑
    - bite YØ4.1- ☑
    - bumping into YØ4.2- ☑
    - sexual (confirmed) T74.2- ☑
      - suspected T76.2- ☑
    - unarmed fight YØ4.Ø- ☑
  - bomb X96.9- ☑
    - antipersonnel X96.Ø- ☑
    - fertilizer X96.3- ☑
    - gasoline X96.1- ☑
    - letter X96.2- ☑
    - petrol X96.1- ☑
    - pipe X96.3- ☑
    - specified NEC X96.8- ☑
  - brawl (hand) (fists) (foot) (unarmed) YØ4.Ø- ☑
  - burning, burns (by fire) NEC X97.- ☑
    - acid YØ8.89- ☑
    - caustic, corrosive substance YØ8.89- ☑
    - chemical from swallowing caustic, corrosive substance — *see* Table of Drugs and Chemicals
    - cigarette(s) X97.- ☑
    - hot object X98.9- ☑
      - fluid NEC X98.2- ☑
      - household appliance X98.3- ☑
      - specified NEC X98.8- ☑
      - steam X98.Ø- ☑
      - tap water X98.1- ☑
      - vapors X98.Ø- ☑
    - scalding — *see* Assault, burning
    - steam X98.Ø- ☑
    - vitriol YØ8.89- ☑
  - caustic, corrosive substance (gas) YØ8.89- ☑
  - crashing of
    - aircraft YØ8.81- ☑
    - motor vehicle YØ3.8- ☑
      - pushed in front of YØ2.Ø- ☑
      - run over YØ3.Ø- ☑
      - specified NEC YØ3.8- ☑
  - cutting or piercing instrument X99.9- ☑
    - dagger X99.2- ☑
    - glass X99.Ø- ☑
    - knife X99.1- ☑
    - specified NEC X99.8- ☑
    - sword X99.2- ☑
  - dagger X99.2- ☑
  - drowning (in) X92.9- ☑
    - bathtub X92.Ø- ☑
- **Assault** — *continued*
  - drowning — *continued*
    - natural water X92.3- ☑
    - specified NEC X92.8- ☑
    - swimming pool X92.1- ☑
      - following fall X92.2- ☑
  - dynamite X96.8- ☑
  - explosive(s) (material) X96.9- ☑
  - fight (hand) (fists) (foot) (unarmed) YØ4.Ø- ☑
    - with weapon — *see* Assault, by type of weapon
  - fire X97.- ☑
  - firearm X95.9- ☑
    - airgun X95.Ø1- ☑
    - handgun X93.- ☑
    - hunting rifle X94.1- ☑
    - larger X94.9- ☑
      - specified NEC X94.8- ☑
    - machine gun X94.2- ☑
    - shotgun X94.Ø- ☑
    - specified NEC X95.8- ☑
  - from high place YØ1.- ☑
  - gunshot (wound) NEC — *see* Assault, firearm, by type
  - incendiary device X97.- ☑
  - injury YØ9
    - to child due to criminal abortion attempt NEC YØ8.89- ☑
  - knife X99.1- ☑
  - late effect of — *see* categories X92-YØ8 with 7th character S
  - placing before moving object NEC YØ2.8- ☑
    - motor vehicle YØ2.Ø- ☑
  - poisoning — *see* categories T36-T65 with 7th character S
  - puncture, any part of body — *see* Assault, cutting or piercing instrument
  - pushing
    - before moving object NEC YØ2.8- ☑
      - motor vehicle YØ2.Ø- ☑
      - subway train YØ2.1- ☑
      - train YØ2.1- ☑
    - from high place YØ1.- ☑
  - rape (confirmed) T74.2- ☑
    - suspected T76.2- ☑
  - scalding — *see* Assault, burning
  - sequelae of — *see* categories X92-YØ8 with 7th character S
  - sexual (by bodily force) T74.2- ☑
    - suspected T76.2- ☑
  - shooting — *see* Assault, firearm
  - specified means NEC YØ8.89- ☑
  - stab, any part of body — *see* Assault, cutting or piercing instrument
  - steam X98.Ø- ☑
  - striking against
    - other person YØ4.2- ☑
    - sports equipment YØ8.Ø9- ☑
      - baseball bat YØ8.Ø2- ☑
      - hockey stick YØ8.Ø1- ☑
  - struck by
    - sports equipment YØ8.Ø9- ☑
      - baseball bat YØ8.Ø2- ☑
      - hockey stick YØ8.Ø1- ☑
  - submersion — *see* Assault, drowning
  - violence YØ9
  - weapon YØ9
    - blunt YØØ.- ☑
    - cutting or piercing — *see* Assault, cutting or piercing instrument
    - firearm — *see* Assault, firearm
  - wound YØ9
    - cutting — *see* Assault, cutting or piercing instrument
    - gunshot — *see* Assault, firearm
    - knife X99.1- ☑
    - piercing — *see* Assault, cutting or piercing instrument
    - puncture — *see* Assault, cutting or piercing instrument
    - stab — *see* Assault, cutting or piercing instrument
- **Attack by mammals NEC** W55.89- ☑
- **Avalanche** — *see* Landslide
- **Aviator's disease** — *see* Air, pressure

## B

- **Barotitis, barodontalgia, barosinusitis, barotrauma** (otitic) (sinus) — *see* Air, pressure
- **Battered** (baby) (child) (person) (syndrome) X58.- ☑
- **Bayonet wound** W26.1- ☑
  - in
    - legal intervention — *see* Legal, intervention, sharp object, bayonet
    - war operations — *see* War operations, combat
  - stated as undetermined whether accidental or intentional Y28.8- ☑
  - suicide (attempt) X78.2- ☑
- **Bean in nose** T17.1- ☑
- **Bed set on fire NEC** — *see* Exposure, fire, uncontrolled, building, bed
- **Beheading** (by guillotine)
  - homicide X99.9- ☑
  - legal execution — *see* Legal, intervention
- **Bending, injury in** (prolonged) (static) X5Ø.1- ☑
- **Bends** — *see* Air, pressure, change
- **Bite, bitten by**
  - alligator W58.Ø1- ☑
  - arthropod (nonvenomous) NEC W57.- ☑
  - bull W55.21- ☑
  - cat W55.Ø1- ☑
  - cow W55.21- ☑
  - crocodile W58.11- ☑
  - dog W54.Ø- ☑
  - goat W55.31- ☑
  - hoof stock NEC W55.31- ☑
  - horse W55.11- ☑
  - human being (accidentally) W5Ø.3- ☑
    - with intent to injure or kill YØ4.1- ☑
    - as, or caused by, a crowd or human stampede (with fall) W52.- ☑
    - assault YØ4.1- ☑
    - homicide (attempt) YØ4.1- ☑
    - in
      - fight YØ4.1- ☑
  - insect (nonvenomous) W57.- ☑
  - lizard (nonvenomous) W59.Ø1- ☑
  - mammal NEC W55.81- ☑
    - marine W56.31- ☑
  - marine animal (nonvenomous) W56.81- ☑
  - millipede W57.- ☑
  - moray eel W56.51- ☑
  - mouse W53.Ø1- ☑
  - person(s) (accidentally) W5Ø.3- ☑
    - with intent to injure or kill YØ4.1- ☑
    - as, or caused by, a crowd or human stampede (with fall) W52.- ☑
    - assault YØ4.1- ☑
    - homicide (attempt) YØ4.1- ☑
    - in
      - fight YØ4.1- ☑
  - pig W55.41- ☑
  - raccoon W55.51- ☑
  - rat W53.11- ☑
  - reptile W59.81- ☑
    - lizard W59.Ø1- ☑
    - snake W59.11- ☑
    - turtle W59.21- ☑
      - terrestrial W59.81- ☑
  - rodent W53.81- ☑
    - mouse W53.Ø1- ☑
    - rat W53.11- ☑
    - specified NEC W53.81- ☑
    - squirrel W53.21- ☑
  - shark W56.41- ☑
  - sheep W55.31- ☑
  - snake (nonvenomous) W59.11- ☑
  - spider (nonvenomous) W57.- ☑
  - squirrel W53.21- ☑
- **Blast** (air) in war operations — *see* War operations, blast
- **Blizzard** X37.2- ☑
- **Blood alcohol level** Y9Ø.9
  - less than 2Ømg/1ØØml Y9Ø.Ø
  - presence in blood, level not specified Y9Ø.9
  - 2Ø-39mg/1ØØml Y9Ø.1
  - 4Ø-59mg/1ØØml Y9Ø.2
  - 6Ø-79mg/1ØØml Y9Ø.3
  - 8Ø-99mg/1ØØml Y9Ø.4
  - 1ØØ-119mg/1ØØml Y9Ø.5
  - 12Ø-199mg/1ØØml Y9Ø.6
  - 2ØØ-239mg/1ØØml Y9Ø.7
- **Blow** X58.- ☑
  - by law-enforcing agent, police (on duty) — *see* Legal, intervention, manhandling
    - blunt object — *see* Legal, intervention, blunt object
- **Blowing up** — *see* Explosion

**Brawl** (hand) (fists) (foot) YØ4.Ø- ☑
**Breakage** (accidental) (part of)
- ladder (causing fall) W11.- ☑
- scaffolding (causing fall) W12.- ☑

**Broken**
- glass, contact with — *see* Contact, with, glass
- power line (causing electric shock) W85.- ☑

**Bumping against, into** (accidentally)
- object NEC W22.8- ☑
  - caused by crowd or human stampede (with fall) W52.- ☑
  - sports equipment W21.9- ☑
  - with fall — *see* Fall, due to, bumping against, object
- person(s) W51.- ☑
  - with fall WØ3.- ☑
    - due to ice or snow WØØ.Ø- ☑
  - assault YØ4.2- ☑
  - caused by, a crowd or human stampede (with fall) W52.- ☑
  - homicide (attempt) YØ4.2- ☑
- sports equipment W21.9- ☑

**Burn, burned, burning** (accidental) (by) (from) (on)
- acid NEC — *see* Table of Drugs and Chemicals
- bed linen — *see* Exposure, fire, uncontrolled, in building, bed
- blowtorch XØ8.8- ☑
  - with ignition of clothing NEC XØ6.2- ☑
    - nightwear XØ5.- ☑
- bonfire, campfire (controlled) — *see also* Exposure, fire, controlled, not in building)
  - uncontrolled — *see* Exposure, fire, uncontrolled, not in building
- candle XØ8.8- ☑
  - with ignition of clothing NEC XØ6.2- ☑
    - nightwear XØ5.- ☑
- caustic liquid, substance (external) (internal) NEC — *see* Table of Drugs and Chemicals
- chemical (external) (internal) — *see also* Table of Drugs and Chemicals
  - in war operations — *see* War operations. fire
- cigar(s) or cigarette(s) XØ8.8- ☑
  - with ignition of clothing NEC XØ6.2- ☑
    - nightwear XØ5.- ☑
- clothes, clothing NEC (from controlled fire) XØ6.2- ☑
  - with conflagration — *see* Exposure, fire, uncontrolled, building
    - not in building or structure — *see* Exposure, fire, uncontrolled, not in building
- cooker (hot) X15.8- ☑
  - stated as undetermined whether accidental or intentional Y27.3- ☑
  - suicide (attempt) X77.3- ☑
- electric blanket X16.- ☑
- engine (hot) X17.- ☑
- fire, flames — *see* Exposure, fire
- flare, Very pistol — *see* Discharge, firearm NEC
- heat
  - from appliance (electrical) (household) X15.8- ☑
    - cooker X15.8- ☑
    - hotplate X15.2- ☑
    - kettle X15.8- ☑
    - light bulb X15.8- ☑
    - saucepan X15.3- ☑
    - skillet X15.3- ☑
    - stated as undetermined whether accidental or intentional Y27.3- ☑
    - stove X15.Ø- ☑
    - suicide (attempt) X77.3- ☑
    - toaster X15.1- ☑
  - in local application or packing during medical or surgical procedure Y63.5
- heating
  - appliance, radiator or pipe X16.- ☑
- homicide (attempt) — *see* Assault, burning
- hot
  - air X14.1- ☑
  - cooker X15.8- ☑
  - drink X1Ø.Ø- ☑
  - engine X17.- ☑
  - fat X1Ø.2- ☑
  - fluid NEC X12.- ☑
  - food X1Ø.1- ☑
  - gases X14.1- ☑
  - heating appliance X16.- ☑
  - household appliance NEC X15.8- ☑
  - kettle X15.8- ☑

**Burn, burned, burning** — *continued*
- hot — *continued*
  - liquid NEC X12.- ☑
  - machinery X17.- ☑
  - metal (molten) (liquid) NEC X18.- ☑
  - object (not producing fire or flames) NEC X19.- ☑
  - oil (cooking) X1Ø.2- ☑
  - pipe(s) X16.- ☑
  - radiator X16.- ☑
  - saucepan (glass) (metal) X15.3- ☑
  - stove (kitchen) X15.Ø- ☑
  - substance NEC X19.- ☑
    - caustic or corrosive NEC — *see* Table of Drugs and Chemicals
  - toaster X15.1- ☑
  - tool X17.- ☑
  - vapor X13.1- ☑
  - water (tap) — *see* Contact, with, hot, tap water
- hotplate X15.2- ☑
  - suicide (attempt) X77.3- ☑
- ignition — *see* Ignition
- in war operations — *see* War operations, fire
- inflicted by other person X97.- ☑
  - by hot objects, hot vapor, and steam — *see* Assault, burning, hot object
- internal, from swallowed caustic, corrosive liquid, substance — *see* Table of Drugs and Chemicals
- iron (hot) X15.8- ☑
  - stated as undetermined whether accidental or intentional Y27.3- ☑
  - suicide (attempt) X77.3- ☑
- kettle (hot) X15.8- ☑
  - stated as undetermined whether accidental or intentional Y27.3- ☑
  - suicide (attempt) X77.3- ☑
- lamp (flame) XØ8.8- ☑
  - with ignition of clothing NEC XØ6.2- ☑
    - nightwear XØ5.- ☑
- lighter (cigar) (cigarette) XØ8.8- ☑
  - with ignition of clothing NEC XØ6.2- ☑
    - nightwear XØ5.- ☑
- lightning — *see* subcategory T75.Ø- ☑
  - causing fire — *see* Exposure, fire
- liquid (boiling) (hot) NEC X12.- ☑
  - stated as undetermined whether accidental or intentional Y27.2- ☑
  - suicide (attempt) X77.2- ☑
- local application of externally applied substance in medical or surgical care Y63.5
- machinery (hot) X17.- ☑
- matches XØ8.8- ☑
  - with ignition of clothing NEC XØ6.2- ☑
    - nightwear XØ5.- ☑
- mattress — *see* Exposure, fire, uncontrolled, building, bed
- medicament, externally applied Y63.5
- metal (hot) (liquid) (molten) NEC X18.- ☑
- nightwear (nightclothes, nightdress, gown, pajamas, robe) XØ5.- ☑
- object (hot) NEC X19.- ☑
- on board watercraft
  - due to
    - accident to watercraft V91.Ø9- ☑
      - powered craft V91.Ø3- ☑
        - ferry boat V91.Ø1- ☑
        - fishing boat V91.Ø2- ☑
        - jetskis V91.Ø3- ☑
        - liner V91.Ø1- ☑
        - merchant ship V91.ØØ- ☑
        - passenger ship V91.Ø1- ☑
      - unpowered craft V91.Ø8- ☑
        - canoe V91.Ø5- ☑
        - inflatable V91.Ø6- ☑
        - kayak V91.Ø5- ☑
        - sailboat V91.Ø4- ☑
        - surf-board V91.Ø8- ☑
        - water skis V91.Ø7- ☑
        - windsurfer V91.Ø8- ☑
    - fire on board V93.Ø9- ☑
      - ferry boat V93.Ø1- ☑
      - fishing boat V93.Ø2- ☑
      - jetskis V93.Ø3- ☑
      - liner V93.Ø1- ☑
      - merchant ship V93.ØØ- ☑
      - passenger ship V93.Ø1- ☑
      - powered craft NEC V93.Ø3- ☑

**Burn, burned, burning** — *continued*
- on board watercraft — *continued*
  - due to — *continued*
    - fire on board — *continued*
      - sailboat V93.Ø4- ☑
    - specified heat source NEC on board V93.19- ☑
      - ferry boat V93.11- ☑
      - fishing boat V93.12- ☑
      - jetskis V93.13- ☑
      - liner V93.11- ☑
      - merchant ship V93.1Ø- ☑
      - passenger ship V93.11- ☑
      - powered craft NEC V93.13- ☑
      - sailboat V93.14- ☑
- pipe (hot) X16.- ☑
  - smoking XØ8.8- ☑
    - with ignition of clothing NEC XØ6.2- ☑
      - nightwear XØ5.- ☑
- powder — *see* Powder burn
- radiator (hot) X16.- ☑
- saucepan (hot) (glass) (metal) X15.3- ☑
  - stated as undetermined whether accidental or intentional Y27.3- ☑
  - suicide (attempt) X77.3- ☑
- self-inflicted X76.- ☑
  - stated as undetermined whether accidental or intentional Y26.- ☑
- stated as undetermined whether accidental or intentional Y27.Ø- ☑
- steam X13.1- ☑
  - pipe X16.- ☑
    - stated as undetermined whether accidental or intentional Y27.8- ☑
  - stated as undetermined whether accidental or intentional Y27.Ø- ☑
  - suicide (attempt) X77.Ø- ☑
- stove (hot) (kitchen) X15.Ø- ☑
  - stated as undetermined whether accidental or intentional Y27.3- ☑
  - suicide (attempt) X77.3- ☑
- substance (hot) NEC X19.- ☑
  - boiling X12.- ☑
    - stated as undetermined whether accidental or intentional Y27.2- ☑
    - suicide (attempt) X77.2- ☑
  - molten (metal) X18.- ☑
- suicide (attempt) NEC X76.- ☑
  - hot
    - household appliance X77.3- ☑
    - object X77.9- ☑
- therapeutic misadventure
  - heat in local application or packing during medical or surgical procedure Y63.5
  - overdose of radiation Y63.2
- toaster (hot) X15.1- ☑
  - stated as undetermined whether accidental or intentional Y27.3- ☑
  - suicide (attempt) X77.3- ☑
- tool (hot) X17.- ☑
- torch, welding XØ8.8- ☑
  - with ignition of clothing NEC XØ6.2- ☑
    - nightwear XØ5.- ☑
- trash fire (controlled) — *see* Exposure, fire, controlled, not in building
  - uncontrolled — *see* Exposure, fire, uncontrolled, not in building
- vapor (hot) X13.1- ☑
  - stated as undetermined whether accidental or intentional Y27.Ø- ☑
  - suicide (attempt) X77.Ø- ☑
- Very pistol — *see* Discharge, firearm NEC

**Butted by animal** W55.82- ☑
- bull W55.22- ☑
- cow W55.22- ☑
- goat W55.32- ☑
- horse W55.12- ☑
- pig W55.42- ☑
- sheep W55.32- ☑

# C

**Caisson disease** — *see* Air, pressure, change
**Campfire** (exposure to) (controlled) — *see also* Exposure, fire, controlled, not in building
- uncontrolled — *see* Exposure, fire, uncontrolled, not in building

- **Capital punishment** (any means) — *see* Legal, intervention
- **Car sickness** T75.3- ☑
- **Casualty** (not due to war) NEC X58.- ☑
  - war — *see* War operations
- **Cat**
  - bite W55.01- ☑
  - scratch W55.03- ☑
- **Cataclysm, cataclysmic** (any injury) NEC — *see* Forces of nature
- **Catching fire** — *see* Exposure, fire
- **Caught**
  - between
    - folding object W23.0- ☑
    - objects (moving) W23.0- ☑
      - and
        - machinery — *see* Contact, with, by type of machine
        - stationary W23.2- ☑
      - stationary W23.1- ☑
        - and moving W23.2- ☑
    - sliding door and door frame W23.0- ☑
  - by, in
    - machinery (moving parts of) — *see* Contact, with, by type of machine
    - washing-machine wringer W23.0- ☑
  - under packing crate (due to losing grip) W23.1- ☑
- **Cave-in caused by cataclysmic earth surface movement or eruption** — *see* Landslide
- **Change**(s) in air pressure — *see* Air, pressure, change
- **Choked, choking** (on) (any object except food or vomitus)
  - food (bone) (seed) — *see* categories T17 and T18.- ☑
  - vomitus T17.81- ☑
- **Civil insurrection** — *see* War operations
- **Cloudburst** (any injury) X37.8- ☑
- **Cold, exposure to** (accidental) (excessive) (extreme) (natural) (place) NEC — *see* Exposure, cold
- **Collapse**
  - building W20.1- ☑
    - burning (uncontrolled fire) X00.2- ☑
  - dam or man-made structure (causing earth movement) X36.0- ☑
  - machinery — *see* Contact, with, by type of machine
  - structure W20.1- ☑
    - burning (uncontrolled fire) X00.2- ☑
- **Collision** (accidental) NEC — *see also* Accident, transport V89.9- ☑
  - pedestrian W51.- ☑
    - with fall W03.- ☑
      - due to ice or snow W00.0- ☑
      - involving pedestrian conveyance — *see* Accident, transport, pedestrian, conveyance
    - and
      - crowd or human stampede (with fall) W52.- ☑
      - object W22.8- ☑
        - with fall — *see* Fall, due to, bumping against, object
  - person(s) — *see* Collision, pedestrian
  - transport vehicle NEC V89.9- ☑
    - and
      - avalanche, fallen or not moving — *see* Accident, transport
        - falling or moving — *see* Landslide
      - landslide, fallen or not moving — *see* Accident, transport
        - falling or moving — *see* Landslide
    - due to cataclysm — *see* Forces of nature, by type
    - intentional, purposeful suicide (attempt) — *see* Suicide, collision
- **Combustion, spontaneous** — *see* Ignition
- **Complication** (delayed) **of or following** (medical or surgical procedure) Y84.9
  - with misadventure — *see* Misadventure
  - amputation of limb(s) Y83.5
  - anastomosis (arteriovenous) (blood vessel) (gastrojejunal) (tendon) (natural or artificial material) Y83.2
  - aspiration (of fluid) Y84.4
    - tissue Y84.8
  - biopsy Y84.8
  - blood
    - sampling Y84.7
    - transfusion
      - procedure Y84.8
  - bypass Y83.2
  - catheterization (urinary) Y84.6
    - cardiac Y84.0
  - colostomy Y83.3
  - cystostomy Y83.3

**Complication** (delayed) **of or following** — *continued*

  - dialysis (kidney) Y84.1
  - drug — *see* Table of Drugs and Chemicals
  - due to misadventure — *see* Misadventure
  - duodenostomy Y83.3
  - electroshock therapy Y84.3
  - external stoma, creation of Y83.3
  - formation of external stoma Y83.3
  - gastrostomy Y83.3
  - graft Y83.2
  - hypothermia (medically-induced) Y84.8
  - implant, implantation (of)
    - artificial
      - internal device (cardiac pacemaker) (electrodes in brain) (heart valve prosthesis) (orthopedic) Y83.1
      - material or tissue (for anastomosis or bypass) Y83.2
        - with creation of external stoma Y83.3
    - natural tissues (for anastomosis or bypass) Y83.2
      - with creation of external stoma Y83.3
  - infusion
    - procedure Y84.8
  - injection — *see* Table of Drugs and Chemicals
    - procedure Y84.8
  - insertion of gastric or duodenal sound Y84.5
  - insulin-shock therapy Y84.3
  - paracentesis (abdominal) (thoracic) (aspirative) Y84.4
  - procedures other than surgical operation — *see* Complication of or following, by type of procedure
  - radiological procedure or therapy Y84.2
  - removal of organ (partial) (total) NEC Y83.6
  - sampling
    - blood Y84.7
    - fluid NEC Y84.4
    - tissue Y84.8
  - shock therapy Y84.3
  - surgical operation NEC — *see also* Complication of or following, by type of operation Y83.9
    - reconstructive NEC Y83.4
      - with
        - anastomosis, bypass or graft Y83.2
        - formation of external stoma Y83.3
    - specified NEC Y83.8
  - transfusion — *see also* Table of Drugs and Chemicals
    - procedure Y84.8
  - transplant, transplantation (heart) (kidney) (liver) (whole organ, any) Y83.0
    - partial organ Y83.4
  - ureterostomy Y83.3
  - vaccination — *see also* Table of Drugs and Chemicals
    - procedure Y84.8
- **Compression**
  - divers' squeeze — *see* Air, pressure, change
  - trachea by
    - food (lodged in esophagus) — *see* categories T17 and T18.- ☑
    - vomitus (lodged in esophagus) T17.81- ☑
- **Conflagration** — *see* Exposure, fire, uncontrolled
- **Constriction** (external)
  - hair W49.01- ☑
  - jewelry W49.04- ☑
  - ring W49.04- ☑
  - rubber band W49.03- ☑
  - specified item NEC W49.09- ☑
  - string W49.02- ☑
  - thread W49.02- ☑
- **Contact** (accidental)
  - with
    - abrasive wheel (metalworking) W31.1- ☑
    - alligator W58.09- ☑
      - bite W58.01- ☑
      - crushing W58.03- ☑
      - strike W58.02- ☑
    - amphibian W62.9- ☑
      - frog W62.0- ☑
      - toad W62.1- ☑
    - animal (nonvenomous) NEC W64.- ☑
      - marine W56.89- ☑
        - bite W56.81- ☑
        - dolphin — *see* Contact, with, dolphin
        - fish NEC — *see* Contact, with, fish
        - mammal — *see* Contact, with, mammal, marine
        - orca — *see* Contact, with, orca
        - sea lion — *see* Contact, with, sea lion
        - shark — *see* Contact, with, shark
        - strike W56.82- ☑
    - animate mechanical force NEC W64.- ☑
    - arrow W21.89- ☑

**Contact** — *continued*

  - with — *continued*
    - arrow — *continued*
      - not thrown, projected or falling W45.8- ☑
    - arthropods (nonvenomous) W57.- ☑
    - axe W27.0- ☑
    - band-saw (industrial) W31.2- ☑
    - bayonet — *see* Bayonet wound
    - bee(s) X58.- ☑
    - bench-saw (industrial) W31.2- ☑
    - bird W61.99- ☑
      - bite W61.91- ☑
      - chicken — *see* Contact, with, chicken
      - duck — *see* Contact, with, duck
      - goose — *see* Contact, with, goose
      - macaw — *see* Contact, with, macaw
      - parrot — *see* Contact, with, parrot
      - psittacine — *see* Contact, with, psittacine
      - strike W61.92- ☑
      - turkey — *see* Contact, with, turkey
    - blender W29.0- ☑
    - boiling water X12.- ☑
      - stated as undetermined whether accidental or intentional Y27.2- ☑
      - suicide (attempt) X77.2- ☑
    - bore, earth-drilling or mining (land) (seabed) W31.0- ☑
    - buffalo — *see* Contact, with, hoof stock NEC
    - bull W55.29- ☑
      - bite W55.21- ☑
      - gored W55.22- ☑
      - strike W55.22- ☑
    - bumper cars W31.81- ☑
    - camel — *see* Contact, with, hoof stock NEC
    - can
      - lid W26.8- ☑
      - opener W27.4- ☑
        - powered W29.0- ☑
    - cat W55.09- ☑
      - bite W55.01- ☑
      - scratch W55.03- ☑
    - caterpillar (venomous) X58.- ☑
    - centipede (venomous) X58.- ☑
    - chain
      - hoist W24.0- ☑
        - agricultural operations W30.89- ☑
      - saw W29.3- ☑
    - chicken W61.39- ☑
      - peck W61.33- ☑
      - strike W61.32- ☑
    - chisel W27.0- ☑
    - circular saw W31.2- ☑
    - cobra X58.- ☑
    - combine (harvester) W30.0- ☑
    - conveyer belt W24.1- ☑
    - cooker (hot) X15.8- ☑
      - stated as undetermined whether accidental or intentional Y27.3- ☑
      - suicide (attempt) X77.3- ☑
    - coral X58.- ☑
    - cotton gin W31.82- ☑
    - cow W55.29- ☑
      - bite W55.21- ☑
      - strike W55.22- ☑
    - crane W24.0- ☑
      - agricultural operations W30.89- ☑
    - crocodile W58.19- ☑
      - bite W58.11- ☑
      - crushing W58.13- ☑
      - strike W58.12- ☑
    - dagger W26.1- ☑
      - stated as undetermined whether accidental or intentional Y28.2- ☑
      - suicide (attempt) X78.2- ☑
    - dairy equipment W31.82- ☑
    - dart W21.89- ☑
      - not thrown, projected or falling W45.8- ☑
    - deer — *see* Contact, with, hoof stock NEC
    - derrick W24.0- ☑
      - agricultural operations W30.89- ☑
        - hay W30.2- ☑
    - dog W54.8- ☑
      - bite W54.0- ☑
      - strike W54.1- ☑
    - dolphin W56.09- ☑
      - bite W56.01- ☑

- **Discharge** — *continued*
  - firearm — *continued*
    - shotgun — *continued*
      - legal intervention — *see* Legal, intervention, firearm, specified NEC
      - stated as undetermined whether accidental or intentional Y23.0- ☑
      - suicide (attempt) X73.0- ☑
    - specified NEC W34.09- ☑
      - assault X95.8- ☑
      - homicide (attempt) X95.8- ☑
      - legal intervention — *see* Legal, intervention, firearm, specified NEC
      - stated as undetermined whether accidental or intentional Y24.8- ☑
      - suicide (attempt) X74.8- ☑
    - stated as undetermined whether accidental or intentional Y24.9- ☑
    - suicide (attempt) X74.9- ☑
    - Very pistol W34.09- ☑
      - assault X95.8- ☑
      - homicide (attempt) X95.8- ☑
      - stated as undetermined whether accidental or intentional Y24.8- ☑
      - suicide (attempt) X74.8- ☑
  - firework(s) W39.- ☑
    - stated as undetermined whether accidental or intentional Y25.- ☑
  - gas-operated gun NEC W34.018- ☑
    - airgun — *see* Discharge, airgun
    - assault X95.09- ☑
    - homicide (attempt) X95.09- ☑
    - paintball gun — *see* Discharge, paintball gun
    - stated as undetermined whether accidental or intentional Y24.8- ☑
    - suicide (attempt) X74.09- ☑
  - gun NEC — *see also* Discharge, firearm NEC
    - air — *see* Discharge, airgun
    - BB — *see* Discharge, airgun
    - for single hand use — *see* Discharge, firearm, handgun
    - hand — *see* Discharge, firearm, handgun
    - machine — *see* Discharge, firearm, machine gun
    - other specified — *see* Discharge, firearm NEC
    - paintball — *see* Discharge, paintball gun
    - pellet — *see* Discharge, airgun
  - handgun — *see* Discharge, firearm, handgun
  - machine gun — *see* Discharge, firearm, machine gun
  - paintball gun W34.011- ☑
    - assault X95.02- ☑
    - homicide (attempt) X95.02- ☑
    - stated as undetermined whether accidental or intentional Y24.8- ☑
    - suicide (attempt) X74.02- ☑
  - pistol — *see* Discharge, firearm, handgun
    - flare — *see* Discharge, firearm, Very pistol
    - pellet — *see* Discharge, airgun
    - Very — *see* Discharge, firearm, Very pistol
  - revolver — *see* Discharge, firearm, handgun
  - rifle (hunting) — *see* Discharge, firearm, hunting rifle
  - shotgun — *see* Discharge, firearm, shotgun
  - spring-operated gun NEC W34.018- ☑
    - assault X95.09- ☑
    - homicide (attempt) X95.09- ☑
    - stated as undetermined whether accidental or intentional Y24.8- ☑
    - suicide (attempt) X74.09- ☑
- **Disease**
  - Andes W94.11- ☑
  - aviator's — *see* Air, pressure
  - range W94.11- ☑
- **Diver's disease, palsy, paralysis, squeeze** — *see* Air, pressure
- **Diving** (into water) — *see* Accident, diving
- **Dog bite** W54.0- ☑
- **Dragged by transport vehicle NEC** — *see also* Accident, transport V09.9- ☑
- **Drinking poison** (accidental) — *see* Table of Drugs and Chemicals
- **Dropped** (accidentally) **while being carried or supported by other person** W04.- ☑
- **Drowning** (accidental) W74.- ☑
  - assault X92.9- ☑
  - due to
    - accident (to)
      - machinery — *see* Contact, with, by type of machine
- **Drowning** — *continued*
  - due to — *continued*
    - accident — *continued*
      - watercraft V90.89- ☑
        - burning V90.29- ☑
          - powered V90.23- ☑
            - fishing boat V90.22- ☑
            - jetskis V90.23- ☑
            - merchant ship V90.20- ☑
            - passenger ship V90.21- ☑
          - unpowered V90.28- ☑
            - canoe V90.25- ☑
            - inflatable V90.26- ☑
            - kayak V90.25- ☑
            - sailboat V90.24- ☑
            - water skis V90.27- ☑
        - crushed V90.39- ☑
          - powered V90.33- ☑
            - fishing boat V90.32- ☑
            - jetskis V90.33- ☑
            - merchant ship V90.30- ☑
            - passenger ship V90.31- ☑
          - unpowered V90.38- ☑
            - canoe V90.35- ☑
            - inflatable V90.36- ☑
            - kayak V90.35- ☑
            - sailboat V90.34- ☑
            - water skis V90.37- ☑
        - overturning V90.09- ☑
          - powered V90.03- ☑
            - fishing boat V90.02- ☑
            - jetskis V90.03- ☑
            - merchant ship V90.00- ☑
            - passenger ship V90.01- ☑
          - unpowered V90.08- ☑
            - canoe V90.05- ☑
            - inflatable V90.06- ☑
            - kayak V90.05- ☑
            - sailboat V90.04- ☑
        - sinking V90.19- ☑
          - powered V90.13- ☑
            - fishing boat V90.12- ☑
            - jetskis V90.13- ☑
            - merchant ship V90.10- ☑
            - passenger ship V90.11- ☑
          - unpowered V90.18- ☑
            - canoe V90.15- ☑
            - inflatable V90.16- ☑
            - kayak V90.15- ☑
            - sailboat V90.14- ☑
        - specified type NEC V90.89- ☑
          - powered V90.83- ☑
            - fishing boat V90.82- ☑
            - jetskis V90.83- ☑
            - merchant ship V90.80- ☑
            - passenger ship V90.81- ☑
          - unpowered V90.88- ☑
            - canoe V90.85- ☑
            - inflatable V90.86- ☑
            - kayak V90.85- ☑
            - sailboat V90.84- ☑
            - water skis V90.87- ☑
    - avalanche — *see* Landslide
    - cataclysmic
      - earth surface movement NEC — *see* Forces of nature, earth movement
      - storm — *see* Forces of nature, cataclysmic storm
    - cloudburst X37.8- ☑
    - cyclone X37.1- ☑
    - fall overboard (from) V92.09- ☑
      - powered craft V92.03- ☑
        - ferry boat V92.01- ☑
        - fishing boat V92.02- ☑
        - jetskis V92.03- ☑
        - liner V92.01- ☑
        - merchant ship V92.00- ☑
        - passenger ship V92.01- ☑
      - resulting from
        - accident to watercraft — *see* Drowning, due to, accident to, watercraft
        - being washed overboard (from) V92.29- ☑
          - powered craft V92.23- ☑
            - ferry boat V92.21- ☑
            - fishing boat V92.22- ☑
            - jetskis V92.23- ☑
- **Drowning** — *continued*
  - due to — *continued*
    - fall overboard — *continued*
      - resulting from — *continued*
        - being washed overboard — *continued*
          - powered craft — *continued*
            - liner V92.21- ☑
            - merchant ship V92.20- ☑
            - passenger ship V92.21- ☑
          - unpowered craft V92.28- ☑
            - canoe V92.25- ☑
            - inflatable V92.26- ☑
            - kayak V92.25- ☑
            - sailboat V92.24- ☑
            - surf-board V92.28- ☑
            - water skis V92.27- ☑
            - windsurfer V92.28- ☑
        - motion of watercraft V92.19- ☑
          - powered craft V92.13- ☑
            - ferry boat V92.11- ☑
            - fishing boat V92.12- ☑
            - jetskis V92.13- ☑
            - liner V92.11- ☑
            - merchant ship V92.10- ☑
            - passenger ship V92.11- ☑
          - unpowered craft
            - canoe V92.15- ☑
            - inflatable V92.16- ☑
            - kayak V92.15- ☑
            - sailboat V92.14- ☑
      - unpowered craft V92.08- ☑
        - canoe V92.05- ☑
        - inflatable V92.06- ☑
        - kayak V92.05- ☑
        - sailboat V92.04- ☑
        - surf-board V92.08- ☑
        - water skis V92.07- ☑
        - windsurfer V92.08- ☑
    - hurricane X37.0- ☑
    - jumping into water from watercraft (involved in accident) — *see also* Drowning, due to, accident to, watercraft
      - without accident to or on watercraft W16.711- ☑
    - tidal wave NEC — *see* Forces of nature, tidal wave
    - torrential rain X37.8- ☑
  - following
    - fall
      - into
        - bathtub W16.211- ☑
        - bucket W16.221- ☑
        - fountain — *see* Drowning, following, fall, into, water, specified NEC
        - quarry — *see* Drowning, following, fall, into, water, specified NEC
        - reservoir — *see* Drowning, following, fall, into, water, specified NEC
        - swimming-pool W16.011- ☑
          - stated as undetermined whether accidental or intentional Y21.3- ☑
          - striking
            - bottom W16.021- ☑
            - wall W16.031- ☑
          - suicide (attempt) X71.2- ☑
        - water NOS W16.41- ☑
          - natural (lake) (open sea) (river) (stream) (pond) W16.111- ☑
            - striking
              - bottom W16.121- ☑
              - side W16.131- ☑
          - specified NEC W16.311- ☑
            - striking
              - bottom W16.321- ☑
              - wall W16.331- ☑
      - overboard NEC — *see* Drowning, due to, fall overboard
    - jump or dive
      - from boat W16.711- ☑
        - striking bottom W16.721- ☑
      - into
        - fountain — *see* Drowning, following, jump or dive, into, water, specified NEC
        - quarry — *see* Drowning, following, jump or dive, into, water, specified NEC
        - reservoir — *see* Drowning, following, jump or dive, into, water, specified NEC
        - swimming-pool W16.511- ☑

- **Drowning** — *continued*
  - following — *continued*
    - jump or dive — *continued*
      - into — *continued*
        - swimming-pool — *continued*
          - striking
            - bottom W16.521- ☑
            - wall W16.531- ☑
          - suicide (attempt) X71.2- ☑
        - water NOS W16.91- ☑
          - natural (lake) (open sea) (river) (stream) (pond) W16.611- ☑
          - specified NEC W16.811- ☑
            - bottom W16.821- ☑
            - striking
              - bottom W16.821- ☑
              - wall W16.831- ☑
          - striking
            - bottom W16.821- ☑
            - wall W16.831- ☑
          - striking bottom W16.621- ☑
  - homicide (attempt) X92.9- ☑
  - in
    - bathtub (accidental) W65.- ☑
      - assault X92.Ø- ☑
      - following fall W16.211- ☑
        - stated as undetermined whether accidental or intentional Y21.1- ☑
      - stated as undetermined whether accidental or intentional Y21.Ø- ☑
      - suicide (attempt) X71.Ø- ☑
    - lake — *see* Drowning, in, natural water
    - natural water (lake) (open sea) (river) (stream) (pond) W69.- ☑
      - assault X92.3- ☑
      - following
        - dive or jump W16.611- ☑
          - striking bottom W16.621- ☑
        - fall W16.111- ☑
          - striking
            - bottom W16.121- ☑
            - side W16.131- ☑
      - stated as undetermined whether accidental or intentional Y21.4- ☑
      - suicide (attempt) X71.3- ☑
    - quarry — *see* Drowning, in, specified place NEC
    - quenching tank — *see* Drowning, in, specified place NEC
    - reservoir — *see* Drowning, in, specified place NEC
    - river — *see* Drowning, in, natural water
    - sea — *see* Drowning, in, natural water
    - specified place NEC W73.- ☑
      - assault X92.8- ☑
      - following
        - dive or jump W16.811- ☑
          - striking
            - bottom W16.821- ☑
            - wall W16.831- ☑
        - fall W16.311- ☑
          - striking
            - bottom W16.321- ☑
            - wall W16.331- ☑
      - stated as undetermined whether accidental or intentional Y21.8- ☑
      - suicide (attempt) X71.8- ☑
    - stream — *see* Drowning, in, natural water
    - swimming-pool W67.- ☑
      - assault X92.1- ☑
        - following fall X92.2- ☑
      - following
        - dive or jump W16.511- ☑
          - striking
            - bottom W16.521- ☑
            - wall W16.531- ☑
        - fall W16.Ø11- ☑
          - striking
            - bottom W16.Ø21- ☑
            - wall W16.Ø31- ☑
      - stated as undetermined whether accidental or intentional Y21.2- ☑
        - following fall Y21.3- ☑
      - suicide (attempt) X71.1- ☑
        - following fall X71.2- ☑
    - war operations — *see* War operations, restriction of airway

- **Drowning** — *continued*
  - resulting from accident to watercraft — *see* Drowning, due to, accident to, watercraft
  - self-inflicted X71.9- ☑
  - stated as undetermined whether accidental or intentional Y21.9- ☑
  - suicide (attempt) X71.9- ☑

# E

- **Earth falling** (on) W2Ø.Ø- ☑
  - caused by cataclysmic earth surface movement or eruption — *see* Landslide
- **Earth** (surface) **movement NEC** — *see* Forces of nature, earth movement
- **Earthquake** (any injury) X34.- ☑
- **Effect**(s) (adverse) **of**
  - air pressure (any) — *see* Air, pressure
  - cold, excessive (exposure to) — *see* Exposure, cold
  - heat (excessive) — *see* Heat
  - hot place (weather) — *see* Heat
  - insolation X3Ø.- ☑
  - late — *see* Sequelae
  - motion — *see* Motion
  - nuclear explosion or weapon in war operations — *see* War operations, nuclear weapon
  - radiation — *see* Radiation
  - travel — *see* Travel
- **Electric shock** (accidental) (by) (in) — *see* Exposure, electric current
- **Electrocution** (accidental) — *see* Exposure, electric current
- **Endotracheal tube wrongly placed during anesthetic procedure**
- **Entanglement**
  - in
    - bed linen, causing suffocation T71.- ☑
    - wheel of pedal cycle V19.88- ☑
- **Entry of foreign body or material** — *see* Foreign body
- **Environmental pollution related condition** — *see* category Z77
- **Execution, legal** (any method) — *see* Legal, intervention
- **Exhaustion**
  - cold — *see* Exposure, cold
  - due to excessive exertion — *see also* Overexertion X5Ø.9- ☑
  - heat — *see* Heat
- **Explosion** (accidental) (of) (with secondary fire) W4Ø.9- ☑
  - acetylene W4Ø.1- ☑
  - aerosol can W36.1- ☑
  - air tank (compressed) (in machinery) W36.2- ☑
  - aircraft (in transit) (powered) NEC V95.9- ☑
    - balloon V96.Ø5- ☑
    - fixed wing NEC (private) V95.25- ☑
      - commercial V95.35- ☑
    - glider V96.25- ☑
      - hang V96.15- ☑
      - powered V95.15- ☑
    - helicopter V95.Ø5- ☑
    - in war operations — *see* War operations, destruction of aircraft
    - microlight V95.15- ☑
    - nonpowered V96.9- ☑
      - specified NEC V96.8- ☑
    - powered NEC V95.8- ☑
    - stated as
      - homicide (attempt) YØ8.81- ☑
      - suicide (attempt) X83.Ø- ☑
    - ultralight V95.15- ☑
  - anesthetic gas in operating room W4Ø.1- ☑
  - antipersonnel bomb W4Ø.8- ☑
    - assault X96.Ø- ☑
    - homicide (attempt) X96.Ø- ☑
    - suicide (attempt) X75.- ☑
  - assault X96.9- ☑
  - bicycle tire W37.Ø- ☑
  - blasting (cap) (materials) W4Ø.Ø- ☑
  - boiler (machinery), not on transport vehicle W35.- ☑
    - on watercraft — *see* Explosion, in, watercraft
  - butane W4Ø.1- ☑
  - caused by other person X96.9- ☑
  - coal gas W4Ø.1- ☑
  - detonator W4Ø.Ø- ☑
  - dump (munitions) W4Ø.8- ☑
  - dynamite W4Ø.Ø- ☑
    - in
      - assault X96.8- ☑

- **Explosion** — *continued*
  - dynamite — *continued*
    - in — *continued*
      - homicide (attempt) X96.8- ☑
      - legal intervention
        - injuring
          - bystander Y35.112- ☑
          - law enforcement personnel Y35.111- ☑
          - suspect Y35.113- ☑
          - unspecified person Y35.119- ☑
      - suicide (attempt) X75.- ☑
  - explosive (material) W4Ø.9- ☑
    - gas W4Ø.1- ☑
    - in blasting operation W4Ø.Ø- ☑
    - specified NEC W4Ø.8- ☑
      - in
        - assault X96.8- ☑
        - homicide (attempt) X96.8- ☑
        - legal intervention
          - injuring
            - bystander Y35.192- ☑
            - law enforcement personnel Y35.191- ☑
            - suspect Y35.193- ☑
            - unspecified person Y35.199- ☑
        - suicide (attempt) X75.- ☑
  - factory (munitions) W4Ø.8- ☑
  - fertilizer bomb W4Ø.8- ☑
    - assault X96.3- ☑
    - homicide (attempt) X96.3- ☑
    - suicide (attempt) X75.- ☑
  - fire-damp W4Ø.1- ☑
  - firearm (parts) NEC W34.19- ☑
    - airgun W34.11Ø- ☑
    - BB gun W34.11Ø- ☑
    - gas, air or spring-operated gun NEC W34.118- ☑
    - handgun W32.1- ☑
    - hunting rifle W33.12- ☑
    - larger firearm W33.1Ø- ☑
      - specified NEC W33.19- ☑
    - machine gun W33.13- ☑
    - paintball gun W34.111- ☑
    - pellet gun W34.11Ø- ☑
    - shotgun W33.11- ☑
    - Very pistol [flare] W34.19- ☑
  - fireworks W39.- ☑
  - gas (coal) (explosive) W4Ø.1- ☑
    - cylinder W36.9- ☑
      - aerosol can W36.1- ☑
      - air tank W36.2- ☑
      - pressurized W36.3- ☑
      - specified NEC W36.8- ☑
  - gasoline (fumes) (tank) not in moving motor vehicle W4Ø.1- ☑
    - bomb W4Ø.8- ☑
      - assault X96.1- ☑
      - homicide (attempt) X96.1- ☑
      - suicide (attempt) X75.- ☑
    - in motor vehicle — *see* Accident, transport, by type of vehicle
  - grain store W4Ø.8- ☑
  - grenade W4Ø.8- ☑
    - in
      - assault X96.8- ☑
      - homicide (attempt) X96.8- ☑
      - legal intervention
        - injuring
          - bystander Y35.192- ☑
          - law enforcement personnel Y35.191- ☑
          - suspect Y35.193- ☑
          - unspecified person Y35.199- ☑
      - suicide (attempt) X75.- ☑
  - handgun (parts) — *see* Explosion, firearm, handgun
  - homicide (attempt) X96.9- ☑
    - antipersonnel bomb — *see* Explosion, antipersonnel bomb
    - fertilizer bomb — *see* Explosion, fertilizer bomb
    - gasoline bomb — *see* Explosion, gasoline bomb
    - letter bomb — *see* Explosion, letter bomb
    - pipe bomb — *see* Explosion, pipe bomb
    - specified NEC X96.8- ☑
  - hose, pressurized W37.8- ☑
  - hot water heater, tank (in machinery) W35.- ☑
    - on watercraft — *see* Explosion, in, watercraft
  - in, on
    - dump W4Ø.8- ☑
    - factory W4Ø.8- ☑

- **Exposure** — *continued*
  - fire, flames — *continued*
    - uncontrolled — *continued*
      - in building or structure — *continued*
        - sofa — *continued*
          - due to — *continued*
            - specified material NEC XØ8.19- ☑
        - specified mode of injury NEC XØØ.8- ☑
      - not in building or structure (any) XØ1.Ø- ☑
        - with
          - fall XØ1.3- ☑
          - smoke inhalation XØ1.1- ☑
        - hit by object XØ1.4- ☑
        - specified mode of injury NEC XØ1.8- ☑
    - undetermined whether accidental or intentional Y26.- ☑
  - forces of nature NEC — *see* Forces of nature
  - G-forces (abnormal) W49.9- ☑
  - gravitational forces (abnormal) W49.9- ☑
  - heat (natural) NEC — *see* Heat
  - high-pressure jet (hydraulic) (pneumatic) W49.9- ☑
  - hydraulic jet W49.9- ☑
  - inanimate mechanical force W49.9- ☑
  - jet, high-pressure (hydraulic) (pneumatic) W49.9- ☑
  - lightning — *see* subcategory T75.Ø- ☑
    - causing fire — *see* Exposure, fire
  - mechanical forces NEC W49.9- ☑
    - animate NEC W64.- ☑
    - inanimate NEC W49.9- ☑
  - noise W42.9- ☑
    - supersonic W42.Ø- ☑
  - noxious substance — *see* Table of Drugs and Chemicals
  - pneumatic jet W49.9- ☑
  - prolonged in deep-freeze unit or refrigerator W93.2- ☑
  - radiation — *see* Radiation
  - smoke — *see also* Exposure, fire
    - tobacco, second hand Z77.22
  - specified factors NEC X58.- ☑
  - sunlight X32.- ☑
    - man-made (sun lamp) W89.8- ☑
      - tanning bed W89.1- ☑
  - supersonic waves W42.Ø- ☑
  - transmission line(s), electric W85.- ☑
  - vibration W49.9- ☑
  - waves
    - infrasound W49.9- ☑
    - sound W42.9- ☑
    - supersonic W42.Ø- ☑
  - weather NEC — *see* Forces of nature
- **External cause status** Y99.9
  - child assisting in compensated work for family Y99.8
  - civilian activity done for financial or other compensation Y99.Ø
  - civilian activity done for income or pay Y99.Ø
  - family member assisting in compensated work for other family member Y99.8
  - hobby not done for income Y99.8
  - leisure activity Y99.8
  - military activity Y99.1
  - off-duty activity of military personnel Y99.8
  - recreation or sport not for income or while a student Y99.8
  - specified NEC Y99.8
  - student activity Y99.8
  - volunteer activity Y99.2

# F

- **Factors, supplemental**
  - alcohol
    - blood level
      - less than 2Ømg/1ØØml Y9Ø.Ø
      - presence in blood, level not specified Y9Ø.9
      - 2Ø-39mg/1ØØml Y9Ø.1
      - 4Ø-59mg/1ØØml Y9Ø.2
      - 6Ø-79mg/1ØØml Y9Ø.3
      - 8Ø-99mg/1ØØml Y9Ø.4
      - 1ØØ-119mg/1ØØml Y9Ø.5
      - 12Ø-199mg/1ØØml Y9Ø.6
      - 2ØØ-239mg/1ØØml Y9Ø.7
      - 24Ømg/1ØØml or more Y9Ø.8
    - presence in blood, but level not specified Y9Ø.9
  - environmental-pollution-related condition- see Z57.- ☑
  - nosocomial condition Y95
  - work-related condition Y99.Ø
- **Failure**
  - in suture or ligature during surgical procedure Y65.2
- **Failure** — *continued*
  - mechanical, of instrument or apparatus (any) (during any medical or surgical procedure) Y65.8
  - sterile precautions (during medical and surgical care) — *see* Misadventure, failure, sterile precautions, by type of procedure
  - to
    - introduce tube or instrument Y65.4
      - endotracheal tube during anesthesia Y65.3
    - make curve (transport vehicle) NEC — *see* Accident, transport
    - remove tube or instrument Y65.4
- **Fall, falling** (accidental) W19.- ☑
  - building W2Ø.1- ☑
    - burning (uncontrolled fire) XØØ.3- ☑
  - down
    - embankment W17.81- ☑
    - escalator W1Ø.Ø- ☑
    - hill W17.81- ☑
    - ladder W11.- ☑
    - ramp W1Ø.2- ☑
    - stairs, steps W1Ø.9- ☑
  - due to
    - bumping against
      - object W18.ØØ- ☑
        - sharp glass W18.Ø2- ☑
        - specified NEC W18.Ø9- ☑
        - sports equipment W18.Ø1- ☑
      - person WØ3.- ☑
        - due to ice or snow WØØ.Ø- ☑
        - on pedestrian conveyance — *see* Accident, transport, pedestrian, conveyance
    - collision with another person WØ3.- ☑
      - due to ice or snow WØØ.Ø- ☑
      - involving pedestrian conveyance — *see* Accident, transport, pedestrian, conveyance
    - grocery cart tipping over W17.82- ☑
    - ice or snow WØØ.9- ☑
      - from one level to another WØØ.2- ☑
        - on stairs or steps WØØ.1- ☑
      - involving pedestrian conveyance — *see* Accident, transport, pedestrian, conveyance
      - on same level WØØ.Ø- ☑
    - slipping (on moving sidewalk) WØ1.Ø- ☑
      - with subsequent striking against object WØ1.1Ø- ☑
        - furniture WØ1.19Ø- ☑
        - sharp object WØ1.119- ☑
          - glass WØ1.11Ø- ☑
          - power tool or machine WØ1.111- ☑
          - specified NEC WØ1.118- ☑
        - specified NEC WØ1.198- ☑
    - striking against
      - object W18.ØØ- ☑
        - sharp glass W18.Ø2- ☑
        - specified NEC W18.Ø9- ☑
        - sports equipment W18.Ø1- ☑
      - person WØ3.- ☑
        - due to ice or snow WØØ.Ø- ☑
        - on pedestrian conveyance — *see* Accident, transport, pedestrian, conveyance
  - earth (with asphyxia or suffocation (by pressure)) — *see* Earth, falling
  - from, off, out of
    - aircraft NEC (with accident to aircraft NEC) V97.Ø- ☑
      - while boarding or alighting V97.1- ☑
    - balcony W13.Ø- ☑
    - bed WØ6.- ☑
    - boat, ship, watercraft NEC (with drowning or submersion) — *see* Drowning, due to, fall overboard
      - with hitting bottom or object V94.Ø- ☑
    - bridge W13.1- ☑
    - building W13.9- ☑
      - burning (uncontrolled fire) XØØ.3- ☑
    - cavity W17.2- ☑
    - chair WØ7.- ☑
    - cherry picker W17.89- ☑
    - cliff W15.- ☑
    - dock W17.4- ☑
    - embankment W17.81- ☑
    - escalator W1Ø.Ø- ☑
    - flagpole W13.8- ☑
    - furniture NEC WØ8.- ☑
    - grocery cart W17.82- ☑
    - haystack W17.89- ☑
    - high place NEC W17.89- ☑
- **Fall, falling** — *continued*
  - from, off, out of — *continued*
    - high place — *continued*
      - stated as undetermined whether accidental or intentional Y3Ø.- ☑
    - hole W17.2- ☑
    - incline W1Ø.2- ☑
    - ladder W11.- ☑
    - lifting device W17.89- ☑
    - machine, machinery — *see also* Contact, with, by type of machine
      - not in operation W17.89- ☑
    - manhole W17.1- ☑
    - mobile elevated work platform [MEWP] W17.89- ☑
    - motorized mobility scooter WØ5.2- ☑
    - one level to another NEC W17.89- ☑
      - intentional, purposeful, suicide (attempt) X8Ø.- ☑
      - stated as undetermined whether accidental or intentional Y3Ø.- ☑
    - pit W17.2- ☑
    - playground equipment WØ9.8- ☑
      - jungle gym WØ9.2- ☑
      - slide WØ9.Ø- ☑
      - swing WØ9.1- ☑
    - quarry W17.89- ☑
    - railing W13.9- ☑
    - ramp W1Ø.2- ☑
    - roof W13.2- ☑
    - scaffolding W12.- ☑
    - scooter (nonmotorized) WØ5.1- ☑
      - motorized mobility WØ5.2- ☑
    - sky lift W17.89- ☑
    - stairs, steps W1Ø.9- ☑
      - curb W1Ø.1- ☑
      - due to ice or snow WØØ.1- ☑
      - escalator W1Ø.Ø- ☑
      - incline W1Ø.2- ☑
      - ramp W1Ø.2- ☑
      - sidewalk curb W1Ø.1- ☑
      - specified NEC W1Ø.8- ☑
      - standing
        - electric scooter VØØ.841- ☑
        - micro-mobility pedestrian conveyance VØØ.848- ☑
    - stepladder W11.- ☑
    - stool WØ8.- ☑
    - storm drain W17.1- ☑
    - streetcar NEC V82.6- ☑
      - while boarding or alighting V82.4- ☑
      - with antecedent collision — *see* Accident, transport, streetcar occupant
    - structure NEC W13.8- ☑
      - burning (uncontrolled fire) XØØ.3- ☑
    - table WØ8.- ☑
    - toilet W18.11- ☑
      - with subsequent striking against object W18.12- ☑
    - train NEC V81.6- ☑
      - during derailment (without antecedent collision) V81.7- ☑
        - with antecedent collision — *see* Accident, transport, railway vehicle occupant
      - while boarding or alighting V81.4- ☑
    - transport vehicle after collision — *see* Accident, transport, by type of vehicle, collision
    - tree W14.- ☑
    - vehicle (in motion) NEC — *see also* Accident, transport V89.9- ☑
      - motor NEC — *see also* Accident, transport, occupant, by type of vehicle V87.8- ☑
      - stationary W17.89- ☑
        - while boarding or alighting — *see* Accident, transport, by type of vehicle, while boarding or alighting
    - viaduct W13.8- ☑
    - wall W13.8- ☑
    - watercraft — *see also* Drowning, due to, fall overboard
      - with hitting bottom or object V94.Ø- ☑
    - well W17.Ø- ☑
    - wheelchair, non-moving WØ5.Ø- ☑
      - powered — *see* Accident, transport, pedestrian, conveyance occupant, specified type NEC
    - window W13.4- ☑
  - in, on
    - aircraft NEC V97.Ø- ☑
      - while boarding or alighting V97.1- ☑

- **Fall, falling** — *continued*
  - in, on — *continued*
    - aircraft — *continued*
      - with accident to aircraft V97.Ø- ☑
    - bathtub (empty) W18.2- ☑
      - filled W16.212- ☑
        - causing drowning W16.211- ☑
    - escalator W1Ø.Ø- ☑
    - incline W1Ø.2- ☑
    - ladder W11.- ☑
    - machine, machinery — *see* Contact, with, by type of machine
    - object, edged, pointed or sharp (with cut) — *see* Fall, by type
    - playground equipment WØ9.8- ☑
      - jungle gym WØ9.2- ☑
      - slide WØ9.Ø- ☑
      - swing WØ9.1- ☑
    - ramp W1Ø.2- ☑
    - scaffolding W12.- ☑
    - shower W18.2- ☑
      - causing drowning W16.211- ☑
    - staircase, stairs, steps W1Ø.9- ☑
      - curb W1Ø.1- ☑
      - due to ice or snow WØØ.1- ☑
      - escalator W1Ø.Ø- ☑
      - incline W1Ø.2- ☑
      - specified NEC W1Ø.8- ☑
    - streetcar (without antecedent collision) V82.5- ☑
      - with antecedent collision — *see* Accident, transport, streetcar occupant
      - while boarding or alighting V82.4- ☑
    - train (without antecedent collision) V81.5- ☑
      - with antecedent collision — *see* Accident, transport, railway vehicle occupant
      - during derailment (without antecedent collision) V81.7- ☑
        - with antecedent collision — *see* Accident, transport, railway vehicle occupant
      - while boarding or alighting V81.4- ☑
    - transport vehicle after collision — *see* Accident, transport, by type of vehicle, collision
    - watercraft V93.39- ☑
      - due to
        - accident to craft V91.29- ☑
          - powered craft V91.23- ☑
            - ferry boat V91.21- ☑
            - fishing boat V91.22- ☑
            - jetskis V91.23- ☑
            - liner V91.21- ☑
            - merchant ship V91.2Ø- ☑
            - passenger ship V91.21- ☑
          - unpowered craft
            - canoe V91.25- ☑
            - inflatable V91.26- ☑
            - kayak V91.25- ☑
            - sailboat V91.24- ☑
      - powered craft V93.33- ☑
        - ferry boat V93.31- ☑
        - fishing boat V93.32- ☑
        - jetskis V93.33- ☑
        - liner V93.31- ☑
        - merchant ship V93.3Ø- ☑
        - passenger ship V93.31- ☑
      - unpowered craft V93.38- ☑
        - canoe V93.35- ☑
        - inflatable V93.36- ☑
        - kayak V93.35- ☑
        - sailboat V93.34- ☑
        - surf-board V93.38- ☑
        - windsurfer V93.38- ☑
  - into
    - cavity W17.2- ☑
    - dock W17.4- ☑
    - fire — *see* Exposure, fire, by type
    - haystack W17.89- ☑
    - hole W17.2- ☑
    - lake — *see* Fall, into, water
    - manhole W17.1- ☑
    - moving part of machinery — *see* Contact, with, by type of machine
    - ocean — *see* Fall, into, water
    - opening in surface NEC W17.89- ☑
    - pit W17.2- ☑
    - pond — *see* Fall, into, water
    - quarry W17.89- ☑

- **Fall, falling** — *continued*
  - into — *continued*
    - river — *see* Fall, into, water
    - shaft W17.89- ☑
    - storm drain W17.1- ☑
    - stream — *see* Fall, into, water
    - swimming pool — *see also* Fall, into, water, in, swimming pool
      - empty W17.3- ☑
    - tank W17.89- ☑
    - water W16.42- ☑
      - causing drowning W16.41- ☑
      - from watercraft — *see* Drowning, due to, fall overboard
      - hitting diving board W21.4- ☑
      - in
        - bathtub W16.212- ☑
          - causing drowning W16.211- ☑
        - bucket W16.222- ☑
          - causing drowning W16.221- ☑
        - natural body of water W16.112- ☑
          - causing drowning W16.111- ☑
          - striking
            - bottom W16.122- ☑
              - causing drowning W16.121- ☑
            - side W16.132- ☑
              - causing drowning W16.131- ☑
        - specified water NEC W16.312- ☑
          - causing drowning W16.311- ☑
          - striking
            - bottom W16.322- ☑
              - causing drowning W16.321- ☑
            - wall W16.332- ☑
              - causing drowning W16.331- ☑
        - swimming pool W16.Ø12- ☑
          - causing drowning W16.Ø11- ☑
          - striking
            - bottom W16.Ø22- ☑
              - causing drowning W16.Ø31- ☑
            - wall W16.Ø32- ☑
              - causing drowning W16.Ø21- ☑
        - utility bucket W16.222- ☑
          - causing drowning W16.221- ☑
    - well W17.Ø- ☑
  - involving
    - bed WØ6.- ☑
    - chair WØ7.- ☑
    - furniture NEC WØ8.- ☑
    - glass — *see* Fall, by type
    - playground equipment WØ9.8- ☑
      - jungle gym WØ9.2- ☑
      - slide WØ9.Ø- ☑
      - swing WØ9.1- ☑
    - roller blades — *see* Accident, transport, pedestrian, conveyance
    - skateboard(s) — *see* Accident, transport, pedestrian, conveyance
    - skates (ice) (in line) (roller) — *see* Accident, transport, pedestrian, conveyance
    - skis — *see* Accident, transport, pedestrian, conveyance
    - table WØ8.- ☑
    - wheelchair, non-moving WØ5.Ø- ☑
      - powered — *see* Accident, transport, pedestrian, conveyance, specified type NEC
  - object — *see* Struck by, object, falling
  - off
    - toilet W18.11- ☑
      - with subsequent striking against object W18.12- ☑
  - on same level W18.3Ø- ☑
    - due to
      - specified NEC W18.39- ☑
      - stepping on an object W18.31- ☑
  - out of
    - bed WØ6.- ☑
    - building NEC W13.8- ☑
    - chair WØ7.- ☑
    - furniture NEC WØ8.- ☑
    - wheelchair, non-moving WØ5.Ø- ☑
      - powered — *see* Accident, transport, pedestrian, conveyance, specified type NEC
    - window W13.4- ☑
  - over
    - animal WØ1.Ø- ☑
    - cliff W15.- ☑

- **Fall, falling** — *continued*
  - over — *continued*
    - embankment W17.81- ☑
    - small object WØ1.Ø- ☑
  - rock W2Ø.8- ☑
  - same level W18.3Ø- ☑
    - from
      - being crushed, pushed, or stepped on by a crowd or human stampede W52.- ☑
      - collision, pushing, shoving, by or with other person WØ3.- ☑
      - slipping, stumbling, tripping WØ1.Ø- ☑
    - involving ice or snow WØØ.Ø- ☑
      - involving skates (ice) (roller), skateboard, skis — *see* Accident, transport, pedestrian, conveyance
  - snowslide (avalanche) — *see* Landslide
  - stone W2Ø.8- ☑
  - structure W2Ø.1- ☑
    - burning (uncontrolled fire) XØØ.3- ☑
  - through
    - bridge W13.1- ☑
    - floor W13.3- ☑
    - roof W13.2- ☑
    - wall W13.8- ☑
    - window W13.4- ☑
  - timber W2Ø.8- ☑
  - tree (caused by lightning) W2Ø.8- ☑
  - while being carried or supported by other person(s) WØ4.- ☑
- **Fallen on by**
  - animal (not being ridden) NEC W55.89- ☑
- **Felo-de-se** — *see* Suicide
- **Fight** (hand) (fists) (foot) — *see* Assault, fight
- **Fire** (accidental) — *see* Exposure, fire
- **Firearm discharge** — *see* Discharge, firearm
- **Fireball effects from nuclear explosion in war operations** — *see* War operations, nuclear weapons
- **Fireworks** (explosion) W39.- ☑
- **Flash burns from explosion** — *see* Explosion
- **Flood** (any injury) (caused by) X38.- ☑
  - collapse of man-made structure causing earth movement X36.Ø- ☑
  - tidal wave — *see* Forces of nature, tidal wave
- **Food** (any type) **in**
  - air passages (with asphyxia, obstruction, or suffocation) — *see* categories T17 and T18.- ☑
  - alimentary tract causing asphyxia (due to compression of trachea) — *see* categories T17 and T18.- ☑
- **Forces of nature** X39.8- ☑
  - avalanche X36.1- ☑
    - causing transport accident — *see* Accident, transport, by type of vehicle
  - blizzard X37.2- ☑
  - cataclysmic storm X37.9- ☑
    - with flood X38.- ☑
    - blizzard X37.2- ☑
    - cloudburst X37.8- ☑
    - cyclone X37.1- ☑
    - dust storm X37.3- ☑
    - hurricane X37.Ø- ☑
    - specified storm NEC X37.8- ☑
    - storm surge X37.Ø- ☑
    - tornado X37.1- ☑
    - twister X37.1- ☑
    - typhoon X37.Ø- ☑
  - cloudburst X37.8- ☑
  - cold (natural) X31.- ☑
  - cyclone X37.1- ☑
  - dam collapse causing earth movement X36.Ø- ☑
  - dust storm X37.3- ☑
  - earth movement X36.1- ☑
    - caused by dam or structure collapse X36.Ø- ☑
    - earthquake X34.- ☑
  - earthquake X34.- ☑
  - flood (caused by) X38.- ☑
    - dam collapse X36.Ø- ☑
    - tidal wave — *see* Forces of nature, tidal wave
  - heat (natural) X3Ø.- ☑
  - hurricane X37.Ø- ☑
  - landslide X36.1- ☑
    - causing transport accident — *see* Accident, transport, by type of vehicle
  - lightning — *see* subcategory T75.Ø- ☑
    - causing fire — *see* Exposure, fire
  - mudslide X36.1- ☑

- **Forces of nature** — *continued*
  - mudslide — *continued*
    - causing transport accident — *see* Accident, transport, by type of vehicle
  - radiation (natural) X39.Ø8- ☑
    - radon X39.Ø1- ☑
  - radon X39.Ø1- ☑
  - specified force NEC X39.8- ☑
  - storm surge X37.Ø- ☑
  - structure collapse causing earth movement X36.Ø- ☑
  - sunlight X32.- ☑
  - tidal wave X37.41- ☑
    - due to
      - earthquake X37.41- ☑
      - landslide X37.43- ☑
      - storm X37.42- ☑
      - volcanic eruption X37.41- ☑
  - tornado X37.1- ☑
  - tsunami X37.41- ☑
  - twister X37.1- ☑
  - typhoon X37.Ø- ☑
  - volcanic eruption X35.- ☑
- **Foreign body**
  - aspiration — *see* Index to Diseases and Injuries, Foreign body, respiratory tract
  - embedded in skin W45.- ☑
  - entering through
    - natural orifice W44.9- ☑
      - audio device W44.G1- ☑
      - battery W44.AØ- ☑
        - button W44.A1- ☑
        - cylindrical W44.A9- ☑
        - other specified NEC W44.A9- ☑
      - bezoar W44.F1- ☑
      - bottle cap W44.E9- ☑
      - can lid W44.E9- ☑
      - combination metal and plastic
        - jewelry W44.G3- ☑
        - toy and toy part W44.G2- ☑
      - dagger W44.H2- ☑
      - dart W44.H1- ☑
      - ear buds W44.G1- ☑
      - food W44.F3- ☑
      - glass W44.CØ- ☑
        - intact W44.C2- ☑
          - bottle W44.C2- ☑
        - shard W44.C1- ☑
        - sharp W44.C1- ☑
      - hearing aids W44.G1- ☑
      - insect W44.F4- ☑
      - knife W44.H2- ☑
      - magnetic metal W44.DØ- ☑
        - bead W44.D1- ☑
        - coin W44.D2- ☑
        - jewelry W44.D4- ☑
        - object specified NEC W44.D9- ☑
        - toy W44.D3- ☑
      - needle (hypodermic) (sewing) W44.H1- ☑
      - non-magnetic metal W44.EØ- ☑
        - bead W44.E1- ☑
        - coin W44.E2- ☑
        - jewelry W44.E4- ☑
        - object specified NEC W44.E9- ☑
        - toy W44.E3- ☑
      - objects of natural or organic material W44.FØ- ☑
        - specified NEC W44.F9- ☑
      - other
        - non-organic objects W44.GØ- ☑
          - specified NEC W44.G9- ☑
        - sharp object unspecified W44.HØ- ☑
      - plastic
        - bead W44.B1- ☑
        - bottle W44.B5- ☑
        - coin W44.B2- ☑
        - jewelry W44.B4- ☑
        - object W44.BØ- ☑
          - specified NEC W44.B9- ☑
        - toy and toy part W44.B3- ☑
      - pull tab W44.E9- ☑
      - rubber band W44.F2- ☑
      - safety pin W44.H1- ☑
      - shard pottery W44.H9- ☑
      - sharp object specified NEC W44.H9- ☑
      - specified NEC W44.8- ☑
      - sword W44.H2- ☑
- **Foreign body** — *continued*
  - entering through — *continued*
    - skin W45.8- ☑
      - can lid W26.8- ☑
      - fishing hook W45.3- ☑
      - nail W45.Ø- ☑
      - paper W26.2- ☑
      - specified NEC W45.8- ☑
      - splinter W45.8- ☑
- **Forest fire** (exposure to) — *see* Exposure, fire, uncontrolled, not in building
- **Found injured** X58.- ☑
  - from exposure (to) — *see* Exposure
  - on
    - highway, road(way), street V89.9- ☑
    - railway right of way V81.9- ☑
- **Fracture** (circumstances unknown or unspecified) X58.- ☑
  - due to specified cause NEC X58.- ☑
- **Freezing** — *see* Exposure, cold
- **Frostbite** X31.- ☑
  - due to man-made conditions — *see* Exposure, cold, man-made
- **Frozen** — *see* Exposure, cold

## G

- **Gored by bull** W55.22- ☑
- **Gunshot wound** — *see also* Discharge, firearm, by type Y24.9- ☑

## H

- **Hailstones, injured by** X39.8- ☑
- **Hanged herself or himself** T71.162- ☑
- **Hanging** (accidental) — *see also* T71.16
  - legal execution — *see* Legal, intervention, specified means NEC
- **Heat** (effects of) (excessive) X3Ø.- ☑
  - due to
    - man-made conditions W92.- ☑
      - on board watercraft V93.29- ☑
        - fishing boat V93.22- ☑
        - merchant ship V93.2Ø- ☑
        - passenger ship V93.21- ☑
        - sailboat V93.24- ☑
        - specified powered craft NEC V93.23- ☑
    - weather (conditions) X3Ø.- ☑
  - from
    - electric heating apparatus causing burning X16.- ☑
    - nuclear explosion in war operations — *see* War operations, nuclear weapons
  - inappropriate in local application or packing in medical or surgical procedure Y63.5
- **Hemorrhage**
  - delayed following medical or surgical treatment without mention of misadventure — *see* Index to Diseases and Injuries, Complication(s)
  - during medical or surgical treatment as misadventure — *see* Index to Diseases and Injuries, Complication(s)
- **High**
  - altitude (effects) — *see* Air, pressure, low
  - level of radioactivity, effects — *see* Radiation
  - pressure (effects) — *see* Air, pressure, high
  - temperature, effects — *see* Heat
- **Hit, hitting** (accidental) by — *see* Struck by
- **Hitting against** — *see* Striking against
- **Homicide** (attempt) (justifiable) — *see* Assault
- **Hot**
  - place, effects — *see also* Heat
  - weather, effects X3Ø.- ☑
- **House fire** (uncontrolled) — *see* Exposure, fire, uncontrolled, building
- **Humidity, causing problem** X39.8- ☑
- **Hunger** X58.- ☑
- **Hurricane** (any injury) X37.Ø- ☑
- **Hypobarism, hypobaropathy** — *see* Air, pressure, low

## I

- **Ictus**
  - caloris — *see also* Heat
  - solaris X3Ø.- ☑
- **Ignition** (accidental) — *see also* Exposure, fire XØ8.8- ☑
  - anesthetic gas in operating room W4Ø.1- ☑
  - apparel XØ6.2- ☑
- **Ignition** — *continued*
  - apparel — *continued*
    - from highly flammable material XØ4.- ☑
    - nightwear XØ5.- ☑
  - bed linen (sheets) (spreads) (pillows) (mattress) — *see* Exposure, fire, uncontrolled, building, bed
  - benzine XØ4.- ☑
  - clothes, clothing NEC (from controlled fire) XØ6.2- ☑
    - from
      - highly flammable material XØ4.- ☑
  - ether XØ4.- ☑
    - in operating room W4Ø.1- ☑
  - explosive material — *see* Explosion
  - gasoline XØ4.- ☑
  - jewelry (plastic) (any) XØ6.Ø- ☑
  - kerosene XØ4.- ☑
  - material
    - explosive — *see* Explosion
    - highly flammable with secondary explosion XØ4.- ☑
  - nightwear XØ5.- ☑
  - paraffin XØ4.- ☑
  - petrol XØ4.- ☑
- **Immersion** (accidental) — *see also* Drowning
  - hand or foot due to cold (excessive) X31.- ☑
- **Implantation of quills of porcupine** W55.89- ☑
- **Inanition** (from) (hunger) X58.- ☑
  - thirst X58.- ☑
- **Inappropriate operation performed**
  - correct operation on wrong side or body part (wrong side) (wrong site) Y65.53
  - operation intended for another patient done on wrong patient Y65.52
  - wrong operation performed on correct patient Y65.51
- **Inattention after, at birth** (homicidal intent) (infanticidal intent) X58.- ☑
- **Incident, adverse**
  - device
    - anesthesiology Y7Ø.8
      - accessory Y7Ø.2
      - diagnostic Y7Ø.Ø
      - miscellaneous Y7Ø.8
      - monitoring Y7Ø.Ø
      - prosthetic Y7Ø.2
      - rehabilitative Y7Ø.1
      - surgical Y7Ø.3
      - therapeutic Y7Ø.1
    - cardiovascular Y71.8
      - accessory Y71.2
      - diagnostic Y71.Ø
      - miscellaneous Y71.8
      - monitoring Y71.Ø
      - prosthetic Y71.2
      - rehabilitative Y71.1
      - surgical Y71.3
      - therapeutic Y71.1
    - gastroenterology Y73.8
      - accessory Y73.2
      - diagnostic Y73.Ø
      - miscellaneous Y73.8
      - monitoring Y73.Ø
      - prosthetic Y73.2
      - rehabilitative Y73.1
      - surgical Y73.3
      - therapeutic Y73.1
    - general
      - hospital Y74.8
        - accessory Y74.2
        - diagnostic Y74.Ø
        - miscellaneous Y74.8
        - monitoring Y74.Ø
        - prosthetic Y74.2
        - rehabilitative Y74.1
        - surgical Y74.3
        - therapeutic Y74.1
      - surgical Y81.8
        - accessory Y81.2
        - diagnostic Y81.Ø
        - miscellaneous Y81.8
        - monitoring Y81.Ø
        - prosthetic Y81.2
        - rehabilitative Y81.1
        - surgical Y81.3
        - therapeutic Y81.1
    - gynecological Y76.8
      - accessory Y76.2
      - diagnostic Y76.Ø
      - miscellaneous Y76.8
      - monitoring Y76.Ø

- **Incident, adverse** — *continued*
  - device — *continued*
    - gynecological — *continued*
      - prosthetic Y76.2
      - rehabilitative Y76.1
      - surgical Y76.3
      - therapeutic Y76.1
    - medical Y82.9
      - specified type NEC Y82.8
    - neurological Y75.8
      - accessory Y75.2
      - diagnostic Y75.Ø
      - miscellaneous Y75.8
      - monitoring Y75.Ø
      - prosthetic Y75.2
      - rehabilitative Y75.1
      - surgical Y75.3
      - therapeutic Y75.1
    - obstetrical Y76.8
      - accessory Y76.2
      - diagnostic Y76.Ø
      - miscellaneous Y76.8
      - monitoring Y76.Ø
      - prosthetic Y76.2
      - rehabilitative Y76.1
      - surgical Y76.3
      - therapeutic Y76.1
    - ophthalmic Y77.8
      - accessory Y77.2
      - contact lens (rigid gas permeable) (soft (hydrophilic)) Y77.11
      - diagnostic Y77.Ø
      - miscellaneous Y77.8
      - monitoring Y77.Ø
      - prosthetic Y77.2
      - rehabilitative Y77.19
      - surgical Y77.3
      - therapeutic Y77.19
    - orthopedic Y79.8
      - accessory Y79.2
      - diagnostic Y79.Ø
      - miscellaneous Y79.8
      - monitoring Y79.Ø
      - prosthetic Y79.2
      - rehabilitative Y79.1
      - surgical Y79.3
      - therapeutic Y79.1
    - otorhinolaryngological Y72.8
      - accessory Y72.2
      - diagnostic Y72.Ø
      - miscellaneous Y72.8
      - monitoring Y72.Ø
      - prosthetic Y72.2
      - rehabilitative Y72.1
      - surgical Y72.3
      - therapeutic Y72.1
    - personal use Y74.8
      - accessory Y74.2
      - diagnostic Y74.Ø
      - miscellaneous Y74.8
      - monitoring Y74.Ø
      - prosthetic Y74.2
      - rehabilitative Y74.1
      - surgical Y74.3
      - therapeutic Y74.1
    - physical medicine Y8Ø.8
      - accessory Y8Ø.2
      - diagnostic Y8Ø.Ø
      - miscellaneous Y8Ø.8
      - monitoring Y8Ø.Ø
      - prosthetic Y8Ø.2
      - rehabilitative Y8Ø.1
      - surgical Y8Ø.3
      - therapeutic Y8Ø.1
    - plastic surgical Y81.8
      - accessory Y81.2
      - diagnostic Y81.Ø
      - miscellaneous Y81.8
      - monitoring Y81.Ø
      - prosthetic Y81.2
      - rehabilitative Y81.1
      - surgical Y81.3
      - therapeutic Y81.1
    - radiological Y78.8
      - accessory Y78.2
      - diagnostic Y78.Ø
      - miscellaneous Y78.8
      - monitoring Y78.Ø
      - prosthetic Y78.2

- **Incident, adverse** — *continued*
  - device — *continued*
    - radiological — *continued*
      - rehabilitative Y78.1
      - surgical Y78.3
      - therapeutic Y78.1
    - urology Y73.8
      - accessory Y73.2
      - diagnostic Y73.Ø
      - miscellaneous Y73.8
      - monitoring Y73.Ø
      - prosthetic Y73.2
      - rehabilitative Y73.1
      - surgical Y73.3
      - therapeutic Y73.1
- **Incineration** (accidental) — *see* Exposure, fire
- **Infanticide** — *see* Assault
- **Infrasound waves** (causing injury) W49.9- ☑
- **Ingestion**
  - foreign body (causing injury) (with obstruction) — *see* Foreign body, alimentary canal
  - poisonous
    - plant(s) X58.- ☑
    - substance NEC — *see* Table of Drugs and Chemicals
- **Inhalation**
  - excessively cold substance, man-made — *see* Exposure, cold, man-made
  - food (any type) (into respiratory tract) (with asphyxia, obstruction respiratory tract, suffocation) T17.92- ☑
  - foreign body — *see* Foreign body, aspiration
  - gastric contents (with asphyxia, obstruction respiratory passage, suffocation) T17.81- ☑
  - hot air or gases X14.Ø- ☑
  - liquid air, hydrogen, nitrogen W93.12- ☑
    - suicide (attempt) X83.2- ☑
  - steam X13.Ø- ☑
    - assault X98.Ø- ☑
    - stated as undetermined whether accidental or intentional Y27.Ø- ☑
    - suicide (attempt) X77.Ø- ☑
  - toxic gas — *see* Table of Drugs and Chemicals
  - vomitus (with asphyxia, obstruction respiratory passage, suffocation) T17.81- ☑
- **Injury, injured** (accidental(ly)) NOS X58.- ☑
  - by, caused by, from
    - assault — *see* Assault
    - law-enforcing agent, police, in course of legal intervention — *see* Legal intervention
    - suicide (attempt) X83.8- ☑
  - due to, in
    - civil insurrection — *see* War operations
    - fight — *see also* Assault, fight YØ4.Ø- ☑
    - war operations — *see* War operations
  - homicide — *see also* Assault YØ9
  - inflicted (by)
    - in course of arrest (attempted), suppression of disturbance, maintenance of order, by law-enforcing agents — *see* Legal intervention
    - other person
      - stated as
        - accidental X58.- ☑
        - intentional, homicide (attempt) — *see* Assault
        - undetermined whether accidental or intentional Y33.- ☑
  - purposely (inflicted) by other person(s) — *see* Assault
  - self-inflicted X83.8- ☑
    - stated as accidental X58.- ☑
  - specified cause NEC X58.- ☑
  - undetermined whether accidental or intentional Y33.- ☑
- **Insolation, effects** X3Ø.- ☑
- **Insufficient nourishment** X58.- ☑
- **Interruption of respiration** (by)
  - food (lodged in esophagus) T18.12Ø- ☑
  - vomitus (lodged in esophagus) T17.81- ☑
- **Intervention, legal** — *see* Legal intervention
- **Intoxication**
  - drug — *see* Table of Drugs and Chemicals
  - poison — *see* Table of Drugs and Chemicals

# J

- **Jammed** (accidentally)
  - between objects (moving) (stationary and moving) W23.Ø- ☑
    - stationary W23.1- ☑
- **Jumped, jumping**
  - before moving object NEC X81.8- ☑
    - motor vehicle X81.Ø- ☑
    - subway train X81.1- ☑
    - train X81.1- ☑
    - undetermined whether accidental or intentional Y31.- ☑
  - from
    - boat (into water) voluntarily, without accident (to or on boat) W16.712- ☑
      - striking bottom W16.722- ☑
        - causing drowning W16.721- ☑
      - with
        - accident to or on boat — *see* Accident, watercraft
        - drowning or submersion W16.711- ☑
          - suicide (attempt) X71.3- ☑
    - building — *see also* Jumped, from, high place W13.9- ☑
      - burning (uncontrolled fire) XØØ.5- ☑
    - high place NEC W17.89- ☑
      - suicide (attempt) X8Ø.- ☑
      - undetermined whether accidental or intentional Y3Ø.- ☑
    - structure — *see also* Jumped, from, high place W13.9- ☑
      - burning (uncontrolled fire) XØØ.5- ☑
  - into water W16.92- ☑
    - causing drowning W16.91- ☑
    - from, off watercraft — *see* Jumped, from, boat
    - in
      - natural body W16.612- ☑
        - causing drowning W16.611- ☑
        - striking bottom W16.622- ☑
          - causing drowning W16.621- ☑
      - specified place NEC W16.812- ☑
        - causing drowning W16.811- ☑
        - striking
          - bottom W16.822- ☑
            - causing drowning W16.821- ☑
          - wall W16.832- ☑
            - causing drowning W16.831- ☑
      - swimming pool W16.512- ☑
        - causing drowning W16.511- ☑
        - striking
          - bottom W16.522- ☑
            - causing drowning W16.521- ☑
          - wall W16.532- ☑
            - causing drowning W16.531- ☑
    - suicide (attempt) X71.3- ☑

# K

- **Kicked by**
  - animal NEC W55.82- ☑
  - person(s) (accidentally) W5Ø.1- ☑
    - with intent to injure or kill YØ4.Ø- ☑
    - as, or caused by, a crowd or human stampede (with fall) W52.- ☑
    - assault YØ4.Ø- ☑
    - homicide (attempt) YØ4.Ø- ☑
    - in
      - fight YØ4.Ø- ☑
      - legal intervention
        - injuring
          - bystander Y35.812- ☑
          - law enforcement personnel Y35.811- ☑
          - suspect Y35.813- ☑
          - unspecified person Y35.819- ☑
- **Kicking**
  - against
    - object W22.8- ☑
      - sports equipment W21.9- ☑
      - stationary W22.Ø9- ☑
        - sports equipment W21.89- ☑
    - person — *see* Striking against, person
    - sports equipment W21.9- ☑
  - carpet stretcher with knee X5Ø.3- ☑
- **Killed, killing** (accidentally) NOS — *see also* Injury X58.- ☑
  - in
    - action — *see* War operations
    - brawl, fight (hand) (fists) (foot) YØ4.Ø- ☑
      - by weapon — *see also* Assault
        - cutting, piercing — *see* Assault, cutting or piercing instrument

**Killed, killing** — *continued*
- in — *continued*
  - brawl, fight — *continued*
    - by weapon — *see also* Assault — *continued*
      - firearm — *see* Discharge, firearm, by type, homicide
- self
  - stated as
    - accident NOS X58.- ☑
    - suicide — *see* Suicide
    - undetermined whether accidental or intentional Y33.- ☑

**Kneeling** (prolonged (static) X5Ø.1- ☑

**Knocked down** (accidentally) (by) NOS X58.- ☑
- animal (not being ridden) NEC — *see also* Struck by, by type of animal
- crowd or human stampede W52.- ☑
- person W51.- ☑
  - in brawl, fight YØ4.Ø- ☑
- transport vehicle NEC — *see also* Accident, transport VØ9.9- ☑

## L

**Laceration NEC** — *see* Injury

**Lack of**
- care (helpless person) (infant) (newborn) X58.- ☑
- food except as result of abandonment or neglect X58.- ☑
  - due to abandonment or neglect X58.- ☑
- water except as result of transport accident X58.- ☑
  - due to transport accident — *see* Accident, transport, by type
  - helpless person, infant, newborn X58.- ☑

**Landslide** (falling on transport vehicle) X36.1- ☑
- caused by collapse of man-made structure X36.Ø- ☑

**Late effect** — *see* Sequelae

**Legal**
- execution (any method) — *see* Legal, intervention
- intervention (by)
  - baton — *see* Legal, intervention, blunt object, baton
  - bayonet — *see* Legal, intervention, sharp object, bayonet
  - blow — *see* Legal, intervention, manhandling
  - blunt object
    - baton
      - injuring
        - bystander Y35.312- ☑
        - law enforcement personnel Y35.311- ☑
        - suspect Y35.313- ☑
        - unspecified person Y35.319- ☑
    - injuring
      - bystander Y35.3Ø2- ☑
      - law enforcement personnel Y35.3Ø1- ☑
      - suspect Y35.3Ø3- ☑
      - unspecified person Y35.3Ø9- ☑
    - specified NEC
      - injuring
        - bystander Y35.392- ☑
        - law enforcement personnel Y35.391- ☑
        - suspect Y35.393- ☑
        - unspecified person Y35.399- ☑
    - stave
      - injuring
        - bystander Y35.392- ☑
        - law enforcement personnel Y35.391- ☑
        - suspect Y35.393- ☑
        - unspecified person Y35.399- ☑
  - bomb — *see* Legal, intervention, explosive
  - conducted energy device
    - injuring
      - bystander Y35.832- ☑
      - law enforcement personnel Y35.831- ☑
      - suspect Y35.833- ☑
      - unspecified person Y35.839- ☑
  - cutting or piercing instrument — *see* Legal, intervention, sharp object
  - dynamite — *see* Legal, intervention, explosive, dynamite
  - electroshock device (taser)
    - injuring
      - bystander Y35.832- ☑
      - law enforcement personnel Y35.831- ☑
      - suspect Y35.833- ☑
      - unspecified person Y35.839- ☑

**Legal** — *continued*
- intervention — *continued*
  - explosive(s)
    - dynamite
      - injuring
        - bystander Y35.112- ☑
        - law enforcement personnel Y35.111- ☑
        - suspect Y35.113- ☑
        - unspecified person Y35.119- ☑
    - grenade
      - injuring
        - bystander Y35.192- ☑
        - law enforcement personnel Y35.191- ☑
        - suspect Y35.193- ☑
        - unspecified person Y35.199- ☑
    - injuring
      - bystander Y35.1Ø2- ☑
      - law enforcement personnel Y35.1Ø1- ☑
      - suspect Y35.1Ø3- ☑
      - unspecified person Y35.1Ø9- ☑
    - mortar bomb
      - injuring
        - bystander Y35.192- ☑
        - law enforcement personnel Y35.191- ☑
        - suspect Y35.193- ☑
        - unspecified person Y35.199- ☑
    - shell
      - injuring
        - bystander Y35.122- ☑
        - law enforcement personnel Y35.121- ☑
        - suspect Y35.123- ☑
        - unspecified person Y35.129- ☑
    - specified NEC
      - injuring
        - bystander Y35.192- ☑
        - law enforcement personnel Y35.191- ☑
        - suspect Y35.193- ☑
        - unspecified person Y35.199- ☑
  - firearm(s) (discharge)
    - handgun
      - injuring
        - bystander Y35.Ø22- ☑
        - law enforcement personnel Y35.Ø21- ☑
        - suspect Y35.Ø23- ☑
        - unspecified person Y35.Ø29- ☑
    - injuring
      - bystander Y35.ØØ2- ☑
      - law enforcement personnel Y35.ØØ1- ☑
      - suspect Y35.ØØ3- ☑
      - unspecified person Y35.ØØ9- ☑
    - machine gun
      - injuring
        - bystander Y35.Ø12- ☑
        - law enforcement personnel Y35.Ø11- ☑
        - suspect Y35.Ø13- ☑
        - unspecified person Y35.Ø19- ☑
    - rifle pellet
      - injuring
        - bystander Y35.Ø32- ☑
        - law enforcement personnel Y35.Ø31- ☑
        - suspect Y35.Ø33- ☑
        - unspecified person Y35.Ø39- ☑
    - rubber bullet
      - injuring
        - bystander Y35.Ø42- ☑
        - law enforcement personnel Y35.Ø41- ☑
        - suspect Y35.Ø43- ☑
        - unspecified person Y35.Ø49- ☑
    - shotgun — *see* Legal, intervention, firearm, specified NEC
    - specified NEC
      - injuring
        - bystander Y35.Ø92- ☑
        - law enforcement personnel Y35.Ø91- ☑
        - suspect Y35.Ø93- ☑
        - unspecified person Y35.Ø99- ☑
  - gas (asphyxiation) (poisoning)
    - injuring
      - bystander Y35.2Ø2- ☑
      - law enforcement personnel Y35.2Ø1- ☑
      - suspect Y35.2Ø3- ☑
      - unspecified person Y35.2Ø9- ☑
    - specified NEC
      - injuring
        - bystander Y35.292- ☑
        - law enforcement personnel Y35.291- ☑

**Legal** — *continued*
- intervention — *continued*
  - gas — *continued*
    - specified — *continued*
      - injuring — *continued*
        - suspect Y35.293- ☑
        - unspecified person Y35.299- ☑
    - tear gas
      - injuring
        - bystander Y35.212- ☑
        - law enforcement personnel Y35.211- ☑
        - suspect Y35.213- ☑
        - unspecified person Y35.219- ☑
  - grenade — *see* Legal, intervention, explosive, grenade
  - injuring
    - bystander Y35.92- ☑
    - law enforcement personnel Y35.91- ☑
    - suspect Y35.93- ☑
    - unspecified person Y35.99- ☑
  - late effect (of) — *see* with 7th character S Y35.- ☑
  - manhandling
    - injuring
      - bystander Y35.812- ☑
      - law enforcement personnel Y35.811- ☑
      - suspect Y35.813- ☑
      - unspecified person Y35.819- ☑
  - sequelae (of) — *see* with 7th character S Y35.- ☑
  - sharp objects
    - bayonet
      - injuring
        - bystander Y35.412- ☑
        - law enforcement personnel Y35.411- ☑
        - suspect Y35.413- ☑
        - unspecified person Y35.419- ☑
    - injuring
      - bystander Y35.4Ø2- ☑
      - law enforcement personnel Y35.4Ø1- ☑
      - suspect Y35.4Ø3- ☑
      - unspecified person Y35.4Ø9- ☑
    - specified NEC
      - injuring
        - bystander Y35.492- ☑
        - law enforcement personnel Y35.491- ☑
        - suspect Y35.493- ☑
        - unspecified person Y35.499- ☑
  - specified means NEC
    - injuring
      - bystander Y35.892- ☑
      - law enforcement personnel Y35.891- ☑
      - suspect Y35.893- ☑
      - unspecified person Y35.899- ☑
  - stabbing — *see* Legal, intervention, sharp object
  - stave — *see* Legal, intervention, blunt object, stave
  - stun gun
    - injuring
      - bystander Y35.832- ☑
      - law enforcement personnel Y35.831- ☑
      - suspect Y35.833- ☑
      - unspecified person Y35.839- ☑
  - taser
    - injuring
      - bystander Y35.832- ☑
      - law enforcement personnel Y35.831- ☑
      - suspect Y35.833- ☑
      - unspecified person Y35.839- ☑
  - tear gas — *see* Legal, intervention, gas, tear gas
  - truncheon — *see* Legal, intervention, blunt object, stave

**Lifting** — *see also* Overexertion
- heavy objects X5Ø.Ø- ☑
- weights X5Ø.Ø- ☑

**Lightning** (shock) (stroke) (struck by) — *see* subcategory T75.Ø- ☑
- causing fire — *see* Exposure, fire

**Loss of control** (transport vehicle) NEC — *see* Accident, transport

**Lost at sea NOS** — *see* Drowning, due to, fall overboard

**Low**
- pressure (effects) — *see* Air, pressure, low
- temperature (effects) — *see* Exposure, cold

**Lying before train, vehicle or other moving object** X81.8- ☑
- subway train X81.1- ☑
- train X81.1- ☑
- undetermined whether accidental or intentional Y31.- ☑

**Lynching** — *see* Assault

# M

- **Malfunction** (mechanism or component) (of)
  - firearm W34.1Ø- ☑
    - airgun W34.11Ø- ☑
    - BB gun W34.11Ø- ☑
    - gas, air or spring-operated gun NEC W34.118- ☑
    - handgun W32.1- ☑
    - hunting rifle W33.12- ☑
    - larger firearm W33.1Ø- ☑
      - specified NEC W33.19- ☑
    - machine gun W33.13- ☑
    - paintball gun W34.111- ☑
    - pellet gun W34.11Ø- ☑
    - shotgun W33.11- ☑
    - specified NEC W34.19- ☑
    - Very pistol [flare] W34.19- ☑
  - handgun — *see* Malfunction, firearm, handgun
- **Maltreatment** — *see* Perpetrator
- **Mangled** (accidentally) NOS X58.- ☑
- **Manhandling** (in brawl, fight) YØ4.Ø- ☑
  - legal intervention — *see* Legal, intervention, manhandling
- **Manslaughter** (nonaccidental) — *see* Assault
- **Mauled by animal NEC** W55.89- ☑
- **Medical procedure, complication of** (delayed or as an abnormal reaction without mention of misadventure) — *see* Complication of or following, by specified type of procedure
  - due to or as a result of misadventure — *see* Misadventure
- **Melting** (due to fire) — *see also* Exposure, fire
  - apparel NEC XØ6.3- ☑
  - clothes, clothing NEC XØ6.3- ☑
    - nightwear XØ5.- ☑
  - fittings or furniture (burning building) (uncontrolled fire) XØØ.8- ☑
  - nightwear XØ5.- ☑
  - plastic jewelry XØ6.1- ☑
- **Mental cruelty** X58.- ☑
- **Military operations** (injuries to military and civilians occuring during peacetime on military property and during routine military exercises and operations) (by) (from) (involving) Y37.9Ø- ☑
  - air blast Y37.2Ø- ☑
  - aircraft
    - destruction — *see* Military operations, destruction of aircraft
  - airway restriction — *see* Military operations, restriction of airways
  - asphyxiation — *see* Military operations, restriction of airways
  - biological weapons Y37.6X- ☑
  - blast Y37.2Ø- ☑
  - blast fragments Y37.2Ø- ☑
  - blast overpressure
    - high level (due to explosion) Y37.A2- ☑
    - low level (due to explosion) Y37.A1- ☑
  - blast wave Y37.2Ø- ☑
  - blast wind Y37.2Ø- ☑
  - bomb Y37.2Ø- ☑
    - dirty Y37.5Ø- ☑
    - gasoline Y37.31- ☑
    - incendiary Y37.31- ☑
    - petrol Y37.31- ☑
  - bullet Y37.43- ☑
    - incendiary Y37.32- ☑
    - rubber Y37.41- ☑
  - chemical weapons Y37.7X- ☑
  - combat
    - hand to hand (unarmed) combat Y37.44- ☑
    - using blunt or piercing object Y37.45- ☑
  - conflagration — *see* Military operations, fire
  - conventional warfare NEC Y37.49- ☑
  - depth-charge Y37.Ø1- ☑
  - destruction of aircraft Y37.1Ø- ☑
    - due to
      - air to air missile Y37.11- ☑
      - collision with other aircraft Y37.12- ☑
      - detonation (accidental) of onboard munitions and explosives Y37.14- ☑
      - enemy fire or explosives Y37.11- ☑
      - explosive placed on aircraft Y37.11- ☑
      - onboard fire Y37.13- ☑
      - rocket propelled grenade [RPG] Y37.11- ☑
      - small arms fire Y37.11- ☑

- **Military operations** — *continued*
  - destruction of aircraft — *continued*
    - due to — *continued*
      - surface to air missile Y37.11- ☑
    - specified NEC Y37.19- ☑
  - detonation (accidental) of
    - onboard marine weapons Y37.Ø5- ☑
    - own munitions or munitions launch device Y37.24- ☑
  - dirty bomb Y37.5Ø- ☑
  - explosion (of) Y37.2Ø- ☑
    - aerial bomb Y37.21- ☑
    - bomb NOS — *see also* Military operations, bomb(s) Y37.2Ø- ☑
    - fragments Y37.2Ø- ☑
    - grenade Y37.29- ☑
    - guided missile Y37.22- ☑
    - improvised explosive device [IED] (person-borne) (roadside) (vehicle-borne) Y37.23- ☑
    - land mine Y37.29- ☑
    - marine mine (at sea) (in harbor) Y37.Ø2- ☑
    - marine weapon Y37.ØØ- ☑
      - specified NEC Y37.Ø9- ☑
    - own munitions or munitions launch device (accidental) Y37.24- ☑
    - sea-based artillery shell Y37.Ø3- ☑
    - specified NEC Y37.29- ☑
    - torpedo Y37.Ø4- ☑
  - fire Y37.3Ø- ☑
    - specified NEC Y37.39- ☑
  - firearms
    - discharge Y37.43- ☑
    - pellets Y37.42- ☑
  - flamethrower Y37.33- ☑
  - fragments (from) (of)
    - improvised explosive device [IED] (person-borne) (roadside) (vehicle-borne) Y37.26- ☑
    - munitions Y37.25- ☑
    - specified NEC Y37.29- ☑
    - weapons Y37.27- ☑
  - friendly fire Y37.92- ☑
  - hand to hand (unarmed) combat Y37.44- ☑
  - HLB overpressure Y37.A2- ☑
  - hot substances — *see* Military operations, fire
  - incendiary bullet Y37.32- ☑
  - LLB overpressure Y37.A1- ☑
  - nuclear weapon (effects of) Y37.5Ø- ☑
    - acute radiation exposure Y37.54- ☑
    - blast pressure Y37.51- ☑
    - direct blast Y37.51- ☑
    - direct heat Y37.53- ☑
    - fallout exposure Y37.54- ☑
    - fireball Y37.53- ☑
    - indirect blast (struck or crushed by blast debris) (being thrown by blast) Y37.52- ☑
    - ionizing radiation (immediate exposure) Y37.54- ☑
    - nuclear radiation Y37.54- ☑
    - radiation
      - ionizing (immediate exposure) Y37.54- ☑
      - nuclear Y37.54- ☑
      - thermal Y37.53- ☑
    - secondary effects Y37.54- ☑
    - specified NEC Y37.59- ☑
    - thermal radiation Y37.53- ☑
  - restriction of air (airway)
    - intentional Y37.46- ☑
    - unintentional Y37.47- ☑
  - rubber bullets Y37.41- ☑
  - shrapnel NOS Y37.29- ☑
  - suffocation — *see* Military operations, restriction of airways
  - unconventional warfare NEC Y37.7X- ☑
  - underwater blast NOS Y37.ØØ- ☑
  - warfare
    - conventional NEC Y37.49- ☑
    - unconventional NEC Y37.7X- ☑
  - weapon of mass destruction [WMD] Y37.91- ☑
  - weapons
    - biological weapons Y37.6X- ☑
    - chemical Y37.7X- ☑
    - nuclear (effects of ) Y37.5Ø- ☑
      - acute radiation exposure Y37.54- ☑
      - blast pressure Y37.51- ☑
      - direct blast Y37.51- ☑
      - direct heat Y37.53- ☑
      - fallout exposure Y37.54- ☑
      - fireball Y37.53- ☑

- **Military operations** — *continued*
  - weapons — *continued*
    - nuclear — *continued*
      - radiation
        - ionizing (immediate exposure) Y37.54- ☑
        - nuclear Y37.54- ☑
        - thermal Y37.53- ☑
      - secondary effects Y37.54- ☑
      - specified NEC Y37.59- ☑
    - of mass destruction [WMD] Y37.91- ☑
- **Misadventure**(s) **to patient**(s) **during surgical or medical care** Y69
  - contaminated medical or biological substance (blood, drug, fluid) Y64.9
    - administered (by) NEC Y64.9
      - immunization Y64.1
      - infusion Y64.Ø
      - injection Y64.1
      - specified means NEC Y64.8
      - transfusion Y64.Ø
      - vaccination Y64.1
  - excessive amount of blood or other fluid during transfusion or infusion Y63.Ø
  - failure
    - in dosage Y63.9
      - electroshock therapy Y63.4
      - inappropriate temperature (too hot or too cold) in local application and packing Y63.5
      - infusion
        - excessive amount of fluid Y63.Ø
        - incorrect dilution of fluid Y63.1
      - insulin-shock therapy Y63.4
      - nonadministration of necessary drug or biological substance Y63.6
      - overdose — *see* Table of Drugs and Chemicals
        - radiation, in therapy Y63.2
      - radiation
        - overdose Y63.2
      - specified procedure NEC Y63.8
      - transfusion
        - excessive amount of blood Y63.Ø
    - mechanical, of instrument or apparatus (any) (during any procedure) Y65.8
    - sterile precautions (during procedure) Y62.9
      - aspiration of fluid or tissue (by puncture or catheterization, except heart) Y62.6
      - biopsy (except needle aspiration) Y62.8
        - needle (aspirating) Y62.6
      - blood sampling Y62.6
      - catheterization Y62.6
        - heart Y62.5
      - dialysis (kidney) Y62.2
      - endoscopic examination Y62.4
      - enema Y62.8
      - immunization Y62.3
      - infusion Y62.1
      - injection Y62.3
      - needle biopsy Y62.6
      - paracentesis (abdominal) (thoracic) Y62.6
      - perfusion Y62.2
      - puncture (lumbar) Y62.6
      - removal of catheter or packing Y62.8
      - specified procedure NEC Y62.8
      - surgical operation Y62.Ø
      - transfusion Y62.1
      - vaccination Y62.3
    - suture or ligature during surgical procedure Y65.2
    - to introduce or to remove tube or instrument — *see* Failure, to
  - hemorrhage — *see* Index to Diseases and Injuries, Complication(s)
  - inadvertent exposure of patient to radiation Y63.3
  - inappropriate
    - operation performed — *see* Inappropriate operation performed
    - temperature (too hot or too cold) in local application or packing Y63.5
  - infusion — *see also* Misadventure, by type, infusion Y69
    - excessive amount of fluid Y63.Ø
    - incorrect dilution of fluid Y63.1
    - wrong fluid Y65.1
  - mismatched blood in transfusion Y65.Ø
  - nonadministration of necessary drug or biological substance Y63.6
  - overdose — *see* Table of Drugs and Chemicals
    - radiation (in therapy) Y63.2
  - perforation — *see* Index to Diseases and Injuries, Complication(s)

External Causes Index
Misadventure — Place of occurrence

- **Place of occurrence** — *continued*
  - residence — *continued*
    - specified residence type — *continued*
      - garage Y92.Ø94
      - garden Y92.Ø96
      - kitchen Y92.Ø9Ø
      - specified NEC Y92.Ø98
      - swimming pool Y92.Ø95
      - yard Y92.Ø96
  - restaurant Y92.511
  - riding school Y92.39
  - river Y92.828
  - road Y92.41Ø
  - rodeo ring Y92.39
  - rugby field Y92.328
  - same day surgery center Y92.53Ø
  - sand pit Y92.64
  - school (private) (public) (state) Y92.219
    - college Y92.214
    - daycare center Y92.21Ø
    - elementary school Y92.211
    - high school Y92.213
    - kindergarten Y92.211
    - middle school Y92.212
    - specified NEC Y92.218
    - trade school Y92.215
    - university Y92.214
    - vocational school Y92.215
  - sea (shore) Y92.832
  - senior citizen center Y92.29
  - service area
    - airport Y92.52Ø
    - bus station Y92.521
    - gas station Y92.524
    - highway rest stop Y92.523
    - railway station Y92.522
  - shipyard Y92.62
  - shop (commercial) Y92.513
  - sidewalk Y92.48Ø
  - silo Y92.79
  - skating rink (roller) Y92.331
    - ice Y92.33Ø
  - slaughter house Y92.86
  - soccer field Y92.322
  - specified place NEC Y92.89
  - sports area Y92.39
    - athletic
      - court Y92.318
        - basketball Y92.31Ø
        - specified NEC Y92.318
        - squash Y92.311
        - tennis Y92.312
      - field Y92.328
        - baseball Y92.32Ø
        - cricket ground Y92.328
        - football Y92.321
        - hockey Y92.328
        - soccer Y92.322
        - specified NEC Y92.328
    - golf course Y92.39
    - gymnasium Y92.39
    - riding school Y92.39
    - skating rink (roller) Y92.331
      - ice Y92.33Ø
    - stadium Y92.39
    - swimming pool Y92.34
  - squash court Y92.311
  - stadium Y92.39
  - steeplechasing course Y92.39
  - store Y92.512
  - stream Y92.828
  - street and highway Y92.41Ø
    - bike path Y92.482
    - freeway Y92.411
    - highway ramp Y92.415
    - interstate highway Y92.411
    - local residential or business street Y92.414
    - motorway Y92.411
    - parking lot Y92.481
    - parkway Y92.412
    - sidewalk Y92.48Ø
    - specified NEC Y92.488
    - state road Y92.413
  - subway car Y92.816
  - supermarket Y92.512
  - swamp Y92.828
  - swimming pool (public) Y92.34
    - private (at) Y92.Ø95
      - boarding house Y92.Ø45

- **Place of occurrence** — *continued*
  - swimming pool — *continued*
    - private — *continued*
      - military base Y92.136
      - mobile home Y92.Ø26
      - nursing home Y92.125
      - orphanage Y92.115
      - prison Y92.146
      - reform school Y92.156
      - single family residence Y92.Ø16
  - synagogue Y92.22
  - tavern Y92.59
  - television station Y92.59
  - tennis court Y92.312
  - theater Y92.254
  - trade area Y92.59
    - bank Y92.51Ø
    - cafe Y92.511
    - casino Y92.59
    - garage Y92.59
    - hotel Y92.59
    - market Y92.512
    - office building Y92.59
    - radio station Y92.59
    - restaurant Y92.511
    - shop Y92.513
    - shopping mall Y92.59
    - store Y92.512
    - supermarket Y92.512
    - television station Y92.59
    - warehouse Y92.59
  - trailer park, residential — *see* Place of occurrence, residence, mobile home
  - trailer site NOS Y92.89
  - train Y92.815
    - station Y92.522
  - truck Y92.812
  - tunnel under construction Y92.69
  - university Y92.214
  - urgent (health) care center Y92.532
  - vehicle (transport) Y92.818
    - airplane Y92.813
    - boat Y92.814
    - bus Y92.811
    - car Y92.81Ø
    - specified NEC Y92.818
    - subway car Y92.816
    - train Y92.815
    - truck Y92.812
  - warehouse Y92.59
  - water reservoir Y92.89
  - wilderness area Y92.828
    - desert Y92.82Ø
    - forest Y92.821
    - marsh Y92.828
    - mountain Y92.828
    - prairie Y92.828
    - specified NEC Y92.828
    - swamp Y92.828
  - workshop Y92.69
  - yard, private Y92.Ø96
    - boarding house Y92.Ø46
    - mobile home Y92.Ø27
    - single family house Y92.Ø17
  - youth center Y92.29
  - zoo (zoological garden) Y92.834
- **Plumbism** — *see* Table of Drugs and Chemicals, lead
- **Poisoning** (accidental) (by) — *see also* Table of Drugs and Chemicals
  - by plant, thorns, spines, sharp leaves or other mechanisms NEC X58.- ☑
  - carbon monoxide
    - generated by
      - motor vehicle — *see* Accident, transport
      - watercraft (in transit) (not in transit) V93.89- ☑
        - ferry boat V93.81- ☑
        - fishing boat V93.82- ☑
        - jet skis V93.83- ☑
        - liner V93.81- ☑
        - merchant ship V93.8Ø- ☑
        - passenger ship V93.81- ☑
        - powered craft NEC V93.83- ☑
  - caused by injection of poisons into skin by plant thorns, spines, sharp leaves X58.- ☑
    - marine or sea plants (venomous) X58.- ☑
  - execution — *see* Legal, intervention, gas
    - intervention
      - by gas — *see* Legal, intervention, gas

- **Poisoning** — *continued*
  - execution — *see* Legal, intervention, gas — *continued*
    - intervention — *continued*
      - other specified means — *see* Legal, intervention, specified means NEC
  - exhaust gas
    - generated by
      - motor vehicle — *see* Accident, transport
      - watercraft (in transit) (not in transit) V93.89- ☑
        - ferry boat V93.81- ☑
        - fishing boat V93.82- ☑
        - jet skis V93.83- ☑
        - liner V93.81- ☑
        - merchant ship V93.8Ø- ☑
        - passenger ship V93.81- ☑
        - powered craft NEC V93.83- ☑
  - fumes or smoke due to
    - explosion — *see also* Explosion W4Ø.9- ☑
    - fire — *see* Exposure, fire
    - ignition — *see* Ignition
  - gas
    - in legal intervention — *see* Legal, intervention, gas
    - legal execution — *see* Legal, intervention, gas
  - in war operations — *see* War operations
  - legal
- **Powder burn** (by) (from)
  - airgun W34.11Ø- ☑
  - BB gun W34.11Ø- ☑
  - firearm NEC W34.19- ☑
  - gas, air or spring-operated gun NEC W34.118- ☑
  - handgun W32.1- ☑
  - hunting rifle W33.12- ☑
  - larger firearm W33.1Ø- ☑
    - specified NEC W33.19- ☑
  - machine gun W33.13- ☑
  - paintball gun W34.111- ☑
  - pellet gun W34.11Ø- ☑
  - shotgun W33.11- ☑
  - Very pistol [flare] W34.19- ☑
- **Premature cessation** (of) **surgical and medical care** Y66
- **Privation** (food) (water) X58.- ☑
- **Procedure** (operation)
  - correct, on wrong side or body part (wrong side) (wrong site) Y65.53
  - intended for another patient done on wrong patient Y65.52
  - performed on patient not scheduled for surgery Y65.52
  - performed on wrong patient Y65.52
  - wrong, performed on correct patient Y65.51
- **Prolonged**
  - sitting in transport vehicle — *see* Sitting
  - stay in
    - high altitude as cause of anoxia, barodontalgia, barotitis or hypoxia W94.11- ☑
    - weightless environment X52.- ☑
- **Pulling, excessive** — *see also* Overexertion X5Ø.9- ☑
- **Puncture, puncturing** — *see also* Contact, with, by type of object or machine
  - by
    - plant thorns, spines, sharp leaves or other mechanisms NEC W6Ø.- ☑
  - during medical or surgical treatment as misadventure — *see* Index to Diseases and Injuries, Complication(s)
- **Pushed, pushing** (accidental) (injury in)
  - by other person(s) (accidental) W51.- ☑
    - as, or caused by, a crowd or human stampede (with fall) W52.- ☑
    - before moving object NEC YØ2.8- ☑
      - motor vehicle YØ2.Ø- ☑
      - subway train YØ2.1- ☑
      - train YØ2.1- ☑
    - from
      - high place NEC
        - in accidental circumstances W17.89- ☑
        - stated as
          - intentional, homicide (attempt) YØ1.- ☑
          - undetermined whether accidental or intentional Y3Ø.- ☑
      - transport vehicle NEC — *see also* Accident, transport V89.9- ☑
        - stated as
          - intentional, homicide (attempt) YØ8.89- ☑
    - with fall WØ3.- ☑
      - due to ice or snow WØØ.Ø- ☑
  - overexertion X5Ø.9- ☑

# R

- **Radiation** (exposure to)
  - arc lamps W89.Ø- ☑
  - atomic power plant (malfunction) NEC W88.1- ☑
  - complication of or abnormal reaction to medical radiotherapy Y84.2
  - electromagnetic, ionizing W88.Ø- ☑
  - gamma rays W88.1- ☑
  - in
    - war operations (from or following nuclear explosion) — *see* War operations
  - inadvertent exposure of patient (receiving test or therapy) Y63.3
  - infrared (heaters and lamps) W9Ø.1- ☑
    - excessive heat from W92.- ☑
  - ionized, ionizing (particles, artificially accelerated)
    - radioisotopes W88.1- ☑
    - specified NEC W88.8- ☑
    - x-rays W88.Ø- ☑
  - isotopes, radioactive — *see* Radiation, radioactive isotopes
  - laser(s) W9Ø.2- ☑
    - in war operations — *see* War operations
    - misadventure in medical care Y63.2
  - light sources (man-made visible and ultraviolet) W89.9- ☑
    - natural X32.- ☑
    - specified NEC W89.8- ☑
    - tanning bed W89.1- ☑
    - welding light W89.Ø- ☑
  - man-made visible light W89.9- ☑
    - specified NEC W89.8- ☑
    - tanning bed W89.1- ☑
    - welding light W89.Ø- ☑
  - microwave W9Ø.8- ☑
  - misadventure in medical or surgical procedure Y63.2
  - natural NEC X39.Ø8- ☑
    - radon X39.Ø1- ☑
  - overdose (in medical or surgical procedure) Y63.2
  - radar W9Ø.Ø- ☑
  - radioactive isotopes (any) W88.1- ☑
    - atomic power plant malfunction W88.1- ☑
    - misadventure in medical or surgical treatment Y63.2
  - radiofrequency W9Ø.Ø- ☑
  - radium NEC W88.1- ☑
  - sun X32.- ☑
  - ultraviolet (light) (man-made) W89.9- ☑
    - natural X32.- ☑
    - specified NEC W89.8- ☑
    - tanning bed W89.1- ☑
    - welding light W89.Ø- ☑
  - welding arc, torch, or light W89.Ø- ☑
    - excessive heat from W92.- ☑
  - x-rays (hard) (soft) W88.Ø- ☑
- **Range disease** W94.11- ☑
- **Rape** (attempted) (confirmed) T74.2- ☑
  - suspected T76.2- ☑
- **Rat bite** W53.11- ☑
- **Reaching** (prolonged) (static) X5Ø.1- ☑
- **Reaction, abnormal to medical procedure** — *see also* Complication of or following, by type of procedure Y84.9
  - biologicals — *see* Table of Drugs and Chemicals
  - drugs — *see* Table of Drugs and Chemicals
  - vaccine — *see* Table of Drugs and Chemicals
  - with misadventure — *see* Misadventure
- **Recoil**
  - airgun W34.11Ø- ☑
  - BB gun W34.11Ø- ☑
  - firearm NEC W34.19- ☑
  - gas, air or spring-operated gun NEC W34.118- ☑
  - handgun W32.1- ☑
  - hunting rifle W33.12- ☑
  - larger firearm W33.1Ø- ☑
    - specified NEC W33.19- ☑
  - machine gun W33.13- ☑
  - paintball gun W34.111- ☑
  - pellet W34.11Ø- ☑
  - shotgun W33.11- ☑
  - Very pistol [flare] W34.19- ☑
- **Reduction in**
  - atmospheric pressure — *see* Air, pressure, change
- **Rock falling on or hitting** (accidentally) (person) W2Ø.8- ☑
  - in cave-in W2Ø.Ø- ☑
- **Run over** (accidentally) (by)
  - animal (not being ridden) NEC W55.89- ☑
  - machinery — *see* Contact, with, by specified type of machine
  - transport vehicle NEC — *see also* Accident, transport VØ9.9- ☑
    - intentional homicide (attempt) YØ3.Ø- ☑
    - motor NEC VØ9.2Ø- ☑
      - intentional homicide (attempt) YØ3.Ø- ☑
- **Running**
  - before moving object X81.8- ☑
    - motor vehicle X81.Ø- ☑
- **Running off, away**
  - animal (being ridden) — *see also* Accident, transport V8Ø.918- ☑
    - not being ridden W55.89- ☑
  - animal-drawn vehicle NEC — *see also* Accident, transport V8Ø.928- ☑
  - highway, road(way), street
    - transport vehicle NEC — *see also* Accident, transport V89.9- ☑
- **Rupture pressurized devices** — *see* Explosion, by type of device

# S

- **Saturnism** — *see* Table of Drugs and Chemicals, lead
- **Scald, scalding** (accidental) (by) (from) (in) X19.- ☑
  - air (hot) X14.1- ☑
  - gases (hot) X14.1- ☑
  - homicide (attempt) — *see* Assault, burning, hot object
  - inflicted by other person
    - stated as intentional, homicide (attempt) — *see* Assault, burning, hot object
  - liquid (boiling) (hot) NEC X12.- ☑
    - stated as undetermined whether accidental or intentional Y27.2- ☑
    - suicide (attempt) X77.2- ☑
  - local application of externally applied substance in medical or surgical care Y63.5
  - metal (molten) (liquid) (hot) NEC X18.- ☑
  - self-inflicted X77.9- ☑
  - stated as undetermined whether accidental or intentional Y27.8- ☑
  - steam X13.1- ☑
    - assault X98.Ø- ☑
    - stated as undetermined whether accidental or intentional Y27.Ø- ☑
    - suicide (attempt) X77.Ø- ☑
  - suicide (attempt) X77.9- ☑
  - vapor (hot) X13.1- ☑
    - assault X98.Ø- ☑
    - stated as undetermined whether accidental or intentional Y27.Ø- ☑
    - suicide (attempt) X77.Ø- ☑
- **Scratched by**
  - cat W55.Ø3- ☑
  - person(s) (accidentally) W5Ø.4- ☑
    - with intent to injure or kill YØ4.Ø- ☑
    - as, or caused by, a crowd or human stampede (with fall) W52.- ☑
    - assault YØ4.Ø- ☑
    - homicide (attempt) YØ4.Ø- ☑
    - in
      - fight YØ4.Ø- ☑
      - legal intervention
        - injuring
          - bystander Y35.892- ☑
          - law enforcement personnel Y35.891- ☑
          - suspect Y35.893- ☑
          - unspecified person Y35.899- ☑
- **Seasickness** T75.3- ☑
- **Self-harm NEC** — *see also* External cause by type, undetermined whether accidental or intentional
  - intentional — *see* Suicide
  - poisoning NEC — *see* Table of Drugs and Chemicals, poisoning, accidental
- **Self-inflicted** (injury) **NEC** — *see also* External cause by type, undetermined whether accidental or intentional
  - intentional — *see* Suicide
  - poisoning NEC — *see* Table of Drugs and Chemicals, poisoning, accidental
- **Sequelae** (of)
  - accident NEC — *see* WØØ-X58 with 7th character S
  - assault (homicidal) (any means) — *see* X92-YØ8 with 7th character S
- **Sequelae** — *continued*
  - homicide, attempt (any means) — *see* X92-YØ8 with 7th character S
  - injury undetermined whether accidentally or purposely inflicted — *see* Y21-Y33 with 7th character S
  - intentional self-harm (classifiable to X71-X83) — *see* X71-X83 with 7th character S
  - legal intervention — *see* with 7th character S Y35.- ☑
  - motor vehicle accident — *see* VØØ-V99 with 7th character S
  - suicide, attempt (any means) — *see* X71-X83 with 7th character S
  - transport accident — *see* VØØ-V99 with 7th character S
  - war operations — *see* War operations
- **Shock**
  - electric — *see* Exposure, electric current
  - from electric appliance (any) (faulty) W86.8- ☑
    - domestic W86.Ø- ☑
    - suicide (attempt) X83.1- ☑
- **Shooting, shot** (accidental(ly)) — *see also* Discharge, firearm, by type
  - herself or himself — *see* Discharge, firearm by type, self-inflicted
  - homicide (attempt) — *see* Discharge, firearm by type, homicide
  - in war operations — *see* War operations
  - inflicted by other person — *see* Discharge, firearm by type, homicide
    - accidental — *see* Discharge, firearm, by type of firearm
  - legal
    - execution — *see* Legal, intervention, firearm
    - intervention — *see* Legal, intervention, firearm
  - self-inflicted — *see* Discharge, firearm by type, suicide
    - accidental — *see* Discharge, firearm, by type of firearm
  - suicide (attempt) — *see* Discharge, firearm by type, suicide
- **Shoving** (accidentally) **by other person** — *see* Pushed, by other person
- **Sickness**
  - alpine W94.11- ☑
  - motion — *see* Motion
  - mountain W94.11- ☑
- **Sinking** (accidental)
  - watercraft (causing drowning, submersion) — *see also* Drowning, due to, accident to, watercraft, sinking
    - causing injury except drowning or submersion — *see* Accident, watercraft, causing, injury NEC
- **Siriasis** X32.- ☑
- **Sitting** (prolonged) (static) X5Ø.1- ☑
- **Slashed wrists** — *see* Cut, self-inflicted
- **Slipping** (accidental) (on same level) (with fall) WØ1.Ø- ☑
  - on
    - ice WØØ.Ø- ☑
      - with skates — *see* Accident, transport, pedestrian, conveyance
    - mud WØ1.Ø- ☑
    - oil WØ1.Ø- ☑
    - snow WØØ.Ø- ☑
      - with skis — *see* Accident, transport, pedestrian, conveyance
    - surface (slippery) (wet) NEC WØ1.Ø- ☑
  - without fall W18.4Ø- ☑
    - due to
      - specified NEC W18.49- ☑
      - stepping from one level to another W18.43- ☑
      - stepping into hole or opening W18.42- ☑
      - stepping on object W18.41- ☑
- **Sliver, wood, contact with** W45.8- ☑
- **Smoldering** (due to fire) — *see* Exposure, fire
- **Sodomy** (attempted) **by force** T74.2- ☑
- **Sound waves** (causing injury) W42.9- ☑
  - supersonic W42.Ø- ☑
- **Splinter, contact with** W45.8- ☑
- **Stab, stabbing** — *see* Cut
- **Standing** (prolonged) (static) X5Ø.1- ☑
- **Starvation** X58.- ☑
- **Status of external cause** Y99.9
  - child assisting in compensated work for family Y99.8
  - civilian activity done for financial or other compensation Y99.Ø
  - civilian activity done for income or pay Y99.Ø
  - family member assisting in compensated work for other family member Y99.8
  - hobby not done for income Y99.8
  - leisure activity Y99.8
  - military activity Y99.1
  - off-duty activity of military personnel Y99.8

- **Status of external cause** — *continued*
  - recreation or sport not for income or while a student Y99.8
  - specified NEC Y99.8
  - student activity Y99.8
  - volunteer activity Y99.2
- **Stepped on**
  - by
    - animal (not being ridden) NEC W55.89- ☑
    - crowd or human stampede W52.- ☑
    - person W50.0- ☑
- **Stepping on**
  - object W22.8- ☑
    - sports equipment W21.9- ☑
    - stationary W22.09- ☑
      - sports equipment W21.89- ☑
    - with fall W18.31- ☑
  - person W51.- ☑
    - by crowd or human stampede W52.- ☑
  - sports equipment W21.9- ☑
- **Sting**
  - arthropod, nonvenomous W57.- ☑
  - insect, nonvenomous W57.- ☑
- **Storm** (cataclysmic) — *see* Forces of nature, cataclysmic storm
- **Straining, excessive** — *see also* Overexertion X50.9- ☑
- **Strangling** — *see* Strangulation
- **Strangulation** (accidental) T71.- ☑
- **Strenuous movements** — *see also* Overexertion X50.9- ☑
- **Striking against**
  - airbag (automobile) W22.10- ☑
    - driver side W22.11- ☑
    - front passenger side W22.12- ☑
    - specified NEC W22.19- ☑
  - bottom when
    - diving or jumping into water (in) W16.822- ☑
      - causing drowning W16.821- ☑
      - from boat W16.722- ☑
        - causing drowning W16.721- ☑
      - natural body W16.622- ☑
        - causing drowning W16.821- ☑
      - swimming pool W16.522- ☑
        - causing drowning W16.521- ☑
    - falling into water (in) W16.322- ☑
      - causing drowning W16.321- ☑
      - fountain — *see* Striking against, bottom when, falling into water, specified NEC
      - natural body W16.122- ☑
        - causing drowning W16.121- ☑
      - reservoir — *see* Striking against, bottom when, falling into water, specified NEC
      - specified NEC W16.322- ☑
        - causing drowning W16.321- ☑
      - swimming pool W16.022- ☑
        - causing drowning W16.021- ☑
  - diving board (swimming-pool) W21.4- ☑
  - object W22.8- ☑
    - caused by crowd or human stampede (with fall) W52.- ☑
    - furniture W22.03- ☑
    - lamppost W22.02- ☑
    - sports equipment W21.9- ☑
    - stationary W22.09- ☑
      - sports equipment W21.89- ☑
    - wall W22.01- ☑
    - with
      - drowning or submersion — *see* Drowning
      - fall — *see* Fall, due to, bumping against, object
  - person(s) W51.- ☑
    - as, or caused by, a crowd or human stampede (with fall) W52.- ☑
    - assault Y04.2- ☑
    - homicide (attempt) Y04.2- ☑
    - with fall W03.- ☑
      - due to ice or snow W00.0- ☑
  - sports equipment W21.9- ☑
  - wall (when) W22.01- ☑
    - diving or jumping into water (in) W16.832- ☑
      - causing drowning W16.831- ☑
      - swimming pool W16.532- ☑
        - causing drowning W16.531- ☑
    - falling into water (in) W16.332- ☑
      - causing drowning W16.331- ☑
      - fountain — *see* Striking against, wall when, falling into water, specified NEC
      - natural body W16.132- ☑

- **Striking against** — *continued*
  - wall — *continued*
    - falling into water — *continued*
      - natural body — *continued*
        - causing drowning W16.131- ☑
      - reservoir — *see* Striking against, wall when, falling into water, specified NEC
      - specified NEC W16.332- ☑
        - causing drowning W16.331- ☑
      - swimming pool W16.032- ☑
        - causing drowning W16.031- ☑
    - swimming pool (when) W22.042- ☑
      - causing drowning W22.041- ☑
      - diving or jumping into water W16.532- ☑
        - causing drowning W16.531- ☑
      - falling into water W16.032- ☑
        - causing drowning W16.031- ☑
- **Struck** (accidentally) **by**
  - airbag (automobile) W22.10- ☑
    - driver side W22.11- ☑
    - front passenger side W22.12- ☑
    - specified NEC W22.19- ☑
  - alligator W58.02- ☑
  - animal (not being ridden) NEC W55.89- ☑
  - avalanche — *see* Landslide
  - ball (hit) (thrown) W21.00- ☑
    - assault Y08.09- ☑
    - baseball W21.03- ☑
    - basketball W21.05- ☑
    - football W21.01- ☑
    - golf ball W21.04- ☑
    - soccer W21.02- ☑
    - softball W21.07- ☑
    - specified NEC W21.09- ☑
    - volleyball W21.06- ☑
  - bat or racquet
    - baseball bat W21.11- ☑
      - assault Y08.02- ☑
    - golf club W21.13- ☑
      - assault Y08.09- ☑
    - specified NEC W21.19- ☑
      - assault Y08.09- ☑
    - tennis racquet W21.12- ☑
      - assault Y08.09- ☑
  - bullet — *see also* Discharge, firearm by type
    - in war operations — *see* War operations
  - crocodile W58.12- ☑
  - dog W54.1- ☑
  - flare, Very pistol — *see* Discharge, firearm NEC
  - hailstones X39.8- ☑
  - hockey (ice)
    - field
      - puck W21.221- ☑
      - stick W21.211- ☑
    - puck W21.220- ☑
    - stick W21.210- ☑
      - assault Y08.01- ☑
  - landslide — *see* Landslide
  - law-enforcement agent (on duty) — *see* Legal, intervention, manhandling
    - with blunt object — *see* Legal, intervention, blunt object
  - lightning T75.0- ☑
    - causing fire — *see* Exposure, fire
  - machine — *see* Contact, with, by type of machine
  - mammal NEC W55.89- ☑
    - marine W56.32- ☑
  - marine animal W56.82- ☑
  - missile
    - firearm — *see* Discharge, firearm by type
    - in war operations — *see* War operations, missile
  - object W22.8- ☑
    - blunt W22.8- ☑
      - assault Y00.- ☑
      - suicide (attempt) X79.- ☑
      - undetermined whether accidental or intentional Y29.- ☑
    - falling W20.8- ☑
      - from, in, on
        - building W20.1- ☑
          - burning (uncontrolled fire) X00.4- ☑
        - cataclysmic
          - earth surface movement NEC — *see* Landslide
          - storm — *see* Forces of nature, cataclysmic storm

- **Struck** (accidentally) **by** — *continued*
  - object — *continued*
    - falling — *continued*
      - from, in, on — *continued*
        - cave-in W20.0- ☑
        - earthquake X34.- ☑
        - machine (in operation) — *see* Contact, with, by type of machine
        - structure W20.1- ☑
          - burning X00.4- ☑
        - transport vehicle (in motion) — *see* Accident, transport, by type of vehicle
        - watercraft V93.49- ☑
          - due to
            - accident to craft V91.39- ☑
              - powered craft V91.33- ☑
                - ferry boat V91.31- ☑
                - fishing boat V91.32- ☑
                - jetskis V91.33- ☑
                - liner V91.31- ☑
                - merchant ship V91.30- ☑
                - passenger ship V91.31- ☑
              - unpowered craft V91.38- ☑
                - canoe V91.35- ☑
                - inflatable V91.36- ☑
                - kayak V91.35- ☑
                - sailboat V91.34- ☑
                - surf-board V91.38- ☑
                - windsurfer V91.38- ☑
          - powered craft V93.43- ☑
            - ferry boat V93.41- ☑
            - fishing boat V93.42- ☑
            - jetskis V93.43- ☑
            - liner V93.41- ☑
            - merchant ship V93.40- ☑
            - passenger ship V93.41- ☑
          - unpowered craft V93.48- ☑
            - sailboat V93.44- ☑
            - surf-board V93.48- ☑
            - windsurfer V93.48- ☑
    - moving NEC W20.8- ☑
    - projected W20.8- ☑
      - assault Y00.- ☑
      - in sports W21.9- ☑
        - assault Y08.09- ☑
        - ball W21.00- ☑
          - baseball W21.03- ☑
          - basketball W21.05- ☑
          - football W21.01- ☑
          - golf ball W21.04- ☑
          - soccer W21.02- ☑
          - softball W21.07- ☑
          - specified NEC W21.09- ☑
          - volleyball W21.06- ☑
        - bat or racquet
          - baseball bat W21.11- ☑
            - assault Y08.02- ☑
          - golf club W21.13- ☑
            - assault Y08.09- ☑
          - specified NEC W21.19- ☑
            - assault Y08.09- ☑
          - tennis racquet W21.12- ☑
            - assault Y08.09- ☑
        - hockey (ice)
          - field
            - puck W21.221- ☑
            - stick W21.211- ☑
          - puck W21.220- ☑
          - stick W21.210- ☑
            - assault Y08.01- ☑
        - specified NEC W21.89- ☑
    - set in motion by explosion — *see* Explosion
    - thrown W20.8- ☑
      - assault Y00.- ☑
      - in sports W21.9- ☑
        - assault Y08.09- ☑
        - ball W21.00- ☑
          - baseball W21.03- ☑
          - basketball W21.05- ☑
          - football W21.01- ☑
          - golf ball W21.04- ☑
          - soccer W21.02- ☑
          - soft ball W21.07- ☑
          - specified NEC W21.09- ☑
          - volleyball W21.06- ☑

- **Struck** (accidentally) **by** — *continued*
  - object — *continued*
    - thrown — *continued*
      - in sports — *continued*
        - bat or racquet
          - baseball bat W21.11- ☑
            - assault YØ8.Ø2- ☑
          - golf club W21.13- ☑
            - assault YØ8.Ø9- ☑
          - specified NEC W21.19- ☑
            - assault YØ8.Ø9- ☑
          - tennis racquet W21.12- ☑
            - assault YØ8.Ø9- ☑
        - hockey (ice)
          - field
            - puck W21.221- ☑
            - stick W21.211- ☑
          - puck W21.22Ø- ☑
          - stick W21.21Ø- ☑
            - assault YØ8.Ø1- ☑
        - specified NEC W21.89- ☑
  - other person(s) W5Ø.Ø- ☑
    - with
      - blunt object W22.8- ☑
        - intentional, homicide (attempt) YØØ.- ☑
        - sports equipment W21.9- ☑
        - undetermined whether accidental or intentional Y29.- ☑
      - fall WØ3.- ☑
        - due to ice or snow WØØ.Ø- ☑
    - as, or caused by, a crowd or human stampede (with fall) W52.- ☑
    - assault YØ4.2- ☑
    - homicide (attempt) YØ4.2- ☑
    - in legal intervention
      - injuring
        - bystander Y35.812- ☑
        - law enforcement personnel Y35.811- ☑
        - suspect Y35.813- ☑
        - unspecified person Y35.819- ☑
    - sports equipment W21.9- ☑
  - police (on duty) — *see* Legal, intervention, manhandling
    - with blunt object — *see* Legal, intervention, blunt object
  - sports equipment W21.9- ☑
    - assault YØ8.Ø9- ☑
    - ball W21.ØØ- ☑
      - baseball W21.Ø3- ☑
      - basketball W21.Ø5- ☑
      - football W21.Ø1- ☑
      - golf ball W21.Ø4- ☑
      - soccer W21.Ø2- ☑
      - soft ball W21.Ø7- ☑
      - specified NEC W21.Ø9- ☑
      - volleyball W21.Ø6- ☑
    - bat or racquet
      - baseball bat W21.11- ☑
        - assault YØ8.Ø2- ☑
      - golf club W21.13- ☑
        - assault YØ8.Ø9- ☑
      - specified NEC W21.19- ☑
      - tennis racquet W21.12- ☑
        - assault YØ8.Ø9- ☑
    - cleats (shoe) W21.31- ☑
    - foot wear NEC W21.39- ☑
    - football helmet W21.81- ☑
    - hockey (ice)
      - field
        - puck W21.221- ☑
        - stick W21.211- ☑
      - puck W21.22Ø- ☑
      - stick W21.21Ø- ☑
        - assault YØ8.Ø1- ☑
    - skate blades W21.32- ☑
    - specified NEC W21.89- ☑
      - assault YØ8.Ø9- ☑
  - thunderbolt — *see* subcategory T75.Ø- ☑
    - causing fire — *see* Exposure, fire
  - transport vehicle NEC — *see also* Accident, transport VØ9.9- ☑
    - intentional, homicide (attempt) YØ3.Ø- ☑
    - motor NEC — *see also* Accident, transport VØ9.2Ø- ☑
      - homicide YØ3.Ø- ☑
  - vehicle (transport) NEC — *see* Accident, transport, by type of vehicle

- **Struck** (accidentally) **by** — *continued*
  - vehicle — *see* Accident, transport, by type of vehicle — *continued*
    - stationary (falling from jack, hydraulic lift, ramp) W2Ø.8- ☑
- **Stumbling**
  - over
    - animal NEC WØ1.Ø- ☑
      - with fall W18.Ø9- ☑
    - carpet, rug or (small) object W22.8- ☑
      - with fall W18.Ø9- ☑
    - person W51.- ☑
      - with fall WØ3.- ☑
        - due to ice or snow WØØ.Ø- ☑
  - without fall W18.4Ø- ☑
    - due to
      - specified NEC W18.49- ☑
      - stepping from one level to another W18.43- ☑
      - stepping into hole or opening W18.42- ☑
      - stepping on object W18.41- ☑
- **Submersion** (accidental) — *see* Drowning
- **Suffocation** (accidental) (by external means) (by pressure) (mechanical) — *see also* category T71.- ☑
  - due to, by
    - avalanche — *see* Landslide
    - explosion — *see* Explosion
    - fire — *see* Exposure, fire
    - food, any type (aspiration) (ingestion) (inhalation) T17.92- ☑
    - ignition — *see* Ignition
    - landslide — *see* Landslide
    - machine(ry) — *see* Contact, with, by type of machine
    - vomitus (aspiration) (inhalation) T17.81- ☑
  - in
    - burning building XØØ.8- ☑
- **Suicide, suicidal** (attempted) (by) X83.8- ☑
  - blunt object X79.- ☑
  - burning, burns X76.- ☑
    - hot object X77.9- ☑
      - fluid NEC X77.2- ☑
      - household appliance X77.3- ☑
      - specified NEC X77.8- ☑
      - steam X77.Ø- ☑
      - tap water X77.1- ☑
      - vapors X77.Ø- ☑
  - caustic substance — *see* Table of Drugs and Chemicals
  - cold, extreme X83.2- ☑
  - collision of motor vehicle with
    - motor vehicle X82.Ø- ☑
    - specified NEC X82.8- ☑
    - train X82.1- ☑
    - tree X82.2- ☑
  - crashing of aircraft X83.Ø- ☑
  - cut (any part of body) X78.9- ☑
  - cutting or piercing instrument X78.9- ☑
    - dagger X78.2- ☑
    - glass X78.Ø- ☑
    - knife X78.1- ☑
    - specified NEC X78.8- ☑
    - sword X78.2- ☑
  - drowning (in) X71.9- ☑
    - bathtub X71.Ø- ☑
    - natural water X71.3- ☑
    - specified NEC X71.8- ☑
    - swimming pool X71.1- ☑
      - following fall X71.2- ☑
  - electrocution X83.1- ☑
  - explosive(s) (material) X75.- ☑
  - fire, flames X76.- ☑
  - firearm X74.9- ☑
    - airgun X74.Ø1- ☑
    - handgun X72.- ☑
    - hunting rifle X73.1- ☑
    - larger X73.9- ☑
      - specified NEC X73.8- ☑
    - machine gun X73.2- ☑
    - shotgun X73.Ø- ☑
    - specified NEC X74.8- ☑
  - hanging X83.8- ☑
  - hot object — *see* Suicide, burning, hot object
  - jumping
    - before moving object X81.8- ☑
      - motor vehicle X81.Ø- ☑
      - subway train X81.1- ☑
      - train X81.1- ☑
    - from high place X8Ø.- ☑

- **Suicide, suicidal** — *continued*
  - late effect of attempt — *see* X71-X83 with 7th character S
  - lying before moving object, train, vehicle X81.8- ☑
  - poisoning — *see* Table of Drugs and Chemicals
  - puncture (any part of body) — *see* Suicide, cutting or piercing instrument
  - scald — *see* Suicide, burning, hot object
  - sequelae of attempt — *see* X71-X83 with 7th character S
  - sharp object (any) — *see* Suicide, cutting or piercing instrument
  - shooting — *see* Suicide, firearm
  - specified means NEC X83.8- ☑
  - stab (any part of body) — *see* Suicide, cutting or piercing instrument
  - steam, hot vapors X77.Ø- ☑
  - strangulation X83.8- ☑
  - submersion — *see* Suicide, drowning
  - suffocation X83.8- ☑
  - wound NEC X83.8- ☑
- **Sunstroke** X32.- ☑
- **Supersonic waves** (causing injury) W42.Ø- ☑
- **Surgical procedure, complication of** (delayed or as an abnormal reaction without mention of misadventure) — *see also* Complication of or following, by type of procedure
  - due to or as a result of misadventure — *see* Misadventure
- **Swallowed, swallowing**
  - foreign body — *see* Foreign body, alimentary canal
  - poison — *see* Table of Drugs and Chemicals
  - substance
    - caustic or corrosive — *see* Table of Drugs and Chemicals
    - poisonous — *see* Table of Drugs and Chemicals

# T

- **Tackle in sport** WØ3.- ☑
- **Terrorism** (involving) Y38.8Ø- ☑
  - biological weapons Y38.6X- ☑
  - chemical weapons Y38.7X- ☑
  - conflagration Y38.3X- ☑
  - drowning and submersion Y38.89- ☑
  - explosion Y38.2X- ☑
    - destruction of aircraft Y38.1X- ☑
    - marine weapons Y38.ØX- ☑
  - fire Y38.3X- ☑
  - firearms Y38.4X- ☑
  - hot substances Y38.3X- ☑
  - lasers Y38.89- ☑
  - nuclear weapons Y38.5X- ☑
  - piercing or stabbing instruments Y38.89- ☑
  - secondary effects Y38.9X- ☑
  - specified method NEC Y38.89- ☑
  - suicide bomber Y38.81- ☑
- **Thirst** X58.- ☑
- **Threat to breathing**
  - aspiration — *see* Aspiration
  - due to cave-in, falling earth or substance NEC T71.- ☑
- **Thrown** (accidentally)
  - against part (any) of or object in transport vehicle (in motion) NEC — *see also* Accident, transport
  - from
    - high place, homicide (attempt) YØ1.- ☑
    - machinery — *see* Contact, with, by type of machine
    - transport vehicle NEC — *see also* Accident, transport V89.9- ☑
  - off — *see* Thrown, from
- **Thunderbolt** — *see* subcategory T75.Ø- ☑
  - causing fire — *see* Exposure, fire
- **Tidal wave** (any injury) **NEC** — *see* Forces of nature, tidal wave
- **Took**
  - overdose (drug) — *see* Table of Drugs and Chemicals
  - poison — *see* Table of Drugs and Chemicals
- **Tornado** (any injury) X37.1- ☑
- **Torrential rain** (any injury) X37.8- ☑
- **Torture** X58.- ☑
- **Trampled by animal NEC** W55.89- ☑
- **Trapped** (accidentally)
  - between objects (moving) (stationary and moving) — *see* Caught
  - by part (any) of
    - electric (assisted) bicycle V29.881- ☑
    - motorcycle V29.888- ☑
    - pedal cycle V19.88- ☑

- **Trapped** — *continued*
  - by part of — *continued*
    - transport vehicle NEC — *see also* Accident, transport V89.9- ☑
- **Travel** (effects) (sickness) T75.3- ☑
- **Tree falling on or hitting** (accidentally) (person) W2Ø.8- ☑
- **Tripping**
  - over
    - animal WØ1.Ø- ☑
      - with fall WØ1.Ø- ☑
    - carpet, rug or (small) object W22.8- ☑
      - with fall W18.Ø9- ☑
    - person W51.- ☑
      - with fall WØ3.- ☑
        - due to ice or snow WØØ.Ø- ☑
  - without fall W18.4Ø- ☑
    - due to
      - specified NEC W18.49- ☑
      - stepping from one level to another W18.43- ☑
      - stepping into hole or opening W18.42- ☑
      - stepping on object W18.41- ☑
- **Twisted by person**(s) (accidentally) W5Ø.2- ☑
  - with intent to injure or kill YØ4.Ø- ☑
  - as, or caused by, a crowd or human stampede (with fall) W52.- ☑
  - assault YØ4.Ø- ☑
  - homicide (attempt) YØ4.Ø- ☑
  - in
    - fight YØ4.Ø- ☑
    - legal intervention — *see* Legal, intervention, manhandling
- **Twisting** (prolonged) (static) X5Ø.1- ☑

# U

- **Underdosing of necessary drugs, medicaments or biological substances** Y63.6
- **Undetermined intent** (contact) (exposure)
  - automobile collision Y32.- ☑
  - blunt object Y29.- ☑
  - drowning (submersion) (in) Y21.9- ☑
    - bathtub Y21.Ø- ☑
      - after fall Y21.1- ☑
    - natural water (lake) (ocean) (pond) (river) (stream) Y21.4- ☑
    - specified place NEC Y21.8- ☑
    - swimming pool Y21.2- ☑
      - after fall Y21.3- ☑
  - explosive material Y25.- ☑
  - fall, jump or push from high place Y3Ø.- ☑
  - falling, lying or running before moving object Y31.- ☑
  - fire Y26.- ☑
  - firearm discharge Y24.9- ☑
    - airgun (BB) (pellet) Y24.Ø- ☑
    - handgun (pistol) (revolver) Y22.- ☑
    - hunting rifle Y23.1- ☑
    - larger Y23.9- ☑
      - hunting rifle Y23.1- ☑
      - machine gun Y23.3- ☑
      - military Y23.2- ☑
      - shotgun Y23.Ø- ☑
      - specified type NEC Y23.8- ☑
    - machine gun Y23.3- ☑
    - military Y23.2- ☑
    - shotgun Y23.Ø- ☑
    - specified type NEC Y24.8- ☑
    - Very pistol Y24.8- ☑
  - hot object Y27.9- ☑
    - fluid NEC Y27.2- ☑
    - household appliance Y27.3- ☑
    - specified object NEC Y27.8- ☑
    - steam Y27.Ø- ☑
    - tap water Y27.1- ☑
    - vapor Y27.Ø- ☑
  - jump, fall or push from high place Y3Ø.- ☑
  - lying, falling or running before moving object Y31.- ☑
  - motor vehicle crash Y32.- ☑
  - push, fall or jump from high place Y3Ø.- ☑
  - running, falling or lying before moving object Y31.- ☑
  - sharp object Y28.9- ☑
    - dagger Y28.2- ☑
    - glass Y28.Ø- ☑
    - knife Y28.1- ☑
    - specified object NEC Y28.8- ☑
    - sword Y28.2- ☑
- **Undetermined intent** — *continued*
  - smoke Y26.- ☑
  - specified event NEC Y33.- ☑
- **Use of hand as hammer** X5Ø.3- ☑

# V

- **Vibration** (causing injury) W49.9- ☑
- **Victim** (of)
  - avalanche — *see* Landslide
  - earth movements NEC — *see* Forces of nature, earth movement
  - earthquake X34.- ☑
  - flood — *see* Flood
  - landslide — *see* Landslide
  - lightning — *see* subcategory T75.Ø- ☑
    - causing fire — *see* Exposure, fire
  - storm (cataclysmic) NEC — *see* Forces of nature, cataclysmic storm
  - volcanic eruption X35.- ☑
- **Volcanic eruption** (any injury) X35.- ☑
- **Vomitus, gastric contents in air passages** (with asphyxia, obstruction or suffocation) T17.81- ☑

# W

- **Walked into stationary object** (any) W22.Ø9- ☑
  - furniture W22.Ø3- ☑
  - lamppost W22.Ø2- ☑
  - wall W22.Ø1- ☑
- **War operations** (injuries to military personnel and civilians during war, civil insurrection and peacekeeping missions) (by) (from) (involving) Y36.9Ø- ☑
  - after cessation of hostilities Y36.89- ☑
    - explosion (of)
      - bomb placed during war operations Y36.82- ☑
      - mine placed during war operations Y36.81- ☑
    - specified NEC Y36.88- ☑
  - air blast Y36.2Ø- ☑
  - aircraft
    - destruction — *see* War operations, destruction of aircraft
  - airway restriction — *see* War operations, restriction of airways
  - asphyxiation — *see* War operations, restriction of airways
  - biological weapons Y36.6X- ☑
  - blast Y36.2Ø- ☑
  - blast fragments Y36.2Ø- ☑
  - blast overpressure
    - high level (due to explosion) Y36.A2- ☑
    - low level (due to explosion) Y36.A1- ☑
  - blast wave Y36.2Ø- ☑
  - blast wind Y36.2Ø- ☑
  - bomb Y36.2Ø- ☑
    - dirty Y36.5Ø- ☑
    - gasoline Y36.31- ☑
    - incendiary Y36.31- ☑
    - petrol Y36.31- ☑
  - bullet Y36.43- ☑
    - incendiary Y36.32- ☑
    - rubber Y36.41- ☑
  - chemical weapons Y36.7X- ☑
  - combat
    - hand to hand (unarmed) combat Y36.44- ☑
    - using blunt or piercing object Y36.45- ☑
  - conflagration — *see* War operations, fire
  - conventional warfare NEC Y36.49- ☑
  - depth-charge Y36.Ø1- ☑
  - destruction of aircraft Y36.1Ø- ☑
    - due to
      - air to air missile Y36.11- ☑
      - collision with other aircraft Y36.12- ☑
      - detonation (accidental) of onboard munitions and explosives Y36.14- ☑
      - enemy fire or explosives Y36.11- ☑
      - explosive placed on aircraft Y36.11- ☑
      - onboard fire Y36.13- ☑
      - rocket propelled grenade [RPG] Y36.11- ☑
      - small arms fire Y36.11- ☑
      - surface to air missile Y36.11- ☑
    - specified NEC Y36.19- ☑
  - detonation (accidental) of
    - onboard marine weapons Y36.Ø5- ☑
    - own munitions or munitions launch device Y36.24- ☑
  - dirty bomb Y36.5Ø- ☑
  - explosion (of) Y36.2Ø- ☑
- **War operations** — *continued*
  - explosion — *continued*
    - aerial bomb Y36.21- ☑
    - after cessation of hostilities
      - bomb placed during war operations Y36.82- ☑
      - mine placed during war operations Y36.81- ☑
    - bomb NOS — *see also* War operations, bomb(s) Y36.2Ø- ☑
    - fragments Y36.2Ø- ☑
    - grenade Y36.29- ☑
    - guided missile Y36.22- ☑
    - improvised explosive device [IED] (person-borne) (roadside) (vehicle-borne) Y36.23- ☑
    - land mine Y36.29- ☑
    - marine mine (at sea) (in harbor) Y36.Ø2- ☑
    - marine weapon Y36.ØØ- ☑
      - specified NEC Y36.Ø9- ☑
    - own munitions or munitions launch device (accidental) Y36.24- ☑
    - sea-based artillery shell Y36.Ø3- ☑
    - specified NEC Y36.29- ☑
    - torpedo Y36.Ø4- ☑
  - fire Y36.3Ø- ☑
    - specified NEC Y36.39- ☑
  - firearms
    - discharge Y36.43- ☑
    - pellets Y36.42- ☑
  - flamethrower Y36.33- ☑
  - fragments (from) (of)
    - improvised explosive device [IED] (person-borne) (roadside) (vehicle-borne) Y36.26- ☑
    - munitions Y36.25- ☑
    - specified NEC Y36.29- ☑
    - weapons Y36.27- ☑
  - friendly fire Y36.92- ☑
  - hand to hand (unarmed) combat Y36.44- ☑
  - HLB overpressure Y36.A2- ☑
  - hot substances — *see* War operations, fire
  - incendiary bullet Y36.32- ☑
  - LLB overpressure Y36.A1- ☑
  - nuclear weapon (effects of) Y36.5Ø- ☑
    - acute radiation exposure Y36.54- ☑
    - blast pressure Y36.51- ☑
    - direct blast Y36.51- ☑
    - direct heat Y36.53- ☑
    - fallout exposure Y36.54- ☑
    - fireball Y36.53- ☑
    - indirect blast (struck or crushed by blast debris) (being thrown by blast) Y36.52- ☑
    - ionizing radiation (immediate exposure) Y36.54- ☑
    - nuclear radiation Y36.54- ☑
    - radiation
      - ionizing (immediate exposure) Y36.54- ☑
      - nuclear Y36.54- ☑
      - thermal Y36.53- ☑
    - secondary effects Y36.54- ☑
    - specified NEC Y36.59- ☑
    - thermal radiation Y36.53- ☑
  - restriction of air (airway)
    - intentional Y36.46- ☑
    - unintentional Y36.47- ☑
  - rubber bullets Y36.41- ☑
  - shrapnel NOS Y36.29- ☑
  - suffocation — *see* War operations, restriction of airways
  - unconventional warfare NEC Y36.7X- ☑
  - underwater blast NOS Y36.ØØ- ☑
  - warfare
    - conventional NEC Y36.49- ☑
    - unconventional NEC Y36.7X- ☑
  - weapon of mass destruction [WMD] Y36.91- ☑
  - weapons
    - biological weapons Y36.6X- ☑
    - chemical Y36.7X- ☑
    - nuclear (effects of) Y36.5Ø- ☑
      - acute radiation exposure Y36.54- ☑
      - blast pressure Y36.51- ☑
      - direct blast Y36.51- ☑
      - direct heat Y36.53- ☑
      - fallout exposure Y36.54- ☑
      - fireball Y36.53- ☑
      - radiation
        - ionizing (immediate exposure) Y36.54- ☑
        - nuclear Y36.54- ☑
        - thermal Y36.53- ☑
      - secondary effects Y36.54- ☑

# ICD-10-CM Tabular List of Diseases and Injuries



## Chapter 1. Certain Infectious and Parasitic Diseases (AØØ–B99), UØ7.1, UØ9.9

### Chapter-specific Guidelines with Coding Examples

The chapter-specific guidelines from the ICD-10-CM Official Guidelines for Coding and Reporting have been provided below. Along with these guidelines are coding examples, contained in the shaded boxes, that have been developed to help illustrate the coding and/or sequencing guidance found in these guidelines.

**a. Human immunodeficiency virus (HIV) infections**

**1) Code only confirmed cases**

Code only confirmed cases of HIV infection/illness. This is an exception to the hospital inpatient guideline Section II, H.

In this context, "confirmation" does not require documentation of positive serology or culture for HIV; the provider's diagnostic statement that the patient is HIV positive or has an HIV-related illness is sufficient.

Patient being seen for hypothyroidism with possible HIV infection

**EØ3.9 Hypothyroidism, unspecified**

*Explanation:* Only the hypothyroidism is coded in this scenario because it has not been confirmed that an HIV infection is present.

**2) Selection and sequencing of HIV codes**

**(a) HIV disease**

If the term "AIDS" or "HIV disease" is documented or if the patient is treated for any HIV-related illness or is described as having any condition(s) resulting from the patient's HIV positive status; code B2Ø, Human immunodeficiency virus [HIV] disease, should be assigned.

**(b) Patient admitted for HIV-related condition**

If a patient is admitted for an HIV-related condition, the principal diagnosis should be B2Ø, Human immunodeficiency virus [HIV] disease followed by additional diagnosis codes for all reported HIV-related conditions.

An exception to this guideline is if the reason for admission is hemolytic-uremic syndrome associated with HIV disease. Assign code D59.31, Infection-associated hemolytic-uremic syndrome, followed by code B2Ø, Human immunodeficiency virus [HIV] disease.

HIV with CMV

**B2Ø Human immunodeficiency virus [HIV] disease**

**B25.9 Cytomegaloviral disease, unspecified**

*Explanation:* Cytomegaloviral infection is an HIV related condition, so the HIV diagnosis code is reported first, followed by the code for the CMV.

**(c) Patient with HIV disease admitted for unrelated condition**

If a patient with HIV disease is admitted for an unrelated condition (such as a traumatic injury), the code for the unrelated condition (e.g., the nature of injury code) should be the principal diagnosis. Code B2Ø would be reported as a secondary diagnosis. Codes for other documented conditions should also be reported as secondary diagnoses.

Sprain of the internal collateral ligament, right ankle; HIV

**S93.491A Sprain of other ligament of right ankle, initial encounter**

**B2Ø Human immunodeficiency virus [HIV] disease**

*Explanation:* The ankle sprain is not related to HIV, so it is the first-listed diagnosis code, and HIV is reported secondarily.

**(d) Patient newly diagnosed with HIV disease**

Whether the patient is newly diagnosed or has had previous admissions/encounters for HIV conditions is irrelevant to the sequencing decision.

Newly diagnosed multiple cutaneous Kaposi's sarcoma lesions in previously diagnosed HIV disease

**B2Ø Human immunodeficiency virus [HIV] disease**

**C46.Ø Kaposi's sarcoma of skin**

*Explanation:* Even though the HIV was diagnosed on a previous encounter, it is still sequenced first when coded with an HIV-related condition. Kaposi's sarcoma is an HIV-related condition.

**(e) Asymptomatic human immunodeficiency virus**

When "HIV positive," "HIV test positive," or similar terminology is documented, and there is no documentation of symptoms or HIV-related illness, code Z21, Asymptomatic human immunodeficiency virus [HIV] infection status, should be assigned.

**(f) Inconclusive HIV serology**

Patients with documentation of inconclusive HIV serology, may be assigned code R75, Inconclusive laboratory evidence of human immunodeficiency virus [HIV].

**(g) Previously diagnosed HIV-related illness**

Patients with documentation of a prior diagnosis of an HIV-related illness should be coded to B2Ø. Once an HIV-related illness has developed, code B2Ø should always be assigned on every subsequent admission/encounter. Patients previously diagnosed with any HIV illness (B2Ø) should never be assigned to R75, Inconclusive laboratory evidence of human immunodeficiency virus [HIV] or Z21, Asymptomatic human immunodeficiency virus [HIV] infection status.

**(h) HIV Infection in pregnancy, childbirth and the puerperium**

When a patient presents during pregnancy, childbirth or the puerperium with documented symptomatic HIV disease or an HIV related illness, assign a code from subcategory O98.7, Human immunodeficiency [HIV] disease complicating pregnancy, childbirth and the puerperium, followed by code B2Ø and additional code(s) for any HIV-related illness(es). Codes from Chapter 15 always take sequencing priority.

When a patient presents during pregnancy, childbirth or the puerperium with documented asymptomatic HIV infection status or is HIV-positive, assign a code from subcategory O98.7 followed by code Z21.

**(i) Encounters for HIV testing**

If a patient without signs or symptoms is tested for HIV, assign code Z11.4, Encounter for screening for human immunodeficiency virus [HIV]. Use additional codes for any associated high-risk behavior, if applicable.

If a patient with signs or symptoms of HIV presents for HIV testing, code the signs and symptoms. An additional counseling code Z71.7, Human immunodeficiency virus [HIV] counseling, may be assigned if counseling is provided during the encounter for the test. Code Z11.4, Encounter for screening for human immunodeficiency virus [HIV], should not be assigned if HIV signs or symptoms are present.

When a patient presents for follow up regarding their HIV test results and the test result is negative, assign code Z71.7, Human immunodeficiency virus [HIV] counseling.

If the results are positive, see previous guidelines and assign codes as appropriate.

**(j) HIV disease or HIV positive status managed by antiretroviral medication**

If a patient with documented HIV disease, HIV-related illness or AIDS is currently managed on antiretroviral medications, assign code B2Ø, Human immunodeficiency virus [HIV] disease.

If a patient with documented HIV positive status is currently managed on antiretroviral medication, assign code Z21, Asymptomatic human immunodeficiency virus [HIV] infection status, in the absence of any additional documentation of HIV disease, HIV-related illness or AIDS.

Code Z79.899, Other long term (current) drug therapy, may be assigned as an additional code to identify the long-term (current) use of antiretroviral medications.

**(k) Encounter for HIV prophylaxis measures**

When a patient is seen for administration of pre-exposure prophylaxis medication for HIV, assign code Z29.81, Encounter for HIV pre-exposure prophylaxis. Pre-exposure prophylaxis (PrEP) is intended to prevent infection in people who are at risk for getting HIV through sex or injection drug use. Any risk factors for HIV should also be coded.

**b. Infectious agents as the cause of diseases classified to other chapters**

Certain infections are classified in chapters other than Chapter 1 and no organism is identified as part of the infection code. In these instances, it is necessary to use an additional code from Chapter 1 to identify the organism. A code from category B95, Streptococcus, Staphylococcus, and Enterococcus as the cause of diseases classified to other chapters, B96, Other bacterial agents as the cause of diseases classified to other chapters, or B97, Viral agents as the cause of diseases classified to other chapters, is to be used as an additional code to identify the organism. An instructional note will be found at the infection code advising that an additional organism code is required.

Acute *E. coli* cystitis

| | |
|---|---|
| **N30.00** | **Acute cystitis without hematuria** |
| **B96.20** | **Unspecified Escherichia coli [E.coli] as the cause of diseases classified elsewhere** |

*Explanation:* An instructional note under the category for the cystitis indicates to code also the specific organism.

**c. Infections resistant to antibiotics**

Many bacterial infections are resistant to current antibiotics. It is necessary to identify all infections documented as antibiotic resistant. Assign a code from category Z16, Resistance to antimicrobial drugs, following the infection code only if the infection code does not identify drug resistance.

Penicillin-resistant *Streptococcus pneumoniae* pneumonia

| | |
|---|---|
| **J13** | **Pneumonia due to Streptococcus pneumoniae** |
| **Z16.11** | **Resistance to penicillins** |

*Explanation:* Code Z16.11 is assigned as a secondary code to represent the penicillin resistance. This code includes resistance to amoxicillin and ampicillin.

**d. Sepsis, severe sepsis, and septic shock infections**

**1) Coding of Sepsis and Severe Sepsis**

**(a) Sepsis**

For a diagnosis of sepsis, assign the appropriate code for the underlying systemic infection. If the type of infection or causal organism is not further specified, assign code A41.9, Sepsis, unspecified organism.

A code from subcategory R65.2, Severe sepsis, should not be assigned unless severe sepsis or an associated acute organ dysfunction is documented.

Gram-negative sepsis

| | |
|---|---|
| **A41.50** | **Gram-negative sepsis, unspecified** |

Staphylococcal sepsis

| | |
|---|---|
| **A41.2** | **Sepsis due to unspecified staphylococcus** |

*Explanation:* In both examples above the organism causing the sepsis is identified, therefore A41.9 Sepsis, unspecified organism, would not be appropriate as this code would not capture the highest degree of specificity found in the documentation. Do not use an additional code for severe sepsis unless an acute organ dysfunction was also documented as "associated with" or "due to" the sepsis or the sepsis was documented as "severe."

**(i) Negative or inconclusive blood cultures and sepsis**

Negative or inconclusive blood cultures do not preclude a diagnosis of sepsis in patients with clinical evidence of the condition; however, the provider should be queried.

**(ii) Urosepsis**

The term urosepsis is a nonspecific term. It is not to be considered synonymous with sepsis. It has no default code in the Alphabetic Index. Should a provider use this term, he/she must be queried for clarification.

**(iii)Sepsis with organ dysfunction**

If a patient has sepsis and associated acute organ dysfunction or multiple organ dysfunction (MOD), follow the instructions for coding severe sepsis.

**(iv) Acute organ dysfunction that is not clearly associated with the sepsis**

If a patient has sepsis and an acute organ dysfunction, but the medical record documentation indicates that the acute organ dysfunction is related to a medical condition other than the sepsis, do not assign a code from subcategory R65.2, Severe sepsis. An acute organ dysfunction must be associated with the sepsis in order to assign the severe sepsis code. If the documentation is not clear as to whether an acute organ dysfunction is related to the sepsis or another medical condition, query the provider.

Sepsis and acute respiratory failure due to COPD exacerbation

| | |
|---|---|
| **A41.9** | **Sepsis, unspecified organism** |
| **J44.1** | **Chronic obstructive pulmonary disease with (acute) exacerbation** |
| **J96.00** | **Acute respiratory failure, unspecified whether with hypoxia or hypercapnia** |

*Explanation:* Although acute organ dysfunction is present in the form of acute respiratory failure, severe sepsis (R65.2) is not coded in this example, as the acute respiratory failure is attributed to the COPD exacerbation rather than the sepsis. Sequencing of these codes would be determined by the reason for the encounter.

**(b) Severe sepsis**

The coding of severe sepsis requires a minimum of 2 codes: first a code for the underlying systemic infection, followed by a code from subcategory R65.2, Severe sepsis. If the causal organism is not documented, assign code A41.9, Sepsis, unspecified organism, for the infection. Additional code(s) for the associated acute organ dysfunction are also required.

Due to the complex nature of severe sepsis, some cases may require querying the provider prior to assignment of the codes.

**2) Septic shock**

Septic shock generally refers to circulatory failure associated with severe sepsis, and therefore, it represents a type of acute organ dysfunction.

For cases of septic shock, the code for the systemic infection should be sequenced first, followed by code R65.21, Severe sepsis with septic shock or code T81.12, Postprocedural septic shock. Any additional codes for the other acute organ dysfunctions should also be assigned. As noted in the sequencing instructions in the Tabular List, the code for septic shock cannot be assigned as a principal diagnosis.

Sepsis with septic shock

| | |
|---|---|
| **A41.9** | **Sepsis, unspecified organism** |
| **R65.21** | **Severe sepsis with septic shock** |

*Explanation*: Documentation of septic shock automatically implies severe sepsis as it is a form of acute organ dysfunction. Septic shock is not coded as the first-listed diagnosis; it is always preceded by the code for the systemic infection.

**3) Sequencing of severe sepsis**

If severe sepsis is present on admission, and meets the definition of principal diagnosis, the underlying systemic infection should be assigned as principal diagnosis followed by the appropriate code from subcategory R65.2 as required by the sequencing rules in the Tabular List. A code from subcategory R65.2 can never be assigned as a principal diagnosis.

When severe sepsis develops during an encounter (it was not present on admission), the underlying systemic infection and the appropriate code from subcategory R65.2 should be assigned as secondary diagnoses.

Severe sepsis may be present on admission, but the diagnosis may not be confirmed until sometime after admission. If the documentation is not clear whether severe sepsis was present on admission, the provider should be queried.

*For infection-associated hemolytic-uremic syndrome with severe sepsis, see guideline I.C.1.d.9.*

**4) Sepsis or severe sepsis with a localized infection**

If the reason for admission is sepsis or severe sepsis and a localized infection, such as pneumonia or cellulitis, a code(s) for the underlying systemic infection should be assigned first and the code for the localized infection should be assigned as a secondary diagnosis. If the patient has severe sepsis, a code from subcategory R65.2 should also be assigned as a secondary diagnosis. If the patient is admitted with a localized infection, such as pneumonia, and sepsis/severe sepsis doesn't develop until after admission, the localized infection should be assigned first, followed by the appropriate sepsis/severe sepsis codes.

*For hemolytic-uremic syndrome associated with sepsis, see guideline I.C.1.d.9.*

Patient presents with acute renal failure due to severe sepsis from *Pseudomonas pneumonia*

| | |
|---|---|
| **A41.52** | **Sepsis due to Pseudomonas** |
| **J15.1** | **Pneumonia due to Pseudomonas** |
| **R65.20** | **Severe sepsis without septic shock** |
| **N17.9** | **Acute kidney failure, unspecified** |

*Explanation:* If all conditions are present, the systemic infection (sepsis) is sequenced first followed by the codes for the localized infection (pneumonia), severe sepsis and any organ dysfunction.

**5) Sepsis due to a postprocedural infection**

**(a) Documentation of causal relationship**

As with all postprocedural complications, code assignment is based on the provider's documentation of the relationship between the infection and the procedure.

**(b) Sepsis due to a postprocedural infection**

For sepsis following a postprocedural wound (surgical site) infection, a code from T81.41 to T81.43, Infection following a procedure, T81.49, Infection following a procedure, other surgical site, or a code from O86.ØØ to O86.Ø3, Infection of obstetric surgical wound, or code O86.Ø9, Infection of obstetric surgical wound, other surgical site, that identifies the site of the infection should be sequenced first, if known. Assign an additional code for sepsis following a procedure (T81.44) or sepsis following an obstetrical procedure (O86.Ø4). Use an additional code to identify the infectious agent. If the patient has severe sepsis, the appropriate code from subcategory R65.2 should also be assigned with the additional code(s) for any acute organ dysfunction.

For infections following infusion, transfusion, therapeutic injection, or immunization, a code from subcategory T8Ø.2, Infections following infusion, transfusion, and therapeutic injection, or code T88.Ø-, Infection following immunization, should be coded first, followed by the code for the specific infection. If the patient has severe sepsis, the appropriate code from subcategory R65.2 should also be assigned, with the additional codes(s) for any acute organ dysfunction.

**(c) Postprocedural infection and postprocedural septic shock**

If a postprocedural infection has resulted in postprocedural septic shock, assign the codes indicated above for sepsis due to a postprocedural infection, followed by code T81.12-, Postprocedural septic shock. Do not assign code R65.21, Severe sepsis with septic shock. Additional code(s) should be assigned for any acute organ dysfunction.

**6) Sepsis and severe sepsis associated with a noninfectious process (condition)**

In some cases, a noninfectious process (condition) such as trauma, may lead to an infection which can result in sepsis or severe sepsis. If sepsis or severe sepsis is documented as associated with a noninfectious condition, such as a burn or serious injury, and this condition meets the definition for principal diagnosis, the code for the noninfectious condition should be sequenced first, followed by the code for the resulting infection. If severe sepsis is present, a code from subcategory R65.2 should also be assigned with any associated organ dysfunction(s) codes. It is not necessary to assign a code from subcategory R65.1, Systemic inflammatory response syndrome (SIRS) of non-infectious origin, for these cases.

If the infection meets the definition of principal diagnosis, it should be sequenced before the non-infectious condition. When both the associated non-infectious condition and the infection meet the definition of principal diagnosis, either may be assigned as principal diagnosis.

Only one code from category R65, Symptoms and signs specifically associated with systemic inflammation and infection, should be assigned. Therefore, when a non-infectious condition leads to an infection resulting in severe sepsis, assign the appropriate code from subcategory R65.2, Severe sepsis. Do not additionally assign a code from subcategory R65.1, Systemic inflammatory response syndrome (SIRS) of non-infectious origin.

*See Section I.C.18. SIRS due to non-infectious process*

**7) Sepsis and septic shock complicating abortion, pregnancy, childbirth, and the puerperium**

*See Section I.C.15. Sepsis and septic shock complicating abortion, pregnancy, childbirth and the puerperium*

**8) Newborn sepsis**

*See Section I.C.16. f. Bacterial sepsis of Newborn*

**9) Hemolytic-uremic syndrome associated with sepsis**

If the reason for admission is hemolytic-uremic syndrome that is associated with sepsis, assign code D59.31, Infection-associated hemolytic-uremic syndrome, as the principal diagnosis. Codes for the underlying systemic infection and any other conditions (such as severe sepsis) should be assigned as secondary diagnoses.

**e. Methicillin resistant Staphylococcus aureus (MRSA) conditions**

**1) Selection and sequencing of MRSA codes**

**(a) Combination codes for MRSA infection**

When a patient is diagnosed with an infection that is due to methicillin resistant *Staphylococcus aureus* (MRSA), and that infection has a combination code that includes the causal organism (e.g., sepsis, pneumonia) assign the appropriate combination code for the condition (e.g., code A41.Ø2, Sepsis due to Methicillin resistant Staphylococcus aureus or code J15.212, Pneumonia due to Methicillin resistant Staphylococcus aureus). Do not assign code B95.62, Methicillin resistant Staphylococcus aureus infection as the cause of diseases classified elsewhere, as an additional code, because the combination code includes the type of infection and the MRSA organism. Do not assign a code from subcategory Z16.11, Resistance to penicillins, as an additional diagnosis.

*See Section C.1. for instructions on coding and sequencing of sepsis and severe sepsis.*

**(b) Other codes for MRSA infection**

When there is documentation of a current infection (e.g., wound infection, stitch abscess, urinary tract infection) due to MRSA, and that infection does not have a combination code that includes the causal organism, assign the appropriate code to identify the condition along with code B95.62, Methicillin resistant Staphylococcus aureus infection as the cause of diseases classified elsewhere for the MRSA infection. Do not assign a code from subcategory Z16.11, Resistance to penicillins.

**(c) Methicillin susceptible Staphylococcus aureus (MSSA) and MRSA colonization**

The condition or state of being colonized or carrying MSSA or MRSA is called colonization or carriage, while an individual person is described as being colonized or being a carrier.

Colonization means that MSSA or MSRA is present on or in the body without necessarily causing illness. A positive MRSA colonization test might be documented by the provider as "MRSA screen positive" or "MRSA nasal swab positive".

Assign code Z22.322, Carrier or suspected carrier of Methicillin resistant Staphylococcus aureus, for patients documented as having MRSA colonization. Assign code Z22.321, Carrier or suspected carrier of Methicillin susceptible Staphylococcus aureus, for patients documented as having MSSA colonization. Colonization is not necessarily indicative of a disease process or as the cause of a specific condition the patient may have unless documented as such by the provider.

**(d) MRSA colonization and infection**

If a patient is documented as having both MRSA colonization and infection during a hospital admission, code Z22.322, Carrier or suspected carrier of Methicillin resistant Staphylococcus aureus, and a code for the MRSA infection may both be assigned.

**f. Zika virus infections**

**1) Code only confirmed cases**

Code only a confirmed diagnosis of Zika virus (A92.5, Zika virus disease) as documented by the provider. This is an exception to the hospital inpatient guideline Section II, H. In this context, "confirmation" does not require documentation of the type of test performed; the provider's diagnostic statement that the condition is confirmed is sufficient. This code should be assigned regardless of the stated mode of transmission.

If the provider documents "suspected", "possible" or "probable" Zika, do not assign code A92.5. Assign a code(s) explaining the reason for encounter (such as fever, rash, or joint pain) or Z2Ø.821, Contact with and (suspected) exposure to Zika virus.

**g. Coronavirus infections**

**1) COVID-19 infection (infection due to SARS-CoV-2)**

**(a) Code only confirmed cases**

Code only a confirmed diagnosis of the 2019 novel coronavirus disease (COVID-19) as documented by the provider. For a confirmed diagnosis, assign code UØ7.1, COVID-19. This is an exception to the hospital inpatient guideline Section II, H. In this context, "confirmation" does not require documentation of a positive test result for COVID-19; the provider's documentation that the individual has COVID-19 is sufficient.

If the provider documents "suspected," "possible," "probable," or "inconclusive" COVID-19, do not assign code UØ7.1. Instead, code the signs and symptoms reported. See guideline I.C.1.g.1.g.

Patient presents with cough and a slight fever and fear they were exposed to the coronavirus. The provider documents cough, temperature of 99.4, lungs clear, rule out COVID-19.

| | |
|---|---|
| **R5Ø.9** | **Fever, unspecified** |
| **RØ5.9** | **Cough, unspecified** |
| **Z2Ø.822** | **Contact with and (suspected) exposure to COVID-19** |

*Explanation*: For patients who have been exposed or fear they have been exposed to coronavirus, report codes for signs and symptoms, followed by the Z code. Report UØ7.1 COVID-19, only when the diagnosis is confirmed through provider documentation.

**(b) Sequencing of codes**

When COVID-19 meets the definition of principal diagnosis, code UØ7.1, COVID-19, should be sequenced first, followed by the appropriate codes for associated manifestations, except when another guideline requires that certain codes be sequenced first, such as obstetrics, sepsis, or transplant complications.

*For a COVID-19 infection that progresses to sepsis, see Section I.C.1.d. Sepsis, Severe Sepsis, and Septic Shock*

*See Section I.C.15.s. for COVID-19 infection in pregnancy, childbirth, and the puerperium*

*See Section I.C.16.h. for COVID-19 infection in newborn*

*For a COVID-19 infection in a lung transplant patient, see Section I.C.19.g.3.a. Transplant complications other than kidney.*

**(c) Acute respiratory manifestations of COVID-19**

When the reason for the encounter/admission is a respiratory manifestation of COVID-19, assign code UØ7.1, COVID-19, as the principal/first-listed diagnosis and assign code(s) for the respiratory manifestation(s) as additional diagnoses.

The following conditions are examples of common respiratory manifestations of COVID-19.

**(i) Pneumonia**

For a patient with pneumonia confirmed as due to COVID-19, assign codes UØ7.1, COVID-19, and J12.82, Pneumonia due to coronavirus disease 2019.

**(ii) Acute bronchitis**

For a patient with acute bronchitis confirmed as due to COVID-19, assign codes UØ7.1, and J2Ø.8, Acute bronchitis due to other specified organisms.

Bronchitis not otherwise specified (NOS) due to COVID-19 should be coded using code UØ7.1 and J4Ø, Bronchitis, not specified as acute or chronic.

**(iii) Lower respiratory infection**

If the COVID-19 is documented as being associated with a lower respiratory infection, not otherwise specified (NOS), or an acute respiratory infection, NOS, codes UØ7.1 and J22, Unspecified acute lower respiratory infection, should be assigned.

If the COVID-19 is documented as being associated with a respiratory infection, NOS, codes UØ7.1 and J98.8, Other specified respiratory disorders, should be assigned.

**(iv) Acute respiratory distress syndrome**

For acute respiratory distress syndrome (ARDS) due to COVID-19, assign codes UØ7.1, and J8Ø, Acute respiratory distress syndrome.

**(v) Acute respiratory failure**

For acute respiratory failure due to COVID-19, assign code UØ7.1, and code J96.Ø-, Acute respiratory failure.

**(d) Non-respiratory manifestations of COVID-19**

When the reason for the encounter/admission is a non-respiratory manifestation (e.g., viral enteritis) of COVID-19, assign code UØ7.1, COVID-19, as the principal/first-listed diagnosis and assign code(s) for the manifestation(s) as additional diagnoses.

**(e) Exposure to COVID-19**

For asymptomatic individuals with actual or suspected exposure to COVID-19, assign code Z2Ø.822, Contact with and (suspected) exposure to COVID-19.

For symptomatic individuals with actual or suspected exposure to COVID-19 and the infection has been ruled out, or test results are inconclusive or unknown, assign code Z2Ø.822, Contact with and (suspected) exposure to COVID-19. See guideline I.C.21.c.1, Contact/Exposure, for additional guidance regarding the use of category Z2Ø codes.

If COVID-19 is confirmed, see guideline I.C.1.g.1.a.

Patient was exposed to COVID-19 by a family member. They are asymptomatic and their test result is negative.

**Z2Ø.822 Contact with and (suspected) exposure to COVID-19**

*Explanation*: Report Z2Ø.822 for patients who have a negative test result but have known exposure to someone who has tested positive for COVID-19.

**(f) Screening for COVID-19**

For screening for COVID-19, including preoperative testing, assign code Z11.52, Encounter for screening for COVID-19.

**(g) Signs and symptoms without definitive diagnosis of COVID-19**

For patients presenting with any signs/symptoms associated with COVID-19 (such as fever, etc.) but a definitive diagnosis has not been established, assign the appropriate code(s) for each of the presenting signs and symptoms such as:

- RØ5.1, Acute cough, or RØ5.9, Cough, unspecified
- RØ6.Ø2, Shortness of breath
- R5Ø.9, Fever, unspecified

If a patient with signs/symptoms associated with COVID-19 also has an actual or suspected contact with or exposure to COVID-19, assign Z2Ø.822, Contact with and (suspected) exposure to COVID19, as an additional code.

**(h) Asymptomatic individuals who test positive for COVID-19**

For asymptomatic individuals who test positive for COVID-19 and there is no provider documentation of a diagnosis of COVID-19, query the provider as to whether or not the individual has COVID-19. A false positive laboratory test is possible, and it is the provider's responsibility to confirm the diagnosis and document accordingly.

**(i) Personal history of COVID-19**

For patients with a history of COVID-19, assign code Z86.16, Personal history of COVID-19.

**(j) Follow-up visits after COVID-19 infection has resolved**

For individuals who previously had COVID-19, without residual symptom(s) or condition(s), and are being seen for follow-up evaluation, and COVID-19 test results are negative, assign codes ZØ9, Encounter for follow-up examination after completed treatment for conditions other than malignant neoplasm, and Z86.16, Personal history of COVID-19.

For follow-up visits for individuals with symptom(s) or condition(s) related to a previous COVID-19 infection, see guideline I.C.1.g.1.m.

*See Section I.C.21.c.8, Factors influencing health states and contact with health services, Follow-up*

**(k) Encounter for antibody testing**

For an encounter for antibody testing that is not being performed to confirm a current COVID-19 infection, nor is a follow-up test after resolution of COVID-19, assign ZØ1.84, Encounter for antibody response examination.

Follow the applicable guidelines above if the individual is being tested to confirm a current COVID-19 infection.

For follow-up testing after a COVID-19 infection, see guideline I.C.1.g.1.j.

**(l) Multisystem inflammatory syndrome**

For individuals with multisystem inflammatory syndrome (MIS) and COVID-19, assign code UØ7.1, COVID-19, as the principal/first-listed diagnosis and assign code M35.81, Multisystem inflammatory syndrome, as an additional diagnosis.

If an individual with a history of COVID-19 develops MIS, assign codes M35.81, Multisystem inflammatory syndrome, and UØ9.9, Post COVID-19 condition, unspecified.

If an individual with a known or suspected exposure to COVID- 19, and no current COVID-19 infection or history of COVID-19, develops MIS, assign codes M35.81, Multisystem inflammatory syndrome, and Z2Ø.822, Contact with and (suspected) exposure to COVID-19.

Additional codes should be assigned for any associated complications of MIS.

**(m)Post COVID-19 condition**

For sequela of COVID-19, or associated symptoms or conditions that develop following a previous COVID-19 infection, assign a code(s) for the specific symptom(s) or condition(s) related to the previous COVID-19 infection, if known, and code UØ9.9, Post COVID-19 condition, unspecified.

Code UØ9.9 should not be assigned for manifestations of an active (current) COVID-19 infection.

If a patient has a condition(s) associated with a previous COVID-19 infection and develops a new active (current) COVID-19 infection, code UØ9.9 may be assigned in conjunction with code UØ7.1, COVID-19, to identify that the patient also has a condition(s) associated with a previous COVID-19 infection. Code(s) for the specific condition(s) associated with the previous COVID-19 infection and code(s) for manifestation(s) of the new active (current) COVID-19 infection should also be assigned.

**(n) Underimmunization for COVID-19 Status**

Code Z28.31Ø, Unvaccinated for COVID-19, may be assigned when the patient has not received a COVID-19 vaccine of any type. Code Z28.311, Partially vaccinated for COVID-19, may be assigned when the patient has been partially vaccinated for COVID-19 as per the recommendations of the Centers for Disease Control and Prevention (CDC) in place at the time of the encounter. For information, visit the CDC's website https://www.cdc.gov/covidschedule.

*See Section I.B.14. for underimmunization documentation by clinicians other than patient's provider.*

# Chapter 1. Certain Infectious and Parasitic Diseases (A00-B99)

INCLUDES diseases generally recognized as communicable or transmissible

Use additional code to identify resistance to antimicrobial drugs (Z16.-)

EXCLUDES 1 ~~*certain localized infections - see body system-related chapters*~~

EXCLUDES 2 *carrier or suspected carrier of infectious disease (Z22.-)*

▶*certain localized infections - see body system-related chapters*◀

*infectious and parasitic diseases complicating pregnancy, childbirth and the puerperium (O98.-)*

*infectious and parasitic diseases specific to the perinatal period (P35-P39)*

*influenza and other acute respiratory infections (J00-J22)*

This chapter contains the following blocks:

| | |
|---|---|
| A00-A09 | Intestinal infectious diseases |
| A15-A19 | Tuberculosis |
| A20-A28 | Certain zoonotic bacterial diseases |
| A30-A49 | Other bacterial diseases |
| A50-A64 | Infections with a predominantly sexual mode of transmission |
| A65-A69 | Other spirochetal diseases |
| A70-A74 | Other diseases caused by chlamydiae |
| A75-A79 | Rickettsioses |
| A80-A89 | Viral and prion infections of the central nervous system |
| A90-A99 | Arthropod-borne viral fevers and viral hemorrhagic fevers |
| B00-B09 | Viral infections characterized by skin and mucous membrane lesions |
| B10 | Other human herpesviruses |
| B15-B19 | Viral hepatitis |
| B20 | Human immunodeficiency virus [HIV] disease |
| B25-B34 | Other viral diseases |
| B35-B49 | Mycoses |
| B50-B64 | Protozoal diseases |
| B65-B83 | Helminthiases |
| B85-B89 | Pediculosis, acariasis and other infestations |
| B90-B94 | Sequelae of infectious and parasitic diseases |
| B95-B97 | Bacterial and viral infectious agents |
| B99 | Other infectious diseases |

## Intestinal infectious diseases (A00-A09)

✓4th **A00 Cholera**

**DEF:** Acute infection of the bowel due to *Vibrio cholerae* that presents with profuse diarrhea, cramps, and vomiting, resulting in severe dehydration, electrolyte imbalance, and death. It is spread through ingestion of food or water contaminated with feces of infected persons.

**A00.0 Cholera due to Vibrio cholerae 01, biovar cholerae**
Classical cholera

**A00.1 Cholera due to Vibrio cholerae 01, biovar eltor**
Cholera eltor

**A00.9 Cholera, unspecified**

✓4th **A01 Typhoid and paratyphoid fevers**

**DEF:** Paratyphoid fever: Prolonged febrile illness, caused by *Salmonella* serotypes other than *S. typhi*, especially *S. enterica* serotypes paratyphi A, B, and C.

**DEF:** Typhoid fever: Acute generalized illness caused by *Salmonella typhi*. Clinical features include fever, headache, abdominal pain, cough, toxemia, leukopenia, abnormal pulse, rose spots on the skin, bacteremia, hyperplasia of intestinal lymph nodes, mesenteric lymphadenopathy, and Peyer's patches in the intestines.

✓5th **A01.0 Typhoid fever**
Infection due to Salmonella typhi

**A01.00 Typhoid fever, unspecified**

**A01.01 Typhoid meningitis** COM

**A01.02 Typhoid fever with heart involvement** COM
Typhoid endocarditis
Typhoid myocarditis

**A01.03 Typhoid pneumonia** ESR

**A01.04 Typhoid arthritis** HCC ESR COM

**A01.05 Typhoid osteomyelitis** HCC ESR COM

**A01.09 Typhoid fever with other complications**

**A01.1 Paratyphoid fever A**

**A01.2 Paratyphoid fever B**

**A01.3 Paratyphoid fever C**

**A01.4 Paratyphoid fever, unspecified**
Infection due to Salmonella paratyphi NOS

✓4th **A02 Other salmonella infections**

INCLUDES infection or foodborne intoxication due to any Salmonella species other than S. typhi and S. paratyphi

**A02.0 Salmonella enteritis**
Salmonellosis

**TIP:** Dehydration (E86.0) is a complication of salmonella enteritis and may be reported separately.

**A02.1 Salmonella sepsis** HCC ESR COM

✓5th **A02.2 Localized salmonella infections**

**A02.20 Localized salmonella infection, unspecified**

**A02.21 Salmonella meningitis** COM

**A02.22 Salmonella pneumonia** ESR

**A02.23 Salmonella arthritis** HCC ESR COM

**A02.24 Salmonella osteomyelitis** HCC ESR COM

**A02.25 Salmonella pyelonephritis**
Salmonella tubulo-interstitial nephropathy

**A02.29 Salmonella with other localized infection**

**A02.8 Other specified salmonella infections**

**A02.9 Salmonella infection, unspecified**

✓4th **A03 Shigellosis**

**DEF:** Infection caused by the genus *Shigella*, of the family *Enterobacteriaceae* that is known to cause an acute dysenteric infection of the bowel with fever, drowsiness, anorexia, nausea, vomiting, bloody diarrhea, abdominal cramps, and distention.

**A03.0 Shigellosis due to Shigella dysenteriae**
Group A shigellosis [Shiga-Kruse dysentery]

**A03.1 Shigellosis due to Shigella flexneri**
Group B shigellosis
**AHA:** 2026,2Q,5

**A03.2 Shigellosis due to Shigella boydii**
Group C shigellosis

**A03.3 Shigellosis due to Shigella sonnei**
Group D shigellosis

**A03.8 Other shigellosis**

**A03.9 Shigellosis, unspecified**
Bacillary dysentery NOS

✓4th **A04 Other bacterial intestinal infections**

EXCLUDES 1 *bacterial foodborne intoxications, NEC (A05.-)*
*tuberculous enteritis (A18.32)*

**DEF:** *Escherichia coli*: Gram-negative, anaerobic bacteria of the family *Enterobacteriaceae* found in the large intestine of warm-blooded animals, generally as a nonpathologic entity aiding in digestion. They become pathogenic when an opportunity to grow somewhere outside this relationship presents itself, such as ingestion of fecal-contaminated food or water.

**A04.0 Enteropathogenic Escherichia coli infection**

**A04.1 Enterotoxigenic Escherichia coli infection**

**A04.2 Enteroinvasive Escherichia coli infection**

**A04.3 Enterohemorrhagic Escherichia coli infection**

**DEF:** *E. coli* infection penetrating the intestinal mucosa, producing microscopic ulceration and bleeding.

**A04.4 Other intestinal Escherichia coli infections**
Escherichia coli enteritis NOS

**A04.5 Campylobacter enteritis**

**TIP:** For Guillain-Barre syndrome occurring as a sequela of *Campylobacter enteritis*, assign code G61.0 as the first-listed diagnosis followed by B94.8 for the sequelae.

**A04.6 Enteritis due to Yersinia enterocolitica**

EXCLUDES 1 *extraintestinal yersiniosis (A28.2)*

✓5th **A04.7 Enterocolitis due to Clostridium difficile**
Clostridioides difficile colitis
Foodborne intoxication by Clostridium difficile
Pseudomembraneous colitis
**AHA:** 2017,4Q,4

**A04.71 Enterocolitis due to Clostridium difficile, recurrent**
**AHA:** 2020,1Q,18

**A04.72 Enterocolitis due to Clostridium difficile, not specified as recurrent**

**A04.8 Other specified bacterial intestinal infections**

**A04.9 Bacterial intestinal infection, unspecified**
Bacterial enteritis NOS

✓4th **A05 Other bacterial foodborne intoxications, not elsewhere classified**

EXCLUDES 1 *Clostridium difficile foodborne intoxication and infection (A04.7-)*
*Escherichia coli infection (A04.0-A04.4)*
*listeriosis (A32.-)*
*salmonella foodborne intoxication and infection (A02.-)*
*toxic effect of noxious foodstuffs (T61-T62)*

**A05.0 Foodborne staphylococcal intoxication**

**TIP:** Assign code A04.8 to report a staphylococcal infection when it is caused by the ingestion of contaminated food but not caused by *S. aureus* toxins.

**A05.1 Botulism food poisoning**
Botulism NOS
Classical foodborne intoxication due to Clostridium botulinum
EXCLUDES 1 *infant botulism (A48.51)*
*wound botulism (A48.52)*
**DEF:** Muscle-paralyzing neurotoxic disease caused by ingesting pre-formed toxin from the bacterium *Clostridium botulinum*. It causes vomiting and diarrhea, vision problems, slurred speech, difficulty swallowing, paralysis, and death.

**A05.2 Foodborne Clostridium perfringens [Clostridium welchii] intoxication**
Enteritis necroticans
Pig-bel

**A05.3 Foodborne Vibrio parahaemolyticus intoxication**

**A05.4 Foodborne Bacillus cereus intoxication**

**A05.5 Foodborne Vibrio vulnificus intoxication**

**A05.8 Other specified bacterial foodborne intoxications**

**A05.9 Bacterial foodborne intoxication, unspecified**

**✓4th A06 Amebiasis**
INCLUDES infection due to Entamoeba histolytica
EXCLUDES 1 *other protozoal intestinal diseases (A07.-)*
EXCLUDES 2 *acanthamebiasis (B60.1-)*
*Naegleriasis (B60.2)*
**DEF:** Infection with a single cell protozoan known as the amoeba. Transmission occurs through ingestion of feces, contaminated food or water, use of human feces as fertilizer, or person-to-person contact.

**A06.0 Acute amebic dysentery**
Acute amebiasis
Intestinal amebiasis NOS

**A06.1 Chronic intestinal amebiasis**

**A06.2 Amebic nondysenteric colitis**

**A06.3 Ameboma of intestine**
Ameboma NOS

**A06.4 Amebic liver abscess** COM
Hepatic amebiasis

**A06.5 Amebic lung abscess** HCC ESR COM
Amebic abscess of lung (and liver)

**A06.6 Amebic brain abscess** COM
Amebic abscess of brain (and liver) (and lung)

**A06.7 Cutaneous amebiasis**

**✓5th A06.8 Amebic infection of other sites**

**A06.81 Amebic cystitis**

**A06.82 Other amebic genitourinary infections**
Amebic balanitis
Amebic vesiculitis
Amebic vulvovaginitis

**A06.89 Other amebic infections**
Amebic appendicitis
Amebic splenic abscess

**A06.9 Amebiasis, unspecified**

**✓4th A07 Other protozoal intestinal diseases**
**DEF:** Protozoa: Group comprised of the simplest, single celled organisms, ranging in size from micro to macroscopic. They can live alone or in colonies, and do not show any differentiation in tissues. Most are motile and can live free in nature, but some are parasitic, causing disease in the variety of hosts they inhabit.

**A07.0 Balantidiasis**
Balantidial dysentery

**A07.1 Giardiasis [lambliasis]**
**DEF:** Infection caused by the flagellate protozoan *Giardia lamblia* causing gastrointestinal problems such as vomiting, chronic diarrhea, and weight loss. The most common parasite in the U.S., this is usually transmitted by ingesting contaminated water while in the cyst state, after which it latches onto the wall of the small intestine.

**A07.2 Cryptosporidiosis** HCC Rx ESR COM
**DEF:** Microscopic parasite found in water and one of the most common causes of waterborne gastrointestinal infectious disease in the United States. It is usually transmitted by ingesting contaminated drinking water or recreational water and causes profuse watery diarrhea, flatulence, abdominal pain, and cramping.

**A07.3 Isosporiasis**
Infection due to Isospora belli and Isospora hominis
Intestinal coccidiosis
Isosporosis

**A07.4 Cyclosporiasis**

**A07.8 Other specified protozoal intestinal diseases**
Intestinal microsporidiosis
Intestinal trichomoniasis
Sarcocystosis
Sarcosporidiosis

**A07.9 Protozoal intestinal disease, unspecified**
Flagellate diarrhea
Protozoal colitis
Protozoal diarrhea
Protozoal dysentery

**✓4th A08 Viral and other specified intestinal infections**
EXCLUDES 1 *influenza with involvement of gastrointestinal tract (J09.X3, J10.2, J11.2)*

**A08.0 Rotaviral enteritis**

**✓5th A08.1 Acute gastroenteropathy due to Norwalk agent and other small round viruses**

**A08.11 Acute gastroenteropathy due to Norwalk agent**
Acute gastroenteropathy due to Norovirus
Acute gastroenteropathy due to Norwalk-like agent

**A08.19 Acute gastroenteropathy due to other small round viruses**
Acute gastroenteropathy due to small round virus [SRV] NOS

**A08.2 Adenoviral enteritis**

**✓5th A08.3 Other viral enteritis**

**A08.31 Calicivirus enteritis**

**A08.32 Astrovirus enteritis**

**A08.39 Other viral enteritis**
Coxsackie virus enteritis
Echovirus enteritis
Enterovirus enteritis NEC
Torovirus enteritis

**A08.4 Viral intestinal infection, unspecified**
Viral enteritis NOS
Viral gastroenteritis NOS
Viral gastroenteropathy NOS
**AHA:** 2016,3Q,12

**A08.8 Other specified intestinal infections**

**A09 Infectious gastroenteritis and colitis, unspecified**
Infectious colitis NOS
Infectious enteritis NOS
Infectious gastroenteritis NOS
EXCLUDES 1 *colitis NOS (K52.9)*
*diarrhea NOS (R19.7)*
*enteritis NOS (K52.9)*
*gastroenteritis NOS (K52.9)*
*noninfective gastroenteritis and colitis, unspecified (K52.9)*
**DEF:** Colitis: Inflammation of mucous membranes of the colon.
**DEF:** Enteritis: Inflammation of mucous membranes of the small intestine.
**DEF:** Gastroenteritis: Inflammation of mucous membranes of the stomach and intestines.

## Tuberculosis (A15-A19)

INCLUDES infections due to Mycobacterium tuberculosis and Mycobacterium bovis

Use additional code, if applicable, for associated cachexia (E88.A)

EXCLUDES 1 *congenital tuberculosis (P37.Ø)*
*nonspecific reaction to test for tuberculosis without active tuberculosis (R76.1-)*
*pneumoconiosis associated with tuberculosis, any type in A15 (J65)*
*positive PPD (R76.11)*
*positive tuberculin skin test without active tuberculosis (R76.11)*
*sequelae of tuberculosis (B9Ø.-)*
*silicotuberculosis (J65)*

**DEF:** Bacterial infection that typically spreads by inhalation of an airborne agent that usually attacks the lungs, but may also affect other organs.

**A15 Respiratory tuberculosis**

**A15.Ø Tuberculosis of lung**
Tuberculous bronchiectasis
Tuberculous fibrosis of lung
Tuberculous pneumonia
Tuberculous pneumothorax

**Tuberculosis of Lung**

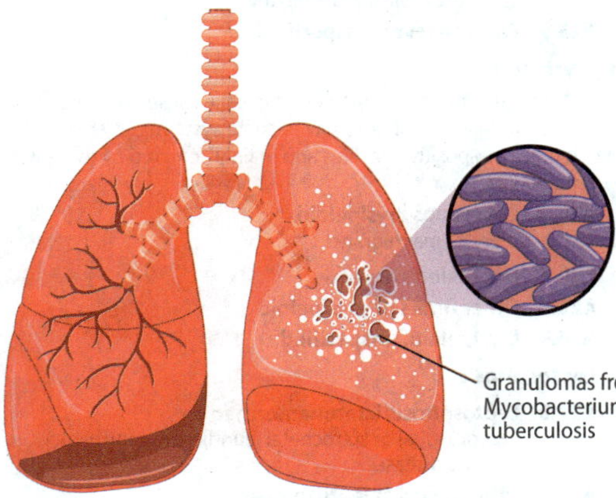


**A15.4 Tuberculosis of intrathoracic lymph nodes**
Tuberculosis of hilar lymph nodes
Tuberculosis of mediastinal lymph nodes
Tuberculosis of tracheobronchial lymph nodes
EXCLUDES 1 *tuberculosis specified as primary (A15.7)*

**A15.5 Tuberculosis of larynx, trachea and bronchus**
Tuberculosis of bronchus
Tuberculosis of glottis
Tuberculosis of larynx
Tuberculosis of trachea

**A15.6 Tuberculous pleurisy**
Tuberculosis of pleura Tuberculous empyema
EXCLUDES 1 *primary respiratory tuberculosis (A15.7)*

**A15.7 Primary respiratory tuberculosis**

**A15.8 Other respiratory tuberculosis**
Mediastinal tuberculosis
Nasopharyngeal tuberculosis
Tuberculosis of nose
Tuberculosis of sinus [any nasal]

**A15.9 Respiratory tuberculosis unspecified**

**A17 Tuberculosis of nervous system**

**A17.Ø Tuberculous meningitis** COM
Tuberculosis of meninges (cerebral)(spinal)
Tuberculous leptomeningitis
EXCLUDES 1 *tuberculous meningoencephalitis (A17.82)*

**A17.1 Meningeal tuberculoma** COM
Tuberculoma of meninges (cerebral) (spinal)
EXCLUDES 2 *tuberculoma of brain and spinal cord (A17.81)*

**A17.8 Other tuberculosis of nervous system**

**A17.81 Tuberculoma of brain and spinal cord** COM
Tuberculous abscess of brain and spinal cord

**A17.82 Tuberculous meningoencephalitis** COM
Tuberculous myelitis

**A17.83 Tuberculous neuritis** COM
Tuberculous mononeuropathy

**A17.89 Other tuberculosis of nervous system** COM
Tuberculous polyneuropathy

**A17.9 Tuberculosis of nervous system, unspecified** COM

**A18 Tuberculosis of other organs**

**A18.Ø Tuberculosis of bones and joints**

**A18.Ø1 Tuberculosis of spine**
Pott's disease or curvature of spine
Tuberculous arthritis
Tuberculous osteomyelitis of spine
Tuberculous spondylitis

**A18.Ø2 Tuberculous arthritis of other joints**
Tuberculosis of hip (joint)
Tuberculosis of knee (joint)

**A18.Ø3 Tuberculosis of other bones**
Tuberculous mastoiditis
Tuberculous osteomyelitis

**A18.Ø9 Other musculoskeletal tuberculosis**
Tuberculous myositis
Tuberculous synovitis
Tuberculous tenosynovitis

**A18.1 Tuberculosis of genitourinary system**

**A18.1Ø Tuberculosis of genitourinary system, unspecified**

**A18.11 Tuberculosis of kidney and ureter**

**A18.12 Tuberculosis of bladder**

**A18.13 Tuberculosis of other urinary organs**
Tuberculous urethritis

**A18.14 Tuberculosis of prostate** A

**A18.15 Tuberculosis of other male genital organs**

**A18.16 Tuberculosis of cervix**

**A18.17 Tuberculous female pelvic inflammatory disease**
Tuberculous endometritis
Tuberculous oophoritis and salpingitis

**A18.18 Tuberculosis of other female genital organs**
Tuberculous ulceration of vulva

**A18.2 Tuberculous peripheral lymphadenopathy**
Tuberculous adenitis
EXCLUDES 2 *tuberculosis of bronchial and mediastinal lymph nodes (A15.4)*
*tuberculosis of mesenteric and retroperitoneal lymph nodes (A18.39)*
*tuberculous tracheobronchial adenopathy (A15.4)*

**A18.3 Tuberculosis of intestines, peritoneum and mesenteric glands**

**A18.31 Tuberculous peritonitis**
Tuberculous ascites
**DEF:** Tuberculous inflammation of the membrane lining the abdomen.

**A18.32 Tuberculous enteritis**
Tuberculosis of anus and rectum
Tuberculosis of intestine (large) (small)

**A18.39 Retroperitoneal tuberculosis**
Tuberculosis of mesenteric glands
Tuberculosis of retroperitoneal (lymph glands)

**A18.4 Tuberculosis of skin and subcutaneous tissue**
Erythema induratum, tuberculous
Lupus exedens
Lupus vulgaris of eyelid
Lupus vulgaris NOS
Scrofuloderma
Tuberculosis of external ear
EXCLUDES 2 *lupus erythematosus (L93.-)*
*systemic lupus erythematosus (M32.-)*

**A18.5 Tuberculosis of eye**
EXCLUDES 2 *lupus vulgaris of eyelid (A18.4)*

**A18.5Ø Tuberculosis of eye, unspecified**

**A18.51 Tuberculous episcleritis**

**A18.52 Tuberculous keratitis**
Tuberculous interstitial keratitis
Tuberculous keratoconjunctivitis (interstitial) (phlyctenular)

**A18.53 Tuberculous chorioretinitis**

**A18.54 Tuberculous iridocyclitis**

**A18.59 Other tuberculosis of eye**
Tuberculous conjunctivitis

**A18.6 Tuberculosis of (inner) (middle) ear**
Tuberculous otitis media
EXCLUDES 2 *tuberculosis of external ear (A18.4)*
*tuberculous mastoiditis (A18.Ø3)*

**A18.7 Tuberculosis of adrenal glands**
Tuberculous Addison's disease

**A18.8 Tuberculosis of other specified organs**

**A18.81 Tuberculosis of thyroid gland**

Chapter 1. Certain Infectious and Parasitic Diseases
A15–A18.81

**A18.82 Tuberculosis of other endocrine glands**
Tuberculosis of pituitary gland
Tuberculosis of thymus gland

**A18.83 Tuberculosis of digestive tract organs, not elsewhere classified**
EXCLUDES 1 *tuberculosis of intestine (A18.32)*

**A18.84 Tuberculosis of heart**
Tuberculous cardiomyopathy
Tuberculous endocarditis
Tuberculous myocarditis
Tuberculous pericarditis

**A18.85 Tuberculosis of spleen**

**A18.89 Tuberculosis of other sites**
Tuberculosis of muscle
Tuberculous cerebral arteritis

**✓4th A19 Miliary tuberculosis**
INCLUDES disseminated tuberculosis
generalized tuberculosis
tuberculous polyserositis

**A19.0 Acute miliary tuberculosis of a single specified site**
**A19.1 Acute miliary tuberculosis of multiple sites**
**A19.2 Acute miliary tuberculosis, unspecified**
**A19.8 Other miliary tuberculosis**
**A19.9 Miliary tuberculosis, unspecified**

## Certain zoonotic bacterial diseases (A20-A28)

**✓4th A20 Plague**
INCLUDES infection due to Yersinia pestis

**A20.0 Bubonic plague**
**A20.1 Cellulocutaneous plague**
**A20.2 Pneumonic plague** ESR
**A20.3 Plague meningitis** COM
**A20.7 Septicemic plague** HCC ESR COM
**A20.8 Other forms of plague**
Abortive plague
Asymptomatic plague
Pestis minor
**A20.9 Plague, unspecified**

**✓4th A21 Tularemia**
INCLUDES deer-fly fever
infection due to Francisella tularensis
rabbit fever

**DEF:** Febrile disease transmitted to humans by the bites of deer flies, fleas, and ticks, by inhaling aerosolized *F. tularensis*, or by ingesting contaminated food or water. Patients quickly develop fever, chills, weakness, headache, backache, and malaise.

**A21.0 Ulceroglandular tularemia**
**A21.1 Oculoglandular tularemia**
Ophthalmic tularemia
**A21.2 Pulmonary tularemia** ESR
**A21.3 Gastrointestinal tularemia**
Abdominal tularemia
**A21.7 Generalized tularemia**
**A21.8 Other forms of tularemia**
**A21.9 Tularemia, unspecified**

**✓4th A22 Anthrax**
INCLUDES infection due to Bacillus anthracis

**A22.0 Cutaneous anthrax**
Malignant carbuncle
Malignant pustule
**A22.1 Pulmonary anthrax** ESR
Inhalation anthrax
Ragpicker's disease
Woolsorter's disease
**A22.2 Gastrointestinal anthrax**
**A22.7 Anthrax sepsis** HCC ESR COM
**A22.8 Other forms of anthrax**
Anthrax meningitis
**A22.9 Anthrax, unspecified**

**✓4th A23 Brucellosis**
INCLUDES Malta fever
Mediterranean fever
undulant fever

**A23.0 Brucellosis due to Brucella melitensis**
**A23.1 Brucellosis due to Brucella abortus**
**A23.2 Brucellosis due to Brucella suis**
**A23.3 Brucellosis due to Brucella canis**
**A23.8 Other brucellosis**
**A23.9 Brucellosis, unspecified**

**✓4th A24 Glanders and melioidosis**

**A24.0 Glanders**
Infection due to Pseudomonas mallei
Malleus
**A24.1 Acute and fulminating melioidosis**
Melioidosis pneumonia
Melioidosis sepsis
**A24.2 Subacute and chronic melioidosis**
**A24.3 Other melioidosis**
**A24.9 Melioidosis, unspecified**
Infection due to Pseudomonas pseudomallei NOS
Whitmore's disease

**✓4th A25 Rat-bite fevers**

**A25.0 Spirillosis**
Sodoku
**A25.1 Streptobacillosis**
Epidemic arthritic erythema
Haverhill fever
Streptobacillary rat-bite fever
**A25.9 Rat-bite fever, unspecified**

**✓4th A26 Erysipeloid**
**DEF:** Acute cutaneous infection typically caused by trauma to the skin. Presenting as cellulitis, it may become systemic, affecting other organs. It is a gram-positive bacillus and mainly acquired by those who routinely handle meat.

**A26.0 Cutaneous erysipeloid**
Erythema migrans
**A26.7 Erysipelothrix sepsis** HCC ESR COM
**A26.8 Other forms of erysipeloid**
**A26.9 Erysipeloid, unspecified**

**✓4th A27 Leptospirosis**

**A27.0 Leptospirosis icterohemorrhagica**
Leptospiral or spirochetal jaundice (hemorrhagic)
Weil's disease
**✓5th A27.8 Other forms of leptospirosis**
**A27.81 Aseptic meningitis in leptospirosis** COM
**A27.89 Other forms of leptospirosis**
**A27.9 Leptospirosis, unspecified**

**✓4th A28 Other zoonotic bacterial diseases, not elsewhere classified**

**A28.0 Pasteurellosis**
**A28.1 Cat-scratch disease**
Cat-scratch fever
**A28.2 Extraintestinal yersiniosis**
EXCLUDES 1 *enteritis due to Yersinia enterocolitica (A04.6)*
*plague (A20.-)*
**A28.8 Other specified zoonotic bacterial diseases, not elsewhere classified**
**A28.9 Zoonotic bacterial disease, unspecified**

## Other bacterial diseases (A30-A49)

**AHA:** 2016,3Q,8-14

**✓4th A30 Leprosy [Hansen's disease]**
INCLUDES infection due to Mycobacterium leprae
EXCLUDES 1 *sequelae of leprosy (B92)*

**A30.0 Indeterminate leprosy**
I leprosy
**A30.1 Tuberculoid leprosy**
TT leprosy
**A30.2 Borderline tuberculoid leprosy**
BT leprosy
**A30.3 Borderline leprosy**
BB leprosy
**A30.4 Borderline lepromatous leprosy**
BL leprosy
**A30.5 Lepromatous leprosy**
LL leprosy
**A30.8 Other forms of leprosy**
**A30.9 Leprosy, unspecified**

**A31 Infection due to other mycobacteria**

EXCLUDES 2 *leprosy (A30.-)*
*tuberculosis (A15-A19)*

**A31.0 Pulmonary mycobacterial infection** HCC Rx ESR COM
Infection due to Mycobacterium avium
Infection due to Mycobacterium intracellulare [Battey bacillus]
Infection due to Mycobacterium kansasii

**A31.1 Cutaneous mycobacterial infection**
Buruli ulcer
Infection due to Mycobacterium marinum
Infection due to Mycobacterium ulcerans

**A31.2 Disseminated mycobacterium avium-intracellulare complex (DMAC)** HCC Rx ESR COM
MAC sepsis

**A31.8 Other mycobacterial infections**

**A31.9 Mycobacterial infection, unspecified**
Atypical mycobacterial infection NOS
Mycobacteriosis NOS

**A32 Listeriosis**

INCLUDES listerial foodborne infection

EXCLUDES 1 *neonatal (disseminated) listeriosis (P37.2)*

**A32.0 Cutaneous listeriosis**

**A32.1 Listerial meningitis and meningoencephalitis**

**A32.11 Listerial meningitis** COM

**A32.12 Listerial meningoencephalitis** COM

**A32.7 Listerial sepsis** HCC ESR COM

**A32.8 Other forms of listeriosis**

**A32.81 Oculoglandular listeriosis**

**A32.82 Listerial endocarditis** COM

**A32.89 Other forms of listeriosis**
Listerial cerebral arteritis

**A32.9 Listeriosis, unspecified**

**A33 Tetanus neonatorum** N

**A34 Obstetrical tetanus** COM M

**A35 Other tetanus** COM
Tetanus NOS

EXCLUDES 1 *obstetrical tetanus (A34)*
*tetanus neonatorum (A33)*

**DEF:** Tetanus: Acute, often fatal, infectious disease caused by the anaerobic, spore-forming bacillus *Clostridium tetani*. The bacillus enters the body through a contaminated wound, burns, surgical wounds, or cutaneous ulcers. Symptoms include lockjaw, spasms, seizures, and paralysis.

**A36 Diphtheria**

**A36.0 Pharyngeal diphtheria**
Diphtheritic membranous angina
Tonsillar diphtheria

**A36.1 Nasopharyngeal diphtheria**

**A36.2 Laryngeal diphtheria**
Diphtheritic laryngotracheitis

**A36.3 Cutaneous diphtheria**

EXCLUDES 2 *erythrasma (L08.1)*

**A36.8 Other diphtheria**

**A36.81 Diphtheritic cardiomyopathy** HCC Rx ESR COM
Diphtheritic myocarditis

**A36.82 Diphtheritic radiculomyelitis**

**A36.83 Diphtheritic polyneuritis**

**A36.84 Diphtheritic tubulo-interstitial nephropathy**

**A36.85 Diphtheritic cystitis**

**A36.86 Diphtheritic conjunctivitis**

**A36.89 Other diphtheritic complications**
Diphtheritic peritonitis

**A36.9 Diphtheria, unspecified**

**A37 Whooping cough**

**DEF:** Acute, highly contagious respiratory tract infection caused by *Bordetella pertussis* and *B. bronchiseptica*. Whooping cough is known by its characteristic paroxysmal cough.

**A37.0 Whooping cough due to Bordetella pertussis**

**A37.00 Whooping cough due to Bordetella pertussis without pneumonia**
Paroxysmal cough due to Bordetella pertussis without pneumonia

**A37.01 Whooping cough due to Bordetella pertussis with pneumonia**
Paroxysmal cough due to Bordetella pertussis with pneumonia

**A37.1 Whooping cough due to Bordetella parapertussis**

**A37.10 Whooping cough due to Bordetella parapertussis without pneumonia**

**A37.11 Whooping cough due to Bordetella parapertussis with pneumonia**

**A37.8 Whooping cough due to other Bordetella species**

**A37.80 Whooping cough due to other Bordetella species without pneumonia**

**A37.81 Whooping cough due to other Bordetella species with pneumonia**

**A37.9 Whooping cough, unspecified species**

**A37.90 Whooping cough, unspecified species without pneumonia**

**A37.91 Whooping cough, unspecified species with pneumonia**

**A38 Scarlet fever**

INCLUDES scarlatina

EXCLUDES 2 *streptococcal sore throat (J02.0)*

**DEF:** Acute contagious disease caused by Group A bacteria, the same bacterium that causes strep throat. Individuals with strep throat can develop scarlet fever particularly if the infection is not treated with antibiotics. It is characterized by a red blush to the skin of the chest and abdomen and swelling of the nose, throat, and mouth.

**A38.0 Scarlet fever with otitis media**

**A38.1 Scarlet fever with myocarditis** COM

**A38.8 Scarlet fever with other complications**

**A38.9 Scarlet fever, uncomplicated**
Scarlet fever, NOS

**A39 Meningococcal infection**

**DEF:** Condition caused by *Neisseria meningitidis*, a bacteria that may invade the spinal cord, brain, heart, joints, optic nerve, or bloodstream.

**A39.0 Meningococcal meningitis** COM

**A39.1 Waterhouse-Friderichsen syndrome** Rx ESR COM
Meningococcal hemorrhagic adrenalitis
Meningococcic adrenal syndrome

**A39.2 Acute meningococcemia** HCC ESR COM

**A39.3 Chronic meningococcemia** HCC ESR COM

**A39.4 Meningococcemia, unspecified** HCC ESR COM

**A39.5 Meningococcal heart disease**

**A39.50 Meningococcal carditis, unspecified** COM

**A39.51 Meningococcal endocarditis** COM

**A39.52 Meningococcal myocarditis** COM

**A39.53 Meningococcal pericarditis** COM

**A39.8 Other meningococcal infections**

**A39.81 Meningococcal encephalitis** COM

**A39.82 Meningococcal retrobulbar neuritis**

**A39.83 Meningococcal arthritis** HCC ESR COM

**A39.84 Postmeningococcal arthritis** HCC ESR COM

**A39.89 Other meningococcal infections**
Meningococcal conjunctivitis

**A39.9 Meningococcal infection, unspecified**
Meningococcal disease NOS

**A40 Streptococcal sepsis**

Code first, if applicable, postprocedural sepsis (T81.44-)
sepsis due to central venous catheter (T80.211-)
streptococcal sepsis during labor (O75.3)
streptococcal sepsis following abortion or ectopic or molar pregnancy (O03.37, O03.87, O04.87, O07.37, O08.82)
streptococcal sepsis following immunization (T88.0-)
streptococcal sepsis following infusion, transfusion or therapeutic injection (T80.22-, T80.29-)

EXCLUDES 1 *neonatal (P36.0-P36.1)*
*puerperal sepsis (O85)*
*sepsis due to Streptococcus, group D (A41.81)*

**AHA:** 2020,2Q,8,28; 2019,4Q,65; 2018,4Q,89; 2018,1Q,16; 2016,1Q,32

**A40.0 Sepsis due to streptococcus, group A** HCC ESR COM

**A40.1 Sepsis due to streptococcus, group B** HCC ESR COM
**AHA:** 2019,1Q,14

**A40.3 Sepsis due to Streptococcus pneumoniae** HCC ESR COM
Pneumococcal sepsis

**A40.8 Other streptococcal sepsis** HCC ESR COM

**A40.9** **Streptococcal sepsis, unspecified** HCC ESR COM

✓4th **A41 Other sepsis**

Code first, if applicable, postprocedural sepsis (T81.44-)
sepsis due to central venous catheter (T80.211-)
sepsis during labor (O75.3)
sepsis following abortion, ectopic or molar pregnancy (O03.37, O03.87, O04.87, O07.37, O08.82)
sepsis following immunization (T88.0-)
sepsis following infusion, transfusion or therapeutic injection (T80.22-, T80.29-)

EXCLUDES 1 *bacteremia NOS (R78.81)*
*neonatal (P36.-)*
*puerperal sepsis (O85)*
*streptococcal sepsis (A40.-)*

EXCLUDES 2 *sepsis (due to) (in) actinomycotic (A42.7)*
*sepsis (due to) (in) anthrax (A22.7)*
*sepsis (due to) (in) candidal (B37.7)*
*sepsis (due to) (in) Erysipelothrix (A26.7)*
*sepsis (due to) (in) extraintestinal yersiniosis (A28.2)*
*sepsis (due to) (in) gonococcal (A54.86)*
*sepsis (due to) (in) herpesviral (B00.7)*
*sepsis (due to) (in) listerial (A32.7)*
*sepsis (due to) (in) melioidosis (A24.1)*
*sepsis (due to) (in) meningococcal (A39.2-A39.4)*
*sepsis (due to) (in) plague (A20.7)*
*sepsis (due to) (in) tularemia (A21.7)*
*toxic shock syndrome (A48.3)*

**AHA:** 2026,1Q,33; 2020,2Q,8,28; 2019,4Q,65; 2019,3Q,17; 2018,4Q,18; 2018,1Q,16; 2016,1Q,32; 2014,2Q,13

✓5th **A41.0 Sepsis due to Staphylococcus aureus**

**A41.01 Sepsis due to Methicillin susceptible Staphylococcus aureus** HCC ESR COM
MSSA sepsis
Staphylococcus aureus sepsis NOS
**AHA:** 2020,2Q,17

**A41.02 Sepsis due to Methicillin resistant Staphylococcus aureus** HCC ESR COM

**A41.1 Sepsis due to other specified staphylococcus** HCC ESR COM
Coagulase negative staphylococcus sepsis
**AHA:** 2024,1Q,19

**A41.2 Sepsis due to unspecified staphylococcus** HCC ESR COM

**A41.3 Sepsis due to Hemophilus influenzae** HCC ESR COM

**A41.4 Sepsis due to anaerobes** HCC ESR COM
EXCLUDES 1 *gas gangrene (A48.0)*

✓5th **A41.5 Sepsis due to other Gram-negative organisms**

**A41.50 Gram-negative sepsis, unspecified** HCC ESR COM
Gram-negative sepsis NOS
**AHA:** 2020,2Q,28

**A41.51 Sepsis due to Escherichia coli [E. coli]** HCC ESR COM
**AHA:** 2020,2Q,17

**A41.52 Sepsis due to Pseudomonas** HCC ESR COM
Pseudomonas aeruginosa

**A41.53 Sepsis due to Serratia** HCC ESR COM

**A41.54 Sepsis due to Acinetobacter baumannii** HCC ESR COM
**AHA:** 2023,4Q,4

**A41.59 Other Gram-negative sepsis** HCC ESR COM
**AHA:** 2026,2Q,5

✓5th **A41.8 Other specified sepsis**

**A41.81 Sepsis due to Enterococcus** HCC ESR COM
**TIP:** *E. faecium,* is a species of *Enterococcus* that is highly resistant to multiple antibiotics. Assign a code from category Z16 when resistance to antimicrobial drugs is documented.

**A41.89 Other specified sepsis** HCC ESR COM
**AHA:** 2020,2Q,8; 2017,1Q,51; 2016,3Q,8-14

**A41.9 Sepsis, unspecified organism** HCC ESR COM
Septicemia NOS
**AHA:** 2022,2Q,5; 2022,1Q,35; 2020,2Q,28

✓4th **A42 Actinomycosis**

EXCLUDES 1 *actinomycetoma (B47.1)*

**A42.0 Pulmonary actinomycosis** ESR

**A42.1 Abdominal actinomycosis**

**A42.2 Cervicofacial actinomycosis**

**A42.7 Actinomycotic sepsis** HCC ESR COM

✓5th **A42.8 Other forms of actinomycosis**

**A42.81 Actinomycotic meningitis** COM

**A42.82 Actinomycotic encephalitis** COM

**A42.89 Other forms of actinomycosis**

**A42.9 Actinomycosis, unspecified**

✓4th **A43 Nocardiosis**

**DEF:** Rare bacterial infection occurring most often in those with weakened immune systems. Can be acquired in soil, decaying plants, or standing water. It typically begins in the lungs and has a tendency to spread to other body systems.

**A43.0 Pulmonary nocardiosis** ESR

**A43.1 Cutaneous nocardiosis**

**A43.8 Other forms of nocardiosis**

**A43.9 Nocardiosis, unspecified**

✓4th **A44 Bartonellosis**

**A44.0 Systemic bartonellosis**
Oroya fever

**A44.1 Cutaneous and mucocutaneous bartonellosis**
Verruga peruana

**A44.8 Other forms of bartonellosis**

**A44.9 Bartonellosis, unspecified**

**A46 Erysipelas**

EXCLUDES 1 *postpartum or puerperal erysipelas (O86.89)*

**DEF:** Skin infection affecting the upper dermis and superficial dermal lymphatics. Lesion edges are well-demarcated with distinct raised borders. It is often caused by group A *Streptococci.*

✓4th **A48 Other bacterial diseases, not elsewhere classified**

EXCLUDES 1 *actinomycetoma (B47.1)*

**A48.0 Gas gangrene** HCC ESR COM
Clostridial cellulitis
Clostridial myonecrosis
**AHA:** 2017,4Q,102

**A48.1 Legionnaires' disease** HCC ESR COM
**DEF:** Severe and often fatal infection by *Legionella pneumophila.* Symptoms include high fever, gastrointestinal pain, headache, myalgia, dry cough, and pneumonia and it is usually transmitted through airborne water droplets via air conditioning systems or hot tubs.

**A48.2 Nonpneumonic Legionnaires' disease [Pontiac fever]**

**A48.3 Toxic shock syndrome** HCC ESR COM
Use additional code to identify the organism (B95, B96)
EXCLUDES 1 *endotoxic shock NOS (R57.8)*
*sepsis NOS (A41.9)*
**AHA:** 2022,1Q,35
**DEF:** Bacteria producing an endotoxin, such as *Staphylococci,* flood the body with the toxins producing a high fever, vomiting and diarrhea, decreasing blood pressure, a skin rash, and shock.
***Synonym(s):*** *TSS.*

**A48.4 Brazilian purpuric fever**
Systemic Hemophilus aegyptius infection

✓5th **A48.5 Other specified botulism**
Non-foodborne intoxication due to toxins of Clostridium botulinum [C. botulinum]
EXCLUDES 1 *food poisoning due to toxins of Clostridium botulinum (A05.1)*

**A48.51 Infant botulism** P

**A48.52 Wound botulism**
Non-foodborne botulism NOS
Use additional code for associated wound

**A48.8 Other specified bacterial diseases**

✓4th **A49 Bacterial infection of unspecified site**

EXCLUDES 1 *bacterial agents as the cause of diseases classified elsewhere (B95-B96)*
~~*chlamydial infection NOS (A74.9)*~~
*meningococcal infection NOS (A39.9)*
*rickettsial infection NOS (A79.9)*
*spirochetal infection NOS (A69.9)*

EXCLUDES 2 ▶*chlamydial infection NOS (A74.9)*◀

✓5th **A49.0 Staphylococcal infection, unspecified site**

**A49.01 Methicillin susceptible Staphylococcus aureus infection, unspecified site**
Methicillin susceptible Staphylococcus aureus (MSSA) infection
Staphylococcus aureus infection NOS

A49.Ø2 **Methicillin resistant Staphylococcus aureus infection, unspecified site**
Methicillin resistant Staphylococcus aureus (MRSA) infection

A49.1 **Streptococcal infection, unspecified site**

A49.2 **Hemophilus influenzae infection, unspecified site**

A49.3 **Mycoplasma infection, unspecified site**

A49.8 **Other bacterial infections of unspecified site**

A49.9 **Bacterial infection, unspecified**
EXCLUDES 1 *bacteremia NOS (R78.81)*

## Infections with a predominantly sexual mode of transmission (A5Ø-A64)

EXCLUDES 1 *nonspecific and nongonococcal urethritis (N34.1)*
*Reiter's disease (MØ2.3-)*
EXCLUDES 2 *human immunodeficiency virus [HIV] disease (B2Ø)*
AHA: 2021,2Q,6

✓4th **A5Ø Congenital syphilis**

✓5th **A5Ø.Ø Early congenital syphilis, symptomatic**
Any congenital syphilitic condition specified as early or manifest less than two years after birth.
- A5Ø.Ø1 **Early congenital syphilitic oculopathy**
- A5Ø.Ø2 **Early congenital syphilitic osteochondropathy**
- A5Ø.Ø3 **Early congenital syphilitic pharyngitis**
  Early congenital syphilitic laryngitis
- A5Ø.Ø4 **Early congenital syphilitic pneumonia** COM
- A5Ø.Ø5 **Early congenital syphilitic rhinitis**
- A5Ø.Ø6 **Early cutaneous congenital syphilis**
- A5Ø.Ø7 **Early mucocutaneous congenital syphilis**
- A5Ø.Ø8 **Early visceral congenital syphilis**
- A5Ø.Ø9 **Other early congenital syphilis, symptomatic**

**A5Ø.1 Early congenital syphilis, latent**
Congenital syphilis without clinical manifestations, with positive serological reaction and negative spinal fluid test, less than two years after birth.

**A5Ø.2 Early congenital syphilis, unspecified**
Congenital syphilis NOS less than two years after birth.

✓5th **A5Ø.3 Late congenital syphilitic oculopathy**
EXCLUDES 1 *Hutchinson's triad (A5Ø.53)*
- A5Ø.3Ø **Late congenital syphilitic oculopathy, unspecified**
- A5Ø.31 **Late congenital syphilitic interstitial keratitis**
- A5Ø.32 **Late congenital syphilitic chorioretinitis**
- A5Ø.39 **Other late congenital syphilitic oculopathy**

✓5th **A5Ø.4 Late congenital neurosyphilis [juvenile neurosyphilis]**
Use additional code to identify any associated mental disorder
EXCLUDES 1 *Hutchinson's triad (A5Ø.53)*
- A5Ø.4Ø **Late congenital neurosyphilis, unspecified** COM
  Juvenile neurosyphilis NOS
- A5Ø.41 **Late congenital syphilitic meningitis** COM
- A5Ø.42 **Late congenital syphilitic encephalitis** COM
- A5Ø.43 **Late congenital syphilitic polyneuropathy** COM
- A5Ø.44 **Late congenital syphilitic optic nerve atrophy** COM
- A5Ø.45 **Juvenile general paresis** COM
  Dementia paralytica juvenilis
  Juvenile taboparetic neurosyphilis
- A5Ø.49 **Other late congenital neurosyphilis** COM
  Juvenile tabes dorsalis

✓5th **A5Ø.5 Other late congenital syphilis, symptomatic**
Any congenital syphilitic condition specified as late or manifest two years or more after birth.
- A5Ø.51 **Clutton's joints**
- A5Ø.52 **Hutchinson's teeth**
- A5Ø.53 **Hutchinson's triad**
- A5Ø.54 **Late congenital cardiovascular syphilis** COM
- A5Ø.55 **Late congenital syphilitic arthropathy** HCC ESR COM
- A5Ø.56 **Late congenital syphilitic osteochondropathy**
- A5Ø.57 **Syphilitic saddle nose**
- A5Ø.59 **Other late congenital syphilis, symptomatic**

**A5Ø.6 Late congenital syphilis, latent**
Congenital syphilis without clinical manifestations, with positive serological reaction and negative spinal fluid test, two years or more after birth.

**A5Ø.7 Late congenital syphilis, unspecified**
Congenital syphilis NOS two years or more after birth.

**A5Ø.9 Congenital syphilis, unspecified**

✓4th **A51 Early syphilis**
DEF: Syphilis: Sexually transmitted disease caused by the *Treponema pallidum* spirochete. Syphilis usually exhibits cutaneous manifestations and may exist for years without symptoms.

**A51.Ø Primary genital syphilis**
Syphilitic chancre NOS

**A51.1 Primary anal syphilis**

**A51.2 Primary syphilis of other sites**

✓5th **A51.3 Secondary syphilis of skin and mucous membranes**
DEF: Transitory or chronic cutaneous eruptions that present within two to 10 weeks following an initial syphilis infection that may include nontender lymphadenopathy along with alopecia and condylomata lata.
- A51.31 **Condyloma latum**
- A51.32 **Syphilitic alopecia**
- A51.39 **Other secondary syphilis of skin**
  Syphilitic leukoderma
  Syphilitic mucous patch
  EXCLUDES 1 *late syphilitic leukoderma (A52.79)*

✓5th **A51.4 Other secondary syphilis**
- A51.41 **Secondary syphilitic meningitis** COM
- A51.42 **Secondary syphilitic female pelvic disease**
- A51.43 **Secondary syphilitic oculopathy**
  Secondary syphilitic chorioretinitis
  Secondary syphilitic iridocyclitis, iritis
  Secondary syphilitic uveitis
- A51.44 **Secondary syphilitic nephritis**
- A51.45 **Secondary syphilitic hepatitis**
- A51.46 **Secondary syphilitic osteopathy**
- A51.49 **Other secondary syphilitic conditions**
  Secondary syphilitic lymphadenopathy
  Secondary syphilitic myositis

**A51.5 Early syphilis, latent**
Syphilis (acquired) without clinical manifestations, with positive serological reaction and negative spinal fluid test, less than two years after infection.

**A51.9 Early syphilis, unspecified**

✓4th **A52 Late syphilis**

✓5th **A52.Ø Cardiovascular and cerebrovascular syphilis**
- A52.ØØ **Cardiovascular syphilis, unspecified** COM
- A52.Ø1 **Syphilitic aneurysm of aorta** COM
- A52.Ø2 **Syphilitic aortitis** COM
- A52.Ø3 **Syphilitic endocarditis** COM
  Syphilitic aortic valve incompetence or stenosis
  Syphilitic mitral valve stenosis
  Syphilitic pulmonary valve regurgitation
- A52.Ø4 **Syphilitic cerebral arteritis**
- A52.Ø5 **Other cerebrovascular syphilis** COM
  Syphilitic cerebral aneurysm (ruptured) (non-ruptured)
  Syphilitic cerebral thrombosis
- A52.Ø6 **Other syphilitic heart involvement** COM
  Syphilitic coronary artery disease
  Syphilitic myocarditis
  Syphilitic pericarditis
- A52.Ø9 **Other cardiovascular syphilis** COM

✓5th **A52.1 Symptomatic neurosyphilis**
- A52.1Ø **Symptomatic neurosyphilis, unspecified** COM
- A52.11 **Tabes dorsalis** COM
  Locomotor ataxia (progressive)
  Tabetic neurosyphilis
- A52.12 **Other cerebrospinal syphilis** COM
- A52.13 **Late syphilitic meningitis** COM
- A52.14 **Late syphilitic encephalitis** COM
- A52.15 **Late syphilitic neuropathy** COM
  Late syphilitic acoustic neuritis
  Late syphilitic optic (nerve) atrophy
  Late syphilitic polyneuropathy
  Late syphilitic retrobulbar neuritis
- A52.16 **Charcôt's arthropathy (tabetic)** COM
  DEF: Progressive neurologic arthropathy in which chronic degeneration of joints in the weight-bearing areas with peripheral hypertrophy occurs as a complication of a neuropathy disorder. Supporting structures relax from a loss of sensation resulting in chronic joint instability.

A52.17 General paresis COM
Dementia paralytica

A52.19 Other symptomatic neurosyphilis COM
Syphilitic parkinsonism

A52.2 Asymptomatic neurosyphilis COM

A52.3 Neurosyphilis, unspecified COM
Gumma (syphilitic)
Syphilis (late)
Syphiloma
AHA: 2021,2Q,6

✓5th A52.7 Other symptomatic late syphilis

A52.71 Late syphilitic oculopathy
Late syphilitic chorioretinitis
Late syphilitic episcleritis

A52.72 Syphilis of lung and bronchus

A52.73 Symptomatic late syphilis of other respiratory organs

A52.74 Syphilis of liver and other viscera
Late syphilitic peritonitis

A52.75 Syphilis of kidney and ureter
Syphilitic glomerular disease

A52.76 Other genitourinary symptomatic late syphilis
Late syphilitic female pelvic inflammatory disease

A52.77 Syphilis of bone and joint

A52.78 Syphilis of other musculoskeletal tissue
Late syphilitic bursitis
Syphilis [stage unspecified] of bursa
Syphilis [stage unspecified] of muscle
Syphilis [stage unspecified] of synovium
Syphilis [stage unspecified] of tendon

A52.79 Other symptomatic late syphilis
Late syphilitic leukoderma
Syphilis of adrenal gland
Syphilis of pituitary gland
Syphilis of thyroid gland
Syphilitic splenomegaly
EXCLUDES 1 *syphilitic leukoderma (secondary) (A51.39)*

A52.8 Late syphilis, latent
Syphilis (acquired) without clinical manifestations, with positive serological reaction and negative spinal fluid test, two years or more after infection

A52.9 Late syphilis, unspecified

✓4th A53 Other and unspecified syphilis

A53.Ø Latent syphilis, unspecified as early or late
Latent syphilis NOS
Positive serological reaction for syphilis

A53.9 Syphilis, unspecified
Infection due to Treponema pallidum NOS
Syphilis (acquired) NOS
EXCLUDES 1 *syphilis NOS under two years of age (A5Ø.2)*

✓4th A54 Gonococcal infection

**DEF:** Sexually transmitted bacterial infection caused by *Neisseria gonorrhoeae*. Women are often asymptomatic, while men tend to develop urinary symptoms quickly.

✓5th A54.Ø Gonococcal infection of lower genitourinary tract without periurethral or accessory gland abscess
EXCLUDES 1 *gonococcal infection with genitourinary gland abscess (A54.1)*
*gonococcal infection with periurethral abscess (A54.1)*

A54.ØØ Gonococcal infection of lower genitourinary tract, unspecified

A54.Ø1 Gonococcal cystitis and urethritis, unspecified

A54.Ø2 Gonococcal vulvovaginitis, unspecified

A54.Ø3 Gonococcal cervicitis, unspecified

A54.Ø9 Other gonococcal infection of lower genitourinary tract

A54.1 Gonococcal infection of lower genitourinary tract with periurethral and accessory gland abscess
Gonococcal Bartholin's gland abscess

✓5th A54.2 Gonococcal pelviperitonitis and other gonococcal genitourinary infection

A54.21 Gonococcal infection of kidney and ureter

A54.22 Gonococcal prostatitis

A54.23 Gonococcal infection of other male genital organs
Gonococcal epididymitis
Gonococcal orchitis

A54.24 Gonococcal female pelvic inflammatory disease
Gonococcal pelviperitonitis
EXCLUDES 1 *gonococcal peritonitis (A54.85)*

A54.29 Other gonococcal genitourinary infections

✓5th A54.3 Gonococcal infection of eye

A54.3Ø Gonococcal infection of eye, unspecified

A54.31 Gonococcal conjunctivitis
Ophthalmia neonatorum due to gonococcus

A54.32 Gonococcal iridocyclitis

A54.33 Gonococcal keratitis

A54.39 Other gonococcal eye infection
Gonococcal endophthalmia

✓5th A54.4 Gonococcal infection of musculoskeletal system

A54.4Ø Gonococcal infection of musculoskeletal system, unspecified HCC ESR COM

A54.41 Gonococcal spondylopathy HCC ESR COM

A54.42 Gonococcal arthritis HCC ESR COM
EXCLUDES 2 *gonococcal infection of spine (A54.41)*

A54.43 Gonococcal osteomyelitis HCC ESR COM
EXCLUDES 2 *gonococcal infection of spine (A54.41)*

A54.49 Gonococcal infection of other musculoskeletal tissue HCC ESR COM
Gonococcal bursitis
Gonococcal myositis
Gonococcal synovitis
Gonococcal tenosynovitis

A54.5 Gonococcal pharyngitis

A54.6 Gonococcal infection of anus and rectum

✓5th A54.8 Other gonococcal infections

A54.81 Gonococcal meningitis COM

A54.82 Gonococcal brain abscess COM

A54.83 Gonococcal heart infection COM
Gonococcal endocarditis
Gonococcal myocarditis
Gonococcal pericarditis

A54.84 Gonococcal pneumonia ESR

A54.85 Gonococcal peritonitis HCC ESR COM
EXCLUDES 1 *gonococcal pelviperitonitis (A54.24)*

A54.86 Gonococcal sepsis HCC ESR COM

A54.89 Other gonococcal infections
Gonococcal keratoderma
Gonococcal lymphadenitis

A54.9 Gonococcal infection, unspecified

A55 Chlamydial lymphogranuloma (venereum)
Climatic or tropical bubo
Durand-Nicolas-Favre disease
Esthiomene
Lymphogranuloma inguinale

✓4th A56 Other sexually transmitted chlamydial diseases
INCLUDES sexually transmitted diseases due to Chlamydia trachomatis
EXCLUDES 1 *neonatal chlamydial conjunctivitis (P39.1)*
*neonatal chlamydial pneumonia (P23.1)*
EXCLUDES 2 *chlamydial lymphogranuloma (A55)*
*conditions classified to A74.-*

**DEF:** *Chlamydia trachomatis*: Bacterium that causes a common venereal disease. Symptoms of chlamydia are usually mild or absent, however, serious complications may cause irreversible damage, including cystitis, pelvic inflammatory disease, and infertility in women and discharge from the penis, prostatitis, and infertility in men. Genital chlamydial infection can cause arthritis, skin lesions, and inflammation of the eye and urethra.
***Synonym(s):*** *Reiter's syndrome.*

✓5th A56.Ø Chlamydial infection of lower genitourinary tract

A56.ØØ Chlamydial infection of lower genitourinary tract, unspecified

A56.Ø1 Chlamydial cystitis and urethritis

A56.Ø2 Chlamydial vulvovaginitis

A56.Ø9 Other chlamydial infection of lower genitourinary tract
Chlamydial cervicitis

✓5th A56.1 Chlamydial infection of pelviperitoneum and other genitourinary organs

A56.11 Chlamydial female pelvic inflammatory disease

A56.19 Other chlamydial genitourinary infection
Chlamydial epididymitis
Chlamydial orchitis

A56.2 Chlamydial infection of genitourinary tract, unspecified

A56.3 Chlamydial infection of anus and rectum

A56.4 Chlamydial infection of pharynx

A56.8 Sexually transmitted chlamydial infection of other sites

**A57 Chancroid**
Ulcus molle
**DEF:** Localized infection by *Haemophilus ducreyi*, causing genital ulcers and infecting the inguinal lymph nodes.

**A58 Granuloma inguinale**
Donovanosis

✓4th **A59 Trichomoniasis**
EXCLUDES 2 *intestinal trichomoniasis (AØ7.8)*
**DEF:** Infection with the parasitic, flagellated protozoa of the genus *Trichomonas*. This protozoon is found in the intestinal and genitourinary tracts of humans and in the mouth around tartar, cavities, and areas of periodontal disease.

✓5th **A59.Ø Urogenital trichomoniasis**
**A59.ØØ Urogenital trichomoniasis, unspecified**
Fluor (vaginalis) due to Trichomonas
Leukorrhea (vaginalis) due to Trichomonas
**A59.Ø1 Trichomonal vulvovaginitis**
**A59.Ø2 Trichomonal prostatitis**
**A59.Ø3 Trichomonal cystitis and urethritis**
**A59.Ø9 Other urogenital trichomoniasis**
Trichomonas cervicitis
**A59.8 Trichomoniasis of other sites**
**A59.9 Trichomoniasis, unspecified**

✓4th **A6Ø Anogenital herpesviral [herpes simplex] infections**
✓5th **A6Ø.Ø Herpesviral infection of genitalia and urogenital tract**
**A6Ø.ØØ Herpesviral infection of urogenital system, unspecified**
**A6Ø.Ø1 Herpesviral infection of penis**
**A6Ø.Ø2 Herpesviral infection of other male genital organs**
**A6Ø.Ø3 Herpesviral cervicitis**
**A6Ø.Ø4 Herpesviral vulvovaginitis**
Herpesviral [herpes simplex] ulceration
Herpesviral [herpes simplex] vaginitis
Herpesviral [herpes simplex] vulvitis
**A6Ø.Ø9 Herpesviral infection of other urogenital tract**
**AHA:** 2020,1Q,20
**A6Ø.1 Herpesviral infection of perianal skin and rectum**
**A6Ø.9 Anogenital herpesviral infection, unspecified**

✓4th **A63 Other predominantly sexually transmitted diseases, not elsewhere classified**
EXCLUDES 2 *molluscum contagiosum (BØ8.1)*
*papilloma of cervix (D26.Ø)*
**A63.Ø Anogenital (venereal) warts**
Anogenital warts due to (human) papillomavirus [HPV]
Condyloma acuminatum
**A63.8 Other specified predominantly sexually transmitted diseases**

**A64 Unspecified sexually transmitted disease**

## Other spirochetal diseases (A65-A69)

EXCLUDES 2 *leptospirosis (A27.-)*
*syphilis (A5Ø-A53)*

**A65 Nonvenereal syphilis**
Bejel
Endemic syphilis
Njovera

✓4th **A66 Yaws**
INCLUDES bouba
frambesia (tropica)
pian
**A66.Ø Initial lesions of yaws**
Chancre of yaws
Frambesia, initial or primary
Initial frambesial ulcer
Mother yaw
**A66.1 Multiple papillomata and wet crab yaws**
Frambesioma
Pianoma
Plantar or palmar papilloma of yaws
**A66.2 Other early skin lesions of yaws**
Cutaneous yaws, less than five years after infection
Early yaws (cutaneous) (macular) (maculopapular) (micropapular) (papular)
Frambeside of early yaws
**A66.3 Hyperkeratosis of yaws**
Ghoul hand
Hyperkeratosis, palmar or plantar (early) (late) due to yaws
Worm-eaten soles
**A66.4 Gummata and ulcers of yaws**
Gummatous frambeside
Nodular late yaws (ulcerated)
**A66.5 Gangosa**
Rhinopharyngitis mutilans
**A66.6 Bone and joint lesions of yaws** HCC ESR COM
Yaws ganglion
Yaws goundou
Yaws gumma, bone
Yaws gummatous osteitis or periostitis
Yaws hydrarthrosis
Yaws osteitis
Yaws periostitis (hypertrophic)
**A66.7 Other manifestations of yaws**
Juxta-articular nodules of yaws
Mucosal yaws
**A66.8 Latent yaws**
Yaws without clinical manifestations, with positive serology
**A66.9 Yaws, unspecified**

✓4th **A67 Pinta [carate]**
**A67.Ø Primary lesions of pinta**
Chancre (primary) of pinta
Papule (primary) of pinta
**A67.1 Intermediate lesions of pinta**
Erythematous plaques of pinta
Hyperchromic lesions of pinta
Hyperkeratosis of pinta
Pintids
**A67.2 Late lesions of pinta**
Achromic skin lesions of pinta
Cicatricial skin lesions of pinta
Dyschromic skin lesions of pinta
**A67.3 Mixed lesions of pinta**
Achromic with hyperchromic skin lesions of pinta [carate]
**A67.9 Pinta, unspecified**

✓4th **A68 Relapsing fevers**
INCLUDES recurrent fever
EXCLUDES 2 *Lyme disease (A69.2-)*
**A68.Ø Louse-borne relapsing fever**
Relapsing fever due to Borrelia recurrentis
**A68.1 Tick-borne relapsing fever**
Relapsing fever due to any Borrelia species other than Borrelia recurrentis
**A68.9 Relapsing fever, unspecified**

✓4th **A69 Other spirochetal infections**
**A69.Ø Necrotizing ulcerative stomatitis**
Cancrum oris
Fusospirochetal gangrene
Noma
Stomatitis gangrenosa
**A69.1 Other Vincent's infections**
Fusospirochetal pharyngitis
Necrotizing ulcerative (acute) gingivitis
Necrotizing ulcerative (acute) gingivostomatitis
Spirochetal stomatitis
Trench mouth
Vincent's angina
Vincent's gingivitis
✓5th **A69.2 Lyme disease**
Erythema chronicum migrans due to Borrelia burgdorferi
**DEF:** Recurrent multisystem disorder through tick bites that begins with lesions of erythema chronicum migrans and is followed by arthritis of the large joints, myalgia, malaise, and neurological and cardiac manifestations.
**A69.2Ø Lyme disease, unspecified**
**AHA:** 2021,4Q,5
**A69.21 Meningitis due to Lyme disease** COM
**A69.22 Other neurologic disorders in Lyme disease**
Cranial neuritis
Meningoencephalitis
Polyneuropathy
**A69.23 Arthritis due to Lyme disease** HCC ESR COM
**A69.29 Other conditions associated with Lyme disease**
Myopericarditis due to Lyme disease
**AHA:** 2016,3Q,12
**A69.8 Other specified spirochetal infections**
**A69.9 Spirochetal infection, unspecified**

## Other diseases caused by chlamydiae (A7Ø-A74)

EXCLUDES 1 *sexually transmitted chlamydial diseases (A55-A56)*

**A7Ø Chlamydia psittaci infections**
Ornithosis
Parrot fever
Psittacosis

✓4th **A71 Trachoma**
EXCLUDES 1 *sequelae of trachoma (B94.Ø)*

**A71.Ø Initial stage of trachoma**
Trachoma dubium

**A71.1 Active stage of trachoma**
Granular conjunctivitis (trachomatous)
Trachomatous follicular conjunctivitis
Trachomatous pannus

**A71.9 Trachoma, unspecified**

✓4th **A74 Other diseases caused by chlamydiae**
EXCLUDES 1 *neonatal chlamydial conjunctivitis (P39.1)*
*neonatal chlamydial pneumonia (P23.1)*
*Reiter's disease (MØ2.3-)*
*sexually transmitted chlamydial diseases (A55-A56)*
EXCLUDES 2 *chlamydial pneumonia (J16.Ø)*

**A74.Ø Chlamydial conjunctivitis**
Paratrachoma

✓5th **A74.8 Other chlamydial diseases**
**A74.81 Chlamydial peritonitis**
**A74.89 Other chlamydial diseases**

**A74.9 Chlamydial infection, unspecified**
Chlamydiosis NOS

## Rickettsioses (A75-A79)

**DEF:** Rickettsia: Condition caused by bacteria that live in lice/ticks transmitted to humans through bites.

✓4th **A75 Typhus fever**
EXCLUDES 1 *rickettsiosis due to Ehrlichia sennetsu (A79.81)*

**A75.Ø Epidemic louse-borne typhus fever due to Rickettsia prowazekii**
Classical typhus (fever)
Epidemic (louse-borne) typhus

**A75.1 Recrudescent typhus [Brill's disease]**
Brill-Zinsser disease

**A75.2 Typhus fever due to Rickettsia typhi**
Murine (flea-borne) typhus

**A75.3 Typhus fever due to Rickettsia tsutsugamushi**
Scrub (mite-borne) typhus
Tsutsugamushi fever
Typhus fever due to Orientia Tsutsugamushi (scrub typhus)

**A75.9 Typhus fever, unspecified**
Typhus (fever) NOS

✓4th **A77 Spotted fever [tick-borne rickettsioses]**

**A77.Ø Spotted fever due to Rickettsia rickettsii**
Rocky Mountain spotted fever
Sao Paulo fever

**A77.1 Spotted fever due to Rickettsia conorii**
African tick typhus
Boutonneuse fever
India tick typhus
Kenya tick typhus
Marseilles fever
Mediterranean tick fever

**A77.2 Spotted fever due to Rickettsia siberica**
North Asian tick fever
Siberian tick typhus

**A77.3 Spotted fever due to Rickettsia australis**
Queensland tick typhus

✓5th **A77.4 Ehrlichiosis**
EXCLUDES 1 *anaplasmosis [A. phagocytophilum] (A79.82)*
*rickettsiosis due to Ehrlichia sennetsu (A79.81)*
**AHA:** 2021,4Q,5

**A77.4Ø Ehrlichiosis, unspecified**
**A77.41 Ehrlichiosis chaffeensis [E. chaffeensis]**
**A77.49 Other ehrlichiosis**
Ehrlichiosis due to E. ewingii
Ehrlichiosis due to E. muris euclairensis

**A77.8 Other spotted fevers**
Rickettsia 364D/R. philipii (Pacific Coast tick fever)
Spotted fever due to Rickettsia africae (African tick bite fever)
Spotted fever due to Rickettsia parkeri

**A77.9 Spotted fever, unspecified**
Tick-borne typhus NOS

**A78 Q fever**
Infection due to Coxiella burnetii
Nine Mile fever
Quadrilateral fever

✓4th **A79 Other rickettsioses**

**A79.Ø Trench fever**
Quintan fever
Wolhynian fever

**A79.1 Rickettsialpox due to Rickettsia akari**
Kew Garden fever
Vesicular rickettsiosis

✓5th **A79.8 Other specified rickettsioses**
**A79.81 Rickettsiosis due to Ehrlichia sennetsu**
Rickettsiosis due to Neorickettsia sennetsu
**A79.82 Anaplasmosis [A. phagocytophilum]**
Transfusion transmitted A. phagocytophilum
**AHA:** 2021,4Q,4-5
**A79.89 Other specified rickettsioses**

**A79.9 Rickettsiosis, unspecified**
Rickettsial infection NOS

## Viral and prion infections of the central nervous system (A8Ø-A89)

EXCLUDES 1 *postpolio syndrome (G14)*
*sequelae of poliomyelitis (B91)*
*sequelae of viral encephalitis (B94.1)*

✓4th **A8Ø Acute poliomyelitis**
EXCLUDES 1 *acute flaccid myelitis (GØ4.82)*

**A8Ø.Ø Acute paralytic poliomyelitis, vaccine-associated** COM
**A8Ø.1 Acute paralytic poliomyelitis, wild virus, imported** COM
**A8Ø.2 Acute paralytic poliomyelitis, wild virus, indigenous** COM
✓5th **A8Ø.3 Acute paralytic poliomyelitis, other and unspecified**
**A8Ø.3Ø Acute paralytic poliomyelitis, unspecified** COM
**A8Ø.39 Other acute paralytic poliomyelitis** COM
**A8Ø.4 Acute nonparalytic poliomyelitis** COM
**A8Ø.9 Acute poliomyelitis, unspecified** COM

✓4th **A81 Atypical virus infections of central nervous system**
INCLUDES diseases of the central nervous system caused by prions
Use additional code, if applicable, to identify:
dementia with anxiety (FØ2.84, FØ2.A4, FØ2.B4, FØ2.C4)
dementia with behavioral disturbance (FØ2.81-, FØ2.A1-, FØ2.B1-, FØ2.C1-)
dementia with mood disturbance (FØ2.83, FØ2.A3, FØ2.B3, FØ2.C3)
dementia with psychotic disturbance (FØ2.82, FØ2.A2, FØ2.B2, FØ2.C2)
dementia without behavioral disturbance (FØ2.8Ø, FØ2.AØ, FØ2.BØ, FØ2.CØ)
mild neurocognitive disorder due to known physiological condition (FØ6.7-)

✓5th **A81.Ø Creutzfeldt-Jakob disease**
**DEF:** Communicable, rare spongiform encephalopathy occurring later in life with progressive destruction of the pyramidal and extrapyramidal systems eventually leading to death. Progressive dementia, wasting of muscles, tremor, and other symptoms are present.

**A81.ØØ Creutzfeldt-Jakob disease, unspecified** HCC Rx ESR
Jakob-Creutzfeldt disease, unspecified
**A81.Ø1 Variant Creutzfeldt-Jakob disease** HCC Rx ESR
vCJD
**A81.Ø9 Other Creutzfeldt-Jakob disease** HCC Rx ESR
CJD
Familial Creutzfeldt-Jakob disease
Iatrogenic Creutzfeldt-Jakob disease
Sporadic Creutzfeldt-Jakob disease
Subacute spongiform encephalopathy (with dementia)

**A81.1 Subacute sclerosing panencephalitis** HCC Rx ESR
Dawson's inclusion body encephalitis
Van Bogaert's sclerosing leukoencephalopathy

**A81.2 Progressive multifocal leukoencephalopathy** HCC Rx ESR
Multifocal leukoencephalopathy NOS

✓5th **A81.8 Other atypical virus infections of central nervous system**
**A81.81 Kuru** HCC Rx ESR

A81.82 **Gerstmann-Straussler-Scheinker syndrome** HCC Rx ESR
GSS syndrome

A81.83 **Fatal familial insomnia** HCC Rx ESR
FFI

A81.89 **Other atypical virus infections of central nervous system** HCC Rx ESR

A81.9 **Atypical virus infection of central nervous system, unspecified** HCC Rx ESR
Prion diseases of the central nervous system NOS

✓4th **A82 Rabies**

A82.Ø **Sylvatic rabies** COM

A82.1 **Urban rabies** COM

A82.9 **Rabies, unspecified** COM

✓4th **A83 Mosquito-borne viral encephalitis**

INCLUDES mosquito-borne viral meningoencephalitis

EXCLUDES 2 *Venezuelan equine encephalitis (A92.2)*
*West Nile fever (A92.3-)*
*West Nile virus (A92.3-)*

A83.Ø **Japanese encephalitis** COM

A83.1 **Western equine encephalitis** COM

A83.2 **Eastern equine encephalitis** COM

A83.3 **St Louis encephalitis** COM

A83.4 **Australian encephalitis** COM
Kunjin virus disease

A83.5 **California encephalitis** COM
California meningoencephalitis
La Crosse encephalitis

A83.6 **Rocio virus disease** COM

A83.8 **Other mosquito-borne viral encephalitis** COM

A83.9 **Mosquito-borne viral encephalitis, unspecified** COM

✓4th **A84 Tick-borne viral encephalitis**

INCLUDES tick-borne viral meningoencephalitis

A84.Ø **Far Eastern tick-borne encephalitis [Russian spring-summer encephalitis]** COM

A84.1 **Central European tick-borne encephalitis** COM

✓5th **A84.8 Other tick-borne viral encephalitis**

**AHA:** 2020,4Q,4-5

A84.81 **Powassan virus disease** COM

A84.89 **Other tick-borne viral encephalitis** COM
Louping ill
Code first, if applicable, transfusion related infection (T8Ø.22-)

A84.9 **Tick-borne viral encephalitis, unspecified** COM

✓4th **A85 Other viral encephalitis, not elsewhere classified**

INCLUDES specified viral encephalomyelitis NEC
specified viral meningoencephalitis NEC

EXCLUDES 1 *encephalitis due to cytomegalovirus (B25.8)*
*encephalitis due to herpesvirus [herpes simplex] (BØØ.4)*
*encephalitis due to herpesvirus NEC (B1Ø.Ø-)*
*encephalitis due to measles virus (BØ5.Ø)*
*encephalitis due to mumps virus (B26.2)*
*encephalitis due to poliomyelitis virus (A8Ø.-)*
*encephalitis due to zoster (BØ2.Ø)*
*lymphocytic choriomeningitis (A87.2)*
*myalgic encephalomyelitis (G93.32)*

A85.Ø **Enteroviral encephalitis** COM
Enteroviral encephalomyelitis

A85.1 **Adenoviral encephalitis** COM
Adenoviral meningoencephalitis

A85.2 **Arthropod-borne viral encephalitis, unspecified** COM

EXCLUDES 1 *West nile virus with encephalitis (A92.31)*

A85.8 **Other specified viral encephalitis** COM
Encephalitis lethargica
Von Economo-Cruchet disease

**A86 Unspecified viral encephalitis** COM
Viral encephalomyelitis NOS
Viral meningoencephalitis NOS

✓4th **A87 Viral meningitis**

EXCLUDES 1 *meningitis due to herpesvirus [herpes simplex] (BØØ.3)*
*meningitis due to measles virus (BØ5.1)*
*meningitis due to mumps virus (B26.1)*
*meningitis due to poliomyelitis virus (A8Ø.-)*
*meningitis due to zoster (BØ2.1)*

**DEF:** Meningitis: Inflammation of the meningeal layers of the brain and spine.

A87.Ø **Enteroviral meningitis** COM
Coxsackievirus meningitis
Echovirus meningitis

A87.1 **Adenoviral meningitis** COM

A87.2 **Lymphocytic choriomeningitis** COM
Lymphocytic meningoencephalitis

A87.8 **Other viral meningitis** COM

A87.9 **Viral meningitis, unspecified** COM

✓4th **A88 Other viral infections of central nervous system, not elsewhere classified**

EXCLUDES 1 *viral encephalitis NOS (A86)*
*viral meningitis NOS (A87.9)*

A88.Ø **Enteroviral exanthematous fever [Boston exanthem]** COM

A88.1 **Epidemic vertigo**

A88.8 **Other specified viral infections of central nervous system** COM

**A89 Unspecified viral infection of central nervous system** COM

## Arthropod-borne viral fevers and viral hemorrhagic fevers (A9Ø-A99)

**A9Ø Dengue fever [classical dengue]**

EXCLUDES 1 *dengue hemorrhagic fever (A91)*

**AHA:** 2016,3Q,13

**A91 Dengue hemorrhagic fever**

✓4th **A92 Other mosquito-borne viral fevers**

EXCLUDES 1 *Ross River disease (B33.1)*

A92.Ø **Chikungunya virus disease**
Chikungunya (hemorrhagic) fever

A92.1 **O'nyong-nyong fever**

A92.2 **Venezuelan equine fever** COM
Venezuelan equine encephalitis
Venezuelan equine encephalomyelitis virus disease

✓5th **A92.3 West Nile virus infection**
West Nile fever

**AHA:** 2016,3Q,12

A92.3Ø **West Nile virus infection, unspecified** COM
West Nile fever NOS
West Nile fever without complications
West Nile virus NOS

A92.31 **West Nile virus infection with encephalitis** COM
West Nile encephalitis
West Nile encephalomyelitis

A92.32 **West Nile virus infection with other neurologic manifestation** COM
Use additional code to specify the neurologic manifestation

A92.39 **West Nile virus infection with other complications** COM
Use additional code to specify the other conditions

A92.4 **Rift Valley fever**

A92.5 **Zika virus disease**
Zika NOS
Zika virus fever
Zika virus infection

EXCLUDES 1 *congenital Zika virus disease (P35.4)*

**AHA:** 2016,4Q,4-7

**DEF:** Virus transmitted via a bite from an infected Aedes species mosquito. Common symptoms of the virus include fever, rash, joint pain, and conjunctivitis; they are usually mild in nature and may last from several days to a week. Most people who have the Zika virus do not require medical attention; however, in pregnant women, the Zika virus can cause a serious birth defect called microcephaly, as well as other severe fetal brain defects.

**TIP:** Assign code Z71.1, when a patient requests testing for Zika virus but in the absence of symptoms or recent exposure to the virus.

**TIP:** Code only confirmed diagnoses of Zika virus; documentation by the physician that the disease is confirmed is sufficient.

A92.8 **Other specified mosquito-borne viral fevers**

**A92.9 Mosquito-borne viral fever, unspecified**

**4th A93 Other arthropod-borne viral fevers, not elsewhere classified**

**A93.0 Oropouche virus disease**
Oropouche fever

**A93.1 Sandfly fever**
Pappataci fever
Phlebotomus fever

**A93.2 Colorado tick fever**

**A93.8 Other specified arthropod-borne viral fevers**
Piry virus disease
Vesicular stomatitis virus disease [Indiana fever]

**A94 Unspecified arthropod-borne viral fever**
Arboviral fever NOS
Arbovirus infection NOS

**4th A95 Yellow fever**

**A95.0 Sylvatic yellow fever**
Jungle yellow fever

**A95.1 Urban yellow fever**

**A95.9 Yellow fever, unspecified**

**4th A96 Arenaviral hemorrhagic fever**

**A96.0 Junin hemorrhagic fever**
Argentinian hemorrhagic fever

**A96.1 Machupo hemorrhagic fever**
Bolivian hemorrhagic fever

**A96.2 Lassa fever**

**A96.8 Other arenaviral hemorrhagic fevers**

**A96.9 Arenaviral hemorrhagic fever, unspecified**

**4th A98 Other viral hemorrhagic fevers, not elsewhere classified**

EXCLUDES 1 *chikungunya hemorrhagic fever (A92.0)*
*dengue hemorrhagic fever (A91)*

**A98.0 Crimean-Congo hemorrhagic fever**
Central Asian hemorrhagic fever

**A98.1 Omsk hemorrhagic fever**

**A98.2 Kyasanur Forest disease**

**A98.3 Marburg virus disease**

**A98.4 Ebola virus disease**

**A98.5 Hemorrhagic fever with renal syndrome**
Epidemic hemorrhagic fever
Hantaan virus disease
Hantavirus disease with renal manifestations
Korean hemorrhagic fever
Nephropathia epidemica
Russian hemorrhagic fever
Songo fever
EXCLUDES 1 *hantavirus (cardio)-pulmonary syndrome (B33.4)*

**A98.8 Other specified viral hemorrhagic fevers**

**A99 Unspecified viral hemorrhagic fever**

## Viral infections characterized by skin and mucous membrane lesions (B00-B09)

**4th B00 Herpesviral [herpes simplex] infections**

EXCLUDES 1 *congenital herpesviral infections (P35.2)*
EXCLUDES 2 *anogenital herpesviral infection (A60.-)*
*gammaherpesviral mononucleosis (B27.0-)*
*herpangina (B08.5)*

**B00.0 Eczema herpeticum**
Kaposi's varicelliform eruption

**B00.1 Herpesviral vesicular dermatitis**
Herpes simplex facialis
Herpes simplex labialis
Herpes simplex otitis externa
Vesicular dermatitis of ear
Vesicular dermatitis of lip

**B00.2 Herpesviral gingivostomatitis and pharyngotonsillitis**
Herpesviral pharyngitis

**B00.3 Herpesviral meningitis** COM

**B00.4 Herpesviral encephalitis** COM
Herpesviral meningoencephalitis
Simian B disease
EXCLUDES 1 *herpesviral encephalitis due to herpesvirus 6 and 7 (B10.01, B10.09)*
*non-simplex herpesviral encephalitis (B10.0-)*

**5th B00.5 Herpesviral ocular disease**

**B00.50 Herpesviral ocular disease, unspecified**

**B00.51 Herpesviral iridocyclitis**
Herpesviral iritis
Herpesviral uveitis, anterior

**B00.52 Herpesviral keratitis**
Herpesviral keratoconjunctivitis

**B00.53 Herpesviral conjunctivitis**

**B00.59 Other herpesviral disease of eye**
Herpesviral dermatitis of eyelid

**B00.7 Disseminated herpesviral disease** HCC ESR COM
Herpesviral sepsis

**5th B00.8 Other forms of herpesviral infections**

**B00.81 Herpesviral hepatitis**

**B00.82 Herpes simplex myelitis** HCC Rx ESR COM

**B00.89 Other herpesviral infection**
Herpesviral whitlow

**B00.9 Herpesviral infection, unspecified**
Herpes simplex infection NOS

**4th B01 Varicella [chickenpox]**

**B01.0 Varicella meningitis** COM

**5th B01.1 Varicella encephalitis, myelitis and encephalomyelitis**
Postchickenpox encephalitis, myelitis and encephalomyelitis

**B01.11 Varicella encephalitis and encephalomyelitis** COM
Postchickenpox encephalitis and encephalomyelitis

**B01.12 Varicella myelitis** HCC Rx ESR COM
Postchickenpox myelitis

**B01.2 Varicella pneumonia**

**5th B01.8 Varicella with other complications**

**B01.81 Varicella keratitis**

**B01.89 Other varicella complications**

**B01.9 Varicella without complication**
Varicella NOS

**4th B02 Zoster [herpes zoster]**

INCLUDES shingles
zona

**B02.0 Zoster encephalitis** COM
Zoster meningoencephalitis

**B02.1 Zoster meningitis** COM
**AHA:** 2019,1Q,18

**5th B02.2 Zoster with other nervous system involvement**

**B02.21 Postherpetic geniculate ganglionitis** Rx

**B02.22 Postherpetic trigeminal neuralgia** Rx

**B02.23 Postherpetic polyneuropathy** Rx

**B02.24 Postherpetic myelitis** HCC Rx ESR COM
Herpes zoster myelitis

**B02.29 Other postherpetic nervous system involvement** Rx
Postherpetic radiculopathy

**5th B02.3 Zoster ocular disease**

**B02.30 Zoster ocular disease, unspecified**

**B02.31 Zoster conjunctivitis**

**B02.32 Zoster iridocyclitis**

**B02.33 Zoster keratitis**
Herpes zoster keratoconjunctivitis

**B02.34 Zoster scleritis**

**B02.39 Other herpes zoster eye disease**
Zoster blepharitis

**B02.7 Disseminated zoster**

**B02.8 Zoster with other complications**
Herpes zoster otitis externa

**B02.9 Zoster without complications**
Zoster NOS

**B03 Smallpox**

NOTE In 1980 the 33rd World Health Assembly declared that smallpox had been eradicated.
The classification is maintained for surveillance purposes.

**B04 Monkeypox**
Mpox
**AHA:** 2022,3Q,3-4

**4th B05 Measles**

INCLUDES morbilli
EXCLUDES 1 *subacute sclerosing panencephalitis (A81.1)*

**B05.0 Measles complicated by encephalitis** COM
Postmeasles encephalitis

**B05.1 Measles complicated by meningitis** COM
Postmeasles meningitis

**B05.2 Measles complicated by pneumonia**
Postmeasles pneumonia

**B05.3 Measles complicated by otitis media**
Postmeasles otitis media

**B05.4 Measles with intestinal complications**

✓5th **B05.8 Measles with other complications**

**B05.81 Measles keratitis and keratoconjunctivitis**

**B05.89 Other measles complications**

**B05.9 Measles without complication**
Measles NOS

✓4th **B06 Rubella [German measles]**

EXCLUDES 1 *congenital rubella (P35.0)*

**DEF:** Highly contagious virus in which the symptoms are mild and short-lived in most people. Rubella during pregnancy, however, can result in abortion, stillbirth, or congenital defects.

✓5th **B06.0 Rubella with neurological complications**

**B06.00 Rubella with neurological complication, unspecified**

**B06.01 Rubella encephalitis** COM
Rubella meningoencephalitis

**B06.02 Rubella meningitis** COM

**B06.09 Other neurological complications of rubella**

✓5th **B06.8 Rubella with other complications**

**B06.81 Rubella pneumonia**

**B06.82 Rubella arthritis** HCC ESR COM

**B06.89 Other rubella complications**

**B06.9 Rubella without complication**
Rubella NOS

✓4th **B07 Viral warts**

INCLUDES verruca simplex
verruca vulgaris
viral warts due to human papillomavirus

EXCLUDES 2 *anogenital (venereal) warts (A63.0)*
*papilloma of bladder (D41.4)*
*papilloma of cervix (D26.0)*
*papilloma larynx (D14.1)*

**B07.0 Plantar wart**
Verruca plantaris

**B07.8 Other viral warts**
Common wart
Flat wart
Verruca plana

**B07.9 Viral wart, unspecified**

✓4th **B08 Other viral infections characterized by skin and mucous membrane lesions, not elsewhere classified**

EXCLUDES 1 *vesicular stomatitis virus disease (A93.8)*

✓5th **B08.0 Other orthopoxvirus infections**

EXCLUDES 2 *monkeypox (B04)*

✓6th **B08.01 Cowpox and vaccinia not from vaccine**

**B08.010 Cowpox**
**DEF:** Disease contracted by milking infected cows. The vesicles usually appear on the fingers, hands, and adjacent areas and usually disappear without scarring. Other symptoms include local edema, lymphangitis, and regional lymphadenitis with or without fever.

**B08.011 Vaccinia not from vaccine**
EXCLUDES 1 *vaccinia (from vaccination) (generalized) (T88.1)*

**B08.02 Orf virus disease**
Contagious pustular dermatitis
Ecthyma contagiosum

**B08.03 Pseudocowpox [milker's node]**

**B08.04 Paravaccinia, unspecified**

**B08.09 Other orthopoxvirus infections**
Orthopoxvirus infection NOS

**B08.1 Molluscum contagiosum**
**DEF:** Benign poxvirus infection causing small bumps on the skin or conjunctiva, transmitted by close contact.

✓5th **B08.2 Exanthema subitum [sixth disease]**
Roseola infantum

**B08.20 Exanthema subitum [sixth disease], unspecified** P
Roseola infantum, unspecified

**B08.21 Exanthema subitum [sixth disease] due to human herpesvirus 6** P
Roseola infantum due to human herpesvirus 6

**B08.22 Exanthema subitum [sixth disease] due to human herpesvirus 7** P
Roseola infantum due to human herpesvirus 7

**B08.3 Erythema infectiosum [fifth disease]**
**DEF:** Infection with human parvovirus B19, mainly occurring in children. Symptoms include a low-grade fever, malaise, or a "cold" a few days before the appearance of a mild rash illness that presents as a "slapped-cheek" rash on the face and a lacy red rash on the trunk and limbs.

**B08.4 Enteroviral vesicular stomatitis with exanthem**
Hand, foot and mouth disease

**B08.5 Enteroviral vesicular pharyngitis**
Herpangina
**DEF:** Acute infectious Coxsackie virus infection causing throat lesions, fever, and vomiting that generally affects children in the summer.

✓5th **B08.6 Parapoxvirus infections**

**B08.60 Parapoxvirus infection, unspecified**

**B08.61 Bovine stomatitis**

**B08.62 Sealpox**

**B08.69 Other parapoxvirus infections**

✓5th **B08.7 Yatapoxvirus infections**

**B08.70 Yatapoxvirus infection, unspecified**

**B08.71 Tanapox virus disease**

**B08.72 Yaba pox virus disease**
Yaba monkey tumor disease

**B08.79 Other yatapoxvirus infections**

**B08.8 Other specified viral infections characterized by skin and mucous membrane lesions**
Enteroviral lymphonodular pharyngitis
Foot-and-mouth disease
Poxvirus NEC

**B09 Unspecified viral infection characterized by skin and mucous membrane lesions**
Viral enanthema NOS
Viral exanthema NOS

## Other human herpesviruses (B10)

✓4th **B10 Other human herpesviruses**

EXCLUDES 2 *cytomegalovirus (B25.9)*
*Epstein-Barr virus (B27.0-)*
*herpes NOS (B00.9)*
*herpes simplex (B00.-)*
*herpes zoster (B02.-)*
*human herpesvirus 1 and 2 (B00.-)*
*human herpesvirus 3 (B01.-, B02.-)*
*human herpesvirus 4 (B27.0-)*
*human herpesvirus 5 (B25.-)*
*human herpesvirus NOS (B00.-)*
*varicella (B01.-)*
*zoster (B02.-)*

✓5th **B10.0 Other human herpesvirus encephalitis**

EXCLUDES 2 *herpes encephalitis NOS (B00.4)*
*herpes simplex encephalitis (B00.4)*
*human herpesvirus encephalitis (B00.4)*
*simian B herpes virus encephalitis (B00.4)*

**B10.01 Human herpesvirus 6 encephalitis** COM

**B10.09 Other human herpesvirus encephalitis** COM
Human herpesvirus 7 encephalitis
**AHA:** 2024,2Q,21

✓5th **B10.8 Other human herpesvirus infection**

**B10.81 Human herpesvirus 6 infection**

**B10.82 Human herpesvirus 7 infection**

**B10.89 Other human herpesvirus infection**
Human herpesvirus 8 infection
Kaposi's sarcoma-associated herpesvirus infection

## Viral hepatitis (B15-B19)

EXCLUDES 1 *sequelae of viral hepatitis (B94.2)*
EXCLUDES 2 *cytomegaloviral hepatitis (B25.1)*
*herpesviral [herpes simplex] hepatitis (B00.81)*

**DEF:** Hepatitis A: HAV infection that is self-limiting with flulike symptoms. Transmission is fecal-oral.
**DEF:** Hepatitis B: HBV infection that can be chronic and systemic. Transmission is bodily fluids.
**DEF:** Hepatitis C: HCV infection that can be chronic and systemic. Transmission is blood transfusion and unidentified agents.
**DEF:** Hepatitis D (delta): HDV that occurs only in the presence of hepatitis B virus. Transmission is contaminated blood in contact with mucous membranes.
**DEF:** Hepatitis E: HEV is an epidemic form. Transmission is fecal-oral, most often from contaminated water.

√4th **B15 Acute hepatitis A**
- **B15.0 Hepatitis A with hepatic coma** COM
- **B15.9 Hepatitis A without hepatic coma**
  - Hepatitis A (acute)(viral) NOS

√4th **B16 Acute hepatitis B**
**AHA:** 2016,3Q,13
- **B16.0 Acute hepatitis B with delta-agent with hepatic coma** COM
- **B16.1 Acute hepatitis B with delta-agent without hepatic coma**
- **B16.2 Acute hepatitis B without delta-agent with hepatic coma** COM
- **B16.9 Acute hepatitis B without delta-agent and without hepatic coma**
  - Hepatitis B (acute) (viral) NOS

√4th **B17 Other acute viral hepatitis**
- **B17.0 Acute delta-(super) infection of hepatitis B carrier**
- √5th **B17.1 Acute hepatitis C**
  - **B17.10 Acute hepatitis C without hepatic coma** Rx
    - Acute hepatitis C NOS
  - **B17.11 Acute hepatitis C with hepatic coma** Rx COM
- **B17.2 Acute hepatitis E**
- **B17.8 Other specified acute viral hepatitis**
  - Hepatitis non-A non-B (acute) (viral) NEC
- **B17.9 Acute viral hepatitis, unspecified**
  - Acute hepatitis NOS
  - Acute infectious hepatitis NOS

√4th **B18 Chronic viral hepatitis**
INCLUDES carrier of viral hepatitis
Use additional code, if applicable, for ascites (R18.8)
**AHA:** 2017,1Q,41
- **B18.0 Chronic viral hepatitis B with delta-agent** HCC Rx ESR COM
- **B18.1 Chronic viral hepatitis B without delta-agent** HCC Rx ESR COM
  - Carrier of viral hepatitis B
  - Chronic (viral) hepatitis B
- **B18.2 Chronic viral hepatitis C** HCC Rx ESR COM
  - Carrier of viral hepatitis C
  - **AHA:** 2018,1Q,4
- **B18.8 Other chronic viral hepatitis** HCC Rx ESR COM
  - Carrier of other viral hepatitis
- **B18.9 Chronic viral hepatitis, unspecified** HCC ESR COM
  - Carrier of unspecified viral hepatitis

√4th **B19 Unspecified viral hepatitis**
- **B19.0 Unspecified viral hepatitis with hepatic coma** COM
- √5th **B19.1 Unspecified viral hepatitis B**
  - **B19.10 Unspecified viral hepatitis B without hepatic coma**
    - Unspecified viral hepatitis B NOS
  - **B19.11 Unspecified viral hepatitis B with hepatic coma** COM
- √5th **B19.2 Unspecified viral hepatitis C**
  - **B19.20 Unspecified viral hepatitis C without hepatic coma** Rx
    - Viral hepatitis C NOS
  - **B19.21 Unspecified viral hepatitis C with hepatic coma** Rx COM
- **B19.9 Unspecified viral hepatitis without hepatic coma**
  - Viral hepatitis NOS

## Human immunodeficiency virus [HIV] disease (B20)

**B20 Human immunodeficiency virus [HIV] disease** HCC Rx ESR COM
INCLUDES acquired immune deficiency syndrome [AIDS]
AIDS-related complex [ARC]
HIV infection, symptomatic
Code first human immunodeficiency virus [HIV] disease complicating pregnancy, childbirth and the puerperium, if applicable (O98.7-)
Use additional code(s) to identify all manifestations of HIV infection
EXCLUDES 1 *asymptomatic human immunodeficiency virus [HIV] infection status (Z21)*
*exposure to HIV virus (Z20.6)*
*inconclusive serologic evidence of HIV (R75)*
**AHA:** 2022,1Q,36; 2021,2Q,6; 2021,1Q,52; 2020,4Q,97; 2020,2Q,12; 2019,1Q,8-11

## Other viral diseases (B25-B34)

√4th **B25 Cytomegaloviral disease**
EXCLUDES 1 *congenital cytomegalovirus infection (P35.1)*
*cytomegaloviral mononucleosis (B27.1-)*
- **B25.0 Cytomegaloviral pneumonitis** HCC Rx ESR COM
- **B25.1 Cytomegaloviral hepatitis** HCC Rx ESR COM
- **B25.2 Cytomegaloviral pancreatitis** HCC Rx ESR COM
- **B25.8 Other cytomegaloviral diseases** HCC Rx ESR COM
  - Cytomegaloviral encephalitis
- **B25.9 Cytomegaloviral disease, unspecified** HCC Rx ESR COM

√4th **B26 Mumps**
INCLUDES epidemic parotitis
infectious parotitis
- **B26.0 Mumps orchitis**
- **B26.1 Mumps meningitis** COM
- **B26.2 Mumps encephalitis** COM
- **B26.3 Mumps pancreatitis** COM
- √5th **B26.8 Mumps with other complications**
  - **B26.81 Mumps hepatitis**
  - **B26.82 Mumps myocarditis** COM
  - **B26.83 Mumps nephritis**
  - **B26.84 Mumps polyneuropathy**
  - **B26.85 Mumps arthritis** HCC ESR COM
  - **B26.89 Other mumps complications**
- **B26.9 Mumps without complication**
  - Mumps NOS
  - Mumps parotitis NOS

√4th **B27 Infectious mononucleosis**
INCLUDES glandular fever
monocytic angina
Pfeiffer's disease
- √5th **B27.0 Gammaherpesviral mononucleosis**
  - Mononucleosis due to Epstein-Barr virus
  - **B27.00 Gammaherpesviral mononucleosis without complication**
  - **B27.01 Gammaherpesviral mononucleosis with polyneuropathy**
  - **B27.02 Gammaherpesviral mononucleosis with meningitis** COM
  - **B27.09 Gammaherpesviral mononucleosis with other complications**
    - Hepatomegaly in gammaherpesviral mononucleosis
    - **AHA:** 2025,2Q,19; 2024,2Q,21
- √5th **B27.1 Cytomegaloviral mononucleosis**
  - **B27.10 Cytomegaloviral mononucleosis without complications**
  - **B27.11 Cytomegaloviral mononucleosis with polyneuropathy**
  - **B27.12 Cytomegaloviral mononucleosis with meningitis** COM
  - **B27.19 Cytomegaloviral mononucleosis with other complication**
    - Hepatomegaly in cytomegaloviral mononucleosis
- √5th **B27.8 Other infectious mononucleosis**
  - **B27.80 Other infectious mononucleosis without complication**
  - **B27.81 Other infectious mononucleosis with polyneuropathy**
  - **B27.82 Other infectious mononucleosis with meningitis** COM

**B27.89 Other infectious mononucleosis with other complication**
Hepatomegaly in other infectious mononucleosis

✓5th **B27.9 Infectious mononucleosis, unspecified**

**B27.9Ø Infectious mononucleosis, unspecified without complication**

**B27.91 Infectious mononucleosis, unspecified with polyneuropathy**

**B27.92 Infectious mononucleosis, unspecified with meningitis** COM

**B27.99 Infectious mononucleosis, unspecified with other complication**
Hepatomegaly in unspecified infectious mononucleosis

✓4th **B3Ø Viral conjunctivitis**

EXCLUDES 1 *herpesviral [herpes simplex] ocular disease (BØØ.5)*
*ocular zoster (BØ2.3)*

**Viral Conjunctivitis**

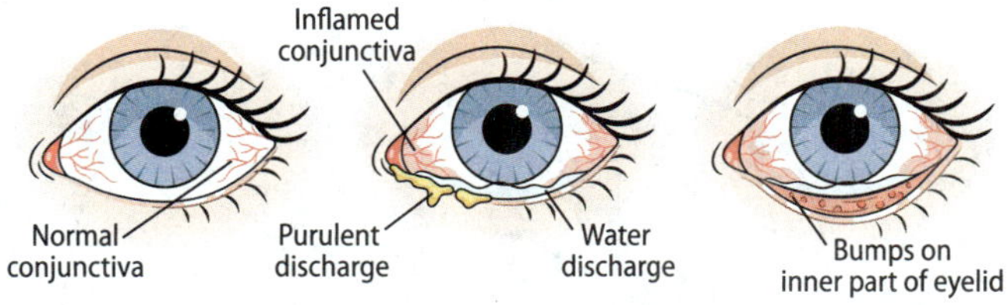


**B3Ø.Ø Keratoconjunctivitis due to adenovirus**
Epidemic keratoconjunctivitis
Shipyard eye

**B3Ø.1 Conjunctivitis due to adenovirus**
Acute adenoviral follicular conjunctivitis
Swimming-pool conjunctivitis

**B3Ø.2 Viral pharyngoconjunctivitis**

**B3Ø.3 Acute epidemic hemorrhagic conjunctivitis (enteroviral)**
Conjunctivitis due to coxsackievirus 24
Conjunctivitis due to enterovirus 7Ø
Hemorrhagic conjunctivitis (acute)(epidemic)

**B3Ø.8 Other viral conjunctivitis**
Newcastle conjunctivitis

**B3Ø.9 Viral conjunctivitis, unspecified**

✓4th **B33 Other viral diseases, not elsewhere classified**

**B33.Ø Epidemic myalgia**
Bornholm disease

**B33.1 Ross River disease**
Epidemic polyarthritis and exanthema
Ross River fever

✓5th **B33.2 Viral carditis**
Coxsackie (virus) carditis

**B33.2Ø Viral carditis, unspecified** COM

**B33.21 Viral endocarditis** COM

**B33.22 Viral myocarditis** COM
AHA: 2025,1Q,34

**B33.23 Viral pericarditis** COM

**B33.24 Viral cardiomyopathy** HCC Rx ESR COM

**B33.3 Retrovirus infections, not elsewhere classified**
Retrovirus infection NOS

**B33.4 Hantavirus (cardio)-pulmonary syndrome [HPS] [HCPS]**
Hantavirus disease with pulmonary manifestations
Sin nombre virus disease
Use additional code to identify any associated acute kidney failure (N17.9)

EXCLUDES 1 *hantavirus disease with renal manifestations (A98.5)*
*hemorrhagic fever with renal manifestations (A98.5)*

**B33.8 Other specified viral diseases**

EXCLUDES 1 *anogenital human papillomavirus infection (A63.Ø)*
*viral warts due to human papillomavirus infection (BØ7)*

✓4th **B34 Viral infection of unspecified site**

EXCLUDES 1 *anogenital human papillomavirus infection (A63.Ø)*
*cytomegaloviral disease NOS (B25.9)*
*herpesvirus [herpes simplex] infection NOS (BØØ.9)*
*retrovirus infection NOS (B33.3)*
*viral agents as the cause of diseases classified elsewhere (B97.-)*
*viral warts due to human papillomavirus infection (BØ7)*

**B34.Ø Adenovirus infection, unspecified**

**B34.1 Enterovirus infection, unspecified**
Coxsackievirus infection NOS
Echovirus infection NOS

**B34.2 Coronavirus infection, unspecified**

EXCLUDES 1 *COVID-19 (UØ7.1)*
*pneumonia due to SARS-associated coronavirus (J12.81)*

AHA: 2020,1Q,34-36

**B34.3 Parvovirus infection, unspecified**

**B34.4 Papovavirus infection, unspecified**

**B34.8 Other viral infections of unspecified site**

**B34.9 Viral infection, unspecified**
Viremia NOS
AHA: 2016,3Q,10

## Mycoses (B35-B49)

EXCLUDES 2 *hypersensitivity pneumonitis due to organic dust (J67.-)*
*mycosis fungoides (C84.Ø-)*

✓4th **B35 Dermatophytosis**

INCLUDES favus
infections due to species of Epidermophyton, Micro-sporum and Trichophyton
tinea, any type except those in B36.-

DEF: Contagious superficial fungal infection of the skin that invades and grows in dead keratin.

**B35.Ø Tinea barbae and tinea capitis**
Beard ringworm
Kerion
Scalp ringworm
Sycosis, mycotic

**B35.1 Tinea unguium**
Dermatophytic onychia
Dermatophytosis of nail
Onychomycosis
Ringworm of nails

**B35.2 Tinea manuum**
Dermatophytosis of hand
Hand ringworm

**B35.3 Tinea pedis**
Athlete's foot
Dermatophytosis of foot
Foot ringworm

**B35.4 Tinea corporis**
Ringworm of the body

**B35.5 Tinea imbricata**
Tokelau

**B35.6 Tinea cruris**
Dhobi itch
Groin ringworm
Jock itch

**B35.8 Other dermatophytoses**
Disseminated dermatophytosis
Granulomatous dermatophytosis

**B35.9 Dermatophytosis, unspecified**
Ringworm NOS

✓4th **B36 Other superficial mycoses**

**B36.Ø Pityriasis versicolor**
Tinea flava
Tinea versicolor

**B36.1 Tinea nigra**
Keratomycosis nigricans palmaris
Microsporosis nigra
Pityriasis nigra

**B36.2 White piedra**
Tinea blanca

**B36.3 Black piedra**

**B36.8 Other specified superficial mycoses**

**B36.9 Superficial mycosis, unspecified**

✓4th **B37 Candidiasis**

INCLUDES candidosis
moniliasis

EXCLUDES 1 *neonatal candidiasis (P37.5)*

DEF: *Candida:* Genus of yeast-like fungi that are commonly found in the mouth, skin, intestinal tract, and vagina. It may cause a white, cheesy discharge.

**B37.Ø Candidal stomatitis**
Oral thrush

B37.1 **Pulmonary candidiasis** HCC Rx ESR COM
Candidal bronchitis
Candidal pneumonia
▶Code also, if applicable:◀
▶pulmonary mycetoma (J4B)◀

B37.2 **Candidiasis of skin and nail**
Candidal onychia
Candidal paronychia
EXCLUDES 2 *diaper dermatitis (L22)*

✓5th B37.3 **Candidiasis of vulva and vagina**
Candidal vulvovaginitis
Monilial vulvovaginitis
Vaginal thrush
**AHA:** 2022,4Q,4-5

B37.31 **Acute candidiasis of vulva and vagina**
Candidiasis of vulva and vagina NOS

B37.32 **Chronic candidiasis of vulva and vagina**
Recurrent candidiasis of vulva and vagina

✓5th B37.4 **Candidiasis of other urogenital sites**

B37.41 **Candidal cystitis and urethritis**

B37.42 **Candidal balanitis**

B37.49 **Other urogenital candidiasis**
Candidal pyelonephritis

B37.5 **Candidal meningitis** COM

B37.6 **Candidal endocarditis** COM

B37.7 **Candidal sepsis** HCC Rx ESR COM
Disseminated candidiasis
Systemic candidiasis
**AHA:** 2024,3Q,13; 2014,4Q,46

✓5th B37.8 **Candidiasis of other sites**

B37.81 **Candidal esophagitis** HCC Rx ESR COM

B37.82 **Candidal enteritis**
Candidal proctitis

B37.83 **Candidal cheilitis**

B37.84 **Candidal otitis externa**

B37.89 **Other sites of candidiasis**
Candidal osteomyelitis

B37.9 **Candidiasis, unspecified**
Thrush NOS

✓4th **B38 Coccidioidomycosis**

B38.Ø **Acute pulmonary coccidioidomycosis** ESR COM
▶Code also, if applicable:◀
▶pulmonary mycetoma (J4B)◀

B38.1 **Chronic pulmonary coccidioidomycosis** ESR COM
▶Code also, if applicable:◀
▶pulmonary mycetoma (J4B)◀

B38.2 **Pulmonary coccidioidomycosis, unspecified** ESR COM
▶Code also, if applicable:◀
▶pulmonary mycetoma (J4B)◀

B38.3 **Cutaneous coccidioidomycosis**

B38.4 **Coccidioidomycosis meningitis** COM
**DEF:** *Coccidioides immitis* infection of the lining of the brain and/or spinal cord.

B38.7 **Disseminated coccidioidomycosis**
Generalized coccidioidomycosis

✓5th B38.8 **Other forms of coccidioidomycosis**

B38.81 **Prostatic coccidioidomycosis**

B38.89 **Other forms of coccidioidomycosis**

B38.9 **Coccidioidomycosis, unspecified**

✓4th **B39 Histoplasmosis**
Code first associated AIDS (B2Ø)
Use additional code for any associated manifestations, such as:
endocarditis (I39)
meningitis (GØ2)
pericarditis (I32)
retinitis (H32)
**DEF:** Type of lung infection caused by breathing in fungal spores often found in the droppings of bats and birds or soil contaminated by their droppings.

**Histoplasmosis**

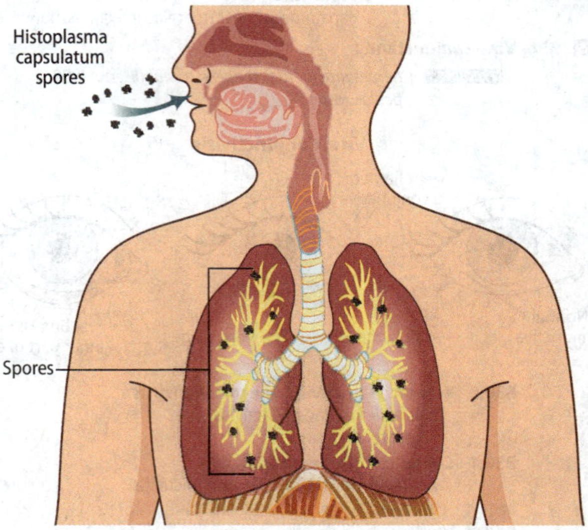


B39.Ø **Acute pulmonary histoplasmosis capsulati** ESR COM

B39.1 **Chronic pulmonary histoplasmosis capsulati** ESR COM

B39.2 **Pulmonary histoplasmosis capsulati, unspecified** ESR COM

B39.3 **Disseminated histoplasmosis capsulati**
Generalized histoplasmosis capsulati

B39.4 **Histoplasmosis capsulati, unspecified**
American histoplasmosis

B39.5 **Histoplasmosis duboisii**
African histoplasmosis

B39.9 **Histoplasmosis, unspecified**

✓4th **B4Ø Blastomycosis**
EXCLUDES 1 *Brazilian blastomycosis (B41.-)*
*keloidal blastomycosis (B48.Ø)*

B4Ø.Ø **Acute pulmonary blastomycosis** ESR COM

B4Ø.1 **Chronic pulmonary blastomycosis** ESR COM

B4Ø.2 **Pulmonary blastomycosis, unspecified** ESR COM

B4Ø.3 **Cutaneous blastomycosis**

B4Ø.7 **Disseminated blastomycosis**
Generalized blastomycosis

✓5th B4Ø.8 **Other forms of blastomycosis**

B4Ø.81 **Blastomycotic meningoencephalitis** COM
Meningomyelitis due to blastomycosis

B4Ø.89 **Other forms of blastomycosis**

B4Ø.9 **Blastomycosis, unspecified**

✓4th **B41 Paracoccidioidomycosis**
INCLUDES Brazilian blastomycosis
Lutz' disease

B41.Ø **Pulmonary paracoccidioidomycosis** ESR COM

B41.7 **Disseminated paracoccidioidomycosis**
Generalized paracoccidioidomycosis

B41.8 **Other forms of paracoccidioidomycosis**

B41.9 **Paracoccidioidomycosis, unspecified**

✓4th **B42 Sporotrichosis**

B42.Ø **Pulmonary sporotrichosis**

B42.1 **Lymphocutaneous sporotrichosis**

B42.7 **Disseminated sporotrichosis**
Generalized sporotrichosis

✓5th B42.8 **Other forms of sporotrichosis**

B42.81 **Cerebral sporotrichosis** COM
Meningitis due to sporotrichosis

B42.82 **Sporotrichosis arthritis** HCC ESR COM

B42.89 **Other forms of sporotrichosis**

B42.9 **Sporotrichosis, unspecified**

✓4th **B43 Chromomycosis and pheomycotic abscess**

B43.Ø **Cutaneous chromomycosis**
Dermatitis verrucosa

B43.1 **Pheomycotic brain abscess** COM
Cerebral chromomycosis

B43.2 **Subcutaneous pheomycotic abscess and cyst**

B43.8 **Other forms of chromomycosis**

B43.9 **Chromomycosis, unspecified**

✓4th **B44 Aspergillosis**

INCLUDES ~~aspergilloma~~

▶Code also, if applicable:◀
▶aspergilloma of other site - code to chronic infection of site◀
▶pulmonary aspergilloma (J4B)◀
▶pulmonary aspergillosis fungal ball (J4B)◀
▶pulmonary mycetoma (J4B)◀
▶sinus aspergilloma (J32.-)◀

B44.Ø **Invasive pulmonary aspergillosis** HCC Rx ESR COM

B44.1 **Other pulmonary aspergillosis** HCC Rx ESR COM

B44.2 **Tonsillar aspergillosis** HCC Rx ESR COM

B44.7 **Disseminated aspergillosis** HCC Rx ESR COM
Generalized aspergillosis

✓5th B44.8 **Other forms of aspergillosis**

B44.81 **Allergic bronchopulmonary aspergillosis** HCC Rx ESR COM

B44.89 **Other forms of aspergillosis** HCC Rx ESR COM

B44.9 **Aspergillosis, unspecified** HCC Rx ESR COM

✓4th **B45 Cryptococcosis**

B45.Ø **Pulmonary cryptococcosis** HCC Rx ESR COM

B45.1 **Cerebral cryptococcosis** HCC Rx ESR COM
Cryptococcal meningitis
Cryptococcosis meningocerebralis

B45.2 **Cutaneous cryptococcosis** HCC Rx ESR COM

B45.3 **Osseous cryptococcosis** HCC Rx ESR COM

B45.7 **Disseminated cryptococcosis** HCC Rx ESR COM
Generalized cryptococcosis

B45.8 **Other forms of cryptococcosis** HCC Rx ESR COM

B45.9 **Cryptococcosis, unspecified** HCC Rx ESR COM

✓4th **B46 Zygomycosis**

B46.Ø **Pulmonary mucormycosis** HCC Rx ESR COM

B46.1 **Rhinocerebral mucormycosis** HCC Rx ESR COM

B46.2 **Gastrointestinal mucormycosis** HCC Rx ESR COM

B46.3 **Cutaneous mucormycosis** HCC Rx ESR COM
Subcutaneous mucormycosis

B46.4 **Disseminated mucormycosis** HCC Rx ESR COM
Generalized mucormycosis

B46.5 **Mucormycosis, unspecified** HCC Rx ESR COM

B46.8 **Other zygomycoses** HCC Rx ESR COM
Entomophthoromycosis

B46.9 **Zygomycosis, unspecified** HCC Rx ESR COM
Phycomycosis NOS

✓4th **B47 Mycetoma**

EXCLUDES 2 ▶*pulmonary mycetoma (J4B)*◀

B47.Ø **Eumycetoma**
Madura foot, mycotic
Maduromycosis

B47.1 **Actinomycetoma**

B47.9 **Mycetoma, unspecified**
Madura foot NOS

✓4th **B48 Other mycoses, not elsewhere classified**

B48.Ø **Lobomycosis**
Keloidal blastomycosis
Lobo's disease

B48.1 **Rhinosporidiosis**

B48.2 **Allescheriasis**
Infection due to Pseudallescheria boydii
EXCLUDES 1 *eumycetoma (B47.Ø)*

B48.3 **Geotrichosis**
Geotrichum stomatitis

B48.4 **Penicillosis** HCC Rx ESR COM
Talaromycosis

B48.8 **Other specified mycoses** HCC Rx ESR COM
Adiaspiromycosis
Infection of tissue and organs by Alternaria
Infection of tissue and organs by Drechslera
Infection of tissue and organs by Fusarium
Infection of tissue and organs by saprophytic fungi NEC
**AHA:** 2014,4Q,46; 2014,2Q,13

**B49 Unspecified mycosis**
Fungemia NOS

## Protozoal diseases (B5Ø-B64)

EXCLUDES 1 *amebiasis (AØ6.-)*
*other protozoal intestinal diseases (AØ7.-)*

✓4th **B5Ø Plasmodium falciparum malaria**

INCLUDES mixed infections of Plasmodium falciparum with any other Plasmodium species

B5Ø.Ø **Plasmodium falciparum malaria with cerebral complications**
Cerebral malaria NOS

B5Ø.8 **Other severe and complicated Plasmodium falciparum malaria**
Severe or complicated Plasmodium falciparum malaria NOS

B5Ø.9 **Plasmodium falciparum malaria, unspecified**

✓4th **B51 Plasmodium vivax malaria**

INCLUDES mixed infections of Plasmodium vivax with other Plasmodium species, except Plasmodium falciparum

EXCLUDES 1 *Plasmodium vivax with Plasmodium falciparum (B5Ø.-)*

B51.Ø **Plasmodium vivax malaria with rupture of spleen**

B51.8 **Plasmodium vivax malaria with other complications**

B51.9 **Plasmodium vivax malaria without complication**
Plasmodium vivax malaria NOS

✓4th **B52 Plasmodium malariae malaria**

INCLUDES mixed infections of Plasmodium malariae with other Plasmodium species, except Plasmodium falciparum and Plasmodium vivax

EXCLUDES 1 *Plasmodium falciparum (B5Ø.-)*
*Plasmodium vivax (B51.-)*

B52.Ø **Plasmodium malariae malaria with nephropathy**

B52.8 **Plasmodium malariae malaria with other complications**

B52.9 **Plasmodium malariae malaria without complication**
Plasmodium malariae malaria NOS

✓4th **B53 Other specified malaria**

B53.Ø **Plasmodium ovale malaria**
EXCLUDES 1 *Plasmodium ovale with Plasmodium falciparum (B5Ø.-)*
*Plasmodium ovale with Plasmodium malariae (B52.-)*
*Plasmodium ovale with Plasmodium vivax (B51.-)*

B53.1 **Malaria due to simian plasmodia**
EXCLUDES 1 *malaria due to simian plasmodia with Plasmodium falciparum (B5Ø.-)*
*malaria due to simian plasmodia with Plasmodium malariae (B52.-)*
*malaria due to simian plasmodia with Plasmodium ovale (B53.Ø)*
*malaria due to simian plasmodia with Plasmodium vivax (B51.-)*

B53.8 **Other malaria, not elsewhere classified**

**B54 Unspecified malaria**

✓4th **B55 Leishmaniasis**

B55.Ø **Visceral leishmaniasis**
Kala-azar
Post-kala-azar dermal leishmaniasis

B55.1 **Cutaneous leishmaniasis**

B55.2 **Mucocutaneous leishmaniasis**

B55.9 **Leishmaniasis, unspecified**

✓4th **B56 African trypanosomiasis**

B56.Ø **Gambiense trypanosomiasis**
Infection due to Trypanosoma brucei gambiense
West African sleeping sickness

B56.1 **Rhodesiense trypanosomiasis**
East African sleeping sickness
Infection due to Trypanosoma brucei rhodesiense

B56.9 **African trypanosomiasis, unspecified**
Sleeping sickness NOS

✓4th **B57 Chagas' disease**

INCLUDES American trypanosomiasis
infection due to Trypanosoma cruzi

**B57.Ø Acute Chagas' disease with heart involvement**
Acute Chagas' disease with myocarditis

**B57.1 Acute Chagas' disease without heart involvement**
Acute Chagas' disease NOS

**B57.2 Chagas' disease (chronic) with heart involvement**
American trypanosomiasis NOS
Chagas' disease (chronic) NOS
Chagas' disease (chronic) with myocarditis
Trypanosomiasis NOS

✓5th **B57.3 Chagas' disease (chronic) with digestive system involvement**

**B57.30 Chagas' disease with digestive system involvement, unspecified**

**B57.31 Megaesophagus in Chagas' disease**

**B57.32 Megacolon in Chagas' disease**

**B57.39 Other digestive system involvement in Chagas' disease**

✓5th **B57.4 Chagas' disease (chronic) with nervous system involvement**

**B57.40 Chagas' disease with nervous system involvement, unspecified**

**B57.41 Meningitis in Chagas' disease** COM

**B57.42 Meningoencephalitis in Chagas' disease** COM

**B57.49 Other nervous system involvement in Chagas' disease**

**B57.5 Chagas' disease (chronic) with other organ involvement**

✓4th **B58 Toxoplasmosis**

INCLUDES infection due to Toxoplasma gondii

EXCLUDES 1 *congenital toxoplasmosis (P37.1)*

✓5th **B58.Ø Toxoplasma oculopathy**

**B58.ØØ Toxoplasma oculopathy, unspecified**

**B58.Ø1 Toxoplasma chorioretinitis**

**B58.Ø9 Other toxoplasma oculopathy**
Toxoplasma uveitis

**B58.1 Toxoplasma hepatitis**

**B58.2 Toxoplasma meningoencephalitis** HCC Rx ESR COM

**B58.3 Pulmonary toxoplasmosis** HCC Rx ESR COM

✓5th **B58.8 Toxoplasmosis with other organ involvement**

**B58.81 Toxoplasma myocarditis** COM

**B58.82 Toxoplasma myositis**

**B58.83 Toxoplasma tubulo-interstitial nephropathy**
Toxoplasma pyelonephritis

**B58.89 Toxoplasmosis with other organ involvement**

**B58.9 Toxoplasmosis, unspecified**

**B59 Pneumocystosis** HCC Rx ESR COM
Pneumonia due to Pneumocystis carinii
Pneumonia due to Pneumocystis jirovecii

✓4th **B6Ø Other protozoal diseases, not elsewhere classified**

EXCLUDES 1 *cryptosporidiosis (AØ7.2)*
*intestinal microsporidiosis (AØ7.8)*
*isosporiasis (AØ7.3)*

✓5th **B6Ø.Ø Babesiosis**

**AHA:** 2020,4Q,5-6

**B6Ø.ØØ Babesiosis, unspecified**
Babesiosis due to unspecified Babesia species
Piroplasmosis, unspecified

**B6Ø.Ø1 Babesiosis due to Babesia microti**
Infection due to B. microti

**B6Ø.Ø2 Babesiosis due to Babesia duncani**
Infection due to B. duncani and B. duncani-type species

**B6Ø.Ø3 Babesiosis due to Babesia divergens**
Babesiosis due to Babesia MO-1
Infection due to B. divergens and B. divergens-like strains

**B6Ø.Ø9 Other babesiosis**
Babesiosis due to Babesia KO-1
Babesiosis due to Babesia venatorum
Infection due to other Babesia species
Infection due to other protozoa of the order Piroplasmida
Other piroplasmosis

✓5th **B6Ø.1 Acanthamebiasis**

**B6Ø.1Ø Acanthamebiasis, unspecified**

**B6Ø.11 Meningoencephalitis due to Acanthamoeba (culbertsoni)** COM

**B6Ø.12 Conjunctivitis due to Acanthamoeba**

**B6Ø.13 Keratoconjunctivitis due to Acanthamoeba**

**B6Ø.19 Other acanthamebic disease**

**B6Ø.2 Naegleriasis**
Primary amebic meningoencephalitis

**B6Ø.8 Other specified protozoal diseases**
Microsporidiosis

**B64 Unspecified protozoal disease**

## Helminthiases (B65-B83)

✓4th **B65 Schistosomiasis [bilharziasis]**

INCLUDES snail fever

**B65.Ø Schistosomiasis due to Schistosoma haematobium [urinary schistosomiasis]**

**B65.1 Schistosomiasis due to Schistosoma mansoni [intestinal schistosomiasis]**

**B65.2 Schistosomiasis due to Schistosoma japonicum**
Asiatic schistosomiasis

**B65.3 Cercarial dermatitis**
Swimmer's itch

**B65.8 Other schistosomiasis**
Infection due to Schistosoma intercalatum
Infection due to Schistosoma mattheei
Infection due to Schistosoma mekongi

**B65.9 Schistosomiasis, unspecified**

✓4th **B66 Other fluke infections**

**B66.Ø Opisthorchiasis**
Infection due to cat liver fluke
Infection due to Opisthorchis (felineus)(viverrini)

**B66.1 Clonorchiasis**
Chinese liver fluke disease
Infection due to Clonorchis sinensis
Oriental liver fluke disease

**B66.2 Dicroceliasis**
Infection due to Dicrocoelium dendriticum
Lancet fluke infection

**B66.3 Fascioliasis**
Infection due to Fasciola gigantica
Infection due to Fasciola hepatica
Infection due to Fasciola indica
Sheep liver fluke disease

**B66.4 Paragonimiasis** ESR COM
Infection due to Paragonimus species
Lung fluke disease
Pulmonary distomiasis

**B66.5 Fasciolopsiasis**
Infection due to Fasciolopsis buski
Intestinal distomiasis

**B66.8 Other specified fluke infections**
Echinostomiasis
Heterophyiasis
Metagonimiasis
Nanophyetiasis
Watsoniasis

**B66.9 Fluke infection, unspecified**

✓4th **B67 Echinococcosis**

INCLUDES hydatidosis

**B67.Ø Echinococcus granulosus infection of liver**

**B67.1 Echinococcus granulosus infection of lung** ESR COM

**B67.2 Echinococcus granulosus infection of bone**

✓5th **B67.3 Echinococcus granulosus infection, other and multiple sites**

**B67.31 Echinococcus granulosus infection, thyroid gland**

**B67.32 Echinococcus granulosus infection, multiple sites**

**B67.39 Echinococcus granulosus infection, other sites**

**B67.4 Echinococcus granulosus infection, unspecified**
Dog tapeworm (infection)

**B67.5 Echinococcus multilocularis infection of liver**

✓5th **B67.6 Echinococcus multilocularis infection, other and multiple sites**

**B67.61 Echinococcus multilocularis infection, multiple sites**

**B67.69 Echinococcus multilocularis infection, other sites**

**B67.7 Echinococcus multilocularis infection, unspecified**

**B67.8 Echinococcosis, unspecified, of liver**

✓5th **B67.9 Echinococcosis, other and unspecified**

**B67.9Ø Echinococcosis, unspecified**
Echinococcosis NOS

**B67.99 Other echinococcosis**

**B68 Taeniasis**

EXCLUDES 1 *cysticercosis (B69.-)*

**B68.0 Taenia solium taeniasis**
Pork tapeworm (infection)

**B68.1 Taenia saginata taeniasis**
Beef tapeworm (infection)
Infection due to adult tapeworm Taenia saginata

**B68.9 Taeniasis, unspecified**

**B69 Cysticercosis**

INCLUDES cysticerciasis infection due to larval form of Taenia solium

**DEF:** Condition that is developed when larvae or eggs of the tapeworm *Taenia solium* are ingested, most commonly in fecally contaminated water or undercooked pork.

**B69.0 Cysticercosis of central nervous system**

**B69.1 Cysticercosis of eye**

**B69.8 Cysticercosis of other sites**

**B69.81 Myositis in cysticercosis**

**B69.89 Cysticercosis of other sites**

**B69.9 Cysticercosis, unspecified**

**B70 Diphyllobothriasis and sparganosis**

**B70.0 Diphyllobothriasis**
Diphyllobothrium (adult) (latum) (pacificum) infection
Fish tapeworm (infection)

EXCLUDES 2 *larval diphyllobothriasis (B70.1)*

**B70.1 Sparganosis**
Infection due to Sparganum (mansoni) (proliferum)
Infection due to Spirometra larva
Larval diphyllobothriasis
Spirometrosis

**B71 Other cestode infections**

**B71.0 Hymenolepiasis**
Dwarf tapeworm infection
Rat tapeworm (infection)

**B71.1 Dipylidiasis**

**B71.8 Other specified cestode infections**
Coenurosis

**B71.9 Cestode infection, unspecified**
Tapeworm (infection) NOS

**B72 Dracunculiasis**

INCLUDES guinea worm infection
infection due to Dracunculus medinensis

**B73 Onchocerciasis**

INCLUDES onchocerca volvulus infection
onchocercosis
river blindness

**B73.0 Onchocerciasis with eye disease**

**B73.00 Onchocerciasis with eye involvement, unspecified**

**B73.01 Onchocerciasis with endophthalmitis**

**B73.02 Onchocerciasis with glaucoma**

**B73.09 Onchocerciasis with other eye involvement**
Infestation of eyelid due to onchocerciasis

**B73.1 Onchocerciasis without eye disease**

**B74 Filariasis**

EXCLUDES 2 *onchocerciasis (B73)*
*tropical (pulmonary) eosinophilia NOS (J82.89)*

**B74.0 Filariasis due to Wuchereria bancrofti**
Bancroftian elephantiasis
Bancroftian filariasis

**B74.1 Filariasis due to Brugia malayi**

**B74.2 Filariasis due to Brugia timori**

**B74.3 Loiasis**
Calabar swelling
Eyeworm disease of Africa
Loa loa infection

**B74.4 Mansonelliasis**
Infection due to Mansonella ozzardi
Infection due to Mansonella perstans
Infection due to Mansonella streptocerca

**B74.8 Other filariases**
Dirofilariasis

**B74.9 Filariasis, unspecified**

**B75 Trichinellosis**

INCLUDES infection due to Trichinella species
trichiniasis

**DEF:** Infection by *Trichinella spiralis,* the smallest of the parasitic nematodes, that is transmitted by eating undercooked pork or bear meat. ***Synonym(s):*** *Trichinosis.*

**B76 Hookworm diseases**

INCLUDES uncinariasis

**B76.0 Ancylostomiasis**
Infection due to Ancylostoma species

**B76.1 Necatoriasis**
Infection due to Necator americanus

**B76.8 Other hookworm diseases**

**B76.9 Hookworm disease, unspecified**
Cutaneous larva migrans NOS

**B77 Ascariasis**

INCLUDES ascaridiasis
roundworm infection

**B77.0 Ascariasis with intestinal complications**

**B77.8 Ascariasis with other complications**

**B77.81 Ascariasis pneumonia**

**B77.89 Ascariasis with other complications**

**B77.9 Ascariasis, unspecified**

**B78 Strongyloidiasis**

EXCLUDES 1 *trichostrongyliasis (B81.2)*

**B78.0 Intestinal strongyloidiasis**

**B78.1 Cutaneous strongyloidiasis**

**B78.7 Disseminated strongyloidiasis**

**B78.9 Strongyloidiasis, unspecified**

**B79 Trichuriasis**

INCLUDES trichocephaliasis
whipworm (disease)(infection)

**B80 Enterobiasis**

INCLUDES oxyuriasis
pinworm infection
threadworm infection

**B81 Other intestinal helminthiases, not elsewhere classified**

EXCLUDES 1 *angiostrongyliasis due to:*
*angiostrongylus cantonensis (B83.2)*
*parastrongylus cantonensis (B83.2)*

**B81.0 Anisakiasis**
Infection due to Anisakis larva

**B81.1 Intestinal capillariasis**
Capillariasis NOS
Infection due to Capillaria philippinensis

EXCLUDES 2 *hepatic capillariasis (B83.8)*

**B81.2 Trichostrongyliasis**

**B81.3 Intestinal angiostrongyliasis**
Angiostrongyliasis due to:
Angiostrongylus costaricensis
Parastrongylus costaricensis

**B81.4 Mixed intestinal helminthiases**
Infection due to intestinal helminths classified to more than one of the categories B65.0-B81.3 and B81.8
Mixed helminthiasis NOS

**B81.8 Other specified intestinal helminthiases**
Infection due to Oesophagostomum species [esophagostomiasis]
Infection due to Ternidens diminutus [ternidensiasis]

**B82 Unspecified intestinal parasitism**

**B82.0 Intestinal helminthiasis, unspecified**

**B82.9 Intestinal parasitism, unspecified**

**B83 Other helminthiases**

EXCLUDES 1 *capillariasis NOS (B81.1)*

EXCLUDES 2 *intestinal capillariasis (B81.1)*

**B83.0 Visceral larva migrans**
Toxocariasis

**B83.1 Gnathostomiasis**
Wandering swelling

**B83.2 Angiostrongyliasis due to Parastrongylus cantonensis**
Eosinophilic meningoencephalitis due to Parastrongylus cantonensis

EXCLUDES 2 *intestinal angiostrongyliasis (B81.3)*

**B83.3 Syngamiasis**
Syngamosis

**B83.4 Internal hirudiniasis**
EXCLUDES 2 *external hirudiniasis (B88.3)*

**B83.8 Other specified helminthiases**
Acanthocephaliasis
Gongylonemiasis
Hepatic capillariasis
Metastrongyliasis
Thelaziasis

**B83.9 Helminthiasis, unspecified**
Worms NOS
EXCLUDES 1 *intestinal helminthiasis NOS (B82.Ø)*

## Pediculosis, acariasis and other infestations (B85-B89)

✓4th **B85 Pediculosis and phthiriasis**

**B85.Ø Pediculosis due to Pediculus humanus capitis**
Head-louse infestation

**B85.1 Pediculosis due to Pediculus humanus corporis**
Body-louse infestation

**B85.2 Pediculosis, unspecified**

**B85.3 Phthiriasis**
Infestation by crab-louse
Infestation by Phthirus pubis

**B85.4 Mixed pediculosis and phthiriasis**
Infestation classifiable to more than one of the categories B85.Ø-B85.3

**B86 Scabies**
Sarcoptic itch
**DEF:** Mite infestation that is caused by *Sarcoptes scabiei*. Scabies causes intense itching and sometimes secondary infection.

✓4th **B87 Myiasis**
INCLUDES infestation by larva of flies

**B87.Ø Cutaneous myiasis**
Creeping myiasis

**B87.1 Wound myiasis**
Traumatic myiasis

**B87.2 Ocular myiasis**

**B87.3 Nasopharyngeal myiasis**
Laryngeal myiasis

**B87.4 Aural myiasis**

✓5th **B87.8 Myiasis of other sites**

**B87.81 Genitourinary myiasis**

**B87.82 Intestinal myiasis**

**B87.89 Myiasis of other sites**

**B87.9 Myiasis, unspecified**

✓4th **B88 Other infestations**

✓5th **B88.Ø Other acariasis**
EXCLUDES 2 *scabies (B86)*

**B88.Ø1 Infestation by Demodex mites**
Demodex brevis infestation
Demodex folliculorum infestation
Code also, if applicable, eyelid inflammation (HØ1.8-)

**B88.Ø9 Other acariasis**
Acarine dermatitis
Dermatitis due to Dermanyssus gallinae
Dermatitis due to Liponyssoides sanguineus
Trombiculosis

**B88.1 Tungiasis [sandflea infestation]**

**B88.2 Other arthropod infestations**
Scarabiasis

**B88.3 External hirudiniasis**
Leech infestation NOS
EXCLUDES 2 *internal hirudiniasis (B83.4)*

**B88.8 Other specified infestations**
Ichthyoparasitism due to Vandellia cirrhosa
Linguatulosis
Porocephaliasis

**B88.9 Infestation, unspecified**
Infestation (skin) NOS
Infestation by mites NOS
Skin parasites NOS

**B89 Unspecified parasitic disease**

## Sequelae of infectious and parasitic diseases (B9Ø-B94)

NOTE Categories B9Ø-B94 are to be used to indicate conditions in categories AØØ-B89 as the cause of sequelae, which are themselves classified elsewhere. The "sequelae" include conditions specified as such; they also include residuals of diseases classifiable to the above categories if there is evidence that the disease itself is no longer present. Codes from these categories are not to be used for chronic infections. Code chronic current infections to active infectious disease as appropriate.

Code first condition resulting from (sequela) the infectious or parasitic disease

✓4th **B9Ø Sequelae of tuberculosis**

**B9Ø.Ø Sequelae of central nervous system tuberculosis**

**B9Ø.1 Sequelae of genitourinary tuberculosis**

**B9Ø.2 Sequelae of tuberculosis of bones and joints**

**B9Ø.8 Sequelae of tuberculosis of other organs**
EXCLUDES 2 *sequelae of respiratory tuberculosis (B9Ø.9)*

**B9Ø.9 Sequelae of respiratory and unspecified tuberculosis**
Sequelae of tuberculosis NOS

**B91 Sequelae of poliomyelitis**
EXCLUDES 1 *postpolio syndrome (G14)*

**B92 Sequelae of leprosy**

✓4th **B94 Sequelae of other and unspecified infectious and parasitic diseases**

**B94.Ø Sequelae of trachoma**

**B94.1 Sequelae of viral encephalitis**

**B94.2 Sequelae of viral hepatitis**

**B94.8 Sequelae of other specified infectious and parasitic diseases**
**AHA:** 2021,1Q,25-30,31-49; 2020,3Q,10-14; 2017,4Q,109

**B94.9 Sequelae of unspecified infectious and parasitic disease**
EXCLUDES 2 *post COVID-19 condition (UØ9.9)*

## Bacterial and viral infectious agents (B95-B97)

NOTE These categories are provided for use as supplementary or additional codes to identify the infectious agent(s) in diseases classified elsewhere.

**AHA:** 2020,2Q,18; 2018,4Q,34; 2018,1Q,16

✓4th **B95 Streptococcus, Staphylococcus, and Enterococcus as the cause of diseases classified elsewhere**

**B95.Ø Streptococcus, group A, as the cause of diseases classified elsewhere** UPD

**B95.1 Streptococcus, group B, as the cause of diseases classified elsewhere** UPD
**AHA:** 2020,1Q,10; 2019,2Q,8-10

**B95.2 Enterococcus as the cause of diseases classified elsewhere** UPD

**B95.3 Streptococcus pneumoniae as the cause of diseases classified elsewhere** UPD

**B95.4 Other streptococcus as the cause of diseases classified elsewhere** UPD
**AHA:** 2025,1Q,20

**B95.5 Unspecified streptococcus as the cause of diseases classified elsewhere** UPD

✓5th **B95.6 Staphylococcus aureus as the cause of diseases classified elsewhere**

**B95.61 Methicillin susceptible Staphylococcus aureus infection as the cause of diseases classified elsewhere** UPD
Methicillin susceptible Staphylococcus aureus (MSSA) infection as the cause of diseases classified elsewhere
Staphylococcus aureus infection NOS as the cause of diseases classified elsewhere

**B95.62 Methicillin resistant Staphylococcus aureus infection as the cause of diseases classified elsewhere** UPD
Methicillin resistant staphylococcus aureus (MRSA) infection as the cause of diseases classified elsewhere
**AHA:** 2016,1Q,12

**B95.7 Other staphylococcus as the cause of diseases classified elsewhere** UPD

**B95.8 Unspecified staphylococcus as the cause of diseases classified elsewhere** UPD

✓4th **B96 Other bacterial agents as the cause of diseases classified elsewhere**

**B96.Ø Mycoplasma pneumoniae [M. pneumoniae] as the cause of diseases classified elsewhere** UPD
Pleuro-pneumonia-like-organism [PPLO]

**B96.1** **Klebsiella pneumoniae [K. pneumoniae] as the cause of diseases classified elsewhere** UPD

✓5th **B96.2** **Escherichia coli [E. coli] as the cause of diseases classified elsewhere**
AHA: 2022,1Q,31

**B96.20** **Unspecified Escherichia coli [E. coli] as the cause of diseases classified elsewhere** UPD
Escherichia coli [E. coli] NOS

**B96.21** **Shiga toxin-producing Escherichia coli [E. coli] [STEC] O157 as the cause of diseases classified elsewhere** UPD
E. coli O157 with confirmation of Shiga toxin when H antigen is unknown, or is not H7
E. coli O157:H- (nonmotile) with confirmation of Shiga toxin
O157:H7 Escherichia coli [E. coli] with or without confirmation of Shiga toxin-production
Shiga toxin-producing Escherichia coli [E. coli] O157:H7 with or without confirmation of Shiga toxin-production
STEC O157:H7 with or without confirmation of Shiga toxin-production

**B96.22** **Other specified Shiga toxin-producing Escherichia coli [E. coli] [STEC] as the cause of diseases classified elsewhere** UPD
Non-O157 Shiga toxin-producing Escherichia coli [E. coli]
Non-O157 Shiga toxin-producing Escherichia coli [E. coli] with known O group

**B96.23** **Unspecified Shiga toxin-producing Escherichia coli [E. coli] [STEC] as the cause of diseases classified elsewhere** UPD
Shiga toxin-producing Escherichia coli [E. coli] with unspecified O group
STEC NOS

**B96.29** **Other Escherichia coli [E. coli] as the cause of diseases classified elsewhere** UPD
Non-Shiga toxin-producing E. coli

**B96.3** **Hemophilus influenzae [H. influenzae] as the cause of diseases classified elsewhere** UPD

**B96.4** **Proteus (mirabilis) (morganii) as the cause of diseases classified elsewhere** UPD

**B96.5** **Pseudomonas (aeruginosa) (mallei) (pseudomallei) as the cause of diseases classified elsewhere** UPD
AHA: 2015,1Q,18

**B96.6** **Bacteroides fragilis [B. fragilis] as the cause of diseases classified elsewhere** UPD

**B96.7** **Clostridium perfringens [C. perfringens] as the cause of diseases classified elsewhere** UPD

✓5th **B96.8** **Other specified bacterial agents as the cause of diseases classified elsewhere**

**B96.81** **Helicobacter pylori [H. pylori] as the cause of diseases classified elsewhere** UPD

**B96.82** **Vibrio vulnificus as the cause of diseases classified elsewhere** UPD

**B96.83** **Acinetobacter baumannii as the cause of diseases classified elsewhere** UPD
AHA: 2023,4Q,4

**B96.89** **Other specified bacterial agents as the cause of diseases classified elsewhere** UPD

✓4th **B97** **Viral agents as the cause of diseases classified elsewhere**
AHA: 2016,3Q,8-10,14

**B97.0** **Adenovirus as the cause of diseases classified elsewhere** UPD

✓5th **B97.1** **Enterovirus as the cause of diseases classified elsewhere**

**B97.10** **Unspecified enterovirus as the cause of diseases classified elsewhere** UPD

**B97.11** **Coxsackievirus as the cause of diseases classified elsewhere** UPD

**B97.12** **Echovirus as the cause of diseases classified elsewhere** UPD

**B97.19** **Other enterovirus as the cause of diseases classified elsewhere** UPD

✓5th **B97.2** **Coronavirus as the cause of diseases classified elsewhere**

**B97.21** **SARS-associated coronavirus as the cause of diseases classified elsewhere** UPD
EXCLUDES 1 *pneumonia due to SARS-associated coronavirus (J12.81)*

**B97.29** **Other coronavirus as the cause of diseases classified elsewhere** UPD
AHA: 2020,2Q,5; 2020,1Q,34-36

✓5th **B97.3** **Retrovirus as the cause of diseases classified elsewhere**
EXCLUDES 1 *human immunodeficiency virus [HIV] disease (B20)*

**B97.30** **Unspecified retrovirus as the cause of diseases classified elsewhere** UPD

**B97.31** **Lentivirus as the cause of diseases classified elsewhere** UPD

**B97.32** **Oncovirus as the cause of diseases classified elsewhere** UPD

**B97.33** **Human T-cell lymphotrophic virus, type I [HTLV-I] as the cause of diseases classified elsewhere** UPD

**B97.34** **Human T-cell lymphotrophic virus, type II [HTLV-II] as the cause of diseases classified elsewhere** UPD

**B97.35** **Human immunodeficiency virus, type 2 [HIV 2] as the cause of diseases classified elsewhere** HCC Rx ESR COM UPD

**B97.39** **Other retrovirus as the cause of diseases classified elsewhere** UPD

**B97.4** **Respiratory syncytial virus as the cause of diseases classified elsewhere** UPD
RSV as the cause of diseases classified elsewhere
Code first related disorders, such as:
otitis media (H65.-)
upper respiratory infection (J06.9)
EXCLUDES 1 *acute bronchiolitis due to respiratory syncytial virus (RSV) (J21.0)*
*acute bronchitis due to respiratory syncytial virus (RSV) (J20.5)*
*respiratory syncytial virus (RSV) pneumonia (J12.1)*
AHA: 2026,2Q,15

**B97.5** **Reovirus as the cause of diseases classified elsewhere** UPD

**B97.6** **Parvovirus as the cause of diseases classified elsewhere** UPD

**B97.7** **Papillomavirus as the cause of diseases classified elsewhere** UPD

✓5th **B97.8** **Other viral agents as the cause of diseases classified elsewhere**

**B97.81** **Human metapneumovirus as the cause of diseases classified elsewhere** UPD

**B97.89** **Other viral agents as the cause of diseases classified elsewhere** UPD

## Other infectious diseases (B99)

✓4th **B99** **Other and unspecified infectious diseases**

**B99.8** **Other infectious disease**

**B99.9** **Unspecified infectious disease**

# Chapter 2. Neoplasms (CØØ–D49)



## Chapter-specific Guidelines with Coding Examples

The chapter-specific guidelines from the ICD-10-CM Official Guidelines for Coding and Reporting have been provided below. Along with these guidelines are coding examples, contained in the shaded boxes, that have been developed to help illustrate the coding and/or sequencing guidance found in these guidelines.

**General guidelines**

Chapter 2 of the ICD-10-CM contains the codes for most benign and all malignant neoplasms. Certain benign neoplasms, such as prostatic adenomas, may be found in the specific body system chapters. To properly code a neoplasm, it is necessary to determine from the record if the neoplasm is benign, in-situ, malignant, or of uncertain histologic behavior. If malignant, any secondary (metastatic) sites should also be determined.

Primary malignant neoplasms overlapping site boundaries

A primary malignant neoplasm that overlaps two or more contiguous (next to each other) sites should be classified to the subcategory/code .8 ('overlapping lesion'), unless the combination is specifically indexed elsewhere. For multiple neoplasms of the same site that are not contiguous such as tumors in different quadrants of the same breast, codes for each site should be assigned.

A 62-year-old female with a malignant lesion of the upper lip that extends from the lipstick area to the labial frenulum

| | |
|---|---|
| **CØØ.8** | **Malignant neoplasm of overlapping sites of lip** |

*Explanation*: Because this is a single lesion that overlaps two contiguous sites, a single code for overlapping sites is assigned.

A 74-year-old male is treated for two distinct malignant lesions, one in the mucosa of the upper lip and a second in the mucosa of the lower lip.

| | |
|---|---|
| **CØØ.3** | **Malignant neoplasm of upper lip, inner aspect** |
| **CØØ.4** | **Malignant neoplasm of lower lip, inner aspect** |

*Explanation*: This patient has two distinct malignant lesions of the upper and lower lips. Because the lesions are not contiguous, two codes are reported.

Malignant neoplasm of ectopic tissue

Malignant neoplasms of ectopic tissue are to be coded to the site of origin mentioned, e.g., ectopic pancreatic malignant neoplasms involving the stomach are coded to malignant neoplasm of pancreas, unspecified (C25.9).

The neoplasm table in the Alphabetic Index should be referenced first. However, if the histological term is documented, that term should be referenced first, rather than going immediately to the Neoplasm Table, in order to determine which column in the Neoplasm Table is appropriate. For example, if the documentation indicates "adenoma," refer to the term in the Alphabetic Index to review the entries under this term and the instructional note to "see also neoplasm, by site, benign." The table provides the proper code based on the type of neoplasm and the site. It is important to select the proper column in the table that corresponds to the type of neoplasm. The Tabular List should then be referenced to verify that the correct code has been selected from the table and that a more specific site code does not exist.

*See Section I.C.21. Factors influencing health status and contact with health services, Status, for information regarding Z15.Ø, codes for genetic susceptibility to cancer.*

**a. Admission/encounter for treatment of primary site**

If the malignancy is chiefly responsible for occasioning the patient admission/encounter and treatment is directed at the primary site, designate the primary malignancy as the principal/first-listed diagnosis.

The only exception to this guideline is if the administration of chemotherapy, immunotherapy or external beam radiation therapy is chiefly responsible for occasioning the admission/encounter. In that case, assign the appropriate Z51.-- code as the first-listed or principal diagnosis, and the underlying diagnosis or problem for which the service is being performed as a secondary diagnosis.

**b. Admission/encounter for treatment of secondary site**

When a patient is admitted because of a primary neoplasm with metastasis and treatment is directed toward the secondary site only, the secondary neoplasm is designated as the principal diagnosis even though the primary malignancy is still present.

Patient with primary prostate cancer with metastasis to lungs presents for wedge resection of mass in right lung

| | |
|---|---|
| **C78.Ø1** | **Secondary malignant neoplasm of right lung** |
| **C61** | **Malignant neoplasm of prostate** |

*Explanation*: Since the encounter is for treatment of the lung metastasis, the secondary lung metastasis is sequenced before the primary prostate cancer.

**c. Coding and sequencing of complications**

Coding and sequencing of complications associated with the malignancies or with the therapy thereof are subject to the following guidelines:

**1) Anemia associated with malignancy**

When admission/encounter is for management of an anemia associated with the malignancy, and the treatment is only for anemia, the appropriate code for the malignancy is sequenced as the principal or first-listed diagnosis followed by the appropriate code for the anemia (such as code D63.Ø, Anemia in neoplastic disease).

Patient is seen for treatment of anemia in advanced primary liver cancer

| | |
|---|---|
| **C22.8** | **Malignant neoplasm of liver, primary, unspecified as to type** |
| **D63.Ø** | **Anemia in neoplastic disease** |

*Explanation*: Even though the admission was solely to treat the anemia, this guideline indicates that the code for the malignancy is sequenced first.

**2) Anemia associated with chemotherapy, immunotherapy and radiation therapy**

When the admission/encounter is for management of an anemia associated with an adverse effect of the administration of chemotherapy or immunotherapy and the only treatment is for the anemia, the anemia code is sequenced first followed by the appropriate codes for the neoplasm and the adverse effect (T45.1X5, Adverse effect of antineoplastic and immunosuppressive drugs).

When the admission/encounter is for management of an anemia associated with an adverse effect of radiotherapy, the anemia code should be sequenced first, followed by the appropriate neoplasm code and code Y84.2, Radiological procedure and radiotherapy as the cause of abnormal reaction of the patient, or of later complication, without mention of misadventure at the time of the procedure.

A 55-year-old male with a large malignant rectal tumor has been receiving external radiation therapy to shrink the tumor prior to planned surgery. He is referred today for a blood transfusion to treat anemia related to radiation therapy.

| | |
|---|---|
| **D64.89** | **Other specified anemias** |
| **C2Ø** | **Malignant neoplasm of rectum** |
| **Y84.2** | **Radiological procedure and radiotherapy as the cause of abnormal reaction of the patient, or of later complication, without mention of misadventure at the time of the procedure** |

*Explanation*: The code for the anemia is sequenced first, followed by the code for the malignancy, and lastly the code for the abnormal reaction due to radiotherapy.

**3) Management of dehydration due to the malignancy**

When the admission/encounter is for management of dehydration due to the malignancy and only the dehydration is being treated (intravenous rehydration), the dehydration is sequenced first, followed by the code(s) for the malignancy.

**4) Treatment of a complication resulting from a surgical procedure**

When the admission/encounter is for treatment of a complication resulting from a surgical procedure, designate the complication as the principal or first-listed diagnosis if treatment is directed at resolving the complication.

**d. Primary malignancy previously excised**

When a primary malignancy has been previously excised or eradicated from its site and there is no further treatment directed to that site and there is no evidence of any existing primary malignancy at that site, a code from category Z85, Personal history of malignant neoplasm, should be used to indicate the former site of the malignancy. Any mention of extension, invasion, or metastasis to another site is coded as a secondary malignant neoplasm to that site. The secondary site may be the principal or first-listed diagnosis with the Z85 code used as a secondary code.

*See section I.C.2.t. Secondary malignant neoplasm of lymphoid tissue.*

History of lung cancer, left upper lobectomy 18 months ago with no current treatment; MRI of the brain shows metastatic disease in the brain

| | |
|---|---|
| **C79.31** | **Secondary malignant neoplasm of brain** |
| **Z85.118** | **Personal history of other malignant neoplasm of bronchus and lung** |

*Explanation*: The patient has undergone a diagnostic procedure that revealed metastatic lung cancer in the brain. The code for the secondary (metastatic) site is sequenced first, followed by a personal history code to identify the former site of the primary malignancy.

**e. Admissions/encounters involving antineoplastic chemotherapy, immunotherapy and radiation therapy**

**1) Episode of care involves surgical removal of neoplasm**

When an episode of care involves the surgical removal of a neoplasm, primary or secondary site, followed by adjunct chemotherapy or radiation treatment during the same episode of care, the code for the neoplasm should be assigned as principal or first-listed diagnosis.

**2) Patient admission/encounter chiefly for administration of antineoplastic chemotherapy, immunotherapy and radiation therapy**

If a patient admission/encounter is chiefly for the administration of chemotherapy, immunotherapy or external beam radiation therapy for the treatment of a neoplasm, assign code Z51.Ø, Encounter for antineoplastic radiation therapy, or Z51.11, Encounter for antineoplastic chemotherapy, or Z51.12, Encounter for antineoplastic immunotherapy as the first-listed or principal diagnosis. If the reason for the encounter is more than one type of antineoplastic therapy, code Z51.Ø and codes from subcategory Z51.1 may be assigned together, in which case one of these codes would be reported as a secondary diagnosis.

The malignancy for which the therapy is being administered should be assigned as a secondary diagnosis.

If a patient admission/encounter is for the insertion or implantation of radioactive elements (e.g., brachytherapy) the appropriate code for the malignancy is sequenced as the principal or first-listed diagnosis. Code Z51.Ø should not be assigned.

Patient presents for second round of rituximab and fludarabine for his chronic B cell lymphocytic leukemia

| | |
|---|---|
| **Z51.11** | **Encounter for antineoplastic chemotherapy** |
| **Z51.12** | **Encounter for antineoplastic immunotherapy** |
| **C91.1Ø** | **Chronic lymphocytic leukemia of B-cell type not having achieved remission** |

*Explanation*: Rituximab is an antineoplastic immunotherapy while fludarabine is an antineoplastic chemotherapy. The two treatments are often used together. The encounter was solely for the purpose of administering this treatment and either can be sequenced first, before the neoplastic condition.

**3) Patient admitted for radiation therapy, chemotherapy or immunotherapy and develops complications**

When a patient is admitted for the purpose of external beam radiotherapy, immunotherapy or chemotherapy and develops complications such as uncontrolled nausea and vomiting or dehydration, the principal or first-listed diagnosis is Z51.Ø, Encounter for antineoplastic radiation therapy, or Z51.11, Encounter for antineoplastic chemotherapy, or Z51.12, Encounter for antineoplastic immunotherapy followed by any codes for the complications.

When a patient is admitted for the purpose of insertion or implantation of radioactive elements (e.g., brachytherapy) and develops complications such as uncontrolled nausea and vomiting or dehydration, the principal or first-listed diagnosis is the appropriate code for the malignancy followed by any codes for the complications.

**f. Admission/encounter to determine extent of malignancy**

When the reason for admission/encounter is to determine the extent of the malignancy, or for a procedure such as paracentesis or thoracentesis, the primary malignancy or appropriate metastatic site is designated as the principal or first-listed diagnosis, even though chemotherapy or radiotherapy is administered.

Patient with left lung cancer with malignant pleural effusion being seen for paracentesis and initiation/administration of chemotherapy

| | |
|---|---|
| **C34.92** | **Malignant neoplasm of unspecified part of left bronchus or lung** |
| **J91.Ø** | **Malignant pleural effusion** |
| **Z51.11** | **Encounter for antineoplastic chemotherapy** |

*Explanation*: The lung cancer is sequenced before the chemotherapy in this instance because the paracentesis for the malignant effusion is also being performed. An instructional note under the malignant effusion instructs that the lung cancer be sequenced first.

**g. Symptoms, signs, and abnormal findings listed in Chapter 18 associated with neoplasms**

Symptoms, signs, and ill-defined conditions listed in Chapter 18 characteristic of, or associated with, an existing primary or secondary site malignancy cannot be used to replace the malignancy as principal or first-listed diagnosis, regardless of the number of admissions or encounters for treatment and care of the neoplasm.

*See Section I.C.21. Factors influencing health status and contact with health services, Encounter for prophylactic organ removal.*

**h. Admission/encounter for pain control/management**

*See Section I.C.6. for information on coding admission/encounter for pain control/management.*

**i. Malignancy in two or more noncontiguous sites**

A patient may have more than one malignant tumor in the same organ. These tumors may represent different primaries or metastatic disease, depending on the site. Should the documentation be unclear, the provider should be queried as to the status of each tumor so that the correct codes can be assigned.

**j. Disseminated malignant neoplasm, unspecified**

Code C8Ø.Ø, Disseminated malignant neoplasm, unspecified, is for use only in those cases where the patient has advanced metastatic disease and no known primary or secondary sites are specified. It should not be used in place of assigning codes for the primary site and all known secondary sites.

**k. Malignant neoplasm without specification of site**

Code C8Ø.1, Malignant (primary) neoplasm, unspecified, equates to Cancer, unspecified. This code should only be used when no determination can be made as to the primary site of a malignancy. This code should rarely be used in the inpatient setting.

Evaluation of painful hip leads to diagnosis of a metastatic bone lesion from an unknown primary neoplasm source

| | |
|---|---|
| **C79.51** | **Secondary malignant neoplasm of bone** |
| **C8Ø.1** | **Malignant (primary) neoplasm, unspecified** |

*Explanation*: If only the secondary site is known, use code C8Ø.1 for the unknown primary site.

**l. Sequencing of neoplasm codes**

**1) Encounter for treatment of primary malignancy**

If the reason for the encounter is for treatment of a primary malignancy, assign the malignancy as the principal/first-listed diagnosis. The primary site is to be sequenced first, followed by any metastatic sites.

**2) Encounter for treatment of secondary malignancy**

When an encounter is for a primary malignancy with metastasis and treatment is directed toward the metastatic (secondary) site(s) only, the metastatic site(s) is designated as the principal/first-listed diagnosis. The primary malignancy is coded as an additional code.

Patient has primary colon cancer with metastasis to rib and is evaluated for possible excision of portion of rib bone

| | |
|---|---|
| **C79.51** | **Secondary malignant neoplasm of bone** |
| **C18.9** | **Malignant neoplasm of colon, unspecified** |

*Explanation*: The treatment for this encounter is focused on the metastasis to the rib bone rather than the primary colon cancer, thus indicating that the bone metastasis is sequenced as the first-listed code.

**3) Malignant neoplasm in a pregnant patient**

When a pregnant patient has a malignant neoplasm, a code from subcategory O9A.1-, Malignant neoplasm complicating pregnancy, childbirth, and the puerperium, should be sequenced first, followed by the appropriate code from Chapter 2 to indicate the type of neoplasm.

> A 30-year-old pregnant female in first trimester evaluated for pituitary gland malignancy
>
> **O9A.111 Malignant neoplasm complicating pregnancy, first trimester**
>
> **C75.1 Malignant neoplasm of pituitary gland**
>
> *Explanation*: Codes from chapter 15 describing complications of pregnancy are sequenced as first-listed codes, further specified by codes from other chapters such as neoplastic, unless the pregnancy is documented as incidental to the condition. See also guideline 1.C.15.a.1.

**4) Encounter for complication associated with a neoplasm**

When an encounter is for management of a complication associated with a neoplasm, such as dehydration, and the treatment is only for the complication, the complication is coded first, followed by the appropriate code(s) for the neoplasm.

The exception to this guideline is anemia. When the admission/encounter is for management of an anemia associated with the malignancy, and the treatment is only for anemia, the appropriate code for the malignancy is sequenced as the principal or first-listed diagnosis followed by code D63.Ø, Anemia in neoplastic disease.

> Patient with pancreatic cancer is seen for initiation of TPN for cancer-related moderate protein-calorie malnutrition
>
> **E44.Ø Moderate protein-calorie malnutrition**
>
> **C25.9 Malignant neoplasm of pancreas, unspecified**
>
> *Explanation*: The encounter is to initiate treatment for malnutrition, a common complication of many types of neoplasms, and is sequenced first.

**5) Complication from surgical procedure for treatment of a neoplasm**

When an encounter is for treatment of a complication resulting from a surgical procedure performed for the treatment of the neoplasm, designate the complication as the principal/first-listed diagnosis. See the guideline regarding the coding of a current malignancy versus personal history to determine if the code for the neoplasm should also be assigned.

**6) Pathologic fracture due to a neoplasm**

When an encounter is for a pathological fracture due to a neoplasm, and the focus of treatment is the fracture, a code from subcategory M84.5, Pathological fracture in neoplastic disease, should be sequenced first, followed by the code for the neoplasm.

If the focus of treatment is the neoplasm with an associated pathological fracture, the neoplasm code should be sequenced first, followed by a code from M84.5 for the pathological fracture.

**m. Current malignancy versus personal history of malignancy**

When a primary malignancy has been excised but further treatment, such as an additional surgery for the malignancy, radiation therapy or chemotherapy is directed to that site, the primary malignancy code should be used until treatment is completed.

> Female patient with ongoing chemotherapy after right mastectomy for breast cancer
>
> **C5Ø.911 Malignant neoplasm of unspecified site of right female breast**
>
> **Z9Ø.11 Acquired absence of right breast and nipple**
>
> *Explanation*: Even though the breast has been removed, the breast cancer is still being treated with chemotherapy and therefore is still coded as a current condition rather than personal history.

When a primary malignancy has been previously excised or eradicated from its site, there is no further treatment (of the malignancy) directed to that site, and there is no evidence of any existing primary malignancy at that site, a code from category Z85, Personal history of malignant neoplasm, should be used to indicate the former site of the malignancy.

Codes from subcategories Z85.Ø – Z85.85 should only be assigned for the former site of a primary malignancy, not the site of a secondary malignancy. Code Z85.89 may be assigned for the former site(s) of either a primary or secondary malignancy.

*See Section I.C.21. Factors influencing health status and contact with health services, History (of)*

**n. Leukemia, multiple myeloma, and malignant plasma cell neoplasms in remission versus personal history**

The categories for leukemia, and category C9Ø, Multiple myeloma and malignant plasma cell neoplasms, have codes indicating whether or not the leukemia has achieved remission. There are also codes Z85.6, Personal history of leukemia, and Z85.79, Personal history of other malignant neoplasms of lymphoid, hematopoietic and related tissues. If the documentation is unclear as to whether the leukemia has achieved remission, the provider should be queried.

*See Section I.C.21. Factors influencing health status and contact with health services, History (of)*

**o. Aftercare following surgery for neoplasm**

*See Section I.C.21. Factors influencing health status and contact with health services, Aftercare*

**p. Follow-up care for completed treatment of a malignancy**

*See Section I.C.21. Factors influencing health status and contact with health services, Follow-up*

**q. Prophylactic organ removal for prevention of malignancy**

*See Section I.C. 21, Factors influencing health status and contact with health services, Prophylactic organ removal*

**r. Malignant neoplasm associated with transplanted organ**

A malignant neoplasm of a transplanted organ should be coded as a transplant complication. Assign first the appropriate code from category T86.-, Complications of transplanted organs and tissue, followed by code C8Ø.2, Malignant neoplasm associated with transplanted organ. Use an additional code for the specific malignancy.

**s. Breast Implant Associated Anaplastic Large Cell Lymphoma**

Breast implant associated anaplastic large cell lymphoma (BIA-ALCL) is a type of lymphoma that can develop around breast implants. Assign code C84.7A, Anaplastic large cell lymphoma, ALK-negative, breast, for BIA-ALCL or C84.7B, Anaplastic large cell lymphoma, ALK-negative, in remission, for BIA-ALCL in remission. Do not assign a complication code from chapter 19.

**t. Secondary malignant neoplasm of lymphoid tissue**

When a malignant neoplasm of lymphoid tissue metastasizes beyond the lymph nodes, a code from categories C81-C85 with a final character identifying "extranodal and solid organ sites" should be assigned rather than a code for the secondary neoplasm of the affected solid organ. For example, for metastasis of diffuse large B-cell lymphoma to the lung, brain and left adrenal gland, assign code C83.398, Diffuse large B-cell lymphoma of other extranodal and solid organ sites.

# Chapter 2. Neoplasms (CØØ-D49)

NOTE

**Functional activity**

All neoplasms are classified in this chapter, whether they are functionally active or not. An additional code from Chapter 4 may be used, to identify functional activity associated with any neoplasm.

**Morphology [Histology]**

Chapter 2 classifies neoplasms primarily by site (topography), with broad groupings for behavior, malignant, in situ, benign, etc. The Table of Neoplasms should be used to identify the correct topography code. In a few cases, such as for malignant melanoma and certain neuroendocrine tumors, the morphology (histologic type) is included in the category and codes.

**Primary malignant neoplasms overlapping site boundaries**

A primary malignant neoplasm that overlaps two or more contiguous (next to each other) sites should be classified to the subcategory/code .8 ("overlapping lesion"), unless the combination is specifically indexed elsewhere. For multiple neoplasms of the same site that are not contiguous, such as tumors in different quadrants of the same breast, codes for each site should be assigned.

**Malignant neoplasm of ectopic tissue**

Malignant neoplasms of ectopic tissue are to be coded to the site mentioned, e.g., ectopic pancreatic malignant neoplasms are coded to pancreas, unspecified (C25.9).

**AHA:** 2024,1Q,24; 2023,2Q,6; 2017,4Q,103; 2017,1Q,4,5-6,8

This chapter contains the following blocks:

| | |
|---|---|
| CØØ-C14 | Malignant neoplasms of lip, oral cavity and pharynx |
| C15-C26 | Malignant neoplasms of digestive organs |
| C3Ø-C39 | Malignant neoplasms of respiratory and intrathoracic organs |
| C4Ø-C41 | Malignant neoplasms of bone and articular cartilage |
| C43-C44 | Melanoma and other malignant neoplasms of skin |
| C45-C49 | Malignant neoplasms of mesothelial and soft tissue |
| C5Ø | Malignant neoplasms of breast |
| C51-C58 | Malignant neoplasms of female genital organs |
| C6Ø-C63 | Malignant neoplasms of male genital organs |
| C64-C68 | Malignant neoplasms of urinary tract |
| C69-C72 | Malignant neoplasms of eye, brain and other parts of central nervous system |
| C73-C75 | Malignant neoplasms of thyroid and other endocrine glands |
| C7A | Malignant neuroendocrine tumors |
| C7B | Secondary neuroendocrine tumors |
| C76-C8Ø | Malignant neoplasms of ill-defined, other secondary and unspecified sites |
| C81-C96 | Malignant neoplasms of lymphoid, hematopoietic and related tissue |
| DØØ-DØ9 | In situ neoplasms |
| D1Ø-D36 | Benign neoplasms, except benign neuroendocrine tumors |
| D3A | Benign neuroendocrine tumors |
| D37-D48 | Neoplasms of uncertain behavior, polycythemia vera and myelodysplastic syndromes |
| D49 | Neoplasms of unspecified behavior |

## MALIGNANT NEOPLASMS (CØØ-C96)

Malignant neoplasms, stated or presumed to be primary (of specified sites), and certain specified histologies, except neuroendocrine, and of lymphoid, hematopoietic and related tissue (CØØ-C75)

**AHA:** 2022,1Q,16

**TIP:** Codes from this code block can be assigned for outpatient encounters based on the diagnosis listed in a pathology or cytology report when authenticated by a pathologist and available at the time of code assignment.

### Malignant neoplasms of lip, oral cavity and pharynx (CØØ-C14)

✓4th **CØØ Malignant neoplasm of lip**

Use additional code to identify:
- alcohol abuse and dependence (F1Ø.-)
- history of tobacco dependence (Z87.891)
- tobacco dependence (F17.-)
- tobacco use (Z72.Ø)

EXCLUDES 1 *malignant melanoma of lip (C43.Ø)*
*Merkel cell carcinoma of lip (C4A.Ø)*
*other and unspecified malignant neoplasm of skin of lip (C44.Ø-)*

**CØØ.Ø Malignant neoplasm of external upper lip**
Malignant neoplasm of lipstick area of upper lip
Malignant neoplasm of upper lip NOS
Malignant neoplasm of vermilion border of upper lip

**CØØ.1 Malignant neoplasm of external lower lip**
Malignant neoplasm of lipstick area of lower lip
Malignant neoplasm of lower lip NOS
Malignant neoplasm of vermilion border of lower lip

**CØØ.2 Malignant neoplasm of external lip, unspecified**
Malignant neoplasm of vermilion border of lip NOS

**CØØ.3 Malignant neoplasm of upper lip, inner aspect**
Malignant neoplasm of buccal aspect of upper lip
Malignant neoplasm of frenulum of upper lip
Malignant neoplasm of mucosa of upper lip
Malignant neoplasm of oral aspect of upper lip

**CØØ.4 Malignant neoplasm of lower lip, inner aspect**
Malignant neoplasm of buccal aspect of lower lip
Malignant neoplasm of frenulum of lower lip
Malignant neoplasm of mucosa of lower lip
Malignant neoplasm of oral aspect of lower lip

**CØØ.5 Malignant neoplasm of lip, unspecified, inner aspect**
Malignant neoplasm of buccal aspect of lip, unspecified
Malignant neoplasm of frenulum of lip, unspecified
Malignant neoplasm of mucosa of lip, unspecified
Malignant neoplasm of oral aspect of lip, unspecified

**CØØ.6 Malignant neoplasm of commissure of lip, unspecified**

**CØØ.8 Malignant neoplasm of overlapping sites of lip**

**CØØ.9 Malignant neoplasm of lip, unspecified**

**CØ1 Malignant neoplasm of base of tongue** HCC Rx ESR COM
Malignant neoplasm of dorsal surface of base of tongue
Malignant neoplasm of fixed part of tongue NOS
Malignant neoplasm of posterior third of tongue

Use additional code to identify:
- alcohol abuse and dependence (F1Ø.-)
- history of tobacco dependence (Z87.891)
- tobacco dependence (F17.-)
- tobacco use (Z72.Ø)

**Malignant Neoplasm of Tongue**

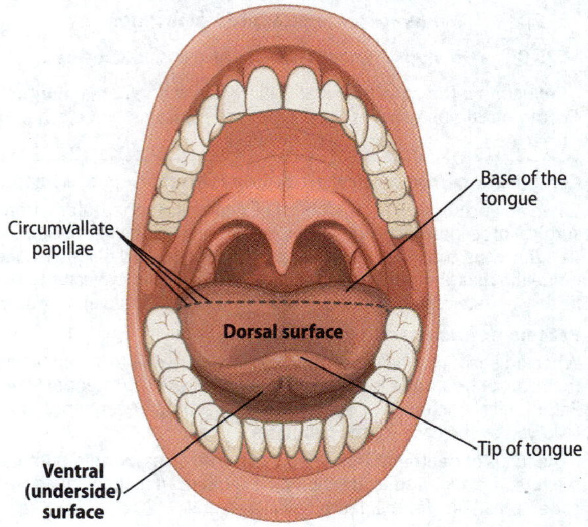


✓4th **CØ2 Malignant neoplasm of other and unspecified parts of tongue**

Use additional code to identify:
- alcohol abuse and dependence (F1Ø.-)
- history of tobacco dependence (Z87.891)
- tobacco dependence (F17.-)
- tobacco use (Z72.Ø)

**CØ2.Ø Malignant neoplasm of dorsal surface of tongue** HCC Rx ESR COM
Malignant neoplasm of anterior two-thirds of tongue, dorsal surface

EXCLUDES 2 *malignant neoplasm of dorsal surface of base of tongue (CØ1)*

**CØ2.1 Malignant neoplasm of border of tongue** HCC Rx ESR COM
Malignant neoplasm of tip of tongue

**CØ2.2 Malignant neoplasm of ventral surface of tongue** HCC Rx ESR COM
Malignant neoplasm of anterior two-thirds of tongue, ventral surface
Malignant neoplasm of frenulum linguae

**CØ2.3 Malignant neoplasm of anterior two-thirds of tongue, part unspecified** HCC Rx ESR COM
Malignant neoplasm of middle third of tongue NOS
Malignant neoplasm of mobile part of tongue NOS

**CØ2.4 Malignant neoplasm of lingual tonsil** HCC Rx ESR COM

EXCLUDES 2 *malignant neoplasm of tonsil NOS (CØ9.9)*

**CØ2.8 Malignant neoplasm of overlapping sites of tongue** HCC Rx ESR COM
Malignant neoplasm of two or more contiguous sites of tongue

**CØ2.9 Malignant neoplasm of tongue, unspecified** HCC Rx ESR COM

**C03 Malignant neoplasm of gum**

INCLUDES malignant neoplasm of alveolar (ridge) mucosa
malignant neoplasm of gingiva

Use additional code to identify:
alcohol abuse and dependence (F10.-)
history of tobacco dependence (Z87.891)
tobacco dependence (F17.-)
tobacco use (Z72.0)

EXCLUDES 2 *malignant odontogenic neoplasms (C41.0-C41.1)*

**C03.0 Malignant neoplasm of upper gum** HCC Rx ESR COM
**C03.1 Malignant neoplasm of lower gum** HCC Rx ESR COM
**C03.9 Malignant neoplasm of gum, unspecified** HCC Rx ESR COM

**C04 Malignant neoplasm of floor of mouth**

Use additional code to identify:
alcohol abuse and dependence (F10.-)
history of tobacco dependence (Z87.891)
tobacco dependence (F17.-)
tobacco use (Z72.0)

**C04.0 Malignant neoplasm of anterior floor of mouth** HCC Rx ESR COM
Malignant neoplasm of anterior to the premolar-canine junction
**C04.1 Malignant neoplasm of lateral floor of mouth** HCC Rx ESR COM
**C04.8 Malignant neoplasm of overlapping sites of floor of mouth** HCC Rx ESR COM
**C04.9 Malignant neoplasm of floor of mouth, unspecified** HCC Rx ESR COM

**C05 Malignant neoplasm of palate**

Use additional code to identify:
alcohol abuse and dependence (F10.-)
history of tobacco dependence (Z87.891)
tobacco dependence (F17.-)
tobacco use (Z72.0)

EXCLUDES 1 *Kaposi's sarcoma of palate (C46.2)*

**C05.0 Malignant neoplasm of hard palate** HCC Rx ESR COM
**C05.1 Malignant neoplasm of soft palate** HCC Rx ESR COM
EXCLUDES 2 *malignant neoplasm of nasopharyngeal surface of soft palate (C11.3)*
**C05.2 Malignant neoplasm of uvula** HCC Rx ESR COM
**C05.8 Malignant neoplasm of overlapping sites of palate** HCC Rx ESR COM
**C05.9 Malignant neoplasm of palate, unspecified** HCC Rx ESR COM
Malignant neoplasm of roof of mouth

**C06 Malignant neoplasm of other and unspecified parts of mouth**

Use additional code to identify:
alcohol abuse and dependence (F10.-)
history of tobacco dependence (Z87.891)
tobacco dependence (F17.-)
tobacco use (Z72.0)

**C06.0 Malignant neoplasm of cheek mucosa** HCC Rx ESR COM
Malignant neoplasm of buccal mucosa NOS
Malignant neoplasm of internal cheek
**C06.1 Malignant neoplasm of vestibule of mouth** HCC Rx ESR COM
Malignant neoplasm of buccal sulcus (upper) (lower)
Malignant neoplasm of labial sulcus (upper) (lower)
**C06.2 Malignant neoplasm of retromolar area** HCC Rx ESR COM
**C06.8 Malignant neoplasm of overlapping sites of other and unspecified parts of mouth**
**C06.80 Malignant neoplasm of overlapping sites of unspecified parts of mouth** HCC Rx ESR COM
**C06.89 Malignant neoplasm of overlapping sites of other parts of mouth** HCC Rx ESR COM
"book leaf" neoplasm [ventral surface of tongue and floor of mouth]
**C06.9 Malignant neoplasm of mouth, unspecified** HCC Rx ESR COM
Malignant neoplasm of minor salivary gland, unspecified site
Malignant neoplasm of oral cavity NOS

**C07 Malignant neoplasm of parotid gland** HCC Rx ESR COM

Use additional code to identify:
alcohol abuse and dependence (F10.-)
exposure to environmental tobacco smoke (Z77.22)
exposure to tobacco smoke in the perinatal period (P96.81)
history of tobacco dependence (Z87.891)
occupational exposure to environmental tobacco smoke (Z57.31)
tobacco dependence (F17.-)
tobacco use (Z72.0)

**C08 Malignant neoplasm of other and unspecified major salivary glands**

INCLUDES malignant neoplasm of salivary ducts

Use additional code to identify:
alcohol abuse and dependence (F10.-)
exposure to environmental tobacco smoke (Z77.22)
exposure to tobacco smoke in the perinatal period (P96.81)
history of tobacco dependence (Z87.891)
occupational exposure to environmental tobacco smoke (Z57.31)
tobacco dependence (F17.-)
tobacco use (Z72.0)

EXCLUDES 1 *malignant neoplasms of specified minor salivary glands which are classified according to their anatomical location*

EXCLUDES 2 *malignant neoplasms of minor salivary glands NOS (C06.9)*
*malignant neoplasm of parotid gland (C07)*

**C08.0 Malignant neoplasm of submandibular gland** HCC Rx ESR COM
Malignant neoplasm of submaxillary gland
**C08.1 Malignant neoplasm of sublingual gland** HCC Rx ESR COM
**C08.9 Malignant neoplasm of major salivary gland, unspecified** HCC Rx ESR COM
Malignant neoplasm of salivary gland (major) NOS

**C09 Malignant neoplasm of tonsil**

Use additional code to identify:
alcohol abuse and dependence (F10.-)
exposure to environmental tobacco smoke (Z77.22)
exposure to tobacco smoke in the perinatal period (P96.81)
history of tobacco dependence (Z87.891)
occupational exposure to environmental tobacco smoke (Z57.31)
tobacco dependence (F17.-)
tobacco use (Z72.0)

EXCLUDES 2 *malignant neoplasm of lingual tonsil (C02.4)*
*malignant neoplasm of pharyngeal tonsil (C11.1)*

**C09.0 Malignant neoplasm of tonsillar fossa** HCC ESR COM
**C09.1 Malignant neoplasm of tonsillar pillar (anterior) (posterior)** HCC ESR COM
**C09.8 Malignant neoplasm of overlapping sites of tonsil** HCC ESR COM
**C09.9 Malignant neoplasm of tonsil, unspecified** HCC ESR COM
Malignant neoplasm of faucial tonsils
Malignant neoplasm of palatine tonsils
Malignant neoplasm of tonsil NOS

**C10 Malignant neoplasm of oropharynx**

Use additional code to identify:
alcohol abuse and dependence (F10.-)
exposure to environmental tobacco smoke (Z77.22)
exposure to tobacco smoke in the perinatal period (P96.81)
history of tobacco dependence (Z87.891)
occupational exposure to environmental tobacco smoke (Z57.31)
tobacco dependence (F17.-)
tobacco use (Z72.0)

EXCLUDES 2 *malignant neoplasm of tonsil (C09.-)*

**DEF:** Oropharynx: Middle portion of pharynx (throat); communicates with the oral cavity, nasopharynx and laryngopharynx.

**C10.0 Malignant neoplasm of vallecula** HCC ESR COM
**C10.1 Malignant neoplasm of anterior surface of epiglottis** HCC ESR COM
Malignant neoplasm of epiglottis, free border [margin]
Malignant neoplasm of glossoepiglottic fold(s)
EXCLUDES 2 *malignant neoplasm of epiglottis (suprahyoid portion) NOS (C32.1)*
**C10.2 Malignant neoplasm of lateral wall of oropharynx** HCC ESR COM
**C10.3 Malignant neoplasm of posterior wall of oropharynx** HCC ESR COM
**C10.4 Malignant neoplasm of branchial cleft** HCC ESR COM
Malignant neoplasm of branchial cyst [site of neoplasm]
**C10.8 Malignant neoplasm of overlapping sites of oropharynx** HCC ESR COM
Malignant neoplasm of junctional region of oropharynx
**C10.9 Malignant neoplasm of oropharynx, unspecified** HCC ESR COM

✓4th **C11 Malignant neoplasm of nasopharynx**
Use additional code to identify:
exposure to environmental tobacco smoke (Z77.22)
exposure to tobacco smoke in the perinatal period (P96.81)
history of tobacco dependence (Z87.891)
occupational exposure to environmental tobacco smoke (Z57.31)
tobacco dependence (F17.-)
tobacco use (Z72.Ø)
**DEF:** Nasopharynx: Upper portion of pharynx (throat); communicates with the nasal cavities, oropharynx and tympanic cavities.

**C11.Ø Malignant neoplasm of superior wall of nasopharynx** HCC ESR COM
Malignant neoplasm of roof of nasopharynx

**C11.1 Malignant neoplasm of posterior wall of nasopharynx** HCC ESR COM
Malignant neoplasm of adenoid
Malignant neoplasm of pharyngeal tonsil

**C11.2 Malignant neoplasm of lateral wall of nasopharynx** HCC ESR COM
Malignant neoplasm of fossa of Rosenmuller
Malignant neoplasm of opening of auditory tube
Malignant neoplasm of pharyngeal recess

**C11.3 Malignant neoplasm of anterior wall of nasopharynx** HCC ESR COM
Malignant neoplasm of floor of nasopharynx
Malignant neoplasm of nasopharyngeal (anterior) (posterior) surface of soft palate
Malignant neoplasm of posterior margin of nasal choana
Malignant neoplasm of posterior margin of nasal septum

**C11.8 Malignant neoplasm of overlapping sites of nasopharynx** HCC ESR COM

**C11.9 Malignant neoplasm of nasopharynx, unspecified** HCC ESR COM
Malignant neoplasm of nasopharyngeal wall NOS

**C12 Malignant neoplasm of pyriform sinus** HCC ESR COM
Malignant neoplasm of pyriform fossa
Use additional code to identify:
exposure to environmental tobacco smoke (Z77.22)
exposure to tobacco smoke in the perinatal period (P96.81)
history of tobacco dependence (Z87.891)
occupational exposure to environmental tobacco smoke (Z57.31)
tobacco dependence (F17.-)
tobacco use (Z72.Ø)

✓4th **C13 Malignant neoplasm of hypopharynx**
Use additional code to identify:
exposure to environmental tobacco smoke (Z77.22)
exposure to tobacco smoke in the perinatal period (P96.81)
history of tobacco dependence (Z87.891)
occupational exposure to environmental tobacco smoke (Z57.31)
tobacco dependence (F17.-)
tobacco use (Z72.Ø)
EXCLUDES 2 *malignant neoplasm of pyriform sinus (C12)*
**DEF:** Hypopharynx: Lower portion of pharynx (throat); communicates with the oropharynx and the esophagus. ***Synonym(s):*** *laryngopharynx.*

**C13.Ø Malignant neoplasm of postcricoid region** HCC ESR COM

**C13.1 Malignant neoplasm of aryepiglottic fold, hypopharyngeal aspect** HCC ESR COM
Malignant neoplasm of aryepiglottic fold NOS
Malignant neoplasm of aryepiglottic fold, marginal zone
Malignant neoplasm of interarytenoid fold NOS
Malignant neoplasm of interarytenoid fold, marginal zone
EXCLUDES 2 *malignant neoplasm of aryepiglottic fold or interarytenoid fold, laryngeal aspect (C32.1)*

**C13.2 Malignant neoplasm of posterior wall of hypopharynx** HCC ESR COM

**C13.8 Malignant neoplasm of overlapping sites of hypopharynx** HCC ESR COM

**C13.9 Malignant neoplasm of hypopharynx, unspecified** HCC ESR COM
Malignant neoplasm of hypopharyngeal wall NOS

✓4th **C14 Malignant neoplasm of other and ill-defined sites in the lip, oral cavity and pharynx**
Use additional code to identify:
alcohol abuse and dependence (F1Ø.-)
exposure to environmental tobacco smoke (Z77.22)
exposure to tobacco smoke in the perinatal period (P96.81)
history of tobacco dependence (Z87.891)
occupational exposure to environmental tobacco smoke (Z57.31)
tobacco dependence (F17.-)
tobacco use (Z72.Ø)
EXCLUDES 1 *malignant neoplasm of oral cavity NOS (CØ6.9)*

**C14.Ø Malignant neoplasm of pharynx, unspecified** HCC ESR COM

**C14.2 Malignant neoplasm of Waldeyer's ring** HCC ESR COM
**DEF:** Waldeyer's ring: Ring of lymphoid tissue that is made up of the two palatine tonsils, the pharyngeal tonsil (adenoid), and the lingual tonsil. It functions as the defense against infection and assists with the development of the immune system.

**C14.8 Malignant neoplasm of overlapping sites of lip, oral cavity and pharynx** HCC ESR COM
Primary malignant neoplasm of two or more contiguous sites of lip, oral cavity and pharynx
EXCLUDES 1 *"book leaf" neoplasm [ventral surface of tongue and floor of mouth] (CØ6.89)*

## Malignant neoplasms of digestive organs (C15-C26)

EXCLUDES 1 *Kaposi's sarcoma of gastrointestinal sites (C46.4)*
EXCLUDES 2 *gastrointestinal stromal tumors (C49.A-)*

✓4th **C15 Malignant neoplasm of esophagus**
Use additional code to identify:
alcohol abuse and dependence (F1Ø.-)
**AHA:** 2022,3Q,10

**C15.3 Malignant neoplasm of upper third of esophagus** HCC ESR COM

**C15.4 Malignant neoplasm of middle third of esophagus** HCC ESR COM

**C15.5 Malignant neoplasm of lower third of esophagus** HCC ESR COM
EXCLUDES 1 *malignant neoplasm of cardio-esophageal junction (C16.Ø)*

**C15.8 Malignant neoplasm of overlapping sites of esophagus** HCC ESR COM

**C15.9 Malignant neoplasm of esophagus, unspecified** HCC ESR COM

✓4th **C16 Malignant neoplasm of stomach**
Use additional code to identify:
alcohol abuse and dependence (F1Ø.-)
EXCLUDES 2 *malignant carcinoid tumor of the stomach (C7A.Ø92)*

**C16.Ø Malignant neoplasm of cardia** HCC Rx ESR COM
Malignant neoplasm of cardiac orifice
Malignant neoplasm of cardio-esophageal junction
Malignant neoplasm of esophagus and stomach
Malignant neoplasm of gastro-esophageal junction

**C16.1 Malignant neoplasm of fundus of stomach** HCC Rx ESR COM

**C16.2 Malignant neoplasm of body of stomach** HCC Rx ESR COM

**C16.3 Malignant neoplasm of pyloric antrum** HCC Rx ESR COM
Malignant neoplasm of gastric antrum

**C16.4 Malignant neoplasm of pylorus** HCC Rx ESR COM
Malignant neoplasm of prepylorus
Malignant neoplasm of pyloric canal

**C16.5 Malignant neoplasm of lesser curvature of stomach, unspecified** HCC Rx ESR COM
Malignant neoplasm of lesser curvature of stomach, not classifiable to C16.1-C16.4

**C16.6 Malignant neoplasm of greater curvature of stomach, unspecified** HCC Rx ESR COM
Malignant neoplasm of greater curvature of stomach, not classifiable to C16.Ø-C16.4

**C16.8 Malignant neoplasm of overlapping sites of stomach** HCC Rx ESR COM

**C16.9 Malignant neoplasm of stomach, unspecified** HCC Rx ESR COM
Gastric cancer NOS

✓4th **C17 Malignant neoplasm of small intestine**
EXCLUDES 1 *malignant carcinoid tumors of the small intestine (C7A.Ø1)*
**AHA:** 2016,1Q,19

**C17.Ø Malignant neoplasm of duodenum** HCC Rx ESR COM

**C17.1 Malignant neoplasm of jejunum** HCC Rx ESR COM

**C17.2 Malignant neoplasm of ileum** HCC Rx ESR COM

EXCLUDES 1 *malignant neoplasm of ileocecal valve (C18.Ø)*

**C17.3 Meckel's diverticulum, malignant** HCC Rx ESR COM

EXCLUDES 1 *Meckel's diverticulum, congenital (Q43.Ø)*

**DEF:** Congenital, abnormal remnant of embryonic digestive system development that leaves a sacculation or outpouching from the wall of the small intestine near the terminal part of the ileum made of acid-secreting tissue as in the stomach.

**C17.8 Malignant neoplasm of overlapping sites of small intestine** HCC Rx ESR COM

**C17.9 Malignant neoplasm of small intestine, unspecified** HCC Rx ESR COM

**C18 Malignant neoplasm of colon**

EXCLUDES 1 *malignant carcinoid tumors of the colon (C7A.Ø2-)*

**Colon**

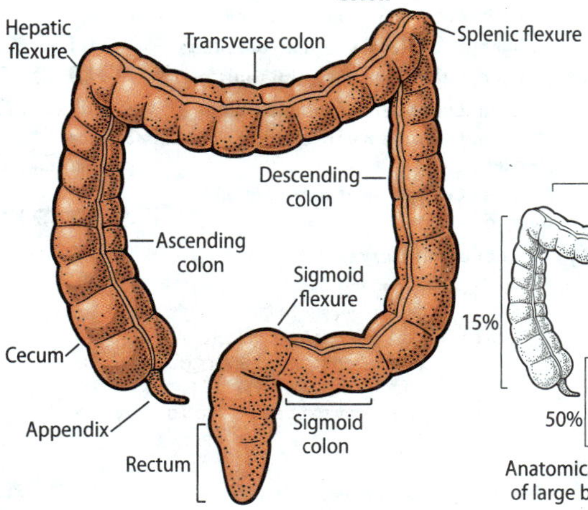


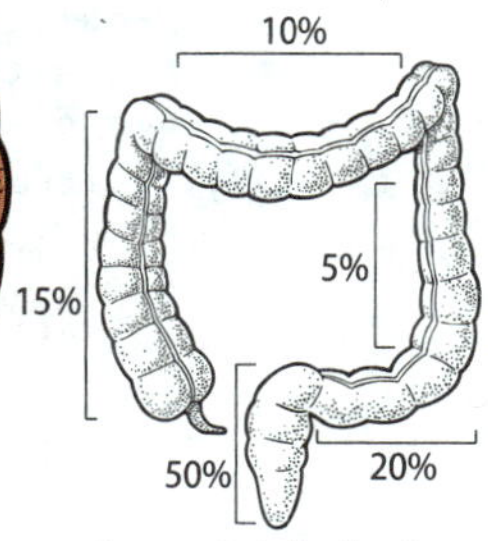


Anatomical distribution of large bowel cancers

**C18.Ø Malignant neoplasm of cecum** HCC ESR COM
Malignant neoplasm of ileocecal valve

**C18.1 Malignant neoplasm of appendix** HCC ESR COM

**C18.2 Malignant neoplasm of ascending colon** HCC ESR COM

**C18.3 Malignant neoplasm of hepatic flexure** HCC ESR COM

**C18.4 Malignant neoplasm of transverse colon** HCC ESR COM

**C18.5 Malignant neoplasm of splenic flexure** HCC ESR COM

**C18.6 Malignant neoplasm of descending colon** HCC ESR COM

**C18.7 Malignant neoplasm of sigmoid colon** HCC ESR COM
Malignant neoplasm of sigmoid (flexure)

EXCLUDES 1 *malignant neoplasm of rectosigmoid junction (C19)*

**C18.8 Malignant neoplasm of overlapping sites of colon** HCC ESR COM

**C18.9 Malignant neoplasm of colon, unspecified** HCC ESR COM
Malignant neoplasm of large intestine NOS

**C19 Malignant neoplasm of rectosigmoid junction** HCC ESR COM
Malignant neoplasm of colon with rectum
Malignant neoplasm of rectosigmoid (colon)

EXCLUDES 1 *malignant carcinoid tumors of the colon (C7A.Ø2-)*

**C2Ø Malignant neoplasm of rectum** HCC ESR COM
Malignant neoplasm of rectal ampulla

EXCLUDES 1 *malignant carcinoid tumor of the rectum (C7A.Ø26)*

**C21 Malignant neoplasm of anus and anal canal**

EXCLUDES 2 *malignant carcinoid tumors of the colon (C7A.Ø2-)*
*malignant melanoma of anal margin (C43.51)*
*malignant melanoma of anal skin (C43.51)*
*malignant melanoma of perianal skin (C43.51)*
*other and unspecified malignant neoplasm of anal margin (C44.5ØØ, C44.51Ø, C44.52Ø, C44.59Ø)*
*other and unspecified malignant neoplasm of anal skin (C44.5ØØ, C44.51Ø, C44.52Ø, C44.59Ø)*
*other and unspecified malignant neoplasm of perianal skin (C44.5ØØ, C44.51Ø, C44.52Ø, C44.59Ø)*

**C21.Ø Malignant neoplasm of anus, unspecified** HCC ESR COM

**C21.1 Malignant neoplasm of anal canal** HCC ESR COM
Malignant neoplasm of anal sphincter

**C21.2 Malignant neoplasm of cloacogenic zone** HCC ESR COM

**C21.8 Malignant neoplasm of overlapping sites of rectum, anus and anal canal** HCC ESR COM
Malignant neoplasm of anorectal junction
Malignant neoplasm of anorectum
Primary malignant neoplasm of two or more contiguous sites of rectum, anus and anal canal

**C22 Malignant neoplasm of liver and intrahepatic bile ducts**

Use additional code to identify:
alcohol abuse and dependence (F1Ø.-)
hepatitis B (B16.-, B18.Ø-B18.1)
hepatitis C (B17.1-, B18.2)

EXCLUDES 1 *malignant neoplasm of biliary tract NOS (C24.9)*
*secondary malignant neoplasm of liver and intrahepatic bile duct (C78.7)*

**C22.Ø Liver cell carcinoma** HCC Rx ESR COM
Hepatocellular carcinoma
Hepatoma
**AHA:** 2016,1Q,18

**C22.1 Intrahepatic bile duct carcinoma** HCC Rx ESR COM
Cholangiocarcinoma

EXCLUDES 1 *malignant neoplasm of hepatic duct (C24.Ø)*

**AHA:** 2023,1Q,24

**C22.2 Hepatoblastoma** HCC Rx ESR COM

**C22.3 Angiosarcoma of liver** HCC Rx ESR COM
Kupffer cell sarcoma

**C22.4 Other sarcomas of liver** HCC Rx ESR COM

**C22.7 Other specified carcinomas of liver** HCC Rx ESR COM

**C22.8 Malignant neoplasm of liver, primary, unspecified as to type** HCC Rx ESR COM

**C22.9 Malignant neoplasm of liver, not specified as primary or secondary** HCC Rx ESR COM

**C23 Malignant neoplasm of gallbladder** HCC Rx ESR COM

**C24 Malignant neoplasm of other and unspecified parts of biliary tract**

EXCLUDES 1 *malignant neoplasm of intrahepatic bile duct (C22.1)*

**C24.Ø Malignant neoplasm of extrahepatic bile duct** HCC Rx ESR COM
Malignant neoplasm of biliary duct or passage NOS
Malignant neoplasm of common bile duct
Malignant neoplasm of cystic duct
Malignant neoplasm of hepatic duct

**C24.1 Malignant neoplasm of ampulla of Vater** HCC Rx ESR COM

**DEF:** Malignant neoplasm in the area of dilation at the juncture of the common bile and pancreatic ducts near the opening into the lumen of the duodenum.

**C24.8 Malignant neoplasm of overlapping sites of biliary tract** HCC Rx ESR COM
Malignant neoplasm involving both intrahepatic and extrahepatic bile ducts
Primary malignant neoplasm of two or more contiguous sites of biliary tract

**C24.9 Malignant neoplasm of biliary tract, unspecified** HCC Rx ESR COM

**✓4th C25 Malignant neoplasm of pancreas**

Code also if applicable exocrine pancreatic insufficiency (K86.81)
Use additional code to identify:
alcohol abuse and dependence (F1Ø.-)

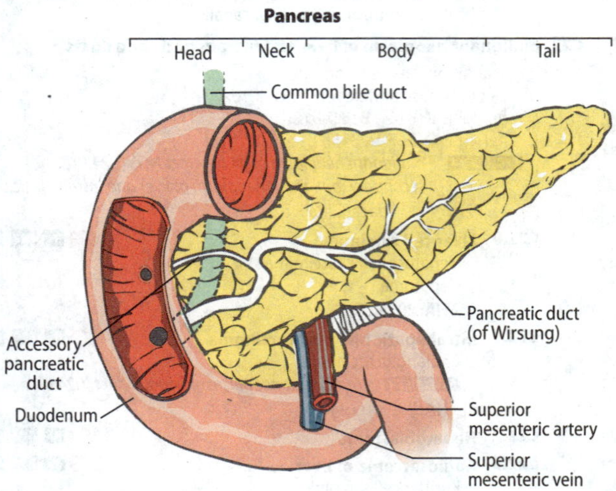


**C25.Ø Malignant neoplasm of head of pancreas** HCC Rx ESR COM

**C25.1 Malignant neoplasm of body of pancreas** HCC Rx ESR COM

**C25.2 Malignant neoplasm of tail of pancreas** HCC Rx ESR COM

**C25.3 Malignant neoplasm of pancreatic duct** HCC Rx ESR COM

**C25.4 Malignant neoplasm of endocrine pancreas** HCC Rx ESR COM
Malignant neoplasm of islets of Langerhans
Use additional code to identify any functional activity

**C25.7 Malignant neoplasm of other parts of pancreas** HCC Rx ESR COM
Malignant neoplasm of neck of pancreas

**C25.8 Malignant neoplasm of overlapping sites of pancreas** HCC Rx ESR COM

**C25.9 Malignant neoplasm of pancreas, unspecified** HCC Rx ESR COM

**✓4th C26 Malignant neoplasm of other and ill-defined digestive organs**

EXCLUDES 1 *malignant neoplasm of peritoneum and retroperitoneum (C48.-)*

**C26.Ø Malignant neoplasm of intestinal tract, part unspecified** HCC ESR COM
Malignant neoplasm of intestine NOS

**C26.1 Malignant neoplasm of spleen** HCC ESR COM
EXCLUDES 1 *Hodgkin lymphoma (C81.-)*
*non-Hodgkin lymphoma (C82-C85)*

**C26.9 Malignant neoplasm of ill-defined sites within the digestive system** HCC ESR COM
Malignant neoplasm of alimentary canal or tract NOS
Malignant neoplasm of gastrointestinal tract NOS
EXCLUDES 1 *malignant neoplasm of abdominal NOS (C76.2)*
*malignant neoplasm of intra-abdominal NOS (C76.2)*

## Malignant neoplasms of respiratory and intrathoracic organs (C3Ø-C39)

INCLUDES malignant neoplasm of middle ear
EXCLUDES 1 *mesothelioma (C45.-)*

**✓4th C3Ø Malignant neoplasm of nasal cavity and middle ear**

**C3Ø.Ø Malignant neoplasm of nasal cavity** HCC Rx ESR COM
Malignant neoplasm of cartilage of nose
Malignant neoplasm of internal nose
Malignant neoplasm of nasal concha
Malignant neoplasm of septum of nose
Malignant neoplasm of vestibule of nose
EXCLUDES 1 *malignant neoplasm of nasal bone (C41.Ø)*
*malignant melanoma of skin of nose (C43.31)*
*malignant neoplasm of nose NOS (C76.Ø)*
*malignant neoplasm of olfactory bulb (C72.2-)*
*malignant neoplasm of posterior margin of nasal septum and choana (C11.3)*
*malignant neoplasm of turbinates (C41.Ø)*
*other and unspecified malignant neoplasm of skin of nose (C44.3Ø1, C44.311, C44.321, C44.391)*

**C3Ø.1 Malignant neoplasm of middle ear** HCC Rx ESR COM
Malignant neoplasm of antrum tympanicum
Malignant neoplasm of auditory tube
Malignant neoplasm of eustachian tube
Malignant neoplasm of inner ear
Malignant neoplasm of mastoid air cells
Malignant neoplasm of tympanic cavity
EXCLUDES 1 *malignant neoplasm of auricular canal (external) (C43.2-,C44.2-)*
*malignant melanoma of skin of (external) ear (C43.2-)*
*malignant neoplasm of bone of ear (meatus) (C41.Ø)*
*malignant neoplasm of cartilage of ear (C49.Ø)*
*other and unspecified malignant neoplasm of skin of (external) ear (C44.2-)*

**✓4th C31 Malignant neoplasm of accessory sinuses**

**C31.Ø Malignant neoplasm of maxillary sinus** HCC Rx ESR COM
Malignant neoplasm of antrum (Highmore) (maxillary)

**C31.1 Malignant neoplasm of ethmoidal sinus** HCC Rx ESR COM

**C31.2 Malignant neoplasm of frontal sinus** HCC Rx ESR COM

**C31.3 Malignant neoplasm of sphenoid sinus** HCC Rx ESR COM

**C31.8 Malignant neoplasm of overlapping sites of accessory sinuses** HCC Rx ESR COM

**C31.9 Malignant neoplasm of accessory sinus, unspecified** HCC Rx ESR COM

**✓4th C32 Malignant neoplasm of larynx**

Use additional code to identify:
alcohol abuse and dependence (F1Ø.-)
exposure to environmental tobacco smoke (Z77.22)
exposure to tobacco smoke in the perinatal period (P96.81)
history of tobacco dependence (Z87.891)
occupational exposure to environmental tobacco smoke (Z57.31)
tobacco dependence (F17.-)
tobacco use (Z72.Ø)

**C32.Ø Malignant neoplasm of glottis** HCC ESR COM
Malignant neoplasm of intrinsic larynx
Malignant neoplasm of laryngeal commissure (anterior)(posterior)
Malignant neoplasm of vocal cord (true) NOS

**C32.1 Malignant neoplasm of supraglottis** HCC ESR COM
Malignant neoplasm of aryepiglottic fold or interarytenoid fold, laryngeal aspect
Malignant neoplasm of epiglottis (suprahyoid portion) NOS
Malignant neoplasm of extrinsic larynx
Malignant neoplasm of false vocal cord
Malignant neoplasm of posterior (laryngeal) surface of epiglottis
Malignant neoplasm of ventricular bands
EXCLUDES 2 *malignant neoplasm of anterior surface of epiglottis (C1Ø.1)*
*malignant neoplasm of aryepiglottic fold or interarytenoid fold NOS (C13.1)*
*malignant neoplasm of aryepiglottic fold or interarytenoid fold, hypopharyngeal aspect (C13.1)*
*malignant neoplasm of aryepiglottic fold or interarytenoid fold, marginal zone (C13.1)*

**C32.2 Malignant neoplasm of subglottis** HCC ESR COM

**C32.3 Malignant neoplasm of laryngeal cartilage** HCC ESR COM

**C32.8 Malignant neoplasm of overlapping sites of larynx** HCC ESR COM

**C32.9 Malignant neoplasm of larynx, unspecified** HCC ESR COM

**C33 Malignant neoplasm of trachea** HCC Rx ESR COM

Use additional code to identify:
exposure to environmental tobacco smoke (Z77.22)
exposure to tobacco smoke in the perinatal period (P96.81)
history of tobacco dependence (Z87.891)
occupational exposure to environmental tobacco smoke (Z57.31)
tobacco dependence (F17.-)
tobacco use (Z72.Ø)

**✓4th C34 Malignant neoplasm of bronchus and lung**

Use additional code to identify:
- exposure to environmental tobacco smoke (Z77.22)
- exposure to tobacco smoke in the perinatal period (P96.81)
- history of tobacco dependence (Z87.891)
- occupational exposure to environmental tobacco smoke (Z57.31)
- tobacco dependence (F17.-)
- tobacco use (Z72.0)

EXCLUDES 1 *Kaposi's sarcoma of lung (C46.5-)*
*malignant carcinoid tumor of the bronchus and lung (C7A.090)*

**AHA:** 2023,1Q,20-21; 2022,4Q,22; 2019,1Q,16

**TIP:** When documented, assign code I31.31 for associated malignant pericardial effusion. The neoplasm code should be sequenced first.

**✓5th C34.0 Malignant neoplasm of main bronchus**

Malignant neoplasm of carina
Malignant neoplasm of hilus (of lung)

**C34.00 Malignant neoplasm of unspecified main bronchus** HCC Rx ESR COM Q

**C34.01 Malignant neoplasm of right main bronchus** HCC Rx ESR COM Q

**C34.02 Malignant neoplasm of left main bronchus** HCC Rx ESR COM Q

**✓5th C34.1 Malignant neoplasm of upper lobe, bronchus or lung**

**C34.10 Malignant neoplasm of upper lobe, unspecified bronchus or lung** HCC Rx ESR COM Q

**C34.11 Malignant neoplasm of upper lobe, right bronchus or lung** HCC Rx ESR COM Q

**C34.12 Malignant neoplasm of upper lobe, left bronchus or lung** HCC Rx ESR COM Q

**C34.2 Malignant neoplasm of middle lobe, bronchus or lung** HCC Rx ESR COM Q

**✓5th C34.3 Malignant neoplasm of lower lobe, bronchus or lung**

**C34.30 Malignant neoplasm of lower lobe, unspecified bronchus or lung** HCC Rx ESR COM Q

**C34.31 Malignant neoplasm of lower lobe, right bronchus or lung** HCC Rx ESR COM Q

**C34.32 Malignant neoplasm of lower lobe, left bronchus or lung** HCC Rx ESR COM Q

**✓5th C34.8 Malignant neoplasm of overlapping sites of bronchus and lung**

**C34.80 Malignant neoplasm of overlapping sites of unspecified bronchus and lung** HCC Rx ESR COM Q

**C34.81 Malignant neoplasm of overlapping sites of right bronchus and lung** HCC Rx ESR COM Q

**C34.82 Malignant neoplasm of overlapping sites of left bronchus and lung** HCC Rx ESR COM Q

**✓5th C34.9 Malignant neoplasm of unspecified part of bronchus or lung**

**C34.90 Malignant neoplasm of unspecified part of unspecified bronchus or lung** HCC Rx ESR COM Q

Lung cancer NOS

**C34.91 Malignant neoplasm of unspecified part of right bronchus or lung** HCC Rx ESR COM Q

**C34.92 Malignant neoplasm of unspecified part of left bronchus or lung** HCC Rx ESR COM Q

**C37 Malignant neoplasm of thymus** HCC Rx ESR COM

EXCLUDES 1 *malignant carcinoid tumor of the thymus (C7A.091)*

**✓4th C38 Malignant neoplasm of heart, mediastinum and pleura**

EXCLUDES 1 *mesothelioma (C45.-)*

**C38.0 Malignant neoplasm of heart** HCC Rx ESR COM

Malignant neoplasm of pericardium

EXCLUDES 1 *malignant neoplasm of great vessels (C49.3)*

**C38.1 Malignant neoplasm of anterior mediastinum** HCC Rx ESR COM

**C38.2 Malignant neoplasm of posterior mediastinum** HCC Rx ESR COM

**C38.3 Malignant neoplasm of mediastinum, part unspecified** HCC Rx ESR COM

**C38.4 Malignant neoplasm of pleura** HCC Rx ESR COM

**C38.8 Malignant neoplasm of overlapping sites of heart, mediastinum and pleura** HCC Rx ESR COM

**✓4th C39 Malignant neoplasm of other and ill-defined sites in the respiratory system and intrathoracic organs**

Use additional code to identify:
- exposure to environmental tobacco smoke (Z77.22)
- exposure to tobacco smoke in the perinatal period (P96.81)
- history of tobacco dependence (Z87.891)
- occupational exposure to environmental tobacco smoke (Z57.31)
- tobacco dependence (F17.-)
- tobacco use (Z72.0)

EXCLUDES 1 *intrathoracic malignant neoplasm NOS (C76.1)*
*thoracic malignant neoplasm NOS (C76.1)*

**C39.0 Malignant neoplasm of upper respiratory tract, part unspecified** HCC Rx ESR COM

**C39.9 Malignant neoplasm of lower respiratory tract, part unspecified** HCC Rx ESR COM

Malignant neoplasm of respiratory tract NOS

## Malignant neoplasms of bone and articular cartilage (C40-C41)

INCLUDES malignant neoplasm of cartilage (articular) (joint)
malignant neoplasm of periosteum

EXCLUDES 1 *malignant neoplasm of bone marrow NOS (C96.9)*
*malignant neoplasm of synovia (C49.-)*

**✓4th C40 Malignant neoplasm of bone and articular cartilage of limbs**

Use additional code to identify major osseous defect, if applicable (M89.7-)

**✓5th C40.0 Malignant neoplasm of scapula and long bones of upper limb**

**C40.00 Malignant neoplasm of scapula and long bones of unspecified upper limb** HCC Rx ESR COM

**C40.01 Malignant neoplasm of scapula and long bones of right upper limb** HCC Rx ESR COM

**C40.02 Malignant neoplasm of scapula and long bones of left upper limb** HCC Rx ESR COM

**✓5th C40.1 Malignant neoplasm of short bones of upper limb**

**C40.10 Malignant neoplasm of short bones of unspecified upper limb** HCC Rx ESR COM

**C40.11 Malignant neoplasm of short bones of right upper limb** HCC Rx ESR COM

**C40.12 Malignant neoplasm of short bones of left upper limb** HCC Rx ESR COM

**✓5th C40.2 Malignant neoplasm of long bones of lower limb**

**C40.20 Malignant neoplasm of long bones of unspecified lower limb** HCC Rx ESR COM

**C40.21 Malignant neoplasm of long bones of right lower limb** HCC Rx ESR COM

**C40.22 Malignant neoplasm of long bones of left lower limb** HCC Rx ESR COM

**✓5th C40.3 Malignant neoplasm of short bones of lower limb**

**C40.30 Malignant neoplasm of short bones of unspecified lower limb** HCC Rx ESR COM

**C40.31 Malignant neoplasm of short bones of right lower limb** HCC Rx ESR COM

**C40.32 Malignant neoplasm of short bones of left lower limb** HCC Rx ESR COM

**✓5th C40.8 Malignant neoplasm of overlapping sites of bone and articular cartilage of limb**

**C40.80 Malignant neoplasm of overlapping sites of bone and articular cartilage of unspecified limb** HCC Rx ESR COM

**C40.81 Malignant neoplasm of overlapping sites of bone and articular cartilage of right limb** HCC Rx ESR COM

**C40.82 Malignant neoplasm of overlapping sites of bone and articular cartilage of left limb** HCC Rx ESR COM

**✓5th C40.9 Malignant neoplasm of unspecified bones and articular cartilage of limb**

**C40.90 Malignant neoplasm of unspecified bones and articular cartilage of unspecified limb** HCC Rx ESR COM

**C40.91 Malignant neoplasm of unspecified bones and articular cartilage of right limb** HCC Rx ESR COM

**C40.92 Malignant neoplasm of unspecified bones and articular cartilage of left limb** HCC Rx ESR COM

✓4th **C41 Malignant neoplasm of bone and articular cartilage of other and unspecified sites**

EXCLUDES 1 *malignant neoplasm of bones of limbs (C4Ø.-)*
*malignant neoplasm of cartilage of ear (C49.Ø)*
*malignant neoplasm of cartilage of eyelid (C49.Ø)*
*malignant neoplasm of cartilage of larynx (C32.3)*
*malignant neoplasm of cartilage of limbs (C4Ø.-)*
*malignant neoplasm of cartilage of nose (C3Ø.Ø)*

**C41.Ø Malignant neoplasm of bones of skull and face** HCC Rx ESR COM
Malignant neoplasm of maxilla (superior)
Malignant neoplasm of orbital bone
EXCLUDES 2 *carcinoma, any type except intraosseous or odontogenic of:*
*malignant neoplasm of jaw bone (lower) (C41.1)*
*maxillary sinus (C31.Ø)*
*upper jaw (CØ3.Ø)*

**C41.1 Malignant neoplasm of mandible** HCC Rx ESR COM
Malignant neoplasm of inferior maxilla
Malignant neoplasm of lower jaw bone
EXCLUDES 2 *carcinoma, any type except intraosseous or odontogenic of:*
*jaw NOS (CØ3.9)*
*lower (CØ3.1)*
*malignant neoplasm of upper jaw bone (C41.Ø)*

**C41.2 Malignant neoplasm of vertebral column** HCC Rx ESR COM
EXCLUDES 1 *malignant neoplasm of sacrum and coccyx (C41.4)*

**C41.3 Malignant neoplasm of ribs, sternum and clavicle** HCC Rx ESR COM

**C41.4 Malignant neoplasm of pelvic bones, sacrum and coccyx** HCC Rx ESR COM

**C41.9 Malignant neoplasm of bone and articular cartilage, unspecified** HCC Rx ESR COM

## Melanoma and other malignant neoplasms of skin (C43-C44)

✓4th **C43 Malignant melanoma of skin**

EXCLUDES 1 *melanoma in situ (DØ3.-)*
EXCLUDES 2 *malignant melanoma of skin of genital organs (C51-C52, C6Ø.-, C63.-)*
*Merkel cell carcinoma (C4A.-)*
*sites other than skin - code to malignant neoplasm of the site*

**C43.Ø Malignant melanoma of lip** HCC Rx ESR COM Q
EXCLUDES 1 *malignant neoplasm of vermilion border of lip (CØØ.Ø-CØØ.2)*

✓5th **C43.1 Malignant melanoma of eyelid, including canthus**
**AHA:** 2018,4Q,4

**C43.10 Malignant melanoma of unspecified eyelid, including canthus** HCC Rx ESR COM

✓6th **C43.11 Malignant melanoma of right eyelid, including canthus**

**C43.111 Malignant melanoma of right upper eyelid, including canthus** HCC Rx ESR COM

**C43.112 Malignant melanoma of right lower eyelid, including canthus** HCC Rx ESR COM

✓6th **C43.12 Malignant melanoma of left eyelid, including canthus**

**C43.121 Malignant melanoma of left upper eyelid, including canthus** HCC Rx ESR COM

**C43.122 Malignant melanoma of left lower eyelid, including canthus** HCC Rx ESR COM

✓5th **C43.2 Malignant melanoma of ear and external auricular canal**

**C43.20 Malignant melanoma of unspecified ear and external auricular canal** HCC Rx ESR COM Q

**C43.21 Malignant melanoma of right ear and external auricular canal** HCC Rx ESR COM Q

**C43.22 Malignant melanoma of left ear and external auricular canal** HCC Rx ESR COM Q

✓5th **C43.3 Malignant melanoma of other and unspecified parts of face**

**C43.30 Malignant melanoma of unspecified part of face** HCC Rx ESR COM Q

**C43.31 Malignant melanoma of nose** HCC Rx ESR COM Q

**C43.39 Malignant melanoma of other parts of face** HCC Rx ESR COM Q

**C43.4 Malignant melanoma of scalp and neck** HCC Rx ESR COM Q

✓5th **C43.5 Malignant melanoma of trunk**
EXCLUDES 2 *malignant neoplasm of anus NOS (C21.Ø)*
*malignant neoplasm of scrotum (C63.2)*

**C43.51 Malignant melanoma of anal skin** HCC Rx ESR COM Q
Malignant melanoma of anal margin
Malignant melanoma of perianal skin

**C43.52 Malignant melanoma of skin of breast** HCC Rx ESR COM Q

**C43.59 Malignant melanoma of other part of trunk** HCC Rx ESR COM Q

✓5th **C43.6 Malignant melanoma of upper limb, including shoulder**

**C43.60 Malignant melanoma of unspecified upper limb, including shoulder** HCC Rx ESR COM Q

**C43.61 Malignant melanoma of right upper limb, including shoulder** HCC Rx ESR COM Q

**C43.62 Malignant melanoma of left upper limb, including shoulder** HCC Rx ESR COM Q

✓5th **C43.7 Malignant melanoma of lower limb, including hip**

**C43.70 Malignant melanoma of unspecified lower limb, including hip** HCC Rx ESR COM Q

**C43.71 Malignant melanoma of right lower limb, including hip** HCC Rx ESR COM Q

**C43.72 Malignant melanoma of left lower limb, including hip** HCC Rx ESR COM Q

**C43.8 Malignant melanoma of overlapping sites of skin** HCC Rx ESR COM Q

**C43.9 Malignant melanoma of skin, unspecified** HCC Rx ESR COM Q
Malignant melanoma of unspecified site of skin
Melanoma (malignant) NOS

✓4th **C4A Merkel cell carcinoma**
**DEF:** Malignant cutaneous cancer predominantly found in elderly patients with sun exposure that usually presents as a flesh-colored or bluish-red lump typically seen on the neck, head, and face.

**C4A.Ø Merkel cell carcinoma of lip** HCC Rx ESR COM
EXCLUDES 1 *malignant neoplasm of vermilion border of lip (CØØ.Ø-CØØ.2)*

✓5th **C4A.1 Merkel cell carcinoma of eyelid, including canthus**
**AHA:** 2018,4Q,4

**C4A.10 Merkel cell carcinoma of unspecified eyelid, including canthus** HCC Rx ESR COM

✓6th **C4A.11 Merkel cell carcinoma of right eyelid, including canthus**

**C4A.111 Merkel cell carcinoma of right upper eyelid, including canthus** HCC Rx ESR COM

**C4A.112 Merkel cell carcinoma of right lower eyelid, including canthus** HCC Rx ESR COM

✓6th **C4A.12 Merkel cell carcinoma of left eyelid, including canthus**

**C4A.121 Merkel cell carcinoma of left upper eyelid, including canthus** HCC Rx ESR COM

**C4A.122 Merkel cell carcinoma of left lower eyelid, including canthus** HCC Rx ESR COM

✓5th **C4A.2 Merkel cell carcinoma of ear and external auricular canal**

**C4A.20 Merkel cell carcinoma of unspecified ear and external auricular canal** HCC Rx ESR COM

**C4A.21 Merkel cell carcinoma of right ear and external auricular canal** HCC Rx ESR COM

**C4A.22 Merkel cell carcinoma of left ear and external auricular canal** HCC Rx ESR COM

✓5th **C4A.3 Merkel cell carcinoma of other and unspecified parts of face**

**C4A.30 Merkel cell carcinoma of unspecified part of face** HCC Rx ESR COM

**C4A.31 Merkel cell carcinoma of nose** HCC Rx ESR COM

**C4A.39 Merkel cell carcinoma of other parts of face** HCC Rx ESR COM

**C4A.4 Merkel cell carcinoma of scalp and neck** HCC Rx ESR COM

✓5th **C4A.5 Merkel cell carcinoma of trunk**
EXCLUDES 2 *malignant neoplasm of anus NOS (C21.Ø)*
*malignant neoplasm of scrotum (C63.2)*

**C4A.51 Merkel cell carcinoma of anal skin** HCC Rx ESR COM
Merkel cell carcinoma of anal margin
Merkel cell carcinoma of perianal skin

**C4A.52 Merkel cell carcinoma of skin of breast** HCC Rx ESR COM

**C4A.59 Merkel cell carcinoma of other part of trunk** HCC Rx ESR COM

✓5th **C4A.6 Merkel cell carcinoma of upper limb, including shoulder**
**C4A.60 Merkel cell carcinoma of unspecified upper limb, including shoulder** HCC Rx ESR COM
**C4A.61 Merkel cell carcinoma of right upper limb, including shoulder** HCC Rx ESR COM
**C4A.62 Merkel cell carcinoma of left upper limb, including shoulder** HCC Rx ESR COM
✓5th **C4A.7 Merkel cell carcinoma of lower limb, including hip**
**C4A.70 Merkel cell carcinoma of unspecified lower limb, including hip** HCC Rx ESR COM
**C4A.71 Merkel cell carcinoma of right lower limb, including hip** HCC Rx ESR COM
**C4A.72 Merkel cell carcinoma of left lower limb, including hip** HCC Rx ESR COM
**C4A.8 Merkel cell carcinoma of overlapping sites** HCC Rx ESR COM
**C4A.9 Merkel cell carcinoma, unspecified** HCC Rx ESR COM
Merkel cell carcinoma NOS
Merkel cell carcinoma of unspecified site

✓4th **C44 Other and unspecified malignant neoplasm of skin**
INCLUDES malignant neoplasm of sebaceous glands
malignant neoplasm of sweat glands
EXCLUDES 1 *Kaposi's sarcoma of skin (C46.Ø)*
*malignant melanoma of skin (C43.-)*
*malignant neoplasm of skin of genital organs (C51-C52, C6Ø.-, C63.2)*
*Merkel cell carcinoma (C4A.-)*

**DEF:** Basal cell carcinoma: Abnormal growth of skin cells that arises from the deepest layer of the epidermis and may present as an open sore, red patches, pink growth, or scar. Typically caused by sun exposure, it is one of the most common forms of skin cancer.

**DEF:** Squamous cell carcinoma: Uncontrolled growth of abnormal skin cells that arises from the outer layers of the skin (epidermis) and may present as an open sore. It is characterized by a firm, red nodule, elevated growth with a central depression, or a flat sore with a scaly crust.

✓5th **C44.Ø Other and unspecified malignant neoplasm of skin of lip**
EXCLUDES 1 *malignant neoplasm of lip (CØØ.-)*
**C44.ØØ Unspecified malignant neoplasm of skin of lip**
**C44.Ø1 Basal cell carcinoma of skin of lip**
**C44.Ø2 Squamous cell carcinoma of skin of lip**
**C44.Ø9 Other specified malignant neoplasm of skin of lip**
✓5th **C44.1 Other and unspecified malignant neoplasm of skin of eyelid, including canthus**
EXCLUDES 1 *connective tissue of eyelid (C49.Ø)*
**AHA:** 2018,4Q,4
✓6th **C44.1Ø Unspecified malignant neoplasm of skin of eyelid, including canthus**
**C44.1Ø1 Unspecified malignant neoplasm of skin of unspecified eyelid, including canthus**
✓7th **C44.1Ø2 Unspecified malignant neoplasm of skin of right eyelid, including canthus**
**C44.1Ø21 Unspecified malignant neoplasm of skin of right upper eyelid, including canthus**
**C44.1Ø22 Unspecified malignant neoplasm of skin of right lower eyelid, including canthus**
✓7th **C44.1Ø9 Unspecified malignant neoplasm of skin of left eyelid, including canthus**
**C44.1Ø91 Unspecified malignant neoplasm of skin of left upper eyelid, including canthus**
**C44.1Ø92 Unspecified malignant neoplasm of skin of left lower eyelid, including canthus**
✓6th **C44.11 Basal cell carcinoma of skin of eyelid, including canthus**
**C44.111 Basal cell carcinoma of skin of unspecified eyelid, including canthus**
✓7th **C44.112 Basal cell carcinoma of skin of right eyelid, including canthus**
**C44.1121 Basal cell carcinoma of skin of right upper eyelid, including canthus**
**C44.1122 Basal cell carcinoma of skin of right lower eyelid, including canthus**
✓7th **C44.119 Basal cell carcinoma of skin of left eyelid, including canthus**
**C44.1191 Basal cell carcinoma of skin of left upper eyelid, including canthus**
**C44.1192 Basal cell carcinoma of skin of left lower eyelid, including canthus**
✓6th **C44.12 Squamous cell carcinoma of skin of eyelid, including canthus**
**C44.121 Squamous cell carcinoma of skin of unspecified eyelid, including canthus**
✓7th **C44.122 Squamous cell carcinoma of skin of right eyelid, including canthus**
**C44.1221 Squamous cell carcinoma of skin of right upper eyelid, including canthus**
**C44.1222 Squamous cell carcinoma of skin of right lower eyelid, including canthus**
✓7th **C44.129 Squamous cell carcinoma of skin of left eyelid, including canthus**
**C44.1291 Squamous cell carcinoma of skin of left upper eyelid, including canthus**
**C44.1292 Squamous cell carcinoma of skin of left lower eyelid, including canthus**
✓6th **C44.13 Sebaceous cell carcinoma of skin of eyelid, including canthus**
**C44.131 Sebaceous cell carcinoma of skin of unspecified eyelid, including canthus**
✓7th **C44.132 Sebaceous cell carcinoma of skin of right eyelid, including canthus**
**C44.1321 Sebaceous cell carcinoma of skin of right upper eyelid, including canthus**
**C44.1322 Sebaceous cell carcinoma of skin of right lower eyelid, including canthus**
✓7th **C44.139 Sebaceous cell carcinoma of skin of left eyelid, including canthus**
**C44.1391 Sebaceous cell carcinoma of skin of left upper eyelid, including canthus**
**C44.1392 Sebaceous cell carcinoma of skin of left lower eyelid, including canthus**
✓6th **C44.19 Other specified malignant neoplasm of skin of eyelid, including canthus**
**C44.191 Other specified malignant neoplasm of skin of unspecified eyelid, including canthus**
✓7th **C44.192 Other specified malignant neoplasm of skin of right eyelid, including canthus**
**C44.1921 Other specified malignant neoplasm of skin of right upper eyelid, including canthus**
**C44.1922 Other specified malignant neoplasm of skin of right lower eyelid, including canthus**
✓7th **C44.199 Other specified malignant neoplasm of skin of left eyelid, including canthus**
**C44.1991 Other specified malignant neoplasm of skin of left upper eyelid, including canthus**
**C44.1992 Other specified malignant neoplasm of skin of left lower eyelid, including canthus**
✓5th **C44.2 Other and unspecified malignant neoplasm of skin of ear and external auricular canal**
EXCLUDES 1 *connective tissue of ear (C49.Ø)*
✓6th **C44.2Ø Unspecified malignant neoplasm of skin of ear and external auricular canal**
**C44.2Ø1 Unspecified malignant neoplasm of skin of unspecified ear and external auricular canal**
**C44.2Ø2 Unspecified malignant neoplasm of skin of right ear and external auricular canal**
**C44.2Ø9 Unspecified malignant neoplasm of skin of left ear and external auricular canal**
✓6th **C44.21 Basal cell carcinoma of skin of ear and external auricular canal**
**C44.211 Basal cell carcinoma of skin of unspecified ear and external auricular canal**
**C44.212 Basal cell carcinoma of skin of right ear and external auricular canal**
**C44.219 Basal cell carcinoma of skin of left ear and external auricular canal**

Chapter 2. Neoplasms

C4A.6–C44.219

✓6th **C44.22 Squamous cell carcinoma of skin of ear and external auricular canal**
- **C44.221 Squamous cell carcinoma of skin of unspecified ear and external auricular canal**
- **C44.222 Squamous cell carcinoma of skin of right ear and external auricular canal**
- **C44.229 Squamous cell carcinoma of skin of left ear and external auricular canal**

✓6th **C44.29 Other specified malignant neoplasm of skin of ear and external auricular canal**
- **C44.291 Other specified malignant neoplasm of skin of unspecified ear and external auricular canal**
- **C44.292 Other specified malignant neoplasm of skin of right ear and external auricular canal**
- **C44.299 Other specified malignant neoplasm of skin of left ear and external auricular canal**

✓5th **C44.3 Other and unspecified malignant neoplasm of skin of other and unspecified parts of face**

✓6th **C44.30 Unspecified malignant neoplasm of skin of other and unspecified parts of face**
- **C44.300 Unspecified malignant neoplasm of skin of unspecified part of face**
- **C44.301 Unspecified malignant neoplasm of skin of nose**
- **C44.309 Unspecified malignant neoplasm of skin of other parts of face**

✓6th **C44.31 Basal cell carcinoma of skin of other and unspecified parts of face**
- **C44.310 Basal cell carcinoma of skin of unspecified parts of face**
- **C44.311 Basal cell carcinoma of skin of nose**
- **C44.319 Basal cell carcinoma of skin of other parts of face**

✓6th **C44.32 Squamous cell carcinoma of skin of other and unspecified parts of face**
- **C44.320 Squamous cell carcinoma of skin of unspecified parts of face**
- **C44.321 Squamous cell carcinoma of skin of nose**
- **C44.329 Squamous cell carcinoma of skin of other parts of face**

✓6th **C44.39 Other specified malignant neoplasm of skin of other and unspecified parts of face**
- **C44.390 Other specified malignant neoplasm of skin of unspecified parts of face**
- **C44.391 Other specified malignant neoplasm of skin of nose**
- **C44.399 Other specified malignant neoplasm of skin of other parts of face**

✓5th **C44.4 Other and unspecified malignant neoplasm of skin of scalp and neck**
- **C44.40 Unspecified malignant neoplasm of skin of scalp and neck**
- **C44.41 Basal cell carcinoma of skin of scalp and neck**
- **C44.42 Squamous cell carcinoma of skin of scalp and neck**
- **C44.49 Other specified malignant neoplasm of skin of scalp and neck**

✓5th **C44.5 Other and unspecified malignant neoplasm of skin of trunk**

EXCLUDES 1 *anus NOS (C21.0)*
*scrotum (C63.2)*

✓6th **C44.50 Unspecified malignant neoplasm of skin of trunk**
- **C44.500 Unspecified malignant neoplasm of anal skin**
  - Unspecified malignant neoplasm of anal margin
  - Unspecified malignant neoplasm of perianal skin
- **C44.501 Unspecified malignant neoplasm of skin of breast**
- **C44.509 Unspecified malignant neoplasm of skin of other part of trunk**

✓6th **C44.51 Basal cell carcinoma of skin of trunk**
- **C44.510 Basal cell carcinoma of anal skin**
  - Basal cell carcinoma of anal margin
  - Basal cell carcinoma of perianal skin
- **C44.511 Basal cell carcinoma of skin of breast**
- **C44.519 Basal cell carcinoma of skin of other part of trunk**

✓6th **C44.52 Squamous cell carcinoma of skin of trunk**
- **C44.520 Squamous cell carcinoma of anal skin**
  - Squamous cell carcinoma of anal margin
  - Squamous cell carcinoma of perianal skin
- **C44.521 Squamous cell carcinoma of skin of breast**
- **C44.529 Squamous cell carcinoma of skin of other part of trunk**

✓6th **C44.59 Other specified malignant neoplasm of skin of trunk**
- **C44.590 Other specified malignant neoplasm of anal skin**
  - Other specified malignant neoplasm of anal margin
  - Other specified malignant neoplasm of perianal skin
- **C44.591 Other specified malignant neoplasm of skin of breast**
- **C44.599 Other specified malignant neoplasm of skin of other part of trunk**

✓5th **C44.6 Other and unspecified malignant neoplasm of skin of upper limb, including shoulder**

✓6th **C44.60 Unspecified malignant neoplasm of skin of upper limb, including shoulder**
- **C44.601 Unspecified malignant neoplasm of skin of unspecified upper limb, including shoulder**
- **C44.602 Unspecified malignant neoplasm of skin of right upper limb, including shoulder**
- **C44.609 Unspecified malignant neoplasm of skin of left upper limb, including shoulder**

✓6th **C44.61 Basal cell carcinoma of skin of upper limb, including shoulder**
- **C44.611 Basal cell carcinoma of skin of unspecified upper limb, including shoulder**
- **C44.612 Basal cell carcinoma of skin of right upper limb, including shoulder**
- **C44.619 Basal cell carcinoma of skin of left upper limb, including shoulder**

✓6th **C44.62 Squamous cell carcinoma of skin of upper limb, including shoulder**
- **C44.621 Squamous cell carcinoma of skin of unspecified upper limb, including shoulder**
- **C44.622 Squamous cell carcinoma of skin of right upper limb, including shoulder**
- **C44.629 Squamous cell carcinoma of skin of left upper limb, including shoulder**

✓6th **C44.69 Other specified malignant neoplasm of skin of upper limb, including shoulder**
- **C44.691 Other specified malignant neoplasm of skin of unspecified upper limb, including shoulder**
- **C44.692 Other specified malignant neoplasm of skin of right upper limb, including shoulder**
- **C44.699 Other specified malignant neoplasm of skin of left upper limb, including shoulder**

✓5th **C44.7 Other and unspecified malignant neoplasm of skin of lower limb, including hip**

✓6th **C44.70 Unspecified malignant neoplasm of skin of lower limb, including hip**
- **C44.701 Unspecified malignant neoplasm of skin of unspecified lower limb, including hip**
- **C44.702 Unspecified malignant neoplasm of skin of right lower limb, including hip**
- **C44.709 Unspecified malignant neoplasm of skin of left lower limb, including hip**

✓6th **C44.71 Basal cell carcinoma of skin of lower limb, including hip**
- **C44.711 Basal cell carcinoma of skin of unspecified lower limb, including hip**
- **C44.712 Basal cell carcinoma of skin of right lower limb, including hip**
- **C44.719 Basal cell carcinoma of skin of left lower limb, including hip**

✓6th **C44.72 Squamous cell carcinoma of skin of lower limb, including hip**
- **C44.721 Squamous cell carcinoma of skin of unspecified lower limb, including hip**
- **C44.722 Squamous cell carcinoma of skin of right lower limb, including hip**
- **C44.729 Squamous cell carcinoma of skin of left lower limb, including hip**

✓6th C44.79 Other specified malignant neoplasm of skin of lower limb, including hip
C44.791 Other specified malignant neoplasm of skin of unspecified lower limb, including hip
C44.792 Other specified malignant neoplasm of skin of right lower limb, including hip
C44.799 Other specified malignant neoplasm of skin of left lower limb, including hip
✓5th C44.8 Other and unspecified malignant neoplasm of overlapping sites of skin
C44.80 Unspecified malignant neoplasm of overlapping sites of skin
C44.81 Basal cell carcinoma of overlapping sites of skin
C44.82 Squamous cell carcinoma of overlapping sites of skin
C44.89 Other specified malignant neoplasm of overlapping sites of skin
✓5th C44.9 Other and unspecified malignant neoplasm of skin, unspecified
C44.90 Unspecified malignant neoplasm of skin, unspecified
Malignant neoplasm of unspecified site of skin
C44.91 Basal cell carcinoma of skin, unspecified
C44.92 Squamous cell carcinoma of skin, unspecified
C44.99 Other specified malignant neoplasm of skin, unspecified

## Malignant neoplasms of mesothelial and soft tissue (C45-C49)

✓4th C45 Mesothelioma
DEF: Rare type of cancer that forms in the thin layer of protective tissue that covers the majority of internal organs (mesothelium).
C45.0 Mesothelioma of pleura HCC Rx ESR COM
EXCLUDES 1 *other malignant neoplasm of pleura (C38.4)*
AHA: 2017,2Q,11
TIP: For pleural mesothelioma that has metastasized to the chest wall, assign this code for the primary site along with C79.89 for metastatic cancer in the chest wall.
C45.1 Mesothelioma of peritoneum HCC Rx ESR COM
Mesothelioma of cul-de-sac
Mesothelioma of mesentery
Mesothelioma of mesocolon
Mesothelioma of omentum
Mesothelioma of peritoneum (parietal) (pelvic)
EXCLUDES 1 *other malignant neoplasm of soft tissue of peritoneum (C48.-)*
C45.2 Mesothelioma of pericardium HCC Rx ESR COM
EXCLUDES 1 *other malignant neoplasm of pericardium (C38.0)*
C45.7 Mesothelioma of other sites HCC Rx ESR COM
C45.9 Mesothelioma, unspecified HCC Rx ESR COM

✓4th C46 Kaposi's sarcoma
Code first any human immunodeficiency virus [HIV] disease (B20)
DEF: Malignant neoplasm that causes patches of abnormal tissue to grow under the skin, in the lining of the mouth, nose, and throat, in lymph nodes, or in other visceral organs. Kaposi's sarcoma is caused by human herpesvirus8 (HHV8).
C46.0 Kaposi's sarcoma of skin HCC Rx ESR COM
C46.1 Kaposi's sarcoma of soft tissue HCC Rx ESR COM
Kaposi's sarcoma of blood vessel
Kaposi's sarcoma of connective tissue
Kaposi's sarcoma of fascia
Kaposi's sarcoma of ligament
Kaposi's sarcoma of lymphatic(s) NEC
Kaposi's sarcoma of muscle
EXCLUDES 2 *Kaposi's sarcoma of lymph glands and nodes (C46.3)*
C46.2 Kaposi's sarcoma of palate HCC Rx ESR COM
C46.3 Kaposi's sarcoma of lymph nodes HCC Rx ESR COM
C46.4 Kaposi's sarcoma of gastrointestinal sites HCC Rx ESR COM
✓5th C46.5 Kaposi's sarcoma of lung
AHA: 2019,1Q,16
TIP: When documented, assign code I31.31 for associated malignant pericardial effusion. The neoplasm code should be sequenced first.
C46.50 Kaposi's sarcoma of unspecified lung HCC Rx ESR COM
C46.51 Kaposi's sarcoma of right lung HCC Rx ESR COM
C46.52 Kaposi's sarcoma of left lung HCC Rx ESR COM
C46.7 Kaposi's sarcoma of other sites HCC Rx ESR COM
C46.9 Kaposi's sarcoma, unspecified HCC Rx ESR COM
Kaposi's sarcoma of unspecified site

✓4th C47 Malignant neoplasm of peripheral nerves and autonomic nervous system
INCLUDES malignant neoplasm of sympathetic and parasympathetic nerves and ganglia
EXCLUDES 1 *Kaposi's sarcoma of soft tissue (C46.1)*
C47.0 Malignant neoplasm of peripheral nerves of head, face and neck HCC Rx ESR COM
EXCLUDES 1 *malignant neoplasm of peripheral nerves of orbit (C69.6-)*
✓5th C47.1 Malignant neoplasm of peripheral nerves of upper limb, including shoulder
C47.10 Malignant neoplasm of peripheral nerves of unspecified upper limb, including shoulder HCC Rx ESR COM
C47.11 Malignant neoplasm of peripheral nerves of right upper limb, including shoulder HCC Rx ESR COM
C47.12 Malignant neoplasm of peripheral nerves of left upper limb, including shoulder HCC Rx ESR COM
✓5th C47.2 Malignant neoplasm of peripheral nerves of lower limb, including hip
C47.20 Malignant neoplasm of peripheral nerves of unspecified lower limb, including hip HCC Rx ESR COM
C47.21 Malignant neoplasm of peripheral nerves of right lower limb, including hip HCC Rx ESR COM
C47.22 Malignant neoplasm of peripheral nerves of left lower limb, including hip HCC Rx ESR COM
C47.3 Malignant neoplasm of peripheral nerves of thorax HCC Rx ESR COM
C47.4 Malignant neoplasm of peripheral nerves of abdomen HCC Rx ESR COM
C47.5 Malignant neoplasm of peripheral nerves of pelvis HCC Rx ESR COM
C47.6 Malignant neoplasm of peripheral nerves of trunk, unspecified HCC Rx ESR COM
Malignant neoplasm of peripheral nerves of unspecified part of trunk
C47.8 Malignant neoplasm of overlapping sites of peripheral nerves and autonomic nervous system HCC Rx ESR COM
C47.9 Malignant neoplasm of peripheral nerves and autonomic nervous system, unspecified HCC Rx ESR COM
Malignant neoplasm of unspecified site of peripheral nerves and autonomic nervous system

✓4th C48 Malignant neoplasm of retroperitoneum and peritoneum
EXCLUDES 1 *Kaposi's sarcoma of connective tissue (C46.1)*
*mesothelioma (C45.-)*
C48.0 Malignant neoplasm of retroperitoneum HCC Rx ESR COM
C48.1 Malignant neoplasm of specified parts of peritoneum HCC Rx ESR COM
Malignant neoplasm of cul-de-sac
Malignant neoplasm of mesentery
Malignant neoplasm of mesocolon
Malignant neoplasm of omentum
Malignant neoplasm of parietal peritoneum
Malignant neoplasm of pelvic peritoneum
C48.2 Malignant neoplasm of peritoneum, unspecified HCC Rx ESR COM
C48.8 Malignant neoplasm of overlapping sites of retroperitoneum and peritoneum HCC Rx ESR COM

✓4th **C49 Malignant neoplasm of other connective and soft tissue**

INCLUDES malignant neoplasm of blood vessel
malignant neoplasm of bursa
malignant neoplasm of cartilage
malignant neoplasm of fascia
malignant neoplasm of fat
malignant neoplasm of ligament, except uterine
malignant neoplasm of lymphatic vessel
malignant neoplasm of muscle
malignant neoplasm of synovia
malignant neoplasm of tendon (sheath)

EXCLUDES 1 *malignant neoplasm of cartilage (of):*
*malignant neoplasm of connective tissue of breast (C5Ø.-)*
*articular (C4Ø-C41)*
*larynx (C32.3)*
*nose (C3Ø.Ø)*

EXCLUDES 2 *Kaposi's sarcoma of soft tissue (C46.1)*
*malignant neoplasm of heart (C38.Ø)*
*malignant neoplasm of peripheral nerves and autonomic nervous system (C47.-)*
*malignant neoplasm of peritoneum (C48.2)*
*malignant neoplasm of retroperitoneum (C48.Ø)*
*malignant neoplasm of uterine ligament (C57.3)*
*mesothelioma (C45.-)*

**C49.Ø Malignant neoplasm of connective and soft tissue of head, face and neck** HCC Rx ESR COM
Malignant neoplasm of connective tissue of ear
Malignant neoplasm of connective tissue of eyelid
EXCLUDES 1 *connective tissue of orbit (C69.6-)*

✓5th **C49.1 Malignant neoplasm of connective and soft tissue of upper limb, including shoulder**
**C49.1Ø Malignant neoplasm of connective and soft tissue of unspecified upper limb, including shoulder** HCC Rx ESR COM
**C49.11 Malignant neoplasm of connective and soft tissue of right upper limb, including shoulder** HCC Rx ESR COM
**C49.12 Malignant neoplasm of connective and soft tissue of left upper limb, including shoulder** HCC Rx ESR COM

✓5th **C49.2 Malignant neoplasm of connective and soft tissue of lower limb, including hip**
**C49.2Ø Malignant neoplasm of connective and soft tissue of unspecified lower limb, including hip** HCC Rx ESR COM
**C49.21 Malignant neoplasm of connective and soft tissue of right lower limb, including hip** HCC Rx ESR COM
**C49.22 Malignant neoplasm of connective and soft tissue of left lower limb, including hip** HCC Rx ESR COM

**C49.3 Malignant neoplasm of connective and soft tissue of thorax** HCC Rx ESR COM
Malignant neoplasm of axilla
Malignant neoplasm of diaphragm
Malignant neoplasm of great vessels
EXCLUDES 1 *malignant neoplasm of breast (C5Ø.-)*
*malignant neoplasm of heart (C38.Ø)*
*malignant neoplasm of mediastinum (C38.1-C38.3)*
*malignant neoplasm of thymus (C37)*
**AHA:** 2015,3Q,19

**C49.4 Malignant neoplasm of connective and soft tissue of abdomen** HCC Rx ESR COM
Malignant neoplasm of abdominal wall
Malignant neoplasm of hypochondrium

**C49.5 Malignant neoplasm of connective and soft tissue of pelvis** HCC Rx ESR COM
Malignant neoplasm of buttock
Malignant neoplasm of groin
Malignant neoplasm of perineum

**C49.6 Malignant neoplasm of connective and soft tissue of trunk, unspecified** HCC Rx ESR COM
Malignant neoplasm of back NOS

**C49.8 Malignant neoplasm of overlapping sites of connective and soft tissue** HCC Rx ESR COM
Primary malignant neoplasm of two or more contiguous sites of connective and soft tissue

**C49.9 Malignant neoplasm of connective and soft tissue, unspecified** HCC Rx ESR COM

✓5th **C49.A Gastrointestinal stromal tumor**
**AHA:** 2016,4Q,8
**DEF:** Uncommon malignant tumor found in the GI tract that originates from interstitial cells of the autonomic nervous system. Most occur in the stomach or small intestine but can originate anywhere in the GI tract.
**C49.AØ Gastrointestinal stromal tumor, unspecified site** HCC Rx ESR COM
**C49.A1 Gastrointestinal stromal tumor of esophagus** HCC Rx ESR COM
**C49.A2 Gastrointestinal stromal tumor of stomach** HCC Rx ESR COM
**C49.A3 Gastrointestinal stromal tumor of small intestine** HCC Rx ESR COM
**C49.A4 Gastrointestinal stromal tumor of large intestine** HCC Rx ESR COM
**C49.A5 Gastrointestinal stromal tumor of rectum** HCC Rx ESR COM
**C49.A9 Gastrointestinal stromal tumor of other sites** HCC Rx ESR COM

## Malignant neoplasms of breast (C5Ø)

✓4th **C5Ø Malignant neoplasm of breast**
INCLUDES connective tissue of breast
Paget's disease of breast
Paget's disease of nipple
Use additional code to identify estrogen, and other hormones and factors receptor status (Z17.-)
EXCLUDES 1 *skin of breast (C44.5Ø1, C44.511, C44.521, C44.591)*
**AHA:** 2017,4Q,19

**Female Breast**

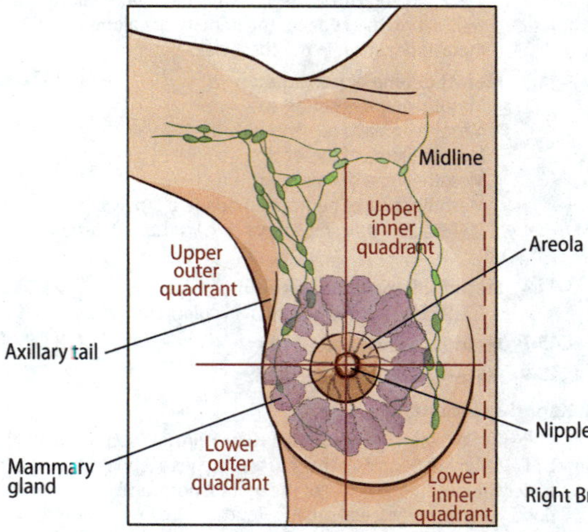


✓5th **C5Ø.Ø Malignant neoplasm of nipple and areola**
✓6th **C5Ø.Ø1 Malignant neoplasm of nipple and areola, female**
**C5Ø.Ø11 Malignant neoplasm of nipple and areola, right female breast** HCC Rx ESR COM
**C5Ø.Ø12 Malignant neoplasm of nipple and areola, left female breast** HCC Rx ESR COM
**C5Ø.Ø19 Malignant neoplasm of nipple and areola, unspecified female breast** HCC Rx ESR COM
✓6th **C5Ø.Ø2 Malignant neoplasm of nipple and areola, male**
**C5Ø.Ø21 Malignant neoplasm of nipple and areola, right male breast** HCC Rx ESR COM
**C5Ø.Ø22 Malignant neoplasm of nipple and areola, left male breast** HCC Rx ESR COM
**C5Ø.Ø29 Malignant neoplasm of nipple and areola, unspecified male breast** HCC Rx ESR COM

✓5th **C5Ø.1 Malignant neoplasm of central portion of breast**
✓6th **C5Ø.11 Malignant neoplasm of central portion of breast, female**
**C5Ø.111 Malignant neoplasm of central portion of right female breast** HCC Rx ESR COM
**C5Ø.112 Malignant neoplasm of central portion of left female breast** HCC Rx ESR COM

C50.119 Malignant neoplasm of central portion of unspecified female breast HCC Rx ESR COM

✓6th C50.12 Malignant neoplasm of central portion of breast, male

C50.121 Malignant neoplasm of central portion of right male breast HCC Rx ESR COM

C50.122 Malignant neoplasm of central portion of left male breast HCC Rx ESR COM

C50.129 Malignant neoplasm of central portion of unspecified male breast HCC Rx ESR COM

✓5th C50.2 Malignant neoplasm of upper-inner quadrant of breast

✓6th C50.21 Malignant neoplasm of upper-inner quadrant of breast, female

C50.211 Malignant neoplasm of upper-inner quadrant of right female breast HCC Rx ESR COM

C50.212 Malignant neoplasm of upper-inner quadrant of left female breast HCC Rx ESR COM

C50.219 Malignant neoplasm of upper-inner quadrant of unspecified female breast HCC Rx ESR COM

✓6th C50.22 Malignant neoplasm of upper-inner quadrant of breast, male

C50.221 Malignant neoplasm of upper-inner quadrant of right male breast HCC Rx ESR COM

C50.222 Malignant neoplasm of upper-inner quadrant of left male breast HCC Rx ESR COM

C50.229 Malignant neoplasm of upper-inner quadrant of unspecified male breast HCC Rx ESR COM

✓5th C50.3 Malignant neoplasm of lower-inner quadrant of breast

✓6th C50.31 Malignant neoplasm of lower-inner quadrant of breast, female

C50.311 Malignant neoplasm of lower-inner quadrant of right female breast HCC Rx ESR COM

C50.312 Malignant neoplasm of lower-inner quadrant of left female breast HCC Rx ESR COM

C50.319 Malignant neoplasm of lower-inner quadrant of unspecified female breast HCC Rx ESR COM

✓6th C50.32 Malignant neoplasm of lower-inner quadrant of breast, male

C50.321 Malignant neoplasm of lower-inner quadrant of right male breast HCC Rx ESR COM

C50.322 Malignant neoplasm of lower-inner quadrant of left male breast HCC Rx ESR COM

C50.329 Malignant neoplasm of lower-inner quadrant of unspecified male breast HCC Rx ESR COM

✓5th C50.4 Malignant neoplasm of upper-outer quadrant of breast

✓6th C50.41 Malignant neoplasm of upper-outer quadrant of breast, female

C50.411 Malignant neoplasm of upper-outer quadrant of right female breast HCC Rx ESR COM

C50.412 Malignant neoplasm of upper-outer quadrant of left female breast HCC Rx ESR COM

C50.419 Malignant neoplasm of upper-outer quadrant of unspecified female breast HCC Rx ESR COM

✓6th C50.42 Malignant neoplasm of upper-outer quadrant of breast, male

C50.421 Malignant neoplasm of upper-outer quadrant of right male breast HCC Rx ESR COM

C50.422 Malignant neoplasm of upper-outer quadrant of left male breast HCC Rx ESR COM

C50.429 Malignant neoplasm of upper-outer quadrant of unspecified male breast HCC Rx ESR COM

✓5th C50.5 Malignant neoplasm of lower-outer quadrant of breast

✓6th C50.51 Malignant neoplasm of lower-outer quadrant of breast, female

C50.511 Malignant neoplasm of lower-outer quadrant of right female breast HCC Rx ESR COM

C50.512 Malignant neoplasm of lower-outer quadrant of left female breast HCC Rx ESR COM

C50.519 Malignant neoplasm of lower-outer quadrant of unspecified female breast HCC Rx ESR COM

✓6th C50.52 Malignant neoplasm of lower-outer quadrant of breast, male

C50.521 Malignant neoplasm of lower-outer quadrant of right male breast HCC Rx ESR COM

C50.522 Malignant neoplasm of lower-outer quadrant of left male breast HCC Rx ESR COM

C50.529 Malignant neoplasm of lower-outer quadrant of unspecified male breast HCC Rx ESR COM

✓5th C50.6 Malignant neoplasm of axillary tail of breast

✓6th C50.61 Malignant neoplasm of axillary tail of breast, female

C50.611 Malignant neoplasm of axillary tail of right female breast HCC Rx ESR COM

C50.612 Malignant neoplasm of axillary tail of left female breast HCC Rx ESR COM

C50.619 Malignant neoplasm of axillary tail of unspecified female breast HCC Rx ESR COM

✓6th C50.62 Malignant neoplasm of axillary tail of breast, male

C50.621 Malignant neoplasm of axillary tail of right male breast HCC Rx ESR COM

C50.622 Malignant neoplasm of axillary tail of left male breast HCC Rx ESR COM

C50.629 Malignant neoplasm of axillary tail of unspecified male breast HCC Rx ESR COM

✓5th C50.8 Malignant neoplasm of overlapping sites of breast

✓6th C50.81 Malignant neoplasm of overlapping sites of breast, female

C50.811 Malignant neoplasm of overlapping sites of right female breast HCC Rx ESR COM

C50.812 Malignant neoplasm of overlapping sites of left female breast HCC Rx ESR COM

C50.819 Malignant neoplasm of overlapping sites of unspecified female breast HCC Rx ESR COM

✓6th C50.82 Malignant neoplasm of overlapping sites of breast, male

C50.821 Malignant neoplasm of overlapping sites of right male breast HCC Rx ESR COM

C50.822 Malignant neoplasm of overlapping sites of left male breast HCC Rx ESR COM

C50.829 Malignant neoplasm of overlapping sites of unspecified male breast HCC Rx ESR COM

✓5th C50.9 Malignant neoplasm of breast of unspecified site

✓6th C50.91 Malignant neoplasm of breast of unspecified site, female

AHA: 2022,3Q,10,14

C50.911 Malignant neoplasm of unspecified site of right female breast HCC Rx ESR COM

C50.912 Malignant neoplasm of unspecified site of left female breast HCC Rx ESR COM

C50.919 Malignant neoplasm of unspecified site of unspecified female breast HCC Rx ESR COM

✓6th C50.92 Malignant neoplasm of breast of unspecified site, male

C50.921 Malignant neoplasm of unspecified site of right male breast HCC Rx ESR COM

C50.922 Malignant neoplasm of unspecified site of left male breast HCC Rx ESR COM

C50.929 Malignant neoplasm of unspecified site of unspecified male breast HCC Rx ESR COM

√5th **C5Ø.A Malignant inflammatory neoplasm of breast**
Inflammatory breast cancer (IBC)
**AHA:** 2025,4Q,5

**C5Ø.AØ Malignant inflammatory neoplasm of unspecified breast** HCC Rx ESR
**C5Ø.A1 Malignant inflammatory neoplasm of right breast** HCC Rx ESR
**C5Ø.A2 Malignant inflammatory neoplasm of left breast** HCC Rx ESR

## Malignant neoplasms of female genital organs (C51-C58)

INCLUDES malignant neoplasm of skin of female genital organs

√4th **C51 Malignant neoplasm of vulva**
EXCLUDES 1 *carcinoma in situ of vulva (DØ7.1)*

**C51.Ø Malignant neoplasm of labium majus** HCC ESR COM
Malignant neoplasm of Bartholin's [greater vestibular] gland
**C51.1 Malignant neoplasm of labium minus** HCC ESR COM
**C51.2 Malignant neoplasm of clitoris** HCC ESR COM
**C51.8 Malignant neoplasm of overlapping sites of vulva** HCC ESR COM
**C51.9 Malignant neoplasm of vulva, unspecified** HCC ESR COM
Malignant neoplasm of external female genitalia NOS
Malignant neoplasm of pudendum

**C52 Malignant neoplasm of vagina** HCC ESR COM
EXCLUDES 1 *carcinoma in situ of vagina (DØ7.2)*

√4th **C53 Malignant neoplasm of cervix uteri**
EXCLUDES 1 *carcinoma in situ of cervix uteri (DØ6.-)*
**AHA:** 2017,4Q,103

**C53.Ø Malignant neoplasm of endocervix** HCC ESR COM
**C53.1 Malignant neoplasm of exocervix** HCC ESR COM
**C53.8 Malignant neoplasm of overlapping sites of cervix uteri** HCC ESR COM
**C53.9 Malignant neoplasm of cervix uteri, unspecified** HCC ESR COM

√4th **C54 Malignant neoplasm of corpus uteri**

**C54.Ø Malignant neoplasm of isthmus uteri** HCC ESR COM
Malignant neoplasm of lower uterine segment
**C54.1 Malignant neoplasm of endometrium** HCC ESR COM
**C54.2 Malignant neoplasm of myometrium** HCC ESR COM
**C54.3 Malignant neoplasm of fundus uteri** HCC ESR COM
**C54.8 Malignant neoplasm of overlapping sites of corpus uteri** HCC ESR COM
**AHA:** 2023,3Q,14
**C54.9 Malignant neoplasm of corpus uteri, unspecified** HCC ESR COM

**C55 Malignant neoplasm of uterus, part unspecified** HCC ESR COM

√4th **C56 Malignant neoplasm of ovary**
Use additional code to identify any functional activity
**AHA:** 2025,3Q,15; 2025,2Q,16

**C56.1 Malignant neoplasm of right ovary** HCC Rx ESR COM
**C56.2 Malignant neoplasm of left ovary** HCC Rx ESR COM
**C56.3 Malignant neoplasm of bilateral ovaries** HCC Rx ESR COM
**C56.9 Malignant neoplasm of unspecified ovary** HCC Rx ESR COM

√4th **C57 Malignant neoplasm of other and unspecified female genital organs**

√5th **C57.Ø Malignant neoplasm of fallopian tube**
Malignant neoplasm of oviduct
Malignant neoplasm of uterine tube

**C57.ØØ Malignant neoplasm of unspecified fallopian tube** HCC Rx ESR COM
**C57.Ø1 Malignant neoplasm of right fallopian tube** HCC Rx ESR COM
**C57.Ø2 Malignant neoplasm of left fallopian tube** HCC Rx ESR COM

√5th **C57.1 Malignant neoplasm of broad ligament**

**C57.1Ø Malignant neoplasm of unspecified broad ligament** HCC Rx ESR COM
**C57.11 Malignant neoplasm of right broad ligament** HCC Rx ESR COM
**C57.12 Malignant neoplasm of left broad ligament** HCC Rx ESR COM

√5th **C57.2 Malignant neoplasm of round ligament**

**C57.2Ø Malignant neoplasm of unspecified round ligament** HCC Rx ESR COM
**C57.21 Malignant neoplasm of right round ligament** HCC Rx ESR COM
**C57.22 Malignant neoplasm of left round ligament** HCC Rx ESR COM

**C57.3 Malignant neoplasm of parametrium** HCC Rx ESR COM
Malignant neoplasm of uterine ligament NOS
**C57.4 Malignant neoplasm of uterine adnexa, unspecified** HCC Rx ESR COM
**C57.7 Malignant neoplasm of other specified female genital organs** HCC ESR COM
Malignant neoplasm of wolffian body or duct
**C57.8 Malignant neoplasm of overlapping sites of female genital organs** HCC ESR COM
Primary malignant neoplasm of two or more contiguous sites of the female genital organs whose point of origin cannot be determined
Primary tubo-ovarian malignant neoplasm whose point of origin cannot be determined
Primary utero-ovarian malignant neoplasm whose point of origin cannot be determined
**C57.9 Malignant neoplasm of female genital organ, unspecified** HCC ESR COM
Malignant neoplasm of female genitourinary tract NOS

**C58 Malignant neoplasm of placenta** HCC Rx ESR COM M
INCLUDES choriocarcinoma NOS
chorionepithelioma NOS
EXCLUDES 1 *chorioadenoma (destruens) (D39.2)*
*hydatidiform mole NOS (OØ1.9)*
*invasive hydatidiform mole (D39.2)*
*male choriocarcinoma NOS (C62.9-)*
*malignant hydatidiform mole (D39.2)*

## Malignant neoplasms of male genital organs (C6Ø-C63)

INCLUDES malignant neoplasm of skin of male genital organs

√4th **C6Ø Malignant neoplasm of penis**

**C6Ø.Ø Malignant neoplasm of prepuce** HCC Rx ESR COM
Malignant neoplasm of foreskin
**C6Ø.1 Malignant neoplasm of glans penis** HCC Rx ESR COM
**C6Ø.2 Malignant neoplasm of body of penis** HCC Rx ESR COM
Malignant neoplasm of corpus cavernosum
**C6Ø.8 Malignant neoplasm of overlapping sites of penis** HCC Rx ESR COM
**C6Ø.9 Malignant neoplasm of penis, unspecified** HCC Rx ESR COM
Malignant neoplasm of skin of penis NOS

**C61 Malignant neoplasm of prostate** HCC Rx ESR COM Q
Use additional code, if applicable, to identify:
hormone sensitivity status (Z19.1-Z19.2)
rising PSA following treatment for malignant neoplasm of prostate (R97.21)
EXCLUDES 1 *malignant neoplasm of seminal vesicle (C63.7)*
**AHA:** 2017,1Q,17

√4th **C62 Malignant neoplasm of testis**
Use additional code to identify any functional activity

√5th **C62.Ø Malignant neoplasm of undescended testis**
Malignant neoplasm of ectopic testis
Malignant neoplasm of retained testis

**C62.ØØ Malignant neoplasm of unspecified undescended testis** HCC Rx ESR COM
**C62.Ø1 Malignant neoplasm of undescended right testis** HCC Rx ESR COM
**C62.Ø2 Malignant neoplasm of undescended left testis** HCC Rx ESR COM

√5th **C62.1 Malignant neoplasm of descended testis**
Malignant neoplasm of scrotal testis

**C62.1Ø Malignant neoplasm of unspecified descended testis** HCC Rx ESR COM
**C62.11 Malignant neoplasm of descended right testis** HCC Rx ESR COM
**C62.12 Malignant neoplasm of descended left testis** HCC Rx ESR COM

√5th **C62.9 Malignant neoplasm of testis, unspecified whether descended or undescended**

**C62.9Ø Malignant neoplasm of unspecified testis, unspecified whether descended or undescended** HCC Rx ESR COM
Malignant neoplasm of testis NOS

C62.91 Malignant neoplasm of right testis, unspecified whether descended or undescended HCC Rx ESR COM

C62.92 Malignant neoplasm of left testis, unspecified whether descended or undescended HCC Rx ESR COM

√4th **C63 Malignant neoplasm of other and unspecified male genital organs**

√5th **C63.Ø Malignant neoplasm of epididymis**

C63.ØØ Malignant neoplasm of unspecified epididymis HCC Rx ESR COM

C63.Ø1 Malignant neoplasm of right epididymis HCC Rx ESR COM

C63.Ø2 Malignant neoplasm of left epididymis HCC Rx ESR COM

√5th **C63.1 Malignant neoplasm of spermatic cord**

C63.1Ø Malignant neoplasm of unspecified spermatic cord HCC Rx ESR COM

C63.11 Malignant neoplasm of right spermatic cord HCC Rx ESR COM

C63.12 Malignant neoplasm of left spermatic cord HCC Rx ESR COM

C63.2 Malignant neoplasm of scrotum HCC Rx ESR COM
Malignant neoplasm of skin of scrotum

C63.7 Malignant neoplasm of other specified male genital organs HCC Rx ESR COM
Malignant neoplasm of seminal vesicle
Malignant neoplasm of tunica vaginalis

C63.8 Malignant neoplasm of overlapping sites of male genital organs HCC Rx ESR COM
Primary malignant neoplasm of two or more contiguous sites of male genital organs whose point of origin cannot be determined

C63.9 Malignant neoplasm of male genital organ, unspecified HCC Rx ESR COM
Malignant neoplasm of male genitourinary tract NOS

## Malignant neoplasms of urinary tract (C64-C68)

√4th **C64 Malignant neoplasm of kidney, except renal pelvis**

EXCLUDES 1 *malignant carcinoid tumor of the kidney (C7A.Ø93)*
*malignant neoplasm of renal calyces (C65.-)*
*malignant neoplasm of renal pelvis (C65.-)*

AHA: 2025,2Q,11

C64.1 Malignant neoplasm of right kidney, except renal pelvis HCC Rx ESR COM

C64.2 Malignant neoplasm of left kidney, except renal pelvis HCC Rx ESR COM

C64.9 Malignant neoplasm of unspecified kidney, except renal pelvis HCC Rx ESR COM

√4th **C65 Malignant neoplasm of renal pelvis**

INCLUDES malignant neoplasm of pelviureteric junction
malignant neoplasm of renal calyces

C65.1 Malignant neoplasm of right renal pelvis HCC Rx ESR COM

C65.2 Malignant neoplasm of left renal pelvis HCC Rx ESR COM

C65.9 Malignant neoplasm of unspecified renal pelvis HCC Rx ESR COM

√4th **C66 Malignant neoplasm of ureter**

EXCLUDES 1 *malignant neoplasm of ureteric orifice of bladder (C67.6)*

C66.1 Malignant neoplasm of right ureter HCC Rx ESR COM

C66.2 Malignant neoplasm of left ureter HCC Rx ESR COM

C66.9 Malignant neoplasm of unspecified ureter HCC Rx ESR COM

√4th **C67 Malignant neoplasm of bladder**

AHA: 2023,3Q,15

C67.Ø Malignant neoplasm of trigone of bladder HCC Rx ESR COM

C67.1 Malignant neoplasm of dome of bladder HCC Rx ESR COM

C67.2 Malignant neoplasm of lateral wall of bladder HCC Rx ESR COM

C67.3 Malignant neoplasm of anterior wall of bladder HCC Rx ESR COM

C67.4 Malignant neoplasm of posterior wall of bladder HCC Rx ESR COM

C67.5 Malignant neoplasm of bladder neck HCC Rx ESR COM
Malignant neoplasm of internal urethral orifice

C67.6 Malignant neoplasm of ureteric orifice HCC Rx ESR COM

C67.7 Malignant neoplasm of urachus HCC Rx ESR COM

C67.8 Malignant neoplasm of overlapping sites of bladder HCC Rx ESR COM

C67.9 Malignant neoplasm of bladder, unspecified HCC Rx ESR COM
AHA: 2016,1Q,19

√4th **C68 Malignant neoplasm of other and unspecified urinary organs**

EXCLUDES 1 *malignant neoplasm of female genitourinary tract NOS (C57.9)*
*malignant neoplasm of male genitourinary tract NOS (C63.9)*

C68.Ø Malignant neoplasm of urethra HCC Rx ESR COM
EXCLUDES 1 *malignant neoplasm of urethral orifice of bladder (C67.5)*

C68.1 Malignant neoplasm of paraurethral glands HCC Rx ESR COM

C68.8 Malignant neoplasm of overlapping sites of urinary organs HCC Rx ESR COM
Primary malignant neoplasm of two or more contiguous sites of urinary organs whose point of origin cannot be determined

C68.9 Malignant neoplasm of urinary organ, unspecified HCC Rx ESR COM
Malignant neoplasm of urinary system NOS

## Malignant neoplasms of eye, brain and other parts of central nervous system (C69-C72)

√4th **C69 Malignant neoplasm of eye and adnexa**

EXCLUDES 1 *malignant neoplasm of connective tissue of eyelid (C49.Ø)*
*malignant neoplasm of eyelid (skin) (C43.1-, C44.1-)*
*malignant neoplasm of optic nerve (C72.3-)*

√5th **C69.Ø Malignant neoplasm of conjunctiva**

C69.ØØ Malignant neoplasm of unspecified conjunctiva HCC Rx ESR COM

C69.Ø1 Malignant neoplasm of right conjunctiva HCC Rx ESR COM

C69.Ø2 Malignant neoplasm of left conjunctiva HCC Rx ESR COM

√5th **C69.1 Malignant neoplasm of cornea**

C69.1Ø Malignant neoplasm of unspecified cornea HCC Rx ESR COM

C69.11 Malignant neoplasm of right cornea HCC Rx ESR COM

C69.12 Malignant neoplasm of left cornea HCC Rx ESR COM

√5th **C69.2 Malignant neoplasm of retina**

EXCLUDES 1 *dark area on retina (D49.81)*
*neoplasm of unspecified behavior of retina and choroid (D49.81)*
*retinal freckle (D49.81)*

C69.2Ø Malignant neoplasm of unspecified retina HCC Rx ESR COM

C69.21 Malignant neoplasm of right retina HCC Rx ESR COM

C69.22 Malignant neoplasm of left retina HCC Rx ESR COM

√5th **C69.3 Malignant neoplasm of choroid**

C69.3Ø Malignant neoplasm of unspecified choroid HCC Rx ESR COM

C69.31 Malignant neoplasm of right choroid HCC Rx ESR COM

C69.32 Malignant neoplasm of left choroid HCC Rx ESR COM

√5th **C69.4 Malignant neoplasm of ciliary body**

C69.4Ø Malignant neoplasm of unspecified ciliary body HCC Rx ESR COM

C69.41 Malignant neoplasm of right ciliary body HCC Rx ESR COM

C69.42 Malignant neoplasm of left ciliary body HCC Rx ESR COM

√5th **C69.5 Malignant neoplasm of lacrimal gland and duct**

Malignant neoplasm of lacrimal sac
Malignant neoplasm of nasolacrimal duct

C69.5Ø Malignant neoplasm of unspecified lacrimal gland and duct HCC Rx ESR COM

C69.51 Malignant neoplasm of right lacrimal gland and duct HCC Rx ESR COM

C69.52 Malignant neoplasm of left lacrimal gland and duct HCC Rx ESR COM

✓5th **C69.6 Malignant neoplasm of orbit**
Malignant neoplasm of connective tissue of orbit
Malignant neoplasm of extraocular muscle
Malignant neoplasm of peripheral nerves of orbit
Malignant neoplasm of retrobulbar tissue
Malignant neoplasm of retro-ocular tissue
EXCLUDES 1 *malignant neoplasm of orbital bone (C41.Ø)*

**C69.6Ø Malignant neoplasm of unspecified orbit** HCC Rx ESR COM
**C69.61 Malignant neoplasm of right orbit** HCC Rx ESR COM
**C69.62 Malignant neoplasm of left orbit** HCC Rx ESR COM

✓5th **C69.8 Malignant neoplasm of overlapping sites of eye and adnexa**
**C69.8Ø Malignant neoplasm of overlapping sites of unspecified eye and adnexa** HCC Rx ESR COM
**C69.81 Malignant neoplasm of overlapping sites of right eye and adnexa** HCC Rx ESR COM
**C69.82 Malignant neoplasm of overlapping sites of left eye and adnexa** HCC Rx ESR COM

✓5th **C69.9 Malignant neoplasm of unspecified site of eye**
Malignant neoplasm of eyeball
**C69.9Ø Malignant neoplasm of unspecified site of unspecified eye** HCC Rx ESR COM
**C69.91 Malignant neoplasm of unspecified site of right eye** HCC Rx ESR COM
**C69.92 Malignant neoplasm of unspecified site of left eye** HCC Rx ESR COM

✓4th **C7Ø Malignant neoplasm of meninges**
**C7Ø.Ø Malignant neoplasm of cerebral meninges** HCC Rx ESR COM
**C7Ø.1 Malignant neoplasm of spinal meninges** HCC Rx ESR COM
**C7Ø.9 Malignant neoplasm of meninges, unspecified** HCC Rx ESR COM

✓4th **C71 Malignant neoplasm of brain**
EXCLUDES 1 *malignant neoplasm of cranial nerves (C72.2-C72.5)*
*retrobulbar malignant neoplasm (C69.6-)*

**Lobes of the Brain**

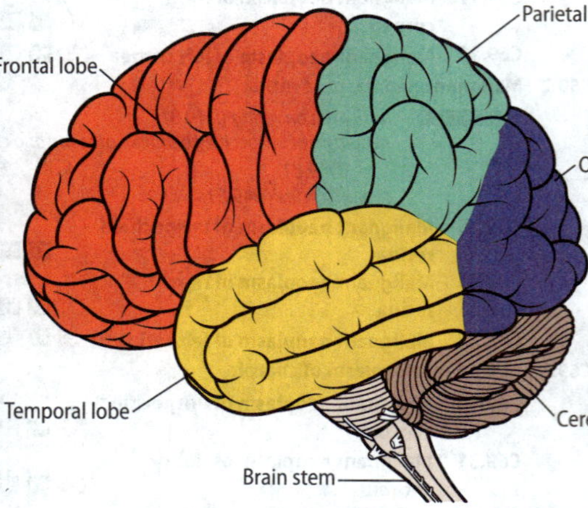


**C71.Ø Malignant neoplasm of cerebrum, except lobes and ventricles** HCC Rx ESR COM
Malignant neoplasm of supratentorial NOS
**C71.1 Malignant neoplasm of frontal lobe** HCC Rx ESR COM
**C71.2 Malignant neoplasm of temporal lobe** HCC Rx ESR COM
**C71.3 Malignant neoplasm of parietal lobe** HCC Rx ESR COM
**C71.4 Malignant neoplasm of occipital lobe** HCC Rx ESR COM
**C71.5 Malignant neoplasm of cerebral ventricle** HCC Rx ESR COM
EXCLUDES 1 *malignant neoplasm of fourth cerebral ventricle (C71.7)*
**C71.6 Malignant neoplasm of cerebellum** HCC Rx ESR COM
**C71.7 Malignant neoplasm of brain stem** HCC Rx ESR COM
Infratentorial malignant neoplasm NOS
Malignant neoplasm of fourth cerebral ventricle
**C71.8 Malignant neoplasm of overlapping sites of brain** HCC Rx ESR COM
**C71.9 Malignant neoplasm of brain, unspecified** HCC Rx ESR COM
**AHA:** 2014,3Q,3

✓4th **C72 Malignant neoplasm of spinal cord, cranial nerves and other parts of central nervous system**
EXCLUDES 1 *malignant neoplasm of meninges (C7Ø.-)*
*malignant neoplasm of peripheral nerves and autonomic nervous system (C47.-)*

**C72.Ø Malignant neoplasm of spinal cord** HCC Rx ESR COM
**C72.1 Malignant neoplasm of cauda equina** HCC Rx ESR COM

✓5th **C72.2 Malignant neoplasm of olfactory nerve**
Malignant neoplasm of olfactory bulb
**C72.2Ø Malignant neoplasm of unspecified olfactory nerve** HCC Rx ESR COM
**C72.21 Malignant neoplasm of right olfactory nerve** HCC Rx ESR COM
**C72.22 Malignant neoplasm of left olfactory nerve** HCC Rx ESR COM

✓5th **C72.3 Malignant neoplasm of optic nerve**
**C72.3Ø Malignant neoplasm of unspecified optic nerve** HCC Rx ESR COM
**C72.31 Malignant neoplasm of right optic nerve** HCC Rx ESR COM
**C72.32 Malignant neoplasm of left optic nerve** HCC Rx ESR COM

✓5th **C72.4 Malignant neoplasm of acoustic nerve**
**C72.4Ø Malignant neoplasm of unspecified acoustic nerve** HCC Rx ESR COM
**C72.41 Malignant neoplasm of right acoustic nerve** HCC Rx ESR COM
**C72.42 Malignant neoplasm of left acoustic nerve** HCC Rx ESR COM

✓5th **C72.5 Malignant neoplasm of other and unspecified cranial nerves**
**C72.5Ø Malignant neoplasm of unspecified cranial nerve** HCC Rx ESR COM
Malignant neoplasm of cranial nerve NOS
**C72.59 Malignant neoplasm of other cranial nerves** HCC Rx ESR COM

**C72.9 Malignant neoplasm of central nervous system, unspecified** HCC Rx ESR COM
Malignant neoplasm of nervous system NOS
Malignant neoplasm of unspecified site of central nervous system

## Malignant neoplasms of thyroid and other endocrine glands (C73-C75)

**C73 Malignant neoplasm of thyroid gland** HCC Rx ESR COM
Use additional code to identify any functional activity

✓4th **C74 Malignant neoplasm of adrenal gland**
**TIP:** If an adrenal gland tumor is described as functioning (producing too much of a hormone), additional codes should be assigned to report the functional activity.

✓5th **C74.Ø Malignant neoplasm of cortex of adrenal gland**
**C74.ØØ Malignant neoplasm of cortex of unspecified adrenal gland** HCC Rx ESR COM
**C74.Ø1 Malignant neoplasm of cortex of right adrenal gland** HCC Rx ESR COM
**C74.Ø2 Malignant neoplasm of cortex of left adrenal gland** HCC Rx ESR COM

✓5th **C74.1 Malignant neoplasm of medulla of adrenal gland**
**C74.1Ø Malignant neoplasm of medulla of unspecified adrenal gland** HCC Rx ESR COM
**C74.11 Malignant neoplasm of medulla of right adrenal gland** HCC Rx ESR COM
**C74.12 Malignant neoplasm of medulla of left adrenal gland** HCC Rx ESR COM

✓5th **C74.9 Malignant neoplasm of unspecified part of adrenal gland**
**C74.9Ø Malignant neoplasm of unspecified part of unspecified adrenal gland** HCC Rx ESR COM
**C74.91 Malignant neoplasm of unspecified part of right adrenal gland** HCC Rx ESR COM
**C74.92 Malignant neoplasm of unspecified part of left adrenal gland** HCC Rx ESR COM

**C75 Malignant neoplasm of other endocrine glands and related structures**

EXCLUDES 1 *malignant carcinoid tumors (C7A.Ø-)*
*malignant neoplasm of adrenal gland (C74.-)*
*malignant neoplasm of endocrine pancreas (C25.4)*
*malignant neoplasm of islets of Langerhans (C25.4)*
*malignant neoplasm of ovary (C56.-)*
*malignant neoplasm of testis (C62.-)*
*malignant neoplasm of thymus (C37)*
*malignant neoplasm of thyroid gland (C73)*
*malignant neuroendocrine tumors (C7A.-)*

**C75.Ø Malignant neoplasm of parathyroid gland** HCC Rx ESR COM
**C75.1 Malignant neoplasm of pituitary gland** HCC Rx ESR COM
**C75.2 Malignant neoplasm of craniopharyngeal duct** HCC Rx ESR COM
**C75.3 Malignant neoplasm of pineal gland** HCC Rx ESR COM
**C75.4 Malignant neoplasm of carotid body** HCC Rx ESR COM
**C75.5 Malignant neoplasm of aortic body and other paraganglia** HCC Rx ESR COM
**C75.8 Malignant neoplasm with pluriglandular involvement, unspecified** HCC Rx ESR COM
**C75.9 Malignant neoplasm of endocrine gland, unspecified** HCC Rx ESR COM

## Malignant neuroendocrine tumors (C7A)

**C7A Malignant neuroendocrine tumors**

Code also any associated multiple endocrine neoplasia [MEN] syndromes (E31.2-)
Use additional code to identify any associated endocrine syndrome, such as:
carcinoid syndrome (E34.ØØ)

EXCLUDES 2 *malignant pancreatic islet cell tumors (C25.4)*
*Merkel cell carcinoma (C4A.-)*

**AHA:** 2019,3Q,7
**DEF:** Tumors comprised of cells that are capable of producing hormonal syndromes in which the normal hormonal balance required to support body system function is adversely affected.

**C7A.Ø Malignant carcinoid tumors**
**AHA:** 2019,3Q,7
**DEF:** Specific type of slow-growing neuroendocrine tumors. Carcinoid tumors occur most commonly in the hormone producing cells of the gastrointestinal tracts and can also occur in the pancreas, testes, ovaries, or lungs.

**C7A.ØØ Malignant carcinoid tumor of unspecified site** HCC Rx ESR COM

**C7A.Ø1 Malignant carcinoid tumors of the small intestine**
**C7A.Ø1Ø Malignant carcinoid tumor of the duodenum** HCC Rx ESR COM
**C7A.Ø11 Malignant carcinoid tumor of the jejunum** HCC Rx ESR COM
**C7A.Ø12 Malignant carcinoid tumor of the ileum** HCC Rx ESR COM
**C7A.Ø19 Malignant carcinoid tumor of the small intestine, unspecified portion** HCC Rx ESR COM

**C7A.Ø2 Malignant carcinoid tumors of the appendix, large intestine, and rectum**
**C7A.Ø2Ø Malignant carcinoid tumor of the appendix** HCC Rx ESR COM
**C7A.Ø21 Malignant carcinoid tumor of the cecum** HCC Rx ESR COM
**C7A.Ø22 Malignant carcinoid tumor of the ascending colon** HCC Rx ESR COM
**C7A.Ø23 Malignant carcinoid tumor of the transverse colon** HCC Rx ESR COM
**C7A.Ø24 Malignant carcinoid tumor of the descending colon** HCC Rx ESR COM
**C7A.Ø25 Malignant carcinoid tumor of the sigmoid colon** HCC Rx ESR COM
**C7A.Ø26 Malignant carcinoid tumor of the rectum** HCC Rx ESR COM
**C7A.Ø29 Malignant carcinoid tumor of the large intestine, unspecified portion** HCC Rx ESR COM
Malignant carcinoid tumor of the colon NOS

**C7A.Ø9 Malignant carcinoid tumors of other sites**
**C7A.Ø9Ø Malignant carcinoid tumor of the bronchus and lung** HCC Rx ESR COM
**AHA:** 2019,1Q,16
**TIP:** When documented, assign code I31.31 for associated malignant pericardial effusion. The neoplasm code should be sequenced first.
**C7A.Ø91 Malignant carcinoid tumor of the thymus** HCC Rx ESR COM
**C7A.Ø92 Malignant carcinoid tumor of the stomach** HCC Rx ESR COM
**C7A.Ø93 Malignant carcinoid tumor of the kidney** HCC Rx ESR COM
**C7A.Ø94 Malignant carcinoid tumor of the foregut, unspecified** HCC Rx ESR COM
**C7A.Ø95 Malignant carcinoid tumor of the midgut, unspecified** HCC Rx ESR COM
**C7A.Ø96 Malignant carcinoid tumor of the hindgut, unspecified** HCC Rx ESR COM
**C7A.Ø98 Malignant carcinoid tumors of other sites** HCC Rx ESR COM

**C7A.1 Malignant poorly differentiated neuroendocrine tumors** HCC Rx ESR COM
High grade neuroendocrine carcinoma, any site
Malignant poorly differentiated neuroendocrine carcinoma, any site
Malignant poorly differentiated neuroendocrine tumor NOS
**AHA:** 2023,1Q,20-21

**C7A.8 Other malignant neuroendocrine tumors** HCC Rx ESR COM
**AHA:** 2019,3Q,7

## Secondary neuroendocrine tumors (C7B)

**C7B Secondary neuroendocrine tumors**

Use additional code to identify any functional activity

**C7B.Ø Secondary carcinoid tumors**
**AHA:** 2019,3Q,7
**DEF:** Specific type of slow-growing neuroendocrine tumors. Carcinoid tumors occur most commonly in the hormone producing cells of the gastrointestinal tracts and can also occur in the pancreas, testes, ovaries, or lungs.

**C7B.ØØ Secondary carcinoid tumors, unspecified site** HCC Rx ESR COM
**C7B.Ø1 Secondary carcinoid tumors of distant lymph nodes** HCC Rx ESR COM
**C7B.Ø2 Secondary carcinoid tumors of liver** HCC Rx ESR COM
**C7B.Ø3 Secondary carcinoid tumors of bone** HCC Rx ESR COM
**C7B.Ø4 Secondary carcinoid tumors of peritoneum** HCC Rx ESR COM
Mesentery metastasis of carcinoid tumor
**C7B.Ø9 Secondary carcinoid tumors of other sites** HCC Rx ESR COM

**C7B.1 Secondary Merkel cell carcinoma** HCC Rx ESR COM
Merkel cell carcinoma nodal presentation
Merkel cell carcinoma visceral metastatic presentation

**C7B.8 Other secondary neuroendocrine tumors** HCC Rx ESR COM
**AHA:** 2024,2Q,10; 2023,1Q,20; 2019,3Q,7

## Malignant neoplasms of ill-defined, other secondary and unspecified sites (C76-C8Ø)

**C76 Malignant neoplasm of other and ill-defined sites**

EXCLUDES 1 *malignant neoplasm of female genitourinary tract NOS (C57.9)*
*malignant neoplasm of lymphoid, hematopoietic and related tissue (C81-C96)*
*malignant neoplasm of male genitourinary tract NOS (C63.9)*
*malignant neoplasm of skin (C44.-)*
*malignant neoplasm of unspecified site NOS (C8Ø.1)*

**C76.Ø Malignant neoplasm of head, face and neck** HCC Rx ESR COM
Malignant neoplasm of cheek NOS
Malignant neoplasm of nose NOS

**C76.1 Malignant neoplasm of thorax** HCC Rx ESR COM
Intrathoracic malignant neoplasm NOS
Malignant neoplasm of axilla NOS
Thoracic malignant neoplasm NOS

**C76.2 Malignant neoplasm of abdomen** HCC Rx ESR COM

C76.3 **Malignant neoplasm of pelvis** HCC Rx ESR COM
Malignant neoplasm of groin NOS
Malignant neoplasm of sites overlapping systems within the pelvis
Rectovaginal (septum) malignant neoplasm
Rectovesical (septum) malignant neoplasm

✓5th C76.4 **Malignant neoplasm of upper limb**
C76.40 **Malignant neoplasm of unspecified upper limb** HCC Rx ESR COM
C76.41 **Malignant neoplasm of right upper limb** HCC Rx ESR COM
C76.42 **Malignant neoplasm of left upper limb** HCC Rx ESR COM

✓5th C76.5 **Malignant neoplasm of lower limb**
C76.50 **Malignant neoplasm of unspecified lower limb** HCC Rx ESR COM
C76.51 **Malignant neoplasm of right lower limb** HCC Rx ESR COM
C76.52 **Malignant neoplasm of left lower limb** HCC Rx ESR COM

C76.8 **Malignant neoplasm of other specified ill-defined sites** HCC Rx ESR COM
Malignant neoplasm of overlapping ill-defined sites

✓4th **C77 Secondary and unspecified malignant neoplasm of lymph nodes**
EXCLUDES 1 *malignant neoplasm of lymph nodes, specified as primary (C81-C86, C88, C96.-)*
*mesentery metastasis of carcinoid tumor (C7B.04)*
*secondary carcinoid tumors of distant lymph nodes (C7B.01)*

C77.0 **Secondary and unspecified malignant neoplasm of lymph nodes of head, face and neck** HCC Rx ESR COM
Secondary and unspecified malignant neoplasm of supraclavicular lymph nodes
**AHA:** 2022,3Q,14

C77.1 **Secondary and unspecified malignant neoplasm of intrathoracic lymph nodes** HCC Rx ESR COM
C77.2 **Secondary and unspecified malignant neoplasm of intra-abdominal lymph nodes** HCC Rx ESR COM
C77.3 **Secondary and unspecified malignant neoplasm of axilla and upper limb lymph nodes** HCC Rx ESR COM
Secondary and unspecified malignant neoplasm of pectoral lymph nodes
C77.4 **Secondary and unspecified malignant neoplasm of inguinal and lower limb lymph nodes** HCC Rx ESR COM
C77.5 **Secondary and unspecified malignant neoplasm of intrapelvic lymph nodes** HCC Rx ESR COM
C77.8 **Secondary and unspecified malignant neoplasm of lymph nodes of multiple regions** HCC Rx ESR COM
C77.9 **Secondary and unspecified malignant neoplasm of lymph node, unspecified** HCC Rx ESR COM

✓4th **C78 Secondary malignant neoplasm of respiratory and digestive organs**
EXCLUDES 1 *secondary carcinoid tumors of liver (C7B.02)*
*secondary carcinoid tumors of peritoneum (C7B.04)*
EXCLUDES 2 *lymph node metastases (C77.0)*
**AHA:** 2023,1Q,22

✓5th C78.0 **Secondary malignant neoplasm of lung**
**AHA:** 2024,2Q,11; 2022,3Q,9; 2019,1Q,16
C78.00 **Secondary malignant neoplasm of unspecified lung** HCC Rx ESR COM
C78.01 **Secondary malignant neoplasm of right lung** HCC Rx ESR COM
C78.02 **Secondary malignant neoplasm of left lung** HCC Rx ESR COM

C78.1 **Secondary malignant neoplasm of mediastinum** HCC Rx ESR COM
C78.2 **Secondary malignant neoplasm of pleura** HCC Rx ESR COM

✓5th C78.3 **Secondary malignant neoplasm of other and unspecified respiratory organs**
C78.30 **Secondary malignant neoplasm of unspecified respiratory organ** HCC Rx ESR COM
● C78.31 **Secondary malignant neoplasm of larynx**
● C78.32 **Secondary malignant neoplasm of pharynx**
C78.39 **Secondary malignant neoplasm of other respiratory organs** HCC Rx ESR COM

C78.4 **Secondary malignant neoplasm of small intestine** HCC Rx ESR COM
C78.5 **Secondary malignant neoplasm of large intestine and rectum** HCC Rx ESR COM
C78.6 **Secondary malignant neoplasm of retroperitoneum and peritoneum** HCC Rx ESR COM
**AHA:** 2025,2Q,16; 2017,2Q,12
C78.7 **Secondary malignant neoplasm of liver and intrahepatic bile duct** HCC Rx ESR COM
**AHA:** 2024,1Q,25; 2022,3Q,14

✓5th C78.8 **Secondary malignant neoplasm of other and unspecified digestive organs**
C78.80 **Secondary malignant neoplasm of unspecified digestive organ** HCC Rx ESR COM
C78.89 **Secondary malignant neoplasm of other digestive organs** HCC Rx ESR COM
Code also exocrine pancreatic insufficiency (K86.81)

✓4th **C79 Secondary malignant neoplasm of other and unspecified sites**
EXCLUDES 1 *secondary carcinoid tumors (C7B.-)*
*secondary neuroendocrine tumors (C7B.-)*
**AHA:** 2023,1Q,22

✓5th C79.0 **Secondary malignant neoplasm of kidney and renal pelvis**
C79.00 **Secondary malignant neoplasm of unspecified kidney and renal pelvis** HCC Rx ESR COM
C79.01 **Secondary malignant neoplasm of right kidney and renal pelvis** HCC Rx ESR COM
C79.02 **Secondary malignant neoplasm of left kidney and renal pelvis** HCC Rx ESR COM

✓5th C79.1 **Secondary malignant neoplasm of bladder and other and unspecified urinary organs**
C79.10 **Secondary malignant neoplasm of unspecified urinary organs** HCC Rx ESR COM
C79.11 **Secondary malignant neoplasm of bladder** HCC Rx ESR COM
EXCLUDES 2 *lymph node metastases (C77.0)*
C79.19 **Secondary malignant neoplasm of other urinary organs** HCC Rx ESR COM

C79.2 **Secondary malignant neoplasm of skin** HCC Rx ESR COM
EXCLUDES 1 *secondary Merkel cell carcinoma (C7B.1)*

✓5th C79.3 **Secondary malignant neoplasm of brain and cerebral meninges**
C79.31 **Secondary malignant neoplasm of brain** HCC Rx ESR COM
**AHA:** 2022,3Q,9-10
C79.32 **Secondary malignant neoplasm of cerebral meninges** HCC Rx ESR COM
**AHA:** 2020,1Q,13

✓5th C79.4 **Secondary malignant neoplasm of other and unspecified parts of nervous system**
C79.40 **Secondary malignant neoplasm of unspecified part of nervous system** HCC Rx ESR COM
C79.49 **Secondary malignant neoplasm of other parts of nervous system** HCC Rx ESR COM

✓5th C79.5 **Secondary malignant neoplasm of bone and bone marrow**
EXCLUDES 1 *secondary carcinoid tumors of bone (C7B.03)*
C79.51 **Secondary malignant neoplasm of bone** HCC Rx ESR COM
**AHA:** 2022,3Q,14
**TIP:** Do not assign in addition to a code from subcategory C90.0 when multiple myeloma is described as metastatic to the bone; bone involvement is integral to multiple myeloma.
C79.52 **Secondary malignant neoplasm of bone marrow** HCC Rx ESR COM

✓5th C79.6 **Secondary malignant neoplasm of ovary**
C79.60 **Secondary malignant neoplasm of unspecified ovary** HCC Rx ESR COM
C79.61 **Secondary malignant neoplasm of right ovary** HCC Rx ESR COM
C79.62 **Secondary malignant neoplasm of left ovary** HCC Rx ESR COM
C79.63 **Secondary malignant neoplasm of bilateral ovaries** HCC Rx ESR COM

✓5th C79.7 **Secondary malignant neoplasm of adrenal gland**
C79.70 **Secondary malignant neoplasm of unspecified adrenal gland** HCC Rx ESR COM
C79.71 **Secondary malignant neoplasm of right adrenal gland** HCC Rx ESR COM
C79.72 **Secondary malignant neoplasm of left adrenal gland** HCC Rx ESR COM

✓5th **C79.8 Secondary malignant neoplasm of other specified sites**

**C79.81 Secondary malignant neoplasm of breast** HCC Rx ESR COM

**C79.82 Secondary malignant neoplasm of genital organs** HCC Rx ESR COM

● **C79.83 Secondary malignant neoplasm of oral cavity**

**C79.89 Secondary malignant neoplasm of other specified sites** HCC Rx ESR COM

AHA: 2017,2Q,11

**C79.9 Secondary malignant neoplasm of unspecified site** HCC Rx ESR COM

Metastatic cancer NOS

Metastatic disease NOS

EXCLUDES 1 *carcinomatosis NOS (C80.0)*

*generalized cancer NOS (C80.0)*

*malignant (primary) neoplasm of unspecified site (C80.1)*

AHA: 2023,2Q,5

✓4th **C80 Malignant neoplasm without specification of site**

EXCLUDES 1 *malignant carcinoid tumor of unspecified site (C7A.00)*

*malignant neoplasm of specified multiple sites - code to each site*

**C80.0 Disseminated malignant neoplasm, unspecified** HCC Rx ESR COM

Carcinomatosis NOS

Generalized cancer, unspecified site (primary) (secondary)

Generalized malignancy, unspecified site (primary) (secondary)

**C80.1 Malignant (primary) neoplasm, unspecified** HCC ESR COM

Cancer NOS

Cancer unspecified site (primary)

Carcinoma unspecified site (primary)

Malignancy unspecified site (primary)

EXCLUDES 1 *secondary malignant neoplasm of unspecified site (C79.9)*

**C80.2 Malignant neoplasm associated with transplanted organ** HCC Rx ESR COM UPD

Code first complication of transplanted organ (T86.-)

Use additional code to identify the specific malignancy

## Malignant neoplasms of lymphoid, hematopoietic and related tissue (C81-C96)

EXCLUDES 2 *Kaposi's sarcoma of lymph nodes (C46.3)*

*secondary and unspecified neoplasm of lymph nodes (C77.-)*

*secondary neoplasm of bone marrow (C79.52)*

*secondary neoplasm of spleen (C78.89)*

✓4th **C81 Hodgkin lymphoma**

EXCLUDES 1 *personal history of Hodgkin lymphoma (Z85.71)*

AHA: 2023,1Q,22

**DEF:** Malignant disorder of lymphoid cells characterized by the presence of progressively swollen lymph nodes and spleen that may also involve the liver. A diagnosis of Hodgkin's lymphoma can be confirmed by the presence of Reed-Sternberg cells. ***Synonym(s):*** *Hodgkin disease.*

✓5th **C81.0 Nodular lymphocyte predominant Hodgkin lymphoma**

**C81.00 Nodular lymphocyte predominant Hodgkin lymphoma, unspecified site** HCC Rx ESR COM

**C81.01 Nodular lymphocyte predominant Hodgkin lymphoma, lymph nodes of head, face, and neck** HCC Rx ESR COM

**C81.02 Nodular lymphocyte predominant Hodgkin lymphoma, intrathoracic lymph nodes** HCC Rx ESR COM

**C81.03 Nodular lymphocyte predominant Hodgkin lymphoma, intra-abdominal lymph nodes** HCC Rx ESR COM

**C81.04 Nodular lymphocyte predominant Hodgkin lymphoma, lymph nodes of axilla and upper limb** HCC Rx ESR COM

**C81.05 Nodular lymphocyte predominant Hodgkin lymphoma, lymph nodes of inguinal region and lower limb** HCC Rx ESR COM

**C81.06 Nodular lymphocyte predominant Hodgkin lymphoma, intrapelvic lymph nodes** HCC Rx ESR COM

**C81.07 Nodular lymphocyte predominant Hodgkin lymphoma, spleen** HCC Rx ESR COM

**C81.08 Nodular lymphocyte predominant Hodgkin lymphoma, lymph nodes of multiple sites** HCC Rx ESR COM

**C81.09 Nodular lymphocyte predominant Hodgkin lymphoma, extranodal and solid organ sites** HCC Rx ESR COM

**C81.0A Nodular lymphocyte predominant Hodgkin lymphoma, in remission** HCC Rx ESR COM

✓5th **C81.1 Nodular sclerosis Hodgkin lymphoma**

Nodular sclerosis classical Hodgkin lymphoma

**C81.10 Nodular sclerosis Hodgkin lymphoma, unspecified site** HCC Rx ESR COM

**C81.11 Nodular sclerosis Hodgkin lymphoma, lymph nodes of head, face, and neck** HCC Rx ESR COM

**C81.12 Nodular sclerosis Hodgkin lymphoma, intrathoracic lymph nodes** HCC Rx ESR COM

**C81.13 Nodular sclerosis Hodgkin lymphoma, intra-abdominal lymph nodes** HCC Rx ESR COM

**C81.14 Nodular sclerosis Hodgkin lymphoma, lymph nodes of axilla and upper limb** HCC Rx ESR COM

**C81.15 Nodular sclerosis Hodgkin lymphoma, lymph nodes of inguinal region and lower limb** HCC Rx ESR COM

**C81.16 Nodular sclerosis Hodgkin lymphoma, intrapelvic lymph nodes** HCC Rx ESR COM

**C81.17 Nodular sclerosis Hodgkin lymphoma, spleen** HCC Rx ESR COM

**C81.18 Nodular sclerosis Hodgkin lymphoma, lymph nodes of multiple sites** HCC Rx ESR COM

**C81.19 Nodular sclerosis Hodgkin lymphoma, extranodal and solid organ sites** HCC Rx ESR COM

**C81.1A Nodular sclerosis Hodgkin lymphoma, in remission** HCC Rx ESR COM

✓5th **C81.2 Mixed cellularity Hodgkin lymphoma**

Mixed cellularity classical Hodgkin lymphoma

**C81.20 Mixed cellularity Hodgkin lymphoma, unspecified site** HCC Rx ESR COM

**C81.21 Mixed cellularity Hodgkin lymphoma, lymph nodes of head, face, and neck** HCC Rx ESR COM

**C81.22 Mixed cellularity Hodgkin lymphoma, intrathoracic lymph nodes** HCC Rx ESR COM

**C81.23 Mixed cellularity Hodgkin lymphoma, intra-abdominal lymph nodes** HCC Rx ESR COM

**C81.24 Mixed cellularity Hodgkin lymphoma, lymph nodes of axilla and upper limb** HCC Rx ESR COM

**C81.25 Mixed cellularity Hodgkin lymphoma, lymph nodes of inguinal region and lower limb** HCC Rx ESR COM

**C81.26 Mixed cellularity Hodgkin lymphoma, intrapelvic lymph nodes** HCC Rx ESR COM

**C81.27 Mixed cellularity Hodgkin lymphoma, spleen** HCC Rx ESR COM

**C81.28 Mixed cellularity Hodgkin lymphoma, lymph nodes of multiple sites** HCC Rx ESR COM

**C81.29 Mixed cellularity Hodgkin lymphoma, extranodal and solid organ sites** HCC Rx ESR COM

**C81.2A Mixed cellularity Hodgkin lymphoma, in remission** HCC Rx ESR COM

✓5th **C81.3 Lymphocyte depleted Hodgkin lymphoma**

Lymphocyte depleted classical Hodgkin lymphoma

**C81.30 Lymphocyte depleted Hodgkin lymphoma, unspecified site** HCC Rx ESR COM

**C81.31 Lymphocyte depleted Hodgkin lymphoma, lymph nodes of head, face, and neck** HCC Rx ESR COM

**C81.32 Lymphocyte depleted Hodgkin lymphoma, intrathoracic lymph nodes** HCC Rx ESR COM

**C81.33 Lymphocyte depleted Hodgkin lymphoma, intra-abdominal lymph nodes** HCC Rx ESR COM

**C81.34 Lymphocyte depleted Hodgkin lymphoma, lymph nodes of axilla and upper limb** HCC Rx ESR COM

**C81.35 Lymphocyte depleted Hodgkin lymphoma, lymph nodes of inguinal region and lower limb** HCC Rx ESR COM

**C81.36 Lymphocyte depleted Hodgkin lymphoma, intrapelvic lymph nodes** HCC Rx ESR COM

**C81.37 Lymphocyte depleted Hodgkin lymphoma, spleen** HCC Rx ESR COM

**C81.38 Lymphocyte depleted Hodgkin lymphoma, lymph nodes of multiple sites** HCC Rx ESR COM

**C81.39 Lymphocyte depleted Hodgkin lymphoma, extranodal and solid organ sites** HCC Rx ESR COM

**C81.3A Lymphocyte depleted Hodgkin lymphoma, in remission** HCC Rx ESR COM

**✓5th C81.4 Lymphocyte-rich Hodgkin lymphoma**
Lymphocyte-rich classical Hodgkin lymphoma
EXCLUDES 1 *nodular lymphocyte predominant Hodgkin lymphoma (C81.0-)*

**C81.40 Lymphocyte-rich Hodgkin lymphoma, unspecified site** HCC Rx ESR COM
**C81.41 Lymphocyte-rich Hodgkin lymphoma, lymph nodes of head, face, and neck** HCC Rx ESR COM
**C81.42 Lymphocyte-rich Hodgkin lymphoma, intrathoracic lymph nodes** HCC Rx ESR COM
**C81.43 Lymphocyte-rich Hodgkin lymphoma, intra-abdominal lymph nodes** HCC Rx ESR COM
**C81.44 Lymphocyte-rich Hodgkin lymphoma, lymph nodes of axilla and upper limb** HCC Rx ESR COM
**C81.45 Lymphocyte-rich Hodgkin lymphoma, lymph nodes of inguinal region and lower limb** HCC Rx ESR COM
**C81.46 Lymphocyte-rich Hodgkin lymphoma, intrapelvic lymph nodes** HCC Rx ESR COM
**C81.47 Lymphocyte-rich Hodgkin lymphoma, spleen** HCC Rx ESR COM
**C81.48 Lymphocyte-rich Hodgkin lymphoma, lymph nodes of multiple sites** HCC Rx ESR COM
**C81.49 Lymphocyte-rich Hodgkin lymphoma, extranodal and solid organ sites** HCC Rx ESR COM
**C81.4A Lymphocyte-rich Hodgkin lymphoma, in remission** HCC Rx ESR COM

**✓5th C81.7 Other Hodgkin lymphoma**
Classical Hodgkin lymphoma NOS
Other classical Hodgkin lymphoma

**C81.70 Other Hodgkin lymphoma, unspecified site** HCC Rx ESR COM
**C81.71 Other Hodgkin lymphoma, lymph nodes of head, face, and neck** HCC Rx ESR COM
**C81.72 Other Hodgkin lymphoma, intrathoracic lymph nodes** HCC Rx ESR COM
**C81.73 Other Hodgkin lymphoma, intra-abdominal lymph nodes** HCC Rx ESR COM
**C81.74 Other Hodgkin lymphoma, lymph nodes of axilla and upper limb** HCC Rx ESR COM
**C81.75 Other Hodgkin lymphoma, lymph nodes of inguinal region and lower limb** HCC Rx ESR COM
**C81.76 Other Hodgkin lymphoma, intrapelvic lymph nodes** HCC Rx ESR COM
**C81.77 Other Hodgkin lymphoma, spleen** HCC Rx ESR COM
**C81.78 Other Hodgkin lymphoma, lymph nodes of multiple sites** HCC Rx ESR COM
**C81.79 Other Hodgkin lymphoma, extranodal and solid organ sites** HCC Rx ESR COM
**C81.7A Other Hodgkin lymphoma, in remission** HCC Rx ESR COM

**✓5th C81.9 Hodgkin lymphoma, unspecified**

**C81.90 Hodgkin lymphoma, unspecified, unspecified site** HCC Rx ESR COM
**C81.91 Hodgkin lymphoma, unspecified, lymph nodes of head, face, and neck** HCC Rx ESR COM
**C81.92 Hodgkin lymphoma, unspecified, intrathoracic lymph nodes** HCC Rx ESR COM
**C81.93 Hodgkin lymphoma, unspecified, intra-abdominal lymph nodes** HCC Rx ESR COM
**C81.94 Hodgkin lymphoma, unspecified, lymph nodes of axilla and upper limb** HCC Rx ESR COM
**C81.95 Hodgkin lymphoma, unspecified, lymph nodes of inguinal region and lower limb** HCC Rx ESR COM
**C81.96 Hodgkin lymphoma, unspecified, intrapelvic lymph nodes** HCC Rx ESR COM
**C81.97 Hodgkin lymphoma, unspecified, spleen** HCC Rx ESR COM
**C81.98 Hodgkin lymphoma, unspecified, lymph nodes of multiple sites** HCC Rx ESR COM
**C81.99 Hodgkin lymphoma, unspecified, extranodal and solid organ sites** HCC Rx ESR COM
**C81.9A Hodgkin lymphoma, unspecified, in remission** HCC Rx ESR COM

**✓4th C82 Follicular lymphoma**
INCLUDES follicular lymphoma with or without diffuse areas
EXCLUDES 1 *mature T/NK-cell lymphomas (C84.-)*
*personal history of non-Hodgkin lymphoma (Z85.72)*
**AHA:** 2023,1Q,22
**DEF:** Most common subgroup of non-Hodgkin lymphomas (NHL), accounting for 20 to 30 percent of all NHLs. NHL is a B-cell lymphoma that is slow growing and characterized by the circular pattern of malignant cell growth with the cells clustered into identifiable nodules or follicles.

**✓5th C82.0 Follicular lymphoma grade I**

**C82.00 Follicular lymphoma grade I, unspecified site** HCC Rx ESR COM
**C82.01 Follicular lymphoma grade I, lymph nodes of head, face, and neck** HCC Rx ESR COM
**C82.02 Follicular lymphoma grade I, intrathoracic lymph nodes** HCC Rx ESR COM
**C82.03 Follicular lymphoma grade I, intra-abdominal lymph nodes** HCC Rx ESR COM
**C82.04 Follicular lymphoma grade I, lymph nodes of axilla and upper limb** HCC Rx ESR COM
**C82.05 Follicular lymphoma grade I, lymph nodes of inguinal region and lower limb** HCC Rx ESR COM
**C82.06 Follicular lymphoma grade I, intrapelvic lymph nodes** HCC Rx ESR COM
**C82.07 Follicular lymphoma grade I, spleen** HCC Rx ESR COM
**C82.08 Follicular lymphoma grade I, lymph nodes of multiple sites** HCC Rx ESR COM
**C82.09 Follicular lymphoma grade I, extranodal and solid organ sites** HCC Rx ESR COM
**C82.0A Follicular lymphoma grade I, in remission** HCC Rx ESR COM

**✓5th C82.1 Follicular lymphoma grade II**

**C82.10 Follicular lymphoma grade II, unspecified site** HCC Rx ESR COM
**C82.11 Follicular lymphoma grade II, lymph nodes of head, face, and neck** HCC Rx ESR COM
**C82.12 Follicular lymphoma grade II, intrathoracic lymph nodes** HCC Rx ESR COM
**C82.13 Follicular lymphoma grade II, intra-abdominal lymph nodes** HCC Rx ESR COM
**C82.14 Follicular lymphoma grade II, lymph nodes of axilla and upper limb** HCC Rx ESR COM
**C82.15 Follicular lymphoma grade II, lymph nodes of inguinal region and lower limb** HCC Rx ESR COM
**C82.16 Follicular lymphoma grade II, intrapelvic lymph nodes** HCC Rx ESR COM
**C82.17 Follicular lymphoma grade II, spleen** HCC Rx ESR COM
**C82.18 Follicular lymphoma grade II, lymph nodes of multiple sites** HCC Rx ESR COM
**C82.19 Follicular lymphoma grade II, extranodal and solid organ sites** HCC Rx ESR COM
**C82.1A Follicular lymphoma grade II, in remission** HCC Rx ESR COM

**✓5th C82.2 Follicular lymphoma grade III, unspecified**

**C82.20 Follicular lymphoma grade III, unspecified, unspecified site** HCC Rx ESR COM
**C82.21 Follicular lymphoma grade III, unspecified, lymph nodes of head, face, and neck** HCC Rx ESR COM
**C82.22 Follicular lymphoma grade III, unspecified, intrathoracic lymph nodes** HCC Rx ESR COM
**C82.23 Follicular lymphoma grade III, unspecified, intra-abdominal lymph nodes** HCC Rx ESR COM
**C82.24 Follicular lymphoma grade III, unspecified, lymph nodes of axilla and upper limb** HCC Rx ESR COM
**C82.25 Follicular lymphoma grade III, unspecified, lymph nodes of inguinal region and lower limb** HCC Rx ESR COM
**C82.26 Follicular lymphoma grade III, unspecified, intrapelvic lymph nodes** HCC Rx ESR COM
**C82.27 Follicular lymphoma grade III, unspecified, spleen** HCC Rx ESR COM
**C82.28 Follicular lymphoma grade III, unspecified, lymph nodes of multiple sites** HCC Rx ESR COM
**C82.29 Follicular lymphoma grade III, unspecified, extranodal and solid organ sites** HCC Rx ESR COM

C82.2A Follicular lymphoma grade III, unspecified, in remission HCC Rx ESR COM

✓5th C82.3 Follicular lymphoma grade IIIa

C82.30 Follicular lymphoma grade IIIa, unspecified site HCC Rx ESR COM

C82.31 Follicular lymphoma grade IIIa, lymph nodes of head, face, and neck HCC Rx ESR COM

C82.32 Follicular lymphoma grade IIIa, intrathoracic lymph nodes HCC Rx ESR COM

C82.33 Follicular lymphoma grade IIIa, intra-abdominal lymph nodes HCC Rx ESR COM

C82.34 Follicular lymphoma grade IIIa, lymph nodes of axilla and upper limb HCC Rx ESR COM

C82.35 Follicular lymphoma grade IIIa, lymph nodes of inguinal region and lower limb HCC Rx ESR COM

C82.36 Follicular lymphoma grade IIIa, intrapelvic lymph nodes HCC Rx ESR COM

C82.37 Follicular lymphoma grade IIIa, spleen HCC Rx ESR COM

C82.38 Follicular lymphoma grade IIIa, lymph nodes of multiple sites HCC Rx ESR COM

C82.39 Follicular lymphoma grade IIIa, extranodal and solid organ sites HCC Rx ESR COM

C82.3A Follicular lymphoma grade IIIa, in remission HCC Rx ESR COM

✓5th C82.4 Follicular lymphoma grade IIIb

C82.40 Follicular lymphoma grade IIIb, unspecified site HCC Rx ESR COM

C82.41 Follicular lymphoma grade IIIb, lymph nodes of head, face, and neck HCC Rx ESR COM

C82.42 Follicular lymphoma grade IIIb, intrathoracic lymph nodes HCC Rx ESR COM

C82.43 Follicular lymphoma grade IIIb, intra-abdominal lymph nodes HCC Rx ESR COM

C82.44 Follicular lymphoma grade IIIb, lymph nodes of axilla and upper limb HCC Rx ESR COM

C82.45 Follicular lymphoma grade IIIb, lymph nodes of inguinal region and lower limb HCC Rx ESR COM

C82.46 Follicular lymphoma grade IIIb, intrapelvic lymph nodes HCC Rx ESR COM

C82.47 Follicular lymphoma grade IIIb, spleen HCC Rx ESR COM

C82.48 Follicular lymphoma grade IIIb, lymph nodes of multiple sites HCC Rx ESR COM

C82.49 Follicular lymphoma grade IIIb, extranodal and solid organ sites HCC Rx ESR COM

C82.4A Follicular lymphoma grade IIIb, in remission HCC Rx ESR COM

✓5th C82.5 Diffuse follicle center lymphoma

C82.50 Diffuse follicle center lymphoma, unspecified site HCC Rx ESR COM

C82.51 Diffuse follicle center lymphoma, lymph nodes of head, face, and neck HCC Rx ESR COM

C82.52 Diffuse follicle center lymphoma, intrathoracic lymph nodes HCC Rx ESR COM

C82.53 Diffuse follicle center lymphoma, intra-abdominal lymph nodes HCC Rx ESR COM

C82.54 Diffuse follicle center lymphoma, lymph nodes of axilla and upper limb HCC Rx ESR COM

C82.55 Diffuse follicle center lymphoma, lymph nodes of inguinal region and lower limb HCC Rx ESR COM

C82.56 Diffuse follicle center lymphoma, intrapelvic lymph nodes HCC Rx ESR COM

C82.57 Diffuse follicle center lymphoma, spleen HCC Rx ESR COM

C82.58 Diffuse follicle center lymphoma, lymph nodes of multiple sites HCC Rx ESR COM

C82.59 Diffuse follicle center lymphoma, extranodal and solid organ sites HCC Rx ESR COM

C82.5A Diffuse follicle center lymphoma, in remission HCC Rx ESR COM

✓5th C82.6 Cutaneous follicle center lymphoma

C82.60 Cutaneous follicle center lymphoma, unspecified site HCC Rx ESR COM

C82.61 Cutaneous follicle center lymphoma, lymph nodes of head, face, and neck HCC Rx ESR COM

C82.62 Cutaneous follicle center lymphoma, intrathoracic lymph nodes HCC Rx ESR COM

C82.63 Cutaneous follicle center lymphoma, intra-abdominal lymph nodes HCC Rx ESR COM

C82.64 Cutaneous follicle center lymphoma, lymph nodes of axilla and upper limb HCC Rx ESR COM

C82.65 Cutaneous follicle center lymphoma, lymph nodes of inguinal region and lower limb HCC Rx ESR COM

C82.66 Cutaneous follicle center lymphoma, intrapelvic lymph nodes HCC Rx ESR COM

C82.67 Cutaneous follicle center lymphoma, spleen HCC Rx ESR COM

C82.68 Cutaneous follicle center lymphoma, lymph nodes of multiple sites HCC Rx ESR COM

C82.69 Cutaneous follicle center lymphoma, extranodal and solid organ sites HCC Rx ESR COM

C82.6A Cutaneous follicle center lymphoma, in remission HCC Rx ESR COM

✓5th C82.8 Other types of follicular lymphoma

C82.80 Other types of follicular lymphoma, unspecified site HCC Rx ESR COM

C82.81 Other types of follicular lymphoma, lymph nodes of head, face, and neck HCC Rx ESR COM

C82.82 Other types of follicular lymphoma, intrathoracic lymph nodes HCC Rx ESR COM

C82.83 Other types of follicular lymphoma, intra-abdominal lymph nodes HCC Rx ESR COM

C82.84 Other types of follicular lymphoma, lymph nodes of axilla and upper limb HCC Rx ESR COM

C82.85 Other types of follicular lymphoma, lymph nodes of inguinal region and lower limb HCC Rx ESR COM

C82.86 Other types of follicular lymphoma, intrapelvic lymph nodes HCC Rx ESR COM

C82.87 Other types of follicular lymphoma, spleen HCC Rx ESR COM

C82.88 Other types of follicular lymphoma, lymph nodes of multiple sites HCC Rx ESR COM

C82.89 Other types of follicular lymphoma, extranodal and solid organ sites HCC Rx ESR COM

C82.8A Other types of follicular lymphoma, in remission HCC Rx ESR COM

✓5th C82.9 Follicular lymphoma, unspecified

C82.90 Follicular lymphoma, unspecified, unspecified site HCC Rx ESR COM

C82.91 Follicular lymphoma, unspecified, lymph nodes of head, face, and neck HCC Rx ESR COM

C82.92 Follicular lymphoma, unspecified, intrathoracic lymph nodes HCC Rx ESR COM

C82.93 Follicular lymphoma, unspecified, intra-abdominal lymph nodes HCC Rx ESR COM

C82.94 Follicular lymphoma, unspecified, lymph nodes of axilla and upper limb HCC Rx ESR COM

C82.95 Follicular lymphoma, unspecified, lymph nodes of inguinal region and lower limb HCC Rx ESR COM

C82.96 Follicular lymphoma, unspecified, intrapelvic lymph nodes HCC Rx ESR COM

C82.97 Follicular lymphoma, unspecified, spleen HCC Rx ESR COM

C82.98 Follicular lymphoma, unspecified, lymph nodes of multiple sites HCC Rx ESR COM

C82.99 Follicular lymphoma, unspecified, extranodal and solid organ sites HCC Rx ESR COM

C82.9A Follicular lymphoma, unspecified, in remission HCC Rx ESR COM

**✓4th C83 Non-follicular lymphoma**

EXCLUDES 1 *personal history of non-Hodgkin lymphoma (Z85.72)*

**AHA:** 2023,1Q,22

**✓5th C83.Ø Small cell B-cell lymphoma**

Lymphoplasmacytic lymphoma
Nodal marginal zone lymphoma
Non-leukemic variant of B-CLL
Splenic marginal zone lymphoma

EXCLUDES 1 *chronic lymphocytic leukemia (C91.1)*
*mature T/NK-cell lymphomas (C84.-)*
*Waldenstrom macroglobulinemia (C88.ØØ)*

**AHA:** 2023,1Q,18

**DEF:** Nonfollicular lymphoma that is rare, slow growing, and usually found in the older population.

**C83.ØØ Small cell B-cell lymphoma, unspecified site** HCC Rx ESR COM

**C83.Ø1 Small cell B-cell lymphoma, lymph nodes of head, face, and neck** HCC Rx ESR COM

**C83.Ø2 Small cell B-cell lymphoma, intrathoracic lymph nodes** HCC Rx ESR COM

**C83.Ø3 Small cell B-cell lymphoma, intra-abdominal lymph nodes** HCC Rx ESR COM

**C83.Ø4 Small cell B-cell lymphoma, lymph nodes of axilla and upper limb** HCC Rx ESR COM

**C83.Ø5 Small cell B-cell lymphoma, lymph nodes of inguinal region and lower limb** HCC Rx ESR COM

**C83.Ø6 Small cell B-cell lymphoma, intrapelvic lymph nodes** HCC Rx ESR COM

**C83.Ø7 Small cell B-cell lymphoma, spleen** HCC Rx ESR COM

**C83.Ø8 Small cell B-cell lymphoma, lymph nodes of multiple sites** HCC Rx ESR COM

**C83.Ø9 Small cell B-cell lymphoma, extranodal and solid organ sites** HCC Rx ESR COM

**C83.ØA Small cell B-cell lymphoma, in remission** HCC Rx ESR COM

**✓5th C83.1 Mantle cell lymphoma**

Centrocytic lymphoma
Malignant lymphomatous polyposis

**DEF:** Rare form of B-cell non-Hodgkin lymphoma named for the location of the tumor cell production, the mantle zone of the lymph nodes.

**C83.1Ø Mantle cell lymphoma, unspecified site** HCC Rx ESR COM

**C83.11 Mantle cell lymphoma, lymph nodes of head, face, and neck** HCC Rx ESR COM

**C83.12 Mantle cell lymphoma, intrathoracic lymph nodes** HCC Rx ESR COM

**C83.13 Mantle cell lymphoma, intra-abdominal lymph nodes** HCC Rx ESR COM

**C83.14 Mantle cell lymphoma, lymph nodes of axilla and upper limb** HCC Rx ESR COM

**C83.15 Mantle cell lymphoma, lymph nodes of inguinal region and lower limb** HCC Rx ESR COM

**C83.16 Mantle cell lymphoma, intrapelvic lymph nodes** HCC Rx ESR COM

**C83.17 Mantle cell lymphoma, spleen** HCC Rx ESR COM

**C83.18 Mantle cell lymphoma, lymph nodes of multiple sites** HCC Rx ESR COM

**C83.19 Mantle cell lymphoma, extranodal and solid organ sites** HCC Rx ESR COM

**C83.1A Mantle cell lymphoma, in remission** HCC Rx ESR COM

Centrocytic lymphoma, in remission

**✓5th C83.3 Diffuse large B-cell lymphoma**

Anaplastic diffuse large B-cell lymphoma
CD3Ø-positive diffuse large B-cell lymphoma
Centroblastic diffuse large B-cell lymphoma
Diffuse large B-cell lymphoma, subtype not specified
Immunoblastic diffuse large B-cell lymphoma
Plasmablastic diffuse large B-cell lymphoma
T-cell rich diffuse large B-cell lymphoma

EXCLUDES 1 *mediastinal (thymic) large B-cell lymphoma (C85.2-)*
*mature T/NK-cell lymphomas (C84.-)*

**DEF:** Nonfollicular lymphoma that is one of the more common types of lymphoma. This cancer is fast growing and affects any age but is found mostly in the older population.

**C83.3Ø Diffuse large B-cell lymphoma, unspecified site** HCC Rx ESR COM

**C83.31 Diffuse large B-cell lymphoma, lymph nodes of head, face, and neck** HCC Rx ESR COM

**C83.32 Diffuse large B-cell lymphoma, intrathoracic lymph nodes** HCC Rx ESR COM

**C83.33 Diffuse large B-cell lymphoma, intra-abdominal lymph nodes** HCC Rx ESR COM

**C83.34 Diffuse large B-cell lymphoma, lymph nodes of axilla and upper limb** HCC Rx ESR COM

**C83.35 Diffuse large B-cell lymphoma, lymph nodes of inguinal region and lower limb** HCC Rx ESR COM

**C83.36 Diffuse large B-cell lymphoma, intrapelvic lymph nodes** HCC Rx ESR COM

**C83.37 Diffuse large B-cell lymphoma, spleen** HCC Rx ESR COM

**C83.38 Diffuse large B-cell lymphoma, lymph nodes of multiple sites** HCC Rx ESR COM

**AHA:** 2023,1Q,22

**✓6th C83.39 Diffuse large B-cell lymphoma, extranodal and solid organ sites**

**AHA:** 2024,4Q,4; 2023,1Q,22

**C83.39Ø Primary central nervous system lymphoma** HCC Rx ESR COM

PCNSL of brain
PCNSL of meninges
PCNSL NOS
PCNSL of spinal cord

EXCLUDES 1 *primary central nervous system lymphoma, Burkitt (C83.79)*
*primary central nervous system lymphoma, lymphoblastic (C83.59)*
*primary central nervous system lymphoma, other (C83.89)*
*primary central nervous system lymphoma, peripheral T-cell (C84.49)*

**C83.398 Diffuse large B-cell lymphoma of other extranodal and solid organ sites** HCC Rx ESR COM

**C83.3A Diffuse large B-cell lymphoma, in remission** HCC Rx ESR COM

**✓5th C83.5 Lymphoblastic (diffuse) lymphoma**

B-precursor lymphoma
Lymphoblastic B-cell lymphoma
Lymphoblastic lymphoma NOS
Lymphoblastic T-cell lymphoma
T-precursor lymphoma

**DEF:** Type of non-Hodgkin lymphoma considered lymphoma or leukemia—the determination is made based on the amount of bone marrow involvement. The cells are small to medium immature T-cells that often originate in the thymus where many of the T-cells are made.

**C83.5Ø Lymphoblastic (diffuse) lymphoma, unspecified site** HCC Rx ESR COM

**C83.51 Lymphoblastic (diffuse) lymphoma, lymph nodes of head, face, and neck** HCC Rx ESR COM

**C83.52 Lymphoblastic (diffuse) lymphoma, intrathoracic lymph nodes** HCC Rx ESR COM

**C83.53 Lymphoblastic (diffuse) lymphoma, intra-abdominal lymph nodes** HCC Rx ESR COM

**C83.54 Lymphoblastic (diffuse) lymphoma, lymph nodes of axilla and upper limb** HCC Rx ESR COM

**C83.55 Lymphoblastic (diffuse) lymphoma, lymph nodes of inguinal region and lower limb** HCC Rx ESR COM

**C83.56 Lymphoblastic (diffuse) lymphoma, intrapelvic lymph nodes** HCC Rx ESR COM

**C83.57 Lymphoblastic (diffuse) lymphoma, spleen** HCC Rx ESR COM

**C83.58 Lymphoblastic (diffuse) lymphoma, lymph nodes of multiple sites** HCC Rx ESR COM

**C83.59 Lymphoblastic (diffuse) lymphoma, extranodal and solid organ sites** HCC Rx ESR COM

**C83.5A Lymphoblastic (diffuse) lymphoma, in remission** HCC Rx ESR COM

**C83.7 Burkitt lymphoma**

Atypical Burkitt lymphoma
Burkitt-like lymphoma

EXCLUDES 1 *mature B-cell leukemia Burkitt type (C91.A-)*

**DEF:** Malignancy of the lymphatic system, most often seen as a large bone-deteriorating lesion within the jaw or as an abdominal mass. It is a form of non-Hodgkin's lymphoma and is recognized as the fastest growing human tumor.

- **C83.70 Burkitt lymphoma, unspecified site** HCC Rx ESR COM
- **C83.71 Burkitt lymphoma, lymph nodes of head, face, and neck** HCC Rx ESR COM
- **C83.72 Burkitt lymphoma, intrathoracic lymph nodes** HCC Rx ESR COM
- **C83.73 Burkitt lymphoma, intra-abdominal lymph nodes** HCC Rx ESR COM
- **C83.74 Burkitt lymphoma, lymph nodes of axilla and upper limb** HCC Rx ESR COM
- **C83.75 Burkitt lymphoma, lymph nodes of inguinal region and lower limb** HCC Rx ESR COM
- **C83.76 Burkitt lymphoma, intrapelvic lymph nodes** HCC Rx ESR COM
- **C83.77 Burkitt lymphoma, spleen** HCC Rx ESR COM
- **C83.78 Burkitt lymphoma, lymph nodes of multiple sites** HCC Rx ESR COM
- **C83.79 Burkitt lymphoma, extranodal and solid organ sites** HCC Rx ESR COM
- **C83.7A Burkitt lymphoma, in remission** HCC Rx ESR COM

**C83.8 Other non-follicular lymphoma**

Intravascular large B-cell lymphoma
Lymphoid granulomatosis
Primary effusion B-cell lymphoma

EXCLUDES 1 *mediastinal (thymic) large B-cell lymphoma (C85.2-)*
*T-cell rich B-cell lymphoma (C83.3-)*

- **C83.80 Other non-follicular lymphoma, unspecified site** HCC Rx ESR COM
- **C83.81 Other non-follicular lymphoma, lymph nodes of head, face, and neck** HCC Rx ESR COM
- **C83.82 Other non-follicular lymphoma, intrathoracic lymph nodes** HCC Rx ESR COM
- **C83.83 Other non-follicular lymphoma, intra-abdominal lymph nodes** HCC Rx ESR COM
- **C83.84 Other non-follicular lymphoma, lymph nodes of axilla and upper limb** HCC Rx ESR COM
- **C83.85 Other non-follicular lymphoma, lymph nodes of inguinal region and lower limb** HCC Rx ESR COM
- **C83.86 Other non-follicular lymphoma, intrapelvic lymph nodes** HCC Rx ESR COM
- **C83.87 Other non-follicular lymphoma, spleen** HCC Rx ESR COM
- **C83.88 Other non-follicular lymphoma, lymph nodes of multiple sites** HCC Rx ESR COM
- **C83.89 Other non-follicular lymphoma, extranodal and solid organ sites** HCC Rx ESR COM
- **C83.8A Other non-follicular lymphoma, in remission** HCC Rx ESR COM

**C83.9 Non-follicular (diffuse) lymphoma, unspecified**

- **C83.90 Non-follicular (diffuse) lymphoma, unspecified, unspecified site** HCC Rx ESR COM
- **C83.91 Non-follicular (diffuse) lymphoma, unspecified, lymph nodes of head, face, and neck** HCC Rx ESR COM
- **C83.92 Non-follicular (diffuse) lymphoma, unspecified, intrathoracic lymph nodes** HCC Rx ESR COM
- **C83.93 Non-follicular (diffuse) lymphoma, unspecified, intra-abdominal lymph nodes** HCC Rx ESR COM
- **C83.94 Non-follicular (diffuse) lymphoma, unspecified, lymph nodes of axilla and upper limb** HCC Rx ESR COM
- **C83.95 Non-follicular (diffuse) lymphoma, unspecified, lymph nodes of inguinal region and lower limb** HCC Rx ESR COM
- **C83.96 Non-follicular (diffuse) lymphoma, unspecified, intrapelvic lymph nodes** HCC Rx ESR COM
- **C83.97 Non-follicular (diffuse) lymphoma, unspecified, spleen** HCC Rx ESR COM
- **C83.98 Non-follicular (diffuse) lymphoma, unspecified, lymph nodes of multiple sites** HCC Rx ESR COM
- **C83.99 Non-follicular (diffuse) lymphoma, unspecified, extranodal and solid organ sites** HCC Rx ESR COM
- **C83.9A Non-follicular (diffuse) lymphoma, unspecified, in remission** HCC Rx ESR COM

## C84 Mature T/NK-cell lymphomas

EXCLUDES 1 *personal history of non-Hodgkin lymphoma (Z85.72)*

**AHA:** 2023,1Q,22

**C84.0 Mycosis fungoides**

EXCLUDES 1 *peripheral T-cell lymphoma, not elsewhere classified (C84.4-)*

**DEF:** Most common form of cutaneous T-cell lymphoma. A type of non-Hodgkin lymphoma in which white blood cells become cancerous and affect the skin and sometimes internal organs.
***Synonym(s):*** *Alibert-Bazin syndrome.*

- **C84.00 Mycosis fungoides, unspecified site** HCC Rx ESR COM
- **C84.01 Mycosis fungoides, lymph nodes of head, face, and neck** HCC Rx ESR COM
- **C84.02 Mycosis fungoides, intrathoracic lymph nodes** HCC Rx ESR COM
- **C84.03 Mycosis fungoides, intra-abdominal lymph nodes** HCC Rx ESR COM
- **C84.04 Mycosis fungoides, lymph nodes of axilla and upper limb** HCC Rx ESR COM
- **C84.05 Mycosis fungoides, lymph nodes of inguinal region and lower limb** HCC Rx ESR COM
- **C84.06 Mycosis fungoides, intrapelvic lymph nodes** HCC Rx ESR COM
- **C84.07 Mycosis fungoides, spleen** HCC Rx ESR COM
- **C84.08 Mycosis fungoides, lymph nodes of multiple sites** HCC Rx ESR COM
- **C84.09 Mycosis fungoides, extranodal and solid organ sites** HCC Rx ESR COM
- **C84.0A Mycosis fungoides, in remission** HCC Rx ESR COM

**C84.1 Sezary disease**

**DEF:** Extension of mycosis fungoides that affects the blood and all of the skin, appearing as sunburn, rather than patches. It spreads to the lymph nodes and is often linked to a weakened immune system.

- **C84.10 Sezary disease, unspecified site** HCC Rx ESR COM
- **C84.11 Sezary disease, lymph nodes of head, face, and neck** HCC Rx ESR COM
- **C84.12 Sezary disease, intrathoracic lymph nodes** HCC Rx ESR COM
- **C84.13 Sezary disease, intra-abdominal lymph nodes** HCC Rx ESR COM
- **C84.14 Sezary disease, lymph nodes of axilla and upper limb** HCC Rx ESR COM
- **C84.15 Sezary disease, lymph nodes of inguinal region and lower limb** HCC Rx ESR COM
- **C84.16 Sezary disease, intrapelvic lymph nodes** HCC Rx ESR COM
- **C84.17 Sezary disease, spleen** HCC Rx ESR COM
- **C84.18 Sezary disease, lymph nodes of multiple sites** HCC Rx ESR COM
- **C84.19 Sezary disease, extranodal and solid organ sites** HCC Rx ESR COM
- **C84.1A Sezary disease, in remission** HCC Rx ESR COM

**C84.4 Peripheral T-cell lymphoma, not elsewhere classified**

Lennert's lymphoma
Lymphoepithelioid lymphoma
Mature T-cell lymphoma, not elsewhere classified

- **C84.40 Peripheral T-cell lymphoma, not elsewhere classified, unspecified site** HCC Rx ESR COM
- **C84.41 Peripheral T-cell lymphoma, not elsewhere classified, lymph nodes of head, face, and neck** HCC Rx ESR COM
- **C84.42 Peripheral T-cell lymphoma, not elsewhere classified, intrathoracic lymph nodes** HCC Rx ESR COM
- **C84.43 Peripheral T-cell lymphoma, not elsewhere classified, intra-abdominal lymph nodes** HCC Rx ESR COM
- **C84.44 Peripheral T-cell lymphoma, not elsewhere classified, lymph nodes of axilla and upper limb** HCC Rx ESR COM
- **C84.45 Peripheral T-cell lymphoma, not elsewhere classified, lymph nodes of inguinal region and lower limb** HCC Rx ESR COM

C84.46 Peripheral T-cell lymphoma, not elsewhere classified, intrapelvic lymph nodes HCC Rx ESR COM
C84.47 Peripheral T-cell lymphoma, not elsewhere classified, spleen HCC Rx ESR COM
C84.48 Peripheral T-cell lymphoma, not elsewhere classified, lymph nodes of multiple sites HCC Rx ESR COM
C84.49 Peripheral T-cell lymphoma, not elsewhere classified, extranodal and solid organ sites HCC Rx ESR COM
C84.4A Peripheral T-cell lymphoma, not elsewhere classified, in remission HCC Rx ESR COM

✓5th C84.6 Anaplastic large cell lymphoma, ALK-positive
Anaplastic large cell lymphoma, CD30-positive
C84.60 Anaplastic large cell lymphoma, ALK-positive, unspecified site HCC Rx ESR COM
C84.61 Anaplastic large cell lymphoma, ALK-positive, lymph nodes of head, face, and neck HCC Rx ESR COM
C84.62 Anaplastic large cell lymphoma, ALK-positive, intrathoracic lymph nodes HCC Rx ESR COM
C84.63 Anaplastic large cell lymphoma, ALK-positive, intra-abdominal lymph nodes HCC Rx ESR COM
C84.64 Anaplastic large cell lymphoma, ALK-positive, lymph nodes of axilla and upper limb HCC Rx ESR COM
C84.65 Anaplastic large cell lymphoma, ALK-positive, lymph nodes of inguinal region and lower limb HCC Rx ESR COM
C84.66 Anaplastic large cell lymphoma, ALK-positive, intrapelvic lymph nodes HCC Rx ESR COM
C84.67 Anaplastic large cell lymphoma, ALK-positive, spleen HCC Rx ESR COM
C84.68 Anaplastic large cell lymphoma, ALK-positive, lymph nodes of multiple sites HCC Rx ESR COM
C84.69 Anaplastic large cell lymphoma, ALK-positive, extranodal and solid organ sites HCC Rx ESR COM
C84.6A Anaplastic large cell lymphoma, ALK-positive, in remission HCC Rx ESR COM

✓5th C84.7 Anaplastic large cell lymphoma, ALK-negative
EXCLUDES 1 *primary cutaneous CD30-positive T-cell proliferations (C86.6-)*
C84.70 Anaplastic large cell lymphoma, ALK-negative, unspecified site HCC Rx ESR COM
C84.71 Anaplastic large cell lymphoma, ALK-negative, lymph nodes of head, face, and neck HCC Rx ESR COM
C84.72 Anaplastic large cell lymphoma, ALK-negative, intrathoracic lymph nodes HCC Rx ESR COM
C84.73 Anaplastic large cell lymphoma, ALK-negative, intra-abdominal lymph nodes HCC Rx ESR COM
C84.74 Anaplastic large cell lymphoma, ALK-negative, lymph nodes of axilla and upper limb HCC Rx ESR COM
C84.75 Anaplastic large cell lymphoma, ALK-negative, lymph nodes of inguinal region and lower limb HCC Rx ESR COM
C84.76 Anaplastic large cell lymphoma, ALK-negative, intrapelvic lymph nodes HCC Rx ESR COM
C84.77 Anaplastic large cell lymphoma, ALK-negative, spleen HCC Rx ESR COM
C84.78 Anaplastic large cell lymphoma, ALK-negative, lymph nodes of multiple sites HCC Rx ESR COM
C84.79 Anaplastic large cell lymphoma, ALK-negative, extranodal and solid organ sites HCC Rx ESR COM
C84.7A Anaplastic large cell lymphoma, ALK-negative, breast HCC Rx ESR COM
Breast implant associated anaplastic large cell lymphoma (BIA-ALCL)
Use additional code to identify:
breast implant status (Z98.82)
personal history of breast implant removal (Z98.86)
AHA: 2021,4Q,6
C84.7B Anaplastic large cell lymphoma, ALK-negative, in remission HCC Rx ESR COM

✓5th C84.A Cutaneous T-cell lymphoma, unspecified
AHA: 2021,2Q,6
C84.A0 Cutaneous T-cell lymphoma, unspecified, unspecified site HCC Rx ESR COM
C84.A1 Cutaneous T-cell lymphoma, unspecified lymph nodes of head, face, and neck HCC Rx ESR COM
C84.A2 Cutaneous T-cell lymphoma, unspecified, intrathoracic lymph nodes HCC Rx ESR COM
C84.A3 Cutaneous T-cell lymphoma, unspecified, intra-abdominal lymph nodes HCC Rx ESR COM
C84.A4 Cutaneous T-cell lymphoma, unspecified, lymph nodes of axilla and upper limb HCC Rx ESR COM
C84.A5 Cutaneous T-cell lymphoma, unspecified, lymph nodes of inguinal region and lower limb HCC Rx ESR COM
C84.A6 Cutaneous T-cell lymphoma, unspecified, intrapelvic lymph nodes HCC Rx ESR COM
C84.A7 Cutaneous T-cell lymphoma, unspecified, spleen HCC Rx ESR COM
C84.A8 Cutaneous T-cell lymphoma, unspecified, lymph nodes of multiple sites HCC Rx ESR COM
C84.A9 Cutaneous T-cell lymphoma, unspecified, extranodal and solid organ sites HCC Rx ESR COM
C84.AA Cutaneous T-cell lymphoma, unspecified, in remission HCC Rx ESR COM

✓5th C84.Z Other mature T/NK-cell lymphomas
NOTE If T-cell lineage or involvement is mentioned in conjunction with a specific lymphoma, code to the more specific description.
EXCLUDES 1 *angioimmunoblastic T-cell lymphoma (C86.50)*
*blastic NK-cell lymphoma (C86.40)*
*enteropathy-type T-cell lymphoma (C86.20)*
*extranodal NK-cell lymphoma, nasal type (C86.00)*
*hepatosplenic T-cell lymphoma (C86.10)*
*primary cutaneous CD30-positive T-cell proliferations (C86.60)*
*subcutaneous panniculitis-like T-cell lymphoma (C86.30)*
*T-cell leukemia (C91.1-)*
C84.Z0 Other mature T/NK-cell lymphomas, unspecified site HCC Rx ESR COM
C84.Z1 Other mature T/NK-cell lymphomas, lymph nodes of head, face, and neck HCC Rx ESR COM
C84.Z2 Other mature T/NK-cell lymphomas, intrathoracic lymph nodes HCC Rx ESR COM
C84.Z3 Other mature T/NK-cell lymphomas, intra-abdominal lymph nodes HCC Rx ESR COM
C84.Z4 Other mature T/NK-cell lymphomas, lymph nodes of axilla and upper limb HCC Rx ESR COM
C84.Z5 Other mature T/NK-cell lymphomas, lymph nodes of inguinal region and lower limb HCC Rx ESR COM
C84.Z6 Other mature T/NK-cell lymphomas, intrapelvic lymph nodes HCC Rx ESR COM
C84.Z7 Other mature T/NK-cell lymphomas, spleen HCC Rx ESR COM
C84.Z8 Other mature T/NK-cell lymphomas, lymph nodes of multiple sites HCC Rx ESR COM
C84.Z9 Other mature T/NK-cell lymphomas, extranodal and solid organ sites HCC Rx ESR COM
C84.ZA Other mature T/NK-cell lymphomas, in remission HCC Rx ESR COM

✓5th C84.9 Mature T/NK-cell lymphomas, unspecified
NK/T cell lymphoma NOS
EXCLUDES 1 *mature T-cell lymphoma, not elsewhere classified (C84.4-)*
C84.90 Mature T/NK-cell lymphomas, unspecified, unspecified site HCC Rx ESR COM
C84.91 Mature T/NK-cell lymphomas, unspecified, lymph nodes of head, face, and neck HCC Rx ESR COM
C84.92 Mature T/NK-cell lymphomas, unspecified, intrathoracic lymph nodes HCC Rx ESR COM
C84.93 Mature T/NK-cell lymphomas, unspecified, intra-abdominal lymph nodes HCC Rx ESR COM
C84.94 Mature T/NK-cell lymphomas, unspecified, lymph nodes of axilla and upper limb HCC Rx ESR COM
C84.95 Mature T/NK-cell lymphomas, unspecified, lymph nodes of inguinal region and lower limb HCC Rx ESR COM
C84.96 Mature T/NK-cell lymphomas, unspecified, intrapelvic lymph nodes HCC Rx ESR COM
C84.97 Mature T/NK-cell lymphomas, unspecified, spleen HCC Rx ESR COM
C84.98 Mature T/NK-cell lymphomas, unspecified, lymph nodes of multiple sites HCC Rx ESR COM
C84.99 Mature T/NK-cell lymphomas, unspecified, extranodal and solid organ sites HCC Rx ESR COM

**C84.9A** **Mature T/NK-cell lymphomas, unspecified, in remission** HCC Rx ESR COM

**C85 Other specified and unspecified types of non-Hodgkin lymphoma**

EXCLUDES 1 *other specified types of T/NK-cell lymphoma (C86.-)*
*personal history of non-Hodgkin lymphoma (Z85.72)*

**AHA:** 2023,1Q,22

**C85.1 Unspecified B-cell lymphoma**

NOTE If B-cell lineage or involvement is mentioned in conjunction with a specific lymphoma, code to the more specific description.

**C85.10** **Unspecified B-cell lymphoma, unspecified site** HCC Rx ESR COM

**C85.11** **Unspecified B-cell lymphoma, lymph nodes of head, face, and neck** HCC Rx ESR COM

**C85.12** **Unspecified B-cell lymphoma, intrathoracic lymph nodes** HCC Rx ESR COM

**C85.13** **Unspecified B-cell lymphoma, intra-abdominal lymph nodes** HCC Rx ESR COM

**C85.14** **Unspecified B-cell lymphoma, lymph nodes of axilla and upper limb** HCC Rx ESR COM

**C85.15** **Unspecified B-cell lymphoma, lymph nodes of inguinal region and lower limb** HCC Rx ESR COM

**C85.16** **Unspecified B-cell lymphoma, intrapelvic lymph nodes** HCC Rx ESR COM

**C85.17** **Unspecified B-cell lymphoma, spleen** HCC Rx ESR COM

**C85.18** **Unspecified B-cell lymphoma, lymph nodes of multiple sites** HCC Rx ESR COM

**C85.19** **Unspecified B-cell lymphoma, extranodal and solid organ sites** HCC Rx ESR COM

**C85.1A** **Unspecified B-cell lymphoma, in remission** HCC Rx ESR COM

**C85.2 Mediastinal (thymic) large B-cell lymphoma**

**C85.20** **Mediastinal (thymic) large B-cell lymphoma, unspecified site** HCC Rx ESR COM

**C85.21** **Mediastinal (thymic) large B-cell lymphoma, lymph nodes of head, face, and neck** HCC Rx ESR COM

**C85.22** **Mediastinal (thymic) large B-cell lymphoma, intrathoracic lymph nodes** HCC Rx ESR COM

**C85.23** **Mediastinal (thymic) large B-cell lymphoma, intra-abdominal lymph nodes** HCC Rx ESR COM

**C85.24** **Mediastinal (thymic) large B-cell lymphoma, lymph nodes of axilla and upper limb** HCC Rx ESR COM

**C85.25** **Mediastinal (thymic) large B-cell lymphoma, lymph nodes of inguinal region and lower limb** HCC Rx ESR COM

**C85.26** **Mediastinal (thymic) large B-cell lymphoma, intrapelvic lymph nodes** HCC Rx ESR COM

**C85.27** **Mediastinal (thymic) large B-cell lymphoma, spleen** HCC Rx ESR COM

**C85.28** **Mediastinal (thymic) large B-cell lymphoma, lymph nodes of multiple sites** HCC Rx ESR COM

**C85.29** **Mediastinal (thymic) large B-cell lymphoma, extranodal and solid organ sites** HCC Rx ESR COM

**C85.2A** **Mediastinal (thymic) large B-cell lymphoma, in remission** HCC Rx ESR COM

**C85.8 Other specified types of non-Hodgkin lymphoma**

**C85.80** **Other specified types of non-Hodgkin lymphoma, unspecified site** HCC Rx ESR COM

**C85.81** **Other specified types of non-Hodgkin lymphoma, lymph nodes of head, face, and neck** HCC Rx ESR COM

**C85.82** **Other specified types of non-Hodgkin lymphoma, intrathoracic lymph nodes** HCC Rx ESR COM

**C85.83** **Other specified types of non-Hodgkin lymphoma, intra-abdominal lymph nodes** HCC Rx ESR COM

**C85.84** **Other specified types of non-Hodgkin lymphoma, lymph nodes of axilla and upper limb** HCC Rx ESR COM

**C85.85** **Other specified types of non-Hodgkin lymphoma, lymph nodes of inguinal region and lower limb** HCC Rx ESR COM

**C85.86** **Other specified types of non-Hodgkin lymphoma, intrapelvic lymph nodes** HCC Rx ESR COM

**C85.87** **Other specified types of non-Hodgkin lymphoma, spleen** HCC Rx ESR COM

**C85.88** **Other specified types of non-Hodgkin lymphoma, lymph nodes of multiple sites** HCC Rx ESR COM

**C85.89** **Other specified types of non-Hodgkin lymphoma, extranodal and solid organ sites** HCC Rx ESR COM

**C85.8A** **Other specified types of non-Hodgkin lymphoma, in remission** HCC Rx ESR COM

**C85.9 Non-Hodgkin lymphoma, unspecified**

Lymphoma NOS
Malignant lymphoma NOS
Non-Hodgkin lymphoma NOS

**C85.90** **Non-Hodgkin lymphoma, unspecified, unspecified site** HCC Rx ESR COM

**C85.91** **Non-Hodgkin lymphoma, unspecified, lymph nodes of head, face, and neck** HCC Rx ESR COM

**C85.92** **Non-Hodgkin lymphoma, unspecified, intrathoracic lymph nodes** HCC Rx ESR COM

**C85.93** **Non-Hodgkin lymphoma, unspecified, intra-abdominal lymph nodes** HCC Rx ESR COM

**C85.94** **Non-Hodgkin lymphoma, unspecified, lymph nodes of axilla and upper limb** HCC Rx ESR COM

**C85.95** **Non-Hodgkin lymphoma, unspecified, lymph nodes of inguinal region and lower limb** HCC Rx ESR COM

**C85.96** **Non-Hodgkin lymphoma, unspecified, intrapelvic lymph nodes** HCC Rx ESR COM

**C85.97** **Non-Hodgkin lymphoma, unspecified, spleen** HCC Rx ESR COM

**C85.98** **Non-Hodgkin lymphoma, unspecified, lymph nodes of multiple sites** HCC Rx ESR COM

**C85.99** **Non-Hodgkin lymphoma, unspecified, extranodal and solid organ sites** HCC Rx ESR COM

**C85.9A** **Non-Hodgkin lymphoma, unspecified, in remission** HCC Rx ESR COM

**C86 Other specified types of T/NK-cell lymphoma**

EXCLUDES 1 *anaplastic large cell lymphoma, ALK negative (C84.7-)*
*anaplastic large cell lymphoma, ALK positive (C84.6-)*
*mature T/NK-cell lymphomas (C84.-)*
*other specified types of non-Hodgkin lymphoma (C85.8-)*

**C86.0 Extranodal NK/T-cell lymphoma, nasal type**

**C86.00** **Extranodal NK/T-cell lymphoma, nasal type not having achieved remission** HCC Rx ESR COM

Extranodal NK/T-cell lymphoma, nasal type NOS
Extranodal NK/T-cell lymphoma, nasal type with failed remission

**C86.01** **Extranodal NK/T-cell lymphoma, nasal type, in remission** HCC Rx ESR COM

**C86.1 Hepatosplenic T-cell lymphoma**

Alpha-beta and gamma delta types

**C86.10** **Hepatosplenic T-cell lymphoma not having achieved remission** HCC Rx ESR COM

Hepatosplenic T-cell lymphoma NOS
Hepatosplenic T-cell lymphoma with failed remission

**C86.11** **Hepatosplenic T-cell lymphoma, in remission** HCC Rx ESR COM

**C86.2 Enteropathy-type (intestinal) T-cell lymphoma**

Enteropathy associated T-cell lymphoma

**C86.20** **Enteropathy-type (intestinal) T-cell lymphoma not having achieved remission** HCC Rx ESR COM

Enteropathy associated T-cell lymphoma NOS
Enteropathy associated T-cell lymphoma not having achieved remission
Enteropathy associated T-cell lymphoma with failed remission
Enteropathy-type (intestinal) T-cell lymphoma NOS
Enteropathy-type (intestinal) T-cell lymphoma with failed remission

**C86.21** **Enteropathy-type (intestinal) T-cell lymphoma, in remission** HCC Rx ESR COM

Enteropathy associated T-cell lymphoma, in remission

**C86.3 Subcutaneous panniculitis-like T-cell lymphoma**

**C86.30** **Subcutaneous panniculitis-like T-cell lymphoma not having achieved remission** HCC Rx ESR COM

Subcutaneous panniculitis-like T-cell lymphoma NOS
Subcutaneous panniculitis-like T-cell lymphoma with failed remission

**C86.31** **Subcutaneous panniculitis-like T-cell lymphoma, in remission** HCC Rx ESR COM

✓5th **C86.4 Blastic NK-cell lymphoma**
Blastic plasmacytoid dendritic cell neoplasm (BPDCN)

**C86.40 Blastic NK-cell lymphoma not having achieved remission** HCC Rx ESR COM
Blastic NK-cell lymphoma NOS
Blastic NK-cell lymphoma with failed remission
Blastic plasmacytoid dendritic cell neoplasm (BPDCN) NOS
Blastic plasmacytoid dendritic cell neoplasm (BPDCN) not having achieved remission
Blastic plasmacytoid dendritic cell neoplasm (BPDCN) with failed remission

**C86.41 Blastic NK-cell lymphoma, in remission** HCC Rx ESR COM
Blastic plasmacytoid dendritic cell neoplasm (BPDCN), in remission

✓5th **C86.5 Angioimmunoblastic T-cell lymphoma**
Angioimmunoblastic lymphadenopathy with dysproteinemia (AILD)

**C86.50 Angioimmunoblastic T-cell lymphoma not having achieved remission** HCC Rx ESR COM
Angioimmunoblastic lymphadenopathy with dysproteinemia (AILD) NOS
Angioimmunoblastic lymphadenopathy with dysproteinemia (AILD) not having achieved remission
Angioimmunoblastic lymphadenopathy with dysproteinemia (AILD) with failed remission
Angioimmunoblastic T-cell lymphoma NOS
Angioimmunoblastic T-cell lymphoma with failed remission

**C86.51 Angioimmunoblastic T-cell lymphoma, in remission** HCC Rx ESR COM
Angioimmunoblastic lymphadenopathy with dysproteinemia (AILD), in remission

✓5th **C86.6 Primary cutaneous CD30-positive T-cell proliferations**
Lymphomatoid papulosis
Primary cutaneous anaplastic large cell lymphoma
Primary cutaneous CD30-positive large T-cell lymphoma

**C86.60 Primary cutaneous CD30-positive T-cell proliferations not having achieved remission** HCC Rx ESR COM
Lymphomatoid papulosis NOS
Lymphomatoid papulosis not having achieved remission
Lymphomatoid papulosis with failed remission
Primary cutaneous anaplastic large cell lymphoma NOS
Primary cutaneous anaplastic large cell lymphoma not having achieved remission
Primary cutaneous anaplastic large cell lymphoma with failed remission
Primary cutaneous CD30-positive large T-cell lymphoma NOS
Primary cutaneous CD30-positive large T-cell lymphoma not having achieved remission
Primary cutaneous CD30-positive large T-cell lymphoma with failed remission
Primary cutaneous CD30-positive T-cell proliferations NOS
Primary cutaneous CD30-positive T-cell proliferations with failed remission

**C86.61 Primary cutaneous CD30-positive T-cell proliferations, in remission** HCC Rx ESR COM

✓4th **C88 Malignant immunoproliferative diseases and certain other B-cell lymphomas**
EXCLUDES 1 *B-cell lymphoma, unspecified (C85.1-)*
*personal history of other malignant neoplasms of lymphoid, hematopoietic and related tissues (Z85.79)*

✓5th **C88.0 Waldenstrom macroglobulinemia**
Lymphoplasmacytic lymphoma with IgM-production
Macroglobulinemia (idiopathic) (primary)
EXCLUDES 1 *small cell B-cell lymphoma (C83.0)*

**C88.00 Waldenstrom macroglobulinemia not having achieved remission** HCC Rx ESR COM
Lymphoplasmacytic lymphoma with IgM-production not having achieved remission
Lymphoplasmacytic lymphoma with IgM-production with failed remission
Lymphoplasmacytic lymphoma with IgM-production, NOS
Macroglobulinemia (idiopathic) (primary) NOS
Macroglobulinemia (idiopathic) (primary) not having achieved remission
Macroglobulinemia (idiopathic) (primary) with failed remission
Waldenstrom macroglobulinemia NOS
Waldenstrom macroglobulinemia with failed remission

**C88.01 Waldenstrom macroglobulinemia, in remission** HCC Rx ESR COM

✓5th **C88.2 Heavy chain disease**
Franklin disease
Gamma heavy chain disease
Mu heavy chain disease

**C88.20 Heavy chain disease not having achieved remission** HCC Rx ESR COM
Franklin disease NOS
Franklin disease not having achieved remission
Franklin disease with failed remission
Gamma heavy chain disease NOS
Gamma heavy chain disease not having achieved remission
Gamma heavy chain disease with failed remission
Heavy chain disease NOS
Heavy chain disease with failed remission
Mu heavy chain disease NOS
Mu heavy chain disease not having achieved remission
Mu heavy chain disease with failed remission

**C88.21 Heavy chain disease, in remission** HCC Rx ESR COM

✓5th **C88.3 Immunoproliferative small intestinal disease**
Alpha heavy chain disease
Mediterranean lymphoma

**C88.30 Immunoproliferative small intestinal disease not having achieved remission** HCC Rx ESR COM
Alpha heavy chain disease NOS
Alpha heavy chain disease not having achieved remission
Alpha heavy chain disease with failed remission
Immunoproliferative small intestinal disease NOS
Immunoproliferative small intestinal disease with failed remission
Mediterranean lymphoma NOS
Mediterranean lymphoma not having achieved remission
Mediterranean lymphoma with failed remission

**C88.31 Immunoproliferative small intestinal disease, in remission** HCC Rx ESR COM

✓5th **C88.4 Extranodal marginal zone B-cell lymphoma of mucosa-associated lymphoid tissue [MALT-lymphoma]**
Lymphoma of bronchial-associated lymphoid tissue [BALT-lymphoma]
Lymphoma of skin-associated lymphoid tissue [SALT-lymphoma]
EXCLUDES 1 *high malignant (diffuse large B-cell) lymphoma (C83.3-)*

**C88.40 Extranodal marginal zone B-cell lymphoma of mucosa-associated lymphoid tissue [MALT-lymphoma] not having achieved remission** HCC Rx ESR COM
Extranodal marginal zone B-cell lymphoma of mucosa-associated lymphoid tissue [MALT-lymphoma] NOS
Extranodal marginal zone B-cell lymphoma of mucosa-associated lymphoid tissue [MALT-lymphoma] with failed remission
Lymphoma of bronchial-associated lymphoid tissue [BALT-lymphoma] NOS
Lymphoma of bronchial-associated lymphoid tissue [BALT-lymphoma] not having achieved remission
Lymphoma of bronchial-associated lymphoid tissue [BALT-lymphoma] with failed remission
Lymphoma of skin-associated lymphoid tissue [SALT-lymphoma] NOS
Lymphoma of skin-associated lymphoid tissue [SALT-lymphoma] not having achieved remission
Lymphoma of skin-associated lymphoid tissue [SALT-lymphoma] with failed remission

**C88.41 Extranodal marginal zone B-cell lymphoma of mucosa-associated lymphoid tissue [MALT-lymphoma], in remission** HCC Rx ESR COM

✓5th **C88.8 Other malignant immunoproliferative diseases**

**C88.80 Other malignant immunoproliferative diseases not having achieved remission** HCC Rx ESR COM
Other malignant immunoproliferative diseases NOS
Other malignant immunoproliferative diseases with failed remission

**C88.81 Other malignant immunoproliferative diseases, in remission** HCC Rx ESR COM

✓5th **C88.9 Malignant immunoproliferative disease, unspecified**
Immunoproliferative disease NOS

**C88.90 Malignant immunoproliferative disease, unspecified not having achieved remission** HCC Rx ESR COM
Immunoproliferative disease NOS
Immunoproliferative disease NOS not having achieved remission
Immunoproliferative disease NOS with failed remission
Malignant immunoproliferative disease, unspecified NOS
Malignant immunoproliferative disease, unspecified with failed remission

**C88.91 Malignant immunoproliferative disease, unspecified, in remission** HCC Rx ESR COM

✓4th **C90 Multiple myeloma and malignant plasma cell neoplasms**
EXCLUDES 1 *personal history of other malignant neoplasms of lymphoid, hematopoietic and related tissues (Z85.79)*
**AHA:** 2019,2Q,30

✓5th **C90.0 Multiple myeloma**
Kahler's disease
Medullary plasmacytoma
Myelomatosis
Plasma cell myeloma
EXCLUDES 1 *solitary myeloma (C90.3-)*
*solitary plasmactyoma (C90.3-)*
**AHA:** 2021,3Q,5
**TIP:** Do not assign an additional code for bone metastasis (C79.51) when multiple myeloma is described as metastatic to the bone; bone involvement is integral to this disease process.
**TIP:** Smoldering multiple myeloma (SMM) is a plasma cell disorder that has not yet progressed to active multiple myeloma. Code D47.2 should be used when only SMM is documented.

**C90.00 Multiple myeloma not having achieved remission** HCC Rx ESR COM
Multiple myeloma NOS
Multiple myeloma with failed remission

**C90.01 Multiple myeloma in remission** HCC Rx ESR COM

**C90.02 Multiple myeloma in relapse** HCC Rx ESR COM

✓5th **C90.1 Plasma cell leukemia**
Plasmacytic leukemia
**AHA:** 2019,2Q,30

**C90.10 Plasma cell leukemia not having achieved remission** HCC Rx ESR COM
Plasma cell leukemia NOS
Plasma cell leukemia with failed remission

**C90.11 Plasma cell leukemia in remission** HCC Rx ESR COM

**C90.12 Plasma cell leukemia in relapse** HCC Rx ESR COM

✓5th **C90.2 Extramedullary plasmacytoma**

**C90.20 Extramedullary plasmacytoma not having achieved remission** HCC Rx ESR COM
Extramedullary plasmacytoma NOS
Extramedullary plasmacytoma with failed remission

**C90.21 Extramedullary plasmacytoma in remission** HCC Rx ESR COM

**C90.22 Extramedullary plasmacytoma in relapse** HCC Rx ESR COM

✓5th **C90.3 Solitary plasmacytoma**
Localized malignant plasma cell tumor NOS
Plasmacytoma NOS
Solitary myeloma

**C90.30 Solitary plasmacytoma not having achieved remission** HCC Rx ESR COM
Solitary plasmacytoma NOS
Solitary plasmacytoma with failed remission

**C90.31 Solitary plasmacytoma in remission** HCC Rx ESR COM

**C90.32 Solitary plasmacytoma in relapse** HCC Rx ESR COM

✓4th **C91 Lymphoid leukemia**
EXCLUDES 1 *personal history of leukemia (Z85.6)*
**AHA:** 2020,1Q,13
**DEF:** Malignant proliferation of immature lymphocytes (white blood cells that make up lymphoid tissue), called lymphoblasts, that originate in the bone marrow. Can be acute (ALL) or chronic (CLL).

✓5th **C91.0 Acute lymphoblastic leukemia [ALL]**
NOTE Codes in subcategory C91.0- should only be used for T-cell and B-cell precursor leukemia

**C91.00 Acute lymphoblastic leukemia not having achieved remission** HCC Rx ESR COM
Acute lymphoblastic leukemia NOS
Acute lymphoblastic leukemia with failed remission

**C91.01 Acute lymphoblastic leukemia, in remission** HCC Rx ESR COM

**C91.02 Acute lymphoblastic leukemia, in relapse** HCC Rx ESR COM

✓5th **C91.1 Chronic lymphocytic leukemia of B-cell type**
Lymphoplasmacytic leukemia
Richter syndrome
EXCLUDES 1 *lymphoplasmacytic lymphoma (C83.0-)*
**AHA:** 2023,1Q,18

**C91.10 Chronic lymphocytic leukemia of B-cell type not having achieved remission** HCC Rx ESR COM
Chronic lymphocytic leukemia of B-cell type NOS
Chronic lymphocytic leukemia of B-cell type with failed remission

**C91.11 Chronic lymphocytic leukemia of B-cell type in remission** HCC Rx ESR COM

**C91.12 Chronic lymphocytic leukemia of B-cell type in relapse** HCC Rx ESR COM

✓5th **C91.3 Prolymphocytic leukemia of B-cell type**

**C91.30 Prolymphocytic leukemia of B-cell type not having achieved remission** HCC Rx ESR COM
Prolymphocytic leukemia of B-cell type NOS
Prolymphocytic leukemia of B-cell type with failed remission

**C91.31 Prolymphocytic leukemia of B-cell type, in remission** HCC Rx ESR COM

**C91.32 Prolymphocytic leukemia of B-cell type, in relapse** HCC Rx ESR COM

✓5th **C91.4 Hairy cell leukemia**
Leukemic reticuloendotheliosis
**DEF:** Rare type of leukemia that is slow growing and often also considered a type of lymphoma. The small B-cell lymphocytes appear with "hairy" projections under a microscope and are found mostly in the bone marrow, spleen, and blood.

**C91.40 Hairy cell leukemia not having achieved remission** HCC Rx ESR COM
Hairy cell leukemia NOS
Hairy cell leukemia with failed remission

**C91.41 Hairy cell leukemia, in remission** HCC Rx ESR COM

**C91.42 Hairy cell leukemia, in relapse** HCC Rx ESR COM

✓5th **C91.5 Adult T-cell lymphoma/leukemia (HTLV-1-associated)**
Acute variant of adult T-cell lymphoma/leukemia (HTLV-1-associated)
Chronic variant of adult T-cell lymphoma/leukemia (HTLV-1-associated)
Lymphomatoid variant of adult T-cell lymphoma/leukemia (HTLV-1-associated)
Smouldering variant of adult T-cell lymphoma/leukemia (HTLV-1-associated)

**C91.50 Adult T-cell lymphoma/leukemia (HTLV-1-associated) not having achieved remission** HCC Rx ESR COM A
Adult T-cell lymphoma/leukemia (HTLV-1-associated) NOS
Adult T-cell lymphoma/leukemia (HTLV-1-associated) with failed remission

**C91.51 Adult T-cell lymphoma/leukemia (HTLV-1-associated), in remission** HCC Rx ESR COM A

**C91.52 Adult T-cell lymphoma/leukemia (HTLV-1-associated), in relapse** HCC Rx ESR COM A

✓5th **C91.6 Prolymphocytic leukemia of T-cell type**

**C91.60 Prolymphocytic leukemia of T-cell type not having achieved remission** HCC Rx ESR COM
Prolymphocytic leukemia of T-cell type NOS
Prolymphocytic leukemia of T-cell type with failed remission

**C91.61 Prolymphocytic leukemia of T-cell type, in remission** HCC Rx ESR COM

**C91.62 Prolymphocytic leukemia of T-cell type, in relapse** HCC Rx ESR COM

✓5th **C91.A Mature B-cell leukemia Burkitt-type**
EXCLUDES 1 *Burkitt lymphoma (C83.7-)*

**C91.A0 Mature B-cell leukemia Burkitt-type not having achieved remission** HCC Rx ESR COM
Mature B-cell leukemia Burkitt-type NOS
Mature B-cell leukemia Burkitt-type with failed remission

**C91.A1 Mature B-cell leukemia Burkitt-type, in remission** HCC Rx ESR COM

**C91.A2 Mature B-cell leukemia Burkitt-type, in relapse** HCC Rx ESR COM

✓5th **C91.Z Other lymphoid leukemia**
T-cell large granular lymphocytic leukemia (associated with rheumatoid arthritis)

**C91.Z0 Other lymphoid leukemia not having achieved remission** HCC Rx ESR COM
Other lymphoid leukemia NOS
Other lymphoid leukemia with failed remission

**C91.Z1 Other lymphoid leukemia, in remission** HCC Rx ESR COM

**C91.Z2 Other lymphoid leukemia, in relapse** HCC Rx ESR COM

✓5th **C91.9 Lymphoid leukemia, unspecified**

**C91.90 Lymphoid leukemia, unspecified not having achieved remission** HCC Rx ESR COM
Lymphoid leukemia NOS
Lymphoid leukemia with failed remission

**C91.91 Lymphoid leukemia, unspecified, in remission** HCC Rx ESR COM

**C91.92 Lymphoid leukemia, unspecified, in relapse** HCC Rx ESR COM

✓4th **C92 Myeloid leukemia**
INCLUDES granulocytic leukemia
myelogenous leukemia
Code also, if applicable, pancytopenia (acquired) (D61.818)
EXCLUDES 1 *personal history of leukemia (Z85.6)*
**AHA:** 2020,1Q,13; 2019,1Q,16
**DEF:** Cancer that develops in immature myelocytes called myeloblasts. These are the cells that become white blood cells (except lymphocytes), red blood cells, or platelet-making cells. Can be acute (AML) or chronic (CML).
**TIP:** Pancytopenia, although common in some types of myeloid leukemias, is not always inherent. When it is documented, code D61.818 can be assigned in addition to a code from this category.

✓5th **C92.0 Acute myeloblastic leukemia**
Acute myeloblastic leukemia (with maturation)
Acute myeloblastic leukemia (without a FAB classification) NOS
Acute myeloblastic leukemia 1/ETO
Acute myeloblastic leukemia M0
Acute myeloblastic leukemia M1
Acute myeloblastic leukemia M2
Acute myeloblastic leukemia with t(8;21)
Acute myeloblastic leukemia, minimal differentiation
Refractory anemia with excess blasts in transformation [RAEBT]
EXCLUDES 1 *acute exacerbation of chronic myeloid leukemia (C92.10)*
*refractory anemia with excess of blasts not in transformation (D46.2-)*
**AHA:** 2018,4Q,87

**C92.00 Acute myeloblastic leukemia, not having achieved remission** HCC Rx ESR COM
Acute myeloblastic leukemia NOS
Acute myeloblastic leukemia with failed remission

**C92.01 Acute myeloblastic leukemia, in remission** HCC Rx ESR COM
**AHA:** 2021,3Q,4

**C92.02 Acute myeloblastic leukemia, in relapse** HCC Rx ESR COM
**AHA:** 2023,1Q,23

✓5th **C92.1 Chronic myeloid leukemia, BCR/ABL-positive**
Chronic myelogenous leukemia with crisis of blast cells
Chronic myelogenous leukemia, Philadelphia chromosome (Ph1) positive
Chronic myelogenous leukemia, t(9;22) (q34;q11)
EXCLUDES 1 *atypical chronic myeloid leukemia BCR/ABL-negative (C92.2-)*
*chronic myelomonocytic leukemia (C93.1-)*
*chronic myeloproliferative disease (D47.1)*

**C92.10 Chronic myeloid leukemia, BCR/ABL-positive, not having achieved remission** HCC Rx ESR COM
Chronic myeloid leukemia, BCR/ABL-positive NOS
Chronic myeloid leukemia, BCR/ABL-positive with failed remission

**C92.11 Chronic myeloid leukemia, BCR/ABL-positive, in remission** HCC Rx ESR COM

**C92.12 Chronic myeloid leukemia, BCR/ABL-positive, in relapse** HCC Rx ESR COM

✓5th **C92.2 Atypical chronic myeloid leukemia, BCR/ABL-negative**

**C92.20 Atypical chronic myeloid leukemia, BCR/ABL-negative, not having achieved remission** HCC Rx ESR COM
Atypical chronic myeloid leukemia, BCR/ABL-negative NOS
Atypical chronic myeloid leukemia, BCR/ABL-negative with failed remission

**C92.21 Atypical chronic myeloid leukemia, BCR/ABL-negative, in remission** HCC Rx ESR COM

**C92.22 Atypical chronic myeloid leukemia, BCR/ABL-negative, in relapse** HCC Rx ESR COM

✓5th **C92.3 Myeloid sarcoma**
A malignant tumor of immature myeloid cells
Chloroma
Granulocytic sarcoma

**C92.30 Myeloid sarcoma, not having achieved remission** HCC Rx ESR COM
Myeloid sarcoma NOS
Myeloid sarcoma with failed remission

**C92.31 Myeloid sarcoma, in remission** HCC Rx ESR COM

**C92.32 Myeloid sarcoma, in relapse** HCC Rx ESR COM

✓5th **C92.4 Acute promyelocytic leukemia**
AML M3
AML Me with t(15;17) and variants

**C92.4Ø Acute promyelocytic leukemia, not having achieved remission** HCC Rx ESR COM
Acute promyelocytic leukemia NOS
Acute promyelocytic leukemia with failed remission

**C92.41 Acute promyelocytic leukemia, in remission** HCC Rx ESR COM

**C92.42 Acute promyelocytic leukemia, in relapse** HCC Rx ESR COM

✓5th **C92.5 Acute myelomonocytic leukemia**
AML M4
AML M4 Eo with inv(16) or t(16;16)

**C92.5Ø Acute myelomonocytic leukemia, not having achieved remission** HCC Rx ESR COM
Acute myelomonocytic leukemia NOS
Acute myelomonocytic leukemia with failed remission

**C92.51 Acute myelomonocytic leukemia, in remission** HCC Rx ESR COM

**C92.52 Acute myelomonocytic leukemia, in relapse** HCC Rx ESR COM

✓5th **C92.6 Acute myeloid leukemia with 11q23-abnormality**
Acute myeloid leukemia with variation of MLL-gene

**C92.6Ø Acute myeloid leukemia with 11q23-abnormality not having achieved remission** HCC Rx ESR COM
Acute myeloid leukemia with 11q23-abnormality NOS
Acute myeloid leukemia with 11q23-abnormality with failed remission

**C92.61 Acute myeloid leukemia with 11q23-abnormality in remission** HCC Rx ESR COM

**C92.62 Acute myeloid leukemia with 11q23-abnormality in relapse** HCC Rx ESR COM

✓5th **C92.A Acute myeloid leukemia with multilineage dysplasia**
Acute myeloid leukemia with dysplasia of remaining hematopoesis and/or myelodysplastic disease in its history

**C92.AØ Acute myeloid leukemia with multilineage dysplasia, not having achieved remission** HCC Rx ESR COM
Acute myeloid leukemia with multilineage dysplasia NOS
Acute myeloid leukemia with multilineage dysplasia with failed remission

**C92.A1 Acute myeloid leukemia with multilineage dysplasia, in remission** HCC Rx ESR COM

**C92.A2 Acute myeloid leukemia with multilineage dysplasia, in relapse** HCC Rx ESR COM

✓5th **C92.Z Other myeloid leukemia**

**C92.ZØ Other myeloid leukemia not having achieved remission** HCC Rx ESR COM
Myeloid leukemia NEC
Myeloid leukemia NEC with failed remission

**C92.Z1 Other myeloid leukemia, in remission** HCC Rx ESR COM

**C92.Z2 Other myeloid leukemia, in relapse** HCC Rx ESR COM

✓5th **C92.9 Myeloid leukemia, unspecified**

**C92.9Ø Myeloid leukemia, unspecified, not having achieved remission** HCC Rx ESR COM
Myeloid leukemia, unspecified NOS
Myeloid leukemia, unspecified with failed remission

**C92.91 Myeloid leukemia, unspecified in remission** HCC Rx ESR COM

**C92.92 Myeloid leukemia, unspecified in relapse** HCC Rx ESR COM

✓4th **C93 Monocytic leukemia**
INCLUDES monocytoid leukemia
EXCLUDES 1 *personal history of leukemia (Z85.6)*
**AHA:** 2020,1Q,13

✓5th **C93.Ø Acute monoblastic/monocytic leukemia**
AML M5
AML M5a
AML M5b

**C93.ØØ Acute monoblastic/monocytic leukemia, not having achieved remission** HCC Rx ESR COM
Acute monoblastic/monocytic leukemia NOS
Acute monoblastic/monocytic leukemia with failed remission

**C93.Ø1 Acute monoblastic/monocytic leukemia, in remission** HCC Rx ESR COM

**C93.Ø2 Acute monoblastic/monocytic leukemia, in relapse** HCC Rx ESR COM

✓5th **C93.1 Chronic myelomonocytic leukemia**
Chronic monocytic leukemia
CMML with eosinophilia
CMML-1
CMML-2
Code also, if applicable, eosinophilia (D72.18)

**C93.1Ø Chronic myelomonocytic leukemia not having achieved remission** HCC Rx ESR COM
Chronic myelomonocytic leukemia NOS
Chronic myelomonocytic leukemia with failed remission

**C93.11 Chronic myelomonocytic leukemia, in remission** HCC Rx ESR COM

**C93.12 Chronic myelomonocytic leukemia, in relapse** HCC Rx ESR COM

✓5th **C93.3 Juvenile myelomonocytic leukemia**

**C93.3Ø Juvenile myelomonocytic leukemia, not having achieved remission** HCC Rx ESR COM P
Juvenile myelomonocytic leukemia NOS
Juvenile myelomonocytic leukemia with failed remission

**C93.31 Juvenile myelomonocytic leukemia, in remission** HCC Rx ESR COM P

**C93.32 Juvenile myelomonocytic leukemia, in relapse** HCC Rx ESR COM P

✓5th **C93.Z Other monocytic leukemia**

**C93.ZØ Other monocytic leukemia, not having achieved remission** HCC Rx ESR COM
Other monocytic leukemia NOS

**C93.Z1 Other monocytic leukemia, in remission** HCC Rx ESR COM

**C93.Z2 Other monocytic leukemia, in relapse** HCC Rx ESR COM

✓5th **C93.9 Monocytic leukemia, unspecified**

**C93.9Ø Monocytic leukemia, unspecified, not having achieved remission** HCC Rx ESR COM
Monocytic leukemia, unspecified NOS
Monocytic leukemia, unspecified with failed remission

**C93.91 Monocytic leukemia, unspecified in remission** HCC Rx ESR COM

**C93.92 Monocytic leukemia, unspecified in relapse** HCC Rx ESR COM

✓4th **C94 Other leukemias of specified cell type**
EXCLUDES 1 *leukemic reticuloendotheliosis (C91.4-)*
*myelodysplastic syndromes (D46.-)*
*personal history of leukemia (Z85.6)*
*plasma cell leukemia (C9Ø.1-)*
**AHA:** 2020,1Q,13

✓5th **C94.Ø Acute erythroid leukemia**
Acute myeloid leukemia M6(a)(b)
Erythroleukemia
**DEF:** Erythroleukemia: Malignant blood dyscrasia (a myeloproliferative disorder).

**C94.ØØ Acute erythroid leukemia, not having achieved remission** HCC Rx ESR COM
Acute erythroid leukemia NOS
Acute erythroid leukemia with failed remission

**C94.Ø1 Acute erythroid leukemia, in remission** HCC Rx ESR COM

**C94.Ø2 Acute erythroid leukemia, in relapse** HCC Rx ESR COM

✓5th **C94.2 Acute megakaryoblastic leukemia**
Acute megakaryocytic leukemia
Acute myeloid leukemia M7

**C94.2Ø Acute megakaryoblastic leukemia not having achieved remission** HCC Rx ESR COM
Acute megakaryoblastic leukemia NOS
Acute megakaryoblastic leukemia with failed remission

**C94.21 Acute megakaryoblastic leukemia, in remission** HCC Rx ESR COM

**C94.22 Acute megakaryoblastic leukemia, in relapse** HCC Rx ESR COM

✓5th **C94.3 Mast cell leukemia**
AHA: 2017,4Q,5

**C94.30 Mast cell leukemia not having achieved remission** HCC Rx ESR COM
Mast cell leukemia NOS
Mast cell leukemia with failed remission

**C94.31 Mast cell leukemia, in remission** HCC Rx ESR COM

**C94.32 Mast cell leukemia, in relapse** HCC Rx ESR COM

✓5th **C94.4 Acute panmyelosis with myelofibrosis**
Acute myelofibrosis
EXCLUDES 1 *myelofibrosis NOS (D75.81)*
*secondary myelofibrosis NOS (D75.81)*

**C94.40 Acute panmyelosis with myelofibrosis not having achieved remission** HCC Rx ESR COM
Acute myelofibrosis NOS
Acute panmyelosis NOS
Acute panmyelosis with myelofibrosis with failed remission

**C94.41 Acute panmyelosis with myelofibrosis, in remission** HCC Rx ESR COM

**C94.42 Acute panmyelosis with myelofibrosis, in relapse** HCC Rx ESR COM

**C94.6 Myelodysplastic disease, not elsewhere classified** HCC Rx ESR COM
Myelodysplastic/myeloproliferative neoplasm, unclassifiable
Myeloproliferative disease, not elsewhere classified

✓5th **C94.8 Other specified leukemias**
Acute basophilic leukemia
Aggressive NK-cell leukemia
Code also, if applicable, eosinophilia (D72.18)

**C94.80 Other specified leukemias not having achieved remission** HCC Rx ESR COM
Other specified leukemia with failed remission
Other specified leukemias NOS

**C94.81 Other specified leukemias, in remission** HCC Rx ESR COM

**C94.82 Other specified leukemias, in relapse** HCC Rx ESR COM

✓4th **C95 Leukemia of unspecified cell type**
EXCLUDES 1 *personal history of leukemia (Z85.6)*
AHA: 2020,1Q,13

✓5th **C95.0 Acute leukemia of unspecified cell type**
Acute bilineal leukemia
Acute mixed lineage leukemia
Biphenotypic acute leukemia
Stem cell leukemia of unclear lineage
EXCLUDES 1 *acute exacerbation of unspecified chronic leukemia (C95.10)*

**C95.00 Acute leukemia of unspecified cell type not having achieved remission** HCC Rx ESR COM
Acute leukemia NOS
Acute leukemia of unspecified cell type with failed remission

**C95.01 Acute leukemia of unspecified cell type, in remission** HCC Rx ESR COM

**C95.02 Acute leukemia of unspecified cell type, in relapse** HCC Rx ESR COM

✓5th **C95.1 Chronic leukemia of unspecified cell type**

**C95.10 Chronic leukemia of unspecified cell type not having achieved remission** HCC Rx ESR COM
Chronic leukemia NOS
Chronic leukemia of unspecified cell type with failed remission

**C95.11 Chronic leukemia of unspecified cell type, in remission** HCC Rx ESR COM

**C95.12 Chronic leukemia of unspecified cell type, in relapse** HCC Rx ESR COM

✓5th **C95.9 Leukemia, unspecified**

**C95.90 Leukemia, unspecified not having achieved remission** HCC Rx ESR COM
Leukemia NOS
Leukemia, unspecified with failed remission

**C95.91 Leukemia, unspecified, in remission** HCC Rx ESR COM

**C95.92 Leukemia, unspecified, in relapse** HCC Rx ESR COM

✓4th **C96 Other and unspecified malignant neoplasms of lymphoid, hematopoietic and related tissue**
EXCLUDES 1 *personal history of other malignant neoplasms of lymphoid, hematopoietic and related tissues (Z85.79)*

**C96.0 Multifocal and multisystemic (disseminated) Langerhans-cell histiocytosis** HCC Rx ESR COM
Histiocytosis X, multisystemic
Letterer-Siwe disease
EXCLUDES 1 *adult pulmonary Langerhans cell histiocytosis (J84.82)*
*multifocal and unisystemic Langerhans-cell histiocytosis (C96.5)*
*unifocal Langerhans-cell histiocytosis (C96.6)*

✓5th **C96.2 Malignant mast cell neoplasm**
EXCLUDES 1 *indolent mastocytosis (D47.02)*
*mast cell leukemia (C94.30)*
*mastocytosis (congenital) (cutaneous) (Q82.2)*
AHA: 2017,4Q,5
DEF: Mast cell: Type of white blood cell found in the loose connective tissue of blood vessels and bronchioles responsible for acute hypersensitivity reactions, including anaphylactic shock. The IgE receptors on these cells bind with allergens causing cell degranulation and diffuse, widespread histamine release that results in airway constriction and vasodilation with decreased systemic blood pressure.

**C96.20 Malignant mast cell neoplasm, unspecified** HCC Rx ESR COM

**C96.21 Aggressive systemic mastocytosis** HCC Rx ESR COM

**C96.22 Mast cell sarcoma** HCC Rx ESR COM

**C96.29 Other malignant mast cell neoplasm** HCC Rx ESR COM

**C96.4 Sarcoma of dendritic cells (accessory cells)** HCC Rx ESR COM
Follicular dendritic cell sarcoma
Interdigitating dendritic cell sarcoma
Langerhans cell sarcoma

**C96.5 Multifocal and unisystemic Langerhans-cell histiocytosis** HCC Rx ESR COM
Hand-Schuller-Christian disease
Histiocytosis X, multifocal
EXCLUDES 1 *multifocal and multisystemic (disseminated) Langerhans-cell histiocytosis (C96.0)*
*unifocal Langerhans-cell histiocytosis (C96.6)*

**C96.6 Unifocal Langerhans-cell histiocytosis** HCC Rx ESR COM
Eosinophilic granuloma
Histiocytosis X NOS
Histiocytosis X, unifocal
Langerhans-cell histiocytosis NOS
EXCLUDES 1 *multifocal and multisysemic (disseminated) Langerhans-cell histiocytosis (C96.0)*
*multifocal and unisystemic Langerhans-cell histiocytosis (C96.5)*

**C96.A Histiocytic sarcoma** HCC Rx ESR COM
Malignant histiocytosis

**C96.Z Other specified malignant neoplasms of lymphoid, hematopoietic and related tissue** HCC Rx ESR COM

**C96.9 Malignant neoplasm of lymphoid, hematopoietic and related tissue, unspecified** HCC Rx ESR COM

## In situ neoplasms (D00-D09)

INCLUDES Bowen's disease
erythroplasia
grade III intraepithelial neoplasia
Queyrat's erythroplasia

AHA: 2023,3Q,15

✓4th **D00 Carcinoma in situ of oral cavity, esophagus and stomach**

EXCLUDES 1 *melanoma in situ (D03.-)*

✓5th **D00.0 Carcinoma in situ of lip, oral cavity and pharynx**

Use additional code to identify:
exposure to environmental tobacco smoke (Z77.22)
exposure to tobacco smoke in the perinatal period (P96.81)
history of tobacco dependence (Z87.891)
occupational exposure to environmental tobacco smoke (Z57.31)
tobacco dependence (F17.-)
tobacco use (Z72.0)

EXCLUDES 1 *carcinoma in situ of aryepiglottic fold or interarytenoid fold, laryngeal aspect (D02.0)*
*carcinoma in situ of epiglottis NOS (D02.0)*
*carcinoma in situ of epiglottis suprahyoid portion (D02.0)*
*carcinoma in situ of skin of lip (D03.0, D04.0)*

**D00.00 Carcinoma in situ of oral cavity, unspecified site**

**D00.01 Carcinoma in situ of labial mucosa and vermilion border**

**D00.02 Carcinoma in situ of buccal mucosa**

**D00.03 Carcinoma in situ of gingiva and edentulous alveolar ridge**

**D00.04 Carcinoma in situ of soft palate**

**D00.05 Carcinoma in situ of hard palate**

**D00.06 Carcinoma in situ of floor of mouth**

**D00.07 Carcinoma in situ of tongue**

**D00.08 Carcinoma in situ of pharynx**

Carcinoma in situ of aryepiglottic fold NOS
Carcinoma in situ of hypopharyngeal aspect of aryepiglottic fold
Carcinoma in situ of marginal zone of aryepiglottic fold

**D00.1 Carcinoma in situ of esophagus**

**D00.2 Carcinoma in situ of stomach**

✓4th **D01 Carcinoma in situ of other and unspecified digestive organs**

EXCLUDES 1 *melanoma in situ (D03.-)*

**D01.0 Carcinoma in situ of colon**

EXCLUDES 1 *carcinoma in situ of rectosigmoid junction (D01.1)*

**D01.1 Carcinoma in situ of rectosigmoid junction**

**D01.2 Carcinoma in situ of rectum**

**D01.3 Carcinoma in situ of anus and anal canal**

Anal intraepithelial neoplasia III [AIN III]
Severe dysplasia of anus

EXCLUDES 1 *anal intraepithelial neoplasia I and II [AIN I and AIN II] (K62.82)*
*carcinoma in situ of anal margin (D04.5)*
*carcinoma in situ of anal skin (D04.5)*
*carcinoma in situ of perianal skin (D04.5)*

✓5th **D01.4 Carcinoma in situ of other and unspecified parts of intestine**

EXCLUDES 1 *carcinoma in situ of ampulla of Vater (D01.5)*

**D01.40 Carcinoma in situ of unspecified part of intestine**

**D01.49 Carcinoma in situ of other parts of intestine**

**D01.5 Carcinoma in situ of liver, gallbladder and bile ducts**

Carcinoma in situ of ampulla of Vater

**D01.7 Carcinoma in situ of other specified digestive organs**

Carcinoma in situ of pancreas

**D01.9 Carcinoma in situ of digestive organ, unspecified**

✓4th **D02 Carcinoma in situ of middle ear and respiratory system**

Use additional code to identify:
exposure to environmental tobacco smoke (Z77.22)
exposure to tobacco smoke in the perinatal period (P96.81)
history of tobacco dependence (Z87.891)
occupational exposure to environmental tobacco smoke (Z57.31)
tobacco dependence (F17.-)
tobacco use (Z72.0)

EXCLUDES 1 *melanoma in situ (D03.-)*

**D02.0 Carcinoma in situ of larynx**

Carcinoma in situ of aryepiglottic fold or interarytenoid fold, laryngeal aspect
Carcinoma in situ of epiglottis (suprahyoid portion)

EXCLUDES 1 *carcinoma in situ of aryepiglottic fold or interarytenoid fold NOS (D00.08)*
*carcinoma in situ of hypopharyngeal aspect (D00.08)*
*carcinoma in situ of marginal zone (D00.08)*

**D02.1 Carcinoma in situ of trachea**

✓5th **D02.2 Carcinoma in situ of bronchus and lung**

**D02.20 Carcinoma in situ of unspecified bronchus and lung**

**D02.21 Carcinoma in situ of right bronchus and lung**

**D02.22 Carcinoma in situ of left bronchus and lung**

**D02.3 Carcinoma in situ of other parts of respiratory system**

Carcinoma in situ of accessory sinuses
Carcinoma in situ of middle ear
Carcinoma in situ of nasal cavities

EXCLUDES 1 *carcinoma in situ of ear (external) (skin) (D04.2-)*
*carcinoma in situ of nose NOS (D09.8)*
*carcinoma in situ of skin of nose (D04.3)*

**D02.4 Carcinoma in situ of respiratory system, unspecified**

✓4th **D03 Melanoma in situ**

**D03.0 Melanoma in situ of lip** HCC Rx ESR COM

✓5th **D03.1 Melanoma in situ of eyelid, including canthus**

AHA: 2018,4Q,4

**D03.10 Melanoma in situ of unspecified eyelid, including canthus** HCC Rx ESR COM

✓6th **D03.11 Melanoma in situ of right eyelid, including canthus**

**D03.111 Melanoma in situ of right upper eyelid, including canthus** HCC Rx ESR COM

**D03.112 Melanoma in situ of right lower eyelid, including canthus** HCC Rx ESR COM

✓6th **D03.12 Melanoma in situ of left eyelid, including canthus**

**D03.121 Melanoma in situ of left upper eyelid, including canthus** HCC Rx ESR COM

**D03.122 Melanoma in situ of left lower eyelid, including canthus** HCC Rx ESR COM

✓5th **D03.2 Melanoma in situ of ear and external auricular canal**

**D03.20 Melanoma in situ of unspecified ear and external auricular canal** HCC Rx ESR COM

**D03.21 Melanoma in situ of right ear and external auricular canal** HCC Rx ESR COM

**D03.22 Melanoma in situ of left ear and external auricular canal** HCC Rx ESR COM

✓5th **D03.3 Melanoma in situ of other and unspecified parts of face**

**D03.30 Melanoma in situ of unspecified part of face** HCC Rx ESR COM

**D03.39 Melanoma in situ of other parts of face** HCC Rx ESR COM

**D03.4 Melanoma in situ of scalp and neck** HCC Rx ESR COM

✓5th **D03.5 Melanoma in situ of trunk**

**D03.51 Melanoma in situ of anal skin** HCC Rx ESR COM

Melanoma in situ of anal margin
Melanoma in situ of perianal skin

**D03.52 Melanoma in situ of breast (skin) (soft tissue)** HCC Rx ESR COM

**D03.59 Melanoma in situ of other part of trunk** HCC Rx ESR COM

✓5th **D03.6 Melanoma in situ of upper limb, including shoulder**

**D03.60 Melanoma in situ of unspecified upper limb, including shoulder** HCC Rx ESR COM

**D03.61 Melanoma in situ of right upper limb, including shoulder** HCC Rx ESR COM

**D03.62 Melanoma in situ of left upper limb, including shoulder** HCC Rx ESR COM

√5th **DØ3.7 Melanoma in situ of lower limb, including hip**
**DØ3.7Ø Melanoma in situ of unspecified lower limb, including hip** HCC Rx ESR COM
**DØ3.71 Melanoma in situ of right lower limb, including hip** HCC Rx ESR COM
**DØ3.72 Melanoma in situ of left lower limb, including hip** HCC Rx ESR COM
**DØ3.8 Melanoma in situ of other sites** HCC Rx ESR COM
Melanoma in situ of scrotum
EXCLUDES 1 *carcinoma in situ of scrotum (DØ7.61)*
**DØ3.9 Melanoma in situ, unspecified** HCC Rx ESR COM

√4th **DØ4 Carcinoma in situ of skin**
EXCLUDES 1 *erythroplasia of Queyrat (penis) NOS (DØ7.4)*
*melanoma in situ (DØ3.-)*
**DØ4.Ø Carcinoma in situ of skin of lip**
EXCLUDES 2 *carcinoma in situ of vermilion border of lip (DØØ.Ø1)*
√5th **DØ4.1 Carcinoma in situ of skin of eyelid, including canthus**
AHA: 2018,4Q,4
**DØ4.1Ø Carcinoma in situ of skin of unspecified eyelid, including canthus**
√6th **DØ4.11 Carcinoma in situ of skin of right eyelid, including canthus**
**DØ4.111 Carcinoma in situ of skin of right upper eyelid, including canthus**
**DØ4.112 Carcinoma in situ of skin of right lower eyelid, including canthus**
√6th **DØ4.12 Carcinoma in situ of skin of left eyelid, including canthus**
**DØ4.121 Carcinoma in situ of skin of left upper eyelid, including canthus**
**DØ4.122 Carcinoma in situ of skin of left lower eyelid, including canthus**
√5th **DØ4.2 Carcinoma in situ of skin of ear and external auricular canal**
**DØ4.2Ø Carcinoma in situ of skin of unspecified ear and external auricular canal**
**DØ4.21 Carcinoma in situ of skin of right ear and external auricular canal**
**DØ4.22 Carcinoma in situ of skin of left ear and external auricular canal**
√5th **DØ4.3 Carcinoma in situ of skin of other and unspecified parts of face**
**DØ4.3Ø Carcinoma in situ of skin of unspecified part of face**
**DØ4.39 Carcinoma in situ of skin of other parts of face**
**DØ4.4 Carcinoma in situ of skin of scalp and neck**
**DØ4.5 Carcinoma in situ of skin of trunk**
Carcinoma in situ of anal margin
Carcinoma in situ of anal skin
Carcinoma in situ of perianal skin
Carcinoma in situ of skin of breast
EXCLUDES 1 *carcinoma in situ of anus NOS (DØ1.3)*
*carcinoma in situ of scrotum (DØ7.61)*
*carcinoma in situ of skin of genital organs (DØ7.-)*
√5th **DØ4.6 Carcinoma in situ of skin of upper limb, including shoulder**
**DØ4.6Ø Carcinoma in situ of skin of unspecified upper limb, including shoulder**
**DØ4.61 Carcinoma in situ of skin of right upper limb, including shoulder**
**DØ4.62 Carcinoma in situ of skin of left upper limb, including shoulder**
√5th **DØ4.7 Carcinoma in situ of skin of lower limb, including hip**
**DØ4.7Ø Carcinoma in situ of skin of unspecified lower limb, including hip**
**DØ4.71 Carcinoma in situ of skin of right lower limb, including hip**
**DØ4.72 Carcinoma in situ of skin of left lower limb, including hip**
**DØ4.8 Carcinoma in situ of skin of other sites**
**DØ4.9 Carcinoma in situ of skin, unspecified**

√4th **DØ5 Carcinoma in situ of breast**
EXCLUDES 1 *carcinoma in situ of skin of breast (DØ4.5)*
▶*malignant neoplasm of breast (C5Ø.-)*◀
*melanoma in situ of breast (skin) (DØ3.5)*
*Paget's disease of breast or nipple (C5Ø.-)*
EXCLUDES 2 ~~*malignant neoplasm of breast (C5Ø.-)*~~
√5th **DØ5.Ø Lobular carcinoma in situ of breast**
**DØ5.ØØ Lobular carcinoma in situ of unspecified breast**
**DØ5.Ø1 Lobular carcinoma in situ of right breast**
**DØ5.Ø2 Lobular carcinoma in situ of left breast**
√5th **DØ5.1 Intraductal carcinoma in situ of breast**
**DØ5.1Ø Intraductal carcinoma in situ of unspecified breast**
**DØ5.11 Intraductal carcinoma in situ of right breast**
**DØ5.12 Intraductal carcinoma in situ of left breast**
√5th **DØ5.8 Other specified type of carcinoma in situ of breast**
**DØ5.8Ø Other specified type of carcinoma in situ of unspecified breast**
**DØ5.81 Other specified type of carcinoma in situ of right breast**
**DØ5.82 Other specified type of carcinoma in situ of left breast**
√5th **DØ5.9 Unspecified type of carcinoma in situ of breast**
**DØ5.9Ø Unspecified type of carcinoma in situ of unspecified breast**
**DØ5.91 Unspecified type of carcinoma in situ of right breast**
**DØ5.92 Unspecified type of carcinoma in situ of left breast**

√4th **DØ6 Carcinoma in situ of cervix uteri**
INCLUDES cervical adenocarcinoma in situ
cervical intraepithelial glandular neoplasia
cervical intraepithelial neoplasia III [CIN III]
severe dysplasia of cervix uteri
EXCLUDES 1 *cervical intraepithelial neoplasia II [CIN II] (N87.1)*
*cytologic evidence of malignancy of cervix without histologic confirmation (R87.614)*
*high grade squamous intraepithelial lesion (HGSIL) of cervix (R87.613)*
*melanoma in situ of cervix (DØ3.5)*
*moderate cervical dysplasia (N87.1)*
**DØ6.Ø Carcinoma in situ of endocervix**
**DØ6.1 Carcinoma in situ of exocervix**
**DØ6.7 Carcinoma in situ of other parts of cervix**
**DØ6.9 Carcinoma in situ of cervix, unspecified**

√4th **DØ7 Carcinoma in situ of other and unspecified genital organs**
EXCLUDES 1 *melanoma in situ of trunk (DØ3.5)*
**DØ7.Ø Carcinoma in situ of endometrium**
**DØ7.1 Carcinoma in situ of vulva**
Severe dysplasia of vulva
Vulvar intraepithelial neoplasia III [VIN III]
EXCLUDES 1 *moderate dysplasia of vulva (N9Ø.1)*
*vulvar intraepithelial neoplasia II [VIN II] (N9Ø.1)*
**DØ7.2 Carcinoma in situ of vagina**
Severe dysplasia of vagina
Vaginal intraepithelial neoplasia III [VAIN III]
EXCLUDES 1 *moderate dysplasia of vagina (N89.1)*
*vaginal intraepithelial neoplasia II [VIN II] (N89.1)*
√5th **DØ7.3 Carcinoma in situ of other and unspecified female genital organs**
**DØ7.3Ø Carcinoma in situ of unspecified female genital organs**
**DØ7.39 Carcinoma in situ of other female genital organs**
**DØ7.4 Carcinoma in situ of penis**
Erythroplasia of Queyrat NOS
**DØ7.5 Carcinoma in situ of prostate**
Prostatic intraepithelial neoplasia III (PIN III)
Severe dysplasia of prostate
EXCLUDES 1 *dysplasia (mild) (moderate) of prostate (N42.3-)*
*prostatic intraepithelial neoplasia II [PIN II] (N42.3-)*
√5th **DØ7.6 Carcinoma in situ of other and unspecified male genital organs**
**DØ7.6Ø Carcinoma in situ of unspecified male genital organs**
**DØ7.61 Carcinoma in situ of scrotum**
**DØ7.69 Carcinoma in situ of other male genital organs**

√4th **DØ9 Carcinoma in situ of other and unspecified sites**
EXCLUDES 1 *melanoma in situ (DØ3.-)*
**DØ9.Ø Carcinoma in situ of bladder**
√5th **DØ9.1 Carcinoma in situ of other and unspecified urinary organs**
**DØ9.1Ø Carcinoma in situ of unspecified urinary organ**
**DØ9.19 Carcinoma in situ of other urinary organs**
√5th **DØ9.2 Carcinoma in situ of eye**
EXCLUDES 1 *carcinoma in situ of skin of eyelid (DØ4.1-)*
**DØ9.2Ø Carcinoma in situ of unspecified eye**
**DØ9.21 Carcinoma in situ of right eye**
**DØ9.22 Carcinoma in situ of left eye**
**DØ9.3 Carcinoma in situ of thyroid and other endocrine glands**
EXCLUDES 1 *carcinoma in situ of endocrine pancreas (DØ1.7)*
*carcinoma in situ of ovary (DØ7.39)*
*carcinoma in situ of testis (DØ7.69)*
**DØ9.8 Carcinoma in situ of other specified sites**
**DØ9.9 Carcinoma in situ, unspecified**

## Benign neoplasms, except benign neuroendocrine tumors (D10-D36)

✓4th **D10 Benign neoplasm of mouth and pharynx**

**D10.0 Benign neoplasm of lip**
Benign neoplasm of lip (frenulum) (inner aspect) (mucosa) (vermilion border)
EXCLUDES 1 *benign neoplasm of skin of lip (D22.0, D23.0)*

**D10.1 Benign neoplasm of tongue**
Benign neoplasm of lingual tonsil

**D10.2 Benign neoplasm of floor of mouth**

✓5th **D10.3 Benign neoplasm of other and unspecified parts of mouth**

**D10.30 Benign neoplasm of unspecified part of mouth**

**D10.39 Benign neoplasm of other parts of mouth**
Benign neoplasm of minor salivary gland NOS
EXCLUDES 1 *benign odontogenic neoplasms (D16.4-D16.5)*
*benign neoplasm of mucosa of lip (D10.0)*
*benign neoplasm of nasopharyngeal surface of soft palate (D10.6)*

**D10.4 Benign neoplasm of tonsil**
Benign neoplasm of tonsil (faucial) (palatine)
EXCLUDES 1 *benign neoplasm of lingual tonsil (D10.1)*
*benign neoplasm of pharyngeal tonsil (D10.6)*
*benign neoplasm of tonsillar fossa (D10.5)*
*benign neoplasm of tonsillar pillars (D10.5)*

**D10.5 Benign neoplasm of other parts of oropharynx**
Benign neoplasm of epiglottis, anterior aspect
Benign neoplasm of tonsillar fossa
Benign neoplasm of tonsillar pillars
Benign neoplasm of vallecula
EXCLUDES 1 *benign neoplasm of epiglottis NOS (D14.1)*
*benign neoplasm of epiglottis, suprahyoid portion (D14.1)*
**DEF:** Oropharynx: Middle portion of pharynx (throat); communicates with the oral cavity, nasopharynx and laryngopharynx.

**D10.6 Benign neoplasm of nasopharynx**
Benign neoplasm of pharyngeal tonsil
Benign neoplasm of posterior margin of septum and choanae
**DEF:** Nasopharynx: Upper portion of pharynx (throat); communicates with the nasal cavities, oropharynx and tympanic cavities.

**D10.7 Benign neoplasm of hypopharynx**
**DEF:** Hypopharynx: Lower portion of pharynx (throat); communicates with the oropharynx and the esophagus.
***Synonym(s):*** *laryngopharynx.*

**D10.9 Benign neoplasm of pharynx, unspecified**

✓4th **D11 Benign neoplasm of major salivary glands**
EXCLUDES 1 *benign neoplasms of specified minor salivary glands which are classified according to their anatomical location*
*benign neoplasms of minor salivary glands NOS (D10.39)*

**D11.0 Benign neoplasm of parotid gland**

**D11.7 Benign neoplasm of other major salivary glands**
Benign neoplasm of sublingual salivary gland
Benign neoplasm of submandibular salivary gland

**D11.9 Benign neoplasm of major salivary gland, unspecified**

✓4th **D12 Benign neoplasm of colon, rectum, anus and anal canal**
EXCLUDES 2 *benign carcinoid tumors of the large intestine, and rectum (D3A.02-)*
*polyp of colon NOS (K63.5)*
**AHA:** 2018,2Q,14; 2017,1Q,15; 2015,2Q,14
**TIP:** Code K63.5 Polyp of colon, is assigned when documentation states hyperplastic colon polyps, regardless of the site in the colon. Slow-growing, hyperplastic polyps are not precancerous and are classified differently from benign or adenomatous polyps.

**D12.0 Benign neoplasm of cecum**
Benign neoplasm of ileocecal valve

**D12.1 Benign neoplasm of appendix**
EXCLUDES 1 *benign carcinoid tumor of the appendix (D3A.020)*

**D12.2 Benign neoplasm of ascending colon**

**D12.3 Benign neoplasm of transverse colon**
Benign neoplasm of hepatic flexure
Benign neoplasm of splenic flexure
**AHA:** 2017,1Q,16

**D12.4 Benign neoplasm of descending colon**

**D12.5 Benign neoplasm of sigmoid colon**

**D12.6 Benign neoplasm of colon, unspecified**
Adenomatosis of colon
Benign neoplasm of large intestine NOS
Polyposis (hereditary) of colon
EXCLUDES 2 *inflammatory polyp of colon (K51.4-)*

**D12.7 Benign neoplasm of rectosigmoid junction**

**D12.8 Benign neoplasm of rectum**
EXCLUDES 1 *benign carcinoid tumor of the rectum (D3A.026)*
**AHA:** 2018,1Q,6

**D12.9 Benign neoplasm of anus and anal canal**
Benign neoplasm of anus NOS
EXCLUDES 1 *benign neoplasm of anal margin (D22.5, D23.5)*
*benign neoplasm of anal skin (D22.5, D23.5)*
*benign neoplasm of perianal skin (D22.5, D23.5)*

✓4th **D13 Benign neoplasm of other and ill-defined parts of digestive system**
EXCLUDES 1 *benign stromal tumors of digestive system (D21.4)*

**D13.0 Benign neoplasm of esophagus**

**D13.1 Benign neoplasm of stomach**
EXCLUDES 1 *benign carcinoid tumor of the stomach (D3A.092)*

**D13.2 Benign neoplasm of duodenum**
EXCLUDES 1 *benign carcinoid tumor of the duodenum (D3A.010)*

✓5th **D13.3 Benign neoplasm of other and unspecified parts of small intestine**
EXCLUDES 1 *benign carcinoid tumors of the small intestine (D3A.01-)*
*benign neoplasm of ileocecal valve (D12.0)*

**D13.30 Benign neoplasm of unspecified part of small intestine**

**D13.39 Benign neoplasm of other parts of small intestine**

**D13.4 Benign neoplasm of liver**
Benign neoplasm of intrahepatic bile ducts

**D13.5 Benign neoplasm of extrahepatic bile ducts**

**D13.6 Benign neoplasm of pancreas**
EXCLUDES 1 *benign neoplasm of endocrine pancreas (D13.7)*

**D13.7 Benign neoplasm of endocrine pancreas**
Benign neoplasm of islets of Langerhans
Islet cell tumor
Use additional code to identify any functional activity

✓5th **D13.9 Benign neoplasm of ill-defined sites within the digestive system**
**AHA:** 2023,4Q,4-5

**D13.91 Familial adenomatous polyposis**
Code also associated conditions, such as:
benign neoplasm of colon (D12.6)
malignant neoplasm of colon (C18.-)

**D13.99 Benign neoplasm of ill-defined sites within the digestive system**
Benign neoplasm of digestive system NOS
Benign neoplasm of intestine NOS
Benign neoplasm of spleen

✓4th **D14 Benign neoplasm of middle ear and respiratory system**

**D14.0 Benign neoplasm of middle ear, nasal cavity and accessory sinuses**
Benign neoplasm of cartilage of nose
EXCLUDES 1 *benign neoplasm of auricular canal (external) (D22.2-, D23.2-)*
*benign neoplasm of bone of ear (D16.4)*
*benign neoplasm of bone of nose (D16.4)*
*benign neoplasm of cartilage of ear (D21.0)*
*benign neoplasm of ear (external)(skin) (D22.2-, D23.2-)*
*benign neoplasm of nose NOS (D36.7)*
*benign neoplasm of olfactory bulb (D33.3)*
*benign neoplasm of posterior margin of septum and choanae (D10.6)*
*benign neoplasm of skin of nose (D22.39, D23.39)*
*polyp of accessory sinus (J33.8)*
*polyp of ear (middle) (H74.4)*
*polyp of nasal (cavity) (J33.-)*

**D14.1 Benign neoplasm of larynx**
Adenomatous polyp of larynx
Benign neoplasm of epiglottis (suprahyoid portion)
EXCLUDES 1 *benign neoplasm of epiglottis, anterior aspect (D10.5)*
*polyp (nonadenomatous) of vocal cord or larynx (J38.1)*

**D14.2 Benign neoplasm of trachea**

✓5th **D14.3 Benign neoplasm of bronchus and lung**
EXCLUDES 1 *benign carcinoid tumor of the bronchus and lung (D3A.090)*

**D14.30 Benign neoplasm of unspecified bronchus and lung**

**D14.31 Benign neoplasm of right bronchus and lung**

D14.32 **Benign neoplasm of left bronchus and lung**

D14.4 **Benign neoplasm of respiratory system, unspecified**

√4th **D15 Benign neoplasm of other and unspecified intrathoracic organs**

EXCLUDES 1 *benign neoplasm of mesothelial tissue (D19.-)*

D15.0 **Benign neoplasm of thymus**

EXCLUDES 1 *benign carcinoid tumor of the thymus (D3A.091)*

D15.1 **Benign neoplasm of heart** COM

EXCLUDES 1 *benign neoplasm of great vessels (D21.3)*

D15.2 **Benign neoplasm of mediastinum**

AHA: 2024,3Q,3

D15.7 **Benign neoplasm of other specified intrathoracic organs**

D15.9 **Benign neoplasm of intrathoracic organ, unspecified**

√4th **D16 Benign neoplasm of bone and articular cartilage**

EXCLUDES 1 *benign neoplasm of connective tissue of ear (D21.0)*
*benign neoplasm of connective tissue of eyelid (D21.0)*
*benign neoplasm of connective tissue of larynx (D14.1)*
*benign neoplasm of connective tissue of nose (D14.0)*
*benign neoplasm of synovia (D21.-)*

√5th D16.0 **Benign neoplasm of scapula and long bones of upper limb**

D16.00 **Benign neoplasm of scapula and long bones of unspecified upper limb**

D16.01 **Benign neoplasm of scapula and long bones of right upper limb**

D16.02 **Benign neoplasm of scapula and long bones of left upper limb**

√5th D16.1 **Benign neoplasm of short bones of upper limb**

D16.10 **Benign neoplasm of short bones of unspecified upper limb**

D16.11 **Benign neoplasm of short bones of right upper limb**

D16.12 **Benign neoplasm of short bones of left upper limb**

√5th D16.2 **Benign neoplasm of long bones of lower limb**

D16.20 **Benign neoplasm of long bones of unspecified lower limb**

D16.21 **Benign neoplasm of long bones of right lower limb**

D16.22 **Benign neoplasm of long bones of left lower limb**

√5th D16.3 **Benign neoplasm of short bones of lower limb**

D16.30 **Benign neoplasm of short bones of unspecified lower limb**

D16.31 **Benign neoplasm of short bones of right lower limb**

D16.32 **Benign neoplasm of short bones of left lower limb**

D16.4 **Benign neoplasm of bones of skull and face**

Benign neoplasm of maxilla (superior)
Benign neoplasm of orbital bone
Keratocyst of maxilla
Keratocystic odontogenic tumor of maxilla

EXCLUDES 2 *benign neoplasm of lower jaw bone (D16.5)*

D16.5 **Benign neoplasm of lower jaw bone**

Keratocyst of mandible
Keratocystic odontogenic tumor of mandible

D16.6 **Benign neoplasm of vertebral column**

EXCLUDES 1 *benign neoplasm of sacrum and coccyx (D16.8)*

D16.7 **Benign neoplasm of ribs, sternum and clavicle**

D16.8 **Benign neoplasm of pelvic bones, sacrum and coccyx**

D16.9 **Benign neoplasm of bone and articular cartilage, unspecified**

√4th **D17 Benign lipomatous neoplasm**

D17.0 **Benign lipomatous neoplasm of skin and subcutaneous tissue of head, face and neck**

D17.1 **Benign lipomatous neoplasm of skin and subcutaneous tissue of trunk**

√5th D17.2 **Benign lipomatous neoplasm of skin and subcutaneous tissue of limb**

D17.20 **Benign lipomatous neoplasm of skin and subcutaneous tissue of unspecified limb**

D17.21 **Benign lipomatous neoplasm of skin and subcutaneous tissue of right arm**

D17.22 **Benign lipomatous neoplasm of skin and subcutaneous tissue of left arm**

D17.23 **Benign lipomatous neoplasm of skin and subcutaneous tissue of right leg**

D17.24 **Benign lipomatous neoplasm of skin and subcutaneous tissue of left leg**

√5th D17.3 **Benign lipomatous neoplasm of skin and subcutaneous tissue of other and unspecified sites**

D17.30 **Benign lipomatous neoplasm of skin and subcutaneous tissue of unspecified sites**

D17.39 **Benign lipomatous neoplasm of skin and subcutaneous tissue of other sites**

D17.4 **Benign lipomatous neoplasm of intrathoracic organs**

D17.5 **Benign lipomatous neoplasm of intra-abdominal organs**

EXCLUDES 1 *benign lipomatous neoplasm of peritoneum and retroperitoneum (D17.79)*

D17.6 **Benign lipomatous neoplasm of spermatic cord**

√5th D17.7 **Benign lipomatous neoplasm of other sites**

D17.71 **Benign lipomatous neoplasm of kidney**

D17.72 **Benign lipomatous neoplasm of other genitourinary organ**

D17.79 **Benign lipomatous neoplasm of other sites**

Benign lipomatous neoplasm of peritoneum
Benign lipomatous neoplasm of retroperitoneum

D17.9 **Benign lipomatous neoplasm, unspecified**

Lipoma NOS

√4th **D18 Hemangioma and lymphangioma, any site**

EXCLUDES 1 ~~*benign neoplasm of glomus jugulare (D35.6)*~~
~~*blue or pigmented nevus (D22.-)*~~
~~*nevus NOS (D22.-)*~~
~~*vascular nevus (Q82.5)*~~

EXCLUDES 2 ▶*benign neoplasm of glomus jugulare (D35.6)*◀
▶*blue or pigmented nevus (D22.-)*◀
▶*nevus NOS (D22.-)*◀
▶*vascular nevus (Q82.5)*◀

√5th D18.0 **Hemangioma**

Angioma NOS
Cavernous nevus

**DEF:** Common benign tumor usually occurring in infancy that is composed of newly formed blood vessels due to malformation of the angioblastic tissue.

D18.00 **Hemangioma unspecified site**

D18.01 **Hemangioma of skin and subcutaneous tissue**

D18.02 **Hemangioma of intracranial structures** HCC Rx ESR COM

D18.03 **Hemangioma of intra-abdominal structures**

D18.09 **Hemangioma of other sites**

D18.1 **Lymphangioma, any site**

AHA: 2018,3Q,31; 2018,2Q,13

√4th **D19 Benign neoplasm of mesothelial tissue**

D19.0 **Benign neoplasm of mesothelial tissue of pleura**

D19.1 **Benign neoplasm of mesothelial tissue of peritoneum**

D19.7 **Benign neoplasm of mesothelial tissue of other sites**

D19.9 **Benign neoplasm of mesothelial tissue, unspecified**

Benign mesothelioma NOS

√4th **D20 Benign neoplasm of soft tissue of retroperitoneum and peritoneum**

EXCLUDES 1 *benign lipomatous neoplasm of peritoneum and retroperitoneum (D17.79)*
*benign neoplasm of mesothelial tissue (D19.-)*

D20.0 **Benign neoplasm of soft tissue of retroperitoneum**

D20.1 **Benign neoplasm of soft tissue of peritoneum**

**D21 Other benign neoplasms of connective and other soft tissue**

INCLUDES benign neoplasm of blood vessel
benign neoplasm of bursa
benign neoplasm of cartilage
benign neoplasm of fascia
benign neoplasm of fat
benign neoplasm of ligament, except uterine
benign neoplasm of lymphatic channel
benign neoplasm of muscle
benign neoplasm of synovia
benign neoplasm of tendon (sheath)
benign stromal tumors

EXCLUDES 1 *benign neoplasm of articular cartilage (D16.-)*
*benign neoplasm of cartilage of larynx (D14.1)*
*benign neoplasm of cartilage of nose (D14.Ø)*
*benign neoplasm of connective tissue of breast (D24.-)*
*benign neoplasm of peripheral nerves and autonomic nervous system (D36.1-)*
*benign neoplasm of peritoneum (D2Ø.1)*
*benign neoplasm of retroperitoneum (D2Ø.Ø)*
*benign neoplasm of uterine ligament, any (D28.2)*
*benign neoplasm of vascular tissue (D18.-)*
*hemangioma (D18.Ø-)*
*lipomatous neoplasm (D17.-)*
*lymphangioma (D18.1)*
*uterine leiomyoma (D25.-)*

**D21.Ø Benign neoplasm of connective and other soft tissue of head, face and neck**
Benign neoplasm of connective tissue of ear
Benign neoplasm of connective tissue of eyelid
EXCLUDES 1 *benign neoplasm of connective tissue of orbit (D31.6-)*

**D21.1 Benign neoplasm of connective and other soft tissue of upper limb, including shoulder**
**D21.1Ø Benign neoplasm of connective and other soft tissue of unspecified upper limb, including shoulder**
**D21.11 Benign neoplasm of connective and other soft tissue of right upper limb, including shoulder**
**D21.12 Benign neoplasm of connective and other soft tissue of left upper limb, including shoulder**

**D21.2 Benign neoplasm of connective and other soft tissue of lower limb, including hip**
**D21.2Ø Benign neoplasm of connective and other soft tissue of unspecified lower limb, including hip**
**D21.21 Benign neoplasm of connective and other soft tissue of right lower limb, including hip**
**D21.22 Benign neoplasm of connective and other soft tissue of left lower limb, including hip**

**D21.3 Benign neoplasm of connective and other soft tissue of thorax**
Benign neoplasm of axilla
Benign neoplasm of diaphragm
Benign neoplasm of great vessels
EXCLUDES 1 *benign neoplasm of heart (D15.1)*
*benign neoplasm of mediastinum (D15.2)*
*benign neoplasm of thymus (D15.Ø)*

**D21.4 Benign neoplasm of connective and other soft tissue of abdomen**
Benign stromal tumors of abdomen

**D21.5 Benign neoplasm of connective and other soft tissue of pelvis**
EXCLUDES 1 *benign neoplasm of any uterine ligament (D28.2)*
*uterine leiomyoma (D25.-)*

**D21.6 Benign neoplasm of connective and other soft tissue of trunk, unspecified**
Benign neoplasm of connective and other soft tissue of back NOS

**D21.9 Benign neoplasm of connective and other soft tissue, unspecified**

**D22 Melanocytic nevi**

INCLUDES atypical nevus
blue hairy pigmented nevus
nevus NOS

**D22.Ø Melanocytic nevi of lip**

**D22.1 Melanocytic nevi of eyelid, including canthus**
AHA: 2018,4Q,4
**D22.1Ø Melanocytic nevi of unspecified eyelid, including canthus**
**D22.11 Melanocytic nevi of right eyelid, including canthus**
**D22.111 Melanocytic nevi of right upper eyelid, including canthus**
**D22.112 Melanocytic nevi of right lower eyelid, including canthus**
**D22.12 Melanocytic nevi of left eyelid, including canthus**
**D22.121 Melanocytic nevi of left upper eyelid, including canthus**
**D22.122 Melanocytic nevi of left lower eyelid, including canthus**

**D22.2 Melanocytic nevi of ear and external auricular canal**
**D22.2Ø Melanocytic nevi of unspecified ear and external auricular canal**
**D22.21 Melanocytic nevi of right ear and external auricular canal**
**D22.22 Melanocytic nevi of left ear and external auricular canal**

**D22.3 Melanocytic nevi of other and unspecified parts of face**
**D22.3Ø Melanocytic nevi of unspecified part of face**
**D22.39 Melanocytic nevi of other parts of face**

**D22.4 Melanocytic nevi of scalp and neck**

**D22.5 Melanocytic nevi of trunk**
Melanocytic nevi of anal margin
Melanocytic nevi of anal skin
Melanocytic nevi of perianal skin
Melanocytic nevi of skin of breast

**D22.6 Melanocytic nevi of upper limb, including shoulder**
**D22.6Ø Melanocytic nevi of unspecified upper limb, including shoulder**
**D22.61 Melanocytic nevi of right upper limb, including shoulder**
**D22.62 Melanocytic nevi of left upper limb, including shoulder**

**D22.7 Melanocytic nevi of lower limb, including hip**
**D22.7Ø Melanocytic nevi of unspecified lower limb, including hip**
**D22.71 Melanocytic nevi of right lower limb, including hip**
**D22.72 Melanocytic nevi of left lower limb, including hip**

**D22.9 Melanocytic nevi, unspecified**

**D23 Other benign neoplasms of skin**

INCLUDES benign neoplasm of hair follicles
benign neoplasm of sebaceous glands
benign neoplasm of sweat glands

EXCLUDES 1 *benign lipomatous neoplasms of skin (D17.Ø-D17.3)*
EXCLUDES 2 *melanocytic nevi (D22.-)*

**D23.Ø Other benign neoplasm of skin of lip**
EXCLUDES 1 *benign neoplasm of vermilion border of lip (D1Ø.Ø)*

**D23.1 Other benign neoplasm of skin of eyelid, including canthus**
AHA: 2018,4Q,4
**D23.1Ø Other benign neoplasm of skin of unspecified eyelid, including canthus**
**D23.11 Other benign neoplasm of skin of right eyelid, including canthus**
**D23.111 Other benign neoplasm of skin of right upper eyelid, including canthus**
**D23.112 Other benign neoplasm of skin of right lower eyelid, including canthus**
**D23.12 Other benign neoplasm of skin of left eyelid, including canthus**
**D23.121 Other benign neoplasm of skin of left upper eyelid, including canthus**
**D23.122 Other benign neoplasm of skin of left lower eyelid, including canthus**

**D23.2 Other benign neoplasm of skin of ear and external auricular canal**
**D23.2Ø Other benign neoplasm of skin of unspecified ear and external auricular canal**
**D23.21 Other benign neoplasm of skin of right ear and external auricular canal**
**D23.22 Other benign neoplasm of skin of left ear and external auricular canal**

**D23.3 Other benign neoplasm of skin of other and unspecified parts of face**
**D23.3Ø Other benign neoplasm of skin of unspecified part of face**
**D23.39 Other benign neoplasm of skin of other parts of face**

**D23.4 Other benign neoplasm of skin of scalp and neck**

**D23.5 Other benign neoplasm of skin of trunk**
Other benign neoplasm of anal margin
Other benign neoplasm of anal skin
Other benign neoplasm of perianal skin
Other benign neoplasm of skin of breast
EXCLUDES 1 *benign neoplasm of anus NOS (D12.9)*

✓5th **D23.6 Other benign neoplasm of skin of upper limb, including shoulder**
- **D23.60 Other benign neoplasm of skin of unspecified upper limb, including shoulder**
- **D23.61 Other benign neoplasm of skin of right upper limb, including shoulder**
- **D23.62 Other benign neoplasm of skin of left upper limb, including shoulder**

✓5th **D23.7 Other benign neoplasm of skin of lower limb, including hip**
- **D23.70 Other benign neoplasm of skin of unspecified lower limb, including hip**
- **D23.71 Other benign neoplasm of skin of right lower limb, including hip**
- **D23.72 Other benign neoplasm of skin of left lower limb, including hip**

**D23.9 Other benign neoplasm of skin, unspecified**

## ✓4th D24 Benign neoplasm of breast

INCLUDES benign neoplasm of connective tissue of breast
benign neoplasm of soft parts of breast
fibroadenoma of breast

EXCLUDES 2 *adenofibrosis of breast (N60.2)*
*benign cyst of breast (N60.-)*
*benign mammary dysplasia (N60.-)*
*benign neoplasm of skin of breast (D22.5, D23.5)*
*fibrocystic disease of breast (N60.-)*

**D24.1 Benign neoplasm of right breast**
**D24.2 Benign neoplasm of left breast**
**D24.9 Benign neoplasm of unspecified breast**

## ✓4th D25 Leiomyoma of uterus

INCLUDES uterine fibroid
uterine fibromyoma
uterine myoma

**Uterine Leiomyomas (Fibroids)**

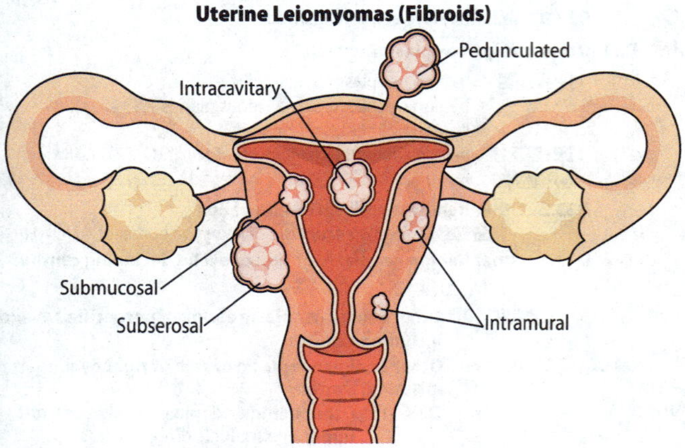


**D25.0 Submucous leiomyoma of uterus**
**D25.1 Intramural leiomyoma of uterus**
Interstitial leiomyoma of uterus
**D25.2 Subserosal leiomyoma of uterus**
Subperitoneal leiomyoma of uterus
**D25.9 Leiomyoma of uterus, unspecified**

## ✓4th D26 Other benign neoplasms of uterus

**D26.0 Other benign neoplasm of cervix uteri**
**D26.1 Other benign neoplasm of corpus uteri**
**D26.7 Other benign neoplasm of other parts of uterus**
**D26.9 Other benign neoplasm of uterus, unspecified**

## ✓4th D27 Benign neoplasm of ovary

Use additional code to identify any functional activity

EXCLUDES 2 *corpus albicans cyst (N83.2-)*
*corpus luteum cyst (N83.1-)*
*endometrial cyst (N80.1-)*
*follicular (atretic) cyst (N83.0-)*
*graafian follicle cyst (N83.0-)*
*ovarian cyst NEC (N83.2-)*
*ovarian retention cyst (N83.2-)*

**D27.0 Benign neoplasm of right ovary**
**D27.1 Benign neoplasm of left ovary**
**D27.9 Benign neoplasm of unspecified ovary**

## ✓4th D28 Benign neoplasm of other and unspecified female genital organs

INCLUDES adenomatous polyp
benign neoplasm of skin of female genital organs
benign teratoma

EXCLUDES 1 *epoophoron cyst (Q50.5)*
*fimbrial cyst (Q50.4)*
*Gartner's duct cyst (Q52.4)*
*parovarian cyst (Q50.5)*

**D28.0 Benign neoplasm of vulva**
**D28.1 Benign neoplasm of vagina**
**D28.2 Benign neoplasm of uterine tubes and ligaments**
Benign neoplasm of fallopian tube
Benign neoplasm of uterine ligament (broad) (round)
**D28.7 Benign neoplasm of other specified female genital organs**
**D28.9 Benign neoplasm of female genital organ, unspecified**

## ✓4th D29 Benign neoplasm of male genital organs

INCLUDES benign neoplasm of skin of male genital organs

**D29.0 Benign neoplasm of penis**
**D29.1 Benign neoplasm of prostate**
EXCLUDES 1 *enlarged prostate (N40.-)*

✓5th **D29.2 Benign neoplasm of testis**
Use additional code to identify any functional activity
- **D29.20 Benign neoplasm of unspecified testis**
- **D29.21 Benign neoplasm of right testis**
- **D29.22 Benign neoplasm of left testis**

✓5th **D29.3 Benign neoplasm of epididymis**
- **D29.30 Benign neoplasm of unspecified epididymis**
- **D29.31 Benign neoplasm of right epididymis**
- **D29.32 Benign neoplasm of left epididymis**

**D29.4 Benign neoplasm of scrotum**
Benign neoplasm of skin of scrotum
**D29.8 Benign neoplasm of other specified male genital organs**
Benign neoplasm of seminal vesicle
Benign neoplasm of spermatic cord
Benign neoplasm of tunica vaginalis
**D29.9 Benign neoplasm of male genital organ, unspecified**

## ✓4th D30 Benign neoplasm of urinary organs

✓5th **D30.0 Benign neoplasm of kidney**
EXCLUDES 1 *benign carcinoid tumor of the kidney (D3A.093)*
*benign neoplasm of renal calyces (D30.1-)*
*benign neoplasm of renal pelvis (D30.1-)*
- **D30.00 Benign neoplasm of unspecified kidney**
- **D30.01 Benign neoplasm of right kidney**
- **D30.02 Benign neoplasm of left kidney**

✓5th **D30.1 Benign neoplasm of renal pelvis**
- **D30.10 Benign neoplasm of unspecified renal pelvis**
- **D30.11 Benign neoplasm of right renal pelvis**
- **D30.12 Benign neoplasm of left renal pelvis**

✓5th **D30.2 Benign neoplasm of ureter**
EXCLUDES 1 *benign neoplasm of ureteric orifice of bladder (D30.3)*
- **D30.20 Benign neoplasm of unspecified ureter**
- **D30.21 Benign neoplasm of right ureter**
- **D30.22 Benign neoplasm of left ureter**

**D30.3 Benign neoplasm of bladder**
Benign neoplasm of ureteric orifice of bladder
Benign neoplasm of urethral orifice of bladder
**D30.4 Benign neoplasm of urethra**
EXCLUDES 1 *benign neoplasm of urethral orifice of bladder (D30.3)*
**D30.8 Benign neoplasm of other specified urinary organs**
Benign neoplasm of paraurethral glands
**D30.9 Benign neoplasm of urinary organ, unspecified**
Benign neoplasm of urinary system NOS

## ✓4th D31 Benign neoplasm of eye and adnexa

EXCLUDES 1 *benign neoplasm of connective tissue of eyelid (D21.0)*
*benign neoplasm of optic nerve (D33.3)*
*benign neoplasm of skin of eyelid (D22.1-, D23.1-)*

✓5th **D31.0 Benign neoplasm of conjunctiva**
- **D31.00 Benign neoplasm of unspecified conjunctiva**
- **D31.01 Benign neoplasm of right conjunctiva**
- **D31.02 Benign neoplasm of left conjunctiva**

✓5th **D31.1 Benign neoplasm of cornea**
- **D31.10 Benign neoplasm of unspecified cornea**
- **D31.11 Benign neoplasm of right cornea**
- **D31.12 Benign neoplasm of left cornea**

**D31.2 Benign neoplasm of retina**

EXCLUDES 1 *dark area on retina (D49.81)*
*hemangioma of retina (D49.81)*
*neoplasm of unspecified behavior of retina and choroid (D49.81)*
*retinal freckle (D49.81)*

**D31.20 Benign neoplasm of unspecified retina**
**D31.21 Benign neoplasm of right retina**
**D31.22 Benign neoplasm of left retina**

**D31.3 Benign neoplasm of choroid**
**D31.30 Benign neoplasm of unspecified choroid**
**D31.31 Benign neoplasm of right choroid**
**D31.32 Benign neoplasm of left choroid**

**D31.4 Benign neoplasm of ciliary body**
**D31.40 Benign neoplasm of unspecified ciliary body**
**D31.41 Benign neoplasm of right ciliary body**
**D31.42 Benign neoplasm of left ciliary body**

**D31.5 Benign neoplasm of lacrimal gland and duct**
Benign neoplasm of lacrimal sac
Benign neoplasm of nasolacrimal duct
**D31.50 Benign neoplasm of unspecified lacrimal gland and duct**
**D31.51 Benign neoplasm of right lacrimal gland and duct**
**D31.52 Benign neoplasm of left lacrimal gland and duct**

**D31.6 Benign neoplasm of unspecified site of orbit**
Benign neoplasm of connective tissue of orbit
Benign neoplasm of extraocular muscle
Benign neoplasm of peripheral nerves of orbit
Benign neoplasm of retrobulbar tissue
Benign neoplasm of retro-ocular tissue
EXCLUDES 1 *benign neoplasm of orbital bone (D16.4)*
**D31.60 Benign neoplasm of unspecified site of unspecified orbit**
**D31.61 Benign neoplasm of unspecified site of right orbit**
**D31.62 Benign neoplasm of unspecified site of left orbit**

**D31.9 Benign neoplasm of unspecified part of eye**
Benign neoplasm of eyeball
**D31.90 Benign neoplasm of unspecified part of unspecified eye**
**D31.91 Benign neoplasm of unspecified part of right eye**
**D31.92 Benign neoplasm of unspecified part of left eye**

**D32 Benign neoplasm of meninges**
**D32.0 Benign neoplasm of cerebral meninges** HCC Rx ESR COM
**D32.1 Benign neoplasm of spinal meninges** HCC Rx ESR COM
**D32.9 Benign neoplasm of meninges, unspecified** HCC Rx ESR COM
Meningioma NOS

**D33 Benign neoplasm of brain and other parts of central nervous system**
EXCLUDES 1 *angioma (D18.0-)*
*benign neoplasm of meninges (D32.-)*
*benign neoplasm of peripheral nerves and autonomic nervous system (D36.1-)*
*hemangioma (D18.0-)*
*neurofibromatosis (Q85.0-)*
*retro-ocular benign neoplasm (D31.6-)*

**D33.0 Benign neoplasm of brain, supratentorial** HCC Rx ESR COM
Benign neoplasm of cerebral ventricle
Benign neoplasm of cerebrum
Benign neoplasm of frontal lobe
Benign neoplasm of occipital lobe
Benign neoplasm of parietal lobe
Benign neoplasm of temporal lobe
EXCLUDES 1 *benign neoplasm of fourth ventricle (D33.1)*

**D33.1 Benign neoplasm of brain, infratentorial** HCC Rx ESR COM
Benign neoplasm of brain stem
Benign neoplasm of cerebellum
Benign neoplasm of fourth ventricle

**D33.2 Benign neoplasm of brain, unspecified** HCC Rx ESR COM
**D33.3 Benign neoplasm of cranial nerves** HCC Rx ESR COM
Benign neoplasm of olfactory bulb
**D33.4 Benign neoplasm of spinal cord** HCC Rx ESR COM
**D33.7 Benign neoplasm of other specified parts of central nervous system** HCC Rx ESR COM
**D33.9 Benign neoplasm of central nervous system, unspecified** HCC Rx ESR COM
Benign neoplasm of nervous system (central) NOS

**D34 Benign neoplasm of thyroid gland**
Use additional code to identify any functional activity

**D35 Benign neoplasm of other and unspecified endocrine glands**
Use additional code to identify any functional activity
EXCLUDES 1 *benign neoplasm of endocrine pancreas (D13.7)*
*benign neoplasm of ovary (D27.-)*
*benign neoplasm of testis (D29.2.-)*
*benign neoplasm of thymus (D15.0)*

**D35.0 Benign neoplasm of adrenal gland**
**D35.00 Benign neoplasm of unspecified adrenal gland**
**D35.01 Benign neoplasm of right adrenal gland**
**D35.02 Benign neoplasm of left adrenal gland**
**D35.1 Benign neoplasm of parathyroid gland**
**D35.2 Benign neoplasm of pituitary gland** HCC Rx ESR COM
**AHA:** 2014,3Q,22
**D35.3 Benign neoplasm of craniopharyngeal duct** HCC Rx ESR COM
**D35.4 Benign neoplasm of pineal gland** HCC Rx ESR COM
**D35.5 Benign neoplasm of carotid body**
**D35.6 Benign neoplasm of aortic body and other paraganglia**
Benign tumor of glomus jugulare
**D35.7 Benign neoplasm of other specified endocrine glands**
**D35.9 Benign neoplasm of endocrine gland, unspecified**
Benign neoplasm of unspecified endocrine gland

**D36 Benign neoplasm of other and unspecified sites**
**D36.0 Benign neoplasm of lymph nodes**
EXCLUDES 1 *lymphangioma (D18.1)*
**D36.1 Benign neoplasm of peripheral nerves and autonomic nervous system**
EXCLUDES 1 *benign neoplasm of peripheral nerves of orbit (D31.6-)*
*neurofibromatosis (Q85.0-)*
**D36.10 Benign neoplasm of peripheral nerves and autonomic nervous system, unspecified**
**D36.11 Benign neoplasm of peripheral nerves and autonomic nervous system of face, head, and neck**
**D36.12 Benign neoplasm of peripheral nerves and autonomic nervous system, upper limb, including shoulder**
**D36.13 Benign neoplasm of peripheral nerves and autonomic nervous system of lower limb, including hip**
**D36.14 Benign neoplasm of peripheral nerves and autonomic nervous system of thorax**
**D36.15 Benign neoplasm of peripheral nerves and autonomic nervous system of abdomen**
**D36.16 Benign neoplasm of peripheral nerves and autonomic nervous system of pelvis**
**D36.17 Benign neoplasm of peripheral nerves and autonomic nervous system of trunk, unspecified**
**D36.7 Benign neoplasm of other specified sites**
Benign neoplasm of back NOS
Benign neoplasm of nose NOS
**D36.9 Benign neoplasm, unspecified site**

## Benign neuroendocrine tumors (D3A)

**D3A Benign neuroendocrine tumors**
Code also any associated multiple endocrine neoplasia [MEN] syndromes (E31.2-)
Use additional code to identify any associated endocrine syndrome, such as:
carcinoid syndrome (E34.00)
EXCLUDES 2 *benign pancreatic islet cell tumors (D13.7)*

**D3A.0 Benign carcinoid tumors**
**DEF:** Specific type of slow-growing neuroendocrine tumors. Carcinoid tumors occur most commonly in the hormone producing cells of the gastrointestinal tracts and can also occur in the pancreas, testes, ovaries, or lungs.
**D3A.00 Benign carcinoid tumor of unspecified site** HCC Rx
Carcinoid tumor NOS
**D3A.01 Benign carcinoid tumors of the small intestine**
**D3A.010 Benign carcinoid tumor of the duodenum** HCC Rx
**D3A.011 Benign carcinoid tumor of the jejunum** HCC Rx
**D3A.012 Benign carcinoid tumor of the ileum** HCC Rx
**D3A.019 Benign carcinoid tumor of the small intestine, unspecified portion** HCC Rx

✓6th **D3A.02 Benign carcinoid tumors of the appendix, large intestine, and rectum**

**D3A.020 Benign carcinoid tumor of the appendix** HCC Rx

**D3A.021 Benign carcinoid tumor of the cecum** HCC Rx

**D3A.022 Benign carcinoid tumor of the ascending colon** HCC Rx

**D3A.023 Benign carcinoid tumor of the transverse colon** HCC Rx

**D3A.024 Benign carcinoid tumor of the descending colon** HCC Rx

**D3A.025 Benign carcinoid tumor of the sigmoid colon** HCC Rx

**D3A.026 Benign carcinoid tumor of the rectum** HCC Rx

**D3A.029 Benign carcinoid tumor of the large intestine, unspecified portion** HCC Rx
Benign carcinoid tumor of the colon NOS

✓6th **D3A.09 Benign carcinoid tumors of other sites**

**D3A.090 Benign carcinoid tumor of the bronchus and lung** HCC Rx

**D3A.091 Benign carcinoid tumor of the thymus** HCC Rx

**D3A.092 Benign carcinoid tumor of the stomach** HCC Rx

**D3A.093 Benign carcinoid tumor of the kidney** HCC Rx

**D3A.094 Benign carcinoid tumor of the foregut, unspecified** HCC Rx

**D3A.095 Benign carcinoid tumor of the midgut, unspecified** HCC Rx

**D3A.096 Benign carcinoid tumor of the hindgut, unspecified** HCC Rx

**D3A.098 Benign carcinoid tumors of other sites** HCC Rx

**D3A.8 Other benign neuroendocrine tumors** HCC Rx
Neuroendocrine tumor NOS

## Neoplasms of uncertain behavior, polycythemia vera and myelodysplastic syndromes (D37-D48)

NOTE Categories D37-D44, and D48 classify by site neoplasms of uncertain behavior, i.e., histologic confirmation whether the neoplasm is malignant or benign cannot be made.

EXCLUDES 1 *neoplasms of unspecified behavior (D49.-)*

✓4th **D37 Neoplasm of uncertain behavior of oral cavity and digestive organs**

EXCLUDES 1 *stromal tumors of uncertain behavior of digestive system (D48.1-)*

✓5th **D37.0 Neoplasm of uncertain behavior of lip, oral cavity and pharynx**

EXCLUDES 1 *neoplasm of uncertain behavior of aryepiglottic fold or interarytenoid fold, laryngeal aspect (D38.0)*
*neoplasm of uncertain behavior of epiglottis NOS (D38.0)*
*neoplasm of uncertain behavior of skin of lip (D48.5)*
*neoplasm of uncertain behavior of suprahyoid portion of epiglottis (D38.0)*

**D37.01 Neoplasm of uncertain behavior of lip**
Neoplasm of uncertain behavior of vermilion border of lip

**D37.02 Neoplasm of uncertain behavior of tongue**

✓6th **D37.03 Neoplasm of uncertain behavior of the major salivary glands**

**D37.030 Neoplasm of uncertain behavior of the parotid salivary glands**

**D37.031 Neoplasm of uncertain behavior of the sublingual salivary glands**

**D37.032 Neoplasm of uncertain behavior of the submandibular salivary glands**

**D37.039 Neoplasm of uncertain behavior of the major salivary glands, unspecified**

**D37.04 Neoplasm of uncertain behavior of the minor salivary glands**
Neoplasm of uncertain behavior of submucosal salivary glands of cheek
Neoplasm of uncertain behavior of submucosal salivary glands of hard palate
Neoplasm of uncertain behavior of submucosal salivary glands of lip
Neoplasm of uncertain behavior of submucosal salivary glands of soft palate

**D37.05 Neoplasm of uncertain behavior of pharynx**
Neoplasm of uncertain behavior of aryepiglottic fold of pharynx NOS
Neoplasm of uncertain behavior of hypopharyngeal aspect of aryepiglottic fold of pharynx
Neoplasm of uncertain behavior of marginal zone of aryepiglottic fold of pharynx

**D37.09 Neoplasm of uncertain behavior of other specified sites of the oral cavity**

**D37.1 Neoplasm of uncertain behavior of stomach**

**D37.2 Neoplasm of uncertain behavior of small intestine**

**D37.3 Neoplasm of uncertain behavior of appendix**

**D37.4 Neoplasm of uncertain behavior of colon**

**D37.5 Neoplasm of uncertain behavior of rectum**
Neoplasm of uncertain behavior of rectosigmoid junction

**D37.6 Neoplasm of uncertain behavior of liver, gallbladder and bile ducts**
Neoplasm of uncertain behavior of ampulla of Vater

**D37.8 Neoplasm of uncertain behavior of other specified digestive organs**
Neoplasm of uncertain behavior of anal canal
Neoplasm of uncertain behavior of anal sphincter
Neoplasm of uncertain behavior of anus NOS
Neoplasm of uncertain behavior of esophagus
Neoplasm of uncertain behavior of intestine NOS
Neoplasm of uncertain behavior of pancreas

EXCLUDES 1 *neoplasm of uncertain behavior of anal margin (D48.5)*
*neoplasm of uncertain behavior of anal skin (D48.5)*
*neoplasm of uncertain behavior of perianal skin (D48.5)*

**D37.9 Neoplasm of uncertain behavior of digestive organ, unspecified**

✓4th **D38 Neoplasm of uncertain behavior of middle ear and respiratory and intrathoracic organs**

EXCLUDES 1 *neoplasm of uncertain behavior of heart (D48.7)*

**D38.0 Neoplasm of uncertain behavior of larynx**
Neoplasm of uncertain behavior of aryepiglottic fold or interarytenoid fold, laryngeal aspect
Neoplasm of uncertain behavior of epiglottis (suprahyoid portion)

EXCLUDES 1 *neoplasm of uncertain behavior of aryepiglottic fold or interarytenoid fold NOS (D37.05)*
*neoplasm of uncertain behavior of hypopharyngeal aspect of aryepiglottic fold (D37.05)*
*neoplasm of uncertain behavior of marginal zone of aryepiglottic fold (D37.05)*

**D38.1 Neoplasm of uncertain behavior of trachea, bronchus and lung**

**D38.2 Neoplasm of uncertain behavior of pleura**

**D38.3 Neoplasm of uncertain behavior of mediastinum**

**D38.4 Neoplasm of uncertain behavior of thymus**

**D38.5 Neoplasm of uncertain behavior of other respiratory organs**
Neoplasm of uncertain behavior of accessory sinuses
Neoplasm of uncertain behavior of cartilage of nose
Neoplasm of uncertain behavior of middle ear
Neoplasm of uncertain behavior of nasal cavities

EXCLUDES 1 *neoplasm of uncertain behavior of ear (external) (skin) (D48.5)*
*neoplasm of uncertain behavior of nose NOS (D48.7)*
*neoplasm of uncertain behavior of skin of nose (D48.5)*

**D38.6 Neoplasm of uncertain behavior of respiratory organ, unspecified**

✓4th **D39 Neoplasm of uncertain behavior of female genital organs**

**D39.0 Neoplasm of uncertain behavior of uterus**

✓5th **D39.1 Neoplasm of uncertain behavior of ovary**
Use additional code to identify any functional activity
**AHA:** 2025,3Q,15

**D39.10 Neoplasm of uncertain behavior of unspecified ovary**

**D39.11 Neoplasm of uncertain behavior of right ovary**

**D39.12 Neoplasm of uncertain behavior of left ovary**

**D39.2 Neoplasm of uncertain behavior of placenta** M
Chorioadenoma destruens
Invasive hydatidiform mole
Malignant hydatidiform mole
EXCLUDES 1 *hydatidiform mole NOS (O01.9)*
**AHA:** 2023,3Q,14

**D39.8 Neoplasm of uncertain behavior of other specified female genital organs**
Neoplasm of uncertain behavior of skin of female genital organs

**D39.9 Neoplasm of uncertain behavior of female genital organ, unspecified**

✓4th **D40 Neoplasm of uncertain behavior of male genital organs**

**D40.0 Neoplasm of uncertain behavior of prostate**

✓5th **D40.1 Neoplasm of uncertain behavior of testis**

**D40.10 Neoplasm of uncertain behavior of unspecified testis**

**D40.11 Neoplasm of uncertain behavior of right testis**

**D40.12 Neoplasm of uncertain behavior of left testis**

**D40.8 Neoplasm of uncertain behavior of other specified male genital organs**
Neoplasm of uncertain behavior of skin of male genital organs

**D40.9 Neoplasm of uncertain behavior of male genital organ, unspecified**

✓4th **D41 Neoplasm of uncertain behavior of urinary organs**

✓5th **D41.0 Neoplasm of uncertain behavior of kidney**
EXCLUDES 1 *neoplasm of uncertain behavior of renal pelvis (D41.1-)*

**D41.00 Neoplasm of uncertain behavior of unspecified kidney**

**D41.01 Neoplasm of uncertain behavior of right kidney**

**D41.02 Neoplasm of uncertain behavior of left kidney**

✓5th **D41.1 Neoplasm of uncertain behavior of renal pelvis**

**D41.10 Neoplasm of uncertain behavior of unspecified renal pelvis**

**D41.11 Neoplasm of uncertain behavior of right renal pelvis**

**D41.12 Neoplasm of uncertain behavior of left renal pelvis**

✓5th **D41.2 Neoplasm of uncertain behavior of ureter**

**D41.20 Neoplasm of uncertain behavior of unspecified ureter**

**D41.21 Neoplasm of uncertain behavior of right ureter**

**D41.22 Neoplasm of uncertain behavior of left ureter**

**D41.3 Neoplasm of uncertain behavior of urethra**

**D41.4 Neoplasm of uncertain behavior of bladder**

**D41.8 Neoplasm of uncertain behavior of other specified urinary organs**

**D41.9 Neoplasm of uncertain behavior of unspecified urinary organ**

✓4th **D42 Neoplasm of uncertain behavior of meninges**

**D42.0 Neoplasm of uncertain behavior of cerebral meninges** HCC Rx ESR COM

**D42.1 Neoplasm of uncertain behavior of spinal meninges** HCC Rx ESR COM

**D42.9 Neoplasm of uncertain behavior of meninges, unspecified** HCC Rx ESR COM

✓4th **D43 Neoplasm of uncertain behavior of brain and central nervous system**
EXCLUDES 1 *neoplasm of uncertain behavior of peripheral nerves and autonomic nervous system (D48.2)*

**D43.0 Neoplasm of uncertain behavior of brain, supratentorial** HCC Rx ESR COM
Neoplasm of uncertain behavior of cerebral ventricle
Neoplasm of uncertain behavior of cerebrum
Neoplasm of uncertain behavior of frontal lobe
Neoplasm of uncertain behavior of occipital lobe
Neoplasm of uncertain behavior of parietal lobe
Neoplasm of uncertain behavior of temporal lobe
EXCLUDES 1 *neoplasm of uncertain behavior of fourth ventricle (D43.1)*

**D43.1 Neoplasm of uncertain behavior of brain, infratentorial** HCC Rx ESR COM
Neoplasm of uncertain behavior of brain stem
Neoplasm of uncertain behavior of cerebellum
Neoplasm of uncertain behavior of fourth ventricle
**AHA:** 2023,2Q,16

**D43.2 Neoplasm of uncertain behavior of brain, unspecified** HCC Rx ESR COM

**D43.3 Neoplasm of uncertain behavior of cranial nerves** HCC Rx ESR COM

**D43.4 Neoplasm of uncertain behavior of spinal cord** HCC Rx ESR COM

**D43.8 Neoplasm of uncertain behavior of other specified parts of central nervous system** HCC Rx ESR COM

**D43.9 Neoplasm of uncertain behavior of central nervous system, unspecified** HCC Rx ESR COM
Neoplasm of uncertain behavior of nervous system (central) NOS

✓4th **D44 Neoplasm of uncertain behavior of endocrine glands**
EXCLUDES 1 *multiple endocrine adenomatosis (E31.2-)*
*multiple endocrine neoplasia (E31.2-)*
*neoplasm of uncertain behavior of endocrine pancreas (D37.8)*
*neoplasm of uncertain behavior of ovary (D39.1-)*
*neoplasm of uncertain behavior of testis (D40.1-)*
*neoplasm of uncertain behavior of thymus (D38.4)*

**D44.0 Neoplasm of uncertain behavior of thyroid gland**
**AHA:** 2024,3Q,3

✓5th **D44.1 Neoplasm of uncertain behavior of adrenal gland**
Use additional code to identify any functional activity

**D44.10 Neoplasm of uncertain behavior of unspecified adrenal gland**

**D44.11 Neoplasm of uncertain behavior of right adrenal gland**

**D44.12 Neoplasm of uncertain behavior of left adrenal gland**

**D44.2 Neoplasm of uncertain behavior of parathyroid gland**

**D44.3 Neoplasm of uncertain behavior of pituitary gland** HCC Rx ESR COM
Use additional code to identify any functional activity

**D44.4 Neoplasm of uncertain behavior of craniopharyngeal duct** HCC Rx ESR COM

**D44.5 Neoplasm of uncertain behavior of pineal gland** HCC Rx ESR COM

**D44.6 Neoplasm of uncertain behavior of carotid body** HCC Rx ESR COM

**D44.7 Neoplasm of uncertain behavior of aortic body and other paraganglia** HCC Rx ESR COM
**AHA:** 2021,2Q,7; 2016,4Q,26

**D44.9 Neoplasm of uncertain behavior of unspecified endocrine gland**

**D45 Polycythemia vera** HCC Rx ESR COM
EXCLUDES 1 *familial polycythemia (D75.0)*
*secondary polycythemia (D75.1)*
**DEF:** Abnormal proliferation of all bone marrow elements, increased red cell mass, and total blood volume. The etiology is unknown, but it is frequently associated with splenomegaly, leukocytosis, and thrombocythemia.

✓4th **D46 Myelodysplastic syndromes**
Use additional code for adverse effect, if applicable, to identify drug (T36-T50 with fifth or sixth character 5)
EXCLUDES 2 *drug-induced aplastic anemia (D61.1)*

**D46.0 Refractory anemia without ring sideroblasts, so stated** HCC Rx ESR COM
Refractory anemia without sideroblasts, without excess of blasts

**D46.1 Refractory anemia with ring sideroblasts** HCC Rx ESR COM
RARS

✓5th **D46.2 Refractory anemia with excess of blasts [RAEB]**

**D46.20 Refractory anemia with excess of blasts, unspecified** HCC Rx ESR COM
RAEB NOS

**D46.21 Refractory anemia with excess of blasts 1** HCC Rx ESR COM
RAEB 1

**D46.22 Refractory anemia with excess of blasts 2** HCC Rx ESR COM
RAEB 2

**D46.A Refractory cytopenia with multilineage dysplasia** HCC Rx ESR COM

**D46.B Refractory cytopenia with multilineage dysplasia and ring sideroblasts** HCC Rx ESR COM
RCMD RS

**D46.C Myelodysplastic syndrome with isolated del(5q) chromosomal abnormality** HCC Rx ESR COM
5q minus syndrome NOS
Myelodysplastic syndrome with 5q deletion

**D46.4 Refractory anemia, unspecified** HCC Rx ESR COM

**D46.Z Other myelodysplastic syndromes** HCC Rx ESR COM
EXCLUDES 1 *chronic myelomonocytic leukemia (C93.1-)*

**D46.9 Myelodysplastic syndrome, unspecified** HCC Rx ESR COM
Myelodysplasia NOS

**√4th D47 Other neoplasms of uncertain behavior of lymphoid, hematopoietic and related tissue**

**√5th D47.Ø Mast cell neoplasms of uncertain behavior**

EXCLUDES 1 *congenital cutaneous mastocytosis (Q82.2)*
*histiocytic neoplasms of uncertain behavior (D47.Z9)*
*malignant mast cell neoplasm (C96.2-)*

**AHA:** 2017,4Q,5

**D47.Ø1 Cutaneous mastocytosis** Rx

Diffuse cutaneous mastocytosis
Maculopapular cutaneous mastocytosis
Solitary mastocytoma
Telangiectasia macularis eruptiva perstans
Urticaria pigmentosa

EXCLUDES 1 *congenital (diffuse) (maculopapular) cutaneous mastocytosis (Q82.2)*
*congenital urticaria pigmentosa (Q82.2)*
*extracutaneous mastocytoma (D47.Ø9)*

**D47.Ø2 Systemic mastocytosis** Rx

Indolent systemic mastocytosis
Isolated bone marrow mastocytosis
Smoldering systemic mastocytosis
Systemic mastocytosis, with an associated hematological non-mast cell lineage disease (SM-AHNMD)

Code also, if applicable, any associated hematological non-mast cell lineage disease, such as:
acute myeloid leukemia (C92.6-, C92.A-)
chronic myelomonocytic leukemia (C93.1-)
essential thrombocytosis (D47.3)
hypereosinophilic syndrome (D72.1)
myelodysplastic syndrome (D46.9)
myeloproliferative syndrome (D47.1)
non-Hodgkin lymphoma (C82-C85)
plasma cell myeloma (C9Ø.Ø-)
polycythemia vera (D45)

EXCLUDES 1 *aggressive systemic mastocytosis (C96.21)*
*mast cell leukemia (C94.3-)*

**D47.Ø9 Other mast cell neoplasms of uncertain behavior** Rx

Extracutaneous mastocytoma
Mast cell tumor NOS
Mastocytoma NOS
Mastocytosis NOS

**D47.1 Chronic myeloproliferative disease** HCC Rx ESR COM

Chronic neutrophilic leukemia
Myeloproliferative disease, unspecified

EXCLUDES 1 *atypical chronic myeloid leukemia BCR/ABL-negative (C92.2-)*
*chronic myeloid leukemia BCR/ABL-positive (C92.1-)*
*myelofibrosis NOS (D75.81)*
*myelophthisic anemia (D61.82)*
*myelophthisis (D61.82)*
*secondary myelofibrosis NOS (D75.81)*

**D47.2 Monoclonal gammopathy**

Monoclonal gammopathy of undetermined significance [MGUS]

**AHA:** 2021,3Q,5

**TIP:** Smoldering multiple myeloma (SMM) is coded here.

**D47.3 Essential (hemorrhagic) thrombocythemia** HCC Rx ESR COM

Essential thrombocytosis
Idiopathic hemorrhagic thrombocythemia
Primary thrombocytosis

EXCLUDES 2 *reactive thrombocytosis (D75.838)*
*secondary thrombocytosis (D75.838)*
*thrombocythemia NOS (D75.839)*
*thrombocytosis NOS (D75.839)*

**DEF:** Chronic myeloproliferative neoplasm involving production of excess blood platelets that may result in abnormal clotting or hemorrhaging.

**D47.4 Osteomyelofibrosis** HCC Rx ESR COM

Chronic idiopathic myelofibrosis
Myelofibrosis (idiopathic) (with myeloid metaplasia)
Myelosclerosis (megakaryocytic) with myeloid metaplasia
Secondary myelofibrosis in myeloproliferative disease

EXCLUDES 1 *acute myelofibrosis (C94.4-)*

**√5th D47.Z Other specified neoplasms of uncertain behavior of lymphoid, hematopoietic and related tissue**

**AHA:** 2016,4Q,8

**D47.Z1 Post-transplant lymphoproliferative disorder (PTLD)** HCC ESR COM UPD

Code first complications of transplanted organs and tissue (T86.-)

**DEF:** Excessive proliferation of B-cell lymphocytes following Epstein-Barr virus infection in organ transplant patients. It may progress to non-Hodgkin lymphoma.

**D47.Z2 Castleman disease** HCC Rx ESR COM

Code also, if applicable, human herpesvirus 8 infection (B1Ø.89)

EXCLUDES 2 *Kaposi's sarcoma (C46.-)*

**DEF:** Rare disease of the lymph nodes and lymphoid tissues that closely mimics lymphoma.

**D47.Z9 Other specified neoplasms of uncertain behavior of lymphoid, hematopoietic and related tissue** HCC Rx ESR COM

Histiocytic tumors of uncertain behavior

**AHA:** 2025,2Q,19

**D47.9 Neoplasm of uncertain behavior of lymphoid, hematopoietic and related tissue, unspecified** HCC Rx ESR COM

Lymphoproliferative disease NOS

**√4th D48 Neoplasm of uncertain behavior of other and unspecified sites**

EXCLUDES 1 *neurofibromatosis (nonmalignant) (Q85.Ø-)*

**D48.Ø Neoplasm of uncertain behavior of bone and articular cartilage**

EXCLUDES 1 *neoplasm of uncertain behavior of cartilage of ear (D48.1-)*
*neoplasm of uncertain behavior of cartilage of larynx (D38.Ø)*
*neoplasm of uncertain behavior of cartilage of nose (D38.5)*
*neoplasm of uncertain behavior of connective tissue of eyelid (D48.1-)*
*neoplasm of uncertain behavior of synovia (D48.1-)*

**√5th D48.1 Neoplasm of uncertain behavior of connective and other soft tissue**

Neoplasm of uncertain behavior of connective tissue of ear
Neoplasm of uncertain behavior of connective tissue of eyelid
Stromal tumors of uncertain behavior of digestive system

EXCLUDES 1 *neoplasm of uncertain behavior of articular cartilage (D48.Ø)*
*neoplasm of uncertain behavior of cartilage of larynx (D38.Ø)*
*neoplasm of uncertain behavior of cartilage of nose (D38.5)*
*neoplasm of uncertain behavior of connective tissue of breast (D48.6-)*

**AHA:** 2023,4Q,5-6

**√6th D48.11 Desmoid tumor**

Aggressive fibromatosis

**D48.11Ø Desmoid tumor of head and neck**
**D48.111 Desmoid tumor of chest wall**
**D48.112 Desmoid tumor, intrathoracic**
**D48.113 Desmoid tumor of abdominal wall**
**D48.114 Desmoid tumor, intraabdominal**
Desmoid tumor of pelvic cavity
Desmoid tumor, peritoneal, retroperitoneal
**D48.115 Desmoid tumor of upper extremity and shoulder girdle**
**D48.116 Desmoid tumor of lower extremity and pelvic girdle**
Desmoid tumor of buttock
**D48.117 Desmoid tumor of back**
**D48.118 Desmoid tumor of other site**
**D48.119 Desmoid tumor of unspecified site**

**D48.19 Other specified neoplasm of uncertain behavior of connective and other soft tissue**

**D48.2 Neoplasm of uncertain behavior of peripheral nerves and autonomic nervous system**

EXCLUDES 1 *neoplasm of uncertain behavior of peripheral nerves of orbit (D48.7)*

**D48.3 Neoplasm of uncertain behavior of retroperitoneum**

**D48.4 Neoplasm of uncertain behavior of peritoneum**

**D48.5 Neoplasm of uncertain behavior of skin**
Neoplasm of uncertain behavior of anal margin
Neoplasm of uncertain behavior of anal skin
Neoplasm of uncertain behavior of perianal skin
Neoplasm of uncertain behavior of skin of breast
EXCLUDES 1 *neoplasm of uncertain behavior of anus NOS (D37.8)*
*neoplasm of uncertain behavior of skin of genital organs (D39.8, D40.8)*
*neoplasm of uncertain behavior of vermilion border of lip (D37.0)*

√5th **D48.6 Neoplasm of uncertain behavior of breast**
Cystosarcoma phyllodes
Neoplasm of uncertain behavior of connective tissue of breast
EXCLUDES 1 *neoplasm of uncertain behavior of skin of breast (D48.5)*

**D48.60 Neoplasm of uncertain behavior of unspecified breast**
**D48.61 Neoplasm of uncertain behavior of right breast**
**D48.62 Neoplasm of uncertain behavior of left breast**

**D48.7 Neoplasm of uncertain behavior of other specified sites**
Neoplasm of uncertain behavior of eye
Neoplasm of uncertain behavior of heart
Neoplasm of uncertain behavior of peripheral nerves of orbit
EXCLUDES 1 *neoplasm of uncertain behavior of connective tissue (D48.1-)*
*neoplasm of uncertain behavior of skin of eyelid (D48.5)*

**D48.9 Neoplasm of uncertain behavior, unspecified**

## Neoplasms of unspecified behavior (D49)

√4th **D49 Neoplasms of unspecified behavior**

NOTE Category D49 classifies by site neoplasms of unspecified morphology and behavior. The term "mass", unless otherwise stated, is not to be regarded as a neoplastic growth.

INCLUDES "growth" NOS
neoplasm NOS
new growth NOS
tumor NOS

EXCLUDES 1 ~~*neoplasms of uncertain behavior (D37-D44, D48)*~~
EXCLUDES 2 ▶*neoplasms of uncertain behavior (D37-D44, D48)*◀

**D49.0 Neoplasm of unspecified behavior of digestive system**
EXCLUDES 1 *neoplasm of unspecified behavior of margin of anus (D49.2)*
*neoplasm of unspecified behavior of perianal skin (D49.2)*
*neoplasm of unspecified behavior of skin of anus (D49.2)*

**D49.1 Neoplasm of unspecified behavior of respiratory system**

**D49.2 Neoplasm of unspecified behavior of bone, soft tissue, and skin**
EXCLUDES 1 *neoplasm of unspecified behavior of anal canal (D49.0)*
*neoplasm of unspecified behavior of anus NOS (D49.0)*
*neoplasm of unspecified behavior of bone marrow (D49.89)*
*neoplasm of unspecified behavior of cartilage of larynx (D49.1)*
*neoplasm of unspecified behavior of cartilage of nose (D49.1)*
*neoplasm of unspecified behavior of connective tissue of breast (D49.3)*
*neoplasm of unspecified behavior of skin of genital organs (D49.59)*
*neoplasm of unspecified behavior of vermilion border of lip (D49.0)*

**D49.3 Neoplasm of unspecified behavior of breast**
EXCLUDES 1 *neoplasm of unspecified behavior of skin of breast (D49.2)*

**D49.4 Neoplasm of unspecified behavior of bladder**

√5th **D49.5 Neoplasm of unspecified behavior of other genitourinary organs**
AHA: 2016,4Q,9

√6th **D49.51 Neoplasm of unspecified behavior of kidney**
**D49.511 Neoplasm of unspecified behavior of right kidney**
**D49.512 Neoplasm of unspecified behavior of left kidney**
**D49.519 Neoplasm of unspecified behavior of unspecified kidney**

**D49.59 Neoplasm of unspecified behavior of other genitourinary organ**

**D49.6 Neoplasm of unspecified behavior of brain** HCC Rx ESR COM
EXCLUDES 1 *neoplasm of unspecified behavior of cerebral meninges (D49.7)*
*neoplasm of unspecified behavior of cranial nerves (D49.7)*

**D49.7 Neoplasm of unspecified behavior of endocrine glands and other parts of nervous system**
EXCLUDES 1 *neoplasm of unspecified behavior of peripheral, sympathetic, and parasympathetic nerves and ganglia (D49.2)*

√5th **D49.8 Neoplasm of unspecified behavior of other specified sites**
EXCLUDES 1 *neoplasm of unspecified behavior of eyelid (skin) (D49.2)*
*neoplasm of unspecified behavior of eyelid cartilage (D49.2)*
*neoplasm of unspecified behavior of great vessels (D49.2)*
*neoplasm of unspecified behavior of optic nerve (D49.7)*

**D49.81 Neoplasm of unspecified behavior of retina and choroid**
Dark area on retina
Retinal freckle

**D49.89 Neoplasm of unspecified behavior of other specified sites**

**D49.9 Neoplasm of unspecified behavior of unspecified site**

# Chapter 3. Disease of the Blood and Blood-Forming Organs and Certain Disorders Involving the Immune Mechanism (D5Ø–D89)



## Chapter-specific Guidelines with Coding Examples

Reserved for future guideline expansion.

# Chapter 3. Diseases of the Blood and Blood-forming Organs and Certain Disorders Involving the Immune Mechanism (D50-D89)

EXCLUDES 2 *autoimmune disease (systemic) NOS (M35.9)*
*certain conditions originating in the perinatal period (P00-P96)*
*complications of pregnancy, childbirth and the puerperium (O00-O9A)*
*congenital malformations, deformations and chromosomal abnormalities (Q00-Q99)*
*endocrine, nutritional and metabolic diseases (E00-E88)*
*human immunodeficiency virus [HIV] disease (B20)*
*injury, poisoning and certain other consequences of external causes (S00-T88)*
*neoplasms (C00-D49)*
*symptoms, signs and abnormal clinical and laboratory findings, not elsewhere classified (R00-R94)*

This chapter contains the following blocks:

| | |
|---|---|
| D50-D53 | Nutritional anemias |
| D55-D59 | Hemolytic anemias |
| D60-D64 | Aplastic and other anemias and other bone marrow failure syndromes |
| D65-D69 | Coagulation defects, purpura and other hemorrhagic conditions |
| D70-D77 | Other disorders of blood and blood-forming organs |
| D78 | Intraoperative and postprocedural complications of the spleen |
| D80-D89 | Certain disorders involving the immune mechanism |

## Nutritional anemias (D50-D53)

**DEF:** Nutritional anemia: The result of inadequate intake or absorption of a vitamin or mineral that impacts the production of red blood cells or causes them to develop abnormally affecting the size and shape.
**TIP:** Documentation must identify a link between anemia and the nutritional deficiency; low levels of a particular nutrient may occur concurrently with anemia but not cause the anemia.

✓4th **D50 Iron deficiency anemia**
INCLUDES asiderotic anemia
hypochromic anemia

**D50.0 Iron deficiency anemia secondary to blood loss (chronic)**
Posthemorrhagic anemia (chronic)
EXCLUDES 1 *acute posthemorrhagic anemia (D62)*
*congenital anemia from fetal blood loss (P61.3)*
**AHA:** 2019,3Q,17

**D50.1 Sideropenic dysphagia**
Kelly-Paterson syndrome
Plummer-Vinson syndrome

**D50.8 Other iron deficiency anemias**
Iron deficiency anemia due to inadequate dietary iron intake

**D50.9 Iron deficiency anemia, unspecified**

✓4th **D51 Vitamin B12 deficiency anemia**
EXCLUDES 1 ~~*vitamin B12 deficiency (E53.8)*~~
EXCLUDES 2 ▶ *deficiency of other B group vitamins (E53-)* ◀

**D51.0 Vitamin B12 deficiency anemia due to intrinsic factor deficiency**
Addison anemia
Biermer anemia
Congenital intrinsic factor deficiency
Pernicious (congenital) anemia
**DEF:** Chronic progressive anemia due to vitamin B12 malabsorption, caused by lack of secretion of intrinsic factor, which is produced by the gastric mucosa of the stomach.

**D51.1 Vitamin B12 deficiency anemia due to selective vitamin B12 malabsorption with proteinuria**
Imerslund (Gräsbeck) syndrome
Megaloblastic hereditary anemia

**D51.2 Transcobalamin II deficiency**

**D51.3 Other dietary vitamin B12 deficiency anemia**
Vegan anemia

**D51.8 Other vitamin B12 deficiency anemias**

**D51.9 Vitamin B12 deficiency anemia, unspecified**

✓4th **D52 Folate deficiency anemia**
EXCLUDES 1 *folate deficiency without anemia (E53.8)*
**DEF:** Deficiency in a B complex vitamin needed for the production of healthy red blood cells. Lack of folate, or folic acid, and other absorption conditions can cause anemia resulting in large, misshapen red blood cells called megaloblasts.

**D52.0 Dietary folate deficiency anemia**
Nutritional megaloblastic anemia
**DEF:** Result of a poor diet with inadequate intake of folate, which is needed to produce healthy red blood cells.

**D52.1 Drug-induced folate deficiency anemia**
Use additional code for adverse effect, if applicable, to identify drug (T36-T50 with fifth or sixth character 5)

**D52.8 Other folate deficiency anemias**

**D52.9 Folate deficiency anemia, unspecified**
Folic acid deficiency anemia NOS

✓4th **D53 Other nutritional anemias**
INCLUDES megaloblastic anemia unresponsive to vitamin B12 or folate therapy

**D53.0 Protein deficiency anemia**
Amino-acid deficiency anemia
Orotaciduric anemia
EXCLUDES 1 *Lesch-Nyhan syndrome (E79.1)*

**D53.1 Other megaloblastic anemias, not elsewhere classified**
Megaloblastic anemia NOS
EXCLUDES 1 *Di Guglielmo's disease (C94.0)*

**D53.2 Scorbutic anemia**
EXCLUDES 1 *scurvy (E54)*

**D53.8 Other specified nutritional anemias**
Anemia associated with deficiency of copper
Anemia associated with deficiency of molybdenum
Anemia associated with deficiency of zinc
EXCLUDES 2 *nutritional deficiencies without anemia, such as:*
*copper deficiency NOS (E61.0)*
*molybdenum deficiency NOS (E61.5)*
*zinc deficiency NOS (E60)*

**D53.9 Nutritional anemia, unspecified**
Simple chronic anemia
EXCLUDES 1 *anemia NOS (D64.9)*
**AHA:** 2018,4Q,88

## Hemolytic anemias (D55-D59)

✓4th **D55 Anemia due to enzyme disorders**
EXCLUDES 1 *drug-induced enzyme deficiency anemia (D59.2)*

**D55.0 Anemia due to glucose-6-phosphate dehydrogenase [G6PD] deficiency** ESR
Favism
G6PD deficiency anemia
EXCLUDES 1 *glucose-6-phosphate dehydrogenase (G6PD) deficiency without anemia (D75.A)*

**D55.1 Anemia due to other disorders of glutathione metabolism** ESR
Anemia (due to) enzyme deficiencies, except G6PD, related to the hexose monophosphate [HMP] shunt pathway
Anemia (due to) hemolytic nonspherocytic (hereditary), type I

✓5th **D55.2 Anemia due to disorders of glycolytic enzymes**
EXCLUDES 1 *disorders of glycolysis not associated with anemia (E74.81-)*
**AHA:** 2021,4Q,6-7

**D55.21 Anemia due to pyruvate kinase deficiency** ESR
PK deficiency anemia
Pyruvate kinase deficiency anemia

**D55.29 Anemia due to other disorders of glycolytic enzymes** ESR
Hexokinase deficiency anemia
Triose-phosphate isomerase deficiency anemia

**D55.3 Anemia due to disorders of nucleotide metabolism** ESR

**D55.8 Other anemias due to enzyme disorders** ESR

**D55.9 Anemia due to enzyme disorder, unspecified** ESR

**✓4th D56 Thalassemia**

EXCLUDES 1 *sickle-cell thalassemia (D57.4-)*

**DEF:** Group of inherited disorders of hemoglobin metabolism causing mild to severe anemia. It is usually found in people of Mediterranean, African, Chinese, or Asian descent.

**Thalassemia**

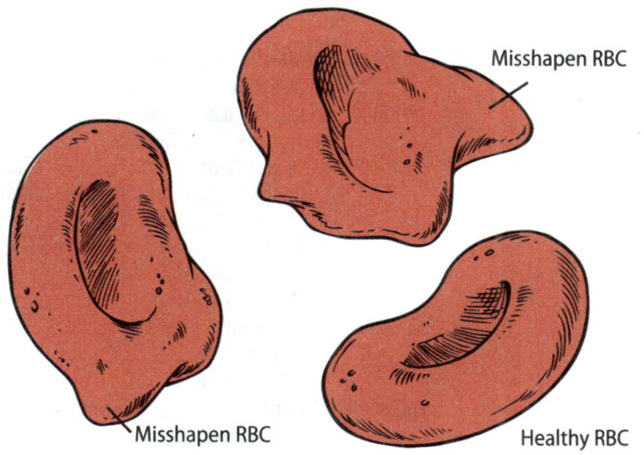


**D56.Ø Alpha thalassemia** ESR

Alpha thalassemia major
Hemoglobin H Constant Spring
Hemoglobin H disease
Hydrops fetalis due to alpha thalassemia
Severe alpha thalassemia
Triple gene defect alpha thalassemia

Use additional code, if applicable, for hydrops fetalis due to alpha thalassemia (P56.99)

EXCLUDES 1 *alpha thalassemia trait or minor (D56.3)*
*asymptomatic alpha thalassemia (D56.3)*
*hydrops fetalis due to isoimmunization (P56.Ø)*
*hydrops fetalis not due to immune hemolysis (P83.2)*

**DEF:** HBA1 and HBA2 genetic variant of chromosome 16 prevalent among those of African and Southeast Asian descent. Alpha thalassemia is associated with a wide spectrum of anemic presentation and includes hemoglobin H disease subtypes.

**D56.1 Beta thalassemia** HCC ESR COM

Beta thalassemia major
Cooley's anemia
Homozygous beta thalassemia
Severe beta thalassemia
Thalassemia intermedia
Thalassemia major

EXCLUDES 1 *beta thalassemia minor (D56.3)*
*beta thalassemia trait (D56.3)*
*delta-beta thalassemia (D56.2)*
*hemoglobin E-beta thalassemia (D56.5)*
*sickle-cell beta thalassemia (D57.4-)*

**D56.2 Delta-beta thalassemia** HCC ESR COM

Homozygous delta-beta thalassemia

EXCLUDES 1 *delta-beta thalassemia minor (D56.3)*
*delta-beta thalassemia trait (D56.3)*

**D56.3 Thalassemia minor**

Alpha thalassemia minor
Alpha thalassemia silent carrier
Alpha thalassemia trait
Beta thalassemia minor
Beta thalassemia trait
Delta-beta thalassemia minor
Delta-beta thalassemia trait
Thalassemia trait NOS

EXCLUDES 1 *alpha thalassemia (D56.Ø)*
*beta thalassemia (D56.1)*
*delta-beta thalassemia (D56.2)*
*hemoglobin E-beta thalassemia (D56.5)*
*sickle-cell trait (D57.3)*

**DEF:** Solitary abnormal gene that identifies a carrier of the disease, yet with an absence of symptoms or a clinically mild anemic presentation.

**D56.4 Hereditary persistence of fetal hemoglobin [HPFH]** ESR

**D56.5 Hemoglobin E-beta thalassemia** HCC ESR COM

EXCLUDES 1 *beta thalassemia (D56.1)*
*beta thalassemia minor (D56.3)*
*beta thalassemia trait (D56.3)*
*delta-beta thalassemia (D56.2)*
*delta-beta thalassemia trait (D56.3)*
*hemoglobin E disease (D58.2)*
*other hemoglobinopathies (D58.2)*
*sickle-cell beta thalassemia (D57.4-)*

**D56.8 Other thalassemias** ESR

Dominant thalassemia
Hemoglobin C thalassemia
Mixed thalassemia
Thalassemia with other hemoglobinopathy

EXCLUDES 1 *hemoglobin C disease (D58.2)*
*hemoglobin E disease (D58.2)*
*other hemoglobinopathies (D58.2)*
*sickle-cell anemia (D57.-)*
*sickle-cell thalassemia (D57.4-)*

**D56.9 Thalassemia, unspecified**

Mediterranean anemia (with other hemoglobinopathy)

**✓4th D57 Sickle-cell disorders**

Use additional code for any associated fever (R5Ø.81)

EXCLUDES 1 *other hemoglobinopathies (D58.-)*

**AHA:** 2023,4Q,6-7; 2022,2Q,28

**DEF:** Severe, chronic inherited diseases caused by a genetic variation in hemoglobin protein of the red blood cell. The gene mutation causes the red blood cell to become hard, sticky, and crescent or sickle shaped, making it harder for red blood cells to travel through the bloodstream, disrupting blood flow and decreasing oxygen transport to tissues.

**Sickle cell**

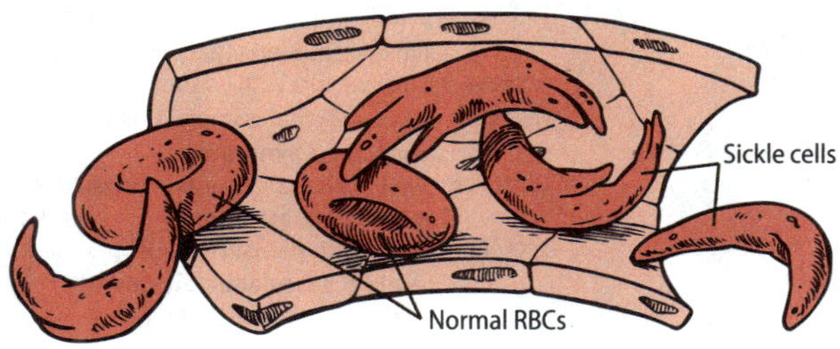


**✓5th D57.Ø Hb-SS disease with crisis**

Hb-SS disease with (vaso-occlusive) pain
Sickle-cell disease with crisis

**AHA:** 2020,4Q,6-7

**D57.ØØ Hb-SS disease with crisis, unspecified** HCC Rx ESR COM

Hb-SS disease with (painful) crisis NOS
Hb-SS disease with (vaso-occlusive) pain NOS

**D57.Ø1 Hb-SS disease with acute chest syndrome** HCC Rx ESR COM

**D57.Ø2 Hb-SS disease with splenic sequestration** HCC Rx ESR COM

**AHA:** 2025,1Q,24

**D57.Ø3 Hb-SS disease with cerebral vascular involvement** HCC Rx ESR COM

Code also, if applicable, cerebral infarction (I63.-)

**D57.Ø4 Hb-SS disease with dactylitis** HCC Rx ESR COM

**D57.Ø9 Hb-SS disease with crisis with other specified complication** HCC Rx ESR COM

Use additional code to identify complications, such as:
cholelithiasis (K8Ø.-)
priapism (N48.32)

**D57.1 Sickle-cell disease without crisis** HCC Rx ESR COM

Hb-SS disease without crisis
Sickle-cell anemia NOS
Sickle-cell disease NOS
Sickle-cell disorder NOS

**✓5th D57.2 Sickle-cell/Hb-C disease**

Hb-S/Hb-C disease
Hb-SC disease

**AHA:** 2020,4Q,6-7

**D57.2Ø Sickle-cell/Hb-C disease without crisis** HCC ESR

**✓6th D57.21 Sickle-cell/Hb-C disease with crisis**

**D57.211 Sickle-cell/Hb-C disease with acute chest syndrome** HCC ESR

**D57.212 Sickle-cell/Hb-C disease with splenic sequestration** HCC ESR

**D57.213 Sickle-cell/Hb-C disease with cerebral vascular involvement** HCC ESR
Code also, if applicable, cerebral infarction (I63.-)

**D57.214 Sickle-cell/Hb-C disease with dactylitis** HCC ESR

**D57.218 Sickle-cell/Hb-C disease with crisis with other specified complication** HCC ESR
Use additional code to identify complications, such as:
cholelithiasis (K8Ø.-)
priapism (N48.32)

**D57.219 Sickle-cell/Hb-C disease with crisis, unspecified** HCC ESR
Sickle-cell/Hb-C disease with (vaso-occlusive) pain NOS
Sickle-cell/Hb-C disease with crisis NOS

**D57.3 Sickle-cell trait** ESR
Hb-S trait
Heterozygous hemoglobin S
**DEF:** Heterozygous genetic makeup characterized by one gene for normal hemoglobin and one for sickle-cell hemoglobin. The clinical disease is rarely present.

✓5th **D57.4 Sickle-cell thalassemia**
Sickle-cell beta thalassemia
Thalassemia Hb-S disease
**AHA:** 2020,4Q,6-7

**D57.4Ø Sickle-cell thalassemia without crisis** HCC ESR
Microdrepanocytosis
Sickle-cell thalassemia NOS

✓6th **D57.41 Sickle-cell thalassemia, unspecified, with crisis**
Sickle-cell thalassemia with (painful) crisis NOS
Sickle-cell thalassemia with (vaso-occlusive) pain NOS

**D57.411 Sickle-cell thalassemia, unspecified, with acute chest syndrome** HCC ESR

**D57.412 Sickle-cell thalassemia, unspecified, with splenic sequestration** HCC ESR

**D57.413 Sickle-cell thalassemia, unspecified, with cerebral vascular involvement** HCC ESR
Code also, if applicable cerebral infarction (I63.-)

**D57.414 Sickle-cell thalassemia, unspecified, with dactylitis** HCC ESR

**D57.418 Sickle-cell thalassemia, unspecified, with crisis with other specified complication** HCC ESR
Use additional code to identify complications, such as:
cholelithiasis (K8Ø.-)
priapism (N48.32)

**D57.419 Sickle-cell thalassemia, unspecified, with crisis** HCC ESR
Sickle-cell thalassemia with (painful) crisis NOS
Sickle-cell thalassemia with (vaso-occlusive) pain NOS

**D57.42 Sickle-cell thalassemia beta zero without crisis** HCC Rx ESR COM
HbS-beta zero without crisis
Sickle-cell beta zero without crisis

✓6th **D57.43 Sickle-cell thalassemia beta zero with crisis**
HbS-beta zero with crisis
Sickle-cell beta zero with crisis

**D57.431 Sickle-cell thalassemia beta zero with acute chest syndrome** HCC Rx ESR COM
HbS-beta zero with acute chest syndrome
Sickle-cell beta zero with acute chest syndrome

**D57.432 Sickle-cell thalassemia beta zero with splenic sequestration** HCC Rx ESR COM
HbS-beta zero with splenic sequestration
Sickle-cell beta zero with splenic sequestration

**D57.433 Sickle-cell thalassemia beta zero with cerebral vascular involvement** HCC Rx ESR COM
HbS-beta zero with cerebral vascular involvement
Sickle-cell beta zero with cerebral vascular involvement
Code also, if applicable cerebral infarction (I63.-)

**D57.434 Sickle-cell thalassemia beta zero with dactylitis** HCC Rx ESR COM

**D57.438 Sickle-cell thalassemia beta zero with crisis with other specified complication** HCC Rx ESR COM
HbS-beta zero with other specified complication
Sickle-cell beta zero with other specified complication
Use additional code to identify complications, such as:
cholelithiasis (K8Ø.-)
priapism (N48.32)

**D57.439 Sickle-cell thalassemia beta zero with crisis, unspecified** HCC Rx ESR COM
HbS-beta zero with other specified complication
Sickle-cell beta zero with crisis unspecified
Sickle-cell thalassemia beta zero with (painful) crisis NOS
Sickle-cell thalassemia beta zero with (vaso-occlusive) pain NOS

**D57.44 Sickle-cell thalassemia beta plus without crisis** HCC ESR
HbS-beta plus without crisis
Sickle-cell beta plus without crisis

✓6th **D57.45 Sickle-cell thalassemia beta plus with crisis**
HbS-beta plus with crisis
Sickle-cell beta plus with crisis

**D57.451 Sickle-cell thalassemia beta plus with acute chest syndrome** HCC ESR
HbS-beta plus with acute chest syndrome
Sickle-cell beta plus with acute chest syndrome

**D57.452 Sickle-cell thalassemia beta plus with splenic sequestration** HCC ESR
HbS-beta plus with splenic sequestration
Sickle-cell beta plus with splenic sequestration

**D57.453 Sickle-cell thalassemia beta plus with cerebral vascular involvement** HCC ESR
HbS-beta plus with cerebral vascular involvement
Sickle-cell beta plus with cerebral vascular involvement
Code also, if applicable cerebral infarction (I63.-)

**D57.454 Sickle-cell thalassemia beta plus with dactylitis** HCC ESR

**D57.458 Sickle-cell thalassemia beta plus with crisis with other specified complication** HCC ESR
HbS-beta plus with crisis with other specified complication
Sickle-cell beta plus with crisis with other specified complication
Use additional code to identify complications, such as:
cholelithiasis (K8Ø.-)
priapism (N48.32)

**D57.459 Sickle-cell thalassemia beta plus with crisis, unspecified** HCC ESR
HbS-beta plus with crisis with unspecified complication
Sickle-cell beta plus with crisis with unspecified complication
Sickle-cell thalassemia beta plus with (painful) crisis NOS
Sickle-cell thalassemia beta plus with (vaso-occlusive) pain NOS

✓5th **D57.8 Other sickle-cell disorders**
Hb-SD disease
Hb-SE disease
**AHA:** 2020,4Q,6-7

**D57.80 Other sickle-cell disorders without crisis** HCC ESR

✓6th **D57.81 Other sickle-cell disorders with crisis**

**D57.811 Other sickle-cell disorders with acute chest syndrome** HCC ESR

**D57.812 Other sickle-cell disorders with splenic sequestration** HCC ESR

**D57.813 Other sickle-cell disorders with cerebral vascular involvement** HCC ESR
Code also, if applicable: cerebral infarction (I63.-)

**D57.814 Other sickle-cell disorders with dactylitis** HCC ESR

**D57.818 Other sickle-cell disorders with crisis with other specified complication** HCC ESR
Use additional code to identify complications, such as:
cholelithiasis (K80.-)
priapism (N48.32)

**D57.819 Other sickle-cell disorders with crisis, unspecified** HCC ESR
Other sickle-cell disorders with (vaso-occlusive) pain NOS
Other sickle-cell disorders with crisis NOS

✓4th **D58 Other hereditary hemolytic anemias**
EXCLUDES 1 *hemolytic anemia of the newborn (P55.-)*

**D58.0 Hereditary spherocytosis** ESR
Acholuric (familial) jaundice
Congenital (spherocytic) hemolytic icterus
Minkowski-Chauffard syndrome
**DEF:** Inherited condition caused by mutations to genes responsible for the production of proteins that form the membranes of red blood cells. The shape and flexibility of the red blood cell membrane is altered, diminishing the cell's ability to traverse the spleen, therefore becoming trapped and destroyed before the red blood cell has reached maturity.

**D58.1 Hereditary elliptocytosis** ESR
Elliptocytosis (congenital)
Ovalocytosis (congenital) (hereditary)

**D58.2 Other hemoglobinopathies** ESR
Abnormal hemoglobin NOS
Congenital Heinz body anemia
Hb-C disease
Hb-D disease
Hb-E disease
Hemoglobinopathy NOS
Unstable hemoglobin hemolytic disease
EXCLUDES 1 *familial polycythemia (D75.0)*
*Hb-M disease (D74.0)*
*hemoglobin E-beta thalassemia (D56.5)*
*hereditary persistence of fetal hemoglobin [HPFH] (D56.4)*
*high-altitude polycythemia (D75.1)*
*methemoglobinemia (D74.-)*
*other hemoglobinopathies with thalassemia (D56.8)*

**D58.8 Other specified hereditary hemolytic anemias** ESR
Stomatocytosis

**D58.9 Hereditary hemolytic anemia, unspecified** ESR

✓4th **D59 Acquired hemolytic anemia**
**DEF:** Non-hereditary anemia characterized by premature destruction of red blood cells caused by infectious organisms, poisons, and physical agents.

**D59.0 Drug-induced autoimmune hemolytic anemia** Rx ESR COM
Use additional code for adverse effect, if applicable, to identify drug (T36-T50 with fifth or sixth character 5)

✓5th **D59.1 Other autoimmune hemolytic anemias**
EXCLUDES 2 *Evans syndrome (D69.41)*
*hemolytic disease of newborn (P55.-)*
*paroxysmal cold hemoglobinuria (D59.6)*
**AHA:** 2020,4Q,7-8

**D59.10 Autoimmune hemolytic anemia, unspecified** HCC Rx ESR COM

**D59.11 Warm autoimmune hemolytic anemia** HCC Rx ESR COM
Warm type (primary) (secondary) (symptomatic) autoimmune hemolytic anemia
Warm type autoimmune hemolytic disease

**D59.12 Cold autoimmune hemolytic anemia** HCC Rx ESR COM
Chronic cold hemagglutinin disease
Cold agglutinin disease
Cold agglutinin hemoglobinuria
Cold type (primary) (secondary) (symptomatic) autoimmune hemolytic anemia
Cold type autoimmune hemolytic disease

**D59.13 Mixed type autoimmune hemolytic anemia** HCC Rx ESR COM
Mixed type autoimmune hemolytic disease
Mixed type, cold and warm, (primary) (secondary) (symptomatic) autoimmune hemolytic anemia

**D59.19 Other autoimmune hemolytic anemia** HCC Rx ESR COM

**D59.2 Drug-induced nonautoimmune hemolytic anemia** Rx ESR COM
Drug-induced enzyme deficiency anemia
Use additional code for adverse effect, if applicable, to identify drug (T36-T50 with fifth or sixth character 5)

✓5th **D59.3 Hemolytic-uremic syndrome**
Code also, if applicable, any associated:
acute kidney failure (N17.-)
chronic kidney disease (N18.-)
**AHA:** 2022,4Q,5-6
**DEF:** Condition typically precipitated by infection causing low platelets and destruction of red blood cells resulting in hemolytic anemia. This cell damage and blockage of renal capillaries lead to kidney failure. Mainly affects children.

**D59.30 Hemolytic-uremic syndrome, unspecified** HCC Rx ESR COM
Hemolytic-uremic syndrome NOS

**D59.31 Infection-associated hemolytic-uremic syndrome** HCC Rx ESR COM
Shiga toxin-producing E. coli [STEC] related hemolytic uremic syndrome
Typical hemolytic uremic syndrome
Use additional code to identify associated infection, such as:
E. coli infection (B96.2-)
human immunodeficiency virus [HIV] disease (B20)
pneumococcal meningitis (G00.1)
pneumococcal pneumonia (J13)
sepsis due to Streptococcus pneumoniae (A40.3)
Shigella dysenteriae (A03.9)
streptococcus pneumoniae as the cause of diseases classified elsewhere (B95.3)

**D59.32 Hereditary hemolytic-uremic syndrome** HCC Rx ESR COM
Atypical hemolytic uremic syndrome with an identified genetic cause
Code also, if applicable:
defects in the complement system (D84.1)
methylmalonic acidemia (E71.120)

**D59.39 Other hemolytic-uremic syndrome** HCC Rx ESR COM
Atypical (nongenetic) hemolytic uremic syndrome
Secondary hemolytic-uremic syndrome
Code first, if applicable, any associated:
complications of heart transplant (T86.2-)
complications of kidney transplant (T86.1-)
complications of liver transplant (T86.4-)
COVID-19 (U07.1)
Code also, if applicable, any associated condition, such as:
hypertensive emergency (I16.1)
malignant neoplasm (C00-C96)
systemic lupus erythematosus (M32.-)
Use additional code, if applicable, for adverse effect to identify drug (T36-T50 with fifth or sixth character 5)
**AHA:** 2022,4Q,6

**D59.4 Other nonautoimmune hemolytic anemias** HCC Rx ESR COM
Mechanical hemolytic anemia
Microangiopathic hemolytic anemia
Toxic hemolytic anemia

**D59.5 Paroxysmal nocturnal hemoglobinuria [Marchiafava-Micheli]** HCC Rx ESR COM
EXCLUDES 1 *hemoglobinuria NOS (R82.3)*

**D59.6 Hemoglobinuria due to hemolysis from other external causes** HCC Rx ESR COM
Hemoglobinuria from exertion
March hemoglobinuria
Paroxysmal cold hemoglobinuria
Use additional code (Chapter 20) to identify external cause
EXCLUDES 1 *hemoglobinuria NOS (R82.3)*

**D59.8 Other acquired hemolytic anemias** HCC Rx ESR COM

**D59.9 Acquired hemolytic anemia, unspecified** HCC Rx ESR COM
Idiopathic hemolytic anemia, chronic

## Aplastic and other anemias and other bone marrow failure syndromes (D60-D64)

**✓4th D60 Acquired pure red cell aplasia [erythroblastopenia]**
INCLUDES red cell aplasia (acquired) (adult) (with thymoma)
EXCLUDES 1 *congenital red cell aplasia (D61.01)*
**DEF:** Bone marrow failure characterized by underproduction of red blood cells while white blood cell and platelet production remains normal.

**D60.0 Chronic acquired pure red cell aplasia** HCC Rx ESR COM

**D60.1 Transient acquired pure red cell aplasia** Rx ESR COM

**D60.8 Other acquired pure red cell aplasias** HCC Rx ESR COM

**D60.9 Acquired pure red cell aplasia, unspecified** HCC Rx ESR COM

**✓4th D61 Other aplastic anemias and other bone marrow failure syndromes**
EXCLUDES 2 *neutropenia (D70.-)*
**AHA:** 2020,3Q,22; 2014,4Q,22
**DEF:** Aplastic anemia: Bone marrow failure characterized by underproduction of red bloods cells, white blood cells and platelets.

**✓5th D61.0 Constitutional aplastic anemia**

**D61.01 Constitutional (pure) red blood cell aplasia** HCC Rx ESR COM
Blackfan-Diamond syndrome
Congenital (pure) red cell aplasia
Familial hypoplastic anemia
Primary (pure) red cell aplasia
Red cell (pure) aplasia of infants
EXCLUDES 1 *acquired red cell aplasia (D60.9)*

**D61.02 Shwachman-Diamond syndrome** HCC Rx ESR COM
Code also, if applicable, associated conditions such as:
acute myeloblastic leukemia (C92.0-)
exocrine pancreatic insufficiency (K86.81)
myelodysplastic syndrome (D46.-)
Use additional code, if applicable, for genetic susceptibility to other malignant neoplasm (Z15.09)
**AHA:** 2023,4Q,8

**D61.03 Fanconi anemia** HCC Rx ESR COM
Fanconi pancytopenia
Fanconi's anemia
EXCLUDES 1 *Fanconi syndrome (E72.0-)*
**AHA:** 2024,4Q,5

**D61.09 Other constitutional aplastic anemia** HCC Rx ESR COM
Pancytopenia with malformations

**D61.1 Drug-induced aplastic anemia** Rx ESR COM
Use additional code for adverse effect, if applicable, to identify drug (T36-T50 with fifth or sixth character 5)

**D61.2 Aplastic anemia due to other external agents** HCC Rx ESR COM
Code first, if applicable, toxic effects of substances chiefly nonmedicinal as to source (T51-T65)

**D61.3 Idiopathic aplastic anemia** HCC Rx ESR COM

**✓5th D61.8 Other specified aplastic anemias and other bone marrow failure syndromes**

**✓6th D61.81 Pancytopenia**
EXCLUDES 1 *pancytopenia (due to) (with) aplastic anemia (D61.9)*
*pancytopenia (due to) (with) bone marrow infiltration (D61.82)*
*pancytopenia (due to) (with) congenital (pure) red cell aplasia (D61.01)*
*pancytopenia (due to) (with) hairy cell leukemia (C91.4-)*
*pancytopenia (due to) (with) human immunodeficiency virus disease (B20)*
*pancytopenia (due to) (with) leukoerythroblastic anemia (D61.82)*
*pancytopenia (due to) (with) myeloproliferative disease (D47.1)*
EXCLUDES 2 *pancytopenia (due to) (with) myelodysplastic syndromes (D46.-)*
**DEF:** Shortage of all three blood cells: white, red, and platelets.

**D61.810 Antineoplastic chemotherapy induced pancytopenia** ESR
EXCLUDES 2 *aplastic anemia due to antineoplastic chemotherapy (D61.1)*
**AHA:** 2020,3Q,22

**D61.811 Other drug-induced pancytopenia** ESR
EXCLUDES 2 *aplastic anemia due to drugs (D61.1)*
**AHA:** 2025,3Q,21; 2023,3Q,4

**D61.818 Other pancytopenia** HCC ESR
**AHA:** 2025,3Q,21; 2023,1Q,23; 2020,3Q,24; 2019,1Q,16
**TIP:** Assign this code in addition to myeloid leukemia codes (C92.-) when pancytopenia is documented. Although common in some types of myeloid leukemia, pancytopenia is not always inherent.

**D61.82 Myelophthisis** HCC Rx ESR COM
Leukoerythroblastic anemia
Myelophthisic anemia
Panmyelophthisis
Code also the underlying disorder, such as:
malignant neoplasm of breast (C50.-)
tuberculosis (A15.-)
EXCLUDES 1 *idiopathic myelofibrosis (D47.1)*
*myelofibrosis NOS (D75.81)*
*myelofibrosis with myeloid metaplasia (D47.4)*
*primary myelofibrosis (D47.1)*
*secondary myelofibrosis (D75.81)*
**DEF:** Condition that occurs when normal hematopoietic tissue in the bone marrow is replaced with abnormal tissue, such as fibrous tissue or tumors. Most commonly seen during the advanced stages of cancer.

**D61.89 Other specified aplastic anemias and other bone marrow failure syndromes** HCC Rx ESR COM

**D61.9 Aplastic anemia, unspecified** Rx ESR COM
Hypoplastic anemia NOS
Medullary hypoplasia

**D62 Acute posthemorrhagic anemia**
EXCLUDES 1 *anemia due to chronic blood loss (D50.0)*
*blood loss anemia NOS (D50.0)*
*congenital anemia from fetal blood loss (P61.3)*
**AHA:** 2023,1Q,15,16; 2019,3Q,11,17

**✓4th D63 Anemia in chronic diseases classified elsewhere**

***D63.0 Anemia in neoplastic disease***
Code first neoplasm (C00-D49)
EXCLUDES 1 *aplastic anemia due to antineoplastic chemotherapy (D61.1)*
EXCLUDES 2 *anemia due to antineoplastic chemotherapy (D64.81)*

***D63.1 Anemia in chronic kidney disease***
Erythropoietin resistant anemia (EPO resistant anemia)
Code first underlying chronic kidney disease (CKD) (N18.-)

**D63.8 Anemia in other chronic diseases classified elsewhere**
Code first underlying disease, such as:
diphyllobothriasis (B7Ø.Ø)
hookworm disease (B76.Ø-B76.9)
hypothyroidism (EØØ.Ø-EØ3.9)
malaria (B5Ø.Ø-B54)
symptomatic late syphilis (A52.79)
tuberculosis (A18.89)

**D64 Other anemias**
EXCLUDES 1 *refractory anemia (D46.-)*
*refractory anemia with excess blasts in transformation [RAEB T] (C92.Ø-)*
**DEF:** Sideroblastic anemia: Hereditary or secondary disorder in which the red blood cells cannot effectively use iron, a nutrient needed to make hemoglobin. Although the iron can enter the red blood cell it is not assimilated into the hemoglobin molecule and builds up ringed sideroblasts around the cell nucleus.

**D64.Ø Hereditary sideroblastic anemia** HCC Rx ESR COM
Sex-linked hypochromic sideroblastic anemia

**D64.1 Secondary sideroblastic anemia due to disease** HCC Rx ESR COM
Code first underlying disease

**D64.2 Secondary sideroblastic anemia due to drugs and toxins** Rx ESR COM
Code first poisoning due to drug or toxin, if applicable (T36-T65 with fifth or sixth character 1-4)
Use additional code for adverse effect, if applicable, to identify drug (T36-T5Ø with fifth or sixth character 5)

**D64.3 Other sideroblastic anemias** HCC Rx ESR COM
Pyridoxine-responsive sideroblastic anemia NEC
Sideroblastic anemia NOS

**D64.4 Congenital dyserythropoietic anemia** HCC
Dyshematopoietic anemia (congenital)
EXCLUDES 1 *Blackfan-Diamond syndrome (D61.Ø1)*
*Di Guglielmo's disease (C94.Ø)*

**D64.8 Other specified anemias**

**D64.81 Anemia due to antineoplastic chemotherapy**
Antineoplastic chemotherapy induced anemia
EXCLUDES 2 *anemia in neoplastic disease (D63.Ø)*
*aplastic anemia due to antineoplastic chemotherapy (D61.1)*
**AHA:** 2023,2Q,17; 2021,3Q,4; 2014,4Q,22

**D64.89 Other specified anemias**
Infantile pseudoleukemia

**D64.9 Anemia, unspecified**
**AHA:** 2020,3Q,24; 2018,4Q,88; 2017,1Q,7

## Coagulation defects, purpura and other hemorrhagic conditions (D65-D69)

**D65 Disseminated intravascular coagulation [defibrination syndrome]** ESR COM
Afibrinogenemia, acquired
Consumption coagulopathy
COVID-19 associated diffuse or disseminated intravascular coagulopathy
Diffuse or disseminated intravascular coagulation [DIC]
Fibrinolytic hemorrhage, acquired
Fibrinolytic purpura
Purpura fulminans
Code also, if applicable, associated condition
EXCLUDES 1 *disseminated intravascular coagulation (complicating):*
~~*abortion or ectopic or molar pregnancy (OØØ-OØ7, OØ8.1)*~~
*in newborn (P6Ø)*
*pregnancy, childbirth and the puerperium (O45.Ø, O46.Ø, O67.Ø, O72.3)*
EXCLUDES 2 ▶*disseminated intravascular coagulation (complicating):*◀
▶*abortion or ectopic or molar pregnancy (OØØ-OØ7, OØ8.1)*◀
**AHA:** 2026,1Q,34; 2021,1Q,39

### Coagulation

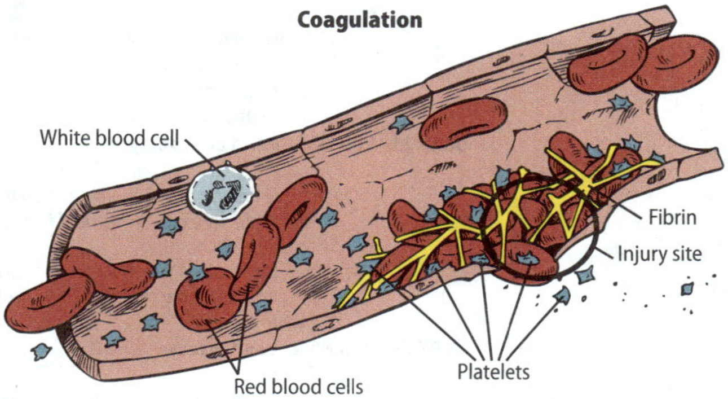


**D66 Hereditary factor VIII deficiency** HCC ESR COM
Classical hemophilia
Deficiency factor VIII (with functional defect)
Hemophilia A
Hemophilia NOS
EXCLUDES 1 *factor VIII deficiency with vascular defect (D68.Ø-)*
**AHA:** 2022,4Q,9
**DEF:** Hereditary, sex-linked lack of antihemophilic globulin (AHG) (factor VIII) that causes abnormal coagulation characterized by increased bleeding; large bruises of skin; bleeding in the mouth, nose, and gastrointestinal tract; and hemorrhages into joints, resulting in swelling and impaired function.
**TIP:** Factor VIII deficiency may also be documented in patients with VWD. Only a code for the VWD should be reported; do not report code D66.

**D67 Hereditary factor IX deficiency** HCC ESR COM
Christmas disease
Factor IX deficiency (with functional defect)
Hemophilia B
Plasma thromboplastin component [PTC] deficiency

**D68 Other coagulation defects**
EXCLUDES 1 *abnormal coagulation profile NOS (R79.1)*
EXCLUDES 2 *coagulation defects complicating abortion or ectopic or molar pregnancy (OØØ-OØ7, OØ8.1)*
*coagulation defects complicating pregnancy, childbirth and the puerperium (O45.Ø, O46.Ø, O67.Ø, O72.3)*
**AHA:** 2016,1Q,14

**D68.Ø Von Willebrand disease**
EXCLUDES 1 *capillary fragility (hereditary) (D69.8)*
*factor VIII deficiency NOS (D66)*
*factor VIII deficiency with functional defect (D66)*
**AHA:** 2022,4Q,7-9
**DEF:** Congenital, abnormal blood coagulation caused by deficient blood factor VII. Symptoms include excess or prolonged bleeding.
**TIP:** Factor VIII deficiency may also be documented in patients with VWD. Only a code for the VWD should be reported; do not report code D66.

**D68.ØØ Von Willebrand disease, unspecified** HCC ESR COM

**D68.01 Von Willebrand disease, type 1** HCC ESR COM
Partial quantitative deficiency of von Willebrand factor
Type 1C von Willebrand disease
**AHA:** 2022,4Q,9

✓6th **D68.02 Von Willebrand disease, type 2**
Qualitative defects of von Willebrand factor

**D68.020 Von Willebrand disease, type 2A** HCC ESR COM
Qualitative defects of von Willebrand factor with decreased platelet adhesion and selective deficiency of high-molecular-weight multimers

**D68.021 Von Willebrand disease, type 2B** HCC ESR COM
Qualitative defects of von Willebrand factor with high-molecular-weight von Willebrand factor loss
Qualitative defects of von Willebrand factor with hyper-adhesive forms
Qualitative defects of von Willebrand factor with increased affinity for platelet glycoprotein Ib

**D68.022 Von Willebrand disease, type 2M** HCC ESR COM
Qualitative defects of von Willebrand factor with defective platelet adhesion with a normal size distribution of von Willebrand factor multimers

**D68.023 Von Willebrand disease, type 2N** HCC ESR COM
Qualitative defects of von Willebrand factor with defective von Willebrand factor to factor VIII binding
Qualitative defects of von Willebrand factor with markedly decreased affinity for factor VIII

**D68.029 Von Willebrand disease, type 2, unspecified** HCC ESR COM
Qualitative defect in von Willebrand factor function, with no further subtyping

**D68.03 Von Willebrand disease, type 3** HCC ESR COM
(Near) complete absence of von Willebrand factor
Total quantitative deficiency of von Willebrand factor

**D68.04 Acquired von Willebrand disease** HCC ESR COM
Acquired von Willebrand syndrome

**D68.09 Other von Willebrand disease** HCC ESR COM
Platelet-type von Willebrand disease
Pseudo-von Willebrand disease
Code also, if applicable, qualitative platelet defects ►(D69.1-)◄

**D68.1 Hereditary factor XI deficiency** HCC ESR COM
Hemophilia C
Plasma thromboplastin antecedent [PTA] deficiency
Rosenthal's disease

**D68.2 Hereditary deficiency of other clotting factors** HCC ESR COM
AC globulin deficiency
Congenital afibrinogenemia
Deficiency of factor I [fibrinogen]
Deficiency of factor II [prothrombin]
Deficiency of factor V [labile]
Deficiency of factor VII [stable]
Deficiency of factor X [Stuart-Prower]
Deficiency of factor XII [Hageman]
Deficiency of factor XIII [fibrin stabilizing]
Dysfibrinogenemia (congenital)
Hypoproconvertinemia
Owren's disease
Proaccelerin deficiency
**AHA:** 2025,2Q,3

✓5th **D68.3 Hemorrhagic disorder due to circulating anticoagulants**

✓6th **D68.31 Hemorrhagic disorder due to intrinsic circulating anticoagulants, antibodies, or inhibitors**

**D68.311 Acquired hemophilia** HCC ESR COM
Autoimmune hemophilia
Autoimmune inhibitors to clotting factors
Secondary hemophilia

**D68.312 Antiphospholipid antibody with hemorrhagic disorder** ESR COM
Lupus anticoagulant (LAC) with hemorrhagic disorder
Systemic lupus erythematosus [SLE] inhibitor with hemorrhagic disorder
EXCLUDES 1 *antiphospholipid antibody, finding without diagnosis (R76.0)*
*lupus anticoagulant (LAC) finding without diagnosis (R76.0)*
*systemic lupus erythematosus [SLE] inhibitor finding without diagnosis (R76.0)*
EXCLUDES 2 *antiphospholipid antibody syndrome (D68.61)*
*antiphospholipid antibody with hypercoagulable state (D68.61)*
*lupus anticoagulant (LAC) with hypercoagulable state (D68.62)*
*systemic lupus erythematosus [SLE] inhibitor with hypercoagulable state (D68.62)*

**D68.318 Other hemorrhagic disorder due to intrinsic circulating anticoagulants, antibodies, or inhibitors** ESR COM
Antithromboplastinemia
Antithromboplastinogenemia
Hemorrhagic disorder due to intrinsic increase in anti-IXa
Hemorrhagic disorder due to intrinsic increase in antithrombin
Hemorrhagic disorder due to intrinsic increase in anti-VIIIa
Hemorrhagic disorder due to intrinsic increase in anti-XIa

**D68.32 Hemorrhagic disorder due to extrinsic circulating anticoagulants** ESR COM
Drug-induced hemorrhagic disorder
Hemorrhagic disorder due to increase in anti-IIa
Hemorrhagic disorder due to increase in anti-Xa
Hyperheparinemia
Use additional code for adverse effect, if applicable, to identify drug (T45.515, T45.525)
**AHA:** 2021,1Q,4; 2016,1Q,14-15
**TIP:** Do not assign to identify routine therapeutic anticoagulation effects; assign only for documented adverse effects.

**D68.4 Acquired coagulation factor deficiency** ESR COM
Deficiency of coagulation factor due to liver disease
Deficiency of coagulation factor due to vitamin K deficiency
EXCLUDES 1 *vitamin K deficiency of newborn (P53)*

✓5th **D68.5 Primary thrombophilia**
Primary hypercoagulable states
EXCLUDES 1 *antiphospholipid syndrome (D68.61)*
*lupus anticoagulant (D68.62)*
*secondary activated protein C resistance (D68.69)*
*secondary antiphospholipid antibody syndrome (D68.69)*
*secondary lupus anticoagulant with hypercoagulable state (D68.69)*
*secondary systemic lupus erythematosus [SLE] inhibitor with hypercoagulable state (D68.69)*
*systemic lupus erythematosus [SLE] inhibitor finding without diagnosis (R76.0)*
*systemic lupus erythematosus [SLE] inhibitor with hemorrhagic disorder (D68.312)*
*thrombotic thrombocytopenic purpura (M31.19)*
**DEF:** Thrombophilia: Increased tendency of the blood to clot, which can lead to thrombus or embolus formation.

**D68.51 Activated protein C resistance** ESR COM
Factor V Leiden mutation
**AHA:** 2025,2Q,3

**D68.52 Prothrombin gene mutation** ESR COM

**D68.59 Other primary thrombophilia** ESR COM
Antithrombin III deficiency
Hypercoagulable state NOS
Primary hypercoagulable state NEC
Primary thrombophilia NEC
Protein C deficiency
Protein S deficiency
Thrombophilia NOS
**AHA:** 2021,2Q,8

✓5th **D68.6 Other thrombophilia**
Other hypercoagulable states
EXCLUDES 1 *diffuse or disseminated intravascular coagulation [DIC] (D65)*
*heparin induced thrombocytopenia (HIT) (D75.82-)*
*hyperhomocysteinemia (E72.11)*

**D68.61 Antiphospholipid syndrome** ESR COM
Anticardiolipin syndrome
Antiphospholipid antibody syndrome
EXCLUDES 1 *anti-phospholipid antibody, finding without diagnosis (R76.Ø)*
EXCLUDES 2 *anti-phospholipid antibody with hemorrhagic disorder (D68.312)*
*lupus anticoagulant syndrome (D68.62)*

**D68.62 Lupus anticoagulant syndrome** ESR COM
Lupus anticoagulant
Presence of systemic lupus erythematosus [SLE] inhibitor
EXCLUDES 1 *lupus anticoagulant (LAC) finding without diagnosis (R76.Ø)*
EXCLUDES 2 *anticardiolipin syndrome (D68.61)*
*antiphospholipid syndrome (D68.61)*
*lupus anticoagulant (LAC) with hemorrhagic disorder (D68.312)*

**D68.69 Other thrombophilia** ESR COM
COVID-19 associated hypercoagulability
Hypercoagulable states NEC
Secondary hypercoagulable state NOS
Code also, if applicable, associated condition
**AHA:** 2021,2Q,8

**D68.8 Other specified coagulation defects** ESR COM
COVID-19 associated coagulopathy
Code also, if applicable, associated condition
EXCLUDES 1 *hemorrhagic disease of newborn (P53)*
**AHA:** 2021,1Q,39

**D68.9 Coagulation defect, unspecified** ESR COM

✓4th **D69 Purpura and other hemorrhagic conditions**
EXCLUDES 1 *benign hypergammaglobulinemic purpura (D89.Ø)*
*cryoglobulinemic purpura (D89.1)*
*essential (hemorrhagic) thrombocythemia (D47.3)*
*hemorrhagic thrombocythemia (D47.3)*
*purpura fulminans (D65)*
*thrombotic thrombocytopenic purpura (M31.19)*
*Waldenstrom hypergammaglobulinemic purpura (D89.Ø)*
**AHA:** 2026,1Q,34

**D69.Ø Allergic purpura** ESR
Allergic vasculitis
Nonthrombocytopenic hemorrhagic purpura
Nonthrombocytopenic idiopathic purpura
Purpura anaphylactoid
Purpura Henoch(-Schonlein)
Purpura rheumatica
Vascular purpura
EXCLUDES 1 *thrombocytopenic hemorrhagic purpura (D69.3)*
**AHA:** 2020,3Q,26
**DEF:** Any hemorrhagic condition, thrombocytic or nonthrombocytopenic in origin, caused by a presumed allergic reaction.

▲ ✓5th **D69.1 Qualitative platelet defects**
~~Bernard-Soulier [giant platelet] syndrome~~
~~Glanzmann's disease~~
~~Grey platelet syndrome~~
~~Thromboasthenia (hemorrhagic) (hereditary)~~
~~Thrombocytopathy~~
EXCLUDES 1 *hemolytic-uremic syndrome (D59.3-)*
EXCLUDES 2 *von Willebrand disease (D68.Ø-)*

● **D69.11 Glanzmann thrombasthenia**
Glanzmann's disease
Thromboasthenia (hemorrhagic) (hereditary)

● **D69.19 Other qualitative platelet defects**
Bernard-Soulier [giant platelet] syndrome
Grey platelet syndrome
Thrombocytopathy

**D69.2 Other nonthrombocytopenic purpura** ESR
Purpura NOS
Purpura simplex
Senile purpura

**D69.3 Immune thrombocytopenic purpura** HCC Rx ESR COM
Hemorrhagic (thrombocytopenic) purpura
Idiopathic thrombocytopenic purpura
Tidal platelet dysgenesis
**DEF:** Tidal platelet dysgenesis: Fluctuation of platelet counts from normal to very low within periods of 20 to 40 days and may involve autoimmune platelet destruction.

✓5th **D69.4 Other primary thrombocytopenia**
EXCLUDES 1 *transient neonatal thrombocytopenia (P61.Ø)*
*Wiskott-Aldrich syndrome (D82.Ø)*

**D69.41 Evans syndrome** HCC ESR COM

**D69.42 Congenital and hereditary thrombocytopenia purpura** HCC ESR COM
Congenital thrombocytopenia
Hereditary thrombocytopenia
Code first congenital or hereditary disorder, such as: thrombocytopenia with absent radius (TAR syndrome) (Q87.2)

**D69.49 Other primary thrombocytopenia** HCC ESR COM
Megakaryocytic hypoplasia
Primary thrombocytopenia NOS

✓5th **D69.5 Secondary thrombocytopenia**
EXCLUDES 1 *heparin induced thrombocytopenia (HIT) (D75.82-)*
*transient thrombocytopenia of newborn (P61.Ø)*

**D69.51 Posttransfusion purpura**
Posttransfusion purpura from whole blood (fresh) or blood products
PTP

**D69.59 Other secondary thrombocytopenia**
**AHA:** 2014,4Q,22

**D69.6 Thrombocytopenia, unspecified** ESR
**AHA:** 2020,3Q,24

**D69.8 Other specified hemorrhagic conditions** ESR
Capillary fragility (hereditary)
Vascular pseudohemophilia

**D69.9 Hemorrhagic condition, unspecified** ESR

## Other disorders of blood and blood-forming organs (D7Ø-D77)

✓4th **D7Ø Neutropenia**
INCLUDES agranulocytosis
decreased absolute neurophile count (ANC)
Code also, if applicable, mucositis (J34.81, K12.3-, K92.81, N76.81)
Use additional code for any associated:
fever (R5Ø.81)
EXCLUDES 1 *neutropenic splenomegaly (D73.81)*
*transient neonatal neutropenia (P61.5)*
**DEF:** Abnormally low number of neutrophils. Neutrophils are phagocytic, meaning they surround and consume harmful pathogens, primarily bacteria. When neutrophil counts decrease the risk of infection increases.

**D7Ø.Ø Congenital agranulocytosis** HCC ESR COM
Congenital neutropenia
Infantile genetic agranulocytosis
Kostmann's disease

**D7Ø.1 Agranulocytosis secondary to cancer chemotherapy** ESR
Code also underlying neoplasm
Use additional code for adverse effect, if applicable, to identify drug (T45.1X5)
**AHA:** 2020,3Q,22; 2014,4Q,22

**D7Ø.2 Other drug-induced agranulocytosis** ESR
Use additional code for adverse effect, if applicable, to identify drug (T36-T5Ø with fifth or sixth character 5)

**D7Ø.3 Neutropenia due to infection** ESR

**D7Ø.4 Cyclic neutropenia** HCC ESR COM
Cyclic hematopoiesis
Periodic neutropenia

**D7Ø.8 Other neutropenia** ESR

**D7Ø.9 Neutropenia, unspecified** ESR
**AHA:** 2020,3Q,24

**✓4th D71 Functional disorders of polymorphonuclear neutrophils**

**D71.1 Leukocyte adhesion deficiency** HCC ESR
LAD-I
LAD-II
LAD-III
Leukocyte adhesion deficiency type I
Leukocyte adhesion deficiency type II
Leukocyte adhesion deficiency type III

**D71.8 Other functional disorders of polymorphonuclear neutrophils** HCC ESR
Cell membrane receptor complex [CR3] defect
Chronic (childhood) granulomatous disease
Congenital dysphagocytosis
Progressive septic granulomatosis

**D71.9 Functional disorders of polymorphonuclear neutrophils, unspecified** HCC ESR

**✓4th D72 Other disorders of white blood cells**
EXCLUDES 1 *basophilia (D72.824)*
~~*neutropenia (D70)*~~
*immunity disorders (D80-D89)*
*preleukemia (syndrome) (D46.9)*
EXCLUDES 2 ▶*neutropenia (D70)*◀

**D72.Ø Genetic anomalies of leukocytes** HCC ESR COM
Alder (granulation) (granulocyte) anomaly
Alder syndrome
Hereditary leukocytic hypersegmentation
Hereditary leukocytic hyposegmentation
Hereditary leukomelanopathy
May-Hegglin (granulation) (granulocyte) anomaly
May-Hegglin syndrome
Pelger-Huet (granulation) (granulocyte) anomaly
Pelger-Huet syndrome
EXCLUDES 1 *Chediak (-Steinbrinck)-Higashi syndrome (E7Ø.33Ø)*

**✓5th D72.1 Eosinophilia**
EXCLUDES 2 *Loffler's syndrome (J82.89)*
*pulmonary eosinophilia (J82.-)*
**AHA:** 2020,4Q,8-10
**DEF:** Abnormally large accumulation or formation of eosinophils (nucleated, granular leukocytes) in the blood, characteristic of allergic states and infection.

**D72.1Ø Eosinophilia, unspecified**

**✓6th D72.11 Hypereosinophilic syndrome [HES]**

**D72.11Ø Idiopathic hypereosinophilic syndrome [IHES]**

**D72.111 Lymphocytic Variant Hypereosinophilic Syndrome [LHES]**
Lymphocyte variant hypereosinophilia
Code also, if applicable, any associated lymphocytic neoplastic disorder

**D72.118 Other hypereosinophilic syndrome**
Episodic angioedema with eosinophilia
Gleich's syndrome

**D72.119 Hypereosinophilic syndrome [HES], unspecified**

**D72.12 Drug rash with eosinophilia and systemic symptoms syndrome**
DRESS syndrome
Use additional code for adverse effect, if applicable, to identify drug (T36-T5Ø with fifth or sixth character 5)

***D72.18 Eosinophilia in diseases classified elsewhere***
Code first underlying disease, such as:
chronic myelomonocytic leukemia (C93.1-)

**D72.19 Other eosinophilia**
Familial eosinophilia
Hereditary eosinophilia

**✓5th D72.8 Other specified disorders of white blood cells**
EXCLUDES 1 *leukemia (C91-C95)*

**✓6th D72.81 Decreased white blood cell count**
EXCLUDES 1 ~~*neutropenia (D7Ø.-)*~~
EXCLUDES 2 ▶*neutropenia (D7Ø)*◀

**D72.81Ø Lymphocytopenia**
Decreased lymphocytes

**D72.818 Other decreased white blood cell count**
Basophilic leukopenia
Eosinophilic leukopenia
Monocytopenia
Other decreased leukocytes
Plasmacytopenia

**D72.819 Decreased white blood cell count, unspecified**
Decreased leukocytes, unspecified
Leukocytopenia, unspecified
Leukopenia
EXCLUDES 1 ~~*malignant leukopenia (D70.9)*~~

**✓6th D72.82 Elevated white blood cell count**
EXCLUDES 1 *eosinophilia (D72.1)*

**D72.82Ø Lymphocytosis (symptomatic)**
Elevated lymphocytes

**D72.821 Monocytosis (symptomatic)**
EXCLUDES 1 *infectious mononucleosis (B27.-)*

**D72.822 Plasmacytosis**

**D72.823 Leukemoid reaction**
Basophilic leukemoid reaction
Leukemoid reaction NOS
Lymphocytic leukemoid reaction
Monocytic leukemoid reaction
Myelocytic leukemoid reaction
Neutrophilic leukemoid reaction

**D72.824 Basophilia**
**DEF:** Increase in the basophils of the blood, a type of white blood cell, often seen in conjunction with neoplastic disorders.

**D72.825 Bandemia**
Bandemia without diagnosis of specific infection
EXCLUDES 1 *confirmed infection - code to infection*
*leukemia (C91.-, C92.-, C93.-, C94.-, C95.-)*
**DEF:** Increase in early neutrophil cells, called band cells, that may indicate infection.

**D72.828 Other elevated white blood cell count**

**D72.829 Elevated white blood cell count, unspecified**
Elevated leukocytes, unspecified
Leukocytosis, unspecified

**D72.89 Other specified disorders of white blood cells**
Abnormality of white blood cells NEC

**D72.9 Disorder of white blood cells, unspecified**
Abnormal leukocyte differential NOS

**✓4th D73 Diseases of spleen**

**D73.Ø Hyposplenism**
Atrophy of spleen
EXCLUDES 1 *asplenia (congenital) (Q89.Ø1)*
*postsurgical absence of spleen (Z9Ø.81)*
**AHA:** 2025,1Q,24

**D73.1 Hypersplenism**
EXCLUDES 1 *neutropenic splenomegaly (D73.81)*
*primary splenic neutropenia (D73.81)*
*splenitis, splenomegaly in late syphilis (A52.79)*
*splenitis, splenomegaly in tuberculosis (A18.85)*
*splenomegaly congenital (Q89.Ø)*
*splenomegaly NOS (R16.1)*

**D73.2 Chronic congestive splenomegaly**

**D73.3 Abscess of spleen**

**D73.4 Cyst of spleen**

**D73.5 Infarction of spleen**
Splenic rupture, nontraumatic
Torsion of spleen
EXCLUDES 1 *rupture of spleen due to Plasmodium vivax malaria (B51.Ø)*
*traumatic rupture of spleen (S36.Ø3-)*

**✓5th D73.8 Other diseases of spleen**

**D73.81 Neutropenic splenomegaly**
Werner-Schultz disease

**D73.89 Other diseases of spleen**
Fibrosis of spleen NOS
Perisplenitis
Splenitis NOS

**D73.9 Disease of spleen, unspecified**

**✓4th D74 Methemoglobinemia**

**D74.Ø Congenital methemoglobinemia**
Congenital NADH-methemoglobin reductase deficiency
Hemoglobin-M [Hb-M] disease
Methemoglobinemia, hereditary

**D74.8 Other methemoglobinemias**
Acquired methemoglobinemia (with sulfhemoglobinemia)
Toxic methemoglobinemia

**D74.9 Methemoglobinemia, unspecified**

✓4th **D75 Other and unspecified diseases of blood and blood-forming organs**
EXCLUDES 2 *acute lymphadenitis (LØ4.-)*
*chronic lymphadenitis (I88.1)*
*enlarged lymph nodes (R59.-)*
*hypergammaglobulinemia NOS (D89.2)*
*lymphadenitis NOS (I88.9)*
*mesenteric lymphadenitis (acute) (chronic) (I88.Ø)*

**D75.Ø Familial erythrocytosis**
Benign polycythemia
Familial polycythemia
EXCLUDES 1 *hereditary ovalocytosis (D58.1)*

**D75.1 Secondary polycythemia**
Acquired polycythemia
Emotional polycythemia
Erythrocytosis NOS
Hypoxemic polycythemia
Nephrogenous polycythemia
Polycythemia due to erythropoietin
Polycythemia due to fall in plasma volume
Polycythemia due to high altitude
Polycythemia due to stress
Polycythemia NOS
Relative polycythemia
EXCLUDES 1 *polycythemia neonatorum (P61.1)*
*polycythemia vera (D45)*
**DEF:** Elevated number of red blood cells in circulating blood as a result of reduced oxygen supply to the tissues.

✓5th **D75.8 Other specified diseases of blood and blood-forming organs**

***D75.81 Myelofibrosis*** HCC Rx ESR COM
Myelofibrosis NOS
Secondary myelofibrosis NOS
Code first the underlying disorder, such as:
malignant neoplasm of breast (C5Ø.-)
Use additional code for adverse effect, if applicable, to identify drug (T45.1X5)
Use additional code, if applicable, for associated therapy-related myelodysplastic syndrome (D46.-)
EXCLUDES 1 *acute myelofibrosis (C94.4-)*
*idiopathic myelofibrosis (D47.1)*
*leukoerythroblastic anemia (D61.82)*
*myelofibrosis with myeloid metaplasia (D47.4)*
*myelophthisic anemia (D61.82)*
*myelophthisis (D61.82)*
*primary myelofibrosis (D47.1)*

✓6th **D75.82 Heparin induced thrombocytopenia (HIT)**
Use additional code, if applicable, for adverse effect of heparin (T45.515-)
**AHA:** 2022,4Q,9-10
**DEF:** Immune-mediated reaction to heparin therapy causing an abrupt fall in platelet count and serious complications such as pulmonary embolism, stroke, AMI, or DVT.

**D75.821 Non-immune heparin-induced thrombocytopenia** ESR COM
Non-immune HIT
Type 1 heparin-induced thrombocytopenia

**D75.822 Immune-mediated heparin-induced thrombocytopenia** ESR COM
Immune-mediated HIT
Type 2 heparin-induced thrombocytopenia

**D75.828 Other heparin-induced thrombocytopenia syndrome** ESR COM
Autoimmune heparin-induced thrombocytopenia syndrome
Delayed-onset heparin-induced thrombocytopenia
Persisting heparin-induced thrombocytopenia

**D75.829 Heparin-induced thrombocytopenia, unspecified** ESR COM

✓6th **D75.83 Thrombocytosis**
EXCLUDES 2 *essential thrombocythemia (D47.3)*
**AHA:** 2021,4Q,7-8

**D75.838 Other thrombocytosis**
Reactive thrombocytosis
Secondary thrombocytosis
Code also underlying condition, if known and applicable

**D75.839 Thrombocytosis, unspecified**
Thrombocythemia NOS
Thrombocytosis NOS

**D75.84 Other platelet-activating anti-PF4 disorders** HCC ESR COM
Spontaneous heparin-induced thrombocytopenia syndrome (without heparin exposure)
Thrombosis with thrombocytopenia syndrome
Vaccine-induced thrombotic thrombocytopenia
Use additional code, if applicable, for adverse effect of other viral vaccine (T5Ø.B95-)
**AHA:** 2022,4Q,9-10

**D75.89 Other specified diseases of blood and blood-forming organs**

**D75.9 Disease of blood and blood-forming organs, unspecified**

**D75.A Glucose-6-phosphate dehydrogenase (G6PD) deficiency without anemia**
EXCLUDES 1 *glucose-6-phosphate dehydrogenase (G6PD) deficiency with anemia (D55.Ø)*
**AHA:** 2019,4Q,4-5

✓4th **D76 Other specified diseases with participation of lymphoreticular and reticulohistiocytic tissue**
EXCLUDES 1 *(Abt-) Letterer-Siwe disease (C96.Ø)*
*eosinophilic granuloma (C96.6)*
*Hand-Schuller-Christian disease (C96.5)*
*histiocytic medullary reticulosis (C96.9)*
*histiocytic sarcoma (C96.A)*
*histiocytosis X, multifocal (C96.5)*
*histiocytosis X, unifocal (C96.6)*
*Langerhans-cell histiocytosis NOS (C96.6)*
*Langerhans-cell histiocytosis, multifocal (C96.5)*
*Langerhans-cell histiocytosis, unifocal (C96.6)*
*leukemic reticuloendotheliosis (C91.4-)*
*lipomelanotic reticulosis (I89.8)*
*malignant histiocytosis (C96.A)*
*malignant reticulosis (C86.Ø)*
*nonlipid reticuloendotheliosis (C96.Ø)*

**D76.1 Hemophagocytic lymphohistiocytosis** HCC ESR COM
Familial hemophagocytic reticulosis
Histiocytoses of mononuclear phagocytes

**D76.2 Hemophagocytic syndrome, infection-associated** ESR COM
Use additional code to identify infectious agent or disease

**D76.3 Other histiocytosis syndromes** HCC ESR COM
Reticulohistiocytoma (giant-cell)
Sinus histiocytosis with massive lymphadenopathy
Xanthogranuloma

***D77 Other disorders of blood and blood-forming organs in diseases classified elsewhere***
Code first underlying disease, such as:
amyloidosis (E85.-)
congenital early syphilis (A5Ø.Ø-)
echinococcosis (B67.Ø-B67.9)
malaria (B5Ø.Ø-B54)
schistosomiasis [bilharziasis] (B65.Ø-B65.9)
vitamin C deficiency (E54)
EXCLUDES 1 *rupture of spleen due to Plasmodium vivax malaria (B51.Ø)*
*splenitis, splenomegaly in late syphilis (A52.79)*
*splenitis, splenomegaly in tuberculosis (A18.85)*

## Intraoperative and postprocedural complications of the spleen (D78)

✓4th **D78 Intraoperative and postprocedural complications of the spleen**
**AHA:** 2016,4Q,9-10

✓5th **D78.Ø Intraoperative hemorrhage and hematoma of the spleen complicating a procedure**
EXCLUDES 1 *intraoperative hemorrhage and hematoma of the spleen due to accidental puncture or laceration during a procedure (D78.1-)*

**D78.Ø1 Intraoperative hemorrhage and hematoma of the spleen complicating a procedure on the spleen**

**D78.Ø2 Intraoperative hemorrhage and hematoma of the spleen complicating other procedure**

✓5th **D78.1 Accidental puncture and laceration of the spleen during a procedure**
- **D78.11 Accidental puncture and laceration of the spleen during a procedure on the spleen**
- **D78.12 Accidental puncture and laceration of the spleen during other procedure**
  - **AHA:** 2022,1Q,22

✓5th **D78.2 Postprocedural hemorrhage of the spleen following a procedure**
- **D78.21 Postprocedural hemorrhage of the spleen following a procedure on the spleen**
- **D78.22 Postprocedural hemorrhage of the spleen following other procedure**

✓5th **D78.3 Postprocedural hematoma and seroma of the spleen following a procedure**
- **D78.31 Postprocedural hematoma of the spleen following a procedure on the spleen**
- **D78.32 Postprocedural hematoma of the spleen following other procedure**
- **D78.33 Postprocedural seroma of the spleen following a procedure on the spleen**
- **D78.34 Postprocedural seroma of the spleen following other procedure**

✓5th **D78.8 Other intraoperative and postprocedural complications of the spleen**
- Use additional code, if applicable, to further specify disorder
- **D78.81 Other intraoperative complications of the spleen**
- **D78.89 Other postprocedural complications of the spleen**

## Certain disorders involving the immune mechanism (D8Ø-D89)

INCLUDES defects in the complement system
immunodeficiency disorders, except human immunodeficiency virus [HIV] disease
sarcoidosis

EXCLUDES 1 *autoimmune disease (systemic) NOS (M35.9)*
*~~human immunodeficiency virus [HIV] disease (B2Ø)~~*
*functional disorders of polymorphonuclear neutrophils (D71-)*

EXCLUDES 2 ▶*human immunodeficiency virus [HIV] disease (B2Ø)*◀

✓4th **D8Ø Immunodeficiency with predominantly antibody defects**
- **D8Ø.Ø Hereditary hypogammaglobulinemia** HCC Rx ESR COM
  - Autosomal recessive agammaglobulinemia (Swiss type)
  - X-linked agammaglobulinemia [Bruton] (with growth hormone deficiency)
- **D8Ø.1 Nonfamilial hypogammaglobulinemia** Rx ESR COM
  - Agammaglobulinemia with immunoglobulin-bearing B-lymphocytes
  - Common variable agammaglobulinemia [CVAgamma]
  - Hypogammaglobulinemia NOS
- **D8Ø.2 Selective deficiency of immunoglobulin A [IgA]** HCC Rx ESR COM
- **D8Ø.3 Selective deficiency of immunoglobulin G [IgG] subclasses** HCC Rx ESR COM
- **D8Ø.4 Selective deficiency of immunoglobulin M [IgM]** HCC Rx ESR COM
- **D8Ø.5 Immunodeficiency with increased immunoglobulin M [IgM]** HCC Rx ESR COM
- **D8Ø.6 Antibody deficiency with near-normal immunoglobulins or with hyperimmunoglobulinemia** Rx ESR COM
- **D8Ø.7 Transient hypogammaglobulinemia of infancy** Rx ESR COM
- **D8Ø.8 Other immunodeficiencies with predominantly antibody defects** Rx ESR COM
  - Kappa light chain deficiency
- **D8Ø.9 Immunodeficiency with predominantly antibody defects, unspecified** Rx ESR COM

✓4th **D81 Combined immunodeficiencies**

EXCLUDES 1 *autosomal recessive agammaglobulinemia (Swiss type) (D8Ø.Ø)*

- **D81.Ø Severe combined immunodeficiency [SCID] with reticular dysgenesis** HCC Rx ESR COM
- **D81.1 Severe combined immunodeficiency [SCID] with low T- and B-cell numbers** HCC Rx ESR COM
- **D81.2 Severe combined immunodeficiency [SCID] with low or normal B-cell numbers** HCC Rx ESR COM

✓5th **D81.3 Adenosine deaminase [ADA] deficiency**
- **AHA:** 2019,4Q,5-6
- **D81.3Ø Adenosine deaminase deficiency, unspecified** HCC Rx ESR COM
  - ADA deficiency NOS
- **D81.31 Severe combined immunodeficiency due to adenosine deaminase deficiency** HCC Rx ESR COM
  - ADA deficiency with SCID
  - Adenosine deaminase [ADA] deficiency with severe combined immunodeficiency
- **D81.32 Adenosine deaminase 2 deficiency** HCC Rx ESR COM
  - ADA2 deficiency
  - Adenosine deaminase deficiency type 2
  - Code also, if applicable, any associated manifestations, such as:
    - polyarteritis nodosa (M3Ø.Ø)
    - stroke (I63.-)
- **D81.39 Other adenosine deaminase deficiency** HCC Rx ESR COM
  - Adenosine deaminase [ADA] deficiency type 1, NOS
  - Adenosine deaminase [ADA] deficiency type 1, without SCID
  - Adenosine deaminase [ADA] deficiency type 1, without severe combined immunodeficiency
  - Partial ADA deficiency (type 1)
  - Partial adenosine deaminase deficiency (type 1)

- **D81.4 Nezelof's syndrome** HCC Rx ESR COM
- **D81.5 Purine nucleoside phosphorylase [PNP] deficiency** HCC Rx ESR COM
- **D81.6 Major histocompatibility complex class I deficiency** HCC Rx ESR COM
  - Bare lymphocyte syndrome
- **D81.7 Major histocompatibility complex class II deficiency** HCC Rx ESR COM

✓5th **D81.8 Other combined immunodeficiencies**

✓6th **D81.81 Biotin-dependent carboxylase deficiency**
- Multiple carboxylase deficiency
- EXCLUDES 1 *biotin-dependent carboxylase deficiency due to dietary deficiency of biotin (E53.8)*
- **D81.81Ø Biotinidase deficiency**
- **D81.818 Other biotin-dependent carboxylase deficiency**
  - Holocarboxylase synthetase deficiency
  - Other multiple carboxylase deficiency
- **D81.819 Biotin-dependent carboxylase deficiency, unspecified**
  - Multiple carboxylase deficiency, unspecified

- **D81.82 Activated Phosphoinositide 3-kinase Delta Syndrome [APDS]** HCC Rx ESR COM
  - p11Ød-activating mutation causing senescent T cells, lymphadenopathy, and immunodeficiency [PASLI] disease
  - Code also, if applicable, any associated manifestations, such as:
    - bronchiectasis (J47.-)
    - herpes virus infections (BØØ.-)
    - other acute respiratory tract infections (JØØ-JØ6; J2Ø-J22)
    - other infections (AØØ-B99)
    - pneumonia (J12-J18)
  - **AHA:** 2022,4Q,11
- **D81.89 Other combined immunodeficiencies** HCC Rx ESR COM

- **D81.9 Combined immunodeficiency, unspecified** HCC Rx ESR COM
  - Severe combined immunodeficiency disorder [SCID] NOS

✓4th **D82 Immunodeficiency associated with other major defects**

EXCLUDES 1 *ataxia telangiectasia [Louis-Bar] (G11.3)*

- **D82.Ø Wiskott-Aldrich syndrome** HCC Rx ESR COM
  - Immunodeficiency with thrombocytopenia and eczema
- **D82.1 Di George's syndrome** HCC Rx ESR COM
  - Pharyngeal pouch syndrome
  - Thymic alymphoplasia
  - Thymic aplasia or hypoplasia with immunodeficiency
  - **AHA:** 2019,3Q,14
- **D82.2 Immunodeficiency with short-limbed stature** Rx ESR COM
- **D82.3 Immunodeficiency following hereditary defective response to Epstein-Barr virus** Rx ESR COM
  - X-linked lymphoproliferative disease
- **D82.4 Hyperimmunoglobulin E [IgE] syndrome** Rx ESR COM
- **D82.8 Immunodeficiency associated with other specified major defects** Rx ESR COM
- **D82.9 Immunodeficiency associated with major defect, unspecified** Rx ESR COM

**D83 Common variable immunodeficiency**

**D83.Ø Common variable immunodeficiency with predominant abnormalities of B-cell numbers and function** HCC Rx ESR COM

**D83.1 Common variable immunodeficiency with predominant immunoregulatory T-cell disorders** HCC Rx ESR COM

**D83.2 Common variable immunodeficiency with autoantibodies to B- or T-cells** HCC Rx ESR COM

**D83.8 Other common variable immunodeficiencies** HCC Rx ESR COM

**D83.9 Common variable immunodeficiency, unspecified** HCC Rx ESR COM

**D84 Other immunodeficiencies**

**D84.Ø Lymphocyte function antigen-1 [LFA-1] defect** Rx ESR COM

**D84.1 Defects in the complement system** HCC Rx ESR COM

C1 esterase inhibitor [C1-INH] deficiency

**D84.8 Other specified immunodeficiencies**

AHA: 2020,4Q,10-12

***D84.81 Immunodeficiency due to conditions classified elsewhere*** Rx ESR COM

Code first underlying condition, such as:
- chromosomal abnormalities (Q9Ø-Q99)
- diabetes mellitus (EØ8-E13)
- malignant neoplasms (CØØ-C96)

EXCLUDES 1 *certain disorders involving the immune mechanism (D8Ø-D83, D84.Ø, D84.1, D84.9)*
*human immunodeficiency virus [HIV] disease (B2Ø)*

AHA: 2021,1Q,52

**D84.82 Immunodeficiency due to drugs and external causes**

**D84.821 Immunodeficiency due to drugs** Rx ESR COM

Immunodeficiency due to (current or past) medication

Use additional code for adverse effect if applicable, to identify adverse effect of drug (T36-T5Ø with fifth or six character 5)

Use additional code, if applicable, for associated long term (current) drug therapy drug or medication such as:
- long term (current) drug therapy systemic steroids (Z79.52)
- other long term (current) drug therapy (Z79.899)

**D84.822 Immunodeficiency due to external causes** Rx ESR COM

Code also, if applicable, radiological procedure and radiotherapy (Y84.2)

Use additional code for external cause such as:
- exposure to ionizing radiation (W88)

**D84.89 Other immunodeficiencies** Rx ESR COM

**D84.9 Immunodeficiency, unspecified** Rx ESR COM

Immunocompromised NOS
Immunodeficient NOS
Immunosuppressed NOS

AHA: 2020,4Q,10

**D86 Sarcoidosis**

DEF: Clustering of immune cells resulting in granuloma formation. Often affects the lungs and lymphatic system but can occur in other body sites.

**D86.Ø Sarcoidosis of lung** Rx ESR COM

**D86.1 Sarcoidosis of lymph nodes**

**D86.2 Sarcoidosis of lung with sarcoidosis of lymph nodes** Rx ESR COM

**D86.3 Sarcoidosis of skin** HCC

**D86.8 Sarcoidosis of other sites**

**D86.81 Sarcoid meningitis** COM

**D86.82 Multiple cranial nerve palsies in sarcoidosis** Rx ESR COM

**D86.83 Sarcoid iridocyclitis**

**D86.84 Sarcoid pyelonephritis**

Tubulo-interstitial nephropathy in sarcoidosis

**D86.85 Sarcoid myocarditis** COM

**D86.86 Sarcoid arthropathy** HCC

Polyarthritis in sarcoidosis

**D86.87 Sarcoid myositis** HCC

**D86.89 Sarcoidosis of other sites**

Hepatic granuloma
Uveoparotid fever [Heerfordt]

**D86.9 Sarcoidosis, unspecified**

**D89 Other disorders involving the immune mechanism, not elsewhere classified**

EXCLUDES 1 *hyperglobulinemia NOS (R77.1)*
*monoclonal gammopathy (of undetermined significance) (D47.2)*

EXCLUDES 2 *transplant failure and rejection (T86.-)*

**D89.Ø Polyclonal hypergammaglobulinemia** Rx

Benign hypergammaglobulinemic purpura
Polyclonal gammopathy NOS

**D89.1 Cryoglobulinemia** Rx ESR

Cryoglobulinemic purpura
Cryoglobulinemic vasculitis
Essential cryoglobulinemia
Idiopathic cryoglobulinemia
Mixed cryoglobulinemia
Primary cryoglobulinemia
Secondary cryoglobulinemia

**D89.2 Hypergammaglobulinemia, unspecified**

**D89.3 Immune reconstitution syndrome** Rx ESR COM

Immune reconstitution inflammatory syndrome [IRIS]

Use additional code for adverse effect, if applicable, to identify drug (T36-T5Ø with fifth or sixth character 5)

**D89.4 Mast cell activation syndrome and related disorders**

EXCLUDES 1 *aggressive systemic mastocytosis (C96.21)*
*(indolent) systemic mastocytosis (D47.Ø2)*
*(non-congenital) cutaneous mastocytosis (D47.Ø1)*
*congenital cutaneous mastocytosis (Q82.2)*
*malignant mast cell neoplasm (C96.2-)*
*malignant mastocytoma (C96.29)*
*mast cell leukemia (C94.3-)*
*mast cell sarcoma (C96.22)*
*mastocytoma NOS (D47.Ø9)*
*other mast cell neoplasms of uncertain behavior (D47.Ø9)*
*systemic mastocytosis associated with a clonal hematologic non-mast cell lineage disease (SM-AHNMD) (D47.Ø2)*

AHA: 2016,4Q,11

**D89.4Ø Mast cell activation, unspecified** Rx ESR COM

Mast cell activation disorder, unspecified
Mast cell activation syndrome, NOS

**D89.41 Monoclonal mast cell activation syndrome** Rx ESR COM

**D89.42 Idiopathic mast cell activation syndrome** Rx ESR COM

**D89.43 Secondary mast cell activation** Rx ESR COM

Secondary mast cell activation syndrome
Code also underlying etiology, if known

**D89.44 Hereditary alpha tryptasemia** Rx ESR COM

Use additional code, if applicable, for:
- allergy status, other than to drugs and biological substances (Z91.Ø-)
- personal history of anaphylaxis (Z87.892)

AHA: 2021,4Q,8

**D89.49 Other mast cell activation disorder** Rx ESR COM

Other mast cell activation syndrome

**D89.8 Other specified disorders involving the immune mechanism, not elsewhere classified**

**D89.81 Graft-versus-host disease**

Code first underlying cause, such as:
- complications of blood transfusion (T8Ø.89)
- complications of transplanted organs and tissue (T86.-)

Use additional code to identify associated manifestations, such as:
- desquamative dermatitis (L3Ø.8)
- diarrhea (R19.7)
- elevated bilirubin (R17)
- hair loss (L65.9)

AHA: 2023,3Q,19

**D89.81Ø Acute graft-versus-host disease** HCC Rx ESR COM UPD

**D89.811 Chronic graft-versus-host disease** HCC Rx ESR COM UPD

**D89.812 Acute on chronic graft-versus-host disease** HCC Rx ESR COM UPD

**D89.813 Graft-versus-host disease, unspecified** HCC Rx ESR COM UPD

**D89.82 Autoimmune lymphoproliferative syndrome [ALPS]** ESR COM

**DEF:** Rare genetic alteration of the Fas protein that impairs normal cellular apoptosis (normal cell death), causing abnormal accumulation of lymphocytes in the lymph glands, liver, and spleen. Symptoms include neutropenia, anemia, and thrombocytopenia.

✓6th **D89.83 Cytokine release syndrome**

Code first underlying cause, such as:
- complications following infusion, transfusion and therapeutic injection (T8Ø.89-)
- complications of transplanted organs and tissue (T86.-)

Use additional code for adverse effect, if applicable, to identify immune checkpoint inhibitors and immunostimulant drugs (T45.AX5)

Use additional code to identify associated manifestations

**AHA:** 2020,4Q,12-15

**DEF:** Form of systemic inflammatory response syndrome (SIRS) in which immune substances (cytokines) are released rapidly and in large amounts from the affected immune cells into the blood. The severity of associated symptoms or manifestations varies based on the underlying cause. This syndrome occurs as a complication of a disease, infection, or drug (often an adverse effect of immunotherapy in the form of treatment receiving monoclonal antibodies or Chimeric Antigen Receptor T [CAR-T] cells).

**D89.831 Cytokine release syndrome, grade 1** UPD

**D89.832 Cytokine release syndrome, grade 2** UPD

**D89.833 Cytokine release syndrome, grade 3** UPD

**D89.834 Cytokine release syndrome, grade 4** UPD

**D89.835 Cytokine release syndrome, grade 5** UPD

**D89.839 Cytokine release syndrome, grade unspecified** UPD

**D89.84 IgG4-related disease** HCC Rx ESR COM

Immunoglobulin G4-related disease

**AHA:** 2023,4Q,9

**D89.89 Other specified disorders involving the immune mechanism, not elsewhere classified** Rx ESR COM

EXCLUDES 1 *human immunodeficiency virus disease (B2Ø)*

**AHA:** 2017,4Q,109

**D89.9 Disorder involving the immune mechanism, unspecified** Rx ESR COM

Immune disease NOS

**AHA:** 2015,3Q,22

# Chapter 4. Endocrine, Nutritional, and Metabolic Diseases (E00–E89)



## Chapter-specific Guidelines with Coding Examples

The chapter-specific guidelines from the ICD-10-CM Official Guidelines for Coding and Reporting have been provided below. Along with these guidelines are coding examples, contained in the shaded boxes, that have been developed to help illustrate the coding and/or sequencing guidance found in these guidelines.

**a. Diabetes mellitus**

The diabetes mellitus codes are combination codes that include the type of diabetes mellitus, the body system affected, and the complications affecting that body system. As many codes within a particular category as are necessary to describe all of the complications of the disease may be used. They should be sequenced based on the reason for a particular encounter. Assign as many codes from categories E08–E13 as needed to identify all of the associated conditions that the patient has.

Patient is seen for uncontrolled diabetes, type 2, with hyperglycemia diabetic nephropathy, and diabetic gastroparesis

| | |
|---|---|
| **E11.65** | **Type 2 diabetes mellitus with hyperglycemia** |
| **E11.21** | **Type 2 diabetes mellitus with diabetic nephropathy** |
| **E11.43** | **Type 2 diabetes mellitus with diabetic autonomic (poly)neuropathy** |
| **K31.84** | **Gastroparesis** |

*Explanation*: Use as many codes to describe the diabetic complications as needed. Many are combination codes that describe more than one condition. Code first the reason for the encounter. The term "uncontrolled" can refer to either hyperglycemia or hypoglycemia. In this case, "uncontrolled" is described as "with hyperglycemia."

**1) Type of diabetes**

The age of a patient is not the sole determining factor, though most type 1 diabetics develop the condition before reaching puberty. For this reason, type 1 diabetes mellitus is also referred to as juvenile diabetes.

**(a) Presymptomatic Type 1 diabetes mellitus**

Codes E10.A-, Type 1 diabetes mellitus, presymptomatic, are assigned for early-stage type 1 diabetes that predates the onset of symptoms.

**(b) Type 2 diabetes mellitus in remission**

Code E11.A, Type 2 diabetes mellitus without complications in remission, is assigned based on provider documentation that the diabetes mellitus is in remission. If the documentation is unclear as to whether the Type 2 diabetes mellitus has achieved remission, the provider should be queried. For example, the term "resolved" is not synonymous with remission.

**2) Type of diabetes mellitus not documented**

If the type of diabetes mellitus is not documented in the medical record the default is E11.-, Type 2 diabetes mellitus.

Office visit lists diabetic retinopathy with macular edema and hypertension on patient problem list

| | |
|---|---|
| **E11.311** | **Type 2 diabetes mellitus with unspecified diabetic retinopathy with macular edema** |
| **I10** | **Essential (primary) hypertension** |

*Explanation*: Since the type of diabetes was not documented, default to category E11.

**3) Diabetes mellitus and the use of insulin, oral hypoglycemics, and injectable non-insulin drugs**

If the documentation in a medical record does not indicate the type of diabetes but does indicate that the patient uses insulin, code E11-, Type 2 diabetes mellitus, should be assigned. Additional code(s) should be assigned from category Z79 to identify the long-term (current) use of insulin, oral hypoglycemic drugs, or injectable non-insulin antidiabetic, as follows:

If the patient is treated with both oral hypoglycemic drugs and insulin, both code Z79.4, Long term (current) use of insulin, and code Z79.84, Long term (current) use of oral hypoglycemic drugs, should be assigned.

If the patient is treated with both insulin and an injectable non-insulin antidiabetic drug, assign codes Z79.4, Long term (current) use of insulin, and Z79.85, Long-term (current) use of injectable non-insulin antidiabetic drugs.

If the patient is treated with both oral hypoglycemic drugs and an injectable non-insulin antidiabetic drug, assign codes Z79.84, Long term (current) use of oral hypoglycemic drugs, and Z79.85, Long-term (current) use of injectable non-insulin antidiabetic drugs.

Code Z79.4 should not be assigned if insulin is given temporarily to bring a type 2 patient's blood sugar under control during an encounter.

Office visit lists chronic diabetes with daily insulin use on patient problem list

| | |
|---|---|
| **E11.9** | **Type 2 diabetes mellitus without complications** |
| **Z79.4** | **Long term (current) use of insulin** |

*Explanation*: Do not assume that a patient on insulin must have type 1 diabetes. The default for diabetes without further specification defaults to type 2. Add the code for long term use of insulin.

**4) Diabetes mellitus in pregnancy and gestational diabetes**

*See Section I.C.15. Diabetes mellitus in pregnancy.*

*See Section I.C.15. Gestational (pregnancy induced) diabetes*

**5) Complications due to insulin pump malfunction**

**(a) Underdose of insulin due to insulin pump failure**

An underdose of insulin due to an insulin pump failure should be assigned to a code from subcategory T85.6, Mechanical complication of other specified internal and external prosthetic devices, implants and grafts, that specifies the type of pump malfunction, as the principal or first-listed code, followed by code T38.3X6-, Underdosing of insulin and oral hypoglycemic [antidiabetic] drugs. Additional codes for the type of diabetes mellitus and any associated complications due to the underdosing should also be assigned.

A 24-year-old type 1 diabetic male treated in for hyperglycemia; insulin pump found to be malfunctioning and underdosing

| | |
|---|---|
| **T85.614A** | **Breakdown (mechanical) of insulin pump, initial encounter** |
| **T38.3X6A** | **Underdosing of insulin and oral hypoglycemic [antidiabetic] drugs, initial encounter** |
| **E10.65** | **Type 1 diabetes mellitus with hyperglycemia** |

*Explanation*: The complication code for the mechanical breakdown of the pump is sequenced first, followed by the underdosing code and type of diabetes with complication. Code all other diabetic complication codes necessary to describe the patient's condition.

**(b) Overdose of insulin due to insulin pump failure**

The principal or first-listed code for an encounter due to an insulin pump malfunction resulting in an overdose of insulin, should also be T85.6-, Mechanical complication of other specified internal and external prosthetic devices, implants and grafts, followed by code T38.3X1-, Poisoning by insulin and oral hypoglycemic [antidiabetic] drugs, accidental (unintentional).

A 24-year-old type 1 diabetic male found down with diabetic coma, brought into ED and treated for hypoglycemia; insulin pump found to be malfunctioning and overdosing

| | |
|---|---|
| **T85.614A** | **Breakdown (mechanical) of insulin pump, initial encounter** |
| **T38.3X1A** | **Poisoning by insulin and oral hypoglycemic [antidiabetic] drugs, accidental (unintentional), initial encounter** |
| **E10.641** | **Type 1 diabetes mellitus with hypoglycemia with coma** |

*Explanation*: The complication code for the mechanical breakdown of the pump is sequenced first, followed by the poisoning code and type of diabetes with complication. All the characters in the combination code must be used to form a valid code and to fully describe the type of diabetes, the hypoglycemia, and the coma.

**6) Secondary diabetes mellitus**

Codes under categories E08, Diabetes mellitus due to underlying condition, E09, Drug or chemical induced diabetes mellitus, and E13, Other specified diabetes mellitus, identify complications/manifestations associated with secondary diabetes mellitus. Secondary diabetes is always caused by another condition or event (e.g., cystic fibrosis, malignant neoplasm of pancreas, pancreatectomy, adverse effect of drug, or poisoning).

**(a) Secondary diabetes mellitus and the use of insulin or oral hypoglycemic drugs**

For patients with secondary diabetes mellitus who routinely use insulin, oral hypoglycemic drugs, or injectable non-insulin drugs, additional code(s) from category Z79 should be assigned to identify the long-term (current) use of insulin, oral hypoglycemic drugs, or non-injectable non-insulin drugs as follows:

If the patient is treated with both oral hypoglycemic drugs and insulin, both code Z79.4, Long term (current) use of insulin, and code Z79.84, Long term (current) use of oral hypoglycemic drugs, should be assigned.

If the patient is treated with both insulin and an injectable non-insulin antidiabetic drug, assign codes Z79.4, Long-term (current) use of insulin, and Z79.85, Long-term (current) use of injectable non-insulin antidiabetic drugs.

If the patient is treated with both oral hypoglycemic drugs and an injectable non-insulin antidiabetic drug, assign codes Z79.84, Long-term (current) use of oral hypoglycemic drugs, and Z79.85, Long-term (current) use of injectable non-insulin antidiabetic drugs.

Code Z79.4 should not be assigned if insulin is given temporarily to bring a secondary diabetic patient's blood sugar under control during an encounter.

Type 2 diabetic with no complications, normally only on oral metformin, is given insulin for three days to maintain glucose control while in the hospital recovering from surgery

**E11.9** **Type 2 diabetes mellitus without complications**

**Z79.84** **Long term (current) use of oral hypoglycemic drugs**

*Explanation*: Although the patient was given insulin for a short time during his hospital stay, the intent was only to maintain the patient's glucose levels while off his regular oral hypoglycemic medication, not for long term use. No code is needed for long term use of insulin, but a Z code for long term use of an oral hypoglycemic should be added to identify the chronic use of this drug.

Type 2 diabetic with diabetic polyneuropathy on insulin

**E11.42** **Type 2 diabetes mellitus with diabetic polyneuropathy**

**Z79.4** **Long term (current) use of insulin**

*Explanation*: Add a Z code for the long term use of insulin and the long term use of metformin because both are taken chronically.

**(b) Assigning and sequencing secondary diabetes codes and its causes**

The sequencing of the secondary diabetes codes in relationship to codes for the cause of the diabetes is based on the Tabular List instructions for categories EØ8, EØ9 and E13.

**(i) Secondary diabetes mellitus due to pancreatectomy**

For postpancreatectomy diabetes mellitus (lack of insulin due to the surgical removal of all or part of the pancreas), assign code E89.1, Postprocedural hypoinsulinemia. Assign a code from category E13 as the principal or first-listed diagnosis and a code from subcategory Z9Ø.41, Acquired absence of pancreas, as an additional code.

**(ii) Secondary diabetes due to drugs**

Secondary diabetes may be caused by an adverse effect of correctly administered medications, poisoning or sequela of poisoning.

*See section I.C.19.e. for coding of adverse effects and poisoning, and section I.C.20 for external cause code reporting.*

Initial encounter for corticosteroid-induced diabetes mellitus

**EØ9.9** **Drug or chemical induced diabetes mellitus without complications**

**T38.ØX5A** **Adverse effect of glucocorticoids and synthetic analogues, initial encounter**

*Explanation*: If the diabetes is caused by an adverse effect of a drug, the diabetic condition is coded first. If it occurs from a poisoning or overdose, the poisoning code causing the diabetes is sequenced first.

**b. Obesity**

The obesity codes in category E66, Overweight and obesity, include codes related to the cause of obesity, such as drug-induced obesity (E66.1), and codes related to effects of obesity, such as code E66.2, Morbid (severe) obesity with alveolar hypoventilation. There are other codes related to obesity in other categories of the classification, such as E88.82, Obesity due to disruption of MC4R pathway; and codes in fifth character subcategory O99.21, Obesity complicating pregnancy, childbirth, and the puerperium.

**1) Obesity class**

The obesity class codes in subcategory E66.81, Obesity class, require a fifth character to convey the severity of obesity. The obesity class should be documented in the medical record by the provider for these codes to be assigned. The obesity class codes can be reported with other obesity codes in the classification found in Chapters 4 and 15 to fully describe the condition. However, if both class 3 obesity and morbid obesity are documented, only a code for class 3 obesity should be assigned as it is more specific.

# Chapter 4. Endocrine, Nutritional and Metabolic Diseases (E00-E89)

**NOTE** All neoplasms, whether functionally active or not, are classified in Chapter 2. Appropriate codes in this chapter (i.e. E05.8, E07.0, E16-E31, E34.-) may be used as additional codes to indicate either functional activity by neoplasms and ectopic endocrine tissue or hyperfunction and hypofunction of endocrine glands associated with neoplasms and other conditions classified elsewhere.

**EXCLUDES 1** *transitory endocrine and metabolic disorders specific to newborn (P70-P74)*

**AHA:** 2018,2Q,6

This chapter contains the following blocks:

| | |
|---|---|
| E00-E07 | Disorders of thyroid gland |
| E08-E13 | Diabetes mellitus |
| E15-E16 | Other disorders of glucose regulation and pancreatic internal secretion |
| E20-E35 | Disorders of other endocrine glands |
| E36 | Intraoperative complications of endocrine system |
| E40-E46 | Malnutrition |
| E50-E64 | Other nutritional deficiencies |
| E65-E68 | Overweight, obesity and other hyperalimentation |
| E70-E88 | Metabolic disorders |
| E89 | Postprocedural endocrine and metabolic complications and disorders, not elsewhere classified |

## Disorders of thyroid gland (E00-E07)

**E00 Congenital iodine-deficiency syndrome**

Use additional code (F70-F79) to identify associated intellectual disabilities

**EXCLUDES 1** *subclinical iodine-deficiency hypothyroidism (E02)*

**E00.0 Congenital iodine-deficiency syndrome, neurological type** Rx
- Endemic cretinism, neurological type

**E00.1 Congenital iodine-deficiency syndrome, myxedematous type** Rx
- Endemic cretinism, myxedematous type
- Endemic hypothyroid cretinism

**E00.2 Congenital iodine-deficiency syndrome, mixed type** Rx
- Endemic cretinism, mixed type

**E00.9 Congenital iodine-deficiency syndrome, unspecified** Rx
- Congenital iodine-deficiency hypothyroidism NOS
- Endemic cretinism NOS

**E01 Iodine-deficiency related thyroid disorders and allied conditions**

**EXCLUDES 1** *congenital iodine-deficiency syndrome (E00.-)*
*subclinical iodine-deficiency hypothyroidism (E02)*

**E01.0 Iodine-deficiency related diffuse (endemic) goiter** Rx

**E01.1 Iodine-deficiency related multinodular (endemic) goiter** Rx
- Iodine-deficiency related nodular goiter

**E01.2 Iodine-deficiency related (endemic) goiter, unspecified** Rx
- Endemic goiter NOS

**E01.8 Other iodine-deficiency related thyroid disorders and allied conditions** Rx
- Acquired iodine-deficiency hypothyroidism NOS

**E02 Subclinical iodine-deficiency hypothyroidism** Rx

**AHA:** 2021,1Q,8

**E03 Other hypothyroidism**

**EXCLUDES 1** *iodine-deficiency related hypothyroidism (E00-E02)*
*postprocedural hypothyroidism (E89.0)*

**AHA:** 2026,1Q,23

**DEF:** Hypothyroidism: Underproduction of thyroid hormone.

**E03.0 Congenital hypothyroidism with diffuse goiter** Rx
- Congenital goiter (nontoxic) NOS
- Congenital parenchymatous goiter (nontoxic)

**EXCLUDES 1** *transitory congenital goiter with normal function (P72.0)*

**E03.1 Congenital hypothyroidism without goiter** Rx
- Aplasia of thyroid (with myxedema)
- Congenital atrophy of thyroid
- Congenital hypothyroidism NOS

**E03.2 Hypothyroidism due to medicaments and other exogenous substances** Rx

Code first poisoning due to drug or toxin, if applicable (T36-T65 with fifth or sixth character 1-4)

Use additional code for adverse effect, if applicable, to identify drug (T36-T50 with fifth or sixth character 5)

**E03.3 Postinfectious hypothyroidism** Rx

**E03.4 Atrophy of thyroid (acquired)** Rx

**EXCLUDES 1** *congenital atrophy of thyroid (E03.1)*

**E03.5 Myxedema coma** HCC Rx ESR COM

**E03.8 Other specified hypothyroidism** Rx

**AHA:** 2021,1Q,8

**E03.9 Hypothyroidism, unspecified** Rx
- Myxedema NOS

**AHA:** 2024,1Q,14

**E04 Other nontoxic goiter**

**EXCLUDES 1** *congenital goiter (NOS) (diffuse) (parenchymatous) (E03.0)*
*iodine-deficiency related goiter (E00-E02)*

**E04.0 Nontoxic diffuse goiter** Rx
- Diffuse (colloid) nontoxic goiter
- Simple nontoxic goiter

**E04.1 Nontoxic single thyroid nodule** Rx
- Colloid nodule (cystic) (thyroid)
- Nontoxic uninodular goiter
- Thyroid (cystic) nodule NOS

**DEF:** Enlarged thyroid, commonly due to decreased thyroid production, with a single nodule. No clinical hypothyroidism.

**E04.2 Nontoxic multinodular goiter** Rx
- Cystic goiter NOS
- Multinodular (cystic) goiter NOS

**DEF:** Enlarged thyroid, commonly due to decreased thyroid production with multiple nodules. No clinical hypothyroidism.

**E04.8 Other specified nontoxic goiter** Rx

**E04.9 Nontoxic goiter, unspecified** Rx
- Goiter NOS
- Nodular goiter (nontoxic) NOS

**E05 Thyrotoxicosis [hyperthyroidism]**

**EXCLUDES 1** *chronic thyroiditis with transient thyrotoxicosis (E06.2)*
*neonatal thyrotoxicosis (P72.1)*

**DEF:** Excessive quantities of hormones from the thyroid gland caused by overproduction or loss of storage ability.

**E05.0 Thyrotoxicosis with diffuse goiter**
- Exophthalmic or toxic goiter NOS
- Graves' disease
- Toxic diffuse goiter

**DEF:** Diffuse thyroid enlargement accompanied by hyperthyroidism, bulging eyes, and dermopathy.

**E05.00 Thyrotoxicosis with diffuse goiter without thyrotoxic crisis or storm** Rx

**E05.01 Thyrotoxicosis with diffuse goiter with thyrotoxic crisis or storm** Rx

**Goiter**

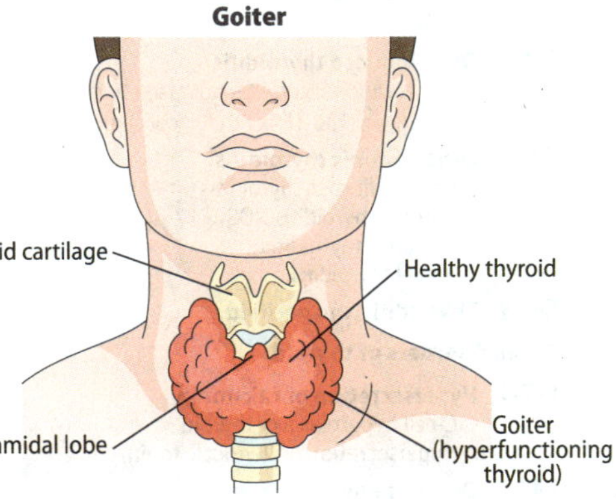


**E05.1 Thyrotoxicosis with toxic single thyroid nodule**
- Thyrotoxicosis with toxic uninodular goiter

**DEF:** Symptomatic hyperthyroidism with a single nodule on the enlarged thyroid gland. Onset of symptoms can be abrupt and include extreme nervousness, insomnia, weight loss, tremors, and psychosis or coma.

**E05.10 Thyrotoxicosis with toxic single thyroid nodule without thyrotoxic crisis or storm** Rx

**E05.11 Thyrotoxicosis with toxic single thyroid nodule with thyrotoxic crisis or storm** Rx

**E05.2 Thyrotoxicosis with toxic multinodular goiter**
- Toxic nodular goiter NOS

**E05.20 Thyrotoxicosis with toxic multinodular goiter without thyrotoxic crisis or storm** Rx

**E05.21 Thyrotoxicosis with toxic multinodular goiter with thyrotoxic crisis or storm** Rx

**E05.3 Thyrotoxicosis from ectopic thyroid tissue**

**E05.30 Thyrotoxicosis from ectopic thyroid tissue without thyrotoxic crisis or storm** Rx

EØ5.31 **Thyrotoxicosis from ectopic thyroid tissue with thyrotoxic crisis or storm** Rx

✓5th EØ5.4 **Thyrotoxicosis factitia**

EØ5.40 **Thyrotoxicosis factitia without thyrotoxic crisis or storm** Rx

EØ5.41 **Thyrotoxicosis factitia with thyrotoxic crisis or storm** Rx

✓5th EØ5.8 **Other thyrotoxicosis**

Overproduction of thyroid-stimulating hormone

EØ5.80 **Other thyrotoxicosis without thyrotoxic crisis or storm** Rx

EØ5.81 **Other thyrotoxicosis with thyrotoxic crisis or storm** Rx

✓5th EØ5.9 **Thyrotoxicosis, unspecified**

Hyperthyroidism NOS

EØ5.90 **Thyrotoxicosis, unspecified without thyrotoxic crisis or storm** Rx

EØ5.91 **Thyrotoxicosis, unspecified with thyrotoxic crisis or storm** Rx

✓4th EØ6 **Thyroiditis**

EXCLUDES 1 *postpartum thyroiditis (O9Ø.5)*

DEF: Inflammation of the thyroid gland.

EØ6.Ø **Acute thyroiditis** Rx

Abscess of thyroid
Pyogenic thyroiditis
Suppurative thyroiditis

Use additional code (B95-B97) to identify infectious agent

EØ6.1 **Subacute thyroiditis** Rx

de Quervain thyroiditis
Giant-cell thyroiditis
Granulomatous thyroiditis
Nonsuppurative thyroiditis
Viral thyroiditis

EXCLUDES 1 *autoimmune thyroiditis (EØ6.3)*

EØ6.2 **Chronic thyroiditis with transient thyrotoxicosis** Rx

EXCLUDES 1 *autoimmune thyroiditis (EØ6.3)*

EØ6.3 **Autoimmune thyroiditis** Rx

Hashimoto's thyroiditis
Hashitoxicosis (transient)
Lymphadenoid goiter
Lymphocytic thyroiditis
Struma lymphomatosa

AHA: 2024,1Q,14

EØ6.4 **Drug-induced thyroiditis** Rx

Use additional code for adverse effect, if applicable, to identify drug (T36-T5Ø with fifth or sixth character 5)

EØ6.5 **Other chronic thyroiditis** Rx

Chronic fibrous thyroiditis
Chronic thyroiditis NOS
Ligneous thyroiditis
Riedel thyroiditis

EØ6.9 **Thyroiditis, unspecified** Rx

✓4th EØ7 **Other disorders of thyroid**

EØ7.Ø **Hypersecretion of calcitonin** Rx

C-cell hyperplasia of thyroid
Hypersecretion of thyrocalcitonin

EØ7.1 **Dyshormogenetic goiter** Rx

Dyshormonogenetic goiter
Familial dyshormogenetic goiter
Familial dyshormonogenetic goiter
Pendred's syndrome

EXCLUDES 1 *transitory congenital goiter with normal function (P72.Ø)*

✓5th EØ7.8 **Other specified disorders of thyroid**

EØ7.81 **Sick-euthyroid syndrome**

Euthyroid sick-syndrome

DEF: Thyroid dysfunction caused by abnormal levels of thyroid hormones T3 and/or T4. This syndrome is often associated with starvation or critical illness.

EØ7.89 **Other specified disorders of thyroid** Rx

Abnormality of thyroid-binding globulin
Hemorrhage of thyroid
Infarction of thyroid

EØ7.9 **Disorder of thyroid, unspecified** Rx

## Diabetes mellitus (EØ8-E13)

AHA: 2020,1Q,12; 2018,2Q,6; 2017,4Q,100-101; 2016,2Q,36; 2016,1Q,11-13; 2013,4Q,114; 2013,3Q,20

**TIP:** There is no default code for diabetes mellitus documented only as uncontrolled. The provider must indicate whether the diabetic patient is hypoglycemic or hyperglycemic to determine the appropriate code.

✓4th EØ8 **Diabetes mellitus due to underlying condition**

Code first the underlying condition, such as:
- congenital rubella (P35.Ø)
- Cushing's syndrome (E24.-)
- cystic fibrosis (E84.-)
- malignant neoplasm (CØØ-C96)
- malnutrition (E4Ø-E46)
- pancreatitis and other diseases of the pancreas (K85-K86.-)

Use additional code to identify control using:
- injectable non-insulin antidiabetic drugs (Z79.85)
- insulin (Z79.4)
- oral antidiabetic drugs (Z79.84)
- oral hypoglycemic drugs (Z79.84)

EXCLUDES 1 *drug or chemical induced diabetes mellitus (EØ9.-)*
*gestational diabetes (O24.4-)*
*neonatal diabetes mellitus (P7Ø.2)*
*postpancreatectomy diabetes mellitus (E13.-)*
*postprocedural diabetes mellitus (E13.-)*
*secondary diabetes mellitus NEC (E13.-)*
*type 1 diabetes mellitus (E1Ø.-)*
*type 2 diabetes mellitus (E11.-)*

✓5th EØ8.Ø **Diabetes mellitus due to underlying condition with hyperosmolarity**

DEF: Diabetic hyperosmolarity: Extremely high levels of glucose in the blood without ketones.

*EØ8.ØØ* ***Diabetes mellitus due to underlying condition with hyperosmolarity without nonketotic hyperglycemic-hyperosmolar coma (NKHHC)*** HCC Rx ESR COM

*EØ8.Ø1* ***Diabetes mellitus due to underlying condition with hyperosmolarity with coma*** HCC Rx ESR COM

✓5th EØ8.1 **Diabetes mellitus due to underlying condition with ketoacidosis**

DEF: Diabetic ketoacidosis: Potentially life-threatening complication due to a shortage of insulin in which the body switches to burning fatty acids and producing acidic ketone bodies.

*EØ8.1Ø* ***Diabetes mellitus due to underlying condition with ketoacidosis without coma*** HCC Rx ESR COM

*EØ8.11* ***Diabetes mellitus due to underlying condition with ketoacidosis with coma*** HCC Rx ESR COM

✓5th EØ8.2 **Diabetes mellitus due to underlying condition with kidney complications**

AHA: 2019,3Q,3; 2018,4Q,88

*EØ8.21* ***Diabetes mellitus due to underlying condition with diabetic nephropathy*** HCC Rx ESR COM

Diabetes mellitus due to underlying condition with intercapillary glomerulosclerosis
Diabetes mellitus due to underlying condition with intracapillary glomerulonephrosis
Diabetes mellitus due to underlying condition with Kimmelstiel-Wilson disease

*EØ8.22* ***Diabetes mellitus due to underlying condition with diabetic chronic kidney disease*** HCC Rx ESR COM

Use additional code to identify stage of chronic kidney disease (N18.1-N18.6)

*EØ8.29* ***Diabetes mellitus due to underlying condition with other diabetic kidney complication*** HCC Rx ESR COM

Renal tubular degeneration in diabetes mellitus due to underlying condition

**E08.3 Diabetes mellitus due to underlying condition with ophthalmic complications**
AHA: 2016,4Q,11-13

One of the following 7th characters is to be assigned to codes in subcategories E08.32, E08.33, E08.34, E08.35, and E08.37 to designate laterality of the disease:
1 right eye
2 left eye
3 bilateral
9 unspecified eye

**E08.31 Diabetes mellitus due to underlying condition with unspecified diabetic retinopathy**
DEF: Diabetic retinopathy: Diabetic complication from damage to the retinal vessels resulting in vision problems that can progress to blindness.

***E08.311 Diabetes mellitus due to underlying condition with unspecified diabetic retinopathy with macular edema*** HCC Rx ESR COM

***E08.319 Diabetes mellitus due to underlying condition with unspecified diabetic retinopathy without macular edema*** HCC Rx ESR COM

**E08.32 Diabetes mellitus due to underlying condition with mild nonproliferative diabetic retinopathy**
Diabetes mellitus due to underlying condition with nonproliferative diabetic retinopathy NOS

***E08.321 Diabetes mellitus due to underlying condition with mild nonproliferative diabetic retinopathy with macular edema*** HCC Rx ESR COM

***E08.329 Diabetes mellitus due to underlying condition with mild nonproliferative diabetic retinopathy without macular edema*** HCC Rx ESR COM

**E08.33 Diabetes mellitus due to underlying condition with moderate nonproliferative diabetic retinopathy**

***E08.331 Diabetes mellitus due to underlying condition with moderate nonproliferative diabetic retinopathy with macular edema*** HCC Rx ESR COM

***E08.339 Diabetes mellitus due to underlying condition with moderate nonproliferative diabetic retinopathy without macular edema*** HCC Rx ESR COM

**E08.34 Diabetes mellitus due to underlying condition with severe nonproliferative diabetic retinopathy**

***E08.341 Diabetes mellitus due to underlying condition with severe nonproliferative diabetic retinopathy with macular edema*** HCC Rx ESR COM

***E08.349 Diabetes mellitus due to underlying condition with severe nonproliferative diabetic retinopathy without macular edema*** HCC Rx ESR COM

**E08.35 Diabetes mellitus due to underlying condition with proliferative diabetic retinopathy**

***E08.351 Diabetes mellitus due to underlying condition with proliferative diabetic retinopathy with macular edema*** HCC Rx ESR COM

***E08.352 Diabetes mellitus due to underlying condition with proliferative diabetic retinopathy with traction retinal detachment involving the macula*** HCC Rx ESR COM

***E08.353 Diabetes mellitus due to underlying condition with proliferative diabetic retinopathy with traction retinal detachment not involving the macula*** HCC Rx ESR COM

***E08.354 Diabetes mellitus due to underlying condition with proliferative diabetic retinopathy with combined traction retinal detachment and rhegmatogenous retinal detachment*** HCC Rx ESR COM

***E08.355 Diabetes mellitus due to underlying condition with stable proliferative diabetic retinopathy*** HCC Rx ESR COM

***E08.359 Diabetes mellitus due to underlying condition with proliferative diabetic retinopathy without macular edema*** HCC Rx ESR COM

***E08.36 Diabetes mellitus due to underlying condition with diabetic cataract*** HCC Rx ESR COM
AHA: 2019,2Q,30-31; 2016,4Q,142

***E08.37 Diabetes mellitus due to underlying condition with diabetic macular edema, resolved following treatment*** HCC Rx ESR COM

***E08.39 Diabetes mellitus due to underlying condition with other diabetic ophthalmic complication*** HCC Rx ESR COM
Use additional code to identify manifestation, such as:
diabetic glaucoma (H40-H42)
AHA: 2023,3Q,19

**E08.4 Diabetes mellitus due to underlying condition with neurological complications**

***E08.40 Diabetes mellitus due to underlying condition with diabetic neuropathy, unspecified*** HCC Rx ESR COM

***E08.41 Diabetes mellitus due to underlying condition with diabetic mononeuropathy*** HCC Rx ESR COM

***E08.42 Diabetes mellitus due to underlying condition with diabetic polyneuropathy*** HCC Rx ESR COM
Diabetes mellitus due to underlying condition with diabetic neuralgia

***E08.43 Diabetes mellitus due to underlying condition with diabetic autonomic (poly)neuropathy*** HCC Rx ESR COM
Diabetes mellitus due to underlying condition with diabetic gastroparesis
AHA: 2013,4Q,114

***E08.44 Diabetes mellitus due to underlying condition with diabetic amyotrophy*** HCC Rx ESR COM

***E08.49 Diabetes mellitus due to underlying condition with other diabetic neurological complication*** HCC Rx ESR COM

**E08.5 Diabetes mellitus due to underlying condition with circulatory complications**

***E08.51 Diabetes mellitus due to underlying condition with diabetic peripheral angiopathy without gangrene*** HCC Rx ESR COM
AHA: 2018,3Q,3-4; 2018,2Q,7

***E08.52 Diabetes mellitus due to underlying condition with diabetic peripheral angiopathy with gangrene*** HCC Rx ESR COM
Diabetes mellitus due to underlying condition with diabetic gangrene
AHA: 2020,2Q,18; 2018,3Q,3; 2018,2Q,7; 2017,4Q,102

***E08.59 Diabetes mellitus due to underlying condition with other circulatory complications*** HCC Rx ESR COM

**E08.6 Diabetes mellitus due to underlying condition with other specified complications**

**E08.61 Diabetes mellitus due to underlying condition with diabetic arthropathy**

***E08.610 Diabetes mellitus due to underlying condition with diabetic neuropathic arthropathy*** HCC Rx ESR COM
Diabetes mellitus due to underlying condition with Charcôt's joints
DEF: Charcot's joint: Progressive neurologic arthropathy in which chronic degeneration of joints in the weight-bearing areas with peripheral hypertrophy occurs as a complication of a neuropathy disorder. Supporting structures relax from a loss of sensation resulting in chronic joint instability.

***E08.618 Diabetes mellitus due to underlying condition with other diabetic arthropathy*** HCC Rx ESR COM
AHA: 2018,2Q,6

**E08.62 Diabetes mellitus due to underlying condition with skin complications**

***E08.620 Diabetes mellitus due to underlying condition with diabetic dermatitis*** HCC Rx ESR COM
Diabetes mellitus due to underlying condition with diabetic necrobiosis lipoidica

*E08.621* ***Diabetes mellitus due to underlying condition with foot ulcer*** HCC Rx ESR COM
Use additional code to identify site of ulcer (L97.4-, L97.5-)
**AHA:** 2020,2Q,19
**TIP:** Do not assign a code for diabetic ulcer when the ulcer is closed/resolved or to report history of diabetic ulcers; Z86.31 Personal history of diabetic foot ulcer, may be assigned.

*E08.622* ***Diabetes mellitus due to underlying condition with other skin ulcer*** HCC Rx ESR COM
Use additional code to identify site of ulcer (L97.1-L97.9, L98.41-L98.49)
**AHA:** 2021,1Q,7; 2017,4Q,17

*E08.628* ***Diabetes mellitus due to underlying condition with other skin complications*** HCC Rx ESR COM

✓6th **E08.63 Diabetes mellitus due to underlying condition with oral complications**

*E08.630* ***Diabetes mellitus due to underlying condition with periodontal disease*** HCC Rx ESR COM

*E08.638* ***Diabetes mellitus due to underlying condition with other oral complications*** HCC Rx ESR COM

✓6th **E08.64 Diabetes mellitus due to underlying condition with hypoglycemia**
Use additional code for hypoglycemia level, if applicable (E16.A-)
**AHA:** 2017,1Q,42

*E08.641* ***Diabetes mellitus due to underlying condition with hypoglycemia with coma*** HCC Rx ESR COM

*E08.649* ***Diabetes mellitus due to underlying condition with hypoglycemia without coma*** HCC Rx ESR COM
**AHA:** 2016,3Q,42; 2015,3Q,21

*E08.65* ***Diabetes mellitus due to underlying condition with hyperglycemia*** HCC Rx ESR COM
**AHA:** 2017,1Q,42; 2013,3Q,20

*E08.69* ***Diabetes mellitus due to underlying condition with other specified complication*** HCC Rx ESR COM
Use additional code to identify complication
**AHA:** 2016,4Q,141; 2016,1Q,13

*E08.8* ***Diabetes mellitus due to underlying condition with unspecified complications*** HCC Rx ESR COM

*E08.9* ***Diabetes mellitus due to underlying condition without complications*** HCC Rx ESR COM
**AHA:** 2023,3Q,19; 2020,2Q,18

✓4th **E09 Drug or chemical induced diabetes mellitus**
Code first poisoning due to drug or toxin, if applicable (T36-T65 with fifth or sixth character 1-4)
Use additional code for adverse effect, if applicable, to identify drug (T36-T50 with fifth or sixth character 5)
Use additional code to identify control using:
injectable non-insulin antidiabetic drugs (Z79.85)
insulin (Z79.4)
oral antidiabetic drugs (Z79.84)
oral hypoglycemic drugs (Z79.84)

**EXCLUDES 1** *diabetes mellitus due to underlying condition (E08.-)*
*gestational diabetes (O24.4-)*
*neonatal diabetes mellitus (P70.2)*
*postpancreatectomy diabetes mellitus (E13.-)*
*postprocedural diabetes mellitus (E13.-)*
*secondary diabetes mellitus NEC (E13.-)*
*type 1 diabetes mellitus (E10.-)*
*type 2 diabetes mellitus (E11.-)*

✓5th **E09.0 Drug or chemical induced diabetes mellitus with hyperosmolarity**
**DEF:** Diabetic hyperosmolarity: Extremely high levels of glucose in the blood without ketones.

**E09.00 Drug or chemical induced diabetes mellitus with hyperosmolarity without nonketotic hyperglycemic-hyperosmolar coma (NKHHC)** Rx ESR COM

**E09.01 Drug or chemical induced diabetes mellitus with hyperosmolarity with coma** Rx ESR COM

✓5th **E09.1 Drug or chemical induced diabetes mellitus with ketoacidosis**
**DEF:** Diabetic ketoacidosis: Potentially life-threatening complication due to a shortage of insulin in which the body switches to burning fatty acids and producing acidic ketone bodies.

**E09.10 Drug or chemical induced diabetes mellitus with ketoacidosis without coma** Rx ESR COM

**E09.11 Drug or chemical induced diabetes mellitus with ketoacidosis with coma** Rx ESR COM

✓5th **E09.2 Drug or chemical induced diabetes mellitus with kidney complications**
**AHA:** 2019,3Q,3; 2018,4Q,88

**E09.21 Drug or chemical induced diabetes mellitus with diabetic nephropathy** Rx ESR COM
Drug or chemical induced diabetes mellitus with intercapillary glomerulosclerosis
Drug or chemical induced diabetes mellitus with intracapillary glomerulonephrosis
Drug or chemical induced diabetes mellitus with Kimmelstiel-Wilson disease

**E09.22 Drug or chemical induced diabetes mellitus with diabetic chronic kidney disease** Rx ESR COM
Use additional code to identify stage of chronic kidney disease (N18.1-N18.6)

**E09.29 Drug or chemical induced diabetes mellitus with other diabetic kidney complication** Rx ESR COM
Drug or chemical induced diabetes mellitus with renal tubular degeneration

✓5th **E09.3 Drug or chemical induced diabetes mellitus with ophthalmic complications**
**AHA:** 2016,4Q,11-13

One of the following 7th characters is to be assigned to codes in subcategories E09.32, E09.33, E09.34, E09.35, and E09.37 to designate laterality of the disease:
1 right eye
2 left eye
3 bilateral
9 unspecified eye

✓6th **E09.31 Drug or chemical induced diabetes mellitus with unspecified diabetic retinopathy**
**DEF:** Diabetic retinopathy: Diabetic complication from damage to the retinal vessels resulting in vision problems that can progress to blindness.

**E09.311 Drug or chemical induced diabetes mellitus with unspecified diabetic retinopathy with macular edema** Rx ESR COM

**E09.319 Drug or chemical induced diabetes mellitus with unspecified diabetic retinopathy without macular edema** Rx ESR COM

✓6th **E09.32 Drug or chemical induced diabetes mellitus with mild nonproliferative diabetic retinopathy**
Drug or chemical induced diabetes mellitus with nonproliferative diabetic retinopathy NOS

✓7th **E09.321 Drug or chemical induced diabetes mellitus with mild nonproliferative diabetic retinopathy with macular edema** Rx ESR COM

✓7th **E09.329 Drug or chemical induced diabetes mellitus with mild nonproliferative diabetic retinopathy without macular edema** Rx ESR COM

✓6th **E09.33 Drug or chemical induced diabetes mellitus with moderate nonproliferative diabetic retinopathy**

✓7th **E09.331 Drug or chemical induced diabetes mellitus with moderate nonproliferative diabetic retinopathy with macular edema** Rx ESR COM

✓7th **E09.339 Drug or chemical induced diabetes mellitus with moderate nonproliferative diabetic retinopathy without macular edema** Rx ESR COM

✓6th **E09.34 Drug or chemical induced diabetes mellitus with severe nonproliferative diabetic retinopathy**

✓7th **E09.341 Drug or chemical induced diabetes mellitus with severe nonproliferative diabetic retinopathy with macular edema** Rx ESR COM

✓7th **E09.349 Drug or chemical induced diabetes mellitus with severe nonproliferative diabetic retinopathy without macular edema** Rx ESR COM

√6th **E09.35 Drug or chemical induced diabetes mellitus with proliferative diabetic retinopathy**

√7th **E09.351 Drug or chemical induced diabetes mellitus with proliferative diabetic retinopathy with macular edema** Rx ESR COM

√7th **E09.352 Drug or chemical induced diabetes mellitus with proliferative diabetic retinopathy with traction retinal detachment involving the macula** Rx ESR COM

√7th **E09.353 Drug or chemical induced diabetes mellitus with proliferative diabetic retinopathy with traction retinal detachment not involving the macula** Rx ESR COM

√7th **E09.354 Drug or chemical induced diabetes mellitus with proliferative diabetic retinopathy with combined traction retinal detachment and rhegmatogenous retinal detachment** Rx ESR COM

√7th **E09.355 Drug or chemical induced diabetes mellitus with stable proliferative diabetic retinopathy** Rx ESR COM

√7th **E09.359 Drug or chemical induced diabetes mellitus with proliferative diabetic retinopathy without macular edema** Rx ESR COM

**E09.36 Drug or chemical induced diabetes mellitus with diabetic cataract** Rx ESR COM

**AHA:** 2019,2Q,30-31; 2016,4Q,142

√x7th **E09.37 Drug or chemical induced diabetes mellitus with diabetic macular edema, resolved following treatment** Rx ESR COM

**E09.39 Drug or chemical induced diabetes mellitus with other diabetic ophthalmic complication** Rx ESR COM

Use additional code to identify manifestation, such as: diabetic glaucoma (H40-H42)

**AHA:** 2023,3Q,19

√5th **E09.4 Drug or chemical induced diabetes mellitus with neurological complications**

**E09.40 Drug or chemical induced diabetes mellitus with neurological complications with diabetic neuropathy, unspecified** Rx ESR COM

**E09.41 Drug or chemical induced diabetes mellitus with neurological complications with diabetic mononeuropathy** Rx ESR COM

**E09.42 Drug or chemical induced diabetes mellitus with neurological complications with diabetic polyneuropathy** Rx ESR COM

Drug or chemical induced diabetes mellitus with diabetic neuralgia

**E09.43 Drug or chemical induced diabetes mellitus with neurological complications with diabetic autonomic (poly)neuropathy** Rx ESR COM

Drug or chemical induced diabetes mellitus with diabetic gastroparesis

**AHA:** 2013,4Q,114

**E09.44 Drug or chemical induced diabetes mellitus with neurological complications with diabetic amyotrophy** Rx ESR COM

**E09.49 Drug or chemical induced diabetes mellitus with neurological complications with other diabetic neurological complication** Rx ESR COM

√5th **E09.5 Drug or chemical induced diabetes mellitus with circulatory complications**

**E09.51 Drug or chemical induced diabetes mellitus with diabetic peripheral angiopathy without gangrene** Rx ESR COM

**AHA:** 2018,3Q,3-4; 2018,2Q,7

**E09.52 Drug or chemical induced diabetes mellitus with diabetic peripheral angiopathy with gangrene** Rx ESR COM

Drug or chemical induced diabetes mellitus with diabetic gangrene

**AHA:** 2020,2Q,18; 2018,3Q,3; 2018,2Q,7; 2017,4Q,102

**E09.59 Drug or chemical induced diabetes mellitus with other circulatory complications** Rx ESR COM

√5th **E09.6 Drug or chemical induced diabetes mellitus with other specified complications**

√6th **E09.61 Drug or chemical induced diabetes mellitus with diabetic arthropathy**

**E09.610 Drug or chemical induced diabetes mellitus with diabetic neuropathic arthropathy** Rx ESR COM

Drug or chemical induced diabetes mellitus with Charcôt's joints

**DEF:** Charcot's joint: Progressive neurologic arthropathy in which chronic degeneration of joints in the weight-bearing areas with peripheral hypertrophy occurs as a complication of a neuropathy disorder. Supporting structures relax from a loss of sensation resulting in chronic joint instability.

**E09.618 Drug or chemical induced diabetes mellitus with other diabetic arthropathy** Rx ESR COM

**AHA:** 2018,2Q,6

√6th **E09.62 Drug or chemical induced diabetes mellitus with skin complications**

**E09.620 Drug or chemical induced diabetes mellitus with diabetic dermatitis** Rx ESR COM

Drug or chemical induced diabetes mellitus with diabetic necrobiosis lipoidica

**E09.621 Drug or chemical induced diabetes mellitus with foot ulcer** Rx ESR COM

Use additional code to identify site of ulcer (L97.4-, L97.5-)

**AHA:** 2020,2Q,19

**TIP:** Do not assign a code for diabetic ulcer when the ulcer is closed/resolved or to report history of diabetic ulcers; Z86.31 Personal history of diabetic foot ulcer, may be assigned.

**E09.622 Drug or chemical induced diabetes mellitus with other skin ulcer** Rx ESR COM

Use additional code to identify site of ulcer (L97.1-L97.9, L98.41-L98.49)

**AHA:** 2021,1Q,7; 2017,4Q,17

**E09.628 Drug or chemical induced diabetes mellitus with other skin complications** Rx ESR COM

√6th **E09.63 Drug or chemical induced diabetes mellitus with oral complications**

**E09.630 Drug or chemical induced diabetes mellitus with periodontal disease** Rx ESR COM

**E09.638 Drug or chemical induced diabetes mellitus with other oral complications** Rx ESR COM

√6th **E09.64 Drug or chemical induced diabetes mellitus with hypoglycemia**

Use additional code for hypoglycemia level, if applicable (E16.A-)

**AHA:** 2017,1Q,42

**E09.641 Drug or chemical induced diabetes mellitus with hypoglycemia with coma** Rx ESR COM

**E09.649 Drug or chemical induced diabetes mellitus with hypoglycemia without coma** Rx ESR COM

**AHA:** 2016,3Q,42; 2015,3Q,21

**E09.65 Drug or chemical induced diabetes mellitus with hyperglycemia** Rx ESR COM

**AHA:** 2017,1Q,42; 2013,3Q,20

**E09.69 Drug or chemical induced diabetes mellitus with other specified complication** Rx ESR COM

Use additional code to identify complication

**AHA:** 2016,4Q,141; 2016,1Q,13

**E09.8 Drug or chemical induced diabetes mellitus with unspecified complications** Rx ESR COM

**E09.9 Drug or chemical induced diabetes mellitus without complications** Rx ESR COM

**AHA:** 2023,3Q,19; 2020,2Q,18

Chapter 4. Endocrine, Nutritional and Metabolic Diseases

E09.35–E09.9

✓4th **E1Ø Type 1 diabetes mellitus**

INCLUDES brittle diabetes (mellitus)
diabetes (mellitus) due to autoimmune process
diabetes (mellitus) due to immune mediated pancreatic islet beta-cell destruction
idiopathic diabetes (mellitus)
juvenile onset diabetes (mellitus)
ketosis-prone diabetes (mellitus)

EXCLUDES 1 *diabetes mellitus due to underlying condition (EØ8.-)*
*drug or chemical induced diabetes mellitus (EØ9.-)*
*gestational diabetes (O24.4-)*
*hyperglycemia NOS (R73.9)*
*neonatal diabetes mellitus (P7Ø.2)*
*postpancreatectomy diabetes mellitus (E13.-)*
*postprocedural diabetes mellitus (E13.-)*
*secondary diabetes mellitus NEC (E13.-)*
*type 2 diabetes mellitus (E11.-)*

**AHA:** 2023,2Q,10; 2020,3Q,30

✓5th **E1Ø.1 Type 1 diabetes mellitus with ketoacidosis**

**AHA:** 2013,3Q,20

**DEF:** Diabetic ketoacidosis: Potentially life-threatening complication due to a shortage of insulin in which the body switches to burning fatty acids and producing acidic ketone bodies.

**E1Ø.1Ø Type 1 diabetes mellitus with ketoacidosis without coma** HCC Rx ESR COM Q

**E1Ø.11 Type 1 diabetes mellitus with ketoacidosis with coma** HCC Rx ESR COM Q

✓5th **E1Ø.2 Type 1 diabetes mellitus with kidney complications**

**AHA:** 2019,3Q,3; 2018,4Q,88

**E1Ø.21 Type 1 diabetes mellitus with diabetic nephropathy** HCC Rx ESR COM Q

Type 1 diabetes mellitus with intercapillary glomerulosclerosis
Type 1 diabetes mellitus with intracapillary glomerulonephrosis
Type 1 diabetes mellitus with Kimmelstiel-Wilson disease

**E1Ø.22 Type 1 diabetes mellitus with diabetic chronic kidney disease** HCC Rx ESR COM Q

Use additional code to identify stage of chronic kidney disease (N18.1-N18.6)

**AHA:** 2024,3Q,12

**E1Ø.29 Type 1 diabetes mellitus with other diabetic kidney complication** HCC Rx ESR COM Q

Type 1 diabetes mellitus with renal tubular degeneration

**AHA:** 2016,1Q,13

✓5th **E1Ø.3 Type 1 diabetes mellitus with ophthalmic complications**

**AHA:** 2016,4Q,11-13

One of the following 7th characters is to be assigned to codes in subcategories E1Ø.32, E1Ø.33, E1Ø.34, E1Ø.35, and E1Ø.37 to designate laterality of the disease:
1 right eye
2 left eye
3 bilateral
9 unspecified eye

✓6th **E1Ø.31 Type 1 diabetes mellitus with unspecified diabetic retinopathy**

**DEF:** Diabetic retinopathy: Diabetic complication from damage to the retinal vessels resulting in vision problems that can progress to blindness.

**E1Ø.311 Type 1 diabetes mellitus with unspecified diabetic retinopathy with macular edema** HCC Rx ESR COM Q

**E1Ø.319 Type 1 diabetes mellitus with unspecified diabetic retinopathy without macular edema** HCC Rx ESR COM Q

✓6th **E1Ø.32 Type 1 diabetes mellitus with mild nonproliferative diabetic retinopathy**

Type 1 diabetes mellitus with nonproliferative diabetic retinopathy NOS

✓7th **E1Ø.321 Type 1 diabetes mellitus with mild nonproliferative diabetic retinopathy with macular edema** HCC Rx ESR COM Q

✓7th **E1Ø.329 Type 1 diabetes mellitus with mild nonproliferative diabetic retinopathy without macular edema** HCC Rx ESR COM Q

✓6th **E1Ø.33 Type 1 diabetes mellitus with moderate nonproliferative diabetic retinopathy**

✓7th **E1Ø.331 Type 1 diabetes mellitus with moderate nonproliferative diabetic retinopathy with macular edema** HCC Rx ESR COM Q

✓7th **E1Ø.339 Type 1 diabetes mellitus with moderate nonproliferative diabetic retinopathy without macular edema** HCC Rx ESR COM Q

✓6th **E1Ø.34 Type 1 diabetes mellitus with severe nonproliferative diabetic retinopathy**

✓7th **E1Ø.341 Type 1 diabetes mellitus with severe nonproliferative diabetic retinopathy with macular edema** HCC Rx ESR COM Q

✓7th **E1Ø.349 Type 1 diabetes mellitus with severe nonproliferative diabetic retinopathy without macular edema** HCC Rx ESR COM Q

✓6th **E1Ø.35 Type 1 diabetes mellitus with proliferative diabetic retinopathy**

✓7th **E1Ø.351 Type 1 diabetes mellitus with proliferative diabetic retinopathy with macular edema** HCC Rx ESR COM Q

✓7th **E1Ø.352 Type 1 diabetes mellitus with proliferative diabetic retinopathy with traction retinal detachment involving the macula** HCC Rx ESR COM Q

✓7th **E1Ø.353 Type 1 diabetes mellitus with proliferative diabetic retinopathy with traction retinal detachment not involving the macula** HCC Rx ESR COM Q

✓7th **E1Ø.354 Type 1 diabetes mellitus with proliferative diabetic retinopathy with combined traction retinal detachment and rhegmatogenous retinal detachment** HCC Rx ESR COM Q

✓7th **E1Ø.355 Type 1 diabetes mellitus with stable proliferative diabetic retinopathy** HCC Rx ESR COM Q

✓7th **E1Ø.359 Type 1 diabetes mellitus with proliferative diabetic retinopathy without macular edema** HCC Rx ESR COM Q

**E1Ø.36 Type 1 diabetes mellitus with diabetic cataract** HCC Rx ESR COM Q

**AHA:** 2019,2Q,30-31; 2016,4Q,142

✓x7th **E1Ø.37 Type 1 diabetes mellitus with diabetic macular edema, resolved following treatment** HCC Rx ESR COM Q

**E1Ø.39 Type 1 diabetes mellitus with other diabetic ophthalmic complication** HCC Rx ESR COM Q

Use additional code to identify manifestation, such as: diabetic glaucoma (H4Ø-H42)

**AHA:** 2023,3Q,19

✓5th **E1Ø.4 Type 1 diabetes mellitus with neurological complications**

**E1Ø.4Ø Type 1 diabetes mellitus with diabetic neuropathy, unspecified** HCC Rx ESR COM Q

**E1Ø.41 Type 1 diabetes mellitus with diabetic mononeuropathy** HCC Rx ESR COM Q

**E1Ø.42 Type 1 diabetes mellitus with diabetic polyneuropathy** HCC Rx ESR COM Q

Type 1 diabetes mellitus with diabetic neuralgia

**E1Ø.43 Type 1 diabetes mellitus with diabetic autonomic (poly)neuropathy** HCC Rx ESR COM Q

Type 1 diabetes mellitus with diabetic gastroparesis

**AHA:** 2013,4Q,114

**E1Ø.44 Type 1 diabetes mellitus with diabetic amyotrophy** HCC Rx ESR COM Q

**E1Ø.49 Type 1 diabetes mellitus with other diabetic neurological complication** HCC Rx ESR COM Q

✓5th **E1Ø.5 Type 1 diabetes mellitus with circulatory complications**

**E1Ø.51 Type 1 diabetes mellitus with diabetic peripheral angiopathy without gangrene** HCC Rx ESR COM Q

**AHA:** 2018,3Q,3-4; 2018,2Q,7

**E1Ø.52 Type 1 diabetes mellitus with diabetic peripheral angiopathy with gangrene** HCC Rx ESR COM Q

Type 1 diabetes mellitus with diabetic gangrene

**AHA:** 2020,2Q,18; 2018,3Q,3; 2018,2Q,7; 2017,4Q,102

**E1Ø.59 Type 1 diabetes mellitus with other circulatory complications** HCC Rx ESR COM Q

✓5th **E10.6 Type 1 diabetes mellitus with other specified complications**

✓6th **E10.61 Type 1 diabetes mellitus with diabetic arthropathy**

**E10.610 Type 1 diabetes mellitus with diabetic neuropathic arthropathy** HCC Rx ESR COM Q

Type 1 diabetes mellitus with Charcôt's joints

**DEF:** Charcot's joint: Progressive neurologic arthropathy in which chronic degeneration of joints in the weight-bearing areas with peripheral hypertrophy occurs as a complication of a neuropathy disorder. Supporting structures relax from a loss of sensation resulting in chronic joint instability.

**E10.618 Type 1 diabetes mellitus with other diabetic arthropathy** HCC Rx ESR COM Q

**AHA:** 2018,2Q,6

✓6th **E10.62 Type 1 diabetes mellitus with skin complications**

**E10.620 Type 1 diabetes mellitus with diabetic dermatitis** HCC Rx ESR COM Q

Type 1 diabetes mellitus with diabetic necrobiosis lipoidica

**AHA:** 2024,3Q,12

**E10.621 Type 1 diabetes mellitus with foot ulcer** HCC Rx ESR COM Q

Use additional code to identify site of ulcer (L97.4-, L97.5-)

**AHA:** 2020,2Q,19

**TIP:** Do not assign a code for diabetic ulcer when the ulcer is closed/resolved or to report history of diabetic ulcers; Z86.31 Personal history of diabetic foot ulcer, may be assigned.

**E10.622 Type 1 diabetes mellitus with other skin ulcer** HCC Rx ESR COM Q

Use additional code to identify site of ulcer (L97.1-L97.9, L98.41-L98.49)

**AHA:** 2021,1Q,7; 2017,4Q,17

**E10.628 Type 1 diabetes mellitus with other skin complications** HCC Rx ESR COM Q

✓6th **E10.63 Type 1 diabetes mellitus with oral complications**

**E10.630 Type 1 diabetes mellitus with periodontal disease** HCC Rx ESR COM Q

**E10.638 Type 1 diabetes mellitus with other oral complications** HCC Rx ESR COM Q

✓6th **E10.64 Type 1 diabetes mellitus with hypoglycemia**

Use additional code for hypoglycemia level, if applicable (E16.A-)

**AHA:** 2017,1Q,42

**E10.641 Type 1 diabetes mellitus with hypoglycemia with coma** HCC Rx ESR COM Q

**E10.649 Type 1 diabetes mellitus with hypoglycemia without coma** HCC Rx ESR COM Q

**AHA:** 2016,3Q,42; 2016,1Q,13; 2015,3Q,21

**E10.65 Type 1 diabetes mellitus with hyperglycemia** HCC Rx ESR COM Q

**AHA:** 2022,1Q,28; 2017,1Q,42; 2013,3Q,20

**E10.69 Type 1 diabetes mellitus with other specified complication** HCC Rx ESR COM Q

Use additional code to identify complication

**AHA:** 2022,1Q,28; 2016,4Q,141; 2016,1Q,13

**E10.8 Type 1 diabetes mellitus with unspecified complications** HCC Rx ESR COM Q

**E10.9 Type 1 diabetes mellitus without complications** HCC Rx ESR COM Q

**AHA:** 2023,3Q,19; 2020,2Q,18

✓5th **E10.A Type 1 diabetes mellitus, presymptomatic**

Early-stage type 1 diabetes mellitus

**AHA:** 2024,4Q,5

**E10.A0 Type 1 diabetes mellitus, presymptomatic, unspecified**

**E10.A1 Type 1 diabetes mellitus, presymptomatic, Stage 1**

Multiple confirmed islet autoantibodies with normoglycemia

**E10.A2 Type 1 diabetes mellitus, presymptomatic, Stage 2** Q

Confirmed islet autoimmunity with dysglycemia

✓4th **E11 Type 2 diabetes mellitus**

INCLUDES diabetes (mellitus) due to insulin secretory defect
diabetes NOS
insulin resistant diabetes (mellitus)

Use additional code to identify control using:
injectable non-insulin antidiabetic drugs (Z79.85)
insulin (Z79.4)
oral antidiabetic drugs (Z79.84)
oral hypoglycemic drugs (Z79.84)

EXCLUDES 1 *diabetes mellitus due to underlying condition (E08.-)*
*drug or chemical induced diabetes mellitus (E09.-)*
*gestational diabetes (O24.4-)*
*neonatal diabetes mellitus (P70.2)*
*postpancreatectomy diabetes mellitus (E13.-)*
*postprocedural diabetes mellitus (E13.-)*
*secondary diabetes mellitus NEC (E13.-)*
*type 1 diabetes mellitus (E10.-)*

**AHA:** 2020,3Q,30; 2020,1Q,12; 2016,2Q,10; 2013,1Q,26

✓5th **E11.0 Type 2 diabetes mellitus with hyperosmolarity**

**DEF:** Diabetic hyperosmolarity: Extremely high levels of glucose in the blood without ketones.

**E11.00 Type 2 diabetes mellitus with hyperosmolarity without nonketotic hyperglycemic-hyperosmolar coma (NKHHC)** HCC Rx ESR COM Q

**AHA:** 2022,1Q,28

**E11.01 Type 2 diabetes mellitus with hyperosmolarity with coma** HCC Rx ESR COM Q

✓5th **E11.1 Type 2 diabetes mellitus with ketoacidosis**

**AHA:** 2017,4Q,6

**DEF:** Diabetic ketoacidosis: Potentially life-threatening complication due to a shortage of insulin in which the body switches to burning fatty acids and producing acidic ketone bodies.

**E11.10 Type 2 diabetes mellitus with ketoacidosis without coma** HCC Rx ESR COM

**E11.11 Type 2 diabetes mellitus with ketoacidosis with coma** HCC Rx ESR COM

✓5th **E11.2 Type 2 diabetes mellitus with kidney complications**

**AHA:** 2019,3Q,3; 2018,4Q,88

**E11.21 Type 2 diabetes mellitus with diabetic nephropathy** HCC Rx ESR COM Q

Type 2 diabetes mellitus with intercapillary glomerulosclerosis

Type 2 diabetes mellitus with intracapillary glomerulonephrosis

Type 2 diabetes mellitus with Kimmelstiel-Wilson disease

**E11.22 Type 2 diabetes mellitus with diabetic chronic kidney disease** HCC Rx ESR COM Q

Use additional code to identify stage of chronic kidney disease (N18.1-N18.6)

**AHA:** 2026,2Q,9; 2025,4Q,7; 2024,3Q,12; 2022,3Q,15

**E11.29 Type 2 diabetes mellitus with other diabetic kidney complication** HCC Rx ESR COM Q

Type 2 diabetes mellitus with renal tubular degeneration

**AHA:** 2025,3Q,4

✓5th **E11.3 Type 2 diabetes mellitus with ophthalmic complications**

**AHA:** 2016,4Q,11-13

One of the following 7th characters is to be assigned to codes in subcategories E11.32, E11.33, E11.34, E11.35, and E11.37 to designate laterality of the disease:
1 right eye
2 left eye
3 bilateral
9 unspecified eye

✓6th **E11.31 Type 2 diabetes mellitus with unspecified diabetic retinopathy**

**DEF:** Diabetic retinopathy: Diabetic complication from damage to the retinal vessels resulting in vision problems that can progress to blindness.

**E11.311 Type 2 diabetes mellitus with unspecified diabetic retinopathy with macular edema** HCC Rx ESR COM Q

**E11.319** Type 2 diabetes mellitus with unspecified diabetic retinopathy without macular edema HCC Rx ESR COM Q

✓6th **E11.32** Type 2 diabetes mellitus with mild nonproliferative diabetic retinopathy
Type 2 diabetes mellitus with nonproliferative diabetic retinopathy NOS

✓7th **E11.321** Type 2 diabetes mellitus with mild nonproliferative diabetic retinopathy with macular edema HCC Rx ESR COM Q

✓7th **E11.329** Type 2 diabetes mellitus with mild nonproliferative diabetic retinopathy without macular edema HCC Rx ESR COM Q

✓6th **E11.33** Type 2 diabetes mellitus with moderate nonproliferative diabetic retinopathy

✓7th **E11.331** Type 2 diabetes mellitus with moderate nonproliferative diabetic retinopathy with macular edema HCC Rx ESR COM Q

✓7th **E11.339** Type 2 diabetes mellitus with moderate nonproliferative diabetic retinopathy without macular edema HCC Rx ESR COM Q

✓6th **E11.34** Type 2 diabetes mellitus with severe nonproliferative diabetic retinopathy

✓7th **E11.341** Type 2 diabetes mellitus with severe nonproliferative diabetic retinopathy with macular edema HCC Rx ESR COM Q

✓7th **E11.349** Type 2 diabetes mellitus with severe nonproliferative diabetic retinopathy without macular edema HCC Rx ESR COM Q

✓6th **E11.35** Type 2 diabetes mellitus with proliferative diabetic retinopathy

✓7th **E11.351** Type 2 diabetes mellitus with proliferative diabetic retinopathy with macular edema HCC Rx ESR COM Q

✓7th **E11.352** Type 2 diabetes mellitus with proliferative diabetic retinopathy with traction retinal detachment involving the macula HCC Rx ESR COM Q

✓7th **E11.353** Type 2 diabetes mellitus with proliferative diabetic retinopathy with traction retinal detachment not involving the macula HCC Rx ESR COM Q

✓7th **E11.354** Type 2 diabetes mellitus with proliferative diabetic retinopathy with combined traction retinal detachment and rhegmatogenous retinal detachment HCC Rx ESR COM Q

✓7th **E11.355** Type 2 diabetes mellitus with stable proliferative diabetic retinopathy HCC Rx ESR COM Q

✓7th **E11.359** Type 2 diabetes mellitus with proliferative diabetic retinopathy without macular edema HCC Rx ESR COM Q

**E11.36** Type 2 diabetes mellitus with diabetic cataract HCC Rx ESR COM Q
**AHA:** 2019,2Q,30-31; 2016,4Q,142

✓x7th **E11.37** Type 2 diabetes mellitus with diabetic macular edema, resolved following treatment HCC Rx ESR COM Q

**E11.39** Type 2 diabetes mellitus with other diabetic ophthalmic complication HCC Rx ESR COM Q
Use additional code to identify manifestation, such as: diabetic glaucoma (H40-H42)
**AHA:** 2023,3Q,19

✓5th **E11.4** Type 2 diabetes mellitus with neurological complications
**AHA:** 2022,3Q,15

**E11.40** Type 2 diabetes mellitus with diabetic neuropathy, unspecified HCC Rx ESR COM Q
**AHA:** 2013,4Q,129

**E11.41** Type 2 diabetes mellitus with diabetic mononeuropathy HCC Rx ESR COM Q

**E11.42** Type 2 diabetes mellitus with diabetic polyneuropathy HCC Rx ESR COM Q
Type 2 diabetes mellitus with diabetic neuralgia
**AHA:** 2020,1Q,12

**E11.43** Type 2 diabetes mellitus with diabetic autonomic (poly)neuropathy HCC Rx ESR COM Q
Type 2 diabetes mellitus with diabetic gastroparesis
**AHA:** 2023,2Q,8; 2013,4Q,114

**E11.44** Type 2 diabetes mellitus with diabetic amyotrophy HCC Rx ESR COM Q

**E11.49** Type 2 diabetes mellitus with other diabetic neurological complication HCC Rx ESR COM Q

✓5th **E11.5** Type 2 diabetes mellitus with circulatory complications

**E11.51** Type 2 diabetes mellitus with diabetic peripheral angiopathy without gangrene HCC Rx ESR COM Q
**AHA:** 2018,3Q,3-4; 2018,2Q,7

**E11.52** Type 2 diabetes mellitus with diabetic peripheral angiopathy with gangrene HCC Rx ESR COM Q
Type 2 diabetes mellitus with diabetic gangrene
**AHA:** 2020,2Q,18; 2018,3Q,3; 2018,2Q,7; 2017,4Q,102

**E11.59** Type 2 diabetes mellitus with other circulatory complications HCC Rx ESR COM Q
**AHA:** 2026,2Q,9

✓5th **E11.6** Type 2 diabetes mellitus with other specified complications

✓6th **E11.61** Type 2 diabetes mellitus with diabetic arthropathy

**E11.610** Type 2 diabetes mellitus with diabetic neuropathic arthropathy HCC Rx ESR COM Q
Type 2 diabetes mellitus with Charcôt's joints
**DEF:** Charcot's joint: Progressive neurologic arthropathy in which chronic degeneration of joints in the weight-bearing areas with peripheral hypertrophy occurs as a complication of a neuropathy disorder. Supporting structures relax from a loss of sensation resulting in chronic joint instability.

**E11.618** Type 2 diabetes mellitus with other diabetic arthropathy HCC Rx ESR COM Q
**AHA:** 2018,2Q,6

✓6th **E11.62** Type 2 diabetes mellitus with skin complications

**E11.620** Type 2 diabetes mellitus with diabetic dermatitis HCC Rx ESR COM Q
Type 2 diabetes mellitus with diabetic necrobiosis lipoidica
**AHA:** 2024,3Q,12

**E11.621** Type 2 diabetes mellitus with foot ulcer HCC Rx ESR COM Q
Use additional code to identify site of ulcer (L97.4-, L97.5-)
**AHA:** 2020,2Q,19; 2020,1Q,12
**TIP:** Do not assign a code for diabetic ulcer when the ulcer is closed/resolved or to report history of diabetic ulcers; Z86.31 Personal history of diabetic foot ulcer, may be assigned.

**E11.622** Type 2 diabetes mellitus with other skin ulcer HCC Rx ESR COM Q
Use additional code to identify site of ulcer (L97.1-L97.9, L98.41-L98.49)
**AHA:** 2021,1Q,7; 2017,4Q,17

**E11.628** Type 2 diabetes mellitus with other skin complications HCC Rx ESR COM Q

✓6th **E11.63** Type 2 diabetes mellitus with oral complications

**E11.630** Type 2 diabetes mellitus with periodontal disease HCC Rx ESR COM Q

**E11.638** Type 2 diabetes mellitus with other oral complications HCC Rx ESR COM Q

✓6th **E11.64** Type 2 diabetes mellitus with hypoglycemia
Use additional code for hypoglycemia level, if applicable (E16.A-)
**AHA:** 2017,1Q,42

**E11.641** Type 2 diabetes mellitus with hypoglycemia with coma HCC Rx ESR COM Q

**E11.649** Type 2 diabetes mellitus with hypoglycemia without coma HCC Rx ESR COM Q
**AHA:** 2016,3Q,42; 2015,3Q,21

**E11.65 Type 2 diabetes mellitus with hyperglycemia** HCC Rx ESR COM Q
AHA: 2026,2Q,9; 2023,2Q,10; 2022,1Q,28; 2017,1Q,42; 2013,3Q,20

**E11.69 Type 2 diabetes mellitus with other specified complication** HCC Rx ESR COM Q
Use additional code to identify complication
AHA: 2025,3Q,3; 2020,1Q,12; 2016,4Q,141; 2016,1Q,13

**E11.8 Type 2 diabetes mellitus with unspecified complications** HCC Rx ESR COM Q

**E11.9 Type 2 diabetes mellitus without complications** HCC Rx ESR COM Q
EXCLUDES 1 *type 2 diabetes mellitus, without complications in remission (E11.A)*
AHA: 2025,1Q,35; 2024,3Q,12; 2023,3Q,19; 2020,2Q,18

**E11.A Type 2 diabetes mellitus without complications in remission**
EXCLUDES 1 *type 2 diabetes mellitus, with complications (E11.Ø-E11.8)*
*type 2 diabetes mellitus, without complications not in remission (E11.9)*
AHA: 2025,4Q,7-8

## ✓4th E13 Other specified diabetes mellitus

INCLUDES diabetes mellitus due to genetic defects of beta-cell function
diabetes mellitus due to genetic defects in insulin action
postpancreatectomy diabetes mellitus
postprocedural diabetes mellitus
secondary diabetes mellitus NEC

Use additional code to identify control using:
injectable non-insulin antidiabetic drugs (Z79.85)
insulin (Z79.4)
oral antidiabetic drugs (Z79.84)
oral hypoglycemic drugs (Z79.84)

EXCLUDES 1 *diabetes (mellitus) due to autoimmune process (E1Ø.-)*
*diabetes (mellitus) due to immune mediated pancreatic islet beta-cell destruction (E1Ø.-)*
*diabetes mellitus due to underlying condition (EØ8.-)*
*drug or chemical induced diabetes mellitus (EØ9.-)*
*gestational diabetes (O24.4-)*
*neonatal diabetes mellitus (P7Ø.2)*
*type 1 diabetes mellitus (E1Ø.-)*

AHA: 2018,3Q,4; 2016,1Q,11-13

TIP: Use this category when the diabetes is documented as diabetes type 1.5. Synonymous terms used in the documentation may also include combined diabetes type 1 and type 2, latent autoimmune diabetes of adults (LADA), slow-progressing type 1 diabetes, or double diabetes.

TIP: When postprocedural or postpancreatectomy hypoinsulinemia (E89.1) is documented with postprocedural or postpancreatectomy diabetes mellitus (E13.-), code E13.- should be sequenced first.

**✓5th E13.Ø Other specified diabetes mellitus with hyperosmolarity**
DEF: Diabetic hyperosmolarity: Extremely high levels of glucose in the blood without ketones.

**E13.ØØ Other specified diabetes mellitus with hyperosmolarity without nonketotic hyperglycemic-hyperosmolar coma (NKHHC)** HCC Rx ESR COM Q

**E13.Ø1 Other specified diabetes mellitus with hyperosmolarity with coma** HCC Rx ESR COM Q

**✓5th E13.1 Other specified diabetes mellitus with ketoacidosis**
AHA: 2016,2Q,10; 2013,1Q,26
DEF: Diabetic ketoacidosis: Potentially life-threatening complication due to a shortage of insulin in which the body switches to burning fatty acids and producing acidic ketone bodies.

**E13.1Ø Other specified diabetes mellitus with ketoacidosis without coma** HCC Rx ESR COM Q

**E13.11 Other specified diabetes mellitus with ketoacidosis with coma** HCC Rx ESR COM Q

**✓5th E13.2 Other specified diabetes mellitus with kidney complications**
AHA: 2019,3Q,3; 2018,4Q,88

**E13.21 Other specified diabetes mellitus with diabetic nephropathy** HCC Rx ESR COM Q
Other specified diabetes mellitus with intercapillary glomerulosclerosis
Other specified diabetes mellitus with intracapillary glomerulonephrosis
Other specified diabetes mellitus with Kimmelstiel-Wilson disease

**E13.22 Other specified diabetes mellitus with diabetic chronic kidney disease** HCC Rx ESR COM Q
Use additional code to identify stage of chronic kidney disease (N18.1-N18.6)

**E13.29 Other specified diabetes mellitus with other diabetic kidney complication** HCC Rx ESR COM Q
Other specified diabetes mellitus with renal tubular degeneration

**✓5th E13.3 Other specified diabetes mellitus with ophthalmic complications**
AHA: 2016,4Q,11-13

One of the following 7th characters is to be assigned to codes in subcategories E13.32, E13.33, E13.34, E13.35, and E13.37 to designate laterality of the disease:
1 right eye
2 left eye
3 bilateral
9 unspecified eye

**✓6th E13.31 Other specified diabetes mellitus with unspecified diabetic retinopathy**
DEF: Diabetic retinopathy: Diabetic complication from damage to the retinal vessels resulting in vision problems that can progress to blindness.

**E13.311 Other specified diabetes mellitus with unspecified diabetic retinopathy with macular edema** HCC Rx ESR COM Q

**E13.319 Other specified diabetes mellitus with unspecified diabetic retinopathy without macular edema** HCC Rx ESR COM Q

**✓6th E13.32 Other specified diabetes mellitus with mild nonproliferative diabetic retinopathy**
Other specified diabetes mellitus with nonproliferative diabetic retinopathy NOS

**✓7th E13.321 Other specified diabetes mellitus with mild nonproliferative diabetic retinopathy with macular edema** HCC Rx ESR COM Q

**✓7th E13.329 Other specified diabetes mellitus with mild nonproliferative diabetic retinopathy without macular edema** HCC Rx ESR COM Q

**✓6th E13.33 Other specified diabetes mellitus with moderate nonproliferative diabetic retinopathy**

**✓7th E13.331 Other specified diabetes mellitus with moderate nonproliferative diabetic retinopathy with macular edema** HCC Rx ESR COM Q

**✓7th E13.339 Other specified diabetes mellitus with moderate nonproliferative diabetic retinopathy without macular edema** HCC Rx ESR COM Q

**✓6th E13.34 Other specified diabetes mellitus with severe nonproliferative diabetic retinopathy**

**✓7th E13.341 Other specified diabetes mellitus with severe nonproliferative diabetic retinopathy with macular edema** HCC Rx ESR COM Q

**✓7th E13.349 Other specified diabetes mellitus with severe nonproliferative diabetic retinopathy without macular edema** HCC Rx ESR COM Q

**✓6th E13.35 Other specified diabetes mellitus with proliferative diabetic retinopathy**

**✓7th E13.351 Other specified diabetes mellitus with proliferative diabetic retinopathy with macular edema** HCC Rx ESR COM Q

**✓7th E13.352 Other specified diabetes mellitus with proliferative diabetic retinopathy with traction retinal detachment involving the macula** HCC Rx ESR COM Q

**✓7th E13.353 Other specified diabetes mellitus with proliferative diabetic retinopathy with traction retinal detachment not involving the macula** HCC Rx ESR COM Q

**✓7th E13.354 Other specified diabetes mellitus with proliferative diabetic retinopathy with combined traction retinal detachment and rhegmatogenous retinal detachment** HCC Rx ESR COM Q

**✓7th E13.355 Other specified diabetes mellitus with stable proliferative diabetic retinopathy** HCC Rx ESR COM Q

✓7th **E13.359 Other specified diabetes mellitus with proliferative diabetic retinopathy without macular edema** HCC Rx ESR COM Q

**E13.36 Other specified diabetes mellitus with diabetic cataract** HCC Rx ESR COM Q
AHA: 2019,2Q,30-31; 2016,4Q,142

✓x7th **E13.37 Other specified diabetes mellitus with diabetic macular edema, resolved following treatment** HCC Rx ESR COM Q

**E13.39 Other specified diabetes mellitus with other diabetic ophthalmic complication** HCC Rx ESR COM Q
Use additional code to identify manifestation, such as:
diabetic glaucoma (H40-H42)
AHA: 2023,3Q,19

✓5th **E13.4 Other specified diabetes mellitus with neurological complications**

**E13.40 Other specified diabetes mellitus with diabetic neuropathy, unspecified** HCC Rx ESR COM Q

**E13.41 Other specified diabetes mellitus with diabetic mononeuropathy** HCC Rx ESR COM Q

**E13.42 Other specified diabetes mellitus with diabetic polyneuropathy** HCC Rx ESR COM Q
Other specified diabetes mellitus with diabetic neuralgia

**E13.43 Other specified diabetes mellitus with diabetic autonomic (poly)neuropathy** HCC Rx ESR COM Q
Other specified diabetes mellitus with diabetic gastroparesis
AHA: 2013,4Q,114

**E13.44 Other specified diabetes mellitus with diabetic amyotrophy** HCC Rx ESR COM Q

**E13.49 Other specified diabetes mellitus with other diabetic neurological complication** HCC Rx ESR COM Q

✓5th **E13.5 Other specified diabetes mellitus with circulatory complications**

**E13.51 Other specified diabetes mellitus with diabetic peripheral angiopathy without gangrene** HCC Rx ESR COM Q
AHA: 2018,3Q,3-4; 2018,2Q,7

**E13.52 Other specified diabetes mellitus with diabetic peripheral angiopathy with gangrene** HCC Rx ESR COM Q
Other specified diabetes mellitus with diabetic gangrene
AHA: 2020,2Q,18; 2018,3Q,3; 2018,2Q,7; 2017,4Q,102

**E13.59 Other specified diabetes mellitus with other circulatory complications** HCC Rx ESR COM Q

✓5th **E13.6 Other specified diabetes mellitus with other specified complications**

✓6th **E13.61 Other specified diabetes mellitus with diabetic arthropathy**

**E13.610 Other specified diabetes mellitus with diabetic neuropathic arthropathy** HCC Rx ESR COM Q
Other specified diabetes mellitus with Charcôt's joints
DEF: Charcot's joint: Progressive neurologic arthropathy in which chronic degeneration of joints in the weight-bearing areas with peripheral hypertrophy occurs as a complication of a neuropathy disorder. Supporting structures relax from a loss of sensation resulting in chronic joint instability.

**E13.618 Other specified diabetes mellitus with other diabetic arthropathy** HCC Rx ESR COM Q
AHA: 2018,2Q,6

✓6th **E13.62 Other specified diabetes mellitus with skin complications**

**E13.620 Other specified diabetes mellitus with diabetic dermatitis** HCC Rx ESR COM Q
Other specified diabetes mellitus with diabetic necrobiosis lipoidica

**E13.621 Other specified diabetes mellitus with foot ulcer** HCC Rx ESR COM Q
Use additional code to identify site of ulcer (L97.4-, L97.5-)
AHA: 2020,2Q,19
TIP: Do not assign a code for diabetic ulcer when the ulcer is closed/resolved or to report history of diabetic ulcers; Z86.31 Personal history of diabetic foot ulcer, may be assigned.

**E13.622 Other specified diabetes mellitus with other skin ulcer** HCC Rx ESR COM Q
Use additional code to identify site of ulcer (L97.1-L97.9, L98.41-L98.49)
AHA: 2021,1Q,7; 2017,4Q,17

**E13.628 Other specified diabetes mellitus with other skin complications** HCC Rx ESR COM Q

✓6th **E13.63 Other specified diabetes mellitus with oral complications**

**E13.630 Other specified diabetes mellitus with periodontal disease** HCC Rx ESR COM Q

**E13.638 Other specified diabetes mellitus with other oral complications** HCC Rx ESR COM Q

✓6th **E13.64 Other specified diabetes mellitus with hypoglycemia**
Use additional code for hypoglycemia level, if applicable (E16.A-)
AHA: 2017,1Q,42

**E13.641 Other specified diabetes mellitus with hypoglycemia with coma** HCC Rx ESR COM Q

**E13.649 Other specified diabetes mellitus with hypoglycemia without coma** HCC Rx ESR COM Q
AHA: 2016,3Q,42; 2015,3Q,21

**E13.65 Other specified diabetes mellitus with hyperglycemia** HCC Rx ESR COM Q
AHA: 2017,1Q,42; 2013,3Q,20

**E13.69 Other specified diabetes mellitus with other specified complication** HCC Rx ESR COM Q
Use additional code to identify complication
AHA: 2016,4Q,141; 2016,1Q,13

**E13.8 Other specified diabetes mellitus with unspecified complications** HCC Rx ESR COM Q

**E13.9 Other specified diabetes mellitus without complications** HCC Rx ESR COM Q
AHA: 2023,3Q,19; 2020,2Q,18

## Other disorders of glucose regulation and pancreatic internal secretion (E15-E16)

**E15 Nondiabetic hypoglycemic coma** ESR COM
INCLUDES drug-induced insulin coma in nondiabetic
hyperinsulinism with hypoglycemic coma
hypoglycemic coma NOS

✓4th **E16 Other disorders of pancreatic internal secretion**

**E16.0 Drug-induced hypoglycemia without coma**
Use additional code for adverse effect, if applicable, to identify drug (T36-T50 with fifth or sixth character 5)
Use additional code for hypoglycemia level, if applicable (E16.A-)
EXCLUDES 1 *diabetes with hypoglycemia without coma (E09.649)*

**E16.1 Other hypoglycemia**
Functional hyperinsulinism
Functional nonhyperinsulinemic hypoglycemia
Hyperinsulinism NOS
Hyperplasia of pancreatic islet beta cells NOS
Use additional code for hypoglycemia level, if applicable (E16.A-)
EXCLUDES 1 *diabetes with hypoglycemia (E08.649, E10.649, E11.649, E13.649)*
*hypoglycemia in infant of diabetic mother (P70.1)*
*neonatal hypoglycemia (P70.4)*
AHA: 2024,2Q,10

**E16.2 Hypoglycemia, unspecified**
Use additional code for hypoglycemia level, if applicable (E16.A-)
EXCLUDES 1 *diabetes with hypoglycemia (EØ8.649, E1Ø.649, E11.649, E13.649)*
AHA: 2024,4Q,7; 2016,3Q,42
TIP: Assign for nondiabetic hypoglycemic encephalopathy not further clarified in the documentation.

**E16.3 Increased secretion of glucagon** Rx
Hyperplasia of pancreatic endocrine cells with glucagon excess

**E16.4 Increased secretion of gastrin** Rx
Hypergastrinemia
Hyperplasia of pancreatic endocrine cells with gastrin excess
Zollinger-Ellison syndrome

**E16.8 Other specified disorders of pancreatic internal secretion** Rx
Increased secretion from endocrine pancreas of growth hormone-releasing hormone
Increased secretion from endocrine pancreas of pancreatic polypeptide
Increased secretion from endocrine pancreas of somatostatin
Increased secretion from endocrine pancreas of vasoactive-intestinal polypeptide

**E16.9 Disorder of pancreatic internal secretion, unspecified** Rx
Islet-cell hyperplasia NOS
Pancreatic endocrine cell hyperplasia NOS

✓5th **E16.A Hypoglycemia level**
AHA: 2024,4Q,6-7

**E16.A1 Hypoglycemia level 1**
Decreased blood glucose level 1

**E16.A2 Hypoglycemia level 2**
Decreased blood glucose level 2

**E16.A3 Hypoglycemia level 3**
Decreased blood glucose level 3

## Disorders of other endocrine glands (E2Ø-E35)

EXCLUDES 1 *galactorrhea (N64.3)*
*gynecomastia (N62)*

✓4th **E2Ø Hypoparathyroidism**
EXCLUDES 1 *Di George's syndrome (D82.1)*
*postprocedural hypoparathyroidism (E89.2)*
*tetany NOS (R29.Ø)*
*transitory neonatal hypoparathyroidism (P71.4)*

**E2Ø.Ø Idiopathic hypoparathyroidism** Rx ESR COM
DEF: Abnormally low secretion of parathyroid hormones, with unknown cause, which triggers decreased calcium and increased phosphorus in the blood that can result in cataracts, muscle cramps, tetany, tingling, or burning in the lips, fingers, and toes.

**E2Ø.1 Pseudohypoparathyroidism**

✓5th **E2Ø.8 Other hypoparathyroidism**

✓6th **E2Ø.81 Hypoparathyroidism due to impaired parathyroid hormone secretion**
AHA: 2023,4Q,9-11

**E2Ø.81Ø Autosomal dominant hypocalcemia** Rx ESR COM
Autosomal dominant hypocalcemia type 1 (ADH1)
Autosomal dominant hypocalcemia type 2 (ADH2)
Code also, if applicable, any associated conditions, such as:
calculus of kidney (N2Ø.Ø)
chronic kidney disease (N18.-)
respiratory distress (J8Ø, RØ6.-)
seizure disorder (G4Ø.-, R56.9)

***E2Ø.811 Secondary hypoparathyroidism in diseases classified elsewhere*** Rx ESR COM
Code first underlying condition, if known

**E2Ø.812 Autoimmune hypoparathyroidism** Rx ESR COM
Code first, if applicable, underlying condition such as:
autoimmune polyglandular failure (E31.Ø)
Schmidt's syndrome (E31.Ø)

**E2Ø.818 Other specified hypoparathyroidism due to impaired parathyroid hormone secretion** Rx ESR COM
Familial isolated hypoparathyroidism

**E2Ø.819 Hypoparathyroidism due to impaired parathyroid hormone secretion, unspecified** Rx ESR COM

**E2Ø.89 Other specified hypoparathyroidism** Rx ESR COM
Familial hypoparathyroidism

**E2Ø.9 Hypoparathyroidism, unspecified** Rx ESR COM
Parathyroid tetany

✓4th **E21 Hyperparathyroidism and other disorders of parathyroid gland**
EXCLUDES 1 *adult osteomalacia (M83.-)*
*ectopic hyperparathyroidism (E34.2)*
*hungry bone syndrome (E83.81)*
*infantile and juvenile osteomalacia (E55.Ø)*
EXCLUDES 2 *familial hypocalciuric hypercalcemia (E83.52)*

**E21.Ø Primary hyperparathyroidism** Rx ESR COM
Hyperplasia of parathyroid
Osteitis fibrosa cystica generalisata [von Recklinghausen's disease of bone]
DEF: Parathyroid dysfunction commonly caused by hyperplasia of two or more glands. Symptoms include hypercalcemia and increased parathyroid hormone levels.

**E21.1 Secondary hyperparathyroidism, not elsewhere classified** Rx ESR COM
EXCLUDES 1 *secondary hyperparathyroidism of renal origin (N25.81)*

**E21.2 Other hyperparathyroidism** Rx ESR COM
Tertiary hyperparathyroidism
EXCLUDES 1 ~~*familial hypocalciuric hypercalcemia (E83.52)*~~
EXCLUDES 2 ▶*familial hypocalciuric hypercalcemia (E83.52)*◀

**E21.3 Hyperparathyroidism, unspecified** Rx ESR COM

**E21.4 Other specified disorders of parathyroid gland** Rx ESR COM

**E21.5 Disorder of parathyroid gland, unspecified** Rx ESR COM

✓4th **E22 Hyperfunction of pituitary gland**
EXCLUDES 1 *Cushing's syndrome (E24.-)*
*Nelson's syndrome (E24.1)*
*overproduction of ACTH not associated with Cushing's disease (E27.Ø)*
*overproduction of pituitary ACTH (E24.Ø)*
*overproduction of thyroid-stimulating hormone (EØ5.8-)*

**E22.Ø Acromegaly and pituitary gigantism** HCC Rx ESR COM
Overproduction of growth hormone
EXCLUDES 1 *constitutional gigantism (E34.4)*
*constitutional tall stature (E34.4)*
*increased secretion from endocrine pancreas of growth hormone-releasing hormone (E16.8)*
DEF: Acromegaly: Chronic condition caused by overproduction of the pituitary growth hormone resulting in enlarged skeletal parts and facial features.

**E22.1 Hyperprolactinemia** Rx ESR COM
Use additional code for adverse effect, if applicable, to identify drug (T36-T5Ø with fifth or sixth character 5)

**E22.2 Syndrome of inappropriate secretion of antidiuretic hormone** Rx ESR COM

**E22.8 Other hyperfunction of pituitary gland** Rx ESR COM
Central precocious puberty

**E22.9 Hyperfunction of pituitary gland, unspecified** Rx ESR COM

✓4th **E23 Hypofunction and other disorders of the pituitary gland**
INCLUDES the listed conditions whether the disorder is in the pituitary or the hypothalamus
EXCLUDES 1 *postprocedural hypopituitarism (E89.3)*
*short stature due to endocrine disorder (E34.3-)*

**E23.Ø Hypopituitarism** Rx ESR COM
Fertile eunuch syndrome
Hypogonadotropic hypogonadism
Idiopathic growth hormone deficiency
Isolated deficiency of gonadotropin
Isolated deficiency of growth hormone
Isolated deficiency of pituitary hormone
Kallmann's syndrome
Lorain-Levi short stature
Necrosis of pituitary gland (postpartum)
Panhypopituitarism
Pituitary cachexia
Pituitary insufficiency NOS
Pituitary short stature
Sheehan's syndrome
Simmonds' disease
Use additional code, if applicable, for associated cachexia (E88.A)
AHA: 2024,1Q,15

**E23.1 Drug-induced hypopituitarism** Rx ESR COM
Use additional code for adverse effect, if applicable, to identify drug (T36-T5Ø with fifth or sixth character 5)

**E23.2 Diabetes insipidus** Rx ESR COM
EXCLUDES 1 *nephrogenic diabetes insipidus (N25.1)*

**E23.3 Hypothalamic dysfunction, not elsewhere classified** Rx ESR COM
EXCLUDES 1 *Prader-Willi syndrome (Q87.11)*
*Russell-Silver syndrome (Q87.19)*
**AHA:** 2024,1Q,15

**E23.6 Other disorders of pituitary gland** Rx ESR COM
Abscess of pituitary
Adiposogenital dystrophy
**AHA:** 2026,2Q,8
**TIP:** Code empty sella syndrome (ESS) here if it is documented. If there is only an imaging finding of an empty sella without pituitary problems, use code R93.0.

**E23.7 Disorder of pituitary gland, unspecified** Rx ESR COM

✓4th **E24 Cushing's syndrome**
EXCLUDES 1 *congenital adrenal hyperplasia (E25.Ø)*
**DEF:** Abdominal striae, acne, hypertension, decreased carbohydrate tolerance, moon face, obesity, protein catabolism, and psychiatric disturbances resulting from increased adrenocortical secretion of cortisol caused by ACTH-dependent adrenocortical hyperplasia or tumor, or by steroid effects.

**E24.Ø Pituitary-dependent Cushing's disease** HCC Rx ESR COM
Overproduction of pituitary ACTH
Pituitary-dependent hypercorticalism

**E24.1 Nelson's syndrome** Rx ESR COM

**E24.2 Drug-induced Cushing's syndrome** Rx ESR COM
Use additional code for adverse effect, if applicable, to identify drug (T36-T5Ø with fifth or sixth character 5)

**E24.3 Ectopic ACTH syndrome** Rx ESR COM

**E24.4 Alcohol-induced pseudo-Cushing's syndrome** Rx ESR COM

**E24.8 Other Cushing's syndrome** Rx ESR COM

**E24.9 Cushing's syndrome, unspecified** Rx ESR COM

✓4th **E25 Adrenogenital disorders**
INCLUDES adrenogenital syndromes, virilizing or feminizing, whether acquired or due to adrenal hyperplasia
consequent on inborn enzyme defects in hormone synthesis
female adrenal pseudohermaphroditism
female heterosexual precocious pseudopuberty
male isosexual precocious pseudopuberty
male macrogenitosomia praecox
male sexual precocity with adrenal hyperplasia
male virilization (female)
EXCLUDES 1 *chromosomal abnormalities (Q9Ø-Q99)*
*indeterminate sex and pseudohermaphroditism (Q56)*

**E25.Ø Congenital adrenogenital disorders associated with enzyme deficiency** Rx ESR COM
21-Hydroxylase deficiency
Congenital adrenal hyperplasia
Salt-losing congenital adrenal hyperplasia

**E25.8 Other adrenogenital disorders** Rx ESR COM
Idiopathic adrenogenital disorder
Use additional code for adverse effect, if applicable, to identify drug (T36-T5Ø with fifth or sixth character 5)

**E25.9 Adrenogenital disorder, unspecified** Rx ESR COM
Adrenogenital syndrome NOS

✓4th **E26 Hyperaldosteronism**

✓5th **E26.Ø Primary hyperaldosteronism**

**E26.Ø1 Conn's syndrome** Rx ESR COM
Code also adrenal adenoma (D35.Ø-)

**E26.Ø2 Glucocorticoid-remediable aldosteronism** Rx ESR COM
Familial aldosteronism type I
**DEF:** Rare autosomal dominant familial form of primary aldosteronism in which the secretion of aldosterone is under the influence of adrenocorticotrophic hormone (ACTH) rather than the renin-angiotensin mechanism. Moderate hypersecretion of aldosterone and suppressed plasma renin activity that are rapidly reversed by administration of glucosteroids. Symptoms include hypertension and mild hypokalemia.

**E26.Ø9 Other primary hyperaldosteronism** Rx ESR COM
Primary aldosteronism due to adrenal hyperplasia (bilateral)

**E26.1 Secondary hyperaldosteronism** Rx ESR COM

✓5th **E26.8 Other hyperaldosteronism**

**E26.81 Bartter's syndrome** Rx ESR COM

**E26.89 Other hyperaldosteronism** Rx ESR COM

**E26.9 Hyperaldosteronism, unspecified** Rx ESR COM
Aldosteronism NOS
Hyperaldosteronism NOS

✓4th **E27 Other disorders of adrenal gland**

**E27.Ø Other adrenocortical overactivity** Rx ESR COM
Overproduction of ACTH, not associated with Cushing's disease
Premature adrenarche
EXCLUDES 1 *Cushing's syndrome (E24.-)*

**E27.1 Primary adrenocortical insufficiency** HCC Rx ESR COM
Addison's disease
Autoimmune adrenalitis
EXCLUDES 1 *Addison only phenotype adrenoleukodystrophy (E71.528)*
*amyloidosis (E85.-)*
*tuberculous Addison's disease (A18.7)*
*Waterhouse-Friderichsen syndrome (A39.1)*

**E27.2 Addisonian crisis** Rx ESR COM
Adrenal crisis
Adrenocortical crisis
**DEF:** Life-threatening condition that occurs when there is not enough cortisol excreted from the adrenal glands. This condition may be due to injury to the adrenal glands or to the pituitary gland, which controls adrenal hormone secretion, or when a patient stops hydrocortisone treatment too quickly or too early.

**E27.3 Drug-induced adrenocortical insufficiency** Rx ESR COM
Use additional code for adverse effect, if applicable, to identify drug (T36-T5Ø with fifth or sixth character 5)

✓5th **E27.4 Other and unspecified adrenocortical insufficiency**
EXCLUDES 1 *adrenoleukodystrophy [Addison-Schilder] (E71.528)*
*Waterhouse-Friderichsen syndrome (A39.1)*

**E27.4Ø Unspecified adrenocortical insufficiency** Rx ESR COM
Adrenocortical insufficiency NOS
Hypoaldosteronism

**E27.49 Other adrenocortical insufficiency** Rx ESR COM
Adrenal hemorrhage
Adrenal infarction
**AHA:** 2024,1Q,15

**E27.5 Adrenomedullary hyperfunction** Rx ESR COM
Adrenomedullary hyperplasia
Catecholamine hypersecretion
Code also, if applicable:
malignant pheochromocytoma (C74.1-)
pheochromocytoma (benign) (D35.Ø-)
secondary hypertension (I15.2)

**E27.8 Other specified disorders of adrenal gland** Rx ESR COM
Abnormality of cortisol-binding globulin

**E27.9 Disorder of adrenal gland, unspecified** Rx ESR COM

✓4th **E28 Ovarian dysfunction**
EXCLUDES 1 *isolated gonadotropin deficiency (E23.Ø)*
*postprocedural ovarian failure (E89.4-)*

**E28.Ø Estrogen excess**
Use additional code for adverse effect, if applicable, to identify drug (T36-T5Ø with fifth or sixth character 5)

**E28.1 Androgen excess**
Hypersecretion of ovarian androgens
Use additional code for adverse effect, if applicable, to identify drug (T36-T5Ø with fifth or sixth character 5)

**E28.2 Polycystic ovarian syndrome**
Sclerocystic ovary syndrome
Stein-Leventhal syndrome
**AHA:** 2022,2Q,16
**DEF:** Common hormonal disorder among women of reproductive age that involves enlarged ovaries with numerous small cysts located along the outer ovarian edge.

✓5th **E28.3 Primary ovarian failure**
EXCLUDES 1 *pure gonadal dysgenesis (Q99.1)*
*Turner's syndrome (Q96.-)*

✓6th **E28.31 Premature menopause**

**E28.31Ø Symptomatic premature menopause** A
Symptoms such as flushing, sleeplessness, headache, lack of concentration, associated with premature menopause

E28.319 **Asymptomatic premature menopause** A
Premature menopause NOS

E28.39 **Other primary ovarian failure**
Decreased estrogen
Resistant ovary syndrome

E28.8 **Other ovarian dysfunction**
Ovarian hyperfunction NOS
EXCLUDES 1 *postprocedural ovarian failure (E89.4-)*

E28.9 **Ovarian dysfunction, unspecified**

✓4th **E29 Testicular dysfunction**
EXCLUDES 1 *androgen insensitivity syndrome (E34.5-)*
*azoospermia or oligospermia NOS (N46.Ø-N46.1)*
*isolated gonadotropin deficiency (E23.Ø)*
*Klinefelter's syndrome (Q98.Ø-Q98.1, Q98.4)*

E29.Ø **Testicular hyperfunction**
Hypersecretion of testicular hormones

E29.1 **Testicular hypofunction**
▶5-Alpha-reductase deficiency (with male pseudohermaphroditism)◀
Defective biosynthesis of testicular androgen NOS
Testicular hypogonadism NOS
Use additional code for adverse effect, if applicable, to identify drug (T36-T5Ø with fifth or sixth character 5)
EXCLUDES 1 *postprocedural testicular hypofunction (E89.5)*

E29.8 **Other testicular dysfunction**

E29.9 **Testicular dysfunction, unspecified**

✓4th **E3Ø Disorders of puberty, not elsewhere classified**

E3Ø.Ø **Delayed puberty**
Constitutional delay of puberty
Delayed sexual development

E3Ø.1 **Precocious puberty** P
Precocious menstruation
EXCLUDES 1 *Albright (-McCune) (-Sternberg) syndrome (Q78.1)*
*central precocious puberty (E22.8)*
*congenital adrenal hyperplasia (E25.Ø)*
*female heterosexual precocious pseudopuberty (E25.-)*
*male isosexual precocious pseudopuberty (E25.-)*

E3Ø.8 **Other disorders of puberty** P
Premature thelarche

E3Ø.9 **Disorder of puberty, unspecified**

✓4th **E31 Polyglandular dysfunction**
EXCLUDES 1 *ataxia telangiectasia [Louis-Bar] (G11.3)*
*dystrophia myotonica [Steinert] (G71.11)*
*pseudohypoparathyroidism (E2Ø.1)*

E31.Ø **Autoimmune polyglandular failure** HCC Rx ESR COM
Schmidt's syndrome

E31.1 **Polyglandular hyperfunction** HCC Rx ESR COM
EXCLUDES 1 *multiple endocrine adenomatosis (E31.2-)*
*multiple endocrine neoplasia (E31.2-)*

✓5th E31.2 **Multiple endocrine neoplasia [MEN] syndromes**
Multiple endocrine adenomatosis
Code also any associated malignancies and other conditions associated with the syndromes
**DEF:** Group of conditions in which several endocrine glands grow excessively (such as in adenomatous hyperplasia) and/or develop benign or malignant tumors. Tumors and hyperplasia associated with MEN often produce excess hormones, which impede normal physiology. There is no comprehensive cure known for MEN syndrome. Treatment is directed at the hyperplasia or tumors in each individual gland. Tumors are usually surgically removed and oral medications or hormonal injections are used to correct hormone imbalances.

E31.2Ø **Multiple endocrine neoplasia [MEN] syndrome, unspecified** HCC Rx ESR COM
Multiple endocrine adenomatosis NOS
Multiple endocrine neoplasia [MEN] syndrome NOS

E31.21 **Multiple endocrine neoplasia [MEN] type I** HCC Rx ESR COM
Wermer's syndrome

E31.22 **Multiple endocrine neoplasia [MEN] type IIA** HCC Rx ESR COM
Sipple's syndrome

E31.23 **Multiple endocrine neoplasia [MEN] type IIB** HCC Rx ESR COM

E31.8 **Other polyglandular dysfunction** HCC Rx ESR COM

E31.9 **Polyglandular dysfunction, unspecified** HCC Rx ESR COM

✓4th **E32 Diseases of thymus**
EXCLUDES 1 *aplasia or hypoplasia of thymus with immunodeficiency (D82.1)*
*myasthenia gravis (G7Ø.Ø)*

E32.Ø **Persistent hyperplasia of thymus** Rx ESR COM
Hypertrophy of thymus

E32.1 **Abscess of thymus** Rx ESR COM

E32.8 **Other diseases of thymus** Rx ESR COM
EXCLUDES 1 *aplasia or hypoplasia with immunodeficiency (D82.1)*
*thymoma (D15.Ø)*

E32.9 **Disease of thymus, unspecified** Rx ESR COM

✓4th **E34 Other endocrine disorders**
EXCLUDES 1 *pseudohypoparathyroidism (E2Ø.1)*

✓5th E34.Ø **Carcinoid syndrome**
Code also the underlying disorder, such as:
primary neuroendocrine tumors (C7A.-)
secondary neuroendocrine tumors (C7B.-)
**AHA:** 2024,4Q,8

E34.ØØ **Carcinoid syndrome, unspecified** HCC Rx ESR COM
Carcinoid disease, unspecified

E34.Ø1 **Carcinoid heart syndrome** HCC Rx ESR COM
Carcinoid heart disease
Hedinger syndrome

E34.Ø9 **Other carcinoid syndrome** HCC Rx ESR COM
Carcinoid disease NEC
Carcinoid syndrome NEC
Other carcinoid disease

E34.1 **Other hypersecretion of intestinal hormones**

E34.2 **Ectopic hormone secretion, not elsewhere classified**
EXCLUDES 1 *ectopic ACTH syndrome (E24.3)*

✓5th E34.3 **Short stature due to endocrine disorder**
EXCLUDES 1 *achondroplastic short stature (Q77.4)*
*hypochondroplastic short stature (Q77.4)*
*nutritional short stature (E45)*
*pituitary short stature (E23.Ø)*
*progeria (E34.8)*
*renal short stature (N25.Ø)*
*Russell-Silver syndrome (Q87.19)*
*short stature (child) (R62.52)*
*short stature in specific dysmorphic syndromes - code to syndrome - see Alphabetical Index*
*short stature NOS (R62.52)*
*short-limbed stature with immunodeficiency (D82.2)*
**AHA:** 2022,4Q,11-13

E34.3Ø **Short stature due to endocrine disorder, unspecified**

E34.31 **Constitutional short stature**
Constitutional delay of growth, puberty, or maturation

✓6th E34.32 **Genetic causes of short stature**

E34.321 **Primary insulin-like growth factor-1 (IGF-1) deficiency**
Acid-labile subunit gene (IGFALS) defect
Growth hormone gene 1 (GH1) defect with growth hormone neutralizing antibodies
Growth hormone insensitivity syndrome (GHIS)
Insulin-like growth factor 1 gene (IGF1) defect
Laron type short stature
Severe primary insulin-like growth factor-1 deficiency (SPIGFD)
Signal transducer and activator of transcription 5B gene (STAT5b) defect

E34.322 **Insulin-like growth factor-1 (IGF-1) resistance**
Genetic syndrome with resistance to insulin-like growth factor-1
Insulin-like growth factor-1 receptor (IGF-1R) defect
Post-insulin-like growth factor-1 receptor signaling defect

E34.328 **Other genetic causes of short stature**
Short stature due to ACAN gene variant
Short stature due to aggrecan deficiency
Short stature due to NPR-2 gene variant

E34.329 **Unspecified genetic causes of short stature**

E34.39 **Other short stature due to endocrine disorder**

E34.4 **Constitutional tall stature** Rx ESR COM
Constitutional gigantism

✓5th **E34.5 Androgen insensitivity syndrome**
**DEF:** X-linked recessive condition in which individuals that are chromosomally male fail to develop normal male external genitalia due to an abnormality on the X chromosome that prohibits the body, completely or in part, from recognizing the androgens produced. ***Synonym(s):*** *AIS*

**E34.50 Androgen insensitivity syndrome, unspecified**
Androgen insensitivity NOS

**E34.51 Complete androgen insensitivity syndrome**
Complete androgen insensitivity
de Quervain syndrome
Goldberg-Maxwell syndrome

**E34.52 Partial androgen insensitivity syndrome**
Partial androgen insensitivity
Reifenstein syndrome

**E34.8 Other specified endocrine disorders**
Pineal gland dysfunction
Progeria
EXCLUDES 2 *pseudohypoparathyroidism (E20.1)*

**E34.9 Endocrine disorder, unspecified**
Endocrine disturbance NOS
Hormone disturbance NOS

***E35 Disorders of endocrine glands in diseases classified elsewhere***
Code first underlying disease, such as:
late congenital syphilis of thymus gland [Dubois disease] (A50.59)
~~Use additional code, if applicable, to identify:~~
~~sequelae of tuberculosis of other organs (B90.8)~~
EXCLUDES 1 *Echinococcus granulosus infection of thyroid gland (B67.3)*
*meningococcal hemorrhagic adrenalitis (A39.1)*
*syphilis of endocrine gland (A52.79)*
*tuberculosis of adrenal gland, except calcification (A18.7)*
*tuberculosis of endocrine gland NEC (A18.82)*
*tuberculosis of thyroid gland (A18.81)*
*Waterhouse-Friderichsen syndrome (A39.1)*

## Intraoperative complications of endocrine system (E36)

✓4th **E36 Intraoperative complications of endocrine system**
EXCLUDES 2 *postprocedural endocrine and metabolic complications and disorders, not elsewhere classified (E89.-)*

✓5th **E36.0 Intraoperative hemorrhage and hematoma of an endocrine system organ or structure complicating a procedure**
EXCLUDES 1 *intraoperative hemorrhage and hematoma of an endocrine system organ or structure due to accidental puncture or laceration during a procedure (E36.1-)*

**E36.01 Intraoperative hemorrhage and hematoma of an endocrine system organ or structure complicating an endocrine system procedure**
**AHA:** 2020,1Q,19

**E36.02 Intraoperative hemorrhage and hematoma of an endocrine system organ or structure complicating other procedure**

✓5th **E36.1 Accidental puncture and laceration of an endocrine system organ or structure during a procedure**

**E36.11 Accidental puncture and laceration of an endocrine system organ or structure during an endocrine system procedure**

**E36.12 Accidental puncture and laceration of an endocrine system organ or structure during other procedure**

**E36.8 Other intraoperative complications of endocrine system**
Use additional code, if applicable, to further specify disorder

## Malnutrition (E40-E46)

EXCLUDES 1 *intestinal malabsorption (K90.-)*
*sequelae of protein-calorie malnutrition (E64.0)*
EXCLUDES 2 *nutritional anemias (D50-D53)*
*starvation (T73.0)*
**AHA:** 2020,1Q,4-7; 2017,4Q,108; 2017,3Q,25
**TIP:** Assign additional code for BMI from category Z68, when documented. BMI can be based on documentation from clinicians who are not the patient's provider.
**TIP:** Malnutrition is not considered integral to cancer; assign the appropriate code in addition to the code for the specific type of cancer.

**E40 Kwashiorkor** ESR COM
Severe malnutrition with nutritional edema with dyspigmentation of skin and hair
EXCLUDES 1 *marasmic kwashiorkor (E42)*

**E41 Nutritional marasmus** ESR COM
Severe malnutrition with marasmus
EXCLUDES 1 *marasmic kwashiorkor (E42)*
**AHA:** 2017,3Q,24
**DEF:** Protein-calorie malabsorption or malnutrition in children characterized by tissue wasting, dehydration, and subcutaneous fat depletion. It may occur with infectious disease.

**E42 Marasmic kwashiorkor** ESR COM
Intermediate form severe protein-calorie malnutrition
Severe protein-calorie malnutrition with signs of both kwashiorkor and marasmus

**E43 Unspecified severe protein-calorie malnutrition** ESR COM
Starvation edema
**AHA:** 2022,1Q,13; 2020,1Q,5,6; 2017,4Q,108

✓4th **E44 Protein-calorie malnutrition of moderate and mild degree**
**AHA:** 2020,1Q,5

**E44.0 Moderate protein-calorie malnutrition** ESR COM
**E44.1 Mild protein-calorie malnutrition** ESR COM

**E45 Retarded development following protein-calorie malnutrition** ESR COM
Nutritional short stature
Nutritional stunting
Physical retardation due to malnutrition

**E46 Unspecified protein-calorie malnutrition** ESR COM
Malnutrition NOS
Protein-calorie imbalance NOS
EXCLUDES 1 *nutritional deficiency NOS (E63.9)*
**AHA:** 2018,4Q,82

## Other nutritional deficiencies (E50-E64)

EXCLUDES 2 *nutritional anemias (D50-D53)*

✓4th **E50 Vitamin A deficiency**
EXCLUDES 1 *sequelae of vitamin A deficiency (E64.1)*

**E50.0 Vitamin A deficiency with conjunctival xerosis**

**E50.1 Vitamin A deficiency with Bitot's spot and conjunctival xerosis**
Bitot's spot in the young child
**DEF:** Vitamin A deficiency with conjunctival dryness and superficial spots of keratinized epithelium.

**E50.2 Vitamin A deficiency with corneal xerosis**

**E50.3 Vitamin A deficiency with corneal ulceration and xerosis**

**E50.4 Vitamin A deficiency with keratomalacia**
**DEF:** Vitamin A deficiency creating corneal dryness that progresses to corneal insensitivity, softness, and necrosis. It is usually bilateral.

**E50.5 Vitamin A deficiency with night blindness**

**E50.6 Vitamin A deficiency with xerophthalmic scars of cornea**

**E50.7 Other ocular manifestations of vitamin A deficiency**
Xerophthalmia NOS

**E50.8 Other manifestations of vitamin A deficiency**
Follicular keratosis
Xeroderma

**E50.9 Vitamin A deficiency, unspecified**
Hypovitaminosis A NOS

✓4th **E51 Thiamine deficiency**
EXCLUDES 1 *sequelae of thiamine deficiency (E64.8)*

✓5th **E51.1 Beriberi**

**E51.11 Dry beriberi**
Beriberi NOS
Beriberi with polyneuropathy

**E51.12 Wet beriberi**
Beriberi with cardiovascular manifestations
Cardiovascular beriberi
Shoshin disease

**E51.2 Wernicke's encephalopathy**
**DEF:** Deficiency of vitamin B1 resulting in a triad of acute mental confusion, ataxia, and ophthalmoplegia; the condition predominatly affects individuals with alcohol dependency.

**E51.8 Other manifestations of thiamine deficiency**

**E51.9 Thiamine deficiency, unspecified**

**E52 Niacin deficiency [pellagra]**
Niacin (-tryptophan) deficiency
Nicotinamide deficiency
Pellagra (alcoholic)
EXCLUDES 1 *sequelae of niacin deficiency (E64.8)*

**E53 Deficiency of other B group vitamins**
EXCLUDES 1 *sequelae of vitamin B deficiency (E64.8)*
**E53.Ø Riboflavin deficiency**
Ariboflavinosis
Vitamin B2 deficiency
**E53.1 Pyridoxine deficiency**
Vitamin B6 deficiency
EXCLUDES 1 *pyridoxine-responsive sideroblastic anemia (D64.3)*
**E53.8 Deficiency of other specified B group vitamins**
Biotin deficiency
Cyanocobalamin deficiency
Folate deficiency
Folic acid deficiency
Pantothenic acid deficiency
Vitamin B12 deficiency
EXCLUDES 1 *folate deficiency anemia (D52.-)*
~~*vitamin B12 deficiency anemia (D51.-)*~~
EXCLUDES 2 ▶*vitamin B12 deficiency anemia (D51.-)*◀
**E53.9 Vitamin B deficiency, unspecified**

**E54 Ascorbic acid deficiency**
Deficiency of vitamin C
Scurvy
EXCLUDES 1 *scorbutic anemia (D53.2)*
*sequelae of vitamin C deficiency (E64.2)*
**DEF:** Vitamin C deficiency causing swollen gums, myalgia, weight loss, and weakness.

**E55 Vitamin D deficiency**
EXCLUDES 1 *adult osteomalacia (M83.-)*
*osteoporosis (M8Ø.-)*
*sequelae of rickets (E64.3)*
**E55.Ø Rickets, active** Rx
Infantile osteomalacia
Juvenile osteomalacia
EXCLUDES 1 *celiac rickets (K9Ø.Ø)*
*Crohn's rickets (K5Ø.-)*
*hereditary vitamin D-dependent rickets (E83.32)*
*inactive rickets (E64.3)*
*renal rickets (N25.Ø)*
*sequelae of rickets (E64.3)*
*vitamin D-resistant rickets (E83.31)*
**DEF:** Rickets: Softening or weakening of the bones due to a lack of vitamin D, calcium, and phosphate.
**E55.9 Vitamin D deficiency, unspecified**
Avitaminosis D

**E56 Other vitamin deficiencies**
EXCLUDES 1 *sequelae of other vitamin deficiencies (E64.8)*
**E56.Ø Deficiency of vitamin E**
**E56.1 Deficiency of vitamin K**
EXCLUDES 1 *deficiency of coagulation factor due to vitamin K deficiency (D68.4)*
*vitamin K deficiency of newborn (P53)*
**E56.8 Deficiency of other vitamins**
**E56.9 Vitamin deficiency, unspecified**

**E58 Dietary calcium deficiency**
EXCLUDES 1 *disorders of calcium metabolism (E83.5-)*
*sequelae of calcium deficiency (E64.8)*

**E59 Dietary selenium deficiency**
Keshan disease
EXCLUDES 1 *sequelae of selenium deficiency (E64.8)*

**E6Ø Dietary zinc deficiency**

**E61 Deficiency of other nutrient elements**
Use additional code for adverse effect, if applicable, to identify drug (T36-T5Ø with fifth or sixth character 5)
EXCLUDES 1 *disorders of mineral metabolism (E83.-)*
*iodine deficiency related thyroid disorders (EØØ-EØ2)*
*sequelae of malnutrition and other nutritional deficiencies (E64.-)*
**E61.Ø Copper deficiency**
**E61.1 Iron deficiency**
EXCLUDES 1 *iron deficiency anemia (D5Ø.-)*
**E61.2 Magnesium deficiency**
**E61.3 Manganese deficiency**
**E61.4 Chromium deficiency**
**E61.5 Molybdenum deficiency**
**E61.6 Vanadium deficiency**
**E61.7 Deficiency of multiple nutrient elements**
**E61.8 Deficiency of other specified nutrient elements**
**E61.9 Deficiency of nutrient element, unspecified**

**E63 Other nutritional deficiencies**
EXCLUDES 2 *dehydration (E86.Ø)*
*failure to thrive, adult (R62.7)*
*failure to thrive, child (R62.51)*
*feeding problems in newborn (P92.-)*
*sequelae of malnutrition and other nutritional deficiencies (E64.-)*
**E63.Ø Essential fatty acid [EFA] deficiency**
**E63.1 Imbalance of constituents of food intake**
**E63.8 Other specified nutritional deficiencies**
**E63.9 Nutritional deficiency, unspecified**

**E64 Sequelae of malnutrition and other nutritional deficiencies**
NOTE This category is to be used to indicate conditions in categories E43, E44, E46, E5Ø-E63 as the cause of sequelae, which are themselves classified elsewhere. The 'sequelae' include conditions specified as such; they also include the late effects of diseases classifiable to the above categories if the disease itself is no longer present
Code first condition resulting from (sequela) of malnutrition and other nutritional deficiencies
**E64.Ø Sequelae of protein-calorie malnutrition** ESR
EXCLUDES 2 *retarded development following protein-calorie malnutrition (E45)*
**E64.1 Sequelae of vitamin A deficiency**
**E64.2 Sequelae of vitamin C deficiency**
**E64.3 Sequelae of rickets**
**E64.8 Sequelae of other nutritional deficiencies**
**E64.9 Sequelae of unspecified nutritional deficiency**

## Overweight, obesity and other hyperalimentation (E65-E68)

**E65 Localized adiposity**
Fat pad

**E66 Overweight and obesity**
Code first obesity complicating pregnancy, childbirth and the puerperium, if applicable (O99.21-)
Use additional code to identify body mass index (BMI), if known, for adults (Z68.1-Z68.45) or pediatrics (Z68.5-)
EXCLUDES 2 *adiposogenital dystrophy (E23.6)*
*lipomatosis dolorosa [Dercum] (E88.2)*
*lipomatosis NOS (E88.2)*
*Prader-Willi syndrome (Q87.11)*
**AHA:** 2025,1Q,4; 2022,3Q,6; 2018,4Q,77,79-80
**TIP:** Do not assign a BMI code (Z68.-) when a pregnant patient is documented as being overweight or obese. Only a code from subcategory O99.21- and a code from this category should be assigned.
**E66.Ø Obesity due to excess calories**
**E66.Ø1 Morbid (severe) obesity due to excess calories** HCC ESR
EXCLUDES 1 *morbid (severe) obesity with alveolar hypoventilation (E66.2)*
**AHA:** 2025,1Q,17; 2022,3Q,6; 2022,2Q,9
**TIP:** If both morbid obesity and class 3 obesity are documented, only the code for class 3 obesity (E66.813) should be assigned.
**E66.Ø9 Other obesity due to excess calories**
**E66.1 Drug-induced obesity**
Use additional code for adverse effect, if applicable, to identify drug (T36-T5Ø with fifth or sixth character 5)
**E66.2 Morbid (severe) obesity with alveolar hypoventilation** HCC ESR
Obesity hypoventilation syndrome (OHS)
Pickwickian syndrome
**E66.3 Overweight**
**AHA:** 2018,4Q,78
**E66.8 Other obesity**
**AHA:** 2024,4Q,8,11
**E66.81 Obesity class**
**AHA:** 2025,1Q,17
**TIP:** Assign a code for the specific class of obesity with any other obesity code within the classification (e.g., E66.1, E88.82, O99.21), except when both morbid obesity (E66.01) and class 3 obesity are documented. In this instance only the code for class 3 obesity should be assigned.
**E66.811 Obesity, class 1**
**E66.812 Obesity, class 2**



Chapter 4. Endocrine, Nutritional and Metabolic Diseases
E53–E66.812

E66.813 **Obesity, class 3** HCC ESR

E66.89 **Other obesity not elsewhere classified**

E66.9 **Obesity, unspecified**
Obesity NOS
**AHA:** 2021,2Q,10

✓4th **E67 Other hyperalimentation**
EXCLUDES 1 *hyperalimentation NOS (R63.2)*
*sequelae of hyperalimentation (E68)*

E67.Ø **Hypervitaminosis A**

E67.1 **Hypercarotenemia**
**DEF:** Elevated blood carotene level as a result of excessive carotenoid ingestion or an inability to convert carotenoids to vitamin A. Characteristics often include yellow discoloration of the skin, which may follow overeating of carotenoid-rich foods such as carrots, sweet potatoes, or squash.

E67.2 **Megavitamin-B6 syndrome**

E67.3 **Hypervitaminosis D**

E67.8 **Other specified hyperalimentation**

**E68 Sequelae of hyperalimentation**
Code first condition resulting from (sequela) of hyperalimentation

## Metabolic disorders (E7Ø-E88)

EXCLUDES 1 *androgen insensitivity syndrome (E34.5-)*
*congenital adrenal hyperplasia (E25.Ø)*
*hemolytic anemias attributable to enzyme disorders (D55.-)*
*Marfan syndrome (Q87.4-)*
*5-alpha-reductase deficiency (E29.1)*
EXCLUDES 2 *Ehlers-Danlos syndromes (Q79.6-)*
**AHA:** 2018,2Q,6

✓4th **E7Ø Disorders of aromatic amino-acid metabolism**

E7Ø.Ø **Classical phenylketonuria** Rx ESR COM

E7Ø.1 **Other hyperphenylalaninemias** Rx ESR COM

✓5th E7Ø.2 **Disorders of tyrosine metabolism**
EXCLUDES 1 *transitory tyrosinemia of newborn (P74.5)*

E7Ø.2Ø **Disorder of tyrosine metabolism, unspecified** Rx ESR COM

E7Ø.21 **Tyrosinemia** Rx ESR COM
Hypertyrosinemia

E7Ø.29 **Other disorders of tyrosine metabolism** Rx ESR COM
Alkaptonuria
Ochronosis

✓5th E7Ø.3 **Albinism**
**DEF:** Absence of pigment in skin, hair, and eyes. This genetic condition is often accompanied by astigmatism, photophobia, and nystagmus.

E7Ø.3Ø **Albinism, unspecified** Rx ESR COM

✓6th E7Ø.31 **Ocular albinism**

E7Ø.31Ø **X-linked ocular albinism** Rx ESR COM

E7Ø.311 **Autosomal recessive ocular albinism** Rx ESR COM

E7Ø.318 **Other ocular albinism** Rx ESR COM

E7Ø.319 **Ocular albinism, unspecified** Rx ESR COM

✓6th E7Ø.32 **Oculocutaneous albinism**
EXCLUDES 1 *Chediak-Higashi syndrome (E7Ø.33Ø)*
*Hermansky-Pudlak syndrome (E7Ø.331)*

E7Ø.32Ø **Tyrosinase negative oculocutaneous albinism** Rx ESR COM
Albinism I
Oculocutaneous albinism ty-neg

E7Ø.321 **Tyrosinase positive oculocutaneous albinism** Rx ESR COM
Albinism II
Oculocutaneous albinism ty-pos

E7Ø.328 **Other oculocutaneous albinism** Rx ESR COM
Cross syndrome

E7Ø.329 **Oculocutaneous albinism, unspecified** Rx ESR COM

✓6th E7Ø.33 **Albinism with hematologic abnormality**

E7Ø.33Ø **Chediak-Higashi syndrome** Rx ESR COM

E7Ø.331 **Hermansky-Pudlak syndrome** Rx ESR COM

E7Ø.338 **Other albinism with hematologic abnormality** Rx ESR COM

E7Ø.339 **Albinism with hematologic abnormality, unspecified** Rx ESR COM

E7Ø.39 **Other specified albinism** Rx ESR COM
Piebaldism

✓5th E7Ø.4 **Disorders of histidine metabolism**

E7Ø.4Ø **Disorders of histidine metabolism, unspecified** Rx ESR COM

E7Ø.41 **Histidinemia** Rx ESR COM

E7Ø.49 **Other disorders of histidine metabolism** Rx ESR COM

E7Ø.5 **Disorders of tryptophan metabolism** Rx ESR COM

✓5th E7Ø.8 **Other disorders of aromatic amino-acid metabolism**
**AHA:** 2020,4Q,15-16

E7Ø.81 **Aromatic L-amino acid decarboxylase deficiency** Rx ESR COM
AADC deficiency

E7Ø.89 **Other disorders of aromatic amino-acid metabolism** Rx ESR COM

E7Ø.9 **Disorder of aromatic amino-acid metabolism, unspecified** Rx ESR COM

✓4th **E71 Disorders of branched-chain amino-acid metabolism and fatty-acid metabolism**

E71.Ø **Maple-syrup-urine disease** Rx ESR COM

✓5th E71.1 **Other disorders of branched-chain amino-acid metabolism**

✓6th E71.11 **Branched-chain organic acidurias**

E71.11Ø **Isovaleric acidemia** Rx ESR COM

E71.111 **3-methylglutaconic aciduria** Rx ESR COM

E71.118 **Other branched-chain organic acidurias** Rx ESR COM

✓6th E71.12 **Disorders of propionate metabolism**

E71.12Ø **Methylmalonic acidemia** Rx ESR COM

E71.121 **Propionic acidemia** Rx ESR COM

E71.128 **Other disorders of propionate metabolism** Rx ESR COM

E71.19 **Other disorders of branched-chain amino-acid metabolism** Rx ESR COM
Hyperleucine-isoleucinemia
Hypervalinemia

E71.2 **Disorder of branched-chain amino-acid metabolism, unspecified** Rx ESR COM

✓5th E71.3 **Disorders of fatty-acid metabolism**
EXCLUDES 1 *peroxisomal disorders (E71.5)*
*Refsum's disease (G6Ø.1)*
*Schilder's disease (G37.Ø)*
EXCLUDES 2 *carnitine deficiency due to inborn error of metabolism (E71.42)*

E71.3Ø **Disorder of fatty-acid metabolism, unspecified** Rx COM

✓6th E71.31 **Disorders of fatty-acid oxidation**

E71.31Ø **Long chain/very long chain acyl CoA dehydrogenase deficiency** Rx ESR COM
LCAD deficiency
VLCAD deficiency

E71.311 **Medium chain acyl CoA dehydrogenase deficiency** Rx ESR COM
MCAD deficiency

E71.312 **Short chain acyl CoA dehydrogenase deficiency** Rx ESR COM
SCAD deficiency

E71.313 **Glutaric aciduria type II** Rx ESR COM
Glutaric aciduria type II A
Glutaric aciduria type II B
Glutaric aciduria type II C
EXCLUDES 1 *glutaric aciduria (type 1) NOS (E72.3)*

E71.314 **Muscle carnitine palmitoyltransferase deficiency** Rx ESR COM

E71.318 **Other disorders of fatty-acid oxidation** Rx ESR COM

E71.32 **Disorders of ketone metabolism** Rx ESR COM

E71.39 **Other disorders of fatty-acid metabolism** Rx ESR COM

✓5th **E71.4 Disorders of carnitine metabolism**
EXCLUDES 1 *muscle carnitine palmitoyltransferase deficiency (E71.314)*
**E71.40 Disorder of carnitine metabolism, unspecified** Rx ESR COM
**E71.41 Primary carnitine deficiency** Rx ESR COM
**E71.42 Carnitine deficiency due to inborn errors of metabolism** Rx ESR COM
Code also associated inborn error or metabolism
**E71.43 Iatrogenic carnitine deficiency** Rx ESR COM
Carnitine deficiency due to hemodialysis
Carnitine deficiency due to Valproic acid therapy
✓6th **E71.44 Other secondary carnitine deficiency**
**E71.440 Ruvalcaba-Myhre-Smith syndrome** Rx ESR COM
**E71.448 Other secondary carnitine deficiency** Rx ESR COM
✓5th **E71.5 Peroxisomal disorders**
EXCLUDES 1 *Schilder's disease (G37.0)*
**E71.50 Peroxisomal disorder, unspecified** Rx ESR COM
✓6th **E71.51 Disorders of peroxisome biogenesis**
Group 1 peroxisomal disorders
EXCLUDES 1 *Refsum's disease (G60.1)*
**E71.510 Zellweger syndrome** Rx ESR COM
**E71.511 Neonatal adrenoleukodystrophy** Rx ESR COM
EXCLUDES 1 *X-linked adrenoleukodystrophy (E71.42-)*
**E71.518 Other disorders of peroxisome biogenesis** Rx ESR COM
✓6th **E71.52 X-linked adrenoleukodystrophy**
**E71.520 Childhood cerebral X-linked adrenoleukodystrophy** Rx ESR COM
**E71.521 Adolescent X-linked adrenoleukodystrophy** Rx ESR COM
**E71.522 Adrenomyeloneuropathy** Rx ESR COM
**E71.528 Other X-linked adrenoleukodystrophy** Rx ESR COM
Addison only phenotype adrenoleukodystrophy
Addison-Schilder adrenoleukodystrophy
**E71.529 X-linked adrenoleukodystrophy, unspecified type** Rx ESR COM
**E71.53 Other group 2 peroxisomal disorders** Rx ESR COM
✓6th **E71.54 Other peroxisomal disorders**
**E71.540 Rhizomelic chondrodysplasia punctata** Rx ESR COM
**E71.541 Zellweger-like syndrome** Rx ESR COM
**E71.542 Other group 3 peroxisomal disorders** Rx ESR COM
**E71.548 Other peroxisomal disorders** Rx ESR COM

✓4th **E72 Other disorders of amino-acid metabolism**
EXCLUDES 1 *disorders of:*
*gout (M1A.-, M10.-)*
*aromatic amino-acid metabolism (E70.-)*
*branched-chain amino-acid metabolism (E71.0-E71.2)*
*fatty-acid metabolism (E71.3)*
*purine and pyrimidine metabolism (E79.-)*
✓5th **E72.0 Disorders of amino-acid transport**
EXCLUDES 1 *disorders of tryptophan metabolism (E70.5)*
**E72.00 Disorders of amino-acid transport, unspecified** Rx ESR COM
**E72.01 Cystinuria** Rx ESR COM
**E72.02 Hartnup's disease** Rx ESR COM
**E72.03 Lowe's syndrome** Rx ESR COM
Use additional code for associated glaucoma (H42)
**E72.04 Cystinosis** Rx ESR COM
Fanconi (-de Toni) (-Debre) syndrome with cystinosis
EXCLUDES 1 *Fanconi (-de Toni) (-Debre) syndrome without cystinosis (E72.09)*
**E72.09 Other disorders of amino-acid transport** Rx ESR COM
Fanconi (-de Toni) (-Debre) syndrome, unspecified
✓5th **E72.1 Disorders of sulfur-bearing amino-acid metabolism**
EXCLUDES 1 *cystinosis (E72.04)*
*cystinuria (E72.01)*
*transcobalamin II deficiency (D51.2)*
**E72.10 Disorders of sulfur-bearing amino-acid metabolism, unspecified** Rx ESR COM
**E72.11 Homocystinuria** Rx ESR COM
Cystathionine synthase deficiency
**AHA:** 2021,4Q,28
**E72.12 Methylenetetrahydrofolate reductase deficiency** Rx ESR COM
**E72.19 Other disorders of sulfur-bearing amino-acid metabolism** Rx ESR COM
Cystathioninuria
Methioninemia
Sulfite oxidase deficiency
✓5th **E72.2 Disorders of urea cycle metabolism**
EXCLUDES 1 *disorders of ornithine metabolism (E72.4)*
**E72.20 Disorder of urea cycle metabolism, unspecified** Rx ESR COM
Hyperammonemia
EXCLUDES 1 *hyperammonemia- hyperornithinemia-homocitrullinemia syndrome E72.4*
*transient hyperammonemia of newborn (P74.6)*
**E72.21 Argininemia** Rx ESR COM
**E72.22 Arginosuccinic aciduria** Rx ESR COM
**E72.23 Citrullinemia** Rx ESR COM
**E72.29 Other disorders of urea cycle metabolism** Rx ESR COM
**E72.3 Disorders of lysine and hydroxylysine metabolism** Rx ESR COM
Glutaric aciduria (type I)
Glutaric aciduria NOS
Hydroxylysinemia
Hyperlysinemia
EXCLUDES 1 *glutaric aciduria type II (E71.313)*
*Refsum's disease (G60.1)*
*Zellweger syndrome (E71.510)*
**E72.4 Disorders of ornithine metabolism** Rx ESR COM
Hyperammonemia-Hyperornithinemia-Homocitrullinemia syndrome
Ornithine transcarbamylase deficiency
Ornithinemia (types I, II)
EXCLUDES 1 *hereditary choroidal dystrophy (H31.2-)*
✓5th **E72.5 Disorders of glycine metabolism**
**E72.50 Disorder of glycine metabolism, unspecified** Rx ESR COM
**E72.51 Non-ketotic hyperglycinemia** Rx ESR COM
**E72.52 Trimethylaminuria** Rx ESR COM
✓6th **E72.53 Primary hyperoxaluria**
Oxalosis
Oxaluria
EXCLUDES 1 *secondary hyperoxaluria (E72.54-)*
**AHA:** 2018,4Q,29
**E72.530 Primary hyperoxaluria, type 1** HCC Rx ESR
**E72.538 Other specified primary hyperoxaluria** HCC Rx ESR
Primary hyperoxaluria, type 2
Primary hyperoxaluria, type 3
**E72.539 Primary hyperoxaluria, unspecified** HCC Rx ESR
✓6th **E72.54 Secondary hyperoxaluria**
EXCLUDES 1 *primary hyperoxaluria (E72.53-)*
**E72.540 Dietary hyperoxaluria**
**E72.541 Enteric hyperoxaluria**
**E72.548 Other secondary hyperoxaluria**
**E72.549 Secondary hyperoxaluria, unspecified**
**E72.59 Other disorders of glycine metabolism** Rx ESR COM
D-glycericacidemia
Hyperhydroxyprolinemia
Hyperprolinemia (types I, II)
Sarcosinemia

√5th **E72.8 Other specified disorders of amino-acid metabolism**
AHA: 2018,4Q,5

**E72.81 Disorders of gamma aminobutyric acid metabolism** Rx ESR COM
4-hydroxybutyric aciduria
Disorders of GABA metabolism
GABA metabolic defect
GABA transaminase deficiency
GABA-T deficiency
Gamma-hydroxybutyric aciduria
SSADHD
Succinic semialdehyde dehydrogenase deficiency

**E72.89 Other specified disorders of amino-acid metabolism** Rx ESR COM
Disorders of beta-amino-acid metabolism
Disorders of gamma-glutamyl cycle

**E72.9 Disorder of amino-acid metabolism, unspecified** Rx ESR COM

√4th **E73 Lactose intolerance**
DEF: Inability to break down sugar in dairy products due to a deficiency in the enzyme lactase.

**E73.0 Congenital lactase deficiency**
**E73.1 Secondary lactase deficiency**
**E73.8 Other lactose intolerance**
**E73.9 Lactose intolerance, unspecified**

√4th **E74 Other disorders of carbohydrate metabolism**
EXCLUDES 1 *diabetes mellitus (E08-E13)*
*hypoglycemia NOS (E16.2)*
*increased secretion of glucagon (E16.3)*
*mucopolysaccharidosis (E76.0-E76.3)*

√5th **E74.0 Glycogen storage disease**

**E74.00 Glycogen storage disease, unspecified** HCC Rx ESR COM

**E74.01 von Gierke disease** HCC Rx ESR COM
Type I glycogen storage disease

**E74.02 Pompe disease** HCC Rx ESR COM
Cardiac glycogenosis
Type II glycogen storage disease

**E74.03 Cori disease** HCC Rx ESR COM
Forbes disease
Type III glycogen storage disease

**E74.04 McArdle disease** HCC Rx ESR COM
Type V glycogen storage disease

**E74.05 Lysosome-associated membrane protein 2 [LAMP2] deficiency** HCC Rx ESR COM
Danon disease
Code also, if applicable, associated manifestations such as:
dilated cardiomyopathy ▶(I42.0-)◀
obstructive hypertrophic cardiomyopathy (I42.1)
AHA: 2023,4Q,11

**E74.09 Other glycogen storage disease** HCC Rx ESR COM
Andersen disease
Glycogen storage disease, types 0, IV, VI-XI
Hers disease
Liver phosphorylase deficiency
Muscle phosphofructokinase deficiency
Tauri disease

√5th **E74.1 Disorders of fructose metabolism**
EXCLUDES 1 *muscle phosphofructokinase deficiency (E74.09)*

**E74.10 Disorder of fructose metabolism, unspecified**

**E74.11 Essential fructosuria**
Fructokinase deficiency

**E74.12 Hereditary fructose intolerance**
Fructosemia

**E74.19 Other disorders of fructose metabolism**
Fructose-1, 6-diphosphatase deficiency

√5th **E74.2 Disorders of galactose metabolism**

**E74.20 Disorders of galactose metabolism, unspecified** Rx ESR COM

**E74.21 Galactosemia** Rx ESR COM
DEF: Any of three genetic disorders caused by a defective galactose metabolism. Symptoms include failure to thrive in infancy, jaundice, liver and spleen damage, cataracts, and mental retardation.

**E74.29 Other disorders of galactose metabolism** Rx ESR COM
Galactokinase deficiency

√5th **E74.3 Other disorders of intestinal carbohydrate absorption**
EXCLUDES 2 *lactose intolerance (E73.-)*

**E74.31 Sucrase-isomaltase deficiency** Rx

**E74.39 Other disorders of intestinal carbohydrate absorption**
Disorder of intestinal carbohydrate absorption NOS
Glucose-galactose malabsorption
Sucrase deficiency

**E74.4 Disorders of pyruvate metabolism and gluconeogenesis** Rx ESR COM
Deficiency of phosphoenolpyruvate carboxykinase
Deficiency of pyruvate carboxylase
Deficiency of pyruvate dehydrogenase
EXCLUDES 1 *disorders of pyruvate metabolism and gluconeogenesis with anemia (D55.-)*
*Leigh's syndrome (G31.82)*

√5th **E74.8 Other specified disorders of carbohydrate metabolism**
AHA: 2020,4Q,16

√6th **E74.81 Disorders of glucose transport, not elsewhere classified**

**E74.810 Glucose transporter protein type 1 deficiency** Rx ESR COM
De Vivo syndrome
Glucose transport defect, blood-brain barrier
Glut1 deficiency
GLUT1 deficiency syndrome 1, infantile onset
GLUT1 deficiency syndrome 2, childhood onset

**E74.818 Other disorders of glucose transport** Rx ESR COM
(Familial) renal glycosuria

**E74.819 Disorders of glucose transport, unspecified** Rx ESR COM

√6th **E74.82 Disorders of citrate metabolism**
AHA: 2024,4Q,10

**E74.820 SLC13A5 Citrate Transporter Disorder** Rx ESR COM

**E74.829 Other disorders of citrate metabolism** Rx ESR COM

**E74.89 Other specified disorders of carbohydrate metabolism** Rx ESR COM
Essential pentosuria
AHA: 2023,3Q,3

**E74.9 Disorder of carbohydrate metabolism, unspecified** Rx ESR COM

√4th **E75 Disorders of sphingolipid metabolism and other lipid storage disorders**
EXCLUDES 1 *mucolipidosis, types I-III (E77.0-E77.1)*
*Refsum's disease (G60.1)*

√5th **E75.0 GM2 gangliosidosis**

**E75.00 GM2 gangliosidosis, unspecified** Rx ESR COM
**E75.01 Sandhoff disease** Rx ESR COM

**E75.Ø2 Tay-Sachs disease** Rx ESR COM
DEF: Genetic mutation of the HEXA gene that inhibits the breakdown of a toxic substance called ganglioside. The accumulation of ganglioside results in destruction of the neurons in the brain and spinal cord.

**Tay-Sachs Disease**

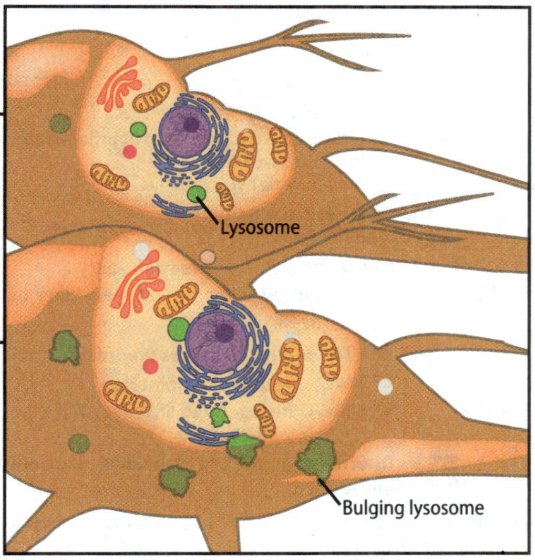


**E75.Ø9 Other GM2 gangliosidosis** Rx ESR COM
Adult GM2 gangliosidosis
Juvenile GM2 gangliosidosis

✓5th **E75.1 Other and unspecified gangliosidosis**

**E75.1Ø Unspecified gangliosidosis** Rx ESR COM
Gangliosidosis NOS

**E75.11 Mucolipidosis IV** Rx ESR COM

**E75.19 Other gangliosidosis** Rx ESR COM
GM1 gangliosidosis
GM3 gangliosidosis

✓5th **E75.2 Other sphingolipidosis**
EXCLUDES 1 *adrenoleukodystrophy [Addison-Schilder] (E71.528)*

**E75.21 Fabry (-Anderson) disease** HCC Rx ESR COM

**E75.22 Gaucher disease** HCC Rx ESR COM

**E75.23 Krabbe disease** Rx ESR COM

✓6th **E75.24 Niemann-Pick disease**
Acid sphingomyelinase deficiency (ASMD)

**E75.24Ø Niemann-Pick disease type A** Rx ESR COM
Acid sphingomyelinase deficiency type A (ASMD type A)
Infantile neurovisceral acid sphingomyelinase deficiency

**E75.241 Niemann-Pick disease type B** Rx ESR COM
Acid sphingomyelinase deficiency type B (ASMD type B)
Chronic visceral acid sphingomyelinase deficiency

**E75.242 Niemann-Pick disease type C** Rx ESR COM

**E75.243 Niemann-Pick disease type D** Rx ESR COM

**E75.244 Niemann-Pick disease type A/B** Rx ESR COM
Acid sphingomyelinase deficiency type A/B (ASMD type A/B)
Chronic neurovisceral acid sphingomyelinase deficiency
AHA: 2021,4Q,8-9

**E75.248 Other Niemann-Pick disease** Rx ESR COM

**E75.249 Niemann-Pick disease, unspecified** Rx ESR COM
Acid sphingomyelinase deficiency (ASMD) NOS

**E75.25 Metachromatic leukodystrophy** Rx ESR COM

**E75.26 Sulfatase deficiency** Rx ESR COM
Multiple sulfatase deficiency (MSD)
AHA: 2018,4Q,5-6

**E75.27 Pelizaeus-Merzbacher disease** Rx ESR COM
AHA: 2023,4Q,12-13

**E75.28 Canavan disease** Rx ESR COM
AHA: 2023,4Q,12-13

**E75.29 Other sphingolipidosis** Rx ESR COM
Farber's syndrome
Sulfatide lipidosis

**E75.3 Sphingolipidosis, unspecified** Rx ESR COM

**E75.4 Neuronal ceroid lipofuscinosis** Rx ESR COM
Batten disease
Bielschowsky-Jansky disease
Kufs disease
Spielmeyer-Vogt disease

**E75.5 Other lipid storage disorders** Rx
Cerebrotendinous cholesterosis [van Bogaert-Scherer-Epstein]
Wolman's disease

**E75.6 Lipid storage disorder, unspecified** Rx

✓4th **E76 Disorders of glycosaminoglycan metabolism**

✓5th **E76.Ø Mucopolysaccharidosis, type I**

**E76.Ø1 Hurler's syndrome** HCC Rx ESR COM

**E76.Ø2 Hurler-Scheie syndrome** HCC Rx ESR COM

**E76.Ø3 Scheie's syndrome** HCC Rx ESR COM

**E76.1 Mucopolysaccharidosis, type II** HCC Rx ESR COM
Hunter's syndrome

✓5th **E76.2 Other mucopolysaccharidoses**

✓6th **E76.21 Morquio mucopolysaccharidoses**

**E76.21Ø Morquio A mucopolysaccharidoses** HCC Rx ESR COM
Classic Morquio syndrome
Morquio syndrome A
Mucopolysaccharidosis, type IVA

**E76.211 Morquio B mucopolysaccharidoses** HCC Rx ESR COM
Morquio syndrome B
Morquio-like mucopolysaccharidoses
Morquio-like syndrome
Mucopolysaccharidosis, type IVB

**E76.219 Morquio mucopolysaccharidoses, unspecified** HCC Rx ESR COM
Morquio syndrome
Mucopolysaccharidosis, type IV

**E76.22 Sanfilippo mucopolysaccharidoses** HCC Rx ESR COM
Mucopolysaccharidosis, type III (A) (B) (C) (D)
Sanfilippo A syndrome
Sanfilippo B syndrome
Sanfilippo C syndrome
Sanfilippo D syndrome

**E76.29 Other mucopolysaccharidoses** HCC Rx ESR COM
beta-Glucuronidase deficiency
Maroteaux-Lamy (mild) (severe) syndrome
Mucopolysaccharidosis, types VI, VII

**E76.3 Mucopolysaccharidosis, unspecified** HCC Rx ESR COM

**E76.8 Other disorders of glucosaminoglycan metabolism** Rx ESR COM

**E76.9 Glucosaminoglycan metabolism disorder, unspecified** Rx ESR COM

✓4th **E77 Disorders of glycoprotein metabolism**

**E77.Ø Defects in post-translational modification of lysosomal enzymes** Rx ESR COM
Mucolipidosis II [I-cell disease]
Mucolipidosis III [pseudo-Hurler polydystrophy]

**E77.1 Defects in glycoprotein degradation** Rx ESR COM
Aspartylglucosaminuria
Fucosidosis
Mannosidosis
Sialidosis [mucolipidosis I]

**E77.8 Other disorders of glycoprotein metabolism** Rx ESR COM

**E77.9 Disorder of glycoprotein metabolism, unspecified** Rx ESR COM

**✓4th E78 Disorders of lipoprotein metabolism and other lipidemias**

EXCLUDES 1 *sphingolipidosis (E75.Ø-E75.3)*

**✓5th E78.Ø Pure hypercholesterolemia**

**AHA:** 2016,4Q,13-14

**E78.ØØ Pure hypercholesterolemia, unspecified** Rx
(Pure) hypercholesterolemia NOS
Fredrickson's hyperlipoproteinemia, type IIa
Hyperbetalipoproteinemia
Low-density-lipoprotein-type [LDL] hyperlipoproteinemia
**AHA:** 2023,2Q,9; 2022,2Q,5-6

**✓6th E78.Ø1 Familial hypercholesterolemia**

**E78.Ø1Ø Homozygous familial hypercholesterolemia [HoFH]** Rx

**E78.Ø11 Heterozygous familial hypercholesterolemia [HeFH]** Rx

**E78.Ø19 Familial hypercholesterolemia, unspecified** Rx
Familial hypercholesterolemia NOS

**E78.1 Pure hyperglyceridemia** Rx
Elevated fasting triglycerides
Endogenous hyperglyceridemia
Fredrickson's hyperlipoproteinemia, type IV
Hyperlipidemia, group B
Hyperprebetalipoproteinemia
Very-low-density-lipoprotein-type [VLDL] hyperlipoproteinemia

**E78.2 Mixed hyperlipidemia** Rx
Broad- or floating-betalipoproteinemia
Combined hyperlipidemia NOS
Elevated cholesterol with elevated triglycerides NEC
Fredrickson's hyperlipoproteinemia, type IIb or III
Hyperbetalipoproteinemia with prebetalipoproteinemia
Hypercholesteremia with endogenous hyperglyceridemia
Hyperlipidemia, group C
Tubo-eruptive xanthoma
Xanthoma tuberosum
EXCLUDES 1 *cerebrotendinous cholesterosis [van Bogaert-Scherer-Epstein] (E75.5)*
*familial combined hyperlipidemia (E78.49)*
**AHA:** 2023,2Q,9; 2022,2Q,6

**E78.3 Hyperchylomicronemia** Rx
Chylomicron retention disease
Fredrickson's hyperlipoproteinemia, type I or V
Hyperlipidemia, group D
Mixed hyperglyceridemia

**✓5th E78.4 Other hyperlipidemia**

**AHA:** 2025,3Q,3; 2018,4Q,6

**E78.41 Elevated Lipoprotein(a)** Rx
Elevated Lp(a)

**E78.49 Other hyperlipidemia** Rx
Familial combined hyperlipidemia

**E78.5 Hyperlipidemia, unspecified** Rx
**AHA:** 2022,2Q,5

**E78.6 Lipoprotein deficiency** Rx
Abetalipoproteinemia
Depressed HDL cholesterol
High-density lipoprotein deficiency
Hypoalphalipoproteinemia
Hypobetalipoproteinemia (familial)
Lecithin cholesterol acyltransferase deficiency
Tangier disease

**✓5th E78.7 Disorders of bile acid and cholesterol metabolism**

EXCLUDES 1 *Niemann-Pick disease type C (E75.242)*

**E78.7Ø Disorder of bile acid and cholesterol metabolism, unspecified** Rx

**E78.71 Barth syndrome** COM

**E78.72 Smith-Lemli-Opitz syndrome** COM

**E78.79 Other disorders of bile acid and cholesterol metabolism** Rx
**AHA:** 2023,1Q,26

**✓5th E78.8 Other disorders of lipoprotein metabolism**

**E78.81 Lipoid dermatoarthritis** Rx

**E78.89 Other lipoprotein metabolism disorders** Rx

**E78.9 Disorder of lipoprotein metabolism, unspecified** Rx

**✓4th E79 Disorders of purine and pyrimidine metabolism**

EXCLUDES 1 *Ataxia-telangiectasia (Q87.19)*
*Bloom's syndrome (Q82.8)*
*calculus of kidney (N2Ø.Ø)*
*Cockayne's syndrome (Q87.19)*
*combined immunodeficiency disorders (D81.-)*
*Fanconi's anemia (D61.Ø9)*
*gout (M1A.-, M1Ø.-)*
*orotaciduric anemia (D53.Ø)*
*progeria (E34.8)*
*Werner's syndrome (E34.8)*
*xeroderma pigmentosum (Q82.1)*

**E79.Ø Hyperuricemia without signs of inflammatory arthritis and tophaceous disease**
Asymptomatic hyperuricemia

**E79.1 Lesch-Nyhan syndrome** HCC Rx ESR COM
HGPRT deficiency

**E79.2 Myoadenylate deaminase deficiency** Rx ESR COM

**✓5th E79.8 Other disorders of purine and pyrimidine metabolism**

**AHA:** 2023,4Q,12-13

**E79.81 Aicardi-Goutieres syndrome** Rx ESR COM

**E79.82 Hereditary xanthinuria** Rx ESR COM

**E79.89 Other specified disorders of purine and pyrimidine metabolism** Rx ESR COM

**E79.9 Disorder of purine and pyrimidine metabolism, unspecified** Rx ESR COM

**✓4th E8Ø Disorders of porphyrin and bilirubin metabolism**

INCLUDES defects of catalase and peroxidase

**E8Ø.Ø Hereditary erythropoietic porphyria** HCC Rx ESR COM
Congenital erythropoietic porphyria
Erythropoietic protoporphyria

**E8Ø.1 Porphyria cutanea tarda** HCC Rx ESR COM

**✓5th E8Ø.2 Other and unspecified porphyria**

**E8Ø.2Ø Unspecified porphyria** HCC Rx ESR COM
Porphyria NOS

**E8Ø.21 Acute intermittent (hepatic) porphyria** HCC Rx ESR COM

**E8Ø.29 Other porphyria** HCC Rx ESR COM
Hereditary coproporphyria

**E8Ø.3 Defects of catalase and peroxidase** HCC Rx ESR COM
Acatalasia [Takahara]

**E8Ø.4 Gilbert syndrome**

**E8Ø.5 Crigler-Najjar syndrome**

**E8Ø.6 Other disorders of bilirubin metabolism**
Dubin-Johnson syndrome
Rotor's syndrome
**AHA:** 2022,3Q,7
**TIP:** Assign codes E80.6 and K76.89 to report benign recurrent intrahepatic cholestasis (BRIC) or progressive familial intrahepatic cholestasis (PFIC).

**E8Ø.7 Disorder of bilirubin metabolism, unspecified**

**✓4th E83 Disorders of mineral metabolism**

EXCLUDES 1 *dietary mineral deficiency (E58-E61)*
*parathyroid disorders (E2Ø-E21)*
*vitamin D deficiency (E55.-)*

**✓5th E83.Ø Disorders of copper metabolism**

**E83.ØØ Disorder of copper metabolism, unspecified** HCC Rx COM

**E83.Ø1 Wilson's disease** HCC Rx COM
Code also associated Kayser Fleischer ring (H18.Ø4-)

**E83.Ø9 Other disorders of copper metabolism** HCC Rx COM
Menkes' (kinky hair) (steely hair) disease

**✓5th E83.1 Disorders of iron metabolism**

EXCLUDES 1 *iron deficiency anemia (D5Ø.-)*
*sideroblastic anemia (D64.Ø-D64.3)*

**E83.1Ø Disorder of iron metabolism, unspecified** Rx

**✓6th E83.11 Hemochromatosis**

EXCLUDES 1 *GALD (P78.84)*
*gestational alloimmune liver disease (P78.84)*
*neonatal hemochromatosis (P78.84)*

**E83.11Ø Hereditary hemochromatosis** Rx ESR
Bronzed diabetes
Pigmentary cirrhosis (of liver)
Primary (hereditary) hemochromatosis

HCC CMS-HCC Rx Rx HCC ESR ESRD HCC COM Commercial HCC N Newborn: 0 P Pediatric: 0-17 M Maternity: 9-64 A Adult: 15-124

E83.111 **Hemochromatosis due to repeated red blood cell transfusions**
Iron overload due to repeated red blood cell transfusions
Transfusion (red blood cell) associated hemochromatosis

E83.118 **Other hemochromatosis** Rx

E83.119 **Hemochromatosis, unspecified** Rx

E83.19 **Other disorders of iron metabolism** Rx
Use additional code, if applicable, for idiopathic pulmonary hemosiderosis (J84.03)

E83.2 **Disorders of zinc metabolism**
Acrodermatitis enteropathica

✓5th E83.3 **Disorders of phosphorus metabolism and phosphatases**
EXCLUDES 1 *adult osteomalacia (M83.-)*
*osteoporosis (M80.-)*
EXCLUDES 2 *disorders of pyrophosphate metabolism (E83.82-)*

E83.30 **Disorder of phosphorus metabolism, unspecified** Rx

E83.31 **Familial hypophosphatemia** HCC Rx
Vitamin D-resistant osteomalacia
Vitamin D-resistant rickets
EXCLUDES 1 *vitamin D-deficiency rickets (E55.0)*

E83.32 **Hereditary vitamin D-dependent rickets (type 1) (type 2)** Rx
25-hydroxyvitamin D 1-alpha-hydroxylase deficiency
Pseudovitamin D deficiency
Vitamin D receptor defect

E83.39 **Other disorders of phosphorus metabolism** Rx
Acid phosphatase deficiency
Hypophosphatasia

✓5th E83.4 **Disorders of magnesium metabolism**

E83.40 **Disorders of magnesium metabolism, unspecified**

E83.41 **Hypermagnesemia**
AHA: 2016,4Q,54

E83.42 **Hypomagnesemia**

E83.49 **Other disorders of magnesium metabolism**

✓5th E83.5 **Disorders of calcium metabolism**
EXCLUDES 1 *autoimmune hypoparathyroidism (E20.812)*
*autosomal dominant hypocalcemia (E20.810)*
*chondrocalcinosis (M11.1-M11.2)*
*hungry bone syndrome (E83.81)*
*hyperparathyroidism (E21.0-E21.3)*
*secondary hypoparathyroidism in diseases classified elsewhere (E20.811)*

E83.50 **Unspecified disorder of calcium metabolism**

E83.51 **Hypocalcemia**

E83.52 **Hypercalcemia**
Familial hypocalciuric hypercalcemia

E83.59 **Other disorders of calcium metabolism**

✓5th E83.8 **Other disorders of mineral metabolism**

E83.81 **Hungry bone syndrome**

✓6th E83.82 **Disorders of pyrophosphate metabolism**

E83.820 **Generalized arterial calcification of infancy with unspecified genetic causality** Rx ESR
Code also, if applicable, associated conditions such as:
heart failure (I50.-)
other secondary hypertension (I15.8)

E83.821 **ENPP1 deficiency causing generalized arterial calcification of infancy** Rx ESR
Code also, if applicable, associated conditions such as:
heart failure (I50.-)
other secondary hypertension (I15.8)

E83.822 **ENPP1 deficiency causing autosomal recessive hypophosphatemic rickets type 2** Rx ESR

E83.823 **ABCC6 deficiency causing generalized arterial calcification of infancy** Rx ESR
Code also, if applicable, associated conditions such as:
heart failure (I50.-)
other secondary hypertension (I15.8)

E83.824 **ABCC6 deficiency causing pseudoxanthoma elasticum** Rx ESR

E83.825 **CD73 deficiency causing arterial calcification** Rx ESR

E83.89 **Other disorders of mineral metabolism**

E83.9 **Disorder of mineral metabolism, unspecified**

✓4th E84 **Cystic fibrosis**
INCLUDES mucoviscidosis
Code also exocrine pancreatic insufficiency (K86.81)
**DEF:** Genetic disorder affecting the respiratory, digestive, and reproductive systems in infants to young adults by disturbing exocrine gland function and causing chronic pulmonary disease with excess mucus production and pancreatic deficiency.

E84.0 **Cystic fibrosis with pulmonary manifestations** HCC Rx ESR COM
Use additional code to identify any infectious organism present, such as:
Pseudomonas (B96.5)
AHA: 2021,1Q,23

✓5th E84.1 **Cystic fibrosis with intestinal manifestations**

E84.11 **Meconium ileus in cystic fibrosis** HCC Rx ESR COM N
EXCLUDES 1 *meconium ileus not due to cystic fibrosis (P76.0)*

E84.19 **Cystic fibrosis with other intestinal manifestations** HCC Rx ESR COM
Distal intestinal obstruction syndrome

E84.8 **Cystic fibrosis with other manifestations** HCC Rx ESR COM

E84.9 **Cystic fibrosis, unspecified** HCC Rx ESR COM

✓4th E85 **Amyloidosis**
EXCLUDES 2 *Alzheimer's disease (G30.0-)*
**DEF:** Conditions of diverse etiologies characterized by the accumulation of insoluble fibrillar proteins (amyloid) in various organs and tissues of the body, compromising vital functions.

E85.0 **Non-neuropathic heredofamilial amyloidosis** HCC ESR COM
Hereditary amyloid nephropathy
Code also associated disorders, such as:
autoinflammatory syndromes (M04.-)
EXCLUDES 2 *transthyretin-related (ATTR) familial amyloid cardiomyopathy (E85.4)*

E85.1 **Neuropathic heredofamilial amyloidosis** HCC ESR COM
Amyloid polyneuropathy (Portuguese)
Transthyretin-related (ATTR) familial amyloid polyneuropathy
AHA: 2012,4Q,99

E85.2 **Heredofamilial amyloidosis, unspecified** HCC ESR COM

E85.3 **Secondary systemic amyloidosis** HCC ESR COM
Hemodialysis-associated amyloidosis

E85.4 **Organ-limited amyloidosis** HCC ESR COM
Localized amyloidosis
Transthyretin-related (ATTR) familial amyloid cardiomyopathy

✓5th E85.8 **Other amyloidosis**
AHA: 2017,4Q,7

E85.81 **Light chain (AL) amyloidosis** HCC ESR COM
AHA: 2024,2Q,9

E85.82 **Wild-type transthyretin-related (ATTR) amyloidosis** HCC ESR COM
Senile systemic amyloidosis (SSA)

E85.89 **Other amyloidosis** HCC ESR COM

E85.9 **Amyloidosis, unspecified** HCC ESR COM

✓4th E86 **Volume depletion**
Use additional code(s) for any associated disorders of electrolyte and acid-base balance (E87.-)
EXCLUDES 1 *dehydration of newborn (P74.1)*
*postprocedural hypovolemic shock (T81.19)*
*traumatic hypovolemic shock (T79.4)*
EXCLUDES 2 *hypovolemic shock NOS (R57.1)*
AHA: 2019,2Q,7; 2018,2Q,6

E86.0 **Dehydration**
AHA: 2019,2Q,7; 2019,1Q,12; 2014,1Q,7
**TIP:** Can be assigned in addition to hypernatremia (E87.0) or hyponatremia (E87.1), when documented.

E86.1 **Hypovolemia**
Depletion of volume of plasma

E86.9 **Volume depletion, unspecified**
**DEF:** Depletion of total body water (dehydration) and/or contraction of total intravascular plasma (hypovolemia).

√4th **E87 Other disorders of fluid, electrolyte and acid-base balance**
EXCLUDES 1 *diabetes insipidus (E23.2)*
*electrolyte imbalance associated with hyperemesis gravidarum (O21.1)*
*electrolyte imbalance following ectopic or molar pregnancy (O08.5)*
*familial periodic paralysis (G72.3)*
*metabolic acidemia in newborn, unspecified (P19.9)*
**AHA:** 2018,2Q,6

**E87.0 Hyperosmolality and hypernatremia**
Sodium [Na] excess
Sodium [Na] overload
EXCLUDES 2 *diabetes with hyperosmolarity (E08, E09, E11, E13 with final characters .00 or .01)*
**AHA:** 2022,1Q,28; 2014,1Q,7
**TIP:** Assign an additional code for dehydration (E86.0), when documented.

**E87.1 Hypo-osmolality and hyponatremia**
Sodium [Na] deficiency
EXCLUDES 1 *syndrome of inappropriate secretion of antidiuretic hormone (E22.2)*
**AHA:** 2014,1Q,7
**TIP:** Assign an additional code for dehydration (E86.0), when documented.

√5th **E87.2 Acidosis**
EXCLUDES 1 *diabetic acidosis - see categories E08-E10, E11, E13 with ketoacidosis*
**AHA:** 2022,4Q,13-14; 2020,3Q,30
**DEF:** Reduction of alkaline in the blood and tissues caused by an increase in acid and decrease in bicarbonate.

**E87.20 Acidosis, unspecified**
Lactic acidosis NOS
Metabolic acidosis NOS
Code also, if applicable, respiratory failure with hypercapnia (J96. with 5th character 2)
**AHA:** 2026,2Q,4

**E87.21 Acute metabolic acidosis**
Acute lactic acidosis
**AHA:** 2024,4Q,16

**E87.22 Chronic metabolic acidosis**
Chronic lactic acidosis
▶Code first, if applicable, underlying etiology◀
**AHA:** 2022,4Q,14

**E87.29 Other acidosis**
Respiratory acidosis NOS
EXCLUDES 2 *acute respiratory acidosis (J96.02)*
*chronic respiratory acidosis (J96.12)*
**AHA:** 2026,1Q,27

**E87.3 Alkalosis**
Alkalosis NOS
Metabolic alkalosis
Respiratory alkalosis

**E87.4 Mixed disorder of acid-base balance**

**E87.5 Hyperkalemia**
Potassium [K] excess
Potassium [K] overload

**E87.6 Hypokalemia**
Potassium [K] deficiency
**AHA:** 2025,4Q,30

√5th **E87.7 Fluid overload**
EXCLUDES 1 *edema NOS (R60.9)*
*fluid retention (R60.9)*

**E87.70 Fluid overload, unspecified**
**AHA:** 2023,1Q,19

**E87.71 Transfusion associated circulatory overload**
Fluid overload due to transfusion (blood) (blood components)
TACO

**E87.79 Other fluid overload**

**E87.8 Other disorders of electrolyte and fluid balance, not elsewhere classified**
Electrolyte imbalance NOS
Hyperchloremia
Hypochloremia

√4th **E88 Other and unspecified metabolic disorders**
Use additional codes for associated conditions
EXCLUDES 1 *histiocytosis X (chronic) (C96.6)*

√5th **E88.0 Disorders of plasma-protein metabolism, not elsewhere classified**
EXCLUDES 1 *monoclonal gammopathy (of undetermined significance) (D47.2)*
*polyclonal hypergammaglobulinemia (D89.0)*
*Waldenstrom macroglobulinemia (C88.00)*
EXCLUDES 2 *disorder of lipoprotein metabolism (E78.-)*

**E88.01 Alpha-1-antitrypsin deficiency** HCC Rx ESR COM
AAT deficiency

**E88.02 Plasminogen deficiency**
Dysplasminogenemia
Hypoplasminogenemia
Type 1 plasminogen deficiency
Type 2 plasminogen deficiency
Code also, if applicable, ligneous conjunctivitis (H10.51-)
Use additional code for associated findings, such as:
hydrocephalus (G91.4)
otitis media (H67.-)
respiratory disorder related to plasminogen deficiency (J99)
**AHA:** 2018,4Q,6-7

**E88.09 Other disorders of plasma-protein metabolism, not elsewhere classified**
Bisalbuminemia

√5th **E88.1 Lipodystrophy, not elsewhere classified**
EXCLUDES 1 *Whipple's disease (K90.81)*

**E88.10 Lipodystrophy, unspecified**
Lipodystrophy NOS

**E88.11 Partial lipodystrophy**
Acquired partial lipodystrophy (APL)
Barraquer-Simons lipodystrophy
Familial partial lipodystrophy (FPLD)

**E88.12 Generalized lipodystrophy**
Acquired generalized lipodystrophy (AGL)
Berardinelli-Siep syndrome
Congenital generalized lipodystrophy (CGL)
Lawrence syndrome

**E88.13 Localized lipodystrophy**
Injection lipodystrophy
Insulin lipodystrophy

**E88.14 HIV-associated lipodystrophy**
Code first any human immunodeficiency virus [HIV] disease (B20)
Use additional code for adverse effect, if applicable, to identify drug (T37.5X5-)

**E88.19 Other lipodystrophy, not elsewhere classified**

**E88.2 Lipomatosis, not elsewhere classified** Rx
Lipomatosis (Check) dolorosa [Dercum]
Lipomatosis NOS
**AHA:** 2025,1Q,26

**E88.3 Tumor lysis syndrome** COM
Tumor lysis syndrome (spontaneous)
Tumor lysis syndrome following antineoplastic drug chemotherapy
Use additional code for adverse effect, if applicable, to identify drug (T45.1X5)
**AHA:** 2020,1Q,37; 2019,2Q,24
**DEF:** Potentially fatal metabolic complication of tumor necrosis caused by spontaneous or treatment-related accumulation of byproducts from dying cancer cells. Symptoms include hyperkalemia, hyperphosphatemia, hypocalcemia, hyperuricemia, and hyperuricosuria.

√5th **E88.4 Mitochondrial metabolism disorders**
EXCLUDES 1 *disorders of pyruvate metabolism (E74.4)*
*Kearns-Sayre syndrome (H49.81)*
*Leber's disease (H47.22)*
*Leigh's encephalopathy (G31.82)*
*mitochondrial myopathy, NEC (G71.3)*
*Reye's syndrome (G93.7)*

**E88.40 Mitochondrial metabolism disorder, unspecified** Rx ESR COM

**E88.41 MELAS syndrome** Rx ESR COM
Mitochondrial myopathy, encephalopathy, lactic acidosis and stroke-like episodes

E88.42 **MERRF syndrome** Rx ESR COM
Myoclonic epilepsy associated with ragged-red fibers
Code also progressive myoclonic epilepsy (G40.3-)

E88.43 **Disorders of mitochondrial tRNA synthetases** Rx ESR COM
ARS2-related mitochondrial disorders
LBSL
Leukoencephalopathy with brainstem - spinal cord involvement - lactate elevation
Leukoencephalopathy with thalamus - brainstem involvement - high lactate
LTBL
Mitochondrial aminoacyl-tRNA synthetase disorders
Code also, if applicable, associated condition such as:
leukoencephalopathy (G93.49)
**AHA:** 2023,4Q,12-13

E88.49 **Other mitochondrial metabolism disorders** Rx ESR COM

✓5th E88.8 **Other specified metabolic disorders**

✓6th E88.81 **Metabolic syndrome and other insulin resistance**
Use additional codes for associated manifestations, such as:
obesity (E66.-)
**AHA:** 2023,4Q,13-14; 2022,3Q,6
**DEF:** Group of health risks that increase the likelihood of developing heart disease, stroke, and diabetes. These risks include certain parameters for blood pressure, cholesterol, and glucose levels.

E88.810 **Metabolic syndrome**
Dysmetabolic syndrome

E88.811 **Insulin resistance syndrome, Type A**

E88.818 **Other insulin resistance**
Insulin resistance syndrome, Type B

E88.819 **Insulin resistance, unspecified**

E88.82 **Obesity due to disruption of MC4R pathway**
Use additional code to identify body mass index (BMI), if known (Z68.-)
Use additional code, if applicable, to identify associated manifestations, such as polyphagia (R63.2)
**AHA:** 2024,4Q,10-11
**TIP:** Assign an additional code for the specific class of obesity (E66.811-E66.813), when documented.

E88.89 **Other specified metabolic disorders** HCC Rx ESR COM
Launois-Bensaude adenolipomatosis
EXCLUDES 1 *adult pulmonary Langerhans cell histiocytosis (J84.82)*

E88.9 **Metabolic disorder, unspecified**

E88.A **Wasting disease (syndrome) due to underlying condition** ESR COM UPD
Cachexia due to underlying condition
Code first underlying condition
EXCLUDES 1 *cachexia NOS (R64)*
*nutritional marasmus (E41)*
EXCLUDES 2 *failure to thrive (R62.51, R62.7)*
**AHA:** 2023,4Q,14-15

## Postprocedural endocrine and metabolic complications and disorders, not elsewhere classified (E89)

✓4th E89 **Postprocedural endocrine and metabolic complications and disorders, not elsewhere classified**
EXCLUDES 2 *intraoperative complications of endocrine system organ or structure (E36.0-, E36.1-, E36.8)*

E89.0 **Postprocedural hypothyroidism** Rx
Postirradiation hypothyroidism
Postsurgical hypothyroidism

E89.1 **Postprocedural hypoinsulinemia**
Postpancreatectomy hyperglycemia
Postsurgical hypoinsulinemia
Code first, if applicable, diabetes mellitus (postpancreatectomy) (postprocedural) (E13.-)
Use additional code, if applicable, to identify:
acquired absence of pancreas (Z90.41-)
insulin use (Z79.4)
EXCLUDES 1 *transient postprocedural hyperglycemia (R73.9)*
*transient postprocedural hypoglycemia (E16.2)*

E89.2 **Postprocedural hypoparathyroidism** Rx ESR COM
Parathyroprival tetany
**AHA:** 2023,3Q,13

E89.3 **Postprocedural hypopituitarism** Rx ESR COM
Postirradiation hypopituitarism

✓5th E89.4 **Postprocedural ovarian failure**

E89.40 **Asymptomatic postprocedural ovarian failure**
Postprocedural ovarian failure NOS

E89.41 **Symptomatic postprocedural ovarian failure**
Symptoms such as flushing, sleeplessness, headache, lack of concentration, associated with postprocedural menopause

E89.5 **Postprocedural testicular hypofunction**

E89.6 **Postprocedural adrenocortical (-medullary) hypofunction** Rx ESR COM

✓5th E89.8 **Other postprocedural endocrine and metabolic complications and disorders**
**AHA:** 2016,4Q,9-10

✓6th E89.81 **Postprocedural hemorrhage of an endocrine system organ or structure following a procedure**

E89.810 **Postprocedural hemorrhage of an endocrine system organ or structure following an endocrine system procedure**

E89.811 **Postprocedural hemorrhage of an endocrine system organ or structure following other procedure**

✓6th E89.82 **Postprocedural hematoma and seroma of an endocrine system organ or structure**

E89.820 **Postprocedural hematoma of an endocrine system organ or structure following an endocrine system procedure**

E89.821 **Postprocedural hematoma of an endocrine system organ or structure following other procedure**

E89.822 **Postprocedural seroma of an endocrine system organ or structure following an endocrine system procedure**

E89.823 **Postprocedural seroma of an endocrine system organ or structure following other procedure**

● ✓6th E89.83 **Postprocedural hypoglycemia following a procedure**
Use additional code, if known, for hypoglycemia level (E16.A-)

● E89.830 **Post bariatric hypoglycemia**

● E89.838 **Other postprocedural hypoglycemia**
Post Nissen fundoplication hypoglycemia

E89.89 **Other postprocedural endocrine and metabolic complications and disorders**
Use additional code, if applicable, to further specify disorder

# Chapter 5. Mental, Behavioral and Neurodevelopmental Disorders (FØ1–F99)

## Chapter-specific Guidelines with Coding Examples

The chapter-specific guidelines from the ICD-10-CM Official Guidelines for Coding and Reporting have been provided below. Along with these guidelines are coding examples, contained in the shaded boxes, that have been developed to help illustrate the coding and/or sequencing guidance found in these guidelines.

### a. Pain disorders related to psychological factors

Assign code F45.41, for pain that is exclusively related to psychological disorders. As indicated by the Excludes 1 note under category G89, a code from category G89 should not be assigned with code F45.41.

> Chest pain determined to be persistent somatoform pain disorder
>
> **F45.41 Pain disorder exclusively related to psychological factors**
>
> *Explanation*: This pain was diagnosed as being exclusively psychological; therefore, no code from category G89 is added.

Code F45.42, Pain disorders with related psychological factors, should be used with a code from category G89, Pain, not elsewhere classified, if there is documentation of a psychological component for a patient with acute or chronic pain.

*See Section I.C.6. Pain*

### b. Mental and behavioral disorders due to psychoactive substance use

#### 1) In remission

Selection of codes describing "in remission" for categories F1Ø-F19, Mental and behavioral disorders due to psychoactive substance use (categories F1Ø-F19 with -.11, -.21, -.91) requires the provider's clinical judgment and are assigned only on the basis of provider documentation (as defined in the Official Guidelines for Coding and Reporting), unless otherwise instructed by the classification.

Mild substance use disorders in early or sustained remission are classified to the appropriate codes for substance abuse in remission, and moderate or severe substance use disorders in early or sustained remission are classified to the appropriate codes for substance dependence in remission.

> Physician documentation indicates the patient is seen to monitor progress on quitting cigarette smoking. The problem list indicates mild tobacco use disorder that is currently in remission.
>
> **F17.211 Nicotine dependence, cigarettes, in remission**
>
> *Explanation*: According to the index, Disorder, tobacco use, cigarettes (mild) (moderate) (severe), in remission (early) (sustained) is categorized to dependence (F17.211). Since the physician clearly documents mild cigarette use "disorder" and that the disorder is in remission, a code for nicotine dependence "in remission" is appropriate.

#### 2) Psychoactive substance use, abuse and dependence

When the provider documentation refers to use, abuse and dependence of the same substance (e.g. alcohol, opioid, cannabis, etc.), only one code should be assigned to identify the pattern of use based on the following hierarchy:

- If both use and abuse are documented, assign only the code for abuse
- If both abuse and dependence are documented, assign only the code for dependence
- If use, abuse and dependence are all documented, assign only the code for dependence
- If both use and dependence are documented, assign only the code for dependence.

> History and physical notes cannabis dependence and ongoing cannabis abuse
>
> **F12.2Ø Cannabis dependence, uncomplicated**
>
> *Explanation*: In the hierarchy, the dependence code is used if both abuse and dependence are documented.

> Current problem list indicates daily opioid use with opioid abuse.
>
> **F11.1Ø Opioid abuse, uncomplicated**
>
> *Explanation*: In the hierarchy, the abuse code is used if both abuse and use are documented.

#### 3) Psychoactive substance use, unspecified

As with all other unspecified diagnoses, the codes for unspecified psychoactive substance use (F1Ø.9-, F11.9-, F12.9-, F13.9-, F14.9-, F15.9-, F16.9-, F18.9-, F19.9-) should only be assigned based on provider documentation and when they meet the definition of a reportable diagnosis (see Section III, Reporting Additional Diagnoses). These codes are to be used only when the psychoactive substance use is associated with a substance related disorder (chapter 5 disorders such as sexual dysfunction, sleep disorder, or a mental or behavioral disorder) or medical condition, and such a relationship is documented by the provider.

#### 4) Medical conditions due to psychoactive substance use, abuse and dependence

Medical conditions due to substance use, abuse, and dependence are not classified as substance-induced disorders. Assign the diagnosis code for the medical condition as directed by the Alphabetical Index along with the appropriate psychoactive substance use, abuse or dependence code. For example, for alcoholic pancreatitis due to alcohol dependence, assign the appropriate code from subcategory K85.2, Alcohol induced acute pancreatitis, and the appropriate code from subcategory F1Ø.2, such as code F1Ø.20, Alcohol dependence, uncomplicated. It would not be appropriate to assign code F1Ø.288, Alcohol dependence with other alcohol-induced disorder.

#### 5) Blood alcohol level

A code from category Y9Ø, Evidence of alcohol involvement determined by blood alcohol level, may be assigned when this information is documented and the patient's provider has documented a condition classifiable to category F1Ø, Alcohol related disorders. The blood alcohol level does not need to be documented by the patient's provider in order for it to be coded.

*See Section I.B.14. for blood alcohol level documentation by clinicians other than patient's provider.*

### c. Factitious disorder

Factitious disorder imposed on self or Munchausen's syndrome is a disorder in which a person falsely reports or causes his or her own physical or psychological signs or symptoms. For patients with documented factitious disorder on self or Munchausen's syndrome, assign the appropriate code from subcategory F68.1-, Factitious disorder imposed on self.

Munchausen's syndrome by proxy (MSBP) is a disorder in which a caregiver (perpetrator) falsely reports or causes an illness or injury in another person (victim) under his or her care, such as a child, an elderly adult, or a person who has a disability. The condition is also referred to as "factitious disorder imposed on another" or "factitious disorder by proxy." The perpetrator, not the victim, receives this diagnosis. Assign code F68.A, Factitious disorder imposed on another, to the perpetrator's record. For the victim of a patient suffering from MSBP, assign the appropriate code from categories T74, Adult and child abuse, neglect and other maltreatment, confirmed, or T76, Adult and child abuse, neglect and other maltreatment, suspected.

*See Section I.C.19.f. Adult and child abuse, neglect and other maltreatment*

### d. Dementia

The ICD-10-CM classifies dementia (categories FØ1, FØ2, and FØ3) on the basis of the etiology and severity (unspecified, mild, moderate or severe). Selection of the appropriate severity level requires the provider's clinical judgment and codes should be assigned only on the basis of provider documentation (as defined in the Official Guidelines for Coding and Reporting), unless otherwise instructed by the classification. If the documentation does not provide information about the severity of the dementia, assign the appropriate code for unspecified severity.

If a patient is admitted to an inpatient acute care hospital or other inpatient facility setting with dementia at one severity level and it progresses to a higher severity level, assign one code for the highest severity level reported during the stay.

# Chapter 5. Mental, Behavioral and Neurodevelopmental Disorders (F01-F99)

INCLUDES disorders of psychological development

EXCLUDES 2 *symptoms, signs and abnormal clinical laboratory findings, not elsewhere classified (R00-R99)*

This chapter contains the following blocks:

F01-F09 Mental disorders due to known physiological conditions
F10-F19 Mental and behavioral disorders due to psychoactive substance use
F20-F29 Schizophrenia, schizotypal, delusional, and other non-mood psychotic disorders
F30-F39 Mood [affective] disorders
F40-F48 Anxiety, dissociative, stress-related, somatoform and other nonpsychotic mental disorders
F50-F59 Behavioral syndromes associated with physiological disturbances and physical factors
F60-F69 Disorders of adult personality and behavior
F70-F79 Intellectual disabilities
F80-F89 Pervasive and specific developmental disorders
F90-F98 Behavioral and emotional disorders with onset usually occurring in childhood and adolescence
F99 Unspecified mental disorder

## Mental disorders due to known physiological conditions (F01-F09)

NOTE This block comprises a range of mental disorders grouped together on the basis of their having in common a demonstrable etiology in cerebral disease, brain injury, or other insult leading to cerebral dysfunction. The dysfunction may be primary, as in diseases, injuries, and insults that affect the brain directly and selectively; or secondary, as in systemic diseases and disorders that attack the brain only as one of the multiple organs or systems of the body that are involved.

✓4th **F01 Vascular dementia**

Vascular dementia as a result of infarction of the brain due to vascular disease, including hypertensive cerebrovascular disease.

INCLUDES arteriosclerotic dementia
major neurocognitive disorder due to vascular disease
multi-infarct dementia

Code first, if applicable, any causal condition

**AHA:** 2022,4Q,14-15

✓5th **F01.5 Vascular dementia, unspecified severity**

**F01.50 Vascular dementia, unspecified severity, without behavioral disturbance, psychotic disturbance, mood disturbance, and anxiety** HCC Rx ESR A

Major neurocognitive disorder due to vascular disease NOS
Vascular dementia NOS

**AHA:** 2021,2Q,4

✓6th **F01.51 Vascular dementia, unspecified severity, with behavioral disturbance**

**F01.511 Vascular dementia, unspecified severity, with agitation** HCC Rx ESR UPD A

Major neurocognitive disorder due to vascular disease, unspecified severity, with aberrant motor behavior such as restlessness, rocking, pacing, or exit-seeking
Major neurocognitive disorder due to vascular disease, unspecified severity, with verbal or physical behaviors such as profanity, shouting, threatening, anger, aggression, combativeness, or violence
Vascular dementia, unspecified severity, with aberrant motor behavior such as restlessness, rocking, pacing, or exit-seeking
Vascular dementia, unspecified severity, with verbal or physical behaviors such as profanity, shouting, threatening, anger, aggression, combativeness, or violence

**F01.518 Vascular dementia, unspecified severity, with other behavioral disturbance** HCC Rx ESR UPD A

Major neurocognitive disorder due to vascular disease, unspecified severity, with behavioral disturbances such as sleep disturbance, social disinhibition, or sexual disinhibition
Vascular dementia, unspecified severity, with behavioral disturbances such as sleep disturbance, social disinhibition, or sexual disinhibition

Use additional code, if applicable, to identify wandering in vascular dementia (Z91.83)

**F01.52 Vascular dementia, unspecified severity, with psychotic disturbance** HCC Rx ESR UPD A

Major neurocognitive disorder due to vascular disease, unspecified severity, with psychotic disturbance such as hallucinations, paranoia, suspiciousness, or delusional state
Vascular dementia, unspecified severity, with psychotic disturbance such as hallucinations, paranoia, suspiciousness, or delusional state

**F01.53 Vascular dementia, unspecified severity, with mood disturbance** HCC Rx ESR UPD A

Major neurocognitive disorder due to vascular disease, unspecified severity, with mood disturbance such as depression, apathy, or anhedonia
Vascular dementia, unspecified severity, with mood disturbance such as depression, apathy, or anhedonia

**F01.54 Vascular dementia, unspecified severity, with anxiety** HCC Rx ESR UPD A

Major neurocognitive disorder due to vascular disease, unspecified severity, with anxiety

✓5th **F01.A Vascular dementia, mild**

EXCLUDES 1 *mild neurocognitive disorder due to known physiological condition with or without behavioral disturbance (F06.7-)*

**F01.A0 Vascular dementia, mild, without behavioral disturbance, psychotic disturbance, mood disturbance, and anxiety** HCC Rx ESR UPD A

Major neurocognitive disorder due to vascular disease, mild, NOS
Vascular dementia, mild, NOS

✓6th **F01.A1 Vascular dementia, mild, with behavioral disturbance**

**F01.A11 Vascular dementia, mild, with agitation** HCC Rx ESR UPD A

Major neurocognitive disorder due to vascular disease, mild, with aberrant motor behavior such as restlessness, rocking, pacing, or exit-seeking
Major neurocognitive disorder due to vascular disease, mild, with verbal or physical behaviors such as profanity, shouting, threatening, anger, aggression, combativeness, or violence
Vascular dementia, mild, with aberrant motor behavior such as restlessness, rocking, pacing, or exit-seeking
Vascular dementia, mild, with verbal or physical behaviors such as profanity, shouting, threatening, anger, aggression, combativeness, or violence

**F01.A18 Vascular dementia, mild, with other behavioral disturbance** HCC Rx ESR UPD A

Major neurocognitive disorder due to vascular disease, mild, with behavioral disturbances such as sleep disturbance, social disinhibition, or sexual disinhibition
Vascular dementia, mild, with behavioral disturbances such as sleep disturbance, social disinhibition, or sexual disinhibition

Use additional code, if applicable, to identify wandering in vascular dementia (Z91.83)

**F01.A2 Vascular dementia, mild, with psychotic disturbance** HCC Rx ESR UPD A
Major neurocognitive disorder due to vascular disease, mild, with psychotic disturbance such as hallucinations, paranoia, suspiciousness, or delusional state
Vascular dementia, mild, with psychotic disturbance such as hallucinations, paranoia, suspiciousness, or delusional state

**F01.A3 Vascular dementia, mild, with mood disturbance** HCC Rx ESR UPD A
Major neurocognitive disorder due to vascular disease, mild, with mood disturbance such as depression, apathy, or anhedonia
Vascular dementia, mild, with mood disturbance such as depression, apathy, or anhedonia

**F01.A4 Vascular dementia, mild, with anxiety** HCC Rx ESR UPD A
Major neurocognitive disorder due to vascular disease, mild, with anxiety

✓5th **F01.B Vascular dementia, moderate**

**F01.B0 Vascular dementia, moderate, without behavioral disturbance, psychotic disturbance, mood disturbance, and anxiety** HCC Rx ESR UPD A
Major neurocognitive disorder due to vascular disease, moderate, NOS
Vascular dementia, moderate, NOS

✓6th **F01.B1 Vascular dementia, moderate, with behavioral disturbance**

**F01.B11 Vascular dementia, moderate, with agitation** HCC Rx ESR UPD A
Major neurocognitive disorder due to vascular disease, moderate, with aberrant motor behavior such as restlessness, rocking, pacing, or exit-seeking
Major neurocognitive disorder due to vascular disease, moderate, with verbal or physical behaviors such as profanity, shouting, threatening, anger, aggression, combativeness, or violence
Vascular dementia, moderate, with aberrant motor behavior such as restlessness, rocking, pacing, or exit-seeking
Vascular dementia, moderate, with verbal or physical behaviors such as profanity, shouting, threatening, anger, aggression, combativeness, or violence

**F01.B18 Vascular dementia, moderate, with other behavioral disturbance** HCC Rx ESR UPD A
Major neurocognitive disorder due to vascular disease, moderate, with behavioral disturbances such as sleep disturbance, social disinhibition, or sexual disinhibition
Vascular dementia, moderate, with behavioral disturbances such as sleep disturbance, social disinhibition, or sexual disinhibition
Use additional code, if applicable, to identify wandering in vascular dementia (Z91.83)

**F01.B2 Vascular dementia, moderate, with psychotic disturbance** HCC Rx ESR UPD A
Major neurocognitive disorder due to vascular disease, moderate, with psychotic disturbance such as hallucinations, paranoia, suspiciousness, or delusional state
Vascular dementia, moderate, with psychotic disturbance such as hallucinations, paranoia, suspiciousness, or delusional state

**F01.B3 Vascular dementia, moderate, with mood disturbance** HCC Rx ESR UPD A
Major neurocognitive disorder due to vascular disease, moderate, with mood disturbance such as depression, apathy, or anhedonia
Vascular dementia, moderate, with mood disturbance such as depression, apathy, or anhedonia

**F01.B4 Vascular dementia, moderate, with anxiety** HCC Rx ESR UPD A
Major neurocognitive disorder due to vascular disease, moderate, with anxiety

✓5th **F01.C Vascular dementia, severe**

**F01.C0 Vascular dementia, severe, without behavioral disturbance, psychotic disturbance, mood disturbance, and anxiety** HCC Rx ESR UPD A
Major neurocognitive disorder due to vascular disease, severe, NOS
Vascular dementia, severe, NOS

✓6th **F01.C1 Vascular dementia, severe, with behavioral disturbance**

**F01.C11 Vascular dementia, severe, with agitation** HCC Rx ESR UPD A
Major neurocognitive disorder due to vascular disease, severe, with aberrant motor behavior such as restlessness, rocking, pacing, or exit-seeking
Major neurocognitive disorder due to vascular disease, severe, with verbal or physical behaviors such as profanity, shouting, threatening, anger, aggression, combativeness, or violence
Vascular dementia, severe, with aberrant motor behavior such as restlessness, rocking, pacing, or exit-seeking
Vascular dementia, severe, with verbal or physical behaviors such as profanity, shouting, threatening, anger, aggression, combativeness, or violence

**F01.C18 Vascular dementia, severe, with other behavioral disturbance** HCC Rx ESR UPD A
Major neurocognitive disorder due to vascular disease, severe, with behavioral disturbances such as sleep disturbance, social disinhibition, or sexual disinhibition
Vascular dementia, severe, with behavioral disturbances such as sleep disturbance, social disinhibition, or sexual disinhibition
Use additional code, if applicable, to identify wandering in vascular dementia (Z91.83)

**F01.C2 Vascular dementia, severe, with psychotic disturbance** HCC Rx ESR UPD A
Major neurocognitive disorder due to vascular disease, severe, with psychotic disturbance such as hallucinations, paranoia, suspiciousness, or delusional state
Vascular dementia, severe, with psychotic disturbance such as hallucinations, paranoia, suspiciousness, or delusional state

**F01.C3 Vascular dementia, severe, with mood disturbance** HCC Rx ESR UPD A
Major neurocognitive disorder due to vascular disease, severe, with mood disturbance such as depression, apathy, or anhedonia
Vascular dementia, severe, with mood disturbance such as depression, apathy, or anhedonia

**F01.C4 Vascular dementia, severe, with anxiety** HCC Rx ESR UPD A
Major neurocognitive disorder due to vascular disease, severe, with anxiety

**FØ2 Dementia in other diseases classified elsewhere**

INCLUDES major neurocognitive disorder in other diseases classified elsewhere

Code first the underlying physiological condition, such as:
- ~~frontotemporal dementia (G31.Ø9)~~
- Alzheimer's (G3Ø.-)
- cerebral lipidosis (E75.4)
- Creutzfeldt-Jakob disease (A81.Ø-)
- epilepsy and recurrent seizures (G4Ø.-)
- hepatolenticular degeneration (E83.Ø1)
- human immunodeficiency virus [HIV] disease (B2Ø)
- Huntington's disease (G1Ø)
- hypercalcemia (E83.52)
- hypothyroidism, acquired (EØØ-EØ3.-)
- intoxications (T36-T65)
- Jakob-Creutzfeldt disease (A81.Ø-)
- multiple sclerosis (G35-)
- neurocognitive disorder with Lewy bodies (G31.83)
- neurosyphilis (A52.17)
- niacin deficiency [pellagra] (E52)
- other frontotemporal neurocognitive disorder ▶(G31.Ø9)◀
- Parkinson's disease (G2Ø.-)
- Pick's disease (G31.Ø1)
- polyarteritis nodosa (M3Ø.Ø)
- prion disease (A81.9)
- systemic lupus erythematosus (M32.-)
- traumatic brain injury (SØ6.-)
- trypanosomiasis (B56.-, B57.-)
- vitamin B deficiency (E53.8)

EXCLUDES 1 *mild neurocognitive disorder due to known physiological condition with or without behavioral disturbance (FØ6.7-)*

EXCLUDES 2 *dementia in alcohol and psychoactive substance disorders (F1Ø-F19, with .17, .27, .97)*
*vascular dementia (FØ1.5-, FØ1.A-, FØ1.B-, FØ1.C-)*

**AHA:** 2022,4Q,14-15

**FØ2.8 Dementia in other diseases classified elsewhere, unspecified severity**

**AHA:** 2024,2Q,8; 2022,4Q,15; 2022,1Q,25; 2017,2Q,7; 2016,4Q,141; 2016,2Q,6

***FØ2.8Ø Dementia in other diseases classified elsewhere, unspecified severity, without behavioral disturbance, psychotic disturbance, mood disturbance, and anxiety*** HCC Rx ESR

Dementia in other diseases classified elsewhere NOS
Major neurocognitive disorder in other diseases classified elsewhere NOS

**AHA:** 2026,1Q,23

**FØ2.81 Dementia in other diseases classified elsewhere, unspecified severity, with behavioral disturbance**

***FØ2.811 Dementia in other diseases classified elsewhere, unspecified severity, with agitation*** HCC Rx ESR

Dementia in other diseases classified elsewhere, unspecified severity, with aberrant motor behavior such as restlessness, rocking, pacing, or exit-seeking
Dementia in other diseases classified elsewhere, unspecified severity, with verbal or physical behaviors such as profanity, shouting, threatening, anger, aggression, combativeness, or violence
Major neurocognitive disorder in other diseases classified elsewhere, unspecified severity, with aberrant motor behavior such as restlessness, rocking, pacing, or exit-seeking
Major neurocognitive disorder in other diseases classified elsewhere, unspecified severity, with verbal or physical behaviors such as profanity, shouting, threatening, anger, aggression, combativeness, or violence

***FØ2.818 Dementia in other diseases classified elsewhere, unspecified severity, with other behavioral disturbance*** HCC Rx ESR

Dementia in other diseases classified elsewhere with sleep disturbance, social disinhibition, or sexual disinhibition
Major neurocognitive disorder in other diseases classified elsewhere with sleep disturbance, social disinhibition, or sexual disinhibition

Use additional code, if applicable, to identify wandering in dementia in conditions classified elsewhere (Z91.83)

***FØ2.82 Dementia in other diseases classified elsewhere, unspecified severity, with psychotic disturbance*** HCC Rx ESR

Dementia in other diseases classified elsewhere, unspecified severity, with psychotic disturbance such as hallucinations, paranoia, suspiciousness, or delusional state
Major neurocognitive disorder in other diseases classified elsewhere, unspecified, with psychotic disturbance such as hallucinations, paranoia, suspiciousness, or delusional state

***FØ2.83 Dementia in other diseases classified elsewhere, unspecified severity, with mood disturbance*** HCC Rx ESR

Dementia in other diseases classified elsewhere, unspecified severity, with mood disturbance such as depression, apathy, or anhedonia
Major neurocognitive disorder in other diseases classified elsewhere unspecified severity,with mood disturbance such as with depression, apathy, or anhedonia

***FØ2.84 Dementia in other diseases classified elsewhere, unspecified severity, with anxiety*** HCC Rx ESR

Major neurocognitive disorder in other diseases classified elsewhere unspecified severity, with anxiety

**FØ2.A Dementia in other diseases classified elsewhere, mild**

EXCLUDES 1 *mild neurocognitive disorder due to known physiological condition with or without behavioral disturbance (FØ6.7-)*

***FØ2.AØ Dementia in other diseases classified elsewhere, mild, without behavioral disturbance, psychotic disturbance, mood disturbance, and anxiety*** HCC Rx ESR

Dementia in other diseases classified elsewhere, mild, NOS
Major neurocognitive disorder in other diseases classified elsewhere, mild, NOS

**FØ2.A1 Dementia in other diseases classified elsewhere, mild, with behavioral disturbance**

***FØ2.A11 Dementia in other diseases classified elsewhere, mild, with agitation*** HCC Rx ESR

Dementia in other diseases classified elsewhere, mild, with aberrant motor behavior such as restlessness, rocking, pacing, or exit-seeking
Dementia in other diseases classified elsewhere, mild, with verbal or physical behaviors such as profanity, shouting, threatening, anger, aggression, combativeness, or violence
Major neurocognitive disorder in other diseases classified elsewhere, mild, with aberrant motor behavior such as restlessness, rocking, pacing, or exit-seeking
Major neurocognitive disorder in other diseases classified elsewhere, mild, with verbal or physical behaviors such as profanity, shouting, threatening, anger, aggression, combativeness, or violence

*F02.A18* ***Dementia in other diseases classified elsewhere, mild, with other behavioral disturbance*** HCC Rx ESR
Dementia in other diseases classified elsewhere, mild, with behavioral disturbances such as sleep disturbance, social disinhibition, or sexual disinhibition
Major neurocognitive disorder in other diseases classified elsewhere, mild, with behavioral disturbances such as sleep disturbance, social disinhibition, or sexual disinhibition
Use additional code, if applicable, to identify wandering in dementia in conditions classified elsewhere (Z91.83)

*F02.A2* ***Dementia in other diseases classified elsewhere, mild, with psychotic disturbance*** HCC Rx ESR
Dementia in other diseases classified elsewhere, mild, with psychotic disturbance such as hallucinations, paranoia, suspiciousness, or delusional state
Major neurocognitive disorder in other diseases classified elsewhere, mild, with psychotic disturbance such as hallucinations, paranoia, suspiciousness, or delusional state

*F02.A3* ***Dementia in other diseases classified elsewhere, mild, with mood disturbance*** HCC Rx ESR
Dementia in other diseases classified elsewhere, mild, with mood disturbance such as depression, apathy, or anhedonia
Major neurocognitive disorder in other diseases classified elsewhere, mild, with mood disturbance such as depression, apathy, or anhedonia

*F02.A4* ***Dementia in other diseases classified elsewhere, mild, with anxiety*** HCC Rx ESR
Major neurocognitive disorder in other diseases classified elsewhere, mild, with anxiety

5th **F02.B Dementia in other diseases classified elsewhere, moderate**

*F02.B0* ***Dementia in other diseases classified elsewhere, moderate, without behavioral disturbance, psychotic disturbance, mood disturbance, and anxiety*** HCC Rx ESR
Dementia in other diseases classified elsewhere, moderate, NOS
Major neurocognitive disorder in other diseases classified elsewhere, moderate, NOS

6th **F02.B1 Dementia in other diseases classified elsewhere, moderate, with behavioral disturbance**

*F02.B11* ***Dementia in other diseases classified elsewhere, moderate, with agitation*** HCC Rx ESR
Dementia in other diseases classified elsewhere, moderate, with aberrant motor behavior such as restlessness, rocking, pacing, or exit-seeking
Dementia in other diseases classified elsewhere, moderate, with verbal or physical behaviors such as profanity, shouting, threatening, anger, aggression, combativeness, or violence
Major neurocognitive disorder in other diseases classified elsewhere, moderate, with aberrant motor behavior such as restlessness, rocking, pacing, or exit-seeking
Major neurocognitive disorder in other diseases classified elsewhere, moderate, with verbal or physical behaviors such as profanity, shouting, threatening, anger, aggression, combativeness, or violence

*F02.B18* ***Dementia in other diseases classified elsewhere, moderate, with other behavioral disturbance*** HCC Rx ESR
Dementia in other diseases classified elsewhere, moderate, with behavioral disturbances such as sleep disturbance, social disinhibition, or sexual disinhibition
Major neurocognitive disorder in other diseases classified elsewhere, moderate, with behavioral disturbance such as sleep disturbance, social disinhibition, or sexual disinhibition
Use additional code, if applicable, to identify wandering in dementia in conditions classified elsewhere (Z91.83)

*F02.B2* ***Dementia in other diseases classified elsewhere, moderate, with psychotic disturbance*** HCC Rx ESR
Dementia in other diseases classified elsewhere, moderate, with psychotic disturbance such as hallucinations, paranoia, suspiciousness, or delusional state
Major neurocognitive disorder in other diseases classified elsewhere, moderate, with psychotic disturbance such as hallucinations, paranoia, suspiciousness, or delusional state

*F02.B3* ***Dementia in other diseases classified elsewhere, moderate, with mood disturbance*** HCC Rx ESR
Dementia in other diseases classified elsewhere, moderate, with mood disturbance such as depression, apathy, or anhedonia
Major neurocognitive disorder in other diseases classified elsewhere, moderate, with mood disturbance such as depression, apathy, or anhedonia

*F02.B4* ***Dementia in other diseases classified elsewhere, moderate, with anxiety*** HCC Rx ESR
Major neurocognitive disorder in other diseases classified elsewhere, moderate, with anxiety

5th **F02.C Dementia in other diseases classified elsewhere, severe**

*F02.C0* ***Dementia in other diseases classified elsewhere, severe, without behavioral disturbance, psychotic disturbance, mood disturbance, and anxiety*** HCC Rx ESR
Dementia in other diseases classified elsewhere, severe, NOS
Major neurocognitive disorder in other diseases classified elsewhere, severe, NOS

6th **F02.C1 Dementia in other diseases classified elsewhere, severe, with behavioral disturbance**

*F02.C11* ***Dementia in other diseases classified elsewhere, severe, with agitation*** HCC Rx ESR
Dementia in other diseases classified elsewhere, severe, with aberrant motor behavior such as restlessness, rocking, pacing, or exit-seeking
Dementia in other diseases classified elsewhere, severe, with verbal or physical behaviors such as profanity, shouting, threatening, anger, aggression, combativeness, or violence
Major neurocognitive disorder in other diseases classified elsewhere, severe, with aberrant motor behavior such as restlessness, rocking, pacing, or exit-seeking
Major neurocognitive disorder in other diseases classified elsewhere, severe, with verbal or physical behaviors such as profanity, shouting, threatening, anger, aggression, combativeness, or violence

FØ2.C18 ***Dementia in other diseases classified elsewhere, severe, with other behavioral disturbance*** HCC Rx ESR
Dementia in other diseases classified elsewhere, severe, with behavioral disturbances such as sleep disturbance, social disinhibition, or sexual disinhibition
Major neurocognitive disorder in other diseases classified elsewhere, severe, with behavioral disturbances such as sleep disturbance, social disinhibition, or sexual disinhibition
Use additional code, if applicable, to identify wandering in dementia in conditions classified elsewhere (Z91.83)

FØ2.C2 ***Dementia in other diseases classified elsewhere, severe, with psychotic disturbance*** HCC Rx ESR
Dementia in other diseases classified elsewhere, severe, with psychotic disturbance such as hallucinations, paranoia, suspiciousness, or delusional state
Major neurocognitive disorder in other diseases classified elsewhere, severe, with psychotic disturbance such as hallucinations, paranoia, suspiciousness, or delusional state

FØ2.C3 ***Dementia in other diseases classified elsewhere, severe, with mood disturbance*** HCC Rx ESR
Dementia in other diseases classified elsewhere, severe, with mood disturbance such as depression, apathy, or anhedonia
Major neurocognitive disorder in other diseases classified elsewhere, severe, with mood disturbance such as depression, apathy, or anhedonia

FØ2.C4 ***Dementia in other diseases classified elsewhere, severe, with anxiety*** HCC Rx ESR
Major neurocognitive disorder in other diseases classified elsewhere, severe, with anxiety

✓4th **FØ3 Unspecified dementia**
Major neurocognitive disorder NOS
Presenile dementia NOS
Presenile psychosis NOS
Primary degenerative dementia NOS
Senile dementia depressed or paranoid type
Senile dementia NOS
Senile psychosis NOS
EXCLUDES 2 *dementia with delirium or acute confusional state (FØ5)*
*mild memory disturbance due to known physiological condition (FØ6.8)*
AHA: 2022,4Q,14-15

✓5th **FØ3.9 Unspecified dementia, unspecified severity**

**FØ3.9Ø Unspecified dementia, unspecified severity, without behavioral disturbance, psychotic disturbance, mood disturbance, and anxiety** HCC Rx ESR A
Dementia NOS
AHA: 2024,2Q,8; 2021,2Q,4; 2012,4Q,92

✓6th **FØ3.91 Unspecified dementia, unspecified severity, with behavioral disturbance**

**FØ3.911 Unspecified dementia, unspecified severity, with agitation** HCC Rx ESR A
Unspecified dementia, unspecified severity, with aberrant motor behavior such as restlessness, rocking, pacing, or exit-seeking
Unspecified dementia, unspecified severity, with verbal or physical behaviors such as profanity, shouting, threatening, anger, aggression, combativeness, or violence

**FØ3.918 Unspecified dementia, unspecified severity, with other behavioral disturbance** HCC Rx ESR A
Unspecified dementia, unspecified severity, with behavioral disturbances such as sleep disturbance, social disinhibition, or sexual disinhibition
Use additional code, if applicable, to identify wandering in unspecified dementia (Z91.83)

**FØ3.92 Unspecified dementia, unspecified severity, with psychotic disturbance** HCC Rx ESR A
Unspecified dementia, unspecified severity, with psychotic disturbance such as hallucinations, paranoia, suspiciousness, or delusional state

**FØ3.93 Unspecified dementia, unspecified severity, with mood disturbance** HCC Rx ESR A
Unspecified dementia, unspecified severity, with mood disturbance such as depression, apathy, or anhedonia
AHA: 2025,3Q,5-6

**FØ3.94 Unspecified dementia, unspecified severity, with anxiety** HCC Rx ESR A
AHA: 2025,3Q,6

✓5th **FØ3.A Unspecified dementia, mild**
EXCLUDES 1 *mild neurocognitive disorder due to known physiological condition with or without behavioral disturbance (FØ6.7-)*

**FØ3.AØ Unspecified dementia, mild, without behavioral disturbance, psychotic disturbance, mood disturbance, and anxiety** HCC Rx ESR A
Dementia, mild, NOS

✓6th **FØ3.A1 Unspecified dementia, mild, with behavioral disturbance**

**FØ3.A11 Unspecified dementia, mild, with agitation** HCC Rx ESR A
Unspecified dementia, mild, with aberrant motor behavior such as restlessness, rocking, pacing, or exit-seeking
Unspecified dementia, mild, with verbal or physical behaviors such as profanity, shouting, threatening, anger, aggression, combativeness, or violence

**FØ3.A18 Unspecified dementia, mild, with other behavioral disturbance** HCC Rx ESR A
Unspecified dementia, mild, with behavioral disturbances such as sleep disturbance, social disinhibition, or sexual disinhibition
Use additional code, if applicable, to identify wandering in unspecified dementia (Z91.83)

**FØ3.A2 Unspecified dementia, mild, with psychotic disturbance** HCC Rx ESR A
Unspecified dementia, mild, with psychotic disturbance such as hallucinations, paranoia, suspiciousness, or delusional state

**FØ3.A3 Unspecified dementia, mild, with mood disturbance** HCC Rx ESR A
Unspecified dementia, mild, with mood disturbance such as depression, apathy, or anhedonia

**FØ3.A4 Unspecified dementia, mild, with anxiety** HCC Rx ESR A

✓5th **FØ3.B Unspecified dementia, moderate**

**FØ3.BØ Unspecified dementia, moderate, without behavioral disturbance, psychotic disturbance, mood disturbance, and anxiety** HCC Rx ESR A
Dementia, moderate, NOS

✓6th **FØ3.B1 Unspecified dementia, moderate, with behavioral disturbance**

**FØ3.B11 Unspecified dementia, moderate, with agitation** HCC Rx ESR A
Unspecified dementia, moderate, with aberrant motor behavior such as restlessness, rocking, pacing, or exit-seeking
Unspecified dementia, moderate, with verbal or physical behaviors such as profanity, shouting, threatening, anger, aggression, combativeness, or violence

**FØ3.B18 Unspecified dementia, moderate, with other behavioral disturbance** HCC Rx ESR A
Unspecified dementia, moderate, with behavioral disturbances such as sleep disturbance, social disinhibition, or sexual disinhibition
Use additional code, if applicable, to identify wandering in unspecified dementia (Z91.83)

**F03.B2 Unspecified dementia, moderate, with psychotic disturbance** HCC Rx ESR A
Unspecified dementia, moderate, with psychotic disturbance such as hallucinations, paranoia, suspiciousness, or delusional state
**AHA:** 2025,3Q,7

**F03.B3 Unspecified dementia, moderate, with mood disturbance** HCC Rx ESR A
Unspecified dementia, moderate, with mood disturbance such as depression, apathy, or anhedonia

**F03.B4 Unspecified dementia, moderate, with anxiety** HCC Rx ESR A

✓5th **F03.C Unspecified dementia, severe**

**F03.C0 Unspecified dementia, severe, without behavioral disturbance, psychotic disturbance, mood disturbance, and anxiety** HCC Rx ESR A
Dementia, severe, NOS

✓6th **F03.C1 Unspecified dementia, severe, with behavioral disturbance**

**F03.C11 Unspecified dementia, severe, with agitation** HCC Rx ESR A
Unspecified dementia, severe, with aberrant motor behavior such as restlessness, rocking, pacing, or exit-seeking
Unspecified dementia, severe, with verbal or physical behaviors such as profanity, shouting, threatening, anger, aggression, combativeness, or violence

**F03.C18 Unspecified dementia, severe, with other behavioral disturbance** HCC Rx ESR A
Unspecified dementia, severe, with behavioral disturbances such as sleep disturbance, social disinhibition, or sexual disinhibition
Use additional code, if applicable, to identify wandering in unspecified dementia (Z91.83)

**F03.C2 Unspecified dementia, severe, with psychotic disturbance** HCC Rx ESR A
Unspecified dementia, severe, with psychotic disturbance such as hallucinations, paranoia, suspiciousness, or delusional state

**F03.C3 Unspecified dementia, severe, with mood disturbance** HCC Rx ESR A
Unspecified dementia, severe, with mood disturbance such as depression, apathy, or anhedonia
**AHA:** 2023,4Q,14

**F03.C4 Unspecified dementia, severe, with anxiety** HCC Rx ESR A

**F04 Amnestic disorder due to known physiological condition** Rx ESR
Korsakov's psychosis or syndrome, nonalcoholic
Code first the underlying physiological condition
EXCLUDES 1 *amnesia NOS (R41.3)*
*anterograde amnesia (R41.1)*
*dissociative amnesia (F44.0)*
*retrograde amnesia (R41.2)*
EXCLUDES 2 *alcohol-induced or unspecified Korsakov's syndrome (F10.26, F10.96)*
*Korsakov's syndrome induced by other psychoactive substances (F13.26, F13.96, F19.16, F19.26, F19.96)*

**F05 Delirium due to known physiological condition** UPD
Acute or subacute brain syndrome
Acute or subacute confusional state (nonalcoholic)
Acute or subacute infective psychosis
Acute or subacute organic reaction
Acute or subacute psycho-organic syndrome
Delirium of mixed etiology
Delirium superimposed on dementia
Sundowning
Code first the underlying physiological condition, such as:
dementia (F03.9-)
EXCLUDES 1 *delirium NOS (R41.0)*
EXCLUDES 2 *delirium tremens alcohol-induced or unspecified (F10.231, F10.921)*
**AHA:** 2019,2Q,34

✓4th **F06 Other mental disorders due to known physiological condition**
INCLUDES mental disorders due to endocrine disorder
mental disorders due to exogenous hormone
mental disorders due to exogenous toxic substance
mental disorders due to primary cerebral disease
mental disorders due to somatic illness
mental disorders due to systemic disease affecting the brain
Code first the underlying physiological condition
EXCLUDES 1 *unspecified dementia (F03.-)*
EXCLUDES 2 *delirium due to known physiological condition (F05)*
*dementia as classified in F01-F02*
*other mental disorders associated with alcohol and other psychoactive substances (F10-F19)*

**F06.0 Psychotic disorder with hallucinations due to known physiological condition**
Organic hallucinatory state (nonalcoholic)
EXCLUDES 2 *hallucinations and perceptual disturbance induced by alcohol and other psychoactive substances (F10-F19 with .151, .251, .951)*
*schizophrenia (F20.-)*

**F06.1 Catatonic disorder due to known physiological condition**
Catatonia associated with another mental disorder
Catatonia NOS
EXCLUDES 1 *catatonic stupor (R40.1)*
*stupor NOS (R40.1)*
EXCLUDES 2 *catatonic schizophrenia (F20.2)*
*dissociative stupor (F44.2)*
**DEF:** Catatonic: Abnormal neuropsychiatric state characterized by stupor, immobility or purposeless movements, or unresponsiveness in a person who otherwise appears awake.

**F06.2 Psychotic disorder with delusions due to known physiological condition**
Paranoid and paranoid-hallucinatory organic states
Schizophrenia-like psychosis in epilepsy
EXCLUDES 2 *alcohol and drug-induced psychotic disorder (F10-F19 with .150, .250, .950)*
*brief psychotic disorder (F23)*
*delusional disorder (F22)*
*schizophrenia (F20.-)*

✓5th **F06.3 Mood disorder due to known physiological condition**
EXCLUDES 2 *mood disorders due to alcohol and other psychoactive substances (F10-F19 with .14, .24, .94)*
*mood disorders, not due to known physiological condition or unspecified (F30-F39)*

**F06.30 Mood disorder due to known physiological condition, unspecified**

**F06.31 Mood disorder due to known physiological condition with depressive features**
Depressive disorder due to known physiological condition, with depressive features

**F06.32 Mood disorder due to known physiological condition with major depressive-like episode**
Depressive disorder due to known physiological condition, with major depressive-like episode

**F06.33 Mood disorder due to known physiological condition with manic features**
Bipolar and related disorder due to a known physiological condition, with manic features
Bipolar and related disorder due to known physiological condition, with manic- or hypomanic-like episodes

**F06.34 Mood disorder due to known physiological condition with mixed features**
Bipolar and related disorder due to known physiological condition, with mixed features
Depressive disorder due to known physiological condition, with mixed features

**F06.4 Anxiety disorder due to known physiological condition**
EXCLUDES 2 *anxiety disorders due to alcohol and other psychoactive substances (F10-F19 with .180, .280, .980)*
*anxiety disorders, not due to known physiological condition or unspecified (F40.-, F41.-)*

√5th **F06.7 Mild neurocognitive disorder due to known physiological condition**
Mild neurocognitive impairment due to a known physiological condition
Code first the underlying physiological condition, such as:
Alzheimer's disease (G30.-)
human immunodeficiency virus [HIV] disease (B20)
Huntington's disease (G10)
neurocognitive disorder with Lewy bodies (G31.83)
other frontotemporal neurocognitive disorder (G31.09)
Parkinson's disease (G20.-)
systemic lupus erythematosus (M32.-)
traumatic brain injury (S06.-)
vitamin B deficiency (E53.-)
EXCLUDES 1 *age related cognitive decline (R41.81)*
*altered mental status (R41.82)*
*cerebral degeneration (G31.9)*
*change in mental status (R41.82)*
*cognitive deficits following (sequelae of) cerebral hemorrhage or infarction (I69.01-I69.11-, I69.21-I69.31-, I69.81-I69.91-)*
*dementia (F01.-, F02.-, F03.-)*
*mild cognitive impairment due to unknown or unspecified etiology (G31.84)*
*neurologic neglect syndrome (R41.4)*
*personality change, nonpsychotic (F68.8)*
**AHA:** 2022,4Q,16

**F06.70 Mild neurocognitive disorder due to known physiological condition without behavioral disturbance** UPD
Mild neurocognitive disorder due to known physiological condition, NOS

**F06.71 Mild neurocognitive disorder due to known physiological condition with behavioral disturbance** UPD

**F06.8 Other specified mental disorders due to known physiological condition**
Epileptic psychosis NOS
Obsessive-compulsive and related disorder due to a known physiological condition
Organic dissociative disorder
Organic emotionally labile [asthenic] disorder

√4th **F07 Personality and behavioral disorders due to known physiological condition**
Code first the underlying physiological condition

**F07.0 Personality change due to known physiological condition** UPD
Frontal lobe syndrome
Limbic epilepsy personality syndrome
Lobotomy syndrome
Organic personality disorder
Organic pseudopsychopathic personality
Organic pseudoretarded personality
Postleucotomy syndrome
EXCLUDES 1 *mild cognitive impairment (G31.84)*
*postconcussional syndrome (F07.81)*
*postencephalitic syndrome (F07.89)*
*signs and symptoms involving emotional state (R45.-)*
EXCLUDES 2 *specific personality disorder (F60.-)*

√5th **F07.8 Other personality and behavioral disorders due to known physiological condition**

**F07.81 Postconcussional syndrome**
Postcontusional syndrome (encephalopathy)
Post-traumatic brain syndrome, nonpsychotic
►Code also, if applicable, sequela of concussion (S06.0X- with seventh character S)◄
Use additional code to identify associated post-traumatic headache, if applicable (G44.3-)
EXCLUDES 1 *current concussion (brain) ►(S06.0X- with seventh character A)◄*
*postencephalitic syndrome (F07.89)*
**DEF:** Concussion symptoms that persist for weeks or months after a head injury. These symptoms may include headache, giddiness, fatigue, insomnia, mood fluctuation, and a subjective feeling of impaired intellectual function with extreme reaction to normal stressors.

**F07.89 Other personality and behavioral disorders due to known physiological condition** UPD
Postencephalitic syndrome
Right hemispheric organic affective disorder

**F07.9 Unspecified personality and behavioral disorder due to known physiological condition** UPD
Organic psychosyndrome

**F09 Unspecified mental disorder due to known physiological condition**
Mental disorder NOS due to known physiological condition
Organic brain syndrome NOS
Organic mental disorder NOS
Organic psychosis NOS
Symptomatic psychosis NOS
Code first the underlying physiological condition
EXCLUDES 1 *mild neurocognitive disorder due to known physiological condition (F06.7-)*
*psychosis NOS (F29)*

## Mental and behavioral disorders due to psychoactive substance use (F10-F19)

**AHA:** 2022,4Q,16-17; 2022,1Q,34; 2020,1Q,9; 2018,4Q,69-70; 2017,4Q,8; 2017,2Q,27
**TIP:** Psychoactive substance withdrawal can occur in individuals who do not have a diagnosis of dependence but who use the substance regularly (i.e., use or abuse) and then reduce or cease the use.

√4th **F10 Alcohol related disorders**
Use additional code for blood alcohol level, if applicable (Y90.-)
**AHA:** 2019,3Q,8

√5th **F10.1 Alcohol abuse**
EXCLUDES 1 *alcohol dependence (F10.2-)*
*alcohol use, unspecified (F10.9-)*
**AHA:** 2018,1Q,16; 2015,2Q,15

**F10.10 Alcohol abuse, uncomplicated**
Alcohol use disorder, mild

**F10.11 Alcohol abuse, in remission**
Alcohol use disorder, mild, in early remission
Alcohol use disorder, mild, in sustained remission
**AHA:** 2022,1Q,25

√6th **F10.12 Alcohol abuse with intoxication**

**F10.120 Alcohol abuse with intoxication, uncomplicated** ESR

**F10.121 Alcohol abuse with intoxication delirium** ESR

**F10.129 Alcohol abuse with intoxication, unspecified** ESR

√6th **F10.13 Alcohol abuse, with withdrawal**
**AHA:** 2020,4Q,16-17

**F10.130 Alcohol abuse with withdrawal, uncomplicated** HCC ESR COM

**F10.131 Alcohol abuse with withdrawal delirium** HCC ESR COM

**F10.132 Alcohol abuse with withdrawal with perceptual disturbance** HCC ESR COM

**F10.139 Alcohol abuse with withdrawal, unspecified** HCC ESR COM

**F10.14 Alcohol abuse with alcohol-induced mood disorder** HCC ESR COM
Alcohol use disorder, mild, with alcohol-induced bipolar or related disorder
Alcohol use disorder, mild, with alcohol-induced depressive disorder

√6th **F10.15 Alcohol abuse with alcohol-induced psychotic disorder**

**F10.150 Alcohol abuse with alcohol-induced psychotic disorder with delusions** HCC ESR COM

**F10.151 Alcohol abuse with alcohol-induced psychotic disorder with hallucinations** HCC ESR COM
**DEF:** Psychosis lasting less than six months with slight or no clouding of consciousness in which auditory hallucinations predominate.

**F10.159 Alcohol abuse with alcohol-induced psychotic disorder, unspecified** HCC ESR COM

√6th **F10.18 Alcohol abuse with other alcohol-induced disorders**
**AHA:** 2022,1Q,33

**F10.180 Alcohol abuse with alcohol-induced anxiety disorder** HCC ESR COM
**AHA:** 2022,1Q,25,33

**F10.181 Alcohol abuse with alcohol-induced sexual dysfunction** HCC ESR COM

F10.182 Alcohol abuse with alcohol-induced sleep disorder HCC ESR COM

F10.188 Alcohol abuse with other alcohol-induced disorder HCC ESR COM
AHA: 2022,1Q,25

F10.19 Alcohol abuse with unspecified alcohol-induced disorder ESR

✓5th F10.2 Alcohol dependence
EXCLUDES 1 *alcohol abuse (F10.1-)*
*alcohol use, unspecified (F10.9-)*
EXCLUDES 2 *toxic effect of alcohol (T51.0-)*

F10.20 Alcohol dependence, uncomplicated HCC ESR COM
Alcohol use disorder, moderate
Alcohol use disorder, severe
AHA: 2020,1Q,9

F10.21 Alcohol dependence, in remission HCC ESR COM
Alcohol use disorder, moderate, in early remission
Alcohol use disorder, moderate, in sustained remission
Alcohol use disorder, severe, in early remission
Alcohol use disorder, severe, in sustained remission

✓6th F10.22 Alcohol dependence with intoxication
Acute drunkenness (in alcoholism)
EXCLUDES 2 *alcohol dependence with withdrawal (F10.23-)*

F10.220 Alcohol dependence with intoxication, uncomplicated HCC ESR COM

F10.221 Alcohol dependence with intoxication delirium HCC ESR COM

F10.229 Alcohol dependence with intoxication, unspecified HCC ESR COM

✓6th F10.23 Alcohol dependence with withdrawal
EXCLUDES 2 *alcohol dependence with intoxication (F10.22-)*
AHA: 2018,1Q,16; 2015,2Q,15

F10.230 Alcohol dependence with withdrawal, uncomplicated HCC ESR COM

F10.231 Alcohol dependence with withdrawal delirium HCC ESR COM

F10.232 Alcohol dependence with withdrawal with perceptual disturbance HCC ESR COM

F10.239 Alcohol dependence with withdrawal, unspecified HCC ESR COM

F10.24 Alcohol dependence with alcohol-induced mood disorder HCC ESR COM
Alcohol use disorder, moderate, with alcohol-induced bipolar or related disorder
Alcohol use disorder, moderate, with alcohol-induced depressive disorder
Alcohol use disorder, severe, with alcohol-induced bipolar or related disorder
Alcohol use disorder, severe, with alcohol-induced depressive disorder

✓6th F10.25 Alcohol dependence with alcohol-induced psychotic disorder

F10.250 Alcohol dependence with alcohol-induced psychotic disorder with delusions HCC ESR COM

F10.251 Alcohol dependence with alcohol-induced psychotic disorder with hallucinations HCC ESR COM

F10.259 Alcohol dependence with alcohol-induced psychotic disorder, unspecified HCC ESR COM

F10.26 Alcohol dependence with alcohol-induced persisting amnestic disorder HCC ESR COM
Alcohol use disorder, moderate, with alcohol-induced major neurocognitive disorder, amnestic-confabulatory type
Alcohol use disorder, severe, with alcohol-induced major neurocognitive disorder, amnestic-confabulatory type
DEF: Prominent and lasting reduced memory span and disordered time appreciation and confabulation that occurs in alcoholics as sequel to acute alcoholic psychosis.

F10.27 Alcohol dependence with alcohol-induced persisting dementia HCC ESR COM
Alcohol use disorder, moderate, with alcohol-induced major neurocognitive disorder, nonamnestic-confabulatory type
Alcohol use disorder, severe, with alcohol-induced major neurocognitive disorder, nonamnestic-confabulatory type

✓6th F10.28 Alcohol dependence with other alcohol-induced disorders

F10.280 Alcohol dependence with alcohol-induced anxiety disorder HCC ESR COM

F10.281 Alcohol dependence with alcohol-induced sexual dysfunction HCC ESR COM

F10.282 Alcohol dependence with alcohol-induced sleep disorder HCC ESR COM

F10.288 Alcohol dependence with other alcohol-induced disorder HCC ESR COM
Alcohol use disorder, moderate, with alcohol-induced mild neurocognitive disorder
Alcohol use disorder, severe, with alcohol-induced mild neurocognitive disorder
AHA: 2020,1Q,9

F10.29 Alcohol dependence with unspecified alcohol-induced disorder HCC ESR COM

✓5th F10.9 Alcohol use, unspecified
EXCLUDES 1 *alcohol abuse (F10.1-)*
*alcohol dependence (F10.2-)*
AHA: 2018,2Q,10-11
TIP: Assign a substance use code only when the provider documents a relationship between the use and an associated physical, mental, or behavioral disorder. As with all diagnoses, substance use codes must meet the definition of a reportable diagnosis.

F10.90 Alcohol use, unspecified, uncomplicated

F10.91 Alcohol use, unspecified, in remission

✓6th F10.92 Alcohol use, unspecified with intoxication

F10.920 Alcohol use, unspecified with intoxication, uncomplicated ESR
AHA: 2018,2Q,10-11

F10.921 Alcohol use, unspecified with intoxication delirium ESR

F10.929 Alcohol use, unspecified with intoxication, unspecified ESR

✓6th F10.93 Alcohol use, unspecified with withdrawal
AHA: 2020,4Q,16-17

F10.930 Alcohol use, unspecified with withdrawal, uncomplicated HCC ESR COM

F10.931 Alcohol use, unspecified with withdrawal delirium HCC ESR COM

F10.932 Alcohol use, unspecified with withdrawal with perceptual disturbance HCC ESR COM

F10.939 Alcohol use, unspecified with withdrawal, unspecified HCC ESR COM

F10.94 Alcohol use, unspecified with alcohol-induced mood disorder HCC ESR COM
Alcohol induced bipolar or related disorder, without use disorder
Alcohol induced depressive disorder, without use disorder

✓6th F10.95 Alcohol use, unspecified with alcohol-induced psychotic disorder

F10.950 Alcohol use, unspecified with alcohol-induced psychotic disorder with delusions HCC ESR COM

F10.951 Alcohol use, unspecified with alcohol-induced psychotic disorder with hallucinations HCC ESR COM

F10.959 Alcohol use, unspecified with alcohol-induced psychotic disorder, unspecified HCC ESR COM
Alcohol-induced psychotic disorder without use disorder

F10.96 Alcohol use, unspecified with alcohol-induced persisting amnestic disorder HCC ESR COM
Alcohol-induced major neurocognitive disorder, amnestic-confabulatory type, without use disorder

F10.97 **Alcohol use, unspecified with alcohol-induced persisting dementia** HCC ESR COM
Alcohol-induced major neurocognitive disorder, nonamnestic-confabulatory type, without use disorder

✓6th F10.98 **Alcohol use, unspecified with other alcohol-induced disorders**

F10.980 **Alcohol use, unspecified with alcohol-induced anxiety disorder** HCC ESR COM
Alcohol induced anxiety disorder, without use disorder

F10.981 **Alcohol use, unspecified with alcohol-induced sexual dysfunction** HCC ESR COM
Alcohol induced sexual dysfunction, without use disorder

F10.982 **Alcohol use, unspecified with alcohol-induced sleep disorder** HCC ESR COM
Alcohol induced sleep disorder, without use disorder

F10.988 **Alcohol use, unspecified with other alcohol-induced disorder** HCC ESR COM
Alcohol induced mild neurocognitive disorder, without use disorder

F10.99 **Alcohol use, unspecified with unspecified alcohol-induced disorder** ESR

✓4th **F11 Opioid related disorders**

✓5th **F11.1 Opioid abuse**

EXCLUDES 1 *opioid dependence (F11.2-)*
*opioid use, unspecified (F11.9-)*

F11.10 **Opioid abuse, uncomplicated** HCC ESR
Opioid use disorder, mild

F11.11 **Opioid abuse, in remission** HCC ESR
Opioid use disorder, mild, in early remission
Opioid use disorder, mild, in sustained remission

✓6th F11.12 **Opioid abuse with intoxication**

F11.120 **Opioid abuse with intoxication, uncomplicated** HCC ESR COM

F11.121 **Opioid abuse with intoxication delirium** HCC ESR COM

F11.122 **Opioid abuse with intoxication with perceptual disturbance** HCC ESR COM

F11.129 **Opioid abuse with intoxication, unspecified** HCC ESR COM

F11.13 **Opioid abuse with withdrawal** HCC ESR COM
**AHA:** 2020,4Q,16-17

F11.14 **Opioid abuse with opioid-induced mood disorder** HCC ESR COM
Opioid use disorder, mild, with opioid-induced depressive disorder

✓6th F11.15 **Opioid abuse with opioid-induced psychotic disorder**

F11.150 **Opioid abuse with opioid-induced psychotic disorder with delusions** HCC ESR COM

F11.151 **Opioid abuse with opioid-induced psychotic disorder with hallucinations** HCC ESR COM

F11.159 **Opioid abuse with opioid-induced psychotic disorder, unspecified** HCC ESR COM

✓6th F11.18 **Opioid abuse with other opioid-induced disorder**

F11.181 **Opioid abuse with opioid-induced sexual dysfunction** HCC ESR COM

F11.182 **Opioid abuse with opioid-induced sleep disorder** HCC ESR COM

F11.188 **Opioid abuse with other opioid-induced disorder** HCC ESR COM
Opioid-associated amnestic syndrome with opioid abuse

F11.19 **Opioid abuse with unspecified opioid-induced disorder** HCC ESR COM

✓5th **F11.2 Opioid dependence**

EXCLUDES 1 *opioid abuse (F11.1-)*
*opioid use, unspecified (F11.9-)*

EXCLUDES 2 *opioid poisoning (T40.0-T40.2-)*

F11.20 **Opioid dependence, uncomplicated** HCC ESR COM
Opioid use disorder, moderate
Opioid use disorder, severe

F11.21 **Opioid dependence, in remission** HCC ESR COM
Opioid use disorder, moderate, in early remission
Opioid use disorder, moderate, in sustained remission
Opioid use disorder, severe, in early remission
Opioid use disorder, severe, in sustained remission

✓6th F11.22 **Opioid dependence with intoxication**

EXCLUDES 1 *opioid dependence with withdrawal (F11.23)*

F11.220 **Opioid dependence with intoxication, uncomplicated** HCC ESR COM

F11.221 **Opioid dependence with intoxication delirium** HCC ESR COM

F11.222 **Opioid dependence with intoxication with perceptual disturbance** HCC ESR COM

F11.229 **Opioid dependence with intoxication, unspecified** HCC ESR COM

F11.23 **Opioid dependence with withdrawal** HCC ESR COM

EXCLUDES 1 *opioid dependence with intoxication (F11.22-)*

F11.24 **Opioid dependence with opioid-induced mood disorder** HCC ESR COM
Opioid use disorder, moderate, with opioid induced depressive disorder

✓6th F11.25 **Opioid dependence with opioid-induced psychotic disorder**

F11.250 **Opioid dependence with opioid-induced psychotic disorder with delusions** HCC ESR COM

F11.251 **Opioid dependence with opioid-induced psychotic disorder with hallucinations** HCC ESR COM

F11.259 **Opioid dependence with opioid-induced psychotic disorder, unspecified** HCC ESR COM

✓6th F11.28 **Opioid dependence with other opioid-induced disorder**

F11.281 **Opioid dependence with opioid-induced sexual dysfunction** HCC ESR COM

F11.282 **Opioid dependence with opioid-induced sleep disorder** HCC ESR COM

F11.288 **Opioid dependence with other opioid-induced disorder** HCC ESR COM
Opioid-associated amnestic syndrome with opioid dependence

F11.29 **Opioid dependence with unspecified opioid-induced disorder** HCC ESR COM

✓5th **F11.9 Opioid use, unspecified**

EXCLUDES 1 *opioid abuse (F11.1-)*
*opioid dependence (F11.2-)*

**TIP:** Assign a substance use code only when the provider documents a relationship between the use and an associated physical, mental, or behavioral disorder. As with all diagnoses, substance use codes must meet the definition of a reportable diagnosis.

F11.90 **Opioid use, unspecified, uncomplicated**
**AHA:** 2018,2Q,10-11

F11.91 **Opioid use, unspecified, in remission**

✓6th F11.92 **Opioid use, unspecified with intoxication**

EXCLUDES 1 *opioid use, unspecified with withdrawal (F11.93)*

F11.920 **Opioid use, unspecified with intoxication, uncomplicated** HCC ESR COM

F11.921 **Opioid use, unspecified with intoxication delirium** HCC ESR COM
Opioid-induced delirium

F11.922 **Opioid use, unspecified with intoxication with perceptual disturbance** HCC ESR COM

F11.929 **Opioid use, unspecified with intoxication, unspecified** HCC ESR COM

F11.93 **Opioid use, unspecified with withdrawal** HCC ESR COM
EXCLUDES 1 *opioid use, unspecified with intoxication (F11.92-)*

F11.94 **Opioid use, unspecified with opioid-induced mood disorder** HCC ESR COM
Opioid induced depressive disorder, without use disorder

✓6th F11.95 **Opioid use, unspecified with opioid-induced psychotic disorder**

F11.950 **Opioid use, unspecified with opioid-induced psychotic disorder with delusions** HCC ESR COM

F11.951 **Opioid use, unspecified with opioid-induced psychotic disorder with hallucinations** HCC ESR COM

F11.959 **Opioid use, unspecified with opioid-induced psychotic disorder, unspecified** HCC ESR COM

✓6th F11.98 **Opioid use, unspecified with other specified opioid-induced disorder**

F11.981 **Opioid use, unspecified with opioid-induced sexual dysfunction** HCC ESR COM
Opioid induced sexual dysfunction, without use disorder

F11.982 **Opioid use, unspecified with opioid-induced sleep disorder** HCC ESR COM
Opioid induced sleep disorder, without use disorder

F11.988 **Opioid use, unspecified with other opioid-induced disorder** HCC ESR COM
Opioid induced anxiety disorder, without use disorder
Opioid-associated amnestic syndrome without use disorder

F11.99 **Opioid use, unspecified with unspecified opioid-induced disorder** HCC ESR COM

✓4th **F12 Cannabis related disorders**
INCLUDES marijuana
**AHA:** 2020,1Q,8

✓5th **F12.1 Cannabis abuse**
EXCLUDES 1 *cannabis dependence (F12.2-)*
*cannabis use, unspecified (F12.9-)*

F12.10 **Cannabis abuse, uncomplicated**
Cannabis use disorder, mild

F12.11 **Cannabis abuse, in remission**
Cannabis use disorder, mild, in early remission
Cannabis use disorder, mild, in sustained remission

✓6th F12.12 **Cannabis abuse with intoxication**

F12.120 **Cannabis abuse with intoxication, uncomplicated** ESR COM

F12.121 **Cannabis abuse with intoxication delirium** ESR COM

F12.122 **Cannabis abuse with intoxication with perceptual disturbance** ESR COM

F12.129 **Cannabis abuse with intoxication, unspecified** ESR COM

F12.13 **Cannabis abuse with withdrawal** HCC ESR COM
**AHA:** 2020,4Q,16-17

✓6th F12.15 **Cannabis abuse with psychotic disorder**

F12.150 **Cannabis abuse with psychotic disorder with delusions** HCC ESR COM

F12.151 **Cannabis abuse with psychotic disorder with hallucinations** HCC ESR COM

F12.159 **Cannabis abuse with psychotic disorder, unspecified** HCC ESR COM

✓6th F12.18 **Cannabis abuse with other cannabis-induced disorder**

F12.180 **Cannabis abuse with cannabis-induced anxiety disorder** HCC ESR COM

F12.188 **Cannabis abuse with other cannabis-induced disorder** HCC ESR COM
Cannabis use disorder, mild, with cannabis-induced sleep disorder

F12.19 **Cannabis abuse with unspecified cannabis-induced disorder** ESR COM

✓5th **F12.2 Cannabis dependence**
EXCLUDES 1 *cannabis abuse (F12.1-)*
*cannabis use, unspecified (F12.9-)*
EXCLUDES 2 *cannabis poisoning (T40.7-)*

F12.20 **Cannabis dependence, uncomplicated** HCC ESR COM
Cannabis use disorder, moderate
Cannabis use disorder, severe

F12.21 **Cannabis dependence, in remission** HCC ESR COM
Cannabis use disorder, moderate, in early remission
Cannabis use disorder, moderate, in sustained remission
Cannabis use disorder, severe, in early remission
Cannabis use disorder, severe, in sustained remission

✓6th F12.22 **Cannabis dependence with intoxication**

F12.220 **Cannabis dependence with intoxication, uncomplicated** HCC ESR COM

F12.221 **Cannabis dependence with intoxication delirium** HCC ESR COM

F12.222 **Cannabis dependence with intoxication with perceptual disturbance** HCC ESR COM

F12.229 **Cannabis dependence with intoxication, unspecified** HCC ESR COM

F12.23 **Cannabis dependence with withdrawal** HCC ESR COM
**AHA:** 2018,4Q,7

✓6th F12.25 **Cannabis dependence with psychotic disorder**

F12.250 **Cannabis dependence with psychotic disorder with delusions** HCC ESR COM

F12.251 **Cannabis dependence with psychotic disorder with hallucinations** HCC ESR COM

F12.259 **Cannabis dependence with psychotic disorder, unspecified** HCC ESR COM

✓6th F12.28 **Cannabis dependence with other cannabis-induced disorder**

F12.280 **Cannabis dependence with cannabis-induced anxiety disorder** HCC ESR COM

F12.288 **Cannabis dependence with other cannabis-induced disorder** HCC ESR COM
Cannabis use disorder, moderate, with cannabis-induced sleep disorder
Cannabis use disorder, severe, with cannabis-induced sleep disorder

F12.29 **Cannabis dependence with unspecified cannabis-induced disorder** HCC ESR COM

✓5th **F12.9 Cannabis use, unspecified**
EXCLUDES 1 *cannabis abuse (F12.1-)*
*cannabis dependence (F12.2-)*
**AHA:** 2025,4Q,30
**TIP:** Assign a substance use code only when the provider documents a relationship between the use and an associated physical, mental, or behavioral disorder. As with all diagnoses, substance use codes must meet the definition of a reportable diagnosis.

F12.90 **Cannabis use, unspecified, uncomplicated**
**AHA:** 2023,3Q,18; 2018,2Q,10-11

F12.91 **Cannabis use, unspecified, in remission**

✓6th F12.92 **Cannabis use, unspecified with intoxication**

F12.920 **Cannabis use, unspecified with intoxication, uncomplicated** ESR COM

F12.921 **Cannabis use, unspecified with intoxication delirium** ESR COM

F12.922 **Cannabis use, unspecified with intoxication with perceptual disturbance** ESR COM

F12.929 **Cannabis use, unspecified with intoxication, unspecified** ESR COM

F12.93 **Cannabis use, unspecified with withdrawal** HCC ESR COM
**AHA:** 2018,4Q,7

✓6th F12.95 **Cannabis use, unspecified with psychotic disorder**

F12.950 **Cannabis use, unspecified with psychotic disorder with delusions** HCC ESR COM

F12.951 **Cannabis use, unspecified with psychotic disorder with hallucinations** HCC ESR COM

**F12.959 Cannabis use, unspecified with psychotic disorder, unspecified** HCC ESR COM
Cannabis induced psychotic disorder, without use disorder

✓6th **F12.98 Cannabis use, unspecified with other cannabis-induced disorder**

**F12.980 Cannabis use, unspecified with anxiety disorder** HCC ESR COM
Cannabis induced anxiety disorder, without use disorder

**F12.988 Cannabis use, unspecified with other cannabis-induced disorder** HCC ESR COM
Cannabis induced sleep disorder, without use disorder

**F12.99 Cannabis use, unspecified with unspecified cannabis-induced disorder** ESR COM

✓4th **F13 Sedative, hypnotic, or anxiolytic related disorders**

✓5th **F13.1 Sedative, hypnotic or anxiolytic-related abuse**
EXCLUDES 1 *sedative, hypnotic or anxiolytic-related dependence (F13.2-)*
*sedative, hypnotic, or anxiolytic use, unspecified (F13.9-)*

**F13.10 Sedative, hypnotic or anxiolytic abuse, uncomplicated** HCC ESR
Sedative, hypnotic, or anxiolytic use disorder, mild

**F13.11 Sedative, hypnotic or anxiolytic abuse, in remission** HCC ESR
Sedative, hypnotic or anxiolytic use disorder, mild, in early remission
Sedative, hypnotic or anxiolytic use disorder, mild, in sustained remission

✓6th **F13.12 Sedative, hypnotic or anxiolytic abuse with intoxication**

**F13.120 Sedative, hypnotic or anxiolytic abuse with intoxication, uncomplicated** HCC ESR COM

**F13.121 Sedative, hypnotic or anxiolytic abuse with intoxication delirium** HCC ESR COM

**F13.129 Sedative, hypnotic or anxiolytic abuse with intoxication, unspecified** HCC ESR COM

✓6th **F13.13 Sedative, hypnotic or anxiolytic abuse with withdrawal**
AHA: 2020,4Q,16-17

**F13.130 Sedative, hypnotic or anxiolytic abuse with withdrawal, uncomplicated** HCC ESR COM

**F13.131 Sedative, hypnotic or anxiolytic abuse with withdrawal delirium** HCC ESR COM

**F13.132 Sedative, hypnotic or anxiolytic abuse with withdrawal with perceptual disturbance** HCC ESR COM

**F13.139 Sedative, hypnotic or anxiolytic abuse with withdrawal, unspecified** HCC ESR COM

**F13.14 Sedative, hypnotic or anxiolytic abuse with sedative, hypnotic or anxiolytic-induced mood disorder** HCC ESR COM
Sedative, hypnotic, or anxiolytic use disorder, mild, with sedative, hypnotic, or anxiolytic-induced bipolar or related disorder
Sedative, hypnotic, or anxiolytic use disorder, mild, with sedative, hypnotic, or anxiolytic-induced depressive disorder

✓6th **F13.15 Sedative, hypnotic or anxiolytic abuse with sedative, hypnotic or anxiolytic-induced psychotic disorder**

**F13.150 Sedative, hypnotic or anxiolytic abuse with sedative, hypnotic or anxiolytic-induced psychotic disorder with delusions** HCC ESR COM

**F13.151 Sedative, hypnotic or anxiolytic abuse with sedative, hypnotic or anxiolytic-induced psychotic disorder with hallucinations** HCC ESR COM

**F13.159 Sedative, hypnotic or anxiolytic abuse with sedative, hypnotic or anxiolytic-induced psychotic disorder, unspecified** HCC ESR COM

✓6th **F13.18 Sedative, hypnotic or anxiolytic abuse with other sedative, hypnotic or anxiolytic-induced disorders**

**F13.180 Sedative, hypnotic or anxiolytic abuse with sedative, hypnotic or anxiolytic-induced anxiety disorder** HCC ESR COM

**F13.181 Sedative, hypnotic or anxiolytic abuse with sedative, hypnotic or anxiolytic-induced sexual dysfunction** HCC ESR COM

**F13.182 Sedative, hypnotic or anxiolytic abuse with sedative, hypnotic or anxiolytic-induced sleep disorder** HCC ESR COM

**F13.188 Sedative, hypnotic or anxiolytic abuse with other sedative, hypnotic or anxiolytic-induced disorder** HCC ESR COM

**F13.19 Sedative, hypnotic or anxiolytic abuse with unspecified sedative, hypnotic or anxiolytic-induced disorder** HCC ESR COM

✓5th **F13.2 Sedative, hypnotic or anxiolytic-related dependence**
EXCLUDES 1 *sedative, hypnotic or anxiolytic-related abuse (F13.1-)*
*sedative, hypnotic, or anxiolytic use, unspecified (F13.9-)*
EXCLUDES 2 *sedative, hypnotic, or anxiolytic poisoning (T42.-)*

**F13.20 Sedative, hypnotic or anxiolytic dependence, uncomplicated** HCC ESR COM

**F13.21 Sedative, hypnotic or anxiolytic dependence, in remission** HCC ESR COM
Sedative, hypnotic or anxiolytic use disorder, moderate, in early remission
Sedative, hypnotic or anxiolytic use disorder, moderate, in sustained remission
Sedative, hypnotic or anxiolytic use disorder, severe, in early remission
Sedative, hypnotic or anxiolytic use disorder, severe, in sustained remission

✓6th **F13.22 Sedative, hypnotic or anxiolytic dependence with intoxication**
EXCLUDES 1 *sedative, hypnotic or anxiolytic dependence with withdrawal (F13.23-)*

**F13.220 Sedative, hypnotic or anxiolytic dependence with intoxication, uncomplicated** HCC ESR COM

**F13.221 Sedative, hypnotic or anxiolytic dependence with intoxication delirium** HCC ESR COM

**F13.229 Sedative, hypnotic or anxiolytic dependence with intoxication, unspecified** HCC ESR COM

✓6th **F13.23 Sedative, hypnotic or anxiolytic dependence with withdrawal**
Sedative, hypnotic, or anxiolytic use disorder, moderate
Sedative, hypnotic, or anxiolytic use disorder, severe
EXCLUDES 1 *sedative, hypnotic or anxiolytic dependence with intoxication (F13.22-)*

**F13.230 Sedative, hypnotic or anxiolytic dependence with withdrawal, uncomplicated** HCC ESR COM

**F13.231 Sedative, hypnotic or anxiolytic dependence with withdrawal delirium** HCC ESR COM

**F13.232 Sedative, hypnotic or anxiolytic dependence with withdrawal with perceptual disturbance** HCC ESR COM
Sedative, hypnotic, or anxiolytic withdrawal with perceptual disturbances

**F13.239 Sedative, hypnotic or anxiolytic dependence with withdrawal, unspecified** HCC ESR COM
Sedative, hypnotic, or anxiolytic withdrawal without perceptual disturbances

**F13.24 Sedative, hypnotic or anxiolytic dependence with sedative, hypnotic or anxiolytic-induced mood disorder** HCC ESR COM
Sedative, hypnotic, or anxiolytic use disorder, moderate, with sedative, hypnotic, or anxiolytic-induced bipolar or related disorder
Sedative, hypnotic, or anxiolytic use disorder, moderate, with sedative, hypnotic, or anxiolytic-induced depressive disorder
Sedative, hypnotic, or anxiolytic use disorder, severe, with sedative, hypnotic, or anxiolytic-induced bipolar or related disorder
Sedative, hypnotic, or anxiolytic use disorder, severe, with sedative, hypnotic, or anxiolytic-induced depressive disorder

✓6th F13.25 **Sedative, hypnotic or anxiolytic dependence with sedative, hypnotic or anxiolytic-induced psychotic disorder**

F13.250 **Sedative, hypnotic or anxiolytic dependence with sedative, hypnotic or anxiolytic-induced psychotic disorder with delusions** HCC ESR COM

F13.251 **Sedative, hypnotic or anxiolytic dependence with sedative, hypnotic or anxiolytic-induced psychotic disorder with hallucinations** HCC ESR COM

F13.259 **Sedative, hypnotic or anxiolytic dependence with sedative, hypnotic or anxiolytic-induced psychotic disorder, unspecified** HCC ESR COM

F13.26 **Sedative, hypnotic or anxiolytic dependence with sedative, hypnotic or anxiolytic-induced persisting amnestic disorder** HCC ESR COM

F13.27 **Sedative, hypnotic or anxiolytic dependence with sedative, hypnotic or anxiolytic-induced persisting dementia** HCC ESR COM

Sedative, hypnotic, or anxiolytic use disorder, moderate, with sedative, hypnotic, or anxiolytic induced major neurocognitive disorder

Sedative, hypnotic, or anxiolytic use disorder, severe, with sedative, hypnotic, or anxiolytic-induced major neurocognitive disorder

✓6th F13.28 **Sedative, hypnotic or anxiolytic dependence with other sedative, hypnotic or anxiolytic-induced disorders**

F13.280 **Sedative, hypnotic or anxiolytic dependence with sedative, hypnotic or anxiolytic-induced anxiety disorder** HCC ESR COM

F13.281 **Sedative, hypnotic or anxiolytic dependence with sedative, hypnotic or anxiolytic-induced sexual dysfunction** HCC ESR COM

F13.282 **Sedative, hypnotic or anxiolytic dependence with sedative, hypnotic or anxiolytic-induced sleep disorder** HCC ESR COM

F13.288 **Sedative, hypnotic or anxiolytic dependence with other sedative, hypnotic or anxiolytic-induced disorder** HCC ESR COM

Sedative, hypnotic, or anxiolytic use disorder, moderate, with sedative, hypnotic, or anxiolytic-induced mild neurocognitive disorder

Sedative, hypnotic, or anxiolytic use disorder, severe, with sedative, hypnotic, or anxiolytic-induced mild neurocognitive disorder

F13.29 **Sedative, hypnotic or anxiolytic dependence with unspecified sedative, hypnotic or anxiolytic-induced disorder** HCC ESR COM

✓5th F13.9 **Sedative, hypnotic or anxiolytic-related use, unspecified**

EXCLUDES 1 *sedative, hypnotic or anxiolytic-related abuse (F13.1-)*
*sedative, hypnotic or anxiolytic-related dependence (F13.2-)*

**TIP:** Assign a substance use code only when the provider documents a relationship between the use and an associated physical, mental, or behavioral disorder. As with all diagnoses, substance use codes must meet the definition of a reportable diagnosis.

F13.90 **Sedative, hypnotic, or anxiolytic use, unspecified, uncomplicated**

**AHA:** 2018,2Q,10-11

F13.91 **Sedative, hypnotic or anxiolytic use, unspecified, in remission**

✓6th F13.92 **Sedative, hypnotic or anxiolytic use, unspecified with intoxication**

EXCLUDES 1 *sedative, hypnotic or anxiolytic use, unspecified with withdrawal (F13.93-)*

F13.920 **Sedative, hypnotic or anxiolytic use, unspecified with intoxication, uncomplicated** HCC ESR COM

F13.921 **Sedative, hypnotic or anxiolytic use, unspecified with intoxication delirium** HCC ESR COM

Sedative, hypnotic, or anxiolytic-induced delirium

F13.929 **Sedative, hypnotic or anxiolytic use, unspecified with intoxication, unspecified** HCC ESR COM

✓6th F13.93 **Sedative, hypnotic or anxiolytic use, unspecified with withdrawal**

EXCLUDES 1 *sedative, hypnotic or anxiolytic use, unspecified with intoxication (F13.92-)*

F13.930 **Sedative, hypnotic or anxiolytic use, unspecified with withdrawal, uncomplicated** HCC ESR COM

F13.931 **Sedative, hypnotic or anxiolytic use, unspecified with withdrawal delirium** HCC ESR COM

F13.932 **Sedative, hypnotic or anxiolytic use, unspecified with withdrawal with perceptual disturbances** HCC ESR COM

F13.939 **Sedative, hypnotic or anxiolytic use, unspecified with withdrawal, unspecified** HCC ESR COM

F13.94 **Sedative, hypnotic or anxiolytic use, unspecified with sedative, hypnotic or anxiolytic-induced mood disorder** HCC ESR COM

Sedative, hypnotic, or anxiolytic-induced bipolar or related disorder, without use disorder

Sedative, hypnotic, or anxiolytic-induced depressive disorder, without use disorder

✓6th F13.95 **Sedative, hypnotic or anxiolytic use, unspecified with sedative, hypnotic or anxiolytic-induced psychotic disorder**

F13.950 **Sedative, hypnotic or anxiolytic use, unspecified with sedative, hypnotic or anxiolytic-induced psychotic disorder with delusions** HCC ESR COM

F13.951 **Sedative, hypnotic or anxiolytic use, unspecified with sedative, hypnotic or anxiolytic-induced psychotic disorder with hallucinations** HCC ESR COM

F13.959 **Sedative, hypnotic or anxiolytic use, unspecified with sedative, hypnotic or anxiolytic-induced psychotic disorder, unspecified** HCC ESR COM

Sedative, hypnotic, or anxiolytic-induced psychotic disorder, without use disorder

F13.96 **Sedative, hypnotic or anxiolytic use, unspecified with sedative, hypnotic or anxiolytic-induced persisting amnestic disorder** HCC ESR COM

F13.97 **Sedative, hypnotic or anxiolytic use, unspecified with sedative, hypnotic or anxiolytic-induced persisting dementia** HCC ESR COM

Sedative, hypnotic, or anxiolytic-induced major neurocognitive disorder, without use disorder

✓6th F13.98 **Sedative, hypnotic or anxiolytic use, unspecified with other sedative, hypnotic or anxiolytic-induced disorders**

F13.980 **Sedative, hypnotic or anxiolytic use, unspecified with sedative, hypnotic or anxiolytic-induced anxiety disorder** HCC ESR COM

Sedative, hypnotic, or anxiolytic-induced anxiety disorder, without use disorder

F13.981 **Sedative, hypnotic or anxiolytic use, unspecified with sedative, hypnotic or anxiolytic-induced sexual dysfunction** HCC ESR COM

Sedative, hypnotic, or anxiolytic-induced sexual dysfunction disorder, without use disorder

F13.982 **Sedative, hypnotic or anxiolytic use, unspecified with sedative, hypnotic or anxiolytic-induced sleep disorder** HCC ESR COM

Sedative, hypnotic, or anxiolytic-induced sleep disorder, without use disorder

**F13.988** **Sedative, hypnotic or anxiolytic use, unspecified with other sedative, hypnotic or anxiolytic-induced disorder** HCC ESR COM
Sedative, hypnotic, or anxiolytic-induced mild neurocognitive disorder

**F13.99** **Sedative, hypnotic or anxiolytic use, unspecified with unspecified sedative, hypnotic or anxiolytic-induced disorder** HCC ESR COM

✓4th **F14 Cocaine related disorders**
EXCLUDES 2 *other stimulant-related disorders (F15.-)*

✓5th **F14.1 Cocaine abuse**
EXCLUDES 1 *cocaine dependence (F14.2-)*
*cocaine use, unspecified (F14.9-)*

**F14.10** **Cocaine abuse, uncomplicated** HCC ESR
Cocaine use disorder, mild

**F14.11** **Cocaine abuse, in remission** HCC ESR
Cocaine use disorder, mild, in early remission
Cocaine use disorder, mild, in sustained remission

✓6th **F14.12** **Cocaine abuse with intoxication**

**F14.120** **Cocaine abuse with intoxication, uncomplicated** HCC ESR COM

**F14.121** **Cocaine abuse with intoxication with delirium** HCC ESR COM

**F14.122** **Cocaine abuse with intoxication with perceptual disturbance** HCC ESR COM

**F14.129** **Cocaine abuse with intoxication, unspecified** HCC ESR COM

**F14.13** **Cocaine abuse, unspecified with withdrawal** HCC ESR COM
**AHA:** 2020,4Q,16-17

**F14.14** **Cocaine abuse with cocaine-induced mood disorder** HCC ESR COM
Cocaine use disorder, mild, with cocaine-induced bipolar or related disorder
Cocaine use disorder, mild, with cocaine-induced depressive disorder

✓6th **F14.15** **Cocaine abuse with cocaine-induced psychotic disorder**

**F14.150** **Cocaine abuse with cocaine-induced psychotic disorder with delusions** HCC ESR COM

**F14.151** **Cocaine abuse with cocaine-induced psychotic disorder with hallucinations** HCC ESR COM

**F14.159** **Cocaine abuse with cocaine-induced psychotic disorder, unspecified** HCC ESR COM

✓6th **F14.18** **Cocaine abuse with other cocaine-induced disorder**

**F14.180** **Cocaine abuse with cocaine-induced anxiety disorder** HCC ESR COM

**F14.181** **Cocaine abuse with cocaine-induced sexual dysfunction** HCC ESR COM

**F14.182** **Cocaine abuse with cocaine-induced sleep disorder** HCC ESR COM

**F14.188** **Cocaine abuse with other cocaine-induced disorder** HCC ESR COM
Cocaine use disorder, mild, with cocaine-induced obsessive compulsive or related disorder

**F14.19** **Cocaine abuse with unspecified cocaine-induced disorder** HCC ESR COM

✓5th **F14.2 Cocaine dependence**
EXCLUDES 1 *cocaine abuse (F14.1-)*
*cocaine use, unspecified (F14.9-)*
EXCLUDES 2 *cocaine poisoning (T40.5-)*

**F14.20** **Cocaine dependence, uncomplicated** HCC ESR COM
Cocaine use disorder, moderate
Cocaine use disorder, severe

**F14.21** **Cocaine dependence, in remission** HCC ESR COM
Cocaine use disorder, moderate, in early remission
Cocaine use disorder, moderate, in sustained remission
Cocaine use disorder, severe, in early remission
Cocaine use disorder, severe, in sustained remission

✓6th **F14.22** **Cocaine dependence with intoxication**
EXCLUDES 1 *cocaine dependence with withdrawal (F14.23)*

**F14.220** **Cocaine dependence with intoxication, uncomplicated** HCC ESR COM

**F14.221** **Cocaine dependence with intoxication delirium** HCC ESR COM

**F14.222** **Cocaine dependence with intoxication with perceptual disturbance** HCC ESR COM

**F14.229** **Cocaine dependence with intoxication, unspecified** HCC ESR COM

**F14.23** **Cocaine dependence with withdrawal** HCC ESR COM
EXCLUDES 1 *cocaine dependence with intoxication (F14.22-)*

**F14.24** **Cocaine dependence with cocaine-induced mood disorder** HCC ESR COM
Cocaine use disorder, moderate, with cocaine-induced bipolar or related disorder
Cocaine use disorder, moderate, with cocaine-induced depressive disorder
Cocaine use disorder, severe, with cocaine-induced bipolar or related disorder
Cocaine use disorder, severe, with cocaine-induced depressive disorder

✓6th **F14.25** **Cocaine dependence with cocaine-induced psychotic disorder**

**F14.250** **Cocaine dependence with cocaine-induced psychotic disorder with delusions** HCC ESR COM

**F14.251** **Cocaine dependence with cocaine-induced psychotic disorder with hallucinations** HCC ESR COM

**F14.259** **Cocaine dependence with cocaine-induced psychotic disorder, unspecified** HCC ESR COM

✓6th **F14.28** **Cocaine dependence with other cocaine-induced disorder**

**F14.280** **Cocaine dependence with cocaine-induced anxiety disorder** HCC ESR COM

**F14.281** **Cocaine dependence with cocaine-induced sexual dysfunction** HCC ESR COM

**F14.282** **Cocaine dependence with cocaine-induced sleep disorder** HCC ESR COM

**F14.288** **Cocaine dependence with other cocaine-induced disorder** HCC ESR COM
Cocaine use disorder, moderate, with cocaine-induced obsessive compulsive or related disorder
Cocaine use disorder, severe, with cocaine-induced obsessive compulsive or related disorder

**F14.29** **Cocaine dependence with unspecified cocaine-induced disorder** HCC ESR COM

✓5th **F14.9 Cocaine use, unspecified**
EXCLUDES 1 *cocaine abuse (F14.1-)*
*cocaine dependence (F14.2-)*
**TIP:** Assign a substance use code only when the provider documents a relationship between the use and an associated physical, mental, or behavioral disorder. As with all diagnoses, substance use codes must meet the definition of a reportable diagnosis.

**F14.90** **Cocaine use, unspecified, uncomplicated**
**AHA:** 2018,2Q,10-11

**F14.91** **Cocaine use, unspecified, in remission**

✓6th **F14.92** **Cocaine use, unspecified with intoxication**

**F14.920** **Cocaine use, unspecified with intoxication, uncomplicated** HCC ESR COM

**F14.921** **Cocaine use, unspecified with intoxication delirium** HCC ESR COM

**F14.922** **Cocaine use, unspecified with intoxication with perceptual disturbance** HCC ESR COM

**F14.929** **Cocaine use, unspecified with intoxication, unspecified** HCC ESR COM

**F14.93** **Cocaine use, unspecified with withdrawal** HCC ESR COM
**AHA:** 2020,4Q,16-17

**F14.94** **Cocaine use, unspecified with cocaine-induced mood disorder** HCC ESR COM
Cocaine induced bipolar or related disorder, without use disorder
Cocaine induced depressive disorder, without use disorder

✓6th **F14.95 Cocaine use, unspecified with cocaine-induced psychotic disorder**

**F14.950 Cocaine use, unspecified with cocaine-induced psychotic disorder with delusions** HCC ESR COM

**F14.951 Cocaine use, unspecified with cocaine-induced psychotic disorder with hallucinations** HCC ESR COM

**F14.959 Cocaine use, unspecified with cocaine-induced psychotic disorder, unspecified** HCC ESR COM
Cocaine induced psychotic disorder, without use disorder

✓6th **F14.98 Cocaine use, unspecified with other specified cocaine-induced disorder**

**F14.980 Cocaine use, unspecified with cocaine-induced anxiety disorder** HCC ESR COM
Cocaine induced anxiety disorder, without use disorder

**F14.981 Cocaine use, unspecified with cocaine-induced sexual dysfunction** HCC ESR COM
Cocaine induced sexual dysfunction, without use disorder

**F14.982 Cocaine use, unspecified with cocaine-induced sleep disorder** HCC ESR COM
Cocaine induced sleep disorder, without use disorder

**F14.988 Cocaine use, unspecified with other cocaine-induced disorder** HCC ESR COM
Cocaine induced obsessive compulsive or related disorder

**F14.99 Cocaine use, unspecified with unspecified cocaine-induced disorder** HCC ESR COM

✓4th **F15 Other stimulant related disorders**

INCLUDES amphetamine-related disorders
caffeine

EXCLUDES 2 *cocaine-related disorders (F14.-)*

✓5th **F15.1 Other stimulant abuse**

EXCLUDES 1 *other stimulant dependence (F15.2-)*
*other stimulant use, unspecified (F15.9-)*

**F15.10 Other stimulant abuse, uncomplicated** HCC ESR
Amphetamine type substance use disorder, mild
Other or unspecified stimulant use disorder, mild

**F15.11 Other stimulant abuse, in remission** HCC ESR
Amphetamine type substance use disorder, mild, in early remission
Amphetamine type substance use disorder, mild, in sustained remission
Other or unspecified stimulant use disorder, mild, in early remission
Other or unspecified stimulant use disorder, mild, in sustained remission
**AHA:** 2021,3Q,8

✓6th **F15.12 Other stimulant abuse with intoxication**

**F15.120 Other stimulant abuse with intoxication, uncomplicated** HCC ESR COM

**F15.121 Other stimulant abuse with intoxication delirium** HCC ESR COM

**F15.122 Other stimulant abuse with intoxication with perceptual disturbance** HCC ESR COM
Amphetamine or other stimulant use disorder, mild, with amphetamine or other stimulant intoxication, with perceptual disturbances

**F15.129 Other stimulant abuse with intoxication, unspecified** HCC ESR COM
Amphetamine or other stimulant use disorder, mild, with amphetamine or other stimulant intoxication, without perceptual disturbances

**F15.13 Other stimulant abuse with withdrawal** HCC ESR COM
**AHA:** 2020,4Q,16-17

**F15.14 Other stimulant abuse with stimulant-induced mood disorder** HCC ESR COM
Amphetamine or other stimulant use disorder, mild, with amphetamine or other stimulant induced bipolar or related disorder
Amphetamine or other stimulant use disorder, mild, with amphetamine or other stimulant induced depressive disorder

✓6th **F15.15 Other stimulant abuse with stimulant-induced psychotic disorder**

**F15.150 Other stimulant abuse with stimulant-induced psychotic disorder with delusions** HCC ESR COM

**F15.151 Other stimulant abuse with stimulant-induced psychotic disorder with hallucinations** HCC ESR COM

**F15.159 Other stimulant abuse with stimulant-induced psychotic disorder, unspecified** HCC ESR COM

✓6th **F15.18 Other stimulant abuse with other stimulant-induced disorder**

**F15.180 Other stimulant abuse with stimulant-induced anxiety disorder** HCC ESR COM

**F15.181 Other stimulant abuse with stimulant-induced sexual dysfunction** HCC ESR COM

**F15.182 Other stimulant abuse with stimulant-induced sleep disorder** HCC ESR COM

**F15.188 Other stimulant abuse with other stimulant-induced disorder** HCC ESR COM
Amphetamine or other stimulant use disorder, mild, with amphetamine or other stimulant induced obsessive-compulsive or related disorder

**F15.19 Other stimulant abuse with unspecified stimulant-induced disorder** HCC ESR COM

✓5th **F15.2 Other stimulant dependence**

EXCLUDES 1 *other stimulant abuse (F15.1-)*
*other stimulant use, unspecified (F15.9-)*

**F15.20 Other stimulant dependence, uncomplicated** HCC ESR COM
Amphetamine type substance use disorder, moderate
Amphetamine type substance use disorder, severe
Other or unspecified stimulant use disorder, moderate
Other or unspecified stimulant use disorder, severe

**F15.21 Other stimulant dependence, in remission** HCC ESR COM
Amphetamine type substance use disorder, moderate, in early remission
Amphetamine type substance use disorder, moderate, in sustained remission
Amphetamine type substance use disorder, severe, in early remission
Amphetamine type substance use disorder, severe, in sustained remission
Other or unspecified stimulant use disorder, moderate, in early remission
Other or unspecified stimulant use disorder, moderate, in sustained remission
Other or unspecified stimulant use disorder, severe, in early remission
Other or unspecified stimulant use disorder, severe, in sustained remission

✓6th **F15.22 Other stimulant dependence with intoxication**

EXCLUDES 1 *other stimulant dependence with withdrawal (F15.23)*

**F15.220 Other stimulant dependence with intoxication, uncomplicated** HCC ESR COM

**F15.221 Other stimulant dependence with intoxication delirium** HCC ESR COM

**F15.222 Other stimulant dependence with intoxication with perceptual disturbance** HCC ESR COM
Amphetamine or other stimulant use disorder, moderate, with amphetamine or other stimulant intoxication, with perceptual disturbances
Amphetamine or other stimulant use disorder, severe, with amphetamine or other stimulant intoxication, with perceptual disturbances

**F15.229 Other stimulant dependence with intoxication, unspecified** HCC ESR COM
Amphetamine or other stimulant use disorder, moderate, with amphetamine or other stimulant intoxication, without perceptual disturbances
Amphetamine or other stimulant use disorder, severe, with amphetamine or other stimulant intoxication, without perceptual disturbances

**F15.23 Other stimulant dependence with withdrawal** HCC ESR COM
Amphetamine or other stimulant withdrawal
EXCLUDES 1 *other stimulant dependence with intoxication (F15.22-)*

**F15.24 Other stimulant dependence with stimulant-induced mood disorder** HCC ESR COM
Amphetamine or other stimulant use disorder, moderate, with amphetamine or other stimulant induced depressive disorder
Amphetamine or other stimulant use disorder, moderate, with amphetamine or other stimulant-induced bipolar or related disorder
Amphetamine or other stimulant use disorder, severe, with amphetamine or other stimulant-induced bipolar or related disorder
Amphetamine or other stimulant use disorder, severe, with amphetamine or other stimulant-induced depressive disorder

✓6th **F15.25 Other stimulant dependence with stimulant-induced psychotic disorder**

**F15.250 Other stimulant dependence with stimulant-induced psychotic disorder with delusions** HCC ESR COM

**F15.251 Other stimulant dependence with stimulant-induced psychotic disorder with hallucinations** HCC ESR COM

**F15.259 Other stimulant dependence with stimulant-induced psychotic disorder, unspecified** HCC ESR COM

✓6th **F15.28 Other stimulant dependence with other stimulant-induced disorder**

**F15.280 Other stimulant dependence with stimulant-induced anxiety disorder** HCC ESR COM

**F15.281 Other stimulant dependence with stimulant-induced sexual dysfunction** HCC ESR COM

**F15.282 Other stimulant dependence with stimulant-induced sleep disorder** HCC ESR COM

**F15.288 Other stimulant dependence with other stimulant-induced disorder** HCC ESR COM
Amphetamine or other stimulant use disorder, moderate, with amphetamine or other stimulant induced obsessive compulsive or related disorder
Amphetamine or other stimulant use disorder, severe, with amphetamine or other stimulant induced obsessive compulsive or related disorder

**F15.29 Other stimulant dependence with unspecified stimulant-induced disorder** HCC ESR COM

✓5th **F15.9 Other stimulant use, unspecified**
EXCLUDES 1 *other stimulant abuse (F15.1-)*
*other stimulant dependence (F15.2-)*

**TIP:** Assign a substance use code only when the provider documents a relationship between the use and an associated physical, mental, or behavioral disorder. As with all diagnoses, substance use codes must meet the definition of a reportable diagnosis.

**F15.90 Other stimulant use, unspecified, uncomplicated**
**AHA:** 2018,2Q,10-11

**F15.91 Other stimulant use, unspecified, in remission**

✓6th **F15.92 Other stimulant use, unspecified with intoxication**
EXCLUDES 1 *other stimulant use, unspecified with withdrawal (F15.93)*

**F15.920 Other stimulant use, unspecified with intoxication, uncomplicated** HCC ESR COM

**F15.921 Other stimulant use, unspecified with intoxication delirium** HCC ESR COM
Amphetamine or other stimulant-induced delirium

**F15.922 Other stimulant use, unspecified with intoxication with perceptual disturbance** HCC ESR COM

**F15.929 Other stimulant use, unspecified with intoxication, unspecified** HCC ESR COM
Caffeine intoxication

**F15.93 Other stimulant use, unspecified with withdrawal** HCC ESR COM
Caffeine withdrawal
EXCLUDES 1 *other stimulant use, unspecified with intoxication (F15.92-)*

**F15.94 Other stimulant use, unspecified with stimulant-induced mood disorder** HCC ESR COM
Amphetamine or other stimulant-induced bipolar or related disorder, without use disorder
Amphetamine or other stimulant-induced depressive disorder, without use disorder

✓6th **F15.95 Other stimulant use, unspecified with stimulant-induced psychotic disorder**

**F15.950 Other stimulant use, unspecified with stimulant-induced psychotic disorder with delusions** HCC ESR COM

**F15.951 Other stimulant use, unspecified with stimulant-induced psychotic disorder with hallucinations** HCC ESR COM

**F15.959 Other stimulant use, unspecified with stimulant-induced psychotic disorder, unspecified** HCC ESR COM
Amphetamine or other stimulant-induced psychotic disorder, without use disorder

✓6th **F15.98 Other stimulant use, unspecified with other stimulant-induced disorder**

**F15.980 Other stimulant use, unspecified with stimulant-induced anxiety disorder** HCC ESR COM
Amphetamine or other stimulant-induced anxiety disorder, without use disorder
Caffeine induced anxiety disorder, without use disorder

**F15.981 Other stimulant use, unspecified with stimulant-induced sexual dysfunction** HCC ESR COM
Amphetamine or other stimulant-induced sexual dysfunction, without use disorder

**F15.982 Other stimulant use, unspecified with stimulant-induced sleep disorder** HCC ESR COM
Amphetamine or other stimulant-induced sleep disorder, without use disorder
Caffeine induced sleep disorder, without use disorder

**F15.988 Other stimulant use, unspecified with other stimulant-induced disorder** HCC ESR COM
Amphetamine or other stimulant-induced obsessive compulsive or related disorder, without use disorder

**F15.99 Other stimulant use, unspecified with unspecified stimulant-induced disorder** HCC ESR COM

**F16 Hallucinogen related disorders**

INCLUDES ecstasy
PCP
phencyclidine

AHA: 2018,4Q,31

**F16.1 Hallucinogen abuse**

EXCLUDES 1 *hallucinogen dependence (F16.2-)*
*hallucinogen use, unspecified (F16.9-)*

**F16.10 Hallucinogen abuse, uncomplicated** HCC ESR
Other hallucinogen use disorder, mild
Phencyclidine use disorder, mild

**F16.11 Hallucinogen abuse, in remission** HCC ESR
Other hallucinogen use disorder, mild, in early remission
Other hallucinogen use disorder, mild, in sustained remission
Phencyclidine use disorder, mild, in early remission
Phencyclidine use disorder, mild, in sustained remission

**F16.12 Hallucinogen abuse with intoxication**

**F16.120 Hallucinogen abuse with intoxication, uncomplicated** HCC ESR COM

**F16.121 Hallucinogen abuse with intoxication with delirium** HCC ESR COM

**F16.122 Hallucinogen abuse with intoxication with perceptual disturbance** HCC ESR COM

**F16.129 Hallucinogen abuse with intoxication, unspecified** HCC ESR COM

**F16.14 Hallucinogen abuse with hallucinogen-induced mood disorder** HCC ESR COM
Other hallucinogen use disorder, mild, with other hallucinogen induced bipolar or related disorder
Other hallucinogen use disorder, mild, with other hallucinogen induced depressive disorder
Phencyclidine use disorder, mild, with phencyclidine induced bipolar or related disorder
Phencyclidine use disorder, mild, with phencyclidine induced depressive disorder

**F16.15 Hallucinogen abuse with hallucinogen-induced psychotic disorder**

**F16.150 Hallucinogen abuse with hallucinogen-induced psychotic disorder with delusions** HCC ESR COM

**F16.151 Hallucinogen abuse with hallucinogen-induced psychotic disorder with hallucinations** HCC ESR COM

**F16.159 Hallucinogen abuse with hallucinogen-induced psychotic disorder, unspecified** HCC ESR COM

**F16.18 Hallucinogen abuse with other hallucinogen-induced disorder**

**F16.180 Hallucinogen abuse with hallucinogen-induced anxiety disorder** HCC ESR COM

**F16.183 Hallucinogen abuse with hallucinogen persisting perception disorder (flashbacks)** HCC ESR COM

**F16.188 Hallucinogen abuse with other hallucinogen-induced disorder** HCC ESR COM

**F16.19 Hallucinogen abuse with unspecified hallucinogen-induced disorder** HCC ESR COM

**F16.2 Hallucinogen dependence**

EXCLUDES 1 *hallucinogen abuse (F16.1-)*
*hallucinogen use, unspecified (F16.9-)*

**F16.20 Hallucinogen dependence, uncomplicated** HCC ESR COM
Other hallucinogen use disorder, moderate
Other hallucinogen use disorder, severe
Phencyclidine use disorder, moderate
Phencyclidine use disorder, severe

**F16.21 Hallucinogen dependence, in remission** HCC ESR COM
Other hallucinogen use disorder, moderate, in early remission
Other hallucinogen use disorder, moderate, in sustained remission
Other hallucinogen use disorder, severe, in early remission
Other hallucinogen use disorder, severe, in sustained remission
Phencyclidine use disorder, moderate, in early remission
Phencyclidine use disorder, moderate, in sustained remission
Phencyclidine use disorder, severe, in early remission
Phencyclidine use disorder, severe, in sustained remission

**F16.22 Hallucinogen dependence with intoxication**

**F16.220 Hallucinogen dependence with intoxication, uncomplicated** HCC ESR COM

**F16.221 Hallucinogen dependence with intoxication with delirium** HCC ESR COM

**F16.229 Hallucinogen dependence with intoxication, unspecified** HCC ESR COM

**F16.24 Hallucinogen dependence with hallucinogen-induced mood disorder** HCC ESR COM
Other hallucinogen use disorder, moderate, with other hallucinogen induced bipolar or related disorder
Other hallucinogen use disorder, moderate, with other hallucinogen induced depressive disorder
Other hallucinogen use disorder, severe, with other hallucinogen-induced bipolar or related disorder
Other hallucinogen use disorder, severe, with other hallucinogen-induced depressive disorder
Phencyclidine use disorder, moderate, with phencyclidine induced bipolar or related disorder
Phencyclidine use disorder, moderate, with phencyclidine induced depressive disorder
Phencyclidine use disorder, severe, with phencyclidine induced bipolar or related disorder
Phencyclidine use disorder, severe, with phencyclidine-induced depressive disorder

**F16.25 Hallucinogen dependence with hallucinogen-induced psychotic disorder**

**F16.250 Hallucinogen dependence with hallucinogen-induced psychotic disorder with delusions** HCC ESR COM

**F16.251 Hallucinogen dependence with hallucinogen-induced psychotic disorder with hallucinations** HCC ESR COM

**F16.259 Hallucinogen dependence with hallucinogen-induced psychotic disorder, unspecified** HCC ESR COM

**F16.28 Hallucinogen dependence with other hallucinogen-induced disorder**

**F16.280 Hallucinogen dependence with hallucinogen-induced anxiety disorder** HCC ESR COM

**F16.283 Hallucinogen dependence with hallucinogen persisting perception disorder (flashbacks)** HCC ESR COM

**F16.288 Hallucinogen dependence with other hallucinogen-induced disorder** HCC ESR COM

**F16.29 Hallucinogen dependence with unspecified hallucinogen-induced disorder** HCC ESR COM

**F16.9 Hallucinogen use, unspecified**

EXCLUDES 1 *hallucinogen abuse (F16.1-)*
*hallucinogen dependence (F16.2-)*

**TIP:** Assign a substance use code only when the provider documents a relationship between the use and an associated physical, mental, or behavioral disorder. As with all diagnoses, substance use codes must meet the definition of a reportable diagnosis.

**F16.90 Hallucinogen use, unspecified, uncomplicated**
AHA: 2018,2Q,10-11

**F16.91 Hallucinogen use, unspecified, in remission**

**F16.92 Hallucinogen use, unspecified with intoxication**

**F16.920 Hallucinogen use, unspecified with intoxication, uncomplicated** HCC ESR COM

**F16.921 Hallucinogen use, unspecified with intoxication with delirium** HCC ESR COM
Other hallucinogen intoxication delirium

**F16.929 Hallucinogen use, unspecified with intoxication, unspecified** HCC ESR COM

**F16.94 Hallucinogen use, unspecified with hallucinogen-induced mood disorder** HCC ESR COM
Other hallucinogen induced bipolar or related disorder, without use disorder
Other hallucinogen induced depressive disorder, without use disorder
Phencyclidine induced bipolar or related disorder, without use disorder
Phencyclidine induced depressive disorder, without use disorder

✓6th **F16.95 Hallucinogen use, unspecified with hallucinogen-induced psychotic disorder**

**F16.950 Hallucinogen use, unspecified with hallucinogen-induced psychotic disorder with delusions** HCC ESR COM

**F16.951 Hallucinogen use, unspecified with hallucinogen-induced psychotic disorder with hallucinations** HCC ESR COM

**F16.959 Hallucinogen use, unspecified with hallucinogen-induced psychotic disorder, unspecified** HCC ESR COM
Other hallucinogen induced psychotic disorder, without use disorder
Phencyclidine induced psychotic disorder, without use disorder

✓6th **F16.98 Hallucinogen use, unspecified with other specified hallucinogen-induced disorder**

**F16.980 Hallucinogen use, unspecified with hallucinogen-induced anxiety disorder** HCC ESR COM
Other hallucinogen-induced anxiety disorder, without use disorder
Phencyclidine induced anxiety disorder, without use disorder

**F16.983 Hallucinogen use, unspecified with hallucinogen persisting perception disorder (flashbacks)** HCC ESR COM

**F16.988 Hallucinogen use, unspecified with other hallucinogen-induced disorder** HCC ESR COM

**F16.99 Hallucinogen use, unspecified with unspecified hallucinogen-induced disorder** HCC ESR COM

✓4th **F17 Nicotine dependence**

EXCLUDES 1 *history of tobacco dependence (Z87.891)*
*tobacco use NOS (Z72.0)*

EXCLUDES 2 *tobacco use (smoking) during pregnancy, childbirth and the puerperium (O99.33-)*
*toxic effect of nicotine (T65.2-)*

**AHA:** 2013,4Q,108-109

✓5th **F17.2 Nicotine dependence**

✓6th **F17.20 Nicotine dependence, unspecified**

**F17.200 Nicotine dependence, unspecified, uncomplicated**
Tobacco use disorder, mild
Tobacco use disorder, moderate
Tobacco use disorder, severe
**AHA:** 2016,1Q,36
**TIP:** Assign when provider documentation indicates "smoker" without further specification.

**F17.201 Nicotine dependence, unspecified, in remission**
Tobacco use disorder, mild, in early remission
Tobacco use disorder, mild, in sustained remission
Tobacco use disorder, moderate, in early remission
Tobacco use disorder, moderate, in sustained remission
Tobacco use disorder, severe, in early remission
Tobacco use disorder, severe, in sustained remission

**F17.203 Nicotine dependence unspecified, with withdrawal**
Tobacco withdrawal

**F17.208 Nicotine dependence, unspecified, with other nicotine-induced disorders**

**F17.209 Nicotine dependence, unspecified, with unspecified nicotine-induced disorders**

✓6th **F17.21 Nicotine dependence, cigarettes**

**F17.210 Nicotine dependence, cigarettes, uncomplicated**
**AHA:** 2017,2Q,28-29

**F17.211 Nicotine dependence, cigarettes, in remission**
Tobacco use disorder, cigarettes, mild, in early remission
Tobacco use disorder, cigarettes, mild, in sustained remission
Tobacco use disorder, cigarettes, moderate, in early remission
Tobacco use disorder, cigarettes, moderate, in sustained remission
Tobacco use disorder, cigarettes, severe, in early remission
Tobacco use disorder, cigarettes, severe, in sustained remission

**F17.213 Nicotine dependence, cigarettes, with withdrawal**

**F17.218 Nicotine dependence, cigarettes, with other nicotine-induced disorders**

**F17.219 Nicotine dependence, cigarettes, with unspecified nicotine-induced disorders**

✓6th **F17.22 Nicotine dependence, chewing tobacco**

**F17.220 Nicotine dependence, chewing tobacco, uncomplicated**

**F17.221 Nicotine dependence, chewing tobacco, in remission**
Tobacco use disorder, chewing tobacco, mild, in early remission
Tobacco use disorder, chewing tobacco, mild, in sustained remission
Tobacco use disorder, chewing tobacco, moderate, in early remission
Tobacco use disorder, chewing tobacco, moderate, in sustained remission
Tobacco use disorder, chewing tobacco, severe, in early remission
Tobacco use disorder, chewing tobacco, severe, in sustained remission

**F17.223 Nicotine dependence, chewing tobacco, with withdrawal**

**F17.228 Nicotine dependence, chewing tobacco, with other nicotine-induced disorders**

**F17.229 Nicotine dependence, chewing tobacco, with unspecified nicotine-induced disorders**

✓6th **F17.29 Nicotine dependence, other tobacco product**

**F17.290 Nicotine dependence, other tobacco product, uncomplicated**
**AHA:** 2017,2Q,28-29

**F17.291 Nicotine dependence, other tobacco product, in remission**
Tobacco use disorder, other tobacco product, mild, in early remission
Tobacco use disorder, other tobacco product, mild, in sustained remission
Tobacco use disorder, other tobacco product, moderate, in early remission
Tobacco use disorder, other tobacco product, moderate, in sustained remission
Tobacco use disorder, other tobacco product, severe, in early remission
Tobacco use disorder, other tobacco product, severe, in sustained remission

**F17.293 Nicotine dependence, other tobacco product, with withdrawal**

**F17.298 Nicotine dependence, other tobacco product, with other nicotine-induced disorders**

**F17.299 Nicotine dependence, other tobacco product, with unspecified nicotine-induced disorders**

**F18 Inhalant related disorders**

INCLUDES volatile solvents

**F18.1 Inhalant abuse**

EXCLUDES 1 *inhalant dependence (F18.2-)*
*inhalant use, unspecified (F18.9-)*

**F18.10 Inhalant abuse, uncomplicated** HCC ESR
Inhalant use disorder, mild

**F18.11 Inhalant abuse, in remission** HCC ESR
Inhalant use disorder, mild, in early remission
Inhalant use disorder, mild, in sustained remission

**F18.12 Inhalant abuse with intoxication**

**F18.120 Inhalant abuse with intoxication, uncomplicated** HCC ESR COM

**F18.121 Inhalant abuse with intoxication delirium** HCC ESR COM

**F18.129 Inhalant abuse with intoxication, unspecified** HCC ESR COM

**F18.14 Inhalant abuse with inhalant-induced mood disorder** HCC ESR COM
Inhalant use disorder, mild, with inhalant induced depressive disorder

**F18.15 Inhalant abuse with inhalant-induced psychotic disorder**

**F18.150 Inhalant abuse with inhalant-induced psychotic disorder with delusions** HCC ESR COM

**F18.151 Inhalant abuse with inhalant-induced psychotic disorder with hallucinations** HCC ESR COM

**F18.159 Inhalant abuse with inhalant-induced psychotic disorder, unspecified** HCC ESR COM

**F18.17 Inhalant abuse with inhalant-induced dementia** HCC ESR COM
Inhalant use disorder, mild, with inhalant induced major neurocognitive disorder

**F18.18 Inhalant abuse with other inhalant-induced disorders**

**F18.180 Inhalant abuse with inhalant-induced anxiety disorder** HCC ESR COM

**F18.188 Inhalant abuse with other inhalant-induced disorder** HCC ESR COM
Inhalant use disorder, mild, with inhalant induced mild neurocognitive disorder

**F18.19 Inhalant abuse with unspecified inhalant-induced disorder** HCC ESR COM

**F18.2 Inhalant dependence**

EXCLUDES 1 *inhalant abuse (F18.1-)*
*inhalant use, unspecified (F18.9-)*

**F18.20 Inhalant dependence, uncomplicated** HCC ESR COM
Inhalant use disorder, moderate
Inhalant use disorder, severe

**F18.21 Inhalant dependence, in remission** HCC ESR COM
Inhalant use disorder, moderate, in early remission
Inhalant use disorder, moderate, in sustained remission
Inhalant use disorder, severe, in early remission
Inhalant use disorder, severe, in sustained remission

**F18.22 Inhalant dependence with intoxication**

**F18.220 Inhalant dependence with intoxication, uncomplicated** HCC ESR COM

**F18.221 Inhalant dependence with intoxication delirium** HCC ESR COM

**F18.229 Inhalant dependence with intoxication, unspecified** HCC ESR COM

**F18.24 Inhalant dependence with inhalant-induced mood disorder** HCC ESR COM
Inhalant use disorder, moderate, with inhalant induced depressive disorder
Inhalant use disorder, severe, with inhalant induced depressive disorder

**F18.25 Inhalant dependence with inhalant-induced psychotic disorder**

**F18.250 Inhalant dependence with inhalant-induced psychotic disorder with delusions** HCC ESR COM

**F18.251 Inhalant dependence with inhalant-induced psychotic disorder with hallucinations** HCC ESR COM

**F18.259 Inhalant dependence with inhalant-induced psychotic disorder, unspecified** HCC ESR COM

**F18.27 Inhalant dependence with inhalant-induced dementia** HCC ESR COM
Inhalant use disorder, moderate, with inhalant induced major neurocognitive disorder
Inhalant use disorder, severe, with inhalant induced major neurocognitive disorder

**F18.28 Inhalant dependence with other inhalant-induced disorders**

**F18.280 Inhalant dependence with inhalant-induced anxiety disorder** HCC ESR COM

**F18.288 Inhalant dependence with other inhalant-induced disorder** HCC ESR COM
Inhalant use disorder, moderate, with inhalant-induced mild neurocognitive disorder
Inhalant use disorder, severe, with inhalant-induced mild neurocognitive disorder

**F18.29 Inhalant dependence with unspecified inhalant-induced disorder** HCC ESR COM

**F18.9 Inhalant use, unspecified**

EXCLUDES 1 *inhalant abuse (F18.1-)*
*inhalant dependence (F18.2-)*

**TIP:** Assign a substance use code only when the provider documents a relationship between the use and an associated physical, mental, or behavioral disorder. As with all diagnoses, substance use codes must meet the definition of a reportable diagnosis.

**F18.90 Inhalant use, unspecified, uncomplicated**
**AHA:** 2018,2Q,10-11

**F18.91 Inhalant use, unspecified, in remission**

**F18.92 Inhalant use, unspecified with intoxication**

**F18.920 Inhalant use, unspecified with intoxication, uncomplicated** HCC ESR COM

**F18.921 Inhalant use, unspecified with intoxication with delirium** HCC ESR COM

**F18.929 Inhalant use, unspecified with intoxication, unspecified** HCC ESR COM

**F18.94 Inhalant use, unspecified with inhalant-induced mood disorder** HCC ESR COM
Inhalant induced depressive disorder

**F18.95 Inhalant use, unspecified with inhalant-induced psychotic disorder**

**F18.950 Inhalant use, unspecified with inhalant-induced psychotic disorder with delusions** HCC ESR COM

**F18.951 Inhalant use, unspecified with inhalant-induced psychotic disorder with hallucinations** HCC ESR COM

**F18.959 Inhalant use, unspecified with inhalant-induced psychotic disorder, unspecified** HCC ESR COM

**F18.97 Inhalant use, unspecified with inhalant-induced persisting dementia** HCC ESR COM
Inhalant-induced major neurocognitive disorder

**F18.98 Inhalant use, unspecified with other inhalant-induced disorders**

**F18.980 Inhalant use, unspecified with inhalant-induced anxiety disorder** HCC ESR COM

**F18.988 Inhalant use, unspecified with other inhalant-induced disorder** HCC ESR COM
Inhalant-induced mild neurocognitive disorder

**F18.99 Inhalant use, unspecified with unspecified inhalant-induced disorder** HCC ESR COM

**F19 Other psychoactive substance related disorders**

INCLUDES polysubstance drug use (indiscriminate drug use)

**F19.1 Other psychoactive substance abuse**

EXCLUDES 1 *other psychoactive substance dependence (F19.2-)*
*other psychoactive substance use, unspecified (F19.9-)*

**F19.10 Other psychoactive substance abuse, uncomplicated** HCC ESR
Other (or unknown) substance use disorder, mild

**F19.11 Other psychoactive substance abuse, in remission** HCC ESR
Other (or unknown) substance use disorder, mild, in early remission
Other (or unknown) substance use disorder, mild, in sustained remission

✓6th **F19.12 Other psychoactive substance abuse with intoxication**

**F19.120 Other psychoactive substance abuse with intoxication, uncomplicated** HCC ESR COM

**F19.121 Other psychoactive substance abuse with intoxication delirium** HCC ESR COM

**F19.122 Other psychoactive substance abuse with intoxication with perceptual disturbances** HCC ESR COM

**F19.129 Other psychoactive substance abuse with intoxication, unspecified** HCC ESR COM

✓6th **F19.13 Other psychoactive substance abuse with withdrawal**
**AHA:** 2020,4Q,16-17

**F19.130 Other psychoactive substance abuse with withdrawal, uncomplicated** HCC ESR COM

**F19.131 Other psychoactive substance abuse with withdrawal delirium** HCC ESR COM

**F19.132 Other psychoactive substance abuse with withdrawal with perceptual disturbance** HCC ESR COM

**F19.139 Other psychoactive substance abuse with withdrawal, unspecified** HCC ESR COM
**AHA:** 2023,3Q,16

**F19.14 Other psychoactive substance abuse with psychoactive substance-induced mood disorder** HCC ESR COM
Other (or unknown) substance use disorder, mild, with other (or unknown) substance-induced bipolar or related disorder
Other (or unknown) substance use disorder, mild, with other (or unknown) substance-induced depressive disorder

✓6th **F19.15 Other psychoactive substance abuse with psychoactive substance-induced psychotic disorder**

**F19.150 Other psychoactive substance abuse with psychoactive substance-induced psychotic disorder with delusions** HCC ESR COM

**F19.151 Other psychoactive substance abuse with psychoactive substance-induced psychotic disorder with hallucinations** HCC ESR COM

**F19.159 Other psychoactive substance abuse with psychoactive substance-induced psychotic disorder, unspecified** HCC ESR COM

**F19.16 Other psychoactive substance abuse with psychoactive substance-induced persisting amnestic disorder** HCC ESR COM

**F19.17 Other psychoactive substance abuse with psychoactive substance-induced persisting dementia** HCC ESR COM
Other (or unknown) substance use disorder, mild, with other (or unknown) substance-induced major neurocognitive disorder

✓6th **F19.18 Other psychoactive substance abuse with other psychoactive substance-induced disorders**

**F19.180 Other psychoactive substance abuse with psychoactive substance-induced anxiety disorder** HCC ESR COM

**F19.181 Other psychoactive substance abuse with psychoactive substance-induced sexual dysfunction** HCC ESR COM

**F19.182 Other psychoactive substance abuse with psychoactive substance-induced sleep disorder** HCC ESR COM

**F19.188 Other psychoactive substance abuse with other psychoactive substance-induced disorder** HCC ESR COM
Other (or unknown) substance use disorder, mild, with other (or unknown) substance induced mild neurocognitive disorder
Other (or unknown) substance use disorder, mild, with other (or unknown) substance induced obsessive-compulsive or related disorder

**F19.19 Other psychoactive substance abuse with unspecified psychoactive substance-induced disorder** HCC ESR COM

✓5th **F19.2 Other psychoactive substance dependence**

EXCLUDES 1 *other psychoactive substance abuse (F19.1-)*
*other psychoactive substance use, unspecified (F19.9-)*

**F19.20 Other psychoactive substance dependence, uncomplicated** HCC ESR COM
Other (or unknown) substance use disorder, moderate
Other (or unknown) substance use disorder, severe

**F19.21 Other psychoactive substance dependence, in remission** HCC ESR COM
Other (or unknown) substance use disorder, moderate, in early remission
Other (or unknown) substance use disorder, moderate, in sustained remission
Other (or unknown) substance use disorder, severe, in early remission
Other (or unknown) substance use disorder, severe, in sustained remission

✓6th **F19.22 Other psychoactive substance dependence with intoxication**

EXCLUDES 1 *other psychoactive substance dependence with withdrawal (F19.23-)*

**F19.220 Other psychoactive substance dependence with intoxication, uncomplicated** HCC ESR COM

**F19.221 Other psychoactive substance dependence with intoxication delirium** HCC ESR COM

**F19.222 Other psychoactive substance dependence with intoxication with perceptual disturbance** HCC ESR COM

**F19.229 Other psychoactive substance dependence with intoxication, unspecified** HCC ESR COM

✓6th **F19.23 Other psychoactive substance dependence with withdrawal**

EXCLUDES 1 *other psychoactive substance dependence with intoxication (F19.22-)*

**F19.230 Other psychoactive substance dependence with withdrawal, uncomplicated** HCC ESR COM

**F19.231 Other psychoactive substance dependence with withdrawal delirium** HCC ESR COM

**F19.232 Other psychoactive substance dependence with withdrawal with perceptual disturbance** HCC ESR COM

**F19.239 Other psychoactive substance dependence with withdrawal, unspecified** HCC ESR COM

**F19.24 Other psychoactive substance dependence with psychoactive substance-induced mood disorder** HCC ESR COM
Other (or unknown) substance use disorder, moderate, with other (or unknown) substance induced bipolar or related disorder
Other (or unknown) substance use disorder, moderate, with other (or unknown) substance induced depressive disorder
Other (or unknown) substance use disorder, severe, with other (or unknown) substance induced bipolar or related disorder
Other (or unknown) substance use disorder, severe, with other (or unknown) substance induced depressive disorder

✓6th **F19.25 Other psychoactive substance dependence with psychoactive substance-induced psychotic disorder**

**F19.250 Other psychoactive substance dependence with psychoactive substance-induced psychotic disorder with delusions** HCC ESR COM

F19.251 **Other psychoactive substance dependence with psychoactive substance-induced psychotic disorder with hallucinations** HCC ESR COM

F19.259 **Other psychoactive substance dependence with psychoactive substance-induced psychotic disorder, unspecified** HCC ESR COM

F19.26 **Other psychoactive substance dependence with psychoactive substance-induced persisting amnestic disorder** HCC ESR COM

F19.27 **Other psychoactive substance dependence with psychoactive substance-induced persisting dementia** HCC ESR COM

Other (or unknown) substance use disorder, moderate, with other (or unknown) substance induced major neurocognitive disorder

Other (or unknown) substance use disorder, severe, with other (or unknown) substance induced major neurocognitive disorder

✓6th F19.28 **Other psychoactive substance dependence with other psychoactive substance-induced disorders**

F19.280 **Other psychoactive substance dependence with psychoactive substance-induced anxiety disorder** HCC ESR COM

F19.281 **Other psychoactive substance dependence with psychoactive substance-induced sexual dysfunction** HCC ESR COM

F19.282 **Other psychoactive substance dependence with psychoactive substance-induced sleep disorder** HCC ESR COM

F19.288 **Other psychoactive substance dependence with other psychoactive substance-induced disorder** HCC ESR COM

Other (or unknown) substance use disorder, moderate, with other (or unknown) substance induced mild neurocognitive disorder

Other (or unknown) substance use disorder, moderate, with other (or unknown) substance induced obsessive compulsive or related disorder

Other (or unknown) substance use disorder, severe, with other (or unknown) substance induced mild neurocognitive disorder

Other (or unknown) substance use disorder, severe, with other (or unknown) substance induced obsessive-compulsive or related disorder

F19.29 **Other psychoactive substance dependence with unspecified psychoactive substance-induced disorder** HCC ESR COM

✓5th F19.9 **Other psychoactive substance use, unspecified**

EXCLUDES 1 *other psychoactive substance abuse (F19.1-)*
*other psychoactive substance dependence (F19.2-)*

**TIP:** Assign a substance use code only when the provider documents a relationship between the use and an associated physical, mental, or behavioral disorder. As with all diagnoses, substance use codes must meet the definition of a reportable diagnosis.

F19.90 **Other psychoactive substance use, unspecified, uncomplicated**

**AHA:** 2018,2Q,10-11

F19.91 **Other psychoactive substance use, unspecified, in remission**

✓6th F19.92 **Other psychoactive substance use, unspecified with intoxication**

EXCLUDES 1 *other psychoactive substance use, unspecified with withdrawal (F19.93)*

F19.920 **Other psychoactive substance use, unspecified with intoxication, uncomplicated** HCC ESR COM

F19.921 **Other psychoactive substance use, unspecified with intoxication with delirium** HCC ESR COM

Other (or unknown) substance-induced delirium

F19.922 **Other psychoactive substance use, unspecified with intoxication with perceptual disturbance** HCC ESR COM

F19.929 **Other psychoactive substance use, unspecified with intoxication, unspecified** HCC ESR COM

✓6th F19.93 **Other psychoactive substance use, unspecified with withdrawal**

EXCLUDES 1 *other psychoactive substance use, unspecified with intoxication (F19.92-)*

F19.930 **Other psychoactive substance use, unspecified with withdrawal, uncomplicated** HCC ESR COM

F19.931 **Other psychoactive substance use, unspecified with withdrawal delirium** HCC ESR COM

F19.932 **Other psychoactive substance use, unspecified with withdrawal with perceptual disturbance** HCC ESR COM

F19.939 **Other psychoactive substance use, unspecified with withdrawal, unspecified** HCC ESR COM

F19.94 **Other psychoactive substance use, unspecified with psychoactive substance-induced mood disorder** HCC ESR COM

Other (or unknown) substance-induced bipolar or related disorder, without use disorder

Other (or unknown) substance-induced depressive disorder, without use disorder

✓6th F19.95 **Other psychoactive substance use, unspecified with psychoactive substance-induced psychotic disorder**

F19.950 **Other psychoactive substance use, unspecified with psychoactive substance-induced psychotic disorder with delusions** HCC ESR COM

F19.951 **Other psychoactive substance use, unspecified with psychoactive substance-induced psychotic disorder with hallucinations** HCC ESR COM

F19.959 **Other psychoactive substance use, unspecified with psychoactive substance-induced psychotic disorder, unspecified** HCC ESR COM

Other or unknown substance-induced psychotic disorder, without use disorder

F19.96 **Other psychoactive substance use, unspecified with psychoactive substance-induced persisting amnestic disorder** HCC ESR COM

F19.97 **Other psychoactive substance use, unspecified with psychoactive substance-induced persisting dementia** HCC ESR COM

Other (or unknown) substance-induced major neurocognitive disorder, without use disorder

✓6th F19.98 **Other psychoactive substance use, unspecified with other psychoactive substance-induced disorders**

F19.980 **Other psychoactive substance use, unspecified with psychoactive substance-induced anxiety disorder** HCC ESR COM

Other (or unknown) substance-induced anxiety disorder, without use disorder

F19.981 **Other psychoactive substance use, unspecified with psychoactive substance-induced sexual dysfunction** HCC ESR COM

Other (or unknown) substance-induced sexual dysfunction, without use disorder

F19.982 **Other psychoactive substance use, unspecified with psychoactive substance-induced sleep disorder** HCC ESR COM

Other (or unknown) substance-induced sleep disorder, without use disorder

F19.988 **Other psychoactive substance use, unspecified with other psychoactive substance-induced disorder** HCC ESR COM

Other (or unknown) substance-induced mild neurocognitive disorder, without use disorder

Other (or unknown) substance-induced obsessive-compulsive or related disorder, without use disorder

**F19.99 Other psychoactive substance use, unspecified with unspecified psychoactive substance-induced disorder** HCC ESR COM

## Schizophrenia, schizotypal, delusional, and other non-mood psychotic disorders (F20-F29)

√4th **F20 Schizophrenia**

Use additional code, if applicable, to identify:
other specified cognitive deficit (R41.84-)

EXCLUDES 1 *brief psychotic disorder (F23)*
*cyclic schizophrenia (F25.0)*
*mood [affective] disorders with psychotic symptoms (F30.2, F31.2, F31.5, F31.64, F32.3, F33.3)*
*schizoaffective disorder (F25.-)*
*schizophrenic reaction NOS (F23)*

EXCLUDES 2 *schizophrenic reaction in:*
*alcoholism (F10.15-, F10.25-, F10.95-)*
*brain disease (F06.2)*
*epilepsy (F06.2)*
*psychoactive drug use (F11-F19 with .15..25, .95)*
*schizotypal disorder (F21)*

**DEF:** Group of disorders with disturbances in thought (delusions, hallucinations), mood (blunted, flattened, inappropriate affect), and sense of self. Schizophrenia also includes bizarre, purposeless behavior, repetitive activity, or inactivity.

**F20.0 Paranoid schizophrenia** HCC Rx ESR COM
Paraphrenic schizophrenia
EXCLUDES 1 *involutional paranoid state (F22)*
*paranoia (F22)*
**DEF:** Preoccupied with delusional suspicions and auditory hallucinations related to a single theme. This type of schizophrenia is usually hostile, grandiose, threatening, persecutory, and occasionally hypochondriacal.

**F20.1 Disorganized schizophrenia** HCC Rx ESR COM
Hebephrenia
Hebephrenic schizophrenia

**F20.2 Catatonic schizophrenia** HCC Rx ESR COM
Schizophrenic catalepsy
Schizophrenic catatonia
Schizophrenic flexibilitas cerea
EXCLUDES 1 *catatonic stupor (R40.1)*
**DEF:** Extreme changes in motor activity. One extreme is a decreased response or reaction to the environment and the other is spontaneous activity.

**F20.3 Undifferentiated schizophrenia** HCC Rx ESR COM
Atypical schizophrenia
EXCLUDES 1 *acute schizophrenia-like psychotic disorder (F23)*
EXCLUDES 2 *post-schizophrenic depression (F32.89)*

**F20.5 Residual schizophrenia** HCC Rx ESR COM
Restzustand (schizophrenic)
Schizophrenic residual state

√5th **F20.8 Other schizophrenia**

**F20.81 Schizophreniform disorder** HCC Rx ESR COM
Schizophreniform psychosis NOS

**F20.89 Other schizophrenia** HCC Rx ESR COM
Cenesthopathic schizophrenia
Simple schizophrenia

**F20.9 Schizophrenia, unspecified** HCC Rx ESR COM
**AHA:** 2019,2Q,32

**F21 Schizotypal disorder** HCC Rx ESR COM
Borderline schizophrenia
Latent schizophrenia
Latent schizophrenic reaction
Prepsychotic schizophrenia
Prodromal schizophrenia
Pseudoneurotic schizophrenia
Pseudopsychopathic schizophrenia
Schizotypal personality disorder
EXCLUDES 2 *Asperger's syndrome (F84.5)*
*schizoid personality disorder (F60.1)*
**DEF:** Disorder characterized by various oddities of thinking, perception, communication, and behavior that may be manifested as magical thinking, ideas of reference, paranoid ideation, recurrent illusions and derealization (depersonalization), or social isolation.

**F22 Delusional disorders** HCC Rx ESR COM
Delusional dysmorphophobia
Involutional paranoid state
Paranoia
Paranoia querulans
Paranoid psychosis
Paranoid state
Paraphrenia (late)
Sensitiver Beziehungswahn
EXCLUDES 1 *mood [affective] disorders with psychotic symptoms (F30.2, F31.2, F31.5, F31.64, F32.3, F33.3)*
*paranoid schizophrenia (F20.0)*
EXCLUDES 2 *paranoid personality disorder (F60.0)*
*paranoid psychosis, psychogenic (F23)*
*paranoid reaction (F23)*

**F23 Brief psychotic disorder** HCC Rx ESR COM
Paranoid reaction
Psychogenic paranoid psychosis
EXCLUDES 2 *mood [affective] disorders with psychotic symptoms (F30.2, F31.2, F31.5, F31.64, F32.3, F33.3)*
**AHA:** 2019,2Q,32

**F24 Shared psychotic disorder** HCC Rx ESR COM
Folie a deux
Induced paranoid disorder
Induced psychotic disorder

√4th **F25 Schizoaffective disorders**
EXCLUDES 1 *mood [affective] disorders with psychotic symptoms (F30.2, F31.2, F31.5, F31.64, F32.3, F33.3)*
*schizophrenia (F20.-)*

**F25.0 Schizoaffective disorder, bipolar type** HCC Rx ESR COM
Cyclic schizophrenia
Schizoaffective disorder, manic type
Schizoaffective disorder, mixed type
Schizoaffective psychosis, bipolar type

**F25.1 Schizoaffective disorder, depressive type** HCC Rx ESR COM
Schizoaffective psychosis, depressive type

**F25.8 Other schizoaffective disorders** HCC Rx ESR COM

**F25.9 Schizoaffective disorder, unspecified** HCC Rx ESR COM
Schizoaffective psychosis NOS

**F28 Other psychotic disorder not due to a substance or known physiological condition** HCC Rx ESR COM
Chronic hallucinatory psychosis
Other specified schizophrenia spectrum and other psychotic disorder

**F29 Unspecified psychosis not due to a substance or known physiological condition** HCC Rx ESR COM
Psychosis NOS
Unspecified schizophrenia spectrum and other psychotic disorder
EXCLUDES 1 *mental disorder NOS (F99)*
*unspecified mental disorder due to known physiological condition (F09)*

## Mood [affective] disorders (F30-F39)

√4th **F30 Manic episode**
INCLUDES bipolar disorder, single manic episode
mixed affective episode
EXCLUDES 1 *bipolar disorder (F31.-)*
*major depressive disorder, recurrent (F33.-)*
*major depressive disorder, single episode (F32.-)*
**DEF:** Mania: Characterized by abnormal states of elation or excitement out of keeping with the individual's circumstances and varying from enhanced liveliness (hypomania) to violent, almost uncontrollable, excitement. Aggression and anger, flight of ideas, distractibility, impaired judgment, and grandiose ideas are common.

√5th **F30.1 Manic episode without psychotic symptoms**

**F30.10 Manic episode without psychotic symptoms, unspecified** HCC Rx ESR COM Q

**F30.11 Manic episode without psychotic symptoms, mild** HCC Rx ESR COM Q

**F30.12 Manic episode without psychotic symptoms, moderate** HCC Rx ESR COM Q

**F30.13 Manic episode, severe, without psychotic symptoms** HCC Rx ESR COM Q

**F30.2 Manic episode, severe with psychotic symptoms** HCC Rx ESR COM Q
Mania with mood-congruent psychotic symptoms
Mania with mood-incongruent psychotic symptoms
Manic stupor

**F30.3 Manic episode in partial remission** HCC Rx ESR COM Q

HCC CMS-HCC   Rx Rx HCC   ESR ESRD HCC   COM Commercial HCC   N Newborn: 0   P Pediatric: 0-17   M Maternity: 9-64   A Adult: 15-124

**F3Ø.4 Manic episode in full remission** Rx ESR COM Q

**F3Ø.8 Other manic episodes** HCC Rx ESR COM Q
Hypomania

**F3Ø.9 Manic episode, unspecified** HCC Rx ESR COM Q
Mania NOS

✓4th **F31 Bipolar disorder**

INCLUDES bipolar I disorder
bipolar type I disorder
manic-depressive illness
manic-depressive psychosis
manic-depressive reaction
seasonal bipolar disorder

EXCLUDES 1 *bipolar disorder, single manic episode (F3Ø.-)*
*major depressive disorder, recurrent (F33.-)*
*major depressive disorder, single episode (F32.-)*

EXCLUDES 2 *cyclothymia (F34.Ø)*

**AHA:** 2020,1Q,23

**F31.Ø Bipolar disorder, current episode hypomanic** HCC Rx ESR COM Q

✓5th **F31.1 Bipolar disorder, current episode manic without psychotic features**

**F31.1Ø Bipolar disorder, current episode manic without psychotic features, unspecified** HCC Rx ESR COM Q

**F31.11 Bipolar disorder, current episode manic without psychotic features, mild** HCC Rx ESR COM Q

**F31.12 Bipolar disorder, current episode manic without psychotic features, moderate** HCC Rx ESR COM Q

**F31.13 Bipolar disorder, current episode manic without psychotic features, severe** HCC Rx ESR COM Q

**F31.2 Bipolar disorder, current episode manic severe with psychotic features** HCC Rx ESR COM Q
Bipolar disorder, current episode manic with mood-congruent psychotic symptoms
Bipolar disorder, current episode manic with mood-incongruent psychotic symptoms
Bipolar I disorder, current or most recent episode manic with psychotic features

✓5th **F31.3 Bipolar disorder, current episode depressed, mild or moderate severity**

**F31.3Ø Bipolar disorder, current episode depressed, mild or moderate severity, unspecified** HCC Rx ESR COM Q

**F31.31 Bipolar disorder, current episode depressed, mild** HCC Rx ESR COM Q

**F31.32 Bipolar disorder, current episode depressed, moderate** HCC Rx ESR COM Q

**F31.4 Bipolar disorder, current episode depressed, severe, without psychotic features** HCC Rx ESR COM Q

**F31.5 Bipolar disorder, current episode depressed, severe, with psychotic features** HCC Rx ESR COM Q
Bipolar disorder, current episode depressed with mood-congruent psychotic symptoms
Bipolar disorder, current episode depressed with mood-incongruent psychotic symptoms
Bipolar I disorder, current or most recent episode depressed, with psychotic features

✓5th **F31.6 Bipolar disorder, current episode mixed**

**F31.6Ø Bipolar disorder, current episode mixed, unspecified** HCC Rx ESR COM Q

**F31.61 Bipolar disorder, current episode mixed, mild** HCC Rx ESR COM Q

**F31.62 Bipolar disorder, current episode mixed, moderate** HCC Rx ESR COM Q

**F31.63 Bipolar disorder, current episode mixed, severe, without psychotic features** HCC Rx ESR COM Q

**F31.64 Bipolar disorder, current episode mixed, severe, with psychotic features** HCC Rx ESR COM Q
Bipolar disorder, current episode mixed with mood-congruent psychotic symptoms
Bipolar disorder, current episode mixed with mood-incongruent psychotic symptoms

✓5th **F31.7 Bipolar disorder, currently in remission**

**F31.7Ø Bipolar disorder, currently in remission, most recent episode unspecified** Rx ESR COM Q

**F31.71 Bipolar disorder, in partial remission, most recent episode hypomanic** HCC Rx ESR COM Q

**F31.72 Bipolar disorder, in full remission, most recent episode hypomanic** Rx ESR COM Q

**F31.73 Bipolar disorder, in partial remission, most recent episode manic** HCC Rx ESR COM Q

**F31.74 Bipolar disorder, in full remission, most recent episode manic** Rx ESR COM Q

**F31.75 Bipolar disorder, in partial remission, most recent episode depressed** HCC Rx ESR COM Q

**F31.76 Bipolar disorder, in full remission, most recent episode depressed** Rx ESR COM Q

**F31.77 Bipolar disorder, in partial remission, most recent episode mixed** HCC Rx ESR COM Q

**F31.78 Bipolar disorder, in full remission, most recent episode mixed** Rx ESR COM Q

✓5th **F31.8 Other bipolar disorders**

**F31.81 Bipolar II disorder** HCC Rx ESR COM Q
Bipolar disorder, type 2

**F31.89 Other bipolar disorder** HCC Rx ESR COM Q
Recurrent manic episodes NOS

**F31.9 Bipolar disorder, unspecified** HCC Rx ESR COM Q
Manic depression
**AHA:** 2020,1Q,23

✓4th **F32 Depressive episode**

INCLUDES single episode of agitated depression
single episode of depressive reaction
single episode of major depression
single episode of psychogenic depression
single episode of reactive depression
single episode of vital depression

EXCLUDES 1 *bipolar disorder (F31.-)*
*manic episode (F3Ø.-)*
*recurrent depressive disorder (F33.-)*

EXCLUDES 2 *adjustment disorder (F43.2)*

**AHA:** 2020,1Q,23

**DEF:** Mood disorder that produces depression that may exhibit as sadness, low self-esteem, or guilt feelings. Other manifestations may be withdrawal from friends and family and interrupted sleep.

**F32.Ø Major depressive disorder, single episode, mild** Rx ESR

**F32.1 Major depressive disorder, single episode, moderate** HCC Rx ESR

**F32.2 Major depressive disorder, single episode, severe without psychotic features** HCC Rx ESR COM
**AHA:** 2024,4Q,14

**F32.3 Major depressive disorder, single episode, severe with psychotic features** HCC Rx ESR COM
Single episode of major depression with mood-congruent psychotic symptoms
Single episode of major depression with mood-incongruent psychotic symptoms
Single episode of major depression with psychotic symptoms
Single episode of psychogenic depressive psychosis
Single episode of psychotic depression
Single episode of reactive depressive psychosis

**F32.4 Major depressive disorder, single episode, in partial remission** Rx ESR

**F32.5 Major depressive disorder, single episode, in full remission** Rx ESR

✓5th **F32.8 Other depressive episodes**
**AHA:** 2016,4Q,14

**F32.81 Premenstrual dysphoric disorder** Rx
EXCLUDES 1 *premenstrual tension syndrome (N94.3)*
**DEF:** Severe manifestation of premenstrual syndrome (PMS) that can be disabling and destructive to day-to-day activities. It can exacerbate pre-existing emotional disorders, like depression and anxiety, and cause feelings of loss of control, fatigue, and irritability.

**F32.89 Other specified depressive episodes** Rx
Atypical depression
Post-schizophrenic depression
Single episode of 'masked' depression NOS

**F32.9 Major depressive disorder, single episode, unspecified** Rx
Major depression NOS
**AHA:** 2021,4Q,10; 2021,1Q,10; 2013,4Q,107

**F32.A Depression, unspecified** Rx
Depression NOS
Depressive disorder NOS
**AHA:** 2025,3Q,5-6; 2021,4Q,9-10

Chapter 5. Mental, Behavioral and Neurodevelopmental Disorders

F3Ø.4–F32.A

**4th F33 Major depressive disorder, recurrent**

INCLUDES recurrent episodes of depressive reaction
recurrent episodes of endogenous depression
recurrent episodes of major depression
recurrent episodes of psychogenic depression
recurrent episodes of reactive depression
recurrent episodes of seasonal affective disorder
recurrent episodes of seasonal depressive disorder
recurrent episodes of vital depression

EXCLUDES 1 *bipolar disorder (F31.-)*
*manic episode (F3Ø.-)*

**AHA:** 2020,1Q,23

**DEF:** Mood disorder that produces depression that may exhibit as sadness, low self-esteem, or guilt feelings. Other manifestations may be withdrawal from friends and family and interrupted sleep.

**F33.Ø Major depressive disorder, recurrent, mild** Rx ESR

**F33.1 Major depressive disorder, recurrent, moderate** HCC Rx ESR

**F33.2 Major depressive disorder, recurrent, severe without psychotic features** HCC Rx ESR COM

**F33.3 Major depressive disorder, recurrent, severe with psychotic symptoms** HCC Rx ESR COM

Endogenous depression with psychotic symptoms
Major depressive disorder, recurrent, with psychotic features
Recurrent severe episodes of major depression with mood-congruent psychotic symptoms
Recurrent severe episodes of major depression with mood-incongruent psychotic symptoms
Recurrent severe episodes of major depression with psychotic symptoms
Recurrent severe episodes of psychogenic depressive psychosis
Recurrent severe episodes of psychotic depression
Recurrent severe episodes of reactive depressive psychosis

**5th F33.4 Major depressive disorder, recurrent, in remission**

**F33.4Ø Major depressive disorder, recurrent, in remission, unspecified** Rx ESR

**F33.41 Major depressive disorder, recurrent, in partial remission** Rx ESR

**F33.42 Major depressive disorder, recurrent, in full remission** Rx ESR

**F33.8 Other recurrent depressive disorders** Rx ESR

Recurrent brief depressive episodes

**F33.9 Major depressive disorder, recurrent, unspecified** Rx ESR

Monopolar depression NOS

**4th F34 Persistent mood [affective] disorders**

**F34.Ø Cyclothymic disorder** Rx

Affective personality disorder
Cycloid personality
Cyclothymia
Cyclothymic personality

**DEF:** Mood disorder characterized by fast and repeated alterations between hypomanic and depressed moods.

**F34.1 Dysthymic disorder** Rx

Depressive neurosis
Depressive personality disorder
Dysthymia
Neurotic depression
Persistent anxiety depression
Persistent depressive disorder

EXCLUDES 2 *anxiety depression (mild or not persistent) (F41.8)*

**DEF:** Depression without psychosis. It is a less severe but persistent depression and is considered a mild to moderate chronic form of depression.

**5th F34.8 Other persistent mood [affective] disorders**

**AHA:** 2016,4Q,14

**F34.81 Disruptive mood dysregulation disorder** Rx ESR COM

**F34.89 Other specified persistent mood disorders** Rx ESR

**F34.9 Persistent mood [affective] disorder, unspecified** Rx ESR

**F39 Unspecified mood [affective] disorder** Rx ESR

Affective psychosis NOS

## Anxiety, dissociative, stress-related, somatoform and other nonpsychotic mental disorders (F4Ø-F48)

**4th F4Ø Phobic anxiety disorders**

**DEF:** Phobia: Broad-range anxiety with abnormally intense dread of certain objects or specific situations that would not normally have that effect.

**5th F4Ø.Ø Agoraphobia**

**DEF:** Profound anxiety or fear of leaving familiar settings like home, or being in unfamiliar locations or with strangers or crowds. Agoraphobia may or may not be preceded by recurrent panic attacks.

**F4Ø.ØØ Agoraphobia, unspecified** Rx

**F4Ø.Ø1 Agoraphobia with panic disorder** Rx

Panic disorder with agoraphobia

EXCLUDES 1 *panic disorder without agoraphobia (F41.Ø)*

**F4Ø.Ø2 Agoraphobia without panic disorder** Rx

**5th F4Ø.1 Social phobias**

Anthropophobia
Social anxiety disorder
Social anxiety disorder of childhood
Social neurosis

**F4Ø.1Ø Social phobia, unspecified** Rx

**F4Ø.11 Social phobia, generalized** Rx

**5th F4Ø.2 Specific (isolated) phobias**

EXCLUDES 2 *dysmorphophobia (nondelusional) (F45.22)*
*nosophobia (F45.22)*

**6th F4Ø.21 Animal type phobia**

**F4Ø.21Ø Arachnophobia** Rx

Fear of spiders

**F4Ø.218 Other animal type phobia** Rx

**6th F4Ø.22 Natural environment type phobia**

**F4Ø.22Ø Fear of thunderstorms** Rx

**F4Ø.228 Other natural environment type phobia** Rx

**6th F4Ø.23 Blood, injection, injury type phobia**

**F4Ø.23Ø Fear of blood** Rx

**F4Ø.231 Fear of injections and transfusions** Rx

**F4Ø.232 Fear of other medical care** Rx

**F4Ø.233 Fear of injury** Rx

**6th F4Ø.24 Situational type phobia**

**F4Ø.24Ø Claustrophobia** Rx

**F4Ø.241 Acrophobia** Rx

**F4Ø.242 Fear of bridges** Rx

**F4Ø.243 Fear of flying** Rx

**F4Ø.248 Other situational type phobia** Rx

**6th F4Ø.29 Other specified phobia**

**F4Ø.29Ø Androphobia** Rx

Fear of men

**F4Ø.291 Gynephobia** Rx

Fear of women

**F4Ø.298 Other specified phobia** Rx

**F4Ø.8 Other phobic anxiety disorders** Rx

Phobic anxiety disorder of childhood

**F4Ø.9 Phobic anxiety disorder, unspecified** Rx

Phobia NOS
Phobic state NOS

**4th F41 Other anxiety disorders**

EXCLUDES 2 *anxiety in:*
*separation anxiety (F93.Ø)*
*acute stress reaction (F43.Ø)*
*neurasthenia (F48.8)*
*psychophysiologic disorders (F45.-)*
*transient adjustment reaction (F43.2)*

**F41.Ø Panic disorder [episodic paroxysmal anxiety]** Rx

Panic attack
Panic state

EXCLUDES 1 *panic disorder with agoraphobia (F4Ø.Ø1)*

**DEF:** Neurotic disorder characterized by recurrent panic or anxiety, apprehension, fear, or terror. Symptoms include shortness of breath, palpitations, dizziness, and shakiness; fear of dying may persist.

**F41.1 Generalized anxiety disorder** Rx
Anxiety neurosis
Anxiety reaction
Anxiety state
Overanxious disorder
EXCLUDES 2 *neurasthenia (F48.8)*

**F41.3 Other mixed anxiety disorders**

**F41.8 Other specified anxiety disorders**
Anxiety depression (mild or not persistent)
Anxiety hysteria
Mixed anxiety and depressive disorder
**AHA:** 2021,1Q,10

**F41.9 Anxiety disorder, unspecified**
Anxiety NOS
**AHA:** 2021,1Q,10

✓4th **F42 Obsessive-compulsive disorder**
EXCLUDES 2 *obsessive-compulsive personality (disorder) (F6Ø.5)*
*obsessive-compulsive symptoms occurring in depression (F32.-, F33.-)*
*obsessive-compulsive symptoms occurring in schizophrenia (F2Ø.-)*
**AHA:** 2016,4Q,14-15

**F42.2 Mixed obsessional thoughts and acts** Rx

**F42.3 Hoarding disorder** Rx

**F42.4 Excoriation (skin-picking) disorder** Rx
EXCLUDES 1 *factitial dermatitis (L98.1)*
*other specified behavioral and emotional disorders with onset usually occurring in early childhood and adolescence (F98.8)*

**F42.8 Other obsessive-compulsive disorder** Rx
Anancastic neurosis
Obsessive-compulsive neurosis

**F42.9 Obsessive-compulsive disorder, unspecified** Rx

✓4th **F43 Reaction to severe stress, and adjustment disorders**

**F43.Ø Acute stress reaction**
Acute crisis reaction
Acute reaction to stress
Combat and operational stress reaction
Combat fatigue
Crisis state
Psychic shock

✓5th **F43.1 Post-traumatic stress disorder (PTSD)**
Traumatic neurosis
**DEF:** Preoccupation with traumatic events beyond normal experience (i.e., rape, personal assault, etc.) that may also include recurring flashbacks of the trauma. Symptoms include difficulty remembering, sleeping, or concentrating, and guilt feelings for surviving.

**F43.1Ø Post-traumatic stress disorder, unspecified** Rx

**F43.11 Post-traumatic stress disorder, acute** Rx

**F43.12 Post-traumatic stress disorder, chronic** Rx

✓5th **F43.2 Adjustment disorders**
Culture shock
Grief reaction
Hospitalism in children
EXCLUDES 2 *separation anxiety disorder of childhood (F93.Ø)*

**F43.2Ø Adjustment disorder, unspecified** Rx

**F43.21 Adjustment disorder with depressed mood** Rx
**AHA:** 2014,1Q,25

**F43.22 Adjustment disorder with anxiety** Rx

**F43.23 Adjustment disorder with mixed anxiety and depressed mood** Rx

**F43.24 Adjustment disorder with disturbance of conduct** Rx

**F43.25 Adjustment disorder with mixed disturbance of emotions and conduct** Rx

**F43.29 Adjustment disorder with other symptoms** Rx

✓5th **F43.8 Other reactions to severe stress**
Other specified trauma and stressor-related disorder
**AHA:** 2022,4Q,17

**F43.81 Prolonged grief disorder**
Complicated grief
Complicated grief disorder
Persistent complex bereavement disorder

**F43.89 Other reactions to severe stress**

**F43.9 Reaction to severe stress, unspecified**
Trauma and stressor-related disorder, NOS
Unspecified trauma and stressor-related disorder

✓4th **F44 Dissociative and conversion disorders**
INCLUDES conversion hysteria
conversion reaction
hysteria
hysterical psychosis
EXCLUDES 2 *malingering [conscious simulation] (Z76.5)*

**F44.Ø Dissociative amnesia** HCC Rx ESR COM
EXCLUDES 1 *amnesia NOS (R41.3)*
*anterograde amnesia (R41.1)*
*dissociative amnesia with dissociative fugue (F44.1)*
*retrograde amnesia (R41.2)*
EXCLUDES 2 *alcohol-or other psychoactive substance-induced amnestic disorder (F1Ø, F13, F19 with .26, .96)*
*amnestic disorder due to known physiological condition (FØ4)*
*postictal amnesia in epilepsy (G4Ø.-)*

**F44.1 Dissociative fugue** HCC Rx ESR COM
Dissociative amnesia with dissociative fugue
EXCLUDES 2 *postictal fugue in epilepsy (G4Ø.-)*
**DEF:** Dissociative hysteria identified by memory loss and flight from familiar surroundings to a completely separate environment. Episodes may last hours or days. Conscious activity is not associated with perception of surroundings and there is no later memory of the episode.

**F44.2 Dissociative stupor** Rx
EXCLUDES 1 *catatonic stupor (R4Ø.1)*
*stupor NOS (R4Ø.1)*
EXCLUDES 2 *catatonic disorder due to known physiological condition (FØ6.1)*
*depressive stupor (F32, F33)*
*manic stupor (F3Ø, F31)*

**F44.4 Conversion disorder with motor symptom or deficit** Rx
Conversion disorder with abnormal movement
Conversion disorder with speech symptoms
Conversion disorder with swallowing symptoms
Conversion disorder with weakness/paralysis
Dissociative motor disorders
Psychogenic aphonia
Psychogenic dysphonia

**F44.5 Conversion disorder with seizures or convulsions** Rx
Conversion disorder with attacks or seizures
Dissociative convulsions
**AHA:** 2021,1Q,3; 2019,1Q,19

**F44.6 Conversion disorder with sensory symptom or deficit** Rx
Conversion disorder with anesthesia or sensory loss
Conversion disorder with special sensory symptoms
Dissociative anesthesia and sensory loss
Psychogenic deafness

**F44.7 Conversion disorder with mixed symptom presentation** Rx

✓5th **F44.8 Other dissociative and conversion disorders**

**F44.81 Dissociative identity disorder** HCC Rx ESR COM
Multiple personality disorder

**F44.89 Other dissociative and conversion disorders** Rx
Ganser's syndrome
Psychogenic confusion
Psychogenic twilight state
Trance and possession disorders

**F44.9 Dissociative and conversion disorder, unspecified** Rx
Dissociative disorder NOS

**√4th F45 Somatoform disorders**

EXCLUDES 2 *dissociative and conversion disorders (F44.-)*
*factitious disorders (F68.1-, F68.A)*
*hair-plucking (F63.3)*
*lalling (F8Ø.Ø)*
*lisping (F8Ø.Ø)*
*malingering [conscious simulation] (Z76.5)*
*nail-biting (F98.8)*
*psychological or behavioral factors associated with disorders or diseases classified elsewhere (F54)*
*sexual dysfunction, not due to a substance or known physiological condition (F52.-)*
*thumb-sucking (F98.8)*
*tic disorders (in childhood and adolescence) (F95.-)*
*Tourette's syndrome (F95.2)*
*trichotillomania (F63.3)*

**DEF:** Types of disorders causing inconsistent physical symptoms that cannot be explained.

**F45.Ø Somatization disorder** Rx
Briquet's disorder
Multiple psychosomatic disorder

**F45.1 Undifferentiated somatoform disorder** Rx
Somatic symptom disorder
Undifferentiated psychosomatic disorder

**√5th F45.2 Hypochondriacal disorders**

EXCLUDES 2 *delusional dysmorphophobia (F22)*
*fixed delusions about bodily functions or shape (F22)*

**F45.2Ø Hypochondriacal disorder, unspecified** Rx

**F45.21 Hypochondriasis** Rx
Hypochondriacal neurosis
Illness anxiety disorder

**F45.22 Body dysmorphic disorder** Rx
Bigorexia
Dysmorphophobia (nondelusional)
Muscle dysmorphia
Nosophobia

**F45.29 Other hypochondriacal disorders** Rx

**√5th F45.4 Pain disorders related to psychological factors**

EXCLUDES 1 *pain NOS (R52)*

**F45.41 Pain disorder exclusively related to psychological factors**
Somatoform pain disorder (persistent)

**F45.42 Pain disorder with related psychological factors**
Code also associated acute or chronic pain (G89.-)

**F45.8 Other somatoform disorders** Rx
Psychogenic dysmenorrhea
Psychogenic dysphagia, including 'globus hystericus'
Psychogenic pruritus
Psychogenic torticollis
Somatoform autonomic dysfunction
Teeth grinding

EXCLUDES 1 *sleep related teeth grinding (G47.63)*

**F45.9 Somatoform disorder, unspecified** Rx
Psychosomatic disorder NOS

**√4th F48 Other nonpsychotic mental disorders**

**F48.1 Depersonalization-derealization syndrome** HCC Rx ESR COM

**F48.2 Pseudobulbar affect**
Involuntary emotional expression disorder
Code first underlying cause, if known, such as:
amyotrophic lateral sclerosis (G12.21)
multiple sclerosis (G35-)
sequelae of cerebrovascular disease (I69.-)
sequelae of traumatic intracranial injury (SØ6.-)

**F48.8 Other specified nonpsychotic mental disorders**
Dhat syndrome
Neurasthenia
Occupational neurosis, including writer's cramp
Psychasthenia
Psychasthenic neurosis
Psychogenic syncope

**F48.9 Nonpsychotic mental disorder, unspecified**
Neurosis NOS

## Behavioral syndromes associated with physiological disturbances and physical factors (F5Ø-F59)

**√4th F5Ø Eating disorders**

EXCLUDES 1 *anorexia NOS (R63.Ø)*
*feeding problems of newborn (P92.-)*
*polyphagia (R63.2)*

EXCLUDES 2 *feeding difficulties (R63.3-)*
*feeding disorder in infancy or childhood (F98.2-)*

**AHA:** 2022,1Q,13; 2018,4Q,82

**TIP:** Assign additional code for BMI from category Z68, when documented. BMI can be based on documentation from clinicians who are not the patient's provider.

**√5th F5Ø.Ø Anorexia nervosa**

EXCLUDES 1 *loss of appetite (R63.Ø)*
*psychogenic loss of appetite (F5Ø.89)*

**AHA:** 2024,4Q,12

**DEF:** Psychological eating disorder characterized by an intense fear of gaining weight and an unrealistic perception of body image that perpetuates the feeling of being fat or having too much fat. Avoidance of food and restrictive or unhealthy eating are common.

**F5Ø.ØØ Anorexia nervosa, unspecified** HCC Rx COM

**√6th F5Ø.Ø1 Anorexia nervosa, restricting type**

**F5Ø.Ø1Ø Anorexia nervosa, restricting type, mild** HCC Rx COM
Anorexia nervosa, restricting type, with a body mass index greater than or equal to 17 kg/m2

**F5Ø.Ø11 Anorexia nervosa, restricting type, moderate** HCC Rx COM
Anorexia nervosa, restricting type, with a body mass index of 16.Ø-16.99 kg/m2

**F5Ø.Ø12 Anorexia nervosa, restricting type, severe** HCC Rx COM
Anorexia nervosa, restricting type, with a body mass index of 15.Ø-15.99 kg/m2
**AHA:** 2024,4Q,12

**F5Ø.Ø13 Anorexia nervosa, restricting type, extreme** HCC Rx COM
Anorexia nervosa, restricting type, with a body mass index of less than 15.Ø kg/m2

**F5Ø.Ø14 Anorexia nervosa, restricting type, in remission** HCC Rx COM
Anorexia nervosa, restricting type, in full remission
Anorexia nervosa, restricting type, in partial remission

**F5Ø.Ø19 Anorexia nervosa, restricting type, unspecified** HCC Rx COM

**√6th F5Ø.Ø2 Anorexia nervosa, binge eating/purging type**

EXCLUDES 1 *bulimia nervosa (F5Ø.2-)*

**F5Ø.Ø2Ø Anorexia nervosa, binge eating/purging type, mild** HCC Rx COM
Anorexia nervosa, binge eating/purging type, with a body mass index greater than or equal to 17 kg/m2

**F5Ø.Ø21 Anorexia nervosa, binge eating/purging type, moderate** HCC Rx COM
Anorexia nervosa, binge eating/purging type, with a body mass index of 16.Ø-16.99 kg/m2

**F5Ø.Ø22 Anorexia nervosa, binge eating/purging type, severe** HCC Rx COM
Anorexia nervosa, binge eating/purging type, with a body mass index of 15.Ø-15.99 kg/m2

**F5Ø.Ø23 Anorexia nervosa, binge eating/purging type, extreme** HCC Rx COM
Anorexia nervosa, binge eating/purging type, with a body mass index of less than 15.Ø kg/m2
**AHA:** 2024,4Q,13

F50.024 **Anorexia nervosa, binge eating/purging type, in remission** HCC Rx COM
Anorexia nervosa, binge eating/purging type, in full remission
Anorexia nervosa, binge eating/purging type, in partial remission

F50.029 **Anorexia nervosa, binge eating/purging type, unspecified** HCC Rx COM

✓5th F50.2 **Bulimia nervosa**
Bulimia NOS
Hyperorexia nervosa
EXCLUDES 1 *anorexia nervosa, binge eating/purging type (F50.02-)*
**AHA:** 2024,4Q,12
**DEF:** Episodic pattern of overeating (binge eating) followed by purging or extreme exercise accompanied by an awareness of the abnormal eating pattern with a fear of not being able to stop eating.

F50.20 **Bulimia nervosa, unspecified** HCC Rx COM

F50.21 **Bulimia nervosa, mild** HCC Rx COM
Bulimia nervosa with 1-3 episodes of inappropriate compensatory behavior per week

F50.22 **Bulimia nervosa, moderate** HCC Rx COM
Bulimia nervosa with 4-7 episodes of inappropriate compensatory behavior per week

F50.23 **Bulimia nervosa, severe** HCC Rx COM
Bulimia nervosa with 8-13 episodes of inappropriate compensatory behavior per week

F50.24 **Bulimia nervosa, extreme** HCC Rx COM
Bulimia nervosa with 14 or more episodes of inappropriate compensatory behavior per week

F50.25 **Bulimia nervosa, in remission** HCC Rx COM
Bulimia nervosa, in full remission
Bulimia nervosa, in partial remission

✓5th F50.8 **Other eating disorders**
**AHA:** 2017,4Q,9; 2016,4Q,15-16

✓6th F50.81 **Binge eating disorder**
**AHA:** 2024,4Q,12

F50.810 **Binge eating disorder, mild** Rx
Binge eating disorder with 1-3 binge eating episodes per week

F50.811 **Binge eating disorder, moderate** Rx
Binge eating disorder with 4-7 binge eating episodes per week

F50.812 **Binge eating disorder, severe** Rx
Binge eating disorder with 8-13 binge eating episodes per week

F50.813 **Binge eating disorder, extreme** Rx
Binge eating disorder with 14 or more eating episodes per week

F50.814 **Binge eating disorder, in remission** Rx
Binge eating disorder, in full remission
Binge eating disorder, in partial remission

F50.819 **Binge eating disorder, unspecified** Rx

F50.82 **Avoidant/restrictive food intake disorder** Rx
Avoidant/restrictive food intake disorder, in remission

F50.83 **Pica in adults** Rx A
Pica in adults, in remission
EXCLUDES 1 *pica in infancy and childhood (F98.3)*
**AHA:** 2024,4Q,14

F50.84 **Rumination disorder in adults** Rx A
Rumination disorder in adults, in remission
EXCLUDES 1 *rumination disorder in infancy and childhood (F98.21)*
**AHA:** 2024,4Q,15

F50.89 **Other specified eating disorder** Rx
Psychogenic loss of appetite

F50.9 **Eating disorder, unspecified** Rx
Atypical anorexia nervosa
Atypical bulimia nervosa
Feeding or eating disorder, unspecified
Other specified feeding disorder

✓4th F51 **Sleep disorders not due to a substance or known physiological condition**
EXCLUDES 2 *organic sleep disorders (G47.-)*

✓5th F51.0 **Insomnia not due to a substance or known physiological condition**
EXCLUDES 2 *alcohol related insomnia (F10.182, F10.282, F10.982)*
*drug-related insomnia (F11.182, F11.282, F11.982, F13.182, F13.282, F13.982, F14.182, F14.282, F14.982, F15.182, F15.282, F15.982, F19.182, F19.282, F19.982)*
*insomnia due to known physiological condition (G47.0-)*
*insomnia NOS (G47.0-)*
*organic insomnia (G47.0-)*
*sleep deprivation (Z72.820)*

F51.01 **Primary insomnia**
Idiopathic insomnia

F51.02 **Adjustment insomnia**

F51.03 **Paradoxical insomnia**

F51.04 **Psychophysiologic insomnia**

F51.05 **Insomnia due to other mental disorder**
Code also associated mental disorder

F51.09 **Other insomnia not due to a substance or known physiological condition**

✓5th F51.1 **Hypersomnia not due to a substance or known physiological condition**
EXCLUDES 2 *alcohol related hypersomnia (F10.182, F10.282, F10.982)*
*drug-related hypersomnia (F11.182, F11.282, F11.982, F13.182, F13.282, F13.982, F14.182, F14.282, F14.982, F15.182, F15.282, F15.982, F19.182, F19.282, F19.982)*
*hypersomnia due to known physiological condition (G47.10)*
*hypersomnia NOS (G47.10)*
*idiopathic hypersomnia (G47.11, G47.12)*
*narcolepsy (G47.4-)*

F51.11 **Primary hypersomnia**

F51.12 **Insufficient sleep syndrome**
EXCLUDES 1 *sleep deprivation (Z72.820)*

F51.13 **Hypersomnia due to other mental disorder**
Code also associated mental disorder

F51.19 **Other hypersomnia not due to a substance or known physiological condition**

F51.3 **Sleepwalking [somnambulism]**
Non-rapid eye movement sleep arousal disorders, sleepwalking type

F51.4 **Sleep terrors [night terrors]**
Non-rapid eye movement sleep arousal disorders, sleep terror type

F51.5 **Nightmare disorder**
Dream anxiety disorder

F51.8 **Other sleep disorders not due to a substance or known physiological condition**

F51.9 **Sleep disorder not due to a substance or known physiological condition, unspecified**
Emotional sleep disorder NOS

✓4th F52 **Sexual dysfunction not due to a substance or known physiological condition**
EXCLUDES 2 *Dhat syndrome (F48.8)*

F52.0 **Hypoactive sexual desire disorder**
Lack or loss of sexual desire
Male hypoactive sexual desire disorder
Sexual anhedonia
EXCLUDES 1 *decreased libido (R68.82)*

F52.1 **Sexual aversion disorder**
Sexual aversion and lack of sexual enjoyment

✓5th F52.2 **Sexual arousal disorders**
Failure of genital response

F52.21 **Male erectile disorder**
Erectile disorder
Psychogenic impotence
EXCLUDES 1 *impotence of organic origin (N52.-)*
*impotence NOS (N52.-)*

F52.22 **Female sexual arousal disorder**
Female sexual interest/arousal disorder

✓5th F52.3 **Orgasmic disorder**
Inhibited orgasm
Psychogenic anorgasmy

F52.31 **Female orgasmic disorder**

**F52.32 Male orgasmic disorder**
Delayed ejaculation

**F52.4 Premature ejaculation**

**F52.5 Vaginismus not due to a substance or known physiological condition**
Psychogenic vaginismus
EXCLUDES 2 *vaginismus (due to a known physiological condition) (N94.2)*
**DEF:** Psychogenic response resulting in painful contractions of the vaginal canal muscles. This condition can be severe enough to prevent sexual intercourse.

**F52.6 Dyspareunia not due to a substance or known physiological condition**
Genito-pelvic pain penetration disorder
Psychogenic dyspareunia
EXCLUDES 2 *dyspareunia (due to a known physiological condition) (N94.1-)*

**F52.8 Other sexual dysfunction not due to a substance or known physiological condition**
Excessive sexual drive
Nymphomania
Satyriasis

**F52.9 Unspecified sexual dysfunction not due to a substance or known physiological condition**
Sexual dysfunction NOS

✓4th **F53 Mental and behavioral disorders associated with the puerperium, not elsewhere classified**
EXCLUDES 1 *mood disorders with psychotic features (F3Ø.2, F31.2, F31.5, F31.64, F32.3, F33.3)*
*postpartum dysphoria (O9Ø.6)*
*psychosis in schizophrenia, schizotypal, delusional, and other psychotic disorders (F2Ø-F29)*
**AHA:** 2018,4Q,8

**F53.Ø Postpartum depression** Rx M
Postnatal depression, NOS
Postpartum depression, NOS

**F53.1 Puerperal psychosis** HCC Rx ESR COM M
Postpartum psychosis
Puerperal psychosis, NOS

***F54 Psychological and behavioral factors associated with disorders or diseases classified elsewhere***
Psychological factors affecting physical conditions
Code first the associated physical disorder, such as:
asthma (J45.-)
dermatitis (L23-L25)
gastric ulcer (K25.-)
mucous colitis (K58.-)
ulcerative colitis (K51.-)
urticaria (L5Ø.-)
EXCLUDES 2 *tension-type headache (G44.2)*

✓4th **F55 Abuse of non-psychoactive substances**
EXCLUDES 2 *abuse of psychoactive substances (F1Ø-F19)*

**F55.Ø Abuse of antacids**

**F55.1 Abuse of herbal or folk remedies**
**AHA:** 2023,3Q,16

**F55.2 Abuse of laxatives**

**F55.3 Abuse of steroids or hormones**

**F55.4 Abuse of vitamins**

**F55.8 Abuse of other non-psychoactive substances**

**F59 Unspecified behavioral syndromes associated with physiological disturbances and physical factors**
Psychogenic physiological dysfunction NOS

## Disorders of adult personality and behavior (F6Ø-F69)

✓4th **F6Ø Specific personality disorders**

**F6Ø.Ø Paranoid personality disorder** HCC Rx ESR COM
Expansive paranoid personality (disorder)
Fanatic personality (disorder)
Paranoid personality (disorder)
Querulant personality (disorder)
Sensitive paranoid personality (disorder)
EXCLUDES 2 *paranoia (F22)*
*paranoia querulans (F22)*
*paranoid psychosis (F22)*
*paranoid schizophrenia (F2Ø.Ø)*
*paranoid state (F22)*

**F6Ø.1 Schizoid personality disorder** HCC Rx ESR COM
EXCLUDES 2 *Asperger's syndrome (F84.5)*
*delusional disorder (F22)*
*schizoid disorder of childhood (F84.5)*
*schizophrenia (F2Ø.-)*
*schizotypal disorder (F21)*

**F6Ø.2 Antisocial personality disorder** HCC Rx ESR COM
Amoral personality (disorder)
Asocial personality (disorder)
Dissocial personality disorder
Psychopathic personality (disorder)
Sociopathic personality (disorder)
EXCLUDES 1 *conduct disorders (F91.-)*
EXCLUDES 2 *borderline personality disorder (F6Ø.3)*

**F6Ø.3 Borderline personality disorder** HCC Rx ESR COM
Aggressive personality (disorder)
Emotionally unstable personality disorder
Explosive personality (disorder)
EXCLUDES 2 *antisocial personality disorder (F6Ø.2)*

**F6Ø.4 Histrionic personality disorder** HCC Rx ESR COM
Hysterical personality (disorder)
Psychoinfantile personality (disorder)

**F6Ø.5 Obsessive-compulsive personality disorder** HCC Rx ESR COM
Anankastic personality (disorder)
Compulsive personality (disorder)
Obsessional personality (disorder)
EXCLUDES 2 *obsessive-compulsive disorder (F42.-)*

**F6Ø.6 Avoidant personality disorder** HCC Rx ESR COM
Anxious personality disorder

**F6Ø.7 Dependent personality disorder** HCC Rx ESR COM
Asthenic personality (disorder)
Inadequate personality (disorder)
Passive personality (disorder)
**DEF:** Lack of self-confidence, fear of abandonment, and an obsessive need to be taken care of.

✓5th **F6Ø.8 Other specific personality disorders**

**F6Ø.81 Narcissistic personality disorder** HCC Rx ESR COM

**F6Ø.89 Other specific personality disorders** HCC Rx ESR COM
"Haltlose" type personality disorder
Eccentric personality disorder
Immature personality disorder
Passive-aggressive personality disorder
Psychoneurotic personality disorder
Self-defeating personality disorder

**F6Ø.9 Personality disorder, unspecified** HCC Rx ESR COM
Character disorder NOS
Character neurosis NOS
Pathological personality NOS

✓4th **F63 Impulse disorders**
EXCLUDES 2 *habitual excessive use of alcohol or psychoactive substances (F1Ø-F19)*
*impulse disorders involving sexual behavior (F65.-)*

**F63.Ø Pathological gambling** Rx
Compulsive gambling
Gambling disorder
EXCLUDES 1 *gambling and betting NOS (Z72.6)*
EXCLUDES 2 *excessive gambling by manic patients (F3Ø, F31)*
*gambling in antisocial personality disorder (F6Ø.2)*

**F63.1 Pyromania** Rx
Pathological fire-setting
EXCLUDES 2 *fire-setting (by) (in):*
*adult with antisocial personality disorder (F6Ø.2)*
*alcohol or psychoactive substance intoxication (F1Ø-F19)*
*conduct disorders (F91.-)*
*mental disorders due to known physiological condition (FØ1-FØ9)*
*schizophrenia (F2Ø.-)*

**F63.2 Kleptomania** Rx
Pathological stealing
EXCLUDES 1 *shoplifting as the reason for observation for suspected mental disorder (ZØ3.8)*
EXCLUDES 2 *depressive disorder with stealing (F31.-, F32.-, F33.-)*
*stealing due to underlying mental condition - code to mental condition*
*stealing in mental disorders due to known physiological condition (FØ1-FØ9)*

**F63.3 Trichotillomania** Rx
Hair plucking
EXCLUDES 2 *other stereotyped movement disorder (F98.4)*

✓5th **F63.8 Other impulse disorders**
**F63.81 Intermittent explosive disorder** Rx
**F63.89 Other impulse disorders** Rx

**F63.9 Impulse disorder, unspecified** Rx
Impulse control disorder NOS

✓4th **F64 Gender identity disorders**
AHA: 2016,4Q,16

**F64.0 Transsexualism**
Gender dysphoria in adolescents and adults
Gender identity disorder in adolescence and adulthood
Gender incongruence in adolescents and adults
Transgender
EXCLUDES 1 *gender identity disorder of childhood (F64.2)*

**F64.1 Dual role transvestism**
Use additional code to identify sex reassignment status ▶(Z87.890-)◀
EXCLUDES 1 *gender identity disorder in childhood (F64.2)*
EXCLUDES 2 *fetishistic transvestism (F65.1)*

**F64.2 Gender identity disorder of childhood** P
Gender dysphoria in children
Gender incongruence of childhood
EXCLUDES 1 *gender identity disorder in adolescence and adulthood (F64.0)*
EXCLUDES 2 *sexual maturation disorder (F66)*

**F64.8 Other gender identity disorders**
Other specified gender dysphoria

**F64.9 Gender identity disorder, unspecified**
Gender dysphoria, unspecified
Gender incongruence, unspecified
Gender-role disorder NOS

● **F64.A Gender identity disorder, in remission**
Gender dysphoria, in remission (desistance)

✓4th **F65 Paraphilias**

**F65.0 Fetishism**
Fetishistic disorder

**F65.1 Transvestic fetishism**
Fetishistic transvestism
Transvestic disorder

**F65.2 Exhibitionism**
Exhibitionistic disorder

**F65.3 Voyeurism**
Voyeuristic disorder

**F65.4 Pedophilia**
Pedophilic disorder

✓5th **F65.5 Sadomasochism**
**F65.50 Sadomasochism, unspecified**
**F65.51 Sexual masochism**
Sexual masochism disorder
**F65.52 Sexual sadism**
Sexual sadism disorder

✓5th **F65.8 Other paraphilias**
**F65.81 Frotteurism**
Frotteuristic disorder
**F65.89 Other paraphilias**
Necrophilia
Other specified paraphilic disorder

**F65.9 Paraphilia, unspecified**
Paraphilic disorder, unspecified
Sexual deviation NOS

**F66 Other sexual disorders**
Sexual maturation disorder
Sexual relationship disorder

✓4th **F68 Other disorders of adult personality and behavior**
AHA: 2018,4Q,9,65

✓5th **F68.1 Factitious disorder imposed on self**
Compensation neurosis
Elaboration of physical symptoms for psychological reasons
Hospital hopper syndrome
Münchausen's syndrome
Peregrinating patient
EXCLUDES 2 *factitial dermatitis (L98.1)*
*person feigning illness (with obvious motivation) (Z76.5)*

**F68.10 Factitious disorder imposed on self, unspecified** Rx
**F68.11 Factitious disorder imposed on self, with predominantly psychological signs and symptoms** Rx
**F68.12 Factitious disorder imposed on self, with predominantly physical signs and symptoms** Rx
**F68.13 Factitious disorder imposed on self, with combined psychological and physical signs and symptoms** Rx

**F68.A Factitious disorder imposed on another** Rx
Factitious disorder by proxy
Münchausen's by proxy

**F68.8 Other specified disorders of adult personality and behavior**

**F69 Unspecified disorder of adult personality and behavior** A

## Intellectual disabilities (F70-F79)

Code first any associated physical or developmental disorders
EXCLUDES 1 *borderline intellectual functioning, IQ above 70 to 84 (R41.83)*

**F70 Mild intellectual disabilities** Rx
IQ level 50-55 to approximately 70
Mild mental subnormality

**F71 Moderate intellectual disabilities** Rx
IQ level 35-40 to 50-55
Moderate mental subnormality

**F72 Severe intellectual disabilities** Rx
IQ 20-25 to 35-40
Severe mental subnormality

**F73 Profound intellectual disabilities** Rx
IQ level below 20-25
Profound mental subnormality

✓4th **F78 Other intellectual disabilities** Rx

✓5th **F78.A Other genetic related intellectual disabilities**
AHA: 2021,4Q,10-11

**F78.A1 SYNGAP1-related intellectual disability** Rx
Code also, if applicable, any associated:
autism spectrum disorder (F84.0)
autistic disorder (F84.0)
encephalopathy (G93.4-)
epilepsy and recurrent seizures (G40.-)
other pervasive developmental disorders (F84.8)
pervasive developmental disorder, NOS (F84.9)

**F78.A9 Other genetic related intellectual disability** Rx
Code also, if applicable, any associated disorders

**F79 Unspecified intellectual disabilities** Rx
Mental deficiency NOS
Mental subnormality NOS

## Pervasive and specific developmental disorders (F80-F89)

**✓4th F80 Specific developmental disorders of speech and language**

**F80.0 Phonological disorder**
Dyslalia
Functional speech articulation disorder
Lalling
Lisping
Phonological developmental disorder
Speech articulation developmental disorder
Speech-sound disorder
EXCLUDES 1 *speech articulation impairment due to aphasia NOS (R47.01)*
*speech articulation impairment due to apraxia (R48.2)*
EXCLUDES 2 *speech articulation impairment due to hearing loss (F80.4)*
*speech articulation impairment due to intellectual disabilities (F70-F79)*
*speech articulation impairment with expressive language developmental disorder (F80.1)*
*speech articulation impairment with mixed receptive expressive language developmental disorder (F80.2)*

**F80.1 Expressive language disorder**
Developmental dysphasia or aphasia, expressive type
EXCLUDES 1 *mixed receptive-expressive language disorder (F80.2)*
*dysphasia and aphasia NOS (R47.-)*
EXCLUDES 2 *acquired aphasia with epilepsy [Landau-Kleffner] (G40.80-)*
*intellectual disabilities (F70-F79)*
*pervasive developmental disorders (F84.-)*
*selective mutism (F94.0)*

**F80.2 Mixed receptive-expressive language disorder**
Developmental dysphasia or aphasia, receptive type
Developmental Wernicke's aphasia
EXCLUDES 1 *central auditory processing disorder (H93.25)*
*dysphasia or aphasia NOS (R47.-)*
*expressive language disorder (F80.1)*
*expressive type dysphasia or aphasia (F80.1)*
*word deafness (H93.25)*
EXCLUDES 2 *acquired aphasia with epilepsy [Landau-Kleffner] (G40.80-)*
*intellectual disabilities (F70-F79)*
*pervasive developmental disorders (F84.-)*
*selective mutism (F94.0)*

**F80.4 Speech and language development delay due to hearing loss**
Code also type of hearing loss (H90.-, H91.-)

**✓5th F80.8 Other developmental disorders of speech and language**
**AHA:** 2017,1Q,27

**F80.81 Childhood onset fluency disorder**
Cluttering NOS
Stuttering NOS
EXCLUDES 1 *adult onset fluency disorder (F98.5)*
*fluency disorder (stuttering) following cerebrovascular disease (I69. with final characters -23)*
*fluency disorder in conditions classified elsewhere (R47.82)*

**F80.82 Social pragmatic communication disorder**
EXCLUDES 1 *Asperger's syndrome (F84.5)*
*autistic disorder (F84.0)*
**AHA:** 2016,4Q,16

**F80.89 Other developmental disorders of speech and language**

**F80.9 Developmental disorder of speech and language, unspecified**
Communication disorder NOS
Language disorder NOS

**✓4th F81 Specific developmental disorders of scholastic skills**

**F81.0 Specific reading disorder**
"Backward reading"
Developmental dyslexia
Specific learning disorder, with impairment in reading
Specific reading retardation
EXCLUDES 1 *alexia NOS (R48.0)*
*dyslexia NOS (R48.0)*
**DEF:** Serious impairment of reading skills unexplained in relation to general intelligence and teaching processes.

**F81.2 Mathematics disorder**
Developmental acalculia
Developmental arithmetical disorder
Developmental Gerstmann's syndrome
Specific learning disorder, with impairment in mathematics
EXCLUDES 1 *acalculia NOS (R48.8)*
EXCLUDES 2 *arithmetical difficulties associated with a reading disorder (F81.0)*
*arithmetical difficulties associated with a spelling disorder (F81.81)*
*arithmetical difficulties due to inadequate teaching (Z55.8)*

**✓5th F81.8 Other developmental disorders of scholastic skills**

**F81.81 Disorder of written expression**
Specific learning disorder, with impairment in written expression
Specific spelling disorder

**F81.89 Other developmental disorders of scholastic skills**

**F81.9 Developmental disorder of scholastic skills, unspecified**
Knowledge acquisition disability NOS
Learning disability NOS
Learning disorder NOS

**F82 Specific developmental disorder of motor function**
Clumsy child syndrome
Developmental coordination disorder
Developmental dyspraxia
EXCLUDES 1 *abnormalities of gait and mobility (R26.-)*
*lack of coordination (R27.-)*
EXCLUDES 2 *lack of coordination secondary to intellectual disabilities (F70-F79)*

**✓4th F84 Pervasive developmental disorders**
Code also any associated medical condition and intellectual disabilities

**F84.0 Autistic disorder** Rx COM
Autism spectrum disorder
Infantile autism
Infantile psychosis
Kanner's syndrome
EXCLUDES 1 *Asperger's syndrome (F84.5)*
**AHA:** 2017,1Q,27
**TIP:** When the encounter is focused on treatment of conditions related to autism spectrum disorder, first assign codes to identify the problem or manifestation receiving therapeutic services.

**F84.2 Rett's syndrome** Rx COM
EXCLUDES 1 *Asperger's syndrome (F84.5)*
*autistic disorder (F84.0)*
*other childhood disintegrative disorder (F84.3)*

**F84.3 Other childhood disintegrative disorder** Rx COM P
Dementia infantilis
Disintegrative psychosis
Heller's syndrome
Symbiotic psychosis
Use additional code to identify any associated neurological condition
EXCLUDES 1 *Asperger's syndrome (F84.5)*
*autistic disorder (F84.0)*
*Rett's syndrome (F84.2)*

**F84.5 Asperger's syndrome** Rx COM
Asperger's disorder
Autistic psychopathy
Schizoid disorder of childhood
**DEF:** High-functioning form of autism. Children with this syndrome usually develop speech on schedule, are generally very intelligent, and communicate well, but have considerable social shortcomings. ***Synonym(s):*** *AS.*

**F84.8 Other pervasive developmental disorders** Rx COM
Overactive disorder associated with intellectual disabilities and stereotyped movements

**F84.9 Pervasive developmental disorder, unspecified** Rx COM
Atypical autism

**F88 Other disorders of psychological development**
Developmental agnosia
Global developmental delay
Other specified neurodevelopmental disorder

**F89 Unspecified disorder of psychological development**
Developmental disorder NOS
Neurodevelopmental disorder NOS

## Behavioral and emotional disorders with onset usually occurring in childhood and adolescence (F90-F98)

NOTE Codes within categories F90-F98 may be used regardless of the age of a patient. These disorders generally have onset within the childhood or adolescent years, but may continue throughout life or not be diagnosed until adulthood

**F90 Attention-deficit hyperactivity disorders**

INCLUDES attention deficit disorder with hyperactivity
attention deficit syndrome with hyperactivity

EXCLUDES 2 *anxiety disorders (F40.-, F41.-)*
*mood [affective] disorders (F30-F39)*
*pervasive developmental disorders (F84.-)*
*schizophrenia (F20.-)*

**F90.0 Attention-deficit hyperactivity disorder, predominantly inattentive type** Rx
Attention-deficit/hyperactivity disorder, predominantly inattentive presentation

**F90.1 Attention-deficit hyperactivity disorder, predominantly hyperactive type** Rx
Attention-deficit/hyperactivity disorder, predominantly hyperactive impulsive presentation

**F90.2 Attention-deficit hyperactivity disorder, combined type** Rx
Attention-deficit/hyperactivity disorder, combined presentation

**F90.8 Attention-deficit hyperactivity disorder, other type** Rx

**F90.9 Attention-deficit hyperactivity disorder, unspecified type** Rx
Attention-deficit hyperactivity disorder of childhood or adolescence NOS
Attention-deficit hyperactivity disorder NOS

**F91 Conduct disorders**

EXCLUDES 1 *antisocial behavior (Z72.81-)*
*antisocial personality disorder (F60.2)*

EXCLUDES 2 *conduct problems associated with attention-deficit hyperactivity disorder (F90.-)*
*mood [affective] disorders (F30-F39)*
*pervasive developmental disorders (F84.-)*
*schizophrenia (F20.-)*

**F91.0 Conduct disorder confined to family context** Rx

**F91.1 Conduct disorder, childhood-onset type** Rx
Conduct disorder, solitary aggressive type
Unsocialized aggressive disorder
Unsocialized conduct disorder

**F91.2 Conduct disorder, adolescent-onset type** Rx
Conduct disorder, group type
Socialized conduct disorder

**F91.3 Oppositional defiant disorder** Rx

**F91.8 Other conduct disorders** Rx
Other specified conduct disorder
Other specified disruptive disorder

**F91.9 Conduct disorder, unspecified** Rx
Behavioral disorder NOS
Conduct disorder NOS
Disruptive behavior disorder NOS
Disruptive disorder NOS

**F93 Emotional disorders with onset specific to childhood**

**F93.0 Separation anxiety disorder of childhood** Rx

EXCLUDES 2 *mood [affective] disorders (F30-F39)*
*nonpsychotic mental disorders (F40-F48)*
*phobic anxiety disorder of childhood (F40.8)*
*social phobia (F40.1)*

**F93.8 Other childhood emotional disorders**
Identity disorder

EXCLUDES 2 *gender identity disorder of childhood (F64.2)*

**F93.9 Childhood emotional disorder, unspecified**

**F94 Disorders of social functioning with onset specific to childhood and adolescence**

**F94.0 Selective mutism**
Elective mutism

EXCLUDES 2 *pervasive developmental disorders (F84.-)*
*schizophrenia (F20.-)*
*specific developmental disorders of speech and language (F80.-)*
*transient mutism as part of separation anxiety in young children (F93.0)*

**F94.1 Reactive attachment disorder of childhood**
Use additional code to identify any associated failure to thrive or growth retardation

EXCLUDES 1 *disinhibited attachment disorder of childhood (F94.2)*
*normal variation in pattern of selective attachment*

EXCLUDES 2 *Asperger's syndrome (F84.5)*
*maltreatment syndromes (T74.-)*
*sexual or physical abuse in childhood, resulting in psychosocial problems (Z62.81-)*

**F94.2 Disinhibited attachment disorder of childhood**
Affectionless psychopathy
Institutional syndrome

EXCLUDES 1 *reactive attachment disorder of childhood (F94.1)*

EXCLUDES 2 *Asperger's syndrome (F84.5)*
*attention-deficit hyperactivity disorders (F90.-)*
*hospitalism in children (F43.2-)*

**F94.8 Other childhood disorders of social functioning**

**F94.9 Childhood disorder of social functioning, unspecified**

**F95 Tic disorder**

**F95.0 Transient tic disorder** Rx
Provisional tic disorder

**F95.1 Chronic motor or vocal tic disorder** Rx

**F95.2 Tourette's disorder** Rx
Combined vocal and multiple motor tic disorder [de la Tourette]
Tourette's syndrome

**F95.8 Other tic disorders** Rx

**F95.9 Tic disorder, unspecified** Rx
Tic NOS

**F98 Other behavioral and emotional disorders with onset usually occurring in childhood and adolescence**

EXCLUDES 2 *breath-holding spells (R06.89)*
*gender identity disorder of childhood (F64.2)*
*Kleine-Levin syndrome (G47.13)*
*obsessive-compulsive disorder (F42.-)*
*sleep disorders not due to a substance or known physiological condition (F51.-)*

**F98.0 Enuresis not due to a substance or known physiological condition**
Enuresis (primary) (secondary) of nonorganic origin
Functional enuresis
Psychogenic enuresis
Urinary incontinence of nonorganic origin

EXCLUDES 1 *enuresis NOS (R32)*

**F98.1 Encopresis not due to a substance or known physiological condition**
Functional encopresis
Incontinence of feces of nonorganic origin
Psychogenic encopresis
Use additional code to identify the cause of any coexisting constipation

EXCLUDES 1 *encopresis NOS (R15.-)*

**F98.2 Other feeding disorders of infancy and childhood**

EXCLUDES 2 *anorexia nervosa and other eating disorders (F50.-)*
*feeding difficulties (R63.3-)*
*feeding problems of newborn (P92.-)*
*pica of infancy or childhood (F98.3)*

**F98.21 Rumination disorder of infancy and childhood** Rx
Rumination disorder in infancy or childhood, in remission

EXCLUDES 1 *rumination disorder in adults (F50.84)*

**F98.29 Other feeding disorders of infancy and early childhood** Rx

**F98.3 Pica of infancy and childhood** Rx
Pica in infancy or childhood, in remission

EXCLUDES 1 *pica in adults (F50.83)*

**F98.4 Stereotyped movement disorders** Rx
Stereotype/habit disorder

EXCLUDES 1 *abnormal involuntary movements (R25.-)*

EXCLUDES 2 *compulsions in obsessive-compulsive disorder (F42.-)*
*hair plucking (F63.3)*
*movement disorders of organic origin (G20-G25)*
*nail-biting (F98.8)*
*nose-picking (F98.8)*
*stereotypies that are part of a broader psychiatric condition (F01-F95)*
*thumb-sucking (F98.8)*
*tic disorders (F95.-)*
*trichotillomania (F63.3)*

**F98.5 Adult onset fluency disorder**

EXCLUDES 1 *childhood onset fluency disorder (F8Ø.81)*
*dysphasia (R47.Ø2)*
*fluency disorder (stuttering) following cerebrovascular disease (I69. with final characters -23)*
*fluency disorder in conditions classified elsewhere (R47.82)*
*tic disorders (F95.-)*

**F98.8 Other specified behavioral and emotional disorders with onset usually occurring in childhood and adolescence**

Excessive masturbation
Nail-biting
Nose-picking
Thumb-sucking

**F98.9 Unspecified behavioral and emotional disorders with onset usually occurring in childhood and adolescence**

## Unspecified mental disorder (F99)

**F99 Mental disorder, not otherwise specified**

Mental illness NOS

EXCLUDES 1 *unspecified mental disorder due to known physiological condition (FØ9)*

# Chapter 6. Diseases of the Nervous System (GØØ–G99)



## Chapter-specific Guidelines with Coding Examples

The chapter-specific guidelines from the ICD-10-CM Official Guidelines for Coding and Reporting have been provided below. Along with these guidelines are coding examples, contained in the shaded boxes, that have been developed to help illustrate the coding and/or sequencing guidance found in these guidelines.

**a. Dominant/nondominant side**

Codes from category G81, Hemiplegia and hemiparesis, and subcategories G83.1, Monoplegia of lower limb, G83.2, Monoplegia of upper limb, and G83.3, Monoplegia, unspecified, identify whether the dominant or nondominant side is affected. Should the affected side be documented, but not specified as dominant or nondominant, and the classification system does not indicate a default, code selection is as follows:

- For ambidextrous patients, the default should be dominant.
- If the left side is affected, the default is non-dominant.
- If the right side is affected, the default is dominant.

> Hemiplegia affecting left side of ambidextrous patient
>
> **G81.92 Hemiplegia, unspecified affecting left dominant side**
>
> *Explanation*: Documentation states that the left side is affected and dominant is used for ambidextrous persons.

> Right spastic hemiplegia, unknown whether patient is right- or left-handed
>
> **G81.11 Spastic hemiplegia affecting right dominant side**
>
> *Explanation*: Since it is unknown whether the patient is right- or left-handed, if the right side is affected, the default is dominant.

**b. Pain—Category G89**

**1) General coding information**

Codes in category G89, Pain, not elsewhere classified, may be used in conjunction with codes from other categories and chapters to provide more detail about acute or chronic pain and neoplasm-related pain, unless otherwise indicated below.

If the pain is not specified as acute or chronic, post-thoracotomy, postprocedural, or neoplasm-related, do not assign codes from category G89.

A code from category G89 should not be assigned if the underlying (definitive) diagnosis is known, unless the reason for the encounter is pain control/ management and not management of the underlying condition.

When an admission or encounter is for a procedure aimed at treating the underlying condition (e.g., spinal fusion, kyphoplasty), a code for the underlying condition (e.g., vertebral fracture, spinal stenosis) should be assigned as the principal diagnosis. No code from category G89 should be assigned.

> Elderly patient with back pain is admitted for outpatient kyphoplasty for age-related osteopathic compression fracture at vertebra T3
>
> **M8Ø.Ø8XA Age-related osteoporosis with current pathological fracture, vertebra(e), initial encounter for fracture**
>
> *Explanation*: No code is assigned for the pain as it is inherent in the underlying condition being treated.

**(a) Category G89 codes as principal or first-listed diagnosis**

Category G89 codes are acceptable as principal diagnosis or the first-listed code:

- When pain control or pain management is the reason for the admission/encounter (e.g., a patient with displaced intervertebral disc, nerve impingement and severe back pain presents for injection of steroid into the spinal canal). The underlying cause of the pain should be reported as an additional diagnosis, if known.

> Patient presents for steroid injection in the right elbow due to chronic pain associated with primary degenerative joint disease.
>
> **G89.29 Other chronic pain**
>
> **M19.Ø21 Primary osteoarthritis, right elbow**
>
> *Explanation*: Since the encounter is for control of pain, not treating the underlying condition, the pain code is sequenced first followed by the underlying condition. The M25 pain code is not necessary as the underlying condition code represents the specific site.

- When a patient is admitted for the insertion of a neurostimulator for pain control, assign the appropriate pain code as the principal or first-listed diagnosis. When an admission or encounter is for a procedure aimed at treating the underlying condition and a neurostimulator is inserted for pain control during the same admission/encounter, a code for the underlying condition should be assigned as the principal diagnosis and the appropriate pain code should be assigned as a secondary diagnosis.

**(b) Use of category G89 codes in conjunction with site specific pain codes**

**(i) Assigning category G89 and site-specific pain codes**

Codes from category G89 may be used in conjunction with codes that identify the site of pain (including codes from chapter 18) if the category G89 code provides additional information. For example, if the code describes the site of the pain, but does not fully describe whether the pain is acute or chronic, then both codes should be assigned.

> Patient is seen to evaluate chronic right knee pain
>
> **M25.561 Pain in right knee**
>
> **G89.29 Other chronic pain**
>
> *Explanation*: No underlying condition has been determined yet so the pain would be the reason for the visit. The M25 pain code in this instance does not fully describe the condition as it does not represent that the pain is chronic. The G89 chronic pain code is assigned to provide specificity.

**(ii) Sequencing of category G89 codes with site-specific pain codes**

The sequencing of category G89 codes with site-specific pain codes (including chapter 18 codes), is dependent on the circumstances of the encounter/admission as follows:

- If the encounter is for pain control or pain management, assign the code from category G89 followed by the code identifying the specific site of pain (e.g., encounter for pain management for acute neck pain from trauma is assigned code G89.11, Acute pain due to trauma, followed by code M54.2, Cervicalgia, to identify the site of pain).

> Management of acute, traumatic left shoulder pain
>
> **G89.11 Acute pain due to trauma**
>
> **M25.512 Pain in left shoulder**
>
> *Explanation*: The reason for the encounter is to manage or control the pain, not to treat or evaluate an underlying condition. The G89 pain code is assigned as the first-listed diagnosis but in this instance does not fully describe the condition as it does not include the site and laterality. The M25 pain code is added to provide this information.

- If the encounter is for any other reason except pain control or pain management, and a related definitive diagnosis has not been established (confirmed) by the provider, assign the code for the specific site of pain first, followed by the appropriate code from category G89.

Tests are performed to investigate the source of the patient's chronic epigastric abdominal pain

**R10.13** **Epigastric pain**

**G89.29** **Other chronic pain**

*Explanation*: In this instance the patient's epigastric pain is not being treated; rather the source of the pain is being investigated. A code from chapter 18 for epigastric pain is sequenced before the additional specificity of the G89 code for the chronic pain.

**2) Pain due to devices, implants and grafts**

*See Section I.C.19. Pain due to medical devices*

**3) Postoperative Pain**

The provider's documentation should be used to guide the coding of postoperative pain, as well as *Section III. Reporting Additional Diagnoses* and *Section IV. Diagnostic Coding and Reporting in the Outpatient Setting.*

The default for post-thoracotomy and other postoperative pain not specified as acute or chronic is the code for the acute form.

Routine or expected postoperative pain immediately after surgery should not be coded.

Pain pump dose is increased for the patient's unexpected, extreme pain post-thoracotomy

**G89.12** **Acute post-thoracotomy pain**

*Explanation*: When acute or chronic is not documented, default to acute. The use of "unexpected, extreme" and the increase of medication dosage indicate that the pain was more than routine or expected.

**(a) Postoperative pain not associated with specific postoperative complication**

Postoperative pain not associated with a specific postoperative complication is assigned to the appropriate postoperative pain code in category G89.

**(b) Postoperative pain associated with specific postoperative complication**

Postoperative pain associated with a specific postoperative complication (such as painful wire sutures) is assigned to the appropriate code(s) found in Chapter 19, Injury, poisoning, and certain other consequences of external causes. If appropriate, use additional code(s) from category G89 to identify acute or chronic pain (G89.18 or G89.28).

**4) Chronic pain**

Chronic pain is classified to subcategory G89.2. There is no time frame defining when pain becomes chronic pain. The provider's documentation should be used to guide use of these codes.

**5) Neoplasm related pain**

Code G89.3 is assigned to pain documented as being related, associated or due to cancer, primary or secondary malignancy, or tumor. This code is assigned regardless of whether the pain is acute or chronic.

This code may be assigned as the principal or first-listed code when the stated reason for the admission/encounter is documented as pain control/pain management. The underlying neoplasm should be reported as an additional diagnosis.

Patient referred today for pain management due to acute pain related to malignancy of the right breast.

**G89.3** **Neoplasm related pain (acute)(chronic)**

**C50.911** **Malignant neoplasm of unspecified site of right female breast**

*Explanation*: Since the encounter was for pain medication management, the pain, rather than the neoplasm, was the reason for the encounter and is sequenced first. This "neoplasm-related pain" code includes both acute and chronic pain.

When the reason for the admission/encounter is management of the neoplasm and the pain associated with the neoplasm is also documented, code G89.3 may be assigned as an additional diagnosis. It is not necessary to assign an additional code for the site of the pain.

*See Section I.C.2. for instructions on the sequencing of neoplasms for all other stated reasons or the admission/encounter (except for pain control/pain management).*

Patient with lung cancer presents with acute hip pain and is evaluated and found to have iliac bone metastasis

**C79.51** **Secondary malignant neoplasm of bone**

**C34.90** **Malignant neoplasm of unspecified part of unspecified bronchus or lung**

**G89.3** **Neoplasm related pain (acute)(chronic)**

*Explanation*: The reason for the encounter was the evaluation and diagnosis of the bone metastasis, whose code would be assigned as first-listed, followed by codes for the primary neoplasm and the pain due to the iliac bone metastasis.

**6) Chronic pain syndrome**

Central pain syndrome (G89.0) and chronic pain syndrome (G89.4) are different than the term "chronic pain," and therefore codes should only be used when the provider has specifically documented this condition.

*See Section I.C.5. Pain disorders related to psychological factors*

# Chapter 6. Diseases of the Nervous System (G00-G99)

EXCLUDES 2 *certain conditions originating in the perinatal period (P04-P96)*
*certain infectious and parasitic diseases (A00-B99)*
*complications of pregnancy, childbirth and the puerperium (O00-O9A)*
*congenital malformations, deformations, and chromosomal abnormalities (Q00-Q99)*
*endocrine, nutritional and metabolic diseases (E00-E88)*
*injury, poisoning and certain other consequences of external causes (S00-T88)*
*neoplasms (C00-D49)*
*symptoms, signs and abnormal clinical and laboratory findings, not elsewhere classified (R00-R94)*

This chapter contains the following blocks:

G00-G09 Inflammatory diseases of the central nervous system
G10-G14 Systemic atrophies primarily affecting the central nervous system
G20-G26 Extrapyramidal and movement disorders
G30-G32 Other degenerative diseases of the nervous system
G35-G37 Demyelinating diseases of the central nervous system
G40-G47 Episodic and paroxysmal disorders
G50-G59 Nerve, nerve root and plexus disorders
G60-G65 Polyneuropathies and other disorders of the peripheral nervous system
G70-G73 Diseases of myoneural junction and muscle
G80-G83 Cerebral palsy and other paralytic syndromes
G89-G99 Other disorders of the nervous system

## Inflammatory diseases of the central nervous system (G00-G09)

✓4th **G00 Bacterial meningitis, not elsewhere classified**

INCLUDES bacterial arachnoiditis
bacterial leptomeningitis
bacterial meningitis
bacterial pachymeningitis

EXCLUDES 1 *bacterial meningoencephalitis (G04.2)*
*bacterial meningomyelitis (G04.2)*

**DEF:** Inflammation of meningeal layers of the brain and spinal cord due to a bacterial infection.

**G00.0 Hemophilus meningitis** COM
Meningitis due to Hemophilus influenzae

**G00.1 Pneumococcal meningitis** COM
Meningitis due to Streptococcal pneumoniae

**G00.2 Streptococcal meningitis** COM
Use additional code to further identify organism (B95.0-B95.5)

**G00.3 Staphylococcal meningitis** COM
Use additional code to further identify organism (B95.61-B95.8)

**G00.8 Other bacterial meningitis** COM
Meningitis due to Escherichia coli
Meningitis due to Friedlander's bacillus
Meningitis due to Klebsiella
Use additional code to further identify organism (B96.-)

**G00.9 Bacterial meningitis, unspecified** COM
Meningitis due to gram-negative bacteria, unspecified
Purulent meningitis NOS
Pyogenic meningitis NOS
Suppurative meningitis NOS

***G01 Meningitis in bacterial diseases classified elsewhere*** COM
Code first underlying disease

EXCLUDES 1 *meningitis (in):*
*meningoencephalitis and meningomyelitis in bacterial diseases classified elsewhere (G05)*
*gonococcal (A54.81)*
*leptospirosis (A27.81)*
*listeriosis (A32.11)*
*Lyme disease (A69.21)*
*meningococcal (A39.0)*
*neurosyphilis (A52.13)*
*tuberculosis (A17.0)*

***G02 Meningitis in other infectious and parasitic diseases classified elsewhere*** COM
Code first underlying disease, such as:
African trypanosomiasis (B56.-)
poliovirus infection (A80.-)

EXCLUDES 1 *candidal meningitis (B37.5)*
*coccidioidomycosis meningitis (B38.4)*
*cryptococcal meningitis (B45.1)*
*herpesviral [herpes simplex] meningitis (B00.3)*
*infectious mononucleosis complicated by meningitis (B27.- with fifth character 2)*
*measles complicated by meningitis (B05.1)*
*meningoencephalitis and meningomyelitis in other infectious and parasitic diseases classified elsewhere (G05)*
*mumps meningitis (B26.1)*
*rubella meningitis (B06.02)*
*varicella [chickenpox] meningitis (B01.0)*
*zoster meningitis (B02.1)*

✓4th **G03 Meningitis due to other and unspecified causes**

INCLUDES arachnoiditis NOS
leptomeningitis NOS
meningitis NOS
pachymeningitis NOS

EXCLUDES 1 *meningoencephalitis (G04.-)*
*meningomyelitis (G04.-)*

**G03.0 Nonpyogenic meningitis** COM
Aseptic meningitis
Nonbacterial meningitis
**DEF:** Type of meningitis where no bacterial, viral, or other infectious source exists that explains the meningitis symptomology.

**G03.1 Chronic meningitis** COM

**G03.2 Benign recurrent meningitis [Mollaret]** COM
**DEF:** Aseptic or noninfectious inflammation of the meninges with the presence of Mollaret cells in the spinal fluid. The patient experiences recurrent bouts of inflammation, lasting anywhere from two to five days.

**G03.8 Meningitis due to other specified causes** COM

**G03.9 Meningitis, unspecified** COM
Arachnoiditis (spinal) NOS

✓4th **G04 Encephalitis, myelitis and encephalomyelitis**

INCLUDES acute ascending myelitis
meningoencephalitis
meningomyelitis

EXCLUDES 1 *encephalopathy NOS (G93.40)*

EXCLUDES 2 *acute transverse myelitis (G37.3)*
*alcoholic encephalopathy (G31.2)*
*multiple sclerosis (G35-)*
*myalgic encephalomyelitis (G93.32)*
*subacute necrotizing myelitis (G37.4)*
*toxic encephalitis (G92.8)*
*toxic encephalopathy (G92.8)*

**DEF:** Encephalitis: Inflammation of the brain, often caused by viral or bacterial infection.
**DEF:** Encephalomyelitis: Inflammatory disease, often viral in nature, that affects the brain and spinal cord.
**DEF:** Myelitis: Inflammation of the spinal cord.

✓5th **G04.0 Acute disseminated encephalitis and encephalomyelitis (ADEM)**

EXCLUDES 1 *acute necrotizing hemorrhagic encephalopathy (G04.3-)*
*other noninfectious acute disseminated encephalomyelitis (noninfectious ADEM) (G04.81)*

**G04.00 Acute disseminated encephalitis and encephalomyelitis, unspecified** COM

**G04.01 Postinfectious acute disseminated encephalitis and encephalomyelitis (postinfectious ADEM)** COM
EXCLUDES 1 *post chickenpox encephalitis (B01.1)*
*post measles encephalitis (B05.0)*
*post measles myelitis (B05.1)*

**G04.02 Postimmunization acute disseminated encephalitis, myelitis and encephalomyelitis** COM
Encephalitis, post immunization
Encephalomyelitis, post immunization
Use additional code to identify the vaccine (T50.A-, T50.B-, T50.Z-)

**G04.1 Tropical spastic paraplegia** HCC Rx ESR COM

**G04.2 Bacterial meningoencephalitis and meningomyelitis, not elsewhere classified** COM

**√5th G04.3 Acute necrotizing hemorrhagic encephalopathy**
EXCLUDES 1 *acute disseminated encephalitis and encephalomyelitis (G04.0-)*

**G04.30 Acute necrotizing hemorrhagic encephalopathy, unspecified** COM

**G04.31 Postinfectious acute necrotizing hemorrhagic encephalopathy** COM

**G04.32 Postimmunization acute necrotizing hemorrhagic encephalopathy** COM
Use additional code to identify the vaccine (T50.A-, T50.B-, T50.Z-)

**G04.39 Other acute necrotizing hemorrhagic encephalopathy** COM
Code also underlying etiology, if applicable

**√5th G04.8 Other encephalitis, myelitis and encephalomyelitis**
Code also any associated seizure (G40.-, R56.9)

**G04.81 Other encephalitis and encephalomyelitis** COM
Noninfectious acute disseminated encephalomyelitis (noninfectious ADEM)

**G04.82 Acute flaccid myelitis** HCC Rx ESR COM
EXCLUDES 1 *transverse myelitis (G37.3)*
**AHA:** 2021,4Q,11

**G04.89 Other myelitis** HCC Rx ESR COM
**AHA:** 2020,1Q,14

**√5th G04.9 Encephalitis, myelitis and encephalomyelitis, unspecified**

**G04.90 Encephalitis and encephalomyelitis, unspecified** COM
Ventriculitis (cerebral) NOS

**G04.91 Myelitis, unspecified** HCC Rx ESR COM

**√4th G05 Encephalitis, myelitis and encephalomyelitis in diseases classified elsewhere**
Code first underlying disease, such as:
- congenital toxoplasmosis encephalitis, myelitis and encephalomyelitis (P37.1)
- cytomegaloviral encephalitis, myelitis and encephalomyelitis (B25.8)
- encephalitis, myelitis and encephalomyelitis (in) systemic lupus erythematosus (M32.19)
- eosinophilic meningoencephalitis (B83.2)
- human immunodeficiency virus [HIV] disease (B20)
- poliovirus (A80.-)
- suppurative otitis media (H66.01-H66.4)
- systemic lupus erythematosus (M32.19)
- trichinellosis (B75)

EXCLUDES 1
*adenoviral encephalitis, myelitis and encephalomyelitis (A85.1)*
*encephalitis, myelitis and encephalomyelitis (in) measles (B05.0)*
*enteroviral encephalitis, myelitis and encephalomyelitis (A85.0)*
*herpesviral [herpes simplex] encephalitis, myelitis and encephalomyelitis (B00.4)*
*listerial encephalitis, myelitis and encephalomyelitis (A32.12)*
*meningococcal encephalitis, myelitis and encephalomyelitis (A39.81)*
*mumps encephalitis, myelitis and encephalomyelitis (B26.2)*
*postchickenpox encephalitis, myelitis and encephalomyelitis (B01.1-)*
*rubella encephalitis, myelitis and encephalomyelitis (B06.01)*
*toxoplasmosis encephalitis, myelitis and encephalomyelitis (B58.2)*
*zoster encephalitis, myelitis and encephalomyelitis (B02.0)*

***G05.3 Encephalitis and encephalomyelitis in diseases classified elsewhere*** COM
Meningoencephalitis in diseases classified elsewhere
Code first underlying disease

***G05.4 Myelitis in diseases classified elsewhere*** HCC Rx ESR COM
Meningomyelitis in diseases classified elsewhere

**√4th G06 Intracranial and intraspinal abscess and granuloma**
Use additional code (B95-B97) to identify infectious agent
**DEF:** Abscess: Circumscribed collection of pus resulting from bacteria, frequently associated with swelling and other signs of inflammation.
**DEF:** Granuloma: Abnormal, dense collections of cells forming a mass or nodule of chronically inflamed tissue with granulations that is usually associated with an infective process.

**G06.0 Intracranial abscess and granuloma** COM
Brain [any part] abscess (embolic)
Cerebellar abscess (embolic)
Cerebral abscess (embolic)
Intracranial epidural abscess or granuloma
Intracranial extradural abscess or granuloma
Intracranial subdural abscess or granuloma
Otogenic abscess (embolic)
EXCLUDES 1 *tuberculous intracranial abscess and granuloma (A17.81)*

**G06.1 Intraspinal abscess and granuloma** COM
Abscess (embolic) of spinal cord [any part]
Intraspinal epidural abscess or granuloma
Intraspinal extradural abscess or granuloma
Intraspinal subdural abscess or granuloma
EXCLUDES 1 *tuberculous intraspinal abscess and granuloma (A17.81)*

**G06.2 Extradural and subdural abscess, unspecified** COM

***G07 Intracranial and intraspinal abscess and granuloma in diseases classified elsewhere*** COM
Code first underlying disease, such as:
- schistosomiasis granuloma of brain (B65.-)

EXCLUDES 1
*abscess of brain:*
*tuberculoma of meninges (A17.1)*
*amebic (A06.6)*
*chromomycotic (B43.1)*
*gonococcal (A54.82)*
*tuberculous (A17.81)*

**G08 Intracranial and intraspinal phlebitis and thrombophlebitis** COM
Septic embolism of intracranial or intraspinal venous sinuses and veins
Septic endophlebitis of intracranial or intraspinal venous sinuses and veins
Septic phlebitis of intracranial or intraspinal venous sinuses and veins
Septic thrombophlebitis of intracranial or intraspinal venous sinuses and veins
Septic thrombosis of intracranial or intraspinal venous sinuses and veins
EXCLUDES 1 *intracranial phlebitis and thrombophlebitis complicating:*
*nonpyogenic intracranial phlebitis and thrombophlebitis (I67.6)*
*abortion, ectopic or molar pregnancy (O00-O07, O08.7)*
*pregnancy, childbirth and the puerperium (O22.5, O87.3)*
EXCLUDES 2 *intracranial phlebitis and thrombophlebitis complicating nonpyogenic intraspinal phlebitis and thrombophlebitis (G95.1)*
**DEF:** Inflammation and formation of a blood clot in a vein within the brain or spine, or their linings.

**G09 Sequelae of inflammatory diseases of central nervous system**
NOTE Category G09 is to be used to indicate conditions whose primary classification is to G00-G08 as the cause of sequelae, themselves classifiable elsewhere. The "sequelae" include conditions specified as residuals.
Code first condition resulting from (sequela) of inflammatory diseases of central nervous system

## Systemic atrophies primarily affecting the central nervous system (G10-G14)

**G10 Huntington's disease** HCC Rx ESR COM
Huntington's chorea
Huntington's dementia
Use additional code, if applicable, to identify:
- dementia with anxiety (F02.84, F02.A4, F02.B4, F02.C4)
- dementia with behavioral disturbance (F02.81-, F02.A1-, F02.B1-, F02.C1-)
- dementia with mood disturbance (F02.83, F02.A3, F02.B3, F02.C3)
- dementia with psychotic disturbance (F02.82, F02.A2, F02.B2, F02.C2)
- dementia without behavioral disturbance (F02.80, F02.A0, F02.B0, F02.C0)
- mild neurocognitive disorder due to known physiological condition (F06.7-)

**DEF:** Genetic disease caused by degeneration of nerve cells in the brain, characterized by chronic progressive mental deterioration. Dementia and death occur within 15 to 20 years of onset.

**G11 Hereditary ataxia**

EXCLUDES 2 *cerebral palsy (G80.-)*
*hereditary and idiopathic neuropathy (G60.-)*
*metabolic disorders (E70-E88)*

**DEF:** Ataxia: Defect in muscular control or coordination due to a central nervous system disorder, particularly when voluntary muscular movements are attempted.

**G11.0 Congenital nonprogressive ataxia** HCC ESR COM

**G11.1 Early-onset cerebellar ataxia**

**AHA:** 2020,4Q,17-18

**G11.10 Early-onset cerebellar ataxia, unspecified** HCC ESR COM

**G11.11 Friedreich ataxia** HCC ESR COM
Autosomal recessive Friedreich ataxia
Friedreich ataxia with retained reflexes

**G11.19 Other early-onset cerebellar ataxia** HCC ESR COM
Early-onset cerebellar ataxia with essential tremor
Early-onset cerebellar ataxia with myoclonus [Hunt's ataxia]
Early-onset cerebellar ataxia with retained tendon reflexes
X-linked recessive spinocerebellar ataxia

**G11.2 Late-onset cerebellar ataxia** HCC ESR COM A

**G11.3 Cerebellar ataxia with defective DNA repair** HCC ESR COM
Ataxia telangiectasia [Louis-Bar]

EXCLUDES 2 *Cockayne's syndrome (Q87.19)*
*other disorders of purine and pyrimidine metabolism (E79.-)*
*xeroderma pigmentosum (Q82.1)*

**G11.4 Hereditary spastic paraplegia** HCC ESR COM

**G11.5 Hypomyelination - hypogonadotropic hypogonadism - hypodontia** HCC ESR COM
4H syndrome
Pol III-related leukodystrophy
**AHA:** 2023,4Q,12-13

**G11.6 Leukodystrophy with vanishing white matter disease** HCC ESR COM
**AHA:** 2023,4Q,12-13

**G11.8 Other hereditary ataxias** HCC ESR COM

**G11.9 Hereditary ataxia, unspecified** HCC ESR COM
Hereditary cerebellar ataxia NOS
Hereditary cerebellar degeneration
Hereditary cerebellar disease
Hereditary cerebellar syndrome

**G12 Spinal muscular atrophy and related syndromes**

**G12.0 Infantile spinal muscular atrophy, type I [Werdnig-Hoffman]** HCC Rx ESR COM

**G12.1 Other inherited spinal muscular atrophy** HCC Rx ESR COM
Adult form spinal muscular atrophy
Childhood form, type II spinal muscular atrophy
Distal spinal muscular atrophy
Juvenile form, type III spinal muscular atrophy [Kugelberg-Welander]
Progressive bulbar palsy of childhood [Fazio-Londe]
Scapuloperoneal form spinal muscular atrophy

**G12.2 Motor neuron disease**

**AHA:** 2017,4Q,9-10

**G12.20 Motor neuron disease, unspecified** HCC Rx ESR COM

**G12.21 Amyotrophic lateral sclerosis** HCC Rx ESR COM A

**G12.22 Progressive bulbar palsy** HCC Rx ESR COM

**G12.23 Primary lateral sclerosis** HCC Rx ESR COM

**G12.24 Familial motor neuron disease** HCC Rx ESR COM

**G12.25 Progressive spinal muscle atrophy** HCC Rx ESR COM

**G12.29 Other motor neuron disease** HCC Rx ESR COM

**G12.8 Other spinal muscular atrophies and related syndromes** HCC Rx ESR COM

**G12.9 Spinal muscular atrophy, unspecified** HCC Rx ESR COM

**G13 Systemic atrophies primarily affecting central nervous system in diseases classified elsewhere**

*G13.0 **Paraneoplastic neuromyopathy and neuropathy*** Rx ESR COM
Carcinomatous neuromyopathy
Sensorial paraneoplastic neuropathy [Denny Brown]
Code first underlying neoplasm (C00-D49)

*G13.1 **Other systemic atrophy primarily affecting central nervous system in neoplastic disease*** Rx ESR COM
Paraneoplastic limbic encephalopathy
Code first underlying neoplasm (C00-D49)

*G13.2 **Systemic atrophy primarily affecting the central nervous system in myxedema*** Rx ESR
Code first underlying disease, such as:
hypothyroidism (E03.-)
myxedematous congenital iodine deficiency (E00.1)

*G13.8 **Systemic atrophy primarily affecting central nervous system in other diseases classified elsewhere*** Rx ESR
Code first underlying disease

**G14 Postpolio syndrome** HCC

INCLUDES postpolio myelitic syndrome

EXCLUDES 1 *sequelae of poliomyelitis (B91)*

## Extrapyramidal and movement disorders (G20-G26)

**G20 Parkinson's disease**

Hemiparkinsonism
Idiopathic Parkinsonism or Parkinson's disease
Paralysis agitans
Primary Parkinsonism or Parkinson's disease
Use additional code, if applicable, to identify:
dementia with anxiety (F02.84, F02.A4, F02.B4, F02.C4)
dementia with behavioral disturbance (F02.81-, F02.A1-, F02.B1-, F02.C1-)
dementia with mood disturbance (F02.83, F02.A3, F02.B3, F02.C3)
dementia with psychotic disturbance (F02.82, F02.A2, F02.B2, F02.C2)
dementia without behavioral disturbance (F02.80, F02.A0, F02.B0, F02.C0)
mild neurocognitive disorder due to known physiological condition (F06.7-)

**AHA:** 2023,4Q,15-17; 2017,2Q,7; 2016,2Q,6

**TIP:** Repeated falls (R29.6) are not integral to Parkinson's disease and can be separately coded.

**G20.A Parkinson's disease without dyskinesia**

**G20.A1 Parkinson's disease without dyskinesia, without mention of fluctuations** HCC Rx ESR COM
Parkinson's disease NOS
Parkinson's disease without dyskinesia, without mention of OFF episodes

**G20.A2 Parkinson's disease without dyskinesia, with fluctuations** HCC Rx ESR COM
Parkinson's disease without dyskinesia, with OFF episodes

**G20.B Parkinson's disease with dyskinesia**

EXCLUDES 1 *drug induced dystonia (G24.0-)*

**G20.B1 Parkinson's disease with dyskinesia, without mention of fluctuations** HCC Rx ESR COM
Parkinson's disease with dyskinesia, without mention of OFF episodes

**G20.B2 Parkinson's disease with dyskinesia, with fluctuations** HCC Rx ESR COM
Parkinson's disease with dyskinesia, with OFF episodes

**G20.C Parkinsonism, unspecified** HCC Rx ESR COM
Parkinsonism, NOS

EXCLUDES 1 *Parkinson's disease NOS (G20.A1)*
*Parkinson's disease with dyskinesia (G20.B-)*
*Parkinson's disease without dyskinesia (G20.A-)*
*secondary parkinsonism (G21.-)*

**G21 Secondary parkinsonism**

EXCLUDES 1 *Huntington's disease (G10)*
*neurocognitive disorder with Lewy bodies (G31.83)*
*Shy-Drager syndrome (G90.3)*
*syphilitic Parkinsonism (A52.19)*

**G21.0 Malignant neuroleptic syndrome**
Use additional code for adverse effect, if applicable, to identify drug (T43.3X5, T43.4X5, T43.505, T43.595)

EXCLUDES 1 *neuroleptic induced parkinsonism (G21.11)*

**G21.1 Other drug-induced secondary parkinsonism**

**G21.11 Neuroleptic induced parkinsonism** Rx ESR COM
Use additional code for adverse effect, if applicable, to identify drug (T43.3X5, T43.4X5, T43.505, T43.595)

EXCLUDES 1 *malignant neuroleptic syndrome (G21.0)*

**G21.19 Other drug induced secondary parkinsonism** HCC Rx ESR COM
Other medication-induced parkinsonism
Use additional code for adverse effect, if applicable, to identify drug (T36-T5Ø with fifth or sixth character 5)

**G21.2 Secondary parkinsonism due to other external agents** Rx ESR COM
Code first (T51-T65) to identify external agent

**G21.3 Postencephalitic parkinsonism** HCC Rx ESR COM

**G21.4 Vascular parkinsonism** HCC Rx ESR COM

**G21.8 Other secondary parkinsonism** HCC Rx ESR COM

**G21.9 Secondary parkinsonism, unspecified** HCC Rx ESR COM

✓4th **G23 Other degenerative diseases of basal ganglia**
EXCLUDES 2 *multi-system degeneration of the autonomic nervous system (G9Ø.3)*

**G23.Ø Hallervorden-Spatz disease** HCC Rx ESR COM
Pigmentary pallidal degeneration

**G23.1 Progressive supranuclear ophthalmoplegia [Steele-Richardson-Olszewski]** HCC Rx ESR COM
Progressive supranuclear palsy

**G23.2 Striatonigral degeneration** HCC Rx ESR COM

**G23.3 Hypomyelination with atrophy of the basal ganglia and cerebellum** HCC Rx ESR COM
H-ABC
TUBB4A-related neurologic disorders
**AHA:** 2023,4Q,12-13

**G23.8 Other specified degenerative diseases of basal ganglia** HCC Rx ESR COM
Calcification of basal ganglia

**G23.9 Degenerative disease of basal ganglia, unspecified** HCC Rx ESR COM

✓4th **G24 Dystonia**
INCLUDES dyskinesia
EXCLUDES 2 *athetoid cerebral palsy (G8Ø.3)*
**DEF:** Disorder of abnormal muscle tone, excessive or inadequate. Involuntary movements and prolonged muscle contractions result in tremors, abnormalities in posture, and twisting body motions that affect an isolated area or the whole body.

✓5th **G24.Ø Drug induced dystonia**
Use additional code for adverse effect, if applicable, to identify drug (T36-T5Ø with fifth or sixth character 5)

**G24.Ø1 Drug induced subacute dyskinesia**
Drug induced blepharospasm
Drug induced orofacial dyskinesia
Neuroleptic induced tardive dyskinesia
Tardive dyskinesia

**G24.Ø2 Drug induced acute dystonia**
Acute dystonic reaction to drugs
Neuroleptic induced acute dystonia

**G24.Ø9 Other drug induced dystonia**

**G24.1 Genetic torsion dystonia**
(Schwalbe-) Ziehen-Oppenheim disease
Dystonia deformans progressiva
Dystonia musculorum deformans
Familial torsion dystonia
Idiopathic (torsion) dystonia NOS
Idiopathic familial dystonia

**G24.2 Idiopathic nonfamilial dystonia**

**G24.3 Spasmodic torticollis**
EXCLUDES 1 *congenital torticollis (Q68.Ø)*
*hysterical torticollis (F44.4)*
*ocular torticollis (R29.891)*
*psychogenic torticollis (F45.8)*
*torticollis NOS (M43.6)*
*traumatic recurrent torticollis (S13.4)*
**DEF:** Twisted, unnatural position of the neck due to contracted cervical muscles that pull the head to one side or cause involuntary shaking of the head.

**G24.4 Idiopathic orofacial dystonia**
Orofacial dyskinesia
EXCLUDES 1 *drug induced orofacial dyskinesia (G24.Ø1)*

**G24.5 Blepharospasm**
EXCLUDES 1 *drug induced blepharospasm (G24.Ø1)*
**DEF:** Involuntary contraction of the orbicularis oculi muscle, resulting in the eyelids being completely closed.

**G24.8 Other dystonia**
Acquired torsion dystonia NOS

**G24.9 Dystonia, unspecified**
Dyskinesia NOS

✓4th **G25 Other extrapyramidal and movement disorders**
EXCLUDES 2 *sleep related movement disorders (G47.6-)*

**G25.Ø Essential tremor**
Familial tremor
EXCLUDES 1 *tremor NOS (R25.1)*

**G25.1 Drug-induced tremor**
Use additional code for adverse effect, if applicable, to identify drug (T36-T5Ø with fifth or sixth character 5)

**G25.2 Other specified forms of tremor**
Intention tremor

**G25.3 Myoclonus**
Drug-induced myoclonus
Palatal myoclonus
Use additional code for adverse effect, if applicable, to identify drug (T36-T5Ø with fifth or sixth character 5)
EXCLUDES 1 *facial myokymia (G51.4)*
*myoclonic epilepsy (G4Ø.-)*
**DEF:** Spasmodic, brief, involuntary muscle contractions that can be due to an undetermined etiology, drug-induced, or caused by a disease process.

**G25.4 Drug-induced chorea**
Use additional code for adverse effect, if applicable, to identify drug (T36-T5Ø with fifth or sixth character 5)

**G25.5 Other chorea**
Chorea NOS
EXCLUDES 1 *chorea NOS with heart involvement (IØ2.Ø)*
*Huntington's chorea (G1Ø)*
*rheumatic chorea (IØ2.-)*
*Sydenham's chorea (IØ2.-)*

✓5th **G25.6 Drug induced tics and other tics of organic origin**

**G25.61 Drug induced tics**
Use additional code for adverse effect, if applicable, to identify drug (T36-T5Ø with fifth or sixth character 5)

**G25.69 Other tics of organic origin**
EXCLUDES 1 *habit spasm (F95.9)*
*tic NOS (F95.9)*
*Tourette's syndrome (F95.2)*

✓5th **G25.7 Other and unspecified drug induced movement disorders**
Use additional code for adverse effect, if applicable, to identify drug (T36-T5Ø with fifth or sixth character 5)

**G25.7Ø Drug induced movement disorder, unspecified**

**G25.71 Drug induced akathisia**
Drug induced acathisia
Neuroleptic induced acute akathisia
Tardive akathisia

**G25.79 Other drug induced movement disorders**

✓5th **G25.8 Other specified extrapyramidal and movement disorders**

**G25.81 Restless legs syndrome**
**DEF:** Neurological disorder of unknown etiology creating an irresistible urge to move the legs, which may temporarily relieve the symptoms. This syndrome is accompanied by motor restlessness and sensations of pain, burning, prickling, or tingling.

**G25.82 Stiff-man syndrome**

**G25.83 Benign shuddering attacks**

**G25.89 Other specified extrapyramidal and movement disorders**

**G25.9 Extrapyramidal and movement disorder, unspecified**

***G26 Extrapyramidal and movement disorders in diseases classified elsewhere***
Code first underlying disease

## Other degenerative diseases of the nervous system (G30-G32)

**G30 Alzheimer's disease**

INCLUDES Alzheimer's dementia senile and presenile forms

Use additional code, if applicable, to identify:
- delirium, if applicable (F05)
- dementia with anxiety (F02.84, F02.A4, F02.B4, F02.C4)
- dementia with behavioral disturbance (F02.81-, F02.A1-, F02.B1-, F02.C1-)
- dementia with mood disturbance (F02.83, F02.A3, F02.B3, F02.C3)
- dementia with psychotic disturbance (F02.82, F02.A2, F02.B2, F02.C2)
- dementia without behavioral disturbance (F02.80, F02.A0, F02.B0, F02.C0)
- mild neurocognitive disorder due to known physiological condition (F06.7-)

EXCLUDES 1 *senile degeneration of brain NEC (G31.1)*
*senile dementia NOS (F03.-)*
*senility NOS (R41.81)*

**AHA:** 2022,4Q,15; 2017,1Q,43

**TIP:** A code from category F02 should always be assigned with a code from this category, even in the absence of documented dementia.

**TIP:** Functional quadriplegia (R53.2) is not integral to Alzheimer's disease and can be coded in addition to codes from category G30.

**G30.0 Alzheimer's disease with early onset** HCC Rx ESR

**G30.1 Alzheimer's disease with late onset** HCC Rx ESR A

**G30.8 Other Alzheimer's disease** HCC Rx ESR

**G30.9 Alzheimer's disease, unspecified** HCC Rx ESR

**AHA:** 2016,2Q,6; 2012,4Q,95

**G31 Other degenerative diseases of nervous system, not elsewhere classified**

Use additional code, if applicable, for codes G31.0-G31.83, G31.85-G31.9, to identify:
- dementia with anxiety (F02.84, F02.A4, F02.B4, F02.C4)
- dementia with behavioral disturbance (F02.81-, F02.A1-, F02.B1-, F02.C1-)
- dementia with mood disturbance (F02.83, F02.A3, F02.B3, F02.C3)
- dementia with psychotic disturbance (F02.82, F02.A2, F02.B2, F02.C2)
- dementia without behavioral disturbance (F02.80, F02.A0, F02.B0, F02.C0)
- mild neurocognitive disorder due to known physiological condition (F06.7-)

EXCLUDES 2 *Reye's syndrome (G93.7)*

**G31.0 Frontotemporal dementia**

**G31.01 Pick's disease** HCC Rx ESR

Primary progressive aphasia
Progressive isolated aphasia

**DEF:** Progressive frontotemporal dementia with asymmetrical atrophy of the frontal and temporal regions of the cerebral cortex and abnormal rounded brain cells called Pick cells with the presence of abnormal staining of protein (called tau). Symptoms include prominent apathy, behavioral changes such as disinhibition and restlessness, echolalia, impairment of language, memory, and intellect, increased carelessness, poor personal hygiene, and decreased attention span.

**G31.09 Other frontotemporal neurocognitive disorder** HCC Rx ESR

Frontal dementia

Use additional code, if applicable, to identify mild neurocognitive disorders due to known physiological condition (F06.7-)

**G31.1 Senile degeneration of brain, not elsewhere classified** Rx ESR

EXCLUDES 1 *Alzheimer's disease (G30.-)*
*senility NOS (R41.81)*

**G31.2 Degeneration of nervous system due to alcohol** Rx ESR

Alcoholic cerebellar ataxia
Alcoholic cerebellar degeneration
Alcoholic cerebral degeneration
Alcoholic encephalopathy
Dysfunction of the autonomic nervous system due to alcohol

Code also associated alcoholism (F10.-)

**G31.8 Other specified degenerative diseases of nervous system**

**G31.80 Leukodystrophy, unspecified** HCC ESR COM

**AHA:** 2023,4Q,12-13

**G31.81 Alpers disease** HCC Rx ESR COM

Grey-matter degeneration

**G31.82 Leigh's disease** HCC Rx ESR COM

Subacute necrotizing encephalopathy

**G31.83 Neurocognitive disorder with Lewy bodies** HCC Rx ESR

Lewy body dementia
Lewy body disease

Use additional code, if applicable, to identify mild neurocognitive disorders due to known physiological condition (F06.7-)

**AHA:** 2017,2Q,7; 2016,4Q,141

**DEF:** Cerebral dementia with neurophysiologic changes, increased hippocampal volume, hypoperfusion in the occipital lobes, beta amyloid deposits with neurofibrillary tangles, and atrophy of the cortex and brainstem. Hallmark neuropsychological characteristics include fluctuating cognition with pronounced variation in attention and alertness, recurrent hallucinations, and Parkinsonism.

**G31.84 Mild cognitive impairment of uncertain or unknown etiology**

Mild cognitive disorder NOS
Mild neurocognitive disorder of uncertain or unknown etiology

Use additional code to identify presence of:
- alcohol abuse and dependence (F10.-)
- exposure to environmental tobacco smoke (Z77.22)
- history of tobacco dependence (Z87.891)
- hypertension (I10-I1A)
- occupational exposure to environmental tobacco smoke (Z57.31)
- tobacco dependence (F17.-)
- tobacco use (Z72.0)

EXCLUDES 1 *age related cognitive decline (R41.81)*
*altered mental status (R41.82)*
*cerebral degeneration (G31.9)*
*cerebrovascular diseases (I60-I69)*
*change in mental status (R41.82)*
*cognitive deficits following (sequelae of) cerebral hemorrhage or infarction (I69.01-, I69.11-, I69.21-, I69.31-, I69.81-, I69.91-)*
*cognitive impairment due to intracranial or head injury (S06.-)*
*dementia (F01.-, F02.-, F03.-)*
*mild neurocognitive disorder due to a known physiological condition (F06.7-)*
*neurologic neglect syndrome (R41.4)*
*personality change, nonpsychotic (F68.8)*

**AHA:** 2021,3Q,3

**G31.85 Corticobasal degeneration** Rx ESR

**G31.86 Alexander disease** HCC Rx ESR COM

**AHA:** 2023,4Q,12-13

**G31.87 Primary progressive apraxia of speech** Rx ESR

**G31.89 Other specified degenerative diseases of nervous system** Rx ESR

**G31.9 Degenerative disease of nervous system, unspecified** Rx ESR

**AHA:** 2021,3Q,3

**G32 Other degenerative disorders of nervous system in diseases classified elsewhere**

***G32.0 Subacute combined degeneration of spinal cord in diseases classified elsewhere*** HCC Rx ESR COM

Dana-Putnam syndrome
Sclerosis of spinal cord (combined) (dorsolateral) (posterolateral)

Code first underlying disease, such as:
- other dietary vitamin B12 deficiency anemia (D51.3)
- vitamin B12 deficiency (E53.8)
- vitamin B12 deficiency anemia due to intrinsic factor deficiency (D51.0)
- vitamin B12 deficiency anemia, unspecified (D51.8)

EXCLUDES 1 *syphilitic combined degeneration of spinal cord (A52.11)*

✓5th **G32.8 Other specified degenerative disorders of nervous system in diseases classified elsewhere**
Code first underlying disease, such as:
amyloidosis cerebral degeneration (E85.-)
cerebral degeneration (due to) hypothyroidism (E00.0-E03.9)
cerebral degeneration (due to) neoplasm (C00-D49)
cerebral degeneration (due to) vitamin B deficiency, except thiamine (E52-E53.-)
EXCLUDES 1 *superior hemorrhagic polioencephalitis [Wernicke's encephalopathy] (E51.2)*

***G32.81 Cerebellar ataxia in diseases classified elsewhere*** HCC ESR COM
Code first underlying disease, such as:
celiac disease (with gluten ataxia) (K90.0)
cerebellar ataxia (in) neoplastic disease (paraneoplastic cerebellar degeneration) (C00-D49)
non-celiac gluten ataxia (M35.9)
EXCLUDES 1 *systemic atrophy primarily affecting the central nervous system in alcoholic cerebellar ataxia (G31.2)*
*systemic atrophy primarily affecting the central nervous system in myxedema (G13.2)*

***G32.89 Other specified degenerative disorders of nervous system in diseases classified elsewhere***
Degenerative encephalopathy in diseases classified elsewhere

## Demyelinating diseases of the central nervous system (G35-G37)

✓4th **G35 Multiple sclerosis**
AHA: 2021,1Q,7

**G35.A Relapsing-remitting multiple sclerosis** HCC Rx ESR
EXCLUDES 1 *demyelinating disease of central nervous system, unspecified (G37.9)*

✓5th **G35.B Primary progressive multiple sclerosis**

**G35.B0 Primary progressive multiple sclerosis, unspecified** HCC Rx ESR

**G35.B1 Active primary progressive multiple sclerosis** HCC Rx ESR
Primary progressive multiple sclerosis with evidence of inflammatory disease activity

**G35.B2 Non-active primary progressive multiple sclerosis** HCC Rx ESR
Primary progressive multiple sclerosis without evidence of inflammatory disease activity

✓5th **G35.C Secondary progressive multiple sclerosis**

**G35.C0 Secondary progressive multiple sclerosis, unspecified** HCC Rx ESR

**G35.C1 Active secondary progressive multiple sclerosis** HCC Rx ESR
Secondary progressive multiple sclerosis with evidence of inflammatory disease activity

**G35.C2 Non-active secondary progressive multiple sclerosis** HCC Rx ESR
Secondary progressive multiple sclerosis without evidence of inflammatory disease activity

**G35.D Multiple sclerosis, unspecified** HCC Rx ESR
Disseminated multiple sclerosis
Generalized multiple sclerosis
Multiple sclerosis of brain stem
Multiple sclerosis of cord
Multiple sclerosis NOS

✓4th **G36 Other acute disseminated demyelination**
EXCLUDES 1 *postinfectious encephalitis and encephalomyelitis NOS (G04.01)*
**DEF:** Demyelination: Abnormal loss of myelin, the protective white matter that insulates nerve endings and facilitates neuroreception and neurotransmission. When this substance is damaged, the nerve is short-circuited, resulting in impaired or loss of function.

**G36.0 Neuromyelitis optica [Devic]** HCC Rx ESR COM
Demyelination in optic neuritis
EXCLUDES 1 ~~*optic neuritis NOS (H46)*~~
EXCLUDES 2 ▶*optic neuritis NOS (H46)*◀

**G36.1 Acute and subacute hemorrhagic leukoencephalitis [Hurst]** HCC ESR

**G36.8 Other specified acute disseminated demyelination** HCC ESR

**G36.9 Acute disseminated demyelination, unspecified** HCC ESR

✓4th **G37 Other demyelinating diseases of central nervous system**

**G37.0 Diffuse sclerosis of central nervous system** HCC Rx ESR COM
Periaxial encephalitis
Schilder's disease
EXCLUDES 1 *X linked adrenoleukodystrophy (E71.52-)*

**G37.1 Central demyelination of corpus callosum** HCC ESR

**G37.2 Central pontine myelinolysis** HCC ESR
AHA: 2022,2Q,10

**G37.3 Acute transverse myelitis in demyelinating disease of central nervous system** HCC Rx ESR COM
Acute transverse myelitis NOS
Acute transverse myelopathy
EXCLUDES 1 *acute flaccid myelitis (G04.82)*
*multiple sclerosis (G35-)*
*neuromyelitis optica [Devic] (G36.0)*

**G37.4 Subacute necrotizing myelitis of central nervous system** HCC Rx ESR COM

**G37.5 Concentric sclerosis [Balo] of central nervous system** HCC Rx ESR COM

✓5th **G37.8 Other specified demyelinating diseases of central nervous system**
AHA: 2023,4Q,18

**G37.81 Myelin oligodendrocyte glycoprotein antibody disease** HCC ESR
MOG antibody disease
Code also associated manifestations, if known, such as:
neuromyelitis optica (G36.0)
noninfectious acute disseminated encephalomyelitis (G04.81)

**G37.89 Other specified demyelinating diseases of central nervous system** HCC ESR

**G37.9 Demyelinating disease of central nervous system, unspecified** HCC ESR
Clinically isolated syndromes

## Episodic and paroxysmal disorders (G40-G47)

✓4th **G40 Epilepsy and recurrent seizures**
NOTE The following terms are to be considered equivalent to intractable: pharmacoresistant (pharmacologically resistant), treatment resistant, refractory (medically) and poorly controlled
EXCLUDES 1 *conversion disorder with seizures (F44.5)*
*convulsions NOS (R56.9)*
*post traumatic seizures (R56.1)*
*seizure (convulsive) NOS (R56.9)*
*seizure of newborn (P90)*
EXCLUDES 2 *hippocampal sclerosis (G93.81)*
*mesial temporal sclerosis (G93.81)*
*temporal sclerosis (G93.81)*
*Todd's paralysis (G83.84)*

✓5th **G40.0 Localization-related (focal) (partial) idiopathic epilepsy and epileptic syndromes with seizures of localized onset**
Benign childhood epilepsy with centrotemporal EEG spikes
Childhood epilepsy with occipital EEG paroxysms
EXCLUDES 1 *adult onset localization-related epilepsy (G40.1-, G40.2-)*

✓6th **G40.00 Localization-related (focal) (partial) idiopathic epilepsy and epileptic syndromes with seizures of localized onset, not intractable**
Localization-related (focal) (partial) idiopathic epilepsy and epileptic syndromes with seizures of localized onset without intractability

**G40.001 Localization-related (focal) (partial) idiopathic epilepsy and epileptic syndromes with seizures of localized onset, not intractable, with status epilepticus** HCC Rx ESR COM

**G40.009 Localization-related (focal) (partial) idiopathic epilepsy and epileptic syndromes with seizures of localized onset, not intractable, without status epilepticus** HCC Rx ESR COM
Localization-related (focal) (partial) idiopathic epilepsy and epileptic syndromes with seizures of localized onset NOS

✓6th **G40.01 Localization-related (focal) (partial) idiopathic epilepsy and epileptic syndromes with seizures of localized onset, intractable**

**G40.011 Localization-related (focal) (partial) idiopathic epilepsy and epileptic syndromes with seizures of localized onset, intractable, with status epilepticus** HCC Rx ESR COM

**G40.019 Localization-related (focal) (partial) idiopathic epilepsy and epileptic syndromes with seizures of localized onset, intractable, without status epilepticus** HCC Rx ESR COM

✓5th **G40.1 Localization-related (focal) (partial) symptomatic epilepsy and epileptic syndromes with simple partial seizures**

Attacks without alteration of consciousness
Epilepsia partialis continua [Kozhevnikof]
Simple partial seizures developing into secondarily generalized seizures

**AHA:** 2023,3Q,4

✓6th **G40.10 Localization-related (focal) (partial) symptomatic epilepsy and epileptic syndromes with simple partial seizures, not intractable**

Localization-related (focal) (partial) symptomatic epilepsy and epileptic syndromes with simple partial seizures without intractability

**G40.101 Localization-related (focal) (partial) symptomatic epilepsy and epileptic syndromes with simple partial seizures, not intractable, with status epilepticus** HCC Rx ESR COM

**G40.109 Localization-related (focal) (partial) symptomatic epilepsy and epileptic syndromes with simple partial seizures, not intractable, without status epilepticus** HCC Rx ESR COM

Localization-related (focal) (partial) symptomatic epilepsy and epileptic syndromes with simple partial seizures NOS

✓6th **G40.11 Localization-related (focal) (partial) symptomatic epilepsy and epileptic syndromes with simple partial seizures, intractable**

**G40.111 Localization-related (focal) (partial) symptomatic epilepsy and epileptic syndromes with simple partial seizures, intractable, with status epilepticus** HCC Rx ESR COM

**G40.119 Localization-related (focal) (partial) symptomatic epilepsy and epileptic syndromes with simple partial seizures, intractable, without status epilepticus** HCC Rx ESR COM

✓5th **G40.2 Localization-related (focal) (partial) symptomatic epilepsy and epileptic syndromes with complex partial seizures**

Attacks with alteration of consciousness, often with automatisms
Complex partial seizures developing into secondarily generalized seizures

✓6th **G40.20 Localization-related (focal) (partial) symptomatic epilepsy and epileptic syndromes with complex partial seizures, not intractable**

Localization-related (focal) (partial) symptomatic epilepsy and epileptic syndromes with complex partial seizures without intractability

**G40.201 Localization-related (focal) (partial) symptomatic epilepsy and epileptic syndromes with complex partial seizures, not intractable, with status epilepticus** HCC Rx ESR COM

**G40.209 Localization-related (focal) (partial) symptomatic epilepsy and epileptic syndromes with complex partial seizures, not intractable, without status epilepticus** HCC Rx ESR COM

Localization-related (focal) (partial) symptomatic epilepsy and epileptic syndromes with complex partial seizures NOS

✓6th **G40.21 Localization-related (focal) (partial) symptomatic epilepsy and epileptic syndromes with complex partial seizures, intractable**

**G40.211 Localization-related (focal) (partial) symptomatic epilepsy and epileptic syndromes with complex partial seizures, intractable, with status epilepticus** HCC Rx ESR COM

**G40.219 Localization-related (focal) (partial) symptomatic epilepsy and epileptic syndromes with complex partial seizures, intractable, without status epilepticus** HCC Rx ESR COM

✓5th **G40.3 Generalized idiopathic epilepsy and epileptic syndromes**

Code also MERRF syndrome, if applicable (E88.42)

✓6th **G40.30 Generalized idiopathic epilepsy and epileptic syndromes, not intractable**

Generalized idiopathic epilepsy and epileptic syndromes without intractability

**G40.301 Generalized idiopathic epilepsy and epileptic syndromes, not intractable, with status epilepticus** HCC Rx ESR COM

**G40.309 Generalized idiopathic epilepsy and epileptic syndromes, not intractable, without status epilepticus** HCC Rx ESR COM

Generalized idiopathic epilepsy and epileptic syndromes NOS

✓6th **G40.31 Generalized idiopathic epilepsy and epileptic syndromes, intractable**

**G40.311 Generalized idiopathic epilepsy and epileptic syndromes, intractable, with status epilepticus** HCC Rx ESR COM

**G40.319 Generalized idiopathic epilepsy and epileptic syndromes, intractable, without status epilepticus** HCC Rx ESR COM

✓5th **G40.A Absence epileptic syndrome**

Absence epileptic syndrome, NOS
Childhood absence epilepsy [pyknolepsy]
Juvenile absence epilepsy

✓6th **G40.A0 Absence epileptic syndrome, not intractable**

**G40.A01 Absence epileptic syndrome, not intractable, with status epilepticus** HCC Rx ESR COM

**G40.A09 Absence epileptic syndrome, not intractable, without status epilepticus** HCC Rx ESR COM

✓6th **G40.A1 Absence epileptic syndrome, intractable**

**G40.A11 Absence epileptic syndrome, intractable, with status epilepticus** HCC Rx ESR COM

**G40.A19 Absence epileptic syndrome, intractable, without status epilepticus** HCC Rx ESR COM

✓5th **G40.B Juvenile myoclonic epilepsy [impulsive petit mal]**

✓6th **G40.B0 Juvenile myoclonic epilepsy, not intractable**

**G40.B01 Juvenile myoclonic epilepsy, not intractable, with status epilepticus** HCC Rx ESR COM

**G40.B09 Juvenile myoclonic epilepsy, not intractable, without status epilepticus** HCC Rx ESR COM

✓6th **G40.B1 Juvenile myoclonic epilepsy, intractable**

**G40.B11 Juvenile myoclonic epilepsy, intractable, with status epilepticus** HCC Rx ESR COM

**G40.B19 Juvenile myoclonic epilepsy, intractable, without status epilepticus** HCC Rx ESR COM

✓5th **G40.C Lafora progressive myoclonus epilepsy**

Lafora body disease
Code also, if applicable, associated conditions such as dementia (F02.8-)

**AHA:** 2023,4Q,18-19

✓6th **G40.C0 Lafora progressive myoclonus epilepsy, not intractable**

**G40.C01 Lafora progressive myoclonus epilepsy, not intractable, with status epilepticus** HCC Rx ESR COM

**G40.C09 Lafora progressive myoclonus epilepsy, not intractable, without status epilepticus** HCC Rx ESR COM
Lafora progressive myoclonus epilepsy NOS

√6th **G40.C1 Lafora progressive myoclonus epilepsy, intractable**

**G40.C11 Lafora progressive myoclonus epilepsy, intractable, with status epilepticus** HCC Rx ESR COM

**G40.C19 Lafora progressive myoclonus epilepsy, intractable, without status epilepticus** HCC Rx ESR COM

√5th **G40.4 Other generalized epilepsy and epileptic syndromes**
Epilepsy with grand mal seizures on awakening
Epilepsy with myoclonic absences
Epilepsy with myoclonic-astatic seizures
Grand mal seizure NOS
Nonspecific atonic epileptic seizures
Nonspecific clonic epileptic seizures
Nonspecific myoclonic epileptic seizures
Nonspecific tonic epileptic seizures
Nonspecific tonic-clonic epileptic seizures
Symptomatic early myoclonic encephalopathy

√6th **G40.40 Other generalized epilepsy and epileptic syndromes, not intractable**
Other generalized epilepsy and epileptic syndromes NOS
Other generalized epilepsy and epileptic syndromes without intractability

**G40.401 Other generalized epilepsy and epileptic syndromes, not intractable, with status epilepticus** HCC Rx ESR COM

**G40.409 Other generalized epilepsy and epileptic syndromes, not intractable, without status epilepticus** HCC Rx ESR COM

√6th **G40.41 Other generalized epilepsy and epileptic syndromes, intractable**

**G40.411 Other generalized epilepsy and epileptic syndromes, intractable, with status epilepticus** HCC Rx ESR COM

**G40.419 Other generalized epilepsy and epileptic syndromes, intractable, without status epilepticus** HCC Rx ESR COM

**G40.42 Cyclin-Dependent Kinase-Like 5 Deficiency Disorder** HCC Rx ESR COM
CDKL5
Use additional code, if known, to identify associated manifestations, such as:
cortical blindness (H47.61-)
global development delay (F88)
**AHA:** 2020,4Q,18-19

√5th **G40.5 Epileptic seizures related to external causes**
Epileptic seizures related to alcohol
Epileptic seizures related to drugs
Epileptic seizures related to hormonal changes
Epileptic seizures related to sleep deprivation
Epileptic seizures related to stress
Code also, if applicable, associated epilepsy and recurrent seizures (G40.-)
Use additional code for adverse effect, if applicable, to identify drug (T36-T50 with fifth or sixth character 5)

√6th **G40.50 Epileptic seizures related to external causes, not intractable**

**G40.501 Epileptic seizures related to external causes, not intractable, with status epilepticus** HCC Rx ESR COM

**G40.509 Epileptic seizures related to external causes, not intractable, without status epilepticus** HCC Rx ESR COM
Epileptic seizures related to external causes, NOS

√5th **G40.8 Other epilepsy and recurrent seizures**
Epilepsies and epileptic syndromes undetermined as to whether they are focal or generalized
Landau-Kleffner syndrome

√6th **G40.80 Other epilepsy**

**G40.801 Other epilepsy, not intractable, with status epilepticus** HCC Rx ESR COM
Other epilepsy without intractability with status epilepticus

**G40.802 Other epilepsy, not intractable, without status epilepticus** HCC Rx ESR COM
Other epilepsy NOS
Other epilepsy without intractability without status epilepticus

**G40.803 Other epilepsy, intractable, with status epilepticus** HCC Rx ESR COM

**G40.804 Other epilepsy, intractable, without status epilepticus** HCC Rx ESR COM

√6th **G40.81 Lennox-Gastaut syndrome**
**DEF:** Severe form of epilepsy with usual onset in early childhood. Seizures are frequent and difficult to treat, causing falls and intellectual impairment.

**G40.811 Lennox-Gastaut syndrome, not intractable, with status epilepticus** HCC Rx ESR COM

**G40.812 Lennox-Gastaut syndrome, not intractable, without status epilepticus** HCC Rx ESR COM

**G40.813 Lennox-Gastaut syndrome, intractable, with status epilepticus** HCC Rx ESR COM

**G40.814 Lennox-Gastaut syndrome, intractable, without status epilepticus** HCC Rx ESR COM

√6th **G40.82 Epileptic spasms**
Infantile spasms
Salaam attacks
West's syndrome

**G40.821 Epileptic spasms, not intractable, with status epilepticus** HCC Rx ESR COM

**G40.822 Epileptic spasms, not intractable, without status epilepticus** HCC Rx ESR COM

**G40.823 Epileptic spasms, intractable, with status epilepticus** HCC Rx ESR COM

**G40.824 Epileptic spasms, intractable, without status epilepticus** HCC Rx ESR COM

√6th **G40.83 Dravet syndrome**
Polymorphic epilepsy in infancy (PMEI)
Severe myoclonic epilepsy in infancy (SMEI)
**AHA:** 2020,4Q,19

**G40.833 Dravet syndrome, intractable, with status epilepticus** HCC Rx ESR COM

**G40.834 Dravet syndrome, intractable, without status epilepticus** HCC Rx ESR COM
Dravet syndrome NOS

√6th **G40.84 KCNQ2-related epilepsy**
**AHA:** 2024,4Q,15

**G40.841 KCNQ2-related epilepsy, not intractable, with status epilepticus** HCC Rx ESR COM

**G40.842 KCNQ2-related epilepsy, not intractable, without status epilepticus** HCC Rx ESR COM
KCNQ2-related epilepsy NOS

**G40.843 KCNQ2-related epilepsy, intractable, with status epilepticus** HCC Rx ESR COM

**G40.844 KCNQ2-related epilepsy, intractable, without status epilepticus** HCC Rx ESR COM

**G40.89 Other seizures** HCC Rx ESR COM
EXCLUDES 1 *post traumatic seizures (R56.1)*
*recurrent seizures NOS (G40.909)*
*seizure NOS (R56.9)*

√5th **G40.9 Epilepsy, unspecified**
**AHA:** 2019,1Q,19

√6th **G40.90 Epilepsy, unspecified, not intractable**
Epilepsy, unspecified, without intractability

**G40.901 Epilepsy, unspecified, not intractable, with status epilepticus** HCC Rx ESR COM

**G40.909 Epilepsy, unspecified, not intractable, without status epilepticus** HCC Rx ESR COM
Epilepsy NOS
Epileptic convulsions NOS
Epileptic fits NOS
Epileptic seizures NOS
Recurrent seizures NOS
Seizure disorder NOS
**AHA:** 2024,2Q,8; 2021,2Q,3; 2021,1Q,3

√6th **G40.91 Epilepsy, unspecified, intractable**
Intractable seizure disorder NOS
**G40.911 Epilepsy, unspecified, intractable, with status epilepticus** HCC Rx ESR COM
**G40.919 Epilepsy, unspecified, intractable, without status epilepticus** HCC Rx ESR COM

√4th **G43 Migraine**

NOTE The following terms are to be considered equivalent to intractable: pharmacoresistant (pharmacologically resistant), treatment resistant, refractory (medically) and poorly controlled

Use additional code for adverse effect, if applicable, to identify drug (T36-T50 with fifth or sixth character 5)

EXCLUDES 1 ~~headache NOS (R51.9)~~
*lower half migraine (G44.00)*

EXCLUDES 2 ▶*headache NOS (R51.9)*◀
*headache syndromes (G44.-)*

**DEF:** Headaches that occur periodically on one or both sides of the head that may be associated with nausea and vomiting, sensitivity to light and sound, dizziness, distorted vision, and cognitive disturbances.

√5th **G43.0 Migraine without aura**
Common migraine
EXCLUDES 1 *chronic migraine without aura (G43.7-)*

√6th **G43.00 Migraine without aura, not intractable**
Migraine without aura without mention of refractory migraine
**G43.001 Migraine without aura, not intractable, with status migrainosus** Rx
**G43.009 Migraine without aura, not intractable, without status migrainosus** Rx
Migraine without aura NOS

√6th **G43.01 Migraine without aura, intractable**
Migraine without aura with refractory migraine
**G43.011 Migraine without aura, intractable, with status migrainosus** Rx
**G43.019 Migraine without aura, intractable, without status migrainosus** Rx

√5th **G43.1 Migraine with aura**
Basilar migraine
Classical migraine
Migraine equivalents
Migraine preceded or accompanied by transient focal neurological phenomena
Migraine triggered seizures
Migraine with acute-onset aura
Migraine with aura without headache (migraine equivalents)
Migraine with prolonged aura
Migraine with typical aura
Retinal migraine
Code also any associated seizure (G40.-, R56.9)
EXCLUDES 1 *chronic migraine with aura (G43.E-)*
*persistent migraine aura (G43.5-, G43.6-)*

√6th **G43.10 Migraine with aura, not intractable**
Migraine with aura without mention of refractory migraine
**G43.101 Migraine with aura, not intractable, with status migrainosus** Rx
**G43.109 Migraine with aura, not intractable, without status migrainosus** Rx
Migraine with aura NOS

√6th **G43.11 Migraine with aura, intractable**
Migraine with aura with refractory migraine
**G43.111 Migraine with aura, intractable, with status migrainosus** Rx
**G43.119 Migraine with aura, intractable, without status migrainosus** Rx

√5th **G43.4 Hemiplegic migraine**
Familial migraine
Sporadic migraine
**AHA:** 2025,2Q,18

√6th **G43.40 Hemiplegic migraine, not intractable**
Hemiplegic migraine without refractory migraine
**G43.401 Hemiplegic migraine, not intractable, with status migrainosus** Rx
**G43.409 Hemiplegic migraine, not intractable, without status migrainosus** Rx
Hemiplegic migraine NOS

√6th **G43.41 Hemiplegic migraine, intractable**
Hemiplegic migraine with refractory migraine
**G43.411 Hemiplegic migraine, intractable, with status migrainosus** Rx
**G43.419 Hemiplegic migraine, intractable, without status migrainosus** Rx

√5th **G43.5 Persistent migraine aura without cerebral infarction**

√6th **G43.50 Persistent migraine aura without cerebral infarction, not intractable**
Persistent migraine aura without cerebral infarction, without refractory migraine
**G43.501 Persistent migraine aura without cerebral infarction, not intractable, with status migrainosus** Rx
**G43.509 Persistent migraine aura without cerebral infarction, not intractable, without status migrainosus** Rx
Persistent migraine aura NOS

√6th **G43.51 Persistent migraine aura without cerebral infarction, intractable**
Persistent migraine aura without cerebral infarction, with refractory migraine
**G43.511 Persistent migraine aura without cerebral infarction, intractable, with status migrainosus** Rx
**G43.519 Persistent migraine aura without cerebral infarction, intractable, without status migrainosus** Rx

√5th **G43.6 Persistent migraine aura with cerebral infarction**
Code also the type of cerebral infarction (I63.-)

√6th **G43.60 Persistent migraine aura with cerebral infarction, not intractable**
Persistent migraine aura with cerebral infarction, without refractory migraine
**G43.601 Persistent migraine aura with cerebral infarction, not intractable, with status migrainosus** Rx
**G43.609 Persistent migraine aura with cerebral infarction, not intractable, without status migrainosus** Rx

√6th **G43.61 Persistent migraine aura with cerebral infarction, intractable**
Persistent migraine aura with cerebral infarction, with refractory migraine
**G43.611 Persistent migraine aura with cerebral infarction, intractable, with status migrainosus** Rx
**G43.619 Persistent migraine aura with cerebral infarction, intractable, without status migrainosus** Rx

√5th **G43.7 Chronic migraine without aura**
Transformed migraine
EXCLUDES 1 *migraine without aura (G43.0-)*

√6th **G43.70 Chronic migraine without aura, not intractable**
Chronic migraine without aura, without refractory migraine
**G43.701 Chronic migraine without aura, not intractable, with status migrainosus** Rx
**G43.709 Chronic migraine without aura, not intractable, without status migrainosus** Rx
Chronic migraine without aura NOS

√6th **G43.71 Chronic migraine without aura, intractable**
Chronic migraine without aura, with refractory migraine
**G43.711 Chronic migraine without aura, intractable, with status migrainosus** Rx
**G43.719 Chronic migraine without aura, intractable, without status migrainosus** Rx

√5th **G43.A Cyclical vomiting**
EXCLUDES 1 *cyclical vomiting syndrome unrelated to migraine (R11.15)*
**AHA:** 2019,4Q,15
**G43.A0 Cyclical vomiting, in migraine, not intractable** Rx
Cyclical vomiting, without refractory migraine
**G43.A1 Cyclical vomiting, in migraine, intractable** Rx
Cyclical vomiting, with refractory migraine

√5th **G43.B Ophthalmoplegic migraine**

**G43.B0 Ophthalmoplegic migraine, not intractable** Rx
Ophthalmoplegic migraine, without refractory migraine

**G43.B1 Ophthalmoplegic migraine, intractable** Rx
Ophthalmoplegic migraine, with refractory migraine

√5th **G43.C Periodic headache syndromes in child or adult**

**G43.C0 Periodic headache syndromes in child or adult, not intractable** Rx
Periodic headache syndromes in child or adult, without refractory migraine

**G43.C1 Periodic headache syndromes in child or adult, intractable** Rx
Periodic headache syndromes in child or adult, with refractory migraine

√5th **G43.D Abdominal migraine**

**G43.D0 Abdominal migraine, not intractable** Rx
Abdominal migraine, without refractory migraine

**G43.D1 Abdominal migraine, intractable** Rx
Abdominal migraine, with refractory migraine

√5th **G43.8 Other migraine**

√6th **G43.80 Other migraine, not intractable**
Other migraine, without refractory migraine

**G43.801 Other migraine, not intractable, with status migrainosus** Rx

**G43.809 Other migraine, not intractable, without status migrainosus** Rx

√6th **G43.81 Other migraine, intractable**
Other migraine, with refractory migraine

**G43.811 Other migraine, intractable, with status migrainosus** Rx

**G43.819 Other migraine, intractable, without status migrainosus** Rx

√6th **G43.82 Menstrual migraine, not intractable**
Menstrual headache, not intractable
Menstrual migraine, without refractory migraine
Menstrually related migraine, not intractable
Pre-menstrual headache, not intractable
Pre-menstrual migraine, not intractable
Pure menstrual migraine, not intractable
Code also associated premenstrual tension syndrome (N94.3)

**G43.821 Menstrual migraine, not intractable, with status migrainosus** Rx

**G43.829 Menstrual migraine, not intractable, without status migrainosus** Rx
Menstrual migraine NOS

√6th **G43.83 Menstrual migraine, intractable**
Menstrual headache, intractable
Menstrual migraine, with refractory migraine
Menstrually related migraine, intractable
Pre-menstrual headache, intractable
Pre-menstrual migraine, intractable
Pure menstrual migraine, intractable
Code also associated premenstrual tension syndrome (N94.3)

**G43.831 Menstrual migraine, intractable, with status migrainosus** Rx

**G43.839 Menstrual migraine, intractable, without status migrainosus** Rx

√5th **G43.9 Migraine, unspecified**

√6th **G43.90 Migraine, unspecified, not intractable**
Migraine, unspecified, without refractory migraine

**G43.901 Migraine, unspecified, not intractable, with status migrainosus** Rx
Status migrainosus NOS

**G43.909 Migraine, unspecified, not intractable, without status migrainosus** Rx
Migraine NOS

√6th **G43.91 Migraine, unspecified, intractable**
Migraine, unspecified, with refractory migraine

**G43.911 Migraine, unspecified, intractable, with status migrainosus** Rx

**G43.919 Migraine, unspecified, intractable, without status migrainosus** Rx

√5th **G43.E Chronic migraine with aura**
EXCLUDES 1 *migraine with aura (G43.1-)*
AHA: 2023,4Q,19-20

√6th **G43.E0 Chronic migraine with aura, not intractable**
Chronic migraine with aura, without refractory migraine

**G43.E01 Chronic migraine with aura, not intractable, with status migrainosus** Rx

**G43.E09 Chronic migraine with aura, not intractable, without status migrainosus** Rx
Chronic migraine with aura NOS

√6th **G43.E1 Chronic migraine with aura, intractable**
Chronic migraine with aura, with refractory migraine

**G43.E11 Chronic migraine with aura, intractable, with status migrainosus** Rx

**G43.E19 Chronic migraine with aura, intractable, without status migrainosus** Rx

√4th **G44 Other headache syndromes**
EXCLUDES 1 *headache NOS (R51.9)*
EXCLUDES 2 *atypical facial pain (G50.1)*
*headache due to lumbar puncture (G97.1)*
*migraines (G43.-)*
*trigeminal neuralgia (G50.0)*

√5th **G44.0 Cluster headaches and other trigeminal autonomic cephalgias (TAC)**
DEF: Cluster headache: Characteristic grouping or clustering of headaches that can last for a number of weeks or months and then completely disappear for months or years. They are typically not associated with gastrointestinal upset or light sensitivity as experienced in migraines.

√6th **G44.00 Cluster headache syndrome, unspecified**
Ciliary neuralgia
Cluster headache NOS
Histamine cephalgia
Lower half migraine
Migrainous neuralgia

**G44.001 Cluster headache syndrome, unspecified, intractable**

**G44.009 Cluster headache syndrome, unspecified, not intractable**
Cluster headache syndrome NOS

√6th **G44.01 Episodic cluster headache**

**G44.011 Episodic cluster headache, intractable**

**G44.019 Episodic cluster headache, not intractable**
Episodic cluster headache NOS

√6th **G44.02 Chronic cluster headache**

**G44.021 Chronic cluster headache, intractable**

**G44.029 Chronic cluster headache, not intractable**
Chronic cluster headache NOS

√6th **G44.03 Episodic paroxysmal hemicrania**
Paroxysmal hemicrania NOS

**G44.031 Episodic paroxysmal hemicrania, intractable**

**G44.039 Episodic paroxysmal hemicrania, not intractable**
Episodic paroxysmal hemicrania NOS

√6th **G44.04 Chronic paroxysmal hemicrania**

**G44.041 Chronic paroxysmal hemicrania, intractable**

**G44.049 Chronic paroxysmal hemicrania, not intractable**
Chronic paroxysmal hemicrania NOS

√6th **G44.05 Short lasting unilateral neuralgiform headache with conjunctival injection and tearing (SUNCT)**

**G44.051 Short lasting unilateral neuralgiform headache with conjunctival injection and tearing (SUNCT), intractable**

**G44.059 Short lasting unilateral neuralgiform headache with conjunctival injection and tearing (SUNCT), not intractable**
Short lasting unilateral neuralgiform headache with conjunctival injection and tearing (SUNCT) NOS

√6th **G44.09 Other trigeminal autonomic cephalgias (TAC)**

**G44.091 Other trigeminal autonomic cephalgias (TAC), intractable**

**G44.099 Other trigeminal autonomic cephalgias (TAC), not intractable**

G44.1 Vascular headache, not elsewhere classified
EXCLUDES 2 *cluster headache (G44.Ø)*
*complicated headache syndromes (G44.5-)*
*drug-induced headache (G44.4-)*
*migraine (G43.-)*
*other specified headache syndromes (G44.8-)*
*post-traumatic headache (G44.3-)*
*tension-type headache (G44.2-)*

✓5th G44.2 Tension-type headache
✓6th G44.2Ø Tension-type headache, unspecified
G44.2Ø1 Tension-type headache, unspecified, intractable
G44.2Ø9 Tension-type headache, unspecified, not intractable
Tension headache NOS
✓6th G44.21 Episodic tension-type headache
G44.211 Episodic tension-type headache, intractable
G44.219 Episodic tension-type headache, not intractable
Episodic tension-type headache NOS
✓6th G44.22 Chronic tension-type headache
G44.221 Chronic tension-type headache, intractable
G44.229 Chronic tension-type headache, not intractable
Chronic tension-type headache NOS

✓5th G44.3 Post-traumatic headache
✓6th G44.3Ø Post-traumatic headache, unspecified
G44.3Ø1 Post-traumatic headache, unspecified, intractable
G44.3Ø9 Post-traumatic headache, unspecified, not intractable
Post-traumatic headache NOS
✓6th G44.31 Acute post-traumatic headache
G44.311 Acute post-traumatic headache, intractable
G44.319 Acute post-traumatic headache, not intractable
Acute post-traumatic headache NOS
✓6th G44.32 Chronic post-traumatic headache
G44.321 Chronic post-traumatic headache, intractable
G44.329 Chronic post-traumatic headache, not intractable
Chronic post-traumatic headache NOS

✓5th G44.4 Drug-induced headache, not elsewhere classified
Medication overuse headache
Use additional code for adverse effect, if applicable, to identify drug (T36-T5Ø with fifth or sixth character 5)
G44.4Ø Drug-induced headache, not elsewhere classified, not intractable
G44.41 Drug-induced headache, not elsewhere classified, intractable

✓5th G44.5 Complicated headache syndromes
G44.51 Hemicrania continua
**DEF:** Persistent primary headache of unknown causation occurring on one side of the face and head. May last for more than three months, with daily and continuous pain of moderate intensity with severe exacerbations.
G44.52 New daily persistent headache (NDPH)
G44.53 Primary thunderclap headache
G44.59 Other complicated headache syndrome

✓5th G44.8 Other specified headache syndromes
EXCLUDES 2 *headache with orthostatic or positional component, not elsewhere classifed (R51.Ø)*
G44.81 Hypnic headache
G44.82 Headache associated with sexual activity
Orgasmic headache
Preorgasmic headache
G44.83 Primary cough headache
G44.84 Primary exertional headache
G44.85 Primary stabbing headache
G44.86 Cervicogenic headache
Code also associated cervical spinal condition, if known
**AHA:** 2021,4Q,11-12
G44.89 Other headache syndrome

✓4th G45 Transient cerebral ischemic attacks and related syndromes
EXCLUDES 1 *neonatal cerebral ischemia (P91.Ø)*
*transient retinal artery occlusion (H34.Ø-)*
**AHA:** 2023,1Q,37; 2018,2Q,9
**DEF:** Transient cerebral ischemic attack: Intermittent or brief cerebral dysfunction from lack of oxygenation with no persistent neurological deficits associated with occlusive vascular disease. TIA may denote an impending cerebrovascular accident.
G45.Ø Vertebro-basilar artery syndrome
G45.1 Carotid artery syndrome (hemispheric)
G45.2 Multiple and bilateral precerebral artery syndromes
G45.3 Amaurosis fugax
G45.4 Transient global amnesia
EXCLUDES 1 *amnesia NOS (R41.3)*
G45.8 Other transient cerebral ischemic attacks and related syndromes
G45.9 Transient cerebral ischemic attack, unspecified
Spasm of cerebral artery
TIA
Transient cerebral ischemia NOS

✓4th G46 Vascular syndromes of brain in cerebrovascular diseases
Code first underlying cerebrovascular disease (I6Ø-I69)
G46.Ø Middle cerebral artery syndrome
G46.1 Anterior cerebral artery syndrome
G46.2 Posterior cerebral artery syndrome
G46.3 Brain stem stroke syndrome
Benedikt syndrome
Claude syndrome
Foville syndrome
Millard-Gubler syndrome
Wallenberg syndrome
Weber syndrome
G46.4 Cerebellar stroke syndrome
G46.5 Pure motor lacunar syndrome
G46.6 Pure sensory lacunar syndrome
G46.7 Other lacunar syndromes
G46.8 Other vascular syndromes of brain in cerebrovascular diseases

✓4th G47 Sleep disorders
EXCLUDES 2 *nightmares (F51.5)*
*nonorganic sleep disorders (F51.-)*
*sleep terrors (F51.4)*
*sleepwalking (F51.3)*
✓5th G47.Ø Insomnia
EXCLUDES 2 *alcohol related insomnia (F1Ø.182, F1Ø.282, F1Ø.982)*
*drug-related insomnia (F11.182, F11.282, F11.982, F13.182, F13.282, F13.982, F14.182, F14.282, F14.982, F15.182, F15.282, F15.982, F19.182, F19.282, F19.982)*
*idiopathic insomnia (F51.Ø1)*
*insomnia due to a mental disorder (F51.Ø5)*
*insomnia not due to a substance or known physiological condition (F51.Ø-)*
*nonorganic insomnia (F51.Ø-)*
*primary insomnia (F51.Ø1)*
*sleep apnea (G47.3-)*
G47.ØØ Insomnia, unspecified
Insomnia NOS
G47.Ø1 Insomnia due to medical condition
Code also associated medical condition
G47.Ø9 Other insomnia
✓5th G47.1 Hypersomnia
EXCLUDES 2 *alcohol-related hypersomnia (F1Ø.182, F1Ø.282, F1Ø.982)*
*drug-related hypersomnia (F11.182, F11.282, F11.982, F13.182, F13.282, F13.982, F14.182, F14.282, F14.982, F15.182, F15.282, F15.982, F19.182, F19.282, F19.982)*
*hypersomnia due to a mental disorder (F51.13)*
*hypersomnia not due to a substance or known physiological condition (F51.1-)*
*primary hypersomnia (F51.11)*
*sleep apnea (G47.3-)*
G47.1Ø Hypersomnia, unspecified
Hypersomnia NOS
G47.11 Idiopathic hypersomnia with long sleep time
Idiopathic hypersomnia NOS
G47.12 Idiopathic hypersomnia without long sleep time

**G47.13** **Recurrent hypersomnia**
Kleine-Levin syndrome
Menstrual related hypersomnia

**G47.14** **Hypersomnia due to medical condition**
Code also associated medical condition

**G47.19** **Other hypersomnia**

✓5th **G47.2** **Circadian rhythm sleep disorders**
Disorders of the sleep wake schedule
Inversion of nyctohemeral rhythm
Inversion of sleep rhythm
**DEF:** Circadian rhythm: Daily cycle (24-hour period) of physical, mental, and behavioral changes. It is largely influenced by environmental cues, such as changes in light or temperature.
***Synonym(s):*** *sleep/wake cycle.*

**G47.20** **Circadian rhythm sleep disorder, unspecified type**
Sleep wake schedule disorder NOS

**G47.21** **Circadian rhythm sleep disorder, delayed sleep phase type**
Delayed sleep phase syndrome

**G47.22** **Circadian rhythm sleep disorder, advanced sleep phase type**

**G47.23** **Circadian rhythm sleep disorder, irregular sleep wake type**
Irregular sleep-wake pattern

**G47.24** **Circadian rhythm sleep disorder, free running type**
Circadian rhythm sleep disorder, non-24-hour sleep-wake type

**G47.25** **Circadian rhythm sleep disorder, jet lag type**

**G47.26** **Circadian rhythm sleep disorder, shift work type**

***G47.27*** ***Circadian rhythm sleep disorder in conditions classified elsewhere***
Code first underlying condition

**G47.29** **Other circadian rhythm sleep disorder**

✓5th **G47.3** **Sleep apnea**
Code also any associated underlying condition
EXCLUDES 1 *apnea NOS (RØ6.81)*
*Cheyne-Stokes breathing (RØ6.3)*
*pickwickian syndrome (E66.2)*
*sleep apnea of newborn (P28.3-)*
**AHA:** 2025,3Q,16

**G47.3Ø** **Sleep apnea, unspecified**
Sleep apnea NOS

**G47.31** **Primary central sleep apnea**
Idiopathic central sleep apnea

**G47.32** **High altitude periodic breathing**

**G47.33** **Obstructive sleep apnea (adult) (pediatric)**
Obstructive sleep apnea hypopnea
EXCLUDES 1 *obstructive sleep apnea of newborn (P28.3-)*

**G47.34** **Idiopathic sleep related nonobstructive alveolar hypoventilation**
Sleep related hypoxia

**G47.35** **Congenital central alveolar hypoventilation syndrome**

***G47.36*** ***Sleep related hypoventilation in conditions classified elsewhere***
Sleep related hypoxemia in conditions classified elsewhere
Code first underlying condition

***G47.37*** ***Central sleep apnea in conditions classified elsewhere***
Code first underlying condition

**G47.39** **Other sleep apnea**

✓5th **G47.4** **Narcolepsy and cataplexy**

✓6th **G47.41** **Narcolepsy**

**G47.411** **Narcolepsy with cataplexy** Rx COM

**G47.419** **Narcolepsy without cataplexy** Rx COM
Narcolepsy NOS

✓6th **G47.42** **Narcolepsy in conditions classified elsewhere**
Code first underlying condition

***G47.421*** ***Narcolepsy in conditions classified elsewhere with cataplexy*** Rx COM

***G47.429*** ***Narcolepsy in conditions classified elsewhere without cataplexy*** Rx COM

✓5th **G47.5** **Parasomnia**
EXCLUDES 1 *alcohol induced parasomnia (F1Ø.182, F1Ø.282, F1Ø.982)*
*drug induced parasomnia (F11.182, F11.282, F11.982, F13.182, F13.282, F13.982, F14.182, F14.282, F14.982, F15.182, F15.282, F15.982, F19.182, F19.282, F19.982)*
*parasomnia not due to a substance or known physiological condition (F51.8)*

**G47.5Ø** **Parasomnia, unspecified**
Parasomnia NOS

**G47.51** **Confusional arousals**

**G47.52** **REM sleep behavior disorder**

**G47.53** **Recurrent isolated sleep paralysis**

***G47.54*** ***Parasomnia in conditions classified elsewhere***
Code first underlying condition

**G47.59** **Other parasomnia**

✓5th **G47.6** **Sleep related movement disorders**
EXCLUDES 2 *restless legs syndrome (G25.81)*

**G47.61** **Periodic limb movement disorder**

**G47.62** **Sleep related leg cramps**

**G47.63** **Sleep related bruxism**
EXCLUDES 1 *psychogenic bruxism (F45.8)*

**G47.69** **Other sleep related movement disorders**

**G47.8** **Other sleep disorders**
Other specified sleep-wake disorder

**G47.9** **Sleep disorder, unspecified**
Sleep disorder NOS
Unspecified sleep-wake disorder

## Nerve, nerve root and plexus disorders (G5Ø-G59)

EXCLUDES 1 *current traumatic nerve, nerve root and plexus disorders - see Injury, nerve by body region*
*neuralgia NOS (M79.2)*
*neuritis NOS (M79.2)*
*peripheral neuritis in pregnancy (O26.82-)*
*radiculitis NOS (M54.1-)*

✓4th **G5Ø** **Disorders of trigeminal nerve**
INCLUDES disorders of 5th cranial nerve

**Trigeminal and Facial Nerve Branches**

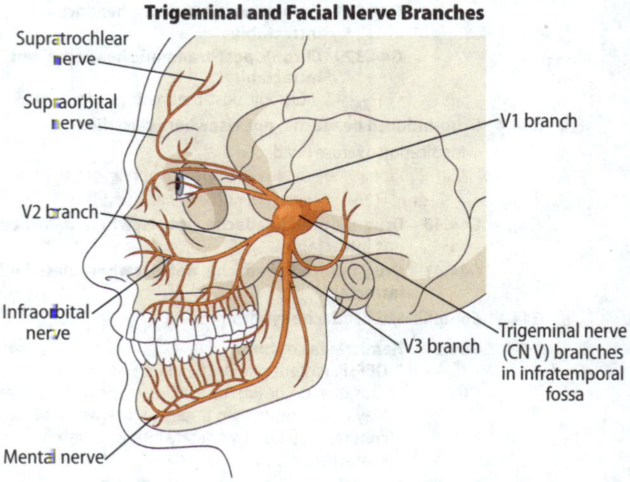


**G5Ø.Ø** **Trigeminal neuralgia** Rx
Syndrome of paroxysmal facial pain
Tic douloureux

**G5Ø.1** **Atypical facial pain** Rx

**G5Ø.8** **Other disorders of trigeminal nerve** Rx

**G5Ø.9** **Disorder of trigeminal nerve, unspecified** Rx

✓4th **G51** **Facial nerve disorders**
INCLUDES disorders of 7th cranial nerve

**G51.Ø** **Bell's palsy**
Facial palsy

**G51.1** **Geniculate ganglionitis**
EXCLUDES 1 *postherpetic geniculate ganglionitis (BØ2.21)*

**G51.2** **Melkersson's syndrome**
Melkersson-Rosenthal syndrome

✓5th **G51.3** **Clonic hemifacial spasm**
**AHA:** 2018,4Q,10

**G51.31** **Clonic hemifacial spasm, right**

G51.32 Clonic hemifacial spasm, left
G51.33 Clonic hemifacial spasm, bilateral
G51.39 Clonic hemifacial spasm, unspecified
G51.4 Facial myokymia
G51.8 Other disorders of facial nerve
G51.9 Disorder of facial nerve, unspecified

**✓4th G52 Disorders of other cranial nerves**
EXCLUDES 2 *disorders of acoustic [8th] nerve (H93.3)*
*disorders of optic [2nd] nerve (H46, H47.0)*
*paralytic strabismus due to nerve palsy (H49.0-H49.2)*

G52.0 Disorders of olfactory nerve
Disorders of 1st cranial nerve
G52.1 Disorders of glossopharyngeal nerve
Disorder of 9th cranial nerve
Glossopharyngeal neuralgia
G52.2 Disorders of vagus nerve
Disorders of pneumogastric [10th] nerve
G52.3 Disorders of hypoglossal nerve
Disorders of 12th cranial nerve
G52.7 Disorders of multiple cranial nerves
Polyneuritis cranialis
G52.8 Disorders of other specified cranial nerves
G52.9 Cranial nerve disorder, unspecified

***G53 Cranial nerve disorders in diseases classified elsewhere***
Code first underlying disease, such as:
neoplasm (C00-D49)
EXCLUDES 1 *multiple cranial nerve palsy in sarcoidosis (D86.82)*
*multiple cranial nerve palsy in syphilis (A52.15)*
*postherpetic geniculate ganglionitis (B02.21)*
*postherpetic trigeminal neuralgia (B02.22)*

**✓4th G54 Nerve root and plexus disorders**
EXCLUDES 1 *current traumatic nerve root and plexus disorders - see nerve injury by body region*
*intervertebral disc disorders (M50-M51)*
*neuralgia or neuritis NOS (M79.2)*
*neuritis or radiculitis brachial NOS (M54.13)*
*neuritis or radiculitis lumbar NOS (M54.16)*
*neuritis or radiculitis lumbosacral NOS (M54.17)*
*neuritis or radiculitis thoracic NOS (M54.14)*
*radiculitis NOS (M54.10)*
*radiculopathy NOS (M54.10)*
*spondylosis (M47.-)*

G54.0 Brachial plexus disorders
Thoracic outlet syndrome
AHA: 2023,2Q,8
DEF: Acquired disorder affecting the spinal nerves that send signals to the shoulder, arm, and hand, causing corresponding motor and sensory dysfunction. This disorder is characterized by regional paresthesia, pain, muscle weakness, and in severe cases paralysis.
G54.1 Lumbosacral plexus disorders
G54.2 Cervical root disorders, not elsewhere classified
G54.3 Thoracic root disorders, not elsewhere classified
G54.4 Lumbosacral root disorders, not elsewhere classified
G54.5 Neuralgic amyotrophy
Parsonage-Aldren-Turner syndrome
Shoulder-girdle neuritis
EXCLUDES 1 *neuralgic amyotrophy in diabetes mellitus (E08-E13 with .44)*
G54.6 Phantom limb syndrome with pain HCC ESR COM
G54.7 Phantom limb syndrome without pain HCC ESR COM
Phantom limb syndrome NOS
G54.8 Other nerve root and plexus disorders
G54.9 Nerve root and plexus disorder, unspecified

***G55 Nerve root and plexus compressions in diseases classified elsewhere***
Code first underlying disease, such as:
neoplasm (C00-D49)
EXCLUDES 1 *nerve root compression (due to) (in) ankylosing spondylitis (M45.-)*
*nerve root compression (due to) (in) dorsopathies (M53.-, M54.-)*
*nerve root compression (due to) (in) intervertebral disc disorders (M50.1.-, M51.1.-)*
*nerve root compression (due to) (in) spondylopathies (M46.-, M48.-)*
*nerve root compression (due to) (in) spondylosis (M47.0-, M47.2-)*

**✓4th G56 Mononeuropathies of upper limb**
EXCLUDES 1 *current traumatic nerve disorder - see nerve injury by body region*
AHA: 2016,4Q,17-18

✓5th G56.0 Carpal tunnel syndrome
DEF: Swelling and inflammation in the tendons or bursa surrounding the median nerve caused by repetitive activity. The resulting compression on the nerve causes pain, numbness, and tingling especially to the palm, index, middle finger, and thumb.
G56.00 Carpal tunnel syndrome, unspecified upper limb
G56.01 Carpal tunnel syndrome, right upper limb
G56.02 Carpal tunnel syndrome, left upper limb
G56.03 Carpal tunnel syndrome, bilateral upper limbs

✓5th G56.1 Other lesions of median nerve
G56.10 Other lesions of median nerve, unspecified upper limb
G56.11 Other lesions of median nerve, right upper limb
G56.12 Other lesions of median nerve, left upper limb
G56.13 Other lesions of median nerve, bilateral upper limbs

✓5th G56.2 Lesion of ulnar nerve
Tardy ulnar nerve palsy
G56.20 Lesion of ulnar nerve, unspecified upper limb
G56.21 Lesion of ulnar nerve, right upper limb
G56.22 Lesion of ulnar nerve, left upper limb
G56.23 Lesion of ulnar nerve, bilateral upper limbs

✓5th G56.3 Lesion of radial nerve
G56.30 Lesion of radial nerve, unspecified upper limb
G56.31 Lesion of radial nerve, right upper limb
G56.32 Lesion of radial nerve, left upper limb
G56.33 Lesion of radial nerve, bilateral upper limbs

✓5th G56.4 Causalgia of upper limb
Complex regional pain syndrome II of upper limb
EXCLUDES 1 *complex regional pain syndrome I of lower limb (G90.52-)*
*complex regional pain syndrome I of upper limb (G90.51-)*
*complex regional pain syndrome II of lower limb (G57.7-)*
*reflex sympathetic dystrophy of lower limb (G90.52-)*
*reflex sympathetic dystrophy of upper limb (G90.51-)*
G56.40 Causalgia of unspecified upper limb
G56.41 Causalgia of right upper limb
G56.42 Causalgia of left upper limb
G56.43 Causalgia of bilateral upper limbs

✓5th G56.8 Other specified mononeuropathies of upper limb
Interdigital neuroma of upper limb
G56.80 Other specified mononeuropathies of unspecified upper limb
G56.81 Other specified mononeuropathies of right upper limb
G56.82 Other specified mononeuropathies of left upper limb
G56.83 Other specified mononeuropathies of bilateral upper limbs

✓5th G56.9 Unspecified mononeuropathy of upper limb
G56.90 Unspecified mononeuropathy of unspecified upper limb
G56.91 Unspecified mononeuropathy of right upper limb
G56.92 Unspecified mononeuropathy of left upper limb
G56.93 Unspecified mononeuropathy of bilateral upper limbs

**✓4th G57 Mononeuropathies of lower limb**
EXCLUDES 1 *current traumatic nerve disorder - see nerve injury by body region*
AHA: 2016,4Q,17-18

✓5th G57.0 Lesion of sciatic nerve
EXCLUDES 1 *sciatica NOS (M54.3-)*
EXCLUDES 2 *sciatica attributed to intervertebral disc disorder (M51.1.-)*
G57.00 Lesion of sciatic nerve, unspecified lower limb
G57.01 Lesion of sciatic nerve, right lower limb
G57.02 Lesion of sciatic nerve, left lower limb
G57.03 Lesion of sciatic nerve, bilateral lower limbs

✓5th G57.1 Meralgia paresthetica
Lateral cutaneous nerve of thigh syndrome
G57.10 Meralgia paresthetica, unspecified lower limb
G57.11 Meralgia paresthetica, right lower limb
G57.12 Meralgia paresthetica, left lower limb

G57.13 Meralgia paresthetica, bilateral lower limbs

✓5th G57.2 Lesion of femoral nerve

G57.20 Lesion of femoral nerve, unspecified lower limb

G57.21 Lesion of femoral nerve, right lower limb

G57.22 Lesion of femoral nerve, left lower limb

G57.23 Lesion of femoral nerve, bilateral lower limbs

✓5th G57.3 Lesion of lateral popliteal nerve

Peroneal nerve palsy

AHA: 2020,3Q,12

G57.30 Lesion of lateral popliteal nerve, unspecified lower limb

G57.31 Lesion of lateral popliteal nerve, right lower limb

G57.32 Lesion of lateral popliteal nerve, left lower limb

G57.33 Lesion of lateral popliteal nerve, bilateral lower limbs

✓5th G57.4 Lesion of medial popliteal nerve

G57.40 Lesion of medial popliteal nerve, unspecified lower limb

G57.41 Lesion of medial popliteal nerve, right lower limb

G57.42 Lesion of medial popliteal nerve, left lower limb

G57.43 Lesion of medial popliteal nerve, bilateral lower limbs

✓5th G57.5 Tarsal tunnel syndrome

G57.50 Tarsal tunnel syndrome, unspecified lower limb

G57.51 Tarsal tunnel syndrome, right lower limb

G57.52 Tarsal tunnel syndrome, left lower limb

G57.53 Tarsal tunnel syndrome, bilateral lower limbs

✓5th G57.6 Lesion of plantar nerve

Morton's metatarsalgia

G57.60 Lesion of plantar nerve, unspecified lower limb

G57.61 Lesion of plantar nerve, right lower limb

G57.62 Lesion of plantar nerve, left lower limb

G57.63 Lesion of plantar nerve, bilateral lower limbs

✓5th G57.7 Causalgia of lower limb

Complex regional pain syndrome II of lower limb

EXCLUDES 1 *complex regional pain syndrome I of lower limb (G9Ø.52-)*
*complex regional pain syndrome I of upper limb (G9Ø.51-)*
*complex regional pain syndrome II of upper limb (G56.4-)*
*reflex sympathetic dystrophy of lower limb (G9Ø.52-)*
*reflex sympathetic dystrophy of upper limb (G9Ø.51-)*

G57.70 Causalgia of unspecified lower limb

G57.71 Causalgia of right lower limb

G57.72 Causalgia of left lower limb

G57.73 Causalgia of bilateral lower limbs

✓5th G57.8 Other specified mononeuropathies of lower limb

Interdigital neuroma of lower limb

G57.80 Other specified mononeuropathies of unspecified lower limb

G57.81 Other specified mononeuropathies of right lower limb

G57.82 Other specified mononeuropathies of left lower limb

G57.83 Other specified mononeuropathies of bilateral lower limbs

✓5th G57.9 Unspecified mononeuropathy of lower limb

G57.90 Unspecified mononeuropathy of unspecified lower limb

G57.91 Unspecified mononeuropathy of right lower limb

G57.92 Unspecified mononeuropathy of left lower limb

G57.93 Unspecified mononeuropathy of bilateral lower limbs

✓4th G58 Other mononeuropathies

G58.Ø Intercostal neuropathy

G58.7 Mononeuritis multiplex

G58.8 Other specified mononeuropathies

G58.9 Mononeuropathy, unspecified

*G59 Mononeuropathy in diseases classified elsewhere*

Code first underlying disease

EXCLUDES 1 *diabetic mononeuropathy (EØ8-E13 with .41)*
*syphilitic nerve paralysis (A52.19)*
*syphilitic neuritis (A52.15)*
*tuberculous mononeuropathy (A17.83)*

## Polyneuropathies and other disorders of the peripheral nervous system (G6Ø-G65)

EXCLUDES 1 *neuralgia NOS (M79.2)*
*neuritis NOS (M79.2)*
*peripheral neuritis in pregnancy (O26.82-)*
*radiculitis NOS (M54.1Ø)*

✓4th G6Ø Hereditary and idiopathic neuropathy

G6Ø.Ø Hereditary motor and sensory neuropathy

Charcôt-Marie-Tooth disease
Dejerine-Sottas disease
Hereditary motor and sensory neuropathy, types I-IV
Hypertrophic neuropathy of infancy
Peroneal muscular atrophy (axonal type) (hypertrophic type)
Roussy-Levy syndrome

G6Ø.1 Refsum's disease

Infantile Refsum disease

DEF: Genetic disorder of the lipid metabolism characterized by retinitis pigmentosa, degenerative nerve disease, ataxia, and dry, rough, scaly skin.

G6Ø.2 Neuropathy in association with hereditary ataxia

G6Ø.3 Idiopathic progressive neuropathy

G6Ø.8 Other hereditary and idiopathic neuropathies

Dominantly inherited sensory neuropathy
Morvan's disease
Nelaton's syndrome
Recessively inherited sensory neuropathy

G6Ø.9 Hereditary and idiopathic neuropathy, unspecified

✓4th G61 Inflammatory polyneuropathy

G61.Ø Guillain-Barre syndrome Rx ESR COM

Acute (post-)infective polyneuritis
Miller Fisher syndrome

AHA: 2020,3Q,12; 2014,2Q,4

DEF: Autoimmune disorder due to an immune response to foreign antigens with paraplegia of limbs, flaccid paralysis, ophthalmoplegia, ataxia, and areflexia. In most cases, this disorder is triggered by a mild viral infection, surgery, or following an immunization.

TIP: Guillain-Barre syndrome can occur as a sequela of *Campylobacter* enteritis. Assign code B94.8 for the sequelae as an additional diagnosis.

G61.1 Serum neuropathy Rx ESR COM

Use additional code for adverse effect, if applicable, to identify serum (T5Ø.-)

✓5th G61.8 Other inflammatory polyneuropathies

G61.81 Chronic inflammatory demyelinating polyneuritis HCC Rx ESR COM

G61.82 Multifocal motor neuropathy HCC Rx ESR COM

MMN

AHA: 2016,4Q,18

G61.89 Other inflammatory polyneuropathies Rx ESR COM

G61.9 Inflammatory polyneuropathy, unspecified Rx ESR COM

✓4th G62 Other and unspecified polyneuropathies

G62.Ø Drug-induced polyneuropathy Rx ESR COM

Use additional code for adverse effect, if applicable, to identify drug (T36-T5Ø with fifth or sixth character 5)

G62.1 Alcoholic polyneuropathy Rx ESR COM

AHA: 2019,3Q,8

G62.2 Polyneuropathy due to other toxic agents Rx ESR COM

Code first (T51-T65) to identify toxic agent

✓5th G62.8 Other specified polyneuropathies

G62.81 Critical illness polyneuropathy Rx ESR COM

Acute motor neuropathy

G62.82 Radiation-induced polyneuropathy Rx ESR COM

Use additional external cause code (W88-W9Ø, X39.Ø-) to identify cause

G62.89 Other specified polyneuropathies

AHA: 2024,3Q,11; 2016,2Q,11

G62.9 Polyneuropathy, unspecified

Neuropathy NOS

**G63 *Polyneuropathy in diseases classified elsewhere*** Rx ESR COM
Code first underlying disease, such as:
amyloidosis (E85.-)
endocrine disease, except diabetes (EØØ-EØ7, E15-E16, E2Ø-E34)
metabolic diseases (E7Ø-E88)
neoplasm (CØØ-D49)
nutritional deficiency (E4Ø-E64)
EXCLUDES 1 *polyneuropathy (in):*
*diabetes mellitus (EØ8-E13 with .42)*
*diphtheria (A36.83)*
*infectious mononucleosis complicated by polyneuropathy (B27.Ø-B27.9 with fifth character 1)*
*Lyme disease (A69.22)*
*mumps (B26.84)*
*postherpetic (BØ2.23)*
*rheumatoid arthritis (MØ5.5-)*
*scleroderma (M34.83)*
*systemic lupus erythematosus (M32.19)*
**AHA:** 2024,3Q,11; 2023,3Q,19; 2021,1Q,7; 2012,4Q,99

**G64 Other disorders of peripheral nervous system**
Disorder of peripheral nervous system NOS

✓4th **G65 Sequelae of inflammatory and toxic polyneuropathies**
Code first condition resulting from (sequela) of inflammatory and toxic polyneuropathies
**G65.Ø Sequelae of Guillain-Barre syndrome** Rx ESR COM
**G65.1 Sequelae of other inflammatory polyneuropathy** Rx ESR COM
**G65.2 Sequelae of toxic polyneuropathy** Rx ESR COM

## Diseases of myoneural junction and muscle (G7Ø-G73)

✓4th **G7Ø Myasthenia gravis and other myoneural disorders**
EXCLUDES 1 *botulism (AØ5.1, A48.51-A48.52)*
*transient neonatal myasthenia gravis (P94.Ø)*

✓5th **G7Ø.Ø Myasthenia gravis**
**AHA:** 2022,3Q,15
**DEF:** Autoimmune neuromuscular disorder caused by antibodies to the acetylcholine receptors at the neuromuscular junction, interfering with proper binding of the neurotransmitter from the neuron to the target muscle, causing muscle weakness, fatigue, and exhaustion, without pain or atrophy.
**G7Ø.ØØ Myasthenia gravis without (acute) exacerbation** HCC Rx ESR COM
Myasthenia gravis NOS
**G7Ø.Ø1 Myasthenia gravis with (acute) exacerbation** HCC Rx ESR COM
Myasthenia gravis in crisis
**G7Ø.1 Toxic myoneural disorders** HCC Rx ESR COM
Code first (T51-T65) to identify toxic agent
**G7Ø.2 Congenital and developmental myasthenia** HCC Rx ESR COM
✓5th **G7Ø.8 Other specified myoneural disorders**
**G7Ø.8Ø Lambert-Eaton syndrome, unspecified** HCC Rx ESR COM
Lambert-Eaton syndrome NOS
**G7Ø.81 *Lambert-Eaton syndrome in disease classified elsewhere*** HCC Rx ESR COM
Code first underlying disease
EXCLUDES 1 *Lambert-Eaton syndrome in neoplastic disease (G73.1)*
**G7Ø.89 Other specified myoneural disorders** HCC Rx ESR COM
**G7Ø.9 Myoneural disorder, unspecified** HCC Rx ESR COM

✓4th **G71 Primary disorders of muscles**
EXCLUDES 2 *arthrogryposis multiplex congenita (Q74.3)*
*metabolic disorders (E7Ø-E88)*
*myositis (M6Ø.-)*

✓5th **G71.Ø Muscular dystrophy**
**AHA:** 2022,4Q,17-18; 2018,4Q,11-12
**G71.ØØ Muscular dystrophy, unspecified** HCC ESR COM
**G71.Ø1 Duchenne or Becker muscular dystrophy** HCC ESR COM
Autosomal recessive, childhood type, muscular dystrophy resembling Duchenne or Becker muscular dystrophy
Benign [Becker] muscular dystrophy
Severe [Duchenne] muscular dystrophy
**G71.Ø2 Facioscapulohumeral muscular dystrophy** HCC ESR COM
Scapulohumeral muscular dystrophy
✓6th **G71.Ø3 Limb girdle muscular dystrophies**
**G71.Ø31 Autosomal dominant limb girdle muscular dystrophy** HCC ESR COM
LGMD D4 calpain-3-related
LGMD D5 collagen 6-related
Limb girdle muscular dystrophy type 1
**G71.Ø32 Autosomal recessive limb girdle muscular dystrophy due to calpain-3 dysfunction** HCC ESR COM
LGMD R1 calpain-3-related
Limb girdle muscular dystrophy type 2A
Primary calpainopathy
**G71.Ø33 Limb girdle muscular dystrophy due to dysferlin dysfunction** HCC ESR COM
Dysferlinopathy
LGMD R2 dysferlin-related
Limb girdle muscular dystrophy type 2B
Miyoshi Myopathy type 1
✓7th **G71.Ø34 Limb girdle muscular dystrophy due to sarcoglycan dysfunction**
**G71.Ø34Ø Limb girdle muscular dystrophy due to sarcoglycan dysfunction, unspecified** HCC ESR COM
Sarcoglycanopathy, NOS
**G71.Ø341 Limb girdle muscular dystrophy due to alpha sarcoglycan dysfunction** HCC ESR COM
Alpha sarcoglycanopathy
Limb girdle muscular dystrophy type 2D
Limb-girdle muscular dystrophy due to alpha-sarcoglycan deficiency
**G71.Ø342 Limb girdle muscular dystrophy due to beta sarcoglycan dysfunction** HCC ESR COM
Beta sarcoglycanopathy
Limb girdle muscular dystrophy due to beta-sarcoglycan deficiency
Limb girdle muscular dystrophy type 2E
**G71.Ø349 Limb girdle muscular dystrophy due to other sarcoglycan dysfunction** HCC ESR COM
Delta sarcoglycanopathy
Delta-sarcoglycan-related LGMD R6
Gamma sarcoglycanopathy
Gamma-sarcoglycan-related LGMD R5
Limb girdle muscular dystrophy type 2C
Limb girdle muscular dystrophy type 2F
**G71.Ø35 Limb girdle muscular dystrophy due to anoctamin-5 dysfunction** HCC ESR COM
Anoctamin-5-related LGMD R12
Anoctaminopathy
Autosomal recessive limb girdle muscular dystrophy type 2L
Miyoshi myopathy type 3
**G71.Ø36 Limb girdle muscular dystrophy due to fukutin related protein dysfunction** HCC ESR
LGMD R9 FKRP-related
Limb girdle muscular dystrophy due to FKRP deficiency
Limb girdle muscular dystrophy type 2I
**G71.Ø38 Other limb girdle muscular dystrophy** HCC ESR COM
LGMD R22 collagen 6-related
Other autosomal recessive limb girdle muscular dystrophy
**G71.Ø39 Limb girdle muscular dystrophy, unspecified** HCC ESR COM

**G71.09 Other specified muscular dystrophies** HCC ESR COM
Benign scapuloperoneal muscular dystrophy with early contractures [Emery-Dreifuss]
Congenital muscular dystrophy NOS
Congenital muscular dystrophy with specific morphological abnormalities of the muscle fiber
Distal muscular dystrophy
Ocular muscular dystrophy
Oculopharyngeal muscular dystrophy
Scapuloperoneal muscular dystrophy

√5th **G71.1 Myotonic disorders**

**G71.11 Myotonic muscular dystrophy** HCC ESR COM
Dystrophia myotonica [Steinert]
Myotonia atrophica
Myotonic dystrophy
Proximal myotonic myopathy (PROMM)
Steinert disease

**G71.12 Myotonia congenita**
Acetazolamide responsive myotonia congenita
Dominant myotonia congenita [Thomsen disease]
Myotonia levior
Recessive myotonia congenita [Becker disease]

**G71.13 Myotonic chondrodystrophy**
Chondrodystrophic myotonia
Congenital myotonic chondrodystrophy
Schwartz-Jampel disease

**G71.14 Drug induced myotonia**
Use additional code for adverse effect, if applicable, to identify drug (T36-T50 with fifth or sixth character 5)

**G71.19 Other specified myotonic disorders**
Myotonia fluctuans
Myotonia permanens
Neuromyotonia [Isaacs]
Paramyotonia congenita (of von Eulenburg)
Pseudomyotonia
Symptomatic myotonia

√5th **G71.2 Congenital myopathies**
EXCLUDES 2 *arthrogryposis multiplex congenita (Q74.3)*
AHA: 2020,4Q,19-21

**G71.20 Congenital myopathy, unspecified** HCC ESR COM

**G71.21 Nemaline myopathy** HCC ESR COM

√6th **G71.22 Centronuclear myopathy**

**G71.220 X-linked myotubular myopathy** HCC ESR COM
Myotubular (centronuclear) myopathy

**G71.228 Other centronuclear myopathy** HCC ESR COM
Autosomal centronuclear myopathy
Autosomal dominant centronuclear myopathy
Autosomal recessive centronuclear myopathy
Centronuclear myopathy, NOS

**G71.29 Other congenital myopathy** HCC ESR COM
Central core disease
Minicore disease
Multicore disease
Multiminicore disease

**G71.3 Mitochondrial myopathy, not elsewhere classified**
EXCLUDES 1 *Kearns-Sayre syndrome (H49.81)*
*Leber's disease (H47.21)*
*Leigh's encephalopathy (G31.82)*
*mitochondrial metabolism disorders (E88.4.-)*
*Reye's syndrome (G93.7)*

**G71.8 Other primary disorders of muscles**

**G71.9 Primary disorder of muscle, unspecified**
Hereditary myopathy NOS

√4th **G72 Other and unspecified myopathies**
EXCLUDES 1 *arthrogryposis multiplex congenita (Q74.3)*
*dermatopolymyositis (M33.-)*
*ischemic infarction of muscle (M62.2-)*
*myositis (M60.-)*
*polymyositis (M33.2.-)*

**G72.0 Drug-induced myopathy**
Use additional code for adverse effect, if applicable, to identify drug (T36-T50 with fifth or sixth character 5)

**G72.1 Alcoholic myopathy**
Use additional code to identify alcoholism (F10.-)

**G72.2 Myopathy due to other toxic agents**
Code first (T51-T65) to identify toxic agent

**G72.3 Periodic paralysis**
Familial periodic paralysis
Hyperkalemic periodic paralysis (familial)
Hypokalemic periodic paralysis (familial)
Myotonic periodic paralysis (familial)
Normokalemic paralysis (familial)
Potassium sensitive periodic paralysis
EXCLUDES 1 *paramyotonia congenita (of von Eulenburg) (G71.19)*

√5th **G72.4 Inflammatory and immune myopathies, not elsewhere classified**

**G72.41 Inclusion body myositis [IBM]** HCC

**G72.49 Other inflammatory and immune myopathies, not elsewhere classified**
Inflammatory myopathy NOS

√5th **G72.8 Other specified myopathies**

**G72.81 Critical illness myopathy**
Acute necrotizing myopathy
Acute quadriplegic myopathy
Intensive care (ICU) myopathy
Myopathy of critical illness
AHA: 2020,3Q,12

**G72.89 Other specified myopathies**

**G72.9 Myopathy, unspecified**

√4th **G73 Disorders of myoneural junction and muscle in diseases classified elsewhere**

**G73.1 *Lambert-Eaton syndrome in neoplastic disease*** HCC Rx ESR COM UPD
Code first underlying neoplasm (C00-D49)
EXCLUDES 1 *Lambert-Eaton syndrome not associated with neoplasm (G70.80-G70.81)*

**G73.3 *Myasthenic syndromes in other diseases classified elsewhere*** HCC Rx ESR COM
Code first underlying disease, such as:
neoplasm (C00-D49)
thyrotoxicosis (E05.-)

**G73.7 *Myopathy in diseases classified elsewhere***
Code first underlying disease, such as:
glycogen storage disease (E74.0-)
hyperparathyroidism (E21.0, E21.3)
hypoparathyroidism (E20.-)
lipid storage disorders (E75.-)
EXCLUDES 1 *myopathy in:*
*rheumatoid arthritis (M05.32)*
*sarcoidosis (D86.87)*
*scleroderma (M34.82)*
*Sjogren syndrome (M35.03)*
*systemic lupus erythematosus (M32.19)*

## Cerebral palsy and other paralytic syndromes (G80-G83)

√4th **G80 Cerebral palsy**
EXCLUDES 1 *hereditary spastic paraplegia (G11.4)*

**G80.0 Spastic quadriplegic cerebral palsy** HCC ESR COM
Congenital spastic paralysis (cerebral)

**G80.1 Spastic diplegic cerebral palsy** HCC ESR COM
Spastic cerebral palsy NOS

**G80.2 Spastic hemiplegic cerebral palsy** HCC ESR COM

**G80.3 Athetoid cerebral palsy** HCC ESR COM
Double athetosis (syndrome)
Dyskinetic cerebral palsy
Dystonic cerebral palsy
Vogt disease

**G80.4 Ataxic cerebral palsy** HCC ESR COM

**G80.8 Other cerebral palsy** HCC ESR COM
Mixed cerebral palsy syndromes

**G80.9 Cerebral palsy, unspecified** HCC ESR COM
Cerebral palsy NOS

## G81 Hemiplegia and hemiparesis

NOTE This category is to be used only when hemiplegia (complete)(incomplete) is reported without further specification, or is stated to be old or longstanding but of unspecified cause. The category is also for use in multiple coding to identify these types of hemiplegia resulting from any cause.

EXCLUDES 1 *congenital cerebral palsy (G8Ø.-)*
*hemiplegia and hemiparesis due to sequela of cerebrovascular disease (I69.Ø5-, I69.15-, I69.25-, I69.35-, I69.85-, I69.95-)*

**AHA:** 2015,1Q,25

**TIP:** If the documentation specifies the affected side but not whether it is the dominant or nondominant side, the default is as follows: for ambidextrous patients, the default is dominant; when the left side is affected, the default is nondominant; and when the right side is affected, the default is dominant.

### G81.Ø Flaccid hemiplegia

- **G81.ØØ Flaccid hemiplegia affecting unspecified side** HCC ESR COM
- **G81.Ø1 Flaccid hemiplegia affecting right dominant side** HCC ESR COM
- **G81.Ø2 Flaccid hemiplegia affecting left dominant side** HCC ESR COM
- **G81.Ø3 Flaccid hemiplegia affecting right nondominant side** HCC ESR COM
- **G81.Ø4 Flaccid hemiplegia affecting left nondominant side** HCC ESR COM

### G81.1 Spastic hemiplegia

- **G81.1Ø Spastic hemiplegia affecting unspecified side** HCC Rx ESR COM
- **G81.11 Spastic hemiplegia affecting right dominant side** HCC Rx ESR COM
- **G81.12 Spastic hemiplegia affecting left dominant side** HCC Rx ESR COM
- **G81.13 Spastic hemiplegia affecting right nondominant side** HCC Rx ESR COM
- **G81.14 Spastic hemiplegia affecting left nondominant side** HCC Rx ESR COM

### G81.9 Hemiplegia, unspecified

**AHA:** 2014,1Q,23

- **G81.9Ø Hemiplegia, unspecified affecting unspecified side** HCC ESR COM
- **G81.91 Hemiplegia, unspecified affecting right dominant side** HCC ESR COM
- **G81.92 Hemiplegia, unspecified affecting left dominant side** HCC ESR COM
- **G81.93 Hemiplegia, unspecified affecting right nondominant side** HCC ESR COM
- **G81.94 Hemiplegia, unspecified affecting left nondominant side** HCC ESR COM

## G82 Paraplegia (paraparesis) and quadriplegia (quadriparesis)

NOTE This category is to be used only when the listed conditions are reported without further specification, or are stated to be old or longstanding but of unspecified cause. The category is also for use in multiple coding to identify these conditions resulting from any cause

EXCLUDES 1 *congenital cerebral palsy (G8Ø.-)*
*functional quadriplegia (R53.2)*
*hysterical paralysis (F44.4)*

### G82.2 Paraplegia

Paralysis of both lower limbs NOS
Paraparesis (lower) NOS
Paraplegia (lower) NOS

**AHA:** 2017,3Q,3

- **G82.2Ø Paraplegia, unspecified** HCC ESR COM
- **G82.21 Paraplegia, complete** HCC ESR COM
- **G82.22 Paraplegia, incomplete** HCC ESR COM

### G82.5 Quadriplegia

**AHA:** 2024,2Q,23

- **G82.5Ø Quadriplegia, unspecified** HCC ESR COM
- **G82.51 Quadriplegia, C1-C4 complete** HCC ESR COM
- **G82.52 Quadriplegia, C1-C4 incomplete** HCC ESR COM
- **G82.53 Quadriplegia, C5-C7 complete** HCC ESR COM
- **G82.54 Quadriplegia, C5-C7 incomplete** HCC ESR COM

## G83 Other paralytic syndromes

NOTE This category is to be used only when the listed conditions are reported without further specification, or are stated to be old or longstanding but of unspecified cause. The category is also for use in multiple coding to identify these conditions resulting from any cause.

INCLUDES paralysis (complete) (incomplete), except as in G8Ø-G82

### G83.Ø Diplegia of upper limbs HCC ESR COM

Diplegia (upper)
Paralysis of both upper limbs

### G83.1 Monoplegia of lower limb

Paralysis of lower limb

EXCLUDES 1 *monoplegia of lower limbs due to sequela of cerebrovascular disease (I69.Ø4-, I69.14-, I69.24-, I69.34-, I69.84-, I69.94-)*

**TIP:** If the documentation specifies the affected side but not whether it is the dominant or nondominant side, the default is as follows: for ambidextrous patients, the default is dominant; when the left side is affected, the default is nondominant; and when the right side is affected, the default is dominant.

- **G83.1Ø Monoplegia of lower limb affecting unspecified side** HCC ESR COM
- **G83.11 Monoplegia of lower limb affecting right dominant side** HCC ESR COM
- **G83.12 Monoplegia of lower limb affecting left dominant side** HCC ESR COM
- **G83.13 Monoplegia of lower limb affecting right nondominant side** HCC ESR COM
- **G83.14 Monoplegia of lower limb affecting left nondominant side** HCC ESR COM

### G83.2 Monoplegia of upper limb

Paralysis of upper limb

EXCLUDES 1 *monoplegia of upper limbs due to sequela of cerebrovascular disease (I69.Ø3-, I69.13-, I69.23-, I69.33-, I69.83-, I69.93-)*

**TIP:** If the documentation specifies the affected side but not whether it is the dominant or nondominant side, the default is as follows: for ambidextrous patients, the default is dominant; when the left side is affected, the default is nondominant; and when the right side is affected, the default is dominant.

- **G83.2Ø Monoplegia of upper limb affecting unspecified side** HCC ESR COM
- **G83.21 Monoplegia of upper limb affecting right dominant side** HCC ESR COM
- **G83.22 Monoplegia of upper limb affecting left dominant side** HCC ESR COM
- **G83.23 Monoplegia of upper limb affecting right nondominant side** HCC ESR COM
- **G83.24 Monoplegia of upper limb affecting left nondominant side** HCC ESR COM

### G83.3 Monoplegia, unspecified

**TIP:** If the documentation specifies the affected side but not whether it is the dominant or nondominant side, the default is as follows: for ambidextrous patients, the default is dominant; when the left side is affected, the default is nondominant; and when the right side is affected, the default is dominant.

- **G83.3Ø Monoplegia, unspecified affecting unspecified side** HCC ESR COM
- **G83.31 Monoplegia, unspecified affecting right dominant side** HCC ESR COM
- **G83.32 Monoplegia, unspecified affecting left dominant side** HCC ESR COM
- **G83.33 Monoplegia, unspecified affecting right nondominant side** HCC ESR COM
- **G83.34 Monoplegia, unspecified affecting left nondominant side** HCC ESR COM

### G83.4 Cauda equina syndrome HCC Rx ESR COM

Neurogenic bladder due to cauda equina syndrome

EXCLUDES 1 *cord bladder NOS (G95.89)*
*neurogenic bladder NOS (N31.9)*

**AHA:** 2024,1Q,17; 2020,3Q,24

**DEF:** Compression of the spinal nerve roots presenting with pain and tingling radiating down the buttocks, back of the thigh and calf, and into the foot in a sciatic manner with aching in the bladder, perineum, and sacrum. Loss of bowel and bladder control may also occur.

**G83.5 Locked-in state** HCC ESR COM
AHA: 2022,2Q,10

✓5th **G83.8 Other specified paralytic syndromes**
EXCLUDES 1 *paralytic syndromes due to current spinal cord injury - code to spinal cord injury (S14, S24, S34)*

**G83.81 Brown-Sequard syndrome** HCC ESR COM
**G83.82 Anterior cord syndrome** HCC ESR COM
**G83.83 Posterior cord syndrome** HCC ESR COM
**G83.84 Todd's paralysis (postepileptic)** HCC ESR COM
**G83.89 Other specified paralytic syndromes** HCC ESR COM

**G83.9 Paralytic syndrome, unspecified** HCC ESR COM

## Other disorders of the nervous system (G89-G99)

✓4th **G89 Pain, not elsewhere classified**
Code also related psychological factors associated with pain (F45.42)
EXCLUDES 1 *generalized pain NOS (R52)*
*pain disorders exclusively related to psychological factors (F45.41)*
*pain NOS (R52)*
EXCLUDES 2 *atypical face pain (G50.1)*
*headache syndromes (G44.-)*
*localized pain, unspecified type - code to pain by site, such as:*
*migraines (G43.-)*
*myalgia (M79.1-)*
*pain from prosthetic devices, implants, and grafts (T82.84, T83.84, T84.84, T85.84-)*
*phantom limb syndrome with pain (G54.6)*
*vulvar vestibulitis (N94.810)*
*vulvodynia (N94.81-)*
*abdomen pain (R10.-)*
*back pain (M54.9)*
*breast pain (N64.4)*
*chest pain (R07.1-R07.9)*
*ear pain (H92.0-)*
*eye pain (H57.1)*
*headache (R51.9)*
*joint pain (M25.5-)*
*limb pain (M79.6-)*
*lumbar region pain (M54.5-)*
*painful urination (R30.9)*
*pelvic and perineal pain (R10.2-)*
*renal colic (N23)*
*shoulder pain (M25.51-)*
*spine pain (M54.-)*
*throat pain (R07.0)*
*tongue pain (K14.6)*
*tooth pain (K08.8)*

**G89.0 Central pain syndrome**
Dejerine-Roussy syndrome
Myelopathic pain syndrome
Thalamic pain syndrome (hyperesthetic)

✓5th **G89.1 Acute pain, not elsewhere classified**
**G89.11 Acute pain due to trauma**
**G89.12 Acute post-thoracotomy pain**
Post-thoracotomy pain NOS
**G89.18 Other acute postprocedural pain**
Postoperative pain NOS
Postprocedural pain NOS

✓5th **G89.2 Chronic pain, not elsewhere classified**
EXCLUDES 1 *causalgia, lower limb (G57.7-)*
*causalgia, upper limb (G56.4-)*
*central pain syndrome (G89.0)*
*chronic pain syndrome (G89.4)*
*complex regional pain syndrome II, lower limb (G57.7-)*
*complex regional pain syndrome II, upper limb (G56.4-)*
*neoplasm related chronic pain (G89.3)*
*reflex sympathetic dystrophy (G90.5-)*
**G89.21 Chronic pain due to trauma**
**G89.22 Chronic post-thoracotomy pain**
**G89.28 Other chronic postprocedural pain**
Other chronic postoperative pain
**G89.29 Other chronic pain**
AHA: 2026,2Q,21; 2023,3Q,17

**G89.3 Neoplasm related pain (acute) (chronic)**
Cancer associated pain
Pain due to malignancy (primary) (secondary)
Tumor associated pain

**G89.4 Chronic pain syndrome**
Chronic pain associated with significant psychosocial dysfunction

✓4th **G90 Disorders of autonomic nervous system**
EXCLUDES 1 *dysfunction of the autonomic nervous system due to alcohol (G31.2)*

✓5th **G90.0 Idiopathic peripheral autonomic neuropathy**
**G90.01 Carotid sinus syncope**
Carotid sinus syndrome
**DEF:** Vagal activation caused by pressure on the carotid sinus baroreceptors. Sympathetic nerve impulses may cause sinus arrest or AV block.
**G90.09 Other idiopathic peripheral autonomic neuropathy**
Idiopathic peripheral autonomic neuropathy NOS

**G90.1 Familial dysautonomia [Riley-Day]** HCC Rx ESR COM

**G90.2 Horner's syndrome**
Bernard(-Horner) syndrome
Cervical sympathetic dystrophy or paralysis

**G90.3 Multi-system degeneration of the autonomic nervous system** HCC Rx ESR COM
Neurogenic orthostatic hypotension [Shy-Drager]
EXCLUDES 1 *orthostatic hypotension NOS (I95.1)*

**G90.4 Autonomic dysreflexia**
Use additional code to identify the cause, such as:
fecal impaction (K56.41)
pressure ulcer (pressure area) (L89.-)
urinary tract infection (N39.0)

✓5th **G90.5 Complex regional pain syndrome I (CRPS I)**
Reflex sympathetic dystrophy
EXCLUDES 1 *causalgia of lower limb (G57.7-)*
*causalgia of upper limb (G56.4-)*
*complex regional pain syndrome II of lower limb (G57.7-)*
*complex regional pain syndrome II of upper limb (G56.4-)*

**G90.50 Complex regional pain syndrome I, unspecified**

✓6th **G90.51 Complex regional pain syndrome I of upper limb**
**G90.511 Complex regional pain syndrome I of right upper limb**
**G90.512 Complex regional pain syndrome I of left upper limb**
**G90.513 Complex regional pain syndrome I of upper limb, bilateral**
**G90.519 Complex regional pain syndrome I of unspecified upper limb**

✓6th **G90.52 Complex regional pain syndrome I of lower limb**
**G90.521 Complex regional pain syndrome I of right lower limb**
**G90.522 Complex regional pain syndrome I of left lower limb**
**G90.523 Complex regional pain syndrome I of lower limb, bilateral**
**G90.529 Complex regional pain syndrome I of unspecified lower limb**

**G90.59 Complex regional pain syndrome I of other specified site**

**✓5th G9Ø.8 Other disorders of autonomic nervous system**

AHA: 2023,2Q,8

**G9Ø.81 Serotonin syndrome**

Serotonin toxicity

Code first poisoning due to drug or toxin, such as:
- linezolid (T36.8X- with sixth character 1-4)
- monoamine oxidase inhibitors (T43.1X with sixth character 1-4)
- selective serotonin and norepinephrine reuptake inhibitors [SSNRI] (T43.21 with sixth character 1-4)
- selective serotonin reuptake inhibitors [SSRI] (T43.22 with sixth character 1-4)

Use additional code for adverse effect, if applicable, to identify drug, such as:

Use additional code, if applicable, to identify:
- disseminated intravascular coagulation (D65)
- hypertensive crisis (I16.-)
- linezolid (T36.8X5)
- metabolic acidosis (E87.2-)
- monoamine oxidase inhibitors (T43.1X5)
- selective serotonin and norepinephrine reuptake inhibitors [SSNRI] (T43.215)
- selective serotonin reuptake inhibitors [SSRI] (T43.225)
- shock, not elsewhere classified (R57.-)
- toxic encephalopathy (G92.-)
- ventricular tachycardia (I47.2-)

AHA: 2024,4Q,16

**G9Ø.89 Other disorders of autonomic nervous system**

**G9Ø.9 Disorder of the autonomic nervous system, unspecified**

**G9Ø.A Postural orthostatic tachycardia syndrome [POTS]**

Chronic orthostatic intolerance
Postural tachycardia syndrome

AHA: 2022,4Q,19-20

**G9Ø.B LMNB1-related autosomal dominant leukodystrophy** HCC ESR COM

AHA: 2023,4Q,12-13

## ✓4th G91 Hydrocephalus

INCLUDES acquired hydrocephalus

EXCLUDES 1 *Arnold-Chiari syndrome with hydrocephalus (QØ7.-)*
*congenital hydrocephalus (QØ3.-)*
*spina bifida with hydrocephalus (QØ5.-)*

DEF: Abnormal buildup of cerebrospinal fluid in the brain causing dilation of the ventricles.

**Hydrocephalus (Acquired)**

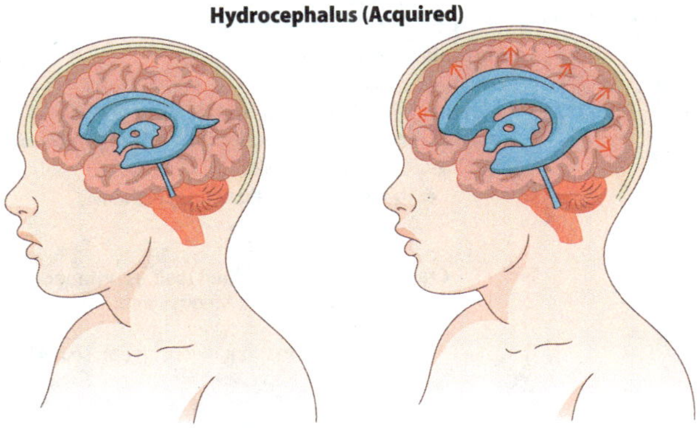

Normal ventricles — Hydrocephalic ventricles

**G91.Ø Communicating hydrocephalus** HCC ESR COM

Secondary normal pressure hydrocephalus

**G91.1 Obstructive hydrocephalus** HCC ESR COM

DEF: Obstruction of the cerebrospinal fluid passage from the brain into the spinal canal characterized by headaches, drowsiness, poor coordination, urinary incontinence, nausea, vomiting, and papilledema.

**G91.2 (Idiopathic) normal pressure hydrocephalus** HCC ESR COM

Normal pressure hydrocephalus NOS

**G91.3 Post-traumatic hydrocephalus, unspecified** HCC ESR COM

***G91.4 Hydrocephalus in diseases classified elsewhere*** HCC ESR COM

Code first underlying condition, such as:
- congenital syphilis (A5Ø.4-)
- neoplasm (CØØ-D49)
- plasminogen deficiency (E88.Ø2)

EXCLUDES 1 *hydrocephalus due to congenital toxoplasmosis (P37.1)*

AHA: 2014,3Q,3

**G91.8 Other hydrocephalus** HCC ESR COM

**G91.9 Hydrocephalus, unspecified** HCC ESR COM

AHA: 2025,3Q,17

## ✓4th G92 Toxic encephalopathy

AHA: 2022,1Q,52; 2021,4Q,12-14; 2021,1Q,13; 2017,1Q,39-40

DEF: Brain tissue degeneration due to a toxic substance.

**✓5th G92.Ø Immune effector cell-associated neurotoxicity syndrome**

Code first underlying cause such as:
- complications of immune effector cellular therapy (T8Ø.82)

Code also, if applicable, associated signs and symptoms, such as:
- cerebral edema (G93.6)
- unspecified convulsions (R56.9)

**G92.ØØ Immune effector cell-associated neurotoxicity syndrome, grade unspecified** UPD

ICANS, grade unspecified

**G92.Ø1 Immune effector cell-associated neurotoxicity syndrome, grade 1** UPD

ICANS, grade 1

**G92.Ø2 Immune effector cell-associated neurotoxicity syndrome, grade 2** UPD

ICANS, grade 2

**G92.Ø3 Immune effector cell-associated neurotoxicity syndrome, grade 3** UPD

ICANS, grade 3

**G92.Ø4 Immune effector cell-associated neurotoxicity syndrome, grade 4** UPD

ICANS, grade 4

**G92.Ø5 Immune effector cell-associated neurotoxicity syndrome, grade 5** UPD

ICANS, grade 5

**G92.8 Other toxic encephalopathy**

Toxic encephalitis
Toxic metabolic encephalopathy

Code first poisoning due to drug or toxin, if applicable, (T36-T65 with fifth or sixth character 1-4)

Use additional code for adverse effect, if applicable, to identify drug (T36-T5Ø with fifth or sixth character 5)

AHA: 2024,4Q,16; 2024,2Q,14; 2022,1Q,52

**G92.9 Unspecified toxic encephalopathy**

Code first poisoning due to drug or toxin, if applicable, (T36-T65 with fifth or sixth character 1-4)

Use additional code for adverse effect, if applicable, to identify drug (T36-T5Ø with fifth or sixth character 5)

## ✓4th G93 Other disorders of brain

**G93.Ø Cerebral cysts**

Arachnoid cyst
Porencephalic cyst, acquired

EXCLUDES 1 *acquired periventricular cysts of newborn (P91.1)*
*congenital cerebral cysts (QØ4.6)*

**G93.1 Anoxic brain damage, not elsewhere classified** HCC ESR COM

EXCLUDES 1 *cerebral anoxia due to anesthesia during labor and delivery (O74.3)*
*cerebral anoxia due to anesthesia during the puerperium (O89.2)*
*neonatal anoxia (P84)*

DEF: Brain injury not resulting from birth trauma that is due to lack of oxygen. Brain cells, when deprived of oxygen, begin to expire after four minutes.

**G93.2 Benign intracranial hypertension**

Pseudotumor

EXCLUDES 1 *hypertensive encephalopathy (I67.4)*
*obstructive hydrocephalus (G91.1)*

**✓5th G93.3 Postviral and related fatigue syndromes**

Use additional code, if applicable, for post COVID-19 condition, unspecified (UØ9.9)

EXCLUDES 1 *chronic fatigue NOS (R53.82)*
*neurasthenia (F48.8)*

AHA: 2022,4Q,20

**G93.31 Postviral fatigue syndrome**

**G93.32 Myalgic encephalomyelitis/chronic fatigue syndrome**
Chronic fatigue syndrome
ME/CFS
Myalgic encephalomyelitis

**G93.39 Other post infection and related fatigue syndromes**

✓5th **G93.4 Other and unspecified encephalopathy**
EXCLUDES 2 *alcoholic encephalopathy (G31.2)*
*encephalopathy in diseases classified elsewhere (G94)*
*hypertensive encephalopathy (I67.4)*
*toxic (metabolic) encephalopathy (G92.8)*

**G93.40 Encephalopathy, unspecified**
**AHA:** 2017,2Q,8

**G93.41 Metabolic encephalopathy**
Septic encephalopathy
**AHA:** 2024,2Q,14; 2017,2Q,8; 2016,3Q,42; 2015,3Q,21
**TIP:** Assign separately when documented with diabetic hypoglycemia (E08.649, E09.649, E10.649, E11.649, E13.649).

**G93.42 Megalencephalic leukoencephalopathy with subcortical cysts** HCC ESR COM
**AHA:** 2023,4Q,12-13

**G93.43 Leukoencephalopathy with calcifications and cysts** HCC ESR COM
**AHA:** 2023,4Q,12-13

**G93.44 Adult-onset leukodystrophy with axonal spheroids** HCC ESR COM A
Adult-onset leukoencephalopathy with axonal spheroids and pigmented glia
**AHA:** 2023,4Q,12-13

**G93.45 Developmental and epileptic encephalopathy** HCC Rx ESR COM
Early infantile epileptic encephalopathy
Code also, if applicable, associated disorders such as:
developmental disorder of speech and language (F80.-)
developmental disorders of scholastic skills (F81.-)
epilepsy, by specific type (G40.-)
intellectual disabilities (F70-F79)
other neurodevelopmental disorder (F88)
pervasive developmental disorders (F84.-)
**AHA:** 2024,4Q,17

**G93.49 Other encephalopathy**
Encephalopathy NEC
**AHA:** 2021,2Q,3; 2018,4Q,16; 2018,2Q,22,24; 2017,2Q,9

**G93.5 Compression of brain** HCC ESR COM
Arnold-Chiari type 1 compression of brain
Compression of brain (stem)
Herniation of brain (stem)
▶Midline shift of brain◀
EXCLUDES 1 *traumatic compression of brain (S06.A-)*
**AHA:** 2020,2Q,31

**G93.6 Cerebral edema** HCC ESR COM
EXCLUDES 1 *cerebral edema due to birth injury (P11.0)*
*traumatic cerebral edema (S06.1-)*
**AHA:** 2022,3Q,9-10

**G93.7 Reye's syndrome** HCC Rx ESR COM P
Code first poisoning due to salicylates, if applicable (T39.0-, with sixth character 1-4)
Use additional code for adverse effect due to salicylates, if applicable (T39.0-, with sixth character 5)
**DEF:** Rare childhood illness often developed after a viral upper respiratory infection. Symptoms include vomiting, elevated serum transaminase, brain swelling, disturbances of consciousness, seizures, and changes in liver and other viscera; it can be fatal.

✓5th **G93.8 Other specified disorders of brain**

**G93.81 Temporal sclerosis**
Hippocampal sclerosis
Mesial temporal sclerosis

**G93.82 Brain death**

**G93.89 Other specified disorders of brain**
Postradiation encephalopathy
**AHA:** 2024,2Q,15; 2020,2Q,24; 2019,3Q,8

**G93.9 Disorder of brain, unspecified**

***G94 Other disorders of brain in diseases classified elsewhere***
Code first underlying disease
EXCLUDES 1 *encephalopathy in congenital syphilis (A50.49)*
*encephalopathy in influenza (J09.X9, J10.81, J11.81)*
*encephalopathy in syphilis (A52.19)*
*hydrocephalus in diseases classified elsewhere (G91.4)*
**AHA:** 2018,2Q,22; 2017,2Q,8-9

✓4th **G95 Other and unspecified diseases of spinal cord**
EXCLUDES 2 *myelitis (G04.-)*

**G95.0 Syringomyelia and syringobulbia** HCC Rx ESR COM

✓5th **G95.1 Vascular myelopathies**
EXCLUDES 2 *intraspinal phlebitis and thrombophlebitis, except non-pyogenic (G08)*

**G95.11 Acute infarction of spinal cord (embolic) (nonembolic)** HCC Rx ESR COM
Anoxia of spinal cord
Arterial thrombosis of spinal cord

**G95.19 Other vascular myelopathies** HCC Rx ESR COM
Edema of spinal cord
Hematomyelia
Nonpyogenic intraspinal phlebitis and thrombophlebitis
Subacute necrotic myelopathy
**AHA:** 2024,3Q,5; 2023,3Q,21

✓5th **G95.2 Other and unspecified cord compression**

**G95.20 Unspecified cord compression** HCC Rx ESR COM

**G95.29 Other cord compression** HCC Rx ESR COM

✓5th **G95.8 Other specified diseases of spinal cord**
EXCLUDES 1 *neurogenic bladder NOS (N31.9)*
*neurogenic bladder due to cauda equina syndrome (G83.4)*
*neuromuscular dysfunction of bladder without spinal cord lesion (N31.-)*

**G95.81 Conus medullaris syndrome** HCC Rx ESR COM

**G95.89 Other specified diseases of spinal cord** HCC Rx ESR COM
Cord bladder NOS
Drug-induced myelopathy
Radiation-induced myelopathy
EXCLUDES 1 *myelopathy NOS (G95.9)*
**AHA:** 2024,3Q,5

**G95.9 Disease of spinal cord, unspecified** HCC Rx ESR COM
Myelopathy NOS
**AHA:** 2025,3Q,18

✓4th **G96 Other disorders of central nervous system**

✓5th **G96.0 Cerebrospinal fluid leak**
Code also if applicable:
intracranial hypotension (G96.81-)
EXCLUDES 1 *cerebrospinal fluid leak from spinal puncture (G97.0)*
**AHA:** 2024,3Q,7; 2020,4Q,21-22; 2018,2Q,13

**G96.00 Cerebrospinal fluid leak, unspecified**
Code also if applicable:
head injury (S00-S09)

**G96.01 Cranial cerebrospinal fluid leak, spontaneous**
Otorrhea due to spontaneous cerebrospinal fluid CSF leak
Rhinorrhea due to spontaneous cerebrospinal fluid CSF leak
Spontaneous cerebrospinal fluid leak from skull base

**G96.02 Spinal cerebrospinal fluid leak, spontaneous**
Spontaneous cerebrospinal fluid leak from spine

**G96.08 Other cranial cerebrospinal fluid leak**
Postoperative cranial cerebrospinal fluid leak
Traumatic cranial cerebrospinal fluid leak
Code also if applicable:
head injury (S00 - S09)
**AHA:** 2024,3Q,7

**G96.09 Other spinal cerebrospinal fluid leak**
Other spinal CSF leak
Postoperative spinal cerebrospinal fluid leak
Traumatic spinal cerebrospinal fluid leak
Code also if applicable:
head injury (S00 - S09)
**AHA:** 2022,3Q,24

**G96.1 Disorders of meninges, not elsewhere classified**

**G96.11 Dural tear**

Code also intracranial hypotension, if applicable (G96.81-)

EXCLUDES 1 *accidental puncture or laceration of dura during a procedure (G97.41)*

**AHA:** 2014,4Q,24

**G96.12 Meningeal adhesions (cerebral) (spinal)**

**G96.19 Other disorders of meninges, not elsewhere classified**

**AHA:** 2020,4Q,22

**G96.191 Perineural cyst**

Cervical nerve root cyst
Lumbar nerve root cyst
Sacral nerve root cyst
Tarlov cyst
Thoracic nerve root cyst

**G96.198 Other disorders of meninges, not elsewhere classified**

**G96.8 Other specified disorders of central nervous system**

**AHA:** 2020,4Q,21,23-24

**G96.81 Intracranial hypotension**

Code also any associated diagnoses, such as:
- brachial amyotrophy (G54.5)
- cerebrospinal fluid leak from spine (G96.Ø2)
- cranial nerve disorders in diseases classified elsewhere (G53)
- nerve root and compressions in diseases classified elsewhere (G55)
- nonpyogenic thrombosis of intracranial venous system (I67.6)
- nontraumatic intracerebral hemorrhage (I61.-)
- nontraumatic subdural hemorrhage (I62.Ø-)
- other and unspecified cord compression (G95.2-)
- other secondary parkinsonism (G21.8)
- reversible cerebrovascular vasoconstriction syndrome (I67.841)
- spinal cord herniation (G95.89)
- stroke (I63.-)
- syringomyelia (G95.Ø)

**DEF:** Central nervous system disorder resulting from a loss of cerebrospinal fluid (CSF) volume. More often associated with CSF leak at the level of the spine rather than the skull base, causes can be spontaneous, iatrogenic or traumatic spinal dura defects or holes, or overdrainage of CSF shunt devices. The most common symptom is headache.

**G96.81Ø Intracranial hypotension, unspecified**

**G96.811 Intracranial hypotension, spontaneous**

**AHA:** 2024,3Q,7

**G96.819 Other intracranial hypotension**

**G96.89 Other specified disorders of central nervous system**

**G96.9 Disorder of central nervous system, unspecified**

**G97 Intraoperative and postprocedural complications and disorders of nervous system, not elsewhere classified**

EXCLUDES 2 *intraoperative and postprocedural cerebrovascular infarction (I97.81-, I97.82-)*

**AHA:** 2016,4Q,9-10

**G97.Ø Cerebrospinal fluid leak from spinal puncture**

Code also any associated diagnoses or complications, such as:
- intracranial hypotension following a procedure (G97.83-G97.84)

**Spinal Puncture**

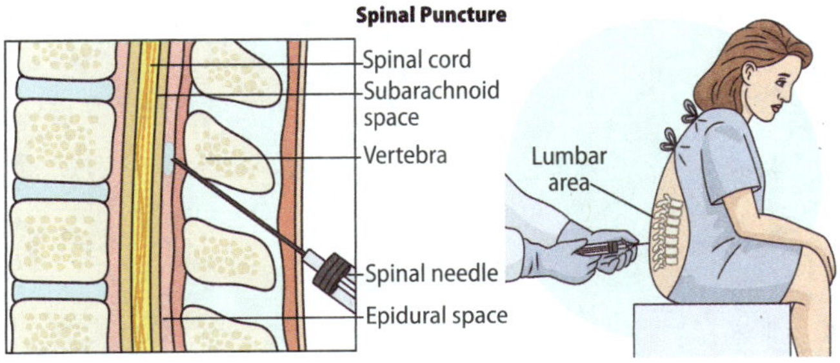


**G97.1 Other reaction to spinal and lumbar puncture**

Headache due to lumbar puncture
Other reaction to spinal dural puncture

Code also, if applicable, any associated headache with orthostatic component (R51.Ø)

**G97.2 Intracranial hypotension following ventricular shunting**

Code also any associated diagnoses or complications

**G97.3 Intraoperative hemorrhage and hematoma of a nervous system organ or structure complicating a procedure**

EXCLUDES 1 *intraoperative hemorrhage and hematoma of a nervous system organ or structure due to accidental puncture and laceration during a procedure (G97.4-)*

**G97.31 Intraoperative hemorrhage and hematoma of a nervous system organ or structure complicating a nervous system procedure**

**G97.32 Intraoperative hemorrhage and hematoma of a nervous system organ or structure complicating other procedure**

**G97.4 Accidental puncture and laceration of a nervous system organ or structure during a procedure**

**G97.41 Accidental puncture or laceration of dura during a procedure**

Incidental (inadvertent) durotomy

Code also any associated diagnoses or complications

**AHA:** 2024,1Q,20-21; 2014,4Q,24

**G97.48 Accidental puncture and laceration of other nervous system organ or structure during a nervous system procedure**

**G97.49 Accidental puncture and laceration of other nervous system organ or structure during other procedure**

**G97.5 Postprocedural hemorrhage of a nervous system organ or structure following a procedure**

**G97.51 Postprocedural hemorrhage of a nervous system organ or structure following a nervous system procedure**

**G97.52 Postprocedural hemorrhage of a nervous system organ or structure following other procedure**

**G97.6 Postprocedural hematoma and seroma of a nervous system organ or structure following a procedure**

**G97.61 Postprocedural hematoma of a nervous system organ or structure following a nervous system procedure**

**AHA:** 2025,2Q,26; 2024,3Q,5; 2020,3Q,24

**G97.62 Postprocedural hematoma of a nervous system organ or structure following other procedure**

**AHA:** 2025,2Q,26

**G97.63 Postprocedural seroma of a nervous system organ or structure following a nervous system procedure**

**G97.64 Postprocedural seroma of a nervous system organ or structure following other procedure**

**G97.8 Other intraoperative and postprocedural complications and disorders of nervous system**

Use additional code to further specify disorder

**AHA:** 2020,4Q,23

**G97.81 Other intraoperative complications of nervous system**

**G97.82 Other postprocedural complications and disorders of nervous system**

**AHA:** 2022,1Q,34

**G97.83 Intracranial hypotension following lumbar cerebrospinal fluid shunting**

Code also any associated diagnoses or complications

**G97.84 Intracranial hypotension following other procedure**

Code also, if applicable:
- accidental puncture or laceration of dura during a procedure (G97.41)
- cerebrospinal fluid leak from spinal puncture (G97.Ø)

**G98 Other disorders of nervous system not elsewhere classified**

INCLUDES nervous system disorder NOS

**G98.Ø Neurogenic arthritis, not elsewhere classified**

Nonsyphilitic neurogenic arthropathy NEC
Nonsyphilitic neurogenic spondylopathy NEC

EXCLUDES 1 *spondylopathy (in):*
- *syringomyelia and syringobulbia (G95.Ø)*
- *tabes dorsalis (A52.11)*

**G98.8 Other disorders of nervous system**

Nervous system disorder NOS

**G99 Other disorders of nervous system in diseases classified elsewhere**

***G99.Ø Autonomic neuropathy in diseases classified elsewhere***

Code first underlying disease, such as:
- amyloidosis (E85.-)
- gout (M1A.-, M1Ø.-)
- hyperthyroidism (EØ5.-)

EXCLUDES 1 *diabetic autonomic neuropathy (EØ8-E13 with .43)*

**G99.2** ***Myelopathy in diseases classified elsewhere*** HCC Rx ESR COM

Code first underlying disease, such as:
neoplasm (CØØ-D49)

EXCLUDES 1 *myelopathy in:*
*intervertebral disease (M5Ø.Ø-, M51.Ø-)*
*spondylosis (M47.Ø-, M47.1-)*

**AHA:** 2018,3Q,18-19

**TIP:** Use this code in addition to a spondylolisthesis code (M43.1-) or a spinal stenosis code (M48.0-) when either of these disorders is documented as the cause of the myelopathy.

**G99.8** ***Other specified disorders of nervous system in diseases classified elsewhere***

Code first underlying disorder, such as:
amyloidosis (E85.-)
avitaminosis (E56.-)

EXCLUDES 1 *nervous system involvement in:*
*cysticercosis (B69.Ø)*
*rubella (BØ6.Ø-)*
*syphilis (A52.1-)*

# Chapter 7. Diseases of the Eye and Adnexa (HØØ–H59)



## Chapter-specific Guidelines with Coding Examples

The chapter-specific guidelines from the ICD-10-CM Official Guidelines for Coding and Reporting have been provided below. Along with these guidelines are coding examples, contained in the shaded boxes, that have been developed to help illustrate the coding and/or sequencing guidance found in these guidelines.

**a. Glaucoma**

**1) Assigning glaucoma codes**

Assign as many codes from category H4Ø, Glaucoma, as needed to identify the type of glaucoma, the affected eye, and the glaucoma stage.

**2) Bilateral glaucoma with same type and stage**

When a patient has bilateral glaucoma and both eyes are documented as being the same type and stage, and there is a code for bilateral glaucoma, report only the code for the type of glaucoma, bilateral, with the seventh character for the stage.

> Bilateral mild stage primary open-angle glaucoma
>
> **H4Ø.1131 Primary open-angle glaucoma, bilateral, mild stage**
>
> *Explanation*: In this scenario, the patient has the same type and stage of glaucoma in both eyes. As this type of glaucoma has a code for bilateral, assign only the code for the bilateral glaucoma with the seventh character for the stage.

When a patient has bilateral glaucoma and both eyes are documented as being the same type and stage, and the classification does not provide a code for bilateral glaucoma (i.e. subcategories H4Ø.1Ø and H4Ø.2Ø) report only one code for the type of glaucoma with the appropriate seventh character for the stage.

> Bilateral open-angle glaucoma, severe stage; not specified as to type
>
> **H4Ø.1ØX3 Unspecified open-angle glaucoma, severe stage**
>
> *Explanation*: In this scenario, the patient has glaucoma of the same type and stage of both eyes, but there is no code specifically for bilateral glaucoma. Only one code is assigned with the appropriate seventh character for the stage.

**3) Bilateral glaucoma stage with different types or stages**

When a patient has bilateral glaucoma and each eye is documented as having a different type or stage, and the classification distinguishes laterality, assign the appropriate code for each eye rather than the code for bilateral glaucoma.

> Bilateral chronic angle-closure glaucoma; right eye is documented as mild stage and left eye as moderate stage
>
> **H4Ø.2211 Chronic angle-closure glaucoma, right eye, mild stage**
>
> **H4Ø.2222 Chronic angle-closure glaucoma, left eye, moderate stage**
>
> *Explanation*: In this scenario the patient has the same type of glaucoma in both eyes, but each eye is at a different stage. Because the subcategory for this condition identifies laterality, one code is assigned for the right eye and one code is assigned for the left eye, each with the appropriate seventh character for the stage appended.

When a patient has bilateral glaucoma and each eye is documented as having a different type, and the classification does not distinguish laterality (i.e. subcategories H4Ø.1Ø and H4Ø.2Ø), assign one code for each type of glaucoma with the appropriate seventh character for the stage.

> Documentation relates mild, unspecified primary angle-closure glaucoma of the left eye with mild unspecified open-angle glaucoma of the right eye
>
> **H4Ø.2ØX1 Unspecified primary angle-closure glaucoma, mild stage**
>
> **H4Ø.1ØX1 Unspecified open-angle glaucoma, mild stage**
>
> *Explanation*: In this scenario the patient has a different type of glaucoma in each eye and the classification does not distinguish laterality. A code for each type of glaucoma is assigned, each with the appropriate seventh character for the stage.

When a patient has bilateral glaucoma and each eye is documented as having the same type, but different stage, and the classification does not distinguish laterality (i.e. subcategories H4Ø.1Ø and H4Ø.2Ø), assign a code for the type of glaucoma for each eye with the seventh character for the specific glaucoma stage documented for each eye.

> Bilateral open-angle glaucoma, not specified as to type; the right eye is documented to be in mild stage and the left eye as being in moderate stage
>
> **H4Ø.1ØX1 Unspecified open-angle glaucoma, mild stage**
>
> **H4Ø.1ØX2 Unspecified open-angle glaucoma, moderate stage**
>
> *Explanation*: In this scenario the patient has the same type of glaucoma in each eye but each eye is at a different stage, and the classification does not distinguish laterality at this subcategory level. Two codes are assigned; both codes represent the same type of glaucoma but each has a different seventh character identifying the appropriate stage for each eye.

**4) Patient admitted with glaucoma and stage evolves during the admission**

If a patient is admitted with glaucoma and the stage progresses during the admission, assign the code for highest stage documented.

**5) Indeterminate stage glaucoma**

Assignment of the seventh character "4" for "indeterminate stage" should be based on the clinical documentation. The seventh character "4" is used for glaucomas whose stage cannot be clinically determined. This seventh character should not be confused with the seventh character "Ø", unspecified, which should be assigned when there is no documentation regarding the stage of the glaucoma.

**b. Blindness**

If "blindness" or "low vision" of both eyes is documented but the visual impairment category is not documented, assign code H54.3, Unqualified visual loss, both eyes. If "blindness" or "low vision" in one eye is documented but the visual impairment category is not documented, assign a code from H54.6-, Unqualified visual loss, one eye. If "blindness" or "visual loss" is documented without any information about whether one or both eyes are affected, assign code H54.7, Unspecified visual loss.

> Patient assessment indicates moderately impaired/low vision in the left eye with no visual impairments in the right eye
>
> **H54.62 Unqualified visual loss, left eye, normal vision right eye**
>
> Report unqualified visual loss when the visual impairment category is not specified. In this case, only the left eye is impacted by visual loss with normal vision of the right eye documented.

# Chapter 7. Diseases of the Eye and Adnexa (HØØ-H59)

**NOTE** Use an external cause code following the code for the eye condition, if applicable, to identify the cause of the eye condition

**EXCLUDES 2** *certain conditions originating in the perinatal period (PØ4-P96)*
*certain infectious and parasitic diseases (AØØ-B99)*
*complications of pregnancy, childbirth and the puerperium (OØØ-O9A)*
*congenital malformations, deformations, and chromosomal abnormalities (QØØ-Q99)*
*diabetes mellitus related eye conditions (EØ9.3-, E1Ø.3-, E11.3-, E13.3-)*
*endocrine, nutritional and metabolic diseases (EØØ-E88)*
*injury (trauma) of eye and orbit (SØ5.-)*
*injury, poisoning and certain other consequences of external causes (SØØ-T88)*
*neoplasms (CØØ-D49)*
*symptoms, signs and abnormal clinical and laboratory findings, not elsewhere classified (RØØ-R94)*
*syphilis related eye disorders (A5Ø.Ø1, A5Ø.3-, A51.43, A52.71)*

This chapter contains the following blocks:

| | |
|---|---|
| HØØ-HØ5 | Disorders of eyelid, lacrimal system and orbit |
| H1Ø-H11 | Disorders of conjunctiva |
| H15-H22 | Disorders of sclera, cornea, iris and ciliary body |
| H25-H28 | Disorders of lens |
| H3Ø-H36 | Disorders of choroid and retina |
| H4Ø-H42 | Glaucoma |
| H43-H44 | Disorders of vitreous body and globe |
| H46-H47 | Disorders of optic nerve and visual pathways |
| H49-H52 | Disorders of ocular muscles, binocular movement, accommodation and refraction |
| H53-H54 | Visual disturbances and blindness |
| H55-H57 | Other disorders of eye and adnexa |
| H59 | Intraoperative and postprocedural complications and disorders of eye and adnexa, not elsewhere classified |

## Disorders of eyelid, lacrimal system and orbit (HØØ-HØ5)

**EXCLUDES 2** *open wound of eyelid (SØ1.1-)*
*superficial injury of eyelid (SØØ.1-, SØØ.2-)*

✓4th **HØØ Hordeolum and chalazion**

✓5th **HØØ.Ø Hordeolum (externum) (internum) of eyelid**

DEF: Acute localized infection of the gland of Zeis (external hordeolum) or Molt or of the meibomian glands (internal hordeolum) of the orbit.

✓6th **HØØ.Ø1 Hordeolum externum**

Hordeolum NOS
Stye

**HØØ.Ø11 Hordeolum externum right upper eyelid**
**HØØ.Ø12 Hordeolum externum right lower eyelid**
**HØØ.Ø13 Hordeolum externum right eye, unspecified eyelid**
**HØØ.Ø14 Hordeolum externum left upper eyelid**
**HØØ.Ø15 Hordeolum externum left lower eyelid**
**HØØ.Ø16 Hordeolum externum left eye, unspecified eyelid**
**HØØ.Ø19 Hordeolum externum unspecified eye, unspecified eyelid**

✓6th **HØØ.Ø2 Hordeolum internum**

Infection of meibomian gland

**HØØ.Ø21 Hordeolum internum right upper eyelid**
**HØØ.Ø22 Hordeolum internum right lower eyelid**
**HØØ.Ø23 Hordeolum internum right eye, unspecified eyelid**
**HØØ.Ø24 Hordeolum internum left upper eyelid**
**HØØ.Ø25 Hordeolum internum left lower eyelid**
**HØØ.Ø26 Hordeolum internum left eye, unspecified eyelid**
**HØØ.Ø29 Hordeolum internum unspecified eye, unspecified eyelid**

✓6th **HØØ.Ø3 Abscess of eyelid**

Furuncle of eyelid

**HØØ.Ø31 Abscess of right upper eyelid**
**HØØ.Ø32 Abscess of right lower eyelid**
**HØØ.Ø33 Abscess of eyelid right eye, unspecified eyelid**
**HØØ.Ø34 Abscess of left upper eyelid**
**HØØ.Ø35 Abscess of left lower eyelid**
**HØØ.Ø36 Abscess of eyelid left eye, unspecified eyelid**
**HØØ.Ø39 Abscess of eyelid unspecified eye, unspecified eyelid**

✓5th **HØØ.1 Chalazion**

Meibomian (gland) cyst

**EXCLUDES 2** *infected meibomian gland (HØØ.Ø2-)*

DEF: Noninfectious, obstructive mass in the oil gland of the eyelid that results in a small chronic lump or inflammation.

**HØØ.11 Chalazion right upper eyelid**
**HØØ.12 Chalazion right lower eyelid**
**HØØ.13 Chalazion right eye, unspecified eyelid**
**HØØ.14 Chalazion left upper eyelid**
**HØØ.15 Chalazion left lower eyelid**
**HØØ.16 Chalazion left eye, unspecified eyelid**
**HØØ.19 Chalazion unspecified eye, unspecified eyelid**

✓4th **HØ1 Other inflammation of eyelid**

✓5th **HØ1.Ø Blepharitis**

**EXCLUDES 1** *blepharoconjunctivitis (H1Ø.5-)*

✓6th **HØ1.ØØ Unspecified blepharitis**

AHA: 2018,4Q,13

**HØ1.ØØ1 Unspecified blepharitis right upper eyelid**
**HØ1.ØØ2 Unspecified blepharitis right lower eyelid**
**HØ1.ØØ3 Unspecified blepharitis right eye, unspecified eyelid**
**HØ1.ØØ4 Unspecified blepharitis left upper eyelid**
**HØ1.ØØ5 Unspecified blepharitis left lower eyelid**
**HØ1.ØØ6 Unspecified blepharitis left eye, unspecified eyelid**
**HØ1.ØØ9 Unspecified blepharitis unspecified eye, unspecified eyelid**
**HØ1.ØØA Unspecified blepharitis right eye, upper and lower eyelids**
**HØ1.ØØB Unspecified blepharitis left eye, upper and lower eyelids**

✓6th **HØ1.Ø1 Ulcerative blepharitis**

AHA: 2018,4Q,13

**HØ1.Ø11 Ulcerative blepharitis right upper eyelid**
**HØ1.Ø12 Ulcerative blepharitis right lower eyelid**
**HØ1.Ø13 Ulcerative blepharitis right eye, unspecified eyelid**
**HØ1.Ø14 Ulcerative blepharitis left upper eyelid**
**HØ1.Ø15 Ulcerative blepharitis left lower eyelid**
**HØ1.Ø16 Ulcerative blepharitis left eye, unspecified eyelid**
**HØ1.Ø19 Ulcerative blepharitis unspecified eye, unspecified eyelid**
**HØ1.Ø1A Ulcerative blepharitis right eye, upper and lower eyelids**
**HØ1.Ø1B Ulcerative blepharitis left eye, upper and lower eyelids**

✓6th **HØ1.Ø2 Squamous blepharitis**

AHA: 2018,4Q,13

**HØ1.Ø21 Squamous blepharitis right upper eyelid**
**HØ1.Ø22 Squamous blepharitis right lower eyelid**
**HØ1.Ø23 Squamous blepharitis right eye, unspecified eyelid**
**HØ1.Ø24 Squamous blepharitis left upper eyelid**
**HØ1.Ø25 Squamous blepharitis left lower eyelid**
**HØ1.Ø26 Squamous blepharitis left eye, unspecified eyelid**
**HØ1.Ø29 Squamous blepharitis unspecified eye, unspecified eyelid**
**HØ1.Ø2A Squamous blepharitis right eye, upper and lower eyelids**
**HØ1.Ø2B Squamous blepharitis left eye, upper and lower eyelids**

✓5th **HØ1.1 Noninfectious dermatoses of eyelid**

✓6th **HØ1.11 Allergic dermatitis of eyelid**

Contact dermatitis of eyelid

**HØ1.111 Allergic dermatitis of right upper eyelid**
**HØ1.112 Allergic dermatitis of right lower eyelid**
**HØ1.113 Allergic dermatitis of right eye, unspecified eyelid**
**HØ1.114 Allergic dermatitis of left upper eyelid**
**HØ1.115 Allergic dermatitis of left lower eyelid**
**HØ1.116 Allergic dermatitis of left eye, unspecified eyelid**
**HØ1.119 Allergic dermatitis of unspecified eye, unspecified eyelid**

✓6th **HØ1.12 Discoid lupus erythematosus of eyelid**

**HØ1.121 Discoid lupus erythematosus of right upper eyelid** Rx

HØ1.122 Discoid lupus erythematosus of right lower eyelid Rx
HØ1.123 Discoid lupus erythematosus of right eye, unspecified eyelid Rx
HØ1.124 Discoid lupus erythematosus of left upper eyelid Rx
HØ1.125 Discoid lupus erythematosus of left lower eyelid Rx
HØ1.126 Discoid lupus erythematosus of left eye, unspecified eyelid Rx
HØ1.129 Discoid lupus erythematosus of unspecified eye, unspecified eyelid Rx

√6th HØ1.13 Eczematous dermatitis of eyelid
HØ1.131 Eczematous dermatitis of right upper eyelid
HØ1.132 Eczematous dermatitis of right lower eyelid
HØ1.133 Eczematous dermatitis of right eye, unspecified eyelid
HØ1.134 Eczematous dermatitis of left upper eyelid
HØ1.135 Eczematous dermatitis of left lower eyelid
HØ1.136 Eczematous dermatitis of left eye, unspecified eyelid
HØ1.139 Eczematous dermatitis of unspecified eye, unspecified eyelid

√6th HØ1.14 Xeroderma of eyelid
HØ1.141 Xeroderma of right upper eyelid
HØ1.142 Xeroderma of right lower eyelid
HØ1.143 Xeroderma of right eye, unspecified eyelid
HØ1.144 Xeroderma of left upper eyelid
HØ1.145 Xeroderma of left lower eyelid
HØ1.146 Xeroderma of left eye, unspecified eyelid
HØ1.149 Xeroderma of unspecified eye, unspecified eyelid

√5th HØ1.8 Other specified inflammations of eyelid
Code also, if applicable, infestation by Demodex mites (B88.Ø1)
HØ1.81 Other specified inflammation of right upper eyelid
HØ1.82 Other specified inflammation of right lower eyelid
HØ1.83 Other specified inflammation of right eye, unspecified eyelid
HØ1.84 Other specified inflammation of left upper eyelid
HØ1.85 Other specified inflammation of left lower eyelid
HØ1.86 Other specified inflammation of left eye, unspecified eyelid
HØ1.89 Other specified inflammation of unspecified eye, unspecified eyelid
HØ1.8A Other specified inflammation of right eye, upper and lower eyelids
HØ1.8B Other specified inflammation of left eye, upper and lower eyelids

HØ1.9 Unspecified inflammation of eyelid
Inflammation of eyelid NOS

√4th **HØ2 Other disorders of eyelid**

EXCLUDES 1 *congenital malformations of eyelid (Q1Ø.Ø-Q1Ø.3)*

√5th HØ2.Ø Entropion and trichiasis of eyelid

**DEF:** Entropion: Inversion of the eyelid, turning the edge in toward the eyeball and causing irritation from contact of the lashes with the surface of the eye.

**DEF:** Trichiasis: Condition wherein the eyelid is in a normal position but lashes are ingrown or misdirected in their growth so that they irritate the tissues of the eye.

**Entropion and Ectropion**

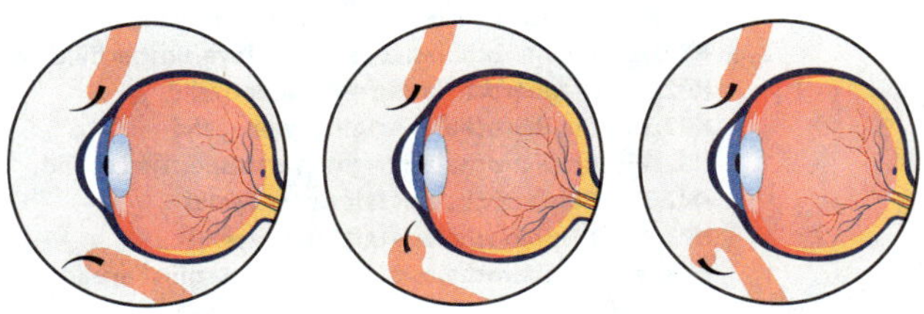

Normal eyelid Entropion Ectropion

√6th HØ2.ØØ Unspecified entropion of eyelid
HØ2.ØØ1 Unspecified entropion of right upper eyelid
HØ2.ØØ2 Unspecified entropion of right lower eyelid
HØ2.ØØ3 Unspecified entropion of right eye, unspecified eyelid
HØ2.ØØ4 Unspecified entropion of left upper eyelid
HØ2.ØØ5 Unspecified entropion of left lower eyelid
HØ2.ØØ6 Unspecified entropion of left eye, unspecified eyelid
HØ2.ØØ9 Unspecified entropion of unspecified eye, unspecified eyelid

√6th HØ2.Ø1 Cicatricial entropion of eyelid
HØ2.Ø11 Cicatricial entropion of right upper eyelid
HØ2.Ø12 Cicatricial entropion of right lower eyelid
HØ2.Ø13 Cicatricial entropion of right eye, unspecified eyelid
HØ2.Ø14 Cicatricial entropion of left upper eyelid
HØ2.Ø15 Cicatricial entropion of left lower eyelid
HØ2.Ø16 Cicatricial entropion of left eye, unspecified eyelid
HØ2.Ø19 Cicatricial entropion of unspecified eye, unspecified eyelid

√6th HØ2.Ø2 Mechanical entropion of eyelid
HØ2.Ø21 Mechanical entropion of right upper eyelid
HØ2.Ø22 Mechanical entropion of right lower eyelid
HØ2.Ø23 Mechanical entropion of right eye, unspecified eyelid
HØ2.Ø24 Mechanical entropion of left upper eyelid
HØ2.Ø25 Mechanical entropion of left lower eyelid
HØ2.Ø26 Mechanical entropion of left eye, unspecified eyelid
HØ2.Ø29 Mechanical entropion of unspecified eye, unspecified eyelid

√6th HØ2.Ø3 Senile entropion of eyelid
HØ2.Ø31 Senile entropion of right upper eyelid A
HØ2.Ø32 Senile entropion of right lower eyelid A
HØ2.Ø33 Senile entropion of right eye, unspecified eyelid A
HØ2.Ø34 Senile entropion of left upper eyelid A
HØ2.Ø35 Senile entropion of left lower eyelid A
HØ2.Ø36 Senile entropion of left eye, unspecified eyelid A
HØ2.Ø39 Senile entropion of unspecified eye, unspecified eyelid A

√6th HØ2.Ø4 Spastic entropion of eyelid
HØ2.Ø41 Spastic entropion of right upper eyelid
HØ2.Ø42 Spastic entropion of right lower eyelid
HØ2.Ø43 Spastic entropion of right eye, unspecified eyelid
HØ2.Ø44 Spastic entropion of left upper eyelid
HØ2.Ø45 Spastic entropion of left lower eyelid
HØ2.Ø46 Spastic entropion of left eye, unspecified eyelid
HØ2.Ø49 Spastic entropion of unspecified eye, unspecified eyelid

√6th HØ2.Ø5 Trichiasis without entropion
HØ2.Ø51 Trichiasis without entropion right upper eyelid
HØ2.Ø52 Trichiasis without entropion right lower eyelid
HØ2.Ø53 Trichiasis without entropion right eye, unspecified eyelid
HØ2.Ø54 Trichiasis without entropion left upper eyelid
HØ2.Ø55 Trichiasis without entropion left lower eyelid
HØ2.Ø56 Trichiasis without entropion left eye, unspecified eyelid
HØ2.Ø59 Trichiasis without entropion unspecified eye, unspecified eyelid

√5th HØ2.1 Ectropion of eyelid

**DEF:** Drooping of the lower eyelid away from the eye or outward turning or eversion of the edge of the eyelid, exposing the palpebral conjunctiva and causing irritation.

√6th HØ2.1Ø Unspecified ectropion of eyelid
HØ2.1Ø1 Unspecified ectropion of right upper eyelid
HØ2.1Ø2 Unspecified ectropion of right lower eyelid
HØ2.1Ø3 Unspecified ectropion of right eye, unspecified eyelid
HØ2.1Ø4 Unspecified ectropion of left upper eyelid
HØ2.1Ø5 Unspecified ectropion of left lower eyelid
HØ2.1Ø6 Unspecified ectropion of left eye, unspecified eyelid

H02.109 Unspecified ectropion of unspecified eye, unspecified eyelid

✓6th H02.11 Cicatricial ectropion of eyelid

H02.111 Cicatricial ectropion of right upper eyelid
H02.112 Cicatricial ectropion of right lower eyelid
H02.113 Cicatricial ectropion of right eye, unspecified eyelid
H02.114 Cicatricial ectropion of left upper eyelid
H02.115 Cicatricial ectropion of left lower eyelid
H02.116 Cicatricial ectropion of left eye, unspecified eyelid
H02.119 Cicatricial ectropion of unspecified eye, unspecified eyelid

✓6th H02.12 Mechanical ectropion of eyelid

H02.121 Mechanical ectropion of right upper eyelid
H02.122 Mechanical ectropion of right lower eyelid
H02.123 Mechanical ectropion of right eye, unspecified eyelid
H02.124 Mechanical ectropion of left upper eyelid
H02.125 Mechanical ectropion of left lower eyelid
H02.126 Mechanical ectropion of left eye, unspecified eyelid
H02.129 Mechanical ectropion of unspecified eye, unspecified eyelid

✓6th H02.13 Senile ectropion of eyelid

H02.131 Senile ectropion of right upper eyelid A
H02.132 Senile ectropion of right lower eyelid A
H02.133 Senile ectropion of right eye, unspecified eyelid A
H02.134 Senile ectropion of left upper eyelid A
H02.135 Senile ectropion of left lower eyelid A
H02.136 Senile ectropion of left eye, unspecified eyelid A
H02.139 Senile ectropion of unspecified eye, unspecified eyelid A

✓6th H02.14 Spastic ectropion of eyelid

H02.141 Spastic ectropion of right upper eyelid
H02.142 Spastic ectropion of right lower eyelid
H02.143 Spastic ectropion of right eye, unspecified eyelid
H02.144 Spastic ectropion of left upper eyelid
H02.145 Spastic ectropion of left lower eyelid
H02.146 Spastic ectropion of left eye, unspecified eyelid
H02.149 Spastic ectropion of unspecified eye, unspecified eyelid

✓6th H02.15 Paralytic ectropion of eyelid

**AHA:** 2018,4Q,13

H02.151 Paralytic ectropion of right upper eyelid
H02.152 Paralytic ectropion of right lower eyelid
H02.153 Paralytic ectropion of right eye, unspecified eyelid
H02.154 Paralytic ectropion of left upper eyelid
H02.155 Paralytic ectropion of left lower eyelid
H02.156 Paralytic ectropion of left eye, unspecified eyelid
H02.159 Paralytic ectropion of unspecified eye, unspecified eyelid

✓5th H02.2 Lagophthalmos

**AHA:** 2018,4Q,14

**DEF:** Condition of the eye that prevents it from closing completely.

✓6th H02.20 Unspecified lagophthalmos

H02.201 Unspecified lagophthalmos right upper eyelid
H02.202 Unspecified lagophthalmos right lower eyelid
H02.203 Unspecified lagophthalmos right eye, unspecified eyelid
H02.204 Unspecified lagophthalmos left upper eyelid
H02.205 Unspecified lagophthalmos left lower eyelid
H02.206 Unspecified lagophthalmos left eye, unspecified eyelid
H02.209 Unspecified lagophthalmos unspecified eye, unspecified eyelid
H02.20A Unspecified lagophthalmos right eye, upper and lower eyelids
H02.20B Unspecified lagophthalmos left eye, upper and lower eyelids
H02.20C Unspecified lagophthalmos, bilateral, upper and lower eyelids

✓6th H02.21 Cicatricial lagophthalmos

H02.211 Cicatricial lagophthalmos right upper eyelid
H02.212 Cicatricial lagophthalmos right lower eyelid
H02.213 Cicatricial lagophthalmos right eye, unspecified eyelid
H02.214 Cicatricial lagophthalmos left upper eyelid
H02.215 Cicatricial lagophthalmos left lower eyelid
H02.216 Cicatricial lagophthalmos left eye, unspecified eyelid
H02.219 Cicatricial lagophthalmos unspecified eye, unspecified eyelid
H02.21A Cicatricial lagophthalmos right eye, upper and lower eyelids
H02.21B Cicatricial lagophthalmos left eye, upper and lower eyelids
H02.21C Cicatricial lagophthalmos, bilateral, upper and lower eyelids

✓6th H02.22 Mechanical lagophthalmos

H02.221 Mechanical lagophthalmos right upper eyelid
H02.222 Mechanical lagophthalmos right lower eyelid
H02.223 Mechanical lagophthalmos right eye, unspecified eyelid
H02.224 Mechanical lagophthalmos left upper eyelid
H02.225 Mechanical lagophthalmos left lower eyelid
H02.226 Mechanical lagophthalmos left eye, unspecified eyelid
H02.229 Mechanical lagophthalmos unspecified eye, unspecified eyelid
H02.22A Mechanical lagophthalmos right eye, upper and lower eyelids
H02.22B Mechanical lagophthalmos left eye, upper and lower eyelids
H02.22C Mechanical lagophthalmos, bilateral, upper and lower eyelids

✓6th H02.23 Paralytic lagophthalmos

H02.231 Paralytic lagophthalmos right upper eyelid
H02.232 Paralytic lagophthalmos right lower eyelid
H02.233 Paralytic lagophthalmos right eye, unspecified eyelid
H02.234 Paralytic lagophthalmos left upper eyelid
H02.235 Paralytic lagophthalmos left lower eyelid
H02.236 Paralytic lagophthalmos left eye, unspecified eyelid
H02.239 Paralytic lagophthalmos unspecified eye, unspecified eyelid
H02.23A Paralytic lagophthalmos right eye, upper and lower eyelids
H02.23B Paralytic lagophthalmos left eye, upper and lower eyelids
H02.23C Paralytic lagophthalmos, bilateral, upper and lower eyelids

✓5th H02.3 Blepharochalasis

Pseudoptosis

**DEF:** Loss of elasticity and relaxation of skin of the eyelid, thickened or indurated skin on the eyelid associated with recurrent episodes of edema, and intracellular atrophy.

H02.30 Blepharochalasis unspecified eye, unspecified eyelid
H02.31 Blepharochalasis right upper eyelid
H02.32 Blepharochalasis right lower eyelid
H02.33 Blepharochalasis right eye, unspecified eyelid
H02.34 Blepharochalasis left upper eyelid
H02.35 Blepharochalasis left lower eyelid
H02.36 Blepharochalasis left eye, unspecified eyelid

✓5th H02.4 Ptosis of eyelid

✓6th H02.40 Unspecified ptosis of eyelid

H02.401 Unspecified ptosis of right eyelid
H02.402 Unspecified ptosis of left eyelid
H02.403 Unspecified ptosis of bilateral eyelids
H02.409 Unspecified ptosis of unspecified eyelid

✓6th **H02.41 Mechanical ptosis of eyelid**
- **H02.411 Mechanical ptosis of right eyelid**
- **H02.412 Mechanical ptosis of left eyelid**
- **H02.413 Mechanical ptosis of bilateral eyelids**
- **H02.419 Mechanical ptosis of unspecified eyelid**

✓6th **H02.42 Myogenic ptosis of eyelid**
- **H02.421 Myogenic ptosis of right eyelid**
- **H02.422 Myogenic ptosis of left eyelid**
- **H02.423 Myogenic ptosis of bilateral eyelids**
- **H02.429 Myogenic ptosis of unspecified eyelid**

✓6th **H02.43 Paralytic ptosis of eyelid**
Neurogenic ptosis of eyelid
- **H02.431 Paralytic ptosis of right eyelid**
- **H02.432 Paralytic ptosis of left eyelid**
- **H02.433 Paralytic ptosis of bilateral eyelids**
- **H02.439 Paralytic ptosis unspecified eyelid**

✓5th **H02.5 Other disorders affecting eyelid function**
EXCLUDES 2 *blepharospasm (G24.5)*
*organic tic (G25.69)*
*psychogenic tic (F95.-)*

✓6th **H02.51 Abnormal innervation syndrome**
- **H02.511 Abnormal innervation syndrome right upper eyelid**
- **H02.512 Abnormal innervation syndrome right lower eyelid**
- **H02.513 Abnormal innervation syndrome right eye, unspecified eyelid**
- **H02.514 Abnormal innervation syndrome left upper eyelid**
- **H02.515 Abnormal innervation syndrome left lower eyelid**
- **H02.516 Abnormal innervation syndrome left eye, unspecified eyelid**
- **H02.519 Abnormal innervation syndrome unspecified eye, unspecified eyelid**

✓6th **H02.52 Blepharophimosis**
Ankyloblepharon
- **H02.521 Blepharophimosis right upper eyelid**
- **H02.522 Blepharophimosis right lower eyelid**
- **H02.523 Blepharophimosis right eye, unspecified eyelid**
- **H02.524 Blepharophimosis left upper eyelid**
- **H02.525 Blepharophimosis left lower eyelid**
- **H02.526 Blepharophimosis left eye, unspecified eyelid**
- **H02.529 Blepharophimosis unspecified eye, unspecified lid**

✓6th **H02.53 Eyelid retraction**
Eyelid lag
- **H02.531 Eyelid retraction right upper eyelid**
- **H02.532 Eyelid retraction right lower eyelid**
- **H02.533 Eyelid retraction right eye, unspecified eyelid**
- **H02.534 Eyelid retraction left upper eyelid**
- **H02.535 Eyelid retraction left lower eyelid**
- **H02.536 Eyelid retraction left eye, unspecified eyelid**
- **H02.539 Eyelid retraction unspecified eye, unspecified lid**

**H02.59 Other disorders affecting eyelid function**
Deficient blink reflex
Sensory disorders

✓5th **H02.6 Xanthelasma of eyelid**
**DEF:** Condition in which there are small yellow tumors that occur on the eyelid, usually appearing near the nose.
- **H02.60 Xanthelasma of unspecified eye, unspecified eyelid**
- **H02.61 Xanthelasma of right upper eyelid**
- **H02.62 Xanthelasma of right lower eyelid**
- **H02.63 Xanthelasma of right eye, unspecified eyelid**
- **H02.64 Xanthelasma of left upper eyelid**
- **H02.65 Xanthelasma of left lower eyelid**
- **H02.66 Xanthelasma of left eye, unspecified eyelid**

✓5th **H02.7 Other and unspecified degenerative disorders of eyelid and periocular area**
- **H02.70 Unspecified degenerative disorders of eyelid and periocular area**

✓6th **H02.71 Chloasma of eyelid and periocular area**
Dyspigmentation of eyelid
Hyperpigmentation of eyelid
- **H02.711 Chloasma of right upper eyelid and periocular area**
- **H02.712 Chloasma of right lower eyelid and periocular area**
- **H02.713 Chloasma of right eye, unspecified eyelid and periocular area**
- **H02.714 Chloasma of left upper eyelid and periocular area**
- **H02.715 Chloasma of left lower eyelid and periocular area**
- **H02.716 Chloasma of left eye, unspecified eyelid and periocular area**
- **H02.719 Chloasma of unspecified eye, unspecified eyelid and periocular area**

✓6th **H02.72 Madarosis of eyelid and periocular area**
Hypotrichosis of eyelid
- **H02.721 Madarosis of right upper eyelid and periocular area**
- **H02.722 Madarosis of right lower eyelid and periocular area**
- **H02.723 Madarosis of right eye, unspecified eyelid and periocular area**
- **H02.724 Madarosis of left upper eyelid and periocular area**
- **H02.725 Madarosis of left lower eyelid and periocular area**
- **H02.726 Madarosis of left eye, unspecified eyelid and periocular area**
- **H02.729 Madarosis of unspecified eye, unspecified eyelid and periocular area**

✓6th **H02.73 Vitiligo of eyelid and periocular area**
Hypopigmentation of eyelid
- **H02.731 Vitiligo of right upper eyelid and periocular area**
- **H02.732 Vitiligo of right lower eyelid and periocular area**
- **H02.733 Vitiligo of right eye, unspecified eyelid and periocular area**
- **H02.734 Vitiligo of left upper eyelid and periocular area**
- **H02.735 Vitiligo of left lower eyelid and periocular area**
- **H02.736 Vitiligo of left eye, unspecified eyelid and periocular area**
- **H02.739 Vitiligo of unspecified eye, unspecified eyelid and periocular area**

**H02.79 Other degenerative disorders of eyelid and periocular area**

✓5th **H02.8 Other specified disorders of eyelid**

✓6th **H02.81 Retained foreign body in eyelid**
Use additional code to identify the type of retained foreign body (Z18.-)
EXCLUDES 1 *laceration of eyelid with foreign body (S01.12-)*
*retained intraocular foreign body (H44.6-, H44.7-)*
*superficial foreign body of eyelid and periocular area (S00.25-)*
- **H02.811 Retained foreign body in right upper eyelid**
- **H02.812 Retained foreign body in right lower eyelid**
- **H02.813 Retained foreign body in right eye, unspecified eyelid**
- **H02.814 Retained foreign body in left upper eyelid**
- **H02.815 Retained foreign body in left lower eyelid**
- **H02.816 Retained foreign body in left eye, unspecified eyelid**
- **H02.819 Retained foreign body in unspecified eye, unspecified eyelid**

✓6th **H02.82 Cysts of eyelid**
Sebaceous cyst of eyelid
- **H02.821 Cysts of right upper eyelid**
- **H02.822 Cysts of right lower eyelid**
- **H02.823 Cysts of right eye, unspecified eyelid**
- **H02.824 Cysts of left upper eyelid**
- **H02.825 Cysts of left lower eyelid**
- **H02.826 Cysts of left eye, unspecified eyelid**
- **H02.829 Cysts of unspecified eye, unspecified eyelid**

✓6th **H02.83 Dermatochalasis of eyelid**

DEF: Acquired form of connective tissue disorder associated with decreased elastic tissue and abnormal elastin formation, resulting in loss of elasticity of the skin of the eyelid. It is generally associated with aging.

**H02.831 Dermatochalasis of right upper eyelid**
**H02.832 Dermatochalasis of right lower eyelid**
**H02.833 Dermatochalasis of right eye, unspecified eyelid**
**H02.834 Dermatochalasis of left upper eyelid**
**H02.835 Dermatochalasis of left lower eyelid**
**H02.836 Dermatochalasis of left eye, unspecified eyelid**
**H02.839 Dermatochalasis of unspecified eye, unspecified eyelid**

✓6th **H02.84 Edema of eyelid**

Hyperemia of eyelid

**H02.841 Edema of right upper eyelid**
**H02.842 Edema of right lower eyelid**
**H02.843 Edema of right eye, unspecified eyelid**
**H02.844 Edema of left upper eyelid**
**H02.845 Edema of left lower eyelid**
**H02.846 Edema of left eye, unspecified eyelid**
**H02.849 Edema of unspecified eye, unspecified eyelid**

✓6th **H02.85 Elephantiasis of eyelid**

**H02.851 Elephantiasis of right upper eyelid**
**H02.852 Elephantiasis of right lower eyelid**
**H02.853 Elephantiasis of right eye, unspecified eyelid**
**H02.854 Elephantiasis of left upper eyelid**
**H02.855 Elephantiasis of left lower eyelid**
**H02.856 Elephantiasis of left eye, unspecified eyelid**
**H02.859 Elephantiasis of unspecified eye, unspecified eyelid**

✓6th **H02.86 Hypertrichosis of eyelid**

**H02.861 Hypertrichosis of right upper eyelid**
**H02.862 Hypertrichosis of right lower eyelid**
**H02.863 Hypertrichosis of right eye, unspecified eyelid**
**H02.864 Hypertrichosis of left upper eyelid**
**H02.865 Hypertrichosis of left lower eyelid**
**H02.866 Hypertrichosis of left eye, unspecified eyelid**
**H02.869 Hypertrichosis of unspecified eye, unspecified eyelid**

✓6th **H02.87 Vascular anomalies of eyelid**

**H02.871 Vascular anomalies of right upper eyelid**
**H02.872 Vascular anomalies of right lower eyelid**
**H02.873 Vascular anomalies of right eye, unspecified eyelid**
**H02.874 Vascular anomalies of left upper eyelid**
**H02.875 Vascular anomalies of left lower eyelid**
**H02.876 Vascular anomalies of left eye, unspecified eyelid**
**H02.879 Vascular anomalies of unspecified eye, unspecified eyelid**

✓6th **H02.88 Meibomian gland dysfunction of eyelid**

AHA: 2018,4Q,14-15

**H02.881 Meibomian gland dysfunction right upper eyelid**
**H02.882 Meibomian gland dysfunction right lower eyelid**
**H02.883 Meibomian gland dysfunction of right eye, unspecified eyelid**
**H02.884 Meibomian gland dysfunction left upper eyelid**
**H02.885 Meibomian gland dysfunction left lower eyelid**
**H02.886 Meibomian gland dysfunction of left eye, unspecified eyelid**
**H02.889 Meibomian gland dysfunction of unspecified eye, unspecified eyelid**
**H02.88A Meibomian gland dysfunction right eye, upper and lower eyelids**
**H02.88B Meibomian gland dysfunction left eye, upper and lower eyelids**

**H02.89 Other specified disorders of eyelid**

Hemorrhage of eyelid

**H02.9 Unspecified disorder of eyelid**

Disorder of eyelid NOS

✓4th **H04 Disorders of lacrimal system**

EXCLUDES 1 *congenital malformations of lacrimal system (Q10.4-Q10.6)*

✓5th **H04.0 Dacryoadenitis**

DEF: Inflammation of the lacrimal gland.

✓6th **H04.00 Unspecified dacryoadenitis**

**H04.001 Unspecified dacryoadenitis, right lacrimal gland**
**H04.002 Unspecified dacryoadenitis, left lacrimal gland**
**H04.003 Unspecified dacryoadenitis, bilateral lacrimal glands**
**H04.009 Unspecified dacryoadenitis, unspecified lacrimal gland**

✓6th **H04.01 Acute dacryoadenitis**

**H04.011 Acute dacryoadenitis, right lacrimal gland**
**H04.012 Acute dacryoadenitis, left lacrimal gland**
**H04.013 Acute dacryoadenitis, bilateral lacrimal glands**
**H04.019 Acute dacryoadenitis, unspecified lacrimal gland**

✓6th **H04.02 Chronic dacryoadenitis**

**H04.021 Chronic dacryoadenitis, right lacrimal gland**
**H04.022 Chronic dacryoadenitis, left lacrimal gland**
**H04.023 Chronic dacryoadenitis, bilateral lacrimal gland**
**H04.029 Chronic dacryoadenitis, unspecified lacrimal gland**

✓6th **H04.03 Chronic enlargement of lacrimal gland**

**H04.031 Chronic enlargement of right lacrimal gland**
**H04.032 Chronic enlargement of left lacrimal gland**
**H04.033 Chronic enlargement of bilateral lacrimal glands**
**H04.039 Chronic enlargement of unspecified lacrimal gland**

✓5th **H04.1 Other disorders of lacrimal gland**

✓6th **H04.11 Dacryops**

**H04.111 Dacryops of right lacrimal gland**
**H04.112 Dacryops of left lacrimal gland**
**H04.113 Dacryops of bilateral lacrimal glands**
**H04.119 Dacryops of unspecified lacrimal gland**

✓6th **H04.12 Dry eye syndrome**

Tear film insufficiency, NOS

**H04.121 Dry eye syndrome of right lacrimal gland**
**H04.122 Dry eye syndrome of left lacrimal gland**
**H04.123 Dry eye syndrome of bilateral lacrimal glands**
**H04.129 Dry eye syndrome of unspecified lacrimal gland**

✓6th **H04.13 Lacrimal cyst**

Lacrimal cystic degeneration

**H04.131 Lacrimal cyst, right lacrimal gland**
**H04.132 Lacrimal cyst, left lacrimal gland**
**H04.133 Lacrimal cyst, bilateral lacrimal glands**
**H04.139 Lacrimal cyst, unspecified lacrimal gland**

✓6th **H04.14 Primary lacrimal gland atrophy**

**H04.141 Primary lacrimal gland atrophy, right lacrimal gland**
**H04.142 Primary lacrimal gland atrophy, left lacrimal gland**
**H04.143 Primary lacrimal gland atrophy, bilateral lacrimal glands**
**H04.149 Primary lacrimal gland atrophy, unspecified lacrimal gland**

✓6th **H04.15 Secondary lacrimal gland atrophy**

**H04.151 Secondary lacrimal gland atrophy, right lacrimal gland**
**H04.152 Secondary lacrimal gland atrophy, left lacrimal gland**
**H04.153 Secondary lacrimal gland atrophy, bilateral lacrimal glands**
**H04.159 Secondary lacrimal gland atrophy, unspecified lacrimal gland**

✓6th **H04.16 Lacrimal gland dislocation**

**H04.161 Lacrimal gland dislocation, right lacrimal gland**

H04.162 Lacrimal gland dislocation, left lacrimal gland
H04.163 Lacrimal gland dislocation, bilateral lacrimal glands
H04.169 Lacrimal gland dislocation, unspecified lacrimal gland
H04.19 Other specified disorders of lacrimal gland

✓5th H04.2 Epiphora

DEF: Excessive tearing or overflow of tears down the cheeks often due to a stricture in the lacrimal passages but can be caused by other conditions.

✓6th H04.20 Unspecified epiphora
H04.201 Unspecified epiphora, right side
H04.202 Unspecified epiphora, left side
H04.203 Unspecified epiphora, bilateral
H04.209 Unspecified epiphora, unspecified side

✓6th H04.21 Epiphora due to excess lacrimation
H04.211 Epiphora due to excess lacrimation, right lacrimal gland
H04.212 Epiphora due to excess lacrimation, left lacrimal gland
H04.213 Epiphora due to excess lacrimation, bilateral lacrimal glands
H04.219 Epiphora due to excess lacrimation, unspecified lacrimal gland

✓6th H04.22 Epiphora due to insufficient drainage
H04.221 Epiphora due to insufficient drainage, right side
H04.222 Epiphora due to insufficient drainage, left side
H04.223 Epiphora due to insufficient drainage, bilateral
H04.229 Epiphora due to insufficient drainage, unspecified side

✓5th H04.3 Acute and unspecified inflammation of lacrimal passages

EXCLUDES 1 *neonatal dacryocystitis (P39.1)*

✓6th H04.30 Unspecified dacryocystitis
H04.301 Unspecified dacryocystitis of right lacrimal passage
H04.302 Unspecified dacryocystitis of left lacrimal passage
H04.303 Unspecified dacryocystitis of bilateral lacrimal passages
H04.309 Unspecified dacryocystitis of unspecified lacrimal passage

✓6th H04.31 Phlegmonous dacryocystitis
H04.311 Phlegmonous dacryocystitis of right lacrimal passage
H04.312 Phlegmonous dacryocystitis of left lacrimal passage
H04.313 Phlegmonous dacryocystitis of bilateral lacrimal passages
H04.319 Phlegmonous dacryocystitis of unspecified lacrimal passage

✓6th H04.32 Acute dacryocystitis
Acute dacryopericystitis
H04.321 Acute dacryocystitis of right lacrimal passage
H04.322 Acute dacryocystitis of left lacrimal passage
H04.323 Acute dacryocystitis of bilateral lacrimal passages
H04.329 Acute dacryocystitis of unspecified lacrimal passage

✓6th H04.33 Acute lacrimal canaliculitis
H04.331 Acute lacrimal canaliculitis of right lacrimal passage
H04.332 Acute lacrimal canaliculitis of left lacrimal passage
H04.333 Acute lacrimal canaliculitis of bilateral lacrimal passages
H04.339 Acute lacrimal canaliculitis of unspecified lacrimal passage

✓5th H04.4 Chronic inflammation of lacrimal passages

✓6th H04.41 Chronic dacryocystitis
H04.411 Chronic dacryocystitis of right lacrimal passage
H04.412 Chronic dacryocystitis of left lacrimal passage
H04.413 Chronic dacryocystitis of bilateral lacrimal passages
H04.419 Chronic dacryocystitis of unspecified lacrimal passage

✓6th H04.42 Chronic lacrimal canaliculitis
H04.421 Chronic lacrimal canaliculitis of right lacrimal passage
H04.422 Chronic lacrimal canaliculitis of left lacrimal passage
H04.423 Chronic lacrimal canaliculitis of bilateral lacrimal passages
H04.429 Chronic lacrimal canaliculitis of unspecified lacrimal passage

✓6th H04.43 Chronic lacrimal mucocele
H04.431 Chronic lacrimal mucocele of right lacrimal passage
H04.432 Chronic lacrimal mucocele of left lacrimal passage
H04.433 Chronic lacrimal mucocele of bilateral lacrimal passages
H04.439 Chronic lacrimal mucocele of unspecified lacrimal passage

✓5th H04.5 Stenosis and insufficiency of lacrimal passages

✓6th H04.51 Dacryolith
H04.511 Dacryolith of right lacrimal passage
H04.512 Dacryolith of left lacrimal passage
H04.513 Dacryolith of bilateral lacrimal passages
H04.519 Dacryolith of unspecified lacrimal passage

✓6th H04.52 Eversion of lacrimal punctum
H04.521 Eversion of right lacrimal punctum
H04.522 Eversion of left lacrimal punctum
H04.523 Eversion of bilateral lacrimal punctum
H04.529 Eversion of unspecified lacrimal punctum

✓6th H04.53 Neonatal obstruction of nasolacrimal duct

EXCLUDES 1 *congenital stenosis and stricture of lacrimal duct (Q10.5)*

H04.531 Neonatal obstruction of right nasolacrimal duct N
H04.532 Neonatal obstruction of left nasolacrimal duct N
H04.533 Neonatal obstruction of bilateral nasolacrimal duct N
H04.539 Neonatal obstruction of unspecified nasolacrimal duct N

✓6th H04.54 Stenosis of lacrimal canaliculi
H04.541 Stenosis of right lacrimal canaliculi
H04.542 Stenosis of left lacrimal canaliculi
H04.543 Stenosis of bilateral lacrimal canaliculi
H04.549 Stenosis of unspecified lacrimal canaliculi

✓6th H04.55 Acquired stenosis of nasolacrimal duct
H04.551 Acquired stenosis of right nasolacrimal duct
H04.552 Acquired stenosis of left nasolacrimal duct
H04.553 Acquired stenosis of bilateral nasolacrimal duct
H04.559 Acquired stenosis of unspecified nasolacrimal duct

✓6th H04.56 Stenosis of lacrimal punctum
H04.561 Stenosis of right lacrimal punctum
H04.562 Stenosis of left lacrimal punctum
H04.563 Stenosis of bilateral lacrimal punctum
H04.569 Stenosis of unspecified lacrimal punctum

✓6th H04.57 Stenosis of lacrimal sac
H04.571 Stenosis of right lacrimal sac
H04.572 Stenosis of left lacrimal sac
H04.573 Stenosis of bilateral lacrimal sac
H04.579 Stenosis of unspecified lacrimal sac

✓5th H04.6 Other changes of lacrimal passages

✓6th H04.61 Lacrimal fistula
H04.611 Lacrimal fistula right lacrimal passage
H04.612 Lacrimal fistula left lacrimal passage
H04.613 Lacrimal fistula bilateral lacrimal passages
H04.619 Lacrimal fistula unspecified lacrimal passage

H04.69 Other changes of lacrimal passages

5th H04.8 Other disorders of lacrimal system
6th H04.81 Granuloma of lacrimal passages
H04.811 Granuloma of right lacrimal passage
H04.812 Granuloma of left lacrimal passage
H04.813 Granuloma of bilateral lacrimal passages
H04.819 Granuloma of unspecified lacrimal passage
H04.89 Other disorders of lacrimal system
H04.9 Disorder of lacrimal system, unspecified

4th H05 Disorders of orbit
EXCLUDES 1 *congenital malformation of orbit (Q10.7)*
5th H05.0 Acute inflammation of orbit
H05.00 Unspecified acute inflammation of orbit
6th H05.01 Cellulitis of orbit
Abscess of orbit
H05.011 Cellulitis of right orbit
H05.012 Cellulitis of left orbit
H05.013 Cellulitis of bilateral orbits
H05.019 Cellulitis of unspecified orbit
6th H05.02 Osteomyelitis of orbit
H05.021 Osteomyelitis of right orbit
H05.022 Osteomyelitis of left orbit
H05.023 Osteomyelitis of bilateral orbits
H05.029 Osteomyelitis of unspecified orbit
6th H05.03 Periostitis of orbit
H05.031 Periostitis of right orbit
H05.032 Periostitis of left orbit
H05.033 Periostitis of bilateral orbits
H05.039 Periostitis of unspecified orbit
6th H05.04 Tenonitis of orbit
H05.041 Tenonitis of right orbit
H05.042 Tenonitis of left orbit
H05.043 Tenonitis of bilateral orbits
H05.049 Tenonitis of unspecified orbit
5th H05.1 Chronic inflammatory disorders of orbit
H05.10 Unspecified chronic inflammatory disorders of orbit
6th H05.11 Granuloma of orbit
Pseudotumor (inflammatory) of orbit
H05.111 Granuloma of right orbit
H05.112 Granuloma of left orbit
H05.113 Granuloma of bilateral orbits
H05.119 Granuloma of unspecified orbit
6th H05.12 Orbital myositis
H05.121 Orbital myositis, right orbit
H05.122 Orbital myositis, left orbit
H05.123 Orbital myositis, bilateral
H05.129 Orbital myositis, unspecified orbit
5th H05.2 Exophthalmic conditions
H05.20 Unspecified exophthalmos
6th H05.21 Displacement (lateral) of globe
H05.211 Displacement (lateral) of globe, right eye
H05.212 Displacement (lateral) of globe, left eye
H05.213 Displacement (lateral) of globe, bilateral
H05.219 Displacement (lateral) of globe, unspecified eye
6th H05.22 Edema of orbit
Orbital congestion
H05.221 Edema of right orbit
H05.222 Edema of left orbit
H05.223 Edema of bilateral orbit
H05.229 Edema of unspecified orbit
6th H05.23 Hemorrhage of orbit
H05.231 Hemorrhage of right orbit
H05.232 Hemorrhage of left orbit
H05.233 Hemorrhage of bilateral orbit
H05.239 Hemorrhage of unspecified orbit
6th H05.24 Constant exophthalmos
H05.241 Constant exophthalmos, right eye
H05.242 Constant exophthalmos, left eye
H05.243 Constant exophthalmos, bilateral
H05.249 Constant exophthalmos, unspecified eye
6th H05.25 Intermittent exophthalmos
H05.251 Intermittent exophthalmos, right eye
H05.252 Intermittent exophthalmos, left eye
H05.253 Intermittent exophthalmos, bilateral
H05.259 Intermittent exophthalmos, unspecified eye
6th H05.26 Pulsating exophthalmos
H05.261 Pulsating exophthalmos, right eye
H05.262 Pulsating exophthalmos, left eye
H05.263 Pulsating exophthalmos, bilateral
H05.269 Pulsating exophthalmos, unspecified eye
5th H05.3 Deformity of orbit
EXCLUDES 1 *congenital deformity of orbit (Q10.7)*
*hypertelorism (Q75.2)*
H05.30 Unspecified deformity of orbit
6th H05.31 Atrophy of orbit
H05.311 Atrophy of right orbit
H05.312 Atrophy of left orbit
H05.313 Atrophy of bilateral orbit
H05.319 Atrophy of unspecified orbit
6th H05.32 Deformity of orbit due to bone disease
Code also associated bone disease
H05.321 Deformity of right orbit due to bone disease
H05.322 Deformity of left orbit due to bone disease
H05.323 Deformity of bilateral orbits due to bone disease
H05.329 Deformity of unspecified orbit due to bone disease
6th H05.33 Deformity of orbit due to trauma or surgery
H05.331 Deformity of right orbit due to trauma or surgery
H05.332 Deformity of left orbit due to trauma or surgery
H05.333 Deformity of bilateral orbits due to trauma or surgery
H05.339 Deformity of unspecified orbit due to trauma or surgery
6th H05.34 Enlargement of orbit
H05.341 Enlargement of right orbit
H05.342 Enlargement of left orbit
H05.343 Enlargement of bilateral orbits
H05.349 Enlargement of unspecified orbit
6th H05.35 Exostosis of orbit
H05.351 Exostosis of right orbit
H05.352 Exostosis of left orbit
H05.353 Exostosis of bilateral orbits
H05.359 Exostosis of unspecified orbit
5th H05.4 Enophthalmos
6th H05.40 Unspecified enophthalmos
H05.401 Unspecified enophthalmos, right eye
H05.402 Unspecified enophthalmos, left eye
H05.403 Unspecified enophthalmos, bilateral
H05.409 Unspecified enophthalmos, unspecified eye
6th H05.41 Enophthalmos due to atrophy of orbital tissue
H05.411 Enophthalmos due to atrophy of orbital tissue, right eye
H05.412 Enophthalmos due to atrophy of orbital tissue, left eye
H05.413 Enophthalmos due to atrophy of orbital tissue, bilateral
H05.419 Enophthalmos due to atrophy of orbital tissue, unspecified eye
6th H05.42 Enophthalmos due to trauma or surgery
H05.421 Enophthalmos due to trauma or surgery, right eye
H05.422 Enophthalmos due to trauma or surgery, left eye
H05.423 Enophthalmos due to trauma or surgery, bilateral
H05.429 Enophthalmos due to trauma or surgery, unspecified eye
5th H05.5 Retained (old) foreign body following penetrating wound of orbit
Retrobulbar foreign body
Use additional code to identify the type of retained foreign body (Z18.-)
EXCLUDES 1 *current penetrating wound of orbit (S05.4-)*
EXCLUDES 2 *retained foreign body of eyelid (H02.81-)*
*retained intraocular foreign body (H44.6-, H44.7-)*
H05.50 Retained (old) foreign body following penetrating wound of unspecified orbit

H05.51 Retained (old) foreign body following penetrating wound of right orbit
H05.52 Retained (old) foreign body following penetrating wound of left orbit
H05.53 Retained (old) foreign body following penetrating wound of bilateral orbits

✓5th H05.8 Other disorders of orbit

✓6th H05.81 Cyst of orbit
Encephalocele of orbit
H05.811 Cyst of right orbit
H05.812 Cyst of left orbit
H05.813 Cyst of bilateral orbits
H05.819 Cyst of unspecified orbit

✓6th H05.82 Myopathy of extraocular muscles
H05.821 Myopathy of extraocular muscles, right orbit
H05.822 Myopathy of extraocular muscles, left orbit
H05.823 Myopathy of extraocular muscles, bilateral
H05.829 Myopathy of extraocular muscles, unspecified orbit

✓6th H05.83 Thyroid orbitopathy
Graves' ophthalmopathy
Graves' orbitopathy
Thyroid eye disease
Code also, if applicable, any associated conditions such as:
autoimmune thyroiditis (E06.3)
thyrotoxicosis with diffuse goiter (E05.0-)
H05.831 Thyroid orbitopathy, right orbit
H05.832 Thyroid orbitopathy, left orbit
H05.833 Thyroid orbitopathy, bilateral
H05.839 Thyroid orbitopathy, unspecified orbit

H05.89 Other disorders of orbit

H05.9 Unspecified disorder of orbit

## Disorders of conjunctiva (H10-H11)

✓4th H10 Conjunctivitis
EXCLUDES 1 *keratoconjunctivitis (H16.2-)*

✓5th H10.0 Mucopurulent conjunctivitis

✓6th H10.01 Acute follicular conjunctivitis
H10.011 Acute follicular conjunctivitis, right eye
H10.012 Acute follicular conjunctivitis, left eye
H10.013 Acute follicular conjunctivitis, bilateral
H10.019 Acute follicular conjunctivitis, unspecified eye

✓6th H10.02 Other mucopurulent conjunctivitis
H10.021 Other mucopurulent conjunctivitis, right eye
H10.022 Other mucopurulent conjunctivitis, left eye
H10.023 Other mucopurulent conjunctivitis, bilateral
H10.029 Other mucopurulent conjunctivitis, unspecified eye

✓5th H10.1 Acute atopic conjunctivitis
Acute papillary conjunctivitis
H10.10 Acute atopic conjunctivitis, unspecified eye
H10.11 Acute atopic conjunctivitis, right eye
H10.12 Acute atopic conjunctivitis, left eye
H10.13 Acute atopic conjunctivitis, bilateral

✓5th H10.2 Other acute conjunctivitis

✓6th H10.21 Acute toxic conjunctivitis
Acute chemical conjunctivitis
Code first (T51-T65) to identify chemical and intent
EXCLUDES 1 *burn and corrosion of eye and adnexa (T26.-)*
H10.211 Acute toxic conjunctivitis, right eye
H10.212 Acute toxic conjunctivitis, left eye
H10.213 Acute toxic conjunctivitis, bilateral
H10.219 Acute toxic conjunctivitis, unspecified eye

✓6th H10.22 Pseudomembranous conjunctivitis
H10.221 Pseudomembranous conjunctivitis, right eye
H10.222 Pseudomembranous conjunctivitis, left eye
H10.223 Pseudomembranous conjunctivitis, bilateral
H10.229 Pseudomembranous conjunctivitis, unspecified eye

✓6th H10.23 Serous conjunctivitis, except viral
EXCLUDES 1 *viral conjunctivitis (B30.-)*
H10.231 Serous conjunctivitis, except viral, right eye
H10.232 Serous conjunctivitis, except viral, left eye
H10.233 Serous conjunctivitis, except viral, bilateral
H10.239 Serous conjunctivitis, except viral, unspecified eye

✓5th H10.3 Unspecified acute conjunctivitis
EXCLUDES 1 *ophthalmia neonatorum NOS (P39.1)*
H10.30 Unspecified acute conjunctivitis, unspecified eye
H10.31 Unspecified acute conjunctivitis, right eye
H10.32 Unspecified acute conjunctivitis, left eye
H10.33 Unspecified acute conjunctivitis, bilateral

✓5th H10.4 Chronic conjunctivitis

✓6th H10.40 Unspecified chronic conjunctivitis
H10.401 Unspecified chronic conjunctivitis, right eye
H10.402 Unspecified chronic conjunctivitis, left eye
H10.403 Unspecified chronic conjunctivitis, bilateral
H10.409 Unspecified chronic conjunctivitis, unspecified eye

✓6th H10.41 Chronic giant papillary conjunctivitis
H10.411 Chronic giant papillary conjunctivitis, right eye
H10.412 Chronic giant papillary conjunctivitis, left eye
H10.413 Chronic giant papillary conjunctivitis, bilateral
H10.419 Chronic giant papillary conjunctivitis, unspecified eye

✓6th H10.42 Simple chronic conjunctivitis
H10.421 Simple chronic conjunctivitis, right eye
H10.422 Simple chronic conjunctivitis, left eye
H10.423 Simple chronic conjunctivitis, bilateral
H10.429 Simple chronic conjunctivitis, unspecified eye

✓6th H10.43 Chronic follicular conjunctivitis
H10.431 Chronic follicular conjunctivitis, right eye
H10.432 Chronic follicular conjunctivitis, left eye
H10.433 Chronic follicular conjunctivitis, bilateral
H10.439 Chronic follicular conjunctivitis, unspecified eye

H10.44 Vernal conjunctivitis
EXCLUDES 1 *vernal keratoconjunctivitis with limbar and corneal involvement (H16.26-)*

H10.45 Other chronic allergic conjunctivitis

✓5th H10.5 Blepharoconjunctivitis

✓6th H10.50 Unspecified blepharoconjunctivitis
H10.501 Unspecified blepharoconjunctivitis, right eye
H10.502 Unspecified blepharoconjunctivitis, left eye
H10.503 Unspecified blepharoconjunctivitis, bilateral
H10.509 Unspecified blepharoconjunctivitis, unspecified eye

✓6th H10.51 Ligneous conjunctivitis
Code also underlying condition if known, such as:
plasminogen deficiency (E88.02)
H10.511 Ligneous conjunctivitis, right eye
H10.512 Ligneous conjunctivitis, left eye
H10.513 Ligneous conjunctivitis, bilateral
H10.519 Ligneous conjunctivitis, unspecified eye

✓6th H10.52 Angular blepharoconjunctivitis
H10.521 Angular blepharoconjunctivitis, right eye
H10.522 Angular blepharoconjunctivitis, left eye
H10.523 Angular blepharoconjunctivitis, bilateral
H10.529 Angular blepharoconjunctivitis, unspecified eye

✓6th H10.53 Contact blepharoconjunctivitis
H10.531 Contact blepharoconjunctivitis, right eye
H10.532 Contact blepharoconjunctivitis, left eye
H10.533 Contact blepharoconjunctivitis, bilateral
H10.539 Contact blepharoconjunctivitis, unspecified eye

**H10.8 Other conjunctivitis**

**H10.81 Pingueculitis**

EXCLUDES 1 *pinguecula (H11.15-)*

**H10.811** Pingueculitis, right eye
**H10.812** Pingueculitis, left eye
**H10.813** Pingueculitis, bilateral
**H10.819** Pingueculitis, unspecified eye

**H10.82 Rosacea conjunctivitis**

Code first underlying rosacea dermatitis (L71.-)

AHA: 2018,4Q,15

**H10.821** Rosacea conjunctivitis, right eye
**H10.822** Rosacea conjunctivitis, left eye
**H10.823** Rosacea conjunctivitis, bilateral
**H10.829** Rosacea conjunctivitis, unspecified eye

**H10.89** Other conjunctivitis

**H10.9** Unspecified conjunctivitis

**H11 Other disorders of conjunctiva**

EXCLUDES 1 *keratoconjunctivitis (H16.2-)*

**H11.0 Pterygium of eye**

EXCLUDES 1 *pseudopterygium (H11.81-)*

DEF: Benign, wedge-shaped, conjunctival thickening that advances from the inner corner of the eye toward the cornea.

**Pterygium**

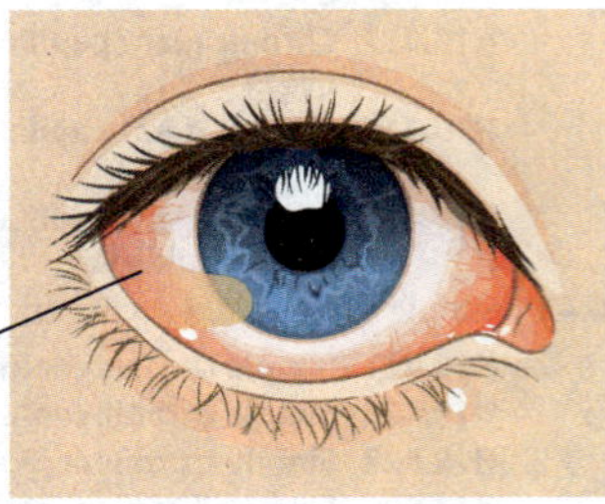


**H11.00 Unspecified pterygium of eye**

**H11.001** Unspecified pterygium of right eye
**H11.002** Unspecified pterygium of left eye
**H11.003** Unspecified pterygium of eye, bilateral
**H11.009** Unspecified pterygium of unspecified eye

**H11.01 Amyloid pterygium**

**H11.011** Amyloid pterygium of right eye
**H11.012** Amyloid pterygium of left eye
**H11.013** Amyloid pterygium of eye, bilateral
**H11.019** Amyloid pterygium of unspecified eye

**H11.02 Central pterygium of eye**

**H11.021** Central pterygium of right eye
**H11.022** Central pterygium of left eye
**H11.023** Central pterygium of eye, bilateral
**H11.029** Central pterygium of unspecified eye

**H11.03 Double pterygium of eye**

**H11.031** Double pterygium of right eye
**H11.032** Double pterygium of left eye
**H11.033** Double pterygium of eye, bilateral
**H11.039** Double pterygium of unspecified eye

**H11.04 Peripheral pterygium of eye, stationary**

**H11.041** Peripheral pterygium, stationary, right eye
**H11.042** Peripheral pterygium, stationary, left eye
**H11.043** Peripheral pterygium, stationary, bilateral
**H11.049** Peripheral pterygium, stationary, unspecified eye

**H11.05 Peripheral pterygium of eye, progressive**

**H11.051** Peripheral pterygium, progressive, right eye
**H11.052** Peripheral pterygium, progressive, left eye
**H11.053** Peripheral pterygium, progressive, bilateral
**H11.059** Peripheral pterygium, progressive, unspecified eye

**H11.06 Recurrent pterygium of eye**

**H11.061** Recurrent pterygium of right eye
**H11.062** Recurrent pterygium of left eye
**H11.063** Recurrent pterygium of eye, bilateral
**H11.069** Recurrent pterygium of unspecified eye

**H11.1 Conjunctival degenerations and deposits**

EXCLUDES 2 *pseudopterygium (H11.81)*

**H11.10** Unspecified conjunctival degenerations

**H11.11 Conjunctival deposits**

**H11.111** Conjunctival deposits, right eye
**H11.112** Conjunctival deposits, left eye
**H11.113** Conjunctival deposits, bilateral
**H11.119** Conjunctival deposits, unspecified eye

**H11.12 Conjunctival concretions**

**H11.121** Conjunctival concretions, right eye
**H11.122** Conjunctival concretions, left eye
**H11.123** Conjunctival concretions, bilateral
**H11.129** Conjunctival concretions, unspecified eye

**H11.13 Conjunctival pigmentations**

Conjunctival argyrosis [argyria]

**H11.131** Conjunctival pigmentations, right eye
**H11.132** Conjunctival pigmentations, left eye
**H11.133** Conjunctival pigmentations, bilateral
**H11.139** Conjunctival pigmentations, unspecified eye

**H11.14 Conjunctival xerosis, unspecified**

EXCLUDES 1 *xerosis of conjunctiva due to vitamin A deficiency (E50.0, E50.1)*

DEF: Abnormal dryness of the conjunctiva due to lack of sufficient tears or conjunctival secretions.

**H11.141** Conjunctival xerosis, unspecified, right eye
**H11.142** Conjunctival xerosis, unspecified, left eye
**H11.143** Conjunctival xerosis, unspecified, bilateral
**H11.149** Conjunctival xerosis, unspecified, unspecified eye

**H11.15 Pinguecula**

EXCLUDES 1 *pingueculitis (H10.81-)*

DEF: Proliferation on the conjunctiva near the sclerocorneal junction, usually of the side of the nose and usually in older patients.

**Pinguecula**

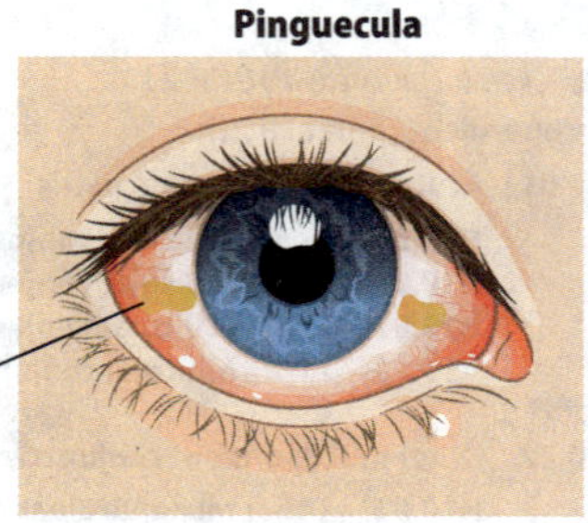


**H11.151** Pinguecula, right eye
**H11.152** Pinguecula, left eye
**H11.153** Pinguecula, bilateral
**H11.159** Pinguecula, unspecified eye

**H11.2 Conjunctival scars**

**H11.21 Conjunctival adhesions and strands (localized)**

**H11.211** Conjunctival adhesions and strands (localized), right eye
**H11.212** Conjunctival adhesions and strands (localized), left eye
**H11.213** Conjunctival adhesions and strands (localized), bilateral
**H11.219** Conjunctival adhesions and strands (localized), unspecified eye

**H11.22 Conjunctival granuloma**

**H11.221** Conjunctival granuloma, right eye
**H11.222** Conjunctival granuloma, left eye
**H11.223** Conjunctival granuloma, bilateral
**H11.229** Conjunctival granuloma, unspecified

**H11.23 Symblepharon**

**H11.231** Symblepharon, right eye
**H11.232** Symblepharon, left eye
**H11.233** Symblepharon, bilateral
**H11.239** Symblepharon, unspecified eye

**H11.24 Scarring of conjunctiva**

**H11.241** Scarring of conjunctiva, right eye
**H11.242** Scarring of conjunctiva, left eye
**H11.243** Scarring of conjunctiva, bilateral
**H11.249** Scarring of conjunctiva, unspecified eye

✓5th **H11.3** Conjunctival hemorrhage
Subconjunctival hemorrhage
- **H11.30** Conjunctival hemorrhage, unspecified eye
- **H11.31** Conjunctival hemorrhage, right eye
- **H11.32** Conjunctival hemorrhage, left eye
- **H11.33** Conjunctival hemorrhage, bilateral

✓5th **H11.4** Other conjunctival vascular disorders and cysts

✓6th **H11.41** Vascular abnormalities of conjunctiva
Conjunctival aneurysm
- **H11.411** Vascular abnormalities of conjunctiva, right eye
- **H11.412** Vascular abnormalities of conjunctiva, left eye
- **H11.413** Vascular abnormalities of conjunctiva, bilateral
- **H11.419** Vascular abnormalities of conjunctiva, unspecified eye

✓6th **H11.42** Conjunctival edema
- **H11.421** Conjunctival edema, right eye
- **H11.422** Conjunctival edema, left eye
- **H11.423** Conjunctival edema, bilateral
- **H11.429** Conjunctival edema, unspecified eye

✓6th **H11.43** Conjunctival hyperemia
- **H11.431** Conjunctival hyperemia, right eye
- **H11.432** Conjunctival hyperemia, left eye
- **H11.433** Conjunctival hyperemia, bilateral
- **H11.439** Conjunctival hyperemia, unspecified eye

✓6th **H11.44** Conjunctival cysts
- **H11.441** Conjunctival cysts, right eye
- **H11.442** Conjunctival cysts, left eye
- **H11.443** Conjunctival cysts, bilateral
- **H11.449** Conjunctival cysts, unspecified eye

✓5th **H11.8** Other specified disorders of conjunctiva

✓6th **H11.81** Pseudopterygium of conjunctiva
- **H11.811** Pseudopterygium of conjunctiva, right eye
- **H11.812** Pseudopterygium of conjunctiva, left eye
- **H11.813** Pseudopterygium of conjunctiva, bilateral
- **H11.819** Pseudopterygium of conjunctiva, unspecified eye

✓6th **H11.82** Conjunctivochalasis
- **H11.821** Conjunctivochalasis, right eye
- **H11.822** Conjunctivochalasis, left eye
- **H11.823** Conjunctivochalasis, bilateral
- **H11.829** Conjunctivochalasis, unspecified eye

**H11.89** Other specified disorders of conjunctiva

**H11.9** Unspecified disorder of conjunctiva

## Disorders of sclera, cornea, iris and ciliary body (H15-H22)

✓4th **H15** Disorders of sclera

✓5th **H15.0** Scleritis

✓6th **H15.00** Unspecified scleritis
- **H15.001** Unspecified scleritis, right eye
- **H15.002** Unspecified scleritis, left eye
- **H15.003** Unspecified scleritis, bilateral
- **H15.009** Unspecified scleritis, unspecified eye

✓6th **H15.01** Anterior scleritis
- **H15.011** Anterior scleritis, right eye
- **H15.012** Anterior scleritis, left eye
- **H15.013** Anterior scleritis, bilateral
- **H15.019** Anterior scleritis, unspecified eye

✓6th **H15.02** Brawny scleritis
- **H15.021** Brawny scleritis, right eye
- **H15.022** Brawny scleritis, left eye
- **H15.023** Brawny scleritis, bilateral
- **H15.029** Brawny scleritis, unspecified eye

✓6th **H15.03** Posterior scleritis
Sclerotenonitis
- **H15.031** Posterior scleritis, right eye
- **H15.032** Posterior scleritis, left eye
- **H15.033** Posterior scleritis, bilateral
- **H15.039** Posterior scleritis, unspecified eye

✓6th **H15.04** Scleritis with corneal involvement
- **H15.041** Scleritis with corneal involvement, right eye
- **H15.042** Scleritis with corneal involvement, left eye
- **H15.043** Scleritis with corneal involvement, bilateral
- **H15.049** Scleritis with corneal involvement, unspecified eye

✓6th **H15.05** Scleromalacia perforans
- **H15.051** Scleromalacia perforans, right eye
- **H15.052** Scleromalacia perforans, left eye
- **H15.053** Scleromalacia perforans, bilateral
- **H15.059** Scleromalacia perforans, unspecified eye

✓6th **H15.09** Other scleritis
Scleral abscess
- **H15.091** Other scleritis, right eye
- **H15.092** Other scleritis, left eye
- **H15.093** Other scleritis, bilateral
- **H15.099** Other scleritis, unspecified eye

✓5th **H15.1** Episcleritis

✓6th **H15.10** Unspecified episcleritis
- **H15.101** Unspecified episcleritis, right eye
- **H15.102** Unspecified episcleritis, left eye
- **H15.103** Unspecified episcleritis, bilateral
- **H15.109** Unspecified episcleritis, unspecified eye

✓6th **H15.11** Episcleritis periodica fugax
- **H15.111** Episcleritis periodica fugax, right eye
- **H15.112** Episcleritis periodica fugax, left eye
- **H15.113** Episcleritis periodica fugax, bilateral
- **H15.119** Episcleritis periodica fugax, unspecified eye

✓6th **H15.12** Nodular episcleritis
- **H15.121** Nodular episcleritis, right eye
- **H15.122** Nodular episcleritis, left eye
- **H15.123** Nodular episcleritis, bilateral
- **H15.129** Nodular episcleritis, unspecified eye

✓5th **H15.8** Other disorders of sclera

EXCLUDES 2 *blue sclera (Q13.5)*
*degenerative myopia (H44.2-)*

✓6th **H15.81** Equatorial staphyloma
- **H15.811** Equatorial staphyloma, right eye
- **H15.812** Equatorial staphyloma, left eye
- **H15.813** Equatorial staphyloma, bilateral
- **H15.819** Equatorial staphyloma, unspecified eye

✓6th **H15.82** Localized anterior staphyloma
- **H15.821** Localized anterior staphyloma, right eye
- **H15.822** Localized anterior staphyloma, left eye
- **H15.823** Localized anterior staphyloma, bilateral
- **H15.829** Localized anterior staphyloma, unspecified eye

✓6th **H15.83** Staphyloma posticum
- **H15.831** Staphyloma posticum, right eye
- **H15.832** Staphyloma posticum, left eye
- **H15.833** Staphyloma posticum, bilateral
- **H15.839** Staphyloma posticum, unspecified eye

✓6th **H15.84** Scleral ectasia
- **H15.841** Scleral ectasia, right eye
- **H15.842** Scleral ectasia, left eye
- **H15.843** Scleral ectasia, bilateral
- **H15.849** Scleral ectasia, unspecified eye

✓6th **H15.85** Ring staphyloma
- **H15.851** Ring staphyloma, right eye
- **H15.852** Ring staphyloma, left eye
- **H15.853** Ring staphyloma, bilateral
- **H15.859** Ring staphyloma, unspecified eye

**H15.89** Other disorders of sclera

**H15.9** Unspecified disorder of sclera

✓4th **H16** Keratitis

DEF: Condition in which the cornea becomes inflamed and irritated.

✓5th **H16.0** Corneal ulcer

✓6th **H16.00** Unspecified corneal ulcer
- **H16.001** Unspecified corneal ulcer, right eye
- **H16.002** Unspecified corneal ulcer, left eye
- **H16.003** Unspecified corneal ulcer, bilateral
- **H16.009** Unspecified corneal ulcer, unspecified eye

✓6th **H16.01** Central corneal ulcer
- **H16.011** Central corneal ulcer, right eye
- **H16.012** Central corneal ulcer, left eye
- **H16.013** Central corneal ulcer, bilateral

H16.019 Central corneal ulcer, unspecified eye

H16.02 Ring corneal ulcer
- H16.021 Ring corneal ulcer, right eye
- H16.022 Ring corneal ulcer, left eye
- H16.023 Ring corneal ulcer, bilateral
- H16.029 Ring corneal ulcer, unspecified eye

H16.03 Corneal ulcer with hypopyon
- H16.031 Corneal ulcer with hypopyon, right eye
- H16.032 Corneal ulcer with hypopyon, left eye
- H16.033 Corneal ulcer with hypopyon, bilateral
- H16.039 Corneal ulcer with hypopyon, unspecified eye

H16.04 Marginal corneal ulcer
- H16.041 Marginal corneal ulcer, right eye
- H16.042 Marginal corneal ulcer, left eye
- H16.043 Marginal corneal ulcer, bilateral
- H16.049 Marginal corneal ulcer, unspecified eye

H16.05 Mooren's corneal ulcer
- H16.051 Mooren's corneal ulcer, right eye
- H16.052 Mooren's corneal ulcer, left eye
- H16.053 Mooren's corneal ulcer, bilateral
- H16.059 Mooren's corneal ulcer, unspecified eye

H16.06 Mycotic corneal ulcer
- H16.061 Mycotic corneal ulcer, right eye
- H16.062 Mycotic corneal ulcer, left eye
- H16.063 Mycotic corneal ulcer, bilateral
- H16.069 Mycotic corneal ulcer, unspecified eye

H16.07 Perforated corneal ulcer
- H16.071 Perforated corneal ulcer, right eye
- H16.072 Perforated corneal ulcer, left eye
- H16.073 Perforated corneal ulcer, bilateral
- H16.079 Perforated corneal ulcer, unspecified eye

## H16.1 Other and unspecified superficial keratitis without conjunctivitis

H16.10 Unspecified superficial keratitis
- H16.101 Unspecified superficial keratitis, right eye
- H16.102 Unspecified superficial keratitis, left eye
- H16.103 Unspecified superficial keratitis, bilateral
- H16.109 Unspecified superficial keratitis, unspecified eye

H16.11 Macular keratitis

Areolar keratitis
Nummular keratitis
Stellate keratitis
Striate keratitis
- H16.111 Macular keratitis, right eye
- H16.112 Macular keratitis, left eye
- H16.113 Macular keratitis, bilateral
- H16.119 Macular keratitis, unspecified eye

H16.12 Filamentary keratitis
- H16.121 Filamentary keratitis, right eye
- H16.122 Filamentary keratitis, left eye
- H16.123 Filamentary keratitis, bilateral
- H16.129 Filamentary keratitis, unspecified eye

H16.13 Photokeratitis

Snow blindness
Welders keratitis
- H16.131 Photokeratitis, right eye
- H16.132 Photokeratitis, left eye
- H16.133 Photokeratitis, bilateral
- H16.139 Photokeratitis, unspecified eye

H16.14 Punctate keratitis
- H16.141 Punctate keratitis, right eye
- H16.142 Punctate keratitis, left eye
- H16.143 Punctate keratitis, bilateral
- H16.149 Punctate keratitis, unspecified eye

## H16.2 Keratoconjunctivitis

H16.20 Unspecified keratoconjunctivitis

Superficial keratitis with conjunctivitis NOS
- H16.201 Unspecified keratoconjunctivitis, right eye
- H16.202 Unspecified keratoconjunctivitis, left eye
- H16.203 Unspecified keratoconjunctivitis, bilateral
- H16.209 Unspecified keratoconjunctivitis, unspecified eye

H16.21 Exposure keratoconjunctivitis
- H16.211 Exposure keratoconjunctivitis, right eye
- H16.212 Exposure keratoconjunctivitis, left eye
- H16.213 Exposure keratoconjunctivitis, bilateral
- H16.219 Exposure keratoconjunctivitis, unspecified eye

H16.22 Keratoconjunctivitis sicca, not specified as Sjögren's

EXCLUDES 1 *Sjögren's syndrome (M35.01)*
- H16.221 Keratoconjunctivitis sicca, not specified as Sjögren's, right eye
- H16.222 Keratoconjunctivitis sicca, not specified as Sjögren's, left eye
- H16.223 Keratoconjunctivitis sicca, not specified as Sjögren's, bilateral
  AHA: 2024,3Q,16
- H16.229 Keratoconjunctivitis sicca, not specified as Sjogren's, unspecified eye

H16.23 Neurotrophic keratoconjunctivitis
- H16.231 Neurotrophic keratoconjunctivitis, right eye
- H16.232 Neurotrophic keratoconjunctivitis, left eye
- H16.233 Neurotrophic keratoconjunctivitis, bilateral
- H16.239 Neurotrophic keratoconjunctivitis, unspecified eye

H16.24 Ophthalmia nodosa
- H16.241 Ophthalmia nodosa, right eye
- H16.242 Ophthalmia nodosa, left eye
- H16.243 Ophthalmia nodosa, bilateral
- H16.249 Ophthalmia nodosa, unspecified eye

H16.25 Phlyctenular keratoconjunctivitis
- H16.251 Phlyctenular keratoconjunctivitis, right eye
- H16.252 Phlyctenular keratoconjunctivitis, left eye
- H16.253 Phlyctenular keratoconjunctivitis, bilateral
- H16.259 Phlyctenular keratoconjunctivitis, unspecified eye

H16.26 Vernal keratoconjunctivitis, with limbar and corneal involvement

EXCLUDES 1 *vernal conjunctivitis without limbar and corneal involvement (H10.44)*
- H16.261 Vernal keratoconjunctivitis, with limbar and corneal involvement, right eye
- H16.262 Vernal keratoconjunctivitis, with limbar and corneal involvement, left eye
- H16.263 Vernal keratoconjunctivitis, with limbar and corneal involvement, bilateral
- H16.269 Vernal keratoconjunctivitis, with limbar and corneal involvement, unspecified eye

H16.29 Other keratoconjunctivitis
- H16.291 Other keratoconjunctivitis, right eye
- H16.292 Other keratoconjunctivitis, left eye
- H16.293 Other keratoconjunctivitis, bilateral
- H16.299 Other keratoconjunctivitis, unspecified eye

## H16.3 Interstitial and deep keratitis

H16.30 Unspecified interstitial keratitis
- H16.301 Unspecified interstitial keratitis, right eye
- H16.302 Unspecified interstitial keratitis, left eye
- H16.303 Unspecified interstitial keratitis, bilateral
- H16.309 Unspecified interstitial keratitis, unspecified eye

H16.31 Corneal abscess
- H16.311 Corneal abscess, right eye
- H16.312 Corneal abscess, left eye
- H16.313 Corneal abscess, bilateral
- H16.319 Corneal abscess, unspecified eye

H16.32 Diffuse interstitial keratitis

Cogan's syndrome
- H16.321 Diffuse interstitial keratitis, right eye
- H16.322 Diffuse interstitial keratitis, left eye
- H16.323 Diffuse interstitial keratitis, bilateral
- H16.329 Diffuse interstitial keratitis, unspecified eye

H16.33 Sclerosing keratitis
- H16.331 Sclerosing keratitis, right eye
- H16.332 Sclerosing keratitis, left eye
- H16.333 Sclerosing keratitis, bilateral
- H16.339 Sclerosing keratitis, unspecified eye

H16.39 Other interstitial and deep keratitis
- H16.391 Other interstitial and deep keratitis, right eye

H16.392 Other interstitial and deep keratitis, left eye
H16.393 Other interstitial and deep keratitis, bilateral
H16.399 Other interstitial and deep keratitis, unspecified eye

√5th H16.4 Corneal neovascularization

√6th H16.4Ø Unspecified corneal neovascularization
H16.4Ø1 Unspecified corneal neovascularization, right eye
H16.4Ø2 Unspecified corneal neovascularization, left eye
H16.4Ø3 Unspecified corneal neovascularization, bilateral
H16.4Ø9 Unspecified corneal neovascularization, unspecified eye

√6th H16.41 Ghost vessels (corneal)
H16.411 Ghost vessels (corneal), right eye
H16.412 Ghost vessels (corneal), left eye
H16.413 Ghost vessels (corneal), bilateral
H16.419 Ghost vessels (corneal), unspecified eye

√6th H16.42 Pannus (corneal)
H16.421 Pannus (corneal), right eye
H16.422 Pannus (corneal), left eye
H16.423 Pannus (corneal), bilateral
H16.429 Pannus (corneal), unspecified eye

√6th H16.43 Localized vascularization of cornea
H16.431 Localized vascularization of cornea, right eye
H16.432 Localized vascularization of cornea, left eye
H16.433 Localized vascularization of cornea, bilateral
H16.439 Localized vascularization of cornea, unspecified eye

√6th H16.44 Deep vascularization of cornea
H16.441 Deep vascularization of cornea, right eye
H16.442 Deep vascularization of cornea, left eye
H16.443 Deep vascularization of cornea, bilateral
H16.449 Deep vascularization of cornea, unspecified eye

H16.8 Other keratitis
H16.9 Unspecified keratitis

## √4th H17 Corneal scars and opacities

√5th H17.Ø Adherent leukoma
H17.ØØ Adherent leukoma, unspecified eye
H17.Ø1 Adherent leukoma, right eye
H17.Ø2 Adherent leukoma, left eye
H17.Ø3 Adherent leukoma, bilateral

√5th H17.1 Central corneal opacity
H17.1Ø Central corneal opacity, unspecified eye
H17.11 Central corneal opacity, right eye
H17.12 Central corneal opacity, left eye
H17.13 Central corneal opacity, bilateral

√5th H17.8 Other corneal scars and opacities

√6th H17.81 Minor opacity of cornea
Corneal nebula
H17.811 Minor opacity of cornea, right eye
H17.812 Minor opacity of cornea, left eye
H17.813 Minor opacity of cornea, bilateral
H17.819 Minor opacity of cornea, unspecified eye

√6th H17.82 Peripheral opacity of cornea
H17.821 Peripheral opacity of cornea, right eye
H17.822 Peripheral opacity of cornea, left eye
H17.823 Peripheral opacity of cornea, bilateral
H17.829 Peripheral opacity of cornea, unspecified eye

H17.89 Other corneal scars and opacities
H17.9 Unspecified corneal scar and opacity

## √4th H18 Other disorders of cornea

√5th H18.Ø Corneal pigmentations and deposits

√6th H18.ØØ Unspecified corneal deposit
H18.ØØ1 Unspecified corneal deposit, right eye
H18.ØØ2 Unspecified corneal deposit, left eye
H18.ØØ3 Unspecified corneal deposit, bilateral
H18.ØØ9 Unspecified corneal deposit, unspecified eye

√6th H18.Ø1 Anterior corneal pigmentations
Staehli's line
H18.Ø11 Anterior corneal pigmentations, right eye
H18.Ø12 Anterior corneal pigmentations, left eye
H18.Ø13 Anterior corneal pigmentations, bilateral
H18.Ø19 Anterior corneal pigmentations, unspecified eye

√6th H18.Ø2 Argentous corneal deposits
H18.Ø21 Argentous corneal deposits, right eye
H18.Ø22 Argentous corneal deposits, left eye
H18.Ø23 Argentous corneal deposits, bilateral
H18.Ø29 Argentous corneal deposits, unspecified eye

√6th H18.Ø3 Corneal deposits in metabolic disorders
Code also associated metabolic disorder
H18.Ø31 Corneal deposits in metabolic disorders, right eye
H18.Ø32 Corneal deposits in metabolic disorders, left eye
H18.Ø33 Corneal deposits in metabolic disorders, bilateral
H18.Ø39 Corneal deposits in metabolic disorders, unspecified eye

√6th H18.Ø4 Kayser-Fleischer ring
Code also associated Wilson's disease (E83.Ø1)
H18.Ø41 Kayser-Fleischer ring, right eye
H18.Ø42 Kayser-Fleischer ring, left eye
H18.Ø43 Kayser-Fleischer ring, bilateral
H18.Ø49 Kayser-Fleischer ring, unspecified eye

√6th H18.Ø5 Posterior corneal pigmentations
Krukenberg's spindle
H18.Ø51 Posterior corneal pigmentations, right eye
H18.Ø52 Posterior corneal pigmentations, left eye
H18.Ø53 Posterior corneal pigmentations, bilateral
H18.Ø59 Posterior corneal pigmentations, unspecified eye

√6th H18.Ø6 Stromal corneal pigmentations
Hematocornea
H18.Ø61 Stromal corneal pigmentations, right eye
H18.Ø62 Stromal corneal pigmentations, left eye
H18.Ø63 Stromal corneal pigmentations, bilateral
H18.Ø69 Stromal corneal pigmentations, unspecified eye

√5th H18.1 Bullous keratopathy
**DEF:** Corneal swelling due to a damaged corneal endothelium. Bullous keratopathy is characterized by recurring, rupturing epithelial blisters causing glaucoma, iridocyclitis, and Fuchs' dystrophy.
H18.1Ø Bullous keratopathy, unspecified eye
H18.11 Bullous keratopathy, right eye
H18.12 Bullous keratopathy, left eye
H18.13 Bullous keratopathy, bilateral

√5th H18.2 Other and unspecified corneal edema
H18.2Ø Unspecified corneal edema

√6th H18.21 Corneal edema secondary to contact lens
EXCLUDES 2 *other corneal disorders due to contact lens (H18.82-)*
H18.211 Corneal edema secondary to contact lens, right eye
H18.212 Corneal edema secondary to contact lens, left eye
H18.213 Corneal edema secondary to contact lens, bilateral
H18.219 Corneal edema secondary to contact lens, unspecified eye

√6th H18.22 Idiopathic corneal edema
H18.221 Idiopathic corneal edema, right eye
H18.222 Idiopathic corneal edema, left eye
H18.223 Idiopathic corneal edema, bilateral
H18.229 Idiopathic corneal edema, unspecified eye

√6th H18.23 Secondary corneal edema
H18.231 Secondary corneal edema, right eye
H18.232 Secondary corneal edema, left eye
H18.233 Secondary corneal edema, bilateral
H18.239 Secondary corneal edema, unspecified eye

✓5th **H18.3 Changes of corneal membranes**

**H18.3Ø Unspecified corneal membrane change**

✓6th **H18.31 Folds and rupture in Bowman's membrane**

**H18.311 Folds and rupture in Bowman's membrane, right eye**

**H18.312 Folds and rupture in Bowman's membrane, left eye**

**H18.313 Folds and rupture in Bowman's membrane, bilateral**

**H18.319 Folds and rupture in Bowman's membrane, unspecified eye**

✓6th **H18.32 Folds in Descemet's membrane**

**H18.321 Folds in Descemet's membrane, right eye**

**H18.322 Folds in Descemet's membrane, left eye**

**H18.323 Folds in Descemet's membrane, bilateral**

**H18.329 Folds in Descemet's membrane, unspecified eye**

✓6th **H18.33 Rupture in Descemet's membrane**

**H18.331 Rupture in Descemet's membrane, right eye**

**H18.332 Rupture in Descemet's membrane, left eye**

**H18.333 Rupture in Descemet's membrane, bilateral**

**H18.339 Rupture in Descemet's membrane, unspecified eye**

✓5th **H18.4 Corneal degeneration**

EXCLUDES 1 *Mooren's ulcer (H16.Ø-)*
*recurrent erosion of cornea (H18.83-)*

**H18.4Ø Unspecified corneal degeneration**

✓6th **H18.41 Arcus senilis**

Senile corneal changes

**H18.411 Arcus senilis, right eye**

**H18.412 Arcus senilis, left eye**

**H18.413 Arcus senilis, bilateral**

**H18.419 Arcus senilis, unspecified eye**

✓6th **H18.42 Band keratopathy**

**H18.421 Band keratopathy, right eye**

**H18.422 Band keratopathy, left eye**

**H18.423 Band keratopathy, bilateral**

**H18.429 Band keratopathy, unspecified eye**

**H18.43 Other calcerous corneal degeneration**

✓6th **H18.44 Keratomalacia**

EXCLUDES 1 *keratomalacia due to vitamin A deficiency (E5Ø.4)*

**H18.441 Keratomalacia, right eye**

**H18.442 Keratomalacia, left eye**

**H18.443 Keratomalacia, bilateral**

**H18.449 Keratomalacia, unspecified eye**

✓6th **H18.45 Nodular corneal degeneration**

**H18.451 Nodular corneal degeneration, right eye**

**H18.452 Nodular corneal degeneration, left eye**

**H18.453 Nodular corneal degeneration, bilateral**

**H18.459 Nodular corneal degeneration, unspecified eye**

✓6th **H18.46 Peripheral corneal degeneration**

**H18.461 Peripheral corneal degeneration, right eye**

**H18.462 Peripheral corneal degeneration, left eye**

**H18.463 Peripheral corneal degeneration, bilateral**

**H18.469 Peripheral corneal degeneration, unspecified eye**

**H18.49 Other corneal degeneration**

✓5th **H18.5 Hereditary corneal dystrophies**

AHA: 2020,4Q,24

✓6th **H18.5Ø Unspecified hereditary corneal dystrophies**

**H18.5Ø1 Unspecified hereditary corneal dystrophies, right eye**

**H18.5Ø2 Unspecified hereditary corneal dystrophies, left eye**

**H18.5Ø3 Unspecified hereditary corneal dystrophies, bilateral**

**H18.5Ø9 Unspecified hereditary corneal dystrophies, unspecified eye**

✓6th **H18.51 Endothelial corneal dystrophy**

Fuchs' dystrophy

**H18.511 Endothelial corneal dystrophy, right eye**

**H18.512 Endothelial corneal dystrophy, left eye**

**H18.513 Endothelial corneal dystrophy, bilateral**

**H18.519 Endothelial corneal dystrophy, unspecified eye**

✓6th **H18.52 Epithelial (juvenile) corneal dystrophy**

**H18.521 Epithelial (juvenile) corneal dystrophy, right eye**

**H18.522 Epithelial (juvenile) corneal dystrophy, left eye**

**H18.523 Epithelial (juvenile) corneal dystrophy, bilateral**

**H18.529 Epithelial (juvenile) corneal dystrophy, unspecified eye**

✓6th **H18.53 Granular corneal dystrophy**

**H18.531 Granular corneal dystrophy, right eye**

**H18.532 Granular corneal dystrophy, left eye**

**H18.533 Granular corneal dystrophy, bilateral**

**H18.539 Granular corneal dystrophy, unspecified eye**

✓6th **H18.54 Lattice corneal dystrophy**

**H18.541 Lattice corneal dystrophy, right eye**

**H18.542 Lattice corneal dystrophy, left eye**

**H18.543 Lattice corneal dystrophy, bilateral**

**H18.549 Lattice corneal dystrophy, unspecified eye**

✓6th **H18.55 Macular corneal dystrophy**

**H18.551 Macular corneal dystrophy, right eye**

**H18.552 Macular corneal dystrophy, left eye**

**H18.553 Macular corneal dystrophy, bilateral**

**H18.559 Macular corneal dystrophy, unspecified eye**

✓6th **H18.59 Other hereditary corneal dystrophies**

**H18.591 Other hereditary corneal dystrophies, right eye**

**H18.592 Other hereditary corneal dystrophies, left eye**

**H18.593 Other hereditary corneal dystrophies, bilateral**

**H18.599 Other hereditary corneal dystrophies, unspecified eye**

✓5th **H18.6 Keratoconus**

✓6th **H18.6Ø Keratoconus, unspecified**

**H18.6Ø1 Keratoconus, unspecified, right eye**

**H18.6Ø2 Keratoconus, unspecified, left eye**

**H18.6Ø3 Keratoconus, unspecified, bilateral**

**H18.6Ø9 Keratoconus, unspecified, unspecified eye**

✓6th **H18.61 Keratoconus, stable**

**H18.611 Keratoconus, stable, right eye**

**H18.612 Keratoconus, stable, left eye**

**H18.613 Keratoconus, stable, bilateral**

**H18.619 Keratoconus, stable, unspecified eye**

✓6th **H18.62 Keratoconus, unstable**

Acute hydrops

**H18.621 Keratoconus, unstable, right eye**

**H18.622 Keratoconus, unstable, left eye**

**H18.623 Keratoconus, unstable, bilateral**

**H18.629 Keratoconus, unstable, unspecified eye**

✓5th **H18.7 Other and unspecified corneal deformities**

EXCLUDES 1 *congenital malformations of cornea (Q13.3-Q13.4)*

**H18.7Ø Unspecified corneal deformity**

✓6th **H18.71 Corneal ectasia**

**H18.711 Corneal ectasia, right eye**

**H18.712 Corneal ectasia, left eye**

**H18.713 Corneal ectasia, bilateral**

**H18.719 Corneal ectasia, unspecified eye**

✓6th **H18.72 Corneal staphyloma**

**H18.721 Corneal staphyloma, right eye**

**H18.722 Corneal staphyloma, left eye**

**H18.723 Corneal staphyloma, bilateral**

**H18.729 Corneal staphyloma, unspecified eye**

✓6th **H18.73 Descemetocele**

**H18.731 Descemetocele, right eye**

**H18.732 Descemetocele, left eye**

**H18.733 Descemetocele, bilateral**

**H18.739 Descemetocele, unspecified eye**

✓6th **H18.79 Other corneal deformities**

**H18.791 Other corneal deformities, right eye**

**H18.792 Other corneal deformities, left eye**

**H18.793 Other corneal deformities, bilateral**

**H18.799 Other corneal deformities, unspecified eye**

√5th **H18.8 Other specified disorders of cornea**

√6th **H18.81 Anesthesia and hypoesthesia of cornea**

**H18.811 Anesthesia and hypoesthesia of cornea, right eye**

**H18.812 Anesthesia and hypoesthesia of cornea, left eye**

**H18.813 Anesthesia and hypoesthesia of cornea, bilateral**

**H18.819 Anesthesia and hypoesthesia of cornea, unspecified eye**

√6th **H18.82 Corneal disorder due to contact lens**

EXCLUDES 2 *corneal edema due to contact lens (H18.21-)*

**H18.821 Corneal disorder due to contact lens, right eye**

**H18.822 Corneal disorder due to contact lens, left eye**

**H18.823 Corneal disorder due to contact lens, bilateral**

**H18.829 Corneal disorder due to contact lens, unspecified eye**

√6th **H18.83 Recurrent erosion of cornea**

**H18.831 Recurrent erosion of cornea, right eye**

**H18.832 Recurrent erosion of cornea, left eye**

**H18.833 Recurrent erosion of cornea, bilateral**

**H18.839 Recurrent erosion of cornea, unspecified eye**

√6th **H18.89 Other specified disorders of cornea**

**H18.891 Other specified disorders of cornea, right eye**

**H18.892 Other specified disorders of cornea, left eye**

**H18.893 Other specified disorders of cornea, bilateral**

**H18.899 Other specified disorders of cornea, unspecified eye**

**H18.9 Unspecified disorder of cornea**

√4th **H2Ø Iridocyclitis**

√5th **H2Ø.Ø Acute and subacute iridocyclitis**

Acute anterior uveitis
Acute cyclitis
Acute iritis
Subacute anterior uveitis
Subacute cyclitis
Subacute iritis

EXCLUDES 1 *iridocyclitis, iritis, uveitis (due to) (in) diabetes mellitus (EØ8-E13 with .39)*
*iridocyclitis, iritis, uveitis (due to) (in) diphtheria (A36.89)*
*iridocyclitis, iritis, uveitis (due to) (in) gonococcal (A54.32)*
*iridocyclitis, iritis, uveitis (due to) (in) herpes (simplex) (BØØ.51)*
*iridocyclitis, iritis, uveitis (due to) (in) herpes zoster (BØ2.32)*
*iridocyclitis, iritis, uveitis (due to) (in) late congenital syphilis (A5Ø.39)*
*iridocyclitis, iritis, uveitis (due to) (in) late syphilis (A52.71)*
*iridocyclitis, iritis, uveitis (due to) (in) sarcoidosis (D86.83)*
*iridocyclitis, iritis, uveitis (due to) (in) syphilis (A51.43)*
*iridocyclitis, iritis, uveitis (due to) (in) toxoplasmosis (B58.Ø9)*
*iridocyclitis, iritis, uveitis (due to) (in) tuberculosis (A18.54)*

**H2Ø.ØØ Unspecified acute and subacute iridocyclitis**

√6th **H2Ø.Ø1 Primary iridocyclitis**

**H2Ø.Ø11 Primary iridocyclitis, right eye**

**H2Ø.Ø12 Primary iridocyclitis, left eye**

**H2Ø.Ø13 Primary iridocyclitis, bilateral**

**H2Ø.Ø19 Primary iridocyclitis, unspecified eye**

√6th **H2Ø.Ø2 Recurrent acute iridocyclitis**

**H2Ø.Ø21 Recurrent acute iridocyclitis, right eye**

**H2Ø.Ø22 Recurrent acute iridocyclitis, left eye**

**H2Ø.Ø23 Recurrent acute iridocyclitis, bilateral**

**H2Ø.Ø29 Recurrent acute iridocyclitis, unspecified eye**

√6th **H2Ø.Ø3 Secondary infectious iridocyclitis**

**H2Ø.Ø31 Secondary infectious iridocyclitis, right eye**

**H2Ø.Ø32 Secondary infectious iridocyclitis, left eye**

**H2Ø.Ø33 Secondary infectious iridocyclitis, bilateral**

**H2Ø.Ø39 Secondary infectious iridocyclitis, unspecified eye**

√6th **H2Ø.Ø4 Secondary noninfectious iridocyclitis**

**H2Ø.Ø41 Secondary noninfectious iridocyclitis, right eye**

**H2Ø.Ø42 Secondary noninfectious iridocyclitis, left eye**

**H2Ø.Ø43 Secondary noninfectious iridocyclitis, bilateral**

**H2Ø.Ø49 Secondary noninfectious iridocyclitis, unspecified eye**

√6th **H2Ø.Ø5 Hypopyon**

**H2Ø.Ø51 Hypopyon, right eye**

**H2Ø.Ø52 Hypopyon, left eye**

**H2Ø.Ø53 Hypopyon, bilateral**

**H2Ø.Ø59 Hypopyon, unspecified eye**

√5th **H2Ø.1 Chronic iridocyclitis**

Use additional code for any associated cataract (H26.21-)

EXCLUDES 2 *posterior cyclitis (H3Ø.2-)*

**H2Ø.1Ø Chronic iridocyclitis, unspecified eye**

**H2Ø.11 Chronic iridocyclitis, right eye**

**H2Ø.12 Chronic iridocyclitis, left eye**

**H2Ø.13 Chronic iridocyclitis, bilateral**

√5th **H2Ø.2 Lens-induced iridocyclitis**

**H2Ø.2Ø Lens-induced iridocyclitis, unspecified eye**

**H2Ø.21 Lens-induced iridocyclitis, right eye**

**H2Ø.22 Lens-induced iridocyclitis, left eye**

**H2Ø.23 Lens-induced iridocyclitis, bilateral**

√5th **H2Ø.8 Other iridocyclitis**

EXCLUDES 2 *glaucomatocyclitis crises (H4Ø.4-)*
*posterior cyclitis (H3Ø.2-)*
*sympathetic uveitis (H44.13-)*

√6th **H2Ø.81 Fuchs' heterochromic cyclitis**

**H2Ø.811 Fuchs' heterochromic cyclitis, right eye**

**H2Ø.812 Fuchs' heterochromic cyclitis, left eye**

**H2Ø.813 Fuchs' heterochromic cyclitis, bilateral**

**H2Ø.819 Fuchs' heterochromic cyclitis, unspecified eye**

√6th **H2Ø.82 Vogt-Koyanagi syndrome**

**H2Ø.821 Vogt-Koyanagi syndrome, right eye**

**H2Ø.822 Vogt-Koyanagi syndrome, left eye**

**H2Ø.823 Vogt-Koyanagi syndrome, bilateral**

**H2Ø.829 Vogt-Koyanagi syndrome, unspecified eye**

**H2Ø.9 Unspecified iridocyclitis**

Uveitis NOS

√4th **H21 Other disorders of iris and ciliary body**

EXCLUDES 2 *sympathetic uveitis (H44.1-)*

√5th **H21.Ø Hyphema**

EXCLUDES 1 *traumatic hyphema (SØ5.1-)*

**Hyphema**

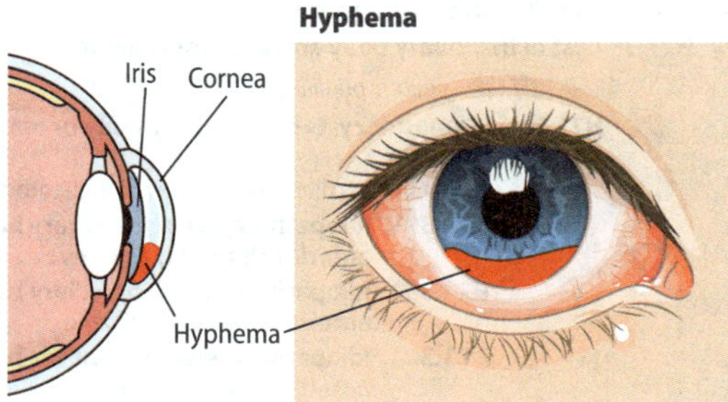


**H21.ØØ Hyphema, unspecified eye**

**H21.Ø1 Hyphema, right eye**

**H21.Ø2 Hyphema, left eye**

**H21.Ø3 Hyphema, bilateral**

√5th **H21.1 Other vascular disorders of iris and ciliary body**

Neovascularization of iris or ciliary body
Rubeosis iridis
Rubeosis of iris

√6th **H21.1X Other vascular disorders of iris and ciliary body**

**H21.1X1 Other vascular disorders of iris and ciliary body, right eye**

H21.1X2 Other vascular disorders of iris and ciliary body, left eye
H21.1X3 Other vascular disorders of iris and ciliary body, bilateral
H21.1X9 Other vascular disorders of iris and ciliary body, unspecified eye

✓5th H21.2 Degeneration of iris and ciliary body

✓6th H21.21 Degeneration of chamber angle
H21.211 Degeneration of chamber angle, right eye
H21.212 Degeneration of chamber angle, left eye
H21.213 Degeneration of chamber angle, bilateral
H21.219 Degeneration of chamber angle, unspecified eye

✓6th H21.22 Degeneration of ciliary body
H21.221 Degeneration of ciliary body, right eye
H21.222 Degeneration of ciliary body, left eye
H21.223 Degeneration of ciliary body, bilateral
H21.229 Degeneration of ciliary body, unspecified eye

✓6th H21.23 Degeneration of iris (pigmentary)
Translucency of iris
H21.231 Degeneration of iris (pigmentary), right eye
H21.232 Degeneration of iris (pigmentary), left eye
H21.233 Degeneration of iris (pigmentary), bilateral
H21.239 Degeneration of iris (pigmentary), unspecified eye

✓6th H21.24 Degeneration of pupillary margin
H21.241 Degeneration of pupillary margin, right eye
H21.242 Degeneration of pupillary margin, left eye
H21.243 Degeneration of pupillary margin, bilateral
H21.249 Degeneration of pupillary margin, unspecified eye

✓6th H21.25 Iridoschisis
H21.251 Iridoschisis, right eye
H21.252 Iridoschisis, left eye
H21.253 Iridoschisis, bilateral
H21.259 Iridoschisis, unspecified eye

✓6th H21.26 Iris atrophy (essential) (progressive)
H21.261 Iris atrophy (essential) (progressive), right eye
H21.262 Iris atrophy (essential) (progressive), left eye
H21.263 Iris atrophy (essential) (progressive), bilateral
H21.269 Iris atrophy (essential) (progressive), unspecified eye

✓6th H21.27 Miotic pupillary cyst
H21.271 Miotic pupillary cyst, right eye
H21.272 Miotic pupillary cyst, left eye
H21.273 Miotic pupillary cyst, bilateral
H21.279 Miotic pupillary cyst, unspecified eye

H21.29 Other iris atrophy

✓5th H21.3 Cyst of iris, ciliary body and anterior chamber
EXCLUDES 2 *miotic pupillary cyst (H21.27-)*

✓6th H21.30 Idiopathic cysts of iris, ciliary body or anterior chamber
Cyst of iris, ciliary body or anterior chamber NOS
H21.301 Idiopathic cysts of iris, ciliary body or anterior chamber, right eye
H21.302 Idiopathic cysts of iris, ciliary body or anterior chamber, left eye
H21.303 Idiopathic cysts of iris, ciliary body or anterior chamber, bilateral
H21.309 Idiopathic cysts of iris, ciliary body or anterior chamber, unspecified eye

✓6th H21.31 Exudative cysts of iris or anterior chamber
H21.311 Exudative cysts of iris or anterior chamber, right eye
H21.312 Exudative cysts of iris or anterior chamber, left eye
H21.313 Exudative cysts of iris or anterior chamber, bilateral
H21.319 Exudative cysts of iris or anterior chamber, unspecified eye

✓6th H21.32 Implantation cysts of iris, ciliary body or anterior chamber
H21.321 Implantation cysts of iris, ciliary body or anterior chamber, right eye
H21.322 Implantation cysts of iris, ciliary body or anterior chamber, left eye
H21.323 Implantation cysts of iris, ciliary body or anterior chamber, bilateral
H21.329 Implantation cysts of iris, ciliary body or anterior chamber, unspecified eye

✓6th H21.33 Parasitic cyst of iris, ciliary body or anterior chamber
H21.331 Parasitic cyst of iris, ciliary body or anterior chamber, right eye
H21.332 Parasitic cyst of iris, ciliary body or anterior chamber, left eye
H21.333 Parasitic cyst of iris, ciliary body or anterior chamber, bilateral
H21.339 Parasitic cyst of iris, ciliary body or anterior chamber, unspecified eye

✓6th H21.34 Primary cyst of pars plana
H21.341 Primary cyst of pars plana, right eye
H21.342 Primary cyst of pars plana, left eye
H21.343 Primary cyst of pars plana, bilateral
H21.349 Primary cyst of pars plana, unspecified eye

✓6th H21.35 Exudative cyst of pars plana
**DEF:** Protein, fatty-filled bullous elevation of the nonpigmented outermost ciliary epithelium of pars plana, due to fluid leak from blood vessels.
H21.351 Exudative cyst of pars plana, right eye
H21.352 Exudative cyst of pars plana, left eye
H21.353 Exudative cyst of pars plana, bilateral
H21.359 Exudative cyst of pars plana, unspecified eye

✓5th H21.4 Pupillary membranes
Iris bombé
Pupillary occlusion
Pupillary seclusion
EXCLUDES 1 *congenital pupillary membranes (Q13.8)*
H21.40 Pupillary membranes, unspecified eye
H21.41 Pupillary membranes, right eye
H21.42 Pupillary membranes, left eye
H21.43 Pupillary membranes, bilateral

✓5th H21.5 Other and unspecified adhesions and disruptions of iris and ciliary body
EXCLUDES 1 *corectopia (Q13.2)*

✓6th H21.50 Unspecified adhesions of iris
Synechia (iris) NOS
H21.501 Unspecified adhesions of iris, right eye
H21.502 Unspecified adhesions of iris, left eye
H21.503 Unspecified adhesions of iris, bilateral
H21.509 Unspecified adhesions of iris and ciliary body, unspecified eye

✓6th H21.51 Anterior synechiae (iris)
H21.511 Anterior synechiae (iris), right eye
H21.512 Anterior synechiae (iris), left eye
H21.513 Anterior synechiae (iris), bilateral
H21.519 Anterior synechiae (iris), unspecified eye

✓6th H21.52 Goniosynechiae
H21.521 Goniosynechiae, right eye
H21.522 Goniosynechiae, left eye
H21.523 Goniosynechiae, bilateral
H21.529 Goniosynechiae, unspecified eye

✓6th H21.53 Iridodialysis
H21.531 Iridodialysis, right eye
H21.532 Iridodialysis, left eye
H21.533 Iridodialysis, bilateral
H21.539 Iridodialysis, unspecified eye

✓6th H21.54 Posterior synechiae (iris)
H21.541 Posterior synechiae (iris), right eye
H21.542 Posterior synechiae (iris), left eye
H21.543 Posterior synechiae (iris), bilateral
H21.549 Posterior synechiae (iris), unspecified eye

✓6th H21.55 Recession of chamber angle
H21.551 Recession of chamber angle, right eye
H21.552 Recession of chamber angle, left eye
H21.553 Recession of chamber angle, bilateral
H21.559 Recession of chamber angle, unspecified eye

**√6th H21.56 Pupillary abnormalities**
Deformed pupil
Ectopic pupil
Rupture of sphincter, pupil
EXCLUDES 1 *congenital deformity of pupil (Q13.2-)*
**H21.561 Pupillary abnormality, right eye**
**H21.562 Pupillary abnormality, left eye**
**H21.563 Pupillary abnormality, bilateral**
**H21.569 Pupillary abnormality, unspecified eye**

**√5th H21.8 Other specified disorders of iris and ciliary body**
**H21.81 Floppy iris syndrome**
Intraoperative floppy iris syndrome (IFIS)
Use additional code for adverse effect, if applicable, to identify drug (T36-T5Ø with fifth or sixth character 5)
**H21.82 Plateau iris syndrome (post-iridectomy) (postprocedural)**
**H21.89 Other specified disorders of iris and ciliary body**

**H21.9 Unspecified disorder of iris and ciliary body**

***H22 Disorders of iris and ciliary body in diseases classified elsewhere***
Code first underlying disease, such as:
gout (M1A.-, M1Ø.-)
leprosy (A3Ø.-)
parasitic disease (B89)

## Disorders of lens (H25-H28)

**√4th H25 Age-related cataract**
Senile cataract
EXCLUDES 2 *capsular glaucoma with pseudoexfoliation of lens (H4Ø.1-)*

**Cataracts**

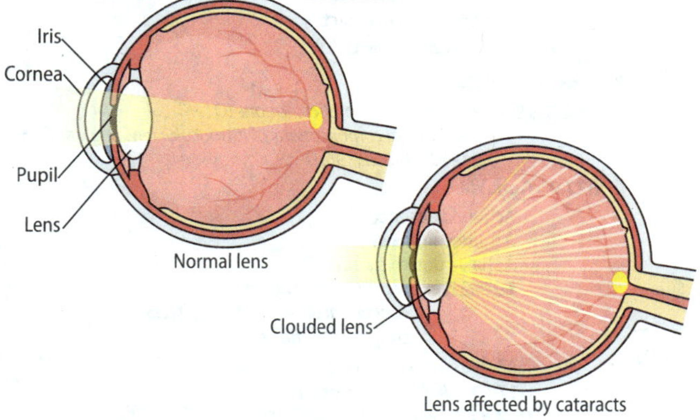


**√5th H25.Ø Age-related incipient cataract**
**√6th H25.Ø1 Cortical age-related cataract**
**H25.Ø11 Cortical age-related cataract, right eye** A
**H25.Ø12 Cortical age-related cataract, left eye** A
**H25.Ø13 Cortical age-related cataract, bilateral** A
**H25.Ø19 Cortical age-related cataract, unspecified eye** A
**√6th H25.Ø3 Anterior subcapsular polar age-related cataract**
**H25.Ø31 Anterior subcapsular polar age-related cataract, right eye** A
**H25.Ø32 Anterior subcapsular polar age-related cataract, left eye** A
**H25.Ø33 Anterior subcapsular polar age-related cataract, bilateral** A
**H25.Ø39 Anterior subcapsular polar age-related cataract, unspecified eye** A
**√6th H25.Ø4 Posterior subcapsular polar age-related cataract**
**H25.Ø41 Posterior subcapsular polar age-related cataract, right eye** A
**H25.Ø42 Posterior subcapsular polar age-related cataract, left eye** A
**H25.Ø43 Posterior subcapsular polar age-related cataract, bilateral** A
**H25.Ø49 Posterior subcapsular polar age-related cataract, unspecified eye** A
**√6th H25.Ø9 Other age-related incipient cataract**
Coronary age-related cataract
Punctate age-related cataract
Water clefts
**H25.Ø91 Other age-related incipient cataract, right eye** A
**H25.Ø92 Other age-related incipient cataract, left eye** A
**H25.Ø93 Other age-related incipient cataract, bilateral** A
**H25.Ø99 Other age-related incipient cataract, unspecified eye** A

**√5th H25.1 Age-related nuclear cataract**
Cataracta brunescens
Nuclear sclerosis cataract
**AHA:** 2019,2Q,31; 2016,1Q,32
**H25.1Ø Age-related nuclear cataract, unspecified eye** A
**H25.11 Age-related nuclear cataract, right eye** A
**H25.12 Age-related nuclear cataract, left eye** A
**H25.13 Age-related nuclear cataract, bilateral** A

**√5th H25.2 Age-related cataract, morgagnian type**
Age-related hypermature cataract
**H25.2Ø Age-related cataract, morgagnian type, unspecified eye** A
**H25.21 Age-related cataract, morgagnian type, right eye** A
**H25.22 Age-related cataract, morgagnian type, left eye** A
**H25.23 Age-related cataract, morgagnian type, bilateral** A

**√5th H25.8 Other age-related cataract**
**√6th H25.81 Combined forms of age-related cataract**
**AHA:** 2019,2Q,30
**H25.811 Combined forms of age-related cataract, right eye** A
**H25.812 Combined forms of age-related cataract, left eye** A
**H25.813 Combined forms of age-related cataract, bilateral** A
**H25.819 Combined forms of age-related cataract, unspecified eye** A
**H25.89 Other age-related cataract** A

**H25.9 Unspecified age-related cataract** A

**√4th H26 Other cataract**
EXCLUDES 1 *congenital cataract (Q12.Ø)*

**√5th H26.Ø Infantile and juvenile cataract**
**√6th H26.ØØ Unspecified infantile and juvenile cataract**
**H26.ØØ1 Unspecified infantile and juvenile cataract, right eye** P
**H26.ØØ2 Unspecified infantile and juvenile cataract, left eye** P
**H26.ØØ3 Unspecified infantile and juvenile cataract, bilateral** P
**H26.ØØ9 Unspecified infantile and juvenile cataract, unspecified eye** P
**√6th H26.Ø1 Infantile and juvenile cortical, lamellar, or zonular cataract**
**H26.Ø11 Infantile and juvenile cortical, lamellar, or zonular cataract, right eye** P
**H26.Ø12 Infantile and juvenile cortical, lamellar, or zonular cataract, left eye** P
**H26.Ø13 Infantile and juvenile cortical, lamellar, or zonular cataract, bilateral** P
**H26.Ø19 Infantile and juvenile cortical, lamellar, or zonular cataract, unspecified eye** P
**√6th H26.Ø3 Infantile and juvenile nuclear cataract**
**H26.Ø31 Infantile and juvenile nuclear cataract, right eye** P
**H26.Ø32 Infantile and juvenile nuclear cataract, left eye** P
**H26.Ø33 Infantile and juvenile nuclear cataract, bilateral** P
**H26.Ø39 Infantile and juvenile nuclear cataract, unspecified eye** P
**√6th H26.Ø4 Anterior subcapsular polar infantile and juvenile cataract**
**H26.Ø41 Anterior subcapsular polar infantile and juvenile cataract, right eye** P

H26.042 Anterior subcapsular polar infantile and juvenile cataract, left eye P
H26.043 Anterior subcapsular polar infantile and juvenile cataract, bilateral P
H26.049 Anterior subcapsular polar infantile and juvenile cataract, unspecified eye P

√6th H26.05 Posterior subcapsular polar infantile and juvenile cataract
H26.051 Posterior subcapsular polar infantile and juvenile cataract, right eye P
H26.052 Posterior subcapsular polar infantile and juvenile cataract, left eye P
H26.053 Posterior subcapsular polar infantile and juvenile cataract, bilateral P
H26.059 Posterior subcapsular polar infantile and juvenile cataract, unspecified eye P

√6th H26.06 Combined forms of infantile and juvenile cataract
H26.061 Combined forms of infantile and juvenile cataract, right eye P
H26.062 Combined forms of infantile and juvenile cataract, left eye P
H26.063 Combined forms of infantile and juvenile cataract, bilateral P
H26.069 Combined forms of infantile and juvenile cataract, unspecified eye P

H26.09 Other infantile and juvenile cataract P

√5th H26.1 Traumatic cataract
Use additional code (Chapter 20) to identify external cause

√6th H26.10 Unspecified traumatic cataract
H26.101 Unspecified traumatic cataract, right eye
H26.102 Unspecified traumatic cataract, left eye
H26.103 Unspecified traumatic cataract, bilateral
H26.109 Unspecified traumatic cataract, unspecified eye

√6th H26.11 Localized traumatic opacities
H26.111 Localized traumatic opacities, right eye
H26.112 Localized traumatic opacities, left eye
H26.113 Localized traumatic opacities, bilateral
H26.119 Localized traumatic opacities, unspecified eye

√6th H26.12 Partially resolved traumatic cataract
H26.121 Partially resolved traumatic cataract, right eye
H26.122 Partially resolved traumatic cataract, left eye
H26.123 Partially resolved traumatic cataract, bilateral
H26.129 Partially resolved traumatic cataract, unspecified eye

√6th H26.13 Total traumatic cataract
H26.131 Total traumatic cataract, right eye
H26.132 Total traumatic cataract, left eye
H26.133 Total traumatic cataract, bilateral
H26.139 Total traumatic cataract, unspecified eye

√5th H26.2 Complicated cataract
H26.20 Unspecified complicated cataract
Cataracta complicata NOS

√6th H26.21 Cataract with neovascularization
Code also, if applicable, associated condition, such as: chronic iridocyclitis (H20.1-)
H26.211 Cataract with neovascularization, right eye
H26.212 Cataract with neovascularization, left eye
H26.213 Cataract with neovascularization, bilateral
H26.219 Cataract with neovascularization, unspecified eye

√6th H26.22 Cataract secondary to ocular disorders (degenerative) (inflammatory)
Code also associated ocular disorder
H26.221 Cataract secondary to ocular disorders (degenerative) (inflammatory), right eye
H26.222 Cataract secondary to ocular disorders (degenerative) (inflammatory), left eye
H26.223 Cataract secondary to ocular disorders (degenerative) (inflammatory), bilateral
H26.229 Cataract secondary to ocular disorders (degenerative) (inflammatory), unspecified eye

√6th H26.23 Glaucomatous flecks (subcapsular)
Code first underlying glaucoma (H40-H42)
H26.231 Glaucomatous flecks (subcapsular), right eye
H26.232 Glaucomatous flecks (subcapsular), left eye
H26.233 Glaucomatous flecks (subcapsular), bilateral
H26.239 Glaucomatous flecks (subcapsular), unspecified eye

√5th H26.3 Drug-induced cataract
Toxic cataract
Use additional code for adverse effect, if applicable, to identify drug (T36-T50 with fifth or sixth character 5)
H26.30 Drug-induced cataract, unspecified eye
H26.31 Drug-induced cataract, right eye
H26.32 Drug-induced cataract, left eye
H26.33 Drug-induced cataract, bilateral

√5th H26.4 Secondary cataract
H26.40 Unspecified secondary cataract

√6th H26.41 Soemmering's ring
H26.411 Soemmering's ring, right eye
H26.412 Soemmering's ring, left eye
H26.413 Soemmering's ring, bilateral
H26.419 Soemmering's ring, unspecified eye

√6th H26.49 Other secondary cataract
AHA: 2018,2Q,14
H26.491 Other secondary cataract, right eye
H26.492 Other secondary cataract, left eye
H26.493 Other secondary cataract, bilateral
H26.499 Other secondary cataract, unspecified eye

H26.8 Other specified cataract
H26.9 Unspecified cataract

√4th H27 Other disorders of lens
EXCLUDES 1 *congenital lens malformations (Q12.-)*
*mechanical complications of intraocular lens implant (T85.2)*
*pseudophakia (Z96.1)*

√5th H27.0 Aphakia
Acquired absence of lens
Acquired aphakia
Aphakia due to trauma
EXCLUDES 1 *cataract extraction status (Z98.4-)*
*congenital absence of lens (Q12.3)*
*congenital aphakia (Q12.3)*
H27.00 Aphakia, unspecified eye
H27.01 Aphakia, right eye
H27.02 Aphakia, left eye
H27.03 Aphakia, bilateral

√5th H27.1 Dislocation of lens
H27.10 Unspecified dislocation of lens

√6th H27.11 Subluxation of lens
H27.111 Subluxation of lens, right eye
H27.112 Subluxation of lens, left eye
H27.113 Subluxation of lens, bilateral
H27.119 Subluxation of lens, unspecified eye

√6th H27.12 Anterior dislocation of lens
H27.121 Anterior dislocation of lens, right eye
H27.122 Anterior dislocation of lens, left eye
H27.123 Anterior dislocation of lens, bilateral
H27.129 Anterior dislocation of lens, unspecified eye

√6th H27.13 Posterior dislocation of lens
H27.131 Posterior dislocation of lens, right eye
H27.132 Posterior dislocation of lens, left eye
H27.133 Posterior dislocation of lens, bilateral
H27.139 Posterior dislocation of lens, unspecified eye

H27.8 Other specified disorders of lens
H27.9 Unspecified disorder of lens

**H28 Cataract in diseases classified elsewhere**
Code first underlying disease, such as:
hypoparathyroidism (E20.-)
myotonia (G71.1-)
myxedema (E03.-)
protein-calorie malnutrition (E40-E46)
EXCLUDES 1 *cataract in diabetes mellitus (E08.36, E09.36, E10.36, E11.36, E13.36)*

## Disorders of choroid and retina (H30-H36)

**H30 Chorioretinal inflammation**

**H30.0 Focal chorioretinal inflammation**
Focal chorioretinitis
Focal choroiditis
Focal retinitis
Focal retinochoroiditis

**H30.00 Unspecified focal chorioretinal inflammation**
Focal chorioretinitis NOS
Focal choroiditis NOS
Focal retinitis NOS
Focal retinochoroiditis NOS
**H30.001** Unspecified focal chorioretinal inflammation, right eye
**H30.002** Unspecified focal chorioretinal inflammation, left eye
**H30.003** Unspecified focal chorioretinal inflammation, bilateral
**H30.009** Unspecified focal chorioretinal inflammation, unspecified eye

**H30.01 Focal chorioretinal inflammation, juxtapapillary**
**H30.011** Focal chorioretinal inflammation, juxtapapillary, right eye
**H30.012** Focal chorioretinal inflammation, juxtapapillary, left eye
**H30.013** Focal chorioretinal inflammation, juxtapapillary, bilateral
**H30.019** Focal chorioretinal inflammation, juxtapapillary, unspecified eye

**H30.02 Focal chorioretinal inflammation of posterior pole**
**H30.021** Focal chorioretinal inflammation of posterior pole, right eye
**H30.022** Focal chorioretinal inflammation of posterior pole, left eye
**H30.023** Focal chorioretinal inflammation of posterior pole, bilateral
**H30.029** Focal chorioretinal inflammation of posterior pole, unspecified eye

**H30.03 Focal chorioretinal inflammation, peripheral**
**H30.031** Focal chorioretinal inflammation, peripheral, right eye
**H30.032** Focal chorioretinal inflammation, peripheral, left eye
**H30.033** Focal chorioretinal inflammation, peripheral, bilateral
**H30.039** Focal chorioretinal inflammation, peripheral, unspecified eye

**H30.04 Focal chorioretinal inflammation, macular or paramacular**
**H30.041** Focal chorioretinal inflammation, macular or paramacular, right eye
**H30.042** Focal chorioretinal inflammation, macular or paramacular, left eye
**H30.043** Focal chorioretinal inflammation, macular or paramacular, bilateral
**H30.049** Focal chorioretinal inflammation, macular or paramacular, unspecified eye

**H30.1 Disseminated chorioretinal inflammation**
Disseminated chorioretinitis
Disseminated choroiditis
Disseminated retinitis
Disseminated retinochoroiditis
EXCLUDES 2 *exudative retinopathy (H35.02-)*

**H30.10 Unspecified disseminated chorioretinal inflammation**
Disseminated chorioretinitis NOS
Disseminated choroiditis NOS
Disseminated retinitis NOS
Disseminated retinochoroiditis NOS
**H30.101** Unspecified disseminated chorioretinal inflammation, right eye
**H30.102** Unspecified disseminated chorioretinal inflammation, left eye
**H30.103** Unspecified disseminated chorioretinal inflammation, bilateral
**H30.109** Unspecified disseminated chorioretinal inflammation, unspecified eye

**H30.11 Disseminated chorioretinal inflammation of posterior pole**
**H30.111** Disseminated chorioretinal inflammation of posterior pole, right eye
**H30.112** Disseminated chorioretinal inflammation of posterior pole, left eye
**H30.113** Disseminated chorioretinal inflammation of posterior pole, bilateral
**H30.119** Disseminated chorioretinal inflammation of posterior pole, unspecified eye

**H30.12 Disseminated chorioretinal inflammation, peripheral**
**H30.121** Disseminated chorioretinal inflammation, peripheral right eye
**H30.122** Disseminated chorioretinal inflammation, peripheral, left eye
**H30.123** Disseminated chorioretinal inflammation, peripheral, bilateral
**H30.129** Disseminated chorioretinal inflammation, peripheral, unspecified eye

**H30.13 Disseminated chorioretinal inflammation, generalized**
**H30.131** Disseminated chorioretinal inflammation, generalized, right eye
**H30.132** Disseminated chorioretinal inflammation, generalized, left eye
**H30.133** Disseminated chorioretinal inflammation, generalized, bilateral
**H30.139** Disseminated chorioretinal inflammation, generalized, unspecified eye

**H30.14 Acute posterior multifocal placoid pigment epitheliopathy**
**H30.141** Acute posterior multifocal placoid pigment epitheliopathy, right eye
**H30.142** Acute posterior multifocal placoid pigment epitheliopathy, left eye
**H30.143** Acute posterior multifocal placoid pigment epitheliopathy, bilateral
**H30.149** Acute posterior multifocal placoid pigment epitheliopathy, unspecified eye

**H30.2 Posterior cyclitis**
Pars planitis
**H30.20** Posterior cyclitis, unspecified eye
**H30.21** Posterior cyclitis, right eye
**H30.22** Posterior cyclitis, left eye
**H30.23** Posterior cyclitis, bilateral

**H30.8 Other chorioretinal inflammations**

**H30.81 Harada's disease**
**H30.811** Harada's disease, right eye
**H30.812** Harada's disease, left eye
**H30.813** Harada's disease, bilateral
**H30.819** Harada's disease, unspecified eye

**H30.89 Other chorioretinal inflammations**
**H30.891** Other chorioretinal inflammations, right eye
**H30.892** Other chorioretinal inflammations, left eye
**H30.893** Other chorioretinal inflammations, bilateral
**H30.899** Other chorioretinal inflammations, unspecified eye

**H30.9 Unspecified chorioretinal inflammation**
Chorioretinitis NOS
Choroiditis NOS
Neuroretinitis NOS
Retinitis NOS
Retinochoroiditis NOS
**H30.90** Unspecified chorioretinal inflammation, unspecified eye
**H30.91** Unspecified chorioretinal inflammation, right eye
**H30.92** Unspecified chorioretinal inflammation, left eye
**H30.93** Unspecified chorioretinal inflammation, bilateral

**H31 Other disorders of choroid**

**H31.0 Chorioretinal scars**
EXCLUDES 2 *postsurgical chorioretinal scars (H59.81-)*

**H31.00 Unspecified chorioretinal scars**
**H31.001** Unspecified chorioretinal scars, right eye

**H31.ØØ2** Unspecified chorioretinal scars, left eye
**H31.ØØ3** Unspecified chorioretinal scars, bilateral
**H31.ØØ9** Unspecified chorioretinal scars, unspecified eye

✓6th **H31.Ø1** Macula scars of posterior pole (postinflammatory) (post-traumatic)

EXCLUDES 1 *postprocedural chorioretinal scar (H59.81-)*

**H31.Ø11** Macula scars of posterior pole (postinflammatory) (post-traumatic), right eye
**H31.Ø12** Macula scars of posterior pole (postinflammatory) (post-traumatic), left eye
**H31.Ø13** Macula scars of posterior pole (postinflammatory) (post-traumatic), bilateral
**H31.Ø19** Macula scars of posterior pole (postinflammatory) (post-traumatic), unspecified eye

✓6th **H31.Ø2** Solar retinopathy

**H31.Ø21** Solar retinopathy, right eye
**H31.Ø22** Solar retinopathy, left eye
**H31.Ø23** Solar retinopathy, bilateral
**H31.Ø29** Solar retinopathy, unspecified eye

✓6th **H31.Ø9** Other chorioretinal scars

**H31.Ø91** Other chorioretinal scars, right eye
**H31.Ø92** Other chorioretinal scars, left eye
**H31.Ø93** Other chorioretinal scars, bilateral
**H31.Ø99** Other chorioretinal scars, unspecified eye

✓5th **H31.1** Choroidal degeneration

EXCLUDES 2 *angioid streaks of macula (H35.33)*

✓6th **H31.1Ø** Unspecified choroidal degeneration

Choroidal sclerosis NOS

**H31.1Ø1** Choroidal degeneration, unspecified, right eye
**H31.1Ø2** Choroidal degeneration, unspecified, left eye
**H31.1Ø3** Choroidal degeneration, unspecified, bilateral
**H31.1Ø9** Choroidal degeneration, unspecified, unspecified eye

✓6th **H31.11** Age-related choroidal atrophy

**H31.111** Age-related choroidal atrophy, right eye A
**H31.112** Age-related choroidal atrophy, left eye A
**H31.113** Age-related choroidal atrophy, bilateral A
**H31.119** Age-related choroidal atrophy, unspecified eye A

✓6th **H31.12** Diffuse secondary atrophy of choroid

**H31.121** Diffuse secondary atrophy of choroid, right eye
**H31.122** Diffuse secondary atrophy of choroid, left eye
**H31.123** Diffuse secondary atrophy of choroid, bilateral
**H31.129** Diffuse secondary atrophy of choroid, unspecified eye

✓5th **H31.2** Hereditary choroidal dystrophy

EXCLUDES 2 *hyperornithinemia (E72.4)*
*ornithinemia (E72.4)*

**H31.2Ø** Hereditary choroidal dystrophy, unspecified
**H31.21** Choroideremia
**H31.22** Choroidal dystrophy (central areolar) (generalized) (peripapillary)
**H31.23** Gyrate atrophy, choroid
**H31.29** Other hereditary choroidal dystrophy

✓5th **H31.3** Choroidal hemorrhage and rupture

✓6th **H31.3Ø** Unspecified choroidal hemorrhage

**H31.3Ø1** Unspecified choroidal hemorrhage, right eye
**H31.3Ø2** Unspecified choroidal hemorrhage, left eye
**H31.3Ø3** Unspecified choroidal hemorrhage, bilateral
**H31.3Ø9** Unspecified choroidal hemorrhage, unspecified eye

✓6th **H31.31** Expulsive choroidal hemorrhage

**H31.311** Expulsive choroidal hemorrhage, right eye
**H31.312** Expulsive choroidal hemorrhage, left eye
**H31.313** Expulsive choroidal hemorrhage, bilateral
**H31.319** Expulsive choroidal hemorrhage, unspecified eye

✓6th **H31.32** Choroidal rupture

**H31.321** Choroidal rupture, right eye
**H31.322** Choroidal rupture, left eye
**H31.323** Choroidal rupture, bilateral
**H31.329** Choroidal rupture, unspecified eye

✓5th **H31.4** Choroidal detachment

✓6th **H31.4Ø** Unspecified choroidal detachment

**H31.4Ø1** Unspecified choroidal detachment, right eye
**H31.4Ø2** Unspecified choroidal detachment, left eye
**H31.4Ø3** Unspecified choroidal detachment, bilateral
**H31.4Ø9** Unspecified choroidal detachment, unspecified eye

✓6th **H31.41** Hemorrhagic choroidal detachment

**H31.411** Hemorrhagic choroidal detachment, right eye
**H31.412** Hemorrhagic choroidal detachment, left eye
**H31.413** Hemorrhagic choroidal detachment, bilateral
**H31.419** Hemorrhagic choroidal detachment, unspecified eye

✓6th **H31.42** Serous choroidal detachment

**H31.421** Serous choroidal detachment, right eye
**H31.422** Serous choroidal detachment, left eye
**H31.423** Serous choroidal detachment, bilateral
**H31.429** Serous choroidal detachment, unspecified eye

**H31.8** Other specified disorders of choroid
**H31.9** Unspecified disorder of choroid

***H32 Chorioretinal disorders in diseases classified elsewhere***

Code first underlying disease, such as:
congenital toxoplasmosis (P37.1)
histoplasmosis (B39.-)
leprosy (A3Ø.-)

EXCLUDES 1 *chorioretinitis (in):*
*toxoplasmosis (acquired) (B58.Ø1)*
*tuberculosis (A18.53)*

✓4th **H33 Retinal detachments and breaks**

EXCLUDES 1 *detachment of retinal pigment epithelium (H35.72-, H35.73-)*

**Retinal Detachment**

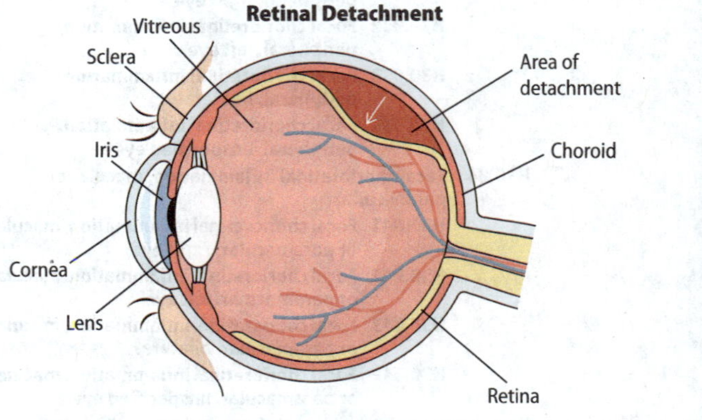


✓5th **H33.Ø** Retinal detachment with retinal break

Rhegmatogenous retinal detachment

EXCLUDES 1 *serous retinal detachment (without retinal break) (H33.2-)*

✓6th **H33.ØØ** Unspecified retinal detachment with retinal break

**H33.ØØ1** Unspecified retinal detachment with retinal break, right eye
**H33.ØØ2** Unspecified retinal detachment with retinal break, left eye
**H33.ØØ3** Unspecified retinal detachment with retinal break, bilateral
**H33.ØØ9** Unspecified retinal detachment with retinal break, unspecified eye

H33.01 Retinal detachment with single break
- H33.011 Retinal detachment with single break, right eye
- H33.012 Retinal detachment with single break, left eye
- H33.013 Retinal detachment with single break, bilateral
- H33.019 Retinal detachment with single break, unspecified eye

H33.02 Retinal detachment with multiple breaks
- H33.021 Retinal detachment with multiple breaks, right eye
- H33.022 Retinal detachment with multiple breaks, left eye
- H33.023 Retinal detachment with multiple breaks, bilateral
- H33.029 Retinal detachment with multiple breaks, unspecified eye

H33.03 Retinal detachment with giant retinal tear
- H33.031 Retinal detachment with giant retinal tear, right eye
- H33.032 Retinal detachment with giant retinal tear, left eye
- H33.033 Retinal detachment with giant retinal tear, bilateral
- H33.039 Retinal detachment with giant retinal tear, unspecified eye

H33.04 Retinal detachment with retinal dialysis
- H33.041 Retinal detachment with retinal dialysis, right eye
- H33.042 Retinal detachment with retinal dialysis, left eye
- H33.043 Retinal detachment with retinal dialysis, bilateral
- H33.049 Retinal detachment with retinal dialysis, unspecified eye

H33.05 Total retinal detachment
- H33.051 Total retinal detachment, right eye
- H33.052 Total retinal detachment, left eye
- H33.053 Total retinal detachment, bilateral
- H33.059 Total retinal detachment, unspecified eye

H33.1 Retinoschisis and retinal cysts

EXCLUDES 1 *congenital retinoschisis (Q14.1)*
*microcystoid degeneration of retina (H35.42-)*

H33.10 Unspecified retinoschisis
- H33.101 Unspecified retinoschisis, right eye
- H33.102 Unspecified retinoschisis, left eye
- H33.103 Unspecified retinoschisis, bilateral
- H33.109 Unspecified retinoschisis, unspecified eye

H33.11 Cyst of ora serrata
- H33.111 Cyst of ora serrata, right eye
- H33.112 Cyst of ora serrata, left eye
- H33.113 Cyst of ora serrata, bilateral
- H33.119 Cyst of ora serrata, unspecified eye

H33.12 Parasitic cyst of retina
- H33.121 Parasitic cyst of retina, right eye
- H33.122 Parasitic cyst of retina, left eye
- H33.123 Parasitic cyst of retina, bilateral
- H33.129 Parasitic cyst of retina, unspecified eye

H33.19 Other retinoschisis and retinal cysts

Pseudocyst of retina
- H33.191 Other retinoschisis and retinal cysts, right eye
- H33.192 Other retinoschisis and retinal cysts, left eye
- H33.193 Other retinoschisis and retinal cysts, bilateral
- H33.199 Other retinoschisis and retinal cysts, unspecified eye

H33.2 Serous retinal detachment

Retinal detachment NOS
Retinal detachment without retinal break

EXCLUDES 1 *central serous chorioretinopathy (H35.71-)*

- H33.20 Serous retinal detachment, unspecified eye
- H33.21 Serous retinal detachment, right eye
- H33.22 Serous retinal detachment, left eye
- H33.23 Serous retinal detachment, bilateral

H33.3 Retinal breaks without detachment

EXCLUDES 1 *chorioretinal scars after surgery for detachment (H59.81-)*

EXCLUDES 2 *peripheral retinal degeneration without break (H35.4-)*

H33.30 Unspecified retinal break
- H33.301 Unspecified retinal break, right eye
- H33.302 Unspecified retinal break, left eye
- H33.303 Unspecified retinal break, bilateral
- H33.309 Unspecified retinal break, unspecified eye

H33.31 Horseshoe tear of retina without detachment

Operculum of retina without detachment
- H33.311 Horseshoe tear of retina without detachment, right eye
- H33.312 Horseshoe tear of retina without detachment, left eye
- H33.313 Horseshoe tear of retina without detachment, bilateral
- H33.319 Horseshoe tear of retina without detachment, unspecified eye

H33.32 Round hole of retina without detachment
- H33.321 Round hole, right eye
- H33.322 Round hole, left eye
- H33.323 Round hole, bilateral
- H33.329 Round hole, unspecified eye

H33.33 Multiple defects of retina without detachment
- H33.331 Multiple defects of retina without detachment, right eye
- H33.332 Multiple defects of retina without detachment, left eye
- H33.333 Multiple defects of retina without detachment, bilateral
- H33.339 Multiple defects of retina without detachment, unspecified eye

H33.4 Traction detachment of retina

Proliferative vitreo-retinopathy with retinal detachment
- H33.40 Traction detachment of retina, unspecified eye
- H33.41 Traction detachment of retina, right eye
- H33.42 Traction detachment of retina, left eye
- H33.43 Traction detachment of retina, bilateral

H33.8 Other retinal detachments

## H34 Retinal vascular occlusions

EXCLUDES 1 *amaurosis fugax (G45.3)*

H34.0 Transient retinal artery occlusion
- H34.00 Transient retinal artery occlusion, unspecified eye
- H34.01 Transient retinal artery occlusion, right eye
- H34.02 Transient retinal artery occlusion, left eye
- H34.03 Transient retinal artery occlusion, bilateral

H34.1 Central retinal artery occlusion
- H34.10 Central retinal artery occlusion, unspecified eye
- H34.11 Central retinal artery occlusion, right eye
- H34.12 Central retinal artery occlusion, left eye
- H34.13 Central retinal artery occlusion, bilateral

H34.2 Other retinal artery occlusions

H34.21 Partial retinal artery occlusion

Hollenhorst's plaque
Retinal microembolism
- H34.211 Partial retinal artery occlusion, right eye
- H34.212 Partial retinal artery occlusion, left eye
- H34.213 Partial retinal artery occlusion, bilateral
- H34.219 Partial retinal artery occlusion, unspecified eye

H34.23 Retinal artery branch occlusion
- H34.231 Retinal artery branch occlusion, right eye
- H34.232 Retinal artery branch occlusion, left eye
- H34.233 Retinal artery branch occlusion, bilateral
- H34.239 Retinal artery branch occlusion, unspecified eye

✓5th **H34.8 Other retinal vascular occlusions**

AHA: 2016,4Q,19

✓6th **H34.81 Central retinal vein occlusion**

One of the following 7th characters is to be assigned to codes in subcategory H34.81 to designate the severity of the occlusion:
0 with macular edema
1 with retinal neovascularization
2 stable/old central retinal vein occlusion

✓7th **H34.811 Central retinal vein occlusion, right eye** HCC
✓7th **H34.812 Central retinal vein occlusion, left eye** HCC
✓7th **H34.813 Central retinal vein occlusion, bilateral** HCC
✓7th **H34.819 Central retinal vein occlusion, unspecified eye** HCC

✓6th **H34.82 Venous engorgement**

Incipient retinal vein occlusion
Partial retinal vein occlusion

**H34.821 Venous engorgement, right eye**
**H34.822 Venous engorgement, left eye**
**H34.823 Venous engorgement, bilateral**
**H34.829 Venous engorgement, unspecified eye**

✓6th **H34.83 Tributary (branch) retinal vein occlusion**

One of the following 7th characters is to be assigned to codes in subcategory H34.83 to designate the severity of the occlusion:
0 with macular edema
1 with retinal neovascularization
2 stable/old tributary (branch) retinal vein occlusion

✓7th **H34.831 Tributary (branch) retinal vein occlusion, right eye** HCC
✓7th **H34.832 Tributary (branch) retinal vein occlusion, left eye** HCC
✓7th **H34.833 Tributary (branch) retinal vein occlusion, bilateral** HCC
✓7th **H34.839 Tributary (branch) retinal vein occlusion, unspecified eye** HCC

**H34.9 Unspecified retinal vascular occlusion**

✓4th **H35 Other retinal disorders**

EXCLUDES 2 *diabetic retinal disorders (E08.311-E08.359, E09.311-E09.359, E10.311-E10.359, E11.311-E11.359, E13.311-E13.359)*

✓5th **H35.0 Background retinopathy and retinal vascular changes**

Code also any associated hypertension (I10)

**H35.00 Unspecified background retinopathy**

✓6th **H35.01 Changes in retinal vascular appearance**

Retinal vascular sheathing

**H35.011 Changes in retinal vascular appearance, right eye**
**H35.012 Changes in retinal vascular appearance, left eye**
**H35.013 Changes in retinal vascular appearance, bilateral**
**H35.019 Changes in retinal vascular appearance, unspecified eye**

✓6th **H35.02 Exudative retinopathy**

Coats retinopathy

**H35.021 Exudative retinopathy, right eye**
**H35.022 Exudative retinopathy, left eye**
**H35.023 Exudative retinopathy, bilateral**
**H35.029 Exudative retinopathy, unspecified eye**

✓6th **H35.03 Hypertensive retinopathy**

**H35.031 Hypertensive retinopathy, right eye**
**H35.032 Hypertensive retinopathy, left eye**
**H35.033 Hypertensive retinopathy, bilateral**
**H35.039 Hypertensive retinopathy, unspecified eye**

✓6th **H35.04 Retinal micro-aneurysms, unspecified**

**H35.041 Retinal micro-aneurysms, unspecified, right eye**
**H35.042 Retinal micro-aneurysms, unspecified, left eye**
**H35.043 Retinal micro-aneurysms, unspecified, bilateral**
**H35.049 Retinal micro-aneurysms, unspecified, unspecified eye**

✓6th **H35.05 Retinal neovascularization, unspecified**

**H35.051 Retinal neovascularization, unspecified, right eye**
**H35.052 Retinal neovascularization, unspecified, left eye**
**H35.053 Retinal neovascularization, unspecified, bilateral**
**H35.059 Retinal neovascularization, unspecified, unspecified eye**

✓6th **H35.06 Retinal vasculitis**

Eales disease
Retinal perivasculitis
**DEF:** Sight-threatening intraocular inflammation of the retinal blood vessels that causes minimal, partial, or even complete blindness.

**H35.061 Retinal vasculitis, right eye**
**H35.062 Retinal vasculitis, left eye**
**H35.063 Retinal vasculitis, bilateral**
**H35.069 Retinal vasculitis, unspecified eye**

✓6th **H35.07 Retinal telangiectasis**

**H35.071 Retinal telangiectasis, right eye**
**H35.072 Retinal telangiectasis, left eye**
**H35.073 Retinal telangiectasis, bilateral**
**H35.079 Retinal telangiectasis, unspecified eye**

**H35.09 Other intraretinal microvascular abnormalities**

Retinal varices

✓5th **H35.1 Retinopathy of prematurity**

✓6th **H35.10 Retinopathy of prematurity, unspecified**

Retinopathy of prematurity NOS

**H35.101 Retinopathy of prematurity, unspecified, right eye**
**H35.102 Retinopathy of prematurity, unspecified, left eye**
**H35.103 Retinopathy of prematurity, unspecified, bilateral**
**H35.109 Retinopathy of prematurity, unspecified, unspecified eye**

✓6th **H35.11 Retinopathy of prematurity, stage 0**

**H35.111 Retinopathy of prematurity, stage 0, right eye**
**H35.112 Retinopathy of prematurity, stage 0, left eye**
**H35.113 Retinopathy of prematurity, stage 0, bilateral**
**H35.119 Retinopathy of prematurity, stage 0, unspecified eye**

✓6th **H35.12 Retinopathy of prematurity, stage 1**

**H35.121 Retinopathy of prematurity, stage 1, right eye**
**H35.122 Retinopathy of prematurity, stage 1, left eye**
**H35.123 Retinopathy of prematurity, stage 1, bilateral**
**H35.129 Retinopathy of prematurity, stage 1, unspecified eye**

✓6th **H35.13 Retinopathy of prematurity, stage 2**

**H35.131 Retinopathy of prematurity, stage 2, right eye**
**H35.132 Retinopathy of prematurity, stage 2, left eye**
**H35.133 Retinopathy of prematurity, stage 2, bilateral**
**H35.139 Retinopathy of prematurity, stage 2, unspecified eye**

✓6th **H35.14 Retinopathy of prematurity, stage 3**

**H35.141 Retinopathy of prematurity, stage 3, right eye**
**H35.142 Retinopathy of prematurity, stage 3, left eye**
**H35.143 Retinopathy of prematurity, stage 3, bilateral**
**H35.149 Retinopathy of prematurity, stage 3, unspecified eye**

✓6th **H35.15 Retinopathy of prematurity, stage 4**

**H35.151 Retinopathy of prematurity, stage 4, right eye**
**H35.152 Retinopathy of prematurity, stage 4, left eye**
**H35.153 Retinopathy of prematurity, stage 4, bilateral**

H35.159 Retinopathy of prematurity, stage 4, unspecified eye

H35.16 Retinopathy of prematurity, stage 5

H35.161 Retinopathy of prematurity, stage 5, right eye

H35.162 Retinopathy of prematurity, stage 5, left eye

H35.163 Retinopathy of prematurity, stage 5, bilateral

H35.169 Retinopathy of prematurity, stage 5, unspecified eye

H35.17 Retrolental fibroplasia

H35.171 Retrolental fibroplasia, right eye

H35.172 Retrolental fibroplasia, left eye

H35.173 Retrolental fibroplasia, bilateral

H35.179 Retrolental fibroplasia, unspecified eye

H35.2 Other non-diabetic proliferative retinopathy

Proliferative vitreo-retinopathy
Thalassemia proliferative retinopathy

EXCLUDES 1 *proliferative vitreo-retinopathy with retinal detachment (H33.4-)*

EXCLUDES 2 *proliferative sickle-cell retinopathy (H36.82-)*

H35.20 Other non-diabetic proliferative retinopathy, unspecified eye

H35.21 Other non-diabetic proliferative retinopathy, right eye

H35.22 Other non-diabetic proliferative retinopathy, left eye

H35.23 Other non-diabetic proliferative retinopathy, bilateral

H35.3 Degeneration of macula and posterior pole

H35.30 Unspecified macular degeneration A

Age-related macular degeneration

H35.31 Nonexudative age-related macular degeneration

Atrophic age-related macular degeneration
Dry age-related macular degeneration

AHA: 2016,4Q,20-21

One of the following 7th characters is to be assigned to each code in subcategory H35.31 to designate the stage of the disease:
- Ø stage unspecified
- 1 early dry stage
- 2 intermediate dry stage
- 3 advanced atrophic without subfoveal involvement/advanced dry stage
- 4 advanced atrophic with subfoveal involvement

H35.311 Nonexudative age-related macular degeneration, right eye A

H35.312 Nonexudative age-related macular degeneration, left eye A

H35.313 Nonexudative age-related macular degeneration, bilateral A

H35.319 Nonexudative age-related macular degeneration, unspecified eye A

H35.32 Exudative age-related macular degeneration

Wet age-related macular degeneration

AHA: 2016,4Q,20-21

One of the following 7th characters is to be assigned to each code in subcategory H35.32 to designate the stage of the disease:
- Ø stage unspecified
- 1 with active choroidal neovascularization
- 2 with inactive choroidal neovascularization/with involuted or regressed neovascularization
- 3 with inactive scar

H35.321 Exudative age-related macular degeneration, right eye HCC ESR COM A

H35.322 Exudative age-related macular degeneration, left eye HCC ESR COM A

H35.323 Exudative age-related macular degeneration, bilateral HCC ESR COM A

H35.329 Exudative age-related macular degeneration, unspecified eye HCC ESR COM A

H35.33 Angioid streaks of macula

DEF: Degeneration of the choroid, characterized by broad, irregular, dark brown streaks radiating from the optic disc; occurs with pseudoxanthoma elasticum or Paget's disease.

H35.34 Macular cyst, hole, or pseudohole

H35.341 Macular cyst, hole, or pseudohole, right eye

H35.342 Macular cyst, hole, or pseudohole, left eye

H35.343 Macular cyst, hole, or pseudohole, bilateral

H35.349 Macular cyst, hole, or pseudohole, unspecified eye

H35.35 Cystoid macular degeneration

EXCLUDES 1 *cystoid macular edema following cataract surgery (H59.Ø3-)*

H35.351 Cystoid macular degeneration, right eye

H35.352 Cystoid macular degeneration, left eye

H35.353 Cystoid macular degeneration, bilateral

H35.359 Cystoid macular degeneration, unspecified eye

H35.36 Drusen (degenerative) of macula

AHA: 2017,1Q,51; 2016,4Q,21

H35.361 Drusen (degenerative) of macula, right eye

H35.362 Drusen (degenerative) of macula, left eye

H35.363 Drusen (degenerative) of macula, bilateral

H35.369 Drusen (degenerative) of macula, unspecified eye

H35.37 Puckering of macula

H35.371 Puckering of macula, right eye

H35.372 Puckering of macula, left eye

H35.373 Puckering of macula, bilateral

H35.379 Puckering of macula, unspecified eye

H35.38 Toxic maculopathy

Code first poisoning due to drug or toxin, if applicable (T36-T65 with fifth or sixth character 1-4)

Use additional code for adverse effect, if applicable, to identify drug (T36-T5Ø with fifth or sixth character 5)

H35.381 Toxic maculopathy, right eye

H35.382 Toxic maculopathy, left eye

H35.383 Toxic maculopathy, bilateral

H35.389 Toxic maculopathy, unspecified eye

H35.4 Peripheral retinal degeneration

EXCLUDES 1 *hereditary retinal degeneration (dystrophy) (H35.5-)*

EXCLUDES 2 *peripheral retinal degeneration with retinal break (H33.3-)*

H35.40 Unspecified peripheral retinal degeneration

H35.41 Lattice degeneration of retina

Palisade degeneration of retina

DEF: Degeneration of the retina, often bilateral, that is usually benign. It is characterized by lines intersecting at irregular intervals in the peripheral retina. Retinal thinning and retinal holes may occur.

H35.411 Lattice degeneration of retina, right eye

H35.412 Lattice degeneration of retina, left eye

H35.413 Lattice degeneration of retina, bilateral

H35.419 Lattice degeneration of retina, unspecified eye

H35.42 Microcystoid degeneration of retina

H35.421 Microcystoid degeneration of retina, right eye

H35.422 Microcystoid degeneration of retina, left eye

H35.423 Microcystoid degeneration of retina, bilateral

H35.429 Microcystoid degeneration of retina, unspecified eye

H35.43 Paving stone degeneration of retina

H35.431 Paving stone degeneration of retina, right eye

H35.432 Paving stone degeneration of retina, left eye

H35.433 Paving stone degeneration of retina, bilateral

H35.439 Paving stone degeneration of retina, unspecified eye

H35.44 Age-related reticular degeneration of retina

H35.441 Age-related reticular degeneration of retina, right eye A

**H35.442** **Age-related reticular degeneration of retina, left eye** A

**H35.443** **Age-related reticular degeneration of retina, bilateral** A

**H35.449** **Age-related reticular degeneration of retina, unspecified eye** A

√6th **H35.45** **Secondary pigmentary degeneration**

**H35.451** **Secondary pigmentary degeneration, right eye**

**H35.452** **Secondary pigmentary degeneration, left eye**

**H35.453** **Secondary pigmentary degeneration, bilateral**

**H35.459** **Secondary pigmentary degeneration, unspecified eye**

√6th **H35.46** **Secondary vitreoretinal degeneration**

**H35.461** **Secondary vitreoretinal degeneration, right eye**

**H35.462** **Secondary vitreoretinal degeneration, left eye**

**H35.463** **Secondary vitreoretinal degeneration, bilateral**

**H35.469** **Secondary vitreoretinal degeneration, unspecified eye**

√5th **H35.5** **Hereditary retinal dystrophy**

EXCLUDES 1 *dystrophies primarily involving Bruch's membrane (H31.1-)*

**H35.5Ø** **Unspecified hereditary retinal dystrophy**

**H35.51** **Vitreoretinal dystrophy**

**H35.52** **Pigmentary retinal dystrophy**

Albipunctate retinal dystrophy
Retinitis pigmentosa
Tapetoretinal dystrophy

**H35.53** **Other dystrophies primarily involving the sensory retina**

Stargardt's disease

**H35.54** **Dystrophies primarily involving the retinal pigment epithelium**

Vitelliform retinal dystrophy

√5th **H35.6** **Retinal hemorrhage**

**H35.6Ø** **Retinal hemorrhage, unspecified eye**

**H35.61** **Retinal hemorrhage, right eye**

**H35.62** **Retinal hemorrhage, left eye**

**H35.63** **Retinal hemorrhage, bilateral**

√5th **H35.7** **Separation of retinal layers**

EXCLUDES 1 *retinal detachment (serous) (H33.2-)*
*rhegmatogenous retinal detachment (H33.Ø-)*

**H35.7Ø** **Unspecified separation of retinal layers**

√6th **H35.71** **Central serous chorioretinopathy**

**H35.711** **Central serous chorioretinopathy, right eye**

**H35.712** **Central serous chorioretinopathy, left eye**

**H35.713** **Central serous chorioretinopathy, bilateral**

**H35.719** **Central serous chorioretinopathy, unspecified eye**

√6th **H35.72** **Serous detachment of retinal pigment epithelium**

**H35.721** **Serous detachment of retinal pigment epithelium, right eye**

**H35.722** **Serous detachment of retinal pigment epithelium, left eye**

**H35.723** **Serous detachment of retinal pigment epithelium, bilateral**

**H35.729** **Serous detachment of retinal pigment epithelium, unspecified eye**

√6th **H35.73** **Hemorrhagic detachment of retinal pigment epithelium**

**H35.731** **Hemorrhagic detachment of retinal pigment epithelium, right eye**

**H35.732** **Hemorrhagic detachment of retinal pigment epithelium, left eye**

**H35.733** **Hemorrhagic detachment of retinal pigment epithelium, bilateral**

**H35.739** **Hemorrhagic detachment of retinal pigment epithelium, unspecified eye**

√5th **H35.8** **Other specified retinal disorders**

EXCLUDES 2 *retinal hemorrhage (H35.6-)*

**H35.81** **Retinal edema**

Retinal cotton wool spots

**H35.82** **Retinal ischemia**

**H35.89** **Other specified retinal disorders**

**H35.9** **Unspecified retinal disorder**

√4th **H36** **Retinal disorders in diseases classified elsewhere**

Code first underlying disease, such as:
lipid storage disorders (E75.-)
sickle-cell disorders (D57.-)

EXCLUDES 1 *arteriosclerotic retinopathy (H35.Ø-)*
*diabetic retinopathy (EØ8.3-, EØ9.3-, E1Ø.3-, E11.3-, E13.3-)*

AHA: 2023,4Q,20-21

√5th **H36.8** **Other retinal disorders in diseases classified elsewhere**

√6th **H36.81** **Nonproliferative sickle-cell retinopathy**

**H36.811** **Nonproliferative sickle-cell retinopathy, right eye** HCC ESR UPD

**H36.812** **Nonproliferative sickle-cell retinopathy, left eye** HCC ESR UPD

**H36.813** **Nonproliferative sickle-cell retinopathy, bilateral** HCC ESR UPD

**H36.819** **Nonproliferative sickle-cell retinopathy, unspecified eye** HCC ESR UPD

√6th **H36.82** **Proliferative sickle-cell retinopathy**

**H36.821** **Proliferative sickle-cell retinopathy, right eye** HCC ESR UPD

**H36.822** **Proliferative sickle-cell retinopathy, left eye** HCC ESR UPD

**H36.823** **Proliferative sickle-cell retinopathy, bilateral** HCC ESR UPD

**H36.829** **Proliferative sickle-cell retinopathy, unspecified eye** HCC ESR UPD

***H36.89*** ***Other retinal disorders in diseases classified elsewhere***

Retinal dystrophy in lipid storage disorders

## Glaucoma (H4Ø-H42)

√4th **H4Ø** **Glaucoma**

EXCLUDES 1 *absolute glaucoma (H44.51-)*
*congenital glaucoma (Q15.Ø)*
*traumatic glaucoma due to birth injury (P15.3)*

**Open Angle/Angle Closure Glaucoma**

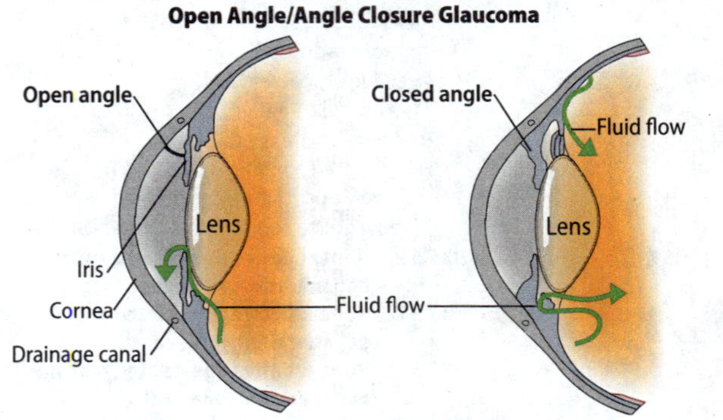


√5th **H4Ø.Ø** **Glaucoma suspect**

√6th **H4Ø.ØØ** **Preglaucoma, unspecified**

**H4Ø.ØØ1** **Preglaucoma, unspecified, right eye**

**H4Ø.ØØ2** **Preglaucoma, unspecified, left eye**

**H4Ø.ØØ3** **Preglaucoma, unspecified, bilateral**

**H4Ø.ØØ9** **Preglaucoma, unspecified, unspecified eye**

√6th **H4Ø.Ø1** **Open angle with borderline findings, low risk**

Open angle, low risk

**H4Ø.Ø11** **Open angle with borderline findings, low risk, right eye**

**H4Ø.Ø12** **Open angle with borderline findings, low risk, left eye**

**H4Ø.Ø13** **Open angle with borderline findings, low risk, bilateral**

**H4Ø.Ø19** **Open angle with borderline findings, low risk, unspecified eye**

√6th **H4Ø.Ø2** **Open angle with borderline findings, high risk**

Open angle, high risk

**H4Ø.Ø21** **Open angle with borderline findings, high risk, right eye**

**H4Ø.Ø22** **Open angle with borderline findings, high risk, left eye**

**H4Ø.Ø23** **Open angle with borderline findings, high risk, bilateral**

**H4Ø.Ø29** **Open angle with borderline findings, high risk, unspecified eye**

√6th **H40.03 Anatomical narrow angle**
Primary angle closure suspect
**H40.031 Anatomical narrow angle, right eye**
**H40.032 Anatomical narrow angle, left eye**
**H40.033 Anatomical narrow angle, bilateral**
**H40.039 Anatomical narrow angle, unspecified eye**

√6th **H40.04 Steroid responder**
**H40.041 Steroid responder, right eye**
**H40.042 Steroid responder, left eye**
**H40.043 Steroid responder, bilateral**
**H40.049 Steroid responder, unspecified eye**

√6th **H40.05 Ocular hypertension**
**H40.051 Ocular hypertension, right eye**
**H40.052 Ocular hypertension, left eye**
**H40.053 Ocular hypertension, bilateral**
**H40.059 Ocular hypertension, unspecified eye**

√6th **H40.06 Primary angle closure without glaucoma damage**
**H40.061 Primary angle closure without glaucoma damage, right eye**
**H40.062 Primary angle closure without glaucoma damage, left eye**
**H40.063 Primary angle closure without glaucoma damage, bilateral**
**H40.069 Primary angle closure without glaucoma damage, unspecified eye**

√5th **H40.1 Open-angle glaucoma**

One of the following 7th characters is to be assigned to each code in subcategories H40.10, H40.11, H40.12, H40.13, and H40.14 to designate the stage of glaucoma.
0 stage unspecified
1 mild stage
2 moderate stage
3 severe stage
4 indeterminate stage

√x7th **H40.10 Unspecified open-angle glaucoma** Rx
**TIP:** Only one code from this subcategory should be assigned when both left and right eyes are the same stage.

√6th **H40.11 Primary open-angle glaucoma**
Chronic simple glaucoma
**AHA:** 2016,4Q,22
√7th **H40.111 Primary open-angle glaucoma, right eye** Rx Q
√7th **H40.112 Primary open-angle glaucoma, left eye** Rx Q
√7th **H40.113 Primary open-angle glaucoma, bilateral** Rx Q
√7th **H40.119 Primary open-angle glaucoma, unspecified eye** Rx

√6th **H40.12 Low-tension glaucoma**
√7th **H40.121 Low-tension glaucoma, right eye** Rx Q
√7th **H40.122 Low-tension glaucoma, left eye** Rx Q
√7th **H40.123 Low-tension glaucoma, bilateral** Rx Q
√7th **H40.129 Low-tension glaucoma, unspecified eye** Rx

√6th **H40.13 Pigmentary glaucoma**
√7th **H40.131 Pigmentary glaucoma, right eye** Rx
√7th **H40.132 Pigmentary glaucoma, left eye** Rx
√7th **H40.133 Pigmentary glaucoma, bilateral** Rx
√7th **H40.139 Pigmentary glaucoma, unspecified eye** Rx

√6th **H40.14 Capsular glaucoma with pseudoexfoliation of lens**
√7th **H40.141 Capsular glaucoma with pseudoexfoliation of lens, right eye** Rx
√7th **H40.142 Capsular glaucoma with pseudoexfoliation of lens, left eye** Rx
√7th **H40.143 Capsular glaucoma with pseudoexfoliation of lens, bilateral** Rx
√7th **H40.149 Capsular glaucoma with pseudoexfoliation of lens, unspecified eye** Rx

√6th **H40.15 Residual stage of open-angle glaucoma**
**H40.151 Residual stage of open-angle glaucoma, right eye** Rx Q
**H40.152 Residual stage of open-angle glaucoma, left eye** Rx Q
**H40.153 Residual stage of open-angle glaucoma, bilateral** Rx Q
**H40.159 Residual stage of open-angle glaucoma, unspecified eye** Rx

√5th **H40.2 Primary angle-closure glaucoma**
EXCLUDES 1 *aqueous misdirection (H40.83-)*
*malignant glaucoma (H40.83-)*

One of the following 7th characters is to be assigned to code H40.20 and H40.22 to designate the stage of glaucoma.
0 stage unspecified
1 mild stage
2 moderate stage
3 severe stage
4 indeterminate stage

√x7th **H40.20 Unspecified primary angle-closure glaucoma** Rx
**TIP:** Only one code from this subcategory should be assigned when both left and right eyes are the same stage.

√6th **H40.21 Acute angle-closure glaucoma**
Acute angle-closure glaucoma attack
Acute angle-closure glaucoma crisis
**H40.211 Acute angle-closure glaucoma, right eye**
**H40.212 Acute angle-closure glaucoma, left eye**
**H40.213 Acute angle-closure glaucoma, bilateral**
**H40.219 Acute angle-closure glaucoma, unspecified eye**

√6th **H40.22 Chronic angle-closure glaucoma**
Chronic primary angle closure glaucoma
√7th **H40.221 Chronic angle-closure glaucoma, right eye** Rx
√7th **H40.222 Chronic angle-closure glaucoma, left eye** Rx
√7th **H40.223 Chronic angle-closure glaucoma, bilateral** Rx
√7th **H40.229 Chronic angle-closure glaucoma, unspecified eye** Rx

√6th **H40.23 Intermittent angle-closure glaucoma**
**H40.231 Intermittent angle-closure glaucoma, right eye** Rx
**H40.232 Intermittent angle-closure glaucoma, left eye** Rx
**H40.233 Intermittent angle-closure glaucoma, bilateral** Rx
**H40.239 Intermittent angle-closure glaucoma, unspecified eye** Rx

√6th **H40.24 Residual stage of angle-closure glaucoma**
**H40.241 Residual stage of angle-closure glaucoma, right eye** Rx
**H40.242 Residual stage of angle-closure glaucoma, left eye** Rx
**H40.243 Residual stage of angle-closure glaucoma, bilateral** Rx
**H40.249 Residual stage of angle-closure glaucoma, unspecified eye** Rx

√5th **H40.3 Glaucoma secondary to eye trauma**
Code also underlying condition

One of the following 7th characters is to be assigned to each code in subcategory H40.3 to designate the stage of glaucoma.
0 stage unspecified
1 mild stage
2 moderate stage
3 severe stage
4 indeterminate stage

√x7th **H40.30 Glaucoma secondary to eye trauma, unspecified eye** Rx
√x7th **H40.31 Glaucoma secondary to eye trauma, right eye** Rx
√x7th **H40.32 Glaucoma secondary to eye trauma, left eye** Rx
√x7th **H40.33 Glaucoma secondary to eye trauma, bilateral** Rx

Chapter 7. Diseases of the Eye and Adnexa
H40.03–H40.33

✓5th **H40.4 Glaucoma secondary to eye inflammation**

Code also underlying condition

One of the following 7th characters is to be assigned to each code in subcategory H40.4 to designate the stage of glaucoma.
- 0 stage unspecified
- 1 mild stage
- 2 moderate stage
- 3 severe stage
- 4 indeterminate stage

✓x7th **H40.40 Glaucoma secondary to eye inflammation, unspecified eye** Rx

✓x7th **H40.41 Glaucoma secondary to eye inflammation, right eye** Rx

✓x7th **H40.42 Glaucoma secondary to eye inflammation, left eye** Rx

✓x7th **H40.43 Glaucoma secondary to eye inflammation, bilateral** Rx

✓5th **H40.5 Glaucoma secondary to other eye disorders**

Code also underlying eye disorder

One of the following 7th characters is to be assigned to each code in subcategory H40.5 to designate the stage of glaucoma.
- 0 stage unspecified
- 1 mild stage
- 2 moderate stage
- 3 severe stage
- 4 indeterminate stage

✓x7th **H40.50 Glaucoma secondary to other eye disorders, unspecified eye** Rx

✓x7th **H40.51 Glaucoma secondary to other eye disorders, right eye** Rx

✓x7th **H40.52 Glaucoma secondary to other eye disorders, left eye** Rx

✓x7th **H40.53 Glaucoma secondary to other eye disorders, bilateral** Rx

✓5th **H40.6 Glaucoma secondary to drugs**

Use additional code for adverse effect, if applicable, to identify drug (T36-T50 with fifth or sixth character 5)

One of the following 7th characters is to be assigned to each code in subcategory H40.6 to designate the stage of glaucoma
- 0 stage unspecified
- 1 mild stage
- 2 moderate stage
- 3 severe stage
- 4 indeterminate stage

✓x7th **H40.60 Glaucoma secondary to drugs, unspecified eye** Rx

✓x7th **H40.61 Glaucoma secondary to drugs, right eye** Rx

✓x7th **H40.62 Glaucoma secondary to drugs, left eye** Rx

✓x7th **H40.63 Glaucoma secondary to drugs, bilateral** Rx

✓5th **H40.8 Other glaucoma**

✓6th **H40.81 Glaucoma with increased episcleral venous pressure**

**H40.811 Glaucoma with increased episcleral venous pressure, right eye** Rx

**H40.812 Glaucoma with increased episcleral venous pressure, left eye** Rx

**H40.813 Glaucoma with increased episcleral venous pressure, bilateral** Rx

**H40.819 Glaucoma with increased episcleral venous pressure, unspecified eye** Rx

✓6th **H40.82 Hypersecretion glaucoma**

**H40.821 Hypersecretion glaucoma, right eye** Rx

**H40.822 Hypersecretion glaucoma, left eye** Rx

**H40.823 Hypersecretion glaucoma, bilateral** Rx

**H40.829 Hypersecretion glaucoma, unspecified eye** Rx

✓6th **H40.83 Aqueous misdirection**

Malignant glaucoma

**H40.831 Aqueous misdirection, right eye** Rx

**H40.832 Aqueous misdirection, left eye** Rx

**H40.833 Aqueous misdirection, bilateral** Rx

**H40.839 Aqueous misdirection, unspecified eye** Rx

✓6th **H40.84 Neovascular secondary angle closure glaucoma**

~~Code first the underlying condition such as:~~
~~central retinal vein occlusion (H34.81)~~
~~diabetes mellitus (E08.39, E09.39, E10.39, E11.39, E13.39)~~
~~retinal ischemia (H35.82)~~

▶Code also the underlying condition such as:◀
- ▶central retinal vein occlusion (H34.81)◀
- ▶diabetes mellitus (E08.39, E09.39, E10.39, E11.39, E13.39)◀
- ▶retinal ischemia (H35.82)◀

**H40.841 Neovascular secondary angle closure glaucoma, right eye** Rx

**H40.842 Neovascular secondary angle closure glaucoma, left eye** Rx

**H40.843 Neovascular secondary angle closure glaucoma, bilateral** Rx

**H40.849 Neovascular secondary angle closure glaucoma, unspecified eye** Rx

**H40.89 Other specified glaucoma** Rx

**H40.9 Unspecified glaucoma** Rx

***H42 Glaucoma in diseases classified elsewhere*** Rx

Code first underlying condition, such as:
- amyloidosis (E85.-)
- aniridia (Q13.1)
- glaucoma (in) diabetes mellitus (E08.39, E09.39, E10.39, E11.39, E13.39)
- Lowe's syndrome (E72.03)
- Rieger anomaly (Q13.81)
- specified metabolic disorder (E70-E88)

EXCLUDES 1 *glaucoma (in) onchocerciasis (B73.02)*
*glaucoma (in) syphilis (A52.71)*
*glaucoma (in) tuberculous (A18.59)*
*neovascular secondary angle closure glaucoma (H40.84-)*

## Disorders of vitreous body and globe (H43-H44)

✓4th **H43 Disorders of vitreous body**

✓5th **H43.0 Vitreous prolapse**

EXCLUDES 1 *traumatic vitreous prolapse (S05.2-)*
*vitreous syndrome following cataract surgery (H59.0-)*

**H43.00 Vitreous prolapse, unspecified eye**

**H43.01 Vitreous prolapse, right eye**

**H43.02 Vitreous prolapse, left eye**

**H43.03 Vitreous prolapse, bilateral**

✓5th **H43.1 Vitreous hemorrhage**

**H43.10 Vitreous hemorrhage, unspecified eye** HCC ESR

**H43.11 Vitreous hemorrhage, right eye** HCC ESR

**H43.12 Vitreous hemorrhage, left eye** HCC ESR

**H43.13 Vitreous hemorrhage, bilateral** HCC ESR

✓5th **H43.2 Crystalline deposits in vitreous body**

**H43.20 Crystalline deposits in vitreous body, unspecified eye**

**H43.21 Crystalline deposits in vitreous body, right eye**

**H43.22 Crystalline deposits in vitreous body, left eye**

**H43.23 Crystalline deposits in vitreous body, bilateral**

✓5th **H43.3 Other vitreous opacities**

✓6th **H43.31 Vitreous membranes and strands**

**H43.311 Vitreous membranes and strands, right eye**

**H43.312 Vitreous membranes and strands, left eye**

**H43.313 Vitreous membranes and strands, bilateral**

**H43.319 Vitreous membranes and strands, unspecified eye**

✓6th **H43.39 Other vitreous opacities**

Vitreous floaters

**H43.391 Other vitreous opacities, right eye**

**H43.392 Other vitreous opacities, left eye**

**H43.393 Other vitreous opacities, bilateral**

**H43.399 Other vitreous opacities, unspecified eye**

✓5th **H43.8 Other disorders of vitreous body**

EXCLUDES 1 *proliferative vitreo-retinopathy with retinal detachment (H33.4-)*

EXCLUDES 2 *vitreous abscess (H44.02-)*

✓6th **H43.81 Vitreous degeneration**

Vitreous detachment

**H43.811 Vitreous degeneration, right eye**

**H43.812 Vitreous degeneration, left eye**

**H43.813 Vitreous degeneration, bilateral**

H43.819 Vitreous degeneration, unspecified eye

✓6th H43.82 Vitreomacular adhesion

Vitreomacular traction

H43.821 Vitreomacular adhesion, right eye A

H43.822 Vitreomacular adhesion, left eye A

H43.823 Vitreomacular adhesion, bilateral A

H43.829 Vitreomacular adhesion, unspecified eye A

H43.89 Other disorders of vitreous body

H43.9 Unspecified disorder of vitreous body

✓4th **H44 Disorders of globe**

INCLUDES disorders affecting multiple structures of eye

✓5th H44.0 Purulent endophthalmitis

Use additional code to identify organism

*EXCLUDES 1 bleb associated endophthalmitis (H59.4-)*

✓6th H44.00 Unspecified purulent endophthalmitis

H44.001 Unspecified purulent endophthalmitis, right eye

H44.002 Unspecified purulent endophthalmitis, left eye

H44.003 Unspecified purulent endophthalmitis, bilateral

H44.009 Unspecified purulent endophthalmitis, unspecified eye

✓6th H44.01 Panophthalmitis (acute)

H44.011 Panophthalmitis (acute), right eye

H44.012 Panophthalmitis (acute), left eye

H44.013 Panophthalmitis (acute), bilateral

H44.019 Panophthalmitis (acute), unspecified eye

✓6th H44.02 Vitreous abscess (chronic)

H44.021 Vitreous abscess (chronic), right eye

H44.022 Vitreous abscess (chronic), left eye

H44.023 Vitreous abscess (chronic), bilateral

H44.029 Vitreous abscess (chronic), unspecified eye

✓5th H44.1 Other endophthalmitis

*EXCLUDES 1 bleb associated endophthalmitis (H59.4-)*

*EXCLUDES 2 ophthalmia nodosa (H16.2-)*

✓6th H44.11 Panuveitis

**DEF:** Inflammation of all layers of the uvea of the eye, including the choroid, iris, and ciliary body. It also typically involves the lens, retina, optic nerve, and vitreous and causes reduced vision or blindness.

H44.111 Panuveitis, right eye

H44.112 Panuveitis, left eye

H44.113 Panuveitis, bilateral

H44.119 Panuveitis, unspecified eye

✓6th H44.12 Parasitic endophthalmitis, unspecified

H44.121 Parasitic endophthalmitis, unspecified, right eye

H44.122 Parasitic endophthalmitis, unspecified, left eye

H44.123 Parasitic endophthalmitis, unspecified, bilateral

H44.129 Parasitic endophthalmitis, unspecified, unspecified eye

✓6th H44.13 Sympathetic uveitis

H44.131 Sympathetic uveitis, right eye

H44.132 Sympathetic uveitis, left eye

H44.133 Sympathetic uveitis, bilateral

H44.139 Sympathetic uveitis, unspecified eye

H44.19 Other endophthalmitis

✓5th H44.2 Degenerative myopia

Malignant myopia

**AHA:** 2017,4Q,10-11

H44.20 Degenerative myopia, unspecified eye

H44.21 Degenerative myopia, right eye

H44.22 Degenerative myopia, left eye

H44.23 Degenerative myopia, bilateral

✓6th H44.2A Degenerative myopia with choroidal neovascularization

Use additional code for any associated choroid disorders (H31.-)

H44.2A1 Degenerative myopia with choroidal neovascularization, right eye

H44.2A2 Degenerative myopia with choroidal neovascularization, left eye

H44.2A3 Degenerative myopia with choroidal neovascularization, bilateral

H44.2A9 Degenerative myopia with choroidal neovascularization, unspecified eye

✓6th H44.2B Degenerative myopia with macular hole

H44.2B1 Degenerative myopia with macular hole, right eye

H44.2B2 Degenerative myopia with macular hole, left eye

H44.2B3 Degenerative myopia with macular hole, bilateral

H44.2B9 Degenerative myopia with macular hole, unspecified eye

✓6th H44.2C Degenerative myopia with retinal detachment

Use additional code to identify the retinal detachment (H33.-)

H44.2C1 Degenerative myopia with retinal detachment, right eye

H44.2C2 Degenerative myopia with retinal detachment, left eye

H44.2C3 Degenerative myopia with retinal detachment, bilateral

H44.2C9 Degenerative myopia with retinal detachment, unspecified eye

✓6th H44.2D Degenerative myopia with foveoschisis

H44.2D1 Degenerative myopia with foveoschisis, right eye

H44.2D2 Degenerative myopia with foveoschisis, left eye

H44.2D3 Degenerative myopia with foveoschisis, bilateral

H44.2D9 Degenerative myopia with foveoschisis, unspecified eye

✓6th H44.2E Degenerative myopia with other maculopathy

H44.2E1 Degenerative myopia with other maculopathy, right eye

H44.2E2 Degenerative myopia with other maculopathy, left eye

H44.2E3 Degenerative myopia with other maculopathy, bilateral

H44.2E9 Degenerative myopia with other maculopathy, unspecified eye

✓5th H44.3 Other and unspecified degenerative disorders of globe

H44.30 Unspecified degenerative disorder of globe

✓6th H44.31 Chalcosis

H44.311 Chalcosis, right eye

H44.312 Chalcosis, left eye

H44.313 Chalcosis, bilateral

H44.319 Chalcosis, unspecified eye

✓6th H44.32 Siderosis of eye

**DEF:** Iron pigment deposits within tissue of the eyeball caused by high iron content of the blood. Symptoms include cataracts, rust-colored anterior subcapsular deposits, iris heterochromia, pupillary mydriasis, and depressed electroretinogram amplitudes.

H44.321 Siderosis of eye, right eye

H44.322 Siderosis of eye, left eye

H44.323 Siderosis of eye, bilateral

H44.329 Siderosis of eye, unspecified eye

✓6th H44.39 Other degenerative disorders of globe

H44.391 Other degenerative disorders of globe, right eye

H44.392 Other degenerative disorders of globe, left eye

H44.393 Other degenerative disorders of globe, bilateral

H44.399 Other degenerative disorders of globe, unspecified eye

✓5th H44.4 Hypotony of eye

H44.40 Unspecified hypotony of eye

✓6th H44.41 Flat anterior chamber hypotony of eye

H44.411 Flat anterior chamber hypotony of right eye

H44.412 Flat anterior chamber hypotony of left eye

H44.413 Flat anterior chamber hypotony of eye, bilateral

H44.419 Flat anterior chamber hypotony of unspecified eye

✓6th H44.42 Hypotony of eye due to ocular fistula

H44.421 Hypotony of right eye due to ocular fistula

H44.422 Hypotony of left eye due to ocular fistula
H44.423 Hypotony of eye due to ocular fistula, bilateral
H44.429 Hypotony of unspecified eye due to ocular fistula

✓6th H44.43 Hypotony of eye due to other ocular disorders
H44.431 Hypotony of eye due to other ocular disorders, right eye
H44.432 Hypotony of eye due to other ocular disorders, left eye
H44.433 Hypotony of eye due to other ocular disorders, bilateral
H44.439 Hypotony of eye due to other ocular disorders, unspecified eye

✓6th H44.44 Primary hypotony of eye
H44.441 Primary hypotony of right eye
H44.442 Primary hypotony of left eye
H44.443 Primary hypotony of eye, bilateral
H44.449 Primary hypotony of unspecified eye

✓5th H44.5 Degenerated conditions of globe
H44.50 Unspecified degenerated conditions of globe

✓6th H44.51 Absolute glaucoma
H44.511 Absolute glaucoma, right eye
H44.512 Absolute glaucoma, left eye
H44.513 Absolute glaucoma, bilateral
H44.519 Absolute glaucoma, unspecified eye

✓6th H44.52 Atrophy of globe
Phthisis bulbi
H44.521 Atrophy of globe, right eye
H44.522 Atrophy of globe, left eye
H44.523 Atrophy of globe, bilateral
H44.529 Atrophy of globe, unspecified eye

✓6th H44.53 Leucocoria
H44.531 Leucocoria, right eye
H44.532 Leucocoria, left eye
H44.533 Leucocoria, bilateral
H44.539 Leucocoria, unspecified eye

✓5th H44.6 Retained (old) intraocular foreign body, magnetic
Use additional code to identify magnetic foreign body (Z18.11)
EXCLUDES 1 *current intraocular foreign body (SØ5.-)*
EXCLUDES 2 *retained foreign body in eyelid (HØ2.81-)*
*retained (old) foreign body following penetrating wound of orbit (HØ5.5-)*
*retained (old) intraocular foreign body, nonmagnetic (H44.7-)*

✓6th H44.60 Unspecified retained (old) intraocular foreign body, magnetic
H44.601 Unspecified retained (old) intraocular foreign body, magnetic, right eye
H44.602 Unspecified retained (old) intraocular foreign body, magnetic, left eye
H44.603 Unspecified retained (old) intraocular foreign body, magnetic, bilateral
H44.609 Unspecified retained (old) intraocular foreign body, magnetic, unspecified eye

✓6th H44.61 Retained (old) magnetic foreign body in anterior chamber
H44.611 Retained (old) magnetic foreign body in anterior chamber, right eye
H44.612 Retained (old) magnetic foreign body in anterior chamber, left eye
H44.613 Retained (old) magnetic foreign body in anterior chamber, bilateral
H44.619 Retained (old) magnetic foreign body in anterior chamber, unspecified eye

✓6th H44.62 Retained (old) magnetic foreign body in iris or ciliary body
H44.621 Retained (old) magnetic foreign body in iris or ciliary body, right eye
H44.622 Retained (old) magnetic foreign body in iris or ciliary body, left eye
H44.623 Retained (old) magnetic foreign body in iris or ciliary body, bilateral
H44.629 Retained (old) magnetic foreign body in iris or ciliary body, unspecified eye

✓6th H44.63 Retained (old) magnetic foreign body in lens
H44.631 Retained (old) magnetic foreign body in lens, right eye
H44.632 Retained (old) magnetic foreign body in lens, left eye
H44.633 Retained (old) magnetic foreign body in lens, bilateral
H44.639 Retained (old) magnetic foreign body in lens, unspecified eye

✓6th H44.64 Retained (old) magnetic foreign body in posterior wall of globe
H44.641 Retained (old) magnetic foreign body in posterior wall of globe, right eye
H44.642 Retained (old) magnetic foreign body in posterior wall of globe, left eye
H44.643 Retained (old) magnetic foreign body in posterior wall of globe, bilateral
H44.649 Retained (old) magnetic foreign body in posterior wall of globe, unspecified eye

✓6th H44.65 Retained (old) magnetic foreign body in vitreous body
H44.651 Retained (old) magnetic foreign body in vitreous body, right eye
H44.652 Retained (old) magnetic foreign body in vitreous body, left eye
H44.653 Retained (old) magnetic foreign body in vitreous body, bilateral
H44.659 Retained (old) magnetic foreign body in vitreous body, unspecified eye

✓6th H44.69 Retained (old) intraocular foreign body, magnetic, in other or multiple sites
H44.691 Retained (old) intraocular foreign body, magnetic, in other or multiple sites, right eye
H44.692 Retained (old) intraocular foreign body, magnetic, in other or multiple sites, left eye
H44.693 Retained (old) intraocular foreign body, magnetic, in other or multiple sites, bilateral
H44.699 Retained (old) intraocular foreign body, magnetic, in other or multiple sites, unspecified eye

✓5th H44.7 Retained (old) intraocular foreign body, nonmagnetic
Use additional code to identify nonmagnetic foreign body (Z18.Ø1-Z18.1Ø, Z18.12, Z18.2-Z18.9)
EXCLUDES 1 *current intraocular foreign body (SØ5.-)*
EXCLUDES 2 *retained foreign body in eyelid (HØ2.81-)*
*retained (old) foreign body following penetrating wound of orbit (HØ5.5-)*
*retained (old) intraocular foreign body, magnetic (H44.6-)*

✓6th H44.7Ø Unspecified retained (old) intraocular foreign body, nonmagnetic
H44.7Ø1 Unspecified retained (old) intraocular foreign body, nonmagnetic, right eye
H44.7Ø2 Unspecified retained (old) intraocular foreign body, nonmagnetic, left eye
H44.7Ø3 Unspecified retained (old) intraocular foreign body, nonmagnetic, bilateral
H44.7Ø9 Unspecified retained (old) intraocular foreign body, nonmagnetic, unspecified eye
Retained (old) intraocular foreign body NOS

✓6th H44.71 Retained (nonmagnetic) (old) foreign body in anterior chamber
H44.711 Retained (nonmagnetic) (old) foreign body in anterior chamber, right eye
H44.712 Retained (nonmagnetic) (old) foreign body in anterior chamber, left eye
H44.713 Retained (nonmagnetic) (old) foreign body in anterior chamber, bilateral
H44.719 Retained (nonmagnetic) (old) foreign body in anterior chamber, unspecified eye

✓6th H44.72 Retained (nonmagnetic) (old) foreign body in iris or ciliary body
H44.721 Retained (nonmagnetic) (old) foreign body in iris or ciliary body, right eye
H44.722 Retained (nonmagnetic) (old) foreign body in iris or ciliary body, left eye
H44.723 Retained (nonmagnetic) (old) foreign body in iris or ciliary body, bilateral
H44.729 Retained (nonmagnetic) (old) foreign body in iris or ciliary body, unspecified eye

✓6th H44.73 Retained (nonmagnetic) (old) foreign body in lens
H44.731 Retained (nonmagnetic) (old) foreign body in lens, right eye

H44.732 Retained (nonmagnetic) (old) foreign body in lens, left eye
H44.733 Retained (nonmagnetic) (old) foreign body in lens, bilateral
H44.739 Retained (nonmagnetic) (old) foreign body in lens, unspecified eye

√6th H44.74 Retained (nonmagnetic) (old) foreign body in posterior wall of globe
H44.741 Retained (nonmagnetic) (old) foreign body in posterior wall of globe, right eye
H44.742 Retained (nonmagnetic) (old) foreign body in posterior wall of globe, left eye
H44.743 Retained (nonmagnetic) (old) foreign body in posterior wall of globe, bilateral
H44.749 Retained (nonmagnetic) (old) foreign body in posterior wall of globe, unspecified eye

√6th H44.75 Retained (nonmagnetic) (old) foreign body in vitreous body
H44.751 Retained (nonmagnetic) (old) foreign body in vitreous body, right eye
H44.752 Retained (nonmagnetic) (old) foreign body in vitreous body, left eye
H44.753 Retained (nonmagnetic) (old) foreign body in vitreous body, bilateral
H44.759 Retained (nonmagnetic) (old) foreign body in vitreous body, unspecified eye

√6th H44.79 Retained (old) intraocular foreign body, nonmagnetic, in other or multiple sites
H44.791 Retained (old) intraocular foreign body, nonmagnetic, in other or multiple sites, right eye
H44.792 Retained (old) intraocular foreign body, nonmagnetic, in other or multiple sites, left eye
H44.793 Retained (old) intraocular foreign body, nonmagnetic, in other or multiple sites, bilateral
H44.799 Retained (old) intraocular foreign body, nonmagnetic, in other or multiple sites, unspecified eye

√5th H44.8 Other disorders of globe

√6th H44.81 Hemophthalmos

DEF: Pool of blood within the eyeball, not from a current injury.

H44.811 Hemophthalmos, right eye
H44.812 Hemophthalmos, left eye
H44.813 Hemophthalmos, bilateral
H44.819 Hemophthalmos, unspecified eye

√6th H44.82 Luxation of globe
H44.821 Luxation of globe, right eye
H44.822 Luxation of globe, left eye
H44.823 Luxation of globe, bilateral
H44.829 Luxation of globe, unspecified eye

H44.89 Other disorders of globe

AHA: 2022,1Q,33

H44.9 Unspecified disorder of globe

## Disorders of optic nerve and visual pathways (H46-H47)

√4th H46 Optic neuritis

EXCLUDES 2 *ischemic optic neuropathy (H47.Ø1-)*
*neuromyelitis optica [Devic] (G36.Ø)*

√5th H46.Ø Optic papillitis
H46.ØØ Optic papillitis, unspecified eye
H46.Ø1 Optic papillitis, right eye
H46.Ø2 Optic papillitis, left eye
H46.Ø3 Optic papillitis, bilateral

√5th H46.1 Retrobulbar neuritis

Retrobulbar neuritis NOS

EXCLUDES 1 *syphilitic retrobulbar neuritis (A52.15)*

H46.1Ø Retrobulbar neuritis, unspecified eye
H46.11 Retrobulbar neuritis, right eye
H46.12 Retrobulbar neuritis, left eye
H46.13 Retrobulbar neuritis, bilateral

H46.2 Nutritional optic neuropathy
H46.3 Toxic optic neuropathy

Code first (T51-T65) to identify cause

H46.8 Other optic neuritis
H46.9 Unspecified optic neuritis

AHA: 2023,3Q,19

√4th H47 Other disorders of optic [2nd] nerve and visual pathways

√5th H47.Ø Disorders of optic nerve, not elsewhere classified

√6th H47.Ø1 Ischemic optic neuropathy
H47.Ø11 Ischemic optic neuropathy, right eye
H47.Ø12 Ischemic optic neuropathy, left eye
H47.Ø13 Ischemic optic neuropathy, bilateral
H47.Ø19 Ischemic optic neuropathy, unspecified eye

√6th H47.Ø2 Hemorrhage in optic nerve sheath
H47.Ø21 Hemorrhage in optic nerve sheath, right eye
H47.Ø22 Hemorrhage in optic nerve sheath, left eye
H47.Ø23 Hemorrhage in optic nerve sheath, bilateral
H47.Ø29 Hemorrhage in optic nerve sheath, unspecified eye

√6th H47.Ø3 Optic nerve hypoplasia
H47.Ø31 Optic nerve hypoplasia, right eye
H47.Ø32 Optic nerve hypoplasia, left eye
H47.Ø33 Optic nerve hypoplasia, bilateral
H47.Ø39 Optic nerve hypoplasia, unspecified eye

√6th H47.Ø9 Other disorders of optic nerve, not elsewhere classified

Compression of optic nerve

H47.Ø91 Other disorders of optic nerve, not elsewhere classified, right eye
H47.Ø92 Other disorders of optic nerve, not elsewhere classified, left eye
H47.Ø93 Other disorders of optic nerve, not elsewhere classified, bilateral
H47.Ø99 Other disorders of optic nerve, not elsewhere classified, unspecified eye

√5th H47.1 Papilledema

DEF: Swelling of the optic papilla, the raised area connected to the optic disk made up of nerves that enter the eyeball. It may be caused by increased intracranial pressure, decreased ocular pressure, or a retinal disorder.

H47.1Ø Unspecified papilledema
H47.11 Papilledema associated with increased intracranial pressure
H47.12 Papilledema associated with decreased ocular pressure
H47.13 Papilledema associated with retinal disorder

√6th H47.14 Foster-Kennedy syndrome
H47.141 Foster-Kennedy syndrome, right eye
H47.142 Foster-Kennedy syndrome, left eye
H47.143 Foster-Kennedy syndrome, bilateral
H47.149 Foster-Kennedy syndrome, unspecified eye

√5th H47.2 Optic atrophy
H47.2Ø Unspecified optic atrophy

√6th H47.21 Primary optic atrophy
H47.211 Primary optic atrophy, right eye
H47.212 Primary optic atrophy, left eye
H47.213 Primary optic atrophy, bilateral
H47.219 Primary optic atrophy, unspecified eye

H47.22 Hereditary optic atrophy

Leber's optic atrophy

√6th H47.23 Glaucomatous optic atrophy
H47.231 Glaucomatous optic atrophy, right eye
H47.232 Glaucomatous optic atrophy, left eye
H47.233 Glaucomatous optic atrophy, bilateral
H47.239 Glaucomatous optic atrophy, unspecified eye

√6th H47.29 Other optic atrophy

Temporal pallor of optic disc

H47.291 Other optic atrophy, right eye
H47.292 Other optic atrophy, left eye
H47.293 Other optic atrophy, bilateral
H47.299 Other optic atrophy, unspecified eye

√5th H47.3 Other disorders of optic disc

√6th H47.31 Coloboma of optic disc
H47.311 Coloboma of optic disc, right eye
H47.312 Coloboma of optic disc, left eye
H47.313 Coloboma of optic disc, bilateral

H47.319 Coloboma of optic disc, unspecified eye

√6th H47.32 Drusen of optic disc
H47.321 Drusen of optic disc, right eye
H47.322 Drusen of optic disc, left eye
H47.323 Drusen of optic disc, bilateral
H47.329 Drusen of optic disc, unspecified eye

√6th H47.33 Pseudopapilledema of optic disc
H47.331 Pseudopapilledema of optic disc, right eye
H47.332 Pseudopapilledema of optic disc, left eye
H47.333 Pseudopapilledema of optic disc, bilateral
H47.339 Pseudopapilledema of optic disc, unspecified eye

√6th H47.39 Other disorders of optic disc
H47.391 Other disorders of optic disc, right eye
H47.392 Other disorders of optic disc, left eye
H47.393 Other disorders of optic disc, bilateral
H47.399 Other disorders of optic disc, unspecified eye

√5th H47.4 Disorders of optic chiasm
Code also underlying condition
H47.41 Disorders of optic chiasm in (due to) inflammatory disorders
H47.42 Disorders of optic chiasm in (due to) neoplasm
H47.43 Disorders of optic chiasm in (due to) vascular disorders
H47.49 Disorders of optic chiasm in (due to) other disorders

√5th H47.5 Disorders of other visual pathways
Disorders of optic tracts, geniculate nuclei and optic radiations
Code also underlying condition

√6th H47.51 Disorders of visual pathways in (due to) inflammatory disorders
H47.511 Disorders of visual pathways in (due to) inflammatory disorders, right side
H47.512 Disorders of visual pathways in (due to) inflammatory disorders, left side
H47.519 Disorders of visual pathways in (due to) inflammatory disorders, unspecified side

√6th H47.52 Disorders of visual pathways in (due to) neoplasm
H47.521 Disorders of visual pathways in (due to) neoplasm, right side
H47.522 Disorders of visual pathways in (due to) neoplasm, left side
H47.529 Disorders of visual pathways in (due to) neoplasm, unspecified side

√6th H47.53 Disorders of visual pathways in (due to) vascular disorders
H47.531 Disorders of visual pathways in (due to) vascular disorders, right side
H47.532 Disorders of visual pathways in (due to) vascular disorders, left side
H47.539 Disorders of visual pathways in (due to) vascular disorders, unspecified side

√5th H47.6 Disorders of visual cortex
Code also underlying condition
EXCLUDES 1 *injury to visual cortex SØ4.Ø4-*

√6th H47.61 Cortical blindness
H47.611 Cortical blindness, right side of brain
H47.612 Cortical blindness, left side of brain
H47.619 Cortical blindness, unspecified side of brain

√6th H47.62 Disorders of visual cortex in (due to) inflammatory disorders
H47.621 Disorders of visual cortex in (due to) inflammatory disorders, right side of brain
H47.622 Disorders of visual cortex in (due to) inflammatory disorders, left side of brain
H47.629 Disorders of visual cortex in (due to) inflammatory disorders, unspecified side of brain

√6th H47.63 Disorders of visual cortex in (due to) neoplasm
H47.631 Disorders of visual cortex in (due to) neoplasm, right side of brain
H47.632 Disorders of visual cortex in (due to) neoplasm, left side of brain
H47.639 Disorders of visual cortex in (due to) neoplasm, unspecified side of brain

√6th H47.64 Disorders of visual cortex in (due to) vascular disorders
H47.641 Disorders of visual cortex in (due to) vascular disorders, right side of brain
H47.642 Disorders of visual cortex in (due to) vascular disorders, left side of brain
H47.649 Disorders of visual cortex in (due to) vascular disorders, unspecified side of brain

H47.9 Unspecified disorder of visual pathways

## Disorders of ocular muscles, binocular movement, accommodation and refraction (H49-H52)

EXCLUDES 2 *nystagmus and other irregular eye movements (H55)*

√4th **H49 Paralytic strabismus**
EXCLUDES 2 *internal ophthalmoplegia (H52.51-)*
*internuclear ophthalmoplegia (H51.2-)*
*progressive supranuclear ophthalmoplegia (G23.1)*

**DEF:** Strabismus: Misalignment of the eyes with the inability to move and focus in the same direction due to conditions affecting the muscles controlling them.

√5th H49.Ø Third [oculomotor] nerve palsy
H49.ØØ Third [oculomotor] nerve palsy, unspecified eye
H49.Ø1 Third [oculomotor] nerve palsy, right eye
H49.Ø2 Third [oculomotor] nerve palsy, left eye
H49.Ø3 Third [oculomotor] nerve palsy, bilateral

√5th H49.1 Fourth [trochlear] nerve palsy
H49.1Ø Fourth [trochlear] nerve palsy, unspecified eye
H49.11 Fourth [trochlear] nerve palsy, right eye
H49.12 Fourth [trochlear] nerve palsy, left eye
H49.13 Fourth [trochlear] nerve palsy, bilateral

√5th H49.2 Sixth [abducent] nerve palsy
H49.2Ø Sixth [abducent] nerve palsy, unspecified eye
H49.21 Sixth [abducent] nerve palsy, right eye
H49.22 Sixth [abducent] nerve palsy, left eye
H49.23 Sixth [abducent] nerve palsy, bilateral

√5th H49.3 Total (external) ophthalmoplegia
H49.3Ø Total (external) ophthalmoplegia, unspecified eye
H49.31 Total (external) ophthalmoplegia, right eye
H49.32 Total (external) ophthalmoplegia, left eye
H49.33 Total (external) ophthalmoplegia, bilateral

√5th H49.4 Progressive external ophthalmoplegia
EXCLUDES 1 *Kearns-Sayre syndrome (H49.81-)*
H49.4Ø Progressive external ophthalmoplegia, unspecified eye
H49.41 Progressive external ophthalmoplegia, right eye
H49.42 Progressive external ophthalmoplegia, left eye
H49.43 Progressive external ophthalmoplegia, bilateral

√5th H49.8 Other paralytic strabismus

√6th H49.81 Kearns-Sayre syndrome
Progressive external ophthalmoplegia with pigmentary retinopathy
Code also, if applicable, other manifestations, such as: heart block (I45.9)
H49.811 Kearns-Sayre syndrome, right eye Rx ESR COM
H49.812 Kearns-Sayre syndrome, left eye Rx ESR COM
H49.813 Kearns-Sayre syndrome, bilateral Rx ESR COM
H49.819 Kearns-Sayre syndrome, unspecified eye Rx ESR COM

√6th H49.88 Other paralytic strabismus
External ophthalmoplegia NOS
H49.881 Other paralytic strabismus, right eye
H49.882 Other paralytic strabismus, left eye
H49.883 Other paralytic strabismus, bilateral
H49.889 Other paralytic strabismus, unspecified eye

H49.9 Unspecified paralytic strabismus

√4th **H5Ø Other strabismus**

**DEF:** Strabismus: Misalignment of the eyes with the inability to move and focus in the same direction due to conditions affecting the muscles controlling them.

√5th H5Ø.Ø Esotropia
Convergent concomitant strabismus
EXCLUDES 1 *intermittent esotropia (H5Ø.31-, H5Ø.32)*
H5Ø.ØØ Unspecified esotropia

√6th H5Ø.Ø1 Monocular esotropia
H5Ø.Ø11 Monocular esotropia, right eye

H5Ø.Ø12 Monocular esotropia, left eye

√6th H5Ø.Ø2 Monocular esotropia with A pattern

H5Ø.Ø21 Monocular esotropia with A pattern, right eye

H5Ø.Ø22 Monocular esotropia with A pattern, left eye

√6th H5Ø.Ø3 Monocular esotropia with V pattern

H5Ø.Ø31 Monocular esotropia with V pattern, right eye

H5Ø.Ø32 Monocular esotropia with V pattern, left eye

√6th H5Ø.Ø4 Monocular esotropia with other noncomitancies

H5Ø.Ø41 Monocular esotropia with other noncomitancies, right eye

H5Ø.Ø42 Monocular esotropia with other noncomitancies, left eye

H5Ø.Ø5 Alternating esotropia

H5Ø.Ø6 Alternating esotropia with A pattern

H5Ø.Ø7 Alternating esotropia with V pattern

H5Ø.Ø8 Alternating esotropia with other noncomitancies

**Eye Muscle Diseases**

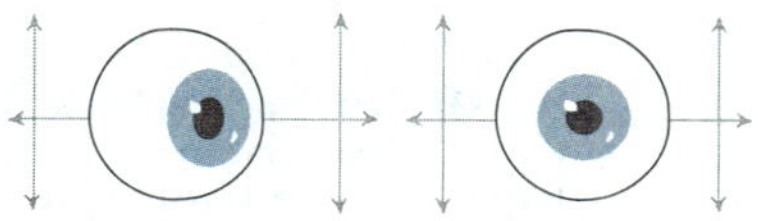

Monocular (one eye only) esotropia (inward)

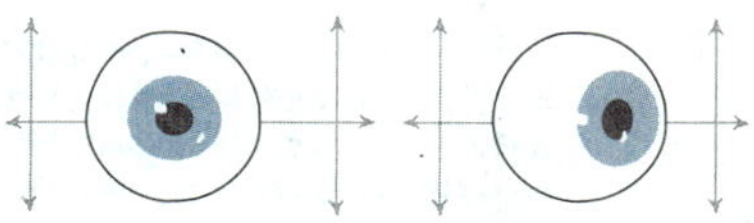
Monocular exotropia (outward)

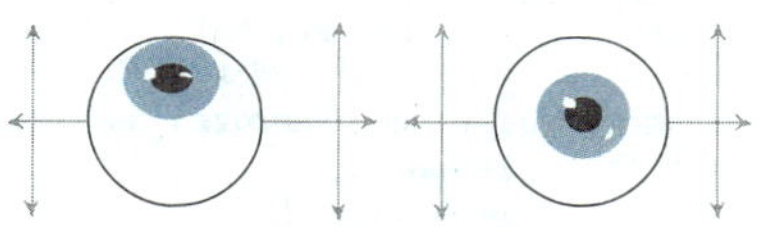
Monocular hypertropia (upward)

√5th H5Ø.1 Exotropia

Divergent concomitant strabismus

EXCLUDES 1 *intermittent exotropia (H5Ø.33-, H5Ø.34)*

H5Ø.1Ø Unspecified exotropia

√6th H5Ø.11 Monocular exotropia

H5Ø.111 Monocular exotropia, right eye

H5Ø.112 Monocular exotropia, left eye

√6th H5Ø.12 Monocular exotropia with A pattern

H5Ø.121 Monocular exotropia with A pattern, right eye

H5Ø.122 Monocular exotropia with A pattern, left eye

√6th H5Ø.13 Monocular exotropia with V pattern

H5Ø.131 Monocular exotropia with V pattern, right eye

H5Ø.132 Monocular exotropia with V pattern, left eye

√6th H5Ø.14 Monocular exotropia with other noncomitancies

H5Ø.141 Monocular exotropia with other noncomitancies, right eye

H5Ø.142 Monocular exotropia with other noncomitancies, left eye

H5Ø.15 Alternating exotropia

H5Ø.16 Alternating exotropia with A pattern

H5Ø.17 Alternating exotropia with V pattern

H5Ø.18 Alternating exotropia with other noncomitancies

√5th H5Ø.2 Vertical strabismus

Hypertropia

H5Ø.21 Vertical strabismus, right eye

H5Ø.22 Vertical strabismus, left eye

√5th H5Ø.3 Intermittent heterotropia

H5Ø.3Ø Unspecified intermittent heterotropia

√6th H5Ø.31 Intermittent monocular esotropia

H5Ø.311 Intermittent monocular esotropia, right eye

H5Ø.312 Intermittent monocular esotropia, left eye

H5Ø.32 Intermittent alternating esotropia

√6th H5Ø.33 Intermittent monocular exotropia

H5Ø.331 Intermittent monocular exotropia, right eye

H5Ø.332 Intermittent monocular exotropia, left eye

H5Ø.34 Intermittent alternating exotropia

√5th H5Ø.4 Other and unspecified heterotropia

H5Ø.4Ø Unspecified heterotropia

√6th H5Ø.41 Cyclotropia

H5Ø.411 Cyclotropia, right eye

H5Ø.412 Cyclotropia, left eye

H5Ø.42 Monofixation syndrome

H5Ø.43 Accommodative component in esotropia

√5th H5Ø.5 Heterophoria

H5Ø.5Ø Unspecified heterophoria

H5Ø.51 Esophoria

H5Ø.52 Exophoria

H5Ø.53 Vertical heterophoria

H5Ø.54 Cyclophoria

H5Ø.55 Alternating heterophoria

√5th H5Ø.6 Mechanical strabismus

AHA: 2023,4Q,21-23

H5Ø.6Ø Mechanical strabismus, unspecified

√6th H5Ø.61 Brown's sheath syndrome

H5Ø.611 Brown's sheath syndrome, right eye

H5Ø.612 Brown's sheath syndrome, left eye

√6th H5Ø.62 Inferior oblique muscle entrapment

H5Ø.621 Inferior oblique muscle entrapment, right eye

H5Ø.622 Inferior oblique muscle entrapment, left eye

H5Ø.629 Inferior oblique muscle entrapment, unspecified eye

√6th H5Ø.63 Inferior rectus muscle entrapment

H5Ø.631 Inferior rectus muscle entrapment, right eye

H5Ø.632 Inferior rectus muscle entrapment, left eye

H5Ø.639 Inferior rectus muscle entrapment, unspecified eye

√6th H5Ø.64 Lateral rectus muscle entrapment

H5Ø.641 Lateral rectus muscle entrapment, right eye

H5Ø.642 Lateral rectus muscle entrapment, left eye

H5Ø.649 Lateral rectus muscle entrapment, unspecified eye

√6th H5Ø.65 Medial rectus muscle entrapment

H5Ø.651 Medial rectus muscle entrapment, right eye

H5Ø.652 Medial rectus muscle entrapment, left eye

H5Ø.659 Medial rectus muscle entrapment, unspecified eye

√6th H5Ø.66 Superior oblique muscle entrapment

H5Ø.661 Superior oblique muscle entrapment, right eye

H5Ø.662 Superior oblique muscle entrapment, left eye

H5Ø.669 Superior oblique muscle entrapment, unspecified eye

√6th H5Ø.67 Superior rectus muscle entrapment

H5Ø.671 Superior rectus muscle entrapment, right eye

H5Ø.672 Superior rectus muscle entrapment, left eye

H5Ø.679 Superior rectus muscle entrapment, unspecified eye

√6th H5Ø.68 Extraocular muscle entrapment, unspecified

H5Ø.681 Extraocular muscle entrapment, unspecified, right eye

H5Ø.682 Extraocular muscle entrapment, unspecified, left eye

H5Ø.689 Extraocular muscle entrapment, unspecified, unspecified eye

H5Ø.69 Other mechanical strabismus

Strabismus due to adhesions

Traumatic limitation of duction of eye muscle

5th H50.8 Other specified strabismus
- 6th H50.81 Duane's syndrome
  - H50.811 Duane's syndrome, right eye
  - H50.812 Duane's syndrome, left eye
- H50.89 Other specified strabismus

H50.9 Unspecified strabismus

4th **H51 Other disorders of binocular movement**

H51.0 Palsy (spasm) of conjugate gaze

5th H51.1 Convergence insufficiency and excess
- H51.11 Convergence insufficiency
- H51.12 Convergence excess

5th H51.2 Internuclear ophthalmoplegia
- H51.20 Internuclear ophthalmoplegia, unspecified eye
- H51.21 Internuclear ophthalmoplegia, right eye
- H51.22 Internuclear ophthalmoplegia, left eye
- H51.23 Internuclear ophthalmoplegia, bilateral

H51.8 Other specified disorders of binocular movement

H51.9 Unspecified disorder of binocular movement

4th **H52 Disorders of refraction and accommodation**

5th H52.0 Hypermetropia
- H52.00 Hypermetropia, unspecified eye
- H52.01 Hypermetropia, right eye
- H52.02 Hypermetropia, left eye
- H52.03 Hypermetropia, bilateral

5th H52.1 Myopia

EXCLUDES 1 *degenerative myopia (H44.2-)*
- H52.10 Myopia, unspecified eye
- H52.11 Myopia, right eye
- H52.12 Myopia, left eye
- H52.13 Myopia, bilateral

5th H52.2 Astigmatism
- 6th H52.20 Unspecified astigmatism
  - H52.201 Unspecified astigmatism, right eye
  - H52.202 Unspecified astigmatism, left eye
  - H52.203 Unspecified astigmatism, bilateral
  - H52.209 Unspecified astigmatism, unspecified eye
- 6th H52.21 Irregular astigmatism
  - H52.211 Irregular astigmatism, right eye
  - H52.212 Irregular astigmatism, left eye
  - H52.213 Irregular astigmatism, bilateral
  - H52.219 Irregular astigmatism, unspecified eye
- 6th H52.22 Regular astigmatism
  - H52.221 Regular astigmatism, right eye
  - H52.222 Regular astigmatism, left eye
  - H52.223 Regular astigmatism, bilateral
  - H52.229 Regular astigmatism, unspecified eye

5th H52.3 Anisometropia and aniseikonia
- H52.31 Anisometropia
- H52.32 Aniseikonia

H52.4 Presbyopia

5th H52.5 Disorders of accommodation
- 6th H52.51 Internal ophthalmoplegia (complete) (total)
  - H52.511 Internal ophthalmoplegia (complete) (total), right eye
  - H52.512 Internal ophthalmoplegia (complete) (total), left eye
  - H52.513 Internal ophthalmoplegia (complete) (total), bilateral
  - H52.519 Internal ophthalmoplegia (complete) (total), unspecified eye
- 6th H52.52 Paresis of accommodation
  - H52.521 Paresis of accommodation, right eye
  - H52.522 Paresis of accommodation, left eye
  - H52.523 Paresis of accommodation, bilateral
  - H52.529 Paresis of accommodation, unspecified eye
- 6th H52.53 Spasm of accommodation
  - H52.531 Spasm of accommodation, right eye
  - H52.532 Spasm of accommodation, left eye
  - H52.533 Spasm of accommodation, bilateral
  - H52.539 Spasm of accommodation, unspecified eye

H52.6 Other disorders of refraction

H52.7 Unspecified disorder of refraction

## Visual disturbances and blindness (H53-H54)

4th **H53 Visual disturbances**

5th H53.0 Amblyopia ex anopsia

EXCLUDES 1 *amblyopia due to vitamin A deficiency (E50.5)*
- 6th H53.00 Unspecified amblyopia
  - H53.001 Unspecified amblyopia, right eye
  - H53.002 Unspecified amblyopia, left eye
  - H53.003 Unspecified amblyopia, bilateral
  - H53.009 Unspecified amblyopia, unspecified eye
- 6th H53.01 Deprivation amblyopia
  - H53.011 Deprivation amblyopia, right eye
  - H53.012 Deprivation amblyopia, left eye
  - H53.013 Deprivation amblyopia, bilateral
  - H53.019 Deprivation amblyopia, unspecified eye
- 6th H53.02 Refractive amblyopia
  - H53.021 Refractive amblyopia, right eye
  - H53.022 Refractive amblyopia, left eye
  - H53.023 Refractive amblyopia, bilateral
  - H53.029 Refractive amblyopia, unspecified eye
- 6th H53.03 Strabismic amblyopia

  EXCLUDES 2 *strabismus (H50.-)*
  - H53.031 Strabismic amblyopia, right eye
  - H53.032 Strabismic amblyopia, left eye
  - H53.033 Strabismic amblyopia, bilateral
  - H53.039 Strabismic amblyopia, unspecified eye
- 6th H53.04 Amblyopia suspect

  AHA: 2016,4Q,22-23
  - H53.041 Amblyopia suspect, right eye
  - H53.042 Amblyopia suspect, left eye
  - H53.043 Amblyopia suspect, bilateral
  - H53.049 Amblyopia suspect, unspecified eye

5th H53.1 Subjective visual disturbances

EXCLUDES 1 *subjective visual disturbances due to vitamin A deficiency (E50.5)*
*visual hallucinations (R44.1)*
- H53.10 Unspecified subjective visual disturbances
- H53.11 Day blindness
  Hemeralopia
- 6th H53.12 Transient visual loss
  Scintillating scotoma

  EXCLUDES 1 *amaurosis fugax (G45.3-)*
  *transient retinal artery occlusion (H34.0-)*

  AHA: 2022,1Q,30
  - H53.121 Transient visual loss, right eye
  - H53.122 Transient visual loss, left eye
  - H53.123 Transient visual loss, bilateral
  - H53.129 Transient visual loss, unspecified eye
- 6th H53.13 Sudden visual loss
  - H53.131 Sudden visual loss, right eye
  - H53.132 Sudden visual loss, left eye
  - H53.133 Sudden visual loss, bilateral
  - H53.139 Sudden visual loss, unspecified eye
- 6th H53.14 Visual discomfort
  Asthenopia
  Photophobia
  - H53.141 Visual discomfort, right eye
  - H53.142 Visual discomfort, left eye
  - H53.143 Visual discomfort, bilateral
  - H53.149 Visual discomfort, unspecified
- H53.15 Visual distortions of shape and size
  Metamorphopsia
- H53.16 Psychophysical visual disturbances
- H53.19 Other subjective visual disturbances
  Visual halos

  AHA: 2022,1Q,30

H53.2 Diplopia
Double vision

5th H53.3 Other and unspecified disorders of binocular vision
- H53.30 Unspecified disorder of binocular vision
- H53.31 Abnormal retinal correspondence
- H53.32 Fusion with defective stereopsis
- H53.33 Simultaneous visual perception without fusion
- H53.34 Suppression of binocular vision

✓5th **H53.4 Visual field defects**

**H53.40 Unspecified visual field defects**

✓6th **H53.41 Scotoma involving central area**

Central scotoma

**AHA:** 2022,1Q,30

**H53.411 Scotoma involving central area, right eye**

**H53.412 Scotoma involving central area, left eye**

**H53.413 Scotoma involving central area, bilateral**

**H53.419 Scotoma involving central area, unspecified eye**

✓6th **H53.42 Scotoma of blind spot area**

Enlarged blind spot

**H53.421 Scotoma of blind spot area, right eye**

**H53.422 Scotoma of blind spot area, left eye**

**H53.423 Scotoma of blind spot area, bilateral**

**H53.429 Scotoma of blind spot area, unspecified eye**

✓6th **H53.43 Sector or arcuate defects**

Arcuate scotoma
Bjerrum scotoma

**H53.431 Sector or arcuate defects, right eye**

**H53.432 Sector or arcuate defects, left eye**

**H53.433 Sector or arcuate defects, bilateral**

**H53.439 Sector or arcuate defects, unspecified eye**

✓6th **H53.45 Other localized visual field defect**

Peripheral visual field defect
Ring scotoma NOS
Scotoma NOS

**H53.451 Other localized visual field defect, right eye**

**H53.452 Other localized visual field defect, left eye**

**H53.453 Other localized visual field defect, bilateral**

**H53.459 Other localized visual field defect, unspecified eye**

✓6th **H53.46 Homonymous bilateral field defects**

Homonymous hemianopia
Homonymous hemianopsia
Quadrant anopia
Quadrant anopsia

**H53.461 Homonymous bilateral field defects, right side**

**H53.462 Homonymous bilateral field defects, left side**

**H53.469 Homonymous bilateral field defects, unspecified side**

Homonymous bilateral field defects NOS

**H53.47 Heteronymous bilateral field defects**

Heteronymous hemianop(s)ia

✓6th **H53.48 Generalized contraction of visual field**

**H53.481 Generalized contraction of visual field, right eye**

**H53.482 Generalized contraction of visual field, left eye**

**H53.483 Generalized contraction of visual field, bilateral**

**H53.489 Generalized contraction of visual field, unspecified eye**

✓5th **H53.5 Color vision deficiencies**

Color blindness

EXCLUDES 2 *day blindness (H53.11)*

**H53.50 Unspecified color vision deficiencies**

Color blindness NOS

**H53.51 Achromatopsia**

**DEF:** Nonprogressive genetic visual disorder characterized by complete color blindness, decreased vision, and light sensitivity.

**H53.52 Acquired color vision deficiency**

**H53.53 Deuteranomaly**

Deuteranopia

**DEF:** Male-only genetic disorder causing difficulty in distinguishing green and red; no shortened spectrum.

**H53.54 Protanomaly**

Protanopia

**H53.55 Tritanomaly**

Tritanopia

**H53.59 Other color vision deficiencies**

✓5th **H53.6 Night blindness**

EXCLUDES 1 *night blindness due to vitamin A deficiency (E50.5)*

**H53.60 Unspecified night blindness**

**H53.61 Abnormal dark adaptation curve**

**H53.62 Acquired night blindness**

**H53.63 Congenital night blindness**

**H53.69 Other night blindness**

✓5th **H53.7 Vision sensitivity deficiencies**

**H53.71 Glare sensitivity**

**H53.72 Impaired contrast sensitivity**

**H53.8 Other visual disturbances**

**H53.9 Unspecified visual disturbance**

✓4th **H54 Blindness and low vision**

NOTE For definition of visual impairment categories see table below

Code first any associated underlying cause of the blindness

EXCLUDES 1 *amaurosis fugax (G45.3)*

**AHA:** 2017,4Q,11-12

✓5th **H54.0 Blindness, both eyes**

Visual impairment categories 3, 4, 5 in both eyes.

✓6th **H54.0X Blindness, both eyes, different category levels**

✓7th **H54.0X3 Blindness right eye, category 3**

**H54.0X33 Blindness right eye category 3, blindness left eye category 3**

**H54.0X34 Blindness right eye category 3, blindness left eye category 4**

**H54.0X35 Blindness right eye category 3, blindness left eye category 5**

✓7th **H54.0X4 Blindness right eye, category 4**

**H54.0X43 Blindness right eye category 4, blindness left eye category 3**

**H54.0X44 Blindness right eye category 4, blindness left eye category 4**

**H54.0X45 Blindness right eye category 4, blindness left eye category 5**

✓7th **H54.0X5 Blindness right eye, category 5**

**H54.0X53 Blindness right eye category 5, blindness left eye category 3**

**H54.0X54 Blindness right eye category 5, blindness left eye category 4**

**H54.0X55 Blindness right eye category 5, blindness left eye category 5**

✓5th **H54.1 Blindness, one eye, low vision other eye**

Visual impairment categories 3, 4, 5 in one eye, with categories 1 or 2 in the other eye.

**H54.10 Blindness, one eye, low vision other eye, unspecified eyes**

✓6th **H54.11 Blindness, right eye, low vision left eye**

✓7th **H54.113 Blindness right eye category 3, low vision left eye**

**H54.1131 Blindness right eye category 3, low vision left eye category 1**

**H54.1132 Blindness right eye category 3, low vision left eye category 2**

✓7th **H54.114 Blindness right eye category 4, low vision left eye**

**H54.1141 Blindness right eye category 4, low vision left eye category 1**

**H54.1142 Blindness right eye category 4, low vision left eye category 2**

✓7th **H54.115 Blindness right eye category 5, low vision left eye**

**H54.1151 Blindness right eye category 5, low vision left eye category 1**

**H54.1152 Blindness right eye category 5, low vision left eye category 2**

✓6th **H54.12 Blindness, left eye, low vision right eye**

✓7th **H54.121 Low vision right eye category 1, blindness left eye**

**H54.1213 Low vision right eye category 1, blindness left eye category 3**

**H54.1214 Low vision right eye category 1, blindness left eye category 4**

**H54.1215 Low vision right eye category 1, blindness left eye category 5**

✓7th **H54.122 Low vision right eye category 2, blindness left eye**

**H54.1223 Low vision right eye category 2, blindness left eye category 3**

**H54.1224 Low vision right eye category 2, blindness left eye category 4**

**H54.1225 Low vision right eye category 2, blindness left eye category 5**

√5th **H54.2 Low vision, both eyes**
Visual impairment categories 1 or 2 in both eyes.
√6th **H54.2X Low vision, both eyes, different category levels**
√7th **H54.2X1 Low vision, right eye, category 1**
**H54.2X11 Low vision right eye category 1, low vision left eye category 1**
**H54.2X12 Low vision right eye category 1, low vision left eye category 2**
√7th **H54.2X2 Low vision, right eye, category 2**
**H54.2X21 Low vision right eye category 2, low vision left eye category 1**
**H54.2X22 Low vision right eye category 2, low vision left eye category 2**

**H54.3 Unqualified visual loss, both eyes**
Visual impairment category 9 in both eyes.
**TIP:** Assign only when both eyes are documented as affected by blindness or low vision but the visual impairment category is not documented.

√5th **H54.4 Blindness, one eye**
Visual impairment categories 3, 4, 5 in one eye [normal vision in other eye]
**H54.40 Blindness, one eye, unspecified eye**
√6th **H54.41 Blindness, right eye, normal vision left eye**
√7th **H54.413 Blindness, right eye, category 3**
**H54.413A Blindness right eye category 3, normal vision left eye**
√7th **H54.414 Blindness, right eye, category 4**
**H54.414A Blindness right eye category 4, normal vision left eye**
√7th **H54.415 Blindness, right eye, category 5**
**H54.415A Blindness right eye category 5, normal vision left eye**
√6th **H54.42 Blindness, left eye, normal vision right eye**
√7th **H54.42A Blindness, left eye, category 3-5**
**H54.42A3 Blindness left eye category 3, normal vision right eye**
**H54.42A4 Blindness left eye category 4, normal vision right eye**
**H54.42A5 Blindness left eye category 5, normal vision right eye**

√5th **H54.5 Low vision, one eye**
Visual impairment categories 1 or 2 in one eye [normal vision in other eye].
**H54.50 Low vision, one eye, unspecified eye**
√6th **H54.51 Low vision, right eye, normal vision left eye**
√7th **H54.511 Low vision, right eye, category 1**
**H54.511A Low vision right eye category 1, normal vision left eye**
√7th **H54.512 Low vision, right eye, category 2**
**H54.512A Low vision right eye category 2, normal vision left eye**
√6th **H54.52 Low vision, left eye, normal vision right eye**
√7th **H54.52A Low vision, left eye, category 1-2**
**H54.52A1 Low vision left eye category 1, normal vision right eye**
**H54.52A2 Low vision left eye category 2, normal vision right eye**

√5th **H54.6 Unqualified visual loss, one eye**
Visual impairment category 9 in one eye [normal vision in other eye].
**TIP:** Assign a code from this category only when one eye is documented as affected by blindness or low vision but the visual impairment category is not documented.
**H54.60 Unqualified visual loss, one eye, unspecified**
**H54.61 Unqualified visual loss, right eye, normal vision left eye**
**H54.62 Unqualified visual loss, left eye, normal vision right eye**

**H54.7 Unspecified visual loss**
Visual impairment category 9 NOS
**TIP:** Assign only when documentation specifies blindness, visual loss, or low vision but not whether one or both eyes are affected or the visual impairment category.

**H54.8 Legal blindness, as defined in USA**
Blindness NOS according to USA definition
EXCLUDES 1 *legal blindness with specification of impairment level (H54.0-H54.7)*

NOTE The table below gives a classification of severity of visual impairment recommended by a WHO Study Group on the Prevention of Blindness, Geneva, 6-10 November 1972.

If the extent of the visual field is taken into account, patients with a field no greater than 10 but greater than 5 around central fixation should be placed in category 3 and patients with a field no greater than 5 around central fixation should be placed in category 4, even if the central acuity is not impaired.

The term "low vision" in category H54 comprises categories 1 and 2 of the table, the term "blindness" categories 3, 4 and 5, and the term "unqualified visual loss" category 9.

| Category of visual impairment | Visual acuity with best possible correction | |
|---|---|---|
| | **Maximum less than:** | **Minimum equal to or better than:** |
| 1 | 6/18<br>3/10 (0.3)<br>20/70 | 6/60<br>1/10 (0.1)<br>20/200 |
| 2 | 6/60<br>1/10 (0.1)<br>20/200 | 3/60<br>1/20 (0.05)<br>20/400 |
| 3 | 3/60<br>1/20 (0.05)<br>20/400 | 1/60 (finger counting at one meter)<br>1/50 (0.02)<br>5/300 (20/1200) |
| 4 | 1/60 (finger counting at one meter)<br>1/50 (0.02)<br>5/300 | Light perception |
| 5 | No light perception | |
| 9 | Undetermined or unspecified | |

## Other disorders of eye and adnexa (H55-H57)

√4th **H55 Nystagmus and other irregular eye movements**
√5th **H55.0 Nystagmus**
**DEF:** Rapid, rhythmic, involuntary movements of the eyeball in vertical, horizontal, rotational, or mixed directions.
**H55.00 Unspecified nystagmus**
**H55.01 Congenital nystagmus**
**H55.02 Latent nystagmus**
**H55.03 Visual deprivation nystagmus**
**H55.04 Dissociated nystagmus**
**H55.09 Other forms of nystagmus**
√5th **H55.8 Other irregular eye movements**
**AHA:** 2020,4Q,25
**H55.81 Deficient saccadic eye movements**
**H55.82 Deficient smooth pursuit eye movements**
**H55.89 Other irregular eye movements**

√4th **H57 Other disorders of eye and adnexa**
√5th **H57.0 Anomalies of pupillary function**
**H57.00 Unspecified anomaly of pupillary function**
**H57.01 Argyll Robertson pupil, atypical**
EXCLUDES 1 *syphilitic Argyll Robertson pupil (A52.19)*
**H57.02 Anisocoria**
**H57.03 Miosis**
**H57.04 Mydriasis**
√6th **H57.05 Tonic pupil**
**H57.051 Tonic pupil, right eye**
**H57.052 Tonic pupil, left eye**
**H57.053 Tonic pupil, bilateral**
**H57.059 Tonic pupil, unspecified eye**
**H57.09 Other anomalies of pupillary function**
√5th **H57.1 Ocular pain**
**H57.10 Ocular pain, unspecified eye**

H57.11 Ocular pain, right eye
H57.12 Ocular pain, left eye
H57.13 Ocular pain, bilateral

✓5th H57.8 Other specified disorders of eye and adnexa
AHA: 2018,4Q,15-16

✓6th H57.81 Brow ptosis
H57.811 Brow ptosis, right
H57.812 Brow ptosis, left
H57.813 Brow ptosis, bilateral
H57.819 Brow ptosis, unspecified

H57.89 Other specified disorders of eye and adnexa

✓6th H57.8A Foreign body sensation eye (ocular)
AHA: 2023,4Q,23
H57.8A1 Foreign body sensation, right eye
H57.8A2 Foreign body sensation, left eye
H57.8A3 Foreign body sensation, bilateral eyes
H57.8A9 Foreign body sensation, unspecified eye

H57.9 Unspecified disorder of eye and adnexa

## Intraoperative and postprocedural complications and disorders of eye and adnexa, not elsewhere classified (H59)

✓4th **H59 Intraoperative and postprocedural complications and disorders of eye and adnexa, not elsewhere classified**
EXCLUDES 1 *mechanical complication of intraocular lens (T85.2)*
*mechanical complication of other ocular prosthetic devices, implants and grafts (T85.3)*
*pseudophakia (Z96.1)*
*secondary cataracts (H26.4-)*

✓5th H59.Ø Disorders of the eye following cataract surgery

✓6th H59.Ø1 Keratopathy (bullous aphakic) following cataract surgery
Vitreal corneal syndrome
Vitreous (touch) syndrome
H59.Ø11 Keratopathy (bullous aphakic) following cataract surgery, right eye
H59.Ø12 Keratopathy (bullous aphakic) following cataract surgery, left eye
H59.Ø13 Keratopathy (bullous aphakic) following cataract surgery, bilateral
H59.Ø19 Keratopathy (bullous aphakic) following cataract surgery, unspecified eye

✓6th H59.Ø2 Cataract (lens) fragments in eye following cataract surgery
H59.Ø21 Cataract (lens) fragments in eye following cataract surgery, right eye
H59.Ø22 Cataract (lens) fragments in eye following cataract surgery, left eye
H59.Ø23 Cataract (lens) fragments in eye following cataract surgery, bilateral
H59.Ø29 Cataract (lens) fragments in eye following cataract surgery, unspecified eye

✓6th H59.Ø3 Cystoid macular edema following cataract surgery
H59.Ø31 Cystoid macular edema following cataract surgery, right eye
H59.Ø32 Cystoid macular edema following cataract surgery, left eye
H59.Ø33 Cystoid macular edema following cataract surgery, bilateral
H59.Ø39 Cystoid macular edema following cataract surgery, unspecified eye

✓6th H59.Ø9 Other disorders of the eye following cataract surgery
H59.Ø91 Other disorders of the right eye following cataract surgery
H59.Ø92 Other disorders of the left eye following cataract surgery
H59.Ø93 Other disorders of the eye following cataract surgery, bilateral
H59.Ø99 Other disorders of unspecified eye following cataract surgery

✓5th H59.1 Intraoperative hemorrhage and hematoma of eye and adnexa complicating a procedure
EXCLUDES 1 *intraoperative hemorrhage and hematoma of eye and adnexa due to accidental puncture or laceration during a procedure (H59.2-)*

✓6th H59.11 Intraoperative hemorrhage and hematoma of eye and adnexa complicating an ophthalmic procedure
H59.111 Intraoperative hemorrhage and hematoma of right eye and adnexa complicating an ophthalmic procedure
H59.112 Intraoperative hemorrhage and hematoma of left eye and adnexa complicating an ophthalmic procedure
H59.113 Intraoperative hemorrhage and hematoma of eye and adnexa complicating an ophthalmic procedure, bilateral
H59.119 Intraoperative hemorrhage and hematoma of unspecified eye and adnexa complicating an ophthalmic procedure

✓6th H59.12 Intraoperative hemorrhage and hematoma of eye and adnexa complicating other procedure
H59.121 Intraoperative hemorrhage and hematoma of right eye and adnexa complicating other procedure
H59.122 Intraoperative hemorrhage and hematoma of left eye and adnexa complicating other procedure
H59.123 Intraoperative hemorrhage and hematoma of eye and adnexa complicating other procedure, bilateral
H59.129 Intraoperative hemorrhage and hematoma of unspecified eye and adnexa complicating other procedure

✓5th H59.2 Accidental puncture and laceration of eye and adnexa during a procedure

✓6th H59.21 Accidental puncture and laceration of eye and adnexa during an ophthalmic procedure
H59.211 Accidental puncture and laceration of right eye and adnexa during an ophthalmic procedure
H59.212 Accidental puncture and laceration of left eye and adnexa during an ophthalmic procedure
H59.213 Accidental puncture and laceration of eye and adnexa during an ophthalmic procedure, bilateral
H59.219 Accidental puncture and laceration of unspecified eye and adnexa during an ophthalmic procedure

✓6th H59.22 Accidental puncture and laceration of eye and adnexa during other procedure
H59.221 Accidental puncture and laceration of right eye and adnexa during other procedure
H59.222 Accidental puncture and laceration of left eye and adnexa during other procedure
H59.223 Accidental puncture and laceration of eye and adnexa during other procedure, bilateral
H59.229 Accidental puncture and laceration of unspecified eye and adnexa during other procedure

✓5th H59.3 Postprocedural hemorrhage, hematoma, and seroma of eye and adnexa following a procedure
AHA: 2016,4Q,9-10

✓6th H59.31 Postprocedural hemorrhage of eye and adnexa following an ophthalmic procedure
H59.311 Postprocedural hemorrhage of right eye and adnexa following an ophthalmic procedure
H59.312 Postprocedural hemorrhage of left eye and adnexa following an ophthalmic procedure
H59.313 Postprocedural hemorrhage of eye and adnexa following an ophthalmic procedure, bilateral
H59.319 Postprocedural hemorrhage of unspecified eye and adnexa following an ophthalmic procedure

✓6th H59.32 Postprocedural hemorrhage of eye and adnexa following other procedure
H59.321 Postprocedural hemorrhage of right eye and adnexa following other procedure
H59.322 Postprocedural hemorrhage of left eye and adnexa following other procedure
H59.323 Postprocedural hemorrhage of eye and adnexa following other procedure, bilateral
H59.329 Postprocedural hemorrhage of unspecified eye and adnexa following other procedure

✓6th H59.33 Postprocedural hematoma of eye and adnexa following an ophthalmic procedure
H59.331 Postprocedural hematoma of right eye and adnexa following an ophthalmic procedure
H59.332 Postprocedural hematoma of left eye and adnexa following an ophthalmic procedure

**H59.333** Postprocedural hematoma of eye and adnexa following an ophthalmic procedure, bilateral

**H59.339** Postprocedural hematoma of unspecified eye and adnexa following an ophthalmic procedure

✓6th **H59.34** Postprocedural hematoma of eye and adnexa following other procedure

**H59.341** Postprocedural hematoma of right eye and adnexa following other procedure

**H59.342** Postprocedural hematoma of left eye and adnexa following other procedure

**H59.343** Postprocedural hematoma of eye and adnexa following other procedure, bilateral

**H59.349** Postprocedural hematoma of unspecified eye and adnexa following other procedure

✓6th **H59.35** Postprocedural seroma of eye and adnexa following an ophthalmic procedure

**H59.351** Postprocedural seroma of right eye and adnexa following an ophthalmic procedure

**H59.352** Postprocedural seroma of left eye and adnexa following an ophthalmic procedure

**H59.353** Postprocedural seroma of eye and adnexa following an ophthalmic procedure, bilateral

**H59.359** Postprocedural seroma of unspecified eye and adnexa following an ophthalmic procedure

✓6th **H59.36** Postprocedural seroma of eye and adnexa following other procedure

**H59.361** Postprocedural seroma of right eye and adnexa following other procedure

**H59.362** Postprocedural seroma of left eye and adnexa following other procedure

**H59.363** Postprocedural seroma of eye and adnexa following other procedure, bilateral

**H59.369** Postprocedural seroma of unspecified eye and adnexa following other procedure

✓5th **H59.4** Inflammation (infection) of postprocedural bleb

Postprocedural blebitis

EXCLUDES 1 *filtering (vitreous) bleb after glaucoma surgery status (Z98.83)*

**H59.40** Inflammation (infection) of postprocedural bleb, unspecified

**H59.41** Inflammation (infection) of postprocedural bleb, stage 1

**H59.42** Inflammation (infection) of postprocedural bleb, stage 2

**H59.43** Inflammation (infection) of postprocedural bleb, stage 3

Bleb endophthalmitis

✓5th **H59.8** Other intraoperative and postprocedural complications and disorders of eye and adnexa, not elsewhere classified

✓6th **H59.81** Chorioretinal scars after surgery for detachment

**H59.811** Chorioretinal scars after surgery for detachment, right eye

**H59.812** Chorioretinal scars after surgery for detachment, left eye

**H59.813** Chorioretinal scars after surgery for detachment, bilateral

**H59.819** Chorioretinal scars after surgery for detachment, unspecified eye

**H59.88** Other intraoperative complications of eye and adnexa, not elsewhere classified

**H59.89** Other postprocedural complications and disorders of eye and adnexa, not elsewhere classified

AHA: 2020,3Q,29

# Chapter 8. Diseases of the Ear and Mastoid Process (H6Ø–H95)



## Chapter-specific Guidelines with Coding Examples

Reserved for future guideline expansion.

# Chapter 8. Diseases of the Ear and Mastoid Process (H60-H95)

NOTE Use an external cause code following the code for the ear condition, if applicable, to identify the cause of the ear condition

EXCLUDES 2 *certain conditions originating in the perinatal period (P04-P96)*
*certain infectious and parasitic diseases (A00-B99)*
*complications of pregnancy, childbirth and the puerperium (O00-O9A)*
*congenital malformations, deformations and chromosomal abnormalities (Q00-Q99)*
*endocrine, nutritional and metabolic diseases (E00-E88)*
*injury, poisoning and certain other consequences of external causes (S00-T88)*
*neoplasms (C00-D49)*
*symptoms, signs and abnormal clinical and laboratory findings, not elsewhere classified (R00-R94)*

This chapter contains the following blocks:

H60-H62 Diseases of external ear
H65-H75 Diseases of middle ear and mastoid
H80-H83 Diseases of inner ear
H90-H94 Other disorders of ear
H95 Intraoperative and postprocedural complications and disorders of ear and mastoid process, not elsewhere classified

## Diseases of external ear (H60-H62)

✓4th **H60 Otitis externa**

✓5th **H60.0 Abscess of external ear**
Boil of external ear
Carbuncle of auricle or external auditory canal
Furuncle of external ear
**H60.00 Abscess of external ear, unspecified ear**
**H60.01 Abscess of right external ear**
**H60.02 Abscess of left external ear**
**H60.03 Abscess of external ear, bilateral**

✓5th **H60.1 Cellulitis of external ear**
Cellulitis of auricle
Cellulitis of external auditory canal
**H60.10 Cellulitis of external ear, unspecified ear**
**H60.11 Cellulitis of right external ear**
**H60.12 Cellulitis of left external ear**
**H60.13 Cellulitis of external ear, bilateral**

✓5th **H60.2 Malignant otitis externa**
**H60.20 Malignant otitis externa, unspecified ear**
**H60.21 Malignant otitis externa, right ear**
**H60.22 Malignant otitis externa, left ear**
**H60.23 Malignant otitis externa, bilateral**

✓5th **H60.3 Other infective otitis externa**

✓6th **H60.31 Diffuse otitis externa**
**H60.311 Diffuse otitis externa, right ear**
**H60.312 Diffuse otitis externa, left ear**
**H60.313 Diffuse otitis externa, bilateral**
**H60.319 Diffuse otitis externa, unspecified ear**

✓6th **H60.32 Hemorrhagic otitis externa**
**H60.321 Hemorrhagic otitis externa, right ear**
**H60.322 Hemorrhagic otitis externa, left ear**
**H60.323 Hemorrhagic otitis externa, bilateral**
**H60.329 Hemorrhagic otitis externa, unspecified ear**

✓6th **H60.33 Swimmer's ear**
**DEF:** Commonly occurs when water gets trapped in the ear after swimming.
**H60.331 Swimmer's ear, right ear**
**H60.332 Swimmer's ear, left ear**
**H60.333 Swimmer's ear, bilateral**
**H60.339 Swimmer's ear, unspecified ear**

✓6th **H60.39 Other infective otitis externa**
**H60.391 Other infective otitis externa, right ear**
**H60.392 Other infective otitis externa, left ear**
**H60.393 Other infective otitis externa, bilateral**
**H60.399 Other infective otitis externa, unspecified ear**

✓5th **H60.4 Cholesteatoma of external ear**
Keratosis obturans of external ear (canal)
EXCLUDES 2 *cholesteatoma of middle ear (H71.-)*
*recurrent cholesteatoma of postmastoidectomy cavity (H95.0-)*
**DEF:** Cholesteatoma: Noncancerous cyst-like mass of cell debris, including cholesterol and epithelial cells resulting from trauma, repeated or improperly healed infections, and congenital enclosure of epidermal cells.
**H60.40 Cholesteatoma of external ear, unspecified ear**
**H60.41 Cholesteatoma of right external ear**
**H60.42 Cholesteatoma of left external ear**
**H60.43 Cholesteatoma of external ear, bilateral**

✓5th **H60.5 Acute noninfective otitis externa**

✓6th **H60.50 Unspecified acute noninfective otitis externa**
Acute otitis externa NOS
**H60.501 Unspecified acute noninfective otitis externa, right ear**
**H60.502 Unspecified acute noninfective otitis externa, left ear**
**H60.503 Unspecified acute noninfective otitis externa, bilateral**
**H60.509 Unspecified acute noninfective otitis externa, unspecified ear**

✓6th **H60.51 Acute actinic otitis externa**
**H60.511 Acute actinic otitis externa, right ear**
**H60.512 Acute actinic otitis externa, left ear**
**H60.513 Acute actinic otitis externa, bilateral**
**H60.519 Acute actinic otitis externa, unspecified ear**

✓6th **H60.52 Acute chemical otitis externa**
**H60.521 Acute chemical otitis externa, right ear**
**H60.522 Acute chemical otitis externa, left ear**
**H60.523 Acute chemical otitis externa, bilateral**
**H60.529 Acute chemical otitis externa, unspecified ear**

✓6th **H60.53 Acute contact otitis externa**
**H60.531 Acute contact otitis externa, right ear**
**H60.532 Acute contact otitis externa, left ear**
**H60.533 Acute contact otitis externa, bilateral**
**H60.539 Acute contact otitis externa, unspecified ear**

✓6th **H60.54 Acute eczematoid otitis externa**
**H60.541 Acute eczematoid otitis externa, right ear**
**H60.542 Acute eczematoid otitis externa, left ear**
**H60.543 Acute eczematoid otitis externa, bilateral**
**H60.549 Acute eczematoid otitis externa, unspecified ear**

✓6th **H60.55 Acute reactive otitis externa**
**H60.551 Acute reactive otitis externa, right ear**
**H60.552 Acute reactive otitis externa, left ear**
**H60.553 Acute reactive otitis externa, bilateral**
**H60.559 Acute reactive otitis externa, unspecified ear**

✓6th **H60.59 Other noninfective acute otitis externa**
**H60.591 Other noninfective acute otitis externa, right ear**
**H60.592 Other noninfective acute otitis externa, left ear**
**H60.593 Other noninfective acute otitis externa, bilateral**
**H60.599 Other noninfective acute otitis externa, unspecified ear**

✓5th **H60.6 Unspecified chronic otitis externa**
**H60.60 Unspecified chronic otitis externa, unspecified ear**
**H60.61 Unspecified chronic otitis externa, right ear**
**H60.62 Unspecified chronic otitis externa, left ear**
**H60.63 Unspecified chronic otitis externa, bilateral**

✓5th **H60.8 Other otitis externa**

✓6th **H60.8X Other otitis externa**
**H60.8X1 Other otitis externa, right ear**
**H60.8X2 Other otitis externa, left ear**
**H60.8X3 Other otitis externa, bilateral**
**H60.8X9 Other otitis externa, unspecified ear**

✓5th **H60.9 Unspecified otitis externa**
**H60.90 Unspecified otitis externa, unspecified ear**
**H60.91 Unspecified otitis externa, right ear**

H60.92 Unspecified otitis externa, left ear
H60.93 Unspecified otitis externa, bilateral

**H61 Other disorders of external ear**

**H61.0 Chondritis and perichondritis of external ear**
Chondrodermatitis nodularis chronica helicis
Perichondritis of auricle
Perichondritis of pinna

H61.00 Unspecified perichondritis of external ear
H61.001 Unspecified perichondritis of right external ear
H61.002 Unspecified perichondritis of left external ear
H61.003 Unspecified perichondritis of external ear, bilateral
H61.009 Unspecified perichondritis of external ear, unspecified ear

H61.01 Acute perichondritis of external ear
H61.011 Acute perichondritis of right external ear
H61.012 Acute perichondritis of left external ear
H61.013 Acute perichondritis of external ear, bilateral
H61.019 Acute perichondritis of external ear, unspecified ear

H61.02 Chronic perichondritis of external ear
H61.021 Chronic perichondritis of right external ear
H61.022 Chronic perichondritis of left external ear
H61.023 Chronic perichondritis of external ear, bilateral
H61.029 Chronic perichondritis of external ear, unspecified ear

H61.03 Chondritis of external ear
Chondritis of auricle
Chondritis of pinna
**AHA:** 2015,1Q,18
**DEF:** Infection that has progressed into the cartilage and presents as indurated and edematous skin over the pinna. Vascular compromise occurs with tissue necrosis and deformity.
H61.031 Chondritis of right external ear
H61.032 Chondritis of left external ear
H61.033 Chondritis of external ear, bilateral
H61.039 Chondritis of external ear, unspecified ear

**H61.1 Noninfective disorders of pinna**
EXCLUDES 2 *cauliflower ear (M95.1-)*
*gouty tophi of ear (M1A.-)*

H61.10 Unspecified noninfective disorders of pinna
Disorder of pinna NOS
H61.101 Unspecified noninfective disorders of pinna, right ear
H61.102 Unspecified noninfective disorders of pinna, left ear
H61.103 Unspecified noninfective disorders of pinna, bilateral
H61.109 Unspecified noninfective disorders of pinna, unspecified ear

H61.11 Acquired deformity of pinna
Acquired deformity of auricle
EXCLUDES 2 *cauliflower ear (M95.1-)*
H61.111 Acquired deformity of pinna, right ear
H61.112 Acquired deformity of pinna, left ear
H61.113 Acquired deformity of pinna, bilateral
H61.119 Acquired deformity of pinna, unspecified ear

H61.12 Hematoma of pinna
Hematoma of auricle
H61.121 Hematoma of pinna, right ear
H61.122 Hematoma of pinna, left ear
H61.123 Hematoma of pinna, bilateral
H61.129 Hematoma of pinna, unspecified ear

H61.19 Other noninfective disorders of pinna
H61.191 Noninfective disorders of pinna, right ear
H61.192 Noninfective disorders of pinna, left ear
H61.193 Noninfective disorders of pinna, bilateral
H61.199 Noninfective disorders of pinna, unspecified ear

**H61.2 Impacted cerumen**
Wax in ear
H61.20 Impacted cerumen, unspecified ear
H61.21 Impacted cerumen, right ear
H61.22 Impacted cerumen, left ear
H61.23 Impacted cerumen, bilateral

**H61.3 Acquired stenosis of external ear canal**
Collapse of external ear canal
EXCLUDES 1 *postprocedural stenosis of external ear canal (H95.81-)*

H61.30 Acquired stenosis of external ear canal, unspecified
H61.301 Acquired stenosis of right external ear canal, unspecified
H61.302 Acquired stenosis of left external ear canal, unspecified
H61.303 Acquired stenosis of external ear canal, unspecified, bilateral
H61.309 Acquired stenosis of external ear canal, unspecified, unspecified ear

H61.31 Acquired stenosis of external ear canal secondary to trauma
H61.311 Acquired stenosis of right external ear canal secondary to trauma
H61.312 Acquired stenosis of left external ear canal secondary to trauma
H61.313 Acquired stenosis of external ear canal secondary to trauma, bilateral
H61.319 Acquired stenosis of external ear canal secondary to trauma, unspecified ear

H61.32 Acquired stenosis of external ear canal secondary to inflammation and infection
**DEF:** Narrowing of the external ear canal due to chronic inflammation or infection.
H61.321 Acquired stenosis of right external ear canal secondary to inflammation and infection
H61.322 Acquired stenosis of left external ear canal secondary to inflammation and infection
H61.323 Acquired stenosis of external ear canal secondary to inflammation and infection, bilateral
H61.329 Acquired stenosis of external ear canal secondary to inflammation and infection, unspecified ear

H61.39 Other acquired stenosis of external ear canal
H61.391 Other acquired stenosis of right external ear canal
H61.392 Other acquired stenosis of left external ear canal
H61.393 Other acquired stenosis of external ear canal, bilateral
H61.399 Other acquired stenosis of external ear canal, unspecified ear

**H61.8 Other specified disorders of external ear**

H61.81 Exostosis of external canal
H61.811 Exostosis of right external canal
H61.812 Exostosis of left external canal
H61.813 Exostosis of external canal, bilateral
H61.819 Exostosis of external canal, unspecified ear

H61.89 Other specified disorders of external ear
H61.891 Other specified disorders of right external ear
H61.892 Other specified disorders of left external ear
H61.893 Other specified disorders of external ear, bilateral
H61.899 Other specified disorders of external ear, unspecified ear

**H61.9 Disorder of external ear, unspecified**
H61.90 Disorder of external ear, unspecified, unspecified ear
H61.91 Disorder of right external ear, unspecified
H61.92 Disorder of left external ear, unspecified
H61.93 Disorder of external ear, unspecified, bilateral

**H62 Disorders of external ear in diseases classified elsewhere**

**H62.4 Otitis externa in other diseases classified elsewhere**
Code first underlying disease, such as:
erysipelas (A46)
impetigo (L01.0-)
EXCLUDES 1 *otitis externa (in):*
*candidiasis (B37.84)*
*herpes viral [herpes simplex] (B00.1)*
*herpes zoster (B02.8)*
H62.40 *Otitis externa in other diseases classified elsewhere, unspecified ear*

Chapter 8. Diseases of the Ear and Mastoid Process
H60.92–H62.40

H62.41 *Otitis externa in other diseases classified elsewhere, right ear*
H62.42 *Otitis externa in other diseases classified elsewhere, left ear*
H62.43 *Otitis externa in other diseases classified elsewhere, bilateral*

√5th **H62.8 Other disorders of external ear in diseases classified elsewhere**
Code first underlying disease, such as:
gout (M1A.-, M10.-)

√6th **H62.8X Other disorders of external ear in diseases classified elsewhere**
H62.8X1 *Other disorders of right external ear in diseases classified elsewhere*
H62.8X2 *Other disorders of left external ear in diseases classified elsewhere*
H62.8X3 *Other disorders of external ear in diseases classified elsewhere, bilateral*
H62.8X9 *Other disorders of external ear in diseases classified elsewhere, unspecified ear*

## Diseases of middle ear and mastoid (H65-H75)

√4th **H65 Nonsuppurative otitis media**
INCLUDES nonsuppurative otitis media with myringitis
Use additional code for any associated perforated tympanic membrane (H72.-)
Use additional code, if applicable, to identify:
exposure to environmental tobacco smoke (Z77.22)
exposure to tobacco smoke in the perinatal period (P96.81)
history of tobacco dependence (Z87.891)
infectious agent (B95-B97)
occupational exposure to environmental tobacco smoke (Z57.31)
tobacco dependence (F17.-)
tobacco use (Z72.0)

√5th **H65.0 Acute serous otitis media**
Acute and subacute secretory otitis
**H65.00 Acute serous otitis media, unspecified ear**
**H65.01 Acute serous otitis media, right ear**
**H65.02 Acute serous otitis media, left ear**
**H65.03 Acute serous otitis media, bilateral**
**H65.04 Acute serous otitis media, recurrent, right ear**
**H65.05 Acute serous otitis media, recurrent, left ear**
**H65.06 Acute serous otitis media, recurrent, bilateral**
**H65.07 Acute serous otitis media, recurrent, unspecified ear**

√5th **H65.1 Other acute nonsuppurative otitis media**
EXCLUDES 1 *otitic barotrauma (T70.0)*
*otitis media (acute) NOS (H66.9)*

√6th **H65.11 Acute and subacute allergic otitis media (mucoid) (sanguinous) (serous)**
**H65.111 Acute and subacute allergic otitis media (mucoid) (sanguinous) (serous), right ear**
**H65.112 Acute and subacute allergic otitis media (mucoid) (sanguinous) (serous), left ear**
**H65.113 Acute and subacute allergic otitis media (mucoid) (sanguinous) (serous), bilateral**
**H65.114 Acute and subacute allergic otitis media (mucoid) (sanguinous) (serous), recurrent, right ear**
**H65.115 Acute and subacute allergic otitis media (mucoid) (sanguinous) (serous), recurrent, left ear**
**H65.116 Acute and subacute allergic otitis media (mucoid) (sanguinous) (serous), recurrent, bilateral**
**H65.117 Acute and subacute allergic otitis media (mucoid) (sanguinous) (serous), recurrent, unspecified ear**
**H65.119 Acute and subacute allergic otitis media (mucoid) (sanguinous) (serous), unspecified ear**

√6th **H65.19 Other acute nonsuppurative otitis media**
Acute and subacute mucoid otitis media
Acute and subacute nonsuppurative otitis media NOS
Acute and subacute sanguinous otitis media
Acute and subacute seromucinous otitis media
**H65.191 Other acute nonsuppurative otitis media, right ear**
**H65.192 Other acute nonsuppurative otitis media, left ear**
**H65.193 Other acute nonsuppurative otitis media, bilateral**
**H65.194 Other acute nonsuppurative otitis media, recurrent, right ear**
**H65.195 Other acute nonsuppurative otitis media, recurrent, left ear**
**H65.196 Other acute nonsuppurative otitis media, recurrent, bilateral**
**H65.197 Other acute nonsuppurative otitis media recurrent, unspecified ear**
**H65.199 Other acute nonsuppurative otitis media, unspecified ear**

√5th **H65.2 Chronic serous otitis media**
Chronic tubotympanal catarrh
**H65.20 Chronic serous otitis media, unspecified ear**
**H65.21 Chronic serous otitis media, right ear**
**H65.22 Chronic serous otitis media, left ear**
**H65.23 Chronic serous otitis media, bilateral**

√5th **H65.3 Chronic mucoid otitis media**
Chronic mucinous otitis media
Chronic secretory otitis media
Chronic transudative otitis media
Glue ear
EXCLUDES 1 *adhesive middle ear disease (H74.1)*
**H65.30 Chronic mucoid otitis media, unspecified ear**
**H65.31 Chronic mucoid otitis media, right ear**
**H65.32 Chronic mucoid otitis media, left ear**
**H65.33 Chronic mucoid otitis media, bilateral**

√5th **H65.4 Other chronic nonsuppurative otitis media**
√6th **H65.41 Chronic allergic otitis media**
**H65.411 Chronic allergic otitis media, right ear**
**H65.412 Chronic allergic otitis media, left ear**
**H65.413 Chronic allergic otitis media, bilateral**
**H65.419 Chronic allergic otitis media, unspecified ear**

√6th **H65.49 Other chronic nonsuppurative otitis media**
Chronic exudative otitis media
Chronic nonsuppurative otitis media NOS
Chronic otitis media with effusion (nonpurulent)
Chronic seromucinous otitis media
**H65.491 Other chronic nonsuppurative otitis media, right ear**
**H65.492 Other chronic nonsuppurative otitis media, left ear**
**H65.493 Other chronic nonsuppurative otitis media, bilateral**
**H65.499 Other chronic nonsuppurative otitis media, unspecified ear**

√5th **H65.9 Unspecified nonsuppurative otitis media**
Allergic otitis media NOS
Catarrhal otitis media NOS
Exudative otitis media NOS
Mucoid otitis media NOS
Otitis media with effusion (nonpurulent) NOS
Secretory otitis media NOS
Seromucinous otitis media NOS
Serous otitis media NOS
Transudative otitis media NOS
**H65.90 Unspecified nonsuppurative otitis media, unspecified ear**
**H65.91 Unspecified nonsuppurative otitis media, right ear**
**H65.92 Unspecified nonsuppurative otitis media, left ear**
**H65.93 Unspecified nonsuppurative otitis media, bilateral**

√4th **H66 Suppurative and unspecified otitis media**
INCLUDES suppurative and unspecified otitis media with myringitis
Use additional code to identify:
exposure to environmental tobacco smoke (Z77.22)
exposure to tobacco smoke in the perinatal period (P96.81)
history of tobacco dependence (Z87.891)
occupational exposure to environmental tobacco smoke (Z57.31)
tobacco dependence (F17.-)
tobacco use (Z72.0)
**AHA:** 2016,1Q,34

√5th **H66.0 Acute suppurative otitis media**
√6th **H66.00 Acute suppurative otitis media without spontaneous rupture of ear drum**
**H66.001 Acute suppurative otitis media without spontaneous rupture of ear drum, right ear**
**H66.002 Acute suppurative otitis media without spontaneous rupture of ear drum, left ear**

H66.ØØ3 Acute suppurative otitis media without spontaneous rupture of ear drum, bilateral
H66.ØØ4 Acute suppurative otitis media without spontaneous rupture of ear drum, recurrent, right ear
H66.ØØ5 Acute suppurative otitis media without spontaneous rupture of ear drum, recurrent, left ear
H66.ØØ6 Acute suppurative otitis media without spontaneous rupture of ear drum, recurrent, bilateral
H66.ØØ7 Acute suppurative otitis media without spontaneous rupture of ear drum, recurrent, unspecified ear
H66.ØØ9 Acute suppurative otitis media without spontaneous rupture of ear drum, unspecified ear

√6th H66.Ø1 Acute suppurative otitis media with spontaneous rupture of ear drum
DEF: Sudden, severe inflammation of the middle ear, causing pressure that perforates the ear drum tissue.
H66.Ø11 Acute suppurative otitis media with spontaneous rupture of ear drum, right ear
H66.Ø12 Acute suppurative otitis media with spontaneous rupture of ear drum, left ear
H66.Ø13 Acute suppurative otitis media with spontaneous rupture of ear drum, bilateral
H66.Ø14 Acute suppurative otitis media with spontaneous rupture of ear drum, recurrent, right ear
H66.Ø15 Acute suppurative otitis media with spontaneous rupture of ear drum, recurrent, left ear
H66.Ø16 Acute suppurative otitis media with spontaneous rupture of ear drum, recurrent, bilateral
H66.Ø17 Acute suppurative otitis media with spontaneous rupture of ear drum, recurrent, unspecified ear
H66.Ø19 Acute suppurative otitis media with spontaneous rupture of ear drum, unspecified ear

√5th H66.1 Chronic tubotympanic suppurative otitis media
Benign chronic suppurative otitis media
Chronic tubotympanic disease
Use additional code for any associated perforated tympanic membrane (H72.-)
H66.1Ø Chronic tubotympanic suppurative otitis media, unspecified
H66.11 Chronic tubotympanic suppurative otitis media, right ear
H66.12 Chronic tubotympanic suppurative otitis media, left ear
H66.13 Chronic tubotympanic suppurative otitis media, bilateral

√5th H66.2 Chronic atticoantral suppurative otitis media
Chronic atticoantral disease
Use additional code for any associated perforated tympanic membrane (H72.-)
H66.2Ø Chronic atticoantral suppurative otitis media, unspecified ear
H66.21 Chronic atticoantral suppurative otitis media, right ear
H66.22 Chronic atticoantral suppurative otitis media, left ear
H66.23 Chronic atticoantral suppurative otitis media, bilateral

√5th H66.3 Other chronic suppurative otitis media
Chronic suppurative otitis media NOS
Use additional code for any associated perforated tympanic membrane (H72.-)
EXCLUDES 1 *tuberculous otitis media (A18.6)*

√6th H66.3X Other chronic suppurative otitis media
H66.3X1 Other chronic suppurative otitis media, right ear
H66.3X2 Other chronic suppurative otitis media, left ear
H66.3X3 Other chronic suppurative otitis media, bilateral
H66.3X9 Other chronic suppurative otitis media, unspecified ear

√5th H66.4 Suppurative otitis media, unspecified
Purulent otitis media NOS
Use additional code for any associated perforated tympanic membrane (H72.-)
H66.4Ø Suppurative otitis media, unspecified, unspecified ear
H66.41 Suppurative otitis media, unspecified, right ear
H66.42 Suppurative otitis media, unspecified, left ear
H66.43 Suppurative otitis media, unspecified, bilateral

√5th H66.9 Otitis media, unspecified
Acute otitis media NOS
Chronic otitis media NOS
Otitis media NOS
Use additional code for any associated perforated tympanic membrane (H72.-)
H66.9Ø Otitis media, unspecified, unspecified ear
H66.91 Otitis media, unspecified, right ear
H66.92 Otitis media, unspecified, left ear
H66.93 Otitis media, unspecified, bilateral

√4th **H67 Otitis media in diseases classified elsewhere**
Code first underlying disease, such as:
plasminogen deficiency (E88.Ø2)
viral disease NEC (BØØ-B34)
Use additional code for any associated perforated tympanic membrane (H72.-)
EXCLUDES 1 *otitis media in:*
*influenza (JØ9.X9, J1Ø.83, J11.83)*
*measles (BØ5.3)*
*scarlet fever (A38.Ø)*
*tuberculosis (A18.6)*
*H67.1 Otitis media in diseases classified elsewhere, right ear*
*H67.2 Otitis media in diseases classified elsewhere, left ear*
*H67.3 Otitis media in diseases classified elsewhere, bilateral*
*H67.9 Otitis media in diseases classified elsewhere, unspecified ear*

√4th **H68 Eustachian salpingitis and obstruction**
DEF: Eustachian tube: Internal channel between the tympanic cavity and the nasopharynx that equalizes internal pressure to the outside pressure and drains mucous production from the middle ear.

√5th H68.Ø Eustachian salpingitis
√6th H68.ØØ Unspecified Eustachian salpingitis
H68.ØØ1 Unspecified Eustachian salpingitis, right ear
H68.ØØ2 Unspecified Eustachian salpingitis, left ear
H68.ØØ3 Unspecified Eustachian salpingitis, bilateral
H68.ØØ9 Unspecified Eustachian salpingitis, unspecified ear
√6th H68.Ø1 Acute Eustachian salpingitis
H68.Ø11 Acute Eustachian salpingitis, right ear
H68.Ø12 Acute Eustachian salpingitis, left ear
H68.Ø13 Acute Eustachian salpingitis, bilateral
H68.Ø19 Acute Eustachian salpingitis, unspecified ear
√6th H68.Ø2 Chronic Eustachian salpingitis
H68.Ø21 Chronic Eustachian salpingitis, right ear
H68.Ø22 Chronic Eustachian salpingitis, left ear
H68.Ø23 Chronic Eustachian salpingitis, bilateral
H68.Ø29 Chronic Eustachian salpingitis, unspecified ear

√5th H68.1 Obstruction of Eustachian tube
Stenosis of Eustachian tube
Stricture of Eustachian tube
√6th H68.1Ø Unspecified obstruction of Eustachian tube
H68.1Ø1 Unspecified obstruction of Eustachian tube, right ear
H68.1Ø2 Unspecified obstruction of Eustachian tube, left ear
H68.1Ø3 Unspecified obstruction of Eustachian tube, bilateral
H68.1Ø9 Unspecified obstruction of Eustachian tube, unspecified ear
√6th H68.11 Osseous obstruction of Eustachian tube
H68.111 Osseous obstruction of Eustachian tube, right ear
H68.112 Osseous obstruction of Eustachian tube, left ear
H68.113 Osseous obstruction of Eustachian tube, bilateral

H68.119 Osseous obstruction of Eustachian tube, unspecified ear

✓6th H68.12 Intrinsic cartilagenous obstruction of Eustachian tube

H68.121 Intrinsic cartilagenous obstruction of Eustachian tube, right ear

H68.122 Intrinsic cartilagenous obstruction of Eustachian tube, left ear

H68.123 Intrinsic cartilagenous obstruction of Eustachian tube, bilateral

H68.129 Intrinsic cartilagenous obstruction of Eustachian tube, unspecified ear

✓6th H68.13 Extrinsic cartilagenous obstruction of Eustachian tube

Compression of Eustachian tube

H68.131 Extrinsic cartilagenous obstruction of Eustachian tube, right ear

H68.132 Extrinsic cartilagenous obstruction of Eustachian tube, left ear

H68.133 Extrinsic cartilagenous obstruction of Eustachian tube, bilateral

H68.139 Extrinsic cartilagenous obstruction of Eustachian tube, unspecified ear

✓4th **H69 Other and unspecified disorders of Eustachian tube**

**DEF:** Eustachian tube: Internal channel between the tympanic cavity and the nasopharynx that equalizes internal pressure to the outside pressure and drains mucous production from the middle ear.

✓5th H69.0 Patulous Eustachian tube

H69.00 Patulous Eustachian tube, unspecified ear

H69.01 Patulous Eustachian tube, right ear

H69.02 Patulous Eustachian tube, left ear

H69.03 Patulous Eustachian tube, bilateral

✓5th H69.8 Other specified disorders of Eustachian tube

H69.80 Other specified disorders of Eustachian tube, unspecified ear

H69.81 Other specified disorders of Eustachian tube, right ear

H69.82 Other specified disorders of Eustachian tube, left ear

H69.83 Other specified disorders of Eustachian tube, bilateral

✓5th H69.9 Unspecified Eustachian tube disorder

H69.90 Unspecified Eustachian tube disorder, unspecified ear

H69.91 Unspecified Eustachian tube disorder, right ear

H69.92 Unspecified Eustachian tube disorder, left ear

H69.93 Unspecified Eustachian tube disorder, bilateral

✓4th **H70 Mastoiditis and related conditions**

✓5th H70.0 Acute mastoiditis

Abscess of mastoid
Empyema of mastoid

✓6th H70.00 Acute mastoiditis without complications

H70.001 Acute mastoiditis without complications, right ear

H70.002 Acute mastoiditis without complications, left ear

H70.003 Acute mastoiditis without complications, bilateral

H70.009 Acute mastoiditis without complications, unspecified ear

✓6th H70.01 Subperiosteal abscess of mastoid

H70.011 Subperiosteal abscess of mastoid, right ear

H70.012 Subperiosteal abscess of mastoid, left ear

H70.013 Subperiosteal abscess of mastoid, bilateral

H70.019 Subperiosteal abscess of mastoid, unspecified ear

✓6th H70.09 Acute mastoiditis with other complications

H70.091 Acute mastoiditis with other complications, right ear

H70.092 Acute mastoiditis with other complications, left ear

H70.093 Acute mastoiditis with other complications, bilateral

H70.099 Acute mastoiditis with other complications, unspecified ear

✓5th H70.1 Chronic mastoiditis

Caries of mastoid
Fistula of mastoid

EXCLUDES 1 *tuberculous mastoiditis (A18.03)*

H70.10 Chronic mastoiditis, unspecified ear

H70.11 Chronic mastoiditis, right ear

H70.12 Chronic mastoiditis, left ear

H70.13 Chronic mastoiditis, bilateral

✓5th H70.2 Petrositis

Inflammation of petrous bone

✓6th H70.20 Unspecified petrositis

H70.201 Unspecified petrositis, right ear

H70.202 Unspecified petrositis, left ear

H70.203 Unspecified petrositis, bilateral

H70.209 Unspecified petrositis, unspecified ear

✓6th H70.21 Acute petrositis

**DEF:** Sudden, severe inflammation of the petrous temporal bone behind the ear, associated with a middle ear infection.

H70.211 Acute petrositis, right ear

H70.212 Acute petrositis, left ear

H70.213 Acute petrositis, bilateral

H70.219 Acute petrositis, unspecified ear

✓6th H70.22 Chronic petrositis

H70.221 Chronic petrositis, right ear

H70.222 Chronic petrositis, left ear

H70.223 Chronic petrositis, bilateral

H70.229 Chronic petrositis, unspecified ear

✓5th H70.8 Other mastoiditis and related conditions

EXCLUDES 1 *preauricular sinus and cyst (Q18.1)*
*sinus, fistula, and cyst of branchial cleft (Q18.0)*

✓6th H70.81 Postauricular fistula

H70.811 Postauricular fistula, right ear

H70.812 Postauricular fistula, left ear

H70.813 Postauricular fistula, bilateral

H70.819 Postauricular fistula, unspecified ear

✓6th H70.89 Other mastoiditis and related conditions

H70.891 Other mastoiditis and related conditions, right ear

H70.892 Other mastoiditis and related conditions, left ear

H70.893 Other mastoiditis and related conditions, bilateral

H70.899 Other mastoiditis and related conditions, unspecified ear

✓5th H70.9 Unspecified mastoiditis

H70.90 Unspecified mastoiditis, unspecified ear

H70.91 Unspecified mastoiditis, right ear

H70.92 Unspecified mastoiditis, left ear

H70.93 Unspecified mastoiditis, bilateral

✓4th **H71 Cholesteatoma of middle ear**

EXCLUDES 2 *cholesteatoma of external ear (H60.4-)*
*recurrent cholesteatoma of postmastoidectomy cavity (H95.0-)*

**AHA:** 2021,3Q,8

**DEF:** Cholesteatoma: Noncancerous cyst-like mass of cell debris, including cholesterol and epithelial cells resulting from trauma, repeated or improperly healed infections, and congenital enclosure of epidermal cells.

**Cholesteatoma of Middle Ear**

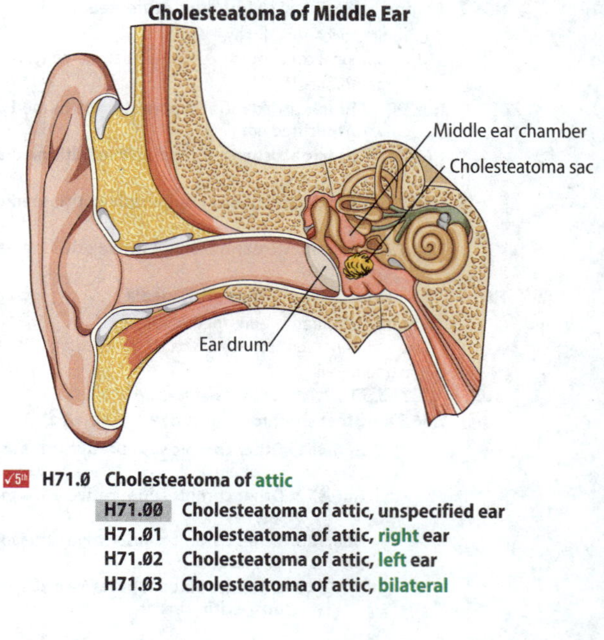


✓5th H71.0 Cholesteatoma of attic

H71.00 Cholesteatoma of attic, unspecified ear

H71.01 Cholesteatoma of attic, right ear

H71.02 Cholesteatoma of attic, left ear

H71.03 Cholesteatoma of attic, bilateral

**H71.1 Cholesteatoma of tympanum**
- H71.10 Cholesteatoma of tympanum, unspecified ear
- H71.11 Cholesteatoma of tympanum, right ear
- H71.12 Cholesteatoma of tympanum, left ear
- H71.13 Cholesteatoma of tympanum, bilateral

**H71.2 Cholesteatoma of mastoid**
- H71.20 Cholesteatoma of mastoid, unspecified ear
- H71.21 Cholesteatoma of mastoid, right ear
- H71.22 Cholesteatoma of mastoid, left ear
- H71.23 Cholesteatoma of mastoid, bilateral

**H71.3 Diffuse cholesteatosis**

AHA: 2021,3Q,8
- H71.30 Diffuse cholesteatosis, unspecified ear
- H71.31 Diffuse cholesteatosis, right ear
- H71.32 Diffuse cholesteatosis, left ear
- H71.33 Diffuse cholesteatosis, bilateral

**H71.9 Unspecified cholesteatoma**
- H71.90 Unspecified cholesteatoma, unspecified ear
- H71.91 Unspecified cholesteatoma, right ear
- H71.92 Unspecified cholesteatoma, left ear
- H71.93 Unspecified cholesteatoma, bilateral

## H72 Perforation of tympanic membrane

INCLUDES persistent post-traumatic perforation of ear drum
postinflammatory perforation of ear drum

Code first any associated otitis media (H65.-, H66.1-, H66.2-, H66.3-, H66.4-, H66.9-, H67.-)

EXCLUDES 1 *acute suppurative otitis media with rupture of the tympanic membrane (H66.01-)*
*traumatic rupture of ear drum (S09.2-)*

**H72.0 Central perforation of tympanic membrane**
- H72.00 Central perforation of tympanic membrane, unspecified ear
- H72.01 Central perforation of tympanic membrane, right ear
- H72.02 Central perforation of tympanic membrane, left ear
- H72.03 Central perforation of tympanic membrane, bilateral

**H72.1 Attic perforation of tympanic membrane**

Perforation of pars flaccida
- H72.10 Attic perforation of tympanic membrane, unspecified ear
- H72.11 Attic perforation of tympanic membrane, right ear
- H72.12 Attic perforation of tympanic membrane, left ear
- H72.13 Attic perforation of tympanic membrane, bilateral

**H72.2 Other marginal perforations of tympanic membrane**

**H72.2X Other marginal perforations of tympanic membrane**
- H72.2X1 Other marginal perforations of tympanic membrane, right ear
- H72.2X2 Other marginal perforations of tympanic membrane, left ear
- H72.2X3 Other marginal perforations of tympanic membrane, bilateral
- H72.2X9 Other marginal perforations of tympanic membrane, unspecified ear

**H72.8 Other perforations of tympanic membrane**

**H72.81 Multiple perforations of tympanic membrane**
- H72.811 Multiple perforations of tympanic membrane, right ear
- H72.812 Multiple perforations of tympanic membrane, left ear
- H72.813 Multiple perforations of tympanic membrane, bilateral
- H72.819 Multiple perforations of tympanic membrane, unspecified ear

**H72.82 Total perforations of tympanic membrane**
- H72.821 Total perforations of tympanic membrane, right ear
- H72.822 Total perforations of tympanic membrane, left ear
- H72.823 Total perforations of tympanic membrane, bilateral
- H72.829 Total perforations of tympanic membrane, unspecified ear

**H72.9 Unspecified perforation of tympanic membrane**
- H72.90 Unspecified perforation of tympanic membrane, unspecified ear
- H72.91 Unspecified perforation of tympanic membrane, right ear
- H72.92 Unspecified perforation of tympanic membrane, left ear
- H72.93 Unspecified perforation of tympanic membrane, bilateral

## H73 Other disorders of tympanic membrane

**H73.0 Acute myringitis**

EXCLUDES 1 *acute myringitis with otitis media (H65, H66)*

**H73.00 Unspecified acute myringitis**

Acute tympanitis NOS
- H73.001 Acute myringitis, right ear
- H73.002 Acute myringitis, left ear
- H73.003 Acute myringitis, bilateral
- H73.009 Acute myringitis, unspecified ear

**H73.01 Bullous myringitis**

DEF: Bacterial or viral otitis media that is characterized by the appearance of serous or hemorrhagic blebs on the ear drum and sudden onset of severe pain in ear.
- H73.011 Bullous myringitis, right ear
- H73.012 Bullous myringitis, left ear
- H73.013 Bullous myringitis, bilateral
- H73.019 Bullous myringitis, unspecified ear

**H73.09 Other acute myringitis**
- H73.091 Other acute myringitis, right ear
- H73.092 Other acute myringitis, left ear
- H73.093 Other acute myringitis, bilateral
- H73.099 Other acute myringitis, unspecified ear

**H73.1 Chronic myringitis**

Chronic tympanitis

EXCLUDES 1 *chronic myringitis with otitis media (H65, H66)*
- H73.10 Chronic myringitis, unspecified ear
- H73.11 Chronic myringitis, right ear
- H73.12 Chronic myringitis, left ear
- H73.13 Chronic myringitis, bilateral

**H73.2 Unspecified myringitis**
- H73.20 Unspecified myringitis, unspecified ear
- H73.21 Unspecified myringitis, right ear
- H73.22 Unspecified myringitis, left ear
- H73.23 Unspecified myringitis, bilateral

**H73.8 Other specified disorders of tympanic membrane**

**H73.81 Atrophic flaccid tympanic membrane**
- H73.811 Atrophic flaccid tympanic membrane, right ear
- H73.812 Atrophic flaccid tympanic membrane, left ear
- H73.813 Atrophic flaccid tympanic membrane, bilateral
- H73.819 Atrophic flaccid tympanic membrane, unspecified ear

**H73.82 Atrophic nonflaccid tympanic membrane**
- H73.821 Atrophic nonflaccid tympanic membrane, right ear
- H73.822 Atrophic nonflaccid tympanic membrane, left ear
- H73.823 Atrophic nonflaccid tympanic membrane, bilateral
- H73.829 Atrophic nonflaccid tympanic membrane, unspecified ear

**H73.89 Other specified disorders of tympanic membrane**
- H73.891 Other specified disorders of tympanic membrane, right ear
- H73.892 Other specified disorders of tympanic membrane, left ear
- H73.893 Other specified disorders of tympanic membrane, bilateral
- H73.899 Other specified disorders of tympanic membrane, unspecified ear

**H73.9 Unspecified disorder of tympanic membrane**
- H73.90 Unspecified disorder of tympanic membrane, unspecified ear
- H73.91 Unspecified disorder of tympanic membrane, right ear
- H73.92 Unspecified disorder of tympanic membrane, left ear
- H73.93 Unspecified disorder of tympanic membrane, bilateral

**H74 Other disorders of middle ear mastoid**

EXCLUDES 2 *mastoiditis (H70.-)*

**H74.0 Tympanosclerosis**

DEF: Calcification of tissue in the ear drum, middle ear bones, and middle ear canal.

**H74.01 Tympanosclerosis, right ear**
**H74.02 Tympanosclerosis, left ear**
**H74.03 Tympanosclerosis, bilateral**
**H74.09 Tympanosclerosis, unspecified ear**

**H74.1 Adhesive middle ear disease**

Adhesive otitis

EXCLUDES 1 *glue ear (H65.3-)*

**H74.11 Adhesive right middle ear disease**
**H74.12 Adhesive left middle ear disease**
**H74.13 Adhesive middle ear disease, bilateral**
**H74.19 Adhesive middle ear disease, unspecified ear**

**H74.2 Discontinuity and dislocation of ear ossicles**

**H74.20 Discontinuity and dislocation of ear ossicles, unspecified ear**
**H74.21 Discontinuity and dislocation of right ear ossicles**
**H74.22 Discontinuity and dislocation of left ear ossicles**
**H74.23 Discontinuity and dislocation of ear ossicles, bilateral**

**H74.3 Other acquired abnormalities of ear ossicles**

**H74.31 Ankylosis of ear ossicles**

**H74.311 Ankylosis of ear ossicles, right ear**
**H74.312 Ankylosis of ear ossicles, left ear**
**H74.313 Ankylosis of ear ossicles, bilateral**
**H74.319 Ankylosis of ear ossicles, unspecified ear**

**H74.32 Partial loss of ear ossicles**

**H74.321 Partial loss of ear ossicles, right ear**
**H74.322 Partial loss of ear ossicles, left ear**
**H74.323 Partial loss of ear ossicles, bilateral**
**H74.329 Partial loss of ear ossicles, unspecified ear**

**H74.39 Other acquired abnormalities of ear ossicles**

**H74.391 Other acquired abnormalities of right ear ossicles**
**H74.392 Other acquired abnormalities of left ear ossicles**
**H74.393 Other acquired abnormalities of ear ossicles, bilateral**
**H74.399 Other acquired abnormalities of ear ossicles, unspecified ear**

**H74.4 Polyp of middle ear**

**H74.40 Polyp of middle ear, unspecified ear**
**H74.41 Polyp of right middle ear**
**H74.42 Polyp of left middle ear**
**H74.43 Polyp of middle ear, bilateral**

**H74.8 Other specified disorders of middle ear and mastoid**

**H74.8X Other specified disorders of middle ear and mastoid**

**H74.8X1 Other specified disorders of right middle ear and mastoid**
**H74.8X2 Other specified disorders of left middle ear and mastoid**
**H74.8X3 Other specified disorders of middle ear and mastoid, bilateral**
**H74.8X9 Other specified disorders of middle ear and mastoid, unspecified ear**

**H74.9 Unspecified disorder of middle ear and mastoid**

**H74.90 Unspecified disorder of middle ear and mastoid, unspecified ear**
**H74.91 Unspecified disorder of right middle ear and mastoid**
**H74.92 Unspecified disorder of left middle ear and mastoid**
**H74.93 Unspecified disorder of middle ear and mastoid, bilateral**

**H75 Other disorders of middle ear and mastoid in diseases classified elsewhere**

Code first underlying disease

**H75.0 Mastoiditis in infectious and parasitic diseases classified elsewhere**

EXCLUDES 1 *mastoiditis (in):*
*syphilis (A52.77)*
*tuberculosis (A18.03)*

***H75.00 Mastoiditis in infectious and parasitic diseases classified elsewhere, unspecified ear***
***H75.01 Mastoiditis in infectious and parasitic diseases classified elsewhere, right ear***
***H75.02 Mastoiditis in infectious and parasitic diseases classified elsewhere, left ear***
***H75.03 Mastoiditis in infectious and parasitic diseases classified elsewhere, bilateral***

**H75.8 Other specified disorders of middle ear and mastoid in diseases classified elsewhere**

***H75.80 Other specified disorders of middle ear and mastoid in diseases classified elsewhere, unspecified ear***
***H75.81 Other specified disorders of right middle ear and mastoid in diseases classified elsewhere***
***H75.82 Other specified disorders of left middle ear and mastoid in diseases classified elsewhere***
***H75.83 Other specified disorders of middle ear and mastoid in diseases classified elsewhere, bilateral***

## Diseases of inner ear (H80-H83)

**H80 Otosclerosis**

INCLUDES otospongiosis

**H80.0 Otosclerosis involving oval window, nonobliterative**

**H80.00 Otosclerosis involving oval window, nonobliterative, unspecified ear**
**H80.01 Otosclerosis involving oval window, nonobliterative, right ear**
**H80.02 Otosclerosis involving oval window, nonobliterative, left ear**
**H80.03 Otosclerosis involving oval window, nonobliterative, bilateral**

**H80.1 Otosclerosis involving oval window, obliterative**

**H80.10 Otosclerosis involving oval window, obliterative, unspecified ear**
**H80.11 Otosclerosis involving oval window, obliterative, right ear**
**H80.12 Otosclerosis involving oval window, obliterative, left ear**
**H80.13 Otosclerosis involving oval window, obliterative, bilateral**

**H80.2 Cochlear otosclerosis**

Otosclerosis involving otic capsule
Otosclerosis involving round window

**H80.20 Cochlear otosclerosis, unspecified ear**
**H80.21 Cochlear otosclerosis, right ear**
**H80.22 Cochlear otosclerosis, left ear**
**H80.23 Cochlear otosclerosis, bilateral**

**H80.8 Other otosclerosis**

**H80.80 Other otosclerosis, unspecified ear**
**H80.81 Other otosclerosis, right ear**
**H80.82 Other otosclerosis, left ear**
**H80.83 Other otosclerosis, bilateral**

**H80.9 Unspecified otosclerosis**

**H80.90 Unspecified otosclerosis, unspecified ear**
**H80.91 Unspecified otosclerosis, right ear**
**H80.92 Unspecified otosclerosis, left ear**
**H80.93 Unspecified otosclerosis, bilateral**

**H81 Disorders of vestibular function**

EXCLUDES 1 *epidemic vertigo (A88.1)*
*vertigo NOS (R42)*

**H81.0 Meniere's disease**

Labyrinthine hydrops
Meniere's syndrome or vertigo

DEF: Distended membranous labyrinth of the middle ear from fluctuating pressure of fluid (hydrops) that causes vertigo, tinnitus, pressure, and hearing loss that may last on and off for several hours. Episodes may occur in clusters or may subside for weeks, months, or even years.

**H81.01 Meniere's disease, right ear**
**H81.02 Meniere's disease, left ear**
**H81.03 Meniere's disease, bilateral**
**H81.09 Meniere's disease, unspecified ear**

**H81.1 Benign paroxysmal vertigo**

**H81.10 Benign paroxysmal vertigo, unspecified ear** Q
**H81.11 Benign paroxysmal vertigo, right ear** Q
**H81.12 Benign paroxysmal vertigo, left ear** Q
**H81.13 Benign paroxysmal vertigo, bilateral** Q

✓5th **H81.2 Vestibular neuronitis**

DEF: Transient benign vertigo caused by inflammation of the vestibular nerve. It is characterized by response to caloric stimulation on one side and nystagmus with rhythmic movement of the eyes. Normal auditory function is present.

**H81.20 Vestibular neuronitis, unspecified ear**
**H81.21 Vestibular neuronitis, right ear**
**H81.22 Vestibular neuronitis, left ear**
**H81.23 Vestibular neuronitis, bilateral**

✓5th **H81.3 Other peripheral vertigo**

✓6th **H81.31 Aural vertigo**

**H81.311 Aural vertigo, right ear**
**H81.312 Aural vertigo, left ear**
**H81.313 Aural vertigo, bilateral**
**H81.319 Aural vertigo, unspecified ear**

✓6th **H81.39 Other peripheral vertigo**

Lermoyez' syndrome
Otogenic vertigo
Peripheral vertigo NOS

**H81.391 Other peripheral vertigo, right ear**
**H81.392 Other peripheral vertigo, left ear**
**H81.393 Other peripheral vertigo, bilateral**
**H81.399 Other peripheral vertigo, unspecified ear**

**H81.4 Vertigo of central origin**

Central positional nystagmus

✓5th **H81.8 Other disorders of vestibular function**

✓6th **H81.8X Other disorders of vestibular function**

**H81.8X1 Other disorders of vestibular function, right ear**
**H81.8X2 Other disorders of vestibular function, left ear**
**H81.8X3 Other disorders of vestibular function, bilateral**
**H81.8X9 Other disorders of vestibular function, unspecified ear**

AHA: 2022,2Q,12

✓5th **H81.9 Unspecified disorder of vestibular function**

Vertiginous syndrome NOS

**H81.90 Unspecified disorder of vestibular function, unspecified ear**
**H81.91 Unspecified disorder of vestibular function, right ear**
**H81.92 Unspecified disorder of vestibular function, left ear**
**H81.93 Unspecified disorder of vestibular function, bilateral**

✓4th **H82 Vertiginous syndromes in diseases classified elsewhere**

Code first underlying disease

EXCLUDES 1 *epidemic vertigo (A88.1)*

*H82.1 Vertiginous syndromes in diseases classified elsewhere, right ear*
*H82.2 Vertiginous syndromes in diseases classified elsewhere, left ear*
*H82.3 Vertiginous syndromes in diseases classified elsewhere, bilateral*
*H82.9 Vertiginous syndromes in diseases classified elsewhere, unspecified ear*

✓4th **H83 Other diseases of inner ear**

✓5th **H83.0 Labyrinthitis**

DEF: Inflammation of the inner ear, or labyrinth, characterized by pus, vertigo, dizziness, nausea, and hearing loss.

**H83.01 Labyrinthitis, right ear**
**H83.02 Labyrinthitis, left ear**
**H83.03 Labyrinthitis, bilateral**
**H83.09 Labyrinthitis, unspecified ear**

✓5th **H83.1 Labyrinthine fistula**

**H83.11 Labyrinthine fistula, right ear**
**H83.12 Labyrinthine fistula, left ear**
**H83.13 Labyrinthine fistula, bilateral**
**H83.19 Labyrinthine fistula, unspecified ear**

✓5th **H83.2 Labyrinthine dysfunction**

Labyrinthine hypersensitivity
Labyrinthine hypofunction
Labyrinthine loss of function

DEF: Decreased function of the labyrinth sensors.

✓6th **H83.2X Labyrinthine dysfunction**

**H83.2X1 Labyrinthine dysfunction, right ear**
**H83.2X2 Labyrinthine dysfunction, left ear**
**H83.2X3 Labyrinthine dysfunction, bilateral**
**H83.2X9 Labyrinthine dysfunction, unspecified ear**

✓5th **H83.3 Noise effects on inner ear**

Acoustic trauma of inner ear
Noise-induced hearing loss of inner ear

✓6th **H83.3X Noise effects on inner ear**

**H83.3X1 Noise effects on right inner ear**
**H83.3X2 Noise effects on left inner ear**
**H83.3X3 Noise effects on inner ear, bilateral**
**H83.3X9 Noise effects on inner ear, unspecified ear**

✓5th **H83.8 Other specified diseases of inner ear**

✓6th **H83.8X Other specified diseases of inner ear**

**H83.8X1 Other specified diseases of right inner ear**
**H83.8X2 Other specified diseases of left inner ear**
**H83.8X3 Other specified diseases of inner ear, bilateral**
**H83.8X9 Other specified diseases of inner ear, unspecified ear**

✓5th **H83.9 Unspecified disease of inner ear**

**H83.90 Unspecified disease of inner ear, unspecified ear**
**H83.91 Unspecified disease of right inner ear**
**H83.92 Unspecified disease of left inner ear**
**H83.93 Unspecified disease of inner ear, bilateral**

## Other disorders of ear (H90-H94)

✓4th **H90 Conductive and sensorineural hearing loss**

EXCLUDES 1 *deaf nonspeaking NEC (H91.3)*
*deafness NOS (H91.9-)*
*hearing loss NOS (H91.9-)*
*noise-induced hearing loss (H83.3-)*
*ototoxic hearing loss (H91.0-)*
*sudden (idiopathic) hearing loss (H91.2-)*

AHA: 2015,2Q,7

DEF: Conductive hearing loss: Hearing loss due to the inability of soundwaves to move from the outer (external) ear to the inner ear.

DEF: Sensorineural hearing loss: Hearing loss that occurs from damage to the hair cells of the inner ear or problems with the nerve pathways from the inner ear to the brain.

**H90.0 Conductive hearing loss, bilateral**

✓5th **H90.1 Conductive hearing loss, unilateral with unrestricted hearing on the contralateral side**

**H90.11 Conductive hearing loss, unilateral, right ear, with unrestricted hearing on the contralateral side**
**H90.12 Conductive hearing loss, unilateral, left ear, with unrestricted hearing on the contralateral side**

**H90.2 Conductive hearing loss, unspecified**

Conductive deafness NOS

**H90.3 Sensorineural hearing loss, bilateral**

✓5th **H90.4 Sensorineural hearing loss, unilateral with unrestricted hearing on the contralateral side**

**H90.41 Sensorineural hearing loss, unilateral, right ear, with unrestricted hearing on the contralateral side**
**H90.42 Sensorineural hearing loss, unilateral, left ear, with unrestricted hearing on the contralateral side**

**H90.5 Unspecified sensorineural hearing loss**

Central hearing loss NOS
Congenital deafness NOS
Neural hearing loss NOS
Perceptive hearing loss NOS
Sensorineural deafness NOS
Sensory hearing loss NOS

EXCLUDES 1 *abnormal auditory perception (H93.2-)*
*psychogenic deafness (F44.6)*

**H90.6 Mixed conductive and sensorineural hearing loss, bilateral**

AHA: 2015,2Q,7

✓5th **H90.7 Mixed conductive and sensorineural hearing loss, unilateral with unrestricted hearing on the contralateral side**

**H90.71 Mixed conductive and sensorineural hearing loss, unilateral, right ear, with unrestricted hearing on the contralateral side**
**H90.72 Mixed conductive and sensorineural hearing loss, unilateral, left ear, with unrestricted hearing on the contralateral side**

**H90.8 Mixed conductive and sensorineural hearing loss, unspecified**

√5th **H90.A Conductive and sensorineural hearing loss with restricted hearing on the contralateral side**
AHA: 2016,4Q,23-25

√6th **H90.A1 Conductive hearing loss, unilateral, with restricted hearing on the contralateral side**
**H90.A11 Conductive hearing loss, unilateral, right ear with restricted hearing on the contralateral side**
**H90.A12 Conductive hearing loss, unilateral, left ear with restricted hearing on the contralateral side**

√6th **H90.A2 Sensorineural hearing loss, unilateral, with restricted hearing on the contralateral side**
**H90.A21 Sensorineural hearing loss, unilateral, right ear, with restricted hearing on the contralateral side**
**H90.A22 Sensorineural hearing loss, unilateral, left ear, with restricted hearing on the contralateral side**

√6th **H90.A3 Mixed conductive and sensorineural hearing loss, unilateral with restricted hearing on the contralateral side**
**H90.A31 Mixed conductive and sensorineural hearing loss, unilateral, right ear with restricted hearing on the contralateral side**
**H90.A32 Mixed conductive and sensorineural hearing loss, unilateral, left ear with restricted hearing on the contralateral side**

√4th **H91 Other and unspecified hearing loss**
EXCLUDES 1 *abnormal auditory perception (H93.2-)*
*hearing loss as classified in H90.-*
*impacted cerumen (H61.2-)*
*noise-induced hearing loss (H83.3-)*
*psychogenic deafness (F44.6)*
*transient ischemic deafness (H93.01-)*

√5th **H91.0 Ototoxic hearing loss**
Code first poisoning due to drug or toxin, if applicable (T36-T65 with fifth or sixth character 1-4)
Use additional code for adverse effect, if applicable, to identify drug (T36-T50 with fifth or sixth character 5)
**H91.01 Ototoxic hearing loss, right ear**
**H91.02 Ototoxic hearing loss, left ear**
**H91.03 Ototoxic hearing loss, bilateral**
**H91.09 Ototoxic hearing loss, unspecified ear**

√5th **H91.1 Presbycusis**
Presbyacusia
**H91.10 Presbycusis, unspecified ear**
**H91.11 Presbycusis, right ear**
**H91.12 Presbycusis, left ear**
**H91.13 Presbycusis, bilateral**

√5th **H91.2 Sudden idiopathic hearing loss**
Sudden hearing loss NOS
**H91.20 Sudden idiopathic hearing loss, unspecified ear**
**H91.21 Sudden idiopathic hearing loss, right ear**
**H91.22 Sudden idiopathic hearing loss, left ear**
**H91.23 Sudden idiopathic hearing loss, bilateral**

**H91.3 Deaf nonspeaking, not elsewhere classified**

√5th **H91.8 Other specified hearing loss**
√6th **H91.8X Other specified hearing loss**
**H91.8X1 Other specified hearing loss, right ear**
**H91.8X2 Other specified hearing loss, left ear**
**H91.8X3 Other specified hearing loss, bilateral**
**H91.8X9 Other specified hearing loss, unspecified ear**

√5th **H91.9 Unspecified hearing loss**
Deafness NOS
High frequency deafness
Low frequency deafness
**H91.90 Unspecified hearing loss, unspecified ear**
**H91.91 Unspecified hearing loss, right ear**
**H91.92 Unspecified hearing loss, left ear**
**H91.93 Unspecified hearing loss, bilateral**

√4th **H92 Otalgia and effusion of ear**
√5th **H92.0 Otalgia**
**H92.01 Otalgia, right ear**
**H92.02 Otalgia, left ear**
**H92.03 Otalgia, bilateral**
**H92.09 Otalgia, unspecified ear**

√5th **H92.1 Otorrhea**
EXCLUDES 1 *leakage of cerebrospinal fluid through ear (G96.0)*
**H92.10 Otorrhea, unspecified ear**
**H92.11 Otorrhea, right ear**
**H92.12 Otorrhea, left ear**
**H92.13 Otorrhea, bilateral**

√5th **H92.2 Otorrhagia**
EXCLUDES 1 *traumatic otorrhagia - code to injury*
**H92.20 Otorrhagia, unspecified ear**
**H92.21 Otorrhagia, right ear**
**H92.22 Otorrhagia, left ear**
**H92.23 Otorrhagia, bilateral**

√4th **H93 Other disorders of ear, not elsewhere classified**
√5th **H93.0 Degenerative and vascular disorders of ear**
EXCLUDES 1 *presbycusis (H91.1)*
√6th **H93.01 Transient ischemic deafness**
**H93.011 Transient ischemic deafness, right ear**
**H93.012 Transient ischemic deafness, left ear**
**H93.013 Transient ischemic deafness, bilateral**
**H93.019 Transient ischemic deafness, unspecified ear**
√6th **H93.09 Unspecified degenerative and vascular disorders of ear**
**H93.091 Unspecified degenerative and vascular disorders of right ear**
**H93.092 Unspecified degenerative and vascular disorders of left ear**
**H93.093 Unspecified degenerative and vascular disorders of ear, bilateral**
**H93.099 Unspecified degenerative and vascular disorders of unspecified ear**

√5th **H93.1 Tinnitus**
**H93.11 Tinnitus, right ear**
**H93.12 Tinnitus, left ear**
**H93.13 Tinnitus, bilateral**
**H93.19 Tinnitus, unspecified ear**

√5th **H93.A Pulsatile tinnitus**
AHA: 2023,2Q,18; 2016,4Q,25-26
**H93.A1 Pulsatile tinnitus, right ear**
**H93.A2 Pulsatile tinnitus, left ear**
**H93.A3 Pulsatile tinnitus, bilateral**
**H93.A9 Pulsatile tinnitus, unspecified ear**

√5th **H93.2 Other abnormal auditory perceptions**
EXCLUDES 2 *auditory hallucinations (R44.0)*
√6th **H93.21 Auditory recruitment**
**H93.211 Auditory recruitment, right ear**
**H93.212 Auditory recruitment, left ear**
**H93.213 Auditory recruitment, bilateral**
**H93.219 Auditory recruitment, unspecified ear**
√6th **H93.22 Diplacusis**
**H93.221 Diplacusis, right ear**
**H93.222 Diplacusis, left ear**
**H93.223 Diplacusis, bilateral**
**H93.229 Diplacusis, unspecified ear**
√6th **H93.23 Hyperacusis**
DEF: Exceptionally acute sense of hearing caused by such conditions as Bell's palsy. This term may also refer to painful sensitivity to sounds.
**H93.231 Hyperacusis, right ear**
**H93.232 Hyperacusis, left ear**
**H93.233 Hyperacusis, bilateral**
**H93.239 Hyperacusis, unspecified ear**
√6th **H93.24 Temporary auditory threshold shift**
**H93.241 Temporary auditory threshold shift, right ear**
**H93.242 Temporary auditory threshold shift, left ear**
**H93.243 Temporary auditory threshold shift, bilateral**
**H93.249 Temporary auditory threshold shift, unspecified ear**
**H93.25 Central auditory processing disorder**
Congenital auditory imperception
Word deafness
EXCLUDES 1 *mixed receptive-expressive language disorder (F80.2)*

✓6th **H93.29 Other abnormal auditory perceptions**
H93.291 Other abnormal auditory perceptions, right ear
H93.292 Other abnormal auditory perceptions, left ear
H93.293 Other abnormal auditory perceptions, bilateral
H93.299 Other abnormal auditory perceptions, unspecified ear

✓5th **H93.3 Disorders of acoustic nerve**
Disorder of 8th cranial nerve
EXCLUDES 1 *acoustic neuroma (D33.3)*
*syphilitic acoustic neuritis (A52.15)*

✓6th **H93.3X Disorders of acoustic nerve**
H93.3X1 Disorders of right acoustic nerve
H93.3X2 Disorders of left acoustic nerve
H93.3X3 Disorders of bilateral acoustic nerves
H93.3X9 Disorders of unspecified acoustic nerve

✓5th **H93.8 Other specified disorders of ear**
✓6th **H93.8X Other specified disorders of ear**
H93.8X1 Other specified disorders of right ear
H93.8X2 Other specified disorders of left ear
H93.8X3 Other specified disorders of ear, bilateral
H93.8X9 Other specified disorders of ear, unspecified ear

✓5th **H93.9 Unspecified disorder of ear**
H93.90 Unspecified disorder of ear, unspecified ear
H93.91 Unspecified disorder of right ear
H93.92 Unspecified disorder of left ear
H93.93 Unspecified disorder of ear, bilateral

✓4th **H94 Other disorders of ear in diseases classified elsewhere**

✓5th **H94.Ø Acoustic neuritis in infectious and parasitic diseases classified elsewhere**
Code first underlying disease, such as:
parasitic disease (B65-B89)
EXCLUDES 1 *acoustic neuritis (in):*
*herpes zoster (BØ2.29)*
*syphilis (A52.15)*

*H94.ØØ Acoustic neuritis in infectious and parasitic diseases classified elsewhere, unspecified ear*
*H94.Ø1 Acoustic neuritis in infectious and parasitic diseases classified elsewhere, right ear*
*H94.Ø2 Acoustic neuritis in infectious and parasitic diseases classified elsewhere, left ear*
*H94.Ø3 Acoustic neuritis in infectious and parasitic diseases classified elsewhere, bilateral*

✓5th **H94.8 Other specified disorders of ear in diseases classified elsewhere**
Code first underlying disease, such as:
congenital syphilis (A5Ø.Ø)
EXCLUDES 1 *aural myiasis (B87.4)*
*syphilitic labyrinthitis (A52.79)*

*H94.8Ø Other specified disorders of ear in diseases classified elsewhere, unspecified ear*
*H94.81 Other specified disorders of right ear in diseases classified elsewhere*
*H94.82 Other specified disorders of left ear in diseases classified elsewhere*
*H94.83 Other specified disorders of ear in diseases classified elsewhere, bilateral*

## Intraoperative and postprocedural complications and disorders of ear and mastoid process, not elsewhere classified (H95)

✓4th **H95 Intraoperative and postprocedural complications and disorders of ear and mastoid process, not elsewhere classified**
AHA: 2016,4Q,9-10

✓5th **H95.Ø Recurrent cholesteatoma of postmastoidectomy cavity**
H95.ØØ Recurrent cholesteatoma of postmastoidectomy cavity, unspecified ear
H95.Ø1 Recurrent cholesteatoma of postmastoidectomy cavity, right ear
H95.Ø2 Recurrent cholesteatoma of postmastoidectomy cavity, left ear
H95.Ø3 Recurrent cholesteatoma of postmastoidectomy cavity, bilateral ears

✓5th **H95.1 Other disorders of ear and mastoid process following mastoidectomy**
✓6th **H95.11 Chronic inflammation of postmastoidectomy cavity**
H95.111 Chronic inflammation of postmastoidectomy cavity, right ear
H95.112 Chronic inflammation of postmastoidectomy cavity, left ear
H95.113 Chronic inflammation of postmastoidectomy cavity, bilateral ears
H95.119 Chronic inflammation of postmastoidectomy cavity, unspecified ear

✓6th **H95.12 Granulation of postmastoidectomy cavity**
H95.121 Granulation of postmastoidectomy cavity, right ear
H95.122 Granulation of postmastoidectomy cavity, left ear
H95.123 Granulation of postmastoidectomy cavity, bilateral ears
H95.129 Granulation of postmastoidectomy cavity, unspecified ear

✓6th **H95.13 Mucosal cyst of postmastoidectomy cavity**
H95.131 Mucosal cyst of postmastoidectomy cavity, right ear
H95.132 Mucosal cyst of postmastoidectomy cavity, left ear
H95.133 Mucosal cyst of postmastoidectomy cavity, bilateral ears
H95.139 Mucosal cyst of postmastoidectomy cavity, unspecified ear

✓6th **H95.19 Other disorders following mastoidectomy**
H95.191 Other disorders following mastoidectomy, right ear
H95.192 Other disorders following mastoidectomy, left ear
H95.193 Other disorders following mastoidectomy, bilateral ears
H95.199 Other disorders following mastoidectomy, unspecified ear

✓5th **H95.2 Intraoperative hemorrhage and hematoma of ear and mastoid process complicating a procedure**
EXCLUDES 1 *intraoperative hemorrhage and hematoma of ear and mastoid process due to accidental puncture or laceration during a procedure (H95.3-)*
H95.21 Intraoperative hemorrhage and hematoma of ear and mastoid process complicating a procedure on the ear and mastoid process
H95.22 Intraoperative hemorrhage and hematoma of ear and mastoid process complicating other procedure

✓5th **H95.3 Accidental puncture and laceration of ear and mastoid process during a procedure**
H95.31 Accidental puncture and laceration of the ear and mastoid process during a procedure on the ear and mastoid process
H95.32 Accidental puncture and laceration of the ear and mastoid process during other procedure

✓5th **H95.4 Postprocedural hemorrhage of ear and mastoid process following a procedure**
H95.41 Postprocedural hemorrhage of ear and mastoid process following a procedure on the ear and mastoid process
H95.42 Postprocedural hemorrhage of ear and mastoid process following other procedure

✓5th **H95.5 Postprocedural hematoma and seroma of ear and mastoid process following a procedure**
H95.51 Postprocedural hematoma of ear and mastoid process following a procedure on the ear and mastoid process
H95.52 Postprocedural hematoma of ear and mastoid process following other procedure
H95.53 Postprocedural seroma of ear and mastoid process following a procedure on the ear and mastoid process
H95.54 Postprocedural seroma of ear and mastoid process following other procedure

✓5th **H95.8 Other intraoperative and postprocedural complications and disorders of the ear and mastoid process, not elsewhere classified**
EXCLUDES 2 *postprocedural complications and disorders following mastoidectomy (H95.Ø-, H95.1-)*

✓6th **H95.81 Postprocedural stenosis of external ear canal**
H95.811 Postprocedural stenosis of right external ear canal

**H95.812** **Postprocedural stenosis of left external ear canal**

**H95.813** **Postprocedural stenosis of external ear canal, bilateral**

**H95.819** **Postprocedural stenosis of unspecified external ear canal**

**H95.88** **Other intraoperative complications and disorders of the ear and mastoid process, not elsewhere classified**

Use additional code, if applicable, to further specify disorder

**H95.89** **Other postprocedural complications and disorders of the ear and mastoid process, not elsewhere classified**

Use additional code, if applicable, to further specify disorder

# Chapter 9. Diseases of the Circulatory System (I00–I99)



## Chapter-specific Guidelines with Coding Examples

The chapter-specific guidelines from the ICD-10-CM Official Guidelines for Coding and Reporting have been provided below. Along with these guidelines are coding examples, contained in the shaded boxes, that have been developed to help illustrate the coding and/or sequencing guidance found in these guidelines.

**a. Hypertension**

The classification presumes a causal relationship between hypertension and heart involvement and between hypertension and kidney involvement, as the two conditions are linked by the term "with" in the Alphabetic Index. These conditions should be coded as related even in the absence of provider documentation explicitly linking them, unless the documentation clearly states the conditions are unrelated.

For hypertension and conditions not specifically linked by relational terms such as "with," "associated with" or "due to" in the classification, provider documentation must link the conditions in order to code them as related.

**1) Hypertension with heart disease**

Hypertension with one or more heart conditions classified to I50.-, Heart failure, I51.4, Myocarditis, unspecified, I51.89, Other ill-defined heart diseases, or I51.9, Heart disease, unspecified, is assigned to a code from category I11, Hypertensive heart disease. Use additional code(s) from category I50, Heart failure, or I51, Complications and ill-defined descriptions of heart disease, to identify the heart condition.

Hypertension with one or more heart conditions classified to I51.5, Myocardial degeneration, or I51.7, Cardiomegaly, is assigned to a code from category I11, Hypertensive heart disease. No additional code is assigned to identify the specific heart condition.

The same heart conditions (I50.-, I51.4-I51.7, I51.89, I51.9) with hypertension are coded separately if the provider has documented they are unrelated to the hypertension. The applicable hypertension code I10, Essential (primary) hypertension, or a code from category I15, Secondary hypertension, should be assigned. Sequence according to the circumstances of the admission/encounter.

**2) Hypertensive chronic kidney disease**

Assign codes from category I12, Hypertensive chronic kidney disease, when both hypertension and a condition classifiable to category N18, Chronic kidney disease (CKD), are present. CKD should not be coded as hypertensive if the provider indicates the CKD is not related to the hypertension.

The appropriate code from category N18 should be used as a secondary code with a code from category I12 to identify the stage of chronic kidney disease.

*See Section I.C.14. Chronic kidney disease.*

If a patient has hypertensive chronic kidney disease and acute renal failure, the acute renal failure should also be coded. Sequence according to the circumstances of the admission/encounter.

**3) Hypertensive heart and chronic kidney disease**

The codes in category I13, Hypertensive heart and chronic kidney disease, are combination codes that include hypertension, heart disease and chronic kidney disease. Assign codes from combination category I13, Hypertensive heart and chronic kidney disease, when there is hypertension with both heart and chronic kidney disease. If heart failure is present, assign an additional code from category I50 to identify the type of heart failure.

The appropriate code from category N18, Chronic kidney disease, should be used as a secondary code with a code from category I13 to identify the stage of chronic kidney disease.

*See Section I.C.14. Chronic kidney disease.*

The Includes note at I13 specifies that the conditions included at I11 and I12 are included together in I13. If a patient has hypertension, heart disease and chronic kidney disease, then a code from I13 should be used, not codes from I11 or I12.

For patients with both acute renal failure and chronic kidney disease, the acute renal failure should also be coded. Sequence according to the circumstances of the admission/encounter.

Hypertensive heart and kidney disease with congestive heart failure and stage 2 chronic kidney disease

| | |
|---|---|
| **I13.0** | **Hypertensive heart and chronic kidney disease with heart failure and stage 1 through stage 4 chronic kidney disease, or unspecified chronic kidney disease** |
| **I50.9** | **Heart failure, unspecified** |
| **N18.2** | **Chronic kidney disease, stage 2 (mild)** |

*Explanation*: Combination codes in category I13 are used to report conditions classifiable to *both* categories I11 and I12. Do not report conditions classifiable to I11 and I12 separately. Use additional codes to report type of heart failure and stage of CKD.

**4) Hypertensive cerebrovascular disease**

For hypertensive cerebrovascular disease, first assign the appropriate code from categories I60-I69, followed by the appropriate hypertension code.

**5) Hypertensive retinopathy**

Subcategory H35.0, Background retinopathy and retinal vascular changes, should be used along with a code from categories I10-I15, in the Hypertensive diseases section, to include the systemic hypertension. The sequencing is based on the reason for the encounter.

**6) Hypertension, secondary**

Secondary hypertension is due to an underlying condition. Two codes are required: one to identify the underlying etiology and one from category I15 to identify the hypertension. Sequencing of codes is determined by the reason for admission/encounter.

Renovascular hypertension due to renal artery atherosclerosis

| | |
|---|---|
| **I15.0** | **Renovascular hypertension** |
| **I70.1** | **Atherosclerosis of renal artery** |

*Explanation*: Secondary hypertension requires two codes: a code to identify the etiology and the appropriate I15 code.

**7) Hypertension, transient**

Assign code R03.0, Elevated blood pressure reading without diagnosis of hypertension, unless patient has an established diagnosis of hypertension. Assign code O13.-, Gestational [pregnancy-induced] hypertension without significant proteinuria, or O14.-, Pre-eclampsia, for transient hypertension of pregnancy.

**8) Hypertension, controlled**

This diagnostic statement usually refers to an existing state of hypertension under control by therapy. Assign the appropriate code from categories I10-I15, Hypertensive diseases.

**9) Hypertension, uncontrolled**

Uncontrolled hypertension may refer to untreated hypertension or hypertension not responding to current therapeutic regimen. In either case, assign the appropriate code from categories I10-I15, Hypertensive diseases.

**10) Hypertensive crisis**

Assign a code from category I16, Hypertensive crisis, for documented hypertensive urgency, hypertensive emergency or unspecified hypertensive crisis. Code also any identified hypertensive disease (I10-I15, **I1A**). The sequencing is based on the reason for the encounter.

**11)Pulmonary hypertension**

Pulmonary hypertension is classified to category I27, Other pulmonary heart diseases. For secondary pulmonary hypertension (I27.1, I27.2-), code also any associated conditions or adverse effects of drugs or toxins. The sequencing is based on the reason for the encounter, except for adverse effects of drugs (See Section I.C.19.e.).

**12)Hypertension, Resistant**

Resistant hypertension refers to blood pressure of a patient with hypertension that remains above goal in spite of the use of antihypertensive medications. Assign code I1A.0, Resistant hypertension, as an additional code when apparent treatment resistant hypertension, treatment resistant hypertension, or true resistant hypertension is documented by the provider. A code for the specific type of existing hypertension is sequenced first, if known.

**b. Atherosclerotic coronary artery disease and angina**

ICD-10-CM has combination codes for atherosclerotic heart disease with angina pectoris. The subcategories for these codes are I25.11, Atherosclerotic heart disease of native coronary artery with angina pectoris and I25.7, Atherosclerosis of coronary artery bypass graft(s) and coronary artery of transplanted heart with angina pectoris.

When using one of these combination codes it is not necessary to use an additional code for angina pectoris. A causal relationship can be assumed in a patient with both atherosclerosis and angina pectoris, unless the documentation indicates the angina is due to something other than the atherosclerosis.

If a patient with coronary artery disease is admitted due to an acute myocardial infarction (AMI), the AMI should be sequenced before the coronary artery disease.

*See Section I.C.9. Acute myocardial infarction (AMI)*

Patient is being seen for spastic angina pectoris. She also has a documented history of progressive coronary artery disease of the native vessels.

**I25.111 Atherosclerotic heart disease of native coronary artery with angina pectoris with documented spasm**

*Explanation*: Report the combination code for atherosclerotic heart disease (coronary artery disease) with angina pectoris. A causal relationship is assumed in a patient with both atherosclerosis and angina pectoris, unless the documentation indicates the angina is due to something other than the atherosclerosis. When using one of these combination codes, it is not necessary to use an additional code for angina pectoris.

**c. Intraoperative and postprocedural cerebrovascular accident**

Medical record documentation should clearly specify the cause- and- effect relationship between the medical intervention and the cerebrovascular accident in order to assign a code for intraoperative or postprocedural cerebrovascular accident.

Proper code assignment depends on whether it was an infarction or hemorrhage and whether it occurred intraoperatively or postoperatively. If it was a cerebral hemorrhage, code assignment depends on the type of procedure performed.

Embolic cerebral infarction of the right middle cerebral artery that occurred during hip replacement surgery. The surgeon documented as due to the surgery.

**I97.811 Intraoperative cerebrovascular infarction during other surgery**

**I63.411 Cerebral infarction due to embolism of right middle cerebral artery**

*Explanation*: Code assignment for intraoperative or postprocedural cerebrovascular accident is based on the provider's documentation of a cause-and-effect relationship between the condition and the procedure. Proper code assignment also depends on whether the cerebrovascular accident was an infarction or hemorrhage, occurred intraoperatively or postoperatively, and the type of procedure performed.

**d. Sequelae of cerebrovascular disease**

**1) Category I69, Sequelae of cerebrovascular disease**

Category I69 is used to indicate conditions classifiable to categories I6Ø-I67 as the causes of sequela (neurologic deficits), themselves classified elsewhere. These "late effects" include neurologic deficits that persist after initial onset of conditions classifiable to categories I6Ø-I67. The neurologic deficits caused by cerebrovascular disease may be present from the onset or may arise at any time after the onset of the condition classifiable to categories I6Ø-I67.

Codes from category I69, Sequelae of cerebrovascular disease, that specify hemiplegia, hemiparesis and monoplegia identify whether the dominant or nondominant side is affected. Should the affected side be documented, but not specified as dominant or nondominant, and the classification system does not indicate a default, code selection is as follows:

- For ambidextrous patients, the default should be dominant.
- If the left side is affected, the default is non-dominant.
- If the right side is affected, the default is dominant.

**2) Codes from category I69 with codes from I60–I67**

Codes from category I69 may be assigned on a health care record with codes from I6Ø-I67, if the patient has a current cerebrovascular disease and deficits from an old cerebrovascular disease.

**3) Codes from category I69 and personal history of transient ischemic attack (TIA) and cerebral infarction (Z86.73)**

Codes from category I69 should not be assigned if the patient does not have neurologic deficits.

*See Section I.C.21. 4. History (of) for use of personal history codes*

**e. Acute myocardial infarction (AMI)**

**1) Type 1 ST elevation myocardial infarction (STEMI) and non-ST elevation myocardial infarction (NSTEMI)**

The ICD-10-CM codes for type 1 acute myocardial infarction (AMI) identify the site, such as anterolateral wall or true posterior wall. Subcategories I21.Ø-I21.2 and code I21.3 are used for type 1 ST elevation myocardial infarction (STEMI). Code I21.4, Non-ST elevation (NSTEMI) myocardial infarction, is used for type 1 non-ST elevation myocardial infarction (NSTEMI) and nontransmural MIs.

If a type 1 NSTEMI evolves to STEMI, assign the STEMI code. If a type 1 STEMI converts to NSTEMI due to thrombolytic therapy, it is still coded as STEMI.

For encounters occurring while the myocardial infarction is equal to, or less than, four weeks old, including transfers to another acute setting or a postacute setting, and the myocardial infarction meets the definition for "other diagnoses" (see Section III, Reporting Additional Diagnoses), codes from category I21 may continue to be reported. For encounters after the 4-week time frame and the patient is still receiving care related to the myocardial infarction, the appropriate aftercare code should be assigned, rather than a code from category I21. For old or healed myocardial infarctions not requiring further care, code I25.2, Old myocardial infarction, may be assigned.

**2) Acute myocardial infarction, unspecified**

Code I21.9, Acute myocardial infarction, unspecified, is the default for unspecified acute myocardial infarction or unspecified type. If only type 1 STEMI or transmural MI without the site is documented, assign code I21.3, ST elevation (STEMI) myocardial infarction of unspecified site.

**3) AMI documented as nontransmural or subendocardial but site provided**

If an AMI is documented as nontransmural or subendocardial, but the site is provided, it is still coded as a subendocardial AMI.

*See Section I.C.21.3.for information on coding status post administration of tPA in a different facility within the last 24 hours.*

**4) Subsequent acute myocardial infarction**

A code from category I22, Subsequent ST elevation (STEMI) and non-ST elevation (NSTEMI) myocardial infarction, is to be used when a patient who has suffered a type 1 or unspecified AMI has a new AMI within the 4-week time frame of the initial AMI. A code from category I22 must be used in conjunction with a code from category I21. The sequencing of the I22 and I21 codes depends on the circumstances of the encounter.

Do not assign code I22 for subsequent myocardial infarctions other than type 1 or unspecified. For subsequent type 2 AMI assign only code I21.A1. For subsequent type 4 or type 5 AMI, assign only code I21.A9.

If a subsequent myocardial infarction of one type occurs within 4 weeks of a myocardial infarction of a different type, assign the appropriate codes from category I21 to identify each type. Do not assign a code from I22. Codes from category I22 should only be assigned if both the initial and subsequent myocardial infarctions are type 1 or unspecified.

Patient suffered an acute NSTEMI 14 days ago and is now seen for an inferior STEMI.

**I22.1 Subsequent ST elevation (STEMI) myocardial infarction of inferior wall**

**I21.4 Non-ST elevation (NSTEMI) myocardial infarction**

*Explanation*: Both MIs were type 1, and the current MI occurred within the four-week time frame; therefore a code for the current/subsequent STEMI (I22.1) is reported as well as a code for the previous NSTEMI (I21.4).

**5) Other types of myocardial infarction**

The ICD-10-CM provides codes for different types of myocardial infarction. Type 1 myocardial infarctions are assigned to codes I21.Ø-I21.4.

Type 2 myocardial infarction (myocardial infarction due to demand ischemia or secondary to ischemic imbalance) is assigned to code I21.A1, Myocardial infarction type 2 with the underlying cause coded first, if applicable. Do not assign code I24.89, Other forms of acute ischemic heart disease, for the demand ischemia. If a type 2 AMI is described as NSTEMI or STEMI, only assign code I21.A1. Codes I21.Ø1-I21.4 should only be assigned for type 1 AMIs.

Acute myocardial infarctions type 3, 4a, 4b, 4c and 5 are assigned to code I21.A9, Other myocardial infarction type.

The "Code also" and "Code first" notes should be followed related to complications, and for coding of postprocedural myocardial infarctions during or following cardiac surgery.

**6) Myocardial infarction with coronary microvascular dysfunction**

Coronary microvascular dysfunction (CMD) is a condition that impacts the microvasculature by restricting microvascular flow and increasing microvascular resistance. Code I21.B, Myocardial infarction with coronary microvascular dysfunction, is assigned for myocardial infarction with coronary microvascular disease, myocardial infarction with coronary microvascular dysfunction, and myocardial infarction with non-obstructive coronary arteries (MINOCA) with microvascular disease.

# Chapter 9. Diseases of the Circulatory System (I00-I99)

EXCLUDES 2 *certain conditions originating in the perinatal period (P04-P96)*
*certain infectious and parasitic diseases (A00-B99)*
*complications of pregnancy, childbirth and the puerperium (O00-O9A)*
*congenital malformations, deformations, and chromosomal abnormalities (Q00-Q99)*
*endocrine, nutritional and metabolic diseases (E00-E88)*
*injury, poisoning and certain other consequences of external causes (S00-T88)*
*neoplasms (C00-D49)*
*symptoms, signs and abnormal clinical and laboratory findings, not elsewhere classified (R00-R94)*
*systemic connective tissue disorders (M30-M36)*
*transient cerebral ischemic attacks and related syndromes (G45.-)*

This chapter contains the following blocks:

| | |
|---|---|
| I00-I02 | Acute rheumatic fever |
| I05-I09 | Chronic rheumatic heart diseases |
| I10-I1A | Hypertensive diseases |
| I20-I25 | Ischemic heart diseases |
| I26-I28 | Pulmonary heart disease and diseases of pulmonary circulation |
| I30-I5A | Other forms of heart disease |
| I60-I69 | Cerebrovascular diseases |
| I70-I79 | Diseases of arteries, arterioles and capillaries |
| I80-I89 | Diseases of veins, lymphatic vessels and lymph nodes, not elsewhere classified |
| I95-I99 | Other and unspecified disorders of the circulatory system |

## Acute rheumatic fever (I00-I02)

**DEF:** Rheumatic fever: Inflammatory disease that can follow a throat infection by group A *streptococci*. Complications can involve the joints (arthritis), subcutaneous tissue (nodules), skin (erythema marginatum), heart (carditis), or brain (chorea).

**I00 Rheumatic fever without heart involvement**
INCLUDES arthritis, rheumatic, acute or subacute
EXCLUDES 1 *rheumatic fever with heart involvement (I01.0-I01.9)*

✓4th **I01 Rheumatic fever with heart involvement**
EXCLUDES 1 *chronic diseases of rheumatic origin (I05-I09) unless rheumatic fever is also present or there is evidence of reactivation or activity of the rheumatic process*

**I01.0 Acute rheumatic pericarditis**
Any condition in I00 with pericarditis
Rheumatic pericarditis (acute)
EXCLUDES 1 *acute pericarditis not specified as rheumatic (I30.-)*

**I01.1 Acute rheumatic endocarditis**
Acute rheumatic valvulitis
Any condition in I00 with endocarditis or valvulitis

**I01.2 Acute rheumatic myocarditis**
Any condition in I00 with myocarditis

**I01.8 Other acute rheumatic heart disease**
Acute rheumatic pancarditis
Any condition in I00 with other or multiple types of heart involvement

**I01.9 Acute rheumatic heart disease, unspecified**
Any condition in I00 with unspecified type of heart involvement
Rheumatic carditis, acute
Rheumatic heart disease, active or acute

✓4th **I02 Rheumatic chorea**
INCLUDES Sydenham's chorea
EXCLUDES 1 *chorea NOS (G25.5)*
*Huntington's chorea (G10)*

**I02.0 Rheumatic chorea with heart involvement**
Chorea NOS with heart involvement
Rheumatic chorea with heart involvement of any type classifiable under I01.-

**I02.9 Rheumatic chorea without heart involvement**
Rheumatic chorea NOS

## Chronic rheumatic heart diseases (I05-I09)

✓4th **I05 Rheumatic mitral valve diseases**
INCLUDES conditions classifiable to both I05.0 and I05.2-I05.9, whether specified as rheumatic or not
EXCLUDES 1 *mitral valve disease specified as nonrheumatic (I34.-)*
*mitral valve disease with aortic and/or tricuspid valve involvement (I08.-)*

**I05.0 Rheumatic mitral stenosis**
Mitral (valve) obstruction (rheumatic)

**I05.1 Rheumatic mitral insufficiency**
Rheumatic mitral incompetence
Rheumatic mitral regurgitation
EXCLUDES 1 *mitral insufficiency not specified as rheumatic (I34.0)*

**I05.2 Rheumatic mitral stenosis with insufficiency**
Rheumatic mitral stenosis with incompetence or regurgitation

**I05.8 Other rheumatic mitral valve diseases**
Rheumatic mitral (valve) failure

**I05.9 Rheumatic mitral valve disease, unspecified**
Rheumatic mitral (valve) disorder (chronic) NOS

✓4th **I06 Rheumatic aortic valve diseases**
EXCLUDES 1 ~~*aortic valve disease not specified as rheumatic (I35.-)*~~
~~*aortic valve disease with mitral and/or tricuspid valve involvement (I08.-)*~~
EXCLUDES 2 ▶*aortic valve disease not specified as rheumatic (I35.-)*◀
▶*aortic valve disease with mitral and/or tricuspid valve involvement (I08.-)*◀

**I06.0 Rheumatic aortic stenosis**
Rheumatic aortic (valve) obstruction

**I06.1 Rheumatic aortic insufficiency**
Rheumatic aortic incompetence
Rheumatic aortic regurgitation

**I06.2 Rheumatic aortic stenosis with insufficiency**
Rheumatic aortic stenosis with incompetence or regurgitation

**I06.8 Other rheumatic aortic valve diseases**

**I06.9 Rheumatic aortic valve disease, unspecified**
Rheumatic aortic (valve) disease NOS

✓4th **I07 Rheumatic tricuspid valve diseases**
INCLUDES rheumatic tricuspid valve diseases specified as rheumatic or unspecified
EXCLUDES 1 *tricuspid valve disease specified as nonrheumatic (I36.-)*
*tricuspid valve disease with aortic and/or mitral valve involvement (I08.-)*

**I07.0 Rheumatic tricuspid stenosis**
Tricuspid (valve) stenosis (rheumatic)

**I07.1 Rheumatic tricuspid insufficiency**
Tricuspid (valve) insufficiency (rheumatic)

**I07.2 Rheumatic tricuspid stenosis and insufficiency**

**I07.8 Other rheumatic tricuspid valve diseases**

**I07.9 Rheumatic tricuspid valve disease, unspecified**
Rheumatic tricuspid valve disorder NOS

✓4th **I08 Multiple valve diseases**
INCLUDES multiple valve diseases specified as rheumatic or unspecified
EXCLUDES 1 *endocarditis, valve unspecified (I38)*
*rheumatic valve disease NOS (I09.1)*
EXCLUDES 2 *multiple valve disease specified as nonrheumatic (I34.-, I35.-, I36.-, I37.-, I38.-, Q22.-, Q23.-,Q24.8-)*

**I08.0 Rheumatic disorders of both mitral and aortic valves**
Involvement of both mitral and aortic valves specified as rheumatic or unspecified
**AHA:** 2025,1Q,19; 2019,2Q,5

**I08.1 Rheumatic disorders of both mitral and tricuspid valves**

**I08.2 Rheumatic disorders of both aortic and tricuspid valves**

**I08.3 Combined rheumatic disorders of mitral, aortic and tricuspid valves**

**I08.8 Other rheumatic multiple valve diseases**

**I08.9 Rheumatic multiple valve disease, unspecified**

✓4th **I09 Other rheumatic heart diseases**

**I09.0 Rheumatic myocarditis**
EXCLUDES 1 *myocarditis not specified as rheumatic (I51.4)*

**I09.1 Rheumatic diseases of endocardium, valve unspecified**
Rheumatic endocarditis (chronic)
Rheumatic valvulitis (chronic)
EXCLUDES 1 *endocarditis, valve unspecified (I38)*

**I09.2 Chronic rheumatic pericarditis**
Adherent pericardium, rheumatic
Chronic rheumatic mediastinopericarditis
Chronic rheumatic myopericarditis
EXCLUDES 1 *chronic pericarditis not specified as rheumatic (I31.-)*

✓5th **I09.8 Other specified rheumatic heart diseases**

**I09.81 Rheumatic heart failure** HCC Rx ESR COM
Use additional code to identify type of heart failure (I50.-)

**I09.89 Other specified rheumatic heart diseases**
Rheumatic disease of pulmonary valve

**IØ9.9 Rheumatic heart disease, unspecified**
Rheumatic carditis
EXCLUDES 1 *rheumatoid carditis (MØ5.31)*

## Hypertensive diseases (I1Ø-I1A)

Use additional code to identify:
exposure to environmental tobacco smoke (Z77.22)
history of tobacco dependence (Z87.891)
occupational exposure to environmental tobacco smoke (Z57.31)
tobacco dependence (F17.-)
tobacco use (Z72.Ø)

EXCLUDES 1 *neonatal hypertension (P29.2)*
*primary pulmonary hypertension (I27.Ø)*
EXCLUDES 2 *hypertensive disease complicating pregnancy, childbirth and the puerperium (O1Ø-O11, O13-O16)*

**I1Ø Essential (primary) hypertension** Rx Q
INCLUDES high blood pressure
hypertension (arterial) (benign) (essential) (malignant) (primary) (systemic)
EXCLUDES 1 *hypertensive disease complicating pregnancy, childbirth and the puerperium (O1Ø-O11, O13-O16)*
EXCLUDES 2 *essential (primary) hypertension involving vessels of brain (I6Ø-I69)*
*essential (primary) hypertension involving vessels of eye (H35.Ø-)*
**AHA:** 2023,4Q,24; 2022,1Q,36; 2020,1Q,12; 2018,2Q,9; 2016,4Q,27

✓4th **I11 Hypertensive heart disease**
INCLUDES any condition in I5Ø.- or I51.4-I51.7, I51.89, I51.9 due to hypertension
**AHA:** 2018,2Q,9
**TIP:** Do not assign a code from this category when provider documentation indicates the heart disease is attributable to another cause.

**I11.Ø Hypertensive heart disease with heart failure** HCC Rx ESR COM
Hypertensive heart failure
Use additional code to identify type of heart failure (I5Ø.-)
**AHA:** 2017,1Q,47

**I11.9 Hypertensive heart disease without heart failure** Rx
Hypertensive heart disease NOS

✓4th **I12 Hypertensive chronic kidney disease**
INCLUDES any condition in N18 and N26 — due to hypertension
arteriosclerosis of kidney
arteriosclerotic nephritis (chronic) (interstitial)
hypertensive nephropathy
nephrosclerosis
EXCLUDES 1 *hypertension due to kidney disease (I15.Ø, I15.1)*
*renovascular hypertension (I15.Ø)*
*secondary hypertension (I15.-)*
EXCLUDES 2 *acute kidney failure (N17.-)*
**AHA:** 2019,3Q,3; 2018,4Q,88; 2016,3Q,22
**TIP:** Do not assign a code from this category when provider documentation indicates the chronic kidney disease (CKD) is attributable to another cause.

**I12.Ø Hypertensive chronic kidney disease with stage 5 chronic kidney disease or end stage renal disease** HCC Rx ESR COM
Use additional code to identify the stage of chronic kidney disease (N18.5, N18.6)

**I12.9 Hypertensive chronic kidney disease with stage 1 through stage 4 chronic kidney disease, or unspecified chronic kidney disease** Rx
Hypertensive chronic kidney disease NOS
Hypertensive renal disease NOS
Use additional code to identify the stage of chronic kidney disease (N18.1-N18.4, N18.9)

✓4th **I13 Hypertensive heart and chronic kidney disease**
INCLUDES any condition in I11.- with any condition in I12.-
cardiorenal disease
cardiovascular renal disease
**TIP:** Do not assign a code from this category when provider documentation indicates the heart and/or chronic kidney disease is attributable to another cause.

**I13.Ø Hypertensive heart and chronic kidney disease with heart failure and stage 1 through stage 4 chronic kidney disease, or unspecified chronic kidney disease** HCC Rx ESR COM
Use additional code to identify stage of chronic kidney disease (N18.1-N18.4, N18.9)
Use additional code to identify type of heart failure (I5Ø.-)

✓5th **I13.1 Hypertensive heart and chronic kidney disease without heart failure**

**I13.1Ø Hypertensive heart and chronic kidney disease without heart failure, with stage 1 through stage 4 chronic kidney disease, or unspecified chronic kidney disease** Rx
Hypertensive heart disease and hypertensive chronic kidney disease NOS
Use additional code to identify the stage of chronic kidney disease (N18.1-N18.4, N18.9)

**I13.11 Hypertensive heart and chronic kidney disease without heart failure, with stage 5 chronic kidney disease, or end stage renal disease** HCC Rx ESR COM
Use additional code to identify the stage of chronic kidney disease (N18.5, N18.6)

**I13.2 Hypertensive heart and chronic kidney disease with heart failure and with stage 5 chronic kidney disease, or end stage renal disease** HCC Rx ESR COM
Use additional code to identify the stage of chronic kidney disease (N18.5, N18.6)
Use additional code to identify type of heart failure (I5Ø.-)

✓4th **I15 Secondary hypertension**
Code also underlying condition
EXCLUDES 1 *postprocedural hypertension (I97.3)*
EXCLUDES 2 *secondary hypertension involving vessels of brain (I6Ø-I69)*
*secondary hypertension involving vessels of eye (H35.Ø-)*

**I15.Ø Renovascular hypertension** Rx
**I15.1 Hypertension secondary to other renal disorders** Rx
**AHA:** 2016,3Q,22
**I15.2 Hypertension secondary to endocrine disorders** Rx
**AHA:** 2026,2Q,9; 2023,2Q,16
**I15.8 Other secondary hypertension** Rx
**I15.9 Secondary hypertension, unspecified** Rx

✓4th **I16 Hypertensive crisis**
Code also any identified hypertensive disease (I1Ø-I15, I1A)
**AHA:** 2016,4Q,26-28

**I16.Ø Hypertensive urgency** Rx
**I16.1 Hypertensive emergency** Rx
▶Code also, if applicable, to identify specific organ dysfunction, such as:◀
▶acute kidney injury (N17.-)◀
▶acute myocardial infarction (I21.-)◀
▶acute pulmonary edema (left and/or right ventricular failure) (J81.Ø, I5Ø.-)◀
▶aortic dissection (I71.Ø-)◀
▶cerebral hemorrhage (I6Ø.-, I61.-, I62.-)◀
▶cerebral infarction (I63.-)◀
▶eclampsia (O15.-)◀
▶hypertensive encephalopathy (I67.4)◀
▶seizure (R56.9)◀
~~Use additional, if applicable, to identify specific organ dysfunction, such as:~~
~~acute kidney injury (N17.-)~~
~~acute myocardial infarction (I21.-)~~
~~acute pulmonary edema (left and/or right ventricular failure) (J81.Ø, I5Ø.-)~~
~~aortic dissection (I71.Ø-)~~
~~cerebral hemorrhage (I6Ø.-, I61.-, I62.-)~~
~~cerebral infarction (I63.-)~~
~~eclampsia (O15.-)~~
~~hypertensive encephalopathy (I67.4)~~
~~seizure (R56.9)~~
**AHA:** 2023,4Q,24

**I16.9 Hypertensive crisis, unspecified** Rx

✓4th **I1A Other hypertension**
**AHA:** 2023,4Q,23-25

**I1A.Ø Resistant hypertension** Rx
Apparent treatment resistant hypertension
Treatment resistant hypertension
True resistant hypertension
Code first specific type of existing hypertension, if known, such as:
essential hypertension (I1Ø)
secondary hypertension (I15.-)

## Ischemic heart diseases (I20-I25)

Code also the presence of hypertension (I10-I1A)

✓4th **I20 Angina pectoris**

Use additional code to identify:
exposure to environmental tobacco smoke (Z77.22)
history of tobacco dependence (Z87.891)
occupational exposure to environmental tobacco smoke (Z57.31)
tobacco dependence (F17.-)
tobacco use (Z72.0)

EXCLUDES 1 *angina pectoris with atherosclerotic heart disease of native coronary arteries (I25.1-)*
*atherosclerosis of coronary artery bypass graft(s) and coronary artery of transplanted heart with angina pectoris (I25.7-)*
*postinfarction angina (I23.7)*

**DEF:** Chest pain due to reduced blood flow resulting in a lack of oxygen to the heart muscles.

**I20.0 Unstable angina** HCC Rx ESR COM
Accelerated angina
Crescendo angina
De novo effort angina
Intermediate coronary syndrome
Preinfarction syndrome
Worsening effort angina

**I20.1 Angina pectoris with documented spasm** Rx ESR
Angiospastic angina
Prinzmetal angina
Spasm-induced angina
Variant angina

**I20.2 Refractory angina pectoris** Rx ESR
**AHA:** 2022,4Q,20-21

✓5th **I20.8 Other forms of angina pectoris**
Use additional code(s) for symptoms associated with angina equivalent
**AHA:** 2023,4Q,25-26

**I20.81 Angina pectoris with coronary microvascular dysfunction** Rx ESR
Angina pectoris with coronary microvascular disease

**I20.89 Other forms of angina pectoris** Rx ESR
Angina of effort
Angina equivalent
Coronary slow flow syndrome
Stable angina
Stenocardia

**I20.9 Angina pectoris, unspecified** Rx ESR
Angina NOS
Anginal syndrome
Cardiac angina
Ischemic chest pain

✓4th **I21 Acute myocardial infarction**

INCLUDES cardiac infarction
coronary (artery) embolism
coronary (artery) occlusion
coronary (artery) rupture
coronary (artery) thrombosis
infarction of heart, myocardium, or ventricle
myocardial infarction specified as acute or with a stated duration of 4 weeks (28 days) or less from onset

Use additional code, if applicable, to identify:
exposure to environmental tobacco smoke (Z77.22)
history of tobacco dependence (Z87.891)
occupational exposure to environmental tobacco smoke (Z57.31)
status post administration of tPA (rtPA) in a different facility within the last 24 hours prior to admission to current facility (Z92.82)
tobacco dependence (F17.-)
tobacco use (Z72.0)

EXCLUDES 2 *old myocardial infarction (I25.2)*
*postmyocardial infarction syndrome (I24.1)*
*subsequent type 1 myocardial infarction (I22.-)*

**AHA:** 2019,2Q,5; 2018,4Q,68; 2018,3Q,5; 2017,4Q,12-14; 2017,1Q,44-45; 2016,4Q,140; 2015,2Q,16; 2013,1Q,25; 2012,4Q,96,102-103

**TIP:** When chronic total occlusion and myocardial infarction are documented as being in different vessels, assign code I25.82 Chronic total occlusion of coronary artery, in addition to the myocardial infarction code.

✓5th **I21.0 ST elevation (STEMI) myocardial infarction of anterior wall**
Type 1 ST elevation myocardial infarction of anterior wall
**DEF:** ST elevation myocardial infarction: Complete obstruction of one or more coronary arteries causing decreased blood flow (ischemia) and necrosis of myocardial muscle cells.

**I21.01 ST elevation (STEMI) myocardial infarction involving left main coronary artery** HCC Rx ESR COM

**I21.02 ST elevation (STEMI) myocardial infarction involving left anterior descending coronary artery** HCC Rx ESR COM
ST elevation (STEMI) myocardial infarction involving diagonal coronary artery
**AHA:** 2013,1Q,25

**I21.09 ST elevation (STEMI) myocardial infarction involving other coronary artery of anterior wall** HCC Rx ESR COM
Acute transmural myocardial infarction of anterior wall
Anteroapical transmural (Q wave) infarction (acute)
Anterolateral transmural (Q wave) infarction (acute)
Anteroseptal transmural (Q wave) infarction (acute)
Transmural (Q wave) infarction (acute) (of) anterior (wall) NOS
**AHA:** 2012,4Q,102-103

✓5th **I21.1 ST elevation (STEMI) myocardial infarction of inferior wall**
Type 1 ST elevation myocardial infarction of inferior wall
**DEF:** ST elevation myocardial infarction: Complete obstruction of one or more coronary arteries causing decreased blood flow (ischemia) and necrosis of myocardial muscle cells.

**I21.11 ST elevation (STEMI) myocardial infarction involving right coronary artery** HCC Rx ESR COM
Inferoposterior transmural (Q wave) infarction (acute)

**I21.19 ST elevation (STEMI) myocardial infarction involving other coronary artery of inferior wall** HCC Rx ESR COM
Acute transmural myocardial infarction of inferior wall
Inferolateral transmural (Q wave) infarction (acute)
Transmural (Q wave) infarction (acute) (of) diaphragmatic wall
Transmural (Q wave) infarction (acute) (of) inferior (wall) NOS
EXCLUDES 2 *ST elevation (STEMI) myocardial infarction involving left circumflex coronary artery (I21.21)*
**AHA:** 2012,4Q,96

✓5th **I21.2 ST elevation (STEMI) myocardial infarction of other sites**
Type 1 ST elevation myocardial infarction of other sites
**DEF:** ST elevation myocardial infarction: Complete obstruction of one or more coronary arteries causing decreased blood flow (ischemia) and necrosis of myocardial muscle cells.

**I21.21 ST elevation (STEMI) myocardial infarction involving left circumflex coronary artery** HCC Rx ESR COM
ST elevation (STEMI) myocardial infarction involving oblique marginal coronary artery

**I21.29 ST elevation (STEMI) myocardial infarction involving other sites** HCC Rx ESR COM
Acute transmural myocardial infarction of other sites
Apical-lateral transmural (Q wave) infarction (acute)
Basal-lateral transmural (Q wave) infarction (acute)
High lateral transmural (Q wave) infarction (acute)
Lateral (wall) NOS transmural (Q wave) infarction (acute)
Posterior (true) transmural (Q wave) infarction (acute)
Posterobasal transmural (Q wave) infarction (acute)
Posterolateral transmural (Q wave) infarction (acute)
Posteroseptal transmural (Q wave) infarction (acute)
Septal transmural (Q wave) infarction (acute) NOS

**I21.3 ST elevation (STEMI) myocardial infarction of unspecified site** HCC Rx ESR COM
Acute transmural myocardial infarction of unspecified site
Transmural (Q wave) myocardial infarction NOS
Type 1 ST elevation myocardial infarction of unspecified site
**DEF:** ST elevation myocardial infarction: Complete obstruction of one or more coronary arteries causing decreased blood flow (ischemia) and necrosis of myocardial muscle cells.

**I21.4 Non-ST elevation (NSTEMI) myocardial infarction** HCC Rx ESR COM
Acute subendocardial myocardial infarction
Non-Q wave myocardial infarction NOS
Nontransmural myocardial infarction NOS
Type 1 non-ST elevation myocardial infarction
**AHA:** 2026,2Q,7; 2026,1Q,35; 2025,2Q,26; 2025,1Q,20; 2024,1Q,28; 2023,2Q,29; 2021,3Q,6; 2019,2Q,33; 2017,1Q,44-45
**DEF:** Partial obstruction of one or more coronary arteries that causes decreased blood flow (ischemia) and may cause partial thickness necrosis of myocardial muscle cells.

**I21.9 Acute myocardial infarction, unspecified** HCC Rx ESR COM
Myocardial infarction (acute) NOS

✓5th **I21.A Other type of myocardial infarction**
**AHA:** 2019,2Q,5

**I21.A1 Myocardial infarction type 2** HCC Rx ESR COM
Myocardial infarction due to demand ischemia
Myocardial infarction secondary to ischemic imbalance
Code first, if applicable, the underlying cause, such as:
- anemia (D5Ø.Ø-D64.9)
- chronic obstructive pulmonary disease (J44.-)
- paroxysmal tachycardia (I47.Ø-I47.9)
- shock (R57.Ø-R57.9)

**AHA:** 2019,4Q,53; 2017,4Q,13-14
**DEF:** Often referred to as due to demand ischemia, myocardial infarction (MI) type 2 refers to an MI due to ischemia and necrosis resulting from an oxygen imbalance to the heart. This mismatch between oxygen decreased supply and increased demand is caused by conditions other than coronary artery disease such as vasospasm, embolism, anemia, hypertension, hypotension, or arrhythmias.

**I21.A9 Other myocardial infarction type** HCC Rx ESR COM
Myocardial infarction associated with revascularization procedure
Myocardial infarction type 3
Myocardial infarction type 4a
Myocardial infarction type 4b
Myocardial infarction type 4c
Myocardial infarction type 5
Code first, if applicable, postprocedural myocardial infarction following cardiac surgery (I97.19Ø), or postprocedural myocardial infarction during cardiac surgery (I97.79Ø)
Code also complication, if known and applicable, such as:
- (acute) stent occlusion (T82.897-)
- (acute) stent stenosis (T82.855-)
- (acute) stent thrombosis (T82.867-)
- cardiac arrest due to underlying cardiac condition (I46.2)
- complication of percutaneous coronary intervention (PCI) (I97.89)
- occlusion of coronary artery bypass graft (T82.218-)

**AHA:** 2026,1Q,35; 2021,3Q,6; 2019,2Q,33

**I21.B Myocardial infarction with coronary microvascular dysfunction** HCC Rx ESR COM
Myocardial infarction with coronary microvascular disease
Myocardial infarction with nonobstructive coronary arteries [MINOCA] with microvascular disease
**AHA:** 2026,2Q,7; 2023,4Q,25-26

✓4th **I22 Subsequent ST elevation (STEMI) and non-ST elevation (NSTEMI) myocardial infarction**
INCLUDES acute myocardial infarction occurring within four weeks (28 days) of a previous acute myocardial infarction, regardless of site
- cardiac infarction
- coronary (artery) embolism
- coronary (artery) occlusion
- coronary (artery) rupture
- coronary (artery) thrombosis
- infarction of heart, myocardium, or ventricle
- recurrent myocardial infarction
- reinfarction of myocardium
- rupture of heart, myocardium, or ventricle
- subsequent type 1 myocardial infarction

Use additional code, if applicable, to identify:
- exposure to environmental tobacco smoke (Z77.22)
- history of tobacco dependence (Z87.891)
- occupational exposure to environmental tobacco smoke (Z57.31)
- status post administration of tPA (rtPA) in a different facility within the last 24 hours prior to admission to current facility (Z92.82)
- tobacco dependence (F17.-)
- tobacco use (Z72.Ø)

EXCLUDES 1 *subsequent myocardial infarction, type 2 (I21.A1)*
*subsequent myocardial infarction of other type (type 3) (type 4) (type 5) (I21.A9)*

**AHA:** 2018,4Q,68; 2018,3Q,5; 2017,4Q,12-13; 2017,2Q,11; 2013,1Q,25; 2012,4Q,97,102-103
**DEF:** Non-ST elevation myocardial infarction: Partial obstruction of one or more coronary arteries that causes decreased blood flow (ischemia) and may cause partial thickness necrosis of myocardial muscle cells.
**DEF:** ST elevation myocardial infarction: Complete obstruction of one or more coronary arteries causing decreased blood flow (ischemia) and necrosis of myocardial muscle cells.
**TIP:** When chronic total occlusion and myocardial infarction are documented as being in different vessels, assign code I25.82 Chronic total occlusion of coronary artery, in addition to the myocardial infarction code.

**I22.Ø Subsequent ST elevation (STEMI) myocardial infarction of anterior wall** HCC Rx ESR COM
Subsequent acute transmural myocardial infarction of anterior wall
Subsequent anteroapical transmural (Q wave) infarction (acute)
Subsequent anterolateral transmural (Q wave) infarction (acute)
Subsequent anteroseptal transmural (Q wave) infarction (acute)
Subsequent transmural (Q wave) infarction (acute)(of) anterior (wall) NOS

**I22.1 Subsequent ST elevation (STEMI) myocardial infarction of inferior wall** HCC Rx ESR COM
Subsequent acute transmural myocardial infarction of inferior wall
Subsequent inferolateral transmural (Q wave) infarction (acute)
Subsequent inferoposterior transmural (Q wave) infarction (acute)
Subsequent transmural (Q wave) infarction (acute)(of) diaphragmatic wall
Subsequent transmural (Q wave) infarction (acute)(of) inferior (wall) NOS
**AHA:** 2012,4Q,102

**I22.2 Subsequent non-ST elevation (NSTEMI) myocardial infarction** HCC Rx ESR COM
Subsequent acute subendocardial myocardial infarction
Subsequent non-Q wave myocardial infarction NOS
Subsequent nontransmural myocardial infarction NOS

**I22.8 Subsequent ST elevation (STEMI) myocardial infarction of other sites** HCC Rx ESR COM
Subsequent acute transmural myocardial infarction of other sites
Subsequent apical-lateral transmural (Q wave) myocardial infarction (acute)
Subsequent basal-lateral transmural (Q wave) myocardial infarction (acute)
Subsequent high lateral transmural (Q wave) myocardial infarction (acute)
Subsequent posterior (true) transmural (Q wave) myocardial infarction (acute)
Subsequent posterobasal transmural (Q wave) myocardial infarction (acute)
Subsequent posterolateral transmural (Q wave) myocardial infarction (acute)
Subsequent posteroseptal transmural (Q wave) myocardial infarction (acute)
Subsequent septal NOS transmural (Q wave) myocardial infarction (acute)
Subsequent transmural (Q wave) myocardial infarction (acute)(of) lateral (wall) NOS

**I22.9 Subsequent ST elevation (STEMI) myocardial infarction of unspecified site** HCC Rx ESR COM
Subsequent acute myocardial infarction of unspecified site
Subsequent myocardial infarction (acute) NOS

✓4th **I23 Certain current complications following ST elevation (STEMI) and non-ST elevation (NSTEMI) myocardial infarction (within the 28 day period)**
**AHA:** 2017,2Q,11
**DEF:** Non-ST elevation myocardial infarction: Partial obstruction of one or more coronary arteries that causes decreased blood flow (ischemia) and may cause partial thickness necrosis of myocardial muscle cells.
**DEF:** ST elevation myocardial infarction: Complete obstruction of one or more coronary arteries causing decreased blood flow (ischemia) and necrosis of myocardial muscle cells.

**I23.Ø Hemopericardium as current complication following acute myocardial infarction** HCC Rx ESR COM A
EXCLUDES 1 *hemopericardium not specified as current complication following acute myocardial infarction (I31.2)*

**I23.1 Atrial septal defect as current complication following acute myocardial infarction** HCC Rx ESR COM A
EXCLUDES 1 *acquired atrial septal defect not specified as current complication following acute myocardial infarction (I51.Ø)*

**I23.2 Ventricular septal defect as current complication following acute myocardial infarction** HCC Rx ESR COM A
EXCLUDES 1 *acquired ventricular septal defect not specified as current complication following acute myocardial infarction (I51.Ø)*

**I23.3 Rupture of cardiac wall without hemopericardium as current complication following acute myocardial infarction** HCC Rx ESR COM A

**I23.4 Rupture of chordae tendineae as current complication following acute myocardial infarction** HCC Rx ESR COM
EXCLUDES 1 *rupture of chordae tendineae not specified as current complication following acute myocardial infarction (I51.1)*

**I23.5 Rupture of papillary muscle as current complication following acute myocardial infarction** HCC Rx ESR COM
EXCLUDES 1 *rupture of papillary muscle not specified as current complication following acute myocardial infarction (I51.2)*

**I23.6 Thrombosis of atrium, auricular appendage, and ventricle as current complications following acute myocardial infarction** HCC Rx ESR COM A
EXCLUDES 1 *thrombosis of atrium, auricular appendage, and ventricle not specified as current complication following acute myocardial infarction (I51.3)*

**I23.7 Postinfarction angina** HCC Rx ESR COM A
**AHA:** 2015,2Q,16
**TIP:** When postinfarction angina occurs with atherosclerotic coronary artery disease, code both I23.7 and I25.118 for atherosclerotic disease with other forms of angina pectoris.

**I23.8 Other current complications following acute myocardial infarction** HCC Rx ESR COM A

✓4th **I24 Other acute ischemic heart diseases**
EXCLUDES 1 *angina pectoris (I2Ø.-)*
*transient myocardial ischemia in newborn (P29.4)*
EXCLUDES 2 *non-ischemic myocardial injury (I5A)*

**I24.Ø Acute coronary thrombosis not resulting in myocardial infarction** HCC Rx ESR COM
Acute coronary (artery) (vein) embolism not resulting in myocardial infarction
Acute coronary (artery) (vein) occlusion not resulting in myocardial infarction
Acute coronary (artery) (vein) thromboembolism not resulting in myocardial infarction
EXCLUDES 1 *atherosclerotic heart disease (I25.1-)*
**AHA:** 2013,1Q,24

**I24.1 Dressler's syndrome** HCC Rx ESR COM
Postmyocardial infarction syndrome
EXCLUDES 1 *postinfarction angina (I23.7)*
**DEF:** Fever, leukocytosis, chest pain, evidence of pericarditis, pleurisy, and pneumonia occurring days or weeks after a myocardial infarction.

✓5th **I24.8 Other forms of acute ischemic heart disease**
EXCLUDES 1 *myocardial infarction due to demand ischemia (I21.A1)*
**AHA:** 2023,4Q,25-26; 2019,4Q,53; 2017,4Q,13

**I24.81 Acute coronary microvascular dysfunction** HCC Rx ESR COM
Acute (presentation of) coronary microvascular disease

**I24.89 Other forms of acute ischemic heart disease** HCC Rx ESR COM

**I24.9 Acute ischemic heart disease, unspecified** HCC Rx ESR COM
EXCLUDES 1 *ischemic heart disease (chronic) NOS (I25.9)*

✓4th **I25 Chronic ischemic heart disease**
Use additional code to identify:
chronic total occlusion of coronary artery (I25.82)
exposure to environmental tobacco smoke (Z77.22)
history of tobacco dependence (Z87.891)
occupational exposure to environmental tobacco smoke (Z57.31)
tobacco dependence (F17.-)
tobacco use (Z72.Ø)
EXCLUDES 2 *non-ischemic myocardial injury (I5A)*
**AHA:** 2025,1Q,20; 2022,4Q,20-21

✓5th **I25.1 Atherosclerotic heart disease of native coronary artery**
Atherosclerotic cardiovascular disease
Coronary (artery) atheroma
Coronary (artery) atherosclerosis
Coronary (artery) disease
Coronary (artery) sclerosis
Use additional code, if applicable, to identify:
coronary atherosclerosis due to calcified coronary lesion (I25.84)
coronary atherosclerosis due to lipid rich plaque (I25.83)
EXCLUDES 2 *atheroembolism (I75.-)*
*atherosclerosis of coronary artery bypass graft(s) and transplanted heart (I25.7-)*

**Atheromas**

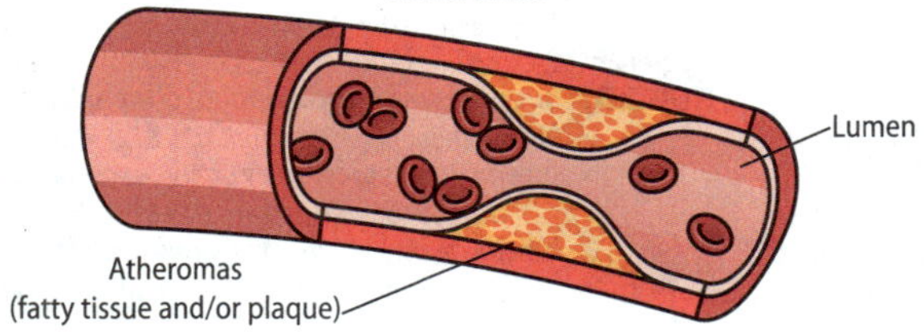


**I25.1Ø Atherosclerotic heart disease of native coronary artery without angina pectoris** Rx A
Atherosclerotic heart disease NOS
**AHA:** 2026,1Q,35; 2024,1Q,28; 2021,3Q,6-7; 2015,2Q,16; 2012,4Q,92

✓6th **I25.11 Atherosclerotic heart disease of native coronary artery with angina pectoris**
**AHA:** 2024,1Q,28

**I25.11Ø Atherosclerotic heart disease of native coronary artery with unstable angina pectoris** HCC Rx ESR COM A
EXCLUDES 1 *unstable angina without atherosclerotic heart disease (I2Ø.Ø)*

**I25.111 Atherosclerotic heart disease of native coronary artery with angina pectoris with documented spasm** Rx ESR A

EXCLUDES 1 *angina pectoris with documented spasm without atherosclerotic heart disease (I2Ø.1)*

**I25.112 Atherosclerotic heart disease of native coronary artery with refractory angina pectoris** Rx ESR A

**I25.118 Atherosclerotic heart disease of native coronary artery with other forms of angina pectoris** Rx ESR A

EXCLUDES 1 *other forms of angina pectoris without atherosclerotic heart disease (I2Ø.8-)*

**AHA:** 2015,2Q,16

**TIP:** When postinfarction angina occurs with atherosclerotic coronary artery disease, code both I23.7 and I25.118 for atherosclerotic disease with other forms of angina pectoris.

**I25.119 Atherosclerotic heart disease of native coronary artery with unspecified angina pectoris** Rx ESR A

Atherosclerotic heart disease with angina NOS

Atherosclerotic heart disease with ischemic chest pain

EXCLUDES 1 *unspecified angina pectoris without atherosclerotic heart disease (I2Ø.9)*

**I25.2 Old myocardial infarction** Rx

Healed myocardial infarction

Past myocardial infarction diagnosed by ECG or other investigation, but currently presenting no symptoms

**I25.3 Aneurysm of heart** Rx

Mural aneurysm

Ventricular aneurysm

✓5th **I25.4 Coronary artery aneurysm and dissection**

**I25.41 Coronary artery aneurysm** Rx

Coronary arteriovenous fistula, acquired

EXCLUDES 1 *congenital coronary (artery) aneurysm (Q24.5)*

**I25.42 Coronary artery dissection** Rx

**DEF:** Tear in the intimal arterial wall of a coronary artery resulting in the sudden intrusion of blood within the layers of the wall.

**I25.5 Ischemic cardiomyopathy** Rx

EXCLUDES 2 *coronary atherosclerosis (I25.1-, I25.7-)*

**AHA:** 2022,3Q,17

**I25.6 Silent myocardial ischemia** Rx

✓5th **I25.7 Atherosclerosis of coronary artery bypass graft(s) and coronary artery of transplanted heart with angina pectoris**

Use additional code, if applicable, to identify:

coronary atherosclerosis due to calcified coronary lesion (I25.84)

coronary atherosclerosis due to lipid rich plaque (I25.83)

EXCLUDES 1 *atherosclerosis of bypass graft(s) of transplanted heart without angina pectoris (I25.812)*

*atherosclerosis of coronary artery bypass graft(s) without angina pectoris (I25.81Ø)*

*atherosclerosis of native coronary artery of transplanted heart without angina pectoris (I25.811)*

✓6th **I25.7Ø Atherosclerosis of coronary artery bypass graft(s), unspecified, with angina pectoris**

**I25.7ØØ Atherosclerosis of coronary artery bypass graft(s), unspecified, with unstable angina pectoris** HCC Rx ESR COM A

EXCLUDES 1 *unstable angina pectoris without atherosclerosis of coronary artery bypass graft (I2Ø.Ø)*

**I25.7Ø1 Atherosclerosis of coronary artery bypass graft(s), unspecified, with angina pectoris with documented spasm** Rx ESR A

EXCLUDES 1 *angina pectoris with documented spasm without atherosclerosis of coronary artery bypass graft (I2Ø.1)*

**I25.7Ø2 Atherosclerosis of coronary artery bypass graft(s), unspecified, with refractory angina pectoris** Rx ESR A

**AHA:** 2022,4Q,21

**I25.7Ø8 Atherosclerosis of coronary artery bypass graft(s), unspecified, with other forms of angina pectoris** Rx ESR A

EXCLUDES 1 *other forms of angina pectoris without atherosclerosis of coronary artery bypass graft (I2Ø.8-)*

**I25.7Ø9 Atherosclerosis of coronary artery bypass graft(s), unspecified, with unspecified angina pectoris** Rx ESR A

EXCLUDES 1 *unspecified angina pectoris without atherosclerosis of coronary artery bypass graft (I2Ø.9)*

✓6th **I25.71 Atherosclerosis of autologous vein coronary artery bypass graft(s) with angina pectoris**

**I25.71Ø Atherosclerosis of autologous vein coronary artery bypass graft(s) with unstable angina pectoris** HCC Rx ESR COM A

EXCLUDES 1 *unstable angina without atherosclerosis of autologous vein coronary artery bypass graft(s) (I2Ø.Ø)*

EXCLUDES 2 *embolism or thrombus of coronary artery bypass graft(s) (T82.8-)*

**I25.711 Atherosclerosis of autologous vein coronary artery bypass graft(s) with angina pectoris with documented spasm** Rx ESR A

EXCLUDES 1 *angina pectoris with documented spasm without atherosclerosis of autologous vein coronary artery bypass graft(s) (I2Ø.1)*

**I25.712 Atherosclerosis of autologous vein coronary artery bypass graft(s) with refractory angina pectoris** Rx ESR A

**I25.718 Atherosclerosis of autologous vein coronary artery bypass graft(s) with other forms of angina pectoris** Rx ESR A

EXCLUDES 1 *other forms of angina pectoris without atherosclerosis of autologous vein coronary artery bypass graft(s) (I2Ø.8-)*

**I25.719 Atherosclerosis of autologous vein coronary artery bypass graft(s) with unspecified angina pectoris** Rx ESR A

EXCLUDES 1 *unspecified angina pectoris without atherosclerosis of autologous vein coronary artery bypass graft(s) (I2Ø.9)*

✓6th **I25.72 Atherosclerosis of autologous artery coronary artery bypass graft(s) with angina pectoris**
Atherosclerosis of internal mammary artery graft with angina pectoris

**I25.720 Atherosclerosis of autologous artery coronary artery bypass graft(s) with unstable angina pectoris** HCC Rx ESR COM A
EXCLUDES 1 *unstable angina without atherosclerosis of autologous artery coronary artery bypass graft(s) (I20.0)*

**I25.721 Atherosclerosis of autologous artery coronary artery bypass graft(s) with angina pectoris with documented spasm** Rx ESR A
EXCLUDES 1 *angina pectoris with documented spasm without atherosclerosis of autologous artery coronary artery bypass graft(s) (I20.1)*

**I25.722 Atherosclerosis of autologous artery coronary artery bypass graft(s) with refractory angina pectoris** Rx ESR A

**I25.728 Atherosclerosis of autologous artery coronary artery bypass graft(s) with other forms of angina pectoris** Rx ESR A
EXCLUDES 1 *other forms of angina pectoris without atherosclerosis of autologous artery coronary artery bypass graft(s) (I20.8-)*

**I25.729 Atherosclerosis of autologous artery coronary artery bypass graft(s) with unspecified angina pectoris** Rx ESR A
EXCLUDES 1 *unspecified angina pectoris without atherosclerosis of autologous artery coronary artery bypass graft(s) (I20.9)*

✓6th **I25.73 Atherosclerosis of nonautologous biological coronary artery bypass graft(s) with angina pectoris**

**I25.730 Atherosclerosis of nonautologous biological coronary artery bypass graft(s) with unstable angina pectoris** HCC Rx ESR COM A
EXCLUDES 1 *unstable angina without atherosclerosis of nonautologous biological coronary artery bypass graft(s) (I20.0)*

**I25.731 Atherosclerosis of nonautologous biological coronary artery bypass graft(s) with angina pectoris with documented spasm** Rx ESR A
EXCLUDES 1 *angina pectoris with documented spasm without atherosclerosis of nonautologous biological coronary artery bypass graft(s) (I20.1)*

**I25.732 Atherosclerosis of nonautologous biological coronary artery bypass graft(s) with refractory angina pectoris** Rx ESR A

**I25.738 Atherosclerosis of nonautologous biological coronary artery bypass graft(s) with other forms of angina pectoris** Rx ESR A
EXCLUDES 1 *other forms of angina pectoris without atherosclerosis of nonautologous biological coronary artery bypass graft(s) (I20.8-)*

**I25.739 Atherosclerosis of nonautologous biological coronary artery bypass graft(s) with unspecified angina pectoris** Rx ESR A
EXCLUDES 1 *unspecified angina pectoris without atherosclerosis of nonautologous biological coronary artery bypass graft(s) (I20.9)*

✓6th **I25.75 Atherosclerosis of native coronary artery of transplanted heart with angina pectoris**
EXCLUDES 1 *atherosclerosis of native coronary artery of transplanted heart without angina pectoris (I25.811)*

**I25.750 Atherosclerosis of native coronary artery of transplanted heart with unstable angina** HCC Rx ESR COM

**I25.751 Atherosclerosis of native coronary artery of transplanted heart with angina pectoris with documented spasm** Rx ESR

**I25.752 Atherosclerosis of native coronary artery of transplanted heart with refractory angina pectoris** Rx ESR A

**I25.758 Atherosclerosis of native coronary artery of transplanted heart with other forms of angina pectoris** Rx ESR

**I25.759 Atherosclerosis of native coronary artery of transplanted heart with unspecified angina pectoris** Rx ESR

✓6th **I25.76 Atherosclerosis of bypass graft of coronary artery of transplanted heart with angina pectoris**
EXCLUDES 1 *atherosclerosis of bypass graft of coronary artery of transplanted heart without angina pectoris (I25.812)*

**I25.760 Atherosclerosis of bypass graft of coronary artery of transplanted heart with unstable angina** HCC Rx ESR COM A

**I25.761 Atherosclerosis of bypass graft of coronary artery of transplanted heart with angina pectoris with documented spasm** Rx ESR A

**I25.762 Atherosclerosis of bypass graft of coronary artery of transplanted heart with refractory angina pectoris** Rx ESR A

**I25.768 Atherosclerosis of bypass graft of coronary artery of transplanted heart with other forms of angina pectoris** Rx ESR A

**I25.769 Atherosclerosis of bypass graft of coronary artery of transplanted heart with unspecified angina pectoris** Rx ESR A

✓6th **I25.79 Atherosclerosis of other coronary artery bypass graft(s) with angina pectoris**

**I25.790 Atherosclerosis of other coronary artery bypass graft(s) with unstable angina pectoris** HCC Rx ESR COM A
EXCLUDES 1 *unstable angina without atherosclerosis of other coronary artery bypass graft(s) (I20.0)*

**I25.791 Atherosclerosis of other coronary artery bypass graft(s) with angina pectoris with documented spasm** Rx ESR A
EXCLUDES 1 *angina pectoris with documented spasm without atherosclerosis of other coronary artery bypass graft(s) (I20.1)*

**I25.792 Atherosclerosis of other coronary artery bypass graft(s) with refractory angina pectoris** Rx ESR A

**I25.798 Atherosclerosis of other coronary artery bypass graft(s) with other forms of angina pectoris** Rx ESR A
EXCLUDES 1 *other forms of angina pectoris without atherosclerosis of other coronary artery bypass graft(s) (I20.8-)*

**I25.799 Atherosclerosis of other coronary artery bypass graft(s) with unspecified angina pectoris** Rx ESR A

EXCLUDES 1 *unspecified angina pectoris without atherosclerosis of other coronary artery bypass graft(s) (I2Ø.9)*

√5th **I25.8 Other forms of chronic ischemic heart disease**

√6th **I25.81 Atherosclerosis of other coronary vessels without angina pectoris**

Use additional code, if applicable, to identify:
coronary atherosclerosis due to calcified coronary lesion (I25.84)
coronary atherosclerosis due to lipid rich plaque (I25.83)

EXCLUDES 2 *atherosclerotic heart disease of native coronary artery without angina pectoris (I25.1Ø)*

**I25.81Ø Atherosclerosis of coronary artery bypass graft(s) without angina pectoris** Rx A

Atherosclerosis of coronary artery bypass graft NOS

EXCLUDES 1 *atherosclerosis of coronary bypass graft(s) with angina pectoris (I25.7Ø-I25.73-, I25.79-)*

**I25.811 Atherosclerosis of native coronary artery of transplanted heart without angina pectoris** Rx

Atherosclerosis of native coronary artery of transplanted heart NOS

EXCLUDES 1 *atherosclerosis of native coronary artery of transplanted heart with angina pectoris (I25.75-)*

**I25.812 Atherosclerosis of bypass graft of coronary artery of transplanted heart without angina pectoris** Rx A

Atherosclerosis of bypass graft of transplanted heart NOS

EXCLUDES 1 *atherosclerosis of bypass graft of transplanted heart with angina pectoris (I25.76)*

**I25.82 Chronic total occlusion of coronary artery** Rx UPD

Complete occlusion of coronary artery
Total occlusion of coronary artery
Code first coronary atherosclerosis (I25.1-, I25.7-, I25.81-)

EXCLUDES 1 *acute coronary occulsion with myocardial infarction (I21.Ø-I21.B, I22.-)*
*acute coronary occlusion without myocardial infarction (I24.Ø)*

**AHA:** 2018,3Q,5

**DEF:** Complete blockage of the coronary artery due to plaque accumulation over an extended period of time, resulting in substantial reduction of blood flow. Symptoms include angina or chest pain.

**TIP:** Report this code in addition to a code from category I21 or I22 when the chronic total occlusion and the myocardial infarction are documented as being in different vessels.

**I25.83 Coronary atherosclerosis due to lipid rich plaque** Rx UPD A

Code first coronary atherosclerosis (I25.1-, I25.7-, I25.81-)

**I25.84 Coronary atherosclerosis due to calcified coronary lesion** Rx UPD

Coronary atherosclerosis due to severely calcified coronary lesion
Code first coronary atherosclerosis (I25.1-, I25.7-, I25.81-)

**I25.85 Chronic coronary microvascular dysfunction** Rx

Chronic (presentation of) coronary microvascular disease
Coronary microvascular dysfunction NOS
**AHA:** 2023,4Q,25-26

**I25.89 Other forms of chronic ischemic heart disease** Rx

**I25.9 Chronic ischemic heart disease, unspecified** Rx

Ischemic heart disease (chronic) NOS

## Pulmonary heart disease and diseases of pulmonary circulation (I26-I28)

√4th **I26 Pulmonary embolism**

INCLUDES pulmonary (acute)(artery)(vein) infarction
pulmonary (acute) (artery)(vein) thromboembolism
pulmonary (acute)(artery)(vein) thrombosis

EXCLUDES 1 *cor pulmonale without embolism (I27.81)*

EXCLUDES 2 *chronic pulmonary embolism (I27.82)*
*personal history of pulmonary embolism (Z86.711)*
*pulmonary embolism complicating abortion, ectopic or molar pregnancy (OØØ-OØ7, OØ8.2)*
*pulmonary embolism complicating pregnancy, childbirth and the puerperium (O88.-)*
*pulmonary embolism due to complications of surgical and medical care (T8Ø.Ø, T81.7-, T82.8-)*
*pulmonary embolism due to trauma (T79.Ø, T79.1)*
*septic (non-pulmonary) arterial embolism (I76)*

**AHA:** 2022,3Q,8

√5th **I26.Ø Pulmonary embolism with acute cor pulmonale**

**DEF:** Cor pulmonale: Heart-lung disease appearing in identifiable forms as chronic or acute. The chronic form of this heart-lung disease is marked by dilation, hypertrophy and failure of the right ventricle due to a disease that has affected the function of the lungs, excluding congenital or left heart diseases and is also called chronic cardiopulmonary disease. The acute form is an overload of the right ventricle from a rapid onset of pulmonary hypertension, usually arising from a pulmonary embolism.

**I26.Ø1 Septic pulmonary embolism with acute cor pulmonale** HCC Rx ESR COM UPD

Code first underlying infection

**I26.Ø2 Saddle embolus of pulmonary artery with acute cor pulmonale** HCC Rx ESR COM

**I26.Ø3 Cement embolism of pulmonary artery with acute cor pulmonale** HCC Rx ESR COM UPD

Code first complication of other artery following a procedure (T81.718)
**AHA:** 2024,4Q,17

**I26.Ø4 Fat embolism of pulmonary artery with acute cor pulmonale** HCC Rx ESR COM

Code first, if applicable:
complication of other artery following a procedure (T81.718)
traumatic fat embolism (T79.1)
**AHA:** 2024,4Q,17

**I26.Ø9 Other pulmonary embolism with acute cor pulmonale** HCC Rx ESR COM

Acute cor pulmonale NOS
Other thrombotic pulmonary embolism with acute cor pulmonale
**AHA:** 2014,4Q,21

√5th **I26.9 Pulmonary embolism without acute cor pulmonale**

**I26.9Ø Septic pulmonary embolism without acute cor pulmonale** HCC Rx ESR COM UPD

Code first underlying infection

**I26.92 Saddle embolus of pulmonary artery without acute cor pulmonale** HCC Rx ESR COM

**I26.93 Single subsegmental thrombotic pulmonary embolism without acute cor pulmonale** HCC Rx ESR COM

Subsegmental pulmonary embolism NOS
**AHA:** 2021,2Q,9; 2019,4Q,6-7

**I26.94 Multiple subsegmental thrombotic pulmonary emboli without acute cor pulmonale** HCC Rx ESR COM

**AHA:** 2022,2Q,13; 2021,2Q,9; 2019,4Q,6-7

**I26.95 Cement embolism of pulmonary artery without acute cor pulmonale** HCC Rx ESR COM UPD

Code first complication of other artery following a procedure (T81.718)
**AHA:** 2024,4Q,17,19

**I26.96 Fat embolism of pulmonary artery without acute cor pulmonale** HCC Rx ESR COM

Code first, if applicable:
complication of other artery following a procedure (T81.718)
traumatic fat embolism (T79.1)
**AHA:** 2024,4Q,17,19

**I26.99 Other pulmonary embolism without acute cor pulmonale** HCC Rx ESR COM
Acute pulmonary embolism NOS
Other thrombotic pulmonary embolism without acute cor pulmonale
Pulmonary embolism NOS
**AHA:** 2022,2Q,13; 2020,3Q,10-11; 2019,2Q,22

√4th **I27 Other pulmonary heart diseases**

**I27.Ø Primary pulmonary hypertension** HCC Rx ESR COM
Heritable pulmonary arterial hypertension
Idiopathic pulmonary arterial hypertension
Primary group 1 pulmonary hypertension
Primary pulmonary arterial hypertension
**EXCLUDES 1** *persistent pulmonary hypertension of newborn (P29.3Ø)*
*pulmonary hypertension NOS (I27.2Ø)*
*secondary pulmonary arterial hypertension (I27.21)*
*secondary pulmonary hypertension (I27.29)*
**DEF:** Condition that occurs when pressure within the pulmonary artery is elevated and vascular resistance is observed in the lungs.

**I27.1 Kyphoscoliotic heart disease** HCC Rx ESR COM

√5th **I27.2 Other secondary pulmonary hypertension**
Code also associated underlying condition
**EXCLUDES 1** *Eisenmenger's syndrome (I27.83)*
**AHA:** 2017,4Q,14-15; 2014,4Q,21
**DEF:** Condition that occurs when pressure within the pulmonary artery is elevated and vascular resistance is observed in the lungs.

**I27.2Ø Pulmonary hypertension, unspecified** HCC Rx ESR COM
Pulmonary hypertension NOS

**I27.21 Secondary pulmonary arterial hypertension** HCC Rx ESR COM
(Associated) (drug-induced) (toxin-induced) (secondary) group 1 pulmonary hypertension
(Associated) (drug-induced) (toxin-induced) pulmonary arterial hypertension NOS
Code also associated conditions if applicable, or adverse effects of drugs or toxins, such as:
adverse effect of appetite depressants (T5Ø.5X5)
congenital heart disease (Q2Ø-Q28)
human immunodeficiency virus [HIV] disease (B2Ø)
polymyositis (M33.2-)
portal hypertension (K76.6)
rheumatoid arthritis (MØ5.-)
schistosomiasis (B65.-)
Sjogren syndrome (M35.Ø-)
systemic sclerosis (M34.-)

**I27.22 Pulmonary hypertension due to left heart disease** HCC Rx ESR COM
Group 2 pulmonary hypertension
Code also associated left heart disease, if known, such as:
multiple valve disease (IØ8.-)
rheumatic aortic valve diseases (IØ6.-)
rheumatic mitral valve diseases (IØ5.-)

**I27.23 Pulmonary hypertension due to lung diseases and hypoxia** HCC Rx ESR COM
Group 3 pulmonary hypertension
Code also associated lung disease, if known, such as:
bronchiectasis (J47.-)
cystic fibrosis with pulmonary manifestations (E84.Ø)
interstitial lung disease (J84.-)
pleural effusion (J9Ø)
sleep apnea (G47.3-)

**I27.24 Chronic thromboembolic pulmonary hypertension** HCC Rx ESR COM
Group 4 pulmonary hypertension
Code also associated pulmonary embolism, if applicable (I26.-, I27.82)

**I27.29 Other secondary pulmonary hypertension** HCC Rx ESR COM
Group 5 pulmonary hypertension
Pulmonary hypertension due to hematologic disorders
Pulmonary hypertension due to metabolic disorders
Pulmonary hypertension due to other systemic disorders
Pulmonary hypertension with unclear multifactorial mechanisms
Code also other associated disorders, if known, such as:
chronic myeloid leukemia (C92.1Ø-C92.22)
essential thrombocythemia (D47.3)
Gaucher disease (E75.22)
hypertensive chronic kidney disease with end stage renal disease (I12.Ø, I13.11, I13.2)
hyperthyroidism (EØ5.-)
hypothyroidism (EØØ-EØ3)
polycythemia vera (D45)
sarcoidosis (D86.-)
**AHA:** 2016,2Q,8

√5th **I27.8 Other specified pulmonary heart diseases**

**I27.81 Cor pulmonale (chronic)** HCC Rx ESR COM
Cor pulmonale NOS
Code also, if applicable, right heart failure (I5Ø.81-)
**EXCLUDES 1** *acute cor pulmonale (I26.Ø-)*
**AHA:** 2014,4Q,21
**DEF:** Heart-lung disease appearing in identifiable forms as chronic or acute. The chronic form of this heart-lung disease is marked by dilation, hypertrophy and failure of the right ventricle due to a disease that has affected the function of the lungs, excluding congenital or left heart diseases and is also called chronic cardiopulmonary disease. The acute form is an overload of the right ventricle from a rapid onset of pulmonary hypertension, usually arising from a pulmonary embolism.

**I27.82 Chronic pulmonary embolism** HCC Rx ESR COM
Use additional code, if applicable, for associated long-term (current) use of anticoagulants (Z79.Ø1)
**EXCLUDES 1** *personal history of pulmonary embolism (Z86.711)*
**AHA:** 2021,2Q,9
**DEF:** Long-standing condition commonly associated with pulmonary hypertension in which small blood clots travel to the lungs repeatedly over many weeks, months, or years, requiring continuation of established anticoagulant or thrombolytic therapy.

**I27.83 Eisenmenger's syndrome** HCC Rx ESR COM
(Irreversible) Eisenmenger's disease
Eisenmenger's complex
Pulmonary hypertension with right to left shunt related to congenital heart disease
Code also underlying heart defect, if known, such as:
atrial septal defect (Q21.1-)
Eisenmenger's defect (Q21.8)
patent ductus arteriosus (Q25.Ø)
ventricular septal defect (Q21.Ø)
**DEF:** Pulmonary hypertension with congenital communication between two circulations resulting in a right to left shunt. This causes reduced oxygen saturation in the arterial blood, leading to cyanosis and organ damage. Once it develops, this life-threating condition is irreversible.

√6th **I27.84 Fontan related circulation**

**I27.84Ø Fontan-associated liver disease [FALD]** Rx

**I27.841 Fontan-associated lymphatic dysfunction** Rx
Code also associated conditions such as:
chylothorax (J94.Ø)
Fontan associated protein-losing enteropathy ►(K9Ø.49)◄
plastic (obstructive) bronchitis (J44.89)

**I27.848 Other Fontan-associated condition** Rx
Use additional code to specify the Fontan associated condition

**I27.849 Fontan related circulation, unspecified** Rx

**I27.89 Other specified pulmonary heart diseases** HCC Rx ESR COM

**I27.9 Pulmonary heart disease, unspecified** HCC Rx ESR COM
Chronic cardiopulmonary disease

✓4th **I28 Other diseases of pulmonary vessels**

**I28.0 Arteriovenous fistula of pulmonary vessels** HCC Rx ESR COM
EXCLUDES 1 *congenital arteriovenous fistula (Q25.72)*

**I28.1 Aneurysm of pulmonary artery** HCC Rx ESR COM
EXCLUDES 1 *congenital aneurysm (Q25.79)*
*congenital arteriovenous aneurysm (Q25.72)*

**I28.8 Other diseases of pulmonary vessels** HCC Rx ESR COM
Pulmonary arteritis
Pulmonary endarteritis
Rupture of pulmonary vessels
Stenosis of pulmonary vessels
Stricture of pulmonary vessels

**I28.9 Disease of pulmonary vessels, unspecified** HCC Rx ESR COM

## Other forms of heart disease (I30-I5A)

✓4th **I30 Acute pericarditis**
INCLUDES acute mediastinopericarditis
acute myopericarditis
acute pericardial effusion
acute pleuropericarditis
acute pneumopericarditis
EXCLUDES 1 *Dressler's syndrome (I24.1)*
*rheumatic pericarditis (acute) (I01.0)*
*viral pericarditis due to Coxsackie virus (B33.23)*
**DEF:** Pericarditis: Inflammation affecting the pericardium, the fibroserous membrane that surrounds the heart.

**I30.0 Acute nonspecific idiopathic pericarditis** COM

**I30.1 Infective pericarditis** COM
Pneumococcal pericarditis
Pneumopyopericardium
Purulent pericarditis
Pyopericarditis
Pyopericardium
Pyopneumopericardium
Staphylococcal pericarditis
Streptococcal pericarditis
Suppurative pericarditis
Viral pericarditis
Use additional code (B95-B97) to identify infectious agent

**I30.8 Other forms of acute pericarditis** COM

**I30.9 Acute pericarditis, unspecified** COM

✓4th **I31 Other diseases of pericardium**
EXCLUDES 1 *diseases of pericardium specified as rheumatic (I09.2)*
*postcardiotomy syndrome (I97.0)*
*traumatic injury to pericardium (S26.-)*

**I31.0 Chronic adhesive pericarditis** COM
Accretio cordis
Adherent pericardium
Adhesive mediastinopericarditis

**I31.1 Chronic constrictive pericarditis** COM
Concretio cordis
Pericardial calcification

**I31.2 Hemopericardium, not elsewhere classified** COM
EXCLUDES 1 *hemopericardium as current complication following acute myocardial infarction (I23.0)*
*malignant pericardial effusion (I31.31)*
**DEF:** Presence of blood in the pericardial sac (pericardium). It can lead to potentially fatal cardiac tamponade if enough blood enters the pericardial cavity.

✓5th **I31.3 Pericardial effusion (noninflammatory)**
EXCLUDES 1 *acute pericardial effusion (I30.9)*
**AHA:** 2022,4Q,22; 2019,1Q,16

***I31.31 Malignant pericardial effusion in diseases classified elsewhere*** HCC COM
Code first underlying neoplasm (C00-D49)
**AHA:** 2022,4Q,22

**I31.39 Other pericardial effusion (noninflammatory)** COM
Chylopericardium

**I31.4 Cardiac tamponade** COM UPD
Code first underlying cause
**DEF:** Life-threatening condition in which fluid or blood accumulates in the space between the muscle of the heart (myocardium) and the outer sac that covers the heart (pericardium), resulting in compression of the heart.

**Cardiac Tamponade**

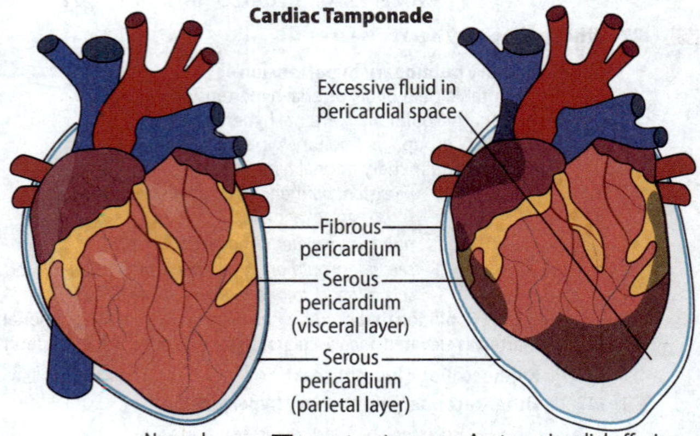


**I31.8 Other specified diseases of pericardium** COM
Epicardial plaques
Focal pericardial adhesions

**I31.9 Disease of pericardium, unspecified** COM
Pericarditis (chronic) NOS

***I32 Pericarditis in diseases classified elsewhere*** COM
Code first underlying disease
EXCLUDES 1 *pericarditis (in):*
*coxsackie (virus) (B33.23)*
*gonococcal (A54.83)*
*meningococcal (A39.53)*
*rheumatoid (arthritis) (M05.31)*
*syphilitic (A52.06)*
*systemic lupus erythematosus (M32.12)*
*tuberculosis (A18.84)*
**DEF:** Pericarditis: Inflammation affecting the pericardium, the fibroserous membrane that surrounds the heart.

✓4th **I33 Acute and subacute endocarditis**
EXCLUDES 1 *acute rheumatic endocarditis (I01.1)*
*endocarditis NOS (I38)*
**DEF:** Endocarditis: Inflammatory disease of the interior lining of the heart chamber and heart valves.

**I33.0 Acute and subacute infective endocarditis** COM
Bacterial endocarditis (acute) (subacute)
Endocarditis lenta (acute) (subacute)
Infective endocarditis (acute) (subacute) NOS
Malignant endocarditis (acute) (subacute)
Purulent endocarditis (acute) (subacute)
Septic endocarditis (acute) (subacute)
Ulcerative endocarditis (acute) (subacute)
Vegetative endocarditis (acute) (subacute)
Use additional code (B95-B97) to identify infectious agent
**AHA:** 2025,1Q,19,20

**I33.9 Acute and subacute endocarditis, unspecified** COM
Acute endocarditis NOS
Acute myoendocarditis NOS
Acute periendocarditis NOS
Subacute endocarditis NOS
Subacute myoendocarditis NOS
Subacute periendocarditis NOS

**I34 Nonrheumatic mitral valve disorders**

EXCLUDES 1 *mitral valve disease (I05.9)*
*mitral valve disorder specified as congenital (Q23.2, Q23.9)*
*mitral valve disorder specified as rheumatic (I05.-)*
*mitral valve disorder of unspecified cause with diseases of aortic and/or tricuspid valve(s) (I08.-)*
*mitral valve disorder of unspecified cause with mitral stenosis or obstruction (I05.0)*
*mitral valve failure (I05.8)*
*mitral valve stenosis (I05.0)*

**I34.0 Nonrheumatic mitral (valve) insufficiency**
Nonrheumatic mitral (valve) incompetence NOS
Nonrheumatic mitral (valve) regurgitation NOS
Code also, if applicable:
nonrheumatic mitral (valve) annulus calcification (I34.81)
**AHA:** 2025,1Q,19

**I34.1 Nonrheumatic mitral (valve) prolapse**
Floppy nonrheumatic mitral valve syndrome
EXCLUDES 1 *Marfan's syndrome (Q87.4-)*

**I34.2 Nonrheumatic mitral (valve) stenosis**
Code also, if applicable:
nonrheumatic mitral (valve) annulus calcification (I34.81)

**I34.8 Other nonrheumatic mitral valve disorders**
**AHA:** 2022,4Q,23

**I34.81 Nonrheumatic mitral (valve) annulus calcification**
Mitral (valve) annulus calcification NOS
Nonrheumatic mitral (valve) annular calcification
Code also, if applicable:
nonrheumatic mitral (valve) insufficiency (I34.0)
nonrheumatic mitral (valve) stenosis (I34.2)

**I34.89 Other nonrheumatic mitral valve disorders**

**I34.9 Nonrheumatic mitral valve disorder, unspecified**

**I35 Nonrheumatic aortic valve disorders**

Code also, if applicable, bicuspid aortic valve (Q23.81)

EXCLUDES 2 *aortic valve disorder of unspecified cause but with diseases of mitral and/or tricuspid valve(s) (I08.-)*
*aortic valve disorder specified as congenital (Q23.0, Q23.1)*
*aortic valve disorder specified as rheumatic (I06.-)*
*hypertrophic subaortic stenosis (I42.1)*

**I35.0 Nonrheumatic aortic (valve) stenosis**
**AHA:** 2024,4Q,26

**I35.1 Nonrheumatic aortic (valve) insufficiency**
Nonrheumatic aortic (valve) incompetence NOS
Nonrheumatic aortic (valve) regurgitation NOS

**I35.2 Nonrheumatic aortic (valve) stenosis with insufficiency**

**I35.8 Other nonrheumatic aortic valve disorders**

**I35.9 Nonrheumatic aortic valve disorder, unspecified**

**I36 Nonrheumatic tricuspid valve disorders**

EXCLUDES 1 *tricuspid valve disorders of unspecified cause (I07.-)*
*tricuspid valve disorders specified as congenital (Q22.4, Q22.8, Q22.9)*
*tricuspid valve disorders specified as rheumatic (I07.-)*
*tricuspid valve disorders with aortic and/or mitral valve involvement (I08.-)*

**I36.0 Nonrheumatic tricuspid (valve) stenosis**

**I36.1 Nonrheumatic tricuspid (valve) insufficiency**
Nonrheumatic tricuspid (valve) incompetence
Nonrheumatic tricuspid (valve) regurgitation

**I36.2 Nonrheumatic tricuspid (valve) stenosis with insufficiency**

**I36.8 Other nonrheumatic tricuspid valve disorders**

**I36.9 Nonrheumatic tricuspid valve disorder, unspecified**

**I37 Nonrheumatic pulmonary valve disorders**

EXCLUDES 1 *pulmonary valve disorder specified as congenital (Q22.1, Q22.2, Q22.3)*
*pulmonary valve disorder specified as rheumatic (I09.89)*

**I37.0 Nonrheumatic pulmonary valve stenosis**

**I37.1 Nonrheumatic pulmonary valve insufficiency**
Nonrheumatic pulmonary valve incompetence
Nonrheumatic pulmonary valve regurgitation

**I37.2 Nonrheumatic pulmonary valve stenosis with insufficiency**

**I37.8 Other nonrheumatic pulmonary valve disorders**

**I37.9 Nonrheumatic pulmonary valve disorder, unspecified**

**I38 Endocarditis, valve unspecified**

INCLUDES endocarditis (chronic) NOS
valvular incompetence NOS
valvular insufficiency NOS
valvular regurgitation NOS
valvular stenosis NOS
valvulitis (chronic) NOS

EXCLUDES 1 *congenital insufficiency of cardiac valve NOS (Q24.8)*
*congenital stenosis of cardiac valve NOS (Q24.8)*
*endocardial fibroelastosis (I42.4)*
*endocarditis specified as rheumatic (I09.1)*

**DEF:** Endocarditis: Inflammatory disease of the interior lining of the heart chamber and heart valves.

***I39 Endocarditis and heart valve disorders in diseases classified elsewhere***

Code first underlying disease, such as:
Q fever (A78)

EXCLUDES 1 *endocardial involvement in:*
*candidiasis (B37.6)*
*gonococcal infection (A54.83)*
*Libman-Sacks disease (M32.11)*
*listerosis (A32.82)*
*meningococcal infection (A39.51)*
*rheumatoid arthritis (M05.31)*
*syphilis (A52.03)*
*tuberculosis (A18.84)*
*typhoid fever (A01.02)*

**DEF:** Endocarditis: Inflammatory disease of the interior lining of the heart chamber and heart valves.

**I40 Acute myocarditis**

INCLUDES subacute myocarditis

EXCLUDES 1 *acute rheumatic myocarditis (I01.2)*

**DEF:** Myocarditis: Inflammation of the middle layer of the heart, which is composed of muscle tissue.

**I40.0 Infective myocarditis** COM
Septic myocarditis
Use additional code (B95-B97) to identify infectious agent

**I40.1 Isolated myocarditis** COM
Fiedler's myocarditis
Giant cell myocarditis
Idiopathic myocarditis

**I40.8 Other acute myocarditis** COM
**AHA:** 2026,1Q,33

**I40.9 Acute myocarditis, unspecified** COM

***I41 Myocarditis in diseases classified elsewhere*** COM

Code first underlying disease, such as:
typhus (A75.0-A75.9)

EXCLUDES 1 *myocarditis (in):*
*acute (B57.0)*
*Chagas' disease (chronic) (B57.2)*
*coxsackie (virus) infection (B33.22)*
*diphtheritic (A36.81)*
*gonococcal (A54.83)*
*influenzal (J09.X9, J10.82, J11.82)*
*meningococcal (A39.52)*
*mumps (B26.82)*
*rheumatoid arthritis (M05.31)*
*sarcoid (D86.85)*
*syphilis (A52.06)*
*toxoplasmosis (B58.81)*
*tuberculous (A18.84)*

**DEF:** Myocarditis: Inflammation of the middle layer of the heart, which is composed of muscle tissue.

**I42 Cardiomyopathy**

INCLUDES myocardiopathy

Code first pre-existing cardiomyopathy complicating pregnancy and puerperium (O99.4)

EXCLUDES 2 *ischemic cardiomyopathy (I25.5)*
*peripartum cardiomyopathy (O90.3)*
*ventricular hypertrophy (I51.7)*

▲ **I42.0 Dilated cardiomyopathy**
~~Congestive cardiomyopathy~~

● **I42.00 Dilated cardiomyopathy, unspecified**
Congestive cardiomyopathy, NOS

● **I42.01 Familial-genetic dilated cardiomyopathy**

● **I42.09 Other dilated cardiomyopathy**
Other nonfamilial dilated cardiomyopathy

Chapter 9. Diseases of the Circulatory System

I34–I42.09

**I42.1 Obstructive hypertrophic cardiomyopathy** HCC Rx ESR COM
Hypertrophic subaortic stenosis (idiopathic)
**DEF:** Cardiomyopathy marked by left ventricle hypertrophy and an enlarged septum that result in obstructed blood flow, arrhythmias, mitral regurgitation, and sudden cardiac death.
**TIP:** When this condition is described as inherited, assign code Q24.8.

**I42.2 Other hypertrophic cardiomyopathy** HCC Rx ESR COM
Nonobstructive hypertrophic cardiomyopathy

**I42.3 Endomyocardial (eosinophilic) disease** HCC Rx ESR COM
Endomyocardial (tropical) fibrosis
Loffler's endocarditis

**I42.4 Endocardial fibroelastosis** HCC Rx ESR COM
Congenital cardiomyopathy
Elastomyofibrosis

**I42.5 Other restrictive cardiomyopathy** HCC Rx ESR COM
Constrictive cardiomyopathy NOS

**I42.6 Alcoholic cardiomyopathy** HCC Rx ESR COM
Code also presence of alcoholism (F1Ø.-)

**I42.7 Cardiomyopathy due to drug and external agent** Rx ESR COM
Code first poisoning due to drug or toxin, if applicable (T36-T65 with fifth or sixth character 1-4)
Use additional code for adverse effect, if applicable, to identify drug (T36-T5Ø with fifth or sixth character 5)
**AHA:** 2021,3Q,8

▲ ✓5th **I42.8 Other cardiomyopathies**
● **I42.81 Arrhythmogenic cardiomyopathy**
● **I42.89 Other cardiomyopathies not elsewhere classified**

**I42.9 Cardiomyopathy, unspecified** HCC Rx ESR COM
Cardiomyopathy (primary) (secondary) NOS

***I43 Cardiomyopathy in diseases classified elsewhere*** HCC Rx ESR COM
Code first underlying disease, such as:
amyloidosis (E85.-)
glycogen storage disease (E74.Ø-)
gout (M1Ø.Ø-)
thyrotoxicosis (EØ5.Ø-EØ5.9-)
EXCLUDES 1 *cardiomyopathy (in):*
*coxsackie (virus) (B33.24)*
*diphtheria (A36.81)*
*sarcoidosis (D86.85)*
*tuberculosis (A18.84)*
**AHA:** 2024,2Q,9

✓4th **I44 Atrioventricular and left bundle-branch block**

**I44.Ø Atrioventricular block, first degree**

**I44.1 Atrioventricular block, second degree**
Atrioventricular block, type I and II
Möbitz block, type I and II
Second degree block, type I and II
Wenckebach's block

**I44.2 Atrioventricular block, complete** HCC ESR COM
Complete heart block NOS
Third degree block
**AHA:** 2025,2Q,4; 2019,2Q,4

✓5th **I44.3 Other and unspecified atrioventricular block**
Atrioventricular block NOS
**I44.3Ø Unspecified atrioventricular block**
**I44.39 Other atrioventricular block**

**I44.4 Left anterior fascicular block**

**I44.5 Left posterior fascicular block**

✓5th **I44.6 Other and unspecified fascicular block**
**I44.6Ø Unspecified fascicular block**
Left bundle-branch hemiblock NOS
**I44.69 Other fascicular block**

**I44.7 Left bundle-branch block, unspecified**

**Conduction Disorders**

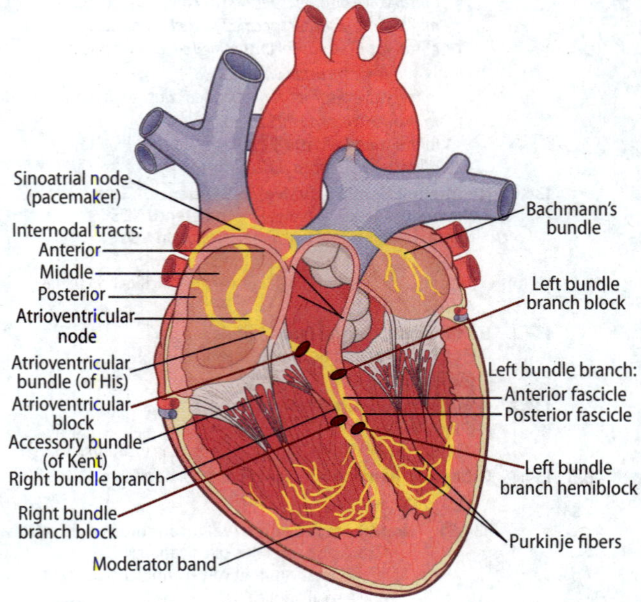


✓4th **I45 Other conduction disorders**

**I45.Ø Right fascicular block**

✓5th **I45.1 Other and unspecified right bundle-branch block**
**I45.1Ø Unspecified right bundle-branch block**
Right bundle-branch block NOS
**I45.19 Other right bundle-branch block**

**I45.2 Bifascicular block**

**I45.3 Trifascicular block**

**I45.4 Nonspecific intraventricular block**
Bundle-branch block NOS

**I45.5 Other specified heart block**
Sinoatrial block
Sinoauricular block
EXCLUDES 1 *heart block NOS (I45.9)*

**I45.6 Pre-excitation syndrome**
Accelerated atrioventricular conduction
Accessory atrioventricular conduction
Anomalous atrioventricular excitation
Lown-Ganong-Levine syndrome
Pre-excitation atrioventricular conduction
Wolff-Parkinson-White syndrome

✓5th **I45.8 Other specified conduction disorders**
**I45.81 Long QT syndrome**
**DEF:** Condition characterized by recurrent syncope, malignant arrhythmias, and sudden death. This syndrome has a characteristic prolonged Q-T interval on an electrocardiogram.
**I45.89 Other specified conduction disorders**
Atrioventricular [AV] dissociation
Interference dissociation
Isorhythmic dissociation
Nonparoxysmal AV nodal tachycardia
**AHA:** 2013,2Q,31

**I45.9 Conduction disorder, unspecified**
Heart block NOS
Stokes-Adams syndrome

✓4th **I46 Cardiac arrest**
EXCLUDES 2 *cardiogenic shock (R57.Ø)*
**AHA:** 2019,2Q,4-5

**I46.2 Cardiac arrest due to underlying cardiac condition** HCC ESR COM UPD
Code first underlying cardiac condition
**AHA:** 2024,1Q,27

**I46.8 Cardiac arrest due to other underlying condition** HCC ESR COM UPD
Code first underlying condition

**I46.9 Cardiac arrest, cause unspecified** HCC ESR COM
**AHA:** 2020,3Q,26

**I47 Paroxysmal tachycardia**

Code first tachycardia complicating:
abortion or ectopic or molar pregnancy (OØØ-OØ7, OØ8.8)
obstetric surgery and procedures (O75.4)

EXCLUDES 1 *tachycardia NOS (RØØ.Ø)*
*sinoauricular tachycardia NOS (RØØ.Ø)*
*sinus [sinusal] tachycardia NOS (RØØ.Ø)*

**I47.Ø Re-entry ventricular arrhythmia** HCC ESR COM

**I47.1 Supraventricular tachycardia**
AHA: 2023,4Q,26-27

**I47.1Ø Supraventricular tachycardia, unspecified** Rx ESR COM

**I47.11 Inappropriate sinus tachycardia, so stated** Rx ESR COM
IST

**I47.19 Other supraventricular tachycardia** Rx ESR COM
Atrial (paroxysmal) tachycardia
Atrioventricular [AV] (paroxysmal) tachycardia
Atrioventricular re-entrant (nodal) tachycardia [AVNRT] [AVRT]
Junctional (paroxysmal) tachycardia
Nodal (paroxysmal) tachycardia

**I47.2 Ventricular tachycardia**
AHA: 2022,4Q,23-24; 2021,3Q,11; 2013,3Q,23

**I47.2Ø Ventricular tachycardia, unspecified** HCC ESR COM

**I47.21 Torsades de pointes** HCC ESR COM
Code also, if applicable, long QT syndrome (I45.81)
Use additional code for adverse effect, if applicable, to identify drug (T36-T5Ø with fifth or sixth character 5)
AHA: 2022,4Q,24
DEF: Torsades de pointes (TdP): Accelerated heart rhythm, anywhere between 150 and 300 beats per minute, that initiates in the lower chambers of the heart (ventricles). Most commonly occurs in the setting of inherited or medication-induced long QT syndrome.

● **I47.22 Catecholaminergic polymorphic ventricular tachycardia [CPVT]**
Familial polymorphic ventricular tachycardia [FPVT]

**I47.29 Other ventricular tachycardia** HCC ESR COM

**I47.9 Paroxysmal tachycardia, unspecified** HCC Rx ESR COM
Bouveret (-Hoffman) syndrome

**I48 Atrial fibrillation and flutter**

**I48.Ø Paroxysmal atrial fibrillation** HCC Rx ESR COM
AHA: 2021,2Q,8; 2018,3Q,6

**I48.1 Persistent atrial fibrillation**
EXCLUDES 1 *permanent atrial fibrillation (I48.21)*
AHA: 2021,2Q,8; 2019,4Q,7; 2019,2Q,3; 2018,3Q,6

**I48.11 Longstanding persistent atrial fibrillation** HCC Rx ESR COM

**I48.19 Other persistent atrial fibrillation** HCC Rx ESR COM
Chronic persistent atrial fibrillation
Persistent atrial fibrillation, NOS
AHA: 2019,4Q,7

**I48.2 Chronic atrial fibrillation**
AHA: 2021,2Q,8; 2019,4Q,7; 2019,2Q,3; 2018,3Q,6

**I48.2Ø Chronic atrial fibrillation, unspecified** HCC Rx ESR COM
EXCLUDES 1 *chronic persistent atrial fibrillation (I48.19)*

**I48.21 Permanent atrial fibrillation** HCC Rx ESR COM

**I48.3 Typical atrial flutter** HCC Rx ESR COM
Type I atrial flutter

**I48.4 Atypical atrial flutter** HCC Rx ESR COM
Type II atrial flutter

**I48.9 Unspecified atrial fibrillation and atrial flutter**

**I48.91 Unspecified atrial fibrillation** HCC Rx ESR COM

**I48.92 Unspecified atrial flutter** HCC Rx ESR COM

**I49 Other cardiac arrhythmias**

Code first cardiac arrhythmia complicating:
abortion or ectopic or molar pregnancy (OØØ-OØ7, OØ8.8)
obstetric surgery and procedures (O75.4)

EXCLUDES 2 *bradycardia NOS (RØØ.1)*
*neonatal dysrhythmia (P29.1-)*
*sinoatrial bradycardia (RØØ.1)*
*sinus bradycardia (RØØ.1)*
*vagal bradycardia (RØØ.1)*

**I49.Ø Ventricular fibrillation and flutter**

**I49.Ø1 Ventricular fibrillation** HCC ESR COM
AHA: 2022,2Q,14

**I49.Ø2 Ventricular flutter** HCC ESR COM

**I49.1 Atrial premature depolarization**
Atrial premature beats

**I49.2 Junctional premature depolarization** HCC Rx ESR COM

**I49.3 Ventricular premature depolarization**
AHA: 2020,2Q,23

**I49.4 Other and unspecified premature depolarization**

**I49.4Ø Unspecified premature depolarization**
Premature beats NOS

**I49.49 Other premature depolarization**
Ectopic beats
Extrasystoles
Extrasystolic arrhythmias
Premature contractions

**I49.5 Sick sinus syndrome** HCC ESR COM
Tachycardia-bradycardia syndrome
AHA: 2019,1Q,33
TIP: The presence of a pacemaker controls but does not cure sick sinus syndrome and therefore is considered a reportable chronic condition. When a pacemaker is evaluated by a provider, this code and code Z95.0 Presence of cardiac pacemaker, should be reported, even in the absence of any notable changes or management.

▲ **I49.8 Other specified cardiac arrhythmias**
~~Brugada syndrome~~
~~Coronary sinus rhythm disorder~~
~~Ectopic rhythm disorder~~
~~Nodal rhythm disorder~~
AHA: 2025,2Q,4

● **I49.81 Brugada syndrome**

● **I49.82 Ventricular bigeminy**
Use additional code, if applicable, for associated symptoms such as:
dizziness (R42)
syncope (R55)

● **I49.89 Other specified cardiac arrhythmias not elsewhere classified**
Coronary sinus rhythm disorder
Ectopic rhythm disorder
Nodal rhythm disorder

**I49.9 Cardiac arrhythmia, unspecified**
Arrhythmia (cardiac) NOS

**I5Ø Heart failure**

Code first:
heart failure complicating abortion or ectopic or molar pregnancy (OØØ-OØ7, OØ8.8)
heart failure due to hypertension (I11.Ø)
heart failure due to hypertension with chronic kidney disease (I13.-)
heart failure following surgery (I97.13-)
obstetric surgery and procedures (O75.4)
rheumatic heart failure (IØ9.81)

EXCLUDES 2 *cardiac arrest (I46.-)*
*neonatal cardiac failure (P29.Ø)*

AHA: 2018,4Q,67; 2018,2Q,9; 2017,1Q,47; 2014,1Q,25; 2013,2Q,33

**I5Ø.1 Left ventricular failure, unspecified** HCC Rx ESR COM
Cardiac asthma
Edema of lung with heart disease NOS
Edema of lung with heart failure
Left heart failure
Pulmonary edema with heart disease NOS
Pulmonary edema with heart failure
EXCLUDES 1 *edema of lung without heart disease or heart failure (J81.-)*
*pulmonary edema without heart disease or failure (J81.-)*

✓5th **I50.2 Systolic (congestive) heart failure**
Heart failure with reduced ejection fraction [HFrEF]
Systolic left ventricular heart failure
Code also end stage heart failure, if applicable (I50.84)
EXCLUDES 1 *combined systolic (congestive) and diastolic (congestive) heart failure (I50.4-)*
**AHA:** 2020,3Q,32; 2017,1Q,46; 2016,1Q,10

**I50.20 Unspecified systolic (congestive) heart failure** HCC Rx ESR COM

**I50.21 Acute systolic (congestive) heart failure** HCC Rx ESR COM

**I50.22 Chronic systolic (congestive) heart failure** HCC Rx ESR COM

**I50.23 Acute on chronic systolic (congestive) heart failure** HCC Rx ESR COM

✓5th **I50.3 Diastolic (congestive) heart failure**
Diastolic left ventricular heart failure
Heart failure with normal ejection fraction
Heart failure with preserved ejection fraction [HFpEF]
Code also end stage heart failure, if applicable (I50.84)
EXCLUDES 1 *combined systolic (congestive) and diastolic (congestive) heart failure (I50.4-)*
**AHA:** 2024,2Q,9; 2020,3Q,32; 2017,1Q,46; 2016,1Q,10

**I50.30 Unspecified diastolic (congestive) heart failure** HCC Rx ESR COM

**I50.31 Acute diastolic (congestive) heart failure** HCC Rx ESR COM
**AHA:** 2025,2Q,5

**I50.32 Chronic diastolic (congestive) heart failure** HCC Rx ESR COM
**AHA:** 2023,3Q,14
**DEF:** HFimpEF: Heart failure with improved ejection fraction
**DEF:** HFrecEF: Heart failure with recovered ejection fraction

**I50.33 Acute on chronic diastolic (congestive) heart failure** HCC Rx ESR COM

✓5th **I50.4 Combined systolic (congestive) and diastolic (congestive) heart failure**
Combined systolic and diastolic left ventricular heart failure
Heart failure with reduced ejection fraction and diastolic dysfunction
Code also end stage heart failure, if applicable (I50.84)
**AHA:** 2017,1Q,46; 2016,1Q,10

**I50.40 Unspecified combined systolic (congestive) and diastolic (congestive) heart failure** HCC Rx ESR COM

**I50.41 Acute combined systolic (congestive) and diastolic (congestive) heart failure** HCC Rx ESR COM

**I50.42 Chronic combined systolic (congestive) and diastolic (congestive) heart failure** HCC Rx ESR COM

**I50.43 Acute on chronic combined systolic (congestive) and diastolic (congestive) heart failure** HCC Rx ESR COM

✓5th **I50.8 Other heart failure**
**AHA:** 2022,3Q,16; 2017,4Q,15-16

✓6th **I50.81 Right heart failure**
Right ventricular failure
**AHA:** 2023,3Q,14

**I50.810 Right heart failure, unspecified** HCC Rx ESR COM
Right heart failure without mention of left heart failure
Right ventricular failure NOS

**I50.811 Acute right heart failure** HCC Rx ESR COM
Acute (isolated) right ventricular failure
Acute isolated right heart failure

**I50.812 Chronic right heart failure** HCC Rx ESR COM
Chronic (isolated) right ventricular failure
Chronic isolated right heart failure

**I50.813 Acute on chronic right heart failure** HCC Rx ESR COM
Acute decompensation of chronic (isolated) right ventricular failure
Acute exacerbation of chronic (isolated) right ventricular failure
Acute on chronic (isolated) right ventricular failure
Acute on chronic isolated right heart failure

**I50.814 Right heart failure due to left heart failure** HCC Rx ESR COM
Right ventricular failure secondary to left ventricular failure
Code also the type of left ventricular failure, if known (I50.2-I50.43)
EXCLUDES 1 *right heart failure with but not due to left heart failure (I50.82)*

**I50.82 Biventricular heart failure** HCC Rx ESR COM
Code also the type of left ventricular failure as systolic, diastolic, or combined, if known (I50.2-I50.43)

**I50.83 High output heart failure** HCC Rx ESR COM
**DEF:** Occurs when the high demand for blood exceeds the capacity of a normally functioning heart to meet the demand.

**I50.84 End stage heart failure** HCC Rx ESR COM
Stage D heart failure
Code also the type of heart failure as systolic, diastolic, or combined, if known (I50.2-I50.43)

**I50.89 Other heart failure** HCC Rx ESR COM

**I50.9 Heart failure, unspecified** HCC Rx ESR COM
Cardiac, heart or myocardial failure NOS
Congestive heart disease
Congestive heart failure NOS
EXCLUDES 2 *fluid overload unrelated to congestive heart failure (E87.70)*
**AHA:** 2017,4Q,15-16; 2017,1Q,45-46; 2014,4Q,21; 2012,4Q,92

✓4th **I51 Complications and ill-defined descriptions of heart disease**
EXCLUDES 2 *heart disease specified as rheumatic (I00-I09)*

**I51.0 Cardiac septal defect, acquired** A
Acquired septal atrial defect (old)
Acquired septal auricular defect (old)
Acquired septal ventricular defect (old)
EXCLUDES 1 *cardiac septal defect as current complication following acute myocardial infarction (I23.1, I23.2)*
**DEF:** Abnormal communication between opposite heart chambers due to a defect of the septum. It is not present at birth.

**I51.1 Rupture of chordae tendineae, not elsewhere classified** HCC Rx ESR COM
EXCLUDES 1 *rupture of chordae tendineae as current complication following acute myocardial infarction (I23.4)*

**I51.2 Rupture of papillary muscle, not elsewhere classified** HCC Rx ESR COM
EXCLUDES 1 *rupture of papillary muscle as current complication following acute myocardial infarction (I23.5)*

**I51.3 Intracardiac thrombosis, not elsewhere classified**
Apical thrombosis (old)
Atrial thrombosis (old)
Auricular thrombosis (old)
Mural thrombosis (old)
Ventricular thrombosis (old)
EXCLUDES 1 *intracardiac thrombosis as current complication following acute myocardial infarction (I23.6)*
**AHA:** 2013,1Q,24

**I51.4 Myocarditis, unspecified** HCC Rx ESR COM
Chronic (interstitial) myocarditis
Myocardial fibrosis
Myocarditis NOS
EXCLUDES 1 *acute or subacute myocarditis (I40.-)*
**AHA:** 2018,4Q,67; 2018,2Q,9

**I51.5 Myocardial degeneration** HCC Rx ESR COM
Fatty degeneration of heart or myocardium
Myocardial disease
Senile degeneration of heart or myocardium
EXCLUDES 1 *myocardial degeneration due to hypertension (I11.-)*
*myocardial degeneration due to hypertension and chronic kidney disease (I13.-)*
**AHA:** 2018,4Q,67; 2018,2Q,9

**I51.7 Cardiomegaly**
Cardiac dilatation
Cardiac hypertrophy
Ventricular dilatation
EXCLUDES 1 *cardiomegaly due to hypertension (I11.-)*
*cardiomegaly due to hypertension and chronic kidney disease (I13.-)*
**AHA:** 2018,4Q,67; 2018,2Q,9

✓5th **I51.8 Other ill-defined heart diseases**
AHA: 2018,2Q,9

**I51.81 Takotsubo syndrome**
Reversible left ventricular dysfunction following sudden emotional stress
Stress induced cardiomyopathy
Takotsubo cardiomyopathy
Transient left ventricular apical ballooning syndrome
AHA: 2025,3Q,14
DEF: Complex of symptoms mimicking myocardial infarct in absence of heart disease, with the majority of cases occurring in postmenopausal women. Heart muscles are temporarily weakened, and a sudden, massive surge of adrenalin stuns the heart, greatly reducing the ability to pump blood.

**I51.89 Other ill-defined heart diseases**
Carditis (acute)(chronic)
Pancarditis (acute)(chronic)
AHA: 2019,2Q,5; 2018,4Q,67

**I51.9 Heart disease, unspecified**
AHA: 2018,4Q,67; 2018,2Q,9

***I52 Other heart disorders in diseases classified elsewhere***
Code first underlying disease, such as:
congenital syphilis (A5Ø.5)
mucopolysaccharidosis (E76.3)
schistosomiasis (B65.Ø-B65.9)
EXCLUDES 1 *heart disease (in):*
*gonococcal infection (A54.83)*
*meningococcal infection (A39.5Ø)*
*rheumatoid arthritis (MØ5.31)*
*syphilis (A52.Ø6)*

**I5A Non-ischemic myocardial injury (non-traumatic)**
Acute (non-ischemic) myocardial injury
Chronic (non-ischemic) myocardial injury
Unspecified (non-ischemic) myocardial injury
Code first the underlying cause, if known and applicable, such as:
acute kidney failure (N17.-)
acute myocarditis (I4Ø.-)
cardiomyopathy (I42.-)
chronic kidney disease (CKD) (N18.-)
heart failure (I5Ø.-)
hypertensive urgency (I16.Ø)
nonrheumatic aortic valve disorders (I35.-)
paroxysmal tachycardia (I47.-)
pulmonary embolism (I26.-)
pulmonary hypertension (I27.Ø, I27.2-)
sepsis (A41.-)
takotsubo syndrome (I51.81)
EXCLUDES 1 *acute myocardial infarction (I21.-)*
*injury of heart (S26.-)*
EXCLUDES 2 *other acute ischemic heart diseases (I24.-)*
AHA: 2025,3Q,14; 2021,4Q,14-15

## Cerebrovascular diseases (I6Ø-I69)

Use additional code to identify presence of:
alcohol abuse and dependence (F1Ø.-)
exposure to environmental tobacco smoke (Z77.22)
history of tobacco dependence (Z87.891)
hypertension (I1Ø-I1A)
occupational exposure to environmental tobacco smoke (Z57.31)
tobacco dependence (F17.-)
tobacco use (Z72.Ø)
EXCLUDES 1 *traumatic intracranial hemorrhage (SØ6.-)*
AHA: 2014,3Q,5; 2012,4Q,91-92

✓4th **I6Ø Nontraumatic subarachnoid hemorrhage**
Use additional code, if known, to indicate National Institutes of Health Stroke Scale (NIHSS) score (R29.7-)
EXCLUDES 1 *syphilitic ruptured cerebral aneurysm (A52.Ø5)*
EXCLUDES 2 *sequelae of subarachnoid hemorrhage (I69.Ø-)*

✓5th **I6Ø.Ø Nontraumatic subarachnoid hemorrhage from carotid siphon and bifurcation**

**I6Ø.ØØ Nontraumatic subarachnoid hemorrhage from unspecified carotid siphon and bifurcation** HCC ESR COM

**I6Ø.Ø1 Nontraumatic subarachnoid hemorrhage from right carotid siphon and bifurcation** HCC ESR COM

**I6Ø.Ø2 Nontraumatic subarachnoid hemorrhage from left carotid siphon and bifurcation** HCC ESR COM

✓5th **I6Ø.1 Nontraumatic subarachnoid hemorrhage from middle cerebral artery**

**I6Ø.1Ø Nontraumatic subarachnoid hemorrhage from unspecified middle cerebral artery** HCC ESR COM

**I6Ø.11 Nontraumatic subarachnoid hemorrhage from right middle cerebral artery** HCC ESR COM

**I6Ø.12 Nontraumatic subarachnoid hemorrhage from left middle cerebral artery** HCC ESR COM

**I6Ø.2 Nontraumatic subarachnoid hemorrhage from anterior communicating artery** HCC ESR COM
AHA: 2025,3Q,17

✓5th **I6Ø.3 Nontraumatic subarachnoid hemorrhage from posterior communicating artery**

**I6Ø.3Ø Nontraumatic subarachnoid hemorrhage from unspecified posterior communicating artery** HCC ESR COM

**I6Ø.31 Nontraumatic subarachnoid hemorrhage from right posterior communicating artery** HCC ESR COM

**I6Ø.32 Nontraumatic subarachnoid hemorrhage from left posterior communicating artery** HCC ESR COM

**I6Ø.4 Nontraumatic subarachnoid hemorrhage from basilar artery** HCC ESR COM

✓5th **I6Ø.5 Nontraumatic subarachnoid hemorrhage from vertebral artery**

**I6Ø.5Ø Nontraumatic subarachnoid hemorrhage from unspecified vertebral artery** HCC ESR COM

**I6Ø.51 Nontraumatic subarachnoid hemorrhage from right vertebral artery** HCC ESR COM

**I6Ø.52 Nontraumatic subarachnoid hemorrhage from left vertebral artery** HCC ESR COM

**I6Ø.6 Nontraumatic subarachnoid hemorrhage from other intracranial arteries** HCC ESR COM

**I6Ø.7 Nontraumatic subarachnoid hemorrhage from unspecified intracranial artery** HCC ESR COM
Ruptured (congenital) berry aneurysm
Ruptured (congenital) cerebral aneurysm
Subarachnoid hemorrhage (nontraumatic) from cerebral artery NOS
Subarachnoid hemorrhage (nontraumatic) from communicating artery NOS
EXCLUDES 1 *berry aneurysm, nonruptured (I67.1)*

**I6Ø.8 Other nontraumatic subarachnoid hemorrhage** HCC ESR COM
Meningeal hemorrhage
Rupture of cerebral arteriovenous malformation

**I6Ø.9 Nontraumatic subarachnoid hemorrhage, unspecified** HCC ESR COM

✓4th **I61 Nontraumatic intracerebral hemorrhage**
Use additional code, if known, to indicate National Institutes of Health Stroke Scale (NIHSS) score (R29.7-)
EXCLUDES 2 *sequelae of intracerebral hemorrhage (I69.1-)*
AHA: 2022,3Q,9-10; 2017,2Q,9-10

**I61.Ø Nontraumatic intracerebral hemorrhage in hemisphere, subcortical** HCC ESR COM
Deep intracerebral hemorrhage (nontraumatic)
AHA: 2016,4Q,27

**I61.1 Nontraumatic intracerebral hemorrhage in hemisphere, cortical** HCC ESR COM
Cerebral lobe hemorrhage (nontraumatic)
Superficial intracerebral hemorrhage (nontraumatic)

**I61.2 Nontraumatic intracerebral hemorrhage in hemisphere, unspecified** HCC ESR COM

**I61.3 Nontraumatic intracerebral hemorrhage in brain stem** HCC ESR COM
AHA: 2023,4Q,42

**I61.4 Nontraumatic intracerebral hemorrhage in cerebellum** HCC ESR COM

**I61.5 Nontraumatic intracerebral hemorrhage, intraventricular** HCC ESR COM

**I61.6 Nontraumatic intracerebral hemorrhage, multiple localized** HCC ESR COM

**I61.8 Other nontraumatic intracerebral hemorrhage** HCC ESR COM
AHA: 2024,2Q,25

**I61.9 Nontraumatic intracerebral hemorrhage, unspecified** HCC ESR COM

✓4th **I62 Other and unspecified nontraumatic intracranial hemorrhage**
Use additional code, if known, to indicate National Institutes of Health Stroke Scale (NIHSS) score (R29.7-)
EXCLUDES 2 *sequelae of intracranial hemorrhage (I69.2)*

✓5th **I62.Ø Nontraumatic subdural hemorrhage**

**I62.ØØ Nontraumatic subdural hemorrhage, unspecified** HCC ESR COM

I62.Ø1 Nontraumatic **acute** subdural hemorrhage HCC ESR COM

I62.Ø2 Nontraumatic **subacute** subdural hemorrhage HCC ESR COM

I62.Ø3 Nontraumatic **chronic** subdural hemorrhage HCC ESR COM

I62.1 Nontraumatic **extradural** hemorrhage HCC ESR COM
Nontraumatic epidural hemorrhage
**AHA:** 2023,3Q,21

I62.9 Nontraumatic intracranial hemorrhage, unspecified HCC ESR COM

√4th **I63 Cerebral infarction**

INCLUDES occlusion and stenosis of cerebral and precerebral arteries, resulting in cerebral infarction

Use additional code, if applicable, to identify status post administration of tPA (rtPA) in a different facility within the last 24 hours prior to admission to current facility (Z92.82)

Use additional code, if known, to indicate National Institutes of Health Stroke Scale (NIHSS) score (R29.7-)

EXCLUDES 1 *neonatal cerebral infarction (P91.82-)*

EXCLUDES 2 *chronic, without residual deficits (sequelae) (Z86.73)*
*sequelae of cerebral infarction (I69.3-)*

**AHA:** 2024,1Q,26; 2017,2Q,9-10; 2016,4Q,28,61-62; 2015,1Q,25; 2014,1Q,23

**TIP:** Weakness on one side of the body documented as secondary to stroke is synonymous with hemiparesis/hemiplegia (G81.-). Weakness of one limb documented as secondary to stroke is synonymous with monoplegia (G83.1-, G83.2-, G83.3-).

√5th I63.Ø Cerebral infarction due to **thrombosis of precerebral** arteries

I63.ØØ Cerebral infarction due to thrombosis of unspecified precerebral artery HCC ESR COM

√6th I63.Ø1 Cerebral infarction due to thrombosis of **vertebral** artery

I63.Ø11 Cerebral infarction due to thrombosis of **right** vertebral artery HCC ESR COM

I63.Ø12 Cerebral infarction due to thrombosis of **left** vertebral artery HCC ESR COM

I63.Ø13 Cerebral infarction due to thrombosis of **bilateral** vertebral arteries HCC ESR COM

I63.Ø19 Cerebral infarction due to thrombosis of unspecified vertebral artery HCC ESR COM

I63.Ø2 Cerebral infarction due to thrombosis of **basilar** artery HCC ESR COM

√6th I63.Ø3 Cerebral infarction due to thrombosis of **carotid** artery

I63.Ø31 Cerebral infarction due to thrombosis of **right** carotid artery HCC ESR COM

I63.Ø32 Cerebral infarction due to thrombosis of **left** carotid artery HCC ESR COM

I63.Ø33 Cerebral infarction due to thrombosis of **bilateral** carotid arteries HCC ESR COM

I63.Ø39 Cerebral infarction due to thrombosis of unspecified carotid artery HCC ESR COM

I63.Ø9 Cerebral infarction due to thrombosis of other precerebral artery HCC ESR COM

√5th I63.1 Cerebral infarction due to **embolism of precerebral** arteries

I63.1Ø Cerebral infarction due to embolism of unspecified precerebral artery HCC ESR COM

√6th I63.11 Cerebral infarction due to embolism of **vertebral** artery

I63.111 Cerebral infarction due to embolism of **right** vertebral artery HCC ESR COM

I63.112 Cerebral infarction due to embolism of **left** vertebral artery HCC ESR COM

I63.113 Cerebral infarction due to embolism of **bilateral** vertebral arteries HCC ESR COM

I63.119 Cerebral infarction due to embolism of unspecified vertebral artery HCC ESR COM

I63.12 Cerebral infarction due to embolism of **basilar** artery HCC ESR COM

√6th I63.13 Cerebral infarction due to embolism of **carotid** artery

I63.131 Cerebral infarction due to embolism of **right** carotid artery HCC ESR COM

I63.132 Cerebral infarction due to embolism of **left** carotid artery HCC ESR COM

I63.133 Cerebral infarction due to embolism of **bilateral** carotid arteries HCC ESR COM

I63.139 Cerebral infarction due to embolism of unspecified carotid artery HCC ESR COM

I63.19 Cerebral infarction due to embolism of other precerebral artery HCC ESR COM

√5th I63.2 Cerebral infarction due to unspecified **occlusion or stenosis of precerebral** arteries
**AHA:** 2020,3Q,27-28

I63.2Ø Cerebral infarction due to unspecified occlusion or stenosis of unspecified precerebral arteries HCC ESR COM

√6th I63.21 Cerebral infarction due to unspecified occlusion or stenosis of **vertebral** arteries

I63.211 Cerebral infarction due to unspecified occlusion or stenosis of **right** vertebral artery HCC ESR COM

I63.212 Cerebral infarction due to unspecified occlusion or stenosis of **left** vertebral artery HCC ESR COM

I63.213 Cerebral infarction due to unspecified occlusion or stenosis of **bilateral** vertebral arteries HCC ESR COM

I63.219 Cerebral infarction due to unspecified occlusion or stenosis of unspecified vertebral artery HCC ESR COM

I63.22 Cerebral infarction due to unspecified occlusion or stenosis of **basilar** artery HCC ESR COM

√6th I63.23 Cerebral infarction due to unspecified occlusion or stenosis of **carotid arteries**

I63.231 Cerebral infarction due to unspecified occlusion or stenosis of **right** carotid arteries HCC ESR COM

I63.232 Cerebral infarction due to unspecified occlusion or stenosis of **left** carotid arteries HCC ESR COM

I63.233 Cerebral infarction due to unspecified occlusion or stenosis of **bilateral** carotid arteries HCC ESR COM

I63.239 Cerebral infarction due to unspecified occlusion or stenosis of unspecified carotid artery HCC ESR COM

I63.29 Cerebral infarction due to unspecified occlusion or stenosis of other precerebral arteries HCC ESR COM

√5th I63.3 Cerebral infarction due to **thrombosis of cerebral** arteries

I63.3Ø Cerebral infarction due to thrombosis of unspecified cerebral artery HCC ESR COM

√6th I63.31 Cerebral infarction due to thrombosis of **middle** cerebral artery

I63.311 Cerebral infarction due to thrombosis of **right** middle cerebral artery HCC ESR COM

I63.312 Cerebral infarction due to thrombosis of **left** middle cerebral artery HCC ESR COM

I63.313 Cerebral infarction due to thrombosis of **bilateral** middle cerebral arteries HCC ESR COM

I63.319 Cerebral infarction due to thrombosis of unspecified middle cerebral artery HCC ESR COM

√6th I63.32 Cerebral infarction due to thrombosis of **anterior** cerebral artery

I63.321 Cerebral infarction due to thrombosis of **right** anterior cerebral artery HCC ESR COM

I63.322 Cerebral infarction due to thrombosis of **left** anterior cerebral artery HCC ESR COM

I63.323 Cerebral infarction due to thrombosis of **bilateral** anterior cerebral arteries HCC ESR COM

I63.329 Cerebral infarction due to thrombosis of unspecified anterior cerebral artery HCC ESR COM

√6th I63.33 Cerebral infarction due to thrombosis of **posterior** cerebral artery

I63.331 Cerebral infarction due to thrombosis of **right** posterior cerebral artery HCC ESR COM

I63.332 Cerebral infarction due to thrombosis of **left** posterior cerebral artery HCC ESR COM

I63.333 Cerebral infarction due to thrombosis of bilateral posterior cerebral arteries HCC ESR COM
I63.339 Cerebral infarction due to thrombosis of unspecified posterior cerebral artery HCC ESR COM

✓6th I63.34 Cerebral infarction due to thrombosis of cerebellar artery
I63.341 Cerebral infarction due to thrombosis of right cerebellar artery HCC ESR COM
I63.342 Cerebral infarction due to thrombosis of left cerebellar artery HCC ESR COM
I63.343 Cerebral infarction due to thrombosis of bilateral cerebellar arteries HCC ESR COM
I63.349 Cerebral infarction due to thrombosis of unspecified cerebellar artery HCC ESR COM

I63.39 Cerebral infarction due to thrombosis of other cerebral artery HCC ESR COM

✓5th I63.4 Cerebral infarction due to embolism of cerebral arteries
I63.40 Cerebral infarction due to embolism of unspecified cerebral artery HCC ESR COM

✓6th I63.41 Cerebral infarction due to embolism of middle cerebral artery
I63.411 Cerebral infarction due to embolism of right middle cerebral artery HCC ESR COM
I63.412 Cerebral infarction due to embolism of left middle cerebral artery HCC ESR COM
I63.413 Cerebral infarction due to embolism of bilateral middle cerebral arteries HCC ESR COM
I63.419 Cerebral infarction due to embolism of unspecified middle cerebral artery HCC ESR COM

✓6th I63.42 Cerebral infarction due to embolism of anterior cerebral artery
I63.421 Cerebral infarction due to embolism of right anterior cerebral artery HCC ESR COM
I63.422 Cerebral infarction due to embolism of left anterior cerebral artery HCC ESR COM
I63.423 Cerebral infarction due to embolism of bilateral anterior cerebral arteries HCC ESR COM
I63.429 Cerebral infarction due to embolism of unspecified anterior cerebral artery HCC ESR COM

✓6th I63.43 Cerebral infarction due to embolism of posterior cerebral artery
I63.431 Cerebral infarction due to embolism of right posterior cerebral artery HCC ESR COM
I63.432 Cerebral infarction due to embolism of left posterior cerebral artery HCC ESR COM
I63.433 Cerebral infarction due to embolism of bilateral posterior cerebral arteries HCC ESR COM
I63.439 Cerebral infarction due to embolism of unspecified posterior cerebral artery HCC ESR COM

✓6th I63.44 Cerebral infarction due to embolism of cerebellar artery
I63.441 Cerebral infarction due to embolism of right cerebellar artery HCC ESR COM
I63.442 Cerebral infarction due to embolism of left cerebellar artery HCC ESR COM
I63.443 Cerebral infarction due to embolism of bilateral cerebellar arteries HCC ESR COM
I63.449 Cerebral infarction due to embolism of unspecified cerebellar artery HCC ESR COM

I63.49 Cerebral infarction due to embolism of other cerebral artery HCC ESR COM

✓5th I63.5 Cerebral infarction due to unspecified occlusion or stenosis of cerebral arteries
I63.50 Cerebral infarction due to unspecified occlusion or stenosis of unspecified cerebral artery HCC ESR COM

✓6th I63.51 Cerebral infarction due to unspecified occlusion or stenosis of middle cerebral artery
I63.511 Cerebral infarction due to unspecified occlusion or stenosis of right middle cerebral artery HCC ESR COM
I63.512 Cerebral infarction due to unspecified occlusion or stenosis of left middle cerebral artery HCC ESR COM
I63.513 Cerebral infarction due to unspecified occlusion or stenosis of bilateral middle cerebral arteries HCC ESR COM
I63.519 Cerebral infarction due to unspecified occlusion or stenosis of unspecified middle cerebral artery HCC ESR COM

✓6th I63.52 Cerebral infarction due to unspecified occlusion or stenosis of anterior cerebral artery
I63.521 Cerebral infarction due to unspecified occlusion or stenosis of right anterior cerebral artery HCC ESR COM
I63.522 Cerebral infarction due to unspecified occlusion or stenosis of left anterior cerebral artery HCC ESR COM
I63.523 Cerebral infarction due to unspecified occlusion or stenosis of bilateral anterior cerebral arteries HCC ESR COM
I63.529 Cerebral infarction due to unspecified occlusion or stenosis of unspecified anterior cerebral artery HCC ESR COM

✓6th I63.53 Cerebral infarction due to unspecified occlusion or stenosis of posterior cerebral artery
I63.531 Cerebral infarction due to unspecified occlusion or stenosis of right posterior cerebral artery HCC ESR COM
I63.532 Cerebral infarction due to unspecified occlusion or stenosis of left posterior cerebral artery HCC ESR COM
I63.533 Cerebral infarction due to unspecified occlusion or stenosis of bilateral posterior cerebral arteries HCC ESR COM
I63.539 Cerebral infarction due to unspecified occlusion or stenosis of unspecified posterior cerebral artery HCC ESR COM

✓6th I63.54 Cerebral infarction due to unspecified occlusion or stenosis of cerebellar artery
I63.541 Cerebral infarction due to unspecified occlusion or stenosis of right cerebellar artery HCC ESR COM
I63.542 Cerebral infarction due to unspecified occlusion or stenosis of left cerebellar artery HCC ESR COM
I63.543 Cerebral infarction due to unspecified occlusion or stenosis of bilateral cerebellar arteries HCC ESR COM
I63.549 Cerebral infarction due to unspecified occlusion or stenosis of unspecified cerebellar artery HCC ESR COM

I63.59 Cerebral infarction due to unspecified occlusion or stenosis of other cerebral artery HCC ESR COM

I63.6 Cerebral infarction due to cerebral venous thrombosis, nonpyogenic HCC ESR COM

✓5th I63.8 Other cerebral infarction
**AHA:** 2018,4Q,16

I63.81 Other cerebral infarction due to occlusion or stenosis of small artery HCC ESR COM
Lacunar infarction
**AHA:** 2025,3Q,18; 2020,3Q,27
**TIP:** Strokes in the corona radiata are a type of lacunar stroke.

I63.89 Other cerebral infarction HCC ESR COM
**AHA:** 2024,1Q,32; 2022,1Q,25

I63.9 Cerebral infarction, unspecified HCC ESR COM
Stroke NOS
EXCLUDES 2 *transient cerebral ischemic attacks and related syndromes (G45.-)*
**AHA:** 2020,2Q,29
**TIP:** When provider documentation does not identify the location of an infarction, imaging reports can be used to pinpoint the location and lead to a more specific infarction code.

**✓4th I65 Occlusion and stenosis of precerebral arteries, not resulting in cerebral infarction**

INCLUDES embolism of precerebral artery
narrowing of precerebral artery
obstruction (complete) (partial) of precerebral artery
thrombosis of precerebral artery

EXCLUDES 1 *insufficiency, NOS, of precerebral artery (G45.-)*
*insufficiency of precerebral arteries causing cerebral infarction (I63.Ø-I63.2)*

**AHA:** 2018,2Q,9

**✓5th I65.Ø Occlusion and stenosis of vertebral artery**
- **I65.Ø1 Occlusion and stenosis of right vertebral artery**
- **I65.Ø2 Occlusion and stenosis of left vertebral artery**
- **I65.Ø3 Occlusion and stenosis of bilateral vertebral arteries**
- **I65.Ø9 Occlusion and stenosis of unspecified vertebral artery**

**I65.1 Occlusion and stenosis of basilar artery**

**✓5th I65.2 Occlusion and stenosis of carotid artery**

**AHA:** 2021,1Q,4; 2020,3Q,28
- **I65.21 Occlusion and stenosis of right carotid artery**
- **I65.22 Occlusion and stenosis of left carotid artery**
- **I65.23 Occlusion and stenosis of bilateral carotid arteries**
- **I65.29 Occlusion and stenosis of unspecified carotid artery**

**I65.8 Occlusion and stenosis of other precerebral arteries**

**I65.9 Occlusion and stenosis of unspecified precerebral artery**
Occlusion and stenosis of precerebral artery NOS

**✓4th I66 Occlusion and stenosis of cerebral arteries, not resulting in cerebral infarction**

INCLUDES embolism of cerebral artery
narrowing of cerebral artery
obstruction (complete) (partial) of cerebral artery
thrombosis of cerebral artery

EXCLUDES 1 *occlusion and stenosis of cerebral artery causing cerebral infarction (I63.3-I63.5)*

**✓5th I66.Ø Occlusion and stenosis of middle cerebral artery**
- **I66.Ø1 Occlusion and stenosis of right middle cerebral artery**
- **I66.Ø2 Occlusion and stenosis of left middle cerebral artery**
- **I66.Ø3 Occlusion and stenosis of bilateral middle cerebral arteries**
- **I66.Ø9 Occlusion and stenosis of unspecified middle cerebral artery**

**✓5th I66.1 Occlusion and stenosis of anterior cerebral artery**
- **I66.11 Occlusion and stenosis of right anterior cerebral artery**
- **I66.12 Occlusion and stenosis of left anterior cerebral artery**
- **I66.13 Occlusion and stenosis of bilateral anterior cerebral arteries**
- **I66.19 Occlusion and stenosis of unspecified anterior cerebral artery**

**✓5th I66.2 Occlusion and stenosis of posterior cerebral artery**
- **I66.21 Occlusion and stenosis of right posterior cerebral artery**
- **I66.22 Occlusion and stenosis of left posterior cerebral artery**
- **I66.23 Occlusion and stenosis of bilateral posterior cerebral arteries**
- **I66.29 Occlusion and stenosis of unspecified posterior cerebral artery**

**I66.3 Occlusion and stenosis of cerebellar arteries**

**I66.8 Occlusion and stenosis of other cerebral arteries**
Occlusion and stenosis of perforating arteries

**I66.9 Occlusion and stenosis of unspecified cerebral artery**

**✓4th I67 Other cerebrovascular diseases**

EXCLUDES 1 *occlusion and stenosis of cerebral artery causing cerebral infarction (I63.3-I63.5-)*
*occlusion and stenosis of precerebral artery causing cerebral infarction (I63.2-)*

EXCLUDES 2 *sequelae of the listed conditions (I69.8)*

**I67.Ø Dissection of cerebral arteries, nonruptured** ESR COM

EXCLUDES 1 *ruptured cerebral arteries (I6Ø.7)*

**AHA:** 2021,3Q,5

**DEF:** Dissecting aneurysm: Tear within an arterial wall that allows blood to accumulate between the outer and middle layers, creating a false lumen.

**I67.1 Cerebral aneurysm, nonruptured** COM
Cerebral aneurysm NOS
Cerebral arteriovenous fistula, acquired
Internal carotid artery aneurysm, intracranial portion
Internal carotid artery aneurysm, NOS

EXCLUDES 1 *congenital cerebral aneurysm, nonruptured (Q28.-)*
*ruptured cerebral aneurysm (I6Ø.7)*

**AHA:** 2021,3Q,5

**TIP:** A diagnosis of dissecting aneurysm should be coded to the dissection code, I67.0. The bulging/aneurysm, although present, occurred secondary to the dissection. The dissection represents the most significant problem.

**Berry Aneurysm**

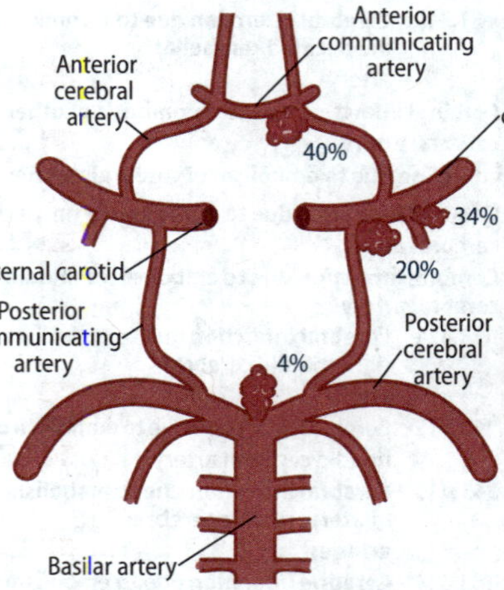


Common sites of berry aneurysms in the circle of Willis arteries

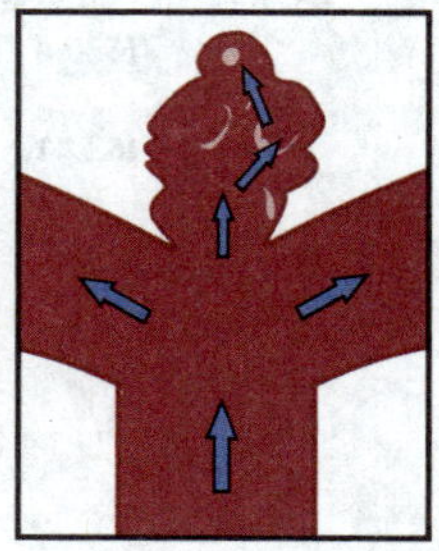

Berry aneurysms form at the site of a weakness in an arterial wall, often at a junction

**I67.2 Cerebral atherosclerosis** A
Atheroma of cerebral and precerebral arteries

**I67.3 Progressive vascular leukoencephalopathy** HCC Rx ESR
Binswanger's disease

**I67.4 Hypertensive encephalopathy** Rx
Code also, if applicable, associated hypertensive conditions such as:
essential (primary) hypertension (I1Ø)
hypertensive chronic kidney disease (I12.-)
hypertensive heart and chronic kidney disease (I13.-)
hypertensive heart disease (I11.-)

EXCLUDES 2 *insufficiency, NOS, of precerebral arteries (G45.2)*

**AHA:** 2023,4Q,24

**I67.5 Moyamoya disease**

**DEF:** Cerebrovascular ischemia. Vessels occlude and rupture, causing tiny hemorrhages at the base of brain. It affects predominantly Japanese people.

**I67.6 Nonpyogenic thrombosis of intracranial venous system**
Nonpyogenic thrombosis of cerebral vein
Nonpyogenic thrombosis of intracranial venous sinus

EXCLUDES 1 *nonpyogenic thrombosis of intracranial venous system causing infarction (I63.6)*

**I67.7 Cerebral arteritis, not elsewhere classified**
Granulomatous angiitis of the nervous system

EXCLUDES 1 *allergic granulomatous angiitis (M3Ø.1)*

**✓5th I67.8 Other specified cerebrovascular diseases**

**I67.81 Acute cerebrovascular insufficiency**
Acute cerebrovascular insufficiency unspecified as to location or reversibility

**I67.82 Cerebral ischemia**
Chronic cerebral ischemia

**I67.83 Posterior reversible encephalopathy syndrome**
PRES

**✓6th I67.84 Cerebral vasospasm and vasoconstriction**

**I67.841 Reversible cerebrovascular vasoconstriction syndrome**
Call-Fleming syndrome
Code first underlying condition, if applicable, such as eclampsia (O15.ØØ-O15.9)

**I67.848 Other cerebrovascular vasospasm and vasoconstriction**

√6th I67.85 **Hereditary cerebrovascular diseases**
AHA: 2018,4Q,17

I67.850 **Cerebral autosomal dominant arteriopathy with subcortical infarcts and leukoencephalopathy**
CADASIL
Code also any associated diagnoses, such as:
epilepsy (G40.-)
stroke (I63.-)
vascular dementia (F01.-)

I67.858 **Other hereditary cerebrovascular disease**

I67.89 **Other cerebrovascular disease**
AHA: 2023,2Q,18

I67.9 **Cerebrovascular disease, unspecified**

√4th **I68 Cerebrovascular disorders in diseases classified elsewhere**

*I68.0* ***Cerebral amyloid angiopathy***
Code first underlying amyloidosis (E85.-)

*I68.2* ***Cerebral arteritis in other diseases classified elsewhere***
Code first underlying disease
EXCLUDES 1 *cerebral arteritis (in):*
*listerosis (A32.89)*
*syphilis (A52.04)*
*systemic lupus erythematosus (M32.19)*
*tuberculosis (A18.89)*

*I68.8* ***Other cerebrovascular disorders in diseases classified elsewhere***
Code first underlying disease
EXCLUDES 1 *syphilitic cerebral aneurysm (A52.05)*

√4th **I69 Sequelae of cerebrovascular disease**

NOTE Category I69 is to be used to indicate conditions in I60-I67 as the cause of sequelae. The "sequelae" include conditions specified as such or as residuals which may occur at any time after the onset of the causal condition

EXCLUDES 1 *personal history of cerebral infarction without residual deficit (Z86.73)*
*personal history of prolonged reversible ischemic neurologic deficit (PRIND) (Z86.73)*
*personal history of reversible ischemic neurologcial deficit (RIND) (Z86.73)*
*sequelae of traumatic intracranial injury (S06.-)*

AHA: 2023,1Q,37; 2020,2Q,29; 2017,1Q,47; 2016,4Q,28; 2015,1Q,25; 2012,4Q,106

TIP: For codes describing hemiplegia, hemiparesis, and monoplegia; if the documentation identifies the affected side but not whether it is the dominant or nondominant side, the default is as follows: for ambidextrous patients, the default is dominant; when the left side is affected, the default is nondominant; and when the right side is affected, the default is dominant.

TIP: Weakness on one side of the body (unilateral weakness) documented as secondary to old cerebrovascular disease is synonymous with hemiparesis/hemiplegia. Weakness of one limb documented as secondary to old cerebrovascular disease is synonymous with monoplegia.

√5th I69.0 **Sequelae of nontraumatic subarachnoid hemorrhage**

I69.00 **Unspecified sequelae of nontraumatic subarachnoid hemorrhage**

√6th I69.01 **Cognitive deficits following nontraumatic subarachnoid hemorrhage**

I69.010 **Attention and concentration deficit following nontraumatic subarachnoid hemorrhage**

I69.011 **Memory deficit following nontraumatic subarachnoid hemorrhage**

I69.012 **Visuospatial deficit and spatial neglect following nontraumatic subarachnoid hemorrhage**

I69.013 **Psychomotor deficit following nontraumatic subarachnoid hemorrhage**

I69.014 **Frontal lobe and executive function deficit following nontraumatic subarachnoid hemorrhage**

I69.015 **Cognitive social or emotional deficit following nontraumatic subarachnoid hemorrhage**

I69.018 **Other symptoms and signs involving cognitive functions following nontraumatic subarachnoid hemorrhage**

I69.019 **Unspecified symptoms and signs involving cognitive functions following nontraumatic subarachnoid hemorrhage**

√6th I69.02 **Speech and language deficits following nontraumatic subarachnoid hemorrhage**

I69.020 **Aphasia following nontraumatic subarachnoid hemorrhage**

I69.021 **Dysphasia following nontraumatic subarachnoid hemorrhage**

I69.022 **Dysarthria following nontraumatic subarachnoid hemorrhage**

I69.023 **Fluency disorder following nontraumatic subarachnoid hemorrhage**
Stuttering following nontraumatic subarachnoid hemorrhage

I69.028 **Other speech and language deficits following nontraumatic subarachnoid hemorrhage**

√6th I69.03 **Monoplegia of upper limb following nontraumatic subarachnoid hemorrhage**
AHA: 2017,1Q,47

I69.031 **Monoplegia of upper limb following nontraumatic subarachnoid hemorrhage affecting right dominant side** HCC ESR COM

I69.032 **Monoplegia of upper limb following nontraumatic subarachnoid hemorrhage affecting left dominant side** HCC ESR COM

I69.033 **Monoplegia of upper limb following nontraumatic subarachnoid hemorrhage affecting right non-dominant side** HCC ESR COM

I69.034 **Monoplegia of upper limb following nontraumatic subarachnoid hemorrhage affecting left non-dominant side** HCC ESR COM

I69.039 **Monoplegia of upper limb following nontraumatic subarachnoid hemorrhage affecting unspecified side** HCC ESR COM

√6th I69.04 **Monoplegia of lower limb following nontraumatic subarachnoid hemorrhage**
AHA: 2017,1Q,47

I69.041 **Monoplegia of lower limb following nontraumatic subarachnoid hemorrhage affecting right dominant side** HCC ESR COM

I69.042 **Monoplegia of lower limb following nontraumatic subarachnoid hemorrhage affecting left dominant side** HCC ESR COM

I69.043 **Monoplegia of lower limb following nontraumatic subarachnoid hemorrhage affecting right non-dominant side** HCC ESR COM

I69.044 **Monoplegia of lower limb following nontraumatic subarachnoid hemorrhage affecting left non-dominant side** HCC ESR COM

I69.049 **Monoplegia of lower limb following nontraumatic subarachnoid hemorrhage affecting unspecified side** HCC ESR COM

√6th I69.05 **Hemiplegia and hemiparesis following nontraumatic subarachnoid hemorrhage**
AHA: 2015,1Q,25

I69.051 **Hemiplegia and hemiparesis following nontraumatic subarachnoid hemorrhage affecting right dominant side** HCC ESR COM

I69.052 **Hemiplegia and hemiparesis following nontraumatic subarachnoid hemorrhage affecting left dominant side** HCC ESR COM

I69.053 **Hemiplegia and hemiparesis following nontraumatic subarachnoid hemorrhage affecting right non-dominant side** HCC ESR COM

I69.054 **Hemiplegia and hemiparesis following nontraumatic subarachnoid hemorrhage affecting left non-dominant side** HCC ESR COM

I69.059 **Hemiplegia and hemiparesis following nontraumatic subarachnoid hemorrhage affecting unspecified side** HCC ESR COM

6th **I69.06 Other paralytic syndrome following nontraumatic subarachnoid hemorrhage**
Use additional code to identify type of paralytic syndrome, such as:
locked-in state (G83.5)
quadriplegia (G82.5-)
EXCLUDES 1 *hemiplegia/hemiparesis following nontraumatic subarachnoid hemorrhage (I69.Ø5-)*
*monoplegia of lower limb following nontraumatic subarachnoid hemorrhage (I69.Ø4-)*
*monoplegia of upper limb following nontraumatic subarachnoid hemorrhage (I69.Ø3-)*

**I69.Ø61 Other paralytic syndrome following nontraumatic subarachnoid hemorrhage affecting right dominant side** HCC ESR COM
**I69.Ø62 Other paralytic syndrome following nontraumatic subarachnoid hemorrhage affecting left dominant side** HCC ESR COM
**I69.Ø63 Other paralytic syndrome following nontraumatic subarachnoid hemorrhage affecting right non-dominant side** HCC ESR COM
**I69.Ø64 Other paralytic syndrome following nontraumatic subarachnoid hemorrhage affecting left non-dominant side** HCC ESR COM
**I69.Ø65 Other paralytic syndrome following nontraumatic subarachnoid hemorrhage, bilateral** HCC ESR COM
**I69.Ø69 Other paralytic syndrome following nontraumatic subarachnoid hemorrhage affecting unspecified side** HCC ESR COM

6th **I69.Ø9 Other sequelae of nontraumatic subarachnoid hemorrhage**
**I69.Ø9Ø Apraxia following nontraumatic subarachnoid hemorrhage**
**I69.Ø91 Dysphagia following nontraumatic subarachnoid hemorrhage**
Use additional code to identify the type of dysphagia, if known (R13.11-R13.19)
**I69.Ø92 Facial weakness following nontraumatic subarachnoid hemorrhage**
Facial droop following nontraumatic subarachnoid hemorrhage
**I69.Ø93 Ataxia following nontraumatic subarachnoid hemorrhage**
**I69.Ø98 Other sequelae following nontraumatic subarachnoid hemorrhage**
Alterations of sensation following nontraumatic subarachnoid hemorrhage
Disturbance of vision following nontraumatic subarachnoid hemorrhage
Use additional code to identify the sequelae

5th **I69.1 Sequelae of nontraumatic intracerebral hemorrhage**
**I69.1Ø Unspecified sequelae of nontraumatic intracerebral hemorrhage**

6th **I69.11 Cognitive deficits following nontraumatic intracerebral hemorrhage**
**I69.11Ø Attention and concentration deficit following nontraumatic intracerebral hemorrhage**
**I69.111 Memory deficit following nontraumatic intracerebral hemorrhage**
**I69.112 Visuospatial deficit and spatial neglect following nontraumatic intracerebral hemorrhage**
**I69.113 Psychomotor deficit following nontraumatic intracerebral hemorrhage**
**I69.114 Frontal lobe and executive function deficit following nontraumatic intracerebral hemorrhage**
**I69.115 Cognitive social or emotional deficit following nontraumatic intracerebral hemorrhage**
**I69.118 Other symptoms and signs involving cognitive functions following nontraumatic intracerebral hemorrhage**
**I69.119 Unspecified symptoms and signs involving cognitive functions following nontraumatic intracerebral hemorrhage**

6th **I69.12 Speech and language deficits following nontraumatic intracerebral hemorrhage**
**I69.12Ø Aphasia following nontraumatic intracerebral hemorrhage**
**I69.121 Dysphasia following nontraumatic intracerebral hemorrhage**
**I69.122 Dysarthria following nontraumatic intracerebral hemorrhage**
**I69.123 Fluency disorder following nontraumatic intracerebral hemorrhage**
Stuttering following nontraumatic intracerebral hemorrhage
**I69.128 Other speech and language deficits following nontraumatic intracerebral hemorrhage**

6th **I69.13 Monoplegia of upper limb following nontraumatic intracerebral hemorrhage**
AHA: 2017,1Q,47
**I69.131 Monoplegia of upper limb following nontraumatic intracerebral hemorrhage affecting right dominant side** HCC ESR COM
**I69.132 Monoplegia of upper limb following nontraumatic intracerebral hemorrhage affecting left dominant side** HCC ESR COM
**I69.133 Monoplegia of upper limb following nontraumatic intracerebral hemorrhage affecting right non-dominant side** HCC ESR COM
**I69.134 Monoplegia of upper limb following nontraumatic intracerebral hemorrhage affecting left non-dominant side** HCC ESR COM
**I69.139 Monoplegia of upper limb following nontraumatic intracerebral hemorrhage affecting unspecified side** HCC ESR COM

6th **I69.14 Monoplegia of lower limb following nontraumatic intracerebral hemorrhage**
AHA: 2017,1Q,47
**I69.141 Monoplegia of lower limb following nontraumatic intracerebral hemorrhage affecting right dominant side** HCC ESR COM
**I69.142 Monoplegia of lower limb following nontraumatic intracerebral hemorrhage affecting left dominant side** HCC ESR COM
**I69.143 Monoplegia of lower limb following nontraumatic intracerebral hemorrhage affecting right non-dominant side** HCC ESR COM
**I69.144 Monoplegia of lower limb following nontraumatic intracerebral hemorrhage affecting left non-dominant side** HCC ESR COM
**I69.149 Monoplegia of lower limb following nontraumatic intracerebral hemorrhage affecting unspecified side** HCC ESR COM

6th **I69.15 Hemiplegia and hemiparesis following nontraumatic intracerebral hemorrhage**
AHA: 2015,1Q,25
**I69.151 Hemiplegia and hemiparesis following nontraumatic intracerebral hemorrhage affecting right dominant side** HCC ESR COM
**I69.152 Hemiplegia and hemiparesis following nontraumatic intracerebral hemorrhage affecting left dominant side** HCC ESR COM
**I69.153 Hemiplegia and hemiparesis following nontraumatic intracerebral hemorrhage affecting right non-dominant side** HCC ESR COM

I69.154 Hemiplegia and hemiparesis following nontraumatic intracerebral hemorrhage affecting left non-dominant side HCC ESR COM

I69.159 Hemiplegia and hemiparesis following nontraumatic intracerebral hemorrhage affecting unspecified side HCC ESR COM

✓6th I69.16 Other paralytic syndrome following nontraumatic intracerebral hemorrhage

Use additional code to identify type of paralytic syndrome, such as:
locked-in state (G83.5)
quadriplegia (G82.5-)

EXCLUDES 1 *hemiplegia/hemiparesis following nontraumatic intracerebral hemorrhage (I69.15-)*
*monoplegia of lower limb following nontraumatic intracerebral hemorrhage (I69.14-)*
*monoplegia of upper limb following nontraumatic intracerebral hemorrhage (I69.13-)*

I69.161 Other paralytic syndrome following nontraumatic intracerebral hemorrhage affecting right dominant side HCC ESR COM

I69.162 Other paralytic syndrome following nontraumatic intracerebral hemorrhage affecting left dominant side HCC ESR COM

I69.163 Other paralytic syndrome following nontraumatic intracerebral hemorrhage affecting right non-dominant side HCC ESR COM

I69.164 Other paralytic syndrome following nontraumatic intracerebral hemorrhage affecting left non-dominant side HCC ESR COM

I69.165 Other paralytic syndrome following nontraumatic intracerebral hemorrhage, bilateral HCC ESR COM

I69.169 Other paralytic syndrome following nontraumatic intracerebral hemorrhage affecting unspecified side HCC ESR COM

✓6th I69.19 Other sequelae of nontraumatic intracerebral hemorrhage

I69.190 Apraxia following nontraumatic intracerebral hemorrhage

I69.191 Dysphagia following nontraumatic intracerebral hemorrhage

Use additional code to identify the type of dysphagia, if known (R13.11-R13.19)

I69.192 Facial weakness following nontraumatic intracerebral hemorrhage

Facial droop following nontraumatic intracerebral hemorrhage

I69.193 Ataxia following nontraumatic intracerebral hemorrhage

I69.198 Other sequelae of nontraumatic intracerebral hemorrhage

Alteration of sensations following nontraumatic intracerebral hemorrhage
Disturbance of vision following nontraumatic intracerebral hemorrhage

Use additional code to identify the sequelae

✓5th I69.2 Sequelae of other nontraumatic intracranial hemorrhage

I69.20 Unspecified sequelae of other nontraumatic intracranial hemorrhage

✓6th I69.21 Cognitive deficits following other nontraumatic intracranial hemorrhage

I69.210 Attention and concentration deficit following other nontraumatic intracranial hemorrhage

I69.211 Memory deficit following other nontraumatic intracranial hemorrhage

I69.212 Visuospatial deficit and spatial neglect following other nontraumatic intracranial hemorrhage

I69.213 Psychomotor deficit following other nontraumatic intracranial hemorrhage

I69.214 Frontal lobe and executive function deficit following other nontraumatic intracranial hemorrhage

I69.215 Cognitive social or emotional deficit following other nontraumatic intracranial hemorrhage

I69.218 Other symptoms and signs involving cognitive functions following other nontraumatic intracranial hemorrhage

I69.219 Unspecified symptoms and signs involving cognitive functions following other nontraumatic intracranial hemorrhage

✓6th I69.22 Speech and language deficits following other nontraumatic intracranial hemorrhage

I69.220 Aphasia following other nontraumatic intracranial hemorrhage

I69.221 Dysphasia following other nontraumatic intracranial hemorrhage

I69.222 Dysarthria following other nontraumatic intracranial hemorrhage

I69.223 Fluency disorder following other nontraumatic intracranial hemorrhage

Stuttering following other nontraumatic intracranial hemorrhage

I69.228 Other speech and language deficits following other nontraumatic intracranial hemorrhage

✓6th I69.23 Monoplegia of upper limb following other nontraumatic intracranial hemorrhage

AHA: 2017,1Q,47

I69.231 Monoplegia of upper limb following other nontraumatic intracranial hemorrhage affecting right dominant side HCC ESR COM

I69.232 Monoplegia of upper limb following other nontraumatic intracranial hemorrhage affecting left dominant side HCC ESR COM

I69.233 Monoplegia of upper limb following other nontraumatic intracranial hemorrhage affecting right non-dominant side HCC ESR COM

I69.234 Monoplegia of upper limb following other nontraumatic intracranial hemorrhage affecting left non-dominant side HCC ESR COM

I69.239 Monoplegia of upper limb following other nontraumatic intracranial hemorrhage affecting unspecified side HCC ESR COM

✓6th I69.24 Monoplegia of lower limb following other nontraumatic intracranial hemorrhage

AHA: 2017,1Q,47

I69.241 Monoplegia of lower limb following other nontraumatic intracranial hemorrhage affecting right dominant side HCC ESR COM

I69.242 Monoplegia of lower limb following other nontraumatic intracranial hemorrhage affecting left dominant side HCC ESR COM

I69.243 Monoplegia of lower limb following other nontraumatic intracranial hemorrhage affecting right non-dominant side HCC ESR COM

I69.244 Monoplegia of lower limb following other nontraumatic intracranial hemorrhage affecting left non-dominant side HCC ESR COM

I69.249 Monoplegia of lower limb following other nontraumatic intracranial hemorrhage affecting unspecified side HCC ESR COM

✓6th I69.25 Hemiplegia and hemiparesis following other nontraumatic intracranial hemorrhage

AHA: 2015,1Q,25

I69.251 Hemiplegia and hemiparesis following other nontraumatic intracranial hemorrhage affecting right dominant side HCC ESR COM

I69.252 Hemiplegia and hemiparesis following other nontraumatic intracranial hemorrhage affecting left dominant side HCC ESR COM

**I69.253 Hemiplegia and hemiparesis following other nontraumatic intracranial hemorrhage affecting right non-dominant side** HCC ESR COM

**I69.254 Hemiplegia and hemiparesis following other nontraumatic intracranial hemorrhage affecting left non-dominant side** HCC ESR COM

**I69.259 Hemiplegia and hemiparesis following other nontraumatic intracranial hemorrhage affecting unspecified side** HCC ESR COM

✓6th **I69.26 Other paralytic syndrome following other nontraumatic intracranial hemorrhage**

Use additional code to identify type of paralytic syndrome, such as:
- locked-in state (G83.5)
- quadriplegia (G82.5-)

EXCLUDES 1 *hemiplegia/hemiparesis following other nontraumatic intracranial hemorrhage (I69.25-)*
*monoplegia of lower limb following other nontraumatic intracranial hemorrhage (I69.24-)*
*monoplegia of upper limb following other nontraumatic intracranial hemorrhage (I69.23-)*

**I69.261 Other paralytic syndrome following other nontraumatic intracranial hemorrhage affecting right dominant side** HCC ESR COM

**I69.262 Other paralytic syndrome following other nontraumatic intracranial hemorrhage affecting left dominant side** HCC ESR COM

**I69.263 Other paralytic syndrome following other nontraumatic intracranial hemorrhage affecting right non-dominant side** HCC ESR COM

**I69.264 Other paralytic syndrome following other nontraumatic intracranial hemorrhage affecting left non-dominant side** HCC ESR COM

**I69.265 Other paralytic syndrome following other nontraumatic intracranial hemorrhage, bilateral** HCC ESR COM

**I69.269 Other paralytic syndrome following other nontraumatic intracranial hemorrhage affecting unspecified side** HCC ESR COM

✓6th **I69.29 Other sequelae of other nontraumatic intracranial hemorrhage**

**I69.290 Apraxia following other nontraumatic intracranial hemorrhage**

**I69.291 Dysphagia following other nontraumatic intracranial hemorrhage**

Use additional code to identify the type of dysphagia, if known (R13.11-R13.19)

**I69.292 Facial weakness following other nontraumatic intracranial hemorrhage**

Facial droop following other nontraumatic intracranial hemorrhage

**I69.293 Ataxia following other nontraumatic intracranial hemorrhage**

**I69.298 Other sequelae of other nontraumatic intracranial hemorrhage**

Alteration of sensation following other nontraumatic intracranial hemorrhage
Disturbance of vision following other nontraumatic intracranial hemorrhage
Use additional code to identify the sequelae

✓5th **I69.3 Sequelae of cerebral infarction**

Sequelae of stroke NOS
**AHA:** 2013,4Q,127-128; 2012,4Q,92,94

**I69.30 Unspecified sequelae of cerebral infarction**

✓6th **I69.31 Cognitive deficits following cerebral infarction**

**I69.310 Attention and concentration deficit following cerebral infarction**

**I69.311 Memory deficit following cerebral infarction**

**I69.312 Visuospatial deficit and spatial neglect following cerebral infarction**

**I69.313 Psychomotor deficit following cerebral infarction**

**I69.314 Frontal lobe and executive function deficit following cerebral infarction**

**I69.315 Cognitive social or emotional deficit following cerebral infarction**

**I69.318 Other symptoms and signs involving cognitive functions following cerebral infarction**

**I69.319 Unspecified symptoms and signs involving cognitive functions following cerebral infarction**

✓6th **I69.32 Speech and language deficits following cerebral infarction**

**I69.320 Aphasia following cerebral infarction**

**I69.321 Dysphasia following cerebral infarction**

**AHA:** 2012,4Q,91

**I69.322 Dysarthria following cerebral infarction**

EXCLUDES 2 *transient ischemic attack (TIA) (G45.9)*

**I69.323 Fluency disorder following cerebral infarction**

Stuttering following cerebral infarction

**I69.328 Other speech and language deficits following cerebral infarction**

✓6th **I69.33 Monoplegia of upper limb following cerebral infarction**

**AHA:** 2017,1Q,47

**I69.331 Monoplegia of upper limb following cerebral infarction affecting right dominant side** HCC ESR COM

**I69.332 Monoplegia of upper limb following cerebral infarction affecting left dominant side** HCC ESR COM

**I69.333 Monoplegia of upper limb following cerebral infarction affecting right non-dominant side** HCC ESR COM

**I69.334 Monoplegia of upper limb following cerebral infarction affecting left non-dominant side** HCC ESR COM

**I69.339 Monoplegia of upper limb following cerebral infarction affecting unspecified side** HCC ESR COM

✓6th **I69.34 Monoplegia of lower limb following cerebral infarction**

**AHA:** 2017,1Q,47

**I69.341 Monoplegia of lower limb following cerebral infarction affecting right dominant side** HCC ESR COM

**I69.342 Monoplegia of lower limb following cerebral infarction affecting left dominant side** HCC ESR COM

**I69.343 Monoplegia of lower limb following cerebral infarction affecting right non-dominant side** HCC ESR COM

**I69.344 Monoplegia of lower limb following cerebral infarction affecting left non-dominant side** HCC ESR COM

**I69.349 Monoplegia of lower limb following cerebral infarction affecting unspecified side** HCC ESR COM

✓6th **I69.35 Hemiplegia and hemiparesis following cerebral infarction**

**AHA:** 2015,1Q,25

**I69.351 Hemiplegia and hemiparesis following cerebral infarction affecting right dominant side** HCC ESR COM

EXCLUDES 2 *transient ischemic attack (TIA) (G45.9)*

**I69.352 Hemiplegia and hemiparesis following cerebral infarction affecting left dominant side** HCC ESR COM

**I69.353 Hemiplegia and hemiparesis following cerebral infarction affecting right non-dominant side** HCC ESR COM

**I69.354 Hemiplegia and hemiparesis following cerebral infarction affecting left non-dominant side** HCC ESR COM

**AHA:** 2012,4Q,91

**I69.359 Hemiplegia and hemiparesis following cerebral infarction affecting unspecified side** HCC ESR COM

√6th **I69.36 Other paralytic syndrome following cerebral infarction**
Use additional code to identify type of paralytic syndrome, such as:
locked-in state (G83.5)
quadriplegia (G82.5-)
EXCLUDES 1 *hemiplegia/hemiparesis following cerebral infarction (I69.35-)*
*monoplegia of lower limb following cerebral infarction (I69.34-)*
*monoplegia of upper limb following cerebral infarction (I69.33-)*

**I69.361 Other paralytic syndrome following cerebral infarction affecting right dominant side** HCC ESR COM
**I69.362 Other paralytic syndrome following cerebral infarction affecting left dominant side** HCC ESR COM
**I69.363 Other paralytic syndrome following cerebral infarction affecting right non-dominant side** HCC ESR COM
**I69.364 Other paralytic syndrome following cerebral infarction affecting left non-dominant side** HCC ESR COM
**I69.365 Other paralytic syndrome following cerebral infarction, bilateral** HCC ESR COM
**I69.369 Other paralytic syndrome following cerebral infarction affecting unspecified side** HCC ESR COM

√6th **I69.39 Other sequelae of cerebral infarction**
**I69.390 Apraxia following cerebral infarction**
**I69.391 Dysphagia following cerebral infarction**
Use additional code to identify the type of dysphagia, if known (R13.11-R13.19)
**I69.392 Facial weakness following cerebral infarction**
Facial droop following cerebral infarction
**AHA:** 2024,2Q,13
**I69.393 Ataxia following cerebral infarction**
**I69.398 Other sequelae of cerebral infarction**
Alteration of sensation following cerebral infarction
Disturbance of vision following cerebral infarction
Use additional code to identify the sequelae
**AHA:** 2024,2Q,13; 2020,2Q,29

√5th **I69.8 Sequelae of other cerebrovascular diseases**
EXCLUDES 1 *sequelae of traumatic intracranial injury (S06.-)*

**I69.80 Unspecified sequelae of other cerebrovascular disease**

√6th **I69.81 Cognitive deficits following other cerebrovascular disease**
**I69.810 Attention and concentration deficit following other cerebrovascular disease**
**I69.811 Memory deficit following other cerebrovascular disease**
**I69.812 Visuospatial deficit and spatial neglect following other cerebrovascular disease**
**I69.813 Psychomotor deficit following other cerebrovascular disease**
**I69.814 Frontal lobe and executive function deficit following other cerebrovascular disease**
**I69.815 Cognitive social or emotional deficit following other cerebrovascular disease**
**I69.818 Other symptoms and signs involving cognitive functions following other cerebrovascular disease**
**I69.819 Unspecified symptoms and signs involving cognitive functions following other cerebrovascular disease**

√6th **I69.82 Speech and language deficits following other cerebrovascular disease**
**I69.820 Aphasia following other cerebrovascular disease**
**I69.821 Dysphasia following other cerebrovascular disease**
**I69.822 Dysarthria following other cerebrovascular disease**
**I69.823 Fluency disorder following other cerebrovascular disease**
Stuttering following other cerebrovascular disease
**I69.828 Other speech and language deficits following other cerebrovascular disease**
**AHA:** 2019,3Q,8

√6th **I69.83 Monoplegia of upper limb following other cerebrovascular disease**
**AHA:** 2017,1Q,47
**I69.831 Monoplegia of upper limb following other cerebrovascular disease affecting right dominant side** HCC ESR COM
**I69.832 Monoplegia of upper limb following other cerebrovascular disease affecting left dominant side** HCC ESR COM
**I69.833 Monoplegia of upper limb following other cerebrovascular disease affecting right non-dominant side** HCC ESR COM
**I69.834 Monoplegia of upper limb following other cerebrovascular disease affecting left non-dominant side** HCC ESR COM
**I69.839 Monoplegia of upper limb following other cerebrovascular disease affecting unspecified side** HCC ESR COM

√6th **I69.84 Monoplegia of lower limb following other cerebrovascular disease**
**AHA:** 2017,1Q,47
**I69.841 Monoplegia of lower limb following other cerebrovascular disease affecting right dominant side** HCC ESR COM
**I69.842 Monoplegia of lower limb following other cerebrovascular disease affecting left dominant side** HCC ESR COM
**I69.843 Monoplegia of lower limb following other cerebrovascular disease affecting right non-dominant side** HCC ESR COM
**I69.844 Monoplegia of lower limb following other cerebrovascular disease affecting left non-dominant side** HCC ESR COM
**I69.849 Monoplegia of lower limb following other cerebrovascular disease affecting unspecified side** HCC ESR COM

√6th **I69.85 Hemiplegia and hemiparesis following other cerebrovascular disease**
**AHA:** 2015,1Q,25
**I69.851 Hemiplegia and hemiparesis following other cerebrovascular disease affecting right dominant side** HCC ESR COM
**I69.852 Hemiplegia and hemiparesis following other cerebrovascular disease affecting left dominant side** HCC ESR COM
**I69.853 Hemiplegia and hemiparesis following other cerebrovascular disease affecting right non-dominant side** HCC ESR COM
**I69.854 Hemiplegia and hemiparesis following other cerebrovascular disease affecting left non-dominant side** HCC ESR COM
**I69.859 Hemiplegia and hemiparesis following other cerebrovascular disease affecting unspecified side** HCC ESR COM

√6th **I69.86 Other paralytic syndrome following other cerebrovascular disease**
Use additional code to identify type of paralytic syndrome, such as:
locked-in state (G83.5)
quadriplegia (G82.5-)
EXCLUDES 1 *hemiplegia/hemiparesis following other cerebrovascular disease (I69.85-)*
*monoplegia of lower limb following other cerebrovascular disease (I69.84-)*
*monoplegia of upper limb following other cerebrovascular disease (I69.83-)*

**I69.861 Other paralytic syndrome following other cerebrovascular disease affecting right dominant side** HCC ESR COM
**I69.862 Other paralytic syndrome following other cerebrovascular disease affecting left dominant side** HCC ESR COM
**I69.863 Other paralytic syndrome following other cerebrovascular disease affecting right non-dominant side** HCC ESR COM

I69.864 Other paralytic syndrome following other cerebrovascular disease affecting left non-dominant side HCC ESR COM

I69.865 Other paralytic syndrome following other cerebrovascular disease, bilateral HCC ESR COM

I69.869 Other paralytic syndrome following other cerebrovascular disease affecting unspecified side HCC ESR COM

✓6th I69.89 Other sequelae of other cerebrovascular disease

I69.890 Apraxia following other cerebrovascular disease

I69.891 Dysphagia following other cerebrovascular disease
Use additional code to identify the type of dysphagia, if known (R13.11-R13.19)

I69.892 Facial weakness following other cerebrovascular disease
Facial droop following other cerebrovascular disease

I69.893 Ataxia following other cerebrovascular disease

I69.898 Other sequelae of other cerebrovascular disease
Alteration of sensation following other cerebrovascular disease
Disturbance of vision following other cerebrovascular disease
Use additional code to identify the sequelae

✓5th I69.9 Sequelae of unspecified cerebrovascular diseases
EXCLUDES 1 *sequelae of stroke (I69.3)*
*sequelae of traumatic intracranial injury (SØ6.-)*

I69.9Ø Unspecified sequelae of unspecified cerebrovascular disease

✓6th I69.91 Cognitive deficits following unspecified cerebrovascular disease

I69.91Ø Attention and concentration deficit following unspecified cerebrovascular disease

I69.911 Memory deficit following unspecified cerebrovascular disease

I69.912 Visuospatial deficit and spatial neglect following unspecified cerebrovascular disease

I69.913 Psychomotor deficit following unspecified cerebrovascular disease

I69.914 Frontal lobe and executive function deficit following unspecified cerebrovascular disease

I69.915 Cognitive social or emotional deficit following unspecified cerebrovascular disease

I69.918 Other symptoms and signs involving cognitive functions following unspecified cerebrovascular disease

I69.919 Unspecified symptoms and signs involving cognitive functions following unspecified cerebrovascular disease

✓6th I69.92 Speech and language deficits following unspecified cerebrovascular disease

I69.92Ø Aphasia following unspecified cerebrovascular disease

I69.921 Dysphasia following unspecified cerebrovascular disease

I69.922 Dysarthria following unspecified cerebrovascular disease

I69.923 Fluency disorder following unspecified cerebrovascular disease
Stuttering following unspecified cerebrovascular disease

I69.928 Other speech and language deficits following unspecified cerebrovascular disease

✓6th I69.93 Monoplegia of upper limb following unspecified cerebrovascular disease
AHA: 2017,1Q,47

I69.931 Monoplegia of upper limb following unspecified cerebrovascular disease affecting right dominant side HCC ESR COM

I69.932 Monoplegia of upper limb following unspecified cerebrovascular disease affecting left dominant side HCC ESR COM

I69.933 Monoplegia of upper limb following unspecified cerebrovascular disease affecting right non-dominant side HCC ESR COM

I69.934 Monoplegia of upper limb following unspecified cerebrovascular disease affecting left non-dominant side HCC ESR COM

I69.939 Monoplegia of upper limb following unspecified cerebrovascular disease affecting unspecified side HCC ESR COM

✓6th I69.94 Monoplegia of lower limb following unspecified cerebrovascular disease
AHA: 2017,1Q,47

I69.941 Monoplegia of lower limb following unspecified cerebrovascular disease affecting right dominant side HCC ESR COM

I69.942 Monoplegia of lower limb following unspecified cerebrovascular disease affecting left dominant side HCC ESR COM

I69.943 Monoplegia of lower limb following unspecified cerebrovascular disease affecting right non-dominant side HCC ESR COM

I69.944 Monoplegia of lower limb following unspecified cerebrovascular disease affecting left non-dominant side HCC ESR COM

I69.949 Monoplegia of lower limb following unspecified cerebrovascular disease affecting unspecified side HCC ESR COM

✓6th I69.95 Hemiplegia and hemiparesis following unspecified cerebrovascular disease
AHA: 2015,1Q,25

I69.951 Hemiplegia and hemiparesis following unspecified cerebrovascular disease affecting right dominant side HCC ESR COM

I69.952 Hemiplegia and hemiparesis following unspecified cerebrovascular disease affecting left dominant side HCC ESR COM

I69.953 Hemiplegia and hemiparesis following unspecified cerebrovascular disease affecting right non-dominant side HCC ESR COM

I69.954 Hemiplegia and hemiparesis following unspecified cerebrovascular disease affecting left non-dominant side HCC ESR COM

I69.959 Hemiplegia and hemiparesis following unspecified cerebrovascular disease affecting unspecified side HCC ESR COM

✓6th I69.96 Other paralytic syndrome following unspecified cerebrovascular disease
Use additional code to identify type of paralytic syndrome, such as:
locked-in state (G83.5)
quadriplegia (G82.5-)
EXCLUDES 1 *hemiplegia/hemiparesis following unspecified cerebrovascular disease (I69.95-)*
*monoplegia of lower limb following unspecified cerebrovascular disease (I69.94-)*
*monoplegia of upper limb following unspecified cerebrovascular disease (I69.93-)*

I69.961 Other paralytic syndrome following unspecified cerebrovascular disease affecting right dominant side HCC ESR COM

I69.962 Other paralytic syndrome following unspecified cerebrovascular disease affecting left dominant side HCC ESR COM

I69.963 Other paralytic syndrome following unspecified cerebrovascular disease affecting right non-dominant side HCC ESR COM

I69.964 Other paralytic syndrome following unspecified cerebrovascular disease affecting left non-dominant side HCC ESR COM

I69.965 Other paralytic syndrome following unspecified cerebrovascular disease, bilateral HCC ESR COM

I69.969 Other paralytic syndrome following unspecified cerebrovascular disease affecting unspecified side HCC ESR COM

✓6th I69.99 Other sequelae of unspecified cerebrovascular disease

I69.990 Apraxia following unspecified cerebrovascular disease

I69.991 Dysphagia following unspecified cerebrovascular disease

Use additional code to identify the type of dysphagia, if known (R13.11-R13.19)

I69.992 Facial weakness following unspecified cerebrovascular disease

Facial droop following unspecified cerebrovascular disease

I69.993 Ataxia following unspecified cerebrovascular disease

I69.998 Other sequelae following unspecified cerebrovascular disease

Alteration in sensation following unspecified cerebrovascular disease

Disturbance of vision following unspecified cerebrovascular disease

Use additional code to identify the sequelae

## Diseases of arteries, arterioles and capillaries (I70-I79)

✓4th **I70 Atherosclerosis**

INCLUDES arterial degeneration
arteriolosclerosis
arteriosclerosis
arteriosclerotic vascular disease
arteriovascular degeneration
atheroma
endarteritis deformans or obliterans
senile arteritis
senile endarteritis
vascular degeneration

Use additional code to identify:
exposure to environmental tobacco smoke (Z77.22)
history of tobacco dependence (Z87.891)
occupational exposure to environmental tobacco smoke (Z57.31)
tobacco dependence (F17.-)
tobacco use (Z72.0)

EXCLUDES 2 *arteriosclerotic cardiovascular disease (I25.1-)*
*arteriosclerotic heart disease (I25.1-)*
*atheroembolism (I75.-)*
*cerebral atherosclerosis (I67.2)*
*coronary atherosclerosis (I25.1-)*
*mesenteric atherosclerosis (K55.1)*
*precerebral atherosclerosis (I67.2)*
*primary pulmonary atherosclerosis (I27.0)*

I70.0 Atherosclerosis of aorta ESR A

I70.1 Atherosclerosis of renal artery ESR A

Goldblatt's kidney

EXCLUDES 2 *atherosclerosis of renal arterioles (I12.-)*

✓5th I70.2 Atherosclerosis of native arteries of the extremities

Monckeberg's (medial) sclerosis

Use additional code, if applicable, to identify chronic total occlusion of artery of extremity (I70.92)

EXCLUDES 2 *atherosclerosis of bypass graft of extremities (I70.30-I70.79)*

AHA: 2020,4Q,98; 2018,3Q,4; 2018,2Q,7

✓6th I70.20 Unspecified atherosclerosis of native arteries of extremities

I70.201 Unspecified atherosclerosis of native arteries of extremities, right leg ESR A

I70.202 Unspecified atherosclerosis of native arteries of extremities, left leg ESR A

I70.203 Unspecified atherosclerosis of native arteries of extremities, bilateral legs ESR A

I70.208 Unspecified atherosclerosis of native arteries of extremities, other extremity ESR A

I70.209 Unspecified atherosclerosis of native arteries of extremities, unspecified extremity ESR A

✓6th I70.21 Atherosclerosis of native arteries of extremities with intermittent claudication

I70.211 Atherosclerosis of native arteries of extremities with intermittent claudication, right leg ESR A

I70.212 Atherosclerosis of native arteries of extremities with intermittent claudication, left leg ESR A

I70.213 Atherosclerosis of native arteries of extremities with intermittent claudication, bilateral legs ESR A

I70.218 Atherosclerosis of native arteries of extremities with intermittent claudication, other extremity ESR A

I70.219 Atherosclerosis of native arteries of extremities with intermittent claudication, unspecified extremity ESR A

✓6th I70.22 Atherosclerosis of native arteries of extremities with rest pain

INCLUDES any condition classifiable to I70.21-
chronic limb-threatening ischemia of native arteries of extremities with rest pain
chronic limb-threatening ischemia NOS of native arteries of extremities
critical limb ischemia of native arteries of extremities with rest pain
critical limb ischemia NOS of native arteries of extremities

I70.221 Atherosclerosis of native arteries of extremities with rest pain, right leg HCC ESR A

I70.222 Atherosclerosis of native arteries of extremities with rest pain, left leg HCC ESR A

I70.223 Atherosclerosis of native arteries of extremities with rest pain, bilateral legs HCC ESR A

I70.228 Atherosclerosis of native arteries of extremities with rest pain, other extremity HCC ESR A

I70.229 Atherosclerosis of native arteries of extremities with rest pain, unspecified extremity HCC ESR A

✓6th I70.23 Atherosclerosis of native arteries of right leg with ulceration

INCLUDES any condition classifiable to I70.211 and I70.221
chronic limb-threatening ischemia of native arteries of right leg with ulceration
critical limb ischemia of native arteries of right leg with ulceration

Use additional code to identify severity of ulcer (L97.-)

I70.231 Atherosclerosis of native arteries of right leg with ulceration of thigh HCC Rx ESR COM A

I70.232 Atherosclerosis of native arteries of right leg with ulceration of calf HCC Rx ESR COM A

I70.233 Atherosclerosis of native arteries of right leg with ulceration of ankle HCC Rx ESR COM A

I70.234 Atherosclerosis of native arteries of right leg with ulceration of heel and midfoot HCC Rx ESR COM A

Atherosclerosis of native arteries of right leg with ulceration of plantar surface of midfoot

**I70.235 Atherosclerosis of native arteries of right leg with ulceration of other part of foot** HCC Rx ESR COM A
Atherosclerosis of native arteries of right leg extremities with ulceration of toe

**I70.238 Atherosclerosis of native arteries of right leg with ulceration of other part of lower leg** HCC Rx ESR COM A

**I70.239 Atherosclerosis of native arteries of right leg with ulceration of unspecified site** HCC Rx ESR COM A

√6th **I70.24 Atherosclerosis of native arteries of left leg with ulceration**
INCLUDES any condition classifiable to I70.212 and I70.222
chronic limb-threatening ischemia of native arteries of left leg with ulceration
critical limb ischemia of native arteries of left leg with ulceration
Use additional code to identify severity of ulcer (L97.-)

**I70.241 Atherosclerosis of native arteries of left leg with ulceration of thigh** HCC Rx ESR COM A

**I70.242 Atherosclerosis of native arteries of left leg with ulceration of calf** HCC Rx ESR COM A

**I70.243 Atherosclerosis of native arteries of left leg with ulceration of ankle** HCC Rx ESR COM A

**I70.244 Atherosclerosis of native arteries of left leg with ulceration of heel and midfoot** HCC Rx ESR COM A
Atherosclerosis of native arteries of left leg with ulceration of plantar surface of midfoot

**I70.245 Atherosclerosis of native arteries of left leg with ulceration of other part of foot** HCC Rx ESR COM A
Atherosclerosis of native arteries of left leg extremities with ulceration of toe

**I70.248 Atherosclerosis of native arteries of left leg with ulceration of other part of lower leg** HCC Rx ESR COM A

**I70.249 Atherosclerosis of native arteries of left leg with ulceration of unspecified site** HCC Rx ESR COM A

**I70.25 Atherosclerosis of native arteries of other extremities with ulceration** HCC Rx ESR COM A
INCLUDES any condition classifiable to I70.218 and I70.228
Use additional code to identify the severity of the ulcer (L98.49-)

√6th **I70.26 Atherosclerosis of native arteries of extremities with gangrene**
INCLUDES any condition classifiable to I70.21-, I70.22-, I70.23-, I70.24-, and I70.25-
chronic limb-threatening ischemia of native arteries of extremities with gangrene
critical limb ischemia of native arteries of extremities with gangrene
Use additional code to identify the severity of any ulcer (L97.-, L98.49-), if applicable

**I70.261 Atherosclerosis of native arteries of extremities with gangrene, right leg** HCC ESR COM A

**I70.262 Atherosclerosis of native arteries of extremities with gangrene, left leg** HCC ESR COM A

**I70.263 Atherosclerosis of native arteries of extremities with gangrene, bilateral legs** HCC ESR COM A

**I70.268 Atherosclerosis of native arteries of extremities with gangrene, other extremity** HCC ESR COM A

**I70.269 Atherosclerosis of native arteries of extremities with gangrene, unspecified extremity** HCC ESR COM A

√6th **I70.29 Other atherosclerosis of native arteries of extremities**

**I70.291 Other atherosclerosis of native arteries of extremities, right leg** ESR A

**I70.292 Other atherosclerosis of native arteries of extremities, left leg** ESR A

**I70.293 Other atherosclerosis of native arteries of extremities, bilateral legs** ESR A

**I70.298 Other atherosclerosis of native arteries of extremities, other extremity** ESR A

**I70.299 Other atherosclerosis of native arteries of extremities, unspecified extremity** ESR A

√5th **I70.3 Atherosclerosis of unspecified type of bypass graft(s) of the extremities**
Use additional code, if applicable, to identify chronic total occlusion of artery of extremity (I70.92)
EXCLUDES 1 *embolism or thrombus of bypass graft(s) of extremities (T82.8-)*
AHA: 2020,4Q,98

√6th **I70.30 Unspecified atherosclerosis of unspecified type of bypass graft(s) of the extremities**

**I70.301 Unspecified atherosclerosis of unspecified type of bypass graft(s) of the extremities, right leg** ESR A

**I70.302 Unspecified atherosclerosis of unspecified type of bypass graft(s) of the extremities, left leg** ESR A

**I70.303 Unspecified atherosclerosis of unspecified type of bypass graft(s) of the extremities, bilateral legs** ESR A

**I70.308 Unspecified atherosclerosis of unspecified type of bypass graft(s) of the extremities, other extremity** ESR A

**I70.309 Unspecified atherosclerosis of unspecified type of bypass graft(s) of the extremities, unspecified extremity** ESR A

√6th **I70.31 Atherosclerosis of unspecified type of bypass graft(s) of the extremities with intermittent claudication**

**I70.311 Atherosclerosis of unspecified type of bypass graft(s) of the extremities with intermittent claudication, right leg** ESR A

**I70.312 Atherosclerosis of unspecified type of bypass graft(s) of the extremities with intermittent claudication, left leg** ESR A

**I70.313 Atherosclerosis of unspecified type of bypass graft(s) of the extremities with intermittent claudication, bilateral legs** ESR A

**I70.318 Atherosclerosis of unspecified type of bypass graft(s) of the extremities with intermittent claudication, other extremity** ESR A

**I70.319 Atherosclerosis of unspecified type of bypass graft(s) of the extremities with intermittent claudication, unspecified extremity** ESR A

√6th **I70.32 Atherosclerosis of unspecified type of bypass graft(s) of the extremities with rest pain**
INCLUDES any condition classifiable to I70.31-
chronic limb-threatening ischemia NOS of unspecified type of bypass graft(s) of the extremities
chronic limb-threatening ischemia of unspecified type of bypass graft(s) of the extremities with rest pain
critical limb ischemia NOS of unspecified type of bypass graft(s) of the extremities
critical limb ischemia of unspecified type of bypass graft(s) of the extremities with rest pain

**I70.321 Atherosclerosis of unspecified type of bypass graft(s) of the extremities with rest pain, right leg** HCC ESR A

**I70.322 Atherosclerosis of unspecified type of bypass graft(s) of the extremities with rest pain, left leg** HCC ESR A

I70.323 Atherosclerosis of unspecified type of bypass graft(s) of the extremities with rest pain, bilateral legs HCC ESR A

I70.328 Atherosclerosis of unspecified type of bypass graft(s) of the extremities with rest pain, other extremity HCC ESR A

I70.329 Atherosclerosis of unspecified type of bypass graft(s) of the extremities with rest pain, unspecified extremity HCC ESR A

6th I70.33 Atherosclerosis of unspecified type of bypass graft(s) of the right leg with ulceration

INCLUDES any condition classifiable to I70.311 and I70.321
chronic limb-threatening ischemia of unspecified type of bypass graft(s) of the right leg with ulceration
critical limb ischemia of unspecified type of bypass graft(s) of the right leg with ulceration

Use additional code to identify severity of ulcer (L97.-)

I70.331 Atherosclerosis of unspecified type of bypass graft(s) of the right leg with ulceration of thigh HCC Rx ESR COM A

I70.332 Atherosclerosis of unspecified type of bypass graft(s) of the right leg with ulceration of calf HCC Rx ESR COM A

I70.333 Atherosclerosis of unspecified type of bypass graft(s) of the right leg with ulceration of ankle HCC Rx ESR COM A

I70.334 Atherosclerosis of unspecified type of bypass graft(s) of the right leg with ulceration of heel and midfoot HCC Rx ESR COM A
Atherosclerosis of unspecified type of bypass graft(s) of right leg with ulceration of plantar surface of midfoot

I70.335 Atherosclerosis of unspecified type of bypass graft(s) of the right leg with ulceration of other part of foot HCC Rx ESR COM A
Atherosclerosis of unspecified type of bypass graft(s) of the right leg with ulceration of toe

I70.338 Atherosclerosis of unspecified type of bypass graft(s) of the right leg with ulceration of other part of lower leg HCC Rx ESR COM A

I70.339 Atherosclerosis of unspecified type of bypass graft(s) of the right leg with ulceration of unspecified site HCC Rx ESR COM A

6th I70.34 Atherosclerosis of unspecified type of bypass graft(s) of the left leg with ulceration

INCLUDES any condition classifiable to I70.312 and I70.322
chronic limb-threatening ischemia of unspecified type of bypass graft(s) of the left leg with ulceration
critical limb ischemia of unspecified type of bypass graft(s) of the left leg with ulceration

Use additional code to identify severity of ulcer (L97.-)

I70.341 Atherosclerosis of unspecified type of bypass graft(s) of the left leg with ulceration of thigh HCC Rx ESR COM A

I70.342 Atherosclerosis of unspecified type of bypass graft(s) of the left leg with ulceration of calf HCC Rx ESR COM A

I70.343 Atherosclerosis of unspecified type of bypass graft(s) of the left leg with ulceration of ankle HCC Rx ESR COM A

I70.344 Atherosclerosis of unspecified type of bypass graft(s) of the left leg with ulceration of heel and midfoot HCC Rx ESR COM A
Atherosclerosis of unspecified type of bypass graft(s) of left leg with ulceration of plantar surface of midfoot

I70.345 Atherosclerosis of unspecified type of bypass graft(s) of the left leg with ulceration of other part of foot HCC Rx ESR COM A
Atherosclerosis of unspecified type of bypass graft(s) of the left leg with ulceration of toe

I70.348 Atherosclerosis of unspecified type of bypass graft(s) of the left leg with ulceration of other part of lower leg HCC Rx ESR COM A

I70.349 Atherosclerosis of unspecified type of bypass graft(s) of the left leg with ulceration of unspecified site HCC Rx ESR COM A

I70.35 Atherosclerosis of unspecified type of bypass graft(s) of other extremity with ulceration HCC Rx ESR COM A

INCLUDES any condition classifiable to I70.318 and I70.328

Use additional code to identify severity of ulcer (L98.49-)

6th I70.36 Atherosclerosis of unspecified type of bypass graft(s) of the extremities with gangrene

INCLUDES any condition classifiable to I70.31-, I70.32-, I70.33-, I70.34-, I70.35
chronic limb-threatening ischemia of unspecified type of bypass graft(s) of the extremities with gangrene
critical limb ischemia of unspecified type of bypass graft(s) of the extremities with gangrene

Use additional code to identify the severity of any ulcer (L97.-, L98.49-), if applicable

I70.361 Atherosclerosis of unspecified type of bypass graft(s) of the extremities with gangrene, right leg HCC ESR COM A

I70.362 Atherosclerosis of unspecified type of bypass graft(s) of the extremities with gangrene, left leg HCC ESR COM A

I70.363 Atherosclerosis of unspecified type of bypass graft(s) of the extremities with gangrene, bilateral legs HCC ESR COM A

I70.368 Atherosclerosis of unspecified type of bypass graft(s) of the extremities with gangrene, other extremity HCC ESR COM A

I70.369 Atherosclerosis of unspecified type of bypass graft(s) of the extremities with gangrene, unspecified extremity HCC ESR COM A

6th I70.39 Other atherosclerosis of unspecified type of bypass graft(s) of the extremities

I70.391 Other atherosclerosis of unspecified type of bypass graft(s) of the extremities, right leg ESR A

I70.392 Other atherosclerosis of unspecified type of bypass graft(s) of the extremities, left leg ESR A

I70.393 Other atherosclerosis of unspecified type of bypass graft(s) of the extremities, bilateral legs ESR A

I70.398 Other atherosclerosis of unspecified type of bypass graft(s) of the extremities, other extremity ESR A

I70.399 Other atherosclerosis of unspecified type of bypass graft(s) of the extremities, unspecified extremity ESR A

5th I70.4 Atherosclerosis of autologous vein bypass graft(s) of the extremities

Use additional code, if applicable, to identify chronic total occlusion of artery of extremity (I70.92)

**AHA:** 2020,4Q,98

6th I70.40 Unspecified atherosclerosis of autologous vein bypass graft(s) of the extremities

I70.401 Unspecified atherosclerosis of autologous vein bypass graft(s) of the extremities, right leg ESR A

I70.402 Unspecified atherosclerosis of autologous vein bypass graft(s) of the extremities, left leg ESR A

**I7Ø.4Ø3** **Unspecified atherosclerosis of autologous vein bypass graft(s) of the extremities, bilateral legs** ESR A

**I7Ø.4Ø8** **Unspecified atherosclerosis of autologous vein bypass graft(s) of the extremities, other extremity** ESR A

**I7Ø.4Ø9** **Unspecified atherosclerosis of autologous vein bypass graft(s) of the extremities, unspecified extremity** ESR A

√6th **I7Ø.41** **Atherosclerosis of autologous vein bypass graft(s) of the extremities with intermittent claudication**

**I7Ø.411** **Atherosclerosis of autologous vein bypass graft(s) of the extremities with intermittent claudication, right leg** ESR A

**I7Ø.412** **Atherosclerosis of autologous vein bypass graft(s) of the extremities with intermittent claudication, left leg** ESR A

**I7Ø.413** **Atherosclerosis of autologous vein bypass graft(s) of the extremities with intermittent claudication, bilateral legs** ESR A

**I7Ø.418** **Atherosclerosis of autologous vein bypass graft(s) of the extremities with intermittent claudication, other extremity** ESR A

**I7Ø.419** **Atherosclerosis of autologous vein bypass graft(s) of the extremities with intermittent claudication, unspecified extremity** ESR A

√6th **I7Ø.42** **Atherosclerosis of autologous vein bypass graft(s) of the extremities with rest pain**

INCLUDES any condition classifiable to I7Ø.41-
chronic limb-threatening ischemia of autologous vein bypass graft(s) of the extremities with rest pain
chronic limb-threatening ischemia NOS of autologous vein bypass graft(s) of the extremities
critical limb ischemia of autologous vein bypass graft(s) of the extremities with rest pain
critical limb ischemia NOS of autologous vein bypass graft(s) of the extremities

**I7Ø.421** **Atherosclerosis of autologous vein bypass graft(s) of the extremities with rest pain, right leg** HCC ESR A

**I7Ø.422** **Atherosclerosis of autologous vein bypass graft(s) of the extremities with rest pain, left leg** HCC ESR A

**I7Ø.423** **Atherosclerosis of autologous vein bypass graft(s) of the extremities with rest pain, bilateral legs** HCC ESR A

**I7Ø.428** **Atherosclerosis of autologous vein bypass graft(s) of the extremities with rest pain, other extremity** HCC ESR A

**I7Ø.429** **Atherosclerosis of autologous vein bypass graft(s) of the extremities with rest pain, unspecified extremity** HCC ESR A

√6th **I7Ø.43** **Atherosclerosis of autologous vein bypass graft(s) of the right leg with ulceration**

INCLUDES any condition classifiable to I7Ø.411 and I7Ø.421
chronic limb-threatening ischemia of autologous vein bypass graft(s) of the right leg with ulceration
critical limb ischemia of autologous vein bypass graft(s) of the right leg with ulceration

Use additional code to identify severity of ulcer (L97.-)

**I7Ø.431** **Atherosclerosis of autologous vein bypass graft(s) of the right leg with ulceration of thigh** HCC Rx ESR COM A

**I7Ø.432** **Atherosclerosis of autologous vein bypass graft(s) of the right leg with ulceration of calf** HCC Rx ESR COM A

**I7Ø.433** **Atherosclerosis of autologous vein bypass graft(s) of the right leg with ulceration of ankle** HCC Rx ESR COM A

**I7Ø.434** **Atherosclerosis of autologous vein bypass graft(s) of the right leg with ulceration of heel and midfoot** HCC Rx ESR COM A
Atherosclerosis of autologous vein bypass graft(s) of right leg with ulceration of plantar surface of midfoot

**I7Ø.435** **Atherosclerosis of autologous vein bypass graft(s) of the right leg with ulceration of other part of foot** HCC Rx ESR COM A
Atherosclerosis of autologous vein bypass graft(s) of right leg with ulceration of toe

**I7Ø.438** **Atherosclerosis of autologous vein bypass graft(s) of the right leg with ulceration of other part of lower leg** HCC Rx ESR COM A

**I7Ø.439** **Atherosclerosis of autologous vein bypass graft(s) of the right leg with ulceration of unspecified site** HCC Rx ESR COM A

√6th **I7Ø.44** **Atherosclerosis of autologous vein bypass graft(s) of the left leg with ulceration**

INCLUDES any condition classifiable to I7Ø.412 and I7Ø.422
chronic limb-threatening ischemia of autologous vein bypass graft(s) of the left leg with ulceration
critical limb ischemia of autologous vein bypass graft(s) of the left leg with ulceration

Use additional code to identify severity of ulcer (L97.-)

**I7Ø.441** **Atherosclerosis of autologous vein bypass graft(s) of the left leg with ulceration of thigh** HCC Rx ESR COM A

**I7Ø.442** **Atherosclerosis of autologous vein bypass graft(s) of the left leg with ulceration of calf** HCC Rx ESR COM A

**I7Ø.443** **Atherosclerosis of autologous vein bypass graft(s) of the left leg with ulceration of ankle** HCC Rx ESR COM A

**I7Ø.444** **Atherosclerosis of autologous vein bypass graft(s) of the left leg with ulceration of heel and midfoot** HCC Rx ESR COM A
Atherosclerosis of autologous vein bypass graft(s) of left leg with ulceration of plantar surface of midfoot

**I7Ø.445** **Atherosclerosis of autologous vein bypass graft(s) of the left leg with ulceration of other part of foot** HCC Rx ESR COM A
Atherosclerosis of autologous vein bypass graft(s) of left leg with ulceration of toe

**I7Ø.448** **Atherosclerosis of autologous vein bypass graft(s) of the left leg with ulceration of other part of lower leg** HCC Rx ESR COM A

**I7Ø.449** **Atherosclerosis of autologous vein bypass graft(s) of the left leg with ulceration of unspecified site** HCC Rx ESR COM A

**I7Ø.45** **Atherosclerosis of autologous vein bypass graft(s) of other extremity with ulceration** HCC Rx ESR COM A

INCLUDES any condition classifiable to I7Ø.418, I7Ø.428, and I7Ø.438

Use additional code to identify severity of ulcer (L98.49)

√6th **I7Ø.46** **Atherosclerosis of autologous vein bypass graft(s) of the extremities with gangrene**

INCLUDES any condition classifiable to I7Ø.41-, I7Ø.42-, and I7Ø.43-, I7Ø.44-, I7Ø.45
chronic limb-threatening ischemia of autologous vein bypass graft(s) of the extremities with gangrene
critical limb ischemia of autologous vein bypass graft(s) of the extremities with gangrene

Use additional code to identify the severity of any ulcer (L97.-, L98.49-), if applicable

**I7Ø.461** **Atherosclerosis of autologous vein bypass graft(s) of the extremities with gangrene, right leg** HCC ESR COM A

**I7Ø.462** **Atherosclerosis of autologous vein bypass graft(s) of the extremities with gangrene, left leg** HCC ESR COM A

I70.463 Atherosclerosis of autologous vein bypass graft(s) of the extremities with gangrene, bilateral legs HCC ESR COM A

I70.468 Atherosclerosis of autologous vein bypass graft(s) of the extremities with gangrene, other extremity HCC ESR COM A

I70.469 Atherosclerosis of autologous vein bypass graft(s) of the extremities with gangrene, unspecified extremity HCC ESR COM A

✓6th I70.49 Other atherosclerosis of autologous vein bypass graft(s) of the extremities

I70.491 Other atherosclerosis of autologous vein bypass graft(s) of the extremities, right leg ESR A

I70.492 Other atherosclerosis of autologous vein bypass graft(s) of the extremities, left leg ESR A

I70.493 Other atherosclerosis of autologous vein bypass graft(s) of the extremities, bilateral legs ESR A

I70.498 Other atherosclerosis of autologous vein bypass graft(s) of the extremities, other extremity ESR A

I70.499 Other atherosclerosis of autologous vein bypass graft(s) of the extremities, unspecified extremity ESR A

✓5th I70.5 Atherosclerosis of nonautologous biological bypass graft(s) of the extremities

Use additional code, if applicable, to identify chronic total occlusion of artery of extremity (I70.92)

AHA: 2020,4Q,98

✓6th I70.50 Unspecified atherosclerosis of nonautologous biological bypass graft(s) of the extremities

I70.501 Unspecified atherosclerosis of nonautologous biological bypass graft(s) of the extremities, right leg ESR A

I70.502 Unspecified atherosclerosis of nonautologous biological bypass graft(s) of the extremities, left leg ESR A

I70.503 Unspecified atherosclerosis of nonautologous biological bypass graft(s) of the extremities, bilateral legs ESR A

I70.508 Unspecified atherosclerosis of nonautologous biological bypass graft(s) of the extremities, other extremity ESR A

I70.509 Unspecified atherosclerosis of nonautologous biological bypass graft(s) of the extremities, unspecified extremity ESR A

✓6th I70.51 Atherosclerosis of nonautologous biological bypass graft(s) of the extremities intermittent claudication

I70.511 Atherosclerosis of nonautologous biological bypass graft(s) of the extremities with intermittent claudication, right leg ESR A

I70.512 Atherosclerosis of nonautologous biological bypass graft(s) of the extremities with intermittent claudication, left leg ESR A

I70.513 Atherosclerosis of nonautologous biological bypass graft(s) of the extremities with intermittent claudication, bilateral legs ESR A

I70.518 Atherosclerosis of nonautologous biological bypass graft(s) of the extremities with intermittent claudication, other extremity ESR A

I70.519 Atherosclerosis of nonautologous biological bypass graft(s) of the extremities with intermittent claudication, unspecified extremity ESR A

✓6th I70.52 Atherosclerosis of nonautologous biological bypass graft(s) of the extremities with rest pain

INCLUDES any condition classifiable to I70.51-
chronic limb-threatening ischemia of nonautologous biological bypass graft(s) of the extremities with rest pain
chronic limb-threatening ischemia NOS of nonautologous biological bypass graft(s) of the extremities
critical limb ischemia of nonautologous biological bypass graft(s) of the extremities with rest pain
critical limb ischemia NOS of nonautologous biological bypass graft(s) of the extremities

I70.521 Atherosclerosis of nonautologous biological bypass graft(s) of the extremities with rest pain, right leg HCC ESR A

I70.522 Atherosclerosis of nonautologous biological bypass graft(s) of the extremities with rest pain, left leg HCC ESR A

I70.523 Atherosclerosis of nonautologous biological bypass graft(s) of the extremities with rest pain, bilateral legs HCC ESR A

I70.528 Atherosclerosis of nonautologous biological bypass graft(s) of the extremities with rest pain, other extremity HCC ESR A

I70.529 Atherosclerosis of nonautologous biological bypass graft(s) of the extremities with rest pain, unspecified extremity HCC ESR A

✓6th I70.53 Atherosclerosis of nonautologous biological bypass graft(s) of the right leg with ulceration

INCLUDES any condition classifiable to I70.511 and I70.521
chronic limb-threatening ischemia of nonautologous biological bypass graft(s) of the right leg with ulceration
critical limb ischemia of nonautologous biological bypass graft(s) of the right leg with ulceration

Use additional code to identify severity of ulcer (L97.-)

I70.531 Atherosclerosis of nonautologous biological bypass graft(s) of the right leg with ulceration of thigh HCC Rx ESR COM A

I70.532 Atherosclerosis of nonautologous biological bypass graft(s) of the right leg with ulceration of calf HCC Rx ESR COM A

I70.533 Atherosclerosis of nonautologous biological bypass graft(s) of the right leg with ulceration of ankle HCC Rx ESR COM A

I70.534 Atherosclerosis of nonautologous biological bypass graft(s) of the right leg with ulceration of heel and midfoot HCC Rx ESR COM A
Atherosclerosis of nonautologous biological bypass graft(s) of right leg with ulceration of plantar surface of midfoot

I70.535 Atherosclerosis of nonautologous biological bypass graft(s) of the right leg with ulceration of other part of foot HCC Rx ESR COM A
Atherosclerosis of nonautologous biological bypass graft(s) of the right leg with ulceration of toe

I70.538 Atherosclerosis of nonautologous biological bypass graft(s) of the right leg with ulceration of other part of lower leg HCC Rx ESR COM A

I70.539 Atherosclerosis of nonautologous biological bypass graft(s) of the right leg with ulceration of unspecified site HCC Rx ESR COM A

✓6th **I7Ø.54 Atherosclerosis of nonautologous biological bypass graft(s) of the left leg with ulceration**
INCLUDES any condition classifiable to I7Ø.512 and I7Ø.522
chronic limb-threatening ischemia of nonautologous biological bypass graft(s) of the left leg with ulceration
critical limb ischemia of nonautologous biological bypass graft(s) of the left leg with ulceration
Use additional code to identify severity of ulcer (L97.-)

**I7Ø.541 Atherosclerosis of nonautologous biological bypass graft(s) of the left leg with ulceration of thigh** HCC Rx ESR COM A

**I7Ø.542 Atherosclerosis of nonautologous biological bypass graft(s) of the left leg with ulceration of calf** HCC Rx ESR COM A

**I7Ø.543 Atherosclerosis of nonautologous biological bypass graft(s) of the left leg with ulceration of ankle** HCC Rx ESR COM A

**I7Ø.544 Atherosclerosis of nonautologous biological bypass graft(s) of the left leg with ulceration of heel and midfoot** HCC Rx ESR COM A
Atherosclerosis of nonautologous biological bypass graft(s) of left leg with ulceration of plantar surface of midfoot

**I7Ø.545 Atherosclerosis of nonautologous biological bypass graft(s) of the left leg with ulceration of other part of foot** HCC Rx ESR COM A
Atherosclerosis of nonautologous biological bypass graft(s) of the left leg with ulceration of toe

**I7Ø.548 Atherosclerosis of nonautologous biological bypass graft(s) of the left leg with ulceration of other part of lower leg** HCC Rx ESR COM A

**I7Ø.549 Atherosclerosis of nonautologous biological bypass graft(s) of the left leg with ulceration of unspecified site** HCC Rx ESR COM A

**I7Ø.55 Atherosclerosis of nonautologous biological bypass graft(s) of other extremity with ulceration** HCC Rx ESR COM A
INCLUDES any condition classifiable to I7Ø.518, I7Ø.528, and I7Ø.538
Use additional code to identify severity of ulcer (L98.49)

✓6th **I7Ø.56 Atherosclerosis of nonautologous biological bypass graft(s) of the extremities with gangrene**
INCLUDES any condition classifiable to I7Ø.51-, I7Ø.52-, and I7Ø.53-, I7Ø.54-, I7Ø.55
chronic limb-threatening ischemia of nonautologous biological bypass graft(s) of the extremities with gangrene
critical limb ischemia of nonautologous biological bypass graft(s) of the extremities with gangrene
Use additional code to identify the severity of any ulcer (L97.-, L98.49-), if applicable

**I7Ø.561 Atherosclerosis of nonautologous biological bypass graft(s) of the extremities with gangrene, right leg** HCC ESR COM A

**I7Ø.562 Atherosclerosis of nonautologous biological bypass graft(s) of the extremities with gangrene, left leg** HCC ESR COM A

**I7Ø.563 Atherosclerosis of nonautologous biological bypass graft(s) of the extremities with gangrene, bilateral legs** HCC ESR COM A

**I7Ø.568 Atherosclerosis of nonautologous biological bypass graft(s) of the extremities with gangrene, other extremity** HCC ESR COM A

**I7Ø.569 Atherosclerosis of nonautologous biological bypass graft(s) of the extremities with gangrene, unspecified extremity** HCC ESR COM A

✓6th **I7Ø.59 Other atherosclerosis of nonautologous biological bypass graft(s) of the extremities**

**I7Ø.591 Other atherosclerosis of nonautologous biological bypass graft(s) of the extremities, right leg** ESR A

**I7Ø.592 Other atherosclerosis of nonautologous biological bypass graft(s) of the extremities, left leg** ESR A

**I7Ø.593 Other atherosclerosis of nonautologous biological bypass graft(s) of the extremities, bilateral legs** ESR A

**I7Ø.598 Other atherosclerosis of nonautologous biological bypass graft(s) of the extremities, other extremity** ESR A

**I7Ø.599 Other atherosclerosis of nonautologous biological bypass graft(s) of the extremities, unspecified extremity** ESR A

✓5th **I7Ø.6 Atherosclerosis of nonbiological bypass graft(s) of the extremities**
Use additional code, if applicable, to identify chronic total occlusion of artery of extremity (I7Ø.92)
**AHA:** 2020,4Q,98

✓6th **I7Ø.6Ø Unspecified atherosclerosis of nonbiological bypass graft(s) of the extremities**

**I7Ø.6Ø1 Unspecified atherosclerosis of nonbiological bypass graft(s) of the extremities, right leg** ESR A

**I7Ø.6Ø2 Unspecified atherosclerosis of nonbiological bypass graft(s) of the extremities, left leg** ESR A

**I7Ø.6Ø3 Unspecified atherosclerosis of nonbiological bypass graft(s) of the extremities, bilateral legs** ESR A

**I7Ø.6Ø8 Unspecified atherosclerosis of nonbiological bypass graft(s) of the extremities, other extremity** ESR A

**I7Ø.6Ø9 Unspecified atherosclerosis of nonbiological bypass graft(s) of the extremities, unspecified extremity** ESR A

✓6th **I7Ø.61 Atherosclerosis of nonbiological bypass graft(s) of the extremities with intermittent claudication**

**I7Ø.611 Atherosclerosis of nonbiological bypass graft(s) of the extremities with intermittent claudication, right leg** ESR A

**I7Ø.612 Atherosclerosis of nonbiological bypass graft(s) of the extremities with intermittent claudication, left leg** ESR A

**I7Ø.613 Atherosclerosis of nonbiological bypass graft(s) of the extremities with intermittent claudication, bilateral legs** ESR A

**I7Ø.618 Atherosclerosis of nonbiological bypass graft(s) of the extremities with intermittent claudication, other extremity** ESR A

**I7Ø.619 Atherosclerosis of nonbiological bypass graft(s) of the extremities with intermittent claudication, unspecified extremity** ESR A

✓6th **I7Ø.62 Atherosclerosis of nonbiological bypass graft(s) of the extremities with rest pain**
INCLUDES any condition classifiable to I7Ø.61-
chronic limb-threatening ischemia of nonbiological bypass graft(s) of the extremities with rest pain
chronic limb-threatening ischemia NOS of nonbiological bypass graft(s) of the extremities
critical limb ischemia of nonbiological bypass graft(s) of the extremities with rest pain
critical limb ischemia NOS of nonbiological bypass graft(s) of the extremities

**I7Ø.621 Atherosclerosis of nonbiological bypass graft(s) of the extremities with rest pain, right leg** HCC ESR A

**I70.622** **Atherosclerosis of nonbiological bypass graft(s) of the extremities with rest pain, left leg** HCC ESR A

**I70.623** **Atherosclerosis of nonbiological bypass graft(s) of the extremities with rest pain, bilateral legs** HCC ESR A

**I70.628** **Atherosclerosis of nonbiological bypass graft(s) of the extremities with rest pain, other extremity** HCC ESR A

**I70.629** **Atherosclerosis of nonbiological bypass graft(s) of the extremities with rest pain, unspecified extremity** HCC ESR A

✓6th **I70.63** **Atherosclerosis of nonbiological bypass graft(s) of the right leg with ulceration**

INCLUDES any condition classifiable to I70.611 and I70.621
chronic limb-threatening ischemia of nonbiological bypass graft(s) of the right leg with ulceration
critical limb ischemia of nonbiological bypass graft(s) of the right leg with ulceration

Use additional code to identify severity of ulcer (L97.-)

**I70.631** **Atherosclerosis of nonbiological bypass graft(s) of the right leg with ulceration of thigh** HCC Rx ESR COM A

**I70.632** **Atherosclerosis of nonbiological bypass graft(s) of the right leg with ulceration of calf** HCC Rx ESR COM A

**I70.633** **Atherosclerosis of nonbiological bypass graft(s) of the right leg with ulceration of ankle** HCC Rx ESR COM A

**I70.634** **Atherosclerosis of nonbiological bypass graft(s) of the right leg with ulceration of heel and midfoot** HCC Rx ESR COM A

Atherosclerosis of nonbiological bypass graft(s) of right leg with ulceration of plantar surface of midfoot

**I70.635** **Atherosclerosis of nonbiological bypass graft(s) of the right leg with ulceration of other part of foot** HCC Rx ESR COM A

Atherosclerosis of nonbiological bypass graft(s) of the right leg with ulceration of toe

**I70.638** **Atherosclerosis of nonbiological bypass graft(s) of the right leg with ulceration of other part of lower leg** HCC Rx ESR COM A

**I70.639** **Atherosclerosis of nonbiological bypass graft(s) of the right leg with ulceration of unspecified site** HCC Rx ESR COM A

✓6th **I70.64** **Atherosclerosis of nonbiological bypass graft(s) of the left leg with ulceration**

INCLUDES any condition classifiable to I70.612 and I70.622
chronic limb-threatening ischemia of nonbiological bypass graft(s) of the left leg with ulceration
critical limb ischemia of nonbiological bypass graft(s) of the left leg with ulceration

Use additional code to identify severity of ulcer (L97.-)

**I70.641** **Atherosclerosis of nonbiological bypass graft(s) of the left leg with ulceration of thigh** HCC Rx ESR COM A

**I70.642** **Atherosclerosis of nonbiological bypass graft(s) of the left leg with ulceration of calf** HCC Rx ESR COM A

**I70.643** **Atherosclerosis of nonbiological bypass graft(s) of the left leg with ulceration of ankle** HCC Rx ESR COM A

**I70.644** **Atherosclerosis of nonbiological bypass graft(s) of the left leg with ulceration of heel and midfoot** HCC Rx ESR COM A

Atherosclerosis of nonbiological bypass graft(s) of left leg with ulceration of plantar surface of midfoot

**I70.645** **Atherosclerosis of nonbiological bypass graft(s) of the left leg with ulceration of other part of foot** HCC Rx ESR COM A

Atherosclerosis of nonbiological bypass graft(s) of the left leg with ulceration of toe

**I70.648** **Atherosclerosis of nonbiological bypass graft(s) of the left leg with ulceration of other part of lower leg** HCC Rx ESR COM A

**I70.649** **Atherosclerosis of nonbiological bypass graft(s) of the left leg with ulceration of unspecified site** HCC Rx ESR COM A

**I70.65** **Atherosclerosis of nonbiological bypass graft(s) of other extremity with ulceration** HCC Rx ESR COM A

INCLUDES any condition classifiable to I70.618 and I70.628

Use additional code to identify severity of ulcer (L98.49)

✓6th **I70.66** **Atherosclerosis of nonbiological bypass graft(s) of the extremities with gangrene**

INCLUDES any condition classifiable to I70.61-, I70.62-, I70.63-, I70.64-, I70.65
chronic limb-threatening ischemia of nonbiological bypass graft(s) of the extremities with gangrene
critical limb ischemia of nonbiological bypass graft(s) of the extremities with gangrene

Use additional code to identify the severity of any ulcer (L97.-, L98.49-), if applicable

**I70.661** **Atherosclerosis of nonbiological bypass graft(s) of the extremities with gangrene, right leg** HCC ESR COM A

**I70.662** **Atherosclerosis of nonbiological bypass graft(s) of the extremities with gangrene, left leg** HCC ESR COM A

**I70.663** **Atherosclerosis of nonbiological bypass graft(s) of the extremities with gangrene, bilateral legs** HCC ESR COM A

**I70.668** **Atherosclerosis of nonbiological bypass graft(s) of the extremities with gangrene, other extremity** HCC ESR COM A

**I70.669** **Atherosclerosis of nonbiological bypass graft(s) of the extremities with gangrene, unspecified extremity** HCC ESR COM A

✓6th **I70.69** **Other atherosclerosis of nonbiological bypass graft(s) of the extremities**

**I70.691** **Other atherosclerosis of nonbiological bypass graft(s) of the extremities, right leg** ESR A

**I70.692** **Other atherosclerosis of nonbiological bypass graft(s) of the extremities, left leg** ESR A

**I70.693** **Other atherosclerosis of nonbiological bypass graft(s) of the extremities, bilateral legs** ESR A

**I70.698** **Other atherosclerosis of nonbiological bypass graft(s) of the extremities, other extremity** ESR A

**I70.699** **Other atherosclerosis of nonbiological bypass graft(s) of the extremities, unspecified extremity** ESR A

✓5th **I70.7** **Atherosclerosis of other type of bypass graft(s) of the extremities**

Use additional code, if applicable, to identify chronic total occlusion of artery of extremity (I70.92)

**AHA:** 2020,4Q,98

✓6th **I70.70** **Unspecified atherosclerosis of other type of bypass graft(s) of the extremities**

**I70.701** **Unspecified atherosclerosis of other type of bypass graft(s) of the extremities, right leg** ESR A

**I70.702** **Unspecified atherosclerosis of other type of bypass graft(s) of the extremities, left leg** ESR A

**I70.703** **Unspecified atherosclerosis of other type of bypass graft(s) of the extremities, bilateral legs** ESR A

**I70.708** **Unspecified atherosclerosis of other type of bypass graft(s) of the extremities, other extremity** ESR A

Chapter 9. Diseases of the Circulatory System

I70.622–I70.708

**I70.709 Unspecified atherosclerosis of other type of bypass graft(s) of the extremities, unspecified extremity** ESR A

✓6th **I70.71 Atherosclerosis of other type of bypass graft(s) of the extremities with intermittent claudication**

**I70.711 Atherosclerosis of other type of bypass graft(s) of the extremities with intermittent claudication, right leg** ESR A

**I70.712 Atherosclerosis of other type of bypass graft(s) of the extremities with intermittent claudication, left leg** ESR A

**I70.713 Atherosclerosis of other type of bypass graft(s) of the extremities with intermittent claudication, bilateral legs** ESR A

**I70.718 Atherosclerosis of other type of bypass graft(s) of the extremities with intermittent claudication, other extremity** ESR A

**I70.719 Atherosclerosis of other type of bypass graft(s) of the extremities with intermittent claudication, unspecified extremity** ESR A

✓6th **I70.72 Atherosclerosis of other type of bypass graft(s) of the extremities with rest pain**

INCLUDES any condition classifiable to I70.71-
chronic limb-threatening ischemia NOS of other type of bypass graft(s) of the extremities
chronic limb-threatening ischemia of other type of bypass graft(s) of the extremities with rest pain
critical limb ischemia NOS of other type of bypass graft(s) of the extremities
critical limb ischemia of other type of bypass graft(s) of the extremities with rest pain

**I70.721 Atherosclerosis of other type of bypass graft(s) of the extremities with rest pain, right leg** HCC ESR A

**I70.722 Atherosclerosis of other type of bypass graft(s) of the extremities with rest pain, left leg** HCC ESR A

**I70.723 Atherosclerosis of other type of bypass graft(s) of the extremities with rest pain, bilateral legs** HCC ESR A

**I70.728 Atherosclerosis of other type of bypass graft(s) of the extremities with rest pain, other extremity** HCC ESR A

**I70.729 Atherosclerosis of other type of bypass graft(s) of the extremities with rest pain, unspecified extremity** HCC ESR A

✓6th **I70.73 Atherosclerosis of other type of bypass graft(s) of the right leg with ulceration**

INCLUDES any condition classifiable to I70.711 and I70.721
chronic limb-threatening ischemia of other type of bypass graft(s) of the right leg with ulceration
critical limb ischemia of other type of bypass graft(s) of the right leg with ulceration

Use additional code to identify severity of ulcer (L97.-)

**I70.731 Atherosclerosis of other type of bypass graft(s) of the right leg with ulceration of thigh** HCC Rx ESR COM A

**I70.732 Atherosclerosis of other type of bypass graft(s) of the right leg with ulceration of calf** HCC Rx ESR COM A

**I70.733 Atherosclerosis of other type of bypass graft(s) of the right leg with ulceration of ankle** HCC Rx ESR COM A

**I70.734 Atherosclerosis of other type of bypass graft(s) of the right leg with ulceration of heel and midfoot** HCC Rx ESR COM A
Atherosclerosis of other type of bypass graft(s) of right leg with ulceration of plantar surface of midfoot

**I70.735 Atherosclerosis of other type of bypass graft(s) of the right leg with ulceration of other part of foot** HCC Rx ESR COM A
Atherosclerosis of other type of bypass graft(s) of right leg with ulceration of toe

**I70.738 Atherosclerosis of other type of bypass graft(s) of the right leg with ulceration of other part of lower leg** HCC Rx ESR COM A

**I70.739 Atherosclerosis of other type of bypass graft(s) of the right leg with ulceration of unspecified site** HCC Rx ESR COM A

✓6th **I70.74 Atherosclerosis of other type of bypass graft(s) of the left leg with ulceration**

INCLUDES any condition classifiable to I70.712 and I70.722
chronic limb-threatening ischemia of other type of bypass graft(s) of the left leg with ulceration
critical limb ischemia of other type of bypass graft(s) of the left leg with ulceration

Use additional code to identify severity of ulcer (L97.-)

**I70.741 Atherosclerosis of other type of bypass graft(s) of the left leg with ulceration of thigh** HCC Rx ESR COM A

**I70.742 Atherosclerosis of other type of bypass graft(s) of the left leg with ulceration of calf** HCC Rx ESR COM A

**I70.743 Atherosclerosis of other type of bypass graft(s) of the left leg with ulceration of ankle** HCC Rx ESR COM A

**I70.744 Atherosclerosis of other type of bypass graft(s) of the left leg with ulceration of heel and midfoot** HCC Rx ESR COM A
Atherosclerosis of other type of bypass graft(s) of left leg with ulceration of plantar surface of midfoot

**I70.745 Atherosclerosis of other type of bypass graft(s) of the left leg with ulceration of other part of foot** HCC Rx ESR COM A
Atherosclerosis of other type of bypass graft(s) of left leg with ulceration of toe

**I70.748 Atherosclerosis of other type of bypass graft(s) of the left leg with ulceration of other part of lower leg** HCC Rx ESR COM A

**I70.749 Atherosclerosis of other type of bypass graft(s) of the left leg with ulceration of unspecified site** HCC Rx ESR COM A

**I70.75 Atherosclerosis of other type of bypass graft(s) of other extremity with ulceration** HCC Rx ESR COM A

INCLUDES any condition classifiable to I70.718 and I70.728

Use additional code to identify severity of ulcer (L98.49)

✓6th **I70.76 Atherosclerosis of other type of bypass graft(s) of the extremities with gangrene**

INCLUDES any condition classifiable to I70.71-, I70.72-, I70.73-, I70.74-, I70.75
chronic limb-threatening ischemia of other type of bypass graft(s) of the extremities with gangrene
critical limb ischemia of other type of bypass graft(s) of the extremities with gangrene

Use additional code to identify the severity of any ulcer (L97.-, L98.49-), if applicable

**I70.761 Atherosclerosis of other type of bypass graft(s) of the extremities with gangrene, right leg** HCC ESR COM A

**I70.762 Atherosclerosis of other type of bypass graft(s) of the extremities with gangrene, left leg** HCC ESR COM A

**I70.763 Atherosclerosis of other type of bypass graft(s) of the extremities with gangrene, bilateral legs** HCC ESR COM A

**I70.768 Atherosclerosis of other type of bypass graft(s) of the extremities with gangrene, other extremity** HCC ESR COM A

I70.769 Atherosclerosis of other type of bypass graft(s) of the extremities with gangrene, unspecified extremity HCC ESR COM A

✓6th I70.79 Other atherosclerosis of other type of bypass graft(s) of the extremities

I70.791 Other atherosclerosis of other type of bypass graft(s) of the extremities, right leg ESR A

I70.792 Other atherosclerosis of other type of bypass graft(s) of the extremities, left leg ESR A

I70.793 Other atherosclerosis of other type of bypass graft(s) of the extremities, bilateral legs ESR A

I70.798 Other atherosclerosis of other type of bypass graft(s) of the extremities, other extremity ESR A

I70.799 Other atherosclerosis of other type of bypass graft(s) of the extremities, unspecified extremity ESR A

I70.8 Atherosclerosis of other arteries A

TIP: Arteriosclerosis of the iliac arteries is coded here.

✓5th I70.9 Other and unspecified atherosclerosis

EXCLUDES 2 *disorders of pyrophosphate metabolism (E83.82-)*

I70.90 Unspecified atherosclerosis A

I70.91 Generalized atherosclerosis A

I70.92 Chronic total occlusion of artery of the extremities ESR UPD A

Complete occlusion of artery of the extremities
Total occlusion of artery of the extremities
Code first atherosclerosis of arteries of the extremities (I70.2-, I70.3-, I70.4-, I70.5-, I70.6-, I70.7-)

## ✓4th I71 Aortic aneurysm and dissection

Code first, if applicable:
syphilitic aortic aneurysm (A52.01)
traumatic aortic aneurysm (S25.09, S35.09)

AHA: 2022,4Q,24-26

TIP: A diagnosis of dissecting aneurysm should be coded to subcategory I71.0 only. The bulging/aneurysm, although present, occurred secondary to the dissection. The dissection represents the most significant problem.

✓5th I71.0 Dissection of aorta

I71.00 Dissection of unspecified site of aorta HCC ESR COM

✓6th I71.01 Dissection of thoracic aorta

AHA: 2024,2Q,17

I71.010 Dissection of ascending aorta HCC ESR COM

I71.011 Dissection of aortic arch HCC ESR COM

I71.012 Dissection of descending thoracic aorta HCC ESR COM

I71.019 Dissection of thoracic aorta, unspecified HCC ESR COM

I71.02 Dissection of abdominal aorta HCC ESR COM

I71.03 Dissection of thoracoabdominal aorta HCC ESR COM

✓5th I71.1 Thoracic aortic aneurysm, ruptured

I71.10 Thoracic aortic aneurysm, ruptured, unspecified HCC ESR COM

I71.11 Aneurysm of the ascending aorta, ruptured HCC ESR COM

I71.12 Aneurysm of the aortic arch, ruptured HCC ESR COM

I71.13 Aneurysm of the descending thoracic aorta, ruptured HCC ESR COM

✓5th I71.2 Thoracic aortic aneurysm, without rupture

I71.20 Thoracic aortic aneurysm, without rupture, unspecified ESR

I71.21 Aneurysm of the ascending aorta, without rupture ESR

I71.22 Aneurysm of the aortic arch, without rupture ESR

I71.23 Aneurysm of the descending thoracic aorta, without rupture ESR

✓5th I71.3 Abdominal aortic aneurysm, ruptured

I71.30 Abdominal aortic aneurysm, ruptured, unspecified HCC ESR COM

I71.31 Pararenal abdominal aortic aneurysm, ruptured HCC ESR COM

I71.32 Juxtarenal abdominal aortic aneurysm, ruptured HCC ESR COM

I71.33 Infrarenal abdominal aortic aneurysm, ruptured HCC ESR COM

✓5th I71.4 Abdominal aortic aneurysm, without rupture

I71.40 Abdominal aortic aneurysm, without rupture, unspecified ESR

I71.41 Pararenal abdominal aortic aneurysm, without rupture ESR

AHA: 2024,2Q,16

I71.42 Juxtarenal abdominal aortic aneurysm, without rupture ESR

I71.43 Infrarenal abdominal aortic aneurysm, without rupture ESR

✓5th I71.5 Thoracoabdominal aortic aneurysm, ruptured

I71.50 Thoracoabdominal aortic aneurysm, ruptured, unspecified HCC ESR COM

I71.51 Supraceliac aneurysm of the thoracoabdominal aorta, ruptured HCC ESR COM

I71.52 Paravisceral aneurysm of the thoracoabdominal aorta, ruptured HCC ESR COM

✓5th I71.6 Thoracoabdominal aortic aneurysm, without rupture

I71.60 Thoracoabdominal aortic aneurysm, without rupture, unspecified ESR

I71.61 Supraceliac aneurysm of the thoracoabdominal aorta, without rupture ESR

I71.62 Paravisceral aneurysm of the thoracoabdominal aorta, without rupture ESR

I71.8 Aortic aneurysm of unspecified site, ruptured HCC ESR COM

Rupture of aorta NOS

I71.9 Aortic aneurysm of unspecified site, without rupture ESR

Aneurysm of aorta
Dilatation of aorta
Hyaline necrosis of aorta

## ✓4th I72 Other aneurysm

INCLUDES aneurysm (cirsoid) (false) (ruptured)

EXCLUDES 2
*acquired aneurysm (I77.0)*
*aneurysm (of) aorta (I71.-)*
*aneurysm (of) arteriovenous NOS (Q27.3-)*
*carotid artery dissection (I77.71)*
*cerebral (nonruptured) aneurysm (I67.1)*
*coronary aneurysm (I25.4)*
*coronary artery dissection (I25.42)*
*dissection of artery NEC (I77.79)*
*dissection of precerebral artery, congenital (nonruptured) (Q28.1)*
*heart aneurysm (I25.3)*
*iliac artery dissection (I77.72)*
*precerebral artery, congential (nonruptured) (Q28.1)*
*pulmonary artery aneurysm (I28.1)*
*renal artery dissection (I77.73)*
*retinal aneurysm (H35.0)*
*ruptured cerebral aneurysm (I60.7)*
*varicose aneurysm (I77.0)*
*vertebral artery dissection (I77.74)*

AHA: 2016,4Q,28-29

I72.0 Aneurysm of carotid artery ESR

Aneurysm of common carotid artery
Aneurysm of external carotid artery
Aneurysm of internal carotid artery, extracranial portion

EXCLUDES 1
*aneurysm of internal carotid artery, intracranial portion (I67.1)*
*aneurysm of internal carotid artery NOS (I67.1)*

I72.1 Aneurysm of artery of upper extremity ESR

I72.2 Aneurysm of renal artery ESR

I72.3 Aneurysm of iliac artery ESR

I72.4 Aneurysm of artery of lower extremity ESR

AHA: 2019,2Q,21

I72.5 Aneurysm of other precerebral arteries ESR

Aneurysm of basilar artery (trunk)

EXCLUDES 2
*aneurysm of carotid artery (I72.0)*
*aneurysm of vertebral artery (I72.6)*
*dissection of carotid artery (I77.71)*
*dissection of other precerebral arteries (I77.75)*
*dissection of vertebral artery (I77.74)*

I72.6 Aneurysm of vertebral artery ESR

EXCLUDES 2 *dissection of vertebral artery (I77.74)*

I72.8 Aneurysm of other specified arteries ESR

**I72.9 Aneurysm of unspecified site** ESR

**Aneurysm**

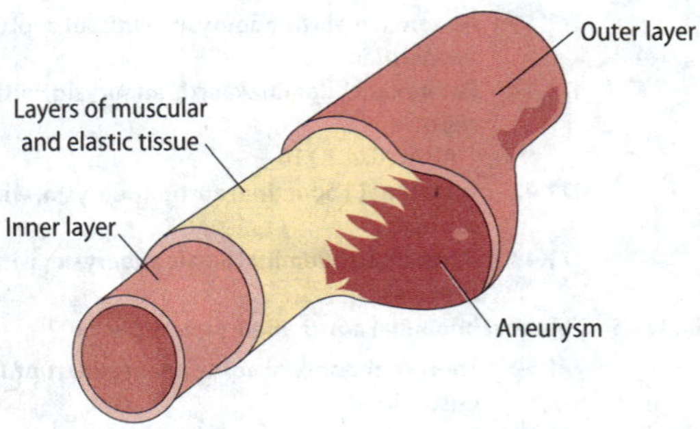


**✓4th I73 Other peripheral vascular diseases**

EXCLUDES 2 *chilblains (T69.1)*
*frostbite (T33-T34)*
*immersion hand or foot (T69.Ø-)*
*spasm of cerebral artery (G45.9)*

**AHA:** 2018,4Q,87

**✓5th I73.Ø Raynaud's syndrome**
Raynaud's disease
Raynaud's phenomenon (secondary)
**DEF:** Constriction of the arteries of the digits caused by cold or by nerve or arterial damage and can be prompted by stress or emotion. Blood cannot reach the skin and soft tissues and the skin turns white with blue mottling.

**I73.ØØ Raynaud's syndrome without gangrene**

**I73.Ø1 Raynaud's syndrome with gangrene** HCC ESR COM

**I73.1 Thromboangiitis obliterans [Buerger's disease]** ESR
**DEF:** Inflammatory disease of the extremity blood vessels, mainly the lower blood vessels. This disease is associated with heavy tobacco use. The arteries are more affected than veins. It occurs primarily in young men and leads to tissue ischemia and gangrene.

**✓5th I73.8 Other specified peripheral vascular diseases**
EXCLUDES 1 *diabetic (peripheral) angiopathy (EØ8-E13 with .51-.52)*

**I73.81 Erythromelalgia** ESR

**I73.89 Other specified peripheral vascular diseases** ESR
Acrocyanosis
Erythrocyanosis
Simple acroparesthesia [Schultze's type]
Vasomotor acroparesthesia [Nothnagel's type]

**I73.9 Peripheral vascular disease, unspecified** ESR
Intermittent claudication
Peripheral angiopathy NOS
Spasm of artery
EXCLUDES 1 *atherosclerosis of the extremities (I7Ø.2-I7Ø.7-)*
**AHA:** 2018,2Q,7

**✓4th I74 Arterial embolism and thrombosis**

INCLUDES embolic infarction
embolic occlusion
thrombotic infarction
thrombotic occlusion

Code first:
embolism and thrombosis complicating abortion or ectopic or molar pregnancy (OØØ-OØ7, OØ8.2)
embolism and thrombosis complicating pregnancy, childbirth and the puerperium (O88.-)

EXCLUDES 2 *atheroembolism (I75.-)*
*basilar embolism and thrombosis (I63.Ø-I63.2, I65.1)*
*carotid embolism and thrombosis (I63.Ø-I63.2, I65.2)*
*cerebral embolism and thrombosis (I63.3-I63.5, I66.-)*
*coronary embolism and thrombosis (I21-I25)*
*mesenteric embolism and thrombosis (K55.Ø-)*
*ophthalmic embolism and thrombosis (H34.-)*
*precerebral embolism and thrombosis NOS (I63.Ø-I63.2, I65.9)*
*pulmonary embolism and thrombosis (I26.-)*
*renal embolism and thrombosis (N28.Ø)*
*retinal embolism and thrombosis (H34.-)*
*septic embolism and thrombosis (I76)*
*vertebral embolism and thrombosis (I63.Ø-I63.2, I65.Ø)*

**AHA:** 2023,2Q,7

**✓5th I74.Ø Embolism and thrombosis of abdominal aorta**

**I74.Ø1 Saddle embolus of abdominal aorta** HCC ESR COM

**I74.Ø9 Other arterial embolism and thrombosis of abdominal aorta** HCC ESR COM
Aortic bifurcation syndrome
Aortoiliac obstruction
Leriche's syndrome

**✓5th I74.1 Embolism and thrombosis of other and unspecified parts of aorta**

**I74.1Ø Embolism and thrombosis of unspecified parts of aorta** HCC ESR COM

**I74.11 Embolism and thrombosis of thoracic aorta** HCC ESR COM

**I74.19 Embolism and thrombosis of other parts of aorta** HCC ESR COM

**I74.2 Embolism and thrombosis of arteries of the upper extremities** HCC ESR COM

**I74.3 Embolism and thrombosis of arteries of the lower extremities** HCC ESR COM

**I74.4 Embolism and thrombosis of arteries of extremities, unspecified** HCC ESR COM
Peripheral arterial embolism NOS

**I74.5 Embolism and thrombosis of iliac artery** HCC ESR COM

**I74.8 Embolism and thrombosis of other arteries** HCC ESR COM

**I74.9 Embolism and thrombosis of unspecified artery** HCC ESR COM

**✓4th I75 Atheroembolism**

INCLUDES atherothrombotic microembolism
cholesterol embolism

**✓5th I75.Ø Atheroembolism of extremities**

**✓6th I75.Ø1 Atheroembolism of upper extremity**

**I75.Ø11 Atheroembolism of right upper extremity** HCC ESR COM

**I75.Ø12 Atheroembolism of left upper extremity** HCC ESR COM

**I75.Ø13 Atheroembolism of bilateral upper extremities** HCC ESR COM

**I75.Ø19 Atheroembolism of unspecified upper extremity** HCC ESR COM

**✓6th I75.Ø2 Atheroembolism of lower extremity**

**I75.Ø21 Atheroembolism of right lower extremity** HCC ESR COM

**I75.Ø22 Atheroembolism of left lower extremity** HCC ESR COM

**I75.Ø23 Atheroembolism of bilateral lower extremities** HCC ESR COM

**I75.Ø29 Atheroembolism of unspecified lower extremity** HCC ESR COM

**✓5th I75.8 Atheroembolism of other sites**

**I75.81 Atheroembolism of kidney** HCC ESR COM
Use additional code for any associated acute kidney failure and chronic kidney disease (N17.-, N18.-)

**I75.89 Atheroembolism of other site** HCC ESR COM

**I76 Septic arterial embolism** HCC ESR COM UPD
Code first underlying infection, such as:
infective endocarditis (I33.Ø)
lung abscess (J85.-)
Use additional code to identify the site of the embolism (I74.-)
EXCLUDES 2 *septic pulmonary embolism (I26.Ø1, I26.9Ø)*

**✓4th I77 Other disorders of arteries and arterioles**

EXCLUDES 2 *collagen (vascular) diseases (M3Ø-M36)*
*hypersensitivity angiitis (M31.Ø)*
*pulmonary artery (I28.-)*

**I77.Ø Arteriovenous fistula, acquired** ESR
Aneurysmal varix
Arteriovenous aneurysm, acquired
EXCLUDES 1 *arteriovenous aneurysm NOS (Q27.3-)*
*presence of arteriovenous shunt (fistula) for dialysis (Z99.2)*
*traumatic - see injury of blood vessel by body region*
EXCLUDES 2 *cerebral (I67.1)*
*coronary (I25.4)*
**DEF:** Communication between an artery and vein caused by trauma or invasive procedures.

**I77.1 Stricture of artery** ESR
Narrowing of artery
**AHA:** 2021,3Q,12

**I77.2 Rupture of artery** ESR
Erosion of artery
Fistula of artery
Ulcer of artery
EXCLUDES 1 *traumatic rupture of artery - see injury of blood vessel by body region*

**I77.3 Arterial fibromuscular dysplasia** ESR
Fibromuscular hyperplasia (of) carotid artery
Fibromuscular hyperplasia (of) renal artery

**I77.4 Celiac artery compression syndrome** ESR
**AHA:** 2021,3Q,12

**I77.5 Necrosis of artery** ESR

**I77.6 Arteritis, unspecified** ESR
Aortitis NOS
Endarteritis NOS
EXCLUDES 1 *arteritis or endarteritis:*
*aortic arch (M31.4)*
*cerebral NEC (I67.7)*
*coronary (I25.89)*
*deformans (I70.-)*
*giant cell (M31.5, M31.6)*
*obliterans (I70.-)*
*senile (I70.-)*

✓5th **I77.7 Other arterial dissection**
EXCLUDES 2 *dissection of aorta (I71.0-)*
*dissection of coronary artery (I25.42)*
**AHA:** 2016,4Q,28-29

**I77.70 Dissection of unspecified artery** ESR COM
**I77.71 Dissection of carotid artery** ESR COM
**I77.72 Dissection of iliac artery** ESR COM
**I77.73 Dissection of renal artery** ESR COM
**I77.74 Dissection of vertebral artery** ESR COM
EXCLUDES 2 *aneurysm of vertebral artery (I72.6)*
**AHA:** 2024,1Q,26
**I77.75 Dissection of other precerebral arteries** ESR COM
Dissection of basilar artery (trunk)
EXCLUDES 2 *aneurysm of carotid artery (I72.0)*
*aneurysm of other precerebral arteries (I72.5)*
*aneurysm of vertebral artery (I72.6)*
*dissection of carotid artery (I77.71)*
*dissection of vertebral artery (I77.74)*
**I77.76 Dissection of artery of upper extremity** ESR COM
**I77.77 Dissection of artery of lower extremity** ESR COM
**I77.79 Dissection of other specified artery** ESR COM

✓5th **I77.8 Other specified disorders of arteries and arterioles**

✓6th **I77.81 Aortic ectasia**
Ectasis aorta
EXCLUDES 1 *aortic aneurysm and dissection (I71.-)*
**I77.810 Thoracic aortic ectasia** ESR
**I77.811 Abdominal aortic ectasia** ESR
**I77.812 Thoracoabdominal aortic ectasia** ESR
**I77.819 Aortic ectasia, unspecified site** ESR

**I77.82 Antineutrophilic cytoplasmic antibody [ANCA] vasculitis** HCC Rx ESR COM
ANCA associated vasculitis
ANCA positive vasculitis
EXCLUDES 2 *eosinophilic granulomatosis with polyangiitis (M30.1)*
*granulomatosis with polyangiitis (M31.3-)*
*microscopic polyangiitis (M31.7)*
**AHA:** 2022,4Q,26-27

**I77.89 Other specified disorders of arteries and arterioles** ESR
**AHA:** 2021,1Q,23

**I77.9 Disorder of arteries and arterioles, unspecified** ESR
**AHA:** 2021,1Q,4; 2018,2Q,7

✓4th **I78 Diseases of capillaries**

**I78.0 Hereditary hemorrhagic telangiectasia** ESR
Rendu-Osler-Weber disease

**I78.1 Nevus, non-neoplastic**
Araneus nevus
Senile nevus
Spider nevus
Stellar nevus
EXCLUDES 1 *nevus NOS (D22.-)*
*vascular NOS (Q82.5)*
EXCLUDES 2 *blue nevus (D22.-)*
*flammeus nevus (Q82.5)*
*hairy nevus (D22.-)*
*melanocytic nevus (D22.-)*
*pigmented nevus (D22.-)*
*portwine nevus (Q82.5)*
*sanguineous nevus (Q82.5)*
*strawberry nevus (Q82.5)*
*verrucous nevus (Q82.5)*
**AHA:** 2019,1Q,21

**I78.8 Other diseases of capillaries**

**I78.9 Disease of capillaries, unspecified**

✓4th **I79 Disorders of arteries, arterioles and capillaries in diseases classified elsewhere**

***I79.0 Aneurysm of aorta in diseases classified elsewhere*** ESR
Code first underlying disease
EXCLUDES 1 *syphilitic aneurysm (A52.01)*

***I79.1 Aortitis in diseases classified elsewhere*** ESR
Code first underlying disease
EXCLUDES 1 *syphilitic aortitis (A52.02)*

***I79.8 Other disorders of arteries, arterioles and capillaries in diseases classified elsewhere*** ESR
Code first underlying disease, such as:
amyloidosis (E85.-)
EXCLUDES 1 *diabetic (peripheral) angiopathy (E08-E13 with .51-.52)*
*syphilitic endarteritis (A52.09)*
*tuberculous endarteritis (A18.89)*

## Diseases of veins, lymphatic vessels and lymph nodes, not elsewhere classified (I80-I89)

✓4th **I80 Phlebitis and thrombophlebitis**
INCLUDES endophlebitis
inflammation, vein
periphlebitis
suppurative phlebitis
Code first, if applicable:
phlebitis and thrombophlebitis complicating abortion, ectopic or molar pregnancy (O00-O07, O08.7)
phlebitis and thrombophlebitis complicating pregnancy, childbirth and the puerperium (O22.-, O87.-)
EXCLUDES 1 *venous embolism and thrombosis of lower extremities (I82.4-, I82.5-, I82.81-)*

✓5th **I80.0 Phlebitis and thrombophlebitis of superficial vessels of lower extremities**
Phlebitis and thrombophlebitis of femoropopliteal vein
**I80.00 Phlebitis and thrombophlebitis of superficial vessels of unspecified lower extremity**
**I80.01 Phlebitis and thrombophlebitis of superficial vessels of right lower extremity**
**I80.02 Phlebitis and thrombophlebitis of superficial vessels of left lower extremity**
**I80.03 Phlebitis and thrombophlebitis of superficial vessels of lower extremities, bilateral**

✓5th **I80.1 Phlebitis and thrombophlebitis of femoral vein**
Phlebitis and thrombophlebitis of common femoral vein
Phlebitis and thrombophlebitis of deep femoral vein
**I80.10 Phlebitis and thrombophlebitis of unspecified femoral vein** HCC Rx ESR COM
**I80.11 Phlebitis and thrombophlebitis of right femoral vein** HCC Rx ESR COM
**I80.12 Phlebitis and thrombophlebitis of left femoral vein** HCC Rx ESR COM
**I80.13 Phlebitis and thrombophlebitis of femoral vein, bilateral** HCC Rx ESR COM

✓5th **I80.2 Phlebitis and thrombophlebitis of other and unspecified deep vessels of lower extremities**

✓6th **I80.20 Phlebitis and thrombophlebitis of unspecified deep vessels of lower extremities**
**I80.201 Phlebitis and thrombophlebitis of unspecified deep vessels of right lower extremity** HCC Rx ESR COM

I80.202 Phlebitis and thrombophlebitis of unspecified deep vessels of left lower extremity HCC Rx ESR COM

I80.203 Phlebitis and thrombophlebitis of unspecified deep vessels of lower extremities, bilateral HCC Rx ESR COM

I80.209 Phlebitis and thrombophlebitis of unspecified deep vessels of unspecified lower extremity HCC Rx ESR COM

✓6th I80.21 Phlebitis and thrombophlebitis of iliac vein

Phlebitis and thrombophlebitis of common iliac vein
Phlebitis and thrombophlebitis of external iliac vein
Phlebitis and thrombophlebitis of internal iliac vein

I80.211 Phlebitis and thrombophlebitis of right iliac vein HCC Rx ESR COM

I80.212 Phlebitis and thrombophlebitis of left iliac vein HCC Rx ESR COM

I80.213 Phlebitis and thrombophlebitis of iliac vein, bilateral HCC Rx ESR COM

I80.219 Phlebitis and thrombophlebitis of unspecified iliac vein HCC Rx ESR COM

✓6th I80.22 Phlebitis and thrombophlebitis of popliteal vein

I80.221 Phlebitis and thrombophlebitis of right popliteal vein HCC Rx ESR COM

I80.222 Phlebitis and thrombophlebitis of left popliteal vein HCC Rx ESR COM

I80.223 Phlebitis and thrombophlebitis of popliteal vein, bilateral HCC Rx ESR COM

I80.229 Phlebitis and thrombophlebitis of unspecified popliteal vein HCC Rx ESR COM

✓6th I80.23 Phlebitis and thrombophlebitis of tibial vein

Phlebitis and thrombophlebitis of anterior tibial vein
Phlebitis and thrombophlebitis of posterior tibial vein

I80.231 Phlebitis and thrombophlebitis of right tibial vein HCC Rx ESR COM

I80.232 Phlebitis and thrombophlebitis of left tibial vein HCC Rx ESR COM

I80.233 Phlebitis and thrombophlebitis of tibial vein, bilateral HCC Rx ESR COM

I80.239 Phlebitis and thrombophlebitis of unspecified tibial vein HCC Rx ESR COM

✓6th I80.24 Phlebitis and thrombophlebitis of peroneal vein

AHA: 2019,4Q,8

I80.241 Phlebitis and thrombophlebitis of right peroneal vein HCC Rx ESR COM

I80.242 Phlebitis and thrombophlebitis of left peroneal vein HCC Rx ESR COM

I80.243 Phlebitis and thrombophlebitis of peroneal vein, bilateral HCC Rx ESR COM

I80.249 Phlebitis and thrombophlebitis of unspecified peroneal vein HCC Rx ESR COM

✓6th I80.25 Phlebitis and thrombophlebitis of calf muscular vein

Phlebitis and thrombophlebitis of calf muscular vein, NOS
Phlebitis and thrombophlebitis of gastrocnemial vein
Phlebitis and thrombophlebitis of soleal vein

AHA: 2019,4Q,8

I80.251 Phlebitis and thrombophlebitis of right calf muscular vein HCC Rx ESR COM

I80.252 Phlebitis and thrombophlebitis of left calf muscular vein HCC Rx ESR COM

I80.253 Phlebitis and thrombophlebitis of calf muscular vein, bilateral HCC Rx ESR COM

I80.259 Phlebitis and thrombophlebitis of unspecified calf muscular vein HCC Rx ESR COM

✓6th I80.29 Phlebitis and thrombophlebitis of other deep vessels of lower extremities

I80.291 Phlebitis and thrombophlebitis of other deep vessels of right lower extremity HCC Rx ESR COM

I80.292 Phlebitis and thrombophlebitis of other deep vessels of left lower extremity HCC Rx ESR COM

I80.293 Phlebitis and thrombophlebitis of other deep vessels of lower extremity, bilateral HCC Rx ESR COM

I80.299 Phlebitis and thrombophlebitis of other deep vessels of unspecified lower extremity HCC Rx ESR COM

I80.3 Phlebitis and thrombophlebitis of lower extremities, unspecified

I80.8 Phlebitis and thrombophlebitis of other sites

I80.9 Phlebitis and thrombophlebitis of unspecified site

**I81 Portal vein thrombosis**

Portal (vein) obstruction

EXCLUDES 2 *hepatic vein thrombosis (I82.0)*
*phlebitis of portal vein (K75.1)*

AHA: 2019,4Q,68

✓4th **I82 Other venous embolism and thrombosis**

Code first venous embolism and thrombosis complicating:
abortion, ectopic or molar pregnancy (O00-O07, O08.7)
pregnancy, childbirth and the puerperium (O22.-, O87.-)

EXCLUDES 2 *venous embolism and thrombosis (of):*
*cerebral (I63.6, I67.6)*
*coronary (I21-I25)*
*intracranial and intraspinal, septic or NOS (G08)*
*intracranial, nonpyogenic (I67.6)*
*intraspinal, nonpyogenic (G95.1)*
*mesenteric (K55.0-)*
*portal (I81)*
*pulmonary (I26.-)*

I82.0 Budd-Chiari syndrome HCC Rx ESR COM

Hepatic vein thrombosis

DEF: Thrombosis or other obstruction of the hepatic veins. Symptoms include an enlarged liver, extensive collateral vessels, intractable ascites, and severe portal hypertension.

I82.1 Thrombophlebitis migrans

✓5th I82.2 Embolism and thrombosis of vena cava and other thoracic veins

✓6th I82.21 Embolism and thrombosis of superior vena cava

I82.210 Acute embolism and thrombosis of superior vena cava HCC Rx ESR COM

Embolism and thrombosis of superior vena cava NOS

I82.211 Chronic embolism and thrombosis of superior vena cava HCC Rx ESR COM

✓6th I82.22 Embolism and thrombosis of inferior vena cava

I82.220 Acute embolism and thrombosis of inferior vena cava HCC Rx ESR COM

Embolism and thrombosis of inferior vena cava NOS

I82.221 Chronic embolism and thrombosis of inferior vena cava HCC Rx ESR COM

✓6th I82.29 Embolism and thrombosis of other thoracic veins

Embolism and thrombosis of brachiocephalic (innominate) vein

I82.290 Acute embolism and thrombosis of other thoracic veins HCC Rx ESR COM

I82.291 Chronic embolism and thrombosis of other thoracic veins HCC Rx ESR COM

I82.3 Embolism and thrombosis of renal vein HCC Rx ESR COM

✓5th I82.4 Acute embolism and thrombosis of deep veins of lower extremity

✓6th I82.40 Acute embolism and thrombosis of unspecified deep veins of lower extremity

Deep vein thrombosis NOS
DVT NOS

EXCLUDES 1 *acute embolism and thrombosis of unspecified deep veins of distal lower extremity (I82.4Z-)*
*acute embolism and thrombosis of unspecified deep veins of proximal lower extremity (I82.4Y-)*

I82.401 Acute embolism and thrombosis of unspecified deep veins of right lower extremity HCC Rx ESR COM

I82.402 Acute embolism and thrombosis of unspecified deep veins of left lower extremity HCC Rx ESR COM

I82.403 Acute embolism and thrombosis of unspecified deep veins of lower extremity, bilateral HCC Rx ESR COM

I82.409 Acute embolism and thrombosis of unspecified deep veins of unspecified lower extremity HCC Rx ESR COM

✓6th **I82.41 Acute embolism and thrombosis of femoral vein**
Acute embolism and thrombosis of common femoral vein
Acute embolism and thrombosis of deep femoral vein
**AHA:** 2023,3Q,12
- **I82.411 Acute embolism and thrombosis of right femoral vein** HCC Rx ESR COM
- **I82.412 Acute embolism and thrombosis of left femoral vein** HCC Rx ESR COM
- **I82.413 Acute embolism and thrombosis of femoral vein, bilateral** HCC Rx ESR COM
- **I82.419 Acute embolism and thrombosis of unspecified femoral vein** HCC Rx ESR COM

✓6th **I82.42 Acute embolism and thrombosis of iliac vein**
Acute embolism and thrombosis of common iliac vein
Acute embolism and thrombosis of external iliac vein
Acute embolism and thrombosis of internal iliac vein
- **I82.421 Acute embolism and thrombosis of right iliac vein** HCC Rx ESR COM
- **I82.422 Acute embolism and thrombosis of left iliac vein** HCC Rx ESR COM
- **I82.423 Acute embolism and thrombosis of iliac vein, bilateral** HCC Rx ESR COM
- **I82.429 Acute embolism and thrombosis of unspecified iliac vein** HCC Rx ESR COM

✓6th **I82.43 Acute embolism and thrombosis of popliteal vein**
- **I82.431 Acute embolism and thrombosis of right popliteal vein** HCC Rx ESR COM
- **I82.432 Acute embolism and thrombosis of left popliteal vein** HCC Rx ESR COM
- **I82.433 Acute embolism and thrombosis of popliteal vein, bilateral** HCC Rx ESR COM
- **I82.439 Acute embolism and thrombosis of unspecified popliteal vein** HCC Rx ESR COM

✓6th **I82.44 Acute embolism and thrombosis of tibial vein**
Acute embolism and thrombosis of anterior tibial vein
Acute embolism and thrombosis of posterior tibial vein
- **I82.441 Acute embolism and thrombosis of right tibial vein** HCC Rx ESR COM
- **I82.442 Acute embolism and thrombosis of left tibial vein** HCC Rx ESR COM
- **I82.443 Acute embolism and thrombosis of tibial vein, bilateral** HCC Rx ESR COM
- **I82.449 Acute embolism and thrombosis of unspecified tibial vein** HCC Rx ESR COM

✓6th **I82.45 Acute embolism and thrombosis of peroneal vein**
**AHA:** 2019,4Q,8-10
- **I82.451 Acute embolism and thrombosis of right peroneal vein** HCC Rx ESR COM
- **I82.452 Acute embolism and thrombosis of left peroneal vein** HCC Rx ESR COM
- **I82.453 Acute embolism and thrombosis of peroneal vein, bilateral** HCC Rx ESR COM
- **I82.459 Acute embolism and thrombosis of unspecified peroneal vein** HCC Rx ESR COM

✓6th **I82.46 Acute embolism and thrombosis of calf muscular vein**
Acute embolism and thrombosis of calf muscular vein, NOS
Acute embolism and thrombosis of gastrocnemial vein
Acute embolism and thrombosis of soleal vein
**AHA:** 2019,4Q,8-10
- **I82.461 Acute embolism and thrombosis of right calf muscular vein** HCC Rx ESR COM
- **I82.462 Acute embolism and thrombosis of left calf muscular vein** HCC Rx ESR COM
- **I82.463 Acute embolism and thrombosis of calf muscular vein, bilateral** HCC Rx ESR COM
- **I82.469 Acute embolism and thrombosis of unspecified calf muscular vein** HCC Rx ESR COM

✓6th **I82.49 Acute embolism and thrombosis of other specified deep vein of lower extremity**
- **I82.491 Acute embolism and thrombosis of other specified deep vein of right lower extremity** HCC Rx ESR COM
- **I82.492 Acute embolism and thrombosis of other specified deep vein of left lower extremity** HCC Rx ESR COM
- **I82.493 Acute embolism and thrombosis of other specified deep vein of lower extremity, bilateral** HCC Rx ESR COM
- **I82.499 Acute embolism and thrombosis of other specified deep vein of unspecified lower extremity** HCC Rx ESR COM

✓6th **I82.4Y Acute embolism and thrombosis of unspecified deep veins of proximal lower extremity**
Acute embolism and thrombosis of deep vein of thigh NOS
Acute embolism and thrombosis of deep vein of upper leg NOS
- **I82.4Y1 Acute embolism and thrombosis of unspecified deep veins of right proximal lower extremity** HCC Rx ESR COM
- **I82.4Y2 Acute embolism and thrombosis of unspecified deep veins of left proximal lower extremity** HCC Rx ESR COM
- **I82.4Y3 Acute embolism and thrombosis of unspecified deep veins of proximal lower extremity, bilateral** HCC Rx ESR COM
- **I82.4Y9 Acute embolism and thrombosis of unspecified deep veins of unspecified proximal lower extremity** HCC Rx ESR COM

✓6th **I82.4Z Acute embolism and thrombosis of unspecified deep veins of distal lower extremity**
Acute embolism and thrombosis of deep vein of calf NOS
Acute embolism and thrombosis of deep vein of lower leg NOS
- **I82.4Z1 Acute embolism and thrombosis of unspecified deep veins of right distal lower extremity** HCC Rx ESR COM
- **I82.4Z2 Acute embolism and thrombosis of unspecified deep veins of left distal lower extremity** HCC Rx ESR COM
- **I82.4Z3 Acute embolism and thrombosis of unspecified deep veins of distal lower extremity, bilateral** HCC Rx ESR COM
- **I82.4Z9 Acute embolism and thrombosis of unspecified deep veins of unspecified distal lower extremity** HCC Rx ESR COM

✓5th **I82.5 Chronic embolism and thrombosis of deep veins of lower extremity**
Use additional code, if applicable, for associated long-term (current) use of anticoagulants (Z79.01)
**EXCLUDES 1** *personal history of venous embolism and thrombosis (Z86.718)*
**AHA:** 2020,2Q,20

✓6th **I82.50 Chronic embolism and thrombosis of unspecified deep veins of lower extremity**
**EXCLUDES 1** *chronic embolism and thrombosis of unspecified deep veins of distal lower extremity (I82.5Z-)*
*chronic embolism and thrombosis of unspecified deep veins of proximal lower extremity (I82.5Y-)*
- **I82.501 Chronic embolism and thrombosis of unspecified deep veins of right lower extremity** HCC Rx ESR COM
- **I82.502 Chronic embolism and thrombosis of unspecified deep veins of left lower extremity** HCC Rx ESR COM
- **I82.503 Chronic embolism and thrombosis of unspecified deep veins of lower extremity, bilateral** HCC Rx ESR COM
- **I82.509 Chronic embolism and thrombosis of unspecified deep veins of unspecified lower extremity** HCC Rx ESR COM

✓6th **I82.51 Chronic embolism and thrombosis of femoral vein**
Chronic embolism and thrombosis of common femoral vein
Chronic embolism and thrombosis of deep femoral vein
- **I82.511 Chronic embolism and thrombosis of right femoral vein** HCC Rx ESR COM
- **I82.512 Chronic embolism and thrombosis of left femoral vein** HCC Rx ESR COM

I82.513 **Chronic embolism and thrombosis of femoral vein, bilateral** HCC Rx ESR COM

I82.519 **Chronic embolism and thrombosis of unspecified femoral vein** HCC Rx ESR COM

√6th I82.52 **Chronic embolism and thrombosis of iliac vein**

Chronic embolism and thrombosis of common iliac vein

Chronic embolism and thrombosis of external iliac vein

Chronic embolism and thrombosis of internal iliac vein

I82.521 **Chronic embolism and thrombosis of right iliac vein** HCC Rx ESR COM

I82.522 **Chronic embolism and thrombosis of left iliac vein** HCC Rx ESR COM

I82.523 **Chronic embolism and thrombosis of iliac vein, bilateral** HCC Rx ESR COM

I82.529 **Chronic embolism and thrombosis of unspecified iliac vein** HCC Rx ESR COM

√6th I82.53 **Chronic embolism and thrombosis of popliteal vein**

I82.531 **Chronic embolism and thrombosis of right popliteal vein** HCC Rx ESR COM

I82.532 **Chronic embolism and thrombosis of left popliteal vein** HCC Rx ESR COM

I82.533 **Chronic embolism and thrombosis of popliteal vein, bilateral** HCC Rx ESR COM

I82.539 **Chronic embolism and thrombosis of unspecified popliteal vein** HCC Rx ESR COM

√6th I82.54 **Chronic embolism and thrombosis of tibial vein**

Chronic embolism and thrombosis of anterior tibial vein

Chronic embolism and thrombosis of posterior tibial vein

I82.541 **Chronic embolism and thrombosis of right tibial vein** HCC Rx ESR COM

I82.542 **Chronic embolism and thrombosis of left tibial vein** HCC Rx ESR COM

I82.543 **Chronic embolism and thrombosis of tibial vein, bilateral** HCC Rx ESR COM

I82.549 **Chronic embolism and thrombosis of unspecified tibial vein** HCC Rx ESR COM

√6th I82.55 **Chronic embolism and thrombosis of peroneal vein**

**AHA:** 2019,4Q,8-10

I82.551 **Chronic embolism and thrombosis of right peroneal vein** HCC Rx ESR COM

I82.552 **Chronic embolism and thrombosis of left peroneal vein** HCC Rx ESR COM

I82.553 **Chronic embolism and thrombosis of peroneal vein, bilateral** HCC Rx ESR COM

I82.559 **Chronic embolism and thrombosis of unspecified peroneal vein** HCC Rx ESR COM

√6th I82.56 **Chronic embolism and thrombosis of calf muscular vein**

Chronic embolism and thrombosis of calf muscular vein NOS

Chronic embolism and thrombosis of gastrocnemial vein

Chronic embolism and thrombosis of soleal vein

**AHA:** 2019,4Q,8-10

I82.561 **Chronic embolism and thrombosis of right calf muscular vein** HCC Rx ESR COM

I82.562 **Chronic embolism and thrombosis of left calf muscular vein** HCC Rx ESR COM

I82.563 **Chronic embolism and thrombosis of calf muscular vein, bilateral** HCC Rx ESR COM

I82.569 **Chronic embolism and thrombosis of unspecified calf muscular vein** HCC Rx ESR COM

√6th I82.59 **Chronic embolism and thrombosis of other specified deep vein of lower extremity**

I82.591 **Chronic embolism and thrombosis of other specified deep vein of right lower extremity** HCC Rx ESR COM

I82.592 **Chronic embolism and thrombosis of other specified deep vein of left lower extremity** HCC Rx ESR COM

I82.593 **Chronic embolism and thrombosis of other specified deep vein of lower extremity, bilateral** HCC Rx ESR COM

I82.599 **Chronic embolism and thrombosis of other specified deep vein of unspecified lower extremity** HCC Rx ESR COM

√6th I82.5Y **Chronic embolism and thrombosis of unspecified deep veins of proximal lower extremity**

Chronic embolism and thrombosis of deep veins of thigh NOS

Chronic embolism and thrombosis of deep veins of upper leg NOS

I82.5Y1 **Chronic embolism and thrombosis of unspecified deep veins of right proximal lower extremity** HCC Rx ESR COM

I82.5Y2 **Chronic embolism and thrombosis of unspecified deep veins of left proximal lower extremity** HCC Rx ESR COM

I82.5Y3 **Chronic embolism and thrombosis of unspecified deep veins of proximal lower extremity, bilateral** HCC Rx ESR COM

I82.5Y9 **Chronic embolism and thrombosis of unspecified deep veins of unspecified proximal lower extremity** HCC Rx ESR COM

√6th I82.5Z **Chronic embolism and thrombosis of unspecified deep veins of distal lower extremity**

Chronic embolism and thrombosis of deep veins of calf NOS

Chronic embolism and thrombosis of deep veins of lower leg NOS

I82.5Z1 **Chronic embolism and thrombosis of unspecified deep veins of right distal lower extremity** HCC Rx ESR COM

I82.5Z2 **Chronic embolism and thrombosis of unspecified deep veins of left distal lower extremity** HCC Rx ESR COM

I82.5Z3 **Chronic embolism and thrombosis of unspecified deep veins of distal lower extremity, bilateral** HCC Rx ESR COM

I82.5Z9 **Chronic embolism and thrombosis of unspecified deep veins of unspecified distal lower extremity** HCC Rx ESR COM

√5th I82.6 **Acute embolism and thrombosis of veins of upper extremity**

√6th I82.60 **Acute embolism and thrombosis of unspecified veins of upper extremity**

I82.601 **Acute embolism and thrombosis of unspecified veins of right upper extremity**

I82.602 **Acute embolism and thrombosis of unspecified veins of left upper extremity**

I82.603 **Acute embolism and thrombosis of unspecified veins of upper extremity, bilateral**

I82.609 **Acute embolism and thrombosis of unspecified veins of unspecified upper extremity**

√6th I82.61 **Acute embolism and thrombosis of superficial veins of upper extremity**

Acute embolism and thrombosis of antecubital vein

Acute embolism and thrombosis of basilic vein

Acute embolism and thrombosis of cephalic vein

I82.611 **Acute embolism and thrombosis of superficial veins of right upper extremity**

I82.612 **Acute embolism and thrombosis of superficial veins of left upper extremity**

I82.613 **Acute embolism and thrombosis of superficial veins of upper extremity, bilateral**

I82.619 **Acute embolism and thrombosis of superficial veins of unspecified upper extremity**

√6th I82.62 **Acute embolism and thrombosis of deep veins of upper extremity**

Acute embolism and thrombosis of brachial vein

Acute embolism and thrombosis of radial vein

Acute embolism and thrombosis of ulnar vein

I82.621 **Acute embolism and thrombosis of deep veins of right upper extremity** HCC Rx ESR COM

I82.622 **Acute embolism and thrombosis of deep veins of left upper extremity** HCC Rx ESR COM

I82.623 **Acute embolism and thrombosis of deep veins of upper extremity, bilateral** HCC Rx ESR COM

I82.629 Acute embolism and thrombosis of deep veins of unspecified upper extremity HCC Rx ESR COM

✓5th I82.7 Chronic embolism and thrombosis of veins of upper extremity
Use additional code, if applicable, for associated long-term (current) use of anticoagulants (Z79.01)
EXCLUDES 1 *personal history of venous embolism and thrombosis (Z86.718)*

✓6th I82.70 Chronic embolism and thrombosis of unspecified veins of upper extremity
I82.701 Chronic embolism and thrombosis of unspecified veins of right upper extremity
I82.702 Chronic embolism and thrombosis of unspecified veins of left upper extremity
I82.703 Chronic embolism and thrombosis of unspecified veins of upper extremity, bilateral
I82.709 Chronic embolism and thrombosis of unspecified veins of unspecified upper extremity

✓6th I82.71 Chronic embolism and thrombosis of superficial veins of upper extremity
Chronic embolism and thrombosis of antecubital vein
Chronic embolism and thrombosis of basilic vein
Chronic embolism and thrombosis of cephalic vein
I82.711 Chronic embolism and thrombosis of superficial veins of right upper extremity
I82.712 Chronic embolism and thrombosis of superficial veins of left upper extremity
I82.713 Chronic embolism and thrombosis of superficial veins of upper extremity, bilateral
I82.719 Chronic embolism and thrombosis of superficial veins of unspecified upper extremity

✓6th I82.72 Chronic embolism and thrombosis of deep veins of upper extremity
Chronic embolism and thrombosis of brachial vein
Chronic embolism and thrombosis of radial vein
Chronic embolism and thrombosis of ulnar vein
I82.721 Chronic embolism and thrombosis of deep veins of right upper extremity HCC Rx ESR COM
I82.722 Chronic embolism and thrombosis of deep veins of left upper extremity HCC Rx ESR COM
I82.723 Chronic embolism and thrombosis of deep veins of upper extremity, bilateral HCC Rx ESR COM
I82.729 Chronic embolism and thrombosis of deep veins of unspecified upper extremity HCC Rx ESR COM

✓5th I82.A Embolism and thrombosis of axillary vein

✓6th I82.A1 Acute embolism and thrombosis of axillary vein
I82.A11 Acute embolism and thrombosis of right axillary vein HCC Rx ESR COM
I82.A12 Acute embolism and thrombosis of left axillary vein HCC Rx ESR COM
I82.A13 Acute embolism and thrombosis of axillary vein, bilateral HCC Rx ESR COM
I82.A19 Acute embolism and thrombosis of unspecified axillary vein HCC Rx ESR COM

✓6th I82.A2 Chronic embolism and thrombosis of axillary vein
I82.A21 Chronic embolism and thrombosis of right axillary vein HCC Rx ESR COM
I82.A22 Chronic embolism and thrombosis of left axillary vein HCC Rx ESR COM
I82.A23 Chronic embolism and thrombosis of axillary vein, bilateral HCC Rx ESR COM
I82.A29 Chronic embolism and thrombosis of unspecified axillary vein HCC Rx ESR COM

✓5th I82.B Embolism and thrombosis of subclavian vein

✓6th I82.B1 Acute embolism and thrombosis of subclavian vein
I82.B11 Acute embolism and thrombosis of right subclavian vein HCC Rx ESR COM
I82.B12 Acute embolism and thrombosis of left subclavian vein HCC Rx ESR COM
I82.B13 Acute embolism and thrombosis of subclavian vein, bilateral HCC Rx ESR COM
I82.B19 Acute embolism and thrombosis of unspecified subclavian vein HCC Rx ESR COM

✓6th I82.B2 Chronic embolism and thrombosis of subclavian vein
I82.B21 Chronic embolism and thrombosis of right subclavian vein HCC Rx ESR COM
I82.B22 Chronic embolism and thrombosis of left subclavian vein HCC Rx ESR COM
I82.B23 Chronic embolism and thrombosis of subclavian vein, bilateral HCC Rx ESR COM
I82.B29 Chronic embolism and thrombosis of unspecified subclavian vein HCC Rx ESR COM

✓5th I82.C Embolism and thrombosis of internal jugular vein

✓6th I82.C1 Acute embolism and thrombosis of internal jugular vein
I82.C11 Acute embolism and thrombosis of right internal jugular vein HCC Rx ESR COM
I82.C12 Acute embolism and thrombosis of left internal jugular vein HCC Rx ESR COM
I82.C13 Acute embolism and thrombosis of internal jugular vein, bilateral HCC Rx ESR COM
I82.C19 Acute embolism and thrombosis of unspecified internal jugular vein HCC Rx ESR COM

✓6th I82.C2 Chronic embolism and thrombosis of internal jugular vein
I82.C21 Chronic embolism and thrombosis of right internal jugular vein HCC Rx ESR COM
I82.C22 Chronic embolism and thrombosis of left internal jugular vein HCC Rx ESR COM
I82.C23 Chronic embolism and thrombosis of internal jugular vein, bilateral HCC Rx ESR COM
I82.C29 Chronic embolism and thrombosis of unspecified internal jugular vein HCC Rx ESR COM

✓5th I82.8 Embolism and thrombosis of other specified veins
Use additional code, if applicable, for associated long-term (current) use of anticoagulants (Z79.01)

✓6th I82.81 Embolism and thrombosis of superficial veins of lower extremities
Embolism and thrombosis of saphenous vein (greater) (lesser)
I82.811 Embolism and thrombosis of superficial veins of right lower extremity
I82.812 Embolism and thrombosis of superficial veins of left lower extremity
I82.813 Embolism and thrombosis of superficial veins of lower extremities, bilateral
I82.819 Embolism and thrombosis of superficial veins of unspecified lower extremity

✓6th I82.89 Embolism and thrombosis of other specified veins
I82.890 Acute embolism and thrombosis of other specified veins
I82.891 Chronic embolism and thrombosis of other specified veins

✓5th I82.9 Embolism and thrombosis of unspecified vein
I82.90 Acute embolism and thrombosis of unspecified vein
Embolism of vein NOS
Thrombosis (vein) NOS
I82.91 Chronic embolism and thrombosis of unspecified vein

✓4th **I83 Varicose veins of lower extremities**
EXCLUDES 2 *varicose veins complicating pregnancy (O22.0-)*
*varicose veins complicating the puerperium (O87.4)*

✓5th I83.0 Varicose veins of lower extremities with ulcer
Use additional code to identify severity of ulcer (L97.-)

✓6th I83.00 Varicose veins of unspecified lower extremity with ulcer
I83.001 Varicose veins of unspecified lower extremity with ulcer of thigh HCC ESR COM A

I83.002 Varicose veins of unspecified lower extremity with ulcer of calf HCC ESR COM A

I83.003 Varicose veins of unspecified lower extremity with ulcer of ankle HCC ESR COM A

I83.004 Varicose veins of unspecified lower extremity with ulcer of heel and midfoot HCC ESR COM A
Varicose veins of unspecified lower extremity with ulcer of plantar surface of midfoot

I83.005 Varicose veins of unspecified lower extremity with ulcer other part of foot HCC ESR COM A
Varicose veins of unspecified lower extremity with ulcer of toe

I83.008 Varicose veins of unspecified lower extremity with ulcer other part of lower leg HCC ESR COM A

I83.009 Varicose veins of unspecified lower extremity with ulcer of unspecified site HCC ESR COM A

✓6th I83.01 Varicose veins of right lower extremity with ulcer

I83.011 Varicose veins of right lower extremity with ulcer of thigh HCC ESR COM A

I83.012 Varicose veins of right lower extremity with ulcer of calf HCC ESR COM A

I83.013 Varicose veins of right lower extremity with ulcer of ankle HCC ESR COM A

I83.014 Varicose veins of right lower extremity with ulcer of heel and midfoot HCC ESR COM A
Varicose veins of right lower extremity with ulcer of plantar surface of midfoot

I83.015 Varicose veins of right lower extremity with ulcer other part of foot HCC ESR COM A
Varicose veins of right lower extremity with ulcer of toe

I83.018 Varicose veins of right lower extremity with ulcer other part of lower leg HCC ESR COM A

I83.019 Varicose veins of right lower extremity with ulcer of unspecified site HCC ESR COM A

✓6th I83.02 Varicose veins of left lower extremity with ulcer

I83.021 Varicose veins of left lower extremity with ulcer of thigh HCC ESR COM A

I83.022 Varicose veins of left lower extremity with ulcer of calf HCC ESR COM A

I83.023 Varicose veins of left lower extremity with ulcer of ankle HCC ESR COM A

I83.024 Varicose veins of left lower extremity with ulcer of heel and midfoot HCC ESR COM A
Varicose veins of left lower extremity with ulcer of plantar surface of midfoot

I83.025 Varicose veins of left lower extremity with ulcer other part of foot HCC ESR COM A
Varicose veins of left lower extremity with ulcer of toe

I83.028 Varicose veins of left lower extremity with ulcer other part of lower leg HCC ESR COM A

I83.029 Varicose veins of left lower extremity with ulcer of unspecified site HCC ESR COM A

✓5th I83.1 Varicose veins of lower extremities with inflammation

I83.10 Varicose veins of unspecified lower extremity with inflammation A

I83.11 Varicose veins of right lower extremity with inflammation A

I83.12 Varicose veins of left lower extremity with inflammation A

✓5th I83.2 Varicose veins of lower extremities with both ulcer and inflammation
Use additional code to identify severity of ulcer (L97.-)

✓6th I83.20 Varicose veins of unspecified lower extremity with both ulcer and inflammation

I83.201 Varicose veins of unspecified lower extremity with both ulcer of thigh and inflammation HCC ESR COM A

I83.202 Varicose veins of unspecified lower extremity with both ulcer of calf and inflammation HCC ESR COM A

I83.203 Varicose veins of unspecified lower extremity with ulcer of ankle and inflammation HCC ESR COM A

I83.204 Varicose veins of unspecified lower extremity with both ulcer of heel and midfoot and inflammation HCC ESR COM A
Varicose veins of unspecified lower extremity with both ulcer of plantar surface of midfoot and inflammation

I83.205 Varicose veins of unspecified lower extremity with both ulcer other part of foot and inflammation HCC ESR COM A
Varicose veins of unspecified lower extremity with both ulcer of toe and inflammation

I83.208 Varicose veins of unspecified lower extremity with both ulcer of other part of lower extremity and inflammation HCC ESR COM A

I83.209 Varicose veins of unspecified lower extremity with both ulcer of unspecified site and inflammation HCC ESR COM A

✓6th I83.21 Varicose veins of right lower extremity with both ulcer and inflammation

I83.211 Varicose veins of right lower extremity with both ulcer of thigh and inflammation HCC ESR COM A

I83.212 Varicose veins of right lower extremity with both ulcer of calf and inflammation HCC ESR COM A

I83.213 Varicose veins of right lower extremity with both ulcer of ankle and inflammation HCC ESR COM A

I83.214 Varicose veins of right lower extremity with both ulcer of heel and midfoot and inflammation HCC ESR COM A
Varicose veins of right lower extremity with both ulcer of plantar surface of midfoot and inflammation

I83.215 Varicose veins of right lower extremity with both ulcer other part of foot and inflammation HCC ESR COM A
Varicose veins of right lower extremity with both ulcer of toe and inflammation

I83.218 Varicose veins of right lower extremity with both ulcer of other part of lower extremity and inflammation HCC ESR COM A

I83.219 Varicose veins of right lower extremity with both ulcer of unspecified site and inflammation HCC ESR COM A

✓6th I83.22 Varicose veins of left lower extremity with both ulcer and inflammation

I83.221 Varicose veins of left lower extremity with both ulcer of thigh and inflammation HCC ESR COM A

I83.222 Varicose veins of left lower extremity with both ulcer of calf and inflammation HCC ESR COM A

I83.223 Varicose veins of left lower extremity with both ulcer of ankle and inflammation HCC ESR COM A

I83.224 Varicose veins of left lower extremity with both ulcer of heel and midfoot and inflammation HCC ESR COM A
Varicose veins of left lower extremity with both ulcer of plantar surface of midfoot and inflammation

I83.225 **Varicose veins of left lower extremity with both ulcer other part of foot and inflammation** HCC ESR COM A
Varicose veins of left lower extremity with both ulcer of toe and inflammation

I83.228 **Varicose veins of left lower extremity with both ulcer of other part of lower extremity and inflammation** HCC ESR COM A

I83.229 **Varicose veins of left lower extremity with both ulcer of unspecified site and inflammation** HCC ESR COM A

√5th I83.8 **Varicose veins of lower extremities with other complications**

√6th I83.81 **Varicose veins of lower extremities with pain**

I83.811 **Varicose veins of right lower extremity with pain** A

I83.812 **Varicose veins of left lower extremity with pain** A

I83.813 **Varicose veins of bilateral lower extremities with pain** A

I83.819 **Varicose veins of unspecified lower extremity with pain** A

√6th I83.89 **Varicose veins of lower extremities with other complications**
Varicose veins of lower extremities with edema
Varicose veins of lower extremities with swelling

I83.891 **Varicose veins of right lower extremity with other complications** A

I83.892 **Varicose veins of left lower extremity with other complications** A

I83.893 **Varicose veins of bilateral lower extremities with other complications** A

I83.899 **Varicose veins of unspecified lower extremity with other complications** A

√5th I83.9 **Asymptomatic varicose veins of lower extremities**
Phlebectasia of lower extremities
Varicose veins of lower extremities
Varix of lower extremities

I83.90 **Asymptomatic varicose veins of unspecified lower extremity** A
Varicose veins NOS

I83.91 **Asymptomatic varicose veins of right lower extremity** A

I83.92 **Asymptomatic varicose veins of left lower extremity** A

I83.93 **Asymptomatic varicose veins of bilateral lower extremities** A

√4th **I85 Esophageal varices**
Use additional code to identify:
alcohol abuse and dependence (F1Ø.-)

√5th I85.Ø **Esophageal varices**
Idiopathic esophageal varices
Primary esophageal varices

I85.ØØ **Esophageal varices without bleeding** HCC ESR COM
Esophageal varices NOS

I85.Ø1 **Esophageal varices with bleeding** HCC ESR COM

√5th I85.1 **Secondary esophageal varices**
Esophageal varices secondary to alcoholic liver disease
Esophageal varices secondary to cirrhosis of liver
Esophageal varices secondary to schistosomiasis
Esophageal varices secondary to toxic liver disease
Code first underlying disease

I85.1Ø **Secondary esophageal varices without bleeding** HCC ESR COM

I85.11 **Secondary esophageal varices with bleeding** HCC ESR COM

√4th **I86 Varicose veins of other sites**
EXCLUDES 1 *varicose veins of unspecified site (I83.9-)*
EXCLUDES 2 *retinal varices (H35.Ø-)*

I86.Ø **Sublingual varices**
**DEF:** Distended, tortuous veins beneath the tongue.

I86.1 **Scrotal varices**
Varicocele

I86.2 **Pelvic varices**

I86.3 **Vulval varices**
EXCLUDES 1 *vulval varices complicating childbirth and the puerperium (O87.8)*
*vulval varices complicating pregnancy (O22.1-)*

I86.4 **Gastric varices**

I86.8 **Varicose veins of other specified sites** A
Varicose ulcer of nasal septum

√4th **I87 Other disorders of veins**

√5th I87.Ø **Postthrombotic syndrome**
Chronic venous hypertension due to deep vein thrombosis
Postphlebitic syndrome
EXCLUDES 1 *chronic venous hypertension without deep vein thrombosis (I87.3-)*

√6th I87.ØØ **Postthrombotic syndrome without complications**
Asymptomatic postthrombotic syndrome

I87.ØØ1 **Postthrombotic syndrome without complications of right lower extremity**

I87.ØØ2 **Postthrombotic syndrome without complications of left lower extremity**

I87.ØØ3 **Postthrombotic syndrome without complications of bilateral lower extremity**

I87.ØØ9 **Postthrombotic syndrome without complications of unspecified extremity**
Postthrombotic syndrome NOS

√6th I87.Ø1 **Postthrombotic syndrome with ulcer**
Use additional code to specify site and severity of ulcer (L97.-)

I87.Ø11 **Postthrombotic syndrome with ulcer of right lower extremity** HCC ESR COM

I87.Ø12 **Postthrombotic syndrome with ulcer of left lower extremity** HCC ESR COM

I87.Ø13 **Postthrombotic syndrome with ulcer of bilateral lower extremity** HCC ESR COM

I87.Ø19 **Postthrombotic syndrome with ulcer of unspecified lower extremity** HCC ESR COM

√6th I87.Ø2 **Postthrombotic syndrome with inflammation**

I87.Ø21 **Postthrombotic syndrome with inflammation of right lower extremity**

I87.Ø22 **Postthrombotic syndrome with inflammation of left lower extremity**

I87.Ø23 **Postthrombotic syndrome with inflammation of bilateral lower extremity**

I87.Ø29 **Postthrombotic syndrome with inflammation of unspecified lower extremity**

√6th I87.Ø3 **Postthrombotic syndrome with ulcer and inflammation**
Use additional code to specify site and severity of ulcer (L97.-)

I87.Ø31 **Postthrombotic syndrome with ulcer and inflammation of right lower extremity** HCC ESR COM

I87.Ø32 **Postthrombotic syndrome with ulcer and inflammation of left lower extremity** HCC ESR COM

I87.Ø33 **Postthrombotic syndrome with ulcer and inflammation of bilateral lower extremity** HCC ESR COM

I87.Ø39 **Postthrombotic syndrome with ulcer and inflammation of unspecified lower extremity** HCC ESR COM

√6th I87.Ø9 **Postthrombotic syndrome with other complications**

I87.Ø91 **Postthrombotic syndrome with other complications of right lower extremity**

I87.Ø92 **Postthrombotic syndrome with other complications of left lower extremity**

I87.Ø93 **Postthrombotic syndrome with other complications of bilateral lower extremity**

I87.Ø99 **Postthrombotic syndrome with other complications of unspecified lower extremity**

I87.1 **Compression of vein**
Stricture of vein
Vena cava syndrome (inferior) (superior)
EXCLUDES 2 *compression of pulmonary vein (I28.8)*
**AHA:** 2023,2Q,8

**I87.2 Venous insufficiency (chronic) (peripheral)**
Stasis dermatitis
Code also, if applicable, associated hypertensive conditions such as:
essential (primary) hypertension (I10)
hypertensive chronic kidney disease (I12.-)
hypertensive heart and chronic kidney disease (I13.-)
hypertensive heart disease (I11.-)
Use additional code, if applicable, to specify site and severity of ulcer (L97.-)
EXCLUDES 1 *stasis dermatitis with varicose veins of lower extremities (I83.1-, I83.2-)*
**AHA:** 2025,1Q,35; 2024,1Q,16
**DEF:** Insufficient drainage of venous blood in any part of the body that results in edema or dermatosis.

✓5th **I87.3 Chronic venous hypertension (idiopathic)**
Stasis edema
EXCLUDES 1 *chronic venous hypertension due to deep vein thrombosis (I87.0-)*
*varicose veins of lower extremities (I83.-)*

✓6th **I87.30 Chronic venous hypertension (idiopathic) without complications**
Asymptomatic chronic venous hypertension (idiopathic)
**I87.301 Chronic venous hypertension (idiopathic) without complications of right lower extremity**
**I87.302 Chronic venous hypertension (idiopathic) without complications of left lower extremity**
**I87.303 Chronic venous hypertension (idiopathic) without complications of bilateral lower extremity**
**I87.309 Chronic venous hypertension (idiopathic) without complications of unspecified lower extremity**
Chronic venous hypertension NOS

✓6th **I87.31 Chronic venous hypertension (idiopathic) with ulcer**
Use additional code to specify site and severity of ulcer (L97.-)
**I87.311 Chronic venous hypertension (idiopathic) with ulcer of right lower extremity** HCC ESR COM
**I87.312 Chronic venous hypertension (idiopathic) with ulcer of left lower extremity** HCC ESR COM
**I87.313 Chronic venous hypertension (idiopathic) with ulcer of bilateral lower extremity** HCC ESR COM
**I87.319 Chronic venous hypertension (idiopathic) with ulcer of unspecified lower extremity** HCC ESR COM

✓6th **I87.32 Chronic venous hypertension (idiopathic) with inflammation**
**I87.321 Chronic venous hypertension (idiopathic) with inflammation of right lower extremity**
**I87.322 Chronic venous hypertension (idiopathic) with inflammation of left lower extremity**
**I87.323 Chronic venous hypertension (idiopathic) with inflammation of bilateral lower extremity**
**I87.329 Chronic venous hypertension (idiopathic) with inflammation of unspecified lower extremity**

✓6th **I87.33 Chronic venous hypertension (idiopathic) with ulcer and inflammation**
Use additional code to specify site and severity of ulcer (L97.-)
**I87.331 Chronic venous hypertension (idiopathic) with ulcer and inflammation of right lower extremity** HCC ESR COM
**I87.332 Chronic venous hypertension (idiopathic) with ulcer and inflammation of left lower extremity** HCC ESR COM
**I87.333 Chronic venous hypertension (idiopathic) with ulcer and inflammation of bilateral lower extremity** HCC ESR COM
**I87.339 Chronic venous hypertension (idiopathic) with ulcer and inflammation of unspecified lower extremity** HCC ESR COM

✓6th **I87.39 Chronic venous hypertension (idiopathic) with other complications**
**I87.391 Chronic venous hypertension (idiopathic) with other complications of right lower extremity**
**I87.392 Chronic venous hypertension (idiopathic) with other complications of left lower extremity**
**I87.393 Chronic venous hypertension (idiopathic) with other complications of bilateral lower extremity**
**I87.399 Chronic venous hypertension (idiopathic) with other complications of unspecified lower extremity**

**I87.8 Other specified disorders of veins**
Phlebosclerosis
Venofibrosis

**I87.9 Disorder of vein, unspecified**

✓4th **I88 Nonspecific lymphadenitis**
EXCLUDES 1 *acute lymphadenitis, except mesenteric (L04.-)*
*enlarged lymph nodes NOS (R59.-)*
*human immunodeficiency virus [HIV] disease resulting in generalized lymphadenopathy (B20)*

**I88.0 Nonspecific mesenteric lymphadenitis**
Mesenteric lymphadenitis (acute)(chronic)

**I88.1 Chronic lymphadenitis, except mesenteric**
Adenitis
Lymphadenitis

**I88.8 Other nonspecific lymphadenitis**

**I88.9 Nonspecific lymphadenitis, unspecified**
Lymphadenitis NOS

✓4th **I89 Other noninfective disorders of lymphatic vessels and lymph nodes**
EXCLUDES 1 *chylocele, tunica vaginalis (nonfilarial) NOS (N50.89)*
*enlarged lymph nodes NOS (R59.-)*
*filarial chylocele (B74.-)*
*hereditary lymphedema (Q82.0)*

**I89.0 Lymphedema, not elsewhere classified**
Elephantiasis (nonfilarial) NOS
Lymphangiectasis
Obliteration, lymphatic vessel
Praecox lymphedema
Secondary lymphedema
EXCLUDES 1 *postmastectomy lymphedema (I97.2)*
**AHA:** 2024,1Q,16

**I89.1 Lymphangitis**
Chronic lymphangitis
Lymphangitis NOS
Subacute lymphangitis
EXCLUDES 1 *acute lymphangitis (L03.-)*

**I89.8 Other specified noninfective disorders of lymphatic vessels and lymph nodes**
Chylocele (nonfilarial)
Chylous ascites
Chylous cyst
Lipomelanotic reticulosis
Lymph node or vessel fistula
Lymph node or vessel infarction
Lymph node or vessel rupture

**I89.9 Noninfective disorder of lymphatic vessels and lymph nodes, unspecified**
Disease of lymphatic vessels NOS

## Other and unspecified disorders of the circulatory system (I95-I99)

✓4th **I95 Hypotension**
EXCLUDES 1 *cardiovascular collapse (R57.9)*
*maternal hypotension syndrome (O26.5-)*
*nonspecific low blood pressure reading NOS (R03.1)*

**I95.0 Idiopathic hypotension**

**I95.1 Orthostatic hypotension**
Hypotension, postural
EXCLUDES 1 *neurogenic orthostatic hypotension [Shy-Drager] (G90.3)*
*orthostatic hypotension due to drugs (I95.2)*
**AHA:** 2023,2Q,8

**I95.2 Hypotension due to drugs**
Orthostatic hypotension due to drugs
Use additional code for adverse effect, if applicable, to identify drug (T36-T50 with fifth or sixth character 5)

I95.3 **Hypotension of hemodialysis**
Intra-dialytic hypotension

✓5th I95.8 **Other hypotension**

I95.81 **Postprocedural hypotension**

I95.89 **Other hypotension**
Chronic hypotension

I95.9 **Hypotension, unspecified**

I96 **Gangrene, not elsewhere classified** HCC ESR COM
Gangrenous cellulitis
EXCLUDES 1 *gangrene in atherosclerosis of native arteries of the extremities (I70.26)*
*gangrene of certain specified sites - see Alphabetical Index*
*gangrene in hernia (K40.1, K40.4, K41.1, K41.4, K42.1, K43.1-, K44.1, K45.1, K46.1)*
*gangrene in other peripheral vascular diseases (I73.-)*
*gas gangrene (A48.0)*
*pyoderma gangrenosum (L88)*
EXCLUDES 2 *gangrene in diabetes mellitus (E08-E13 with .52)*
**AHA:** 2022,3Q,13; 2018,4Q,87; 2018,3Q,3; 2017,3Q,6; 2013,2Q,34

✓4th I97 **Intraoperative and postprocedural complications and disorders of circulatory system, not elsewhere classified**
EXCLUDES 2 *postprocedural shock (T81.1-)*
**AHA:** 2021,1Q,13; 2019,2Q,21

I97.0 **Postcardiotomy syndrome**

✓5th I97.1 **Other postprocedural cardiac functional disturbances**
EXCLUDES 2 *acute pulmonary insufficiency following thoracic surgery (J95.1)*
*intraoperative cardiac functional disturbances (I97.7-)*

✓6th I97.11 **Postprocedural cardiac insufficiency**

I97.110 **Postprocedural cardiac insufficiency following cardiac surgery**

I97.111 **Postprocedural cardiac insufficiency following other surgery**

✓6th I97.12 **Postprocedural cardiac arrest**

I97.120 **Postprocedural cardiac arrest following cardiac surgery**

I97.121 **Postprocedural cardiac arrest following other surgery**

✓6th I97.13 **Postprocedural heart failure**
Use additional code to identify the heart failure (I50.-)

I97.130 **Postprocedural heart failure following cardiac surgery**

I97.131 **Postprocedural heart failure following other surgery**

✓6th I97.19 **Other postprocedural cardiac functional disturbances**
Use additional code, if applicable, to further specify disorder

I97.190 **Other postprocedural cardiac functional disturbances following cardiac surgery**
Use additional code, if applicable, for type 4 or type 5 myocardial infarction, to further specify disorder
**AHA:** 2019,2Q,33

I97.191 **Other postprocedural cardiac functional disturbances following other surgery**

I97.2 **Postmastectomy lymphedema syndrome** A
Elephantiasis due to mastectomy
Obliteration of lymphatic vessels

I97.3 **Postprocedural hypertension**

✓5th I97.4 **Intraoperative hemorrhage and hematoma of a circulatory system organ or structure complicating a procedure**
EXCLUDES 1 *intraoperative hemorrhage and hematoma of a circulatory system organ or structure due to accidental puncture and laceration during a procedure (I97.5-)*
EXCLUDES 2 *intraoperative cerebrovascular hemorrhage complicating a procedure (G97.3-)*

✓6th I97.41 **Intraoperative hemorrhage and hematoma of a circulatory system organ or structure complicating a circulatory system procedure**

I97.410 **Intraoperative hemorrhage and hematoma of a circulatory system organ or structure complicating a cardiac catheterization**

I97.411 **Intraoperative hemorrhage and hematoma of a circulatory system organ or structure complicating a cardiac bypass**

I97.418 **Intraoperative hemorrhage and hematoma of a circulatory system organ or structure complicating other circulatory system procedure**

I97.42 **Intraoperative hemorrhage and hematoma of a circulatory system organ or structure complicating other procedure**
**AHA:** 2020,1Q,19

✓5th I97.5 **Accidental puncture and laceration of a circulatory system organ or structure during a procedure**
EXCLUDES 2 *accidental puncture and laceration of brain during a procedure (G97.4-)*

I97.51 **Accidental puncture and laceration of a circulatory system organ or structure during a circulatory system procedure**
**AHA:** 2019,2Q,24

I97.52 **Accidental puncture and laceration of a circulatory system organ or structure during other procedure**

✓5th I97.6 **Postprocedural hemorrhage, hematoma and seroma of a circulatory system organ or structure following a procedure**
EXCLUDES 2 *postprocedural cerebrovascular hemorrhage complicating a procedure (G97.5-)*
**AHA:** 2016,4Q,9-10

✓6th I97.61 **Postprocedural hemorrhage of a circulatory system organ or structure following a circulatory system procedure**

I97.610 **Postprocedural hemorrhage of a circulatory system organ or structure following a cardiac catheterization**

I97.611 **Postprocedural hemorrhage of a circulatory system organ or structure following cardiac bypass**

I97.618 **Postprocedural hemorrhage of a circulatory system organ or structure following other circulatory system procedure**

✓6th I97.62 **Postprocedural hemorrhage, hematoma and seroma of a circulatory system organ or structure following other procedure**

I97.620 **Postprocedural hemorrhage of a circulatory system organ or structure following other procedure**

I97.621 **Postprocedural hematoma of a circulatory system organ or structure following other procedure**

I97.622 **Postprocedural seroma of a circulatory system organ or structure following other procedure**

✓6th I97.63 **Postprocedural hematoma of a circulatory system organ or structure following a circulatory system procedure**

I97.630 **Postprocedural hematoma of a circulatory system organ or structure following a cardiac catheterization**

I97.631 **Postprocedural hematoma of a circulatory system organ or structure following cardiac bypass**

I97.638 **Postprocedural hematoma of a circulatory system organ or structure following other circulatory system procedure**

✓6th I97.64 **Postprocedural seroma of a circulatory system organ or structure following a circulatory system procedure**

I97.640 **Postprocedural seroma of a circulatory system organ or structure following a cardiac catheterization**

I97.641 **Postprocedural seroma of a circulatory system organ or structure following cardiac bypass**

I97.648 **Postprocedural seroma of a circulatory system organ or structure following other circulatory system procedure**

✓5th I97.7 **Intraoperative cardiac functional disturbances**
EXCLUDES 2 *acute pulmonary insufficiency following thoracic surgery (J95.1)*
*postprocedural cardiac functional disturbances (I97.1-)*

✓6th I97.71 **Intraoperative cardiac arrest**

I97.710 **Intraoperative cardiac arrest during cardiac surgery**

I97.711 **Intraoperative cardiac arrest during other surgery**

6th **I97.79 Other intraoperative cardiac functional disturbances**
Use additional code, if applicable, to further specify disorder

**I97.790 Other intraoperative cardiac functional disturbances during cardiac surgery**

**I97.791 Other intraoperative cardiac functional disturbances during other surgery**

5th **I97.8 Other intraoperative and postprocedural complications and disorders of the circulatory system, not elsewhere classified**
Use additional code, if applicable, to further specify disorder

6th **I97.81 Intraoperative cerebrovascular infarction**

**I97.810 Intraoperative cerebrovascular infarction during cardiac surgery** ESR

**I97.811 Intraoperative cerebrovascular infarction during other surgery** ESR

6th **I97.82 Postprocedural cerebrovascular infarction**

**I97.820 Postprocedural cerebrovascular infarction following cardiac surgery** ESR

**I97.821 Postprocedural cerebrovascular infarction following other surgery** ESR

**I97.88 Other intraoperative complications of the circulatory system, not elsewhere classified**

**I97.89 Other postprocedural complications and disorders of the circulatory system, not elsewhere classified**
**AHA:** 2025,2Q,5; 2024,1Q,26; 2021,3Q,33; 2020,3Q,3-8; 2019,2Q,33

4th **I99 Other and unspecified disorders of circulatory system**

**I99.8 Other disorder of circulatory system**
**AHA:** 2020,4Q,98

**I99.9 Unspecified disorder of circulatory system**

# Chapter 10. Diseases of the Respiratory System (JØØ–J99), UØ7.Ø

## Chapter-specific Guidelines with Coding Examples

The chapter-specific guidelines from the ICD-10-CM Official Guidelines for Coding and Reporting have been provided below. Along with these guidelines are coding examples, contained in the shICD-1Ø-CM 2Ø27aded boxes, that have been developed to help illustrate the coding and/or sequencing guidance found in these guidelines.

### a. Chronic obstructive pulmonary disease [COPD] and asthma

#### 1) Acute exacerbation of chronic obstructive bronchitis and asthma

The codes in categories J44 and J45 distinguish between uncomplicated cases and those in acute exacerbation. An acute exacerbation is a worsening or a decompensation of a chronic condition. An acute exacerbation is not equivalent to an infection superimposed on a chronic condition, though an exacerbation may be triggered by an infection.

Acute streptococcal bronchitis with acute exacerbation of COPD

**J2Ø.2** **Acute bronchitis due to streptococcus**

**J44.Ø** **Chronic obstructive pulmonary disease with (acute) lower respiratory infection**

**J44.1** **Chronic obstructive pulmonary disease with (acute) exacerbation**

*Explanation*: ICD-10-CM uses combination codes to create organism-specific classifications for acute bronchitis. Category J44 codes include combination codes with severity components, which differentiate between COPD with acute lower respiratory infection (acute bronchitis), COPD with acute exacerbation, and COPD without mention of a complication (unspecified).

An acute exacerbation is a worsening or a decompensation of a chronic condition. An acute exacerbation is not equivalent to an infection superimposed on a chronic condition, though an exacerbation may be triggered by an infection, as in this example.

Exacerbation of moderate persistent asthma with status asthmaticus

**J45.42** **Moderate persistent asthma with status asthmaticus**

*Explanation*: Category J45 Asthma includes severity-specific subcategories and fifth-character codes to distinguish between uncomplicated cases, those in acute exacerbation, and those with status asthmaticus.

### b. Acute respiratory failure

#### 1) Acute respiratory failure as principal diagnosis

A code from subcategory J96.Ø, Acute respiratory failure, or subcategory J96.2, Acute and chronic respiratory failure, may be assigned as a principal diagnosis when it is the condition established after study to be chiefly responsible for occasioning the admission to the hospital, and the selection is supported by the Alphabetic Index and Tabular List. However, chapter-specific coding guidelines (such as obstetrics, poisoning, HIV, newborn) that provide sequencing direction take precedence.

Acute hypoxic respiratory failure due to exacerbation of chronic obstructive bronchitis

**J96.Ø1** **Acute respiratory failure with hypoxia**

**J44.1** **Chronic obstructive pulmonary disease with (acute) exacerbation**

*Explanation*: Category J96 classifies respiratory failure with combination codes that designate the severity and the presence of hypoxia and hypercapnia. Code J96.Ø1 is sequenced as the first-listed diagnosis, as the reason for the encounter. Respiratory failure may be assigned as a principal diagnosis when it is the condition established after study to be chiefly responsible for occasioning the encounter and the selection is supported by the Alphabetic Index and Tabular List.

#### 2) Acute respiratory failure as secondary diagnosis

Respiratory failure may be listed as a secondary diagnosis if it occurs after admission, or if it is present on admission, but does not meet the definition of principal diagnosis.

Acute respiratory failure due to accidental oxycodone overdose

**T4Ø.2X1A** **Poisoning by other opioids, accidental (unintentional), initial encounter**

**J96.ØØ** **Acute respiratory failure, unspecified whether with hypoxia or hypercapnia**

*Explanation*: Respiratory failure may be assigned as a principal diagnosis when it is the condition established after study to be chiefly responsible for occasioning the encounter, and the selection is supported by the Alphabetic Index and Tabular List. However, chapter-specific coding guidelines, such as poisoning, that provide sequencing direction take precedence. When coding a poisoning or reaction to the improper use of a medication (e.g., overdose, wrong substance given or taken in error, wrong route of administration), first assign the appropriate code from categories T36–T5Ø. Use additional code(s) for all manifestations of the poisoning. In this instance, the respiratory failure is a manifestation of the poisoning and is sequenced as a secondary diagnosis.

#### 3) Sequencing of acute respiratory failure and another acute condition

When a patient is admitted with respiratory failure and another acute condition, (e.g., myocardial infarction, cerebrovascular accident, aspiration pneumonia), the principal diagnosis will not be the same in every situation. This applies whether the other acute condition is a respiratory or nonrespiratory condition. Selection of the principal diagnosis will be dependent on the circumstances of admission. If both the respiratory failure and the other acute condition are equally responsible for occasioning the admission to the hospital, and there are no chapter-specific sequencing rules, the guideline regarding two or more diagnoses that equally meet the definition for principal diagnosis (*Section II, C.*) may be applied in these situations.

If the documentation is not clear as to whether acute respiratory failure and another condition are equally responsible for occasioning the admission, query the provider for clarification.

Patient presents with acute pneumococcal pneumonia and acute respiratory failure

**J96.ØØ** **Acute respiratory failure, unspecified whether with hypoxia or hypercapnia**

**J13** **Pneumonia due to Streptococcus pneumoniae**

*Explanation*: When a patient is seen for respiratory failure and another acute condition, such as a bacterial pneumonia, the principal or first-listed diagnosis is not the same in every situation. This applies whether the other acute condition is a respiratory or nonrespiratory condition. The principal diagnosis depends on the problem chiefly responsible for the encounter.

### c. Influenza due to certain identified influenza viruses

Code only confirmed cases of influenza due to certain identified influenza viruses (category JØ9), and due to other identified influenza virus (category J1Ø). This is an exception to the hospital inpatient guideline Section II, H. (Uncertain Diagnosis).

In this context, "confirmation" does not require documentation of positive laboratory testing specific for avian or other novel influenza A or other identified influenza virus. However, coding should be based on the provider's diagnostic statement that the patient has avian influenza, or other novel influenza A, for category JØ9, or has another particular identified strain of influenza, such as H1N1 or H3N2, but not identified as novel or variant, for category J1Ø.

If the provider records "suspected" or "possible" or "probable" avian influenza, or novel influenza, or other identified influenza, then the appropriate influenza code from category J11, Influenza due to unidentified influenza virus, should be assigned. A code from category JØ9, Influenza due to certain identified influenza viruses, should not be assigned nor should a code from category J1Ø, Influenza due to other identified influenza virus.

Influenza due to avian influenza virus with pneumonia

**JØ9.X1 Influenza due to identified novel influenza A virus with pneumonia**

*Explanation*: Codes in category JØ9 Influenza due to certain identified influenza viruses should be assigned only for confirmed cases. "Confirmation" does not require positive laboratory testing of a specific influenza virus but does need to be based on the provider's diagnostic statement, which should not include terms such as "possible," "probable," or "suspected."

**d. Ventilator associated pneumonia**

**1) Documentation of ventilator associated pneumonia**

As with all procedural or postprocedural complications, code assignment is based on the provider's documentation of the relationship between the condition and the procedure.

Code J95.851, Ventilator associated pneumonia, should be assigned only when the provider has documented ventilator associated pneumonia (VAP). An additional code to identify the organism (e.g., Pseudomonas aeruginosa, code B96.5) should also be assigned. Do not assign an additional code from categories J12-J18 to identify the type of pneumonia.

Code J95.851 should not be assigned for cases where the patient has pneumonia and is on a mechanical ventilator and the provider has not specifically stated that the pneumonia is ventilator-associated pneumonia. If the documentation is unclear as to whether the patient has a pneumonia that is a complication attributable to the mechanical ventilator, query the provider.

**2) Ventilator associated pneumonia develops after admission**

A patient may be admitted with one type of pneumonia (e.g., code J13, Pneumonia due to Streptococcus pneumonia) and subsequently develop VAP. In this instance, the principal diagnosis would be the appropriate code from categories J12-J18 for the pneumonia diagnosed at the time of admission. Code J95.851, Ventilator associated pneumonia, would be assigned as an additional diagnosis when the provider has also documented the presence of ventilator associated pneumonia.

**e. Vaping-related disorders**

For patients presenting with condition(s) related to vaping, assign code UØ7.Ø, Vaping-related disorder, as the principal diagnosis. For lung injury due to vaping, assign only code UØ7.Ø. Assign additional codes for other manifestations, such as acute respiratory failure (subcategory J96.Ø-) or pneumonitis (code J68.Ø).

Associated respiratory signs and symptoms due to vaping, such as cough, shortness of breath, etc., are not coded separately, when a definitive diagnosis has been established. However, it would be appropriate to code separately any gastrointestinal symptoms, such as diarrhea and abdominal pain.

*See Section I.C.1.g.1.c.i. for Pneumonia confirmed as due to COVID-19*

# Chapter 10. Diseases of the Respiratory System (J00-J99)

NOTE When a respiratory condition is described as occurring in more than one site and is not specifically indexed, it should be classified to the lower anatomic site (e.g., tracheobronchitis to bronchitis in J40).

Use additional code, where applicable, to identify:
exposure to environmental tobacco smoke (Z77.22)
exposure to tobacco smoke in the perinatal period (P96.81)
history of tobacco dependence (Z87.891)
occupational exposure to environmental tobacco smoke (Z57.31)
tobacco dependence (F17.-)
tobacco use (Z72.0)

EXCLUDES 2 *certain conditions originating in the perinatal period (P04-P96)*
*certain infectious and parasitic diseases (A00-B99)*
*complications of pregnancy, childbirth and the puerperium (O00-O9A)*
*congenital malformations, deformations and chromosomal abnormalities (Q00-Q99)*
*endocrine, nutritional and metabolic diseases (E00-E88)*
*injury, poisoning and certain other consequences of external causes (S00-T88)*
*neoplasms (C00-D49)*
*smoke inhalation (T59.81-)*
*symptoms, signs and abnormal clinical and laboratory findings, not elsewhere classified (R00-R94)*

This chapter contains the following blocks:

| | |
|---|---|
| J00-J06 | Acute upper respiratory infections |
| J09-J18 | Influenza and pneumonia |
| J20-J22 | Other acute lower respiratory infections |
| J30-J39 | Other diseases of upper respiratory tract |
| J40-J4B | Chronic lower respiratory diseases |
| J60-J70 | Lung diseases due to external agents |
| J80-J84 | Other respiratory diseases principally affecting the interstitium |
| J85-J86 | Suppurative and necrotic conditions of the lower respiratory tract |
| J90-J94 | Other diseases of the pleura |
| J95 | Intraoperative and postprocedural complications and disorders of respiratory system, not elsewhere classified |
| J96-J99 | Other diseases of the respiratory system |

## Acute upper respiratory infections (J00-J06)

EXCLUDES 1 *chronic obstructive pulmonary disease with acute lower respiratory infection (J44.0)*

**J00 Acute nasopharyngitis [common cold]**
Acute rhinitis
Coryza (acute)
Infective nasopharyngitis NOS
Infective rhinitis
Nasal catarrh, acute
Nasopharyngitis NOS
EXCLUDES 1 *acute pharyngitis (J02.-)*
*acute sore throat NOS (J02.9)*
*influenza virus with other respiratory manifestations (J09.X2, J10.1, J11.1)*
*pharyngitis NOS (J02.9)*
*rhinitis NOS (J31.0)*
*sore throat NOS (J02.9)*
EXCLUDES 2 *allergic rhinitis (J30.1-J30.9)*
*chronic pharyngitis (J31.2)*
*chronic rhinitis (J31.0)*
*chronic sore throat (J31.2)*
*nasopharyngitis, chronic (J31.1)*
*vasomotor rhinitis (J30.0)*

✓4th **J01 Acute sinusitis**
INCLUDES acute abscess of sinus
acute empyema of sinus
acute infection of sinus
acute inflammation of sinus
acute suppuration of sinus
Use additional code (B95-B97) to identify infectious agent
EXCLUDES 1 *sinusitis NOS (J32.9)*
EXCLUDES 2 *chronic sinusitis (J32.0-J32.8)*

✓5th **J01.0 Acute maxillary sinusitis**
Acute antritis
**J01.00 Acute maxillary sinusitis, unspecified**
**J01.01 Acute recurrent maxillary sinusitis**

✓5th **J01.1 Acute frontal sinusitis**
**J01.10 Acute frontal sinusitis, unspecified**
**J01.11 Acute recurrent frontal sinusitis**

✓5th **J01.2 Acute ethmoidal sinusitis**
**J01.20 Acute ethmoidal sinusitis, unspecified**
**J01.21 Acute recurrent ethmoidal sinusitis**

✓5th **J01.3 Acute sphenoidal sinusitis**
**J01.30 Acute sphenoidal sinusitis, unspecified**
**J01.31 Acute recurrent sphenoidal sinusitis**

✓5th **J01.4 Acute pansinusitis**
**J01.40 Acute pansinusitis, unspecified**
**J01.41 Acute recurrent pansinusitis**

✓5th **J01.8 Other acute sinusitis**
**J01.80 Other acute sinusitis**
Acute sinusitis involving more than one sinus but not pansinusitis
**J01.81 Other acute recurrent sinusitis**
Acute recurrent sinusitis involving more than one sinus but not pansinusitis

✓5th **J01.9 Acute sinusitis, unspecified**
**J01.90 Acute sinusitis, unspecified**
**J01.91 Acute recurrent sinusitis, unspecified**

✓4th **J02 Acute pharyngitis**
INCLUDES acute sore throat
EXCLUDES 1 *acute laryngopharyngitis (J06.0)*
*peritonsillar abscess (J36)*
*pharyngeal abscess (J39.1)*
*retropharyngeal abscess (J39.0)*
EXCLUDES 2 *chronic pharyngitis (J31.2)*

**J02.0 Streptococcal pharyngitis**
Septic pharyngitis
Streptococcal sore throat
EXCLUDES 2 *scarlet fever (A38.-)*

**J02.8 Acute pharyngitis due to other specified organisms**
Use additional code (B95-B97) to identify infectious agent
EXCLUDES 1 *acute pharyngitis due to coxsackie virus (B08.5)*
*acute pharyngitis due to gonococcus (A54.5)*
*acute pharyngitis due to herpes [simplex] virus (B00.2)*
*acute pharyngitis due to infectious mononucleosis (B27.-)*
*enteroviral vesicular pharyngitis (B08.5)*

**J02.9 Acute pharyngitis, unspecified**
Gangrenous pharyngitis (acute)
Infective pharyngitis (acute) NOS
Pharyngitis (acute) NOS
Sore throat (acute) NOS
Suppurative pharyngitis (acute)
Ulcerative pharyngitis (acute)
EXCLUDES 1 *influenza virus with other respiratory manifestations (J09.X2, J10.1, J11.1)*

✓4th **J03 Acute tonsillitis**
EXCLUDES 1 *acute sore throat (J02.-)*
*hypertrophy of tonsils (J35.1)*
*peritonsillar abscess (J36)*
*sore throat NOS (J02.9)*
*streptococcal sore throat (J02.0)*
EXCLUDES 2 *chronic tonsillitis (J35.0)*

✓5th **J03.0 Streptococcal tonsillitis**
**J03.00 Acute streptococcal tonsillitis, unspecified**
**J03.01 Acute recurrent streptococcal tonsillitis**

✓5th **J03.8 Acute tonsillitis due to other specified organisms**
Use additional code (B95-B97) to identify infectious agent
EXCLUDES 1 *diphtheritic tonsillitis (A36.0)*
*herpesviral pharyngotonsillitis (B00.2)*
*streptococcal tonsillitis (J03.0)*
*tuberculous tonsillitis (A15.8)*
*Vincent's tonsillitis (A69.1)*
**J03.80 Acute tonsillitis due to other specified organisms**
**J03.81 Acute recurrent tonsillitis due to other specified organisms**

✓5th **J03.9 Acute tonsillitis, unspecified**
Follicular tonsillitis (acute)
Gangrenous tonsillitis (acute)
Infective tonsillitis (acute)
Tonsillitis (acute) NOS
Ulcerative tonsillitis (acute)
EXCLUDES 1 *influenza virus with other respiratory manifestations (J09.X2, J10.1, J11.1)*
**J03.90 Acute tonsillitis, unspecified**
**J03.91 Acute recurrent tonsillitis, unspecified**

√4th **J04 Acute laryngitis and tracheitis**

Code also influenza, if present, such as:
influenza due to identified novel influenza A virus with other respiratory manifestations (J09.X2)
influenza due to other identified influenza virus with other respiratory manifestations (J10.1)
influenza due to unidentified influenza virus with other respiratory manifestations (J11.1)
Use additional code (B95-B97) to identify infectious agent

EXCLUDES 1 *acute obstructive laryngitis [croup] and epiglottitis (J05.-)*
EXCLUDES 2 *laryngismus (stridulus) (J38.5)*

**J04.0 Acute laryngitis**
Edematous laryngitis (acute)
Laryngitis (acute) NOS
Subglottic laryngitis (acute)
Suppurative laryngitis (acute)
Ulcerative laryngitis (acute)
EXCLUDES 1 *acute obstructive laryngitis (J05.0)*
EXCLUDES 2 *chronic laryngitis (J37.0)*

√5th **J04.1 Acute tracheitis**
Acute viral tracheitis
Catarrhal tracheitis (acute)
Tracheitis (acute) NOS
EXCLUDES 2 *chronic tracheitis (J42)*

**J04.10 Acute tracheitis without obstruction**
**J04.11 Acute tracheitis with obstruction**

**J04.2 Acute laryngotracheitis**
Laryngotracheitis NOS
Tracheitis (acute) with laryngitis (acute)
EXCLUDES 1 *acute obstructive laryngotracheitis (J05.0)*
EXCLUDES 2 *chronic laryngotracheitis (J37.1)*

√5th **J04.3 Supraglottitis, unspecified**
**J04.30 Supraglottitis, unspecified, without obstruction**
**J04.31 Supraglottitis, unspecified, with obstruction**

√4th **J05 Acute obstructive laryngitis [croup] and epiglottitis**

Code also, influenza, if present, such as:
influenza due to identified novel influenza A virus with other respiratory manifestations (J09.X2)
influenza due to other identified influenza virus with other respiratory manifestations (J10.1)
influenza due to unidentified influenza virus with other respiratory manifestations (J11.1)
Use additional code (B95-B97) to identify infectious agent

**J05.0 Acute obstructive laryngitis [croup]**
Obstructive laryngitis (acute) NOS
Obstructive laryngotracheitis NOS
**DEF:** Acute laryngeal obstruction due to allergies, foreign bodies, or in the majority of cases a viral infection. Symptoms include a harsh, barking cough, hoarseness, and a persistent, high-pitched respiratory sound (stridor).

√5th **J05.1 Acute epiglottitis**
EXCLUDES 2 *epiglottitis, chronic (J37.0)*

**J05.10 Acute epiglottitis without obstruction**
Epiglottitis NOS
**J05.11 Acute epiglottitis with obstruction**

√4th **J06 Acute upper respiratory infections of multiple and unspecified sites**

EXCLUDES 1 *acute respiratory infection NOS (J22)*
*influenza virus with other respiratory manifestations (J09.X2, J10.1, J11.1)*
*streptococcal pharyngitis (J02.0)*

**J06.0 Acute laryngopharyngitis**

**J06.9 Acute upper respiratory infection, unspecified**
Upper respiratory disease, acute
Upper respiratory infection NOS
Use additional code (B95-B97) to identify infectious agent, if known, such as:
respiratory syncytial virus (RSV) (B97.4)
**AHA:** 2020,1Q,22

## Influenza and pneumonia (J09-J18)

Use additional code, if applicable, to identify resistance to antimicrobial drugs (Z16.-)

EXCLUDES 2 *allergic or eosinophilic pneumonia (J82)*
*aspiration pneumonia NOS (J69.0)*
*meconium pneumonia (P24.01)*
*neonatal aspiration pneumonia (P24.-)*
*pneumonia due to solids and liquids (J69.-)*
*congenital pneumonia (P23.9)*
*lipid pneumonia (J69.1)*
*rheumatic pneumonia (I00)*
*ventilator associated pneumonia (J95.851)*

**AHA:** 2017,4Q,96

√4th **J09 Influenza due to certain identified influenza viruses**

EXCLUDES 1 *influenza A/H1N1 (J10.-)*
*influenza due to other identified influenza virus (J10.-)*
*influenza due to unidentified influenza virus (J11.-)*
*seasonal influenza due to other identified influenza virus (J10.-)*
*seasonal influenza due to unidentified influenza virus (J11.-)*

√5th **J09.X Influenza due to identified novel influenza A virus**
Avian influenza
Bird influenza
Influenza A/H5N1
Influenza of other animal origin, not bird or swine
Swine influenza virus (viruses that normally cause infections in pigs)
**AHA:** 2016,3Q,10

**J09.X1 Influenza due to identified novel influenza A virus with pneumonia**
Code also, if applicable, associated:
lung abscess (J85.1)
other specified type of pneumonia

**J09.X2 Influenza due to identified novel influenza A virus with other respiratory manifestations**
Influenza due to identified novel influenza A virus NOS
Influenza due to identified novel influenza A virus with laryngitis
Influenza due to identified novel influenza A virus with pharyngitis
Influenza due to identified novel influenza A virus with upper respiratory symptoms
Use additional code, if applicable, for associated:
pleural effusion (J91.8)
sinusitis (J01.-)

**J09.X3 Influenza due to identified novel influenza A virus with gastrointestinal manifestations**
Influenza due to identified novel influenza A virus gastroenteritis
EXCLUDES 1 *'intestinal flu' [viral gastroenteritis] (A08.-)*

**J09.X9 Influenza due to identified novel influenza A virus with other manifestations**
Influenza due to identified novel influenza A virus with encephalopathy
Influenza due to identified novel influenza A virus with myocarditis
Influenza due to identified novel influenza A virus with otitis media
Use additional code to identify manifestation

√4th **J10 Influenza due to other identified influenza virus**

INCLUDES influenza A (non-novel)
influenza B
influenza C

EXCLUDES 1 *influenza due to avian influenza virus (J09.X-)*
*influenza due to swine flu (J09.X-)*
*influenza due to unidentifed influenza virus (J11.-)*

√5th **J10.0 Influenza due to other identified influenza virus with pneumonia**
Code also associated lung abscess, if applicable (J85.1)

**J10.00 Influenza due to other identified influenza virus with unspecified type of pneumonia**
**J10.01 Influenza due to other identified influenza virus with the same other identified influenza virus pneumonia**
**J10.08 Influenza due to other identified influenza virus with other specified pneumonia**
Code also other specified type of pneumonia

**J10.1 Influenza due to other identified influenza virus with other respiratory manifestations**
Influenza due to other identified influenza virus NOS
Influenza due to other identified influenza virus with laryngitis
Influenza due to other identified influenza virus with pharyngitis
Influenza due to other identified influenza virus with upper respiratory symptoms
Use additional code for associated pleural effusion, if applicable (J91.8)
Use additional code for associated sinusitis, if applicable (J01.-)
**AHA:** 2016,3Q,10-11

**J10.2 Influenza due to other identified influenza virus with gastrointestinal manifestations**
Influenza due to other identified influenza virus gastroenteritis
EXCLUDES 1 *"intestinal flu" [viral gastroenteritis] (A08.-)*

✓5th **J10.8 Influenza due to other identified influenza virus with other manifestations**

**J10.81 Influenza due to other identified influenza virus with encephalopathy**

**J10.82 Influenza due to other identified influenza virus with myocarditis**

**J10.83 Influenza due to other identified influenza virus with otitis media**
Use additional code for any associated perforated tympanic membrane (H72.-)

**J10.89 Influenza due to other identified influenza virus with other manifestations**
Use additional codes to identify the manifestations

✓4th **J11 Influenza due to unidentified influenza virus**

✓5th **J11.0 Influenza due to unidentified influenza virus with pneumonia**
Code also associated lung abscess, if applicable (J85.1)
**AHA:** 2016,3Q,11

**J11.00 Influenza due to unidentified influenza virus with unspecified type of pneumonia**
Influenza with pneumonia NOS

**J11.08 Influenza due to unidentified influenza virus with specified pneumonia**
Code also other specified type of pneumonia

**J11.1 Influenza due to unidentified influenza virus with other respiratory manifestations**
Influenza NOS
Influenza with upper respiratory symptoms NOS
Influenzal laryngitis NOS
Influenzal pharyngitis NOS
Use additional code for associated pleural effusion, if applicable (J91.8)
Use additional code for associated sinusitis, if applicable (J01.-)

**J11.2 Influenza due to unidentified influenza virus with gastrointestinal manifestations**
Influenza gastroenteritis NOS
EXCLUDES 1 *"intestinal flu" [viral gastroenteritis] (A08.-)*

✓5th **J11.8 Influenza due to unidentified influenza virus with other manifestations**

**J11.81 Influenza due to unidentified influenza virus with encephalopathy**
Influenzal encephalopathy NOS

**J11.82 Influenza due to unidentified influenza virus with myocarditis**
Influenzal myocarditis NOS

**J11.83 Influenza due to unidentified influenza virus with otitis media**
Influenzal otitis media NOS
Use additional code for any associated perforated tympanic membrane (H72.-)

**J11.89 Influenza due to unidentified influenza virus with other manifestations**
Use additional codes to identify the manifestations

✓4th **J12 Viral pneumonia, not elsewhere classified**
INCLUDES bronchopneumonia due to viruses other than influenza viruses
Code first associated influenza, if applicable (J09.X1, J10.0-, J11.0-)
Code also associated abscess, if applicable (J85.1)
EXCLUDES 2 *aspiration pneumonia due to anesthesia during labor and delivery (O74.0)*
*aspiration pneumonia due to anesthesia during pregnancy (O29)*
*aspiration pneumonia due to anesthesia during puerperium (O89.0)*
*aspiration pneumonia due to solids and liquids (J69.-)*
*aspiration pneumonia NOS (J69.0)*
*congenital pneumonia (P23.0)*
*congenital rubella pneumonitis (P35.0)*
*interstitial pneumonia NOS (J84.9)*
*lipid pneumonia (J69.1)*
*neonatal aspiration pneumonia (P24.-)*
**AHA:** 2020,2Q,28; 2019,1Q,35; 2018,3Q,24; 2016,3Q,15; 2013,4Q,118

**J12.0 Adenoviral pneumonia**

**J12.1 Respiratory syncytial virus pneumonia**
RSV pneumonia

**J12.2 Parainfluenza virus pneumonia**

**J12.3 Human metapneumovirus pneumonia**

✓5th **J12.8 Other viral pneumonia**

**J12.81 Pneumonia due to SARS-associated coronavirus**
Severe acute respiratory syndrome NOS
**DEF:** Inflammation of the lungs with consolidation, caused by the severe adult respiratory syndrome (SARS)-associated coronavirus or SARS-CoV. This pneumonia should not be confused with that caused by SARS-CoV-2 (COVID-19).

**J12.82 Pneumonia due to coronavirus disease 2019** UPD
Pneumonia due to 2019 novel coronavirus (SARS-CoV-2)
Pneumonia due to COVID-19
Code first COVID-19 (U07.1)
**AHA:** 2021,1Q,25-30,31-49

**J12.89 Other viral pneumonia**
**AHA:** 2021,1Q,33-34; 2020,2Q,8,11; 2020,1Q,34-36

**J12.9 Viral pneumonia, unspecified**

**J13 Pneumonia due to Streptococcus pneumoniae** ESR
Bronchopneumonia due to S. pneumoniae
Code first, if applicable, associated influenza (J09.X1, J10.0-, J11.0-)
Code also, if applicable, any associated condition such as:
abscess (J85.1)
aspiration pneumonia (J69.-)
EXCLUDES 1 *congenital pneumonia due to S. pneumoniae (P23.6)*
*lobar pneumonia, unspecified organism (J18.1)*
*pneumonia due to other streptococci (J15.3-J15.4)*
**AHA:** 2020,2Q,28; 2019,1Q,35; 2018,3Q,24; 2016,3Q,15; 2013,4Q,118

**J14 Pneumonia due to Hemophilus influenzae** ESR
Bronchopneumonia due to H. influenzae
Code first, if applicable, associated influenza (J09.X1, J10.0-, J11.0-)
Code also, if applicable, any associated condition such as:
abscess (J85.1)
aspiration pneumonia (J69.-)
EXCLUDES 1 *congenital pneumonia due to H. influenzae (P23.6)*
**AHA:** 2020,2Q,28; 2019,1Q,35; 2018,3Q,24; 2016,3Q,15; 2013,4Q,118

✓4th **J15 Bacterial pneumonia, not elsewhere classified**
INCLUDES Bronchopneumonia due to bacteria other than S. pneumoniae and H. influenzae
Code first, if applicable, associated influenza (J09.X1, J10.0-, J11.0-)
Code also, if applicable, any associated condition such as:
abscess (J85.1)
aspiration pneumonia (J69.-)
EXCLUDES 1 *chlamydial pneumonia (J16.0)*
*congenital pneumonia (P23.-)*
*Legionnaires' disease (A48.1)*
*spirochetal pneumonia (A69.8)*
**AHA:** 2020,2Q,28; 2019,1Q,35; 2018,3Q,24; 2016,3Q,15; 2013,4Q,118

**J15.0 Pneumonia due to Klebsiella pneumoniae** HCC ESR COM

**J15.1 Pneumonia due to Pseudomonas** HCC ESR COM

✓5th **J15.2 Pneumonia due to staphylococcus**

**J15.20 Pneumonia due to staphylococcus, unspecified** HCC ESR COM

√6th **J15.21 Pneumonia due to Staphylococcus aureus**

**J15.211 Pneumonia due to methicillin susceptible Staphylococcus aureus** HCC ESR COM
MSSA pneumonia
Pneumonia due to Staphylococcus aureus NOS

**J15.212 Pneumonia due to methicillin resistant Staphylococcus aureus** HCC ESR COM

**J15.29 Pneumonia due to other staphylococcus** HCC ESR COM

**J15.3 Pneumonia due to streptococcus, group B** ESR

**J15.4 Pneumonia due to other streptococci** ESR
EXCLUDES 1 *pneumonia due to streptococcus, group B (J15.3)*
*pneumonia due to Streptococcus pneumoniae (J13)*

**J15.5 Pneumonia due to Escherichia coli** HCC ESR COM

√5th **J15.6 Pneumonia due to other Gram-negative bacteria**
**AHA:** 2023,4Q,27; 2020,2Q,28

**J15.61 Pneumonia due to Acinetobacter baumannii** HCC ESR COM

**J15.69 Pneumonia due to other Gram-negative bacteria** HCC ESR COM
Pneumonia due to other aerobic Gram-negative bacteria
Pneumonia due to Serratia marcescens

**J15.7 Pneumonia due to Mycoplasma pneumoniae**

**J15.8 Pneumonia due to other specified bacteria** HCC ESR COM

**J15.9 Unspecified bacterial pneumonia**
Pneumonia due to gram-positive bacteria

√4th **J16 Pneumonia due to other infectious organisms, not elsewhere classified**
Code first, if applicable, associated influenza (J09.X1, J10.0-, J11.0-)
Code also, if applicable, any associated condition such as:
abscess (J85.1)
aspiration pneumonia (J69.-)
EXCLUDES 1 *congenital pneumonia (P23.-)*
*ornithosis (A70)*
*pneumocystosis (B59)*
*pneumonia NOS (J18.9)*
**AHA:** 2020,2Q,28; 2019,1Q,35; 2018,3Q,24; 2016,3Q,15; 2013,4Q,118

**J16.0 Chlamydial pneumonia**

**J16.8 Pneumonia due to other specified infectious organisms**

***J17 Pneumonia in diseases classified elsewhere***
Code first underlying disease, such as:
Q fever (A78)
rheumatic fever (I00)
schistosomiasis (B65.0-B65.9)
Code also, if applicable, any associated condition such as:
abscess (J85.1)
aspiration pneumonia (J69.-)
EXCLUDES 1 *candidial pneumonia (B37.1)*
*chlamydial pneumonia (J16.0)*
*gonorrheal pneumonia (A54.84)*
*histoplasmosis pneumonia (B39.0-B39.2)*
*measles pneumonia (B05.2)*
*nocardiosis pneumonia (A43.0)*
*pneumocystosis (B59)*
*pneumonia due to Pneumocystis carinii (B59)*
*pneumonia due to Pneumocystis jirovecii (B59)*
*pneumonia in actinomycosis (A42.0)*
*pneumonia in anthrax (A22.1)*
*pneumonia in ascariasis (B77.81)*
*pneumonia in aspergillosis (B44.0-B44.1)*
*pneumonia in coccidioidomycosis (B38.0-B38.2)*
*pneumonia in cytomegalovirus disease (B25.0)*
*pneumonia in toxoplasmosis (B58.3)*
*rubella pneumonia (B06.81)*
*salmonella pneumonia (A02.22)*
*spirochetal infection NEC with pneumonia (A69.8)*
*tularemia pneumonia (A21.2)*
*typhoid fever with pneumonia (A01.03)*
*varicella pneumonia (B01.2)*
*whooping cough with pneumonia (A37 with fifth character 1)*
**AHA:** 2020,2Q,28; 2019,1Q,35; 2016,3Q,15; 2013,4Q,118

√4th **J18 Pneumonia, unspecified organism**
Code first, if applicable, associated influenza (J09.X1, J10.0-, J11.0-)
Code also, if applicable, any associated condition such as:
aspiration pneumonia (J69.-)
EXCLUDES 1 *congenital pneumonia (P23.0)*
*drug-induced interstitial lung disorder (J70.2-J70.4)*
*interstitial pneumonia NOS (J84.9)*
*neonatal aspiration pneumonia (P24.-)*
*pneumonitis due to fumes and vapors (J68.0)*
*usual interstitial pneumonia (J84.178)*
EXCLUDES 2 *abscess of lung with pneumonia (J85.1)*
*aspiration pneumonia due to anesthesia during labor and delivery (O74.0)*
*aspiration pneumonia due to anesthesia during pregnancy (O29)*
*aspiration pneumonia due to anesthesia during puerperium (O89.0)*
*aspiration pneumonia due to solids and liquids (J69.-)*
*aspiration pneumonia NOS (J69.0)*
*lipid pneumonia (J69.1)*
*pneumonitis due to external agents (J67-J70)*
**AHA:** 2020,2Q,28; 2019,1Q,35; 2016,3Q,15; 2013,4Q,118

**J18.0 Bronchopneumonia, unspecified organism**
EXCLUDES 1 *hypostatic bronchopneumonia (J18.2)*
*lipid pneumonia (J69.1)*
EXCLUDES 2 *acute bronchiolitis (J21.-)*
*chronic bronchiolitis (J44.89)*
*other specified chronic obstructive pulmonary disease (J44.89)*

**J18.1 Lobar pneumonia, unspecified organism** ESR
**AHA:** 2019,3Q,37; 2018,3Q,24
**DEF:** Lobar pneumonia is characterized by consolidated inflammation confined or localized to only one or a few lobes of the lung. The consolidation affects primarily the alveolar air spaces, unlike bronchopneumonia, which arises from the bronchi or bronchioles and affects a wide area without any localization.
**TIP:** Documentation of right upper lobe, left upper lobe, right lower lobe, left lower lobe, or right middle lobe pneumonia alone is not synonymous with "lobar pneumonia," nor should a diagnosis of lobar pneumonia be assumed based on an imaging report that identifies pneumonia in a specific lobe. Assign J18.1 only when the provider specifically documents "lobar pneumonia" without specifying a causal organism.

**J18.2 Hypostatic pneumonia, unspecified organism** COM
Hypostatic bronchopneumonia
Passive pneumonia

**J18.8 Other pneumonia, unspecified organism**

**J18.9 Pneumonia, unspecified organism**
**AHA:** 2020,2Q,28; 2019,3Q,15; 2019,2Q,28; 2014,3Q,4; 2013,4Q,119; 2012,4Q,94

## Other acute lower respiratory infections (J20-J22)

EXCLUDES 2 *chronic obstructive pulmonary disease with acute lower respiratory infection (J44.0)*

√4th **J20 Acute bronchitis**

INCLUDES acute and subacute bronchitis (with) bronchospasm
acute and subacute bronchitis (with) tracheitis
acute and subacute bronchitis (with) tracheobronchitis, acute
acute and subacute fibrinous bronchitis
acute and subacute membranous bronchitis
acute and subacute purulent bronchitis
acute and subacute septic bronchitis

EXCLUDES 1 *bronchitis NOS (J40)*
*tracheobronchitis NOS (J40)*

EXCLUDES 2 *acute bronchitis with bronchiectasis (J47.0)*
*acute bronchitis with chronic obstructive asthma (J44.0)*
*acute bronchitis with chronic obstructive pulmonary disease (J44.0)*
*allergic bronchitis NOS (J45.909)*
*bronchitis due to chemicals, fumes and vapors (J68.0)*
*chronic bronchitis NOS (J42)*
*chronic mucopurulent bronchitis (J41.1)*
*chronic obstructive bronchitis (J44.-)*
*chronic obstructive tracheobronchitis (J44.-)*
*chronic simple bronchitis (J41.0)*
*chronic tracheobronchitis (J42)*

**AHA:** 2019,1Q,35; 2016,3Q,10,16

**DEF:** Acute inflammation of the main branches of the bronchial tree due to infectious or irritant agents. Symptoms include cough with a varied production of sputum, fever, substernal soreness, and lung rales. Bronchitis usually lasts three to 10 days.

**J20.0 Acute bronchitis due to Mycoplasma pneumoniae**

**J20.1 Acute bronchitis due to Hemophilus influenzae**

**J20.2 Acute bronchitis due to streptococcus**

**J20.3 Acute bronchitis due to coxsackievirus**

**J20.4 Acute bronchitis due to parainfluenza virus**

**J20.5 Acute bronchitis due to respiratory syncytial virus**
Acute bronchitis due to RSV

**J20.6 Acute bronchitis due to rhinovirus**

**J20.7 Acute bronchitis due to echovirus**

**J20.8 Acute bronchitis due to other specified organisms**
**AHA:** 2020,1Q,34-36

**J20.9 Acute bronchitis, unspecified**

√4th **J21 Acute bronchiolitis**

INCLUDES acute bronchiolitis with bronchospasm

EXCLUDES 2 *respiratory bronchiolitis interstitial lung disease (J84.115)*

**J21.0 Acute bronchiolitis due to respiratory syncytial virus**
Acute bronchiolitis due to RSV

**J21.1 Acute bronchiolitis due to human metapneumovirus**

**J21.8 Acute bronchiolitis due to other specified organisms**

**J21.9 Acute bronchiolitis, unspecified**
Bronchiolitis (acute)
EXCLUDES 1 *chronic bronchiolitis (J44.89)*

**J22 Unspecified acute lower respiratory infection**
Acute (lower) respiratory (tract) infection NOS
EXCLUDES 1 *upper respiratory infection (acute) (J06.9)*
**AHA:** 2020,1Q,22,34-36

## Other diseases of upper respiratory tract (J30-J39)

√4th **J30 Vasomotor and allergic rhinitis**

INCLUDES spasmodic rhinorrhea

EXCLUDES 1 *allergic rhinitis with asthma (bronchial) (J45.909)*
*rhinitis NOS (J31.0)*

**J30.0 Vasomotor rhinitis**
**DEF:** Noninfectious and nonallergic type of rhinitis for which the cause is often unknown. Symptoms often mimic those of allergic rhinitis with a diagnosis of vasomotor rhinitis typically made after ruling out allergens as the cause.

**J30.1 Allergic rhinitis due to pollen**
Allergy NOS due to pollen
Hay fever
Pollinosis

**J30.2 Other seasonal allergic rhinitis**

**J30.5 Allergic rhinitis due to food**

√5th **J30.8 Other allergic rhinitis**

**J30.81 Allergic rhinitis due to animal (cat) (dog) hair and dander**

**J30.89 Other allergic rhinitis**
Perennial allergic rhinitis

**J30.9 Allergic rhinitis, unspecified**

√4th **J31 Chronic rhinitis, nasopharyngitis and pharyngitis**

**J31.0 Chronic rhinitis**
Atrophic rhinitis (chronic)
Granulomatous rhinitis (chronic)
Hypertrophic rhinitis (chronic)
Obstructive rhinitis (chronic)
Ozena
Purulent rhinitis (chronic)
Rhinitis (chronic) NOS
Ulcerative rhinitis (chronic)
EXCLUDES 1 *allergic rhinitis (J30.1-J30.9)*
*vasomotor rhinitis (J30.0)*
**DEF:** Persistent inflammation of the mucous membranes of the nose, characterized by a postnasal drip.

**J31.1 Chronic nasopharyngitis**
EXCLUDES 2 *acute nasopharyngitis (J00)*
**DEF:** Persistent inflammation of the mucous membranes extending from the nares to the pharynx. It is characterized by constant irritation in the nasopharynx and postnasal drip.

**J31.2 Chronic pharyngitis**
Atrophic pharyngitis (chronic)
Chronic sore throat
Granular pharyngitis (chronic)
Hypertrophic pharyngitis (chronic)
EXCLUDES 2 *acute pharyngitis (J02.9)*

√4th **J32 Chronic sinusitis**

INCLUDES sinus abscess
sinus empyema
sinus infection
sinus suppuration

Use additional code to identify:
infectious agent (B95-B97)

EXCLUDES 2 *acute sinusitis (J01.-)*

**J32.0 Chronic maxillary sinusitis**
Antritis (chronic)
Maxillary sinusitis NOS

**J32.1 Chronic frontal sinusitis**
Frontal sinusitis NOS

**J32.2 Chronic ethmoidal sinusitis**
Ethmoidal sinusitis NOS
EXCLUDES 1 *Woakes' ethmoiditis (J33.1)*

**J32.3 Chronic sphenoidal sinusitis**
Sphenoidal sinusitis NOS

**J32.4 Chronic pansinusitis**
Pansinusitis NOS

**J32.8 Other chronic sinusitis**
Sinusitis (chronic) involving more than one sinus but not pansinusitis

**J32.9 Chronic sinusitis, unspecified**
Sinusitis (chronic) NOS

√4th **J33 Nasal polyp**

EXCLUDES 1 *adenomatous polyps (D14.0)*

**J33.0 Polyp of nasal cavity**
Choanal polyp
Nasopharyngeal polyp

**J33.1 Polypoid sinus degeneration**
Woakes' syndrome or ethmoiditis

**J33.8 Other polyp of sinus**
Accessory polyp of sinus
Ethmoidal polyp of sinus
Maxillary polyp of sinus
Sphenoidal polyp of sinus

**J33.9 Nasal polyp, unspecified**

√4th **J34 Other and unspecified disorders of nose and nasal sinuses**

EXCLUDES 2 *varicose ulcer of nasal septum (I86.8)*

**J34.0 Abscess, furuncle and carbuncle of nose**
Cellulitis of nose
Necrosis of nose
Ulceration of nose

**J34.1 Cyst and mucocele of nose and nasal sinus**

**J34.2 Deviated nasal septum**
Deflection or deviation of septum (nasal) (acquired)
EXCLUDES 1 *congenital deviated nasal septum (Q67.4)*
**DEF:** Condition in which the nasal septum, a thin wall composed of cartilage and bone that separates the two nostrils, is crooked or displaced from the midline.

**J34.3 Hypertrophy of nasal turbinates**
**DEF:** Overgrowth of bones within the nasal turbinate, which are ridges of bone and soft tissue that project from the sidewalls of the nasal passages. Hypertrophy can cause obstruction of the nasal passages.

✓5th **J34.8 Other specified disorders of nose and nasal sinuses**

**J34.81 Nasal mucositis (ulcerative)**
Code also type of associated therapy, such as:
antineoplastic and immunosuppressive drugs (T45.1X-)
radiological procedure and radiotherapy (Y84.2)
EXCLUDES 2 *gastrointestinal mucositis (ulcerative) (K92.81)*
*mucositis (ulcerative) of vagina and vulva (N76.81)*
*oral mucositis (ulcerative) (K12.3-)*

✓6th **J34.82 Nasal valve collapse**
Nasal valve compromise
Nasal valve stenosis
Code first underlying cause, such as:
deviated nasal septum (J34.2)
**AHA:** 2024,4Q,20

✓7th **J34.820 Internal nasal valve collapse**
**J34.8200 Internal nasal valve collapse, unspecified**
**J34.8201 Internal nasal valve collapse, static**
Narrowing of the septum, head of the inferior turbinate and the upper lateral cartilage
**J34.8202 Internal nasal valve collapse, dynamic**
Collapse or falling of the upper, middle sidewall of the nose on inspiration

✓7th **J34.821 External nasal valve collapse**
**J34.8210 External nasal valve collapse, unspecified**
**J34.8211 External nasal valve collapse, static**
Fixed narrowing of the caudal septum, lower lateral cartilage, alar rim and nasal sill
**J34.8212 External nasal valve collapse, dynamic**
Collapse or falling of the lower sidewall or nostril of the nose on inspiration

**J34.829 Nasal valve collapse, unspecified**
Nasal valve collapse, NOS

● ✓6th **J34.83 Odontogenic sinusitis**
● **J34.830 Odontogenic sinusitis, maxillary sinus**
● **J34.831 Odontogenic sinusitis, ethmoid sinus**
● **J34.832 Odontogenic sinusitis, frontal sinus**
● **J34.833 Odontogenic sinusitis, sphenoid sinus**
● **J34.839 Odontogenic sinusitis, unspecified**
Odontogenic sinusitis NOS

**J34.89 Other specified disorders of nose and nasal sinuses**
Perforation of nasal septum NOS
Rhinolith

**J34.9 Unspecified disorder of nose and nasal sinuses**

✓4th **J35 Chronic diseases of tonsils and adenoids**

✓5th **J35.0 Chronic tonsillitis and adenoiditis**
EXCLUDES 2 *acute tonsillitis (J03.-)*
**J35.01 Chronic tonsillitis**
**J35.02 Chronic adenoiditis**
**J35.03 Chronic tonsillitis and adenoiditis**

**J35.1 Hypertrophy of tonsils**
Enlargement of tonsils
EXCLUDES 1 *hypertrophy of tonsils with tonsillitis (J35.0-)*

**J35.2 Hypertrophy of adenoids**
Enlargement of adenoids
EXCLUDES 1 *hypertrophy of adenoids with adenoiditis (J35.0-)*

**J35.3 Hypertrophy of tonsils with hypertrophy of adenoids**
EXCLUDES 1 *hypertrophy of tonsils and adenoids with tonsillitis and adenoiditis (J35.03)*

**J35.8 Other chronic diseases of tonsils and adenoids**
Adenoid vegetations
Amygdalolith
Calculus, tonsil
Cicatrix of tonsil (and adenoid)
Tonsillar tag
Ulcer of tonsil

**J35.9 Chronic disease of tonsils and adenoids, unspecified**
Disease (chronic) of tonsils and adenoids NOS

**J36 Peritonsillar abscess**
INCLUDES abscess of tonsil
peritonsillar cellulitis
quinsy
Use additional code (B95-B97) to identify infectious agent
EXCLUDES 1 *acute tonsillitis (J03.-)*
*chronic tonsillitis (J35.0)*
*retropharyngeal abscess (J39.0)*
*tonsillitis NOS (J03.9-)*

✓4th **J37 Chronic laryngitis and laryngotracheitis**
Use additional code to identify:
exposure to environmental tobacco smoke (Z77.22)
exposure to tobacco smoke in the perinatal period (P96.81)
history of tobacco dependence (Z87.891)
infectious agent (B95-B97)
occupational exposure to environmental tobacco smoke (Z57.31)
tobacco dependence (F17.-)
tobacco use (Z72.0)

**J37.0 Chronic laryngitis**
Catarrhal laryngitis
Hypertrophic laryngitis
Sicca laryngitis
EXCLUDES 2 *acute laryngitis (J04.0)*
*obstructive (acute) laryngitis (J05.0)*

**J37.1 Chronic laryngotracheitis**
Laryngitis, chronic, with tracheitis (chronic)
Tracheitis, chronic, with laryngitis
EXCLUDES 1 *chronic tracheitis (J42)*
EXCLUDES 2 *acute laryngotracheitis (J04.2)*
*acute tracheitis (J04.1)*

✓4th **J38 Diseases of vocal cords and larynx, not elsewhere classified**
EXCLUDES 1 *congenital laryngeal stridor (P28.89)*
*obstructive laryngitis (acute) (J05.0)*
*postprocedural subglottic stenosis (J95.5)*
*stridor (R06.1)*
*ulcerative laryngitis (J04.0)*

✓5th **J38.0 Paralysis of vocal cords and larynx**
Laryngoplegia
Paralysis of glottis
**J38.00 Paralysis of vocal cords and larynx, unspecified**
**J38.01 Paralysis of vocal cords and larynx, unilateral**
**AHA:** 2025,1Q,27
**J38.02 Paralysis of vocal cords and larynx, bilateral**

**J38.1 Polyp of vocal cord and larynx**
EXCLUDES 1 *adenomatous polyps (D14.1)*

**J38.2 Nodules of vocal cords**
Chorditis (fibrinous)(nodosa)(tuberosa)
Singer's nodes
Teacher's nodes

**J38.3 Other diseases of vocal cords**
Abscess of vocal cords
Cellulitis of vocal cords
Granuloma of vocal cords
Leukokeratosis of vocal cords
Leukoplakia of vocal cords

**J38.4 Edema of larynx**
Edema (of) glottis
Subglottic edema
Supraglottic edema
EXCLUDES 1 *acute obstructive laryngitis [croup] (J05.0)*
*edematous laryngitis (J04.0)*

**J38.5 Laryngeal spasm**
Laryngismus (stridulus)

**J38.6 Stenosis of larynx**

**J38.7 Other diseases of larynx**
Abscess of larynx
Cellulitis of larynx
Disease of larynx NOS
Necrosis of larynx
Pachyderma of larynx
Perichondritis of larynx
Ulcer of larynx

**✓4th J39 Other diseases of upper respiratory tract**
EXCLUDES 1 *acute respiratory infection NOS (J22)*
*acute upper respiratory infection (J06.9)*
*upper respiratory inflammation due to chemicals, gases, fumes or vapors (J68.2)*

**J39.0 Retropharyngeal and parapharyngeal abscess**
Peripharyngeal abscess
EXCLUDES 1 *peritonsillar abscess (J36)*
**DEF:** Purulent infection behind the pharynx and the front of the precerebral fascia, characterized by neck stiffness, cervical lymphadenopathy, sore throat, fever, and stridor.

**J39.1 Other abscess of pharynx**
Cellulitis of pharynx
Nasopharyngeal abscess

**J39.2 Other diseases of pharynx**
Cyst of pharynx
Edema of pharynx
EXCLUDES 2 *chronic pharyngitis (J31.2)*
*ulcerative pharyngitis (J02.9)*

**J39.3 Upper respiratory tract hypersensitivity reaction, site unspecified**
EXCLUDES 1 *hypersensitivity reaction of upper respiratory tract, such as:*
*extrinsic allergic alveolitis (J67.9)*
*pneumoconiosis (J60-J67.9)*

**J39.8 Other specified diseases of upper respiratory tract**
**AHA:** 2023,1Q,30

**J39.9 Disease of upper respiratory tract, unspecified**

## Chronic lower respiratory diseases ▶(J40-J4B)◀

EXCLUDES 1 *bronchitis due to chemicals, gases, fumes and vapors (J68.0)*
EXCLUDES 2 *cystic fibrosis (E84.-)*

**J40 Bronchitis, not specified as acute or chronic**
Bronchitis NOS
Bronchitis with tracheitis NOS
Catarrhal bronchitis
Tracheobronchitis NOS
Use additional code to identify:
exposure to environmental tobacco smoke (Z77.22)
exposure to tobacco smoke in the perinatal period (P96.81)
history of tobacco dependence (Z87.891)
occupational exposure to environmental tobacco smoke (Z57.31)
tobacco dependence (F17.-)
tobacco use (Z72.0)
EXCLUDES 1 *acute bronchitis (J20.-)*
*allergic bronchitis NOS (J45.909)*
*asthmatic bronchitis NOS (J45.9-)*
*bronchitis due to chemicals, gases, fumes and vapors (J68.0)*
**AHA:** 2020,1Q,34-36

**✓4th J41 Simple and mucopurulent chronic bronchitis**
Use additional code to identify:
exposure to environmental tobacco smoke (Z77.22)
exposure to tobacco smoke in the perinatal period (P96.81)
history of tobacco dependence (Z87.891)
occupational exposure to environmental tobacco smoke (Z57.31)
tobacco dependence (F17.-)
tobacco use (Z72.0)
EXCLUDES 2 *chronic bronchitis NOS (J42)*
*chronic obstructive bronchitis (J44.-)*

**J41.0 Simple chronic bronchitis** HCC Rx ESR COM
**J41.1 Mucopurulent chronic bronchitis** HCC Rx ESR COM
**J41.8 Mixed simple and mucopurulent chronic bronchitis** HCC Rx ESR COM

**J42 Unspecified chronic bronchitis** HCC Rx ESR COM
Chronic bronchitis NOS
Chronic tracheitis
Chronic tracheobronchitis
▶Code also, if applicable, chronic respiratory conditions due to chemicals, gases, fumes and vapors (J68.4)◀
Use additional code to identify:
exposure to environmental tobacco smoke (Z77.22)
exposure to tobacco smoke in the perinatal period (P96.81)
history of tobacco dependence (Z87.891)
occupational exposure to environmental tobacco smoke (Z57.31)
tobacco dependence (F17.-)
tobacco use (Z72.0)
EXCLUDES 1 *bronchiolitis obliterans and bronchiolitis obliterans syndrome (J44.81)*
*chronic asthmatic bronchitis (J44.-)*
*chronic bronchitis with airways obstruction (J44.-)*
*chronic emphysematous bronchitis (J44.-)*
*chronic obstructive pulmonary disease NOS (J44.9)*
*simple and mucopurulent chronic bronchitis (J41.-)*

**✓4th J43 Emphysema**
EXCLUDES 1 *compensatory emphysema (J98.3)*
*interstitial emphysema (J98.2)*
*mediastinal emphysema (J98.2)*
*neonatal interstitial emphysema (P25.0)*
*surgical (subcutaneous) emphysema (T81.82)*
EXCLUDES 2 *emphysema due to inhalation of chemicals, gases, fumes or vapors (J68.4)*
*emphysema with chronic (obstructive) bronchitis (J44.-)*
*emphysematous (obstructive) bronchitis (J44.-)*
*traumatic subcutaneous emphysema (T79.7)*
**DEF:** Pathological condition in which there is destructive enlargement of the air sacs in the lungs resulting in damage and lack of elasticity to the alveolar walls, commonly seen in long-term smokers.

**Emphysema**

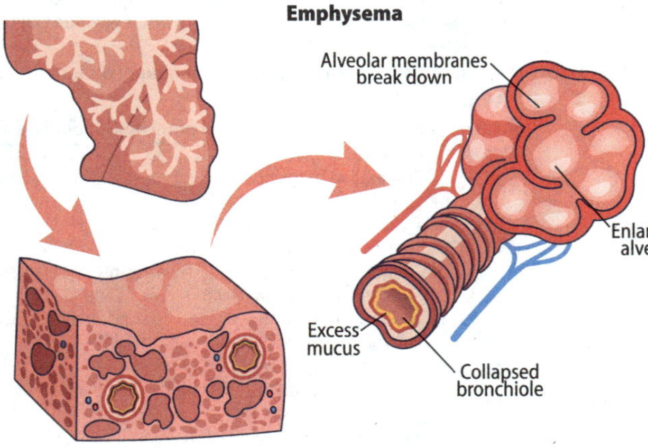


**J43.0 Unilateral pulmonary emphysema [MacLeod's syndrome]** HCC Rx ESR COM
Swyer-James syndrome
Unilateral emphysema
Unilateral hyperlucent lung
Unilateral pulmonary artery functional hypoplasia
Unilateral transparency of lung

**J43.1 Panlobular emphysema** HCC Rx ESR COM
Panacinar emphysema

**J43.2 Centrilobular emphysema** HCC Rx ESR COM

**J43.8 Other emphysema** HCC Rx ESR COM

**J43.9 Emphysema, unspecified** HCC Rx ESR COM
Bullous emphysema (lung)(pulmonary)
Emphysema (lung)(pulmonary) NOS
Emphysematous bleb
Vesicular emphysema (lung)(pulmonary)
**AHA:** 2024,2Q,4; 2019,1Q,34-36; 2017,4Q,97-98

**✓4th J44 Other chronic obstructive pulmonary disease**

INCLUDES asthma with chronic obstructive pulmonary disease
chronic asthmatic (obstructive) bronchitis
chronic bronchitis with airway obstruction
chronic bronchitis with emphysema
chronic emphysematous bronchitis
chronic obstructive asthma
chronic obstructive bronchitis
chronic obstructive tracheobronchitis

Code also type of asthma, if applicable (J45.-)

EXCLUDES 2 *bronchiectasis (J47.-)*
*chronic bronchitis NOS (J42)*
*chronic simple and mucopurulent bronchitis (J41.-)*
*chronic tracheitis (J42)*
*chronic tracheobronchitis (J42)*
*emphysema without chronic bronchitis (J43.-)*

**AHA:** 2024,2Q,3-5; 2019,1Q,34-36; 2017,4Q,97-98; 2017,1Q,25-26; 2016,3Q,15-16; 2013,4Q,109

**J44.Ø Chronic obstructive pulmonary disease with (acute) lower respiratory infection** HCC Rx ESR COM

Code also to identify the infection

**AHA:** 2019,1Q,35; 2017,4Q,96; 2017,1Q,24-25

**TIP:** Do not assign when only aspiration pneumonia is present. Aspiration pneumonia is not classified as a respiratory infection.

**J44.1 Chronic obstructive pulmonary disease with (acute) exacerbation** HCC Rx ESR COM

Decompensated COPD
Decompensated COPD with (acute) exacerbation

EXCLUDES 2 *chronic obstructive pulmonary disease [COPD] with acute bronchitis (J44.Ø)*
*lung diseases due to external agents (J6Ø-J7Ø)*

**AHA:** 2019,1Q,34; 2017,4Q,96; 2017,1Q,26; 2016,1Q,36

**TIP:** Assign J43.9 when COPD exacerbation with emphysema is documented.

**TIP:** Exacerbation of COPD should not be assumed based upon worsening of a concomitant respiratory disease or when COPD is described as end-stage.

**✓5th J44.8 Other specified chronic obstructive pulmonary disease**

**AHA:** 2023,4Q,27

**J44.81 Bronchiolitis obliterans and bronchiolitis obliterans syndrome** HCC Rx ESR COM

Obliterative bronchiolitis

Code first, if applicable:
complication of bone marrow transplant (T86.Ø9)
lung transplant rejection (T86.81Ø)
other complications of heart-lung transplant (T86.39)
other complications of lung transplant (T86.818)

Code also, if applicable, associated conditions, such as:
chronic graft-versus-host disease (D89.811)
chronic lung allograft dysfunction (J4A.-)
chronic respiratory conditions due to chemicals, gases, fumes and vapors (J68.4)
complication of stem cell transplant (T86.5)
heart-lung transplant rejection (T86.31)

**J44.89 Other specified chronic obstructive pulmonary disease** HCC Rx ESR COM

Chronic asthmatic (obstructive) bronchitis
Chronic emphysematous bronchitis

**J44.9 Chronic obstructive pulmonary disease, unspecified** HCC Rx ESR COM

Chronic obstructive airway disease NOS
Chronic obstructive lung disease NOS

EXCLUDES 2 *lung diseases due to external agents (J6Ø-J7Ø)*

**AHA:** 2019,1Q,36; 2017,4Q,96-97; 2016,1Q,36; 2014,4Q,21; 2013,4Q,109

**✓4th J4A Chronic lung allograft dysfunction**

Code first, if applicable:
heart-lung transplant rejection (T86.31)
lung transplant rejection (T86.81Ø)
other complications of heart-lung transplant (T86.39)
other complications of lung transplant (T86.818)

Code also, if applicable, bronchiolitis obliterans syndrome (J44.81)

**AHA:** 2023,4Q,28

**J4A.Ø Restrictive allograft syndrome** HCC Rx ESR COM

Code also, if applicable, for mixed chronic lung allograft dysfunction, bronchiolitis obliterans syndrome (J44.81)

**J4A.8 Other chronic lung allograft dysfunction** HCC Rx ESR COM

**J4A.9 Chronic lung allograft dysfunction, unspecified** HCC Rx ESR COM

● **J4B Pulmonary mycetoma**

Pulmonary fungal ball

Code also, if known, associated infection, such as:
aspergillosis (B44.-)
chronic pulmonary coccidioidomycosis (B38.1)
pulmonary candidiasis (B37.1)

**✓4th J45 Asthma**

INCLUDES allergic (predominantly) asthma
allergic bronchitis NOS
allergic rhinitis with asthma
atopic asthma
extrinsic allergic asthma
hay fever with asthma
idiosyncratic asthma
intrinsic nonallergic asthma
nonallergic asthma

Use additional code to identify:
eosinophilic asthma (J82.83)
exposure to environmental tobacco smoke (Z77.22)
exposure to tobacco smoke in the perinatal period (P96.81)
history of tobacco dependence (Z87.891)
occupational exposure to environmental tobacco smoke (Z57.31)
tobacco dependence (F17.-)
tobacco use (Z72.Ø)

EXCLUDES 1 *detergent asthma (J69.8)*
*miner's asthma (J6Ø)*
*wheezing NOS (RØ6.2)*
*wood asthma (J67.8)*

EXCLUDES 2 *asthma with chronic obstructive pulmonary disease (J44.89)*
*chronic asthmatic (obstructive) bronchitis (J44.89)*
*chronic obstructive asthma (J44.89)*
*other specified chronic obstructive pulmonary disease (J44.89)*

**AHA:** 2024,2Q,3; 2023,1Q,17; 2019,1Q,36; 2017,1Q,25-26; 2012,4Q,99

**DEF:** Status asthmaticus: Severe, intractable episode of asthma that is unresponsive to normal therapeutic measures.

**Asthma**

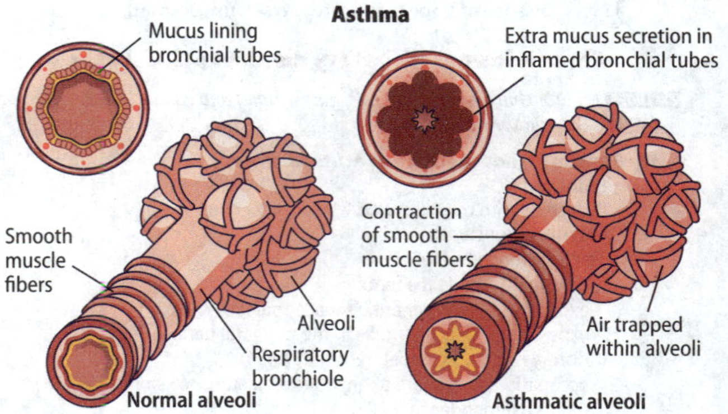


**✓5th J45.2 Mild intermittent asthma**

**J45.2Ø Mild intermittent asthma, uncomplicated** Rx COM

Mild intermittent asthma NOS

**J45.21 Mild intermittent asthma with (acute) exacerbation** Rx COM

**J45.22 Mild intermittent asthma with status asthmaticus** Rx COM

**✓5th J45.3 Mild persistent asthma**

**J45.3Ø Mild persistent asthma, uncomplicated** Rx COM

Mild persistent asthma NOS

**J45.31 Mild persistent asthma with (acute) exacerbation** Rx COM

**AHA:** 2016,1Q,35

**J45.32 Mild persistent asthma with status asthmaticus** Rx COM

**✓5th J45.4 Moderate persistent asthma**

**AHA:** 2026,2Q,21; 2025,3Q,11

**J45.4Ø Moderate persistent asthma, uncomplicated** Rx COM

Moderate persistent asthma NOS

**J45.41 Moderate persistent asthma with (acute) exacerbation** Rx COM

**AHA:** 2025,3Q,11; 2017,1Q,26

**J45.42 Moderate persistent asthma with status asthmaticus** Rx COM

√5th **J45.5 Severe persistent asthma**

**J45.50 Severe persistent asthma, uncomplicated** HCC Rx COM
Severe persistent asthma NOS

**J45.51 Severe persistent asthma with (acute) exacerbation** HCC Rx COM

**J45.52 Severe persistent asthma with status asthmaticus** HCC Rx COM

√5th **J45.9 Other and unspecified asthma**

√6th **J45.90 Unspecified asthma**
Asthmatic bronchitis NOS
Childhood asthma NOS
Late onset asthma
**AHA:** 2017,4Q,96; 2017,1Q,25

**J45.901 Unspecified asthma with (acute) exacerbation** Rx COM

**J45.902 Unspecified asthma with status asthmaticus** Rx COM

**J45.909 Unspecified asthma, uncomplicated** Rx COM
Asthma NOS
EXCLUDES 2 *lung diseases due to external agents (J60-J70)*
**AHA:** 2017,1Q,25

√6th **J45.99 Other asthma**

**J45.990 Exercise induced bronchospasm** Rx COM

**J45.991 Cough variant asthma** Rx COM

**J45.998 Other asthma** Rx COM

√4th **J47 Bronchiectasis**

INCLUDES bronchiolectasis

Use additional code to identify:
- exposure to environmental tobacco smoke (Z77.22)
- exposure to tobacco smoke in the perinatal period (P96.81)
- history of tobacco dependence (Z87.891)
- occupational exposure to environmental tobacco smoke (Z57.31)
- tobacco dependence (F17.-)
- tobacco use (Z72.0)

EXCLUDES 1 *congenital bronchiectasis (Q33.4)*
*tuberculous bronchiectasis (current disease) (A15.0)*

**DEF:** Dilation of the bronchi with mucus production and persistent cough due to infection or chronic conditions that causes diminished lung capacity and frequent infections of the lung.

**J47.0 Bronchiectasis with acute lower respiratory infection** HCC Rx ESR COM
Bronchiectasis with acute bronchitis
Code also to identify infection, if applicable

**J47.1 Bronchiectasis with (acute) exacerbation** HCC Rx ESR COM
**AHA:** 2021,1Q,23

**J47.9 Bronchiectasis, uncomplicated** HCC Rx ESR COM
Bronchiectasis NOS
**AHA:** 2024,2Q,5

## Lung diseases due to external agents (J60-J70)

EXCLUDES 2 *asthma (J45.-)*
*malignant neoplasm of bronchus and lung (C34.-)*

**DEF:** Pneumoconiosis: Condition caused by inhaling inorganic dust particles, typically associated with occupations that require regular exposure to mineral dusts. A form of interstitial lung disease that contributes to the inflammation of the air sacs, causing the lung tissue to harden.

**J60 Coalworker's pneumoconiosis** HCC ESR COM A
Anthracosilicosis
Anthracosis
Black lung disease
Coalworker's lung
EXCLUDES 1 *coalworker pneumoconiosis with tuberculosis, any type in A15 (J65)*

**J61 Pneumoconiosis due to asbestos and other mineral fibers** HCC ESR COM A
Asbestosis
EXCLUDES 1 *pleural plaque with asbestosis (J92.0)*
*pneumoconiosis with tuberculosis, any type in A15 (J65)*

√4th **J62 Pneumoconiosis due to dust containing silica**

INCLUDES silicotic fibrosis (massive) of lung
EXCLUDES 1 *pneumoconiosis with tuberculosis, any type in A15 (J65)*

**J62.0 Pneumoconiosis due to talc dust** HCC ESR COM

**J62.8 Pneumoconiosis due to other dust containing silica** HCC ESR COM
Silicosis NOS

√4th **J63 Pneumoconiosis due to other inorganic dusts**

EXCLUDES 1 *pneumoconiosis with tuberculosis, any type in A15 (J65)*

**J63.0 Aluminosis (of lung)** HCC ESR COM

**J63.1 Bauxite fibrosis (of lung)** HCC ESR COM

**J63.2 Berylliosis** HCC ESR COM

**J63.3 Graphite fibrosis (of lung)** HCC ESR COM

**J63.4 Siderosis** HCC ESR COM
**AHA:** 2019,3Q,8

**J63.5 Stannosis** HCC ESR COM

**J63.6 Pneumoconiosis due to other specified inorganic dusts** HCC ESR COM

**J64 Unspecified pneumoconiosis** HCC ESR COM
EXCLUDES 1 *pneumonoconiosis with tuberculosis, any type in A15 (J65)*

**J65 Pneumoconiosis associated with tuberculosis** HCC ESR COM
Any condition in J60-J64 with tuberculosis, any type in A15
Silicotuberculosis
Use additional code, if applicable, for associated cachexia (E88.A)

√4th **J66 Airway disease due to specific organic dust**

EXCLUDES 2 *allergic alveolitis (J67.-)*
*asbestosis (J61)*
*bagassosis (J67.1)*
*farmer's lung (J67.0)*
*hypersensitivity pneumonitis due to organic dust (J67.-)*
*reactive airways dysfunction syndrome (J68.3)*

**J66.0 Byssinosis** HCC ESR COM
Airway disease due to cotton dust

**J66.1 Flax-dressers' disease** HCC ESR COM

**J66.2 Cannabinosis** HCC ESR COM

**J66.8 Airway disease due to other specific organic dusts** HCC ESR COM

√4th **J67 Hypersensitivity pneumonitis due to organic dust**

INCLUDES allergic alveolitis and pneumonitis due to inhaled organic dust and particles of fungal, actinomycetic or other origin
EXCLUDES 1 *pneumonitis due to inhalation of chemicals, gases, fumes or vapors (J68.0)*

**J67.0 Farmer's lung** HCC ESR COM
Harvester's lung
Haymaker's lung
Moldy hay disease

**J67.1 Bagassosis** HCC ESR COM
Bagasse disease
Bagasse pneumonitis

**J67.2 Bird fancier's lung** HCC ESR COM
Budgerigar fancier's disease or lung
Pigeon fancier's disease or lung

**J67.3 Suberosis** HCC ESR COM
Corkhandler's disease or lung
Corkworker's disease or lung

**J67.4 Maltworker's lung** HCC ESR COM
Alveolitis due to Aspergillus clavatus

**J67.5 Mushroom-worker's lung** HCC ESR COM

**J67.6 Maple-bark-stripper's lung** HCC ESR COM
Alveolitis due to Cryptostroma corticale
Cryptostromosis

**J67.7 Air conditioner and humidifier lung** HCC ESR COM
Allergic alveolitis due to fungal, thermophilic actinomycetes and other organisms growing in ventilation [air conditioning] systems

**J67.8 Hypersensitivity pneumonitis due to other organic dusts** HCC ESR COM
Cheese-washer's lung
Coffee-worker's lung
Fish-meal worker's lung
Furrier's lung
Sequoiosis

**J67.9 Hypersensitivity pneumonitis due to unspecified organic dust** HCC ESR COM
Allergic alveolitis (extrinsic) NOS
Hypersensitivity pneumonitis NOS

✓4th **J68 Respiratory conditions due to inhalation of chemicals, gases, fumes and vapors**
Code first (T51-T65) to identify cause
Use additional code to identify associated respiratory conditions, such as:
acute respiratory failure (J96.Ø-)

**J68.Ø Bronchitis and pneumonitis due to chemicals, gases, fumes and vapors** HCC ESR COM
Chemical bronchitis (acute)
**AHA:** 2019,2Q,31

**J68.1 Pulmonary edema due to chemicals, gases, fumes and vapors** HCC ESR COM
Chemical pulmonary edema (acute) (chronic)
EXCLUDES 1 *pulmonary edema (acute) (chronic) NOS (J81.-)*

**J68.2 Upper respiratory inflammation due to chemicals, gases, fumes and vapors, not elsewhere classified** HCC ESR COM

**J68.3 Other acute and subacute respiratory conditions due to chemicals, gases, fumes and vapors** HCC ESR COM
Reactive airways dysfunction syndrome

**J68.4 Chronic respiratory conditions due to chemicals, gases, fumes and vapors** HCC ESR COM
Code also, if applicable, chronic conditions, such as:
▶chronic bronchitis (J42)◀
emphysema (J43.-)
obliterative bronchiolitis (J44.81)
pulmonary fibrosis (J84.1Ø)
EXCLUDES 1 *chronic pulmonary edema due to chemicals, gases, fumes and vapors (J68.1)*

**J68.8 Other respiratory conditions due to chemicals, gases, fumes and vapors** HCC ESR COM

**J68.9 Unspecified respiratory condition due to chemicals, gases, fumes and vapors** HCC ESR COM

✓4th **J69 Pneumonitis due to solids and liquids**
▶Code also, if applicable, other types of pneumonias, such as:◀
▶bacterial pneumonia (J13-J15.-)◀
▶viral pneumonia (J12.-)◀
EXCLUDES 1 *neonatal aspiration syndromes (P24.-)*
*postprocedural pneumonitis (J95.4)*
**AHA:** 2017,1Q,24
**DEF:** Pneumonitis: Noninfectious inflammation of the walls of the alveoli in the lung tissue due to inhalation of food, vomit, oils, essences, or other solids or liquids.

**J69.Ø Pneumonitis due to inhalation of food and vomit** HCC ESR COM
Aspiration pneumonia (due to) food (regurgitated)
Aspiration pneumonia (due to) gastric secretions
Aspiration pneumonia (due to) milk
Aspiration pneumonia (due to) vomit
Aspiration pneumonia NOS
Code also any associated foreign body in respiratory tract (T17.-)
EXCLUDES 1 *chemical pneumonitis due to anesthesia (J95.4)*
*obstetric aspiration pneumonitis (O74.Ø)*
**AHA:** 2020,2Q,11,28; 2019,3Q,17; 2019,2Q,6,31

**J69.1 Pneumonitis due to inhalation of oils and essences** HCC ESR COM
Exogenous lipoid pneumonia
Lipid pneumonia NOS
Code first (T51-T65) to identify substance
EXCLUDES 1 *endogenous lipoid pneumonia (J84.89)*

**J69.8 Pneumonitis due to inhalation of other solids and liquids** HCC ESR COM
Pneumonitis due to aspiration of blood
Pneumonitis due to aspiration of detergent
Code first (T51-T65) to identify substance

✓4th **J7Ø Respiratory conditions due to other external agents**

**J7Ø.Ø Acute pulmonary manifestations due to radiation** ESR COM
Radiation pneumonitis
Use additional code (W88-W9Ø, X39.Ø-) to identify the external cause

**J7Ø.1 Chronic and other pulmonary manifestations due to radiation** ESR COM
Fibrosis of lung following radiation
Use additional code (W88-W9Ø, X39.Ø-) to identify the external cause

**J7Ø.2 Acute drug-induced interstitial lung disorders** ESR
Use additional code for adverse effect, if applicable, to identify drug (T36-T5Ø with fifth or sixth character 5)
EXCLUDES 1 *interstitial pneumonia NOS (J84.9)*
*lymphoid interstitial pneumonia (J84.2)*
**AHA:** 2019,2Q,28

**J7Ø.3 Chronic drug-induced interstitial lung disorders** ESR
Use additional code for adverse effect, if applicable, to identify drug (T36-T5Ø with fifth or sixth character 5)
EXCLUDES 1 *interstitial pneumonia NOS (J84.9)*
*lymphoid interstitial pneumonia (J84.2)*

**J7Ø.4 Drug-induced interstitial lung disorders, unspecified** ESR
Use additional code for adverse effect, if applicable, to identify drug (T36-T5Ø with fifth or sixth character 5)
EXCLUDES 1 *interstitial pneumonia NOS (J84.9)*
*lymphoid interstitial pneumonia (J84.2)*
**AHA:** 2019,2Q,28

**J7Ø.5 Respiratory conditions due to smoke inhalation** ESR
Code first smoke inhalation (T59.81-)
EXCLUDES 2 *smoke inhalation due to chemicals, gases, fumes and vapors (J68.9)*
**AHA:** 2013,4Q,121

**J7Ø.8 Respiratory conditions due to other specified external agents** ESR
Code first (T51-T65) to identify the external agent

**J7Ø.9 Respiratory conditions due to unspecified external agent** ESR
Code first (T51-T65) to identify the external agent

## Other respiratory diseases principally affecting the interstitium (J8Ø-J84)

**J8Ø Acute respiratory distress syndrome** HCC ESR COM
Acute respiratory distress syndrome in adult or child
Adult hyaline membrane disease
EXCLUDES 1 *respiratory distress syndrome in newborn (perinatal) (P22.Ø)*
**AHA:** 2021,1Q,23; 2020,4Q,96; 2020,1Q,34-36; 2017,1Q,26
**DEF:** Lung inflammation or injury resulting in a build-up of fluid in the air sacs, preventing the passage of oxygen from the air into the bloodstream.

✓4th **J81 Pulmonary edema**
Use additional code to identify:
exposure to environmental tobacco smoke (Z77.22)
history of tobacco dependence (Z87.891)
occupational exposure to environmental tobacco smoke (Z57.31)
tobacco dependence (F17.-)
tobacco use (Z72.Ø)
EXCLUDES 1 *chemical (acute) pulmonary edema (J68.1)*
*hypostatic pneumonia (J18.2)*
*passive pneumonia (J18.2)*
*pulmonary edema due to external agents (J6Ø-J7Ø)*
*pulmonary edema with heart disease NOS (I5Ø.1)*
*pulmonary edema with heart failure (I5Ø.1)*
**DEF:** Accumulation of fluid in the air sacs of the lungs, making it difficult to breathe.

**J81.Ø Acute pulmonary edema** HCC ESR COM
Acute edema of lung
**AHA:** 2023,1Q,25; 2020,3Q,27

**J81.1 Chronic pulmonary edema** COM
Pulmonary congestion (chronic) (passive)
Pulmonary edema NOS

✓4th **J82 Pulmonary eosinophilia, not elsewhere classified**
EXCLUDES 2 *pulmonary eosinophilia due to aspergillosis (B44.-)*
*pulmonary eosinophilia due to drugs (J7Ø.2-J7Ø.4)*
*pulmonary eosinophilia due to specified parasitic infection (B5Ø-B83)*
*pulmonary eosinophilia due to systemic connective tissue disorders (M3Ø-M36)*
*pulmonary infiltrate NOS (R91.8)*
**DEF:** Infiltration of eosinophils (white blood cells of the immune system) into the parenchyma of the lungs, resulting in cough, fever, and dyspnea.

✓5th **J82.8 Pulmonary eosinophilia, not elsewhere classified**
**AHA:** 2020,4Q,25-27

**J82.81 Chronic eosinophilic pneumonia** HCC Rx ESR COM
Eosinophilic pneumonia, NOS

**J82.82 Acute eosinophilic pneumonia**

**J82.83 Eosinophilic asthma** Rx COM
Code first asthma, by type, such as:
mild intermittent asthma (J45.2-)
mild persistent asthma (J45.3-)
moderate persistent asthma (J45.4-)
severe persistent asthma (J45.5-)

**J82.89 Other pulmonary eosinophilia, not elsewhere classified** ESR COM
Allergic pneumonia
Loffler's pneumonia
Tropical (pulmonary) eosinophilia NOS

✓4th **J84 Other interstitial pulmonary diseases**
Code also, if applicable, associated condition
EXCLUDES 1 *drug-induced interstitial lung disorders (J7Ø.2-J7Ø.4)*
*interstitial emphysema (J98.2)*
EXCLUDES 2 *lung diseases due to external agents (J6Ø-J7Ø)*
**DEF:** Interstitial: Within the small spaces or gaps occurring in tissue or organs.

✓5th **J84.Ø Alveolar and parieto-alveolar conditions**

**J84.Ø1 Alveolar proteinosis** HCC Rx ESR COM
**DEF:** Reduced ventilation due to proteinaceous deposits on alveoli. Symptoms include dyspnea, cough, chest pain, weakness, weight loss, and hemoptysis.

**J84.Ø2 Pulmonary alveolar microlithiasis** HCC Rx ESR COM

***J84.Ø3 Idiopathic pulmonary hemosiderosis*** HCC Rx ESR COM
Essential brown induration of lung
Code first underlying disease, such as:
disorders of iron metabolism (E83.1-)
EXCLUDES 1 *acute idiopathic pulmonary hemorrhage in infants [AIPHI] (RØ4.81)*
**DEF:** Fibrosis of the alveolar walls marked by abnormal accumulation of iron as hemosiderin in the lungs. It primarily affects children and symptoms include anemia, fluid in the lungs, and blood in the sputum. Etiology is unknown.

**J84.Ø9 Other alveolar and parieto-alveolar conditions** HCC Rx ESR COM

✓5th **J84.1 Other interstitial pulmonary diseases with fibrosis**
Code also, if applicable, pulmonary fibrosis (chronic) due to inhalation of chemicals, gases, fumes or vapors (J68.4)
EXCLUDES 1 *pulmonary fibrosis (chronic) following radiation (J7Ø.1)*

**J84.1Ø Pulmonary fibrosis, unspecified** HCC Rx ESR COM
Capillary fibrosis of lung
Cirrhosis of lung (chronic) NOS
Fibrosis of lung (atrophic) (chronic) (confluent) (massive) (perialveolar) (peribronchial) NOS
Induration of lung (chronic) NOS
Postinflammatory pulmonary fibrosis
**AHA:** 2024,2Q,20

✓6th **J84.11 Idiopathic interstitial pneumonia**
EXCLUDES 1 *lymphoid interstitial pneumonia (J84.2)*
*pneumocystis pneumonia (B59)*

**J84.111 Idiopathic interstitial pneumonia, not otherwise specified** HCC Rx ESR COM

**J84.112 Idiopathic pulmonary fibrosis** HCC Rx ESR COM
Cryptogenic fibrosing alveolitis
Idiopathic fibrosing alveolitis

**J84.113 Idiopathic non-specific interstitial pneumonitis** HCC Rx ESR COM
EXCLUDES 1 *non-specific interstitial pneumonia NOS, or due to known underlying cause (J84.89)*

**J84.114 Acute interstitial pneumonitis** HCC Rx ESR COM
Hamman-Rich syndrome
EXCLUDES 1 *pneumocystis pneumonia (B59)*

**J84.115 Respiratory bronchiolitis interstitial lung disease** HCC Rx ESR COM

**J84.116 Cryptogenic organizing pneumonia** HCC Rx ESR COM
EXCLUDES 1 *organizing pneumonia NOS, or due to known underlying cause (J84.89)*

**J84.117 Desquamative interstitial pneumonia** HCC Rx ESR COM

✓6th **J84.17 Other interstitial pulmonary diseases with fibrosis in diseases classified elsewhere**
**AHA:** 2020,4Q,27-28

***J84.17Ø Interstitial lung disease with progressive fibrotic phenotype in diseases classified elsewhere*** HCC Rx ESR COM
Progressive fibrotic interstitial lung disease
Code first underlying disease, such as:
lung diseases due to external agents (J6Ø-J7Ø)
rheumatoid arthritis (MØ5.ØØ-MØ6.9)
sarcoidosis (D86.-)
systemic connective tissue disorders (M3Ø-M36)

***J84.178 Other interstitial pulmonary diseases with fibrosis in diseases classified elsewhere*** HCC Rx ESR COM
Interstitial pneumonia (nonspecific) (usual) due to collagen vascular disease
Interstitial pneumonia (nonspecific) (usual) in diseases classified elsewhere
Organizing pneumonia due to collagen vascular disease
Organizing pneumonia in diseases classified elsewhere
Code first underlying disease, such as:
progressive systemic sclerosis (M34.Ø)
rheumatoid arthritis (MØ5.ØØ-MØ6.9)
systemic lupus erythematosis (M32.Ø-M32.9)

**J84.2 Lymphoid interstitial pneumonia** HCC Rx ESR COM
Lymphoid interstitial pneumonitis

✓5th **J84.8 Other specified interstitial pulmonary diseases**
EXCLUDES 1 *exogenous lipoid pneumonia (J69.1)*
*unspecified lipoid pneumonia (J69.1)*

**J84.81 Lymphangioleiomyomatosis** HCC Rx ESR COM
Lymphangiomyomatosis

**J84.82 Adult pulmonary Langerhans cell histiocytosis** HCC Rx ESR COM A
Adult PLCH

**J84.83 Surfactant mutations of the lung** Rx ESR COM
**DEF:** Genetic disorder resulting in insufficient secretion of a complex mixture of phospholipids and proteins that reduce surface tension in the alveoli following the onset of breathing to facilitate lung expansion in the newborn. It is the leading indication for pediatric lung transplantation.

✓6th **J84.84 Other interstitial lung diseases of childhood**

**J84.841 Neuroendocrine cell hyperplasia of infancy** Rx ESR COM

**J84.842 Pulmonary interstitial glycogenosis** Rx ESR COM

**J84.843 Alveolar capillary dysplasia with vein misalignment** Rx ESR COM

**J84.848 Other interstitial lung diseases of childhood** Rx ESR COM

**J84.89 Other specified interstitial pulmonary diseases** HCC Rx ESR COM
Endogenous lipoid pneumonia
Interstitial pneumonitis
Non-specific interstitial pneumonitis NOS
Organizing pneumonia NOS
Code first, if applicable:
poisoning due to drug or toxin (T51-T65 with fifth or sixth character to indicate intent), for toxic pneumonopathy
underlying cause of pneumonopathy, if known
Use additional code, for adverse effect, to identify drug (T36-T5Ø with fifth or sixth character 5), if drug-induced
EXCLUDES 1 *cryptogenic organizing pneumonia (J84.116)*
*idiopathic non-specific interstitial pneumonitis (J84.113)*
*lipoid pneumonia, exogenous or unspecified (J69.1)*
*lymphoid interstitial pneumonia (J84.2)*
**AHA:** 2021,4Q,106; 2021,1Q,48; 2019,2Q,28

**J84.9 Interstitial pulmonary disease, unspecified** HCC Rx ESR COM
Interstitial pneumonia NOS

## Suppurative and necrotic conditions of the lower respiratory tract (J85-J86)

✓4th **J85 Abscess of lung and mediastinum**

Use additional code (B95-B97) to identify infectious agent

**J85.Ø Gangrene and necrosis of lung** HCC ESR COM

**J85.1 Abscess of lung with pneumonia** HCC ESR COM

Code also the type of pneumonia

**J85.2 Abscess of lung without pneumonia** HCC ESR COM

Abscess of lung NOS

**J85.3 Abscess of mediastinum** HCC ESR COM

✓4th **J86 Pyothorax**

Use additional code (B95-B97) to identify infectious agent

EXCLUDES 1 *abscess of lung (J85.-)*
*pyothorax due to tuberculosis (A15.6)*

**DEF:** Collection of pus in the pleural space that is commonly caused by an infection that spreads from the lung, such as bacterial pneumonia or a lung abscess.

**J86.Ø Pyothorax with fistula** HCC ESR COM

Any condition classifiable to J86.9 with fistula
Bronchocutaneous fistula
Bronchopleural fistula
Hepatopleural fistula
Mediastinal fistula
Pleural fistula
Thoracic fistula

Code also, if applicable, disruption of internal operation (surgical) wound (T81.32-)

**AHA:** 2024,3Q,4

**DEF:** Purulent infection of the respiratory cavity, with communication from a cavity to another structure.

**J86.9 Pyothorax without fistula** HCC ESR COM

Abscess of pleura
Abscess of thorax
Empyema (chest) (lung) (pleura)
Fibrinopurulent pleurisy
Purulent pleurisy
Pyopneumothorax
Septic pleurisy
Seropurulent pleurisy
Suppurative pleurisy

## Other diseases of the pleura (J9Ø-J94)

**J9Ø Pleural effusion, not elsewhere classified**

Encysted pleurisy
Pleural effusion NOS
Pleurisy with effusion (exudative) (serous)

EXCLUDES 1 *chylous (pleural) effusion (J94.Ø)*
*malignant pleural effusion (J91.Ø)*
*pleurisy NOS (RØ9.1)*
*tuberculous pleural effusion (A15.6)*

**DEF:** Collection of lymph and other fluid within the pleural space.

✓4th **J91 Pleural effusion in conditions classified elsewhere**

EXCLUDES 2 *pleural effusion in heart failure (I5Ø.-)*
*pleural effusion in systemic lupus erythematosus (M32.13)*

**DEF:** Collection of lymph and other fluid within the pleural space.

***J91.Ø Malignant pleural effusion*** HCC

Code first underlying neoplasm (CØØ-D49)

**AHA:** 2024,2Q,11; 2022,3Q,14

***J91.8 Pleural effusion in other conditions classified elsewhere***

Code first underlying disease, such as:
filariasis (B74.Ø-B74.9)
influenza (JØ9.X2, J1Ø.1, J11.1)

**AHA:** 2024,3Q,4; 2015,2Q,15

**TIP:** Assign this code as a secondary diagnosis to congestive heart failure (I5Ø.-) only if pleural effusion is specifically evaluated or treated.

**Pleural Effusion**

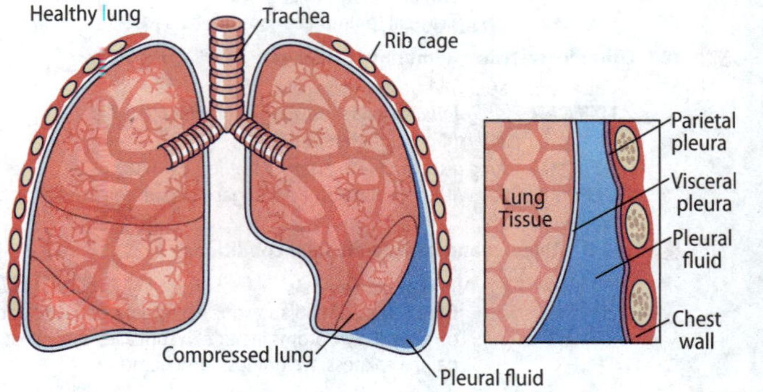


✓4th **J92 Pleural plaque**

INCLUDES pleural thickening

**DEF:** Areas of fibrous thickening that form on the parietal or visceral pleura, the membranes that line the ribs and lungs.

**J92.Ø Pleural plaque with presence of asbestos**

**J92.9 Pleural plaque without asbestos**

Pleural plaque NOS

✓4th **J93 Pneumothorax and air leak**

EXCLUDES 1 *congenital or perinatal pneumothorax (P25.1)*
*postprocedural air leak (J95.812)*
*postprocedural pneumothorax (J95.811)*
*pyopneumothorax (J86.-)*
*traumatic pneumothorax (S27.Ø)*
*tuberculous (current disease) pneumothorax (A15.-)*

**DEF:** Pneumothorax: Lung displacement due to abnormal leakage of air or gas that is trapped in the pleural space formed by the membrane that encloses the lungs and lines the thoracic cavity.

**J93.Ø Spontaneous tension pneumothorax**

**DEF:** Leaking air from the lung into the lining, causing collapse.

✓5th **J93.1 Other spontaneous pneumothorax**

**J93.11 Primary spontaneous pneumothorax**

**J93.12 Secondary spontaneous pneumothorax** UPD

Code first underlying condition, such as:
catamenial pneumothorax due to endometriosis (N8Ø.B-)
cystic fibrosis (E84.-)
eosinophilic pneumonia (J82.81-J82.82)
lymphangioleiomyomatosis (J84.81)
malignant neoplasm of bronchus and lung (C34.-)
Marfan syndrome (Q87.4-)
pneumonia due to Pneumocystis carinii (B59)
secondary malignant neoplasm of lung (C78.Ø-)
spontaneous rupture of the esophagus (K22.3)

✓5th **J93.8 Other pneumothorax and air leak**

**J93.81 Chronic pneumothorax**

**J93.82 Other air leak**

Persistent air leak

**J93.83 Other pneumothorax**

Acute pneumothorax
Spontaneous pneumothorax NOS

**AHA:** 2020,3Q,9-10

**J93.9 Pneumothorax, unspecified**

Pneumothorax NOS

✓4th **J94 Other pleural conditions**

EXCLUDES 1 *pleurisy NOS (RØ9.1)*
*traumatic hemopneumothorax (S27.2)*
*traumatic hemothorax (S27.1)*
*tuberculous pleural conditions (current disease) (A15.-)*

**J94.Ø Chylous effusion**

Chyliform effusion

**DEF:** Fluid within the pleural space due to the leaking of lymph contents into the space, usually as a result of thoracic duct damage or injury or mediastinal lymphoma.

**J94.1 Fibrothorax**
**DEF:** Fibrosis within the pleural lining of the lungs commonly seen as a stiff layer surrounding the lung typically attributed to traumatic hemothorax or pleural effusion.

**J94.2 Hemothorax**
Hemopneumothorax

**J94.8 Other specified pleural conditions**
Hydropneumothorax
Hydrothorax
**AHA:** 2024,3Q,4; 2021,1Q,48

**J94.9 Pleural condition, unspecified**

## Intraoperative and postprocedural complications and disorders of respiratory system, not elsewhere classified (J95)

✓4th **J95 Intraoperative and postprocedural complications and disorders of respiratory system, not elsewhere classified**
EXCLUDES 2 *aspiration pneumonia (J69.-)*
*emphysema (subcutaneous) resulting from a procedure (T81.82)*
*hypostatic pneumonia (J18.2)*
*pulmonary manifestations due to radiation (J70.0-J70.1)*

✓5th **J95.0 Tracheostomy complications**
**DEF:** Tracheostomy: Formation of a tracheal opening on the neck surface with tube insertion to allow for respiration in cases of obstruction or decreased patency. A tracheostomy may be planned or performed on an emergency basis for temporary or long-term use.

**Tracheostomy**

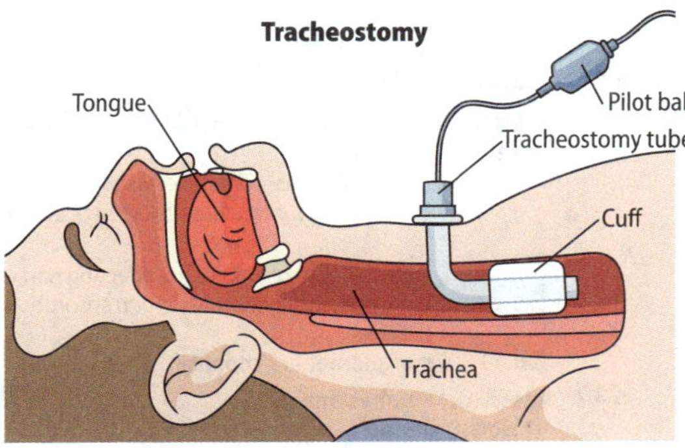


**J95.00 Unspecified tracheostomy complication** HCC ESR COM

**J95.01 Hemorrhage from tracheostomy stoma** HCC ESR COM

**J95.02 Infection of tracheostomy stoma** HCC ESR COM
Use additional code to identify type of infection, such as:
cellulitis of neck (L03.221)
sepsis (A40, A41.-)

**J95.03 Malfunction of tracheostomy stoma** HCC ESR COM
Mechanical complication of tracheostomy stoma
Obstruction of tracheostomy airway
Tracheal stenosis due to tracheostomy

**J95.04 Tracheo-esophageal fistula following tracheostomy** HCC ESR COM

**J95.09 Other tracheostomy complication** HCC ESR COM

**J95.1 Acute pulmonary insufficiency following thoracic surgery** ESR
EXCLUDES 2 *functional disturbances following cardiac surgery (I97.0, I97.1-)*

**J95.2 Acute pulmonary insufficiency following nonthoracic surgery** ESR
EXCLUDES 2 *functional disturbances following cardiac surgery (I97.0, I97.1-)*

**J95.3 Chronic pulmonary insufficiency following surgery** ESR
EXCLUDES 2 *functional disturbances following cardiac surgery (I97.0, I97.1-)*

**J95.4 Chemical pneumonitis due to anesthesia**
Mendelson's syndrome
Postprocedural aspiration pneumonia
Use additional code for adverse effect, if applicable, to identify drug (T41.- with fifth or sixth character 5)
EXCLUDES 1 *aspiration pneumonitis due to anesthesia complicating labor and delivery (O74.0)*
*aspiration pneumonitis due to anesthesia complicating pregnancy (O29)*
*aspiration pneumonitis due to anesthesia complicating the puerperium (O89.01)*

**J95.5 Postprocedural subglottic stenosis**

✓5th **J95.6 Intraoperative hemorrhage and hematoma of a respiratory system organ or structure complicating a procedure**
EXCLUDES 1 *intraoperative hemorrhage and hematoma of a respiratory system organ or structure due to accidental puncture and laceration during procedure (J95.7-)*

**J95.61 Intraoperative hemorrhage and hematoma of a respiratory system organ or structure complicating a respiratory system procedure**

**J95.62 Intraoperative hemorrhage and hematoma of a respiratory system organ or structure complicating other procedure**

✓5th **J95.7 Accidental puncture and laceration of a respiratory system organ or structure during a procedure**
EXCLUDES 2 *postprocedural pneumothorax (J95.811)*

**J95.71 Accidental puncture and laceration of a respiratory system organ or structure during a respiratory system procedure**

**J95.72 Accidental puncture and laceration of a respiratory system organ or structure during other procedure**

✓5th **J95.8 Other intraoperative and postprocedural complications and disorders of respiratory system, not elsewhere classified**
**AHA:** 2016,4Q,9-10

✓6th **J95.81 Postprocedural pneumothorax and air leak**

**J95.811 Postprocedural pneumothorax**
**AHA:** 2021,1Q,48

**J95.812 Postprocedural air leak**

✓6th **J95.82 Postprocedural respiratory failure**
EXCLUDES 1 ~~*respiratory failure in other conditions (J96.-)*~~
EXCLUDES 2 ►*respiratory failure in other conditions (J96.-)*◄

**J95.821 Acute postprocedural respiratory failure** ESR
Postprocedural respiratory failure NOS
**AHA:** 2024,4Q,19

**J95.822 Acute and chronic postprocedural respiratory failure** ESR

✓6th **J95.83 Postprocedural hemorrhage of a respiratory system organ or structure following a procedure**
**AHA:** 2023,2Q,28

**J95.830 Postprocedural hemorrhage of a respiratory system organ or structure following a respiratory system procedure**

**J95.831 Postprocedural hemorrhage of a respiratory system organ or structure following other procedure**

**J95.84 Transfusion-related acute lung injury (TRALI)**
**DEF:** Relatively rare, but serious, pulmonary complication of blood transfusion, with acute respiratory distress, noncardiogenic pulmonary edema, cyanosis, hypoxemia, hypotension, fever, and chills.

✓6th **J95.85 Complication of respirator [ventilator]**

**J95.850 Mechanical complication of respirator** HCC ESR COM
EXCLUDES 1 *encounter for respirator [ventilator] dependence during power failure (Z99.12)*

**J95.851 Ventilator associated pneumonia** HCC ESR
Ventilator associated pneumonitis
Use additional code to identify the organism, if known (B95.-, B96.-, B97.-)
EXCLUDES 1 *ventilator lung in newborn (P27.8)*
**AHA:** 2020,2Q,17; 2017,1Q,25

J95.859 Other complication of respirator [ventilator] HCC ESR COM
AHA: 2021,1Q,48

✓6th J95.86 Postprocedural hematoma and seroma of a respiratory system organ or structure following a procedure

J95.860 Postprocedural hematoma of a respiratory system organ or structure following a respiratory system procedure

J95.861 Postprocedural hematoma of a respiratory system organ or structure following other procedure

J95.862 Postprocedural seroma of a respiratory system organ or structure following a respiratory system procedure

J95.863 Postprocedural seroma of a respiratory system organ or structure following other procedure

J95.87 Transfusion-associated dyspnea (TAD)
EXCLUDES 1 *transfusion associated circulatory overload (TACO) (E87.71)*
*transfusion-related acute lung injury (TRALI) (J95.84)*
AHA: 2022,4Q,27

J95.88 Other intraoperative complications of respiratory system, not elsewhere classified

J95.89 Other postprocedural complications and disorders of respiratory system, not elsewhere classified
Use additional code to identify disorder, such as:
aspiration pneumonia (J69.-)
bacterial or viral pneumonia (J12-J18)
EXCLUDES 2 *acute pulmonary insufficiency following thoracic surgery (J95.1)*
*postprocedural subglottic stenosis (J95.5)*

## Other diseases of the respiratory system (J96-J99)

✓4th **J96 Respiratory failure, not elsewhere classified**
EXCLUDES 1 *acute respiratory distress syndrome (J80)*
*cardiorespiratory failure (R09.2)*
*newborn respiratory distress syndrome (P22.0)*
*postprocedural respiratory failure (J95.82-)*
*respiratory arrest (R09.2)*
*respiratory arrest of newborn (P28.81)*
*respiratory failure of newborn (P28.5)*
AHA: 2021,1Q,27,44-45; 2020,4Q,96

✓5th J96.0 Acute respiratory failure

J96.00 Acute respiratory failure, unspecified whether with hypoxia or hypercapnia HCC ESR COM
AHA: 2016,3Q,14; 2013,4Q,121

J96.01 Acute respiratory failure with hypoxia HCC ESR COM
AHA: 2025,3Q,11; 2024,2Q,11; 2020,3Q,12

J96.02 Acute respiratory failure with hypercapnia HCC ESR COM
Acute respiratory acidosis

✓5th J96.1 Chronic respiratory failure

J96.10 Chronic respiratory failure, unspecified whether with hypoxia or hypercapnia HCC ESR COM
AHA: 2016,1Q,38; 2015,1Q,21

J96.11 Chronic respiratory failure with hypoxia HCC ESR COM
AHA: 2013,4Q,129

J96.12 Chronic respiratory failure with hypercapnia HCC ESR COM
Chronic respiratory acidosis

✓5th J96.2 Acute and chronic respiratory failure
Acute on chronic respiratory failure
AHA: 2026,1Q,28

J96.20 Acute and chronic respiratory failure, unspecified whether with hypoxia or hypercapnia HCC ESR COM

J96.21 Acute and chronic respiratory failure with hypoxia HCC ESR COM

J96.22 Acute and chronic respiratory failure with hypercapnia HCC ESR COM

✓5th J96.9 Respiratory failure, unspecified

J96.90 Respiratory failure, unspecified, unspecified whether with hypoxia or hypercapnia HCC ESR COM

J96.91 Respiratory failure, unspecified with hypoxia HCC ESR COM

J96.92 Respiratory failure, unspecified with hypercapnia HCC ESR COM

✓4th **J98 Other respiratory disorders**
Use additional code to identify:
exposure to environmental tobacco smoke (Z77.22)
exposure to tobacco smoke in the perinatal period (P96.81)
history of tobacco dependence (Z87.891)
occupational exposure to environmental tobacco smoke (Z57.31)
tobacco dependence (F17.-)
tobacco use (Z72.0)
EXCLUDES 1 *newborn apnea (P28.4-)*
*newborn sleep apnea (P28.3-)*
EXCLUDES 2 *apnea NOS (R06.81)*
*sleep apnea (G47.3-)*

✓5th J98.0 Diseases of bronchus, not elsewhere classified

J98.01 Acute bronchospasm
EXCLUDES 1 *acute bronchiolitis with bronchospasm (J21.-)*
*acute bronchitis with bronchospasm (J20.-)*
*asthma (J45.-)*
*exercise induced bronchospasm (J45.990)*

J98.09 Other diseases of bronchus, not elsewhere classified
Broncholithiasis
Calcification of bronchus
Stenosis of bronchus
Tracheobronchial collapse
Tracheobronchial dyskinesia
Ulcer of bronchus
AHA: 2022,3Q,8

✓5th J98.1 Pulmonary collapse
EXCLUDES 1 *therapeutic collapse of lung status (Z98.3)*

J98.11 Atelectasis
EXCLUDES 1 *newborn atelectasis*
*tuberculous atelectasis (current disease) (A15)*
DEF: Collapse of lung tissue affecting part or all of one lung, preventing normal oxygen absorption to healthy tissues.

J98.19 Other pulmonary collapse

J98.2 Interstitial emphysema HCC Rx ESR COM
Mediastinal emphysema
EXCLUDES 1 *emphysema NOS (J43.9)*
*emphysema in newborn (P25.0)*
*surgical emphysema (subcutaneous) (T81.82)*
*traumatic subcutaneous emphysema (T79.7)*

J98.3 Compensatory emphysema HCC Rx ESR COM
DEF: Distention of all or part of the lung caused by disease processes or surgical intervention that decreased volume in another part of the lung, causing an overcompensation reaction. Compensatory emphysema occurs in association with pneumonias, pleural effusions, atelectasis, empyema, and pneumothorax.

J98.4 Other disorders of lung
Calcification of lung
Cystic lung disease (acquired)
Lung disease NOS
Pulmolithiasis
EXCLUDES 1 *acute interstitial pneumonitis (J84.114)*
*pulmonary insufficiency following surgery (J95.1-J95.2)*
AHA: 2025,3Q,13; 2024,2Q,20

✓5th J98.5 Diseases of mediastinum, not elsewhere classified
EXCLUDES 2 *abscess of mediastinum (J85.3)*
AHA: 2016,4Q,29

J98.51 Mediastinitis
Code first underlying condition, if applicable, such as postoperative mediastinitis (T81.-)

J98.59 Other diseases of mediastinum, not elsewhere classified
Fibrosis of mediastinum
Hernia of mediastinum
Retraction of mediastinum

J98.6 Disorders of diaphragm
Diaphragmatitis
Paralysis of diaphragm
Relaxation of diaphragm
EXCLUDES 1 *congenital malformation of diaphragm NEC (Q79.1)*
*congenital diaphragmatic hernia (Q79.0)*
EXCLUDES 2 *diaphragmatic hernia (K44.-)*

**J98.8 Other specified respiratory disorders**
AHA: 2025,2Q,7; 2020,1Q,34-36

**J98.9 Respiratory disorder, unspecified**
Respiratory disease (chronic) NOS

***J99 Respiratory disorders in diseases classified elsewhere*** HCC Rx ESR COM
Code first underlying disease, such as:
amyloidosis (E85.-)
ankylosing spondylitis (M45.-)
▶bronchomycosis (B49)◀
congenital syphilis (A5Ø.-)
cryoglobulinemia (D89.1)
early congenital syphilis (A5Ø.Ø-)
plasminogen deficiency (E88.Ø2)
schistosomiasis (B65.Ø-B65.9)

EXCLUDES 1 *respiratory disorders in:*
*amebiasis (AØ6.5)*
*blastomycosis (B4Ø.Ø-B4Ø.2)*
*candidiasis (B37.1)*
*coccidioidomycosis (B38.Ø-B38.2)*
*cystic fibrosis with pulmonary manifestations (E84.Ø)*
*dermatomyositis (M33.Ø1, M33.11)*
*histoplasmosis (B39.Ø-B39.2)*
*late syphilis (A52.72, A52.73)*
*polymyositis (M33.21)*
*Sjogren syndrome (M35.Ø2)*
*systemic lupus erythematosus (M32.13)*
*systemic sclerosis (M34.81)*
*Wegener's granulomatosis (M31.3Ø-M31.31)*

# Chapter 11. Diseases of the Digestive System (KØØ–K95)

## Chapter-specific Guidelines with Coding Examples

Reserved for future guideline expansion.

# Chapter 11. Diseases of the Digestive System (K00-K95)

EXCLUDES 2 *certain conditions originating in the perinatal period (P04-P96)*
*certain infectious and parasitic diseases (A00-B99)*
*complications of pregnancy, childbirth and the puerperium (O00-O9A)*
*congenital malformations, deformations and chromosomal abnormalities (Q00-Q99)*
*endocrine, nutritional and metabolic diseases (E00-E88)*
*injury, poisoning and certain other consequences of external causes (S00-T88)*
*neoplasms (C00-D49)*
*symptoms, signs and abnormal clinical and laboratory findings, not elsewhere classified (R00-R94)*

This chapter contains the following blocks:

K00-K14 Diseases of oral cavity and salivary glands
K20-K31 Diseases of esophagus, stomach and duodenum
K35-K38 Diseases of appendix
K40-K46 Hernia
K50-K52 Noninfective enteritis and colitis
K55-K64 Other diseases of intestines
K65-K6A Diseases of peritoneum, retroperitoneum and pelvis
K70-K77 Diseases of liver
K80-K87 Disorders of gallbladder, biliary tract and pancreas
K90-K95 Other diseases of the digestive system

## Diseases of oral cavity and salivary glands (K00-K14)

✓4th **K00 Disorders of tooth development and eruption**
EXCLUDES 2 *embedded and impacted teeth (K01.-)*

**K00.0 Anodontia**
Hypodontia
Oligodontia
EXCLUDES 1 *acquired absence of teeth (K08.1-)*
**DEF:** Partial or complete absence of teeth due to a congenital defect involving the tooth bud.

**K00.1 Supernumerary teeth**
Distomolar
Fourth molar
Mesiodens
Paramolar
Supplementary teeth
EXCLUDES 2 *supernumerary roots (K00.2)*

**K00.2 Abnormalities of size and form of teeth**
Concrescence of teeth
Dens evaginatus
Dens in dente
Dens invaginatus
Enamel pearls
Fusion of teeth
Gemination of teeth
Macrodontia
Microdontia
Peg-shaped [conical] teeth
Supernumerary roots
Taurodontism
Tuberculum paramolare
EXCLUDES 1 *abnormalities of teeth due to congenital syphilis (A50.5)*
*tuberculum Carabelli, which is regarded as a normal variation and should not be coded*

**K00.3 Mottled teeth**
Dental fluorosis
Mottling of enamel
Nonfluoride enamel opacities
EXCLUDES 2 *deposits [accretions] on teeth (K03.6)*

**K00.4 Disturbances in tooth formation**
Aplasia and hypoplasia of cementum
Dilaceration of tooth
Enamel hypoplasia (neonatal) (postnatal) (prenatal)
Regional odontodysplasia
Turner's tooth
EXCLUDES 1 *Hutchinson's teeth and mulberry molars in congenital syphilis (A50.5)*
EXCLUDES 2 *mottled teeth (K00.3)*

**K00.5 Hereditary disturbances in tooth structure, not elsewhere classified**
Amelogenesis imperfecta
Dentinal dysplasia
Dentinogenesis imperfecta
Odontogenesis imperfecta
Shell teeth

**K00.6 Disturbances in tooth eruption**
Dentia praecox
Natal tooth
Neonatal tooth
Premature eruption of tooth
Premature shedding of primary [deciduous] tooth
Prenatal teeth
Retained [persistent] primary tooth
EXCLUDES 2 *embedded and impacted teeth (K01.-)*

**K00.7 Teething syndrome**

**K00.8 Other disorders of tooth development**
Color changes during tooth formation
Intrinsic staining of teeth NOS
EXCLUDES 2 *posteruptive color changes (K03.7)*

**K00.9 Disorder of tooth development, unspecified**
Disorder of odontogenesis NOS

✓4th **K01 Embedded and impacted teeth**
EXCLUDES 1 *abnormal position of fully erupted teeth (M26.3-)*

**K01.0 Embedded teeth**

**K01.1 Impacted teeth**

✓4th **K02 Dental caries**
INCLUDES caries of dentine
dental cavities
early childhood caries
pre-eruptive caries
recurrent caries (dentino enamel junction) (enamel) (to the pulp)
tooth decay

**Tooth Anatomy**

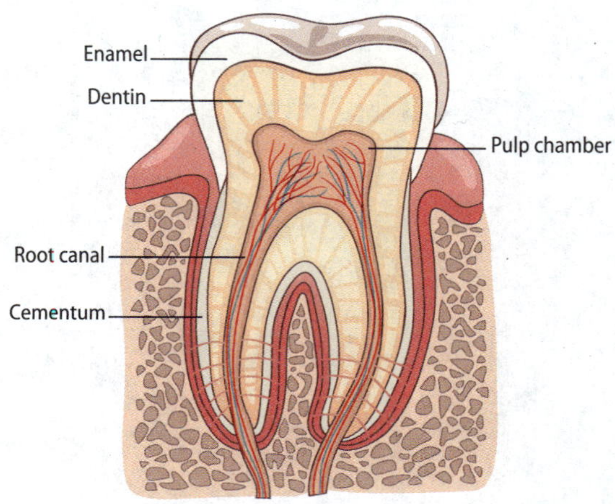


**K02.3 Arrested dental caries**
Arrested coronal and root caries

✓5th **K02.5 Dental caries on pit and fissure surface**
Dental caries on chewing surface of tooth

**K02.51 Dental caries on pit and fissure surface limited to enamel**
White spot lesions [initial caries] on pit and fissure surface of tooth

**K02.52 Dental caries on pit and fissure surface penetrating into dentin**
Primary dental caries, cervical origin

**K02.53 Dental caries on pit and fissure surface penetrating into pulp**

✓5th **K02.6 Dental caries on smooth surface**

**K02.61 Dental caries on smooth surface limited to enamel**
White spot lesions [initial caries] on smooth surface of tooth

**K02.62 Dental caries on smooth surface penetrating into dentin**

**K02.63 Dental caries on smooth surface penetrating into pulp**

**K02.7 Dental root caries**

**K02.9 Dental caries, unspecified**

**KØ3 Other diseases of hard tissues of teeth**

EXCLUDES 2 *bruxism (F45.8)*
*dental caries (KØ2.-)*
*teeth-grinding NOS (F45.8)*

**KØ3.Ø Excessive attrition of teeth**
Approximal wear of teeth
Occlusal wear of teeth
**DEF:** Attrition: In dentistry, wearing away or erosion of tooth surface from abrasive food or grinding teeth.

**KØ3.1 Abrasion of teeth**
Dentifrice abrasion of teeth
Habitual abrasion of teeth
Occupational abrasion of teeth
Ritual abrasion of teeth
Traditional abrasion of teeth
Wedge defect NOS

**KØ3.2 Erosion of teeth**
Erosion of teeth due to diet
Erosion of teeth due to drugs and medicaments
Erosion of teeth due to persistent vomiting
Erosion of teeth NOS
Idiopathic erosion of teeth
Occupational erosion of teeth

**KØ3.3 Pathological resorption of teeth**
Internal granuloma of pulp
Resorption of teeth (external)

**KØ3.4 Hypercementosis**
Cementation hyperplasia

**KØ3.5 Ankylosis of teeth**

**KØ3.6 Deposits [accretions] on teeth**
Betel deposits [accretions] on teeth
Black deposits [accretions] on teeth
Extrinsic staining of teeth NOS
Green deposits [accretions] on teeth
Materia alba deposits [accretions] on teeth
Orange deposits [accretions] on teeth
Staining of teeth NOS
Subgingival dental calculus
Supragingival dental calculus
Tobacco deposits [accretions] on teeth

**KØ3.7 Posteruptive color changes of dental hard tissues**
EXCLUDES 2 *deposits [accretions] on teeth (KØ3.6)*

**KØ3.8 Other specified diseases of hard tissues of teeth**

**KØ3.81 Cracked tooth**
EXCLUDES 1 *asymptomatic craze lines in enamel - omit code*
*broken or fractured tooth due to trauma (SØ2.5)*

**KØ3.89 Other specified diseases of hard tissues of teeth**

**KØ3.9 Disease of hard tissues of teeth, unspecified**

**KØ4 Diseases of pulp and periapical tissues**
**AHA:** 2016,4Q,29-30

**KØ4.Ø Pulpitis**
Acute pulpitis
Chronic (hyperplastic) (ulcerative) pulpitis

**KØ4.Ø1 Reversible pulpitis**

**KØ4.Ø2 Irreversible pulpitis**

**KØ4.1 Necrosis of pulp**
Pulpal gangrene

**KØ4.2 Pulp degeneration**
Denticles
Pulpal calcifications
Pulpal stones

**KØ4.3 Abnormal hard tissue formation in pulp**
Secondary or irregular dentine

**KØ4.4 Acute apical periodontitis of pulpal origin**
Acute apical periodontitis NOS
EXCLUDES 1 *acute periodontitis (KØ5.2-)*
**DEF:** Severe inflammation of the area surrounding the tip of a tooth's root that is often secondary to infection or trauma.

**KØ4.5 Chronic apical periodontitis**
Apical or periapical granuloma
Apical periodontitis NOS
EXCLUDES 1 *chronic periodontitis (KØ5.3-)*

**KØ4.6 Periapical abscess with sinus**
Dental abscess with sinus
Dentoalveolar abscess with sinus

**KØ4.7 Periapical abscess without sinus**
Dental abscess without sinus
Dentoalveolar abscess without sinus

**KØ4.8 Radicular cyst**
Apical (periodontal) cyst
Periapical cyst
Residual radicular cyst
EXCLUDES 2 *lateral periodontal cyst (KØ9.Ø)*
**DEF:** Most common odontogenic cyst in tissue around the tooth apex due to chronic inflammation of dental pulp.

**KØ4.9 Other and unspecified diseases of pulp and periapical tissues**

**KØ4.9Ø Unspecified diseases of pulp and periapical tissues**

**KØ4.99 Other diseases of pulp and periapical tissues**

**KØ5 Gingivitis and periodontal diseases**
Use additional code to identify:
alcohol abuse and dependence (F1Ø.-)
exposure to environmental tobacco smoke (Z77.22)
exposure to tobacco smoke in the perinatal period (P96.81)
history of tobacco dependence (Z87.891)
occupational exposure to environmental tobacco smoke (Z57.31)
tobacco dependence (F17.-)
tobacco use (Z72.Ø)
**AHA:** 2016,4Q,29-30

**KØ5.Ø Acute gingivitis**
EXCLUDES 1 *acute necrotizing ulcerative gingivitis (A69.1)*
*herpesviral [herpes simplex] gingivostomatitis (BØØ.2)*

**KØ5.ØØ Acute gingivitis, plaque induced**
Acute gingivitis NOS
Plaque induced gingival disease

**KØ5.Ø1 Acute gingivitis, non-plaque induced**

**KØ5.1 Chronic gingivitis**
Desquamative gingivitis (chronic)
Gingivitis (chronic) NOS
Hyperplastic gingivitis (chronic)
Pregnancy associated gingivitis
Simple marginal gingivitis (chronic)
Ulcerative gingivitis (chronic)
Code first, if applicable, diseases of the digestive system complicating pregnacy (O99.61-)

**KØ5.1Ø Chronic gingivitis, plaque induced**
Chronic gingivitis NOS
Gingivitis NOS

**KØ5.11 Chronic gingivitis, non-plaque induced**

**KØ5.2 Aggressive periodontitis**
Acute pericoronitis
EXCLUDES 1 *acute apical periodontitis (KØ4.4)*
*periapical abscess (KØ4.7)*
*periapical abscess with sinus (KØ4.6)*

**KØ5.2Ø Aggressive periodontitis, unspecified**

**KØ5.21 Aggressive periodontitis, localized**
Periodontal abscess

**KØ5.211 Aggressive periodontitis, localized, slight**

**KØ5.212 Aggressive periodontitis, localized, moderate**

**KØ5.213 Aggressive periodontitis, localized, severe**

**KØ5.219 Aggressive periodontitis, localized, unspecified severity**

**KØ5.22 Aggressive periodontitis, generalized**

**KØ5.221 Aggressive periodontitis, generalized, slight**

**KØ5.222 Aggressive periodontitis, generalized, moderate**

**KØ5.223 Aggressive periodontitis, generalized, severe**

**KØ5.229 Aggressive periodontitis, generalized, unspecified severity**

**KØ5.3 Chronic periodontitis**
Chronic pericoronitis
Complex periodontitis
Periodontitis NOS
Simplex periodontitis
EXCLUDES 1 *chronic apical periodontitis (KØ4.5)*

**KØ5.3Ø Chronic periodontitis, unspecified**

**KØ5.31 Chronic periodontitis, localized**

**KØ5.311 Chronic periodontitis, localized, slight**

**KØ5.312 Chronic periodontitis, localized, moderate**

**KØ5.313 Chronic periodontitis, localized, severe**

**KØ5.319 Chronic periodontitis, localized, unspecified severity**

✓6th KØ5.32 **Chronic periodontitis, generalized**
- KØ5.321 **Chronic periodontitis, generalized, slight**
- KØ5.322 **Chronic periodontitis, generalized, moderate**
- KØ5.323 **Chronic periodontitis, generalized, severe**
- KØ5.329 **Chronic periodontitis, generalized, unspecified severity**

KØ5.4 **Periodontosis**
Juvenile periodontosis

KØ5.5 **Other periodontal diseases**
Combined periodontic-endodontic lesion
Narrow gingival width (of periodontal soft tissue)
EXCLUDES 2 *leukoplakia of gingiva (K13.21)*

KØ5.6 **Periodontal disease, unspecified**

✓4th **KØ6 Other disorders of gingiva and edentulous alveolar ridge**

EXCLUDES 2 *acute gingivitis (KØ5.Ø)*
*atrophy of edentulous alveolar ridge (KØ8.2)*
*chronic gingivitis (KØ5.1)*
*gingivitis NOS (KØ5.1)*

AHA: 2016,4Q,29-30

✓5th KØ6.Ø **Gingival recession**
Gingival recession (postinfective) (postprocedural)
AHA: 2017,4Q,16

✓6th KØ6.Ø1 **Gingival recession, localized**
- KØ6.Ø1Ø **Localized gingival recession, unspecified**
  Localized gingival recession, NOS
- KØ6.Ø11 **Localized gingival recession, minimal**
- KØ6.Ø12 **Localized gingival recession, moderate**
- KØ6.Ø13 **Localized gingival recession, severe**

✓6th KØ6.Ø2 **Gingival recession, generalized**
- KØ6.Ø2Ø **Generalized gingival recession, unspecified**
  Generalized gingival recession, NOS
- KØ6.Ø21 **Generalized gingival recession, minimal**
- KØ6.Ø22 **Generalized gingival recession, moderate**
- KØ6.Ø23 **Generalized gingival recession, severe**

KØ6.1 **Gingival enlargement**
Gingival fibromatosis

KØ6.2 **Gingival and edentulous alveolar ridge lesions associated with trauma**
Irritative hyperplasia of edentulous ridge [denture hyperplasia]
Use additional code (Chapter 2Ø) to identify external cause or denture status (Z97.2)

KØ6.3 **Horizontal alveolar bone loss**

KØ6.8 **Other specified disorders of gingiva and edentulous alveolar ridge**
Fibrous epulis
Flabby alveolar ridge
Giant cell epulis
Peripheral giant cell granuloma of gingiva
Pyogenic granuloma of gingiva
Vertical ridge deficiency
EXCLUDES 2 *gingival cyst (KØ9.Ø)*

KØ6.9 **Disorder of gingiva and edentulous alveolar ridge, unspecified**

✓4th **KØ8 Other disorders of teeth and supporting structures**

EXCLUDES 2 *dentofacial anomalies [including malocclusion] (M26.-)*
*disorders of jaw (M27.-)*

AHA: 2016,4Q,29-30

KØ8.Ø **Exfoliation of teeth due to systemic causes**
Code also underlying systemic condition

✓5th KØ8.1 **Complete loss of teeth**
Acquired loss of teeth, complete
EXCLUDES 1 *congenital absence of teeth (KØØ.Ø)*
*exfoliation of teeth due to systemic causes (KØ8.Ø)*
*partial loss of teeth (KØ8.4-)*

✓6th KØ8.1Ø **Complete loss of teeth, unspecified cause**
- KØ8.1Ø1 **Complete loss of teeth, unspecified cause, class I**
- KØ8.1Ø2 **Complete loss of teeth, unspecified cause, class II**
- KØ8.1Ø3 **Complete loss of teeth, unspecified cause, class III**
- KØ8.1Ø4 **Complete loss of teeth, unspecified cause, class IV**
- KØ8.1Ø9 **Complete loss of teeth, unspecified cause, unspecified class**
  Edentulism NOS

✓6th KØ8.11 **Complete loss of teeth due to trauma**
- KØ8.111 **Complete loss of teeth due to trauma, class I**
- KØ8.112 **Complete loss of teeth due to trauma, class II**
- KØ8.113 **Complete loss of teeth due to trauma, class III**
- KØ8.114 **Complete loss of teeth due to trauma, class IV**
- KØ8.119 **Complete loss of teeth due to trauma, unspecified class**

✓6th KØ8.12 **Complete loss of teeth due to periodontal diseases**
- KØ8.121 **Complete loss of teeth due to periodontal diseases, class I**
- KØ8.122 **Complete loss of teeth due to periodontal diseases, class II**
- KØ8.123 **Complete loss of teeth due to periodontal diseases, class III**
- KØ8.124 **Complete loss of teeth due to periodontal diseases, class IV**
- KØ8.129 **Complete loss of teeth due to periodontal diseases, unspecified class**

✓6th KØ8.13 **Complete loss of teeth due to caries**
- KØ8.131 **Complete loss of teeth due to caries, class I**
- KØ8.132 **Complete loss of teeth due to caries, class II**
- KØ8.133 **Complete loss of teeth due to caries, class III**
- KØ8.134 **Complete loss of teeth due to caries, class IV**
- KØ8.139 **Complete loss of teeth due to caries, unspecified class**

✓6th KØ8.19 **Complete loss of teeth due to other specified cause**
- KØ8.191 **Complete loss of teeth due to other specified cause, class I**
- KØ8.192 **Complete loss of teeth due to other specified cause, class II**
- KØ8.193 **Complete loss of teeth due to other specified cause, class III**
- KØ8.194 **Complete loss of teeth due to other specified cause, class IV**
- KØ8.199 **Complete loss of teeth due to other specified cause, unspecified class**

✓5th KØ8.2 **Atrophy of edentulous alveolar ridge**
- KØ8.2Ø **Unspecified atrophy of edentulous alveolar ridge**
  Atrophy of the mandible NOS
  Atrophy of the maxilla NOS
- KØ8.21 **Minimal atrophy of the mandible**
  Minimal atrophy of the edentulous mandible
- KØ8.22 **Moderate atrophy of the mandible**
  Moderate atrophy of the edentulous mandible
- KØ8.23 **Severe atrophy of the mandible**
  Severe atrophy of the edentulous mandible
- KØ8.24 **Minimal atrophy of maxilla**
  Minimal atrophy of the edentulous maxilla
- KØ8.25 **Moderate atrophy of the maxilla**
  Moderate atrophy of the edentulous maxilla
- KØ8.26 **Severe atrophy of the maxilla**
  Severe atrophy of the edentulous maxilla

KØ8.3 **Retained dental root**

✓5th KØ8.4 **Partial loss of teeth**
Acquired loss of teeth, partial
EXCLUDES 1 *complete loss of teeth (KØ8.1-)*
*congenital absence of teeth (KØØ.Ø)*
EXCLUDES 2 *exfoliation of teeth due to systemic causes (KØ8.Ø)*

✓6th KØ8.4Ø **Partial loss of teeth, unspecified cause**
- KØ8.4Ø1 **Partial loss of teeth, unspecified cause, class I**
- KØ8.4Ø2 **Partial loss of teeth, unspecified cause, class II**
- KØ8.4Ø3 **Partial loss of teeth, unspecified cause, class III**
- KØ8.4Ø4 **Partial loss of teeth, unspecified cause, class IV**
- KØ8.4Ø9 **Partial loss of teeth, unspecified cause, unspecified class**
  Tooth extraction status NOS

✓6th KØ8.41 **Partial loss of teeth due to trauma**
- KØ8.411 **Partial loss of teeth due to trauma, class I**

K08.412 **Partial loss of teeth due to trauma, class II**
K08.413 **Partial loss of teeth due to trauma, class III**
K08.414 **Partial loss of teeth due to trauma, class IV**
K08.419 **Partial loss of teeth due to trauma, unspecified class**

✓6th K08.42 **Partial loss of teeth due to periodontal diseases**
K08.421 **Partial loss of teeth due to periodontal diseases, class I**
K08.422 **Partial loss of teeth due to periodontal diseases, class II**
K08.423 **Partial loss of teeth due to periodontal diseases, class III**
K08.424 **Partial loss of teeth due to periodontal diseases, class IV**
K08.429 **Partial loss of teeth due to periodontal diseases, unspecified class**

✓6th K08.43 **Partial loss of teeth due to caries**
K08.431 **Partial loss of teeth due to caries, class I**
K08.432 **Partial loss of teeth due to caries, class II**
K08.433 **Partial loss of teeth due to caries, class III**
K08.434 **Partial loss of teeth due to caries, class IV**
K08.439 **Partial loss of teeth due to caries, unspecified class**

✓6th K08.49 **Partial loss of teeth due to other specified cause**
K08.491 **Partial loss of teeth due to other specified cause, class I**
K08.492 **Partial loss of teeth due to other specified cause, class II**
K08.493 **Partial loss of teeth due to other specified cause, class III**
K08.494 **Partial loss of teeth due to other specified cause, class IV**
K08.499 **Partial loss of teeth due to other specified cause, unspecified class**

✓5th K08.5 **Unsatisfactory restoration of tooth**
Defective bridge, crown, filling
Defective dental restoration
EXCLUDES 1 *dental restoration status (Z98.811)*
EXCLUDES 2 *endosseous dental implant failure (M27.6-)*
*unsatisfactory endodontic treatment (M27.5-)*

K08.50 **Unsatisfactory restoration of tooth, unspecified**
Defective dental restoration NOS
K08.51 **Open restoration margins of tooth**
Dental restoration failure of marginal integrity
Open margin on tooth restoration
Poor gingival margin to tooth restoration
K08.52 **Unrepairable overhanging of dental restorative materials**
Overhanging of tooth restoration

✓6th K08.53 **Fractured dental restorative material**
EXCLUDES 1 *cracked tooth (K03.81)*
*traumatic fracture of tooth (S02.5)*
K08.530 **Fractured dental restorative material without loss of material**
K08.531 **Fractured dental restorative material with loss of material**
K08.539 **Fractured dental restorative material, unspecified**

K08.54 **Contour of existing restoration of tooth biologically incompatible with oral health**
Dental restoration failure of periodontal anatomical integrity
Unacceptable contours of existing restoration of tooth
Unacceptable morphology of existing restoration of tooth
K08.55 **Allergy to existing dental restorative material**
Use additional code to identify the specific type of allergy
K08.56 **Poor aesthetic of existing restoration of tooth**
Dental restoration aesthetically inadequate or displeasing
K08.59 **Other unsatisfactory restoration of tooth**
Other defective dental restoration

✓5th K08.8 **Other specified disorders of teeth and supporting structures**
K08.81 **Primary occlusal trauma**
K08.82 **Secondary occlusal trauma**
K08.89 **Other specified disorders of teeth and supporting structures**
Enlargement of alveolar ridge NOS
Insufficient anatomic crown height
Insufficient clinical crown length
Irregular alveolar process
Toothache NOS

K08.9 **Disorder of teeth and supporting structures, unspecified**

✓4th K09 **Cysts of oral region, not elsewhere classified**
INCLUDES lesions showing histological features both of aneurysmal cyst and of another fibro-osseous lesion
EXCLUDES 2 *cysts of jaw (M27.0-, M27.4-)*
*radicular cyst (K04.8)*

K09.0 **Developmental odontogenic cysts**
Dentigerous cyst
Eruption cyst
Follicular cyst
Gingival cyst
Lateral periodontal cyst
Primordial cyst
EXCLUDES 2 *keratocysts (D16.4, D16.5)*
*odontogenic keratocystic tumors (D16.4, D16.5)*
K09.1 **Developmental (nonodontogenic) cysts of oral region**
Cyst (of) incisive canal
Cyst (of) palatine of papilla
Globulomaxillary cyst
Median palatal cyst
Nasoalveolar cyst
Nasolabial cyst
Nasopalatine duct cyst
K09.8 **Other cysts of oral region, not elsewhere classified**
Dermoid cyst
Epidermoid cyst
Epstein's pearl
Lymphoepithelial cyst
K09.9 **Cyst of oral region, unspecified**

✓4th K11 **Diseases of salivary glands**
Use additional code to identify:
alcohol abuse and dependence (F10.-)
exposure to environmental tobacco smoke (Z77.22)
exposure to tobacco smoke in the perinatal period (P96.81)
history of tobacco dependence (Z87.891)
occupational exposure to environmental tobacco smoke (Z57.31)
tobacco dependence (F17.-)
tobacco use (Z72.0)

K11.0 **Atrophy of salivary gland**
K11.1 **Hypertrophy of salivary gland**
**DEF:** Overgrowth of or enlarged salivary gland tissue caused by infection, salivary duct blockage, autoimmune diseases, and benign and malignant tumors.

✓5th K11.2 **Sialoadenitis**
Parotitis
EXCLUDES 1 *epidemic parotitis (B26.-)*
*mumps (B26.-)*
*uveoparotid fever [Heerfordt] (D86.89)*
**DEF:** Inflammation of the salivary gland.
K11.20 **Sialoadenitis, unspecified**
K11.21 **Acute sialoadenitis**
EXCLUDES 1 *acute recurrent sialoadenitis (K11.22)*
K11.22 **Acute recurrent sialoadenitis**
K11.23 **Chronic sialoadenitis**

K11.3 **Abscess of salivary gland**
K11.4 **Fistula of salivary gland**
EXCLUDES 1 *congenital fistula of salivary gland (Q38.4)*
K11.5 **Sialolithiasis**
Calculus of salivary gland or duct
Stone of salivary gland or duct
K11.6 **Mucocele of salivary gland**
Mucous extravasation cyst of salivary gland
Mucous retention cyst of salivary gland
Ranula
K11.7 **Disturbances of salivary secretion**
Hypoptyalism
Ptyalism
Xerostomia
EXCLUDES 2 *dry mouth NOS (R68.2)*

**K11.8 Other diseases of salivary glands**
Benign lymphoepithelial lesion of salivary gland
Mikulicz' disease
Necrotizing sialometaplasia
Sialectasia
Stenosis of salivary duct
Stricture of salivary duct
EXCLUDES 1 *Sjogren syndrome (M35.Ø-)*

**K11.9 Disease of salivary gland, unspecified**
Sialoadenopathy NOS

**✓4th K12 Stomatitis and related lesions**
Use additional code to identify:
alcohol abuse and dependence (F1Ø.-)
exposure to environmental tobacco smoke (Z77.22)
exposure to tobacco smoke in the perinatal period (P96.81)
history of tobacco dependence (Z87.891)
occupational exposure to environmental tobacco smoke (Z57.31)
tobacco dependence (F17.-)
tobacco use (Z72.Ø)
EXCLUDES 1 *cancrum oris (A69.Ø)*
*cheilitis (K13.Ø)*
*gangrenous stomatitis (A69.Ø)*
*herpesviral [herpes simplex] gingivostomatitis (BØØ.2)*
*noma (A69.Ø)*

**K12.Ø Recurrent oral aphthae**
Aphthous stomatitis (major) (minor)
Bednar's aphthae
Periadenitis mucosa necrotica recurrens
Recurrent aphthous ulcer
Stomatitis herpetiformis
**DEF:** Disorder of unknown etiology with small oval or round painful ulcers of the mouth marked by a grayish exudate and a red halo effect.

**K12.1 Other forms of stomatitis**
Denture stomatitis
Stomatitis NOS
Ulcerative stomatitis
Vesicular stomatitis
EXCLUDES 1 *acute necrotizing ulcerative stomatitis (A69.1)*
*Vincent's stomatitis (A69.1)*

**K12.2 Cellulitis and abscess of mouth**
Cellulitis of mouth (floor)
Submandibular abscess
EXCLUDES 2 *abscess of salivary gland (K11.3)*
*abscess of tongue (K14.Ø)*
*periapical abscess (KØ4.6-KØ4.7)*
*periodontal abscess (KØ5.21)*
*peritonsillar abscess (J36)*

**✓5th K12.3 Oral mucositis (ulcerative)**
Mucositis (oral) (oropharyneal)
EXCLUDES 2 *gastrointestinal mucositis (ulcerative) (K92.81)*
*mucositis (ulcerative) of vagina and vulva (N76.81)*
*nasal mucositis (ulcerative) (J34.81)*

**K12.3Ø Oral mucositis (ulcerative), unspecified**

**K12.31 Oral mucositis (ulcerative) due to antineoplastic therapy**
Use additional code for adverse effect, if applicable, to identify antineoplastic and immunosuppressive drugs (T45.1X5)
Use additional code for other antineoplastic therapy, such as:
radiological procedure and radiotherapy (Y84.2)

**K12.32 Oral mucositis (ulcerative) due to other drugs**
Use additional code for adverse effect, if applicable, to identify drug (T36-T5Ø with fifth or sixth character 5)

**K12.33 Oral mucositis (ulcerative) due to radiation**
Use additional external cause code (W88-W9Ø, X39.Ø-) to identify cause

**K12.39 Other oral mucositis (ulcerative)**
Viral oral mucositis (ulcerative)

**✓4th K13 Other diseases of lip and oral mucosa**
INCLUDES epithelial disturbances of tongue
Use additional code to identify:
alcohol abuse and dependence (F1Ø.-)
exposure to environmental tobacco smoke (Z77.22)
exposure to tobacco smoke in the perinatal period (P96.81)
history of tobacco dependence (Z87.891)
occupational exposure to environmental tobacco smoke (Z57.31)
tobacco dependence (F17.-)
tobacco use (Z72.Ø)
EXCLUDES 2 *certain disorders of gingiva and edentulous alveolar ridge (KØ5-KØ6)*
*cysts of oral region (KØ9.-)*
*diseases of tongue (K14.-)*
*stomatitis and related lesions (K12.-)*

**K13.Ø Diseases of lips**
Abscess of lips
Angular cheilitis
Cellulitis of lips
Cheilitis NOS
Cheilodynia
Cheilosis
Exfoliative cheilitis
Fistula of lips
Glandular cheilitis
Hypertrophy of lips
Perlèche NEC
EXCLUDES 1 *ariboflavinosis (E53.Ø)*
*cheilitis due to radiation-related disorders (L55-L59)*
*congenital fistula of lips (Q38.Ø)*
*congenital hypertrophy of lips (Q18.6)*
*perlèche due to candidiasis (B37.83)*
*perlèche due to riboflavin deficiency (E53.Ø)*

**K13.1 Cheek and lip biting**

**✓5th K13.2 Leukoplakia and other disturbances of oral epithelium, including tongue**
EXCLUDES 1 *carcinoma in situ of oral epithelium (DØØ.Ø-)*
*hairy leukoplakia (K13.3)*
**DEF:** Leukoplakia: Thickened white patches or lesions appearing on a mucous membrane, such as oral mucosa or tongue.

**K13.21 Leukoplakia of oral mucosa, including tongue**
Leukokeratosis of oral mucosa
Leukoplakia of gingiva, lips, tongue
EXCLUDES 1 *hairy leukoplakia (K13.3)*
*leukokeratosis nicotina palati (K13.24)*

**K13.22 Minimal keratinized residual ridge mucosa**
Minimal keratinization of alveolar ridge mucosa

**K13.23 Excessive keratinized residual ridge mucosa**
Excessive keratinization of alveolar ridge mucosa

**K13.24 Leukokeratosis nicotina palati**
Smoker's palate

**K13.29 Other disturbances of oral epithelium, including tongue**
Erythroplakia of mouth or tongue
Focal epithelial hyperplasia of mouth or tongue
Leukoedema of mouth or tongue
Other oral epithelium disturbances

**K13.3 Hairy leukoplakia**

**K13.4 Granuloma and granuloma-like lesions of oral mucosa**
Eosinophilic granuloma
Granuloma pyogenicum
Verrucous xanthoma

**K13.5 Oral submucous fibrosis**
Submucous fibrosis of tongue

**K13.6 Irritative hyperplasia of oral mucosa**
EXCLUDES 2 *irritative hyperplasia of edentulous ridge [denture hyperplasia] (KØ6.2)*

**✓5th K13.7 Other and unspecified lesions of oral mucosa**

**K13.7Ø Unspecified lesions of oral mucosa**

**K13.79 Other lesions of oral mucosa**
Focal oral mucinosis
**AHA:** 2022,2Q,7

**K14 Diseases of tongue**

Use additional code to identify:
alcohol abuse and dependence (F10.-)
exposure to environmental tobacco smoke (Z77.22)
history of tobacco dependence (Z87.891)
occupational exposure to environmental tobacco smoke (Z57.31)
tobacco dependence (F17.-)
tobacco use (Z72.0)

EXCLUDES 2 *erythroplakia (K13.29)*
*focal epithelial hyperplasia (K13.29)*
*hairy leukoplakia (K13.3)*
*leukoedema of tongue (K13.29)*
*leukoplakia of tongue (K13.21)*
*macroglossia (congenital) (Q38.2)*
*submucous fibrosis of tongue (K13.5)*

**K14.0 Glossitis**
Abscess of tongue
Ulceration (traumatic) of tongue
EXCLUDES 1 *atrophic glossitis (K14.4)*
**DEF:** Inflammation and swelling of the tongue that may be associated with infection, adverse drug reactions, smoking, or injury.

**K14.1 Geographic tongue**
Benign migratory glossitis
Glossitis areata exfoliativa

**K14.2 Median rhomboid glossitis**

**K14.3 Hypertrophy of tongue papillae**
Black hairy tongue
Coated tongue
Hypertrophy of foliate papillae
Lingua villosa nigra

**K14.4 Atrophy of tongue papillae**
Atrophic glossitis

**K14.5 Plicated tongue**
Fissured tongue
Furrowed tongue
Scrotal tongue
EXCLUDES 1 *fissured tongue, congenital (Q38.3)*

**K14.6 Glossodynia**
Glossopyrosis
Painful tongue

**K14.8 Other diseases of tongue**
Atrophy of tongue
Crenated tongue
Enlargement of tongue
Glossocele
Glossoptosis
Hypertrophy of tongue

**K14.9 Disease of tongue, unspecified**
Glossopathy NOS

## Diseases of esophagus, stomach and duodenum (K20-K31)

EXCLUDES 2 *hiatus hernia (K44.-)*

**K20 Esophagitis**

Use additional code to identify:
alcohol abuse and dependence (F10.-)

EXCLUDES 1 *erosion of esophagus (K22.1-)*
*esophagitis with gastro-esophageal reflux disease (K21.0-)*
*reflux esophagitis (K21.0-)*
*ulcerative esophagitis (K22.1-)*

EXCLUDES 2 *eosinophilic gastritis or gastroenteritis (K52.81)*

**AHA:** 2023,1Q,20

**K20.0 Eosinophilic esophagitis**
**AHA:** 2020,4Q,9

**K20.8 Other esophagitis**
**AHA:** 2020,4Q,28-29

**K20.80 Other esophagitis without bleeding**
Abscess of esophagus
Other esophagitis NOS

**K20.81 Other esophagitis with bleeding**

**K20.9 Esophagitis, unspecified**
**AHA:** 2020,4Q,28-29

**K20.90 Esophagitis, unspecified without bleeding**
Esophagitis NOS

**K20.91 Esophagitis, unspecified with bleeding**

**K21 Gastro-esophageal reflux disease**

EXCLUDES 1 *newborn esophageal reflux (P78.83)*

**K21.0 Gastro-esophageal reflux disease with esophagitis**
**AHA:** 2020,4Q,28-29

**K21.00 Gastro-esophageal reflux disease with esophagitis, without bleeding**
Reflux esophagitis

**K21.01 Gastro-esophageal reflux disease with esophagitis, with bleeding**

**K21.9 Gastro-esophageal reflux disease without esophagitis**
Esophageal reflux NOS
**AHA:** 2016,1Q,18

**K22 Other diseases of esophagus**

EXCLUDES 2 *esophageal varices (I85.-)*

**K22.0 Achalasia of cardia**
Achalasia NOS
Cardiospasm
EXCLUDES 1 *congenital cardiospasm (Q39.5)*
**DEF:** Esophageal motility disorder that is caused by absence of the esophageal peristalsis and impaired relaxation of the lower esophageal sphincter. It is characterized by dysphagia, regurgitation, and heartburn.

**K22.1 Ulcer of esophagus**
Barrett's ulcer
Erosion of esophagus
Fungal ulcer of esophagus
Peptic ulcer of esophagus
Ulcer of esophagus due to ingestion of chemicals
Ulcer of esophagus due to ingestion of drugs and medicaments
Ulcerative esophagitis
Code first poisoning due to drug or toxin, if applicable (T36-T65 with fifth or sixth character 1-4)
Use additional code for adverse effect, if applicable, to identify drug (T36-T50 with fifth or sixth character 5)
EXCLUDES 1 *Barrett's esophagus (K22.7-)*
**AHA:** 2018,3Q,22; 2017,3Q,27
**TIP:** Assign a code for "with bleeding" when an esophageal ulcer and bleeding (hematemesis) are documented. The ICD-10-CM classification assumes the two are related without the provider linking the two conditions. Evidence of bleeding during a procedure is not required.

**K22.10 Ulcer of esophagus without bleeding**
Ulcer of esophagus NOS

**K22.11 Ulcer of esophagus with bleeding**
EXCLUDES 2 *bleeding esophageal varices (I85.01, I85.11)*
**AHA:** 2023,1Q,20
**TIP:** For bleeding esophageal ulcers resulting from anticoagulant therapy, assign this code, code D68.32 Hemorrhagic disorder due to extrinsic circulating anticoagulant, and adverse effect code T45.515- with the appropriate seventh character.

**K22.2 Esophageal obstruction**
Compression of esophagus
Constriction of esophagus
Stenosis of esophagus
Stricture of esophagus
EXCLUDES 1 *congenital stenosis or stricture of esophagus (Q39.3)*

**K22.3 Perforation of esophagus**
Rupture of esophagus
EXCLUDES 1 *traumatic perforation of (thoracic) esophagus (S27.8-)*

**K22.4 Dyskinesia of esophagus**
Corkscrew esophagus
Diffuse esophageal spasm
Spasm of esophagus
EXCLUDES 1 *cardiospasm (K22.0)*
**AHA:** 2025,2Q,17

**K22.5 Diverticulum of esophagus, acquired**
Esophageal pouch, acquired
EXCLUDES 1 *diverticulum of esophagus (congenital) (Q39.6)*

**K22.6 Gastro-esophageal laceration-hemorrhage syndrome**
Mallory-Weiss syndrome

✓5th **K22.7 Barrett's esophagus**
Barrett's disease
Barrett's syndrome
EXCLUDES 1 *Barrett's ulcer (K22.1)*
*malignant neoplasm of esophagus (C15.-)*
**DEF:** Metaplastic disorder in which specialized columnar epithelial cells replace the normal squamous epithelial cells. Secondary to chronic gastroesophageal reflux damage to the mucosa, this disorder increases the risk of developing adenocarcinoma.

**K22.70 Barrett's esophagus without dysplasia** Q
Barrett's esophagus NOS

✓6th **K22.71 Barrett's esophagus with dysplasia**
**K22.710 Barrett's esophagus with low grade dysplasia** Q
**K22.711 Barrett's esophagus with high grade dysplasia** Q
**K22.719 Barrett's esophagus with dysplasia, unspecified** Q

✓5th **K22.8 Other specified diseases of esophagus**
EXCLUDES 2 *esophageal varices (I85.-)*
*Paterson-Kelly syndrome (D50.1)*
**AHA:** 2021,4Q,15; 2020,1Q,16

**K22.81 Esophageal polyp**
EXCLUDES 1 *benign neoplasm of esophagus (D13.0)*

**K22.82 Esophagogastric junction polyp**
EXCLUDES 1 *benign neoplasm of stomach (D13.1)*

**K22.89 Other specified disease of esophagus**
Hemorrhage of esophagus NOS
**AHA:** 2026,2Q,16; 2024,2Q,26
**TIP:** Use this code to report lichen planus of esophagus (ELP).

**K22.9 Disease of esophagus, unspecified**

***K23 Disorders of esophagus in diseases classified elsewhere***
Code first underlying disease, such as:
congenital syphilis (A50.5)
EXCLUDES 1 *late syphilis (A52.79)*
*megaesophagus due to Chagas' disease (B57.31)*
*tuberculosis (A18.83)*

✓4th **K25 Gastric ulcer**
INCLUDES erosion (acute) of stomach
pylorus ulcer (peptic)
stomach ulcer (peptic)
Use additional code to identify:
alcohol abuse and dependence (F10.-)
EXCLUDES 1 *acute gastritis (K29.0-)*
*peptic ulcer NOS (K27.-)*
**AHA:** 2021,1Q,9,11; 2017,3Q,27
**TIP:** Assign a code for "with hemorrhage" when a gastric ulcer and GI bleeding are documented. The ICD-10-CM classification assumes the two are related without the provider linking the two conditions. Evidence of bleeding during a procedure is not required.
**TIP:** For bleeding ulcers resulting from anticoagulant therapy, assign the appropriate "with hemorrhage" ulcer code from this category, code D68.32 Hemorrhagic disorder due to extrinsic circulating anticoagulant, and adverse effect code T45.515- with the appropriate seventh character.

**K25.0 Acute gastric ulcer with hemorrhage**
**AHA:** 2023,1Q,16
**K25.1 Acute gastric ulcer with perforation** HCC ESR COM
**K25.2 Acute gastric ulcer with both hemorrhage and perforation** HCC ESR COM
**K25.3 Acute gastric ulcer without hemorrhage or perforation**
**K25.4 Chronic or unspecified gastric ulcer with hemorrhage**
**K25.5 Chronic or unspecified gastric ulcer with perforation** HCC ESR COM
**K25.6 Chronic or unspecified gastric ulcer with both hemorrhage and perforation** HCC ESR COM
**K25.7 Chronic gastric ulcer without hemorrhage or perforation**
**K25.9 Gastric ulcer, unspecified as acute or chronic, without hemorrhage or perforation**

**Gastrointestinal Ulcers**

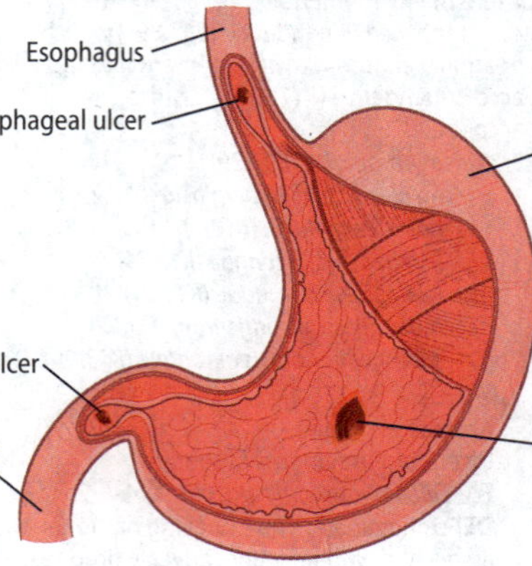


✓4th **K26 Duodenal ulcer**
INCLUDES duodenum ulcer (peptic)
erosion (acute) of duodenum
postpyloric ulcer (peptic)
Use additional code to identify:
alcohol abuse and dependence (F10.-)
EXCLUDES 1 *peptic ulcer NOS (K27.-)*
**AHA:** 2023,2Q,11; 2017,3Q,27
**TIP:** Assign a code for "with hemorrhage" when a duodenal ulcer and GI bleeding are documented. The ICD-10-CM classification assumes the two are related without the provider linking the two conditions. Evidence of bleeding during a procedure is not required.
**TIP:** For bleeding ulcers resulting from anticoagulant therapy, assign the appropriate "with hemorrhage" ulcer code from this category, code D68.32 Hemorrhagic disorder due to extrinsic circulating anticoagulant, and adverse effect code T45.515- with the appropriate seventh character.

**K26.0 Acute duodenal ulcer with hemorrhage**
**K26.1 Acute duodenal ulcer with perforation** HCC ESR COM
**K26.2 Acute duodenal ulcer with both hemorrhage and perforation** HCC ESR COM
**K26.3 Acute duodenal ulcer without hemorrhage or perforation**
**K26.4 Chronic or unspecified duodenal ulcer with hemorrhage**
**AHA:** 2016,1Q,14
**K26.5 Chronic or unspecified duodenal ulcer with perforation** HCC ESR COM
**K26.6 Chronic or unspecified duodenal ulcer with both hemorrhage and perforation** HCC ESR COM
**K26.7 Chronic duodenal ulcer without hemorrhage or perforation**
**K26.9 Duodenal ulcer, unspecified as acute or chronic, without hemorrhage or perforation**

✓4th **K27 Peptic ulcer, site unspecified**
INCLUDES gastroduodenal ulcer NOS
peptic ulcer NOS
Use additional code to identify:
alcohol abuse and dependence (F10.-)
EXCLUDES 1 *peptic ulcer of newborn (P78.82)*
**AHA:** 2017,3Q,27
**TIP:** Assign a code for "with hemorrhage" when a peptic ulcer and GI bleeding are documented. The ICD-10-CM classification assumes the two are related without the provider linking the two conditions. Evidence of bleeding during a procedure is not required.
**TIP:** For bleeding ulcers resulting from anticoagulant therapy, assign the appropriate "with hemorrhage" ulcer code from this category, code D68.32 Hemorrhagic disorder due to extrinsic circulating anticoagulant, and adverse effect code T45.515- with the appropriate seventh character.

**K27.0 Acute peptic ulcer, site unspecified, with hemorrhage**
**K27.1 Acute peptic ulcer, site unspecified, with perforation** HCC ESR COM
**K27.2 Acute peptic ulcer, site unspecified, with both hemorrhage and perforation** HCC ESR COM
**K27.3 Acute peptic ulcer, site unspecified, without hemorrhage or perforation**
**K27.4 Chronic or unspecified peptic ulcer, site unspecified, with hemorrhage**
**K27.5 Chronic or unspecified peptic ulcer, site unspecified, with perforation** HCC ESR COM
**K27.6 Chronic or unspecified peptic ulcer, site unspecified, with both hemorrhage and perforation** HCC ESR COM

K27.7 Chronic peptic ulcer, site unspecified, without hemorrhage or perforation

K27.9 Peptic ulcer, site unspecified, unspecified as acute or chronic, without hemorrhage or perforation

✓4th **K28 Gastrojejunal ulcer**

INCLUDES anastomotic ulcer (peptic) or erosion
gastrocolic ulcer (peptic) or erosion
gastrointestinal ulcer (peptic) or erosion
gastrojejunal ulcer (peptic) or erosion
jejunal ulcer (peptic) or erosion
marginal ulcer (peptic) or erosion
stomal ulcer (peptic) or erosion

Use additional code to identify:
alcohol abuse and dependence (F10.-)

EXCLUDES 1 *primary ulcer of small intestine (K63.3)*

**AHA:** 2017,3Q,27

**TIP:** Assign a code for "with hemorrhage" when a gastrojejunal ulcer and GI bleeding are documented. The ICD-10-CM classification assumes the two are related without the provider linking the two conditions. Evidence of bleeding during a procedure is not required.

**TIP:** For bleeding ulcers resulting from anticoagulant therapy, assign the appropriate "with hemorrhage" ulcer code from this category, code D68.32 Hemorrhagic disorder due to extrinsic circulating anticoagulant, and adverse effect code T45.515- with the appropriate seventh character.

K28.0 Acute gastrojejunal ulcer with hemorrhage

K28.1 Acute gastrojejunal ulcer with perforation HCC ESR COM

K28.2 Acute gastrojejunal ulcer with both hemorrhage and perforation HCC ESR COM

K28.3 Acute gastrojejunal ulcer without hemorrhage or perforation

K28.4 Chronic or unspecified gastrojejunal ulcer with hemorrhage
**AHA:** 2023,3Q,10

K28.5 Chronic or unspecified gastrojejunal ulcer with perforation HCC ESR COM

K28.6 Chronic or unspecified gastrojejunal ulcer with both hemorrhage and perforation HCC ESR COM

K28.7 Chronic gastrojejunal ulcer without hemorrhage or perforation

K28.9 Gastrojejunal ulcer, unspecified as acute or chronic, without hemorrhage or perforation

✓4th **K29 Gastritis and duodenitis**

EXCLUDES 1 *eosinophilic gastritis or gastroenteritis (K52.81)*
*Zollinger-Ellison syndrome (E16.4)*

**AHA:** 2018,3Q,22

**TIP:** Assign a code for "with bleeding" when gastritis or duodenitis and GI bleeding are documented. The ICD-10-CM classification assumes the two are related without the provider linking the two conditions. Evidence of bleeding during a procedure is not required.

**TIP:** For bleeding ulcers resulting from anticoagulant therapy, assign the appropriate "with hemorrhage" ulcer code from this category, code D68.32 Hemorrhagic disorder due to extrinsic circulating anticoagulant, and adverse effect code T45.515- with the appropriate seventh character.

✓5th K29.0 Acute gastritis
Use additional code to identify:
alcohol abuse and dependence (F10.-)
EXCLUDES 1 *erosion (acute) of stomach (K25.-)*

K29.00 Acute gastritis without bleeding
K29.01 Acute gastritis with bleeding

✓5th K29.2 Alcoholic gastritis
Use additional code to identify:
alcohol abuse and dependence (F10.-)

K29.20 Alcoholic gastritis without bleeding
K29.21 Alcoholic gastritis with bleeding

✓5th K29.3 Chronic superficial gastritis
K29.30 Chronic superficial gastritis without bleeding
K29.31 Chronic superficial gastritis with bleeding

✓5th K29.4 Chronic atrophic gastritis
Gastric atrophy
K29.40 Chronic atrophic gastritis without bleeding
K29.41 Chronic atrophic gastritis with bleeding

✓5th K29.5 Unspecified chronic gastritis
Chronic antral gastritis
Chronic fundal gastritis
K29.50 Unspecified chronic gastritis without bleeding
K29.51 Unspecified chronic gastritis with bleeding

✓5th K29.6 Other gastritis
Giant hypertrophic gastritis
Granulomatous gastritis
Menetrier's disease
K29.60 Other gastritis without bleeding
K29.61 Other gastritis with bleeding

✓5th K29.7 Gastritis, unspecified
K29.70 Gastritis, unspecified, without bleeding
K29.71 Gastritis, unspecified, with bleeding

✓5th K29.8 Duodenitis
K29.80 Duodenitis without bleeding
**AHA:** 2025,2Q,5
K29.81 Duodenitis with bleeding

✓5th K29.9 Gastroduodenitis, unspecified
K29.90 Gastroduodenitis, unspecified, without bleeding
K29.91 Gastroduodenitis, unspecified, with bleeding

**K30 Functional dyspepsia**
Indigestion
EXCLUDES 1 *dyspepsia NOS (R10.13)*
*heartburn (R12)*
*nervous dyspepsia (F45.8)*
*neurotic dyspepsia (F45.8)*
*psychogenic dyspepsia (F45.8)*

✓4th **K31 Other diseases of stomach and duodenum**

INCLUDES functional disorders of stomach

EXCLUDES 2 *diabetic gastroparesis (E08.43, E09.43, E10.43, E11.43, E13.43)*
*diverticulum of duodenum (K57.00-K57.13)*

K31.0 Acute dilatation of stomach
Acute distention of stomach

K31.1 Adult hypertrophic pyloric stenosis COM A
▶Acquired hypertrophic pyloric stenosis◀
▶Adult pyloric stenosis◀
Pyloric stenosis NOS
EXCLUDES 1 ▶*congenital pyloric stenosis*◀ *(Q40.0)*
**AHA:** 2023,3Q,11

● K31.B Hypertrophic pyloric stenosis, in childhood
Infantile hypertrophic pyloric stenosis
Pediatric hypertrophic pyloric stenosis
Pediatric pyloric stenosis
EXCLUDES 1 *congenital pyloric stenosis (Q40.0)*

K31.2 Hourglass stricture and stenosis of stomach
EXCLUDES 1 *congenital hourglass stomach (Q40.2)*
*hourglass contraction of stomach (K31.89)*

K31.3 Pylorospasm, not elsewhere classified COM
EXCLUDES 1 *congenital or infantile pylorospasm (Q40.0)*
*neurotic pylorospasm (F45.8)*
*psychogenic pylorospasm (F45.8)*

K31.4 Gastric diverticulum
EXCLUDES 1 *congenital diverticulum of stomach (Q40.2)*

K31.5 Obstruction of duodenum COM
Constriction of duodenum
Duodenal ileus (chronic)
Stenosis of duodenum
Stricture of duodenum
Volvulus of duodenum
EXCLUDES 1 *congenital stenosis of duodenum (Q41.0)*

K31.6 Fistula of stomach and duodenum
Gastrocolic fistula
Gastrojejunocolic fistula
Code also, if applicable, disruption of internal operation (surgical) wound (T81.32-)

K31.7 Polyp of stomach and duodenum
EXCLUDES 1 *adenomatous polyp of stomach (D13.1)*
**AHA:** 2020,1Q,16

✓5th K31.8 Other specified diseases of stomach and duodenum

✓6th K31.81 Angiodysplasia of stomach and duodenum
**TIP:** Assign a code for "with bleeding" when angiodysplasia of the stomach or the duodenum and GI bleeding are documented. The ICD-10-CM classification assumes the two are related without the provider linking the two conditions. Evidence of bleeding during a procedure is not required.

K31.811 Angiodysplasia of stomach and duodenum with bleeding
**AHA:** 2023,1Q,16

K31.819 Angiodysplasia of stomach and duodenum without bleeding
Angiodysplasia of stomach and duodenum NOS

**K31.82 Dieulafoy lesion (hemorrhagic) of stomach and duodenum**
EXCLUDES 2 *Dieulafoy lesion of intestine (K63.81)*
**DEF:** Abnormally large submucosal artery protruding through a defect in the stomach mucosa or intestines that can cause massive and life-threatening hemorrhaging.

**K31.83 Achlorhydria**
**DEF:** Absence of hydrochloric acid in gastric secretions due to gastric mucosa atrophy. Achlorhydria is unresponsive to histamines.

**K31.84 Gastroparesis**
Gastroparalysis
Code first underlying disease, if known, such as:
anorexia nervosa (F50.0-)
diabetes mellitus (E08.43, E09.43, E10.43, E11.43, E13.43)
scleroderma (M34.-)
**AHA:** 2026,1Q,25; 2013,4Q,114

**K31.89 Other diseases of stomach and duodenum**
**AHA:** 2024,2Q,26; 2020,1Q,15; 2017,1Q,28

**K31.9 Disease of stomach and duodenum, unspecified**

✓5th **K31.A Gastric intestinal metaplasia**
**AHA:** 2021,4Q,15-16

**K31.A0 Gastric intestinal metaplasia, unspecified**
Gastric intestinal metaplasia indefinite for dysplasia
Gastric intestinal metaplasia NOS

✓6th **K31.A1 Gastric intestinal metaplasia without dysplasia**
**K31.A11 Gastric intestinal metaplasia without dysplasia, involving the antrum**
**K31.A12 Gastric intestinal metaplasia without dysplasia, involving the body (corpus)**
**K31.A13 Gastric intestinal metaplasia without dysplasia, involving the fundus**
**K31.A14 Gastric intestinal metaplasia without dysplasia, involving the cardia**
**K31.A15 Gastric intestinal metaplasia without dysplasia, involving multiple sites**
**K31.A19 Gastric intestinal metaplasia without dysplasia, unspecified site**

✓6th **K31.A2 Gastric intestinal metaplasia with dysplasia**
**K31.A21 Gastric intestinal metaplasia with low grade dysplasia**
**K31.A22 Gastric intestinal metaplasia with high grade dysplasia**
**K31.A29 Gastric intestinal metaplasia with dysplasia, unspecified**

## Diseases of appendix (K35-K38)

✓4th **K35 Acute appendicitis**
**AHA:** 2018,4Q,17-18

✓5th **K35.2 Acute appendicitis with generalized peritonitis**
**AHA:** 2023,4Q,28-29

✓6th **K35.20 Acute appendicitis with generalized peritonitis, without abscess**
**K35.200 Acute appendicitis with generalized peritonitis, without perforation or abscess**
(Acute) appendicitis with generalized peritonitis without rupture or perforation of appendix NOS
**K35.201 Acute appendicitis with generalized peritonitis, with perforation, without abscess**
Appendicitis (acute) with generalized (diffuse) peritonitis following rupture or perforation of appendix NOS
**K35.209 Acute appendicitis with generalized peritonitis, without abscess, unspecified as to perforation**
(Acute) appendicitis with generalized peritonitis NOS

✓6th **K35.21 Acute appendicitis with generalized peritonitis, with abscess**
**K35.210 Acute appendicitis with generalized peritonitis, without perforation, with abscess**
(Acute) appendicitis with generalized peritonitis without rupture or perforation of appendix, with abscess
**K35.211 Acute appendicitis with generalized peritonitis, with perforation and abscess**
Appendicitis (acute) with generalized (diffuse) peritonitis following rupture or perforation of appendix, with abscess
**K35.219 Acute appendicitis with generalized peritonitis, with abscess, unspecified as to perforation**
(Acute) appendicitis with generalized peritonitis and abscess NOS

✓5th **K35.3 Acute appendicitis with localized peritonitis**
**K35.30 Acute appendicitis with localized peritonitis, without perforation or gangrene**
Acute appendicitis with localized peritonitis NOS
**K35.31 Acute appendicitis with localized peritonitis and gangrene, without perforation**
**K35.32 Acute appendicitis with perforation, localized peritonitis, and gangrene, without abscess**
(Acute) appendicitis with perforation NOS
Perforated appendix NOS
Ruptured appendix (with localized peritonitis) NOS
**AHA:** 2020,1Q,16
**K35.33 Acute appendicitis with perforation, localized peritonitis, and gangrene, with abscess**
(Acute) appendicitis with (peritoneal) abscess NOS
Ruptured appendix with localized peritonitis and abscess

✓5th **K35.8 Other and unspecified acute appendicitis**
**K35.80 Unspecified acute appendicitis**
Acute appendicitis NOS
Acute appendicitis without (localized) (generalized) peritonitis

✓6th **K35.89 Other acute appendicitis**
**AHA:** 2020,1Q,16
**K35.890 Other acute appendicitis without perforation or gangrene**
**K35.891 Other acute appendicitis without perforation, with gangrene**
(Acute) appendicitis with gangrene NOS

**K36 Other appendicitis**
Chronic appendicitis
Recurrent appendicitis

**K37 Unspecified appendicitis**
EXCLUDES 1 *unspecified appendicitis with peritonitis (K35.2-, K35.3-)*

✓4th **K38 Other diseases of appendix**
**K38.0 Hyperplasia of appendix**
**K38.1 Appendicular concretions**
Fecalith of appendix
Stercolith of appendix
**K38.2 Diverticulum of appendix**
**K38.3 Fistula of appendix**
**K38.8 Other specified diseases of appendix**
Intussusception of appendix
**K38.9 Disease of appendix, unspecified**

## Hernia (K40-K46)

NOTE Hernia with both gangrene and obstruction is classified to hernia with gangrene.

INCLUDES acquired hernia
congenital [except diaphragmatic or hiatus] hernia
recurrent hernia

**AHA:** 2021,3Q,30-31

**TIP:** Do not assign a code for bilateral hernia when the right and left sides have differing pathology. For example, two codes would be assigned for bilateral femoral hernia in which the left side is incarcerated (with obstruction) but the right side is not incarcerated; the code for bilateral would not apply in this case.

### ✓4th K40 Inguinal hernia

INCLUDES bubonocele
direct inguinal hernia
double inguinal hernia
indirect inguinal hernia
inguinal hernia NOS
oblique inguinal hernia
scrotal hernia

**DEF:** Within the groin region.

✓5th **K40.0 Bilateral inguinal hernia, with obstruction, without gangrene**
Incarcerated inguinal hernia (bilateral) without gangrene
Inguinal hernia (bilateral) causing obstruction without gangrene
Irreducible inguinal hernia (bilateral) without gangrene
Strangulated inguinal hernia (bilateral) without gangrene

**K40.00 Bilateral inguinal hernia, with obstruction, without gangrene, not specified as recurrent**
Bilateral inguinal hernia, with obstruction, without gangrene NOS

**K40.01 Bilateral inguinal hernia, with obstruction, without gangrene, recurrent**

✓5th **K40.1 Bilateral inguinal hernia, with gangrene**

**K40.10 Bilateral inguinal hernia, with gangrene, not specified as recurrent**
Bilateral inguinal hernia, with gangrene NOS

**K40.11 Bilateral inguinal hernia, with gangrene, recurrent**

✓5th **K40.2 Bilateral inguinal hernia, without obstruction or gangrene**

**K40.20 Bilateral inguinal hernia, without obstruction or gangrene, not specified as recurrent**
Bilateral inguinal hernia NOS

**K40.21 Bilateral inguinal hernia, without obstruction or gangrene, recurrent**

✓5th **K40.3 Unilateral inguinal hernia, with obstruction, without gangrene**
Incarcerated inguinal hernia (unilateral) without gangrene
Inguinal hernia (unilateral) causing obstruction without gangrene
Irreducible inguinal hernia (unilateral) without gangrene
Strangulated inguinal hernia (unilateral) without gangrene

**K40.30 Unilateral inguinal hernia, with obstruction, without gangrene, not specified as recurrent**
Inguinal hernia, with obstruction NOS
Unilateral inguinal hernia, with obstruction, without gangrene NOS

**K40.31 Unilateral inguinal hernia, with obstruction, without gangrene, recurrent**

✓5th **K40.4 Unilateral inguinal hernia, with gangrene**

**K40.40 Unilateral inguinal hernia, with gangrene, not specified as recurrent**
Inguinal hernia with gangrene NOS
Unilateral inguinal hernia with gangrene NOS

**K40.41 Unilateral inguinal hernia, with gangrene, recurrent**

✓5th **K40.9 Unilateral inguinal hernia, without obstruction or gangrene**

**K40.90 Unilateral inguinal hernia, without obstruction or gangrene, not specified as recurrent**
Inguinal hernia NOS
Unilateral inguinal hernia NOS

**K40.91 Unilateral inguinal hernia, without obstruction or gangrene, recurrent**

**Hernia Sites**

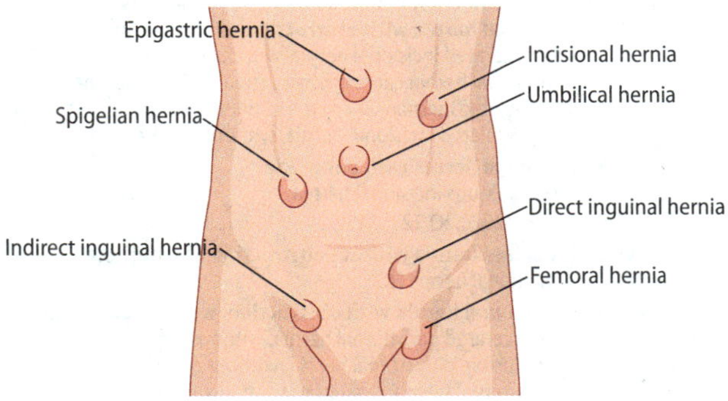


### ✓4th K41 Femoral hernia

✓5th **K41.0 Bilateral femoral hernia, with obstruction, without gangrene**
Femoral hernia (bilateral) causing obstruction, without gangrene
Incarcerated femoral hernia (bilateral), without gangrene
Irreducible femoral hernia (bilateral), without gangrene
Strangulated femoral hernia (bilateral), without gangrene

**K41.00 Bilateral femoral hernia, with obstruction, without gangrene, not specified as recurrent**
Bilateral femoral hernia, with obstruction, without gangrene NOS

**K41.01 Bilateral femoral hernia, with obstruction, without gangrene, recurrent**

✓5th **K41.1 Bilateral femoral hernia, with gangrene**

**K41.10 Bilateral femoral hernia, with gangrene, not specified as recurrent**
Bilateral femoral hernia, with gangrene NOS

**K41.11 Bilateral femoral hernia, with gangrene, recurrent**

✓5th **K41.2 Bilateral femoral hernia, without obstruction or gangrene**

**K41.20 Bilateral femoral hernia, without obstruction or gangrene, not specified as recurrent**
Bilateral femoral hernia NOS

**K41.21 Bilateral femoral hernia, without obstruction or gangrene, recurrent**

✓5th **K41.3 Unilateral femoral hernia, with obstruction, without gangrene**
Femoral hernia (unilateral) causing obstruction, without gangrene
Incarcerated femoral hernia (unilateral), without gangrene
Irreducible femoral hernia (unilateral), without gangrene
Strangulated femoral hernia (unilateral), without gangrene

**K41.30 Unilateral femoral hernia, with obstruction, without gangrene, not specified as recurrent**
Femoral hernia, with obstruction NOS
Unilateral femoral hernia, with obstruction NOS

**K41.31 Unilateral femoral hernia, with obstruction, without gangrene, recurrent**

✓5th **K41.4 Unilateral femoral hernia, with gangrene**

**K41.40 Unilateral femoral hernia, with gangrene, not specified as recurrent**
Femoral hernia, with gangrene NOS
Unilateral femoral hernia, with gangrene NOS

**K41.41 Unilateral femoral hernia, with gangrene, recurrent**

✓5th **K41.9 Unilateral femoral hernia, without obstruction or gangrene**

**K41.90 Unilateral femoral hernia, without obstruction or gangrene, not specified as recurrent**
Femoral hernia NOS
Unilateral femoral hernia NOS

**K41.91 Unilateral femoral hernia, without obstruction or gangrene, recurrent**

### ✓4th K42 Umbilical hernia

INCLUDES paraumbilical hernia
EXCLUDES 1 *omphalocele (Q79.2)*

**K42.0 Umbilical hernia with obstruction, without gangrene**
Incarcerated umbilical hernia, without gangrene
Irreducible umbilical hernia, without gangrene
Strangulated umbilical hernia, without gangrene
Umbilical hernia causing obstruction, without gangrene

**K42.1 Umbilical hernia with gangrene**
Gangrenous umbilical hernia

**K42.9 Umbilical hernia without obstruction or gangrene**
Umbilical hernia NOS

✓4th **K43 Ventral hernia**

**DEF:** Condition in which a loop of bowel protrudes through a weakness in the abdominal wall muscles that may occur as a birth defect, past surgical site (incisional), or form at a stomal site (parastomal).

**K43.Ø Incisional hernia with obstruction, without gangrene**
- Incarcerated incisional hernia, without gangrene
- Incisional hernia causing obstruction, without gangrene
- Irreducible incisional hernia, without gangrene
- Strangulated incisional hernia, without gangrene

**K43.1 Incisional hernia with gangrene**
- Gangrenous incisional hernia
- **AHA:** 2020,2Q,22

**K43.2 Incisional hernia without obstruction or gangrene**
- Incisional hernia NOS

**K43.3 Parastomal hernia with obstruction, without gangrene**
- Incarcerated parastomal hernia, without gangrene
- Irreducible parastomal hernia, without gangrene
- Parastomal hernia causing obstruction, without gangrene
- Strangulated parastomal hernia, without gangrene

**K43.4 Parastomal hernia with gangrene**
- Gangrenous parastomal hernia

**K43.5 Parastomal hernia without obstruction or gangrene**
- Parastomal hernia NOS

**K43.6 Other and unspecified ventral hernia with obstruction, without gangrene**
- Epigastric hernia causing obstruction, without gangrene
- Hypogastric hernia causing obstruction, without gangrene
- Incarcerated epigastric hernia without gangrene
- Incarcerated hypogastric hernia without gangrene
- Incarcerated midline hernia without gangrene
- Incarcerated spigelian hernia without gangrene
- Incarcerated subxiphoid hernia without gangrene
- Irreducible epigastric hernia without gangrene
- Irreducible hypogastric hernia without gangrene
- Irreducible midline hernia without gangrene
- Irreducible spigelian hernia without gangrene
- Irreducible subxiphoid hernia without gangrene
- Midline hernia causing obstruction, without gangrene
- Spigelian hernia causing obstruction, without gangrene
- Strangulated epigastric hernia without gangrene
- Strangulated hypogastric hernia without gangrene
- Strangulated midline hernia without gangrene
- Strangulated spigelian hernia without gangrene
- Strangulated subxiphoid hernia without gangrene
- Subxiphoid hernia causing obstruction, without gangrene

**K43.7 Other and unspecified ventral hernia with gangrene**
- Any condition listed under K43.6 specified as gangrenous

**K43.9 Ventral hernia without obstruction or gangrene**
- Epigastric hernia
- Ventral hernia NOS

✓4th **K44 Diaphragmatic hernia**

INCLUDES hiatus hernia (esophageal) (sliding)
paraesophageal hernia

EXCLUDES 1 *congenital diaphragmatic hernia (Q79.Ø)*
*congenital hiatus hernia (Q4Ø.1)*

**DEF:** Protrusion of an abdominal organ, usually the stomach, through the esophageal opening within the diaphragm and occurring in two types: the sliding hiatal hernia and the paraesophageal hernia.

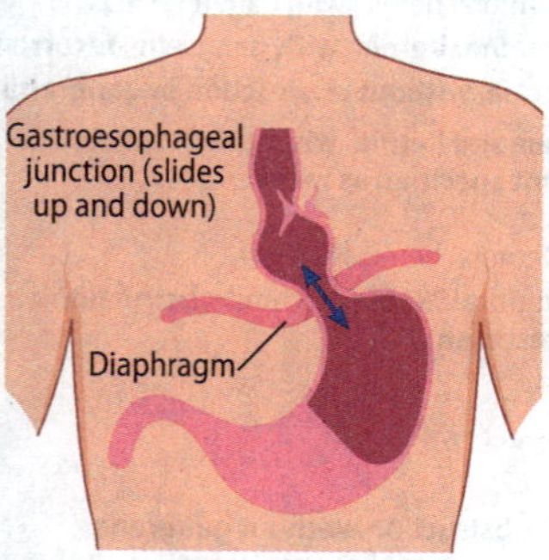

Sliding hiatal hernia

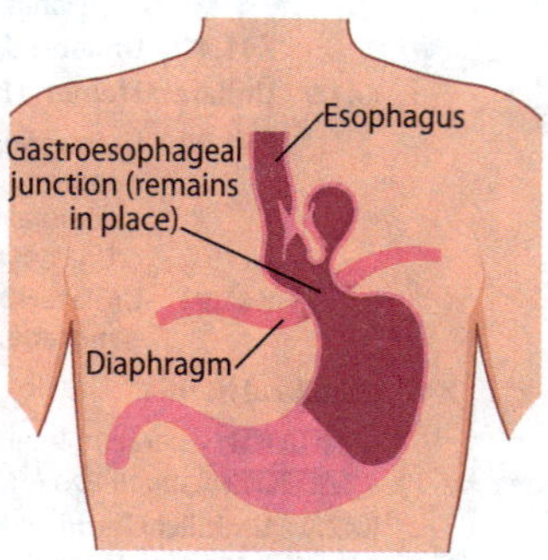

Paraesophageal hiatal hernia

**K44.Ø Diaphragmatic hernia with obstruction, without gangrene**
- Diaphragmatic hernia causing obstruction
- Incarcerated diaphragmatic hernia
- Irreducible diaphragmatic hernia
- Strangulated diaphragmatic hernia
- **AHA:** 2022,2Q,13

**K44.1 Diaphragmatic hernia with gangrene**
- Gangrenous diaphragmatic hernia

**K44.9 Diaphragmatic hernia without obstruction or gangrene**
- Diaphragmatic hernia NOS

✓4th **K45 Other abdominal hernia**

INCLUDES abdominal hernia, specified site NEC
lumbar hernia
obturator hernia
pudendal hernia
retroperitoneal hernia
sciatic hernia

**K45.Ø Other specified abdominal hernia with obstruction, without gangrene**
- Other specified abdominal hernia causing obstruction
- Other specified incarcerated abdominal hernia
- Other specified irreducible abdominal hernia
- Other specified strangulated abdominal hernia

**K45.1 Other specified abdominal hernia with gangrene**
- Any condition listed under K45 specified as gangrenous
- **AHA:** 2024,2Q,22

**K45.8 Other specified abdominal hernia without obstruction or gangrene**

✓4th **K46 Unspecified abdominal hernia**

INCLUDES enterocele
epiplocele
hernia NOS
interstitial hernia
intestinal hernia
intra-abdominal hernia

EXCLUDES 1 *vaginal enterocele (N81.5)*

**K46.Ø Unspecified abdominal hernia with obstruction, without gangrene**
- Unspecified abdominal hernia causing obstruction
- Unspecified incarcerated abdominal hernia
- Unspecified irreducible abdominal hernia
- Unspecified strangulated abdominal hernia

**K46.1 Unspecified abdominal hernia with gangrene**
- Any condition listed under K46 specified as gangrenous

**K46.9 Unspecified abdominal hernia without obstruction or gangrene**
- Abdominal hernia NOS

## Noninfective enteritis and colitis (K5Ø-K52)

INCLUDES noninfective inflammatory bowel disease

EXCLUDES 1 *irritable bowel syndrome (K58.-)*
*megacolon (K59.3-)*

✓4th **K5Ø Crohn's disease [regional enteritis]**

INCLUDES granulomatous enteritis

Use additional code to identify any associated fistulas, if applicable:
Use additional code to identify manifestations, such as:
- anal fistula (K6Ø.3-)
- anorectal fistula (K6Ø.5-)
- pyoderma gangrenosum (L88)
- rectal fistula (K6Ø.4-)

EXCLUDES 1 *ulcerative colitis (K51.-)*

**AHA:** 2026,2Q,9; 2019,3Q,5; 2012,4Q,104

**DEF:** Chronic inflammation of the gastrointestinal tract characterized by chronic granulomatous disease, most commonly affecting the intestines and the terminal ileum.

✓5th **K5Ø.Ø Crohn's disease of small intestine**
- Crohn's disease [regional enteritis] of duodenum
- Crohn's disease [regional enteritis] of ileum
- Crohn's disease [regional enteritis] of jejunum
- Regional ileitis
- Terminal ileitis

EXCLUDES 1 *Crohn's disease of both small and large intestine (K5Ø.8-)*

**K5Ø.ØØ Crohn's disease of small intestine without complications** HCC Rx ESR COM

✓6th **K5Ø.Ø1 Crohn's disease of small intestine with complications**

**K5Ø.Ø11 Crohn's disease of small intestine with rectal bleeding** HCC Rx ESR COM

**K5Ø.Ø12 Crohn's disease of small intestine with intestinal obstruction** HCC Rx ESR COM

**K5Ø.Ø13 Crohn's disease of small intestine with fistula** HCC Rx ESR COM

**K5Ø.Ø14 Crohn's disease of small intestine with abscess** HCC Rx ESR COM
- **AHA:** 2012,4Q,104

K50.018 Crohn's disease of small intestine with other complication HCC Rx ESR COM

K50.019 Crohn's disease of small intestine with unspecified complications HCC Rx ESR COM

✓5th K50.1 Crohn's disease of large intestine

Crohn's disease [regional enteritis] of colon
Crohn's disease [regional enteritis] of large bowel
Crohn's disease [regional enteritis] of rectum
Granulomatous colitis
Regional colitis

EXCLUDES 1 *Crohn's disease of both small and large intestine (K50.8)*

K50.10 Crohn's disease of large intestine without complications HCC Rx ESR COM

✓6th K50.11 Crohn's disease of large intestine with complications

K50.111 Crohn's disease of large intestine with rectal bleeding HCC Rx ESR COM

K50.112 Crohn's disease of large intestine with intestinal obstruction HCC Rx ESR COM

K50.113 Crohn's disease of large intestine with fistula HCC Rx ESR COM

K50.114 Crohn's disease of large intestine with abscess HCC Rx ESR COM

K50.118 Crohn's disease of large intestine with other complication HCC Rx ESR COM

K50.119 Crohn's disease of large intestine with unspecified complications HCC Rx ESR COM

✓5th K50.8 Crohn's disease of both small and large intestine

K50.80 Crohn's disease of both small and large intestine without complications HCC Rx ESR COM

✓6th K50.81 Crohn's disease of both small and large intestine with complications

K50.811 Crohn's disease of both small and large intestine with rectal bleeding HCC Rx ESR COM

K50.812 Crohn's disease of both small and large intestine with intestinal obstruction HCC Rx ESR COM

K50.813 Crohn's disease of both small and large intestine with fistula HCC Rx ESR COM

K50.814 Crohn's disease of both small and large intestine with abscess HCC Rx ESR COM

K50.818 Crohn's disease of both small and large intestine with other complication HCC Rx ESR COM

K50.819 Crohn's disease of both small and large intestine with unspecified complications HCC Rx ESR COM

✓5th K50.9 Crohn's disease, unspecified

K50.90 Crohn's disease, unspecified, without complications HCC Rx ESR COM

Crohn's disease NOS
Regional enteritis NOS

✓6th K50.91 Crohn's disease, unspecified, with complications

K50.911 Crohn's disease, unspecified, with rectal bleeding HCC Rx ESR COM

K50.912 Crohn's disease, unspecified, with intestinal obstruction HCC Rx ESR COM

K50.913 Crohn's disease, unspecified, with fistula HCC Rx ESR COM

K50.914 Crohn's disease, unspecified, with abscess HCC Rx ESR COM

K50.918 Crohn's disease, unspecified, with other complication HCC Rx ESR COM

K50.919 Crohn's disease, unspecified, with unspecified complications HCC Rx ESR COM

✓4th K51 Ulcerative colitis

Use additional code to identify any associated fistulas, if applicable:
Use additional code to identify manifestations, such as:
anal fistula (K60.3-)
anorectal fistula (K60.5-)
pyoderma gangrenosum (L88)
rectal fistula (K60.4-)

EXCLUDES 1 *Crohn's disease [regional enteritis] (K50.-)*

✓5th K51.0 Ulcerative (chronic) pancolitis

Backwash ileitis

K51.00 Ulcerative (chronic) pancolitis without complications HCC Rx ESR COM

Ulcerative (chronic) pancolitis NOS

✓6th K51.01 Ulcerative (chronic) pancolitis with complications

K51.011 Ulcerative (chronic) pancolitis with rectal bleeding HCC Rx ESR COM

K51.012 Ulcerative (chronic) pancolitis with intestinal obstruction HCC Rx ESR COM

K51.013 Ulcerative (chronic) pancolitis with fistula HCC Rx ESR COM

K51.014 Ulcerative (chronic) pancolitis with abscess HCC Rx ESR COM

K51.018 Ulcerative (chronic) pancolitis with other complication HCC Rx ESR COM

K51.019 Ulcerative (chronic) pancolitis with unspecified complications HCC Rx ESR COM

✓5th K51.2 Ulcerative (chronic) proctitis

K51.20 Ulcerative (chronic) proctitis without complications HCC Rx ESR COM

Ulcerative (chronic) proctitis NOS

✓6th K51.21 Ulcerative (chronic) proctitis with complications

K51.211 Ulcerative (chronic) proctitis with rectal bleeding HCC Rx ESR COM

K51.212 Ulcerative (chronic) proctitis with intestinal obstruction HCC Rx ESR COM

K51.213 Ulcerative (chronic) proctitis with fistula HCC Rx ESR COM

K51.214 Ulcerative (chronic) proctitis with abscess HCC Rx ESR COM

K51.218 Ulcerative (chronic) proctitis with other complication HCC Rx ESR COM

K51.219 Ulcerative (chronic) proctitis with unspecified complications HCC Rx ESR COM

✓5th K51.3 Ulcerative (chronic) rectosigmoiditis

K51.30 Ulcerative (chronic) rectosigmoiditis without complications HCC Rx ESR COM

Ulcerative (chronic) rectosigmoiditis NOS

✓6th K51.31 Ulcerative (chronic) rectosigmoiditis with complications

K51.311 Ulcerative (chronic) rectosigmoiditis with rectal bleeding HCC Rx ESR COM

K51.312 Ulcerative (chronic) rectosigmoiditis with intestinal obstruction HCC Rx ESR COM

K51.313 Ulcerative (chronic) rectosigmoiditis with fistula HCC Rx ESR COM

K51.314 Ulcerative (chronic) rectosigmoiditis with abscess HCC Rx ESR COM

K51.318 Ulcerative (chronic) rectosigmoiditis with other complication HCC Rx ESR COM

K51.319 Ulcerative (chronic) rectosigmoiditis with unspecified complications HCC Rx ESR COM

✓5th K51.4 Inflammatory polyps of colon

EXCLUDES 2 *adenomatous polyp of colon (D12.6)*
*polyposis of colon (D12.6)*
*polyps of colon NOS (K63.5)*

K51.40 Inflammatory polyps of colon without complications HCC Rx ESR COM

Inflammatory polyps of colon NOS

✓6th K51.41 Inflammatory polyps of colon with complications

K51.411 Inflammatory polyps of colon with rectal bleeding HCC Rx ESR COM

K51.412 Inflammatory polyps of colon with intestinal obstruction HCC Rx ESR COM

K51.413 Inflammatory polyps of colon with fistula HCC Rx ESR COM

K51.414 **Inflammatory polyps of colon with abscess** HCC Rx ESR COM

K51.418 **Inflammatory polyps of colon with other complication** HCC Rx ESR COM

K51.419 **Inflammatory polyps of colon with unspecified complications** HCC Rx ESR COM

✓5th **K51.5 Left sided colitis**

Left hemicolitis

K51.50 **Left sided colitis without complications** HCC Rx ESR COM

Left sided colitis NOS

✓6th **K51.51 Left sided colitis with complications**

K51.511 **Left sided colitis with rectal bleeding** HCC Rx ESR COM

K51.512 **Left sided colitis with intestinal obstruction** HCC Rx ESR COM

K51.513 **Left sided colitis with fistula** HCC Rx ESR COM

K51.514 **Left sided colitis with abscess** HCC Rx ESR COM

K51.518 **Left sided colitis with other complication** HCC Rx ESR COM

K51.519 **Left sided colitis with unspecified complications** HCC Rx ESR COM

✓5th **K51.8 Other ulcerative colitis**

K51.80 **Other ulcerative colitis without complications** HCC Rx ESR COM

✓6th **K51.81 Other ulcerative colitis with complications**

K51.811 **Other ulcerative colitis with rectal bleeding** HCC Rx ESR COM

K51.812 **Other ulcerative colitis with intestinal obstruction** HCC Rx ESR COM

K51.813 **Other ulcerative colitis with fistula** HCC Rx ESR COM

K51.814 **Other ulcerative colitis with abscess** HCC Rx ESR COM

K51.818 **Other ulcerative colitis with other complication** HCC Rx ESR COM

K51.819 **Other ulcerative colitis with unspecified complications** HCC Rx ESR COM

✓5th **K51.9 Ulcerative colitis, unspecified**

K51.90 **Ulcerative colitis, unspecified, without complications** HCC Rx ESR COM

✓6th **K51.91 Ulcerative colitis, unspecified, with complications**

K51.911 **Ulcerative colitis, unspecified with rectal bleeding** HCC Rx ESR COM

K51.912 **Ulcerative colitis, unspecified with intestinal obstruction** HCC Rx ESR COM

K51.913 **Ulcerative colitis, unspecified with fistula** HCC Rx ESR COM

K51.914 **Ulcerative colitis, unspecified with abscess** HCC Rx ESR COM

K51.918 **Ulcerative colitis, unspecified with other complication** HCC Rx ESR COM

K51.919 **Ulcerative colitis, unspecified with unspecified complications** HCC Rx ESR COM

✓4th **K52 Other and unspecified noninfective gastroenteritis and colitis**

**AHA:** 2016,4Q,30-31

**K52.0 Gastroenteritis and colitis due to radiation**

**K52.1 Toxic gastroenteritis and colitis**

Drug-induced gastroenteritis and colitis

Code first (T51-T65) to identify toxic agent

Use additional code for adverse effect, if applicable, to identify drug (T36-T50 with fifth or sixth character 5)

**AHA:** 2019,1Q,17

✓5th **K52.2 Allergic and dietetic gastroenteritis and colitis**

Food hypersensitivity gastroenteritis or colitis

Use additional code to identify type of food allergy (Z91.01-, Z91.02-)

EXCLUDES 2 *allergic eosinophilic colitis (K52.82)*
*allergic eosinophilic esophagitis (K20.0)*
*allergic eosinophilic gastritis (K52.81)*
*allergic eosinophilic gastroenteritis (K52.81)*

**DEF:** True immunoglobulin E (IgE)-mediated allergic reaction of the lining of the stomach, intestines, or colon to food proteins. It causes nausea, vomiting, diarrhea, and abdominal cramping.

K52.21 **Food protein-induced enterocolitis syndrome**

FPIES

Use additional code for hypovolemic shock, if present (R57.1)

K52.22 **Food protein-induced enteropathy**

K52.29 **Other allergic and dietetic gastroenteritis and colitis**

Allergic proctocolitis
Food hypersensitivity gastroenteritis or colitis
Food protein-induced proctocolitis
Food-induced eosinophilic proctocolitis
Immediate gastrointestinal hypersensitivity
Milk protein-induced proctocolitis

**K52.3 Indeterminate colitis**

Colonic inflammatory bowel disease unclassified (IBDU)

EXCLUDES 1 *unspecified colitis (K52.9)*

✓5th **K52.8 Other specified noninfective gastroenteritis and colitis**

K52.81 **Eosinophilic gastritis or gastroenteritis**

Eosinophilic enteritis

EXCLUDES 2 *eosinophilic esophagitis (K20.0)*

**DEF:** Disorder involving the accumulation of eosinophil in the lining of the stomach or multiple levels of the gastrointestinal tract, but without a known cause such as connective tissue disease, drug reaction, malignancy, or parasitic infection.

K52.82 **Eosinophilic colitis**

EXCLUDES 2 *allergic proctocolitis (K52.29)*
*food protein-induced enterocolitis syndrome (FPIES) (K52.21)*
*food protein-induced proctocolitis (K52.29)*
*food-induced eosinophilic proctocolitis (K52.29)*
*milk protein-induced proctocolitis (K52.29)*

**DEF:** Disorder involving the accumulation of eosinophil in the tissues lining the colon, but without a known cause such as connective tissue disease, drug reaction, malignancy, or parasitic infection. The resultant inflammation may cause extreme abdominal pain, diarrhea, or bloody stool.

✓6th K52.83 **Microscopic colitis**

K52.831 **Collagenous colitis** Rx

K52.832 **Lymphocytic colitis** Rx

K52.838 **Other microscopic colitis** Rx

K52.839 **Microscopic colitis, unspecified** Rx

K52.89 **Other specified noninfective gastroenteritis and colitis**

**AHA:** 2019,1Q,20

**K52.9 Noninfective gastroenteritis and colitis, unspecified**

Colitis NOS
Enteritis NOS
Gastroenteritis NOS
Ileitis NOS
Jejunitis NOS
Sigmoiditis NOS

EXCLUDES 1 *diarrhea NOS (R19.7)*
*functional diarrhea (K59.1)*
*infectious gastroenteritis and colitis NOS (A09)*
*neonatal diarrhea (noninfective) (P78.3)*
*psychogenic diarrhea (F45.8)*

**AHA:** 2021,3Q,3

## Other diseases of intestines (K55-K64)

✓4th **K55 Vascular disorders of intestine**

EXCLUDES 1 *necrotizing enterocolitis of newborn (P77.-)*

EXCLUDES 2 *angioectasia (angiodysplasia) duodenum (K31.81-)*

**AHA:** 2016,4Q,32

✓5th **K55.Ø Acute vascular disorders of intestine**

Infarction of appendices epiploicae
Mesenteric (artery) (vein) embolism
Mesenteric (artery) (vein) infarction
Mesenteric (artery) (vein) thrombosis

**AHA:** 2019,4Q,68

✓6th **K55.Ø1 Acute (reversible) ischemia of small intestine**

**K55.Ø11 Focal (segmental) acute (reversible) ischemia of small intestine** ESR COM

**K55.Ø12 Diffuse acute (reversible) ischemia of small intestine** ESR COM

**K55.Ø19 Acute (reversible) ischemia of small intestine, extent unspecified** ESR COM

✓6th **K55.Ø2 Acute infarction of small intestine**

Gangrene of small intestine
Necrosis of small intestine

**K55.Ø21 Focal (segmental) acute infarction of small intestine** ESR COM

**K55.Ø22 Diffuse acute infarction of small intestine** ESR COM

**K55.Ø29 Acute infarction of small intestine, extent unspecified** ESR COM

✓6th **K55.Ø3 Acute (reversible) ischemia of large intestine**

Acute fulminant ischemic colitis
Subacute ischemic colitis

**K55.Ø31 Focal (segmental) acute (reversible) ischemia of large intestine** ESR COM

**K55.Ø32 Diffuse acute (reversible) ischemia of large intestine** ESR COM

**K55.Ø39 Acute (reversible) ischemia of large intestine, extent unspecified** ESR COM

**AHA:** 2019,4Q,68

✓6th **K55.Ø4 Acute infarction of large intestine**

Gangrene of large intestine
Necrosis of large intestine

**K55.Ø41 Focal (segmental) acute infarction of large intestine** ESR COM

**K55.Ø42 Diffuse acute infarction of large intestine** ESR COM

**K55.Ø49 Acute infarction of large intestine, extent unspecified** ESR COM

✓6th **K55.Ø5 Acute (reversible) ischemia of intestine, part unspecified**

**K55.Ø51 Focal (segmental) acute (reversible) ischemia of intestine, part unspecified** ESR COM

**K55.Ø52 Diffuse acute (reversible) ischemia of intestine, part unspecified** ESR COM

**K55.Ø59 Acute (reversible) ischemia of intestine, part and extent unspecified** ESR COM

✓6th **K55.Ø6 Acute infarction of intestine, part unspecified**

Acute intestinal infarction
Gangrene of intestine
Necrosis of intestine

**K55.Ø61 Focal (segmental) acute infarction of intestine, part unspecified** ESR COM

**K55.Ø62 Diffuse acute infarction of intestine, part unspecified** ESR COM

**K55.Ø69 Acute infarction of intestine, part and extent unspecified** ESR COM

**K55.1 Chronic vascular disorders of intestine** ESR COM

Chronic ischemic colitis
Chronic ischemic enteritis
Chronic ischemic enterocolitis
Ischemic stricture of intestine
Mesenteric atherosclerosis
Mesenteric vascular insufficiency

✓5th **K55.2 Angiodysplasia of colon**

**AHA:** 2018,3Q,21

**TIP:** Assign a code for "with hemorrhage" when angiodysplasia and GI bleeding are documented. The ICD-10-CM classification assumes the two are related without the provider linking the two conditions. Evidence of bleeding during a procedure is not required.

**K55.2Ø Angiodysplasia of colon without hemorrhage**

**K55.21 Angiodysplasia of colon with hemorrhage**

**DEF:** Small vascular abnormalities due to fragile blood vessels in the colon, resulting in blood loss from the gastrointestinal (GI) tract.

✓5th **K55.3 Necrotizing enterocolitis**

EXCLUDES 1 *necrotizing enterocolitis of newborn (P77.-)*

EXCLUDES 2 *necrotizing enterocolitis due to Clostridium difficile (AØ4.7-)*

**K55.3Ø Necrotizing enterocolitis, unspecified** ESR COM

Necrotizing enterocolitis, NOS

**K55.31 Stage 1 necrotizing enterocolitis** ESR COM

Necrotizing enterocolitis without pneumatosis, without perforation

**K55.32 Stage 2 necrotizing enterocolitis** ESR COM

Necrotizing enterocolitis with pneumatosis, without perforation

**K55.33 Stage 3 necrotizing enterocolitis** ESR COM

Necrotizing enterocolitis with perforation
Necrotizing enterocolitis with pneumatosis and perforation

**K55.8 Other vascular disorders of intestine** ESR COM

**K55.9 Vascular disorder of intestine, unspecified** ESR COM

Ischemic colitis
Ischemic enteritis
Ischemic enterocolitis

✓4th **K56 Paralytic ileus and intestinal obstruction without hernia**

EXCLUDES 1 *congenital stricture or stenosis of intestine (Q41-Q42)*
*cystic fibrosis with meconium ileus (E84.11)*
*ischemic stricture of intestine (K55.1)*
*meconium ileus NOS (P76.Ø)*
*neonatal intestinal obstructions classifiable to P76.-*
*obstruction of duodenum (K31.5)*
*postprocedural intestinal obstruction (K91.3-)*

EXCLUDES 2 *stenosis of anus or rectum (K62.4)*

**K56.Ø Paralytic ileus** HCC ESR COM

Paralysis of bowel
Paralysis of colon
Paralysis of intestine

EXCLUDES 1 *gallstone ileus (K56.3)*
*ileus NOS (K56.7)*
*obstructive ileus NOS (K56.69-)*

**DEF:** Intestinal obstruction due to paralysis of bowel motility or peristalsis.

**K56.1 Intussusception** HCC ESR COM

Intussusception or invagination of bowel
Intussusception or invagination of colon
Intussusception or invagination of intestine
Intussusception or invagination of rectum

EXCLUDES 2 *intussusception of appendix (K38.8)*

**AHA:** 2023,3Q,11

**DEF:** Intestinal obstruction due to prolapse of a bowel section into an adjacent section. It occurs primarily in children and symptoms include acute abdominal pain, vomiting, and passage of blood and mucus from the rectum.

**K56.2 Volvulus** HCC ESR COM

Strangulation of colon or intestine
Torsion of colon or intestine
Twist of colon or intestine

EXCLUDES 2 *volvulus of duodenum (K31.5)*

**AHA:** 2024,2Q,22

**DEF:** Twisting, knotting, or entanglement of the bowel on itself that may quickly compromise oxygen supply to the intestinal tissues. A volvulus usually occurs at the sigmoid and ileocecal areas of the intestines.

**Volvulus**

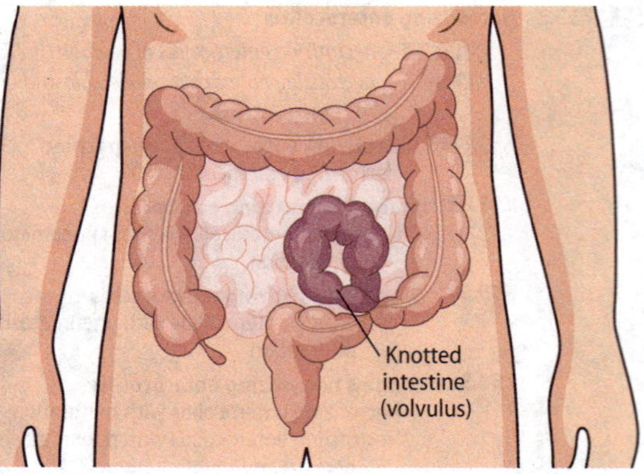


**K56.3 Gallstone ileus** HCC ESR COM

Obstruction of intestine by gallstone

√5th **K56.4 Other impaction of intestine**

**K56.41 Fecal impaction** HCC ESR COM

EXCLUDES 2 *incomplete defecation (R15.Ø)*

**AHA:** 2024,2Q,6

**K56.49 Other impaction of intestine** HCC ESR COM

√5th **K56.5 Intestinal adhesions [bands] with obstruction (postinfection)**

Abdominal hernia due to adhesions with obstruction
Peritoneal adhesions [bands] with intestinal obstruction (postinfection)

**AHA:** 2017,4Q,16-17

**K56.5Ø Intestinal adhesions [bands], unspecified as to partial versus complete obstruction** HCC ESR COM

Intestinal adhesions with obstruction NOS

**K56.51 Intestinal adhesions [bands], with partial obstruction** HCC ESR COM

Intestinal adhesions with incomplete obstruction

**K56.52 Intestinal adhesions [bands] with complete obstruction** HCC ESR COM

√5th **K56.6 Other and unspecified intestinal obstruction**

**AHA:** 2017,4Q,16-17; 2017,2Q,12

√6th **K56.6Ø Unspecified intestinal obstruction**

**K56.6ØØ Partial intestinal obstruction, unspecified as to cause** HCC ESR COM

Incomplete intestinal obstruction, NOS

**K56.6Ø1 Complete intestinal obstruction, unspecified as to cause** HCC ESR COM

**K56.6Ø9 Unspecified intestinal obstruction, unspecified as to partial versus complete obstruction** HCC ESR COM

Intestinal obstruction NOS

√6th **K56.69 Other intestinal obstruction**

Enterostenosis NOS
Obstructive ileus NOS
Occlusion of colon or intestine NOS
Stenosis of colon or intestine NOS
Stricture of colon or intestine NOS

**K56.69Ø Other partial intestinal obstruction** HCC ESR COM

Other incomplete intestinal obstruction

**K56.691 Other complete intestinal obstruction** HCC ESR COM

**K56.699 Other intestinal obstruction unspecified as to partial versus complete obstruction** HCC ESR COM

Other intestinal obstruction, NEC

**AHA:** 2023,3Q,10

**K56.7 Ileus, unspecified** HCC ESR COM

EXCLUDES 1 *obstructive ileus (K56.69-)*

EXCLUDES 2 *intestinal obstruction with hernia (K4Ø-K46)*

**AHA:** 2017,1Q,40

√4th **K57 Diverticular disease of intestine**

▶Code also if applicable:◀
▶pelvic abscess (K6A.Ø-)◀
▶peritonitis (K65.-)◀

EXCLUDES 1 *congenital diverticulum of intestine (Q43.8)*
*Meckel's diverticulum (Q43.Ø)*

EXCLUDES 2 *diverticulum of appendix (K38.2)*

**AHA:** 2022,1Q,26-27; 2021,1Q,9,11; 2018,3Q,21

**TIP:** Assign a code for "with bleeding" when diverticular disease of the intestine and GI bleeding are documented. The ICD-10-CM classification assumes the two are related without the provider linking the two conditions. Evidence of bleeding during a procedure is not required.

√5th **K57.Ø Diverticulitis of small intestine with perforation and abscess**

EXCLUDES 1 *diverticulitis of both small and large intestine with perforation and abscess (K57.4-)*

**K57.ØØ Diverticulitis of small intestine with perforation and abscess without bleeding**

**K57.Ø1 Diverticulitis of small intestine with perforation and abscess with bleeding**

√5th **K57.1 Diverticular disease of small intestine without perforation or abscess**

EXCLUDES 1 *diverticular disease of both small and large intestine without perforation or abscess (K57.5-)*

**K57.1Ø Diverticulosis of small intestine without perforation or abscess without bleeding**

Diverticular disease of small intestine NOS

**K57.11 Diverticulosis of small intestine without perforation or abscess with bleeding**

**K57.12 Diverticulitis of small intestine without perforation or abscess without bleeding**

**K57.13 Diverticulitis of small intestine without perforation or abscess with bleeding**

√5th **K57.2 Diverticulitis of large intestine with perforation and abscess**

EXCLUDES 1 *diverticulitis of both small and large intestine with perforation and abscess (K57.4-)*

**K57.2Ø Diverticulitis of large intestine with perforation and abscess without bleeding**

**AHA:** 2026,2Q,12; 2025,2Q,6

**K57.21 Diverticulitis of large intestine with perforation and abscess with bleeding**

√5th **K57.3 Diverticular disease of large intestine without perforation or abscess**

EXCLUDES 1 *diverticular disease of both small and large intestine without perforation or abscess (K57.5-)*

**K57.3Ø Diverticulosis of large intestine without perforation or abscess without bleeding**

Diverticular disease of colon NOS

**K57.31 Diverticulosis of large intestine without perforation or abscess with bleeding**

**K57.32 Diverticulitis of large intestine without perforation or abscess without bleeding**

**K57.33 Diverticulitis of large intestine without perforation or abscess with bleeding**

√5th **K57.4 Diverticulitis of both small and large intestine with perforation and abscess**

**K57.4Ø Diverticulitis of both small and large intestine with perforation and abscess without bleeding**

**K57.41 Diverticulitis of both small and large intestine with perforation and abscess with bleeding**

√5th **K57.5 Diverticular disease of both small and large intestine without perforation or abscess**

**K57.5Ø Diverticulosis of both small and large intestine without perforation or abscess without bleeding**

Diverticular disease of both small and large intestine NOS

**K57.51 Diverticulosis of both small and large intestine without perforation or abscess with bleeding**

**K57.52 Diverticulitis of both small and large intestine without perforation or abscess without bleeding**

**K57.53 Diverticulitis of both small and large intestine without perforation or abscess with bleeding**

√5th **K57.8 Diverticulitis of intestine, part unspecified, with perforation and abscess**

**K57.8Ø Diverticulitis of intestine, part unspecified, with perforation and abscess without bleeding**

K57.81 **Diverticulitis of intestine, part unspecified, with perforation and abscess with bleeding**

K57.9 **Diverticular disease of intestine, part unspecified, without perforation or abscess**

K57.90 **Diverticulosis of intestine, part unspecified, without perforation or abscess without bleeding**
Diverticular disease of intestine NOS

K57.91 **Diverticulosis of intestine, part unspecified, without perforation or abscess with bleeding**

K57.92 **Diverticulitis of intestine, part unspecified, without perforation or abscess without bleeding**

K57.93 **Diverticulitis of intestine, part unspecified, without perforation or abscess with bleeding**

## K58 Irritable bowel syndrome

INCLUDES irritable colon
spastic colon

AHA: 2016,4Q,32-33

K58.0 **Irritable bowel syndrome with diarrhea**
K58.1 **Irritable bowel syndrome with constipation**
K58.2 **Mixed irritable bowel syndrome**
K58.8 **Other irritable bowel syndrome**
K58.9 **Irritable bowel syndrome, unspecified**
Irritable bowel syndrome NOS

## K59 Other functional intestinal disorders

EXCLUDES 1 *change in bowel habit NOS (R19.4)*
*intestinal malabsorption (K90.-)*
*psychogenic intestinal disorders (F45.8)*

EXCLUDES 2 *functional disorders of stomach (K31.-)*

K59.0 **Constipation**

EXCLUDES 1 *fecal impaction (K56.41)*

EXCLUDES 2 *incomplete defecation (R15.0)*

AHA: 2024,2Q,6; 2016,4Q,33

K59.00 **Constipation, unspecified**

K59.01 **Slow transit constipation**
DEF: Delay in the transit of fecal material through the colon secondary to smooth muscle dysfunction or decreased peristaltic contractions along the colon.

K59.02 **Outlet dysfunction constipation**
AHA: 2023,1Q,24
TIP: Report this code for documented pelvic floor dyssynergia, outlet type constipation, or anismus.

K59.03 **Drug induced constipation**
Use additional code for adverse effect, if applicable, to identify drug (T36-T50 with fifth or sixth character 5)

K59.04 **Chronic idiopathic constipation**
Functional constipation

K59.09 **Other constipation**
Chronic constipation

K59.1 **Functional diarrhea**

EXCLUDES 1 *diarrhea NOS (R19.7)*
*irritable bowel syndrome with diarrhea (K58.0)*

K59.2 **Neurogenic bowel, not elsewhere classified**
DEF: Disorder of bowel due to a spinal cord lesion because of injury or as a complication of conditions such as multiple sclerosis (MS) or spina bifida. Loss of bowel control is the primary symptom, manifested as constipation or bowel incontinence.

K59.3 **Megacolon, not elsewhere classified**
Dilatation of colon
Code first, if applicable (T51-T65) to identify toxic agent

EXCLUDES 1 *congenital megacolon (aganglionic) (Q43.1)*
*megacolon (due to) (in) Chagas' disease (B57.32)*
*megacolon (due to) (in) Clostridium difficile (A04.7-)*
*megacolon (due to) (in) Hirschsprung's disease (Q43.1)*

AHA: 2016,4Q,33-34

K59.31 **Toxic megacolon** HCC ESR COM

K59.39 **Other megacolon**
Megacolon NOS

K59.4 **Anal spasm**
Proctalgia fugax

K59.8 **Other specified functional intestinal disorders**
AHA: 2020,4Q,29-30

K59.81 **Ogilvie syndrome**
Acute colonic pseudo-obstruction (ACPO)

K59.89 **Other specified functional intestinal disorders**
Atony of colon
Pseudo-obstruction (acute) (chronic) of intestine

K59.9 **Functional intestinal disorder, unspecified**

## K60 Fissure and fistula of anal and rectal regions

EXCLUDES 1 ~~*fissure and fistula of anal and rectal regions with abscess or cellulitis (K61.-)*~~

EXCLUDES 2 *abscess or cellulitis of anal and rectal regions (K61.-)*
*anal sphincter tear (healed) (nontraumatic) (old) (K62.81)*

AHA: 2024,4Q,21

K60.0 **Acute anal fissure**
K60.1 **Chronic anal fissure**
K60.2 **Anal fissure, unspecified**

K60.3 **Anal fistula**
Code first, if applicable:
Crohn's disease (K50.-)
ulcerative colitis (K51.-)

EXCLUDES 1 *congenital fistula (Q43.6)*

K60.30 **Anal fistula, unspecified**
Anal fistula NOS

K60.31 **Anal fistula, simple**
Low intersphincteric anal fistula
Superficial anal fistula

K60.311 **Anal fistula, simple, initial**
Anal fistula, simple, new

K60.312 **Anal fistula, simple, persistent**
Anal fistula, simple, chronic

K60.313 **Anal fistula, simple, recurrent**
Anal fistula simple, occurring following complete healing

K60.319 **Anal fistula, simple, unspecified**

K60.32 **Anal fistula, complex**
Extrasphincteric anal fistula
High intersphincteric anal fistula
Suprasphincteric anal fistula
Transsphincteric anal fistula
Code also, if applicable:
perianal abscess (K61.0)
rectovaginal fistula (N82.3)
stenosis of anus and rectum (K62.4)

K60.321 **Anal fistula, complex, initial**
Anal fistula, complex, new

K60.322 **Anal fistula, complex, persistent**
Anal fistula, complex, chronic

K60.323 **Anal fistula, complex, recurrent**
Anal fistula complex, occurring following complete healing

K60.329 **Anal fistula, complex, unspecified**

K60.4 **Rectal fistula**
Fistula of rectum to skin
Code first, if applicable:
Crohn's disease (K50.-)
ulcerative colitis (K51.-)

EXCLUDES 1 *congenital fistula (Q43.6)*
*rectovaginal fistula (N82.3)*
*vesicorectal fistual (N32.1)*

K60.40 **Rectal fistula, unspecified**
Rectal fistula NOS

K60.41 **Rectal fistula, simple**
Low intersphincteric rectal fistula
Superficial rectal fistula

K60.411 **Rectal fistula, simple, initial**
Rectal, fistula, simple, new

K60.412 **Rectal fistula, simple, persistent**
Rectal fistula, simple, chronic

K60.413 **Rectal fistula, simple, recurrent**
Rectal fistula simple, occurring following complete healing

K60.419 **Rectal fistula, simple, unspecified**

K60.42 **Rectal fistula, complex**
Extrasphincteric rectal fistula
High intersphincteric rectal fistula
Suprasphincteric rectal fistula
Transsphincteric rectal fistula
Code also, if applicable:
perianal abscess (K61.0)
rectovaginal fistula (N82.3)
stenosis of anus and rectum (K62.4)

K60.421 **Rectal fistula, complex, initial**
Rectal fistula, complex, new

K60.422 **Rectal fistula, complex, persistent**
Rectal fistula, complex, chronic

K60.423 **Rectal fistula, complex, recurrent**
Rectal fistula complex occurring following complete healing

K60.429 **Rectal fistula, complex, unspecified**

✓5th K60.5 **Anorectal fistula**
Code first, if applicable:
Crohn's disease (K50.-)
ulcerative colitis (K51.-)
EXCLUDES 1 *congenital fistula (Q43.6)*

K60.50 **Anorectal fistula, unspecified**
Anorectal fistula NOS

✓6th K60.51 **Anorectal fistula, simple**
Low intersphincteric anorectal fistula
Superficial anorectal fistula

K60.511 **Anorectal fistula, simple, initial**
Anorectal fistula, simple, new

K60.512 **Anorectal fistula, simple, persistent**
Anorectal fistula, simple, chronic

K60.513 **Anorectal fistula, simple, recurrent**
Anorectal fistula simple, occurring following complete healing

K60.519 **Anorectal fistula, simple, unspecified**

✓6th K60.52 **Anorectal fistula, complex**
Extrasphincteric anorectal fistula
High intersphincteric anorectal fistula
Suprasphincteric anorectal fistula
Transsphincteric anorectal fistula
Code also, if applicable:
perianal abscess (K61.0)
rectovaginal fistula (N82.3)
stenosis of anus and rectum (K62.4)

K60.521 **Anorectal fistula, complex, initial**
Anorectal fistula, complex, new

K60.522 **Anorectal fistula, complex, persistent**
Anorectal fistula, complex, chronic

K60.523 **Anorectal fistula, complex, recurrent**
Anorectal fistula complex, occurring following complete healing

K60.529 **Anorectal fistula, complex, unspecified**

✓4th K61 **Abscess of anal and rectal regions**
INCLUDES abscess of anal and rectal regions
cellulitis of anal and rectal regions

K61.0 **Anal abscess**
Perianal abscess
EXCLUDES 2 *intrasphincteric abscess (K61.4)*

K61.1 **Rectal abscess**
Perirectal abscess
EXCLUDES 1 *ischiorectal abscess (K61.39)*
**AHA:** 2012,4Q,104

K61.2 **Anorectal abscess**

✓5th K61.3 **Ischiorectal abscess**
**AHA:** 2018,4Q,19

K61.31 **Horseshoe abscess**

K61.39 **Other ischiorectal abscess**
Abscess of ischiorectal fossa
Ischiorectal abscess, NOS

K61.4 **Intrasphincteric abscess**
Intersphincteric abscess

K61.5 **Supralevator abscess**
**AHA:** 2018,4Q,19

✓4th K62 **Other diseases of anus and rectum**
INCLUDES anal canal
EXCLUDES 2 *colostomy and enterostomy malfunction (K94.0-, K94.1-)*
*fecal incontinence (R15.-)*
*hemorrhoids (K64.-)*

K62.0 **Anal polyp**

K62.1 **Rectal polyp**
EXCLUDES 1 *adenomatous polyp (D12.8)*
**AHA:** 2018,1Q,6

K62.2 **Anal prolapse**
Prolapse of anal canal

K62.3 **Rectal prolapse**
Prolapse of rectal mucosa

K62.4 **Stenosis of anus and rectum**
Stricture of anus (sphincter)
**AHA:** 2019,2Q,13

K62.5 **Hemorrhage of anus and rectum**
EXCLUDES 1 *gastrointestinal bleeding NOS (K92.2)*
*melena (K92.1)*
*neonatal rectal hemorrhage (P54.2)*
**AHA:** 2019,1Q,21

K62.6 **Ulcer of anus and rectum**
Solitary ulcer of anus and rectum
Stercoral ulcer of anus and rectum
EXCLUDES 1 *fissure and fistula of anus and rectum (K60.-)*
*ulcerative colitis (K51.-)*

K62.7 **Radiation proctitis**
Use additional code to identify the type of radiation (W88.-) or radiation therapy (Y84.2)
**AHA:** 2019,1Q,21

✓5th K62.8 **Other specified diseases of anus and rectum**
EXCLUDES 2 *ulcerative proctitis (K51.2)*

K62.81 **Anal sphincter tear (healed) (nontraumatic) (old)**
Tear of anus, nontraumatic
Use additional code for any associated fecal incontinence (R15.-)
EXCLUDES 2 *anal fissure (K60.-)*
*anal sphincter tear (healed) (old) complicating delivery (O34.7-)*
*traumatic tear of anal sphincter (S31.831)*

K62.82 **Dysplasia of anus**
Anal intraepithelial neoplasia I and II (AIN I and II) (histologically confirmed)
Dysplasia of anus NOS
Mild and moderate dysplasia of anus (histologically confirmed)
EXCLUDES 1 *abnormal results from anal cytologic examination without histologic confirmation (R85.61-)*
*anal intraepithelial neoplasia III (D01.3)*
*carcinoma in situ of anus (D01.3)*
*HGSIL of anus (R85.613)*
*severe dysplasia of anus (D01.3)*

K62.89 **Other specified diseases of anus and rectum**
Proctitis NOS
Use additional code for any associated fecal incontinence (R15.-)

K62.9 **Disease of anus and rectum, unspecified**

✓4th K63 **Other diseases of intestine**

K63.0 **Abscess of intestine**
EXCLUDES 1 *abscess of intestine with Crohn's disease (K50.014, K50.114, K50.814, K50.914)*
*abscess of intestine with diverticular disease (K57.0, K57.2, K57.4, K57.8)*
*abscess of intestine with ulcerative colitis (K51.014, K51.214, K51.314, K51.414, K51.514, K51.814, K51.914)*
EXCLUDES 2 *abscess of anal and rectal regions (K61.-)*
*abscess of appendix (K35.3-)*

K63.1 **Perforation of intestine (nontraumatic)** HCC ESR COM
Perforation (nontraumatic) of rectum
EXCLUDES 1 *perforation (nontraumatic) of duodenum (K26.-)*
*perforation (nontraumatic) of intestine with diverticular disease (K57.0, K57.2, K57.4, K57.8)*
EXCLUDES 2 *perforation (nontraumatic) of appendix (K35.2-, K35.3-)*
**AHA:** 2025,2Q,8; 2020,2Q,22

K63.2 **Fistula of intestine**
Code also, if applicable, disruption of internal operation (surgical) wound (T81.32-)
EXCLUDES 1 *fistula of duodenum (K31.6)*
*fistula of intestine with Crohn's disease (K50.013, K50.113, K50.813, K50.913)*
*fistula of intestine with ulcerative colitis (K51.013, K51.213, K51.313, K51.413, K51.513, K51.813, K51.913)*
EXCLUDES 2 *fistula of anal and rectal regions (K60.-)*
*fistula of appendix (K38.3)*
*intestinal-genital fistula, female (N82.2-N82.4)*
*vesicointestinal fistula (N32.1)*
**AHA:** 2017,3Q,4

**K63.3 Ulcer of intestine**
Primary ulcer of small intestine
EXCLUDES 1 *duodenal ulcer (K26.-)*
*gastrointestinal ulcer (K28.-)*
*gastrojejunal ulcer (K28.-)*
*jejunal ulcer (K28.-)*
*peptic ulcer, site unspecified (K27.-)*
*ulcer of anus or rectum (K62.6)*
*ulcer of intestine with perforation (K63.1)*
*ulcerative colitis (K51.-)*

**K63.4 Enteroptosis**

**K63.5 Polyp of colon**
EXCLUDES 2 *adenomatous polyp of colon (D12.-)*
*inflammatory polyp of colon (K51.4-)*
*polyposis of colon (D12.6)*
**AHA:** 2019,1Q,33; 2018,2Q,14; 2017,1Q,15; 2015,2Q,14
**TIP:** Assign this code when documentation states hyperplastic colon polyp regardless of the site in the colon. Slow-growing, hyperplastic polyps are not precancerous and are classified differently from benign or adenomatous polyps.

√5th **K63.8 Other specified diseases of intestine**

**K63.81 Dieulafoy lesion of intestine**
EXCLUDES 2 *Dieulafoy lesion of stomach and duodenum (K31.82)*
**DEF:** Abnormally large submucosal artery protruding through a defect in the stomach mucosa or intestines that can cause massive and life-threatening hemorrhaging.

√6th **K63.82 Intestinal microbial overgrowth**
**AHA:** 2023,4Q,29-30

√7th **K63.821 Small intestinal bacterial overgrowth**

**K63.8211 Small intestinal bacterial overgrowth, hydrogen-subtype**

**K63.8212 Small intestinal bacterial overgrowth, hydrogen sulfide-subtype**

**K63.8219 Small intestinal bacterial overgrowth, unspecified**

**K63.822 Small intestinal fungal overgrowth**

**K63.829 Intestinal methanogen overgrowth, unspecified**

**K63.89 Other specified diseases of intestine**
**AHA:** 2013,2Q,31

**K63.9 Disease of intestine, unspecified**

√4th **K64 Hemorrhoids and perianal venous thrombosis**
INCLUDES piles
EXCLUDES 1 *hemorrhoids complicating childbirth and the puerperium (O87.2)*
*hemorrhoids complicating pregnancy (O22.4)*

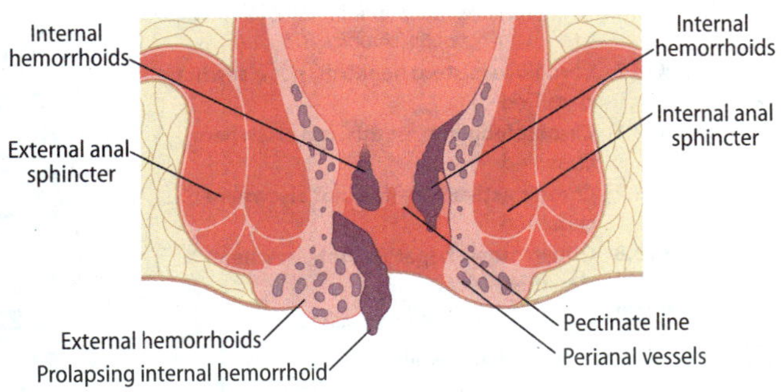


**K64.0 First degree hemorrhoids**
Grade/stage I hemorrhoids
Hemorrhoids (bleeding) without prolapse outside of anal canal

**K64.1 Second degree hemorrhoids**
Grade/stage II hemorrhoids
Hemorrhoids (bleeding) that prolapse with straining, but retract spontaneously

**K64.2 Third degree hemorrhoids**
Grade/stage III hemorrhoids
Hemorrhoids (bleeding) that prolapse with straining and require manual replacement back inside anal canal

**K64.3 Fourth degree hemorrhoids**
Grade/stage IV hemorrhoids
Hemorrhoids (bleeding) with prolapsed tissue that cannot be manually replaced

**K64.4 Residual hemorrhoidal skin tags**
External hemorrhoids, NOS
Skin tags of anus

**K64.5 Perianal venous thrombosis**
External hemorrhoids with thrombosis
Perianal hematoma
Thrombosed hemorrhoids NOS

**K64.8 Other hemorrhoids**
Internal hemorrhoids, without mention of degree
Prolapsed hemorrhoids, degree not specified

**K64.9 Unspecified hemorrhoids**
Hemorrhoids (bleeding) NOS
Hemorrhoids (bleeding) without mention of degree

## ▶Diseases of peritoneum, retroperitoneum and pelvis (K65-K6A)◀

√4th **K65 Peritonitis**
Code also if applicable diverticular disease of intestine (K57.-)
Use additional code (B95-B97), to identify infectious agent, if known
EXCLUDES 1 *acute appendicitis with generalized peritonitis (K35.2-)*
*aseptic peritonitis (T81.6)*
*benign paroxysmal peritonitis (E85.0)*
*chemical peritonitis (T81.6)*
*gonococcal peritonitis (A54.85)*
*neonatal peritonitis (P78.0-P78.1)*
*pelvic peritonitis, female (N73.3-N73.5)*
*periodic familial peritonitis (E85.0)*
*peritonitis due to talc or other foreign substance (T81.6)*
*peritonitis in chlamydia (A74.81)*
*peritonitis in diphtheria (A36.89)*
*peritonitis in syphilis (late) (A52.74)*
*peritonitis in tuberculosis (A18.31)*
*peritonitis with or following abortion or ectopic or molar pregnancy (O00-O07, O08.0)*
*peritonitis with or following appendicitis (K35.-)*
*puerperal peritonitis (O85)*
*retroperitoneal infections (K68.-)*

**K65.0 Generalized (acute) peritonitis** HCC ESR COM
Pelvic peritonitis (acute), male
Subphrenic peritonitis (acute)
Suppurative peritonitis (acute)

**K65.1 Peritoneal abscess** HCC ESR COM
Abdominopelvic abscess
Abscess (of) omentum
Abscess (of) peritoneum
Mesenteric abscess
Retrocecal abscess
Subdiaphragmatic abscess
Subhepatic abscess
Subphrenic abscess
EXCLUDES 2 ▶*pelvic abscess (extraperitoneal) (K6A.0-)*◀
**AHA:** 2026,2Q,12; 2024,1Q,20; 2022,1Q,26; 2019,1Q,15

**K65.2 Spontaneous bacterial peritonitis** HCC ESR COM
EXCLUDES 1 *bacterial peritonitis NOS (K65.9)*

**K65.3 Choleperitonitis** HCC ESR COM
Peritonitis due to bile
**DEF:** Inflammation of the peritoneum due to leakage of bile into the peritoneal cavity resulting from rupture of the bile passages or gallbladder.

**K65.4 Sclerosing mesenteritis** HCC ESR COM
(Idiopathic) sclerosing mesenteric fibrosis
Fat necrosis of peritoneum
Mesenteric lipodystrophy
Mesenteric panniculitis
Retractile mesenteritis

**K65.8 Other peritonitis** HCC ESR COM
Chronic proliferative peritonitis
Peritonitis due to urine

**K65.9 Peritonitis, unspecified** HCC ESR COM
Bacterial peritonitis NOS
**AHA:** 2022,1Q,27; 2013,2Q,31

● ✓4th **K6A Diseases of the pelvis, not elsewhere classified**

● ✓5th **K6A.Ø Pelvic abscess**

Code also, if applicable:
diverticular disease of intestine (K57.-)
female pelvic inflammatory disease (N73.-)
Use additional code (B95-B97), to identify infectious agent, if known

EXCLUDES 2 *peritoneal abscess (K65.1)*
*retroperitoneal abscess (K68.1-)*

● **K6A.Ø1 Prevesical abscess**
Retropubic abscess

● **K6A.Ø9 Other pelvic abscess**
Pelvic abscess, unspecified

● **K6A.8 Other diseases of the pelvis, not elsewhere classified**

## Diseases of liver (K7Ø-K77)

EXCLUDES 1 *jaundice NOS (R17)*
EXCLUDES 2 *hemochromatosis (E83.11-)*
*Reye's syndrome (G93.7)*
*viral hepatitis (B15-B19)*
*Wilson's disease (E83.Ø1)*

✓4th **K7Ø Alcoholic liver disease**

Use additional code to identify:
alcohol abuse and dependence (F1Ø.-)

**K7Ø.Ø Alcoholic fatty liver** A

✓5th **K7Ø.1 Alcoholic hepatitis**

**K7Ø.1Ø Alcoholic hepatitis without ascites** HCC COM A

**K7Ø.11 Alcoholic hepatitis with ascites** HCC COM A

**K7Ø.2 Alcoholic fibrosis and sclerosis of liver** A

✓5th **K7Ø.3 Alcoholic cirrhosis of liver**
Alcoholic cirrhosis NOS

**K7Ø.3Ø Alcoholic cirrhosis of liver without ascites** HCC ESR COM A

**K7Ø.31 Alcoholic cirrhosis of liver with ascites** HCC ESR COM A
AHA: 2018,1Q,4

✓5th **K7Ø.4 Alcoholic hepatic failure**
Acute alcoholic hepatic failure
Alcoholic hepatic failure NOS
Chronic alcoholic hepatic failure
Subacute alcoholic hepatic failure

**K7Ø.4Ø Alcoholic hepatic failure without coma** HCC ESR COM A

**K7Ø.41 Alcoholic hepatic failure with coma** HCC ESR COM A

**K7Ø.9 Alcoholic liver disease, unspecified** ESR A

✓4th **K71 Toxic liver disease**

INCLUDES drug-induced idiosyncratic (unpredictable) liver disease
drug-induced toxic (predictable) liver disease

Code first poisoning due to drug or toxin, if applicable (T36-T65 with fifth or sixth character 1-4)
Use additional code for adverse effect, if applicable, to identify drug (T36-T5Ø with fifth or sixth character 5)

EXCLUDES 2 *alcoholic liver disease (K7Ø.-)*
*Budd-Chiari syndrome (I82.Ø)*

**K71.Ø Toxic liver disease with cholestasis**
"Pure" cholestasis
Cholestasis with hepatocyte injury

✓5th **K71.1 Toxic liver disease with hepatic necrosis**
Hepatic failure (acute) (chronic) due to drugs

**K71.1Ø Toxic liver disease with hepatic necrosis, without coma** COM

**K71.11 Toxic liver disease with hepatic necrosis, with coma** ESR COM

**K71.2 Toxic liver disease with acute hepatitis**

**K71.3 Toxic liver disease with chronic persistent hepatitis** HCC COM

**K71.4 Toxic liver disease with chronic lobular hepatitis** HCC COM

✓5th **K71.5 Toxic liver disease with chronic active hepatitis**
Toxic liver disease with lupoid hepatitis

**K71.5Ø Toxic liver disease with chronic active hepatitis without ascites** HCC COM

**K71.51 Toxic liver disease with chronic active hepatitis with ascites** HCC COM
AHA: 2018,1Q,4

**K71.6 Toxic liver disease with hepatitis, not elsewhere classified**

**K71.7 Toxic liver disease with fibrosis and cirrhosis of liver** HCC COM

**K71.8 Toxic liver disease with other disorders of liver**
Toxic liver disease with focal nodular hyperplasia
Toxic liver disease with hepatic granulomas
Toxic liver disease with peliosis hepatis
Toxic liver disease with veno-occlusive disease of liver
AHA: 2024,1Q,25; 2015,2Q,17

**K71.9 Toxic liver disease, unspecified**

✓4th **K72 Hepatic failure, not elsewhere classified**

INCLUDES fulminant hepatitis NEC, with hepatic failure
liver (cell) necrosis with hepatic failure
malignant hepatitis NEC, with hepatic failure
yellow liver atrophy or dystrophy

Use additional code, if applicable, for ascites (R18.8)

EXCLUDES 1 *alcoholic hepatic failure (K7Ø.4)*
*hepatic failure with toxic liver disease (K71.1-)*
*icterus of newborn (P55-P59)*
*postprocedural hepatic failure (K91.82)*
EXCLUDES 2 *hepatic failure complicating abortion or ectopic or molar pregnancy (OØØ-OØ7, OØ8.8)*
*hepatic failure complicating pregnancy, childbirth and the puerperium (O26.6-)*
*viral hepatitis with hepatic coma (B15-B19)*

AHA: 2017,1Q,41

✓5th **K72.Ø Acute and subacute hepatic failure**
Acute non-viral hepatitis NOS
AHA: 2015,2Q,17; 2014,2Q,13

**K72.ØØ Acute and subacute hepatic failure without coma** COM
AHA: 2021,1Q,13

**K72.Ø1 Acute and subacute hepatic failure with coma** ESR COM

✓5th **K72.1 Chronic hepatic failure**
End stage liver disease

**K72.1Ø Chronic hepatic failure without coma** HCC ESR COM
AHA: 2021,1Q,13

**K72.11 Chronic hepatic failure with coma** HCC ESR COM

✓5th **K72.9 Hepatic failure, unspecified**

**K72.9Ø Hepatic failure, unspecified without coma** HCC ESR COM
AHA: 2022,1Q,52; 2018,4Q,20; 2016,2Q,35

**K72.91 Hepatic failure, unspecified with coma** HCC ESR COM
Hepatic coma NOS

✓4th **K73 Chronic hepatitis, not elsewhere classified**

Use additional code, if applicable, for ascites (R18.8)

EXCLUDES 1 *alcoholic hepatitis (chronic) (K7Ø.1-)*
*drug-induced hepatitis (chronic) (K71.-)*
*granulomatous hepatitis (chronic) NEC (K75.3)*
*reactive, nonspecific hepatitis (chronic) (K75.2)*
*viral hepatitis (chronic) (B15-B19)*

**K73.Ø Chronic persistent hepatitis, not elsewhere classified** HCC ESR COM

**K73.1 Chronic lobular hepatitis, not elsewhere classified** HCC ESR COM

**K73.2 Chronic active hepatitis, not elsewhere classified** HCC ESR COM

**K73.8 Other chronic hepatitis, not elsewhere classified** HCC ESR COM

**K73.9 Chronic hepatitis, unspecified** HCC ESR COM

✓4th **K74 Fibrosis and cirrhosis of liver**

Code also, if applicable, viral hepatitis (acute) (chronic) (B15-B19)

EXCLUDES 1 *alcoholic cirrhosis (of liver) (K7Ø.3)*
*alcoholic fibrosis of liver (K7Ø.2)*
*cardiac sclerosis of liver (K76.1)*
*cirrhosis (of liver) with toxic liver disease (K71.7)*
*congenital cirrhosis (of liver) (P78.81)*
*pigmentary cirrhosis (of liver) (E83.11Ø)*

✓5th **K74.Ø Hepatic fibrosis**
Code first underlying liver disease, such as:
nonalcoholic steatohepatitis (NASH) (K75.81)
AHA: 2020,4Q,30-31

**K74.ØØ Hepatic fibrosis, unspecified**

**K74.Ø1 Hepatic fibrosis, early fibrosis**
▶Hepatic fibrosis, stage F1◀
▶Mild hepatic fibrosis◀

● **K74.ØA Hepatic fibrosis, moderate fibrosis**
Hepatic fibrosis, stage F2
Moderate hepatic fibrosis

**K74.Ø2 Hepatic fibrosis, advanced fibrosis**
Hepatic fibrosis, stage F3
EXCLUDES 1 *cirrhosis of liver (K74.6-)*
*hepatic fibrosis, stage F4 (K74.6-)*

**K74.1 Hepatic sclerosis**

**K74.2 Hepatic fibrosis with hepatic sclerosis**

**K74.3 Primary biliary cirrhosis** HCC Rx ESR COM
Chronic nonsuppurative destructive cholangitis
Primary biliary cholangitis
EXCLUDES 2 *primary sclerosing cholangitis (K83.Ø1)*

**K74.4 Secondary biliary cirrhosis** HCC ESR COM

**K74.5 Biliary cirrhosis, unspecified** HCC ESR COM

✓5th **K74.6 Other and unspecified cirrhosis of liver**
AHA: 2026,1Q,29-30; 2020,4Q,30-31

**K74.6Ø Unspecified cirrhosis of liver** HCC ESR COM
Cirrhosis (of liver) NOS
AHA: 2025,3Q,20; 2018,1Q,4

**K74.69 Other cirrhosis of liver** HCC ESR COM
Cryptogenic cirrhosis (of liver)
Macronodular cirrhosis (of liver)
Micronodular cirrhosis (of liver)
Mixed type cirrhosis (of liver)
Portal cirrhosis (of liver)
Postnecrotic cirrhosis (of liver)

✓4th **K75 Other inflammatory liver diseases**
EXCLUDES 2 *toxic liver disease (K71.-)*

**K75.Ø Abscess of liver** COM
Cholangitic hepatic abscess
Hematogenic hepatic abscess
Hepatic abscess NOS
Lymphogenic hepatic abscess
Pylephlebitic hepatic abscess
EXCLUDES 1 *amebic liver abscess (AØ6.4)*
*cholangitis without liver abscess (K83.Ø9)*
*pylephlebitis without liver abscess (K75.1)*
EXCLUDES 2 *acute or subacute hepatitis NOS (B17.9)*
*acute or subacute non-viral hepatitis (K72.Ø)*
*chronic hepatitis NEC (K73.8)*

**K75.1 Phlebitis of portal vein** COM
Pylephlebitis
EXCLUDES 1 *pylephlebitic liver abscess (K75.Ø)*
DEF: Inflammation of the portal vein or branches due to diverticulitis, perforated appendicitis, or peritonitis. Symptoms include fever, chills, jaundice, sweating, and abscess in various body parts.

**K75.2 Nonspecific reactive hepatitis**
EXCLUDES 1 *acute or subacute hepatitis (K72.Ø-)*
*chronic hepatitis NEC (K73.-)*
*viral hepatitis (B15-B19)*

**K75.3 Granulomatous hepatitis, not elsewhere classified**
EXCLUDES 1 *acute or subacute hepatitis (K72.Ø-)*
*chronic hepatitis NEC (K73.-)*
*viral hepatitis (B15-B19)*

**K75.4 Autoimmune hepatitis** HCC ESR COM
Lupoid hepatitis NEC

✓5th **K75.8 Other specified inflammatory liver diseases**

**K75.81 Nonalcoholic steatohepatitis (NASH)**
Metabolic dysfunction-associated steatohepatitis (MASH)
Use additional code, if applicable, hepatic fibrosis (K74.Ø-)
AHA: 2026,1Q,29

**K75.89 Other specified inflammatory liver diseases**

**K75.9 Inflammatory liver disease, unspecified**
Hepatitis NOS
EXCLUDES 1 *acute or subacute hepatitis (K72.Ø-)*
*chronic hepatitis NEC (K73.-)*
*viral hepatitis (B15-B19)*
AHA: 2015,2Q,17

✓4th **K76 Other diseases of liver**
EXCLUDES 2 *alcoholic liver disease (K7Ø.-)*
*amyloid degeneration of liver (E85.-)*
*cystic disease of liver (congenital) (Q44.6)*
*hepatic vein thrombosis (I82.Ø)*
*hepatomegaly NOS (R16.Ø)*
*pigmentary cirrhosis (of liver) (E83.11Ø)*
*portal vein thrombosis (I81)*
*toxic liver disease (K71.-)*

**K76.Ø Fatty (change of) liver, not elsewhere classified**
Metabolic dysfunction-associated steatotic liver disease (MASLD)
Nonalcoholic fatty liver disease (NAFLD)
EXCLUDES 1 *nonalcoholic steatohepatitis (NASH) (K75.81)*

**K76.1 Chronic passive congestion of liver**
Cardiac cirrhosis
Cardiac sclerosis

**K76.2 Central hemorrhagic necrosis of liver** COM
EXCLUDES 1 *liver necrosis with hepatic failure (K72.-)*

**K76.3 Infarction of liver** COM

**K76.4 Peliosis hepatis**
Hepatic angiomatosis

**K76.5 Hepatic veno-occlusive disease**
EXCLUDES 1 *Budd-Chiari syndrome (I82.Ø)*

**K76.6 Portal hypertension** HCC ESR COM
Use additional code for any associated complications, such as:
portal hypertensive gastropathy (K31.89)
AHA: 2020,1Q,15

**K76.7 Hepatorenal syndrome** HCC ESR COM
EXCLUDES 1 *hepatorenal syndrome following labor and delivery (O9Ø.41)*
*postprocedural hepatorenal syndrome (K91.83)*
AHA: 2025,1Q,26

✓5th **K76.8 Other specified diseases of liver**

**K76.81 Hepatopulmonary syndrome** HCC ESR COM
Code first underlying liver disease, such as:
alcoholic cirrhosis of liver (K7Ø.3-)
cirrhosis of liver without mention of alcohol (K74.6-)

**K76.82 Hepatic encephalopathy** HCC ESR COM
Hepatic encephalopathy without coma
Hepatic encephalopathy, NOS
Hepatocerebral intoxication
Portal-systemic encephalopathy
Code also underlying liver disease, such as:
acute and subacute hepatic failure without coma (K72.ØØ)
alcoholic hepatic failure without coma (K7Ø.4Ø)
chronic hepatic failure without coma (K72.1Ø)
hepatic failure with toxic liver disease without coma (K71.1Ø)
hepatic failure without coma (K72.9Ø)
icterus of newborn (P55-P59)
postprocedural hepatic failure (K91.82)
viral hepatitis without hepatic coma (B15.9, B16.1, B16.9, B17.1Ø, B19.1Ø, B19.2Ø, B19.9)
EXCLUDES 1 *acute and subacute hepatic failure with coma (K72.Ø1)*
*alcoholic hepatic failure with coma (K7Ø.41)*
*chronic hepatic failure with coma (K72.11)*
*hepatic failure with coma (K72.91)*
AHA: 2022,4Q,27-28

● **K76.83 Intestinal failure-associated liver disease**
IFALD
EXCLUDES 1 *intestinal failure (K9Ø.83)*

**K76.89 Other specified diseases of liver**
Cyst (simple) of liver
Focal nodular hyperplasia of liver
Hepatoptosis
AHA: 2023,1Q,26; 2022,3Q,7
TIP: Assign codes E80.6 and K76.89 to report benign recurrent intrahepatic cholestasis (BRIC) or progressive familial intrahepatic cholestasis (PFIC).

**K76.9 Liver disease, unspecified**

**K77 *Liver disorders in diseases classified elsewhere***

Code first underlying disease, such as:
- amyloidosis (E85.-)
- congenital syphilis (A50.0, A50.5)
- congenital toxoplasmosis (P37.1)
- infectious mononucleosis with liver disease (B27.0-B27.9 with fifth character 9)
- schistosomiasis (B65.0-B65.9)

EXCLUDES 1
- *alcoholic hepatitis (K70.1-)*
- *alcoholic liver disease (K70.-)*
- *cytomegaloviral hepatitis (B25.1)*
- *herpesviral [herpes simplex] hepatitis (B00.81)*
- *mumps hepatitis (B26.81)*
- *sarcoidosis with liver disease (D86.89)*
- *secondary syphilis with liver disease (A51.45)*
- *syphilis (late) with liver disease (A52.74)*
- *toxoplasmosis (acquired) hepatitis (B58.1)*
- *tuberculosis with liver disease (A18.83)*

## Disorders of gallbladder, biliary tract and pancreas (K80-K87)

✓4th **K80 Cholelithiasis**

EXCLUDES 1 *retained cholelithiasis following cholecystectomy (K91.86)*

**AHA:** 2018,4Q,20

**DEF:** Presence or formation of concretions (calculi or "gallstones") in the gallbladder. The stones contain cholesterol, calcium carbonate, or calcium bilirubinate in pure forms or in various combinations.

**Cholelithiasis**

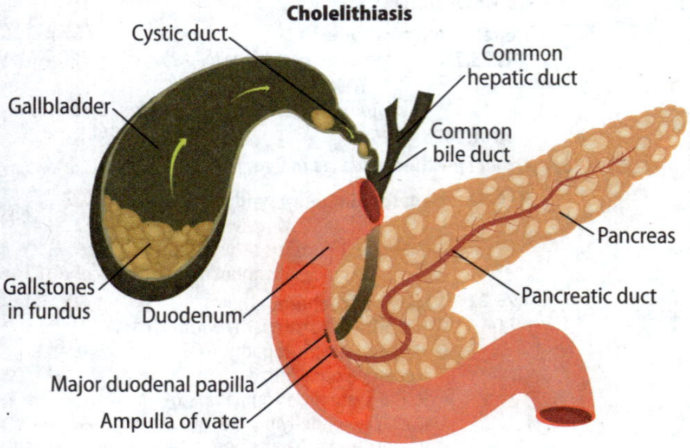


✓5th **K80.0 Calculus of gallbladder with acute cholecystitis**

Any condition listed in K80.2 with acute cholecystitis

Use additional code if applicable for associated gangrene of gallbladder (K82.A1), or perforation of gallbladder (K82.A2)

- **K80.00 Calculus of gallbladder with acute cholecystitis without obstruction**
  - **AHA:** 2023,2Q,11
- **K80.01 Calculus of gallbladder with acute cholecystitis with obstruction**

✓5th **K80.1 Calculus of gallbladder with other cholecystitis**

Use additional code if applicable for associated gangrene of gallbladder (K82.A1), or perforation of gallbladder (K82.A2)

- **K80.10 Calculus of gallbladder with chronic cholecystitis without obstruction**
  - Cholelithiasis with cholecystitis NOS
- **K80.11 Calculus of gallbladder with chronic cholecystitis with obstruction**
- **K80.12 Calculus of gallbladder with acute and chronic cholecystitis without obstruction**
- **K80.13 Calculus of gallbladder with acute and chronic cholecystitis with obstruction**
- **K80.18 Calculus of gallbladder with other cholecystitis without obstruction**
- **K80.19 Calculus of gallbladder with other cholecystitis with obstruction**

✓5th **K80.2 Calculus of gallbladder without cholecystitis**

Cholecystolithiasis without cholecystitis
Cholelithiasis (without cholecystitis)
Colic (recurrent) of gallbladder (without cholecystitis)
Gallstone (impacted) of cystic duct (without cholecystitis)
Gallstone (impacted) of gallbladder (without cholecystitis)

- **K80.20 Calculus of gallbladder without cholecystitis without obstruction**
- **K80.21 Calculus of gallbladder without cholecystitis with obstruction**

✓5th **K80.3 Calculus of bile duct with cholangitis**

Any condition listed in K80.5 with cholangitis

**DEF:** Cholangitis: Inflammation of the bile ducts.

- **K80.30 Calculus of bile duct with cholangitis, unspecified, without obstruction**
- **K80.31 Calculus of bile duct with cholangitis, unspecified, with obstruction**
- **K80.32 Calculus of bile duct with acute cholangitis without obstruction**
- **K80.33 Calculus of bile duct with acute cholangitis with obstruction**
- **K80.34 Calculus of bile duct with chronic cholangitis without obstruction**
- **K80.35 Calculus of bile duct with chronic cholangitis with obstruction**
- **K80.36 Calculus of bile duct with acute and chronic cholangitis without obstruction**
- **K80.37 Calculus of bile duct with acute and chronic cholangitis with obstruction**

✓5th **K80.4 Calculus of bile duct with cholecystitis**

Any condition listed in K80.5 with cholecystitis (with cholangitis)

Code also, if applicable, fistula of bile duct (K83.3)

Use additional code if applicable for associated gangrene of gallbladder (K82.A1), or perforation of gallbladder (K82.A2)

**AHA:** 2019,1Q,17

- **K80.40 Calculus of bile duct with cholecystitis, unspecified, without obstruction**
- **K80.41 Calculus of bile duct with cholecystitis, unspecified, with obstruction**
  - **AHA:** 2019,1Q,17
- **K80.42 Calculus of bile duct with acute cholecystitis without obstruction**
- **K80.43 Calculus of bile duct with acute cholecystitis with obstruction**
- **K80.44 Calculus of bile duct with chronic cholecystitis without obstruction**
- **K80.45 Calculus of bile duct with chronic cholecystitis with obstruction**
- **K80.46 Calculus of bile duct with acute and chronic cholecystitis without obstruction**
- **K80.47 Calculus of bile duct with acute and chronic cholecystitis with obstruction**

✓5th **K80.5 Calculus of bile duct without cholangitis or cholecystitis**

Choledocholithiasis (without cholangitis or cholecystitis)
Gallstone (impacted) of bile duct NOS (without cholangitis or cholecystitis)
Gallstone (impacted) of common duct (without cholangitis or cholecystitis)
Gallstone (impacted) of hepatic duct (without cholangitis or cholecystitis)
Hepatic cholelithiasis (without cholangitis or cholecystitis)
Hepatic colic (recurrent) (without cholangitis or cholecystitis)

**DEF:** Cholangitis: Inflammation of the bile ducts.

- **K80.50 Calculus of bile duct without cholangitis or cholecystitis without obstruction**
- **K80.51 Calculus of bile duct without cholangitis or cholecystitis with obstruction**

✓5th **K80.6 Calculus of gallbladder and bile duct with cholecystitis**

Use additional code if applicable for associated gangrene of gallbladder (K82.A1), or perforation of gallbladder (K82.A2)

- **K80.60 Calculus of gallbladder and bile duct with cholecystitis, unspecified, without obstruction**
- **K80.61 Calculus of gallbladder and bile duct with cholecystitis, unspecified, with obstruction**
- **K80.62 Calculus of gallbladder and bile duct with acute cholecystitis without obstruction**
- **K80.63 Calculus of gallbladder and bile duct with acute cholecystitis with obstruction**
- **K80.64 Calculus of gallbladder and bile duct with chronic cholecystitis without obstruction**
- **K80.65 Calculus of gallbladder and bile duct with chronic cholecystitis with obstruction**
- **K80.66 Calculus of gallbladder and bile duct with acute and chronic cholecystitis without obstruction**
- **K80.67 Calculus of gallbladder and bile duct with acute and chronic cholecystitis with obstruction**

✓5th **K80.7 Calculus of gallbladder and bile duct without cholecystitis**

- **K80.70 Calculus of gallbladder and bile duct without cholecystitis without obstruction**
- **K80.71 Calculus of gallbladder and bile duct without cholecystitis with obstruction**

✓5th **K80.8 Other cholelithiasis**

**K80.80 Other cholelithiasis without obstruction**

**K80.81 Other cholelithiasis with obstruction**

✓4th **K81 Cholecystitis**

Use additional code if applicable for associated gangrene of gallbladder (K82.A1), or perforation of gallbladder (K82.A2)

EXCLUDES 1 *cholecystitis with cholelithiasis (K80.-)*

**AHA:** 2018,4Q,20

**K81.0 Acute cholecystitis**

Abscess of gallbladder
Angiocholecystitis
Emphysematous (acute) cholecystitis
Empyema of gallbladder
Gangrene of gallbladder
Gangrenous cholecystitis
Suppurative cholecystitis

**K81.1 Chronic cholecystitis**

**K81.2 Acute cholecystitis with chronic cholecystitis**

**K81.9 Cholecystitis, unspecified**

✓4th **K82 Other diseases of gallbladder**

EXCLUDES 1 *nonvisualization of gallbladder (R93.2)*
*postcholecystectomy syndrome (K91.5)*

**K82.0 Obstruction of gallbladder**

Occlusion of cystic duct or gallbladder without cholelithiasis
Stenosis of cystic duct or gallbladder without cholelithiasis
Stricture of cystic duct or gallbladder without cholelithiasis

EXCLUDES 1 *obstruction of gallbladder with cholelithiasis (K80.-)*

**K82.1 Hydrops of gallbladder**

Mucocele of gallbladder

**K82.2 Perforation of gallbladder**

Rupture of cystic duct or gallbladder

EXCLUDES 1 *perforation of gallbladder in cholecystitis (K82.A2)*

**K82.3 Fistula of gallbladder**

Cholecystocolic fistula
Cholecystoduodenal fistula

Code also, if applicable, disruption of internal operation (surgical) wound (T81.32-)

**K82.4 Cholesterolosis of gallbladder**

Strawberry gallbladder

EXCLUDES 1 *cholesterolosis of gallbladder with cholecystitis (K81.-)*
*cholesterolosis of gallbladder with cholelithiasis (K80.-)*

**K82.8 Other specified diseases of gallbladder**

Adhesions of cystic duct or gallbladder
Atrophy of cystic duct or gallbladder
Cyst of cystic duct or gallbladder
Dyskinesia of cystic duct or gallbladder
Hypertrophy of cystic duct or gallbladder
Nonfunctioning of cystic duct or gallbladder
Ulcer of cystic duct or gallbladder

**K82.9 Disease of gallbladder, unspecified**

✓5th **K82.A Disorders of gallbladder in diseases classified elsewhere**

Code first the type of cholecystitis (K81.-), or cholelithiasis with cholecystitis (K80.00-K80.19, K80.40-K80.47, K80.60-K80.67)

**AHA:** 2018,4Q,19-20

***K82.A1 Gangrene of gallbladder in cholecystitis***

***K82.A2 Perforation of gallbladder in cholecystitis***

✓4th **K83 Other diseases of biliary tract**

EXCLUDES 1 *postcholecystectomy syndrome (K91.5)*

EXCLUDES 2 *conditions involving the cystic duct (K81-K82)*
*conditions involving the gallbladder (K81-K82)*

✓5th **K83.0 Cholangitis**

EXCLUDES 1 *cholangitic liver abscess (K75.0)*
*cholangitis with choledocholithiasis (K80.3-, K80.4-)*

EXCLUDES 2 *chronic nonsuppurative destructive cholangitis (K74.3)*
*primary biliary cholangitis (K74.3)*
*primary biliary cirrhosis (K74.3)*

**AHA:** 2018,4Q,20

**K83.01 Primary sclerosing cholangitis** HCC

**K83.09 Other cholangitis** HCC

Ascending cholangitis
Cholangitis NOS
Primary cholangitis
Recurrent cholangitis
Sclerosing cholangitis
Secondary cholangitis
Stenosing cholangitis
Suppurative cholangitis

**K83.1 Obstruction of bile duct** HCC

Occlusion of bile duct without cholelithiasis
Stenosis of bile duct without cholelithiasis
Stricture of bile duct without cholelithiasis

EXCLUDES 1 *congenital obstruction of bile duct (Q44.3)*
*obstruction of bile duct with cholelithiasis (K80.-)*

**AHA:** 2023,1Q,26; 2016,1Q,18

**K83.2 Perforation of bile duct**

Rupture of bile duct

**K83.3 Fistula of bile duct**

Choledochoduodenal fistula

**AHA:** 2019,1Q,17

**K83.4 Spasm of sphincter of Oddi**

**K83.5 Biliary cyst**

**K83.8 Other specified diseases of biliary tract**

Adhesions of biliary tract
Atrophy of biliary tract
Hypertrophy of biliary tract
Ulcer of biliary tract

**K83.9 Disease of biliary tract, unspecified**

✓4th **K85 Acute pancreatitis**

INCLUDES acute (recurrent) pancreatitis
subacute pancreatitis

**AHA:** 2016,4Q,34

✓5th **K85.0 Idiopathic acute pancreatitis**

**K85.00 Idiopathic acute pancreatitis without necrosis or infection** COM

**K85.01 Idiopathic acute pancreatitis with uninfected necrosis** COM

**K85.02 Idiopathic acute pancreatitis with infected necrosis** COM

✓5th **K85.1 Biliary acute pancreatitis**

Gallstone pancreatitis

**AHA:** 2023,2Q,11

**K85.10 Biliary acute pancreatitis without necrosis or infection** COM

**K85.11 Biliary acute pancreatitis with uninfected necrosis** COM

**K85.12 Biliary acute pancreatitis with infected necrosis** COM

✓5th **K85.2 Alcohol induced acute pancreatitis**

EXCLUDES 2 *alcohol induced chronic pancreatitis (K86.0)*

**K85.20 Alcohol induced acute pancreatitis without necrosis or infection** COM

**AHA:** 2020,1Q,9

**K85.21 Alcohol induced acute pancreatitis with uninfected necrosis** COM

**K85.22 Alcohol induced acute pancreatitis with infected necrosis** COM

✓5th **K85.3 Drug induced acute pancreatitis**

Use additional code for adverse effect, if applicable, to identify drug (T36-T50 with fifth or sixth character 5)

Use additional code to identify drug abuse and dependence (F11.-F17.-)

**K85.30 Drug induced acute pancreatitis without necrosis or infection** COM

**AHA:** 2026,1Q,24

**K85.31 Drug induced acute pancreatitis with uninfected necrosis** COM

**K85.32 Drug induced acute pancreatitis with infected necrosis** COM

✓5th **K85.8 Other acute pancreatitis**

**K85.80 Other acute pancreatitis without necrosis or infection** COM

**K85.81 Other acute pancreatitis with uninfected necrosis** COM

**K85.82 Other acute pancreatitis with infected necrosis** COM

✓5th **K85.9 Acute pancreatitis, unspecified**

Pancreatitis NOS

**K85.90 Acute pancreatitis without necrosis or infection, unspecified** COM

**K85.91 Acute pancreatitis with uninfected necrosis, unspecified** COM

**K85.92 Acute pancreatitis with infected necrosis, unspecified** COM

**K86 Other diseases of pancreas**

EXCLUDES 2 *fibrocystic disease of pancreas (E84.-)*
*islet cell tumor (of pancreas) (D13.7)*
*pancreatic steatorrhea (K90.3)*

**K86.0 Alcohol-induced chronic pancreatitis** HCC Rx ESR COM
Code also exocrine pancreatic insufficiency (K86.81)
Use additional code to identify:
alcohol abuse and dependence (F10.-)
EXCLUDES 2 *alcohol induced acute pancreatitis (K85.2-)*

**K86.1 Other chronic pancreatitis** HCC Rx ESR COM
Chronic pancreatitis NOS
Infectious chronic pancreatitis
Recurrent chronic pancreatitis
Relapsing chronic pancreatitis
Code also exocrine pancreatic insufficiency (K86.81)

**K86.2 Cyst of pancreas** Rx

**K86.3 Pseudocyst of pancreas** Rx

**K86.8 Other specified diseases of pancreas**
**AHA:** 2016,4Q,34-35

**K86.81 Exocrine pancreatic insufficiency** Rx

**K86.89 Other specified diseases of pancreas** Rx
Aseptic pancreatic necrosis, unrelated to acute pancreatitis
Atrophy of pancreas
Calculus of pancreas
Cirrhosis of pancreas
Fibrosis of pancreas
Pancreatic fat necrosis, unrelated to acute pancreatitis
Pancreatic infantilism
Pancreatic necrosis NOS, unrelated to acute pancreatitis
**AHA:** 2024,3Q,4

**K86.9 Disease of pancreas, unspecified** Rx

***K87 Disorders of gallbladder, biliary tract and pancreas in diseases classified elsewhere*** Rx
Code first underlying disease
EXCLUDES 1 *cytomegaloviral pancreatitis (B25.2)*
*mumps pancreatitis (B26.3)*
*syphilitic gallbladder (A52.74)*
*syphilitic pancreas (A52.74)*
*tuberculosis of gallbladder (A18.83)*
*tuberculosis of pancreas (A18.83)*

## Other diseases of the digestive system (K90-K95)

**K90 Intestinal malabsorption**

EXCLUDES 1 *intestinal malabsorption following gastrointestinal surgery (K91.2)*
**AHA:** 2017,4Q,108

**K90.0 Celiac disease** Rx
Celiac disease with steatorrhea
Celiac gluten-sensitive enteropathy
Nontropical sprue
Code also exocrine pancreatic insufficiency (K86.81)
Use additional code for associated disorders including:
dermatitis herpetiformis (L13.0)
gluten ataxia (G32.81)
**DEF:** Malabsorption syndrome due to gluten consumption. Symptoms include fetid, bulky, frothy, oily stools; a distended abdomen; gas; asthenia; electrolyte depletion; and vitamin B, D, and K deficiency.

**K90.1 Tropical sprue** Rx
Sprue NOS
Tropical steatorrhea

**K90.2 Blind loop syndrome, not elsewhere classified** Rx
Blind loop syndrome NOS
EXCLUDES 1 *congenital blind loop syndrome (Q43.8)*
*postsurgical blind loop syndrome (K91.2)*

**K90.3 Pancreatic steatorrhea** Rx

**K90.4 Other malabsorption due to intolerance**
EXCLUDES 2 *celiac gluten-sensitive enteropathy (K90.0)*
*lactose intolerance (E73.-)*
**AHA:** 2016,4Q,35-36

**K90.41 Non-celiac gluten sensitivity**
Gluten sensitivity NOS
Non-celiac gluten sensitive enteropathy

**K90.49 Malabsorption due to intolerance, not elsewhere classified** Rx
Malabsorption due to intolerance to carbohydrate
Malabsorption due to intolerance to fat
Malabsorption due to intolerance to protein
Malabsorption due to intolerance to starch

**K90.8 Other intestinal malabsorption**
**AHA:** 2023,4Q,31-33

**K90.81 Whipple's disease** Rx

**K90.82 Short bowel syndrome**
Short gut syndrome
EXCLUDES 1 *postsurgical malabsorption, not elsewhere classified (K91.2)*

**K90.821 Short bowel syndrome with colon in continuity** Rx
Short bowel syndrome with colonic continuity

**K90.822 Short bowel syndrome without colon in continuity** Rx
Short bowel syndrome without colonic continuity
Use additional code, if applicable, for colostomy status (Z93.3)

**K90.829 Short bowel syndrome, unspecified** Rx

**K90.83 Intestinal failure** Rx

**K90.89 Other intestinal malabsorption** Rx

**K90.9 Intestinal malabsorption, unspecified** Rx

**K91 Intraoperative and postprocedural complications and disorders of digestive system, not elsewhere classified**

EXCLUDES 2 *complications of artificial opening of digestive system (K94.-)*
*complications of bariatric procedures (K95.-)*
*gastrojejunal ulcer (K28.-)*
*postprocedural (radiation) retroperitoneal abscess (K68.11)*
*radiation colitis (K52.0)*
*radiation gastroenteritis (K52.0)*
*radiation proctitis (K62.7)*
**AHA:** 2016,4Q,9-10

**K91.0 Vomiting following gastrointestinal surgery**

**K91.1 Postgastric surgery syndromes**
Dumping syndrome
Postgastrectomy syndrome
Postvagotomy syndrome

**K91.2 Postsurgical malabsorption, not elsewhere classified** Rx
Postsurgical blind loop syndrome
EXCLUDES 1 *malabsorption osteomalacia in adults (M83.2)*
*malabsorption osteoporosis, postsurgical (M80.8-, M81.8)*

**K91.3 Postprocedural intestinal obstruction**
**AHA:** 2017,4Q,16-17; 2017,1Q,40

**K91.30 Postprocedural intestinal obstruction, unspecified as to partial versus complete**
Postprocedural intestinal obstruction NOS

**K91.31 Postprocedural partial intestinal obstruction**
Postprocedural incomplete intestinal obstruction

**K91.32 Postprocedural complete intestinal obstruction**

**K91.5 Postcholecystectomy syndrome**

**K91.6 Intraoperative hemorrhage and hematoma of a digestive system organ or structure complicating a procedure**
EXCLUDES 1 *intraoperative hemorrhage and hematoma of a digestive system organ or structure due to accidental puncture and laceration during a procedure (K91.7-)*

**K91.61 Intraoperative hemorrhage and hematoma of a digestive system organ or structure complicating a digestive system procedure**
**AHA:** 2020,1Q,19

**K91.62 Intraoperative hemorrhage and hematoma of a digestive system organ or structure complicating other procedure**

**K91.7 Accidental puncture and laceration of a digestive system organ or structure during a procedure**
**AHA:** 2022,1Q,51

**K91.71 Accidental puncture and laceration of a digestive system organ or structure during a digestive system procedure**
**AHA:** 2021,2Q,11

K91.72 **Accidental puncture and laceration of a digestive system organ or structure during other procedure**
AHA: 2019,2Q,23

✓5th K91.8 **Other intraoperative and postprocedural complications and disorders of digestive system**

K91.81 **Other intraoperative complications of digestive system**

K91.82 **Postprocedural hepatic failure**

K91.83 **Postprocedural hepatorenal syndrome**

✓6th K91.84 **Postprocedural hemorrhage of a digestive system organ or structure following a procedure**

K91.840 **Postprocedural hemorrhage of a digestive system organ or structure following a digestive system procedure**
AHA: 2016,1Q,15

K91.841 **Postprocedural hemorrhage of a digestive system organ or structure following other procedure**

✓6th K91.85 **Complications of intestinal pouch**

K91.850 **Pouchitis** HCC ESR COM
Inflammation of internal ileoanal pouch
DEF: Inflammatory complication of an existing surgically created ileoanal pouch, resulting in multiple GI complaints, including diarrhea, abdominal pain, rectal bleeding, fecal urgency, or incontinence.

K91.858 **Other complications of intestinal pouch** HCC ESR COM
AHA: 2019,2Q,13

K91.86 **Retained cholelithiasis following cholecystectomy**

✓6th K91.87 **Postprocedural hematoma and seroma of a digestive system organ or structure following a procedure**

K91.870 **Postprocedural hematoma of a digestive system organ or structure following a digestive system procedure**
AHA: 2022,1Q,24

K91.871 **Postprocedural hematoma of a digestive system organ or structure following other procedure**

K91.872 **Postprocedural seroma of a digestive system organ or structure following a digestive system procedure**

K91.873 **Postprocedural seroma of a digestive system organ or structure following other procedure**

K91.89 **Other postprocedural complications and disorders of digestive system**
Use additional code, if applicable, to further specify disorder
EXCLUDES 2 *postprocedural retroperitoneal abscess (K68.11)*
AHA: 2020,2Q,22; 2017,1Q,40

✓4th **K92 Other diseases of digestive system**
EXCLUDES 1 *neonatal gastrointestinal hemorrhage (P54.Ø-P54.3)*

K92.Ø **Hematemesis**

K92.1 **Melena**
EXCLUDES 1 *occult blood in feces (R19.5)*

K92.2 **Gastrointestinal hemorrhage, unspecified**
Gastric hemorrhage NOS
Intestinal hemorrhage NOS
EXCLUDES 1 *acute hemorrhagic gastritis (K29.Ø1)*
*angiodysplasia of stomach with hemorrhage (K31.811)*
*diverticular disease with hemorrhage (K57.-)*
*gastritis and duodenitis with hemorrhage (K29.-)*
*hemorrhage of anus and rectum (K62.5)*
*peptic ulcer with hemorrhage (K25-K28)*
AHA: 2021,1Q,11

✓5th K92.8 **Other specified diseases of the digestive system**

K92.81 **Gastrointestinal mucositis (ulcerative)**
Code also type of associated therapy, such as:
antineoplastic and immunosuppressive drugs (T45.1X-)
radiological procedure and radiotherapy (Y84.2)
EXCLUDES 2 *mucositis (ulcerative) of vagina and vulva (N76.81)*
*nasal mucositis (ulcerative) (J34.81)*
*oral mucositis (ulcerative) (K12.3-)*

K92.89 **Other specified diseases of the digestive system**

K92.9 **Disease of digestive system, unspecified**

✓4th **K94 Complications of artificial openings of the digestive system**

✓5th K94.Ø **Colostomy complications**

K94.ØØ **Colostomy complication, unspecified** HCC ESR COM

K94.Ø1 **Colostomy hemorrhage** HCC ESR COM

K94.Ø2 **Colostomy infection** HCC ESR COM
Use additional code to specify type of infection, such as:
cellulitis of abdominal wall (LØ3.311)
sepsis (A4Ø.-, A41.-)

K94.Ø3 **Colostomy malfunction** HCC ESR COM
Mechanical complication of colostomy

K94.Ø9 **Other complications of colostomy** HCC ESR COM

✓5th K94.1 **Enterostomy complications**

K94.1Ø **Enterostomy complication, unspecified** HCC ESR COM

K94.11 **Enterostomy hemorrhage** HCC ESR COM

K94.12 **Enterostomy infection** HCC ESR COM
Use additional code to specify type of infection, such as:
cellulitis of abdominal wall (LØ3.311)
sepsis (A4Ø.-, A41.-)

K94.13 **Enterostomy malfunction** HCC ESR COM
Mechanical complication of enterostomy

K94.19 **Other complications of enterostomy** HCC ESR COM

✓5th K94.2 **Gastrostomy complications**

K94.2Ø **Gastrostomy complication, unspecified** HCC ESR COM

K94.21 **Gastrostomy hemorrhage** HCC ESR COM

K94.22 **Gastrostomy infection** HCC ESR COM
Use additional code to specify type of infection, such as:
cellulitis of abdominal wall (LØ3.311)
sepsis (A4Ø.-, A41.-)

K94.23 **Gastrostomy malfunction** HCC ESR COM
Mechanical complication of gastrostomy
AHA: 2019,1Q,26

K94.29 **Other complications of gastrostomy** HCC ESR COM

✓5th K94.3 **Esophagostomy complications**

K94.3Ø **Esophagostomy complications, unspecified** HCC ESR COM

K94.31 **Esophagostomy hemorrhage** HCC ESR COM

K94.32 **Esophagostomy infection** HCC ESR COM
Use additional code to identify the infection

K94.33 **Esophagostomy malfunction** HCC ESR COM
Mechanical complication of esophagostomy

K94.39 **Other complications of esophagostomy** HCC ESR COM

✓4th **K95 Complications of bariatric procedures**

✓5th K95.Ø **Complications of gastric band procedure**

K95.Ø1 **Infection due to gastric band procedure**
Use additional code to specify type of infection or organism, such as:
bacterial and viral infectious agents (B95.-, B96.-)
cellulitis of abdominal wall (LØ3.311)
sepsis (A4Ø.-, A41.-)

K95.Ø9 **Other complications of gastric band procedure**
Use additional code, if applicable, to further specify complication

✓5th K95.8 **Complications of other bariatric procedure**
EXCLUDES 1 *complications of gastric band surgery (K95.Ø-)*

K95.81 **Infection due to other bariatric procedure**
Use additional code to specify type of infection or organism, such as:
bacterial and viral infectious agents (B95.-, B96.-)
cellulitis of abdominal wall (LØ3.311)
sepsis (A4Ø.-, A41.-)

K95.89 **Other complications of other bariatric procedure**
Use additional code, if applicable, to further specify complication

# Chapter 12. Diseases of the Skin and Subcutaneous Tissue (LØØ–L99)



## Chapter-specific Guidelines with Coding Examples

The chapter-specific guidelines from the ICD-10-CM Official Guidelines for Coding and Reporting have been provided below. Along with these guidelines are coding examples, contained in the shaded boxes, that have been developed to help illustrate the coding and/or sequencing guidance found in these guidelines.

**a. Pressure ulcer stage codes**

**1) Pressure ulcer stages**

Codes in category L89, Pressure ulcer, identify the site and stage of the pressure ulcer.

The ICD-10-CM classifies pressure ulcer stages based on severity, which is designated by stages 1-4, deep tissue pressure injury, unspecified stage, and unstageable.

Assign as many codes from category L89 as needed to identify all the pressure ulcers the patient has, if applicable.

*See Section I.B.14. for pressure ulcer stage documentation by clinicians other than patient's provider.*

Stage 3 pressure ulcer left ankle, 6 x 7 cm that invades the fascia; stage 2 pressure ulcer of left hip

**L89.523** **Pressure ulcer of left ankle, stage 3**

**L89.222** **Pressure ulcer of left hip, stage 2**

*Explanation:* Patient has a left ankle pressure ulcer documented as stage 3 and a left hip pressure ulcer documented as stage 2. Combination codes from category L89 Pressure ulcer, identify the site of the pressure ulcer as well as the stage. Assign as many codes from category L89 as needed to identify all the pressure ulcers the patient has.

**2) Unstageable pressure ulcers**

Assignment of the code for unstageable pressure ulcer (L89.--Ø) should be based on the clinical documentation. These codes are used for pressure ulcers whose stage cannot be clinically determined (e.g., the ulcer is covered by eschar or has been treated with a skin or muscle graft). This code should not be confused with the codes for unspecified stage (L89.--9). When there is no documentation regarding the stage of the pressure ulcer, assign the appropriate code for unspecified stage (L89.--9).

Pressure ulcer of the right lower back documented as unstageable due to the presence of thick eschar covering the ulcer

**L89.13Ø** **Pressure ulcer of right lower back, unstageable**

*Explanation:* Codes for unstageable pressure ulcers are assigned when the stage cannot be clinically determined (e.g., the ulcer is covered by eschar or has been treated with a skin or muscle graft).

If during an encounter, the stage of an unstageable pressure ulcer is revealed after debridement, assign only the code for the stage revealed following debridement.

**3) Documented pressure ulcer stage**

Assignment of the pressure ulcer stage code should be guided by clinical documentation of the stage or documentation of the terms found in the Alphabetic Index. For clinical terms describing the stage that are not found in the Alphabetic Index, and there is no documentation of the stage, the provider should be queried.

Left heel pressure ulcer with partial thickness skin loss involving the dermis

**L89.622** **Pressure ulcer of left heel, stage 2**

*Explanation:* Code assignment for the pressure ulcer stage should be guided by either the clinical documentation of the stage or the documentation of terms found in the Alphabetic Index. The clinical documentation describing the left heel pressure ulcer "partial thickness skin loss involving the dermis" matches the ICD-10-CM index parenthetical description for stage 2 "(abrasion, blister, partial thickness skin loss involving epidermis and/or dermis)."

**4) Patients admitted with pressure ulcers documented as healed**

No code is assigned if the documentation states that the pressure ulcer is completely healed at the time of admission.

Patient receiving follow-up examination of a completely healed pressure ulcer of the foot

**ZØ9** **Encounter for follow-up examination after completed treatment for conditions other than malignant neoplasm**

**Z87.2** **Personal history of diseases of the skin and subcutaneous tissue**

*Explanation:* Assign only codes for the reason for the encounter and the personal history of the pressure ulcer. Personal history code Z87.2 includes conditions classifiable to LØØ–L99 such as pressure ulcer. No code is assigned for a pressure ulcer documented as completely healed.

**5) Pressure ulcers documented as healing**

Pressure ulcers described as healing should be assigned the appropriate pressure ulcer stage code based on the documentation in the medical record. If the documentation does not provide information about the stage of the healing pressure ulcer, assign the appropriate code for unspecified stage.

If the documentation is unclear as to whether the patient has a current (new) pressure ulcer or if the patient is being treated for a healing pressure ulcer, query the provider.

For ulcers that were present on admission but healed at the time of discharge, assign the code for the site and stage of the pressure ulcer at the time of admission.

**6) Patient admitted with pressure ulcer evolving into another stage during the admission**

If a patient is admitted to an inpatient hospital with a pressure ulcer at one stage and it progresses to a higher stage, two separate codes should be assigned: one code for the site and stage of the ulcer on admission and a second code for the same ulcer site and the highest stage reported during the stay.

**7) Pressure-induced deep tissue damage**

For pressure-induced deep tissue damage or deep tissue pressure injury, assign only the appropriate code for pressure-induced deep tissue damage (L89.--6).

**b. Non-pressure chronic ulcers**

**1) Patients admitted with non-pressure ulcers documented as healed**

No code is assigned if the documentation states that the non-pressure ulcer is completely healed at the time of admission.

**2) Non-pressure ulcers documented as healing**

Non-pressure ulcers described as healing should be assigned the appropriate non-pressure ulcer code based on the documentation in the medical record. If the documentation does not provide information about the severity of the healing non-pressure ulcer, assign the appropriate code for unspecified severity.

If the documentation is unclear as to whether the patient has a current (new) non-pressure ulcer or if the patient is being treated for a healing non-pressure ulcer, query the provider.

For ulcers that were present on admission but healed at the time of discharge, assign the code for the site and severity of the non-pressure ulcer at the time of admission.

**3) Patient admitted with non-pressure ulcer that progresses to another severity level during the admission**

If a patient is admitted to an inpatient hospital with a non-pressure ulcer at one severity level and it progresses to a higher severity level, two separate codes should be assigned: one code for the site and severity level of the ulcer on admission and a second code for the same ulcer site and the highest severity level reported during the stay.

*See Section I.B.14. for pressure ulcer stage documentation by clinicians other than patient's provider.*

# Chapter 12. Diseases of the Skin and Subcutaneous Tissue (LØØ-L99)

EXCLUDES 2 *certain conditions originating in the perinatal period (PØ4-P96)*
*certain infectious and parasitic diseases (AØØ-B99)*
*complications of pregnancy, childbirth and the puerperium (OØØ-O9A)*
*congenital malformations, deformations, and chromosomal abnormalities (QØØ-Q99)*
*endocrine, nutritional and metabolic diseases (EØØ-E88)*
*lipomelanotic reticulosis (I89.8)*
*neoplasms (CØØ-D49)*
*symptoms, signs and abnormal clinical and laboratory findings, not elsewhere classified (RØØ-R94)*
*systemic connective tissue disorders (M3Ø-M36)*
*viral warts (BØ7.-)*

**AHA:** 2022,2Q,7

This chapter contains the following blocks:

| | |
|---|---|
| LØØ-LØ8 | Infections of the skin and subcutaneous tissue |
| L1Ø-L14 | Bullous disorders |
| L2Ø-L3Ø | Dermatitis and eczema |
| L4Ø-L45 | Papulosquamous disorders |
| L49-L54 | Urticaria and erythema |
| L55-L59 | Radiation-related disorders of the skin and subcutaneous tissue |
| L6Ø-L75 | Disorders of skin appendages |
| L76 | Intraoperative and postprocedural complications of skin and subcutaneous tissue |
| L8Ø-L99 | Other disorders of the skin and subcutaneous tissue |

## Infections of the skin and subcutaneous tissue (LØØ-LØ8)

Use additional code (B95-B97) to identify infectious agent

EXCLUDES 2 *hordeolum (HØØ.Ø)*
*infective dermatitis (L3Ø.3)*
*local infections of skin classified in Chapter 1*
*lupus panniculitis (L93.2)*
*panniculitis NOS (M79.3)*
*panniculitis of neck and back (M54.Ø-)*
*perlèche NOS (K13.Ø)*
*perlèche due to candidiasis (B37.Ø)*
*perlèche due to riboflavin deficiency (E53.Ø)*
*pyogenic granuloma (L98.Ø)*
*relapsing panniculitis [Weber-Christian] (M35.6)*
*viral warts (BØ7.-)*
*zoster (BØ2.-)*

**LØØ Staphylococcal scaled skin syndrome** COM
Ritter's disease
Use additional code to identify percentage of skin exfoliation (L49.-)
EXCLUDES 1 *bullous impetigo (LØ1.Ø3)*
*pemphigus neonatorum (LØ1.Ø3)*
*toxic epidermal necrolysis [Lyell] (L51.2)*
**DEF:** Infectious skin disease of children younger than 5 years marked by eruptions ranging from a few localized blisters to widespread, easily ruptured, fine vesicles and bullae affecting almost the entire body. It results in exfoliation of large planes of skin and leaves raw areas.

✓4th **LØ1 Impetigo**
EXCLUDES 1 *impetigo herpetiformis (L4Ø.1)*
**DEF:** Acute, superficial, highly contagious skin infection commonly occurring in children. Skin lesions usually appear on the face and consist of vesicles and bullae that burst and form yellow crusts.

✓5th **LØ1.Ø Impetigo**
Impetigo contagiosa
Impetigo vulgaris

**LØ1.ØØ Impetigo, unspecified**
Impetigo NOS

**LØ1.Ø1 Non-bullous impetigo**

**LØ1.Ø2 Bockhart's impetigo**
Impetigo follicularis
Perifolliculitis NOS
Superficial pustular perifolliculitis
**DEF:** Superficial inflammation of the hair follicles commonly caused by *Staphylococcus aureus* that manifests as rounded, sphere-shaped, pustular eruptions in the areas of the scalp, beard, underarms, extremities, and buttocks.

**LØ1.Ø3 Bullous impetigo**
Impetigo neonatorum
Pemphigus neonatorum

**LØ1.Ø9 Other impetigo**
Ulcerative impetigo

**LØ1.1 Impetiginization of other dermatoses**

✓4th **LØ2 Cutaneous abscess, furuncle and carbuncle**
Use additional code to identify organism (B95-B96)
EXCLUDES 2 *abscess of anus and rectal regions (K61.-)*
*abscess of female genital organs (external) (N76.4)*
*abscess of male genital organs (external) (N48.2, N49.-)*
**DEF:** Carbuncle: Infection of the skin that arises from a collection of interconnected infected boils or furuncles, usually from hair follicles infected by *Staphylococcus*. This condition can produce pus and form drainage cavities.
**DEF:** Furuncle: Inflamed, painful abscess, cyst, or nodule on the skin caused by bacteria, often *Staphylococcus*, entering along the hair follicle.

✓5th **LØ2.Ø Cutaneous abscess, furuncle and carbuncle of face**
EXCLUDES 2 *abscess of ear, external (H6Ø.Ø)*
*abscess of eyelid (HØØ.Ø)*
*abscess of head [any part, except face] (LØ2.8)*
*abscess of lacrimal gland (HØ4.Ø)*
*abscess of lacrimal passages (HØ4.3)*
*abscess of mouth (K12.2)*
*abscess of nose (J34.Ø)*
*abscess of orbit (HØ5.Ø)*
*submandibular abscess (K12.2)*

**LØ2.Ø1 Cutaneous abscess of face**

**LØ2.Ø2 Furuncle of face**
Boil of face
Folliculitis of face

**LØ2.Ø3 Carbuncle of face**

✓5th **LØ2.1 Cutaneous abscess, furuncle and carbuncle of neck**

**LØ2.11 Cutaneous abscess of neck**

**LØ2.12 Furuncle of neck**
Boil of neck
Folliculitis of neck

**LØ2.13 Carbuncle of neck**

✓5th **LØ2.2 Cutaneous abscess, furuncle and carbuncle of trunk**
EXCLUDES 1 *non-newborn omphalitis (LØ8.82)*
*omphalitis of newborn (P38.-)*
EXCLUDES 2 *abscess of breast (N61.1)*
*abscess of buttocks ▶(LØ2.31)◀*
*abscess of female external genital organs (N76.4)*
*abscess of hip (LØ2.4)*
*abscess of male external genital organs (N48.2, N49.-)*

✓6th **LØ2.21 Cutaneous abscess of trunk**

**LØ2.211 Cutaneous abscess of abdominal wall**
**LØ2.212 Cutaneous abscess of back [any part, except buttock and flank]**
**LØ2.213 Cutaneous abscess of chest wall**
**LØ2.214 Cutaneous abscess of groin**
**LØ2.215 Cutaneous abscess of perineum**
**LØ2.216 Cutaneous abscess of umbilicus**
**LØ2.217 Cutaneous abscess of flank**
**LØ2.219 Cutaneous abscess of trunk, unspecified**

✓6th **LØ2.22 Furuncle of trunk**
Boil of trunk
Folliculitis of trunk

**LØ2.221 Furuncle of abdominal wall**
**LØ2.222 Furuncle of back [any part, except buttock and flank]**
**LØ2.223 Furuncle of chest wall**
**LØ2.224 Furuncle of groin**
**LØ2.225 Furuncle of perineum**
**LØ2.226 Furuncle of umbilicus**
**LØ2.227 Furuncle of flank**
**LØ2.229 Furuncle of trunk, unspecified**

✓6th **LØ2.23 Carbuncle of trunk**

**LØ2.231 Carbuncle of abdominal wall**
▲ **LØ2.232 Carbuncle of back [any part, except buttock and flank]**
**LØ2.233 Carbuncle of chest wall**
**LØ2.234 Carbuncle of groin**
**LØ2.235 Carbuncle of perineum**
**LØ2.236 Carbuncle of umbilicus**
● **LØ2.237 Carbuncle of flank**
**LØ2.239 Carbuncle of trunk, unspecified**

✓5th **LØ2.3 Cutaneous abscess, furuncle and carbuncle of buttock**
EXCLUDES 1 *pilonidal cyst with abscess (LØ5.Ø1)*

**LØ2.31 Cutaneous abscess of buttock**
Cutaneous abscess of gluteal region

**L02.32 Furuncle of buttock**
Boil of buttock
Folliculitis of buttock
Furuncle of gluteal region

**L02.33 Carbuncle of buttock**
Carbuncle of gluteal region

**L02.4 Cutaneous abscess, furuncle and carbuncle of limb**
EXCLUDES 2 *cutaneous abscess, furuncle and carbuncle of foot (L02.6-)*
*cutaneous abscess, furuncle and carbuncle of groin (L02.214, L02.224, L02.234)*
*cutaneous abscess, furuncle and carbuncle of hand (L02.5-)*

**L02.41 Cutaneous abscess of limb**
**L02.411 Cutaneous abscess of right axilla**
**L02.412 Cutaneous abscess of left axilla**
**L02.413 Cutaneous abscess of right upper limb**
**L02.414 Cutaneous abscess of left upper limb**
**L02.415 Cutaneous abscess of right lower limb**
**L02.416 Cutaneous abscess of left lower limb**
**L02.419 Cutaneous abscess of limb, unspecified**

**L02.42 Furuncle of limb**
Boil of limb
Folliculitis of limb
**L02.421 Furuncle of right axilla**
**L02.422 Furuncle of left axilla**
**L02.423 Furuncle of right upper limb**
**L02.424 Furuncle of left upper limb**
**L02.425 Furuncle of right lower limb**
**L02.426 Furuncle of left lower limb**
**L02.429 Furuncle of limb, unspecified**

**L02.43 Carbuncle of limb**
**L02.431 Carbuncle of right axilla**
**L02.432 Carbuncle of left axilla**
**L02.433 Carbuncle of right upper limb**
**L02.434 Carbuncle of left upper limb**
**L02.435 Carbuncle of right lower limb**
**L02.436 Carbuncle of left lower limb**
**L02.439 Carbuncle of limb, unspecified**

**L02.5 Cutaneous abscess, furuncle and carbuncle of hand**

**L02.51 Cutaneous abscess of hand**
**L02.511 Cutaneous abscess of right hand**
**L02.512 Cutaneous abscess of left hand**
**L02.519 Cutaneous abscess of unspecified hand**

**L02.52 Furuncle hand**
Boil of hand
Folliculitis of hand
**L02.521 Furuncle right hand**
**L02.522 Furuncle left hand**
**L02.529 Furuncle unspecified hand**

**L02.53 Carbuncle of hand**
**L02.531 Carbuncle of right hand**
**L02.532 Carbuncle of left hand**
**L02.539 Carbuncle of unspecified hand**

**L02.6 Cutaneous abscess, furuncle and carbuncle of foot**

**L02.61 Cutaneous abscess of foot**
**L02.611 Cutaneous abscess of right foot**
**L02.612 Cutaneous abscess of left foot**
**L02.619 Cutaneous abscess of unspecified foot**

**L02.62 Furuncle of foot**
Boil of foot
Folliculitis of foot
**L02.621 Furuncle of right foot**
**L02.622 Furuncle of left foot**
**L02.629 Furuncle of unspecified foot**

**L02.63 Carbuncle of foot**
**L02.631 Carbuncle of right foot**
**L02.632 Carbuncle of left foot**
**L02.639 Carbuncle of unspecified foot**

**L02.8 Cutaneous abscess, furuncle and carbuncle of other sites**

**L02.81 Cutaneous abscess of other sites**
**L02.811 Cutaneous abscess of head [any part, except face]**
**L02.818 Cutaneous abscess of other sites**

**L02.82 Furuncle of other sites**
Boil of other sites
Folliculitis of other sites
**L02.821 Furuncle of head [any part, except face]**
**L02.828 Furuncle of other sites**

**L02.83 Carbuncle of other sites**
**L02.831 Carbuncle of head [any part, except face]**
**L02.838 Carbuncle of other sites**

**L02.9 Cutaneous abscess, furuncle and carbuncle, unspecified**
**L02.91 Cutaneous abscess, unspecified**
**L02.92 Furuncle, unspecified**
Boil NOS
Furunculosis NOS
**L02.93 Carbuncle, unspecified**

**L03 Cellulitis and acute lymphangitis**
EXCLUDES 2 *cellulitis of anal and rectal region (K61.-)*
*cellulitis of external auditory canal (H60.1)*
*cellulitis of eyelid (H00.0)*
*cellulitis of female external genital organs (N76.4)*
*cellulitis of lacrimal apparatus (H04.3)*
*cellulitis of male external genital organs (N48.2, N49.-)*
*cellulitis of mouth (K12.2)*
*cellulitis of nose (J34.0)*
*eosinophilic cellulitis [Wells] (L98.3)*
*febrile neutrophilic dermatosis [Sweet] (L98.2)*
*lymphangitis (chronic) (subacute) (I89.1)*

**AHA:** 2017,4Q,100
**DEF:** Cellulitis: Infection of the skin and subcutaneous tissues, most often caused by *Staphylococcus* or *Streptococcus* bacteria secondary to a cutaneous lesion. Progression of the inflammation may lead to abscess and tissue death, or even systemic infection-like bacteremia.
**DEF:** Lymphangitis: Inflammation of the lymph channels most often caused by *Streptococcus*.

**L03.0 Cellulitis and acute lymphangitis of finger and toe**
Infection of nail
Onychia
Paronychia
Perionychia

**L03.01 Cellulitis of finger**
Felon
Whitlow
EXCLUDES 1 *herpetic whitlow (B00.89)*
**DEF:** Felon: Superficial bacterial skin infection at the tip of the finger.
**L03.011 Cellulitis of right finger**
**L03.012 Cellulitis of left finger**
**L03.019 Cellulitis of unspecified finger**

**L03.02 Acute lymphangitis of finger**
Hangnail with lymphangitis of finger
**L03.021 Acute lymphangitis of right finger**
**L03.022 Acute lymphangitis of left finger**
**L03.029 Acute lymphangitis of unspecified finger**

**L03.03 Cellulitis of toe**
**L03.031 Cellulitis of right toe**
**L03.032 Cellulitis of left toe**
**L03.039 Cellulitis of unspecified toe**

**L03.04 Acute lymphangitis of toe**
Hangnail with lymphangitis of toe
**L03.041 Acute lymphangitis of right toe**
**L03.042 Acute lymphangitis of left toe**
**L03.049 Acute lymphangitis of unspecified toe**

**L03.1 Cellulitis and acute lymphangitis of other parts of limb**

**L03.11 Cellulitis of other parts of limb**
EXCLUDES 2 *cellulitis of fingers (L03.01-)*
*cellulitis of toes (L03.03-)*
*groin (L03.314)*
**L03.111 Cellulitis of right axilla**
**L03.112 Cellulitis of left axilla**
**L03.113 Cellulitis of right upper limb**
**L03.114 Cellulitis of left upper limb**
**L03.115 Cellulitis of right lower limb**
**L03.116 Cellulitis of left lower limb**
**L03.119 Cellulitis of unspecified part of limb**

**L03.12 Acute lymphangitis of other parts of limb**
EXCLUDES 2 *acute lymphangitis of fingers (L03.2-)*
*acute lymphangitis of groin (L03.324)*
*acute lymphangitis of toes (L03.04-)*
**L03.121 Acute lymphangitis of right axilla**

**LØ3.122** Acute lymphangitis of left axilla
**LØ3.123** Acute lymphangitis of right upper limb
**LØ3.124** Acute lymphangitis of left upper limb
**LØ3.125** Acute lymphangitis of right lower limb
**LØ3.126** Acute lymphangitis of left lower limb
**LØ3.129** Acute lymphangitis of unspecified part of limb

✓5th **LØ3.2 Cellulitis and acute lymphangitis of face and neck**

✓6th **LØ3.21 Cellulitis and acute lymphangitis of face**

**LØ3.211 Cellulitis of face**
EXCLUDES 2 *abscess of orbit (HØ5.Ø1-)*
*cellulitis of ear (H6Ø.1-)*
*cellulitis of eyelid (HØØ.Ø-)*
*cellulitis of head (LØ3.81)*
*cellulitis of lacrimal apparatus (HØ4.3)*
*cellulitis of lip (K13.Ø)*
*cellulitis of mouth (K12.2)*
*cellulitis of nose (internal) (J34.Ø)*
*cellulitis of orbit (HØ5.Ø1-)*
*cellulitis of scalp (LØ3.81)*
**AHA:** 2013,4Q,123

**LØ3.212 Acute lymphangitis of face**
**LØ3.213 Periorbital cellulitis**
Preseptal cellulitis
**AHA:** 2016,4Q,36

✓6th **LØ3.22 Cellulitis and acute lymphangitis of neck**

**LØ3.221 Cellulitis of neck**
**LØ3.222 Acute lymphangitis of neck**

✓5th **LØ3.3 Cellulitis and acute lymphangitis of trunk**

✓6th **LØ3.31 Cellulitis of trunk**
EXCLUDES 2 *cellulitis of anal and rectal regions (K61.-)*
*cellulitis of breast NOS (N61.Ø)*
*cellulitis of female external genital organs (N76.4)*
*cellulitis of male external genital organs (N48.2, N49.-)*
*omphalitis of newborn (P38.-)*
*puerperal cellulitis of breast (O91.2)*

**LØ3.311 Cellulitis of abdominal wall**
EXCLUDES 2 *cellulitis of umbilicus (LØ3.316)*
*cellulitis of groin (LØ3.314)*
▲ **LØ3.312 Cellulitis of back [any part except buttock and flank]**
**LØ3.313 Cellulitis of chest wall**
**LØ3.314 Cellulitis of groin**
**LØ3.315 Cellulitis of perineum**
**LØ3.316 Cellulitis of umbilicus**
**LØ3.317 Cellulitis of buttock**
**LØ3.319 Cellulitis of trunk, unspecified**
**LØ3.31A Cellulitis of flank**

✓6th **LØ3.32 Acute lymphangitis of trunk**

**LØ3.321 Acute lymphangitis of abdominal wall**
▲ **LØ3.322 Acute lymphangitis of back [any part except buttock and flank]**
**LØ3.323 Acute lymphangitis of chest wall**
**LØ3.324 Acute lymphangitis of groin**
**LØ3.325 Acute lymphangitis of perineum**
**LØ3.326 Acute lymphangitis of umbilicus**
**LØ3.327 Acute lymphangitis of buttock**
**LØ3.329 Acute lymphangitis of trunk, unspecified**
**LØ3.32A Acute lymphangitis of flank**

✓5th **LØ3.8 Cellulitis and acute lymphangitis of other sites**

✓6th **LØ3.81 Cellulitis of other sites**

**LØ3.811 Cellulitis of head [any part, except face]**
Cellulitis of scalp
EXCLUDES 2 *cellulitis of face (LØ3.211)*
**LØ3.818 Cellulitis of other sites**

✓6th **LØ3.89 Acute lymphangitis of other sites**

**LØ3.891 Acute lymphangitis of head [any part, except face]**
**LØ3.898 Acute lymphangitis of other sites**

✓5th **LØ3.9 Cellulitis and acute lymphangitis, unspecified**

**LØ3.9Ø Cellulitis, unspecified**
**LØ3.91 Acute lymphangitis, unspecified**
EXCLUDES 1 *lymphangitis NOS (I89.1)*

✓4th **LØ4 Acute lymphadenitis**

INCLUDES abscess (acute) of lymph nodes, except mesenteric
acute lymphadenitis, except mesenteric
EXCLUDES 1 *chronic or subacute lymphadenitis, except mesenteric (I88.1)*
*enlarged lymph nodes (R59.-)*
*human immunodeficiency virus [HIV] disease resulting in generalized lymphadenopathy (B2Ø)*
*lymphadenitis NOS (I88.9)*
*nonspecific mesenteric lymphadenitis (I88.Ø)*
**DEF:** Inflammation or enlargement of the lymph nodes.

**LØ4.Ø Acute lymphadenitis of face, head and neck**
**LØ4.1 Acute lymphadenitis of trunk**
**LØ4.2 Acute lymphadenitis of upper limb**
Acute lymphadenitis of axilla
Acute lymphadenitis of shoulder
**LØ4.3 Acute lymphadenitis of lower limb**
Acute lymphadenitis of hip
EXCLUDES 2 *acute lymphadenitis of groin (LØ4.1)*
**LØ4.8 Acute lymphadenitis of other sites**
**LØ4.9 Acute lymphadenitis, unspecified**

✓4th **LØ5 Pilonidal cyst and sinus**

**DEF:** Pilonidal cyst: Sac or sinus cavity of trapped epithelial tissues in the sacrococcygeal region, usually associated with ingrown hair.
**DEF:** Pilonidal sinus: Fistula, tract, or channel that extends from an infected area of ingrown hair to another site within the skin or out to the skin surface.

**Pilonidal Cyst**

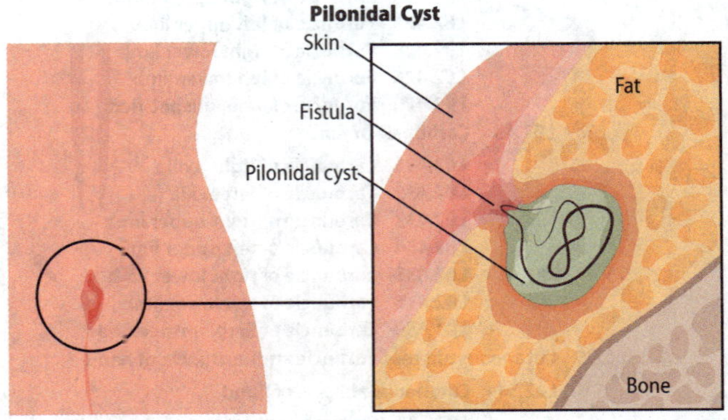


✓5th **LØ5.Ø Pilonidal cyst and sinus with abscess**

**LØ5.Ø1 Pilonidal cyst with abscess**
Pilonidal abscess
Pilonidal dimple with abscess
Postanal dimple with abscess
EXCLUDES 2 *congenital sacral dimple (Q82.6)*
*parasacral dimple (Q82.6)*
**LØ5.Ø2 Pilonidal sinus with abscess**
Coccygeal fistula with abscess
Coccygeal sinus with abscess
Pilonidal fistula with abscess

✓5th **LØ5.9 Pilonidal cyst and sinus without abscess**

**LØ5.91 Pilonidal cyst without abscess**
Pilonidal cyst NOS
Pilonidal dimple
Postanal dimple
EXCLUDES 2 *congenital sacral dimple (Q82.6)*
*parasacral dimple (Q82.6)*
**LØ5.92 Pilonidal sinus without abscess**
Coccygeal fistula
Coccygeal sinus without abscess
Pilonidal fistula

✓4th **LØ8 Other local infections of skin and subcutaneous tissue**

**LØ8.Ø Pyoderma**
Dermatitis gangrenosa
Purulent dermatitis
Septic dermatitis
Suppurative dermatitis
EXCLUDES 1 *pyoderma gangrenosum (L88)*
*pyoderma vegetans (LØ8.81)*
**DEF:** Any superficial skin disease commonly characterized by the discharging of pus not attributed to another condition.
**LØ8.1 Erythrasma**
**DEF:** Chronic, superficial skin infection of brown scaly patches, commonly found in skin folds most prevalent in the overweight or diabetic population.

√5th L08.8 **Other specified local infections of the skin and subcutaneous tissue**

L08.81 **Pyoderma vegetans**

EXCLUDES 1 *pyoderma gangrenosum (L88)*
*pyoderma NOS (L08.0)*

L08.82 **Omphalitis not of newborn**

EXCLUDES 1 *omphalitis of newborn (P38.-)*

L08.89 **Other specified local infections of the skin and subcutaneous tissue**

L08.9 **Local infection of the skin and subcutaneous tissue, unspecified**

## Bullous disorders (L10-L14)

EXCLUDES 1 *benign familial pemphigus [Hailey-Hailey] (Q82.8)*
*staphylococcal scalded skin syndrome (L00)*
*toxic epidermal necrolysis [Lyell] (L51.2)*

√4th L10 **Pemphigus**

EXCLUDES 1 *pemphigus neonatorum (L01.03)*

L10.0 **Pemphigus vulgaris** HCC Rx COM
L10.1 **Pemphigus vegetans** HCC Rx COM
L10.2 **Pemphigus foliaceous** HCC Rx COM
L10.3 **Brazilian pemphigus [fogo selvagem]** HCC Rx COM
L10.4 **Pemphigus erythematosus** HCC Rx COM
Senear-Usher syndrome
L10.5 **Drug-induced pemphigus** Rx COM
Use additional code for adverse effect, if applicable, to identify drug (T36-T50 with fifth or sixth character 5)

√5th L10.8 **Other pemphigus**

L10.81 **Paraneoplastic pemphigus** HCC Rx COM
L10.89 **Other pemphigus** HCC Rx COM

L10.9 **Pemphigus, unspecified** HCC Rx COM

√4th L11 **Other acantholytic disorders**

L11.0 **Acquired keratosis follicularis**
EXCLUDES 1 *keratosis follicularis (congenital) [Darier-White] (Q82.8)*
**AHA:** 2021,3Q,10
L11.1 **Transient acantholytic dermatosis [Grover]**
L11.8 **Other specified acantholytic disorders**
L11.9 **Acantholytic disorder, unspecified**

√4th L12 **Pemphigoid**

EXCLUDES 1 *herpes gestationis (O26.4-)*
*impetigo herpetiformis (L40.1)*

L12.0 **Bullous pemphigoid** HCC Rx COM
L12.1 **Cicatricial pemphigoid** HCC Rx COM
Benign mucous membrane pemphigoid
**DEF:** Chronic autoimmune disease characterized by subepidermal blistering lesions of the mucosa, including the conjunctiva. It is seen predominantly in the elderly and produces adhesions and scarring.
L12.2 **Chronic bullous disease of childhood** Rx P
Juvenile dermatitis herpetiformis

√5th L12.3 **Acquired epidermolysis bullosa**

EXCLUDES 1 *epidermolysis bullosa (congenital) (Q81.-)*

L12.30 **Acquired epidermolysis bullosa, unspecified** ESR COM
L12.31 **Epidermolysis bullosa due to drug** ESR COM
Use additional code for adverse effect, if applicable, to identify drug (T36-T50 with fifth or sixth character 5)
L12.35 **Other acquired epidermolysis bullosa** ESR COM

L12.8 **Other pemphigoid** HCC Rx COM
L12.9 **Pemphigoid, unspecified** HCC Rx COM

√4th L13 **Other bullous disorders**

L13.0 **Dermatitis herpetiformis** Rx
Duhring's disease
Hydroa herpetiformis
EXCLUDES 1 *juvenile dermatitis herpetiformis (L12.2)*
*senile dermatitis herpetiformis (L12.0)*
**DEF:** Skin disease to which people are genetically predisposed resulting from an immunological response to gluten. Dermatitis herpetiformis is an extremely pruritic eruption of various lesions that frequently heal, leaving hyperpigmentation or hypopigmentation and occasionally scarring. It is usually associated with asymptomatic gluten-sensitive enteropathy.
L13.1 **Subcorneal pustular dermatitis** Rx
Sneddon-Wilkinson disease
L13.8 **Other specified bullous disorders** Rx
L13.9 **Bullous disorder, unspecified** Rx

L14 ***Bullous disorders in diseases classified elsewhere*** Rx
Code first underlying disease

## Dermatitis and eczema (L20-L30)

NOTE In this block the terms dermatitis and eczema are used synonymously and interchangeably.

EXCLUDES 2 *chronic (childhood) granulomatous disease (D71-)*
*dermatitis gangrenosa (L08.0)*
*dermatitis herpetiformis (L13.0)*
*dry skin dermatitis (L85.3)*
*factitial dermatitis (L98.1)*
*perioral dermatitis (L71.0)*
*radiation-related disorders of the skin and subcutaneous tissue (L55-L59)*
*stasis dermatitis (I87.2)*

√4th L20 **Atopic dermatitis**

L20.0 **Besnier's prurigo**

√5th L20.8 **Other atopic dermatitis**

EXCLUDES 2 *circumscribed neurodermatitis (L28.0)*

L20.81 **Atopic neurodermatitis**
Diffuse neurodermatitis
L20.82 **Flexural eczema**
L20.83 **Infantile (acute) (chronic) eczema** P
L20.84 **Intrinsic (allergic) eczema**
L20.89 **Other atopic dermatitis**

L20.9 **Atopic dermatitis, unspecified**

√4th L21 **Seborrheic dermatitis**

EXCLUDES 2 *infective dermatitis (L30.3)*
*seborrheic keratosis (L82.-)*

L21.0 **Seborrhea capitis**
Cradle cap
**AHA:** 2018,1Q,6
**TIP:** Assign for dandruff in an adult patient.
L21.1 **Seborrheic infantile dermatitis** P
L21.8 **Other seborrheic dermatitis**
L21.9 **Seborrheic dermatitis, unspecified**
Seborrhea NOS

L22 **Diaper dermatitis**
Diaper erythema
Diaper rash
Psoriasiform diaper rash
**AHA:** 2021,4Q,18

√4th L23 **Allergic contact dermatitis**

EXCLUDES 1 *allergy NOS (T78.40)*
*contact dermatitis NOS (L25.9)*
*dermatitis NOS (L30.9)*

EXCLUDES 2 *dermatitis due to substances taken internally (L27.-)*
*dermatitis of eyelid (H01.1-)*
*diaper dermatitis (L22)*
*eczema of external ear (H60.5-)*
*irritant contact dermatitis (L24.-)*
*perioral dermatitis (L71.0)*
*radiation-related disorders of the skin and subcutaneous tissue (L55-L59)*

L23.0 **Allergic contact dermatitis due to metals**
Allergic contact dermatitis due to chromium
Allergic contact dermatitis due to nickel
L23.1 **Allergic contact dermatitis due to adhesives**
L23.2 **Allergic contact dermatitis due to cosmetics**
L23.3 **Allergic contact dermatitis due to drugs in contact with skin**
Use additional code for adverse effect, if applicable, to identify drug (T36-T50 with fifth or sixth character 5)
EXCLUDES 2 *dermatitis due to ingested drugs and medicaments (L27.0-L27.1)*
L23.4 **Allergic contact dermatitis due to dyes**
L23.5 **Allergic contact dermatitis due to other chemical products**
Allergic contact dermatitis due to cement
Allergic contact dermatitis due to insecticide
Allergic contact dermatitis due to plastic
Allergic contact dermatitis due to rubber
L23.6 **Allergic contact dermatitis due to food in contact with the skin**
EXCLUDES 2 *dermatitis due to ingested food (L27.2)*
L23.7 **Allergic contact dermatitis due to plants, except food**
EXCLUDES 2 *allergy NOS due to pollen (J30.1)*

**L23.8 Allergic contact dermatitis due to other agents**

**L23.81 Allergic contact dermatitis due to animal (cat) (dog) dander**

Allergic contact dermatitis due to animal (cat) (dog) hair

**L23.89 Allergic contact dermatitis due to other agents**

**L23.9 Allergic contact dermatitis, unspecified cause**

Allergic contact eczema NOS

**L24 Irritant contact dermatitis**

EXCLUDES 1 *allergy NOS (T78.40)*
*contact dermatitis NOS (L25.9)*
*dermatitis NOS (L30.9)*

EXCLUDES 2 *allergic contact dermatitis (L23.-)*
*dermatitis due to substances taken internally (L27.-)*
*dermatitis of eyelid (H01.1-)*
*diaper dermatitis (L22)*
*eczema of external ear (H60.5-)*
*perioral dermatitis (L71.0)*
*radiation-related disorders of the skin and subcutaneous tissue (L55-L59)*

**L24.0 Irritant contact dermatitis due to detergents**

**L24.1 Irritant contact dermatitis due to oils and greases**

**L24.2 Irritant contact dermatitis due to solvents**

Irritant contact dermatitis due to chlorocompound
Irritant contact dermatitis due to cyclohexane
Irritant contact dermatitis due to ester
Irritant contact dermatitis due to glycol
Irritant contact dermatitis due to hydrocarbon
Irritant contact dermatitis due to ketone

**L24.3 Irritant contact dermatitis due to cosmetics**

**L24.4 Irritant contact dermatitis due to drugs in contact with skin**

Use additional code for adverse effect, if applicable, to identify drug (T36-T50 with fifth or sixth character 5)

**L24.5 Irritant contact dermatitis due to other chemical products**

Irritant contact dermatitis due to cement
Irritant contact dermatitis due to insecticide
Irritant contact dermatitis due to plastic
Irritant contact dermatitis due to rubber

**L24.6 Irritant contact dermatitis due to food in contact with skin**

EXCLUDES 2 *dermatitis due to ingested food (L27.2)*

**L24.7 Irritant contact dermatitis due to plants, except food**

EXCLUDES 2 *allergy NOS to pollen (J30.1)*

**L24.8 Irritant contact dermatitis due to other agents**

**L24.81 Irritant contact dermatitis due to metals**

Irritant contact dermatitis due to chromium
Irritant contact dermatitis due to nickel

**L24.89 Irritant contact dermatitis due to other agents**

Irritant contact dermatitis due to dyes

**L24.9 Irritant contact dermatitis, unspecified cause**

Irritant contact eczema NOS

**L24.A Irritant contact dermatitis due to friction or contact with body fluids**

EXCLUDES 1 *irritant contact dermatitis related to stoma or fistula (L24.B-)*

EXCLUDES 2 *erythema intertrigo (L30.4)*

AHA: 2021,4Q,16-18

**L24.A0 Irritant contact dermatitis due to friction or contact with body fluids, unspecified**

**L24.A1 Irritant contact dermatitis due to saliva**

**L24.A2 Irritant contact dermatitis due to fecal, urinary or dual incontinence**

EXCLUDES 1 *diaper dermatitis (L22)*

**L24.A9 Irritant contact dermatitis due friction or contact with other specified body fluids**

Irritant contact dermatitis related to endotracheal tube
Wound fluids, exudate

**L24.B Irritant contact dermatitis related to stoma or fistula**

Use additional code to identify any artificial opening status (Z93.-), if applicable, for contact dermatitis related to stoma secretions

AHA: 2021,4Q,16-18

**L24.B0 Irritant contact dermatitis related to unspecified stoma or fistula**

Irritant contact dermatitis related to fistula NOS
Irritant contact dermatitis related to stoma NOS

**L24.B1 Irritant contact dermatitis related to digestive stoma or fistula**

Irritant contact dermatitis related to gastrostomy
Irritant contact dermatitis related to jejunostomy
Irritant contact dermatitis related to saliva or spit fistula

**L24.B2 Irritant contact dermatitis related to respiratory stoma or fistula**

Irritant contact dermatitis related to tracheostomy

**L24.B3 Irritant contact dermatitis related to fecal or urinary stoma or fistula**

Irritant contact dermatitis related to colostomy
Irritant contact dermatitis related to enterocutaneous fistula
Irritant contact dermatitis related to ileostomy

**L25 Unspecified contact dermatitis**

EXCLUDES 1 *allergic contact dermatitis (L23.-)*
*allergy NOS (T78.40)*
*dermatitis NOS (L30.9)*
*irritant contact dermatitis (L24.-)*

EXCLUDES 2 *dermatitis due to ingested substances (L27.-)*
*dermatitis of eyelid (H01.1-)*
*eczema of external ear (H60.5-)*
*perioral dermatitis (L71.0)*
*radiation-related disorders of the skin and subcutaneous tissue (L55-L59)*

**L25.0 Unspecified contact dermatitis due to cosmetics**

**L25.1 Unspecified contact dermatitis due to drugs in contact with skin**

Use additional code for adverse effect, if applicable, to identify drug (T36-T50 with fifth or sixth character 5)

EXCLUDES 2 *dermatitis due to ingested drugs and medicaments (L27.0-L27.1)*

**L25.2 Unspecified contact dermatitis due to dyes**

**L25.3 Unspecified contact dermatitis due to other chemical products**

Unspecified contact dermatitis due to cement
Unspecified contact dermatitis due to insecticide

**L25.4 Unspecified contact dermatitis due to food in contact with skin**

EXCLUDES 2 *dermatitis due to ingested food (L27.2)*

**L25.5 Unspecified contact dermatitis due to plants, except food**

EXCLUDES 1 *nettle rash (L50.9)*

EXCLUDES 2 *allergy NOS due to pollen (J30.1)*

**L25.8 Unspecified contact dermatitis due to other agents**

**L25.9 Unspecified contact dermatitis, unspecified cause**

Contact dermatitis (occupational) NOS
Contact eczema (occupational) NOS

**L26 Exfoliative dermatitis**

Hebra's pityriasis

EXCLUDES 1 *Ritter's disease (L00)*

**L27 Dermatitis due to substances taken internally**

EXCLUDES 1 *allergy NOS (T78.40)*

EXCLUDES 2 *adverse food reaction, except dermatitis (T78.0-T78.1)*
*contact dermatitis (L23-L25)*
*drug photoallergic response (L56.1)*
*drug phototoxic response (L56.0)*
*urticaria (L50.-)*

**L27.0 Generalized skin eruption due to drugs and medicaments taken internally**

Use additional code for adverse effect, if applicable, to identify drug (T36-T50 with fifth or sixth character 5)

**L27.1 Localized skin eruption due to drugs and medicaments taken internally**

Use additional code for adverse effect, if applicable, to identify drug (T36-T50 with fifth or sixth character 5)

**L27.2 Dermatitis due to ingested food**

EXCLUDES 2 *dermatitis due to food in contact with skin (L23.6, L24.6, L25.4)*

**L27.8 Dermatitis due to other substances taken internally**

**L27.9 Dermatitis due to unspecified substance taken internally**

**L28 Lichen simplex chronicus and prurigo**

**L28.0 Lichen simplex chronicus**

Circumscribed neurodermatitis
Lichen NOS

**L28.1 Prurigo nodularis**

**L28.2 Other prurigo**

Prurigo Hebra
Prurigo mitis
Prurigo NOS
Urticaria papulosa

✓4th **L29 Pruritus**

EXCLUDES 1 *neurotic excoriation (L98.1)*
*psychogenic pruritus (F45.8)*

**L29.Ø Pruritus ani**
**L29.1 Pruritus scroti**
**L29.2 Pruritus vulvae**
**L29.3 Anogenital pruritus, unspecified**
✓5th **L29.8 Other pruritus**
**L29.81 Cholestatic pruritus**
Code also, if applicable, type of liver disease
Use additional code for adverse effect, if applicable, to identify drug (T36-T5Ø with fifth or sixth character 5)
**AHA:** 2024,4Q,22
**L29.89 Other pruritus**
**L29.9 Pruritus, unspecified**
Itch NOS

✓4th **L3Ø Other and unspecified dermatitis**

EXCLUDES 2 *contact dermatitis (L23-L25)*
*dry skin dermatitis (L85.3)*
*small plaque parapsoriasis (L41.3)*
*stasis dermatitis (I87.2)*

**L3Ø.Ø Nummular dermatitis**
**L3Ø.1 Dyshidrosis [pompholyx]**
**L3Ø.2 Cutaneous autosensitization**
Candidid [levurid]
Dermatophytid
Eczematid
**L3Ø.3 Infective dermatitis**
Infectious eczematoid dermatitis
**L3Ø.4 Erythema intertrigo**
**L3Ø.5 Pityriasis alba**
**AHA:** 2018,1Q,6
**L3Ø.8 Other specified dermatitis**
**L3Ø.9 Dermatitis, unspecified**
Eczema NOS

## Papulosquamous disorders (L4Ø-L45)

✓4th **L4Ø Psoriasis**

**DEF:** Chronic autoimmune condition that speeds up skin cell growth, causing excessive immature skin cells to form raised, rounded erythematous lesions covered by dry, silvery scaling patches. Most commonly found on the scalp, elbows, knees, hands, feet, and genitals, it can also affect the joints with stiffness and swelling.

**L4Ø.Ø Psoriasis vulgaris** Rx
Nummular psoriasis
Plaque psoriasis
**L4Ø.1 Generalized pustular psoriasis** Rx
Impetigo herpetiformis
Von Zumbusch's disease
**L4Ø.2 Acrodermatitis continua** Rx
**L4Ø.3 Pustulosis palmaris et plantaris** Rx
**L4Ø.4 Guttate psoriasis** Rx
✓5th **L4Ø.5 Arthropathic psoriasis**
**L4Ø.5Ø Arthropathic psoriasis, unspecified** HCC Rx ESR COM
**L4Ø.51 Distal interphalangeal psoriatic arthropathy** HCC Rx ESR COM
**L4Ø.52 Psoriatic arthritis mutilans** HCC Rx ESR COM
**L4Ø.53 Psoriatic spondylitis** HCC Rx ESR COM
**L4Ø.54 Psoriatic juvenile arthropathy** HCC Rx ESR COM
**L4Ø.59 Other psoriatic arthropathy** HCC Rx ESR COM
**L4Ø.8 Other psoriasis** Rx
Flexural psoriasis
**L4Ø.9 Psoriasis, unspecified** Rx

✓4th **L41 Parapsoriasis**

EXCLUDES 1 *poikiloderma vasculare atrophicans (L94.5)*

**L41.Ø Pityriasis lichenoides et varioliformis acuta** Rx
Mucha-Habermann disease
**L41.1 Pityriasis lichenoides chronica** Rx
**L41.3 Small plaque parapsoriasis** Rx
**L41.4 Large plaque parapsoriasis** Rx
**L41.5 Retiform parapsoriasis** Rx
**L41.8 Other parapsoriasis** Rx
**L41.9 Parapsoriasis, unspecified** Rx

**L42 Pityriasis rosea**

✓4th **L43 Lichen planus**

EXCLUDES 1 *lichen planopilaris (L66.1-)*

**L43.Ø Hypertrophic lichen planus**
**L43.1 Bullous lichen planus**
**L43.2 Lichenoid drug reaction**
Use additional code for adverse effect, if applicable, to identify drug (T36-T5Ø with fifth or sixth character 5)
**L43.3 Subacute (active) lichen planus**
Lichen planus tropicus
**L43.8 Other lichen planus**
**L43.9 Lichen planus, unspecified**
**AHA:** 2026,2Q,16

✓4th **L44 Other papulosquamous disorders**

**L44.Ø Pityriasis rubra pilaris**
**L44.1 Lichen nitidus**
**DEF:** Chronic, inflammatory, asymptomatic skin disorder, characterized by numerous glistening, flat-topped, discrete, skin-colored micropapules, most often on the penis, lower abdomen, inner thighs, wrists, forearms, breasts, and buttocks.
**L44.2 Lichen striatus**
**L44.3 Lichen ruber moniliformis**
**L44.4 Infantile papular acrodermatitis [Gianotti-Crosti]** P
**L44.8 Other specified papulosquamous disorders**
**L44.9 Papulosquamous disorder, unspecified**

***L45 Papulosquamous disorders in diseases classified elsewhere***
Code first underlying disease

## Urticaria and erythema (L49-L54)

EXCLUDES 1 *Lyme disease (A69.2-)*
*rosacea (L71.-)*

✓4th **L49 Exfoliation due to erythematous conditions according to extent of body surface involved**

Code first erythematous condition causing exfoliation, such as:
(Staphylococcal) scalded skin syndrome (LØØ)
Ritter's disease (LØØ)
Stevens-Johnson syndrome (L51.1)
Stevens-Johnson syndrome-toxic epidermal necrolysis overlap syndrome (L51.3)
toxic epidermal necrolysis (L51.2)
**DEF:** Exfoliation: Falling or sloughing off skin in layers.

**L49.Ø Exfoliation due to erythematous condition involving less than 1Ø percent of body surface** UPD
Exfoliation due to erythematous condition NOS
**L49.1 Exfoliation due to erythematous condition involving 1Ø-19 percent of body surface** COM UPD
**L49.2 Exfoliation due to erythematous condition involving 2Ø-29 percent of body surface** COM UPD
**L49.3 Exfoliation due to erythematous condition involving 3Ø-39 percent of body surface** COM UPD
**L49.4 Exfoliation due to erythematous condition involving 4Ø-49 percent of body surface** COM UPD
**L49.5 Exfoliation due to erythematous condition involving 5Ø-59 percent of body surface** COM UPD
**L49.6 Exfoliation due to erythematous condition involving 6Ø-69 percent of body surface** COM UPD
**L49.7 Exfoliation due to erythematous condition involving 7Ø-79 percent of body surface** COM UPD
**L49.8 Exfoliation due to erythematous condition involving 8Ø-89 percent of body surface** COM UPD
**L49.9 Exfoliation due to erythematous condition involving 9Ø or more percent of body surface** COM UPD

✓4th **L5Ø Urticaria**

EXCLUDES 1 *allergic contact dermatitis (L23.-)*
*angioneurotic edema (T78.3)*
*giant urticaria (T78.3)*
*hereditary angio-edema (D84.1)*
*Quincke's edema (T78.3)*
*serum urticaria (T8Ø.6-)*
*solar urticaria (L56.3)*
*urticaria neonatorum (P83.8)*
*urticaria papulosa (L28.2)*
*urticaria pigmentosa (D47.Ø1)*

**DEF:** Eruption of itching edema of the skin. ***Synonym(s):*** *hives.*

**L5Ø.Ø Allergic urticaria**
**L5Ø.1 Idiopathic urticaria**

**L5Ø.2 Urticaria due to cold and heat**

EXCLUDES 2 *familial cold urticaria (MØ4.2)*

**L5Ø.3 Dermatographic urticaria**

**L5Ø.4 Vibratory urticaria**

**L5Ø.5 Cholinergic urticaria**

**L5Ø.6 Contact urticaria**

**L5Ø.8 Other urticaria**

Chronic urticaria

Recurrent periodic urticaria

**L5Ø.9 Urticaria, unspecified**

✓4th **L51 Erythema multiforme**

Use additional code for adverse effect, if applicable, to identify drug (T36-T5Ø with fifth or sixth character 5)

Use additional code to identify associated manifestations, such as:

Use additional code to identify percentage of skin exfoliation (L49.-)

arthropathy associated with dermatological disorders (M14.8-)

conjunctival edema (H11.42)

conjunctivitis (H1Ø.22-)

corneal scars and opacities (H17.-)

corneal ulcer (H16.Ø-)

edema of eyelid (HØ2.84-)

inflammation of eyelid (HØ1.8-)

keratoconjunctivitis sicca (H16.22-)

mechanical lagophthalmos (HØ2.22-)

stomatitis (K12.-)

symblepharon (H11.23-)

EXCLUDES 1 *staphylococcal scalded skin syndrome (LØØ)*

*Ritter's disease (LØØ)*

**DEF:** Acute complex of symptoms with a varied pattern of skin eruptions, such as macular, bullous, papular, nodose, or vesicular lesions on the neck, face, and legs. Erythema (redness of skin and mucous membranes) multiforme (multiple forms) is a hypersensitivity (allergic) reaction that can occur at any age but primarily affects children or young adults.

**L51.Ø Nonbullous erythema multiforme**

**L51.1 Stevens-Johnson syndrome** ESR COM

**L51.2 Toxic epidermal necrolysis [Lyell]** ESR COM

**L51.3 Stevens-Johnson syndrome-toxic epidermal necrolysis overlap syndrome** ESR COM

SJS-TEN overlap syndrome

**L51.8 Other erythema multiforme**

**L51.9 Erythema multiforme, unspecified**

Erythema iris

Erythema multiforme major NOS

Erythema multiforme minor NOS

Herpes iris

**L52 Erythema nodosum**

EXCLUDES 1 *tuberculous erythema nodosum (A18.4)*

**DEF:** Form of panniculitis (inflammation of the fat layer beneath the skin) most often occurring in women. Commonly seen as a hypersensitivity reaction to infections, drugs, sarcoidosis, and specific enteropathies. The acute stage is associated with fever, malaise, and arthralgia. The lesions are pink to blue in color as tender nodules and are found on the front of the legs below the knees.

✓4th **L53 Other erythematous conditions**

EXCLUDES 1 *erythema ab igne (L59.Ø)*

*erythema due to external agents in contact with skin (L23-L25)*

*erythema intertrigo (L3Ø.4)*

**L53.Ø Toxic erythema**

Code first poisoning due to drug or toxin, if applicable (T36-T65 with fifth or sixth character 1-4)

Use additional code for adverse effect, if applicable, to identify drug (T36-T5Ø with fifth or sixth character 5)

EXCLUDES 1 *neonatal erythema toxicum (P83.1)*

**L53.1 Erythema annulare centrifugum**

**L53.2 Erythema marginatum**

**L53.3 Other chronic figurate erythema**

**L53.8 Other specified erythematous conditions**

**L53.9 Erythematous condition, unspecified**

Erythema NOS

Erythroderma NOS

***L54 Erythema in diseases classified elsewhere***

Code first underlying disease

## Radiation-related disorders of the skin and subcutaneous tissue (L55-L59)

✓4th **L55 Sunburn**

**L55.Ø Sunburn of first degree**

**L55.1 Sunburn of second degree**

**L55.2 Sunburn of third degree** COM

**L55.9 Sunburn, unspecified**

✓4th **L56 Other acute skin changes due to ultraviolet radiation**

Use additional code to identify the source of the ultraviolet radiation (W89, X32)

**L56.Ø Drug phototoxic response**

Use additional code for adverse effect, if applicable, to identify drug (T36-T5Ø with fifth or sixth character 5)

**L56.1 Drug photoallergic response**

Use additional code for adverse effect, if applicable, to identify drug (T36-T5Ø with fifth or sixth character 5)

**L56.2 Photocontact dermatitis [berloque dermatitis]**

**L56.3 Solar urticaria**

**L56.4 Polymorphous light eruption**

**L56.5 Disseminated superficial actinic porokeratosis (DSAP)**

**DEF:** Autosomal dominant skin condition occurring in sun-exposed areas of the skin (particularly the arms and legs), characterized by superficial annular, keratotic, brownish-red spots or thickenings with depressed centers and sharp, ridged borders. It may evolve into squamous cell carcinoma.

**L56.8 Other specified acute skin changes due to ultraviolet radiation**

**L56.9 Acute skin change due to ultraviolet radiation, unspecified**

✓4th **L57 Skin changes due to chronic exposure to nonionizing radiation**

Use additional code to identify the source of the ultraviolet radiation (W89), or other nonionizing radiation (W9Ø)

**L57.Ø Actinic keratosis**

Keratosis NOS

Senile keratosis

Solar keratosis

**L57.1 Actinic reticuloid**

**L57.2 Cutis rhomboidalis nuchae**

**L57.3 Poikiloderma of Civatte**

**L57.4 Cutis laxa senilis**

Elastosis senilis

**L57.5 Actinic granuloma**

**L57.8 Other skin changes due to chronic exposure to nonionizing radiation**

Farmer's skin

Sailor's skin

Solar dermatitis

**L57.9 Skin changes due to chronic exposure to nonionizing radiation, unspecified**

✓4th **L58 Radiodermatitis**

Use additional code to identify the source of the radiation (W88, W9Ø)

**L58.Ø Acute radiodermatitis**

**L58.1 Chronic radiodermatitis**

**L58.9 Radiodermatitis, unspecified**

✓4th **L59 Other disorders of skin and subcutaneous tissue related to radiation**

**L59.Ø Erythema ab igne [dermatitis ab igne]**

**L59.8 Other specified disorders of the skin and subcutaneous tissue related to radiation**

**AHA:** 2017,1Q,33

**L59.9 Disorder of the skin and subcutaneous tissue related to radiation, unspecified**

## Disorders of skin appendages (L6Ø-L75)

**EXCLUDES 1** *congenital malformations of integument (Q84.-)*

✓4th **L6Ø Nail disorders**

**EXCLUDES 2** *clubbing of nails (R68.3)*
*onychia and paronychia (LØ3.Ø-)*

**Nail Disorders**

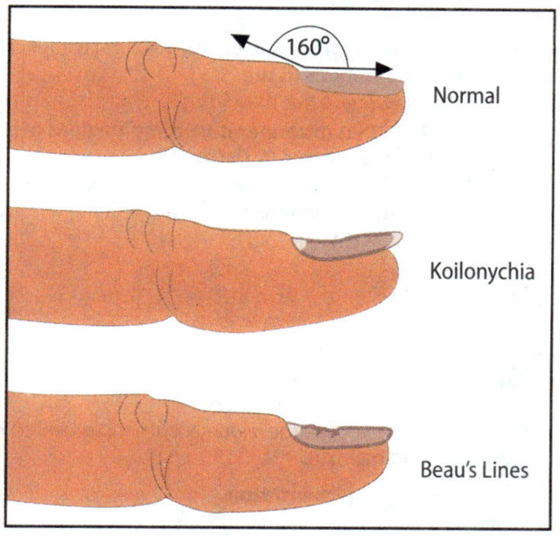


**L6Ø.Ø Ingrowing nail**
**L6Ø.1 Onycholysis**
**L6Ø.2 Onychogryphosis**
**L6Ø.3 Nail dystrophy**
**L6Ø.4 Beau's lines**
**L6Ø.5 Yellow nail syndrome**
**L6Ø.8 Other nail disorders**
**L6Ø.9 Nail disorder, unspecified**

***L62 Nail disorders in diseases classified elsewhere***
Code first underlying disease, such as:
pachydermoperiostosis (M89.4-)

✓4th **L63 Alopecia areata**
**L63.Ø Alopecia (capitis) totalis**
**L63.1 Alopecia universalis**
**L63.2 Ophiasis**
**L63.8 Other alopecia areata**
**L63.9 Alopecia areata, unspecified**

✓4th **L64 Androgenic alopecia**
**INCLUDES** male-pattern baldness
**L64.Ø Drug-induced androgenic alopecia**
Use additional code for adverse effect, if applicable, to identify drug (T36-T5Ø with fifth or sixth character 5)
**L64.8 Other androgenic alopecia**
**L64.9 Androgenic alopecia, unspecified**

✓4th **L65 Other nonscarring hair loss**
Use additional code for adverse effect, if applicable, to identify drug (T36-T5Ø with fifth or sixth character 5)
**EXCLUDES 1** *trichotillomania (F63.3)*
**L65.Ø Telogen effluvium**
**DEF:** Form of nonscarring alopecia characterized by shedding of hair from premature telogen development in follicles due to stress, including shock, childbirth, surgery, drugs, or weight loss.
**L65.1 Anagen effluvium**
**L65.2 Alopecia mucinosa**
**L65.8 Other specified nonscarring hair loss**
**L65.9 Nonscarring hair loss, unspecified**
Alopecia NOS

✓4th **L66 Cicatricial alopecia [scarring hair loss]**
**L66.Ø Pseudopelade**
✓5th **L66.1 Lichen planopilaris**
**AHA:** 2024,4Q,23
**L66.1Ø Lichen planopilaris, unspecified**
**L66.11 Classic lichen planopilaris**
Follicular lichen planus
**L66.12 Frontal fibrosing alopecia**
FFA
**L66.19 Other lichen planopilaris**
Lassueur Graham-Little Piccardi syndrome
**L66.2 Folliculitis decalvans**
**L66.3 Perifolliculitis capitis abscedens**
**L66.4 Folliculitis ulerythematosa reticulata**
✓5th **L66.8 Other cicatricial alopecia**
**AHA:** 2024,4Q,23; 2015,1Q,19
**L66.81 Central centrifugal cicatricial alopecia**
CCCA
**L66.89 Other cicatricial alopecia**
**L66.9 Cicatricial alopecia, unspecified**

✓4th **L67 Hair color and hair shaft abnormalities**
**EXCLUDES 1** *monilethrix (Q84.1)*
*pili annulati (Q84.1)*
*telogen effluvium (L65.Ø)*
**L67.Ø Trichorrhexis nodosa**
**L67.1 Variations in hair color**
Canities
Greyness, hair (premature)
Heterochromia of hair
Poliosis circumscripta, acquired
Poliosis NOS
**L67.8 Other hair color and hair shaft abnormalities**
Fragilitas crinium
**L67.9 Hair color and hair shaft abnormality, unspecified**

✓4th **L68 Hypertrichosis**
**INCLUDES** excess hair
**EXCLUDES 1** *congenital hypertrichosis (Q84.2)*
*persistent lanugo (Q84.2)*
**L68.Ø Hirsutism**
**L68.1 Acquired hypertrichosis lanuginosa**
**L68.2 Localized hypertrichosis**
**L68.3 Polytrichia**
**L68.8 Other hypertrichosis**
**L68.9 Hypertrichosis, unspecified**

✓4th **L7Ø Acne**
**EXCLUDES 2** *acne keloid (L73.Ø)*
**L7Ø.Ø Acne vulgaris**
**L7Ø.1 Acne conglobata**
**L7Ø.2 Acne varioliformis**
Acne necrotica miliaris
**DEF:** Rare form of acne characterized by development of persistent brown papulopustules followed by scar formation. This type of acne usually presents on the brow and temporoparietal part of the scalp.
**L7Ø.3 Acne tropica**
**L7Ø.4 Infantile acne** P
**L7Ø.5 Acné excoriée**
Acné excoriée des jeunes filles
Picker's acne
**L7Ø.8 Other acne**
**L7Ø.9 Acne, unspecified**

✓4th **L71 Rosacea**
Use additional code for adverse effect, if applicable, to identify drug (T36-T5Ø with fifth or sixth character 5)
**L71.Ø Perioral dermatitis**
**L71.1 Rhinophyma**
**L71.8 Other rosacea**
**AHA:** 2018,4Q,15
**L71.9 Rosacea, unspecified**

✓4th **L72 Follicular cysts of skin and subcutaneous tissue**
**L72.Ø Epidermal cyst**
✓5th **L72.1 Pilar and trichodermal cyst**
**L72.11 Pilar cyst**
**L72.12 Trichodermal cyst**
Trichilemmal (proliferating) cyst
**L72.2 Steatocystoma multiplex**
**L72.3 Sebaceous cyst**
**EXCLUDES 2** *pilar cyst (L72.11)*
*trichilemmal (proliferating) cyst (L72.12)*
**L72.8 Other follicular cysts of the skin and subcutaneous tissue**
**L72.9 Follicular cyst of the skin and subcutaneous tissue, unspecified**

✓4th **L73 Other follicular disorders**
**L73.Ø Acne keloid**
**L73.1 Pseudofolliculitis barbae**

**L73.2 Hidradenitis suppurativa**

**L73.8 Other specified follicular disorders**
Sycosis barbae

**L73.9 Follicular disorder, unspecified**

√4th **L74 Eccrine sweat disorders**
EXCLUDES 2 *generalized hyperhidrosis (R61)*
**DEF:** Eccrine sweat glands: Glands found in the dermal and hypodermal layer of the skin throughout the body, particularly on the forehead, scalp, axillae, palms, and soles. These glands produce watery and neutral or slightly acidic sweat.

**L74.Ø Miliaria rubra**

**L74.1 Miliaria crystallina**

**L74.2 Miliaria profunda**
Miliaria tropicalis

**L74.3 Miliaria, unspecified**

**L74.4 Anhidrosis**
Hypohidrosis
**DEF:** Inability to sweat normally. When the body can't cool itself through perspiration it can lead to heatstroke, a life-threatening condition.

√5th **L74.5 Focal hyperhidrosis**

√6th **L74.51 Primary focal hyperhidrosis**

**L74.51Ø Primary focal hyperhidrosis, axilla**

**L74.511 Primary focal hyperhidrosis, face**

**L74.512 Primary focal hyperhidrosis, palms**

**L74.513 Primary focal hyperhidrosis, soles**

**L74.519 Primary focal hyperhidrosis, unspecified**

**L74.52 Secondary focal hyperhidrosis**
Frey's syndrome

**L74.8 Other eccrine sweat disorders**

**L74.9 Eccrine sweat disorder, unspecified**
Sweat gland disorder NOS

√4th **L75 Apocrine sweat disorders**
EXCLUDES 1 *dyshidrosis (L3Ø.1)*
*hidradenitis suppurativa (L73.2)*
**DEF:** Apocrine sweat glands: Found in the axilla, areola, and circumanal region, these glands begin to function in puberty and produce viscid milky secretions in response to external stimuli.

**L75.Ø Bromhidrosis**

**L75.1 Chromhidrosis**

**L75.2 Apocrine miliaria**
Fox-Fordyce disease
**DEF:** Chronic, usually pruritic disease evidenced by small follicular papular eruptions, especially in the axillary and pubic areas. Apocrine miliaria develops from the closure and rupture of the affected apocrine glands' intraepidermal portion of the ducts.

**L75.8 Other apocrine sweat disorders**

**L75.9 Apocrine sweat disorder, unspecified**

## Intraoperative and postprocedural complications of skin and subcutaneous tissue (L76)

√4th **L76 Intraoperative and postprocedural complications of skin and subcutaneous tissue**
**AHA:** 2016,4Q,9-10

√5th **L76.Ø Intraoperative hemorrhage and hematoma of skin and subcutaneous tissue complicating a procedure**
EXCLUDES 1 *intraoperative hemorrhage and hematoma of skin and subcutaneous tissue due to accidental puncture and laceration during a procedure (L76.1-)*

**L76.Ø1 Intraoperative hemorrhage and hematoma of skin and subcutaneous tissue complicating a dermatologic procedure**

**L76.Ø2 Intraoperative hemorrhage and hematoma of skin and subcutaneous tissue complicating other procedure**

√5th **L76.1 Accidental puncture and laceration of skin and subcutaneous tissue during a procedure**

**L76.11 Accidental puncture and laceration of skin and subcutaneous tissue during a dermatologic procedure**

**L76.12 Accidental puncture and laceration of skin and subcutaneous tissue during other procedure**

√5th **L76.2 Postprocedural hemorrhage of skin and subcutaneous tissue following a procedure**

**L76.21 Postprocedural hemorrhage of skin and subcutaneous tissue following a dermatologic procedure**

**L76.22 Postprocedural hemorrhage of skin and subcutaneous tissue following other procedure**

√5th **L76.3 Postprocedural hematoma and seroma of skin and subcutaneous tissue following a procedure**

**L76.31 Postprocedural hematoma of skin and subcutaneous tissue following a dermatologic procedure**

**L76.32 Postprocedural hematoma of skin and subcutaneous tissue following other procedure**

**L76.33 Postprocedural seroma of skin and subcutaneous tissue following a dermatologic procedure**

**L76.34 Postprocedural seroma of skin and subcutaneous tissue following other procedure**

√5th **L76.8 Other intraoperative and postprocedural complications of skin and subcutaneous tissue**
Use additional code, if applicable, to further specify disorder

**L76.81 Other intraoperative complications of skin and subcutaneous tissue**

**L76.82 Other postprocedural complications of skin and subcutaneous tissue**
**AHA:** 2017,3Q,6

## Other disorders of the skin and subcutaneous tissue (L8Ø-L99)

**L8Ø Vitiligo**
EXCLUDES 2 *vitiligo of eyelids (HØ2.73-)*
*vitiligo of vulva (N9Ø.89)*
**DEF:** Persistent, progressive development of nonpigmented white patches on otherwise normal skin.

√4th **L81 Other disorders of pigmentation**
EXCLUDES 1 *birthmark NOS (Q82.5)*
*Peutz-Jeghers syndrome (Q85.89)*
EXCLUDES 2 *nevus - see Alphabetical Index*

**L81.Ø Postinflammatory hyperpigmentation**

**L81.1 Chloasma**

**L81.2 Freckles**

**L81.3 Cafe au lait spots**

**L81.4 Other melanin hyperpigmentation**
Lentigo

**L81.5 Leukoderma, not elsewhere classified**

**L81.6 Other disorders of diminished melanin formation**

**L81.7 Pigmented purpuric dermatosis**
Angioma serpiginosum

**L81.8 Other specified disorders of pigmentation**
Iron pigmentation
Tattoo pigmentation

**L81.9 Disorder of pigmentation, unspecified**

√4th **L82 Seborrheic keratosis**
INCLUDES basal cell papilloma
dermatosis papulosa nigra
Leser-Trélat disease
EXCLUDES 2 *seborrheic dermatitis (L21.-)*
**DEF:** Common, benign, noninvasive, lightly pigmented, warty growth composed of basaloid cells that usually appear at middle age as soft, easily crumbling plaques on the face, trunk, and extremities.

**L82.Ø Inflamed seborrheic keratosis**
**AHA:** 2023,2Q,12; 2021,3Q,10

**L82.1 Other seborrheic keratosis**
Seborrheic keratosis NOS

**L83 Acanthosis nigricans**
Confluent and reticulated papillomatosis
**DEF:** Diffuse, velvety hyperplasia of the spinous skin layer of the axilla and other body folds marked by gray, brown, or black pigmentation. In adult form, it is often associated with malignant acanthosis nigricans in a benign, nevoid form relatively generalized.

**L84 Corns and callosities**
Callus
Clavus

√4th **L85 Other epidermal thickening**
EXCLUDES 2 *hypertrophic disorders of the skin (L91.-)*

**L85.Ø Acquired ichthyosis**
EXCLUDES 1 *congenital ichthyosis (Q8Ø.-)*

**L85.1 Acquired keratosis [keratoderma] palmaris et plantaris**
EXCLUDES 1 *inherited keratosis palmaris et plantaris (Q82.8)*

**L85.2 Keratosis punctata (palmaris et plantaris)**

**L85.3 Xerosis cutis**
Dry skin dermatitis

**L85.8 Other specified epidermal thickening**
Cutaneous horn

**L85.9 Epidermal thickening, unspecified**

**L86 Keratoderma in diseases classified elsewhere**

Code first underlying disease, such as:
Reiter's disease (M02.3-)

EXCLUDES 1 *gonococcal keratoderma (A54.89)*
*gonococcal keratosis (A54.89)*
*keratoderma due to vitamin A deficiency (E50.8)*
*keratosis due to vitamin A deficiency (E50.8)*
*xeroderma due to vitamin A deficiency (E50.8)*

√4th **L87 Transepidermal elimination disorders**

EXCLUDES 1 *granuloma annulare (perforating) (L92.0)*

**L87.0 Keratosis follicularis et parafollicularis in cutem penetrans**
Hyperkeratosis follicularis penetrans
Kyrle disease

**L87.1 Reactive perforating collagenosis**

**L87.2 Elastosis perforans serpiginosa**

**L87.8 Other transepidermal elimination disorders**

**L87.9 Transepidermal elimination disorder, unspecified**

**L88 Pyoderma gangrenosum** HCC Rx COM
Phagedenic pyoderma

EXCLUDES 1 *dermatitis gangrenosa (L08.0)*

**DEF:** Persistent debilitating skin disease characterized by irregular, boggy, blue-red ulcerations, with central healing and undermined edges.

√4th **L89 Pressure ulcer**

INCLUDES bed sore
decubitus ulcer
plaster ulcer
pressure area
pressure sore

Code first any associated gangrene (I96)

EXCLUDES 2 *decubitus (trophic) ulcer of cervix (uteri) (N86)*
*diabetic ulcers (E08.621, E08.622, E09.621, E09.622, E10.621, E10.622, E11.621, E11.622, E13.621, E13.622)*
*non-pressure chronic ulcer of skin (L97.-)*
*skin infections (L00-L08)*
*varicose ulcer (I83.0, I83.2)*

**AHA:** 2022,2Q,8; 2021,1Q,24; 2019,4Q,10-11,54; 2018,4Q,69; 2018,3Q,3; 2018,2Q,21; 2017,4Q,109; 2017,1Q,49; 2016,4Q,143

**TIP:** The stage of a diagnosed pressure ulcer can be based on documentation from clinicians who are not the patient's provider.

**Four Stages of Pressure Ulcer**

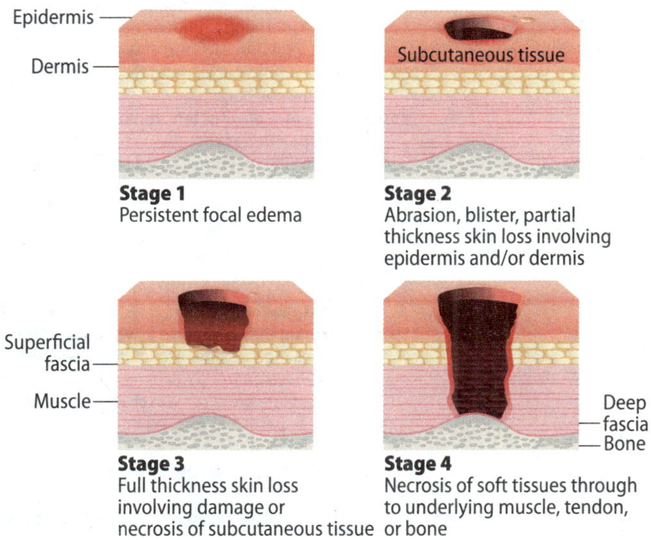


√5th **L89.0 Pressure ulcer of elbow**

√6th **L89.00 Pressure ulcer of unspecified elbow**

**L89.000 Pressure ulcer of unspecified elbow, unstageable** HCC ESR

**L89.001 Pressure ulcer of unspecified elbow, stage 1**
Healing pressure ulcer of unspecified elbow, stage 1
Pressure pre-ulcer skin changes limited to persistent focal edema, unspecified elbow

**L89.002 Pressure ulcer of unspecified elbow, stage 2** HCC ESR
Healing pressure ulcer of unspecified elbow, stage 2
Pressure ulcer with abrasion, blister, partial thickness skin loss involving epidermis and/or dermis, unspecified elbow

**L89.003 Pressure ulcer of unspecified elbow, stage 3** HCC ESR
Healing pressure ulcer of unspecified elbow, stage 3
Pressure ulcer with full thickness skin loss involving damage or necrosis of subcutaneous tissue, unspecified elbow

**L89.004 Pressure ulcer of unspecified elbow, stage 4** HCC ESR
Healing pressure ulcer of unspecified elbow, stage 4
Pressure ulcer with necrosis of soft tissues through to underlying muscle, tendon, or bone, unspecified elbow

**L89.006 Pressure-induced deep tissue damage of unspecified elbow**

**L89.009 Pressure ulcer of unspecified elbow, unspecified stage**
Healing pressure ulcer of elbow NOS
Healing pressure ulcer of unspecified elbow, unspecified stage

√6th **L89.01 Pressure ulcer of right elbow**

**L89.010 Pressure ulcer of right elbow, unstageable** HCC ESR

**L89.011 Pressure ulcer of right elbow, stage 1**
Healing pressure ulcer of right elbow, stage 1
Pressure pre-ulcer skin changes limited to persistent focal edema, right elbow

**L89.012 Pressure ulcer of right elbow, stage 2** HCC ESR
Healing pressure ulcer of right elbow, stage 2
Pressure ulcer with abrasion, blister, partial thickness skin loss involving epidermis and/or dermis, right elbow

**L89.013 Pressure ulcer of right elbow, stage 3** HCC ESR
Healing pressure ulcer of right elbow, stage 3
Pressure ulcer with full thickness skin loss involving damage or necrosis of subcutaneous tissue, right elbow

**L89.014 Pressure ulcer of right elbow, stage 4** HCC ESR
Healing pressure ulcer of right elbow, stage 4
Pressure ulcer with necrosis of soft tissues through to underlying muscle, tendon, or bone, right elbow

**L89.016 Pressure-induced deep tissue damage of right elbow**

**L89.019 Pressure ulcer of right elbow, unspecified stage**
Healing pressure ulcer of right elbow NOS

√6th **L89.02 Pressure ulcer of left elbow**

**L89.020 Pressure ulcer of left elbow, unstageable** HCC ESR

**L89.021 Pressure ulcer of left elbow, stage 1**
Healing pressure ulcer of left elbow, stage 1
Pressure pre-ulcer skin changes limited to persistent focal edema, left elbow

**L89.022 Pressure ulcer of left elbow, stage 2** HCC ESR
Healing pressure ulcer of left elbow, stage 2
Pressure ulcer with abrasion, blister, partial thickness skin loss involving epidermis and/or dermis, left elbow

**L89.023 Pressure ulcer of left elbow, stage 3** HCC ESR
Healing pressure ulcer of left elbow, stage 3
Pressure ulcer with full thickness skin loss involving damage or necrosis of subcutaneous tissue, left elbow

**L89.024 Pressure ulcer of left elbow, stage 4** HCC ESR
Healing pressure ulcer of left elbow, stage 4
Pressure ulcer with necrosis of soft tissues through to underlying muscle, tendon, or bone, left elbow

**L89.026 Pressure-induced deep tissue damage of left elbow**

**L89.029 Pressure ulcer of left elbow, unspecified stage**
Healing pressure ulcer of left elbow NOS

√5th **L89.1 Pressure ulcer of back**

√6th **L89.10 Pressure ulcer of unspecified part of back**

**L89.100 Pressure ulcer of unspecified part of back, unstageable** HCC ESR

**L89.101 Pressure ulcer of unspecified part of back, stage 1**
Healing pressure ulcer of unspecified part of back, stage 1
Pressure pre-ulcer skin changes limited to persistent focal edema, unspecified part of back

**L89.102 Pressure ulcer of unspecified part of back, stage 2** HCC ESR
Healing pressure ulcer of unspecified part of back, stage 2
Pressure ulcer with abrasion, blister, partial thickness skin loss involving epidermis and/or dermis, unspecified part of back

**L89.103 Pressure ulcer of unspecified part of back, stage 3** HCC ESR
Healing pressure ulcer of unspecified part of back, stage 3
Pressure ulcer with full thickness skin loss involving damage or necrosis of subcutaneous tissue, unspecified part of back

**L89.104 Pressure ulcer of unspecified part of back, stage 4** HCC ESR
Healing pressure ulcer of unspecified part of back, stage 4
Pressure ulcer with necrosis of soft tissues through to underlying muscle, tendon, or bone, unspecified part of back

**L89.106 Pressure-induced deep tissue damage of unspecified part of back**

**L89.109 Pressure ulcer of unspecified part of back, unspecified stage**
Healing pressure ulcer of unspecified part of back NOS
Healing pressure ulcer of unspecified part of back, unspecified stage

√6th **L89.11 Pressure ulcer of right upper back**
Pressure ulcer of right shoulder blade
**AHA:** 2026,2Q,6

**L89.110 Pressure ulcer of right upper back, unstageable** HCC ESR

**L89.111 Pressure ulcer of right upper back, stage 1**
Healing pressure ulcer of right upper back, stage 1
Pressure pre-ulcer skin changes limited to persistent focal edema, right upper back

**L89.112 Pressure ulcer of right upper back, stage 2** HCC ESR
Healing pressure ulcer of right upper back, stage 2
Pressure ulcer with abrasion, blister, partial thickness skin loss involving epidermis and/or dermis, right upper back

**L89.113 Pressure ulcer of right upper back, stage 3** HCC ESR
Healing pressure ulcer of right upper back, stage 3
Pressure ulcer with full thickness skin loss involving damage or necrosis of subcutaneous tissue, right upper back

**L89.114 Pressure ulcer of right upper back, stage 4** HCC ESR
Healing pressure ulcer of right upper back, stage 4
Pressure ulcer with necrosis of soft tissues through to underlying muscle, tendon, or bone, right upper back

**L89.116 Pressure-induced deep tissue damage of right upper back**

**L89.119 Pressure ulcer of right upper back, unspecified stage**
Healing pressure ulcer of right upper back NOS
Healing pressure ulcer of right upper back, unspecified stage

√6th **L89.12 Pressure ulcer of left upper back**
Pressure ulcer of left shoulder blade
**AHA:** 2026,2Q,6

**L89.120 Pressure ulcer of left upper back, unstageable** HCC ESR

**L89.121 Pressure ulcer of left upper back, stage 1**
Healing pressure ulcer of left upper back, stage 1
Pressure pre-ulcer skin changes limited to persistent focal edema, left upper back

**L89.122 Pressure ulcer of left upper back, stage 2** HCC ESR
Healing pressure ulcer of left upper back, stage 2
Pressure ulcer with abrasion, blister, partial thickness skin loss involving epidermis and/or dermis, left upper back

**L89.123 Pressure ulcer of left upper back, stage 3** HCC ESR
Healing pressure ulcer of left upper back, stage 3
Pressure ulcer with full thickness skin loss involving damage or necrosis of subcutaneous tissue, left upper back

**L89.124 Pressure ulcer of left upper back, stage 4** HCC ESR
Healing pressure ulcer of left upper back, stage 4
Pressure ulcer with necrosis of soft tissues through to underlying muscle, tendon, or bone, left upper back

**L89.126 Pressure-induced deep tissue damage of left upper back**

**L89.129 Pressure ulcer of left upper back, unspecified stage**
Healing pressure ulcer of left upper back NOS
Healing pressure ulcer of left upper back, unspecified stage

√6th **L89.13 Pressure ulcer of right lower back**

**L89.130 Pressure ulcer of right lower back, unstageable** HCC ESR

**L89.131 Pressure ulcer of right lower back, stage 1**
Healing pressure ulcer of right lower back, stage 1
Pressure pre-ulcer skin changes limited to persistent focal edema, right lower back

**L89.132 Pressure ulcer of right lower back, stage 2** HCC ESR
Healing pressure ulcer of right lower back, stage 2
Pressure ulcer with abrasion, blister, partial thickness skin loss involving epidermis and/or dermis, right lower back

**L89.133 Pressure ulcer of right lower back, stage 3** HCC ESR
Healing pressure ulcer of right lower back, stage 3
Pressure ulcer with full thickness skin loss involving damage or necrosis of subcutaneous tissue, right lower back

L89.134 **Pressure ulcer of right lower back, stage 4** HCC ESR
Healing pressure ulcer of right lower back, stage 4
Pressure ulcer with necrosis of soft tissues through to underlying muscle, tendon, or bone, right lower back

L89.136 **Pressure-induced deep tissue damage of right lower back**

L89.139 **Pressure ulcer of right lower back, unspecified stage**
Healing pressure ulcer of right lower back NOS
Healing pressure ulcer of right lower back, unspecified stage

✓6th L89.14 **Pressure ulcer of left lower back**

L89.140 **Pressure ulcer of left lower back, unstageable** HCC ESR

L89.141 **Pressure ulcer of left lower back, stage 1**
Healing pressure ulcer of left lower back, stage 1
Pressure pre-ulcer skin changes limited to persistent focal edema, left lower back

L89.142 **Pressure ulcer of left lower back, stage 2** HCC ESR
Healing pressure ulcer of left lower back, stage 2
Pressure ulcer with abrasion, blister, partial thickness skin loss involving epidermis and/or dermis, left lower back

L89.143 **Pressure ulcer of left lower back, stage 3** HCC ESR
Healing pressure ulcer of left lower back, stage 3
Pressure ulcer with full thickness skin loss involving damage or necrosis of subcutaneous tissue, left lower back

L89.144 **Pressure ulcer of left lower back, stage 4** HCC ESR
Healing pressure ulcer of left lower back, stage 4
Pressure ulcer with necrosis of soft tissues through to underlying muscle, tendon, or bone, left lower back

L89.146 **Pressure-induced deep tissue damage of left lower back**

L89.149 **Pressure ulcer of left lower back, unspecified stage**
Healing pressure ulcer of left lower back NOS
Healing pressure ulcer of left lower back, unspecified stage

✓6th L89.15 **Pressure ulcer of sacral region**
Pressure ulcer of coccyx
Pressure ulcer of tailbone
AHA: 2021,3Q,10

L89.150 **Pressure ulcer of sacral region, unstageable** HCC ESR

L89.151 **Pressure ulcer of sacral region, stage 1**
Healing pressure ulcer of sacral region, stage 1
Pressure pre-ulcer skin changes limited to persistent focal edema, sacral region

L89.152 **Pressure ulcer of sacral region, stage 2** HCC ESR
Healing pressure ulcer of sacral region, stage 2
Pressure ulcer with abrasion, blister, partial thickness skin loss involving epidermis and/or dermis, sacral region

L89.153 **Pressure ulcer of sacral region, stage 3** HCC ESR
Healing pressure ulcer of sacral region, stage 3
Pressure ulcer with full thickness skin loss involving damage or necrosis of subcutaneous tissue, sacral region

L89.154 **Pressure ulcer of sacral region, stage 4** HCC ESR
Healing pressure ulcer of sacral region, stage 4
Pressure ulcer with necrosis of soft tissues through to underlying muscle, tendon, or bone, sacral region
AHA: 2022,2Q,8

L89.156 **Pressure-induced deep tissue damage of sacral region**

L89.159 **Pressure ulcer of sacral region, unspecified stage**
Healing pressure ulcer of sacral region NOS
Healing pressure ulcer of sacral region, unspecified stage

✓5th L89.2 **Pressure ulcer of hip**

✓6th L89.20 **Pressure ulcer of unspecified hip**

L89.200 **Pressure ulcer of unspecified hip, unstageable** HCC ESR

L89.201 **Pressure ulcer of unspecified hip, stage 1**
Healing pressure ulcer of unspecified hip back, stage 1
Pressure pre-ulcer skin changes limited to persistent focal edema, unspecified hip

L89.202 **Pressure ulcer of unspecified hip, stage 2** HCC ESR
Healing pressure ulcer of unspecified hip, stage 2
Pressure ulcer with abrasion, blister, partial thickness skin loss involving epidermis and/or dermis, unspecified hip

L89.203 **Pressure ulcer of unspecified hip, stage 3** HCC ESR
Healing pressure ulcer of unspecified hip, stage 3
Pressure ulcer with full thickness skin loss involving damage or necrosis of subcutaneous tissue, unspecified hip

L89.204 **Pressure ulcer of unspecified hip, stage 4** HCC ESR
Healing pressure ulcer of unspecified hip, stage 4
Pressure ulcer with necrosis of soft tissues through to underlying muscle, tendon, or bone, unspecified hip

L89.206 **Pressure-induced deep tissue damage of unspecified hip**

L89.209 **Pressure ulcer of unspecified hip, unspecified stage**
Healing pressure ulcer of unspecified hip NOS
Healing pressure ulcer of unspecified hip, unspecified stage

✓6th L89.21 **Pressure ulcer of right hip**

L89.210 **Pressure ulcer of right hip, unstageable** HCC ESR

L89.211 **Pressure ulcer of right hip, stage 1**
Healing pressure ulcer of right hip back, stage 1
Pressure pre-ulcer skin changes limited to persistent focal edema, right hip

L89.212 **Pressure ulcer of right hip, stage 2** HCC ESR
Healing pressure ulcer of right hip, stage 2
Pressure ulcer with abrasion, blister, partial thickness skin loss involving epidermis and/or dermis, right hip

L89.213 **Pressure ulcer of right hip, stage 3** HCC ESR
Healing pressure ulcer of right hip, stage 3
Pressure ulcer with full thickness skin loss involving damage or necrosis of subcutaneous tissue, right hip

L89.214 **Pressure ulcer of right hip, stage 4** HCC ESR
Healing pressure ulcer of right hip, stage 4
Pressure ulcer with necrosis of soft tissues through to underlying muscle, tendon, or bone, right hip

L89.216 **Pressure-induced deep tissue damage of right hip**

**L89.219 Pressure ulcer of right hip, unspecified stage**
Healing pressure ulcer of right hip NOS
Healing pressure ulcer of right hip, unspecified stage

✓6th **L89.22 Pressure ulcer of left hip**

**L89.220 Pressure ulcer of left hip, unstageable** HCC ESR

**L89.221 Pressure ulcer of left hip, stage 1**
Healing pressure ulcer of left hip back, stage 1
Pressure pre-ulcer skin changes limited to persistent focal edema, left hip

**L89.222 Pressure ulcer of left hip, stage 2** HCC ESR
Healing pressure ulcer of left hip, stage 2
Pressure ulcer with abrasion, blister, partial thickness skin loss involving epidermis and/or dermis, left hip

**L89.223 Pressure ulcer of left hip, stage 3** HCC ESR
Healing pressure ulcer of left hip, stage 3
Pressure ulcer with full thickness skin loss involving damage or necrosis of subcutaneous tissue, left hip

**L89.224 Pressure ulcer of left hip, stage 4** HCC ESR
Healing pressure ulcer of left hip, stage 4
Pressure ulcer with necrosis of soft tissues through to underlying muscle, tendon, or bone, left hip

**L89.226 Pressure-induced deep tissue damage of left hip**

**L89.229 Pressure ulcer of left hip, unspecified stage**
Healing pressure ulcer of left hip NOS
Healing pressure ulcer of left hip, unspecified stage

✓5th **L89.3 Pressure ulcer of buttock**
AHA: 2021,3Q,10

✓6th **L89.30 Pressure ulcer of unspecified buttock**

**L89.300 Pressure ulcer of unspecified buttock, unstageable** HCC ESR

**L89.301 Pressure ulcer of unspecified buttock, stage 1**
Healing pressure ulcer of unspecified buttock, stage 1
Pressure pre-ulcer skin changes limited to persistent focal edema, unspecified buttock

**L89.302 Pressure ulcer of unspecified buttock, stage 2** HCC ESR
Healing pressure ulcer of unspecified buttock, stage 2
Pressure ulcer with abrasion, blister, partial thickness skin loss involving epidermis and/or dermis, unspecified buttock

**L89.303 Pressure ulcer of unspecified buttock, stage 3** HCC ESR
Healing pressure ulcer of unspecified buttock, stage 3
Pressure ulcer with full thickness skin loss involving damage or necrosis of subcutaneous tissue, unspecified buttock

**L89.304 Pressure ulcer of unspecified buttock, stage 4** HCC ESR
Healing pressure ulcer of unspecified buttock, stage 4
Pressure ulcer with necrosis of soft tissues through to underlying muscle, tendon, or bone, unspecified buttock

**L89.306 Pressure-induced deep tissue damage of unspecified buttock**

**L89.309 Pressure ulcer of unspecified buttock, unspecified stage**
Healing pressure ulcer of unspecified buttock NOS
Healing pressure ulcer of unspecified buttock, unspecified stage

✓6th **L89.31 Pressure ulcer of right buttock**

**L89.310 Pressure ulcer of right buttock, unstageable** HCC ESR

**L89.311 Pressure ulcer of right buttock, stage 1**
Healing pressure ulcer of right buttock, stage 1
Pressure pre-ulcer skin changes limited to persistent focal edema, right buttock

**L89.312 Pressure ulcer of right buttock, stage 2** HCC ESR
Healing pressure ulcer of right buttock, stage 2
Pressure ulcer with abrasion, blister, partial thickness skin loss involving epidermis and/or dermis, right buttock

**L89.313 Pressure ulcer of right buttock, stage 3** HCC ESR
Healing pressure ulcer of right buttock, stage 3
Pressure ulcer with full thickness skin loss involving damage or necrosis of subcutaneous tissue, right buttock

**L89.314 Pressure ulcer of right buttock, stage 4** HCC ESR
Healing pressure ulcer of right buttock, stage 4
Pressure ulcer with necrosis of soft tissues through to underlying muscle, tendon, or bone, right buttock

**L89.316 Pressure-induced deep tissue damage of right buttock**

**L89.319 Pressure ulcer of right buttock, unspecified stage**
Healing pressure ulcer of right buttock NOS
Healing pressure ulcer of right buttock, unspecified stage

✓6th **L89.32 Pressure ulcer of left buttock**

**L89.320 Pressure ulcer of left buttock, unstageable** HCC ESR

**L89.321 Pressure ulcer of left buttock, stage 1**
Healing pressure ulcer of left buttock, stage 1
Pressure pre-ulcer skin changes limited to persistent focal edema, left buttock

**L89.322 Pressure ulcer of left buttock, stage 2** HCC ESR
Healing pressure ulcer of left buttock, stage 2
Pressure ulcer with abrasion, blister, partial thickness skin loss involving epidermis and/or dermis, left buttock

**L89.323 Pressure ulcer of left buttock, stage 3** HCC ESR
Healing pressure ulcer of left buttock, stage 3
Pressure ulcer with full thickness skin loss involving damage or necrosis of subcutaneous tissue, left buttock

**L89.324 Pressure ulcer of left buttock, stage 4** HCC ESR
Healing pressure ulcer of left buttock, stage 4
Pressure ulcer with necrosis of soft tissues through to underlying muscle, tendon, or bone, left buttock

**L89.326 Pressure-induced deep tissue damage of left buttock**

**L89.329 Pressure ulcer of left buttock, unspecified stage**
Healing pressure ulcer of left buttock NOS
Healing pressure ulcer of left buttock, unspecified stage

✓5th **L89.4 Pressure ulcer of contiguous site of back, buttock and hip**

**L89.40 Pressure ulcer of contiguous site of back, buttock and hip, unspecified stage**
Healing pressure ulcer of contiguous site of back, buttock and hip NOS
Healing pressure ulcer of contiguous site of back, buttock and hip, unspecified stage

L89.41 **Pressure ulcer of contiguous site of back, buttock and hip, stage 1**
Healing pressure ulcer of contiguous site of back, buttock and hip, stage 1
Pressure pre-ulcer skin changes limited to persistent focal edema, contiguous site of back, buttock and hip

L89.42 **Pressure ulcer of contiguous site of back, buttock and hip, stage 2** HCC ESR
Healing pressure ulcer of contiguous site of back, buttock and hip, stage 2
Pressure ulcer with abrasion, blister, partial thickness skin loss involving epidermis and/or dermis, contiguous site of back, buttock and hip

L89.43 **Pressure ulcer of contiguous site of back, buttock and hip, stage 3** HCC ESR
Healing pressure ulcer of contiguous site of back, buttock and hip, stage 3
Pressure ulcer with full thickness skin loss involving damage or necrosis of subcutaneous tissue, contiguous site of back, buttock and hip

L89.44 **Pressure ulcer of contiguous site of back, buttock and hip, stage 4** HCC ESR
Healing pressure ulcer of contiguous site of back, buttock and hip, stage 4
Pressure ulcer with necrosis of soft tissues through to underlying muscle, tendon, or bone, contiguous site of back, buttock and hip

L89.45 **Pressure ulcer of contiguous site of back, buttock and hip, unstageable** HCC ESR

L89.46 **Pressure-induced deep tissue damage of contiguous site of back, buttock and hip**

√5th L89.5 **Pressure ulcer of ankle**

√6th L89.50 **Pressure ulcer of unspecified ankle**

L89.500 **Pressure ulcer of unspecified ankle, unstageable** HCC ESR

L89.501 **Pressure ulcer of unspecified ankle, stage 1**
Healing pressure ulcer of unspecified ankle, stage 1
Pressure pre-ulcer skin changes limited to persistent focal edema, unspecified ankle

L89.502 **Pressure ulcer of unspecified ankle, stage 2** HCC ESR
Healing pressure ulcer of unspecified ankle, stage 2
Pressure ulcer with abrasion, blister, partial thickness skin loss involving epidermis and/or dermis, unspecified ankle

L89.503 **Pressure ulcer of unspecified ankle, stage 3** HCC ESR
Healing pressure ulcer of unspecified ankle, stage 3
Pressure ulcer with full thickness skin loss involving damage or necrosis of subcutaneous tissue, unspecified ankle

L89.504 **Pressure ulcer of unspecified ankle, stage 4** HCC ESR
Healing pressure ulcer of unspecified ankle, stage 4
Pressure ulcer with necrosis of soft tissues through to underlying muscle, tendon, or bone, unspecified ankle

L89.506 **Pressure-induced deep tissue damage of unspecified ankle**

L89.509 **Pressure ulcer of unspecified ankle, unspecified stage**
Healing pressure ulcer of unspecified ankle NOS
Healing pressure ulcer of unspecified ankle, unspecified stage

√6th L89.51 **Pressure ulcer of right ankle**

L89.510 **Pressure ulcer of right ankle, unstageable** HCC ESR

L89.511 **Pressure ulcer of right ankle, stage 1**
Healing pressure ulcer of right ankle, stage 1
Pressure pre-ulcer skin changes limited to persistent focal edema, right ankle

L89.512 **Pressure ulcer of right ankle, stage 2** HCC ESR
Healing pressure ulcer of right ankle, stage 2
Pressure ulcer with abrasion, blister, partial thickness skin loss involving epidermis and/or dermis, right ankle

L89.513 **Pressure ulcer of right ankle, stage 3** HCC ESR
Healing pressure ulcer of right ankle, stage 3
Pressure ulcer with full thickness skin loss involving damage or necrosis of subcutaneous tissue, right ankle

L89.514 **Pressure ulcer of right ankle, stage 4** HCC ESR
Healing pressure ulcer of right ankle, stage 4
Pressure ulcer with necrosis of soft tissues through to underlying muscle, tendon, or bone, right ankle

L89.516 **Pressure-induced deep tissue damage of right ankle**

L89.519 **Pressure ulcer of right ankle, unspecified stage**
Healing pressure ulcer of right ankle NOS
Healing pressure ulcer of right ankle, unspecified stage

√6th L89.52 **Pressure ulcer of left ankle**

L89.520 **Pressure ulcer of left ankle, unstageable** HCC ESR

L89.521 **Pressure ulcer of left ankle, stage 1**
Healing pressure ulcer of left ankle, stage 1
Pressure pre-ulcer skin changes limited to persistent focal edema, left ankle

L89.522 **Pressure ulcer of left ankle, stage 2** HCC ESR
Healing pressure ulcer of left ankle, stage 2
Pressure ulcer with abrasion, blister, partial thickness skin loss involving epidermis and/or dermis, left ankle

L89.523 **Pressure ulcer of left ankle, stage 3** HCC ESR
Healing pressure ulcer of left ankle, stage 3
Pressure ulcer with full thickness skin loss involving damage or necrosis of subcutaneous tissue, left ankle

L89.524 **Pressure ulcer of left ankle, stage 4** HCC ESR
Healing pressure ulcer of left ankle, stage 4
Pressure ulcer with necrosis of soft tissues through to underlying muscle, tendon, or bone, left ankle

L89.526 **Pressure-induced deep tissue damage of left ankle**

L89.529 **Pressure ulcer of left ankle, unspecified stage**
Healing pressure ulcer of left ankle NOS
Healing pressure ulcer of left ankle, unspecified stage

√5th L89.6 **Pressure ulcer of heel**

√6th L89.60 **Pressure ulcer of unspecified heel**

L89.600 **Pressure ulcer of unspecified heel, unstageable** HCC ESR

L89.601 **Pressure ulcer of unspecified heel, stage 1**
Healing pressure ulcer of unspecified heel, stage 1
Pressure pre-ulcer skin changes limited to persistent focal edema, unspecified heel

L89.602 **Pressure ulcer of unspecified heel, stage 2** HCC ESR
Healing pressure ulcer of unspecified heel, stage 2
Pressure ulcer with abrasion, blister, partial thickness skin loss involving epidermis and/or dermis, unspecified heel

L89.603 **Pressure ulcer of unspecified heel, stage 3** HCC ESR
Healing pressure ulcer of unspecified heel, stage 3
Pressure ulcer with full thickness skin loss involving damage or necrosis of subcutaneous tissue, unspecified heel

**L89.604 Pressure ulcer of unspecified heel, stage 4** HCC ESR
Healing pressure ulcer of unspecified heel, stage 4
Pressure ulcer with necrosis of soft tissues through to underlying muscle, tendon, or bone, unspecified heel

**L89.606 Pressure-induced deep tissue damage of unspecified heel**

**L89.609 Pressure ulcer of unspecified heel, unspecified stage**
Healing pressure ulcer of unspecified heel NOS
Healing pressure ulcer of unspecified heel, unspecified stage

√6th **L89.61 Pressure ulcer of right heel**

**L89.610 Pressure ulcer of right heel, unstageable** HCC ESR

**L89.611 Pressure ulcer of right heel, stage 1**
Healing pressure ulcer of right heel, stage 1
Pressure pre-ulcer skin changes limited to persistent focal edema, right heel

**L89.612 Pressure ulcer of right heel, stage 2** HCC ESR
Healing pressure ulcer of right heel, stage 2
Pressure ulcer with abrasion, blister, partial thickness skin loss involving epidermis and/or dermis, right heel

**L89.613 Pressure ulcer of right heel, stage 3** HCC ESR
Healing pressure ulcer of right heel, stage 3
Pressure ulcer with full thickness skin loss involving damage or necrosis of subcutaneous tissue, right heel

**L89.614 Pressure ulcer of right heel, stage 4** HCC ESR
Healing pressure ulcer of right heel, stage 4
Pressure ulcer with necrosis of soft tissues through to underlying muscle, tendon, or bone, right heel

**L89.616 Pressure-induced deep tissue damage of right heel**

**L89.619 Pressure ulcer of right heel, unspecified stage**
Healing pressure ulcer of right heel NOS
Healing pressure ulcer of right heel, unspecified stage

√6th **L89.62 Pressure ulcer of left heel**

**L89.620 Pressure ulcer of left heel, unstageable** HCC ESR

**L89.621 Pressure ulcer of left heel, stage 1**
Healing pressure ulcer of left heel, stage 1
Pressure pre-ulcer skin changes limited to persistent focal edema, left heel

**L89.622 Pressure ulcer of left heel, stage 2** HCC ESR
Healing pressure ulcer of left heel, stage 2
Pressure ulcer with abrasion, blister, partial thickness skin loss involving epidermis and/or dermis, left heel

**L89.623 Pressure ulcer of left heel, stage 3** HCC ESR
Healing pressure ulcer of left heel, stage 3
Pressure ulcer with full thickness skin loss involving damage or necrosis of subcutaneous tissue, left heel

**L89.624 Pressure ulcer of left heel, stage 4** HCC ESR
Healing pressure ulcer of left heel, stage 4
Pressure ulcer with necrosis of soft tissues through to underlying muscle, tendon, or bone, left heel

**L89.626 Pressure-induced deep tissue damage of left heel**

**L89.629 Pressure ulcer of left heel, unspecified stage**
Healing pressure ulcer of left heel NOS
Healing pressure ulcer of left heel, unspecified stage

√5th **L89.8 Pressure ulcer of other site**

√6th **L89.81 Pressure ulcer of head**
Pressure ulcer of face

**L89.810 Pressure ulcer of head, unstageable** HCC ESR

**L89.811 Pressure ulcer of head, stage 1**
Healing pressure ulcer of head, stage 1
Pressure pre-ulcer skin changes limited to persistent focal edema, head

**L89.812 Pressure ulcer of head, stage 2** HCC ESR
Healing pressure ulcer of head, stage 2
Pressure ulcer with abrasion, blister, partial thickness skin loss involving epidermis and/or dermis, head

**L89.813 Pressure ulcer of head, stage 3** HCC ESR
Healing pressure ulcer of head, stage 3
Pressure ulcer with full thickness skin loss involving damage or necrosis of subcutaneous tissue, head

**L89.814 Pressure ulcer of head, stage 4** HCC ESR
Healing pressure ulcer of head, stage 4
Pressure ulcer with necrosis of soft tissues through to underlying muscle, tendon, or bone, head

**L89.816 Pressure-induced deep tissue damage of head**

**L89.819 Pressure ulcer of head, unspecified stage**
Healing pressure ulcer of head NOS
Healing pressure ulcer of head, unspecified stage

√6th **L89.89 Pressure ulcer of other site**

**L89.890 Pressure ulcer of other site, unstageable** HCC ESR

**L89.891 Pressure ulcer of other site, stage 1**
Healing pressure ulcer of other site, stage 1
Pressure pre-ulcer skin changes limited to persistent focal edema, other site

**L89.892 Pressure ulcer of other site, stage 2** HCC ESR
Healing pressure ulcer of other site, stage 2
Pressure ulcer with abrasion, blister, partial thickness skin loss involving epidermis and/or dermis, other site

**L89.893 Pressure ulcer of other site, stage 3** HCC ESR
Healing pressure ulcer of other site, stage 3
Pressure ulcer with full thickness skin loss involving damage or necrosis of subcutaneous tissue, other site

**L89.894 Pressure ulcer of other site, stage 4** HCC ESR
Healing pressure ulcer of other site, stage 4
Pressure ulcer with necrosis of soft tissues through to underlying muscle, tendon, or bone, other site

**L89.896 Pressure-induced deep tissue damage of other site**

**L89.899 Pressure ulcer of other site, unspecified stage**
Healing pressure ulcer of other site NOS
Healing pressure ulcer of other site, unspecified stage

√5th **L89.9 Pressure ulcer of unspecified site**

**L89.90 Pressure ulcer of unspecified site, unspecified stage**
Healing pressure ulcer of unspecified site NOS
Healing pressure ulcer of unspecified site, unspecified stage

**L89.91 Pressure ulcer of unspecified site, stage 1**
Healing pressure ulcer of unspecified site, stage 1
Pressure pre-ulcer skin changes limited to persistent focal edema, unspecified site

**L89.92 Pressure ulcer of unspecified site, stage 2** HCC ESR
Healing pressure ulcer of unspecified site, stage 2
Pressure ulcer with abrasion, blister, partial thickness skin loss involving epidermis and/or dermis, unspecified site

**L89.93 Pressure ulcer of unspecified site, stage 3** HCC ESR
Healing pressure ulcer of unspecified site, stage 3
Pressure ulcer with full thickness skin loss involving damage or necrosis of subcutaneous tissue, unspecified site

**L89.94 Pressure ulcer of unspecified site, stage 4** HCC ESR
Healing pressure ulcer of unspecified site, stage 4
Pressure ulcer with necrosis of soft tissues through to underlying muscle, tendon, or bone, unspecified site

**L89.95 Pressure ulcer of unspecified site, unstageable** HCC ESR

**L89.96 Pressure-induced deep tissue damage of unspecified site**

**✓4th L90 Atrophic disorders of skin**

**L90.0 Lichen sclerosus et atrophicus**
EXCLUDES 2 *lichen sclerosus of external female genital organs (N90.4)*
*lichen sclerosus of external male genital organs (N48.0)*

**L90.1 Anetoderma of Schweninger-Buzzi**

**L90.2 Anetoderma of Jadassohn-Pellizzari**

**L90.3 Atrophoderma of Pasini and Pierini**

**L90.4 Acrodermatitis chronica atrophicans**

**L90.5 Scar conditions and fibrosis of skin**
Adherent scar (skin)
Cicatrix
Disfigurement of skin due to scar
Fibrosis of skin NOS
Scar NOS
EXCLUDES 2 *hypertrophic scar (L91.0)*
*keloid scar (L91.0)*
**AHA:** 2016,2Q,5; 2015,1Q,19

**L90.6 Striae atrophicae**

**L90.8 Other atrophic disorders of skin**

**L90.9 Atrophic disorder of skin, unspecified**

**✓4th L91 Hypertrophic disorders of skin**

**L91.0 Hypertrophic scar**
Keloid
Keloid scar
EXCLUDES 2 *acne keloid (L73.0)*
*scar NOS (L90.5)*
**DEF:** Overgrowth of scar tissue due to excess amounts of collagen during connective tissue repair, occurring mainly on the upper trunk and face.

**L91.8 Other hypertrophic disorders of the skin**

**L91.9 Hypertrophic disorder of the skin, unspecified**

**✓4th L92 Granulomatous disorders of skin and subcutaneous tissue**
EXCLUDES 2 *actinic granuloma (L57.5)*

**L92.0 Granuloma annulare**
Perforating granuloma annulare

**L92.1 Necrobiosis lipoidica, not elsewhere classified**
EXCLUDES 1 *necrobiosis lipoidica associated with diabetes mellitus (E08-E13 with .620)*

**L92.2 Granuloma faciale [eosinophilic granuloma of skin]**

**L92.3 Foreign body granuloma of the skin and subcutaneous tissue**
Use additional code to identify the type of retained foreign body (Z18.-)

**L92.8 Other granulomatous disorders of the skin and subcutaneous tissue**

**L92.9 Granulomatous disorder of the skin and subcutaneous tissue, unspecified**
EXCLUDES 2 *umbilical granuloma (P83.81)*
**AHA:** 2017,4Q,21-22

**✓4th L93 Lupus erythematosus**
Use additional code for adverse effect, if applicable, to identify drug (T36-T50 with fifth or sixth character 5)
EXCLUDES 1 *lupus exedens (A18.4)*
*lupus vulgaris (A18.4)*
*scleroderma (M34.-)*
*systemic lupus erythematosus (M32.-)*
**DEF:** Inflammatory, autoimmune skin condition in which the body's autoimmune system attacks healthy tissue of the integumentary system.

**L93.0 Discoid lupus erythematosus** Rx
Lupus erythematosus NOS

**L93.1 Subacute cutaneous lupus erythematosus** Rx

**L93.2 Other local lupus erythematosus** Rx
Lupus erythematosus profundus
Lupus panniculitis

**✓4th L94 Other localized connective tissue disorders**
EXCLUDES 1 *systemic connective tissue disorders (M30-M36)*

**L94.0 Localized scleroderma [morphea]**
Circumscribed scleroderma

**L94.1 Linear scleroderma**
En coup de sabre lesion

**L94.2 Calcinosis cutis**

**L94.3 Sclerodactyly**

**L94.4 Gottron's papules**

**L94.5 Poikiloderma vasculare atrophicans** Rx

**L94.6 Ainhum**

**L94.8 Other specified localized connective tissue disorders**

**L94.9 Localized connective tissue disorder, unspecified**

**✓4th L95 Vasculitis limited to skin, not elsewhere classified**
EXCLUDES 1 *angioma serpiginosum (L81.7)*
*Henoch(-Schonlein) purpura (D69.0)*
*hypersensitivity angiitis (M31.0)*
*lupus panniculitis (L93.2)*
*panniculitis of neck and back (M54.0-)*
*panniculitis NOS (M79.3)*
*polyarteritis nodosa (M30.0)*
*relapsing panniculitis (M35.6)*
*rheumatoid vasculitis (M05.2)*
*serum sickness (T80.6-)*
*urticaria (L50.-)*
*Wegener's granulomatosis (M31.3-)*

**L95.0 Livedoid vasculitis**
Atrophie blanche (en plaque)

**L95.1 Erythema elevatum diutinum**

**L95.8 Other vasculitis limited to the skin**

**L95.9 Vasculitis limited to the skin, unspecified**

**✓4th L97 Non-pressure chronic ulcer of lower limb, not elsewhere classified**
INCLUDES chronic ulcer of skin of lower limb NOS
non-healing ulcer of skin
non-infected sinus of skin
trophic ulcer NOS
tropical ulcer NOS
ulcer of skin of lower limb NOS
Code first any associated underlying condition, such as:
any associated gangrene (I96)
atherosclerosis of the lower extremities (I70.23-, I70.24-, I70.33-, I70.34-, I70.43-, I70.44-, I70.53-, I70.54-, I70.63-, I70.64-, I70.73-, I70.74-)
chronic venous hypertension (I87.31-, I87.33-)
diabetic ulcers (E08.621, E08.622, E09.621, E09.622, E10.621, E10.622, E11.621, E11.622, E13.621, E13.622)
postphlebitic syndrome (I87.01-, I87.03-)
postthrombotic syndrome (I87.01-, I87.03-)
varicose ulcer (I83.0-, I83.2-)
EXCLUDES 2 *pressure ulcer (pressure area) (L89.-)*
*skin infections (L00-L08)*
*specific infections classified to A00-B99*
**AHA:** 2021,1Q,7; 2020,2Q,19; 2018,4Q,69; 2017,4Q,17
**TIP:** The depth and/or severity of a diagnosed nonpressure ulcer can be determined based on medical record documentation from clinicians who are not the patient's provider.

**✓5th L97.1 Non-pressure chronic ulcer of thigh**

**✓6th L97.10 Non-pressure chronic ulcer of unspecified thigh**

**L97.101 Non-pressure chronic ulcer of unspecified thigh limited to breakdown of skin** HCC Rx ESR COM

**L97.102 Non-pressure chronic ulcer of unspecified thigh with fat layer exposed** HCC Rx ESR COM

**L97.103 Non-pressure chronic ulcer of unspecified thigh with necrosis of muscle** HCC Rx ESR COM

**L97.104 Non-pressure chronic ulcer of unspecified thigh with necrosis of bone** HCC Rx ESR COM

**L97.105 Non-pressure chronic ulcer of unspecified thigh with muscle involvement without evidence of necrosis** HCC Rx ESR COM

**L97.106 Non-pressure chronic ulcer of unspecified thigh with bone involvement without evidence of necrosis** HCC Rx ESR COM

**L97.108 Non-pressure chronic ulcer of unspecified thigh with other specified severity** HCC Rx ESR COM

L97.109 Non-pressure chronic ulcer of unspecified thigh with unspecified severity HCC Rx ESR COM

✓6th L97.11 Non-pressure chronic ulcer of right thigh

L97.111 Non-pressure chronic ulcer of right thigh limited to breakdown of skin HCC Rx ESR COM

L97.112 Non-pressure chronic ulcer of right thigh with fat layer exposed HCC Rx ESR COM

L97.113 Non-pressure chronic ulcer of right thigh with necrosis of muscle HCC Rx ESR COM

L97.114 Non-pressure chronic ulcer of right thigh with necrosis of bone HCC Rx ESR COM

L97.115 Non-pressure chronic ulcer of right thigh with muscle involvement without evidence of necrosis HCC Rx ESR COM

L97.116 Non-pressure chronic ulcer of right thigh with bone involvement without evidence of necrosis HCC Rx ESR COM

L97.118 Non-pressure chronic ulcer of right thigh with other specified severity HCC Rx ESR COM

L97.119 Non-pressure chronic ulcer of right thigh with unspecified severity HCC Rx ESR COM

✓6th L97.12 Non-pressure chronic ulcer of left thigh

L97.121 Non-pressure chronic ulcer of left thigh limited to breakdown of skin HCC Rx ESR COM

L97.122 Non-pressure chronic ulcer of left thigh with fat layer exposed HCC Rx ESR COM

L97.123 Non-pressure chronic ulcer of left thigh with necrosis of muscle HCC Rx ESR COM

L97.124 Non-pressure chronic ulcer of left thigh with necrosis of bone HCC Rx ESR COM

L97.125 Non-pressure chronic ulcer of left thigh with muscle involvement without evidence of necrosis HCC Rx ESR COM

L97.126 Non-pressure chronic ulcer of left thigh with bone involvement without evidence of necrosis HCC Rx ESR COM

L97.128 Non-pressure chronic ulcer of left thigh with other specified severity HCC Rx ESR COM

L97.129 Non-pressure chronic ulcer of left thigh with unspecified severity HCC Rx ESR COM

✓5th L97.2 Non-pressure chronic ulcer of calf

Non-pressure chronic ulcer of shin

**AHA:** 2024,1Q,16

✓6th L97.20 Non-pressure chronic ulcer of unspecified calf

L97.201 Non-pressure chronic ulcer of unspecified calf limited to breakdown of skin HCC Rx ESR COM

L97.202 Non-pressure chronic ulcer of unspecified calf with fat layer exposed HCC Rx ESR COM

L97.203 Non-pressure chronic ulcer of unspecified calf with necrosis of muscle HCC Rx ESR COM

L97.204 Non-pressure chronic ulcer of unspecified calf with necrosis of bone HCC Rx ESR COM

L97.205 Non-pressure chronic ulcer of unspecified calf with muscle involvement without evidence of necrosis HCC Rx ESR COM

L97.206 Non-pressure chronic ulcer of unspecified calf with bone involvement without evidence of necrosis HCC Rx ESR COM

L97.208 Non-pressure chronic ulcer of unspecified calf with other specified severity HCC Rx ESR COM

L97.209 Non-pressure chronic ulcer of unspecified calf with unspecified severity HCC Rx ESR COM

✓6th L97.21 Non-pressure chronic ulcer of right calf

L97.211 Non-pressure chronic ulcer of right calf limited to breakdown of skin HCC Rx ESR COM

L97.212 Non-pressure chronic ulcer of right calf with fat layer exposed HCC Rx ESR COM

L97.213 Non-pressure chronic ulcer of right calf with necrosis of muscle HCC Rx ESR COM

L97.214 Non-pressure chronic ulcer of right calf with necrosis of bone HCC Rx ESR COM

L97.215 Non-pressure chronic ulcer of right calf with muscle involvement without evidence of necrosis HCC Rx ESR COM

L97.216 Non-pressure chronic ulcer of right calf with bone involvement without evidence of necrosis HCC Rx ESR COM

L97.218 Non-pressure chronic ulcer of right calf with other specified severity HCC Rx ESR COM

L97.219 Non-pressure chronic ulcer of right calf with unspecified severity HCC Rx ESR COM

✓6th L97.22 Non-pressure chronic ulcer of left calf

L97.221 Non-pressure chronic ulcer of left calf limited to breakdown of skin HCC Rx ESR COM

L97.222 Non-pressure chronic ulcer of left calf with fat layer exposed HCC Rx ESR COM

L97.223 Non-pressure chronic ulcer of left calf with necrosis of muscle HCC Rx ESR COM

L97.224 Non-pressure chronic ulcer of left calf with necrosis of bone HCC Rx ESR COM

L97.225 Non-pressure chronic ulcer of left calf with muscle involvement without evidence of necrosis HCC Rx ESR COM

L97.226 Non-pressure chronic ulcer of left calf with bone involvement without evidence of necrosis HCC Rx ESR COM

L97.228 Non-pressure chronic ulcer of left calf with other specified severity HCC Rx ESR COM

L97.229 Non-pressure chronic ulcer of left calf with unspecified severity HCC Rx ESR COM

✓5th L97.3 Non-pressure chronic ulcer of ankle

✓6th L97.30 Non-pressure chronic ulcer of unspecified ankle

L97.301 Non-pressure chronic ulcer of unspecified ankle limited to breakdown of skin HCC Rx ESR COM

L97.302 Non-pressure chronic ulcer of unspecified ankle with fat layer exposed HCC Rx ESR COM

L97.303 Non-pressure chronic ulcer of unspecified ankle with necrosis of muscle HCC Rx ESR COM

L97.304 Non-pressure chronic ulcer of unspecified ankle with necrosis of bone HCC Rx ESR COM

L97.305 Non-pressure chronic ulcer of unspecified ankle with muscle involvement without evidence of necrosis HCC Rx ESR COM

L97.306 Non-pressure chronic ulcer of unspecified ankle with bone involvement without evidence of necrosis HCC Rx ESR COM

L97.308 Non-pressure chronic ulcer of unspecified ankle with other specified severity HCC Rx ESR COM

L97.309 Non-pressure chronic ulcer of unspecified ankle with unspecified severity HCC Rx ESR COM

✓6th L97.31 Non-pressure chronic ulcer of right ankle

L97.311 Non-pressure chronic ulcer of right ankle limited to breakdown of skin HCC Rx ESR COM

L97.312 Non-pressure chronic ulcer of right ankle with fat layer exposed HCC Rx ESR COM

L97.313 Non-pressure chronic ulcer of right ankle with necrosis of muscle HCC Rx ESR COM

L97.314 Non-pressure chronic ulcer of right ankle with necrosis of bone HCC Rx ESR COM

L97.315 Non-pressure chronic ulcer of right ankle with muscle involvement without evidence of necrosis HCC Rx ESR COM

L97.316 Non-pressure chronic ulcer of right ankle with bone involvement without evidence of necrosis HCC Rx ESR COM

L97.318 Non-pressure chronic ulcer of right ankle with other specified severity HCC Rx ESR COM

L97.319 Non-pressure chronic ulcer of right ankle with unspecified severity HCC Rx ESR COM

✓6th L97.32 Non-pressure chronic ulcer of left ankle

L97.321 Non-pressure chronic ulcer of left ankle limited to breakdown of skin HCC Rx ESR COM

L97.322 Non-pressure chronic ulcer of left ankle with fat layer exposed HCC Rx ESR COM

L97.323 Non-pressure chronic ulcer of left ankle with necrosis of muscle HCC Rx ESR COM

L97.324 Non-pressure chronic ulcer of left ankle with necrosis of bone HCC Rx ESR COM

L97.325 Non-pressure chronic ulcer of left ankle with muscle involvement without evidence of necrosis HCC Rx ESR COM

L97.326 Non-pressure chronic ulcer of left ankle with bone involvement without evidence of necrosis HCC Rx ESR COM

L97.328 Non-pressure chronic ulcer of left ankle with other specified severity HCC Rx ESR COM

L97.329 Non-pressure chronic ulcer of left ankle with unspecified severity HCC Rx ESR COM

✓5th L97.4 Non-pressure chronic ulcer of heel and midfoot

Non-pressure chronic ulcer of plantar surface of midfoot

✓6th L97.40 Non-pressure chronic ulcer of unspecified heel and midfoot

L97.401 Non-pressure chronic ulcer of unspecified heel and midfoot limited to breakdown of skin HCC Rx ESR COM

L97.402 Non-pressure chronic ulcer of unspecified heel and midfoot with fat layer exposed HCC Rx ESR COM

L97.403 Non-pressure chronic ulcer of unspecified heel and midfoot with necrosis of muscle HCC Rx ESR COM

L97.404 Non-pressure chronic ulcer of unspecified heel and midfoot with necrosis of bone HCC Rx ESR COM

L97.405 Non-pressure chronic ulcer of unspecified heel and midfoot with muscle involvement without evidence of necrosis HCC Rx ESR COM

L97.406 Non-pressure chronic ulcer of unspecified heel and midfoot with bone involvement without evidence of necrosis HCC Rx ESR COM

L97.408 Non-pressure chronic ulcer of unspecified heel and midfoot with other specified severity HCC Rx ESR COM

L97.409 Non-pressure chronic ulcer of unspecified heel and midfoot with unspecified severity HCC Rx ESR COM

✓6th L97.41 Non-pressure chronic ulcer of right heel and midfoot

L97.411 Non-pressure chronic ulcer of right heel and midfoot limited to breakdown of skin HCC Rx ESR COM

L97.412 Non-pressure chronic ulcer of right heel and midfoot with fat layer exposed HCC Rx ESR COM

AHA: 2020,2Q,19

L97.413 Non-pressure chronic ulcer of right heel and midfoot with necrosis of muscle HCC Rx ESR COM

L97.414 Non-pressure chronic ulcer of right heel and midfoot with necrosis of bone HCC Rx ESR COM

L97.415 Non-pressure chronic ulcer of right heel and midfoot with muscle involvement without evidence of necrosis HCC Rx ESR COM

L97.416 Non-pressure chronic ulcer of right heel and midfoot with bone involvement without evidence of necrosis HCC Rx ESR COM

L97.418 Non-pressure chronic ulcer of right heel and midfoot with other specified severity HCC Rx ESR COM

L97.419 Non-pressure chronic ulcer of right heel and midfoot with unspecified severity HCC Rx ESR COM

✓6th L97.42 Non-pressure chronic ulcer of left heel and midfoot

L97.421 Non-pressure chronic ulcer of left heel and midfoot limited to breakdown of skin HCC Rx ESR COM

AHA: 2016,1Q,12

L97.422 Non-pressure chronic ulcer of left heel and midfoot with fat layer exposed HCC Rx ESR COM

AHA: 2020,2Q,19

L97.423 Non-pressure chronic ulcer of left heel and midfoot with necrosis of muscle HCC Rx ESR COM

L97.424 Non-pressure chronic ulcer of left heel and midfoot with necrosis of bone HCC Rx ESR COM

L97.425 Non-pressure chronic ulcer of left heel and midfoot with muscle involvement without evidence of necrosis HCC Rx ESR COM

L97.426 Non-pressure chronic ulcer of left heel and midfoot with bone involvement without evidence of necrosis HCC Rx ESR COM

L97.428 Non-pressure chronic ulcer of left heel and midfoot with other specified severity HCC Rx ESR COM

L97.429 Non-pressure chronic ulcer of left heel and midfoot with unspecified severity HCC Rx ESR COM

✓5th L97.5 Non-pressure chronic ulcer of other part of foot

Non-pressure chronic ulcer of toe

✓6th L97.50 Non-pressure chronic ulcer of other part of unspecified foot

L97.501 Non-pressure chronic ulcer of other part of unspecified foot limited to breakdown of skin HCC Rx ESR COM

L97.502 Non-pressure chronic ulcer of other part of unspecified foot with fat layer exposed HCC Rx ESR COM

L97.503 Non-pressure chronic ulcer of other part of unspecified foot with necrosis of muscle HCC Rx ESR COM

L97.504 Non-pressure chronic ulcer of other part of unspecified foot with necrosis of bone HCC Rx ESR COM

L97.505 Non-pressure chronic ulcer of other part of unspecified foot with muscle involvement without evidence of necrosis HCC Rx ESR COM

L97.506 Non-pressure chronic ulcer of other part of unspecified foot with bone involvement without evidence of necrosis HCC Rx ESR COM

L97.508 Non-pressure chronic ulcer of other part of unspecified foot with other specified severity HCC Rx ESR COM

L97.509 Non-pressure chronic ulcer of other part of unspecified foot with unspecified severity HCC Rx ESR COM

✓6th L97.51 Non-pressure chronic ulcer of other part of right foot

AHA: 2020,1Q,12

L97.511 Non-pressure chronic ulcer of other part of right foot limited to breakdown of skin HCC Rx ESR COM

L97.512 Non-pressure chronic ulcer of other part of right foot with fat layer exposed HCC Rx ESR COM

AHA: 2020,2Q,19

L97.513 Non-pressure chronic ulcer of other part of right foot with necrosis of muscle HCC Rx ESR COM

L97.514 Non-pressure chronic ulcer of other part of right foot with necrosis of bone HCC Rx ESR COM

L97.515 Non-pressure chronic ulcer of other part of right foot with muscle involvement without evidence of necrosis HCC Rx ESR COM

L97.516 Non-pressure chronic ulcer of other part of right foot with bone involvement without evidence of necrosis HCC Rx ESR COM

L97.518 Non-pressure chronic ulcer of other part of right foot with other specified severity HCC Rx ESR COM

L97.519 Non-pressure chronic ulcer of other part of right foot with unspecified severity HCC Rx ESR COM

6th L97.52 Non-pressure chronic ulcer of other part of left foot

AHA: 2020,1Q,12

L97.521 Non-pressure chronic ulcer of other part of left foot limited to breakdown of skin HCC Rx ESR COM

L97.522 Non-pressure chronic ulcer of other part of left foot with fat layer exposed HCC Rx ESR COM

AHA: 2020,2Q,19

L97.523 Non-pressure chronic ulcer of other part of left foot with necrosis of muscle HCC Rx ESR COM

L97.524 Non-pressure chronic ulcer of other part of left foot with necrosis of bone HCC Rx ESR COM

L97.525 Non-pressure chronic ulcer of other part of left foot with muscle involvement without evidence of necrosis HCC Rx ESR COM

L97.526 Non-pressure chronic ulcer of other part of left foot with bone involvement without evidence of necrosis HCC Rx ESR COM

L97.528 Non-pressure chronic ulcer of other part of left foot with other specified severity HCC Rx ESR COM

L97.529 Non-pressure chronic ulcer of other part of left foot with unspecified severity HCC Rx ESR COM

5th L97.8 Non-pressure chronic ulcer of other part of lower leg

6th L97.80 Non-pressure chronic ulcer of other part of unspecified lower leg

L97.801 Non-pressure chronic ulcer of other part of unspecified lower leg limited to breakdown of skin HCC Rx ESR COM

L97.802 Non-pressure chronic ulcer of other part of unspecified lower leg with fat layer exposed HCC Rx ESR COM

L97.803 Non-pressure chronic ulcer of other part of unspecified lower leg with necrosis of muscle HCC Rx ESR COM

L97.804 Non-pressure chronic ulcer of other part of unspecified lower leg with necrosis of bone HCC Rx ESR COM

L97.805 Non-pressure chronic ulcer of other part of unspecified lower leg with muscle involvement without evidence of necrosis HCC Rx ESR COM

L97.806 Non-pressure chronic ulcer of other part of unspecified lower leg with bone involvement without evidence of necrosis HCC Rx ESR COM

L97.808 Non-pressure chronic ulcer of other part of unspecified lower leg with other specified severity HCC Rx ESR COM

L97.809 Non-pressure chronic ulcer of other part of unspecified lower leg with unspecified severity HCC Rx ESR COM

6th L97.81 Non-pressure chronic ulcer of other part of right lower leg

L97.811 Non-pressure chronic ulcer of other part of right lower leg limited to breakdown of skin HCC Rx ESR COM

L97.812 Non-pressure chronic ulcer of other part of right lower leg with fat layer exposed HCC Rx ESR COM

L97.813 Non-pressure chronic ulcer of other part of right lower leg with necrosis of muscle HCC Rx ESR COM

L97.814 Non-pressure chronic ulcer of other part of right lower leg with necrosis of bone HCC Rx ESR COM

L97.815 Non-pressure chronic ulcer of other part of right lower leg with muscle involvement without evidence of necrosis HCC Rx ESR COM

L97.816 Non-pressure chronic ulcer of other part of right lower leg with bone involvement without evidence of necrosis HCC Rx ESR COM

L97.818 Non-pressure chronic ulcer of other part of right lower leg with other specified severity HCC Rx ESR COM

L97.819 Non-pressure chronic ulcer of other part of right lower leg with unspecified severity HCC Rx ESR COM

6th L97.82 Non-pressure chronic ulcer of other part of left lower leg

L97.821 Non-pressure chronic ulcer of other part of left lower leg limited to breakdown of skin HCC Rx ESR COM

L97.822 Non-pressure chronic ulcer of other part of left lower leg with fat layer exposed HCC Rx ESR COM

L97.823 Non-pressure chronic ulcer of other part of left lower leg with necrosis of muscle HCC Rx ESR COM

L97.824 Non-pressure chronic ulcer of other part of left lower leg with necrosis of bone HCC Rx ESR COM

L97.825 Non-pressure chronic ulcer of other part of left lower leg with muscle involvement without evidence of necrosis HCC Rx ESR COM

L97.826 Non-pressure chronic ulcer of other part of left lower leg with bone involvement without evidence of necrosis HCC Rx ESR COM

L97.828 Non-pressure chronic ulcer of other part of left lower leg with other specified severity HCC Rx ESR COM

L97.829 Non-pressure chronic ulcer of other part of left lower leg with unspecified severity HCC Rx ESR COM

5th L97.9 Non-pressure chronic ulcer of unspecified part of lower leg

AHA: 2025,1Q,35

6th L97.90 Non-pressure chronic ulcer of unspecified part of unspecified lower leg

L97.901 Non-pressure chronic ulcer of unspecified part of unspecified lower leg limited to breakdown of skin HCC Rx ESR COM

L97.902 Non-pressure chronic ulcer of unspecified part of unspecified lower leg with fat layer exposed HCC Rx ESR COM

L97.903 Non-pressure chronic ulcer of unspecified part of unspecified lower leg with necrosis of muscle HCC Rx ESR COM

L97.904 Non-pressure chronic ulcer of unspecified part of unspecified lower leg with necrosis of bone HCC Rx ESR COM

L97.905 Non-pressure chronic ulcer of unspecified part of unspecified lower leg with muscle involvement without evidence of necrosis HCC Rx ESR COM

L97.906 Non-pressure chronic ulcer of unspecified part of unspecified lower leg with bone involvement without evidence of necrosis HCC Rx ESR COM

L97.908 Non-pressure chronic ulcer of unspecified part of unspecified lower leg with other specified severity HCC Rx ESR COM

L97.909 Non-pressure chronic ulcer of unspecified part of unspecified lower leg with unspecified severity HCC Rx ESR COM

6th L97.91 Non-pressure chronic ulcer of unspecified part of right lower leg

L97.911 Non-pressure chronic ulcer of unspecified part of right lower leg limited to breakdown of skin HCC Rx ESR COM

L97.912 Non-pressure chronic ulcer of unspecified part of right lower leg with fat layer exposed HCC Rx ESR COM

L97.913 Non-pressure chronic ulcer of unspecified part of right lower leg with necrosis of muscle HCC Rx ESR COM

L97.914 Non-pressure chronic ulcer of unspecified part of right lower leg with necrosis of bone HCC Rx ESR COM

L97.915 Non-pressure chronic ulcer of unspecified part of right lower leg with muscle involvement without evidence of necrosis HCC Rx ESR COM

L97.916 Non-pressure chronic ulcer of unspecified part of right lower leg with bone involvement without evidence of necrosis HCC Rx ESR COM

L97.918 Non-pressure chronic ulcer of unspecified part of right lower leg with other specified severity HCC Rx ESR COM

L97.919 Non-pressure chronic ulcer of unspecified part of right lower leg with unspecified severity HCC Rx ESR COM

✓6th L97.92 Non-pressure chronic ulcer of unspecified part of left lower leg

L97.921 Non-pressure chronic ulcer of unspecified part of left lower leg limited to breakdown of skin HCC Rx ESR COM

L97.922 Non-pressure chronic ulcer of unspecified part of left lower leg with fat layer exposed HCC Rx ESR COM

L97.923 Non-pressure chronic ulcer of unspecified part of left lower leg with necrosis of muscle HCC Rx ESR COM

L97.924 Non-pressure chronic ulcer of unspecified part of left lower leg with necrosis of bone HCC Rx ESR COM

L97.925 Non-pressure chronic ulcer of unspecified part of left lower leg with muscle involvement without evidence of necrosis HCC Rx ESR COM

L97.926 Non-pressure chronic ulcer of unspecified part of left lower leg with bone involvement without evidence of necrosis HCC Rx ESR COM

L97.928 Non-pressure chronic ulcer of unspecified part of left lower leg with other specified severity HCC Rx ESR COM

L97.929 Non-pressure chronic ulcer of unspecified part of left lower leg with unspecified severity HCC Rx ESR COM

✓4th **L98 Other disorders of skin and subcutaneous tissue, not elsewhere classified**

**L98.Ø Pyogenic granuloma**

EXCLUDES 2 *pyogenic granuloma of gingiva (KØ6.8)*
*pyogenic granuloma of maxillary alveolar ridge (KØ4.5)*
*pyogenic granuloma of oral mucosa (K13.4)*

**DEF:** Solitary polypoid capillary hemangioma often associated with local irritation, trauma, and superimposed inflammation. Located on the skin and gingival or oral mucosa, they bleed easily and may ulcerate and form crusted sores.

**L98.1 Factitial dermatitis**

Neurotic excoriation

EXCLUDES 1 *excoriation (skin-picking) disorder (F42.4)*

**AHA:** 2016,4Q,15

**DEF:** Self-inflicted skin lesions to satisfy an unconscious psychological or emotional need. Methods used to injure the skin include deep excoriations with a sharp instrument, scarification with a knife, or the application of caustic chemicals and burning, sometimes with a cigarette.

**L98.2 Febrile neutrophilic dermatosis [Sweet]**

**L98.3 Eosinophilic cellulitis [Wells]**

✓5th **L98.4 Non-pressure chronic ulcer of skin, not elsewhere classified**

Chronic ulcer of skin NOS
Tropical ulcer NOS
Ulcer of skin NOS

EXCLUDES 2 *gangrene (I96)*
*pressure ulcer (pressure area) (L89.-)*
*skin infections (LØØ-LØ8)*
*specific infections classified to AØØ-B99*
*ulcer of lower limb NEC (L97.-)*
*varicose ulcer (I83.Ø-I83.93)*

**AHA:** 2017,4Q,17

**TIP:** The depth and/or severity of a diagnosed nonpressure ulcer can be determined based on medical record documentation from clinicians who are not the patient's provider.

✓6th L98.41 Non-pressure chronic ulcer of buttock

L98.411 Non-pressure chronic ulcer of buttock limited to breakdown of skin HCC Rx ESR COM

L98.412 Non-pressure chronic ulcer of buttock with fat layer exposed HCC Rx ESR COM

L98.413 Non-pressure chronic ulcer of buttock with necrosis of muscle HCC Rx ESR COM

L98.414 Non-pressure chronic ulcer of buttock with necrosis of bone HCC Rx ESR COM

L98.415 Non-pressure chronic ulcer of buttock with muscle involvement without evidence of necrosis HCC Rx ESR COM

L98.416 Non-pressure chronic ulcer of buttock with bone involvement without evidence of necrosis HCC Rx ESR COM

L98.418 Non-pressure chronic ulcer of buttock with other specified severity HCC Rx ESR COM

L98.419 Non-pressure chronic ulcer of buttock with unspecified severity HCC Rx ESR COM

✓6th L98.42 Non-pressure chronic ulcer of back

L98.421 Non-pressure chronic ulcer of back limited to breakdown of skin HCC Rx ESR COM

L98.422 Non-pressure chronic ulcer of back with fat layer exposed HCC Rx ESR COM

L98.423 Non-pressure chronic ulcer of back with necrosis of muscle HCC Rx ESR COM

L98.424 Non-pressure chronic ulcer of back with necrosis of bone HCC Rx ESR COM

L98.425 Non-pressure chronic ulcer of back with muscle involvement without evidence of necrosis HCC Rx ESR COM

L98.426 Non-pressure chronic ulcer of back with bone involvement without evidence of necrosis HCC Rx ESR COM

L98.428 Non-pressure chronic ulcer of back with other specified severity HCC Rx ESR COM

L98.429 Non-pressure chronic ulcer of back with unspecified severity HCC Rx ESR COM

✓6th L98.43 Non-pressure chronic ulcer of abdomen

L98.431 Non-pressure chronic ulcer of abdomen limited to breakdown of skin HCC Rx ESR

L98.432 Non-pressure chronic ulcer of abdomen with fat layer exposed HCC Rx ESR

L98.433 Non-pressure chronic ulcer of abdomen with necrosis of muscle HCC Rx ESR

L98.434 Non-pressure chronic ulcer of abdomen with necrosis of bone HCC Rx ESR

L98.435 Non-pressure chronic ulcer of abdomen with muscle involvement without evidence of necrosis HCC Rx ESR

L98.436 Non-pressure chronic ulcer of abdomen with bone involvement without evidence of necrosis HCC Rx ESR

L98.438 Non-pressure chronic ulcer of abdomen with other specified severity HCC Rx ESR

L98.439 Non-pressure chronic ulcer of abdomen with unspecified severity HCC Rx ESR

✓6th L98.44 Non-pressure chronic ulcer of chest

L98.441 Non-pressure chronic ulcer of chest limited to breakdown of skin HCC Rx ESR

L98.442 Non-pressure chronic ulcer of chest with fat layer exposed HCC Rx ESR

L98.443 Non-pressure chronic ulcer of chest with necrosis of muscle HCC Rx ESR

L98.444 Non-pressure chronic ulcer of chest with necrosis of bone HCC Rx ESR

L98.445 Non-pressure chronic ulcer of chest with muscle involvement without evidence of necrosis HCC Rx ESR

L98.446 Non-pressure chronic ulcer of chest with bone involvement without evidence of necrosis HCC Rx ESR

L98.448 Non-pressure chronic ulcer of chest with other specified severity HCC Rx ESR

L98.449 Non-pressure chronic ulcer of chest with unspecified severity HCC Rx ESR

√6th L98.45 Non-pressure chronic ulcer of neck

L98.451 Non-pressure chronic ulcer of neck limited to breakdown of skin HCC Rx ESR

L98.452 Non-pressure chronic ulcer of neck with fat layer exposed HCC Rx ESR

L98.453 Non-pressure chronic ulcer of neck with necrosis of muscle HCC Rx ESR

L98.454 Non-pressure chronic ulcer of neck with necrosis of bone HCC Rx ESR

L98.455 Non-pressure chronic ulcer of neck with muscle involvement without evidence of necrosis HCC Rx ESR

L98.456 Non-pressure chronic ulcer of neck with bone involvement without evidence of necrosis HCC Rx ESR

L98.458 Non-pressure chronic ulcer of neck with other specified severity HCC Rx ESR

L98.459 Non-pressure chronic ulcer of neck with unspecified severity HCC Rx ESR

√6th L98.46 Non-pressure chronic ulcer of face

L98.461 Non-pressure chronic ulcer of face limited to breakdown of skin HCC Rx ESR

L98.462 Non-pressure chronic ulcer of face with fat layer exposed HCC Rx ESR

L98.463 Non-pressure chronic ulcer of face with necrosis of muscle HCC Rx ESR

L98.464 Non-pressure chronic ulcer of face with necrosis of bone HCC Rx ESR

L98.465 Non-pressure chronic ulcer of face with muscle involvement without evidence of necrosis HCC Rx ESR

L98.466 Non-pressure chronic ulcer of face with bone involvement without evidence of necrosis HCC Rx ESR

L98.468 Non-pressure chronic ulcer of face with other specified severity HCC Rx ESR

L98.469 Non-pressure chronic ulcer of face with unspecified severity HCC Rx ESR

√6th L98.47 Non-pressure chronic ulcer of groin

L98.471 Non-pressure chronic ulcer of groin limited to breakdown of skin HCC Rx ESR

L98.472 Non-pressure chronic ulcer of groin with fat layer exposed HCC Rx ESR

L98.473 Non-pressure chronic ulcer of groin with necrosis of muscle HCC Rx ESR

L98.474 Non-pressure chronic ulcer of groin with necrosis of bone HCC Rx ESR

L98.475 Non-pressure chronic ulcer of groin with muscle involvement without evidence of necrosis HCC Rx ESR

L98.476 Non-pressure chronic ulcer of groin with bone involvement without evidence of necrosis HCC Rx ESR

L98.478 Non-pressure chronic ulcer of groin with other specified severity HCC Rx ESR

L98.479 Non-pressure chronic ulcer of groin with unspecified severity HCC Rx ESR

√6th L98.49 Non-pressure chronic ulcer of skin of other sites

Non-pressure chronic ulcer of skin NOS

L98.491 Non-pressure chronic ulcer of skin of other sites limited to breakdown of skin HCC Rx ESR COM

L98.492 Non-pressure chronic ulcer of skin of other sites with fat layer exposed HCC Rx ESR COM

L98.493 Non-pressure chronic ulcer of skin of other sites with necrosis of muscle HCC Rx ESR COM

L98.494 Non-pressure chronic ulcer of skin of other sites with necrosis of bone HCC Rx ESR COM

L98.495 Non-pressure chronic ulcer of skin of other sites with muscle involvement without evidence of necrosis HCC Rx ESR COM

L98.496 Non-pressure chronic ulcer of skin of other sites with bone involvement without evidence of necrosis HCC Rx ESR COM

L98.498 Non-pressure chronic ulcer of skin of other sites with other specified severity HCC Rx ESR COM

L98.499 Non-pressure chronic ulcer of skin of other sites with unspecified severity HCC Rx ESR COM

√5th L98.A Non-pressure chronic ulcer of upper limb, not elsewhere classified

Chronic ulcer of upper limb NOS
Non-healing ulcer of upper limb
Ulcer of upper limb NEC

EXCLUDES 2 *gangrene (I96)*
*pressure ulcer (pressure area) (L89.-)*
*skin infections (LØØ-LØ8)*
*specific infections classified to AØØ-B99*
*ulcer of lower limb NEC (L97.-)*
*varicose ulcer (I83.Ø-I83.93)*

**AHA:** 2025,4Q,38

√6th L98.A1 Non-pressure chronic ulcer of upper arm

Non-pressure chronic ulcer of axilla

√7th L98.A11 Non-pressure chronic ulcer of right upper arm

L98.A111 Non-pressure chronic ulcer of right upper arm limited to breakdown of skin HCC Rx ESR

L98.A112 Non-pressure chronic ulcer of right upper arm with fat layer exposed HCC Rx ESR

L98.A113 Non-pressure chronic ulcer of right upper arm with necrosis of muscle HCC Rx ESR

L98.A114 Non-pressure chronic ulcer of right upper arm with necrosis of bone HCC Rx ESR

L98.A115 Non-pressure chronic ulcer of right upper arm with muscle involvement without evidence of necrosis HCC Rx ESR

L98.A116 Non-pressure chronic ulcer of right upper arm with bone involvement without evidence of necrosis HCC Rx ESR

L98.A118 Non-pressure chronic ulcer of right upper arm with other specified severity HCC Rx ESR

L98.A119 Non-pressure chronic ulcer of right upper arm with unspecified severity HCC Rx ESR

√7th L98.A12 Non-pressure chronic ulcer of left upper arm

L98.A121 Non-pressure chronic ulcer of left upper arm limited to breakdown of skin HCC Rx ESR

L98.A122 Non-pressure chronic ulcer of left upper arm with fat layer exposed HCC Rx ESR

L98.A123 Non-pressure chronic ulcer of left upper arm with necrosis of muscle HCC Rx ESR

L98.A124 Non-pressure chronic ulcer of left upper arm with necrosis of bone HCC Rx ESR

L98.A125 Non-pressure chronic ulcer of left upper arm with muscle involvement without evidence of necrosis HCC Rx ESR

L98.A126 Non-pressure chronic ulcer of left upper arm with bone involvement without evidence of necrosis HCC Rx ESR
L98.A128 Non-pressure chronic ulcer of left upper arm with other specified severity HCC Rx ESR
L98.A129 Non-pressure chronic ulcer of left upper arm with unspecified severity HCC Rx ESR

✓7th L98.A19 Non-pressure chronic ulcer of unspecified upper arm
L98.A191 Non-pressure chronic ulcer of unspecified upper arm limited to breakdown of skin HCC Rx ESR
L98.A192 Non-pressure chronic ulcer of unspecified upper arm with fat layer exposed HCC Rx ESR
L98.A193 Non-pressure chronic ulcer of unspecified upper arm with necrosis of muscle HCC Rx ESR
L98.A194 Non-pressure chronic ulcer of unspecified upper arm with necrosis of bone HCC Rx ESR
L98.A195 Non-pressure chronic ulcer of unspecified upper arm with muscle involvement without evidence of necrosis HCC Rx ESR
L98.A196 Non-pressure chronic ulcer of unspecified upper arm with bone involvement without evidence of necrosis HCC Rx ESR
L98.A198 Non-pressure chronic ulcer of unspecified upper arm with other specified severity HCC Rx ESR
L98.A199 Non-pressure chronic ulcer of unspecified upper arm with unspecified severity HCC Rx ESR

✓6th L98.A2 Non-pressure chronic ulcer of forearm

✓7th L98.A21 Non-pressure chronic ulcer of right forearm
L98.A211 Non-pressure chronic ulcer of right forearm limited to breakdown of skin HCC Rx ESR
L98.A212 Non-pressure chronic ulcer of right forearm with fat layer exposed HCC Rx ESR
L98.A213 Non-pressure chronic ulcer of right forearm with necrosis of muscle HCC Rx ESR
L98.A214 Non-pressure chronic ulcer of right forearm with necrosis of bone HCC Rx ESR
L98.A215 Non-pressure chronic ulcer of right forearm with muscle involvement without evidence of necrosis HCC Rx ESR
L98.A216 Non-pressure chronic ulcer of right forearm with bone involvement without evidence of necrosis HCC Rx ESR
L98.A218 Non-pressure chronic ulcer of right forearm with other specified severity HCC Rx ESR
L98.A219 Non-pressure chronic ulcer of right forearm with unspecified severity HCC Rx ESR

✓7th L98.A22 Non-pressure chronic ulcer of left forearm
L98.A221 Non-pressure chronic ulcer of left forearm limited to breakdown of skin HCC Rx ESR
L98.A222 Non-pressure chronic ulcer of left forearm with fat layer exposed HCC Rx ESR
L98.A223 Non-pressure chronic ulcer of left forearm with necrosis of muscle HCC Rx ESR
L98.A224 Non-pressure chronic ulcer of left forearm with necrosis of bone HCC Rx ESR
L98.A225 Non-pressure chronic ulcer of left forearm with muscle involvement without evidence of necrosis HCC Rx ESR
L98.A226 Non-pressure chronic ulcer of left forearm with bone involvement without evidence of necrosis HCC Rx ESR
L98.A228 Non-pressure chronic ulcer of left forearm with other specified severity HCC Rx ESR
L98.A229 Non-pressure chronic ulcer of left forearm with unspecified severity HCC Rx ESR

✓7th L98.A29 Non-pressure chronic ulcer of unspecified forearm
L98.A291 Non-pressure chronic ulcer of unspecified forearm limited to breakdown of skin HCC Rx ESR
L98.A292 Non-pressure chronic ulcer of unspecified forearm with fat layer exposed HCC Rx ESR
L98.A293 Non-pressure chronic ulcer of unspecified forearm with necrosis of muscle HCC Rx ESR
L98.A294 Non-pressure chronic ulcer of unspecified forearm with necrosis of bone HCC Rx ESR
L98.A295 Non-pressure chronic ulcer of unspecified forearm with muscle involvement without evidence of necrosis HCC Rx ESR
L98.A296 Non-pressure chronic ulcer of unspecified forearm with bone involvement without evidence of necrosis HCC Rx ESR
L98.A298 Non-pressure chronic ulcer of unspecified forearm with other specified severity HCC Rx ESR
L98.A299 Non-pressure chronic ulcer of unspecified forearm with unspecified severity HCC Rx ESR

✓6th L98.A3 Non-pressure chronic ulcer of hand

✓7th L98.A31 Non-pressure chronic ulcer of right hand
L98.A311 Non-pressure chronic ulcer of right hand limited to breakdown of skin HCC Rx ESR
L98.A312 Non-pressure chronic ulcer of right hand with fat layer exposed HCC Rx ESR
L98.A313 Non-pressure chronic ulcer of right hand with necrosis of muscle HCC Rx ESR
L98.A314 Non-pressure chronic ulcer of right hand with necrosis of bone HCC Rx ESR
L98.A315 Non-pressure chronic ulcer of right hand with muscle involvement without evidence of necrosis HCC Rx ESR
L98.A316 Non-pressure chronic ulcer of right hand with bone involvement without evidence of necrosis HCC Rx ESR
L98.A318 Non-pressure chronic ulcer of right hand with other specified severity HCC Rx ESR
L98.A319 Non-pressure chronic ulcer of right hand with unspecified severity HCC Rx ESR

✓7th L98.A32 Non-pressure chronic ulcer of left hand

L98.A321 Non-pressure chronic ulcer of left hand limited to breakdown of skin HCC Rx ESR

L98.A322 Non-pressure chronic ulcer of left hand with fat layer exposed HCC Rx ESR

L98.A323 Non-pressure chronic ulcer of left hand with necrosis of muscle HCC Rx ESR

L98.A324 Non-pressure chronic ulcer of left hand with necrosis of bone HCC Rx ESR

L98.A325 Non-pressure chronic ulcer of left hand with muscle involvement without evidence of necrosis HCC Rx ESR

L98.A326 Non-pressure chronic ulcer of left hand with bone involvement without evidence of necrosis HCC Rx ESR

L98.A328 Non-pressure chronic ulcer of left hand with other specified severity HCC Rx ESR

L98.A329 Non-pressure chronic ulcer of left hand with unspecified severity HCC Rx ESR

√7th **L98.A39 Non-pressure chronic ulcer of unspecified hand**

L98.A391 Non-pressure chronic ulcer of unspecified hand limited to breakdown of skin HCC Rx ESR

L98.A392 Non-pressure chronic ulcer of unspecified hand with fat layer exposed HCC Rx ESR

L98.A393 Non-pressure chronic ulcer of unspecified hand with necrosis of muscle HCC Rx ESR

L98.A394 Non-pressure chronic ulcer of unspecified hand with necrosis of bone HCC Rx ESR

L98.A395 Non-pressure chronic ulcer of unspecified hand with muscle involvement without evidence of necrosis HCC Rx ESR

L98.A396 Non-pressure chronic ulcer of unspecified hand with bone involvement without evidence of necrosis HCC Rx ESR

L98.A398 Non-pressure chronic ulcer of unspecified hand with other specified severity HCC Rx ESR

L98.A399 Non-pressure chronic ulcer of unspecified hand with unspecified severity HCC Rx ESR

**L98.5 Mucinosis of the skin**

Focal mucinosis
Lichen myxedematosus
Reticular erythematous mucinosis

EXCLUDES 1 *focal oral mucinosis (K13.79)*
*myxedema (EØ3.9)*

**L98.6 Other infiltrative disorders of the skin and subcutaneous tissue**

EXCLUDES 1 *hyalinosis cutis et mucosae (E78.89)*

**L98.7 Excessive and redundant skin and subcutaneous tissue**

Loose or sagging skin following dietary weight loss
Loose or sagging skin, following bariatric surgery weight loss
Loose or sagging skin, NOS

EXCLUDES 2 *acquired excess or redundant skin of eyelid (HØ2.3-)*
*congenital excess or redundant skin of eyelid (Q1Ø.3)*
*skin changes due to chronic exposure to nonionizing radiation (L57.-)*

**AHA:** 2022,3Q,11; 2016,4Q,36

**L98.8 Other specified disorders of the skin and subcutaneous tissue**

**AHA:** 2013,2Q,32

**L98.9 Disorder of the skin and subcutaneous tissue, unspecified**

***L99 Other disorders of skin and subcutaneous tissue in diseases classified elsewhere***

Code first underlying disease, such as:
amyloidosis (E85.-)

EXCLUDES 1 *skin disorders in diabetes (EØ8-E13 with .62-)*
*skin disorders in gonorrhea (A54.89)*
*skin disorders in syphilis (A51.31, A52.79)*

**AHA:** 2021,1Q,39

# Chapter 13. Diseases of the Musculoskeletal System and Connective Tissue (MØØ–M99)

## Chapter-specific Guidelines with Coding Examples

The chapter-specific guidelines from the ICD-10-CM Official Guidelines for Coding and Reporting have been provided below. Along with these guidelines are coding examples, contained in the shaded boxes, that have been developed to help illustrate the coding and/or sequencing guidance found in these guidelines.

**a. Site and laterality**

Most of the codes within Chapter 13 have site and laterality designations. The site represents the bone, joint or the muscle involved.

**1) Bone versus joint**

For certain conditions, the bone may be affected at the upper or lower end, (e.g., avascular necrosis of bone, M87, Osteoporosis, M8Ø, M81). Though the portion of the bone affected may be at the joint, the site designation will be the bone, not the joint.

> Idiopathic avascular necrosis of the femoral head of the left hip joint
>
> **M87.Ø52 Idiopathic aseptic necrosis of left femur**
>
> *Explanation:* For certain conditions such as avascular necrosis, the bone may be affected at the joint, but the site designation is the bone, not the joint.

**2) Multiple sites**

Codes describing specified sites are assigned individually by site when documented. When the specified site(s) are not documented, assign the appropriate code for "multiple sites."

**b. Acute traumatic versus chronic or recurrent musculoskeletal conditions**

Many musculoskeletal conditions are a result of previous injury or trauma to a site, or are recurrent conditions. Bone, joint or muscle conditions that are the result of a healed injury are usually found in chapter 13. Recurrent bone, joint or muscle conditions are also usually found in chapter 13. Any current, acute injury should be coded to the appropriate injury code from chapter 19. Chronic or recurrent conditions should generally be coded with a code from chapter 13. If it is difficult to determine from the documentation in the record which code is best to describe a condition, query the provider.

> Acute traumatic bucket handle tear of right medial meniscus
>
> **S83.211A Bucket-handle tear of medial meniscus, current injury, right knee, initial encounter**
>
> *Explanation:* Any current, acute injury is not coded in chapter 13. It should instead be coded to the appropriate injury code from chapter 19.

> Old bucket handle tear of right medial meniscus
>
> **M23.2Ø3 Derangement of unspecified medial meniscus due to old tear or injury, right knee**
>
> *Explanation:* Chronic or recurrent conditions should generally be coded with a code from chapter 13.

**c. Coding of Pathologic Fractures**

7th character A is for use as long as the patient is receiving active treatment for the fracture. Examples of active treatment are: surgical treatment, emergency department encounter, evaluation and continuing treatment by the same or a different physician. While the patient may be seen by a new or different provider over the course of treatment for a pathological fracture, assignment of the 7th character is based on whether the patient is undergoing active treatment and not whether the provider is seeing the patient for the first time.

> Pathologic fracture of left foot, unknown cause, currently under active treatment by a follow-up provider
>
> **M84.475A Pathological fracture, left foot, initial encounter for fracture**
>
> *Explanation:* Seventh character A is for use as long as the patient is receiving active treatment for a pathologic fracture. Examples of active treatment are surgical treatment, emergency department encounter, evaluation, and continuing treatment by the same or a different physician.
>
> The seventh character is based on whether the patient is undergoing active treatment and not whether the provider is seeing the patient for the first time.

7th character D is to be used for encounters after the patient has completed active treatment for the fracture and is receiving routine care for the fracture during the healing or recovery phase. The other 7th characters, listed under each subcategory in the Tabular List, are to be used for subsequent encounters for treatment of problems associated with the healing, such as malunions, nonunions, and sequelae.

Care for complications of surgical treatment for fracture repairs during the healing or recovery phase should be coded with the appropriate complication codes.

*See Section I.C.19. Coding of traumatic fractures.*

**d. Osteoporosis**

Osteoporosis is a systemic condition, meaning that all bones of the musculoskeletal system are affected. Therefore, site is not a component of the codes under category M81, Osteoporosis without current pathological fracture. The site codes under category M8Ø, Osteoporosis with current pathological fracture, identify the site of the fracture, not the osteoporosis.

**1) Osteoporosis without pathological fracture**

Category M81, Osteoporosis without current pathological fracture, is for use for patients with osteoporosis who do not currently have a pathologic fracture due to the osteoporosis, even if they have had a fracture in the past. For patients with a history of osteoporosis fractures, status code Z87.31Ø, Personal history of (healed) osteoporosis fracture, should follow the code from M81.

> Age-related osteoporosis with healed osteoporotic fracture of the lumbar vertebra
>
> **M81.Ø Age-related osteoporosis without current pathological fracture**
>
> **Z87.31Ø Personal history of (healed) osteoporosis fracture**
>
> *Explanation:* Category M81 is used for patients with osteoporosis who do not currently have a pathologic fracture due to the osteoporosis. To report a previous (healed) fracture, status code Z87.31Ø Personal history of (healed) osteoporosis fracture, should follow the code from M81.

**2) Osteoporosis with current pathological fracture**

Category M8Ø, Osteoporosis with current pathological fracture, is for patients who have a current pathologic fracture at the time of an encounter. The codes under M8Ø identify the site of the fracture. A code from category M8Ø, not a traumatic fracture code, should be used for any patient with known osteoporosis who suffers a fracture, even if the patient had a minor fall or trauma, if that fall or trauma would not usually break a normal, healthy bone.

> Disuse osteoporosis with current fracture of right shoulder sustained lifting a grocery bag, initial encounter
>
> **M8Ø.811A Other osteoporosis with current pathological fracture, right shoulder, initial encounter for fracture**
>
> *Explanation:* A code from category M8Ø, not a traumatic fracture code, should be used for any patient with known osteoporosis who suffers a fracture, even if the patient had a minor fall or trauma, if that fall or trauma would not usually break a normal, healthy bone.

**e. Multisystem inflammatory syndrome**

*See Section I.C.1.g.1.l. for Multisystem Inflammatory Syndrome*

# Muscle/Tendon Table

ICD-10-CM categorizes certain muscles and tendons in the upper and lower extremities by their action (e.g., extension, flexion), their anatomical location (e.g., posterior, anterior), and/or whether they are intrinsic or extrinsic to a certain anatomical area. The Muscle/Tendon Table is provided at the beginning of chapters 13 and 19 as a resource to help users when code selection depends on one or more of these characteristics. A **TIP** has been placed at those categories and/or subcategories that relate to this table. Please note that this table is not all-inclusive, and proper code assignment should be based on the provider's documentation.

| Body Region | Muscle | Extensor Tendon | Flexor Tendon | Other Tendon |
|---|---|---|---|---|
| **Shoulder** | | | | |
| | Deltoid | Posterior deltoid | Anterior deltoid | |
| | Rotator cuff | | | |
| | Infraspinatus | | | Infraspinatus |
| | Subscapularis | | | Subscapularis |
| | Supraspinatus | | | Supraspinatus |
| | Teres minor | | | Teres minor |
| | Teres major | Teres major | | |
| **Upper arm** | | | | |
| | Anterior muscles | | | |
| | Biceps brachii — long head | | Biceps brachii — long head | |
| | Biceps brachii — short head | | Biceps brachii — short head | |
| | Brachialis | | Brachialis | |
| | Coracobrachialis | | Coracobrachialis | |
| | Posterior muscles | | | |
| | Triceps brachii | Triceps brachii | | |
| **Forearm** | | | | |
| | Anterior muscles | | | |
| | Flexors | | | |
| | Deep | | | |
| | Flexor digitorum profundus | | Flexor digitorum profundus | |
| | Flexor pollicis longus | | Flexor pollicis longus | |
| | Intermediate | | | |
| | Flexor digitorum superficialis | | Flexor digitorum superficialis | |
| | Superficial | | | |
| | Flexor carpi radialis | | Flexor carpi radialis | |
| | Flexor carpi ulnaris | | Flexor carpi ulnaris | |
| | Palmaris longus | | Palmaris longus | |
| | Pronators | | | |
| | Pronator quadratus | | | Pronator quadratus |
| | Pronator teres | | | Pronator teres |
| | Posterior muscles | | | |
| | Extensors | | | |
| | Deep | | | |
| | Abductor pollicis longus | | | Abductor pollicis longus |
| | Extensor indicis | Extensor indicis | | |
| | Extensor pollicis brevis | Extensor pollicis brevis | | |
| | Extensor pollicis longus | Extensor pollicis longus | | |
| | Superficial | | | |
| | Brachioradialis | | | Brachioradialis |
| | Extensor carpi radialis brevis | Extensor carpi radialis brevis | | |
| | Extensor carpi radialis longus | Extensor carpi radialis longus | | |
| | Extensor carpi ulnaris | Extensor carpi ulnaris | | |
| | Extensor digiti minimi | Extensor digiti minimi | | |
| | Extensor digitorum | Extensor digitorum | | |
| | Anconeus | Anconeus | | |
| | Supinator | | | Supinator |

| Body Region | Muscle | Extensor Tendon | Flexor Tendon | Other Tendon |
|---|---|---|---|---|
| **Hand** | | | | |
| Extrinsic — attach to a site in the forearm as well as a site in the hand with action related to hand movement at the wrist | | | | |
| | Extensor carpi radialis brevis | Extensor carpi radialis brevis | | |
| | Extensor carpi radialis longus | Extensor carpi radialis longus | | |
| | Extensor carpi ulnaris | Extensor carpi ulnaris | | |
| | Flexor carpi radialis | | Flexor carpi radialis | |
| | Flexor carpi ulnaris | | Flexor carpi ulnaris | |
| | Flexor digitorum superficialis | | Flexor digitorum superficialis | |
| | Palmaris longus | | Palmaris longus | |
| Extrinsic — attach to a site in the forearm as well as a site in the hand with action in the hand related to finger movement | | | | |
| | Adductor pollicis longus | | | Adductor pollicis longus |
| | Extensor digiti minimi | Extensor digiti minimi | | |
| | Extensor digitorum | Extensor digitorum | | |
| | Extensor indicis | Extensor indicis | | |
| | Flexor digitorum profundus | | Flexor digitorum profundus | |
| | Flexor digitorum superficialis | | Flexor digitorum superficialis | |
| Extrinsic — attach to a site in the forearm as well as a site in the hand with action in the hand related to thumb movement | | | | |
| | Extensor pollicis brevis | Extensor pollicis brevis | | |
| | Extensor pollicis longus | Extensor pollicis longus | | |
| | Flexor pollicis longus | | Flexor pollicis longus | |
| Intrinsic — found within the hand only | | | | |
| | Adductor pollicis | | | Adductor pollicis |
| | Dorsal interossei | Dorsal interossei | Dorsal interossei | |
| | Lumbricals | Lumbricals | Lumbricals | |
| | Palmaris brevis | | | Palmaris brevis |
| | Palmar interossei | Palmar interossei | Palmar interossei | |
| | Hypothenar muscles | | | |
| | Abductor digiti minimi | | | Abductor digiti minimi |
| | Flexor digiti minimi brevis | | Flexor digiti minimi brevis | |
| | Opponens digiti minimi | | Opponens digiti minimi | |
| | Thenar muscles | | | |
| | Abductor pollicis brevis | | | Abductor pollicis brevis |
| | Flexor pollicis brevis | | Flexor pollicis brevis | |
| | Opponens pollicis | | Opponens pollicis | |
| **Thigh** | | | | |
| | Anterior muscles | | | |
| | Iliopsoas | | Iliopsoas | |
| | Pectineus | | Pectineus | |
| | Quadriceps | Quadriceps | | |
| | Rectus femoris | Rectus femoris — Extends knee | Rectus femoris — Flexes hip | |
| | Vastus intermedius | Vastus intermedius | | |
| | Vastus lateralis | Vastus lateralis | | |
| | Vastus medialis | Vastus medialis | | |
| | Sartorius | | Sartorius | |
| | Medial muscles | | | |
| | Adductor brevis | | | Adductor brevis |
| | Adductor longus | | | Adductor longus |
| | Adductor magnus | | | Adductor magnus |
| | Gracilis | | | Gracilis |
| | Obturator externus | | | Obturator externus |
| | Posterior muscles | | | |
| | Hamstring | Hamstring — Extends hip | Hamstring — Flexes knee | |
| | Biceps femoris | Biceps femoris | Biceps femoris | |
| | Semimembranosus | Semimembranosus | Semimembranosus | |
| | Semitendinosus | Semitendinosus | Semitendinosus | |

| Body Region | Muscle | Extensor Tendon | Flexor Tendon | Other Tendon |
|---|---|---|---|---|
| **Lower leg** | | | | |
| | Anterior muscles | | | |
| | Extensor digitorum longus | Extensor digitorum longus | | |
| | Extensor hallucis longus | Extensor hallucis longus | | |
| | Fibularis (peroneus) tertius | Fibularis (peroneus) tertius | | |
| | Tibialis anterior | Tibialis anterior | | Tibialis anterior |
| | Lateral muscles | | | |
| | Fibularis (peroneus) brevis | | Fibularis (peroneus) brevis | |
| | Fibularis (peroneus) longus | | Fibularis (peroneus) longus | |
| | Posterior muscles | | | |
| | Deep | | | |
| | Flexor digitorum longus | | Flexor digitorum longus | |
| | Flexor hallucis longus | | Flexor hallucis longus | |
| | Popliteus | | Popliteus | |
| | Tibialis posterior | | Tibialis posterior | |
| | Superficial | | | |
| | Gastrocnemius | | Gastrocnemius | |
| | Plantaris | | Plantaris | |
| | Soleus | | Soleus | |
| | | | | Calcaneal (Achilles) |
| **Ankle/Foot** | | | | |
| Extrinsic — attach to a site in the lower leg as well as a site in the foot with action related to foot movement at the ankle | | | | |
| | Plantaris | | Plantaris | |
| | Soleus | | Soleus | |
| | Tibialis anterior | Tibialis anterior | | |
| | Tibialis posterior | | Tibialis posterior | |
| Extrinsic — attach to a site in the lower leg as well as a site in the foot with action in the foot related to toe movement | | | | |
| | Extensor digitorum longus | Extensor digitorum longus | | |
| | Extensor hallucis longus | Extensor hallucis longus | | |
| | Flexor digitorum longus | | Flexor digitorum longus | |
| | Flexor hallucis longus | | Flexor hallucis longus | |
| Intrinsic — found within the ankle/foot only | | | | |
| | Dorsal muscles | | | |
| | Extensor digitorum brevis | Extensor digitorum brevis | | |
| | Extensor hallucis brevis | Extensor hallucis brevis | | |
| | Plantar muscles | | | |
| | Abductor digiti minimi | | Abductor digiti minimi | |
| | Abductor hallucis | | Abductor hallucis | |
| | Dorsal interossei | Dorsal interossei | Dorsal interossei | |
| | Flexor digiti minimi brevis | | Flexor digiti minimi brevis | |
| | Flexor digitorum brevis | | Flexor digitorum brevis | |
| | Flexor hallucis brevis | | Flexor hallucis brevis | |
| | Lumbricals | Lumbricals | Lumbricals | |
| | Quadratus plantae | | Quadratus plantae | |
| | Plantar interossei | Plantar interossei | Plantar interossei | |

# Chapter 13. Diseases of the Musculoskeletal System and Connective Tissue (MØØ-M99)

**NOTE** Use an external cause code following the code for the musculoskeletal condition, if applicable, to identify the cause of the musculoskeletal condition

**EXCLUDES 2** *arthropathic psoriasis (L4Ø.5-)*
*certain conditions originating in the perinatal period (PØ4-P96)*
*certain infectious and parasitic diseases (AØØ-B99)*
*compartment syndrome (traumatic) (T79.A-)*
*complications of pregnancy, childbirth and the puerperium (OØØ-O9A)*
*congenital malformations, deformations, and chromosomal abnormalities (QØØ-Q99)*
*endocrine, nutritional and metabolic diseases (EØØ-E88)*
*injury, poisoning and certain other consequences of external causes (SØØ-T88)*
*neoplasms (CØØ-D49)*
*symptoms, signs and abnormal clinical and laboratory findings, not elsewhere classified (RØØ-R94)*

This chapter contains the following blocks:

MØØ-MØ2 Infectious arthropathies
MØ4 Autoinflammatory syndromes
MØ5-M14 Inflammatory polyarthropathies
M15-M19 Osteoarthritis
M2Ø-M25 Other joint disorders
M26-M27 Dentofacial anomalies [including malocclusion] and other disorders of jaw
M3Ø-M36 Systemic connective tissue disorders
M4Ø-M43 Deforming dorsopathies
M45-M49 Spondylopathies
M5Ø-M54 Other dorsopathies
M6Ø-M63 Disorders of muscles
M65-M67 Disorders of synovium and tendon
M7Ø-M79 Other soft tissue disorders
M8Ø-M85 Disorders of bone density and structure
M86-M9Ø Other osteopathies
M91-M94 Chondropathies
M95 Other disorders of the musculoskeletal system and connective tissue
M96 Intraoperative and postprocedural complications and disorders of musculoskeletal system, not elsewhere classified
M97 Periprosthetic fracture around internal prosthetic joint
M99 Biomechanical lesions, not elsewhere classified

## ARTHROPATHIES (MØØ-M25)

**INCLUDES** disorders affecting predominantly peripheral (limb) joints

### Infectious arthropathies (MØØ-MØ2)

**NOTE** This block comprises arthropathies due to microbiological agents. Distinction is made between the following types of etiological relationship:

a) direct infection of joint, where organisms invade synovial tissue and microbial antigen is present in the joint;

b) indirect infection, which may be of two types: a reactive arthropathy, where microbial infection of the body is established but neither organisms nor antigens can be identified in the joint, and a postinfective arthropathy, where microbial antigen is present but recovery of an organism is inconstant and evidence of local multiplication is lacking.

**AHA:** 2019,3Q,16

✓4th **MØØ Pyogenic arthritis**

**EXCLUDES 2** *infection and inflammatory reaction due to internal joint prosthesis (T84.5-)*

**AHA:** 2022,1Q,31

**DEF:** Pyogenic: Relating to or involving pus production, often referred to as suppurative or purulent.

✓5th **MØØ.Ø Staphylococcal arthritis and polyarthritis**

Use additional code (B95.61-B95.8) to identify bacterial agent

**MØØ.ØØ Staphylococcal arthritis, unspecified joint** HCC ESR COM

✓6th **MØØ.Ø1 Staphylococcal arthritis, shoulder**

**MØØ.Ø11 Staphylococcal arthritis, right shoulder** HCC ESR COM
**MØØ.Ø12 Staphylococcal arthritis, left shoulder** HCC ESR COM
**MØØ.Ø19 Staphylococcal arthritis, unspecified shoulder** HCC ESR COM

✓6th **MØØ.Ø2 Staphylococcal arthritis, elbow**

**MØØ.Ø21 Staphylococcal arthritis, right elbow** HCC ESR COM
**MØØ.Ø22 Staphylococcal arthritis, left elbow** HCC ESR COM
**MØØ.Ø29 Staphylococcal arthritis, unspecified elbow** HCC ESR COM

✓6th **MØØ.Ø3 Staphylococcal arthritis, wrist**

Staphylococcal arthritis of carpal bones

**MØØ.Ø31 Staphylococcal arthritis, right wrist** HCC ESR COM
**MØØ.Ø32 Staphylococcal arthritis, left wrist** HCC ESR COM
**MØØ.Ø39 Staphylococcal arthritis, unspecified wrist** HCC ESR COM

✓6th **MØØ.Ø4 Staphylococcal arthritis, hand**

Staphylococcal arthritis of metacarpus and phalanges

**MØØ.Ø41 Staphylococcal arthritis, right hand** HCC ESR COM
**MØØ.Ø42 Staphylococcal arthritis, left hand** HCC ESR COM
**MØØ.Ø49 Staphylococcal arthritis, unspecified hand** HCC ESR COM

✓6th **MØØ.Ø5 Staphylococcal arthritis, hip**

**MØØ.Ø51 Staphylococcal arthritis, right hip** HCC ESR COM
**MØØ.Ø52 Staphylococcal arthritis, left hip** HCC ESR COM
**MØØ.Ø59 Staphylococcal arthritis, unspecified hip** HCC ESR COM

✓6th **MØØ.Ø6 Staphylococcal arthritis, knee**

**MØØ.Ø61 Staphylococcal arthritis, right knee** HCC ESR COM
**MØØ.Ø62 Staphylococcal arthritis, left knee** HCC ESR COM
**MØØ.Ø69 Staphylococcal arthritis, unspecified knee** HCC ESR COM

✓6th **MØØ.Ø7 Staphylococcal arthritis, ankle and foot**

Staphylococcal arthritis, tarsus, metatarsus and phalanges

**MØØ.Ø71 Staphylococcal arthritis, right ankle and foot** HCC ESR COM
**MØØ.Ø72 Staphylococcal arthritis, left ankle and foot** HCC ESR COM
**MØØ.Ø79 Staphylococcal arthritis, unspecified ankle and foot** HCC ESR COM

**MØØ.Ø8 Staphylococcal arthritis, vertebrae** HCC ESR COM
**MØØ.Ø9 Staphylococcal polyarthritis** HCC ESR COM

✓5th **MØØ.1 Pneumococcal arthritis and polyarthritis**

**MØØ.1Ø Pneumococcal arthritis, unspecified joint** HCC ESR COM

✓6th **MØØ.11 Pneumococcal arthritis, shoulder**

**MØØ.111 Pneumococcal arthritis, right shoulder** HCC ESR COM
**MØØ.112 Pneumococcal arthritis, left shoulder** HCC ESR COM
**MØØ.119 Pneumococcal arthritis, unspecified shoulder** HCC ESR COM

✓6th **MØØ.12 Pneumococcal arthritis, elbow**

**MØØ.121 Pneumococcal arthritis, right elbow** HCC ESR COM
**MØØ.122 Pneumococcal arthritis, left elbow** HCC ESR COM
**MØØ.129 Pneumococcal arthritis, unspecified elbow** HCC ESR COM

✓6th **MØØ.13 Pneumococcal arthritis, wrist**

Pneumococcal arthritis of carpal bones

**MØØ.131 Pneumococcal arthritis, right wrist** HCC ESR COM
**MØØ.132 Pneumococcal arthritis, left wrist** HCC ESR COM
**MØØ.139 Pneumococcal arthritis, unspecified wrist** HCC ESR COM

✓6th **MØØ.14 Pneumococcal arthritis, hand**

Pneumococcal arthritis of metacarpus and phalanges

**MØØ.141 Pneumococcal arthritis, right hand** HCC ESR COM
**MØØ.142 Pneumococcal arthritis, left hand** HCC ESR COM
**MØØ.149 Pneumococcal arthritis, unspecified hand** HCC ESR COM

√6th **MØØ.15 Pneumococcal arthritis, hip**
- **MØØ.151 Pneumococcal arthritis, right hip** HCC ESR COM
- **MØØ.152 Pneumococcal arthritis, left hip** HCC ESR COM
- **MØØ.159 Pneumococcal arthritis, unspecified hip** HCC ESR COM

√6th **MØØ.16 Pneumococcal arthritis, knee**
- **MØØ.161 Pneumococcal arthritis, right knee** HCC ESR COM
- **MØØ.162 Pneumococcal arthritis, left knee** HCC ESR COM
- **MØØ.169 Pneumococcal arthritis, unspecified knee** HCC ESR COM

√6th **MØØ.17 Pneumococcal arthritis, ankle and foot**
Pneumococcal arthritis, tarsus, metatarsus and phalanges
- **MØØ.171 Pneumococcal arthritis, right ankle and foot** HCC ESR COM
- **MØØ.172 Pneumococcal arthritis, left ankle and foot** HCC ESR COM
- **MØØ.179 Pneumococcal arthritis, unspecified ankle and foot** HCC ESR COM

**MØØ.18 Pneumococcal arthritis, vertebrae** HCC ESR COM
**MØØ.19 Pneumococcal polyarthritis** HCC ESR COM

√5th **MØØ.2 Other streptococcal arthritis and polyarthritis**
Use additional code (B95.Ø-B95.2, B95.4-B95.5) to identify bacterial agent

**MØØ.2Ø Other streptococcal arthritis, unspecified joint** HCC ESR COM

√6th **MØØ.21 Other streptococcal arthritis, shoulder**
- **MØØ.211 Other streptococcal arthritis, right shoulder** HCC ESR COM
- **MØØ.212 Other streptococcal arthritis, left shoulder** HCC ESR COM
- **MØØ.219 Other streptococcal arthritis, unspecified shoulder** HCC ESR COM

√6th **MØØ.22 Other streptococcal arthritis, elbow**
- **MØØ.221 Other streptococcal arthritis, right elbow** HCC ESR COM
- **MØØ.222 Other streptococcal arthritis, left elbow** HCC ESR COM
- **MØØ.229 Other streptococcal arthritis, unspecified elbow** HCC ESR COM

√6th **MØØ.23 Other streptococcal arthritis, wrist**
Other streptococcal arthritis of carpal bones
- **MØØ.231 Other streptococcal arthritis, right wrist** HCC ESR COM
- **MØØ.232 Other streptococcal arthritis, left wrist** HCC ESR COM
- **MØØ.239 Other streptococcal arthritis, unspecified wrist** HCC ESR COM

√6th **MØØ.24 Other streptococcal arthritis, hand**
Other streptococcal arthritis metacarpus and phalanges
- **MØØ.241 Other streptococcal arthritis, right hand** HCC ESR COM
- **MØØ.242 Other streptococcal arthritis, left hand** HCC ESR COM
- **MØØ.249 Other streptococcal arthritis, unspecified hand** HCC ESR COM

√6th **MØØ.25 Other streptococcal arthritis, hip**
- **MØØ.251 Other streptococcal arthritis, right hip** HCC ESR COM
- **MØØ.252 Other streptococcal arthritis, left hip** HCC ESR COM
- **MØØ.259 Other streptococcal arthritis, unspecified hip** HCC ESR COM

√6th **MØØ.26 Other streptococcal arthritis, knee**
- **MØØ.261 Other streptococcal arthritis, right knee** HCC ESR COM
- **MØØ.262 Other streptococcal arthritis, left knee** HCC ESR COM
- **MØØ.269 Other streptococcal arthritis, unspecified knee** HCC ESR COM

√6th **MØØ.27 Other streptococcal arthritis, ankle and foot**
Other streptococcal arthritis, tarsus, metatarsus and phalanges
- **MØØ.271 Other streptococcal arthritis, right ankle and foot** HCC ESR COM
- **MØØ.272 Other streptococcal arthritis, left ankle and foot** HCC ESR COM
- **MØØ.279 Other streptococcal arthritis, unspecified ankle and foot** HCC ESR COM

**MØØ.28 Other streptococcal arthritis, vertebrae** HCC ESR COM
**MØØ.29 Other streptococcal polyarthritis** HCC ESR COM

√5th **MØØ.8 Arthritis and polyarthritis due to other bacteria**
Use additional code (B96) to identify bacteria

**MØØ.8Ø Arthritis due to other bacteria, unspecified joint** HCC ESR COM

√6th **MØØ.81 Arthritis due to other bacteria, shoulder**
- **MØØ.811 Arthritis due to other bacteria, right shoulder** HCC ESR COM
- **MØØ.812 Arthritis due to other bacteria, left shoulder** HCC ESR COM
- **MØØ.819 Arthritis due to other bacteria, unspecified shoulder** HCC ESR COM

√6th **MØØ.82 Arthritis due to other bacteria, elbow**
- **MØØ.821 Arthritis due to other bacteria, right elbow** HCC ESR COM
- **MØØ.822 Arthritis due to other bacteria, left elbow** HCC ESR COM
- **MØØ.829 Arthritis due to other bacteria, unspecified elbow** HCC ESR COM

√6th **MØØ.83 Arthritis due to other bacteria, wrist**
Arthritis due to other bacteria, carpal bones
- **MØØ.831 Arthritis due to other bacteria, right wrist** HCC ESR COM
- **MØØ.832 Arthritis due to other bacteria, left wrist** HCC ESR COM
- **MØØ.839 Arthritis due to other bacteria, unspecified wrist** HCC ESR COM

√6th **MØØ.84 Arthritis due to other bacteria, hand**
Arthritis due to other bacteria, metacarpus and phalanges
- **MØØ.841 Arthritis due to other bacteria, right hand** HCC ESR COM
- **MØØ.842 Arthritis due to other bacteria, left hand** HCC ESR COM
- **MØØ.849 Arthritis due to other bacteria, unspecified hand** HCC ESR COM

√6th **MØØ.85 Arthritis due to other bacteria, hip**
- **MØØ.851 Arthritis due to other bacteria, right hip** HCC ESR COM
- **MØØ.852 Arthritis due to other bacteria, left hip** HCC ESR COM
- **MØØ.859 Arthritis due to other bacteria, unspecified hip** HCC ESR COM

√6th **MØØ.86 Arthritis due to other bacteria, knee**
AHA: 2019,3Q,16
- **MØØ.861 Arthritis due to other bacteria, right knee** HCC ESR COM
- **MØØ.862 Arthritis due to other bacteria, left knee** HCC ESR COM
- **MØØ.869 Arthritis due to other bacteria, unspecified knee** HCC ESR COM

√6th **MØØ.87 Arthritis due to other bacteria, ankle and foot**
Arthritis due to other bacteria, tarsus, metatarsus, and phalanges
- **MØØ.871 Arthritis due to other bacteria, right ankle and foot** HCC ESR COM
- **MØØ.872 Arthritis due to other bacteria, left ankle and foot** HCC ESR COM
- **MØØ.879 Arthritis due to other bacteria, unspecified ankle and foot** HCC ESR COM

**MØØ.88 Arthritis due to other bacteria, vertebrae** HCC ESR COM
**MØØ.89 Polyarthritis due to other bacteria** HCC ESR COM

**MØØ.9 Pyogenic arthritis, unspecified** HCC ESR COM
Infective arthritis NOS

**M01 Direct infections of joint in infectious and parasitic diseases classified elsewhere**

Code first underlying disease, such as:
- leprosy [Hansen's disease] (A30.-)
- mycoses (B35-B49)
- O'nyong-nyong fever (A92.1)
- paratyphoid fever (A01.1-A01.4)

EXCLUDES 1
- *arthropathy in Lyme disease (A69.23)*
- *gonococcal arthritis (A54.42)*
- *meningococcal arthritis (A39.83)*
- *mumps arthritis (B26.85)*
- *postinfective arthropathy (M02.-)*
- *postmeningococcal arthritis (A39.84)*
- *reactive arthritis (M02.3)*
- *rubella arthritis (B06.82)*
- *sarcoidosis arthritis (D86.86)*
- *tuberculosis arthritis (A18.01-A18.02)*
- *typhoid fever arthritis (A01.04)*

**M01.X Direct infection of joint in infectious and parasitic diseases classified elsewhere**

*M01.X0 Direct infection of unspecified joint in infectious and parasitic diseases classified elsewhere* HCC ESR COM

**M01.X1 Direct infection of shoulder joint in infectious and parasitic diseases classified elsewhere**

*M01.X11 Direct infection of right shoulder in infectious and parasitic diseases classified elsewhere* HCC ESR COM

*M01.X12 Direct infection of left shoulder in infectious and parasitic diseases classified elsewhere* HCC ESR COM

*M01.X19 Direct infection of unspecified shoulder in infectious and parasitic diseases classified elsewhere* HCC ESR COM

**M01.X2 Direct infection of elbow in infectious and parasitic diseases classified elsewhere**

*M01.X21 Direct infection of right elbow in infectious and parasitic diseases classified elsewhere* HCC ESR COM

*M01.X22 Direct infection of left elbow in infectious and parasitic diseases classified elsewhere* HCC ESR COM

*M01.X29 Direct infection of unspecified elbow in infectious and parasitic diseases classified elsewhere* HCC ESR COM

**M01.X3 Direct infection of wrist in infectious and parasitic diseases classified elsewhere**

Direct infection of carpal bones in infectious and parasitic diseases classified elsewhere

*M01.X31 Direct infection of right wrist in infectious and parasitic diseases classified elsewhere* HCC ESR COM

*M01.X32 Direct infection of left wrist in infectious and parasitic diseases classified elsewhere* HCC ESR COM

*M01.X39 Direct infection of unspecified wrist in infectious and parasitic diseases classified elsewhere* HCC ESR COM

**M01.X4 Direct infection of hand in infectious and parasitic diseases classified elsewhere**

Direct infection of metacarpus and phalanges in infectious and parasitic diseases classified elsewhere

*M01.X41 Direct infection of right hand in infectious and parasitic diseases classified elsewhere* HCC ESR COM

*M01.X42 Direct infection of left hand in infectious and parasitic diseases classified elsewhere* HCC ESR COM

*M01.X49 Direct infection of unspecified hand in infectious and parasitic diseases classified elsewhere* HCC ESR COM

**M01.X5 Direct infection of hip in infectious and parasitic diseases classified elsewhere**

*M01.X51 Direct infection of right hip in infectious and parasitic diseases classified elsewhere* HCC ESR COM

*M01.X52 Direct infection of left hip in infectious and parasitic diseases classified elsewhere* HCC ESR COM

*M01.X59 Direct infection of unspecified hip in infectious and parasitic diseases classified elsewhere* HCC ESR COM

**M01.X6 Direct infection of knee in infectious and parasitic diseases classified elsewhere**

*M01.X61 Direct infection of right knee in infectious and parasitic diseases classified elsewhere* HCC ESR COM

*M01.X62 Direct infection of left knee in infectious and parasitic diseases classified elsewhere* HCC ESR COM

*M01.X69 Direct infection of unspecified knee in infectious and parasitic diseases classified elsewhere* HCC ESR COM

**M01.X7 Direct infection of ankle and foot in infectious and parasitic diseases classified elsewhere**

Direct infection of tarsus, metatarsus and phalanges in infectious and parasitic diseases classified elsewhere

*M01.X71 Direct infection of right ankle and foot in infectious and parasitic diseases classified elsewhere* HCC ESR COM

*M01.X72 Direct infection of left ankle and foot in infectious and parasitic diseases classified elsewhere* HCC ESR COM

*M01.X79 Direct infection of unspecified ankle and foot in infectious and parasitic diseases classified elsewhere* HCC ESR COM

*M01.X8 Direct infection of vertebrae in infectious and parasitic diseases classified elsewhere* HCC ESR COM

*M01.X9 Direct infection of multiple joints in infectious and parasitic diseases classified elsewhere* HCC ESR COM

**M02 Postinfective and reactive arthropathies**

Code first underlying disease, such as:
- congenital syphilis [Clutton's joints] (A50.5)
- enteritis due to Yersinia enterocolitica (A04.6)
- infective endocarditis (I33.0)
- viral hepatitis (B15-B19)

EXCLUDES 1
- *Behcet's disease (M35.2)*
- *direct infections of joint in infectious and parasitic diseases classified elsewhere (M01.-)*
- *mumps arthritis (B26.85)*
- *postmeningococcal arthritis (A39.84)*
- *rheumatic fever (I00)*
- *rubella arthritis (B06.82)*
- *syphilis arthritis (late) (A52.77)*
- *tabetic arthropathy [Charcôt's] (A52.16)*

**M02.0 Arthropathy following intestinal bypass**

**M02.00 Arthropathy following intestinal bypass, unspecified site**

**M02.01 Arthropathy following intestinal bypass, shoulder**

**M02.011 Arthropathy following intestinal bypass, right shoulder**

**M02.012 Arthropathy following intestinal bypass, left shoulder**

**M02.019 Arthropathy following intestinal bypass, unspecified shoulder**

**M02.02 Arthropathy following intestinal bypass, elbow**

**M02.021 Arthropathy following intestinal bypass, right elbow**

**M02.022 Arthropathy following intestinal bypass, left elbow**

**M02.029 Arthropathy following intestinal bypass, unspecified elbow**

**M02.03 Arthropathy following intestinal bypass, wrist**

Arthropathy following intestinal bypass, carpal bones

**M02.031 Arthropathy following intestinal bypass, right wrist**

**M02.032 Arthropathy following intestinal bypass, left wrist**

**M02.039 Arthropathy following intestinal bypass, unspecified wrist**

**M02.04 Arthropathy following intestinal bypass, hand**

Arthropathy following intestinal bypass, metacarpals and phalanges

**M02.041 Arthropathy following intestinal bypass, right hand**

**M02.042 Arthropathy following intestinal bypass, left hand**

**M02.049 Arthropathy following intestinal bypass, unspecified hand**

**M02.05 Arthropathy following intestinal bypass, hip**

**M02.051 Arthropathy following intestinal bypass, right hip**

**MØ2.Ø52** Arthropathy following intestinal bypass, left hip

**MØ2.Ø59** Arthropathy following intestinal bypass, unspecified hip

✓6th **MØ2.Ø6** Arthropathy following intestinal bypass, knee

**MØ2.Ø61** Arthropathy following intestinal bypass, right knee

**MØ2.Ø62** Arthropathy following intestinal bypass, left knee

**MØ2.Ø69** Arthropathy following intestinal bypass, unspecified knee

✓6th **MØ2.Ø7** Arthropathy following intestinal bypass, ankle and foot

Arthropathy following intestinal bypass, tarsus, metatarsus and phalanges

**MØ2.Ø71** Arthropathy following intestinal bypass, right ankle and foot

**MØ2.Ø72** Arthropathy following intestinal bypass, left ankle and foot

**MØ2.Ø79** Arthropathy following intestinal bypass, unspecified ankle and foot

**MØ2.Ø8** Arthropathy following intestinal bypass, vertebrae

**MØ2.Ø9** Arthropathy following intestinal bypass, multiple sites

✓5th **MØ2.1** Postdysenteric arthropathy

**MØ2.1Ø** Postdysenteric arthropathy, unspecified site HCC ESR COM

✓6th **MØ2.11** Postdysenteric arthropathy, shoulder

**MØ2.111** Postdysenteric arthropathy, right shoulder HCC ESR COM

**MØ2.112** Postdysenteric arthropathy, left shoulder HCC ESR COM

**MØ2.119** Postdysenteric arthropathy, unspecified shoulder HCC ESR COM

✓6th **MØ2.12** Postdysenteric arthropathy, elbow

**MØ2.121** Postdysenteric arthropathy, right elbow HCC ESR COM

**MØ2.122** Postdysenteric arthropathy, left elbow HCC ESR COM

**MØ2.129** Postdysenteric arthropathy, unspecified elbow HCC ESR COM

✓6th **MØ2.13** Postdysenteric arthropathy, wrist

Postdysenteric arthropathy, carpal bones

**MØ2.131** Postdysenteric arthropathy, right wrist HCC ESR COM

**MØ2.132** Postdysenteric arthropathy, left wrist HCC ESR COM

**MØ2.139** Postdysenteric arthropathy, unspecified wrist HCC ESR COM

✓6th **MØ2.14** Postdysenteric arthropathy, hand

Postdysenteric arthropathy, metacarpus and phalanges

**MØ2.141** Postdysenteric arthropathy, right hand HCC ESR COM

**MØ2.142** Postdysenteric arthropathy, left hand HCC ESR COM

**MØ2.149** Postdysenteric arthropathy, unspecified hand HCC ESR COM

✓6th **MØ2.15** Postdysenteric arthropathy, hip

**MØ2.151** Postdysenteric arthropathy, right hip HCC ESR COM

**MØ2.152** Postdysenteric arthropathy, left hip HCC ESR COM

**MØ2.159** Postdysenteric arthropathy, unspecified hip HCC ESR COM

✓6th **MØ2.16** Postdysenteric arthropathy, knee

**MØ2.161** Postdysenteric arthropathy, right knee HCC ESR COM

**MØ2.162** Postdysenteric arthropathy, left knee HCC ESR COM

**MØ2.169** Postdysenteric arthropathy, unspecified knee HCC ESR COM

✓6th **MØ2.17** Postdysenteric arthropathy, ankle and foot

Postdysenteric arthropathy, tarsus, metatarsus and phalanges

**MØ2.171** Postdysenteric arthropathy, right ankle and foot HCC ESR COM

**MØ2.172** Postdysenteric arthropathy, left ankle and foot HCC ESR COM

**MØ2.179** Postdysenteric arthropathy, unspecified ankle and foot HCC ESR COM

**MØ2.18** Postdysenteric arthropathy, vertebrae HCC ESR COM

**MØ2.19** Postdysenteric arthropathy, multiple sites HCC ESR COM

✓5th **MØ2.2** Postimmunization arthropathy

**MØ2.2Ø** Postimmunization arthropathy, unspecified site

✓6th **MØ2.21** Postimmunization arthropathy, shoulder

**MØ2.211** Postimmunization arthropathy, right shoulder

**MØ2.212** Postimmunization arthropathy, left shoulder

**MØ2.219** Postimmunization arthropathy, unspecified shoulder

✓6th **MØ2.22** Postimmunization arthropathy, elbow

**MØ2.221** Postimmunization arthropathy, right elbow

**MØ2.222** Postimmunization arthropathy, left elbow

**MØ2.229** Postimmunization arthropathy, unspecified elbow

✓6th **MØ2.23** Postimmunization arthropathy, wrist

Postimmunization arthropathy, carpal bones

**MØ2.231** Postimmunization arthropathy, right wrist

**MØ2.232** Postimmunization arthropathy, left wrist

**MØ2.239** Postimmunization arthropathy, unspecified wrist

✓6th **MØ2.24** Postimmunization arthropathy, hand

Postimmunization arthropathy, metacarpus and phalanges

**MØ2.241** Postimmunization arthropathy, right hand

**MØ2.242** Postimmunization arthropathy, left hand

**MØ2.249** Postimmunization arthropathy, unspecified hand

✓6th **MØ2.25** Postimmunization arthropathy, hip

**MØ2.251** Postimmunization arthropathy, right hip

**MØ2.252** Postimmunization arthropathy, left hip

**MØ2.259** Postimmunization arthropathy, unspecified hip

✓6th **MØ2.26** Postimmunization arthropathy, knee

**MØ2.261** Postimmunization arthropathy, right knee

**MØ2.262** Postimmunization arthropathy, left knee

**MØ2.269** Postimmunization arthropathy, unspecified knee

✓6th **MØ2.27** Postimmunization arthropathy, ankle and foot

Postimmunization arthropathy, tarsus, metatarsus and phalanges

**MØ2.271** Postimmunization arthropathy, right ankle and foot

**MØ2.272** Postimmunization arthropathy, left ankle and foot

**MØ2.279** Postimmunization arthropathy, unspecified ankle and foot

**MØ2.28** Postimmunization arthropathy, vertebrae

**MØ2.29** Postimmunization arthropathy, multiple sites

✓5th **MØ2.3** Reiter's disease

Reactive arthritis

**DEF:** Arthritis, iridocyclitis, and urethritis, sometimes with diarrhea. While symptoms may recur, arthritis is constant.

**MØ2.3Ø** Reiter's disease, unspecified site HCC Rx ESR COM

✓6th **MØ2.31** Reiter's disease, shoulder

**MØ2.311** Reiter's disease, right shoulder HCC Rx ESR COM

**MØ2.312** Reiter's disease, left shoulder HCC Rx ESR COM

**MØ2.319** Reiter's disease, unspecified shoulder HCC Rx ESR COM

✓6th **MØ2.32** Reiter's disease, elbow

**MØ2.321** Reiter's disease, right elbow HCC Rx ESR COM

**MØ2.322** Reiter's disease, left elbow HCC Rx ESR COM

**MØ2.329** Reiter's disease, unspecified elbow HCC Rx ESR COM

✓6th **MØ2.33** Reiter's disease, wrist

Reiter's disease, carpal bones

**MØ2.331** Reiter's disease, right wrist HCC Rx ESR COM

M02.332 Reiter's disease, left wrist HCC Rx ESR COM
M02.339 Reiter's disease, unspecified wrist HCC Rx ESR COM

✓6th M02.34 Reiter's disease, hand
Reiter's disease, metacarpus and phalanges
M02.341 Reiter's disease, right hand HCC Rx ESR COM
M02.342 Reiter's disease, left hand HCC Rx ESR COM
M02.349 Reiter's disease, unspecified hand HCC Rx ESR COM

✓6th M02.35 Reiter's disease, hip
M02.351 Reiter's disease, right hip HCC Rx ESR COM
M02.352 Reiter's disease, left hip HCC Rx ESR COM
M02.359 Reiter's disease, unspecified hip HCC Rx ESR COM

✓6th M02.36 Reiter's disease, knee
M02.361 Reiter's disease, right knee HCC Rx ESR COM
M02.362 Reiter's disease, left knee HCC Rx ESR COM
M02.369 Reiter's disease, unspecified knee HCC Rx ESR COM

✓6th M02.37 Reiter's disease, ankle and foot
Reiter's disease, tarsus, metatarsus and phalanges
M02.371 Reiter's disease, right ankle and foot HCC Rx ESR COM
M02.372 Reiter's disease, left ankle and foot HCC Rx ESR COM
M02.379 Reiter's disease, unspecified ankle and foot HCC Rx ESR COM

M02.38 Reiter's disease, vertebrae HCC Rx ESR COM
M02.39 Reiter's disease, multiple sites HCC Rx ESR COM

✓5th M02.8 Other reactive arthropathies
*M02.80 Other reactive arthropathies, unspecified site* HCC ESR COM

✓6th M02.81 Other reactive arthropathies, shoulder
*M02.811 Other reactive arthropathies, right shoulder* HCC ESR COM
*M02.812 Other reactive arthropathies, left shoulder* HCC ESR COM
*M02.819 Other reactive arthropathies, unspecified shoulder* HCC ESR COM

✓6th M02.82 Other reactive arthropathies, elbow
*M02.821 Other reactive arthropathies, right elbow* HCC ESR COM
*M02.822 Other reactive arthropathies, left elbow* HCC ESR COM
*M02.829 Other reactive arthropathies, unspecified elbow* HCC ESR COM

✓6th M02.83 Other reactive arthropathies, wrist
Other reactive arthropathies, carpal bones
*M02.831 Other reactive arthropathies, right wrist* HCC ESR COM
*M02.832 Other reactive arthropathies, left wrist* HCC ESR COM
*M02.839 Other reactive arthropathies, unspecified wrist* HCC ESR COM

✓6th M02.84 Other reactive arthropathies, hand
Other reactive arthropathies, metacarpus and phalanges
*M02.841 Other reactive arthropathies, right hand* HCC ESR COM
*M02.842 Other reactive arthropathies, left hand* HCC ESR COM
*M02.849 Other reactive arthropathies, unspecified hand* HCC ESR COM

✓6th M02.85 Other reactive arthropathies, hip
*M02.851 Other reactive arthropathies, right hip* HCC ESR COM
*M02.852 Other reactive arthropathies, left hip* HCC ESR COM
*M02.859 Other reactive arthropathies, unspecified hip* HCC ESR COM

✓6th M02.86 Other reactive arthropathies, knee
*M02.861 Other reactive arthropathies, right knee* HCC ESR COM
*M02.862 Other reactive arthropathies, left knee* HCC ESR COM
*M02.869 Other reactive arthropathies, unspecified knee* HCC ESR COM

✓6th M02.87 Other reactive arthropathies, ankle and foot
Other reactive arthropathies, tarsus, metatarsus and phalanges
*M02.871 Other reactive arthropathies, right ankle and foot* HCC ESR COM
*M02.872 Other reactive arthropathies, left ankle and foot* HCC ESR COM
*M02.879 Other reactive arthropathies, unspecified ankle and foot* HCC ESR COM

*M02.88 Other reactive arthropathies, vertebrae* HCC ESR COM
*M02.89 Other reactive arthropathies, multiple sites* HCC ESR COM

*M02.9 Reactive arthropathy, unspecified* HCC ESR COM

## Autoinflammatory syndromes (M04)

✓4th **M04 Autoinflammatory syndromes**
EXCLUDES 2 *Crohn's disease (K50.-)*
AHA: 2016,4Q,37

**M04.1 Periodic fever syndromes** HCC Rx ESR COM
Familial Mediterranean fever
Hyperimmunoglobin D syndrome
Mevalonate kinase deficiency
Tumor necrosis factor receptor associated periodic syndrome [TRAPS]

**M04.2 Cryopyrin-associated periodic syndromes** HCC Rx ESR COM
Chronic infantile neurological, cutaneous and articular syndrome [CINCA]
Familial cold autoinflammatory syndrome
Familial cold urticaria
Muckle-Wells syndrome
Neonatal onset multisystemic inflammatory disorder [NOMID]

● **M04.3 VEXAS syndrome**
Vacuoles, E1 ubiquitin-activating enzyme, X-linked, autoinflammatory, somatic syndrome
Code also any associated conditions

**M04.8 Other autoinflammatory syndromes** HCC Rx ESR COM
Blau syndrome
Deficiency of interleukin 1 receptor antagonist [DIRA]
Majeed syndrome
Periodic fever, aphthous stomatitis, pharyngitis, and adenopathy syndrome [PFAPA]
Pyogenic arthritis, pyoderma gangrenosum, and acne syndrome [PAPA]

**M04.9 Autoinflammatory syndrome, unspecified** HCC Rx ESR COM

## Inflammatory polyarthropathies (M05-M14)

✓4th **M05 Rheumatoid arthritis with rheumatoid factor**
EXCLUDES 1 *juvenile rheumatoid arthritis (M08.-)*
*rheumatic fever (I00)*
*rheumatoid arthritis of spine (M45.-)*
AHA: 2020,4Q,31-32
DEF: Rheumatoid arthritis: Autoimmune systemic disease that causes chronic inflammation of the joints and other areas of the body, manifested by inflammatory changes in articular structures and synovial membranes, atrophy, and loss in bone density.

✓5th M05.0 Felty's syndrome
Rheumatoid arthritis with splenoadenomegaly and leukopenia
M05.00 Felty's syndrome, unspecified site HCC Rx ESR COM

✓6th M05.01 Felty's syndrome, shoulder
M05.011 Felty's syndrome, right shoulder HCC Rx ESR COM
M05.012 Felty's syndrome, left shoulder HCC Rx ESR COM
M05.019 Felty's syndrome, unspecified shoulder HCC Rx ESR COM

✓6th M05.02 Felty's syndrome, elbow
M05.021 Felty's syndrome, right elbow HCC Rx ESR COM

M05.022 Felty's syndrome, left elbow HCC Rx ESR COM
M05.029 Felty's syndrome, unspecified elbow HCC Rx ESR COM
✓6th M05.03 Felty's syndrome, wrist
Felty's syndrome, carpal bones
M05.031 Felty's syndrome, right wrist HCC Rx ESR COM
M05.032 Felty's syndrome, left wrist HCC Rx ESR COM
M05.039 Felty's syndrome, unspecified wrist HCC Rx ESR COM
✓6th M05.04 Felty's syndrome, hand
Felty's syndrome, metacarpus and phalanges
M05.041 Felty's syndrome, right hand HCC Rx ESR COM
M05.042 Felty's syndrome, left hand HCC Rx ESR COM
M05.049 Felty's syndrome, unspecified hand HCC Rx ESR COM
✓6th M05.05 Felty's syndrome, hip
M05.051 Felty's syndrome, right hip HCC Rx ESR COM
M05.052 Felty's syndrome, left hip HCC Rx ESR COM
M05.059 Felty's syndrome, unspecified hip HCC Rx ESR COM
✓6th M05.06 Felty's syndrome, knee
M05.061 Felty's syndrome, right knee HCC Rx ESR COM
M05.062 Felty's syndrome, left knee HCC Rx ESR COM
M05.069 Felty's syndrome, unspecified knee HCC Rx ESR COM
✓6th M05.07 Felty's syndrome, ankle and foot
Felty's syndrome, tarsus, metatarsus and phalanges
M05.071 Felty's syndrome, right ankle and foot HCC Rx ESR COM
M05.072 Felty's syndrome, left ankle and foot HCC Rx ESR COM
M05.079 Felty's syndrome, unspecified ankle and foot HCC Rx ESR COM
M05.09 Felty's syndrome, multiple sites HCC Rx ESR COM
✓5th M05.1 Rheumatoid lung disease with rheumatoid arthritis
M05.10 Rheumatoid lung disease with rheumatoid arthritis of unspecified site HCC Rx ESR COM
✓6th M05.11 Rheumatoid lung disease with rheumatoid arthritis of shoulder
M05.111 Rheumatoid lung disease with rheumatoid arthritis of right shoulder HCC Rx ESR COM
M05.112 Rheumatoid lung disease with rheumatoid arthritis of left shoulder HCC Rx ESR COM
M05.119 Rheumatoid lung disease with rheumatoid arthritis of unspecified shoulder HCC Rx ESR COM
✓6th M05.12 Rheumatoid lung disease with rheumatoid arthritis of elbow
M05.121 Rheumatoid lung disease with rheumatoid arthritis of right elbow HCC Rx ESR COM
M05.122 Rheumatoid lung disease with rheumatoid arthritis of left elbow HCC Rx ESR COM
M05.129 Rheumatoid lung disease with rheumatoid arthritis of unspecified elbow HCC Rx ESR COM
✓6th M05.13 Rheumatoid lung disease with rheumatoid arthritis of wrist
Rheumatoid lung disease with rheumatoid arthritis, carpal bones
M05.131 Rheumatoid lung disease with rheumatoid arthritis of right wrist HCC Rx ESR COM
M05.132 Rheumatoid lung disease with rheumatoid arthritis of left wrist HCC Rx ESR COM
M05.139 Rheumatoid lung disease with rheumatoid arthritis of unspecified wrist HCC Rx ESR COM
✓6th M05.14 Rheumatoid lung disease with rheumatoid arthritis of hand
Rheumatoid lung disease with rheumatoid arthritis, metacarpus and phalanges
M05.141 Rheumatoid lung disease with rheumatoid arthritis of right hand HCC Rx ESR COM
M05.142 Rheumatoid lung disease with rheumatoid arthritis of left hand HCC Rx ESR COM
M05.149 Rheumatoid lung disease with rheumatoid arthritis of unspecified hand HCC Rx ESR COM
✓6th M05.15 Rheumatoid lung disease with rheumatoid arthritis of hip
M05.151 Rheumatoid lung disease with rheumatoid arthritis of right hip HCC Rx ESR COM
M05.152 Rheumatoid lung disease with rheumatoid arthritis of left hip HCC Rx ESR COM
M05.159 Rheumatoid lung disease with rheumatoid arthritis of unspecified hip HCC Rx ESR COM
✓6th M05.16 Rheumatoid lung disease with rheumatoid arthritis of knee
M05.161 Rheumatoid lung disease with rheumatoid arthritis of right knee HCC Rx ESR COM
M05.162 Rheumatoid lung disease with rheumatoid arthritis of left knee HCC Rx ESR COM
M05.169 Rheumatoid lung disease with rheumatoid arthritis of unspecified knee HCC Rx ESR COM
✓6th M05.17 Rheumatoid lung disease with rheumatoid arthritis of ankle and foot
Rheumatoid lung disease with rheumatoid arthritis, tarsus, metatarsus and phalanges
M05.171 Rheumatoid lung disease with rheumatoid arthritis of right ankle and foot HCC Rx ESR COM
M05.172 Rheumatoid lung disease with rheumatoid arthritis of left ankle and foot HCC Rx ESR COM
M05.179 Rheumatoid lung disease with rheumatoid arthritis of unspecified ankle and foot HCC Rx ESR COM
M05.19 Rheumatoid lung disease with rheumatoid arthritis of multiple sites HCC Rx ESR COM
✓5th M05.2 Rheumatoid vasculitis with rheumatoid arthritis
M05.20 Rheumatoid vasculitis with rheumatoid arthritis of unspecified site HCC Rx ESR COM
✓6th M05.21 Rheumatoid vasculitis with rheumatoid arthritis of shoulder
M05.211 Rheumatoid vasculitis with rheumatoid arthritis of right shoulder HCC Rx ESR COM
M05.212 Rheumatoid vasculitis with rheumatoid arthritis of left shoulder HCC Rx ESR COM
M05.219 Rheumatoid vasculitis with rheumatoid arthritis of unspecified shoulder HCC Rx ESR COM
✓6th M05.22 Rheumatoid vasculitis with rheumatoid arthritis of elbow
M05.221 Rheumatoid vasculitis with rheumatoid arthritis of right elbow HCC Rx ESR COM
M05.222 Rheumatoid vasculitis with rheumatoid arthritis of left elbow HCC Rx ESR COM
M05.229 Rheumatoid vasculitis with rheumatoid arthritis of unspecified elbow HCC Rx ESR COM
✓6th M05.23 Rheumatoid vasculitis with rheumatoid arthritis of wrist
Rheumatoid vasculitis with rheumatoid arthritis, carpal bones
M05.231 Rheumatoid vasculitis with rheumatoid arthritis of right wrist HCC Rx ESR COM
M05.232 Rheumatoid vasculitis with rheumatoid arthritis of left wrist HCC Rx ESR COM
M05.239 Rheumatoid vasculitis with rheumatoid arthritis of unspecified wrist HCC Rx ESR COM

✓6th **MØ5.24 Rheumatoid vasculitis with rheumatoid arthritis of hand**
Rheumatoid vasculitis with rheumatoid arthritis, metacarpus and phalanges
**MØ5.241 Rheumatoid vasculitis with rheumatoid arthritis of right hand** HCC Rx ESR COM
**MØ5.242 Rheumatoid vasculitis with rheumatoid arthritis of left hand** HCC Rx ESR COM
**MØ5.249 Rheumatoid vasculitis with rheumatoid arthritis of unspecified hand** HCC Rx ESR COM

✓6th **MØ5.25 Rheumatoid vasculitis with rheumatoid arthritis of hip**
**MØ5.251 Rheumatoid vasculitis with rheumatoid arthritis of right hip** HCC Rx ESR COM
**MØ5.252 Rheumatoid vasculitis with rheumatoid arthritis of left hip** HCC Rx ESR COM
**MØ5.259 Rheumatoid vasculitis with rheumatoid arthritis of unspecified hip** HCC Rx ESR COM

✓6th **MØ5.26 Rheumatoid vasculitis with rheumatoid arthritis of knee**
**MØ5.261 Rheumatoid vasculitis with rheumatoid arthritis of right knee** HCC Rx ESR COM
**MØ5.262 Rheumatoid vasculitis with rheumatoid arthritis of left knee** HCC Rx ESR COM
**MØ5.269 Rheumatoid vasculitis with rheumatoid arthritis of unspecified knee** HCC Rx ESR COM

✓6th **MØ5.27 Rheumatoid vasculitis with rheumatoid arthritis of ankle and foot**
Rheumatoid vasculitis with rheumatoid arthritis, tarsus, metatarsus and phalanges
**MØ5.271 Rheumatoid vasculitis with rheumatoid arthritis of right ankle and foot** HCC Rx ESR COM
**MØ5.272 Rheumatoid vasculitis with rheumatoid arthritis of left ankle and foot** HCC Rx ESR COM
**MØ5.279 Rheumatoid vasculitis with rheumatoid arthritis of unspecified ankle and foot** HCC Rx ESR COM

**MØ5.29 Rheumatoid vasculitis with rheumatoid arthritis of multiple sites** HCC Rx ESR COM

✓5th **MØ5.3 Rheumatoid heart disease with rheumatoid arthritis**
Rheumatoid carditis
Rheumatoid endocarditis
Rheumatoid myocarditis
Rheumatoid pericarditis

**MØ5.30 Rheumatoid heart disease with rheumatoid arthritis of unspecified site** HCC Rx ESR COM

✓6th **MØ5.31 Rheumatoid heart disease with rheumatoid arthritis of shoulder**
**MØ5.311 Rheumatoid heart disease with rheumatoid arthritis of right shoulder** HCC Rx ESR COM
**MØ5.312 Rheumatoid heart disease with rheumatoid arthritis of left shoulder** HCC Rx ESR COM
**MØ5.319 Rheumatoid heart disease with rheumatoid arthritis of unspecified shoulder** HCC Rx ESR COM

✓6th **MØ5.32 Rheumatoid heart disease with rheumatoid arthritis of elbow**
**MØ5.321 Rheumatoid heart disease with rheumatoid arthritis of right elbow** HCC Rx ESR COM
**MØ5.322 Rheumatoid heart disease with rheumatoid arthritis of left elbow** HCC Rx ESR COM
**MØ5.329 Rheumatoid heart disease with rheumatoid arthritis of unspecified elbow** HCC Rx ESR COM

✓6th **MØ5.33 Rheumatoid heart disease with rheumatoid arthritis of wrist**
Rheumatoid heart disease with rheumatoid arthritis, carpal bones
**MØ5.331 Rheumatoid heart disease with rheumatoid arthritis of right wrist** HCC Rx ESR COM
**MØ5.332 Rheumatoid heart disease with rheumatoid arthritis of left wrist** HCC Rx ESR COM
**MØ5.339 Rheumatoid heart disease with rheumatoid arthritis of unspecified wrist** HCC Rx ESR COM

✓6th **MØ5.34 Rheumatoid heart disease with rheumatoid arthritis of hand**
Rheumatoid heart disease with rheumatoid arthritis, metacarpus and phalanges
**MØ5.341 Rheumatoid heart disease with rheumatoid arthritis of right hand** HCC Rx ESR COM
**MØ5.342 Rheumatoid heart disease with rheumatoid arthritis of left hand** HCC Rx ESR COM
**MØ5.349 Rheumatoid heart disease with rheumatoid arthritis of unspecified hand** HCC Rx ESR COM

✓6th **MØ5.35 Rheumatoid heart disease with rheumatoid arthritis of hip**
**MØ5.351 Rheumatoid heart disease with rheumatoid arthritis of right hip** HCC Rx ESR COM
**MØ5.352 Rheumatoid heart disease with rheumatoid arthritis of left hip** HCC Rx ESR COM
**MØ5.359 Rheumatoid heart disease with rheumatoid arthritis of unspecified hip** HCC Rx ESR COM

✓6th **MØ5.36 Rheumatoid heart disease with rheumatoid arthritis of knee**
**MØ5.361 Rheumatoid heart disease with rheumatoid arthritis of right knee** HCC Rx ESR COM
**MØ5.362 Rheumatoid heart disease with rheumatoid arthritis of left knee** HCC Rx ESR COM
**MØ5.369 Rheumatoid heart disease with rheumatoid arthritis of unspecified knee** HCC Rx ESR COM

✓6th **MØ5.37 Rheumatoid heart disease with rheumatoid arthritis of ankle and foot**
Rheumatoid heart disease with rheumatoid arthritis, tarsus, metatarsus and phalanges
**MØ5.371 Rheumatoid heart disease with rheumatoid arthritis of right ankle and foot** HCC Rx ESR COM
**MØ5.372 Rheumatoid heart disease with rheumatoid arthritis of left ankle and foot** HCC Rx ESR COM
**MØ5.379 Rheumatoid heart disease with rheumatoid arthritis of unspecified ankle and foot** HCC Rx ESR COM

**MØ5.39 Rheumatoid heart disease with rheumatoid arthritis of multiple sites** HCC Rx ESR COM

✓5th **MØ5.4 Rheumatoid myopathy with rheumatoid arthritis**

**MØ5.40 Rheumatoid myopathy with rheumatoid arthritis of unspecified site** HCC Rx ESR COM

✓6th **MØ5.41 Rheumatoid myopathy with rheumatoid arthritis of shoulder**
**MØ5.411 Rheumatoid myopathy with rheumatoid arthritis of right shoulder** HCC Rx ESR COM
**MØ5.412 Rheumatoid myopathy with rheumatoid arthritis of left shoulder** HCC Rx ESR COM
**MØ5.419 Rheumatoid myopathy with rheumatoid arthritis of unspecified shoulder** HCC Rx ESR COM

✓6th **MØ5.42 Rheumatoid myopathy with rheumatoid arthritis of elbow**
**MØ5.421 Rheumatoid myopathy with rheumatoid arthritis of right elbow** HCC Rx ESR COM
**MØ5.422 Rheumatoid myopathy with rheumatoid arthritis of left elbow** HCC Rx ESR COM
**MØ5.429 Rheumatoid myopathy with rheumatoid arthritis of unspecified elbow** HCC Rx ESR COM

√6th **MØ5.43 Rheumatoid myopathy with rheumatoid arthritis of wrist**
Rheumatoid myopathy with rheumatoid arthritis, carpal bones
**MØ5.431 Rheumatoid myopathy with rheumatoid arthritis of right wrist** HCC Rx ESR COM
**MØ5.432 Rheumatoid myopathy with rheumatoid arthritis of left wrist** HCC Rx ESR COM
**MØ5.439 Rheumatoid myopathy with rheumatoid arthritis of unspecified wrist** HCC Rx ESR COM

√6th **MØ5.44 Rheumatoid myopathy with rheumatoid arthritis of hand**
Rheumatoid myopathy with rheumatoid arthritis, metacarpus and phalanges
**MØ5.441 Rheumatoid myopathy with rheumatoid arthritis of right hand** HCC Rx ESR COM
**MØ5.442 Rheumatoid myopathy with rheumatoid arthritis of left hand** HCC Rx ESR COM
**MØ5.449 Rheumatoid myopathy with rheumatoid arthritis of unspecified hand** HCC Rx ESR COM

√6th **MØ5.45 Rheumatoid myopathy with rheumatoid arthritis of hip**
**MØ5.451 Rheumatoid myopathy with rheumatoid arthritis of right hip** HCC Rx ESR COM
**MØ5.452 Rheumatoid myopathy with rheumatoid arthritis of left hip** HCC Rx ESR COM
**MØ5.459 Rheumatoid myopathy with rheumatoid arthritis of unspecified hip** HCC Rx ESR COM

√6th **MØ5.46 Rheumatoid myopathy with rheumatoid arthritis of knee**
**MØ5.461 Rheumatoid myopathy with rheumatoid arthritis of right knee** HCC Rx ESR COM
**MØ5.462 Rheumatoid myopathy with rheumatoid arthritis of left knee** HCC Rx ESR COM
**MØ5.469 Rheumatoid myopathy with rheumatoid arthritis of unspecified knee** HCC Rx ESR COM

√6th **MØ5.47 Rheumatoid myopathy with rheumatoid arthritis of ankle and foot**
Rheumatoid myopathy with rheumatoid arthritis, tarsus, metatarsus and phalanges
**MØ5.471 Rheumatoid myopathy with rheumatoid arthritis of right ankle and foot** HCC Rx ESR COM
**MØ5.472 Rheumatoid myopathy with rheumatoid arthritis of left ankle and foot** HCC Rx ESR COM
**MØ5.479 Rheumatoid myopathy with rheumatoid arthritis of unspecified ankle and foot** HCC Rx ESR COM

**MØ5.49 Rheumatoid myopathy with rheumatoid arthritis of multiple sites** HCC Rx ESR COM

√5th **MØ5.5 Rheumatoid polyneuropathy with rheumatoid arthritis**
**MØ5.5Ø Rheumatoid polyneuropathy with rheumatoid arthritis of unspecified site** HCC Rx ESR COM

√6th **MØ5.51 Rheumatoid polyneuropathy with rheumatoid arthritis of shoulder**
**MØ5.511 Rheumatoid polyneuropathy with rheumatoid arthritis of right shoulder** HCC Rx ESR COM
**MØ5.512 Rheumatoid polyneuropathy with rheumatoid arthritis of left shoulder** HCC Rx ESR COM
**MØ5.519 Rheumatoid polyneuropathy with rheumatoid arthritis of unspecified shoulder** HCC Rx ESR COM

√6th **MØ5.52 Rheumatoid polyneuropathy with rheumatoid arthritis of elbow**
**MØ5.521 Rheumatoid polyneuropathy with rheumatoid arthritis of right elbow** HCC Rx ESR COM
**MØ5.522 Rheumatoid polyneuropathy with rheumatoid arthritis of left elbow** HCC Rx ESR COM
**MØ5.529 Rheumatoid polyneuropathy with rheumatoid arthritis of unspecified elbow** HCC Rx ESR COM

√6th **MØ5.53 Rheumatoid polyneuropathy with rheumatoid arthritis of wrist**
Rheumatoid polyneuropathy with rheumatoid arthritis, carpal bones
**MØ5.531 Rheumatoid polyneuropathy with rheumatoid arthritis of right wrist** HCC Rx ESR COM
**MØ5.532 Rheumatoid polyneuropathy with rheumatoid arthritis of left wrist** HCC Rx ESR COM
**MØ5.539 Rheumatoid polyneuropathy with rheumatoid arthritis of unspecified wrist** HCC Rx ESR COM

√6th **MØ5.54 Rheumatoid polyneuropathy with rheumatoid arthritis of hand**
Rheumatoid polyneuropathy with rheumatoid arthritis, metacarpus and phalanges
**MØ5.541 Rheumatoid polyneuropathy with rheumatoid arthritis of right hand** HCC Rx ESR COM
**MØ5.542 Rheumatoid polyneuropathy with rheumatoid arthritis of left hand** HCC Rx ESR COM
**MØ5.549 Rheumatoid polyneuropathy with rheumatoid arthritis of unspecified hand** HCC Rx ESR COM

√6th **MØ5.55 Rheumatoid polyneuropathy with rheumatoid arthritis of hip**
**MØ5.551 Rheumatoid polyneuropathy with rheumatoid arthritis of right hip** HCC Rx ESR COM
**MØ5.552 Rheumatoid polyneuropathy with rheumatoid arthritis of left hip** HCC Rx ESR COM
**MØ5.559 Rheumatoid polyneuropathy with rheumatoid arthritis of unspecified hip** HCC Rx ESR COM

√6th **MØ5.56 Rheumatoid polyneuropathy with rheumatoid arthritis of knee**
**MØ5.561 Rheumatoid polyneuropathy with rheumatoid arthritis of right knee** HCC Rx ESR COM
**MØ5.562 Rheumatoid polyneuropathy with rheumatoid arthritis of left knee** HCC Rx ESR COM
**MØ5.569 Rheumatoid polyneuropathy with rheumatoid arthritis of unspecified knee** HCC Rx ESR COM

√6th **MØ5.57 Rheumatoid polyneuropathy with rheumatoid arthritis of ankle and foot**
Rheumatoid polyneuropathy with rheumatoid arthritis, tarsus, metatarsus and phalanges
**MØ5.571 Rheumatoid polyneuropathy with rheumatoid arthritis of right ankle and foot** HCC Rx ESR COM
**MØ5.572 Rheumatoid polyneuropathy with rheumatoid arthritis of left ankle and foot** HCC Rx ESR COM
**MØ5.579 Rheumatoid polyneuropathy with rheumatoid arthritis of unspecified ankle and foot** HCC Rx ESR COM

**MØ5.59 Rheumatoid polyneuropathy with rheumatoid arthritis of multiple sites** HCC Rx ESR COM

√5th **MØ5.6 Rheumatoid arthritis with involvement of other organs and systems**
**MØ5.6Ø Rheumatoid arthritis of unspecified site with involvement of other organs and systems** HCC Rx ESR COM

√6th **MØ5.61 Rheumatoid arthritis of shoulder with involvement of other organs and systems**
**MØ5.611 Rheumatoid arthritis of right shoulder with involvement of other organs and systems** HCC Rx ESR COM
**MØ5.612 Rheumatoid arthritis of left shoulder with involvement of other organs and systems** HCC Rx ESR COM
**MØ5.619 Rheumatoid arthritis of unspecified shoulder with involvement of other organs and systems** HCC Rx ESR COM

✓6th **M05.62** Rheumatoid arthritis of elbow with involvement of other organs and systems
- **M05.621** Rheumatoid arthritis of right elbow with involvement of other organs and systems HCC Rx ESR COM
- **M05.622** Rheumatoid arthritis of left elbow with involvement of other organs and systems HCC Rx ESR COM
- **M05.629** Rheumatoid arthritis of unspecified elbow with involvement of other organs and systems HCC Rx ESR COM

✓6th **M05.63** Rheumatoid arthritis of wrist with involvement of other organs and systems
Rheumatoid arthritis of carpal bones with involvement of other organs and systems
- **M05.631** Rheumatoid arthritis of right wrist with involvement of other organs and systems HCC Rx ESR COM
- **M05.632** Rheumatoid arthritis of left wrist with involvement of other organs and systems HCC Rx ESR COM
- **M05.639** Rheumatoid arthritis of unspecified wrist with involvement of other organs and systems HCC Rx ESR COM

✓6th **M05.64** Rheumatoid arthritis of hand with involvement of other organs and systems
Rheumatoid arthritis of metacarpus and phalanges with involvement of other organs and systems
- **M05.641** Rheumatoid arthritis of right hand with involvement of other organs and systems HCC Rx ESR COM
- **M05.642** Rheumatoid arthritis of left hand with involvement of other organs and systems HCC Rx ESR COM
- **M05.649** Rheumatoid arthritis of unspecified hand with involvement of other organs and systems HCC Rx ESR COM

✓6th **M05.65** Rheumatoid arthritis of hip with involvement of other organs and systems
- **M05.651** Rheumatoid arthritis of right hip with involvement of other organs and systems HCC Rx ESR COM
- **M05.652** Rheumatoid arthritis of left hip with involvement of other organs and systems HCC Rx ESR COM
- **M05.659** Rheumatoid arthritis of unspecified hip with involvement of other organs and systems HCC Rx ESR COM

✓6th **M05.66** Rheumatoid arthritis of knee with involvement of other organs and systems
- **M05.661** Rheumatoid arthritis of right knee with involvement of other organs and systems HCC Rx ESR COM
- **M05.662** Rheumatoid arthritis of left knee with involvement of other organs and systems HCC Rx ESR COM
- **M05.669** Rheumatoid arthritis of unspecified knee with involvement of other organs and systems HCC Rx ESR COM

✓6th **M05.67** Rheumatoid arthritis of ankle and foot with involvement of other organs and systems
Rheumatoid arthritis of tarsus, metatarsus and phalanges with involvement of other organs and systems
- **M05.671** Rheumatoid arthritis of right ankle and foot with involvement of other organs and systems HCC Rx ESR COM
- **M05.672** Rheumatoid arthritis of left ankle and foot with involvement of other organs and systems HCC Rx ESR COM
- **M05.679** Rheumatoid arthritis of unspecified ankle and foot with involvement of other organs and systems HCC Rx ESR COM

**M05.69** Rheumatoid arthritis of multiple sites with involvement of other organs and systems HCC Rx ESR COM

✓5th **M05.7** Rheumatoid arthritis with rheumatoid factor without organ or systems involvement

**M05.70** Rheumatoid arthritis with rheumatoid factor of unspecified site without organ or systems involvement HCC Rx ESR COM

✓6th **M05.71** Rheumatoid arthritis with rheumatoid factor of shoulder without organ or systems involvement
- **M05.711** Rheumatoid arthritis with rheumatoid factor of right shoulder without organ or systems involvement HCC Rx ESR COM
- **M05.712** Rheumatoid arthritis with rheumatoid factor of left shoulder without organ or systems involvement HCC Rx ESR COM
- **M05.719** Rheumatoid arthritis with rheumatoid factor of unspecified shoulder without organ or systems involvement HCC Rx ESR COM

✓6th **M05.72** Rheumatoid arthritis with rheumatoid factor of elbow without organ or systems involvement
- **M05.721** Rheumatoid arthritis with rheumatoid factor of right elbow without organ or systems involvement HCC Rx ESR COM
- **M05.722** Rheumatoid arthritis with rheumatoid factor of left elbow without organ or systems involvement HCC Rx ESR COM
- **M05.729** Rheumatoid arthritis with rheumatoid factor of unspecified elbow without organ or systems involvement HCC Rx ESR COM

✓6th **M05.73** Rheumatoid arthritis with rheumatoid factor of wrist without organ or systems involvement
- **M05.731** Rheumatoid arthritis with rheumatoid factor of right wrist without organ or systems involvement HCC Rx ESR COM
- **M05.732** Rheumatoid arthritis with rheumatoid factor of left wrist without organ or systems involvement HCC Rx ESR COM
- **M05.739** Rheumatoid arthritis with rheumatoid factor of unspecified wrist without organ or systems involvement HCC Rx ESR COM

✓6th **M05.74** Rheumatoid arthritis with rheumatoid factor of hand without organ or systems involvement
- **M05.741** Rheumatoid arthritis with rheumatoid factor of right hand without organ or systems involvement HCC Rx ESR COM
- **M05.742** Rheumatoid arthritis with rheumatoid factor of left hand without organ or systems involvement HCC Rx ESR COM
- **M05.749** Rheumatoid arthritis with rheumatoid factor of unspecified hand without organ or systems involvement HCC Rx ESR COM

✓6th **M05.75** Rheumatoid arthritis with rheumatoid factor of hip without organ or systems involvement
- **M05.751** Rheumatoid arthritis with rheumatoid factor of right hip without organ or systems involvement HCC Rx ESR COM
- **M05.752** Rheumatoid arthritis with rheumatoid factor of left hip without organ or systems involvement HCC Rx ESR COM
- **M05.759** Rheumatoid arthritis with rheumatoid factor of unspecified hip without organ or systems involvement HCC Rx ESR COM

✓6th **M05.76** Rheumatoid arthritis with rheumatoid factor of knee without organ or systems involvement
- **M05.761** Rheumatoid arthritis with rheumatoid factor of right knee without organ or systems involvement HCC Rx ESR COM
- **M05.762** Rheumatoid arthritis with rheumatoid factor of left knee without organ or systems involvement HCC Rx ESR COM
- **M05.769** Rheumatoid arthritis with rheumatoid factor of unspecified knee without organ or systems involvement HCC Rx ESR COM

✓6th **M05.77** Rheumatoid arthritis with rheumatoid factor of ankle and foot without organ or systems involvement
- **M05.771** Rheumatoid arthritis with rheumatoid factor of right ankle and foot without organ or systems involvement HCC Rx ESR COM
- **M05.772** Rheumatoid arthritis with rheumatoid factor of left ankle and foot without organ or systems involvement HCC Rx ESR COM
- **M05.779** Rheumatoid arthritis with rheumatoid factor of unspecified ankle and foot without organ or systems involvement HCC Rx ESR COM

**MØ5.79** Rheumatoid arthritis with rheumatoid factor of multiple sites without organ or systems involvement HCC Rx ESR COM

**MØ5.7A** Rheumatoid arthritis with rheumatoid factor of other specified site without organ or systems involvement HCC Rx ESR COM

✓5th **MØ5.8** Other rheumatoid arthritis with rheumatoid factor

**MØ5.8Ø** Other rheumatoid arthritis with rheumatoid factor of unspecified site HCC Rx ESR COM

✓6th **MØ5.81** Other rheumatoid arthritis with rheumatoid factor of shoulder

**MØ5.811** Other rheumatoid arthritis with rheumatoid factor of right shoulder HCC Rx ESR COM

**MØ5.812** Other rheumatoid arthritis with rheumatoid factor of left shoulder HCC Rx ESR COM

**MØ5.819** Other rheumatoid arthritis with rheumatoid factor of unspecified shoulder HCC Rx ESR COM

✓6th **MØ5.82** Other rheumatoid arthritis with rheumatoid factor of elbow

**MØ5.821** Other rheumatoid arthritis with rheumatoid factor of right elbow HCC Rx ESR COM

**MØ5.822** Other rheumatoid arthritis with rheumatoid factor of left elbow HCC Rx ESR COM

**MØ5.829** Other rheumatoid arthritis with rheumatoid factor of unspecified elbow HCC Rx ESR COM

✓6th **MØ5.83** Other rheumatoid arthritis with rheumatoid factor of wrist

**MØ5.831** Other rheumatoid arthritis with rheumatoid factor of right wrist HCC Rx ESR COM

**MØ5.832** Other rheumatoid arthritis with rheumatoid factor of left wrist HCC Rx ESR COM

**MØ5.839** Other rheumatoid arthritis with rheumatoid factor of unspecified wrist HCC Rx ESR COM

✓6th **MØ5.84** Other rheumatoid arthritis with rheumatoid factor of hand

**MØ5.841** Other rheumatoid arthritis with rheumatoid factor of right hand HCC Rx ESR COM

**MØ5.842** Other rheumatoid arthritis with rheumatoid factor of left hand HCC Rx ESR COM

**MØ5.849** Other rheumatoid arthritis with rheumatoid factor of unspecified hand HCC Rx ESR COM

✓6th **MØ5.85** Other rheumatoid arthritis with rheumatoid factor of hip

**MØ5.851** Other rheumatoid arthritis with rheumatoid factor of right hip HCC Rx ESR COM

**MØ5.852** Other rheumatoid arthritis with rheumatoid factor of left hip HCC Rx ESR COM

**MØ5.859** Other rheumatoid arthritis with rheumatoid factor of unspecified hip HCC Rx ESR COM

✓6th **MØ5.86** Other rheumatoid arthritis with rheumatoid factor of knee

**MØ5.861** Other rheumatoid arthritis with rheumatoid factor of right knee HCC Rx ESR COM

**MØ5.862** Other rheumatoid arthritis with rheumatoid factor of left knee HCC Rx ESR COM

**MØ5.869** Other rheumatoid arthritis with rheumatoid factor of unspecified knee HCC Rx ESR COM

✓6th **MØ5.87** Other rheumatoid arthritis with rheumatoid factor of ankle and foot

**MØ5.871** Other rheumatoid arthritis with rheumatoid factor of right ankle and foot HCC Rx ESR COM

**MØ5.872** Other rheumatoid arthritis with rheumatoid factor of left ankle and foot HCC Rx ESR COM

**MØ5.879** Other rheumatoid arthritis with rheumatoid factor of unspecified ankle and foot HCC Rx ESR COM

**MØ5.89** Other rheumatoid arthritis with rheumatoid factor of multiple sites HCC Rx ESR COM

**MØ5.8A** Other rheumatoid arthritis with rheumatoid factor of other specified site HCC Rx ESR COM

**MØ5.9** Rheumatoid arthritis with rheumatoid factor, unspecified HCC Rx ESR COM

**MØ5.A** Abnormal rheumatoid factor and anti-citrullinated protein antibody with rheumatoid arthritis HCC Rx ESR

Code first rheumatoid arthritis with rheumatoid factor by site, if known (MØ5.ØØ-MØ5.8A)

✓4th **MØ6 Other rheumatoid arthritis**

**AHA:** 2020,4Q,31-32

**DEF:** Rheumatoid arthritis: Autoimmune systemic disease that causes chronic inflammation of the joints and other areas of the body, manifested by inflammatory changes in articular structures and synovial membranes, atrophy, and loss in bone density.

✓5th **MØ6.Ø** Rheumatoid arthritis without rheumatoid factor

**MØ6.ØØ** Rheumatoid arthritis without rheumatoid factor, unspecified site HCC Rx ESR COM

✓6th **MØ6.Ø1** Rheumatoid arthritis without rheumatoid factor, shoulder

**MØ6.Ø11** Rheumatoid arthritis without rheumatoid factor, right shoulder HCC Rx ESR COM

**MØ6.Ø12** Rheumatoid arthritis without rheumatoid factor, left shoulder HCC Rx ESR COM

**MØ6.Ø19** Rheumatoid arthritis without rheumatoid factor, unspecified shoulder HCC Rx ESR COM

✓6th **MØ6.Ø2** Rheumatoid arthritis without rheumatoid factor, elbow

**MØ6.Ø21** Rheumatoid arthritis without rheumatoid factor, right elbow HCC Rx ESR COM

**MØ6.Ø22** Rheumatoid arthritis without rheumatoid factor, left elbow HCC Rx ESR COM

**MØ6.Ø29** Rheumatoid arthritis without rheumatoid factor, unspecified elbow HCC Rx ESR COM

✓6th **MØ6.Ø3** Rheumatoid arthritis without rheumatoid factor, wrist

**MØ6.Ø31** Rheumatoid arthritis without rheumatoid factor, right wrist HCC Rx ESR COM

**MØ6.Ø32** Rheumatoid arthritis without rheumatoid factor, left wrist HCC Rx ESR COM

**MØ6.Ø39** Rheumatoid arthritis without rheumatoid factor, unspecified wrist HCC Rx ESR COM

✓6th **MØ6.Ø4** Rheumatoid arthritis without rheumatoid factor, hand

**MØ6.Ø41** Rheumatoid arthritis without rheumatoid factor, right hand HCC Rx ESR COM

**MØ6.Ø42** Rheumatoid arthritis without rheumatoid factor, left hand HCC Rx ESR COM

**MØ6.Ø49** Rheumatoid arthritis without rheumatoid factor, unspecified hand HCC Rx ESR COM

✓6th **MØ6.Ø5** Rheumatoid arthritis without rheumatoid factor, hip

**MØ6.Ø51** Rheumatoid arthritis without rheumatoid factor, right hip HCC Rx ESR COM

**MØ6.Ø52** Rheumatoid arthritis without rheumatoid factor, left hip HCC Rx ESR COM

**MØ6.Ø59** Rheumatoid arthritis without rheumatoid factor, unspecified hip HCC Rx ESR COM

✓6th **MØ6.Ø6** Rheumatoid arthritis without rheumatoid factor, knee

**MØ6.Ø61** Rheumatoid arthritis without rheumatoid factor, right knee HCC Rx ESR COM

**MØ6.Ø62** Rheumatoid arthritis without rheumatoid factor, left knee HCC Rx ESR COM

**MØ6.Ø69** Rheumatoid arthritis without rheumatoid factor, unspecified knee HCC Rx ESR COM

✓6th **MØ6.Ø7** Rheumatoid arthritis without rheumatoid factor, ankle and foot

**MØ6.Ø71** Rheumatoid arthritis without rheumatoid factor, right ankle and foot HCC Rx ESR COM

M06.072 Rheumatoid arthritis without rheumatoid factor, left ankle and foot HCC Rx ESR COM
M06.079 Rheumatoid arthritis without rheumatoid factor, unspecified ankle and foot HCC Rx ESR COM
M06.08 Rheumatoid arthritis without rheumatoid factor, vertebrae HCC Rx ESR COM
M06.09 Rheumatoid arthritis without rheumatoid factor, multiple sites HCC Rx ESR COM
M06.0A Rheumatoid arthritis without rheumatoid factor, other specified site HCC Rx ESR COM

M06.1 Adult-onset Still's disease HCC Rx ESR COM A
EXCLUDES 1 *Still's disease NOS (M08.2-)*
**DEF:** Type of systemic arthritis characterized by a transient rash and spiking fevers. This condition may resolve or develop into a chronic condition and may affect internal organs, as well as joints.
***Synonym(s):*** *AOSD*

✓5th M06.2 Rheumatoid bursitis
M06.20 Rheumatoid bursitis, unspecified site HCC Rx ESR COM
✓6th M06.21 Rheumatoid bursitis, shoulder
M06.211 Rheumatoid bursitis, right shoulder HCC Rx ESR COM
M06.212 Rheumatoid bursitis, left shoulder HCC Rx ESR COM
M06.219 Rheumatoid bursitis, unspecified shoulder HCC Rx ESR COM
✓6th M06.22 Rheumatoid bursitis, elbow
M06.221 Rheumatoid bursitis, right elbow HCC Rx ESR COM
M06.222 Rheumatoid bursitis, left elbow HCC Rx ESR COM
M06.229 Rheumatoid bursitis, unspecified elbow HCC Rx ESR COM
✓6th M06.23 Rheumatoid bursitis, wrist
M06.231 Rheumatoid bursitis, right wrist HCC Rx ESR COM
M06.232 Rheumatoid bursitis, left wrist HCC Rx ESR COM
M06.239 Rheumatoid bursitis, unspecified wrist HCC Rx ESR COM
✓6th M06.24 Rheumatoid bursitis, hand
M06.241 Rheumatoid bursitis, right hand HCC Rx ESR COM
M06.242 Rheumatoid bursitis, left hand HCC Rx ESR COM
M06.249 Rheumatoid bursitis, unspecified hand HCC Rx ESR COM
✓6th M06.25 Rheumatoid bursitis, hip
M06.251 Rheumatoid bursitis, right hip HCC Rx ESR COM
M06.252 Rheumatoid bursitis, left hip HCC Rx ESR COM
M06.259 Rheumatoid bursitis, unspecified hip HCC Rx ESR COM
✓6th M06.26 Rheumatoid bursitis, knee
M06.261 Rheumatoid bursitis, right knee HCC Rx ESR COM
M06.262 Rheumatoid bursitis, left knee HCC Rx ESR COM
M06.269 Rheumatoid bursitis, unspecified knee HCC Rx ESR COM
✓6th M06.27 Rheumatoid bursitis, ankle and foot
M06.271 Rheumatoid bursitis, right ankle and foot HCC Rx ESR COM
M06.272 Rheumatoid bursitis, left ankle and foot HCC Rx ESR COM
M06.279 Rheumatoid bursitis, unspecified ankle and foot HCC Rx ESR COM
M06.28 Rheumatoid bursitis, vertebrae HCC Rx ESR COM
M06.29 Rheumatoid bursitis, multiple sites HCC Rx ESR COM

✓5th M06.3 Rheumatoid nodule
M06.30 Rheumatoid nodule, unspecified site HCC Rx ESR COM
✓6th M06.31 Rheumatoid nodule, shoulder
M06.311 Rheumatoid nodule, right shoulder HCC Rx ESR COM
M06.312 Rheumatoid nodule, left shoulder HCC Rx ESR COM
M06.319 Rheumatoid nodule, unspecified shoulder HCC Rx ESR COM
✓6th M06.32 Rheumatoid nodule, elbow
M06.321 Rheumatoid nodule, right elbow HCC Rx ESR COM
M06.322 Rheumatoid nodule, left elbow HCC Rx ESR COM
M06.329 Rheumatoid nodule, unspecified elbow HCC Rx ESR COM
✓6th M06.33 Rheumatoid nodule, wrist
M06.331 Rheumatoid nodule, right wrist HCC Rx ESR COM
M06.332 Rheumatoid nodule, left wrist HCC Rx ESR COM
M06.339 Rheumatoid nodule, unspecified wrist HCC Rx ESR COM
✓6th M06.34 Rheumatoid nodule, hand
M06.341 Rheumatoid nodule, right hand HCC Rx ESR COM
M06.342 Rheumatoid nodule, left hand HCC Rx ESR COM
M06.349 Rheumatoid nodule, unspecified hand HCC Rx ESR COM
✓6th M06.35 Rheumatoid nodule, hip
M06.351 Rheumatoid nodule, right hip HCC Rx ESR COM
M06.352 Rheumatoid nodule, left hip HCC Rx ESR COM
M06.359 Rheumatoid nodule, unspecified hip HCC Rx ESR COM
✓6th M06.36 Rheumatoid nodule, knee
M06.361 Rheumatoid nodule, right knee HCC Rx ESR COM
M06.362 Rheumatoid nodule, left knee HCC Rx ESR COM
M06.369 Rheumatoid nodule, unspecified knee HCC Rx ESR COM
✓6th M06.37 Rheumatoid nodule, ankle and foot
M06.371 Rheumatoid nodule, right ankle and foot HCC Rx ESR COM
M06.372 Rheumatoid nodule, left ankle and foot HCC Rx ESR COM
M06.379 Rheumatoid nodule, unspecified ankle and foot HCC Rx ESR COM
M06.38 Rheumatoid nodule, vertebrae HCC Rx ESR COM
M06.39 Rheumatoid nodule, multiple sites HCC Rx ESR COM

M06.4 Inflammatory polyarthropathy HCC Rx ESR COM
EXCLUDES 1 *polyarthritis NOS (M13.0)*
**AHA:** 2025,2Q,9-10; 2024,1Q,17

✓5th M06.8 Other specified rheumatoid arthritis
M06.80 Other specified rheumatoid arthritis, unspecified site HCC Rx ESR COM
✓6th M06.81 Other specified rheumatoid arthritis, shoulder
M06.811 Other specified rheumatoid arthritis, right shoulder HCC Rx ESR COM
M06.812 Other specified rheumatoid arthritis, left shoulder HCC Rx ESR COM
M06.819 Other specified rheumatoid arthritis, unspecified shoulder HCC Rx ESR COM
✓6th M06.82 Other specified rheumatoid arthritis, elbow
M06.821 Other specified rheumatoid arthritis, right elbow HCC Rx ESR COM
M06.822 Other specified rheumatoid arthritis, left elbow HCC Rx ESR COM
M06.829 Other specified rheumatoid arthritis, unspecified elbow HCC Rx ESR COM
✓6th M06.83 Other specified rheumatoid arthritis, wrist
M06.831 Other specified rheumatoid arthritis, right wrist HCC Rx ESR COM
M06.832 Other specified rheumatoid arthritis, left wrist HCC Rx ESR COM

M06.839 Other specified rheumatoid arthritis, unspecified wrist HCC Rx ESR COM

✓6th M06.84 Other specified rheumatoid arthritis, hand

M06.841 Other specified rheumatoid arthritis, right hand HCC Rx ESR COM

M06.842 Other specified rheumatoid arthritis, left hand HCC Rx ESR COM

M06.849 Other specified rheumatoid arthritis, unspecified hand HCC Rx ESR COM

✓6th M06.85 Other specified rheumatoid arthritis, hip

M06.851 Other specified rheumatoid arthritis, right hip HCC Rx ESR COM

M06.852 Other specified rheumatoid arthritis, left hip HCC Rx ESR COM

M06.859 Other specified rheumatoid arthritis, unspecified hip HCC Rx ESR COM

✓6th M06.86 Other specified rheumatoid arthritis, knee

M06.861 Other specified rheumatoid arthritis, right knee HCC Rx ESR COM

M06.862 Other specified rheumatoid arthritis, left knee HCC Rx ESR COM

M06.869 Other specified rheumatoid arthritis, unspecified knee HCC Rx ESR COM

✓6th M06.87 Other specified rheumatoid arthritis, ankle and foot

M06.871 Other specified rheumatoid arthritis, right ankle and foot HCC Rx ESR COM

M06.872 Other specified rheumatoid arthritis, left ankle and foot HCC Rx ESR COM

M06.879 Other specified rheumatoid arthritis, unspecified ankle and foot HCC Rx ESR COM

M06.88 Other specified rheumatoid arthritis, vertebrae HCC Rx ESR COM

M06.89 Other specified rheumatoid arthritis, multiple sites HCC Rx ESR COM

M06.8A Other specified rheumatoid arthritis, other specified site HCC Rx ESR COM

M06.9 Rheumatoid arthritis, unspecified HCC Rx ESR COM

AHA: 2024,1Q,17

✓4th **M07 Enteropathic arthropathies**

Code also associated enteropathy, such as:
regional enteritis [Crohn's disease] (K50.-)
ulcerative colitis (K51.-)

EXCLUDES 1 *psoriatic arthropathies (L40.5-)*

✓5th M07.6 Enteropathic arthropathies

M07.60 Enteropathic arthropathies, unspecified site

✓6th M07.61 Enteropathic arthropathies, shoulder

M07.611 Enteropathic arthropathies, right shoulder

M07.612 Enteropathic arthropathies, left shoulder

M07.619 Enteropathic arthropathies, unspecified shoulder

✓6th M07.62 Enteropathic arthropathies, elbow

M07.621 Enteropathic arthropathies, right elbow

M07.622 Enteropathic arthropathies, left elbow

M07.629 Enteropathic arthropathies, unspecified elbow

✓6th M07.63 Enteropathic arthropathies, wrist

M07.631 Enteropathic arthropathies, right wrist

M07.632 Enteropathic arthropathies, left wrist

M07.639 Enteropathic arthropathies, unspecified wrist

✓6th M07.64 Enteropathic arthropathies, hand

M07.641 Enteropathic arthropathies, right hand

M07.642 Enteropathic arthropathies, left hand

M07.649 Enteropathic arthropathies, unspecified hand

✓6th M07.65 Enteropathic arthropathies, hip

M07.651 Enteropathic arthropathies, right hip

M07.652 Enteropathic arthropathies, left hip

M07.659 Enteropathic arthropathies, unspecified hip

✓6th M07.66 Enteropathic arthropathies, knee

M07.661 Enteropathic arthropathies, right knee

M07.662 Enteropathic arthropathies, left knee

M07.669 Enteropathic arthropathies, unspecified knee

✓6th M07.67 Enteropathic arthropathies, ankle and foot

M07.671 Enteropathic arthropathies, right ankle and foot

M07.672 Enteropathic arthropathies, left ankle and foot

M07.679 Enteropathic arthropathies, unspecified ankle and foot

M07.68 Enteropathic arthropathies, vertebrae

M07.69 Enteropathic arthropathies, multiple sites

✓4th **M08 Juvenile arthritis**

Code also any associated underlying condition, such as:
regional enteritis [Crohn's disease] (K50.-)
ulcerative colitis (K51.-)

EXCLUDES 1 *arthropathy in Whipple's disease (M14.8)*
*Felty's syndrome (M05.0)*
*juvenile dermatomyositis (M33.0-)*
*psoriatic juvenile arthropathy (L40.54)*

AHA: 2020,4Q,31-32

✓5th M08.0 Unspecified juvenile rheumatoid arthritis

Juvenile rheumatoid arthritis with or without rheumatoid factor

M08.00 Unspecified juvenile rheumatoid arthritis of unspecified site HCC Rx ESR COM

✓6th M08.01 Unspecified juvenile rheumatoid arthritis, shoulder

M08.011 Unspecified juvenile rheumatoid arthritis, right shoulder HCC Rx ESR COM

M08.012 Unspecified juvenile rheumatoid arthritis, left shoulder HCC Rx ESR COM

M08.019 Unspecified juvenile rheumatoid arthritis, unspecified shoulder HCC Rx ESR COM

✓6th M08.02 Unspecified juvenile rheumatoid arthritis of elbow

M08.021 Unspecified juvenile rheumatoid arthritis, right elbow HCC Rx ESR COM

M08.022 Unspecified juvenile rheumatoid arthritis, left elbow HCC Rx ESR COM

M08.029 Unspecified juvenile rheumatoid arthritis, unspecified elbow HCC Rx ESR COM

✓6th M08.03 Unspecified juvenile rheumatoid arthritis, wrist

M08.031 Unspecified juvenile rheumatoid arthritis, right wrist HCC Rx ESR COM

M08.032 Unspecified juvenile rheumatoid arthritis, left wrist HCC Rx ESR COM

M08.039 Unspecified juvenile rheumatoid arthritis, unspecified wrist HCC Rx ESR COM

✓6th M08.04 Unspecified juvenile rheumatoid arthritis, hand

M08.041 Unspecified juvenile rheumatoid arthritis, right hand HCC Rx ESR COM

M08.042 Unspecified juvenile rheumatoid arthritis, left hand HCC Rx ESR COM

M08.049 Unspecified juvenile rheumatoid arthritis, unspecified hand HCC Rx ESR COM

✓6th M08.05 Unspecified juvenile rheumatoid arthritis, hip

M08.051 Unspecified juvenile rheumatoid arthritis, right hip HCC Rx ESR COM

M08.052 Unspecified juvenile rheumatoid arthritis, left hip HCC Rx ESR COM

M08.059 Unspecified juvenile rheumatoid arthritis, unspecified hip HCC Rx ESR COM

✓6th M08.06 Unspecified juvenile rheumatoid arthritis, knee

M08.061 Unspecified juvenile rheumatoid arthritis, right knee HCC Rx ESR COM

M08.062 Unspecified juvenile rheumatoid arthritis, left knee HCC Rx ESR COM

M08.069 Unspecified juvenile rheumatoid arthritis, unspecified knee HCC Rx ESR COM

✓6th M08.07 Unspecified juvenile rheumatoid arthritis, ankle and foot

M08.071 Unspecified juvenile rheumatoid arthritis, right ankle and foot HCC Rx ESR COM

M08.072 Unspecified juvenile rheumatoid arthritis, left ankle and foot HCC Rx ESR COM

M08.079 Unspecified juvenile rheumatoid arthritis, unspecified ankle and foot HCC Rx ESR COM

M08.08 Unspecified juvenile rheumatoid arthritis, vertebrae HCC Rx ESR COM

M08.09 Unspecified juvenile rheumatoid arthritis, multiple sites HCC Rx ESR COM

M08.0A Unspecified juvenile rheumatoid arthritis, other specified site HCC Rx ESR COM

M08.1 Juvenile ankylosing spondylitis HCC Rx ESR COM

EXCLUDES 1 *ankylosing spondylitis in adults (M45.0-)*

✓5th M08.2 Juvenile rheumatoid arthritis with systemic onset

Still's disease NOS

EXCLUDES 1 *adult-onset Still's disease (M06.1-)*

**DEF:** Systemic juvenile rheumatoid arthritis characterized by a transient rash and spiking fevers that may affect internal organs, as well as joints.

M08.20 Juvenile rheumatoid arthritis with systemic onset, unspecified site HCC Rx ESR COM

✓6th M08.21 Juvenile rheumatoid arthritis with systemic onset, shoulder

M08.211 Juvenile rheumatoid arthritis with systemic onset, right shoulder HCC Rx ESR COM

M08.212 Juvenile rheumatoid arthritis with systemic onset, left shoulder HCC Rx ESR COM

M08.219 Juvenile rheumatoid arthritis with systemic onset, unspecified shoulder HCC Rx ESR COM

✓6th M08.22 Juvenile rheumatoid arthritis with systemic onset, elbow

M08.221 Juvenile rheumatoid arthritis with systemic onset, right elbow HCC Rx ESR COM

M08.222 Juvenile rheumatoid arthritis with systemic onset, left elbow HCC Rx ESR COM

M08.229 Juvenile rheumatoid arthritis with systemic onset, unspecified elbow HCC Rx ESR COM

✓6th M08.23 Juvenile rheumatoid arthritis with systemic onset, wrist

M08.231 Juvenile rheumatoid arthritis with systemic onset, right wrist HCC Rx ESR COM

M08.232 Juvenile rheumatoid arthritis with systemic onset, left wrist HCC Rx ESR COM

M08.239 Juvenile rheumatoid arthritis with systemic onset, unspecified wrist HCC Rx ESR COM

✓6th M08.24 Juvenile rheumatoid arthritis with systemic onset, hand

M08.241 Juvenile rheumatoid arthritis with systemic onset, right hand HCC Rx ESR COM

M08.242 Juvenile rheumatoid arthritis with systemic onset, left hand HCC Rx ESR COM

M08.249 Juvenile rheumatoid arthritis with systemic onset, unspecified hand HCC Rx ESR COM

✓6th M08.25 Juvenile rheumatoid arthritis with systemic onset, hip

M08.251 Juvenile rheumatoid arthritis with systemic onset, right hip HCC Rx ESR COM

M08.252 Juvenile rheumatoid arthritis with systemic onset, left hip HCC Rx ESR COM

M08.259 Juvenile rheumatoid arthritis with systemic onset, unspecified hip HCC Rx ESR COM

✓6th M08.26 Juvenile rheumatoid arthritis with systemic onset, knee

M08.261 Juvenile rheumatoid arthritis with systemic onset, right knee HCC Rx ESR COM

M08.262 Juvenile rheumatoid arthritis with systemic onset, left knee HCC Rx ESR COM

M08.269 Juvenile rheumatoid arthritis with systemic onset, unspecified knee HCC Rx ESR COM

✓6th M08.27 Juvenile rheumatoid arthritis with systemic onset, ankle and foot

M08.271 Juvenile rheumatoid arthritis with systemic onset, right ankle and foot HCC Rx ESR COM

M08.272 Juvenile rheumatoid arthritis with systemic onset, left ankle and foot HCC Rx ESR COM

M08.279 Juvenile rheumatoid arthritis with systemic onset, unspecified ankle and foot HCC Rx ESR COM

M08.28 Juvenile rheumatoid arthritis with systemic onset, vertebrae HCC Rx ESR COM

M08.29 Juvenile rheumatoid arthritis with systemic onset, multiple sites HCC Rx ESR COM

M08.2A Juvenile rheumatoid arthritis with systemic onset, other specified site HCC Rx ESR COM

M08.3 Juvenile rheumatoid polyarthritis (seronegative) HCC Rx ESR COM

✓5th M08.4 Pauciarticular juvenile rheumatoid arthritis

M08.40 Pauciarticular juvenile rheumatoid arthritis, unspecified site HCC Rx ESR COM

✓6th M08.41 Pauciarticular juvenile rheumatoid arthritis, shoulder

M08.411 Pauciarticular juvenile rheumatoid arthritis, right shoulder HCC Rx ESR COM

M08.412 Pauciarticular juvenile rheumatoid arthritis, left shoulder HCC Rx ESR COM

M08.419 Pauciarticular juvenile rheumatoid arthritis, unspecified shoulder HCC Rx ESR COM

✓6th M08.42 Pauciarticular juvenile rheumatoid arthritis, elbow

M08.421 Pauciarticular juvenile rheumatoid arthritis, right elbow HCC Rx ESR COM

M08.422 Pauciarticular juvenile rheumatoid arthritis, left elbow HCC Rx ESR COM

M08.429 Pauciarticular juvenile rheumatoid arthritis, unspecified elbow HCC Rx ESR COM

✓6th M08.43 Pauciarticular juvenile rheumatoid arthritis, wrist

M08.431 Pauciarticular juvenile rheumatoid arthritis, right wrist HCC Rx ESR COM

M08.432 Pauciarticular juvenile rheumatoid arthritis, left wrist HCC Rx ESR COM

M08.439 Pauciarticular juvenile rheumatoid arthritis, unspecified wrist HCC Rx ESR COM

✓6th M08.44 Pauciarticular juvenile rheumatoid arthritis, hand

M08.441 Pauciarticular juvenile rheumatoid arthritis, right hand HCC Rx ESR COM

M08.442 Pauciarticular juvenile rheumatoid arthritis, left hand HCC Rx ESR COM

M08.449 Pauciarticular juvenile rheumatoid arthritis, unspecified hand HCC Rx ESR COM

✓6th M08.45 Pauciarticular juvenile rheumatoid arthritis, hip

M08.451 Pauciarticular juvenile rheumatoid arthritis, right hip HCC Rx ESR COM

M08.452 Pauciarticular juvenile rheumatoid arthritis, left hip HCC Rx ESR COM

M08.459 Pauciarticular juvenile rheumatoid arthritis, unspecified hip HCC Rx ESR COM

✓6th M08.46 Pauciarticular juvenile rheumatoid arthritis, knee

M08.461 Pauciarticular juvenile rheumatoid arthritis, right knee HCC Rx ESR COM

M08.462 Pauciarticular juvenile rheumatoid arthritis, left knee HCC Rx ESR COM

M08.469 Pauciarticular juvenile rheumatoid arthritis, unspecified knee HCC Rx ESR COM

✓6th M08.47 Pauciarticular juvenile rheumatoid arthritis, ankle and foot

M08.471 Pauciarticular juvenile rheumatoid arthritis, right ankle and foot HCC Rx ESR COM

M08.472 Pauciarticular juvenile rheumatoid arthritis, left ankle and foot HCC Rx ESR COM

**MØ8.479** Pauciarticular juvenile rheumatoid arthritis, unspecified ankle and foot HCC Rx ESR COM

**MØ8.48** Pauciarticular juvenile rheumatoid arthritis, vertebrae HCC Rx ESR COM

**MØ8.4A** Pauciarticular juvenile rheumatoid arthritis, other specified site HCC Rx ESR COM

√5th **MØ8.8 Other juvenile arthritis**

**MØ8.8Ø** Other juvenile arthritis, unspecified site HCC Rx ESR COM

√6th **MØ8.81** Other juvenile arthritis, shoulder

**MØ8.811** Other juvenile arthritis, right shoulder HCC Rx ESR COM

**MØ8.812** Other juvenile arthritis, left shoulder HCC Rx ESR COM

**MØ8.819** Other juvenile arthritis, unspecified shoulder HCC Rx ESR COM

√6th **MØ8.82** Other juvenile arthritis, elbow

**MØ8.821** Other juvenile arthritis, right elbow HCC Rx ESR COM

**MØ8.822** Other juvenile arthritis, left elbow HCC Rx ESR COM

**MØ8.829** Other juvenile arthritis, unspecified elbow HCC Rx ESR COM

√6th **MØ8.83** Other juvenile arthritis, wrist

**MØ8.831** Other juvenile arthritis, right wrist HCC Rx ESR COM

**MØ8.832** Other juvenile arthritis, left wrist HCC Rx ESR COM

**MØ8.839** Other juvenile arthritis, unspecified wrist HCC Rx ESR COM

√6th **MØ8.84** Other juvenile arthritis, hand

**MØ8.841** Other juvenile arthritis, right hand HCC Rx ESR COM

**MØ8.842** Other juvenile arthritis, left hand HCC Rx ESR COM

**MØ8.849** Other juvenile arthritis, unspecified hand HCC Rx ESR COM

√6th **MØ8.85** Other juvenile arthritis, hip

**MØ8.851** Other juvenile arthritis, right hip HCC Rx ESR COM

**MØ8.852** Other juvenile arthritis, left hip HCC Rx ESR COM

**MØ8.859** Other juvenile arthritis, unspecified hip HCC Rx ESR COM

√6th **MØ8.86** Other juvenile arthritis, knee

**MØ8.861** Other juvenile arthritis, right knee HCC Rx ESR COM

**MØ8.862** Other juvenile arthritis, left knee HCC Rx ESR COM

**MØ8.869** Other juvenile arthritis, unspecified knee HCC Rx ESR COM

√6th **MØ8.87** Other juvenile arthritis, ankle and foot

**MØ8.871** Other juvenile arthritis, right ankle and foot HCC Rx ESR COM

**MØ8.872** Other juvenile arthritis, left ankle and foot HCC Rx ESR COM

**MØ8.879** Other juvenile arthritis, unspecified ankle and foot HCC Rx ESR COM

**MØ8.88** Other juvenile arthritis, other specified site HCC Rx ESR COM
Other juvenile arthritis, vertebrae

**MØ8.89** Other juvenile arthritis, multiple sites HCC Rx ESR COM

√5th **MØ8.9 Juvenile arthritis, unspecified**

EXCLUDES 1 *juvenile rheumatoid arthritis, unspecified (MØ8.Ø-)*

**MØ8.9Ø** Juvenile arthritis, unspecified, unspecified site HCC Rx ESR COM

√6th **MØ8.91** Juvenile arthritis, unspecified, shoulder

**MØ8.911** Juvenile arthritis, unspecified, right shoulder HCC Rx ESR COM

**MØ8.912** Juvenile arthritis, unspecified, left shoulder HCC Rx ESR COM

**MØ8.919** Juvenile arthritis, unspecified, unspecified shoulder HCC Rx ESR COM

√6th **MØ8.92** Juvenile arthritis, unspecified, elbow

**MØ8.921** Juvenile arthritis, unspecified, right elbow HCC Rx ESR COM

**MØ8.922** Juvenile arthritis, unspecified, left elbow HCC Rx ESR COM

**MØ8.929** Juvenile arthritis, unspecified, unspecified elbow HCC Rx ESR COM

√6th **MØ8.93** Juvenile arthritis, unspecified, wrist

**MØ8.931** Juvenile arthritis, unspecified, right wrist HCC Rx ESR COM

**MØ8.932** Juvenile arthritis, unspecified, left wrist HCC Rx ESR COM

**MØ8.939** Juvenile arthritis, unspecified, unspecified wrist HCC Rx ESR COM

√6th **MØ8.94** Juvenile arthritis, unspecified, hand

**MØ8.941** Juvenile arthritis, unspecified, right hand HCC Rx ESR COM

**MØ8.942** Juvenile arthritis, unspecified, left hand HCC Rx ESR COM

**MØ8.949** Juvenile arthritis, unspecified, unspecified hand HCC Rx ESR COM

√6th **MØ8.95** Juvenile arthritis, unspecified, hip

**MØ8.951** Juvenile arthritis, unspecified, right hip HCC Rx ESR COM

**MØ8.952** Juvenile arthritis, unspecified, left hip HCC Rx ESR COM

**MØ8.959** Juvenile arthritis, unspecified, unspecified hip HCC Rx ESR COM

√6th **MØ8.96** Juvenile arthritis, unspecified, knee

**MØ8.961** Juvenile arthritis, unspecified, right knee HCC Rx ESR COM

**MØ8.962** Juvenile arthritis, unspecified, left knee HCC Rx ESR COM

**MØ8.969** Juvenile arthritis, unspecified, unspecified knee HCC Rx ESR COM

√6th **MØ8.97** Juvenile arthritis, unspecified, ankle and foot

**MØ8.971** Juvenile arthritis, unspecified, right ankle and foot HCC Rx ESR COM

**MØ8.972** Juvenile arthritis, unspecified, left ankle and foot HCC Rx ESR COM

**MØ8.979** Juvenile arthritis, unspecified, unspecified ankle and foot HCC Rx ESR COM

**MØ8.98** Juvenile arthritis, unspecified, vertebrae HCC Rx ESR COM

**MØ8.99** Juvenile arthritis, unspecified, multiple sites HCC Rx ESR COM

**MØ8.9A** Juvenile arthritis, unspecified, other specified site HCC Rx ESR COM

√4th **M1A Chronic gout**

Use additional code to identify:
- autonomic neuropathy in diseases classified elsewhere (G99.Ø)
- calculus of urinary tract in diseases classified elsewhere (N22)
- cardiomyopathy in diseases classified elsewhere (I43)
- disorders of external ear in diseases classified elsewhere (H61.1-, H62.8-)
- disorders of iris and ciliary body in diseases classified elsewhere (H22)
- glomerular disorders in diseases classified elsewhere (NØ8)

EXCLUDES 1 *gout NOS (M1Ø.-)*

EXCLUDES 2 *acute gout (M1Ø.-)*

The appropriate 7th character is to be added to each code from category M1A.
Ø without tophus (tophi)
1 with tophus (tophi)

√5th **M1A.Ø Idiopathic chronic gout**
Chronic gouty bursitis
Primary chronic gout

√x7th **M1A.ØØ** Idiopathic chronic gout, unspecified site

√6th **M1A.Ø1** Idiopathic chronic gout, shoulder

√7th **M1A.Ø11** Idiopathic chronic gout, right shoulder

√7th **M1A.Ø12** Idiopathic chronic gout, left shoulder

√7th **M1A.Ø19** Idiopathic chronic gout, unspecified shoulder

√6th **M1A.Ø2** Idiopathic chronic gout, elbow

√7th **M1A.Ø21** Idiopathic chronic gout, right elbow

√7th **M1A.Ø22** Idiopathic chronic gout, left elbow

√7th **M1A.Ø29** Idiopathic chronic gout, unspecified elbow

- M1A.03 Idiopathic chronic gout, wrist
  - M1A.031 Idiopathic chronic gout, right wrist
  - M1A.032 Idiopathic chronic gout, left wrist
  - M1A.039 Idiopathic chronic gout, unspecified wrist
- M1A.04 Idiopathic chronic gout, hand
  - M1A.041 Idiopathic chronic gout, right hand
  - M1A.042 Idiopathic chronic gout, left hand
  - M1A.049 Idiopathic chronic gout, unspecified hand
- M1A.05 Idiopathic chronic gout, hip
  - M1A.051 Idiopathic chronic gout, right hip
  - M1A.052 Idiopathic chronic gout, left hip
  - M1A.059 Idiopathic chronic gout, unspecified hip
- M1A.06 Idiopathic chronic gout, knee
  - M1A.061 Idiopathic chronic gout, right knee
  - M1A.062 Idiopathic chronic gout, left knee
  - M1A.069 Idiopathic chronic gout, unspecified knee
- M1A.07 Idiopathic chronic gout, ankle and foot
  - M1A.071 Idiopathic chronic gout, right ankle and foot
  - M1A.072 Idiopathic chronic gout, left ankle and foot
  - M1A.079 Idiopathic chronic gout, unspecified ankle and foot
- M1A.08 Idiopathic chronic gout, vertebrae
- M1A.09 Idiopathic chronic gout, multiple sites

M1A.1 Lead-induced chronic gout

Code first toxic effects of lead and its compounds (T56.0-)

- M1A.10 Lead-induced chronic gout, unspecified site
- M1A.11 Lead-induced chronic gout, shoulder
  - M1A.111 Lead-induced chronic gout, right shoulder
  - M1A.112 Lead-induced chronic gout, left shoulder
  - M1A.119 Lead-induced chronic gout, unspecified shoulder
- M1A.12 Lead-induced chronic gout, elbow
  - M1A.121 Lead-induced chronic gout, right elbow
  - M1A.122 Lead-induced chronic gout, left elbow
  - M1A.129 Lead-induced chronic gout, unspecified elbow
- M1A.13 Lead-induced chronic gout, wrist
  - M1A.131 Lead-induced chronic gout, right wrist
  - M1A.132 Lead-induced chronic gout, left wrist
  - M1A.139 Lead-induced chronic gout, unspecified wrist
- M1A.14 Lead-induced chronic gout, hand
  - M1A.141 Lead-induced chronic gout, right hand
  - M1A.142 Lead-induced chronic gout, left hand
  - M1A.149 Lead-induced chronic gout, unspecified hand
- M1A.15 Lead-induced chronic gout, hip
  - M1A.151 Lead-induced chronic gout, right hip
  - M1A.152 Lead-induced chronic gout, left hip
  - M1A.159 Lead-induced chronic gout, unspecified hip
- M1A.16 Lead-induced chronic gout, knee
  - M1A.161 Lead-induced chronic gout, right knee
  - M1A.162 Lead-induced chronic gout, left knee
  - M1A.169 Lead-induced chronic gout, unspecified knee
- M1A.17 Lead-induced chronic gout, ankle and foot
  - M1A.171 Lead-induced chronic gout, right ankle and foot
  - M1A.172 Lead-induced chronic gout, left ankle and foot
  - M1A.179 Lead-induced chronic gout, unspecified ankle and foot
- M1A.18 Lead-induced chronic gout, vertebrae
- M1A.19 Lead-induced chronic gout, multiple sites

M1A.2 Drug-induced chronic gout

Use additional code for adverse effect, if applicable, to identify drug (T36-T50 with fifth or sixth character 5)

- M1A.20 Drug-induced chronic gout, unspecified site
- M1A.21 Drug-induced chronic gout, shoulder
  - M1A.211 Drug-induced chronic gout, right shoulder
  - M1A.212 Drug-induced chronic gout, left shoulder
  - M1A.219 Drug-induced chronic gout, unspecified shoulder
- M1A.22 Drug-induced chronic gout, elbow
  - M1A.221 Drug-induced chronic gout, right elbow
  - M1A.222 Drug-induced chronic gout, left elbow
  - M1A.229 Drug-induced chronic gout, unspecified elbow
- M1A.23 Drug-induced chronic gout, wrist
  - M1A.231 Drug-induced chronic gout, right wrist
  - M1A.232 Drug-induced chronic gout, left wrist
  - M1A.239 Drug-induced chronic gout, unspecified wrist
- M1A.24 Drug-induced chronic gout, hand
  - M1A.241 Drug-induced chronic gout, right hand
  - M1A.242 Drug-induced chronic gout, left hand
  - M1A.249 Drug-induced chronic gout, unspecified hand
- M1A.25 Drug-induced chronic gout, hip
  - M1A.251 Drug-induced chronic gout, right hip
  - M1A.252 Drug-induced chronic gout, left hip
  - M1A.259 Drug-induced chronic gout, unspecified hip
- M1A.26 Drug-induced chronic gout, knee
  - M1A.261 Drug-induced chronic gout, right knee
  - M1A.262 Drug-induced chronic gout, left knee
  - M1A.269 Drug-induced chronic gout, unspecified knee
- M1A.27 Drug-induced chronic gout, ankle and foot
  - M1A.271 Drug-induced chronic gout, right ankle and foot
  - M1A.272 Drug-induced chronic gout, left ankle and foot
  - M1A.279 Drug-induced chronic gout, unspecified ankle and foot
- M1A.28 Drug-induced chronic gout, vertebrae
- M1A.29 Drug-induced chronic gout, multiple sites

M1A.3 Chronic gout due to renal impairment

Code first associated renal disease

- M1A.30 Chronic gout due to renal impairment, unspecified site
- M1A.31 Chronic gout due to renal impairment, shoulder
  - M1A.311 Chronic gout due to renal impairment, right shoulder
  - M1A.312 Chronic gout due to renal impairment, left shoulder
  - M1A.319 Chronic gout due to renal impairment, unspecified shoulder
- M1A.32 Chronic gout due to renal impairment, elbow
  - M1A.321 Chronic gout due to renal impairment, right elbow
  - M1A.322 Chronic gout due to renal impairment, left elbow
  - M1A.329 Chronic gout due to renal impairment, unspecified elbow
- M1A.33 Chronic gout due to renal impairment, wrist
  - M1A.331 Chronic gout due to renal impairment, right wrist
  - M1A.332 Chronic gout due to renal impairment, left wrist
  - M1A.339 Chronic gout due to renal impairment, unspecified wrist
- M1A.34 Chronic gout due to renal impairment, hand
  - M1A.341 Chronic gout due to renal impairment, right hand
  - M1A.342 Chronic gout due to renal impairment, left hand
  - M1A.349 Chronic gout due to renal impairment, unspecified hand
- M1A.35 Chronic gout due to renal impairment, hip
  - M1A.351 Chronic gout due to renal impairment, right hip
  - M1A.352 Chronic gout due to renal impairment, left hip

**M1A.359** Chronic gout due to renal impairment, unspecified hip
**M1A.36** Chronic gout due to renal impairment, knee
**M1A.361** Chronic gout due to renal impairment, right knee
**M1A.362** Chronic gout due to renal impairment, left knee
**M1A.369** Chronic gout due to renal impairment, unspecified knee
**M1A.37** Chronic gout due to renal impairment, ankle and foot
**M1A.371** Chronic gout due to renal impairment, right ankle and foot
**M1A.372** Chronic gout due to renal impairment, left ankle and foot
**M1A.379** Chronic gout due to renal impairment, unspecified ankle and foot
**M1A.38** Chronic gout due to renal impairment, vertebrae
**M1A.39** Chronic gout due to renal impairment, multiple sites
**M1A.4** Other secondary chronic gout
Code first associated condition
**M1A.40** Other secondary chronic gout, unspecified site
**M1A.41** Other secondary chronic gout, shoulder
**M1A.411** Other secondary chronic gout, right shoulder
**M1A.412** Other secondary chronic gout, left shoulder
**M1A.419** Other secondary chronic gout, unspecified shoulder
**M1A.42** Other secondary chronic gout, elbow
**M1A.421** Other secondary chronic gout, right elbow
**M1A.422** Other secondary chronic gout, left elbow
**M1A.429** Other secondary chronic gout, unspecified elbow
**M1A.43** Other secondary chronic gout, wrist
**M1A.431** Other secondary chronic gout, right wrist
**M1A.432** Other secondary chronic gout, left wrist
**M1A.439** Other secondary chronic gout, unspecified wrist
**M1A.44** Other secondary chronic gout, hand
**M1A.441** Other secondary chronic gout, right hand
**M1A.442** Other secondary chronic gout, left hand
**M1A.449** Other secondary chronic gout, unspecified hand
**M1A.45** Other secondary chronic gout, hip
**M1A.451** Other secondary chronic gout, right hip
**M1A.452** Other secondary chronic gout, left hip
**M1A.459** Other secondary chronic gout, unspecified hip
**M1A.46** Other secondary chronic gout, knee
**M1A.461** Other secondary chronic gout, right knee
**M1A.462** Other secondary chronic gout, left knee
**M1A.469** Other secondary chronic gout, unspecified knee
**M1A.47** Other secondary chronic gout, ankle and foot
**M1A.471** Other secondary chronic gout, right ankle and foot
**M1A.472** Other secondary chronic gout, left ankle and foot
**M1A.479** Other secondary chronic gout, unspecified ankle and foot
**M1A.48** Other secondary chronic gout, vertebrae
**M1A.49** Other secondary chronic gout, multiple sites
**M1A.9** Chronic gout, unspecified

**M1Ø** **Gout**
Acute gout
Gout attack
Gout flare
Podagra
Use additional code to identify:
autonomic neuropathy in diseases classified elsewhere (G99.Ø)
calculus of urinary tract in diseases classified elsewhere (N22)
cardiomyopathy in diseases classified elsewhere (I43)
disorders of external ear in diseases classified elsewhere (H61.1-, H62.8-)
disorders of iris and ciliary body in diseases classified elsewhere (H22)
glomerular disorders in diseases classified elsewhere (NØ8)
EXCLUDES 2 *chronic gout (M1A.-)*
**DEF:** Purine and pyrimidine metabolic disorders, manifested by hyperuricemia and recurrent acute inflammatory arthritis. Monosodium urate or monohydrate crystals may be deposited in and around the joints, leading to joint destruction and severe crippling.

**M1Ø.Ø** Idiopathic gout
Gouty bursitis
Primary gout
**M1Ø.ØØ** Idiopathic gout, unspecified site
**M1Ø.Ø1** Idiopathic gout, shoulder
**M1Ø.Ø11** Idiopathic gout, right shoulder
**M1Ø.Ø12** Idiopathic gout, left shoulder
**M1Ø.Ø19** Idiopathic gout, unspecified shoulder
**M1Ø.Ø2** Idiopathic gout, elbow
**M1Ø.Ø21** Idiopathic gout, right elbow
**M1Ø.Ø22** Idiopathic gout, left elbow
**M1Ø.Ø29** Idiopathic gout, unspecified elbow
**M1Ø.Ø3** Idiopathic gout, wrist
**M1Ø.Ø31** Idiopathic gout, right wrist
**M1Ø.Ø32** Idiopathic gout, left wrist
**M1Ø.Ø39** Idiopathic gout, unspecified wrist
**M1Ø.Ø4** Idiopathic gout, hand
**M1Ø.Ø41** Idiopathic gout, right hand
**M1Ø.Ø42** Idiopathic gout, left hand
**M1Ø.Ø49** Idiopathic gout, unspecified hand
**M1Ø.Ø5** Idiopathic gout, hip
**M1Ø.Ø51** Idiopathic gout, right hip
**M1Ø.Ø52** Idiopathic gout, left hip
**M1Ø.Ø59** Idiopathic gout, unspecified hip
**M1Ø.Ø6** Idiopathic gout, knee
**M1Ø.Ø61** Idiopathic gout, right knee
**M1Ø.Ø62** Idiopathic gout, left knee
**M1Ø.Ø69** Idiopathic gout, unspecified knee
**M1Ø.Ø7** Idiopathic gout, ankle and foot
**M1Ø.Ø71** Idiopathic gout, right ankle and foot
**M1Ø.Ø72** Idiopathic gout, left ankle and foot
**M1Ø.Ø79** Idiopathic gout, unspecified ankle and foot
**M1Ø.Ø8** Idiopathic gout, vertebrae
**M1Ø.Ø9** Idiopathic gout, multiple sites
**M1Ø.1** Lead-induced gout
Code first toxic effects of lead and its compounds (T56.Ø-)
**M1Ø.1Ø** Lead-induced gout, unspecified site
**M1Ø.11** Lead-induced gout, shoulder
**M1Ø.111** Lead-induced gout, right shoulder
**M1Ø.112** Lead-induced gout, left shoulder
**M1Ø.119** Lead-induced gout, unspecified shoulder
**M1Ø.12** Lead-induced gout, elbow
**M1Ø.121** Lead-induced gout, right elbow
**M1Ø.122** Lead-induced gout, left elbow
**M1Ø.129** Lead-induced gout, unspecified elbow
**M1Ø.13** Lead-induced gout, wrist
**M1Ø.131** Lead-induced gout, right wrist
**M1Ø.132** Lead-induced gout, left wrist
**M1Ø.139** Lead-induced gout, unspecified wrist
**M1Ø.14** Lead-induced gout, hand
**M1Ø.141** Lead-induced gout, right hand
**M1Ø.142** Lead-induced gout, left hand
**M1Ø.149** Lead-induced gout, unspecified hand
**M1Ø.15** Lead-induced gout, hip
**M1Ø.151** Lead-induced gout, right hip
**M1Ø.152** Lead-induced gout, left hip
**M1Ø.159** Lead-induced gout, unspecified hip
**M1Ø.16** Lead-induced gout, knee
**M1Ø.161** Lead-induced gout, right knee
**M1Ø.162** Lead-induced gout, left knee

M10.169 Lead-induced gout, unspecified knee
✓6th M10.17 Lead-induced gout, ankle and foot
M10.171 Lead-induced gout, right ankle and foot
M10.172 Lead-induced gout, left ankle and foot
M10.179 Lead-induced gout, unspecified ankle and foot
M10.18 Lead-induced gout, vertebrae
M10.19 Lead-induced gout, multiple sites
✓5th M10.2 Drug-induced gout
Use additional code for adverse effect, if applicable, to identify drug (T36-T50 with fifth or sixth character 5)
M10.20 Drug-induced gout, unspecified site
✓6th M10.21 Drug-induced gout, shoulder
M10.211 Drug-induced gout, right shoulder
M10.212 Drug-induced gout, left shoulder
M10.219 Drug-induced gout, unspecified shoulder
✓6th M10.22 Drug-induced gout, elbow
M10.221 Drug-induced gout, right elbow
M10.222 Drug-induced gout, left elbow
M10.229 Drug-induced gout, unspecified elbow
✓6th M10.23 Drug-induced gout, wrist
M10.231 Drug-induced gout, right wrist
M10.232 Drug-induced gout, left wrist
M10.239 Drug-induced gout, unspecified wrist
✓6th M10.24 Drug-induced gout, hand
M10.241 Drug-induced gout, right hand
M10.242 Drug-induced gout, left hand
M10.249 Drug-induced gout, unspecified hand
✓6th M10.25 Drug-induced gout, hip
M10.251 Drug-induced gout, right hip
M10.252 Drug-induced gout, left hip
M10.259 Drug-induced gout, unspecified hip
✓6th M10.26 Drug-induced gout, knee
M10.261 Drug-induced gout, right knee
M10.262 Drug-induced gout, left knee
M10.269 Drug-induced gout, unspecified knee
✓6th M10.27 Drug-induced gout, ankle and foot
M10.271 Drug-induced gout, right ankle and foot
M10.272 Drug-induced gout, left ankle and foot
M10.279 Drug-induced gout, unspecified ankle and foot
M10.28 Drug-induced gout, vertebrae
M10.29 Drug-induced gout, multiple sites
✓5th M10.3 Gout due to renal impairment
Code first associated renal disease
M10.30 Gout due to renal impairment, unspecified site
✓6th M10.31 Gout due to renal impairment, shoulder
M10.311 Gout due to renal impairment, right shoulder
M10.312 Gout due to renal impairment, left shoulder
M10.319 Gout due to renal impairment, unspecified shoulder
✓6th M10.32 Gout due to renal impairment, elbow
M10.321 Gout due to renal impairment, right elbow
M10.322 Gout due to renal impairment, left elbow
M10.329 Gout due to renal impairment, unspecified elbow
✓6th M10.33 Gout due to renal impairment, wrist
M10.331 Gout due to renal impairment, right wrist
M10.332 Gout due to renal impairment, left wrist
M10.339 Gout due to renal impairment, unspecified wrist
✓6th M10.34 Gout due to renal impairment, hand
M10.341 Gout due to renal impairment, right hand
M10.342 Gout due to renal impairment, left hand
M10.349 Gout due to renal impairment, unspecified hand
✓6th M10.35 Gout due to renal impairment, hip
M10.351 Gout due to renal impairment, right hip
M10.352 Gout due to renal impairment, left hip
M10.359 Gout due to renal impairment, unspecified hip
✓6th M10.36 Gout due to renal impairment, knee
M10.361 Gout due to renal impairment, right knee
M10.362 Gout due to renal impairment, left knee
M10.369 Gout due to renal impairment, unspecified knee
✓6th M10.37 Gout due to renal impairment, ankle and foot
M10.371 Gout due to renal impairment, right ankle and foot
M10.372 Gout due to renal impairment, left ankle and foot
M10.379 Gout due to renal impairment, unspecified ankle and foot
M10.38 Gout due to renal impairment, vertebrae
M10.39 Gout due to renal impairment, multiple sites
✓5th M10.4 Other secondary gout
Code first associated condition
M10.40 Other secondary gout, unspecified site
✓6th M10.41 Other secondary gout, shoulder
M10.411 Other secondary gout, right shoulder
M10.412 Other secondary gout, left shoulder
M10.419 Other secondary gout, unspecified shoulder
✓6th M10.42 Other secondary gout, elbow
M10.421 Other secondary gout, right elbow
M10.422 Other secondary gout, left elbow
M10.429 Other secondary gout, unspecified elbow
✓6th M10.43 Other secondary gout, wrist
M10.431 Other secondary gout, right wrist
M10.432 Other secondary gout, left wrist
M10.439 Other secondary gout, unspecified wrist
✓6th M10.44 Other secondary gout, hand
M10.441 Other secondary gout, right hand
M10.442 Other secondary gout, left hand
M10.449 Other secondary gout, unspecified hand
✓6th M10.45 Other secondary gout, hip
M10.451 Other secondary gout, right hip
M10.452 Other secondary gout, left hip
M10.459 Other secondary gout, unspecified hip
✓6th M10.46 Other secondary gout, knee
M10.461 Other secondary gout, right knee
M10.462 Other secondary gout, left knee
M10.469 Other secondary gout, unspecified knee
✓6th M10.47 Other secondary gout, ankle and foot
M10.471 Other secondary gout, right ankle and foot
M10.472 Other secondary gout, left ankle and foot
M10.479 Other secondary gout, unspecified ankle and foot
M10.48 Other secondary gout, vertebrae
M10.49 Other secondary gout, multiple sites
M10.9 Gout, unspecified
Gout NOS

✓4th **M11 Other crystal arthropathies**
✓5th M11.0 Hydroxyapatite deposition disease
**DEF:** Disease caused by deposits of calcium phosphate crystals in the soft tissues close to the joint (especially tendons) or in the joints. These calcifications can be mono or polyarticular and can cause destruction of the joint involved.
M11.00 Hydroxyapatite deposition disease, unspecified site
✓6th M11.01 Hydroxyapatite deposition disease, shoulder
M11.011 Hydroxyapatite deposition disease, right shoulder
M11.012 Hydroxyapatite deposition disease, left shoulder
M11.019 Hydroxyapatite deposition disease, unspecified shoulder
✓6th M11.02 Hydroxyapatite deposition disease, elbow
M11.021 Hydroxyapatite deposition disease, right elbow
M11.022 Hydroxyapatite deposition disease, left elbow
M11.029 Hydroxyapatite deposition disease, unspecified elbow
✓6th M11.03 Hydroxyapatite deposition disease, wrist
M11.031 Hydroxyapatite deposition disease, right wrist
M11.032 Hydroxyapatite deposition disease, left wrist
M11.039 Hydroxyapatite deposition disease, unspecified wrist

√6th M11.04 Hydroxyapatite deposition disease, hand
M11.041 Hydroxyapatite deposition disease, right hand
M11.042 Hydroxyapatite deposition disease, left hand
M11.049 Hydroxyapatite deposition disease, unspecified hand
√6th M11.05 Hydroxyapatite deposition disease, hip
M11.051 Hydroxyapatite deposition disease, right hip
M11.052 Hydroxyapatite deposition disease, left hip
M11.059 Hydroxyapatite deposition disease, unspecified hip
√6th M11.06 Hydroxyapatite deposition disease, knee
M11.061 Hydroxyapatite deposition disease, right knee
M11.062 Hydroxyapatite deposition disease, left knee
M11.069 Hydroxyapatite deposition disease, unspecified knee
√6th M11.07 Hydroxyapatite deposition disease, ankle and foot
M11.071 Hydroxyapatite deposition disease, right ankle and foot
M11.072 Hydroxyapatite deposition disease, left ankle and foot
M11.079 Hydroxyapatite deposition disease, unspecified ankle and foot
M11.08 Hydroxyapatite deposition disease, vertebrae
M11.09 Hydroxyapatite deposition disease, multiple sites
√5th M11.1 Familial chondrocalcinosis
M11.10 Familial chondrocalcinosis, unspecified site
√6th M11.11 Familial chondrocalcinosis, shoulder
M11.111 Familial chondrocalcinosis, right shoulder
M11.112 Familial chondrocalcinosis, left shoulder
M11.119 Familial chondrocalcinosis, unspecified shoulder
√6th M11.12 Familial chondrocalcinosis, elbow
M11.121 Familial chondrocalcinosis, right elbow
M11.122 Familial chondrocalcinosis, left elbow
M11.129 Familial chondrocalcinosis, unspecified elbow
√6th M11.13 Familial chondrocalcinosis, wrist
M11.131 Familial chondrocalcinosis, right wrist
M11.132 Familial chondrocalcinosis, left wrist
M11.139 Familial chondrocalcinosis, unspecified wrist
√6th M11.14 Familial chondrocalcinosis, hand
M11.141 Familial chondrocalcinosis, right hand
M11.142 Familial chondrocalcinosis, left hand
M11.149 Familial chondrocalcinosis, unspecified hand
√6th M11.15 Familial chondrocalcinosis, hip
M11.151 Familial chondrocalcinosis, right hip
M11.152 Familial chondrocalcinosis, left hip
M11.159 Familial chondrocalcinosis, unspecified hip
√6th M11.16 Familial chondrocalcinosis, knee
M11.161 Familial chondrocalcinosis, right knee
M11.162 Familial chondrocalcinosis, left knee
M11.169 Familial chondrocalcinosis, unspecified knee
√6th M11.17 Familial chondrocalcinosis, ankle and foot
M11.171 Familial chondrocalcinosis, right ankle and foot
M11.172 Familial chondrocalcinosis, left ankle and foot
M11.179 Familial chondrocalcinosis, unspecified ankle and foot
M11.18 Familial chondrocalcinosis, vertebrae
M11.19 Familial chondrocalcinosis, multiple sites
√5th M11.2 Other chondrocalcinosis
Chondrocalcinosis NOS
**AHA:** 2018,3Q,20
**TIP:** Pseudogout is captured with codes in this subcategory.
M11.20 Other chondrocalcinosis, unspecified site
√6th M11.21 Other chondrocalcinosis, shoulder
M11.211 Other chondrocalcinosis, right shoulder
M11.212 Other chondrocalcinosis, left shoulder
M11.219 Other chondrocalcinosis, unspecified shoulder
√6th M11.22 Other chondrocalcinosis, elbow
M11.221 Other chondrocalcinosis, right elbow
M11.222 Other chondrocalcinosis, left elbow
M11.229 Other chondrocalcinosis, unspecified elbow
√6th M11.23 Other chondrocalcinosis, wrist
M11.231 Other chondrocalcinosis, right wrist
M11.232 Other chondrocalcinosis, left wrist
M11.239 Other chondrocalcinosis, unspecified wrist
√6th M11.24 Other chondrocalcinosis, hand
M11.241 Other chondrocalcinosis, right hand
M11.242 Other chondrocalcinosis, left hand
M11.249 Other chondrocalcinosis, unspecified hand
√6th M11.25 Other chondrocalcinosis, hip
M11.251 Other chondrocalcinosis, right hip
M11.252 Other chondrocalcinosis, left hip
M11.259 Other chondrocalcinosis, unspecified hip
√6th M11.26 Other chondrocalcinosis, knee
M11.261 Other chondrocalcinosis, right knee
M11.262 Other chondrocalcinosis, left knee
M11.269 Other chondrocalcinosis, unspecified knee
√6th M11.27 Other chondrocalcinosis, ankle and foot
M11.271 Other chondrocalcinosis, right ankle and foot
M11.272 Other chondrocalcinosis, left ankle and foot
M11.279 Other chondrocalcinosis, unspecified ankle and foot
M11.28 Other chondrocalcinosis, vertebrae
M11.29 Other chondrocalcinosis, multiple sites
√5th M11.8 Other specified crystal arthropathies
M11.80 Other specified crystal arthropathies, unspecified site
√6th M11.81 Other specified crystal arthropathies, shoulder
M11.811 Other specified crystal arthropathies, right shoulder
M11.812 Other specified crystal arthropathies, left shoulder
M11.819 Other specified crystal arthropathies, unspecified shoulder
√6th M11.82 Other specified crystal arthropathies, elbow
M11.821 Other specified crystal arthropathies, right elbow
M11.822 Other specified crystal arthropathies, left elbow
M11.829 Other specified crystal arthropathies, unspecified elbow
√6th M11.83 Other specified crystal arthropathies, wrist
M11.831 Other specified crystal arthropathies, right wrist
M11.832 Other specified crystal arthropathies, left wrist
M11.839 Other specified crystal arthropathies, unspecified wrist
√6th M11.84 Other specified crystal arthropathies, hand
M11.841 Other specified crystal arthropathies, right hand
M11.842 Other specified crystal arthropathies, left hand
M11.849 Other specified crystal arthropathies, unspecified hand
√6th M11.85 Other specified crystal arthropathies, hip
M11.851 Other specified crystal arthropathies, right hip
M11.852 Other specified crystal arthropathies, left hip
M11.859 Other specified crystal arthropathies, unspecified hip
√6th M11.86 Other specified crystal arthropathies, knee
M11.861 Other specified crystal arthropathies, right knee
M11.862 Other specified crystal arthropathies, left knee
M11.869 Other specified crystal arthropathies, unspecified knee

√6th M11.87 Other specified crystal arthropathies, ankle and foot
- M11.871 Other specified crystal arthropathies, right ankle and foot
- M11.872 Other specified crystal arthropathies, left ankle and foot
- M11.879 Other specified crystal arthropathies, unspecified ankle and foot

M11.88 Other specified crystal arthropathies, vertebrae

M11.89 Other specified crystal arthropathies, multiple sites

M11.9 Crystal arthropathy, unspecified

## √4th M12 Other and unspecified arthropathy

EXCLUDES 1 *arthrosis (M15-M19)*
*cricoarytenoid arthropathy (J38.7)*

### √5th M12.0 Chronic postrheumatic arthropathy [Jaccoud]

M12.00 Chronic postrheumatic arthropathy [Jaccoud], unspecified site HCC Rx ESR COM

√6th M12.01 Chronic postrheumatic arthropathy [Jaccoud], shoulder
- M12.011 Chronic postrheumatic arthropathy [Jaccoud], right shoulder HCC Rx ESR COM
- M12.012 Chronic postrheumatic arthropathy [Jaccoud], left shoulder HCC Rx ESR COM
- M12.019 Chronic postrheumatic arthropathy [Jaccoud], unspecified shoulder HCC Rx ESR COM

√6th M12.02 Chronic postrheumatic arthropathy [Jaccoud], elbow
- M12.021 Chronic postrheumatic arthropathy [Jaccoud], right elbow HCC Rx ESR COM
- M12.022 Chronic postrheumatic arthropathy [Jaccoud], left elbow HCC Rx ESR COM
- M12.029 Chronic postrheumatic arthropathy [Jaccoud], unspecified elbow HCC Rx ESR COM

√6th M12.03 Chronic postrheumatic arthropathy [Jaccoud], wrist
- M12.031 Chronic postrheumatic arthropathy [Jaccoud], right wrist HCC Rx ESR COM
- M12.032 Chronic postrheumatic arthropathy [Jaccoud], left wrist HCC Rx ESR COM
- M12.039 Chronic postrheumatic arthropathy [Jaccoud], unspecified wrist HCC Rx ESR COM

√6th M12.04 Chronic postrheumatic arthropathy [Jaccoud], hand
- M12.041 Chronic postrheumatic arthropathy [Jaccoud], right hand HCC Rx ESR COM
- M12.042 Chronic postrheumatic arthropathy [Jaccoud], left hand HCC Rx ESR COM
- M12.049 Chronic postrheumatic arthropathy [Jaccoud], unspecified hand HCC Rx ESR COM

√6th M12.05 Chronic postrheumatic arthropathy [Jaccoud], hip
- M12.051 Chronic postrheumatic arthropathy [Jaccoud], right hip HCC Rx ESR COM
- M12.052 Chronic postrheumatic arthropathy [Jaccoud], left hip HCC Rx ESR COM
- M12.059 Chronic postrheumatic arthropathy [Jaccoud], unspecified hip HCC Rx ESR COM

√6th M12.06 Chronic postrheumatic arthropathy [Jaccoud], knee
- M12.061 Chronic postrheumatic arthropathy [Jaccoud], right knee HCC Rx ESR COM
- M12.062 Chronic postrheumatic arthropathy [Jaccoud], left knee HCC Rx ESR COM
- M12.069 Chronic postrheumatic arthropathy [Jaccoud], unspecified knee HCC Rx ESR COM

√6th M12.07 Chronic postrheumatic arthropathy [Jaccoud], ankle and foot
- M12.071 Chronic postrheumatic arthropathy [Jaccoud], right ankle and foot HCC Rx ESR COM
- M12.072 Chronic postrheumatic arthropathy [Jaccoud], left ankle and foot HCC Rx ESR COM
- M12.079 Chronic postrheumatic arthropathy [Jaccoud], unspecified ankle and foot HCC Rx ESR COM

M12.08 Chronic postrheumatic arthropathy [Jaccoud], other specified site HCC Rx ESR COM
Chronic postrheumatic arthropathy [Jaccoud], vertebrae

M12.09 Chronic postrheumatic arthropathy [Jaccoud], multiple sites HCC Rx ESR COM

### √5th M12.1 Kaschin-Beck disease

Osteochondroarthrosis deformans endemica

M12.10 Kaschin-Beck disease, unspecified site

√6th M12.11 Kaschin-Beck disease, shoulder
- M12.111 Kaschin-Beck disease, right shoulder
- M12.112 Kaschin-Beck disease, left shoulder
- M12.119 Kaschin-Beck disease, unspecified shoulder

√6th M12.12 Kaschin-Beck disease, elbow
- M12.121 Kaschin-Beck disease, right elbow
- M12.122 Kaschin-Beck disease, left elbow
- M12.129 Kaschin-Beck disease, unspecified elbow

√6th M12.13 Kaschin-Beck disease, wrist
- M12.131 Kaschin-Beck disease, right wrist
- M12.132 Kaschin-Beck disease, left wrist
- M12.139 Kaschin-Beck disease, unspecified wrist

√6th M12.14 Kaschin-Beck disease, hand
- M12.141 Kaschin-Beck disease, right hand
- M12.142 Kaschin-Beck disease, left hand
- M12.149 Kaschin-Beck disease, unspecified hand

√6th M12.15 Kaschin-Beck disease, hip
- M12.151 Kaschin-Beck disease, right hip
- M12.152 Kaschin-Beck disease, left hip
- M12.159 Kaschin-Beck disease, unspecified hip

√6th M12.16 Kaschin-Beck disease, knee
- M12.161 Kaschin-Beck disease, right knee
- M12.162 Kaschin-Beck disease, left knee
- M12.169 Kaschin-Beck disease, unspecified knee

√6th M12.17 Kaschin-Beck disease, ankle and foot
- M12.171 Kaschin-Beck disease, right ankle and foot
- M12.172 Kaschin-Beck disease, left ankle and foot
- M12.179 Kaschin-Beck disease, unspecified ankle and foot

M12.18 Kaschin-Beck disease, vertebrae

M12.19 Kaschin-Beck disease, multiple sites

### √5th M12.2 Villonodular synovitis (pigmented)

M12.20 Villonodular synovitis (pigmented), unspecified site

√6th M12.21 Villonodular synovitis (pigmented), shoulder
- M12.211 Villonodular synovitis (pigmented), right shoulder
- M12.212 Villonodular synovitis (pigmented), left shoulder
- M12.219 Villonodular synovitis (pigmented), unspecified shoulder

√6th M12.22 Villonodular synovitis (pigmented), elbow
- M12.221 Villonodular synovitis (pigmented), right elbow
- M12.222 Villonodular synovitis (pigmented), left elbow
- M12.229 Villonodular synovitis (pigmented), unspecified elbow

√6th M12.23 Villonodular synovitis (pigmented), wrist
- M12.231 Villonodular synovitis (pigmented), right wrist
- M12.232 Villonodular synovitis (pigmented), left wrist
- M12.239 Villonodular synovitis (pigmented), unspecified wrist

√6th M12.24 Villonodular synovitis (pigmented), hand
- M12.241 Villonodular synovitis (pigmented), right hand
- M12.242 Villonodular synovitis (pigmented), left hand
- M12.249 Villonodular synovitis (pigmented), unspecified hand

√6th M12.25 Villonodular synovitis (pigmented), hip
- M12.251 Villonodular synovitis (pigmented), right hip
- M12.252 Villonodular synovitis (pigmented), left hip
- M12.259 Villonodular synovitis (pigmented), unspecified hip

✓6th **M12.26 Villonodular synovitis (pigmented), knee**
- **M12.261 Villonodular synovitis (pigmented), right knee**
- **M12.262 Villonodular synovitis (pigmented), left knee**
- **M12.269 Villonodular synovitis (pigmented), unspecified knee**

✓6th **M12.27 Villonodular synovitis (pigmented), ankle and foot**
- **M12.271 Villonodular synovitis (pigmented), right ankle and foot**
- **M12.272 Villonodular synovitis (pigmented), left ankle and foot**
- **M12.279 Villonodular synovitis (pigmented), unspecified ankle and foot**

**M12.28 Villonodular synovitis (pigmented), other specified site**
Villonodular synovitis (pigmented), vertebrae

**M12.29 Villonodular synovitis (pigmented), multiple sites**

✓5th **M12.3 Palindromic rheumatism**

**DEF:** Sudden and recurring attacks of moderate to severe joint pain and swelling generally occurring in the hands or feet of unknown etiology. After the attack subsides, the joints appear normal again.

**M12.30 Palindromic rheumatism, unspecified site**

✓6th **M12.31 Palindromic rheumatism, shoulder**
- **M12.311 Palindromic rheumatism, right shoulder**
- **M12.312 Palindromic rheumatism, left shoulder**
- **M12.319 Palindromic rheumatism, unspecified shoulder**

✓6th **M12.32 Palindromic rheumatism, elbow**
- **M12.321 Palindromic rheumatism, right elbow**
- **M12.322 Palindromic rheumatism, left elbow**
- **M12.329 Palindromic rheumatism, unspecified elbow**

✓6th **M12.33 Palindromic rheumatism, wrist**
- **M12.331 Palindromic rheumatism, right wrist**
- **M12.332 Palindromic rheumatism, left wrist**
- **M12.339 Palindromic rheumatism, unspecified wrist**

✓6th **M12.34 Palindromic rheumatism, hand**
- **M12.341 Palindromic rheumatism, right hand**
- **M12.342 Palindromic rheumatism, left hand**
- **M12.349 Palindromic rheumatism, unspecified hand**

✓6th **M12.35 Palindromic rheumatism, hip**
- **M12.351 Palindromic rheumatism, right hip**
- **M12.352 Palindromic rheumatism, left hip**
- **M12.359 Palindromic rheumatism, unspecified hip**

✓6th **M12.36 Palindromic rheumatism, knee**
- **M12.361 Palindromic rheumatism, right knee**
- **M12.362 Palindromic rheumatism, left knee**
- **M12.369 Palindromic rheumatism, unspecified knee**

✓6th **M12.37 Palindromic rheumatism, ankle and foot**
- **M12.371 Palindromic rheumatism, right ankle and foot**
- **M12.372 Palindromic rheumatism, left ankle and foot**
- **M12.379 Palindromic rheumatism, unspecified ankle and foot**

**M12.38 Palindromic rheumatism, other specified site**
Palindromic rheumatism, vertebrae

**M12.39 Palindromic rheumatism, multiple sites**

✓5th **M12.4 Intermittent hydrarthrosis**

**M12.40 Intermittent hydrarthrosis, unspecified site**

✓6th **M12.41 Intermittent hydrarthrosis, shoulder**
- **M12.411 Intermittent hydrarthrosis, right shoulder**
- **M12.412 Intermittent hydrarthrosis, left shoulder**
- **M12.419 Intermittent hydrarthrosis, unspecified shoulder**

✓6th **M12.42 Intermittent hydrarthrosis, elbow**
- **M12.421 Intermittent hydrarthrosis, right elbow**
- **M12.422 Intermittent hydrarthrosis, left elbow**
- **M12.429 Intermittent hydrarthrosis, unspecified elbow**

✓6th **M12.43 Intermittent hydrarthrosis, wrist**
- **M12.431 Intermittent hydrarthrosis, right wrist**
- **M12.432 Intermittent hydrarthrosis, left wrist**
- **M12.439 Intermittent hydrarthrosis, unspecified wrist**

✓6th **M12.44 Intermittent hydrarthrosis, hand**
- **M12.441 Intermittent hydrarthrosis, right hand**
- **M12.442 Intermittent hydrarthrosis, left hand**
- **M12.449 Intermittent hydrarthrosis, unspecified hand**

✓6th **M12.45 Intermittent hydrarthrosis, hip**
- **M12.451 Intermittent hydrarthrosis, right hip**
- **M12.452 Intermittent hydrarthrosis, left hip**
- **M12.459 Intermittent hydrarthrosis, unspecified hip**

✓6th **M12.46 Intermittent hydrarthrosis, knee**
- **M12.461 Intermittent hydrarthrosis, right knee**
- **M12.462 Intermittent hydrarthrosis, left knee**
- **M12.469 Intermittent hydrarthrosis, unspecified knee**

✓6th **M12.47 Intermittent hydrarthrosis, ankle and foot**
- **M12.471 Intermittent hydrarthrosis, right ankle and foot**
- **M12.472 Intermittent hydrarthrosis, left ankle and foot**
- **M12.479 Intermittent hydrarthrosis, unspecified ankle and foot**

**M12.48 Intermittent hydrarthrosis, other site**

**M12.49 Intermittent hydrarthrosis, multiple sites**

✓5th **M12.5 Traumatic arthropathy**

**EXCLUDES 1**
*current injury-see Alphabetic Index*
*post-traumatic osteoarthritis of first carpometacarpal joint (M18.2-M18.3)*
*post-traumatic osteoarthritis of hip (M16.4-M16.5)*
*post-traumatic osteoarthritis of knee (M17.2-M17.3)*
*post-traumatic osteoarthritis NOS (M19.1-)*
*post-traumatic osteoarthritis of other single joints (M19.1-)*

**AHA:** 2015,1Q,17

**M12.50 Traumatic arthropathy, unspecified site**

✓6th **M12.51 Traumatic arthropathy, shoulder**
- **M12.511 Traumatic arthropathy, right shoulder**
- **M12.512 Traumatic arthropathy, left shoulder**
- **M12.519 Traumatic arthropathy, unspecified shoulder**

✓6th **M12.52 Traumatic arthropathy, elbow**
- **M12.521 Traumatic arthropathy, right elbow**
- **M12.522 Traumatic arthropathy, left elbow**
- **M12.529 Traumatic arthropathy, unspecified elbow**

✓6th **M12.53 Traumatic arthropathy, wrist**
- **M12.531 Traumatic arthropathy, right wrist**
- **M12.532 Traumatic arthropathy, left wrist**
- **M12.539 Traumatic arthropathy, unspecified wrist**

✓6th **M12.54 Traumatic arthropathy, hand**
- **M12.541 Traumatic arthropathy, right hand**
- **M12.542 Traumatic arthropathy, left hand**
- **M12.549 Traumatic arthropathy, unspecified hand**

✓6th **M12.55 Traumatic arthropathy, hip**
- **M12.551 Traumatic arthropathy, right hip**
- **M12.552 Traumatic arthropathy, left hip**
- **M12.559 Traumatic arthropathy, unspecified hip**

✓6th **M12.56 Traumatic arthropathy, knee**
- **M12.561 Traumatic arthropathy, right knee**
- **M12.562 Traumatic arthropathy, left knee**
- **M12.569 Traumatic arthropathy, unspecified knee**

✓6th **M12.57 Traumatic arthropathy, ankle and foot**
- **M12.571 Traumatic arthropathy, right ankle and foot**
- **M12.572 Traumatic arthropathy, left ankle and foot**
- **M12.579 Traumatic arthropathy, unspecified ankle and foot**

**M12.58 Traumatic arthropathy, other specified site**
Traumatic arthropathy, vertebrae

**M12.59 Traumatic arthropathy, multiple sites**

✓5th **M12.8 Other specific arthropathies, not elsewhere classified**
Transient arthropathy

**M12.80 Other specific arthropathies, not elsewhere classified, unspecified site**

✓6th **M12.81 Other specific arthropathies, not elsewhere classified, shoulder**
- **M12.811 Other specific arthropathies, not elsewhere classified, right shoulder**

M12.812 Other specific arthropathies, not elsewhere classified, left shoulder
M12.819 Other specific arthropathies, not elsewhere classified, unspecified shoulder

M12.82 Other specific arthropathies, not elsewhere classified, elbow
M12.821 Other specific arthropathies, not elsewhere classified, right elbow
M12.822 Other specific arthropathies, not elsewhere classified, left elbow
M12.829 Other specific arthropathies, not elsewhere classified, unspecified elbow

M12.83 Other specific arthropathies, not elsewhere classified, wrist
M12.831 Other specific arthropathies, not elsewhere classified, right wrist
M12.832 Other specific arthropathies, not elsewhere classified, left wrist
M12.839 Other specific arthropathies, not elsewhere classified, unspecified wrist

M12.84 Other specific arthropathies, not elsewhere classified, hand
M12.841 Other specific arthropathies, not elsewhere classified, right hand
M12.842 Other specific arthropathies, not elsewhere classified, left hand
M12.849 Other specific arthropathies, not elsewhere classified, unspecified hand

M12.85 Other specific arthropathies, not elsewhere classified, hip
M12.851 Other specific arthropathies, not elsewhere classified, right hip
M12.852 Other specific arthropathies, not elsewhere classified, left hip
M12.859 Other specific arthropathies, not elsewhere classified, unspecified hip

M12.86 Other specific arthropathies, not elsewhere classified, knee
M12.861 Other specific arthropathies, not elsewhere classified, right knee
M12.862 Other specific arthropathies, not elsewhere classified, left knee
M12.869 Other specific arthropathies, not elsewhere classified, unspecified knee

M12.87 Other specific arthropathies, not elsewhere classified, ankle and foot
M12.871 Other specific arthropathies, not elsewhere classified, right ankle and foot
M12.872 Other specific arthropathies, not elsewhere classified, left ankle and foot
M12.879 Other specific arthropathies, not elsewhere classified, unspecified ankle and foot

M12.88 Other specific arthropathies, not elsewhere classified, other specified site
Other specific arthropathies, not elsewhere classified, vertebrae

M12.89 Other specific arthropathies, not elsewhere classified, multiple sites

M12.9 Arthropathy, unspecified

## M13 Other arthritis

EXCLUDES 1 *arthrosis (M15-M19)*
*osteoarthritis (M15-M19)*

M13.Ø Polyarthritis, unspecified

M13.1 Monoarthritis, not elsewhere classified

M13.1Ø Monoarthritis, not elsewhere classified, unspecified site

M13.11 Monoarthritis, not elsewhere classified, shoulder
M13.111 Monoarthritis, not elsewhere classified, right shoulder
M13.112 Monoarthritis, not elsewhere classified, left shoulder
M13.119 Monoarthritis, not elsewhere classified, unspecified shoulder

M13.12 Monoarthritis, not elsewhere classified, elbow
M13.121 Monoarthritis, not elsewhere classified, right elbow
M13.122 Monoarthritis, not elsewhere classified, left elbow
M13.129 Monoarthritis, not elsewhere classified, unspecified elbow

M13.13 Monoarthritis, not elsewhere classified, wrist
M13.131 Monoarthritis, not elsewhere classified, right wrist
M13.132 Monoarthritis, not elsewhere classified, left wrist
M13.139 Monoarthritis, not elsewhere classified, unspecified wrist

M13.14 Monoarthritis, not elsewhere classified, hand
M13.141 Monoarthritis, not elsewhere classified, right hand
M13.142 Monoarthritis, not elsewhere classified, left hand
M13.149 Monoarthritis, not elsewhere classified, unspecified hand

M13.15 Monoarthritis, not elsewhere classified, hip
M13.151 Monoarthritis, not elsewhere classified, right hip
M13.152 Monoarthritis, not elsewhere classified, left hip
M13.159 Monoarthritis, not elsewhere classified, unspecified hip

M13.16 Monoarthritis, not elsewhere classified, knee
M13.161 Monoarthritis, not elsewhere classified, right knee
M13.162 Monoarthritis, not elsewhere classified, left knee
M13.169 Monoarthritis, not elsewhere classified, unspecified knee

M13.17 Monoarthritis, not elsewhere classified, ankle and foot
M13.171 Monoarthritis, not elsewhere classified, right ankle and foot
M13.172 Monoarthritis, not elsewhere classified, left ankle and foot
M13.179 Monoarthritis, not elsewhere classified, unspecified ankle and foot

M13.8 Other specified arthritis
Allergic arthritis
EXCLUDES 1 *osteoarthritis (M15-M19)*

M13.8Ø Other specified arthritis, unspecified site
AHA: 2025,2Q,9

M13.81 Other specified arthritis, shoulder
M13.811 Other specified arthritis, right shoulder
M13.812 Other specified arthritis, left shoulder
M13.819 Other specified arthritis, unspecified shoulder

M13.82 Other specified arthritis, elbow
M13.821 Other specified arthritis, right elbow
M13.822 Other specified arthritis, left elbow
M13.829 Other specified arthritis, unspecified elbow

M13.83 Other specified arthritis, wrist
M13.831 Other specified arthritis, right wrist
M13.832 Other specified arthritis, left wrist
M13.839 Other specified arthritis, unspecified wrist

M13.84 Other specified arthritis, hand
M13.841 Other specified arthritis, right hand
M13.842 Other specified arthritis, left hand
M13.849 Other specified arthritis, unspecified hand

M13.85 Other specified arthritis, hip
M13.851 Other specified arthritis, right hip
M13.852 Other specified arthritis, left hip
M13.859 Other specified arthritis, unspecified hip

M13.86 Other specified arthritis, knee
M13.861 Other specified arthritis, right knee
M13.862 Other specified arthritis, left knee
M13.869 Other specified arthritis, unspecified knee

M13.87 Other specified arthritis, ankle and foot
M13.871 Other specified arthritis, right ankle and foot
M13.872 Other specified arthritis, left ankle and foot
M13.879 Other specified arthritis, unspecified ankle and foot

M13.88 Other specified arthritis, other site
M13.89 Other specified arthritis, multiple sites
AHA: 2025,2Q,10

**M14 Arthropathies in other diseases classified elsewhere**

EXCLUDES 1 *arthropathy in:*
*enteropathic arthropathies (M07.-)*
*juvenile psoriatic arthropathy (L40.54)*
*lipoid dermatoarthritis (E78.81)*
*diabetes mellitus (E08-E13 with .61-)*
*hematological disorders (M36.2-M36.3)*
*hypersensitivity reactions (M36.4)*
*neoplastic disease (M36.1)*
*neurosyphillis (A52.16)*
*sarcoidosis (D86.86)*

**M14.6 Charcot's joint**
Neuropathic arthropathy
EXCLUDES 1 *Charcôt's joint in diabetes mellitus (E08-E13 with .610)*
*Charcôt's joint in tabes dorsalis (A52.16)*
**DEF:** Progressive neurologic arthropathy in which chronic degeneration of joints in the weight-bearing areas with peripheral hypertrophy occurs as a complication of a neuropathy disorder. Supporting structures relax from a loss of sensation resulting in chronic joint instability.

**M14.60 Charcot's joint, unspecified site**
**M14.61 Charcot's joint, shoulder**
**M14.611 Charcot's joint, right shoulder**
**M14.612 Charcot's joint, left shoulder**
**M14.619 Charcot's joint, unspecified shoulder**
**M14.62 Charcot's joint, elbow**
**M14.621 Charcot's joint, right elbow**
**M14.622 Charcot's joint, left elbow**
**M14.629 Charcot's joint, unspecified elbow**
**M14.63 Charcot's joint, wrist**
**M14.631 Charcot's joint, right wrist**
**M14.632 Charcot's joint, left wrist**
**M14.639 Charcot's joint, unspecified wrist**
**M14.64 Charcot's joint, hand**
**M14.641 Charcot's joint, right hand**
**M14.642 Charcot's joint, left hand**
**M14.649 Charcot's joint, unspecified hand**
**M14.65 Charcot's joint, hip**
**M14.651 Charcot's joint, right hip**
**M14.652 Charcot's joint, left hip**
**M14.659 Charcot's joint, unspecified hip**
**M14.66 Charcot's joint, knee**
**M14.661 Charcot's joint, right knee**
**M14.662 Charcot's joint, left knee**
**M14.669 Charcot's joint, unspecified knee**
**M14.67 Charcot's joint, ankle and foot**
**M14.671 Charcot's joint, right ankle and foot**
**M14.672 Charcot's joint, left ankle and foot**
**M14.679 Charcot's joint, unspecified ankle and foot**
**M14.68 Charcot's joint, vertebrae**
**M14.69 Charcot's joint, multiple sites**

**M14.8 Arthropathies in other specified diseases classified elsewhere**
Code first underlying disease, such as:
amyloidosis (E85.-)
erythema multiforme (L51.-)
erythema nodosum (L52)
hemochromatosis (E83.11-)
hyperparathyroidism (E21.-)
hypothyroidism (E00-E03)
sickle-cell disorders (D57.-)
thyrotoxicosis [hyperthyroidism] (E05.-)
Whipple's disease (K90.81)

***M14.80 Arthropathies in other specified diseases classified elsewhere, unspecified site***
**M14.81 Arthropathies in other specified diseases classified elsewhere, shoulder**
***M14.811 Arthropathies in other specified diseases classified elsewhere, right shoulder***
***M14.812 Arthropathies in other specified diseases classified elsewhere, left shoulder***
***M14.819 Arthropathies in other specified diseases classified elsewhere, unspecified shoulder***
**M14.82 Arthropathies in other specified diseases classified elsewhere, elbow**
***M14.821 Arthropathies in other specified diseases classified elsewhere, right elbow***
***M14.822 Arthropathies in other specified diseases classified elsewhere, left elbow***
***M14.829 Arthropathies in other specified diseases classified elsewhere, unspecified elbow***
**M14.83 Arthropathies in other specified diseases classified elsewhere, wrist**
***M14.831 Arthropathies in other specified diseases classified elsewhere, right wrist***
***M14.832 Arthropathies in other specified diseases classified elsewhere, left wrist***
***M14.839 Arthropathies in other specified diseases classified elsewhere, unspecified wrist***
**M14.84 Arthropathies in other specified diseases classified elsewhere, hand**
***M14.841 Arthropathies in other specified diseases classified elsewhere, right hand***
***M14.842 Arthropathies in other specified diseases classified elsewhere, left hand***
***M14.849 Arthropathies in other specified diseases classified elsewhere, unspecified hand***
**M14.85 Arthropathies in other specified diseases classified elsewhere, hip**
***M14.851 Arthropathies in other specified diseases classified elsewhere, right hip***
***M14.852 Arthropathies in other specified diseases classified elsewhere, left hip***
***M14.859 Arthropathies in other specified diseases classified elsewhere, unspecified hip***
**M14.86 Arthropathies in other specified diseases classified elsewhere, knee**
***M14.861 Arthropathies in other specified diseases classified elsewhere, right knee***
***M14.862 Arthropathies in other specified diseases classified elsewhere, left knee***
***M14.869 Arthropathies in other specified diseases classified elsewhere, unspecified knee***
**M14.87 Arthropathies in other specified diseases classified elsewhere, ankle and foot**
***M14.871 Arthropathies in other specified diseases classified elsewhere, right ankle and foot***
***M14.872 Arthropathies in other specified diseases classified elsewhere, left ankle and foot***
***M14.879 Arthropathies in other specified diseases classified elsewhere, unspecified ankle and foot***
***M14.88 Arthropathies in other specified diseases classified elsewhere, vertebrae***
***M14.89 Arthropathies in other specified diseases classified elsewhere, multiple sites***

## Osteoarthritis (M15-M19)

EXCLUDES 2 *osteoarthritis of spine (M47.-)*
**AHA:** 2020,2Q,14; 2016,4Q,147
**TIP:** Assign a primary osteoarthritis code when the site of the osteoarthritis is documented but the type of osteoarthritis — primary, secondary, generalized, or post-traumatic — is not documented. Primary is considered the default.

**M15 Polyosteoarthritis**
INCLUDES arthritis of multiple sites
EXCLUDES 1 *bilateral involvement of single joint (M16-M19)*

**M15.0 Primary generalized (osteo)arthritis**
**M15.1 Heberden's nodes (with arthropathy)**
Interphalangeal distal osteoarthritis
**M15.2 Bouchard's nodes (with arthropathy)**
Juxtaphalangeal distal osteoarthritis
**M15.3 Secondary multiple arthritis**
Post-traumatic polyosteoarthritis
**M15.4 Erosive (osteo)arthritis**
**M15.8 Other polyosteoarthritis**
**M15.9 Polyosteoarthritis, unspecified**
Generalized osteoarthritis NOS

**M16 Osteoarthritis of hip**
**AHA:** 2016,4Q,146
**M16.0 Bilateral primary osteoarthritis of hip**
**AHA:** 2018,2Q,15
**M16.1 Unilateral primary osteoarthritis of hip**
Primary osteoarthritis of hip NOS
**AHA:** 2018,2Q,15
**M16.10 Unilateral primary osteoarthritis, unspecified hip**
**M16.11 Unilateral primary osteoarthritis, right hip**
**M16.12 Unilateral primary osteoarthritis, left hip**
**M16.2 Bilateral osteoarthritis resulting from hip dysplasia**

✓5th **M16.3 Unilateral osteoarthritis resulting from hip dysplasia**
Dysplastic osteoarthritis of hip NOS
**M16.30 Unilateral osteoarthritis resulting from hip dysplasia, unspecified hip**
**M16.31 Unilateral osteoarthritis resulting from hip dysplasia, right hip**
**M16.32 Unilateral osteoarthritis resulting from hip dysplasia, left hip**
**M16.4 Bilateral post-traumatic osteoarthritis of hip**
✓5th **M16.5 Unilateral post-traumatic osteoarthritis of hip**
Post-traumatic osteoarthritis of hip NOS
**M16.50 Unilateral post-traumatic osteoarthritis, unspecified hip**
**M16.51 Unilateral post-traumatic osteoarthritis, right hip**
**M16.52 Unilateral post-traumatic osteoarthritis, left hip**
**M16.6 Other bilateral secondary osteoarthritis of hip**
**M16.7 Other unilateral secondary osteoarthritis of hip**
Secondary osteoarthritis of hip NOS
**M16.9 Osteoarthritis of hip, unspecified**

✓4th **M17 Osteoarthritis of knee**
AHA: 2016,4Q,146-147
**M17.0 Bilateral primary osteoarthritis of knee**
AHA: 2018,2Q,15
✓5th **M17.1 Unilateral primary osteoarthritis of knee**
Primary osteoarthritis of knee NOS
AHA: 2018,2Q,15
**M17.10 Unilateral primary osteoarthritis, unspecified knee**
**M17.11 Unilateral primary osteoarthritis, right knee**
**M17.12 Unilateral primary osteoarthritis, left knee**
**M17.2 Bilateral post-traumatic osteoarthritis of knee**
✓5th **M17.3 Unilateral post-traumatic osteoarthritis of knee**
Post-traumatic osteoarthritis of knee NOS
**M17.30 Unilateral post-traumatic osteoarthritis, unspecified knee**
**M17.31 Unilateral post-traumatic osteoarthritis, right knee**
**M17.32 Unilateral post-traumatic osteoarthritis, left knee**
**M17.4 Other bilateral secondary osteoarthritis of knee**
**M17.5 Other unilateral secondary osteoarthritis of knee**
Secondary osteoarthritis of knee NOS
**M17.9 Osteoarthritis of knee, unspecified**

✓4th **M18 Osteoarthritis of first carpometacarpal joint**
**M18.0 Bilateral primary osteoarthritis of first carpometacarpal joints**
✓5th **M18.1 Unilateral primary osteoarthritis of first carpometacarpal joint**
Primary osteoarthritis of first carpometacarpal joint NOS
**M18.10 Unilateral primary osteoarthritis of first carpometacarpal joint, unspecified hand**
**M18.11 Unilateral primary osteoarthritis of first carpometacarpal joint, right hand**
**M18.12 Unilateral primary osteoarthritis of first carpometacarpal joint, left hand**
**M18.2 Bilateral post-traumatic osteoarthritis of first carpometacarpal joints**
✓5th **M18.3 Unilateral post-traumatic osteoarthritis of first carpometacarpal joint**
Post-traumatic osteoarthritis of first carpometacarpal joint NOS
**M18.30 Unilateral post-traumatic osteoarthritis of first carpometacarpal joint, unspecified hand**
**M18.31 Unilateral post-traumatic osteoarthritis of first carpometacarpal joint, right hand**
**M18.32 Unilateral post-traumatic osteoarthritis of first carpometacarpal joint, left hand**
**M18.4 Other bilateral secondary osteoarthritis of first carpometacarpal joints**
✓5th **M18.5 Other unilateral secondary osteoarthritis of first carpometacarpal joint**
Secondary osteoarthritis of first carpometacarpal joint NOS
**M18.50 Other unilateral secondary osteoarthritis of first carpometacarpal joint, unspecified hand**
**M18.51 Other unilateral secondary osteoarthritis of first carpometacarpal joint, right hand**
**M18.52 Other unilateral secondary osteoarthritis of first carpometacarpal joint, left hand**
**M18.9 Osteoarthritis of first carpometacarpal joint, unspecified**

✓4th **M19 Other and unspecified osteoarthritis**
EXCLUDES 1 *polyarthritis (M15.-)*
EXCLUDES 2 *arthrosis of spine (M47.-)*
*hallux rigidus (M20.2)*
*osteoarthritis of spine (M47.-)*
AHA: 2020,4Q,31-32
✓5th **M19.0 Primary osteoarthritis of other joints**
AHA: 2018,2Q,15; 2016,4Q,145
✓6th **M19.01 Primary osteoarthritis, shoulder**
**M19.011 Primary osteoarthritis, right shoulder**
**M19.012 Primary osteoarthritis, left shoulder**
**M19.019 Primary osteoarthritis, unspecified shoulder**
✓6th **M19.02 Primary osteoarthritis, elbow**
**M19.021 Primary osteoarthritis, right elbow**
**M19.022 Primary osteoarthritis, left elbow**
**M19.029 Primary osteoarthritis, unspecified elbow**
✓6th **M19.03 Primary osteoarthritis, wrist**
**M19.031 Primary osteoarthritis, right wrist**
**M19.032 Primary osteoarthritis, left wrist**
**M19.039 Primary osteoarthritis, unspecified wrist**
✓6th **M19.04 Primary osteoarthritis, hand**
EXCLUDES 2 *primary osteoarthritis of first carpometacarpal joint (M18.0-, M18.1-)*
**M19.041 Primary osteoarthritis, right hand**
**M19.042 Primary osteoarthritis, left hand**
**M19.049 Primary osteoarthritis, unspecified hand**
✓6th **M19.07 Primary osteoarthritis ankle and foot**
**M19.071 Primary osteoarthritis, right ankle and foot**
**M19.072 Primary osteoarthritis, left ankle and foot**
**M19.079 Primary osteoarthritis, unspecified ankle and foot**
**M19.09 Primary osteoarthritis, other specified site**
✓5th **M19.1 Post-traumatic osteoarthritis of other joints**
✓6th **M19.11 Post-traumatic osteoarthritis, shoulder**
**M19.111 Post-traumatic osteoarthritis, right shoulder**
**M19.112 Post-traumatic osteoarthritis, left shoulder**
**M19.119 Post-traumatic osteoarthritis, unspecified shoulder**
✓6th **M19.12 Post-traumatic osteoarthritis, elbow**
**M19.121 Post-traumatic osteoarthritis, right elbow**
**M19.122 Post-traumatic osteoarthritis, left elbow**
**M19.129 Post-traumatic osteoarthritis, unspecified elbow**
✓6th **M19.13 Post-traumatic osteoarthritis, wrist**
**M19.131 Post-traumatic osteoarthritis, right wrist**
**M19.132 Post-traumatic osteoarthritis, left wrist**
**M19.139 Post-traumatic osteoarthritis, unspecified wrist**
✓6th **M19.14 Post-traumatic osteoarthritis, hand**
EXCLUDES 2 *post-traumatic osteoarthritis of first carpometacarpal joint (M18.2-, M18.3-)*
**M19.141 Post-traumatic osteoarthritis, right hand**
**M19.142 Post-traumatic osteoarthritis, left hand**
**M19.149 Post-traumatic osteoarthritis, unspecified hand**
✓6th **M19.17 Post-traumatic osteoarthritis, ankle and foot**
**M19.171 Post-traumatic osteoarthritis, right ankle and foot**
**M19.172 Post-traumatic osteoarthritis, left ankle and foot**
**M19.179 Post-traumatic osteoarthritis, unspecified ankle and foot**
**M19.19 Post-traumatic osteoarthritis, other specified site**
✓5th **M19.2 Secondary osteoarthritis of other joints**
✓6th **M19.21 Secondary osteoarthritis, shoulder**
**M19.211 Secondary osteoarthritis, right shoulder**
**M19.212 Secondary osteoarthritis, left shoulder**
**M19.219 Secondary osteoarthritis, unspecified shoulder**
✓6th **M19.22 Secondary osteoarthritis, elbow**
**M19.221 Secondary osteoarthritis, right elbow**
**M19.222 Secondary osteoarthritis, left elbow**

**M19.229 Secondary osteoarthritis, unspecified elbow**

6th **M19.23 Secondary osteoarthritis, wrist**

**M19.231 Secondary osteoarthritis, right wrist**

**M19.232 Secondary osteoarthritis, left wrist**

**M19.239 Secondary osteoarthritis, unspecified wrist**

6th **M19.24 Secondary osteoarthritis, hand**

**M19.241 Secondary osteoarthritis, right hand**

**M19.242 Secondary osteoarthritis, left hand**

**M19.249 Secondary osteoarthritis, unspecified hand**

6th **M19.27 Secondary osteoarthritis, ankle and foot**

**M19.271 Secondary osteoarthritis, right ankle and foot**

**M19.272 Secondary osteoarthritis, left ankle and foot**

**M19.279 Secondary osteoarthritis, unspecified ankle and foot**

**M19.29 Secondary osteoarthritis, other specified site**

5th **M19.9 Osteoarthritis, unspecified site**

**TIP:** Assign M19.90 when neither the site nor the type of osteoarthritis — primary, secondary, or post-traumatic — is documented.

**M19.90 Unspecified osteoarthritis, unspecified site**
Arthritis NOS
Arthrosis NOS
Osteoarthritis NOS
**AHA:** 2016,4Q,145-147

**M19.91 Primary osteoarthritis, unspecified site**
Primary osteoarthritis NOS

**M19.92 Post-traumatic osteoarthritis, unspecified site**
Post-traumatic osteoarthritis NOS

**M19.93 Secondary osteoarthritis, unspecified site**
Secondary osteoarthritis NOS

## Other joint disorders (M2Ø-M25)

EXCLUDES 2 *joints of the spine (M4Ø-M54)*

4th **M2Ø Acquired deformities of fingers and toes**

EXCLUDES 1 *acquired absence of fingers and toes (Z89.-)*
*congenital absence of fingers and toes (Q71.3-, Q72.3-)*
*congenital deformities and malformations of fingers and toes (Q66.-, Q68-Q7Ø, Q74.-)*

5th **M2Ø.Ø Deformity of finger(s)**

EXCLUDES 1 *clubbing of fingers (R68.3)*
*palmar fascial fibromatosis [Dupuytren] (M72.Ø)*
*trigger finger (M65.3)*

6th **M2Ø.ØØ Unspecified deformity of finger(s)**

**M2Ø.ØØ1 Unspecified deformity of right finger(s)**

**M2Ø.ØØ2 Unspecified deformity of left finger(s)**

**M2Ø.ØØ9 Unspecified deformity of unspecified finger(s)**

6th **M2Ø.Ø1 Mallet finger**

**M2Ø.Ø11 Mallet finger of right finger(s)**

**M2Ø.Ø12 Mallet finger of left finger(s)**

**M2Ø.Ø19 Mallet finger of unspecified finger(s)**

6th **M2Ø.Ø2 Boutonnière deformity**

**DEF:** Deformity of the finger caused by flexion of the proximal interphalangeal joint and hyperextension of the distal joint. The deformity results from rheumatoid arthritis, osteoarthritis, or injury.

**M2Ø.Ø21 Boutonniere deformity of right finger(s)**

**M2Ø.Ø22 Boutonniere deformity of left finger(s)**

**M2Ø.Ø29 Boutonniere deformity of unspecified finger(s)**

6th **M2Ø.Ø3 Swan-neck deformity**

**DEF:** Flexed distal and hyperextended proximal interphalangeal joint most commonly caused by rheumatoid arthritis.

**M2Ø.Ø31 Swan-neck deformity of right finger(s)**

**M2Ø.Ø32 Swan-neck deformity of left finger(s)**

**M2Ø.Ø39 Swan-neck deformity of unspecified finger(s)**

6th **M2Ø.Ø9 Other deformity of finger(s)**

**M2Ø.Ø91 Other deformity of right finger(s)**

**M2Ø.Ø92 Other deformity of left finger(s)**

**M2Ø.Ø99 Other deformity of finger(s), unspecified finger(s)**

5th **M2Ø.1 Hallux valgus (acquired)**

EXCLUDES 2 *bunion (M21.6-)*

**AHA:** 2016,4Q,38

**DEF:** Deformity in which the great toe deviates toward the other toes and may even be positioned over or under the second toe.

**Hallux Valgus**

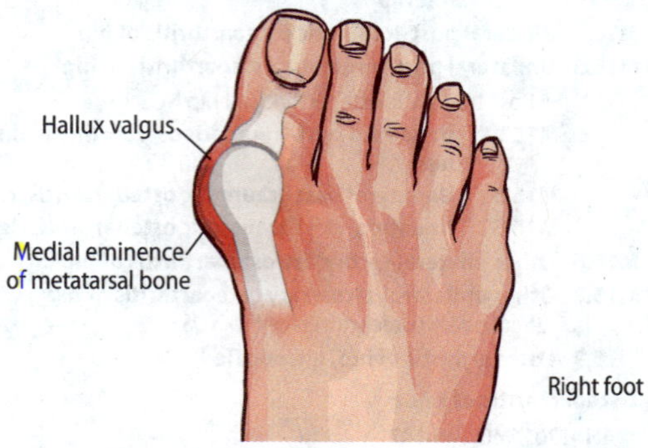


**M2Ø.1Ø Hallux valgus (acquired), unspecified foot**

**M2Ø.11 Hallux valgus (acquired), right foot**

**M2Ø.12 Hallux valgus (acquired), left foot**

5th **M2Ø.2 Hallux rigidus**

**M2Ø.2Ø Hallux rigidus, unspecified foot**

**M2Ø.21 Hallux rigidus, right foot**

**M2Ø.22 Hallux rigidus, left foot**

5th **M2Ø.3 Hallux varus (acquired)**

**DEF:** Deformity in which the great toe deviates away from the other toes.

**M2Ø.3Ø Hallux varus (acquired), unspecified foot**

**M2Ø.31 Hallux varus (acquired), right foot**

**M2Ø.32 Hallux varus (acquired), left foot**

5th **M2Ø.4 Other hammer toe(s) (acquired)**

**M2Ø.4Ø Other hammer toe(s) (acquired), unspecified foot**

**M2Ø.41 Other hammer toe(s) (acquired), right foot**

**M2Ø.42 Other hammer toe(s) (acquired), left foot**

5th **M2Ø.5 Other deformities of toe(s) (acquired)**

6th **M2Ø.5X Other deformities of toe(s) (acquired)**

**M2Ø.5X1 Other deformities of toe(s) (acquired), right foot**

**M2Ø.5X2 Other deformities of toe(s) (acquired), left foot**

**M2Ø.5X9 Other deformities of toe(s) (acquired), unspecified foot**

5th **M2Ø.6 Acquired deformities of toe(s), unspecified**

**M2Ø.6Ø Acquired deformities of toe(s), unspecified, unspecified foot**

**M2Ø.61 Acquired deformities of toe(s), unspecified, right foot**

**M2Ø.62 Acquired deformities of toe(s), unspecified, left foot**

4th **M21 Other acquired deformities of limbs**

EXCLUDES 1 *acquired absence of limb (Z89.-)*
*congenital absence of limbs (Q71-Q73)*
*congenital deformities and malformations of limbs (Q65-Q66, Q68-Q74)*

EXCLUDES 2 *acquired deformities of fingers or toes (M2Ø.-)*
*coxa plana (M91.2)*

5th **M21.Ø Valgus deformity, not elsewhere classified**

EXCLUDES 1 *metatarsus valgus (Q66.6)*
*talipes calcaneovalgus (Q66.4-)*

**M21.ØØ Valgus deformity, not elsewhere classified, unspecified site**

6th **M21.Ø2 Valgus deformity, not elsewhere classified, elbow**
Cubitus valgus

**M21.Ø21 Valgus deformity, not elsewhere classified, right elbow**

**M21.Ø22 Valgus deformity, not elsewhere classified, left elbow**

**M21.Ø29 Valgus deformity, not elsewhere classified, unspecified elbow**

6th **M21.Ø5 Valgus deformity, not elsewhere classified, hip**

**M21.Ø51 Valgus deformity, not elsewhere classified, right hip**

**M21.Ø52 Valgus deformity, not elsewhere classified, left hip**

**M21.Ø59** **Valgus deformity, not elsewhere classified, unspecified hip**

✓6th **M21.Ø6** **Valgus deformity, not elsewhere classified, knee**

Genu valgum
Knock knee
**DEF:** Genu valga/valgum: Condition in which the thighs slant inward, causing the knees to be angled abnormally close together, leaving the space between the ankles wider than normal.

**Genu Valga (knock-knee)**

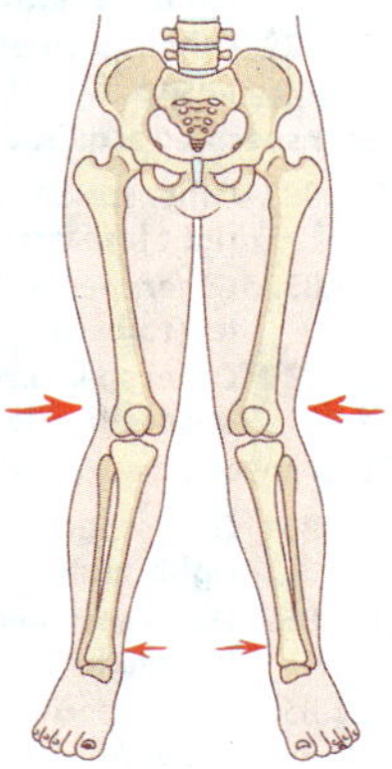

**M21.Ø61** **Valgus deformity, not elsewhere classified, right knee**
**M21.Ø62** **Valgus deformity, not elsewhere classified, left knee**
**M21.Ø69** **Valgus deformity, not elsewhere classified, unspecified knee**

✓6th **M21.Ø7** **Valgus deformity, not elsewhere classified, ankle**

**M21.Ø71** **Valgus deformity, not elsewhere classified, right ankle**
**M21.Ø72** **Valgus deformity, not elsewhere classified, left ankle**
**M21.Ø79** **Valgus deformity, not elsewhere classified, unspecified ankle**

✓5th **M21.1** **Varus deformity, not elsewhere classified**

EXCLUDES 1 *metatarsus varus (Q66.22-)*
*tibia vara (M92.51-)*

**M21.1Ø** **Varus deformity, not elsewhere classified, unspecified site**

✓6th **M21.12** **Varus deformity, not elsewhere classified, elbow**

Cubitus varus, elbow

**M21.121** **Varus deformity, not elsewhere classified, right elbow**
**M21.122** **Varus deformity, not elsewhere classified, left elbow**
**M21.129** **Varus deformity, not elsewhere classified, unspecified elbow**

✓6th **M21.15** **Varus deformity, not elsewhere classified, hip**

**M21.151** **Varus deformity, not elsewhere classified, right hip**
**M21.152** **Varus deformity, not elsewhere classified, left hip**
**M21.159** **Varus deformity, not elsewhere classified, unspecified hip**

✓6th **M21.16** **Varus deformity, not elsewhere classified, knee**

Bow leg
Genu varum
**DEF:** Genu varus/varum: Condition in which the thighs and/or legs are bowed in an outward curve with an abnormally increased space between the knees.

**Genu Varus (bowleg)**

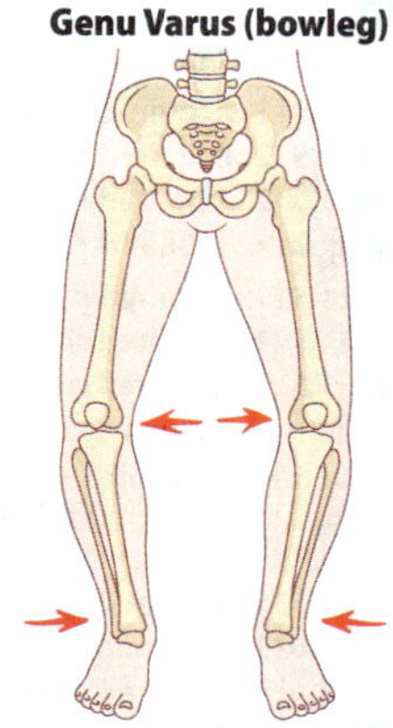

**M21.161** **Varus deformity, not elsewhere classified, right knee**
**M21.162** **Varus deformity, not elsewhere classified, left knee**
**M21.169** **Varus deformity, not elsewhere classified, unspecified knee**

✓6th **M21.17** **Varus deformity, not elsewhere classified, ankle**

**M21.171** **Varus deformity, not elsewhere classified, right ankle**
**M21.172** **Varus deformity, not elsewhere classified, left ankle**
**M21.179** **Varus deformity, not elsewhere classified, unspecified ankle**

✓5th **M21.2** **Flexion deformity**

**M21.2Ø** **Flexion deformity, unspecified site**

✓6th **M21.21** **Flexion deformity, shoulder**

**M21.211** **Flexion deformity, right shoulder**
**M21.212** **Flexion deformity, left shoulder**
**M21.219** **Flexion deformity, unspecified shoulder**

✓6th **M21.22** **Flexion deformity, elbow**

**M21.221** **Flexion deformity, right elbow**
**M21.222** **Flexion deformity, left elbow**
**M21.229** **Flexion deformity, unspecified elbow**

✓6th **M21.23** **Flexion deformity, wrist**

**M21.231** **Flexion deformity, right wrist**
**M21.232** **Flexion deformity, left wrist**
**M21.239** **Flexion deformity, unspecified wrist**

✓6th **M21.24** **Flexion deformity, finger joints**

**M21.241** **Flexion deformity, right finger joints**
**M21.242** **Flexion deformity, left finger joints**
**M21.249** **Flexion deformity, unspecified finger joints**

✓6th **M21.25** **Flexion deformity, hip**

**M21.251** **Flexion deformity, right hip**
**M21.252** **Flexion deformity, left hip**
**M21.259** **Flexion deformity, unspecified hip**

✓6th **M21.26** **Flexion deformity, knee**

**M21.261** **Flexion deformity, right knee**
**M21.262** **Flexion deformity, left knee**
**M21.269** **Flexion deformity, unspecified knee**

✓6th **M21.27** **Flexion deformity, ankle and toes**

**M21.271** **Flexion deformity, right ankle and toes**
**M21.272** **Flexion deformity, left ankle and toes**
**M21.279** **Flexion deformity, unspecified ankle and toes**

✓5th **M21.3** **Wrist or foot drop (acquired)**

✓6th **M21.33** **Wrist drop (acquired)**

**M21.331** **Wrist drop, right wrist**
**M21.332** **Wrist drop, left wrist**
**M21.339** **Wrist drop, unspecified wrist**

✓6th **M21.37** **Foot drop (acquired)**

**M21.371** **Foot drop, right foot**
**M21.372** **Foot drop, left foot**
**M21.379** **Foot drop, unspecified foot**

√5th M21.4 Flat foot [pes planus] (acquired)
EXCLUDES 1 *congenital pes planus (Q66.5-)*
M21.40 Flat foot [pes planus] (acquired), unspecified foot
M21.41 Flat foot [pes planus] (acquired), right foot
M21.42 Flat foot [pes planus] (acquired), left foot

√5th M21.5 Acquired clawhand, clubhand, clawfoot and clubfoot
EXCLUDES 1 *clubfoot, not specified as acquired (Q66.89)*

√6th M21.51 Acquired clawhand
M21.511 Acquired clawhand, right hand
M21.512 Acquired clawhand, left hand
M21.519 Acquired clawhand, unspecified hand

√6th M21.52 Acquired clubhand
M21.521 Acquired clubhand, right hand
M21.522 Acquired clubhand, left hand
M21.529 Acquired clubhand, unspecified hand

√6th M21.53 Acquired clawfoot
DEF: High foot arch with hyperextended toes at the metatarsophalangeal joint and flexed toes at the distal joints.
M21.531 Acquired clawfoot, right foot
M21.532 Acquired clawfoot, left foot
M21.539 Acquired clawfoot, unspecified foot

√6th M21.54 Acquired clubfoot
DEF: Acquired anomaly of the foot with the heel elevated and rotated outward and the toes pointing inward.
M21.541 Acquired clubfoot, right foot
M21.542 Acquired clubfoot, left foot
M21.549 Acquired clubfoot, unspecified foot

√5th M21.6 Other acquired deformities of foot
EXCLUDES 2 *deformities of toe (acquired) (M20.1-M20.6-)*
AHA: 2016,4Q,38

√6th M21.61 Bunion
M21.611 Bunion of right foot
M21.612 Bunion of left foot
M21.619 Bunion of unspecified foot

√6th M21.62 Bunionette
M21.621 Bunionette of right foot
M21.622 Bunionette of left foot
M21.629 Bunionette of unspecified foot

√6th M21.6X Other acquired deformities of foot
AHA: 2023,3Q,20
M21.6X1 Other acquired deformities of right foot
M21.6X2 Other acquired deformities of left foot
M21.6X9 Other acquired deformities of unspecified foot

√5th M21.7 Unequal limb length (acquired)
NOTE The site used should correspond to the shorter limb
M21.70 Unequal limb length (acquired), unspecified site

√6th M21.72 Unequal limb length (acquired), humerus
M21.721 Unequal limb length (acquired), right humerus
M21.722 Unequal limb length (acquired), left humerus
M21.729 Unequal limb length (acquired), unspecified humerus

√6th M21.73 Unequal limb length (acquired), ulna and radius
M21.731 Unequal limb length (acquired), right ulna
M21.732 Unequal limb length (acquired), left ulna
M21.733 Unequal limb length (acquired), right radius
M21.734 Unequal limb length (acquired), left radius
M21.739 Unequal limb length (acquired), unspecified ulna and radius

√6th M21.75 Unequal limb length (acquired), femur
M21.751 Unequal limb length (acquired), right femur
M21.752 Unequal limb length (acquired), left femur
M21.759 Unequal limb length (acquired), unspecified femur

√6th M21.76 Unequal limb length (acquired), tibia and fibula
M21.761 Unequal limb length (acquired), right tibia
M21.762 Unequal limb length (acquired), left tibia
M21.763 Unequal limb length (acquired), right fibula
M21.764 Unequal limb length (acquired), left fibula
M21.769 Unequal limb length (acquired), unspecified tibia and fibula

√5th M21.8 Other specified acquired deformities of limbs
EXCLUDES 2 *coxa plana (M91.2)*
M21.80 Other specified acquired deformities of unspecified limb

√6th M21.82 Other specified acquired deformities of upper arm
M21.821 Other specified acquired deformities of right upper arm
M21.822 Other specified acquired deformities of left upper arm
M21.829 Other specified acquired deformities of unspecified upper arm

√6th M21.83 Other specified acquired deformities of forearm
M21.831 Other specified acquired deformities of right forearm
M21.832 Other specified acquired deformities of left forearm
M21.839 Other specified acquired deformities of unspecified forearm

√6th M21.85 Other specified acquired deformities of thigh
M21.851 Other specified acquired deformities of right thigh
M21.852 Other specified acquired deformities of left thigh
M21.859 Other specified acquired deformities of unspecified thigh

√6th M21.86 Other specified acquired deformities of lower leg
M21.861 Other specified acquired deformities of right lower leg
M21.862 Other specified acquired deformities of left lower leg
M21.869 Other specified acquired deformities of unspecified lower leg

√5th M21.9 Unspecified acquired deformity of limb and hand
M21.90 Unspecified acquired deformity of unspecified limb

√6th M21.92 Unspecified acquired deformity of upper arm
M21.921 Unspecified acquired deformity of right upper arm
M21.922 Unspecified acquired deformity of left upper arm
M21.929 Unspecified acquired deformity of unspecified upper arm

√6th M21.93 Unspecified acquired deformity of forearm
M21.931 Unspecified acquired deformity of right forearm
M21.932 Unspecified acquired deformity of left forearm
M21.939 Unspecified acquired deformity of unspecified forearm

√6th M21.94 Unspecified acquired deformity of hand
M21.941 Unspecified acquired deformity of hand, right hand
M21.942 Unspecified acquired deformity of hand, left hand
M21.949 Unspecified acquired deformity of hand, unspecified hand

√6th M21.95 Unspecified acquired deformity of thigh
M21.951 Unspecified acquired deformity of right thigh
M21.952 Unspecified acquired deformity of left thigh
M21.959 Unspecified acquired deformity of unspecified thigh

√6th M21.96 Unspecified acquired deformity of lower leg
M21.961 Unspecified acquired deformity of right lower leg
M21.962 Unspecified acquired deformity of left lower leg
M21.969 Unspecified acquired deformity of unspecified lower leg

√4th **M22 Disorder of patella**
EXCLUDES 2 *traumatic dislocation of patella (S83.0-)*

√5th M22.0 Recurrent dislocation of patella
AHA: 2026,2Q,3
M22.00 Recurrent dislocation of patella, unspecified knee
M22.01 Recurrent dislocation of patella, right knee
M22.02 Recurrent dislocation of patella, left knee

✓5th **M22.1 Recurrent subluxation of patella**
Incomplete dislocation of patella
**M22.1Ø Recurrent subluxation of patella, unspecified knee**
**M22.11 Recurrent subluxation of patella, right knee**
**M22.12 Recurrent subluxation of patella, left knee**

✓5th **M22.2 Patellofemoral disorders**
✓6th **M22.2X Patellofemoral disorders**
**M22.2X1 Patellofemoral disorders, right knee**
**M22.2X2 Patellofemoral disorders, left knee**
**M22.2X9 Patellofemoral disorders, unspecified knee**

✓5th **M22.3 Other derangements of patella**
✓6th **M22.3X Other derangements of patella**
**M22.3X1 Other derangements of patella, right knee**
**M22.3X2 Other derangements of patella, left knee**
**M22.3X9 Other derangements of patella, unspecified knee**

✓5th **M22.4 Chondromalacia patellae**
**M22.4Ø Chondromalacia patellae, unspecified knee**
**M22.41 Chondromalacia patellae, right knee**
**M22.42 Chondromalacia patellae, left knee**

✓5th **M22.8 Other disorders of patella**
✓6th **M22.8X Other disorders of patella**
**M22.8X1 Other disorders of patella, right knee**
**M22.8X2 Other disorders of patella, left knee**
**M22.8X9 Other disorders of patella, unspecified knee**

✓5th **M22.9 Unspecified disorder of patella**
**M22.9Ø Unspecified disorder of patella, unspecified knee**
**M22.91 Unspecified disorder of patella, right knee**
**M22.92 Unspecified disorder of patella, left knee**

✓4th **M23 Internal derangement of knee**
EXCLUDES 1 *ankylosis (M24.66)*
*deformity of knee (M21.-)*
*osteochondritis dissecans (M93.2)*
EXCLUDES 2 *current injury - see injury of knee and lower leg (S8Ø-S89)*
*recurrent dislocation or subluxation of joints (M24.4)*
*recurrent dislocation or subluxation of patella (M22.Ø-M22.1)*

✓5th **M23.Ø Cystic meniscus**
✓6th **M23.ØØ Cystic meniscus, unspecified meniscus**
Cystic meniscus, unspecified lateral meniscus
Cystic meniscus, unspecified medial meniscus
**M23.ØØØ Cystic meniscus, unspecified lateral meniscus, right knee**
**M23.ØØ1 Cystic meniscus, unspecified lateral meniscus, left knee**
**M23.ØØ2 Cystic meniscus, unspecified lateral meniscus, unspecified knee**
**M23.ØØ3 Cystic meniscus, unspecified medial meniscus, right knee**
**M23.ØØ4 Cystic meniscus, unspecified medial meniscus, left knee**
**M23.ØØ5 Cystic meniscus, unspecified medial meniscus, unspecified knee**
**M23.ØØ6 Cystic meniscus, unspecified meniscus, right knee**
**M23.ØØ7 Cystic meniscus, unspecified meniscus, left knee**
**M23.ØØ9 Cystic meniscus, unspecified meniscus, unspecified knee**

✓6th **M23.Ø1 Cystic meniscus, anterior horn of medial meniscus**
**M23.Ø11 Cystic meniscus, anterior horn of medial meniscus, right knee**
**M23.Ø12 Cystic meniscus, anterior horn of medial meniscus, left knee**
**M23.Ø19 Cystic meniscus, anterior horn of medial meniscus, unspecified knee**

✓6th **M23.Ø2 Cystic meniscus, posterior horn of medial meniscus**
**M23.Ø21 Cystic meniscus, posterior horn of medial meniscus, right knee**
**M23.Ø22 Cystic meniscus, posterior horn of medial meniscus, left knee**
**M23.Ø29 Cystic meniscus, posterior horn of medial meniscus, unspecified knee**

✓6th **M23.Ø3 Cystic meniscus, other medial meniscus**
**M23.Ø31 Cystic meniscus, other medial meniscus, right knee**
**M23.Ø32 Cystic meniscus, other medial meniscus, left knee**
**M23.Ø39 Cystic meniscus, other medial meniscus, unspecified knee**

✓6th **M23.Ø4 Cystic meniscus, anterior horn of lateral meniscus**
**M23.Ø41 Cystic meniscus, anterior horn of lateral meniscus, right knee**
**M23.Ø42 Cystic meniscus, anterior horn of lateral meniscus, left knee**
**M23.Ø49 Cystic meniscus, anterior horn of lateral meniscus, unspecified knee**

✓6th **M23.Ø5 Cystic meniscus, posterior horn of lateral meniscus**
**M23.Ø51 Cystic meniscus, posterior horn of lateral meniscus, right knee**
**M23.Ø52 Cystic meniscus, posterior horn of lateral meniscus, left knee**
**M23.Ø59 Cystic meniscus, posterior horn of lateral meniscus, unspecified knee**

✓6th **M23.Ø6 Cystic meniscus, other lateral meniscus**
**M23.Ø61 Cystic meniscus, other lateral meniscus, right knee**
**M23.Ø62 Cystic meniscus, other lateral meniscus, left knee**
**M23.Ø69 Cystic meniscus, other lateral meniscus, unspecified knee**

✓5th **M23.2 Derangement of meniscus due to old tear or injury**
Old bucket-handle tear
**AHA:** 2019,2Q,26

**Derangement of Meniscus**

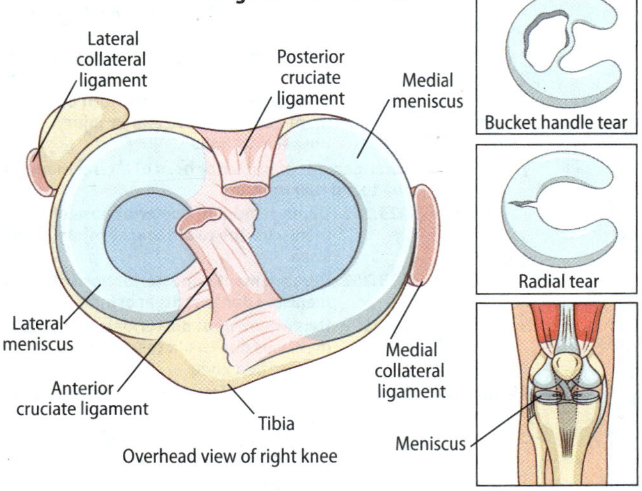


✓6th **M23.2Ø Derangement of unspecified meniscus due to old tear or injury**
Derangement of unspecified lateral meniscus due to old tear or injury
Derangement of unspecified medial meniscus due to old tear or injury
**M23.2ØØ Derangement of unspecified lateral meniscus due to old tear or injury, right knee**
**M23.2Ø1 Derangement of unspecified lateral meniscus due to old tear or injury, left knee**
**M23.2Ø2 Derangement of unspecified lateral meniscus due to old tear or injury, unspecified knee**
**M23.2Ø3 Derangement of unspecified medial meniscus due to old tear or injury, right knee**
**M23.2Ø4 Derangement of unspecified medial meniscus due to old tear or injury, left knee**
**M23.2Ø5 Derangement of unspecified medial meniscus due to old tear or injury, unspecified knee**
**M23.2Ø6 Derangement of unspecified meniscus due to old tear or injury, right knee**
**M23.2Ø7 Derangement of unspecified meniscus due to old tear or injury, left knee**
**M23.2Ø9 Derangement of unspecified meniscus due to old tear or injury, unspecified knee**

√6th M23.21 Derangement of anterior horn of medial meniscus due to old tear or injury
M23.211 Derangement of anterior horn of medial meniscus due to old tear or injury, right knee
M23.212 Derangement of anterior horn of medial meniscus due to old tear or injury, left knee
M23.219 Derangement of anterior horn of medial meniscus due to old tear or injury, unspecified knee

√6th M23.22 Derangement of posterior horn of medial meniscus due to old tear or injury
M23.221 Derangement of posterior horn of medial meniscus due to old tear or injury, right knee
M23.222 Derangement of posterior horn of medial meniscus due to old tear or injury, left knee
M23.229 Derangement of posterior horn of medial meniscus due to old tear or injury, unspecified knee

√6th M23.23 Derangement of other medial meniscus due to old tear or injury
M23.231 Derangement of other medial meniscus due to old tear or injury, right knee
M23.232 Derangement of other medial meniscus due to old tear or injury, left knee
M23.239 Derangement of other medial meniscus due to old tear or injury, unspecified knee

√6th M23.24 Derangement of anterior horn of lateral meniscus due to old tear or injury
M23.241 Derangement of anterior horn of lateral meniscus due to old tear or injury, right knee
M23.242 Derangement of anterior horn of lateral meniscus due to old tear or injury, left knee
M23.249 Derangement of anterior horn of lateral meniscus due to old tear or injury, unspecified knee

√6th M23.25 Derangement of posterior horn of lateral meniscus due to old tear or injury
M23.251 Derangement of posterior horn of lateral meniscus due to old tear or injury, right knee
M23.252 Derangement of posterior horn of lateral meniscus due to old tear or injury, left knee
M23.259 Derangement of posterior horn of lateral meniscus due to old tear or injury, unspecified knee

√6th M23.26 Derangement of other lateral meniscus due to old tear or injury
M23.261 Derangement of other lateral meniscus due to old tear or injury, right knee
M23.262 Derangement of other lateral meniscus due to old tear or injury, left knee
M23.269 Derangement of other lateral meniscus due to old tear or injury, unspecified knee

√5th M23.3 Other meniscus derangements
Degenerate meniscus
Detached meniscus
Retained meniscus

√6th M23.30 Other meniscus derangements, unspecified meniscus
Other meniscus derangements, unspecified lateral meniscus
Other meniscus derangements, unspecified medial meniscus
M23.300 Other meniscus derangements, unspecified lateral meniscus, right knee
M23.301 Other meniscus derangements, unspecified lateral meniscus, left knee
M23.302 Other meniscus derangements, unspecified lateral meniscus, unspecified knee
M23.303 Other meniscus derangements, unspecified medial meniscus, right knee
M23.304 Other meniscus derangements, unspecified medial meniscus, left knee
M23.305 Other meniscus derangements, unspecified medial meniscus, unspecified knee
M23.306 Other meniscus derangements, unspecified meniscus, right knee
M23.307 Other meniscus derangements, unspecified meniscus, left knee
M23.309 Other meniscus derangements, unspecified meniscus, unspecified knee

√6th M23.31 Other meniscus derangements, anterior horn of medial meniscus
M23.311 Other meniscus derangements, anterior horn of medial meniscus, right knee
M23.312 Other meniscus derangements, anterior horn of medial meniscus, left knee
M23.319 Other meniscus derangements, anterior horn of medial meniscus, unspecified knee

√6th M23.32 Other meniscus derangements, posterior horn of medial meniscus
M23.321 Other meniscus derangements, posterior horn of medial meniscus, right knee
M23.322 Other meniscus derangements, posterior horn of medial meniscus, left knee
M23.329 Other meniscus derangements, posterior horn of medial meniscus, unspecified knee

√6th M23.33 Other meniscus derangements, other medial meniscus
M23.331 Other meniscus derangements, other medial meniscus, right knee
M23.332 Other meniscus derangements, other medial meniscus, left knee
M23.339 Other meniscus derangements, other medial meniscus, unspecified knee

√6th M23.34 Other meniscus derangements, anterior horn of lateral meniscus
M23.341 Other meniscus derangements, anterior horn of lateral meniscus, right knee
M23.342 Other meniscus derangements, anterior horn of lateral meniscus, left knee
M23.349 Other meniscus derangements, anterior horn of lateral meniscus, unspecified knee

√6th M23.35 Other meniscus derangements, posterior horn of lateral meniscus
M23.351 Other meniscus derangements, posterior horn of lateral meniscus, right knee
M23.352 Other meniscus derangements, posterior horn of lateral meniscus, left knee
M23.359 Other meniscus derangements, posterior horn of lateral meniscus, unspecified knee

√6th M23.36 Other meniscus derangements, other lateral meniscus
M23.361 Other meniscus derangements, other lateral meniscus, right knee
M23.362 Other meniscus derangements, other lateral meniscus, left knee
M23.369 Other meniscus derangements, other lateral meniscus, unspecified knee

√5th M23.4 Loose body in knee
M23.40 Loose body in knee, unspecified knee
M23.41 Loose body in knee, right knee
M23.42 Loose body in knee, left knee

√5th M23.5 Chronic instability of knee
M23.50 Chronic instability of knee, unspecified knee
M23.51 Chronic instability of knee, right knee
M23.52 Chronic instability of knee, left knee

√5th M23.6 Other spontaneous disruption of ligament(s) of knee

√6th M23.60 Other spontaneous disruption of unspecified ligament of knee
M23.601 Other spontaneous disruption of unspecified ligament of right knee
M23.602 Other spontaneous disruption of unspecified ligament of left knee
M23.609 Other spontaneous disruption of unspecified ligament of unspecified knee

√6th M23.61 Other spontaneous disruption of anterior cruciate ligament of knee
M23.611 Other spontaneous disruption of anterior cruciate ligament of right knee
M23.612 Other spontaneous disruption of anterior cruciate ligament of left knee
M23.619 Other spontaneous disruption of anterior cruciate ligament of unspecified knee

√6th M23.62 Other spontaneous disruption of posterior cruciate ligament of knee
M23.621 Other spontaneous disruption of posterior cruciate ligament of right knee
M23.622 Other spontaneous disruption of posterior cruciate ligament of left knee
M23.629 Other spontaneous disruption of posterior cruciate ligament of unspecified knee

✓6th M23.63 Other spontaneous disruption of medial collateral ligament of knee
M23.631 Other spontaneous disruption of medial collateral ligament of right knee
M23.632 Other spontaneous disruption of medial collateral ligament of left knee
M23.639 Other spontaneous disruption of medial collateral ligament of unspecified knee
✓6th M23.64 Other spontaneous disruption of lateral collateral ligament of knee
M23.641 Other spontaneous disruption of lateral collateral ligament of right knee
M23.642 Other spontaneous disruption of lateral collateral ligament of left knee
M23.649 Other spontaneous disruption of lateral collateral ligament of unspecified knee
✓6th M23.67 Other spontaneous disruption of capsular ligament of knee
M23.671 Other spontaneous disruption of capsular ligament of right knee
M23.672 Other spontaneous disruption of capsular ligament of left knee
M23.679 Other spontaneous disruption of capsular ligament of unspecified knee
✓5th M23.8 Other internal derangements of knee
Laxity of ligament of knee
Snapping knee
✓6th M23.8X Other internal derangements of knee
M23.8X1 Other internal derangements of right knee
M23.8X2 Other internal derangements of left knee
M23.8X9 Other internal derangements of unspecified knee
✓5th M23.9 Unspecified internal derangement of knee
M23.90 Unspecified internal derangement of unspecified knee
M23.91 Unspecified internal derangement of right knee
M23.92 Unspecified internal derangement of left knee

✓4th **M24 Other specific joint derangements**
EXCLUDES 1 *current injury - see injury of joint by body region*
EXCLUDES 2 *ganglion (M67.4)*
*snapping knee (M23.8-)*
*temporomandibular joint disorders (M26.6-)*
AHA: 2020,4Q,31-32
✓5th M24.0 Loose body in joint
EXCLUDES 2 *loose body in knee (M23.4)*
M24.00 Loose body in unspecified joint
✓6th M24.01 Loose body in shoulder
M24.011 Loose body in right shoulder
M24.012 Loose body in left shoulder
M24.019 Loose body in unspecified shoulder
✓6th M24.02 Loose body in elbow
M24.021 Loose body in right elbow
M24.022 Loose body in left elbow
M24.029 Loose body in unspecified elbow
✓6th M24.03 Loose body in wrist
M24.031 Loose body in right wrist
M24.032 Loose body in left wrist
M24.039 Loose body in unspecified wrist
✓6th M24.04 Loose body in finger joints
M24.041 Loose body in right finger joint(s)
M24.042 Loose body in left finger joint(s)
M24.049 Loose body in unspecified finger joint(s)
✓6th M24.05 Loose body in hip
M24.051 Loose body in right hip
M24.052 Loose body in left hip
M24.059 Loose body in unspecified hip
✓6th M24.07 Loose body in ankle and toe joints
M24.071 Loose body in right ankle
M24.072 Loose body in left ankle
M24.073 Loose body in unspecified ankle
M24.074 Loose body in right toe joint(s)
M24.075 Loose body in left toe joint(s)
M24.076 Loose body in unspecified toe joint(s)
M24.08 Loose body, other site
✓5th M24.1 Other articular cartilage disorders
EXCLUDES 2 *chondrocalcinosis (M11.1-, M11.2-)*
*internal derangement of knee (M23.-)*
*metastatic calcification (E83.59)*
*ochronosis (E70.29)*
M24.10 Other articular cartilage disorders, unspecified site
✓6th M24.11 Other articular cartilage disorders, shoulder
M24.111 Other articular cartilage disorders, right shoulder
M24.112 Other articular cartilage disorders, left shoulder
M24.119 Other articular cartilage disorders, unspecified shoulder
✓6th M24.12 Other articular cartilage disorders, elbow
M24.121 Other articular cartilage disorders, right elbow
M24.122 Other articular cartilage disorders, left elbow
M24.129 Other articular cartilage disorders, unspecified elbow
✓6th M24.13 Other articular cartilage disorders, wrist
M24.131 Other articular cartilage disorders, right wrist
M24.132 Other articular cartilage disorders, left wrist
M24.139 Other articular cartilage disorders, unspecified wrist
✓6th M24.14 Other articular cartilage disorders, hand
M24.141 Other articular cartilage disorders, right hand
M24.142 Other articular cartilage disorders, left hand
M24.149 Other articular cartilage disorders, unspecified hand
✓6th M24.15 Other articular cartilage disorders, hip
M24.151 Other articular cartilage disorders, right hip
M24.152 Other articular cartilage disorders, left hip
M24.159 Other articular cartilage disorders, unspecified hip
✓6th M24.17 Other articular cartilage disorders, ankle and foot
M24.171 Other articular cartilage disorders, right ankle
M24.172 Other articular cartilage disorders, left ankle
M24.173 Other articular cartilage disorders, unspecified ankle
M24.174 Other articular cartilage disorders, right foot
M24.175 Other articular cartilage disorders, left foot
M24.176 Other articular cartilage disorders, unspecified foot
M24.19 Other articular cartilage disorders, other specified site
✓5th M24.2 Disorder of ligament
Instability secondary to old ligament injury
Ligamentous laxity NOS
EXCLUDES 1 *familial ligamentous laxity (M35.7)*
EXCLUDES 2 *internal derangement of knee (M23.5-M23.8X9)*
M24.20 Disorder of ligament, unspecified site
✓6th M24.21 Disorder of ligament, shoulder
M24.211 Disorder of ligament, right shoulder
M24.212 Disorder of ligament, left shoulder
M24.219 Disorder of ligament, unspecified shoulder
✓6th M24.22 Disorder of ligament, elbow
M24.221 Disorder of ligament, right elbow
M24.222 Disorder of ligament, left elbow
M24.229 Disorder of ligament, unspecified elbow
✓6th M24.23 Disorder of ligament, wrist
M24.231 Disorder of ligament, right wrist
M24.232 Disorder of ligament, left wrist
M24.239 Disorder of ligament, unspecified wrist
✓6th M24.24 Disorder of ligament, hand
M24.241 Disorder of ligament, right hand
M24.242 Disorder of ligament, left hand
M24.249 Disorder of ligament, unspecified hand
✓6th M24.25 Disorder of ligament, hip
M24.251 Disorder of ligament, right hip

M24.252 Disorder of ligament, left hip
M24.259 Disorder of ligament, unspecified hip
√6th M24.27 Disorder of ligament, ankle and foot
M24.271 Disorder of ligament, right ankle
M24.272 Disorder of ligament, left ankle
M24.273 Disorder of ligament, unspecified ankle
M24.274 Disorder of ligament, right foot
M24.275 Disorder of ligament, left foot
M24.276 Disorder of ligament, unspecified foot
M24.28 Disorder of ligament, vertebrae
AHA: 2023,2Q,13
M24.29 Disorder of ligament, other specified site
√5th M24.3 Pathological dislocation of joint, not elsewhere classified
EXCLUDES 1 *congenital dislocation or displacement of joint - see congenital malformations and deformations of the musculoskeletal system (Q65-Q79)*
*current injury - see injury of joints and ligaments by body region*
*recurrent dislocation of joint (M24.4-)*
M24.3Ø Pathological dislocation of unspecified joint, not elsewhere classified
√6th M24.31 Pathological dislocation of shoulder, not elsewhere classified
M24.311 Pathological dislocation of right shoulder, not elsewhere classified
M24.312 Pathological dislocation of left shoulder, not elsewhere classified
M24.319 Pathological dislocation of unspecified shoulder, not elsewhere classified
√6th M24.32 Pathological dislocation of elbow, not elsewhere classified
M24.321 Pathological dislocation of right elbow, not elsewhere classified
M24.322 Pathological dislocation of left elbow, not elsewhere classified
M24.329 Pathological dislocation of unspecified elbow, not elsewhere classified
√6th M24.33 Pathological dislocation of wrist, not elsewhere classified
M24.331 Pathological dislocation of right wrist, not elsewhere classified
M24.332 Pathological dislocation of left wrist, not elsewhere classified
M24.339 Pathological dislocation of unspecified wrist, not elsewhere classified
√6th M24.34 Pathological dislocation of hand, not elsewhere classified
M24.341 Pathological dislocation of right hand, not elsewhere classified
M24.342 Pathological dislocation of left hand, not elsewhere classified
M24.349 Pathological dislocation of unspecified hand, not elsewhere classified
√6th M24.35 Pathological dislocation of hip, not elsewhere classified
AHA: 2022,1Q,32
M24.351 Pathological dislocation of right hip, not elsewhere classified
M24.352 Pathological dislocation of left hip, not elsewhere classified
M24.359 Pathological dislocation of unspecified hip, not elsewhere classified
√6th M24.36 Pathological dislocation of knee, not elsewhere classified
M24.361 Pathological dislocation of right knee, not elsewhere classified
M24.362 Pathological dislocation of left knee, not elsewhere classified
M24.369 Pathological dislocation of unspecified knee, not elsewhere classified
√6th M24.37 Pathological dislocation of ankle and foot, not elsewhere classified
M24.371 Pathological dislocation of right ankle, not elsewhere classified
M24.372 Pathological dislocation of left ankle, not elsewhere classified
M24.373 Pathological dislocation of unspecified ankle, not elsewhere classified
M24.374 Pathological dislocation of right foot, not elsewhere classified
M24.375 Pathological dislocation of left foot, not elsewhere classified
M24.376 Pathological dislocation of unspecified foot, not elsewhere classified
M24.39 Pathological dislocation of other specified joint, not elsewhere classified
√5th M24.4 Recurrent dislocation of joint
Recurrent subluxation of joint
EXCLUDES 2 *recurrent dislocation of patella (M22.Ø-M22.1)*
*recurrent vertebral dislocation (M43.3-, M43.4, M43.5-)*
M24.4Ø Recurrent dislocation, unspecified joint
√6th M24.41 Recurrent dislocation, shoulder
M24.411 Recurrent dislocation, right shoulder
M24.412 Recurrent dislocation, left shoulder
M24.419 Recurrent dislocation, unspecified shoulder
√6th M24.42 Recurrent dislocation, elbow
M24.421 Recurrent dislocation, right elbow
M24.422 Recurrent dislocation, left elbow
M24.429 Recurrent dislocation, unspecified elbow
√6th M24.43 Recurrent dislocation, wrist
M24.431 Recurrent dislocation, right wrist
M24.432 Recurrent dislocation, left wrist
M24.439 Recurrent dislocation, unspecified wrist
√6th M24.44 Recurrent dislocation, hand and finger(s)
M24.441 Recurrent dislocation, right hand
M24.442 Recurrent dislocation, left hand
M24.443 Recurrent dislocation, unspecified hand
M24.444 Recurrent dislocation, right finger
M24.445 Recurrent dislocation, left finger
M24.446 Recurrent dislocation, unspecified finger
√6th M24.45 Recurrent dislocation, hip
M24.451 Recurrent dislocation, right hip
M24.452 Recurrent dislocation, left hip
M24.459 Recurrent dislocation, unspecified hip
√6th M24.46 Recurrent dislocation, knee
M24.461 Recurrent dislocation, right knee
M24.462 Recurrent dislocation, left knee
M24.469 Recurrent dislocation, unspecified knee
√6th M24.47 Recurrent dislocation, ankle, foot and toes
M24.471 Recurrent dislocation, right ankle
M24.472 Recurrent dislocation, left ankle
M24.473 Recurrent dislocation, unspecified ankle
M24.474 Recurrent dislocation, right foot
M24.475 Recurrent dislocation, left foot
M24.476 Recurrent dislocation, unspecified foot
M24.477 Recurrent dislocation, right toe(s)
M24.478 Recurrent dislocation, left toe(s)
M24.479 Recurrent dislocation, unspecified toe(s)
M24.49 Recurrent dislocation, other specified joint
√5th M24.5 Contracture of joint
EXCLUDES 1 *contracture of muscle without contracture of joint (M62.4-)*
*contracture of tendon (sheath) without contracture of joint (M62.4-)*
*Dupuytren's contracture (M72.Ø)*
EXCLUDES 2 *acquired deformities of limbs (M2Ø-M21)*
AHA: 2016,2Q,6
M24.5Ø Contracture, unspecified joint
√6th M24.51 Contracture, shoulder
M24.511 Contracture, right shoulder
M24.512 Contracture, left shoulder
M24.519 Contracture, unspecified shoulder
√6th M24.52 Contracture, elbow
M24.521 Contracture, right elbow
M24.522 Contracture, left elbow
M24.529 Contracture, unspecified elbow
√6th M24.53 Contracture, wrist
M24.531 Contracture, right wrist
M24.532 Contracture, left wrist
M24.539 Contracture, unspecified wrist
√6th M24.54 Contracture, hand
M24.541 Contracture, right hand
M24.542 Contracture, left hand
M24.549 Contracture, unspecified hand
√6th M24.55 Contracture, hip
M24.551 Contracture, right hip
M24.552 Contracture, left hip

M24.559 Contracture, unspecified hip

✓6th M24.56 Contracture, knee

M24.561 Contracture, right knee
M24.562 Contracture, left knee
M24.569 Contracture, unspecified knee

✓6th M24.57 Contracture, ankle and foot

M24.571 Contracture, right ankle
M24.572 Contracture, left ankle
M24.573 Contracture, unspecified ankle
M24.574 Contracture, right foot
M24.575 Contracture, left foot
M24.576 Contracture, unspecified foot

M24.59 Contracture, other specified joint

✓5th **M24.6 Ankylosis of joint**

EXCLUDES 1 *stiffness of joint without ankylosis (M25.6-)*
EXCLUDES 2 *spine (M43.2-)*

**AHA:** 2025,1Q,25

**DEF:** Ankylosis: Abnormal union or fusion of bones in a joint, which is normally moveable.

M24.6Ø Ankylosis, unspecified joint

✓6th M24.61 Ankylosis, shoulder

M24.611 Ankylosis, right shoulder
M24.612 Ankylosis, left shoulder
M24.619 Ankylosis, unspecified shoulder

✓6th M24.62 Ankylosis, elbow

M24.621 Ankylosis, right elbow
M24.622 Ankylosis, left elbow
M24.629 Ankylosis, unspecified elbow

✓6th M24.63 Ankylosis, wrist

M24.631 Ankylosis, right wrist
M24.632 Ankylosis, left wrist
M24.639 Ankylosis, unspecified wrist

✓6th M24.64 Ankylosis, hand

M24.641 Ankylosis, right hand
M24.642 Ankylosis, left hand
M24.649 Ankylosis, unspecified hand

✓6th M24.65 Ankylosis, hip

M24.651 Ankylosis, right hip
M24.652 Ankylosis, left hip
M24.659 Ankylosis, unspecified hip

✓6th M24.66 Ankylosis, knee

M24.661 Ankylosis, right knee
M24.662 Ankylosis, left knee
M24.669 Ankylosis, unspecified knee

✓6th M24.67 Ankylosis, ankle and foot

M24.671 Ankylosis, right ankle
M24.672 Ankylosis, left ankle
M24.673 Ankylosis, unspecified ankle
M24.674 Ankylosis, right foot
M24.675 Ankylosis, left foot
M24.676 Ankylosis, unspecified foot

M24.69 Ankylosis, other specified joint

**M24.7 Protrusio acetabuli**

**DEF:** Intrapelvic protrusion of the acetabulum characterized by the sinking of the floor of the acetabulum, causing the femoral head to protrude. It limits hip movement and is of unknown etiology. ***Synonym(s):*** *Otto's pelvis.*

✓5th **M24.8 Other specific joint derangements, not elsewhere classified**

EXCLUDES 2 *iliotibial band syndrome (M76.3)*

M24.8Ø Other specific joint derangements of unspecified joint, not elsewhere classified

✓6th M24.81 Other specific joint derangements of shoulder, not elsewhere classified

M24.811 Other specific joint derangements of right shoulder, not elsewhere classified
M24.812 Other specific joint derangements of left shoulder, not elsewhere classified
M24.819 Other specific joint derangements of unspecified shoulder, not elsewhere classified

✓6th M24.82 Other specific joint derangements of elbow, not elsewhere classified

M24.821 Other specific joint derangements of right elbow, not elsewhere classified
M24.822 Other specific joint derangements of left elbow, not elsewhere classified
M24.829 Other specific joint derangements of unspecified elbow, not elsewhere classified

✓6th M24.83 Other specific joint derangements of wrist, not elsewhere classified

M24.831 Other specific joint derangements of right wrist, not elsewhere classified
M24.832 Other specific joint derangements of left wrist, not elsewhere classified
M24.839 Other specific joint derangements of unspecified wrist, not elsewhere classified

✓6th M24.84 Other specific joint derangements of hand, not elsewhere classified

M24.841 Other specific joint derangements of right hand, not elsewhere classified
M24.842 Other specific joint derangements of left hand, not elsewhere classified
M24.849 Other specific joint derangements of unspecified hand, not elsewhere classified

✓6th M24.85 Other specific joint derangements of hip, not elsewhere classified

Irritable hip

M24.851 Other specific joint derangements of right hip, not elsewhere classified
M24.852 Other specific joint derangements of left hip, not elsewhere classified
M24.859 Other specific joint derangements of unspecified hip, not elsewhere classified

✓6th M24.87 Other specific joint derangements of ankle and foot, not elsewhere classified

M24.871 Other specific joint derangements of right ankle, not elsewhere classified
M24.872 Other specific joint derangements of left ankle, not elsewhere classified
M24.873 Other specific joint derangements of unspecified ankle, not elsewhere classified
M24.874 Other specific joint derangements of right foot, not elsewhere classified
M24.875 Other specific joint derangements left foot, not elsewhere classified
M24.876 Other specific joint derangements of unspecified foot, not elsewhere classified

M24.89 Other specific joint derangement of other specified joint, not elsewhere classified

M24.9 Joint derangement, unspecified

✓4th **M25 Other joint disorder, not elsewhere classified**

EXCLUDES 2 *abnormality of gait and mobility (R26.-)*
*acquired deformities of limb (M2Ø-M21)*
*calcification of bursa (M71.4-)*
*calcification of shoulder (joint) (M75.3)*
*calcification of tendon (M65.2-)*
*difficulty in walking (R26.2)*
*temporomandibular joint disorder (M26.6-)*

**AHA:** 2020,4Q,31-32

✓5th **M25.Ø Hemarthrosis**

EXCLUDES 1 *current injury - see injury of joint by body region*
*hemophilic arthropathy (M36.2)*

M25.ØØ Hemarthrosis, unspecified joint

✓6th M25.Ø1 Hemarthrosis, shoulder

M25.Ø11 Hemarthrosis, right shoulder
M25.Ø12 Hemarthrosis, left shoulder
M25.Ø19 Hemarthrosis, unspecified shoulder

✓6th M25.Ø2 Hemarthrosis, elbow

M25.Ø21 Hemarthrosis, right elbow
M25.Ø22 Hemarthrosis, left elbow
M25.Ø29 Hemarthrosis, unspecified elbow

✓6th M25.Ø3 Hemarthrosis, wrist

M25.Ø31 Hemarthrosis, right wrist
M25.Ø32 Hemarthrosis, left wrist
M25.Ø39 Hemarthrosis, unspecified wrist

✓6th M25.Ø4 Hemarthrosis, hand

M25.Ø41 Hemarthrosis, right hand
M25.Ø42 Hemarthrosis, left hand
M25.Ø49 Hemarthrosis, unspecified hand

✓6th M25.Ø5 Hemarthrosis, hip

M25.Ø51 Hemarthrosis, right hip
M25.Ø52 Hemarthrosis, left hip
M25.Ø59 Hemarthrosis, unspecified hip

✓6th M25.Ø6 Hemarthrosis, knee

M25.Ø61 Hemarthrosis, right knee
M25.Ø62 Hemarthrosis, left knee
M25.Ø69 Hemarthrosis, unspecified knee

6th M25.07 Hemarthrosis, ankle and foot
M25.071 Hemarthrosis, right ankle
M25.072 Hemarthrosis, left ankle
M25.073 Hemarthrosis, unspecified ankle
M25.074 Hemarthrosis, right foot
M25.075 Hemarthrosis, left foot
M25.076 Hemarthrosis, unspecified foot
M25.08 Hemarthrosis, other specified site
Hemarthrosis, vertebrae

5th M25.1 Fistula of joint
M25.10 Fistula, unspecified joint
6th M25.11 Fistula, shoulder
M25.111 Fistula, right shoulder
M25.112 Fistula, left shoulder
M25.119 Fistula, unspecified shoulder
6th M25.12 Fistula, elbow
M25.121 Fistula, right elbow
M25.122 Fistula, left elbow
M25.129 Fistula, unspecified elbow
6th M25.13 Fistula, wrist
M25.131 Fistula, right wrist
M25.132 Fistula, left wrist
M25.139 Fistula, unspecified wrist
6th M25.14 Fistula, hand
M25.141 Fistula, right hand
M25.142 Fistula, left hand
M25.149 Fistula, unspecified hand
6th M25.15 Fistula, hip
M25.151 Fistula, right hip
M25.152 Fistula, left hip
M25.159 Fistula, unspecified hip
6th M25.16 Fistula, knee
M25.161 Fistula, right knee
M25.162 Fistula, left knee
M25.169 Fistula, unspecified knee
6th M25.17 Fistula, ankle and foot
M25.171 Fistula, right ankle
M25.172 Fistula, left ankle
M25.173 Fistula, unspecified ankle
M25.174 Fistula, right foot
M25.175 Fistula, left foot
M25.176 Fistula, unspecified foot
M25.18 Fistula, other specified site
Fistula, vertebrae

5th M25.2 Flail joint
**DEF:** Hinged joint that exhibits an abnormal or excessive degree of range and mobility.
M25.20 Flail joint, unspecified joint
6th M25.21 Flail joint, shoulder
M25.211 Flail joint, right shoulder
M25.212 Flail joint, left shoulder
M25.219 Flail joint, unspecified shoulder
6th M25.22 Flail joint, elbow
M25.221 Flail joint, right elbow
M25.222 Flail joint, left elbow
M25.229 Flail joint, unspecified elbow
6th M25.23 Flail joint, wrist
M25.231 Flail joint, right wrist
M25.232 Flail joint, left wrist
M25.239 Flail joint, unspecified wrist
6th M25.24 Flail joint, hand
M25.241 Flail joint, right hand
M25.242 Flail joint, left hand
M25.249 Flail joint, unspecified hand
6th M25.25 Flail joint, hip
M25.251 Flail joint, right hip
M25.252 Flail joint, left hip
M25.259 Flail joint, unspecified hip
6th M25.26 Flail joint, knee
M25.261 Flail joint, right knee
M25.262 Flail joint, left knee
M25.269 Flail joint, unspecified knee
6th M25.27 Flail joint, ankle and foot
M25.271 Flail joint, right ankle and foot
M25.272 Flail joint, left ankle and foot
M25.279 Flail joint, unspecified ankle and foot
M25.28 Flail joint, other site

5th M25.3 Other instability of joint
EXCLUDES 1 *instability of joint secondary to old ligament injury (M24.2-)*
*instability of joint secondary to removal of joint prosthesis (M96.8-)*
EXCLUDES 2 *spinal instabilities (M53.2-)*
M25.30 Other instability, unspecified joint
6th M25.31 Other instability, shoulder
M25.311 Other instability, right shoulder
M25.312 Other instability, left shoulder
M25.319 Other instability, unspecified shoulder
6th M25.32 Other instability, elbow
M25.321 Other instability, right elbow
M25.322 Other instability, left elbow
M25.329 Other instability, unspecified elbow
6th M25.33 Other instability, wrist
M25.331 Other instability, right wrist
M25.332 Other instability, left wrist
M25.339 Other instability, unspecified wrist
6th M25.34 Other instability, hand
M25.341 Other instability, right hand
M25.342 Other instability, left hand
M25.349 Other instability, unspecified hand
6th M25.35 Other instability, hip
M25.351 Other instability, right hip
M25.352 Other instability, left hip
M25.359 Other instability, unspecified hip
6th M25.36 Other instability, knee
M25.361 Other instability, right knee
M25.362 Other instability, left knee
M25.369 Other instability, unspecified knee
6th M25.37 Other instability, ankle and foot
M25.371 Other instability, right ankle
M25.372 Other instability, left ankle
M25.373 Other instability, unspecified ankle
M25.374 Other instability, right foot
M25.375 Other instability, left foot
M25.376 Other instability, unspecified foot
M25.39 Other instability, other specified joint

5th M25.4 Effusion of joint
EXCLUDES 1 *hydrarthrosis in yaws (A66.6)*
*intermittent hydrarthrosis (M12.4-)*
*other infective (teno)synovitis (M65.1-)*
M25.40 Effusion, unspecified joint
6th M25.41 Effusion, shoulder
M25.411 Effusion, right shoulder
M25.412 Effusion, left shoulder
M25.419 Effusion, unspecified shoulder
6th M25.42 Effusion, elbow
M25.421 Effusion, right elbow
M25.422 Effusion, left elbow
M25.429 Effusion, unspecified elbow
6th M25.43 Effusion, wrist
M25.431 Effusion, right wrist
M25.432 Effusion, left wrist
M25.439 Effusion, unspecified wrist
6th M25.44 Effusion, hand
M25.441 Effusion, right hand
M25.442 Effusion, left hand
M25.449 Effusion, unspecified hand
6th M25.45 Effusion, hip
M25.451 Effusion, right hip
M25.452 Effusion, left hip
M25.459 Effusion, unspecified hip
6th M25.46 Effusion, knee
M25.461 Effusion, right knee
M25.462 Effusion, left knee
M25.469 Effusion, unspecified knee
6th M25.47 Effusion, ankle and foot
M25.471 Effusion, right ankle
M25.472 Effusion, left ankle
M25.473 Effusion, unspecified ankle
M25.474 Effusion, right foot

M25.475 Effusion, left foot
M25.476 Effusion, unspecified foot
M25.48 Effusion, other site
✓5th M25.5 Pain in joint
EXCLUDES 2 *pain in fingers (M79.64-)*
*pain in foot (M79.67-)*
*pain in hand (M79.64-)*
*pain in limb (M79.6-)*
*pain in toes (M79.67-)*
M25.50 Pain in unspecified joint
✓6th M25.51 Pain in shoulder
M25.511 Pain in right shoulder
M25.512 Pain in left shoulder
M25.519 Pain in unspecified shoulder
✓6th M25.52 Pain in elbow
M25.521 Pain in right elbow
M25.522 Pain in left elbow
M25.529 Pain in unspecified elbow
✓6th M25.53 Pain in wrist
M25.531 Pain in right wrist
M25.532 Pain in left wrist
M25.539 Pain in unspecified wrist
✓6th M25.54 Pain in joints of hand
AHA: 2016,4Q,38
M25.541 Pain in joints of right hand
M25.542 Pain in joints of left hand
M25.549 Pain in joints of unspecified hand
Pain in joints of hand NOS
✓6th M25.55 Pain in hip
M25.551 Pain in right hip
M25.552 Pain in left hip
M25.559 Pain in unspecified hip
✓6th M25.56 Pain in knee
M25.561 Pain in right knee
M25.562 Pain in left knee
M25.569 Pain in unspecified knee
✓6th M25.57 Pain in ankle and joints of foot
M25.571 Pain in right ankle and joints of right foot
M25.572 Pain in left ankle and joints of left foot
M25.579 Pain in unspecified ankle and joints of unspecified foot
M25.59 Pain in other specified joint
✓5th M25.6 Stiffness of joint, not elsewhere classified
EXCLUDES 1 *ankylosis of joint (M24.6-)*
*contracture of joint (M24.5-)*
M25.60 Stiffness of unspecified joint, not elsewhere classified
✓6th M25.61 Stiffness of shoulder, not elsewhere classified
M25.611 Stiffness of right shoulder, not elsewhere classified
M25.612 Stiffness of left shoulder, not elsewhere classified
M25.619 Stiffness of unspecified shoulder, not elsewhere classified
✓6th M25.62 Stiffness of elbow, not elsewhere classified
M25.621 Stiffness of right elbow, not elsewhere classified
M25.622 Stiffness of left elbow, not elsewhere classified
M25.629 Stiffness of unspecified elbow, not elsewhere classified
✓6th M25.63 Stiffness of wrist, not elsewhere classified
M25.631 Stiffness of right wrist, not elsewhere classified
M25.632 Stiffness of left wrist, not elsewhere classified
M25.639 Stiffness of unspecified wrist, not elsewhere classified
✓6th M25.64 Stiffness of hand, not elsewhere classified
M25.641 Stiffness of right hand, not elsewhere classified
M25.642 Stiffness of left hand, not elsewhere classified
M25.649 Stiffness of unspecified hand, not elsewhere classified
✓6th M25.65 Stiffness of hip, not elsewhere classified
M25.651 Stiffness of right hip, not elsewhere classified
M25.652 Stiffness of left hip, not elsewhere classified
M25.659 Stiffness of unspecified hip, not elsewhere classified
✓6th M25.66 Stiffness of knee, not elsewhere classified
M25.661 Stiffness of right knee, not elsewhere classified
M25.662 Stiffness of left knee, not elsewhere classified
M25.669 Stiffness of unspecified knee, not elsewhere classified
✓6th M25.67 Stiffness of ankle and foot, not elsewhere classified
M25.671 Stiffness of right ankle, not elsewhere classified
M25.672 Stiffness of left ankle, not elsewhere classified
M25.673 Stiffness of unspecified ankle, not elsewhere classified
M25.674 Stiffness of right foot, not elsewhere classified
M25.675 Stiffness of left foot, not elsewhere classified
M25.676 Stiffness of unspecified foot, not elsewhere classified
M25.69 Stiffness of other specified joint, not elsewhere classified
✓5th M25.7 Osteophyte
M25.70 Osteophyte, unspecified joint
✓6th M25.71 Osteophyte, shoulder
M25.711 Osteophyte, right shoulder
M25.712 Osteophyte, left shoulder
M25.719 Osteophyte, unspecified shoulder
✓6th M25.72 Osteophyte, elbow
M25.721 Osteophyte, right elbow
M25.722 Osteophyte, left elbow
M25.729 Osteophyte, unspecified elbow
✓6th M25.73 Osteophyte, wrist
M25.731 Osteophyte, right wrist
M25.732 Osteophyte, left wrist
M25.739 Osteophyte, unspecified wrist
✓6th M25.74 Osteophyte, hand
M25.741 Osteophyte, right hand
M25.742 Osteophyte, left hand
M25.749 Osteophyte, unspecified hand
✓6th M25.75 Osteophyte, hip
M25.751 Osteophyte, right hip
M25.752 Osteophyte, left hip
M25.759 Osteophyte, unspecified hip
✓6th M25.76 Osteophyte, knee
M25.761 Osteophyte, right knee
M25.762 Osteophyte, left knee
M25.769 Osteophyte, unspecified knee
✓6th M25.77 Osteophyte, ankle and foot
M25.771 Osteophyte, right ankle
M25.772 Osteophyte, left ankle
M25.773 Osteophyte, unspecified ankle
M25.774 Osteophyte, right foot
M25.775 Osteophyte, left foot
M25.776 Osteophyte, unspecified foot
M25.78 Osteophyte, vertebrae
✓5th M25.8 Other specified joint disorders
M25.80 Other specified joint disorders, unspecified joint
✓6th M25.81 Other specified joint disorders, shoulder
AHA: 2022,3Q,18
M25.811 Other specified joint disorders, right shoulder
M25.812 Other specified joint disorders, left shoulder
M25.819 Other specified joint disorders, unspecified shoulder
✓6th M25.82 Other specified joint disorders, elbow
M25.821 Other specified joint disorders, right elbow
M25.822 Other specified joint disorders, left elbow
M25.829 Other specified joint disorders, unspecified elbow
✓6th M25.83 Other specified joint disorders, wrist
M25.831 Other specified joint disorders, right wrist

M25.832 Other specified joint disorders, left wrist
M25.839 Other specified joint disorders, unspecified wrist
✓6th M25.84 Other specified joint disorders, hand
M25.841 Other specified joint disorders, right hand
M25.842 Other specified joint disorders, left hand
M25.849 Other specified joint disorders, unspecified hand
✓6th M25.85 Other specified joint disorders, hip
AHA: 2014,4Q,25
M25.851 Other specified joint disorders, right hip
M25.852 Other specified joint disorders, left hip
M25.859 Other specified joint disorders, unspecified hip
✓6th M25.86 Other specified joint disorders, knee
M25.861 Other specified joint disorders, right knee
M25.862 Other specified joint disorders, left knee
M25.869 Other specified joint disorders, unspecified knee
✓6th M25.87 Other specified joint disorders, ankle and foot
M25.871 Other specified joint disorders, right ankle and foot
M25.872 Other specified joint disorders, left ankle and foot
M25.879 Other specified joint disorders, unspecified ankle and foot
M25.9 Joint disorder, unspecified

## Dentofacial anomalies [including malocclusion] and other disorders of jaw (M26-M27)

EXCLUDES 1 *hemifacial atrophy or hypertrophy (Q67.4)*
*unilateral condylar hyperplasia or hypoplasia (M27.8)*

✓4th **M26 Dentofacial anomalies [including malocclusion]**
✓5th M26.0 Major anomalies of jaw size
EXCLUDES 1 *acromegaly (E22.0)*
*Robin's syndrome (Q87.0)*
M26.00 Unspecified anomaly of jaw size
M26.01 Maxillary hyperplasia
M26.02 Maxillary hypoplasia
AHA: 2014,3Q,23
M26.03 Mandibular hyperplasia
M26.04 Mandibular hypoplasia
M26.05 Macrogenia
M26.06 Microgenia
M26.07 Excessive tuberosity of jaw
Entire maxillary tuberosity
M26.09 Other specified anomalies of jaw size
✓5th M26.1 Anomalies of jaw-cranial base relationship
M26.10 Unspecified anomaly of jaw-cranial base relationship
M26.11 Maxillary asymmetry
M26.12 Other jaw asymmetry
M26.19 Other specified anomalies of jaw-cranial base relationship
AHA: 2020,1Q,21
✓5th M26.2 Anomalies of dental arch relationship
M26.20 Unspecified anomaly of dental arch relationship
✓6th M26.21 Malocclusion, Angle's class
M26.211 Malocclusion, Angle's class I
Neutro-occlusion
M26.212 Malocclusion, Angle's class II
Disto-occlusion Division I
Disto-occlusion Division II
M26.213 Malocclusion, Angle's class III
Mesio-occlusion
M26.219 Malocclusion, Angle's class, unspecified
✓6th M26.22 Open occlusal relationship
M26.220 Open anterior occlusal relationship
Anterior open bite
M26.221 Open posterior occlusal relationship
Posterior open bite
M26.23 Excessive horizontal overlap
Excessive horizontal overjet
M26.24 Reverse articulation
Crossbite (anterior) (posterior)
M26.25 Anomalies of interarch distance
M26.29 Other anomalies of dental arch relationship
Midline deviation of dental arch
Overbite (excessive) deep
Overbite (excessive) horizontal
Overbite (excessive) vertical
Posterior lingual occlusion of mandibular teeth
✓5th M26.3 Anomalies of tooth position of fully erupted tooth or teeth
EXCLUDES 2 *embedded and impacted teeth (K01.-)*
M26.30 Unspecified anomaly of tooth position of fully erupted tooth or teeth
Abnormal spacing of fully erupted tooth or teeth NOS
Displacement of fully erupted tooth or teeth NOS
Transposition of fully erupted tooth or teeth NOS
M26.31 Crowding of fully erupted teeth
M26.32 Excessive spacing of fully erupted teeth
Diastema of fully erupted tooth or teeth NOS
M26.33 Horizontal displacement of fully erupted tooth or teeth
Tipped tooth or teeth
Tipping of fully erupted tooth
M26.34 Vertical displacement of fully erupted tooth or teeth
Extruded tooth
Infraeruption of tooth or teeth
Supraeruption of tooth or teeth
M26.35 Rotation of fully erupted tooth or teeth
M26.36 Insufficient interocclusal distance of fully erupted teeth (ridge)
Lack of adequate intermaxillary vertical dimension of fully erupted teeth
M26.37 Excessive interocclusal distance of fully erupted teeth
Excessive intermaxillary vertical dimension of fully erupted teeth
Loss of occlusal vertical dimension of fully erupted teeth
M26.39 Other anomalies of tooth position of fully erupted tooth or teeth
M26.4 Malocclusion, unspecified
✓5th M26.5 Dentofacial functional abnormalities
EXCLUDES 1 *bruxism (F45.8)*
*teeth-grinding NOS (F45.8)*
M26.50 Dentofacial functional abnormalities, unspecified
M26.51 Abnormal jaw closure
M26.52 Limited mandibular range of motion
M26.53 Deviation in opening and closing of the mandible
M26.54 Insufficient anterior guidance
Insufficient anterior occlusal guidance
M26.55 Centric occlusion maximum intercuspation discrepancy
EXCLUDES 1 *centric occlusion NOS (M26.59)*
M26.56 Non-working side interference
Balancing side interference
M26.57 Lack of posterior occlusal support
M26.59 Other dentofacial functional abnormalities
Centric occlusion (of teeth) NOS
Malocclusion due to abnormal swallowing
Malocclusion due to mouth breathing
Malocclusion due to tongue, lip or finger habits

**M26.6 Temporomandibular joint disorders**

EXCLUDES 2 *current temporomandibular joint dislocation (S03.0)*
*current temporomandibular joint sprain (S03.4)*

AHA: 2016,4Q,38-39

**Temporomandibular Joint**

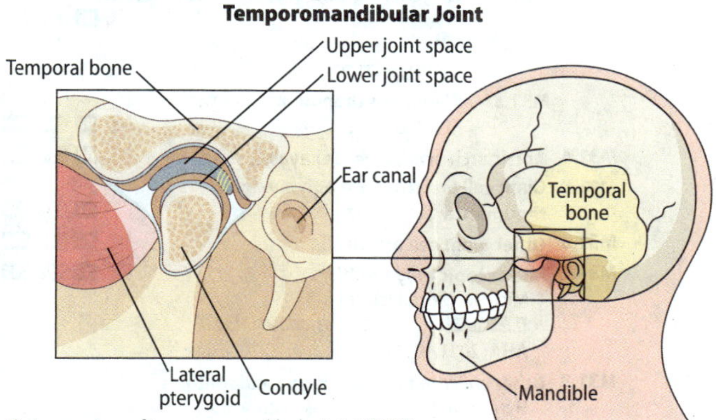


Cutaway view of temporomandibular joint (TMJ)

**M26.60 Temporomandibular joint disorder, unspecified**
- **M26.601 Right temporomandibular joint disorder, unspecified**
- **M26.602 Left temporomandibular joint disorder, unspecified**
- **M26.603 Bilateral temporomandibular joint disorder, unspecified**
- **M26.609 Unspecified temporomandibular joint disorder, unspecified side**
  Temporomandibular joint disorder NOS

**M26.61 Adhesions and ankylosis of temporomandibular joint**
- **M26.611 Adhesions and ankylosis of right temporomandibular joint**
- **M26.612 Adhesions and ankylosis of left temporomandibular joint**
- **M26.613 Adhesions and ankylosis of bilateral temporomandibular joint**
- **M26.619 Adhesions and ankylosis of temporomandibular joint, unspecified side**

**M26.62 Arthralgia of temporomandibular joint**
- **M26.621 Arthralgia of right temporomandibular joint**
- **M26.622 Arthralgia of left temporomandibular joint**
- **M26.623 Arthralgia of bilateral temporomandibular joint**
- **M26.629 Arthralgia of temporomandibular joint, unspecified side**

**M26.63 Articular disc disorder of temporomandibular joint**
- **M26.631 Articular disc disorder of right temporomandibular joint**
- **M26.632 Articular disc disorder of left temporomandibular joint**
- **M26.633 Articular disc disorder of bilateral temporomandibular joint**
- **M26.639 Articular disc disorder of temporomandibular joint, unspecified side**

**M26.64 Arthritis of temporomandibular joint**

AHA: 2020,4Q,32

- **M26.641 Arthritis of right temporomandibular joint**
- **M26.642 Arthritis of left temporomandibular joint**
- **M26.643 Arthritis of bilateral temporomandibular joint**
- **M26.649 Arthritis of unspecified temporomandibular joint**

**M26.65 Arthropathy of temporomandibular joint**

AHA: 2020,4Q,32

- **M26.651 Arthropathy of right temporomandibular joint**
- **M26.652 Arthropathy of left temporomandibular joint**
- **M26.653 Arthropathy of bilateral temporomandibular joint**
- **M26.659 Arthropathy of unspecified temporomandibular joint**

**M26.69 Other specified disorders of temporomandibular joint**

**M26.7 Dental alveolar anomalies**
- **M26.70 Unspecified alveolar anomaly**
- **M26.71 Alveolar maxillary hyperplasia**
- **M26.72 Alveolar mandibular hyperplasia**
- **M26.73 Alveolar maxillary hypoplasia**
- **M26.74 Alveolar mandibular hypoplasia**
- **M26.79 Other specified alveolar anomalies**

**M26.8 Other dentofacial anomalies**
- **M26.81 Anterior soft tissue impingement**
  Anterior soft tissue impingement on teeth
- **M26.82 Posterior soft tissue impingement**
  Posterior soft tissue impingement on teeth
- **M26.89 Other dentofacial anomalies**

**M26.9 Dentofacial anomaly, unspecified**

## M27 Other diseases of jaws

**M27.0 Developmental disorders of jaws**
Latent bone cyst of jaw
Stafne's cyst
Torus mandibularis
Torus palatinus

**M27.1 Giant cell granuloma, central**
Giant cell granuloma NOS
EXCLUDES 1 *peripheral giant cell granuloma (K06.8)*

**M27.2 Inflammatory conditions of jaws**
Osteitis of jaw(s)
Osteomyelitis (neonatal) jaw(s)
Osteoradionecrosis jaw(s)
Periostitis jaw(s)
Sequestrum of jaw bone
Use additional code (W88-W90, X39.0) to identify radiation, if radiation-induced
EXCLUDES 2 *osteonecrosis of jaw due to drug (M87.180)*

**M27.3 Alveolitis of jaws**
Alveolar osteitis
Dry socket

**M27.4 Other and unspecified cysts of jaw**
EXCLUDES 1 *cysts of oral region (K09.-)*
*latent bone cyst of jaw (M27.0)*
*Stafne's cyst (M27.0)*

- **M27.40 Unspecified cyst of jaw**
  Cyst of jaw NOS
- **M27.49 Other cysts of jaw**
  Aneurysmal cyst of jaw
  Hemorrhagic cyst of jaw
  Traumatic cyst of jaw

**M27.5 Periradicular pathology associated with previous endodontic treatment**
- **M27.51 Perforation of root canal space due to endodontic treatment**
- **M27.52 Endodontic overfill**
- **M27.53 Endodontic underfill**
- **M27.59 Other periradicular pathology associated with previous endodontic treatment**

**M27.6 Endosseous dental implant failure**
- **M27.61 Osseointegration failure of dental implant**
  Hemorrhagic complications of dental implant placement
  Iatrogenic osseointegration failure of dental implant
  Osseointegration failure of dental implant due to complications of systemic disease
  Osseointegration failure of dental implant due to poor bone quality
  Pre-integration failure of dental implant NOS
  Pre-osseointegration failure of dental implant
- **M27.62 Post-osseointegration biological failure of dental implant**
  Failure of dental implant due to lack of attached gingiva
  Failure of dental implant due to occlusal trauma (caused by poor prosthetic design)
  Failure of dental implant due to parafunctional habits
  Failure of dental implant due to periodontal infection (peri-implantitis)
  Failure of dental implant due to poor oral hygiene
  Iatrogenic post-osseointegration failure of dental implant
  Post-osseointegration failure of dental implant due to complications of systemic disease

M27.63 **Post-osseointegration mechanical failure of dental implant**
Failure of dental prosthesis causing loss of dental implant
Fracture of dental implant
EXCLUDES 2 *cracked tooth (KØ3.81)*
*fractured dental restorative material with loss of material (KØ8.531)*
*fractured dental restorative material without loss of material (KØ8.53Ø)*
*fractured tooth (SØ2.5)*

M27.69 **Other endosseous dental implant failure**
Dental implant failure NOS

M27.8 **Other specified diseases of jaws**
Cherubism
Exostosis
Fibrous dysplasia
Unilateral condylar hyperplasia
Unilateral condylar hypoplasia
EXCLUDES 1 *jaw pain (R68.84)*

M27.9 **Disease of jaws, unspecified**

## Systemic connective tissue disorders (MØ-M36)

INCLUDES autoimmune disease NOS
collagen (vascular) disease NOS
systemic autoimmune disease
systemic collagen (vascular) disease
EXCLUDES 1 *autoimmune disease, single organ or single cell-type -code to relevant condition category*

✓4th **M3Ø Polyarteritis nodosa and related conditions**
EXCLUDES 1 *microscopic polyarteritis (M31.7)*

M3Ø.Ø **Polyarteritis nodosa** HCC Rx ESR COM

M3Ø.1 **Polyarteritis with lung involvement [Churg-Strauss]** HCC Rx ESR COM
Allergic granulomatous angiitis
Eosinophilic granulomatosis with polyangiitis [EGPA]
AHA: 2021,1Q,23

M3Ø.2 **Juvenile polyarteritis** HCC Rx ESR COM

M3Ø.3 **Mucocutaneous lymph node syndrome [Kawasaki]** HCC Rx ESR COM

M3Ø.8 **Other conditions related to polyarteritis nodosa** HCC Rx ESR COM
Polyangiitis overlap syndrome

✓4th **M31 Other necrotizing vasculopathies**

M31.Ø **Hypersensitivity angiitis** HCC Rx ESR COM
Goodpasture's syndrome

✓5th M31.1 **Thrombotic microangiopathy**
AHA: 2021,4Q,19

M31.1Ø **Thrombotic microangiopathy, unspecified** HCC Rx ESR COM

M31.11 **Hematopoietic stem cell transplantation-associated thrombotic microangiopathy [HSCT-TMA]** HCC Rx ESR COM
Transplant-associated thrombotic microangiopathy [TA-TMA]
Code first if applicable:
complications of bone marrow transplant (T86.Ø-)
complications of stem cell transplant (T86.5)
Use additional code to identify specific organ dysfunction, such as:
acute kidney failure (N17.-)
acute respiratory distress syndrome (J8Ø)
capillary leak syndrome (I78.8)
diffuse alveolar hemorrhage (RØ4.89)
encephalopathy (metabolic) (septic) (G93.41)
fluid overload, unspecified (E87.7Ø)
graft versus host disease (D89.81-)
hemolytic uremic syndrome (D59.3-)
hepatic failure (K72.-)
hepatic veno-occlusive disease (K76.5)
idiopathic interstitial pneumonia (J84.11-)
sinusoidal obstruction syndrome (K76.5)

M31.19 **Other thrombotic microangiopathy** HCC Rx ESR COM
Thrombotic thrombocytopenic purpura

M31.2 **Lethal midline granuloma** HCC Rx ESR COM

✓5th M31.3 **Wegener's granulomatosis**
Granulomatosis with polyangiitis
Necrotizing respiratory granulomatosis
AHA: 2021,1Q,23

M31.3Ø **Wegener's granulomatosis without renal involvement** HCC Rx ESR COM
Wegener's granulomatosis NOS
AHA: 2021,2Q,10

M31.31 **Wegener's granulomatosis with renal involvement** HCC Rx ESR COM

M31.4 **Aortic arch syndrome [Takayasu]** HCC Rx ESR COM

M31.5 **Giant cell arteritis with polymyalgia rheumatica** HCC Rx ESR COM

M31.6 **Other giant cell arteritis** HCC Rx ESR COM

M31.7 **Microscopic polyangiitis** HCC Rx ESR COM
Microscopic polyarteritis
EXCLUDES 1 *polyarteritis nodosa (M3Ø.Ø)*
AHA: 2021,1Q,23

M31.8 **Other specified necrotizing vasculopathies** HCC ESR
Hypocomplementemic vasculitis
Septic vasculitis

M31.9 **Necrotizing vasculopathy, unspecified** HCC ESR

✓4th **M32 Systemic lupus erythematosus (SLE)**
EXCLUDES 1 *lupus erythematosus (discoid) (NOS) (L93.Ø)*
AHA: 2020,4Q,11; 2018,3Q,14
TIP: There is no default code for "lupus NOS." Query the provider for the specific type of lupus in order to assign the appropriate code.

M32.Ø **Drug-induced systemic lupus erythematosus** Rx ESR COM
Use additional code for adverse effect, if applicable, to identify drug (T36-T5Ø with fifth or sixth character 5)

✓5th M32.1 **Systemic lupus erythematosus with organ or system involvement**

M32.1Ø **Systemic lupus erythematosus, organ or system involvement unspecified** HCC Rx ESR COM

M32.11 **Endocarditis in systemic lupus erythematosus** HCC Rx ESR COM
Libman-Sacks disease

M32.12 **Pericarditis in systemic lupus erythematosus** HCC Rx ESR COM
Lupus pericarditis

M32.13 **Lung involvement in systemic lupus erythematosus** HCC Rx ESR COM
Pleural effusion due to systemic lupus erythematosus

M32.14 **Glomerular disease in systemic lupus erythematosus** HCC Rx ESR COM
Lupus renal disease NOS
AHA: 2013,4Q,125

M32.15 **Tubulo-interstitial nephropathy in systemic lupus erythematosus** HCC Rx ESR COM

M32.19 **Other organ or system involvement in systemic lupus erythematosus** HCC Rx ESR COM
Use additional code(s) to identify organ or system involvement, such as encephalitis (GØ5.3)
AHA: 2026,1Q,33

M32.8 **Other forms of systemic lupus erythematosus** HCC Rx ESR COM

M32.9 **Systemic lupus erythematosus, unspecified** HCC Rx ESR COM
SLE NOS
Systemic lupus erythematosus NOS
Systemic lupus erythematosus without organ involvement

✓4th **M33 Dermatopolymyositis**
AHA: 2017,4Q,18

✓5th M33.Ø **Juvenile dermatomyositis**

M33.ØØ **Juvenile dermatomyositis, organ involvement unspecified** HCC Rx ESR COM

M33.Ø1 **Juvenile dermatomyositis with respiratory involvement** HCC Rx ESR COM

M33.Ø2 **Juvenile dermatomyositis with myopathy** HCC Rx ESR COM

M33.Ø3 **Juvenile dermatomyositis without myopathy** HCC Rx ESR COM

M33.Ø9 **Juvenile dermatomyositis with other organ involvement** HCC Rx ESR COM

✓5th M33.1 **Other dermatomyositis**
Adult dermatomyositis

M33.1Ø **Other dermatomyositis, organ involvement unspecified** HCC Rx ESR COM

M33.11 Other dermatomyositis with respiratory involvement HCC Rx ESR COM
M33.12 Other dermatomyositis with myopathy HCC Rx ESR COM
M33.13 Other dermatomyositis without myopathy HCC Rx ESR COM
Dermatomyositis NOS
M33.19 Other dermatomyositis with other organ involvement HCC Rx ESR COM

M33.2 Polymyositis
M33.20 Polymyositis, organ involvement unspecified HCC Rx ESR COM
M33.21 Polymyositis with respiratory involvement HCC Rx ESR COM
M33.22 Polymyositis with myopathy HCC Rx ESR COM
M33.29 Polymyositis with other organ involvement HCC Rx ESR COM

M33.9 Dermatopolymyositis, unspecified
M33.90 Dermatopolymyositis, unspecified, organ involvement unspecified HCC Rx ESR COM
M33.91 Dermatopolymyositis, unspecified with respiratory involvement HCC Rx ESR COM
M33.92 Dermatopolymyositis, unspecified with myopathy HCC Rx ESR COM
M33.93 Dermatopolymyositis, unspecified without myopathy HCC Rx ESR COM
M33.99 Dermatopolymyositis, unspecified with other organ involvement HCC Rx ESR COM

## M34 Systemic sclerosis [scleroderma]
EXCLUDES 1 *circumscribed scleroderma (L94.Ø)*
*neonatal scleroderma (P83.88)*

M34.Ø Progressive systemic sclerosis HCC Rx ESR COM
M34.1 CR(E)ST syndrome HCC Rx ESR COM
Combination of calcinosis, Raynaud's phenomenon, esophageal dysfunction, sclerodactyly, telangiectasia
M34.2 Systemic sclerosis induced by drug and chemical Rx ESR COM
Code first poisoning due to drug or toxin, if applicable (T36-T65 with fifth or sixth character 1-4)
Use additional code for adverse effect, if applicable, to identify drug (T36-T5Ø with fifth or sixth character 5)

M34.8 Other forms of systemic sclerosis
M34.81 Systemic sclerosis with lung involvement HCC Rx ESR COM
Code also if applicable:
other interstitial pulmonary diseases (J84.89)
secondary pulmonary arterial hypertension (I27.21)
M34.82 Systemic sclerosis with myopathy HCC Rx ESR COM
M34.83 Systemic sclerosis with polyneuropathy HCC Rx ESR COM
M34.89 Other systemic sclerosis HCC Rx ESR COM
M34.9 Systemic sclerosis, unspecified HCC Rx ESR COM

## M35 Other systemic involvement of connective tissue
EXCLUDES 1 *reactive perforating collagenosis (L87.1)*

M35.Ø Sjogren syndrome
Sicca syndrome
Use additional code to identify associated manifestations
EXCLUDES 1 *dry mouth, unspecified (R68.2)*
**AHA:** 2024,3Q,16; 2021,4Q,20
**DEF:** Autoimmune disease associated with keratoconjunctivitis, laryngopharyngitis, rhinitis, dry mouth, enlarged parotid gland, and chronic polyarthritis.
M35.ØØ Sjogren syndrome, unspecified Rx ESR COM
M35.Ø1 Sjogren syndrome with keratoconjunctivitis Rx ESR COM
M35.Ø2 Sjogren syndrome with lung involvement HCC Rx ESR COM
M35.Ø3 Sjogren syndrome with myopathy Rx ESR COM
M35.Ø4 Sjogren syndrome with tubulo-interstitial nephropathy Rx ESR COM
Renal tubular acidosis in sicca syndrome
M35.Ø5 Sjogren syndrome with inflammatory arthritis Rx ESR COM
M35.Ø6 Sjogren syndrome with peripheral nervous system involvement Rx ESR COM
M35.Ø7 Sjogren syndrome with central nervous system involvement Rx ESR COM
M35.Ø8 Sjogren syndrome with gastrointestinal involvement Rx ESR COM
M35.ØA Sjogren syndrome with glomerular disease Rx ESR COM
M35.ØB Sjogren syndrome with vasculitis Rx ESR COM
M35.ØC Sjogren syndrome with dental involvement Rx ESR COM
M35.Ø9 Sjogren syndrome with other organ involvement Rx ESR COM

M35.1 Other overlap syndromes Rx ESR COM
Mixed connective tissue disease
EXCLUDES 1 *polyangiitis overlap syndrome (M3Ø.8)*
M35.2 Behcet's disease HCC Rx ESR COM
M35.3 Polymyalgia rheumatica ESR COM
EXCLUDES 1 *polymyalgia rheumatica with giant cell arteritis (M31.5)*
M35.4 Diffuse (eosinophilic) fasciitis
M35.5 Multifocal fibrosclerosis Rx ESR COM
M35.6 Relapsing panniculitis [Weber-Christian]
EXCLUDES 1 *lupus panniculitis (L93.2)*
*panniculitis NOS (M79.3-)*
M35.7 Hypermobility syndrome
Familial ligamentous laxity
EXCLUDES 1 *ligamentous laxity, NOS (M24.2-)*
EXCLUDES 2 *Ehlers-Danlos syndromes (Q79.6-)*

M35.8 Other specified systemic involvement of connective tissue
**AHA:** 2021,1Q,36; 2020,3Q,13-14
M35.81 Multisystem inflammatory syndrome HCC ESR COM
MIS-A
MIS-C
Multisystem inflammatory syndrome in adults
Multisystem inflammatory syndrome in children
Pediatric inflammatory multisystem syndrome
PIMS
Code first, if applicable, COVID-19 (UØ7.1)
Code also any associated complications such as:
acute hepatic failure (K72.Ø-)
acute kidney failure (N17.-)
acute myocarditis (I4Ø.-)
acute respiratory distress syndrome (J8Ø)
cardiac arrhythmia (I47-I49.-)
pneumonia due to COVID-19 (J12.82)
severe sepsis (R65.2-)
viral cardiomyopathy (B33.24)
viral pericarditis (B33.23)
Use additional code, if applicable, for:
exposure to COVID-19 or SARS-CoV-2 infection (Z2Ø.822)
personal history of COVID-19 (Z86.16)
post COVID-19 condition (UØ9.9)
**AHA:** 2021,4Q,102; 2021,1Q,29,36,41
**DEF:** Hyperinflammatory condition that seems to be largely associated with past or present coronavirus disease 2019 (COVID-19) infection. Predominantly occurring in children, with less frequent occurrences in adults, symptoms often include fever, laboratory evidence of inflammation, and evidence of clinically severe illness requiring hospitalization with multisystem (two or more) organ involvement. ***Synonym(s):*** *MIS, MIS-C.*
M35.89 Other specified systemic involvement of connective tissue Rx ESR COM
M35.9 Systemic involvement of connective tissue, unspecified Rx ESR COM
Autoimmune disease (systemic) NOS
Collagen (vascular) disease NOS

## M36 Systemic disorders of connective tissue in diseases classified elsewhere
EXCLUDES 2 *arthropathies in diseases classified elsewhere (M14.-)*
*M36.Ø* *Dermato(poly)myositis in neoplastic disease* HCC Rx ESR COM
Code first underlying neoplasm (CØØ-D49)
*M36.1* *Arthropathy in neoplastic disease*
Code first underlying neoplasm, such as:
leukemia (C91-C95)
malignant histiocytosis (C96.A)
multiple myeloma (C9Ø.Ø)

*M36.2* ***Hemophilic arthropathy***
Hemarthrosis in hemophilic arthropathy
Code first underlying disease, such as:
factor IX deficiency (D67)
factor VIII deficiency (D66)
hemophilia (classical) (D66)
hemophilia B (D67)
hemophilia C (D68.1)
with vascular defect (D68.Ø-)

*M36.3* ***Arthropathy in other blood disorders***
Code first underlying disease, such as:
disease of blood and blood-forming organs, unspecified (D75.9)
other hemoglobinopathies (D58.2)
thalassemia (D56.-)

*M36.4* ***Arthropathy in hypersensitivity reactions classified elsewhere***
Code first underlying disease, such as:
Henoch (-Schonlein) purpura (D69.Ø)
serum sickness (T8Ø.6-)

*M36.8* ***Systemic disorders of connective tissue in other diseases classified elsewhere*** Rx ESR COM
Code first underlying disease, such as:
alkaptonuria (E7Ø.29)
hypogammaglobulinemia (D8Ø.-)
ochronosis (E7Ø.29)

## DORSOPATHIES (M4Ø-M54)

### Deforming dorsopathies (M4Ø-M43)

✓4th **M4Ø Kyphosis and lordosis**
Code first underlying disease
EXCLUDES 1 *congenital kyphosis and lordosis (Q76.4)*
*kyphoscoliosis (M41.-)*
*postprocedural kyphosis and lordosis (M96.-)*

**Kyphosis and Lordosis**

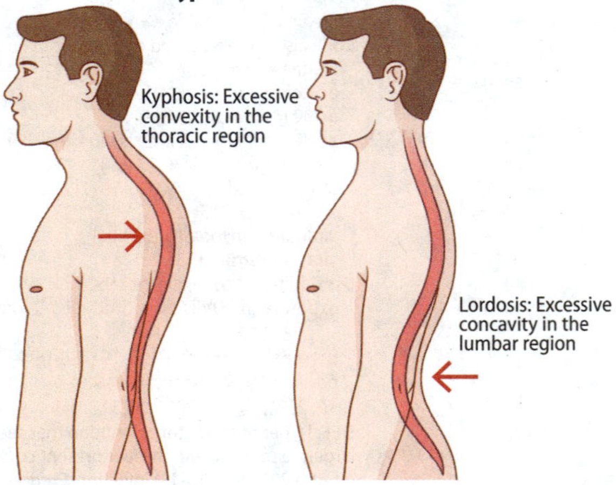


✓5th **M4Ø.Ø Postural kyphosis**
EXCLUDES 1 *osteochondrosis of spine (M42.-)*
**M4Ø.ØØ Postural kyphosis, site unspecified**
**M4Ø.Ø3 Postural kyphosis, cervicothoracic region**
**M4Ø.Ø4 Postural kyphosis, thoracic region**
**M4Ø.Ø5 Postural kyphosis, thoracolumbar region**

✓5th **M4Ø.1 Other secondary kyphosis**
**M4Ø.1Ø Other secondary kyphosis, site unspecified** UPD
**M4Ø.12 Other secondary kyphosis, cervical region** UPD
**M4Ø.13 Other secondary kyphosis, cervicothoracic region** UPD
**M4Ø.14 Other secondary kyphosis, thoracic region** UPD
**M4Ø.15 Other secondary kyphosis, thoracolumbar region** UPD

✓5th **M4Ø.2 Other and unspecified kyphosis**
✓6th **M4Ø.2Ø Unspecified kyphosis**
**M4Ø.2Ø2 Unspecified kyphosis, cervical region**
**M4Ø.2Ø3 Unspecified kyphosis, cervicothoracic region**
**M4Ø.2Ø4 Unspecified kyphosis, thoracic region**
**M4Ø.2Ø5 Unspecified kyphosis, thoracolumbar region**
**M4Ø.2Ø9 Unspecified kyphosis, site unspecified**
✓6th **M4Ø.29 Other kyphosis**
**M4Ø.292 Other kyphosis, cervical region**
**M4Ø.293 Other kyphosis, cervicothoracic region**
**M4Ø.294 Other kyphosis, thoracic region**
**M4Ø.295 Other kyphosis, thoracolumbar region**
**M4Ø.299 Other kyphosis, site unspecified**

✓5th **M4Ø.3 Flatback syndrome**
**M4Ø.3Ø Flatback syndrome, site unspecified**
**M4Ø.35 Flatback syndrome, thoracolumbar region**
**M4Ø.36 Flatback syndrome, lumbar region**
**M4Ø.37 Flatback syndrome, lumbosacral region**

✓5th **M4Ø.4 Postural lordosis**
Acquired lordosis
**M4Ø.4Ø Postural lordosis, site unspecified**
**M4Ø.45 Postural lordosis, thoracolumbar region**
**M4Ø.46 Postural lordosis, lumbar region**
**M4Ø.47 Postural lordosis, lumbosacral region**

✓5th **M4Ø.5 Lordosis, unspecified**
**M4Ø.5Ø Lordosis, unspecified, site unspecified**
**M4Ø.55 Lordosis, unspecified, thoracolumbar region**
**M4Ø.56 Lordosis, unspecified, lumbar region**
**M4Ø.57 Lordosis, unspecified, lumbosacral region**

✓4th **M41 Scoliosis**
INCLUDES kyphoscoliosis
EXCLUDES 1 *congenital scoliosis due to bony malformation (Q76.3)*
*congenital scoliosis NOS (Q67.5)*
*kyphoscoliotic heart disease (I27.1)*
*postural congenital scoliosis (Q67.5)*
EXCLUDES 2 *postprocedural scoliosis (M96.89)*
*postradiation scoliosis (M96.5)*
AHA: 2022,1Q,30

**Scoliosis**

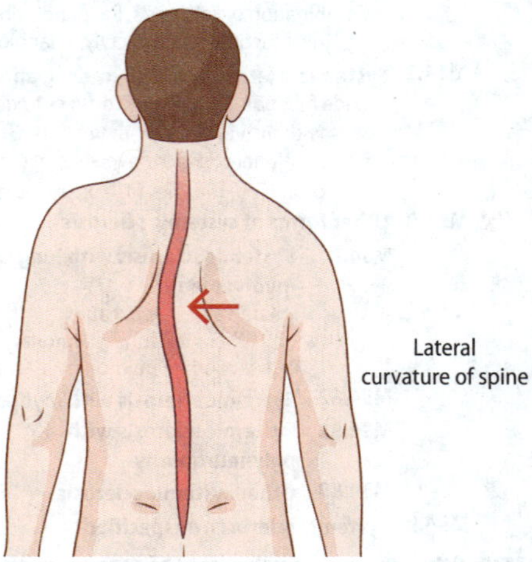


✓5th **M41.Ø Infantile idiopathic scoliosis**
AHA: 2014,4Q,26
**M41.ØØ Infantile idiopathic scoliosis, site unspecified**
**M41.Ø2 Infantile idiopathic scoliosis, cervical region**
**M41.Ø3 Infantile idiopathic scoliosis, cervicothoracic region**
**M41.Ø4 Infantile idiopathic scoliosis, thoracic region**
**M41.Ø5 Infantile idiopathic scoliosis, thoracolumbar region**
**M41.Ø6 Infantile idiopathic scoliosis, lumbar region**
**M41.Ø7 Infantile idiopathic scoliosis, lumbosacral region**
**M41.Ø8 Infantile idiopathic scoliosis, sacral and sacrococcygeal region**

✓5th **M41.1 Juvenile and adolescent idiopathic scoliosis**
✓6th **M41.11 Juvenile idiopathic scoliosis**
AHA: 2014,4Q,28
**M41.112 Juvenile idiopathic scoliosis, cervical region**
**M41.113 Juvenile idiopathic scoliosis, cervicothoracic region**
**M41.114 Juvenile idiopathic scoliosis, thoracic region**
**M41.115 Juvenile idiopathic scoliosis, thoracolumbar region**
**M41.116 Juvenile idiopathic scoliosis, lumbar region**

M41.117 Juvenile idiopathic scoliosis, lumbosacral region

M41.119 Juvenile idiopathic scoliosis, site unspecified

√6th M41.12 Adolescent idiopathic scoliosis

AHA: 2024,1Q,23

M41.122 Adolescent idiopathic scoliosis, cervical region

M41.123 Adolescent idiopathic scoliosis, cervicothoracic region

M41.124 Adolescent idiopathic scoliosis, thoracic region

AHA: 2024,3Q,13

M41.125 Adolescent idiopathic scoliosis, thoracolumbar region

M41.126 Adolescent idiopathic scoliosis, lumbar region

M41.127 Adolescent idiopathic scoliosis, lumbosacral region

M41.129 Adolescent idiopathic scoliosis, site unspecified

√5th M41.2 Other idiopathic scoliosis

M41.20 Other idiopathic scoliosis, site unspecified

M41.22 Other idiopathic scoliosis, cervical region

M41.23 Other idiopathic scoliosis, cervicothoracic region

M41.24 Other idiopathic scoliosis, thoracic region

M41.25 Other idiopathic scoliosis, thoracolumbar region

M41.26 Other idiopathic scoliosis, lumbar region

M41.27 Other idiopathic scoliosis, lumbosacral region

√5th M41.3 Thoracogenic scoliosis

M41.30 Thoracogenic scoliosis, site unspecified

M41.34 Thoracogenic scoliosis, thoracic region

M41.35 Thoracogenic scoliosis, thoracolumbar region

√5th M41.4 Neuromuscular scoliosis

Scoliosis secondary to cerebral palsy, Friedreich's ataxia, poliomyelitis and other neuromuscular disorders

Code also underlying condition

AHA: 2014,4Q,27

M41.40 Neuromuscular scoliosis, site unspecified

M41.41 Neuromuscular scoliosis, occipito-atlanto-axial region

M41.42 Neuromuscular scoliosis, cervical region

M41.43 Neuromuscular scoliosis, cervicothoracic region

M41.44 Neuromuscular scoliosis, thoracic region

M41.45 Neuromuscular scoliosis, thoracolumbar region

M41.46 Neuromuscular scoliosis, lumbar region

M41.47 Neuromuscular scoliosis, lumbosacral region

√5th M41.5 Other secondary scoliosis

Code first underlying disease

AHA: 2019,1Q,19

M41.50 Other secondary scoliosis, site unspecified UPD

M41.52 Other secondary scoliosis, cervical region UPD

M41.53 Other secondary scoliosis, cervicothoracic region UPD

M41.54 Other secondary scoliosis, thoracic region UPD

M41.55 Other secondary scoliosis, thoracolumbar region UPD

M41.56 Other secondary scoliosis, lumbar region UPD

M41.57 Other secondary scoliosis, lumbosacral region UPD

√5th M41.8 Other forms of scoliosis

AHA: 2022,1Q,30

M41.80 Other forms of scoliosis, site unspecified

M41.82 Other forms of scoliosis, cervical region

M41.83 Other forms of scoliosis, cervicothoracic region

M41.84 Other forms of scoliosis, thoracic region

M41.85 Other forms of scoliosis, thoracolumbar region

M41.86 Other forms of scoliosis, lumbar region

M41.87 Other forms of scoliosis, lumbosacral region

M41.9 Scoliosis, unspecified

AHA: 2022,1Q,30

√4th **M42 Spinal osteochondrosis**

√5th M42.0 Juvenile osteochondrosis of spine

Calve's disease

Scheuermann's disease

EXCLUDES 1 *postural kyphosis (M40.0)*

M42.00 Juvenile osteochondrosis of spine, site unspecified COM

M42.01 Juvenile osteochondrosis of spine, occipito-atlanto-axial region COM

M42.02 Juvenile osteochondrosis of spine, cervical region COM

M42.03 Juvenile osteochondrosis of spine, cervicothoracic region COM

M42.04 Juvenile osteochondrosis of spine, thoracic region COM

M42.05 Juvenile osteochondrosis of spine, thoracolumbar region COM

M42.06 Juvenile osteochondrosis of spine, lumbar region COM

M42.07 Juvenile osteochondrosis of spine, lumbosacral region COM

M42.08 Juvenile osteochondrosis of spine, sacral and sacrococcygeal region COM

M42.09 Juvenile osteochondrosis of spine, multiple sites in spine COM

√5th M42.1 Adult osteochondrosis of spine

M42.10 Adult osteochondrosis of spine, site unspecified A

M42.11 Adult osteochondrosis of spine, occipito-atlanto-axial region A

M42.12 Adult osteochondrosis of spine, cervical region A

M42.13 Adult osteochondrosis of spine, cervicothoracic region A

M42.14 Adult osteochondrosis of spine, thoracic region A

M42.15 Adult osteochondrosis of spine, thoracolumbar region A

M42.16 Adult osteochondrosis of spine, lumbar region A

M42.17 Adult osteochondrosis of spine, lumbosacral region A

M42.18 Adult osteochondrosis of spine, sacral and sacrococcygeal region A

M42.19 Adult osteochondrosis of spine, multiple sites in spine A

M42.9 Spinal osteochondrosis, unspecified

√4th **M43 Other deforming dorsopathies**

EXCLUDES 1 *congenital spondylolysis and spondylolisthesis (Q76.2)*
*hemivertebra (Q76.3-Q76.4)*
*Klippel-Feil syndrome (Q76.1)*
*lumbarization and sacralization (Q76.4)*
*platyspondylisis (Q76.4)*
*spina bifida occulta (Q76.0)*
*spinal curvature in osteoporosis (M80.-)*
*spinal curvature in Paget's disease of bone [osteitis deformans] (M88.-)*

√5th M43.0 Spondylolysis

EXCLUDES 1 *congenital spondylolysis (Q76.2)*
*spondylolisthesis (M43.1)*

AHA: 2023,3Q,20

M43.00 Spondylolysis, site unspecified

M43.01 Spondylolysis, occipito-atlanto-axial region

M43.02 Spondylolysis, cervical region

M43.03 Spondylolysis, cervicothoracic region

M43.04 Spondylolysis, thoracic region

M43.05 Spondylolysis, thoracolumbar region

M43.06 Spondylolysis, lumbar region

M43.07 Spondylolysis, lumbosacral region

M43.08 Spondylolysis, sacral and sacrococcygeal region

M43.09 Spondylolysis, multiple sites in spine

√5th M43.1 Spondylolisthesis

EXCLUDES 1 *acute traumatic of lumbosacral region (S33.1)*
*acute traumatic of sites other than lumbosacral - code to Fracture, vertebra, by region*
*congenital spondylolisthesis (Q76.2)*

AHA: 2023,3Q,20; 2020,2Q,21; 2018,3Q,18

DEF: anterolisthesis: Forward displacement of one vertebra slipping over another. This condition can cause compression of the nerve roots exiting the spine.

DEF: retrolisthesis: Backward displacement of one vertebra slipping over another. This condition can cause compression of the nerve roots exiting the spine.

TIP: Code also any associated radiculopathy (M54.1-) and/or myelopathy (G99.2).

M43.10 Spondylolisthesis, site unspecified

M43.11 Spondylolisthesis, occipito-atlanto-axial region

M43.12 Spondylolisthesis, cervical region

**M43.13 Spondylolisthesis, cervicothoracic region**
**M43.14 Spondylolisthesis, thoracic region**
**M43.15 Spondylolisthesis, thoracolumbar region**
**M43.16 Spondylolisthesis, lumbar region**
AHA: 2024,1Q,17
**M43.17 Spondylolisthesis, lumbosacral region**
**M43.18 Spondylolisthesis, sacral and sacrococcygeal region**
**M43.19 Spondylolisthesis, multiple sites in spine**

5th **M43.2 Fusion of spine**
Ankylosis of spinal joint
EXCLUDES 1 *ankylosing spondylitis (M45.Ø-)*
*congenital fusion of spine (Q76.4)*
EXCLUDES 2 *arthrodesis status (Z98.1)*
*pseudoarthrosis after fusion or arthrodesis (M96.Ø)*
**M43.2Ø Fusion of spine, site unspecified**
**M43.21 Fusion of spine, occipito-atlanto-axial region**
**M43.22 Fusion of spine, cervical region**
**M43.23 Fusion of spine, cervicothoracic region**
**M43.24 Fusion of spine, thoracic region**
**M43.25 Fusion of spine, thoracolumbar region**
**M43.26 Fusion of spine, lumbar region**
**M43.27 Fusion of spine, lumbosacral region**
**M43.28 Fusion of spine, sacral and sacrococcygeal region**

**M43.3 Recurrent atlantoaxial dislocation with myelopathy**
**M43.4 Other recurrent atlantoaxial dislocation**

5th **M43.5 Other recurrent vertebral dislocation**
EXCLUDES 1 *biomechanical lesions NEC (M99.-)*
6th **M43.5X Other recurrent vertebral dislocation**
**M43.5X2 Other recurrent vertebral dislocation, cervical region**
**M43.5X3 Other recurrent vertebral dislocation, cervicothoracic region**
**M43.5X4 Other recurrent vertebral dislocation, thoracic region**
**M43.5X5 Other recurrent vertebral dislocation, thoracolumbar region**
**M43.5X6 Other recurrent vertebral dislocation, lumbar region**
**M43.5X7 Other recurrent vertebral dislocation, lumbosacral region**
**M43.5X8 Other recurrent vertebral dislocation, sacral and sacrococcygeal region**
**M43.5X9 Other recurrent vertebral dislocation, site unspecified**

**M43.6 Torticollis**
EXCLUDES 1 *congenital (sternomastoid) torticollis (Q68.Ø)*
*current injury - see Injury, of spine, by body region*
*ocular torticollis (R29.891)*
*psychogenic torticollis (F45.8)*
*spasmodic torticollis (G24.3)*
*torticollis due to birth injury (P15.2)*
DEF: Twisted, unnatural position of the neck due to contracted cervical muscles that pull the head to one side.

5th **M43.8 Other specified deforming dorsopathies**
EXCLUDES 2 *kyphosis and lordosis (M4Ø.-)*
*scoliosis (M41.-)*
6th **M43.8X Other specified deforming dorsopathies**
**M43.8X1 Other specified deforming dorsopathies, occipito-atlanto-axial region**
**M43.8X2 Other specified deforming dorsopathies, cervical region**
**M43.8X3 Other specified deforming dorsopathies, cervicothoracic region**
**M43.8X4 Other specified deforming dorsopathies, thoracic region**
**M43.8X5 Other specified deforming dorsopathies, thoracolumbar region**
**M43.8X6 Other specified deforming dorsopathies, lumbar region**
**M43.8X7 Other specified deforming dorsopathies, lumbosacral region**
**M43.8X8 Other specified deforming dorsopathies, sacral and sacrococcygeal region**
**M43.8X9 Other specified deforming dorsopathies, site unspecified**

**M43.9 Deforming dorsopathy, unspecified**
Curvature of spine NOS

## Spondylopathies (M45-M49)

4th **M45 Ankylosing spondylitis**
Rheumatoid arthritis of spine
EXCLUDES 1 *arthropathy in Reiter's disease (MØ2.3-)*
*juvenile (ankylosing) spondylitis (MØ8.1)*
EXCLUDES 2 *Behcet's disease (M35.2)*
**M45.Ø Ankylosing spondylitis of multiple sites in spine** HCC Rx ESR COM
**M45.1 Ankylosing spondylitis of occipito-atlanto-axial region** HCC Rx ESR COM
**M45.2 Ankylosing spondylitis of cervical region** HCC Rx ESR COM
**M45.3 Ankylosing spondylitis of cervicothoracic region** HCC Rx ESR COM
**M45.4 Ankylosing spondylitis of thoracic region** HCC Rx ESR COM
**M45.5 Ankylosing spondylitis of thoracolumbar region** HCC Rx ESR COM
**M45.6 Ankylosing spondylitis lumbar region** HCC Rx ESR COM
**M45.7 Ankylosing spondylitis of lumbosacral region** HCC Rx ESR COM
**M45.8 Ankylosing spondylitis sacral and sacrococcygeal region** HCC Rx ESR COM
**M45.9 Ankylosing spondylitis of unspecified sites in spine** HCC Rx ESR COM

5th **M45.A Non-radiographic axial spondyloarthritis**
AHA: 2021,4Q,21-22
**M45.AØ Non-radiographic axial spondyloarthritis of unspecified sites in spine** HCC Rx ESR COM
**M45.A1 Non-radiographic axial spondyloarthritis of occipito-atlanto-axial region** HCC Rx ESR COM
**M45.A2 Non-radiographic axial spondyloarthritis of cervical region** HCC Rx ESR COM
**M45.A3 Non-radiographic axial spondyloarthritis of cervicothoracic region** HCC Rx ESR COM
**M45.A4 Non-radiographic axial spondyloarthritis of thoracic region** HCC Rx ESR COM
**M45.A5 Non-radiographic axial spondyloarthritis of thoracolumbar region** HCC Rx ESR COM
**M45.A6 Non-radiographic axial spondyloarthritis of lumbar region** HCC Rx ESR COM
**M45.A7 Non-radiographic axial spondyloarthritis of lumbosacral region** HCC Rx ESR COM
**M45.A8 Non-radiographic axial spondyloarthritis of sacral and sacrococcygeal region** HCC Rx ESR COM
**M45.AB Non-radiographic axial spondyloarthritis of multiple sites in spine** HCC Rx ESR COM

4th **M46 Other inflammatory spondylopathies**
5th **M46.Ø Spinal enthesopathy**
Disorder of ligamentous or muscular attachments of spine
**M46.ØØ Spinal enthesopathy, site unspecified** ESR
**M46.Ø1 Spinal enthesopathy, occipito-atlanto-axial region** ESR
**M46.Ø2 Spinal enthesopathy, cervical region** ESR
**M46.Ø3 Spinal enthesopathy, cervicothoracic region** ESR
**M46.Ø4 Spinal enthesopathy, thoracic region** ESR
**M46.Ø5 Spinal enthesopathy, thoracolumbar region** ESR
**M46.Ø6 Spinal enthesopathy, lumbar region** ESR
**M46.Ø7 Spinal enthesopathy, lumbosacral region** ESR
**M46.Ø8 Spinal enthesopathy, sacral and sacrococcygeal region** ESR
**M46.Ø9 Spinal enthesopathy, multiple sites in spine** ESR
**M46.1 Sacroiliitis, not elsewhere classified** ESR
AHA: 2020,2Q,14
DEF: Inflammation of the sacroiliac joint (situated at the juncture of the sacrum and hip). Symptoms include pain in the buttocks or lower back that can extend down one or both legs.
5th **M46.2 Osteomyelitis of vertebra**
**M46.2Ø Osteomyelitis of vertebra, site unspecified** HCC ESR COM
**M46.21 Osteomyelitis of vertebra, occipito-atlanto-axial region** HCC ESR COM
**M46.22 Osteomyelitis of vertebra, cervical region** HCC ESR COM
**M46.23 Osteomyelitis of vertebra, cervicothoracic region** HCC ESR COM

M46.24 Osteomyelitis of vertebra, thoracic region HCC ESR COM
M46.25 Osteomyelitis of vertebra, thoracolumbar region HCC ESR COM
M46.26 Osteomyelitis of vertebra, lumbar region HCC ESR COM
M46.27 Osteomyelitis of vertebra, lumbosacral region HCC ESR COM
M46.28 Osteomyelitis of vertebra, sacral and sacrococcygeal region HCC ESR COM

✓5th M46.3 Infection of intervertebral disc (pyogenic)
Use additional code (B95-B97) to identify infectious agent
M46.30 Infection of intervertebral disc (pyogenic), site unspecified HCC ESR COM
M46.31 Infection of intervertebral disc (pyogenic), occipito-atlanto-axial region HCC ESR COM
M46.32 Infection of intervertebral disc (pyogenic), cervical region HCC ESR COM
M46.33 Infection of intervertebral disc (pyogenic), cervicothoracic region HCC ESR COM
M46.34 Infection of intervertebral disc (pyogenic), thoracic region HCC ESR COM
M46.35 Infection of intervertebral disc (pyogenic), thoracolumbar region HCC ESR COM
M46.36 Infection of intervertebral disc (pyogenic), lumbar region HCC ESR COM
M46.37 Infection of intervertebral disc (pyogenic), lumbosacral region HCC ESR COM
M46.38 Infection of intervertebral disc (pyogenic), sacral and sacrococcygeal region HCC ESR COM
M46.39 Infection of intervertebral disc (pyogenic), multiple sites in spine HCC ESR COM

✓5th M46.4 Discitis, unspecified
M46.40 Discitis, unspecified, site unspecified
M46.41 Discitis, unspecified, occipito-atlanto-axial region
M46.42 Discitis, unspecified, cervical region
M46.43 Discitis, unspecified, cervicothoracic region
M46.44 Discitis, unspecified, thoracic region
M46.45 Discitis, unspecified, thoracolumbar region
M46.46 Discitis, unspecified, lumbar region
M46.47 Discitis, unspecified, lumbosacral region
M46.48 Discitis, unspecified, sacral and sacrococcygeal region
M46.49 Discitis, unspecified, multiple sites in spine

✓5th M46.5 Other infective spondylopathies
M46.50 Other infective spondylopathies, site unspecified ESR
M46.51 Other infective spondylopathies, occipito-atlanto-axial region ESR
M46.52 Other infective spondylopathies, cervical region ESR
M46.53 Other infective spondylopathies, cervicothoracic region ESR
M46.54 Other infective spondylopathies, thoracic region ESR
M46.55 Other infective spondylopathies, thoracolumbar region ESR
M46.56 Other infective spondylopathies, lumbar region ESR
M46.57 Other infective spondylopathies, lumbosacral region ESR
M46.58 Other infective spondylopathies, sacral and sacrococcygeal region ESR
M46.59 Other infective spondylopathies, multiple sites in spine ESR

✓5th M46.8 Other specified inflammatory spondylopathies
M46.80 Other specified inflammatory spondylopathies, site unspecified ESR
M46.81 Other specified inflammatory spondylopathies, occipito-atlanto-axial region ESR
M46.82 Other specified inflammatory spondylopathies, cervical region ESR
M46.83 Other specified inflammatory spondylopathies, cervicothoracic region ESR
M46.84 Other specified inflammatory spondylopathies, thoracic region ESR
M46.85 Other specified inflammatory spondylopathies, thoracolumbar region ESR
M46.86 Other specified inflammatory spondylopathies, lumbar region ESR
M46.87 Other specified inflammatory spondylopathies, lumbosacral region ESR
M46.88 Other specified inflammatory spondylopathies, sacral and sacrococcygeal region ESR
M46.89 Other specified inflammatory spondylopathies, multiple sites in spine ESR

✓5th M46.9 Unspecified inflammatory spondylopathy
M46.90 Unspecified inflammatory spondylopathy, site unspecified ESR
M46.91 Unspecified inflammatory spondylopathy, occipito-atlanto-axial region ESR
M46.92 Unspecified inflammatory spondylopathy, cervical region ESR
AHA: 2019,3Q,10
M46.93 Unspecified inflammatory spondylopathy, cervicothoracic region ESR
M46.94 Unspecified inflammatory spondylopathy, thoracic region ESR
M46.95 Unspecified inflammatory spondylopathy, thoracolumbar region ESR
M46.96 Unspecified inflammatory spondylopathy, lumbar region ESR
M46.97 Unspecified inflammatory spondylopathy, lumbosacral region ESR
M46.98 Unspecified inflammatory spondylopathy, sacral and sacrococcygeal region ESR
M46.99 Unspecified inflammatory spondylopathy, multiple sites in spine ESR

✓4th M47 Spondylosis
INCLUDES arthrosis or osteoarthritis of spine
degeneration of facet joints
AHA: 2020,1Q,17; 2019,3Q,10-11; 2016,4Q,147

✓5th M47.0 Anterior spinal and vertebral artery compression syndromes
✓6th M47.01 Anterior spinal artery compression syndromes
M47.011 Anterior spinal artery compression syndromes, occipito-atlanto-axial region
M47.012 Anterior spinal artery compression syndromes, cervical region
AHA: 2023,1Q,37
M47.013 Anterior spinal artery compression syndromes, cervicothoracic region
M47.014 Anterior spinal artery compression syndromes, thoracic region
M47.015 Anterior spinal artery compression syndromes, thoracolumbar region
M47.016 Anterior spinal artery compression syndromes, lumbar region
M47.019 Anterior spinal artery compression syndromes, site unspecified
✓6th M47.02 Vertebral artery compression syndromes
M47.021 Vertebral artery compression syndromes, occipito-atlanto-axial region
M47.022 Vertebral artery compression syndromes, cervical region
AHA: 2023,1Q,37
M47.029 Vertebral artery compression syndromes, site unspecified

✓5th M47.1 Other spondylosis with myelopathy
Spondylogenic compression of spinal cord
*EXCLUDES 1 vertebral subluxation (M43.3-M43.5X9)*
AHA: 2020,1Q,17
M47.10 Other spondylosis with myelopathy, site unspecified
M47.11 Other spondylosis with myelopathy, occipito-atlanto-axial region
M47.12 Other spondylosis with myelopathy, cervical region
M47.13 Other spondylosis with myelopathy, cervicothoracic region
M47.14 Other spondylosis with myelopathy, thoracic region
M47.15 Other spondylosis with myelopathy, thoracolumbar region
M47.16 Other spondylosis with myelopathy, lumbar region

✓5th M47.2 Other spondylosis with radiculopathy
AHA: 2020,1Q,17
M47.20 Other spondylosis with radiculopathy, site unspecified

M47.21 Other spondylosis with radiculopathy, occipito-atlanto-axial region
M47.22 Other spondylosis with radiculopathy, cervical region
M47.23 Other spondylosis with radiculopathy, cervicothoracic region
M47.24 Other spondylosis with radiculopathy, thoracic region
M47.25 Other spondylosis with radiculopathy, thoracolumbar region
M47.26 Other spondylosis with radiculopathy, lumbar region
M47.27 Other spondylosis with radiculopathy, lumbosacral region
M47.28 Other spondylosis with radiculopathy, sacral and sacrococcygeal region

√5th M47.8 Other spondylosis

√6th M47.81 Spondylosis without myelopathy or radiculopathy
AHA: 2025,3Q,19; 2019,3Q,10-11; 2018,2Q,14
M47.811 Spondylosis without myelopathy or radiculopathy, occipito-atlanto-axial region
M47.812 Spondylosis without myelopathy or radiculopathy, cervical region
M47.813 Spondylosis without myelopathy or radiculopathy, cervicothoracic region
M47.814 Spondylosis without myelopathy or radiculopathy, thoracic region
M47.815 Spondylosis without myelopathy or radiculopathy, thoracolumbar region
M47.816 Spondylosis without myelopathy or radiculopathy, lumbar region
M47.817 Spondylosis without myelopathy or radiculopathy, lumbosacral region
M47.818 Spondylosis without myelopathy or radiculopathy, sacral and sacrococcygeal region
M47.819 Spondylosis without myelopathy or radiculopathy, site unspecified

√6th M47.89 Other spondylosis
M47.891 Other spondylosis, occipito-atlanto-axial region
M47.892 Other spondylosis, cervical region
M47.893 Other spondylosis, cervicothoracic region
M47.894 Other spondylosis, thoracic region
M47.895 Other spondylosis, thoracolumbar region
M47.896 Other spondylosis, lumbar region
M47.897 Other spondylosis, lumbosacral region
M47.898 Other spondylosis, sacral and sacrococcygeal region
M47.899 Other spondylosis, site unspecified

M47.9 Spondylosis, unspecified

## √4th M48 Other spondylopathies

√5th M48.Ø Spinal stenosis
Caudal stenosis
AHA: 2020,1Q,17; 2018,3Q,18-19
TIP: Code also any associated radiculopathy (M54.1-) and/or myelopathy (G99.2).
M48.ØØ Spinal stenosis, site unspecified
M48.Ø1 Spinal stenosis, occipito-atlanto-axial region
M48.Ø2 Spinal stenosis, cervical region
M48.Ø3 Spinal stenosis, cervicothoracic region
M48.Ø4 Spinal stenosis, thoracic region
M48.Ø5 Spinal stenosis, thoracolumbar region

√6th M48.Ø6 Spinal stenosis, lumbar region
AHA: 2018,3Q,19; 2017,4Q,18-19
M48.Ø61 Spinal stenosis, lumbar region without neurogenic claudication
Spinal stenosis, lumbar region NOS
M48.Ø62 Spinal stenosis, lumbar region with neurogenic claudication

M48.Ø7 Spinal stenosis, lumbosacral region
M48.Ø8 Spinal stenosis, sacral and sacrococcygeal region

√5th M48.1 Ankylosing hyperostosis [Forestier]
Diffuse idiopathic skeletal hyperostosis [DISH]
M48.1Ø Ankylosing hyperostosis [Forestier], site unspecified
M48.11 Ankylosing hyperostosis [Forestier], occipito-atlanto-axial region
M48.12 Ankylosing hyperostosis [Forestier], cervical region
M48.13 Ankylosing hyperostosis [Forestier], cervicothoracic region
M48.14 Ankylosing hyperostosis [Forestier], thoracic region
M48.15 Ankylosing hyperostosis [Forestier], thoracolumbar region
M48.16 Ankylosing hyperostosis [Forestier], lumbar region
M48.17 Ankylosing hyperostosis [Forestier], lumbosacral region
M48.18 Ankylosing hyperostosis [Forestier], sacral and sacrococcygeal region
M48.19 Ankylosing hyperostosis [Forestier], multiple sites in spine

√5th M48.2 Kissing spine
M48.2Ø Kissing spine, site unspecified
M48.21 Kissing spine, occipito-atlanto-axial region
M48.22 Kissing spine, cervical region
M48.23 Kissing spine, cervicothoracic region
M48.24 Kissing spine, thoracic region
M48.25 Kissing spine, thoracolumbar region
M48.26 Kissing spine, lumbar region
M48.27 Kissing spine, lumbosacral region

√5th M48.3 Traumatic spondylopathy
M48.3Ø Traumatic spondylopathy, site unspecified
M48.31 Traumatic spondylopathy, occipito-atlanto-axial region
M48.32 Traumatic spondylopathy, cervical region
M48.33 Traumatic spondylopathy, cervicothoracic region
M48.34 Traumatic spondylopathy, thoracic region
M48.35 Traumatic spondylopathy, thoracolumbar region
M48.36 Traumatic spondylopathy, lumbar region
M48.37 Traumatic spondylopathy, lumbosacral region
M48.38 Traumatic spondylopathy, sacral and sacrococcygeal region

√5th M48.4 Fatigue fracture of vertebra
Stress fracture of vertebra
EXCLUDES 1 *pathological fracture NOS (M84.4-)*
*pathological fracture of vertebra due to neoplasm (M84.58)*
*pathological fracture of vertebra due to osteoporosis (M8Ø.-)*
*pathological fracture of vertebra due to other diagnosis (M84.68)*
*traumatic fracture of vertebrae (S12.Ø-S12.3-, S22.Ø-, S32.Ø-)*

The appropriate 7th character is to be added to each code from subcategory M48.4.
A initial encounter for fracture
D subsequent encounter for fracture with routine healing
G subsequent encounter for fracture with delayed healing
S sequela of fracture

√x7th M48.4Ø Fatigue fracture of vertebra, site unspecified Q
√x7th M48.41 Fatigue fracture of vertebra, occipito-atlanto-axial region Q
√x7th M48.42 Fatigue fracture of vertebra, cervical region Q
√x7th M48.43 Fatigue fracture of vertebra, cervicothoracic region Q
√x7th M48.44 Fatigue fracture of vertebra, thoracic region Q
√x7th M48.45 Fatigue fracture of vertebra, thoracolumbar region Q
√x7th M48.46 Fatigue fracture of vertebra, lumbar region Q
√x7th M48.47 Fatigue fracture of vertebra, lumbosacral region Q
√x7th M48.48 Fatigue fracture of vertebra, sacral and sacrococcygeal region Q

**M48.5 Collapsed vertebra, not elsewhere classified**

Collapsed vertebra NOS
Compression fracture of vertebra NOS
Wedging of vertebra NOS

EXCLUDES 1 *current injury - see Injury of spine, by body region*
*fatigue fracture of vertebra (M48.4)*
*pathological fracture NOS (M84.4-)*
*pathological fracture of vertebra due to neoplasm (M84.58)*
*pathological fracture of vertebra due to osteoporosis (M80.-)*
*pathological fracture of vertebra due to other diagnosis (M84.68)*
*stress fracture of vertebra (M48.4-)*
*traumatic fracture of vertebra (S12.-, S22.-, S32.-)*

The appropriate 7th character is to be added to each code from subcategory M48.5.
A initial encounter for fracture
D subsequent encounter for fracture with routine healing
G subsequent encounter for fracture with delayed healing
S sequela of fracture

**M48.50 Collapsed vertebra, not elsewhere classified, site unspecified** HCC Rx ESR COM
**M48.51 Collapsed vertebra, not elsewhere classified, occipito-atlanto-axial region** HCC Rx ESR COM
**M48.52 Collapsed vertebra, not elsewhere classified, cervical region** HCC Rx ESR COM
**M48.53 Collapsed vertebra, not elsewhere classified, cervicothoracic region** HCC Rx ESR COM
**M48.54 Collapsed vertebra, not elsewhere classified, thoracic region** HCC Rx ESR COM
**M48.55 Collapsed vertebra, not elsewhere classified, thoracolumbar region** HCC Rx ESR COM
**M48.56 Collapsed vertebra, not elsewhere classified, lumbar region** HCC Rx ESR COM
**M48.57 Collapsed vertebra, not elsewhere classified, lumbosacral region** HCC Rx ESR COM
**M48.58 Collapsed vertebra, not elsewhere classified, sacral and sacrococcygeal region** HCC Rx ESR COM

**M48.8 Other specified spondylopathies**

Ossification of posterior longitudinal ligament

**M48.8X Other specified spondylopathies**

**M48.8X1 Other specified spondylopathies, occipito-atlanto-axial region** HCC Rx ESR COM
**M48.8X2 Other specified spondylopathies, cervical region** HCC Rx ESR COM
**M48.8X3 Other specified spondylopathies, cervicothoracic region** HCC Rx ESR COM
**M48.8X4 Other specified spondylopathies, thoracic region** HCC Rx ESR COM
**M48.8X5 Other specified spondylopathies, thoracolumbar region** HCC Rx ESR COM
**M48.8X6 Other specified spondylopathies, lumbar region** HCC Rx ESR COM
**M48.8X7 Other specified spondylopathies, lumbosacral region** HCC Rx ESR COM
**M48.8X8 Other specified spondylopathies, sacral and sacrococcygeal region** HCC Rx ESR COM
**M48.8X9 Other specified spondylopathies, site unspecified** HCC Rx ESR COM

**M48.9 Spondylopathy, unspecified**

**M49 Spondylopathies in diseases classified elsewhere**

INCLUDES curvature of spine in diseases classified elsewhere
deformity of spine in diseases classified elsewhere
kyphosis in diseases classified elsewhere
scoliosis in diseases classified elsewhere
spondylopathy in diseases classified elsewhere

Code first underlying disease, such as:
brucellosis (A23.-)
Charcôt-Marie-Tooth disease (G60.0)
enterobacterial infections (A01-A04)
osteitis fibrosa cystica (E21.0)

EXCLUDES 1 *curvature of spine in tuberculosis [Pott's] (A18.01)*
*enteropathic arthropathies (M07.-)*
*gonococcal spondylitis (A54.41)*
*neuropathic [tabes dorsalis] spondylitis (A52.11)*
*neuropathic spondylopathy in syringomyelia (G95.0)*
*neuropathic spondylopathy in tabes dorsalis (A52.11)*
*nonsyphilitic neuropathic spondylopathy NEC (G98.0)*
*spondylitis in syphilis (acquired) (A52.77)*
*tuberculous spondylitis (A18.01)*
*typhoid fever spondylitis (A01.05)*

**M49.8 Spondylopathy in diseases classified elsewhere**

***M49.80 Spondylopathy in diseases classified elsewhere, site unspecified*** ESR
***M49.81 Spondylopathy in diseases classified elsewhere, occipito-atlanto-axial region*** ESR
***M49.82 Spondylopathy in diseases classified elsewhere, cervical region*** ESR
***M49.83 Spondylopathy in diseases classified elsewhere, cervicothoracic region*** ESR
***M49.84 Spondylopathy in diseases classified elsewhere, thoracic region*** ESR
***M49.85 Spondylopathy in diseases classified elsewhere, thoracolumbar region*** ESR
***M49.86 Spondylopathy in diseases classified elsewhere, lumbar region*** ESR
***M49.87 Spondylopathy in diseases classified elsewhere, lumbosacral region*** ESR
***M49.88 Spondylopathy in diseases classified elsewhere, sacral and sacrococcygeal region*** ESR
***M49.89 Spondylopathy in diseases classified elsewhere, multiple sites in spine*** ESR

## Other dorsopathies (M50-M54)

EXCLUDES 1 *current injury - see injury of spine by body region*
*discitis NOS (M46.4-)*

**M50 Cervical disc disorders**

INCLUDES cervicothoracic disc disorders
cervicothoracic disc disorders with cervicalgia

**AHA:** 2016,4Q,39-40; 2016,1Q,17

**M50.0 Cervical disc disorder with myelopathy**

**AHA:** 2018,3Q,19

**M50.00 Cervical disc disorder with myelopathy, unspecified cervical region**

**M50.01 Cervical disc disorder with myelopathy, high cervical region**
C2-C3 disc disorder with myelopathy
C3-C4 disc disorder with myelopathy

**M50.02 Cervical disc disorder with myelopathy, mid-cervical region**

**M50.020 Cervical disc disorder with myelopathy, mid-cervical region, unspecified level**

**M50.021 Cervical disc disorder at C4-C5 level with myelopathy**
C4-C5 disc disorder with myelopathy

**M50.022 Cervical disc disorder at C5-C6 level with myelopathy**
C5-C6 disc disorder with myelopathy

**M50.023 Cervical disc disorder at C6-C7 level with myelopathy**
C6-C7 disc disorder with myelopathy

**M50.03 Cervical disc disorder with myelopathy, cervicothoracic region**
C7-T1 disc disorder with myelopathy

**M50.1 Cervical disc disorder with radiculopathy**

EXCLUDES 2 *brachial radiculitis NOS (M54.13)*

**AHA:** 2018,3Q,19

**M50.10 Cervical disc disorder with radiculopathy, unspecified cervical region**

**M5Ø.11 Cervical disc disorder with radiculopathy, high cervical region**
C2-C3 disc disorder with radiculopathy
C3 radiculopathy due to disc disorder
C3-C4 disc disorder with radiculopathy
C4 radiculopathy due to disc disorder

√6th **M5Ø.12 Cervical disc disorder with radiculopathy, mid-cervical region**

**M5Ø.12Ø Mid-cervical disc disorder, unspecified level**

**M5Ø.121 Cervical disc disorder at C4-C5 level with radiculopathy**
C4-C5 disc disorder with radiculopathy
C5 radiculopathy due to disc disorder

**M5Ø.122 Cervical disc disorder at C5-C6 level with radiculopathy**
C5-C6 disc disorder with radiculopathy
C6 radiculopathy due to disc disorder

**M5Ø.123 Cervical disc disorder at C6-C7 level with radiculopathy**
C6-C7 disc disorder with radiculopathy
C7 radiculopathy due to disc disorder

**M5Ø.13 Cervical disc disorder with radiculopathy, cervicothoracic region**
C7-T1 disc disorder with radiculopathy
C8 radiculopathy due to disc disorder

√5th **M5Ø.2 Other cervical disc displacement**

**M5Ø.2Ø Other cervical disc displacement, unspecified cervical region**

**M5Ø.21 Other cervical disc displacement, high cervical region**
Other C2-C3 cervical disc displacement
Other C3-C4 cervical disc displacement

√6th **M5Ø.22 Other cervical disc displacement, mid-cervical region**

**M5Ø.22Ø Other cervical disc displacement, mid-cervical region, unspecified level**

**M5Ø.221 Other cervical disc displacement at C4-C5 level**
Other C4-C5 cervical disc displacement

**M5Ø.222 Other cervical disc displacement at C5-C6 level**
Other C5-C6 cervical disc displacement

**M5Ø.223 Other cervical disc displacement at C6-C7 level**
Other C6-C7 cervical disc displacement

**M5Ø.23 Other cervical disc displacement, cervicothoracic region**
Other C7-T1 cervical disc displacement

√5th **M5Ø.3 Other cervical disc degeneration**

**M5Ø.3Ø Other cervical disc degeneration, unspecified cervical region**

**M5Ø.31 Other cervical disc degeneration, high cervical region**
Other C2-C3 cervical disc degeneration
Other C3-C4 cervical disc degeneration

√6th **M5Ø.32 Other cervical disc degeneration, mid-cervical region**

**M5Ø.32Ø Other cervical disc degeneration, mid-cervical region, unspecified level**

**M5Ø.321 Other cervical disc degeneration at C4-C5 level**
Other C4-C5 cervical disc degeneration

**M5Ø.322 Other cervical disc degeneration at C5-C6 level**
Other C5-C6 cervical disc degeneration

**M5Ø.323 Other cervical disc degeneration at C6-C7 level**
Other C6-C7 cervical disc degeneration

**M5Ø.33 Other cervical disc degeneration, cervicothoracic region**
Other C7-T1 cervical disc degeneration

√5th **M5Ø.8 Other cervical disc disorders**

**M5Ø.8Ø Other cervical disc disorders, unspecified cervical region**

**M5Ø.81 Other cervical disc disorders, high cervical region**
Other C2-C3 cervical disc disorders
Other C3-C4 cervical disc disorders

√6th **M5Ø.82 Other cervical disc disorders, mid-cervical region**

**M5Ø.82Ø Other cervical disc disorders, mid-cervical region, unspecified level**

**M5Ø.821 Other cervical disc disorders at C4-C5 level**
Other C4-C5 cervical disc disorders

**M5Ø.822 Other cervical disc disorders at C5-C6 level**
Other C5-C6 cervical disc disorders

**M5Ø.823 Other cervical disc disorders at C6-C7 level**
Other C6-C7 cervical disc disorders

**M5Ø.83 Other cervical disc disorders, cervicothoracic region**
Other C7-T1 cervical disc disorders

√5th **M5Ø.9 Cervical disc disorder, unspecified**

**M5Ø.9Ø Cervical disc disorder, unspecified, unspecified cervical region**

**M5Ø.91 Cervical disc disorder, unspecified, high cervical region**
C2-C3 cervical disc disorder, unspecified
C3-C4 cervical disc disorder, unspecified

√6th **M5Ø.92 Cervical disc disorder, unspecified, mid-cervical region**

**M5Ø.92Ø Unspecified cervical disc disorder, mid-cervical region, unspecified level**

**M5Ø.921 Unspecified cervical disc disorder at C4-C5 level**
Unspecified C4-C5 cervical disc disorder

**M5Ø.922 Unspecified cervical disc disorder at C5-C6 level**
Unspecified C5-C6 cervical disc disorder

**M5Ø.923 Unspecified cervical disc disorder at C6-C7 level**
Unspecified C6-C7 cervical disc disorder

**M5Ø.93 Cervical disc disorder, unspecified, cervicothoracic region**
C7-T1 cervical disc disorder, unspecified

√4th **M51 Thoracic, thoracolumbar, and lumbosacral intervertebral disc disorders**

EXCLUDES 2 *cervical and cervicothoracic disc disorders (M5Ø.-)*
*sacral and sacrococcygeal disorders (M53.3)*

√5th **M51.Ø Thoracic, thoracolumbar and lumbosacral intervertebral disc disorders with myelopathy**

**M51.Ø4 Intervertebral disc disorders with myelopathy, thoracic region**

**M51.Ø5 Intervertebral disc disorders with myelopathy, thoracolumbar region**

**M51.Ø6 Intervertebral disc disorders with myelopathy, lumbar region**

√5th **M51.1 Thoracic, thoracolumbar and lumbosacral intervertebral disc disorders with radiculopathy**
Sciatica due to intervertebral disc disorder
EXCLUDES 1 *lumbar radiculitis NOS (M54.16)*
*sciatica NOS (M54.3)*
**AHA:** 2018,3Q,18

**M51.14 Intervertebral disc disorders with radiculopathy, thoracic region**

**M51.15 Intervertebral disc disorders with radiculopathy, thoracolumbar region**

**M51.16 Intervertebral disc disorders with radiculopathy, lumbar region**

**M51.17 Intervertebral disc disorders with radiculopathy, lumbosacral region**

√5th **M51.2 Other thoracic, thoracolumbar and lumbosacral intervertebral disc displacement**
Lumbago due to displacement of intervertebral disc
**AHA:** 2022,1Q,26

**Displacement Intervertebral Disc**

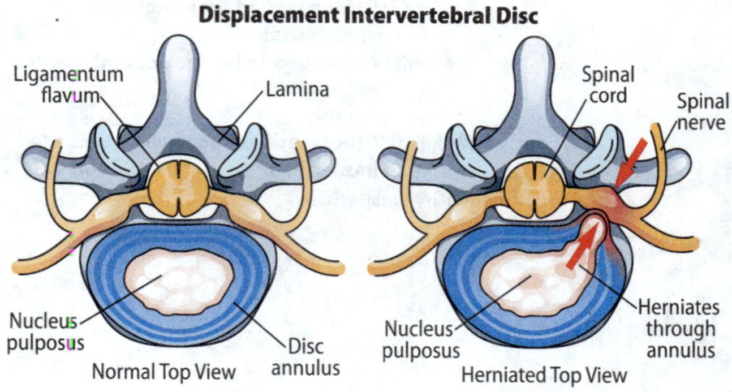


**M51.24 Other intervertebral disc displacement, thoracic region**

**M51.25 Other intervertebral disc displacement, thoracolumbar region**

**M51.26 Other intervertebral disc displacement, lumbar region**

**M51.27 Other intervertebral disc displacement, lumbosacral region**

✓5th **M51.3 Other thoracic, thoracolumbar and lumbosacral intervertebral disc degeneration**
AHA: 2022,1Q,26; 2018,2Q,15; 2013,3Q,22

**M51.34 Other intervertebral disc degeneration, thoracic region**

**M51.35 Other intervertebral disc degeneration, thoracolumbar region**

✓6th **M51.36 Other intervertebral disc degeneration, lumbar region**
AHA: 2024,4Q,24

**M51.360 Other intervertebral disc degeneration, lumbar region with discogenic back pain only**
Other intervertebral disc degeneration, lumbar region with axial back pain only

**M51.361 Other intervertebral disc degeneration, lumbar region with lower extremity pain only**
Other intervertebral disc degeneration, lumbar region with leg pain only
Other intervertebral disc degeneration, lumbar region with referred sclerotomal pain only

**M51.362 Other intervertebral disc degeneration, lumbar region with discogenic back pain and lower extremity pain**
Other intervertebral disc degeneration, lumbar region with axial back pain and referred sclerotomal pain
Other intervertebral disc degeneration, lumbar region with discogenic back pain and leg pain

**M51.369 Other intervertebral disc degeneration, lumbar region without mention of lumbar back pain or lower extremity pain**
Other intervertebral disc degeneration, lumbar region without mention of lumbar back pain or leg pain
Other intervertebral disc degeneration, lumbar region, NOS

✓6th **M51.37 Other intervertebral disc degeneration, lumbosacral region**
AHA: 2024,4Q,24

**M51.370 Other intervertebral disc degeneration, lumbosacral region with discogenic back pain only**
Other intervertebral disc degeneration, lumbosacral region with axial back pain only

**M51.371 Other intervertebral disc degeneration, lumbosacral region with lower extremity pain only**
Other intervertebral disc degeneration, lumbosacral region with leg pain only
Other intervertebral disc degeneration, lumbosacral region with referred sclerotomal pain only

**M51.372 Other intervertebral disc degeneration, lumbosacral region with discogenic back pain and lower extremity pain**
Other intervertebral disc degeneration, lumbosacral region with axial back pain and referred sclerotomal pain
Other intervertebral disc degeneration, lumbosacral region with discogenic back pain and leg pain

**M51.379 Other intervertebral disc degeneration, lumbosacral region without mention of lumbar back pain or lower extremity pain**
Other intervertebral disc degeneration, lumbosacral region without mention of lumbar back pain or leg pain
Other intervertebral disc degeneration, lumbosacral region, NOS

✓5th **M51.4 Schmorl's nodes**
DEF: Irregular bone defect in the margin of the vertebral body that causes herniation into the end plate of the vertebral body.

**M51.44 Schmorl's nodes, thoracic region**

**M51.45 Schmorl's nodes, thoracolumbar region**

**M51.46 Schmorl's nodes, lumbar region**

**M51.47 Schmorl's nodes, lumbosacral region**

✓5th **M51.8 Other thoracic, thoracolumbar and lumbosacral intervertebral disc disorders**

**M51.84 Other intervertebral disc disorders, thoracic region**

**M51.85 Other intervertebral disc disorders, thoracolumbar region**

**M51.86 Other intervertebral disc disorders, lumbar region**

**M51.87 Other intervertebral disc disorders, lumbosacral region**

**M51.9 Unspecified thoracic, thoracolumbar and lumbosacral intervertebral disc disorder**

✓5th **M51.A Other lumbar and lumbosacral annulus fibrosus disc defects**
AHA: 2022,4Q,28-29

**M51.A0 Intervertebral annulus fibrosus defect, lumbar region, unspecified size**
Code first, if applicable, lumbar disc herniation (M51.06, M51.16, M51.26)

**M51.A1 Intervertebral annulus fibrosus defect, small, lumbar region**
Code first, if applicable, lumbar disc herniation (M51.06, M51.16, M51.26)

**M51.A2 Intervertebral annulus fibrosus defect, large, lumbar region**
Code first, if applicable, lumbar disc herniation (M51.06, M51.16, M51.26)

**M51.A3 Intervertebral annulus fibrosus defect, lumbosacral region, unspecified size**
Code first, if applicable, lumbosacral disc herniation (M51.17, M51.27)

**M51.A4 Intervertebral annulus fibrosus defect, small, lumbosacral region**
Code first, if applicable, lumbosacral disc herniation (M51.17, M51.27)

**M51.A5 Intervertebral annulus fibrosus defect, large, lumbosacral region**
Code first, if applicable, lumbosacral disc herniation (M51.17, M51.27)

✓4th **M53 Other and unspecified dorsopathies, not elsewhere classified**

**M53.0 Cervicocranial syndrome**
Posterior cervical sympathetic syndrome

**M53.1 Cervicobrachial syndrome**
EXCLUDES 2 *cervical disc disorder (M50.-)*
*thoracic outlet syndrome (G54.0)*

✓5th **M53.2 Spinal instabilities**

✓6th **M53.2X Spinal instabilities**

**M53.2X1 Spinal instabilities, occipito-atlanto-axial region**

**M53.2X2 Spinal instabilities, cervical region**

**M53.2X3 Spinal instabilities, cervicothoracic region**

**M53.2X4 Spinal instabilities, thoracic region**

**M53.2X5 Spinal instabilities, thoracolumbar region**

**M53.2X6 Spinal instabilities, lumbar region**

**M53.2X7 Spinal instabilities, lumbosacral region**

**M53.2X8 Spinal instabilities, sacral and sacrococcygeal region**

**M53.2X9 Spinal instabilities, site unspecified**

**M53.3 Sacrococcygeal disorders, not elsewhere classified**
Coccygodynia

✓5th **M53.8 Other specified dorsopathies**

**M53.80 Other specified dorsopathies, site unspecified**

**M53.81 Other specified dorsopathies, occipito-atlanto-axial region**

**M53.82 Other specified dorsopathies, cervical region**

**M53.83 Other specified dorsopathies, cervicothoracic region**

**M53.84 Other specified dorsopathies, thoracic region**

**M53.85 Other specified dorsopathies, thoracolumbar region**

**M53.86 Other specified dorsopathies, lumbar region**

**M53.87 Other specified dorsopathies, lumbosacral region**

**M53.88 Other specified dorsopathies, sacral and sacrococcygeal region**

**M53.9 Dorsopathy, unspecified**

✓4th **M54 Dorsalgia**
EXCLUDES 1 *psychogenic dorsalgia (F45.41)*

✓5th **M54.0 Panniculitis affecting regions of neck and back**
EXCLUDES 1 *lupus panniculitis (L93.2)*
*panniculitis NOS (M79.3)*
*relapsing [Weber-Christian] panniculitis (M35.6)*

**M54.00 Panniculitis affecting regions of neck and back, site unspecified**

**M54.01 Panniculitis affecting regions of neck and back, occipito-atlanto-axial region**

**M54.02** **Panniculitis affecting regions of neck and back, cervical region**
**M54.03** **Panniculitis affecting regions of neck and back, cervicothoracic region**
**M54.04** **Panniculitis affecting regions of neck and back, thoracic region**
**M54.05** **Panniculitis affecting regions of neck and back, thoracolumbar region**
**M54.06** **Panniculitis affecting regions of neck and back, lumbar region**
**M54.07** **Panniculitis affecting regions of neck and back, lumbosacral region**
**M54.08** **Panniculitis affecting regions of neck and back, sacral and sacrococcygeal region**
**M54.09** **Panniculitis affecting regions, neck and back, multiple sites in spine**

✓5th **M54.1 Radiculopathy**
Brachial neuritis or radiculitis NOS
Lumbar neuritis or radiculitis NOS
Lumbosacral neuritis or radiculitis NOS
Radiculitis NOS
Thoracic neuritis or radiculitis NOS
EXCLUDES 1 *neuralgia and neuritis NOS (M79.2)*
*radiculopathy with cervical disc disorder (M50.1)*
*radiculopathy with lumbar and other intervertebral disc disorder (M51.1-)*
*radiculopathy with spondylosis (M47.2-)*
**AHA:** 2018,3Q,18
**TIP:** A code from this subcategory can be used in addition to a spondylolisthesis code (M43.1-) or a spinal stenosis code (M48.0-) when either condition is documented as the cause of the radiculopathy.
**M54.10** **Radiculopathy, site unspecified**
**M54.11** **Radiculopathy, occipito-atlanto-axial region**
**M54.12** **Radiculopathy, cervical region**
**M54.13** **Radiculopathy, cervicothoracic region**
**M54.14** **Radiculopathy, thoracic region**
**M54.15** **Radiculopathy, thoracolumbar region**
**M54.16** **Radiculopathy, lumbar region**
**M54.17** **Radiculopathy, lumbosacral region**
**M54.18** **Radiculopathy, sacral and sacrococcygeal region**

**M54.2 Cervicalgia**
EXCLUDES 1 *cervicalgia due to intervertebral cervical disc disorder (M50.-)*

✓5th **M54.3 Sciatica**
EXCLUDES 1 *intervertebral disc degeneration, lumbar region with lower extremity pain only (M51.361)*
*intervertebral disc degeneration, lumbosacral region with lower extremity pain only (M51.371)*
*lesion of sciatic nerve (G57.0)*
*sciatica due to intervertebral disc disorder (M51.1-)*
*sciatica with lumbago (M54.4-)*
**M54.30** **Sciatica, unspecified side**
**M54.31** **Sciatica, right side**
**M54.32** **Sciatica, left side**

✓5th **M54.4 Lumbago with sciatica**
EXCLUDES 1 *intervertebral disc degeneration, lumbar region with discogenic back pain and lower extremity pain (M51.362)*
*intervertebral disc degeneration, lumbosacral region with discogenic back pain and lower extremity pain (M51.372)*
*lumbago with sciatica due to intervertebral disc disorder (M51.1-)*
**AHA:** 2016,2Q,7
**M54.40** **Lumbago with sciatica, unspecified side**
**M54.41** **Lumbago with sciatica, right side**
**M54.42** **Lumbago with sciatica, left side**

✓5th **M54.5 Low back pain**
EXCLUDES 1 *intervertebral disc degeneration, lumbar region with discogenic back pain only (M51.360)*
*intervertebral disc degeneration, lumbosacral region with discogenic back pain only (M51.370)*
*low back strain (S39.012)*
*lumbago due to intervertebral disc displacement (M51.2-)*
*lumbago with sciatica (M54.4-)*
**AHA:** 2026,1Q,32; 2021,4Q,22
**M54.50** **Low back pain, unspecified**
Loin pain
Lumbago NOS
**M54.51** **Vertebrogenic low back pain**
Low back vertebral endplate pain
**M54.59** **Other low back pain**

**M54.6 Pain in thoracic spine**
EXCLUDES 1 *pain in thoracic spine due to intervertebral disc disorder (M51.-)*

✓5th **M54.8 Other dorsalgia**
EXCLUDES 1 *dorsalgia in thoracic region (M54.6)*
*low back pain (M54.5-)*
**M54.81** **Occipital neuralgia**
**M54.89** **Other dorsalgia**

**M54.9 Dorsalgia, unspecified**
Back pain NOS
Backache NOS

## SOFT TISSUE DISORDERS (M60-M79)

### Disorders of muscles (M60-M63)

EXCLUDES 1 *dermatopolymyositis (M33.-)*
*myopathy in amyloidosis (E85.-)*
*myopathy in polyarteritis nodosa (M30.0)*
*myopathy in rheumatoid arthritis (M05.32)*
*myopathy in scleroderma (M34.-)*
*myopathy in Sjögren's syndrome (M35.03)*
*myopathy in systemic lupus erythematosus (M32.-)*
EXCLUDES 2 *muscular dystrophies and myopathies (G71-G72)*

✓4th **M60 Myositis**
EXCLUDES 2 *inclusion body myositis [IBM] (G72.41)*

✓5th **M60.0 Infective myositis**
Tropical pyomyositis
Use additional code (B95-B97) to identify infectious agent

✓6th **M60.00 Infective myositis, unspecified site**
**M60.000** **Infective myositis, unspecified right arm**
Infective myositis, right upper limb NOS
**M60.001** **Infective myositis, unspecified left arm**
Infective myositis, left upper limb NOS
**M60.002** **Infective myositis, unspecified arm**
Infective myositis, upper limb NOS
**M60.003** **Infective myositis, unspecified right leg**
Infective myositis, right lower limb NOS
**M60.004** **Infective myositis, unspecified left leg**
Infective myositis, left lower limb NOS
**M60.005** **Infective myositis, unspecified leg**
Infective myositis, lower limb NOS
**M60.009** **Infective myositis, unspecified site**

✓6th **M60.01 Infective myositis, shoulder**
**M60.011** **Infective myositis, right shoulder**
**M60.012** **Infective myositis, left shoulder**
**M60.019** **Infective myositis, unspecified shoulder**

✓6th **M60.02 Infective myositis, upper arm**
**M60.021** **Infective myositis, right upper arm**
**M60.022** **Infective myositis, left upper arm**
**M60.029** **Infective myositis, unspecified upper arm**

✓6th **M60.03 Infective myositis, forearm**
**M60.031** **Infective myositis, right forearm**
**M60.032** **Infective myositis, left forearm**
**M60.039** **Infective myositis, unspecified forearm**

✓6th **M60.04 Infective myositis, hand and fingers**
**M60.041** **Infective myositis, right hand**
**M60.042** **Infective myositis, left hand**
**M60.043** **Infective myositis, unspecified hand**
**M60.044** **Infective myositis, right finger(s)**
**M60.045** **Infective myositis, left finger(s)**
**M60.046** **Infective myositis, unspecified finger(s)**

M60.05 Infective myositis, thigh
M60.051 Infective myositis, right thigh
M60.052 Infective myositis, left thigh
M60.059 Infective myositis, unspecified thigh
M60.06 Infective myositis, lower leg
M60.061 Infective myositis, right lower leg
M60.062 Infective myositis, left lower leg
M60.069 Infective myositis, unspecified lower leg
M60.07 Infective myositis, ankle, foot and toes
M60.070 Infective myositis, right ankle
M60.071 Infective myositis, left ankle
M60.072 Infective myositis, unspecified ankle
M60.073 Infective myositis, right foot
M60.074 Infective myositis, left foot
M60.075 Infective myositis, unspecified foot
M60.076 Infective myositis, right toe(s)
M60.077 Infective myositis, left toe(s)
M60.078 Infective myositis, unspecified toe(s)
M60.08 Infective myositis, other site
M60.09 Infective myositis, multiple sites

M60.1 Interstitial myositis
M60.10 Interstitial myositis of unspecified site
M60.11 Interstitial myositis, shoulder
M60.111 Interstitial myositis, right shoulder
M60.112 Interstitial myositis, left shoulder
M60.119 Interstitial myositis, unspecified shoulder
M60.12 Interstitial myositis, upper arm
M60.121 Interstitial myositis, right upper arm
M60.122 Interstitial myositis, left upper arm
M60.129 Interstitial myositis, unspecified upper arm
M60.13 Interstitial myositis, forearm
M60.131 Interstitial myositis, right forearm
M60.132 Interstitial myositis, left forearm
M60.139 Interstitial myositis, unspecified forearm
M60.14 Interstitial myositis, hand
M60.141 Interstitial myositis, right hand
M60.142 Interstitial myositis, left hand
M60.149 Interstitial myositis, unspecified hand
M60.15 Interstitial myositis, thigh
M60.151 Interstitial myositis, right thigh
M60.152 Interstitial myositis, left thigh
M60.159 Interstitial myositis, unspecified thigh
M60.16 Interstitial myositis, lower leg
M60.161 Interstitial myositis, right lower leg
M60.162 Interstitial myositis, left lower leg
M60.169 Interstitial myositis, unspecified lower leg
M60.17 Interstitial myositis, ankle and foot
M60.171 Interstitial myositis, right ankle and foot
M60.172 Interstitial myositis, left ankle and foot
M60.179 Interstitial myositis, unspecified ankle and foot
M60.18 Interstitial myositis, other site
M60.19 Interstitial myositis, multiple sites

M60.2 Foreign body granuloma of soft tissue, not elsewhere classified
Use additional code to identify the type of retained foreign body (Z18.-)
EXCLUDES 1 *foreign body granuloma of skin and subcutaneous tissue (L92.3)*
M60.20 Foreign body granuloma of soft tissue, not elsewhere classified, unspecified site
M60.21 Foreign body granuloma of soft tissue, not elsewhere classified, shoulder
M60.211 Foreign body granuloma of soft tissue, not elsewhere classified, right shoulder
M60.212 Foreign body granuloma of soft tissue, not elsewhere classified, left shoulder
M60.219 Foreign body granuloma of soft tissue, not elsewhere classified, unspecified shoulder
M60.22 Foreign body granuloma of soft tissue, not elsewhere classified, upper arm
M60.221 Foreign body granuloma of soft tissue, not elsewhere classified, right upper arm
M60.222 Foreign body granuloma of soft tissue, not elsewhere classified, left upper arm
M60.229 Foreign body granuloma of soft tissue, not elsewhere classified, unspecified upper arm
M60.23 Foreign body granuloma of soft tissue, not elsewhere classified, forearm
M60.231 Foreign body granuloma of soft tissue, not elsewhere classified, right forearm
M60.232 Foreign body granuloma of soft tissue, not elsewhere classified, left forearm
M60.239 Foreign body granuloma of soft tissue, not elsewhere classified, unspecified forearm
M60.24 Foreign body granuloma of soft tissue, not elsewhere classified, hand
M60.241 Foreign body granuloma of soft tissue, not elsewhere classified, right hand
M60.242 Foreign body granuloma of soft tissue, not elsewhere classified, left hand
M60.249 Foreign body granuloma of soft tissue, not elsewhere classified, unspecified hand
M60.25 Foreign body granuloma of soft tissue, not elsewhere classified, thigh
M60.251 Foreign body granuloma of soft tissue, not elsewhere classified, right thigh
M60.252 Foreign body granuloma of soft tissue, not elsewhere classified, left thigh
M60.259 Foreign body granuloma of soft tissue, not elsewhere classified, unspecified thigh
M60.26 Foreign body granuloma of soft tissue, not elsewhere classified, lower leg
M60.261 Foreign body granuloma of soft tissue, not elsewhere classified, right lower leg
M60.262 Foreign body granuloma of soft tissue, not elsewhere classified, left lower leg
M60.269 Foreign body granuloma of soft tissue, not elsewhere classified, unspecified lower leg
M60.27 Foreign body granuloma of soft tissue, not elsewhere classified, ankle and foot
M60.271 Foreign body granuloma of soft tissue, not elsewhere classified, right ankle and foot
M60.272 Foreign body granuloma of soft tissue, not elsewhere classified, left ankle and foot
M60.279 Foreign body granuloma of soft tissue, not elsewhere classified, unspecified ankle and foot
M60.28 Foreign body granuloma of soft tissue, not elsewhere classified, other site

M60.8 Other myositis
M60.80 Other myositis, unspecified site
M60.81 Other myositis shoulder
M60.811 Other myositis, right shoulder
M60.812 Other myositis, left shoulder
M60.819 Other myositis, unspecified shoulder
M60.82 Other myositis, upper arm
M60.821 Other myositis, right upper arm
M60.822 Other myositis, left upper arm
M60.829 Other myositis, unspecified upper arm
M60.83 Other myositis, forearm
M60.831 Other myositis, right forearm
M60.832 Other myositis, left forearm
M60.839 Other myositis, unspecified forearm
M60.84 Other myositis, hand
M60.841 Other myositis, right hand
M60.842 Other myositis, left hand
M60.849 Other myositis, unspecified hand
M60.85 Other myositis, thigh
M60.851 Other myositis, right thigh
M60.852 Other myositis, left thigh
M60.859 Other myositis, unspecified thigh
M60.86 Other myositis, lower leg
M60.861 Other myositis, right lower leg
M60.862 Other myositis, left lower leg
M60.869 Other myositis, unspecified lower leg
M60.87 Other myositis, ankle and foot
M60.871 Other myositis, right ankle and foot
M60.872 Other myositis, left ankle and foot
M60.879 Other myositis, unspecified ankle and foot
M60.88 Other myositis, other site
M60.89 Other myositis, multiple sites

M60.9 Myositis, unspecified

**√4th M61 Calcification and ossification of muscle**

**√5th M61.0 Myositis ossificans traumatica**

**M61.00 Myositis ossificans traumatica, unspecified site**

**√6th M61.01 Myositis ossificans traumatica, shoulder**

**M61.011 Myositis ossificans traumatica, right shoulder**

**M61.012 Myositis ossificans traumatica, left shoulder**

**M61.019 Myositis ossificans traumatica, unspecified shoulder**

**√6th M61.02 Myositis ossificans traumatica, upper arm**

**M61.021 Myositis ossificans traumatica, right upper arm**

**M61.022 Myositis ossificans traumatica, left upper arm**

**M61.029 Myositis ossificans traumatica, unspecified upper arm**

**√6th M61.03 Myositis ossificans traumatica, forearm**

**M61.031 Myositis ossificans traumatica, right forearm**

**M61.032 Myositis ossificans traumatica, left forearm**

**M61.039 Myositis ossificans traumatica, unspecified forearm**

**√6th M61.04 Myositis ossificans traumatica, hand**

**M61.041 Myositis ossificans traumatica, right hand**

**M61.042 Myositis ossificans traumatica, left hand**

**M61.049 Myositis ossificans traumatica, unspecified hand**

**√6th M61.05 Myositis ossificans traumatica, thigh**

**M61.051 Myositis ossificans traumatica, right thigh**

**M61.052 Myositis ossificans traumatica, left thigh**

**M61.059 Myositis ossificans traumatica, unspecified thigh**

**√6th M61.06 Myositis ossificans traumatica, lower leg**

**M61.061 Myositis ossificans traumatica, right lower leg**

**M61.062 Myositis ossificans traumatica, left lower leg**

**M61.069 Myositis ossificans traumatica, unspecified lower leg**

**√6th M61.07 Myositis ossificans traumatica, ankle and foot**

**M61.071 Myositis ossificans traumatica, right ankle and foot**

**M61.072 Myositis ossificans traumatica, left ankle and foot**

**M61.079 Myositis ossificans traumatica, unspecified ankle and foot**

**M61.08 Myositis ossificans traumatica, other site**

**M61.09 Myositis ossificans traumatica, multiple sites**

**√5th M61.1 Myositis ossificans progressiva**

Fibrodysplasia ossificans progressiva

**M61.10 Myositis ossificans progressiva, unspecified site**

**√6th M61.11 Myositis ossificans progressiva, shoulder**

**M61.111 Myositis ossificans progressiva, right shoulder**

**M61.112 Myositis ossificans progressiva, left shoulder**

**M61.119 Myositis ossificans progressiva, unspecified shoulder**

**√6th M61.12 Myositis ossificans progressiva, upper arm**

**M61.121 Myositis ossificans progressiva, right upper arm**

**M61.122 Myositis ossificans progressiva, left upper arm**

**M61.129 Myositis ossificans progressiva, unspecified upper arm**

**√6th M61.13 Myositis ossificans progressiva, forearm**

**M61.131 Myositis ossificans progressiva, right forearm**

**M61.132 Myositis ossificans progressiva, left forearm**

**M61.139 Myositis ossificans progressiva, unspecified forearm**

**√6th M61.14 Myositis ossificans progressiva, hand and finger(s)**

**M61.141 Myositis ossificans progressiva, right hand**

**M61.142 Myositis ossificans progressiva, left hand**

**M61.143 Myositis ossificans progressiva, unspecified hand**

**M61.144 Myositis ossificans progressiva, right finger(s)**

**M61.145 Myositis ossificans progressiva, left finger(s)**

**M61.146 Myositis ossificans progressiva, unspecified finger(s)**

**√6th M61.15 Myositis ossificans progressiva, thigh**

**M61.151 Myositis ossificans progressiva, right thigh**

**M61.152 Myositis ossificans progressiva, left thigh**

**M61.159 Myositis ossificans progressiva, unspecified thigh**

**√6th M61.16 Myositis ossificans progressiva, lower leg**

**M61.161 Myositis ossificans progressiva, right lower leg**

**M61.162 Myositis ossificans progressiva, left lower leg**

**M61.169 Myositis ossificans progressiva, unspecified lower leg**

**√6th M61.17 Myositis ossificans progressiva, ankle, foot and toe(s)**

**M61.171 Myositis ossificans progressiva, right ankle**

**M61.172 Myositis ossificans progressiva, left ankle**

**M61.173 Myositis ossificans progressiva, unspecified ankle**

**M61.174 Myositis ossificans progressiva, right foot**

**M61.175 Myositis ossificans progressiva, left foot**

**M61.176 Myositis ossificans progressiva, unspecified foot**

**M61.177 Myositis ossificans progressiva, right toe(s)**

**M61.178 Myositis ossificans progressiva, left toe(s)**

**M61.179 Myositis ossificans progressiva, unspecified toe(s)**

**M61.18 Myositis ossificans progressiva, other site**

**M61.19 Myositis ossificans progressiva, multiple sites**

**√5th M61.2 Paralytic calcification and ossification of muscle**

Myositis ossificans associated with quadriplegia or paraplegia

**M61.20 Paralytic calcification and ossification of muscle, unspecified site**

**√6th M61.21 Paralytic calcification and ossification of muscle, shoulder**

**M61.211 Paralytic calcification and ossification of muscle, right shoulder**

**M61.212 Paralytic calcification and ossification of muscle, left shoulder**

**M61.219 Paralytic calcification and ossification of muscle, unspecified shoulder**

**√6th M61.22 Paralytic calcification and ossification of muscle, upper arm**

**M61.221 Paralytic calcification and ossification of muscle, right upper arm**

**M61.222 Paralytic calcification and ossification of muscle, left upper arm**

**M61.229 Paralytic calcification and ossification of muscle, unspecified upper arm**

**√6th M61.23 Paralytic calcification and ossification of muscle, forearm**

**M61.231 Paralytic calcification and ossification of muscle, right forearm**

**M61.232 Paralytic calcification and ossification of muscle, left forearm**

**M61.239 Paralytic calcification and ossification of muscle, unspecified forearm**

**√6th M61.24 Paralytic calcification and ossification of muscle, hand**

**M61.241 Paralytic calcification and ossification of muscle, right hand**

**M61.242 Paralytic calcification and ossification of muscle, left hand**

**M61.249 Paralytic calcification and ossification of muscle, unspecified hand**

**√6th M61.25 Paralytic calcification and ossification of muscle, thigh**

**M61.251 Paralytic calcification and ossification of muscle, right thigh**

**M61.252 Paralytic calcification and ossification of muscle, left thigh**

**M61.259 Paralytic calcification and ossification of muscle, unspecified thigh**

**√6th M61.26 Paralytic calcification and ossification of muscle, lower leg**

**M61.261 Paralytic calcification and ossification of muscle, right lower leg**

M61.262 Paralytic calcification and ossification of muscle, left lower leg
M61.269 Paralytic calcification and ossification of muscle, unspecified lower leg
✓6th M61.27 Paralytic calcification and ossification of muscle, ankle and foot
M61.271 Paralytic calcification and ossification of muscle, right ankle and foot
M61.272 Paralytic calcification and ossification of muscle, left ankle and foot
M61.279 Paralytic calcification and ossification of muscle, unspecified ankle and foot
M61.28 Paralytic calcification and ossification of muscle, other site
M61.29 Paralytic calcification and ossification of muscle, multiple sites
✓5th M61.3 Calcification and ossification of muscles associated with burns
Myositis ossificans associated with burns
M61.30 Calcification and ossification of muscles associated with burns, unspecified site
✓6th M61.31 Calcification and ossification of muscles associated with burns, shoulder
M61.311 Calcification and ossification of muscles associated with burns, right shoulder
M61.312 Calcification and ossification of muscles associated with burns, left shoulder
M61.319 Calcification and ossification of muscles associated with burns, unspecified shoulder
✓6th M61.32 Calcification and ossification of muscles associated with burns, upper arm
M61.321 Calcification and ossification of muscles associated with burns, right upper arm
M61.322 Calcification and ossification of muscles associated with burns, left upper arm
M61.329 Calcification and ossification of muscles associated with burns, unspecified upper arm
✓6th M61.33 Calcification and ossification of muscles associated with burns, forearm
M61.331 Calcification and ossification of muscles associated with burns, right forearm
M61.332 Calcification and ossification of muscles associated with burns, left forearm
M61.339 Calcification and ossification of muscles associated with burns, unspecified forearm
✓6th M61.34 Calcification and ossification of muscles associated with burns, hand
M61.341 Calcification and ossification of muscles associated with burns, right hand
M61.342 Calcification and ossification of muscles associated with burns, left hand
M61.349 Calcification and ossification of muscles associated with burns, unspecified hand
✓6th M61.35 Calcification and ossification of muscles associated with burns, thigh
M61.351 Calcification and ossification of muscles associated with burns, right thigh
M61.352 Calcification and ossification of muscles associated with burns, left thigh
M61.359 Calcification and ossification of muscles associated with burns, unspecified thigh
✓6th M61.36 Calcification and ossification of muscles associated with burns, lower leg
M61.361 Calcification and ossification of muscles associated with burns, right lower leg
M61.362 Calcification and ossification of muscles associated with burns, left lower leg
M61.369 Calcification and ossification of muscles associated with burns, unspecified lower leg
✓6th M61.37 Calcification and ossification of muscles associated with burns, ankle and foot
M61.371 Calcification and ossification of muscles associated with burns, right ankle and foot
M61.372 Calcification and ossification of muscles associated with burns, left ankle and foot
M61.379 Calcification and ossification of muscles associated with burns, unspecified ankle and foot
M61.38 Calcification and ossification of muscles associated with burns, other site
M61.39 Calcification and ossification of muscles associated with burns, multiple sites
✓5th M61.4 Other calcification of muscle
EXCLUDES 1 *calcific tendinitis NOS (M65.2-)*
*calcific tendinitis of shoulder (M75.3)*
M61.40 Other calcification of muscle, unspecified site
✓6th M61.41 Other calcification of muscle, shoulder
M61.411 Other calcification of muscle, right shoulder
M61.412 Other calcification of muscle, left shoulder
M61.419 Other calcification of muscle, unspecified shoulder
✓6th M61.42 Other calcification of muscle, upper arm
M61.421 Other calcification of muscle, right upper arm
M61.422 Other calcification of muscle, left upper arm
M61.429 Other calcification of muscle, unspecified upper arm
✓6th M61.43 Other calcification of muscle, forearm
M61.431 Other calcification of muscle, right forearm
M61.432 Other calcification of muscle, left forearm
M61.439 Other calcification of muscle, unspecified forearm
✓6th M61.44 Other calcification of muscle, hand
M61.441 Other calcification of muscle, right hand
M61.442 Other calcification of muscle, left hand
M61.449 Other calcification of muscle, unspecified hand
✓6th M61.45 Other calcification of muscle, thigh
M61.451 Other calcification of muscle, right thigh
M61.452 Other calcification of muscle, left thigh
M61.459 Other calcification of muscle, unspecified thigh
✓6th M61.46 Other calcification of muscle, lower leg
M61.461 Other calcification of muscle, right lower leg
M61.462 Other calcification of muscle, left lower leg
M61.469 Other calcification of muscle, unspecified lower leg
✓6th M61.47 Other calcification of muscle, ankle and foot
M61.471 Other calcification of muscle, right ankle and foot
M61.472 Other calcification of muscle, left ankle and foot
M61.479 Other calcification of muscle, unspecified ankle and foot
M61.48 Other calcification of muscle, other site
M61.49 Other calcification of muscle, multiple sites
✓5th M61.5 Other ossification of muscle
M61.50 Other ossification of muscle, unspecified site
✓6th M61.51 Other ossification of muscle, shoulder
M61.511 Other ossification of muscle, right shoulder
M61.512 Other ossification of muscle, left shoulder
M61.519 Other ossification of muscle, unspecified shoulder
✓6th M61.52 Other ossification of muscle, upper arm
M61.521 Other ossification of muscle, right upper arm
M61.522 Other ossification of muscle, left upper arm
M61.529 Other ossification of muscle, unspecified upper arm
✓6th M61.53 Other ossification of muscle, forearm
M61.531 Other ossification of muscle, right forearm
M61.532 Other ossification of muscle, left forearm
M61.539 Other ossification of muscle, unspecified forearm
✓6th M61.54 Other ossification of muscle, hand
M61.541 Other ossification of muscle, right hand
M61.542 Other ossification of muscle, left hand
M61.549 Other ossification of muscle, unspecified hand
✓6th M61.55 Other ossification of muscle, thigh
M61.551 Other ossification of muscle, right thigh
M61.552 Other ossification of muscle, left thigh
**AHA:** 2024,3Q,14
M61.559 Other ossification of muscle, unspecified thigh

6th M61.56 Other ossification of muscle, lower leg
M61.561 Other ossification of muscle, right lower leg
M61.562 Other ossification of muscle, left lower leg
M61.569 Other ossification of muscle, unspecified lower leg
6th M61.57 Other ossification of muscle, ankle and foot
M61.571 Other ossification of muscle, right ankle and foot
M61.572 Other ossification of muscle, left ankle and foot
M61.579 Other ossification of muscle, unspecified ankle and foot
M61.58 Other ossification of muscle, other site
M61.59 Other ossification of muscle, multiple sites
M61.9 Calcification and ossification of muscle, unspecified

4th **M62 Other disorders of muscle**
EXCLUDES 1 *alcoholic myopathy (G72.1)*
*cramp and spasm (R25.2)*
*drug-induced myopathy (G72.Ø)*
*myalgia (M79.1-)*
*stiff-man syndrome (G25.82)*
EXCLUDES 2 *nontraumatic hematoma of muscle (M79.81)*

5th M62.Ø Separation of muscle (nontraumatic)
Diastasis of muscle
EXCLUDES 1 *diastasis recti complicating pregnancy, labor and delivery (O71.8)*
*traumatic separation of muscle - see strain of muscle by body region*
M62.ØØ Separation of muscle (nontraumatic), unspecified site
6th M62.Ø1 Separation of muscle (nontraumatic), shoulder
M62.Ø11 Separation of muscle (nontraumatic), right shoulder
M62.Ø12 Separation of muscle (nontraumatic), left shoulder
M62.Ø19 Separation of muscle (nontraumatic), unspecified shoulder
6th M62.Ø2 Separation of muscle (nontraumatic), upper arm
M62.Ø21 Separation of muscle (nontraumatic), right upper arm
M62.Ø22 Separation of muscle (nontraumatic), left upper arm
M62.Ø29 Separation of muscle (nontraumatic), unspecified upper arm
6th M62.Ø3 Separation of muscle (nontraumatic), forearm
M62.Ø31 Separation of muscle (nontraumatic), right forearm
M62.Ø32 Separation of muscle (nontraumatic), left forearm
M62.Ø39 Separation of muscle (nontraumatic), unspecified forearm
6th M62.Ø4 Separation of muscle (nontraumatic), hand
M62.Ø41 Separation of muscle (nontraumatic), right hand
M62.Ø42 Separation of muscle (nontraumatic), left hand
M62.Ø49 Separation of muscle (nontraumatic), unspecified hand
6th M62.Ø5 Separation of muscle (nontraumatic), thigh
M62.Ø51 Separation of muscle (nontraumatic), right thigh
M62.Ø52 Separation of muscle (nontraumatic), left thigh
M62.Ø59 Separation of muscle (nontraumatic), unspecified thigh
6th M62.Ø6 Separation of muscle (nontraumatic), lower leg
M62.Ø61 Separation of muscle (nontraumatic), right lower leg
M62.Ø62 Separation of muscle (nontraumatic), left lower leg
M62.Ø69 Separation of muscle (nontraumatic), unspecified lower leg
6th M62.Ø7 Separation of muscle (nontraumatic), ankle and foot
M62.Ø71 Separation of muscle (nontraumatic), right ankle and foot
M62.Ø72 Separation of muscle (nontraumatic), left ankle and foot
M62.Ø79 Separation of muscle (nontraumatic), unspecified ankle and foot
M62.Ø8 Separation of muscle (nontraumatic), other site

5th M62.1 Other rupture of muscle (nontraumatic)
EXCLUDES 1 *traumatic rupture of muscle - see strain of muscle by body region*
EXCLUDES 2 *rupture of tendon (M66.-)*
M62.1Ø Other rupture of muscle (nontraumatic), unspecified site
6th M62.11 Other rupture of muscle (nontraumatic), shoulder
M62.111 Other rupture of muscle (nontraumatic), right shoulder
M62.112 Other rupture of muscle (nontraumatic), left shoulder
M62.119 Other rupture of muscle (nontraumatic), unspecified shoulder
6th M62.12 Other rupture of muscle (nontraumatic), upper arm
M62.121 Other rupture of muscle (nontraumatic), right upper arm
M62.122 Other rupture of muscle (nontraumatic), left upper arm
M62.129 Other rupture of muscle (nontraumatic), unspecified upper arm
6th M62.13 Other rupture of muscle (nontraumatic), forearm
M62.131 Other rupture of muscle (nontraumatic), right forearm
M62.132 Other rupture of muscle (nontraumatic), left forearm
M62.139 Other rupture of muscle (nontraumatic), unspecified forearm
6th M62.14 Other rupture of muscle (nontraumatic), hand
M62.141 Other rupture of muscle (nontraumatic), right hand
M62.142 Other rupture of muscle (nontraumatic), left hand
M62.149 Other rupture of muscle (nontraumatic), unspecified hand
6th M62.15 Other rupture of muscle (nontraumatic), thigh
M62.151 Other rupture of muscle (nontraumatic), right thigh
M62.152 Other rupture of muscle (nontraumatic), left thigh
M62.159 Other rupture of muscle (nontraumatic), unspecified thigh
6th M62.16 Other rupture of muscle (nontraumatic), lower leg
M62.161 Other rupture of muscle (nontraumatic), right lower leg
M62.162 Other rupture of muscle (nontraumatic), left lower leg
M62.169 Other rupture of muscle (nontraumatic), unspecified lower leg
6th M62.17 Other rupture of muscle (nontraumatic), ankle and foot
M62.171 Other rupture of muscle (nontraumatic), right ankle and foot
M62.172 Other rupture of muscle (nontraumatic), left ankle and foot
M62.179 Other rupture of muscle (nontraumatic), unspecified ankle and foot
M62.18 Other rupture of muscle (nontraumatic), other site

5th M62.2 Nontraumatic ischemic infarction of muscle
EXCLUDES 1 *compartment syndrome (traumatic) (T79.A-)*
*nontraumatic compartment syndrome (M79.A-)*
*rhabdomyolysis (M62.82)*
*traumatic ischemia of muscle (T79.6)*
*Volkmann's ischemic contracture (T79.6)*
M62.2Ø Nontraumatic ischemic infarction of muscle, unspecified site
6th M62.21 Nontraumatic ischemic infarction of muscle, shoulder
M62.211 Nontraumatic ischemic infarction of muscle, right shoulder
M62.212 Nontraumatic ischemic infarction of muscle, left shoulder
M62.219 Nontraumatic ischemic infarction of muscle, unspecified shoulder
6th M62.22 Nontraumatic ischemic infarction of muscle, upper arm
M62.221 Nontraumatic ischemic infarction of muscle, right upper arm

M62.222 Nontraumatic ischemic infarction of muscle, left upper arm
M62.229 Nontraumatic ischemic infarction of muscle, unspecified upper arm
✓6th M62.23 Nontraumatic ischemic infarction of muscle, forearm
M62.231 Nontraumatic ischemic infarction of muscle, right forearm
M62.232 Nontraumatic ischemic infarction of muscle, left forearm
M62.239 Nontraumatic ischemic infarction of muscle, unspecified forearm
✓6th M62.24 Nontraumatic ischemic infarction of muscle, hand
M62.241 Nontraumatic ischemic infarction of muscle, right hand
M62.242 Nontraumatic ischemic infarction of muscle, left hand
M62.249 Nontraumatic ischemic infarction of muscle, unspecified hand
✓6th M62.25 Nontraumatic ischemic infarction of muscle, thigh
M62.251 Nontraumatic ischemic infarction of muscle, right thigh
M62.252 Nontraumatic ischemic infarction of muscle, left thigh
M62.259 Nontraumatic ischemic infarction of muscle, unspecified thigh
✓6th M62.26 Nontraumatic ischemic infarction of muscle, lower leg
M62.261 Nontraumatic ischemic infarction of muscle, right lower leg
M62.262 Nontraumatic ischemic infarction of muscle, left lower leg
M62.269 Nontraumatic ischemic infarction of muscle, unspecified lower leg
✓6th M62.27 Nontraumatic ischemic infarction of muscle, ankle and foot
M62.271 Nontraumatic ischemic infarction of muscle, right ankle and foot
M62.272 Nontraumatic ischemic infarction of muscle, left ankle and foot
M62.279 Nontraumatic ischemic infarction of muscle, unspecified ankle and foot
M62.28 Nontraumatic ischemic infarction of muscle, other site
M62.3 Immobility syndrome (paraplegic)
✓5th M62.4 Contracture of muscle
Contracture of tendon (sheath)
EXCLUDES 1 *contracture of joint (M24.5-)*
M62.4Ø Contracture of muscle, unspecified site
✓6th M62.41 Contracture of muscle, shoulder
M62.411 Contracture of muscle, right shoulder
M62.412 Contracture of muscle, left shoulder
M62.419 Contracture of muscle, unspecified shoulder
✓6th M62.42 Contracture of muscle, upper arm
M62.421 Contracture of muscle, right upper arm
M62.422 Contracture of muscle, left upper arm
M62.429 Contracture of muscle, unspecified upper arm
✓6th M62.43 Contracture of muscle, forearm
M62.431 Contracture of muscle, right forearm
M62.432 Contracture of muscle, left forearm
M62.439 Contracture of muscle, unspecified forearm
✓6th M62.44 Contracture of muscle, hand
M62.441 Contracture of muscle, right hand
M62.442 Contracture of muscle, left hand
M62.449 Contracture of muscle, unspecified hand
✓6th M62.45 Contracture of muscle, thigh
M62.451 Contracture of muscle, right thigh
M62.452 Contracture of muscle, left thigh
M62.459 Contracture of muscle, unspecified thigh
✓6th M62.46 Contracture of muscle, lower leg
AHA: 2023,2Q,14
M62.461 Contracture of muscle, right lower leg
M62.462 Contracture of muscle, left lower leg
M62.469 Contracture of muscle, unspecified lower leg
✓6th M62.47 Contracture of muscle, ankle and foot
M62.471 Contracture of muscle, right ankle and foot
M62.472 Contracture of muscle, left ankle and foot
M62.479 Contracture of muscle, unspecified ankle and foot
M62.48 Contracture of muscle, other site
M62.49 Contracture of muscle, multiple sites
✓5th M62.5 Muscle wasting and atrophy, not elsewhere classified
Disuse atrophy NEC
EXCLUDES 1 *neuralgic amyotrophy (G54.5)*
*progressive muscular atrophy (G12.21)*
*sarcopenia (M62.84)*
EXCLUDES 2 *pelvic muscle wasting (N81.84)*
M62.5Ø Muscle wasting and atrophy, not elsewhere classified, unspecified site
✓6th M62.51 Muscle wasting and atrophy, not elsewhere classified, shoulder
M62.511 Muscle wasting and atrophy, not elsewhere classified, right shoulder
M62.512 Muscle wasting and atrophy, not elsewhere classified, left shoulder
M62.519 Muscle wasting and atrophy, not elsewhere classified, unspecified shoulder
✓6th M62.52 Muscle wasting and atrophy, not elsewhere classified, upper arm
M62.521 Muscle wasting and atrophy, not elsewhere classified, right upper arm
M62.522 Muscle wasting and atrophy, not elsewhere classified, left upper arm
M62.529 Muscle wasting and atrophy, not elsewhere classified, unspecified upper arm
✓6th M62.53 Muscle wasting and atrophy, not elsewhere classified, forearm
M62.531 Muscle wasting and atrophy, not elsewhere classified, right forearm
M62.532 Muscle wasting and atrophy, not elsewhere classified, left forearm
M62.539 Muscle wasting and atrophy, not elsewhere classified, unspecified forearm
✓6th M62.54 Muscle wasting and atrophy, not elsewhere classified, hand
M62.541 Muscle wasting and atrophy, not elsewhere classified, right hand
M62.542 Muscle wasting and atrophy, not elsewhere classified, left hand
M62.549 Muscle wasting and atrophy, not elsewhere classified, unspecified hand
✓6th M62.55 Muscle wasting and atrophy, not elsewhere classified, thigh
M62.551 Muscle wasting and atrophy, not elsewhere classified, right thigh
M62.552 Muscle wasting and atrophy, not elsewhere classified, left thigh
M62.559 Muscle wasting and atrophy, not elsewhere classified, unspecified thigh
✓6th M62.56 Muscle wasting and atrophy, not elsewhere classified, lower leg
M62.561 Muscle wasting and atrophy, not elsewhere classified, right lower leg
M62.562 Muscle wasting and atrophy, not elsewhere classified, left lower leg
M62.569 Muscle wasting and atrophy, not elsewhere classified, unspecified lower leg
✓6th M62.57 Muscle wasting and atrophy, not elsewhere classified, ankle and foot
M62.571 Muscle wasting and atrophy, not elsewhere classified, right ankle and foot
M62.572 Muscle wasting and atrophy, not elsewhere classified, left ankle and foot
M62.579 Muscle wasting and atrophy, not elsewhere classified, unspecified ankle and foot
M62.58 Muscle wasting and atrophy, not elsewhere classified, other site
M62.59 Muscle wasting and atrophy, not elsewhere classified, multiple sites
✓6th M62.5A Muscle wasting and atrophy, not elsewhere classified, back
AHA: 2022,4Q,29
M62.5AØ Muscle wasting and atrophy, not elsewhere classified, back, cervical
M62.5A1 Muscle wasting and atrophy, not elsewhere classified, back, thoracic
M62.5A2 Muscle wasting and atrophy, not elsewhere classified, back, lumbosacral
M62.5A9 Muscle wasting and atrophy, not elsewhere classified, back, unspecified level

✓5th **M62.8 Other specified disorders of muscle**
EXCLUDES 2 *nontraumatic hematoma of muscle (M79.81)*
**M62.81 Muscle weakness (generalized)**
EXCLUDES 1 *muscle weakness in sarcopenia (M62.84)*
**M62.82 Rhabdomyolysis**
EXCLUDES 1 *traumatic rhabdomyolysis (T79.6)*
**AHA:** 2024,4Q,16; 2019,2Q,12
**DEF:** Rapid disintegration or destruction of skeletal muscle caused by direct or indirect injury, resulting in the excretion of muscle protein myoglobin into the urine.
✓6th **M62.83 Muscle spasm**
**M62.83Ø Muscle spasm of back**
**M62.831 Muscle spasm of calf**
Charley-horse
**M62.838 Other muscle spasm**
**M62.84 Sarcopenia**
Age-related sarcopenia
Code first underlying disease, if applicable, such as:
disorders of myoneural junction and muscle disease in diseases classified elsewhere (G73.-)
other and unspecified myopathies (G72.-)
primary disorders of muscles (G71.-)
**AHA:** 2016,4Q,41
**M62.85 Dysfunction of the multifidus muscles, lumbar region**
**AHA:** 2024,4Q,25
**M62.89 Other specified disorders of muscle**
Muscle (sheath) hernia
**M62.9 Disorder of muscle, unspecified**

✓4th **M63 Disorders of muscle in diseases classified elsewhere**
Code first underlying disease, such as:
leprosy (A3Ø.-)
neoplasm (C49.-, C79.89, D21.-, D48.1-)
schistosomiasis (B65.-)
trichinellosis (B75)
EXCLUDES 1 *myopathy in cysticercosis (B69.81)*
*myopathy in endocrine diseases (G73.7)*
*myopathy in metabolic diseases (G73.7)*
*myopathy in sarcoidosis (D86.87)*
*myopathy in secondary syphilis (A51.49)*
*myopathy in syphilis (late) (A52.78)*
*myopathy in toxoplasmosis (B58.82)*
*myopathy in tuberculosis (A18.Ø9)*
✓5th **M63.8 Disorders of muscle in diseases classified elsewhere**
***M63.8Ø Disorders of muscle in diseases classified elsewhere, unspecified site***
✓6th **M63.81 Disorders of muscle in diseases classified elsewhere, shoulder**
***M63.811 Disorders of muscle in diseases classified elsewhere, right shoulder***
***M63.812 Disorders of muscle in diseases classified elsewhere, left shoulder***
***M63.819 Disorders of muscle in diseases classified elsewhere, unspecified shoulder***
✓6th **M63.82 Disorders of muscle in diseases classified elsewhere, upper arm**
***M63.821 Disorders of muscle in diseases classified elsewhere, right upper arm***
***M63.822 Disorders of muscle in diseases classified elsewhere, left upper arm***
***M63.829 Disorders of muscle in diseases classified elsewhere, unspecified upper arm***
✓6th **M63.83 Disorders of muscle in diseases classified elsewhere, forearm**
***M63.831 Disorders of muscle in diseases classified elsewhere, right forearm***
***M63.832 Disorders of muscle in diseases classified elsewhere, left forearm***
***M63.839 Disorders of muscle in diseases classified elsewhere, unspecified forearm***
✓6th **M63.84 Disorders of muscle in diseases classified elsewhere, hand**
***M63.841 Disorders of muscle in diseases classified elsewhere, right hand***
***M63.842 Disorders of muscle in diseases classified elsewhere, left hand***
***M63.849 Disorders of muscle in diseases classified elsewhere, unspecified hand***
✓6th **M63.85 Disorders of muscle in diseases classified elsewhere, thigh**
***M63.851 Disorders of muscle in diseases classified elsewhere, right thigh***
***M63.852 Disorders of muscle in diseases classified elsewhere, left thigh***
***M63.859 Disorders of muscle in diseases classified elsewhere, unspecified thigh***
✓6th **M63.86 Disorders of muscle in diseases classified elsewhere, lower leg**
***M63.861 Disorders of muscle in diseases classified elsewhere, right lower leg***
***M63.862 Disorders of muscle in diseases classified elsewhere, left lower leg***
***M63.869 Disorders of muscle in diseases classified elsewhere, unspecified lower leg***
✓6th **M63.87 Disorders of muscle in diseases classified elsewhere, ankle and foot**
***M63.871 Disorders of muscle in diseases classified elsewhere, right ankle and foot***
***M63.872 Disorders of muscle in diseases classified elsewhere, left ankle and foot***
***M63.879 Disorders of muscle in diseases classified elsewhere, unspecified ankle and foot***
***M63.88 Disorders of muscle in diseases classified elsewhere, other site***
***M63.89 Disorders of muscle in diseases classified elsewhere, multiple sites***

## Disorders of synovium and tendon (M65-M67)

✓4th **M65 Synovitis and tenosynovitis**
EXCLUDES 1 *chronic crepitant synovitis of hand and wrist (M7Ø.Ø-)*
*current injury - see injury of ligament or tendon by body region*
*soft tissue disorders related to use, overuse and pressure (M7Ø.-)*
✓5th **M65.Ø Abscess of tendon sheath**
Use additional code (B95-B96) to identify bacterial agent.
**M65.ØØ Abscess of tendon sheath, unspecified site**
✓6th **M65.Ø1 Abscess of tendon sheath, shoulder**
**M65.Ø11 Abscess of tendon sheath, right shoulder**
**M65.Ø12 Abscess of tendon sheath, left shoulder**
**M65.Ø19 Abscess of tendon sheath, unspecified shoulder**
✓6th **M65.Ø2 Abscess of tendon sheath, upper arm**
**M65.Ø21 Abscess of tendon sheath, right upper arm**
**M65.Ø22 Abscess of tendon sheath, left upper arm**
**M65.Ø29 Abscess of tendon sheath, unspecified upper arm**
✓6th **M65.Ø3 Abscess of tendon sheath, forearm**
**M65.Ø31 Abscess of tendon sheath, right forearm**
**M65.Ø32 Abscess of tendon sheath, left forearm**
**M65.Ø39 Abscess of tendon sheath, unspecified forearm**
✓6th **M65.Ø4 Abscess of tendon sheath, hand**
**M65.Ø41 Abscess of tendon sheath, right hand**
**M65.Ø42 Abscess of tendon sheath, left hand**
**M65.Ø49 Abscess of tendon sheath, unspecified hand**
✓6th **M65.Ø5 Abscess of tendon sheath, thigh**
**M65.Ø51 Abscess of tendon sheath, right thigh**
**M65.Ø52 Abscess of tendon sheath, left thigh**
**M65.Ø59 Abscess of tendon sheath, unspecified thigh**
✓6th **M65.Ø6 Abscess of tendon sheath, lower leg**
**M65.Ø61 Abscess of tendon sheath, right lower leg**
**M65.Ø62 Abscess of tendon sheath, left lower leg**
**M65.Ø69 Abscess of tendon sheath, unspecified lower leg**
✓6th **M65.Ø7 Abscess of tendon sheath, ankle and foot**
**M65.Ø71 Abscess of tendon sheath, right ankle and foot**
**M65.Ø72 Abscess of tendon sheath, left ankle and foot**
**M65.Ø79 Abscess of tendon sheath, unspecified ankle and foot**
**M65.Ø8 Abscess of tendon sheath, other site**
✓5th **M65.1 Other infective (teno)synovitis**
**M65.1Ø Other infective (teno)synovitis, unspecified site**

√6th M65.11 Other infective (teno)synovitis, shoulder
M65.111 Other infective (teno)synovitis, right shoulder
M65.112 Other infective (teno)synovitis, left shoulder
M65.119 Other infective (teno)synovitis, unspecified shoulder
√6th M65.12 Other infective (teno)synovitis, elbow
M65.121 Other infective (teno)synovitis, right elbow
M65.122 Other infective (teno)synovitis, left elbow
M65.129 Other infective (teno)synovitis, unspecified elbow
√6th M65.13 Other infective (teno)synovitis, wrist
M65.131 Other infective (teno)synovitis, right wrist
M65.132 Other infective (teno)synovitis, left wrist
M65.139 Other infective (teno)synovitis, unspecified wrist
√6th M65.14 Other infective (teno)synovitis, hand
M65.141 Other infective (teno)synovitis, right hand
M65.142 Other infective (teno)synovitis, left hand
M65.149 Other infective (teno)synovitis, unspecified hand
√6th M65.15 Other infective (teno)synovitis, hip
M65.151 Other infective (teno)synovitis, right hip
M65.152 Other infective (teno)synovitis, left hip
M65.159 Other infective (teno)synovitis, unspecified hip
√6th M65.16 Other infective (teno)synovitis, knee
M65.161 Other infective (teno)synovitis, right knee
M65.162 Other infective (teno)synovitis, left knee
M65.169 Other infective (teno)synovitis, unspecified knee
√6th M65.17 Other infective (teno)synovitis, ankle and foot
M65.171 Other infective (teno)synovitis, right ankle and foot
M65.172 Other infective (teno)synovitis, left ankle and foot
M65.179 Other infective (teno)synovitis, unspecified ankle and foot
M65.18 Other infective (teno)synovitis, other site
M65.19 Other infective (teno)synovitis, multiple sites
√5th M65.2 Calcific tendinitis
EXCLUDES 1 *tendinitis as classified in M75-M77*
*calcified tendinitis of shoulder (M75.3)*
M65.20 Calcific tendinitis, unspecified site
√6th M65.22 Calcific tendinitis, upper arm
M65.221 Calcific tendinitis, right upper arm
M65.222 Calcific tendinitis, left upper arm
M65.229 Calcific tendinitis, unspecified upper arm
√6th M65.23 Calcific tendinitis, forearm
M65.231 Calcific tendinitis, right forearm
M65.232 Calcific tendinitis, left forearm
M65.239 Calcific tendinitis, unspecified forearm
√6th M65.24 Calcific tendinitis, hand
M65.241 Calcific tendinitis, right hand
M65.242 Calcific tendinitis, left hand
M65.249 Calcific tendinitis, unspecified hand
√6th M65.25 Calcific tendinitis, thigh
M65.251 Calcific tendinitis, right thigh
M65.252 Calcific tendinitis, left thigh
M65.259 Calcific tendinitis, unspecified thigh
√6th M65.26 Calcific tendinitis, lower leg
M65.261 Calcific tendinitis, right lower leg
M65.262 Calcific tendinitis, left lower leg
M65.269 Calcific tendinitis, unspecified lower leg
√6th M65.27 Calcific tendinitis, ankle and foot
M65.271 Calcific tendinitis, right ankle and foot
M65.272 Calcific tendinitis, left ankle and foot
M65.279 Calcific tendinitis, unspecified ankle and foot
M65.28 Calcific tendinitis, other site
M65.29 Calcific tendinitis, multiple sites
√5th M65.3 Trigger finger
Nodular tendinous disease
M65.30 Trigger finger, unspecified finger
√6th M65.31 Trigger thumb
M65.311 Trigger thumb, right thumb
M65.312 Trigger thumb, left thumb
M65.319 Trigger thumb, unspecified thumb
√6th M65.32 Trigger finger, index finger
M65.321 Trigger finger, right index finger
M65.322 Trigger finger, left index finger
M65.329 Trigger finger, unspecified index finger
√6th M65.33 Trigger finger, middle finger
M65.331 Trigger finger, right middle finger
M65.332 Trigger finger, left middle finger
M65.339 Trigger finger, unspecified middle finger
√6th M65.34 Trigger finger, ring finger
M65.341 Trigger finger, right ring finger
M65.342 Trigger finger, left ring finger
M65.349 Trigger finger, unspecified ring finger
√6th M65.35 Trigger finger, little finger
M65.351 Trigger finger, right little finger
M65.352 Trigger finger, left little finger
M65.359 Trigger finger, unspecified little finger
M65.4 Radial styloid tenosynovitis [de Quervain]
√5th M65.8 Other synovitis and tenosynovitis
M65.80 Other synovitis and tenosynovitis, unspecified site
√6th M65.81 Other synovitis and tenosynovitis, shoulder
M65.811 Other synovitis and tenosynovitis, right shoulder
M65.812 Other synovitis and tenosynovitis, left shoulder
M65.819 Other synovitis and tenosynovitis, unspecified shoulder
√6th M65.82 Other synovitis and tenosynovitis, upper arm
M65.821 Other synovitis and tenosynovitis, right upper arm
M65.822 Other synovitis and tenosynovitis, left upper arm
M65.829 Other synovitis and tenosynovitis, unspecified upper arm
√6th M65.83 Other synovitis and tenosynovitis, forearm
M65.831 Other synovitis and tenosynovitis, right forearm
M65.832 Other synovitis and tenosynovitis, left forearm
M65.839 Other synovitis and tenosynovitis, unspecified forearm
√6th M65.84 Other synovitis and tenosynovitis, hand
M65.841 Other synovitis and tenosynovitis, right hand
M65.842 Other synovitis and tenosynovitis, left hand
M65.849 Other synovitis and tenosynovitis, unspecified hand
√6th M65.85 Other synovitis and tenosynovitis, thigh
M65.851 Other synovitis and tenosynovitis, right thigh
M65.852 Other synovitis and tenosynovitis, left thigh
M65.859 Other synovitis and tenosynovitis, unspecified thigh
√6th M65.86 Other synovitis and tenosynovitis, lower leg
M65.861 Other synovitis and tenosynovitis, right lower leg
M65.862 Other synovitis and tenosynovitis, left lower leg
M65.869 Other synovitis and tenosynovitis, unspecified lower leg
√6th M65.87 Other synovitis and tenosynovitis, ankle and foot
M65.871 Other synovitis and tenosynovitis, right ankle and foot
M65.872 Other synovitis and tenosynovitis, left ankle and foot
M65.879 Other synovitis and tenosynovitis, unspecified ankle and foot
M65.88 Other synovitis and tenosynovitis, other site
M65.89 Other synovitis and tenosynovitis, multiple sites
√5th M65.9 Synovitis and tenosynovitis, unspecified
AHA: 2024,4Q,25
M65.90 Unspecified synovitis and tenosynovitis, unspecified site

✓6th M65.91 Unspecified synovitis and tenosynovitis, shoulder
M65.911 Unspecified synovitis and tenosynovitis, right shoulder
M65.912 Unspecified synovitis and tenosynovitis, left shoulder
M65.919 Unspecified synovitis and tenosynovitis, unspecified shoulder
✓6th M65.92 Unspecified synovitis and tenosynovitis, upper arm
M65.921 Unspecified synovitis and tenosynovitis, right upper arm
M65.922 Unspecified synovitis and tenosynovitis, left upper arm
M65.929 Unspecified synovitis and tenosynovitis, unspecified upper arm
✓6th M65.93 Unspecified synovitis and tenosynovitis, forearm
M65.931 Unspecified synovitis and tenosynovitis, right forearm
M65.932 Unspecified synovitis and tenosynovitis, left forearm
M65.939 Unspecified synovitis and tenosynovitis, unspecified forearm
✓6th M65.94 Unspecified synovitis and tenosynovitis, hand
M65.941 Unspecified synovitis and tenosynovitis, right hand
M65.942 Unspecified synovitis and tenosynovitis, left hand
M65.949 Unspecified synovitis and tenosynovitis, unspecified hand
✓6th M65.95 Unspecified synovitis and tenosynovitis, thigh
M65.951 Unspecified synovitis and tenosynovitis, right thigh
M65.952 Unspecified synovitis and tenosynovitis, left thigh
M65.959 Unspecified synovitis and tenosynovitis, unspecified thigh
✓6th M65.96 Unspecified synovitis and tenosynovitis, lower leg
M65.961 Unspecified synovitis and tenosynovitis, right lower leg
M65.962 Unspecified synovitis and tenosynovitis, left lower leg
M65.969 Unspecified synovitis and tenosynovitis, unspecified lower leg
✓6th M65.97 Unspecified synovitis and tenosynovitis, ankle and foot
M65.971 Unspecified synovitis and tenosynovitis, right ankle and foot
M65.972 Unspecified synovitis and tenosynovitis, left ankle and foot
M65.979 Unspecified synovitis and tenosynovitis, unspecified ankle and foot
M65.98 Unspecified synovitis and tenosynovitis, other site
M65.99 Unspecified synovitis and tenosynovitis, multiple sites

✓4th **M66 Spontaneous rupture of synovium and tendon**

INCLUDES rupture that occurs when a normal force is applied to tissues that are inferred to have less than normal strength

EXCLUDES 2 *rotator cuff syndrome (M75.1-)*
*rupture where an abnormal force is applied to normal tissue - see injury of tendon by body region*

M66.Ø Rupture of popliteal cyst
✓5th M66.1 Rupture of synovium
Rupture of synovial cyst
EXCLUDES 2 *rupture of popliteal cyst (M66.Ø)*
M66.1Ø Rupture of synovium, unspecified joint
✓6th M66.11 Rupture of synovium, shoulder
M66.111 Rupture of synovium, right shoulder
M66.112 Rupture of synovium, left shoulder
M66.119 Rupture of synovium, unspecified shoulder
✓6th M66.12 Rupture of synovium, elbow
M66.121 Rupture of synovium, right elbow
M66.122 Rupture of synovium, left elbow
M66.129 Rupture of synovium, unspecified elbow
✓6th M66.13 Rupture of synovium, wrist
M66.131 Rupture of synovium, right wrist
M66.132 Rupture of synovium, left wrist
M66.139 Rupture of synovium, unspecified wrist
✓6th M66.14 Rupture of synovium, hand and fingers
M66.141 Rupture of synovium, right hand
M66.142 Rupture of synovium, left hand
M66.143 Rupture of synovium, unspecified hand
M66.144 Rupture of synovium, right finger(s)
M66.145 Rupture of synovium, left finger(s)
M66.146 Rupture of synovium, unspecified finger(s)
✓6th M66.15 Rupture of synovium, hip
M66.151 Rupture of synovium, right hip
M66.152 Rupture of synovium, left hip
M66.159 Rupture of synovium, unspecified hip
✓6th M66.17 Rupture of synovium, ankle, foot and toes
M66.171 Rupture of synovium, right ankle
M66.172 Rupture of synovium, left ankle
M66.173 Rupture of synovium, unspecified ankle
M66.174 Rupture of synovium, right foot
M66.175 Rupture of synovium, left foot
M66.176 Rupture of synovium, unspecified foot
M66.177 Rupture of synovium, right toe(s)
M66.178 Rupture of synovium, left toe(s)
M66.179 Rupture of synovium, unspecified toe(s)
M66.18 Rupture of synovium, other site
✓5th M66.2 Spontaneous rupture of extensor tendons
**TIP:** Refer to the Muscle/Tendon table at the beginning of this chapter.
M66.2Ø Spontaneous rupture of extensor tendons, unspecified site
✓6th M66.21 Spontaneous rupture of extensor tendons, shoulder
M66.211 Spontaneous rupture of extensor tendons, right shoulder
M66.212 Spontaneous rupture of extensor tendons, left shoulder
M66.219 Spontaneous rupture of extensor tendons, unspecified shoulder
✓6th M66.22 Spontaneous rupture of extensor tendons, upper arm
M66.221 Spontaneous rupture of extensor tendons, right upper arm
M66.222 Spontaneous rupture of extensor tendons, left upper arm
M66.229 Spontaneous rupture of extensor tendons, unspecified upper arm
✓6th M66.23 Spontaneous rupture of extensor tendons, forearm
M66.231 Spontaneous rupture of extensor tendons, right forearm
M66.232 Spontaneous rupture of extensor tendons, left forearm
M66.239 Spontaneous rupture of extensor tendons, unspecified forearm
✓6th M66.24 Spontaneous rupture of extensor tendons, hand
M66.241 Spontaneous rupture of extensor tendons, right hand
M66.242 Spontaneous rupture of extensor tendons, left hand
M66.249 Spontaneous rupture of extensor tendons, unspecified hand
✓6th M66.25 Spontaneous rupture of extensor tendons, thigh
M66.251 Spontaneous rupture of extensor tendons, right thigh
M66.252 Spontaneous rupture of extensor tendons, left thigh
M66.259 Spontaneous rupture of extensor tendons, unspecified thigh
✓6th M66.26 Spontaneous rupture of extensor tendons, lower leg
M66.261 Spontaneous rupture of extensor tendons, right lower leg
M66.262 Spontaneous rupture of extensor tendons, left lower leg
M66.269 Spontaneous rupture of extensor tendons, unspecified lower leg
✓6th M66.27 Spontaneous rupture of extensor tendons, ankle and foot
M66.271 Spontaneous rupture of extensor tendons, right ankle and foot
M66.272 Spontaneous rupture of extensor tendons, left ankle and foot
M66.279 Spontaneous rupture of extensor tendons, unspecified ankle and foot
M66.28 Spontaneous rupture of extensor tendons, other site
M66.29 Spontaneous rupture of extensor tendons, multiple sites

✓5th M66.3 Spontaneous rupture of flexor tendons
TIP: Refer to the Muscle/Tendon table at the beginning of this chapter.
M66.30 Spontaneous rupture of flexor tendons, unspecified site
✓6th M66.31 Spontaneous rupture of flexor tendons, shoulder
M66.311 Spontaneous rupture of flexor tendons, right shoulder
M66.312 Spontaneous rupture of flexor tendons, left shoulder
M66.319 Spontaneous rupture of flexor tendons, unspecified shoulder
✓6th M66.32 Spontaneous rupture of flexor tendons, upper arm
M66.321 Spontaneous rupture of flexor tendons, right upper arm
M66.322 Spontaneous rupture of flexor tendons, left upper arm
M66.329 Spontaneous rupture of flexor tendons, unspecified upper arm
✓6th M66.33 Spontaneous rupture of flexor tendons, forearm
M66.331 Spontaneous rupture of flexor tendons, right forearm
M66.332 Spontaneous rupture of flexor tendons, left forearm
M66.339 Spontaneous rupture of flexor tendons, unspecified forearm
✓6th M66.34 Spontaneous rupture of flexor tendons, hand
M66.341 Spontaneous rupture of flexor tendons, right hand
M66.342 Spontaneous rupture of flexor tendons, left hand
M66.349 Spontaneous rupture of flexor tendons, unspecified hand
✓6th M66.35 Spontaneous rupture of flexor tendons, thigh
M66.351 Spontaneous rupture of flexor tendons, right thigh
M66.352 Spontaneous rupture of flexor tendons, left thigh
M66.359 Spontaneous rupture of flexor tendons, unspecified thigh
✓6th M66.36 Spontaneous rupture of flexor tendons, lower leg
M66.361 Spontaneous rupture of flexor tendons, right lower leg
M66.362 Spontaneous rupture of flexor tendons, left lower leg
M66.369 Spontaneous rupture of flexor tendons, unspecified lower leg
✓6th M66.37 Spontaneous rupture of flexor tendons, ankle and foot
M66.371 Spontaneous rupture of flexor tendons, right ankle and foot
M66.372 Spontaneous rupture of flexor tendons, left ankle and foot
M66.379 Spontaneous rupture of flexor tendons, unspecified ankle and foot
M66.38 Spontaneous rupture of flexor tendons, other site
M66.39 Spontaneous rupture of flexor tendons, multiple sites
✓5th M66.8 Spontaneous rupture of other tendons
TIP: Refer to the Muscle/Tendon table at the beginning of this chapter.
M66.80 Spontaneous rupture of other tendons, unspecified site
✓6th M66.81 Spontaneous rupture of other tendons, shoulder
M66.811 Spontaneous rupture of other tendons, right shoulder
M66.812 Spontaneous rupture of other tendons, left shoulder
M66.819 Spontaneous rupture of other tendons, unspecified shoulder
✓6th M66.82 Spontaneous rupture of other tendons, upper arm
M66.821 Spontaneous rupture of other tendons, right upper arm
M66.822 Spontaneous rupture of other tendons, left upper arm
M66.829 Spontaneous rupture of other tendons, unspecified upper arm
✓6th M66.83 Spontaneous rupture of other tendons, forearm
M66.831 Spontaneous rupture of other tendons, right forearm
M66.832 Spontaneous rupture of other tendons, left forearm
M66.839 Spontaneous rupture of other tendons, unspecified forearm
✓6th M66.84 Spontaneous rupture of other tendons, hand
M66.841 Spontaneous rupture of other tendons, right hand
M66.842 Spontaneous rupture of other tendons, left hand
M66.849 Spontaneous rupture of other tendons, unspecified hand
✓6th M66.85 Spontaneous rupture of other tendons, thigh
M66.851 Spontaneous rupture of other tendons, right thigh
M66.852 Spontaneous rupture of other tendons, left thigh
M66.859 Spontaneous rupture of other tendons, unspecified thigh
✓6th M66.86 Spontaneous rupture of other tendons, lower leg
M66.861 Spontaneous rupture of other tendons, right lower leg
M66.862 Spontaneous rupture of other tendons, left lower leg
M66.869 Spontaneous rupture of other tendons, unspecified lower leg
✓6th M66.87 Spontaneous rupture of other tendons, ankle and foot
M66.871 Spontaneous rupture of other tendons, right ankle and foot
M66.872 Spontaneous rupture of other tendons, left ankle and foot
M66.879 Spontaneous rupture of other tendons, unspecified ankle and foot
M66.88 Spontaneous rupture of other tendons, other sites
M66.89 Spontaneous rupture of other tendons, multiple sites
M66.9 Spontaneous rupture of unspecified tendon
Rupture at musculotendinous junction, nontraumatic

✓4th **M67 Other disorders of synovium and tendon**
EXCLUDES 1 *palmar fascial fibromatosis [Dupuytren] (M72.0)*
*tendinitis NOS (M77.9-)*
*xanthomatosis localized to tendons (E78.2)*
✓5th M67.0 Short Achilles tendon (acquired)
M67.00 Short Achilles tendon (acquired), unspecified ankle
M67.01 Short Achilles tendon (acquired), right ankle
M67.02 Short Achilles tendon (acquired), left ankle
✓5th M67.2 Synovial hypertrophy, not elsewhere classified
EXCLUDES 1 *villonodular synovitis (pigmented) (M12.2-)*
M67.20 Synovial hypertrophy, not elsewhere classified, unspecified site
✓6th M67.21 Synovial hypertrophy, not elsewhere classified, shoulder
M67.211 Synovial hypertrophy, not elsewhere classified, right shoulder
M67.212 Synovial hypertrophy, not elsewhere classified, left shoulder
M67.219 Synovial hypertrophy, not elsewhere classified, unspecified shoulder
✓6th M67.22 Synovial hypertrophy, not elsewhere classified, upper arm
M67.221 Synovial hypertrophy, not elsewhere classified, right upper arm
M67.222 Synovial hypertrophy, not elsewhere classified, left upper arm
M67.229 Synovial hypertrophy, not elsewhere classified, unspecified upper arm
✓6th M67.23 Synovial hypertrophy, not elsewhere classified, forearm
M67.231 Synovial hypertrophy, not elsewhere classified, right forearm
M67.232 Synovial hypertrophy, not elsewhere classified, left forearm
M67.239 Synovial hypertrophy, not elsewhere classified, unspecified forearm
✓6th M67.24 Synovial hypertrophy, not elsewhere classified, hand
M67.241 Synovial hypertrophy, not elsewhere classified, right hand
M67.242 Synovial hypertrophy, not elsewhere classified, left hand
M67.249 Synovial hypertrophy, not elsewhere classified, unspecified hand

√6th **M67.25 Synovial hypertrophy, not elsewhere classified, thigh**
- **M67.251 Synovial hypertrophy, not elsewhere classified, right thigh**
- **M67.252 Synovial hypertrophy, not elsewhere classified, left thigh**
- **M67.259 Synovial hypertrophy, not elsewhere classified, unspecified thigh**

√6th **M67.26 Synovial hypertrophy, not elsewhere classified, lower leg**
- **M67.261 Synovial hypertrophy, not elsewhere classified, right lower leg**
- **M67.262 Synovial hypertrophy, not elsewhere classified, left lower leg**
- **M67.269 Synovial hypertrophy, not elsewhere classified, unspecified lower leg**

√6th **M67.27 Synovial hypertrophy, not elsewhere classified, ankle and foot**
- **M67.271 Synovial hypertrophy, not elsewhere classified, right ankle and foot**
- **M67.272 Synovial hypertrophy, not elsewhere classified, left ankle and foot**
- **M67.279 Synovial hypertrophy, not elsewhere classified, unspecified ankle and foot**

**M67.28 Synovial hypertrophy, not elsewhere classified, other site**

**M67.29 Synovial hypertrophy, not elsewhere classified, multiple sites**

√5th **M67.3 Transient synovitis**

Toxic synovitis

EXCLUDES 1 *palindromic rheumatism (M12.3-)*

**M67.30 Transient synovitis, unspecified site**

√6th **M67.31 Transient synovitis, shoulder**
- **M67.311 Transient synovitis, right shoulder**
- **M67.312 Transient synovitis, left shoulder**
- **M67.319 Transient synovitis, unspecified shoulder**

√6th **M67.32 Transient synovitis, elbow**
- **M67.321 Transient synovitis, right elbow**
- **M67.322 Transient synovitis, left elbow**
- **M67.329 Transient synovitis, unspecified elbow**

√6th **M67.33 Transient synovitis, wrist**
- **M67.331 Transient synovitis, right wrist**
- **M67.332 Transient synovitis, left wrist**
- **M67.339 Transient synovitis, unspecified wrist**

√6th **M67.34 Transient synovitis, hand**
- **M67.341 Transient synovitis, right hand**
- **M67.342 Transient synovitis, left hand**
- **M67.349 Transient synovitis, unspecified hand**

√6th **M67.35 Transient synovitis, hip**
- **M67.351 Transient synovitis, right hip**
- **M67.352 Transient synovitis, left hip**
- **M67.359 Transient synovitis, unspecified hip**

√6th **M67.36 Transient synovitis, knee**
- **M67.361 Transient synovitis, right knee**
- **M67.362 Transient synovitis, left knee**
- **M67.369 Transient synovitis, unspecified knee**

√6th **M67.37 Transient synovitis, ankle and foot**
- **M67.371 Transient synovitis, right ankle and foot**
- **M67.372 Transient synovitis, left ankle and foot**
- **M67.379 Transient synovitis, unspecified ankle and foot**

**M67.38 Transient synovitis, other site**

**M67.39 Transient synovitis, multiple sites**

√5th **M67.4 Ganglion**

Ganglion of joint or tendon (sheath)

EXCLUDES 1 *ganglion in yaws (A66.6)*

EXCLUDES 2 *cyst of bursa (M71.2-M71.3)*
*cyst of synovium (M71.2-M71.3)*

**DEF:** Fluid-filled, benign cyst appearing on a tendon sheath or aponeurosis, frequently connecting to an underlying joint.

**M67.40 Ganglion, unspecified site**

√6th **M67.41 Ganglion, shoulder**
- **M67.411 Ganglion, right shoulder**
- **M67.412 Ganglion, left shoulder**
- **M67.419 Ganglion, unspecified shoulder**

√6th **M67.42 Ganglion, elbow**
- **M67.421 Ganglion, right elbow**
- **M67.422 Ganglion, left elbow**
- **M67.429 Ganglion, unspecified elbow**

√6th **M67.43 Ganglion, wrist**

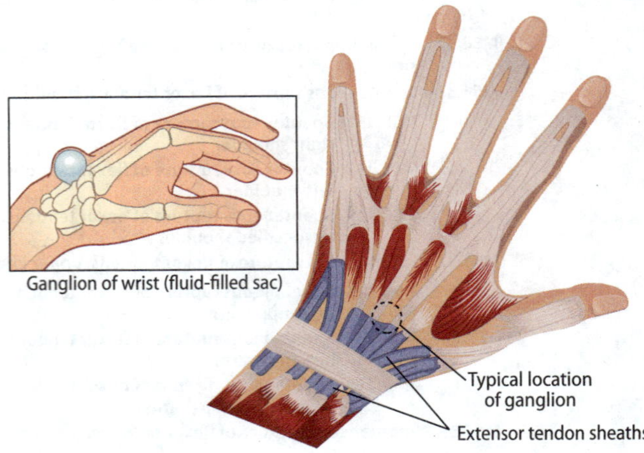


- **M67.431 Ganglion, right wrist**
- **M67.432 Ganglion, left wrist**
- **M67.439 Ganglion, unspecified wrist**

√6th **M67.44 Ganglion, hand**
- **M67.441 Ganglion, right hand**
- **M67.442 Ganglion, left hand**
- **M67.449 Ganglion, unspecified hand**

√6th **M67.45 Ganglion, hip**
- **M67.451 Ganglion, right hip**
- **M67.452 Ganglion, left hip**
- **M67.459 Ganglion, unspecified hip**

√6th **M67.46 Ganglion, knee**
- **M67.461 Ganglion, right knee**
- **M67.462 Ganglion, left knee**
- **M67.469 Ganglion, unspecified knee**

√6th **M67.47 Ganglion, ankle and foot**
- **M67.471 Ganglion, right ankle and foot**
- **M67.472 Ganglion, left ankle and foot**
- **M67.479 Ganglion, unspecified ankle and foot**

**M67.48 Ganglion, other site**

**M67.49 Ganglion, multiple sites**

√5th **M67.5 Plica syndrome**

Plica knee

**M67.50 Plica syndrome, unspecified knee**

**M67.51 Plica syndrome, right knee**

**M67.52 Plica syndrome, left knee**

√5th **M67.8 Other specified disorders of synovium and tendon**

**M67.80 Other specified disorders of synovium and tendon, unspecified site**

√6th **M67.81 Other specified disorders of synovium and tendon, shoulder**
- **M67.811 Other specified disorders of synovium, right shoulder**
- **M67.812 Other specified disorders of synovium, left shoulder**
- **M67.813 Other specified disorders of tendon, right shoulder**
- **M67.814 Other specified disorders of tendon, left shoulder**
- **M67.819 Other specified disorders of synovium and tendon, unspecified shoulder**

√6th **M67.82 Other specified disorders of synovium and tendon, elbow**
- **M67.821 Other specified disorders of synovium, right elbow**
- **M67.822 Other specified disorders of synovium, left elbow**
- **M67.823 Other specified disorders of tendon, right elbow**
- **M67.824 Other specified disorders of tendon, left elbow**
- **M67.829 Other specified disorders of synovium and tendon, unspecified elbow**

√6th **M67.83 Other specified disorders of synovium and tendon, wrist**
- **M67.831 Other specified disorders of synovium, right wrist**

M67.832 Other specified disorders of synovium, left wrist
M67.833 Other specified disorders of tendon, right wrist
M67.834 Other specified disorders of tendon, left wrist
M67.839 Other specified disorders of synovium and tendon, unspecified wrist

√6th M67.84 Other specified disorders of synovium and tendon, hand
M67.841 Other specified disorders of synovium, right hand
M67.842 Other specified disorders of synovium, left hand
M67.843 Other specified disorders of tendon, right hand
M67.844 Other specified disorders of tendon, left hand
M67.849 Other specified disorders of synovium and tendon, unspecified hand

√6th M67.85 Other specified disorders of synovium and tendon, hip
M67.851 Other specified disorders of synovium, right hip
M67.852 Other specified disorders of synovium, left hip
M67.853 Other specified disorders of tendon, right hip
M67.854 Other specified disorders of tendon, left hip
M67.859 Other specified disorders of synovium and tendon, unspecified hip

√6th M67.86 Other specified disorders of synovium and tendon, knee
M67.861 Other specified disorders of synovium, right knee
M67.862 Other specified disorders of synovium, left knee
M67.863 Other specified disorders of tendon, right knee
M67.864 Other specified disorders of tendon, left knee
M67.869 Other specified disorders of synovium and tendon, unspecified knee

√6th M67.87 Other specified disorders of synovium and tendon, ankle and foot
M67.871 Other specified disorders of synovium, right ankle and foot
M67.872 Other specified disorders of synovium, left ankle and foot
M67.873 Other specified disorders of tendon, right ankle and foot
M67.874 Other specified disorders of tendon, left ankle and foot
M67.879 Other specified disorders of synovium and tendon, unspecified ankle and foot

M67.88 Other specified disorders of synovium and tendon, other site
M67.89 Other specified disorders of synovium and tendon, multiple sites

√5th M67.9 Unspecified disorder of synovium and tendon
M67.90 Unspecified disorder of synovium and tendon, unspecified site

√6th M67.91 Unspecified disorder of synovium and tendon, shoulder
M67.911 Unspecified disorder of synovium and tendon, right shoulder
M67.912 Unspecified disorder of synovium and tendon, left shoulder
M67.919 Unspecified disorder of synovium and tendon, unspecified shoulder

√6th M67.92 Unspecified disorder of synovium and tendon, upper arm
M67.921 Unspecified disorder of synovium and tendon, right upper arm
M67.922 Unspecified disorder of synovium and tendon, left upper arm
M67.929 Unspecified disorder of synovium and tendon, unspecified upper arm

√6th M67.93 Unspecified disorder of synovium and tendon, forearm
M67.931 Unspecified disorder of synovium and tendon, right forearm
M67.932 Unspecified disorder of synovium and tendon, left forearm
M67.939 Unspecified disorder of synovium and tendon, unspecified forearm

√6th M67.94 Unspecified disorder of synovium and tendon, hand
M67.941 Unspecified disorder of synovium and tendon, right hand
M67.942 Unspecified disorder of synovium and tendon, left hand
M67.949 Unspecified disorder of synovium and tendon, unspecified hand

√6th M67.95 Unspecified disorder of synovium and tendon, thigh
M67.951 Unspecified disorder of synovium and tendon, right thigh
M67.952 Unspecified disorder of synovium and tendon, left thigh
M67.959 Unspecified disorder of synovium and tendon, unspecified thigh

√6th M67.96 Unspecified disorder of synovium and tendon, lower leg
M67.961 Unspecified disorder of synovium and tendon, right lower leg
M67.962 Unspecified disorder of synovium and tendon, left lower leg
M67.969 Unspecified disorder of synovium and tendon, unspecified lower leg

√6th M67.97 Unspecified disorder of synovium and tendon, ankle and foot
M67.971 Unspecified disorder of synovium and tendon, right ankle and foot
M67.972 Unspecified disorder of synovium and tendon, left ankle and foot
M67.979 Unspecified disorder of synovium and tendon, unspecified ankle and foot

M67.98 Unspecified disorder of synovium and tendon, other site
M67.99 Unspecified disorder of synovium and tendon, multiple sites

● √5th M67.A Plantar fasciitis
● √6th M67.A0 Plantar fasciitis, foot
● M67.A01 Plantar fasciitis, right foot
● M67.A02 Plantar fasciitis, left foot
● M67.A09 Plantar fasciitis, unspecified foot
Plantar fasciitis NOS

## Other soft tissue disorders (M70-M79)

√4th **M70 Soft tissue disorders related to use, overuse and pressure**

INCLUDES soft tissue disorders of occupational origin

Use additional external cause code to identify activity causing disorder (Y93.-)

EXCLUDES 1 *bursitis NOS (M71.9-)*

EXCLUDES 2 *bursitis of shoulder (M75.5)*
*enthesopathies (M76-M77)*
*pressure ulcer (pressure area) (L89.-)*

√5th M70.0 Crepitant synovitis (acute) (chronic) of hand and wrist

√6th M70.03 Crepitant synovitis (acute) (chronic), wrist
M70.031 Crepitant synovitis (acute) (chronic), right wrist
M70.032 Crepitant synovitis (acute) (chronic), left wrist
M70.039 Crepitant synovitis (acute) (chronic), unspecified wrist

√6th M70.04 Crepitant synovitis (acute) (chronic), hand
M70.041 Crepitant synovitis (acute) (chronic), right hand
M70.042 Crepitant synovitis (acute) (chronic), left hand
M70.049 Crepitant synovitis (acute) (chronic), unspecified hand

√5th M70.1 Bursitis of hand
M70.10 Bursitis, unspecified hand
M70.11 Bursitis, right hand
M70.12 Bursitis, left hand

√5th M70.2 Olecranon bursitis
M70.20 Olecranon bursitis, unspecified elbow
M70.21 Olecranon bursitis, right elbow
M70.22 Olecranon bursitis, left elbow

✓5th M70.3 Other bursitis of elbow
- M70.30 Other bursitis of elbow, unspecified elbow
- M70.31 Other bursitis of elbow, right elbow
- M70.32 Other bursitis of elbow, left elbow

✓5th M70.4 Prepatellar bursitis
- M70.40 Prepatellar bursitis, unspecified knee
- M70.41 Prepatellar bursitis, right knee
- M70.42 Prepatellar bursitis, left knee

**Knee Bursae**

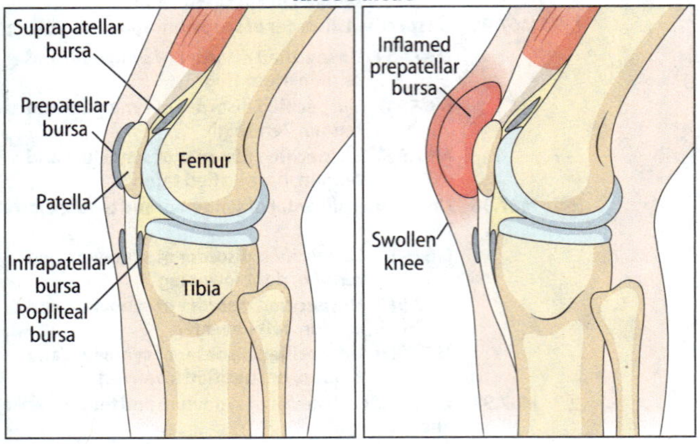


✓5th M70.5 Other bursitis of knee
- M70.50 Other bursitis of knee, unspecified knee
- M70.51 Other bursitis of knee, right knee
- M70.52 Other bursitis of knee, left knee

✓5th M70.6 Trochanteric bursitis

Trochanteric tendinitis
- M70.60 Trochanteric bursitis, unspecified hip
- M70.61 Trochanteric bursitis, right hip
- M70.62 Trochanteric bursitis, left hip

✓5th M70.7 Other bursitis of hip

Ischial bursitis
- M70.70 Other bursitis of hip, unspecified hip
- M70.71 Other bursitis of hip, right hip
- M70.72 Other bursitis of hip, left hip

✓5th M70.8 Other soft tissue disorders related to use, overuse and pressure
- M70.80 Other soft tissue disorders related to use, overuse and pressure of unspecified site

✓6th M70.81 Other soft tissue disorders related to use, overuse and pressure of shoulder
- M70.811 Other soft tissue disorders related to use, overuse and pressure, right shoulder
- M70.812 Other soft tissue disorders related to use, overuse and pressure, left shoulder
- M70.819 Other soft tissue disorders related to use, overuse and pressure, unspecified shoulder

✓6th M70.82 Other soft tissue disorders related to use, overuse and pressure of upper arm
- M70.821 Other soft tissue disorders related to use, overuse and pressure, right upper arm
- M70.822 Other soft tissue disorders related to use, overuse and pressure, left upper arm
- M70.829 Other soft tissue disorders related to use, overuse and pressure, unspecified upper arms

✓6th M70.83 Other soft tissue disorders related to use, overuse and pressure of forearm
- M70.831 Other soft tissue disorders related to use, overuse and pressure, right forearm
- M70.832 Other soft tissue disorders related to use, overuse and pressure, left forearm
- M70.839 Other soft tissue disorders related to use, overuse and pressure, unspecified forearm

✓6th M70.84 Other soft tissue disorders related to use, overuse and pressure of hand
- M70.841 Other soft tissue disorders related to use, overuse and pressure, right hand
- M70.842 Other soft tissue disorders related to use, overuse and pressure, left hand
- M70.849 Other soft tissue disorders related to use, overuse and pressure, unspecified hand

✓6th M70.85 Other soft tissue disorders related to use, overuse and pressure of thigh
- M70.851 Other soft tissue disorders related to use, overuse and pressure, right thigh
- M70.852 Other soft tissue disorders related to use, overuse and pressure, left thigh
- M70.859 Other soft tissue disorders related to use, overuse and pressure, unspecified thigh

✓6th M70.86 Other soft tissue disorders related to use, overuse and pressure lower leg
- M70.861 Other soft tissue disorders related to use, overuse and pressure, right lower leg
- M70.862 Other soft tissue disorders related to use, overuse and pressure, left lower leg
- M70.869 Other soft tissue disorders related to use, overuse and pressure, unspecified leg

✓6th M70.87 Other soft tissue disorders related to use, overuse and pressure of ankle and foot
- M70.871 Other soft tissue disorders related to use, overuse and pressure, right ankle and foot
- M70.872 Other soft tissue disorders related to use, overuse and pressure, left ankle and foot
- M70.879 Other soft tissue disorders related to use, overuse and pressure, unspecified ankle and foot

M70.88 Other soft tissue disorders related to use, overuse and pressure other site

M70.89 Other soft tissue disorders related to use, overuse and pressure multiple sites

✓5th M70.9 Unspecified soft tissue disorder related to use, overuse and pressure
- M70.90 Unspecified soft tissue disorder related to use, overuse and pressure of unspecified site

✓6th M70.91 Unspecified soft tissue disorder related to use, overuse and pressure of shoulder
- M70.911 Unspecified soft tissue disorder related to use, overuse and pressure, right shoulder
- M70.912 Unspecified soft tissue disorder related to use, overuse and pressure, left shoulder
- M70.919 Unspecified soft tissue disorder related to use, overuse and pressure, unspecified shoulder

✓6th M70.92 Unspecified soft tissue disorder related to use, overuse and pressure of upper arm
- M70.921 Unspecified soft tissue disorder related to use, overuse and pressure, right upper arm
- M70.922 Unspecified soft tissue disorder related to use, overuse and pressure, left upper arm
- M70.929 Unspecified soft tissue disorder related to use, overuse and pressure, unspecified upper arm

✓6th M70.93 Unspecified soft tissue disorder related to use, overuse and pressure of forearm
- M70.931 Unspecified soft tissue disorder related to use, overuse and pressure, right forearm
- M70.932 Unspecified soft tissue disorder related to use, overuse and pressure, left forearm
- M70.939 Unspecified soft tissue disorder related to use, overuse and pressure, unspecified forearm

✓6th M70.94 Unspecified soft tissue disorder related to use, overuse and pressure of hand
- M70.941 Unspecified soft tissue disorder related to use, overuse and pressure, right hand
- M70.942 Unspecified soft tissue disorder related to use, overuse and pressure, left hand
- M70.949 Unspecified soft tissue disorder related to use, overuse and pressure, unspecified hand

✓6th M70.95 Unspecified soft tissue disorder related to use, overuse and pressure of thigh
- M70.951 Unspecified soft tissue disorder related to use, overuse and pressure, right thigh
- M70.952 Unspecified soft tissue disorder related to use, overuse and pressure, left thigh
- M70.959 Unspecified soft tissue disorder related to use, overuse and pressure, unspecified thigh

✓6th M70.96 Unspecified soft tissue disorder related to use, overuse and pressure lower leg
- M70.961 Unspecified soft tissue disorder related to use, overuse and pressure, right lower leg
- M70.962 Unspecified soft tissue disorder related to use, overuse and pressure, left lower leg

M7Ø.969 Unspecified soft tissue disorder related to use, overuse and pressure, unspecified lower leg

✓6th M7Ø.97 Unspecified soft tissue disorder related to use, overuse and pressure of ankle and foot

M7Ø.971 Unspecified soft tissue disorder related to use, overuse and pressure, right ankle and foot

M7Ø.972 Unspecified soft tissue disorder related to use, overuse and pressure, left ankle and foot

M7Ø.979 Unspecified soft tissue disorder related to use, overuse and pressure, unspecified ankle and foot

M7Ø.98 Unspecified soft tissue disorder related to use, overuse and pressure other

M7Ø.99 Unspecified soft tissue disorder related to use, overuse and pressure multiple sites

✓4th **M71 Other bursopathies**

EXCLUDES 1 *bunion (M2Ø.1)*
*bursitis related to use, overuse or pressure (M7Ø.-)*
*enthesopathies (M76-M77)*

✓5th **M71.Ø Abscess of bursa**

Use additional code (B95.-, B96.-) to identify causative organism

M71.ØØ Abscess of bursa, unspecified site

✓6th M71.Ø1 Abscess of bursa, shoulder

M71.Ø11 Abscess of bursa, right shoulder
M71.Ø12 Abscess of bursa, left shoulder
M71.Ø19 Abscess of bursa, unspecified shoulder

✓6th M71.Ø2 Abscess of bursa, elbow

M71.Ø21 Abscess of bursa, right elbow
M71.Ø22 Abscess of bursa, left elbow
M71.Ø29 Abscess of bursa, unspecified elbow

✓6th M71.Ø3 Abscess of bursa, wrist

M71.Ø31 Abscess of bursa, right wrist
M71.Ø32 Abscess of bursa, left wrist
M71.Ø39 Abscess of bursa, unspecified wrist

✓6th M71.Ø4 Abscess of bursa, hand

M71.Ø41 Abscess of bursa, right hand
M71.Ø42 Abscess of bursa, left hand
M71.Ø49 Abscess of bursa, unspecified hand

✓6th M71.Ø5 Abscess of bursa, hip

M71.Ø51 Abscess of bursa, right hip
M71.Ø52 Abscess of bursa, left hip
M71.Ø59 Abscess of bursa, unspecified hip

✓6th M71.Ø6 Abscess of bursa, knee

M71.Ø61 Abscess of bursa, right knee
M71.Ø62 Abscess of bursa, left knee
M71.Ø69 Abscess of bursa, unspecified knee

✓6th M71.Ø7 Abscess of bursa, ankle and foot

M71.Ø71 Abscess of bursa, right ankle and foot
M71.Ø72 Abscess of bursa, left ankle and foot
M71.Ø79 Abscess of bursa, unspecified ankle and foot

M71.Ø8 Abscess of bursa, other site
M71.Ø9 Abscess of bursa, multiple sites

✓5th **M71.1 Other infective bursitis**

Use additional code (B95.-, B96.-) to identify causative organism

M71.1Ø Other infective bursitis, unspecified site

✓6th M71.11 Other infective bursitis, shoulder

M71.111 Other infective bursitis, right shoulder
M71.112 Other infective bursitis, left shoulder
M71.119 Other infective bursitis, unspecified shoulder

✓6th M71.12 Other infective bursitis, elbow

M71.121 Other infective bursitis, right elbow
M71.122 Other infective bursitis, left elbow
M71.129 Other infective bursitis, unspecified elbow

✓6th M71.13 Other infective bursitis, wrist

M71.131 Other infective bursitis, right wrist
M71.132 Other infective bursitis, left wrist
M71.139 Other infective bursitis, unspecified wrist

✓6th M71.14 Other infective bursitis, hand

M71.141 Other infective bursitis, right hand
M71.142 Other infective bursitis, left hand
M71.149 Other infective bursitis, unspecified hand

✓6th M71.15 Other infective bursitis, hip

M71.151 Other infective bursitis, right hip
M71.152 Other infective bursitis, left hip
M71.159 Other infective bursitis, unspecified hip

✓6th M71.16 Other infective bursitis, knee

M71.161 Other infective bursitis, right knee
M71.162 Other infective bursitis, left knee
M71.169 Other infective bursitis, unspecified knee

✓6th M71.17 Other infective bursitis, ankle and foot

M71.171 Other infective bursitis, right ankle and foot
M71.172 Other infective bursitis, left ankle and foot
M71.179 Other infective bursitis, unspecified ankle and foot

M71.18 Other infective bursitis, other site
M71.19 Other infective bursitis, multiple sites

✓5th **M71.2 Synovial cyst of popliteal space [Baker]**

EXCLUDES 1 *synovial cyst of popliteal space with rupture (M66.Ø)*

**DEF:** Sac filled with clear synovial fluid in adults, usually secondary to disease inside the joint, located on the back of the knee in the popliteal fossa area. In children, the cyst usually represents a ganglion of one of the tendons in the knee.

**Baker's Cyst**

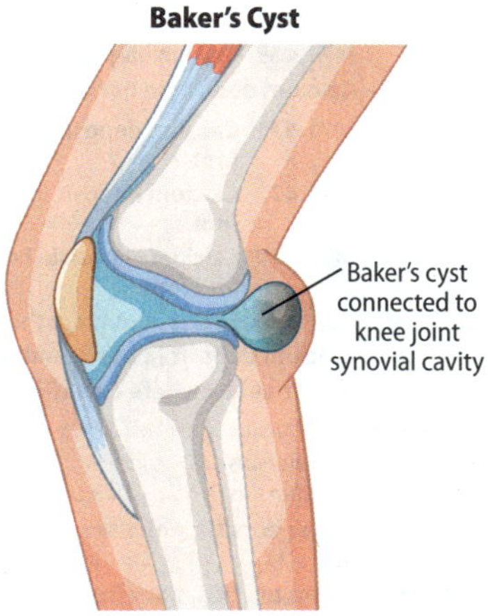


M71.2Ø Synovial cyst of popliteal space [Baker], unspecified knee
M71.21 Synovial cyst of popliteal space [Baker], right knee
M71.22 Synovial cyst of popliteal space [Baker], left knee

✓5th **M71.3 Other bursal cyst**

Synovial cyst NOS

EXCLUDES 1 *synovial cyst with rupture (M66.1-)*

M71.3Ø Other bursal cyst, unspecified site

✓6th M71.31 Other bursal cyst, shoulder

M71.311 Other bursal cyst, right shoulder
M71.312 Other bursal cyst, left shoulder
M71.319 Other bursal cyst, unspecified shoulder

✓6th M71.32 Other bursal cyst, elbow

M71.321 Other bursal cyst, right elbow
M71.322 Other bursal cyst, left elbow
M71.329 Other bursal cyst, unspecified elbow

✓6th M71.33 Other bursal cyst, wrist

M71.331 Other bursal cyst, right wrist
M71.332 Other bursal cyst, left wrist
M71.339 Other bursal cyst, unspecified wrist

✓6th M71.34 Other bursal cyst, hand

M71.341 Other bursal cyst, right hand
M71.342 Other bursal cyst, left hand
M71.349 Other bursal cyst, unspecified hand

✓6th M71.35 Other bursal cyst, hip

M71.351 Other bursal cyst, right hip
M71.352 Other bursal cyst, left hip
M71.359 Other bursal cyst, unspecified hip

✓6th M71.37 Other bursal cyst, ankle and foot

M71.371 Other bursal cyst, right ankle and foot
M71.372 Other bursal cyst, left ankle and foot
M71.379 Other bursal cyst, unspecified ankle and foot

M71.38 Other bursal cyst, other site
M71.39 Other bursal cyst, multiple sites

✓5th **M71.4 Calcium deposit in bursa**

EXCLUDES 2 *calcium deposit in bursa of shoulder (M75.3)*

**M71.40 Calcium deposit in bursa, unspecified site**

✓6th **M71.42 Calcium deposit in bursa, elbow**

**M71.421 Calcium deposit in bursa, right elbow**

**M71.422 Calcium deposit in bursa, left elbow**

**M71.429 Calcium deposit in bursa, unspecified elbow**

✓6th **M71.43 Calcium deposit in bursa, wrist**

**M71.431 Calcium deposit in bursa, right wrist**

**M71.432 Calcium deposit in bursa, left wrist**

**M71.439 Calcium deposit in bursa, unspecified wrist**

✓6th **M71.44 Calcium deposit in bursa, hand**

**M71.441 Calcium deposit in bursa, right hand**

**M71.442 Calcium deposit in bursa, left hand**

**M71.449 Calcium deposit in bursa, unspecified hand**

✓6th **M71.45 Calcium deposit in bursa, hip**

**M71.451 Calcium deposit in bursa, right hip**

**M71.452 Calcium deposit in bursa, left hip**

**M71.459 Calcium deposit in bursa, unspecified hip**

✓6th **M71.46 Calcium deposit in bursa, knee**

**M71.461 Calcium deposit in bursa, right knee**

**M71.462 Calcium deposit in bursa, left knee**

**M71.469 Calcium deposit in bursa, unspecified knee**

✓6th **M71.47 Calcium deposit in bursa, ankle and foot**

**M71.471 Calcium deposit in bursa, right ankle and foot**

**M71.472 Calcium deposit in bursa, left ankle and foot**

**M71.479 Calcium deposit in bursa, unspecified ankle and foot**

**M71.48 Calcium deposit in bursa, other site**

**M71.49 Calcium deposit in bursa, multiple sites**

✓5th **M71.5 Other bursitis, not elsewhere classified**

EXCLUDES 1 *bursitis NOS (M71.9-)*

EXCLUDES 2 *bursitis of shoulder (M75.5)*

*bursitis of tibial collateral [Pellegrini-Stieda] (M76.4-)*

**M71.50 Other bursitis, not elsewhere classified, unspecified site**

✓6th **M71.52 Other bursitis, not elsewhere classified, elbow**

**M71.521 Other bursitis, not elsewhere classified, right elbow**

**M71.522 Other bursitis, not elsewhere classified, left elbow**

**M71.529 Other bursitis, not elsewhere classified, unspecified elbow**

✓6th **M71.53 Other bursitis, not elsewhere classified, wrist**

**M71.531 Other bursitis, not elsewhere classified, right wrist**

**M71.532 Other bursitis, not elsewhere classified, left wrist**

**M71.539 Other bursitis, not elsewhere classified, unspecified wrist**

✓6th **M71.54 Other bursitis, not elsewhere classified, hand**

**M71.541 Other bursitis, not elsewhere classified, right hand**

**M71.542 Other bursitis, not elsewhere classified, left hand**

**M71.549 Other bursitis, not elsewhere classified, unspecified hand**

✓6th **M71.55 Other bursitis, not elsewhere classified, hip**

**M71.551 Other bursitis, not elsewhere classified, right hip**

**M71.552 Other bursitis, not elsewhere classified, left hip**

**M71.559 Other bursitis, not elsewhere classified, unspecified hip**

✓6th **M71.56 Other bursitis, not elsewhere classified, knee**

**M71.561 Other bursitis, not elsewhere classified, right knee**

**M71.562 Other bursitis, not elsewhere classified, left knee**

**M71.569 Other bursitis, not elsewhere classified, unspecified knee**

✓6th **M71.57 Other bursitis, not elsewhere classified, ankle and foot**

**M71.571 Other bursitis, not elsewhere classified, right ankle and foot**

**M71.572 Other bursitis, not elsewhere classified, left ankle and foot**

**M71.579 Other bursitis, not elsewhere classified, unspecified ankle and foot**

**M71.58 Other bursitis, not elsewhere classified, other site**

✓5th **M71.8 Other specified bursopathies**

**M71.80 Other specified bursopathies, unspecified site**

✓6th **M71.81 Other specified bursopathies, shoulder**

**M71.811 Other specified bursopathies, right shoulder**

**M71.812 Other specified bursopathies, left shoulder**

**M71.819 Other specified bursopathies, unspecified shoulder**

✓6th **M71.82 Other specified bursopathies, elbow**

**M71.821 Other specified bursopathies, right elbow**

**M71.822 Other specified bursopathies, left elbow**

**M71.829 Other specified bursopathies, unspecified elbow**

✓6th **M71.83 Other specified bursopathies, wrist**

**M71.831 Other specified bursopathies, right wrist**

**M71.832 Other specified bursopathies, left wrist**

**M71.839 Other specified bursopathies, unspecified wrist**

✓6th **M71.84 Other specified bursopathies, hand**

**M71.841 Other specified bursopathies, right hand**

**M71.842 Other specified bursopathies, left hand**

**M71.849 Other specified bursopathies, unspecified hand**

✓6th **M71.85 Other specified bursopathies, hip**

**M71.851 Other specified bursopathies, right hip**

**M71.852 Other specified bursopathies, left hip**

**M71.859 Other specified bursopathies, unspecified hip**

✓6th **M71.86 Other specified bursopathies, knee**

**M71.861 Other specified bursopathies, right knee**

**M71.862 Other specified bursopathies, left knee**

**M71.869 Other specified bursopathies, unspecified knee**

✓6th **M71.87 Other specified bursopathies, ankle and foot**

**M71.871 Other specified bursopathies, right ankle and foot**

**M71.872 Other specified bursopathies, left ankle and foot**

**M71.879 Other specified bursopathies, unspecified ankle and foot**

**M71.88 Other specified bursopathies, other site**

**M71.89 Other specified bursopathies, multiple sites**

**M71.9 Bursopathy, unspecified**

Bursitis NOS

✓4th **M72 Fibroblastic disorders**

EXCLUDES 2 *retroperitoneal fibromatosis (D48.3)*

**M72.0 Palmar fascial fibromatosis [Dupuytren]** A

**DEF:** Dupuytren's contracture: Flexion deformity of a finger, due to shortened, thickened fibrosing of palmar fascia. The cause is unknown, but it is associated with long-standing epilepsy.

**M72.1 Knuckle pads**

▲ ✓5th **M72.2 Plantar fascial fibromatosis**

~~Plantar fasciitis~~

▶Ledderhose disease◀

**DEF:** Rapid-growing and multiplanar nodular swellings and pain in the foot that is not associated with contractures.

● **M72.20 Plantar fascial fibromatosis, unspecified foot**

● **M72.21 Plantar fascial fibromatosis, right foot**

● **M72.22 Plantar fascial fibromatosis, left foot**

**M72.4 Pseudosarcomatous fibromatosis**

Nodular fasciitis

**M72.6 Necrotizing fasciitis** HCC ESR COM

Use additional code (B95.-, B96.-) to identify causative organism

**M72.8 Other fibroblastic disorders**
Abscess of fascia
Fasciitis NEC
Other infective fasciitis
Use additional code to (B95.-, B96.-) identify causative organism
EXCLUDES 1 *diffuse (eosinophilic) fasciitis (M35.4)*
*necrotizing fasciitis (M72.6)*
*nodular fasciitis (M72.4)*
*perirenal fasciitis NOS (N13.5)*
*perirenal fasciitis with infection (N13.6)*
*plantar fasciitis ►(M67.A0-)◄*
AHA: 2025,1Q,31

**M72.9 Fibroblastic disorder, unspecified**
Fasciitis NOS
Fibromatosis NOS

**✓4th M75 Shoulder lesions**
EXCLUDES 2 *shoulder-hand syndrome (M89.0-)*

**✓5th M75.0 Adhesive capsulitis of shoulder**
Frozen shoulder
Periarthritis of shoulder
AHA: 2015,2Q,23
**M75.00** Adhesive capsulitis of unspecified shoulder
**M75.01** Adhesive capsulitis of right shoulder
**M75.02** Adhesive capsulitis of left shoulder

**✓5th M75.1 Rotator cuff tear or rupture, not specified as traumatic**
Rotator cuff syndrome
Supraspinatus syndrome
Supraspinatus tear or rupture, not specified as traumatic
EXCLUDES 1 *tear of rotator cuff, traumatic (S46.01-)*
**✓6th M75.10 Unspecified rotator cuff tear or rupture, not specified as traumatic**
**M75.100** Unspecified rotator cuff tear or rupture of unspecified shoulder, not specified as traumatic
**M75.101** Unspecified rotator cuff tear or rupture of right shoulder, not specified as traumatic
**M75.102** Unspecified rotator cuff tear or rupture of left shoulder, not specified as traumatic
**✓6th M75.11 Incomplete rotator cuff tear or rupture not specified as traumatic**
**M75.110** Incomplete rotator cuff tear or rupture of unspecified shoulder, not specified as traumatic
**M75.111** Incomplete rotator cuff tear or rupture of right shoulder, not specified as traumatic
**M75.112** Incomplete rotator cuff tear or rupture of left shoulder, not specified as traumatic
**✓6th M75.12 Complete rotator cuff tear or rupture not specified as traumatic**
**M75.120** Complete rotator cuff tear or rupture of unspecified shoulder, not specified as traumatic
**M75.121** Complete rotator cuff tear or rupture of right shoulder, not specified as traumatic
**M75.122** Complete rotator cuff tear or rupture of left shoulder, not specified as traumatic

**✓5th M75.2 Bicipital tendinitis**
**M75.20** Bicipital tendinitis, unspecified shoulder
**M75.21** Bicipital tendinitis, right shoulder
**M75.22** Bicipital tendinitis, left shoulder

**✓5th M75.3 Calcific tendinitis of shoulder**
Calcified bursa of shoulder
**M75.30** Calcific tendinitis of unspecified shoulder
**M75.31** Calcific tendinitis of right shoulder
**M75.32** Calcific tendinitis of left shoulder

**✓5th M75.4 Impingement syndrome of shoulder**
AHA: 2022,3Q,18
**M75.40** Impingement syndrome of unspecified shoulder
**M75.41** Impingement syndrome of right shoulder
**M75.42** Impingement syndrome of left shoulder

**✓5th M75.5 Bursitis of shoulder**
**M75.50** Bursitis of unspecified shoulder
**M75.51** Bursitis of right shoulder
**M75.52** Bursitis of left shoulder

**✓5th M75.8 Other shoulder lesions**
**M75.80** Other shoulder lesions, unspecified shoulder
**M75.81** Other shoulder lesions, right shoulder
**M75.82** Other shoulder lesions, left shoulder

**✓5th M75.9 Shoulder lesion, unspecified**
**M75.90** Shoulder lesion, unspecified, unspecified shoulder
**M75.91** Shoulder lesion, unspecified, right shoulder
**M75.92** Shoulder lesion, unspecified, left shoulder

**✓4th M76 Enthesopathies, lower limb, excluding foot**
EXCLUDES 2 *bursitis due to use, overuse and pressure (M70.-)*
*enthesopathies of ankle and foot (M77.5-)*

**✓5th M76.0 Gluteal tendinitis**
**M76.00** Gluteal tendinitis, unspecified hip
**M76.01** Gluteal tendinitis, right hip
**M76.02** Gluteal tendinitis, left hip

**✓5th M76.1 Psoas tendinitis**
**M76.10** Psoas tendinitis, unspecified hip
**M76.11** Psoas tendinitis, right hip
**M76.12** Psoas tendinitis, left hip

**✓5th M76.2 Iliac crest spur**
**M76.20** Iliac crest spur, unspecified hip
**M76.21** Iliac crest spur, right hip
**M76.22** Iliac crest spur, left hip

**✓5th M76.3 Iliotibial band syndrome**
**M76.30** Iliotibial band syndrome, unspecified leg
**M76.31** Iliotibial band syndrome, right leg
**M76.32** Iliotibial band syndrome, left leg

**✓5th M76.4 Tibial collateral bursitis [Pellegrini-Stieda]**
**M76.40** Tibial collateral bursitis [Pellegrini-Stieda], unspecified leg
**M76.41** Tibial collateral bursitis [Pellegrini-Stieda], right leg
**M76.42** Tibial collateral bursitis [Pellegrini-Stieda], left leg

**✓5th M76.5 Patellar tendinitis**
**M76.50** Patellar tendinitis, unspecified knee
**M76.51** Patellar tendinitis, right knee
**M76.52** Patellar tendinitis, left knee

**✓5th M76.6 Achilles tendinitis**
Achilles bursitis
**M76.60** Achilles tendinitis, unspecified leg
**M76.61** Achilles tendinitis, right leg
**M76.62** Achilles tendinitis, left leg

**✓5th M76.7 Peroneal tendinitis**
**M76.70** Peroneal tendinitis, unspecified leg
**M76.71** Peroneal tendinitis, right leg
**M76.72** Peroneal tendinitis, left leg

**✓5th M76.8 Other specified enthesopathies of lower limb, excluding foot**
**✓6th M76.81 Anterior tibial syndrome**
**M76.811** Anterior tibial syndrome, right leg
**M76.812** Anterior tibial syndrome, left leg
**M76.819** Anterior tibial syndrome, unspecified leg
**✓6th M76.82 Posterior tibial tendinitis**
**M76.821** Posterior tibial tendinitis, right leg
**M76.822** Posterior tibial tendinitis, left leg
**M76.829** Posterior tibial tendinitis, unspecified leg
**✓6th M76.89 Other specified enthesopathies of lower limb, excluding foot**
**M76.891** Other specified enthesopathies of right lower limb, excluding foot
**M76.892** Other specified enthesopathies of left lower limb, excluding foot
**M76.899** Other specified enthesopathies of unspecified lower limb, excluding foot

**M76.9 Unspecified enthesopathy, lower limb, excluding foot**

**✓4th M77 Other enthesopathies**
EXCLUDES 1 *bursitis NOS (M71.9-)*
EXCLUDES 2 *bursitis due to use, overuse and pressure (M70.-)*
*osteophyte (M25.7)*
*spinal enthesopathy (M46.0-)*

**✓5th M77.0 Medial epicondylitis**
**M77.00** Medial epicondylitis, unspecified elbow
**M77.01** Medial epicondylitis, right elbow
**M77.02** Medial epicondylitis, left elbow

**✓5th M77.1 Lateral epicondylitis**
Tennis elbow
**M77.10** Lateral epicondylitis, unspecified elbow
**M77.11** Lateral epicondylitis, right elbow
**M77.12** Lateral epicondylitis, left elbow

✓5th **M77.2 Periarthritis of wrist**
- **M77.20 Periarthritis, unspecified wrist**
- **M77.21 Periarthritis, right wrist**
- **M77.22 Periarthritis, left wrist**

✓5th **M77.3 Calcaneal spur**

**DEF:** Overgrowth of calcaneus bone on the underside of the heel that causes pain on walking. Calcaneal spur is due to a chronic avulsion injury of the plantar fascia from the calcaneus.

- **M77.30 Calcaneal spur, unspecified foot**
- **M77.31 Calcaneal spur, right foot**
- **M77.32 Calcaneal spur, left foot**

✓5th **M77.4 Metatarsalgia**

EXCLUDES 1 *Morton's metatarsalgia (G57.6)*

- **M77.40 Metatarsalgia, unspecified foot**
- **M77.41 Metatarsalgia, right foot**
- **M77.42 Metatarsalgia, left foot**

✓5th **M77.5 Other enthesopathy of foot and ankle**
- **M77.50 Other enthesopathy of unspecified foot and ankle**
- **M77.51 Other enthesopathy of right foot and ankle**
- **M77.52 Other enthesopathy of left foot and ankle**

**M77.8 Other enthesopathies, not elsewhere classified**

**M77.9 Enthesopathy, unspecified**

Bone spur NOS
Capsulitis NOS
Periarthritis NOS
Tendinitis NOS

✓4th **M79 Other and unspecified soft tissue disorders, not elsewhere classified**

EXCLUDES 1 *psychogenic rheumatism (F45.8)*
*soft tissue pain, psychogenic (F45.41)*

**M79.0 Rheumatism, unspecified**

EXCLUDES 1 *fibromyalgia (M79.7)*
*palindromic rheumatism (M12.3-)*

✓5th **M79.1 Myalgia**

Myofascial pain syndrome

EXCLUDES 1 *fibromyalgia (M79.7)*
*myositis (M60.-)*

**AHA:** 2018,4Q,21

- **M79.10 Myalgia, unspecified site**
- **M79.11 Myalgia of mastication muscle**
- **M79.12 Myalgia of auxiliary muscles, head and neck**
- **M79.18 Myalgia, other site**

**M79.2 Neuralgia and neuritis, unspecified**

EXCLUDES 1 *brachial radiculitis NOS (M54.1)*
*lumbosacral radiculitis NOS (M54.1)*
*mononeuropathies (G56-G58)*
*radiculitis NOS (M54.1)*
*sciatica (M54.3-M54.4)*

**TIP:** Assign for documented neuropathic pain.

**M79.3 Panniculitis, unspecified**

EXCLUDES 1 *lupus panniculitis (L93.2)*
*neck and back panniculitis (M54.0-)*
*relapsing [Weber-Christian] panniculitis (M35.6)*

**AHA:** 2024,1Q,16

**M79.4 Hypertrophy of (infrapatellar) fat pad**

**M79.5 Residual foreign body in soft tissue**

EXCLUDES 1 *foreign body granuloma of skin and subcutaneous tissue (L92.3)*
*foreign body granuloma of soft tissue (M60.2-)*

**AHA:** 2023,2Q,27

✓5th **M79.6 Pain in limb, hand, foot, fingers and toes**

EXCLUDES 2 *pain in joint (M25.5-)*

✓6th **M79.60 Pain in limb, unspecified**
- **M79.601 Pain in right arm**
  Pain in right upper limb NOS
- **M79.602 Pain in left arm**
  Pain in left upper limb NOS
- **M79.603 Pain in arm, unspecified**
  Pain in upper limb NOS
- **M79.604 Pain in right leg**
  Pain in right lower limb NOS
- **M79.605 Pain in left leg**
  Pain in left lower limb NOS
- **M79.606 Pain in leg, unspecified**
  Pain in lower limb NOS
- **M79.609 Pain in unspecified limb**
  Pain in limb NOS

✓6th **M79.62 Pain in upper arm**

Pain in axillary region

- **M79.621 Pain in right upper arm**
- **M79.622 Pain in left upper arm**
- **M79.629 Pain in unspecified upper arm**

✓6th **M79.63 Pain in forearm**
- **M79.631 Pain in right forearm**
- **M79.632 Pain in left forearm**
- **M79.639 Pain in unspecified forearm**

✓6th **M79.64 Pain in hand and fingers**
- **M79.641 Pain in right hand**
- **M79.642 Pain in left hand**
- **M79.643 Pain in unspecified hand**
- **M79.644 Pain in right finger(s)**
- **M79.645 Pain in left finger(s)**
- **M79.646 Pain in unspecified finger(s)**

✓6th **M79.65 Pain in thigh**
- **M79.651 Pain in right thigh**
- **M79.652 Pain in left thigh**
- **M79.659 Pain in unspecified thigh**

✓6th **M79.66 Pain in lower leg**
- **M79.661 Pain in right lower leg**
- **M79.662 Pain in left lower leg**
- **M79.669 Pain in unspecified lower leg**

✓6th **M79.67 Pain in foot and toes**
- **M79.671 Pain in right foot**
- **M79.672 Pain in left foot**
- **M79.673 Pain in unspecified foot**
- **M79.674 Pain in right toe(s)**
- **M79.675 Pain in left toe(s)**
- **M79.676 Pain in unspecified toe(s)**

**M79.7 Fibromyalgia**

Fibromyositis
Fibrositis
Myofibrositis

✓5th **M79.A Nontraumatic compartment syndrome**

Code first, if applicable, associated postprocedural complication

EXCLUDES 1 *compartment syndrome NOS (T79.A-)*
*fibromyalgia (M79.7)*
*nontraumatic ischemic infarction of muscle (M62.2-)*
*traumatic compartment syndrome (T79.A-)*

✓6th **M79.A1 Nontraumatic compartment syndrome of upper extremity**

Nontraumatic compartment syndrome of shoulder, arm, forearm, wrist, hand, and fingers

- **M79.A11 Nontraumatic compartment syndrome of right upper extremity**
- **M79.A12 Nontraumatic compartment syndrome of left upper extremity**
- **M79.A19 Nontraumatic compartment syndrome of unspecified upper extremity**

✓6th **M79.A2 Nontraumatic compartment syndrome of lower extremity**

Nontraumatic compartment syndrome of hip, buttock, thigh, leg, foot, and toes

- **M79.A21 Nontraumatic compartment syndrome of right lower extremity**
- **M79.A22 Nontraumatic compartment syndrome of left lower extremity**
- **M79.A29 Nontraumatic compartment syndrome of unspecified lower extremity**

**M79.A3 Nontraumatic compartment syndrome of abdomen**

**M79.A9 Nontraumatic compartment syndrome of other sites**

✓5th **M79.8 Other specified soft tissue disorders**
- **M79.81 Nontraumatic hematoma of soft tissue**
  Nontraumatic hematoma of muscle
  Nontraumatic seroma of muscle and soft tissue
- **M79.89 Other specified soft tissue disorders**
  Polyalgia

**M79.9 Soft tissue disorder, unspecified**

## OSTEOPATHIES AND CHONDROPATHIES (M8Ø-M94)

### Disorders of bone density and structure (M8Ø-M85)

✓4th **M8Ø Osteoporosis with current pathological fracture**

INCLUDES osteoporosis with current fragility fracture

Use additional code to identify major osseous defect, if applicable (M89.7-)

EXCLUDES 1 *collapsed vertebra NOS (M48.5)*
*pathological fracture NOS (M84.4)*
*wedging of vertebra NOS (M48.5)*

EXCLUDES 2 *personal history of (healed) osteoporosis fracture (Z87.31Ø)*

**AHA:** 2018,2Q,12

**TIP:** The site codes in this category identify the site of the fracture, not the site of the osteoporosis.

The appropriate 7th character is to be added to each code from category M8Ø:
- A initial encounter for fracture
- D subsequent encounter for fracture with routine healing
- G subsequent encounter for fracture with delayed healing
- K subsequent encounter for fracture with nonunion
- P subsequent encounter for fracture with malunion
- S sequela

✓5th **M8Ø.Ø Age-related osteoporosis with current pathological fracture**
Involutional osteoporosis with current pathological fracture
Osteoporosis NOS with current pathological fracture
Postmenopausal osteoporosis with current pathological fracture
Senile osteoporosis with current pathological fracture

√x7th **M8Ø.ØØ Age-related osteoporosis with current pathological fracture, unspecified site** Rx Q A

✓6th **M8Ø.Ø1 Age-related osteoporosis with current pathological fracture, shoulder**

✓7th **M8Ø.Ø11 Age-related osteoporosis with current pathological fracture, right shoulder** Rx Q A

✓7th **M8Ø.Ø12 Age-related osteoporosis with current pathological fracture, left shoulder** Rx Q A

✓7th **M8Ø.Ø19 Age-related osteoporosis with current pathological fracture, unspecified shoulder** Rx Q A

✓6th **M8Ø.Ø2 Age-related osteoporosis with current pathological fracture, humerus**

✓7th **M8Ø.Ø21 Age-related osteoporosis with current pathological fracture, right humerus** Rx Q A

✓7th **M8Ø.Ø22 Age-related osteoporosis with current pathological fracture, left humerus** Rx Q A

✓7th **M8Ø.Ø29 Age-related osteoporosis with current pathological fracture, unspecified humerus** Rx Q A

✓6th **M8Ø.Ø3 Age-related osteoporosis with current pathological fracture, forearm**
Age-related osteoporosis with current pathological fracture of wrist

✓7th **M8Ø.Ø31 Age-related osteoporosis with current pathological fracture, right forearm** Rx Q A

✓7th **M8Ø.Ø32 Age-related osteoporosis with current pathological fracture, left forearm** Rx Q A

✓7th **M8Ø.Ø39 Age-related osteoporosis with current pathological fracture, unspecified forearm** Rx Q A

✓6th **M8Ø.Ø4 Age-related osteoporosis with current pathological fracture, hand**

✓7th **M8Ø.Ø41 Age-related osteoporosis with current pathological fracture, right hand** Rx Q A

✓7th **M8Ø.Ø42 Age-related osteoporosis with current pathological fracture, left hand** Rx Q A

✓7th **M8Ø.Ø49 Age-related osteoporosis with current pathological fracture, unspecified hand** Rx Q A

✓6th **M8Ø.Ø5 Age-related osteoporosis with current pathological fracture, femur**
Age-related osteoporosis with current pathological fracture of hip

✓7th **M8Ø.Ø51 Age-related osteoporosis with current pathological fracture, right femur** HCC Rx ESR COM Q A

✓7th **M8Ø.Ø52 Age-related osteoporosis with current pathological fracture, left femur** HCC Rx ESR COM Q A

✓7th **M8Ø.Ø59 Age-related osteoporosis with current pathological fracture, unspecified femur** HCC Rx ESR COM Q A

✓6th **M8Ø.Ø6 Age-related osteoporosis with current pathological fracture, lower leg**

✓7th **M8Ø.Ø61 Age-related osteoporosis with current pathological fracture, right lower leg** Rx Q A

✓7th **M8Ø.Ø62 Age-related osteoporosis with current pathological fracture, left lower leg** Rx Q A

✓7th **M8Ø.Ø69 Age-related osteoporosis with current pathological fracture, unspecified lower leg** Rx Q A

✓6th **M8Ø.Ø7 Age-related osteoporosis with current pathological fracture, ankle and foot**

✓7th **M8Ø.Ø71 Age-related osteoporosis with current pathological fracture, right ankle and foot** Rx Q A

✓7th **M8Ø.Ø72 Age-related osteoporosis with current pathological fracture, left ankle and foot** Rx Q A

✓7th **M8Ø.Ø79 Age-related osteoporosis with current pathological fracture, unspecified ankle and foot** Rx Q A

√x7th **M8Ø.Ø8 Age-related osteoporosis with current pathological fracture, vertebra(e)** HCC Rx ESR COM Q A

√x7th **M8Ø.ØA Age-related osteoporosis with current pathological fracture, other site** Rx Q A
**AHA:** 2020,4Q,32-33

✓6th **M8Ø.ØB Age-related osteoporosis with current pathological fracture, pelvis**
**AHA:** 2023,4Q,33-34

✓7th **M8Ø.ØB1 Age-related osteoporosis with current pathological fracture, right pelvis** Rx Q A

✓7th **M8Ø.ØB2 Age-related osteoporosis with current pathological fracture, left pelvis** Rx Q A

✓7th **M8Ø.ØB9 Age-related osteoporosis with current pathological fracture, unspecified pelvis** Rx Q A

✓5th **M8Ø.8 Other osteoporosis with current pathological fracture**
Drug-induced osteoporosis with current pathological fracture
Idiopathic osteoporosis with current pathological fracture
Osteoporosis of disuse with current pathological fracture
Postoophorectomy osteoporosis with current pathological fracture
Postsurgical malabsorption osteoporosis with current pathological fracture
Post-traumatic osteoporosis with current pathological fracture
Use additional code for adverse effect, if applicable, to identify drug (T36-T5Ø with fifth or sixth character 5)

√x7th **M8Ø.8Ø Other osteoporosis with current pathological fracture, unspecified site** Rx Q

✓6th **M8Ø.81 Other osteoporosis with pathological fracture, shoulder**

✓7th **M8Ø.811 Other osteoporosis with current pathological fracture, right shoulder** Rx Q

✓7th **M8Ø.812 Other osteoporosis with current pathological fracture, left shoulder** Rx Q

✓7th **M8Ø.819 Other osteoporosis with current pathological fracture, unspecified shoulder** Rx Q

✓6th **M8Ø.82 Other osteoporosis with current pathological fracture, humerus**

✓7th **M8Ø.821 Other osteoporosis with current pathological fracture, right humerus** Rx Q

7th **M80.822 Other osteoporosis with current pathological fracture, left humerus** Rx Q

7th **M80.829 Other osteoporosis with current pathological fracture, unspecified humerus** Rx Q

6th **M80.83 Other osteoporosis with current pathological fracture, forearm**

Other osteoporosis with current pathological fracture of wrist

7th **M80.831 Other osteoporosis with current pathological fracture, right forearm** Rx Q

7th **M80.832 Other osteoporosis with current pathological fracture, left forearm** Rx Q

7th **M80.839 Other osteoporosis with current pathological fracture, unspecified forearm** Rx Q

6th **M80.84 Other osteoporosis with current pathological fracture, hand**

7th **M80.841 Other osteoporosis with current pathological fracture, right hand** Rx Q

7th **M80.842 Other osteoporosis with current pathological fracture, left hand** Rx Q

7th **M80.849 Other osteoporosis with current pathological fracture, unspecified hand** Rx Q

6th **M80.85 Other osteoporosis with current pathological fracture, femur**

Other osteoporosis with current pathological fracture of hip

7th **M80.851 Other osteoporosis with current pathological fracture, right femur** HCC Rx ESR COM Q

7th **M80.852 Other osteoporosis with current pathological fracture, left femur** HCC Rx ESR COM Q

7th **M80.859 Other osteoporosis with current pathological fracture, unspecified femur** HCC Rx ESR COM Q

6th **M80.86 Other osteoporosis with current pathological fracture, lower leg**

7th **M80.861 Other osteoporosis with current pathological fracture, right lower leg** Rx Q

7th **M80.862 Other osteoporosis with current pathological fracture, left lower leg** Rx Q

7th **M80.869 Other osteoporosis with current pathological fracture, unspecified lower leg** Rx Q

6th **M80.87 Other osteoporosis with current pathological fracture, ankle and foot**

7th **M80.871 Other osteoporosis with current pathological fracture, right ankle and foot** Rx Q

7th **M80.872 Other osteoporosis with current pathological fracture, left ankle and foot** Rx Q

7th **M80.879 Other osteoporosis with current pathological fracture, unspecified ankle and foot** Rx Q

x7th **M80.88 Other osteoporosis with current pathological fracture, vertebra(e)** HCC Rx ESR COM Q

x7th **M80.8A Other osteoporosis with current pathological fracture, other site** Rx Q

**AHA:** 2020,4Q,32

6th **M80.8B Other osteoporosis with current pathological fracture, pelvis**

**AHA:** 2023,4Q,33-34

7th **M80.8B1 Other osteoporosis with current pathological fracture, right pelvis** Rx Q

7th **M80.8B2 Other osteoporosis with current pathological fracture, left pelvis** Rx Q

7th **M80.8B9 Other osteoporosis with current pathological fracture, unspecified pelvis** Rx Q

4th **M81 Osteoporosis without current pathological fracture**

Use additional code to identify:
- major osseous defect, if applicable (M89.7-)
- personal history of (healed) osteoporosis fracture, if applicable (Z87.310)

EXCLUDES 1 *osteoporosis with current pathological fracture (M80.-)*
*Sudeck's atrophy (M89.0)*

**M81.0 Age-related osteoporosis without current pathological fracture** Rx Q A

Involutional osteoporosis without current pathological fracture
Osteoporosis NOS
Postmenopausal osteoporosis without current pathological fracture
Senile osteoporosis without current pathological fracture

**M81.6 Localized osteoporosis [Lequesne]** Rx Q

EXCLUDES 1 *Sudeck's atrophy (M89.0)*

**M81.8 Other osteoporosis without current pathological fracture** Rx Q

Drug-induced osteoporosis without current pathological fracture
Idiopathic osteoporosis without current pathological fracture
Osteoporosis of disuse without current pathological fracture
Postoophorectomy osteoporosis without current pathological fracture
Postsurgical malabsorption osteoporosis without current pathological fracture
Post-traumatic osteoporosis without current pathological fracture
Use additional code for adverse effect, if applicable, to identify drug (T36-T50 with fifth or sixth character 5)

4th **M83 Adult osteomalacia**

EXCLUDES 1 *infantile and juvenile osteomalacia (E55.0)*
*renal osteodystrophy (N25.0)*
*rickets (active) (E55.0)*
*rickets (active) sequelae (E64.3)*
*vitamin D-resistant osteomalacia (E83.31)*
*vitamin D-resistant rickets (active) (E83.31)*

**M83.0 Puerperal osteomalacia** Rx M

**M83.1 Senile osteomalacia** Rx A

**M83.2 Adult osteomalacia due to malabsorption** Rx A

Postsurgical malabsorption osteomalacia in adults

**M83.3 Adult osteomalacia due to malnutrition** Rx A

**M83.4 Aluminum bone disease** Rx

**M83.5 Other drug-induced osteomalacia in adults** Rx A

Use additional code for adverse effect, if applicable, to identify drug (T36-T50 with fifth or sixth character 5)

**M83.8 Other adult osteomalacia** Rx A

**M83.9 Adult osteomalacia, unspecified** Rx A

4th **M84 Disorder of continuity of bone**

EXCLUDES 2 *traumatic fracture of bone-see fracture, by site*

5th **M84.3 Stress fracture**

Fatigue fracture
March fracture
Stress fracture NOS
Stress reaction
Use additional external cause code(s) to identify the cause of the stress fracture

EXCLUDES 1 *pathological fracture due to osteoporosis (M80.-)*
*pathological fracture NOS (M84.4.-)*
*traumatic fracture (S12.-, S22.-, S32.-, S42.-, S52.-, S62.-, S72.-, S82.-, S92.-)*

EXCLUDES 2 *personal history of (healed) stress (fatigue) fracture (Z87.312)*
*stress fracture of vertebra (M48.4-)*

The appropriate 7th character is to be added to each code from subcategory M84.3.
- A initial encounter for fracture
- D subsequent encounter for fracture with routine healing
- G subsequent encounter for fracture with delayed healing
- K subsequent encounter for fracture with nonunion
- P subsequent encounter for fracture with malunion
- S sequela

x7th **M84.30 Stress fracture, unspecified site**

6th **M84.31 Stress fracture, shoulder**

7th **M84.311 Stress fracture, right shoulder** Q

7th **M84.312 Stress fracture, left shoulder** Q

7th **M84.319 Stress fracture, unspecified shoulder** Q

6th **M84.32 Stress fracture, humerus**

7th **M84.321 Stress fracture, right humerus** Q

M84.322 Stress fracture, left humerus Q
M84.329 Stress fracture, unspecified humerus Q
M84.33 Stress fracture, ulna and radius
M84.331 Stress fracture, right ulna Q
M84.332 Stress fracture, left ulna Q
M84.333 Stress fracture, right radius Q
M84.334 Stress fracture, left radius Q
M84.339 Stress fracture, unspecified ulna and radius Q
M84.34 Stress fracture, hand and fingers
M84.341 Stress fracture, right hand Q
M84.342 Stress fracture, left hand Q
M84.343 Stress fracture, unspecified hand Q
M84.344 Stress fracture, right finger(s)
M84.345 Stress fracture, left finger(s)
M84.346 Stress fracture, unspecified finger(s)
M84.35 Stress fracture, pelvis and femur
Stress fracture, hip
M84.350 Stress fracture, pelvis Q
M84.351 Stress fracture, right femur Q
M84.352 Stress fracture, left femur Q
M84.353 Stress fracture, unspecified femur Q
M84.359 Stress fracture, hip, unspecified Q
M84.36 Stress fracture, tibia and fibula
M84.361 Stress fracture, right tibia Q
M84.362 Stress fracture, left tibia Q
M84.363 Stress fracture, right fibula Q
M84.364 Stress fracture, left fibula Q
M84.369 Stress fracture, unspecified tibia and fibula Q
M84.37 Stress fracture, ankle, foot and toes
M84.371 Stress fracture, right ankle Q
M84.372 Stress fracture, left ankle Q
M84.373 Stress fracture, unspecified ankle Q
M84.374 Stress fracture, right foot Q
M84.375 Stress fracture, left foot Q
M84.376 Stress fracture, unspecified foot Q
M84.377 Stress fracture, right toe(s)
M84.378 Stress fracture, left toe(s)
M84.379 Stress fracture, unspecified toe(s)
M84.38 Stress fracture, other site Q
EXCLUDES 2 *stress fracture of vertebra (M48.4-)*

M84.4 Pathological fracture, not elsewhere classified
Chronic fracture
Pathological fracture NOS
EXCLUDES 1 *collapsed vertebra NEC (M48.5)*
*pathological fracture in neoplastic disease (M84.5-)*
*pathological fracture in osteoporosis (M80.-)*
*pathological fracture in other disease (M84.6-)*
*stress fracture (M84.3-)*
*traumatic fracture (S12.-, S22.-, S32.-, S42.-, S52.-, S62.-, S72.-, S82.-, S92.-)*
EXCLUDES 2 *personal history of (healed) pathological fracture (Z87.311)*

The appropriate 7th character is to be added to each code from subcategory M84.4.
A initial encounter for fracture
D subsequent encounter for fracture with routine healing
G subsequent encounter for fracture with delayed healing
K subsequent encounter for fracture with nonunion
P subsequent encounter for fracture with malunion
S sequela

M84.40 Pathological fracture, unspecified site Rx
M84.41 Pathological fracture, shoulder
M84.411 Pathological fracture, right shoulder Rx
M84.412 Pathological fracture, left shoulder Rx
M84.419 Pathological fracture, unspecified shoulder Rx
M84.42 Pathological fracture, humerus
M84.421 Pathological fracture, right humerus Rx
M84.422 Pathological fracture, left humerus Rx
M84.429 Pathological fracture, unspecified humerus Rx
M84.43 Pathological fracture, ulna and radius
M84.431 Pathological fracture, right ulna Rx
M84.432 Pathological fracture, left ulna Rx
M84.433 Pathological fracture, right radius Rx
M84.434 Pathological fracture, left radius Rx
M84.439 Pathological fracture, unspecified ulna and radius Rx
M84.44 Pathological fracture, hand and fingers
M84.441 Pathological fracture, right hand Rx
M84.442 Pathological fracture, left hand Rx
M84.443 Pathological fracture, unspecified hand Rx
M84.444 Pathological fracture, right finger(s) Rx
M84.445 Pathological fracture, left finger(s) Rx
M84.446 Pathological fracture, unspecified finger(s) Rx
M84.45 Pathological fracture, femur and pelvis
AHA: 2016,4Q,43
M84.451 Pathological fracture, right femur HCC Rx ESR COM
M84.452 Pathological fracture, left femur HCC Rx ESR COM
M84.453 Pathological fracture, unspecified femur HCC Rx ESR COM
M84.454 Pathological fracture, pelvis Rx
M84.459 Pathological fracture, hip, unspecified HCC Rx ESR COM
M84.46 Pathological fracture, tibia and fibula
M84.461 Pathological fracture, right tibia Rx
M84.462 Pathological fracture, left tibia Rx
M84.463 Pathological fracture, right fibula Rx
M84.464 Pathological fracture, left fibula Rx
M84.469 Pathological fracture, unspecified tibia and fibula Rx
M84.47 Pathological fracture, ankle, foot and toes
M84.471 Pathological fracture, right ankle Rx
M84.472 Pathological fracture, left ankle Rx
M84.473 Pathological fracture, unspecified ankle Rx
M84.474 Pathological fracture, right foot Rx
M84.475 Pathological fracture, left foot Rx
M84.476 Pathological fracture, unspecified foot Rx
M84.477 Pathological fracture, right toe(s) Rx
M84.478 Pathological fracture, left toe(s) Rx
M84.479 Pathological fracture, unspecified toe(s) Rx
M84.48 Pathological fracture, other site Rx

M84.5 Pathological fracture in neoplastic disease
Code also underlying neoplasm

The appropriate 7th character is to be added to each code from subcategory M84.5.
A initial encounter for fracture
D subsequent encounter for fracture with routine healing
G subsequent encounter for fracture with delayed healing
K subsequent encounter for fracture with nonunion
P subsequent encounter for fracture with malunion
S sequela

M84.50 Pathological fracture in neoplastic disease, unspecified site Rx
M84.51 Pathological fracture in neoplastic disease, shoulder
M84.511 Pathological fracture in neoplastic disease, right shoulder Rx
M84.512 Pathological fracture in neoplastic disease, left shoulder Rx
M84.519 Pathological fracture in neoplastic disease, unspecified shoulder Rx

√6th **M84.52** Pathological fracture in neoplastic disease, humerus
- √7th **M84.521** Pathological fracture in neoplastic disease, right humerus Rx
- √7th **M84.522** Pathological fracture in neoplastic disease, left humerus Rx
- √7th **M84.529** Pathological fracture in neoplastic disease, unspecified humerus Rx

√6th **M84.53** Pathological fracture in neoplastic disease, ulna and radius
- √7th **M84.531** Pathological fracture in neoplastic disease, right ulna Rx
- √7th **M84.532** Pathological fracture in neoplastic disease, left ulna Rx
- √7th **M84.533** Pathological fracture in neoplastic disease, right radius Rx
- √7th **M84.534** Pathological fracture in neoplastic disease, left radius Rx
- √7th **M84.539** Pathological fracture in neoplastic disease, unspecified ulna and radius Rx

√6th **M84.54** Pathological fracture in neoplastic disease, hand
- √7th **M84.541** Pathological fracture in neoplastic disease, right hand Rx
- √7th **M84.542** Pathological fracture in neoplastic disease, left hand Rx
- √7th **M84.549** Pathological fracture in neoplastic disease, unspecified hand Rx

√6th **M84.55** Pathological fracture in neoplastic disease, pelvis and femur
- √7th **M84.550** Pathological fracture in neoplastic disease, pelvis Rx
- √7th **M84.551** Pathological fracture in neoplastic disease, right femur HCC Rx ESR COM
- √7th **M84.552** Pathological fracture in neoplastic disease, left femur HCC Rx ESR COM
- √7th **M84.553** Pathological fracture in neoplastic disease, unspecified femur HCC Rx ESR COM
- √7th **M84.559** Pathological fracture in neoplastic disease, hip, unspecified HCC Rx ESR COM

√6th **M84.56** Pathological fracture in neoplastic disease, tibia and fibula
- √7th **M84.561** Pathological fracture in neoplastic disease, right tibia Rx
- √7th **M84.562** Pathological fracture in neoplastic disease, left tibia Rx
- √7th **M84.563** Pathological fracture in neoplastic disease, right fibula Rx
- √7th **M84.564** Pathological fracture in neoplastic disease, left fibula Rx
- √7th **M84.569** Pathological fracture in neoplastic disease, unspecified tibia and fibula Rx

√6th **M84.57** Pathological fracture in neoplastic disease, ankle and foot
- √7th **M84.571** Pathological fracture in neoplastic disease, right ankle Rx
- √7th **M84.572** Pathological fracture in neoplastic disease, left ankle Rx
- √7th **M84.573** Pathological fracture in neoplastic disease, unspecified ankle Rx
- √7th **M84.574** Pathological fracture in neoplastic disease, right foot Rx
- √7th **M84.575** Pathological fracture in neoplastic disease, left foot Rx
- √7th **M84.576** Pathological fracture in neoplastic disease, unspecified foot Rx

√x7th **M84.58** Pathological fracture in neoplastic disease, other specified site Rx
  Pathological fracture in neoplastic disease, vertebrae

√5th **M84.6** Pathological fracture in other disease

Code also underlying condition

**EXCLUDES 1** *pathological fracture in osteoporosis (M8Ø.-)*

The appropriate 7th character is to be added to each code from subcategory M84.6.
- A initial encounter for fracture
- D subsequent encounter for fracture with routine healing
- G subsequent encounter for fracture with delayed healing
- K subsequent encounter for fracture with nonunion
- P subsequent encounter for fracture with malunion
- S sequela

√x7th **M84.6Ø** Pathological fracture in other disease, unspecified site Rx

√6th **M84.61** Pathological fracture in other disease, shoulder
- √7th **M84.611** Pathological fracture in other disease, right shoulder Rx
- √7th **M84.612** Pathological fracture in other disease, left shoulder Rx
- √7th **M84.619** Pathological fracture in other disease, unspecified shoulder Rx

√6th **M84.62** Pathological fracture in other disease, humerus
- √7th **M84.621** Pathological fracture in other disease, right humerus Rx
- √7th **M84.622** Pathological fracture in other disease, left humerus Rx
- √7th **M84.629** Pathological fracture in other disease, unspecified humerus Rx

√6th **M84.63** Pathological fracture in other disease, ulna and radius
- √7th **M84.631** Pathological fracture in other disease, right ulna Rx
- √7th **M84.632** Pathological fracture in other disease, left ulna Rx
- √7th **M84.633** Pathological fracture in other disease, right radius Rx
- √7th **M84.634** Pathological fracture in other disease, left radius Rx
- √7th **M84.639** Pathological fracture in other disease, unspecified ulna and radius Rx

√6th **M84.64** Pathological fracture in other disease, hand
- √7th **M84.641** Pathological fracture in other disease, right hand Rx
- √7th **M84.642** Pathological fracture in other disease, left hand Rx
- √7th **M84.649** Pathological fracture in other disease, unspecified hand Rx

√6th **M84.65** Pathological fracture in other disease, pelvis and femur
- √7th **M84.65Ø** Pathological fracture in other disease, pelvis Rx
- √7th **M84.651** Pathological fracture in other disease, right femur HCC Rx ESR COM
- √7th **M84.652** Pathological fracture in other disease, left femur HCC Rx ESR COM
- √7th **M84.653** Pathological fracture in other disease, unspecified femur HCC Rx ESR COM
- √7th **M84.659** Pathological fracture in other disease, hip, unspecified HCC Rx ESR COM

√6th **M84.66** Pathological fracture in other disease, tibia and fibula
- √7th **M84.661** Pathological fracture in other disease, right tibia Rx
- √7th **M84.662** Pathological fracture in other disease, left tibia Rx
- √7th **M84.663** Pathological fracture in other disease, right fibula Rx
- √7th **M84.664** Pathological fracture in other disease, left fibula Rx
- √7th **M84.669** Pathological fracture in other disease, unspecified tibia and fibula Rx

√6th **M84.67** Pathological fracture in other disease, ankle and foot
- √7th **M84.671** Pathological fracture in other disease, right ankle Rx
- √7th **M84.672** Pathological fracture in other disease, left ankle Rx
- √7th **M84.673** Pathological fracture in other disease, unspecified ankle Rx
- √7th **M84.674** Pathological fracture in other disease, right foot Rx

√7th M84.675 Pathological fracture in other disease, left foot Rx

√7th M84.676 Pathological fracture in other disease, unspecified foot Rx

√x7th M84.68 Pathological fracture in other disease, other site Rx

√5th M84.7 Nontraumatic fracture, not elsewhere classified

√6th M84.75 Atypical femoral fracture

AHA: 2016,4Q,41-42

The appropriate 7th character is to be added to each code from M84.75.
- A initial encounter for fracture
- D subsequent encounter for fracture with routine healing
- G subsequent encounter for fracture with delayed healing
- K subsequent encounter for fracture with nonunion
- P subsequent encounter for fracture with malunion
- S sequela

√7th M84.750 Atypical femoral fracture, unspecified Q

√7th M84.751 Incomplete atypical femoral fracture, right leg Q

√7th M84.752 Incomplete atypical femoral fracture, left leg Q

√7th M84.753 Incomplete atypical femoral fracture, unspecified leg Q

√7th M84.754 Complete transverse atypical femoral fracture, right leg HCC ESR COM Q

√7th M84.755 Complete transverse atypical femoral fracture, left leg HCC ESR COM Q

√7th M84.756 Complete transverse atypical femoral fracture, unspecified leg HCC ESR COM Q

√7th M84.757 Complete oblique atypical femoral fracture, right leg HCC ESR COM Q

√7th M84.758 Complete oblique atypical femoral fracture, left leg HCC ESR COM

√7th M84.759 Complete oblique atypical femoral fracture, unspecified leg HCC ESR COM Q

√5th M84.8 Other disorders of continuity of bone

M84.80 Other disorders of continuity of bone, unspecified site

√6th M84.81 Other disorders of continuity of bone, shoulder

M84.811 Other disorders of continuity of bone, right shoulder

M84.812 Other disorders of continuity of bone, left shoulder

M84.819 Other disorders of continuity of bone, unspecified shoulder

√6th M84.82 Other disorders of continuity of bone, humerus

M84.821 Other disorders of continuity of bone, right humerus

M84.822 Other disorders of continuity of bone, left humerus

M84.829 Other disorders of continuity of bone, unspecified humerus

√6th M84.83 Other disorders of continuity of bone, ulna and radius

M84.831 Other disorders of continuity of bone, right ulna

M84.832 Other disorders of continuity of bone, left ulna

M84.833 Other disorders of continuity of bone, right radius

M84.834 Other disorders of continuity of bone, left radius

M84.839 Other disorders of continuity of bone, unspecified ulna and radius

√6th M84.84 Other disorders of continuity of bone, hand

M84.841 Other disorders of continuity of bone, right hand

M84.842 Other disorders of continuity of bone, left hand

M84.849 Other disorders of continuity of bone, unspecified hand

√6th M84.85 Other disorders of continuity of bone, pelvic region and thigh

M84.851 Other disorders of continuity of bone, right pelvic region and thigh

M84.852 Other disorders of continuity of bone, left pelvic region and thigh

M84.859 Other disorders of continuity of bone, unspecified pelvic region and thigh

√6th M84.86 Other disorders of continuity of bone, tibia and fibula

M84.861 Other disorders of continuity of bone, right tibia

M84.862 Other disorders of continuity of bone, left tibia

M84.863 Other disorders of continuity of bone, right fibula

M84.864 Other disorders of continuity of bone, left fibula

M84.869 Other disorders of continuity of bone, unspecified tibia and fibula

√6th M84.87 Other disorders of continuity of bone, ankle and foot

M84.871 Other disorders of continuity of bone, right ankle and foot

M84.872 Other disorders of continuity of bone, left ankle and foot

M84.879 Other disorders of continuity of bone, unspecified ankle and foot

M84.88 Other disorders of continuity of bone, other site

M84.9 Disorder of continuity of bone, unspecified

√4th **M85 Other disorders of bone density and structure**

EXCLUDES 1 *osteogenesis imperfecta (Q78.0)*
*osteopetrosis (Q78.2)*
*osteopoikilosis (Q78.8)*
*polyostotic fibrous dysplasia (Q78.1)*

√5th M85.0 Fibrous dysplasia (monostotic)

EXCLUDES 2 *fibrous dysplasia of jaw (M27.8)*

M85.00 Fibrous dysplasia (monostotic), unspecified site

√6th M85.01 Fibrous dysplasia (monostotic), shoulder

M85.011 Fibrous dysplasia (monostotic), right shoulder

M85.012 Fibrous dysplasia (monostotic), left shoulder

M85.019 Fibrous dysplasia (monostotic), unspecified shoulder

√6th M85.02 Fibrous dysplasia (monostotic), upper arm

M85.021 Fibrous dysplasia (monostotic), right upper arm

M85.022 Fibrous dysplasia (monostotic), left upper arm

M85.029 Fibrous dysplasia (monostotic), unspecified upper arm

√6th M85.03 Fibrous dysplasia (monostotic), forearm

M85.031 Fibrous dysplasia (monostotic), right forearm

M85.032 Fibrous dysplasia (monostotic), left forearm

M85.039 Fibrous dysplasia (monostotic), unspecified forearm

√6th M85.04 Fibrous dysplasia (monostotic), hand

M85.041 Fibrous dysplasia (monostotic), right hand

M85.042 Fibrous dysplasia (monostotic), left hand

M85.049 Fibrous dysplasia (monostotic), unspecified hand

√6th M85.05 Fibrous dysplasia (monostotic), thigh

M85.051 Fibrous dysplasia (monostotic), right thigh

M85.052 Fibrous dysplasia (monostotic), left thigh

M85.059 Fibrous dysplasia (monostotic), unspecified thigh

√6th M85.06 Fibrous dysplasia (monostotic), lower leg

M85.061 Fibrous dysplasia (monostotic), right lower leg

M85.062 Fibrous dysplasia (monostotic), left lower leg

M85.069 Fibrous dysplasia (monostotic), unspecified lower leg

√6th M85.07 Fibrous dysplasia (monostotic), ankle and foot

M85.071 Fibrous dysplasia (monostotic), right ankle and foot

M85.072 Fibrous dysplasia (monostotic), left ankle and foot

M85.079 Fibrous dysplasia (monostotic), unspecified ankle and foot

M85.08 Fibrous dysplasia (monostotic), other site

M85.09 Fibrous dysplasia (monostotic), multiple sites

✓5th **M85.1 Skeletal fluorosis**
M85.10 Skeletal fluorosis, unspecified site
✓6th M85.11 Skeletal fluorosis, shoulder
M85.111 Skeletal fluorosis, right shoulder
M85.112 Skeletal fluorosis, left shoulder
M85.119 Skeletal fluorosis, unspecified shoulder
✓6th M85.12 Skeletal fluorosis, upper arm
M85.121 Skeletal fluorosis, right upper arm
M85.122 Skeletal fluorosis, left upper arm
M85.129 Skeletal fluorosis, unspecified upper arm
✓6th M85.13 Skeletal fluorosis, forearm
M85.131 Skeletal fluorosis, right forearm
M85.132 Skeletal fluorosis, left forearm
M85.139 Skeletal fluorosis, unspecified forearm
✓6th M85.14 Skeletal fluorosis, hand
M85.141 Skeletal fluorosis, right hand
M85.142 Skeletal fluorosis, left hand
M85.149 Skeletal fluorosis, unspecified hand
✓6th M85.15 Skeletal fluorosis, thigh
M85.151 Skeletal fluorosis, right thigh
M85.152 Skeletal fluorosis, left thigh
M85.159 Skeletal fluorosis, unspecified thigh
✓6th M85.16 Skeletal fluorosis, lower leg
M85.161 Skeletal fluorosis, right lower leg
M85.162 Skeletal fluorosis, left lower leg
M85.169 Skeletal fluorosis, unspecified lower leg
✓6th M85.17 Skeletal fluorosis, ankle and foot
M85.171 Skeletal fluorosis, right ankle and foot
M85.172 Skeletal fluorosis, left ankle and foot
M85.179 Skeletal fluorosis, unspecified ankle and foot
M85.18 Skeletal fluorosis, other site
M85.19 Skeletal fluorosis, multiple sites

**M85.2 Hyperostosis of skull**
**DEF:** Abnormal bone growth on the inner aspect of the cranial bones.

✓5th **M85.3 Osteitis condensans**
M85.30 Osteitis condensans, unspecified site
✓6th M85.31 Osteitis condensans, shoulder
M85.311 Osteitis condensans, right shoulder
M85.312 Osteitis condensans, left shoulder
M85.319 Osteitis condensans, unspecified shoulder
✓6th M85.32 Osteitis condensans, upper arm
M85.321 Osteitis condensans, right upper arm
M85.322 Osteitis condensans, left upper arm
M85.329 Osteitis condensans, unspecified upper arm
✓6th M85.33 Osteitis condensans, forearm
M85.331 Osteitis condensans, right forearm
M85.332 Osteitis condensans, left forearm
M85.339 Osteitis condensans, unspecified forearm
✓6th M85.34 Osteitis condensans, hand
M85.341 Osteitis condensans, right hand
M85.342 Osteitis condensans, left hand
M85.349 Osteitis condensans, unspecified hand
✓6th M85.35 Osteitis condensans, thigh
M85.351 Osteitis condensans, right thigh
M85.352 Osteitis condensans, left thigh
M85.359 Osteitis condensans, unspecified thigh
✓6th M85.36 Osteitis condensans, lower leg
M85.361 Osteitis condensans, right lower leg
M85.362 Osteitis condensans, left lower leg
M85.369 Osteitis condensans, unspecified lower leg
✓6th M85.37 Osteitis condensans, ankle and foot
M85.371 Osteitis condensans, right ankle and foot
M85.372 Osteitis condensans, left ankle and foot
M85.379 Osteitis condensans, unspecified ankle and foot
M85.38 Osteitis condensans, other site
M85.39 Osteitis condensans, multiple sites

✓5th **M85.4 Solitary bone cyst**
EXCLUDES 2 *solitary cyst of jaw (M27.4)*
M85.40 Solitary bone cyst, unspecified site
✓6th M85.41 Solitary bone cyst, shoulder
M85.411 Solitary bone cyst, right shoulder
M85.412 Solitary bone cyst, left shoulder
M85.419 Solitary bone cyst, unspecified shoulder
✓6th M85.42 Solitary bone cyst, humerus
M85.421 Solitary bone cyst, right humerus
M85.422 Solitary bone cyst, left humerus
M85.429 Solitary bone cyst, unspecified humerus
✓6th M85.43 Solitary bone cyst, ulna and radius
M85.431 Solitary bone cyst, right ulna and radius
M85.432 Solitary bone cyst, left ulna and radius
M85.439 Solitary bone cyst, unspecified ulna and radius
✓6th M85.44 Solitary bone cyst, hand
M85.441 Solitary bone cyst, right hand
M85.442 Solitary bone cyst, left hand
M85.449 Solitary bone cyst, unspecified hand
✓6th M85.45 Solitary bone cyst, pelvis
M85.451 Solitary bone cyst, right pelvis
M85.452 Solitary bone cyst, left pelvis
M85.459 Solitary bone cyst, unspecified pelvis
✓6th M85.46 Solitary bone cyst, tibia and fibula
M85.461 Solitary bone cyst, right tibia and fibula
M85.462 Solitary bone cyst, left tibia and fibula
M85.469 Solitary bone cyst, unspecified tibia and fibula
✓6th M85.47 Solitary bone cyst, ankle and foot
M85.471 Solitary bone cyst, right ankle and foot
M85.472 Solitary bone cyst, left ankle and foot
M85.479 Solitary bone cyst, unspecified ankle and foot
M85.48 Solitary bone cyst, other site

✓5th **M85.5 Aneurysmal bone cyst**
EXCLUDES 2 *aneurysmal cyst of jaw (M27.4)*
**DEF:** Solitary bone lesion that bulges into the periosteum and is marked by a calcified rim.
M85.50 Aneurysmal bone cyst, unspecified site
✓6th M85.51 Aneurysmal bone cyst, shoulder
M85.511 Aneurysmal bone cyst, right shoulder
M85.512 Aneurysmal bone cyst, left shoulder
M85.519 Aneurysmal bone cyst, unspecified shoulder
✓6th M85.52 Aneurysmal bone cyst, upper arm
M85.521 Aneurysmal bone cyst, right upper arm
M85.522 Aneurysmal bone cyst, left upper arm
M85.529 Aneurysmal bone cyst, unspecified upper arm
✓6th M85.53 Aneurysmal bone cyst, forearm
M85.531 Aneurysmal bone cyst, right forearm
M85.532 Aneurysmal bone cyst, left forearm
M85.539 Aneurysmal bone cyst, unspecified forearm
✓6th M85.54 Aneurysmal bone cyst, hand
M85.541 Aneurysmal bone cyst, right hand
M85.542 Aneurysmal bone cyst, left hand
M85.549 Aneurysmal bone cyst, unspecified hand
✓6th M85.55 Aneurysmal bone cyst, thigh
M85.551 Aneurysmal bone cyst, right thigh
M85.552 Aneurysmal bone cyst, left thigh
M85.559 Aneurysmal bone cyst, unspecified thigh
✓6th M85.56 Aneurysmal bone cyst, lower leg
M85.561 Aneurysmal bone cyst, right lower leg
M85.562 Aneurysmal bone cyst, left lower leg
M85.569 Aneurysmal bone cyst, unspecified lower leg
✓6th M85.57 Aneurysmal bone cyst, ankle and foot
M85.571 Aneurysmal bone cyst, right ankle and foot
M85.572 Aneurysmal bone cyst, left ankle and foot
M85.579 Aneurysmal bone cyst, unspecified ankle and foot
M85.58 Aneurysmal bone cyst, other site
M85.59 Aneurysmal bone cyst, multiple sites

✓5th **M85.6 Other cyst of bone**
EXCLUDES 1 *cyst of jaw NEC (M27.4)*
*osteitis fibrosa cystica generalisata [von Recklinghausen's disease of bone] (E21.0)*
M85.60 Other cyst of bone, unspecified site
✓6th M85.61 Other cyst of bone, shoulder
M85.611 Other cyst of bone, right shoulder

M85.612 Other cyst of bone, left shoulder
M85.619 Other cyst of bone, unspecified shoulder

M85.62 Other cyst of bone, upper arm
M85.621 Other cyst of bone, right upper arm
M85.622 Other cyst of bone, left upper arm
M85.629 Other cyst of bone, unspecified upper arm

M85.63 Other cyst of bone, forearm
M85.631 Other cyst of bone, right forearm
M85.632 Other cyst of bone, left forearm
M85.639 Other cyst of bone, unspecified forearm

M85.64 Other cyst of bone, hand
M85.641 Other cyst of bone, right hand
M85.642 Other cyst of bone, left hand
M85.649 Other cyst of bone, unspecified hand

M85.65 Other cyst of bone, thigh
M85.651 Other cyst of bone, right thigh
M85.652 Other cyst of bone, left thigh
M85.659 Other cyst of bone, unspecified thigh

M85.66 Other cyst of bone, lower leg
M85.661 Other cyst of bone, right lower leg
M85.662 Other cyst of bone, left lower leg
M85.669 Other cyst of bone, unspecified lower leg

M85.67 Other cyst of bone, ankle and foot
M85.671 Other cyst of bone, right ankle and foot
M85.672 Other cyst of bone, left ankle and foot
M85.679 Other cyst of bone, unspecified ankle and foot

M85.68 Other cyst of bone, other site
M85.69 Other cyst of bone, multiple sites

M85.8 Other specified disorders of bone density and structure
Hyperostosis of bones, except skull
Osteosclerosis, acquired
EXCLUDES 1 *diffuse idiopathic skeletal hyperostosis [DISH] (M48.1)*
*osteosclerosis congenita (Q77.4)*
*osteosclerosis fragilitas (generalista) (Q78.2)*
*osteosclerosis myelofibrosis (D75.81)*

M85.80 Other specified disorders of bone density and structure, unspecified site

M85.81 Other specified disorders of bone density and structure, shoulder
M85.811 Other specified disorders of bone density and structure, right shoulder
M85.812 Other specified disorders of bone density and structure, left shoulder
M85.819 Other specified disorders of bone density and structure, unspecified shoulder

M85.82 Other specified disorders of bone density and structure, upper arm
M85.821 Other specified disorders of bone density and structure, right upper arm
M85.822 Other specified disorders of bone density and structure, left upper arm
M85.829 Other specified disorders of bone density and structure, unspecified upper arm

M85.83 Other specified disorders of bone density and structure, forearm
M85.831 Other specified disorders of bone density and structure, right forearm
M85.832 Other specified disorders of bone density and structure, left forearm
M85.839 Other specified disorders of bone density and structure, unspecified forearm

M85.84 Other specified disorders of bone density and structure, hand
M85.841 Other specified disorders of bone density and structure, right hand
M85.842 Other specified disorders of bone density and structure, left hand
M85.849 Other specified disorders of bone density and structure, unspecified hand

M85.85 Other specified disorders of bone density and structure, thigh
M85.851 Other specified disorders of bone density and structure, right thigh
M85.852 Other specified disorders of bone density and structure, left thigh
M85.859 Other specified disorders of bone density and structure, unspecified thigh

M85.86 Other specified disorders of bone density and structure, lower leg
M85.861 Other specified disorders of bone density and structure, right lower leg
M85.862 Other specified disorders of bone density and structure, left lower leg
M85.869 Other specified disorders of bone density and structure, unspecified lower leg

M85.87 Other specified disorders of bone density and structure, ankle and foot
M85.871 Other specified disorders of bone density and structure, right ankle and foot
M85.872 Other specified disorders of bone density and structure, left ankle and foot
M85.879 Other specified disorders of bone density and structure, unspecified ankle and foot

M85.88 Other specified disorders of bone density and structure, other site
M85.89 Other specified disorders of bone density and structure, multiple sites

M85.9 Disorder of bone density and structure, unspecified
AHA: 2021,3Q,11

## Other osteopathies (M86-M90)

EXCLUDES 1 *postprocedural osteopathies (M96.-)*

**M86 Osteomyelitis**
Use additional code (B95-B97) to identify infectious agent
Use additional code to identify major osseous defect, if applicable (M89.7-)
EXCLUDES 1 *osteomyelitis due to:*
*echinococcus (B67.2)*
*gonococcus (A54.43)*
*salmonella (A02.24)*
EXCLUDES 2 *ostemyelitis of:*
*orbit (H05.0-)*
*petrous bone (H70.2-)*
*vertebra (M46.2-)*
AHA: 2025,2Q,13

M86.0 Acute hematogenous osteomyelitis
M86.00 Acute hematogenous osteomyelitis, unspecified site HCC ESR COM

M86.01 Acute hematogenous osteomyelitis, shoulder
M86.011 Acute hematogenous osteomyelitis, right shoulder HCC ESR COM
M86.012 Acute hematogenous osteomyelitis, left shoulder HCC ESR COM
M86.019 Acute hematogenous osteomyelitis, unspecified shoulder HCC ESR COM

M86.02 Acute hematogenous osteomyelitis, humerus
M86.021 Acute hematogenous osteomyelitis, right humerus HCC ESR COM
M86.022 Acute hematogenous osteomyelitis, left humerus HCC ESR COM
M86.029 Acute hematogenous osteomyelitis, unspecified humerus HCC ESR COM

M86.03 Acute hematogenous osteomyelitis, radius and ulna
M86.031 Acute hematogenous osteomyelitis, right radius and ulna HCC ESR COM
M86.032 Acute hematogenous osteomyelitis, left radius and ulna HCC ESR COM
M86.039 Acute hematogenous osteomyelitis, unspecified radius and ulna HCC ESR COM

M86.04 Acute hematogenous osteomyelitis, hand
M86.041 Acute hematogenous osteomyelitis, right hand HCC ESR COM
M86.042 Acute hematogenous osteomyelitis, left hand HCC ESR COM
M86.049 Acute hematogenous osteomyelitis, unspecified hand HCC ESR COM

M86.05 Acute hematogenous osteomyelitis, femur
M86.051 Acute hematogenous osteomyelitis, right femur HCC ESR COM
M86.052 Acute hematogenous osteomyelitis, left femur HCC ESR COM
M86.059 Acute hematogenous osteomyelitis, unspecified femur HCC ESR COM

√6th M86.06 Acute hematogenous osteomyelitis, tibia and fibula
M86.061 Acute hematogenous osteomyelitis, right tibia and fibula HCC ESR COM
M86.062 Acute hematogenous osteomyelitis, left tibia and fibula HCC ESR COM
M86.069 Acute hematogenous osteomyelitis, unspecified tibia and fibula HCC ESR COM
√6th M86.07 Acute hematogenous osteomyelitis, ankle and foot
M86.071 Acute hematogenous osteomyelitis, right ankle and foot HCC ESR COM
M86.072 Acute hematogenous osteomyelitis, left ankle and foot HCC ESR COM
M86.079 Acute hematogenous osteomyelitis, unspecified ankle and foot HCC ESR COM
M86.08 Acute hematogenous osteomyelitis, other sites HCC ESR COM
M86.09 Acute hematogenous osteomyelitis, multiple sites HCC ESR COM
√5th M86.1 Other acute osteomyelitis
M86.10 Other acute osteomyelitis, unspecified site HCC ESR COM
√6th M86.11 Other acute osteomyelitis, shoulder
M86.111 Other acute osteomyelitis, right shoulder HCC ESR COM
M86.112 Other acute osteomyelitis, left shoulder HCC ESR COM
M86.119 Other acute osteomyelitis, unspecified shoulder HCC ESR COM
√6th M86.12 Other acute osteomyelitis, humerus
M86.121 Other acute osteomyelitis, right humerus HCC ESR COM
M86.122 Other acute osteomyelitis, left humerus HCC ESR COM
M86.129 Other acute osteomyelitis, unspecified humerus HCC ESR COM
√6th M86.13 Other acute osteomyelitis, radius and ulna
M86.131 Other acute osteomyelitis, right radius and ulna HCC ESR COM
M86.132 Other acute osteomyelitis, left radius and ulna HCC ESR COM
M86.139 Other acute osteomyelitis, unspecified radius and ulna HCC ESR COM
√6th M86.14 Other acute osteomyelitis, hand
M86.141 Other acute osteomyelitis, right hand HCC ESR COM
M86.142 Other acute osteomyelitis, left hand HCC ESR COM
M86.149 Other acute osteomyelitis, unspecified hand HCC ESR COM
√6th M86.15 Other acute osteomyelitis, femur
M86.151 Other acute osteomyelitis, right femur HCC ESR COM
M86.152 Other acute osteomyelitis, left femur HCC ESR COM
M86.159 Other acute osteomyelitis, unspecified femur HCC ESR COM
√6th M86.16 Other acute osteomyelitis, tibia and fibula
M86.161 Other acute osteomyelitis, right tibia and fibula HCC ESR COM
M86.162 Other acute osteomyelitis, left tibia and fibula HCC ESR COM
M86.169 Other acute osteomyelitis, unspecified tibia and fibula HCC ESR COM
√6th M86.17 Other acute osteomyelitis, ankle and foot
AHA: 2020,1Q,12
M86.171 Other acute osteomyelitis, right ankle and foot HCC ESR COM
M86.172 Other acute osteomyelitis, left ankle and foot HCC ESR COM
M86.179 Other acute osteomyelitis, unspecified ankle and foot HCC ESR COM
M86.18 Other acute osteomyelitis, other site HCC ESR COM
M86.19 Other acute osteomyelitis, multiple sites HCC ESR COM

√5th M86.2 Subacute osteomyelitis
M86.20 Subacute osteomyelitis, unspecified site HCC ESR COM
√6th M86.21 Subacute osteomyelitis, shoulder
M86.211 Subacute osteomyelitis, right shoulder HCC ESR COM
M86.212 Subacute osteomyelitis, left shoulder HCC ESR COM
M86.219 Subacute osteomyelitis, unspecified shoulder HCC ESR COM
√6th M86.22 Subacute osteomyelitis, humerus
M86.221 Subacute osteomyelitis, right humerus HCC ESR COM
M86.222 Subacute osteomyelitis, left humerus HCC ESR COM
M86.229 Subacute osteomyelitis, unspecified humerus HCC ESR COM
√6th M86.23 Subacute osteomyelitis, radius and ulna
M86.231 Subacute osteomyelitis, right radius and ulna HCC ESR COM
M86.232 Subacute osteomyelitis, left radius and ulna HCC ESR COM
M86.239 Subacute osteomyelitis, unspecified radius and ulna HCC ESR COM
√6th M86.24 Subacute osteomyelitis, hand
M86.241 Subacute osteomyelitis, right hand HCC ESR COM
M86.242 Subacute osteomyelitis, left hand HCC ESR COM
M86.249 Subacute osteomyelitis, unspecified hand HCC ESR COM
√6th M86.25 Subacute osteomyelitis, femur
M86.251 Subacute osteomyelitis, right femur HCC ESR COM
M86.252 Subacute osteomyelitis, left femur HCC ESR COM
M86.259 Subacute osteomyelitis, unspecified femur HCC ESR COM
√6th M86.26 Subacute osteomyelitis, tibia and fibula
M86.261 Subacute osteomyelitis, right tibia and fibula HCC ESR COM
M86.262 Subacute osteomyelitis, left tibia and fibula HCC ESR COM
M86.269 Subacute osteomyelitis, unspecified tibia and fibula HCC ESR COM
√6th M86.27 Subacute osteomyelitis, ankle and foot
M86.271 Subacute osteomyelitis, right ankle and foot HCC ESR COM
M86.272 Subacute osteomyelitis, left ankle and foot HCC ESR COM
M86.279 Subacute osteomyelitis, unspecified ankle and foot HCC ESR COM
M86.28 Subacute osteomyelitis, other site HCC ESR COM
M86.29 Subacute osteomyelitis, multiple sites HCC ESR COM
√5th M86.3 Chronic multifocal osteomyelitis
M86.30 Chronic multifocal osteomyelitis, unspecified site HCC ESR COM
√6th M86.31 Chronic multifocal osteomyelitis, shoulder
M86.311 Chronic multifocal osteomyelitis, right shoulder HCC ESR COM
M86.312 Chronic multifocal osteomyelitis, left shoulder HCC ESR COM
M86.319 Chronic multifocal osteomyelitis, unspecified shoulder HCC ESR COM
√6th M86.32 Chronic multifocal osteomyelitis, humerus
M86.321 Chronic multifocal osteomyelitis, right humerus HCC ESR COM
M86.322 Chronic multifocal osteomyelitis, left humerus HCC ESR COM
M86.329 Chronic multifocal osteomyelitis, unspecified humerus HCC ESR COM
√6th M86.33 Chronic multifocal osteomyelitis, radius and ulna
M86.331 Chronic multifocal osteomyelitis, right radius and ulna HCC ESR COM

M86.332 Chronic multifocal osteomyelitis, left radius and ulna HCC ESR COM
M86.339 Chronic multifocal osteomyelitis, unspecified radius and ulna HCC ESR COM
✓6th M86.34 Chronic multifocal osteomyelitis, hand
M86.341 Chronic multifocal osteomyelitis, right hand HCC ESR COM
M86.342 Chronic multifocal osteomyelitis, left hand HCC ESR COM
M86.349 Chronic multifocal osteomyelitis, unspecified hand HCC ESR COM
✓6th M86.35 Chronic multifocal osteomyelitis, femur
M86.351 Chronic multifocal osteomyelitis, right femur HCC ESR COM
M86.352 Chronic multifocal osteomyelitis, left femur HCC ESR COM
M86.359 Chronic multifocal osteomyelitis, unspecified femur HCC ESR COM
✓6th M86.36 Chronic multifocal osteomyelitis, tibia and fibula
M86.361 Chronic multifocal osteomyelitis, right tibia and fibula HCC ESR COM
M86.362 Chronic multifocal osteomyelitis, left tibia and fibula HCC ESR COM
M86.369 Chronic multifocal osteomyelitis, unspecified tibia and fibula HCC ESR COM
✓6th M86.37 Chronic multifocal osteomyelitis, ankle and foot
M86.371 Chronic multifocal osteomyelitis, right ankle and foot HCC ESR COM
M86.372 Chronic multifocal osteomyelitis, left ankle and foot HCC ESR COM
M86.379 Chronic multifocal osteomyelitis, unspecified ankle and foot HCC ESR COM
M86.38 Chronic multifocal osteomyelitis, other site HCC ESR COM
M86.39 Chronic multifocal osteomyelitis, multiple sites HCC ESR COM
✓5th M86.4 Chronic osteomyelitis with draining sinus
M86.40 Chronic osteomyelitis with draining sinus, unspecified site HCC ESR COM
✓6th M86.41 Chronic osteomyelitis with draining sinus, shoulder
M86.411 Chronic osteomyelitis with draining sinus, right shoulder HCC ESR COM
M86.412 Chronic osteomyelitis with draining sinus, left shoulder HCC ESR COM
M86.419 Chronic osteomyelitis with draining sinus, unspecified shoulder HCC ESR COM
✓6th M86.42 Chronic osteomyelitis with draining sinus, humerus
M86.421 Chronic osteomyelitis with draining sinus, right humerus HCC ESR COM
M86.422 Chronic osteomyelitis with draining sinus, left humerus HCC ESR COM
M86.429 Chronic osteomyelitis with draining sinus, unspecified humerus HCC ESR COM
✓6th M86.43 Chronic osteomyelitis with draining sinus, radius and ulna
M86.431 Chronic osteomyelitis with draining sinus, right radius and ulna HCC ESR COM
M86.432 Chronic osteomyelitis with draining sinus, left radius and ulna HCC ESR COM
M86.439 Chronic osteomyelitis with draining sinus, unspecified radius and ulna HCC ESR COM
✓6th M86.44 Chronic osteomyelitis with draining sinus, hand
M86.441 Chronic osteomyelitis with draining sinus, right hand HCC ESR COM
M86.442 Chronic osteomyelitis with draining sinus, left hand HCC ESR COM
M86.449 Chronic osteomyelitis with draining sinus, unspecified hand HCC ESR COM
✓6th M86.45 Chronic osteomyelitis with draining sinus, femur
M86.451 Chronic osteomyelitis with draining sinus, right femur HCC ESR COM
M86.452 Chronic osteomyelitis with draining sinus, left femur HCC ESR COM
M86.459 Chronic osteomyelitis with draining sinus, unspecified femur HCC ESR COM
✓6th M86.46 Chronic osteomyelitis with draining sinus, tibia and fibula
M86.461 Chronic osteomyelitis with draining sinus, right tibia and fibula HCC ESR COM
M86.462 Chronic osteomyelitis with draining sinus, left tibia and fibula HCC ESR COM
M86.469 Chronic osteomyelitis with draining sinus, unspecified tibia and fibula HCC ESR COM
✓6th M86.47 Chronic osteomyelitis with draining sinus, ankle and foot
M86.471 Chronic osteomyelitis with draining sinus, right ankle and foot HCC ESR COM
M86.472 Chronic osteomyelitis with draining sinus, left ankle and foot HCC ESR COM
M86.479 Chronic osteomyelitis with draining sinus, unspecified ankle and foot HCC ESR COM
M86.48 Chronic osteomyelitis with draining sinus, other site HCC ESR COM
M86.49 Chronic osteomyelitis with draining sinus, multiple sites HCC ESR COM
✓5th M86.5 Other chronic hematogenous osteomyelitis
M86.50 Other chronic hematogenous osteomyelitis, unspecified site HCC ESR COM
✓6th M86.51 Other chronic hematogenous osteomyelitis, shoulder
M86.511 Other chronic hematogenous osteomyelitis, right shoulder HCC ESR COM
M86.512 Other chronic hematogenous osteomyelitis, left shoulder HCC ESR COM
M86.519 Other chronic hematogenous osteomyelitis, unspecified shoulder HCC ESR COM
✓6th M86.52 Other chronic hematogenous osteomyelitis, humerus
M86.521 Other chronic hematogenous osteomyelitis, right humerus HCC ESR COM
M86.522 Other chronic hematogenous osteomyelitis, left humerus HCC ESR COM
M86.529 Other chronic hematogenous osteomyelitis, unspecified humerus HCC ESR COM
✓6th M86.53 Other chronic hematogenous osteomyelitis, radius and ulna
M86.531 Other chronic hematogenous osteomyelitis, right radius and ulna HCC ESR COM
M86.532 Other chronic hematogenous osteomyelitis, left radius and ulna HCC ESR COM
M86.539 Other chronic hematogenous osteomyelitis, unspecified radius and ulna HCC ESR COM
✓6th M86.54 Other chronic hematogenous osteomyelitis, hand
M86.541 Other chronic hematogenous osteomyelitis, right hand HCC ESR COM
M86.542 Other chronic hematogenous osteomyelitis, left hand HCC ESR COM
M86.549 Other chronic hematogenous osteomyelitis, unspecified hand HCC ESR COM
✓6th M86.55 Other chronic hematogenous osteomyelitis, femur
M86.551 Other chronic hematogenous osteomyelitis, right femur HCC ESR COM
M86.552 Other chronic hematogenous osteomyelitis, left femur HCC ESR COM
M86.559 Other chronic hematogenous osteomyelitis, unspecified femur HCC ESR COM
✓6th M86.56 Other chronic hematogenous osteomyelitis, tibia and fibula
M86.561 Other chronic hematogenous osteomyelitis, right tibia and fibula HCC ESR COM
M86.562 Other chronic hematogenous osteomyelitis, left tibia and fibula HCC ESR COM

M86.569 Other chronic hematogenous osteomyelitis, unspecified tibia and fibula HCC ESR COM

✓6th M86.57 Other chronic hematogenous osteomyelitis, ankle and foot
- M86.571 Other chronic hematogenous osteomyelitis, right ankle and foot HCC ESR COM
- M86.572 Other chronic hematogenous osteomyelitis, left ankle and foot HCC ESR COM
- M86.579 Other chronic hematogenous osteomyelitis, unspecified ankle and foot HCC ESR COM

M86.58 Other chronic hematogenous osteomyelitis, other site HCC ESR COM

M86.59 Other chronic hematogenous osteomyelitis, multiple sites HCC ESR COM

✓5th M86.6 Other chronic osteomyelitis

M86.6Ø Other chronic osteomyelitis, unspecified site HCC ESR COM

✓6th M86.61 Other chronic osteomyelitis, shoulder
- M86.611 Other chronic osteomyelitis, right shoulder HCC ESR COM
- M86.612 Other chronic osteomyelitis, left shoulder HCC ESR COM
- M86.619 Other chronic osteomyelitis, unspecified shoulder HCC ESR COM

✓6th M86.62 Other chronic osteomyelitis, humerus
- M86.621 Other chronic osteomyelitis, right humerus HCC ESR COM
- M86.622 Other chronic osteomyelitis, left humerus HCC ESR COM
- M86.629 Other chronic osteomyelitis, unspecified humerus HCC ESR COM

✓6th M86.63 Other chronic osteomyelitis, radius and ulna
- M86.631 Other chronic osteomyelitis, right radius and ulna HCC ESR COM
- M86.632 Other chronic osteomyelitis, left radius and ulna HCC ESR COM
- M86.639 Other chronic osteomyelitis, unspecified radius and ulna HCC ESR COM

✓6th M86.64 Other chronic osteomyelitis, hand
- M86.641 Other chronic osteomyelitis, right hand HCC ESR COM
- M86.642 Other chronic osteomyelitis, left hand HCC ESR COM
- M86.649 Other chronic osteomyelitis, unspecified hand HCC ESR COM

✓6th M86.65 Other chronic osteomyelitis, thigh
- M86.651 Other chronic osteomyelitis, right thigh HCC ESR COM
- M86.652 Other chronic osteomyelitis, left thigh HCC ESR COM
- M86.659 Other chronic osteomyelitis, unspecified thigh HCC ESR COM

✓6th M86.66 Other chronic osteomyelitis, tibia and fibula
- M86.661 Other chronic osteomyelitis, right tibia and fibula HCC ESR COM
- M86.662 Other chronic osteomyelitis, left tibia and fibula HCC ESR COM
- M86.669 Other chronic osteomyelitis, unspecified tibia and fibula HCC ESR COM

✓6th M86.67 Other chronic osteomyelitis, ankle and foot
- M86.671 Other chronic osteomyelitis, right ankle and foot HCC ESR COM
  AHA: 2016,1Q,13
- M86.672 Other chronic osteomyelitis, left ankle and foot HCC ESR COM
- M86.679 Other chronic osteomyelitis, unspecified ankle and foot HCC ESR COM

M86.68 Other chronic osteomyelitis, other site HCC ESR COM

M86.69 Other chronic osteomyelitis, multiple sites HCC ESR COM

✓5th M86.8 Other osteomyelitis
Brodie's abscess
AHA: 2022,1Q,31

✓6th M86.8X Other osteomyelitis

M86.8XØ Other osteomyelitis, multiple sites HCC ESR COM

▲ ✓7th M86.8X1 Other osteomyelitis, shoulder
- ● M86.8X11 Other osteomyelitis, right shoulder
- ● M86.8X12 Other osteomyelitis, left shoulder
- ● M86.8X19 Other osteomyelitis, unspecified shoulder

▲ ✓7th M86.8X2 Other osteomyelitis, upper arm
- ● M86.8X21 Other osteomyelitis, right upper arm
- ● M86.8X22 Other osteomyelitis, left upper arm
- ● M86.8X29 Other osteomyelitis, unspecified upper arm

▲ ✓7th M86.8X3 Other osteomyelitis, forearm
- ● M86.8X31 Other osteomyelitis, right forearm
- ● M86.8X32 Other osteomyelitis, left forearm
- ● M86.8X39 Other osteomyelitis, unspecified forearm

▲ ✓7th M86.8X4 Other osteomyelitis, hand
- ● M86.8X41 Other osteomyelitis, right hand
- ● M86.8X42 Other osteomyelitis, left hand
- ● M86.8X49 Other osteomyelitis, unspecified hand

▲ ✓7th M86.8X5 Other osteomyelitis, thigh
- ● M86.8X51 Other osteomyelitis, right thigh
- ● M86.8X52 Other osteomyelitis, left thigh
- ● M86.8X59 Other osteomyelitis, unspecified thigh

▲ ✓7th M86.8X6 Other osteomyelitis, lower leg
- ● M86.8X61 Other osteomyelitis, right lower leg
- ● M86.8X62 Other osteomyelitis, left lower leg
- ● M86.8X69 Other osteomyelitis, unspecified lower leg

▲ ✓7th M86.8X7 Other osteomyelitis, ankle and foot
- ● M86.8X71 Other osteomyelitis, right ankle and foot
- ● M86.8X72 Other osteomyelitis, left ankle and foot
- ● M86.8X79 Other osteomyelitis, unspecified ankle and foot

▲ ✓7th M86.8X8 Other osteomyelitis, other site
- ● M86.8X8Ø Other osteomyelitis, skull
- ● M86.8X81 Other osteomyelitis, face and sinuses
  Pott's puffy tumor
- ● M86.8X89 Other osteomyelitis, other site

M86.8X9 Other osteomyelitis, unspecified sites HCC ESR COM

M86.9 Osteomyelitis, unspecified HCC ESR COM
Infection of bone NOS
Periostitis without osteomyelitis

✓4th M87 Osteonecrosis

INCLUDES avascular necrosis of bone

Use additional code to identify major osseous defect, if applicable (M89.7-)

EXCLUDES 1 *juvenile osteonecrosis (M91-M92)*
*osteochondropathies (M9Ø-M93)*

✓5th M87.Ø Idiopathic aseptic necrosis of bone

M87.ØØ Idiopathic aseptic necrosis of unspecified bone HCC Rx ESR COM

✓6th M87.Ø1 Idiopathic aseptic necrosis of shoulder
Idiopathic aseptic necrosis of clavicle and scapula
- M87.Ø11 Idiopathic aseptic necrosis of right shoulder HCC Rx ESR COM
- M87.Ø12 Idiopathic aseptic necrosis of left shoulder HCC Rx ESR COM

M87.019 Idiopathic aseptic necrosis of unspecified shoulder HCC Rx ESR COM

✓6th M87.02 Idiopathic aseptic necrosis of humerus

M87.021 Idiopathic aseptic necrosis of right humerus HCC Rx ESR COM

M87.022 Idiopathic aseptic necrosis of left humerus HCC Rx ESR COM

M87.029 Idiopathic aseptic necrosis of unspecified humerus HCC Rx ESR COM

✓6th M87.03 Idiopathic aseptic necrosis of radius, ulna and carpus

M87.031 Idiopathic aseptic necrosis of right radius HCC Rx ESR COM

M87.032 Idiopathic aseptic necrosis of left radius HCC Rx ESR COM

M87.033 Idiopathic aseptic necrosis of unspecified radius HCC Rx ESR COM

M87.034 Idiopathic aseptic necrosis of right ulna HCC Rx ESR COM

M87.035 Idiopathic aseptic necrosis of left ulna HCC Rx ESR COM

M87.036 Idiopathic aseptic necrosis of unspecified ulna HCC Rx ESR COM

M87.037 Idiopathic aseptic necrosis of right carpus HCC Rx ESR COM

M87.038 Idiopathic aseptic necrosis of left carpus HCC Rx ESR COM

M87.039 Idiopathic aseptic necrosis of unspecified carpus HCC Rx ESR COM

✓6th M87.04 Idiopathic aseptic necrosis of hand and fingers

Idiopathic aseptic necrosis of metacarpals and phalanges of hands

M87.041 Idiopathic aseptic necrosis of right hand HCC Rx ESR COM

M87.042 Idiopathic aseptic necrosis of left hand HCC Rx ESR COM

M87.043 Idiopathic aseptic necrosis of unspecified hand HCC Rx ESR COM

M87.044 Idiopathic aseptic necrosis of right finger(s) HCC Rx ESR COM

M87.045 Idiopathic aseptic necrosis of left finger(s) HCC Rx ESR COM

M87.046 Idiopathic aseptic necrosis of unspecified finger(s) HCC Rx ESR COM

✓6th M87.05 Idiopathic aseptic necrosis of pelvis and femur

M87.050 Idiopathic aseptic necrosis of pelvis HCC Rx ESR COM

M87.051 Idiopathic aseptic necrosis of right femur HCC Rx ESR COM

M87.052 Idiopathic aseptic necrosis of left femur HCC Rx ESR COM

M87.059 Idiopathic aseptic necrosis of unspecified femur HCC Rx ESR COM

✓6th M87.06 Idiopathic aseptic necrosis of tibia and fibula

M87.061 Idiopathic aseptic necrosis of right tibia HCC Rx ESR COM

M87.062 Idiopathic aseptic necrosis of left tibia HCC Rx ESR COM

M87.063 Idiopathic aseptic necrosis of unspecified tibia HCC Rx ESR COM

M87.064 Idiopathic aseptic necrosis of right fibula HCC Rx ESR COM

M87.065 Idiopathic aseptic necrosis of left fibula HCC Rx ESR COM

M87.066 Idiopathic aseptic necrosis of unspecified fibula HCC Rx ESR COM

✓6th M87.07 Idiopathic aseptic necrosis of ankle, foot and toes

Idiopathic aseptic necrosis of metatarsus, tarsus, and phalanges of toes

M87.071 Idiopathic aseptic necrosis of right ankle HCC Rx ESR COM

M87.072 Idiopathic aseptic necrosis of left ankle HCC Rx ESR COM

M87.073 Idiopathic aseptic necrosis of unspecified ankle HCC Rx ESR COM

M87.074 Idiopathic aseptic necrosis of right foot HCC Rx ESR COM

M87.075 Idiopathic aseptic necrosis of left foot HCC Rx ESR COM

M87.076 Idiopathic aseptic necrosis of unspecified foot HCC Rx ESR COM

M87.077 Idiopathic aseptic necrosis of right toe(s) HCC Rx ESR COM

M87.078 Idiopathic aseptic necrosis of left toe(s) HCC Rx ESR COM

M87.079 Idiopathic aseptic necrosis of unspecified toe(s) HCC Rx ESR COM

M87.08 Idiopathic aseptic necrosis of bone, other site HCC Rx ESR COM

M87.09 Idiopathic aseptic necrosis of bone, multiple sites HCC Rx ESR COM

✓5th M87.1 Osteonecrosis due to drugs

Use additional code for adverse effect, if applicable, to identify drug (T36-T50 with fifth or sixth character 5)

M87.10 Osteonecrosis due to drugs, unspecified bone Rx ESR COM

✓6th M87.11 Osteonecrosis due to drugs, shoulder

M87.111 Osteonecrosis due to drugs, right shoulder Rx ESR COM

M87.112 Osteonecrosis due to drugs, left shoulder Rx ESR COM

M87.119 Osteonecrosis due to drugs, unspecified shoulder Rx ESR COM

✓6th M87.12 Osteonecrosis due to drugs, humerus

M87.121 Osteonecrosis due to drugs, right humerus Rx ESR COM

M87.122 Osteonecrosis due to drugs, left humerus Rx ESR COM

M87.129 Osteonecrosis due to drugs, unspecified humerus Rx ESR COM

✓6th M87.13 Osteonecrosis due to drugs of radius, ulna and carpus

M87.131 Osteonecrosis due to drugs of right radius Rx ESR COM

M87.132 Osteonecrosis due to drugs of left radius Rx ESR COM

M87.133 Osteonecrosis due to drugs of unspecified radius Rx ESR COM

M87.134 Osteonecrosis due to drugs of right ulna Rx ESR COM

M87.135 Osteonecrosis due to drugs of left ulna Rx ESR COM

M87.136 Osteonecrosis due to drugs of unspecified ulna Rx ESR COM

M87.137 Osteonecrosis due to drugs of right carpus Rx ESR COM

M87.138 Osteonecrosis due to drugs of left carpus Rx ESR COM

M87.139 Osteonecrosis due to drugs of unspecified carpus Rx ESR COM

✓6th M87.14 Osteonecrosis due to drugs, hand and fingers

M87.141 Osteonecrosis due to drugs, right hand Rx ESR COM

M87.142 Osteonecrosis due to drugs, left hand Rx ESR COM

M87.143 Osteonecrosis due to drugs, unspecified hand Rx ESR COM

M87.144 Osteonecrosis due to drugs, right finger(s) Rx ESR COM

M87.145 Osteonecrosis due to drugs, left finger(s) Rx ESR COM

M87.146 Osteonecrosis due to drugs, unspecified finger(s) Rx ESR COM

✓6th M87.15 Osteonecrosis due to drugs, pelvis and femur

M87.150 Osteonecrosis due to drugs, pelvis Rx ESR COM

M87.151 Osteonecrosis due to drugs, right femur Rx ESR COM

M87.152 Osteonecrosis due to drugs, left femur Rx ESR COM

M87.159 Osteonecrosis due to drugs, unspecified femur Rx ESR COM

✓6th M87.16 Osteonecrosis due to drugs, tibia and fibula

M87.161 Osteonecrosis due to drugs, right tibia Rx ESR COM

M87.162 Osteonecrosis due to drugs, left tibia Rx ESR COM

M87.163 Osteonecrosis due to drugs, unspecified tibia Rx ESR COM
M87.164 Osteonecrosis due to drugs, right fibula Rx ESR COM
M87.165 Osteonecrosis due to drugs, left fibula Rx ESR COM
M87.166 Osteonecrosis due to drugs, unspecified fibula Rx ESR COM

✓6th M87.17 Osteonecrosis due to drugs, ankle, foot and toes
M87.171 Osteonecrosis due to drugs, right ankle Rx ESR COM
M87.172 Osteonecrosis due to drugs, left ankle Rx ESR COM
M87.173 Osteonecrosis due to drugs, unspecified ankle Rx ESR COM
M87.174 Osteonecrosis due to drugs, right foot Rx ESR COM
M87.175 Osteonecrosis due to drugs, left foot Rx ESR COM
M87.176 Osteonecrosis due to drugs, unspecified foot Rx ESR COM
M87.177 Osteonecrosis due to drugs, right toe(s) Rx ESR COM
M87.178 Osteonecrosis due to drugs, left toe(s) Rx ESR COM
M87.179 Osteonecrosis due to drugs, unspecified toe(s) Rx ESR COM

✓6th M87.18 Osteonecrosis due to drugs, other site
M87.180 Osteonecrosis due to drugs, jaw Rx ESR COM
M87.188 Osteonecrosis due to drugs, other site Rx ESR COM

M87.19 Osteonecrosis due to drugs, multiple sites Rx ESR COM

✓5th M87.2 Osteonecrosis due to previous trauma
M87.20 Osteonecrosis due to previous trauma, unspecified bone HCC Rx ESR COM

✓6th M87.21 Osteonecrosis due to previous trauma, shoulder
M87.211 Osteonecrosis due to previous trauma, right shoulder HCC Rx ESR COM
M87.212 Osteonecrosis due to previous trauma, left shoulder HCC Rx ESR COM
M87.219 Osteonecrosis due to previous trauma, unspecified shoulder HCC Rx ESR COM

✓6th M87.22 Osteonecrosis due to previous trauma, humerus
M87.221 Osteonecrosis due to previous trauma, right humerus HCC Rx ESR COM
M87.222 Osteonecrosis due to previous trauma, left humerus HCC Rx ESR COM
M87.229 Osteonecrosis due to previous trauma, unspecified humerus HCC Rx ESR COM

✓6th M87.23 Osteonecrosis due to previous trauma of radius, ulna and carpus
M87.231 Osteonecrosis due to previous trauma of right radius HCC Rx ESR COM
M87.232 Osteonecrosis due to previous trauma of left radius HCC Rx ESR COM
M87.233 Osteonecrosis due to previous trauma of unspecified radius HCC Rx ESR COM
M87.234 Osteonecrosis due to previous trauma of right ulna HCC Rx ESR COM
M87.235 Osteonecrosis due to previous trauma of left ulna HCC Rx ESR COM
M87.236 Osteonecrosis due to previous trauma of unspecified ulna HCC Rx ESR COM
M87.237 Osteonecrosis due to previous trauma of right carpus HCC Rx ESR COM
M87.238 Osteonecrosis due to previous trauma of left carpus HCC Rx ESR COM
M87.239 Osteonecrosis due to previous trauma of unspecified carpus HCC Rx ESR COM

✓6th M87.24 Osteonecrosis due to previous trauma, hand and fingers
M87.241 Osteonecrosis due to previous trauma, right hand HCC Rx ESR COM
M87.242 Osteonecrosis due to previous trauma, left hand HCC Rx ESR COM
M87.243 Osteonecrosis due to previous trauma, unspecified hand HCC Rx ESR COM
M87.244 Osteonecrosis due to previous trauma, right finger(s) HCC Rx ESR COM
M87.245 Osteonecrosis due to previous trauma, left finger(s) HCC Rx ESR COM
M87.246 Osteonecrosis due to previous trauma, unspecified finger(s) HCC Rx ESR COM

✓6th M87.25 Osteonecrosis due to previous trauma, pelvis and femur
M87.250 Osteonecrosis due to previous trauma, pelvis HCC Rx ESR COM
M87.251 Osteonecrosis due to previous trauma, right femur HCC Rx ESR COM
M87.252 Osteonecrosis due to previous trauma, left femur HCC Rx ESR COM
M87.256 Osteonecrosis due to previous trauma, unspecified femur HCC Rx ESR COM

✓6th M87.26 Osteonecrosis due to previous trauma, tibia and fibula
M87.261 Osteonecrosis due to previous trauma, right tibia HCC Rx ESR COM
M87.262 Osteonecrosis due to previous trauma, left tibia HCC Rx ESR COM
M87.263 Osteonecrosis due to previous trauma, unspecified tibia HCC Rx ESR COM
M87.264 Osteonecrosis due to previous trauma, right fibula HCC Rx ESR COM
M87.265 Osteonecrosis due to previous trauma, left fibula HCC Rx ESR COM
M87.266 Osteonecrosis due to previous trauma, unspecified fibula HCC Rx ESR COM

✓6th M87.27 Osteonecrosis due to previous trauma, ankle, foot and toes
M87.271 Osteonecrosis due to previous trauma, right ankle HCC Rx ESR COM
M87.272 Osteonecrosis due to previous trauma, left ankle HCC Rx ESR COM
M87.273 Osteonecrosis due to previous trauma, unspecified ankle HCC Rx ESR COM
M87.274 Osteonecrosis due to previous trauma, right foot HCC Rx ESR COM
M87.275 Osteonecrosis due to previous trauma, left foot HCC Rx ESR COM
M87.276 Osteonecrosis due to previous trauma, unspecified foot HCC Rx ESR COM
M87.277 Osteonecrosis due to previous trauma, right toe(s) HCC Rx ESR COM
M87.278 Osteonecrosis due to previous trauma, left toe(s) HCC Rx ESR COM
M87.279 Osteonecrosis due to previous trauma, unspecified toe(s) HCC Rx ESR COM

M87.28 Osteonecrosis due to previous trauma, other site HCC Rx ESR COM
M87.29 Osteonecrosis due to previous trauma, multiple sites HCC Rx ESR COM

✓5th M87.3 Other secondary osteonecrosis
M87.30 Other secondary osteonecrosis, unspecified bone HCC Rx ESR COM

✓6th M87.31 Other secondary osteonecrosis, shoulder
M87.311 Other secondary osteonecrosis, right shoulder HCC Rx ESR COM
M87.312 Other secondary osteonecrosis, left shoulder HCC Rx ESR COM
M87.319 Other secondary osteonecrosis, unspecified shoulder HCC Rx ESR COM

✓6th M87.32 Other secondary osteonecrosis, humerus
M87.321 Other secondary osteonecrosis, right humerus HCC Rx ESR COM
M87.322 Other secondary osteonecrosis, left humerus HCC Rx ESR COM
M87.329 Other secondary osteonecrosis, unspecified humerus HCC Rx ESR COM

✓6th M87.33 Other secondary osteonecrosis of radius, ulna and carpus
M87.331 Other secondary osteonecrosis of right radius HCC Rx ESR COM

M87.332 Other secondary osteonecrosis of left radius HCC Rx ESR COM
M87.333 Other secondary osteonecrosis of unspecified radius HCC Rx ESR COM
M87.334 Other secondary osteonecrosis of right ulna HCC Rx ESR COM
M87.335 Other secondary osteonecrosis of left ulna HCC Rx ESR COM
M87.336 Other secondary osteonecrosis of unspecified ulna HCC Rx ESR COM
M87.337 Other secondary osteonecrosis of right carpus HCC Rx ESR COM
M87.338 Other secondary osteonecrosis of left carpus HCC Rx ESR COM
M87.339 Other secondary osteonecrosis of unspecified carpus HCC Rx ESR COM

√6th M87.34 Other secondary osteonecrosis, hand and fingers
M87.341 Other secondary osteonecrosis, right hand HCC Rx ESR COM
M87.342 Other secondary osteonecrosis, left hand HCC Rx ESR COM
M87.343 Other secondary osteonecrosis, unspecified hand HCC Rx ESR COM
M87.344 Other secondary osteonecrosis, right finger(s) HCC Rx ESR COM
M87.345 Other secondary osteonecrosis, left finger(s) HCC Rx ESR COM
M87.346 Other secondary osteonecrosis, unspecified finger(s) HCC Rx ESR COM

√6th M87.35 Other secondary osteonecrosis, pelvis and femur
M87.350 Other secondary osteonecrosis, pelvis HCC Rx ESR COM
M87.351 Other secondary osteonecrosis, right femur HCC Rx ESR COM
M87.352 Other secondary osteonecrosis, left femur HCC Rx ESR COM
M87.353 Other secondary osteonecrosis, unspecified femur HCC Rx ESR COM

√6th M87.36 Other secondary osteonecrosis, tibia and fibula
M87.361 Other secondary osteonecrosis, right tibia HCC Rx ESR COM
M87.362 Other secondary osteonecrosis, left tibia HCC Rx ESR COM
M87.363 Other secondary osteonecrosis, unspecified tibia HCC Rx ESR COM
M87.364 Other secondary osteonecrosis, right fibula HCC Rx ESR COM
M87.365 Other secondary osteonecrosis, left fibula HCC Rx ESR COM
M87.366 Other secondary osteonecrosis, unspecified fibula HCC Rx ESR COM

√6th M87.37 Other secondary osteonecrosis, ankle and foot
M87.371 Other secondary osteonecrosis, right ankle HCC Rx ESR COM
M87.372 Other secondary osteonecrosis, left ankle HCC Rx ESR COM
M87.373 Other secondary osteonecrosis, unspecified ankle HCC Rx ESR COM
M87.374 Other secondary osteonecrosis, right foot HCC Rx ESR COM
M87.375 Other secondary osteonecrosis, left foot HCC Rx ESR COM
M87.376 Other secondary osteonecrosis, unspecified foot HCC Rx ESR COM
M87.377 Other secondary osteonecrosis, right toe(s) HCC Rx ESR COM
M87.378 Other secondary osteonecrosis, left toe(s) HCC Rx ESR COM
M87.379 Other secondary osteonecrosis, unspecified toe(s) HCC Rx ESR COM

M87.38 Other secondary osteonecrosis, other site HCC Rx ESR COM
M87.39 Other secondary osteonecrosis, multiple sites HCC Rx ESR COM

√5th M87.8 Other osteonecrosis
M87.80 Other osteonecrosis, unspecified bone HCC Rx ESR COM

√6th M87.81 Other osteonecrosis, shoulder
M87.811 Other osteonecrosis, right shoulder HCC Rx ESR COM
M87.812 Other osteonecrosis, left shoulder HCC Rx ESR COM
M87.819 Other osteonecrosis, unspecified shoulder HCC Rx ESR COM

√6th M87.82 Other osteonecrosis, humerus
M87.821 Other osteonecrosis, right humerus HCC Rx ESR COM
M87.822 Other osteonecrosis, left humerus HCC Rx ESR COM
M87.829 Other osteonecrosis, unspecified humerus HCC Rx ESR COM

√6th M87.83 Other osteonecrosis of radius, ulna and carpus
M87.831 Other osteonecrosis of right radius HCC Rx ESR COM
M87.832 Other osteonecrosis of left radius HCC Rx ESR COM
M87.833 Other osteonecrosis of unspecified radius HCC Rx ESR COM
M87.834 Other osteonecrosis of right ulna HCC Rx ESR COM
M87.835 Other osteonecrosis of left ulna HCC Rx ESR COM
M87.836 Other osteonecrosis of unspecified ulna HCC Rx ESR COM
M87.837 Other osteonecrosis of right carpus HCC Rx ESR COM
M87.838 Other osteonecrosis of left carpus HCC Rx ESR COM
M87.839 Other osteonecrosis of unspecified carpus HCC Rx ESR COM

√6th M87.84 Other osteonecrosis, hand and fingers
M87.841 Other osteonecrosis, right hand HCC Rx ESR COM
M87.842 Other osteonecrosis, left hand HCC Rx ESR COM
M87.843 Other osteonecrosis, unspecified hand HCC Rx ESR COM
M87.844 Other osteonecrosis, right finger(s) HCC Rx ESR COM
M87.845 Other osteonecrosis, left finger(s) HCC Rx ESR COM
M87.849 Other osteonecrosis, unspecified finger(s) HCC Rx ESR COM

√6th M87.85 Other osteonecrosis, pelvis and femur
M87.850 Other osteonecrosis, pelvis HCC Rx ESR COM
M87.851 Other osteonecrosis, right femur HCC Rx ESR COM
M87.852 Other osteonecrosis, left femur HCC Rx ESR COM
M87.859 Other osteonecrosis, unspecified femur HCC Rx ESR COM

√6th M87.86 Other osteonecrosis, tibia and fibula
M87.861 Other osteonecrosis, right tibia HCC Rx ESR COM
M87.862 Other osteonecrosis, left tibia HCC Rx ESR COM
M87.863 Other osteonecrosis, unspecified tibia HCC Rx ESR COM
M87.864 Other osteonecrosis, right fibula HCC Rx ESR COM
M87.865 Other osteonecrosis, left fibula HCC Rx ESR COM
M87.869 Other osteonecrosis, unspecified fibula HCC Rx ESR COM

√6th M87.87 Other osteonecrosis, ankle, foot and toes
M87.871 Other osteonecrosis, right ankle HCC Rx ESR COM
M87.872 Other osteonecrosis, left ankle HCC Rx ESR COM
M87.873 Other osteonecrosis, unspecified ankle HCC Rx ESR COM
M87.874 Other osteonecrosis, right foot HCC Rx ESR COM

M87.875 Other osteonecrosis, left foot HCC Rx ESR COM
M87.876 Other osteonecrosis, unspecified foot HCC Rx ESR COM
M87.877 Other osteonecrosis, right toe(s) HCC Rx ESR COM
M87.878 Other osteonecrosis, left toe(s) HCC Rx ESR COM
M87.879 Other osteonecrosis, unspecified toe(s) HCC Rx ESR COM
M87.88 Other osteonecrosis, other site HCC Rx ESR COM
M87.89 Other osteonecrosis, multiple sites HCC Rx ESR COM
M87.9 Osteonecrosis, unspecified HCC Rx ESR COM
Necrosis of bone NOS

**√4th M88 Osteitis deformans [Paget's disease of bone]**
EXCLUDES 1 *osteitis deformans in neoplastic disease (M9Ø.6)*
DEF: Bone disease characterized by numerous cycles of bone resorption by the body. Resorption is followed by accelerated repair attempts, causing bone deformities and bowing, with associated fractures and pain.
M88.Ø Osteitis deformans of skull
M88.1 Osteitis deformans of vertebrae
√5th M88.8 Osteitis deformans of other bones
√6th M88.81 Osteitis deformans of shoulder
M88.811 Osteitis deformans of right shoulder
M88.812 Osteitis deformans of left shoulder
M88.819 Osteitis deformans of unspecified shoulder
√6th M88.82 Osteitis deformans of upper arm
M88.821 Osteitis deformans of right upper arm
M88.822 Osteitis deformans of left upper arm
M88.829 Osteitis deformans of unspecified upper arm
√6th M88.83 Osteitis deformans of forearm
M88.831 Osteitis deformans of right forearm
M88.832 Osteitis deformans of left forearm
M88.839 Osteitis deformans of unspecified forearm
√6th M88.84 Osteitis deformans of hand
M88.841 Osteitis deformans of right hand
M88.842 Osteitis deformans of left hand
M88.849 Osteitis deformans of unspecified hand
√6th M88.85 Osteitis deformans of thigh
M88.851 Osteitis deformans of right thigh
M88.852 Osteitis deformans of left thigh
M88.859 Osteitis deformans of unspecified thigh
√6th M88.86 Osteitis deformans of lower leg
M88.861 Osteitis deformans of right lower leg
M88.862 Osteitis deformans of left lower leg
M88.869 Osteitis deformans of unspecified lower leg
√6th M88.87 Osteitis deformans of ankle and foot
M88.871 Osteitis deformans of right ankle and foot
M88.872 Osteitis deformans of left ankle and foot
M88.879 Osteitis deformans of unspecified ankle and foot
M88.88 Osteitis deformans of other bones
EXCLUDES 2 *osteitis deformans of skull (M88.Ø)*
*osteitis deformans of vertebrae (M88.1)*
M88.89 Osteitis deformans of multiple sites
M88.9 Osteitis deformans of unspecified bone

**√4th M89 Other disorders of bone**
√5th M89.Ø Algoneurodystrophy
Shoulder-hand syndrome
Sudeck's atrophy
EXCLUDES 1 *causalgia, lower limb (G57.7-)*
*causalgia, upper limb (G56.4-)*
*complex regional pain syndrome II, lower limb (G57.7-)*
*complex regional pain syndrome II, upper limb (G56.4-)*
*reflex sympathetic dystrophy (G9Ø.5-)*
M89.ØØ Algoneurodystrophy, unspecified site
√6th M89.Ø1 Algoneurodystrophy, shoulder
M89.Ø11 Algoneurodystrophy, right shoulder
M89.Ø12 Algoneurodystrophy, left shoulder
M89.Ø19 Algoneurodystrophy, unspecified shoulder
√6th M89.Ø2 Algoneurodystrophy, upper arm
M89.Ø21 Algoneurodystrophy, right upper arm
M89.Ø22 Algoneurodystrophy, left upper arm
M89.Ø29 Algoneurodystrophy, unspecified upper arm
√6th M89.Ø3 Algoneurodystrophy, forearm
M89.Ø31 Algoneurodystrophy, right forearm
M89.Ø32 Algoneurodystrophy, left forearm
M89.Ø39 Algoneurodystrophy, unspecified forearm
√6th M89.Ø4 Algoneurodystrophy, hand
M89.Ø41 Algoneurodystrophy, right hand
M89.Ø42 Algoneurodystrophy, left hand
M89.Ø49 Algoneurodystrophy, unspecified hand
√6th M89.Ø5 Algoneurodystrophy, thigh
M89.Ø51 Algoneurodystrophy, right thigh
M89.Ø52 Algoneurodystrophy, left thigh
M89.Ø59 Algoneurodystrophy, unspecified thigh
√6th M89.Ø6 Algoneurodystrophy, lower leg
M89.Ø61 Algoneurodystrophy, right lower leg
M89.Ø62 Algoneurodystrophy, left lower leg
M89.Ø69 Algoneurodystrophy, unspecified lower leg
√6th M89.Ø7 Algoneurodystrophy, ankle and foot
M89.Ø71 Algoneurodystrophy, right ankle and foot
M89.Ø72 Algoneurodystrophy, left ankle and foot
M89.Ø79 Algoneurodystrophy, unspecified ankle and foot
M89.Ø8 Algoneurodystrophy, other site
M89.Ø9 Algoneurodystrophy, multiple sites
√5th M89.1 Physeal arrest
Arrest of growth plate
Epiphyseal arrest
Growth plate arrest
√6th M89.12 Physeal arrest, humerus
M89.121 Complete physeal arrest, right proximal humerus
M89.122 Complete physeal arrest, left proximal humerus
M89.123 Partial physeal arrest, right proximal humerus
M89.124 Partial physeal arrest, left proximal humerus
M89.125 Complete physeal arrest, right distal humerus
M89.126 Complete physeal arrest, left distal humerus
M89.127 Partial physeal arrest, right distal humerus
M89.128 Partial physeal arrest, left distal humerus
M89.129 Physeal arrest, humerus, unspecified
√6th M89.13 Physeal arrest, forearm
M89.131 Complete physeal arrest, right distal radius
M89.132 Complete physeal arrest, left distal radius
M89.133 Partial physeal arrest, right distal radius
M89.134 Partial physeal arrest, left distal radius
M89.138 Other physeal arrest of forearm
M89.139 Physeal arrest, forearm, unspecified
√6th M89.15 Physeal arrest, femur
M89.151 Complete physeal arrest, right proximal femur
M89.152 Complete physeal arrest, left proximal femur
M89.153 Partial physeal arrest, right proximal femur
M89.154 Partial physeal arrest, left proximal femur
M89.155 Complete physeal arrest, right distal femur
M89.156 Complete physeal arrest, left distal femur
M89.157 Partial physeal arrest, right distal femur
M89.158 Partial physeal arrest, left distal femur
M89.159 Physeal arrest, femur, unspecified
√6th M89.16 Physeal arrest, lower leg
M89.16Ø Complete physeal arrest, right proximal tibia
M89.161 Complete physeal arrest, left proximal tibia
M89.162 Partial physeal arrest, right proximal tibia
M89.163 Partial physeal arrest, left proximal tibia
M89.164 Complete physeal arrest, right distal tibia
M89.165 Complete physeal arrest, left distal tibia
M89.166 Partial physeal arrest, right distal tibia
M89.167 Partial physeal arrest, left distal tibia
M89.168 Other physeal arrest of lower leg
M89.169 Physeal arrest, lower leg, unspecified
M89.18 Physeal arrest, other site

✓5th M89.2 Other disorders of bone development and growth
M89.20 Other disorders of bone development and growth, unspecified site
✓6th M89.21 Other disorders of bone development and growth, shoulder
M89.211 Other disorders of bone development and growth, right shoulder
M89.212 Other disorders of bone development and growth, left shoulder
M89.219 Other disorders of bone development and growth, unspecified shoulder
✓6th M89.22 Other disorders of bone development and growth, humerus
M89.221 Other disorders of bone development and growth, right humerus
M89.222 Other disorders of bone development and growth, left humerus
M89.229 Other disorders of bone development and growth, unspecified humerus
✓6th M89.23 Other disorders of bone development and growth, ulna and radius
M89.231 Other disorders of bone development and growth, right ulna
M89.232 Other disorders of bone development and growth, left ulna
M89.233 Other disorders of bone development and growth, right radius
M89.234 Other disorders of bone development and growth, left radius
M89.239 Other disorders of bone development and growth, unspecified ulna and radius
✓6th M89.24 Other disorders of bone development and growth, hand
M89.241 Other disorders of bone development and growth, right hand
M89.242 Other disorders of bone development and growth, left hand
M89.249 Other disorders of bone development and growth, unspecified hand
✓6th M89.25 Other disorders of bone development and growth, femur
M89.251 Other disorders of bone development and growth, right femur
M89.252 Other disorders of bone development and growth, left femur
M89.259 Other disorders of bone development and growth, unspecified femur
✓6th M89.26 Other disorders of bone development and growth, tibia and fibula
M89.261 Other disorders of bone development and growth, right tibia
M89.262 Other disorders of bone development and growth, left tibia
M89.263 Other disorders of bone development and growth, right fibula
M89.264 Other disorders of bone development and growth, left fibula
M89.269 Other disorders of bone development and growth, unspecified lower leg
✓6th M89.27 Other disorders of bone development and growth, ankle and foot
M89.271 Other disorders of bone development and growth, right ankle and foot
M89.272 Other disorders of bone development and growth, left ankle and foot
M89.279 Other disorders of bone development and growth, unspecified ankle and foot
M89.28 Other disorders of bone development and growth, other site
M89.29 Other disorders of bone development and growth, multiple sites
✓5th M89.3 Hypertrophy of bone
M89.30 Hypertrophy of bone, unspecified site
✓6th M89.31 Hypertrophy of bone, shoulder
M89.311 Hypertrophy of bone, right shoulder
M89.312 Hypertrophy of bone, left shoulder
M89.319 Hypertrophy of bone, unspecified shoulder
✓6th M89.32 Hypertrophy of bone, humerus
M89.321 Hypertrophy of bone, right humerus
M89.322 Hypertrophy of bone, left humerus
M89.329 Hypertrophy of bone, unspecified humerus
✓6th M89.33 Hypertrophy of bone, ulna and radius
M89.331 Hypertrophy of bone, right ulna
M89.332 Hypertrophy of bone, left ulna
M89.333 Hypertrophy of bone, right radius
M89.334 Hypertrophy of bone, left radius
M89.339 Hypertrophy of bone, unspecified ulna and radius
✓6th M89.34 Hypertrophy of bone, hand
M89.341 Hypertrophy of bone, right hand
M89.342 Hypertrophy of bone, left hand
M89.349 Hypertrophy of bone, unspecified hand
✓6th M89.35 Hypertrophy of bone, femur
M89.351 Hypertrophy of bone, right femur
M89.352 Hypertrophy of bone, left femur
M89.359 Hypertrophy of bone, unspecified femur
✓6th M89.36 Hypertrophy of bone, tibia and fibula
M89.361 Hypertrophy of bone, right tibia
M89.362 Hypertrophy of bone, left tibia
M89.363 Hypertrophy of bone, right fibula
M89.364 Hypertrophy of bone, left fibula
M89.369 Hypertrophy of bone, unspecified tibia and fibula
✓6th M89.37 Hypertrophy of bone, ankle and foot
M89.371 Hypertrophy of bone, right ankle and foot
M89.372 Hypertrophy of bone, left ankle and foot
M89.379 Hypertrophy of bone, unspecified ankle and foot
M89.38 Hypertrophy of bone, other site
M89.39 Hypertrophy of bone, multiple sites
✓5th M89.4 Other hypertrophic osteoarthropathy
Marie-Bamberger disease
Pachydermoperiostosis
M89.40 Other hypertrophic osteoarthropathy, unspecified site
✓6th M89.41 Other hypertrophic osteoarthropathy, shoulder
M89.411 Other hypertrophic osteoarthropathy, right shoulder
M89.412 Other hypertrophic osteoarthropathy, left shoulder
M89.419 Other hypertrophic osteoarthropathy, unspecified shoulder
✓6th M89.42 Other hypertrophic osteoarthropathy, upper arm
M89.421 Other hypertrophic osteoarthropathy, right upper arm
M89.422 Other hypertrophic osteoarthropathy, left upper arm
M89.429 Other hypertrophic osteoarthropathy, unspecified upper arm
✓6th M89.43 Other hypertrophic osteoarthropathy, forearm
M89.431 Other hypertrophic osteoarthropathy, right forearm
M89.432 Other hypertrophic osteoarthropathy, left forearm
M89.439 Other hypertrophic osteoarthropathy, unspecified forearm
✓6th M89.44 Other hypertrophic osteoarthropathy, hand
M89.441 Other hypertrophic osteoarthropathy, right hand
M89.442 Other hypertrophic osteoarthropathy, left hand
M89.449 Other hypertrophic osteoarthropathy, unspecified hand
✓6th M89.45 Other hypertrophic osteoarthropathy, thigh
M89.451 Other hypertrophic osteoarthropathy, right thigh
M89.452 Other hypertrophic osteoarthropathy, left thigh
M89.459 Other hypertrophic osteoarthropathy, unspecified thigh
✓6th M89.46 Other hypertrophic osteoarthropathy, lower leg
M89.461 Other hypertrophic osteoarthropathy, right lower leg
M89.462 Other hypertrophic osteoarthropathy, left lower leg
M89.469 Other hypertrophic osteoarthropathy, unspecified lower leg
✓6th M89.47 Other hypertrophic osteoarthropathy, ankle and foot
M89.471 Other hypertrophic osteoarthropathy, right ankle and foot

M89.472 Other hypertrophic osteoarthropathy, left ankle and foot
M89.479 Other hypertrophic osteoarthropathy, unspecified ankle and foot
M89.48 Other hypertrophic osteoarthropathy, other site
M89.49 Other hypertrophic osteoarthropathy, multiple sites

√5th **M89.5 Osteolysis**
Use additional code to identify major osseous defect, if applicable (M89.7-)
EXCLUDES 2 *periprosthetic osteolysis of internal prosthetic joint (T84.Ø5-)*
M89.5Ø Osteolysis, unspecified site
√6th M89.51 Osteolysis, shoulder
M89.511 Osteolysis, right shoulder
M89.512 Osteolysis, left shoulder
M89.519 Osteolysis, unspecified shoulder
√6th M89.52 Osteolysis, upper arm
M89.521 Osteolysis, right upper arm
M89.522 Osteolysis, left upper arm
M89.529 Osteolysis, unspecified upper arm
√6th M89.53 Osteolysis, forearm
M89.531 Osteolysis, right forearm
M89.532 Osteolysis, left forearm
M89.539 Osteolysis, unspecified forearm
√6th M89.54 Osteolysis, hand
M89.541 Osteolysis, right hand
M89.542 Osteolysis, left hand
M89.549 Osteolysis, unspecified hand
√6th M89.55 Osteolysis, thigh
M89.551 Osteolysis, right thigh
M89.552 Osteolysis, left thigh
M89.559 Osteolysis, unspecified thigh
√6th M89.56 Osteolysis, lower leg
M89.561 Osteolysis, right lower leg
M89.562 Osteolysis, left lower leg
M89.569 Osteolysis, unspecified lower leg
√6th M89.57 Osteolysis, ankle and foot
M89.571 Osteolysis, right ankle and foot
M89.572 Osteolysis, left ankle and foot
M89.579 Osteolysis, unspecified ankle and foot
M89.58 Osteolysis, other site
M89.59 Osteolysis, multiple sites

√5th **M89.6 Osteopathy after poliomyelitis**
Use additional code (B91) to identify previous poliomyelitis
EXCLUDES 1 *postpolio syndrome (G14)*
M89.6Ø Osteopathy after poliomyelitis, unspecified site HCC ESR COM
√6th M89.61 Osteopathy after poliomyelitis, shoulder
M89.611 Osteopathy after poliomyelitis, right shoulder HCC ESR COM
M89.612 Osteopathy after poliomyelitis, left shoulder HCC ESR COM
M89.619 Osteopathy after poliomyelitis, unspecified shoulder HCC ESR COM
√6th M89.62 Osteopathy after poliomyelitis, upper arm
M89.621 Osteopathy after poliomyelitis, right upper arm HCC ESR COM
M89.622 Osteopathy after poliomyelitis, left upper arm HCC ESR COM
M89.629 Osteopathy after poliomyelitis, unspecified upper arm HCC ESR COM
√6th M89.63 Osteopathy after poliomyelitis, forearm
M89.631 Osteopathy after poliomyelitis, right forearm HCC ESR COM
M89.632 Osteopathy after poliomyelitis, left forearm HCC ESR COM
M89.639 Osteopathy after poliomyelitis, unspecified forearm HCC ESR COM
√6th M89.64 Osteopathy after poliomyelitis, hand
M89.641 Osteopathy after poliomyelitis, right hand HCC ESR COM
M89.642 Osteopathy after poliomyelitis, left hand HCC ESR COM
M89.649 Osteopathy after poliomyelitis, unspecified hand HCC ESR COM
√6th M89.65 Osteopathy after poliomyelitis, thigh
M89.651 Osteopathy after poliomyelitis, right thigh HCC ESR COM
M89.652 Osteopathy after poliomyelitis, left thigh HCC ESR COM
M89.659 Osteopathy after poliomyelitis, unspecified thigh HCC ESR COM
√6th M89.66 Osteopathy after poliomyelitis, lower leg
M89.661 Osteopathy after poliomyelitis, right lower leg HCC ESR COM
M89.662 Osteopathy after poliomyelitis, left lower leg HCC ESR COM
M89.669 Osteopathy after poliomyelitis, unspecified lower leg HCC ESR COM
√6th M89.67 Osteopathy after poliomyelitis, ankle and foot
M89.671 Osteopathy after poliomyelitis, right ankle and foot HCC ESR COM
M89.672 Osteopathy after poliomyelitis, left ankle and foot HCC ESR COM
M89.679 Osteopathy after poliomyelitis, unspecified ankle and foot HCC ESR COM
M89.68 Osteopathy after poliomyelitis, other site HCC ESR COM
M89.69 Osteopathy after poliomyelitis, multiple sites HCC ESR COM

√5th **M89.7 Major osseous defect**
Code first underlying disease, if known, such as:
aseptic necrosis of bone (M87.-)
malignant neoplasm of bone (C4Ø.-)
osteolysis (M89.5-)
osteomyelitis (M86.-)
osteonecrosis (M87.-)
osteoporosis (M8Ø.-, M81.-)
periprosthetic osteolysis (T84.Ø5-)
M89.7Ø Major osseous defect, unspecified site
√6th M89.71 Major osseous defect, shoulder region
Major osseous defect clavicle or scapula
M89.711 Major osseous defect, right shoulder region
M89.712 Major osseous defect, left shoulder region
M89.719 Major osseous defect, unspecified shoulder region
√6th M89.72 Major osseous defect, humerus
M89.721 Major osseous defect, right humerus
M89.722 Major osseous defect, left humerus
M89.729 Major osseous defect, unspecified humerus
√6th M89.73 Major osseous defect, forearm
Major osseous defect of radius and ulna
M89.731 Major osseous defect, right forearm
M89.732 Major osseous defect, left forearm
M89.739 Major osseous defect, unspecified forearm
√6th M89.74 Major osseous defect, hand
Major osseous defect of carpus, fingers, metacarpus
M89.741 Major osseous defect, right hand
M89.742 Major osseous defect, left hand
M89.749 Major osseous defect, unspecified hand
√6th M89.75 Major osseous defect, pelvic region and thigh
Major osseous defect of femur and pelvis
M89.751 Major osseous defect, right pelvic region and thigh
M89.752 Major osseous defect, left pelvic region and thigh
M89.759 Major osseous defect, unspecified pelvic region and thigh
√6th M89.76 Major osseous defect, lower leg
Major osseous defect of fibula and tibia
M89.761 Major osseous defect, right lower leg
M89.762 Major osseous defect, left lower leg
M89.769 Major osseous defect, unspecified lower leg
√6th M89.77 Major osseous defect, ankle and foot
Major osseous defect of metatarsus, tarsus, toes
M89.771 Major osseous defect, right ankle and foot
M89.772 Major osseous defect, left ankle and foot
M89.779 Major osseous defect, unspecified ankle and foot
M89.78 Major osseous defect, other site
M89.79 Major osseous defect, multiple sites

M89.8 Other specified disorders of bone
Infantile cortical hyperostoses
Post-traumatic subperiosteal ossification
AHA: 2022,2Q,10

M89.8X Other specified disorders of bone
M89.8X0 Other specified disorders of bone, multiple sites
M89.8X1 Other specified disorders of bone, shoulder
M89.8X2 Other specified disorders of bone, upper arm
M89.8X3 Other specified disorders of bone, forearm
AHA: 2019,3Q,9
M89.8X4 Other specified disorders of bone, hand
M89.8X5 Other specified disorders of bone, thigh
M89.8X6 Other specified disorders of bone, lower leg
M89.8X7 Other specified disorders of bone, ankle and foot
M89.8X8 Other specified disorders of bone, other site
AHA: 2025,2Q,13; 2023,2Q,18
M89.8X9 Other specified disorders of bone, unspecified site

M89.9 Disorder of bone, unspecified

M90 Osteopathies in diseases classified elsewhere
EXCLUDES 1 *osteochondritis, osteomyelitis, and osteopathy (in):*
*cryptococcosis (B45.3)*
*diabetes mellitus (E08-E13 with .69-)*
*gonococcal (A54.43)*
*neurogenic syphilis (A52.11)*
*renal osteodystrophy (N25.0)*
*salmonellosis (A02.24)*
*secondary syphilis (A51.46)*
*syphilis (late) (A52.77)*

M90.5 Osteonecrosis in diseases classified elsewhere
Code first underlying disease, such as:
caisson disease (T70.3)
hemoglobinopathy (D50-D64)

*M90.50 Osteonecrosis in diseases classified elsewhere, unspecified site* HCC Rx ESR COM

M90.51 Osteonecrosis in diseases classified elsewhere, shoulder
*M90.511 Osteonecrosis in diseases classified elsewhere, right shoulder* HCC Rx ESR COM
*M90.512 Osteonecrosis in diseases classified elsewhere, left shoulder* HCC Rx ESR COM
*M90.519 Osteonecrosis in diseases classified elsewhere, unspecified shoulder* HCC Rx ESR COM

M90.52 Osteonecrosis in diseases classified elsewhere, upper arm
*M90.521 Osteonecrosis in diseases classified elsewhere, right upper arm* HCC Rx ESR COM
*M90.522 Osteonecrosis in diseases classified elsewhere, left upper arm* HCC Rx ESR COM
*M90.529 Osteonecrosis in diseases classified elsewhere, unspecified upper arm* HCC Rx ESR COM

M90.53 Osteonecrosis in diseases classified elsewhere, forearm
*M90.531 Osteonecrosis in diseases classified elsewhere, right forearm* HCC Rx ESR COM
*M90.532 Osteonecrosis in diseases classified elsewhere, left forearm* HCC Rx ESR COM
*M90.539 Osteonecrosis in diseases classified elsewhere, unspecified forearm* HCC Rx ESR COM

M90.54 Osteonecrosis in diseases classified elsewhere, hand
*M90.541 Osteonecrosis in diseases classified elsewhere, right hand* HCC Rx ESR COM
*M90.542 Osteonecrosis in diseases classified elsewhere, left hand* HCC Rx ESR COM
*M90.549 Osteonecrosis in diseases classified elsewhere, unspecified hand* HCC Rx ESR COM

M90.55 Osteonecrosis in diseases classified elsewhere, thigh
*M90.551 Osteonecrosis in diseases classified elsewhere, right thigh* HCC Rx ESR COM
*M90.552 Osteonecrosis in diseases classified elsewhere, left thigh* HCC Rx ESR COM
*M90.559 Osteonecrosis in diseases classified elsewhere, unspecified thigh* HCC Rx ESR COM

M90.56 Osteonecrosis in diseases classified elsewhere, lower leg
*M90.561 Osteonecrosis in diseases classified elsewhere, right lower leg* HCC Rx ESR COM
*M90.562 Osteonecrosis in diseases classified elsewhere, left lower leg* HCC Rx ESR COM
*M90.569 Osteonecrosis in diseases classified elsewhere, unspecified lower leg* HCC Rx ESR COM

M90.57 Osteonecrosis in diseases classified elsewhere, ankle and foot
*M90.571 Osteonecrosis in diseases classified elsewhere, right ankle and foot* HCC Rx ESR COM
*M90.572 Osteonecrosis in diseases classified elsewhere, left ankle and foot* HCC Rx ESR COM
*M90.579 Osteonecrosis in diseases classified elsewhere, unspecified ankle and foot* HCC Rx ESR COM

*M90.58 Osteonecrosis in diseases classified elsewhere, other site* HCC Rx ESR COM
*M90.59 Osteonecrosis in diseases classified elsewhere, multiple sites* HCC Rx ESR COM

M90.6 Osteitis deformans in neoplastic diseases
Osteitis deformans in malignant neoplasm of bone
Code first the neoplasm (C40.-, C41.-)
EXCLUDES 1 *osteitis deformans [Paget's disease of bone] (M88.-)*

*M90.60 Osteitis deformans in neoplastic diseases, unspecified site*

M90.61 Osteitis deformans in neoplastic diseases, shoulder
*M90.611 Osteitis deformans in neoplastic diseases, right shoulder*
*M90.612 Osteitis deformans in neoplastic diseases, left shoulder*
*M90.619 Osteitis deformans in neoplastic diseases, unspecified shoulder*

M90.62 Osteitis deformans in neoplastic diseases, upper arm
*M90.621 Osteitis deformans in neoplastic diseases, right upper arm*
*M90.622 Osteitis deformans in neoplastic diseases, left upper arm*
*M90.629 Osteitis deformans in neoplastic diseases, unspecified upper arm*

M90.63 Osteitis deformans in neoplastic diseases, forearm
*M90.631 Osteitis deformans in neoplastic diseases, right forearm*
*M90.632 Osteitis deformans in neoplastic diseases, left forearm*
*M90.639 Osteitis deformans in neoplastic diseases, unspecified forearm*

M90.64 Osteitis deformans in neoplastic diseases, hand
*M90.641 Osteitis deformans in neoplastic diseases, right hand*
*M90.642 Osteitis deformans in neoplastic diseases, left hand*
*M90.649 Osteitis deformans in neoplastic diseases, unspecified hand*

M90.65 Osteitis deformans in neoplastic diseases, thigh
*M90.651 Osteitis deformans in neoplastic diseases, right thigh*
*M90.652 Osteitis deformans in neoplastic diseases, left thigh*
*M90.659 Osteitis deformans in neoplastic diseases, unspecified thigh*

M90.66 Osteitis deformans in neoplastic diseases, lower leg
*M90.661 Osteitis deformans in neoplastic diseases, right lower leg*
*M90.662 Osteitis deformans in neoplastic diseases, left lower leg*

*M90.669 Osteitis deformans in neoplastic diseases, unspecified lower leg*

✓6th M90.67 Osteitis deformans in neoplastic diseases, ankle and foot

*M90.671 Osteitis deformans in neoplastic diseases, right ankle and foot*

*M90.672 Osteitis deformans in neoplastic diseases, left ankle and foot*

*M90.679 Osteitis deformans in neoplastic diseases, unspecified ankle and foot*

*M90.68 Osteitis deformans in neoplastic diseases, other site*

*M90.69 Osteitis deformans in neoplastic diseases, multiple sites*

✓5th M90.8 Osteopathy in diseases classified elsewhere

Code first underlying disease, such as:
rickets (E55.0)
vitamin-D-resistant rickets (E83.31)

*M90.80 Osteopathy in diseases classified elsewhere, unspecified site*

✓6th M90.81 Osteopathy in diseases classified elsewhere, shoulder

*M90.811 Osteopathy in diseases classified elsewhere, right shoulder*

*M90.812 Osteopathy in diseases classified elsewhere, left shoulder*

*M90.819 Osteopathy in diseases classified elsewhere, unspecified shoulder*

✓6th M90.82 Osteopathy in diseases classified elsewhere, upper arm

*M90.821 Osteopathy in diseases classified elsewhere, right upper arm*

*M90.822 Osteopathy in diseases classified elsewhere, left upper arm*

*M90.829 Osteopathy in diseases classified elsewhere, unspecified upper arm*

✓6th M90.83 Osteopathy in diseases classified elsewhere, forearm

*M90.831 Osteopathy in diseases classified elsewhere, right forearm*

*M90.832 Osteopathy in diseases classified elsewhere, left forearm*

*M90.839 Osteopathy in diseases classified elsewhere, unspecified forearm*

✓6th M90.84 Osteopathy in diseases classified elsewhere, hand

*M90.841 Osteopathy in diseases classified elsewhere, right hand*

*M90.842 Osteopathy in diseases classified elsewhere, left hand*

*M90.849 Osteopathy in diseases classified elsewhere, unspecified hand*

✓6th M90.85 Osteopathy in diseases classified elsewhere, thigh

*M90.851 Osteopathy in diseases classified elsewhere, right thigh*

*M90.852 Osteopathy in diseases classified elsewhere, left thigh*

*M90.859 Osteopathy in diseases classified elsewhere, unspecified thigh*

✓6th M90.86 Osteopathy in diseases classified elsewhere, lower leg

*M90.861 Osteopathy in diseases classified elsewhere, right lower leg*

*M90.862 Osteopathy in diseases classified elsewhere, left lower leg*

*M90.869 Osteopathy in diseases classified elsewhere, unspecified lower leg*

✓6th M90.87 Osteopathy in diseases classified elsewhere, ankle and foot

*M90.871 Osteopathy in diseases classified elsewhere, right ankle and foot*

*M90.872 Osteopathy in diseases classified elsewhere, left ankle and foot*

*M90.879 Osteopathy in diseases classified elsewhere, unspecified ankle and foot*

*M90.88 Osteopathy in diseases classified elsewhere, other site*

*M90.89 Osteopathy in diseases classified elsewhere, multiple sites*

## Chondropathies (M91-M94)

EXCLUDES 1 *postprocedural chondropathies (M96.-)*

✓4th **M91 Juvenile osteochondrosis of hip and pelvis**

EXCLUDES 1 *slipped upper femoral epiphysis (nontraumatic) (M93.0-)*

M91.0 Juvenile osteochondrosis of pelvis COM

Osteochondrosis (juvenile) of acetabulum
Osteochondrosis (juvenile) of iliac crest [Buchanan]
Osteochondrosis (juvenile) of ischiopubic synchondrosis [van Neck]
Osteochondrosis (juvenile) of symphysis pubis [Pierson]

✓5th M91.1 Juvenile osteochondrosis of head of femur [Legg-Calve-Perthes]

M91.10 Juvenile osteochondrosis of head of femur [Legg-Calve-Perthes], unspecified leg COM

M91.11 Juvenile osteochondrosis of head of femur [Legg-Calve-Perthes], right leg COM

M91.12 Juvenile osteochondrosis of head of femur [Legg-Calve-Perthes], left leg COM

✓5th M91.2 Coxa plana

Hip deformity due to previous juvenile osteochondrosis

M91.20 Coxa plana, unspecified hip COM

M91.21 Coxa plana, right hip COM

M91.22 Coxa plana, left hip COM

✓5th M91.3 Pseudocoxalgia

M91.30 Pseudocoxalgia, unspecified hip COM

M91.31 Pseudocoxalgia, right hip COM

M91.32 Pseudocoxalgia, left hip COM

✓5th M91.4 Coxa magna

M91.40 Coxa magna, unspecified hip COM

M91.41 Coxa magna, right hip COM

M91.42 Coxa magna, left hip COM

✓5th M91.8 Other juvenile osteochondrosis of hip and pelvis

Juvenile osteochondrosis after reduction of congenital dislocation of hip

M91.80 Other juvenile osteochondrosis of hip and pelvis, unspecified leg COM

M91.81 Other juvenile osteochondrosis of hip and pelvis, right leg COM

M91.82 Other juvenile osteochondrosis of hip and pelvis, left leg COM

✓5th M91.9 Juvenile osteochondrosis of hip and pelvis, unspecified

M91.90 Juvenile osteochondrosis of hip and pelvis, unspecified, unspecified leg COM

M91.91 Juvenile osteochondrosis of hip and pelvis, unspecified, right leg COM

M91.92 Juvenile osteochondrosis of hip and pelvis, unspecified, left leg COM

✓4th **M92 Other juvenile osteochondrosis**

✓5th M92.0 Juvenile osteochondrosis of humerus

Osteochondrosis (juvenile) of capitulum of humerus [Panner]
Osteochondrosis (juvenile) of head of humerus [Haas]

M92.00 Juvenile osteochondrosis of humerus, unspecified arm

M92.01 Juvenile osteochondrosis of humerus, right arm

M92.02 Juvenile osteochondrosis of humerus, left arm

✓5th M92.1 Juvenile osteochondrosis of radius and ulna

Osteochondrosis (juvenile) of lower ulna [Burns]
Osteochondrosis (juvenile) of radial head [Brailsford]

M92.10 Juvenile osteochondrosis of radius and ulna, unspecified arm

M92.11 Juvenile osteochondrosis of radius and ulna, right arm

M92.12 Juvenile osteochondrosis of radius and ulna, left arm

✓5th M92.2 Juvenile osteochondrosis, hand

✓6th M92.20 Unspecified juvenile osteochondrosis, hand

M92.201 Unspecified juvenile osteochondrosis, right hand

M92.202 Unspecified juvenile osteochondrosis, left hand

M92.209 Unspecified juvenile osteochondrosis, unspecified hand

√6th **M92.21 Osteochondrosis (juvenile) of carpal lunate [Kienbock]**
- **M92.211 Osteochondrosis (juvenile) of carpal lunate [Kienbock], right hand**
- **M92.212 Osteochondrosis (juvenile) of carpal lunate [Kienbock], left hand**
- **M92.219 Osteochondrosis (juvenile) of carpal lunate [Kienbock], unspecified hand**

√6th **M92.22 Osteochondrosis (juvenile) of metacarpal heads [Mauclaire]**
- **M92.221 Osteochondrosis (juvenile) of metacarpal heads [Mauclaire], right hand**
- **M92.222 Osteochondrosis (juvenile) of metacarpal heads [Mauclaire], left hand**
- **M92.229 Osteochondrosis (juvenile) of metacarpal heads [Mauclaire], unspecified hand**

√6th **M92.29 Other juvenile osteochondrosis, hand**
- **M92.291 Other juvenile osteochondrosis, right hand**
- **M92.292 Other juvenile osteochondrosis, left hand**
- **M92.299 Other juvenile osteochondrosis, unspecified hand**

√5th **M92.3 Other juvenile osteochondrosis, upper limb**
- **M92.30 Other juvenile osteochondrosis, unspecified upper limb**
- **M92.31 Other juvenile osteochondrosis, right upper limb**
- **M92.32 Other juvenile osteochondrosis, left upper limb**

√5th **M92.4 Juvenile osteochondrosis of patella**

Osteochondrosis (juvenile) of primary patellar center [Kohler]
Osteochondrosis (juvenile) of secondary patellar centre [Sinding Larsen]

- **M92.40 Juvenile osteochondrosis of patella, unspecified knee**
- **M92.41 Juvenile osteochondrosis of patella, right knee**
- **M92.42 Juvenile osteochondrosis of patella, left knee**

√5th **M92.5 Juvenile osteochondrosis of tibia and fibula**

**AHA:** 2020,4Q,33-34

√6th **M92.50 Unspecified juvenile osteochondrosis of tibia and fibula**
- **M92.501 Unspecified juvenile osteochondrosis, right leg**
- **M92.502 Unspecified juvenile osteochondrosis, left leg**
- **M92.503 Unspecified juvenile osteochondrosis, bilateral leg**
- **M92.509 Unspecified juvenile osteochondrosis, unspecified leg**

√6th **M92.51 Juvenile osteochondrosis of proximal tibia**

Blount disease
Tibia vara

- **M92.511 Juvenile osteochondrosis of proximal tibia, right leg**
- **M92.512 Juvenile osteochondrosis of proximal tibia, left leg**
- **M92.513 Juvenile osteochondrosis of proximal tibia, bilateral**
- **M92.519 Juvenile osteochondrosis of proximal tibia, unspecified leg**

√6th **M92.52 Juvenile osteochondrosis of tibia tubercle**

Osgood-Schlatter disease

- **M92.521 Juvenile osteochondrosis of tibia tubercle, right leg**
- **M92.522 Juvenile osteochondrosis of tibia tubercle, left leg**
- **M92.523 Juvenile osteochondrosis of tibia tubercle, bilateral**
- **M92.529 Juvenile osteochondrosis of tibia tubercle, unspecified leg**

√6th **M92.59 Other juvenile osteochondrosis of tibia and fibula**
- **M92.591 Other juvenile osteochondrosis of tibia and fibula, right leg**
- **M92.592 Other juvenile osteochondrosis of tibia and fibula, left leg**
- **M92.593 Other juvenile osteochondrosis of tibia and fibula, bilateral**
- **M92.599 Other juvenile osteochondrosis of tibia and fibula, unspecified leg**

√5th **M92.6 Juvenile osteochondrosis of tarsus**

Osteochondrosis (juvenile) of calcaneum [Sever]
Osteochondrosis (juvenile) of os tibiale externum [Haglund]
Osteochondrosis (juvenile) of talus [Diaz]
Osteochondrosis (juvenile) of tarsal navicular [Kohler]

- **M92.60 Juvenile osteochondrosis of tarsus, unspecified ankle**
- **M92.61 Juvenile osteochondrosis of tarsus, right ankle**
- **M92.62 Juvenile osteochondrosis of tarsus, left ankle**

√5th **M92.7 Juvenile osteochondrosis of metatarsus**

Osteochondrosis (juvenile) of fifth metatarsus [Iselin]
Osteochondrosis (juvenile) of second metatarsus [Freiberg]

- **M92.70 Juvenile osteochondrosis of metatarsus, unspecified foot**
- **M92.71 Juvenile osteochondrosis of metatarsus, right foot**
- **M92.72 Juvenile osteochondrosis of metatarsus, left foot**

**M92.8 Other specified juvenile osteochondrosis**

**DEF:** Calcaneal apophysitis: Inflammation of the calcaneus at the point of Achilles tendon insertion usually occurring in boys ages 8 to 14. Pain, tenderness, and localized swelling are present.

**M92.9 Juvenile osteochondrosis, unspecified**

Juvenile apophysitis NOS
Juvenile epiphysitis NOS
Juvenile osteochondritis NOS
Juvenile osteochondrosis NOS

√4th **M93 Other osteochondropathies**

EXCLUDES 2 *osteochondrosis of spine (M42.-)*

√5th **M93.0 Slipped upper femoral epiphysis (nontraumatic)**

Slipped capital femoral epiphysis (SCFE)
Slipped upper femoral epiphysis (SUFE)
Use additional code for associated chondrolysis (M94.3)

**AHA:** 2022,4Q,30-31

√6th **M93.00 Unspecified slipped upper femoral epiphysis (nontraumatic)**
- **M93.001 Unspecified slipped upper femoral epiphysis (nontraumatic), right hip** COM
- **M93.002 Unspecified slipped upper femoral epiphysis (nontraumatic), left hip** COM
- **M93.003 Unspecified slipped upper femoral epiphysis (nontraumatic), unspecified hip** COM
- **M93.004 Unspecified slipped upper femoral epiphysis (nontraumatic), bilateral hips** COM

√6th **M93.01 Acute slipped upper femoral epiphysis, stable (nontraumatic)**
- **M93.011 Acute slipped upper femoral epiphysis, stable (nontraumatic), right hip** COM
- **M93.012 Acute slipped upper femoral epiphysis, stable (nontraumatic), left hip** COM
- **M93.013 Acute slipped upper femoral epiphysis, stable (nontraumatic), unspecified hip** COM
- **M93.014 Acute slipped upper femoral epiphysis, stable (nontraumatic), bilateral hips** COM

√6th **M93.02 Chronic slipped upper femoral epiphysis, stable (nontraumatic)**
- **M93.021 Chronic slipped upper femoral epiphysis, stable (nontraumatic), right hip** COM
- **M93.022 Chronic slipped upper femoral epiphysis, stable (nontraumatic), left hip** COM
- **M93.023 Chronic slipped upper femoral epiphysis, stable (nontraumatic), unspecified hip** COM
- **M93.024 Chronic slipped upper femoral epiphysis, stable (nontraumatic), bilateral hips** COM

√6th **M93.03 Acute on chronic slipped upper femoral epiphysis, stable (nontraumatic)**
- **M93.031 Acute on chronic slipped upper femoral epiphysis, stable (nontraumatic), right hip** COM
- **M93.032 Acute on chronic slipped upper femoral epiphysis, stable (nontraumatic), left hip** COM
- **M93.033 Acute on chronic slipped upper femoral epiphysis, stable (nontraumatic), unspecified hip** COM

M93.034 Acute on chronic slipped upper femoral epiphysis, stable (nontraumatic), bilateral hips COM

✓6th M93.04 Acute slipped upper femoral epiphysis, unstable (nontraumatic)

M93.041 Acute slipped upper femoral epiphysis, unstable (nontraumatic), right hip COM

M93.042 Acute slipped upper femoral epiphysis, unstable (nontraumatic), left hip COM

M93.043 Acute slipped upper femoral epiphysis, unstable (nontraumatic), unspecified hip COM

M93.044 Acute slipped upper femoral epiphysis, unstable (nontraumatic), bilateral hips COM

✓6th M93.05 Acute on chronic slipped upper femoral epiphysis, unstable (nontraumatic)

M93.051 Acute on chronic slipped upper femoral epiphysis, unstable (nontraumatic), right hip COM

M93.052 Acute on chronic slipped upper femoral epiphysis, unstable (nontraumatic), left hip COM

M93.053 Acute on chronic slipped upper femoral epiphysis, unstable (nontraumatic), unspecified hip COM

M93.054 Acute on chronic slipped upper femoral epiphysis, unstable (nontraumatic), bilateral hips COM

✓6th M93.06 Acute slipped upper femoral epiphysis, unspecified stability (nontraumatic)

M93.061 Acute slipped upper femoral epiphysis, unspecified stability (nontraumatic), right hip COM

M93.062 Acute slipped upper femoral epiphysis, unspecified stability (nontraumatic), left hip COM

M93.063 Acute slipped upper femoral epiphysis, unspecified stability (nontraumatic), unspecified hip COM

M93.064 Acute slipped upper femoral epiphysis, unspecified stability (nontraumatic), bilateral hips COM

✓6th M93.07 Acute on chronic slipped upper femoral epiphysis, unspecified stability (nontraumatic)

M93.071 Acute on chronic slipped upper femoral epiphysis, unspecified stability (nontraumatic), right hip COM

M93.072 Acute on chronic slipped upper femoral epiphysis, unspecified stability (nontraumatic), left hip COM

M93.073 Acute on chronic slipped upper femoral epiphysis, unspecified stability (nontraumatic), unspecified hip COM

M93.074 Acute on chronic slipped upper femoral epiphysis, unspecified stability (nontraumatic), bilateral hips COM

M93.1 Kienbock's disease of adults A

Adult osteochondrosis of carpal lunates

✓5th M93.2 Osteochondritis dissecans

**DEF:** Avascular necrosis caused by lack of blood flow to the bone and cartilage of a joint causing the bone to die. This can result in splinters or pieces of cartilage breaking off in the joint.

M93.20 Osteochondritis dissecans of unspecified site

✓6th M93.21 Osteochondritis dissecans of shoulder

M93.211 Osteochondritis dissecans, right shoulder

M93.212 Osteochondritis dissecans, left shoulder

M93.219 Osteochondritis dissecans, unspecified shoulder

✓6th M93.22 Osteochondritis dissecans of elbow

M93.221 Osteochondritis dissecans, right elbow

M93.222 Osteochondritis dissecans, left elbow

M93.229 Osteochondritis dissecans, unspecified elbow

✓6th M93.23 Osteochondritis dissecans of wrist

M93.231 Osteochondritis dissecans, right wrist

M93.232 Osteochondritis dissecans, left wrist

M93.239 Osteochondritis dissecans, unspecified wrist

✓6th M93.24 Osteochondritis dissecans of joints of hand

M93.241 Osteochondritis dissecans, joints of right hand

M93.242 Osteochondritis dissecans, joints of left hand

M93.249 Osteochondritis dissecans, joints of unspecified hand

✓6th M93.25 Osteochondritis dissecans of hip

M93.251 Osteochondritis dissecans, right hip

M93.252 Osteochondritis dissecans, left hip

M93.259 Osteochondritis dissecans, unspecified hip

✓6th M93.26 Osteochondritis dissecans knee

M93.261 Osteochondritis dissecans, right knee

M93.262 Osteochondritis dissecans, left knee

M93.269 Osteochondritis dissecans, unspecified knee

✓6th M93.27 Osteochondritis dissecans of ankle and joints of foot

M93.271 Osteochondritis dissecans, right ankle and joints of right foot

M93.272 Osteochondritis dissecans, left ankle and joints of left foot

M93.279 Osteochondritis dissecans, unspecified ankle and joints of foot

M93.28 Osteochondritis dissecans other site

M93.29 Osteochondritis dissecans multiple sites

✓5th M93.8 Other specified osteochondropathies

M93.80 Other specified osteochondropathies of unspecified site

✓6th M93.81 Other specified osteochondropathies of shoulder

M93.811 Other specified osteochondropathies, right shoulder

M93.812 Other specified osteochondropathies, left shoulder

M93.819 Other specified osteochondropathies, unspecified shoulder

✓6th M93.82 Other specified osteochondropathies of upper arm

M93.821 Other specified osteochondropathies, right upper arm

M93.822 Other specified osteochondropathies, left upper arm

M93.829 Other specified osteochondropathies, unspecified upper arm

✓6th M93.83 Other specified osteochondropathies of forearm

M93.831 Other specified osteochondropathies, right forearm

M93.832 Other specified osteochondropathies, left forearm

M93.839 Other specified osteochondropathies, unspecified forearm

✓6th M93.84 Other specified osteochondropathies of hand

M93.841 Other specified osteochondropathies, right hand

M93.842 Other specified osteochondropathies, left hand

M93.849 Other specified osteochondropathies, unspecified hand

✓6th M93.85 Other specified osteochondropathies of thigh

M93.851 Other specified osteochondropathies, right thigh

M93.852 Other specified osteochondropathies, left thigh

M93.859 Other specified osteochondropathies, unspecified thigh

✓6th M93.86 Other specified osteochondropathies lower leg

M93.861 Other specified osteochondropathies, right lower leg

M93.862 Other specified osteochondropathies, left lower leg

M93.869 Other specified osteochondropathies, unspecified lower leg

✓6th M93.87 Other specified osteochondropathies of ankle and foot

M93.871 Other specified osteochondropathies, right ankle and foot

M93.872 Other specified osteochondropathies, left ankle and foot

M93.879 Other specified osteochondropathies, unspecified ankle and foot

M93.88 Other specified osteochondropathies other

M93.89 Other specified osteochondropathies multiple sites

**M93.9 Osteochondropathy, unspecified**
Apophysitis NOS
Epiphysitis NOS
Osteochondritis NOS
Osteochondrosis NOS
**M93.90 Osteochondropathy, unspecified of unspecified site**
**M93.91 Osteochondropathy, unspecified of shoulder**
**M93.911 Osteochondropathy, unspecified, right shoulder**
**M93.912 Osteochondropathy, unspecified, left shoulder**
**M93.919 Osteochondropathy, unspecified, unspecified shoulder**
**M93.92 Osteochondropathy, unspecified of upper arm**
**M93.921 Osteochondropathy, unspecified, right upper arm**
**M93.922 Osteochondropathy, unspecified, left upper arm**
**M93.929 Osteochondropathy, unspecified, unspecified upper arm**
**M93.93 Osteochondropathy, unspecified of forearm**
**M93.931 Osteochondropathy, unspecified, right forearm**
**M93.932 Osteochondropathy, unspecified, left forearm**
**M93.939 Osteochondropathy, unspecified, unspecified forearm**
**M93.94 Osteochondropathy, unspecified of hand**
**M93.941 Osteochondropathy, unspecified, right hand**
**M93.942 Osteochondropathy, unspecified, left hand**
**M93.949 Osteochondropathy, unspecified, unspecified hand**
**M93.95 Osteochondropathy, unspecified of thigh**
**M93.951 Osteochondropathy, unspecified, right thigh**
**M93.952 Osteochondropathy, unspecified, left thigh**
**M93.959 Osteochondropathy, unspecified, unspecified thigh**
**M93.96 Osteochondropathy, unspecified lower leg**
**M93.961 Osteochondropathy, unspecified, right lower leg**
**M93.962 Osteochondropathy, unspecified, left lower leg**
**M93.969 Osteochondropathy, unspecified, unspecified lower leg**
**M93.97 Osteochondropathy, unspecified of ankle and foot**
**M93.971 Osteochondropathy, unspecified, right ankle and foot**
**M93.972 Osteochondropathy, unspecified, left ankle and foot**
**M93.979 Osteochondropathy, unspecified, unspecified ankle and foot**
**M93.98 Osteochondropathy, unspecified other**
**M93.99 Osteochondropathy, unspecified multiple sites**

**M94 Other disorders of cartilage**
**M94.0 Chondrocostal junction syndrome [Tietze]**
Costochondritis
**M94.1 Relapsing polychondritis**
**M94.2 Chondromalacia**
EXCLUDES 1 *chondromalacia patellae (M22.4)*
**M94.20 Chondromalacia, unspecified site**
**M94.21 Chondromalacia, shoulder**
**M94.211 Chondromalacia, right shoulder**
**M94.212 Chondromalacia, left shoulder**
**M94.219 Chondromalacia, unspecified shoulder**
**M94.22 Chondromalacia, elbow**
**M94.221 Chondromalacia, right elbow**
**M94.222 Chondromalacia, left elbow**
**M94.229 Chondromalacia, unspecified elbow**
**M94.23 Chondromalacia, wrist**
**M94.231 Chondromalacia, right wrist**
**M94.232 Chondromalacia, left wrist**
**M94.239 Chondromalacia, unspecified wrist**
**M94.24 Chondromalacia, joints of hand**
**M94.241 Chondromalacia, joints of right hand**
**M94.242 Chondromalacia, joints of left hand**
**M94.249 Chondromalacia, joints of unspecified hand**
**M94.25 Chondromalacia, hip**
**M94.251 Chondromalacia, right hip**
**M94.252 Chondromalacia, left hip**
**M94.259 Chondromalacia, unspecified hip**
**M94.26 Chondromalacia, knee**
**AHA:** 2026,2Q,6
**M94.261 Chondromalacia, right knee**
**M94.262 Chondromalacia, left knee**
**M94.269 Chondromalacia, unspecified knee**
**M94.27 Chondromalacia, ankle and joints of foot**
**M94.271 Chondromalacia, right ankle and joints of right foot**
**M94.272 Chondromalacia, left ankle and joints of left foot**
**M94.279 Chondromalacia, unspecified ankle and joints of foot**
**M94.28 Chondromalacia, other site**
**M94.29 Chondromalacia, multiple sites**
**M94.3 Chondrolysis**
Code first any associated slipped upper femoral epiphysis (nontraumatic) (M93.0-)
**M94.35 Chondrolysis, hip**
**M94.351 Chondrolysis, right hip**
**M94.352 Chondrolysis, left hip**
**M94.359 Chondrolysis, unspecified hip**
**M94.8 Other specified disorders of cartilage**
**M94.8X Other specified disorders of cartilage**
**M94.8X0 Other specified disorders of cartilage, multiple sites**
**M94.8X1 Other specified disorders of cartilage, shoulder**
**M94.8X2 Other specified disorders of cartilage, upper arm**
**M94.8X3 Other specified disorders of cartilage, forearm**
**M94.8X4 Other specified disorders of cartilage, hand**
**M94.8X5 Other specified disorders of cartilage, thigh**
**M94.8X6 Other specified disorders of cartilage, lower leg**
**M94.8X7 Other specified disorders of cartilage, ankle and foot**
**M94.8X8 Other specified disorders of cartilage, other site**
**M94.8X9 Other specified disorders of cartilage, unspecified sites**
**M94.9 Disorder of cartilage, unspecified**

## Other disorders of the musculoskeletal system and connective tissue (M95)

**M95 Other acquired deformities of musculoskeletal system and connective tissue**
EXCLUDES 2 *acquired absence of limbs and organs (Z89-Z90)*
*acquired deformities of limbs (M20-M21)*
*congenital malformations and deformations of the musculoskeletal system (Q65-Q79)*
*deforming dorsopathies (M40-M43)*
*dentofacial anomalies [including malocclusion] (M26.-)*
*postprocedural musculoskeletal disorders (M96.-)*
**M95.0 Acquired deformity of nose**
EXCLUDES 2 *deviated nasal septum (J34.2)*
**M95.1 Cauliflower ear**
EXCLUDES 2 *other acquired deformities of ear (H61.1)*
**DEF:** Acquired deformity of the external ear due to injury or subsequent perichondritis.
**M95.10 Cauliflower ear, unspecified ear**
**M95.11 Cauliflower ear, right ear**
**M95.12 Cauliflower ear, left ear**
**M95.2 Other acquired deformity of head**
**AHA:** 2023,1Q,30; 2022,1Q,34
**M95.3 Acquired deformity of neck**
**M95.4 Acquired deformity of chest and rib**
**AHA:** 2022,2Q,14; 2014,4Q,26-27

M95.5 Acquired deformity of pelvis
EXCLUDES 1 *maternal care for known or suspected disproportion (O33.-)*

M95.8 Other specified acquired deformities of musculoskeletal system

M95.9 Acquired deformity of musculoskeletal system, unspecified

## Intraoperative and postprocedural complications and disorders of musculoskeletal system, not elsewhere classified (M96)

✓4th **M96 Intraoperative and postprocedural complications and disorders of musculoskeletal system, not elsewhere classified**
EXCLUDES 2 *arthropathy following intestinal bypass (M02.Ø-)*
*complications of internal orthopedic prosthetic devices, implants and grafts (T84.-)*
*disorders associated with osteoporosis (M8Ø)*
*periprosthetic fracture around internal prosthetic joint (M97.-)*
*presence of functional implants and other devices (Z96-Z97)*

M96.Ø Pseudarthrosis after fusion or arthrodesis

M96.1 Postlaminectomy syndrome, not elsewhere classified
AHA: 2025,3Q,18; 2024,1Q,17

M96.2 Postradiation kyphosis

M96.3 Postlaminectomy kyphosis

M96.4 Postsurgical lordosis

M96.5 Postradiation scoliosis

✓5th M96.6 Fracture of bone following insertion of orthopedic implant, joint prosthesis, or bone plate
Intraoperative fracture of bone during insertion of orthopedic implant, joint prosthesis, or bone plate
EXCLUDES 2 *complication of internal orthopedic devices, implants or grafts (T84.-)*

✓6th M96.62 Fracture of humerus following insertion of orthopedic implant, joint prosthesis, or bone plate
M96.621 Fracture of humerus following insertion of orthopedic implant, joint prosthesis, or bone plate, right arm ESR
M96.622 Fracture of humerus following insertion of orthopedic implant, joint prosthesis, or bone plate, left arm ESR
M96.629 Fracture of humerus following insertion of orthopedic implant, joint prosthesis, or bone plate, unspecified arm ESR

✓6th M96.63 Fracture of radius or ulna following insertion of orthopedic implant, joint prosthesis, or bone plate
M96.631 Fracture of radius or ulna following insertion of orthopedic implant, joint prosthesis, or bone plate, right arm ESR
M96.632 Fracture of radius or ulna following insertion of orthopedic implant, joint prosthesis, or bone plate, left arm ESR
M96.639 Fracture of radius or ulna following insertion of orthopedic implant, joint prosthesis, or bone plate, unspecified arm ESR

M96.65 Fracture of pelvis following insertion of orthopedic implant, joint prosthesis, or bone plate ESR

✓6th M96.66 Fracture of femur following insertion of orthopedic implant, joint prosthesis, or bone plate
M96.661 Fracture of femur following insertion of orthopedic implant, joint prosthesis, or bone plate, right leg ESR
M96.662 Fracture of femur following insertion of orthopedic implant, joint prosthesis, or bone plate, left leg ESR
M96.669 Fracture of femur following insertion of orthopedic implant, joint prosthesis, or bone plate, unspecified leg ESR

✓6th M96.67 Fracture of tibia or fibula following insertion of orthopedic implant, joint prosthesis, or bone plate
M96.671 Fracture of tibia or fibula following insertion of orthopedic implant, joint prosthesis, or bone plate, right leg ESR
M96.672 Fracture of tibia or fibula following insertion of orthopedic implant, joint prosthesis, or bone plate, left leg ESR
M96.679 Fracture of tibia or fibula following insertion of orthopedic implant, joint prosthesis, or bone plate, unspecified leg ESR

M96.69 Fracture of other bone following insertion of orthopedic implant, joint prosthesis, or bone plate ESR

✓5th M96.8 Other intraoperative and postprocedural complications and disorders of musculoskeletal system, not elsewhere classified
AHA: 2016,4Q,9-10

✓6th M96.81 Intraoperative hemorrhage and hematoma of a musculoskeletal structure complicating a procedure
EXCLUDES 1 *intraoperative hemorrhage and hematoma of a musculoskeletal structure due to accidental puncture and laceration during a procedure (M96.82-)*
M96.81Ø Intraoperative hemorrhage and hematoma of a musculoskeletal structure complicating a musculoskeletal system procedure
M96.811 Intraoperative hemorrhage and hematoma of a musculoskeletal structure complicating other procedure

✓6th M96.82 Accidental puncture and laceration of a musculoskeletal structure during a procedure
M96.82Ø Accidental puncture and laceration of a musculoskeletal structure during a musculoskeletal system procedure
M96.821 Accidental puncture and laceration of a musculoskeletal structure during other procedure

✓6th M96.83 Postprocedural hemorrhage of a musculoskeletal structure following a procedure
M96.83Ø Postprocedural hemorrhage of a musculoskeletal structure following a musculoskeletal system procedure
M96.831 Postprocedural hemorrhage of a musculoskeletal structure following other procedure

✓6th M96.84 Postprocedural hematoma and seroma of a musculoskeletal structure following a procedure
M96.84Ø Postprocedural hematoma of a musculoskeletal structure following a musculoskeletal system procedure
M96.841 Postprocedural hematoma of a musculoskeletal structure following other procedure
AHA: 2016,4Q,10
M96.842 Postprocedural seroma of a musculoskeletal structure following a musculoskeletal system procedure
M96.843 Postprocedural seroma of a musculoskeletal structure following other procedure
AHA: 2023,2Q,13; 2018,3Q,6

M96.89 Other intraoperative and postprocedural complications and disorders of the musculoskeletal system
Instability of joint secondary to removal of joint prosthesis
Use additional code, if applicable, to further specify disorder
AHA: 2024,1Q,17,23; 2023,2Q,14; 2022,2Q,14; 2021,1Q,5

✓5th M96.A Fracture of ribs, sternum and thorax associated with compression of the chest and cardiopulmonary resuscitation
AHA: 2022,4Q,31-33

M96.A1 Fracture of sternum associated with chest compression and cardiopulmonary resuscitation
Fracture of xiphoid process associated with chest compression and cardiopulmonary resuscitation

M96.A2 Fracture of one rib associated with chest compression and cardiopulmonary resuscitation

M96.A3 Multiple fractures of ribs associated with chest compression and cardiopulmonary resuscitation
AHA: 2022,4Q,32

M96.A4 Flail chest associated with chest compression and cardiopulmonary resuscitation

M96.A9 Other fracture associated with chest compression and cardiopulmonary resuscitation

## Periprosthetic fractures around internal prosthetic joint (M97)

**M97 Periprosthetic fracture around internal prosthetic joint**

Code first, if known, the specific type and cause of fracture, such as traumatic or pathological

EXCLUDES 2 *fracture of bone following insertion of orthopedic implant, joint prosthesis or bone plate (M96.6-)*
*breakage (fracture) of prosthetic joint (T84.01-)*

AHA: 2016,4Q,42-43

The appropriate 7th character is to be added to each code from category M97.
A initial encounter
D subsequent encounter
S sequela

**M97.0 Periprosthetic fracture around internal prosthetic hip joint**
AHA: 2018,1Q,21; 2016,4Q,42
- M97.01 Periprosthetic fracture around internal prosthetic right hip joint HCC ESR Q
- M97.02 Periprosthetic fracture around internal prosthetic left hip joint HCC ESR Q

**M97.1 Periprosthetic fracture around internal prosthetic knee joint**
- M97.11 Periprosthetic fracture around internal prosthetic right knee joint Q
- M97.12 Periprosthetic fracture around internal prosthetic left knee joint Q

**M97.2 Periprosthetic fracture around internal prosthetic ankle joint**
- M97.21 Periprosthetic fracture around internal prosthetic right ankle joint Q
- M97.22 Periprosthetic fracture around internal prosthetic left ankle joint Q

**M97.3 Periprosthetic fracture around internal prosthetic shoulder joint**
- M97.31 Periprosthetic fracture around internal prosthetic right shoulder joint Q
- M97.32 Periprosthetic fracture around internal prosthetic left shoulder joint Q

**M97.4 Periprosthetic fracture around internal prosthetic elbow joint**
- M97.41 Periprosthetic fracture around internal prosthetic right elbow joint Q
- M97.42 Periprosthetic fracture around internal prosthetic left elbow joint Q

**M97.8 Periprosthetic fracture around other internal prosthetic joint**
Periprosthetic fracture around internal prosthetic finger joint
Periprosthetic fracture around internal prosthetic spinal joint
Periprosthetic fracture around internal prosthetic toe joint
Periprosthetic fracture around internal prosthetic wrist joint
Use additional code to identify the joint (Z96.6-)

**M97.9 Periprosthetic fracture around unspecified internal prosthetic joint**

## Biomechanical lesions, not elsewhere classified (M99)

**M99 Biomechanical lesions, not elsewhere classified**

NOTE This category should not be used if the condition can be classified elsewhere.

DEF: Biomechanical lesion: Term used by osteopathic and chiropractic physicians to describe musculoskeletal conditions treated that are not more appropriately classified elsewhere.

**M99.0 Segmental and somatic dysfunction**
- M99.00 Segmental and somatic dysfunction of head region
- M99.01 Segmental and somatic dysfunction of cervical region
- M99.02 Segmental and somatic dysfunction of thoracic region
- M99.03 Segmental and somatic dysfunction of lumbar region
- M99.04 Segmental and somatic dysfunction of sacral region
- M99.05 Segmental and somatic dysfunction of pelvic region
- M99.06 Segmental and somatic dysfunction of lower extremity
- M99.07 Segmental and somatic dysfunction of upper extremity
- M99.08 Segmental and somatic dysfunction of rib cage
- M99.09 Segmental and somatic dysfunction of abdomen and other regions

**M99.1 Subluxation complex (vertebral)**
- M99.10 Subluxation complex (vertebral) of head region
- M99.11 Subluxation complex (vertebral) of cervical region
- M99.12 Subluxation complex (vertebral) of thoracic region
- M99.13 Subluxation complex (vertebral) of lumbar region
- M99.14 Subluxation complex (vertebral) of sacral region
- M99.15 Subluxation complex (vertebral) of pelvic region
- M99.16 Subluxation complex (vertebral) of lower extremity
- M99.17 Subluxation complex (vertebral) of upper extremity
- M99.18 Subluxation complex (vertebral) of rib cage
- M99.19 Subluxation complex (vertebral) of abdomen and other regions

**M99.2 Subluxation stenosis of neural canal**
- M99.20 Subluxation stenosis of neural canal of head region
- M99.21 Subluxation stenosis of neural canal of cervical region
- M99.22 Subluxation stenosis of neural canal of thoracic region
- M99.23 Subluxation stenosis of neural canal of lumbar region
- M99.24 Subluxation stenosis of neural canal of sacral region
- M99.25 Subluxation stenosis of neural canal of pelvic region
- M99.26 Subluxation stenosis of neural canal of lower extremity
- M99.27 Subluxation stenosis of neural canal of upper extremity
- M99.28 Subluxation stenosis of neural canal of rib cage
- M99.29 Subluxation stenosis of neural canal of abdomen and other regions

**M99.3 Osseous stenosis of neural canal**
- M99.30 Osseous stenosis of neural canal of head region
- M99.31 Osseous stenosis of neural canal of cervical region
- M99.32 Osseous stenosis of neural canal of thoracic region
- M99.33 Osseous stenosis of neural canal of lumbar region
- M99.34 Osseous stenosis of neural canal of sacral region
- M99.35 Osseous stenosis of neural canal of pelvic region
- M99.36 Osseous stenosis of neural canal of lower extremity
- M99.37 Osseous stenosis of neural canal of upper extremity
- M99.38 Osseous stenosis of neural canal of rib cage
- M99.39 Osseous stenosis of neural canal of abdomen and other regions

**M99.4 Connective tissue stenosis of neural canal**
- M99.40 Connective tissue stenosis of neural canal of head region
- M99.41 Connective tissue stenosis of neural canal of cervical region
- M99.42 Connective tissue stenosis of neural canal of thoracic region
- M99.43 Connective tissue stenosis of neural canal of lumbar region
- M99.44 Connective tissue stenosis of neural canal of sacral region
- M99.45 Connective tissue stenosis of neural canal of pelvic region
- M99.46 Connective tissue stenosis of neural canal of lower extremity
- M99.47 Connective tissue stenosis of neural canal of upper extremity
- M99.48 Connective tissue stenosis of neural canal of rib cage
- M99.49 Connective tissue stenosis of neural canal of abdomen and other regions

**M99.5 Intervertebral disc stenosis of neural canal**
- M99.50 Intervertebral disc stenosis of neural canal of head region
- M99.51 Intervertebral disc stenosis of neural canal of cervical region
- M99.52 Intervertebral disc stenosis of neural canal of thoracic region
- M99.53 Intervertebral disc stenosis of neural canal of lumbar region
- M99.54 Intervertebral disc stenosis of neural canal of sacral region
- M99.55 Intervertebral disc stenosis of neural canal of pelvic region
- M99.56 Intervertebral disc stenosis of neural canal of lower extremity
- M99.57 Intervertebral disc stenosis of neural canal of upper extremity
- M99.58 Intervertebral disc stenosis of neural canal of rib cage
- M99.59 Intervertebral disc stenosis of neural canal of abdomen and other regions

**M99.6 Osseous and subluxation stenosis of intervertebral foramina**
- M99.60 Osseous and subluxation stenosis of intervertebral foramina of head region

M99.61 Osseous and subluxation stenosis of intervertebral foramina of cervical region
M99.62 Osseous and subluxation stenosis of intervertebral foramina of thoracic region
M99.63 Osseous and subluxation stenosis of intervertebral foramina of lumbar region
M99.64 Osseous and subluxation stenosis of intervertebral foramina of sacral region
M99.65 Osseous and subluxation stenosis of intervertebral foramina of pelvic region
M99.66 Osseous and subluxation stenosis of intervertebral foramina of lower extremity
M99.67 Osseous and subluxation stenosis of intervertebral foramina of upper extremity
M99.68 Osseous and subluxation stenosis of intervertebral foramina of rib cage
M99.69 Osseous and subluxation stenosis of intervertebral foramina of abdomen and other regions

✓5th **M99.7 Connective tissue and disc stenosis of intervertebral foramina**

M99.70 Connective tissue and disc stenosis of intervertebral foramina of head region
M99.71 Connective tissue and disc stenosis of intervertebral foramina of cervical region
M99.72 Connective tissue and disc stenosis of intervertebral foramina of thoracic region
M99.73 Connective tissue and disc stenosis of intervertebral foramina of lumbar region
M99.74 Connective tissue and disc stenosis of intervertebral foramina of sacral region
M99.75 Connective tissue and disc stenosis of intervertebral foramina of pelvic region
M99.76 Connective tissue and disc stenosis of intervertebral foramina of lower extremity
M99.77 Connective tissue and disc stenosis of intervertebral foramina of upper extremity
M99.78 Connective tissue and disc stenosis of intervertebral foramina of rib cage
M99.79 Connective tissue and disc stenosis of intervertebral foramina of abdomen and other regions

✓5th **M99.8 Other biomechanical lesions**

M99.80 Other biomechanical lesions of head region
M99.81 Other biomechanical lesions of cervical region
M99.82 Other biomechanical lesions of thoracic region
M99.83 Other biomechanical lesions of lumbar region
M99.84 Other biomechanical lesions of sacral region
M99.85 Other biomechanical lesions of pelvic region
M99.86 Other biomechanical lesions of lower extremity
M99.87 Other biomechanical lesions of upper extremity
M99.88 Other biomechanical lesions of rib cage
M99.89 Other biomechanical lesions of abdomen and other regions

**M99.9 Biomechanical lesion, unspecified**

# Chapter 14. Diseases of Genitourinary System (NØØ–N99)



## Chapter-specific Guidelines with Coding Examples

The chapter-specific guidelines from the ICD-10-CM Official Guidelines for Coding and Reporting have been provided below. Along with these guidelines are coding examples, contained in the shaded boxes, that have been developed to help illustrate the coding and/or sequencing guidance found in these guidelines.

**a. Chronic kidney disease**

**1) Stages of chronic kidney disease (CKD)**

The ICD-10-CM classifies CKD based on severity. The severity of CKD is designated by stages 1-5. Stage 2, code N18.2, equates to mild CKD; stage 3, codes N18.3Ø-N18.32, equate to moderate CKD; and stage 4, code N18.4, equates to severe CKD. Code N18.6, End stage renal disease (ESRD), is assigned when the provider has documented end-stage renal disease (ESRD).

If both a stage of CKD and ESRD are documented, assign code N18.6 only.

Stage 5 chronic kidney disease with ESRD requiring chronic dialysis

| | |
|---|---|
| **N18.6** | **End stage renal disease** |
| **Z99.2** | **Dependence on renal dialysis** |

*Explanation:* The diagnostic statement indicates the patient has chronic kidney disease, documented both as stage 5 and as ESRD requiring chronic dialysis. Code N18.6 End stage renal disease (ESRD), is assigned when the provider has documented end-stage-renal disease (ESRD). If both a stage of CKD and ESRD are documented, assign code N18.6 only.

**2) Chronic kidney disease and kidney transplant status**

Patients who have undergone kidney transplant may still have some form of chronic kidney disease (CKD) because the kidney transplant may not fully restore kidney function. Therefore, the presence of CKD alone does not constitute a transplant complication. Assign the appropriate N18 code for the patient's stage of CKD and code Z94.Ø, Kidney transplant status. If a transplant complication such as failure or rejection or other transplant complication is documented, see section I.C.19.g for information on coding complications of a kidney transplant. If the documentation is unclear as to whether the patient has a complication of the transplant, query the provider.

Patient with residual chronic kidney disease stage 1 after kidney transplant

| | |
|---|---|
| **N18.1** | **Chronic kidney disease, stage 1** |
| **Z94.Ø** | **Kidney transplant status** |

*Explanation:* Patients who have undergone kidney transplant may still have some form of chronic kidney disease (CKD) because the kidney transplant may not fully restore kidney function. The presence of CKD alone does not constitute a transplant complication. Assign the appropriate N18 code for the patient's stage of CKD and code Z94.Ø Kidney transplant status.

**3) Chronic kidney disease with other conditions**

Patients with CKD may also suffer from other serious conditions, most commonly diabetes mellitus and hypertension. The sequencing of the CKD code in relationship to codes for other contributing conditions is based on the conventions in the Tabular List.

*See I.C.9. Hypertensive chronic kidney disease.*

*See I.C.19. Chronic kidney disease and kidney transplant complications.*

Type 1 diabetic chronic kidney disease, stage 2

| | |
|---|---|
| **E1Ø.22** | **Type 1 diabetes mellitus with diabetic chronic kidney disease** |
| **N18.2** | **Chronic kidney disease, stage 2 (mild)** |

*Explanation:* Patients with CKD may also suffer from other serious conditions such as diabetes mellitus. The sequencing of the CKD code in relationship to codes for other contributing conditions is based on the conventions in the Tabular List. Diabetic CKD code E1Ø.22 includes an instructional note to "Use additional code to identify stage of chronic kidney disease (N18.1–N18.6)," thus providing sequencing direction.

# Chapter 14. Diseases of the Genitourinary System (NØØ-N99)

EXCLUDES 2 *certain conditions originating in the perinatal period (PØ4-P96)*
*certain infectious and parasitic diseases (AØØ-B99)*
*complications of pregnancy, childbirth and the puerperium (OØØ-O9A)*
*congenital malformations, deformations and chromosomal abnormalities (QØØ-Q99)*
*endocrine, nutritional and metabolic diseases (EØØ-E88)*
*injury, poisoning and certain other consequences of external causes (SØØ-T88)*
*neoplasms (CØØ-D49)*
*symptoms, signs and abnormal clinical and laboratory findings, not elsewhere classified (RØØ-R94)*

This chapter contains the following blocks:

NØØ-NØ8 Glomerular diseases
N1Ø-N16 Renal tubulo-interstitial diseases
N17-N19 Acute kidney failure and chronic kidney disease
N2Ø-N23 Urolithiasis
N25-N29 Other disorders of kidney and ureter
N3Ø-N39 Other diseases of the urinary system
N4Ø-N53 Diseases of male genital organs
N6Ø-N65 Disorders of breast
N7Ø-N77 Inflammatory diseases of female pelvic organs
N8Ø-N98 Noninflammatory disorders of female genital tract
N99 Intraoperative and postprocedural complications and disorders of genitourinary system, not elsewhere classified

## Glomerular diseases (NØØ-NØ8)

Code also any associated kidney failure (N17-N19)
EXCLUDES 1 *hypertensive chronic kidney disease (I12.-)*
**AHA:** 2020,4Q,34-35
**DEF:** Glomeruli: Clusters of microscopic blood vessels located within the kidneys containing small pores through which waste products are filtered from the blood and urine is formed.
**DEF:** Glomerulonephritis: Disease of the kidney with diffuse inflammation of the capillary loops of the glomeruli.

✓4th **NØØ Acute nephritic syndrome**
INCLUDES acute glomerular disease
acute glomerulonephritis
acute nephritis
EXCLUDES 1 *acute tubulo-interstitial nephritis (N1Ø)*
*nephritic syndrome NOS (NØ5.-)*
**AHA:** 2021,1Q,23

**NØØ.Ø Acute nephritic syndrome with minor glomerular abnormality**
Acute nephritic syndrome with minimal change lesion

**NØØ.1 Acute nephritic syndrome with focal and segmental glomerular lesions**
Acute nephritic syndrome with focal and segmental hyalinosis
Acute nephritic syndrome with focal and segmental sclerosis
Acute nephritic syndrome with focal glomerulonephritis

**NØØ.2 Acute nephritic syndrome with diffuse membranous glomerulonephritis**

**NØØ.3 Acute nephritic syndrome with diffuse mesangial proliferative glomerulonephritis**

**NØØ.4 Acute nephritic syndrome with diffuse endocapillary proliferative glomerulonephritis**

**NØØ.5 Acute nephritic syndrome with diffuse mesangiocapillary glomerulonephritis**
EXCLUDES 1 *acute nephritic syndrome with C3 glomerulonephritis (NØØ.A)*
*acute nephritic syndrome with C3 glomerulopathy (NØØ.A)*

**NØØ.6 Acute nephritic syndrome with dense deposit disease**
Acute nephritic syndrome with C3 glomerulopathy with dense deposit disease
Acute nephritic syndrome with membranoproliferative glomerulonephritis, type 2

**NØØ.7 Acute nephritic syndrome with diffuse crescentic glomerulonephritis**
Acute nephritic syndrome with extracapillary glomerulonephritis

**NØØ.8 Acute nephritic syndrome with other morphologic changes**
Acute nephritic syndrome with proliferative glomerulonephritis NOS

**NØØ.9 Acute nephritic syndrome with unspecified morphologic changes**

**NØØ.A Acute nephritic syndrome with C3 glomerulonephritis**
Acute nephritic syndrome with C3 glomerulopathy, NOS
EXCLUDES 1 *acute nephritic syndrome (with C3 glomerulopathy) with dense deposit disease (NØØ.6)*

✓5th **NØØ.B Acute nephritic syndrome with immune complex membranoproliferative glomerulonephritis**

**NØØ.B1 Acute nephritic syndrome with idiopathic immune membranoproliferative glomerulonephritis (IC-MPGN)**

**NØØ.B2 Acute nephritic syndrome with secondary immune complex membranoproliferative glomerulonephritis (IC-MPGN)**

✓4th **NØ1 Rapidly progressive nephritic syndrome**
INCLUDES rapidly progressive glomerular disease
rapidly progressive glomerulonephritis
rapidly progressive nephritis
EXCLUDES 1 *nephritic syndrome NOS (NØ5.-)*
**AHA:** 2021,1Q,23

**NØ1.Ø Rapidly progressive nephritic syndrome with minor glomerular abnormality**
Rapidly progressive nephritic syndrome with minimal change lesion

**NØ1.1 Rapidly progressive nephritic syndrome with focal and segmental glomerular lesions**
Rapidly progressive nephritic syndrome with focal and segmental hyalinosis
Rapidly progressive nephritic syndrome with focal and segmental sclerosis
Rapidly progressive nephritic syndrome with focal glomerulonephritis

**NØ1.2 Rapidly progressive nephritic syndrome with diffuse membranous glomerulonephritis**

**NØ1.3 Rapidly progressive nephritic syndrome with diffuse mesangial proliferative glomerulonephritis**

**NØ1.4 Rapidly progressive nephritic syndrome with diffuse endocapillary proliferative glomerulonephritis**

**NØ1.5 Rapidly progressive nephritic syndrome with diffuse mesangiocapillary glomerulonephritis**
Rapidly progressive nephritic syndrome with membranoproliferative glomerulonephritis, types 1 and 3, or NOS
EXCLUDES 1 *rapidly progressive nephritic syndrome with C3 glomerulonephritis (NØ1.A)*
*rapidly progressive nephritic syndrome with C3 glomerulopathy (NØ1.A)*

**NØ1.6 Rapidly progressive nephritic syndrome with dense deposit disease**
Rapidly progressive nephritic syndrome with C3 glomerulopathy with dense deposit disease
Rapidly progressive nephritic syndrome with membranoproliferative glomerulonephritis, type 2

**NØ1.7 Rapidly progressive nephritic syndrome with diffuse crescentic glomerulonephritis**
Rapidly progressive nephritic syndrome with extracapillary glomerulonephritis

**NØ1.8 Rapidly progressive nephritic syndrome with other morphologic changes**
Rapidly progressive nephritic syndrome with proliferative glomerulonephritis NOS

**NØ1.9 Rapidly progressive nephritic syndrome with unspecified morphologic changes**

**NØ1.A Rapidly progressive nephritic syndrome with C3 glomerulonephritis**
Rapidly progressive nephritic syndrome with C3 glomerulopathy, NOS
EXCLUDES 1 *rapidly progressive nephritic syndrome (with C3 glomerulopathy) with dense deposit disease (NØ1.6)*

✓4th **NØ2 Recurrent and persistent hematuria**
EXCLUDES 1 *acute cystitis with hematuria (N3Ø.Ø1)*
*hematuria NOS (R31.9)*
*hematuria not associated with specified morphologic lesions (R31.-)*

**NØ2.Ø Recurrent and persistent hematuria with minor glomerular abnormality**
Recurrent and persistent hematuria with minimal change lesion

**NØ2.1 Recurrent and persistent hematuria with focal and segmental glomerular lesions**
Recurrent and persistent hematuria with focal and segmental hyalinosis
Recurrent and persistent hematuria with focal and segmental sclerosis
Recurrent and persistent hematuria with focal glomerulonephritis

**NØ2.2 Recurrent and persistent hematuria with diffuse membranous glomerulonephritis**

**NØ2.3 Recurrent and persistent hematuria with diffuse mesangial proliferative glomerulonephritis**

**NØ2.4 Recurrent and persistent hematuria with diffuse endocapillary proliferative glomerulonephritis**

**NØ2.5 Recurrent and persistent hematuria with diffuse mesangiocapillary glomerulonephritis**
Recurrent and persistent hematuria with membranoproliferative glomerulonephritis, types 1 and 3, or NOS
EXCLUDES 1 *recurrent and persistent hematuria with C3 glomerulonephritis (NØ2.A)*
*recurrent and persistent hematuria with C3 glomerulopathy (NØ2.A)*

**NØ2.6 Recurrent and persistent hematuria with dense deposit disease**
Recurrent and persistent hematuria with C3 glomerulopathy with dense deposit disease
Recurrent and persistent hematuria with membranoproliferative glomerulonephritis, type 2

**NØ2.7 Recurrent and persistent hematuria with diffuse crescentic glomerulonephritis**
Recurrent and persistent hematuria with extracapillary glomerulonephritis

**NØ2.8 Recurrent and persistent hematuria with other morphologic changes**
Recurrent and persistent hematuria with proliferative glomerulonephritis NOS

**NØ2.9 Recurrent and persistent hematuria with unspecified morphologic changes**
AHA: 2017,2Q,5

**NØ2.A Recurrent and persistent hematuria with C3 glomerulonephritis**
Recurrent and persistent hematuria with C3 glomerulopathy
EXCLUDES 1 *recurrent and persistent hematuria (with C3 glomerulopathy) with dense deposit disease (NØ2.6)*

√5th **NØ2.B Recurrent and persistent immunoglobulin A nephropathy**
AHA: 2023,4Q,34-35

**NØ2.B1 Recurrent and persistent immunoglobulin A nephropathy with glomerular lesion**

**NØ2.B2 Recurrent and persistent immunoglobulin A nephropathy with focal and segmental glomerular lesion**
Recurrent and persistent immunoglobulin A nephropathy with focal and segmental hyalinosis or sclerosis

**NØ2.B3 Recurrent and persistent immunoglobulin A nephropathy with diffuse membranoproliferative glomerulonephritis**

**NØ2.B4 Recurrent and persistent immunoglobulin A nephropathy with diffuse membranous glomerulonephritis**

**NØ2.B5 Recurrent and persistent immunoglobulin A nephropathy with diffuse mesangial proliferative glomerulonephritis**

**NØ2.B6 Recurrent and persistent immunoglobulin A nephropathy with diffuse mesangiocapillary glomerulonephritis**

**NØ2.B9 Other recurrent and persistent immunoglobulin A nephropathy**

√4th **NØ3 Chronic nephritic syndrome**
INCLUDES chronic glomerular disease
chronic glomerulonephritis
chronic nephritis
EXCLUDES 1 *chronic tubulo-interstitial nephritis (N11.-)*
*diffuse sclerosing glomerulonephritis (NØ5.8-)*
*nephritic syndrome NOS (NØ5.-)*
AHA: 2021,1Q,23
DEF: Slow, progressive type of nephritis characterized by inflammation of the capillary loops in the glomeruli of the kidney, which leads to renal failure.

**NØ3.Ø Chronic nephritic syndrome with minor glomerular abnormality**
Chronic nephritic syndrome with minimal change lesion

**NØ3.1 Chronic nephritic syndrome with focal and segmental glomerular lesions**
Chronic nephritic syndrome with focal and segmental hyalinosis
Chronic nephritic syndrome with focal and segmental sclerosis
Chronic nephritic syndrome with focal glomerulonephritis

**NØ3.2 Chronic nephritic syndrome with diffuse membranous glomerulonephritis**

**NØ3.3 Chronic nephritic syndrome with diffuse mesangial proliferative glomerulonephritis**

**NØ3.4 Chronic nephritic syndrome with diffuse endocapillary proliferative glomerulonephritis**

**NØ3.5 Chronic nephritic syndrome with diffuse mesangiocapillary glomerulonephritis**
Chronic nephritic syndrome with membranoproliferative glomerulonephritis, types 1 and 3, or NOS
EXCLUDES 1 *chronic nephritic syndrome with C3 glomerulonephritis (NØ3.A)*
*chronic nephritic syndrome with C3 glomerulopathy (NØ3.A)*

**NØ3.6 Chronic nephritic syndrome with dense deposit disease**
Chronic nephritic syndrome with C3 glomerulopathy with dense deposit disease
Chronic nephritic syndrome with membranoproliferative glomerulonephritis, type 2

**NØ3.7 Chronic nephritic syndrome with diffuse crescentic glomerulonephritis**
Chronic nephritic syndrome with extracapillary glomerulonephritis

**NØ3.8 Chronic nephritic syndrome with other morphologic changes**
Chronic nephritic syndrome with proliferative glomerulonephritis NOS

**NØ3.9 Chronic nephritic syndrome with unspecified morphologic changes**

**NØ3.A Chronic nephritic syndrome with C3 glomerulonephritis**
Chronic nephritic syndrome with C3 glomerulopathy
EXCLUDES 1 *chronic nephritic syndrome (with C3 glomerulopathy) with dense deposit disease (NØ3.6)*

√4th **NØ4 Nephrotic syndrome**
INCLUDES congenital nephrotic syndrome
lipoid nephrosis

**NØ4.Ø Nephrotic syndrome with minor glomerular abnormality**
Nephrotic syndrome with minimal change lesion
AHA: 2024,3Q,14-15

**NØ4.1 Nephrotic syndrome with focal and segmental glomerular lesions**
Nephrotic syndrome with focal and segmental hyalinosis
Nephrotic syndrome with focal and segmental sclerosis
Nephrotic syndrome with focal glomerulonephritis

√5th **NØ4.2 Nephrotic syndrome with diffuse membranous glomerulonephritis**
AHA: 2023,4Q,35-36

**NØ4.2Ø Nephrotic syndrome with diffuse membranous glomerulonephritis, unspecified**
Membranous nephropathy NOS with nephrotic syndrome

**NØ4.21 Primary membranous nephropathy with nephrotic syndrome**
Idiopathic membranous nephropathy with nephrotic syndrome

**NØ4.22 Secondary membranous nephropathy with nephrotic syndrome**
Code first, if applicable, other disease or disorder or poisoning causing membranous nephropathy
Use additional code, if applicable, for adverse effect of drug causing membranous nephropathy

**NØ4.29 Other nephrotic syndrome with diffuse membranous glomerulonephritis**

**NØ4.3 Nephrotic syndrome with diffuse mesangial proliferative glomerulonephritis**

**NØ4.4 Nephrotic syndrome with diffuse endocapillary proliferative glomerulonephritis**

**NØ4.5 Nephrotic syndrome with diffuse mesangiocapillary glomerulonephritis**
EXCLUDES 1 *nephrotic syndrome with C3 glomerulonephritis (NØ4.A)*
*nephrotic syndrome with C3 glomerulopathy (NØ4.A)*

**NØ4.6 Nephrotic syndrome with dense deposit disease**
Nephrotic syndrome with C3 glomerulopathy with dense deposit disease
Nephrotic syndrome with membranoproliferative glomerulonephritis, type 2

**NØ4.7 Nephrotic syndrome with diffuse crescentic glomerulonephritis**
Nephrotic syndrome with extracapillary glomerulonephritis

**NØ4.8 Nephrotic syndrome with other morphologic changes**
Nephrotic syndrome with proliferative glomerulonephritis NOS

**NØ4.9 Nephrotic syndrome with unspecified morphologic changes**

**NØ4.A Nephrotic syndrome with C3 glomerulonephritis**
Nephrotic syndrome with C3 glomerulopathy
EXCLUDES 1 *nephrotic syndrome (with C3 glomerulopathy) with dense deposit disease (NØ4.6)*

√5th **NØ4.B Nephrotic syndrome with immune complex membranoproliferative glomerulonephritis (IC-MPGN)**

**NØ4.B1 Nephrotic syndrome with idiopathic immune complex membranoproliferative glomerulonephritis (IC-MPGN)**

**NØ4.B2 Nephrotic syndrome with secondary immune complex membranoproliferative glomerulonephritis (IC-MPGN)**

√4th **NØ5 Unspecified nephritic syndrome**

INCLUDES glomerular disease NOS
glomerulonephritis NOS
nephritis NOS
nephropathy NOS and renal disease NOS with morphological lesion specified in .Ø-.8

EXCLUDES 1 *nephropathy NOS with no stated morphological lesion (N28.9)*
*renal disease NOS with no stated morphological lesion (N28.9)*
*tubulo-interstitial nephritis NOS (N12)*

**NØ5.Ø Unspecified nephritic syndrome with minor glomerular abnormality**
Unspecified nephritic syndrome with minimal change lesion

**NØ5.1 Unspecified nephritic syndrome with focal and segmental glomerular lesions**
Unspecified nephritic syndrome with focal and segmental hyalinosis
Unspecified nephritic syndrome with focal and segmental sclerosis
Unspecified nephritic syndrome with focal glomerulonephritis

**NØ5.2 Unspecified nephritic syndrome with diffuse membranous glomerulonephritis**

**NØ5.3 Unspecified nephritic syndrome with diffuse mesangial proliferative glomerulonephritis**

**NØ5.4 Unspecified nephritic syndrome with diffuse endocapillary proliferative glomerulonephritis**

**NØ5.5 Unspecified nephritic syndrome with diffuse mesangiocapillary glomerulonephritis**
Unspecified nephritic syndrome with membranoproliferative glomerulonephritis, types 1 and 3, or NOS
EXCLUDES 1 *unspecified nephritic syndrome with C3 glomerulonephritis (NØ5.A)*
*unspecified nephritic syndrome with C3 glomerulopathy (NØ5.A)*

**NØ5.6 Unspecified nephritic syndrome with dense deposit disease**
Unspecified nephritic syndrome with C3 glomerulopathy with dense deposit disease
Unspecified nephritic syndrome with membranoproliferative glomerulonephritis, type 2

**NØ5.7 Unspecified nephritic syndrome with diffuse crescentic glomerulonephritis**
Unspecified nephritic syndrome with extracapillary glomerulonephritis

**NØ5.8 Unspecified nephritic syndrome with other morphologic changes**
Unspecified nephritic syndrome with proliferative glomerulonephritis NOS

**NØ5.9 Unspecified nephritic syndrome with unspecified morphologic changes**

**NØ5.A Unspecified nephritic syndrome with C3 glomerulonephritis**
Unspecified nephritic syndrome with C3 glomerulopathy
EXCLUDES 1 *unspecified nephritic syndrome (with C3 glomerulopathy) with dense deposit disease (NØ5.6)*

√4th **NØ6 Isolated proteinuria with specified morphological lesion**

EXCLUDES 1 *proteinuria not associated with specific morphologic lesions (R8Ø.Ø)*

**NØ6.Ø Isolated proteinuria with minor glomerular abnormality**
Isolated proteinuria with minimal change lesion

**NØ6.1 Isolated proteinuria with focal and segmental glomerular lesions**
Isolated proteinuria with focal and segmental hyalinosis
Isolated proteinuria with focal and segmental sclerosis
Isolated proteinuria with focal glomerulonephritis

√5th **NØ6.2 Isolated proteinuria with diffuse membranous glomerulonephritis**
**AHA:** 2023,4Q,35-36

**NØ6.2Ø Isolated proteinuria with diffuse membranous glomerulonephritis, unspecified**
Membranous nephropathy, NOS
EXCLUDES 1 *membranous nephropathy NOS with nephrotic syndrome (NØ4.2Ø)*

**NØ6.21 Primary membranous nephropathy with isolated proteinuria**
Idiopathic membranous nephropathy (with isolated proteinuria)
Primary membranous nephropathy, NOS
EXCLUDES 1 *primary membranous nephropathy with nephrotic syndrome (NØ4.21)*

**NØ6.22 Secondary membranous nephropathy with isolated proteinuria**
Secondary membranous nephropathy, NOS
Code first, if applicable, other disease or disorder or poisoning causing membranous nephropathy
Use additional code, if applicable, for adverse effect of drug causing membranous nephropathy
EXCLUDES 1 *secondary membranous nephropathy with nephrotic syndrome (NØ4.22)*

**NØ6.29 Other isolated proteinuria with diffuse membranous glomerulonephritis**

**NØ6.3 Isolated proteinuria with diffuse mesangial proliferative glomerulonephritis**

**NØ6.4 Isolated proteinuria with diffuse endocapillary proliferative glomerulonephritis**

**NØ6.5 Isolated proteinuria with diffuse mesangiocapillary glomerulonephritis**
Isolated proteinuria with membranoproliferative glomerulonephritis, types 1 and 3, or NOS
EXCLUDES 1 *isolated proteinuria with C3 glomerulonephritis (NØ6.A)*
*isolated proteinuria with C3 glomerulopathy (NØ6.A)*

**NØ6.6 Isolated proteinuria with dense deposit disease**
Isolated proteinuria with C3 glomerulopathy with dense deposit disease
Isolated proteinuria with membranoproliferative glomerulonephritis, type 2

**NØ6.7 Isolated proteinuria with diffuse crescentic glomerulonephritis**
Isolated proteinuria with extracapillary glomerulonephritis

**NØ6.8 Isolated proteinuria with other morphologic lesion**
Isolated proteinuria with proliferative glomerulonephritis NOS

**NØ6.9 Isolated proteinuria with unspecified morphologic lesion**

**NØ6.A Isolated proteinuria with C3 glomerulonephritis**
Isolated proteinuria with C3 glomerulopathy
EXCLUDES 1 *isolated proteinuria (with C3 glomerulopathy) with dense deposit disease (NØ6.6)*

√4th **NØ7 Hereditary nephropathy, not elsewhere classified**

EXCLUDES 2 *Alport's syndrome (Q87.81-)*
*hereditary amyloid nephropathy (E85.-)*
*nail patella syndrome (Q87.2)*
*non-neuropathic heredofamilial amyloidosis (E85.-)*

**NØ7.Ø Hereditary nephropathy, not elsewhere classified with minor glomerular abnormality**
Hereditary nephropathy, not elsewhere classified with minimal change lesion

**NØ7.1 Hereditary nephropathy, not elsewhere classified with focal and segmental glomerular lesions**
Hereditary nephropathy, not elsewhere classified with focal and segmental hyalinosis
Hereditary nephropathy, not elsewhere classified with focal and segmental sclerosis
Hereditary nephropathy, not elsewhere classified with focal glomerulonephritis

**NØ7.2 Hereditary nephropathy, not elsewhere classified with diffuse membranous glomerulonephritis**

**NØ7.3 Hereditary nephropathy, not elsewhere classified with diffuse mesangial proliferative glomerulonephritis**

**NØ7.4 Hereditary nephropathy, not elsewhere classified with diffuse endocapillary proliferative glomerulonephritis**

**NØ7.5 Hereditary nephropathy, not elsewhere classified with diffuse mesangiocapillary glomerulonephritis**
Hereditary nephropathy, not elsewhere classified with membranoproliferative glomerulonephritis, types 1 and 3, or NOS
EXCLUDES 1 *hereditary nephropathy, not elsewhere classified with C3 glomerulonephritis (NØ7.A)*
*hereditary nephropathy, not elsewhere classified with C3 glomerulopathy (NØ7.A)*

**NØ7.6 Hereditary nephropathy, not elsewhere classified with dense deposit disease**
Hereditary nephropathy, not elsewhere classified with C3 glomerulopathy with dense deposit disease
Hereditary nephropathy, not elsewhere classified with membranoproliferative glomerulonephritis, type 2

**N07.7 Hereditary nephropathy, not elsewhere classified with diffuse crescentic glomerulonephritis**
Hereditary nephropathy, not elsewhere classified with extracapillary glomerulonephritis

**N07.8 Hereditary nephropathy, not elsewhere classified with other morphologic lesions**
Hereditary nephropathy, not elsewhere classified with proliferative glomerulonephritis NOS

**N07.9 Hereditary nephropathy, not elsewhere classified with unspecified morphologic lesions**

**N07.A Hereditary nephropathy, not elsewhere classified with C3 glomerulonephritis**
Hereditary nephropathy, not elsewhere classified with C3 glomerulopathy
EXCLUDES 1 *hereditary nephropathy, not elsewhere classified (with C3 glomerulopathy) with dense deposit disease (N07.6)*

**N07.B Hereditary nephropathy, not elsewhere classified with APOL1-mediated kidney disease [AMKD]**
AMKD (with glomerulonephritis)
AMKD (with glomerulosclerosis)

***N08 Glomerular disorders in diseases classified elsewhere***
Glomerulonephritis
Nephritis
Nephropathy
Code first underlying disease, such as:
amyloidosis (E85.-)
congenital syphilis (A50.5)
cryoglobulinemia (D89.1)
disseminated intravascular coagulation (D65)
gout (M1A.-, M10.-)
microscopic polyangiitis (M31.7)
multiple myeloma (C90.0-)
sepsis (A40.0-A41.9)
sickle-cell disease (D57.0-D57.8)
EXCLUDES 1 *glomerulonephritis, nephritis and nephropathy (in):*
*pyelonephritis in diseases classified elsewhere (N16)*
*renal tubulo-interstitial disorders classified elsewhere (N16)*
*antiglomerular basement membrane disease (M31.0)*
*diabetes (E08-E13 with .21)*
*gonococcal (A54.21)*
*Goodpasture's syndrome (M31.0)*
*hemolytic-uremic syndrome (D59.3-)*
*lupus (M32.14)*
*mumps (B26.83)*
*syphilis (A52.75)*
*systemic lupus erythematosus (M32.14)*
*Wegener's granulomatosis (M31.31)*

## Renal tubulo-interstitial diseases (N10-N16)

INCLUDES pyelonephritis
EXCLUDES 1 *pyeloureteritis cystica (N28.85)*

**N10 Acute pyelonephritis**
Acute infectious interstitial nephritis
Acute pyelitis
Acute tubulo-interstitial nephritis
Hemoglobin nephrosis
Myoglobin nephrosis
Use additional code (B95-B97), to identify infectious agent
**AHA:** 2020,3Q,25; 2019,3Q,13

✓4th **N11 Chronic tubulo-interstitial nephritis**
INCLUDES chronic infectious interstitial nephritis
chronic pyelitis
chronic pyelonephritis
Use additional code (B95-B97), to identify infectious agent

**N11.0 Nonobstructive reflux-associated chronic pyelonephritis**
Pyelonephritis (chronic) associated with (vesicoureteral) reflux
EXCLUDES 1 *vesicoureteral reflux NOS (N13.70)*

**N11.1 Chronic obstructive pyelonephritis**
Pyelonephritis (chronic) associated with anomaly of pelviureteric junction
Pyelonephritis (chronic) associated with anomaly of pyeloureteric junction
Pyelonephritis (chronic) associated with crossing of vessel
Pyelonephritis (chronic) associated with kinking of ureter
Pyelonephritis (chronic) associated with obstruction of ureter
Pyelonephritis (chronic) associated with stricture of pelviureteric junction
Pyelonephritis (chronic) associated with stricture of ureter
EXCLUDES 1 *calculous pyelonephritis (N20.9)*
*obstructive uropathy (N13.-)*

**N11.8 Other chronic tubulo-interstitial nephritis**
Nonobstructive chronic pyelonephritis NOS

**N11.9 Chronic tubulo-interstitial nephritis, unspecified**
Chronic interstitial nephritis NOS
Chronic pyelitis NOS
Chronic pyelonephritis NOS

**N12 Tubulo-interstitial nephritis, not specified as acute or chronic**
Interstitial nephritis NOS
Pyelitis NOS
Pyelonephritis NOS
EXCLUDES 1 *calculous pyelonephritis (N20.9)*

✓4th **N13 Obstructive and reflux uropathy**
EXCLUDES 2 *calculus of kidney and ureter without hydronephrosis (N20.-)*
*congenital obstructive defects of renal pelvis and ureter (Q62.0-Q62.3)*
*hydronephrosis with ureteropelvic junction obstruction (Q62.11)*
*obstructive pyelonephritis (N11.1)*
**DEF:** Hydronephrosis: Distension of the kidney caused by an accumulation of urine that cannot flow out due to an obstruction that may be caused by conditions such as kidney stones or vesicoureteral reflux.

**N13.0 Hydronephrosis with ureteropelvic junction obstruction**
Hydronephrosis due to acquired occlusion of ureteropelvic junction
EXCLUDES 2 *hydronephrosis with ureteropelvic junction obstruction due to calculus (N13.2)*
**AHA:** 2016,4Q,43

**Hydronephrosis/UPJ Obstruction**

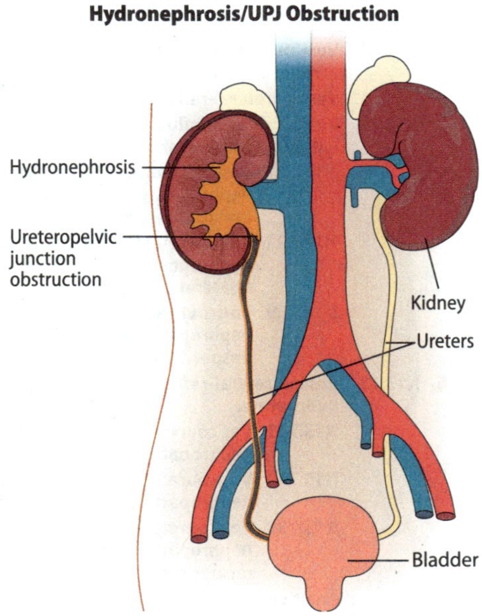


**N13.1 Hydronephrosis with ureteral stricture, not elsewhere classified**
EXCLUDES 1 *hydronephrosis with ureteral stricture with infection (N13.6)*

**N13.2 Hydronephrosis with renal and ureteral calculous obstruction**
EXCLUDES 1 *hydronephrosis with renal and ureteral calculous obstruction with infection (N13.6)*

✓5th **N13.3 Other and unspecified hydronephrosis**
EXCLUDES 1 *hydronephrosis with infection (N13.6)*

**N13.30 Unspecified hydronephrosis**
**N13.39 Other hydronephrosis**

**N13.4 Hydroureter**
EXCLUDES 1 *congenital hydroureter (Q62.3-)*
*hydroureter with infection (N13.6)*
*vesicoureteral-reflux with hydroureter (N13.73-)*
**DEF:** Abnormal enlargement or distension of the ureter with water or urine caused by an obstruction.

**N13.5 Crossing vessel and stricture of ureter without hydronephrosis**
Kinking and stricture of ureter without hydronephrosis
EXCLUDES 1 *crossing vessel and stricture of ureter without hydronephrosis with infection (N13.6)*

**N13.6 Pyonephrosis**
Conditions in N13.Ø-N13.5 with infection
Obstructive uropathy with infection
Use additional code (B95-B97), to identify infectious agent
**AHA:** 2018,2Q,21

✓5th **N13.7 Vesicoureteral-reflux**
EXCLUDES 1 *reflux-associated pyelonephritis (N11.Ø)*
**DEF:** Urine passage from the bladder flows backward up into the ureter and kidneys that can lead to bacterial infection and an increase in hydrostatic pressure, causing kidney damage.

**Vesicoureteral Reflux**

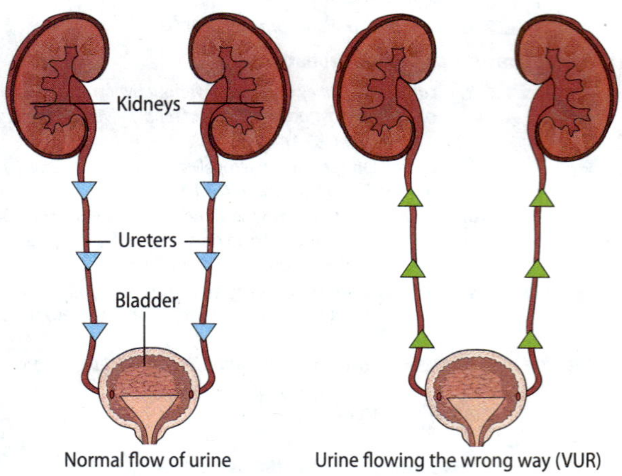


**N13.7Ø Vesicoureteral-reflux, unspecified**
Vesicoureteral-reflux NOS

**N13.71 Vesicoureteral-reflux without reflux nephropathy**

✓6th **N13.72 Vesicoureteral-reflux with reflux nephropathy without hydroureter**

**N13.721 Vesicoureteral-reflux with reflux nephropathy without hydroureter, unilateral**

**N13.722 Vesicoureteral-reflux with reflux nephropathy without hydroureter, bilateral**

**N13.729 Vesicoureteral-reflux with reflux nephropathy without hydroureter, unspecified**

✓6th **N13.73 Vesicoureteral-reflux with reflux nephropathy with hydroureter**

**N13.731 Vesicoureteral-reflux with reflux nephropathy with hydroureter, unilateral**

**N13.732 Vesicoureteral-reflux with reflux nephropathy with hydroureter, bilateral**

**N13.739 Vesicoureteral-reflux with reflux nephropathy with hydroureter, unspecified**

**N13.8 Other obstructive and reflux uropathy**
Urinary tract obstruction due to specified cause
Code first, if applicable, any causal condition, such as:
enlarged prostate (N4Ø.1)

**N13.9 Obstructive and reflux uropathy, unspecified**
Urinary tract obstruction NOS

✓4th **N14 Drug- and heavy-metal-induced tubulo-interstitial and tubular conditions**
Code first poisoning due to drug or toxin, if applicable (T36-T65 with fifth or sixth character 1-4)
Use additional code for adverse effect, if applicable, to identify drug (T36-T5Ø with fifth or sixth character 5)

**N14.Ø Analgesic nephropathy**

✓5th **N14.1 Nephropathy induced by other drugs, medicaments and biological substances**
**AHA:** 2022,4Q,33; 2021,3Q,9-10

**N14.11 Contrast-induced nephropathy**
Contrast medium, radiography nephropathy
EXCLUDES 2 *acute kidney failure (N17.-)*

**N14.19 Nephropathy induced by other drugs, medicaments and biological substances**

**N14.2 Nephropathy induced by unspecified drug, medicament or biological substance**

**N14.3 Nephropathy induced by heavy metals**

**N14.4 Toxic nephropathy, not elsewhere classified**

✓4th **N15 Other renal tubulo-interstitial diseases**

**N15.Ø Balkan nephropathy**
Balkan endemic nephropathy

**N15.1 Renal and perinephric abscess**

**N15.8 Other specified renal tubulo-interstitial diseases**

**N15.9 Renal tubulo-interstitial disease, unspecified**
Infection of kidney NOS
EXCLUDES 1 *urinary tract infection NOS (N39.Ø)*

***N16 Renal tubulo-interstitial disorders in diseases classified elsewhere***
Pyelonephritis
Tubulo-interstitial nephritis
Code first underlying disease, such as:
brucellosis (A23.Ø-A23.9)
cryoglobulinemia (D89.1)
glycogen storage disease (E74.Ø-)
leukemia (C91-C95)
lymphoma (C81.Ø-C85.9, C96.Ø-C96.9)
multiple myeloma (C9Ø.Ø-)
sepsis (A4Ø.Ø-A41.9)
Wilson's disease (E83.Ø1)
EXCLUDES 1 *diphtheritic pyelonephritis and tubulo-interstitial nephritis (A36.84)*
*pyelonephritis and tubulo-interstitial nephritis in candidiasis (B37.49)*
*pyelonephritis and tubulo-interstitial nephritis in cystinosis (E72.Ø4)*
*pyelonephritis and tubulo-interstitial nephritis in salmonella infection (AØ2.25)*
*pyelonephritis and tubulo-interstitial nephritis in sarcoidosis (D86.84)*
*pyelonephritis and tubulo-interstitial nephritis in Sjogren syndrome (M35.Ø4)*
*pyelonephritis and tubulo-interstitial nephritis in systemic lupus erythematosus (M32.15)*
*pyelonephritis and tubulo-interstitial nephritis in toxoplasmosis (B58.83)*
*renal tubular degeneration in diabetes (EØ8-E13 with .29)*
*syphilitic pyelonephritis and tubulo-interstitial nephritis (A52.75)*

## Acute kidney failure and chronic kidney disease (N17-N19)

EXCLUDES 2 *congenital renal failure (P96.Ø)*
*drug- and heavy-metal-induced tubulo-interstitial and tubular conditions (N14.-)*
*extrarenal uremia (R39.2)*
*hemolytic-uremic syndrome (D59.3-)*
*hepatorenal syndrome (K76.7)*
*postpartum hepatorenal syndrome (O9Ø.41)*
*posttraumatic renal failure (T79.5)*
*prerenal uremia (R39.2)*
*renal failure complicating abortion or ectopic or molar pregnancy (OØØ-OØ7, OØ8.4)*
*renal failure following labor and delivery (O9Ø.41)*
*renal failure postprocedural (N99.Ø)*

✓4th **N17 Acute kidney failure**
Code also associated underlying condition
EXCLUDES 1 *posttraumatic renal failure (T79.5)*
**AHA:** 2020,3Q,22; 2019,2Q,7; 2019,1Q,12; 2013,4Q,124

**N17.Ø Acute kidney failure with tubular necrosis** ESR
Acute tubular necrosis
Renal tubular necrosis
Tubular necrosis NOS
**AHA:** 2026,2Q,5; 2025,3Q,22; 2024,3Q,15; 2022,4Q,33; 2021,3Q,10

**N17.1 Acute kidney failure with acute cortical necrosis** ESR
Acute cortical necrosis
Cortical necrosis NOS
Renal cortical necrosis

**N17.2 Acute kidney failure with medullary necrosis** ESR
Acute medullary [papillary] necrosis
Medullary [papillary] necrosis NOS
Renal medullary [papillary] necrosis

**N17.8 Other acute kidney failure** ESR
**AHA:** 2026,1Q,30-31; 2025,1Q,26

**N17.9 Acute kidney failure, unspecified** ESR
Acute kidney injury (nontraumatic)
EXCLUDES 2 *traumatic kidney injury (S37.Ø-)*

**✓4th N18 Chronic kidney disease (CKD)**
Code first any associated:
diabetic chronic kidney disease (EØ8.22, EØ9.22, E1Ø.22, E11.22, E13.22)
hypertensive chronic kidney disease (I12.-, I13.-)
Use additional code, if applicable, to identify:
associated cachexia (E88.A)
kidney transplant status (Z94.Ø)
**AHA:** 2026,2Q,9; 2025,4Q,7; 2025,2Q,8; 2023,1Q,17; 2022,4Q,14; 2019,3Q,3; 2018,4Q,88; 2013,1Q,24
**TIP:** CKD/ESRD occurring in an individual with a history of kidney transplant should not be assumed to be a transplant complication unless specifically indicated as such by provider documentation.

**N18.1 Chronic kidney disease, stage 1**
**N18.2 Chronic kidney disease, stage 2 (mild)**
**✓5th N18.3 Chronic kidney disease, stage 3 (moderate)**
**AHA:** 2020,4Q,35
**N18.30 Chronic kidney disease, stage 3 unspecified** HCC ESR
**N18.31 Chronic kidney disease, stage 3a** HCC ESR
**N18.32 Chronic kidney disease, stage 3b** HCC ESR
**N18.4 Chronic kidney disease, stage 4 (severe)** HCC Rx ESR COM
**N18.5 Chronic kidney disease, stage 5** HCC Rx ESR COM
EXCLUDES 1 *chronic kidney disease, stage 5 requiring chronic dialysis (N18.6)*
**DEF:** End-stage renal disease (ESRD) with a GFR value of 15 ml/min or less not yet requiring chronic dialysis.
**TIP:** When both ESRD and CKD 5 are documented, code only for ESRD.

**N18.6 End stage renal disease** HCC Rx ESR COM
Chronic kidney disease requiring chronic dialysis
Use additional code to identify dialysis status (Z99.2)
**AHA:** 2023,1Q,19; 2022,3Q,15; 2016,3Q,22; 2016,1Q,12; 2013,4Q,124-125
**TIP:** When both ESRD and CKD 5 are documented, code only for ESRD.

**N18.9 Chronic kidney disease, unspecified**
Chronic renal disease
Chronic renal failure NOS
Chronic renal insufficiency
Chronic uremia NOS
Diffuse sclerosing glomerulonephritis NOS

**N19 Unspecified kidney failure**
Uremia NOS
EXCLUDES 1 *acute kidney failure (N17.-)*
*chronic kidney disease (N18.-)*
*chronic uremia (N18.9)*
*extrarenal uremia (R39.2)*
*prerenal uremia (R39.2)*
*renal insufficiency (acute) (N28.9)*
*uremia of newborn (P96.Ø)*

## Urolithiasis (N2Ø-N23)

**AHA:** 2017,1Q,5; 2015,2Q,8
**TIP:** Codes from this code block can be assigned based on the diagnosis listed in a radiology report when authenticated by a radiologist and available at the time of code assignment.

**✓4th N2Ø Calculus of kidney and ureter**
Calculous pyelonephritis
EXCLUDES 1 *nephrocalcinosis (E83.59)*
*that with hydronephrosis (N13.2)*
**AHA:** 2019,3Q,13

**N2Ø.Ø Calculus of kidney**
Nephrolithiasis NOS
Renal calculus
Renal stone
Staghorn calculus
Stone in kidney
**AHA:** 2019,3Q,13

**N2Ø.1 Calculus of ureter**
Calculus of the ureteropelvic junction
Ureteric stone
**AHA:** 2016,3Q,22

**N2Ø.2 Calculus of kidney with calculus of ureter**
**N2Ø.9 Urinary calculus, unspecified**

**✓4th N21 Calculus of lower urinary tract**
INCLUDES calculus of lower urinary tract with cystitis and urethritis

**N21.Ø Calculus in bladder**
Calculus in diverticulum of bladder
Urinary bladder stone
EXCLUDES 2 *staghorn calculus (N2Ø.Ø)*

**N21.1 Calculus in urethra**
EXCLUDES 2 *calculus of prostate (N42.Ø)*

**N21.8 Other lower urinary tract calculus**
**N21.9 Calculus of lower urinary tract, unspecified**
EXCLUDES 1 *calculus of urinary tract NOS (N2Ø.9)*

***N22 Calculus of urinary tract in diseases classified elsewhere***
Code first underlying disease, such as:
gout (M1A.-, M1Ø.-)
schistosomiasis (B65.Ø-B65.9)

**N23 Unspecified renal colic**

## Other disorders of kidney and ureter (N25-N29)

EXCLUDES 2 *disorders of kidney and ureter with urolithiasis (N2Ø-N23)*

**✓4th N25 Disorders resulting from impaired renal tubular function**

**N25.Ø Renal osteodystrophy** Rx
Azotemic osteodystrophy
Phosphate-losing tubular disorders
Renal rickets
Renal short stature
EXCLUDES 2 *metabolic disorders classifiable to E7Ø-E88*
**DEF:** Various bone diseases occurring when kidney function is impaired or fails. Abnormal levels of phosphorous and calcium can lead to osteomalacia, osteoporosis, or osteosclerosis.

**N25.1 Nephrogenic diabetes insipidus** Rx ESR COM
EXCLUDES 1 *diabetes insipidus NOS (E23.2)*
**DEF:** Type of diabetes due to the inability of renal tubules to reabsorb water back into the body. It is not responsive to vasopressin (antidiuretic hormone) and it is characterized by excessive thirst and excessive urine production. It may develop into chronic renal insufficiency.

**✓5th N25.8 Other disorders resulting from impaired renal tubular function**
**N25.81 Secondary hyperparathyroidism of renal origin** Rx ESR COM
EXCLUDES 1 *secondary hyperparathyroidism, non-renal (E21.1)*
EXCLUDES 2 *metabolic disorders classifiable to E7Ø-E88*
**DEF:** Parathyroid dysfunction caused by chronic renal failure. Phosphate clearance and vitamin D production is impaired resulting in lowered calcium blood levels and an excessive production of parathyroid hormone.
**N25.89 Other disorders resulting from impaired renal tubular function**
Hypokalemic nephropathy
Lightwood-Albright syndrome
Renal tubular acidosis NOS

**N25.9 Disorder resulting from impaired renal tubular function, unspecified**

**✓4th N26 Unspecified contracted kidney**
EXCLUDES 1 *contracted kidney due to hypertension (I12.-)*
*diffuse sclerosing glomerulonephritis (NØ5.8.-)*
*hypertensive nephrosclerosis (arteriolar) (arteriosclerotic) (I12.-)*
*small kidney of unknown cause (N27.-)*

**N26.1 Atrophy of kidney (terminal)**
**N26.2 Page kidney** Rx
**N26.9 Renal sclerosis, unspecified**

**✓4th N27 Small kidney of unknown cause**
INCLUDES oligonephronia
**N27.Ø Small kidney, unilateral**
**N27.1 Small kidney, bilateral**
**N27.9 Small kidney, unspecified**

√4th **N28 Other disorders of kidney and ureter, not elsewhere classified**

**N28.Ø Ischemia and infarction of kidney** ESR COM

Renal artery embolism
Renal artery obstruction
Renal artery occlusion
Renal artery thrombosis
Renal infarct

EXCLUDES 1 *atherosclerosis of renal artery (extrarenal part) (I7Ø.1)*
*congenital stenosis of renal artery (Q27.1)*
*Goldblatt's kidney (I7Ø.1)*

**N28.1 Cyst of kidney, acquired**

Cyst (multiple) (solitary) of kidney (acquired)

EXCLUDES 1 *cystic kidney disease (congenital) (Q61.-)*

√5th **N28.8 Other specified disorders of kidney and ureter**

EXCLUDES 1 *hydroureter (N13.4)*
*ureteric stricture with hydronephrosis (N13.1)*
*ureteric stricture without hydronephrosis (N13.5)*

**N28.81 Hypertrophy of kidney**
**N28.82 Megaloureter**
**N28.83 Nephroptosis**
**N28.84 Pyelitis cystica**
**N28.85 Pyeloureteritis cystica**
**N28.86 Ureteritis cystica**
**N28.89 Other specified disorders of kidney and ureter**

**AHA:** 2025,2Q,8; 2023,3Q,5

**N28.9 Disorder of kidney and ureter, unspecified**

Nephropathy NOS
Renal disease (acute) NOS
Renal insufficiency (acute)

EXCLUDES 1 *chronic renal insufficiency (N18.9)*
*unspecified nephritic syndrome (NØ5.-)*

**AHA:** 2016,1Q,13

***N29 Other disorders of kidney and ureter in diseases classified elsewhere***

Code first underlying disease, such as:
amyloidosis (E85.-)
nephrocalcinosis (E83.59)
schistosomiasis (B65.Ø-B65.9)

EXCLUDES 1 *disorders of kidney and ureter in:*
*cystinosis (E72.Ø)*
*gonorrhea (A54.21)*
*syphilis (A52.75)*
*tuberculosis (A18.11)*

## Other diseases of the urinary system (N3Ø-N39)

EXCLUDES 2 *urinary infection (complicating):*
*abortion or ectopic or molar pregnancy (OØØ-OØ7, OØ8.8)*
*pregnancy, childbirth and the puerperium (O23.-, O75.3, O86.2-)*

√4th **N3Ø Cystitis**

Use additional code to identify infectious agent (B95-B97)

EXCLUDES 1 *prostatocystitis (N41.3)*

**AHA:** 2017,1Q,6

**DEF:** Inflammation of the urinary bladder. Symptoms include dysuria, frequency of urination, urgency, and hematuria.

√5th **N3Ø.Ø Acute cystitis**

EXCLUDES 1 *irradiation cystitis (N3Ø.4-)*
*trigonitis (N3Ø.3-)*

**N3Ø.ØØ Acute cystitis without hematuria**
**N3Ø.Ø1 Acute cystitis with hematuria**

√5th **N3Ø.1 Interstitial cystitis (chronic)**

**N3Ø.1Ø Interstitial cystitis (chronic) without hematuria**
**N3Ø.11 Interstitial cystitis (chronic) with hematuria**

√5th **N3Ø.2 Other chronic cystitis**

**N3Ø.2Ø Other chronic cystitis without hematuria**
**N3Ø.21 Other chronic cystitis with hematuria**

√5th **N3Ø.3 Trigonitis**

Urethrotrigonitis

**N3Ø.3Ø Trigonitis without hematuria**
**N3Ø.31 Trigonitis with hematuria**

√5th **N3Ø.4 Irradiation cystitis**

**N3Ø.4Ø Irradiation cystitis without hematuria**
**N3Ø.41 Irradiation cystitis with hematuria**

√5th **N3Ø.8 Other cystitis**

Abscess of bladder

**N3Ø.8Ø Other cystitis without hematuria**
**N3Ø.81 Other cystitis with hematuria**

√5th **N3Ø.9 Cystitis, unspecified**

**N3Ø.9Ø Cystitis, unspecified without hematuria**
**N3Ø.91 Cystitis, unspecified with hematuria**

√4th **N31 Neuromuscular dysfunction of bladder, not elsewhere classified**

Use additional code to identify any associated urinary incontinence (N39.3-N39.4-)

EXCLUDES 1 *cord bladder NOS (G95.89)*
*neurogenic bladder due to cauda equina syndrome (G83.4)*
*neuromuscular dysfunction due to spinal cord lesion (G95.89)*

**N31.Ø Uninhibited neuropathic bladder, not elsewhere classified**
**N31.1 Reflex neuropathic bladder, not elsewhere classified**
**N31.2 Flaccid neuropathic bladder, not elsewhere classified**

Atonic (motor) (sensory) neuropathic bladder
Autonomous neuropathic bladder
Nonreflex neuropathic bladder

**N31.8 Other neuromuscular dysfunction of bladder**
**N31.9 Neuromuscular dysfunction of bladder, unspecified**

Neurogenic bladder dysfunction NOS

√4th **N32 Other disorders of bladder**

EXCLUDES 2 *calculus of bladder (N21.Ø)*
*cystocele (N81.1-)*
*hernia or prolapse of bladder, female (N81.1-)*

**N32.Ø Bladder-neck obstruction**

Bladder-neck stenosis (acquired)

EXCLUDES 1 *congenital bladder-neck obstruction (Q64.3-)*

**DEF:** Bladder outlet and vesicourethral obstruction that occurs as a consequence of benign prostatic hypertrophy or prostatic cancer. It may also occur in either sex due to strictures, radiation, cystoscopy, catheterization, injury, infection, blood clots, bladder cancer, impaction, or other disease that compresses the bladder neck.

**N32.1 Vesicointestinal fistula**

Vesicorectal fistula

**AHA:** 2025,2Q,6

**N32.2 Vesical fistula, not elsewhere classified**

EXCLUDES 1 *fistula between bladder and female genital tract (N82.Ø-N82.1)*

**N32.3 Diverticulum of bladder**

EXCLUDES 1 *congenital diverticulum of bladder (Q64.6)*
*diverticulitis of bladder (N3Ø.8-)*

√5th **N32.8 Other specified disorders of bladder**

**N32.81 Overactive bladder**

Detrusor muscle hyperactivity

EXCLUDES 1 *frequent urination due to specified bladder condition — code to condition*

**DEF:** Sudden involuntary contractions of the muscular wall of the bladder that results in a sudden, strong urge to urinate.

**N32.89 Other specified disorders of bladder**

Bladder hemorrhage
Bladder hypertrophy
Calcified bladder
Contracted bladder

**N32.9 Bladder disorder, unspecified**

***N33 Bladder disorders in diseases classified elsewhere***

Code first underlying disease, such as:
schistosomiasis (B65.Ø-B65.9)

EXCLUDES 1 *bladder disorder in syphilis (A52.76)*
*bladder disorder in tuberculosis (A18.12)*
*candidal cystitis (B37.41)*
*chlamydial cystitis (A56.Ø1)*
*cystitis in gonorrhea (A54.Ø1)*
*cystitis in neurogenic bladder (N31.-)*
*diphtheritic cystitis (A36.85)*
*neurogenic bladder (N31.-)*
*syphilitic cystitis (A52.76)*
*trichomonal cystitis (A59.Ø3)*

√4th **N34 Urethritis and urethral syndrome**

Use additional code (B95-B97), to identify infectious agent

EXCLUDES 2 *Reiter's disease (MØ2.3-)*
*urethritis in diseases with a predominantly sexual mode of transmission (A5Ø-A64)*
*urethrotrigonitis (N3Ø.3-)*

**AHA:** 2017,1Q,6

**N34.Ø Urethral abscess**

Abscess (of) Cowper's gland
Abscess (of) Littre's gland
Abscess (of) urethral (gland)
Periurethral abscess

EXCLUDES 1 *urethral caruncle (N36.2)*

**N34.1 Nonspecific urethritis**
Nongonococcal urethritis
Nonvenereal urethritis

**N34.2 Other urethritis**
Meatitis, urethral
Postmenopausal urethritis
Ulcer of urethra (meatus)
Urethritis NOS

**N34.3 Urethral syndrome, unspecified**

✓4th **N35 Urethral stricture**
EXCLUDES 1 *congenital urethral stricture (Q64.3-)*
*postprocedural urethral stricture (N99.1-)*
AHA: 2018,4Q,21-22

✓5th **N35.Ø Post-traumatic urethral stricture**
Urethral stricture due to injury
EXCLUDES 1 *postprocedural urethral stricture (N99.1-)*

✓6th **N35.Ø1 Post-traumatic urethral stricture, male**
**N35.Ø1Ø Post-traumatic urethral stricture, male, meatal**
**N35.Ø11 Post-traumatic bulbous urethral stricture**
**N35.Ø12 Post-traumatic membranous urethral stricture**
**N35.Ø13 Post-traumatic anterior urethral stricture**
**N35.Ø14 Post-traumatic urethral stricture, male, unspecified**
**N35.Ø16 Post-traumatic urethral stricture, male, overlapping sites**

✓6th **N35.Ø2 Post-traumatic urethral stricture, female**
**N35.Ø21 Urethral stricture due to childbirth**
**N35.Ø28 Other post-traumatic urethral stricture, female**

✓5th **N35.1 Postinfective urethral stricture, not elsewhere classified**
EXCLUDES 1 *gonococcal urethral stricture (A54.Ø1)*
*syphilitic urethral stricture (A52.76)*
*urethral stricture associated with schistosomiasis (B65.-, N29)*

✓6th **N35.11 Postinfective urethral stricture, not elsewhere classified, male**
**N35.111 Postinfective urethral stricture, not elsewhere classified, male, meatal**
**N35.112 Postinfective bulbous urethral stricture, not elsewhere classified, male**
**N35.113 Postinfective membranous urethral stricture, not elsewhere classified, male**
**N35.114 Postinfective anterior urethral stricture, not elsewhere classified, male**
**N35.116 Postinfective urethral stricture, not elsewhere classified, male, overlapping sites**
**N35.119 Postinfective urethral stricture, not elsewhere classified, male, unspecified**

**N35.12 Postinfective urethral stricture, not elsewhere classified, female**

✓5th **N35.8 Other urethral stricture**
EXCLUDES 1 *postprocedural urethral stricture (N99.1-)*

✓6th **N35.81 Other urethral stricture, male**
**N35.811 Other urethral stricture, male, meatal**
**N35.812 Other bulbous urethral stricture, male**
**N35.813 Other membranous urethral stricture, male**
**N35.814 Other anterior urethral stricture, male**
**N35.816 Other urethral stricture, male, overlapping sites**
**N35.819 Other urethral stricture, male, unspecified site**

**N35.82 Other urethral stricture, female**

✓5th **N35.9 Urethral stricture, unspecified**

✓6th **N35.91 Urethral stricture, unspecified, male**
**N35.911 Unspecified urethral stricture, male, meatal**
**N35.912 Unspecified bulbous urethral stricture, male**
**N35.913 Unspecified membranous urethral stricture, male**
**N35.914 Unspecified anterior urethral stricture, male**
**N35.916 Unspecified urethral stricture, male, overlapping sites**
**N35.919 Unspecified urethral stricture, male, unspecified site**
Pinhole meatus NOS
Urethral stricture NOS

**N35.92 Unspecified urethral stricture, female**

✓4th **N36 Other disorders of urethra**

**N36.Ø Urethral fistula**
Urethroperineal fistula
Urethrorectal fistula
Urinary fistula NOS
EXCLUDES 1 *urethroscrotal fistula (N5Ø.89)*
*urethrovaginal fistula (N82.1)*
*urethrovesicovaginal fistula (N82.1)*

**N36.1 Urethral diverticulum**

**N36.2 Urethral caruncle**

✓5th **N36.4 Urethral functional and muscular disorders**
Use additional code to identify associated urinary stress incontinence (N39.3)
**N36.41 Hypermobility of urethra**
**N36.42 Intrinsic sphincter deficiency (ISD)**
**N36.43 Combined hypermobility of urethra and intrinsic sphincter deficiency**
**N36.44 Muscular disorders of urethra**
Bladder sphincter dyssynergy

**N36.5 Urethral false passage**

**N36.8 Other specified disorders of urethra**
EXCLUDES 1 *congenital urethrocele (Q64.7)*
*female urethrocele (N81.Ø)*
AHA: 2022,2Q,7

**N36.9 Urethral disorder, unspecified**

***N37 Urethral disorders in diseases classified elsewhere***
Code first underlying disease
EXCLUDES 1 *urethritis (in):*
*candidal infection (B37.41)*
*chlamydial (A56.Ø1)*
*gonorrhea (A54.Ø1)*
*syphilis (A52.76)*
*trichomonal infection (A59.Ø3)*
*tuberculosis (A18.13)*

✓4th **N39 Other disorders of urinary system**
EXCLUDES 2 *hematuria NOS (R31.-)*
*proteinuria NOS (R8Ø.-)*
*recurrent or persistent hematuria (NØ2.-)*
*recurrent or persistent hematuria with specified morphological lesion (NØ2.-)*

**N39.Ø Urinary tract infection, site not specified**
Use additional code (B95-B97), to identify infectious agent
EXCLUDES 1 *candidiasis of urinary tract (B37.4-)*
*neonatal urinary tract infection (P39.3)*
*pyuria (R82.81)*
*urinary tract infection of specified site, such as:*
*cystitis (N3Ø.-)*
*pyonephrosis (N13.6)*
*urethritis (N34.-)*
AHA: 2019,3Q,17; 2018,2Q,21,22; 2018,1Q,16; 2017,1Q,6; 2012,4Q,94

**N39.3 Stress incontinence (female) (male)**
Code also any associated overactive bladder (N32.81)
EXCLUDES 1 *mixed incontinence (N39.46)*

✓5th **N39.4 Other specified urinary incontinence**
Code also any associated overactive bladder (N32.81)
EXCLUDES 1 *enuresis NOS (R32)*
*functional urinary incontinence (R39.81)*
*urinary incontinence associated with cognitive impairment (R39.81)*
*urinary incontinence of nonorganic origin (F98.Ø)*
*urinary incontinence NOS (R32)*
**N39.41 Urge incontinence**
EXCLUDES 1 *mixed incontinence (N39.46)*
**N39.42 Incontinence without sensory awareness**
Insensible (urinary) incontinence
**N39.43 Post-void dribbling**
**N39.44 Nocturnal enuresis**
EXCLUDES 2 *nocturnal polyuria (R35.81)*
**N39.45 Continuous leakage**
**N39.46 Mixed incontinence**
Urge and stress incontinence

✓6th **N39.49 Other specified urinary incontinence**

**AHA:** 2016,4Q,44

**N39.490 Overflow incontinence**

**N39.491 Coital incontinence**

**N39.492 Postural (urinary) incontinence**

**N39.498 Other specified urinary incontinence**

Reflex incontinence

Total incontinence

**N39.8 Other specified disorders of urinary system**

**N39.9 Disorder of urinary system, unspecified**

## Diseases of male genital organs (NØØ-N53)

## Diseases of male genital organs (N4Ø-N53)

✓4th **N4Ø Benign prostatic hyperplasia**

INCLUDES adenofibromatous hypertrophy of prostate
benign hypertrophy of the prostate
benign prostatic hypertrophy
BPH
enlarged prostate
nodular prostate
polyp of prostate

EXCLUDES 1 *benign neoplasms of prostate (adenoma, benign) (fibroadenoma) (fibroma) (myoma) (D29.1)*

EXCLUDES 2 *malignant neoplasm of prostate (C61)*

**DEF:** Enlargement of the prostate gland due to an abnormal proliferation of fibrostromal tissue in the paraurethral glands. This condition causes impingement of the urethra resulting in obstructed urinary flow.

**N4Ø.Ø Benign prostatic hyperplasia without lower urinary tract symptoms** A

Enlarged prostate NOS

Enlarged prostate without LUTS

**N4Ø.1 Benign prostatic hyperplasia with lower urinary tract symptoms** A

Enlarged prostate with LUTS

Use additional code for associated symptoms, when specified:
- incomplete bladder emptying (R39.14)
- nocturia (R35.1)
- straining on urination (R39.16)
- urinary frequency (R35.Ø)
- urinary hesitancy (R39.11)
- urinary incontinence (N39.4-)
- urinary obstruction (N13.8)
- urinary retention (R33.8)
- urinary urgency (R39.15)
- weak urinary stream (R39.12)

**AHA:** 2018,4Q,55

**N4Ø.2 Nodular prostate without lower urinary tract symptoms** A

Nodular prostate without LUTS

**N4Ø.3 Nodular prostate with lower urinary tract symptoms** A

Use additional code for associated symptoms, when specified:
- incomplete bladder emptying (R39.14)
- nocturia (R35.1)
- straining on urination (R39.16)
- urinary frequency (R35.Ø)
- urinary hesitancy (R39.11)
- urinary incontinence (N39.4-)
- urinary obstruction (N13.8)
- urinary retention (R33.8)
- urinary urgency (R39.15)
- weak urinary stream (R39.12)

✓4th **N41 Inflammatory diseases of prostate**

Use additional code (B95-B97), to identify infectious agent

**N41.Ø Acute prostatitis** A

**AHA:** 2024,1Q,16

**N41.1 Chronic prostatitis** A

**N41.2 Abscess of prostate** A

**N41.3 Prostatocystitis** A

**AHA:** 2024,1Q,16

**N41.4 Granulomatous prostatitis** A

**N41.8 Other inflammatory diseases of prostate** A

**N41.9 Inflammatory disease of prostate, unspecified** A

Prostatitis NOS

✓4th **N42 Other and unspecified disorders of prostate**

**N42.Ø Calculus of prostate** A

Prostatic stone

**DEF:** Formation of a small, solid stone often composed of calcium carbonate or calcium phosphate in the prostate gland.

**N42.1 Congestion and hemorrhage of prostate** A

EXCLUDES 1 *enlarged prostate (N4Ø.-)*
*hematuria (R31.-)*
*hyperplasia of prostate (N4Ø.-)*
*inflammatory diseases of prostate (N41.-)*

✓5th **N42.3 Dysplasia of prostate**

**AHA:** 2016,4Q,44

**N42.3Ø Unspecified dysplasia of prostate**

**N42.31 Prostatic intraepithelial neoplasia**

PIN

Prostatic intraepithelial neoplasia I (PIN I)

Prostatic intraepithelial neoplasia II (PIN II)

EXCLUDES 1 *prostatic intraepithelial neoplasia III (PIN III) (DØ7.5)*

**DEF:** Abnormality of shape and size of the intraepithelial tissues of the prostate. It is a premalignant condition characterized by stalks and absence of a basilar cell layer.

**N42.32 Atypical small acinar proliferation of prostate**

**N42.39 Other dysplasia of prostate**

✓5th **N42.8 Other specified disorders of prostate**

**N42.81 Prostatodynia syndrome** A

Painful prostate syndrome

**N42.82 Prostatosis syndrome** A

**N42.83 Cyst of prostate** A

**N42.89 Other specified disorders of prostate** A

**N42.9 Disorder of prostate, unspecified** A

✓4th **N43 Hydrocele and spermatocele**

INCLUDES hydrocele of spermatic cord, testis or tunica vaginalis

EXCLUDES 1 *congenital hydrocele (P83.5)*

**DEF:** Hydrocele: Serous fluid that collects in the tunica vaginalis of the scrotum along the spermatic cord in males.

**N43.Ø Encysted hydrocele**

**N43.1 Infected hydrocele**

Use additional code (B95-B97), to identify infectious agent

**N43.2 Other hydrocele**

**Hydrocele**

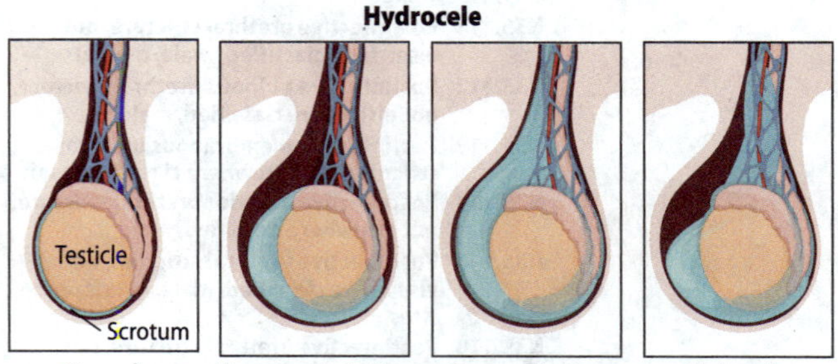


Normal | Noncommunicating hydrocele | Communicating hydrocele | Hydrocele of the cord

**N43.3 Hydrocele, unspecified**

✓5th **N43.4 Spermatocele of epididymis**

Spermatic cyst

**DEF:** Spermatocele: Noncancerous accumulation of fluid and dead sperm cells normally located at the head of the epididymis that exhibits itself as a hard, smooth scrotal mass and do not normally require treatment unless they become enlarged or cause pain.

**N43.4Ø Spermatocele of epididymis, unspecified**

**N43.41 Spermatocele of epididymis, single**

**N43.42 Spermatocele of epididymis, multiple**

✓4th **N44 Noninflammatory disorders of testis**

✓5th **N44.Ø Torsion of testis**

**N44.ØØ Torsion of testis, unspecified**

**N44.Ø1 Extravaginal torsion of spermatic cord**

**DEF:** Torsion of the spermatic cord just below the tunica vaginalis attachments.

**N44.Ø2 Intravaginal torsion of spermatic cord**

Torsion of spermatic cord NOS

**N44.Ø3 Torsion of appendix testis**

**N44.Ø4 Torsion of appendix epididymis**

**N44.1 Cyst of tunica albuginea testis**

**N44.2 Benign cyst of testis**

**N44.8 Other noninflammatory disorders of the testis**

**N45 Orchitis and epididymitis**
Use additional code (B95-B97), to identify infectious agent
**N45.1 Epididymitis**
**N45.2 Orchitis**
**N45.3 Epididymo-orchitis**
**N45.4 Abscess of epididymis or testis**

**N46 Male infertility**
EXCLUDES 1 *vasectomy status (Z98.52)*
**N46.Ø Azoospermia**
Absolute male infertility
Male infertility due to germinal (cell) aplasia
Male infertility due to spermatogenic arrest (complete)
**DEF:** Failure of the development of sperm or the absence of sperm in semen.
**N46.Ø1 Organic azoospermia** A
Azoospermia NOS
**N46.Ø2 Azoospermia due to extratesticular causes**
Code also associated cause
**N46.Ø21 Azoospermia due to drug therapy** A
**N46.Ø22 Azoospermia due to infection** A
**N46.Ø23 Azoospermia due to obstruction of efferent ducts** A
**N46.Ø24 Azoospermia due to radiation** A
**N46.Ø25 Azoospermia due to systemic disease** A
**N46.Ø29 Azoospermia due to other extratesticular causes** A
**N46.1 Oligospermia**
Male infertility due to germinal cell desquamation
Male infertility due to hypospermatogenesis
Male infertility due to incomplete spermatogenic arrest
**DEF:** Insufficient production of sperm in semen.
**N46.11 Organic oligospermia** A
Oligospermia NOS
**N46.12 Oligospermia due to extratesticular causes**
Code also associated cause
**N46.121 Oligospermia due to drug therapy** A
**N46.122 Oligospermia due to infection** A
**N46.123 Oligospermia due to obstruction of efferent ducts** A
**N46.124 Oligospermia due to radiation** A
**N46.125 Oligospermia due to systemic disease** A
**N46.129 Oligospermia due to other extratesticular causes** A
**N46.8 Other male infertility** A
**N46.9 Male infertility, unspecified** A

**N47 Disorders of prepuce**
**N47.Ø Adherent prepuce, newborn** N
**N47.1 Phimosis**
**DEF:** Condition in which the foreskin is contracted and cannot be drawn back behind the glans penis.
**N47.2 Paraphimosis**
**N47.3 Deficient foreskin**
**N47.4 Benign cyst of prepuce**
**N47.5 Adhesions of prepuce and glans penis**
**N47.6 Balanoposthitis**
Use additional code (B95-B97), to identify infectious agent
EXCLUDES 1 *balanitis (N48.1)*
**N47.7 Other inflammatory diseases of prepuce**
Use additional code (B95-B97), to identify infectious agent
**N47.8 Other disorders of prepuce**

**N48 Other disorders of penis**
**N48.Ø Leukoplakia of penis**
Balanitis xerotica obliterans
Kraurosis of penis
Lichen sclerosus of external male genital organs
EXCLUDES 1 *carcinoma in situ of penis (DØ7.4)*
**N48.1 Balanitis**
Use additional code (B95-B97), to identify infectious agent
EXCLUDES 1 *amebic balanitis (AØ6.8)*
*balanitis xerotica obliterans (N48.Ø)*
*candidal balanitis (B37.42)*
*gonococcal balanitis (A54.23)*
*herpesviral [herpes simplex] balanitis (A6Ø.Ø1)*
**DEF:** Inflammation of the glans penis, most often affecting uncircumcised males.
**N48.2 Other inflammatory disorders of penis**
Use additional code (B95-B97), to identify infectious agent
EXCLUDES 1 *balanitis (N48.1)*
*balanitis xerotica obliterans (N48.Ø)*
*balanoposthitis (N47.6)*
**N48.21 Abscess of corpus cavernosum and penis**
**N48.22 Cellulitis of corpus cavernosum and penis**
**N48.29 Other inflammatory disorders of penis**
**N48.3 Priapism**
Painful erection
Code first underlying cause
**N48.3Ø Priapism, unspecified**
**N48.31 Priapism due to trauma**
***N48.32 Priapism due to disease classified elsewhere***
**N48.33 Priapism, drug-induced**
**N48.39 Other priapism**
**N48.5 Ulcer of penis**
**N48.6 Induration penis plastica**
Peyronie's disease
Plastic induration of penis
**N48.8 Other specified disorders of penis**
**N48.81 Thrombosis of superficial vein of penis**
**N48.82 Acquired torsion of penis**
Acquired torsion of penis NOS
EXCLUDES 1 *congenital torsion of penis (Q55.63)*
**N48.83 Acquired buried penis**
EXCLUDES 1 *congenital hidden penis (Q55.64)*
**N48.89 Other specified disorders of penis**
**N48.9 Disorder of penis, unspecified**

**N49 Inflammatory disorders of male genital organs, not elsewhere classified**
Use additional code (B95-B97), to identify infectious agent
EXCLUDES 1 *inflammation of penis (N48.1, N48.2-)*
*orchitis and epididymitis (N45.-)*
**N49.Ø Inflammatory disorders of seminal vesicle**
Vesiculitis NOS
**N49.1 Inflammatory disorders of spermatic cord, tunica vaginalis and vas deferens**
Vasitis
**N49.2 Inflammatory disorders of scrotum**
**N49.3 Fournier gangrene** HCC COM
**AHA:** 2020,2Q,18
**N49.8 Inflammatory disorders of other specified male genital organs**
Inflammation of multiple sites in male genital organs
**N49.9 Inflammatory disorder of unspecified male genital organ**
Abscess of unspecified male genital organ
Boil of unspecified male genital organ
Carbuncle of unspecified male genital organ
Cellulitis of unspecified male genital organ

**N5Ø Other and unspecified disorders of male genital organs**
EXCLUDES 2 *torsion of testis (N44.Ø-)*
**N5Ø.Ø Atrophy of testis**
**N5Ø.1 Vascular disorders of male genital organs**
Hematocele, NOS, of male genital organs
Hemorrhage of male genital organs
Thrombosis of male genital organs
**N5Ø.3 Cyst of epididymis**
**N5Ø.8 Other specified disorders of male genital organs**
**AHA:** 2016,4Q,45
**N5Ø.81 Testicular pain**
**N5Ø.811 Right testicular pain**
**N5Ø.812 Left testicular pain**
**N5Ø.819 Testicular pain, unspecified**
**N5Ø.82 Scrotal pain**

**N50.89 Other specified disorders of the male genital organs**
Atrophy of scrotum, seminal vesicle, spermatic cord, tunica vaginalis and vas deferens
Chylocele, tunica vaginalis (nonfilarial) NOS
Edema of scrotum, seminal vesicle, spermatic cord, tunica vaginalis and vas deferens
Hypertrophy of scrotum, seminal vesicle, spermatic cord, tunica vaginalis and vas deferens
Stricture of spermatic cord, tunica vaginalis, and vas deferens
Ulcer of scrotum, seminal vesicle, spermatic cord, testis, tunica vaginalis and vas deferens
Urethroscrotal fistula

**N50.9 Disorder of male genital organs, unspecified**

***N51 Disorders of male genital organs in diseases classified elsewhere***
Code first underlying disease, such as:
filariasis (B74.0-B74.9)
EXCLUDES 1 *amebic balanitis (A06.8)*
*candidal balanitis (B37.42)*
*gonococcal balanitis (A54.23)*
*gonococcal prostatitis (A54.22)*
*herpesviral [herpes simplex] balanitis (A60.01)*
*trichomonal prostatitis (A59.02)*
*tuberculous prostatitis (A18.14)*

✓4th **N52 Male erectile dysfunction**
EXCLUDES 1 *psychogenic impotence (F52.21)*

✓5th **N52.0 Vasculogenic erectile dysfunction**
**N52.01 Erectile dysfunction due to arterial insufficiency** A
**N52.02 Corporo-venous occlusive erectile dysfunction** A
**N52.03 Combined arterial insufficiency and corporo-venous occlusive erectile dysfunction** A

***N52.1 Erectile dysfunction due to diseases classified elsewhere*** A
Code first underlying disease

**N52.2 Drug-induced erectile dysfunction** A

✓5th **N52.3 Postprocedural erectile dysfunction**
AHA: 2016,4Q,45
**N52.31 Erectile dysfunction following radical prostatectomy** A
**N52.32 Erectile dysfunction following radical cystectomy** A
**N52.33 Erectile dysfunction following urethral surgery** A
**N52.34 Erectile dysfunction following simple prostatectomy** A
**N52.35 Erectile dysfunction following radiation therapy** A
**N52.36 Erectile dysfunction following interstitial seed therapy** A
**N52.37 Erectile dysfunction following prostate ablative therapy** A
Erectile dysfunction following cryotherapy
Erectile dysfunction following other prostate ablative therapies
Erectile dysfunction following ultrasound ablative therapies
**N52.39 Other and unspecified postprocedural erectile dysfunction** A

**N52.8 Other male erectile dysfunction** A

**N52.9 Male erectile dysfunction, unspecified** A
Impotence NOS

✓4th **N53 Other male sexual dysfunction**
EXCLUDES 1 *psychogenic sexual dysfunction (F52.-)*

✓5th **N53.1 Ejaculatory dysfunction**
EXCLUDES 1 *premature ejaculation (F52.4)*
**N53.11 Retarded ejaculation**
**N53.12 Painful ejaculation**
**N53.13 Anejaculatory orgasm**
**N53.14 Retrograde ejaculation**
DEF: Form of male sexual dysfunction in which the semen enters the bladder instead of going out through the urethra during ejaculation.
**N53.19 Other ejaculatory dysfunction**
Ejaculatory dysfunction NOS

**N53.8 Other male sexual dysfunction**

**N53.9 Unspecified male sexual dysfunction**

## Disorders of breast (N60-N65)

EXCLUDES 1 *disorders of breast associated with childbirth (O91-O92)*

✓4th **N60 Benign mammary dysplasia**
INCLUDES fibrocystic mastopathy

✓5th **N60.0 Solitary cyst of breast**
Cyst of breast
**N60.01 Solitary cyst of right breast**
**N60.02 Solitary cyst of left breast**
**N60.09 Solitary cyst of unspecified breast**

✓5th **N60.1 Diffuse cystic mastopathy**
Cystic breast
Fibrocystic disease of breast
EXCLUDES 1 *diffuse cystic mastopathy with epithelial proliferation (N60.3-)*
**N60.11 Diffuse cystic mastopathy of right breast** A
**N60.12 Diffuse cystic mastopathy of left breast** A
**N60.19 Diffuse cystic mastopathy of unspecified breast** A

✓5th **N60.2 Fibroadenosis of breast**
Adenofibrosis of breast
EXCLUDES 2 *fibroadenoma of breast (D24.-)*
**N60.21 Fibroadenosis of right breast**
**N60.22 Fibroadenosis of left breast**
**N60.29 Fibroadenosis of unspecified breast**

✓5th **N60.3 Fibrosclerosis of breast**
Cystic mastopathy with epithelial proliferation
**N60.31 Fibrosclerosis of right breast**
**N60.32 Fibrosclerosis of left breast**
**N60.39 Fibrosclerosis of unspecified breast**

✓5th **N60.4 Mammary duct ectasia**
**N60.41 Mammary duct ectasia of right breast**
**N60.42 Mammary duct ectasia of left breast**
**N60.49 Mammary duct ectasia of unspecified breast**

✓5th **N60.8 Other benign mammary dysplasias**
**N60.81 Other benign mammary dysplasias of right breast**
**N60.82 Other benign mammary dysplasias of left breast**
**N60.89 Other benign mammary dysplasias of unspecified breast**

✓5th **N60.9 Unspecified benign mammary dysplasia**
**N60.91 Unspecified benign mammary dysplasia of right breast**
**N60.92 Unspecified benign mammary dysplasia of left breast**
**N60.99 Unspecified benign mammary dysplasia of unspecified breast**

✓4th **N61 Inflammatory disorders of breast**
EXCLUDES 1 *inflammatory carcinoma of breast (C50.A-)*
*inflammatory disorder of breast associated with childbirth (O91.-)*
*neonatal infective mastitis (P39.0)*
*thrombophlebitis of breast [Mondor's disease] (I80.8)*

**N61.0 Mastitis without abscess**
Cellulitis (acute) (nonpuerperal) (subacute) of breast NOS
Cellulitis (acute) (nonpuerperal) (subacute) of nipple NOS
Infective mastitis (acute) (nonpuerperal) (subacute)
Mastitis (acute) (nonpuerperal) (subacute) NOS

**N61.1 Abscess of the breast and nipple**
Abscess (acute) (chronic) (nonpuerperal) of areola
Abscess (acute) (chronic) (nonpuerperal) of breast
Carbuncle of breast
Mastitis with abscess

✓5th **N61.2 Granulomatous mastitis**
AHA: 2020,4Q,35
**N61.20 Granulomatous mastitis, unspecified breast**
**N61.21 Granulomatous mastitis, right breast**
**N61.22 Granulomatous mastitis, left breast**
**N61.23 Granulomatous mastitis, bilateral breast**

**N62 Hypertrophy of breast**
Gynecomastia
Hypertrophy of breast NOS
Massive pubertal hypertrophy of breast
EXCLUDES 1 *breast engorgement of newborn (P83.4)*
*disproportion of reconstructed breast (N65.1)*
AHA: 2023,3Q,22

**N63 Unspecified lump in breast**
Nodule(s) NOS in breast
AHA: 2022,3Q,8; 2019,4Q,12; 2017,4Q,19

**N63.Ø Unspecified lump in unspecified breast**

**N63.1 Unspecified lump in the right breast**
- **N63.1Ø** Unspecified lump in the right breast, unspecified quadrant
- **N63.11** Unspecified lump in the right breast, upper outer quadrant
- **N63.12** Unspecified lump in the right breast, upper inner quadrant
- **N63.13** Unspecified lump in the right breast, lower outer quadrant
- **N63.14** Unspecified lump in the right breast, lower inner quadrant
- **N63.15** Unspecified lump in the right breast, overlapping quadrants

**N63.2 Unspecified lump in the left breast**
- **N63.2Ø** Unspecified lump in the left breast, unspecified quadrant
- **N63.21** Unspecified lump in the left breast, upper outer quadrant
- **N63.22** Unspecified lump in the left breast, upper inner quadrant
- **N63.23** Unspecified lump in the left breast, lower outer quadrant
- **N63.24** Unspecified lump in the left breast, lower inner quadrant
- **N63.25** Unspecified lump in the left breast, overlapping quadrants

**N63.3 Unspecified lump in axillary tail**
- **N63.31** Unspecified lump in axillary tail of the right breast
- **N63.32** Unspecified lump in axillary tail of the left breast

**N63.4 Unspecified lump in breast, subareolar**
- **N63.41** Unspecified lump in right breast, subareolar
- **N63.42** Unspecified lump in left breast, subareolar

**N64 Other disorders of breast**
EXCLUDES 2 *mechanical complication of breast prosthesis and implant (T85.4-)*

**N64.Ø Fissure and fistula of nipple**

**N64.1 Fat necrosis of breast**
Fat necrosis (segmental) of breast
Code first breast necrosis due to breast graft (T85.898)

**N64.2 Atrophy of breast**

**N64.3 Galactorrhea not associated with childbirth**

**N64.4 Mastodynia**

**N64.5 Other signs and symptoms in breast**
EXCLUDES 2 *abnormal findings on diagnostic imaging of breast (R92.-)*
- **N64.51** Induration of breast
- **N64.52** Nipple discharge
  EXCLUDES 1 *abnormal findings in nipple discharge (R89.-)*
- **N64.53** Retraction of nipple
- **N64.59** Other signs and symptoms in breast

**N64.8 Other specified disorders of breast**
- **N64.81** Ptosis of breast [A]
  EXCLUDES 1 *ptosis of native breast in relation to reconstructed breast (N65.1)*
- **N64.82** Hypoplasia of breast [A]
  Micromastia
  EXCLUDES 1 *congenital absence of breast (Q83.Ø)*
  *hypoplasia of native breast in relation to reconstructed breast (N65.1)*
- **N64.89** Other specified disorders of breast
  Galactocele
  Subinvolution of breast (postlactational)
  AHA: 2019,1Q,32; 2018,1Q,3

**N64.9 Disorder of breast, unspecified**

**N65 Deformity and disproportion of reconstructed breast**

**N65.Ø Deformity of reconstructed breast** [A]
Contour irregularity in reconstructed breast
Excess tissue in reconstructed breast
Misshapen reconstructed breast

**N65.1 Disproportion of reconstructed breast** [A]
Breast asymmetry between native breast and reconstructed breast
Disproportion between native breast and reconstructed breast
AHA: 2025,3Q,23

## Inflammatory diseases of female pelvic organs (N7Ø-N77)

▶Code also, if applicable, pelvic abscess (K6A.Ø-)◀
EXCLUDES 1 *inflammatory diseases of female pelvic organs complicating:*
*abortion or ectopic or molar pregnancy (OØØ-OØ7, OØ8.Ø)*
*pregnancy, childbirth and the puerperium (O23.-, O75.3, O85, O86.-)*

**N7Ø Salpingitis and oophoritis**
INCLUDES abscess (of) fallopian tube
abscess (of) ovary
pyosalpinx
salpingo-oophoritis
tubo-ovarian abscess
tubo-ovarian inflammatory disease
Use additional code (B95-B97), to identify infectious agent
EXCLUDES 1 *gonococcal infection (A54.24)*
*tuberculous infection (A18.17)*

**N7Ø.Ø Acute salpingitis and oophoritis**
- **N7Ø.Ø1** Acute salpingitis
- **N7Ø.Ø2** Acute oophoritis
- **N7Ø.Ø3** Acute salpingitis and oophoritis

**N7Ø.1 Chronic salpingitis and oophoritis**
Hydrosalpinx
- **N7Ø.11** Chronic salpingitis
- **N7Ø.12** Chronic oophoritis
- **N7Ø.13** Chronic salpingitis and oophoritis

**N7Ø.9 Salpingitis and oophoritis, unspecified**
- **N7Ø.91** Salpingitis, unspecified
- **N7Ø.92** Oophoritis, unspecified
- **N7Ø.93** Salpingitis and oophoritis, unspecified

**N71 Inflammatory disease of uterus, except cervix**
INCLUDES endo (myo) metritis
metritis
myometritis
pyometra
uterine abscess
Use additional code (B95-B97), to identify infectious agent
EXCLUDES 1 *hyperplastic endometritis (N85.Ø-)*
*infection of uterus following delivery (O85, O86.-)*

**N71.Ø Acute inflammatory disease of uterus**

**N71.1 Chronic inflammatory disease of uterus**

**N71.9 Inflammatory disease of uterus, unspecified**

**N72 Inflammatory disease of cervix uteri**
INCLUDES cervicitis (with or without erosion or ectropion)
endocervicitis (with or without erosion or ectropion)
exocervicitis (with or without erosion or ectropion)
Use additional code (B95-B97), to identify infectious agent
EXCLUDES 1 *erosion and ectropion of cervix without cervicitis (N86)*

**N73 Other female pelvic inflammatory diseases**
Use additional code (B95-B97), to identify infectious agent

**N73.Ø Acute parametritis and pelvic cellulitis**
Abscess of broad ligament
Abscess of parametrium
Pelvic cellulitis, female
DEF: Parametritis: Inflammation of the parametrium.

**N73.1 Chronic parametritis and pelvic cellulitis**
Any condition in N73.Ø specified as chronic
EXCLUDES 1 *tuberculous parametritis and pelvic cellultis (A18.17)*

**N73.2 Unspecified parametritis and pelvic cellulitis**
Any condition in N73.Ø unspecified whether acute or chronic

**N73.3 Female acute pelvic peritonitis**
AHA: 2026,2Q,12

**N73.4 Female chronic pelvic peritonitis**
EXCLUDES 1 *tuberculous pelvic (female) peritonitis (A18.17)*

**N73.5 Female pelvic peritonitis, unspecified**

**N73.6 Female pelvic peritoneal adhesions (postinfective)**
EXCLUDES 2 *postprocedural pelvic peritoneal adhesions (N99.4)*
AHA: 2014,1Q,6

**N73.8 Other specified female pelvic inflammatory diseases**

**N73.9 Female pelvic inflammatory disease, unspecified**
Female pelvic infection or inflammation NOS

**N74 Female pelvic inflammatory disorders in diseases classified elsewhere**
Code first underlying disease
EXCLUDES 1 chlamydial cervicitis (A56.02)
chlamydial pelvic inflammatory disease (A56.11)
gonococcal cervicitis (A54.03)
gonococcal pelvic inflammatory disease (A54.24)
herpesviral [herpes simplex] cervicitis (A60.03)
herpesviral [herpes simplex] pelvic inflammatory disease (A60.09)
syphilitic cervicitis (A52.76)
syphilitic pelvic inflammatory disease (A52.76)
trichomonal cervicitis (A59.09)
tuberculous cervicitis (A18.16)
tuberculous pelvic inflammatory disease (A18.17)

**N75 Diseases of Bartholin's gland**
DEF: Bartholin's gland: Mucous-producing gland found in the vestibular bulbs on either side of the vaginal orifice and connected to the mucosal membrane at the opening by a duct.
**N75.0 Cyst of Bartholin's gland**
**N75.1 Abscess of Bartholin's gland**
AHA: 2025,1Q,22
**N75.8 Other diseases of Bartholin's gland**
Bartholinitis
**N75.9 Disease of Bartholin's gland, unspecified**

**N76 Other inflammation of vagina and vulva**
Use additional code (B95-B97), to identify infectious agent
EXCLUDES 2 senile (atrophic) vaginitis (N95.2)
vulvar vestibulitis (N94.810)
**N76.0 Acute vaginitis**
Acute vulvovaginitis
Vaginitis NOS
Vulvovaginitis NOS
**N76.1 Subacute and chronic vaginitis**
Chronic vulvovaginitis
Subacute vulvovaginitis
**N76.2 Acute vulvitis**
Vulvitis NOS
**N76.3 Subacute and chronic vulvitis**
**N76.4 Abscess of vulva**
Furuncle of vulva
**N76.5 Ulceration of vagina**
**N76.6 Ulceration of vulva**
**N76.8 Other specified inflammation of vagina and vulva**
**N76.81 Mucositis (ulcerative) of vagina and vulva**
Code also type of associated therapy, such as:
antineoplastic and immunosuppressive drugs (T45.1X-)
radiological procedure and radiotherapy (Y84.2)
EXCLUDES 2 gastrointestinal mucositis (ulcerative) (K92.81)
nasal mucositis (ulcerative) (J34.81)
oral mucositis (ulcerative) (K12.3-)
**N76.82 Fournier disease of vagina and vulva** HCC ESR COM
Fournier gangrene of vagina and vulva
Code also, if applicable, diabetes mellitus (E08-E13 with .9)
EXCLUDES 1 gangrene in diabetes mellitus (E08-E13 with .52)
AHA: 2022,4Q,34
**N76.89 Other specified inflammation of vagina and vulva**

**N77 Vulvovaginal ulceration and inflammation in diseases classified elsewhere**
**N77.0 Ulceration of vulva in diseases classified elsewhere**
Code first underlying disease, such as:
Behcet's disease (M35.2)
EXCLUDES 1 ulceration of vulva in gonococcal infection (A54.02)
ulceration of vulva in herpesviral [herpes simplex] infection (A60.04)
ulceration of vulva in syphilis (A51.0)
ulceration of vulva in tuberculosis (A18.18)
**N77.1 Vaginitis, vulvitis and vulvovaginitis in diseases classified elsewhere**
Code first underlying disease, such as:
pinworm (B80)
EXCLUDES 1 candidal vulvovaginitis (B37.3-)
chlamydial vulvovaginitis (A56.02)
gonococcal vulvovaginitis (A54.02)
herpesviral [herpes simplex] vulvovaginitis (A60.04)
trichomonal vulvovaginitis (A59.01)
tuberculous vulvovaginitis (A18.18)
vulvovaginitis in early syphilis (A51.0)
vulvovaginitis in late syphilis (A52.76)

## Noninflammatory disorders of female genital tract (N80-N98)

**N80 Endometriosis**
AHA: 2022,4Q,34-36
DEF: Aberrant uterine mucosal tissue appearing in areas of the pelvic cavity outside of its normal location, lining the uterus, and inflaming surrounding tissues often resulting in infertility or spontaneous abortion.
**N80.0 Endometriosis of uterus**
Endometriosis of the cervix
EXCLUDES 1 stromal endometriosis (D39.0)
**N80.00 Endometriosis of the uterus, unspecified**
**N80.01 Superficial endometriosis of the uterus**
**N80.02 Deep endometriosis of the uterus**
Deep retrocervical endometriosis
**N80.03 Adenomyosis of the uterus**
Adenomyosis NOS
**N80.1 Endometriosis of ovary**
**N80.10 Endometriosis of ovary, unspecified depth**
**N80.101 Endometriosis of right ovary, unspecified depth**
**N80.102 Endometriosis of left ovary, unspecified depth**
**N80.103 Endometriosis of bilateral ovaries, unspecified depth**
**N80.109 Endometriosis of ovary, unspecified side, unspecified depth**
Endometriosis of ovary NOS
**N80.11 Superficial endometriosis of the ovary**
**N80.111 Superficial endometriosis of right ovary**
AHA: 2022,4Q,35
**N80.112 Superficial endometriosis of left ovary**
**N80.113 Superficial endometriosis of bilateral ovaries**
**N80.119 Superficial endometriosis of ovary, unspecified ovary**
**N80.12 Deep endometriosis of ovary**
Deep ovarian endometriosis
Endometrioma
**N80.121 Deep endometriosis of right ovary**
**N80.122 Deep endometriosis of left ovary**
**N80.123 Deep endometriosis of bilateral ovaries**
**N80.129 Deep endometriosis of ovary, unspecified ovary**
**N80.2 Endometriosis of fallopian tube**
**N80.20 Endometriosis of fallopian tube, unspecified depth**
**N80.201 Endometriosis of right fallopian tube, unspecified depth**
**N80.202 Endometriosis of left fallopian tube, unspecified depth**
**N80.203 Endometriosis of bilateral fallopian tubes, unspecified depth**
**N80.209 Endometriosis of unspecified fallopian tube, unspecified depth**
Endometriosis fallopian tube NOS
**N80.21 Superficial endometriosis of fallopian tube**
**N80.211 Superficial endometriosis of right fallopian tube**
**N80.212 Superficial endometriosis of left fallopian tube**
**N80.213 Superficial endometriosis of bilateral fallopian tubes**
**N80.219 Superficial endometriosis of unspecified fallopian tube**
**N80.22 Deep endometriosis of the fallopian tube**
Deep endometriosis involving muscular wall of fallopian tube
**N80.221 Deep endometriosis of right fallopian tube**

N80.222 Deep endometriosis of left fallopian tube
N80.223 Deep endometriosis of bilateral fallopian tubes
N80.229 Deep endometriosis of unspecified fallopian tube

N80.3 Endometriosis of pelvic peritoneum
N80.30 Endometriosis of pelvic peritoneum, unspecified
Endometriosis of the retroperitoneum NOS
N80.31 Endometriosis of the anterior cul-de-sac
N80.311 Superficial endometriosis of the anterior cul-de-sac
N80.312 Deep endometriosis of the anterior cul-de-sac
N80.319 Endometriosis of the anterior cul-de-sac, unspecified depth
Endometriosis of the anterior cul-de-sac NOS
N80.32 Endometriosis of the posterior cul-de-sac
N80.321 Superficial endometriosis of the posterior cul-de-sac
N80.322 Deep endometriosis of the posterior cul-de-sac
N80.329 Endometriosis of the posterior cul-de-sac, unspecified depth
Endometriosis of the posterior cul-de-sac NOS
N80.33 Superficial endometriosis of the pelvic sidewall
N80.331 Superficial endometriosis of the right pelvic sidewall
N80.332 Superficial endometriosis of the left pelvic sidewall
N80.333 Superficial endometriosis of bilateral pelvic sidewall
N80.339 Superficial endometriosis of pelvic sidewall, unspecified side
N80.34 Deep endometriosis of the pelvic sidewall
N80.341 Deep endometriosis of the right pelvic sidewall
N80.342 Deep endometriosis of the left pelvic sidewall
N80.343 Deep endometriosis of the bilateral pelvic sidewall
N80.349 Deep endometriosis of the pelvic sidewall, unspecified side
AHA: 2022,4Q,36
N80.35 Endometriosis of the pelvic sidewall, unspecified depth
N80.351 Endometriosis of the right pelvic sidewall, unspecified depth
N80.352 Endometriosis of the left pelvic sidewall, unspecified depth
N80.353 Endometriosis of bilateral pelvic sidewall, unspecified depth
N80.359 Endometriosis of pelvic sidewall, unspecified side, unspecified depth
Endometriosis of the pelvic sidewall NOS
N80.36 Superficial endometriosis of the pelvic brim
N80.361 Superficial endometriosis of the right pelvic brim
N80.362 Superficial endometriosis of the left pelvic brim
N80.363 Superficial endometriosis of bilateral pelvic brim
N80.369 Superficial endometriosis of the pelvic brim, unspecified side
N80.37 Deep endometriosis of the pelvic brim
N80.371 Deep endometriosis of the right pelvic brim
N80.372 Deep endometriosis of the left pelvic brim
N80.373 Deep endometriosis of bilateral pelvic brim
N80.379 Deep endometriosis of the pelvic brim, unspecified side
N80.38 Endometriosis of the pelvic brim, unspecified depth
N80.381 Endometriosis of the right pelvic brim, unspecified depth
N80.382 Endometriosis of the left pelvic brim, unspecified depth
N80.383 Endometriosis of bilateral pelvic brim, unspecified depth
N80.389 Endometriosis of the pelvic brim, unspecified side, unspecified depth
Endometriosis of the pelvic brim NOS
N80.3A Superficial endometriosis of the uterosacral ligament(s)
N80.3A1 Superficial endometriosis of the right uterosacral ligament
N80.3A2 Superficial endometriosis of the left uterosacral ligament
N80.3A3 Superficial endometriosis of the bilateral uterosacral ligament(s)
N80.3A9 Superficial endometriosis of the uterosacral ligament(s), unspecified side
N80.3B Deep endometriosis of the uterosacral ligament(s)
N80.3B1 Deep endometriosis of the right uterosacral ligament
N80.3B2 Deep endometriosis of the left uterosacral ligament
N80.3B3 Deep endometriosis of bilateral uterosacral ligament(s)
N80.3B9 Deep endometriosis of the uterosacral ligament(s), unspecified side
N80.3C Endometriosis of the uterosacral ligament(s), unspecified depth
N80.3C1 Endometriosis of the right uterosacral ligament, unspecified depth
N80.3C2 Endometriosis of the left uterosacral ligament, unspecified depth
N80.3C3 Endometriosis of bilateral uterosacral ligament(s), unspecified depth
N80.3C9 Endometriosis of the uterosacral ligament(s), unspecified side, unspecified depth
Endometriosis of the uterosacral ligament(s) NOS
N80.39 Endometriosis of other pelvic peritoneum
N80.391 Superficial endometriosis of the pelvic peritoneum, other specified sites
N80.392 Deep endometriosis of the pelvic peritoneum, other specified sites
N80.399 Endometriosis of the pelvic peritoneum, other specified sites, unspecified depth

N80.4 Endometriosis of rectovaginal septum and vagina
N80.40 Endometriosis of rectovaginal septum, unspecified involvement of vagina
Endometriosis of the rectovaginal septum, NOS
N80.41 Endometriosis of rectovaginal septum without involvement of vagina
N80.42 Endometriosis of rectovaginal septum with involvement of vagina

N80.5 Endometriosis of intestine
N80.50 Endometriosis of intestine, unspecified
N80.51 Endometriosis of the rectum
N80.511 Superficial endometriosis of the rectum
N80.512 Deep endometriosis of the rectum
Deep endometriosis of the rectum, multifocal
N80.519 Endometriosis of the rectum, unspecified depth
Endometriosis of the rectum NOS
N80.52 Endometriosis of the sigmoid colon
N80.521 Superficial endometriosis of the sigmoid colon
N80.522 Deep endometriosis of the sigmoid colon
N80.529 Endometriosis of the sigmoid colon, unspecified depth
Endometriosis of the sigmoid colon NOS
N80.53 Endometriosis of the cecum
N80.531 Superficial endometriosis of the cecum
N80.532 Deep endometriosis of the cecum
N80.539 Endometriosis of the cecum, unspecified depth
Endometriosis of the cecum NOS
N80.54 Endometriosis of the appendix
N80.541 Superficial endometriosis of the appendix
N80.542 Deep endometriosis of the appendix
N80.549 Endometriosis of the appendix, unspecified depth
Endometriosis of the appendix NOS

✓6th **N8Ø.55 Endometriosis of other parts of the colon**
Endometriosis of descending colon
Endometriosis of transverse colon

**N8Ø.551 Superficial endometriosis of other parts of the colon**

**N8Ø.552 Deep endometriosis of other parts of the colon**

**N8Ø.559 Endometriosis of other parts of the colon, unspecified depth**
Endometriosis of colon NOS

✓6th **N8Ø.56 Endometriosis of the small intestine**

**N8Ø.561 Superficial endometriosis of the small intestine**

**N8Ø.562 Deep endometriosis of the small intestine**
Deep endometriosis of the small intestine, multifocal

**N8Ø.569 Endometriosis of the small intestine, unspecified depth**
Endometriosis of the small intestine NOS

**N8Ø.6 Endometriosis in cutaneous scar**

✓5th **N8Ø.A Endometriosis of bladder and ureters**

**N8Ø.AØ Endometriosis of bladder, unspecified depth**
Endometriosis of bladder NOS

**N8Ø.A1 Superficial endometriosis of bladder**

**N8Ø.A2 Deep endometriosis of bladder**

✓6th **N8Ø.A4 Superficial endometriosis of ureter**
Extrinsic endometriosis of ureter
Code also, if applicable, obstructive and reflux uropathy (N13.-)

**N8Ø.A41 Superficial endometriosis of right ureter**

**N8Ø.A42 Superficial endometriosis of left ureter**

**N8Ø.A43 Superficial endometriosis of bilateral ureters**

**N8Ø.A49 Superficial endometriosis of unspecified ureter**

✓6th **N8Ø.A5 Deep endometriosis of ureter**
Intrinsic endometriosis of ureter
Code also, if applicable, obstructive and reflux uropathy (N13.-)

**N8Ø.A51 Deep endometriosis of right ureter**

**N8Ø.A52 Deep endometriosis of left ureter**

**N8Ø.A53 Deep endometriosis of bilateral ureters**

**N8Ø.A59 Deep endometriosis of unspecified ureter**

✓6th **N8Ø.A6 Endometriosis of ureter, unspecified depth**
Code also, if applicable, obstructive and reflux uropathy (N13.-)

**N8Ø.A61 Endometriosis of right ureter, unspecified depth**

**N8Ø.A62 Endometriosis of left ureter, unspecified depth**

**N8Ø.A63 Endometriosis of bilateral ureters, unspecified depth**

**N8Ø.A69 Endometriosis of unspecified ureter, unspecified depth**

✓5th **N8Ø.B Endometriosis of cardiothoracic space**
Endometriosis of thorax
Code also, if applicable:
catamenial hemothorax (J94.2)
catamenial pneumothorax (J93.12)

**N8Ø.B1 Endometriosis of pleura**

**N8Ø.B2 Endometriosis of lung**

✓6th **N8Ø.B3 Endometriosis of diaphragm**

**N8Ø.B31 Superficial endometriosis of diaphragm**

**N8Ø.B32 Deep endometriosis of diaphragm**

**N8Ø.B39 Endometriosis of diaphragm, unspecified depth**
Endometriosis of the diaphragm NOS

**N8Ø.B4 Endometriosis of the pericardial space**

**N8Ø.B5 Endometriosis of the mediastinal space**

**N8Ø.B6 Endometriosis of cardiothoracic space**

✓5th **N8Ø.C Endometriosis of the abdomen**

**N8Ø.CØ Endometriosis of the abdomen, unspecified**
Endometriosis of the abdomen NOS

✓6th **N8Ø.C1 Endometriosis of the anterior abdominal wall**

**N8Ø.C1Ø Endometriosis of the anterior abdominal wall, subcutaneous tissue**

**N8Ø.C11 Endometriosis of the anterior abdominal wall, fascia and muscular layers**

**N8Ø.C19 Endometriosis of the anterior abdominal wall, unspecified depth**
Endometriosis of the anterior abdominal wall NOS

**N8Ø.C2 Endometriosis of the umbilicus**

**N8Ø.C3 Endometriosis of the inguinal canal**

**N8Ø.C4 Endometriosis of extra-pelvic abdominal peritoneum**

**N8Ø.C9 Endometriosis of other site of abdomen**

✓5th **N8Ø.D Endometriosis of the pelvic nerves**
Endometriosis of the nerves of the retroperitoneum

**N8Ø.DØ Endometriosis of the pelvic nerves, unspecified**
Endometriosis of nerve of the retroperitoneum, NOS

**N8Ø.D1 Endometriosis of the sacral splanchnic nerves**
Endometriosis of the pelvic splanchnic nerves

**N8Ø.D2 Endometriosis of the sacral nerve roots**

**N8Ø.D3 Endometriosis of the obturator nerve**

**N8Ø.D4 Endometriosis of the sciatic nerve**

**N8Ø.D5 Endometriosis of the pudendal nerve**

**N8Ø.D6 Endometriosis of the femoral nerve**

**N8Ø.D9 Endometriosis of other pelvic nerve**
Endometriosis of the other nerves of the retroperitoneum

**N8Ø.8 Other endometriosis**
Endometriosis of other site

**N8Ø.9 Endometriosis, unspecified**

✓4th **N81 Female genital prolapse**

EXCLUDES 1 *genital prolapse complicating pregnancy, labor or delivery (O34.5-)*
*prolapse and hernia of ovary and fallopian tube (N83.4-)*
*prolapse of vaginal vault after hysterectomy (N99.3)*

**Types of Pelvic Organ Prolapse**

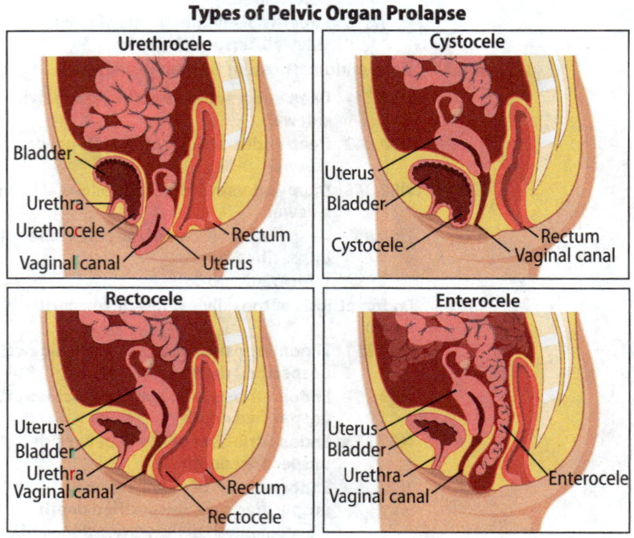


**N81.Ø Urethrocele**

EXCLUDES 1 *urethrocele with cystocele (N81.1-)*
*urethrocele with prolapse of uterus (N81.2-N81.4)*

✓5th **N81.1 Cystocele**
Cystocele with urethrocele
Cystourethrocele

EXCLUDES 1 *cystocele with prolapse of uterus (N81.2-N81.4)*

**N81.1Ø Cystocele, unspecified** Q
Prolapse of (anterior) vaginal wall NOS

**N81.11 Cystocele, midline** Q

**N81.12 Cystocele, lateral** Q
Paravaginal cystocele
**DEF:** Detachment of the lateral support connections of the vagina at the arcus tendineus fasciae pelvis (ATFP) that results in bladder drop. The bladder herniates into the vagina laterally.

**N81.2 Incomplete uterovaginal prolapse** Q
First degree uterine prolapse
Prolapse of cervix NOS
Second degree uterine prolapse

EXCLUDES 1 *cervical stump prolapse (N81.85)*

**N81.3 Complete uterovaginal prolapse** Q
Procidentia (uteri) NOS
Third degree uterine prolapse

**N81.4 Uterovaginal prolapse, unspecified** Q
Prolapse of uterus NOS

**N81.5 Vaginal enterocele**
EXCLUDES 1 *enterocele with prolapse of uterus (N81.2-N81.4)*

**N81.6 Rectocele**
Prolapse of posterior vaginal wall
Use additional code for any associated fecal incontinence, if applicable (R15.-)
EXCLUDES 1 *rectocele with prolapse of uterus (N81.2-N81.4)*
EXCLUDES 2 *perineocele (N81.81)*
*rectal prolapse (K62.3)*

√5th **N81.8 Other female genital prolapse**
**N81.81 Perineocele**
**N81.82 Incompetence or weakening of pubocervical tissue**
**N81.83 Incompetence or weakening of rectovaginal tissue**
**N81.84 Pelvic muscle wasting**
Disuse atrophy of pelvic muscles and anal sphincter
**N81.85 Cervical stump prolapse**
**N81.89 Other female genital prolapse** Q
Deficient perineum
Old laceration of muscles of pelvic floor

**N81.9 Female genital prolapse, unspecified** Q

√4th **N82 Fistulae involving female genital tract**
EXCLUDES 1 *vesicointestinal fistulae (N32.1)*

**N82.Ø Vesicovaginal fistula**
**N82.1 Other female urinary-genital tract fistulae**
Cervicovesical fistula
Ureterovaginal fistula
Urethrovaginal fistula
Uteroureteric fistula
Uterovesical fistula
**AHA:** 2017,3Q,3
**N82.2 Fistula of vagina to small intestine**
**N82.3 Fistula of vagina to large intestine**
Rectovaginal fistula
**N82.4 Other female intestinal-genital tract fistulae**
Intestinouterine fistula
**N82.5 Female genital tract-skin fistulae**
Uterus to abdominal wall fistula
Vaginoperineal fistula
**N82.8 Other female genital tract fistulae**
**N82.9 Female genital tract fistula, unspecified**

√4th **N83 Noninflammatory disorders of ovary, fallopian tube and broad ligament**
EXCLUDES 2 *hydrosalpinx (N7Ø.1-)*
**AHA:** 2016,4Q,46

√5th **N83.Ø Follicular cyst of ovary**
Cyst of graafian follicle
Hemorrhagic follicular cyst (of ovary)
**N83.ØØ Follicular cyst of ovary, unspecified side**
**N83.Ø1 Follicular cyst of right ovary**
**N83.Ø2 Follicular cyst of left ovary**

√5th **N83.1 Corpus luteum cyst**
Hemorrhagic corpus luteum cyst
**AHA:** 2022,1Q,23
**N83.1Ø Corpus luteum cyst of ovary, unspecified side**
**N83.11 Corpus luteum cyst of right ovary**
**N83.12 Corpus luteum cyst of left ovary**

√5th **N83.2 Other and unspecified ovarian cysts**
EXCLUDES 1 *developmental ovarian cyst (Q5Ø.1)*
*neoplastic ovarian cyst (D27.-)*
*polycystic ovarian syndrome (E28.2)*
*Stein-Leventhal syndrome (E28.2)*
**AHA:** 2026,1Q,32; 2022,1Q,23

√6th **N83.2Ø Unspecified ovarian cysts**
**N83.2Ø1 Unspecified ovarian cyst, right side**
**N83.2Ø2 Unspecified ovarian cyst, left side**
**N83.2Ø9 Unspecified ovarian cyst, unspecified side**
Ovarian cyst, NOS

√6th **N83.29 Other ovarian cysts**
Retention cyst of ovary
Simple cyst of ovary
**N83.291 Other ovarian cyst, right side**
**N83.292 Other ovarian cyst, left side**
**N83.299 Other ovarian cyst, unspecified side**

√5th **N83.3 Acquired atrophy of ovary and fallopian tube**
√6th **N83.31 Acquired atrophy of ovary**
**N83.311 Acquired atrophy of right ovary**
**N83.312 Acquired atrophy of left ovary**
**N83.319 Acquired atrophy of ovary, unspecified side**
Acquired atrophy of ovary, NOS
√6th **N83.32 Acquired atrophy of fallopian tube**
**N83.321 Acquired atrophy of right fallopian tube**
**N83.322 Acquired atrophy of left fallopian tube**
**N83.329 Acquired atrophy of fallopian tube, unspecified side**
Acquired atrophy of fallopian tube, NOS
√6th **N83.33 Acquired atrophy of ovary and fallopian tube**
**N83.331 Acquired atrophy of right ovary and fallopian tube**
**N83.332 Acquired atrophy of left ovary and fallopian tube**
**N83.339 Acquired atrophy of ovary and fallopian tube, unspecified side**
Acquired atrophy of ovary and fallopian tube, NOS

√5th **N83.4 Prolapse and hernia of ovary and fallopian tube**
**N83.4Ø Prolapse and hernia of ovary and fallopian tube, unspecified side**
Prolapse and hernia of ovary and fallopian tube, NOS
**N83.41 Prolapse and hernia of right ovary and fallopian tube**
**N83.42 Prolapse and hernia of left ovary and fallopian tube**

√5th **N83.5 Torsion of ovary, ovarian pedicle and fallopian tube**
Torsion of accessory tube
√6th **N83.51 Torsion of ovary and ovarian pedicle**
**N83.511 Torsion of right ovary and ovarian pedicle**
**N83.512 Torsion of left ovary and ovarian pedicle**
**N83.519 Torsion of ovary and ovarian pedicle, unspecified side**
Torsion of ovary and ovarian pedicle, NOS
√6th **N83.52 Torsion of fallopian tube**
Torsion of hydatid of Morgagni
**N83.521 Torsion of right fallopian tube**
**N83.522 Torsion of left fallopian tube**
**N83.529 Torsion of fallopian tube, unspecified side**
Torsion of fallopian tube, NOS
**N83.53 Torsion of ovary, ovarian pedicle and fallopian tube**

**N83.6 Hematosalpinx**
EXCLUDES 1 *hematosalpinx (with) (in):*
*hematocolpos (N89.7)*
*hematometra (N85.7)*
*tubal pregnancy (OØØ.1-)*
**N83.7 Hematoma of broad ligament**
**N83.8 Other noninflammatory disorders of ovary, fallopian tube and broad ligament**
Broad ligament laceration syndrome [Allen-Masters]
**N83.9 Noninflammatory disorder of ovary, fallopian tube and broad ligament, unspecified**

√4th **N84 Polyp of female genital tract**
EXCLUDES 1 *adenomatous polyp (D28.-)*
*placental polyp (O9Ø.89)*

**N84.Ø Polyp of corpus uteri**
Polyp of endometrium
Polyp of uterus NOS
EXCLUDES 1 *polypoid endometrial hyperplasia (N85.Ø-)*
**N84.1 Polyp of cervix uteri**
Mucous polyp of cervix
**N84.2 Polyp of vagina**
**N84.3 Polyp of vulva**
Polyp of labia
**N84.8 Polyp of other parts of female genital tract**
**N84.9 Polyp of female genital tract, unspecified**

**✓4th N85 Other noninflammatory disorders of uterus, except cervix**
EXCLUDES 1 *endometriosis (N8Ø.-)*
*inflammatory diseases of uterus (N71.-)*
*noninflammatory disorders of cervix, except malposition (N86-N88)*
*polyp of corpus uteri (N84.Ø)*
*uterine prolapse (N81.-)*

**✓5th N85.Ø Endometrial hyperplasia**

**N85.ØØ Endometrial hyperplasia, unspecified**
Hyperplasia (adenomatous) (cystic) (glandular) of endometrium
Hyperplastic endometritis

**N85.Ø1 Benign endometrial hyperplasia**
Endometrial hyperplasia (complex) (simple) without atypia

**N85.Ø2 Endometrial intraepithelial neoplasia [EIN]**
Endometrial hyperplasia with atypia
EXCLUDES 1 *malignant neoplasm of endometrium (with endometrial intraepithelial neoplasia [EIN]) (C54.1)*

**N85.2 Hypertrophy of uterus**
Bulky or enlarged uterus
EXCLUDES 1 *puerperal hypertrophy of uterus (O9Ø.89)*

**N85.3 Subinvolution of uterus**
EXCLUDES 1 *puerperal subinvolution of uterus (O9Ø.89)*

**N85.4 Malposition of uterus**
Anteversion of uterus
Retroflexion of uterus
Retroversion of uterus
EXCLUDES 1 *malposition of uterus complicating pregnancy, labor or delivery (O34.5-, O65.5)*

**N85.5 Inversion of uterus**
EXCLUDES 1 *current obstetric trauma (O71.2)*
*postpartum inversion of uterus (O71.2)*
**DEF:** Abnormality in which the uterus turns inside out.

**Inversion of Uterus**

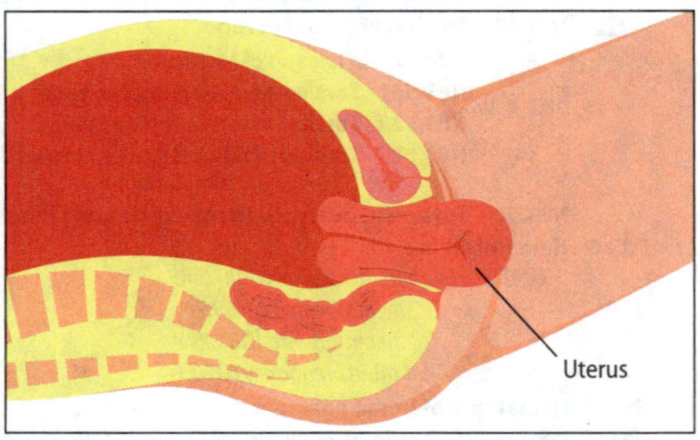


**N85.6 Intrauterine synechiae**

**N85.7 Hematometra**
Hematosalpinx with hematometra
EXCLUDES 1 *hematometra with hematocolpos (N89.7)*
**DEF:** Accumulation of blood within the uterus.

**N85.8 Other specified noninflammatory disorders of uterus**
Atrophy of uterus, acquired
Fibrosis of uterus NOS

**N85.9 Noninflammatory disorder of uterus, unspecified**
Disorder of uterus NOS

**N85.A Isthmocele**
Isthmocele (non-pregnant state)
Code also any associated conditions such as:
abnormal uterine and vaginal bleeding, unspecified (N93.9)
female infertility of uterine origin (N97.2)
pelvic and perineal pain (R1Ø.2-)
EXCLUDES 1 *maternal care for cesarean scar defect (isthmocele) (O34.22)*
**AHA:** 2022,4Q,36-37

**N86 Erosion and ectropion of cervix uteri**
Decubitus (trophic) ulcer of cervix
Eversion of cervix
EXCLUDES 1 *erosion and ectropion of cervix with cervicitis (N72)*

**✓4th N87 Dysplasia of cervix uteri**
EXCLUDES 1 *abnormal results from cervical cytologic examination without histologic confirmation (R87.61-)*
*carcinoma in situ of cervix uteri (DØ6.-)*
*cervical intraepithelial neoplasia III [CIN III] (DØ6.-)*
*HGSIL of cervix (R87.613)*
*severe dysplasia of cervix uteri (DØ6.-)*

**N87.Ø Mild cervical dysplasia**
Cervical intraepithelial neoplasia I [CIN I]

**N87.1 Moderate cervical dysplasia**
Cervical intraepithelial neoplasia II [CIN II]

**N87.9 Dysplasia of cervix uteri, unspecified**
Anaplasia of cervix
Cervical atypism
Cervical dysplasia NOS

**✓4th N88 Other noninflammatory disorders of cervix uteri**
EXCLUDES 2 *inflammatory disease of cervix (N72)*
*polyp of cervix (N84.1)*

**N88.Ø Leukoplakia of cervix uteri**

**N88.1 Old laceration of cervix uteri**
Adhesions of cervix
EXCLUDES 1 *current obstetric trauma (O71.3)*

**N88.2 Stricture and stenosis of cervix uteri**
EXCLUDES 1 *stricture and stenosis of cervix uteri complicating labor (O65.5)*

**N88.3 Incompetence of cervix uteri**
Investigation and management of (suspected) cervical incompetence in a nonpregnant woman
EXCLUDES 1 *cervical incompetence complicating pregnancy (O34.3-)*
**DEF:** Inadequate functioning of the cervix marked by abnormal widening during pregnancy and causing premature birth or miscarriage.

**N88.4 Hypertrophic elongation of cervix uteri**

**N88.8 Other specified noninflammatory disorders of cervix uteri**
EXCLUDES 1 *current obstetric trauma (O71.3)*

**N88.9 Noninflammatory disorder of cervix uteri, unspecified**

**✓4th N89 Other noninflammatory disorders of vagina**
EXCLUDES 1 *abnormal results from vaginal cytologic examination without histologic confirmation (R87.62-)*
*~~senile (atrophic) vaginitis (N95.2)~~*
*carcinoma in situ of vagina (DØ7.2)*
*HGSIL of vagina (R87.623)*
*inflammation of vagina (N76.-)*
*severe dysplasia of vagina (DØ7.2)*
*trichomonal leukorrhea (A59.ØØ)*
*vaginal intraepithelial neoplasia [VAIN], grade III (DØ7.2)*
EXCLUDES 2 ►*senile (atrophic) vaginitis (N95.2)*◄

**N89.Ø Mild vaginal dysplasia**
Vaginal intraepithelial neoplasia [VAIN], grade I

**N89.1 Moderate vaginal dysplasia**
Vaginal intraepithelial neoplasia [VAIN], grade II

**N89.3 Dysplasia of vagina, unspecified**

**N89.4 Leukoplakia of vagina**

**N89.5 Stricture and atresia of vagina**
Vaginal adhesions
Vaginal stenosis
EXCLUDES 1 *congenital atresia or stricture (Q52.4)*
*postprocedural adhesions of vagina (N99.2)*

**N89.6 Tight hymenal ring**
Rigid hymen
Tight introitus
EXCLUDES 1 *imperforate hymen (Q52.3)*

**N89.7 Hematocolpos**
Hematocolpos with hematometra or hematosalpinx
**AHA:** 2016,4Q,58

**N89.8 Other specified noninflammatory disorders of vagina**
Leukorrhea NOS
Old vaginal laceration
Pessary ulcer of vagina
EXCLUDES 1 *current obstetric trauma (O7Ø.-, O71.4, O71.7-O71.8)*
*old laceration involving muscles of pelvic floor (N81.8)*

**N89.9 Noninflammatory disorder of vagina, unspecified**

**N90 Other noninflammatory disorders of vulva and perineum**

EXCLUDES 1 *anogenital (venereal) warts (A63.0)*
*carcinoma in situ of vulva (D07.1)*
*condyloma acuminatum (A63.0)*
*current obstetric trauma (O70.-, O71.7-O71.8)*
*inflammation of vulva (N76.-)*
*severe dysplasia of vulva (D07.1)*
*vulvar intraepithelial neoplasm III [VIN III] (D07.1)*

**N90.0 Mild vulvar dysplasia**
Vulvar intraepithelial neoplasia [VIN], grade I

**N90.1 Moderate vulvar dysplasia**
Vulvar intraepithelial neoplasia [VIN], grade II

**N90.3 Dysplasia of vulva, unspecified**

**N90.4 Leukoplakia of vulva**
Dystrophy of vulva
Kraurosis of vulva
Lichen sclerosus of external female genital organs

**N90.5 Atrophy of vulva**
Stenosis of vulva

**N90.6 Hypertrophy of vulva**
AHA: 2016,4Q,46

**N90.60 Unspecified hypertrophy of vulva**
Unspecified hypertrophy of labia

**N90.61 Childhood asymmetric labium majus enlargement**
CALME

**N90.69 Other specified hypertrophy of vulva**
Other specified hypertrophy of labia

**N90.7 Vulvar cyst**

**N90.8 Other specified noninflammatory disorders of vulva and perineum**

**N90.81 Female genital mutilation status**
Female genital cutting status

**N90.810 Female genital mutilation status, unspecified**
Female genital cutting status, unspecified
Female genital mutilation status NOS

**N90.811 Female genital mutilation Type I status**
Clitorectomy status
Female genital cutting Type I status

**N90.812 Female genital mutilation Type II status**
Clitorectomy with excision of labia minora status
Female genital cutting Type II status

**N90.813 Female genital mutilation Type III status**
Female genital cutting Type III status
Infibulation status

**N90.818 Other female genital mutilation status**
Female genital cutting Type IV status
Female genital mutilation Type IV status
Other female genital cutting status

**N90.89 Other specified noninflammatory disorders of vulva and perineum**
Adhesions of vulva
Hypertrophy of clitoris

**N90.9 Noninflammatory disorder of vulva and perineum, unspecified**

**N91 Absent, scanty and rare menstruation**

EXCLUDES 1 *ovarian dysfunction (E28.-)*

**N91.0 Primary amenorrhea**

**N91.1 Secondary amenorrhea**

**N91.2 Amenorrhea, unspecified**

**N91.3 Primary oligomenorrhea**

**N91.4 Secondary oligomenorrhea**

**N91.5 Oligomenorrhea, unspecified**
Hypomenorrhea NOS

**N92 Excessive, frequent and irregular menstruation**

EXCLUDES 1 *postmenopausal bleeding (N95.0)*
*precocious puberty (menstruation) (E30.1)*

**N92.0 Excessive and frequent menstruation with regular cycle**
Heavy periods NOS
Menorrhagia NOS
Polymenorrhea

**N92.1 Excessive and frequent menstruation with irregular cycle**
Irregular intermenstrual bleeding
Irregular, shortened intervals between menstrual bleeding
Menometrorrhagia
Metrorrhagia

**N92.2 Excessive menstruation at puberty** P
Excessive bleeding associated with onset of menstrual periods
Pubertal menorrhagia
Puberty bleeding

**N92.3 Ovulation bleeding**
Regular intermenstrual bleeding

**N92.4 Excessive bleeding in the premenopausal period**
Climacteric menorrhagia or metrorrhagia
Menopausal menorrhagia or metrorrhagia
Perimenopausal bleeding
Perimenopausal menorrhagia or metrorrhagia
Preclimacteric menorrhagia or metrorrhagia
Premenopausal menorrhagia or metrorrhagia

**N92.5 Other specified irregular menstruation**

**N92.6 Irregular menstruation, unspecified**
Irregular bleeding NOS
Irregular periods NOS

EXCLUDES 1 *irregular menstruation with:*
*lengthened intervals or scanty bleeding (N91.3-N91.5)*
*shortened intervals or excessive bleeding (N92.1)*

**N93 Other abnormal uterine and vaginal bleeding**

EXCLUDES 1 *neonatal vaginal hemorrhage (P54.6)*
*precocious puberty (menstruation) (E30.1)*
*pseudomenses (P54.6)*

**N93.0 Postcoital and contact bleeding**

**N93.1 Pre-pubertal vaginal bleeding**
AHA: 2016,4Q,47

**N93.8 Other specified abnormal uterine and vaginal bleeding**
Dysfunctional or functional uterine or vaginal bleeding NOS

**N93.9 Abnormal uterine and vaginal bleeding, unspecified**

**N94 Pain and other conditions associated with female genital organs and menstrual cycle**

**N94.0 Mittelschmerz**
DEF: One-sided, lower abdominal pain occurring between menstrual periods that is associated with ovulation.

**N94.1 Dyspareunia**

EXCLUDES 1 *psychogenic dyspareunia (F52.6)*

AHA: 2016,4Q,47

**N94.10 Unspecified dyspareunia**

**N94.11 Superficial (introital) dyspareunia**

**N94.12 Deep dyspareunia**

**N94.19 Other specified dyspareunia**

**N94.2 Vaginismus**

EXCLUDES 1 *psychogenic vaginismus (F52.5)*

DEF: Spontaneous contractions of the muscles surrounding the vagina, causing it to constrict or close.

**N94.3 Premenstrual tension syndrome**
Code also associated menstrual migraine (G43.82-, G43.83-)

EXCLUDES 1 *premenstrual dysphoric disorder (F32.81)*

**N94.4 Primary dysmenorrhea**

**N94.5 Secondary dysmenorrhea**

**N94.6 Dysmenorrhea, unspecified**

EXCLUDES 1 *psychogenic dysmenorrhea (F45.8)*

**N94.8 Other specified conditions associated with female genital organs and menstrual cycle**

**N94.81 Vulvodynia**

**N94.810 Vulvar vestibulitis**

**N94.818 Other vulvodynia**

**N94.819 Vulvodynia, unspecified**
Vulvodynia NOS

**N94.89 Other specified conditions associated with female genital organs and menstrual cycle**
DEF: Hydrocele: Serous fluid that collects in the canal of Nuck in females.

**N94.9 Unspecified condition associated with female genital organs and menstrual cycle**

Chapter 14. Diseases of the Genitourinary System

N90–N94.9

✓4th **N95 Menopausal and other perimenopausal disorders**
Menopausal and other perimenopausal disorders due to naturally occurring (age-related) menopause and perimenopause
EXCLUDES 1 *excessive bleeding in the premenopausal period (N92.4)*
*menopausal and perimenopausal disorders due to artificial or premature menopause (E89.4-, E28.31-)*
*premature menopause (E28.31-)*
EXCLUDES 2 *postmenopausal osteoporosis (M81.Ø-)*
*postmenopausal osteoporosis with current pathological fracture (M8Ø.Ø-)*
*postmenopausal urethritis (N34.2)*

**N95.Ø Postmenopausal bleeding**

**N95.1 Menopausal and female climacteric states**
Symptoms such as flushing, sleeplessness, headache, lack of concentration, associated with natural (age-related) menopause
Use additional code for associated symptoms
EXCLUDES 1 *asymptomatic menopausal state (Z78.Ø)*
*symptoms associated with artificial menopause (E89.41)*
*symptoms associated with premature menopause (E28.31Ø)*

**N95.2 Postmenopausal atrophic vaginitis**
Senile (atrophic) vaginitis

**N95.8 Other specified menopausal and perimenopausal disorders**

**N95.9 Unspecified menopausal and perimenopausal disorder**

**N96 Recurrent pregnancy loss**
Investigation or care in a nonpregnant woman with history of recurrent pregnancy loss
EXCLUDES 1 *recurrent pregnancy loss with current pregnancy (O26.2-)*

✓4th **N97 Female infertility**
INCLUDES inability to achieve a pregnancy
sterility, female NOS
EXCLUDES 2 *female infertility associated with:*
*hypopituitarism (E23.Ø)*
*incompetence of cervix uteri (N88.3)*
*Stein-Leventhal syndrome (E28.2)*

**DEF:** Infertility: Inability to conceive for at least one year with regular intercourse.
**DEF:** Primary infertility: Infertility occurring in patients who have never conceived.
**DEF:** Secondary infertility: Infertility occurring in patients who have previously conceived.

**N97.Ø Female infertility associated with anovulation**
**AHA:** 2022,2Q,16

**N97.1 Female infertility of tubal origin**
Female infertility associated with congenital anomaly of tube
Female infertility due to tubal block
Female infertility due to tubal occlusion
Female infertility due to tubal stenosis

**N97.2 Female infertility of uterine origin**
Female infertility associated with congenital anomaly of uterus
Female infertility due to nonimplantation of ovum

**N97.8 Female infertility of other origin**
**AHA:** 2022,2Q,15

**N97.9 Female infertility, unspecified**

✓4th **N98 Complications associated with artificial fertilization**

**N98.Ø Infection associated with artificial insemination**

**N98.1 Hyperstimulation of ovaries**
Hyperstimulation of ovaries associated with induced ovulation
Hyperstimulation of ovaries NOS

**N98.2 Complications of attempted introduction of fertilized ovum following in vitro fertilization**

**N98.3 Complications of attempted introduction of embryo in embryo transfer**

**N98.8 Other complications associated with artificial fertilization**

**N98.9 Complication associated with artificial fertilization, unspecified**

## Intraoperative and postprocedural complications and disorders of genitourinary system, not elsewhere classified (N99)

✓4th **N99 Intraoperative and postprocedural complications and disorders of genitourinary system, not elsewhere classified**
EXCLUDES 2 *irradiation cystitis (N3Ø.4-)*
*postoophorectomy osteoporosis with current pathological fracture (M8Ø.8-)*
*postoophorectomy osteoporosis without current pathological fracture (M81.8)*

**N99.Ø Postprocedural (acute) (chronic) kidney failure**
Use additional code to type of kidney disease

✓5th **N99.1 Postprocedural urethral stricture**
Postcatheterization urethral stricture

✓6th **N99.11 Postprocedural urethral stricture, male**
**AHA:** 2016,4Q,47-48

**N99.11Ø Postprocedural urethral stricture, male, meatal**
**N99.111 Postprocedural bulbous urethral stricture, male**
**N99.112 Postprocedural membranous urethral stricture, male**
**N99.113 Postprocedural anterior bulbous urethral stricture, male**
**N99.114 Postprocedural urethral stricture, male, unspecified**
**N99.115 Postprocedural fossa navicularis urethral stricture**
**N99.116 Postprocedural urethral stricture, male, overlapping sites**

**N99.12 Postprocedural urethral stricture, female**

**N99.2 Postprocedural adhesions of vagina**

**N99.3 Prolapse of vaginal vault after hysterectomy**

**N99.4 Postprocedural pelvic peritoneal adhesions**
EXCLUDES 2 *pelvic peritoneal adhesions NOS (N73.6)*
*postinfective pelvic peritoneal adhesions (N73.6)*

✓5th **N99.5 Complications of stoma of urinary tract**
EXCLUDES 2 *mechanical complication of urinary catheter (T83.Ø-)*
**AHA:** 2016,4Q,48

✓6th **N99.51 Complication of cystostomy**
**N99.51Ø Cystostomy hemorrhage** ESR
**N99.511 Cystostomy infection** ESR
**N99.512 Cystostomy malfunction** ESR
**N99.518 Other cystostomy complication** ESR

✓6th **N99.52 Complication of incontinent external stoma of urinary tract**
**N99.52Ø Hemorrhage of incontinent external stoma of urinary tract** ESR
**N99.521 Infection of incontinent external stoma of urinary tract** ESR
**N99.522 Malfunction of incontinent external stoma of urinary tract** ESR
**N99.523 Herniation of incontinent stoma of urinary tract** ESR
**N99.524 Stenosis of incontinent stoma of urinary tract** ESR
**N99.528 Other complication of incontinent external stoma of urinary tract** ESR

✓6th **N99.53 Complication of continent stoma of urinary tract**
**N99.53Ø Hemorrhage of continent stoma of urinary tract** ESR
**N99.531 Infection of continent stoma of urinary tract** ESR
**N99.532 Malfunction of continent stoma of urinary tract** ESR
**N99.533 Herniation of continent stoma of urinary tract** ESR
**N99.534 Stenosis of continent stoma of urinary tract** ESR
**N99.538 Other complication of continent stoma of urinary tract** ESR

✓5th **N99.6 Intraoperative hemorrhage and hematoma of a genitourinary system organ or structure complicating a procedure**

EXCLUDES 1 *intraoperative hemorrhage and hematoma of a genitourinary system organ or structure due to accidental puncture or laceration during a procedure (N99.7-)*

**N99.61 Intraoperative hemorrhage and hematoma of a genitourinary system organ or structure complicating a genitourinary system procedure**

**N99.62 Intraoperative hemorrhage and hematoma of a genitourinary system organ or structure complicating other procedure**

✓5th **N99.7 Accidental puncture and laceration of a genitourinary system organ or structure during a procedure**

**N99.71 Accidental puncture and laceration of a genitourinary system organ or structure during a genitourinary system procedure**

**N99.72 Accidental puncture and laceration of a genitourinary system organ or structure during other procedure**

✓5th **N99.8 Other intraoperative and postprocedural complications and disorders of genitourinary system**

AHA: 2016,4Q,9-10

**N99.81 Other intraoperative complications of genitourinary system**

✓6th **N99.82 Postprocedural hemorrhage of a genitourinary system organ or structure following a procedure**

**N99.820 Postprocedural hemorrhage of a genitourinary system organ or structure following a genitourinary system procedure**

AHA: 2025,2Q,20-21

**N99.821 Postprocedural hemorrhage of a genitourinary system organ or structure following other procedure**

**N99.83 Residual ovary syndrome**

✓6th **N99.84 Postprocedural hematoma and seroma of a genitourinary system organ or structure following a procedure**

**N99.840 Postprocedural hematoma of a genitourinary system organ or structure following a genitourinary system procedure**

**N99.841 Postprocedural hematoma of a genitourinary system organ or structure following other procedure**

**N99.842 Postprocedural seroma of a genitourinary system organ or structure following a genitourinary system procedure**

**N99.843 Postprocedural seroma of a genitourinary system organ or structure following other procedure**

**N99.85 Post endometrial ablation syndrome**

AHA: 2019,4Q,12

● ✓6th **N99.86 Intraoperative and postprocedural complications and disorders of breast**

● **N99.860 Intraoperative and postprocedural nipple ischemia**

● **N99.861 Intraoperative and postprocedural nipple necrosis**

**N99.89 Other postprocedural complications and disorders of genitourinary system**

# Chapter 15. Pregnancy, Childbirth, and the Puerperium (O00–O9A)

## Chapter-specific Guidelines with Coding Examples

The chapter-specific guidelines from the ICD-10-CM Official Guidelines for Coding and Reporting have been provided below. Along with these guidelines are coding examples, contained in the shaded boxes, that have been developed to help illustrate the coding and/or sequencing guidance found in these guidelines.

### a. General rules for obstetric cases

**1) Codes from Chapter 15 and sequencing priority**

Obstetric cases require codes from chapter 15, codes in the range O00-O9A, Pregnancy, Childbirth, and the Puerperium. Chapter 15 codes have sequencing priority over codes from other chapters. Additional codes from other chapters may be used in conjunction with chapter 15 codes to further specify conditions. Should the provider document that the pregnancy is incidental to the encounter, then code Z33.1, Pregnant state, incidental, should be used in place of any chapter 15 codes. It is the provider's responsibility to state that the condition being treated is not affecting the pregnancy.

> Bladder abscess in pregnant patient at 25 weeks' gestation
>
> **O23.12 Infections of bladder in pregnancy, second trimester**
>
> **N30.80 Other cystitis without hematuria**
>
> **Z3A.25 25 weeks gestation of pregnancy**
>
> *Explanation:* The documentation does not indicate that the pregnancy is incidental or in any way unaffected by the bladder abscess; therefore, an obstetrics code should be sequenced first. An additional code was provided to identify the specific bladder condition as this information is not called out specifically in the obstetrics code.

**2) Chapter 15 codes used only on the maternal record**

Chapter 15 codes are to be used only on the maternal record, never on the record of the newborn.

**3) Final character for trimester**

The majority of codes in Chapter 15 have a final character indicating the trimester of pregnancy. The timeframes for the trimesters are indicated at the beginning of the chapter. If trimester is not a component of a code, it is because the condition always occurs in a specific trimester, or the concept of trimester of pregnancy is not applicable. Certain codes have characters for only certain trimesters because the condition does not occur in all trimesters, but it may occur in more than just one. Assignment of the final character for trimester should be based on the provider's documentation of the trimester (or number of weeks) for the current admission/encounter. This applies to the assignment of trimester for pre-existing conditions as well as those that develop during or are due to the pregnancy. The provider's documentation of the number of weeks may be used to assign the appropriate code identifying the trimester.

> Pregnant patient at 21 weeks' gestation admitted with excessive vomiting
>
> **O21.2 Late vomiting of pregnancy**
>
> **Z3A.21 21 weeks gestation of pregnancy**
>
> *Explanation:* Category O21 classifies vomiting in pregnancy. Although code selection is based on whether the vomiting is before or after 20 completed weeks, these codes are not further classified by trimester. If vomiting only in the second trimester was documented, the provider should be queried for the specific week of gestation, as this will affect code selection.

Whenever delivery occurs during the current admission, and there is an "in childbirth" option for the obstetric complication being coded, the "in childbirth" code should be assigned. When the classification does not provide an obstetric code with an "in childbirth" option, it is appropriate to assign a code describing the current trimester.

**4) Selection of trimester for inpatient admissions that encompass more than one trimester**

In instances when a patient is admitted to a hospital for complications of pregnancy during one trimester and remains in the hospital into a subsequent trimester, the trimester character for the antepartum complication code should be assigned on the basis of the trimester when the complication developed, not the trimester of the discharge. If the condition developed prior to the current admission/encounter or represents a pre-existing condition, the trimester character for the trimester at the time of the admission/encounter should be assigned.

**5) Unspecified trimester**

Each category that includes codes for trimester has a code for "unspecified trimester." The "unspecified trimester" code should rarely be used, such as when the documentation in the record is insufficient to determine the trimester and it is not possible to obtain clarification.

**6) 7th character for fetus identification**

Where applicable, a 7th character is to be assigned for certain categories (O31, O32, O33.3 - O33.6, O35, O36, O40, O41, O60.1, O60.2, O64, and O69) to identify the fetus for which the complication code applies.

Assign 7th character "0":

- For single gestations.
- When the documentation in the record is insufficient to determine the fetus affected and it is not possible to obtain clarification.
- When it is not possible to clinically determine which fetus is affected.

> Maternal patient with twin gestations is seen after ultrasound identifies fetus B to be in breech presentation
>
> **O32.1XX2 Maternal care for breech presentation, fetus 2**
>
> *Explanation:* The documentation indicates that although there are two fetuses, only one fetus is determined to be in breech presentation. Whether fetus 2 or fetus B is used, the coder can assign the seventh character of 2 to identify the second fetus as the one in breech.

**7) Completed weeks of gestation**

In ICD-10-CM, "completed" weeks of gestation refers to full weeks. For example, if the provider documents gestation at 39 weeks and 6 days, the code for 39 weeks of gestation should be assigned, as the patient has not yet reached 40 completed weeks.

### b. Selection of OB principal or first-listed diagnosis

**1) Routine outpatient prenatal visits**

For routine outpatient prenatal visits when no complications are present, a code from category Z34, Encounter for supervision of normal pregnancy, should be used as the first-listed diagnosis. These codes should not be used in conjunction with chapter 15 codes.

**2) Supervision of high-risk pregnancy**

Codes from category O09, Supervision of high-risk pregnancy, are intended for use only during the prenatal period. For complications during the labor or delivery episode as a result of a high-risk pregnancy, assign the applicable complication codes from Chapter 15. If there are no complications during the labor or delivery episode, assign code O80, Encounter for full-term uncomplicated delivery.

For routine prenatal outpatient visits for patients with high-risk pregnancies, a code from category O09, Supervision of high-risk pregnancy, should be used as the first-listed diagnosis. Secondary chapter 15 codes may be used in conjunction with these codes if appropriate.

> 36-year-old seen in labor with second child at 39 weeks' gestation, delivered a healthy baby, delivery complicated by tear of fourchette that was repaired
>
> **O70.0 First degree perineal laceration during delivery**
>
> **Z3A.39 39 weeks gestation of pregnancy**
>
> **Z37.0 Single live birth**
>
> Explanation: Although this patient is over 35 and having her second child (elderly multigravida), do not append a code from subcategory O09.52-. A code describing the tear of the fourchette, which complicated the delivery, should be used in addition to the applicable Z codes.

**3) Episodes when no delivery occurs**

In episodes when no delivery occurs, the principal diagnosis should correspond to the principal complication of the pregnancy which necessitated the encounter. Should more than one complication exist, all of which are treated or monitored, any of the complication codes may be sequenced first.

**4) When a delivery occurs**

When an obstetric patient is admitted and delivers during that admission, the condition that prompted the admission should be sequenced as the principal diagnosis. If multiple conditions prompted the admission, sequence the one most related to the delivery as the principal diagnosis. A code for any complication of the delivery should be assigned as an additional diagnosis. In cases of cesarean delivery, if the patient was admitted with a condition that resulted in the performance of a cesarean procedure, that condition should be selected as the principal diagnosis. If the reason for the admission was unrelated to the condition resulting in the cesarean delivery, the condition related to the reason for the admission should be selected as the principal diagnosis.

Maternal patient with diet-controlled gestational diabetes was seen at 38 weeks' gestation in obstructed labor due to footling presentation; cesarean performed for the malpresentation

| | |
|---|---|
| **O64.8XXØ** | **Obstructed labor due to other malposition and malpresentation, not applicable or unspecified** |
| **O24.42Ø** | **Gestational diabetes mellitus in childbirth, diet controlled** |
| **Z3A.38** | **38 weeks gestation of pregnancy** |
| **Z37.Ø** | **Single live birth** |

*Explanation:* The obstructed labor necessitated the cesarean procedure.

**5) Outcome of delivery**

A code from category Z37, Outcome of delivery, should be included on every maternal record when a delivery has occurred. These codes are not to be used on subsequent records or on the newborn record.

**c. Pre-existing conditions versus conditions due to the pregnancy**

Certain categories in Chapter 15 distinguish between conditions of the mother that existed prior to pregnancy (pre-existing) and those that are a direct result of pregnancy. When assigning codes from Chapter 15, it is important to assess if a condition was pre-existing prior to pregnancy or developed during or due to the pregnancy in order to assign the correct code.

Categories that do not distinguish between pre-existing and pregnancy-related conditions may be used for either. It is acceptable to use codes specifically for the puerperium with codes complicating pregnancy and childbirth if a condition arises postpartum during the delivery encounter.

Type 2 diabetic patient presents at 19 weeks gestation for glucose check. Patient has been taking oral metformin for several years and currently is experiencing no diabetic complications.

| | |
|---|---|
| **O24.112** | **Pre-existing type 2 diabetes mellitus, in pregnancy, second trimester** |
| **E11.9** | **Type 2 diabetes mellitus without complications** |
| **Z79.84** | **Long term (current) use of oral hypoglycemic drugs** |

*Explanation:* The documentation states that the patient has been on a diabetic medication (oral metformin) for several years, indicating the patient was diabetic prior to becoming pregnant. Reporting pre-existing Type 2 diabetes in a pregnant patient requires two codes to capture the condition, a code from category O24 and a code from category E11. A note at E11 indicates that the code for long-term use of oral hypoglycemic drugs should also be reported.

**d. Pre-existing hypertension in pregnancy**

Category O1Ø, Pre-existing hypertension complicating pregnancy, childbirth and the puerperium, includes codes for hypertensive heart and hypertensive chronic kidney disease. When assigning one of the O1Ø codes that includes hypertensive heart disease or hypertensive chronic kidney disease, it is necessary to add a secondary code from the appropriate hypertension category to specify the type of heart failure or chronic kidney disease.

*See Section I.C.9. Hypertension.*

**e. Fetal conditions affecting the management of the mother**

**1) Codes from categories O35 and O36**

Codes from categories O35, Maternal care for known or suspected fetal abnormality and damage, and O36, Maternal care for other fetal problems, are assigned only when the fetal condition is actually responsible for modifying the management of the mother, i.e., by requiring diagnostic studies, additional observation, special care, or termination of pregnancy. The fact that the fetal condition exists does not justify assigning a code from this series to the mother's record.

A patient with twin gestation is seen for spotting 15 weeks into her pregnancy; the doctors also suspect fetal hydrocephalus. Patient is instructed to return in one week for additional diagnostic testing, sooner if the problem worsens.

| | |
|---|---|
| **O35.ØØXØ** | **Maternal care for (suspected) central nervous system malformation or damage in fetus, unspecified, not applicable or unspecified** |
| **O26.852** | **Spotting complicating pregnancy, second trimester** |
| **Z3A.15** | **15 weeks gestation of pregnancy** |

*Explanation:* Whether the fetal hydrocephalus was suspected or confirmed, an additional code is warranted for this condition since documentation indicates the patient is to return sooner than her routine visit for further testing.

**2) In utero surgery**

In cases when surgery is performed on the fetus, a diagnosis code from category O35, Maternal care for known or suspected fetal abnormality and damage, should be assigned identifying the fetal condition. Assign the appropriate procedure code for the procedure performed.

No code from Chapter 16, the perinatal codes, should be used on the mother's record to identify fetal conditions. Surgery performed in utero on a fetus is still to be coded as an obstetric encounter.

**f. HIV infection in pregnancy, childbirth and the puerperium**

During pregnancy, childbirth or the puerperium, a patient admitted because of an HIV-related illness should receive a principal diagnosis from subcategory O98.7-, Human immunodeficiency [HIV] disease complicating pregnancy, childbirth and the puerperium, followed by the code(s) for the HIV-related illness(es).

Patients with asymptomatic HIV infection status admitted during pregnancy, childbirth, or the puerperium should receive codes of O98.7- and Z21, Asymptomatic human immunodeficiency virus [HIV] infection status.

A previously asymptomatic HIV patient who is 13 weeks pregnant is evaluated for HIV-related candidal bronchitis

| | |
|---|---|
| **O98.711** | **Human immunodeficiency virus [HIV] disease complicating pregnancy, first trimester** |
| **B2Ø** | **Human immunodeficiency virus [HIV] disease** |
| **B37.1** | **Pulmonary candidiasis** |
| **Z3A.13** | **13 weeks gestation of pregnancy** |

*Explanation:* Because candidal bronchitis is an AIDS-related condition, this patient is now considered to have HIV disease. An obstetrics code indicating that HIV is complicating the pregnancy is coded first, followed by B2Ø for HIV disease as well as a code for the candidal bronchitis.

**g. Diabetes mellitus in pregnancy**

Diabetes mellitus is a significant complicating factor in pregnancy. Pregnant patients who are diabetic should be assigned a code from category O24, Diabetes mellitus in pregnancy, childbirth, and the puerperium, first, followed by the appropriate diabetes code(s) (EØ8-E13) from Chapter 4.

**h. Long term use of insulin and oral hypoglycemics**

*See section I.C.4.a.3 for information on the long term-use of insulin and oral hypoglycemics.*

**i. Gestational (pregnancy induced) diabetes**

Gestational (pregnancy induced) diabetes can occur during the second and third trimester of pregnancy in patients who were not diabetic prior to pregnancy. Gestational diabetes can cause complications in the pregnancy similar to those of pre-existing diabetes mellitus. It also puts the patient at greater risk of developing diabetes after the pregnancy.

Codes for gestational diabetes are in subcategory O24.4, Gestational diabetes mellitus. No other code from category O24, Diabetes mellitus in pregnancy, childbirth, and the puerperium, should be used with a code from O24.4.

The codes under subcategory O24.4 include diet controlled, insulin controlled, and controlled by oral hypoglycemic drugs. If a patient with gestational diabetes is treated with both diet and insulin, only the code for insulin-controlled is required. If a patient with gestational diabetes is treated with both diet and oral hypoglycemic medications, only the code for "controlled by oral hypoglycemic drugs" is required. Codes Z79.4, Long-term (current) use of insulin, Z79.84, Long-term (current) use of oral hypoglycemic drugs, and Z79.85, Long-term (current) use of injectable non-insulin antidiabetic drugs, should not be assigned with codes from subcategory O24.4.

An abnormal glucose tolerance in pregnancy is assigned a code from subcategory O99.81, Abnormal glucose complicating pregnancy, childbirth, and the puerperium.

**j. Sepsis and septic shock complicating abortion, pregnancy, childbirth and the puerperium**

When assigning a chapter 15 code for sepsis complicating abortion, pregnancy, childbirth, and the puerperium, a code for the specific type of infection should be assigned as an additional diagnosis. If severe sepsis is present, a code from subcategory R65.2, Severe sepsis, and code(s) for associated organ dysfunction(s) should also be assigned as additional diagnoses.

> Patient is seen several days after a miscarriage with sepsis; cultures return MSSA
>
> **O03.87** **Sepsis following complete or unspecified spontaneous abortion**
>
> **B95.61** **Methicillin susceptible Staphylococcus aureus infection as the cause of diseases classified elsewhere**
>
> *Explanation:* The type of infection that caused this patient to become septic was methicillin susceptible *Staphylococcus aureus* (MSSA), which as a secondary code helps capture all aspects related to this patient's septic condition.

**k. Puerperal sepsis**

Code O85, Puerperal sepsis, should be assigned with a secondary code to identify the causal organism (e.g., for a bacterial infection, assign a code from category B95-B96, Bacterial infections in conditions classified elsewhere). A code from category A40, Streptococcal sepsis, or A41, Other sepsis, should not be used for puerperal sepsis. If applicable, use additional codes to identify severe sepsis (R65.2-) and any associated acute organ dysfunction.

Code O85 should not be assigned for sepsis following an obstetrical procedure (See Section I.C.1.d.5.b., Sepsis due to a postprocedural infection).

**l. Alcohol, tobacco and drug use during pregnancy, childbirth and the puerperium**

**1) Alcohol use during pregnancy, childbirth and the puerperium**

Codes under subcategory O99.31, Alcohol use complicating pregnancy, childbirth, and the puerperium, should be assigned for any pregnancy case when a patient uses alcohol during the pregnancy or postpartum. A secondary code from category F10, Alcohol related disorders, should also be assigned to identify manifestations of the alcohol use.

**2) Tobacco use during pregnancy, childbirth and the puerperium**

Codes under subcategory O99.33, Smoking (tobacco) complicating pregnancy, childbirth, and the puerperium, should be assigned for any pregnancy case when a patient uses any type of tobacco product during the pregnancy or postpartum.

A secondary code from category F17, Nicotine dependence, should also be assigned to identify the type of nicotine dependence.

**3) Drug use during pregnancy, childbirth and the puerperium**

Codes under subcategory O99.32, Drug use complicating pregnancy, childbirth, and the puerperium, should be assigned for any pregnancy case when a patient uses drugs during the pregnancy or postpartum. This can involve illegal drugs, or inappropriate use or abuse of prescription drugs. Secondary code(s) from categories F11-F16 and F18-F19 should also be assigned to identify manifestations of the drug use.

**m. Poisoning, toxic effects, adverse effects and underdosing in a pregnant patient**

A code from subcategory O9A.2, Injury, poisoning and certain other consequences of external causes complicating pregnancy, childbirth, and the puerperium, should be sequenced first, followed by the appropriate injury, poisoning, toxic effect, adverse effect or underdosing code, and then the additional code(s) that specifies the condition caused by the poisoning, toxic effect, adverse effect or underdosing.

*See Section I.C.19. Adverse effects, poisoning, underdosing and toxic effects.*

> Patient treated for accidental carbon monoxide poisoning from a gas heating implement; the patient is 18 weeks' pregnant
>
> **O9A.212** **Injury, poisoning and certain other consequences of external causes complicating pregnancy, second trimester**
>
> **T58.11XA** **Toxic effect of carbon monoxide from utility gas, accidental (unintentional), initial encounter**
>
> **Z3A.18** **18 weeks gestation of pregnancy**
>
> *Explanation:* Although the carbon monoxide poisoning is the reason for the encounter, a code from the obstetrics chapter must be sequenced first. Chapter 15 codes have sequencing priority over codes from other chapters.

**n. Normal delivery, code O80**

**1) Encounter for full term uncomplicated delivery**

Code O80 should be assigned when a patient is admitted for a full-term normal delivery and delivers a single, healthy infant without any complications antepartum, during the delivery, or postpartum during the delivery episode. Code O80 is always a principal diagnosis. It is not to be used if any other code from chapter 15 is needed to describe a current complication of the antenatal, delivery, or postnatal period. Additional codes from other chapters may be used with code O80 if they are not related to or are in any way complicating the pregnancy.

**2) Uncomplicated delivery with resolved antepartum complication**

Code O80 may be used if the patient had a complication at some point during the pregnancy, but the complication is not present at the time of the admission for delivery.

> Patient presents in labor at 39 weeks' gestation and delivers a healthy newborn; patient had abnormal glucose levels in her first trimester, which have since resolved
>
> **O80** **Encounter for full-term uncomplicated delivery**
>
> **Z37.0** **Single live birth**
>
> *Explanation:* The abnormal glucose levels during the first trimester cannot be coded if they are not affecting the patient's current trimester. Without additional complications associated with the pregnancy, fetus, or mother, code O80 is appropriate.

**3) Outcome of delivery for O80**

Z37.0, Single live birth, is the only outcome of delivery code appropriate for use with O80.

**o. The peripartum and postpartum periods**

**1) Peripartum and postpartum periods**

The postpartum period begins immediately after delivery and continues for six weeks following delivery. The peripartum period is defined as the last month of pregnancy to five months postpartum.

**2) Peripartum and postpartum complication**

A postpartum complication is any complication occurring within the six-week period.

**3) Pregnancy-related complications after 6-week period**

Chapter 15 codes may also be used to describe pregnancy-related complications after the peripartum or postpartum period if the provider documents that a condition is pregnancy related.

> Patient referred for varicose veins. She had a baby boy three months ago; the varicose veins started to appear one month ago. The doctor attributes the patient's pregnancy as the cause of the varicose veins, which continue to be painful and bother the patient. She is seeking surgical relief.
>
> **O87.4** **Varicose veins of the lower extremity in the puerperium**
>
> *Explanation:* Although the varicose veins occurred several months after the delivery of the newborn, the doctor attributed the varicose veins to pregnancy and therefore a code from chapter 15 is appropriate.

**4) Admission for routine postpartum care following delivery outside hospital**

When the mother delivers outside the hospital prior to admission and is admitted for routine postpartum care and no complications are noted, code Z39.Ø, Encounter for care and examination of mother immediately after delivery, should be assigned as the principal diagnosis.

**5) Pregnancy associated cardiomyopathy**

Pregnancy associated cardiomyopathy, code O9Ø.3, is unique in that it may be diagnosed in the third trimester of pregnancy but may continue to progress months after delivery. For this reason, it is referred to as peripartum cardiomyopathy. Code O9Ø.3 is only for use when the cardiomyopathy develops as a result of pregnancy in a patient who did not have pre-existing heart disease.

**p. Code O94, Sequelae of complication of pregnancy, childbirth, and the puerperium**

**1) Code O94**

Code O94, Sequelae of complication of pregnancy, childbirth, and the puerperium, is for use in those cases when an initial complication of a pregnancy develops a sequela or sequelae requiring care or treatment at a future date.

**2) After the initial postpartum period**

This code may be used at any time after the initial postpartum period.

**3) Sequencing of code O94**

This code, like all sequela codes, is to be sequenced following the code describing the sequelae of the complication.

**q. Termination of pregnancy and spontaneous abortions**

**1) Abortion with liveborn fetus**

When an attempted termination of pregnancy results in a liveborn fetus, assign code Z33.2, Encounter for elective termination of pregnancy and a code from category Z37, Outcome of Delivery.

**2) Retained products of conception following an abortion**

Subsequent encounters for retained products of conception following a spontaneous abortion or elective termination of pregnancy, without complications are assigned OØ3.4, Incomplete spontaneous abortion without complication, or code OØ7.4, Failed attempted termination of pregnancy without complication. This advice is appropriate even when the patient was discharged previously with a discharge diagnosis of complete abortion. If the patient has a specific complication associated with the spontaneous abortion or elective termination of pregnancy in addition to retained products of conception, assign the appropriate complication code (e.g., OØ3.-, OØ4.-, OØ7.-) instead of code OØ3.4 or OØ7.4.

> Patient was seen two days ago for complete spontaneous abortion but returns today for urinary tract infection (UTI) with ultrasound showing retained products of conception
>
> **OØ3.38 Urinary tract infection following incomplete spontaneous abortion**
>
> *Explanation:* Although the diagnosis from the patient's previous stay indicated that the patient had a complete abortion, it is now determined that there were actually retained products of conception (POC). An abortion with retained POC is considered incomplete and in this case resulted in the patient developing a UTI.

**3) Complications leading to abortion**

Codes from Chapter 15 may be used as additional codes to identify any documented complications of the pregnancy in conjunction with codes in categories in OØ4, OØ7 and OØ8.

**4) Hemorrhage following elective abortion**

For hemorrhage post elective abortion, assign code OØ4.6, Delayed or excessive hemorrhage following (induced) termination of pregnancy. Do not assign code O72.1, Other immediate postpartum hemorrhage, as this code should not be assigned for post abortion conditions.

**r. Abuse in a pregnant patient**

For suspected or confirmed cases of abuse of a pregnant patient, a code(s) from subcategories O9A.3, Physical abuse complicating pregnancy, childbirth, and the puerperium, O9A.4, Sexual abuse complicating pregnancy, childbirth, and the puerperium, and O9A.5, Psychological abuse complicating pregnancy, childbirth, and the puerperium, should be sequenced first, followed by the appropriate codes (if applicable) to identify any associated current injury due to physical abuse, sexual abuse, and the perpetrator of abuse.

*See Section I.C.19. Adult and child abuse, neglect and other maltreatment.*

**s. COVID-19 infection in pregnancy, childbirth, and the puerperium**

During pregnancy, childbirth or the puerperium, when COVID-19 is the reason for admission/encounter, code O98.5-, Other viral diseases complicating pregnancy, childbirth and the puerperium, should be sequenced as the principal/first-listed diagnosis, and code UØ7.1, COVID-19, and the appropriate codes for associated manifestation(s) should be assigned as additional diagnoses. Codes from Chapter 15 always take sequencing priority.

If the reason for admission/encounter is unrelated to COVID-19 but the patient has been diagnosed with COVID-19 during the admission/encounter, the appropriate code for the reason for admission/encounter should be sequenced as the principal/first-listed diagnosis, and codes O98.5- and UØ7.1, as well as the appropriate codes for associated COVID-19 manifestations, should be assigned as additional diagnoses.

# Chapter 15. Pregnancy, Childbirth and the Puerperium (OØØ-O9A)

**NOTE** CODES FROM THIS CHAPTER ARE FOR USE ONLY ON MATERNAL RECORDS, NEVER ON NEWBORN RECORDS

Codes from this chapter are for use for conditions related to or aggravated by the pregnancy, childbirth, or by the puerperium (maternal causes or obstetric causes)

**NOTE** Trimesters are counted from the first day of the last menstrual period. They are defined as follows:

1st trimester- less than 14 weeks Ø days

2nd trimester- 14 weeks Ø days to less than 28 weeks Ø days

3rd trimester- 28 weeks Ø days until delivery

Use additional code, if applicable, from category Z3A, Weeks of gestation, to identify the specific week of the pregnancy, if known.

**EXCLUDES 1** *supervision of normal pregnancy (Z34.-)*

**EXCLUDES 2** *mental and behavioral disorders associated with the puerperium (F53.-)*
*obstetrical tetanus (A34)*
*postpartum necrosis of pituitary gland (E23.Ø)*
*puerperal osteomalacia (M83.Ø)*

**AHA:** 2025,3Q,21; 2016,1Q,3-5; 2014,3Q,17

This chapter contains the following blocks:

OØØ-OØ8 Pregnancy with abortive outcome
OØ9 Supervision of high risk pregnancy
O1Ø-O16 Edema, proteinuria and hypertensive disorders in pregnancy, childbirth and the puerperium
O2Ø-O29 Other maternal disorders predominantly related to pregnancy
O3Ø-O48 Maternal care related to the fetus and amniotic cavity and possible delivery problems
O6Ø-O77 Complications of labor and delivery
O8Ø-O82 Encounter for delivery
O85-O92 Complications predominantly related to the puerperium
O94-O9A Other obstetric conditions, not elsewhere classified

## Pregnancy with abortive outcome (OØØ-OØ8)

**EXCLUDES 1** *continuing pregnancy in multiple gestation after abortion of one fetus or more (O31.1-, O31.3-)*

**TIP:** Do not assign a code from category Z3A with codes in this code block.

**✓4th OØØ Ectopic pregnancy**

**INCLUDES** ruptured ectopic pregnancy

Use additional code from category OØ8 to identify any associated complication

**AHA:** 2016,4Q,48-50; 2014,3Q,17

**DEF:** Implantation of a fertilized egg outside the uterus, usually in the fallopian tube or abdomen that requires emergency treatment.

**Ectopic Pregnancy**

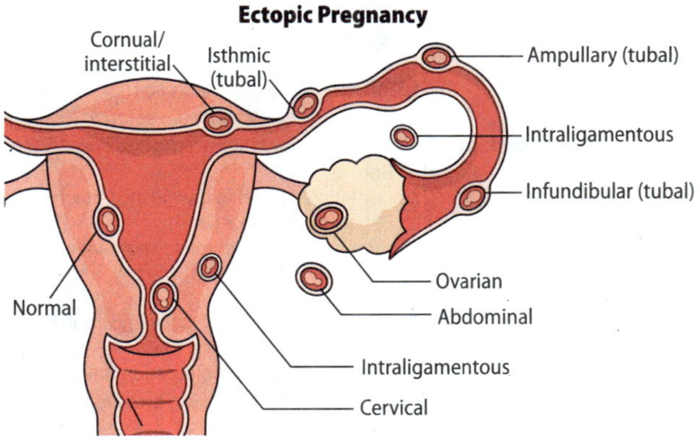


**✓5th OØØ.Ø Abdominal pregnancy**

**EXCLUDES 1** *maternal care for viable fetus in abdominal pregnancy (O36.7-)*

**OØØ.ØØ Abdominal pregnancy without intrauterine pregnancy** COM M
Abdominal pregnancy NOS

**OØØ.Ø1 Abdominal pregnancy with intrauterine pregnancy** COM M

**✓5th OØØ.1 Tubal pregnancy**
Fallopian pregnancy
Rupture of (fallopian) tube due to pregnancy
Tubal abortion
**AHA:** 2017,4Q,20

**✓6th OØØ.1Ø Tubal pregnancy without intrauterine pregnancy**
Tubal pregnancy NOS

**OØØ.1Ø1 Right tubal pregnancy without intrauterine pregnancy** COM M

**OØØ.1Ø2 Left tubal pregnancy without intrauterine pregnancy** COM M

**OØØ.1Ø9 Unspecified tubal pregnancy without intrauterine pregnancy** COM M

**✓6th OØØ.11 Tubal pregnancy with intrauterine pregnancy**

**OØØ.111 Right tubal pregnancy with intrauterine pregnancy** COM M

**OØØ.112 Left tubal pregnancy with intrauterine pregnancy** COM M

**OØØ.119 Unspecified tubal pregnancy with intrauterine pregnancy** COM M

**✓6th OØØ.12 Interstitial ectopic pregnancy without intrauterine pregnancy**

**OØØ.121 Right interstitial ectopic pregnancy without intrauterine pregnancy**

**OØØ.122 Left interstitial ectopic pregnancy without intrauterine pregnancy**

**OØØ.129 Unspecified interstitial ectopic pregnancy without intrauterine pregnancy**

**✓6th OØØ.13 Interstitial ectopic pregnancy with intrauterine pregnancy**

**OØØ.131 Right interstitial ectopic pregnancy with intrauterine pregnancy**

**OØØ.132 Left interstitial ectopic pregnancy with intrauterine pregnancy**

**OØØ.139 Unspecified interstitial ectopic pregnancy with intrauterine pregnancy**

**✓5th OØØ.2 Ovarian pregnancy**
**AHA:** 2017,4Q,20

**✓6th OØØ.2Ø Ovarian pregnancy without intrauterine pregnancy**
Ovarian pregnancy NOS

**OØØ.2Ø1 Right ovarian pregnancy without intrauterine pregnancy** COM M

**OØØ.2Ø2 Left ovarian pregnancy without intrauterine pregnancy** COM M

**OØØ.2Ø9 Unspecified ovarian pregnancy without intrauterine pregnancy** COM M

**✓6th OØØ.21 Ovarian pregnancy with intrauterine pregnancy**

**OØØ.211 Right ovarian pregnancy with intrauterine pregnancy** COM M

**OØØ.212 Left ovarian pregnancy with intrauterine pregnancy** COM M

**OØØ.219 Unspecified ovarian pregnancy with intrauterine pregnancy** COM M

**✓5th OØØ.3 Cesarean scar ectopic pregnancy**

**OØØ.31 Cesarean scar ectopic pregnancy without intrauterine pregnancy**

**OØØ.32 Cesarean scar ectopic pregnancy with intrauterine pregnancy**

**✓5th OØØ.4 Cervical ectopic pregnancy**

**OØØ.41 Cervical ectopic pregnancy without intrauterine pregnancy**

**OØØ.42 Cervical ectopic pregnancy with intrauterine pregnancy**

**✓5th OØØ.5 Cornual ectopic pregnancy**

**✓6th OØØ.51 Cornual ectopic pregnancy without intrauterine pregnancy**

**OØØ.511 Right cornual ectopic pregnancy without intrauterine pregnancy**

**OØØ.512 Left cornual ectopic pregnancy without intrauterine pregnancy**

**OØØ.519 Unspecified cornual ectopic pregnancy without intrauterine pregnancy**

**✓6th OØØ.52 Cornual ectopic pregnancy with intrauterine pregnancy**

**OØØ.521 Right cornual ectopic pregnancy with intrauterine pregnancy**

**OØØ.522 Left cornual ectopic pregnancy with intrauterine pregnancy**

**OØØ.529 Unspecified cornual ectopic pregnancy with intrauterine pregnancy**

✓5th **O00.8 Other ectopic pregnancy**

~~Cervical pregnancy~~
~~Cornual pregnancy~~
Intraligamentous pregnancy
Mural pregnancy

**O00.80 Other ectopic pregnancy without intrauterine pregnancy** COM M
Other ectopic pregnancy NOS

**O00.81 Other ectopic pregnancy with intrauterine pregnancy** COM M

✓5th **O00.9 Ectopic pregnancy, unspecified**

**O00.90 Unspecified ectopic pregnancy without intrauterine pregnancy** COM M
Ectopic pregnancy NOS

**O00.91 Unspecified ectopic pregnancy with intrauterine pregnancy** COM M

✓4th **O01 Hydatidiform mole**

Use additional code from category O08 to identify any associated complication

EXCLUDES 1 *chorioadenoma (destruens) (D39.2)*
*malignant hydatidiform mole (D39.2)*

**AHA:** 2014,3Q,17

**DEF:** Abnormal product of pregnancy, marked by a mass of cysts resembling a bunch of grapes due to chorionic villi proliferation and dissolution. It must be surgically removed.

**O01.0 Classical hydatidiform mole** COM M
Complete hydatidiform mole

**O01.1 Incomplete and partial hydatidiform mole** COM M

**O01.9 Hydatidiform mole, unspecified** COM M
Trophoblastic disease NOS
Vesicular mole NOS

✓4th **O02 Other abnormal products of conception**

Use additional code from category O08 to identify any associated complication

EXCLUDES 1 *papyraceous fetus (O31.0-)*

**AHA:** 2014,3Q,17

**O02.0 Blighted ovum and nonhydatidiform mole** COM M
Carneous mole
Fleshy mole
Intrauterine mole NOS
Molar pregnancy NEC
Pathological ovum

**O02.1 Missed abortion** COM M
Early fetal death, before completion of 20 weeks of gestation, with retention of dead fetus

EXCLUDES 1 *failed induced abortion (O07.-)*
*fetal death (intrauterine) (late) (O36.4)*
*missed abortion with blighted ovum (O02.0)*
*missed abortion with hydatidiform mole (O01.-)*
*missed abortion with nonhydatidiform (O02.0)*
*missed abortion with other abnormal products of conception (O02.8-)*
*missed delivery (O36.4)*
*stillbirth (P95)*

**AHA:** 2025,1Q,18; 2022,2Q,3; 2019,3Q,11

✓5th **O02.8 Other specified abnormal products of conception**

EXCLUDES 1 *abnormal products of conception with blighted ovum (O02.0)*
*abnormal products of conception with hydatidiform mole (O01.-)*
*abnormal products of conception with nonhydatidiform mole (O02.0)*

**O02.81 Inappropriate change in quantitative human chorionic gonadotropin (hCG) in early pregnancy** COM M
Biochemical pregnancy
Chemical pregnancy
Inappropriate level of quantitative human chorionic gonadotropin (hCG) for gestational age in early pregnancy

**O02.89 Other abnormal products of conception** COM M

**O02.9 Abnormal product of conception, unspecified** COM M

✓4th **O03 Spontaneous abortion**

NOTE Incomplete abortion includes retained products of conception following spontaneous abortion

INCLUDES miscarriage

**AHA:** 2025,1Q,18; 2023,1Q,17

**O03.0 Genital tract and pelvic infection following incomplete spontaneous abortion** COM M
Endometritis following incomplete spontaneous abortion
Oophoritis following incomplete spontaneous abortion
Parametritis following incomplete spontaneous abortion
Pelvic peritonitis following incomplete spontaneous abortion
Salpingitis following incomplete spontaneous abortion
Salpingo-oophoritis following incomplete spontaneous abortion

EXCLUDES 1 *sepsis following incomplete spontaneous abortion (O03.37)*
*urinary tract infection following incomplete spontaneous abortion (O03.38)*

**O03.1 Delayed or excessive hemorrhage following incomplete spontaneous abortion** COM M
Afibrinogenemia following incomplete spontaneous abortion
Defibrination syndrome following incomplete spontaneous abortion
Hemolysis following incomplete spontaneous abortion
Intravascular coagulation following incomplete spontaneous abortion

**AHA:** 2022,1Q,19

**O03.2 Embolism following incomplete spontaneous abortion** COM M
Air embolism following incomplete spontaneous abortion
Amniotic fluid embolism following incomplete spontaneous abortion
Blood-clot embolism following incomplete spontaneous abortion
Embolism NOS following incomplete spontaneous abortion
Fat embolism following incomplete spontaneous abortion
Pulmonary embolism following incomplete spontaneous abortion
Pyemic embolism following incomplete spontaneous abortion
Septic or septicopyemic embolism following incomplete spontaneous abortion
Soap embolism following incomplete spontaneous abortion

✓5th **O03.3 Other and unspecified complications following incomplete spontaneous abortion**

**O03.30 Unspecified complication following incomplete spontaneous abortion** COM M

**O03.31 Shock following incomplete spontaneous abortion** COM M
Circulatory collapse following incomplete spontaneous abortion
Shock (postprocedural) following incomplete spontaneous abortion

EXCLUDES 1 *shock due to infection following incomplete spontaneous abortion (O03.37)*

**O03.32 Renal failure following incomplete spontaneous abortion** COM M
Kidney failure (acute) following incomplete spontaneous abortion
Oliguria following incomplete spontaneous abortion
Renal shutdown following incomplete spontaneous abortion
Renal tubular necrosis following incomplete spontaneous abortion
Uremia following incomplete spontaneous abortion

**O03.33 Metabolic disorder following incomplete spontaneous abortion** COM M

**O03.34 Damage to pelvic organs following incomplete spontaneous abortion** COM M
Laceration, perforation, tear or chemical damage of bladder following incomplete spontaneous abortion
Laceration, perforation, tear or chemical damage of bowel following incomplete spontaneous abortion
Laceration, perforation, tear or chemical damage of broad ligament following incomplete spontaneous abortion
Laceration, perforation, tear or chemical damage of cervix following incomplete spontaneous abortion
Laceration, perforation, tear or chemical damage of periurethral tissue following incomplete spontaneous abortion
Laceration, perforation, tear or chemical damage of uterus following incomplete spontaneous abortion
Laceration, perforation, tear or chemical damage of vagina following incomplete spontaneous abortion

**O03.35 Other venous complications following incomplete spontaneous abortion** COM M

**O03.36 Cardiac arrest following incomplete spontaneous abortion** COM M

**O03.37 Sepsis following incomplete spontaneous abortion** COM M
Use additional code to identify infectious agent (B95-B97)
Use additional code to identify severe sepsis, if applicable (R65.2-)
EXCLUDES 1 *septic or septicopyemic embolism following incomplete spontaneous abortion (O03.2)*

**O03.38 Urinary tract infection following incomplete spontaneous abortion** COM M
Cystitis following incomplete spontaneous abortion

**O03.39 Incomplete spontaneous abortion with other complications** COM M

**O03.4 Incomplete spontaneous abortion without complication** COM M

**O03.5 Genital tract and pelvic infection following complete or unspecified spontaneous abortion** COM M
Endometritis following complete or unspecified spontaneous abortion
Oophoritis following complete or unspecified spontaneous abortion
Parametritis following complete or unspecified spontaneous abortion
Pelvic peritonitis following complete or unspecified spontaneous abortion
Salpingitis following complete or unspecified spontaneous abortion
Salpingo-oophoritis following complete or unspecified spontaneous abortion
EXCLUDES 1 *sepsis following complete or unspecified spontaneous abortion (O03.87)*
*urinary tract infection following complete or unspecified spontaneous abortion (O03.88)*

**O03.6 Delayed or excessive hemorrhage following complete or unspecified spontaneous abortion** COM M
Afibrinogenemia following complete or unspecified spontaneous abortion
Defibrination syndrome following complete or unspecified spontaneous abortion
Hemolysis following complete or unspecified spontaneous abortion
Intravascular coagulation following complete or unspecified spontaneous abortion
**AHA:** 2022,1Q,19

**O03.7 Embolism following complete or unspecified spontaneous abortion** COM M
Air embolism following complete or unspecified spontaneous abortion
Amniotic fluid embolism following complete or unspecified spontaneous abortion
Blood-clot embolism following complete or unspecified spontaneous abortion
Embolism NOS following complete or unspecified spontaneous abortion
Fat embolism following complete or unspecified spontaneous abortion
Pulmonary embolism following complete or unspecified spontaneous abortion
Pyemic embolism following complete or unspecified spontaneous abortion
Septic or septicopyemic embolism following complete or unspecified spontaneous abortion
Soap embolism following complete or unspecified spontaneous abortion

√5th **O03.8 Other and unspecified complications following complete or unspecified spontaneous abortion**

**O03.80 Unspecified complication following complete or unspecified spontaneous abortion** COM M

**O03.81 Shock following complete or unspecified spontaneous abortion** COM M
Circulatory collapse following complete or unspecified spontaneous abortion
Shock (postprocedural) following complete or unspecified spontaneous abortion
EXCLUDES 1 *shock due to infection following complete or unspecified spontaneous abortion (O03.87)*

**O03.82 Renal failure following complete or unspecified spontaneous abortion** COM M
Kidney failure (acute) following complete or unspecified spontaneous abortion
Oliguria following complete or unspecified spontaneous abortion
Renal shutdown following complete or unspecified spontaneous abortion
Renal tubular necrosis following complete or unspecified spontaneous abortion
Uremia following complete or unspecified spontaneous abortion

**O03.83 Metabolic disorder following complete or unspecified spontaneous abortion** COM M

**O03.84 Damage to pelvic organs following complete or unspecified spontaneous abortion** COM M
Laceration, perforation, tear or chemical damage of bladder following complete or unspecified spontaneous abortion
Laceration, perforation, tear or chemical damage of bowel following complete or unspecified spontaneous abortion
Laceration, perforation, tear or chemical damage of broad ligament following complete or unspecified spontaneous abortion
Laceration, perforation, tear or chemical damage of cervix following complete or unspecified spontaneous abortion
Laceration, perforation, tear or chemical damage of periurethral tissue following complete or unspecified spontaneous abortion
Laceration, perforation, tear or chemical damage of uterus following complete or unspecified spontaneous abortion
Laceration, perforation, tear or chemical damage of vagina following complete or unspecified spontaneous abortion

**O03.85 Other venous complications following complete or unspecified spontaneous abortion** COM M

**O03.86 Cardiac arrest following complete or unspecified spontaneous abortion** COM M

**O03.87 Sepsis following complete or unspecified spontaneous abortion** COM M

Use additional code to identify infectious agent (B95-B97)

Use additional code to identify severe sepsis, if applicable (R65.2-)

EXCLUDES 1 *septic or septicopyemic embolism following complete or unspecified spontaneous abortion (O03.7)*

**O03.88 Urinary tract infection following complete or unspecified spontaneous abortion** COM M

Cystitis following complete or unspecified spontaneous abortion

**O03.89 Complete or unspecified spontaneous abortion with other complications** COM M

**O03.9 Complete or unspecified spontaneous abortion without complication** COM M

Miscarriage NOS

Spontaneous abortion NOS

**✓4th O04 Complications following (induced) termination of pregnancy**

INCLUDES complications following (induced) termination of pregnancy

EXCLUDES 2 *encounter for elective termination of pregnancy (Z33.2)*

*failed attempted termination of pregnancy (O07.-)*

**O04.5 Genital tract and pelvic infection following (induced) termination of pregnancy** M

Endometritis following (induced) termination of pregnancy

Oophoritis following (induced) termination of pregnancy

Parametritis following (induced) termination of pregnancy

Pelvic peritonitis following (induced) termination of pregnancy

Salpingitis following (induced) termination of pregnancy

Salpingo-oophoritis following (induced) termination of pregnancy

EXCLUDES 1 *sepsis following (induced) termination of pregnancy (O04.87)*

*urinary tract infection following (induced) termination of pregnancy (O04.88)*

**O04.6 Delayed or excessive hemorrhage following (induced) termination of pregnancy** M

Afibrinogenemia following (induced) termination of pregnancy

Defibrination syndrome following (induced) termination of pregnancy

Hemolysis following (induced) termination of pregnancy

Intravascular coagulation following (induced) termination of pregnancy

**AHA:** 2025,1Q,18; 2023,2Q,15; 2019,3Q,11

**O04.7 Embolism following (induced) termination of pregnancy** M

Air embolism following (induced) termination of pregnancy

Amniotic fluid embolism following (induced) termination of pregnancy

Blood-clot embolism following (induced) termination of pregnancy

Embolism NOS following (induced) termination of pregnancy

Fat embolism following (induced) termination of pregnancy

Pulmonary embolism following (induced) termination of pregnancy

Pyemic embolism following (induced) termination of pregnancy

Septic or septicopyemic embolism following (induced) termination of pregnancy

Soap embolism following (induced) termination of pregnancy

**✓5th O04.8 (Induced) termination of pregnancy with other and unspecified complications**

**O04.80 (Induced) termination of pregnancy with unspecified complications** M

**O04.81 Shock following (induced) termination of pregnancy** M

Circulatory collapse following (induced) termination of pregnancy

Shock (postprocedural) following (induced) termination of pregnancy

EXCLUDES 1 *shock due to infection following (induced) termination of pregnancy (O04.87)*

**O04.82 Renal failure following (induced) termination of pregnancy** M

Kidney failure (acute) following (induced) termination of pregnancy

Oliguria following (induced) termination of pregnancy

Renal shutdown following (induced) termination of pregnancy

Renal tubular necrosis following (induced) termination of pregnancy

Uremia following (induced) termination of pregnancy

**O04.83 Metabolic disorder following (induced) termination of pregnancy** M

**O04.84 Damage to pelvic organs following (induced) termination of pregnancy** M

Laceration, perforation, tear or chemical damage of bladder following (induced) termination of pregnancy

Laceration, perforation, tear or chemical damage of bowel following (induced) termination of pregnancy

Laceration, perforation, tear or chemical damage of broad ligament following (induced) termination of pregnancy

Laceration, perforation, tear or chemical damage of cervix following (induced) termination of pregnancy

Laceration, perforation, tear or chemical damage of periurethral tissue following (induced) termination of pregnancy

Laceration, perforation, tear or chemical damage of uterus following (induced) termination of pregnancy

Laceration, perforation, tear or chemical damage of vagina following (induced) termination of pregnancy

**O04.85 Other venous complications following (induced) termination of pregnancy** M

**O04.86 Cardiac arrest following (induced) termination of pregnancy** M

**O04.87 Sepsis following (induced) termination of pregnancy** M

Use additional code to identify infectious agent (B95-B97)

Use additional code to identify severe sepsis, if applicable (R65.2-)

EXCLUDES 1 *septic or septicopyemic embolism following (induced) termination of pregnancy (O04.7)*

**O04.88 Urinary tract infection following (induced) termination of pregnancy** M

Cystitis following (induced) termination of pregnancy

**O04.89 (Induced) termination of pregnancy with other complications** M

**✓4th O07 Failed attempted termination of pregnancy**

INCLUDES failure of attempted induction of termination of pregnancy

incomplete elective abortion

EXCLUDES 1 *incomplete spontaneous abortion (O03.0-)*

**O07.0 Genital tract and pelvic infection following failed attempted termination of pregnancy** M

Endometritis following failed attempted termination of pregnancy

Oophoritis following failed attempted termination of pregnancy

Parametritis following failed attempted termination of pregnancy

Pelvic peritonitis following failed attempted termination of pregnancy

Salpingitis following failed attempted termination of pregnancy

Salpingo-oophoritis following failed attempted termination of pregnancy

EXCLUDES 1 *sepsis following failed attempted termination of pregnancy (O07.37)*

*urinary tract infection following failed attempted termination of pregnancy (O07.38)*

**O07.1 Delayed or excessive hemorrhage following failed attempted termination of pregnancy** M

Afibrinogenemia following failed attempted termination of pregnancy

Defibrination syndrome following failed attempted termination of pregnancy

Hemolysis following failed attempted termination of pregnancy

Intravascular coagulation following failed attempted termination of pregnancy

**O07.2 Embolism following failed attempted termination of pregnancy** M
Air embolism following failed attempted termination of pregnancy
Amniotic fluid embolism following failed attempted termination of pregnancy
Blood-clot embolism following failed attempted termination of pregnancy
Embolism NOS following failed attempted termination of pregnancy
Fat embolism following failed attempted termination of pregnancy
Pulmonary embolism following failed attempted termination of pregnancy
Pyemic embolism following failed attempted termination of pregnancy
Septic or septicopyemic embolism following failed attempted termination of pregnancy
Soap embolism following failed attempted termination of pregnancy

✓5th **O07.3 Failed attempted termination of pregnancy with other and unspecified complications**

**O07.30 Failed attempted termination of pregnancy with unspecified complications** M

**O07.31 Shock following failed attempted termination of pregnancy** M
Circulatory collapse following failed attempted termination of pregnancy
Shock (postprocedural) following failed attempted termination of pregnancy
EXCLUDES 1 *shock due to infection following failed attempted termination of pregnancy (O07.37)*

**O07.32 Renal failure following failed attempted termination of pregnancy** M
Kidney failure (acute) following failed attempted termination of pregnancy
Oliguria following failed attempted termination of pregnancy
Renal shutdown following failed attempted termination of pregnancy
Renal tubular necrosis following failed attempted termination of pregnancy
Uremia following failed attempted termination of pregnancy

**O07.33 Metabolic disorder following failed attempted termination of pregnancy** M

**O07.34 Damage to pelvic organs following failed attempted termination of pregnancy** M
Laceration, perforation, tear or chemical damage of bladder following failed attempted termination of pregnancy
Laceration, perforation, tear or chemical damage of bowel following failed attempted termination of pregnancy
Laceration, perforation, tear or chemical damage of broad ligament following failed attempted termination of pregnancy
Laceration, perforation, tear or chemical damage of cervix following failed attempted termination of pregnancy
Laceration, perforation, tear or chemical damage of periurethral tissue following failed attempted termination of pregnancy
Laceration, perforation, tear or chemical damage of uterus following failed attempted termination of pregnancy
Laceration, perforation, tear or chemical damage of vagina following failed attempted termination of pregnancy

**O07.35 Other venous complications following failed attempted termination of pregnancy** M

**O07.36 Cardiac arrest following failed attempted termination of pregnancy** M

**O07.37 Sepsis following failed attempted termination of pregnancy** M
Use additional code (B95-B97), to identify infectious agent
Use additional code (R65.2-) to identify severe sepsis, if applicable
EXCLUDES 1 *septic or septicopyemic embolism following failed attempted termination of pregnancy (O07.2)*

**O07.38 Urinary tract infection following failed attempted termination of pregnancy** M
Cystitis following failed attempted termination of pregnancy

**O07.39 Failed attempted termination of pregnancy with other complications** M

**O07.4 Failed attempted termination of pregnancy without complication** M

✓4th **O08 Complications following ectopic and molar pregnancy**
This category is for use with categories O00-O02 to identify any associated complications
AHA: 2025,1Q,18

**O08.0 Genital tract and pelvic infection following ectopic and molar pregnancy** COM M
Endometritis following ectopic and molar pregnancy
Oophoritis following ectopic and molar pregnancy
Parametritis following ectopic and molar pregnancy
Pelvic peritonitis following ectopic and molar pregnancy
Salpingitis following ectopic and molar pregnancy
Salpingo-oophoritis following ectopic and molar pregnancy
EXCLUDES 1 *sepsis following ectopic and molar pregnancy (O08.82)*
*urinary tract infection (O08.83)*

**O08.1 Delayed or excessive hemorrhage following ectopic and molar pregnancy** COM M
Afibrinogenemia following ectopic and molar pregnancy
Defibrination syndrome following ectopic and molar pregnancy
Hemolysis following ectopic and molar pregnancy
Intravascular coagulation following ectopic and molar pregnancy
EXCLUDES 1 *delayed or excessive hemorrhage due to incomplete abortion (O03.1)*

**O08.2 Embolism following ectopic and molar pregnancy** COM M
Air embolism following ectopic and molar pregnancy
Amniotic fluid embolism following ectopic and molar pregnancy
Blood-clot embolism following ectopic and molar pregnancy
Embolism NOS following ectopic and molar pregnancy
Fat embolism following ectopic and molar pregnancy
Pulmonary embolism following ectopic and molar pregnancy
Pyemic embolism following ectopic and molar pregnancy
Septic or septicopyemic embolism following ectopic and molar pregnancy
Soap embolism following ectopic and molar pregnancy

**O08.3 Shock following ectopic and molar pregnancy** COM M
Circulatory collapse following ectopic and molar pregnancy
Shock (postprocedural) following ectopic and molar pregnancy
EXCLUDES 1 *shock due to infection following ectopic and molar pregnancy (O08.82)*

**O08.4 Renal failure following ectopic and molar pregnancy** COM M
Kidney failure (acute) following ectopic and molar pregnancy
Oliguria following ectopic and molar pregnancy
Renal shutdown following ectopic and molar pregnancy
Renal tubular necrosis following ectopic and molar pregnancy
Uremia following ectopic and molar pregnancy

**O08.5 Metabolic disorders following an ectopic and molar pregnancy** COM M

**O08.6 Damage to pelvic organs and tissues following an ectopic and molar pregnancy** COM M
Laceration, perforation, tear or chemical damage of bladder following an ectopic and molar pregnancy
Laceration, perforation, tear or chemical damage of bowel following an ectopic and molar pregnancy
Laceration, perforation, tear or chemical damage of broad ligament following an ectopic and molar pregnancy
Laceration, perforation, tear or chemical damage of cervix following an ectopic and molar pregnancy
Laceration, perforation, tear or chemical damage of periurethral tissue following an ectopic and molar pregnancy
Laceration, perforation, tear or chemical damage of uterus following an ectopic and molar pregnancy
Laceration, perforation, tear or chemical damage of vagina following an ectopic and molar pregnancy

**O08.7 Other venous complications following an ectopic and molar pregnancy** COM M

✓5th **O08.8 Other complications following an ectopic and molar pregnancy**

**O08.81 Cardiac arrest following an ectopic and molar pregnancy** COM M

**O08.82 Sepsis following ectopic and molar pregnancy** COM M
Use additional code (B95-B97), to identify infectious agent
Use additional code (R65.2-) to identify severe sepsis, if applicable
EXCLUDES 1 *septic or septicopyemic embolism following ectopic and molar pregnancy (O08.2)*

**O08.83 Urinary tract infection following an ectopic and molar pregnancy** COM M
Cystitis following an ectopic and molar pregnancy

**O08.89 Other complications following an ectopic and molar pregnancy** COM M

**O08.9 Unspecified complication following an ectopic and molar pregnancy** COM M

## Supervision of high risk pregnancy (O09)

**✓4th O09 Supervision of high risk pregnancy**
AHA: 2019,3Q,5; 2016,4Q,48-50,150

**✓5th O09.0 Supervision of pregnancy with history of infertility**
- **O09.00 Supervision of pregnancy with history of infertility, unspecified trimester** COM M
- **O09.01 Supervision of pregnancy with history of infertility, first trimester** COM M
- **O09.02 Supervision of pregnancy with history of infertility, second trimester** COM M
- **O09.03 Supervision of pregnancy with history of infertility, third trimester** COM M

**✓5th O09.1 Supervision of pregnancy with history of ectopic pregnancy**
- **O09.10 Supervision of pregnancy with history of ectopic pregnancy, unspecified trimester** COM M
- **O09.11 Supervision of pregnancy with history of ectopic pregnancy, first trimester** COM M
- **O09.12 Supervision of pregnancy with history of ectopic pregnancy, second trimester** COM M
- **O09.13 Supervision of pregnancy with history of ectopic pregnancy, third trimester** COM M

**✓5th O09.A Supervision of pregnancy with history of molar pregnancy**
DEF: Molar pregnancy: Trophoblastic neoplasm that mimics pregnancy by proliferating from a pathologic ovum and resulting only in a mass of cysts resembling grapes, 80 percent of which are benign, but require surgical removal.
- **O09.A0 Supervision of pregnancy with history of molar pregnancy, unspecified trimester** COM M
- **O09.A1 Supervision of pregnancy with history of molar pregnancy, first trimester** COM M
- **O09.A2 Supervision of pregnancy with history of molar pregnancy, second trimester** COM M
- **O09.A3 Supervision of pregnancy with history of molar pregnancy, third trimester** COM M

**✓5th O09.2 Supervision of pregnancy with other poor reproductive or obstetric history**
EXCLUDES 2 *pregnancy care for patient with history of recurrent pregnancy loss (O26.2-)*

**✓6th O09.21 Supervision of pregnancy with history of pre-term labor**
- **O09.211 Supervision of pregnancy with history of pre-term labor, first trimester** COM M
- **O09.212 Supervision of pregnancy with history of pre-term labor, second trimester** COM M
- **O09.213 Supervision of pregnancy with history of pre-term labor, third trimester** COM M
- **O09.219 Supervision of pregnancy with history of pre-term labor, unspecified trimester** COM M

**✓6th O09.29 Supervision of pregnancy with other poor reproductive or obstetric history**
Supervision of pregnancy with history of neonatal death
Supervision of pregnancy with history of stillbirth
- **O09.291 Supervision of pregnancy with other poor reproductive or obstetric history, first trimester** COM M
- **O09.292 Supervision of pregnancy with other poor reproductive or obstetric history, second trimester** COM M
- **O09.293 Supervision of pregnancy with other poor reproductive or obstetric history, third trimester** COM M
- **O09.299 Supervision of pregnancy with other poor reproductive or obstetric history, unspecified trimester** COM M

**✓5th O09.3 Supervision of pregnancy with insufficient antenatal care**
Supervision of concealed pregnancy
Supervision of hidden pregnancy
- **O09.30 Supervision of pregnancy with insufficient antenatal care, unspecified trimester** COM M
- **O09.31 Supervision of pregnancy with insufficient antenatal care, first trimester** COM M
- **O09.32 Supervision of pregnancy with insufficient antenatal care, second trimester** COM M
- **O09.33 Supervision of pregnancy with insufficient antenatal care, third trimester** COM M

**✓5th O09.4 Supervision of pregnancy with grand multiparity**
- **O09.40 Supervision of pregnancy with grand multiparity, unspecified trimester** COM M
- **O09.41 Supervision of pregnancy with grand multiparity, first trimester** COM M
- **O09.42 Supervision of pregnancy with grand multiparity, second trimester** COM M
- **O09.43 Supervision of pregnancy with grand multiparity, third trimester** COM M

**✓5th O09.5 Supervision of elderly primigravida and multigravida**
Pregnancy for a female 35 years and older at expected date of delivery

**✓6th O09.51 Supervision of elderly primigravida**
- **O09.511 Supervision of elderly primigravida, first trimester** COM M
- **O09.512 Supervision of elderly primigravida, second trimester** COM M
- **O09.513 Supervision of elderly primigravida, third trimester** COM M
- **O09.519 Supervision of elderly primigravida, unspecified trimester** COM M

**✓6th O09.52 Supervision of elderly multigravida**
- **O09.521 Supervision of elderly multigravida, first trimester** COM M
- **O09.522 Supervision of elderly multigravida, second trimester** COM M
- **O09.523 Supervision of elderly multigravida, third trimester** COM M
- **O09.529 Supervision of elderly multigravida, unspecified trimester** COM M

**✓5th O09.6 Supervision of young primigravida and multigravida**
Supervision of pregnancy for a female less than 16 years old at expected date of delivery

**✓6th O09.61 Supervision of young primigravida**
- **O09.611 Supervision of young primigravida, first trimester** COM M
- **O09.612 Supervision of young primigravida, second trimester** COM M
- **O09.613 Supervision of young primigravida, third trimester** COM M
- **O09.619 Supervision of young primigravida, unspecified trimester** COM M

**✓6th O09.62 Supervision of young multigravida**
- **O09.621 Supervision of young multigravida, first trimester** COM M
- **O09.622 Supervision of young multigravida, second trimester** COM M
- **O09.623 Supervision of young multigravida, third trimester** COM M
- **O09.629 Supervision of young multigravida, unspecified trimester** COM M

**✓5th O09.7 Supervision of high risk pregnancy due to social problems**
- **O09.70 Supervision of high risk pregnancy due to social problems, unspecified trimester** COM M
- **O09.71 Supervision of high risk pregnancy due to social problems, first trimester** COM M
- **O09.72 Supervision of high risk pregnancy due to social problems, second trimester** COM M
- **O09.73 Supervision of high risk pregnancy due to social problems, third trimester** COM M

**O09.8 Supervision of other high risk pregnancies**

**O09.81 Supervision of pregnancy resulting from assisted reproductive technology**

Supervision of pregnancy resulting from in-vitro fertilization

EXCLUDES 2 *gestational carrier status (Z33.3)*

**O09.811 Supervision of pregnancy resulting from assisted reproductive technology, first trimester** COM M

**O09.812 Supervision of pregnancy resulting from assisted reproductive technology, second trimester** COM M

**O09.813 Supervision of pregnancy resulting from assisted reproductive technology, third trimester** COM M

**O09.819 Supervision of pregnancy resulting from assisted reproductive technology, unspecified trimester** COM M

**O09.82 Supervision of pregnancy with history of in utero procedure during previous pregnancy**

**O09.821 Supervision of pregnancy with history of in utero procedure during previous pregnancy, first trimester** COM M

**O09.822 Supervision of pregnancy with history of in utero procedure during previous pregnancy, second trimester** COM M

**O09.823 Supervision of pregnancy with history of in utero procedure during previous pregnancy, third trimester** COM M

**O09.829 Supervision of pregnancy with history of in utero procedure during previous pregnancy, unspecified trimester** COM M

EXCLUDES 1 *supervision of pregnancy affected by in utero procedure during current pregnancy (O35.7)*

**O09.89 Supervision of other high risk pregnancies**

**O09.891 Supervision of other high risk pregnancies, first trimester** COM M

**O09.892 Supervision of other high risk pregnancies, second trimester** COM M

**O09.893 Supervision of other high risk pregnancies, third trimester** COM M

**O09.899 Supervision of other high risk pregnancies, unspecified trimester** COM M

**O09.9 Supervision of high risk pregnancy, unspecified**

**O09.90 Supervision of high risk pregnancy, unspecified, unspecified trimester** COM M

**O09.91 Supervision of high risk pregnancy, unspecified, first trimester** COM M

**O09.92 Supervision of high risk pregnancy, unspecified, second trimester** COM M

**O09.93 Supervision of high risk pregnancy, unspecified, third trimester** COM M

## Edema, proteinuria and hypertensive disorders in pregnancy, childbirth and the puerperium (O10-O16)

**AHA:** 2016,4Q,50

**O10 Pre-existing hypertension complicating pregnancy, childbirth and the puerperium**

INCLUDES pre-existing hypertension with pre-existing proteinuria complicating pregnancy, childbirth and the puerperium

EXCLUDES 2 *pre-existing hypertension with superimposed pre-eclampsia complicating pregnancy, childbirth and the puerperium (O11.-)*

**AHA:** 2025,2Q,17

**O10.0 Pre-existing essential hypertension complicating pregnancy, childbirth and the puerperium**

Any condition in I10 specified as a reason for obstetric care during pregnancy, childbirth or the puerperium

**O10.01 Pre-existing essential hypertension complicating pregnancy**

**O10.011 Pre-existing essential hypertension complicating pregnancy, first trimester** COM M

**O10.012 Pre-existing essential hypertension complicating pregnancy, second trimester** COM M

**O10.013 Pre-existing essential hypertension complicating pregnancy, third trimester** COM M

**O10.019 Pre-existing essential hypertension complicating pregnancy, unspecified trimester** COM M

**O10.02 Pre-existing essential hypertension complicating childbirth** COM M

**O10.03 Pre-existing essential hypertension complicating the puerperium** COM M

**O10.1 Pre-existing hypertensive heart disease complicating pregnancy, childbirth and the puerperium**

Any condition in I11 specified as a reason for obstetric care during pregnancy, childbirth or the puerperium

Use additional code from I11 to identify the type of hypertensive heart disease

**O10.11 Pre-existing hypertensive heart disease complicating pregnancy**

**O10.111 Pre-existing hypertensive heart disease complicating pregnancy, first trimester** COM M

**O10.112 Pre-existing hypertensive heart disease complicating pregnancy, second trimester** COM M

**O10.113 Pre-existing hypertensive heart disease complicating pregnancy, third trimester** COM M

**O10.119 Pre-existing hypertensive heart disease complicating pregnancy, unspecified trimester** COM M

**O10.12 Pre-existing hypertensive heart disease complicating childbirth** COM M

**O10.13 Pre-existing hypertensive heart disease complicating the puerperium** COM M

**O10.2 Pre-existing hypertensive chronic kidney disease complicating pregnancy, childbirth and the puerperium**

Any condition in I12 specified as a reason for obstetric care during pregnancy, childbirth or the puerperium

Use additional code from I12 to identify the type of hypertensive chronic kidney disease

**O10.21 Pre-existing hypertensive chronic kidney disease complicating pregnancy**

**O10.211 Pre-existing hypertensive chronic kidney disease complicating pregnancy, first trimester** COM M

**O10.212 Pre-existing hypertensive chronic kidney disease complicating pregnancy, second trimester** COM M

**O10.213 Pre-existing hypertensive chronic kidney disease complicating pregnancy, third trimester** COM M

**O10.219 Pre-existing hypertensive chronic kidney disease complicating pregnancy, unspecified trimester** COM M

**O10.22 Pre-existing hypertensive chronic kidney disease complicating childbirth** COM M

**O10.23 Pre-existing hypertensive chronic kidney disease complicating the puerperium** COM M

**O10.3 Pre-existing hypertensive heart and chronic kidney disease complicating pregnancy, childbirth and the puerperium**

Any condition in I13 specified as a reason for obstetric care during pregnancy, childbirth or the puerperium

Use additional code from I13 to identify the type of hypertensive heart and chronic kidney disease

**O10.31 Pre-existing hypertensive heart and chronic kidney disease complicating pregnancy**

**O10.311 Pre-existing hypertensive heart and chronic kidney disease complicating pregnancy, first trimester** COM M

**O10.312 Pre-existing hypertensive heart and chronic kidney disease complicating pregnancy, second trimester** COM M

**O10.313 Pre-existing hypertensive heart and chronic kidney disease complicating pregnancy, third trimester** COM M

**O10.319 Pre-existing hypertensive heart and chronic kidney disease complicating pregnancy, unspecified trimester** COM M

**O10.32 Pre-existing hypertensive heart and chronic kidney disease complicating childbirth** COM M

O10.33 Pre-existing hypertensive heart and chronic kidney disease complicating the puerperium COM M

✓5th O10.4 Pre-existing secondary hypertension complicating pregnancy, childbirth and the puerperium
Any condition in I15 specified as a reason for obstetric care during pregnancy, childbirth or the puerperium
Use additional code from I15 to identify the type of secondary hypertension

✓6th O10.41 Pre-existing secondary hypertension complicating pregnancy
O10.411 Pre-existing secondary hypertension complicating pregnancy, first trimester COM M
O10.412 Pre-existing secondary hypertension complicating pregnancy, second trimester COM M
O10.413 Pre-existing secondary hypertension complicating pregnancy, third trimester COM M
O10.419 Pre-existing secondary hypertension complicating pregnancy, unspecified trimester COM M

O10.42 Pre-existing secondary hypertension complicating childbirth COM M
O10.43 Pre-existing secondary hypertension complicating the puerperium COM M

✓5th O10.9 Unspecified pre-existing hypertension complicating pregnancy, childbirth and the puerperium

✓6th O10.91 Unspecified pre-existing hypertension complicating pregnancy
AHA: 2025,2Q,17
O10.911 Unspecified pre-existing hypertension complicating pregnancy, first trimester COM M
O10.912 Unspecified pre-existing hypertension complicating pregnancy, second trimester COM M
O10.913 Unspecified pre-existing hypertension complicating pregnancy, third trimester COM M
O10.919 Unspecified pre-existing hypertension complicating pregnancy, unspecified trimester COM M

O10.92 Unspecified pre-existing hypertension complicating childbirth COM M
O10.93 Unspecified pre-existing hypertension complicating the puerperium COM M

✓4th O11 Pre-existing hypertension with pre-eclampsia
INCLUDES conditions in O10 complicated by pre-eclampsia
pre-eclampsia superimposed pre-existing in hypertension
Use additional code from O10 to identify the type of hypertension
**DEF:** Complication of pregnancy manifesting in the development of borderline hypertension, protein in the urine, and unresponsive swelling between the 20th week of pregnancy and the end of the first week following birth in mild to moderate cases. Severe preeclampsia presents with hypertension, associated with marked swelling, proteinuria, abdominal pain, and/or visual changes.

O11.1 Pre-existing hypertension with pre-eclampsia, first trimester COM M
O11.2 Pre-existing hypertension with pre-eclampsia, second trimester COM M
O11.3 Pre-existing hypertension with pre-eclampsia, third trimester COM M
O11.4 Pre-existing hypertension with pre-eclampsia, complicating childbirth COM M
O11.5 Pre-existing hypertension with pre-eclampsia, complicating the puerperium COM M
O11.9 Pre-existing hypertension with pre-eclampsia, unspecified trimester COM M

✓4th O12 Gestational [pregnancy-induced] edema and proteinuria without hypertension

✓5th O12.0 Gestational edema
O12.00 Gestational edema, unspecified trimester COM M
O12.01 Gestational edema, first trimester COM M
O12.02 Gestational edema, second trimester COM M
O12.03 Gestational edema, third trimester COM M
O12.04 Gestational edema, complicating childbirth COM M
O12.05 Gestational edema, complicating the puerperium COM M

✓5th O12.1 Gestational proteinuria
O12.10 Gestational proteinuria, unspecified trimester COM M
O12.11 Gestational proteinuria, first trimester COM M
O12.12 Gestational proteinuria, second trimester COM M
O12.13 Gestational proteinuria, third trimester COM M
O12.14 Gestational proteinuria, complicating childbirth COM M
O12.15 Gestational proteinuria, complicating the puerperium COM M

✓5th O12.2 Gestational edema with proteinuria
O12.20 Gestational edema with proteinuria, unspecified trimester COM M
O12.21 Gestational edema with proteinuria, first trimester COM M
O12.22 Gestational edema with proteinuria, second trimester COM M
O12.23 Gestational edema with proteinuria, third trimester COM M
O12.24 Gestational edema with proteinuria, complicating childbirth COM M
O12.25 Gestational edema with proteinuria, complicating the puerperium COM M

✓4th O13 Gestational [pregnancy-induced] hypertension without significant proteinuria
INCLUDES gestational hypertension NOS
transient hypertension of pregnancy
AHA: 2016,1Q,5

O13.1 Gestational [pregnancy-induced] hypertension without significant proteinuria, first trimester COM M
O13.2 Gestational [pregnancy-induced] hypertension without significant proteinuria, second trimester COM M
O13.3 Gestational [pregnancy-induced] hypertension without significant proteinuria, third trimester COM M
O13.4 Gestational [pregnancy-induced] hypertension without significant proteinuria, complicating childbirth COM M
O13.5 Gestational [pregnancy-induced] hypertension without significant proteinuria, complicating the puerperium COM M
O13.9 Gestational [pregnancy-induced] hypertension without significant proteinuria, unspecified trimester COM M

✓4th O14 Pre-eclampsia
*EXCLUDES 1* *pre-existing hypertension with pre-eclampsia (O11)*
**DEF:** Complication of pregnancy manifesting in the development of borderline hypertension, protein in the urine, and unresponsive swelling between the 20th week of pregnancy and the end of the first week following birth in mild to moderate cases. Severe preeclampsia presents with hypertension, associated with marked swelling, proteinuria, abdominal pain, and/or visual changes.

✓5th O14.0 Mild to moderate pre-eclampsia
AHA: 2019,3Q,12; 2019,2Q,8
O14.00 Mild to moderate pre-eclampsia, unspecified trimester COM M
O14.02 Mild to moderate pre-eclampsia, second trimester COM M
O14.03 Mild to moderate pre-eclampsia, third trimester COM M
O14.04 Mild to moderate pre-eclampsia, complicating childbirth COM M
AHA: 2019,2Q,8
O14.05 Mild to moderate pre-eclampsia, complicating the puerperium COM M

✓5th O14.1 Severe pre-eclampsia
*EXCLUDES 1* *HELLP syndrome (O14.2-)*
AHA: 2019,3Q,12
O14.10 Severe pre-eclampsia, unspecified trimester COM M
O14.12 Severe pre-eclampsia, second trimester COM M
O14.13 Severe pre-eclampsia, third trimester COM M
O14.14 Severe pre-eclampsia complicating childbirth COM M
O14.15 Severe pre-eclampsia, complicating the puerperium COM M

**O14.2 HELLP syndrome**
Severe pre-eclampsia with hemolysis, elevated liver enzymes and low platelet count (HELLP)
**AHA:** 2019,3Q,12

- **O14.20 HELLP syndrome (HELLP), unspecified trimester** COM M
- **O14.22 HELLP syndrome (HELLP), second trimester** COM M
- **O14.23 HELLP syndrome (HELLP), third trimester** COM M
- **O14.24 HELLP syndrome, complicating childbirth** COM M
- **O14.25 HELLP syndrome, complicating the puerperium** COM M

**O14.9 Unspecified pre-eclampsia**

- **O14.90 Unspecified pre-eclampsia, unspecified trimester** COM M
- **O14.92 Unspecified pre-eclampsia, second trimester** COM M
- **O14.93 Unspecified pre-eclampsia, third trimester** COM M
- **O14.94 Unspecified pre-eclampsia, complicating childbirth** COM M
- **O14.95 Unspecified pre-eclampsia, complicating the puerperium** COM M

**O15 Eclampsia**
INCLUDES convulsions following conditions in O10-O14 and O16
**DEF:** Tetany and toxemia producing seizure activity or coma in a pregnant patient who most often has presented with prior preeclampsia (i.e., hypertension, albuminuria, and edema).

**O15.0 Eclampsia complicating pregnancy**

- **O15.00 Eclampsia complicating pregnancy, unspecified trimester** COM M
- **O15.02 Eclampsia complicating pregnancy, second trimester** COM M
- **O15.03 Eclampsia complicating pregnancy, third trimester** COM M

**O15.1 Eclampsia complicating labor** COM M
**O15.2 Eclampsia complicating the puerperium** COM M
**O15.9 Eclampsia, unspecified as to time period** COM M
Eclampsia NOS

**O16 Unspecified maternal hypertension**

- **O16.1 Unspecified maternal hypertension, first trimester** COM M
- **O16.2 Unspecified maternal hypertension, second trimester** COM M
- **O16.3 Unspecified maternal hypertension, third trimester** COM M
- **O16.4 Unspecified maternal hypertension, complicating childbirth** COM M
- **O16.5 Unspecified maternal hypertension, complicating the puerperium** COM M
- **O16.9 Unspecified maternal hypertension, unspecified trimester** COM M

## Other maternal disorders predominantly related to pregnancy (O20-O29)

EXCLUDES 2 *maternal care related to the fetus and amniotic cavity and possible delivery problems (O30-O48)*
*maternal diseases classifiable elsewhere but complicating pregnancy, labor and delivery, and the puerperium (O98-O99)*

**O20 Hemorrhage in early pregnancy**
INCLUDES hemorrhage before completion of 20 weeks gestation
EXCLUDES 1 *pregnancy with abortive outcome (O00-O08)*

**O20.0 Threatened abortion** COM M
Hemorrhage specified as due to threatened abortion
**DEF:** Bloody discharge during pregnancy. The cervix may be dilated and pregnancy threatened, but the pregnancy is not terminated.

**O20.8 Other hemorrhage in early pregnancy** COM M
**AHA:** 2023,3Q,18

**O20.9 Hemorrhage in early pregnancy, unspecified** COM M

**O21 Excessive vomiting in pregnancy**

**O21.0 Mild hyperemesis gravidarum** COM M
Hyperemesis gravidarum, mild or unspecified, starting before the end of the 20th week of gestation

**O21.1 Hyperemesis gravidarum with metabolic disturbance** COM M
Hyperemesis gravidarum, starting before the end of the 20th week of gestation, with metabolic disturbance such as carbohydrate depletion
Hyperemesis gravidarum, starting before the end of the 20th week of gestation, with metabolic disturbance such as dehydration
Hyperemesis gravidarum, starting before the end of the 20th week of gestation, with metabolic disturbance such as electrolyte imbalance

**O21.2 Late vomiting of pregnancy** COM M
Excessive vomiting starting after 20 completed weeks of gestation

**O21.8 Other vomiting complicating pregnancy** COM M
Vomiting due to diseases classified elsewhere, complicating pregnancy
Use additional code, to identify cause

**O21.9 Vomiting of pregnancy, unspecified** COM M

**O22 Venous complications and hemorrhoids in pregnancy**
EXCLUDES 1 *venous complications of:*
*abortion NOS (O03.9)*
*ectopic or molar pregnancy (O08.7)*
*failed attempted abortion (O07.35)*
*induced abortion (O04.85)*
*spontaneous abortion (O03.89)*
EXCLUDES 2 *obstetric pulmonary embolism (O88.-)*
*venous complications and hemorrhoids of childbirth and the puerperium (O87.-)*

**O22.0 Varicose veins of lower extremity in pregnancy**
Varicose veins NOS in pregnancy
**DEF:** Distended, tortuous veins of the lower extremities associated with pregnancy.

- **O22.00 Varicose veins of lower extremity in pregnancy, unspecified trimester** COM M
- **O22.01 Varicose veins of lower extremity in pregnancy, first trimester** COM M
- **O22.02 Varicose veins of lower extremity in pregnancy, second trimester** COM M
- **O22.03 Varicose veins of lower extremity in pregnancy, third trimester** COM M

**O22.1 Genital varices in pregnancy**
Perineal varices in pregnancy
Vaginal varices in pregnancy
Vulval varices in pregnancy

- **O22.10 Genital varices in pregnancy, unspecified trimester** COM M
- **O22.11 Genital varices in pregnancy, first trimester** COM M
- **O22.12 Genital varices in pregnancy, second trimester** COM M
- **O22.13 Genital varices in pregnancy, third trimester** COM M

**O22.2 Superficial thrombophlebitis in pregnancy**
Phlebitis in pregnancy NOS
Thrombophlebitis of legs in pregnancy
Thrombosis in pregnancy NOS
Use additional code to identify the superficial thrombophlebitis (I80.0-)

- **O22.20 Superficial thrombophlebitis in pregnancy, unspecified trimester** COM M
- **O22.21 Superficial thrombophlebitis in pregnancy, first trimester** COM M
- **O22.22 Superficial thrombophlebitis in pregnancy, second trimester** COM M
- **O22.23 Superficial thrombophlebitis in pregnancy, third trimester** COM M

**O22.3 Deep phlebothrombosis in pregnancy**
Deep vein thrombosis, antepartum
Use additional code to identify the deep vein thrombosis (I82.4-, I82.5-, I82.62-, I82.72-)
Use additional code, if applicable, for associated long-term (current) use of anticoagulants (Z79.01)

- **O22.30 Deep phlebothrombosis in pregnancy, unspecified trimester** COM M
- **O22.31 Deep phlebothrombosis in pregnancy, first trimester** COM M
- **O22.32 Deep phlebothrombosis in pregnancy, second trimester** COM M
- **O22.33 Deep phlebothrombosis in pregnancy, third trimester** COM M

√5th **O22.4 Hemorrhoids in pregnancy**

**O22.40 Hemorrhoids in pregnancy, unspecified trimester** COM M

**O22.41 Hemorrhoids in pregnancy, first trimester** COM M

**O22.42 Hemorrhoids in pregnancy, second trimester** COM M

**O22.43 Hemorrhoids in pregnancy, third trimester** COM M

√5th **O22.5 Cerebral venous thrombosis in pregnancy**

Cerebrovenous sinus thrombosis in pregnancy

**O22.50 Cerebral venous thrombosis in pregnancy, unspecified trimester** COM M

**O22.51 Cerebral venous thrombosis in pregnancy, first trimester** COM M

**O22.52 Cerebral venous thrombosis in pregnancy, second trimester** COM M

**O22.53 Cerebral venous thrombosis in pregnancy, third trimester** COM M

√5th **O22.8 Other venous complications in pregnancy**

√6th **O22.8X Other venous complications in pregnancy**

**O22.8X1 Other venous complications in pregnancy, first trimester** COM M

**O22.8X2 Other venous complications in pregnancy, second trimester** COM M

**O22.8X3 Other venous complications in pregnancy, third trimester** COM M

**O22.8X9 Other venous complications in pregnancy, unspecified trimester** COM M

√5th **O22.9 Venous complication in pregnancy, unspecified**

Gestational phlebitis NOS
Gestational phlebopathy NOS
Gestational thrombosis NOS

**O22.90 Venous complication in pregnancy, unspecified, unspecified trimester** COM M

**O22.91 Venous complication in pregnancy, unspecified, first trimester** COM M

**O22.92 Venous complication in pregnancy, unspecified, second trimester** COM M

**O22.93 Venous complication in pregnancy, unspecified, third trimester** COM M

√4th **O23 Infections of genitourinary tract in pregnancy**

Use additional code to identify organism (B95.-, B96.-)

EXCLUDES 2 *gonococcal infections complicating pregnancy, childbirth and the puerperium (O98.2)*
*infections with a predominantly sexual mode of transmission NOS complicating pregnancy, childbirth and the puerperium (O98.3)*
*syphilis complicating pregnancy, childbirth and the puerperium (O98.1)*
*tuberculosis of genitourinary system complicating pregnancy, childbirth and the puerperium (O98.0)*
*venereal disease NOS complicating pregnancy, childbirth and the puerperium (O98.3)*

**AHA:** 2018,2Q,20

√5th **O23.0 Infections of kidney in pregnancy**

Pyelonephritis in pregnancy

**O23.00 Infections of kidney in pregnancy, unspecified trimester** COM M

**O23.01 Infections of kidney in pregnancy, first trimester** COM M

**O23.02 Infections of kidney in pregnancy, second trimester** COM M

**O23.03 Infections of kidney in pregnancy, third trimester** COM M

√5th **O23.1 Infections of bladder in pregnancy**

**O23.10 Infections of bladder in pregnancy, unspecified trimester** COM M

**O23.11 Infections of bladder in pregnancy, first trimester** COM M

**O23.12 Infections of bladder in pregnancy, second trimester** COM M

**O23.13 Infections of bladder in pregnancy, third trimester** COM M

√5th **O23.2 Infections of urethra in pregnancy**

**O23.20 Infections of urethra in pregnancy, unspecified trimester** COM M

**O23.21 Infections of urethra in pregnancy, first trimester** COM M

**O23.22 Infections of urethra in pregnancy, second trimester** COM M

**O23.23 Infections of urethra in pregnancy, third trimester** COM M

√5th **O23.3 Infections of other parts of urinary tract in pregnancy**

**O23.30 Infections of other parts of urinary tract in pregnancy, unspecified trimester** COM M

**O23.31 Infections of other parts of urinary tract in pregnancy, first trimester** COM M

**O23.32 Infections of other parts of urinary tract in pregnancy, second trimester** COM M

**O23.33 Infections of other parts of urinary tract in pregnancy, third trimester** COM M

√5th **O23.4 Unspecified infection of urinary tract in pregnancy**

**O23.40 Unspecified infection of urinary tract in pregnancy, unspecified trimester** COM M

**O23.41 Unspecified infection of urinary tract in pregnancy, first trimester** COM M

**O23.42 Unspecified infection of urinary tract in pregnancy, second trimester** COM M

**O23.43 Unspecified infection of urinary tract in pregnancy, third trimester** COM M

√5th **O23.5 Infections of the genital tract in pregnancy**

√6th **O23.51 Infection of cervix in pregnancy**

**O23.511 Infections of cervix in pregnancy, first trimester** COM M

**O23.512 Infections of cervix in pregnancy, second trimester** COM M

**O23.513 Infections of cervix in pregnancy, third trimester** COM M

**O23.519 Infections of cervix in pregnancy, unspecified trimester** COM M

√6th **O23.52 Salpingo-oophoritis in pregnancy**

Oophoritis in pregnancy
Salpingitis in pregnancy

**O23.521 Salpingo-oophoritis in pregnancy, first trimester** COM M

**O23.522 Salpingo-oophoritis in pregnancy, second trimester** COM M

**O23.523 Salpingo-oophoritis in pregnancy, third trimester** COM M

**O23.529 Salpingo-oophoritis in pregnancy, unspecified trimester** COM M

√6th **O23.59 Infection of other part of genital tract in pregnancy**

**AHA:** 2025,1Q,22; 2022,1Q,20

**O23.591 Infection of other part of genital tract in pregnancy, first trimester** COM M

**O23.592 Infection of other part of genital tract in pregnancy, second trimester** COM M

**O23.593 Infection of other part of genital tract in pregnancy, third trimester** COM M

**O23.599 Infection of other part of genital tract in pregnancy, unspecified trimester** COM M

√5th **O23.9 Unspecified genitourinary tract infection in pregnancy**

Genitourinary tract infection in pregnancy NOS

**AHA:** 2025,1Q,22

**O23.90 Unspecified genitourinary tract infection in pregnancy, unspecified trimester** COM M

**O23.91 Unspecified genitourinary tract infection in pregnancy, first trimester** COM M

**O23.92 Unspecified genitourinary tract infection in pregnancy, second trimester** COM M

**O23.93 Unspecified genitourinary tract infection in pregnancy, third trimester** COM M

**O24 Diabetes mellitus in pregnancy, childbirth and the puerperium**

**O24.0 Pre-existing type 1 diabetes mellitus, in pregnancy, childbirth and the puerperium**
Juvenile onset diabetes mellitus, in pregnancy, childbirth and the puerperium
Ketosis-prone diabetes mellitus in pregnancy, childbirth and the puerperium
Use additional code from category E10 to further identify any manifestations

**O24.01 Pre-existing type 1 diabetes mellitus, in pregnancy**
- **O24.011 Pre-existing type 1 diabetes mellitus, in pregnancy, first trimester** COM Q M
- **O24.012 Pre-existing type 1 diabetes mellitus, in pregnancy, second trimester** COM Q M
- **O24.013 Pre-existing type 1 diabetes mellitus, in pregnancy, third trimester** COM Q M
- **O24.019 Pre-existing type 1 diabetes mellitus, in pregnancy, unspecified trimester** COM Q M

**O24.02 Pre-existing type 1 diabetes mellitus, in childbirth** COM Q M
**O24.03 Pre-existing type 1 diabetes mellitus, in the puerperium** COM Q M

**O24.1 Pre-existing type 2 diabetes mellitus, in pregnancy, childbirth and the puerperium**
Insulin-resistant diabetes mellitus in pregnancy, childbirth and the puerperium
Use additional code (for):
from category E11 to further identify any manifestations
injectable non-insulin antidiabetic drugs (Z79.85)
long-term (current) use of insulin (Z79.4)

**O24.11 Pre-existing type 2 diabetes mellitus, in pregnancy**
- **O24.111 Pre-existing type 2 diabetes mellitus, in pregnancy, first trimester** COM Q M
- **O24.112 Pre-existing type 2 diabetes mellitus, in pregnancy, second trimester** COM Q M
- **O24.113 Pre-existing type 2 diabetes mellitus, in pregnancy, third trimester** COM Q M
- **O24.119 Pre-existing type 2 diabetes mellitus, in pregnancy, unspecified trimester** COM Q M

**O24.12 Pre-existing type 2 diabetes mellitus, in childbirth** COM Q M
**O24.13 Pre-existing type 2 diabetes mellitus, in the puerperium** COM Q M

**O24.3 Unspecified pre-existing diabetes mellitus in pregnancy, childbirth and the puerperium**
Use additional code (for):
from category E11 to further identify any manifestation
injectable non-insulin antidiabetic drugs (Z79.85)
long-term (current) use of insulin (Z79.4)

**O24.31 Unspecified pre-existing diabetes mellitus in pregnancy**
- **O24.311 Unspecified pre-existing diabetes mellitus in pregnancy, first trimester** COM Q M
- **O24.312 Unspecified pre-existing diabetes mellitus in pregnancy, second trimester** COM Q M
- **O24.313 Unspecified pre-existing diabetes mellitus in pregnancy, third trimester** COM Q M
- **O24.319 Unspecified pre-existing diabetes mellitus in pregnancy, unspecified trimester** COM Q M

**O24.32 Unspecified pre-existing diabetes mellitus in childbirth** COM Q M
**O24.33 Unspecified pre-existing diabetes mellitus in the puerperium** COM Q M

**O24.4 Gestational diabetes mellitus**
Diabetes mellitus arising in pregnancy
Gestational diabetes mellitus NOS
**AHA:** 2020,3Q,30; 2016,4Q,50; 2015,4Q,34

**O24.41 Gestational diabetes mellitus in pregnancy**
- **O24.410 Gestational diabetes mellitus in pregnancy, diet controlled** COM M
- **O24.414 Gestational diabetes mellitus in pregnancy, insulin controlled** COM M
- **O24.415 Gestational diabetes mellitus in pregnancy, controlled by oral hypoglycemic drugs** COM M
  Gestational diabetes mellitus in pregnancy, controlled by oral antidiabetic drugs
- **O24.419 Gestational diabetes mellitus in pregnancy, unspecified control** COM M

**O24.42 Gestational diabetes mellitus in childbirth**
**AHA:** 2016,1Q,5
- **O24.420 Gestational diabetes mellitus in childbirth, diet controlled** COM M
- **O24.424 Gestational diabetes mellitus in childbirth, insulin controlled** COM M
- **O24.425 Gestational diabetes mellitus in childbirth, controlled by oral hypoglycemic drugs** COM M
  Gestational diabetes mellitus in childbirth, controlled by oral antidiabetic drugs
- **O24.429 Gestational diabetes mellitus in childbirth, unspecified control** COM M

**O24.43 Gestational diabetes mellitus in the puerperium**
- **O24.430 Gestational diabetes mellitus in the puerperium, diet controlled** COM M
- **O24.434 Gestational diabetes mellitus in the puerperium, insulin controlled** COM M
- **O24.435 Gestational diabetes mellitus in puerperium, controlled by oral hypoglycemic drugs** COM M
  Gestational diabetes mellitus in puerperium, controlled by oral antidiabetic drugs
- **O24.439 Gestational diabetes mellitus in the puerperium, unspecified control** COM M

**O24.8 Other pre-existing diabetes mellitus in pregnancy, childbirth, and the puerperium**
Use additional code (for):
from categories E08, E09 and E13 to further identify any manifestation
injectable non-insulin antidiabetic drugs (Z79.85)
long-term (current) use of insulin (Z79.4)

**O24.81 Other pre-existing diabetes mellitus in pregnancy**
- **O24.811 Other pre-existing diabetes mellitus in pregnancy, first trimester** COM Q M
- **O24.812 Other pre-existing diabetes mellitus in pregnancy, second trimester** COM Q M
- **O24.813 Other pre-existing diabetes mellitus in pregnancy, third trimester** COM Q M
- **O24.819 Other pre-existing diabetes mellitus in pregnancy, unspecified trimester** COM Q M

**O24.82 Other pre-existing diabetes mellitus in childbirth** COM Q M
**O24.83 Other pre-existing diabetes mellitus in the puerperium** COM Q M

**O24.9 Unspecified diabetes mellitus in pregnancy, childbirth and the puerperium**
Use additional code (for):
from categories E08, E09 and E13 to further identify any manifestation
injectable non-insulin antidiabetic drugs (Z79.85)
long-term (current) use of insulin (Z79.4)

**O24.91 Unspecified diabetes mellitus in pregnancy**
- **O24.911 Unspecified diabetes mellitus in pregnancy, first trimester** COM M
- **O24.912 Unspecified diabetes mellitus in pregnancy, second trimester** COM M
- **O24.913 Unspecified diabetes mellitus in pregnancy, third trimester** COM M
- **O24.919 Unspecified diabetes mellitus in pregnancy, unspecified trimester** COM M

**O24.92 Unspecified diabetes mellitus in childbirth** COM M
**O24.93 Unspecified diabetes mellitus in the puerperium** COM M

**O25 Malnutrition in pregnancy, childbirth and the puerperium**

**O25.1 Malnutrition in pregnancy**
- **O25.10 Malnutrition in pregnancy, unspecified trimester** COM M
- **O25.11 Malnutrition in pregnancy, first trimester** COM M

O25.12 Malnutrition in pregnancy, second trimester COM M
O25.13 Malnutrition in pregnancy, third trimester COM M
O25.2 Malnutrition in childbirth COM M
O25.3 Malnutrition in the puerperium COM M

✓4th **O26 Maternal care for other conditions predominantly related to pregnancy**

✓5th O26.Ø Excessive weight gain in pregnancy
EXCLUDES 2 *gestational edema (O12.Ø, O12.2)*
O26.ØØ Excessive weight gain in pregnancy, unspecified trimester COM M
O26.Ø1 Excessive weight gain in pregnancy, first trimester COM M
O26.Ø2 Excessive weight gain in pregnancy, second trimester COM M
O26.Ø3 Excessive weight gain in pregnancy, third trimester COM M

✓5th O26.1 Low weight gain in pregnancy
O26.1Ø Low weight gain in pregnancy, unspecified trimester COM M
O26.11 Low weight gain in pregnancy, first trimester COM M
O26.12 Low weight gain in pregnancy, second trimester COM M
O26.13 Low weight gain in pregnancy, third trimester COM M

✓5th O26.2 Pregnancy care for patient with recurrent pregnancy loss
O26.2Ø Pregnancy care for patient with recurrent pregnancy loss, unspecified trimester COM M
O26.21 Pregnancy care for patient with recurrent pregnancy loss, first trimester COM M
O26.22 Pregnancy care for patient with recurrent pregnancy loss, second trimester COM M
O26.23 Pregnancy care for patient with recurrent pregnancy loss, third trimester COM M

✓5th O26.3 Retained intrauterine contraceptive device in pregnancy
O26.3Ø Retained intrauterine contraceptive device in pregnancy, unspecified trimester COM M
O26.31 Retained intrauterine contraceptive device in pregnancy, first trimester COM M
O26.32 Retained intrauterine contraceptive device in pregnancy, second trimester COM M
O26.33 Retained intrauterine contraceptive device in pregnancy, third trimester COM M

✓5th O26.4 Herpes gestationis
**DEF:** Rare skin disorder of unknown origin that appears on the abdomen in the second and third trimester as intensely itchy blisters that spread to other sites.
O26.4Ø Herpes gestationis, unspecified trimester COM M
O26.41 Herpes gestationis, first trimester COM M
O26.42 Herpes gestationis, second trimester COM M
O26.43 Herpes gestationis, third trimester COM M

✓5th O26.5 Maternal hypotension syndrome
Supine hypotensive syndrome
O26.5Ø Maternal hypotension syndrome, unspecified trimester COM M
O26.51 Maternal hypotension syndrome, first trimester COM M
O26.52 Maternal hypotension syndrome, second trimester COM M
O26.53 Maternal hypotension syndrome, third trimester COM M

✓5th O26.6 Liver and biliary tract disorders in pregnancy, childbirth and the puerperium
Use additional code to identify the specific disorder
EXCLUDES 2 *hepatorenal syndrome following labor and delivery (O9Ø.41)*

✓6th O26.61 Liver and biliary tract disorders in pregnancy
O26.611 Liver and biliary tract disorders in pregnancy, first trimester COM M
O26.612 Liver and biliary tract disorders in pregnancy, second trimester COM M
O26.613 Liver and biliary tract disorders in pregnancy, third trimester COM M
O26.619 Liver and biliary tract disorders in pregnancy, unspecified trimester COM M
O26.62 Liver and biliary tract disorders in childbirth COM M
**AHA:** 2023,1Q,26
O26.63 Liver and biliary tract disorders in the puerperium COM M

✓6th O26.64 Intrahepatic cholestasis of pregnancy
Use additional code for hepatic obstruction (K76.89)
**AHA:** 2023,4Q,36-37
O26.641 Intrahepatic cholestasis of pregnancy, first trimester COM M
O26.642 Intrahepatic cholestasis of pregnancy, second trimester COM M
O26.643 Intrahepatic cholestasis of pregnancy, third trimester COM M
O26.649 Intrahepatic cholestasis of pregnancy, unspecified trimester COM M

✓5th O26.7 Subluxation of symphysis (pubis) in pregnancy, childbirth and the puerperium
EXCLUDES 1 *traumatic separation of symphysis (pubis) during childbirth (O71.6)*

✓6th O26.71 Subluxation of symphysis (pubis) in pregnancy
O26.711 Subluxation of symphysis (pubis) in pregnancy, first trimester COM M
O26.712 Subluxation of symphysis (pubis) in pregnancy, second trimester COM M
O26.713 Subluxation of symphysis (pubis) in pregnancy, third trimester COM M
O26.719 Subluxation of symphysis (pubis) in pregnancy, unspecified trimester COM M
O26.72 Subluxation of symphysis (pubis) in childbirth COM M
O26.73 Subluxation of symphysis (pubis) in the puerperium COM M

✓5th O26.8 Other specified pregnancy related conditions

✓6th O26.81 Pregnancy related exhaustion and fatigue
O26.811 Pregnancy related exhaustion and fatigue, first trimester COM M
O26.812 Pregnancy related exhaustion and fatigue, second trimester COM M
O26.813 Pregnancy related exhaustion and fatigue, third trimester COM M
O26.819 Pregnancy related exhaustion and fatigue, unspecified trimester COM M

✓6th O26.82 Pregnancy related peripheral neuritis
O26.821 Pregnancy related peripheral neuritis, first trimester COM M
O26.822 Pregnancy related peripheral neuritis, second trimester COM M
O26.823 Pregnancy related peripheral neuritis, third trimester COM M
O26.829 Pregnancy related peripheral neuritis, unspecified trimester COM M

✓6th O26.83 Pregnancy related renal disease
Use additional code to identify the specific disorder
O26.831 Pregnancy related renal disease, first trimester COM M
O26.832 Pregnancy related renal disease, second trimester COM M
O26.833 Pregnancy related renal disease, third trimester COM M
O26.839 Pregnancy related renal disease, unspecified trimester COM M

✓6th O26.84 Uterine size-date discrepancy complicating pregnancy
EXCLUDES 1 *encounter for suspected problem with fetal growth ruled out (ZØ3.74)*
O26.841 Uterine size-date discrepancy, first trimester COM M
O26.842 Uterine size-date discrepancy, second trimester COM M
O26.843 Uterine size-date discrepancy, third trimester COM M
O26.849 Uterine size-date discrepancy, unspecified trimester COM M

✓6th **O26.85 Spotting complicating pregnancy**

**O26.851 Spotting complicating pregnancy, first trimester** COM M

**O26.852 Spotting complicating pregnancy, second trimester** COM M

**O26.853 Spotting complicating pregnancy, third trimester** COM M

**O26.859 Spotting complicating pregnancy, unspecified trimester** COM M

**O26.86 Pruritic urticarial papules and plaques of pregnancy (PUPPP)** COM M

Polymorphic eruption of pregnancy

✓6th **O26.87 Cervical shortening**

EXCLUDES 1 *encounter for suspected cervical shortening ruled out (Z03.75)*

**DEF:** Cervix that has shortened to less than 25 mm before the 24th week of pregnancy. A shortened cervix is a warning sign for impending premature delivery and is treated by cervical cerclage placement or progesterone.

**O26.872 Cervical shortening, second trimester** COM M

**O26.873 Cervical shortening, third trimester** COM M

**O26.879 Cervical shortening, unspecified trimester** COM M

✓6th **O26.89 Other specified pregnancy related conditions**

Use additional code, if applicable, to identify specific condition such as insulin resistance (E88.81-)

**AHA:** 2015,3Q,40

**O26.891 Other specified pregnancy related conditions, first trimester** COM M

**O26.892 Other specified pregnancy related conditions, second trimester** COM M

**O26.893 Other specified pregnancy related conditions, third trimester** COM M

**O26.899 Other specified pregnancy related conditions, unspecified trimester** COM M

✓5th **O26.9 Pregnancy related conditions, unspecified**

**O26.90 Pregnancy related conditions, unspecified, unspecified trimester** COM M

**O26.91 Pregnancy related conditions, unspecified, first trimester** COM M

**O26.92 Pregnancy related conditions, unspecified, second trimester** COM M

**O26.93 Pregnancy related conditions, unspecified, third trimester** COM M

✓4th **O28 Abnormal findings on antenatal screening of mother**

EXCLUDES 1 *diagnostic findings classified elsewhere - see Alphabetical Index*

**O28.0 Abnormal hematological finding on antenatal screening of mother** M

**O28.1 Abnormal biochemical finding on antenatal screening of mother** M

**O28.2 Abnormal cytological finding on antenatal screening of mother** M

**O28.3 Abnormal ultrasonic finding on antenatal screening of mother** M

**O28.4 Abnormal radiological finding on antenatal screening of mother** M

**O28.5 Abnormal chromosomal and genetic finding on antenatal screening of mother** M

**O28.8 Other abnormal findings on antenatal screening of mother** M

**O28.9 Unspecified abnormal findings on antenatal screening of mother** M

✓4th **O29 Complications of anesthesia during pregnancy**

INCLUDES maternal complications arising from the administration of a general, regional or local anesthetic, analgesic or other sedation during pregnancy

Use additional code, if necessary, to identify the complication

EXCLUDES 2 *complications of anesthesia during labor and delivery (O74.-)*
*complications of anesthesia during the puerperium (O89.-)*

✓5th **O29.0 Pulmonary complications of anesthesia during pregnancy**

✓6th **O29.01 Aspiration pneumonitis due to anesthesia during pregnancy**

Inhalation of stomach contents or secretions NOS due to anesthesia during pregnancy

Mendelson's syndrome due to anesthesia during pregnancy

**O29.011 Aspiration pneumonitis due to anesthesia during pregnancy, first trimester** COM M

**O29.012 Aspiration pneumonitis due to anesthesia during pregnancy, second trimester** COM M

**O29.013 Aspiration pneumonitis due to anesthesia during pregnancy, third trimester** COM M

**O29.019 Aspiration pneumonitis due to anesthesia during pregnancy, unspecified trimester** COM M

✓6th **O29.02 Pressure collapse of lung due to anesthesia during pregnancy**

**O29.021 Pressure collapse of lung due to anesthesia during pregnancy, first trimester** COM M

**O29.022 Pressure collapse of lung due to anesthesia during pregnancy, second trimester** COM M

**O29.023 Pressure collapse of lung due to anesthesia during pregnancy, third trimester** COM M

**O29.029 Pressure collapse of lung due to anesthesia during pregnancy, unspecified trimester** COM M

✓6th **O29.09 Other pulmonary complications of anesthesia during pregnancy**

**O29.091 Other pulmonary complications of anesthesia during pregnancy, first trimester** COM M

**O29.092 Other pulmonary complications of anesthesia during pregnancy, second trimester** COM M

**O29.093 Other pulmonary complications of anesthesia during pregnancy, third trimester** COM M

**O29.099 Other pulmonary complications of anesthesia during pregnancy, unspecified trimester** COM M

✓5th **O29.1 Cardiac complications of anesthesia during pregnancy**

✓6th **O29.11 Cardiac arrest due to anesthesia during pregnancy**

**O29.111 Cardiac arrest due to anesthesia during pregnancy, first trimester** COM M

**O29.112 Cardiac arrest due to anesthesia during pregnancy, second trimester** COM M

**O29.113 Cardiac arrest due to anesthesia during pregnancy, third trimester** COM M

**O29.119 Cardiac arrest due to anesthesia during pregnancy, unspecified trimester** COM M

✓6th **O29.12 Cardiac failure due to anesthesia during pregnancy**

**O29.121 Cardiac failure due to anesthesia during pregnancy, first trimester** COM M

**O29.122 Cardiac failure due to anesthesia during pregnancy, second trimester** COM M

**O29.123 Cardiac failure due to anesthesia during pregnancy, third trimester** COM M

**O29.129 Cardiac failure due to anesthesia during pregnancy, unspecified trimester** COM M

✓6th **O29.19 Other cardiac complications of anesthesia during pregnancy**

**O29.191 Other cardiac complications of anesthesia during pregnancy, first trimester** COM M

**O29.192 Other cardiac complications of anesthesia during pregnancy, second trimester** COM M

O29.193 Other cardiac complications of anesthesia during pregnancy, third trimester COM M

O29.199 Other cardiac complications of anesthesia during pregnancy, unspecified trimester COM M

√5th O29.2 Central nervous system complications of anesthesia during pregnancy

√6th O29.21 Cerebral anoxia due to anesthesia during pregnancy

O29.211 Cerebral anoxia due to anesthesia during pregnancy, first trimester COM M

O29.212 Cerebral anoxia due to anesthesia during pregnancy, second trimester COM M

O29.213 Cerebral anoxia due to anesthesia during pregnancy, third trimester COM M

O29.219 Cerebral anoxia due to anesthesia during pregnancy, unspecified trimester COM M

√6th O29.29 Other central nervous system complications of anesthesia during pregnancy

O29.291 Other central nervous system complications of anesthesia during pregnancy, first trimester COM M

O29.292 Other central nervous system complications of anesthesia during pregnancy, second trimester COM M

O29.293 Other central nervous system complications of anesthesia during pregnancy, third trimester COM M

O29.299 Other central nervous system complications of anesthesia during pregnancy, unspecified trimester COM M

√5th O29.3 Toxic reaction to local anesthesia during pregnancy

√6th O29.3X Toxic reaction to local anesthesia during pregnancy

O29.3X1 Toxic reaction to local anesthesia during pregnancy, first trimester COM M

O29.3X2 Toxic reaction to local anesthesia during pregnancy, second trimester COM M

O29.3X3 Toxic reaction to local anesthesia during pregnancy, third trimester COM M

O29.3X9 Toxic reaction to local anesthesia during pregnancy, unspecified trimester COM M

√5th O29.4 Spinal and epidural anesthesia induced headache during pregnancy

O29.4Ø Spinal and epidural anesthesia induced headache during pregnancy, unspecified trimester COM M

O29.41 Spinal and epidural anesthesia induced headache during pregnancy, first trimester COM M

O29.42 Spinal and epidural anesthesia induced headache during pregnancy, second trimester COM M

O29.43 Spinal and epidural anesthesia induced headache during pregnancy, third trimester COM M

√5th O29.5 Other complications of spinal and epidural anesthesia during pregnancy

√6th O29.5X Other complications of spinal and epidural anesthesia during pregnancy

O29.5X1 Other complications of spinal and epidural anesthesia during pregnancy, first trimester COM M

O29.5X2 Other complications of spinal and epidural anesthesia during pregnancy, second trimester COM M

O29.5X3 Other complications of spinal and epidural anesthesia during pregnancy, third trimester COM M

O29.5X9 Other complications of spinal and epidural anesthesia during pregnancy, unspecified trimester COM M

√5th O29.6 Failed or difficult intubation for anesthesia during pregnancy

O29.6Ø Failed or difficult intubation for anesthesia during pregnancy, unspecified trimester COM M

O29.61 Failed or difficult intubation for anesthesia during pregnancy, first trimester COM M

O29.62 Failed or difficult intubation for anesthesia during pregnancy, second trimester COM M

O29.63 Failed or difficult intubation for anesthesia during pregnancy, third trimester COM M

√5th O29.8 Other complications of anesthesia during pregnancy

√6th O29.8X Other complications of anesthesia during pregnancy

O29.8X1 Other complications of anesthesia during pregnancy, first trimester COM M

O29.8X2 Other complications of anesthesia during pregnancy, second trimester COM M

O29.8X3 Other complications of anesthesia during pregnancy, third trimester COM M

O29.8X9 Other complications of anesthesia during pregnancy, unspecified trimester COM M

√5th O29.9 Unspecified complication of anesthesia during pregnancy

O29.9Ø Unspecified complication of anesthesia during pregnancy, unspecified trimester COM M

O29.91 Unspecified complication of anesthesia during pregnancy, first trimester COM M

O29.92 Unspecified complication of anesthesia during pregnancy, second trimester COM M

O29.93 Unspecified complication of anesthesia during pregnancy, third trimester COM M

## Maternal care related to the fetus and amniotic cavity and possible delivery problems (O3Ø-O48)

√4th **O3Ø Multiple gestation**

Code also any complications specific to multiple gestation

AHA: 2016,4Q,51

√5th O3Ø.Ø Twin pregnancy

√6th O3Ø.ØØ Twin pregnancy, unspecified number of placenta and unspecified number of amniotic sacs

O3Ø.ØØ1 Twin pregnancy, unspecified number of placenta and unspecified number of amniotic sacs, first trimester COM M

O3Ø.ØØ2 Twin pregnancy, unspecified number of placenta and unspecified number of amniotic sacs, second trimester COM M

O3Ø.ØØ3 Twin pregnancy, unspecified number of placenta and unspecified number of amniotic sacs, third trimester COM M

O3Ø.ØØ9 Twin pregnancy, unspecified number of placenta and unspecified number of amniotic sacs, unspecified trimester COM M

√6th O3Ø.Ø1 Twin pregnancy, monochorionic/monoamniotic

Twin pregnancy, one placenta, one amniotic sac

EXCLUDES 1 *conjoined twins (O3Ø.Ø2-)*

O3Ø.Ø11 Twin pregnancy, monochorionic/monoamniotic, first trimester COM M

O3Ø.Ø12 Twin pregnancy, monochorionic/monoamniotic, second trimester COM M

O3Ø.Ø13 Twin pregnancy, monochorionic/monoamniotic, third trimester COM M

O3Ø.Ø19 Twin pregnancy, monochorionic/monoamniotic, unspecified trimester COM M

√6th O3Ø.Ø2 Conjoined twin pregnancy

O3Ø.Ø21 Conjoined twin pregnancy, first trimester COM M

O3Ø.Ø22 Conjoined twin pregnancy, second trimester COM M

O3Ø.Ø23 Conjoined twin pregnancy, third trimester COM M

O3Ø.Ø29 Conjoined twin pregnancy, unspecified trimester COM M

√6th O3Ø.Ø3 Twin pregnancy, monochorionic/diamniotic

Twin pregnancy, one placenta, two amniotic sacs

O3Ø.Ø31 Twin pregnancy, monochorionic/diamniotic, first trimester COM M

O3Ø.Ø32 Twin pregnancy, monochorionic/diamniotic, second trimester COM M

O3Ø.Ø33 Twin pregnancy, monochorionic/diamniotic, third trimester COM M

O30.039 Twin pregnancy, monochorionic/diamniotic, unspecified trimester COM M

✓6th O30.04 Twin pregnancy, dichorionic/diamniotic
Twin pregnancy, two placentae, two amniotic sacs

O30.041 Twin pregnancy, dichorionic/diamniotic, first trimester COM M

O30.042 Twin pregnancy, dichorionic/diamniotic, second trimester COM M

O30.043 Twin pregnancy, dichorionic/diamniotic, third trimester COM M

O30.049 Twin pregnancy, dichorionic/diamniotic, unspecified trimester COM M

✓6th O30.09 Twin pregnancy, unable to determine number of placenta and number of amniotic sacs

O30.091 Twin pregnancy, unable to determine number of placenta and number of amniotic sacs, first trimester COM M

O30.092 Twin pregnancy, unable to determine number of placenta and number of amniotic sacs, second trimester COM M

O30.093 Twin pregnancy, unable to determine number of placenta and number of amniotic sacs, third trimester COM M

O30.099 Twin pregnancy, unable to determine number of placenta and number of amniotic sacs, unspecified trimester COM M

✓5th O30.1 Triplet pregnancy

✓6th O30.10 Triplet pregnancy, unspecified number of placenta and unspecified number of amniotic sacs
AHA: 2016,2Q,8

O30.101 Triplet pregnancy, unspecified number of placenta and unspecified number of amniotic sacs, first trimester COM M

O30.102 Triplet pregnancy, unspecified number of placenta and unspecified number of amniotic sacs, second trimester COM M

O30.103 Triplet pregnancy, unspecified number of placenta and unspecified number of amniotic sacs, third trimester COM M

O30.109 Triplet pregnancy, unspecified number of placenta and unspecified number of amniotic sacs, unspecified trimester COM M

✓6th O30.11 Triplet pregnancy with two or more monochorionic fetuses

O30.111 Triplet pregnancy with two or more monochorionic fetuses, first trimester COM M

O30.112 Triplet pregnancy with two or more monochorionic fetuses, second trimester COM M

O30.113 Triplet pregnancy with two or more monochorionic fetuses, third trimester COM M

O30.119 Triplet pregnancy with two or more monochorionic fetuses, unspecified trimester COM M

✓6th O30.12 Triplet pregnancy with two or more monoamniotic fetuses

O30.121 Triplet pregnancy with two or more monoamniotic fetuses, first trimester COM M

O30.122 Triplet pregnancy with two or more monoamniotic fetuses, second trimester COM M

O30.123 Triplet pregnancy with two or more monoamniotic fetuses, third trimester COM M

O30.129 Triplet pregnancy with two or more monoamniotic fetuses, unspecified trimester COM M

✓6th O30.13 Triplet pregnancy, trichorionic/triamniotic
AHA: 2018,4Q,22

O30.131 Triplet pregnancy, trichorionic/triamniotic, first trimester COM M

O30.132 Triplet pregnancy, trichorionic/triamniotic, second trimester COM M

O30.133 Triplet pregnancy, trichorionic/triamniotic, third trimester COM M

O30.139 Triplet pregnancy, trichorionic/triamniotic, unspecified trimester COM M

✓6th O30.19 Triplet pregnancy, unable to determine number of placenta and number of amniotic sacs

O30.191 Triplet pregnancy, unable to determine number of placenta and number of amniotic sacs, first trimester COM M

O30.192 Triplet pregnancy, unable to determine number of placenta and number of amniotic sacs, second trimester COM M

O30.193 Triplet pregnancy, unable to determine number of placenta and number of amniotic sacs, third trimester COM M

O30.199 Triplet pregnancy, unable to determine number of placenta and number of amniotic sacs, unspecified trimester COM M

✓5th O30.2 Quadruplet pregnancy

✓6th O30.20 Quadruplet pregnancy, unspecified number of placenta and unspecified number of amniotic sacs

O30.201 Quadruplet pregnancy, unspecified number of placenta and unspecified number of amniotic sacs, first trimester COM M

O30.202 Quadruplet pregnancy, unspecified number of placenta and unspecified number of amniotic sacs, second trimester COM M

O30.203 Quadruplet pregnancy, unspecified number of placenta and unspecified number of amniotic sacs, third trimester COM M

O30.209 Quadruplet pregnancy, unspecified number of placenta and unspecified number of amniotic sacs, unspecified trimester COM M

✓6th O30.21 Quadruplet pregnancy with two or more monochorionic fetuses

O30.211 Quadruplet pregnancy with two or more monochorionic fetuses, first trimester COM M

O30.212 Quadruplet pregnancy with two or more monochorionic fetuses, second trimester COM M

O30.213 Quadruplet pregnancy with two or more monochorionic fetuses, third trimester COM M

O30.219 Quadruplet pregnancy with two or more monochorionic fetuses, unspecified trimester COM M

✓6th O30.22 Quadruplet pregnancy with two or more monoamniotic fetuses

O30.221 Quadruplet pregnancy with two or more monoamniotic fetuses, first trimester COM M

O30.222 Quadruplet pregnancy with two or more monoamniotic fetuses, second trimester COM M

O30.223 Quadruplet pregnancy with two or more monoamniotic fetuses, third trimester COM M

O30.229 Quadruplet pregnancy with two or more monoamniotic fetuses, unspecified trimester COM M

✓6th O30.23 Quadruplet pregnancy, quadrachorionic/quadra-amniotic
AHA: 2018,4Q,22

O30.231 Quadruplet pregnancy, quadrachorionic/quadra-amniotic, first trimester COM M

O30.232 Quadruplet pregnancy, quadrachorionic/quadra-amniotic, second trimester COM M

O30.233 Quadruplet pregnancy, quadrachorionic/quadra-amniotic, third trimester COM M

O30.239 Quadruplet pregnancy, quadrachorionic/quadra-amniotic, unspecified trimester COM M

√6th O30.29 Quadruplet pregnancy, unable to determine number of placenta and number of amniotic sacs
- O30.291 Quadruplet pregnancy, unable to determine number of placenta and number of amniotic sacs, first trimester COM M
- O30.292 Quadruplet pregnancy, unable to determine number of placenta and number of amniotic sacs, second trimester COM M
- O30.293 Quadruplet pregnancy, unable to determine number of placenta and number of amniotic sacs, third trimester COM M
- O30.299 Quadruplet pregnancy, unable to determine number of placenta and number of amniotic sacs, unspecified trimester COM M

√5th O30.8 Other specified multiple gestation

Multiple gestation pregnancy greater then quadruplets

√6th O30.80 Other specified multiple gestation, unspecified number of placenta and unspecified number of amniotic sacs
- O30.801 Other specified multiple gestation, unspecified number of placenta and unspecified number of amniotic sacs, first trimester COM M
- O30.802 Other specified multiple gestation, unspecified number of placenta and unspecified number of amniotic sacs, second trimester COM M
- O30.803 Other specified multiple gestation, unspecified number of placenta and unspecified number of amniotic sacs, third trimester COM M
- O30.809 Other specified multiple gestation, unspecified number of placenta and unspecified number of amniotic sacs, unspecified trimester COM M

√6th O30.81 Other specified multiple gestation with two or more monochorionic fetuses
- O30.811 Other specified multiple gestation with two or more monochorionic fetuses, first trimester COM M
- O30.812 Other specified multiple gestation with two or more monochorionic fetuses, second trimester COM M
- O30.813 Other specified multiple gestation with two or more monochorionic fetuses, third trimester COM M
- O30.819 Other specified multiple gestation with two or more monochorionic fetuses, unspecified trimester COM M

√6th O30.82 Other specified multiple gestation with two or more monoamniotic fetuses
- O30.821 Other specified multiple gestation with two or more monoamniotic fetuses, first trimester COM M
- O30.822 Other specified multiple gestation with two or more monoamniotic fetuses, second trimester COM M
- O30.823 Other specified multiple gestation with two or more monoamniotic fetuses, third trimester COM M
- O30.829 Other specified multiple gestation with two or more monoamniotic fetuses, unspecified trimester COM M

√6th O30.83 Other specified multiple gestation, number of chorions and amnions are both equal to the number of fetuses

Heptachorionic, hepta-amniotic pregnancy (septuplets)
Hexachorionic, hexa-amniotic pregnancy (sextuplets)
Pentachorionic, penta-amniotic pregnancy (quintuplets)

**AHA:** 2018,4Q,22
- O30.831 Other specified multiple gestation, number of chorions and amnions are both equal to the number of fetuses, first trimester COM M
- O30.832 Other specified multiple gestation, number of chorions and amnions are both equal to the number of fetuses, second trimester COM M
- O30.833 Other specified multiple gestation, number of chorions and amnions are both equal to the number of fetuses, third trimester COM M
- O30.839 Other specified multiple gestation, number of chorions and amnions are both equal to the number of fetuses, unspecified trimester COM M

√6th O30.89 Other specified multiple gestation, unable to determine number of placenta and number of amniotic sacs
- O30.891 Other specified multiple gestation, unable to determine number of placenta and number of amniotic sacs, first trimester COM M
- O30.892 Other specified multiple gestation, unable to determine number of placenta and number of amniotic sacs, second trimester COM M
- O30.893 Other specified multiple gestation, unable to determine number of placenta and number of amniotic sacs, third trimester COM M
- O30.899 Other specified multiple gestation, unable to determine number of placenta and number of amniotic sacs, unspecified trimester COM M

√5th O30.9 Multiple gestation, unspecified

Multiple pregnancy NOS
- O30.90 Multiple gestation, unspecified, unspecified trimester COM M
- O30.91 Multiple gestation, unspecified, first trimester COM M
- O30.92 Multiple gestation, unspecified, second trimester COM M
- O30.93 Multiple gestation, unspecified, third trimester COM M

## √4th O31 Complications specific to multiple gestation

EXCLUDES 2 *delayed delivery of second twin, triplet, etc. (O63.2)*
*malpresentation of one fetus or more (O32.9)*
*placental transfusion syndromes (O43.0-)*

**AHA:** 2012,4Q,107

One of the following 7th characters is to be assigned to each code under category O31. 7th character 0 is for single gestations and multiple gestations where the fetus is unspecified. 7th characters 1 through 9 are for cases of multiple gestations to identify the fetus for which the code applies. The appropriate code from category O30, Multiple gestation, must also be assigned when assigning a code from category O31 that has a 7th character of 1 through 9.

0 not applicable or unspecified
1 fetus 1
2 fetus 2
3 fetus 3
4 fetus 4
5 fetus 5
9 other fetus

√5th O31.0 Papyraceous fetus

Fetus compressus

**DEF:** Fetus that has died, but remains in utero for weeks before delivery, becoming compacted and mummified in appearance, with skin resembling parchment. Occurs most commonly in multigestational pregnancies. ***Synonym(s):*** *paper doll fetus.*

- √x7th O31.00 Papyraceous fetus, unspecified trimester COM M
- √x7th O31.01 Papyraceous fetus, first trimester COM M
- √x7th O31.02 Papyraceous fetus, second trimester COM M
- √x7th O31.03 Papyraceous fetus, third trimester COM M

√5th O31.1 Continuing pregnancy after spontaneous abortion of one fetus or more
- √x7th O31.10 Continuing pregnancy after spontaneous abortion of one fetus or more, unspecified trimester COM M
- √x7th O31.11 Continuing pregnancy after spontaneous abortion of one fetus or more, first trimester COM M
- √x7th O31.12 Continuing pregnancy after spontaneous abortion of one fetus or more, second trimester COM M
- √x7th O31.13 Continuing pregnancy after spontaneous abortion of one fetus or more, third trimester COM M

√5th **O31.2 Continuing pregnancy after intrauterine death of one fetus or more**

√x7th **O31.2Ø Continuing pregnancy after intrauterine death of one fetus or more, unspecified trimester** COM M

√x7th **O31.21 Continuing pregnancy after intrauterine death of one fetus or more, first trimester** COM M

√x7th **O31.22 Continuing pregnancy after intrauterine death of one fetus or more, second trimester** COM M

√x7th **O31.23 Continuing pregnancy after intrauterine death of one fetus or more, third trimester** COM M

√5th **O31.3 Continuing pregnancy after elective fetal reduction of one fetus or more**

Continuing pregnancy after selective termination of one fetus or more

√x7th **O31.3Ø Continuing pregnancy after elective fetal reduction of one fetus or more, unspecified trimester** COM M

√x7th **O31.31 Continuing pregnancy after elective fetal reduction of one fetus or more, first trimester** COM M

√x7th **O31.32 Continuing pregnancy after elective fetal reduction of one fetus or more, second trimester** COM M

√x7th **O31.33 Continuing pregnancy after elective fetal reduction of one fetus or more, third trimester** COM M

● √5th **O31.4 Continuing pregnancy after vanishing twin syndrome of one fetus or more**

● √x7th **O31.4Ø Continuing pregnancy after vanishing twin syndrome of one fetus or more, unspecified trimester**

● √x7th **O31.41 Continuing pregnancy after vanishing twin syndrome of one fetus or more, first trimester**

● √x7th **O31.42 Continuing pregnancy after vanishing twin syndrome of one fetus or more, second trimester**

● √x7th **O31.43 Continuing pregnancy after vanishing twin syndrome of one fetus or more, third trimester**

√5th **O31.8 Other complications specific to multiple gestation** COM

√6th **O31.8X Other complications specific to multiple gestation**

√7th **O31.8X1 Other complications specific to multiple gestation, first trimester** M

√7th **O31.8X2 Other complications specific to multiple gestation, second trimester** M

√7th **O31.8X3 Other complications specific to multiple gestation, third trimester** M

√7th **O31.8X9 Other complications specific to multiple gestation, unspecified trimester** M

√4th **O32 Maternal care for malpresentation of fetus**

INCLUDES the listed conditions as a reason for observation, hospitalization or other obstetric care of the mother, or for cesarean delivery before onset of labor

EXCLUDES 1 *malpresentation of fetus with obstructed labor (O64.-)*

**AHA:** 2026,2Q,11; 2012,4Q,107

One of the following 7th characters is to be assigned to each code under category O32. 7th character Ø is for single gestations and multiple gestations where the fetus is unspecified. 7th characters 1 through 9 are for cases of multiple gestations to identify the fetus for which the code applies. The appropriate code from category O3Ø, Multiple gestation, must also be assigned when assigning a code from category O32 that has a 7th character of 1 through 9.

Ø not applicable or unspecified
1 fetus 1
2 fetus 2
3 fetus 3
4 fetus 4
5 fetus 5
9 other fetus

**Fetal Malpresentation**

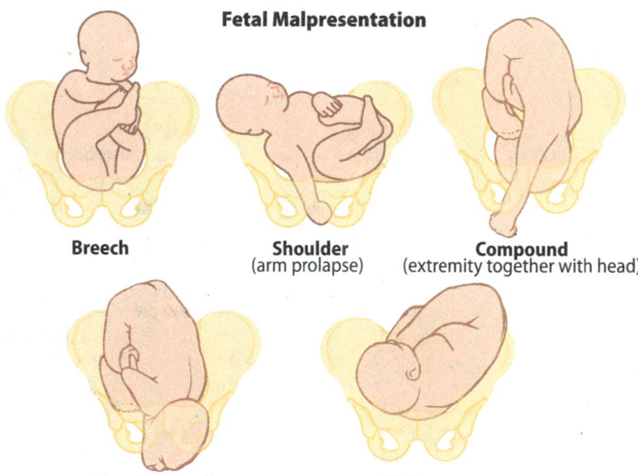


√x7th **O32.Ø Maternal care for unstable lie** COM M

√x7th **O32.1 Maternal care for breech presentation** COM M

Maternal care for buttocks presentation
Maternal care for complete breech
Maternal care for frank breech

EXCLUDES 1 *footling presentation (O32.8)*
*incomplete breech (O32.8)*

**DEF:** Fetus presentation in a longitudinal lie with the buttocks or feet closest to birth canal that may require external cephalic version or cesarean delivery.

√x7th **O32.2 Maternal care for transverse and oblique lie** COM M

Maternal care for oblique presentation
Maternal care for transverse presentation

√x7th **O32.3 Maternal care for face, brow and chin presentation** COM M

√x7th **O32.4 Maternal care for high head at term** COM M

Maternal care for failure of head to enter pelvic brim

√x7th **O32.6 Maternal care for compound presentation** COM M

√x7th **O32.8 Maternal care for other malpresentation of fetus** COM M

Maternal care for footling presentation
Maternal care for incomplete breech

**AHA:** 2026,2Q,10,12

√x7th **O32.9 Maternal care for malpresentation of fetus, unspecified** COM M

√4th **O33 Maternal care for disproportion**

INCLUDES the listed conditions as a reason for observation, hospitalization or other obstetric care of the mother, or for cesarean delivery before onset of labor

EXCLUDES 1 *disproportion with obstructed labor (O65-O66)*

**O33.Ø Maternal care for disproportion due to deformity of maternal pelvic bones** COM M

Maternal care for disproportion due to pelvic deformity causing disproportion NOS

**O33.1 Maternal care for disproportion due to generally contracted pelvis** COM M

Maternal care for disproportion due to contracted pelvis NOS causing disproportion

**O33.2 Maternal care for disproportion due to inlet contraction of pelvis** COM M

Maternal care for disproportion due to inlet contraction (pelvis) causing disproportion

√x7th **O33.3 Maternal care for disproportion due to outlet contraction of pelvis** COM M

Maternal care for disproportion due to mid-cavity contraction (pelvis)

Maternal care for disproportion due to outlet contraction (pelvis)

One of the following 7th characters is to be assigned to code O33.3. 7th character Ø is for single gestations and multiple gestations where the fetus is unspecified. 7th characters 1 through 9 are for cases of multiple gestations to identify the fetus for which the code applies. The appropriate code from category O3Ø, Multiple gestation, must also be assigned when assigning code O33.3 with a 7th character of 1 through 9.

- Ø not applicable or unspecified
- 1 fetus 1
- 2 fetus 2
- 3 fetus 3
- 4 fetus 4
- 5 fetus 5
- 9 other fetus

√x7th **O33.4 Maternal care for disproportion of mixed maternal and fetal origin** COM M

One of the following 7th characters is to be assigned to code O33.4. 7th character Ø is for single gestations and multiple gestations where the fetus is unspecified. 7th characters 1 through 9 are for cases of multiple gestations to identify the fetus for which the code applies. The appropriate code from category O3Ø, Multiple gestation, must also be assigned when assigning code O33.4 with a 7th character of 1 through 9.

- Ø not applicable or unspecified
- 1 fetus 1
- 2 fetus 2
- 3 fetus 3
- 4 fetus 4
- 5 fetus 5
- 9 other fetus

√x7th **O33.5 Maternal care for disproportion due to unusually large fetus** COM M

Maternal care for disproportion due to disproportion of fetal origin with normally formed fetus

Maternal care for disproportion due to fetal disproportion NOS

One of the following 7th characters is to be assigned to code O33.5. 7th character Ø is for single gestations and multiple gestations where the fetus is unspecified. 7th characters 1 through 9 are for cases of multiple gestations to identify the fetus for which the code applies. The appropriate code from category O3Ø, Multiple gestation, must also be assigned when assigning code O33.5 with a 7th character of 1 through 9.

- Ø not applicable or unspecified
- 1 fetus 1
- 2 fetus 2
- 3 fetus 3
- 4 fetus 4
- 5 fetus 5
- 9 other fetus

√x7th **O33.6 Maternal care for disproportion due to hydrocephalic fetus** COM M

One of the following 7th characters is to be assigned to code O33.6. 7th character Ø is for single gestations and multiple gestations where the fetus is unspecified. 7th characters 1 through 9 are for cases of multiple gestations to identify the fetus for which the code applies. The appropriate code from category O3Ø, Multiple gestation, must also be assigned when assigning code O33.6 with a 7th character of 1 through 9.

- Ø not applicable or unspecified
- 1 fetus 1
- 2 fetus 2
- 3 fetus 3
- 4 fetus 4
- 5 fetus 5
- 9 other fetus

√x7th **O33.7 Maternal care for disproportion due to other fetal deformities** COM M

Maternal care for disproportion due to fetal ascites

Maternal care for disproportion due to fetal hydrops

Maternal care for disproportion due to fetal meningomyelocele

Maternal care for disproportion due to fetal sacral teratoma

Maternal care for disproportion due to fetal tumor

EXCLUDES 1 *obstructed labor due to other fetal deformities (O66.3)*

**AHA:** 2016,4Q,51

One of the following 7th characters is to be assigned to code O33.7. 7th character Ø is for single gestations and multiple gestations where the fetus is unspecified. 7th characters 1 through 9 are for cases of multiple gestations to identify the fetus for which the code applies. The appropriate code from category O3Ø, Multiple gestation, must also be assigned when assigning code O33.7 with a 7th character of 1 through 9.

- Ø not applicable or unspecified
- 1 fetus 1
- 2 fetus 2
- 3 fetus 3
- 4 fetus 4
- 5 fetus 5
- 9 other fetus

**O33.8 Maternal care for disproportion of other origin** COM M

**O33.9 Maternal care for disproportion, unspecified** COM M

Maternal care for disproportion due to cephalopelvic disproportion NOS

Maternal care for disproportion due to fetopelvic disproportion NOS

√4th **O34 Maternal care for abnormality of pelvic organs**

INCLUDES the listed conditions as a reason for hospitalization or other obstetric care of the mother, or for cesarean delivery before onset of labor

Code first any associated obstructed labor (O65.5)

Use additional code for specific condition

√5th **O34.Ø Maternal care for congenital malformation of uterus**

Maternal care for double uterus

Maternal care for uterus bicornis

**O34.ØØ Maternal care for unspecified congenital malformation of uterus, unspecified trimester** COM M

**O34.Ø1 Maternal care for unspecified congenital malformation of uterus, first trimester** COM M

**O34.Ø2 Maternal care for unspecified congenital malformation of uterus, second trimester** COM M

**O34.Ø3 Maternal care for unspecified congenital malformation of uterus, third trimester** COM M

√5th **O34.1 Maternal care for benign tumor of corpus uteri**

EXCLUDES 2 *maternal care for benign tumor of cervix (O34.4-)*
*maternal care for malignant neoplasm of uterus (O9A.1-)*

**O34.1Ø Maternal care for benign tumor of corpus uteri, unspecified trimester** COM M

**O34.11 Maternal care for benign tumor of corpus uteri, first trimester** COM M

**O34.12 Maternal care for benign tumor of corpus uteri, second trimester** COM M

**O34.13 Maternal care for benign tumor of corpus uteri, third trimester** COM M

**O34.2 Maternal care due to uterine scar from previous surgery**
AHA: 2020,4Q,36; 2016,4Q,76

**O34.21 Maternal care for scar from previous cesarean delivery**
AHA: 2018,3Q,23; 2016,4Q,51-52

**O34.211 Maternal care for low transverse scar from previous cesarean delivery** COM M

**O34.212 Maternal care for vertical scar from previous cesarean delivery** COM M
Maternal care for classical scar from previous cesarean delivery

**O34.218 Maternal care for other type scar from previous cesarean delivery** COM M
Mid-transverse T incision

**O34.219 Maternal care for unspecified type scar from previous cesarean delivery** COM M

**O34.22 Maternal care for cesarean scar defect (isthmocele)** COM M

**O34.29 Maternal care due to uterine scar from other previous surgery** COM M
Maternal care due to uterine scar from other transmural uterine incision

**O34.3 Maternal care for cervical incompetence**
Maternal care for cerclage with or without cervical incompetence
Maternal care for Shirodkar suture with or without cervical incompetence
DEF: Inadequate functioning of the cervix marked by abnormal widening during pregnancy and causing premature birth or miscarriage.

**O34.30 Maternal care for cervical incompetence, unspecified trimester** COM M

**O34.31 Maternal care for cervical incompetence, first trimester** COM M

**O34.32 Maternal care for cervical incompetence, second trimester** COM M

**O34.33 Maternal care for cervical incompetence, third trimester** COM M

**O34.4 Maternal care for other abnormalities of cervix**

**O34.40 Maternal care for other abnormalities of cervix, unspecified trimester** COM M

**O34.41 Maternal care for other abnormalities of cervix, first trimester** COM M

**O34.42 Maternal care for other abnormalities of cervix, second trimester** COM M

**O34.43 Maternal care for other abnormalities of cervix, third trimester** COM M

**O34.5 Maternal care for other abnormalities of gravid uterus**

**O34.51 Maternal care for incarceration of gravid uterus**

**O34.511 Maternal care for incarceration of gravid uterus, first trimester** COM M

**O34.512 Maternal care for incarceration of gravid uterus, second trimester** COM M

**O34.513 Maternal care for incarceration of gravid uterus, third trimester** COM M

**O34.519 Maternal care for incarceration of gravid uterus, unspecified trimester** COM M

**O34.52 Maternal care for prolapse of gravid uterus**

**O34.521 Maternal care for prolapse of gravid uterus, first trimester** COM M

**O34.522 Maternal care for prolapse of gravid uterus, second trimester** COM M

**O34.523 Maternal care for prolapse of gravid uterus, third trimester** COM M

**O34.529 Maternal care for prolapse of gravid uterus, unspecified trimester** COM M

**O34.53 Maternal care for retroversion of gravid uterus**

**O34.531 Maternal care for retroversion of gravid uterus, first trimester** COM M

**O34.532 Maternal care for retroversion of gravid uterus, second trimester** COM M

**O34.533 Maternal care for retroversion of gravid uterus, third trimester** COM M

**O34.539 Maternal care for retroversion of gravid uterus, unspecified trimester** COM M

**O34.59 Maternal care for other abnormalities of gravid uterus**

**O34.591 Maternal care for other abnormalities of gravid uterus, first trimester** COM M

**O34.592 Maternal care for other abnormalities of gravid uterus, second trimester** COM M

**O34.593 Maternal care for other abnormalities of gravid uterus, third trimester** COM M

**O34.599 Maternal care for other abnormalities of gravid uterus, unspecified trimester** COM M

**O34.6 Maternal care for abnormality of vagina**
EXCLUDES 2 *maternal care for vaginal varices in pregnancy (O22.1-)*

**O34.60 Maternal care for abnormality of vagina, unspecified trimester** COM M

**O34.61 Maternal care for abnormality of vagina, first trimester** COM M

**O34.62 Maternal care for abnormality of vagina, second trimester** COM M

**O34.63 Maternal care for abnormality of vagina, third trimester** COM M

**O34.7 Maternal care for abnormality of vulva and perineum**
EXCLUDES 2 *maternal care for perineal and vulval varices in pregnancy (O22.1-)*

**O34.70 Maternal care for abnormality of vulva and perineum, unspecified trimester** COM M

**O34.71 Maternal care for abnormality of vulva and perineum, first trimester** COM M

**O34.72 Maternal care for abnormality of vulva and perineum, second trimester** COM M

**O34.73 Maternal care for abnormality of vulva and perineum, third trimester** COM M

**O34.8 Maternal care for other abnormalities of pelvic organs**

**O34.80 Maternal care for other abnormalities of pelvic organs, unspecified trimester** COM M

**O34.81 Maternal care for other abnormalities of pelvic organs, first trimester** COM M

**O34.82 Maternal care for other abnormalities of pelvic organs, second trimester** COM M

**O34.83 Maternal care for other abnormalities of pelvic organs, third trimester** COM M

**O34.9 Maternal care for abnormality of pelvic organ, unspecified**

**O34.90 Maternal care for abnormality of pelvic organ, unspecified, unspecified trimester** COM M

**O34.91 Maternal care for abnormality of pelvic organ, unspecified, first trimester** COM M

**O34.92 Maternal care for abnormality of pelvic organ, unspecified, second trimester** COM M

**O34.93 Maternal care for abnormality of pelvic organ, unspecified, third trimester** COM M

**O35 Maternal care for known or suspected fetal abnormality and damage**
INCLUDES the listed conditions in the fetus as a reason for hospitalization or other obstetric care to the mother, or for termination of pregnancy
Code also any associated maternal condition
EXCLUDES 1 *encounter for suspected maternal and fetal conditions ruled out (Z03.7-)*
AHA: 2022,4Q,37

One of the following 7th characters is to be assigned to each code under category O35. 7th character 0 is for single gestations and multiple gestations where the fetus is unspecified. 7th characters 1 through 9 are for cases of multiple gestations to identify the fetus for which the code applies. The appropriate code from category O30, Multiple gestation, must also be assigned when assigning a code from category O35 that has a 7th character of 1 through 9.
0 not applicable or unspecified
1 fetus 1
2 fetus 2
3 fetus 3
4 fetus 4
5 fetus 5
9 other fetus

**O35.0 Maternal care for (suspected) central nervous system malformation in fetus**
EXCLUDES 2 *chromosomal abnormality in fetus (O35.1-)*

**O35.00 Maternal care for (suspected) central nervous system malformation or damage in fetus, unspecified** COM M

**O35.01 Maternal care for (suspected) central nervous system malformation or damage in fetus, agenesis of the corpus callosum** COM M

√x7th **O35.02 Maternal care for (suspected) central nervous system malformation or damage in fetus, anencephaly** COM M

√x7th **O35.03 Maternal care for (suspected) central nervous system malformation or damage in fetus, choroid plexus cysts** COM M

√x7th **O35.04 Maternal care for (suspected) central nervous system malformation or damage in fetus, encephalocele** COM M

√x7th **O35.05 Maternal care for (suspected) central nervous system malformation or damage in fetus, holoprosencephaly** COM M

**AHA:** 2024,3Q,9

√x7th **O35.06 Maternal care for (suspected) central nervous system malformation or damage in fetus, hydrocephaly** COM M

Maternal care for fetal hydrocephalus

√x7th **O35.07 Maternal care for (suspected) central nervous system malformation or damage in fetus, microcephaly** COM M

√x7th **O35.08 Maternal care for (suspected) central nervous system malformation or damage in fetus, spina bifida** COM M

√x7th **O35.09 Maternal care for (suspected) other central nervous system malformation or damage in fetus** COM M

√5th **O35.1 Maternal care for (suspected) chromosomal abnormality in fetus**

**AHA:** 2023,2Q,15

√x7th **O35.10 Maternal care for (suspected) chromosomal abnormality in fetus, unspecified** COM M

√x7th **O35.11 Maternal care for (suspected) chromosomal abnormality in fetus, Trisomy 13** COM M

▶Maternal care for (suspected) chromosomal abnormality in fetus, Patau syndrome◀

√x7th **O35.12 Maternal care for (suspected) chromosomal abnormality in fetus, Trisomy 18** COM M

▶Maternal care for (suspected) chromosomal abnormality in fetus, Edwards syndrome◀

√x7th **O35.13 Maternal care for (suspected) chromosomal abnormality in fetus, Trisomy 21** COM M

▶Maternal care for (suspected) chromosomal abnormality in fetus, Down syndrome◀

**AHA:** 2025,3Q,21

√x7th **O35.14 Maternal care for (suspected) chromosomal abnormality in fetus, Turner Syndrome** COM M

√x7th **O35.15 Maternal care for (suspected) chromosomal abnormality in fetus, sex chromosome abnormality** COM M

▶Maternal care for (suspected) chromosomal abnormality in fetus, Klinefelter syndrome◀

▶Maternal care for (suspected) chromosomal abnormality in fetus, Trisomy X◀

▶Maternal care for (suspected) chromosomal abnormality in fetus, XYY syndrome◀

√x7th **O35.19 Maternal care for (suspected) chromosomal abnormality in fetus, other chromosomal abnormality** COM M

√x7th **O35.A Maternal care for other (suspected) fetal abnormality and damage, fetal facial anomalies** COM M

√x7th **O35.B Maternal care for other (suspected) fetal abnormality and damage, fetal cardiac anomalies** COM M

√x7th **O35.C Maternal care for other (suspected) fetal abnormality and damage, fetal pulmonary anomalies** COM M

√x7th **O35.D Maternal care for other (suspected) fetal abnormality and damage, fetal gastrointestinal anomalies** COM M

√x7th **O35.E Maternal care for other (suspected) fetal abnormality and damage, fetal genitourinary anomalies** COM M

√x7th **O35.F Maternal care for other (suspected) fetal abnormality and damage, fetal musculoskeletal anomalies of trunk** COM M

EXCLUDES 2 *maternal care for other (suspected) fetal abnormality and damage, fetal lower extremities anomalies (O35.H)*

*maternal care for other (suspected) fetal abnormality and damage, fetal upper extremities anomalies (O35.G)*

√x7th **O35.G Maternal care for other (suspected) fetal abnormality and damage, fetal upper extremities anomalies** COM M

√x7th **O35.H Maternal care for other (suspected) fetal abnormality and damage, fetal lower extremities anomalies** COM M

√x7th **O35.2 Maternal care for (suspected) hereditary disease in fetus** COM M

EXCLUDES 2 *chromosomal abnormality in fetus (O35.1-)*

√x7th **O35.3 Maternal care for (suspected) damage to fetus from viral disease in mother** COM M

Maternal care for damage to fetus from maternal cytomegalovirus infection

Maternal care for damage to fetus from maternal rubella

√x7th **O35.4 Maternal care for (suspected) damage to fetus from alcohol** COM M

√x7th **O35.5 Maternal care for (suspected) damage to fetus by drugs** COM M

Maternal care for damage to fetus from drug addiction

√x7th **O35.6 Maternal care for (suspected) damage to fetus by radiation** COM M

√x7th **O35.7 Maternal care for (suspected) damage to fetus by other medical procedures** COM M

Maternal care for damage to fetus by amniocentesis

Maternal care for damage to fetus by biopsy procedures

Maternal care for damage to fetus by hematological investigation

Maternal care for damage to fetus by intrauterine contraceptive device

Maternal care for damage to fetus by intrauterine surgery

√x7th **O35.8 Maternal care for other (suspected) fetal abnormality and damage** COM M

Maternal care for damage to fetus from maternal listeriosis

Maternal care for damage to fetus from maternal toxoplasmosis

√x7th **O35.9 Maternal care for (suspected) fetal abnormality and damage, unspecified** COM M

√4th **O36 Maternal care for other fetal problems**

INCLUDES the listed conditions in the fetus as a reason for hospitalization or other obstetric care of the mother, or for termination of pregnancy

EXCLUDES 1 *encounter for suspected maternal and fetal conditions ruled out (Z03.7-)*

*placental transfusion syndromes (O43.0-)*

EXCLUDES 2 *labor and delivery complicated by fetal stress (O77.-)*

**AHA:** 2015,3Q,40

One of the following 7th characters is to be assigned to each code under category O36. 7th character 0 is for single gestations and multiple gestations where the fetus is unspecified. 7th characters 1 through 9 are for cases of multiple gestations to identify the fetus for which the code applies. The appropriate code from category O30, Multiple gestation, must also be assigned when assigning a code from category O36 that has a 7th character of 1 through 9.

0 not applicable or unspecified
1 fetus 1
2 fetus 2
3 fetus 3
4 fetus 4
5 fetus 5
9 other fetus

√5th **O36.0 Maternal care for rhesus isoimmunization**

Maternal care for Rh incompatibility (with hydrops fetalis)

√6th **O36.01 Maternal care for anti-D [Rh] antibodies**

**AHA:** 2014,4Q,17

√7th **O36.011 Maternal care for anti-D [Rh] antibodies, first trimester** COM M

√7th **O36.012 Maternal care for anti-D [Rh] antibodies, second trimester** COM M

√7th **O36.013 Maternal care for anti-D [Rh] antibodies, third trimester** COM M

√7th **O36.019 Maternal care for anti-D [Rh] antibodies, unspecified trimester** COM M

√6th **O36.09 Maternal care for other rhesus isoimmunization**

√7th **O36.091 Maternal care for other rhesus isoimmunization, first trimester** COM M

√7th **O36.092 Maternal care for other rhesus isoimmunization, second trimester** COM M

√7th **O36.093 Maternal care for other rhesus isoimmunization, third trimester** COM M

√7th **O36.099 Maternal care for other rhesus isoimmunization, unspecified trimester** COM M

√5th **O36.1 Maternal care for other isoimmunization**
Maternal care for ABO isoimmunization

√6th **O36.11 Maternal care for Anti-A sensitization**
Maternal care for isoimmunization NOS (with hydrops fetalis)

√7th **O36.111 Maternal care for Anti-A sensitization, first trimester** COM M

√7th **O36.112 Maternal care for Anti-A sensitization, second trimester** COM M

√7th **O36.113 Maternal care for Anti-A sensitization, third trimester** COM M

√7th **O36.119 Maternal care for Anti-A sensitization, unspecified trimester** COM M

√6th **O36.19 Maternal care for other isoimmunization**
Maternal care for Anti-B sensitization

√7th **O36.191 Maternal care for other isoimmunization, first trimester** COM M

√7th **O36.192 Maternal care for other isoimmunization, second trimester** COM M

√7th **O36.193 Maternal care for other isoimmunization, third trimester** COM M

√7th **O36.199 Maternal care for other isoimmunization, unspecified trimester** COM M

√5th **O36.2 Maternal care for hydrops fetalis**
Maternal care for hydrops fetalis NOS
Maternal care for hydrops fetalis not associated with isoimmunization

EXCLUDES 1 *hydrops fetalis associated with ABO isoimmunization (O36.1-)*
*hydrops fetalis associated with rhesus isoimmunization (O36.Ø-)*

**DEF:** Hydrops fetalis: Abnormal fluid buildup in at least two of the following fetal organ spaces: the skin (edema), abdomen (ascites), around the heart (pericardia effusion), and around the lung (pleural effusion). Fluid accumulation may also occur in the mother as polyhydramnios and edema of the placenta.

√x7th **O36.2Ø Maternal care for hydrops fetalis, unspecified trimester** COM M

√x7th **O36.21 Maternal care for hydrops fetalis, first trimester** COM M

√x7th **O36.22 Maternal care for hydrops fetalis, second trimester** COM M

√x7th **O36.23 Maternal care for hydrops fetalis, third trimester** COM M

√x7th **O36.4 Maternal care for intrauterine death** COM M
Maternal care for intrauterine fetal death after completion of 2Ø weeks of gestation
Maternal care for intrauterine fetal death NOS
Maternal care for late fetal death
Maternal care for missed delivery

EXCLUDES 1 *missed abortion (OØ2.1)*
*stillbirth (P95)*

**AHA:** 2022,2Q,3

√5th **O36.5 Maternal care for known or suspected poor fetal growth**

√6th **O36.51 Maternal care for known or suspected placental insufficiency**

√7th **O36.511 Maternal care for known or suspected placental insufficiency, first trimester** COM M

√7th **O36.512 Maternal care for known or suspected placental insufficiency, second trimester** COM M

√7th **O36.513 Maternal care for known or suspected placental insufficiency, third trimester** COM M

√7th **O36.519 Maternal care for known or suspected placental insufficiency, unspecified trimester** COM M

√6th **O36.59 Maternal care for other known or suspected poor fetal growth**
Maternal care for known or suspected light-for-dates NOS
Maternal care for known or suspected small-for-dates NOS

√7th **O36.591 Maternal care for other known or suspected poor fetal growth, first trimester** COM M

√7th **O36.592 Maternal care for other known or suspected poor fetal growth, second trimester** COM M

√7th **O36.593 Maternal care for other known or suspected poor fetal growth, third trimester** COM M
**AHA:** 2024,3Q,10

√7th **O36.599 Maternal care for other known or suspected poor fetal growth, unspecified trimester** COM M

√5th **O36.6 Maternal care for excessive fetal growth**
Maternal care for known or suspected large-for-dates

√x7th **O36.6Ø Maternal care for excessive fetal growth, unspecified trimester** COM M

√x7th **O36.61 Maternal care for excessive fetal growth, first trimester** COM M

√x7th **O36.62 Maternal care for excessive fetal growth, second trimester** COM M

√x7th **O36.63 Maternal care for excessive fetal growth, third trimester** COM M

√5th **O36.7 Maternal care for viable fetus in abdominal pregnancy**

√x7th **O36.7Ø Maternal care for viable fetus in abdominal pregnancy, unspecified trimester** COM M

√x7th **O36.71 Maternal care for viable fetus in abdominal pregnancy, first trimester** COM M

√x7th **O36.72 Maternal care for viable fetus in abdominal pregnancy, second trimester** COM M

√x7th **O36.73 Maternal care for viable fetus in abdominal pregnancy, third trimester** COM M

√5th **O36.8 Maternal care for other specified fetal problems**

√x7th **O36.8Ø Pregnancy with inconclusive fetal viability** COM M
Encounter to determine fetal viability of pregnancy
**AHA:** 2019,2Q,29

√6th **O36.81 Decreased fetal movements**

√7th **O36.812 Decreased fetal movements, second trimester** COM M

√7th **O36.813 Decreased fetal movements, third trimester** COM M

√7th **O36.819 Decreased fetal movements, unspecified trimester** COM M

√6th **O36.82 Fetal anemia and thrombocytopenia**

√7th **O36.821 Fetal anemia and thrombocytopenia, first trimester** COM M

√7th **O36.822 Fetal anemia and thrombocytopenia, second trimester** COM M

√7th **O36.823 Fetal anemia and thrombocytopenia, third trimester** COM M

√7th **O36.829 Fetal anemia and thrombocytopenia, unspecified trimester** COM M

√6th **O36.83 Maternal care for abnormalities of the fetal heart rate or rhythm**
Maternal care for depressed fetal heart rate tones
Maternal care for fetal bradycardia
Maternal care for fetal heart rate abnormal variability
Maternal care for fetal heart rate decelerations
Maternal care for fetal heart rate irregularity
Maternal care for fetal tachycardia
Maternal care for non-reassuring fetal heart rate or rhythm

**AHA:** 2017,4Q,20

**TIP:** Assign for documented fetal tachycardia, bradycardia, decelerations, or loss of variability detected during antenatal testing.

√7th **O36.831 Maternal care for abnormalities of the fetal heart rate or rhythm, first trimester** COM M

√7th **O36.832 Maternal care for abnormalities of the fetal heart rate or rhythm, second trimester** COM M

√7th **O36.833 Maternal care for abnormalities of the fetal heart rate or rhythm, third trimester** COM M

√7th **O36.839 Maternal care for abnormalities of the fetal heart rate or rhythm, unspecified trimester** COM M

√6th **O36.89 Maternal care for other specified fetal problems**

√7th **O36.891 Maternal care for other specified fetal problems, first trimester** COM M

√7th **O36.892 Maternal care for other specified fetal problems, second trimester** COM M

√7th **O36.893 Maternal care for other specified fetal problems, third trimester** COM M

√7th **O36.899 Maternal care for other specified fetal problems, unspecified trimester** COM M

√5th **O36.9 Maternal care for fetal problem, unspecified**

√x7th **O36.90 Maternal care for fetal problem, unspecified, unspecified trimester** COM M

√x7th **O36.91 Maternal care for fetal problem, unspecified, first trimester** COM M

√x7th **O36.92 Maternal care for fetal problem, unspecified, second trimester** COM M

√x7th **O36.93 Maternal care for fetal problem, unspecified, third trimester** COM M

√4th **O4Ø Polyhydramnios**

INCLUDES hydramnios

EXCLUDES 1 *encounter for suspected maternal and fetal conditions ruled out (ZØ3.7-)*

**AHA:** 2016,1Q,4

**DEF:** Excess amniotic fluid surrounding the fetus, typically defined as a total fluid volume of greater than 24 cm.

One of the following 7th characters is to be assigned to each code under category O4Ø. 7th character Ø is for single gestations and multiple gestations where the fetus is unspecified. 7th characters 1 through 9 are for cases of multiple gestations to identify the fetus for which the code applies. The appropriate code from category O3Ø, Multiple gestation, must also be assigned when assigning a code from category O4Ø that has a 7th character of 1 through 9.

Ø not applicable or unspecified
1 fetus 1
2 fetus 2
3 fetus 3
4 fetus 4
5 fetus 5
9 other fetus

√x7th **O4Ø.1 Polyhydramnios, first trimester** COM M

√x7th **O4Ø.2 Polyhydramnios, second trimester** COM M

√x7th **O4Ø.3 Polyhydramnios, third trimester** COM M

√x7th **O4Ø.9 Polyhydramnios, unspecified trimester** COM M

√4th **O41 Other disorders of amniotic fluid and membranes**

EXCLUDES 1 *encounter for suspected maternal and fetal conditions ruled out (ZØ3.7-)*

One of the following 7th characters is to be assigned to each code under category O41. 7th character Ø is for single gestations and multiple gestations where the fetus is unspecified. 7th characters 1 through 9 are for cases of multiple gestations to identify the fetus for which the code applies. The appropriate code from category O3Ø, Multiple gestation, must also be assigned when assigning a code from category O41 that has a 7th character of 1 through 9.

Ø not applicable or unspecified
1 fetus 1
2 fetus 2
3 fetus 3
4 fetus 4
5 fetus 5
9 other fetus

√5th **O41.Ø Oligohydramnios**

Oligohydramnios without rupture of membranes

**DEF:** Low amniotic fluid, occurring most frequently in the last trimester.

√x7th **O41.ØØ Oligohydramnios, unspecified trimester** COM M

√x7th **O41.Ø1 Oligohydramnios, first trimester** COM M

√x7th **O41.Ø2 Oligohydramnios, second trimester** COM M

√x7th **O41.Ø3 Oligohydramnios, third trimester** COM M

√5th **O41.1 Infection of amniotic sac and membranes**

√6th **O41.1Ø Infection of amniotic sac and membranes, unspecified**

√7th **O41.1Ø1 Infection of amniotic sac and membranes, unspecified, first trimester** COM M

√7th **O41.1Ø2 Infection of amniotic sac and membranes, unspecified, second trimester** COM M

√7th **O41.1Ø3 Infection of amniotic sac and membranes, unspecified, third trimester** COM M

√7th **O41.1Ø9 Infection of amniotic sac and membranes, unspecified, unspecified trimester** COM M

√6th **O41.12 Chorioamnionitis**

**AHA:** 2019,2Q,34

√7th **O41.121 Chorioamnionitis, first trimester** COM M

√7th **O41.122 Chorioamnionitis, second trimester** COM M

√7th **O41.123 Chorioamnionitis, third trimester** COM M

√7th **O41.129 Chorioamnionitis, unspecified trimester** COM M

√6th **O41.14 Placentitis**

√7th **O41.141 Placentitis, first trimester** COM M

√7th **O41.142 Placentitis, second trimester** COM M

√7th **O41.143 Placentitis, third trimester** COM M

√7th **O41.149 Placentitis, unspecified trimester** COM M

√5th **O41.8 Other specified disorders of amniotic fluid and membranes**

√6th **O41.8X Other specified disorders of amniotic fluid and membranes**

**AHA:** 2024,1Q,13

√7th **O41.8X1 Other specified disorders of amniotic fluid and membranes, first trimester** COM M

√7th **O41.8X2 Other specified disorders of amniotic fluid and membranes, second trimester** COM M

√7th **O41.8X3 Other specified disorders of amniotic fluid and membranes, third trimester** COM M

√7th **O41.8X9 Other specified disorders of amniotic fluid and membranes, unspecified trimester** COM M

√5th **O41.9 Disorder of amniotic fluid and membranes, unspecified**

√x7th **O41.9Ø Disorder of amniotic fluid and membranes, unspecified, unspecified trimester** COM M

√x7th **O41.91 Disorder of amniotic fluid and membranes, unspecified, first trimester** COM M

√x7th **O41.92 Disorder of amniotic fluid and membranes, unspecified, second trimester** COM M

√x7th **O41.93 Disorder of amniotic fluid and membranes, unspecified, third trimester** COM M

√4th **O42 Premature rupture of membranes**

**AHA:** 2023,3Q,17; 2016,1Q,3

√5th **O42.Ø Premature rupture of membranes, onset of labor within 24 hours of rupture**

**O42.ØØ Premature rupture of membranes, onset of labor within 24 hours of rupture, unspecified weeks of gestation** COM M

√6th **O42.Ø1 Preterm premature rupture of membranes, onset of labor within 24 hours of rupture**

Premature rupture of membranes before 37 completed weeks of gestation

**O42.Ø11 Preterm premature rupture of membranes, onset of labor within 24 hours of rupture, first trimester** COM M

**O42.Ø12 Preterm premature rupture of membranes, onset of labor within 24 hours of rupture, second trimester** COM M

**O42.Ø13 Preterm premature rupture of membranes, onset of labor within 24 hours of rupture, third trimester** COM M

**O42.Ø19 Preterm premature rupture of membranes, onset of labor within 24 hours of rupture, unspecified trimester** COM M

**O42.Ø2 Full-term premature rupture of membranes, onset of labor within 24 hours of rupture** COM M

Premature rupture of membranes at or after 37 completed weeks of gestation, onset of labor within 24 hours of rupture

√5th **O42.1 Premature rupture of membranes, onset of labor more than 24 hours following rupture**

**AHA:** 2016,1Q,5

**O42.1Ø Premature rupture of membranes, onset of labor more than 24 hours following rupture, unspecified weeks of gestation** COM M

✓6th **O42.11 Preterm premature rupture of membranes, onset of labor more than 24 hours following rupture**
Premature rupture of membranes before 37 completed weeks of gestation
**O42.111 Preterm premature rupture of membranes, onset of labor more than 24 hours following rupture, first trimester** COM M
**O42.112 Preterm premature rupture of membranes, onset of labor more than 24 hours following rupture, second trimester** COM M
**O42.113 Preterm premature rupture of membranes, onset of labor more than 24 hours following rupture, third trimester** COM M
**O42.119 Preterm premature rupture of membranes, onset of labor more than 24 hours following rupture, unspecified trimester** COM M
**O42.12 Full-term premature rupture of membranes, onset of labor more than 24 hours following rupture** COM M
Premature rupture of membranes at or after 37 completed weeks of gestation, onset of labor more than 24 hours following rupture

✓5th **O42.9 Premature rupture of membranes, unspecified as to length of time between rupture and onset of labor**
**O42.90 Premature rupture of membranes, unspecified as to length of time between rupture and onset of labor, unspecified weeks of gestation** COM M
✓6th **O42.91 Preterm premature rupture of membranes, unspecified as to length of time between rupture and onset of labor**
Premature rupture of membranes before 37 completed weeks of gestation
**O42.911 Preterm premature rupture of membranes, unspecified as to length of time between rupture and onset of labor, first trimester** COM M
**O42.912 Preterm premature rupture of membranes, unspecified as to length of time between rupture and onset of labor, second trimester** COM M
**O42.913 Preterm premature rupture of membranes, unspecified as to length of time between rupture and onset of labor, third trimester** COM M
**O42.919 Preterm premature rupture of membranes, unspecified as to length of time between rupture and onset of labor, unspecified trimester** COM M
**O42.92 Full-term premature rupture of membranes, unspecified as to length of time between rupture and onset of labor** COM M
Premature rupture of membranes at or after 37 completed weeks of gestation, unspecified as to length of time between rupture and onset of labor

✓4th **O43 Placental disorders**
EXCLUDES 2 *maternal care for poor fetal growth due to placental insufficiency (O36.5-)*
*placenta previa (O44.-)*
*placental polyp (O90.89)*
*placentitis (O41.14-)*
*premature separation of placenta [abruptio placentae] (O45.-)*

✓5th **O43.0 Placental transfusion syndromes**
✓6th **O43.01 Fetomaternal placental transfusion syndrome**
Maternofetal placental transfusion syndrome
**O43.011 Fetomaternal placental transfusion syndrome, first trimester** COM M
**O43.012 Fetomaternal placental transfusion syndrome, second trimester** COM M
**O43.013 Fetomaternal placental transfusion syndrome, third trimester** COM M
**O43.019 Fetomaternal placental transfusion syndrome, unspecified trimester** COM M
✓6th **O43.02 Fetus-to-fetus placental transfusion syndrome**
**DEF:** Condition in which an imbalance in amniotic fluid occurs due to uneven blood flow between twins sharing a placenta.

**Twin to Twin Transfusion Syndrome (TTTS)**

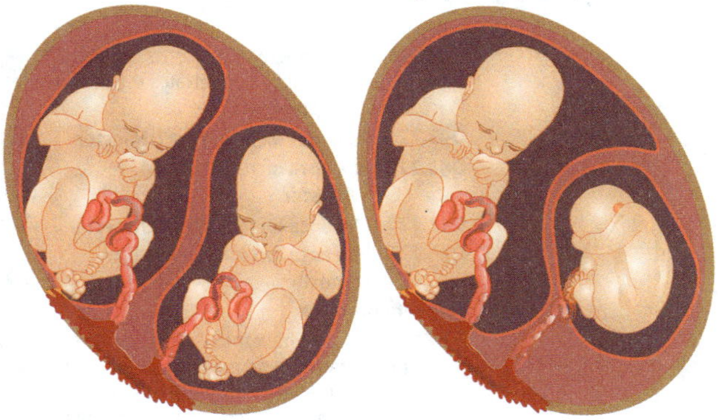


**O43.021 Fetus-to-fetus placental transfusion syndrome, first trimester** COM M
**O43.022 Fetus-to-fetus placental transfusion syndrome, second trimester** COM M
**O43.023 Fetus-to-fetus placental transfusion syndrome, third trimester** COM M
**O43.029 Fetus-to-fetus placental transfusion syndrome, unspecified trimester** COM M

✓5th **O43.1 Malformation of placenta**
✓6th **O43.10 Malformation of placenta, unspecified**
Abnormal placenta NOS
**O43.101 Malformation of placenta, unspecified, first trimester** COM M
**O43.102 Malformation of placenta, unspecified, second trimester** COM M
**O43.103 Malformation of placenta, unspecified, third trimester** COM M
**O43.109 Malformation of placenta, unspecified, unspecified trimester** COM M
✓6th **O43.11 Circumvallate placenta**
**O43.111 Circumvallate placenta, first trimester** COM M
**O43.112 Circumvallate placenta, second trimester** COM M
**O43.113 Circumvallate placenta, third trimester** COM M
**O43.119 Circumvallate placenta, unspecified trimester** COM M
✓6th **O43.12 Velamentous insertion of umbilical cord**
**O43.121 Velamentous insertion of umbilical cord, first trimester** COM M
**O43.122 Velamentous insertion of umbilical cord, second trimester** COM M
**O43.123 Velamentous insertion of umbilical cord, third trimester** COM M
**O43.129 Velamentous insertion of umbilical cord, unspecified trimester** COM M
✓6th **O43.19 Other malformation of placenta**
**O43.191 Other malformation of placenta, first trimester** COM M
**O43.192 Other malformation of placenta, second trimester** COM M
**O43.193 Other malformation of placenta, third trimester** COM M
**O43.199 Other malformation of placenta, unspecified trimester** COM M

✓5th **O43.2 Morbidly adherent placenta**
Code also associated third stage postpartum hemorrhage, if applicable (O72.0)
EXCLUDES 1 *retained placenta (O73.-)*
✓6th **O43.21 Placenta accreta**
**DEF:** Condition where the placenta adheres too deeply to the uterine wall; often associated with placenta previa.
**O43.211 Placenta accreta, first trimester** COM M

O43.212 Placenta accreta, second trimester COM M
O43.213 Placenta accreta, third trimester COM M
O43.219 Placenta accreta, unspecified trimester COM M

√6th O43.22 Placenta increta
AHA: 2022,1Q,20
DEF: Condition where the placenta adheres too deeply to the uterine wall and penetrates the muscle; often associated with placenta previa.
O43.221 Placenta increta, first trimester COM M
O43.222 Placenta increta, second trimester COM M
O43.223 Placenta increta, third trimester COM M
O43.229 Placenta increta, unspecified trimester COM M

√6th O43.23 Placenta percreta
DEF: Condition where the placenta attaches through the uterine muscle and may invade other organs, resulting in antenatal complications, premature delivery, retention of all or a portion of the placenta, or postpartum bleeding.
O43.231 Placenta percreta, first trimester COM M
O43.232 Placenta percreta, second trimester COM M
O43.233 Placenta percreta, third trimester COM M
O43.239 Placenta percreta, unspecified trimester COM M

√5th O43.8 Other placental disorders
√6th O43.81 Placental infarction
O43.811 Placental infarction, first trimester COM M
O43.812 Placental infarction, second trimester COM M
O43.813 Placental infarction, third trimester COM M
O43.819 Placental infarction, unspecified trimester COM M

√6th O43.89 Other placental disorders
Placental dysfunction
O43.891 Other placental disorders, first trimester COM M
O43.892 Other placental disorders, second trimester COM M
O43.893 Other placental disorders, third trimester COM M
O43.899 Other placental disorders, unspecified trimester COM M

√5th O43.9 Unspecified placental disorder
O43.9Ø Unspecified placental disorder, unspecified trimester COM M
O43.91 Unspecified placental disorder, first trimester COM M
O43.92 Unspecified placental disorder, second trimester COM M
O43.93 Unspecified placental disorder, third trimester COM M

√4th O44 Placenta previa
AHA: 2016,4Q,52-53
DEF: Placenta implanted in the lower segment of the uterus, which commonly causes hemorrhage in the last trimester of pregnancy.

√5th O44.Ø Complete placenta previa NOS or without hemorrhage
Placenta previa NOS
O44.ØØ Complete placenta previa NOS or without hemorrhage, unspecified trimester COM M
O44.Ø1 Complete placenta previa NOS or without hemorrhage, first trimester COM M
O44.Ø2 Complete placenta previa NOS or without hemorrhage, second trimester COM M
O44.Ø3 Complete placenta previa NOS or without hemorrhage, third trimester COM M

√5th O44.1 Complete placenta previa with hemorrhage
EXCLUDES 1 *labor and delivery complicated by hemorrhage from vasa previa (O69.4)*
O44.1Ø Complete placenta previa with hemorrhage, unspecified trimester COM M
O44.11 Complete placenta previa with hemorrhage, first trimester COM M
O44.12 Complete placenta previa with hemorrhage, second trimester COM M
O44.13 Complete placenta previa with hemorrhage, third trimester COM M

√5th O44.2 Partial placenta previa without hemorrhage
Marginal placenta previa, NOS or without hemorrhage
O44.2Ø Partial placenta previa NOS or without hemorrhage, unspecified trimester COM M
O44.21 Partial placenta previa NOS or without hemorrhage, first trimester COM M
O44.22 Partial placenta previa NOS or without hemorrhage, second trimester COM M
O44.23 Partial placenta previa NOS or without hemorrhage, third trimester COM M

√5th O44.3 Partial placenta previa with hemorrhage
Marginal placenta previa with hemorrhage
O44.3Ø Partial placenta previa with hemorrhage, unspecified trimester COM M
O44.31 Partial placenta previa with hemorrhage, first trimester COM M
O44.32 Partial placenta previa with hemorrhage, second trimester COM M
O44.33 Partial placenta previa with hemorrhage, third trimester COM M

√5th O44.4 Low lying placenta NOS or without hemorrhage
Low implantation of placenta NOS or without hemorrhage
O44.4Ø Low lying placenta NOS or without hemorrhage, unspecified trimester COM M
O44.41 Low lying placenta NOS or without hemorrhage, first trimester COM M
O44.42 Low lying placenta NOS or without hemorrhage, second trimester COM M
O44.43 Low lying placenta NOS or without hemorrhage, third trimester COM M

√5th O44.5 Low lying placenta with hemorrhage
Low implantation of placenta with hemorrhage
O44.5Ø Low lying placenta with hemorrhage, unspecified trimester COM M
O44.51 Low lying placenta with hemorrhage, first trimester COM M
O44.52 Low lying placenta with hemorrhage, second trimester COM M
O44.53 Low lying placenta with hemorrhage, third trimester COM M

√4th O45 Premature separation of placenta [abruptio placentae]
√5th O45.Ø Premature separation of placenta with coagulation defect
√6th O45.ØØ Premature separation of placenta with coagulation defect, unspecified
O45.ØØ1 Premature separation of placenta with coagulation defect, unspecified, first trimester COM M
O45.ØØ2 Premature separation of placenta with coagulation defect, unspecified, second trimester COM M
O45.ØØ3 Premature separation of placenta with coagulation defect, unspecified, third trimester COM M
O45.ØØ9 Premature separation of placenta with coagulation defect, unspecified, unspecified trimester COM M

√6th O45.Ø1 Premature separation of placenta with afibrinogenemia
Premature separation of placenta with hypofibrinogenemia
O45.Ø11 Premature separation of placenta with afibrinogenemia, first trimester COM M
O45.Ø12 Premature separation of placenta with afibrinogenemia, second trimester COM M
O45.Ø13 Premature separation of placenta with afibrinogenemia, third trimester COM M
O45.Ø19 Premature separation of placenta with afibrinogenemia, unspecified trimester COM M

O45.02 Premature separation of placenta with disseminated intravascular coagulation
- O45.021 Premature separation of placenta with disseminated intravascular coagulation, first trimester COM M
- O45.022 Premature separation of placenta with disseminated intravascular coagulation, second trimester COM M
- O45.023 Premature separation of placenta with disseminated intravascular coagulation, third trimester COM M
- O45.029 Premature separation of placenta with disseminated intravascular coagulation, unspecified trimester COM M

O45.09 Premature separation of placenta with other coagulation defect
- O45.091 Premature separation of placenta with other coagulation defect, first trimester COM M
- O45.092 Premature separation of placenta with other coagulation defect, second trimester COM M
- O45.093 Premature separation of placenta with other coagulation defect, third trimester COM M
- O45.099 Premature separation of placenta with other coagulation defect, unspecified trimester COM M

O45.8 Other premature separation of placenta

O45.8X Other premature separation of placenta
- O45.8X1 Other premature separation of placenta, first trimester COM M
- O45.8X2 Other premature separation of placenta, second trimester COM M
- O45.8X3 Other premature separation of placenta, third trimester COM M
- O45.8X9 Other premature separation of placenta, unspecified trimester COM M

O45.9 Premature separation of placenta, unspecified

Abruptio placentae NOS
- O45.90 Premature separation of placenta, unspecified, unspecified trimester COM M
- O45.91 Premature separation of placenta, unspecified, first trimester COM M
- O45.92 Premature separation of placenta, unspecified, second trimester COM M
- O45.93 Premature separation of placenta, unspecified, third trimester COM M

## O46 Antepartum hemorrhage, not elsewhere classified

EXCLUDES 1 *hemorrhage in early pregnancy (O20.-)*
*intrapartum hemorrhage NEC (O67.-)*
*placenta previa (O44.-)*
*premature separation of placenta [abruptio placentae] (O45.-)*

**DEF:** Uterine hemorrhage prior to delivery that is not related to placenta previa or abruptio placentae.

O46.0 Antepartum hemorrhage with coagulation defect

O46.00 Antepartum hemorrhage with coagulation defect, unspecified
- O46.001 Antepartum hemorrhage with coagulation defect, unspecified, first trimester COM M
- O46.002 Antepartum hemorrhage with coagulation defect, unspecified, second trimester COM M
- O46.003 Antepartum hemorrhage with coagulation defect, unspecified, third trimester COM M
- O46.009 Antepartum hemorrhage with coagulation defect, unspecified, unspecified trimester COM M

O46.01 Antepartum hemorrhage with afibrinogenemia

Antepartum hemorrhage with hypofibrinogenemia
- O46.011 Antepartum hemorrhage with afibrinogenemia, first trimester COM M
- O46.012 Antepartum hemorrhage with afibrinogenemia, second trimester COM M
- O46.013 Antepartum hemorrhage with afibrinogenemia, third trimester COM M
- O46.019 Antepartum hemorrhage with afibrinogenemia, unspecified trimester COM M

O46.02 Antepartum hemorrhage with disseminated intravascular coagulation
- O46.021 Antepartum hemorrhage with disseminated intravascular coagulation, first trimester COM M
- O46.022 Antepartum hemorrhage with disseminated intravascular coagulation, second trimester COM M
- O46.023 Antepartum hemorrhage with disseminated intravascular coagulation, third trimester COM M
- O46.029 Antepartum hemorrhage with disseminated intravascular coagulation, unspecified trimester COM M

O46.09 Antepartum hemorrhage with other coagulation defect
- O46.091 Antepartum hemorrhage with other coagulation defect, first trimester COM M
- O46.092 Antepartum hemorrhage with other coagulation defect, second trimester COM M
- O46.093 Antepartum hemorrhage with other coagulation defect, third trimester COM M
- O46.099 Antepartum hemorrhage with other coagulation defect, unspecified trimester COM M

O46.8 Other antepartum hemorrhage

O46.8X Other antepartum hemorrhage
- O46.8X1 Other antepartum hemorrhage, first trimester COM M
- O46.8X2 Other antepartum hemorrhage, second trimester COM M
- O46.8X3 Other antepartum hemorrhage, third trimester COM M
- O46.8X9 Other antepartum hemorrhage, unspecified trimester COM M

O46.9 Antepartum hemorrhage, unspecified
- O46.90 Antepartum hemorrhage, unspecified, unspecified trimester COM M
- O46.91 Antepartum hemorrhage, unspecified, first trimester COM M
- O46.92 Antepartum hemorrhage, unspecified, second trimester COM M
- O46.93 Antepartum hemorrhage, unspecified, third trimester COM M

## O47 False labor

INCLUDES Braxton Hicks contractions
threatened labor

EXCLUDES 1 *preterm labor (O60.-)*

**AHA:** 2021,1Q,10

O47.0 False labor before 37 completed weeks of gestation
- O47.00 False labor before 37 completed weeks of gestation, unspecified trimester COM M
- O47.02 False labor before 37 completed weeks of gestation, second trimester COM M
- O47.03 False labor before 37 completed weeks of gestation, third trimester COM M

O47.1 False labor at or after 37 completed weeks of gestation COM M

O47.9 False labor, unspecified COM M

## O48 Late pregnancy

**AHA:** 2022,2Q,3

O48.0 Post-term pregnancy COM M

Pregnancy over 40 completed weeks to 42 completed weeks gestation

O48.1 Prolonged pregnancy COM M

Pregnancy which has advanced beyond 42 completed weeks gestation

**AHA:** 2016,1Q,5

Chapter 15. Pregnancy, Childbirth and the Puerperium

## Complications of labor and delivery (O60-O77)

✓4th **O60 Preterm labor**

INCLUDES onset (spontaneous) of labor before 37 completed weeks of gestation

EXCLUDES 1 *false labor (O47.0-)*
*threatened labor NOS (O47.0-)*

✓5th **O60.0 Preterm labor without delivery**

**O60.00 Preterm labor without delivery, unspecified trimester** COM M

**O60.02 Preterm labor without delivery, second trimester** COM M

**O60.03 Preterm labor without delivery, third trimester** COM M

✓5th **O60.1 Preterm labor with preterm delivery**

**AHA:** 2016,2Q,10

One of the following 7th characters is to be assigned to each code under subcategory O60.1. 7th character 0 is for single gestations and multiple gestations where the fetus is unspecified. 7th characters 1 through 9 are for cases of multiple gestations to identify the fetus for which the code applies. The appropriate code from category O30, Multiple gestation, must also be assigned when assigning a code from subcategory O60.1 that has a 7th character of 1 through 9.

0 not applicable or unspecified
1 fetus 1
2 fetus 2
3 fetus 3
4 fetus 4
5 fetus 5
9 other fetus

√x7th **O60.10 Preterm labor with preterm delivery, unspecified trimester** COM M
Preterm labor with delivery NOS

√x7th **O60.12 Preterm labor second trimester with preterm delivery second trimester** COM M

√x7th **O60.13 Preterm labor second trimester with preterm delivery third trimester** COM M

√x7th **O60.14 Preterm labor third trimester with preterm delivery third trimester** COM M

✓5th **O60.2 Term delivery with preterm labor**

One of the following 7th characters is to be assigned to each code under subcategory O60.2. 7th character 0 is for single gestations and multiple gestations where the fetus is unspecified. 7th characters 1 through 9 are for cases of multiple gestations to identify the fetus for which the code applies. The appropriate code from category O30, Multiple gestation, must also be assigned when assigning a code from subcategory O60.2 that has a 7th character of 1 through 9.

0 not applicable or unspecified
1 fetus 1
2 fetus 2
3 fetus 3
4 fetus 4
5 fetus 5
9 other fetus

√x7th **O60.20 Term delivery with preterm labor, unspecified trimester** COM M

√x7th **O60.22 Term delivery with preterm labor, second trimester** COM M

√x7th **O60.23 Term delivery with preterm labor, third trimester** COM M

✓4th **O61 Failed induction of labor**

**O61.0 Failed medical induction of labor** COM M
Failed induction (of labor) by oxytocin
Failed induction (of labor) by prostaglandins

**O61.1 Failed instrumental induction of labor** COM M
Failed mechanical induction (of labor)
Failed surgical induction (of labor)

**O61.8 Other failed induction of labor** COM M

**O61.9 Failed induction of labor, unspecified** COM M

✓4th **O62 Abnormalities of forces of labor**

**DEF:** Uterine inertia: Weak or poorly coordinated contractions of the uterus during labor.

**O62.0 Primary inadequate contractions** COM M
Failure of cervical dilatation
Primary hypotonic uterine dysfunction
Uterine inertia during latent phase of labor
**AHA:** 2024,1Q,13

**O62.1 Secondary uterine inertia** COM M
Arrested active phase of labor
Secondary hypotonic uterine dysfunction
**AHA:** 2026,2Q,11

**O62.2 Other uterine inertia** COM M
Atony of uterus NOS
Atony of uterus without hemorrhage
Desultory labor
Hypotonic uterine dysfunction NOS
Irregular labor
Poor contractions
Slow slope active phase of labor
Uterine inertia NOS

EXCLUDES 1 *atony of uterus with hemorrhage (postpartum) (O72.1)*
*postpartum atony of uterus without hemorrhage (O75.89)*

**DEF:** Uterine atony: Failure of the uterine muscles to contract after the fetus and placenta are delivered.

**O62.3 Precipitate labor** COM M
**DEF:** Rapid labor with delivery occurring in three hours or less from the onset of contractions.

**O62.4 Hypertonic, incoordinate, and prolonged uterine contractions** COM M
Cervical spasm
Contraction ring dystocia
Dyscoordinate labor
Hour-glass contraction of uterus
Hypertonic uterine dysfunction
Incoordinate uterine action
Tetanic contractions
Uterine dystocia NOS
Uterine spasm

EXCLUDES 1 *dystocia (fetal) (maternal) NOS (O66.9)*

**O62.8 Other abnormalities of forces of labor** COM M

**O62.9 Abnormality of forces of labor, unspecified** COM M

✓4th **O63 Long labor**

**O63.0 Prolonged first stage (of labor)** COM M

**O63.1 Prolonged second stage (of labor)** COM M

**O63.2 Delayed delivery of second twin, triplet, etc.** COM M

**O63.9 Long labor, unspecified** COM M
Prolonged labor NOS

O60–O63.9

**√4th O64 Obstructed labor due to malposition and malpresentation of fetus**

One of the following 7th characters is to be assigned to each code under category O64. 7th character Ø is for single gestations and multiple gestations where the fetus is unspecified. 7th characters 1 through 9 are for cases of multiple gestations to identify the fetus for which the code applies. The appropriate code from category O3Ø, Multiple gestation, must also be assigned when assigning a code from category O64 that has a 7th character of 1 through 9.

Ø not applicable or unspecified
1 fetus 1
2 fetus 2
3 fetus 3
4 fetus 4
5 fetus 5
9 other fetus

**Fetal Malposition**

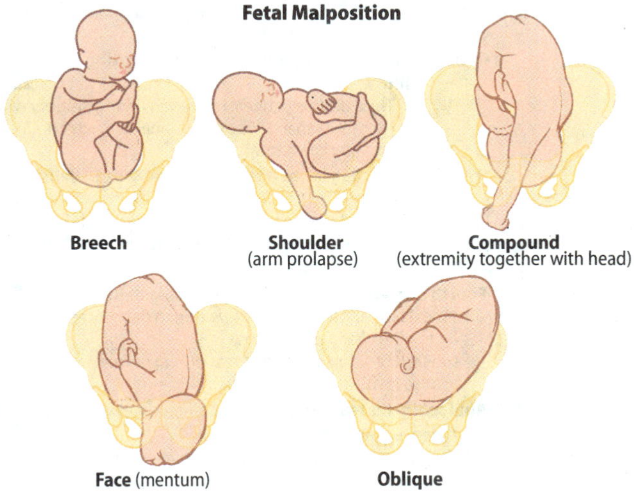


√x7th **O64.Ø Obstructed labor due to incomplete rotation of fetal head** COM M
Deep transverse arrest
Obstructed labor due to persistent occipitoiliac (position)
Obstructed labor due to persistent occipitoposterior (position)
Obstructed labor due to persistent occipitosacral (position)
Obstructed labor due to persistent occipitotransverse (position)

√x7th **O64.1 Obstructed labor due to breech presentation** COM M
Obstructed labor due to buttocks presentation
Obstructed labor due to complete breech presentation
Obstructed labor due to frank breech presentation

√x7th **O64.2 Obstructed labor due to face presentation** COM M
Obstructed labor due to chin presentation

√x7th **O64.3 Obstructed labor due to brow presentation** COM M

√x7th **O64.4 Obstructed labor due to shoulder presentation** COM M
Prolapsed arm
EXCLUDES 1 *impacted shoulders (O66.Ø)*
*shoulder dystocia (O66.Ø)*

√x7th **O64.5 Obstructed labor due to compound presentation** COM M

√x7th **O64.8 Obstructed labor due to other malposition and malpresentation** COM M
Obstructed labor due to footling presentation
Obstructed labor due to incomplete breech presentation

√x7th **O64.9 Obstructed labor due to malposition and malpresentation, unspecified** COM M

**√4th O65 Obstructed labor due to maternal pelvic abnormality**

**O65.Ø Obstructed labor due to deformed pelvis** COM M

**O65.1 Obstructed labor due to generally contracted pelvis** COM M

**O65.2 Obstructed labor due to pelvic inlet contraction** COM M

**O65.3 Obstructed labor due to pelvic outlet and mid-cavity contraction** COM M

**O65.4 Obstructed labor due to fetopelvic disproportion, unspecified** COM M
EXCLUDES 1 *dystocia due to abnormality of fetus (O66.2-O66.3)*

**O65.5 Obstructed labor due to abnormality of maternal pelvic organs** COM M
Obstructed labor due to conditions listed in O34.-
Use additional code to identify abnormality of pelvic organs O34.-

**O65.8 Obstructed labor due to other maternal pelvic abnormalities** COM M

**O65.9 Obstructed labor due to maternal pelvic abnormality, unspecified** COM M

**√4th O66 Other obstructed labor**

**O66.Ø Obstructed labor due to shoulder dystocia** COM M
Impacted shoulders
**DEF:** Obstructed labor due to impacted fetal shoulders. It is an emergency condition that may require cesarean section, forceps delivery, vacuum extraction, or symphysiotomy.

**O66.1 Obstructed labor due to locked twins** COM M

**O66.2 Obstructed labor due to unusually large fetus** COM M

**O66.3 Obstructed labor due to other abnormalities of fetus** COM M
Dystocia due to fetal ascites
Dystocia due to fetal hydrops
Dystocia due to fetal meningomyelocele
Dystocia due to fetal sacral teratoma
Dystocia due to fetal tumor
Dystocia due to hydrocephalic fetus
Use additional code to identify cause of obstruction

√5th **O66.4 Failed trial of labor**

**O66.4Ø Failed trial of labor, unspecified** COM M

**O66.41 Failed attempted vaginal birth after previous cesarean delivery** COM M
Code first rupture of uterus, if applicable (O71.Ø-, O71.1)

**O66.5 Attempted application of vacuum extractor and forceps** COM M
Attempted application of vacuum or forceps, with subsequent delivery by forceps or cesarean delivery

**O66.6 Obstructed labor due to other multiple fetuses** COM M

**O66.8 Other specified obstructed labor** COM M
Use additional code to identify cause of obstruction

**O66.9 Obstructed labor, unspecified** COM M
Dystocia NOS
Fetal dystocia NOS
Maternal dystocia NOS

**√4th O67 Labor and delivery complicated by intrapartum hemorrhage, not elsewhere classified**
EXCLUDES 1 *antepartum hemorrhage NEC (O46.-)*
*placenta previa (O44.-)*
*premature separation of placenta [abruptio placentae] (O45.-)*
EXCLUDES 2 *postpartum hemorrhage (O72.-)*

**O67.Ø Intrapartum hemorrhage with coagulation defect** COM M
Intrapartum hemorrhage (excessive) associated with afibrinogenemia
Intrapartum hemorrhage (excessive) associated with disseminated intravascular coagulation
Intrapartum hemorrhage (excessive) associated with hyperfibrinolysis
Intrapartum hemorrhage (excessive) associated with hypofibrinogenemia

**O67.8 Other intrapartum hemorrhage** COM M
Excessive intrapartum hemorrhage

**O67.9 Intrapartum hemorrhage, unspecified** COM M

**O68 Labor and delivery complicated by abnormality of fetal acid-base balance** COM M
Fetal acidemia complicating labor and delivery
Fetal acidosis complicating labor and delivery
Fetal alkalosis complicating labor and delivery
Fetal metabolic acidemia complicating labor and delivery
EXCLUDES 1 *fetal stress NOS (O77.9)*
*labor and delivery complicated by electrocardiographic evidence of fetal stress (O77.8)*
*labor and delivery complicated by ultrasonic evidence of fetal stress (O77.8)*
EXCLUDES 2 *abnormality in fetal heart rate or rhythm (O76)*
*labor and delivery complicated by meconium in amniotic fluid (O77.Ø)*

Chapter 15. Pregnancy, Childbirth and the Puerperium

O64–O68

**√4th O69 Labor and delivery complicated by umbilical cord complications**

AHA: 2016,1Q,5

One of the following 7th characters is to be assigned to each code under category O69. 7th character Ø is for single gestations and multiple gestations where the fetus is unspecified. 7th characters 1 through 9 are for cases of multiple gestations to identify the fetus for which the code applies. The appropriate code from category O3Ø, Multiple gestation, must also be assigned when assigning a code from category O69 that has a 7th character of 1 through 9.

Ø not applicable or unspecified
1 fetus 1
2 fetus 2
3 fetus 3
4 fetus 4
5 fetus 5
9 other fetus

√x7th **O69.Ø Labor and delivery complicated by prolapse of cord** COM M

DEF: Abnormal presentation of the fetus marked by a protruding umbilical cord during labor. It can cause fetal death.

√x7th **O69.1 Labor and delivery complicated by cord around neck, with compression** COM M

EXCLUDES 1 *labor and delivery complicated by cord around neck, without compression (O69.81)*

√x7th **O69.2 Labor and delivery complicated by other cord entanglement, with compression** COM M

Labor and delivery complicated by compression of cord NOS
Labor and delivery complicated by entanglement of cords of twins in monoamniotic sac
Labor and delivery complicated by knot in cord

EXCLUDES 1 *labor and delivery complicated by other cord entanglement, without compression (O69.82)*

√x7th **O69.3 Labor and delivery complicated by short cord** COM M

√x7th **O69.4 Labor and delivery complicated by vasa previa** COM M

Labor and delivery complicated by hemorrhage from vasa previa

√x7th **O69.5 Labor and delivery complicated by vascular lesion of cord** COM M

Labor and delivery complicated by cord bruising
Labor and delivery complicated by cord hematoma
Labor and delivery complicated by thrombosis of umbilical vessels

√5th **O69.8 Labor and delivery complicated by other cord complications**

√x7th **O69.81 Labor and delivery complicated by cord around neck, without compression** COM M

AHA: 2016,1Q,5

√x7th **O69.82 Labor and delivery complicated by other cord entanglement, without compression** COM M

√x7th **O69.89 Labor and delivery complicated by other cord complications** COM M

AHA: 2023,2Q,29

√x7th **O69.9 Labor and delivery complicated by cord complication, unspecified** COM M

**√4th O7Ø Perineal laceration during delivery**

INCLUDES episiotomy extended by laceration

EXCLUDES 1 *obstetric high vaginal laceration alone (O71.4)*

AHA: 2016,2Q,34; 2016,1Q,3-4,5

**O7Ø.Ø First degree perineal laceration during delivery** COM M

Perineal laceration, rupture or tear involving fourchette during delivery
Perineal laceration, rupture or tear involving labia during delivery
Perineal laceration, rupture or tear involving skin during delivery
Perineal laceration, rupture or tear involving vagina during delivery
Perineal laceration, rupture or tear involving vulva during delivery
Slight perineal laceration, rupture or tear during delivery

**O7Ø.1 Second degree perineal laceration during delivery** COM M

Perineal laceration, rupture or tear during delivery as in O7Ø.Ø, also involving pelvic floor
Perineal laceration, rupture or tear during delivery as in O7Ø.Ø, also involving perineal muscles
Perineal laceration, rupture or tear during delivery as in O7Ø.Ø, also involving vaginal muscles

EXCLUDES 1 *perineal laceration involving anal sphincter (O7Ø.2-)*

√5th **O7Ø.2 Third degree perineal laceration during delivery**

Perineal laceration, rupture or tear during delivery as in O7Ø.1, also involving anal sphincter
Perineal laceration, rupture or tear during delivery as in O7Ø.1, also involving rectovaginal septum
Perineal laceration, rupture or tear during delivery as in O7Ø.1, also involving sphincter NOS

EXCLUDES 1 *anal sphincter tear during delivery without third degree perineal laceration (O7Ø.4)*
*perineal laceration involving anal or rectal mucosa (O7Ø.3)*

AHA: 2016,4Q,53-54

**O7Ø.2Ø Third degree perineal laceration during delivery, unspecified** COM M

**O7Ø.21 Third degree perineal laceration during delivery, IIIa** COM M

Third degree perineal laceration during delivery with less than 5Ø% of external anal sphincter (EAS) thickness torn

**O7Ø.22 Third degree perineal laceration during delivery, IIIb** COM M

Third degree perineal laceration during delivery with more than 5Ø% external anal sphincter (EAS) thickness torn

**O7Ø.23 Third degree perineal laceration during delivery, IIIc** COM M

Third degree perineal laceration during delivery with both external anal sphincter (EAS) and internal anal sphincter (IAS) torn

**O7Ø.3 Fourth degree perineal laceration during delivery** COM M

Perineal laceration, rupture or tear during delivery as in O7Ø.2, also involving anal mucosa
Perineal laceration, rupture or tear during delivery as in O7Ø.2, also involving rectal mucosa

**O7Ø.4 Anal sphincter tear complicating delivery, not associated with third degree laceration** COM M

EXCLUDES 1 *anal sphincter tear with third degree perineal laceration (O7Ø.2-)*

**O7Ø.9 Perineal laceration during delivery, unspecified** COM M

**√4th O71 Other obstetric trauma**

INCLUDES obstetric damage from instruments

√5th **O71.Ø Rupture of uterus (spontaneous) before onset of labor**

EXCLUDES 1 *disruption of (current) cesarean delivery wound (O9Ø.Ø)*
*laceration of uterus, NEC (O71.81)*

**O71.ØØ Rupture of uterus before onset of labor, unspecified trimester** COM M

**O71.Ø2 Rupture of uterus before onset of labor, second trimester** COM M

**O71.Ø3 Rupture of uterus before onset of labor, third trimester** COM M

**O71.1 Rupture of uterus during labor** COM M

Rupture of uterus not stated as occurring before onset of labor

EXCLUDES 1 *disruption of cesarean delivery wound (O9Ø.Ø)*
*laceration of uterus, NEC (O71.81)*

**O71.2 Postpartum inversion of uterus** COM M

**O71.3 Obstetric laceration of cervix** COM M

Annular detachment of cervix

**O71.4 Obstetric high vaginal laceration alone** COM M

Laceration of vaginal wall without perineal laceration

EXCLUDES 1 *obstetric high vaginal laceration with perineal laceration (O7Ø.-)*

AHA: 2016,1Q,5

**O71.5 Other obstetric injury to pelvic organs** COM M

Obstetric injury to bladder
Obstetric injury to urethra

EXCLUDES 2 *obstetric periurethral trauma (O71.82)*

AHA: 2014,4Q,18

**O71.6 Obstetric damage to pelvic joints and ligaments** COM M

Obstetric avulsion of inner symphyseal cartilage
Obstetric damage to coccyx
Obstetric traumatic separation of symphysis (pubis)

**O71.7 Obstetric hematoma of pelvis** COM M

Obstetric hematoma of perineum
Obstetric hematoma of vagina
Obstetric hematoma of vulva

✓5th **O71.8 Other specified obstetric trauma**

**O71.81 Laceration of uterus, not elsewhere classified** COM M
AHA: 2025,1Q,21

**O71.82 Other specified trauma to perineum and vulva** COM M
Obstetric periurethral trauma
AHA: 2016,1Q,4; 2014,4Q,18

**O71.89 Other specified obstetric trauma** COM M

**O71.9 Obstetric trauma, unspecified** COM M

✓4th **O72 Postpartum hemorrhage**

INCLUDES hemorrhage after delivery of fetus or infant

**O72.Ø Third-stage hemorrhage** COM M
Hemorrhage associated with retained, trapped or adherent placenta
Retained placenta NOS
Code also type of adherent placenta (O43.2-)
AHA: 2019,3Q,11

**O72.1 Other immediate postpartum hemorrhage** COM M
Hemorrhage following delivery of placenta
Postpartum hemorrhage (atonic) NOS
Uterine atony with hemorrhage
EXCLUDES 1 *uterine atony NOS (O62.2)*
*postpartum atony of uterus without hemorrhage (O75.89)*
*uterine atony without hemorrhage (O62.2)*
AHA: 2023,2Q,15; 2016,1Q,4
DEF: Uterine atony: Failure of the uterine muscles to contract after the fetus and placenta are delivered.

**O72.2 Delayed and secondary postpartum hemorrhage** COM M
Hemorrhage associated with retained portions of placenta or membranes after the first 24 hours following delivery of placenta
Retained products of conception NOS, following delivery

**O72.3 Postpartum coagulation defects** COM M
Postpartum afibrinogenemia
Postpartum fibrinolysis

✓4th **O73 Retained placenta and membranes, without hemorrhage**

EXCLUDES 1 *placenta accreta (O43.21-)*
*placenta increta (O43.22-)*
*placenta percreta (O43.23-)*

DEF: Postpartum condition resulting from failure to expel placental membrane tissues due to failed contractions of the uterine wall.

**O73.Ø Retained placenta without hemorrhage** COM M
Adherent placenta, without hemorrhage
Trapped placenta without hemorrhage

**O73.1 Retained portions of placenta and membranes, without hemorrhage** COM M
Retained products of conception following delivery, without hemorrhage

✓4th **O74 Complications of anesthesia during labor and delivery**

INCLUDES maternal complications arising from the administration of a general, regional or local anesthetic, analgesic or other sedation during labor and delivery

Use additional code, if applicable, to identify specific complication

**O74.Ø Aspiration pneumonitis due to anesthesia during labor and delivery** COM M
Inhalation of stomach contents or secretions NOS due to anesthesia during labor and delivery
Mendelson's syndrome due to anesthesia during labor and delivery

**O74.1 Other pulmonary complications of anesthesia during labor and delivery** COM M

**O74.2 Cardiac complications of anesthesia during labor and delivery** COM M

**O74.3 Central nervous system complications of anesthesia during labor and delivery** COM M

**O74.4 Toxic reaction to local anesthesia during labor and delivery** COM M

**O74.5 Spinal and epidural anesthesia-induced headache during labor and delivery** COM M

**O74.6 Other complications of spinal and epidural anesthesia during labor and delivery** COM M

**O74.7 Failed or difficult intubation for anesthesia during labor and delivery** COM M

**O74.8 Other complications of anesthesia during labor and delivery** COM M

**O74.9 Complication of anesthesia during labor and delivery, unspecified** COM M

✓4th **O75 Other complications of labor and delivery, not elsewhere classified**

EXCLUDES 2 *puerperal (postpartum) infection (O86.-)*
*puerperal (postpartum) sepsis (O85)*

**O75.Ø Maternal distress during labor and delivery** COM M

**O75.1 Shock during or following labor and delivery** COM M
Obstetric shock following labor and delivery

**O75.2 Pyrexia during labor, not elsewhere classified** COM M

**O75.3 Other infection during labor** COM M
Sepsis during labor
Use additional code (B95-B97), to identify infectious agent
AHA: 2025,1Q,22

**O75.4 Other complications of obstetric surgery and procedures** COM M
Cardiac arrest following obstetric surgery or procedures
Cardiac failure following obstetric surgery or procedures
Cerebral anoxia following obstetric surgery or procedures
Pulmonary edema following obstetric surgery or procedures
Use additional code to identify specific complication
EXCLUDES 2 *complications of anesthesia during labor and delivery (O74.-)*
*disruption of obstetrical (surgical) wound (O9Ø.Ø-O9Ø.1)*
*hematoma of obstetrical (surgical) wound (O9Ø.2)*
*infection of obstetrical (surgical) wound (O86.Ø-)*
AHA: 2025,1Q,21

**O75.5 Delayed delivery after artificial rupture of membranes** COM M

✓5th **O75.8 Other specified complications of labor and delivery**

**O75.81 Maternal exhaustion complicating labor and delivery** COM M

**O75.82 Onset (spontaneous) of labor after 37 completed weeks of gestation but before 39 completed weeks gestation, with delivery by (planned) cesarean section** COM UPD M
Delivery by (planned) cesarean section occurring after 37 completed weeks of gestation but before 39 completed weeks gestation due to (spontaneous) onset of labor
Code first to specify reason for planned cesarean section such as:
cephalopelvic disproportion (normally formed fetus) (O33.9)
previous cesarean delivery (O34.21-)
AHA: 2022,2Q,3

**O75.89 Other specified complications of labor and delivery** COM M

**O75.9 Complication of labor and delivery, unspecified** COM M

**O76 Abnormality in fetal heart rate and rhythm complicating labor and delivery** COM M
Depressed fetal heart rate tones complicating labor and delivery
Fetal bradycardia complicating labor and delivery
Fetal heart rate abnormal variability complicating labor and delivery
Fetal heart rate decelerations complicating labor and delivery
Fetal heart rate irregularity complicating labor and delivery
Fetal tachycardia complicating labor and delivery
Non-reassuring fetal heart rate or rhythm complicating labor and delivery
EXCLUDES 1 *fetal stress NOS (O77.9)*
*labor and delivery complicated by electrocardiographic evidence of fetal stress (O77.8)*
*labor and delivery complicated by ultrasonic evidence of fetal stress (O77.8)*
EXCLUDES 2 *fetal metabolic acidemia (O68)*
*other fetal stress (O77.Ø-O77.1)*
AHA: 2013,4Q,118

✓4th **O77 Other fetal stress complicating labor and delivery**

**O77.Ø Labor and delivery complicated by meconium in amniotic fluid** COM M
AHA: 2022,2Q,16; 2013,4Q,117-118

**O77.1 Fetal stress in labor or delivery due to drug administration** COM M

**O77.8 Labor and delivery complicated by other evidence of fetal stress** COM M
Labor and delivery complicated by electrocardiographic evidence of fetal stress
Labor and delivery complicated by ultrasonic evidence of fetal stress
EXCLUDES 1 *abnormality of fetal acid-base balance (O68)*
*abnormality in fetal heart rate or rhythm (O76)*
*fetal metabolic acidemia (O68)*

**O77.9 Labor and delivery complicated by fetal stress, unspecified** COM M
EXCLUDES 1 *abnormality of fetal acid-base balance (O68)*
*abnormality in fetal heart rate or rhythm (O76)*
*fetal metabolic acidemia (O68)*

## Encounter for delivery (O80-O82)

**O80 Encounter for full-term uncomplicated delivery** COM M
NOTE Delivery requiring minimal or no assistance, with or without episiotomy, without fetal manipulation [e.g., rotation version] or instrumentation [forceps] of a spontaneous, cephalic, vaginal, full-term, single, live-born infant. This code is for use as a single diagnosis code and is not to be used with any other code from chapter 15.
Use additional code to indicate outcome of delivery (Z37.0)
**AHA:** 2016,4Q,150; 2014,2Q,9

**O82 Encounter for cesarean delivery without indication** COM M
Use additional code to indicate outcome of delivery (Z37.0)
**AHA:** 2026,1Q,27-28

## Complications predominantly related to the puerperium (O85-O92)

EXCLUDES 2 *mental and behavioral disorders associated with the puerperium (F53.-)*
*obstetrical tetanus (A34)*
*puerperal osteomalacia (M83.0)*

**O85 Puerperal sepsis** COM M
Postpartum sepsis
Puerperal peritonitis
Puerperal pyemia
Use additional code (B95-B97), to identify infectious agent
Use additional code (R65.2-) to identify severe sepsis, if applicable
EXCLUDES 1 *fever of unknown origin following delivery (O86.4)*
*obstetric pyemic and septic embolism (O88.3-)*
*puerperal septic thrombophlebitis (O86.81)*
EXCLUDES 2 *genital tract infection following delivery (O86.1-)*
*sepsis during labor (O75.3)*
*urinary tract infection following delivery (O86.2-)*
**AHA:** 2022,2Q,5; 2020,2Q,32; 2019,2Q,39; 2018,4Q,23

✓4th **O86 Other puerperal infections**
Use additional code (B95-B97), to identify infectious agent
EXCLUDES 2 *infection during labor (O75.3)*
*obstetrical tetanus (A34)*

✓5th **O86.0 Infection of obstetric surgical wound**
Infected cesarean delivery wound following delivery
Infected perineal repair following delivery
EXCLUDES 1 *complications of procedures, not elsewhere classified (T81.4-)*
*postprocedural fever NOS (R50.82)*
*postprocedural retroperitoneal abscess (K68.11)*
**AHA:** 2020,2Q,32; 2018,4Q,22-23,62

**O86.00 Infection of obstetric surgical wound, unspecified** COM M

**O86.01 Infection of obstetric surgical wound, superficial incisional site** COM M
Stitch abscess following an obstetrical procedure
Subcutaneous abscess following an obstetrical procedure

**O86.02 Infection of obstetric surgical wound, deep incisional site** COM M
Intramuscular abscess following an obstetrical procedure
Sub-fascial abscess following an obstetrical procedure
**AHA:** 2020,2Q,32

**O86.03 Infection of obstetric surgical wound, organ and space site** COM M
Intraabdominal abscess following an obstetrical procedure
Subphrenic abscess following an obstetrical procedure

**O86.04 Sepsis following an obstetrical procedure** COM M
Use additional code to identify the sepsis
**AHA:** 2020,2Q,32; 2019,2Q,39

**O86.09 Infection of obstetric surgical wound, other surgical site** COM M

✓5th **O86.1 Other infection of genital tract following delivery**

**O86.11 Cervicitis following delivery** COM M

**O86.12 Endometritis following delivery** COM M

**O86.13 Vaginitis following delivery** COM M

**O86.19 Other infection of genital tract following delivery** COM M

✓5th **O86.2 Urinary tract infection following delivery**

**O86.20 Urinary tract infection following delivery, unspecified** COM M
Puerperal urinary tract infection NOS
**AHA:** 2022,2Q,5

**O86.21 Infection of kidney following delivery** COM M

**O86.22 Infection of bladder following delivery** COM M
Infection of urethra following delivery

**O86.29 Other urinary tract infection following delivery** COM M

**O86.4 Pyrexia of unknown origin following delivery** COM M
Puerperal infection NOS following delivery
Puerperal pyrexia NOS following delivery
EXCLUDES 2 *pyrexia during labor (O75.2)*
**DEF:** Fever of unknown origin experienced by the mother after childbirth.

✓5th **O86.8 Other specified puerperal infections**

**O86.81 Puerperal septic thrombophlebitis** COM M

**O86.89 Other specified puerperal infections** COM M

✓4th **O87 Venous complications and hemorrhoids in the puerperium**
INCLUDES venous complications in labor, delivery and the puerperium
EXCLUDES 2 *obstetric embolism (O88.-)*
*puerperal septic thrombophlebitis (O86.81)*
*venous complications in pregnancy (O22.-)*

**O87.0 Superficial thrombophlebitis in the puerperium** COM M
Puerperal phlebitis NOS
Puerperal thrombosis NOS
Use additional code, if applicable, to identify the superficial vein thrombosis, such as thrombosis of superficial vessels of lower extremities (I80.0-)

**O87.1 Deep phlebothrombosis in the puerperium** COM M
Deep vein thrombosis, postpartum
Pelvic thrombophlebitis, postpartum
Use additional code to identify the deep vein thrombosis (I82.4-, I82.5-, I82.62-, I82.72-)
Use additional code, if applicable, for associated long-term (current) use of anticoagulants (Z79.01)

**O87.2 Hemorrhoids in the puerperium** COM M

**O87.3 Cerebral venous thrombosis in the puerperium** COM M
Cerebrovenous sinus thrombosis in the puerperium

**O87.4 Varicose veins of lower extremity in the puerperium** COM M

**O87.8 Other venous complications in the puerperium** COM M
Genital varices in the puerperium

**O87.9 Venous complication in the puerperium, unspecified** COM M
Puerperal phlebopathy NOS

✓4th **O88 Obstetric embolism**
EXCLUDES 1 *embolism complicating abortion NOS (O03.2)*
*embolism complicating ectopic or molar pregnancy (O08.2)*
*embolism complicating failed attempted abortion (O07.2)*
*embolism complicating induced abortion (O04.7)*
*embolism complicating spontaneous abortion (O03.2, O03.7)*

✓5th **O88.0 Obstetric air embolism**
**DEF:** Sudden blocking of the pulmonary artery or right ventricle with air or nitrogen bubbles.

✓6th **O88.01 Obstetric air embolism in pregnancy**

**O88.011 Air embolism in pregnancy, first trimester** COM M

**O88.012 Air embolism in pregnancy, second trimester** COM M

**O88.013 Air embolism in pregnancy, third trimester** COM M

**O88.019 Air embolism in pregnancy, unspecified trimester** COM M

**O88.02 Air embolism in childbirth** COM M

O88.Ø3 Air embolism in the puerperium COM M

✓5th O88.1 Amniotic fluid embolism
Anaphylactoid syndrome in pregnancy

✓6th O88.11 Amniotic fluid embolism in pregnancy
O88.111 Amniotic fluid embolism in pregnancy, first trimester COM M
O88.112 Amniotic fluid embolism in pregnancy, second trimester COM M
O88.113 Amniotic fluid embolism in pregnancy, third trimester COM M
O88.119 Amniotic fluid embolism in pregnancy, unspecified trimester COM M

O88.12 Amniotic fluid embolism in childbirth COM M
O88.13 Amniotic fluid embolism in the puerperium COM M

✓5th O88.2 Obstetric thromboembolism

✓6th O88.21 Thromboembolism in pregnancy
Obstetric (pulmonary) embolism NOS
O88.211 Thromboembolism in pregnancy, first trimester COM M
O88.212 Thromboembolism in pregnancy, second trimester COM M
O88.213 Thromboembolism in pregnancy, third trimester COM M
O88.219 Thromboembolism in pregnancy, unspecified trimester COM M

O88.22 Thromboembolism in childbirth COM M
O88.23 Thromboembolism in the puerperium COM M
Puerperal (pulmonary) embolism NOS

✓5th O88.3 Obstetric pyemic and septic embolism

✓6th O88.31 Pyemic and septic embolism in pregnancy
O88.311 Pyemic and septic embolism in pregnancy, first trimester COM M
O88.312 Pyemic and septic embolism in pregnancy, second trimester COM M
O88.313 Pyemic and septic embolism in pregnancy, third trimester COM M
O88.319 Pyemic and septic embolism in pregnancy, unspecified trimester COM M

O88.32 Pyemic and septic embolism in childbirth COM M
O88.33 Pyemic and septic embolism in the puerperium COM M

✓5th O88.8 Other obstetric embolism
Obstetric fat embolism

✓6th O88.81 Other embolism in pregnancy
O88.811 Other embolism in pregnancy, first trimester COM M
O88.812 Other embolism in pregnancy, second trimester COM M
O88.813 Other embolism in pregnancy, third trimester COM M
O88.819 Other embolism in pregnancy, unspecified trimester COM M

O88.82 Other embolism in childbirth COM M
O88.83 Other embolism in the puerperium COM M

✓4th **O89 Complications of anesthesia during the puerperium**

INCLUDES maternal complications arising from the administration of a general, regional or local anesthetic, analgesic or other sedation during the puerperium

Use additional code, if applicable, to identify specific complication

✓5th O89.Ø Pulmonary complications of anesthesia during the puerperium
O89.Ø1 Aspiration pneumonitis due to anesthesia during the puerperium COM M
Inhalation of stomach contents or secretions NOS due to anesthesia during the puerperium
Mendelson's syndrome due to anesthesia during the puerperium
O89.Ø9 Other pulmonary complications of anesthesia during the puerperium COM M

O89.1 Cardiac complications of anesthesia during the puerperium COM M
O89.2 Central nervous system complications of anesthesia during the puerperium COM M
O89.3 Toxic reaction to local anesthesia during the puerperium COM M
O89.4 Spinal and epidural anesthesia-induced headache during the puerperium COM M
O89.5 Other complications of spinal and epidural anesthesia during the puerperium COM M
O89.6 Failed or difficult intubation for anesthesia during the puerperium COM M
O89.8 Other complications of anesthesia during the puerperium COM M
O89.9 Complication of anesthesia during the puerperium, unspecified COM M

✓4th **O9Ø Complications of the puerperium, not elsewhere classified**

O9Ø.Ø Disruption of cesarean delivery wound COM M
Dehiscence of cesarean delivery wound
EXCLUDES 1 *rupture of uterus (spontaneous) before onset of labor (O71.Ø-)*
*rupture of uterus during labor (O71.1)*

O9Ø.1 Disruption of perineal obstetric wound COM M
Disruption of wound of episiotomy
Disruption of wound of perineal laceration
Secondary perineal tear

O9Ø.2 Hematoma of obstetric wound COM M

O9Ø.3 Peripartum cardiomyopathy COM M
Conditions in I42- arising during pregnancy and the puerperium
EXCLUDES 1 *pre-existing heart disease complicating pregnancy and the puerperium (O99.4-)*
**AHA:** 2022,3Q,16-17
**DEF:** Any structural or functional abnormality of the ventricular myocardium. It is a noninflammatory disease of obscure or unknown etiology with onset during the postpartum period.

✓5th O9Ø.4 Postpartum acute kidney failure
EXCLUDES 1 *anuria and oliguria (R34)*
**AHA:** 2023,4Q,37
O9Ø.41 Hepatorenal syndrome following labor and delivery COM M
O9Ø.49 Other postpartum acute kidney failure COM M
Postpartum acute kidney failure
Puerperal anuria
Puerperal oliguria

O9Ø.5 Postpartum thyroiditis COM M

O9Ø.6 Postpartum mood disturbance COM M
Postpartum blues
Postpartum dysphoria
Postpartum sadness
EXCLUDES 1 *postpartum depression (F53.Ø)*
*puerperal psychosis (F53.1)*

✓5th O9Ø.8 Other complications of the puerperium, not elsewhere classified
O9Ø.81 Anemia of the puerperium COM M
Postpartum anemia NOS
EXCLUDES 1 *pre-existing anemia complicating the puerperium (O99.Ø3)*
**AHA:** 2019,3Q,11
O9Ø.89 Other complications of the puerperium, not elsewhere classified COM M
Placental polyp

O9Ø.9 Complication of the puerperium, unspecified COM M

✓4th **O91 Infections of breast associated with pregnancy, the puerperium and lactation**
Use additional code to identify infection

✓5th O91.Ø Infection of nipple associated with pregnancy, the puerperium and lactation

✓6th O91.Ø1 Infection of nipple associated with pregnancy
Gestational abscess of nipple
O91.Ø11 Infection of nipple associated with pregnancy, first trimester COM M
O91.Ø12 Infection of nipple associated with pregnancy, second trimester COM M
O91.Ø13 Infection of nipple associated with pregnancy, third trimester COM M
O91.Ø19 Infection of nipple associated with pregnancy, unspecified trimester COM M

O91.Ø2 Infection of nipple associated with the puerperium M
Puerperal abscess of nipple
O91.Ø3 Infection of nipple associated with lactation M
Abscess of nipple associated with lactation

√5th **O91.1 Abscess of breast associated with pregnancy, the puerperium and lactation**

√6th **O91.11 Abscess of breast associated with pregnancy**
Gestational mammary abscess
Gestational purulent mastitis
Gestational subareolar abscess

**O91.111 Abscess of breast associated with pregnancy, first trimester** COM M

**O91.112 Abscess of breast associated with pregnancy, second trimester** COM M

**O91.113 Abscess of breast associated with pregnancy, third trimester** COM M

**O91.119 Abscess of breast associated with pregnancy, unspecified trimester** COM M

**O91.12 Abscess of breast associated with the puerperium** M
Puerperal mammary abscess
Puerperal purulent mastitis
Puerperal subareolar abscess

**O91.13 Abscess of breast associated with lactation** M
Mammary abscess associated with lactation
Purulent mastitis associated with lactation
Subareolar abscess associated with lactation

√5th **O91.2 Nonpurulent mastitis associated with pregnancy, the puerperium and lactation**

√6th **O91.21 Nonpurulent mastitis associated with pregnancy**
Gestational interstitial mastitis
Gestational lymphangitis of breast
Gestational mastitis NOS
Gestational parenchymatous mastitis

**O91.211 Nonpurulent mastitis associated with pregnancy, first trimester** COM M

**O91.212 Nonpurulent mastitis associated with pregnancy, second trimester** COM M

**O91.213 Nonpurulent mastitis associated with pregnancy, third trimester** COM M

**O91.219 Nonpurulent mastitis associated with pregnancy, unspecified trimester** COM M

**O91.22 Nonpurulent mastitis associated with the puerperium** M
Puerperal interstitial mastitis
Puerperal lymphangitis of breast
Puerperal mastitis NOS
Puerperal parenchymatous mastitis

**O91.23 Nonpurulent mastitis associated with lactation** M
Interstitial mastitis associated with lactation
Lymphangitis of breast associated with lactation
Mastitis NOS associated with lactation
Parenchymatous mastitis associated with lactation

√4th **O92 Other disorders of breast and disorders of lactation associated with pregnancy and the puerperium**

√5th **O92.Ø Retracted nipple associated with pregnancy, the puerperium, and lactation**

√6th **O92.Ø1 Retracted nipple associated with pregnancy**

**O92.Ø11 Retracted nipple associated with pregnancy, first trimester** COM M

**O92.Ø12 Retracted nipple associated with pregnancy, second trimester** COM M

**O92.Ø13 Retracted nipple associated with pregnancy, third trimester** COM M

**O92.Ø19 Retracted nipple associated with pregnancy, unspecified trimester** COM M

**O92.Ø2 Retracted nipple associated with the puerperium** M

**O92.Ø3 Retracted nipple associated with lactation** M

√5th **O92.1 Cracked nipple associated with pregnancy, the puerperium, and lactation**
Fissure of nipple, gestational or puerperal

√6th **O92.11 Cracked nipple associated with pregnancy**

**O92.111 Cracked nipple associated with pregnancy, first trimester** COM M

**O92.112 Cracked nipple associated with pregnancy, second trimester** COM M

**O92.113 Cracked nipple associated with pregnancy, third trimester** COM M

**O92.119 Cracked nipple associated with pregnancy, unspecified trimester** COM M

**O92.12 Cracked nipple associated with the puerperium** M

**O92.13 Cracked nipple associated with lactation** M

√5th **O92.2 Other and unspecified disorders of breast associated with pregnancy and the puerperium**

**O92.2Ø Unspecified disorder of breast associated with pregnancy and the puerperium** M

**O92.29 Other disorders of breast associated with pregnancy and the puerperium** M

**O92.3 Agalactia** M
Primary agalactia
EXCLUDES 1 *elective agalactia (O92.5)*
*secondary agalactia (O92.5)*
*therapeutic agalactia (O92.5)*
**DEF:** Absence of milk secretion in a female after delivery.

**O92.4 Hypogalactia** M

**O92.5 Suppressed lactation** M
Elective agalactia
Secondary agalactia
Therapeutic agalactia
EXCLUDES 1 *primary agalactia (O92.3)*

**O92.6 Galactorrhea** M
**DEF:** Excessive or persistent milk secretion by the breast that may occur in the absence of nursing.

√5th **O92.7 Other and unspecified disorders of lactation**

**O92.7Ø Unspecified disorders of lactation** M

**O92.79 Other disorders of lactation** M
Puerperal galactocele

## Other obstetric conditions, not elsewhere classified (O94-O9A)

**O94 Sequelae of complication of pregnancy, childbirth, and the puerperium** UPD M

NOTE This category is to be used to indicate conditions in OØØ-O77.-, O85-O94 and O98-O9A.- as the cause of late effects. The sequelae include conditions specified as such, or as late effects, which may occur at any time after the puerperium

Code first condition resulting from (sequela) of complication of pregnancy, childbirth, and the puerperium

**AHA:** 2022,3Q,16-17

√4th **O98 Maternal infectious and parasitic diseases classifiable elsewhere but complicating pregnancy, childbirth and the puerperium**

INCLUDES the listed conditions when complicating the pregnant state, when aggravated by the pregnancy, or as a reason for obstetric care

Use additional code (Chapter 1), to identify specific infectious or parasitic disease

EXCLUDES 2 *herpes gestationis (O26.4-)*
*infectious carrier state (O99.82-, O99.83-)*
*obstetrical tetanus (A34)*
*puerperal infection (O86.-)*
*puerperal sepsis (O85)*
*when the reason for maternal care is that the disease is known or suspected to have affected the fetus (O35-O36)*

√5th **O98.Ø Tuberculosis complicating pregnancy, childbirth and the puerperium**
Conditions in A15-A19

√6th **O98.Ø1 Tuberculosis complicating pregnancy**

**O98.Ø11 Tuberculosis complicating pregnancy, first trimester** COM M

**O98.Ø12 Tuberculosis complicating pregnancy, second trimester** COM M

**O98.Ø13 Tuberculosis complicating pregnancy, third trimester** COM M

**O98.Ø19 Tuberculosis complicating pregnancy, unspecified trimester** COM M

**O98.Ø2 Tuberculosis complicating childbirth** COM M

**O98.Ø3 Tuberculosis complicating the puerperium** COM M

√5th **O98.1 Syphilis complicating pregnancy, childbirth and the puerperium**
Conditions in A5Ø-A53

√6th **O98.11 Syphilis complicating pregnancy**

**O98.111 Syphilis complicating pregnancy, first trimester** COM M

**O98.112 Syphilis complicating pregnancy, second trimester** COM M

**O98.113 Syphilis complicating pregnancy, third trimester** COM M

O98.119 Syphilis complicating pregnancy, unspecified trimester COM M

O98.12 Syphilis complicating childbirth COM M

O98.13 Syphilis complicating the puerperium COM M

✓5th O98.2 Gonorrhea complicating pregnancy, childbirth and the puerperium

Conditions in A54.-

✓6th O98.21 Gonorrhea complicating pregnancy

O98.211 Gonorrhea complicating pregnancy, first trimester COM M

O98.212 Gonorrhea complicating pregnancy, second trimester COM M

O98.213 Gonorrhea complicating pregnancy, third trimester COM M

O98.219 Gonorrhea complicating pregnancy, unspecified trimester COM M

O98.22 Gonorrhea complicating childbirth COM M

O98.23 Gonorrhea complicating the puerperium COM M

✓5th O98.3 Other infections with a predominantly sexual mode of transmission complicating pregnancy, childbirth and the puerperium

Conditions in A55-A64

AHA: 2020,1Q,20

✓6th O98.31 Other infections with a predominantly sexual mode of transmission complicating pregnancy

O98.311 Other infections with a predominantly sexual mode of transmission complicating pregnancy, first trimester COM M

O98.312 Other infections with a predominantly sexual mode of transmission complicating pregnancy, second trimester COM M

O98.313 Other infections with a predominantly sexual mode of transmission complicating pregnancy, third trimester COM M

O98.319 Other infections with a predominantly sexual mode of transmission complicating pregnancy, unspecified trimester COM M

O98.32 Other infections with a predominantly sexual mode of transmission complicating childbirth COM M

O98.33 Other infections with a predominantly sexual mode of transmission complicating the puerperium COM M

✓5th O98.4 Viral hepatitis complicating pregnancy, childbirth and the puerperium

Conditions in B15-B19

✓6th O98.41 Viral hepatitis complicating pregnancy

O98.411 Viral hepatitis complicating pregnancy, first trimester COM M

O98.412 Viral hepatitis complicating pregnancy, second trimester COM M

O98.413 Viral hepatitis complicating pregnancy, third trimester COM M

O98.419 Viral hepatitis complicating pregnancy, unspecified trimester COM M

O98.42 Viral hepatitis complicating childbirth COM M

O98.43 Viral hepatitis complicating the puerperium COM M

✓5th O98.5 Other viral diseases complicating pregnancy, childbirth and the puerperium

Conditions in A8Ø-BØ9, B25-B34, R87.81-, R87.82-

EXCLUDES 1 *human immunodeficiency virus [HIV] disease complicating pregnancy, childbirth and the puerperium (O98.7-)*

**TIP:** Assign a code from this subcategory as the principal or first-listed diagnosis for a patient admitted/presenting during pregnancy, childbirth, or the puerperium because of COVID-19; assign U07.1 and codes for associated manifestations as secondary codes.

✓6th O98.51 Other viral diseases complicating pregnancy

O98.511 Other viral diseases complicating pregnancy, first trimester COM M

O98.512 Other viral diseases complicating pregnancy, second trimester COM M

O98.513 Other viral diseases complicating pregnancy, third trimester COM M

O98.519 Other viral diseases complicating pregnancy, unspecified trimester COM M

O98.52 Other viral diseases complicating childbirth COM M

O98.53 Other viral diseases complicating the puerperium COM M

✓5th O98.6 Protozoal diseases complicating pregnancy, childbirth and the puerperium

Conditions in B5Ø-B64

✓6th O98.61 Protozoal diseases complicating pregnancy

O98.611 Protozoal diseases complicating pregnancy, first trimester COM M

O98.612 Protozoal diseases complicating pregnancy, second trimester COM M

O98.613 Protozoal diseases complicating pregnancy, third trimester COM M

O98.619 Protozoal diseases complicating pregnancy, unspecified trimester COM M

O98.62 Protozoal diseases complicating childbirth COM M

O98.63 Protozoal diseases complicating the puerperium COM M

✓5th O98.7 Human immunodeficiency virus [HIV] disease complicating pregnancy, childbirth and the puerperium

Use additional code to identify the type of HIV disease:
- acquired immune deficiency syndrome (AIDS) (B2Ø)
- asymptomatic HIV status (Z21)
- HIV positive NOS (Z21)
- symptomatic HIV disease (B2Ø)

✓6th O98.71 Human immunodeficiency virus [HIV] disease complicating pregnancy

O98.711 Human immunodeficiency virus [HIV] disease complicating pregnancy, first trimester COM M

O98.712 Human immunodeficiency virus [HIV] disease complicating pregnancy, second trimester COM M

O98.713 Human immunodeficiency virus [HIV] disease complicating pregnancy, third trimester COM M

O98.719 Human immunodeficiency virus [HIV] disease complicating pregnancy, unspecified trimester COM M

O98.72 Human immunodeficiency virus [HIV] disease complicating childbirth COM M

O98.73 Human immunodeficiency virus [HIV] disease complicating the puerperium COM M

✓5th O98.8 Other maternal infectious and parasitic diseases complicating pregnancy, childbirth and the puerperium

AHA: 2020,1Q,10

✓6th O98.81 Other maternal infectious and parasitic diseases complicating pregnancy

O98.811 Other maternal infectious and parasitic diseases complicating pregnancy, first trimester COM M

O98.812 Other maternal infectious and parasitic diseases complicating pregnancy, second trimester COM M

O98.813 Other maternal infectious and parasitic diseases complicating pregnancy, third trimester COM M

O98.819 Other maternal infectious and parasitic diseases complicating pregnancy, unspecified trimester COM M

O98.82 Other maternal infectious and parasitic diseases complicating childbirth COM M

O98.83 Other maternal infectious and parasitic diseases complicating the puerperium COM M

AHA: 2022,2Q,5

✓5th O98.9 Unspecified maternal infectious and parasitic disease complicating pregnancy, childbirth and the puerperium

✓6th O98.91 Unspecified maternal infectious and parasitic disease complicating pregnancy

O98.911 Unspecified maternal infectious and parasitic disease complicating pregnancy, first trimester COM M

O98.912 Unspecified maternal infectious and parasitic disease complicating pregnancy, second trimester COM M

O98.913 Unspecified maternal infectious and parasitic disease complicating pregnancy, third trimester COM M

O98.919 Unspecified maternal infectious and parasitic disease complicating pregnancy, unspecified trimester COM M

O98.92 Unspecified maternal infectious and parasitic disease complicating childbirth COM M

O98.93 Unspecified maternal infectious and parasitic disease complicating the puerperium COM M

**✓4th O99 Other maternal diseases classifiable elsewhere but complicating pregnancy, childbirth and the puerperium**

INCLUDES conditions which complicate the pregnant state, are aggravated by the pregnancy or are a main reason for obstetric care

Use additional code to identify specific condition

EXCLUDES 2 *when the reason for maternal care is that the condition is known or suspected to have affected the fetus (O35-O36)*

**✓5th O99.0 Anemia complicating pregnancy, childbirth and the puerperium**

Conditions in D50-D64

EXCLUDES 1 *anemia arising in the puerperium (O90.81)*
*postpartum anemia NOS (O90.81)*

**AHA:** 2019,3Q,11

**✓6th O99.01 Anemia complicating pregnancy**

**AHA:** 2016,1Q,4

O99.011 Anemia complicating pregnancy, first trimester COM M

O99.012 Anemia complicating pregnancy, second trimester COM M

O99.013 Anemia complicating pregnancy, third trimester COM M

O99.019 Anemia complicating pregnancy, unspecified trimester COM M

O99.02 Anemia complicating childbirth COM M

O99.03 Anemia complicating the puerperium COM M

EXCLUDES 1 *postpartum anemia not pre-existing prior to delivery (O90.81)*

**✓5th O99.1 Other diseases of the blood and blood-forming organs and certain disorders involving the immune mechanism complicating pregnancy, childbirth and the puerperium**

Conditions in D65-D89

EXCLUDES 1 *hemorrhage with coagulation defects (O45.-, O46.0-, O67.0, O72.3)*

**✓6th O99.11 Other diseases of the blood and blood-forming organs and certain disorders involving the immune mechanism complicating pregnancy**

O99.111 Other diseases of the blood and blood-forming organs and certain disorders involving the immune mechanism complicating pregnancy, first trimester COM M

O99.112 Other diseases of the blood and blood-forming organs and certain disorders involving the immune mechanism complicating pregnancy, second trimester COM M

O99.113 Other diseases of the blood and blood-forming organs and certain disorders involving the immune mechanism complicating pregnancy, third trimester COM M

O99.119 Other diseases of the blood and blood-forming organs and certain disorders involving the immune mechanism complicating pregnancy, unspecified trimester COM M

O99.12 Other diseases of the blood and blood-forming organs and certain disorders involving the immune mechanism complicating childbirth COM M

O99.13 Other diseases of the blood and blood-forming organs and certain disorders involving the immune mechanism complicating the puerperium COM M

**✓5th O99.2 Endocrine, nutritional and metabolic diseases complicating pregnancy, childbirth and the puerperium**

Conditions in E00-E89

EXCLUDES 2 *diabetes mellitus (O24.-)*
*malnutrition (O25.-)*
*postpartum thyroiditis (O90.5)*

**✓6th O99.21 Obesity complicating pregnancy, childbirth, and the puerperium**

Use additional code to identify the type of obesity (E66.-)

**AHA:** 2021,2Q,10; 2018,4Q,80

**TIP:** Do not assign a BMI code (Z68.-) for obese or overweight patients who are pregnant.

O99.210 Obesity complicating pregnancy, unspecified trimester COM M

O99.211 Obesity complicating pregnancy, first trimester COM M

O99.212 Obesity complicating pregnancy, second trimester COM M

O99.213 Obesity complicating pregnancy, third trimester COM M

O99.214 Obesity complicating childbirth COM M

O99.215 Obesity complicating the puerperium COM M

**✓6th O99.28 Other endocrine, nutritional and metabolic diseases complicating pregnancy, childbirth and the puerperium**

**AHA:** 2021,1Q,8

O99.280 Endocrine, nutritional and metabolic diseases complicating pregnancy, unspecified trimester COM M

O99.281 Endocrine, nutritional and metabolic diseases complicating pregnancy, first trimester COM M

O99.282 Endocrine, nutritional and metabolic diseases complicating pregnancy, second trimester COM M

O99.283 Endocrine, nutritional and metabolic diseases complicating pregnancy, third trimester COM M

O99.284 Endocrine, nutritional and metabolic diseases complicating childbirth COM M

O99.285 Endocrine, nutritional and metabolic diseases complicating the puerperium COM M

**✓5th O99.3 Mental disorders and diseases of the nervous system complicating pregnancy, childbirth and the puerperium**

**✓6th O99.31 Alcohol use complicating pregnancy, childbirth, and the puerperium**

Use additional code(s) from F10 to identify manifestations of the alcohol use

O99.310 Alcohol use complicating pregnancy, unspecified trimester COM M

O99.311 Alcohol use complicating pregnancy, first trimester COM M

O99.312 Alcohol use complicating pregnancy, second trimester COM M

O99.313 Alcohol use complicating pregnancy, third trimester COM M

O99.314 Alcohol use complicating childbirth COM M

O99.315 Alcohol use complicating the puerperium COM M

**✓6th O99.32 Drug use complicating pregnancy, childbirth, and the puerperium**

Use additional code(s) from F11-F16 and F18-F19 to identify manifestations of the drug use

**AHA:** 2018,4Q,69-70; 2018,2Q,10

**TIP:** When drug use is documented during pregnancy, assign first a code from this subcategory followed by an additional code from F11-F16 and F18-F19 identifying the specific drug use even if not documented as associated with a physical, mental, or behavioral disorder. According to chapter 15 guidelines, it is the provider's responsibility to state that the condition being treated is *not* affecting the pregnancy.

O99.320 Drug use complicating pregnancy, unspecified trimester COM M

O99.321 Drug use complicating pregnancy, first trimester COM M

O99.322 **Drug use complicating pregnancy, second trimester** COM M

O99.323 **Drug use complicating pregnancy, third trimester** COM M

O99.324 **Drug use complicating childbirth** COM M

O99.325 **Drug use complicating the puerperium** COM M

✓6th **O99.33 Tobacco use disorder complicating pregnancy, childbirth, and the puerperium**

Smoking complicating pregnancy, childbirth, and the puerperium

Use additional code from category F17 to identify type of tobacco nicotine dependence

O99.330 **Smoking (tobacco) complicating pregnancy, unspecified trimester** COM M

O99.331 **Smoking (tobacco) complicating pregnancy, first trimester** COM M

O99.332 **Smoking (tobacco) complicating pregnancy, second trimester** COM M

O99.333 **Smoking (tobacco) complicating pregnancy, third trimester** COM M

O99.334 **Smoking (tobacco) complicating childbirth** COM M

O99.335 **Smoking (tobacco) complicating the puerperium** COM M

✓6th **O99.34 Other mental disorders complicating pregnancy, childbirth, and the puerperium**

Conditions in F01-F09, F20-F52 and F54-F99

EXCLUDES 2 *postpartum mood disturbance (O90.6)*
*postnatal psychosis (F53.1)*
*puerperal psychosis (F53.1)*

O99.340 **Other mental disorders complicating pregnancy, unspecified trimester** COM M

O99.341 **Other mental disorders complicating pregnancy, first trimester** COM M

O99.342 **Other mental disorders complicating pregnancy, second trimester** COM M

O99.343 **Other mental disorders complicating pregnancy, third trimester** COM M

O99.344 **Other mental disorders complicating childbirth** COM M

O99.345 **Other mental disorders complicating the puerperium** COM M

**AHA:** 2018,4Q,8

✓6th **O99.35 Diseases of the nervous system complicating pregnancy, childbirth, and the puerperium**

Conditions in G00-G99

EXCLUDES 2 *pregnancy related peripheral neuritis (O26.8-)*

**AHA:** 2026,2Q,21

O99.350 **Diseases of the nervous system complicating pregnancy, unspecified trimester** COM M

O99.351 **Diseases of the nervous system complicating pregnancy, first trimester** COM M

O99.352 **Diseases of the nervous system complicating pregnancy, second trimester** COM M

O99.353 **Diseases of the nervous system complicating pregnancy, third trimester** COM M

O99.354 **Diseases of the nervous system complicating childbirth** COM M

O99.355 **Diseases of the nervous system complicating the puerperium** COM M

**AHA:** 2025,3Q,17

✓5th **O99.4 Diseases of the circulatory system complicating pregnancy, childbirth and the puerperium**

Conditions in I00-I99

EXCLUDES 1 *peripartum cardiomyopathy (O90.3)*

EXCLUDES 2 *hypertensive disorders (O10-O16)*
*obstetric embolism (O88.-)*
*venous complications and cerebrovenous sinus thrombosis in labor, childbirth and the puerperium (O87.-)*
*venous complications and cerebrovenous sinus thrombosis in pregnancy (O22.-)*

**AHA:** 2016,2Q,8

✓6th **O99.41 Diseases of the circulatory system complicating pregnancy**

O99.411 **Diseases of the circulatory system complicating pregnancy, first trimester** COM M

O99.412 **Diseases of the circulatory system complicating pregnancy, second trimester** COM M

O99.413 **Diseases of the circulatory system complicating pregnancy, third trimester** COM M

O99.419 **Diseases of the circulatory system complicating pregnancy, unspecified trimester** COM M

**O99.42 Diseases of the circulatory system complicating childbirth** COM M

**O99.43 Diseases of the circulatory system complicating the puerperium** COM M

**AHA:** 2025,3Q,17

✓5th **O99.5 Diseases of the respiratory system complicating pregnancy, childbirth and the puerperium**

Conditions in J00-J99

✓6th **O99.51 Diseases of the respiratory system complicating pregnancy**

O99.511 **Diseases of the respiratory system complicating pregnancy, first trimester** COM M

O99.512 **Diseases of the respiratory system complicating pregnancy, second trimester** COM M

O99.513 **Diseases of the respiratory system complicating pregnancy, third trimester** COM M

O99.519 **Diseases of the respiratory system complicating pregnancy, unspecified trimester** COM M

**O99.52 Diseases of the respiratory system complicating childbirth** COM M

**O99.53 Diseases of the respiratory system complicating the puerperium** COM M

✓5th **O99.6 Diseases of the digestive system complicating pregnancy, childbirth and the puerperium**

Conditions in K00-K93

EXCLUDES 2 *hemorrhoids in pregnancy (O22.4-)*
*liver and biliary tract disorders in pregnancy, childbirth and the puerperium (O26.6-)*

✓6th **O99.61 Diseases of the digestive system complicating pregnancy**

**AHA:** 2016,1Q,4

O99.611 **Diseases of the digestive system complicating pregnancy, first trimester** COM M

O99.612 **Diseases of the digestive system complicating pregnancy, second trimester** COM M

O99.613 **Diseases of the digestive system complicating pregnancy, third trimester** COM M

O99.619 **Diseases of the digestive system complicating pregnancy, unspecified trimester** COM M

**O99.62 Diseases of the digestive system complicating childbirth** COM M

**O99.63 Diseases of the digestive system complicating the puerperium** COM M

√5th **O99.7 Diseases of the skin and subcutaneous tissue complicating pregnancy, childbirth and the puerperium**
Conditions in LØØ-L99
EXCLUDES 2 *herpes gestationis (O26.4)*
*pruritic urticarial papules and plaques of pregnancy (PUPPP) (O26.86)*

√6th **O99.71 Diseases of the skin and subcutaneous tissue complicating pregnancy**
**O99.711 Diseases of the skin and subcutaneous tissue complicating pregnancy, first trimester** COM M
**O99.712 Diseases of the skin and subcutaneous tissue complicating pregnancy, second trimester** COM M
**O99.713 Diseases of the skin and subcutaneous tissue complicating pregnancy, third trimester** COM M
**O99.719 Diseases of the skin and subcutaneous tissue complicating pregnancy, unspecified trimester** COM M

**O99.72 Diseases of the skin and subcutaneous tissue complicating childbirth** COM M
**O99.73 Diseases of the skin and subcutaneous tissue complicating the puerperium** COM M

√5th **O99.8 Other specified diseases and conditions complicating pregnancy, childbirth and the puerperium**
Conditions in DØØ-D48, HØØ-H95, MØØ-N99, and QØØ-Q99
Use additional code to identify condition
EXCLUDES 2 *genitourinary infections in pregnancy (O23.-)*
*infection of genitourinary tract following delivery (O86.1-O86.4)*
*malignant neoplasm complicating pregnancy, childbirth and the puerperium (O9A.1-)*
*maternal care for known or suspected abnormality of maternal pelvic organs (O34.-)*
*postpartum acute kidney failure (O9Ø.49)*
*traumatic injuries in pregnancy (O9A.2-)*

√6th **O99.81 Abnormal glucose complicating pregnancy, childbirth and the puerperium**
EXCLUDES 1 *gestational diabetes (O24.4-)*
**O99.81Ø Abnormal glucose complicating pregnancy** COM M
**O99.814 Abnormal glucose complicating childbirth** COM M
**O99.815 Abnormal glucose complicating the puerperium** COM M

√6th **O99.82 Streptococcus B carrier state complicating pregnancy, childbirth and the puerperium**
EXCLUDES 1 *carrier of streptococcus group B (GBS) in a nonpregnant woman (Z22.33Ø)*
**DEF:** *Streptococcus* group B colonization: Bacteria normally found in the vagina or lower intestine of many healthy adult women that may infect the fetus during childbirth, causing mental or physical handicaps or death. Women who test positive for *Streptococcus* group B during pregnancy are considered a "colonized" status and are treated with IV antibiotics at the time of delivery and may also be treated with oral antibiotics during the pregnancy.
**O99.82Ø Streptococcus B carrier state complicating pregnancy** COM M
**O99.824 Streptococcus B carrier state complicating childbirth** COM M
**AHA:** 2019,2Q,8
**O99.825 Streptococcus B carrier state complicating the puerperium** COM M

√6th **O99.83 Other infection carrier state complicating pregnancy, childbirth and the puerperium**
Use additional code to identify the carrier state (Z22.-)
**O99.83Ø Other infection carrier state complicating pregnancy** COM M
**O99.834 Other infection carrier state complicating childbirth** COM M
**O99.835 Other infection carrier state complicating the puerperium** COM M

√6th **O99.84 Bariatric surgery status complicating pregnancy, childbirth and the puerperium**
Gastric banding status complicating pregnancy, childbirth and the puerperium
Gastric bypass status for obesity complicating pregnancy, childbirth and the puerperium
Obesity surgery status complicating pregnancy, childbirth and the puerperium
**O99.84Ø Bariatric surgery status complicating pregnancy, unspecified trimester** COM M
**O99.841 Bariatric surgery status complicating pregnancy, first trimester** COM M
**O99.842 Bariatric surgery status complicating pregnancy, second trimester** COM M
**O99.843 Bariatric surgery status complicating pregnancy, third trimester** COM M
**O99.844 Bariatric surgery status complicating childbirth** COM M
**O99.845 Bariatric surgery status complicating the puerperium** COM M

√6th **O99.89 Other specified diseases and conditions complicating pregnancy, childbirth and the puerperium**
**AHA:** 2026,2Q,21; 2023,3Q,17; 2020,4Q,36-37
**O99.891 Other specified diseases and conditions complicating pregnancy** COM M
**O99.892 Other specified diseases and conditions complicating childbirth** COM M
**O99.893 Other specified diseases and conditions complicating puerperium** COM M

√4th **O9A Maternal malignant neoplasms, traumatic injuries and abuse classifiable elsewhere but complicating pregnancy, childbirth and the puerperium**

√5th **O9A.1 Malignant neoplasm complicating pregnancy, childbirth and the puerperium**
Conditions in CØØ-C96
Use additional code to identify neoplasm
EXCLUDES 2 *maternal care for benign tumor of corpus uteri (O34.1-)*
*maternal care for benign tumor of cervix (O34.4-)*
**AHA:** 2015,3Q,19

√6th **O9A.11 Malignant neoplasm complicating pregnancy**
**O9A.111 Malignant neoplasm complicating pregnancy, first trimester** COM M
**O9A.112 Malignant neoplasm complicating pregnancy, second trimester** COM M
**O9A.113 Malignant neoplasm complicating pregnancy, third trimester** COM M
**O9A.119 Malignant neoplasm complicating pregnancy, unspecified trimester** COM M

**O9A.12 Malignant neoplasm complicating childbirth** COM M
**O9A.13 Malignant neoplasm complicating the puerperium** COM M

√5th **O9A.2 Injury, poisoning and certain other consequences of external causes complicating pregnancy, childbirth and the puerperium**
Conditions in SØØ-T88, except T74 and T76
Use additional code(s) to identify the injury or poisoning
EXCLUDES 2 *physical, sexual and psychological abuse complicating pregnancy, childbirth and the puerperium (O9A.3-, O9A.4-, O9A.5-)*

√6th **O9A.21 Injury, poisoning and certain other consequences of external causes complicating pregnancy**
**O9A.211 Injury, poisoning and certain other consequences of external causes complicating pregnancy, first trimester** COM M
**O9A.212 Injury, poisoning and certain other consequences of external causes complicating pregnancy, second trimester** COM M
**O9A.213 Injury, poisoning and certain other consequences of external causes complicating pregnancy, third trimester** COM M
**O9A.219 Injury, poisoning and certain other consequences of external causes complicating pregnancy, unspecified trimester** COM M

**O9A.22 Injury, poisoning and certain other consequences of external causes complicating childbirth** COM M

**O9A.23** Injury, poisoning and certain other consequences of external causes complicating the puerperium COM M

✓5th **O9A.3** Physical abuse complicating pregnancy, childbirth and the puerperium

Conditions in T74.11 or T76.11

Use additional code (if applicable):

to identify any associated current injury due to physical abuse

to identify the perpetrator of abuse (YØ7.-)

EXCLUDES 2 *sexual abuse complicating pregnancy, childbirth and the puerperium (O9A.4)*

✓6th **O9A.31** Physical abuse complicating pregnancy

**O9A.311** Physical abuse complicating pregnancy, first trimester COM M

**O9A.312** Physical abuse complicating pregnancy, second trimester COM M

**O9A.313** Physical abuse complicating pregnancy, third trimester COM M

**O9A.319** Physical abuse complicating pregnancy, unspecified trimester COM M

**O9A.32** Physical abuse complicating childbirth COM M

**O9A.33** Physical abuse complicating the puerperium COM M

✓5th **O9A.4** Sexual abuse complicating pregnancy, childbirth and the puerperium

Conditions in T74.21 or T76.21

Use additional code (if applicable):

to identify any associated current injury due to sexual abuse

to identify the perpetrator of abuse (YØ7.-)

✓6th **O9A.41** Sexual abuse complicating pregnancy

**O9A.411** Sexual abuse complicating pregnancy, first trimester COM M

**O9A.412** Sexual abuse complicating pregnancy, second trimester COM M

**O9A.413** Sexual abuse complicating pregnancy, third trimester COM M

**O9A.419** Sexual abuse complicating pregnancy, unspecified trimester COM M

**O9A.42** Sexual abuse complicating childbirth COM M

**O9A.43** Sexual abuse complicating the puerperium COM M

✓5th **O9A.5** Psychological abuse complicating pregnancy, childbirth and the puerperium

Conditions in T74.31 or T76.31

Use additional code to identify the perpetrator of abuse (YØ7.-)

✓6th **O9A.51** Psychological abuse complicating pregnancy

**O9A.511** Psychological abuse complicating pregnancy, first trimester COM M

**O9A.512** Psychological abuse complicating pregnancy, second trimester COM M

**O9A.513** Psychological abuse complicating pregnancy, third trimester COM M

**O9A.519** Psychological abuse complicating pregnancy, unspecified trimester COM M

**O9A.52** Psychological abuse complicating childbirth COM M

**O9A.53** Psychological abuse complicating the puerperium COM M

# Chapter 16. Certain Conditions Originating in the Perinatal Period (PØØ–P96)



## Chapter-specific Guidelines with Coding Examples

The chapter-specific guidelines from the ICD-10-CM Official Guidelines for Coding and Reporting have been provided below. Along with these guidelines are coding examples, contained in the shaded boxes, that have been developed to help illustrate the coding and/or sequencing guidance found in these guidelines.

For coding and reporting purposes the perinatal period is defined as before birth through the 28th day following birth. The following guidelines are provided for reporting purposes

**a. General perinatal rules**

**1) Use of Chapter 16 codes**

Codes in this chapter are never for use on the maternal record. Codes from Chapter 15, the obstetric chapter, are never permitted on the newborn record. Chapter 16 codes may be used throughout the life of the patient if the condition is still present.

**2) Principal diagnosis for birth record**

When coding the birth episode in a newborn record, assign a code from category Z38, Liveborn infants according to place of birth and type of delivery, as the principal diagnosis. A code from category Z38 is assigned only once, to a newborn at the time of birth. If a newborn is transferred to another institution, a code from category Z38 should not be used at the receiving hospital.

A code from category Z38 is used only on the newborn record, not on the mother's record.

**3) Use of codes from other chapters with codes from Chapter 16**

Codes from other chapters may be used with codes from chapter 16 if the codes from the other chapters provide more specific detail. Codes for signs and symptoms may be assigned when a definitive diagnosis has not been established. If the reason for the encounter is a perinatal condition, the code from chapter 16 should be sequenced first.

**4) Use of Chapter 16 codes after the perinatal period**

Should a condition originate in the perinatal period, and continue throughout the life of the patient, the perinatal code should continue to be used regardless of the patient's age.

> A 7-year-old patient with history of birth injury that resulted in Erb's palsy is seen for subscapularis release
>
> **P14.Ø** **Erb's paralysis due to birth injury**
>
> *Explanation:* Although in this instance Erb's palsy is specifically related to a birth injury, it has not resolved and continues to be a health concern. A perinatal code is appropriate even though this patient is beyond the perinatal period.

**5) Birth process or community acquired conditions**

If a newborn has a condition that may be either due to the birth process or community acquired and the documentation does not indicate which it is, the default is due to the birth process and the code from Chapter 16 should be used. If the condition is community-acquired, a code from Chapter 16 should not be assigned.

*For COVID-19 infection in a newborn, see guideline I.C.16.h.*

**6) Code all clinically significant conditions**

All clinically significant conditions noted on routine newborn examination should be coded. A condition is clinically significant if it requires:

clinical evaluation; or

therapeutic treatment; or

diagnostic procedures; or

extended length of hospital stay; or

increased nursing care and/or monitoring; or

has implications for future health care needs

Note: The perinatal guidelines listed above are the same as the general coding guidelines for "additional diagnoses", except for the final point regarding implications for future health care needs. Codes should be assigned for conditions that have been specified by the provider as having implications for future health care needs.

**b. Observation and evaluation of newborns for suspected conditions not found**

**1) Use of Z05 codes**

Assign a code from category ZØ5, Observation and evaluation of newborn for suspected diseases and conditions ruled out, to identify those instances when a healthy newborn is evaluated for a suspected condition/disease that is determined after study not to be present. Do not use a code from category ZØ5 when the patient is documented to have signs or symptoms of a suspected problem; in such cases code the sign or symptom.

**2) Z05 on other than the birth record**

A code from category ZØ5 may also be assigned as a principal or first-listed code for readmissions or encounters when the code from category Z38 no longer applies. Codes from category ZØ5 are for use only for healthy newborns and infants for which no condition **is found to be present after study.**

**3) Z05 on a birth record**

A code from category ZØ5 is to be used as a secondary code after the code from category Z38, Liveborn infants according to place of birth and type of delivery.

> Newborn delivered via vaginal delivery; previous ultrasounds showed what appeared to be an abnormality of the right kidney. Kidney function tests were performed and ultrasounds taken and any genitourinary conditions ruled out.
>
> **Z38.ØØ** **Single liveborn infant, delivered vaginally**
>
> **ZØ5.6** **Observation and evaluation of newborn for suspected genitourinary condition ruled out**
>
> *Explanation:* The newborn had no signs or symptoms of kidney or other genitourinary condition but was evaluated after delivery due to the abnormal prenatal ultrasound findings. A Z code describing the type and place of birth should be coded first, followed by a ZØ5 category code for the work performed to rule out a suspected genitourinary condition.

**c. Coding additional perinatal diagnoses**

**1) Assigning codes for conditions that require treatment**

Assign codes for conditions that require treatment or further investigation, prolong the length of stay, or require resource utilization.

**2) Codes for conditions specified as having implications for future health care needs**

Assign codes for conditions that have been specified by the provider as having implications for future health care needs.

Note: This guideline should not be used for adult patients.

> An abnormal noise was heard in the left hip of a post-term newborn during a physical examination. The pediatrician would like to follow the patient after discharge as a hip click can be an early sign of hip dysplasia. The newborn was delivered via cesarean at 41 weeks.
>
> **Z38.Ø1** **Single liveborn infant, delivered by cesarean**
>
> **PØ8.21** **Post-term newborn**
>
> **R29.4** **Clicking hip**
>
> *Explanation:* The abnormal hip noise or click is appended as a secondary diagnosis not only because it is an abnormal finding upon examination, but also due to its potential to be part of a bigger health issue. The hip dysplasia has not yet been diagnosed and does not warrant a code at this time.

**d. Prematurity and fetal growth retardation**

Providers utilize different criteria in determining prematurity. A code for prematurity should not be assigned unless it is documented. Assignment of codes in categories PØ5, Disorders of newborn related to slow fetal growth and fetal malnutrition, and PØ7, Disorders of newborn related to short gestation and low birth weight, not elsewhere classified, should be based on the recorded birth weight and estimated gestational age.

When both birth weight and gestational age are available, two codes from category PØ7 should be assigned, with the code for birth weight sequenced before the code for gestational age.

**e. Low birth weight and immaturity status**

Codes from category PØ7, Disorders of newborn related to short gestation and low birth weight, not elsewhere classified, are for use for a child or adult who was premature or had a low birth weight as a newborn and this is affecting the patient's current health status.

*See Section I.C.21. Factors influencing health status and contact with health services, Status.*

A 35-year-old patient, who weighed 659 grams at birth, is seen for heart disease documented as being a consequence of the low birth weight

| | |
|---|---|
| **I51.9** | **Heart disease, unspecified** |
| **PØ7.Ø2** | **Extremely low birth weight newborn, 5ØØ–749 grams** |

*Explanation:* A code from subcategories PØ7.Ø- and PØ7.1- is appropriate, regardless of the age of the patient, as long as the documentation provides a clear link between the patient's current illness and the low birth weight.

**f. Bacterial sepsis of newborn**

Category P36, Bacterial sepsis of newborn, includes congenital sepsis. If a perinate is documented as having sepsis without documentation of congenital or community acquired, the default is congenital and a code from category P36 should be assigned. If the P36 code includes the causal organism, an additional code from category B95, Streptococcus, Staphylococcus, and Enterococcus as the cause of diseases classified elsewhere, or B96, Other bacterial agents as the cause of diseases classified elsewhere, should not be assigned. If the P36 code does not include the causal organism, assign an additional code from category B96. If applicable, use additional codes to identify severe sepsis (R65.2-) and any associated acute organ dysfunction.

A full-term infant develops severe sepsis 24 hours after discharge from the hospital and is readmitted; cultures identified *E. coli* as the infective agent

| | |
|---|---|
| **P36.4** | **Sepsis of newborn due to Escherichia coli** |
| **R65.2Ø** | **Severe sepsis without septic shock** |

*Explanation:* Even though this newborn was discharged and could have acquired *E. coli* from his/her external environment, due to the lack of documentation specifying specifically how this pathogen was acquired, the default is to code the *E. coli* sepsis as congenital. A code from chapter 1, "Certain Infectious and Parasitic Diseases," is not required because the perinatal sepsis code identifies both the sepsis and the bacteria causing the sepsis.

**g. Stillbirth**

Code P95, Stillbirth, is only for use in institutions that maintain separate records for stillbirths. No other code should be used with P95. Code P95 should not be used on the mother's record.

**h. COVID-19 infection in newborn**

For a newborn that tests positive for COVID-19, assign code UØ7.1, COVID-19, and the appropriate codes for associated manifestation(s) in neonates/newborns in the absence of documentation indicating a specific type of transmission. For a newborn that tests positive for COVID-19 and the provider documents the condition was contracted in utero or during the birth process, assign codes P35.8, Other congenital viral diseases, and UØ7.1, COVID-19. When coding the birth episode in a newborn record, the appropriate code from category Z38, Liveborn infants according to place of birth and type of delivery, should be assigned as the principal diagnosis.

# Chapter 16. Certain Conditions Originating in the Perinatal Period (P00-P96)

**NOTE** Codes from this chapter are for use on newborn records only, never on maternal records

**INCLUDES** conditions that have their origin in the fetal or perinatal period (before birth through the first 28 days after birth) even if morbidity occurs later

**EXCLUDES 2** *congenital malformations, deformations and chromosomal abnormalities (Q00-Q99)*
*endocrine, nutritional and metabolic diseases (E00-E88)*
*injury, poisoning and certain other consequences of external causes (S00-T88)*
*neoplasms (C00-D49)*
*tetanus neonatorum (A33)*

This chapter contains the following blocks:



## Newborn affected by maternal factors and by complications of pregnancy, labor, and delivery (P00-P04)

**NOTE** These codes are for use when the listed maternal conditions are specified as the cause of confirmed morbidity or potential morbidity which have their origin in the perinatal period (before birth through the first 28 days after birth).

**AHA:** 2016,4Q,54-55

✓4th **P00 Newborn affected by maternal conditions that may be unrelated to present pregnancy**
Code first any current condition in newborn
**EXCLUDES 2** *encounter for observation of newborn for suspected diseases and conditions ruled out (Z05.-)*
*newborn affected by maternal complications of pregnancy (P01.-)*
*newborn affected by maternal endocrine and metabolic disorders (P70-P74)*
*newborn affected by noxious substances transmitted via placenta or breast milk (P04.-)*

**P00.0 Newborn affected by maternal hypertensive disorders**
Newborn affected by maternal conditions classifiable to O10-O11, O13-O16

**P00.1 Newborn affected by maternal renal and urinary tract diseases**
Newborn affected by maternal conditions classifiable to N00-N39

**P00.2 Newborn affected by maternal infectious and parasitic diseases**
Newborn affected by maternal infectious disease classifiable to A00-B99, J09 and J10
**EXCLUDES 1** *maternal genital tract or other localized infections (P00.8)*
**EXCLUDES 2** *infections specific to the perinatal period (P35-P39)*
*newborn affected by (positive) maternal group B streptococcus (GBS) colonization (P00.82)*
**AHA:** 2019,2Q,10; 2015,3Q,20

**P00.3 Newborn affected by other maternal circulatory and respiratory diseases**
Newborn affected by maternal conditions classifiable to I00-I99, J00-J99, Q20-Q34 and not included in P00.0, P00.2

**P00.4 Newborn affected by maternal nutritional disorders**
Maternal malnutrition NOS
Newborn affected by maternal disorders classifiable to E40-E64

**P00.5 Newborn affected by maternal injury**
Newborn affected by maternal conditions classifiable to O9A.2-

**P00.6 Newborn affected by surgical procedure on mother**
Newborn affected by amniocentesis
**EXCLUDES 1** *Cesarean delivery for present delivery (P03.4)*
*damage to placenta from amniocentesis, Cesarean delivery or surgical induction (P02.1)*
*previous surgery to uterus or pelvic organs (P03.89)*
**EXCLUDES 2** *newborn affected by complication of (fetal) intrauterine procedure (P96.5)*

**P00.7 Newborn affected by other medical procedures on mother, not elsewhere classified**
Newborn affected by radiation to mother
**EXCLUDES 1** *damage to placenta from amniocentesis, cesarean delivery or surgical induction (P02.1)*
*newborn affected by other complications of labor and delivery (P03.-)*

✓5th **P00.8 Newborn affected by other maternal conditions**

**P00.81 Newborn affected by periodontal disease in mother**

**P00.82 Newborn affected by (positive) maternal group B streptococcus (GBS) colonization**
Contact with positive maternal group B streptococcus
**AHA:** 2021,4Q,23

**P00.89 Newborn affected by other maternal conditions**
Newborn affected by conditions classifiable to T80-T88
Newborn affected by maternal genital tract or other localized infections
Newborn affected by maternal systemic lupus erythematosus
Use additional code to identify infectious agent, if known
**EXCLUDES 2** *newborn affected by positive maternal group B streptococcus (GBS) colonization (P00.82)*
**AHA:** 2019,2Q,9

**P00.9 Newborn affected by unspecified maternal condition**

✓4th **P01 Newborn affected by maternal complications of pregnancy**
Code first any current condition in newborn
**EXCLUDES 2** *encounter for observation of newborn for suspected diseases and conditions ruled out (Z05.-)*

**P01.0 Newborn affected by incompetent cervix**

**P01.1 Newborn affected by premature rupture of membranes**

**P01.2 Newborn affected by oligohydramnios**
**EXCLUDES 1** *oligohydramnios due to premature rupture of membranes (P01.1)*
**DEF:** Low amniotic fluid level, resulting in underdeveloped organs in the fetus.

**P01.3 Newborn affected by polyhydramnios**
Newborn affected by hydramnios
**DEF:** Excess amniotic fluid surrounding the fetus, typically defined as a total fluid volume of greater than 24 cm.

**P01.4 Newborn affected by ectopic pregnancy**
Newborn affected by abdominal pregnancy

**P01.5 Newborn affected by multiple pregnancy**
Newborn affected by triplet (pregnancy)
Newborn affected by twin (pregnancy)

**P01.6 Newborn affected by maternal death**

**P01.7 Newborn affected by malpresentation before labor**
Newborn affected by breech presentation before labor
Newborn affected by external version before labor
Newborn affected by face presentation before labor
Newborn affected by transverse lie before labor
Newborn affected by unstable lie before labor
**AHA:** 2025,1Q,23

**P01.8 Newborn affected by other maternal complications of pregnancy**

**P01.9 Newborn affected by maternal complication of pregnancy, unspecified**

✓4th **P02 Newborn affected by complications of placenta, cord and membranes**
Code first any current condition in newborn
**EXCLUDES 2** *encounter for observation of newborn for suspected diseases and conditions ruled out (Z05.-)*

**P02.0 Newborn affected by placenta previa**
**DEF:** Placenta developed in the lower segment of the uterus that can cause hemorrhaging leading to preterm delivery.

**P02.1 Newborn affected by other forms of placental separation and hemorrhage**
Newborn affected by abruptio placenta
Newborn affected by accidental hemorrhage
Newborn affected by antepartum hemorrhage
Newborn affected by damage to placenta from amniocentesis, cesarean delivery or surgical induction
Newborn affected by maternal blood loss
Newborn affected by premature separation of placenta

✓5th **P02.2 Newborn affected by other and unspecified morphological and functional abnormalities of placenta**

**P02.20 Newborn affected by unspecified morphological and functional abnormalities of placenta**

**P02.29 Newborn affected by other morphological and functional abnormalities of placenta**
Newborn affected by placental dysfunction
Newborn affected by placental infarction
Newborn affected by placental insufficiency

**P02.3 Newborn affected by placental transfusion syndromes**
Newborn affected by placental and cord abnormalities resulting in twin-to-twin or other transplacental transfusion

**P02.4 Newborn affected by prolapsed cord**

**P02.5 Newborn affected by other compression of umbilical cord**
Newborn affected by entanglement of umbilical cord
Newborn affected by knot in umbilical cord
Newborn affected by umbilical cord (tightly) around neck
**AHA:** 2026,2Q,13; 2022,1Q,22

✓5th **P02.6 Newborn affected by other and unspecified conditions of umbilical cord**

**P02.60 Newborn affected by unspecified conditions of umbilical cord**

**P02.69 Newborn affected by other conditions of umbilical cord**
Newborn affected by short umbilical cord
Newborn affected by vasa previa
EXCLUDES 1 *newborn affected by single umbilical artery (Q27.0)*

✓5th **P02.7 Newborn affected by chorioamnionitis**
**AHA:** 2018,4Q,23-24
**DEF:** Inflammation of the fetal membranes due to maternal infection characterized by fetal tachycardia, respiratory distress, apnea, weak cries, and poor sucking.

**P02.70 Newborn affected by fetal inflammatory response syndrome** HCC ESR COM
Newborn affected by FIRS

**P02.78 Newborn affected by other conditions from chorioamnionitis**
Newborn affected by amnionitis
Newborn affected by membranitis
Newborn affected by placentitis

**P02.8 Newborn affected by other abnormalities of membranes**

**P02.9 Newborn affected by abnormality of membranes, unspecified**

✓4th **P03 Newborn affected by other complications of labor and delivery**
Code first any current condition in newborn
EXCLUDES 2 *encounter for observation of newborn for suspected diseases and conditions ruled out (Z05.-)*

**P03.0 Newborn affected by breech delivery and extraction**

**P03.1 Newborn affected by other malpresentation, malposition and disproportion during labor and delivery**
Newborn affected by transverse lie
Newborn affected by conditions classifiable to O64-O66
Newborn affected by contracted pelvis
Newborn affected by persistent occipitoposterior

**P03.2 Newborn affected by forceps delivery**

**Forceps-Assisted Birth**

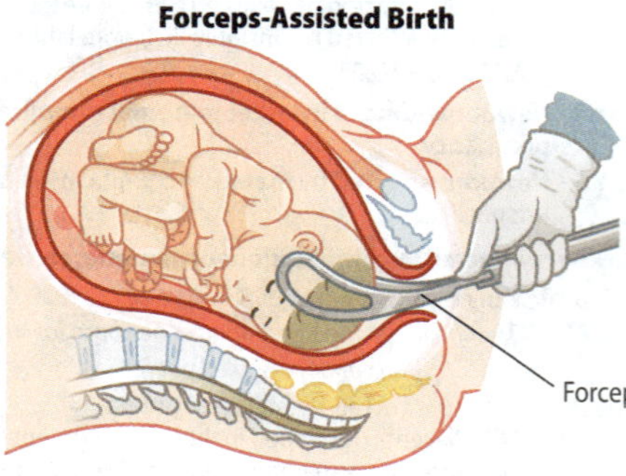


**P03.3 Newborn affected by delivery by vacuum extractor [ventouse]**

**Vacuum-Assisted Birth**

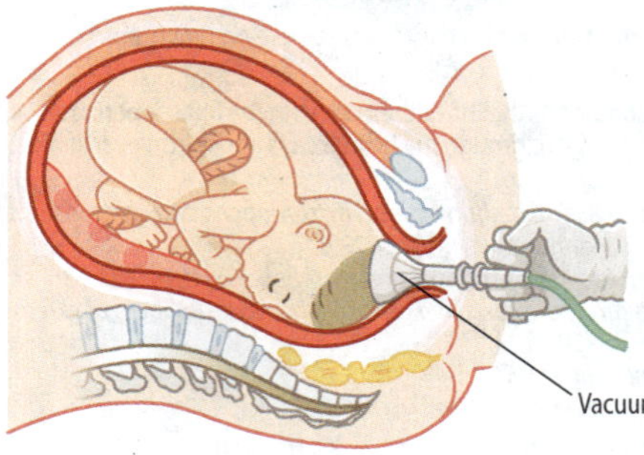


**P03.4 Newborn affected by Cesarean delivery**

**P03.5 Newborn affected by precipitate delivery**
Newborn affected by rapid second stage

**P03.6 Newborn affected by abnormal uterine contractions**
Newborn affected by conditions classifiable to O62.-, except O62.3
Newborn affected by hypertonic labor
Newborn affected by uterine inertia

✓5th **P03.8 Newborn affected by other specified complications of labor and delivery**

✓6th **P03.81 Newborn affected by abnormality in fetal (intrauterine) heart rate or rhythm**
EXCLUDES 1 *neonatal cardiac dysrhythmia (P29.1-)*

**P03.810 Newborn affected by abnormality in fetal (intrauterine) heart rate or rhythm before the onset of labor**

**P03.811 Newborn affected by abnormality in fetal (intrauterine) heart rate or rhythm during labor**

**P03.819 Newborn affected by abnormality in fetal (intrauterine) heart rate or rhythm, unspecified as to time of onset**

**P03.82 Meconium passage during delivery**
EXCLUDES 1 *meconium aspiration (P24.00, P24.01)*
*meconium staining (P96.83)*
**DEF:** Fetal intestinal activity that increases in response to a fetomaternal distressed state during delivery. The anal sphincter relaxes and meconium is passed into the amniotic fluid.

**P03.89 Newborn affected by other specified complications of labor and delivery**
Newborn affected by abnormality of maternal soft tissues
Newborn affected by conditions classifiable to O60-O75 and by procedures used in labor and delivery not included in P02.- and P03.0-P03.6
Newborn affected by induction of labor

**P03.9 Newborn affected by complication of labor and delivery, unspecified**

✓4th **P04 Newborn affected by noxious substances transmitted via placenta or breast milk**
INCLUDES nonteratogenic effects of substances transmitted via placenta
Code first any current condition in newborn, if applicable
EXCLUDES 2 *congenital malformations (Q00-Q99)*
*encounter for observation of newborn for suspected diseases and conditions ruled out (Z05.-)*
*neonatal jaundice from excessive hemolysis due to drugs or toxins transmitted from mother (P58.4)*
*newborn in contact with and (suspected) exposures hazardous to health not transmitted via placenta or breast milk (Z77.-)*

**P04.0 Newborn affected by maternal anesthesia and analgesia in pregnancy, labor and delivery** HCC COM
Newborn affected by reactions and intoxications from maternal opiates and tranquilizers administered for procedures during pregnancy or labor and delivery
EXCLUDES 2 *newborn affected by other maternal medication (P04.1-)*

**P04.1 Newborn affected by other maternal medication**

Code first, if applicable, withdrawal symptoms from maternal use of drugs of addiction (P96.1)

withdrawal symptoms from therapeutic use of drugs in newborn (P96.2)

EXCLUDES 1 *dysmorphism due to warfarin (Q86.2)*
*fetal hydantoin syndrome (Q86.1)*

EXCLUDES 2 *maternal anesthesia and analgesia in pregnancy, labor and delivery (P04.0)*
*maternal use of drugs of addiction (P04.4-)*

AHA: 2018,4Q,24-25

**P04.11 Newborn affected by maternal antineoplastic chemotherapy** HCC COM

**P04.12 Newborn affected by maternal cytotoxic drugs** HCC COM

**P04.13 Newborn affected by maternal use of anticonvulsants** HCC COM

**P04.14 Newborn affected by maternal use of opiates** HCC COM

**P04.15 Newborn affected by maternal use of antidepressants** HCC COM

**P04.16 Newborn affected by maternal use of amphetamines** HCC COM

**P04.17 Newborn affected by maternal use of sedative-hypnotics** HCC COM

**P04.1A Newborn affected by maternal use of anxiolytics** HCC COM

**P04.18 Newborn affected by other maternal medication** HCC COM

**P04.19 Newborn affected by maternal use of unspecified medication** HCC COM

**P04.2 Newborn affected by maternal use of tobacco** HCC COM

Newborn affected by exposure in utero to tobacco smoke

EXCLUDES 2 *newborn exposure to environmental tobacco smoke (P96.81)*

**P04.3 Newborn affected by maternal use of alcohol** HCC COM

EXCLUDES 1 *fetal alcohol syndrome (Q86.0)*

**P04.4 Newborn affected by maternal use of drugs of addiction**

AHA: 2018,4Q,25

**P04.40 Newborn affected by maternal use of unspecified drugs of addiction** HCC COM

**P04.41 Newborn affected by maternal use of cocaine** HCC COM

**P04.42 Newborn affected by maternal use of hallucinogens** HCC COM

EXCLUDES 2 *newborn affected by other maternal medication (P04.1-)*

**P04.49 Newborn affected by maternal use of other drugs of addiction** HCC COM

EXCLUDES 2 *newborn affected by maternal anesthesia and analgesia (P04.0)*
*withdrawal symptoms from maternal use of drugs of addiction (P96.1)*

**P04.5 Newborn affected by maternal use of nutritional chemical substances** HCC COM

**P04.6 Newborn affected by maternal exposure to environmental chemical substances** HCC COM

**P04.8 Newborn affected by other maternal noxious substances**

AHA: 2018,4Q,25

**P04.81 Newborn affected by maternal use of cannabis** HCC COM

**P04.89 Newborn affected by other maternal noxious substances** HCC COM

**P04.9 Newborn affected by maternal noxious substance, unspecified** HCC COM

## Disorders of newborn related to length of gestation and fetal growth (P05-P08)

**P05 Disorders of newborn related to slow fetal growth and fetal malnutrition**

AHA: 2016,4Q,55-56

**P05.0 Newborn light for gestational age**

Newborn light-for-dates

Weight below but length above 10th percentile for gestational age

**P05.00 Newborn light for gestational age, unspecified weight** COM

**P05.01 Newborn light for gestational age, less than 500 grams** COM

**P05.02 Newborn light for gestational age, 500-749 grams** COM

**P05.03 Newborn light for gestational age, 750-999 grams** COM

**P05.04 Newborn light for gestational age, 1000-1249 grams** COM

**P05.05 Newborn light for gestational age, 1250-1499 grams** COM

**P05.06 Newborn light for gestational age, 1500-1749 grams** COM

**P05.07 Newborn light for gestational age, 1750-1999 grams** COM

**P05.08 Newborn light for gestational age, 2000-2499 grams** COM

**P05.09 Newborn light for gestational age, 2500 grams and over** COM

Newborn light for gestational age, other

**P05.1 Newborn small for gestational age**

Newborn small-and-light-for-dates

Newborn small-for-dates

Weight and length below 10th percentile for gestational age

**P05.10 Newborn small for gestational age, unspecified weight** COM

**P05.11 Newborn small for gestational age, less than 500 grams** COM

**P05.12 Newborn small for gestational age, 500-749 grams** COM

**P05.13 Newborn small for gestational age, 750-999 grams** COM

**P05.14 Newborn small for gestational age, 1000-1249 grams** COM

**P05.15 Newborn small for gestational age, 1250-1499 grams** COM

**P05.16 Newborn small for gestational age, 1500-1749 grams** COM

**P05.17 Newborn small for gestational age, 1750-1999 grams** COM

**P05.18 Newborn small for gestational age, 2000-2499 grams** COM

**P05.19 Newborn small for gestational age, other** COM

Newborn small for gestational age, 2500 grams and over

**P05.2 Newborn affected by fetal (intrauterine) malnutrition not light or small for gestational age** COM

Infant, not light or small for gestational age, showing signs of fetal malnutrition, such as dry, peeling skin and loss of subcutaneous tissue

EXCLUDES 1 *newborn affected by fetal malnutrition with light for gestational age (P05.0-)*
*newborn affected by fetal malnutrition with small for gestational age (P05.1-)*

**P05.9 Newborn affected by slow intrauterine growth, unspecified** COM

Newborn affected by fetal growth retardation NOS

**P07 Disorders of newborn related to short gestation and low birth weight, not elsewhere classified**

NOTE When both birth weight and gestational age of the newborn are available, both should be coded with birth weight sequenced before gestational age

INCLUDES the listed conditions, without further specification, as the cause of morbidity or additional care, in newborn

**P07.0 Extremely low birth weight newborn**

Newborn birth weight 999 g. or less

EXCLUDES 1 *low birth weight due to slow fetal growth and fetal malnutrition (P05.-)*

**P07.00 Extremely low birth weight newborn, unspecified weight** COM

**P07.01 Extremely low birth weight newborn, less than 500 grams** COM

**P07.02 Extremely low birth weight newborn, 500-749 grams** COM

**P07.03 Extremely low birth weight newborn, 750-999 grams** COM

**P07.1 Other low birth weight newborn**
Newborn birth weight 1000-2499 g.
EXCLUDES 1 *low birth weight due to slow fetal growth and fetal malnutrition (P05.-)*

**P07.10 Other low birth weight newborn, unspecified weight** COM
**P07.14 Other low birth weight newborn, 1000-1249 grams** COM
**P07.15 Other low birth weight newborn, 1250-1499 grams** COM
**P07.16 Other low birth weight newborn, 1500-1749 grams** COM
**P07.17 Other low birth weight newborn, 1750-1999 grams** COM
**P07.18 Other low birth weight newborn, 2000-2499 grams** COM

**P07.2 Extreme immaturity of newborn**
Less than 28 completed weeks (less than 196 completed days) of gestation.

**P07.20 Extreme immaturity of newborn, unspecified weeks of gestation** COM
Gestational age less than 28 completed weeks NOS
**P07.21 Extreme immaturity of newborn, gestational age less than 23 completed weeks** COM
Extreme immaturity of newborn, gestational age less than 23 weeks, 0 days
**P07.22 Extreme immaturity of newborn, gestational age 23 completed weeks** COM
Extreme immaturity of newborn, gestational age 23 weeks, 0 days through 23 weeks, 6 days
**P07.23 Extreme immaturity of newborn, gestational age 24 completed weeks** COM
Extreme immaturity of newborn, gestational age 24 weeks, 0 days through 24 weeks, 6 days
**P07.24 Extreme immaturity of newborn, gestational age 25 completed weeks** COM
Extreme immaturity of newborn, gestational age 25 weeks, 0 days through 25 weeks, 6 days
**P07.25 Extreme immaturity of newborn, gestational age 26 completed weeks** COM
Extreme immaturity of newborn, gestational age 26 weeks, 0 days through 26 weeks, 6 days
**P07.26 Extreme immaturity of newborn, gestational age 27 completed weeks** COM
Extreme immaturity of newborn, gestational age 27 weeks, 0 days through 27 weeks, 6 days

**P07.3 Preterm [premature] newborn [other]**
28 completed weeks or more but less than 37 completed weeks (196 completed days but less than 259 completed days) of gestation
Prematurity NOS
**AHA:** 2017,3Q,26

**P07.30 Preterm newborn, unspecified weeks of gestation** COM
**P07.31 Preterm newborn, gestational age 28 completed weeks** COM
Preterm newborn, gestational age 28 weeks, 0 days through 28 weeks, 6 days
**P07.32 Preterm newborn, gestational age 29 completed weeks** COM
Preterm newborn, gestational age 29 weeks, 0 days through 29 weeks, 6 days
**P07.33 Preterm newborn, gestational age 30 completed weeks** COM
Preterm newborn, gestational age 30 weeks, 0 days through 30 weeks, 6 days
**P07.34 Preterm newborn, gestational age 31 completed weeks** COM
Preterm newborn, gestational age 31 weeks, 0 days through 31 weeks, 6 days
**P07.35 Preterm newborn, gestational age 32 completed weeks** COM
Preterm newborn, gestational age 32 weeks, 0 days through 32 weeks, 6 days
**P07.36 Preterm newborn, gestational age 33 completed weeks** COM
Preterm newborn, gestational age 33 weeks, 0 days through 33 weeks, 6 days
**P07.37 Preterm newborn, gestational age 34 completed weeks** COM
Preterm newborn, gestational age 34 weeks, 0 days through 34 weeks, 6 days
**P07.38 Preterm newborn, gestational age 35 completed weeks** COM
Preterm newborn, gestational age 35 weeks, 0 days through 35 weeks, 6 days
**P07.39 Preterm newborn, gestational age 36 completed weeks** COM
Preterm newborn, gestational age 36 weeks, 0 days through 36 weeks, 6 days

**P08 Disorders of newborn related to long gestation and high birth weight**
NOTE When both birth weight and gestational age of the newborn are available, priority of assignment should be given to birth weight
INCLUDES the listed conditions, without further specification, as causes of morbidity or additional care, in newborn

**P08.0 Exceptionally large newborn baby** COM
Usually implies a birth weight of 4500 g. or more
EXCLUDES 1 *syndrome of infant of diabetic mother (P70.1)*
*syndrome of infant of mother with gestational diabetes (P70.0)*

**P08.1 Other heavy for gestational age newborn** COM
Other newborn heavy- or large-for-dates regardless of period of gestation
Usually implies a birth weight of 4000 g. to 4499 g.
EXCLUDES 1 *newborn with a birth weight of 4500 or more (P08.0)*
*syndrome of infant of diabetic mother (P70.1)*
*syndrome of infant of mother with gestational diabetes (P70.0)*

**P08.2 Late newborn, not heavy for gestational age**
**AHA:** 2014,1Q,14

**P08.21 Post-term newborn** COM
Newborn with gestation period over 40 completed weeks to 42 completed weeks
**P08.22 Prolonged gestation of newborn** COM
Newborn with gestation period over 42 completed weeks (294 days or more), not heavy- or large-for-dates.
Postmaturity NOS

## Abnormal findings on neonatal screening (P09)

**P09 Abnormal findings on neonatal screening**
INCLUDES abnormal findings on state mandated newborn screens
failed newborn screening
EXCLUDES 2 *nonspecific serologic evidence of human immunodeficiency virus [HIV] (R75)*
**AHA:** 2021,4Q,24

**P09.1 Abnormal findings on neonatal screening for inborn errors of metabolism**
**P09.2 Abnormal findings on neonatal screening for congenital endocrine disease**
Abnormal findings on neonatal screening for congenital adrenal hyperplasia
Abnormal findings on neonatal screening for hypothyroidism screen
**P09.3 Abnormal findings on neonatal screening for congenital hematologic disorders**
Abnormal findings for hemoglobinopathy screening
Abnormal findings on red cell membrane defects screen
Abnormal findings on sickle cell screen
**P09.4 Abnormal findings on neonatal screening for cystic fibrosis**
**P09.5 Abnormal findings on neonatal screening for critical congenital heart disease**
Neonatal congenital heart disease screening failure
**P09.6 Abnormal findings on neonatal hearing screening**
EXCLUDES 2 *encounter for hearing examination following failed hearing screening (Z01.110)*
**P09.8 Other abnormal findings on neonatal screening**
**P09.9 Abnormal findings on neonatal screening, unspecified**

## Birth trauma (P10-P15)

✓4th **P10 Intracranial laceration and hemorrhage due to birth injury**
EXCLUDES 1 *intracranial hemorrhage of newborn NOS (P52.9)*
*intracranial hemorrhage of newborn due to anoxia or hypoxia (P52.-)*
*nontraumatic intracranial hemorrhage of newborn (P52.-)*

**P10.0 Subdural hemorrhage due to birth injury** HCC COM
Subdural hematoma (localized) due to birth injury
EXCLUDES 1 *subdural hemorrhage accompanying tentorial tear (P10.4)*

**P10.1 Cerebral hemorrhage due to birth injury** HCC COM

**P10.2 Intraventricular hemorrhage due to birth injury** HCC COM

**P10.3 Subarachnoid hemorrhage due to birth injury** HCC COM

**P10.4 Tentorial tear due to birth injury** HCC COM

**P10.8 Other intracranial lacerations and hemorrhages due to birth injury** HCC COM

**P10.9 Unspecified intracranial laceration and hemorrhage due to birth injury** HCC COM

✓4th **P11 Other birth injuries to central nervous system**

**P11.0 Cerebral edema due to birth injury** HCC COM

**P11.1 Other specified brain damage due to birth injury** HCC COM

**P11.2 Unspecified brain damage due to birth injury** HCC COM

**P11.3 Birth injury to facial nerve**
Facial palsy due to birth injury

**P11.4 Birth injury to other cranial nerves**

**P11.5 Birth injury to spine and spinal cord** HCC COM
Fracture of spine due to birth injury

**P11.9 Birth injury to central nervous system, unspecified**

✓4th **P12 Birth injury to scalp**

**Birth Injuries to Scalp**

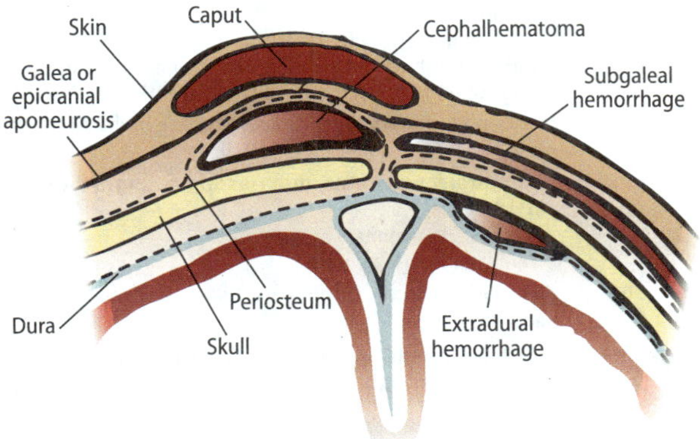


**P12.0 Cephalhematoma due to birth injury**
**DEF:** Condition that occurs in a neonate when blood vessels between the skull and periosteum rupture and blood collects in the subperiosteal space (below the periosteum). It is typically caused by prolonged labor or trauma due to instrument-assisted delivery (e.g., forceps, vacuum extraction), although in rare circumstances, it may indicate a linear skull fracture with intracranial hemorrhage.

**P12.1 Chignon (from vacuum extraction) due to birth injury**
**DEF:** Artificial swelling of the scalp that occurs when a collection of interstitial fluid and blood forms in the area of the scalp where the suction cup was applied during a vacuum-assisted delivery.

**P12.2 Epicranial subaponeurotic hemorrhage due to birth injury** HCC
Subgaleal hemorrhage

**P12.3 Bruising of scalp due to birth injury**

**P12.4 Injury of scalp of newborn due to monitoring equipment**
Sampling incision of scalp of newborn
Scalp clip (electrode) injury of newborn

✓5th **P12.8 Other birth injuries to scalp**

**P12.81 Caput succedaneum**
**DEF:** Swelling of the scalp as a result of pressure being exerted on the head from the vaginal walls, uterus, or instrumentation used in assisting a delivery (e.g., vacuum).

**P12.89 Other birth injuries to scalp**

**P12.9 Birth injury to scalp, unspecified**

✓4th **P13 Birth injury to skeleton**
EXCLUDES 2 *birth injury to spine (P11.5)*

**P13.0 Fracture of skull due to birth injury**

**P13.1 Other birth injuries to skull**
EXCLUDES 1 *cephalhematoma (P12.0)*

**P13.2 Birth injury to femur**

**P13.3 Birth injury to other long bones**

**P13.4 Fracture of clavicle due to birth injury**

**P13.8 Birth injuries to other parts of skeleton**

**P13.9 Birth injury to skeleton, unspecified**

✓4th **P14 Birth injury to peripheral nervous system**

**P14.0 Erb's paralysis due to birth injury**
**DEF:** Erb's paralysis: Most common type of brachial plexus (peripheral nerve) injury in a neonate that involves nerve damage at the level of C5-C6. ***Synonym(s):*** *Erb's palsy*

**P14.1 Klumpke's paralysis due to birth injury**

**P14.2 Phrenic nerve paralysis due to birth injury**

**P14.3 Other brachial plexus birth injuries**

**P14.8 Birth injuries to other parts of peripheral nervous system**

**P14.9 Birth injury to peripheral nervous system, unspecified**

✓4th **P15 Other birth injuries**

**P15.0 Birth injury to liver**
Rupture of liver due to birth injury

**P15.1 Birth injury to spleen**
Rupture of spleen due to birth injury

**P15.2 Sternomastoid injury due to birth injury**

**P15.3 Birth injury to eye**
Subconjunctival hemorrhage due to birth injury
Traumatic glaucoma due to birth injury

**P15.4 Birth injury to face**
Facial congestion due to birth injury

**P15.5 Birth injury to external genitalia**

**P15.6 Subcutaneous fat necrosis due to birth injury**

**P15.8 Other specified birth injuries**

**P15.9 Birth injury, unspecified**

## Respiratory and cardiovascular disorders specific to the perinatal period (P19-P29)

✓4th **P19 Metabolic acidemia in newborn**
INCLUDES metabolic acidemia in newborn

**P19.0 Metabolic acidemia in newborn first noted before onset of labor**

**P19.1 Metabolic acidemia in newborn first noted during labor**

**P19.2 Metabolic acidemia noted at birth**

**P19.9 Metabolic acidemia in newborn, unspecified**

✓4th **P22 Respiratory distress of newborn**
**AHA:** 2019,2Q,29

**P22.0 Respiratory distress syndrome of newborn** HCC COM
Cardiorespiratory distress syndrome of newborn
Hyaline membrane disease
Idiopathic respiratory distress syndrome [IRDS or RDS] of newborn
Pulmonary hypoperfusion syndrome
Respiratory distress syndrome, type I
EXCLUDES 2 *respiratory arrest of newborn (P28.81)*
*respiratory failure of newborn NOS (P28.5)*
**AHA:** 2019,2Q,29
**DEF:** Severe chest contractions upon air intake and expiratory grunting. The infant appears blue due to oxygen deficiency and has a rapid respiratory rate, formerly called hyaline membrane disease.

**P22.1 Transient tachypnea of newborn**
Idiopathic tachypnea of newborn
Respiratory distress syndrome, type II
Wet lung syndrome
**DEF:** Rapid, labored breathing of a newborn. It is a short-term problem that begins after birth and lasts about three days.

**P22.8 Other respiratory distress of newborn**
EXCLUDES 1 *respiratory arrest of newborn (P28.81)*
*respiratory failure of newborn NOS (P28.5)*

**P22.9 Respiratory distress of newborn, unspecified**
EXCLUDES 1 *respiratory arrest of newborn (P28.81)*
*respiratory failure of newborn NOS (P28.5)*

**✓4th P23 Congenital pneumonia**

INCLUDES infective pneumonia acquired in utero or during birth

EXCLUDES 1 *neonatal pneumonia resulting from aspiration (P24.-)*

**P23.Ø Congenital pneumonia due to viral agent** COM
Use additional code (B97) to identify organism
EXCLUDES 1 *congenital rubella pneumonitis (P35.Ø)*

**P23.1 Congenital pneumonia due to Chlamydia** COM

**P23.2 Congenital pneumonia due to staphylococcus** COM

**P23.3 Congenital pneumonia due to streptococcus, group B** COM

**P23.4 Congenital pneumonia due to Escherichia coli** COM

**P23.5 Congenital pneumonia due to Pseudomonas** COM

**P23.6 Congenital pneumonia due to other bacterial agents** COM
Congenital pneumonia due to Hemophilus influenzae
Congenital pneumonia due to Klebsiella pneumoniae
Congenital pneumonia due to Mycoplasma
Congenital pneumonia due to Streptococcus, except group B
Use additional code (B95-B96) to identify organism

**P23.8 Congenital pneumonia due to other organisms** COM

**P23.9 Congenital pneumonia, unspecified** COM

**✓4th P24 Neonatal aspiration**

INCLUDES aspiration in utero and during delivery

**✓5th P24.Ø Meconium aspiration**
EXCLUDES 1 *meconium passage (without aspiration) during delivery (PØ3.82)*
*meconium staining (P96.83)*
**DEF:** Meconium in the trachea or seen on chest x-ray after birth.

**P24.ØØ Meconium aspiration without respiratory symptoms**
Meconium aspiration NOS

**P24.Ø1 Meconium aspiration with respiratory symptoms** COM
Meconium aspiration pneumonia
Meconium aspiration pneumonitis
Meconium aspiration syndrome NOS
Use additional code to identify any secondary pulmonary hypertension, if applicable (I27.2-)
**DEF:** Aspiration of fetal intestinal material during or prior to delivery. It is usually a complication of placental insufficiency, causing pneumonitis and bronchial obstruction (inflammatory reaction of lungs).

**✓5th P24.1 Neonatal aspiration of (clear) amniotic fluid and mucus**
Neonatal aspiration of liquor (amnii)

**P24.1Ø Neonatal aspiration of (clear) amniotic fluid and mucus without respiratory symptoms**
Neonatal aspiration of amniotic fluid and mucus NOS

**P24.11 Neonatal aspiration of (clear) amniotic fluid and mucus with respiratory symptoms** COM
Neonatal aspiration of amniotic fluid and mucus with pneumonia
Neonatal aspiration of amniotic fluid and mucus with pneumonitis
Use additional code to identify any secondary pulmonary hypertension, if applicable (I27.2-)

**✓5th P24.2 Neonatal aspiration of blood**

**P24.2Ø Neonatal aspiration of blood without respiratory symptoms**
Neonatal aspiration of blood NOS

**P24.21 Neonatal aspiration of blood with respiratory symptoms** COM
Neonatal aspiration of blood with pneumonia
Neonatal aspiration of blood with pneumonitis
Use additional code to identify any secondary pulmonary hypertension, if applicable (I27.2-)

**✓5th P24.3 Neonatal aspiration of milk and regurgitated food**
Neonatal aspiration of stomach contents

**P24.3Ø Neonatal aspiration of milk and regurgitated food without respiratory symptoms**
Neonatal aspiration of milk and regurgitated food NOS

**P24.31 Neonatal aspiration of milk and regurgitated food with respiratory symptoms** COM
Neonatal aspiration of milk and regurgitated food with pneumonia
Neonatal aspiration of milk and regurgitated food with pneumonitis
Use additional code to identify any secondary pulmonary hypertension, if applicable (I27.2-)

**✓5th P24.8 Other neonatal aspiration**

**P24.8Ø Other neonatal aspiration without respiratory symptoms**
Neonatal aspiration NEC

**P24.81 Other neonatal aspiration with respiratory symptoms** COM
Neonatal aspiration pneumonia NEC
Neonatal aspiration with pneumonia NOS
Neonatal aspiration with pneumonitis NEC
Neonatal aspiration with pneumonitis NOS
Use additional code to identify any secondary pulmonary hypertension, if applicable (I27.2-)

**P24.9 Neonatal aspiration, unspecified**

**✓4th P25 Interstitial emphysema and related conditions originating in the perinatal period**

**P25.Ø Interstitial emphysema originating in the perinatal period**

**P25.1 Pneumothorax originating in the perinatal period**

**P25.2 Pneumomediastinum originating in the perinatal period**

**P25.3 Pneumopericardium originating in the perinatal period**

**P25.8 Other conditions related to interstitial emphysema originating in the perinatal period**

**✓4th P26 Pulmonary hemorrhage originating in the perinatal period**

EXCLUDES 1 *acute idiopathic hemorrhage in infants over 28 days old (RØ4.81)*

**P26.Ø Tracheobronchial hemorrhage originating in the perinatal period** HCC COM

**P26.1 Massive pulmonary hemorrhage originating in the perinatal period** HCC COM

**P26.8 Other pulmonary hemorrhages originating in the perinatal period** HCC COM

**P26.9 Unspecified pulmonary hemorrhage originating in the perinatal period** HCC COM

**✓4th P27 Chronic respiratory disease originating in the perinatal period**

EXCLUDES 2 *respiratory distress of newborn (P22.Ø-P22.9)*

**P27.Ø Wilson-Mikity syndrome** HCC COM
Pulmonary dysmaturity
**DEF:** Pulmonary insufficiency in newborn babies, especially those with low birth weight. Rapid onset of hypercapnia and cyanosis occur during the first month of life frequently resulting in death.

**P27.1 Bronchopulmonary dysplasia originating in the perinatal period** HCC COM

**P27.8 Other chronic respiratory diseases originating in the perinatal period** HCC COM
Congenital pulmonary fibrosis
Ventilator lung in newborn

**P27.9 Unspecified chronic respiratory disease originating in the perinatal period** HCC COM

**✓4th P28 Other respiratory conditions originating in the perinatal period**

Code also, if applicable, congenital malformations of the respiratory system (Q3Ø-Q34)

**P28.Ø Primary atelectasis of newborn** HCC COM
Primary failure to expand terminal respiratory units
Pulmonary hypoplasia associated with short gestation
Pulmonary immaturity NOS

**✓5th P28.1 Other and unspecified atelectasis of newborn**

**P28.1Ø Unspecified atelectasis of newborn** HCC COM
Atelectasis of newborn NOS

**P28.11 Resorption atelectasis without respiratory distress syndrome** HCC COM
EXCLUDES 1 *resorption atelectasis with respiratory distress syndrome (P22.Ø)*

**P28.19 Other atelectasis of newborn** HCC COM
Partial atelectasis of newborn
Secondary atelectasis of newborn

**P28.2 Cyanotic attacks of newborn**
EXCLUDES 1 *apnea of newborn (P28.3- - P28.4-)*

**✓5th P28.3 Primary sleep apnea of newborn**
Sleep apnea of newborn NOS
EXCLUDES 2 *other apnea of newborn (P28.4-)*
**AHA:** 2022,4Q,38-39
**DEF:** Unexplained cessation of breathing when a neonate makes no respiratory effort for 20 seconds or longer or when a neonate's breathing cessation is accompanied by cyanosis, bradycardia, or hypotonia.

**P28.3Ø Primary sleep apnea of newborn, unspecified**
Transient oxygen desaturation spells of newborn during sleep

**P28.31 Primary central sleep apnea of newborn**

P28.32 **Primary obstructive sleep apnea of newborn**
P28.33 **Primary mixed sleep apnea of newborn**
P28.39 **Other primary sleep apnea of newborn**

√5th P28.4 **Other apnea of newborn**
EXCLUDES 2 *primary sleep apnea of newborn (P28.3-)*
**AHA:** 2022,4Q,38-39

P28.40 **Unspecified apnea of newborn**
Apnea of newborn, NOS
Transient oxygen desaturation spells of newborn
P28.41 **Central neonatal apnea of newborn**
P28.42 **Obstructive apnea of newborn**
P28.43 **Mixed neonatal apnea of newborn**
P28.49 **Other apnea of newborn**
Apnea of prematurity

P28.5 **Respiratory failure of newborn** HCC COM
EXCLUDES 2 *respiratory arrest of newborn (P28.81)*
*respiratory distress of newborn (P22.Ø)*
**AHA:** 2026,2Q,13; 2019,2Q,29

√5th P28.8 **Other specified respiratory conditions of newborn**
P28.81 **Respiratory arrest of newborn** HCC COM
P28.89 **Other specified respiratory conditions of newborn**
Congenital laryngeal stridor
Sniffles in newborn
Snuffles in newborn
EXCLUDES 1 *early congenital syphilitic rhinitis (A5Ø.Ø5)*

P28.9 **Respiratory condition of newborn, unspecified**
Respiratory depression in newborn
**AHA:** 2026,2Q,13

√4th **P29 Cardiovascular disorders originating in the perinatal period**
EXCLUDES 2 *congenital malformations of the circulatory system (Q2Ø-Q28)*

P29.Ø **Neonatal cardiac failure** HCC COM
Code also associated underlying condition

√5th P29.1 **Neonatal cardiac dysrhythmia**
P29.11 **Neonatal tachycardia**
P29.12 **Neonatal bradycardia**

P29.2 **Neonatal hypertension**

√5th P29.3 **Persistent fetal circulation**
**AHA:** 2017,4Q,20-21
P29.3Ø **Pulmonary hypertension of newborn** COM
Persistent pulmonary hypertension of newborn
**DEF:** Condition that occurs when pressure within the pulmonary artery is elevated and vascular resistance is observed in the lungs.
P29.38 **Other persistent fetal circulation** COM
Delayed closure of ductus arteriosus

P29.4 **Transient myocardial ischemia in newborn**

√5th P29.8 **Other cardiovascular disorders originating in the perinatal period**
P29.81 **Cardiac arrest of newborn** HCC COM
P29.89 **Other cardiovascular disorders originating in the perinatal period**
**AHA:** 2014,4Q,23

P29.9 **Cardiovascular disorder originating in the perinatal period, unspecified**

## Infections specific to the perinatal period (P35-P39)

Infections acquired in utero, during birth via the umbilicus, or during the first 28 days after birth

EXCLUDES 2 *asymptomatic human immunodeficiency virus [HIV] infection status (Z21)*
*congenital gonococcal infection (A54.-)*
*congenital pneumonia (P23.-)*
*congenital syphilis (A5Ø.-)*
*human immunodeficiency virus [HIV] disease (B2Ø)*
*infant botulism (A48.51)*
*infectious diseases not specific to the perinatal period (AØØ-B99, JØ9, J1Ø.-)*
*intestinal infectious disease (AØØ-AØ9)*
*laboratory evidence of human immunodeficiency virus [HIV] (R75)*
*tetanus neonatorum (A33)*

√4th **P35 Congenital viral diseases**
INCLUDES infections acquired in utero or during birth

P35.Ø **Congenital rubella syndrome**
Congenital rubella pneumonitis
P35.1 **Congenital cytomegalovirus infection** COM
P35.2 **Congenital herpesviral [herpes simplex] infection**
P35.3 **Congenital viral hepatitis**
P35.4 **Congenital Zika virus disease**
Use additional code to identify manifestations of congenital Zika virus disease
**AHA:** 2018,4Q,25-26
P35.8 **Other congenital viral diseases**
Congenital varicella [chickenpox]
**AHA:** 2020,2Q,13
P35.9 **Congenital viral disease, unspecified**

√4th **P36 Bacterial sepsis of newborn**
INCLUDES congenital sepsis
Use additional code(s), if applicable, to identify severe sepsis (R65.2-) and associated acute organ dysfunction(s)

P36.Ø **Sepsis of newborn due to streptococcus, group B** HCC ESR COM

√5th P36.1 **Sepsis of newborn due to other and unspecified streptococci**
P36.1Ø **Sepsis of newborn due to unspecified streptococci** HCC ESR COM
P36.19 **Sepsis of newborn due to other streptococci** HCC ESR COM

P36.2 **Sepsis of newborn due to Staphylococcus aureus** HCC ESR COM

√5th P36.3 **Sepsis of newborn due to other and unspecified staphylococci**
P36.3Ø **Sepsis of newborn due to unspecified staphylococci** HCC ESR COM
P36.39 **Sepsis of newborn due to other staphylococci** HCC ESR COM

P36.4 **Sepsis of newborn due to Escherichia coli** HCC ESR COM
P36.5 **Sepsis of newborn due to anaerobes** HCC ESR COM
P36.8 **Other bacterial sepsis of newborn** HCC ESR COM
Use additional code from category B96 to identify organism
P36.9 **Bacterial sepsis of newborn, unspecified** HCC ESR COM

√4th **P37 Other congenital infectious and parasitic diseases**
EXCLUDES 2 *congenital syphilis (A5Ø.-)*
*infectious neonatal diarrhea (AØØ-AØ9)*
*necrotizing enterocolitis in newborn (P77.-)*
*noninfectious neonatal diarrhea (P78.3)*
*ophthalmia neonatorum due to gonococcus (A54.31)*
*tetanus neonatorum (A33)*

P37.Ø **Congenital tuberculosis**
P37.1 **Congenital toxoplasmosis**
Hydrocephalus due to congenital toxoplasmosis
P37.2 **Neonatal (disseminated) listeriosis**
P37.3 **Congenital falciparum malaria**
P37.4 **Other congenital malaria**
P37.5 **Neonatal candidiasis**
P37.8 **Other specified congenital infectious and parasitic diseases**
P37.9 **Congenital infectious or parasitic disease, unspecified**

√4th **P38 Omphalitis of newborn**
EXCLUDES 1 *omphalitis not of newborn (LØ8.82)*
*tetanus omphalitis (A33)*
*umbilical hemorrhage of newborn (P51.-)*
**DEF:** Omphalitis: Infection and inflammation of the umbilical stump, often due to bacteria that can spread beyond the umbilical stump to the fascia, muscle, or even the umbilical vessels.

P38.1 **Omphalitis with mild hemorrhage**
P38.9 **Omphalitis without hemorrhage**
Omphalitis of newborn NOS

√4th **P39 Other infections specific to the perinatal period**
Use additional code to identify organism or specific infection

P39.Ø **Neonatal infective mastitis**
EXCLUDES 1 *breast engorgement of newborn (P83.4)*
*noninfective mastitis of newborn (P83.4)*
P39.1 **Neonatal conjunctivitis and dacryocystitis**
Neonatal chlamydial conjunctivitis
Ophthalmia neonatorum NOS
EXCLUDES 1 *gonococcal conjunctivitis (A54.31)*
P39.2 **Intra-amniotic infection affecting newborn, not elsewhere classified**
P39.3 **Neonatal urinary tract infection**
P39.4 **Neonatal skin infection**
Neonatal pyoderma
EXCLUDES 1 *pemphigus neonatorum (LØØ)*
*staphylococcal scalded skin syndrome (LØØ)*
P39.8 **Other specified infections specific to the perinatal period**
P39.9 **Infection specific to the perinatal period, unspecified**

## Hemorrhagic and hematological disorders of newborn (P5Ø-P61)

EXCLUDES 1 *congenital stenosis and stricture of bile ducts (Q44.3)*
*Crigler-Najjar syndrome (E8Ø.5)*
*Dubin-Johnson syndrome (E8Ø.6)*
*Gilbert syndrome (E8Ø.4)*
*hereditary hemolytic anemias (D55-D58)*

✓4th **P5Ø Newborn affected by intrauterine (fetal) blood loss**
EXCLUDES 1 *congenital anemia from intrauterine (fetal) blood loss (P61.3)*
**P5Ø.Ø Newborn affected by intrauterine (fetal) blood loss from vasa previa**
**P5Ø.1 Newborn affected by intrauterine (fetal) blood loss from ruptured cord**
**P5Ø.2 Newborn affected by intrauterine (fetal) blood loss from placenta**
**P5Ø.3 Newborn affected by hemorrhage into co-twin**
**P5Ø.4 Newborn affected by hemorrhage into maternal circulation**
**P5Ø.5 Newborn affected by intrauterine (fetal) blood loss from cut end of co-twin's cord**
**P5Ø.8 Newborn affected by other intrauterine (fetal) blood loss**
**P5Ø.9 Newborn affected by intrauterine (fetal) blood loss, unspecified**
Newborn affected by fetal hemorrhage NOS

✓4th **P51 Umbilical hemorrhage of newborn**
EXCLUDES 1 *omphalitis with mild hemorrhage (P38.1)*
*umbilical hemorrhage from cut end of co-twins cord (P5Ø.5)*
**P51.Ø Massive umbilical hemorrhage of newborn**
**P51.8 Other umbilical hemorrhages of newborn**
Slipped umbilical ligature NOS
**P51.9 Umbilical hemorrhage of newborn, unspecified**

✓4th **P52 Intracranial nontraumatic hemorrhage of newborn**
INCLUDES intracranial hemorrhage due to anoxia or hypoxia
EXCLUDES 1 *intracranial hemorrhage due to birth injury (P1Ø.-)*
*intracranial hemorrhage due to other injury (SØ6.-)*
**P52.Ø Intraventricular (nontraumatic) hemorrhage, grade 1, of newborn** HCC COM
Bleeding into germinal matrix
Subependymal hemorrhage (without intraventricular extension)
**P52.1 Intraventricular (nontraumatic) hemorrhage, grade 2, of newborn** HCC COM
Bleeding into ventricle
Subependymal hemorrhage with intraventricular extension
✓5th **P52.2 Intraventricular (nontraumatic) hemorrhage, grade 3 and grade 4, of newborn**
**P52.21 Intraventricular (nontraumatic) hemorrhage, grade 3, of newborn** HCC COM
Subependymal hemorrhage with intraventricular extension with enlargement of ventricle
**P52.22 Intraventricular (nontraumatic) hemorrhage, grade 4, of newborn** HCC COM
Bleeding into cerebral cortex
Subependymal hemorrhage with intracerebral extension
**P52.3 Unspecified intraventricular (nontraumatic) hemorrhage of newborn** HCC COM
**P52.4 Intracerebral (nontraumatic) hemorrhage of newborn** HCC COM
**P52.5 Subarachnoid (nontraumatic) hemorrhage of newborn** HCC COM
**P52.6 Cerebellar (nontraumatic) and posterior fossa hemorrhage of newborn** HCC COM
**P52.8 Other intracranial (nontraumatic) hemorrhages of newborn** HCC COM
**P52.9 Intracranial (nontraumatic) hemorrhage of newborn, unspecified** HCC COM

**P53 Hemorrhagic disease of newborn** COM
Vitamin K deficiency of newborn

✓4th **P54 Other neonatal hemorrhages**
EXCLUDES 1 *newborn affected by (intrauterine) blood loss (P5Ø.-)*
*pulmonary hemorrhage originating in the perinatal period (P26.-)*
**P54.Ø Neonatal hematemesis**
EXCLUDES 1 *neonatal hematemesis due to swallowed maternal blood (P78.2)*
**P54.1 Neonatal melena**
EXCLUDES 1 *neonatal melena due to swallowed maternal blood (P78.2)*
**P54.2 Neonatal rectal hemorrhage**
**P54.3 Other neonatal gastrointestinal hemorrhage**
**P54.4 Neonatal adrenal hemorrhage**
**P54.5 Neonatal cutaneous hemorrhage**
Neonatal bruising
Neonatal ecchymoses
Neonatal petechiae
Neonatal superficial hematomata
EXCLUDES 2 *bruising of scalp due to birth injury (P12.3)*
*cephalhematoma due to birth injury (P12.Ø)*
**P54.6 Neonatal vaginal hemorrhage**
Neonatal pseudomenses
**P54.8 Other specified neonatal hemorrhages**
**P54.9 Neonatal hemorrhage, unspecified**

✓4th **P55 Hemolytic disease of newborn**
**P55.Ø Rh isoimmunization of newborn** HCC COM
**DEF:** Incompatible Rh fetal-maternal blood grouping that prematurely destroys red blood cells. Symptoms include jaundice, asphyxia, pulmonary hypertension, edema, respiratory distress, kernicterus, and coagulopathies. It is detected by a Coombs test.
**TIP:** A positive Coombs test without documentation of associated Rh isoimmunization should be coded to R79.89 Other specified abnormal findings of blood chemistry.
**P55.1 ABO isoimmunization of newborn** HCC COM
**AHA:** 2015,3Q,20
**P55.8 Other hemolytic diseases of newborn** HCC COM
**AHA:** 2018,3Q,24
**P55.9 Hemolytic disease of newborn, unspecified** HCC COM

✓4th **P56 Hydrops fetalis due to hemolytic disease**
EXCLUDES 1 *hydrops fetalis NOS (P83.2)*
**P56.Ø Hydrops fetalis due to isoimmunization** HCC COM
✓5th **P56.9 Hydrops fetalis due to other and unspecified hemolytic disease**
**P56.90 Hydrops fetalis due to unspecified hemolytic disease** HCC COM
**P56.99 Hydrops fetalis due to other hemolytic disease** HCC COM

✓4th **P57 Kernicterus**
**P57.Ø Kernicterus due to isoimmunization** HCC COM
**DEF:** Complication of erythroblastosis fetalis associated with severe neural symptoms, high blood bilirubin levels, and nerve cell destruction. It results in bilirubin-pigmented gray matter of the central nervous system.
**P57.8 Other specified kernicterus** HCC COM
EXCLUDES 1 *Crigler-Najjar syndrome (E8Ø.5)*
**P57.9 Kernicterus, unspecified** HCC COM

✓4th **P58 Neonatal jaundice due to other excessive hemolysis**
EXCLUDES 1 *jaundice due to isoimmunization (P55-P57)*
**P58.Ø Neonatal jaundice due to bruising**
**P58.1 Neonatal jaundice due to bleeding**
**P58.2 Neonatal jaundice due to infection**
**P58.3 Neonatal jaundice due to polycythemia**
✓5th **P58.4 Neonatal jaundice due to drugs or toxins transmitted from mother or given to newborn**
Code first poisoning due to drug or toxin, if applicable (T36-T65 with fifth or sixth character 1-4)
Use additional code for adverse effect, if applicable, to identify drug (T36-T5Ø with fifth or sixth character 5)
**P58.41 Neonatal jaundice due to drugs or toxins transmitted from mother**
**P58.42 Neonatal jaundice due to drugs or toxins given to newborn**
**P58.5 Neonatal jaundice due to swallowed maternal blood**
**P58.8 Neonatal jaundice due to other specified excessive hemolysis**
**P58.9 Neonatal jaundice due to excessive hemolysis, unspecified**

✓4th **P59 Neonatal jaundice from other and unspecified causes**
EXCLUDES 1 *jaundice due to inborn errors of metabolism (E7Ø-E88)*
*kernicterus (P57.-)*
**P59.Ø Neonatal jaundice associated with preterm delivery**
Hyperbilirubinemia of prematurity
Jaundice due to delayed conjugation associated with preterm delivery
**AHA:** 2025,1Q,24

P59.1 Inspissated bile syndrome COM
DEF: Biliary obstruction in newborn resulting from obstruction of outflow tract.

✓5th P59.2 Neonatal jaundice from other and unspecified hepatocellular damage
EXCLUDES 1 *congenital viral hepatitis (P35.3)*

P59.20 Neonatal jaundice from unspecified hepatocellular damage COM

P59.29 Neonatal jaundice from other hepatocellular damage COM
Neonatal (idiopathic) hepatitis
Neonatal giant cell hepatitis

P59.3 Neonatal jaundice from breast milk inhibitor

P59.8 Neonatal jaundice from other specified causes

P59.9 Neonatal jaundice, unspecified
Neonatal physiological jaundice (intense)(prolonged) NOS
AHA: 2015,3Q,20

P60 Disseminated intravascular coagulation of newborn COM
Defibrination syndrome of newborn

✓4th P61 Other perinatal hematological disorders
EXCLUDES 1 *transient hypogammaglobulinemia of infancy (D80.7)*

P61.0 Transient neonatal thrombocytopenia COM
Neonatal thrombocytopenia due to exchange transfusion
Neonatal thrombocytopenia due to idiopathic maternal thrombocytopenia
Neonatal thrombocytopenia due to isoimmunization
DEF: Temporary decrease in blood platelets of a newborn that is secondary to placental insufficiency.

P61.1 Polycythemia neonatorum
DEF: Abnormal increase of total red blood cells of a newborn that results in hyperviscosity, which slows the flow of blood through small blood vessels.

P61.2 Anemia of prematurity

P61.3 Congenital anemia from fetal blood loss

P61.4 Other congenital anemias, not elsewhere classified
Congenital anemia NOS

P61.5 Transient neonatal neutropenia COM
EXCLUDES 1 *congenital neutropenia (nontransient) (D70.0)*
DEF: Low blood neutrophil counts of newborn that occurs due to maternal hypertension, sepsis, twin-twin transfusion, alloimmunization, and hemolytic disease.

P61.6 Other transient neonatal disorders of coagulation COM

P61.8 Other specified perinatal hematological disorders

P61.9 Perinatal hematological disorder, unspecified

## Transitory endocrine and metabolic disorders specific to newborn (P70-P74)

INCLUDES transitory endocrine and metabolic disturbances caused by the infant's response to maternal endocrine and metabolic factors, or its adjustment to extrauterine environment

AHA: 2018,2Q,6

✓4th P70 Transitory disorders of carbohydrate metabolism specific to newborn

P70.0 Syndrome of infant of mother with gestational diabetes
Newborn (with hypoglycemia) affected by maternal gestational diabetes
EXCLUDES 1 *newborn (with hypoglycemia) affected by maternal (pre-existing) diabetes mellitus (P70.1)*
*syndrome of infant of a diabetic mother (P70.1)*

P70.1 Syndrome of infant of a diabetic mother
Newborn (with hypoglycemia) affected by maternal (pre-existing) diabetes mellitus
EXCLUDES 1 *newborn (with hypoglycemia) affected by maternal gestational diabetes (P70.0)*
*syndrome of infant of mother with gestational diabetes (P70.0)*

P70.2 Neonatal diabetes mellitus

P70.3 Iatrogenic neonatal hypoglycemia

P70.4 Other neonatal hypoglycemia
Transitory neonatal hypoglycemia

P70.8 Other transitory disorders of carbohydrate metabolism of newborn

P70.9 Transitory disorder of carbohydrate metabolism of newborn, unspecified

✓4th P71 Transitory neonatal disorders of calcium and magnesium metabolism

P71.0 Cow's milk hypocalcemia in newborn

P71.1 Other neonatal hypocalcemia
EXCLUDES 1 *neonatal hypoparathyroidism (P71.4)*

P71.2 Neonatal hypomagnesemia

P71.3 Neonatal tetany without calcium or magnesium deficiency
Neonatal tetany NOS

P71.4 Transitory neonatal hypoparathyroidism

P71.8 Other transitory neonatal disorders of calcium and magnesium metabolism
AHA: 2016,4Q,54

P71.9 Transitory neonatal disorder of calcium and magnesium metabolism, unspecified

✓4th P72 Other transitory neonatal endocrine disorders
EXCLUDES 1 *congenital hypothyroidism with or without goiter (E03.0-E03.1)*
*dyshormogenetic goiter (E07.1)*
*dyshormonogenetic goiter (E07.1)*
*Pendred's syndrome (E07.1)*

P72.0 Neonatal goiter, not elsewhere classified
Transitory congenital goiter with normal functioning

P72.1 Transitory neonatal hyperthyroidism
Neonatal thyrotoxicosis

P72.2 Other transitory neonatal disorders of thyroid function, not elsewhere classified
Transitory neonatal hypothyroidism

P72.8 Other specified transitory neonatal endocrine disorders

P72.9 Transitory neonatal endocrine disorder, unspecified

✓4th P74 Other transitory neonatal electrolyte and metabolic disturbances
AHA: 2018,4Q,26-27

P74.0 Late metabolic acidosis of newborn
EXCLUDES 1 *(fetal) metabolic acidosis of newborn (P19)*

P74.1 Dehydration of newborn

✓5th P74.2 Disturbances of sodium balance of newborn

P74.21 Hypernatremia of newborn

P74.22 Hyponatremia of newborn

✓5th P74.3 Disturbances of potassium balance of newborn

P74.31 Hyperkalemia of newborn

P74.32 Hypokalemia of newborn

✓5th P74.4 Other transitory electrolyte disturbances of newborn

P74.41 Alkalosis of newborn
Hyperbicarbonatemia

✓6th P74.42 Disturbances of chlorine balance of newborn

P74.421 Hyperchloremia of newborn
Hyperchloremic metabolic acidosis
EXCLUDES 2 *late metabolic acidosis of the newborn (P74.0)*

P74.422 Hypochloremia of newborn

P74.49 Other transitory electrolyte disturbance of newborn

P74.5 Transitory tyrosinemia of newborn

P74.6 Transitory hyperammonemia of newborn

P74.8 Other transitory metabolic disturbances of newborn
Amino-acid metabolic disorders described as transitory

P74.9 Transitory metabolic disturbance of newborn, unspecified

## Digestive system disorders of newborn (P76-P78)

✓4th P76 Other intestinal obstruction of newborn

P76.0 Meconium plug syndrome
Meconium ileus NOS
EXCLUDES 1 *meconium ileus in cystic fibrosis (E84.11)*
DEF: Meconium obstruction of a newborn's intestines, resulting from unusually thick or hard meconium.

P76.1 Transitory ileus of newborn
EXCLUDES 1 *Hirschsprung's disease (Q43.1)*

P76.2 Intestinal obstruction due to inspissated milk

P76.8 Other specified intestinal obstruction of newborn
EXCLUDES 1 *intestinal obstruction classifiable to K56.-*

P76.9 Intestinal obstruction of newborn, unspecified

✓4th P77 Necrotizing enterocolitis of newborn
DEF: Serious intestinal infection and inflammation in preterm infants. Severity is measured by stages and may progress to life-threatening perforation or peritonitis. Resection surgical treatment may be necessary.

P77.1 Stage 1 necrotizing enterocolitis in newborn HCC COM
Necrotizing enterocolitis without pneumatosis, without perforation
DEF: Broad-spectrum symptoms with nonspecific signs, including feeding intolerance, abdominal distention, bradycardia, and metabolic abnormalities.

**P77.2 Stage 2 necrotizing enterocolitis in newborn** HCC COM
Necrotizing enterocolitis with pneumatosis, without perforation
**DEF:** Radiographic confirmation of necrotizing enterocolitis showing intestinal dilatation, fixed loops of bowels, pneumatosis intestinalis, metabolic acidosis, and thrombocytopenia.

**P77.3 Stage 3 necrotizing enterocolitis in newborn** HCC COM
Necrotizing enterocolitis with perforation
Necrotizing enterocolitis with pneumatosis and perforation
**DEF:** Advanced stage in which an infant demonstrates signs of bowel perforation, septic shock, metabolic acidosis, ascites, disseminated intravascular coagulopathy, and neutropenia.

**P77.9 Necrotizing enterocolitis in newborn, unspecified** HCC COM
Necrotizing enterocolitis in newborn, NOS

✓4th **P78 Other perinatal digestive system disorders**
EXCLUDES 1 *cystic fibrosis (E84.0-E84.9)*
*neonatal gastrointestinal hemorrhages (P54.0-P54.3)*

**P78.0 Perinatal intestinal perforation** HCC COM
Meconium peritonitis

**P78.1 Other neonatal peritonitis**
Neonatal peritonitis NOS

**P78.2 Neonatal hematemesis and melena due to swallowed maternal blood**

**P78.3 Noninfective neonatal diarrhea**
Neonatal diarrhea NOS

✓5th **P78.8 Other specified perinatal digestive system disorders**

**P78.81 Congenital cirrhosis (of liver)**

**P78.82 Peptic ulcer of newborn**

**P78.83 Newborn esophageal reflux**
Neonatal esophageal reflux

**P78.84 Gestational alloimmune liver disease** COM
GALD
Neonatal hemochromatosis
EXCLUDES 1 *hemochromatosis (E83.11-)*
**AHA:** 2017,4Q,21
**DEF:** Severe hepatic injury with onset during fetal development with manifestations beginning during fetal life. It is due to maternal antibodies to fetal hepatic cells (hepatocytes) that cross the placenta into the fetal circulation, causing hepatic cell necrosis.

**P78.89 Other specified perinatal digestive system disorders**

**P78.9 Perinatal digestive system disorder, unspecified**

## Conditions involving the integument and temperature regulation of newborn (P80-P83)

✓4th **P80 Hypothermia of newborn**
**DEF:** Decrease in newborn body temperature due to their larger ratio of surface area to body weight, thin skin with blood vessels close to the surface, and a limited amount of subcutaneous fat.

**P80.0 Cold injury syndrome**
Severe and usually chronic hypothermia associated with a pink flushed appearance, edema and neurological and biochemical abnormalities.
EXCLUDES 1 *mild hypothermia of newborn (P80.8)*

**P80.8 Other hypothermia of newborn**
Mild hypothermia of newborn

**P80.9 Hypothermia of newborn, unspecified**

✓4th **P81 Other disturbances of temperature regulation of newborn**

**P81.0 Environmental hyperthermia of newborn**

**P81.8 Other specified disturbances of temperature regulation of newborn**

**P81.9 Disturbance of temperature regulation of newborn, unspecified**
Fever of newborn NOS

✓4th **P83 Other conditions of integument specific to newborn**
EXCLUDES 1 *congenital malformations of skin and integument (Q80-Q84)*
*hydrops fetalis due to hemolytic disease (P56.-)*
*neonatal skin infection (P39.4)*
*staphylococcal scalded skin syndrome (L00)*
EXCLUDES 2 *cradle cap (L21.0)*
*diaper [napkin] dermatitis (L22)*

**P83.0 Sclerema neonatorum**
**DEF:** Diffuse, rapidly progressing white, waxy, nonpitting hardening of tissue, usually of legs and feet that is life-threatening. It is found in preterm or debilitated infants. Etiology is unknown.

**P83.1 Neonatal erythema toxicum**

**P83.2 Hydrops fetalis not due to hemolytic disease**
Hydrops fetalis NOS
**DEF:** Severe, life-threatening problem of a newborn characterized by severe edema of the entire body. It is unrelated to immune response.

✓5th **P83.3 Other and unspecified edema specific to newborn**

**P83.30 Unspecified edema specific to newborn**

**P83.39 Other edema specific to newborn**

**P83.4 Breast engorgement of newborn**
Noninfective mastitis of newborn

**P83.5 Congenital hydrocele**
**DEF:** Hydrocele: Serous fluid that collects in the tunica vaginalis of the scrotum along the spermatic cord in males.

**P83.6 Umbilical polyp of newborn**

✓5th **P83.8 Other specified conditions of integument specific to newborn**
**AHA:** 2017,4Q,21-22

**P83.81 Umbilical granuloma**
EXCLUDES 2 *granulomatous disorder of the skin and subcutaneous tissue, unspecified (L92.9)*

**P83.88 Other specified conditions of integument specific to newborn**
Bronze baby syndrome
Neonatal scleroderma
Urticaria neonatorum

**P83.9 Condition of the integument specific to newborn, unspecified**

## Other problems with newborn (P84)

**P84 Other problems with newborn**
Acidemia of newborn
Acidosis of newborn
Anoxia of newborn NOS
Asphyxia of newborn NOS
Hypercapnia of newborn
Hypoxemia of newborn
Hypoxia of newborn NOS
Mixed metabolic and respiratory acidosis of newborn
EXCLUDES 1 *intracranial hemorrhage due to anoxia or hypoxia (P52.-)*
*hypoxic ischemic encephalopathy [HIE] (P91.6-)*
*late metabolic acidosis of newborn (P74.0)*

## Other disorders originating in the perinatal period (P90-P96)

**P90 Convulsions of newborn** HCC COM
EXCLUDES 1 *benign myoclonic epilepsy in infancy (G40.3-)*
*benign neonatal convulsions (familial) (G40.3-)*

✓4th **P91 Other disturbances of cerebral status of newborn**

**P91.0 Neonatal cerebral ischemia** HCC COM
EXCLUDES 1 *neonatal cerebral infarction (P91.82-)*

**P91.1 Acquired periventricular cysts of newborn** HCC COM

**P91.2 Neonatal cerebral leukomalacia** HCC COM
Periventricular leukomalacia

**P91.3 Neonatal cerebral irritability** HCC COM

**P91.4 Neonatal cerebral depression** HCC COM

**P91.5 Neonatal coma** HCC COM

✓5th **P91.6 Hypoxic ischemic encephalopathy [HIE]**
EXCLUDES 1 *neonatal cerebral depression (P91.4)*
*neonatal cerebral irritability (P91.3)*
*neonatal coma (P91.5)*
**AHA:** 2017,4Q,22

**P91.60 Hypoxic ischemic encephalopathy [HIE], unspecified** HCC COM

**P91.61 Mild hypoxic ischemic encephalopathy [HIE]** HCC COM

**P91.62 Moderate hypoxic ischemic encephalopathy [HIE]** HCC COM

**P91.63 Severe hypoxic ischemic encephalopathy [HIE]** HCC COM

√5th **P91.8 Other specified disturbances of cerebral status of newborn**
AHA: 2017,4Q,22

√6th **P91.81 Neonatal encephalopathy**

*P91.811* ***Neonatal encephalopathy in diseases classified elsewhere*** HCC COM
Code first underlying condition, if known, such as:
congenital cirrhosis (of liver) (P78.81)
intracranial nontraumatic hemorrhage of newborn (P52.-)
kernicterus (P57.-)

**P91.819 Neonatal encephalopathy, unspecified** HCC COM

√6th **P91.82 Neonatal cerebral infarction**
Neonatal stroke
Perinatal arterial ischemic stroke
Perinatal cerebral infarction
EXCLUDES 1 *cerebral infarction (I63.-)*
EXCLUDES 2 *intracranial hemorrhage of newborn (P52.-)*
AHA: 2020,4Q,37-38

**P91.821 Neonatal cerebral infarction, right side of brain** HCC ESR COM

**P91.822 Neonatal cerebral infarction, left side of brain** HCC ESR COM

**P91.823 Neonatal cerebral infarction, bilateral** HCC ESR COM

**P91.829 Neonatal cerebral infarction, unspecified side** HCC ESR COM

**P91.88 Other specified disturbances of cerebral status of newborn** HCC COM

**P91.9 Disturbance of cerebral status of newborn, unspecified** HCC COM

√4th **P92 Feeding problems of newborn**
EXCLUDES 1 *eating disorders (F50.-)*
EXCLUDES 2 *feeding problems in child over 28 days old (R63.3-)*
AHA: 2016,3Q,19

√5th **P92.0 Vomiting of newborn**
EXCLUDES 1 *vomiting of child over 28 days old (R11.-)*

**P92.01 Bilious vomiting of newborn**
EXCLUDES 1 *bilious vomiting in child over 28 days old (R11.14)*

**P92.09 Other vomiting of newborn**
EXCLUDES 1 *regurgitation of food in newborn (P92.1)*

**P92.1 Regurgitation and rumination of newborn**

**P92.2 Slow feeding of newborn**

**P92.3 Underfeeding of newborn**

**P92.4 Overfeeding of newborn**

**P92.5 Neonatal difficulty in feeding at breast**
AHA: 2017,1Q,28

**P92.6 Failure to thrive in newborn**
EXCLUDES 1 *failure to thrive in child over 28 days old (R62.51)*

**P92.8 Other feeding problems of newborn**

**P92.9 Feeding problem of newborn, unspecified**

√4th **P93 Reactions and intoxications due to drugs administered to newborn**
INCLUDES reactions and intoxications due to drugs administered to fetus affecting newborn
EXCLUDES 1 *jaundice due to drugs or toxins transmitted from mother or given to newborn (P58.4-)*
*reactions and intoxications from maternal opiates, tranquilizers and other medication (P04.0-P04.1, P04.4-)*
*withdrawal symptoms from maternal use of drugs of addiction (P96.1)*
*withdrawal symptoms from therapeutic use of drugs in newborn (P96.2)*

**P93.0 Grey baby syndrome** HCC COM
Grey syndrome from chloramphenicol administration in newborn

**P93.8 Other reactions and intoxications due to drugs administered to newborn** HCC COM
Use additional code for adverse effect, if applicable, to identify drug (T36-T50 with fifth or sixth character 5)

√4th **P94 Disorders of muscle tone of newborn**

**P94.0 Transient neonatal myasthenia gravis**
EXCLUDES 1 *myasthenia gravis (G70.0)*

**P94.1 Congenital hypertonia**

**P94.2 Congenital hypotonia**
Floppy baby syndrome, unspecified

**P94.8 Other disorders of muscle tone of newborn**

**P94.9 Disorder of muscle tone of newborn, unspecified**

**P95 Stillbirth**
Deadborn fetus NOS
Fetal death of unspecified cause
Stillbirth NOS
EXCLUDES 1 *maternal care for intrauterine death (O36.4)*
*missed abortion (O02.1)*
*outcome of delivery, stillbirth (Z37.1, Z37.3, Z37.4, Z37.7)*

√4th **P96 Other conditions originating in the perinatal period**

**P96.0 Congenital renal failure**
Uremia of newborn

**P96.1 Neonatal withdrawal symptoms from maternal use of drugs of addiction** HCC COM
Drug withdrawal syndrome in infant of dependent mother
Neonatal abstinence syndrome
EXCLUDES 1 *reactions and intoxications from maternal opiates and tranquilizers administered during labor and delivery (P04.0)*
AHA: 2018,4Q,24-25

**P96.2 Withdrawal symptoms from therapeutic use of drugs in newborn** HCC COM

**P96.3 Wide cranial sutures of newborn**
Neonatal craniotabes

**P96.5 Complication to newborn due to (fetal) intrauterine procedure**
EXCLUDES 2 *newborn affected by amniocentesis (P00.6)*

√5th **P96.8 Other specified conditions originating in the perinatal period**

**P96.81 Exposure to (parental) (environmental) tobacco smoke in the perinatal period**
EXCLUDES 2 *exposure to environmental tobacco smoke after the perinatal period (Z77.22)*
*newborn affected by in utero exposure to tobacco (P04.2)*

**P96.82 Delayed separation of umbilical cord**

**P96.83 Meconium staining**
EXCLUDES 1 *meconium aspiration (P24.00, P24.01)*
*meconium passage during delivery (P03.82)*
DEF: Meconium passed in utero causing discoloration on the fetal skin and nails or on the umbilicus. This staining may be incidental or may be an indicator of significant fetal stress that could affect outcomes.

**P96.89 Other specified conditions originating in the perinatal period**
Use additional code to specify condition
AHA: 2023,3Q,3

**P96.9 Condition originating in the perinatal period, unspecified**
Congenital debility NOS

Chapter 16. Certain Conditions Originating in the Perinatal Period

P91.8–P96.9

# Chapter 17. Congenital Malformations, Deformations, Chromosomal Abnormalities, and *Genetic Disorders* (QØØ–*QA1*)

## Chapter-specific Guidelines with Coding Examples

The chapter-specific guidelines from the ICD-10-CM Official Guidelines for Coding and Reporting have been provided below. Along with these guidelines are coding examples, contained in the shaded boxes, that have been developed to help illustrate the coding and/or sequencing guidance found in these guidelines.

Assign an appropriate code(s) from categories QØØ-**QA1**, Congenital malformations, deformations, chromosomal abnormalities, **and genetic disorders** when a malformation/deformation, chromosomal abnormality, **or genetic disorder** is documented. A malformation/deformation/chromosomal abnormality, **or genetic disorder** may be the principal/first-listed diagnosis or secondary diagnosis on a record.

When a malformation/deformation, chromosomal abnormality, **or genetic disorder** does not have a unique code assignment, assign additional code(s) for any manifestations that may be present.

When the code assignment specifically identifies the malformation/deformation, chromosomal abnormality, **or genetic disorder,** manifestations that are an inherent component of the anomaly should not be coded separately. Additional codes should be assigned for manifestations that are not an inherent component.

8-day-old infant with tetralogy of Fallot and pulmonary stenosis

**Q21.3 Tetralogy of Fallot**

*Explanation:* Pulmonary stenosis is inherent in the disease process of tetralogy of Fallot. When the code assignment specifically identifies the malformation/deformation/or chromosomal abnormality, manifestations that are inherent components of the anomaly should not be coded separately.

7-month-old infant with Down syndrome and common atrioventricular canal

**Q9Ø.9 Down syndrome, unspecified**

**Q21.23 Complete atrioventricular septal defect**

*Explanation:* While a common atrioventricular canal is often associated with patients with Down syndrome, this manifestation is not an inherent component and may be reported separately. When the code assignment specifically identifies the anomaly, manifestations that are inherent components of the condition should not be coded separately. Additional codes should be assigned for manifestations that are not inherent components.

Codes from Chapter 17 may be used throughout the life of the patient. If a congenital malformation or deformity has been corrected, a personal history code should be used to identify the history of the malformation or deformity. Although present at birth, a malformation/deformation, chromosomal abnormality, **or genetic disorder** may not be identified until later in life. Whenever the condition is diagnosed by the provider, it is appropriate to assign a code from categories QØØ-**QA1**. For the birth admission, the appropriate code from category Z38, Liveborn infants, according to place of birth and type of delivery, should be sequenced as the principal diagnosis, followed by any congenital anomaly codes in categories QØØ-**QA1**.

Three-year-old with history of corrected ventricular septal defect

**Z87.74 Personal history of (corrected) congenital malformations of heart and circulatory system**

*Explanation:* If a congenital malformation or deformity has been corrected, a personal history code should be used to identify the history of the malformation or deformity.

Forty-year-old man with headaches diagnosed with congenital arteriovenous malformation of cerebral vessels by brain scan

**Q28.2 Arteriovenous malformation of cerebral vessels**

*Explanation:* Although present at birth, malformations may not be identified until later in life. Whenever a congenital condition is diagnosed by the physician, it is appropriate to assign a code from this chapter.

# Chapter 17. Congenital malformations, deformations, chromosomal abnormalities, and genetic disorders (Q00-QA1)

NOTE Codes from this chapter are not for use on maternal records

EXCLUDES 2 *inborn errors of metabolism (E70-E88)*

This chapter contains the following blocks:



## Congenital malformations of the nervous system (Q00-Q07)

✓4th **Q00 Anencephaly and similar malformations**

**Q00.0 Anencephaly** HCC Rx ESR COM
Acephaly
Acrania
Amyelencephaly
Hemianencephaly
Hemicephaly

**Q00.1 Craniorachischisis** HCC Rx ESR COM

**Q00.2 Iniencephaly** HCC Rx ESR COM

✓4th **Q01 Encephalocele**

INCLUDES Arnold-Chiari syndrome, type III
encephalocystocele
encephalomyelocele
hydroencephalocele
hydromeningocele, cranial
meningocele, cerebral
meningoencephalocele

EXCLUDES 1 *Meckel-Gruber syndrome (Q61.9)*

**DEF:** Congenital protrusion of brain tissue through a defect in the skull.

**Q01.0 Frontal encephalocele** HCC Rx ESR COM

**Q01.1 Nasofrontal encephalocele** HCC Rx ESR COM

**Q01.2 Occipital encephalocele** HCC Rx ESR COM

**Q01.8 Encephalocele of other sites** HCC Rx ESR COM

**Q01.9 Encephalocele, unspecified** HCC Rx ESR COM

**Q02 Microcephaly** HCC Rx ESR COM

INCLUDES hydromicrocephaly
micrencephalon

Code first, if applicable, congenital Zika virus disease

EXCLUDES 1 *Meckel-Gruber syndrome (Q61.9)*

**AHA:** 2018,4Q,26

**DEF:** Congenital disorder in which the head circumference is more than two standard deviations below the mean for age, sex, race, and gestation and associated with a decreased life expectancy.

✓4th **Q03 Congenital hydrocephalus**

INCLUDES hydrocephalus in newborn

EXCLUDES 1 *acquired hydrocephalus (G91.-)*
*Arnold-Chiari syndrome, type II (Q07.0-)*
*hydrocephalus due to congenital toxoplasmosis (P37.1)*
*hydrocephalus with spina bifida (Q05.0-Q05.4)*

**DEF:** Hydrocephalus: Abnormal buildup of cerebrospinal fluid in the brain causing dilation of the ventricles.

**Congenital Hydrocephalus**

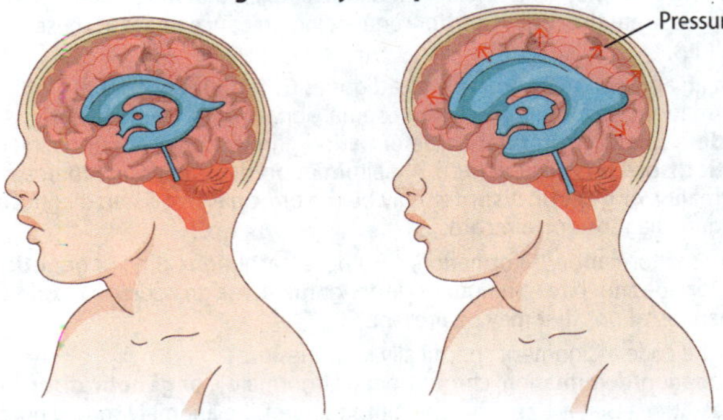


**Q03.0 Malformations of aqueduct of Sylvius** HCC Rx ESR COM
Anomaly of aqueduct of Sylvius
Obstruction of aqueduct of Sylvius, congenital
Stenosis of aqueduct of Sylvius

**Q03.1 Atresia of foramina of Magendie and Luschka** HCC Rx ESR COM
Dandy-Walker syndrome

**Q03.8 Other congenital hydrocephalus** HCC Rx ESR COM

**Q03.9 Congenital hydrocephalus, unspecified** HCC Rx ESR COM

✓4th **Q04 Other congenital malformations of brain**

EXCLUDES 1 *cyclopia (Q87.0)*
*macrocephaly (Q75.3)*

**Q04.0 Congenital malformations of corpus callosum** HCC Rx ESR COM
Agenesis of corpus callosum

**Q04.1 Arhinencephaly** HCC Rx ESR COM

**Q04.2 Holoprosencephaly** HCC Rx ESR COM

**Q04.3 Other reduction deformities of brain** HCC Rx ESR COM
Absence of part of brain
Agenesis of part of brain
Agyria
Aplasia of part of brain
Hydranencephaly
Hypoplasia of part of brain
Lissencephaly
Microgyria
Pachygyria

EXCLUDES 1 *congenital malformations of corpus callosum (Q04.0)*

**Q04.4 Septo-optic dysplasia of brain** HCC Rx ESR COM

**Q04.5 Megalencephaly** HCC Rx ESR COM

**Q04.6 Congenital cerebral cysts** HCC Rx ESR COM
Porencephaly
Schizencephaly

EXCLUDES 1 *acquired porencephalic cyst (G93.0)*

**Q04.8 Other specified congenital malformations of brain** HCC Rx ESR COM
Arnold-Chiari syndrome, type IV
Macrogyria

**Q04.9 Congenital malformation of brain, unspecified** HCC Rx ESR COM
Congenital anomaly NOS of brain
Congenital deformity NOS of brain
Congenital disease or lesion NOS of brain
Multiple anomalies NOS of brain, congenital

**✓4th Q05 Spina bifida**

INCLUDES hydromeningocele (spinal)
meningocele (spinal)
meningomyelocele
myelocele
myelomeningocele
rachischisis
spina bifida (aperta)(cystica)
syringomyelocele

Use additional code for any associated paraplegia (paraparesis) (G82.2-)

EXCLUDES 1 *Arnold-Chiari syndrome, type II (Q07.0-)*
*spina bifida occulta (Q76.0)*

**DEF:** Lack of closure in the vertebral column with protrusion of the spinal cord through the defect, often in the lumbosacral area. This condition can be recognized by the presence of alpha-fetoproteins in the amniotic fluid.

**Spina Bifida**

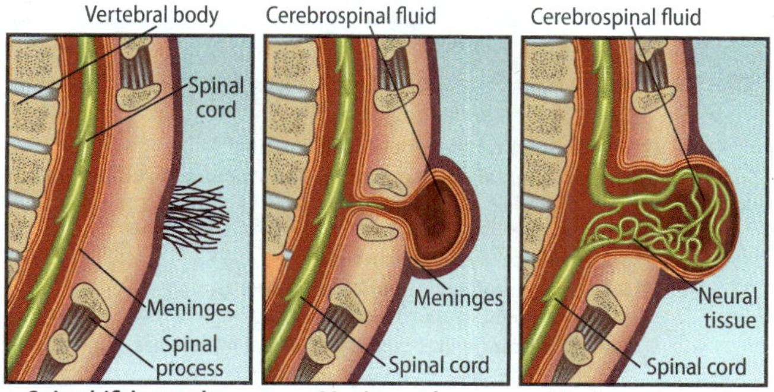


Spina bifida occulta | Meningocele | Myelomeningocele

**Q05.0 Cervical spina bifida with hydrocephalus** HCC Rx ESR COM

**Q05.1 Thoracic spina bifida with hydrocephalus** HCC Rx ESR COM
Dorsal spina bifida with hydrocephalus
Thoracolumbar spina bifida with hydrocephalus

**Q05.2 Lumbar spina bifida with hydrocephalus** HCC Rx ESR COM
Lumbosacral spina bifida with hydrocephalus

**Q05.3 Sacral spina bifida with hydrocephalus** HCC Rx ESR COM

**Q05.4 Unspecified spina bifida with hydrocephalus** HCC Rx ESR COM

**Q05.5 Cervical spina bifida without hydrocephalus** HCC Rx ESR COM

**Q05.6 Thoracic spina bifida without hydrocephalus** HCC Rx ESR COM
Dorsal spina bifida NOS
Thoracolumbar spina bifida NOS

**Q05.7 Lumbar spina bifida without hydrocephalus** HCC Rx ESR COM
Lumbosacral spina bifida NOS

**Q05.8 Sacral spina bifida without hydrocephalus** HCC Rx ESR COM

**Q05.9 Spina bifida, unspecified** HCC Rx ESR COM

**✓4th Q06 Other congenital malformations of spinal cord**

**Q06.0 Amyelia** HCC Rx ESR COM

**Q06.1 Hypoplasia and dysplasia of spinal cord** HCC Rx ESR COM
Atelomyelia
Myelatelia
Myelodysplasia of spinal cord

**Q06.2 Diastematomyelia** HCC Rx ESR COM
**DEF:** Rare congenital anomaly often associated with spina bifida. The spinal cord is separated into longitudinal halves by a bony, cartilaginous or fibrous septum, each half surrounded by a dural sac.

**Q06.3 Other congenital cauda equina malformations** HCC Rx ESR COM

**Q06.4 Hydromyelia** HCC Rx ESR COM
Hydrorachis

**Q06.8 Other specified congenital malformations of spinal cord** HCC Rx ESR COM

**Q06.9 Congenital malformation of spinal cord, unspecified** HCC Rx ESR COM
Congenital anomaly NOS of spinal cord
Congenital deformity NOS of spinal cord
Congenital disease or lesion NOS of spinal cord

**✓4th Q07 Other congenital malformations of nervous system**

EXCLUDES 2 *congenital central alveolar hypoventilation syndrome (G47.35)*
*familial dysautonomia [Riley-Day] (G90.1)*
*neurofibromatosis (nonmalignant) (Q85.0-)*

**✓5th Q07.0 Arnold-Chiari syndrome**
Arnold-Chiari syndrome, type II
EXCLUDES 1 *Arnold-Chiari syndrome, type III (Q01.-)*
*Arnold-Chiari syndrome, type IV (Q04.8)*
**DEF:** Congenital malformation of the brain in which the cerebellum protrudes through the foramen magnum into the spinal canal.

**Q07.00 Arnold-Chiari syndrome without spina bifida or hydrocephalus** HCC Rx ESR COM

**Q07.01 Arnold-Chiari syndrome with spina bifida** HCC Rx ESR COM

**Q07.02 Arnold-Chiari syndrome with hydrocephalus** HCC Rx ESR COM

**Q07.03 Arnold-Chiari syndrome with spina bifida and hydrocephalus** HCC Rx ESR COM

**Q07.8 Other specified congenital malformations of nervous system** HCC Rx ESR COM
Agenesis of nerve
Displacement of brachial plexus
Jaw-winking syndrome
Marcus Gunn's syndrome

**Q07.9 Congenital malformation of nervous system, unspecified** HCC Rx ESR COM
Congenital anomaly NOS of nervous system
Congenital deformity NOS of nervous system
Congenital disease or lesion NOS of nervous system

## Congenital malformations of eye, ear, face and neck (Q10-Q18)

EXCLUDES 2 *cleft lip and cleft palate (Q35-Q37)*
*congenital malformation of cervical spine (Q05.0, Q05.5, Q67.5, Q76.0-Q76.4)*
*congenital malformation of larynx (Q31.-)*
*congenital malformation of lip NEC (Q38.0)*
*congenital malformation of nose (Q30.-)*
*congenital malformation of parathyroid gland (Q89.2)*
*congenital malformation of thyroid gland (Q89.2)*

**✓4th Q10 Congenital malformations of eyelid, lacrimal apparatus and orbit**

EXCLUDES 1 *cryptophthalmos NOS (Q11.2)*
*cryptophthalmos syndrome (Q87.0)*

**Q10.0 Congenital ptosis**
**DEF:** Congenital drooping of the eyelid. Ptosis is mostly idiopathic, but may occur genetically.

**Q10.1 Congenital ectropion**

**Q10.2 Congenital entropion**

**Q10.3 Other congenital malformations of eyelid**
Ablepharon
Blepharophimosis, congenital
Coloboma of eyelid
Congenital absence or agenesis of cilia
Congenital absence or agenesis of eyelid
Congenital accessory eye muscle
Congenital accessory eyelid
Congenital malformation of eyelid NOS

**Q10.4 Absence and agenesis of lacrimal apparatus**
Congenital absence of punctum lacrimale

**Q10.5 Congenital stenosis and stricture of lacrimal duct**

**Q10.6 Other congenital malformations of lacrimal apparatus**
Congenital malformation of lacrimal apparatus NOS

**Q10.7 Congenital malformation of orbit**

**✓4th Q11 Anophthalmos, microphthalmos and macrophthalmos**

**Q11.0 Cystic eyeball**

**Q11.1 Other anophthalmos**
Agenesis of eye
Anophthalmos NOS
Aplasia of eye

**Q11.2 Microphthalmos**
Cryptophthalmos NOS
Dysplasia of eye
Hypoplasia of eye
Rudimentary eye
EXCLUDES 1 *cryptophthalmos syndrome (Q87.0)*

**Q11.3 Macrophthalmos**
EXCLUDES 1 *macrophthalmos in congenital glaucoma (Q15.0)*

**✓4th Q12 Congenital lens malformations**

**Q12.0 Congenital cataract**

**Q12.1** **Congenital displaced lens**

**Q12.2** **Coloboma of lens**

**Coloboma of Lens**

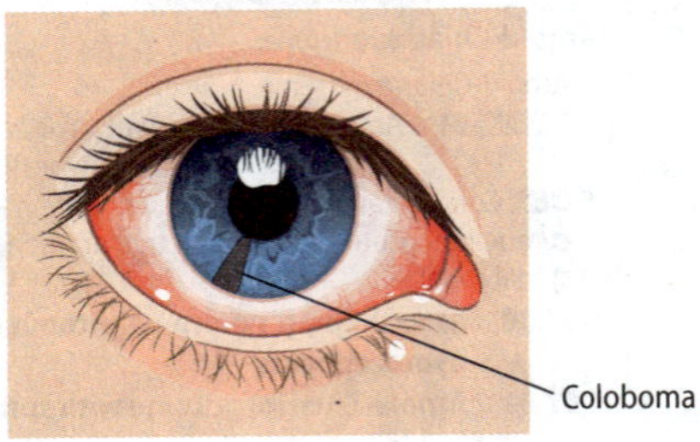


**Q12.3** **Congenital aphakia**

**Q12.4** **Spherophakia**

**Q12.8** **Other congenital lens malformations**
- Microphakia

**Q12.9** **Congenital lens malformation, unspecified**

✓4th **Q13** **Congenital malformations of anterior segment of eye**

**Q13.Ø** **Coloboma of iris**
- Coloboma NOS
- **DEF:** Defective or absent section of ocular tissue that may present as mild cupping or a small pit in the ocular disc due to extensive defects in the iris, ciliary body, choroids, and retina.

**Q13.1** **Absence of iris**
- Aniridia
- Use additional code for associated glaucoma (H42)
- **DEF:** Incompletely formed or absent iris. It affects both eyes and is a dominant trait.

**Q13.2** **Other congenital malformations of iris**
- Anisocoria, congenital
- Atresia of pupil
- Congenital malformation of iris NOS
- Corectopia

**Q13.3** **Congenital corneal opacity**

**Q13.4** **Other congenital corneal malformations**
- Congenital malformation of cornea NOS
- Microcornea
- Peter's anomaly

**Q13.5** **Blue sclera**

✓5th **Q13.8** **Other congenital malformations of anterior segment of eye**

**Q13.81** **Rieger anomaly**
- Axenfeld-Rieger syndrome
- Code also any other associated congenital malformations such as cardiac defects
- Use additional code for associated glaucoma (H42)

**Q13.89** **Other congenital malformations of anterior segment of eye**

**Q13.9** **Congenital malformation of anterior segment of eye, unspecified**

✓4th **Q14** **Congenital malformations of posterior segment of eye**

EXCLUDES 2 *optic nerve hypoplasia (H47.Ø3-)*

**Q14.Ø** **Congenital malformation of vitreous humor**
- Congenital vitreous opacity

**Q14.1** **Congenital malformation of retina**
- Congenital retinal aneurysm

**Q14.2** **Congenital malformation of optic disc**
- Coloboma of optic disc

**Q14.3** **Congenital malformation of choroid**

**Q14.8** **Other congenital malformations of posterior segment of eye**
- Coloboma of the fundus

**Q14.9** **Congenital malformation of posterior segment of eye, unspecified**

✓4th **Q15** **Other congenital malformations of eye**

EXCLUDES 1 *congenital nystagmus (H55.Ø1)*
*ocular albinism (E7Ø.31-)*
*optic nerve hypoplasia (H47.Ø3-)*
*retinitis pigmentosa (H35.52)*

**Q15.Ø** **Congenital glaucoma**
- Axenfeld's anomaly
- Buphthalmos
- Glaucoma of childhood
- Glaucoma of newborn
- Hydrophthalmos
- Keratoglobus, congenital, with glaucoma
- Macrocornea with glaucoma
- Macrophthalmos in congenital glaucoma
- Megalocornea with glaucoma

**Q15.8** **Other specified congenital malformations of eye**

**Q15.9** **Congenital malformation of eye, unspecified**
- Congenital anomaly of eye
- Congenital deformity of eye

✓4th **Q16** **Congenital malformations of ear causing impairment of hearing**

EXCLUDES 1 *congenital deafness (H9Ø.-)*

**Q16.Ø** **Congenital absence of (ear) auricle**

**Q16.1** **Congenital absence, atresia and stricture of auditory canal (external)**
- Congenital atresia or stricture of osseous meatus

**Q16.2** **Absence of eustachian tube**

**Q16.3** **Congenital malformation of ear ossicles**
- Congenital fusion of ear ossicles

**Q16.4** **Other congenital malformations of middle ear**
- Congenital malformation of middle ear NOS

**Q16.5** **Congenital malformation of inner ear**
- Congenital anomaly of membranous labyrinth
- Congenital anomaly of organ of Corti

**Q16.9** **Congenital malformation of ear causing impairment of hearing, unspecified**
- Congenital absence of ear NOS

✓4th **Q17** **Other congenital malformations of ear**

EXCLUDES 1 *congenital malformations of ear with impairment of hearing (Q16.Ø-Q16.9)*
*preauricular sinus (Q18.1)*

**Q17.Ø** **Accessory auricle**
- Accessory tragus
- Polyotia
- Preauricular appendage or tag
- Supernumerary ear
- Supernumerary lobule

**Q17.1** **Macrotia**
- **DEF:** Birth defect characterized by abnormal enlargement of the pinna of the ear.

**Q17.2** **Microtia**

**Q17.3** **Other misshapen ear**
- Pointed ear

**Q17.4** **Misplaced ear**
- Low-set ears
- EXCLUDES 1 *cervical auricle (Q18.2)*

**Q17.5** **Prominent ear**
- Bat ear

**Q17.8** **Other specified congenital malformations of ear**
- Congenital absence of lobe of ear

**Q17.9** **Congenital malformation of ear, unspecified**
- Congenital anomaly of ear NOS

✓4th **Q18** **Other congenital malformations of face and neck**

EXCLUDES 1 *cleft lip and cleft palate (Q35-Q37)*
*conditions classified to Q67.Ø-Q67.4*
*congenital malformations of skull and face bones (Q75.-)*
*cyclopia (Q87.Ø)*
*dentofacial anomalies [including malocclusion] (M26.-)*
*malformation syndromes affecting facial appearance (Q87.Ø)*
*persistent thyroglossal duct (Q89.2)*

**Q18.Ø** **Sinus, fistula and cyst of branchial cleft**
- Branchial vestige

**Q18.1** **Preauricular sinus and cyst**
- Cervicoaural fistula
- Fistula of auricle, congenital

**Q18.2** **Other branchial cleft malformations**
- Branchial cleft malformation NOS
- Cervical auricle
- Otocephaly

**Q18.3 Webbing of neck**
Pterygium colli
**DEF:** Congenital malformation characterized by a thick, triangular skinfold that stretches from the lateral side of the neck across the shoulder. It is associated with genetic conditions such as Turner's and Noonan's syndromes.

**Q18.4 Macrostomia**
**DEF:** Rare congenital craniofacial bilateral or unilateral anomaly of the mouth due to malformed maxillary and mandibular processes. It results in an abnormally large mouth extending toward the ear.

**Q18.5 Microstomia**

**Q18.6 Macrocheilia**
Hypertrophy of lip, congenital

**Q18.7 Microcheilia**

**Q18.8 Other specified congenital malformations of face and neck**
Medial cyst of face and neck
Medial fistula of face and neck
Medial sinus of face and neck

**Q18.9 Congenital malformation of face and neck, unspecified**
Congenital anomaly NOS of face and neck

## Congenital malformations of the circulatory system (Q2Ø-Q28)

✓4th **Q2Ø Congenital malformations of cardiac chambers and connections**
EXCLUDES 1 *dextrocardia with situs inversus (Q89.3)*
*mirror-image atrial arrangement with situs inversus (Q89.3)*

**Q2Ø.Ø Common arterial trunk** Rx COM
Persistent truncus arteriosus
EXCLUDES 1 *aortic septal defect (Q21.4)*

**Q2Ø.1 Double outlet right ventricle** Rx COM
Taussig-Bing syndrome

**Q2Ø.2 Double outlet left ventricle** Rx COM

**Q2Ø.3 Discordant ventriculoarterial connection** Rx COM
Dextrotransposition of aorta
Transposition of great vessels (complete)

**Q2Ø.4 Double inlet ventricle** Rx COM
Common ventricle
Cor triloculare biatriatum
Single ventricle

**Q2Ø.5 Discordant atrioventricular connection** Rx COM
Corrected transposition
Levotransposition
Ventricular inversion

**Q2Ø.6 Isomerism of atrial appendages** COM
Isomerism of atrial appendages with asplenia or polysplenia

**Q2Ø.8 Other congenital malformations of cardiac chambers and connections** Rx COM
Cor binoculare

**Q2Ø.9 Congenital malformation of cardiac chambers and connections, unspecified** COM

✓4th **Q21 Congenital malformations of cardiac septa**
EXCLUDES 1 *acquired cardiac septal defect (I51.Ø)*

**Q21.Ø Ventricular septal defect** Rx COM
Roger's disease

**Ventricular Septal Defect**

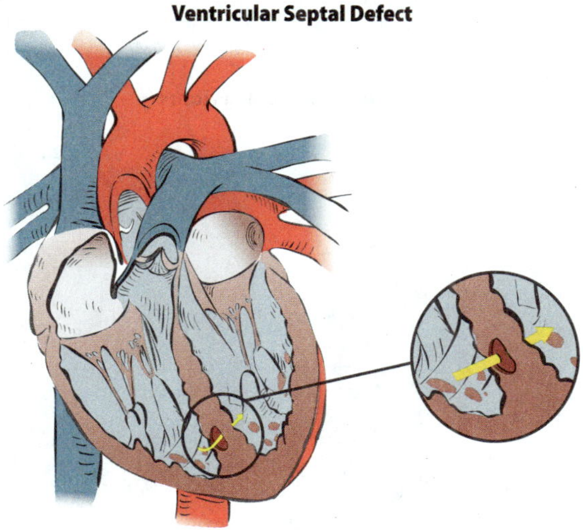

✓5th **Q21.1 Atrial septal defect**
EXCLUDES 2 *ostium primum atrial septal defect (type I) (Q21.2Ø)*
**AHA:** 2022,4Q,39-40

**Atrial Septal Defect**

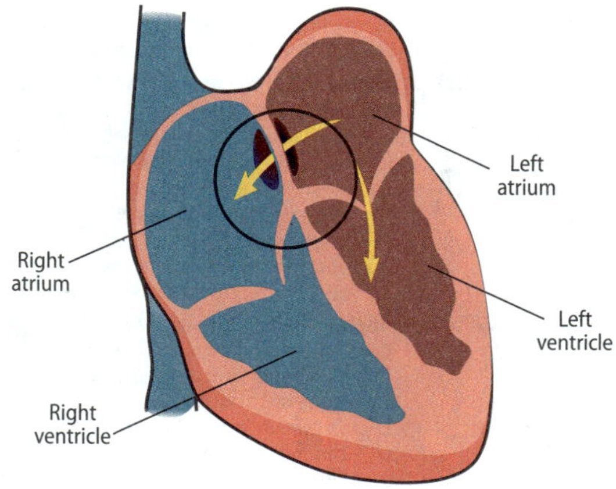


**Q21.1Ø Atrial septal defect, unspecified** COM

**Q21.11 Secundum atrial septal defect** COM
Fenestrated atrial septum
Patent or persistent ostium secundum defect (type II)

**Q21.12 Patent foramen ovale** COM
Persistent foramen ovale

**Q21.13 Coronary sinus atrial septal defect** COM
Coronary sinus defect
Unroofed coronary sinus

**Q21.14 Superior sinus venosus atrial septal defect** COM
Superior vena cava type atrial septal defect

**Q21.15 Inferior sinus venosus atrial septal defect** COM
Inferior vena cava type atrial septal defect

**Q21.16 Sinus venosus atrial septal defect, unspecified** COM
Sinus venosus defect, NOS

**Q21.19 Other specified atrial septal defect** COM
Common atrium
Other specified atrial septal abnormality

✓5th **Q21.2 Atrioventricular septal defect**
Atrioventricular canal defect
Endocardial cushion defect
Ostium primum atrial septal defect (type I)
**AHA:** 2022,4Q,39-40

**Atrioventricular Septal Defect**

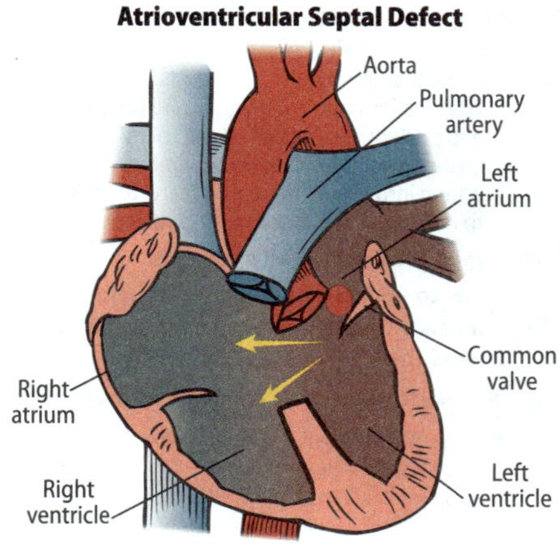


**Q21.2Ø Atrioventricular septal defect, unspecified as to partial or complete** Rx COM
Atrioventricular canal, NOS
Endocardial cushion defect NOS
Ostium primum atrial septal defect (type I) NOS

**Q21.21 Partial atrioventricular septal defect** Rx COM
Incomplete atrioventricular canal
Incomplete atrioventricular septal defect
Incomplete endocardial cushion defect
Ostium primum atrial septal defect (type I) with separate atrioventricular valves
Partial atrioventricular canal
Partial endocardial cushion defect

**Q21.22 Transitional atrioventricular septal defect** Rx COM
Intermediate atrioventricular canal
Intermediate atrioventricular septal defect
Intermediate endocardial cushion defect
Ostium primum atrial septal defect (type I) with separate atrioventricular valves and a small or restrictive inlet VSD
Transitional atrioventricular canal
Transitional endocardial cushion defect

**Q21.23 Complete atrioventricular septal defect** Rx COM
Common atrioventricular canal
Common atrioventricular septal defect
Common endocardial cushion defect
Ostium primum atrial septal defect (type I) with common atrioventricular valve and a moderate or larger inlet VSD

**Q21.3 Tetralogy of Fallot** Rx COM
Ventricular septal defect with pulmonary stenosis or atresia, dextroposition of aorta and hypertrophy of right ventricle.
**AHA:** 2014,3Q,16

**Q21.4 Aortopulmonary septal defect** COM
Aortic septal defect
Aortopulmonary window

**Q21.8 Other congenital malformations of cardiac septa** COM
Eisenmenger's defect
Pentalogy of Fallot
Code also, if applicable:
Eisenmenger's complex (I27.83)
Eisenmenger's syndrome (I27.83)

**Q21.9 Congenital malformation of cardiac septum, unspecified** COM
Septal (heart) defect NOS

✓4th **Q22 Congenital malformations of pulmonary and tricuspid valves**

**Q22.Ø Pulmonary valve atresia** Rx COM

**Q22.1 Congenital pulmonary valve stenosis** COM

**Q22.2 Congenital pulmonary valve insufficiency** COM
Congenital pulmonary valve regurgitation
**AHA:** 2022,4Q,39-40

**Q22.3 Other congenital malformations of pulmonary valve** COM
Congenital malformation of pulmonary valve NOS
Supernumerary cusps of pulmonary valve

**Q22.4 Congenital tricuspid stenosis** COM
Congenital tricuspid atresia

**Q22.5 Ebstein's anomaly** COM
**DEF:** Malformation of the tricuspid valve characterized by septal and posterior leaflets attaching to the wall of the right ventricle. Ebstein's anomaly causes the right ventricle to fuse with the atrium into a large right atrium and a small ventricle and leads to heart failure and abnormal cardiac rhythm.

**Q22.6 Hypoplastic right heart syndrome** COM

**Q22.8 Other congenital malformations of tricuspid valve** COM

**Q22.9 Congenital malformation of tricuspid valve, unspecified** COM

✓4th **Q23 Congenital malformations of aortic and mitral valves**

**Q23.Ø Congenital stenosis of aortic valve** COM
Congenital aortic atresia
Congenital aortic stenosis NOS
EXCLUDES 1 *congenital stenosis of aortic valve in hypoplastic left heart syndrome (Q23.4)*
*congenital subaortic stenosis (Q24.4)*
*supravalvular aortic stenosis (congenital) (Q25.3)*

**Q23.1 Congenital insufficiency of aortic valve** COM
Congenital aortic insufficiency

**Q23.2 Congenital mitral stenosis** COM
Congenital mitral atresia

**Q23.3 Congenital mitral insufficiency** COM

**Q23.4 Hypoplastic left heart syndrome** Rx COM

✓5th **Q23.8 Other congenital malformations of aortic and mitral valves**
**AHA:** 2024,4Q,26

**Q23.81 Bicuspid aortic valve** COM
Congenital bicuspid aortic valve
Unicuspid (congenital) aortic valve (at birth)
Code also, if applicable, acquired aortic valve disorders, such as:
aortic (valve) insufficiency (nonrheumatic) (I35.1)
aortic (valve) stenosis (nonrheumatic) (I35.Ø)
aortic (valve) stenosis with insufficiency (nonrheumatic) (I35.2)

**Q23.82 Congenital mitral valve cleft leaflet**
Cleft mitral valve leaflet at birth

**Q23.88 Other congenital malformations of aortic and mitral valves** COM

**Q23.9 Congenital malformation of aortic and mitral valves, unspecified** COM

✓4th **Q24 Other congenital malformations of heart**
EXCLUDES 1 *endocardial fibroelastosis (I42.4)*

**Q24.Ø Dextrocardia** COM
EXCLUDES 1 *dextrocardia with situs inversus (Q89.3)*
*isomerism of atrial appendages (with asplenia or polysplenia) (Q2Ø.6)*
*mirror-image atrial arrangement with situs inversus (Q89.3)*
**DEF:** Congenital condition in which the heart is located on the right side of the chest rather than in its normal position on the left.

**Q24.1 Levocardia** COM

**Q24.2 Cor triatriatum** COM

**Q24.3 Pulmonary infundibular stenosis** COM
Subvalvular pulmonic stenosis

**Q24.4 Congenital subaortic stenosis** COM
**DEF:** Congenital heart defect characterized by stenosis of the left ventricular outflow tract due to a fibrous tissue ring or septal hypertrophy below the aortic valve.

**Q24.5 Malformation of coronary vessels** Rx COM
Congenital coronary (artery) aneurysm
**AHA:** 2026,2Q,7

**Q24.6 Congenital heart block** COM

**Q24.8 Other specified congenital malformations of heart** COM
Congenital diverticulum of left ventricle
Congenital malformation of myocardium
Congenital malformation of pericardium
Malposition of heart
Uhl's disease

**Q24.9 Congenital malformation of heart, unspecified** COM
Congenital anomaly of heart
Congenital disease of heart

✓4th **Q25 Congenital malformations of great arteries**

**Q25.Ø Patent ductus arteriosus** Rx COM
Patent ductus Botallo
Persistent ductus arteriosus
**DEF:** Condition in which the normal channel between the pulmonary artery and the aorta fails to close at birth, causing arterial blood to recirculate in the lungs and inhibiting the blood supply to the aorta. ***Synonym(s):*** *PDA.*

**Patent Ductus Arteriosus**

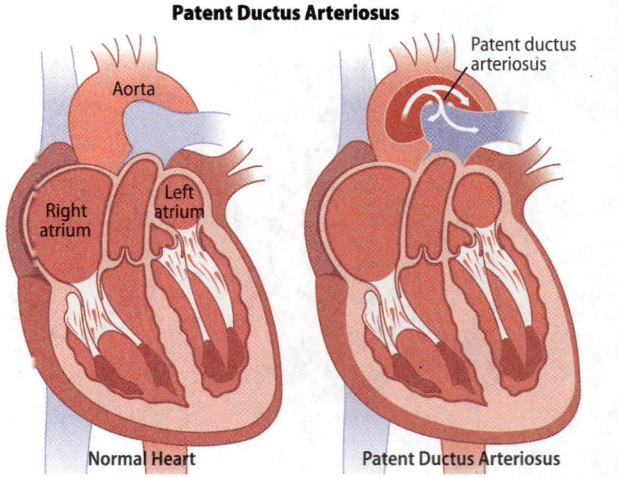

**Q25.1 Coarctation of aorta** COM
Coarctation of aorta (preductal) (postductal)
Stenosis of aorta
**AHA:** 2016,4Q,56-57

✓5th **Q25.2 Atresia of aorta**
**AHA:** 2016,4Q,56-57

**Q25.21 Interruption of aortic arch** COM
Atresia of aortic arch

**Q25.29 Other atresia of aorta** COM
Atresia of aorta

**Q25.3 Supravalvular aortic stenosis** COM
EXCLUDES 1 *congenital aortic stenosis NOS (Q23.Ø)*
*congenital stenosis of aortic valve (Q23.Ø)*

✓5th **Q25.4 Other congenital malformations of aorta**
EXCLUDES 1 *hypoplasia of aorta in hypoplastic left heart syndrome (Q23.4)*
**AHA:** 2016,4Q,57

**Q25.4Ø Congenital malformation of aorta unspecified** COM

**Q25.41 Absence and aplasia of aorta** COM

**Q25.42 Hypoplasia of aorta** COM

**Q25.43 Congenital aneurysm of aorta** COM
Congenital aneurysm of aortic root
Congenital aneurysm of aortic sinus

**Q25.44 Congenital dilation of aorta** COM

**Q25.45 Double aortic arch** COM
Vascular ring of aorta

**Aortic Arch Anomalies**

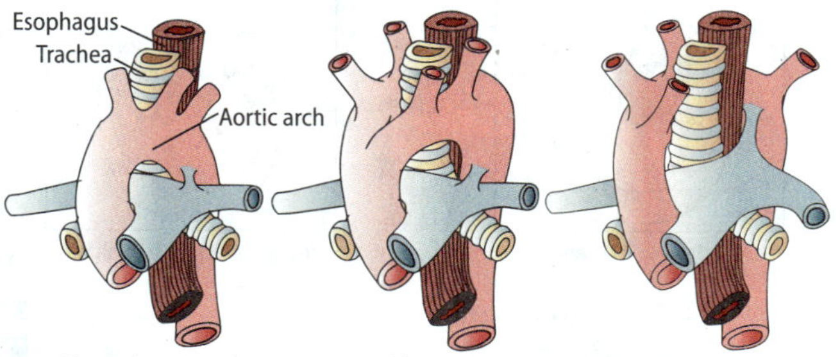

Normal aortic arch — Double aortic arch — Right aortic arch

**Q25.46 Tortuous aortic arch** COM
Persistent convolutions of aortic arch

**Q25.47 Right aortic arch** COM
Persistent right aortic arch

**Q25.48 Anomalous origin of subclavian artery** COM

**Q25.49 Other congenital malformations of aorta** COM
Aortic arch
Bovine arch

**Q25.5 Atresia of pulmonary artery** Rx COM

**Q25.6 Stenosis of pulmonary artery** COM
Supravalvular pulmonary stenosis

✓5th **Q25.7 Other congenital malformations of pulmonary artery**

**Q25.71 Coarctation of pulmonary artery** Rx COM

**Q25.72 Congenital pulmonary arteriovenous malformation** COM
Congenital pulmonary arteriovenous aneurysm

**Q25.79 Other congenital malformations of pulmonary artery** COM
Aberrant pulmonary artery
Agenesis of pulmonary artery
Congenital aneurysm of pulmonary artery
Congenital anomaly of pulmonary artery
Hypoplasia of pulmonary artery

**Q25.8 Other congenital malformations of other great arteries** COM

**Q25.9 Congenital malformation of great arteries, unspecified** COM

✓4th **Q26 Congenital malformations of great veins**

**Q26.Ø Congenital stenosis of vena cava** Rx COM
Congenital stenosis of vena cava (inferior)(superior)

**Q26.1 Persistent left superior vena cava** Rx COM

**Q26.2 Total anomalous pulmonary venous connection** Rx COM
Total anomalous pulmonary venous return [TAPVR], subdiaphragmatic
Total anomalous pulmonary venous return [TAPVR], supradiaphragmatic

**Q26.3 Partial anomalous pulmonary venous connection** Rx COM
Partial anomalous pulmonary venous return

**Q26.4 Anomalous pulmonary venous connection, unspecified** Rx COM

**Q26.5 Anomalous portal venous connection** COM

**Q26.6 Portal vein-hepatic artery fistula** COM

**Q26.8 Other congenital malformations of great veins** Rx COM
Absence of vena cava (inferior) (superior)
Azygos continuation of inferior vena cava
Persistent left posterior cardinal vein
Scimitar syndrome

**Q26.9 Congenital malformation of great vein, unspecified** Rx COM
Congenital anomaly of vena cava (inferior) (superior) NOS

✓4th **Q27 Other congenital malformations of peripheral vascular system**
EXCLUDES 2 *anomalies of cerebral and precerebral vessels (Q28.Ø-Q28.3)*
*anomalies of coronary vessels (Q24.5)*
*anomalies of pulmonary artery (Q25.5-Q25.7)*
*congenital retinal aneurysm (Q14.1)*
*hemangioma and lymphangioma (D18.-)*

**Q27.Ø Congenital absence and hypoplasia of umbilical artery** COM
Single umbilical artery

**Q27.1 Congenital renal artery stenosis** COM

**Q27.2 Other congenital malformations of renal artery** COM
Congenital malformation of renal artery NOS
Multiple renal arteries

✓5th **Q27.3 Arteriovenous malformation (peripheral)**
Arteriovenous aneurysm
EXCLUDES 1 *acquired arteriovenous aneurysm (I77.Ø)*
EXCLUDES 2 *arteriovenous malformation of cerebral vessels (Q28.2)*
*arteriovenous malformation of precerebral vessels (Q28.Ø)*
**DEF:** Arteriovenous malformation: Connecting passage between an artery and a vein.

**Q27.3Ø Arteriovenous malformation, site unspecified** COM

**Q27.31 Arteriovenous malformation of vessel of upper limb** COM

**Q27.32 Arteriovenous malformation of vessel of lower limb** COM

**Q27.33 Arteriovenous malformation of digestive system vessel** COM
**AHA:** 2018,3Q,21

**Q27.34 Arteriovenous malformation of renal vessel** COM

**Q27.39 Arteriovenous malformation, other site** COM

**Q27.4 Congenital phlebectasia** COM

**Q27.8 Other specified congenital malformations of peripheral vascular system** COM
Absence of peripheral vascular system
Atresia of peripheral vascular system
Congenital aneurysm (peripheral)
Congenital stricture, artery
Congenital varix
EXCLUDES 1 *arteriovenous malformation (Q27.3-)*

**Q27.9 Congenital malformation of peripheral vascular system, unspecified** COM
Anomaly of artery or vein NOS

✓4th **Q28 Other congenital malformations of circulatory system**
EXCLUDES 1 *congenital aneurysm NOS (Q27.8)*
*congenital coronary aneurysm (Q24.5)*
*ruptured cerebral arteriovenous malformation (I6Ø.8)*
*ruptured malformation of precerebral vessels (I72.Ø)*
EXCLUDES 2 *congenital peripheral aneurysm (Q27.8)*
*congenital pulmonary aneurysm (Q25.79)*
*congenital retinal aneurysm (Q14.1)*

**Q28.Ø Arteriovenous malformation of precerebral vessels** COM
Congenital arteriovenous precerebral aneurysm (nonruptured)

**Q28.1 Other malformations of precerebral vessels** COM
Congenital malformation of precerebral vessels NOS
Congenital precerebral aneurysm (nonruptured)

**Q28.2 Arteriovenous malformation of cerebral vessels** COM
Arteriovenous malformation of brain NOS
Congenital arteriovenous cerebral aneurysm (nonruptured)

**Q28.3 Other malformations of cerebral vessels** COM
Congenital cerebral aneurysm (nonruptured)
Congenital malformation of cerebral vessels NOS
Developmental venous anomaly

**Q28.8 Other specified congenital malformations of circulatory system** COM
Congenital aneurysm, specified site NEC
Spinal vessel anomaly
EXCLUDES 2 *disorders of pyrophosphate metabolism (E83.82-)*

**Q28.9 Congenital malformation of circulatory system, unspecified** COM

## Congenital malformations of the respiratory system (Q30-Q34)

✓4th **Q30 Congenital malformations of nose**
EXCLUDES 1 *congenital deviation of nasal septum (Q67.4)*

**Q30.0 Choanal atresia**
Atresia of nares (anterior) (posterior)
Congenital stenosis of nares (anterior) (posterior)

**Q30.1 Agenesis and underdevelopment of nose**
Congenital absent of nose

**Q30.2 Fissured, notched and cleft nose**

**Q30.3 Congenital perforated nasal septum**

**Q30.8 Other congenital malformations of nose**
Accessory nose
Congenital anomaly of nasal sinus wall
**AHA:** 2022,2Q,17

**Q30.9 Congenital malformation of nose, unspecified**

✓4th **Q31 Congenital malformations of larynx**
EXCLUDES 1 *congenital laryngeal stridor NOS (P28.89)*

**Q31.0 Web of larynx**
Glottic web of larynx
Subglottic web of larynx
Web of larynx NOS
**DEF:** Congenital malformation of the larynx marked by thin, translucent, or thick fibrotic membrane-like structure between the vocal folds. It is characterized by shortness of breath and stridor.

**Q31.1 Congenital subglottic stenosis**

**Q31.2 Laryngeal hypoplasia**

**Q31.3 Laryngocele**

**Q31.5 Congenital laryngomalacia**

**Q31.8 Other congenital malformations of larynx**
Absence of larynx
Agenesis of larynx
Atresia of larynx
Congenital cleft thyroid cartilage
Congenital fissure of epiglottis
Congenital stenosis of larynx NEC
Posterior cleft of cricoid cartilage

**Q31.9 Congenital malformation of larynx, unspecified**

✓4th **Q32 Congenital malformations of trachea and bronchus**
EXCLUDES 1 *congenital bronchiectasis (Q33.4)*

**Q32.0 Congenital tracheomalacia**

**Q32.1 Other congenital malformations of trachea**
Atresia of trachea
Congenital anomaly of tracheal cartilage
Congenital dilatation of trachea
Congenital malformation of trachea
Congenital stenosis of trachea
Congenital tracheocele

**Q32.2 Congenital bronchomalacia**

**Q32.3 Congenital stenosis of bronchus**

**Q32.4 Other congenital malformations of bronchus**
Absence of bronchus
Agenesis of bronchus
Atresia of bronchus
Congenital diverticulum of bronchus
Congenital malformation of bronchus NOS

✓4th **Q33 Congenital malformations of lung**

**Q33.0 Congenital cystic lung**
Congenital cystic lung disease
Congenital honeycomb lung
Congenital polycystic lung disease
EXCLUDES 1 *cystic fibrosis (E84.0)*
*cystic lung disease, acquired or unspecified (J98.4)*

**Q33.1 Accessory lobe of lung**
Azygos lobe (fissured), lung

**Q33.2 Sequestration of lung**

**Q33.3 Agenesis of lung**
Congenital absence of lung (lobe)

**Q33.4 Congenital bronchiectasis**

**Q33.5 Ectopic tissue in lung**

**Q33.6 Congenital hypoplasia and dysplasia of lung**
EXCLUDES 1 *pulmonary hypoplasia associated with short gestation (P28.0)*

**Q33.8 Other congenital malformations of lung**

**Q33.9 Congenital malformation of lung, unspecified**

✓4th **Q34 Other congenital malformations of respiratory system**
EXCLUDES 2 *congenital central alveolar hypoventilation syndrome (G47.35)*

**Q34.0 Anomaly of pleura**

**Q34.1 Congenital cyst of mediastinum**

**Q34.8 Other specified congenital malformations of respiratory system**
Atresia of nasopharynx

**Q34.9 Congenital malformation of respiratory system, unspecified**
Congenital absence of respiratory system
Congenital anomaly of respiratory system NOS

## Cleft lip and cleft palate (Q35-Q37)

EXCLUDES 2 *Robin's syndrome (Q87.0)*
Use additional code to identify associated malformation of the nose (Q30.2)

✓4th **Q35 Cleft palate**
INCLUDES fissure of palate
palatoschisis
EXCLUDES 1 *cleft palate with cleft lip (Q37.-)*
**DEF:** Congenital fissure or defect of the roof of the mouth opening to the nasal cavity due to failure of embryonic cells to fuse completely.

**Cleft Palate**

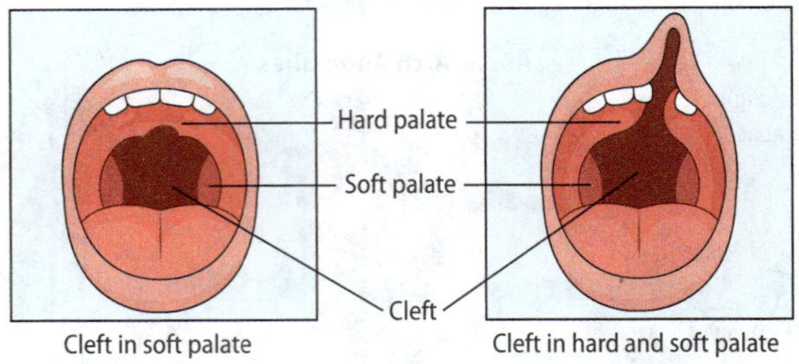


**Q35.1 Cleft hard palate** COM

**Q35.3 Cleft soft palate** COM

**Q35.5 Cleft hard palate with cleft soft palate** COM

**Q35.7 Cleft uvula** COM

**Q35.9 Cleft palate, unspecified** COM
Cleft palate NOS

✓4th **Q36 Cleft lip**
INCLUDES cheiloschisis
congenital fissure of lip
harelip
labium leporinum
EXCLUDES 1 *cleft lip with cleft palate (Q37.-)*
**DEF:** Congenital fissure or opening in the upper lip due to failure of embryonic cells to fuse completely.

**Cleft Lip**

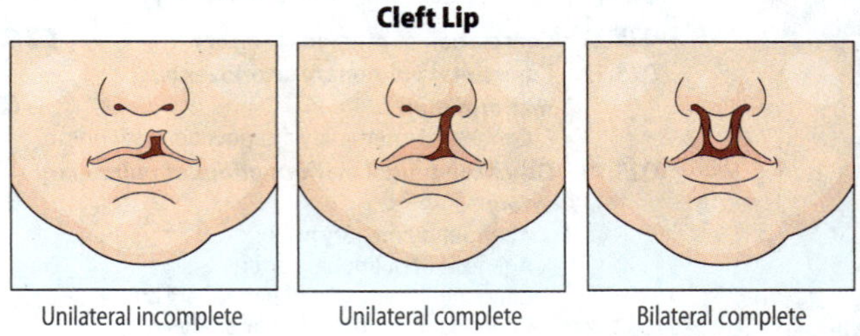


**Q36.0 Cleft lip, bilateral** COM

**Q36.1 Cleft lip, median** COM

**Q36.9 Cleft lip, unilateral** COM
Cleft lip NOS

✓4th **Q37 Cleft palate with cleft lip**
INCLUDES cheilopalatoschisis

**Q37.0 Cleft hard palate with bilateral cleft lip** COM

**Q37.1 Cleft hard palate with unilateral cleft lip** COM
Cleft hard palate with cleft lip NOS

**Q37.2 Cleft soft palate with bilateral cleft lip** COM

**Q37.3** **Cleft soft palate with unilateral cleft lip** COM
Cleft soft palate with cleft lip NOS

**Q37.4** **Cleft hard and soft palate with bilateral cleft lip** COM

**Q37.5** **Cleft hard and soft palate with unilateral cleft lip** COM
Cleft hard and soft palate with cleft lip NOS

**Q37.8** **Unspecified cleft palate with bilateral cleft lip** COM

**Q37.9** **Unspecified cleft palate with unilateral cleft lip** COM
Cleft palate with cleft lip NOS

## Other congenital malformations of the digestive system (Q38-Q45)

✓4th **Q38 Other congenital malformations of tongue, mouth and pharynx**
EXCLUDES 1 *dentofacial anomalies (M26.-)*
*macrostomia (Q18.4)*
*microstomia (Q18.5)*

**Q38.0** **Congenital malformations of lips, not elsewhere classified**
Congenital fistula of lip
Congenital malformation of lip NOS
Van der Woude's syndrome
EXCLUDES 1 *cleft lip (Q36.-)*
*cleft lip with cleft palate (Q37.-)*
*macrocheilia (Q18.6)*
*microcheilia (Q18.7)*

**Q38.1** **Ankyloglossia**
Tongue tie

**Q38.2** **Macroglossia**
Congenital hypertrophy of tongue

**Q38.3** **Other congenital malformations of tongue**
Aglossia
Bifid tongue
Congenital adhesion of tongue
Congenital fissure of tongue
Congenital malformation of tongue NOS
Double tongue
Hypoglossia
Hypoplasia of tongue
Microglossia

**Q38.4** **Congenital malformations of salivary glands and ducts**
Atresia of salivary glands and ducts
Congenital absence of salivary glands and ducts
Congenital accessory salivary glands and ducts
Congenital fistula of salivary gland

**Q38.5** **Congenital malformations of palate, not elsewhere classified**
Congenital absence of uvula
Congenital high arched palate
Congenital malformation of palate NOS
EXCLUDES 1 *cleft palate (Q35.-)*
*cleft palate with cleft lip (Q37.-)*

**Q38.6** **Other congenital malformations of mouth**
Congenital malformation of mouth NOS

**Q38.7** **Congenital pharyngeal pouch**
Congenital diverticulum of pharynx
EXCLUDES 1 *pharyngeal pouch syndrome (D82.1)*

**Q38.8** **Other congenital malformations of pharynx**
Congenital malformation of pharynx NOS
Imperforate pharynx

✓4th **Q39 Congenital malformations of esophagus**

**Q39.0** **Atresia of esophagus without fistula** COM
Atresia of esophagus NOS

**Q39.1** **Atresia of esophagus with tracheo-esophageal fistula** COM
Atresia of esophagus with broncho-esophageal fistula

**Q39.2** **Congenital tracheo-esophageal fistula without atresia** COM
Congenital tracheo-esophageal fistula NOS

**Q39.3** **Congenital stenosis and stricture of esophagus** COM

**Q39.4** **Esophageal web** COM

**Q39.5** **Congenital dilatation of esophagus**
Congenital cardiospasm

**Q39.6** **Congenital diverticulum of esophagus**
Congenital esophageal pouch

**Q39.8** **Other congenital malformations of esophagus**
Congenital absence of esophagus
Congenital displacement of esophagus
Congenital duplication of esophagus

**Q39.9** **Congenital malformation of esophagus, unspecified**

✓4th **Q40 Other congenital malformations of upper alimentary tract**

**Q40.0** **Congenital hypertrophic pyloric stenosis** HCC COM
▶Congenital constriction◀
▶Congenital hypertrophy◀
▶Congenital spasm◀
▶Congenital stenosis◀
▶Congenital stricture◀

**Q40.1** **Congenital hiatus hernia**
Congenital displacement of cardia through esophageal hiatus
EXCLUDES 1 *congenital diaphragmatic hernia (Q79.0)*

**Q40.2** **Other specified congenital malformations of stomach**
Congenital displacement of stomach
Congenital diverticulum of stomach
Congenital duplication of stomach
Congenital hourglass stomach
Megalogastria
Microgastria

**Q40.3** **Congenital malformation of stomach, unspecified**

**Q40.8** **Other specified congenital malformations of upper alimentary tract**

**Q40.9** **Congenital malformation of upper alimentary tract, unspecified**
Congenital anomaly of upper alimentary tract
Congenital deformity of upper alimentary tract

✓4th **Q41 Congenital absence, atresia and stenosis of small intestine**
INCLUDES congenital obstruction, occlusion or stricture of small intestine or intestine NOS
EXCLUDES 1 *cystic fibrosis with intestinal manifestation (E84.11)*
*meconium ileus NOS (without cystic fibrosis) (P76.0)*

**Q41.0** **Congenital absence, atresia and stenosis of duodenum** HCC COM

**Q41.1** **Congenital absence, atresia and stenosis of jejunum** HCC COM
Apple peel syndrome
Imperforate jejunum

**Q41.2** **Congenital absence, atresia and stenosis of ileum** HCC COM

**Q41.8** **Congenital absence, atresia and stenosis of other specified parts of small intestine** HCC COM

**Q41.9** **Congenital absence, atresia and stenosis of small intestine, part unspecified** HCC COM
Congenital absence, atresia and stenosis of intestine NOS

✓4th **Q42 Congenital absence, atresia and stenosis of large intestine**
INCLUDES congenital obstruction, occlusion and stricture of large intestine

**Q42.0** **Congenital absence, atresia and stenosis of rectum with fistula** HCC COM

**Q42.1** **Congenital absence, atresia and stenosis of rectum without fistula** HCC COM
Imperforate rectum

**Q42.2** **Congenital absence, atresia and stenosis of anus with fistula** HCC COM

**Q42.3** **Congenital absence, atresia and stenosis of anus without fistula** HCC COM
Imperforate anus

**Q42.8** **Congenital absence, atresia and stenosis of other parts of large intestine** HCC COM

**Q42.9** **Congenital absence, atresia and stenosis of large intestine, part unspecified** HCC COM

✓4th **Q43 Other congenital malformations of intestine**

**Q43.0** **Meckel's diverticulum (displaced) (hypertrophic)**
Persistent omphalomesenteric duct
Persistent vitelline duct
**DEF:** Congenital, abnormal remnant of embryonic digestive system development that leaves a sacculation or outpouching from the wall of the small intestine near the terminal part of the ileum made of acid-secreting tissue as in the stomach.

**Q43.1** **Hirschsprung's disease** HCC COM
Aganglionosis
Congenital (aganglionic) megacolon
**DEF:** Congenital enlargement or dilation of the colon, with the absence of nerve cells in a segment of colon distally that causes the inability to defecate.

**Q43.2** **Other congenital functional disorders of colon** HCC COM
Congenital dilatation of colon

**Q43.3 Congenital malformations of intestinal fixation** HCC COM
Congenital omental, anomalous adhesions [bands]
Congenital peritoneal adhesions [bands]
Incomplete rotation of cecum and colon
Insufficient rotation of cecum and colon
Jackson's membrane
Malrotation of colon
Rotation failure of cecum and colon
Universal mesentery

**Q43.4 Duplication of intestine**

**Q43.5 Ectopic anus**

**Q43.6 Congenital fistula of rectum and anus**
EXCLUDES 1 *congenital fistula of anus with absence, atresia and stenosis (Q42.2)*
*congenital fistula of rectum with absence, atresia and stenosis (Q42.Ø)*
*congenital rectovaginal fistula (Q52.2)*
*congenital urethrorectal fistula (Q64.73)*
*pilonidal fistula or sinus (LØ5.-)*

**Q43.7 Persistent cloaca**
Cloaca NOS

**Q43.8 Other specified congenital malformations of intestine**
Congenital blind loop syndrome
Congenital diverticulitis, colon
Congenital diverticulum, intestine
Dolichocolon
Megaloappendix
Megaloduodenum
Microcolon
Transposition of appendix
Transposition of colon
Transposition of intestine
**AHA:** 2013,2Q,31

**Q43.9 Congenital malformation of intestine, unspecified**

✓4th **Q44 Congenital malformations of gallbladder, bile ducts and liver**

**Q44.Ø Agenesis, aplasia and hypoplasia of gallbladder**
Congenital absence of gallbladder

**Q44.1 Other congenital malformations of gallbladder**
Congenital malformation of gallbladder NOS
Intrahepatic gallbladder

**Q44.2 Atresia of bile ducts** HCC

**Q44.3 Congenital stenosis and stricture of bile ducts** HCC

**Q44.4 Choledochal cyst**

**Q44.5 Other congenital malformations of bile ducts**
Accessory hepatic duct
Biliary duct duplication
Congenital malformation of bile duct NOS
Cystic duct duplication

**Q44.6 Cystic disease of liver**
Fibrocystic disease of liver

✓5th **Q44.7 Other congenital malformations of liver**
Code also, if applicable, associated malformations affecting other systems
**AHA:** 2023,4Q,37-38

**Q44.7Ø Other congenital malformation of liver, unspecified**
Congenital malformation of liver, NOS

**Q44.71 Alagille syndrome** HCC
Alagille-Watson syndrome

**Q44.79 Other congenital malformations of liver**
Accessory liver
Congenital absence of liver
Congenital hepatomegaly

✓4th **Q45 Other congenital malformations of digestive system**
EXCLUDES 2 *congenital diaphragmatic hernia (Q79.Ø)*
*congenital hiatus hernia (Q4Ø.1)*

**Q45.Ø Agenesis, aplasia and hypoplasia of pancreas**
Congenital absence of pancreas

**Q45.1 Annular pancreas**

**Q45.2 Congenital pancreatic cyst**

**Q45.3 Other congenital malformations of pancreas and pancreatic duct**
Accessory pancreas
Congenital malformation of pancreas or pancreatic duct NOS
EXCLUDES 1 *congenital diabetes mellitus (E1Ø.-)*
*cystic fibrosis (E84.Ø-E84.9)*
*fibrocystic disease of pancreas (E84.-)*
*neonatal diabetes mellitus (P7Ø.2)*

**Q45.8 Other specified congenital malformations of digestive system**
Absence (complete) (partial) of alimentary tract NOS
Duplication of digestive system
Malposition, congenital of digestive system

**Q45.9 Congenital malformation of digestive system, unspecified**
Congenital anomaly of digestive system
Congenital deformity of digestive system

## Congenital malformations of genital organs (Q5Ø-Q56)

EXCLUDES 1 *androgen insensitivity syndrome (E34.5-)*
*syndromes associated with anomalies in the number and form of chromosomes (Q9Ø-Q99)*

✓4th **Q5Ø Congenital malformations of ovaries, fallopian tubes and broad ligaments**

✓5th **Q5Ø.Ø Congenital absence of ovary**
EXCLUDES 1 *Turner's syndrome (Q96.-)*

**Q5Ø.Ø1 Congenital absence of ovary, unilateral**

**Q5Ø.Ø2 Congenital absence of ovary, bilateral**

**Q5Ø.1 Developmental ovarian cyst**

**Q5Ø.2 Congenital torsion of ovary**

✓5th **Q5Ø.3 Other congenital malformations of ovary**

**Q5Ø.31 Accessory ovary**

**Q5Ø.32 Ovarian streak**
46, XX with streak gonads

**Q5Ø.39 Other congenital malformation of ovary**
Congenital malformation of ovary NOS

**Q5Ø.4 Embryonic cyst of fallopian tube**
Fimbrial cyst

**Q5Ø.5 Embryonic cyst of broad ligament**
Epoophoron cyst
Parovarian cyst

**Q5Ø.6 Other congenital malformations of fallopian tube and broad ligament**
Absence of fallopian tube and broad ligament
Accessory fallopian tube and broad ligament
Atresia of fallopian tube and broad ligament
Congenital malformation of fallopian tube or broad ligament NOS

✓4th **Q51 Congenital malformations of uterus and cervix**

**Q51.Ø Agenesis and aplasia of uterus**
Congenital absence of uterus

✓5th **Q51.1 Doubling of uterus with doubling of cervix and vagina**

**Q51.1Ø Doubling of uterus with doubling of cervix and vagina without obstruction**
Doubling of uterus with doubling of cervix and vagina NOS

**Q51.11 Doubling of uterus with doubling of cervix and vagina with obstruction**

✓5th **Q51.2 Other doubling of uterus**
Doubling of uterus NOS
Septate uterus
**AHA:** 2018,4Q,27

**Q51.21 Complete doubling of uterus**
Complete septate uterus

**Q51.22 Partial doubling of uterus**
Partial septate uterus

**Q51.28 Other and unspecified doubling of uterus**
Septate uterus NOS

**Q51.3 Bicornate uterus**
Bicornate uterus, complete or partial

**Q51.4 Unicornate uterus**
Unicornate uterus with or without a separate uterine horn
Uterus with only one functioning horn

**Q51.5 Agenesis and aplasia of cervix**
Congenital absence of cervix

**Q51.6 Embryonic cyst of cervix**

**Q51.7 Congenital fistulae between uterus and digestive and urinary tracts**

✓5th **Q51.8 Other congenital malformations of uterus and cervix**

✓6th **Q51.81 Other congenital malformations of uterus**

**Q51.81Ø Arcuate uterus**
Arcuatus uterus

**Q51.811 Hypoplasia of uterus**

**Q51.818 Other congenital malformations of uterus**
Mullerian anomaly of uterus NEC

✓6th **Q51.82 Other congenital malformations of cervix**

**Q51.82Ø Cervical duplication**

**Q51.821 Hypoplasia of cervix**

**Q51.828 Other congenital malformations of cervix**

**Q51.9 Congenital malformation of uterus and cervix, unspecified**

**Q52 Other congenital malformations of female genitalia**

**Q52.0 Congenital absence of vagina**
Vaginal agenesis, total or partial

**Q52.1 Doubling of vagina**
EXCLUDES 1 *doubling of vagina with doubling of uterus and cervix (Q51.1-)*

**Q52.10 Doubling of vagina, unspecified**
Septate vagina NOS

**Q52.11 Transverse vaginal septum**

**Q52.12 Longitudinal vaginal septum**
AHA: 2016,4Q,58-59

**Q52.120 Longitudinal vaginal septum, nonobstructing**

**Q52.121 Longitudinal vaginal septum, obstructing, right side**

**Q52.122 Longitudinal vaginal septum, obstructing, left side**

**Q52.123 Longitudinal vaginal septum, microperforate, right side**

**Q52.124 Longitudinal vaginal septum, microperforate, left side**

**Q52.129 Other and unspecified longitudinal vaginal septum**

**Q52.2 Congenital rectovaginal fistula**
EXCLUDES 1 *cloaca (Q43.7)*

**Q52.3 Imperforate hymen**
DEF: Obstructive anomaly of vagina, characterized by complete closure of the membranous fold around the external opening of the vagina, obstructing the vaginal introitus.

**Q52.4 Other congenital malformations of vagina**
Canal of Nuck cyst, congenital
Congenital malformation of vagina NOS
Embryonic vaginal cyst
Gartner's duct cyst
AHA: 2022,2Q,15

**Q52.5 Fusion of labia**

**Q52.6 Congenital malformation of clitoris**

**Q52.7 Other and unspecified congenital malformations of vulva**

**Q52.70 Unspecified congenital malformations of vulva**
Congenital malformation of vulva NOS

**Q52.71 Congenital absence of vulva**

**Q52.79 Other congenital malformations of vulva**
Congenital cyst of vulva

**Q52.8 Other specified congenital malformations of female genitalia**

**Q52.9 Congenital malformation of female genitalia, unspecified**

**Q53 Undescended and ectopic testicle**

**Q53.0 Ectopic testis**

**Q53.00 Ectopic testis, unspecified**

**Q53.01 Ectopic testis, unilateral**

**Q53.02 Ectopic testes, bilateral**

**Q53.1 Undescended testicle, unilateral**
AHA: 2017,4Q,22-23

**Q53.10 Unspecified undescended testicle, unilateral**

**Q53.11 Abdominal testis, unilateral**

**Q53.111 Unilateral intraabdominal testis**

**Q53.112 Unilateral inguinal testis**

**Q53.12 Ectopic perineal testis, unilateral**

**Q53.13 Unilateral high scrotal testis**

**Q53.2 Undescended testicle, bilateral**
AHA: 2017,4Q,22-23

**Q53.20 Undescended testicle, unspecified, bilateral**

**Q53.21 Abdominal testis, bilateral**

**Q53.211 Bilateral intraabdominal testes**

**Q53.212 Bilateral inguinal testes**

**Q53.22 Ectopic perineal testis, bilateral**

**Q53.23 Bilateral high scrotal testes**

**Q53.9 Undescended testicle, unspecified**
Cryptorchism NOS

**Q54 Hypospadias**
EXCLUDES 1 *epispadias (Q64.0)*
DEF: Abnormal opening of the urethra on the ventral (underside) surface of the penis.

**Hypospadias**

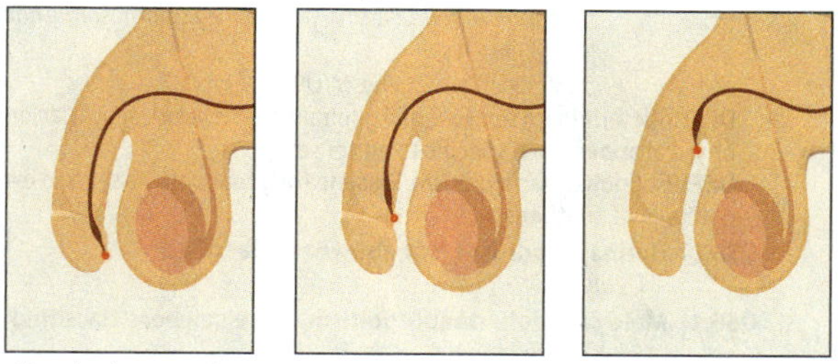

Glanular hypospadias | Coronal hypospadias | Penile hypospadias

**Q54.0 Hypospadias, balanic**
Hypospadias, coronal
Hypospadias, glandular

**Q54.1 Hypospadias, penile**

**Q54.2 Hypospadias, penoscrotal**

**Q54.3 Hypospadias, perineal**

**Q54.4 Congenital chordee**
Chordee without hypospadias

**Q54.8 Other hypospadias**
Hypospadias with intersex state

**Q54.9 Hypospadias, unspecified**

**Q55 Other congenital malformations of male genital organs**
EXCLUDES 1 *congenital hydrocele (P83.5)*
*hypospadias (Q54.-)*

**Q55.0 Absence and aplasia of testis**
Monorchism

**Q55.1 Hypoplasia of testis and scrotum**
Fusion of testes

**Q55.2 Other and unspecified congenital malformations of testis and scrotum**

**Q55.20 Unspecified congenital malformations of testis and scrotum**
Congenital malformation of testis or scrotum NOS

**Q55.21 Polyorchism**
DEF: Congenital anomaly in which there are more than two testes.

**Q55.22 Retractile testis**

**Q55.23 Scrotal transposition**

**Q55.29 Other congenital malformations of testis and scrotum**

**Q55.3 Atresia of vas deferens**
Code first any associated cystic fibrosis (E84.-)

**Q55.4 Other congenital malformations of vas deferens, epididymis, seminal vesicles and prostate**
Absence or aplasia of prostate
Absence or aplasia of spermatic cord
Congenital malformation of vas deferens, epididymis, seminal vesicles or prostate NOS

**Q55.5 Congenital absence and aplasia of penis**

**Q55.6 Other congenital malformations of penis**

**Q55.61 Curvature of penis (lateral)**

**Q55.62 Hypoplasia of penis**
Micropenis

**Q55.63 Congenital torsion of penis**
EXCLUDES 1 *acquired torsion of penis (N48.82)*

**Q55.64 Hidden penis**
Buried penis
Concealed penis
EXCLUDES 1 *acquired buried penis (N48.83)*

**Q55.69 Other congenital malformation of penis**
Congenital malformation of penis NOS

**Q55.7 Congenital vasocutaneous fistula**

**Q55.8 Other specified congenital malformations of male genital organs**

**Q55.9 Congenital malformation of male genital organ, unspecified**
Congenital anomaly of male genital organ
Congenital deformity of male genital organ

Chapter 17. Congenital Malformations, Deformations, Chromosomal Abnormalities, and Genetic Disorders

**✓4th Q56 Indeterminate sex and pseudohermaphroditism**

EXCLUDES 1 *46, XX true hermaphrodite (Q99.1)*
*androgen insensitivity syndrome (E34.5-)*
*chimera 46, XX/46, XY true hermaphrodite (Q99.Ø)*
*female pseudohermaphroditism with adrenocortical disorder (E25.-)*
*pseudohermaphroditism with specified chromosomal anomaly (Q96-Q99)*
*pure gonadal dysgenesis (Q99.1)*

**DEF:** Indeterminate sex: External genitalia that is nondescript, lacking the physical appearance specific to either sex.
**DEF:** Pseudohermaphroditism: Presence of gonads of one sex and external genitalia of another sex.

**Q56.Ø Hermaphroditism, not elsewhere classified**
Ovotestis

**Q56.1 Male pseudohermaphroditism, not elsewhere classified**
46, XY with streak gonads
Male pseudohermaphroditism NOS

**Q56.2 Female pseudohermaphroditism, not elsewhere classified**
Female pseudohermaphroditism NOS

**Q56.3 Pseudohermaphroditism, unspecified**

**Q56.4 Indeterminate sex, unspecified**
Ambiguous genitalia

## Congenital malformations of the urinary system (Q6Ø-Q64)

**✓4th Q6Ø Renal agenesis and other reduction defects of kidney**

INCLUDES congenital absence of kidney
congenital atrophy of kidney
infantile atrophy of kidney

**Q6Ø.Ø Renal agenesis, unilateral**
**Q6Ø.1 Renal agenesis, bilateral**
**Q6Ø.2 Renal agenesis, unspecified**
**Q6Ø.3 Renal hypoplasia, unilateral**
**Q6Ø.4 Renal hypoplasia, bilateral**
**Q6Ø.5 Renal hypoplasia, unspecified**
**Q6Ø.6 Potter's syndrome**

**✓4th Q61 Cystic kidney disease**

EXCLUDES 1 *acquired cyst of kidney (N28.1)*
*Potter's syndrome (Q6Ø.6)*

**✓5th Q61.Ø Congenital renal cyst**

**Q61.ØØ Congenital renal cyst, unspecified**
Cyst of kidney NOS (congenital)

**Q61.Ø1 Congenital single renal cyst**

**Q61.Ø2 Congenital multiple renal cysts**

**✓5th Q61.1 Polycystic kidney, infantile type**
Polycystic kidney, autosomal recessive

**Q61.11 Cystic dilatation of collecting ducts** COM

**Q61.19 Other polycystic kidney, infantile type** COM

**Q61.2 Polycystic kidney, adult type**
Polycystic kidney, autosomal dominant

**Q61.3 Polycystic kidney, unspecified**
**AHA:** 2016,3Q,22

**Q61.4 Renal dysplasia**
Multicystic dysplastic kidney
Multicystic kidney (development)
Multicystic kidney disease
Multicystic renal dysplasia
EXCLUDES 1 *polycystic kidney disease (Q61.11-Q61.3)*

**Q61.5 Medullary cystic kidney**
Nephronophthisis
Sponge kidney NOS
**DEF:** Sponge kidney: Dilated collecting tubules that are usually asymptomatic. Calcinosis in tubules may cause renal insufficiency.

**Q61.8 Other cystic kidney diseases**
Fibrocystic kidney
Fibrocystic renal degeneration or disease

**Q61.9 Cystic kidney disease, unspecified**
Meckel-Gruber syndrome

**✓4th Q62 Congenital obstructive defects of renal pelvis and congenital malformations of ureter**

**Q62.Ø Congenital hydronephrosis**

**✓5th Q62.1 Congenital occlusion of ureter**
Atresia and stenosis of ureter

**Q62.1Ø Congenital occlusion of ureter, unspecified**

**Q62.11 Congenital occlusion of ureteropelvic junction**

**Q62.12 Congenital occlusion of ureterovesical orifice**

**Q62.2 Congenital megaureter**
Congenital dilatation of ureter

**✓5th Q62.3 Other obstructive defects of renal pelvis and ureter**

**Q62.31 Congenital ureterocele, orthotopic**

**Q62.32 Cecoureterocele**
Ectopic ureterocele

**Q62.39 Other obstructive defects of renal pelvis and ureter**
Ureteropelvic junction obstruction NOS

**Q62.4 Agenesis of ureter**
Congenital absence ureter

**Q62.5 Duplication of ureter**
Accessory ureter
Double ureter

**✓5th Q62.6 Malposition of ureter**

**Q62.6Ø Malposition of ureter, unspecified**
**Q62.61 Deviation of ureter**
**Q62.62 Displacement of ureter**
**Q62.63 Anomalous implantation of ureter**
Ectopia of ureter
Ectopic ureter
**Q62.69 Other malposition of ureter**

**Q62.7 Congenital vesico-uretero-renal reflux**

**Q62.8 Other congenital malformations of ureter**
Anomaly of ureter NOS

**✓4th Q63 Other congenital malformations of kidney**

EXCLUDES 1 *congenital nephrotic syndrome (NØ4.-)*

**Q63.Ø Accessory kidney**

**Q63.1 Lobulated, fused and horseshoe kidney**

**Q63.2 Ectopic kidney**
Congenital displaced kidney
Malrotation of kidney

**Q63.3 Hyperplastic and giant kidney**
Compensatory hypertrophy of kidney

**Q63.8 Other specified congenital malformations of kidney**
Congenital renal calculi

**Q63.9 Congenital malformation of kidney, unspecified**

**✓4th Q64 Other congenital malformations of urinary system**

**Q64.Ø Epispadias**
EXCLUDES 1 *hypospadias (Q54.-)*

**Epispadias**

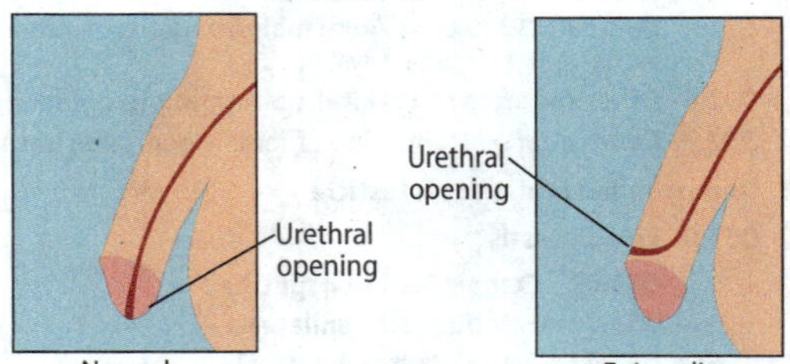


Normal Epispadias

**✓5th Q64.1 Exstrophy of urinary bladder**

**Q64.1Ø Exstrophy of urinary bladder, unspecified** COM
Ectopia vesicae

**Q64.11 Supravesical fissure of urinary bladder** COM

**Q64.12 Cloacal exstrophy of urinary bladder** COM

**Q64.19 Other exstrophy of urinary bladder** COM
Extroversion of bladder

**Q64.2 Congenital posterior urethral valves**

**✓5th Q64.3 Other atresia and stenosis of urethra and bladder neck**

**Q64.31 Congenital bladder neck obstruction**
Congenital obstruction of vesicourethral orifice

**Q64.32 Congenital stricture of urethra**

**Q64.33 Congenital stricture of urinary meatus**

**Q64.39 Other atresia and stenosis of urethra and bladder neck**
Atresia and stenosis of urethra and bladder neck NOS

**Q64.4 Malformation of urachus**
Cyst of urachus
Patent urachus
Prolapse of urachus

**Q64.5 Congenital absence of bladder and urethra**

**Q64.6 Congenital diverticulum of bladder**

✓5th **Q64.7 Other and unspecified congenital malformations of bladder and urethra**
EXCLUDES 1 *congenital prolapse of bladder (mucosa) (Q79.4)*
**Q64.70 Unspecified congenital malformation of bladder and urethra**
Malformation of bladder or urethra NOS
**Q64.71 Congenital prolapse of urethra**
**Q64.72 Congenital prolapse of urinary meatus**
**Q64.73 Congenital urethrorectal fistula**
**Q64.74 Double urethra**
**Q64.75 Double urinary meatus**
**Q64.79 Other congenital malformations of bladder and urethra**
**Q64.8 Other specified congenital malformations of urinary system**
**Q64.9 Congenital malformation of urinary system, unspecified**
Congenital anomaly NOS of urinary system
Congenital deformity NOS of urinary system

## Congenital malformations and deformations of the musculoskeletal system (Q65-Q79)

✓4th **Q65 Congenital deformities of hip**
EXCLUDES 1 *clicking hip (R29.4)*
✓5th **Q65.0 Congenital dislocation of hip, unilateral**
**Q65.00 Congenital dislocation of unspecified hip, unilateral** COM
**Q65.01 Congenital dislocation of right hip, unilateral** COM
**Q65.02 Congenital dislocation of left hip, unilateral** COM
**Q65.1 Congenital dislocation of hip, bilateral** COM
**Q65.2 Congenital dislocation of hip, unspecified** COM
✓5th **Q65.3 Congenital partial dislocation of hip, unilateral**
**Q65.30 Congenital partial dislocation of unspecified hip, unilateral** COM
**Q65.31 Congenital partial dislocation of right hip, unilateral** COM
**Q65.32 Congenital partial dislocation of left hip, unilateral** COM
**Q65.4 Congenital partial dislocation of hip, bilateral** COM
**Q65.5 Congenital partial dislocation of hip, unspecified** COM
**Q65.6 Congenital unstable hip** COM
Congenital dislocatable hip
✓5th **Q65.8 Other congenital deformities of hip**
**Q65.81 Congenital coxa valga** COM
**Q65.82 Congenital coxa vara** COM
**Q65.89 Other specified congenital deformities of hip** COM
Anteversion of femoral neck
Congenital acetabular dysplasia
**Q65.9 Congenital deformity of hip, unspecified** COM

✓4th **Q66 Congenital deformities of feet**
EXCLUDES 1 *reduction defects of feet (Q72.-)*
*valgus deformities (acquired) (M21.0-)*
*varus deformities (acquired) (M21.1-)*
**AHA:** 2019,4Q,13
✓5th **Q66.0 Congenital talipes equinovarus**
**Q66.00 Congenital talipes equinovarus, unspecified foot**
**Q66.01 Congenital talipes equinovarus, right foot**
**Q66.02 Congenital talipes equinovarus, left foot**
✓5th **Q66.1 Congenital talipes calcaneovarus**
**Q66.10 Congenital talipes calcaneovarus, unspecified foot**
**Q66.11 Congenital talipes calcaneovarus, right foot**
**Q66.12 Congenital talipes calcaneovarus, left foot**
✓5th **Q66.2 Congenital metatarsus (primus) varus**
**AHA:** 2016,4Q,59
✓6th **Q66.21 Congenital metatarsus primus varus**
**Q66.211 Congenital metatarsus primus varus, right foot**
**Q66.212 Congenital metatarsus primus varus, left foot**
**Q66.219 Congenital metatarsus primus varus, unspecified foot**
✓6th **Q66.22 Congenital metatarsus adductus**
Congenital metatarsus varus
**Q66.221 Congenital metatarsus adductus, right foot**
**Q66.222 Congenital metatarsus adductus, left foot**
**Q66.229 Congenital metatarsus adductus, unspecified foot**
✓5th **Q66.3 Other congenital varus deformities of feet**
Hallux varus, congenital
**AHA:** 2023,3Q,20
**Q66.30 Other congenital varus deformities of feet, unspecified foot**
**Q66.31 Other congenital varus deformities of feet, right foot**
**Q66.32 Other congenital varus deformities of feet, left foot**
✓5th **Q66.4 Congenital talipes calcaneovalgus**
**Q66.40 Congenital talipes calcaneovalgus, unspecified foot**
**Q66.41 Congenital talipes calcaneovalgus, right foot**
**Q66.42 Congenital talipes calcaneovalgus, left foot**
✓5th **Q66.5 Congenital pes planus**
Congenital flat foot
Congenital rigid flat foot
Congenital spastic (everted) flat foot
EXCLUDES 1 *pes planus, acquired (M21.4)*
**Q66.50 Congenital pes planus, unspecified foot**
**Q66.51 Congenital pes planus, right foot**
**Q66.52 Congenital pes planus, left foot**
**Q66.6 Other congenital valgus deformities of feet**
Congenital metatarsus valgus
✓5th **Q66.7 Congenital pes cavus**
**Q66.70 Congenital pes cavus, unspecified foot**
**Q66.71 Congenital pes cavus, right foot**
**Q66.72 Congenital pes cavus, left foot**
✓5th **Q66.8 Other congenital deformities of feet**
**Q66.80 Congenital vertical talus deformity, unspecified foot**
**Q66.81 Congenital vertical talus deformity, right foot**
**Q66.82 Congenital vertical talus deformity, left foot**
**Q66.89 Other specified congenital deformities of feet**
Congenital asymmetric talipes
Congenital clubfoot NOS
Congenital talipes NOS
Congenital tarsal coalition
Hammer toe, congenital
**DEF:** Clubfoot: Congenital anomaly of the foot with the heel elevated and rotated outward and the toes pointing inward.
✓5th **Q66.9 Congenital deformity of feet, unspecified**
**Q66.90 Congenital deformity of feet, unspecified, unspecified foot**
**Q66.91 Congenital deformity of feet, unspecified, right foot**
**Q66.92 Congenital deformity of feet, unspecified, left foot**

✓4th **Q67 Congenital musculoskeletal deformities of head, face, spine and chest**
EXCLUDES 1 *congenital malformation syndromes classified to Q87.-*
*Potter's syndrome (Q60.6)*
**Q67.0 Congenital facial asymmetry**
**Q67.1 Congenital compression facies**
**Q67.2 Dolichocephaly**
EXCLUDES 1 *sagittal craniosynostosis (Q75.01)*
**Q67.3 Plagiocephaly**
EXCLUDES 1 *coronal craniosynostosis (Q75.02-)*
*lambdoid craniosynostosis (Q75.04-)*
**Q67.4 Other congenital deformities of skull, face and jaw**
Congenital depressions in skull
Congenital hemifacial atrophy or hypertrophy
Deviation of nasal septum, congenital
Squashed or bent nose, congenital
EXCLUDES 1 *dentofacial anomalies [including malocclusion] (M26.-)*
*syphilitic saddle nose (A50.5)*
**DEF:** Deviated septum: Condition in which the nasal septum, a thin wall composed of cartilage and bone that separates the two nostrils, is crooked or displaced from the midline.
**Q67.5 Congenital deformity of spine**
Congenital postural scoliosis
Congenital scoliosis NOS
EXCLUDES 1 *infantile idiopathic scoliosis (M41.0)*
*scoliosis due to congenital bony malformation (Q76.3)*
**AHA:** 2014,4Q,26
**Q67.6 Pectus excavatum**
Congenital funnel chest
**Q67.7 Pectus carinatum**
Congenital pigeon chest
**Q67.8 Other congenital deformities of chest**
Congenital deformity of chest wall NOS

**Q68 Other congenital musculoskeletal deformities**

EXCLUDES 1 *reduction defects of limb(s) (Q71-Q73)*

EXCLUDES 2 *congenital myotonic chondrodystrophy (G71.13)*

**Q68.Ø Congenital deformity of sternocleidomastoid muscle**
Congenital (sternomastoid) torticollis
Congenital contracture of sternocleidomastoid (muscle)
Sternomastoid tumor (congenital)

**Q68.1 Congenital deformity of finger(s) and hand**
Congenital clubfinger
Spade-like hand (congenital)

**Q68.2 Congenital deformity of knee**
Congenital dislocation of knee
Congenital genu recurvatum

**Q68.3 Congenital bowing of femur**
EXCLUDES 1 *anteversion of femur (neck) (Q65.89)*

**Q68.4 Congenital bowing of tibia and fibula**

**Q68.5 Congenital bowing of long bones of leg, unspecified**

**Q68.6 Discoid meniscus**

**Q68.8 Other specified congenital musculoskeletal deformities**
Congenital deformity of clavicle
Congenital deformity of elbow
Congenital deformity of forearm
Congenital deformity of scapula
Congenital deformity of wrist
Congenital dislocation of elbow
Congenital dislocation of shoulder
Congenital dislocation of wrist

**Q69 Polydactyly**

**Q69.Ø Accessory finger(s)**

**Q69.1 Accessory thumb(s)**

**Q69.2 Accessory toe(s)**
Accessory hallux

**Q69.9 Polydactyly, unspecified**
Supernumerary digit(s) NOS

**Q7Ø Syndactyly**

**Q7Ø.Ø Fused fingers**
Complex syndactyly of fingers with synostosis

**Q7Ø.ØØ Fused fingers, unspecified hand**
**Q7Ø.Ø1 Fused fingers, right hand**
**Q7Ø.Ø2 Fused fingers, left hand**
**Q7Ø.Ø3 Fused fingers, bilateral**

**Q7Ø.1 Webbed fingers**
Simple syndactyly of fingers without synostosis

**Q7Ø.1Ø Webbed fingers, unspecified hand**
**Q7Ø.11 Webbed fingers, right hand**
**Q7Ø.12 Webbed fingers, left hand**
**Q7Ø.13 Webbed fingers, bilateral**

**Q7Ø.2 Fused toes**
Complex syndactyly of toes with synostosis

**Q7Ø.2Ø Fused toes, unspecified foot**
**Q7Ø.21 Fused toes, right foot**
**Q7Ø.22 Fused toes, left foot**
**Q7Ø.23 Fused toes, bilateral**

**Q7Ø.3 Webbed toes**
Simple syndactyly of toes without synostosis

**Q7Ø.3Ø Webbed toes, unspecified foot**
**Q7Ø.31 Webbed toes, right foot**
**Q7Ø.32 Webbed toes, left foot**
**Q7Ø.33 Webbed toes, bilateral**

**Q7Ø.4 Polysyndactyly, unspecified**
EXCLUDES 1 *specified syndactyly of hand and feet - code to specified conditions (Q7Ø.Ø-Q7Ø.3-)*

**Q7Ø.9 Syndactyly, unspecified**
Symphalangy NOS

**Q71 Reduction defects of upper limb**

**Q71.Ø Congenital complete absence of upper limb**

**Q71.ØØ Congenital complete absence of unspecified upper limb**
**Q71.Ø1 Congenital complete absence of right upper limb**
**Q71.Ø2 Congenital complete absence of left upper limb**
**Q71.Ø3 Congenital complete absence of upper limb, bilateral**

**Q71.1 Congenital absence of upper arm and forearm with hand present**

**Q71.1Ø Congenital absence of unspecified upper arm and forearm with hand present**
**Q71.11 Congenital absence of right upper arm and forearm with hand present**
**Q71.12 Congenital absence of left upper arm and forearm with hand present**
**Q71.13 Congenital absence of upper arm and forearm with hand present, bilateral**

**Q71.2 Congenital absence of both forearm and hand**

**Q71.2Ø Congenital absence of both forearm and hand, unspecified upper limb**
**Q71.21 Congenital absence of both forearm and hand, right upper limb**
**Q71.22 Congenital absence of both forearm and hand, left upper limb**
**Q71.23 Congenital absence of both forearm and hand, bilateral**

**Q71.3 Congenital absence of hand and finger**

**Q71.3Ø Congenital absence of unspecified hand and finger**
**Q71.31 Congenital absence of right hand and finger**
**Q71.32 Congenital absence of left hand and finger**
**Q71.33 Congenital absence of hand and finger, bilateral**

**Q71.4 Longitudinal reduction defect of radius**
Clubhand (congenital)
Radial clubhand

**Q71.4Ø Longitudinal reduction defect of unspecified radius**
**Q71.41 Longitudinal reduction defect of right radius**
**Q71.42 Longitudinal reduction defect of left radius**
**Q71.43 Longitudinal reduction defect of radius, bilateral**

**Q71.5 Longitudinal reduction defect of ulna**

**Q71.5Ø Longitudinal reduction defect of unspecified ulna**
**Q71.51 Longitudinal reduction defect of right ulna**
**Q71.52 Longitudinal reduction defect of left ulna**
**Q71.53 Longitudinal reduction defect of ulna, bilateral**

**Q71.6 Lobster-claw hand**

**Q71.6Ø Lobster-claw hand, unspecified hand**
**Q71.61 Lobster-claw right hand**
**Q71.62 Lobster-claw left hand**
**Q71.63 Lobster-claw hand, bilateral**

**Q71.8 Other reduction defects of upper limb**

**Q71.81 Congenital shortening of upper limb**

**Q71.811 Congenital shortening of right upper limb**
**Q71.812 Congenital shortening of left upper limb**
**Q71.813 Congenital shortening of upper limb, bilateral**
**Q71.819 Congenital shortening of unspecified upper limb**

**Q71.89 Other reduction defects of upper limb**

**Q71.891 Other reduction defects of right upper limb**
**Q71.892 Other reduction defects of left upper limb**
**Q71.893 Other reduction defects of upper limb, bilateral**
**Q71.899 Other reduction defects of unspecified upper limb**

**Q71.9 Unspecified reduction defect of upper limb**

**Q71.9Ø Unspecified reduction defect of unspecified upper limb**
**Q71.91 Unspecified reduction defect of right upper limb**
**Q71.92 Unspecified reduction defect of left upper limb**
**Q71.93 Unspecified reduction defect of upper limb, bilateral**

**Q72 Reduction defects of lower limb**

**Q72.Ø Congenital complete absence of lower limb**

**Q72.ØØ Congenital complete absence of unspecified lower limb**
**Q72.Ø1 Congenital complete absence of right lower limb**
**Q72.Ø2 Congenital complete absence of left lower limb**
**Q72.Ø3 Congenital complete absence of lower limb, bilateral**

**Q72.1 Congenital absence of thigh and lower leg with foot present**

**Q72.1Ø Congenital absence of unspecified thigh and lower leg with foot present**
**Q72.11 Congenital absence of right thigh and lower leg with foot present**
**Q72.12 Congenital absence of left thigh and lower leg with foot present**
**Q72.13 Congenital absence of thigh and lower leg with foot present, bilateral**

**Q72.2 Congenital absence of both lower leg and foot**

**Q72.2Ø Congenital absence of both lower leg and foot, unspecified lower limb**
**Q72.21 Congenital absence of both lower leg and foot, right lower limb**

Q72.22 **Congenital absence of both lower leg and foot, left lower limb**
Q72.23 **Congenital absence of both lower leg and foot, bilateral**

Q72.3 **Congenital absence of foot and toe(s)**
Q72.30 **Congenital absence of unspecified foot and toe(s)**
Q72.31 **Congenital absence of right foot and toe(s)**
Q72.32 **Congenital absence of left foot and toe(s)**
Q72.33 **Congenital absence of foot and toe(s), bilateral**

Q72.4 **Longitudinal reduction defect of femur**
Proximal femoral focal deficiency
Q72.40 **Longitudinal reduction defect of unspecified femur**
Q72.41 **Longitudinal reduction defect of right femur**
Q72.42 **Longitudinal reduction defect of left femur**
Q72.43 **Longitudinal reduction defect of femur, bilateral**

Q72.5 **Longitudinal reduction defect of tibia**
Q72.50 **Longitudinal reduction defect of unspecified tibia**
Q72.51 **Longitudinal reduction defect of right tibia**
Q72.52 **Longitudinal reduction defect of left tibia**
Q72.53 **Longitudinal reduction defect of tibia, bilateral**

Q72.6 **Longitudinal reduction defect of fibula**
Q72.60 **Longitudinal reduction defect of unspecified fibula**
Q72.61 **Longitudinal reduction defect of right fibula**
Q72.62 **Longitudinal reduction defect of left fibula**
Q72.63 **Longitudinal reduction defect of fibula, bilateral**

Q72.7 **Split foot**
Q72.70 **Split foot, unspecified lower limb**
Q72.71 **Split foot, right lower limb**
Q72.72 **Split foot, left lower limb**
Q72.73 **Split foot, bilateral**

Q72.8 **Other reduction defects of lower limb**
Q72.81 **Congenital shortening of lower limb**
Q72.811 **Congenital shortening of right lower limb**
Q72.812 **Congenital shortening of left lower limb**
Q72.813 **Congenital shortening of lower limb, bilateral**
Q72.819 **Congenital shortening of unspecified lower limb**
Q72.89 **Other reduction defects of lower limb**
Q72.891 **Other reduction defects of right lower limb**
Q72.892 **Other reduction defects of left lower limb**
Q72.893 **Other reduction defects of lower limb, bilateral**
Q72.899 **Other reduction defects of unspecified lower limb**

Q72.9 **Unspecified reduction defect of lower limb**
Q72.90 **Unspecified reduction defect of unspecified lower limb**
Q72.91 **Unspecified reduction defect of right lower limb**
Q72.92 **Unspecified reduction defect of left lower limb**
Q72.93 **Unspecified reduction defect of lower limb, bilateral**

## Q73 Reduction defects of unspecified limb

Q73.0 **Congenital absence of unspecified limb(s)**
Amelia NOS
Q73.1 **Phocomelia, unspecified limb(s)**
Phocomelia NOS
Q73.8 **Other reduction defects of unspecified limb(s)**
Ectromelia of limb NOS
Hemimelia of limb NOS
Longitudinal reduction deformity of unspecified limb(s)
Reduction defect of limb NOS

## Q74 Other congenital malformations of limb(s)

EXCLUDES 1 *polydactyly (Q69.-)*
*reduction defect of limb (Q71-Q73)*
*syndactyly (Q70.-)*

Q74.0 **Other congenital malformations of upper limb(s), including shoulder girdle**
Accessory carpal bones
Cleidocranial dysostosis
Congenital pseudarthrosis of clavicle
Macrodactylia (fingers)
Madelung's deformity
Radioulnar synostosis
Sprengel's deformity
Triphalangeal thumb

Q74.1 **Congenital malformation of knee**
Congenital absence of patella
Congenital dislocation of patella
Congenital genu valgum
Congenital genu varum
Rudimentary patella
EXCLUDES 1 *congenital dislocation of knee (Q68.2)*
*congenital genu recurvatum (Q68.2)*
*nail patella syndrome (Q87.2)*

Q74.2 **Other congenital malformations of lower limb(s), including pelvic girdle**
Congenital fusion of sacroiliac joint
Congenital malformation of ankle joint
Congenital malformation of sacroiliac joint
EXCLUDES 1 *anteversion of femur (neck) (Q65.89)*

Q74.3 **Arthrogryposis multiplex congenita**
Q74.8 **Other specified congenital malformations of limb(s)**
Q74.9 **Unspecified congenital malformation of limb(s)**
Congenital anomaly of limb(s) NOS

## Q75 Other congenital malformations of skull and face bones

EXCLUDES 1 *congenital malformation of face NOS (Q18.-)*
*congenital malformation syndromes classified to Q87.-*
*dentofacial anomalies [including malocclusion] (M26.-)*
*musculoskeletal deformities of head and face (Q67.0-Q67.4)*
*skull defects associated with congenital anomalies of brain such as:*
*anencephaly (Q00.0)*
*encephalocele (Q01.-)*
*hydrocephalus (Q03.-)*
*microcephaly (Q02)*

Q75.0 **Craniosynostosis**
**AHA:** 2023,4Q,38-39
**DEF:** Congenital condition in which one or more of the cranial sutures fuse prematurely, creating a deformed or aberrant head shape.
Q75.00 **Craniosynostosis, unspecified**
Craniosynostosis NOS
Q75.001 **Craniosynostosis, unspecified type, unilateral**
Q75.002 **Craniosynostosis, unspecified type, bilateral**
Q75.009 **Craniosynostosis, unspecified**
Imperfect fusion of skull
Q75.01 **Sagittal craniosynostosis**
Non-deformational dolichocephaly
Non-deformational scaphocephaly
EXCLUDES 1 *plagiocephaly (Q67.3)*
Q75.02 **Coronal craniosynostosis**
EXCLUDES 1 *dolichocephaly (Q67.2)*
Q75.021 **Coronal craniosynostosis, unilateral**
Non-deformational anterior plagiocephaly
Q75.022 **Coronal craniosynostosis, bilateral**
Non-deformational brachycephaly
Q75.029 **Coronal craniosynostosis, unspecified**
Q75.03 **Metopic craniosynostosis**
Trigonocephaly
Q75.04 **Lambdoid craniosynostosis**
Non-deformational posterior plagiocephaly
EXCLUDES 1 *dolichocephaly (Q67.2)*
Q75.041 **Lambdoid craniosynostosis, unilateral**
Q75.042 **Lambdoid craniosynostosis, bilateral**
Q75.049 **Lambdoid craniosynostosis, unspecified**
Q75.05 **Multi-suture craniosynostosis**
Q75.051 **Cloverleaf skull**
Kleeblattschaedel skull
Q75.052 **Pansynostosis**
Q75.058 **Other multi-suture craniosynostosis**
EXCLUDES 1 *coronal craniosynostosis, bilateral (Q75.022)*
*lambdoid craniosynostosis, bilateral (Q75.042)*
Q75.08 **Other single-suture craniosynostosis**

Q75.1 **Craniofacial dysostosis**
Crouzon's disease
Q75.2 **Hypertelorism**
Q75.3 **Macrocephaly**

**Q75.4 Mandibulofacial dysostosis**
Franceschetti syndrome
Treacher Collins syndrome

**Q75.5 Oculomandibular dysostosis**

**Q75.8 Other specified congenital malformations of skull and face bones**
Absence of skull bone, congenital
Congenital deformity of forehead
Platybasia

**Q75.9 Congenital malformation of skull and face bones, unspecified**
Congenital anomaly of face bones NOS
Congenital anomaly of skull NOS

✓4th **Q76 Congenital malformations of spine and bony thorax**
EXCLUDES 1 *congenital musculoskeletal deformities of spine and chest (Q67.5-Q67.8)*

**Q76.Ø Spina bifida occulta**
EXCLUDES 1 *meningocele (spinal) (QØ5.-)*
*spina bifida (aperta) (cystica) (QØ5.-)*

**Q76.1 Klippel-Feil syndrome**
Cervical fusion syndrome

**Q76.2 Congenital spondylolisthesis**
Congenital spondylolysis
EXCLUDES 1 *spondylolisthesis (acquired) (M43.1-)*
*spondylolysis (acquired) (M43.Ø-)*

**Q76.3 Congenital scoliosis due to congenital bony malformation**
Hemivertebra fusion or failure of segmentation with scoliosis

✓5th **Q76.4 Other congenital malformations of spine, not associated with scoliosis**

✓6th **Q76.41 Congenital kyphosis**
**Q76.411 Congenital kyphosis, occipito-atlanto-axial region**
**Q76.412 Congenital kyphosis, cervical region**
**Q76.413 Congenital kyphosis, cervicothoracic region**
**Q76.414 Congenital kyphosis, thoracic region**
**Q76.415 Congenital kyphosis, thoracolumbar region**
**Q76.419 Congenital kyphosis, unspecified region**

✓6th **Q76.42 Congenital lordosis**
**Q76.425 Congenital lordosis, thoracolumbar region**
**Q76.426 Congenital lordosis, lumbar region**
**Q76.427 Congenital lordosis, lumbosacral region**
**Q76.428 Congenital lordosis, sacral and sacrococcygeal region**
**Q76.429 Congenital lordosis, unspecified region**

**Q76.49 Other congenital malformations of spine, not associated with scoliosis**
Congenital absence of vertebra NOS
Congenital fusion of spine NOS
Congenital malformation of lumbosacral (joint) (region) NOS
Congenital malformation of spine NOS
Hemivertebra NOS
Malformation of spine NOS
Platyspondylisis NOS
Supernumerary vertebra NOS

**Q76.5 Cervical rib**
Supernumerary rib in cervical region

**Q76.6 Other congenital malformations of ribs**
Accessory rib
Congenital absence of rib
Congenital fusion of ribs
Congenital malformation of ribs NOS
EXCLUDES 1 *short rib syndrome (Q77.2)*

**Q76.7 Congenital malformation of sternum**
Congenital absence of sternum
Sternum bifidum

**Q76.8 Other congenital malformations of bony thorax**

**Q76.9 Congenital malformation of bony thorax, unspecified**

✓4th **Q77 Osteochondrodysplasia with defects of growth of tubular bones and spine**
EXCLUDES 1 *mucopolysaccharidosis (E76.Ø-E76.3)*
EXCLUDES 2 *congenital myotonic chondrodystrophy (G71.13)*

**Q77.Ø Achondrogenesis** COM
Hypochondrogenesis

**Q77.1 Thanatophoric short stature** COM

**Q77.2 Short rib syndrome** COM
Asphyxiating thoracic dysplasia [Jeune]

**Q77.3 Chondrodysplasia punctata** COM
EXCLUDES 1 *Rhizomelic chondrodysplasia punctata (E71.54Ø)*

**Q77.4 Achondroplasia** COM
Hypochondroplasia
Osteosclerosis congenita

**Q77.5 Diastrophic dysplasia** COM

**Q77.6 Chondroectodermal dysplasia** COM
Ellis-van Creveld syndrome

**Q77.7 Spondyloepiphyseal dysplasia** COM

**Q77.8 Other osteochondrodysplasia with defects of growth of tubular bones and spine** COM

**Q77.9 Osteochondrodysplasia with defects of growth of tubular bones and spine, unspecified** COM

✓4th **Q78 Other osteochondrodysplasias**
EXCLUDES 2 *congenital myotonic chondrodystrophy (G71.13)*

**Q78.Ø Osteogenesis imperfecta** COM
Fragilitas ossium
Osteopsathyrosis

**Q78.1 Polyostotic fibrous dysplasia** COM
Albright(-McCune)(-Sternberg) syndrome

**Q78.2 Osteopetrosis** COM
Albers-Schonberg syndrome
Osteosclerosis NOS
**DEF:** Rare congenital condition in which the bones are excessively dense, resulting from a discrepancy in the formation and breakdown of bone.

**Q78.3 Progressive diaphyseal dysplasia** COM
Camurati-Engelmann syndrome

**Q78.4 Enchondromatosis** COM
Maffucci's syndrome
Ollier's disease

**Q78.5 Metaphyseal dysplasia** COM
Pyle's syndrome

**Q78.6 Multiple congenital exostoses** COM
Diaphyseal aclasis

**Q78.8 Other specified osteochondrodysplasias** COM
Osteopoikilosis

**Q78.9 Osteochondrodysplasia, unspecified** COM
Chondrodystrophy NOS
Osteodystrophy NOS

✓4th **Q79 Congenital malformations of musculoskeletal system, not elsewhere classified**
EXCLUDES 2 *congenital (sternomastoid) torticollis (Q68.Ø)*

**Q79.Ø Congenital diaphragmatic hernia** COM
EXCLUDES 1 *congenital hiatus hernia (Q4Ø.1)*

**Q79.1 Other congenital malformations of diaphragm** COM
Absence of diaphragm
Congenital malformation of diaphragm NOS
Eventration of diaphragm

**Q79.2 Exomphalos** COM
Omphalocele
EXCLUDES 1 *umbilical hernia (K42.-)*

**Q79.3 Gastroschisis** COM

**Gastroschisis**

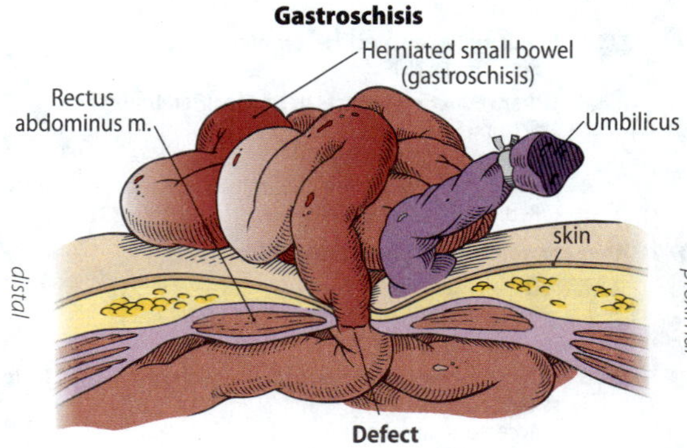


**Q79.4 Prune belly syndrome** COM
Congenital prolapse of bladder mucosa
Eagle-Barrett syndrome

✓5th **Q79.5 Other congenital malformations of abdominal wall**
EXCLUDES 1 *umbilical hernia (K42.-)*

**Q79.51 Congenital hernia of bladder** COM
**Q79.59 Other congenital malformations of abdominal wall**

√5th **Q79.6 Ehlers-Danlos syndromes**
AHA: 2019,4Q,13-14
DEF: Connective tissue disorder that causes hyperextended skin and joints and results in fragile blood vessels with bleeding, poor wound healing, and subcutaneous pseudotumors.

**Q79.60 Ehlers-Danlos syndrome, unspecified** Rx COM

**Q79.61 Classical Ehlers-Danlos syndrome** Rx COM
Classical EDS (cEDS)

**Q79.62 Hypermobile Ehlers-Danlos syndrome** Rx COM
Hypermobile EDS (hEDS)

**Q79.63 Vascular Ehlers-Danlos syndrome** Rx COM
Vascular EDS (vEDS)

**Q79.69 Other Ehlers-Danlos syndromes** Rx COM

**Q79.8 Other congenital malformations of musculoskeletal system**
Absence of muscle
Absence of tendon
Accessory muscle
Amyotrophia congenita
Congenital constricting bands
Congenital shortening of tendon
Poland syndrome

**Q79.9 Congenital malformation of musculoskeletal system, unspecified**
Congenital anomaly of musculoskeletal system NOS
Congenital deformity of musculoskeletal system NOS

## Other congenital malformations (Q8Ø-Q89)

√4th **Q8Ø Congenital ichthyosis**
EXCLUDES 1 *Refsum's disease (G6Ø.1)*
DEF: Excessive production of skin cells resulting in red, dry, scaly skin.

**Q8Ø.Ø Ichthyosis vulgaris**
**Q8Ø.1 X-linked ichthyosis**
**Q8Ø.2 Lamellar ichthyosis**
Collodion baby
**Q8Ø.3 Congenital bullous ichthyosiform erythroderma**
**Q8Ø.4 Harlequin fetus**
**Q8Ø.8 Other congenital ichthyosis**
**Q8Ø.9 Congenital ichthyosis, unspecified**

√4th **Q81 Epidermolysis bullosa**

**Q81.Ø Epidermolysis bullosa simplex** COM
EXCLUDES 1 *Cockayne's syndrome (Q87.19)*

**Q81.1 Epidermolysis bullosa letalis** COM
Herlitz' syndrome

**Q81.2 Epidermolysis bullosa dystrophica** COM
**Q81.8 Other epidermolysis bullosa** COM
**Q81.9 Epidermolysis bullosa, unspecified** COM

√4th **Q82 Other congenital malformations of skin**
EXCLUDES 1 *acrodermatitis enteropathica (E83.2)*
*congenital erythropoietic porphyria (E8Ø.Ø)*
*pilonidal cyst or sinus (LØ5.-)*
*Sturge-Weber (-Dimitri) syndrome (Q85.89)*

**Q82.Ø Hereditary lymphedema**
**Q82.1 Xeroderma pigmentosum**
**Q82.2 Congenital cutaneous mastocytosis**
Congenital diffuse cutaneous mastocytosis
Congenital maculopapular cutaneous mastocytosis
Congenital urticaria pigmentosa
EXCLUDES 1 *cutaneous mastocytosis NOS (D47.Ø1)*
*diffuse cutaneous mastocytosis (with onset after newborn period) (D47.Ø1)*
*malignant mastocytosis (C96.2-)*
*systemic mastocytosis (D47.Ø2)*
*urticaria pigmentosa (non-congenital) (with onset after newborn period) (D47.Ø1)*
AHA: 2017,4Q,5

**Q82.3 Incontinentia pigmenti**
**Q82.4 Ectodermal dysplasia (anhidrotic)**
EXCLUDES 1 *Ellis-van Creveld syndrome (Q77.6)*

**Q82.5 Congenital non-neoplastic nevus**
Birthmark NOS
Flammeus Nevus
Portwine Nevus
Sanguineous Nevus
Strawberry Nevus
Vascular Nevus NOS
Verrucous Nevus
EXCLUDES 2 *araneus nevus (I78.1)*
*Cafe au lait spots (L81.3)*
*lentigo (L81.4)*
*melanocytic nevus (D22.-)*
*nevus NOS (D22.-)*
*pigmented nevus (D22.-)*
*spider nevus (I78.1)*
*stellar nevus (I78.1)*
AHA: 2024,3Q,5

**Q82.6 Congenital sacral dimple**
Parasacral dimple
EXCLUDES 2 *pilonidal cyst with abscess (LØ5.Ø1)*
*pilonidal cyst without abscess (LØ5.91)*
AHA: 2016,4Q,60

**Q82.8 Other specified congenital malformations of skin**
Abnormal palmar creases
Accessory skin tags
Benign familial pemphigus [Hailey-Hailey]
Congenital poikiloderma
Cutis laxa (hyperelastica)
Dermatoglyphic anomalies
Inherited keratosis palmaris et plantaris
Keratosis follicularis [Darier-White]
EXCLUDES 1 *Ehlers-Danlos syndromes (Q79.6-)*
EXCLUDES 2 *disorders of pyrophosphate metabolism (E83.82-)*
AHA: 2021,3Q,10; 2016,1Q,17

**Q82.9 Congenital malformation of skin, unspecified**

√4th **Q83 Congenital malformations of breast**
EXCLUDES 2 *absence of pectoral muscle (Q79.8)*
*hypoplasia of breast (N64.82)*
*micromastia (N64.82)*

**Q83.Ø Congenital absence of breast with absent nipple**
**Q83.1 Accessory breast**
Supernumerary breast
**Q83.2 Absent nipple**
**Q83.3 Accessory nipple**
Supernumerary nipple
**Q83.8 Other congenital malformations of breast**
**Q83.9 Congenital malformation of breast, unspecified**

√4th **Q84 Other congenital malformations of integument**

**Q84.Ø Congenital alopecia**
Congenital atrichosis
**Q84.1 Congenital morphological disturbances of hair, not elsewhere classified**
Beaded hair
Monilethrix
Pili annulati
EXCLUDES 1 *Menkes' kinky hair syndrome (E83.Ø9)*
**Q84.2 Other congenital malformations of hair**
Congenital hypertrichosis
Congenital malformation of hair NOS
Persistent lanugo
**Q84.3 Anonychia**
EXCLUDES 1 *nail patella syndrome (Q87.2)*
**Q84.4 Congenital leukonychia**
**Q84.5 Enlarged and hypertrophic nails**
Congenital onychauxis
Pachyonychia
**Q84.6 Other congenital malformations of nails**
Congenital clubnail
Congenital koilonychia
Congenital malformation of nail NOS
**Q84.8 Other specified congenital malformations of integument**
Aplasia cutis congenita
**Q84.9 Congenital malformation of integument, unspecified**
Congenital anomaly of integument NOS
Congenital deformity of integument NOS

**✓4th Q85 Phakomatoses, not elsewhere classified**
EXCLUDES 1 *ataxia telangiectasia [Louis-Bar] (G11.3)*
*familial dysautonomia [Riley-Day] (G90.1)*

**✓5th Q85.0 Neurofibromatosis (nonmalignant)**

**Q85.00 Neurofibromatosis, unspecified** HCC ESR COM

**Q85.01 Neurofibromatosis, type 1** HCC ESR COM
Von Recklinghausen disease

**Q85.02 Neurofibromatosis, type 2** HCC ESR COM
Acoustic neurofibromatosis
**DEF:** Inherited condition with cutaneous lesions, benign tumors of peripheral nerves, and bilateral 8th nerve masses.

**Q85.03 Schwannomatosis** HCC ESR COM
**DEF:** Genetic mutation (SMARCB1/INI1) causing multiple benign tumors along the nerve pathways, except on the 8th cranial (vestibular) nerve.

**Q85.09 Other neurofibromatosis** HCC ESR COM

**Q85.1 Tuberous sclerosis** HCC Rx ESR COM
Bourneville's disease
Epiloia

**✓5th Q85.8 Other phakomatoses, not elsewhere classified**
EXCLUDES 1 *Meckel-Gruber syndrome (Q61.9)*
**AHA:** 2022,4Q,40-41; 2021,3Q,12

**Q85.81 PTEN hamartoma tumor syndrome** HCC Rx ESR COM
PHTS
PTEN related Cowden syndrome
Code also, if applicable, genetic susceptibility to malignant neoplasm (Z15.0-)
**AHA:** 2022,4Q,41
**TIP:** PTEN hamartoma tumor syndrome (PHTS) manifests differently in each patient. Separate codes should be assigned in addition to code Q85.81 for any manifestations of PHTS, such as macrocephaly, autism, or learning delays.

**Q85.82 Other Cowden syndrome** HCC Rx ESR COM

**Q85.83 Von Hippel-Lindau syndrome** HCC Rx ESR COM
Code also manifestations
**AHA:** 2023,2Q,16

**Q85.89 Other phakomatoses, not elsewhere classified** HCC Rx ESR COM
Peutz-Jeghers syndrome
Sturge-Weber(-Dimitri) syndrome

**Q85.9 Phakomatosis, unspecified** HCC Rx ESR COM
Hamartosis NOS

**✓4th Q86 Congenital malformation syndromes due to known exogenous causes, not elsewhere classified**
EXCLUDES 2 *iodine-deficiency-related hypothyroidism (E00-E02)*
*nonteratogenic effects of substances transmitted via placenta or breast milk (P04.-)*

**Q86.0 Fetal alcohol syndrome (dysmorphic)** COM

**Q86.1 Fetal hydantoin syndrome** COM
Meadow's syndrome

**Q86.2 Dysmorphism due to warfarin** COM

**Q86.8 Other congenital malformation syndromes due to known exogenous causes** COM

**✓4th Q87 Other specified congenital malformation syndromes affecting multiple systems**
Use additional code(s) to identify all associated manifestations

**Q87.0 Congenital malformation syndromes predominantly affecting facial appearance**
Acrocephalopolysyndactyly
Acrocephalosyndactyly [Apert]
Cryptophthalmos syndrome
Cyclopia
Goldenhar syndrome
Moebius syndrome
Oro-facial-digital syndrome
Robin syndrome
Whistling face

**✓5th Q87.1 Congenital malformation syndromes predominantly associated with short stature**
EXCLUDES 1 *Ellis-van Creveld syndrome (Q77.6)*
*Smith-Lemli-Opitz syndrome (E78.72)*
**AHA:** 2019,4Q,14-15

**Q87.11 Prader-Willi syndrome** Rx COM
**AHA:** 2024,4Q,11

**Q87.19 Other congenital malformation syndromes predominantly associated with short stature** COM
Aarskog syndrome
Cockayne syndrome
De Lange syndrome
Dubowitz syndrome
Noonan syndrome
Robinow-Silverman-Smith syndrome
Russell-Silver syndrome
Seckel syndrome

**Q87.2 Congenital malformation syndromes predominantly involving limbs** COM
Holt-Oram syndrome
Klippel-Trenaunay-Weber syndrome
Nail patella syndrome
Rubinstein-Taybi syndrome
Sirenomelia syndrome
Thrombocytopenia with absent radius [TAR] syndrome
VATER syndrome

**Q87.3 Congenital malformation syndromes involving early overgrowth** COM
Beckwith-Wiedemann syndrome
Sotos syndrome
Weaver syndrome

**✓5th Q87.4 Marfan syndrome**
**DEF:** Disorder that affects the connective tissue of multiple systems, including disproportionally long or abnormal bone structure and eye and cardiovascular complications.

**Q87.40 Marfan syndrome, unspecified** Rx COM

**✓6th Q87.41 Marfan syndrome with cardiovascular manifestations**

**Q87.410 Marfan syndrome with aortic dilation** Rx COM

**Q87.418 Marfan syndrome with other cardiovascular manifestations** Rx COM

**Q87.42 Marfan syndrome with ocular manifestations** Rx COM

**Q87.43 Marfan syndrome with skeletal manifestation** Rx COM

**Q87.5 Other congenital malformation syndromes with other skeletal changes** COM

**✓5th Q87.8 Other specified congenital malformation syndromes, not elsewhere classified**
EXCLUDES 1 *Zellweger syndrome (E71.510)*
**AHA:** 2023,4Q,39-40

**Q87.81 Alport syndrome** COM
Use additional code to identify stage of chronic kidney disease (N18.1-N18.6)

**Q87.82 Arterial tortuosity syndrome** Rx COM
**AHA:** 2016,4Q,60-61

**Q87.83 Bardet-Biedl syndrome** COM

**Q87.84 Laurence-Moon syndrome** COM

**Q87.85 MED13L syndrome** COM
Asadollahi-Rauch syndrome
Mediator complex subunit 13L syndrome
Code also, if applicable, any associated manifestations such as:
autism spectrum disorder (F84.0-)
congenital malformations of cardiac septa (Q21.-)
epilepsy and recurrent seizures (G40.-)
intellectual disability (F70-F79)

**Q87.86 Kleefstra syndrome** Rx COM
**AHA:** 2024,4Q,27

**Q87.87 Hao-Fountain Syndrome**
HAFOUS
Use additional code, if applicable, for associated conditions such as:
autism spectrum disorder (F84.0)
developmental speech disorder (F80.-)
epilepsy, by specific type (G40.-)
intellectual disabilities (F70-F79)
pervasive developmental disorders (F84.-)

Q87.88 CTNNB1 syndrome
Use additional code, if applicable, for associated conditions such as:
cerebral palsy (G80.-)
congenital heart malformations (Q20.0-Q24.9)
developmental disorder of speech and language (F80.-)
exudative retinopathy (H35.02-)
intellectual disability (F70-F79)
microcephaly (Q02)

Q87.89 Other specified congenital malformation syndromes, not elsewhere classified COM

● Q87.A Loeys-Dietz syndrome
EXCLUDES 1 *arterial tortuosity syndrome (Q87.82)*
*Ehlers-Danlos syndrome (Q79.6)*
*Marfan syndrome (Q87.40-Q87.43)*
*other systemic involvement of connective tissue (M35)*

**Q89 Other congenital malformations, not elsewhere classified**

Q89.0 Congenital absence and malformations of spleen
EXCLUDES 1 *isomerism of atrial appendages (with asplenia or polysplenia) (Q20.6)*

Q89.01 Asplenia (congenital)
AHA: 2025,1Q,24

Q89.09 Congenital malformations of spleen
Congenital splenomegaly

Q89.1 Congenital malformations of adrenal gland
EXCLUDES 1 *adrenogenital disorders (E25.-)*
*congenital adrenal hyperplasia (E25.0)*

Q89.2 Congenital malformations of other endocrine glands
Congenital malformation of parathyroid or thyroid gland
Persistent thyroglossal duct
Thyroglossal cyst
EXCLUDES 1 *congenital goiter (E03.0)*
*congenital hypothyroidism (E03.1)*

Q89.3 Situs inversus COM
Dextrocardia with situs inversus
Mirror-image atrial arrangement with situs inversus
Situs inversus or transversus abdominalis
Situs inversus or transversus thoracis
Transposition of abdominal viscera
Transposition of thoracic viscera
EXCLUDES 1 *dextrocardia NOS (Q24.0)*
DEF: Congenital anomaly in which the internal thoracic and abdominal organs are transposed laterally and found on the opposite side from the normal position.

Q89.4 Conjoined twins COM
Craniopagus
Dicephaly
Pygopagus
Thoracopagus

Q89.7 Multiple congenital malformations, not elsewhere classified
Multiple congenital anomalies NOS
Multiple congenital deformities NOS
EXCLUDES 1 *congenital malformation syndromes affecting multiple systems (Q87.-)*

Q89.8 Other specified congenital malformations
Use additional code(s) to identify all associated manifestations
AHA: 2021,3Q,12

Q89.81 Kabuki syndrome
Kabuki syndrome, type 1, due to KMT2D mutation
Kabuki syndrome, type 2, due to KDM6A mutation
Niikawa-Kuroki syndrome

Q89.89 Other specified congenital malformations

Q89.9 Congenital malformation, unspecified
Congenital anomaly NOS
Congenital deformity NOS

## Chromosomal abnormalities, not elsewhere classified (Q90-Q99)

EXCLUDES 2 *mitochondrial metabolic disorders (E88.4-)*

**Q90 Down syndrome**
Code also associated physical condition(s), such as atrioventricular septal defect (Q21.2-)
Use additional code(s) to identify any associated degree of intellectual disabilities (F70-F79)

Q90.0 Trisomy 21, nonmosaicism (meiotic nondisjunction) COM
Q90.1 Trisomy 21, mosaicism (mitotic nondisjunction) COM
Q90.2 Trisomy 21, translocation COM
Q90.9 Down syndrome, unspecified COM
Trisomy 21 NOS

**Q91 Trisomy 18 and Trisomy 13**

Q91.0 Trisomy 18, nonmosaicism (meiotic nondisjunction) Rx COM
Q91.1 Trisomy 18, mosaicism (mitotic nondisjunction) Rx COM
Q91.2 Trisomy 18, translocation Rx COM
Q91.3 Trisomy 18, unspecified Rx COM
Q91.4 Trisomy 13, nonmosaicism (meiotic nondisjunction) Rx COM
Q91.5 Trisomy 13, mosaicism (mitotic nondisjunction) Rx COM
Q91.6 Trisomy 13, translocation Rx COM
Q91.7 Trisomy 13, unspecified Rx COM

**Q92 Other trisomies and partial trisomies of the autosomes, not elsewhere classified**
INCLUDES unbalanced translocations and insertions
EXCLUDES 1 *trisomies of chromosomes 13, 18, 21 (Q90-Q91)*

Q92.0 Whole chromosome trisomy, nonmosaicism (meiotic nondisjunction) Rx COM
Q92.1 Whole chromosome trisomy, mosaicism (mitotic nondisjunction) Rx COM
Q92.2 Partial trisomy Rx COM
Less than whole arm duplicated
Whole arm or more duplicated
EXCLUDES 1 *partial trisomy due to unbalanced translocation (Q92.5)*

Q92.5 Duplications with other complex rearrangements Rx COM
Partial trisomy due to unbalanced translocations
Code also any associated deletions due to unbalanced translocations, inversions and insertions (Q93.7)

Q92.6 Marker chromosomes
Individual with marker heterochromatin
Trisomies due to dicentrics
Trisomies due to extra rings
Trisomies due to isochromosomes

Q92.61 Marker chromosomes in normal individual Rx COM
Q92.62 Marker chromosomes in abnormal individual Rx COM

Q92.7 Triploidy and polyploidy Rx COM
Q92.8 Other specified trisomies and partial trisomies of autosomes Rx COM
Duplications identified by fluorescence in situ hybridization (FISH)
Duplications identified by in situ hybridization (ISH)
Duplications seen only at prometaphase
Q92.9 Trisomy and partial trisomy of autosomes, unspecified Rx COM

**Q93 Monosomies and deletions from the autosomes, not elsewhere classified**

Q93.0 Whole chromosome monosomy, nonmosaicism (meiotic nondisjunction) Rx COM
Q93.1 Whole chromosome monosomy, mosaicism (mitotic nondisjunction) Rx COM
Q93.2 Chromosome replaced with ring, dicentric or isochromosome Rx COM
Q93.3 Deletion of short arm of chromosome 4 Rx COM
Wolff-Hirschorn syndrome
Q93.4 Deletion of short arm of chromosome 5 Rx COM
Cri-du-chat syndrome
Q93.5 Other deletions of part of a chromosome
AHA: 2018,4Q,28

Q93.51 Angelman syndrome Rx COM
Q93.52 Phelan-McDermid syndrome Rx COM
22q13.3 deletion syndrome
Use additional code(s) to identify any associated conditions, such as:
autism spectrum disorder (F84.0)
degree of intellectual disabilities (F70-F79)
epilepsy and recurrent seizures (G40.-)
lymphedema (I89.0)
AHA: 2023,4Q,40-41
Q93.59 Other deletions of part of a chromosome Rx COM

Q93.7 Deletions with other complex rearrangements Rx COM
Deletions due to unbalanced translocations, inversions and insertions
Code also any associated duplications due to unbalanced translocations, inversions and insertions (Q92.5)

√5th **Q93.8 Other deletions from the autosomes**

**Q93.81 Velo-cardio-facial syndrome** Rx COM
Deletion 22q11.2
**AHA:** 2019,3Q,14
**DEF:** Microdeletion syndrome affecting multiple organs characterized by a cleft palate, heart defects, an elongated face with almond-shaped eyes, wide nose, small ears, weak immune system, weak musculature, hypothyroidism, short stature, and scoliosis. The deletion occurs at q11.2 on the long arm of the chromosome 22.

**Q93.82 Williams syndrome** Rx COM
**AHA:** 2018,4Q,28-29

**Q93.88 Other microdeletions** Rx COM
Miller-Dieker syndrome
Smith-Magenis syndrome

**Q93.89 Other deletions from the autosomes** Rx COM
Deletions identified by fluorescence in situ hybridization (FISH)
Deletions identified by in situ hybridization (ISH)
Deletions seen only at prometaphase

**Q93.9 Deletion from autosomes, unspecified** Rx COM

√4th **Q95 Balanced rearrangements and structural markers, not elsewhere classified**
INCLUDES Robertsonian and balanced reciprocal translocations and insertions

**Q95.Ø Balanced translocation and insertion in normal individual**
**Q95.1 Chromosome inversion in normal individual**
**Q95.2 Balanced autosomal rearrangement in abnormal individual** Rx COM
**Q95.3 Balanced sex/autosomal rearrangement in abnormal individual** Rx COM
**Q95.5 Individual with autosomal fragile site**
**Q95.8 Other balanced rearrangements and structural markers**
**Q95.9 Balanced rearrangement and structural marker, unspecified**

√4th **Q96 Turner's syndrome**
EXCLUDES 1 *Noonan syndrome (Q87.19)*

**Q96.Ø Karyotype 45, X** COM
**Q96.1 Karyotype 46, X iso (Xq)** COM
Karyotype 46, isochromosome Xq
**Q96.2 Karyotype 46, X with abnormal sex chromosome, except iso (Xq)** COM
Karyotype 46, X with abnormal sex chromosome, except isochromosome Xq
**Q96.3 Mosaicism, 45, X/46, XX or XY** COM
**Q96.4 Mosaicism, 45, X/other cell line(s) with abnormal sex chromosome** COM
**Q96.8 Other variants of Turner's syndrome** COM
**Q96.9 Turner's syndrome, unspecified** COM

√4th **Q97 Other sex chromosome abnormalities, female phenotype, not elsewhere classified**
EXCLUDES 1 *Turner's syndrome (Q96.-)*

**Q97.Ø Karyotype 47, XXX** COM
**Q97.1 Female with more than three X chromosomes** COM
**Q97.2 Mosaicism, lines with various numbers of X chromosomes** COM
**Q97.3 Female with 46, XY karyotype** COM
**Q97.8 Other specified sex chromosome abnormalities, female phenotype** COM
**Q97.9 Sex chromosome abnormality, female phenotype, unspecified** COM

√4th **Q98 Other sex chromosome abnormalities, male phenotype, not elsewhere classified**

**Q98.Ø Klinefelter syndrome karyotype 47, XXY** COM
**Q98.1 Klinefelter syndrome, male with more than two X chromosomes** COM
**Q98.3 Other male with 46, XX karyotype** COM
**Q98.4 Klinefelter syndrome, unspecified** COM
**Q98.5 Karyotype 47, XYY** COM
**Q98.6 Male with structurally abnormal sex chromosome** COM
**Q98.7 Male with sex chromosome mosaicism** COM
**Q98.8 Other specified sex chromosome abnormalities, male phenotype** COM
**Q98.9 Sex chromosome abnormality, male phenotype, unspecified** COM

√4th **Q99 Other chromosome abnormalities, not elsewhere classified**

**Q99.Ø Chimera 46, XX/46, XY** COM
Chimera 46, XX/46, XY true hermaphrodite
**Q99.1 46, XX true hermaphrodite** COM
46, XX with streak gonads
46, XY with streak gonads
Pure gonadal dysgenesis
**Q99.2 Fragile X chromosome** Rx COM
Fragile X syndrome

√5th **Q99.8 Other specified chromosome abnormalities**

√6th **Q99.81 Usher syndrome**
Use additional code to identify any auditory and visual manifestations

**Q99.811 Usher syndrome, type 1**
**Q99.812 Usher syndrome, type 2**
**Q99.813 Usher syndrome, type 3**
**Q99.818 Other Usher syndrome**
Usher syndrome, type 4
**Q99.819 Usher syndrome, unspecified**

**Q99.89 Other specified chromosome abnormalities**

**Q99.9 Chromosomal abnormality, unspecified** COM

## Genetic disorders, not elsewhere classified ▶(QAØ-QA1)◀

√4th **QAØ Neurodevelopmental disorders related to specific genetic pathogenic variants**
Code also, if applicable, any associated conditions, such as:
attention-deficit hyperactivity disorders (F9Ø.-)
autism spectrum disorder (F84.Ø)
developmental and epileptic encephalopathy (G93.45)
epilepsy, by specific type (G4Ø.-)
intellectual disabilities (F7Ø-F79)
pervasive developmental disorders (F84.-)

√5th **QAØ.Ø Neurodevelopmental disorders related to pathogenic variants in specific genes**

√6th **QAØ.Ø1 Neurodevelopmental disorders related to pathogenic variants in certain specific genes**

√7th **QAØ.Ø1Ø Neurodevelopmental disorders, related to pathogenic variants in ion channel genes**

**QAØ.Ø1Ø1 SCN2A-related neurodevelopmental disorder**
**QAØ.Ø1Ø2 CACNA1A-related neurodevelopmental disorder**
**QAØ.Ø1Ø9 Neurodevelopmental disorder related to pathogenic variant in other ion channel gene**
SCN8A-related neurodevelopmental disorder

**QAØ.Ø11 Neurodevelopmental disorders, related to pathogenic variants in glutamate receptor genes**

**QAØ.Ø12 Neurodevelopmental disorders, related to pathogenic variants in other receptor genes**

√7th **QAØ.Ø13 Neurodevelopmental disorders, related to pathogenic variants in other transporter and solute carrier genes**

**QAØ.Ø131 SLC6A1-related disorder**
GABA transporter 1 deficiency
**QAØ.Ø139 Neurodevelopmental disorder, related to pathogenic variant in other transporter or solute carrier gene**

√7th **QAØ.Ø14 Neurodevelopmental disorders, related to pathogenic variants in synapse related genes**

**QAØ.Ø141 Syntaxin-binding protein 1-related disorder**
STXBP1-related disorders
**QAØ.Ø142 DLG4-related synaptopathy**
**QAØ.Ø149 Neurodevelopmental disorder, related to pathogenic variant in other synapse related gene**
Other genetic synaptopathy

√7th **QAØ.Ø15 Neurodevelopmental disorders, related to genes associated with transcription and gene expression**

**QAØ.Ø151 FOXG1 syndrome**
FOXG1-related disorder
FOXG1-related encephalopathy
FOXG1-related neurodevelopmental disorder

**QAØ.Ø159 Neurodevelopmental disorder, related to other genes associated with transcription and gene expression**

**QAØ.8 Other neurodevelopmental disorders related to pathogenic variants in other specific genes**

● ✓4th **QA1 Genetic disorders associated with neoplasms, not elsewhere classified**
Code also, if applicable, any associated conditions, such as:
genetic susceptibility to malignant neoplasm by site (Z15.Ø-)
malignant neoplasms (CØØ.Ø-C96.9)
personal history of malignant neoplasm (Z85.-)
EXCLUDES 2 *multiple endocrine neoplasia [MEN] syndromes (E31.2-)*

● ✓5th **QA1.7 Inherited neoplasm predisposition syndromes involving multiple systems, not elsewhere classified**

● **QA1.71 Lynch syndrome**
Hereditary nonpolyposis colorectal cancer susceptibility
Lynch syndrome due to EPCAM
Lynch syndrome due to MLH1
Lynch syndrome due to MSH2
Lynch syndrome due to MSH6
Lynch syndrome due to PMS2

● ✓6th **QA1.79 Other inherited neoplasm predisposition syndrome of multiple systems**

● **QA1.79Ø Familial cancer syndrome with pathogenic BRCA1 mutation**
BRCA1-cancer predisposition syndrome
Hereditary breast and ovarian cancer syndrome with pathogenic BRCA1 mutation

● **QA1.791 Familial cancer syndrome with pathogenic BRCA2 mutation**
BRCA2-cancer predisposition syndrome
Hereditary breast and ovarian cancer syndrome with pathogenic BRCA2 mutation

● **QA1.792 Li Fraumeni syndrome**

● **QA1.798 Other inherited neoplasm predisposition syndrome of multiple systems**

# Chapter 18. Symptoms, Signs, and Abnormal Clinical and Laboratory Findings, Not Elsewhere Classified (RØØ–R99)

## Chapter-specific Guidelines with Coding Examples

The chapter-specific guidelines from the ICD-10-CM Official Guidelines for Coding and Reporting have been provided below. Along with these guidelines are coding examples, contained in the shaded boxes, that have been developed to help illustrate the coding and/or sequencing guidance found in these guidelines.

Chapter 18 includes symptoms, signs, abnormal results of clinical or other investigative procedures, and ill-defined conditions which no diagnosis classifiable elsewhere is recorded. Signs and symptoms that point to a specific diagnosis have been assigned to a category in other chapters of the classification.

**a. Use of symptom codes**

Codes that describe symptoms and signs are acceptable for reporting purposes when a related definitive diagnosis has not been established (confirmed) by the provider.

**b. Use of a symptom code with a definitive diagnosis code**

Codes for signs and symptoms may be reported in addition to a related definitive diagnosis when the sign or symptom is not routinely associated with that diagnosis, such as the various signs and symptoms associated with complex syndromes. The definitive diagnosis code should be sequenced before the symptom code.

Signs or symptoms that are associated routinely with a disease process should not be assigned as additional codes, unless otherwise instructed by the classification.

> Pneumonia with hemoptysis
>
> **J18.9** **Pneumonia, unspecified organism**
>
> **RØ4.2** **Hemoptysis**
>
> *Explanation:* Codes for signs and symptoms may be reported in addition to a related definitive diagnosis when the sign or symptom is not routinely associated with that diagnosis.

**c. Combination codes that include symptoms**

ICD-10-CM contains a number of combination codes that identify both the definitive diagnosis and common symptoms of that diagnosis. When using one of these combination codes, an additional code should not be assigned for the symptom.

> IBS with diarrhea
>
> **K58.Ø** **Irritable bowel syndrome with diarrhea**
>
> *Explanation:* When a combination code identifies both the definitive diagnosis and the symptom, an additional code should not be assigned for the symptom.

**d. Repeated falls**

Code R29.6, Repeated falls, is for use for encounters when a patient has recently fallen and the reason for the fall is being investigated.

Code Z91.81, History of falling, is for use when a patient has fallen in the past and is at risk for future falls. When appropriate, both codes R29.6 and Z91.81 may be assigned together.

**e. Coma**

Code R4Ø.2Ø, Unspecified coma, should be assigned when the underlying cause of the coma is not known, or the cause is a traumatic brain injury and the coma scale is not documented in the medical record.

Do not report codes for unspecified coma, individual or total Glasgow coma scale scores for a patient with a medically induced coma or a sedated patient.

**1) Coma scale**

The coma scale codes (R4Ø.21- to R4Ø.24-) can be used in conjunction with traumatic brain injury codes. These codes cannot be used with R4Ø.2A, Nontraumatic coma due to underlying condition. They are primarily for use by trauma registries, but they may be used in any setting where this information is collected. The coma scale codes should be sequenced after the diagnosis code(s).

These codes, one from each subcategory, are needed to complete the scale. The 7th character indicates when the scale was recorded. The 7th character should match for all three codes.

At a minimum, report the initial score documented on presentation at your facility. This may be a score from the emergency medicine technician (EMT) or in the emergency department. If desired, a facility may choose to capture multiple coma scale scores.

Assign code R4Ø.24-, Glasgow coma scale, total score, when only the total score is documented in the medical record and not the individual score(s).

If multiple coma scores are captured within the first 24 hours after hospital admission, assign only the code for the score at the time of admission. ICD-1Ø-CM does not classify coma scores that are reported after admission but less than 24 hours later.

*See Section I.B.14. for coma scale documentation by clinicians other than patient's provider*

> 36-year-old man found down after unknown injury with skull fracture and with concussion and loss of consciousness of unknown duration. Upon hospital admission, the patient was evaluated with the following Glasgow coma scores:
>
> Eye-opening response—3: eyes open to speech
>
> Verbal response—3: random speech with no conversational exchange
>
> Motor response—4: pulls limb away from painful stimulus
>
> **SØ2.ØXXA** **Fracture of vault of skull, initial encounter for closed fracture**
>
> **SØ6.ØX9A** **Concussion with loss of consciousness of unspecified duration, initial encounter**
>
> **R4Ø.2133** **Coma scale, eyes open, to sound, at hospital admission**
>
> **R4Ø.2233** **Coma scale, best verbal response, inappropriate words, at hospital admission**
>
> **R4Ø.2343** **Coma scale, best motor response, flexion withdrawal, at hospital admission**
>
> *Explanation:* When individual scores for the Glasgow coma scale are documented, one code from each category is needed to complete the scale. The seventh character indicates when the scale was recorded and should match for all three codes. Assign a code from subcategory R4Ø.24- Glasgow coma scale, total score, when only the total and not the individual score(s) is documented.

**f. Functional quadriplegia**

GUIDELINE HAS BEEN DELETED EFFECTIVE OCTOBER 1, 2017

**g. SIRS due to non-infectious process**

The systemic inflammatory response syndrome (SIRS) can develop as a result of certain non-infectious disease processes, such as trauma, malignant neoplasm, or pancreatitis. When SIRS is documented with a noninfectious condition, and no subsequent infection is documented, the code for the underlying condition, such as an injury, should be assigned, followed by code R65.1Ø, Systemic inflammatory response syndrome (SIRS) of non-infectious origin without acute organ dysfunction, or code R65.11, Systemic inflammatory response syndrome (SIRS) of non-infectious origin with acute organ dysfunction. If an associated acute organ dysfunction is documented, the appropriate code(s) for the specific type of organ dysfunction(s) should be assigned in addition to code R65.11. If acute organ dysfunction is documented, but it cannot be determined if the acute organ dysfunction is associated with SIRS or due to another condition (e.g., directly due to the trauma), the provider should be queried.

> Systemic inflammatory response syndrome (SIRS) due to acute gallstone pancreatitis
>
> **K85.1Ø** **Biliary acute pancreatitis without necrosis or infection**
>
> **R65.1Ø** **Systemic inflammatory response syndrome [SIRS] of non-infectious origin without acute organ dysfunction**
>
> *Explanation:* When SIRS is documented with a non-infectious condition without subsequent infection documented, the code for the underlying condition such as pancreatitis should be assigned followed by the appropriate code for SIRS of noninfectious origin, either with or without associated organ dysfunction.

**h. Death NOS**

Code R99, Ill-defined and unknown cause of mortality, is only for use in the very limited circumstance when a patient who has already died is brought into an emergency department or other healthcare facility and is pronounced dead upon arrival. It does not represent the discharge disposition of death.

**i. NIHSS stroke scale**

The NIH stroke scale (NIHSS) codes (R29.7- -) can be used in conjunction with acute stroke codes (I6Ø-I63) to idenICD-1Ø-CM 2Ø27tify the patient's neurological status and the severity of the stroke. The stroke scale codes should be sequenced after the acute stroke diagnosis code(s).

At a minimum, report the initial score documented. If desired, a facility may choose to capture multiple stroke scale scores.

*See Section I.B.14. for NIHSS stroke scale documentation by clinicians other than patient's provider*

# Chapter 18. Symptoms, Signs and Abnormal Clinical and Laboratory Findings, Not Elsewhere Classified (RØØ-R99)

**NOTE** This chapter includes symptoms, signs, abnormal results of clinical or other investigative procedures, and ill-defined conditions regarding which no diagnosis classifiable elsewhere is recorded.

Signs and symptoms that point rather definitely to a given diagnosis have been assigned to a category in other chapters of the classification. In general, categories in this chapter include the less well-defined conditions and symptoms that, without the necessary study of the case to establish a final diagnosis, point perhaps equally to two or more diseases or to two or more systems of the body. Practically all categories in the chapter could be designated 'not otherwise specified', 'unknown etiology' or 'transient'. The Alphabetical Index should be consulted to determine which symptoms and signs are to be allocated here and which to other chapters. The residual subcategories, numbered .8, are generally provided for other relevant symptoms that cannot be allocated elsewhere in the classification.

The conditions and signs or symptoms included in categories RØØ-R94 consist of:

(a) cases for which no more specific diagnosis can be made even after all the facts bearing on the case have been investigated;

(b) signs or symptoms existing at the time of initial encounter that proved to be transient and whose causes could not be determined;

(c) provisional diagnosis in a patient who failed to return for further investigation or care;

(d) cases referred elsewhere for investigation or treatment before the diagnosis was made;

(e) cases in which a more precise diagnosis was not available for any other reason;

(f) certain symptoms, for which supplementary information is provided, that represent important problems in medical care in their own right.

**EXCLUDES 2** *abnormal findings on antenatal screening of mother (O28.-)*
*certain conditions originating in the perinatal period (PØ4-P96)*
*signs and symptoms classified in the body system chapters*
*signs and symptoms of breast (N63, N64.5)*

**AHA:** 2017,1Q,6,7

This chapter contains the following blocks:

RØØ-RØ9 Symptoms and signs involving the circulatory and respiratory systems
R1Ø-R19 Symptoms and signs involving the digestive system and abdomen
R2Ø-R23 Symptoms and signs involving the skin and subcutaneous tissue
R25-R29 Symptoms and signs involving the nervous and musculoskeletal systems
R3Ø-R39 Symptoms and signs involving the genitourinary system
R4Ø-R46 Symptoms and signs involving cognition, perception, emotional state and behavior
R47-R49 Symptoms and signs involving speech and voice
R5Ø-R69 General symptoms and signs
R7Ø-R79 Abnormal findings on examination of blood, without diagnosis
R8Ø-R82 Abnormal findings on examination of urine, without diagnosis
R83-R89 Abnormal findings on examination of other body fluids, substances and tissues, without diagnosis
R9Ø-R94 Abnormal findings on diagnostic imaging and in function studies, without diagnosis
R97 Abnormal tumor markers
R99 Ill-defined and unknown cause of mortality

## Symptoms and signs involving the circulatory and respiratory systems (RØØ-RØ9)

✓4th **RØØ Abnormalities of heart beat**
**EXCLUDES 1** *abnormalities originating in the perinatal period (P29.1-)*
**EXCLUDES 2** *specified arrhythmias (I47-I49)*

**RØØ.Ø Tachycardia, unspecified**
Rapid heart beat
Sinoauricular tachycardia NOS
Sinus [sinusal] tachycardia NOS
**EXCLUDES 1** *inappropriate sinus tachycardia, so stated (I47.11)*
*neonatal tachycardia (P29.11)*
*paroxysmal tachycardia (I47.-)*
**AHA:** 2022,4Q,46
**DEF:** Excessively rapid heart rate of more than 100 beats per minute.

**RØØ.1 Bradycardia, unspecified**
Sinoatrial bradycardia
Sinus bradycardia
Slow heart beat
Vagal bradycardia
Use additional code for adverse effect, if applicable, to identify drug (T36-T5Ø with fifth or sixth character 5)
**EXCLUDES 1** *neonatal bradycardia (P29.12)*
**AHA:** 2020,2Q,23
**DEF:** Slowed heartbeat, usually defined as a rate fewer than 60 beats per minute. Heart rhythm may be slow as a result of a congenital defect or an acquired problem.

**RØØ.2 Palpitations**
Awareness of heart beat

**RØØ.8 Other abnormalities of heart beat**

**RØØ.9 Unspecified abnormalities of heart beat**

✓4th **RØ1 Cardiac murmurs and other cardiac sounds**
**EXCLUDES 1** *cardiac murmurs and sounds originating in the perinatal period (P29.8)*

**RØ1.Ø Benign and innocent cardiac murmurs**
Functional cardiac murmur

**RØ1.1 Cardiac murmur, unspecified**
Cardiac bruit NOS
Heart murmur NOS
Systolic murmur NOS

**RØ1.2 Other cardiac sounds**
Cardiac dullness, increased or decreased
Precordial friction

✓4th **RØ3 Abnormal blood-pressure reading, without diagnosis**

**RØ3.Ø Elevated blood-pressure reading, without diagnosis of hypertension**
**NOTE** This category is to be used to record an episode of elevated blood pressure in a patient in whom no formal diagnosis of hypertension has been made, or as an isolated incidental finding.

**RØ3.1 Nonspecific low blood-pressure reading**
**EXCLUDES 1** *hypotension (I95.-)*
*maternal hypotension syndrome (O26.5-)*
*neurogenic orthostatic hypotension (G9Ø.3)*

✓4th **RØ4 Hemorrhage from respiratory passages**

**RØ4.Ø Epistaxis**
Hemorrhage from nose
Nosebleed
**AHA:** 2023,2Q,28

**RØ4.1 Hemorrhage from throat**
**EXCLUDES 2** *hemoptysis (RØ4.2)*

**RØ4.2 Hemoptysis**
Blood-stained sputum
Cough with hemorrhage
**AHA:** 2013,4Q,118

✓5th **RØ4.8 Hemorrhage from other sites in respiratory passages**

**RØ4.81 Acute idiopathic pulmonary hemorrhage in infants** P
Acute idiopathic hemorrhage in infants over 28 days old
AIPHI
**EXCLUDES 1** *perinatal pulmonary hemorrhage (P26.-)*
*von Willebrand disease (D68.Ø-)*

**RØ4.89 Hemorrhage from other sites in respiratory passages**
Pulmonary hemorrhage NOS

**RØ4.9 Hemorrhage from respiratory passages, unspecified**

✓4th **RØ5 Cough**
**EXCLUDES 1** *paroxysmal cough due to Bordetella pertussis (A37.Ø-)*
*smoker's cough (J41.Ø)*
**EXCLUDES 2** *cough with hemorrhage (RØ4.2)*
**AHA:** 2021,4Q,24-25; 2016,2Q,33

**RØ5.1 Acute cough**

**RØ5.2 Subacute cough**

**RØ5.3 Chronic cough**
Persistent cough
Refractory cough
Unexplained cough

**RØ5.4 Cough syncope** UPD
Code first syncope and collapse (R55)

**RØ5.8 Other specified cough**

**RØ5.9 Cough, unspecified**

**✓4th RØ6 Abnormalities of breathing**

EXCLUDES 1 *acute respiratory distress syndrome (J8Ø)*
*respiratory arrest (RØ9.2)*
*respiratory arrest of newborn (P28.81)*
*respiratory distress syndrome of newborn (P22.-)*
*respiratory failure (J96.-)*
*respiratory failure of newborn (P28.5)*

**✓5th RØ6.Ø Dyspnea**

EXCLUDES 1 *tachypnea NOS (RØ6.82)*
*transient tachypnea of newborn (P22.1)*

**RØ6.ØØ Dyspnea, unspecified**
**AHA:** 2017,1Q,26

**RØ6.Ø1 Orthopnea**

**RØ6.Ø2 Shortness of breath**

**RØ6.Ø3 Acute respiratory distress**
**AHA:** 2017,4Q,23

**RØ6.Ø9 Other forms of dyspnea**

**RØ6.1 Stridor**

EXCLUDES 1 *congenital laryngeal stridor (P28.89)*
*laryngismus (stridulus) (J38.5)*

**DEF:** Certain type of wheezing described as a loud, constant, musical sound produced when breathing with an obstructed airway, like the inspiratory sound heard when laryngeal or esophageal obstruction is present.

**RØ6.2 Wheezing**

EXCLUDES 1 *asthma (J45.-)*

**AHA:** 2016,2Q,33
**DEF:** High-pitched whistling sound during breathing due to stenosis of the respiratory passageway. Wheezing is associated with asthma, sleep apnea, bronchiectasis, bronchiolitis, COPD, and pleural effusion.

**RØ6.3 Periodic breathing**
Cheyne-Stokes breathing

**RØ6.4 Hyperventilation**

EXCLUDES 1 *psychogenic hyperventilation (F45.8)*

**RØ6.5 Mouth breathing**

EXCLUDES 2 *dry mouth NOS (R68.2)*

**RØ6.6 Hiccough**

EXCLUDES 1 *psychogenic hiccough (F45.8)*

**RØ6.7 Sneezing**

**✓5th RØ6.8 Other abnormalities of breathing**

**RØ6.81 Apnea, not elsewhere classified**
Apnea NOS

EXCLUDES 1 *apnea (of) newborn (P28.4-)*
*sleep apnea (G47.3-)*
*sleep apnea of newborn (primary) (P28.3-)*

**RØ6.82 Tachypnea, not elsewhere classified**
Tachypnea NOS

EXCLUDES 1 *transitory tachypnea of newborn (P22.1)*

**RØ6.83 Snoring**

**RØ6.89 Other abnormalities of breathing**
Breath-holding (spells)
Sighing

**RØ6.9 Unspecified abnormalities of breathing**

**✓4th RØ7 Pain in throat and chest**

EXCLUDES 1 *epidemic myalgia (B33.Ø)*

EXCLUDES 2 *jaw pain R68.84*
*pain in breast (N64.4)*

**RØ7.Ø Pain in throat**

EXCLUDES 1 *chronic sore throat (J31.2)*
*sore throat (acute) NOS (JØ2.9)*

EXCLUDES 2 *dysphagia (R13.1-)*
*pain in neck (M54.2)*

**RØ7.1 Chest pain on breathing**
Painful respiration

**RØ7.2 Precordial pain**
**DEF:** Pain felt in the anterior (front) chest wall over the region of the heart. This type of pain is generally felt slightly to the left of the sternum, but may also extend into the surrounding chest wall region.

**✓5th RØ7.8 Other chest pain**
**AHA:** 2024,3Q,16

**RØ7.81 Pleurodynia**
Pleurodynia NOS

EXCLUDES 1 *epidemic pleurodynia (B33.Ø)*

**RØ7.82 Intercostal pain**

**RØ7.89 Other chest pain**
Anterior chest-wall pain NOS
**AHA:** 2021,1Q,42

**RØ7.9 Chest pain, unspecified**

**✓4th RØ9 Other symptoms and signs involving the circulatory and respiratory system**

EXCLUDES 1 *acute respiratory distress syndrome (J8Ø)*
*respiratory arrest of newborn (P28.81)*
*respiratory distress syndrome of newborn (P22.Ø)*
*respiratory failure (J96.-)*
*respiratory failure of newborn (P28.5)*

**✓5th RØ9.Ø Asphyxia and hypoxemia**

EXCLUDES 1 *asphyxia due to carbon monoxide (T58.-)*
*asphyxia due to foreign body in respiratory tract (T17.-)*
*birth (intrauterine) asphyxia (P84)*
*hyperventilation (RØ6.4)*
*traumatic asphyxia (T71.-)*

EXCLUDES 2 *hypercapnia (RØ6.89)*

**RØ9.Ø1 Asphyxia**
**DEF:** Interference of oxygen intake due to obstruction or injury of airways resulting in a lack of oxygen perfusion to the tissues or excessive carbon dioxide in the blood. Can cause unconsciousness or death.

**RØ9.Ø2 Hypoxemia**
**AHA:** 2019,3Q,15
**DEF:** Insufficient oxygen in the arterial blood resulting in inadequate delivery of oxygen to the body tissues.

**RØ9.1 Pleurisy**

EXCLUDES 1 *pleurisy with effusion (J9Ø)*

**RØ9.2 Respiratory arrest** HCC ESR COM
Cardiorespiratory failure

EXCLUDES 1 *cardiac arrest (I46.-)*
*respiratory arrest of newborn (P28.81)*
*respiratory distress of newborn (P22.Ø)*
*respiratory failure (J96.-)*
*respiratory failure of newborn (P28.5)*
*respiratory insufficiency (RØ6.89)*
*respiratory insufficiency of newborn (P28.5)*

**RØ9.3 Abnormal sputum**
Abnormal amount of sputum
Abnormal color of sputum
Abnormal odor of sputum
Excessive sputum

EXCLUDES 1 *blood-stained sputum (RØ4.2)*

**✓5th RØ9.8 Other specified symptoms and signs involving the circulatory and respiratory systems**

**RØ9.81 Nasal congestion**

**RØ9.82 Postnasal drip**

**RØ9.89 Other specified symptoms and signs involving the circulatory and respiratory systems**
Abnormal chest percussion
Bruit (arterial)
Chest tympany
Choking sensation
Friction sounds in chest
Rales
Weak pulse

EXCLUDES 2 *foreign body in throat (T17.2-)*
*wheezing (RØ6.2)*

**AHA:** 2021,1Q,42

**✓5th RØ9.A Foreign body sensation of the circulatory and respiratory system**
**AHA:** 2023,4Q,41-42

**RØ9.AØ Foreign body sensation, unspecified**

**RØ9.A1 Foreign body sensation, nose**

**RØ9.A2 Foreign body sensation, throat**
Foreign body sensation globus

**RØ9.A9 Foreign body sensation, other site**

## Symptoms and signs involving the digestive system and abdomen (R1Ø-R19)

EXCLUDES 2 *congenital or infantile pylorospasm (Q4Ø.Ø)*
*gastrointestinal hemorrhage (K92.Ø-K92.2)*
*intestinal obstruction (K56.-)*
*newborn gastrointestinal hemorrhage (P54.Ø-P54.3)*
*newborn intestinal obstruction (P76.-)*
*pylorospasm (K31.3)*
*signs and symptoms involving the urinary system (R3Ø-R39)*
*symptoms referable to female genital organs (N94.-)*
*symptoms referable to male genital organs (N48-N5Ø)*

✓4th **R1Ø Abdominal and pelvic pain**
EXCLUDES 1 *renal colic (N23)*
EXCLUDES 2 *costovertebral (angle) tenderness (R39.85)*
*dorsalgia (M54.-)*
*flatulence and related conditions (R14.-)*

**R1Ø.Ø Acute abdomen**
Severe abdominal pain (generalized) (with abdominal rigidity)
EXCLUDES 1 *abdominal rigidity NOS (R19.3)*
*generalized abdominal pain NOS (R1Ø.84)*
*localized abdominal pain (R1Ø.1-R1Ø.3-)*

✓5th **R1Ø.1 Pain localized to upper abdomen**
EXCLUDES 2 *pain localized to flank (R1Ø.A-)*
*pelvic and perineal pain (R1Ø.2-)*

**R1Ø.1Ø Upper abdominal pain, unspecified**
**R1Ø.11 Right upper quadrant pain**
**R1Ø.12 Left upper quadrant pain**
**R1Ø.13 Epigastric pain**
Dyspepsia
EXCLUDES 1 *functional dyspepsia (K3Ø)*

**Abdominal Pain**

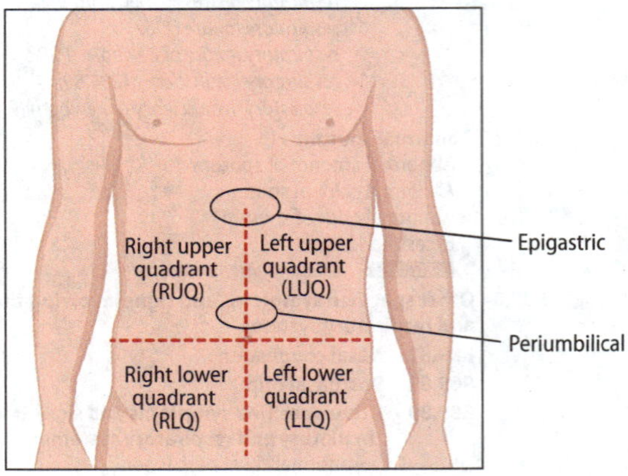


✓5th **R1Ø.2 Pelvic and perineal pain**
EXCLUDES 1 *vulvodynia (N94.81)*
EXCLUDES 2 *pain localized to other parts of lower abdomen (R1Ø.3-)*
*pain localized to upper abdomen (R1Ø.1-)*

**R1Ø.2Ø Pelvic and perineal pain unspecified side**
**R1Ø.21 Pelvic and perineal pain right side**
**R1Ø.22 Pelvic and perineal pain left side**
**R1Ø.23 Pelvic and perineal pain bilateral**
**R1Ø.24 Suprapubic pain**

✓5th **R1Ø.3 Pain localized to other parts of lower abdomen**
EXCLUDES 2 *pain localized to flank (R1Ø.A-)*
*pelvic and perineal pain (R1Ø.2-)*
**AHA:** 2025,4Q,28

**R1Ø.3Ø Lower abdominal pain, unspecified**
**R1Ø.31 Right lower quadrant pain**
**R1Ø.32 Left lower quadrant pain**
**R1Ø.33 Periumbilical pain**

✓5th **R1Ø.8 Other abdominal pain**

✓6th **R1Ø.81 Abdominal tenderness**
Abdominal tenderness NOS
EXCLUDES 2 *pain localized to other parts of lower abdomen (R1Ø.3-)*
*pain localized to upper abdomen (R1Ø.1-)*

**R1Ø.811 Right upper quadrant abdominal tenderness**
**R1Ø.812 Left upper quadrant abdominal tenderness**
**R1Ø.813 Right lower quadrant abdominal tenderness**
**R1Ø.814 Left lower quadrant abdominal tenderness**
**R1Ø.815 Periumbilic abdominal tenderness**
**R1Ø.816 Epigastric abdominal tenderness**
**R1Ø.817 Generalized abdominal tenderness**
**R1Ø.819 Abdominal tenderness, unspecified site**

✓6th **R1Ø.82 Rebound abdominal tenderness**
EXCLUDES 2 *pain localized to other parts of lower abdomen (R1Ø.3-)*
*pain localized to upper abdomen (R1Ø.1-)*

**R1Ø.821 Right upper quadrant rebound abdominal tenderness**
**R1Ø.822 Left upper quadrant rebound abdominal tenderness**
**R1Ø.823 Right lower quadrant rebound abdominal tenderness**
**R1Ø.824 Left lower quadrant rebound abdominal tenderness**
**R1Ø.825 Periumbilic rebound abdominal tenderness**
**R1Ø.826 Epigastric rebound abdominal tenderness**
**R1Ø.827 Generalized rebound abdominal tenderness**
**R1Ø.829 Rebound abdominal tenderness, unspecified site**

**R1Ø.83 Colic** P
Colic NOS
Infantile colic
EXCLUDES 1 *colic in adult and child over 12 months old (R1Ø.84)*
**DEF:** Inconsolable crying in an otherwise well-fed and healthy infant for more than three hours a day, three days a week, for more than three weeks.

**R1Ø.84 Generalized abdominal pain**
EXCLUDES 1 *generalized abdominal pain associated with acute abdomen (R1Ø.Ø)*

**R1Ø.85 Abdominal pain of multiple sites**
EXCLUDES 1 *abdominal rigidity NOS (R19.3)*
*generalized abdominal pain associated with acute abdomen (R1Ø.Ø)*
*generalized abdominal pain NOS (R1Ø.84)*
*localized abdominal pain ►(R1Ø.1-R1Ø.3-)◄*

✓6th **R1Ø.8A Flank tenderness**
**AHA:** 2025,4Q,28-29

**R1Ø.8A1 Right flank tenderness**
**R1Ø.8A2 Left flank tenderness**
**R1Ø.8A3 Suprapubic tenderness**
**R1Ø.8A9 Flank tenderness, unspecified**
Flank tenderness NOS

**R1Ø.9 Unspecified abdominal pain**

✓5th **R1Ø.A Pain localized to flank**
Lateral abdomen pain
Lateral flank pain
Latus region pain
EXCLUDES 2 *pain localized to other parts of lower abdomen (R1Ø.3-)*
*pain localized to upper abdomen (R1Ø.1-)*
**AHA:** 2025,4Q,28

**R1Ø.AØ Flank pain, unspecified side**
**R1Ø.A1 Flank pain, right side**
**R1Ø.A2 Flank pain, left side**
**R1Ø.A3 Flank pain, bilateral**

✓4th **R11 Nausea and vomiting**
EXCLUDES 1 *cyclical vomiting associated with migraine (G43.A-)*
*excessive vomiting in pregnancy (O21.-)*
*hematemesis (K92.Ø)*
*neonatal hematemesis (P54.Ø)*
*newborn vomiting (P92.Ø-)*
*psychogenic vomiting (F5Ø.89)*
*vomiting associated with bulimia nervosa (F5Ø.2-)*
*vomiting following gastrointestinal surgery (K91.Ø)*
**AHA:** 2017,1Q,28

**R11.Ø Nausea**
Nausea NOS
Nausea without vomiting

✓5th **R11.1 Vomiting**

**R11.1Ø Vomiting, unspecified**
Vomiting NOS
**R11.11 Vomiting without nausea**

**R11.12 Projectile vomiting**

**R11.13 Vomiting of fecal matter**

**R11.14 Bilious vomiting**

Bilious emesis

**R11.15 Cyclical vomiting syndrome unrelated to migraine**

Cyclic vomiting syndrome NOS

Persistent vomiting

EXCLUDES 1 *cyclical vomiting in migraine (G43.A-)*

EXCLUDES 2 *bulimia nervosa (F5Ø.2Ø)*

*diabetes mellitus due to underlying condition (EØ8.-)*

**AHA:** 2019,4Q,15

**R11.16 Cannabis hyperemesis syndrome** HCC ESR

Cannabinoid hyperemesis syndrome

Code also:

cannabis abuse (F12.1-)

cannabis dependence (F12.2-)

cannabis use, unspecified (F12.92-, F12.93, F12.95-, F12.98-, F12.99)

Code also manifestations, such as:

dehydration (E86.Ø)

electrolyte imbalance (E87.8)

**AHA:** 2025,4Q,30

**R11.2 Nausea with vomiting, unspecified**

Persistent nausea with vomiting NOS

**AHA:** 2020,1Q,8

**R12 Heartburn**

EXCLUDES 1 ~~*dyspepsia NOS (R1Ø.13)*~~

*functional dyspepsia (K3Ø)*

EXCLUDES 2 ▶*dyspepsia NOS (R1Ø.13)*◀

√4th **R13 Aphagia and dysphagia**

**R13.Ø Aphagia**

Inability to swallow

EXCLUDES 1 *psychogenic aphagia (F5Ø.9)*

√5th **R13.1 Dysphagia**

Code first, if applicable, dysphagia following cerebrovascular disease (I69. with final characters -91)

EXCLUDES 1 *psychogenic dysphagia (F45.8)*

**Swallowing Function**

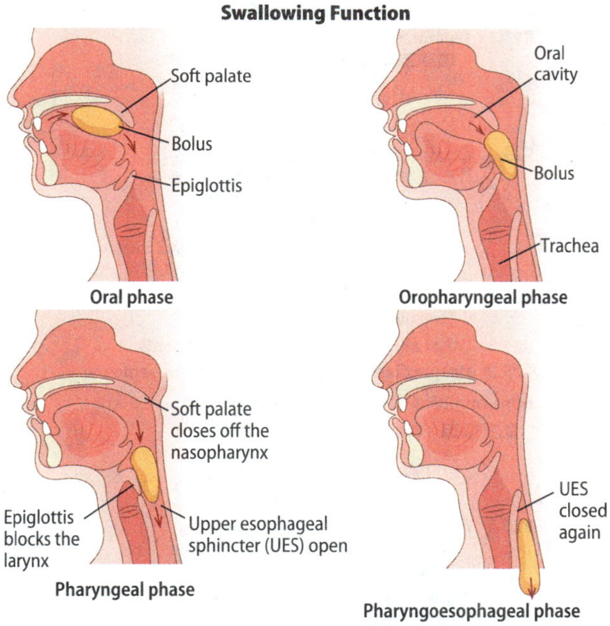


**R13.1Ø Dysphagia, unspecified**

Difficulty in swallowing NOS

**R13.11 Dysphagia, oral phase**

**R13.12 Dysphagia, oropharyngeal phase**

**R13.13 Dysphagia, pharyngeal phase**

**R13.14 Dysphagia, pharyngoesophageal phase**

**R13.19 Other dysphagia**

Cervical dysphagia

Neurogenic dysphagia

√4th **R14 Flatulence and related conditions**

EXCLUDES 1 *psychogenic aerophagy (F45.8)*

**R14.Ø Abdominal distension (gaseous)**

Bloating

Tympanites (abdominal) (intestinal)

**R14.1 Gas pain**

**R14.2 Eructation**

**R14.3 Flatulence**

√4th **R15 Fecal incontinence**

INCLUDES encopresis NOS

EXCLUDES 1 *fecal incontinence of nonorganic origin (F98.1)*

**R15.Ø Incomplete defecation**

EXCLUDES 2 *constipation (K59.Ø-)*

*fecal impaction (K56.41)*

**R15.1 Fecal smearing**

Fecal soiling

**R15.2 Fecal urgency**

**R15.9 Full incontinence of feces**

Fecal incontinence NOS

√4th **R16 Hepatomegaly and splenomegaly, not elsewhere classified**

**R16.Ø Hepatomegaly, not elsewhere classified**

Hepatomegaly NOS

**R16.1 Splenomegaly, not elsewhere classified**

Splenomegaly NOS

**R16.2 Hepatomegaly with splenomegaly, not elsewhere classified**

Hepatosplenomegaly NOS

**R17 Unspecified jaundice**

EXCLUDES 1 *neonatal jaundice (P55, P57-P59)*

√4th **R18 Ascites**

INCLUDES fluid in peritoneal cavity

EXCLUDES 1 *ascites in alcoholic cirrhosis (K7Ø.31)*

*ascites in alcoholic hepatitis (K7Ø.11)*

*ascites in toxic liver disease with chronic active hepatitis (K71.51)*

**DEF:** Abnormal accumulation of free fluid in the abdominal cavity, causing distention and tightness in addition to shortness of breath as the fluid accumulates. Ascites is usually an underlying disorder and can be a manifestation of any number of diseases.

**R18.Ø Malignant ascites** HCC UPD

Code first malignancy, such as:

malignant neoplasm of ovary (C56.-)

secondary malignant neoplasm of retroperitoneum and peritoneum (C78.6)

**R18.8 Other ascites**

Ascites NOS

Peritoneal effusion (chronic)

**AHA:** 2018,1Q,4

√4th **R19 Other symptoms and signs involving the digestive system and abdomen**

EXCLUDES 1 *acute abdomen (R1Ø.Ø)*

√5th **R19.Ø Intra-abdominal and pelvic swelling, mass and lump**

EXCLUDES 1 *abdominal distension (gaseous) (R14.-)*

*ascites (R18.-)*

**R19.ØØ Intra-abdominal and pelvic swelling, mass and lump, unspecified site**

**R19.Ø1 Right upper quadrant abdominal swelling, mass and lump**

**R19.Ø2 Left upper quadrant abdominal swelling, mass and lump**

**R19.Ø3 Right lower quadrant abdominal swelling, mass and lump**

**R19.Ø4 Left lower quadrant abdominal swelling, mass and lump**

**R19.Ø5 Periumbilic swelling, mass or lump**

Diffuse or generalized umbilical swelling or mass

**R19.Ø6 Epigastric swelling, mass or lump**

**R19.Ø7 Generalized intra-abdominal and pelvic swelling, mass and lump**

Diffuse or generalized intra-abdominal swelling or mass NOS

Diffuse or generalized pelvic swelling or mass NOS

**R19.Ø9 Other intra-abdominal and pelvic swelling, mass and lump**

√5th **R19.1 Abnormal bowel sounds**

**R19.11 Absent bowel sounds**

**R19.12 Hyperactive bowel sounds**

**R19.15 Other abnormal bowel sounds**

Abnormal bowel sounds NOS

**R19.2 Visible peristalsis**
Hyperperistalsis
**DEF:** Visible movements of muscular attempts to move food through the digestive tract due to pyloric obstruction, stomach obstruction, or intestinal obstruction.

√5th **R19.3 Abdominal rigidity**
EXCLUDES 1 *abdominal rigidity with severe abdominal pain (R1Ø.Ø)*

**R19.3Ø Abdominal rigidity, unspecified site**
**R19.31 Right upper quadrant abdominal rigidity**
**R19.32 Left upper quadrant abdominal rigidity**
**R19.33 Right lower quadrant abdominal rigidity**
**R19.34 Left lower quadrant abdominal rigidity**
**R19.35 Periumbilic abdominal rigidity**
**R19.36 Epigastric abdominal rigidity**
**R19.37 Generalized abdominal rigidity**

**R19.4 Change in bowel habit**
EXCLUDES 1 *constipation (K59.Ø-)*
*functional diarrhea (K59.1)*

**R19.5 Other fecal abnormalities**
Abnormal stool color
Bulky stools
Mucus in stools
Occult blood in feces
Occult blood in stools
EXCLUDES 1 *melena (K92.1)*
*neonatal melena (P54.1)*
**AHA:** 2021,1Q,9; 2019,1Q,32

**R19.6 Halitosis**

**R19.7 Diarrhea, unspecified**
Diarrhea NOS
EXCLUDES 1 *functional diarrhea (K59.1)*
*neonatal diarrhea (P78.3)*
*psychogenic diarrhea (F45.8)*
**AHA:** 2021,3Q,3

**R19.8 Other specified symptoms and signs involving the digestive system and abdomen**

## Symptoms and signs involving the skin and subcutaneous tissue (R2Ø-R23)

EXCLUDES 2 *symptoms relating to breast (N64.4-N64.5)*

√4th **R2Ø Disturbances of skin sensation**
EXCLUDES 1 *dissociative anesthesia and sensory loss (F44.6)*
*psychogenic disturbances (F45.8)*

**R2Ø.Ø Anesthesia of skin**
**R2Ø.1 Hypoesthesia of skin**
**R2Ø.2 Paresthesia of skin**
Formication
Pins and needles
Tingling skin
EXCLUDES 1 *acroparesthesia (I73.8)*
**R2Ø.3 Hyperesthesia**
**R2Ø.8 Other disturbances of skin sensation**
**R2Ø.9 Unspecified disturbances of skin sensation**

**R21 Rash and other nonspecific skin eruption**
INCLUDES rash NOS
EXCLUDES 1 *specified type of rash - code to condition*
*vesicular eruption (R23.8)*

√4th **R22 Localized swelling, mass and lump of skin and subcutaneous tissue**
INCLUDES subcutaneous nodules (localized)(superficial)
EXCLUDES 1 *abnormal findings on diagnostic imaging (R9Ø-R93)*
*edema (R6Ø.-)*
*enlarged lymph nodes (R59.-)*
*localized adiposity (E65)*
*swelling of joint (M25.4-)*

**R22.Ø Localized swelling, mass and lump, head**
**R22.1 Localized swelling, mass and lump, neck**
**R22.2 Localized swelling, mass and lump, trunk**
EXCLUDES 1 *intra-abdominal or pelvic mass and lump (R19.Ø-)*
*intra-abdominal or pelvic swelling (R19.Ø-)*
EXCLUDES 2 *breast mass and lump (N63)*
**AHA:** 2022,3Q,8

√5th **R22.3 Localized swelling, mass and lump, upper limb**
**R22.3Ø Localized swelling, mass and lump, unspecified upper limb**
**R22.31 Localized swelling, mass and lump, right upper limb**
**R22.32 Localized swelling, mass and lump, left upper limb**
**R22.33 Localized swelling, mass and lump, upper limb, bilateral**

√5th **R22.4 Localized swelling, mass and lump, lower limb**
**R22.4Ø Localized swelling, mass and lump, unspecified lower limb**
**R22.41 Localized swelling, mass and lump, right lower limb**
**R22.42 Localized swelling, mass and lump, left lower limb**
**R22.43 Localized swelling, mass and lump, lower limb, bilateral**

**R22.9 Localized swelling, mass and lump, unspecified**

√4th **R23 Other skin changes**
**R23.Ø Cyanosis**
EXCLUDES 1 *acrocyanosis (I73.8)*
*cyanotic attacks of newborn (P28.2)*
**DEF:** Bluish or purplish discoloration of the skin due to an inadequate oxygen blood level.

**R23.1 Pallor**
Clammy skin

**R23.2 Flushing**
Excessive blushing
Code first, if applicable, menopausal and female climacteric states (N95.1)

**R23.3 Spontaneous ecchymoses**
Petechiae
EXCLUDES 1 *ecchymoses of newborn (P54.5)*
*purpura (D69.-)*

**R23.4 Changes in skin texture**
Desquamation of skin
Induration of skin
Scaling of skin
EXCLUDES 1 *epidermal thickening NOS (L85.9)*

**R23.8 Other skin changes**
**R23.9 Unspecified skin changes**

## Symptoms and signs involving the nervous and musculoskeletal systems (R25-R29)

√4th **R25 Abnormal involuntary movements**
EXCLUDES 1 *specific movement disorders (G2Ø-G26)*
*stereotyped movement disorders (F98.4)*
*tic disorders (F95.-)*

**R25.Ø Abnormal head movements**
**R25.1 Tremor, unspecified**
EXCLUDES 1 *chorea NOS (G25.5)*
*essential tremor (G25.Ø)*
*hysterical tremor (F44.4)*
*intention tremor (G25.2)*

**R25.2 Cramp and spasm**
EXCLUDES 2 *carpopedal spasm (R29.Ø)*
*charley-horse (M62.831)*
*infantile spasms (G4Ø.4-)*
*muscle spasm of back (M62.83Ø)*
*muscle spasm of calf (M62.831)*

**R25.3 Fasciculation**
Twitching NOS
**R25.8 Other abnormal involuntary movements**
**R25.9 Unspecified abnormal involuntary movements**

√4th **R26 Abnormalities of gait and mobility**
EXCLUDES 1 *ataxia NOS (R27.Ø)*
*hereditary ataxia (G11.-)*
*immobility syndrome (paraplegic) (M62.3)*
*locomotor (syphilitic) ataxia (A52.11)*

**R26.Ø Ataxic gait**
Staggering gait
**AHA:** 2022,2Q,12

**R26.1 Paralytic gait**
Spastic gait

**R26.2 Difficulty in walking, not elsewhere classified**
EXCLUDES 1 *falling (R29.6)*
~~*unsteadiness on feet (R26.81)*~~
EXCLUDES 2 ▶*unsteadiness on feet (R26.81)*◀
**AHA:** 2016,2Q,7

√5th **R26.8 Other abnormalities of gait and mobility**
**R26.81 Unsteadiness on feet**
**R26.89 Other abnormalities of gait and mobility**
**AHA:** 2020,2Q,29

**R26.9 Unspecified abnormalities of gait and mobility**

**R27 Other lack of coordination**
EXCLUDES 1 *ataxic gait (R26.Ø)*
*hereditary ataxia (G11.-)*
*vertigo NOS (R42)*

**R27.Ø Ataxia, unspecified**
EXCLUDES 1 *ataxia following cerebrovascular disease (I69. with final characters -93)*

**R27.8 Other lack of coordination**

**R27.9 Unspecified lack of coordination**

**R29 Other symptoms and signs involving the nervous and musculoskeletal systems**

**R29.Ø Tetany**
Carpopedal spasm
EXCLUDES 1 *hysterical tetany (F44.5)*
*neonatal tetany (P71.3)*
*parathyroid tetany (E2Ø.9)*
*post-thyroidectomy tetany (E89.2)*
**DEF:** Calcium or other mineral imbalance causing voluntary muscles such as hands, feet, or larynx to spasm rhythmically.

**R29.1 Meningismus**

**R29.2 Abnormal reflex**
EXCLUDES 2 *abnormal pupillary reflex (H57.Ø)*
*hyperactive gag reflex (J39.2)*
*vasovagal reaction or syncope (R55)*

**R29.3 Abnormal posture**

**R29.4 Clicking hip**
EXCLUDES 1 *congenital deformities of hip (Q65.-)*

**R29.5 Transient paralysis**
Code first any associated spinal cord injury (S14.Ø, S14.1-, S24.Ø, S24.1-, S34.Ø-, S34.1-)
EXCLUDES 1 *transient ischemic attack (G45.9)*

**R29.6 Repeated falls**
Falling
Tendency to fall
EXCLUDES 2 *at risk for falling (Z91.81)*
*history of falling (Z91.81)*
**AHA:** 2016,2Q,6

**R29.7 National Institutes of Health Stroke Scale (NIHSS) score**
Code first the type of cerebral infarction ▶(I6Ø.-, I61.-, I62.-, I63.-)◀
**AHA:** 2016,4Q,61-62
**TIP:** Codes from this subcategory may be assigned based on medical record documentation from clinicians who are not the patient's provider.

**R29.7Ø NIHSS score Ø-9**
- **R29.7ØØ NIHSS score Ø** UPD
- **R29.7Ø1 NIHSS score 1** UPD
- **R29.7Ø2 NIHSS score 2** UPD
- **R29.7Ø3 NIHSS score 3** UPD
- **R29.7Ø4 NIHSS score 4** UPD
- **R29.7Ø5 NIHSS score 5** UPD
- **R29.7Ø6 NIHSS score 6** UPD
- **R29.7Ø7 NIHSS score 7** UPD
- **R29.7Ø8 NIHSS score 8** UPD
- **R29.7Ø9 NIHSS score 9** UPD

**R29.71 NIHSS score 1Ø-19**
- **R29.71Ø NIHSS score 1Ø** UPD
- **R29.711 NIHSS score 11** UPD
- **R29.712 NIHSS score 12** UPD
- **R29.713 NIHSS score 13** UPD
- **R29.714 NIHSS score 14** UPD
- **R29.715 NIHSS score 15** UPD
- **R29.716 NIHSS score 16** UPD
- **R29.717 NIHSS score 17** UPD
- **R29.718 NIHSS score 18** UPD
- **R29.719 NIHSS score 19** UPD

**R29.72 NIHSS score 2Ø-29**
- **R29.72Ø NIHSS score 2Ø** UPD
- **R29.721 NIHSS score 21** UPD
- **R29.722 NIHSS score 22** UPD
- **R29.723 NIHSS score 23** UPD
- **R29.724 NIHSS score 24** UPD
- **R29.725 NIHSS score 25** UPD
- **R29.726 NIHSS score 26** UPD
- **R29.727 NIHSS score 27** UPD
- **R29.728 NIHSS score 28** UPD
- **R29.729 NIHSS score 29** UPD

**R29.73 NIHSS score 3Ø-39**
- **R29.73Ø NIHSS score 3Ø** UPD
- **R29.731 NIHSS score 31** UPD
- **R29.732 NIHSS score 32** UPD
- **R29.733 NIHSS score 33** UPD
- **R29.734 NIHSS score 34** UPD
- **R29.735 NIHSS score 35** UPD
- **R29.736 NIHSS score 36** UPD
- **R29.737 NIHSS score 37** UPD
- **R29.738 NIHSS score 38** UPD
- **R29.739 NIHSS score 39** UPD

**R29.74 NIHSS score 4Ø-42**
- **R29.74Ø NIHSS score 4Ø** UPD
- **R29.741 NIHSS score 41** UPD
- **R29.742 NIHSS score 42** UPD

**R29.8 Other symptoms and signs involving the nervous and musculoskeletal systems**

**R29.81 Other symptoms and signs involving the nervous system**

**R29.81Ø Facial weakness**
Facial droop
EXCLUDES 1 *Bell's palsy (G51.Ø)*
*facial weakness following cerebrovascular disease (I69. with final characters -92)*

**R29.818 Other symptoms and signs involving the nervous system**

**R29.89 Other symptoms and signs involving the musculoskeletal system**
EXCLUDES 2 *pain in limb (M79.6-)*

**R29.89Ø Loss of height**
EXCLUDES 1 *osteoporosis (M8Ø-M81)*

**R29.891 Ocular torticollis**
EXCLUDES 1 *congenital (sternomastoid) torticollis Q68.Ø*
*psychogenic torticollis (F45.8)*
*spasmodic torticollis (G24.3)*
*torticollis due to birth injury (P15.8)*
*torticollis NOS M43.6*
**DEF:** Abnormal head posture as a result of a contracted state of cervical muscles to correct a visual disturbance, either double vision or a visual field defect.

**R29.898 Other symptoms and signs involving the musculoskeletal system**

**R29.9 Unspecified symptoms and signs involving the nervous and musculoskeletal systems**

**R29.9Ø Unspecified symptoms and signs involving the nervous system**

**R29.91 Unspecified symptoms and signs involving the musculoskeletal system**

## Symptoms and signs involving the genitourinary system (R3Ø-R39)

**R3Ø Pain associated with micturition**
EXCLUDES 1 *psychogenic pain associated with micturition (F45.8)*

**R3Ø.Ø Dysuria**
Strangury

**R3Ø.1 Vesical tenesmus**
**DEF:** Feeling of a full bladder even when there is little or no urine in the bladder.

**R3Ø.9 Painful micturition, unspecified**
Painful urination NOS

**R31 Hematuria**
EXCLUDES 1 *hematuria included with underlying conditions, such as:*
*acute cystitis with hematuria (N3Ø.Ø1)*
*recurrent and persistent hematuria in glomerular diseases (NØ2.-)*
**AHA:** 2025,2Q,20-21; 2017,1Q,17

**R31.Ø Gross hematuria**

**R31.1 Benign essential microscopic hematuria**

√5th **R31.2 Other microscopic hematuria**
AHA: 2016,4Q,62
**R31.21 Asymptomatic microscopic hematuria**
AMH
**R31.29 Other microscopic hematuria**
**R31.9 Hematuria, unspecified**

**R32 Unspecified urinary incontinence**
Enuresis NOS
EXCLUDES 1 *functional urinary incontinence (R39.81)*
*nonorganic enuresis (F98.0)*
*stress incontinence and other specified urinary incontinence (N39.3-N39.4-)*
*urinary incontinence associated with cognitive impairment (R39.81)*

√4th **R33 Retention of urine**
EXCLUDES 1 *psychogenic retention of urine (F45.8)*
**R33.0 Drug induced retention of urine**
Use additional code for adverse effect, if applicable, to identify drug (T36-T50 with fifth or sixth character 5)
**R33.8 Other retention of urine**
Code first, if applicable, any causal condition, such as:
enlarged prostate (N40.1)
AHA: 2018,4Q,55
**R33.9 Retention of urine, unspecified**

**R34 Anuria and oliguria**
EXCLUDES 1 *anuria and oliguria complicating abortion or ectopic or molar pregnancy (O00-O07, O08.4)*
*anuria and oliguria complicating pregnancy (O26.83-)*
*anuria and oliguria complicating the puerperium (O90.49)*

√4th **R35 Polyuria**
Code first, if applicable, any causal condition, such as:
enlarged prostate (N40.1)
EXCLUDES 1 *psychogenic polyuria (F45.8)*
**R35.0 Frequency of micturition**
**R35.1 Nocturia**
√5th **R35.8 Other polyuria**
AHA: 2021,4Q,26
**R35.81 Nocturnal polyuria**
EXCLUDES 2 *nocturnal enuresis (N39.44)*
**R35.89 Other polyuria**
Polyuria NOS

√4th **R36 Urethral discharge**
**R36.0 Urethral discharge without blood**
**R36.1 Hematospermia**
**R36.9 Urethral discharge, unspecified**
Penile discharge NOS
Urethrorrhea

**R37 Sexual dysfunction, unspecified**

√4th **R39 Other and unspecified symptoms and signs involving the genitourinary system**
**R39.0 Extravasation of urine**
√5th **R39.1 Other difficulties with micturition**
Code first, if applicable, any causal condition, such as:
enlarged prostate (N40.1)
**R39.11 Hesitancy of micturition**
**R39.12 Poor urinary stream**
Weak urinary stream
**R39.13 Splitting of urinary stream**
**R39.14 Feeling of incomplete bladder emptying**
**R39.15 Urgency of urination**
EXCLUDES 1 *urge incontinence (N39.41, N39.46)*
**R39.16 Straining to void**
√6th **R39.19 Other difficulties with micturition**
AHA: 2016,4Q,63
**R39.191 Need to immediately re-void**
**R39.192 Position dependent micturition**
**R39.198 Other difficulties with micturition**
**R39.2 Extrarenal uremia**
Prerenal uremia
EXCLUDES 1 *uremia NOS (N19)*

√5th **R39.8 Other symptoms and signs involving the genitourinary system**
AHA: 2017,4Q,22-23
**R39.81 Functional urinary incontinence**
Urinary incontinence due to cognitive impairment, or severe physical disability or immobility
EXCLUDES 1 *stress incontinence and other specified urinary incontinence (N39.3-N39.4-)*
*urinary incontinence NOS (R32)*
**R39.82 Chronic bladder pain**
AHA: 2016,4Q,64
**R39.83 Unilateral non-palpable testicle**
**R39.84 Bilateral non-palpable testicles**
√6th **R39.85 Costovertebral (angle) tenderness**
EXCLUDES 2 *abdominal and pelvic pain (R10.-)*
**R39.851 Costovertebral (angle) tenderness, right side**
**R39.852 Costovertebral (angle) tenderness, left side**
**R39.853 Costovertebral (angle) tenderness, bilateral**
**R39.859 Costovertebral (angle) tenderness, unspecified side**
**R39.89 Other symptoms and signs involving the genitourinary system**
**R39.9 Unspecified symptoms and signs involving the genitourinary system**

## Symptoms and signs involving cognition, perception, emotional state and behavior (R40-R46)

EXCLUDES 2 *symptoms and signs constituting part of a pattern of mental disorder (F01-F99)*

√4th **R40 Somnolence, stupor and coma**
EXCLUDES 1 *neonatal coma (P91.5)*
*somnolence, stupor and coma in diabetes (E08-E13)*
*somnolence, stupor and coma in hepatic failure (K72.-)*
*somnolence, stupor and coma in hypoglycemia (nondiabetic) (E15)*
**R40.0 Somnolence**
Drowsiness
EXCLUDES 1 *coma (R40.2-)*
**R40.1 Stupor**
Catatonic stupor
Semicoma
EXCLUDES 1 *catatonic schizophrenia (F20.2)*
*coma (R40.2-)*
*depressive stupor (F31.-, F32.-, F33.-)*
*dissociative stupor (F44.2)*
*manic stupor (F30.2)*
√5th **R40.2 Coma**
NOTE One code from each subcategory, R40.21-R40.23, is required to complete the coma scale
Code first any associated:
fracture of skull (S02.-)
intracranial injury (S06.-)
AHA: 2020,3Q,46; 2019,2Q,12; 2018,4Q,70; 2017,4Q,23-25,95; 2015,2Q,17; 2014,1Q,19
TIP: Codes for individual (R40.21-, R40.22-, R40.23-) or total (R40.24-) coma scale scores may be assigned based on medical record documentation from clinicians who are not the patient's provider.
TIP: It is not appropriate to assign individual (R40.21-, R40.22-, R40.23-) or total (R40.24-) coma scale score codes for patients who are sedated or in medically induced comas, nor in conjunction with code R40.2A.
**R40.20 Unspecified coma** HCC ESR COM
Coma NOS
Unconsciousness NOS
AHA: 2021,4Q,112-113; 2021,2Q,5

**R40.21 Coma scale, eyes open**

The following appropriate 7th character is to be added to subcategory R40.21-, R40.22-, R40.23-, and R40.24-.
- 0 unspecified time
- 1 in the field [EMT or ambulance]
- 2 at arrival to emergency department
- 3 at hospital admission
- 4 24 hours or more after hospital admission

**R40.211 Coma scale, eyes open, never** HCC ESR COM UPD
Coma scale eye opening score of 1

**R40.212 Coma scale, eyes open, to pain** HCC ESR COM UPD
Coma scale eye opening score of 2

**R40.213 Coma scale, eyes open, to sound** UPD
Coma scale eye opening score of 3

**R40.214 Coma scale, eyes open, spontaneous** UPD
Coma scale eye opening score of 4

**R40.22 Coma scale, best verbal response**

**R40.221 Coma scale, best verbal response, none** HCC ESR COM UPD
Coma scale verbal score of 1

**R40.222 Coma scale, best verbal response, incomprehensible words** HCC ESR COM UPD
Coma scale verbal score of 2
Incomprehensible sounds (2-5 years of age)
Moans/grunts to pain; restless (< 2 years old)

**R40.223 Coma scale, best verbal response, inappropriate words** UPD
Coma scale verbal score of 3
Inappropriate crying or screaming (< 2 years of age)
Screaming (2-5 years of age)

**R40.224 Coma scale, best verbal response, confused conversation** UPD
Coma scale verbal score of 4
Inappropriate words (2-5 years of age)
Irritable cries (< 2 years of age)

**R40.225 Coma scale, best verbal response, oriented** UPD
Coma scale verbal score of 5
Cooing or babbling or crying appropriately (< 2 years of age)
Uses appropriate words (2-5 years of age)

**R40.23 Coma scale, best motor response**

**R40.231 Coma scale, best motor response, none** HCC ESR COM UPD
Coma scale motor score of 1

**R40.232 Coma scale, best motor response, extension** HCC ESR COM UPD
Abnormal extensor posturing to pain or noxious stimuli (< 2 years of age)
Coma scale motor score of 2
Extensor posturing to pain or noxious stimuli (2-5 years of age)

**R40.233 Coma scale, best motor response, abnormal flexion** UPD
Abnormal flexure posturing to pain or noxious stimuli (2-5 years of age)
Coma scale motor score of 3
Flexion/decorticate posturing (< 2 years of age)

**R40.234 Coma scale, best motor response, flexion withdrawal** ESR COM UPD
Coma scale motor score of 4
Withdraws from pain or noxious stimuli (2-5 years of age)

**R40.235 Coma scale, best motor response, localizes pain** UPD
Coma scale motor score of 5
Localizes pain (2-5 years of age)
Withdraws to touch (< 2 years of age)

**R40.236 Coma scale, best motor response, obeys commands** UPD
Coma scale motor score of 6
Normal or spontaneous movement (< 2 years of age)
Obeys commands (2-5 years of age)

**R40.24 Glasgow coma scale, total score**

NOTE Assign a code from subcategory R40.24, when only the total coma score is documented

AHA: 2021,2Q,4; 2016,4Q,64-65

**R40.241 Glasgow coma scale score 13-15** UPD

**R40.242 Glasgow coma scale score 9-12** UPD

**R40.243 Glasgow coma scale score 3-8** HCC ESR COM UPD

**R40.244 Other coma, without documented Glasgow coma scale score, or with partial score reported** HCC ESR COM UPD

**R40.2A Nontraumatic coma due to underlying condition** HCC ESR COM UPD
Secondary coma
Code first underlying condition
EXCLUDES 1 *coma scale, best motor response (R40.24.-)*
*coma scale, best verbal response (R40.22.-)*
*coma scale, eyes open (R40.21.-)*
*Glasgow coma scale, total score (R40.23.-)*

AHA: 2023,4Q,42

**R40.3 Persistent vegetative state** HCC ESR COM
DEF: Persistent wakefulness without consciousness due to a nonfunctioning cerebral cortex.

**R40.4 Transient alteration of awareness**
AHA: 2020,2Q,24

**R41 Other symptoms and signs involving cognitive functions and awareness**
EXCLUDES 1 *dissociative [conversion] disorders (F44.-)*
*mild cognitive impairment of uncertain or unknown etiology) (G31.84)*

**R41.0 Disorientation, unspecified**
Confusion NOS
Delirium NOS
EXCLUDES 1 *delirium due to known physiological condition (F05)*
AHA: 2022,2Q,11; 2019,2Q,34

**R41.1 Anterograde amnesia**

**R41.2 Retrograde amnesia**

**R41.3 Other amnesia**
Amnesia NOS
Memory loss NOS
EXCLUDES 1 *amnestic disorder due to known physiologic condition (F04)*
*amnestic syndrome due to psychoactive substance use (F10-F19 with 5th character .6)*
*mild memory disturbance due to known physiological condition (F06.8)*
*transient global amnesia (G45.4)*

**R41.4 Neurologic neglect syndrome**
Asomatognosia
Hemi-akinesia
Hemi-inattention
Hemispatial neglect
Left-sided neglect
Sensory neglect
Visuospatial neglect
EXCLUDES 1 *visuospatial deficit (R41.842)*

**R41.8 Other symptoms and signs involving cognitive functions and awareness**

**R41.81 Age-related cognitive decline** A
Senility NOS

**R41.82 Altered mental status, unspecified**
Change in mental status NOS
EXCLUDES 1 *altered level of consciousness (R40.-)*
*altered mental status due to known condition - code to condition*
*delirium NOS (R41.0)*
AHA: 2012,4Q,97

**R41.83 Borderline intellectual functioning**
IQ level 71 to 84
EXCLUDES 1 *intellectual disabilities (F70-F79)*

√6th **R41.84 Other specified cognitive deficit**
Code first the underlying condition, if known, such as:
schizophrenia (F2Ø.-)
EXCLUDES 1 *cognitive deficits as sequelae of cerebrovascular disease (I69.Ø1-, I69.11-, I69.21-, I69.31-, I69.81-, I69.91-)*

**R41.84Ø Attention and concentration deficit**
EXCLUDES 1 *attention-deficit hyperactivity disorders (F9Ø.-)*

**R41.841 Cognitive communication deficit**

**R41.842 Visuospatial deficit**

**R41.843 Psychomotor deficit**

**R41.844 Frontal lobe and executive function deficit**

**R41.85 Anosognosia**
AHA: 2024,4Q,27

**R41.89 Other symptoms and signs involving cognitive functions and awareness**

**R41.9 Unspecified symptoms and signs involving cognitive functions and awareness**
Unspecified neurocognitive disorder

**R42 Dizziness and giddiness** Q
Light-headedness
Vertigo NOS
EXCLUDES 1 *vertiginous syndromes (H81.-)*
*vertigo from infrasound (T75.23)*

√4th **R43 Disturbances of smell and taste**

**R43.Ø Anosmia**
DEF: Permanent or transient absence of smell that may be congenital or acquired.

**R43.1 Parosmia**
DEF: Abnormal perception of smell usually triggered by environmental odors.

**R43.2 Parageusia**
DEF: Abnormal perception of taste.

**R43.8 Other disturbances of smell and taste**
Mixed disturbance of smell and taste

**R43.9 Unspecified disturbances of smell and taste**

√4th **R44 Other symptoms and signs involving general sensations and perceptions**
EXCLUDES 1 *alcoholic hallucinations (F1Ø.151, F1Ø.251, F1Ø.951)*
*hallucinations in drug psychosis (F11-F19 with fifth to sixth characters 51)*
*hallucinations in mood disorders with psychotic symptoms (F3Ø.2, F31.5, F32.3, F33.3)*
*hallucinations in schizophrenia, schizotypal and delusional disorders (F2Ø-F29)*
EXCLUDES 2 *disturbances of skin sensation (R2Ø.-)*

**R44.Ø Auditory hallucinations**

**R44.1 Visual hallucinations**

**R44.2 Other hallucinations**

**R44.3 Hallucinations, unspecified**
AHA: 2025,3Q,7; 2022,2Q,11

**R44.8 Other symptoms and signs involving general sensations and perceptions**

**R44.9 Unspecified symptoms and signs involving general sensations and perceptions**

√4th **R45 Symptoms and signs involving emotional state**

**R45.Ø Nervousness**
Nervous tension

**R45.1 Restlessness and agitation**

**R45.2 Unhappiness**

**R45.3 Demoralization and apathy**
EXCLUDES 1 *anhedonia (R45.84)*

**R45.4 Irritability and anger**

**R45.5 Hostility**

**R45.6 Violent behavior**

**R45.7 State of emotional shock and stress, unspecified**

√5th **R45.8 Other symptoms and signs involving emotional state**

**R45.81 Low self-esteem**

**R45.82 Worries**

**R45.83 Excessive crying of child, adolescent or adult**
EXCLUDES 1 *excessive crying of infant (baby) R68.11*

**R45.84 Anhedonia**

√6th **R45.85 Homicidal and suicidal ideations**
EXCLUDES 1 *suicide attempt (T14.91)*

**R45.85Ø Homicidal ideations**

**R45.851 Suicidal ideations**
AHA: 2022,1Q,29
DEF: Thoughts of committing suicide but no actual attempt of suicide has been made.

**R45.86 Emotional lability**

**R45.87 Impulsiveness**

**R45.88 Nonsuicidal self-harm** HCC Rx ESR COM
Nonsuicidal self-injury
Nonsuicidal self-mutilation
Self-inflicted injury without suicidal intent
Code also injury, if known
AHA: 2021,4Q,26-27

**R45.89 Other symptoms and signs involving emotional state**
Flat affect
Loneliness

√4th **R46 Symptoms and signs involving appearance and behavior**
EXCLUDES 1 *appearance and behavior in schizophrenia, schizotypal and delusional disorders (F2Ø-F29)*
*mental and behavioral disorders (FØ1-F99)*

**R46.Ø Very low level of personal hygiene**

**R46.1 Bizarre personal appearance**

**R46.2 Strange and inexplicable behavior**

**R46.3 Overactivity**

**R46.4 Slowness and poor responsiveness**
EXCLUDES 1 *stupor (R4Ø.1)*

**R46.5 Suspiciousness and marked evasiveness**

**R46.6 Undue concern and preoccupation with stressful events**

**R46.7 Verbosity and circumstantial detail obscuring reason for contact**

√5th **R46.8 Other symptoms and signs involving appearance and behavior**

**R46.81 Obsessive-compulsive behavior**
EXCLUDES 1 *obsessive-compulsive disorder (F42.-)*

**R46.89 Other symptoms and signs involving appearance and behavior**

## Symptoms and signs involving speech and voice (R47-R49)

√4th **R47 Speech disturbances, not elsewhere classified**
EXCLUDES 1 *autism (F84.Ø)*
*cluttering (F8Ø.81)*
*specific developmental disorders of speech and language (F8Ø.-)*
*stuttering (F8Ø.81)*

√5th **R47.Ø Dysphasia and aphasia**

**R47.Ø1 Aphasia**
EXCLUDES 1 *aphasia following cerebrovascular disease (I69. with final characters -2Ø)*
*progressive isolated aphasia (G31.Ø1)*

**R47.Ø2 Dysphasia**
EXCLUDES 1 *dysphasia following cerebrovascular disease (I69. with final characters -21)*

**R47.1 Dysarthria and anarthria**
EXCLUDES 1 *dysarthria following cerebrovascular disease (I69. with final characters -22)*

√5th **R47.8 Other speech disturbances**
EXCLUDES 1 *dysarthria following cerebrovascular disease (I69. with final characters -28)*

**R47.81 Slurred speech**

***R47.82 Fluency disorder in conditions classified elsewhere***
Stuttering in conditions classified elsewhere
Code first underlying disease or condition, such as:
Parkinson's disease (G2Ø.-)
EXCLUDES 1 *adult onset fluency disorder (F98.5)*
*childhood onset fluency disorder (F8Ø.81)*
*fluency disorder (stuttering) following cerebrovascular disease (I69. with final characters -23)*

**R47.89 Other speech disturbances**

**R47.9 Unspecified speech disturbances**

√4th **R48 Dyslexia and other symbolic dysfunctions, not elsewhere classified**
EXCLUDES 1 *specific developmental disorders of scholastic skills (F81.-)*

**R48.Ø Dyslexia and alexia**

**R48.1 Agnosia**
Astereognosia (astereognosis)
Autotopagnosia
EXCLUDES 1 *visual object agnosia (R48.3)*
DEF: Inability to recognize common things such as faces, objects, smells, or voices.

**R48.2 Apraxia**
EXCLUDES 1 *apraxia following cerebrovascular disease (I69. with final characters -9Ø)*

**R48.3 Visual agnosia**
Prosopagnosia
Simultanagnosia (asimultagnosia)

**R48.8 Other symbolic dysfunctions**
Acalculia
Agraphia
AHA: 2017,1Q,27

**R48.9 Unspecified symbolic dysfunctions**

✓4th **R49 Voice and resonance disorders**
EXCLUDES 1 *psychogenic voice and resonance disorders (F44.4)*

**R49.Ø Dysphonia**
Hoarseness

**R49.1 Aphonia**
Loss of voice

✓5th **R49.2 Hypernasality and hyponasality**

**R49.21 Hypernasality**

**R49.22 Hyponasality**

**R49.8 Other voice and resonance disorders**

**R49.9 Unspecified voice and resonance disorder**
Change in voice NOS
Resonance disorder NOS

## General symptoms and signs (R5Ø-R69)

✓4th **R5Ø Fever of other and unknown origin**
EXCLUDES 1 *chills without fever (R68.83)*
*febrile convulsions (R56.Ø-)*
*fever of unknown origin during labor (O75.2)*
*fever of unknown origin in newborn (P81.9)*
*hypothermia due to illness (R68.Ø)*
*malignant hyperthermia due to anesthesia (T88.3)*
*puerperal pyrexia NOS (O86.4)*

**R5Ø.2 Drug induced fever**
Use additional code for adverse effect, if applicable, to identify drug (T36-T5Ø with fifth or sixth character 5)
EXCLUDES 1 *postvaccination (postimmunization) fever (R5Ø.83)*

✓5th **R5Ø.8 Other specified fever**

***R5Ø.81 Fever presenting with conditions classified elsewhere***
Code first underlying condition when associated fever is present, such as with:
leukemia (C91-C95)
neutropenia (D7Ø.-)
sickle-cell disease (D57.-)
AHA: 2020,3Q,22; 2014,4Q,22

**R5Ø.82 Postprocedural fever**
EXCLUDES 1 *postprocedural infection (T81.4-)*
*posttransfusion fever (R5Ø.84)*
*postvaccination (postimmunization) fever (R5Ø.83)*

**R5Ø.83 Postvaccination fever**
Postimmunization fever

**R5Ø.84 Febrile nonhemolytic transfusion reaction**
FNHTR
Posttransfusion fever

**R5Ø.9 Fever, unspecified**
Fever NOS
Fever of unknown origin [FUO]
Fever with chills
Fever with rigors
Hyperpyrexia NOS
Persistent fever
Pyrexia NOS

✓4th **R51 Headache**
EXCLUDES 2 *atypical face pain (G5Ø.1)*
*migraine and other headache syndromes (G43-G44)*
*trigeminal neuralgia (G5Ø.Ø)*
AHA: 2020,4Q,38-39

**R51.Ø Headache with orthostatic component, not elsewhere classified**
Headache with positional component, not elsewhere classified

**R51.9 Headache, unspecified**
Facial pain NOS

**R52 Pain, unspecified**
Acute pain NOS
Generalized pain NOS
Pain NOS
EXCLUDES 1 *acute and chronic pain, not elsewhere classified (G89.-)*
*localized pain, unspecified type - code to pain by site, such as:*
*pain disorders exclusively related to psychological factors (F45.41)*
*abdomen pain (R1Ø.-)*
*back pain (M54.9)*
*breast pain (N64.4)*
*chest pain (RØ7.1-RØ7.9)*
*ear pain (H92.Ø-)*
*eye pain (H57.1)*
*headache (R51.9)*
*joint pain (M25.5-)*
*limb pain (M79.6-)*
*lumbar region pain (M54.5-)*
*pelvic and perineal pain (R1Ø.2-)*
*renal colic (N23)*
*shoulder pain (M25.51-)*
*spine pain (M54.-)*
*throat pain (RØ7.Ø)*
*tongue pain (K14.6)*
*tooth pain (KØ8.8)*

✓4th **R53 Malaise and fatigue**

**R53.Ø Neoplastic (malignant) related fatigue**
Code first associated neoplasm

**R53.1 Weakness**
Asthenia NOS
EXCLUDES 1 *age-related weakness (R54)*
*muscle weakness (generalized) (M62.81)*
*sarcopenia (M62.84)*
*senile asthenia (R54)*
AHA: 2017,1Q,7; 2015,1Q,25

**R53.2 Functional quadriplegia** HCC ESR COM
Complete immobility due to severe physical disability or frailty
EXCLUDES 1 *frailty NOS (R54)*
*hysterical paralysis (F44.4)*
*immobility syndrome (M62.3)*
*neurologic quadriplegia (G82.5-)*
*quadriplegia (G82.5Ø)*
AHA: 2022,4Q,15; 2016,2Q,6
DEF: Inability to move due to a nonphysiological condition, such as dementia. The patient has no mental ability to move independently.

✓5th **R53.8 Other malaise and fatigue**
EXCLUDES 1 *combat exhaustion and fatigue (F43.Ø)*
*congenital debility (P96.9)*
*exhaustion and fatigue due to excessive exertion (T73.3)*
*exhaustion and fatigue due to exposure (T73.2)*
*exhaustion and fatigue due to heat (T67.-)*
*exhaustion and fatigue due to pregnancy (O26.8-)*
*exhaustion and fatigue due to recurrent depressive episode (F33-)*
*exhaustion and fatigue due to senile debility (R54)*

**R53.81 Other malaise**
Chronic debility
Debility NOS
General physical deterioration
Malaise NOS
Nervous debility
EXCLUDES 1 *age-related physical debility (R54)*
AHA: 2021,1Q,43

**R53.82 Chronic fatigue, unspecified**
EXCLUDES 1 *chronic fatigue syndrome (G93.32)*
*myalgic encephalomyelitis (G93.32)*
*other post infection and related fatigue syndromes (G93.39)*
*postviral fatigue syndrome (G93.31)*

**R53.83 Other fatigue**
Fatigue NOS
Lack of energy
Lethargy
Tiredness
EXCLUDES 2 *exhaustion and fatigue due to depressive episode (F32.-)*

**R54 Age-related physical debility** A
Frailty
Old age
Senescence
Senile asthenia
Senile debility
EXCLUDES 1 *age-related cognitive decline (R41.81)*
*sarcopenia (M62.84)*
*senile psychosis (F03.-)*
*senility NOS (R41.81)*

**R55 Syncope and collapse**
Blackout
Fainting
Vasovagal attack
EXCLUDES 1 *cardiogenic shock (R57.0)*
*carotid sinus syncope (G90.01)*
*heat syncope (T67.1)*
*neurocirculatory asthenia (F45.8)*
*neurogenic orthostatic hypotension (G90.3)*
*orthostatic hypotension (I95.1)*
*postprocedural shock (T81.1-)*
*psychogenic syncope (F48.8)*
*shock complicating or following abortion or ectopic or molar pregnancy (O00-O07, O08.3)*
*shock complicating or following labor and delivery (O75.1)*
*shock NOS (R57.9)*
*Stokes-Adams attack (I45.9)*
*unconsciousness NOS (R40.2-)*

✓4th **R56 Convulsions, not elsewhere classified**
EXCLUDES 1 *dissociative convulsions and seizures (F44.5)*
*epileptic convulsions and seizures (G40.-)*
*newborn convulsions and seizures (P90)*

✓5th **R56.0 Febrile convulsions**

**R56.00 Simple febrile convulsions** HCC ESR COM
Febrile convulsion NOS
Febrile seizure NOS

**R56.01 Complex febrile convulsions** HCC ESR COM
Atypical febrile seizure
Complex febrile seizure
Complicated febrile seizure
EXCLUDES 1 *status epilepticus (G40.901)*

**R56.1 Post traumatic seizures** HCC ESR COM
EXCLUDES 1 *post traumatic epilepsy (G40.-)*

**R56.9 Unspecified convulsions** HCC ESR COM
Convulsion disorder
Fit NOS
Recurrent convulsions
Seizure(s) (convulsive) NOS
**AHA:** 2022,4Q,46; 2021,1Q,3; 2019,1Q,19

✓4th **R57 Shock, not elsewhere classified**
EXCLUDES 1 *anaphylactic shock NOS (T78.2)*
*anaphylactic reaction or shock due to adverse food reaction (T78.0-)*
*anaphylactic shock due to adverse effect of correct drug or medicament properly administered (T88.6)*
*anaphylactic shock due to serum (T80.5-)*
*electric shock (T75.4)*
*obstetric shock (O75.1)*
*postprocedural shock (T81.1-)*
*psychic shock (F43.0)*
*shock complicating or following ectopic or molar pregnancy (O00-O07, O08.3)*
*shock due to anesthesia (T88.2)*
*shock due to lightning (T75.01)*
*toxic shock syndrome (A48.3)*
*traumatic shock (T79.4)*

**R57.0 Cardiogenic shock** HCC ESR COM
EXCLUDES 2 *septic shock (R65.21)*
**AHA:** 2020,3Q,26
**DEF:** Associated with myocardial infarction, cardiac tamponade, and massive pulmonary embolism. Symptoms include mental confusion, reduced blood pressure, tachycardia, pallor, and cold, clammy skin.

**R57.1 Hypovolemic shock** HCC ESR COM
**AHA:** 2019,2Q,7

**R57.8 Other shock** HCC ESR COM
**AHA:** 2026,2Q,8

**R57.9 Shock, unspecified** HCC ESR COM
Failure of peripheral circulation NOS

**R58 Hemorrhage, not elsewhere classified**
Hemorrhage NOS
EXCLUDES 1 *hemorrhage included with underlying conditions, such as:*
*acute duodenal ulcer with hemorrhage (K26.0)*
*acute gastritis with bleeding (K29.01)*
*ulcerative enterocolitis with rectal bleeding (K51.01)*

✓4th **R59 Enlarged lymph nodes**
INCLUDES swollen glands
EXCLUDES 1 *acute lymphadenitis (L04.-)*
*chronic lymphadenitis (I88.1)*
*lymphadenitis NOS (I88.9)*
*mesenteric (acute) (chronic) lymphadenitis (I88.0)*

**R59.0 Localized enlarged lymph nodes**

**R59.1 Generalized enlarged lymph nodes**
Lymphadenopathy NOS

**R59.9 Enlarged lymph nodes, unspecified**

✓4th **R60 Edema, not elsewhere classified**
EXCLUDES 1 *angioneurotic edema (T78.3)*
*ascites (R18.-)*
*cerebral edema (G93.6)*
*cerebral edema due to birth injury (P11.0)*
*edema of larynx (J38.4)*
*edema of nasopharynx (J39.2)*
*edema of pharynx (J39.2)*
*gestational edema (O12.0-)*
*hereditary edema (Q82.0)*
*hydrops fetalis NOS (P83.2)*
*hydrothorax (J94.8)*
*newborn edema (P83.3)*
*pulmonary edema (J81.-)*

**R60.0 Localized edema**

**R60.1 Generalized edema**
EXCLUDES 2 *nutritional edema (E40-E46)*

**R60.9 Edema, unspecified**
Fluid retention NOS

**R61 Generalized hyperhidrosis**
Excessive sweating
Night sweats
Secondary hyperhidrosis
Code first, if applicable, menopausal and female climacteric states (N95.1)
EXCLUDES 1 *focal (primary) (secondary) hyperhidrosis (L74.5-)*
*Frey's syndrome (L74.52)*
*localized (primary) (secondary) hyperhidrosis (L74.5-)*

✓4th **R62 Lack of expected normal physiological development in childhood and adults**
EXCLUDES 1 *delayed puberty (E30.0)*
*gonadal dysgenesis (Q99.1)*
*hypopituitarism (E23.0)*

**R62.0 Delayed milestone in childhood** P
Delayed attainment of expected physiological developmental stage
Late talker
Late walker

✓5th **R62.5 Other and unspecified lack of expected normal physiological development in childhood**
EXCLUDES 1 *HIV disease resulting in failure to thrive (B20)*
*physical retardation due to malnutrition (E45)*

**R62.50 Unspecified lack of expected normal physiological development in childhood**
Infantilism NOS

**R62.51 Failure to thrive (child)** P
Failure to gain weight
Faltering growth
EXCLUDES 1 *failure to thrive in child under 28 days old (P92.6)*
**AHA:** 2018,4Q,82
**DEF:** Nonorganic failure to thrive (FTT): Symptom of neglect or abuse.
**DEF:** Organic failure to thrive (FTT): Acute or chronic illness that interferes with nutritional intake, absorption, metabolism excretion, and energy requirements.

**R62.52 Short stature (child)**
Lack of growth
Physical retardation
Short stature NOS
EXCLUDES 1 *short stature due to endocrine disorder (E34.3-)*

R62.59 **Other lack of expected normal physiological development in childhood**

R62.7 **Adult failure to thrive** A

✓4th **R63 Symptoms and signs concerning food and fluid intake**

EXCLUDES 1 *bulimia NOS (F5Ø.2-)*

R63.Ø **Anorexia**

Loss of appetite

EXCLUDES 1 *anorexia nervosa (F5Ø.Ø-)*
*loss of appetite of nonorganic origin (F5Ø.89)*

**AHA:** 2018,4Q,82

**TIP:** Assign an additional code from category Z68 when BMI is documented. BMI can be based on documentation from clinicians who are not the patient's provider.

R63.1 **Polydipsia**

Excessive thirst

R63.2 **Polyphagia**

Excessive eating
Hyperalimentation NOS

✓5th R63.3 **Feeding difficulties**

EXCLUDES 2 *eating disorders (F5Ø.-)*
*feeding problems of newborn (P92.-)*
*infant feeding disorder of nonorganic origin (F98.2-)*

**AHA:** 2021,4Q,27-28; 2017,1Q,28; 2016,3Q,19

R63.3Ø **Feeding difficulties, unspecified**

R63.31 **Pediatric feeding disorder, acute** P

Pediatric feeding dysfunction, acute

Code also, if applicable, associated conditions such as:
aspiration pneumonia (J69.Ø)
dysphagia (R13.1-)
gastro-esophageal reflux disease (K21.-)
malnutrition (E4Ø-E46)

R63.32 **Pediatric feeding disorder, chronic** P

Pediatric feeding dysfunction, chronic

Code also, if applicable, associated conditions such as:
aspiration pneumonia (J69.Ø)
dysphagia (R13.1-)
gastro-esophageal reflux disease (K21.-)
malnutrition (E4Ø-E46)

R63.39 **Other feeding difficulties**

Feeding problem (elderly) (infant) NOS
Picky eater

R63.4 **Abnormal weight loss**

**AHA:** 2018,4Q,82

**TIP:** Assign an additional code from category Z68 when BMI is documented. BMI can be based on documentation from clinicians who are not the patient's provider.

R63.5 **Abnormal weight gain**

EXCLUDES 1 *excessive weight gain in pregnancy (O26.Ø-)*
*obesity (E66.-)*

**AHA:** 2018,4Q,82

**TIP:** Assign an additional code from category Z68 when BMI is documented. BMI can be based on documentation from clinicians who are not the patient's provider.

R63.6 **Underweight**

Use additional code to identify body mass index (BMI), if known (Z68.-)

EXCLUDES 1 *abnormal weight loss (R63.4)*
*anorexia nervosa (F5Ø.Ø-)*
*malnutrition (E4Ø-E46)*

**AHA:** 2018,4Q,82

R63.8 **Other symptoms and signs concerning food and fluid intake**

**R64 Cachexia** ESR COM

EXCLUDES 1 *abnormal weight loss (R63.4)*
*cachexia due to underlying condition (E88.A)*
*nutritional marasmus (E41)*

**AHA:** 2018,4Q,82; 2017,3Q,24

✓4th **R65 Symptoms and signs specifically associated with systemic inflammation and infection**

**AHA:** 2019,2Q,38

**TIP:** When documentation states SIRS with an infection, assign only a code for the infection. ICD-10-CM does not offer a code for SIRS due to infectious process. If sepsis is suspected, query the provider.

✓5th R65.1 **Systemic inflammatory response syndrome [SIRS] of non-infectious origin**

Code first underlying condition, such as:
heatstroke (T67.Ø-)
injury and trauma (SØØ-T88)

EXCLUDES 1 *sepsis - code to infection*
*severe sepsis (R65.2)*

R65.1Ø **Systemic inflammatory response syndrome [SIRS] of non-infectious origin without acute organ dysfunction** HCC ESR COM UPD

Systemic inflammatory response syndrome (SIRS) NOS

**AHA:** 2019,2Q,24

R65.11 **Systemic inflammatory response syndrome [SIRS] of non-infectious origin with acute organ dysfunction** HCC ESR COM UPD

Use additional code to identify specific acute organ dysfunction, such as:
acute kidney failure (N17.-)
acute respiratory failure (J96.Ø-)
critical illness myopathy (G72.81)
critical illness polyneuropathy (G62.81)
disseminated intravascular coagulopathy [DIC] (D65)
encephalopathy (metabolic) (septic) (G93.41)
hepatic failure (K72.Ø-)

✓5th R65.2 **Severe sepsis**

Infection with associated acute organ dysfunction
Sepsis with acute organ dysfunction
Sepsis with multiple organ dysfunction
Systemic inflammatory response syndrome due to infectious process with acute organ dysfunction

Code first underlying infection, such as:
infection following a procedure (T81.4-)
infections following infusion, transfusion and therapeutic injection (T8Ø.2-)
puerperal sepsis (O85)
sepsis following (induced) termination of pregnancy (OØ4.87)
sepsis following complete or unspecified spontaneous abortion (OØ3.87)
sepsis following ectopic and molar pregnancy (OØ8.82)
sepsis following incomplete spontaneous abortion (OØ3.37)
sepsis NOS (A41.9)

Use additional code to identify specific acute organ dysfunction, such as:
acute kidney failure (N17.-)
acute respiratory failure (J96.Ø-)
critical illness myopathy (G72.81)
critical illness polyneuropathy (G62.81)
disseminated intravascular coagulopathy [DIC] (D65)
encephalopathy (metabolic) (septic) (G93.41)
hepatic failure (K72.Ø-)

**AHA:** 2020,2Q,17; 2018,4Q,62-63; 2017,4Q,98-99; 2016,3Q,8

R65.2Ø **Severe sepsis without septic shock** HCC ESR COM UPD

Severe sepsis NOS

**AHA:** 2020,2Q,17; 2016,3Q,14; 2013,4Q,119

R65.21 **Severe sepsis with septic shock** HCC ESR COM UPD

EXCLUDES 1 *postprocedural septic shock (T81.12-)*

**AHA:** 2018,4Q,63

✓4th **R68 Other general symptoms and signs**

R68.Ø **Hypothermia, not associated with low environmental temperature**

EXCLUDES 1 *hypothermia NOS (accidental) (T68)*
*hypothermia due to anesthesia (T88.51)*
*hypothermia due to low environmental temperature (T68)*
*newborn hypothermia (P8Ø.-)*

✓5th R68.1 **Nonspecific symptoms peculiar to infancy**

EXCLUDES 1 *colic, infantile (R1Ø.83)*
*neonatal cerebral irritability (P91.3)*
*teething syndrome (KØØ.7)*

R68.11 **Excessive crying of infant (baby)** P

EXCLUDES 1 *excessive crying of child, adolescent, or adult (R45.83)*

**R68.12 Fussy infant (baby)** P
Irritable infant

**R68.13 Apparent life threatening event in infant (ALTE)** P
Apparent life threatening event in newborn
Brief resolved unexplained event (BRUE)
Code first confirmed diagnosis, if known
Use additional code(s) for associated signs and symptoms if no confirmed diagnosis established, or if signs and symptoms are not associated routinely with confirmed diagnosis, or provide additional information for cause of ALTE

**R68.19 Other nonspecific symptoms peculiar to infancy** P

**R68.2 Dry mouth, unspecified**
EXCLUDES 1 *dry mouth due to dehydration (E86.Ø)*
*dry mouth due to Sjogren syndrome (M35.Ø-)*
EXCLUDES 2 *salivary gland hyposecretion (K11.7)*

**R68.3 Clubbing of fingers**
Clubbing of nails
EXCLUDES 1 *congenital clubfinger (Q68.1)*
**DEF:** Enlarged soft tissue of the distal fingers that usually occurs in heart and lung diseases.

✓5th **R68.8 Other general symptoms and signs**

**R68.81 Early satiety**
**DEF:** Premature feeling of being full after eating only a small amount of food. The mechanism of satiety is multifactorial.

**R68.82 Decreased libido** A
Decreased sexual desire

**R68.83 Chills (without fever)**
Chills NOS
EXCLUDES 1 *chills with fever (R5Ø.9)*

**R68.84 Jaw pain**
Mandibular pain
Maxilla pain
EXCLUDES 1 *temporomandibular joint arthralgia (M26.62-)*

**R68.89 Other general symptoms and signs**

**R69 Illness, unspecified**
Unknown and unspecified causes of morbidity

## Abnormal findings on examination of blood, without diagnosis (R7Ø-R79)

EXCLUDES 2 *abnormal findings on antenatal screening of mother (O28.-)*
*abnormalities of lipids (E78.-)*
*abnormalities of platelets and thrombocytes (D69.-)*
*abnormalities of white blood cells classified elsewhere (D7Ø-D72)*
*coagulation hemorrhagic disorders (D65-D68)*
*diagnostic abnormal findings classified elsewhere - see Alphabetical Index*
*hemorrhagic and hematological disorders of newborn (P5Ø-P61)*

✓4th **R7Ø Elevated erythrocyte sedimentation rate and abnormality of plasma viscosity**

**R7Ø.Ø Elevated erythrocyte sedimentation rate**

**R7Ø.1 Abnormal plasma viscosity**

✓4th **R71 Abnormality of red blood cells**
EXCLUDES 1 *anemias (D5Ø-D64)*
*anemia of premature infant (P61.2)*
*benign (familial) polycythemia (D75.Ø)*
*congenital anemias (P61.2-P61.4)*
*newborn anemia due to isoimmunization (P55.-)*
*polycythemia neonatorum (P61.1)*
*polycythemia NOS (D75.1)*
*polycythemia vera (D45)*
*secondary polycythemia (D75.1)*

**R71.Ø Precipitous drop in hematocrit**
Drop (precipitous) in hemoglobin
Drop in hematocrit

**R71.8 Other abnormality of red blood cells**
Abnormal red-cell morphology NOS
Abnormal red-cell volume NOS
Anisocytosis
Poikilocytosis

✓4th **R73 Elevated blood glucose level**
EXCLUDES 1 *diabetes mellitus (EØ8-E13)*
*diabetes mellitus in pregnancy, childbirth and the puerperium (O24.-)*
*neonatal disorders (P7Ø.Ø-P7Ø.2)*
*postsurgical hypoinsulinemia (E89.1)*

✓5th **R73.Ø Abnormal glucose**
EXCLUDES 1 *abnormal glucose in pregnancy (O99.81-)*
*diabetes mellitus (EØ8-E13)*
*dysmetabolic syndrome X (E88.81-)*
*gestational diabetes (O24.4-)*
*glycosuria (R81)*
*hypoglycemia (E16.2)*
*type 1 diabetes mellitus, presymptomatic (E1Ø.A-)*

**R73.Ø1 Impaired fasting glucose**
Elevated fasting glucose

**R73.Ø2 Impaired glucose tolerance (oral)**
Elevated glucose tolerance

**R73.Ø3 Prediabetes**
Latent diabetes
**AHA:** 2026,1Q,24; 2024,3Q,11; 2016,4Q,65

**R73.Ø9 Other abnormal glucose**
Abnormal glucose NOS
Abnormal non-fasting glucose tolerance

**R73.9 Hyperglycemia, unspecified**

✓4th **R74 Abnormal serum enzyme levels**

✓5th **R74.Ø Nonspecific elevation of levels of transaminase and lactic acid dehydrogenase [LDH]**
**AHA:** 2020,4Q,39

**R74.Ø1 Elevation of levels of liver transaminase levels**
Elevation of levels of alanine transaminase (ALT)
Elevation of levels of aspartate transaminase (AST)

**R74.Ø2 Elevation of levels of lactic acid dehydrogenase [LDH]**

**R74.8 Abnormal levels of other serum enzymes**
Abnormal level of acid phosphatase
Abnormal level of alkaline phosphatase
Abnormal level of amylase
Abnormal level of lipase [triacylglycerol lipase]
**AHA:** 2019,2Q,6

**R74.9 Abnormal serum enzyme level, unspecified**

**R75 Inconclusive laboratory evidence of human immunodeficiency virus [HIV]**
Nonconclusive HIV-test finding in infants
EXCLUDES 1 *asymptomatic human immunodeficiency virus [HIV] infection status (Z21)*
*human immunodeficiency virus [HIV] disease (B2Ø)*

✓4th **R76 Other abnormal immunological findings in serum**

**R76.Ø Raised antibody titer**
EXCLUDES 1 *isoimmunization in pregnancy (O36.Ø-O36.1)*
*isoimmunization affecting newborn (P55.-)*
**AHA:** 2021,1Q,6

✓5th **R76.1 Nonspecific reaction to test for tuberculosis**

**R76.11 Nonspecific reaction to tuberculin skin test without active tuberculosis**
Abnormal result of Mantoux test
PPD positive
Tuberculin (skin test) positive
Tuberculin (skin test) reactor
EXCLUDES 1 *nonspecific reaction to cell mediated immunity measurement of gamma interferon antigen response without active tuberculosis (R76.12)*

**R76.12 Nonspecific reaction to cell mediated immunity measurement of gamma interferon antigen response without active tuberculosis**
Nonspecific reaction to QuantiFERON-TB test (QFT) without active tuberculosis
EXCLUDES 1 *nonspecific reaction to tuberculin skin test without active tuberculosis (R76.11)*
*positive tuberculin skin test (R76.11)*

✓5th **R76.8 Other specified abnormal immunological findings in serum**
AHA: 2021,1Q,6

**R76.81 Abnormal rheumatoid factor and anti-citrullinated protein antibody without rheumatoid arthritis**
Abnormal anti-CCP
Abnormal anti-cyclic citrullinated protein antibody and rheumatoid factor
EXCLUDES 1 *rheumatoid arthritis with rheumatoid factor (MØ5.-)*

**R76.89 Other specified abnormal immunological findings in serum**
Raised level of immunoglobulins NOS

**R76.9 Abnormal immunological finding in serum, unspecified**

✓4th **R77 Other abnormalities of plasma proteins**
EXCLUDES 1 *disorders of plasma-protein metabolism (E88.Ø-)*

**R77.Ø Abnormality of albumin**

**R77.1 Abnormality of globulin**
Hyperglobulinemia NOS

**R77.2 Abnormality of alphafetoprotein**

**R77.8 Other specified abnormalities of plasma proteins**

**R77.9 Abnormality of plasma protein, unspecified**
AHA: 2019,2Q,6

✓4th **R78 Findings of drugs and other substances, not normally found in blood**
▶Use additional code to identify any retained foreign body, if applicable◀ (Z18.-)
EXCLUDES 2 *mental or behavioral disorders due to psychoactive substance use (F1Ø-F19)*

**R78.Ø Finding of alcohol in blood**
Use additional external cause code (Y9Ø.-), for detail regarding alcohol level

**R78.1 Finding of opiate drug in blood**

**R78.2 Finding of cocaine in blood**

**R78.3 Finding of hallucinogen in blood**

**R78.4 Finding of other drugs of addictive potential in blood**

**R78.5 Finding of other psychotropic drug in blood**

**R78.6 Finding of steroid agent in blood**

✓5th **R78.7 Finding of abnormal level of heavy metals in blood**

**R78.71 Abnormal lead level in blood**
EXCLUDES 1 *lead poisoning (T56.Ø-)*

● **R78.72 Abnormal gadolinium level in blood**
EXCLUDES 1 *toxic effect of gadolinium (T56.82-)*

**R78.79 Finding of abnormal level of heavy metals in blood**

✓5th **R78.8 Finding of other specified substances, not normally found in blood**

**R78.81 Bacteremia**
EXCLUDES 1 *sepsis — code to specified infection*
AHA: 2025,1Q,20
DEF: Laboratory finding of bacteria in the blood in the absence of two or more signs of sepsis. Transient in nature, it can progress to septicemia with a severe infectious process.

**R78.89 Finding of other specified substances, not normally found in blood**
Finding of abnormal level of lithium in blood

**R78.9 Finding of unspecified substance, not normally found in blood**

✓4th **R79 Other abnormal findings of blood chemistry**
Use additional code to identify any retained foreign body, if applicable (Z18.-)
EXCLUDES 1 *asymptomatic hyperuricemia (E79.Ø)*
~~*hyperglycemia NOS (R73.9)*~~
*hypoglycemia NOS (E16.2)*
*neonatal hypoglycemia (P7Ø.3-P7Ø.4)*
*specific findings indicating disorder of amino-acid metabolism (E7Ø-E72)*
*specific findings indicating disorder of carbohydrate metabolism (E73-E74)*
*specific findings indicating disorder of lipid metabolism (E75.-)*
EXCLUDES 2 ▶*hyperglycemia NOS (R73.9)*◀

**R79.Ø Abnormal level of blood mineral**
Abnormal blood level of cobalt
Abnormal blood level of copper
Abnormal blood level of iron
Abnormal blood level of magnesium
Abnormal blood level of mineral NEC
Abnormal blood level of zinc
EXCLUDES 1 *abnormal level of lithium (R78.89)*
*disorders of mineral metabolism (E83.-)*
*neonatal hypomagnesemia (P71.2)*
*nutritional mineral deficiency (E58-E61)*

**R79.1 Abnormal coagulation profile**
Abnormal or prolonged bleeding time
Abnormal or prolonged coagulation time
Abnormal or prolonged partial thromboplastin time [PTT]
Abnormal or prolonged prothrombin time [PT]
Low von Willebrand factor
EXCLUDES 1 *coagulation defects (D68.-)*
EXCLUDES 2 *abnormality of fluid, electrolyte or acid-base balance (E86-E87)*

✓5th **R79.8 Other specified abnormal findings of blood chemistry**

**R79.81 Abnormal blood-gas level**

**R79.82 Elevated C-reactive protein [CRP]**

**R79.83 Abnormal findings of blood amino-acid level**
Homocysteinemia
EXCLUDES 1 *disorders of amino-acid metabolism (E7Ø-E72)*
AHA: 2021,4Q,28

**R79.89 Other specified abnormal findings of blood chemistry**
AHA: 2026,2Q,4; 2019,2Q,6
TIP: Assign for positive Coombs test when not further clarified in the documentation.

**R79.9 Abnormal finding of blood chemistry, unspecified**

## Abnormal findings on examination of urine, without diagnosis (R8Ø-R82)

EXCLUDES 1 *abnormal findings on antenatal screening of mother (O28.-)*
*diagnostic abnormal findings classified elsewhere - see Alphabetical Index*
*specific findings indicating disorder of amino-acid metabolism (E7Ø-E72)*
*specific findings indicating disorder of carbohydrate metabolism (E73-E74)*

✓4th **R8Ø Proteinuria**
EXCLUDES 1 *gestational proteinuria (O12.1-)*

**R8Ø.Ø Isolated proteinuria**
Idiopathic proteinuria
EXCLUDES 1 *isolated proteinuria with specific morphological lesion (NØ6.-)*

**R8Ø.1 Persistent proteinuria, unspecified**

**R8Ø.2 Orthostatic proteinuria, unspecified**
Postural proteinuria

**R8Ø.3 Bence Jones proteinuria**

**R8Ø.8 Other proteinuria**
AHA: 2025,3Q,4

**R8Ø.9 Proteinuria, unspecified**
Albuminuria NOS

**R81 Glycosuria**
EXCLUDES 1 *renal glycosuria (E74.818)*

✓4th **R82 Other and unspecified abnormal findings in urine**
INCLUDES chromoabnormalities in urine
Use additional code to identify any retained foreign body, if applicable (Z18.-)
EXCLUDES 2 *hematuria (R31.-)*

**R82.Ø Chyluria**
EXCLUDES 1 *filarial chyluria (B74.-)*

**R82.1 Myoglobinuria**

**R82.2 Biliuria**

**R82.3 Hemoglobinuria**

EXCLUDES 1 *hemoglobinuria due to hemolysis from external causes NEC (D59.6)*
*hemoglobinuria due to paroxysmal nocturnal [Marchiafava-Micheli] (D59.5)*

**DEF:** Free hemoglobin in blood due to rapid hemolysis of red blood cells. Causes include burns, crushed injury, sickle cell anemia, thalassemia, parasitic infections, or kidney infections.

**R82.4 Acetonuria**

Ketonuria

**DEF:** Excessive excretion of acetone in urine that commonly occurs in diabetic acidosis.

**R82.5 Elevated urine levels of drugs, medicaments and biological substances**

Elevated urine levels of 17-ketosteroids
Elevated urine levels of catecholamines
Elevated urine levels of indoleacetic acid
Elevated urine levels of steroids

**R82.6 Abnormal urine levels of substances chiefly nonmedicinal as to source**

Abnormal urine level of heavy metals

√5th **R82.7 Abnormal findings on microbiological examination of urine**

EXCLUDES 1 *colonization status (Z22.-)*

**AHA:** 2016,4Q,65

**R82.71 Bacteriuria**

**R82.79 Other abnormal findings on microbiological examination of urine**

Positive culture findings of urine

√5th **R82.8 Abnormal findings on cytological and histological examination of urine**

**AHA:** 2019,4Q,16

**R82.81 Pyuria**

Sterile pyuria

**R82.89 Other abnormal findings on cytological and histological examination of urine**

√5th **R82.9 Other and unspecified abnormal findings in urine**

**R82.9Ø Unspecified abnormal findings in urine**

**R82.91 Other chromoabnormalities of urine**

Chromoconversion (dipstick)
Idiopathic dipstick converts positive for blood with no cellular forms in sediment

EXCLUDES 1 *hemoglobinuria (R82.3)*
*myoglobinuria (R82.1)*

√6th **R82.99 Other abnormal findings in urine**

**AHA:** 2018,4Q,29-30

**R82.991 Hypocitraturia**

**R82.992 Hyperoxaluria**

EXCLUDES 1 *primary hyperoxaluria (E72.53-)*
*secondary hyperoxaluria (E72.54-)*

**R82.993 Hyperuricosuria**

**R82.994 Hypercalciuria**

Idiopathic hypercalciuria

**R82.998 Other abnormal findings in urine**

Cells and casts in urine
Crystalluria
Melanuria

## Abnormal findings on examination of other body fluids, substances and tissues, without diagnosis (R83-R89)

EXCLUDES 1 *abnormal findings on antenatal screening of mother (O28.-)*
*diagnostic abnormal findings classified elsewhere - see Alphabetical Index*

EXCLUDES 2 *abnormal findings on examination of blood, without diagnosis (R7Ø-R79)*
*abnormal findings on examination of urine, without diagnosis (R8Ø-R82)*
*abnormal tumor markers (R97.-)*

√4th **R83 Abnormal findings in cerebrospinal fluid**

**R83.Ø Abnormal level of enzymes in cerebrospinal fluid**

**R83.1 Abnormal level of hormones in cerebrospinal fluid**

**R83.2 Abnormal level of other drugs, medicaments and biological substances in cerebrospinal fluid**

**R83.3 Abnormal level of substances chiefly nonmedicinal as to source in cerebrospinal fluid**

**R83.4 Abnormal immunological findings in cerebrospinal fluid**

**R83.5 Abnormal microbiological findings in cerebrospinal fluid**

Positive culture findings in cerebrospinal fluid

EXCLUDES 1 *colonization status (Z22.-)*

**R83.6 Abnormal cytological findings in cerebrospinal fluid**

**R83.8 Other abnormal findings in cerebrospinal fluid**

Abnormal chromosomal findings in cerebrospinal fluid

**R83.9 Unspecified abnormal finding in cerebrospinal fluid**

√4th **R84 Abnormal findings in specimens from respiratory organs and thorax**

INCLUDES abnormal findings in bronchial washings
abnormal findings in nasal secretions
abnormal findings in pleural fluid
abnormal findings in sputum
abnormal findings in throat scrapings

EXCLUDES 1 *blood-stained sputum (RØ4.2)*

**R84.Ø Abnormal level of enzymes in specimens from respiratory organs and thorax**

**R84.1 Abnormal level of hormones in specimens from respiratory organs and thorax**

**R84.2 Abnormal level of other drugs, medicaments and biological substances in specimens from respiratory organs and thorax**

**R84.3 Abnormal level of substances chiefly nonmedicinal as to source in specimens from respiratory organs and thorax**

**R84.4 Abnormal immunological findings in specimens from respiratory organs and thorax**

**R84.5 Abnormal microbiological findings in specimens from respiratory organs and thorax**

Positive culture findings in specimens from respiratory organs and thorax

EXCLUDES 1 *colonization status (Z22.-)*

**R84.6 Abnormal cytological findings in specimens from respiratory organs and thorax**

**R84.7 Abnormal histological findings in specimens from respiratory organs and thorax**

**R84.8 Other abnormal findings in specimens from respiratory organs and thorax**

Abnormal chromosomal findings in specimens from respiratory organs and thorax

**R84.9 Unspecified abnormal finding in specimens from respiratory organs and thorax**

√4th **R85 Abnormal findings in specimens from digestive organs and abdominal cavity**

INCLUDES abnormal findings in peritoneal fluid
abnormal findings in saliva

EXCLUDES 1 *cloudy peritoneal dialysis effluent (R88.Ø)*
*fecal abnormalities (R19.5)*

**R85.Ø Abnormal level of enzymes in specimens from digestive organs and abdominal cavity**

**R85.1 Abnormal level of hormones in specimens from digestive organs and abdominal cavity**

**R85.2 Abnormal level of other drugs, medicaments and biological substances in specimens from digestive organs and abdominal cavity**

**R85.3 Abnormal level of substances chiefly nonmedicinal as to source in specimens from digestive organs and abdominal cavity**

**R85.4 Abnormal immunological findings in specimens from digestive organs and abdominal cavity**

**R85.5 Abnormal microbiological findings in specimens from digestive organs and abdominal cavity**

Positive culture findings in specimens from digestive organs and abdominal cavity

EXCLUDES 1 *colonization status (Z22.-)*

**R85.6 Abnormal cytological findings in specimens from digestive organs and abdominal cavity**

**R85.61 Abnormal cytologic smear of anus**

EXCLUDES 1 *abnormal cytological findings in specimens from other digestive organs and abdominal cavity (R85.69)*
*anal intraepithelial neoplasia I [AIN I] (K62.82)*
*anal intraepithelial neoplasia II [AIN II] (K62.82)*
*anal intraepithelial neoplasia III [AIN III] (DØ1.3)*
*carcinoma in situ of anus (histologically confirmed) (DØ1.3)*
*dysplasia (mild) (moderate) of anus (histologically confirmed) (K62.82)*
*severe dysplasia of anus (histologically confirmed) (DØ1.3)*

EXCLUDES 2 *anal high risk human papillomavirus (HPV) DNA test positive (R85.81)*
*anal low risk human papillomavirus (HPV) DNA test positive (R85.82)*

**R85.61Ø Atypical squamous cells of undetermined significance on cytologic smear of anus [ASC-US]**

**R85.611 Atypical squamous cells cannot exclude high grade squamous intraepithelial lesion on cytologic smear of anus [ASC-H]**

**R85.612 Low grade squamous intraepithelial lesion on cytologic smear of anus [LGSIL]**

**R85.613 High grade squamous intraepithelial lesion on cytologic smear of anus [HGSIL]**

**R85.614 Cytologic evidence of malignancy on smear of anus**

**R85.615 Unsatisfactory cytologic smear of anus**
Inadequate sample of cytologic smear of anus

**R85.616 Satisfactory anal smear but lacking transformation zone**

**R85.618 Other abnormal cytological findings on specimens from anus**

**R85.619 Unspecified abnormal cytological findings in specimens from anus**
Abnormal anal cytology NOS
Atypical glandular cells of anus NOS

**R85.69 Abnormal cytological findings in specimens from other digestive organs and abdominal cavity**

**R85.7 Abnormal histological findings in specimens from digestive organs and abdominal cavity**

**R85.8 Other abnormal findings in specimens from digestive organs and abdominal cavity**

**R85.81 Anal high risk human papillomavirus [HPV] DNA test positive**

EXCLUDES 1 *anogenital warts due to human papillomavirus (HPV) (A63.Ø)*
*condyloma acuminatum (A63.Ø)*

**R85.82 Anal low risk human papillomavirus [HPV] DNA test positive**
Use additional code for associated human papillomavirus (B97.7)

**R85.89 Other abnormal findings in specimens from digestive organs and abdominal cavity**
Abnormal chromosomal findings in specimens from digestive organs and abdominal cavity

**R85.9 Unspecified abnormal finding in specimens from digestive organs and abdominal cavity**

## R86 Abnormal findings in specimens from male genital organs

INCLUDES abnormal findings in prostatic secretions
abnormal findings in semen, seminal fluid
abnormal spermatozoa

EXCLUDES 1 *azoospermia (N46.Ø-)*
*oligospermia (N46.1-)*

**R86.Ø Abnormal level of enzymes in specimens from male genital organs**

**R86.1 Abnormal level of hormones in specimens from male genital organs**

**R86.2 Abnormal level of other drugs, medicaments and biological substances in specimens from male genital organs**

**R86.3 Abnormal level of substances chiefly nonmedicinal as to source in specimens from male genital organs**

**R86.4 Abnormal immunological findings in specimens from male genital organs**

**R86.5 Abnormal microbiological findings in specimens from male genital organs**
Positive culture findings in specimens from male genital organs

EXCLUDES 1 *colonization status (Z22.-)*

**R86.6 Abnormal cytological findings in specimens from male genital organs**

**R86.7 Abnormal histological findings in specimens from male genital organs**

**R86.8 Other abnormal findings in specimens from male genital organs**
Abnormal chromosomal findings in specimens from male genital organs

**R86.9 Unspecified abnormal finding in specimens from male genital organs**

## R87 Abnormal findings in specimens from female genital organs

INCLUDES abnormal findings in secretion and smears from cervix uteri
abnormal findings in secretion and smears from vagina
abnormal findings in secretion and smears from vulva

**R87.Ø Abnormal level of enzymes in specimens from female genital organs**

**R87.1 Abnormal level of hormones in specimens from female genital organs**

**R87.2 Abnormal level of other drugs, medicaments and biological substances in specimens from female genital organs**

**R87.3 Abnormal level of substances chiefly nonmedicinal as to source in specimens from female genital organs**

**R87.4 Abnormal immunological findings in specimens from female genital organs**

**R87.5 Abnormal microbiological findings in specimens from female genital organs**
Positive culture findings in specimens from female genital organs

EXCLUDES 1 *colonization status (Z22.-)*

**R87.6 Abnormal cytological findings in specimens from female genital organs**

**R87.61 Abnormal cytological findings in specimens from cervix uteri**

EXCLUDES 1 *abnormal cytological findings in specimens from other female genital organs (R87.69)*
*abnormal cytological findings in specimens from vagina (R87.62-)*
*carcinoma in situ of cervix uteri (histologically confirmed) (DØ6.-)*
*cervical intraepithelial neoplasia I [CIN I] (N87.Ø)*
*cervical intraepithelial neoplasia II [CIN II] (N87.1)*
*cervical intraepithelial neoplasia III [CIN III] (DØ6.-)*
*dysplasia (mild) (moderate) of cervix uteri (histologically confirmed) (N87.-)*
*severe dysplasia of cervix uteri (histologically confirmed) (DØ6.-)*

EXCLUDES 2 *cervical high risk human papillomavirus (HPV) DNA test positive (R87.81Ø)*
*cervical low risk human papillomavirus (HPV) DNA test positive (R87.82Ø)*

**R87.61Ø Atypical squamous cells of undetermined significance on cytologic smear of cervix [ASC-US]**

**R87.611 Atypical squamous cells cannot exclude high grade squamous intraepithelial lesion on cytologic smear of cervix [ASC-H]**

**R87.612 Low grade squamous intraepithelial lesion on cytologic smear of cervix [LGSIL]**

**R87.613 High grade squamous intraepithelial lesion on cytologic smear of cervix [HGSIL]**

**R87.614 Cytologic evidence of malignancy on smear of cervix**

**R87.615 Unsatisfactory cytologic smear of cervix**
Inadequate sample of cytologic smear of cervix

**R87.616 Satisfactory cervical smear but lacking transformation zone**

**R87.618 Other abnormal cytological findings on specimens from cervix uteri**

**R87.619 Unspecified abnormal cytological findings in specimens from cervix uteri**
Abnormal cervical cytology NOS
Abnormal Papanicolaou smear of cervix NOS
Abnormal thin preparation smear of cervix NOS
Atypical endocervical cells of cervix NOS
Atypical endometrial cells of cervix NOS
Atypical glandular cells of cervix NOS

√6th **R87.62 Abnormal cytological findings in specimens from vagina**
Use additional code to identify acquired absence of uterus and cervix, if applicable (Z90.71-)
EXCLUDES 1 *abnormal cytological findings in specimens from cervix uteri (R87.61-)*
*abnormal cytological findings in specimens from other female genital organs (R87.69)*
*carcinoma in situ of vagina (histologically confirmed) (D07.2)*
*dysplasia (mild) (moderate) of vagina (histologically confirmed) (N89.-)*
*severe dysplasia of vagina (histologically confirmed) (D07.2)*
*vaginal intraepithelial neoplasia I [VAIN I] (N89.0)*
*vaginal intraepithelial neoplasia II [VAIN II] (N89.1)*
*vaginal intraepithelial neoplasia III [VAIN III] (D07.2)*
EXCLUDES 2 *vaginal high risk human papillomavirus (HPV) DNA test positive (R87.811)*
*vaginal low risk human papillomavirus (HPV) DNA test positive (R87.821)*

**R87.620 Atypical squamous cells of undetermined significance on cytologic smear of vagina [ASC-US]**

**R87.621 Atypical squamous cells cannot exclude high grade squamous intraepithelial lesion on cytologic smear of vagina [ASC-H]**

**R87.622 Low grade squamous intraepithelial lesion on cytologic smear of vagina [LGSIL]**

**R87.623 High grade squamous intraepithelial lesion on cytologic smear of vagina [HGSIL]**

**R87.624 Cytologic evidence of malignancy on smear of vagina**

**R87.625 Unsatisfactory cytologic smear of vagina**
Inadequate sample of cytologic smear of vagina

**R87.628 Other abnormal cytological findings on specimens from vagina**

**R87.629 Unspecified abnormal cytological findings in specimens from vagina**
Abnormal Papanicolaou smear of vagina NOS
Abnormal thin preparation smear of vagina NOS
Abnormal vaginal cytology NOS
Atypical endocervical cells of vagina NOS
Atypical endometrial cells of vagina NOS
Atypical glandular cells of vagina NOS

**R87.69 Abnormal cytological findings in specimens from other female genital organs**
Abnormal cytological findings in specimens from female genital organs NOS
EXCLUDES 1 *dysplasia of vulva (histologically confirmed) (N90.0-N90.3)*

**R87.7 Abnormal histological findings in specimens from female genital organs**
EXCLUDES 1 *carcinoma in situ (histologically confirmed) of female genital organs (D06-D07.3)*
*cervical intraepithelial neoplasia I [CIN I] (N87.0)*
*cervical intraepithelial neoplasia II [CIN II] (N87.1)*
*cervical intraepithelial neoplasia III [CIN III] (D06.-)*
*dysplasia (mild) (moderate) of cervix uteri (histologically confirmed) (N87.-)*
*dysplasia (mild) (moderate) of vagina (histologically confirmed) (N89.-)*
*severe dysplasia of cervix uteri (histologically confirmed) (D06.-)*
*severe dysplasia of vagina (histologically confirmed) (D07.2)*
*vaginal intraepithelial neoplasia I [VAIN I] (N89.0)*
*vaginal intraepithelial neoplasia II [VAIN II] (N89.1)*
*vaginal intraepithelial neoplasia III [VAIN III] (D07.2)*

√5th **R87.8 Other abnormal findings in specimens from female genital organs**

√6th **R87.81 High risk human papillomavirus [HPV] DNA test positive from female genital organs**
EXCLUDES 1 *anogenital warts due to human papillomavirus (HPV) (A63.0)*
*condyloma acuminatum (A63.0)*

**R87.810 Cervical high risk human papillomavirus [HPV] DNA test positive**

**R87.811 Vaginal high risk human papillomavirus [HPV] DNA test positive**

√6th **R87.82 Low risk human papillomavirus [HPV] DNA test positive from female genital organs**
Use additional code for associated human papillomavirus (B97.7)

**R87.820 Cervical low risk human papillomavirus [HPV] DNA test positive**

**R87.821 Vaginal low risk human papillomavirus [HPV] DNA test positive**

**R87.89 Other abnormal findings in specimens from female genital organs**
Abnormal chromosomal findings in specimens from female genital organs

**R87.9 Unspecified abnormal finding in specimens from female genital organs**

√4th **R88 Abnormal findings in other body fluids and substances**

**R88.0 Cloudy (hemodialysis) (peritoneal) dialysis effluent**

**R88.8 Abnormal findings in other body fluids and substances**

√4th **R89 Abnormal findings in specimens from other organs, systems and tissues**
INCLUDES abnormal findings in nipple discharge
abnormal findings in synovial fluid
abnormal findings in wound secretions

**R89.0 Abnormal level of enzymes in specimens from other organs, systems and tissues**

**R89.1 Abnormal level of hormones in specimens from other organs, systems and tissues**

**R89.2 Abnormal level of other drugs, medicaments and biological substances in specimens from other organs, systems and tissues**

**R89.3 Abnormal level of substances chiefly nonmedicinal as to source in specimens from other organs, systems and tissues**

**R89.4 Abnormal immunological findings in specimens from other organs, systems and tissues**

**R89.5 Abnormal microbiological findings in specimens from other organs, systems and tissues**
Positive culture findings in specimens from other organs, systems and tissues
EXCLUDES 1 *colonization status (Z22.-)*

**R89.6 Abnormal cytological findings in specimens from other organs, systems and tissues**

**R89.7 Abnormal histological findings in specimens from other organs, systems and tissues**
**AHA:** 2025,2Q,5

**R89.8 Other abnormal findings in specimens from other organs, systems and tissues**
Abnormal chromosomal findings in specimens from other organs, systems and tissues

**R89.9 Unspecified abnormal finding in specimens from other organs, systems and tissues**

## Abnormal findings on diagnostic imaging and in function studies, without diagnosis (R90-R94)

**INCLUDES** nonspecific abnormal findings on diagnostic imaging by computerized axial tomography [CAT scan]
nonspecific abnormal findings on diagnostic imaging by magnetic resonance imaging [MRI][NMR]
nonspecific abnormal findings on diagnostic imaging by positron emission tomography [PET scan]
nonspecific abnormal findings on diagnostic imaging by thermography
nonspecific abnormal findings on diagnostic imaging by ultrasound [echogram]
nonspecific abnormal findings on diagnostic imaging by X-ray examination

**EXCLUDES 1** *abnormal findings on antenatal screening of mother (O28.-)*
*diagnostic abnormal findings classified elsewhere - see Alphabetical Index*

✓4th **R90 Abnormal findings on diagnostic imaging of central nervous system**

**R90.0 Intracranial space-occupying lesion found on diagnostic imaging of central nervous system**

✓5th **R90.8 Other abnormal findings on diagnostic imaging of central nervous system**

**R90.81 Abnormal echoencephalogram**

**R90.82 White matter disease, unspecified**

**R90.89 Other abnormal findings on diagnostic imaging of central nervous system**
Other cerebrovascular abnormality found on diagnostic imaging of central nervous system

✓4th **R91 Abnormal findings on diagnostic imaging of lung**

**R91.1 Solitary pulmonary nodule**
Coin lesion lung
Solitary pulmonary nodule, subsegmental branch of the bronchial tree

**R91.8 Other nonspecific abnormal finding of lung field**
Lung mass NOS found on diagnostic imaging of lung
Pulmonary infiltrate NOS
Shadow, lung

✓4th **R92 Abnormal and inconclusive findings on diagnostic imaging of breast**

**R92.0 Mammographic microcalcification found on diagnostic imaging of breast**
**EXCLUDES 2** *mammographic calcification (calculus) found on diagnostic imaging of breast (R92.1)*
**DEF:** Calcium and cellular debris deposits in the breast that cannot be felt but can be detected on a mammogram. The deposits can be a sign of cancer, benign conditions, or changes in the breast tissue as a result of inflammation, injury, or an obstructed duct.

**R92.1 Mammographic calcification found on diagnostic imaging of breast**
Mammographic calculus found on diagnostic imaging of breast

**R92.2 Inconclusive mammogram**
Inconclusive mammogram NEC
Inconclusive mammography NEC
**AHA:** 2015,1Q,24

✓5th **R92.3 Mammographic density found on imaging of breast**
Code also, if applicable, inconclusive mammogram (R92.2)
**AHA:** 2023,4Q,42-44

**R92.30 Dense breasts, unspecified**
Dense breasts NOS
Low density

✓6th **R92.31 Mammographic fatty tissue density of breast**
~~Breast Imaging Reporting and Data System (BI-RADS): 1~~
▶Breast density category within Imaging Reporting and Data System (BI-RADS): A◀

**R92.311 Mammographic fatty tissue density, right breast**

**R92.312 Mammographic fatty tissue density, left breast**

**R92.313 Mammographic fatty tissue density, bilateral breasts**

✓6th **R92.32 Mammographic fibroglandular density of breast**
~~Breast Imaging Reporting and Data System (BI-RADS): 2~~
▶Breast density category within Imaging Reporting and Data System (BI-RADS): B◀

**R92.321 Mammographic fibroglandular density, right breast**

**R92.322 Mammographic fibroglandular density, left breast**

**R92.323 Mammographic fibroglandular density, bilateral breasts**

✓6th **R92.33 Mammographic heterogeneous density of breast**
~~Breast Imaging Reporting and Data System (BI-RADS): 3~~
▶Breast density category within Imaging Reporting and Data System (BI-RADS): C◀

**R92.331 Mammographic heterogeneous density, right breast**

**R92.332 Mammographic heterogeneous density, left breast**

**R92.333 Mammographic heterogeneous density, bilateral breasts**

✓6th **R92.34 Mammographic extreme density of breast**
~~Breast Imaging Reporting and Data System (BI-RADS): 4~~
▶Breast density category within Imaging Reporting and Data System (BI-RADS): D◀

**R92.341 Mammographic extreme density, right breast**

**R92.342 Mammographic extreme density, left breast**

**R92.343 Mammographic extreme density, bilateral breasts**

**R92.8 Other abnormal and inconclusive findings on diagnostic imaging of breast**

✓4th **R93 Abnormal findings on diagnostic imaging of other body structures**

**R93.0 Abnormal findings on diagnostic imaging of skull and head, not elsewhere classified**
**EXCLUDES 1** *intracranial space-occupying lesion found on diagnostic imaging (R90.0)*
**AHA:** 2026,2Q,8

**R93.1 Abnormal findings on diagnostic imaging of heart and coronary circulation**
Abnormal echocardiogram NOS
Abnormal heart shadow

**R93.2 Abnormal findings on diagnostic imaging of liver and biliary tract**
Nonvisualization of gallbladder

**R93.3 Abnormal findings on diagnostic imaging of other parts of digestive tract**

✓5th **R93.4 Abnormal findings on diagnostic imaging of urinary organs**
**EXCLUDES 2** *hypertrophy of kidney (N28.81)*
**AHA:** 2016,4Q,66

**R93.41 Abnormal radiologic findings on diagnostic imaging of renal pelvis, ureter, or bladder**
Filling defect of bladder found on diagnostic imaging
Filling defect of renal pelvis found on diagnostic imaging
Filling defect of ureter found on diagnostic imaging

✓6th **R93.42 Abnormal radiologic findings on diagnostic imaging of kidney**

**R93.421 Abnormal radiologic findings on diagnostic imaging of right kidney**

**R93.422 Abnormal radiologic findings on diagnostic imaging of left kidney**

**R93.429 Abnormal radiologic findings on diagnostic imaging of unspecified kidney**

**R93.49 Abnormal radiologic findings on diagnostic imaging of other urinary organs**

**R93.5 Abnormal findings on diagnostic imaging of other abdominal regions, including retroperitoneum**

**R93.6 Abnormal findings on diagnostic imaging of limbs**
**EXCLUDES 2** *abnormal finding in skin and subcutaneous tissue (R93.8-)*
**AHA:** 2020,1Q,14

**R93.7 Abnormal findings on diagnostic imaging of other parts of musculoskeletal system**
**EXCLUDES 2** *abnormal findings on diagnostic imaging of skull (R93.0)*

✓5th **R93.8 Abnormal findings on diagnostic imaging of other specified body structures**
**AHA:** 2018,4Q,30

✓6th **R93.81 Abnormal radiologic findings on diagnostic imaging of testis**

**R93.811 Abnormal radiologic findings on diagnostic imaging of right testicle**

**R93.812 Abnormal radiologic findings on diagnostic imaging of left testicle**

**R93.813 Abnormal radiologic findings on diagnostic imaging of testicles, bilateral**

**R93.819 Abnormal radiologic findings on diagnostic imaging of unspecified testicle**

**R93.89 Abnormal findings on diagnostic imaging of other specified body structures**
Abnormal finding by radioisotope localization of placenta
Abnormal radiological finding in skin and subcutaneous tissue
Mediastinal shift

**R93.9 Diagnostic imaging inconclusive due to excess body fat of patient**

√4th **R94 Abnormal results of function studies**
INCLUDES abnormal results of radionuclide [radioisotope] uptake studies
abnormal results of scintigraphy

√5th **R94.0 Abnormal results of function studies of central nervous system**
**R94.01 Abnormal electroencephalogram [EEG]**
**R94.02 Abnormal brain scan**
**R94.09 Abnormal results of other function studies of central nervous system**

√5th **R94.1 Abnormal results of function studies of peripheral nervous system and special senses**
√6th **R94.11 Abnormal results of function studies of eye**
**R94.110 Abnormal electro-oculogram [EOG]**
**R94.111 Abnormal electroretinogram [ERG]**
Abnormal retinal function study
**R94.112 Abnormal visually evoked potential [VEP]**
**R94.113 Abnormal oculomotor study**
**R94.118 Abnormal results of other function studies of eye**

√6th **R94.12 Abnormal results of function studies of ear and other special senses**
AHA: 2016,3Q,17
**R94.120 Abnormal auditory function study**
**R94.121 Abnormal vestibular function study**
**R94.128 Abnormal results of other function studies of ear and other special senses**

√6th **R94.13 Abnormal results of function studies of peripheral nervous system**
**R94.130 Abnormal response to nerve stimulation, unspecified**
**R94.131 Abnormal electromyogram [EMG]**
EXCLUDES 1 *electromyogram of eye (R94.113)*
**R94.138 Abnormal results of other function studies of peripheral nervous system**

**R94.2 Abnormal results of pulmonary function studies**
Reduced ventilatory capacity
Reduced vital capacity

√5th **R94.3 Abnormal results of cardiovascular function studies**
**R94.30 Abnormal result of cardiovascular function study, unspecified**
**R94.31 Abnormal electrocardiogram [ECG] [EKG]**
EXCLUDES 1 *long QT syndrome (I45.81)*
**R94.39 Abnormal result of other cardiovascular function study**
Abnormal electrophysiological intracardiac studies
Abnormal phonocardiogram
Abnormal vectorcardiogram
AHA: 2023,1Q,25

**R94.4 Abnormal results of kidney function studies**
Abnormal renal function test
**R94.5 Abnormal results of liver function studies**
**R94.6 Abnormal results of thyroid function studies**
**R94.7 Abnormal results of other endocrine function studies**
EXCLUDES 2 *abnormal glucose (R73.0-)*
**R94.8 Abnormal results of function studies of other organs and systems**
Abnormal basal metabolic rate [BMR]
Abnormal bladder function test
Abnormal splenic function test

## Abnormal tumor markers (R97)

√4th **R97 Abnormal tumor markers**
Elevated tumor associated antigens [TAA]
Elevated tumor specific antigens [TSA]

**R97.0 Elevated carcinoembryonic antigen [CEA]**
**R97.1 Elevated cancer antigen 125 [CA 125]**
√5th **R97.2 Elevated prostate specific antigen [PSA]**
AHA: 2016,4Q,66
**R97.20 Elevated prostate specific antigen [PSA]** A
**R97.21 Rising PSA following treatment for malignant neoplasm of prostate** A
AHA: 2023,2Q,5
**R97.8 Other abnormal tumor markers**

## Ill-defined and unknown cause of mortality (R99)

**R99 Ill-defined and unknown cause of mortality**
Death (unexplained) NOS
Unspecified cause of mortality

# Chapter 19. Injury, Poisoning, and Certain Other Consequences of External Causes (SØØ–T88)



## Chapter-specific Guidelines with Coding Examples

The chapter-specific guidelines from the ICD-10-CM Official Guidelines for Coding and Reporting have been provided below. Along with these guidelines are coding examples, contained in the shaded boxes, that have been developed to help illustrate the coding and/or sequencing guidance found in these guidelines.

**a. Application of 7th characters in Chapter 19**

Most categories in chapter 19 have a 7th character requirement for each applicable code. Most categories in this chapter have three 7th character values (with the exception of fractures): A, initial encounter, D, subsequent encounter and S, sequela. Categories for traumatic fractures have additional 7th character values. While the patient may be seen by a new or different provider over the course of treatment for an injury, assignment of the 7th character is based on whether the patient is undergoing active treatment and not whether the provider is seeing the patient for the first time.

For complication codes, active treatment refers to treatment for the condition described by the code, even though it may be related to an earlier precipitating problem. For example, code T84.50XA, Infection and inflammatory reaction due to unspecified internal joint prosthesis, initial encounter, is used when active treatment is provided for the infection, even though the condition relates to the prosthetic device, implant or graft that was placed at a previous encounter.

7th character "A", initial encounter is used for each encounter where the patient is receiving active treatment for the condition.

Patient evaluated after fall from a skateboard onto the sidewalk, x-rays identify a nondisplaced fracture to the distal pole of the right scaphoid bone. The patient is placed in a cast.

| | |
|---|---|
| **S62.Ø14A** | **Nondisplaced fracture of distal pole of navicular [scaphoid] bone of right wrist, initial encounter for closed fracture** |
| **VØØ.131A** | **Fall from skateboard, initial encounter** |
| **Y93.51** | **Activity, roller skating (inline) and skateboarding** |
| **Y92.48Ø** | **Sidewalk as the place of occurrence of the external cause** |
| **Y99.8** | **Other external cause status** |

*Explanation:* This fracture would be coded with a seventh character A for initial encounter because the patient received x-rays to identify the site of the fracture and treatment was rendered; this would be considered active treatment.

7th character "D" subsequent encounter is used for encounters after the patient has completed active treatment of the condition and is receiving routine care for the condition during the healing or recovery phase.

Patient seen in follow-up after fall from a skateboard onto the sidewalk resulted in casting of the right arm. X-rays are taken to evaluate how well the nondisplaced fracture to the distal pole of the right scaphoid bone is healing. The physician feels the fracture is healing appropriately; no adjustments to the cast are made.

| | |
|---|---|
| **S62.Ø14D** | **Nondisplaced fracture of distal pole of navicular [scaphoid] bone of right wrist, subsequent encounter for fracture with routine healing** |
| **VØØ.131D** | **Fall from skateboard, subsequent encounter** |

*Explanation:* This fracture would be coded with a seventh character D for subsequent encounter, whether the same physician who provided the initial cast application or a different physician is now seeing the patient. Although the patient received x-rays, the intent of the x-rays was to assess how the fracture was healing. There was no active treatment rendered and the visit is therefore considered a subsequent encounter.

The aftercare Z codes should not be used for aftercare for conditions such as injuries or poisonings, where 7th characters are provided to identify subsequent care. For example, for aftercare of an injury, assign the acute injury code with the 7th character "D" (subsequent encounter).

7th character "S", sequela, is for use for complications or conditions that arise as a direct result of a condition, such as scar formation after a burn. The scars are sequelae of the burn. When using 7th character "S", it is necessary to use both the injury code that precipitated the sequela and the code for the sequela itself. The "S" is added only to the injury code, not the sequela code. The 7th character "S" identifies the injury responsible for the sequela. The specific type of sequela (e.g. scar) is sequenced first, followed by the injury code.

*See Section I.B.10. Sequelae, (Late Effects)*

Patient with a history of a nondisplaced fracture to the distal pole of the right scaphoid bone due to a fall from a skateboard is seen for evaluation of arthritis to the right wrist that has developed as a consequence of the traumatic fracture.

| | |
|---|---|
| **M12.531** | **Traumatic arthropathy, right wrist** |
| **S62.Ø14S** | **Nondisplaced fracture of distal pole of navicular [scaphoid] bone of right wrist, sequela** |
| **VØØ.131S** | **Fall from skateboard, sequela** |

*Explanation:* The code identifying the specific sequela condition (traumatic arthritis) should be coded first followed by the injury that instigated the development of the sequela (fracture). The scaphoid fracture injury code is given a 7th character S for sequela to represent its role as the inciting injury. The fracture has healed and is not being managed or treated on this admit and therefore is not applicable as a first listed or principal diagnosis. However, it is directly related to the development of the arthritis and should be appended as a secondary code to signify this cause and effect relationship.

**b. Coding of injuries**

When coding injuries, assign separate codes for each injury unless a combination code is provided, in which case the combination code is assigned. Codes from category TØ7, Unspecified multiple injuries should not be assigned in the inpatient setting unless information for a more specific code is not available. Traumatic injury codes (SØØ-T14.9) are not to be used for normal, healing surgical wounds or to identify complications of surgical wounds.

11-year-old girl fell from her horse, resulting in a laceration to her right forearm with several large pieces of wooden fragments embedded in the wound as well as abrasions to her right ear; in addition, her right shoulder was dislocated.

| | |
|---|---|
| **S43.ØØ4A** | **Unspecified dislocation of right shoulder joint, initial encounter** |
| **S51.821A** | **Laceration with foreign body of right forearm, initial encounter** |
| **SØØ.411A** | **Abrasion of right ear, initial encounter** |
| **V8Ø.Ø1ØA** | **Animal-rider injured by fall from or being thrown from horse in noncollision accident, initial encounter** |
| **Y93.52** | **Activity, horseback riding** |

*Explanation:* Each separate injury should be reported. The patient's injury to the forearm is reported with one combination code that captures both the laceration and the foreign body.

The code for the most serious injury, as determined by the provider and the focus of treatment, is sequenced first.

**1) Superficial injuries**

Superficial injuries such as abrasions or contusions are not coded when associated with more severe injuries of the same site.

**2) Primary injury with damage to nerves/blood vessels**

When a primary injury results in minor damage to peripheral nerves or blood vessels, the primary injury is sequenced first with additional code(s) for injuries to nerves and spinal cord (such as category SØ4), and/or injury to blood vessels (such as category S15). When the primary injury is to the blood vessels or nerves, that injury should be sequenced first.

**3) Iatrogenic injuries**

Injury codes from Chapter 19 should not be assigned for injuries that occur during, or as a result of, a medical intervention. Assign the appropriate complication code(s).

**c. Coding of traumatic fractures**

The principles of multiple coding of injuries should be followed in coding fractures. Fractures of specified sites are coded individually by site in accordance with both the provisions within categories SØ2, S12, S22, S32, S42, S49, S52, S59, S62, S72, S79, S82, S89, S92 and the level of detail furnished by medical record content.

A fracture not indicated as open or closed should be coded to closed. A fracture not indicated whether displaced or not displaced should be coded to displaced.

More specific guidelines are as follows:

**1) Initial vs. subsequent encounter for fractures**

Traumatic fractures are coded using the appropriate 7th character for initial encounter (A, B, C) for each encounter where the patient is receiving active treatment for the fracture. The appropriate 7th character for initial encounter should also be assigned for a patient who delayed seeking treatment for the fracture or nonunion.

Fractures are coded using the appropriate 7th character for subsequent care for encounters after the patient has completed active treatment of the fracture and is receiving routine care for the fracture during the healing or recovery phase.

Care for complications of surgical treatment for fracture repairs during the healing or recovery phase should be coded with the appropriate complication codes.

Care of complications of fractures, such as malunion and nonunion, should be reported with the appropriate 7th character for subsequent care with nonunion (K, M, N,) or subsequent care with malunion (P, Q, R).

Malunion/nonunion: The appropriate 7th character for initial encounter should also be assigned for a patient who delayed seeking treatment for the fracture or nonunion.

Female patient fell during a forest hiking excursion almost six months ago and until recently did not feel she needed to seek medical attention for her left ankle pain; x-rays show nonunion of lateral malleolus and surgery has been scheduled

| | |
|---|---|
| **S82.62XA** | **Displaced fracture of lateral malleolus of left fibula, initial encounter for closed fracture** |
| **WØ1.ØXXA** | **Fall on same level from slipping, tripping and stumbling without subsequent striking against object, initial encounter** |
| **Y92.821** | **Forest as place of occurrence of the external cause** |
| **Y93.Ø1** | **Activity, walking, marching and hiking** |
| **Y99.8** | **Other external cause status** |

*Explanation:* A seventh character of A is used for the lateral malleolus nonunion fracture to signify that the fracture is receiving active treatment. The delayed care for the fracture has resulted in a nonunion, but capturing the nonunion in the seventh character is trumped by the provision of active care.

The open fracture designations in the assignment of the 7th character for fractures of the forearm, femur and lower leg, including ankle are based on the Gustilo open fracture classification. When the Gustilo classification type is not specified for an open fracture, the 7th character for open fracture type I or II should be assigned (B, E, H, M, Q).

A code from category M8Ø, not a traumatic fracture code, should be used for any patient with known osteoporosis who suffers a fracture, even if the patient had a minor fall or trauma, if that fall or trauma would not usually break a normal, healthy bone.

*See Section I.C.13. Osteoporosis.*

The aftercare Z codes should not be used for aftercare for traumatic fractures. For aftercare of a traumatic fracture, assign the acute fracture code with the appropriate 7th character.

**2) Multiple fractures sequencing**

Multiple fractures are sequenced in accordance with the severity of the fracture.

**3) Physeal fractures**

For physeal fractures, assign only the code identifying the type of physeal fracture. Do not assign a separate code to identify the specific bone that is fractured.

**d. Coding of burns and corrosions**

The ICD-1Ø-CM makes a distinction between burns and corrosions. The burn codes are for thermal burns, except sunburns, that come from a heat source, such as a fire or hot appliance. The burn codes are also for burns resulting from electricity and radiation. Corrosions are burns due to chemicals. The guidelines are the same for burns and corrosions.

Current burns (T20-T25) are classified by depth, extent and by agent (X code). Burns are classified by depth as first degree (erythema), second degree (blistering), and third degree (full-thickness involvement). Burns of the eye and internal organs (T26-T28) are classified by site, but not by degree.

**1) Sequencing of burn and related condition codes**

Sequence first the code that reflects the highest degree of burn when more than one burn is present.

a. When the reason for the admission or encounter is for treatment of external multiple burns, sequence first the code that reflects the burn of the highest degree.

b. When a patient has both internal and external burns, the circumstances of admission govern the selection of the principal diagnosis or first-listed diagnosis.

c. When a patient is admitted for burn injuries and other related conditions such as smoke inhalation and/or respiratory failure, the circumstances of admission govern the selection of the principal or first-listed diagnosis.

Patient referred for minor first-degree burns to multiple sites of her right and left hands as well as severe smoke inhalation. While she was sleeping at home, a candle on her dresser lit the bedroom curtains on fire.

| | |
|---|---|
| **T59.811A** | **Toxic effect of smoke, accidental (unintentional), initial encounter** |
| **J7Ø.5** | **Respiratory conditions due to smoke inhalation** |
| **T23.191A** | **Burn of first degree of multiple sites of right wrist and hand, initial encounter** |
| **T23.192A** | **Burn of first degree of multiple sites of left wrist and hand, initial encounter** |
| **XØ8.8XXA** | **Exposure to other specified smoke, fire and flames, initial encounter** |
| **Y99.8** | **Other external cause status** |
| **Y92.ØØ3** | **Bedroom of unspecified non-institutional (private) residence as the place of occurrence of the external cause** |
| **Y93.84** | **Activity, sleeping** |

*Explanation:* Based on the documentation, the inhalation injury is more severe than the first-degree burns and is sequenced first. The burns to the hands are appended as secondary diagnoses.

**2) Burns of the same anatomic site**

Classify burns of the same anatomic site and on the same side but of different degrees to the subcategory identifying the highest degree recorded in the diagnosis (e.g., for second and third degree burns of right thigh, assign only code T24.311-).

**3) Non-healing burns**

Non-healing burns are coded as acute burns.

Necrosis of burned skin should be coded as a non-healed burn.

**4) Infected burn**

For any documented infected burn site, use an additional code for the infection.

**5) Assign separate codes for each burn site**

When coding burns, assign separate codes for each burn site. Category T3Ø, Burn and corrosion, body region unspecified is extremely vague and should rarely be used.

Codes for burns of "multiple sites" should only be assigned when the medical record documentation does not specify the individual sites.

**6) Burns and corrosions classified according to extent of body surface involved**

Assign codes from category T31, Burns classified according to extent of body surface involved, or T32, Corrosions classified according to extent of body surface involved, for acute burns or corrosions when the site of the burn or corrosion is not specified or when there is a need for additional data. It is advisable to use category T31 as additional coding when needed to provide data for evaluating burn mortality, such as that needed by burn units. It is also advisable to use category T31 as an additional code for reporting purposes when there is mention of a third-degree burn involving 2Ø percent or more of the body surface. Codes from categories T31 and T32 should not be used for sequelae of burns or corrosions.

Categories T31 and T32 are based on the classic "rule of nines" in estimating body surface involved: head and neck are assigned nine percent, each arm nine percent, each leg 18 percent, the anterior trunk 18 percent, posterior trunk 18 percent, and genitalia one percent. Providers may change these percentage assignments where necessary to accommodate infants and children who have proportionately larger heads than adults, and patients who have large buttocks, thighs, or abdomen that involve burns.

Patient seen for dressing change after he accidentally spilled acetic acid on himself two days ago. The second-degree burns to his right thigh, covering about 3 percent of his body surface, are healing appropriately.

**T54.2X1D** **Toxic effect of corrosive acids and acid-like substances, accidental (unintentional), subsequent encounter**

**T24.611D** **Corrosion of second degree of right thigh, subsequent encounter**

**T32.Ø** **Corrosions involving less than 1Ø% of body surface**

*Explanation:* Code T32.Ø provides additional information as to how much of the patient's body was affected by the corrosive substance.

**7) Encounters for treatment of sequela of burns**

Encounters for the treatment of the late effects of burns or corrosions (i.e., scars or joint contractures) should be coded with a burn or corrosion code with the 7th character "S" for sequela.

**8) Sequelae with a late effect code and current burn**

When appropriate, both a code for a current burn or corrosion with 7th character "A" or "D" and a burn or corrosion code with 7th character "S" may be assigned on the same record (when both a current burn and sequelae of an old burn exist). Burns and corrosions do not heal at the same rate and a current healing wound may still exist with sequela of a healed burn or corrosion.

*See Section I.B.10. Sequela (Late Effects)*

Female patient seen for second-degree burn to the left ear; she also has significant scarring on her left elbow from a third-degree burn from childhood

**T2Ø.212A** **Burn of second degree of left ear [any part, except ear drum], initial encounter**

**L9Ø.5** **Scar conditions and fibrosis of skin**

**T22.322S** **Burn of third degree of left elbow, sequela**

*Explanation:* The patient is being seen for management of a current second-degree burn, which is reflected in the code by appending the seventh character of A, indicating active treatment or management of this burn. The elbow scarring is a sequela of a previous third-degree burn. The sequela condition precedes the original burn injury, which is appended with a seventh character of S.

**9) Use of an external cause code with burns and corrosions**

An external cause code should be used with burns and corrosions to identify the source and intent of the burn, as well as the place where it occurred.

**e. Adverse effects, poisoning, underdosing and toxic effects**

Codes in categories T36-T65 are combination codes that include the substance that was taken as well as the intent. No additional external cause code is required for poisonings, toxic effects, adverse effects and underdosing codes.

**1) Do not code directly from the Table of Drugs**

Do not code directly from the Table of Drugs and Chemicals. Always refer back to the Tabular List.

**2) Use as many codes as necessary to describe**

Use as many codes as necessary to describe completely all drugs, medicinal or biological substances.

**3) If the same code would describe the causative agent**

If the same code would describe the causative agent for more than one adverse reaction, poisoning, toxic effect or underdosing, assign the code only once.

**4) If two or more drugs, medicinal or biological substances**

If two or more drugs, medicinal or biological substances are taken, code each individually unless a combination code is listed in the Table of Drugs and Chemicals.

If multiple unspecified drugs, medicinal or biological substances were taken, assign the appropriate code from subcategory T5Ø.91, Poisoning by, adverse effect of and underdosing of multiple unspecified drugs, medicaments and biological substances.

**5) The occurrence of drug toxicity is classified in ICD-10-CM as follows:**

**(a) Adverse effect**

When coding an adverse effect of a drug that has been correctly prescribed and properly administered, assign the appropriate code for the nature of the adverse effect followed by the appropriate code for the adverse effect of the drug (T36-T5Ø). The code for the drug should have a 5th or 6th character "5" (for example T36.ØX5-) Examples of the nature of an adverse effect are tachycardia, delirium, gastrointestinal hemorrhaging, vomiting, hypokalemia, hepatitis, renal failure, or respiratory failure.

**(b) Poisoning**

When coding a poisoning or reaction to the improper use of a medication (e.g., overdose, wrong substance given or taken in error, wrong route of administration), first assign the appropriate code from categories T36-T5Ø. The poisoning codes have an associated intent as their 5th or 6th character (accidental, intentional self-harm, assault and undetermined). If the intent of the poisoning is unknown or unspecified, code the intent as accidental intent. The undetermined intent is only for use if the documentation in the record specifies that the intent cannot be determined. Use additional code(s) for all manifestations of poisonings.

If there is also a diagnosis of abuse or dependence of the substance, the abuse or dependence is assigned as an additional code.

Examples of poisoning include:

(i) Error was made in drug prescription
Errors made in drug prescription or in the administration of the drug by provider, nurse, patient, or other person.

(ii Overdose of a drug intentionally taken
If an overdose of a drug was intentionally taken or administered and resulted in drug toxicity, it would be coded as a poisoning.

(iii) Nonprescribed drug taken with correctly prescribed and properly administered drug
If a nonprescribed drug or medicinal agent was taken in combination with a correctly prescribed and properly administered drug, any drug toxicity or other reaction resulting from the interaction of the two drugs would be classified as a poisoning.

(iv) Interaction of drug(s) and alcohol
When a reaction results from the interaction of a drug(s) and alcohol, this would be classified as poisoning.

*See Section I.C.4. if poisoning is the result of insulin pump malfunctions.*

*For Sequela (Late Effects) see Section I.B.1Ø.*

**(c) Underdosing**

Underdosing refers to taking less of a medication than is prescribed by a provider or a manufacturer's instruction. Discontinuing the use of a prescribed medication on the patient's own initiative (not directed by the patient's provider) is also classified as an underdosing. For underdosing, assign the code from categories T36-T5Ø (fifth or sixth character "6"). Documentation of a change in the patient's condition is not required in order to assign an underdosing code. Documentation that the patient is taking less of a medication than is prescribed or discontinued the prescribed medication is sufficient for code assignment.

Codes for underdosing should never be assigned as principal or first-listed codes. If a patient has a relapse or exacerbation of the medical condition for which the drug is prescribed because of the reduction in dose, then the medical condition itself should be coded.

Noncompliance (Z91.12-, Z91.13-, Z91.14- and Z91.A4-) or complication of care (Y63.6-Y63.9) codes are to be used with an underdosing code to indicate intent, if known.

Patient referred for atrial fibrillation with history of chronic atrial fibrillation for which she is prescribed amiodarone. Financial concerns have left the patient unable to pay for her prescriptions and she has been skipping her amiodarone dose every other day to offset the cost.

**I48.2Ø** **Chronic atrial fibrillation, unspecified**

**T46.2X6A** **Underdosing of other antidysrhythmic drugs, initial encounter**

**Z91.12Ø** **Patient's intentional underdosing of medication regimen due to financial hardship**

*Explanation:* By skipping her amiodarone pill every other day, the patient's atrial fibrillation returned. The condition for which the drug was being taken is reported first, followed by an underdosing code to show that the patient was not adhering to her prescription regiment. The Z code helps elaborate on the patient's social and/or economic circumstances that led to the patient taking less then what she was prescribed.



Chapter 19. Injury, Poisoning, and Certain Other Consequences of External Causes

**(d) Toxic effects**

When a harmful substance is ingested or comes in contact with a person, this is classified as a toxic effect. The toxic effect codes are in categories T51–T65. When coding a toxic effect, assign the toxic effect code first, followed by codes for all associated manifestations of the toxic effect.

Toxic effect codes have an associated intent: accidental, intentional self-harm, assault and undetermined.

*For Sequela (Late Effects) see Section I.B.10. Sequela*

**f. Adult and child abuse, neglect and other maltreatment**

Sequence first the appropriate code from categories T74, Adult and child abuse, neglect and other maltreatment, confirmed, or T76, Adult and child abuse, neglect and other maltreatment, suspected, for abuse, neglect and other maltreatment, followed by any accompanying mental health or injury code(s).

If the documentation in the medical record states abuse or neglect, it is coded as confirmed (T74.-). It is coded as suspected if it is documented as suspected (T76.-).

For cases of confirmed abuse or neglect an external cause code from the assault section (X92-Y09) should be added to identify the cause of any physical injuries. A perpetrator code (Y07) should be added when the perpetrator of the abuse is known. For suspected cases of abuse or neglect, do not report external cause or perpetrator code.

If a suspected case of abuse, neglect or mistreatment is ruled out during an encounter code Z04.71, Encounter for examination and observation following alleged physical adult abuse, ruled out, or code Z04.72, Encounter for examination and observation following alleged child physical abuse, ruled out, should be used, not a code from T76.

If a suspected case of alleged rape or sexual abuse is ruled out during an encounter code Z04.41, Encounter for examination and observation following alleged adult rape or code Z04.42, Encounter for examination and observation following alleged child rape, should be used, not a code from T76.

If a suspected case of forced sexual exploitation or forced labor exploitation is ruled out during an encounter, code Z04.81, Encounter for examination and observation of victim following forced sexual exploitation, or code Z04.82, Encounter for examination and observation of victim following forced labor exploitation, should be used, not a code from T76.

*See Section I.C.15. Abuse in a pregnant patient.*

**g. Complications of care**

**1) General guidelines for complications of care**

**(a) Documentation of complications of care**

*See Section I.B.16. for information on documentation of complications of care.*

**2) Pain due to medical devices**

Pain associated with devices, implants or grafts left in a surgical site (for example painful hip prosthesis) is assigned to the appropriate code(s) found in Chapter 19, Injury, poisoning, and certain other consequences of external causes. Specific codes for pain due to medical devices are found in the T code section of the ICD-10-CM. Use additional code(s) from category G89 to identify acute or chronic pain due to presence of the device, implant or graft (G89.18 or G89.28).

Chronic left breast pain secondary to breast implant

| | |
|---|---|
| **T85.848A** | **Pain due to other internal prosthetic devices, implants and grafts, initial encounter** |
| **N64.4** | **Mastodynia** |
| **G89.28** | **Other chronic postprocedural pain** |

*Explanation:* As the pain is a complication related to the breast implant, the complication code is sequenced first. The T code does not describe the site or type of pain, so additional codes may be appended to indicate that the patient is experiencing chronic pain in the breast.

**3) Transplant complications**

**(a) Transplant complications other than kidney**

Codes under category T86, Complications of transplanted organs and tissues, are for use for both complications and rejection of transplanted organs. A transplant complication code is only assigned if the complication affects the function of the transplanted organ. Two codes are required to fully describe a transplant complication: the appropriate code from category T86 and a secondary code that identifies the complication.

Pre-existing conditions or conditions that develop after the transplant are not coded as complications unless they affect the function of the transplanted organs.

*See I.C.21. for transplant organ removal status*

*See I.C.2. for malignant neoplasm associated with transplanted organ.*

*See I.C.1.d.4. for sequencing of sepsis due to infection in transplanted organ*

**(b) Kidney transplant complications**

Patients who have undergone kidney transplant may still have some form of chronic kidney disease (CKD) because the kidney transplant may not fully restore kidney function. Code T86.1- should be assigned for documented complications of a kidney transplant, such as transplant failure or rejection or other transplant complication. Code T86.1- should not be assigned for post kidney transplant patients who have chronic kidney (CKD) unless a transplant complication such as transplant failure or rejection is documented. If the documentation is unclear as to whether the patient has a complication of the transplant, query the provider.

Conditions that affect the function of the transplanted kidney, other than CKD, should be assigned a code from subcategory T86.1, Complications of transplanted organ, Kidney, and a secondary code that identifies the complication.

For patients with CKD following a kidney transplant, but who do not have a complication such as failure or rejection, *see section I.C.14. Chronic kidney disease and kidney transplant status.*

*See I.C.1.d.4. for sequencing of sepsis due to infection in transplanted organ*

Patient seen for chronic kidney disease stage 2; history of successful kidney transplant with no complications identified

| | |
|---|---|
| **N18.2** | **Chronic kidney disease, stage 2 (mild)** |
| **Z94.0** | **Kidney transplant status** |

*Explanation:* This patient's stage 2 CKD is not indicated as being due to the transplanted kidney but instead is just the residual disease the patient had prior to the transplant.

**4) Complication codes that include the external cause**

As with certain other T codes, some of the complications of care codes have the external cause included in the code. The code includes the nature of the complication as well as the type of procedure that caused the complication. No external cause code indicating the type of procedure is necessary for these codes.

**5) Complications of care codes within the body system chapters**

Intraoperative and postprocedural complication codes are found within the body system chapters with codes specific to the organs and structures of that body system. These codes should be sequenced first, followed by a code(s) for the specific complication, if applicable.

Postprocedural ischemic infarction of the left middle cerebral artery due to cardiac surgery

| | |
|---|---|
| **I97.820** | **Postprocedural cerebrovascular infarction following cardiac surgery** |
| **I63.512** | **Cerebral infarction due to unspecified occlusion or stenosis of left middle cerebral artery** |

*Explanation:* The infarction was caused by the cardiac procedure and is coded as a postprocedural complication. The postprocedural cerebrovascular infarction is the first-listed diagnosis, followed by the code for the infarction itself.

Complication codes from the body system chapters should be assigned for intraoperative and postprocedural complications (e.g., the appropriate complication code from chapter 9 would be assigned for a vascular intraoperative or postprocedural complication) unless the complication is specifically indexed to a T code in chapter 19.

# Muscle/Tendon Table

ICD-10-CM categorizes certain muscles and tendons in the upper and lower extremities by their action (e.g., extension, flexion), their anatomical location (e.g., posterior, anterior), and/or whether they are intrinsic or extrinsic to a certain anatomical area. The Muscle/Tendon Table is provided at the beginning of chapters 13 and 19 as a resource to help users when code selection depends on one or more of these characteristics. A **TIP** has been placed at those categories and/or subcategories that relate to this table. Please note that this table is not all-inclusive, and proper code assignment should be based on the provider's documentation.

| Body Region | Muscle | Extensor Tendon | Flexor Tendon | Other Tendon |
|---|---|---|---|---|
| **Shoulder** | | | | |
| | Deltoid | Posterior deltoid | Anterior deltoid | |
| | Rotator cuff | | | |
| | Infraspinatus | | | Infraspinatus |
| | Subscapularis | | | Subscapularis |
| | Supraspinatus | | | Supraspinatus |
| | Teres minor | | | Teres minor |
| | Teres major | Teres major | | |
| **Upper arm** | | | | |
| | Anterior muscles | | | |
| | Biceps brachii — long head | | Biceps brachii — long head | |
| | Biceps brachii — short head | | Biceps brachii — short head | |
| | Brachialis | | Brachialis | |
| | Coracobrachialis | | Coracobrachialis | |
| | Posterior muscles | | | |
| | Triceps brachii | Triceps brachii | | |
| **Forearm** | | | | |
| | Anterior muscles | | | |
| | Flexors | | | |
| | Deep | | | |
| | Flexor digitorum profundus | | Flexor digitorum profundus | |
| | Flexor pollicis longus | | Flexor pollicis longus | |
| | Intermediate | | | |
| | Flexor digitorum superficialis | | Flexor digitorum superficialis | |
| | Superficial | | | |
| | Flexor carpi radialis | | Flexor carpi radialis | |
| | Flexor carpi ulnaris | | Flexor carpi ulnaris | |
| | Palmaris longus | | Palmaris longus | |
| | Pronators | | | |
| | Pronator quadratus | | | Pronator quadratus |
| | Pronator teres | | | Pronator teres |
| | Posterior muscles | | | |
| | Extensors | | | |
| | Deep | | | |
| | Abductor pollicis longus | | | Abductor pollicis longus |
| | Extensor indicis | Extensor indicis | | |
| | Extensor pollicis brevis | Extensor pollicis brevis | | |
| | Extensor pollicis longus | Extensor pollicis longus | | |
| | Superficial | | | |
| | Brachioradialis | | | Brachioradialis |
| | Extensor carpi radialis brevis | Extensor carpi radialis brevis | | |
| | Extensor carpi radialis longus | Extensor carpi radialis longus | | |
| | Extensor carpi ulnaris | Extensor carpi ulnaris | | |
| | Extensor digiti minimi | Extensor digiti minimi | | |
| | Extensor digitorum | Extensor digitorum | | |
| | Anconeus | Anconeus | | |
| | Supinator | | | Supinator |

| Body Region | Muscle | Extensor Tendon | Flexor Tendon | Other Tendon |
|---|---|---|---|---|
| **Hand** | | | | |
| Extrinsic — attach to a site in the forearm as well as a site in the hand with action related to hand movement at the wrist | | | | |
| | Extensor carpi radialis brevis | Extensor carpi radialis brevis | | |
| | Extensor carpi radialis longus | Extensor carpi radialis longus | | |
| | Extensor carpi ulnaris | Extensor carpi ulnaris | | |
| | Flexor carpi radialis | | Flexor carpi radialis | |
| | Flexor carpi ulnaris | | Flexor carpi ulnaris | |
| | Flexor digitorum superficialis | | Flexor digitorum superficialis | |
| | Palmaris longus | | Palmaris longus | |
| Extrinsic — attach to a site in the forearm as well as a site in the hand with action in the hand related to finger movement | | | | |
| | Adductor pollicis longus | | | Adductor pollicis longus |
| | Extensor digiti minimi | Extensor digiti minimi | | |
| | Extensor digitorum | Extensor digitorum | | |
| | Extensor indicis | Extensor indicis | | |
| | Flexor digitorum profundus | | Flexor digitorum profundus | |
| | Flexor digitorum superficialis | | Flexor digitorum superficialis | |
| Extrinsic — attach to a site in the forearm as well as a site in the hand with action in the hand related to thumb movement | | | | |
| | Extensor pollicis brevis | Extensor pollicis brevis | | |
| | Extensor pollicis longus | Extensor pollicis longus | | |
| | Flexor pollicis longus | | Flexor pollicis longus | |
| Intrinsic — found within the hand only | | | | |
| | Adductor pollicis | | | Adductor pollicis |
| | Dorsal interossei | Dorsal interossei | Dorsal interossei | |
| | Lumbricals | Lumbricals | Lumbricals | |
| | Palmaris brevis | | | Palmaris brevis |
| | Palmar interossei | Palmar interossei | Palmar interossei | |
| | Hypothenar muscles | | | |
| | Abductor digiti minimi | | | Abductor digiti minimi |
| | Flexor digiti minimi brevis | | Flexor digiti minimi brevis | |
| | Opponens digiti minimi | | Opponens digiti minimi | |
| | Thenar muscles | | | |
| | Abductor pollicis brevis | | | Abductor pollicis brevis |
| | Flexor pollicis brevis | | Flexor pollicis brevis | |
| | Opponens pollicis | | Opponens pollicis | |
| **Thigh** | | | | |
| | Anterior muscles | | | |
| | Iliopsoas | | Iliopsoas | |
| | Pectineus | | Pectineus | |
| | Quadriceps | Quadriceps | | |
| | Rectus femoris | Rectus femoris — Extends knee | Rectus femoris — Flexes hip | |
| | Vastus intermedius | Vastus intermedius | | |
| | Vastus lateralis | Vastus lateralis | | |
| | Vastus medialis | Vastus medialis | | |
| | Sartorius | | Sartorius | |
| | Medial muscles | | | |
| | Adductor brevis | | | Adductor brevis |
| | Adductor longus | | | Adductor longus |
| | Adductor magnus | | | Adductor magnus |
| | Gracilis | | | Gracilis |
| | Obturator externus | | | Obturator externus |
| | Posterior muscles | | | |
| | Hamstring | Hamstring — Extends hip | Hamstring — Flexes knee | |
| | Biceps femoris | Biceps femoris | Biceps femoris | |
| | Semimembranosus | Semimembranosus | Semimembranosus | |
| | Semitendinosus | Semitendinosus | Semitendinosus | |

| Body Region | Muscle | Extensor Tendon | Flexor Tendon | Other Tendon |
|---|---|---|---|---|
| **Lower leg** | | | | |
| | Anterior muscles | | | |
| | Extensor digitorum longus | Extensor digitorum longus | | |
| | Extensor hallucis longus | Extensor hallucis longus | | |
| | Fibularis (peroneus) tertius | Fibularis (peroneus) tertius | | |
| | Tibialis anterior | Tibialis anterior | | Tibialis anterior |
| | Lateral muscles | | | |
| | Fibularis (peroneus) brevis | | Fibularis (peroneus) brevis | |
| | Fibularis (peroneus) longus | | Fibularis (peroneus) longus | |
| | Posterior muscles | | | |
| | Deep | | | |
| | Flexor digitorum longus | | Flexor digitorum longus | |
| | Flexor hallucis longus | | Flexor hallucis longus | |
| | Popliteus | | Popliteus | |
| | Tibialis posterior | | Tibialis posterior | |
| | Superficial | | | |
| | Gastrocnemius | | Gastrocnemius | |
| | Plantaris | | Plantaris | |
| | Soleus | | Soleus | |
| | | | | Calcaneal (Achilles) |
| **Ankle/Foot** | | | | |
| Extrinsic — attach to a site in the lower leg as well as a site in the foot with action related to foot movement at the ankle | | | | |
| | Plantaris | | Plantaris | |
| | Soleus | | Soleus | |
| | Tibialis anterior | Tibialis anterior | | |
| | Tibialis posterior | | Tibialis posterior | |
| Extrinsic — attach to a site in the lower leg as well as a site in the foot with action in the foot related to toe movement | | | | |
| | Extensor digitorum longus | Extensor digitorum longus | | |
| | Extensor hallucis longus | Extensor hallucis longus | | |
| | Flexor digitorum longus | | Flexor digitorum longus | |
| | Flexor hallucis longus | | Flexor hallucis longus | |
| Intrinsic — found within the ankle/foot only | | | | |
| | Dorsal muscles | | | |
| | Extensor digitorum brevis | Extensor digitorum brevis | | |
| | Extensor hallucis brevis | Extensor hallucis brevis | | |
| | Plantar muscles | | | |
| | Abductor digiti minimi | | Abductor digiti minimi | |
| | Abductor hallucis | | Abductor hallucis | |
| | Dorsal interossei | Dorsal interossei | Dorsal interossei | |
| | Flexor digiti minimi brevis | | Flexor digiti minimi brevis | |
| | Flexor digitorum brevis | | Flexor digitorum brevis | |
| | Flexor hallucis brevis | | Flexor hallucis brevis | |
| | Lumbricals | Lumbricals | Lumbricals | |
| | Quadratus plantae | | Quadratus plantae | |
| | Plantar interossei | Plantar interossei | Plantar interossei | |

# Chapter 19. Injury, Poisoning and Certain Other Consequences of External Causes (SØØ-T88)

NOTE Use secondary code(s) from Chapter 20, External causes of morbidity, to indicate cause of injury. Codes within the T section that include the external cause do not require an additional external cause code.

Use additional code to identify any retained foreign body, if applicable (Z18.-)

EXCLUDES 2 *birth trauma (P1Ø-P15)*
*obstetric trauma (O7Ø-O71)*

NOTE The chapter uses the S-section for coding different types of injuries related to single body regions and the T-section to cover injuries to unspecified body regions as well as poisoning and certain other consequences of external causes.

**AHA:** 2016,2Q,3-7; 2015,4Q,35-38; 2015,3Q,37-39,40; 2015,2Q,6; 2015,1Q,3-21

**TIP:** The specific site of an injury can be determined from the radiology report when authenticated by a radiologist and available at the time of code assignment.

This chapter contains the following blocks:

| | |
|---|---|
| SØØ-SØ9 | Injuries to the head |
| S1Ø-S19 | Injuries to the neck |
| S2Ø-S29 | Injuries to the thorax |
| S3Ø-S39 | Injuries to the abdomen, lower back, lumbar spine, pelvis and external genitals |
| S4Ø-S49 | Injuries to the shoulder and upper arm |
| S5Ø-S59 | Injuries to the elbow and forearm |
| S6Ø-S69 | Injuries to the wrist, hand and fingers |
| S7Ø-S79 | Injuries to the hip and thigh |
| S8Ø-S89 | Injuries to the knee and lower leg |
| S9Ø-S99 | Injuries to the ankle and foot |
| TØ7 | Injuries involving multiple body regions |
| T14 | Injury of unspecified body region |
| T15-T19 | Effects of foreign body entering through natural orifice |
| T2Ø-T25 | Burns and corrosions of external body surface, specified by site |
| T26-T28 | Burns and corrosions confined to eye and internal organs |
| T3Ø-T32 | Burns and corrosions of multiple and unspecified body regions |
| T33-T34 | Frostbite |
| T36-T5Ø | Poisoning by, adverse effect of and underdosing of drugs, medicaments and biological substances |
| T51-T65 | Toxic effects of substances chiefly nonmedicinal as to source |
| T66-T78 | Other and unspecified effects of external causes |
| T79 | Certain early complications of trauma |
| T8Ø-T88 | Complications of surgical and medical care, not elsewhere classified |

## Injuries to the head (SØØ-SØ9)

INCLUDES injuries of ear
injuries of eye
injuries of face [any part]
injuries of gum
injuries of jaw
injuries of oral cavity
injuries of palate
injuries of periocular area
injuries of scalp
injuries of temporomandibular joint area
injuries of tongue
injuries of tooth

Code also for any associated infection

EXCLUDES 2 *burns and corrosions (T2Ø-T32)*
*effects of foreign body in ear (T16)*
*effects of foreign body in larynx (T17.3)*
*effects of foreign body in mouth NOS (T18.Ø)*
*effects of foreign body in nose (T17.Ø-T17.1)*
*effects of foreign body in pharynx (T17.2)*
*effects of foreign body on external eye (T15.-)*
*frostbite (T33-T34)*
*insect bite or sting, venomous (T63.4)*

4th **SØØ Superficial injury of head**

EXCLUDES 1 *diffuse cerebral contusion (SØ6.2-)*
*focal cerebral contusion (SØ6.3-)*
*injury of eye and orbit (SØ5.-)*
*open wound of head (SØ1.-)*

The appropriate 7th character is to be added to each code from category SØØ.
A initial encounter
D subsequent encounter
S sequela

5th **SØØ.Ø Superficial injury of scalp**

x7th **SØØ.ØØ Unspecified superficial injury of scalp**
x7th **SØØ.Ø1 Abrasion of scalp**
x7th **SØØ.Ø2 Blister (nonthermal) of scalp**
x7th **SØØ.Ø3 Contusion of scalp**
Bruise of scalp
Hematoma of scalp
x7th **SØØ.Ø4 External constriction of part of scalp**
x7th **SØØ.Ø5 Superficial foreign body of scalp**
Splinter in the scalp
x7th **SØØ.Ø6 Insect bite (nonvenomous) of scalp**
x7th **SØØ.Ø7 Other superficial bite of scalp**
EXCLUDES 1 *open bite of scalp (SØ1.Ø5)*

5th **SØØ.1 Contusion of eyelid and periocular area**
Black eye
EXCLUDES 2 *contusion of eyeball and orbital tissues (SØ5.1-)*

x7th **SØØ.1Ø Contusion of unspecified eyelid and periocular area**
x7th **SØØ.11 Contusion of right eyelid and periocular area**
x7th **SØØ.12 Contusion of left eyelid and periocular area**

5th **SØØ.2 Other and unspecified superficial injuries of eyelid and periocular area**
EXCLUDES 2 *superficial injury of conjunctiva and cornea (SØ5.Ø-)*

6th **SØØ.2Ø Unspecified superficial injury of eyelid and periocular area**
7th **SØØ.2Ø1 Unspecified superficial injury of right eyelid and periocular area**
7th **SØØ.2Ø2 Unspecified superficial injury of left eyelid and periocular area**
7th **SØØ.2Ø9 Unspecified superficial injury of unspecified eyelid and periocular area**

6th **SØØ.21 Abrasion of eyelid and periocular area**
7th **SØØ.211 Abrasion of right eyelid and periocular area**
7th **SØØ.212 Abrasion of left eyelid and periocular area**
7th **SØØ.219 Abrasion of unspecified eyelid and periocular area**

6th **SØØ.22 Blister (nonthermal) of eyelid and periocular area**
7th **SØØ.221 Blister (nonthermal) of right eyelid and periocular area**
7th **SØØ.222 Blister (nonthermal) of left eyelid and periocular area**
7th **SØØ.229 Blister (nonthermal) of unspecified eyelid and periocular area**

6th **SØØ.24 External constriction of eyelid and periocular area**
7th **SØØ.241 External constriction of right eyelid and periocular area**
7th **SØØ.242 External constriction of left eyelid and periocular area**
7th **SØØ.249 External constriction of unspecified eyelid and periocular area**

6th **SØØ.25 Superficial foreign body of eyelid and periocular area**
Splinter of eyelid and periocular area
EXCLUDES 2 *retained foreign body in eyelid (HØ2.81-)*
7th **SØØ.251 Superficial foreign body of right eyelid and periocular area**
7th **SØØ.252 Superficial foreign body of left eyelid and periocular area**
7th **SØØ.259 Superficial foreign body of unspecified eyelid and periocular area**

6th **SØØ.26 Insect bite (nonvenomous) of eyelid and periocular area**
7th **SØØ.261 Insect bite (nonvenomous) of right eyelid and periocular area**
7th **SØØ.262 Insect bite (nonvenomous) of left eyelid and periocular area**
7th **SØØ.269 Insect bite (nonvenomous) of unspecified eyelid and periocular area**

6th **SØØ.27 Other superficial bite of eyelid and periocular area**
EXCLUDES 1 *open bite of eyelid and periocular area (SØ1.15)*
7th **SØØ.271 Other superficial bite of right eyelid and periocular area**
7th **SØØ.272 Other superficial bite of left eyelid and periocular area**
7th **SØØ.279 Other superficial bite of unspecified eyelid and periocular area**

5th **SØØ.3 Superficial injury of nose**

x7th **SØØ.3Ø Unspecified superficial injury of nose**
x7th **SØØ.31 Abrasion of nose**
x7th **SØØ.32 Blister (nonthermal) of nose**
x7th **SØØ.33 Contusion of nose**
Bruise of nose
Hematoma of nose
x7th **SØØ.34 External constriction of nose**

S00.35 Superficial foreign body of nose
Splinter in the nose
S00.36 Insect bite (nonvenomous) of nose
S00.37 Other superficial bite of nose
EXCLUDES 1 *open bite of nose (S01.25)*

S00.4 Superficial injury of ear
S00.40 Unspecified superficial injury of ear
S00.401 Unspecified superficial injury of right ear
S00.402 Unspecified superficial injury of left ear
S00.409 Unspecified superficial injury of unspecified ear
S00.41 Abrasion of ear
S00.411 Abrasion of right ear
S00.412 Abrasion of left ear
S00.419 Abrasion of unspecified ear
S00.42 Blister (nonthermal) of ear
S00.421 Blister (nonthermal) of right ear
S00.422 Blister (nonthermal) of left ear
S00.429 Blister (nonthermal) of unspecified ear
S00.43 Contusion of ear
Bruise of ear
Hematoma of ear
S00.431 Contusion of right ear
S00.432 Contusion of left ear
S00.439 Contusion of unspecified ear
S00.44 External constriction of ear
S00.441 External constriction of right ear
S00.442 External constriction of left ear
S00.449 External constriction of unspecified ear
S00.45 Superficial foreign body of ear
Splinter in the ear
S00.451 Superficial foreign body of right ear
S00.452 Superficial foreign body of left ear
S00.459 Superficial foreign body of unspecified ear
S00.46 Insect bite (nonvenomous) of ear
S00.461 Insect bite (nonvenomous) of right ear
S00.462 Insect bite (nonvenomous) of left ear
S00.469 Insect bite (nonvenomous) of unspecified ear
S00.47 Other superficial bite of ear
EXCLUDES 1 *open bite of ear (S01.35)*
S00.471 Other superficial bite of right ear
S00.472 Other superficial bite of left ear
S00.479 Other superficial bite of unspecified ear

S00.5 Superficial injury of lip and oral cavity
S00.50 Unspecified superficial injury of lip and oral cavity
S00.501 Unspecified superficial injury of lip
S00.502 Unspecified superficial injury of oral cavity
S00.51 Abrasion of lip and oral cavity
S00.511 Abrasion of lip
S00.512 Abrasion of oral cavity
S00.52 Blister (nonthermal) of lip and oral cavity
S00.521 Blister (nonthermal) of lip
S00.522 Blister (nonthermal) of oral cavity
S00.53 Contusion of lip and oral cavity
S00.531 Contusion of lip
Bruise of lip
Hematoma of lip
S00.532 Contusion of oral cavity
Bruise of oral cavity
Hematoma of oral cavity
S00.54 External constriction of lip and oral cavity
S00.541 External constriction of lip
S00.542 External constriction of oral cavity
S00.55 Superficial foreign body of lip and oral cavity
S00.551 Superficial foreign body of lip
Splinter of lip and oral cavity
S00.552 Superficial foreign body of oral cavity
Splinter of lip and oral cavity
S00.56 Insect bite (nonvenomous) of lip and oral cavity
S00.561 Insect bite (nonvenomous) of lip
S00.562 Insect bite (nonvenomous) of oral cavity
S00.57 Other superficial bite of lip and oral cavity
S00.571 Other superficial bite of lip
EXCLUDES 1 *open bite of lip (S01.551)*
S00.572 Other superficial bite of oral cavity
EXCLUDES 1 *open bite of oral cavity (S01.552)*

S00.8 Superficial injury of other parts of head
Superficial injuries of face [any part]
S00.80 Unspecified superficial injury of other part of head
S00.81 Abrasion of other part of head
S00.82 Blister (nonthermal) of other part of head
S00.83 Contusion of other part of head
Bruise of other part of head
Hematoma of other part of head
S00.84 External constriction of other part of head
S00.85 Superficial foreign body of other part of head
Splinter in other part of head
S00.86 Insect bite (nonvenomous) of other part of head
S00.87 Other superficial bite of other part of head
EXCLUDES 1 *open bite of other part of head (S01.85)*

S00.9 Superficial injury of unspecified part of head
S00.90 Unspecified superficial injury of unspecified part of head
S00.91 Abrasion of unspecified part of head
S00.92 Blister (nonthermal) of unspecified part of head
S00.93 Contusion of unspecified part of head
Bruise of head
Hematoma of head
S00.94 External constriction of unspecified part of head
S00.95 Superficial foreign body of unspecified part of head
Splinter of head
S00.96 Insect bite (nonvenomous) of unspecified part of head
S00.97 Other superficial bite of unspecified part of head
EXCLUDES 1 *open bite of head (S01.95)*

## S01 Open wound of head

Code also any associated:
injury of cranial nerve (S04.-)
injury of muscle and tendon of head (S09.1-)
intracranial injury (S06.-)
wound infection

EXCLUDES 1 *open skull fracture (S02.- with 7th character B)*
EXCLUDES 2 *injury of eye and orbit (S05.-)*
*traumatic amputation of part of head (S08.-)*

The appropriate 7th character is to be added to each code from category S01.
A initial encounter
D subsequent encounter
S sequela

S01.0 Open wound of scalp
EXCLUDES 1 *avulsion of scalp (S08.0-)*
S01.00 Unspecified open wound of scalp
S01.01 Laceration without foreign body of scalp
S01.02 Laceration with foreign body of scalp
S01.03 Puncture wound without foreign body of scalp
S01.04 Puncture wound with foreign body of scalp
S01.05 Open bite of scalp
Bite of scalp NOS
EXCLUDES 1 *superficial bite of scalp (S00.06, S00.07-)*

S01.1 Open wound of eyelid and periocular area
Open wound of eyelid and periocular area with or without involvement of lacrimal passages
S01.10 Unspecified open wound of eyelid and periocular area
S01.101 Unspecified open wound of right eyelid and periocular area
S01.102 Unspecified open wound of left eyelid and periocular area

√7th **S01.109** Unspecified open wound of unspecified eyelid and periocular area

√6th **S01.11** Laceration without foreign body of eyelid and periocular area

√7th S01.111 Laceration without foreign body of right eyelid and periocular area

√7th S01.112 Laceration without foreign body of left eyelid and periocular area

√7th **S01.119** Laceration without foreign body of unspecified eyelid and periocular area

√6th **S01.12** Laceration with foreign body of eyelid and periocular area

√7th S01.121 Laceration with foreign body of right eyelid and periocular area

√7th S01.122 Laceration with foreign body of left eyelid and periocular area

√7th **S01.129** Laceration with foreign body of unspecified eyelid and periocular area

√6th **S01.13** Puncture wound without foreign body of eyelid and periocular area

√7th S01.131 Puncture wound without foreign body of right eyelid and periocular area

√7th S01.132 Puncture wound without foreign body of left eyelid and periocular area

√7th **S01.139** Puncture wound without foreign body of unspecified eyelid and periocular area

√6th **S01.14** Puncture wound with foreign body of eyelid and periocular area

√7th S01.141 Puncture wound with foreign body of right eyelid and periocular area

√7th S01.142 Puncture wound with foreign body of left eyelid and periocular area

√7th **S01.149** Puncture wound with foreign body of unspecified eyelid and periocular area

√6th **S01.15** Open bite of eyelid and periocular area

Bite of eyelid and periocular area NOS

EXCLUDES 1 *superficial bite of eyelid and periocular area (S00.26, S00.27)*

√7th S01.151 Open bite of right eyelid and periocular area

√7th S01.152 Open bite of left eyelid and periocular area

√7th **S01.159** Open bite of unspecified eyelid and periocular area

√5th **S01.2 Open wound of nose**

√x7th **S01.20** Unspecified open wound of nose

√x7th S01.21 Laceration without foreign body of nose

√x7th S01.22 Laceration with foreign body of nose

√x7th S01.23 Puncture wound without foreign body of nose

√x7th S01.24 Puncture wound with foreign body of nose

√x7th S01.25 Open bite of nose

Bite of nose NOS

EXCLUDES 1 *superficial bite of nose (S00.36, S00.37)*

√5th **S01.3 Open wound of ear**

√6th **S01.30** Unspecified open wound of ear

√7th **S01.301** Unspecified open wound of right ear

√7th **S01.302** Unspecified open wound of left ear

√7th **S01.309** Unspecified open wound of unspecified ear

√6th **S01.31** Laceration without foreign body of ear

√7th S01.311 Laceration without foreign body of right ear

√7th S01.312 Laceration without foreign body of left ear

√7th **S01.319** Laceration without foreign body of unspecified ear

√6th **S01.32** Laceration with foreign body of ear

√7th S01.321 Laceration with foreign body of right ear

√7th S01.322 Laceration with foreign body of left ear

√7th **S01.329** Laceration with foreign body of unspecified ear

√6th **S01.33** Puncture wound without foreign body of ear

√7th S01.331 Puncture wound without foreign body of right ear

√7th S01.332 Puncture wound without foreign body of left ear

√7th **S01.339** Puncture wound without foreign body of unspecified ear

√6th **S01.34** Puncture wound with foreign body of ear

√7th S01.341 Puncture wound with foreign body of right ear

√7th S01.342 Puncture wound with foreign body of left ear

√7th **S01.349** Puncture wound with foreign body of unspecified ear

√6th **S01.35** Open bite of ear

Bite of ear NOS

EXCLUDES 1 *superficial bite of ear (S00.46, S00.47)*

√7th S01.351 Open bite of right ear

√7th S01.352 Open bite of left ear

√7th **S01.359** Open bite of unspecified ear

√5th **S01.4 Open wound of cheek and temporomandibular area**

√6th **S01.40** Unspecified open wound of cheek and temporomandibular area

√7th **S01.401** Unspecified open wound of right cheek and temporomandibular area

√7th **S01.402** Unspecified open wound of left cheek and temporomandibular area

√7th **S01.409** Unspecified open wound of unspecified cheek and temporomandibular area

√6th **S01.41** Laceration without foreign body of cheek and temporomandibular area

√7th S01.411 Laceration without foreign body of right cheek and temporomandibular area

√7th S01.412 Laceration without foreign body of left cheek and temporomandibular area

√7th **S01.419** Laceration without foreign body of unspecified cheek and temporomandibular area

√6th **S01.42** Laceration with foreign body of cheek and temporomandibular area

√7th S01.421 Laceration with foreign body of right cheek and temporomandibular area

√7th S01.422 Laceration with foreign body of left cheek and temporomandibular area

√7th **S01.429** Laceration with foreign body of unspecified cheek and temporomandibular area

√6th **S01.43** Puncture wound without foreign body of cheek and temporomandibular area

√7th S01.431 Puncture wound without foreign body of right cheek and temporomandibular area

√7th S01.432 Puncture wound without foreign body of left cheek and temporomandibular area

√7th **S01.439** Puncture wound without foreign body of unspecified cheek and temporomandibular area

√6th **S01.44** Puncture wound with foreign body of cheek and temporomandibular area

√7th S01.441 Puncture wound with foreign body of right cheek and temporomandibular area

√7th S01.442 Puncture wound with foreign body of left cheek and temporomandibular area

√7th **S01.449** Puncture wound with foreign body of unspecified cheek and temporomandibular area

√6th **S01.45** Open bite of cheek and temporomandibular area

Bite of cheek and temporomandibular area NOS

EXCLUDES 2 *superficial bite of cheek and temporomandibular area (S00.86, S00.87)*

√7th S01.451 Open bite of right cheek and temporomandibular area

√7th S01.452 Open bite of left cheek and temporomandibular area

√7th **S01.459** Open bite of unspecified cheek and temporomandibular area

√5th **S01.5 Open wound of lip and oral cavity**

EXCLUDES 2 *tooth dislocation (S03.2)*
*tooth fracture (S02.5)*

√6th **S01.50** Unspecified open wound of lip and oral cavity

√7th **S01.501** Unspecified open wound of lip

√7th **S01.502** Unspecified open wound of oral cavity

√6th **S01.51** Laceration of lip and oral cavity without foreign body

√7th S01.511 Laceration without foreign body of lip

√7th S01.512 Laceration without foreign body of oral cavity

√6th S01.52 Laceration of lip and oral cavity with foreign body
√7th S01.521 Laceration with foreign body of lip
√7th S01.522 Laceration with foreign body of oral cavity
√6th S01.53 Puncture wound of lip and oral cavity without foreign body
√7th S01.531 Puncture wound without foreign body of lip
√7th S01.532 Puncture wound without foreign body of oral cavity
√6th S01.54 Puncture wound of lip and oral cavity with foreign body
√7th S01.541 Puncture wound with foreign body of lip
√7th S01.542 Puncture wound with foreign body of oral cavity
√6th S01.55 Open bite of lip and oral cavity
√7th S01.551 Open bite of lip
Bite of lip NOS
EXCLUDES 1 *superficial bite of lip (S00.571)*
√7th S01.552 Open bite of oral cavity
Bite of oral cavity NOS
EXCLUDES 1 *superficial bite of oral cavity (S00.572)*
√5th S01.8 Open wound of other parts of head
√x7th S01.80 Unspecified open wound of other part of head
√x7th S01.81 Laceration without foreign body of other part of head
√x7th S01.82 Laceration with foreign body of other part of head
√x7th S01.83 Puncture wound without foreign body of other part of head
√x7th S01.84 Puncture wound with foreign body of other part of head
√x7th S01.85 Open bite of other part of head
Bite of other part of head NOS
EXCLUDES 1 *superficial bite of other part of head (S00.87)*
√5th S01.9 Open wound of unspecified part of head
√x7th S01.90 Unspecified open wound of unspecified part of head
√x7th S01.91 Laceration without foreign body of unspecified part of head
√x7th S01.92 Laceration with foreign body of unspecified part of head
√x7th S01.93 Puncture wound without foreign body of unspecified part of head
√x7th S01.94 Puncture wound with foreign body of unspecified part of head
√x7th S01.95 Open bite of unspecified part of head
Bite of head NOS
EXCLUDES 1 *superficial bite of head NOS (S00.97)*

√4th **S02 Fracture of skull and facial bones**

NOTE A fracture not indicated as open or closed should be coded to closed.

Code also any associated intracranial injury (S06.-)

**AHA:** 2021,1Q,6; 2017,1Q,42; 2016,4Q,66-67

The appropriate 7th character is to be added to each code from category S02.
A initial encounter for closed fracture
B initial encounter for open fracture
D subsequent encounter for fracture with routine healing
G subsequent encounter for fracture with delayed healing
K subsequent encounter for fracture with nonunion
S sequela

√x7th S02.0 Fracture of vault of skull HCC ESR
Fracture of frontal bone
Fracture of parietal bone
√5th S02.1 Fracture of base of skull
EXCLUDES 2 *lateral orbital wall (S02.84-)*
*medial orbital wall (S02.83-)*
*orbital floor (S02.3-)*
**AHA:** 2019,4Q,16-17
√6th S02.10 Unspecified fracture of base of skull
√7th S02.101 Fracture of base of skull, right side HCC ESR
√7th S02.102 Fracture of base of skull, left side HCC ESR
√7th S02.109 Fracture of base of skull, unspecified side HCC ESR
√6th S02.11 Fracture of occiput
√7th S02.110 Type I occipital condyle fracture, unspecified side HCC ESR
√7th S02.111 Type II occipital condyle fracture, unspecified side HCC ESR
√7th S02.112 Type III occipital condyle fracture, unspecified side HCC ESR
√7th S02.113 Unspecified occipital condyle fracture HCC ESR
√7th S02.118 Other fracture of occiput, unspecified side HCC ESR
√7th S02.119 Unspecified fracture of occiput HCC ESR
√7th S02.11A Type I occipital condyle fracture, right side HCC ESR
√7th S02.11B Type I occipital condyle fracture, left side HCC ESR
√7th S02.11C Type II occipital condyle fracture, right side HCC ESR
√7th S02.11D Type II occipital condyle fracture, left side HCC ESR
√7th S02.11E Type III occipital condyle fracture, right side HCC ESR
√7th S02.11F Type III occipital condyle fracture, left side HCC ESR
√7th S02.11G Other fracture of occiput, right side HCC ESR
√7th S02.11H Other fracture of occiput, left side HCC ESR
√6th S02.12 Fracture of orbital roof
**AHA:** 2019,4Q,16-17
√7th S02.121 Fracture of orbital roof, right side HCC ESR
√7th S02.122 Fracture of orbital roof, left side HCC ESR
√7th S02.129 Fracture of orbital roof, unspecified side HCC ESR
√x7th S02.19 Other fracture of base of skull HCC ESR
Fracture of anterior fossa of base of skull
Fracture of ethmoid sinus
Fracture of frontal sinus
Fracture of middle fossa of base of skull
Fracture of posterior fossa of base of skull
Fracture of sphenoid
Fracture of temporal bone
√x7th S02.2 Fracture of nasal bones
√5th S02.3 Fracture of orbital floor
Fracture of inferior orbital wall
EXCLUDES 1 *orbit NOS (S02.85)*
EXCLUDES 2 *lateral orbital wall (S02.84-)*
*medial orbital wall (S02.83-)*
*orbital roof (S02.1-)*
√x7th S02.30 Fracture of orbital floor, unspecified side HCC ESR
√x7th S02.31 Fracture of orbital floor, right side HCC ESR
√x7th S02.32 Fracture of orbital floor, left side HCC ESR
√5th S02.4 Fracture of malar, maxillary and zygoma bones
Fracture of superior maxilla
Fracture of upper jaw (bone)
Fracture of zygomatic process of temporal bone
√6th S02.40 Fracture of malar, maxillary and zygoma bones, unspecified
√7th S02.400 Malar fracture, unspecified side HCC ESR
√7th S02.401 Maxillary fracture, unspecified side HCC ESR
√7th S02.402 Zygomatic fracture, unspecified side HCC ESR
√7th S02.40A Malar fracture, right side HCC ESR
√7th S02.40B Malar fracture, left side HCC ESR
√7th S02.40C Maxillary fracture, right side HCC ESR
√7th S02.40D Maxillary fracture, left side HCC ESR
√7th S02.40E Zygomatic fracture, right side HCC ESR
√7th S02.40F Zygomatic fracture, left side HCC ESR

√6th **SØ2.41 LeFort fracture**

**DEF:** Named for Rene Le Fort, these fractures describe different combinations of multiple fractures that occur from significant force to the midface. A common denominator in all three types of LeFort fractures is fracture of the pterygoid processes, which are two bony plates resembling wings that extend downward from the sphenoid bone.

**LeFort Fracture Types**

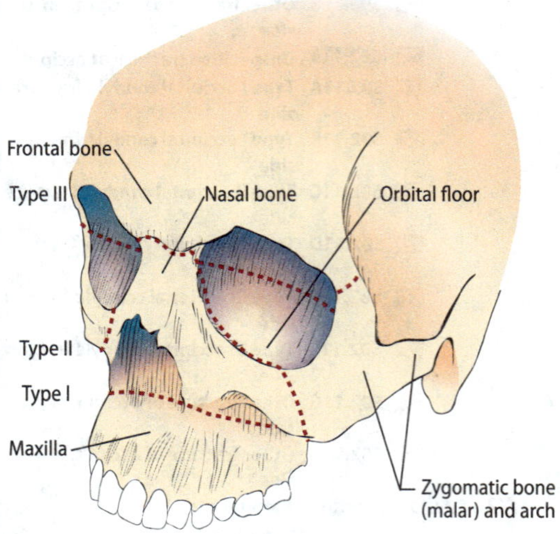


√7th **SØ2.411 LeFort I fracture** HCC ESR

√7th **SØ2.412 LeFort II fracture** HCC ESR

√7th **SØ2.413 LeFort III fracture** HCC ESR

√x7th **SØ2.42 Fracture of alveolus of maxilla** HCC ESR

√x7th **SØ2.5 Fracture of tooth (traumatic)**

Broken tooth

EXCLUDES 1 *cracked tooth (nontraumatic) (KØ3.81)*

√5th **SØ2.6 Fracture of mandible**

Fracture of lower jaw (bone)

√6th **SØ2.6Ø Fracture of mandible, unspecified**

√7th **SØ2.6ØØ Fracture of unspecified part of body of mandible, unspecified side** HCC ESR

√7th **SØ2.6Ø1 Fracture of unspecified part of body of right mandible** HCC ESR

√7th **SØ2.6Ø2 Fracture of unspecified part of body of left mandible** HCC ESR

√7th **SØ2.6Ø9 Fracture of mandible, unspecified** HCC ESR

√6th **SØ2.61 Fracture of condylar process of mandible**

√7th **SØ2.61Ø Fracture of condylar process of mandible, unspecified side** HCC ESR

√7th **SØ2.611 Fracture of condylar process of right mandible** HCC ESR

√7th **SØ2.612 Fracture of condylar process of left mandible** HCC ESR

√6th **SØ2.62 Fracture of subcondylar process of mandible**

√7th **SØ2.62Ø Fracture of subcondylar process of mandible, unspecified side** HCC ESR

√7th **SØ2.621 Fracture of subcondylar process of right mandible** HCC ESR

√7th **SØ2.622 Fracture of subcondylar process of left mandible** HCC ESR

√6th **SØ2.63 Fracture of coronoid process of mandible**

√7th **SØ2.63Ø Fracture of coronoid process of mandible, unspecified side** HCC ESR

√7th **SØ2.631 Fracture of coronoid process of right mandible** HCC ESR

√7th **SØ2.632 Fracture of coronoid process of left mandible** HCC ESR

√6th **SØ2.64 Fracture of ramus of mandible**

√7th **SØ2.64Ø Fracture of ramus of mandible, unspecified side** HCC ESR

√7th **SØ2.641 Fracture of ramus of right mandible** HCC ESR

√7th **SØ2.642 Fracture of ramus of left mandible** HCC ESR

√6th **SØ2.65 Fracture of angle of mandible**

√7th **SØ2.65Ø Fracture of angle of mandible, unspecified side** HCC ESR

√7th **SØ2.651 Fracture of angle of right mandible** HCC ESR

√7th **SØ2.652 Fracture of angle of left mandible** HCC ESR

√x7th **SØ2.66 Fracture of symphysis of mandible** HCC ESR

√6th **SØ2.67 Fracture of alveolus of mandible**

√7th **SØ2.67Ø Fracture of alveolus of mandible, unspecified side** HCC ESR

√7th **SØ2.671 Fracture of alveolus of right mandible** HCC ESR

√7th **SØ2.672 Fracture of alveolus of left mandible** HCC ESR

√x7th **SØ2.69 Fracture of mandible of other specified site** HCC ESR

√5th **SØ2.8 Fractures of other specified skull and facial bones**

Fracture of palate

EXCLUDES 2 *fracture of orbital floor (SØ2.3-)*
*fracture of orbital roof (SØ2.12-)*

√x7th **SØ2.8Ø Fracture of other specified skull and facial bones, unspecified side** HCC ESR

√x7th **SØ2.81 Fracture of other specified skull and facial bones, right side** HCC ESR

√x7th **SØ2.82 Fracture of other specified skull and facial bones, left side** HCC ESR

√6th **SØ2.83 Fracture of medial orbital wall**

EXCLUDES 2 *orbital floor (SØ2.3-)*
*orbital roof (SØ2.12-)*

**AHA:** 2019,4Q,16-17

√7th **SØ2.831 Fracture of medial orbital wall, right side** HCC ESR

√7th **SØ2.832 Fracture of medial orbital wall, left side** HCC ESR

√7th **SØ2.839 Fracture of medial orbital wall, unspecified side** HCC ESR

√6th **SØ2.84 Fracture of lateral orbital wall**

EXCLUDES 2 *orbital floor (SØ2.3-)*
*orbital roof (SØ2.12-)*

**AHA:** 2019,4Q,16-17

√7th **SØ2.841 Fracture of lateral orbital wall, right side** HCC ESR

√7th **SØ2.842 Fracture of lateral orbital wall, left side** HCC ESR

√7th **SØ2.849 Fracture of lateral orbital wall, unspecified side** HCC ESR

√x7th **SØ2.85 Fracture of orbit, unspecified** HCC ESR

Fracture of orbit NOS
Fracture of orbit wall NOS

EXCLUDES 1 *lateral orbital wall (SØ2.84-)*
*medial orbital wall (SØ2.83-)*
*orbital floor (SØ2.3-)*
*orbital roof (SØ2.12-)*

√5th **SØ2.9 Fracture of unspecified skull and facial bones**

√x7th **SØ2.91 Unspecified fracture of skull** HCC ESR

**AHA:** 2020,2Q,24

√x7th **SØ2.92 Unspecified fracture of facial bones** HCC ESR

**S03 Dislocation and sprain of joints and ligaments of head**

INCLUDES avulsion of joint (capsule) or ligament of head
laceration of cartilage, joint (capsule) or ligament of head
sprain of cartilage, joint (capsule) or ligament of head
traumatic hemarthrosis of joint or ligament of head
traumatic rupture of joint or ligament of head
traumatic subluxation of joint or ligament of head
traumatic tear of joint or ligament of head

Code also any associated open wound

EXCLUDES 2 *strain of muscle or tendon of head (S09.1)*

The appropriate 7th character is to be added to each code from category S03.
A initial encounter
D subsequent encounter
S sequela

**S03.0 Dislocation of jaw**
Dislocation of jaw (cartilage) (meniscus)
Dislocation of mandible
Dislocation of temporomandibular (joint)
**AHA:** 2016,4Q,67

**S03.00 Dislocation of jaw, unspecified side**
**S03.01 Dislocation of jaw, right side**
**S03.02 Dislocation of jaw, left side**
**S03.03 Dislocation of jaw, bilateral**

**S03.1 Dislocation of septal cartilage of nose**
**S03.2 Dislocation of tooth**
**S03.4 Sprain of jaw**
Sprain of temporomandibular (joint) (ligament)
**AHA:** 2016,4Q,67

**S03.40 Sprain of jaw, unspecified side**
**S03.41 Sprain of jaw, right side**
**S03.42 Sprain of jaw, left side**
**S03.43 Sprain of jaw, bilateral**

**S03.8 Sprain of joints and ligaments of other parts of head**
**S03.9 Sprain of joints and ligaments of unspecified parts of head**

**S04 Injury of cranial nerve**

The selection of side should be based on the side of the body being affected

Code first any associated intracranial injury (S06.-)
Code also any associated:
open wound of head (S01.-)
skull fracture (S02.-)

The appropriate 7th character is to be added to each code from category S04.
A initial encounter
D subsequent encounter
S sequela

**S04.0 Injury of optic nerve and pathways**
Use additional code to identify any visual field defect or blindness (H53.4-, H54.-)

**S04.01 Injury of optic nerve**
Injury of 2nd cranial nerve
**S04.011 Injury of optic nerve, right eye**
**S04.012 Injury of optic nerve, left eye**
**S04.019 Injury of optic nerve, unspecified eye**
Injury of optic nerve NOS

**S04.02 Injury of optic chiasm**

**S04.03 Injury of optic tract and pathways**
Injury of optic radiation
**S04.031 Injury of optic tract and pathways, right side**
**S04.032 Injury of optic tract and pathways, left side**
**S04.039 Injury of optic tract and pathways, unspecified side**
Injury of optic tract and pathways NOS

**S04.04 Injury of visual cortex**
**S04.041 Injury of visual cortex, right side**
**S04.042 Injury of visual cortex, left side**
**S04.049 Injury of visual cortex, unspecified side**
Injury of visual cortex NOS

**S04.1 Injury of oculomotor nerve**
Injury of 3rd cranial nerve
**S04.10 Injury of oculomotor nerve, unspecified side**
**S04.11 Injury of oculomotor nerve, right side**
**S04.12 Injury of oculomotor nerve, left side**

**S04.2 Injury of trochlear nerve**
Injury of 4th cranial nerve
**S04.20 Injury of trochlear nerve, unspecified side**
**S04.21 Injury of trochlear nerve, right side**
**S04.22 Injury of trochlear nerve, left side**

**S04.3 Injury of trigeminal nerve**
Injury of 5th cranial nerve
**S04.30 Injury of trigeminal nerve, unspecified side**
**S04.31 Injury of trigeminal nerve, right side**
**S04.32 Injury of trigeminal nerve, left side**

**S04.4 Injury of abducent nerve**
Injury of 6th cranial nerve
**S04.40 Injury of abducent nerve, unspecified side**
**S04.41 Injury of abducent nerve, right side**
**S04.42 Injury of abducent nerve, left side**

**S04.5 Injury of facial nerve**
Injury of 7th cranial nerve
**S04.50 Injury of facial nerve, unspecified side**
**S04.51 Injury of facial nerve, right side**
**S04.52 Injury of facial nerve, left side**

**S04.6 Injury of acoustic nerve**
Injury of 8th cranial nerve
Injury of auditory nerve
**S04.60 Injury of acoustic nerve, unspecified side**
**S04.61 Injury of acoustic nerve, right side**
**S04.62 Injury of acoustic nerve, left side**

**S04.7 Injury of accessory nerve**
Injury of 11th cranial nerve
**S04.70 Injury of accessory nerve, unspecified side**
**S04.71 Injury of accessory nerve, right side**
**S04.72 Injury of accessory nerve, left side**

**S04.8 Injury of other cranial nerves**

**S04.81 Injury of olfactory [1st] nerve**
**S04.811 Injury of olfactory [1st] nerve, right side**
**S04.812 Injury of olfactory [1st] nerve, left side**
**S04.819 Injury of olfactory [1st] nerve, unspecified side**

**S04.89 Injury of other cranial nerves**
Injury of vagus [10th] nerve
**S04.891 Injury of other cranial nerves, right side**
**S04.892 Injury of other cranial nerves, left side**
**S04.899 Injury of other cranial nerves, unspecified side**

**S04.9 Injury of unspecified cranial nerve**

**S05 Injury of eye and orbit**

INCLUDES open wound of eye and orbit

EXCLUDES 2 *2nd cranial [optic] nerve injury (S04.0-)*
*3rd cranial [oculomotor] nerve injury (S04.1-)*
*open wound of eyelid and periocular area (S01.1-)*
*orbital bone fracture (S02.1-, S02.3-, S02.8-)*
*superficial injury of eyelid (S00.1-S00.2)*

The appropriate 7th character is to be added to each code from category S05.
A initial encounter
D subsequent encounter
S sequela

**S05.0 Injury of conjunctiva and corneal abrasion without foreign body**
EXCLUDES 1 *foreign body in conjunctival sac (T15.1)*
*foreign body in cornea (T15.0)*

**S05.00 Injury of conjunctiva and corneal abrasion without foreign body, unspecified eye**
**S05.01 Injury of conjunctiva and corneal abrasion without foreign body, right eye**
**S05.02 Injury of conjunctiva and corneal abrasion without foreign body, left eye**

√5th **S05.1 Contusion of eyeball and orbital tissues**
Traumatic hyphema
EXCLUDES 2 *black eye NOS (S00.1)*
*contusion of eyelid and periocular area (S00.1)*
√x7th **S05.10 Contusion of eyeball and orbital tissues, unspecified eye**
√x7th **S05.11 Contusion of eyeball and orbital tissues, right eye**
√x7th **S05.12 Contusion of eyeball and orbital tissues, left eye**

√5th **S05.2 Ocular laceration and rupture with prolapse or loss of intraocular tissue**
√x7th **S05.20 Ocular laceration and rupture with prolapse or loss of intraocular tissue, unspecified eye**
√x7th **S05.21 Ocular laceration and rupture with prolapse or loss of intraocular tissue, right eye**
√x7th **S05.22 Ocular laceration and rupture with prolapse or loss of intraocular tissue, left eye**

√5th **S05.3 Ocular laceration without prolapse or loss of intraocular tissue**
Laceration of eye NOS
**AHA:** 2022,1Q,33
**DEF:** Tear in ocular tissue without displacing structures that is due to blunt trauma. It is characterized by pain, redness, and decreased vision.
√x7th **S05.30 Ocular laceration without prolapse or loss of intraocular tissue, unspecified eye**
√x7th **S05.31 Ocular laceration without prolapse or loss of intraocular tissue, right eye**
√x7th **S05.32 Ocular laceration without prolapse or loss of intraocular tissue, left eye**

√5th **S05.4 Penetrating wound of orbit with or without foreign body**
EXCLUDES 2 *retained (old) foreign body following penetrating wound in orbit (H05.5-)*
√x7th **S05.40 Penetrating wound of orbit with or without foreign body, unspecified eye**
√x7th **S05.41 Penetrating wound of orbit with or without foreign body, right eye**
√x7th **S05.42 Penetrating wound of orbit with or without foreign body, left eye**

√5th **S05.5 Penetrating wound with foreign body of eyeball**
EXCLUDES 2 *retained (old) intraocular foreign body (H44.6-, H44.7)*
√x7th **S05.50 Penetrating wound with foreign body of unspecified eyeball**
√x7th **S05.51 Penetrating wound with foreign body of right eyeball**
√x7th **S05.52 Penetrating wound with foreign body of left eyeball**

√5th **S05.6 Penetrating wound without foreign body of eyeball**
Ocular penetration NOS
√x7th **S05.60 Penetrating wound without foreign body of unspecified eyeball**
√x7th **S05.61 Penetrating wound without foreign body of right eyeball**
√x7th **S05.62 Penetrating wound without foreign body of left eyeball**

√5th **S05.7 Avulsion of eye**
Traumatic enucleation
√x7th **S05.70 Avulsion of unspecified eye**
√x7th **S05.71 Avulsion of right eye**
√x7th **S05.72 Avulsion of left eye**

√5th **S05.8 Other injuries of eye and orbit**
Lacrimal duct injury
√6th **S05.8X Other injuries of eye and orbit**
√7th **S05.8X1 Other injuries of right eye and orbit**
√7th **S05.8X2 Other injuries of left eye and orbit**
√7th **S05.8X9 Other injuries of unspecified eye and orbit**

√5th **S05.9 Unspecified injury of eye and orbit**
Injury of eye NOS
√x7th **S05.90 Unspecified injury of unspecified eye and orbit**
√x7th **S05.91 Unspecified injury of right eye and orbit**
√x7th **S05.92 Unspecified injury of left eye and orbit**

√4th **S06 Intracranial injury**
NOTE 7th characters D and S do not apply to codes in category S06 with 6th character 7 – death due to brain injury prior to regaining consciousness, or 8 – death due to other cause prior to regaining consciousness.
INCLUDES traumatic brain injury
Code also any associated:
open wound of head (S01.-)
skull fracture (S02.-)
Use additional code, if applicable, to identify mild neurocognitive disorders due to known physiological condition (F06.7-)
EXCLUDES 1 *head injury NOS (S09.90)*
**AHA:** 2022,4Q,42-45; 2017,4Q,25; 2017,1Q,42; 2015,3Q,37
**TIP:** Do not assign Z87.820 Personal history of traumatic brain injury, when residual conditions persist after an intracranial injury. The codes for the residual conditions should be first listed, followed by a code from category S06 using seventh character S to identify sequelae.

The appropriate 7th character is to be added to each code from category S06, except as described in the NOTE above.
A initial encounter
D subsequent encounter
S sequela

√5th **S06.0 Concussion**
Commotio cerebri
EXCLUDES 1 *concussion with other intracranial injuries classified in subcategories S06.1- to S06.6-, and S06.81- to S06.89-, code to specified intracranial injury*
**AHA:** 2016,4Q,67-68
√6th **S06.0X Concussion**
√7th **S06.0X0 Concussion without loss of consciousness** ESR
√7th **S06.0X1 Concussion with loss of consciousness of 30 minutes or less** ESR
Concussion with brief loss of consciousness
√7th **S06.0XA Concussion with loss of consciousness status unknown** ESR
Concussion NOS
√7th **S06.0X9 Concussion with loss of consciousness of unspecified duration** ESR

√5th **S06.1 Traumatic cerebral edema**
Diffuse traumatic cerebral edema
Focal traumatic cerebral edema
**AHA:** 2019,3Q,35; 2015,1Q,12-13
√6th **S06.1X Traumatic cerebral edema**
√7th **S06.1X0 Traumatic cerebral edema without loss of consciousness** HCC ESR
√7th **S06.1X1 Traumatic cerebral edema with loss of consciousness of 30 minutes or less** HCC ESR
Traumatic cerebral edema with brief loss of consciousness
√7th **S06.1X2 Traumatic cerebral edema with loss of consciousness of 31 minutes to 59 minutes** HCC ESR
√7th **S06.1X3 Traumatic cerebral edema with loss of consciousness of 1 hour to 5 hours 59 minutes** HCC ESR COM
√7th **S06.1X4 Traumatic cerebral edema with loss of consciousness of 6 hours to 24 hours** HCC ESR COM
√7th **S06.1X5 Traumatic cerebral edema with loss of consciousness greater than 24 hours with return to pre-existing conscious level** HCC ESR COM
√7th **S06.1X6 Traumatic cerebral edema with loss of consciousness greater than 24 hours without return to pre-existing conscious level with patient surviving** HCC ESR COM
√7th **S06.1X7 Traumatic cerebral edema with loss of consciousness of any duration with death due to brain injury prior to regaining consciousness**
√7th **S06.1X8 Traumatic cerebral edema with loss of consciousness of any duration with death due to other cause prior to regaining consciousness**

√7th **S06.1XA Traumatic cerebral edema with loss of consciousness status unknown** HCC ESR
Traumatic cerebral edema NOS

√7th **S06.1X9 Traumatic cerebral edema with loss of consciousness of unspecified duration** HCC ESR

√5th **S06.2 Diffuse traumatic brain injury**
Diffuse axonal brain injury
Use additional code, if applicable, for traumatic brain compression or herniation (S06.A-)
EXCLUDES 1 *traumatic diffuse cerebral edema (S06.1X-)*
**AHA:** 2020,3Q,46

√6th **S06.2X Diffuse traumatic brain injury**

√7th **S06.2X0 Diffuse traumatic brain injury without loss of consciousness** HCC ESR

√7th **S06.2X1 Diffuse traumatic brain injury with loss of consciousness of 30 minutes or less** HCC ESR
Diffuse traumatic brain injury with brief loss of consciousness

√7th **S06.2X2 Diffuse traumatic brain injury with loss of consciousness of 31 minutes to 59 minutes** HCC ESR

√7th **S06.2X3 Diffuse traumatic brain injury with loss of consciousness of 1 hour to 5 hours 59 minutes** HCC ESR COM

√7th **S06.2X4 Diffuse traumatic brain injury with loss of consciousness of 6 hours to 24 hours** HCC ESR COM

√7th **S06.2X5 Diffuse traumatic brain injury with loss of consciousness greater than 24 hours with return to pre-existing conscious levels** HCC ESR COM

√7th **S06.2X6 Diffuse traumatic brain injury with loss of consciousness greater than 24 hours without return to pre-existing conscious level with patient surviving** HCC ESR COM

√7th **S06.2X7 Diffuse traumatic brain injury with loss of consciousness of any duration with death due to brain injury prior to regaining consciousness**

√7th **S06.2X8 Diffuse traumatic brain injury with loss of consciousness of any duration with death due to other cause prior to regaining consciousness**

√7th **S06.2XA Diffuse traumatic brain injury with loss of consciousness status unknown** HCC ESR
Diffuse traumatic brain injury NOS

√7th **S06.2X9 Diffuse traumatic brain injury with loss of consciousness of unspecified duration** HCC ESR

√5th **S06.3 Focal traumatic brain injury**
Use additional code, if applicable, for traumatic brain compression or herniation (S06.A-)
EXCLUDES 2 *any condition classifiable to S06.4-S06.6*
*focal cerebral edema (S06.1)*
**AHA:** 2020,3Q,46; 2019,3Q,35; 2015,1Q,12-13

√6th **S06.30 Unspecified focal traumatic brain injury**

√7th **S06.300 Unspecified focal traumatic brain injury without loss of consciousness** HCC ESR

√7th **S06.301 Unspecified focal traumatic brain injury with loss of consciousness of 30 minutes or less** HCC ESR
Unspecified focal traumatic brain injury with brief loss of consciousness

√7th **S06.302 Unspecified focal traumatic brain injury with loss of consciousness of 31 minutes to 59 minutes** HCC ESR

√7th **S06.303 Unspecified focal traumatic brain injury with loss of consciousness of 1 hour to 5 hours 59 minutes** HCC ESR COM

√7th **S06.304 Unspecified focal traumatic brain injury with loss of consciousness of 6 hours to 24 hours** HCC ESR COM

√7th **S06.305 Unspecified focal traumatic brain injury with loss of consciousness greater than 24 hours with return to pre-existing conscious level** HCC ESR COM

√7th **S06.306 Unspecified focal traumatic brain injury with loss of consciousness greater than 24 hours without return to pre-existing conscious level with patient surviving** HCC ESR COM

√7th **S06.307 Unspecified focal traumatic brain injury with loss of consciousness of any duration with death due to brain injury prior to regaining consciousness**

√7th **S06.308 Unspecified focal traumatic brain injury with loss of consciousness of any duration with death due to other cause prior to regaining consciousness**

√7th **S06.30A Unspecified focal traumatic brain injury with loss of consciousness status unknown** HCC ESR
Unspecified focal traumatic brain injury NOS

√7th **S06.309 Unspecified focal traumatic brain injury with loss of consciousness of unspecified duration** HCC ESR

√6th **S06.31 Contusion and laceration of right cerebrum**

√7th **S06.310 Contusion and laceration of right cerebrum without loss of consciousness** HCC ESR

√7th **S06.311 Contusion and laceration of right cerebrum with loss of consciousness of 30 minutes or less** HCC ESR
Contusion and laceration of right cerebrum with brief loss of consciousness

√7th **S06.312 Contusion and laceration of right cerebrum with loss of consciousness of 31 minutes to 59 minutes** HCC ESR

√7th **S06.313 Contusion and laceration of right cerebrum with loss of consciousness of 1 hour to 5 hours 59 minutes** HCC ESR COM

√7th **S06.314 Contusion and laceration of right cerebrum with loss of consciousness of 6 hours to 24 hours** HCC ESR COM

√7th **S06.315 Contusion and laceration of right cerebrum with loss of consciousness greater than 24 hours with return to pre-existing conscious level** HCC ESR COM

√7th **S06.316 Contusion and laceration of right cerebrum with loss of consciousness greater than 24 hours without return to pre-existing conscious level with patient surviving** HCC ESR COM

√7th **S06.317 Contusion and laceration of right cerebrum with loss of consciousness of any duration with death due to brain injury prior to regaining consciousness**

√7th **S06.318 Contusion and laceration of right cerebrum with loss of consciousness of any duration with death due to other cause prior to regaining consciousness**

√7th **S06.31A Contusion and laceration of right cerebrum with loss of consciousness status unknown** HCC ESR
Contusion and laceration of right cerebrum NOS

√7th **S06.319 Contusion and laceration of right cerebrum with loss of consciousness of unspecified duration** HCC ESR

√6th **S06.32 Contusion and laceration of left cerebrum**

√7th **S06.320 Contusion and laceration of left cerebrum without loss of consciousness** HCC ESR

√7th **S06.321 Contusion and laceration of left cerebrum with loss of consciousness of 30 minutes or less** HCC ESR
Contusion and laceration of left cerebrum with brief loss of consciousness

√7th **S06.322 Contusion and laceration of left cerebrum with loss of consciousness of 31 minutes to 59 minutes** HCC ESR

√7th **S06.323 Contusion and laceration of left cerebrum with loss of consciousness of 1 hour to 5 hours 59 minutes** HCC ESR COM

√7th **S06.324 Contusion and laceration of left cerebrum with loss of consciousness of 6 hours to 24 hours** HCC ESR COM

√7th **S06.325 Contusion and laceration of left cerebrum with loss of consciousness greater than 24 hours with return to pre-existing conscious level** HCC ESR COM

7th **S06.326 Contusion and laceration of left cerebrum with loss of consciousness greater than 24 hours without return to pre-existing conscious level with patient surviving** HCC ESR COM

7th **S06.327 Contusion and laceration of left cerebrum with loss of consciousness of any duration with death due to brain injury prior to regaining consciousness**

7th **S06.328 Contusion and laceration of left cerebrum with loss of consciousness of any duration with death due to other cause prior to regaining consciousness**

7th **S06.32A Contusion and laceration of left cerebrum with loss of consciousness status unknown** HCC ESR

Contusion and laceration of left cerebrum NOS

7th **S06.329 Contusion and laceration of left cerebrum with loss of consciousness of unspecified duration** HCC ESR

6th **S06.33 Contusion and laceration of cerebrum, unspecified**

7th **S06.330 Contusion and laceration of cerebrum, unspecified, without loss of consciousness** HCC ESR

7th **S06.331 Contusion and laceration of cerebrum, unspecified, with loss of consciousness of 30 minutes or less** HCC ESR

Contusion and laceration of cerebrum, unspecified, with brief loss of consciousness

7th **S06.332 Contusion and laceration of cerebrum, unspecified, with loss of consciousness of 31 minutes to 59 minutes** HCC ESR

7th **S06.333 Contusion and laceration of cerebrum, unspecified, with loss of consciousness of 1 hour to 5 hours 59 minutes** HCC ESR COM

7th **S06.334 Contusion and laceration of cerebrum, unspecified, with loss of consciousness of 6 hours to 24 hours** HCC ESR COM

7th **S06.335 Contusion and laceration of cerebrum, unspecified, with loss of consciousness greater than 24 hours with return to pre-existing conscious level** HCC ESR COM

7th **S06.336 Contusion and laceration of cerebrum, unspecified, with loss of consciousness greater than 24 hours without return to pre-existing conscious level with patient surviving** HCC ESR COM

7th **S06.337 Contusion and laceration of cerebrum, unspecified, with loss of consciousness of any duration with death due to brain injury prior to regaining consciousness**

7th **S06.338 Contusion and laceration of cerebrum, unspecified, with loss of consciousness of any duration with death due to other cause prior to regaining consciousness**

7th **S06.33A Contusion and laceration of cerebrum, unspecified, with loss of consciousness status unknown** HCC ESR

Contusion and laceration of cerebrum NOS

7th **S06.339 Contusion and laceration of cerebrum, unspecified, with loss of consciousness of unspecified duration** HCC ESR

6th **S06.34 Traumatic hemorrhage of right cerebrum**

Traumatic intracerebral hemorrhage and hematoma of right cerebrum

7th **S06.340 Traumatic hemorrhage of right cerebrum without loss of consciousness** HCC ESR

7th **S06.341 Traumatic hemorrhage of right cerebrum with loss of consciousness of 30 minutes or less** HCC ESR

Traumatic hemorrhage of right cerebrum with brief loss of consciousness

7th **S06.342 Traumatic hemorrhage of right cerebrum with loss of consciousness of 31 minutes to 59 minutes** HCC ESR

7th **S06.343 Traumatic hemorrhage of right cerebrum with loss of consciousness of 1 hours to 5 hours 59 minutes** HCC ESR COM

7th **S06.344 Traumatic hemorrhage of right cerebrum with loss of consciousness of 6 hours to 24 hours** HCC ESR COM

7th **S06.345 Traumatic hemorrhage of right cerebrum with loss of consciousness greater than 24 hours with return to pre-existing conscious level** HCC ESR COM

7th **S06.346 Traumatic hemorrhage of right cerebrum with loss of consciousness greater than 24 hours without return to pre-existing conscious level with patient surviving** HCC ESR COM

7th **S06.347 Traumatic hemorrhage of right cerebrum with loss of consciousness of any duration with death due to brain injury prior to regaining consciousness**

7th **S06.348 Traumatic hemorrhage of right cerebrum with loss of consciousness of any duration with death due to other cause prior to regaining consciousness**

7th **S06.34A Traumatic hemorrhage of right cerebrum with loss of consciousness status unknown** HCC ESR

Traumatic hemorrhage of right cerebrum NOS

7th **S06.349 Traumatic hemorrhage of right cerebrum with loss of consciousness of unspecified duration** HCC ESR

6th **S06.35 Traumatic hemorrhage of left cerebrum**

Traumatic intracerebral hemorrhage and hematoma of left cerebrum

7th **S06.350 Traumatic hemorrhage of left cerebrum without loss of consciousness** HCC ESR

7th **S06.351 Traumatic hemorrhage of left cerebrum with loss of consciousness of 30 minutes or less** HCC ESR

Traumatic hemorrhage of left cerebrum with brief loss of consciousness

7th **S06.352 Traumatic hemorrhage of left cerebrum with loss of consciousness of 31 minutes to 59 minutes** HCC ESR

7th **S06.353 Traumatic hemorrhage of left cerebrum with loss of consciousness of 1 hours to 5 hours 59 minutes** HCC ESR COM

7th **S06.354 Traumatic hemorrhage of left cerebrum with loss of consciousness of 6 hours to 24 hours** HCC ESR COM

7th **S06.355 Traumatic hemorrhage of left cerebrum with loss of consciousness greater than 24 hours with return to pre-existing conscious level** HCC ESR COM

7th **S06.356 Traumatic hemorrhage of left cerebrum with loss of consciousness greater than 24 hours without return to pre-existing conscious level with patient surviving** HCC ESR COM

7th **S06.357 Traumatic hemorrhage of left cerebrum with loss of consciousness of any duration with death due to brain injury prior to regaining consciousness**

7th **S06.358 Traumatic hemorrhage of left cerebrum with loss of consciousness of any duration with death due to other cause prior to regaining consciousness**

7th **S06.35A Traumatic hemorrhage of left cerebrum with loss of consciousness status unknown** HCC ESR

Traumatic hemorrhage of left cerebrum NOS

7th **S06.359 Traumatic hemorrhage of left cerebrum with loss of consciousness of unspecified duration** HCC ESR

6th **S06.36 Traumatic hemorrhage of cerebrum, unspecified**

Traumatic intracerebral hemorrhage and hematoma, unspecified

7th **S06.360 Traumatic hemorrhage of cerebrum, unspecified, without loss of consciousness** HCC ESR

**S06.361** Traumatic hemorrhage of cerebrum, unspecified, with loss of consciousness of 30 minutes or less HCC ESR
Traumatic hemorrhage of cerebrum, unspecified, with brief loss of consciousness

**S06.362** Traumatic hemorrhage of cerebrum, unspecified, with loss of consciousness of 31 minutes to 59 minutes HCC ESR

**S06.363** Traumatic hemorrhage of cerebrum, unspecified, with loss of consciousness of 1 hours to 5 hours 59 minutes HCC ESR COM

**S06.364** Traumatic hemorrhage of cerebrum, unspecified, with loss of consciousness of 6 hours to 24 hours HCC ESR COM

**S06.365** Traumatic hemorrhage of cerebrum, unspecified, with loss of consciousness greater than 24 hours with return to pre-existing conscious level HCC ESR COM

**S06.366** Traumatic hemorrhage of cerebrum, unspecified, with loss of consciousness greater than 24 hours without return to pre-existing conscious level with patient surviving HCC ESR COM

**S06.367** Traumatic hemorrhage of cerebrum, unspecified, with loss of consciousness of any duration with death due to brain injury prior to regaining consciousness

**S06.368** Traumatic hemorrhage of cerebrum, unspecified, with loss of consciousness of any duration with death due to other cause prior to regaining consciousness

**S06.36A** Traumatic hemorrhage of cerebrum, unspecified, with loss of consciousness status unknown HCC ESR
Traumatic hemorrhage of cerebrum NOS

**S06.369** Traumatic hemorrhage of cerebrum, unspecified, with loss of consciousness of unspecified duration HCC ESR

**S06.37 Contusion, laceration, and hemorrhage of cerebellum**

**S06.370** Contusion, laceration, and hemorrhage of cerebellum without loss of consciousness HCC ESR

**S06.371** Contusion, laceration, and hemorrhage of cerebellum with loss of consciousness of 30 minutes or less HCC ESR
Contusion, laceration, and hemorrhage of cerebellum with brief loss of consciousness

**S06.372** Contusion, laceration, and hemorrhage of cerebellum with loss of consciousness of 31 minutes to 59 minutes HCC ESR

**S06.373** Contusion, laceration, and hemorrhage of cerebellum with loss of consciousness of 1 hour to 5 hours 59 minutes HCC ESR COM

**S06.374** Contusion, laceration, and hemorrhage of cerebellum with loss of consciousness of 6 hours to 24 hours HCC ESR COM

**S06.375** Contusion, laceration, and hemorrhage of cerebellum with loss of consciousness greater than 24 hours with return to pre-existing conscious level HCC ESR COM

**S06.376** Contusion, laceration, and hemorrhage of cerebellum with loss of consciousness greater than 24 hours without return to pre-existing conscious level with patient surviving HCC ESR COM

**S06.377** Contusion, laceration, and hemorrhage of cerebellum with loss of consciousness of any duration with death due to brain injury prior to regaining consciousness

**S06.378** Contusion, laceration, and hemorrhage of cerebellum with loss of consciousness of any duration with death due to other cause prior to regaining consciousness

**S06.37A** Contusion, laceration, and hemorrhage of cerebellum with loss of consciousness status unknown HCC ESR
Contusion, laceration, and hemorrhage of cerebellum NOS

**S06.379** Contusion, laceration, and hemorrhage of cerebellum with loss of consciousness of unspecified duration HCC ESR

**S06.38 Contusion, laceration, and hemorrhage of brainstem**

**S06.380** Contusion, laceration, and hemorrhage of brainstem without loss of consciousness HCC ESR

**S06.381** Contusion, laceration, and hemorrhage of brainstem with loss of consciousness of 30 minutes or less HCC ESR
Contusion, laceration, and hemorrhage of brainstem with brief loss of consciousness

**S06.382** Contusion, laceration, and hemorrhage of brainstem with loss of consciousness of 31 minutes to 59 minutes HCC ESR

**S06.383** Contusion, laceration, and hemorrhage of brainstem with loss of consciousness of 1 hour to 5 hours 59 minutes HCC ESR COM

**S06.384** Contusion, laceration, and hemorrhage of brainstem with loss of consciousness of 6 hours to 24 hours HCC ESR COM

**S06.385** Contusion, laceration, and hemorrhage of brainstem with loss of consciousness greater than 24 hours with return to pre-existing conscious level HCC ESR COM

**S06.386** Contusion, laceration, and hemorrhage of brainstem with loss of consciousness greater than 24 hours without return to pre-existing conscious level with patient surviving HCC ESR COM

**S06.387** Contusion, laceration, and hemorrhage of brainstem with loss of consciousness of any duration with death due to brain injury prior to regaining consciousness

**S06.388** Contusion, laceration, and hemorrhage of brainstem with loss of consciousness of any duration with death due to other cause prior to regaining consciousness

**S06.38A** Contusion, laceration, and hemorrhage of brainstem with loss of consciousness status unknown HCC ESR
Contusion, laceration, and hemorrhage of brainstem NOS

**S06.389** Contusion, laceration, and hemorrhage of brainstem with loss of consciousness of unspecified duration HCC ESR

**S06.4 Epidural hemorrhage**
Extradural hemorrhage (traumatic)
Extradural hemorrhage NOS
**DEF:** Epidural space: Space between the endosteum of the cranium (skull) and the dura mater, the outermost layer of a three-layer membrane that covers the brain.

**S06.4X Epidural hemorrhage**

**S06.4X0** Epidural hemorrhage without loss of consciousness HCC ESR

**S06.4X1** Epidural hemorrhage with loss of consciousness of 30 minutes or less HCC ESR
Epidural hemorrhage with brief loss of consciousness

**S06.4X2** Epidural hemorrhage with loss of consciousness of 31 minutes to 59 minutes HCC ESR

**S06.4X3** Epidural hemorrhage with loss of consciousness of 1 hour to 5 hours 59 minutes HCC ESR COM

**S06.4X4** Epidural hemorrhage with loss of consciousness of 6 hours to 24 hours HCC ESR COM

**S06.4X5** Epidural hemorrhage with loss of consciousness greater than 24 hours with return to pre-existing conscious level HCC ESR COM

7th **S06.4X6** **Epidural hemorrhage with loss of consciousness greater than 24 hours without return to pre-existing conscious level with patient surviving** HCC ESR COM

7th **S06.4X7** **Epidural hemorrhage with loss of consciousness of any duration with death due to brain injury prior to regaining consciousness**

7th **S06.4X8** **Epidural hemorrhage with loss of consciousness of any duration with death due to other causes prior to regaining consciousness**

7th **S06.4XA** **Epidural hemorrhage with loss of consciousness status unknown** HCC ESR
Epidural hemorrhage NOS

7th **S06.4X9** **Epidural hemorrhage with loss of consciousness of unspecified duration** HCC ESR

5th **S06.5** **Traumatic subdural hemorrhage**
Use additional code, if applicable, for traumatic brain compression or herniation (S06.A-)
**AHA:** 2021,2Q,5; 2021,1Q,4
**DEF:** Subdural: Potential space between the dura mater and arachnoid membrane around the brain.

6th **S06.5X** **Traumatic subdural hemorrhage**

7th **S06.5X0** **Traumatic subdural hemorrhage without loss of consciousness** HCC ESR

7th **S06.5X1** **Traumatic subdural hemorrhage with loss of consciousness of 30 minutes or less** HCC ESR
Traumatic subdural hemorrhage with brief loss of consciousness

7th **S06.5X2** **Traumatic subdural hemorrhage with loss of consciousness of 31 minutes to 59 minutes** HCC ESR

7th **S06.5X3** **Traumatic subdural hemorrhage with loss of consciousness of 1 hour to 5 hours 59 minutes** HCC ESR COM

7th **S06.5X4** **Traumatic subdural hemorrhage with loss of consciousness of 6 hours to 24 hours** HCC ESR COM

7th **S06.5X5** **Traumatic subdural hemorrhage with loss of consciousness greater than 24 hours with return to pre-existing conscious level** HCC ESR COM

7th **S06.5X6** **Traumatic subdural hemorrhage with loss of consciousness greater than 24 hours without return to pre-existing conscious level with patient surviving** HCC ESR COM

7th **S06.5X7** **Traumatic subdural hemorrhage with loss of consciousness of any duration with death due to brain injury before regaining consciousness**

7th **S06.5X8** **Traumatic subdural hemorrhage with loss of consciousness of any duration with death due to other cause before regaining consciousness**

7th **S06.5XA** **Traumatic subdural hemorrhage with loss of consciousness status unknown** HCC ESR
Traumatic subdural hemorrhage NOS
**AHA:** 2022,4Q,44

7th **S06.5X9** **Traumatic subdural hemorrhage with loss of consciousness of unspecified duration** HCC ESR

5th **S06.6** **Traumatic subarachnoid hemorrhage**
Use additional code, if applicable, for traumatic brain compression or herniation (S06.A-)
**AHA:** 2021,2Q,5; 2021,1Q,4
**DEF:** Subarachnoid: Space located between the arachnoid membrane and the pia mater that contains cerebrospinal fluid.

6th **S06.6X** **Traumatic subarachnoid hemorrhage**

7th **S06.6X0** **Traumatic subarachnoid hemorrhage without loss of consciousness** HCC ESR

7th **S06.6X1** **Traumatic subarachnoid hemorrhage with loss of consciousness of 30 minutes or less** HCC ESR
Traumatic subarachnoid hemorrhage with brief loss of consciousness

7th **S06.6X2** **Traumatic subarachnoid hemorrhage with loss of consciousness of 31 minutes to 59 minutes** HCC ESR

7th **S06.6X3** **Traumatic subarachnoid hemorrhage with loss of consciousness of 1 hour to 5 hours 59 minutes** HCC ESR COM

7th **S06.6X4** **Traumatic subarachnoid hemorrhage with loss of consciousness of 6 hours to 24 hours** HCC ESR COM

7th **S06.6X5** **Traumatic subarachnoid hemorrhage with loss of consciousness greater than 24 hours with return to pre-existing conscious level** HCC ESR COM

7th **S06.6X6** **Traumatic subarachnoid hemorrhage with loss of consciousness greater than 24 hours without return to pre-existing conscious level with patient surviving** HCC ESR COM

7th **S06.6X7** **Traumatic subarachnoid hemorrhage with loss of consciousness of any duration with death due to brain injury prior to regaining consciousness**

7th **S06.6X8** **Traumatic subarachnoid hemorrhage with loss of consciousness of any duration with death due to other cause prior to regaining consciousness**

7th **S06.6XA** **Traumatic subarachnoid hemorrhage with loss of consciousness status unknown** HCC ESR
Traumatic subarachnoid hemorrhage NOS
**AHA:** 2022,4Q,44

7th **S06.6X9** **Traumatic subarachnoid hemorrhage with loss of consciousness of unspecified duration** HCC ESR

5th **S06.8** **Other specified intracranial injuries**

6th **S06.81** **Injury of right internal carotid artery, intracranial portion, not elsewhere classified**

7th **S06.810** **Injury of right internal carotid artery, intracranial portion, not elsewhere classified without loss of consciousness** HCC ESR

7th **S06.811** **Injury of right internal carotid artery, intracranial portion, not elsewhere classified with loss of consciousness of 30 minutes or less** HCC ESR
Injury of right internal carotid artery, intracranial portion, not elsewhere classified with brief loss of consciousness

7th **S06.812** **Injury of right internal carotid artery, intracranial portion, not elsewhere classified with loss of consciousness of 31 minutes to 59 minutes** HCC ESR

7th **S06.813** **Injury of right internal carotid artery, intracranial portion, not elsewhere classified with loss of consciousness of 1 hour to 5 hours 59 minutes** HCC ESR COM

7th **S06.814** **Injury of right internal carotid artery, intracranial portion, not elsewhere classified with loss of consciousness of 6 hours to 24 hours** HCC ESR COM

7th **S06.815** **Injury of right internal carotid artery, intracranial portion, not elsewhere classified with loss of consciousness greater than 24 hours with return to pre-existing conscious level** HCC ESR COM

7th **S06.816** **Injury of right internal carotid artery, intracranial portion, not elsewhere classified with loss of consciousness greater than 24 hours without return to pre-existing conscious level with patient surviving** HCC ESR COM

7th **S06.817** **Injury of right internal carotid artery, intracranial portion, not elsewhere classified with loss of consciousness of any duration with death due to brain injury prior to regaining consciousness**

7th **S06.818** **Injury of right internal carotid artery, intracranial portion, not elsewhere classified with loss of consciousness of any duration with death due to other cause prior to regaining consciousness**

√7th **S06.81A Injury of right internal carotid artery, intracranial portion, not elsewhere classified with loss of consciousness status unknown** HCC ESR
Injury of right internal carotid artery, intracranial portion, not elsewhere classified NOS

√7th **S06.819 Injury of right internal carotid artery, intracranial portion, not elsewhere classified with loss of consciousness of unspecified duration** HCC ESR

√6th **S06.82 Injury of left internal carotid artery, intracranial portion, not elsewhere classified**

√7th **S06.820 Injury of left internal carotid artery, intracranial portion, not elsewhere classified without loss of consciousness** HCC ESR

√7th **S06.821 Injury of left internal carotid artery, intracranial portion, not elsewhere classified with loss of consciousness of 30 minutes or less** HCC ESR
Injury of left internal carotid artery, intracranial portion, not elsewhere classified with brief loss of consciousness

√7th **S06.822 Injury of left internal carotid artery, intracranial portion, not elsewhere classified with loss of consciousness of 31 minutes to 59 minutes** HCC ESR

√7th **S06.823 Injury of left internal carotid artery, intracranial portion, not elsewhere classified with loss of consciousness of 1 hour to 5 hours 59 minutes** HCC ESR COM

√7th **S06.824 Injury of left internal carotid artery, intracranial portion, not elsewhere classified with loss of consciousness of 6 hours to 24 hours** HCC ESR COM

√7th **S06.825 Injury of left internal carotid artery, intracranial portion, not elsewhere classified with loss of consciousness greater than 24 hours with return to pre-existing conscious level** HCC ESR COM

√7th **S06.826 Injury of left internal carotid artery, intracranial portion, not elsewhere classified with loss of consciousness greater than 24 hours without return to pre-existing conscious level with patient surviving** HCC ESR COM

√7th **S06.827 Injury of left internal carotid artery, intracranial portion, not elsewhere classified with loss of consciousness of any duration with death due to brain injury prior to regaining consciousness**

√7th **S06.828 Injury of left internal carotid artery, intracranial portion, not elsewhere classified with loss of consciousness of any duration with death due to other cause prior to regaining consciousness**

√7th **S06.82A Injury of left internal carotid artery, intracranial portion, not elsewhere classified with loss of consciousness status unknown** HCC ESR
Injury of left internal carotid artery, intracranial portion, not elsewhere classified NOS

√7th **S06.829 Injury of left internal carotid artery, intracranial portion, not elsewhere classified with loss of consciousness of unspecified duration** HCC ESR

√6th **S06.8A Primary blast injury of brain, not elsewhere classified**
Code also, if applicable, focal traumatic brain injury (S06.3-)
EXCLUDES 2 *traumatic cerebral edema (S06.1)*

√7th **S06.8A0 Primary blast injury of brain, not elsewhere classified without loss of consciousness** HCC ESR

√7th **S06.8A1 Primary blast injury of brain, not elsewhere classified with loss of consciousness of 30 minutes or less** HCC ESR
Primary blast injury of brain, not elsewhere classified with brief loss of consciousness

√7th **S06.8A2 Primary blast injury of brain, not elsewhere classified with loss of consciousness of 31 minutes to 59 minutes** HCC ESR

√7th **S06.8A3 Primary blast injury of brain, not elsewhere classified with loss of consciousness of 1 hour to 5 hours 59 minutes** HCC ESR COM

√7th **S06.8A4 Primary blast injury of brain, not elsewhere classified with loss of consciousness of 6 hours to 24 hours** HCC ESR COM

√7th **S06.8A5 Primary blast injury of brain, not elsewhere classified with loss of consciousness greater than 24 hours with return to pre-existing conscious level** HCC ESR COM

√7th **S06.8A6 Primary blast injury of brain, not elsewhere classified with loss of consciousness greater than 24 hours without return to pre-existing conscious level with patient surviving** HCC ESR COM

√7th **S06.8A7 Primary blast injury of brain, not elsewhere classified with loss of consciousness of any duration with death due to brain injury prior to regaining consciousness**

√7th **S06.8A8 Primary blast injury of brain, not elsewhere classified with loss of consciousness of any duration with death due to other cause prior to regaining consciousness**

√7th **S06.8AA Primary blast injury of brain, not elsewhere classified with loss of consciousness status unknown** HCC ESR
Primary blast injury of brain NOS

√7th **S06.8A9 Primary blast injury of brain, not elsewhere classified with loss of consciousness of unspecified duration** HCC ESR

√6th **S06.89 Other specified intracranial injury**
EXCLUDES 1 *concussion (S06.0X-)*
AHA: 2024,2Q,15

√7th **S06.890 Other specified intracranial injury without loss of consciousness** HCC ESR

√7th **S06.891 Other specified intracranial injury with loss of consciousness of 30 minutes or less** HCC ESR
Other specified intracranial injury with brief loss of consciousness

√7th **S06.892 Other specified intracranial injury with loss of consciousness of 31 minutes to 59 minutes** HCC ESR

√7th **S06.893 Other specified intracranial injury with loss of consciousness of 1 hour to 5 hours 59 minutes** HCC ESR COM

√7th **S06.894 Other specified intracranial injury with loss of consciousness of 6 hours to 24 hours** HCC ESR COM

√7th **S06.895 Other specified intracranial injury with loss of consciousness greater than 24 hours with return to pre-existing conscious level** HCC ESR COM

√7th **S06.896 Other specified intracranial injury with loss of consciousness greater than 24 hours without return to pre-existing conscious level with patient surviving** HCC ESR COM

√7th **S06.897 Other specified intracranial injury with loss of consciousness of any duration with death due to brain injury prior to regaining consciousness**

√7th **S06.898 Other specified intracranial injury with loss of consciousness of any duration with death due to other cause prior to regaining consciousness**

√7th **S06.89A Other specified intracranial injury with loss of consciousness status unknown** HCC ESR

√7th **S06.899 Other specified intracranial injury with loss of consciousness of unspecified duration** HCC ESR

**S06.9 Unspecified intracranial injury**
Brain injury NOS
Head injury NOS with loss of consciousness
Traumatic brain injury NOS
EXCLUDES 1 *conditions classifiable to S06.0- to S06.8- code to specified intracranial injury*
*head injury NOS (S09.90)*
AHA: 2020,3Q,46; 2020,2Q,31

**S06.9X Unspecified intracranial injury**
**S06.9X0 Unspecified intracranial injury without loss of consciousness** HCC ESR
**S06.9X1 Unspecified intracranial injury with loss of consciousness of 30 minutes or less** HCC ESR
Unspecified intracranial injury with brief loss of consciousness
**S06.9X2 Unspecified intracranial injury with loss of consciousness of 31 minutes to 59 minutes** HCC ESR
**S06.9X3 Unspecified intracranial injury with loss of consciousness of 1 hour to 5 hours 59 minutes** HCC ESR COM
**S06.9X4 Unspecified intracranial injury with loss of consciousness of 6 hours to 24 hours** HCC ESR COM
**S06.9X5 Unspecified intracranial injury with loss of consciousness greater than 24 hours with return to pre-existing conscious level** HCC ESR COM
**S06.9X6 Unspecified intracranial injury with loss of consciousness greater than 24 hours without return to pre-existing conscious level with patient surviving** HCC ESR COM
**S06.9X7 Unspecified intracranial injury with loss of consciousness of any duration with death due to brain injury prior to regaining consciousness**
**S06.9X8 Unspecified intracranial injury with loss of consciousness of any duration with death due to other cause prior to regaining consciousness**
**S06.9XA Unspecified intracranial injury with loss of consciousness status unknown** HCC ESR
**S06.9X9 Unspecified intracranial injury with loss of consciousness of unspecified duration** HCC ESR

**S06.A Traumatic brain compression and herniation**
Traumatic cerebral compression
▶Traumatic midline shift of brain◀
Code first the underlying traumatic brain injury, such as:
diffuse traumatic brain injury (S06.2-)
focal traumatic brain injury (S06.3-)
traumatic subarachnoid hemorrhage (S06.6-)
traumatic subdural hemorrhage (S06.5-)
AHA: 2021,4Q,29

**S06.A0 Traumatic brain compression without herniation** HCC ESR UPD
Traumatic brain compression NOS
Traumatic cerebral compression NOS
**S06.A1 Traumatic brain compression with herniation** HCC ESR UPD
Traumatic brain herniation
Traumatic brainstem compression with herniation
Traumatic cerebellar compression with herniation
Traumatic cerebral compression with herniation

**S07 Crushing injury of head**
Use additional code for all associated injuries, such as:
intracranial injuries (S06.-)
skull fractures (S02.-)

The appropriate 7th character is to be added to each code from category S07.
A initial encounter
D subsequent encounter
S sequela

**S07.0 Crushing injury of face**
**S07.1 Crushing injury of skull**
**S07.8 Crushing injury of other parts of head**
**S07.9 Crushing injury of head, part unspecified**

**S08 Avulsion and traumatic amputation of part of head**
An amputation not identified as partial or complete should be coded to complete

The appropriate 7th character is to be added to each code from category S08.
A initial encounter
D subsequent encounter
S sequela

**S08.0 Avulsion of scalp**
**S08.1 Traumatic amputation of ear**
**S08.11 Complete traumatic amputation of ear**
**S08.111 Complete traumatic amputation of right ear**
**S08.112 Complete traumatic amputation of left ear**
**S08.119 Complete traumatic amputation of unspecified ear**
**S08.12 Partial traumatic amputation of ear**
**S08.121 Partial traumatic amputation of right ear**
**S08.122 Partial traumatic amputation of left ear**
**S08.129 Partial traumatic amputation of unspecified ear**
**S08.8 Traumatic amputation of other parts of head**
**S08.81 Traumatic amputation of nose**
**S08.811 Complete traumatic amputation of nose**
**S08.812 Partial traumatic amputation of nose**
**S08.89 Traumatic amputation of other parts of head**

**S09 Other and unspecified injuries of head**

The appropriate 7th character is to be added to each code from category S09.
A initial encounter
D subsequent encounter
S sequela

**S09.0 Injury of blood vessels of head, not elsewhere classified**
EXCLUDES 1 *injury of cerebral blood vessels (S06.-)*
*injury of precerebral blood vessels (S15.-)*
**S09.1 Injury of muscle and tendon of head**
Code also any associated open wound (S01.-)
EXCLUDES 2 *sprain to joints and ligament of head (S03.9)*
**S09.10 Unspecified injury of muscle and tendon of head**
Injury of muscle and tendon of head NOS
**S09.11 Strain of muscle and tendon of head**
**S09.12 Laceration of muscle and tendon of head**
**S09.19 Other specified injury of muscle and tendon of head**
**S09.2 Traumatic rupture of ear drum**
EXCLUDES 1 *traumatic rupture of ear drum due to blast injury (S09.31-)*
**S09.20 Traumatic rupture of unspecified ear drum**
**S09.21 Traumatic rupture of right ear drum**
**S09.22 Traumatic rupture of left ear drum**
**S09.3 Other specified and unspecified injury of middle and inner ear**
EXCLUDES 1 *injury to ear NOS (S09.91-)*
EXCLUDES 2 *injury to external ear (S00.4-, S01.3-, S08.1-)*
**S09.30 Unspecified injury of middle and inner ear**
**S09.301 Unspecified injury of right middle and inner ear**
**S09.302 Unspecified injury of left middle and inner ear**
**S09.309 Unspecified injury of unspecified middle and inner ear**
**S09.31 Primary blast injury of ear**
Blast injury of ear NOS
**S09.311 Primary blast injury of right ear**
**S09.312 Primary blast injury of left ear**
**S09.313 Primary blast injury of ear, bilateral**
**S09.319 Primary blast injury of unspecified ear**
**S09.39 Other specified injury of middle and inner ear**
Secondary blast injury to ear
**S09.391 Other specified injury of right middle and inner ear**
**S09.392 Other specified injury of left middle and inner ear**

HCC CMS-HCC Rx Rx HCC ESR ESRD HCC COM Commercial HCC N Newborn: 0 P Pediatric: 0-17 M Maternity: 9-64 A Adult: 15-124

✓7th **S09.399 Other specified injury of unspecified middle and inner ear**

✓x7th **S09.8 Other specified injuries of head**

✓5th **S09.9 Unspecified injury of face and head**

✓x7th **S09.90 Unspecified injury of head**
Head injury NOS
EXCLUDES 1 *brain injury NOS (S06.9-)*
*head injury NOS with loss of consciousness (S06.9-)*
*intracranial injury NOS (S06.9-)*

✓x7th **S09.91 Unspecified injury of ear**
Injury of ear NOS

✓x7th **S09.92 Unspecified injury of nose**
Injury of nose NOS

✓x7th **S09.93 Unspecified injury of face**
Injury of face NOS
**AHA:** 2019,2Q,23

## Injuries to the neck (S10-S19)

INCLUDES injuries of nape
injuries of supraclavicular region
injuries of throat

EXCLUDES 2 *burns and corrosions (T20-T32)*
*effects of foreign body in esophagus (T18.1)*
*effects of foreign body in larynx (T17.3)*
*effects of foreign body in pharynx (T17.2)*
*effects of foreign body in trachea (T17.4)*
*frostbite (T33-T34)*
*insect bite or sting, venomous (T63.4)*

✓4th **S10 Superficial injury of neck**

The appropriate 7th character is to be added to each code from category S10.
A initial encounter
D subsequent encounter
S sequela

✓x7th **S10.0 Contusion of throat**
Contusion of cervical esophagus
Contusion of larynx
Contusion of pharynx
Contusion of trachea

✓5th **S10.1 Other and unspecified superficial injuries of throat**

✓x7th **S10.10 Unspecified superficial injuries of throat**

✓x7th **S10.11 Abrasion of throat**

✓x7th **S10.12 Blister (nonthermal) of throat**

✓x7th **S10.14 External constriction of part of throat**

✓x7th **S10.15 Superficial foreign body of throat**
Splinter in the throat

✓x7th **S10.16 Insect bite (nonvenomous) of throat**

✓x7th **S10.17 Other superficial bite of throat**
EXCLUDES 1 *open bite of throat (S11.85)*

✓5th **S10.8 Superficial injury of other specified parts of neck**

✓x7th **S10.80 Unspecified superficial injury of other specified part of neck**

✓x7th **S10.81 Abrasion of other specified part of neck**

✓x7th **S10.82 Blister (nonthermal) of other specified part of neck**

✓x7th **S10.83 Contusion of other specified part of neck**

✓x7th **S10.84 External constriction of other specified part of neck**

✓x7th **S10.85 Superficial foreign body of other specified part of neck**
Splinter in other specified part of neck

✓x7th **S10.86 Insect bite of other specified part of neck**

✓x7th **S10.87 Other superficial bite of other specified part of neck**
EXCLUDES 1 *open bite of other specified parts of neck (S11.85)*

✓5th **S10.9 Superficial injury of unspecified part of neck**

✓x7th **S10.90 Unspecified superficial injury of unspecified part of neck**

✓x7th **S10.91 Abrasion of unspecified part of neck**

✓x7th **S10.92 Blister (nonthermal) of unspecified part of neck**

✓x7th **S10.93 Contusion of unspecified part of neck**

✓x7th **S10.94 External constriction of unspecified part of neck**

✓x7th **S10.95 Superficial foreign body of unspecified part of neck**

✓x7th **S10.96 Insect bite of unspecified part of neck**

✓x7th **S10.97 Other superficial bite of unspecified part of neck**

✓4th **S11 Open wound of neck**

Code also any associated:
spinal cord injury (S14.0, S14.1-)
wound infection

EXCLUDES 2 *open fracture of vertebra (S12.- with 7th character B)*

The appropriate 7th character is to be added to each code from category S11.
A initial encounter
D subsequent encounter
S sequela

✓5th **S11.0 Open wound of larynx and trachea**

✓6th **S11.01 Open wound of larynx**
EXCLUDES 2 *open wound of vocal cord (S11.03)*

✓7th **S11.011 Laceration without foreign body of larynx**

✓7th **S11.012 Laceration with foreign body of larynx**

✓7th **S11.013 Puncture wound without foreign body of larynx**

✓7th **S11.014 Puncture wound with foreign body of larynx**

✓7th **S11.015 Open bite of larynx**
Bite of larynx NOS

✓7th **S11.019 Unspecified open wound of larynx**

✓6th **S11.02 Open wound of trachea**
Open wound of cervical trachea
Open wound of trachea NOS
EXCLUDES 2 *open wound of thoracic trachea (S27.5-)*

✓7th **S11.021 Laceration without foreign body of trachea**

✓7th **S11.022 Laceration with foreign body of trachea**

✓7th **S11.023 Puncture wound without foreign body of trachea**

✓7th **S11.024 Puncture wound with foreign body of trachea**

✓7th **S11.025 Open bite of trachea**
Bite of trachea NOS

✓7th **S11.029 Unspecified open wound of trachea**

✓6th **S11.03 Open wound of vocal cord**

✓7th **S11.031 Laceration without foreign body of vocal cord**

✓7th **S11.032 Laceration with foreign body of vocal cord**

✓7th **S11.033 Puncture wound without foreign body of vocal cord**

✓7th **S11.034 Puncture wound with foreign body of vocal cord**

✓7th **S11.035 Open bite of vocal cord**
Bite of vocal cord NOS

✓7th **S11.039 Unspecified open wound of vocal cord**

✓5th **S11.1 Open wound of thyroid gland**

✓x7th **S11.10 Unspecified open wound of thyroid gland**

✓x7th **S11.11 Laceration without foreign body of thyroid gland**

✓x7th **S11.12 Laceration with foreign body of thyroid gland**

✓x7th **S11.13 Puncture wound without foreign body of thyroid gland**

✓x7th **S11.14 Puncture wound with foreign body of thyroid gland**

✓x7th **S11.15 Open bite of thyroid gland**
Bite of thyroid gland NOS

✓5th **S11.2 Open wound of pharynx and cervical esophagus**
EXCLUDES 1 *open wound of esophagus NOS (S27.8-)*

✓x7th **S11.20 Unspecified open wound of pharynx and cervical esophagus**

✓x7th **S11.21 Laceration without foreign body of pharynx and cervical esophagus**

✓x7th **S11.22 Laceration with foreign body of pharynx and cervical esophagus**

✓x7th **S11.23 Puncture wound without foreign body of pharynx and cervical esophagus**

✓x7th **S11.24 Puncture wound with foreign body of pharynx and cervical esophagus**

✓x7th **S11.25 Open bite of pharynx and cervical esophagus**
Bite of pharynx and cervical esophagus NOS

✓5th **S11.8 Open wound of other specified parts of neck**

✓x7th **S11.80 Unspecified open wound of other specified part of neck**

✓x7th **S11.81 Laceration without foreign body of other specified part of neck**

√x7th S11.82 **Laceration with foreign body of other specified part of neck**

√x7th S11.83 **Puncture wound without foreign body of other specified part of neck**

√x7th S11.84 **Puncture wound with foreign body of other specified part of neck**

√x7th S11.85 **Open bite of other specified part of neck**
Bite of other specified part of neck NOS
EXCLUDES 1 *superficial bite of other specified part of neck (S1Ø.87)*

√x7th S11.89 **Other open wound of other specified part of neck**

√5th S11.9 **Open wound of unspecified part of neck**

√x7th S11.9Ø **Unspecified open wound of unspecified part of neck**

√x7th S11.91 **Laceration without foreign body of unspecified part of neck**

√x7th S11.92 **Laceration with foreign body of unspecified part of neck**

√x7th S11.93 **Puncture wound without foreign body of unspecified part of neck**

√x7th S11.94 **Puncture wound with foreign body of unspecified part of neck**

√x7th S11.95 **Open bite of unspecified part of neck**
Bite of neck NOS
EXCLUDES 1 *superficial bite of neck (S1Ø.97)*

√4th **S12 Fracture of cervical vertebra and other parts of neck**

NOTE A fracture not indicated as displaced or nondisplaced should be coded to displaced.

A fracture not indicated as open or closed should be coded to closed.

INCLUDES fracture of cervical neural arch
fracture of cervical spine
fracture of cervical spinous process
fracture of cervical transverse process
fracture of cervical vertebral arch
fracture of neck

Code first any associated cervical spinal cord injury (S14.Ø, S14.1-)

**AHA:** 2024,2Q,23; 2021,1Q,6; 2018,2Q,12; 2015,3Q,37-39

The appropriate 7th character is to be added to all codes from subcategories S12.Ø-S12.6.
A initial encounter for closed fracture
B initial encounter for open fracture
D subsequent encounter for fracture with routine healing
G subsequent encounter for fracture with delayed healing
K subsequent encounter for fracture with nonunion
S sequela

√5th S12.Ø **Fracture of first cervical vertebra**
Atlas

√6th S12.ØØ **Unspecified fracture of first cervical vertebra**

√7th S12.ØØØ **Unspecified displaced fracture of first cervical vertebra** HCC ESR COM Q

√7th S12.ØØ1 **Unspecified nondisplaced fracture of first cervical vertebra** HCC ESR COM Q

√x7th S12.Ø1 **Stable burst fracture of first cervical vertebra** HCC ESR COM Q

√x7th S12.Ø2 **Unstable burst fracture of first cervical vertebra** HCC ESR COM Q

√6th S12.Ø3 **Posterior arch fracture of first cervical vertebra**

√7th S12.Ø3Ø **Displaced posterior arch fracture of first cervical vertebra** HCC ESR COM Q

√7th S12.Ø31 **Nondisplaced posterior arch fracture of first cervical vertebra** HCC ESR COM Q

√6th S12.Ø4 **Lateral mass fracture of first cervical vertebra**

√7th S12.Ø4Ø **Displaced lateral mass fracture of first cervical vertebra** HCC ESR COM Q

√7th S12.Ø41 **Nondisplaced lateral mass fracture of first cervical vertebra** HCC ESR COM Q

√6th S12.Ø9 **Other fracture of first cervical vertebra**

√7th S12.Ø9Ø **Other displaced fracture of first cervical vertebra** HCC ESR COM Q

√7th S12.Ø91 **Other nondisplaced fracture of first cervical vertebra** HCC ESR COM Q

√5th S12.1 **Fracture of second cervical vertebra**
Axis

√6th S12.1Ø **Unspecified fracture of second cervical vertebra**

√7th S12.1ØØ **Unspecified displaced fracture of second cervical vertebra** HCC ESR COM Q

√7th S12.1Ø1 **Unspecified nondisplaced fracture of second cervical vertebra** HCC ESR COM Q

√6th S12.11 **Type II dens fracture**

√7th S12.11Ø **Anterior displaced Type II dens fracture** HCC ESR COM Q

√7th S12.111 **Posterior displaced Type II dens fracture** HCC ESR COM Q

√7th S12.112 **Nondisplaced Type II dens fracture** HCC ESR COM Q

√6th S12.12 **Other dens fracture**

√7th S12.12Ø **Other displaced dens fracture** HCC ESR COM Q

√7th S12.121 **Other nondisplaced dens fracture** HCC ESR COM Q

√6th S12.13 **Unspecified traumatic spondylolisthesis of second cervical vertebra**

√7th S12.13Ø **Unspecified traumatic displaced spondylolisthesis of second cervical vertebra** HCC ESR COM Q

√7th S12.131 **Unspecified traumatic nondisplaced spondylolisthesis of second cervical vertebra** HCC ESR COM Q

√x7th S12.14 **Type III traumatic spondylolisthesis of second cervical vertebra** HCC ESR COM Q

√6th S12.15 **Other traumatic spondylolisthesis of second cervical vertebra**

√7th S12.15Ø **Other traumatic displaced spondylolisthesis of second cervical vertebra** HCC ESR COM Q

√7th S12.151 **Other traumatic nondisplaced spondylolisthesis of second cervical vertebra** HCC ESR COM Q

√6th S12.19 **Other fracture of second cervical vertebra**

√7th S12.19Ø **Other displaced fracture of second cervical vertebra** HCC ESR COM Q

√7th S12.191 **Other nondisplaced fracture of second cervical vertebra** HCC ESR COM Q

√5th S12.2 **Fracture of third cervical vertebra**

√6th S12.2Ø **Unspecified fracture of third cervical vertebra**

√7th S12.2ØØ **Unspecified displaced fracture of third cervical vertebra** HCC ESR COM Q

√7th S12.2Ø1 **Unspecified nondisplaced fracture of third cervical vertebra** HCC ESR COM Q

√6th S12.23 **Unspecified traumatic spondylolisthesis of third cervical vertebra**

√7th S12.23Ø **Unspecified traumatic displaced spondylolisthesis of third cervical vertebra** HCC ESR COM Q

√7th S12.231 **Unspecified traumatic nondisplaced spondylolisthesis of third cervical vertebra** HCC ESR COM Q

√x7th S12.24 **Type III traumatic spondylolisthesis of third cervical vertebra** HCC ESR COM Q

√6th S12.25 **Other traumatic spondylolisthesis of third cervical vertebra**

√7th S12.25Ø **Other traumatic displaced spondylolisthesis of third cervical vertebra** HCC ESR COM Q

√7th S12.251 **Other traumatic nondisplaced spondylolisthesis of third cervical vertebra** HCC ESR COM Q

√6th S12.29 **Other fracture of third cervical vertebra**

√7th S12.29Ø **Other displaced fracture of third cervical vertebra** HCC ESR COM Q

√7th S12.291 **Other nondisplaced fracture of third cervical vertebra** HCC ESR COM Q

√5th S12.3 **Fracture of fourth cervical vertebra**

√6th S12.3Ø **Unspecified fracture of fourth cervical vertebra**

√7th S12.3ØØ **Unspecified displaced fracture of fourth cervical vertebra** HCC ESR COM Q

√7th S12.3Ø1 **Unspecified nondisplaced fracture of fourth cervical vertebra** HCC ESR COM Q

√6th S12.33 **Unspecified traumatic spondylolisthesis of fourth cervical vertebra**

√7th S12.33Ø **Unspecified traumatic displaced spondylolisthesis of fourth cervical vertebra** HCC ESR COM Q

√7th S12.331 Unspecified traumatic nondisplaced spondylolisthesis of fourth cervical vertebra HCC ESR COM Q

√x7th S12.34 Type III traumatic spondylolisthesis of fourth cervical vertebra HCC ESR COM Q

√6th S12.35 Other traumatic spondylolisthesis of fourth cervical vertebra

√7th S12.350 Other traumatic displaced spondylolisthesis of fourth cervical vertebra HCC ESR COM Q

√7th S12.351 Other traumatic nondisplaced spondylolisthesis of fourth cervical vertebra HCC ESR COM Q

√6th S12.39 Other fracture of fourth cervical vertebra

√7th S12.390 Other displaced fracture of fourth cervical vertebra HCC ESR COM Q

√7th S12.391 Other nondisplaced fracture of fourth cervical vertebra HCC ESR COM Q

√5th S12.4 Fracture of fifth cervical vertebra

√6th S12.40 Unspecified fracture of fifth cervical vertebra

√7th S12.400 Unspecified displaced fracture of fifth cervical vertebra HCC ESR COM Q

√7th S12.401 Unspecified nondisplaced fracture of fifth cervical vertebra HCC ESR COM Q

√6th S12.43 Unspecified traumatic spondylolisthesis of fifth cervical vertebra

√7th S12.430 Unspecified traumatic displaced spondylolisthesis of fifth cervical vertebra HCC ESR COM Q

√7th S12.431 Unspecified traumatic nondisplaced spondylolisthesis of fifth cervical vertebra HCC ESR COM Q

√x7th S12.44 Type III traumatic spondylolisthesis of fifth cervical vertebra HCC ESR COM Q

√6th S12.45 Other traumatic spondylolisthesis of fifth cervical vertebra

√7th S12.450 Other traumatic displaced spondylolisthesis of fifth cervical vertebra HCC ESR COM Q

√7th S12.451 Other traumatic nondisplaced spondylolisthesis of fifth cervical vertebra HCC ESR COM Q

√6th S12.49 Other fracture of fifth cervical vertebra

√7th S12.490 Other displaced fracture of fifth cervical vertebra HCC ESR COM Q

√7th S12.491 Other nondisplaced fracture of fifth cervical vertebra HCC ESR COM Q

√5th S12.5 Fracture of sixth cervical vertebra

√6th S12.50 Unspecified fracture of sixth cervical vertebra

√7th S12.500 Unspecified displaced fracture of sixth cervical vertebra HCC ESR COM Q

√7th S12.501 Unspecified nondisplaced fracture of sixth cervical vertebra HCC ESR COM Q

√6th S12.53 Unspecified traumatic spondylolisthesis of sixth cervical vertebra

√7th S12.530 Unspecified traumatic displaced spondylolisthesis of sixth cervical vertebra HCC ESR COM Q

√7th S12.531 Unspecified traumatic nondisplaced spondylolisthesis of sixth cervical vertebra HCC ESR COM Q

√x7th S12.54 Type III traumatic spondylolisthesis of sixth cervical vertebra HCC ESR COM Q

√6th S12.55 Other traumatic spondylolisthesis of sixth cervical vertebra

√7th S12.550 Other traumatic displaced spondylolisthesis of sixth cervical vertebra HCC ESR COM Q

√7th S12.551 Other traumatic nondisplaced spondylolisthesis of sixth cervical vertebra HCC ESR COM Q

√6th S12.59 Other fracture of sixth cervical vertebra

√7th S12.590 Other displaced fracture of sixth cervical vertebra HCC ESR COM Q

√7th S12.591 Other nondisplaced fracture of sixth cervical vertebra HCC ESR COM Q

√5th S12.6 Fracture of seventh cervical vertebra

√6th S12.60 Unspecified fracture of seventh cervical vertebra

√7th S12.600 Unspecified displaced fracture of seventh cervical vertebra HCC ESR COM Q

√7th S12.601 Unspecified nondisplaced fracture of seventh cervical vertebra HCC ESR COM Q

√6th S12.63 Unspecified traumatic spondylolisthesis of seventh cervical vertebra

√7th S12.630 Unspecified traumatic displaced spondylolisthesis of seventh cervical vertebra HCC ESR COM Q

√7th S12.631 Unspecified traumatic nondisplaced spondylolisthesis of seventh cervical vertebra HCC ESR COM Q

√x7th S12.64 Type III traumatic spondylolisthesis of seventh cervical vertebra HCC ESR COM Q

√6th S12.65 Other traumatic spondylolisthesis of seventh cervical vertebra

√7th S12.650 Other traumatic displaced spondylolisthesis of seventh cervical vertebra HCC ESR COM Q

√7th S12.651 Other traumatic nondisplaced spondylolisthesis of seventh cervical vertebra HCC ESR COM Q

√6th S12.69 Other fracture of seventh cervical vertebra

√7th S12.690 Other displaced fracture of seventh cervical vertebra HCC ESR COM Q

√7th S12.691 Other nondisplaced fracture of seventh cervical vertebra HCC ESR COM Q

√x7th S12.8 Fracture of other parts of neck HCC ESR COM Q

Fracture of hyoid bone
Fracture of larynx
Fracture of thyroid cartilage
Fracture of trachea

The appropriate 7th character is to be added to code S12.8.
A initial encounter
D subsequent encounter
S sequela

√x7th S12.9 Fracture of neck, unspecified HCC ESR COM Q

Fracture of cervical spine NOS
Fracture of cervical vertebra NOS
Fracture of neck NOS

The appropriate 7th character is to be added to code S12.9.
A initial encounter
D subsequent encounter
S sequela

√4th **S13 Dislocation and sprain of joints and ligaments at neck level**

INCLUDES avulsion of joint or ligament at neck level
laceration of cartilage, joint or ligament at neck level
sprain of cartilage, joint or ligament at neck level
traumatic hemarthrosis of joint or ligament at neck level
traumatic rupture of joint or ligament at neck level
traumatic subluxation of joint or ligament at neck level
traumatic tear of joint or ligament at neck level

Code also any associated open wound

EXCLUDES 2 *strain of muscle or tendon at neck level (S16.1)*

The appropriate 7th character is to be added to each code from category S13.
A initial encounter
D subsequent encounter
S sequela

√x7th S13.0 Traumatic rupture of cervical intervertebral disc

EXCLUDES 1 *rupture or displacement (nontraumatic) of cervical intervertebral disc NOS (M50.-)*

√5th S13.1 Subluxation and dislocation of cervical vertebrae

Code also any associated:
open wound of neck (S11.-)
spinal cord injury (S14.1-)

EXCLUDES 2 *fracture of cervical vertebrae (S12.0-S12.3-)*

√6th S13.10 Subluxation and dislocation of unspecified cervical vertebrae

√7th S13.100 Subluxation of unspecified cervical vertebrae

√7th S13.101 Dislocation of unspecified cervical vertebrae

Chapter 19. Injury, Poisoning and Certain Other Consequences of External Causes

S12.331–S13.101

√6th S13.11 Subluxation and dislocation of CØ/C1 cervical vertebrae
Subluxation and dislocation of atlantooccipital joint
Subluxation and dislocation of atloidooccipital joint
Subluxation and dislocation of occipitoatloid joint
√7th S13.11Ø Subluxation of CØ/C1 cervical vertebrae
√7th S13.111 Dislocation of CØ/C1 cervical vertebrae
√6th S13.12 Subluxation and dislocation of C1/C2 cervical vertebrae
Subluxation and dislocation of atlantoaxial joint
√7th S13.12Ø Subluxation of C1/C2 cervical vertebrae
√7th S13.121 Dislocation of C1/C2 cervical vertebrae
√6th S13.13 Subluxation and dislocation of C2/C3 cervical vertebrae
√7th S13.13Ø Subluxation of C2/C3 cervical vertebrae
√7th S13.131 Dislocation of C2/C3 cervical vertebrae
√6th S13.14 Subluxation and dislocation of C3/C4 cervical vertebrae
√7th S13.14Ø Subluxation of C3/C4 cervical vertebrae
√7th S13.141 Dislocation of C3/C4 cervical vertebrae
√6th S13.15 Subluxation and dislocation of C4/C5 cervical vertebrae
√7th S13.15Ø Subluxation of C4/C5 cervical vertebrae
√7th S13.151 Dislocation of C4/C5 cervical vertebrae
√6th S13.16 Subluxation and dislocation of C5/C6 cervical vertebrae
√7th S13.16Ø Subluxation of C5/C6 cervical vertebrae
√7th S13.161 Dislocation of C5/C6 cervical vertebrae
√6th S13.17 Subluxation and dislocation of C6/C7 cervical vertebrae
√7th S13.17Ø Subluxation of C6/C7 cervical vertebrae
√7th S13.171 Dislocation of C6/C7 cervical vertebrae
√6th S13.18 Subluxation and dislocation of C7/T1 cervical vertebrae
√7th S13.18Ø Subluxation of C7/T1 cervical vertebrae
√7th S13.181 Dislocation of C7/T1 cervical vertebrae
√5th S13.2 Dislocation of other and unspecified parts of neck
√x7th S13.2Ø Dislocation of unspecified parts of neck
√x7th S13.29 Dislocation of other parts of neck
√x7th S13.4 Sprain of ligaments of cervical spine
Sprain of anterior longitudinal (ligament), cervical
Sprain of atlanto-axial (joints)
Sprain of atlanto-occipital (joints)
Whiplash injury of cervical spine
√x7th S13.5 Sprain of thyroid region
Sprain of cricoarytenoid (joint) (ligament)
Sprain of cricothyroid (joint) (ligament)
Sprain of thyroid cartilage
√x7th S13.8 Sprain of joints and ligaments of other parts of neck
√x7th S13.9 Sprain of joints and ligaments of unspecified parts of neck

√4th **S14 Injury of nerves and spinal cord at neck level**

NOTE Code to highest level of cervical cord injury

Code also any associated:
fracture of cervical vertebra (S12.Ø- — S12.6.-)
open wound of neck (S11.-)
transient paralysis (R29.5)

AHA: 2024,2Q,23

The appropriate 7th character is to be added to each code from category S14.
A initial encounter
D subsequent encounter
S sequela

√x7th S14.Ø Concussion and edema of cervical spinal cord HCC ESR COM
√5th S14.1 Other and unspecified injuries of cervical spinal cord
√6th S14.1Ø Unspecified injury of cervical spinal cord
√7th S14.1Ø1 Unspecified injury at C1 level of cervical spinal cord HCC ESR COM
√7th S14.1Ø2 Unspecified injury at C2 level of cervical spinal cord HCC ESR COM
√7th S14.1Ø3 Unspecified injury at C3 level of cervical spinal cord HCC ESR COM
√7th S14.1Ø4 Unspecified injury at C4 level of cervical spinal cord HCC ESR COM
√7th S14.1Ø5 Unspecified injury at C5 level of cervical spinal cord HCC ESR COM
√7th S14.1Ø6 Unspecified injury at C6 level of cervical spinal cord HCC ESR COM
√7th S14.1Ø7 Unspecified injury at C7 level of cervical spinal cord HCC ESR COM
√7th S14.1Ø8 Unspecified injury at C8 level of cervical spinal cord HCC ESR COM
√7th S14.1Ø9 Unspecified injury at unspecified level of cervical spinal cord HCC ESR COM
Injury of cervical spinal cord NOS
√6th S14.11 Complete lesion of cervical spinal cord
√7th S14.111 Complete lesion at C1 level of cervical spinal cord HCC ESR COM
√7th S14.112 Complete lesion at C2 level of cervical spinal cord HCC ESR COM
√7th S14.113 Complete lesion at C3 level of cervical spinal cord HCC ESR COM
√7th S14.114 Complete lesion at C4 level of cervical spinal cord HCC ESR COM
√7th S14.115 Complete lesion at C5 level of cervical spinal cord HCC ESR COM
√7th S14.116 Complete lesion at C6 level of cervical spinal cord HCC ESR COM
√7th S14.117 Complete lesion at C7 level of cervical spinal cord HCC ESR COM
√7th S14.118 Complete lesion at C8 level of cervical spinal cord HCC ESR COM
√7th S14.119 Complete lesion at unspecified level of cervical spinal cord HCC ESR COM
√6th S14.12 Central cord syndrome of cervical spinal cord
√7th S14.121 Central cord syndrome at C1 level of cervical spinal cord HCC ESR COM
√7th S14.122 Central cord syndrome at C2 level of cervical spinal cord HCC ESR COM
√7th S14.123 Central cord syndrome at C3 level of cervical spinal cord HCC ESR COM
√7th S14.124 Central cord syndrome at C4 level of cervical spinal cord HCC ESR COM
√7th S14.125 Central cord syndrome at C5 level of cervical spinal cord HCC ESR COM
√7th S14.126 Central cord syndrome at C6 level of cervical spinal cord HCC ESR COM
√7th S14.127 Central cord syndrome at C7 level of cervical spinal cord HCC ESR COM
√7th S14.128 Central cord syndrome at C8 level of cervical spinal cord HCC ESR COM
√7th S14.129 Central cord syndrome at unspecified level of cervical spinal cord HCC ESR COM
√6th S14.13 Anterior cord syndrome of cervical spinal cord
√7th S14.131 Anterior cord syndrome at C1 level of cervical spinal cord HCC ESR COM
√7th S14.132 Anterior cord syndrome at C2 level of cervical spinal cord HCC ESR COM
√7th S14.133 Anterior cord syndrome at C3 level of cervical spinal cord HCC ESR COM
√7th S14.134 Anterior cord syndrome at C4 level of cervical spinal cord HCC ESR COM
√7th S14.135 Anterior cord syndrome at C5 level of cervical spinal cord HCC ESR COM
√7th S14.136 Anterior cord syndrome at C6 level of cervical spinal cord HCC ESR COM
√7th S14.137 Anterior cord syndrome at C7 level of cervical spinal cord HCC ESR COM
√7th S14.138 Anterior cord syndrome at C8 level of cervical spinal cord HCC ESR COM
√7th S14.139 Anterior cord syndrome at unspecified level of cervical spinal cord HCC ESR COM
√6th S14.14 Brown-Sequard syndrome of cervical spinal cord
√7th S14.141 Brown-Sequard syndrome at C1 level of cervical spinal cord HCC ESR COM
√7th S14.142 Brown-Sequard syndrome at C2 level of cervical spinal cord HCC ESR COM
√7th S14.143 Brown-Sequard syndrome at C3 level of cervical spinal cord HCC ESR COM
√7th S14.144 Brown-Sequard syndrome at C4 level of cervical spinal cord HCC ESR COM

✓7th S14.145 Brown-Sequard syndrome at C5 level of cervical spinal cord HCC ESR COM
✓7th S14.146 Brown-Sequard syndrome at C6 level of cervical spinal cord HCC ESR COM
✓7th S14.147 Brown-Sequard syndrome at C7 level of cervical spinal cord HCC ESR COM
✓7th S14.148 Brown-Sequard syndrome at C8 level of cervical spinal cord HCC ESR COM
✓7th S14.149 Brown-Sequard syndrome at unspecified level of cervical spinal cord HCC ESR COM

✓6th S14.15 Other incomplete lesions of cervical spinal cord
Incomplete lesion of cervical spinal cord NOS
Posterior cord syndrome of cervical spinal cord
✓7th S14.151 Other incomplete lesion at C1 level of cervical spinal cord HCC ESR COM
✓7th S14.152 Other incomplete lesion at C2 level of cervical spinal cord HCC ESR COM
✓7th S14.153 Other incomplete lesion at C3 level of cervical spinal cord HCC ESR COM
✓7th S14.154 Other incomplete lesion at C4 level of cervical spinal cord HCC ESR COM
✓7th S14.155 Other incomplete lesion at C5 level of cervical spinal cord HCC ESR COM
✓7th S14.156 Other incomplete lesion at C6 level of cervical spinal cord HCC ESR COM
✓7th S14.157 Other incomplete lesion at C7 level of cervical spinal cord HCC ESR COM
✓7th S14.158 Other incomplete lesion at C8 level of cervical spinal cord HCC ESR COM
✓7th S14.159 Other incomplete lesion at unspecified level of cervical spinal cord HCC ESR COM

✓x7th S14.2 Injury of nerve root of cervical spine
✓x7th S14.3 Injury of brachial plexus
✓x7th S14.4 Injury of peripheral nerves of neck
✓x7th S14.5 Injury of cervical sympathetic nerves
✓x7th S14.8 Injury of other specified nerves of neck
✓x7th S14.9 Injury of unspecified nerves of neck

## ✓4th S15 Injury of blood vessels at neck level

Code also any associated open wound (S11.-)

The appropriate 7th character is to be added to each code from category S15.
A initial encounter
D subsequent encounter
S sequela

✓5th S15.0 Injury of carotid artery of neck
Injury of carotid artery (common) (external) (internal, extracranial portion)
Injury of carotid artery NOS
EXCLUDES 1 *injury of internal carotid artery, intracranial portion (S06.8)*

✓6th S15.00 Unspecified injury of carotid artery
✓7th S15.001 Unspecified injury of right carotid artery
✓7th S15.002 Unspecified injury of left carotid artery
✓7th S15.009 Unspecified injury of unspecified carotid artery

✓6th S15.01 Minor laceration of carotid artery
Incomplete transection of carotid artery
Laceration of carotid artery NOS
Superficial laceration of carotid artery
✓7th S15.011 Minor laceration of right carotid artery
✓7th S15.012 Minor laceration of left carotid artery
✓7th S15.019 Minor laceration of unspecified carotid artery

✓6th S15.02 Major laceration of carotid artery
Complete transection of carotid artery
Traumatic rupture of carotid artery
✓7th S15.021 Major laceration of right carotid artery
✓7th S15.022 Major laceration of left carotid artery
✓7th S15.029 Major laceration of unspecified carotid artery

✓6th S15.09 Other specified injury of carotid artery
✓7th S15.091 Other specified injury of right carotid artery
✓7th S15.092 Other specified injury of left carotid artery
✓7th S15.099 Other specified injury of unspecified carotid artery

✓5th S15.1 Injury of vertebral artery

✓6th S15.10 Unspecified injury of vertebral artery
✓7th S15.101 Unspecified injury of right vertebral artery
✓7th S15.102 Unspecified injury of left vertebral artery
✓7th S15.109 Unspecified injury of unspecified vertebral artery

✓6th S15.11 Minor laceration of vertebral artery
Incomplete transection of vertebral artery
Laceration of vertebral artery NOS
Superficial laceration of vertebral artery
✓7th S15.111 Minor laceration of right vertebral artery
✓7th S15.112 Minor laceration of left vertebral artery
✓7th S15.119 Minor laceration of unspecified vertebral artery

✓6th S15.12 Major laceration of vertebral artery
Complete transection of vertebral artery
Traumatic rupture of vertebral artery
✓7th S15.121 Major laceration of right vertebral artery
✓7th S15.122 Major laceration of left vertebral artery
✓7th S15.129 Major laceration of unspecified vertebral artery

✓6th S15.19 Other specified injury of vertebral artery
✓7th S15.191 Other specified injury of right vertebral artery
✓7th S15.192 Other specified injury of left vertebral artery
✓7th S15.199 Other specified injury of unspecified vertebral artery

✓5th S15.2 Injury of external jugular vein

✓6th S15.20 Unspecified injury of external jugular vein
✓7th S15.201 Unspecified injury of right external jugular vein
✓7th S15.202 Unspecified injury of left external jugular vein
✓7th S15.209 Unspecified injury of unspecified external jugular vein

✓6th S15.21 Minor laceration of external jugular vein
Incomplete transection of external jugular vein
Laceration of external jugular vein NOS
Superficial laceration of external jugular vein
✓7th S15.211 Minor laceration of right external jugular vein
✓7th S15.212 Minor laceration of left external jugular vein
✓7th S15.219 Minor laceration of unspecified external jugular vein

✓6th S15.22 Major laceration of external jugular vein
Complete transection of external jugular vein
Traumatic rupture of external jugular vein
✓7th S15.221 Major laceration of right external jugular vein
✓7th S15.222 Major laceration of left external jugular vein
✓7th S15.229 Major laceration of unspecified external jugular vein

✓6th S15.29 Other specified injury of external jugular vein
✓7th S15.291 Other specified injury of right external jugular vein
✓7th S15.292 Other specified injury of left external jugular vein
✓7th S15.299 Other specified injury of unspecified external jugular vein

✓5th S15.3 Injury of internal jugular vein

✓6th S15.30 Unspecified injury of internal jugular vein
✓7th S15.301 Unspecified injury of right internal jugular vein
✓7th S15.302 Unspecified injury of left internal jugular vein
✓7th S15.309 Unspecified injury of unspecified internal jugular vein

✓6th S15.31 Minor laceration of internal jugular vein
Incomplete transection of internal jugular vein
Laceration of internal jugular vein NOS
Superficial laceration of internal jugular vein
✓7th S15.311 Minor laceration of right internal jugular vein

√7th **S15.312 Minor laceration of left internal jugular vein**

√7th **S15.319 Minor laceration of unspecified internal jugular vein**

√6th **S15.32 Major laceration of internal jugular vein**

Complete transection of internal jugular vein
Traumatic rupture of internal jugular vein

√7th **S15.321 Major laceration of right internal jugular vein**

√7th **S15.322 Major laceration of left internal jugular vein**

√7th **S15.329 Major laceration of unspecified internal jugular vein**

√6th **S15.39 Other specified injury of internal jugular vein**

√7th **S15.391 Other specified injury of right internal jugular vein**

√7th **S15.392 Other specified injury of left internal jugular vein**

√7th **S15.399 Other specified injury of unspecified internal jugular vein**

√x7th **S15.8 Injury of other specified blood vessels at neck level**

√x7th **S15.9 Injury of unspecified blood vessel at neck level**

√4th **S16 Injury of muscle, fascia and tendon at neck level**

Code also any associated open wound (S11.-)

EXCLUDES 2 *sprain of joint or ligament at neck level (S13.9)*

The appropriate 7th character is to be added to each code from category S16.
A initial encounter
D subsequent encounter
S sequela

√x7th **S16.1 Strain of muscle, fascia and tendon at neck level**

√x7th **S16.2 Laceration of muscle, fascia and tendon at neck level**

√x7th **S16.8 Other specified injury of muscle, fascia and tendon at neck level**

√x7th **S16.9 Unspecified injury of muscle, fascia and tendon at neck level**

√4th **S17 Crushing injury of neck**

Use additional code for all associated injuries, such as:
injury of blood vessels (S15.-)
open wound of neck (S11.-)
spinal cord injury (S14.Ø, S14.1-)
vertebral fracture (S12.Ø- — S12.3-)

The appropriate 7th character is to be added to each code from category S17.
A initial encounter
D subsequent encounter
S sequela

√x7th **S17.Ø Crushing injury of larynx and trachea**

√x7th **S17.8 Crushing injury of other specified parts of neck**

√x7th **S17.9 Crushing injury of neck, part unspecified**

√4th **S19 Other specified and unspecified injuries of neck**

The appropriate 7th character is to be added to each code from category S19.
A initial encounter
D subsequent encounter
S sequela

√5th **S19.8 Other specified injuries of neck**

√x7th **S19.8Ø Other specified injuries of unspecified part of neck**

√x7th **S19.81 Other specified injuries of larynx**

√x7th **S19.82 Other specified injuries of cervical trachea**

EXCLUDES 2 *other specified injury of thoracic trachea (S27.5-)*

√x7th **S19.83 Other specified injuries of vocal cord**

√x7th **S19.84 Other specified injuries of thyroid gland**

√x7th **S19.85 Other specified injuries of pharynx and cervical esophagus**

**AHA:** 2022,1Q,27

√x7th **S19.89 Other specified injuries of other specified part of neck**

√x7th **S19.9 Unspecified injury of neck**

## Injuries to the thorax (S2Ø-S29)

INCLUDES injuries of breast
injuries of chest (wall)
injuries of interscapular area

EXCLUDES 2 *burns and corrosions (T2Ø-T32)*
*effects of foreign body in bronchus (T17.5)*
*effects of foreign body in esophagus (T18.1)*
*effects of foreign body in lung (T17.8)*
*effects of foreign body in trachea (T17.4)*
*frostbite (T33-T34)*
*injuries of axilla*
*injuries of clavicle*
*injuries of scapular region*
*injuries of shoulder*
*insect bite or sting, venomous (T63.4)*

√4th **S2Ø Superficial injury of thorax**

**AHA:** 2020,4Q,39

The appropriate 7th character is to be added to each code from category S2Ø.
A initial encounter
D subsequent encounter
S sequela

√5th **S2Ø.Ø Contusion of breast**

√x7th **S2Ø.ØØ Contusion of breast, unspecified breast**

√x7th **S2Ø.Ø1 Contusion of right breast**

√x7th **S2Ø.Ø2 Contusion of left breast**

√5th **S2Ø.1 Other and unspecified superficial injuries of breast**

√6th **S2Ø.1Ø Unspecified superficial injuries of breast**

√7th **S2Ø.1Ø1 Unspecified superficial injuries of breast, right breast**

√7th **S2Ø.1Ø2 Unspecified superficial injuries of breast, left breast**

√7th **S2Ø.1Ø9 Unspecified superficial injuries of breast, unspecified breast**

√6th **S2Ø.11 Abrasion of breast**

√7th **S2Ø.111 Abrasion of breast, right breast**

√7th **S2Ø.112 Abrasion of breast, left breast**

√7th **S2Ø.119 Abrasion of breast, unspecified breast**

√6th **S2Ø.12 Blister (nonthermal) of breast**

√7th **S2Ø.121 Blister (nonthermal) of breast, right breast**

√7th **S2Ø.122 Blister (nonthermal) of breast, left breast**

√7th **S2Ø.129 Blister (nonthermal) of breast, unspecified breast**

√6th **S2Ø.14 External constriction of part of breast**

√7th **S2Ø.141 External constriction of part of breast, right breast**

√7th **S2Ø.142 External constriction of part of breast, left breast**

√7th **S2Ø.149 External constriction of part of breast, unspecified breast**

√6th **S2Ø.15 Superficial foreign body of breast**

Splinter in the breast

√7th **S2Ø.151 Superficial foreign body of breast, right breast**

√7th **S2Ø.152 Superficial foreign body of breast, left breast**

√7th **S2Ø.159 Superficial foreign body of breast, unspecified breast**

√6th **S2Ø.16 Insect bite (nonvenomous) of breast**

√7th **S2Ø.161 Insect bite (nonvenomous) of breast, right breast**

√7th **S2Ø.162 Insect bite (nonvenomous) of breast, left breast**

√7th **S2Ø.169 Insect bite (nonvenomous) of breast, unspecified breast**

√6th **S2Ø.17 Other superficial bite of breast**

EXCLUDES 1 *open bite of breast (S21.Ø5-)*

√7th **S2Ø.171 Other superficial bite of breast, right breast**

√7th **S2Ø.172 Other superficial bite of breast, left breast**

√7th **S2Ø.179 Other superficial bite of breast, unspecified breast**

√5th **S2Ø.2 Contusion of thorax**

√x7th **S2Ø.2Ø Contusion of thorax, unspecified**

√6th **S2Ø.21 Contusion of front wall of thorax**

√7th **S2Ø.211 Contusion of right front wall of thorax**

S20.212 Contusion of left front wall of thorax
S20.213 Contusion of bilateral front wall of thorax
S20.214 Contusion of middle front wall of thorax
S20.219 Contusion of unspecified front wall of thorax
S20.22 Contusion of back wall of thorax
S20.221 Contusion of right back wall of thorax
S20.222 Contusion of left back wall of thorax
S20.223 Contusion of bilateral back wall of thorax
S20.224 Contusion of middle back wall of thorax
S20.229 Contusion of unspecified back wall of thorax
S20.3 Other and unspecified superficial injuries of front wall of thorax
S20.30 Unspecified superficial injuries of front wall of thorax
S20.301 Unspecified superficial injuries of right front wall of thorax
S20.302 Unspecified superficial injuries of left front wall of thorax
S20.303 Unspecified superficial injuries of bilateral front wall of thorax
S20.304 Unspecified superficial injuries of middle front wall of thorax
S20.309 Unspecified superficial injuries of unspecified front wall of thorax
S20.31 Abrasion of front wall of thorax
S20.311 Abrasion of right front wall of thorax
S20.312 Abrasion of left front wall of thorax
S20.313 Abrasion of bilateral front wall of thorax
S20.314 Abrasion of middle front wall of thorax
S20.319 Abrasion of unspecified front wall of thorax
S20.32 Blister (nonthermal) of front wall of thorax
S20.321 Blister (nonthermal) of right front wall of thorax
S20.322 Blister (nonthermal) of left front wall of thorax
S20.323 Blister (nonthermal) of bilateral front wall of thorax
S20.324 Blister (nonthermal) of middle front wall of thorax
S20.329 Blister (nonthermal) of unspecified front wall of thorax
S20.34 External constriction of front wall of thorax
S20.341 External constriction of right front wall of thorax
S20.342 External constriction of left front wall of thorax
S20.343 External constriction of bilateral front wall of thorax
S20.344 External constriction of middle front wall of thorax
S20.349 External constriction of unspecified front wall of thorax
S20.35 Superficial foreign body of front wall of thorax
Splinter in front wall of thorax
S20.351 Superficial foreign body of right front wall of thorax
S20.352 Superficial foreign body of left front wall of thorax
S20.353 Superficial foreign body of bilateral front wall of thorax
S20.354 Superficial foreign body of middle front wall of thorax
S20.359 Superficial foreign body of unspecified front wall of thorax
S20.36 Insect bite (nonvenomous) of front wall of thorax
S20.361 Insect bite (nonvenomous) of right front wall of thorax
S20.362 Insect bite (nonvenomous) of left front wall of thorax
S20.363 Insect bite (nonvenomous) of bilateral front wall of thorax
S20.364 Insect bite (nonvenomous) of middle front wall of thorax
S20.369 Insect bite (nonvenomous) of unspecified front wall of thorax
S20.37 Other superficial bite of front wall of thorax
EXCLUDES 1 *open bite of front wall of thorax (S21.15)*
S20.371 Other superficial bite of right front wall of thorax
S20.372 Other superficial bite of left front wall of thorax
S20.373 Other superficial bite of bilateral front wall of thorax
S20.374 Other superficial bite of middle front wall of thorax
S20.379 Other superficial bite of unspecified front wall of thorax
S20.4 Other and unspecified superficial injuries of back wall of thorax
S20.40 Unspecified superficial injuries of back wall of thorax
S20.401 Unspecified superficial injuries of right back wall of thorax
S20.402 Unspecified superficial injuries of left back wall of thorax
S20.409 Unspecified superficial injuries of unspecified back wall of thorax
S20.41 Abrasion of back wall of thorax
S20.411 Abrasion of right back wall of thorax
S20.412 Abrasion of left back wall of thorax
S20.419 Abrasion of unspecified back wall of thorax
S20.42 Blister (nonthermal) of back wall of thorax
S20.421 Blister (nonthermal) of right back wall of thorax
S20.422 Blister (nonthermal) of left back wall of thorax
S20.429 Blister (nonthermal) of unspecified back wall of thorax
S20.44 External constriction of back wall of thorax
S20.441 External constriction of right back wall of thorax
S20.442 External constriction of left back wall of thorax
S20.449 External constriction of unspecified back wall of thorax
S20.45 Superficial foreign body of back wall of thorax
Splinter of back wall of thorax
S20.451 Superficial foreign body of right back wall of thorax
S20.452 Superficial foreign body of left back wall of thorax
S20.459 Superficial foreign body of unspecified back wall of thorax
S20.46 Insect bite (nonvenomous) of back wall of thorax
S20.461 Insect bite (nonvenomous) of right back wall of thorax
S20.462 Insect bite (nonvenomous) of left back wall of thorax
S20.469 Insect bite (nonvenomous) of unspecified back wall of thorax
S20.47 Other superficial bite of back wall of thorax
EXCLUDES 1 *open bite of back wall of thorax (S21.25)*
S20.471 Other superficial bite of right back wall of thorax
S20.472 Other superficial bite of left back wall of thorax
S20.479 Other superficial bite of unspecified back wall of thorax
S20.9 Superficial injury of unspecified parts of thorax
EXCLUDES 1 *contusion of thorax NOS (S20.20)*
S20.90 Unspecified superficial injury of unspecified parts of thorax
Superficial injury of thoracic wall NOS
S20.91 Abrasion of unspecified parts of thorax
S20.92 Blister (nonthermal) of unspecified parts of thorax
S20.94 External constriction of unspecified parts of thorax
S20.95 Superficial foreign body of unspecified parts of thorax
Splinter in thorax NOS
S20.96 Insect bite (nonvenomous) of unspecified parts of thorax
S20.97 Other superficial bite of unspecified parts of thorax
EXCLUDES 1 *open bite of thorax NOS (S21.95)*

4th **S21 Open wound of thorax**

Code also any associated injury, such as:
- injury of heart (S26.-)
- injury of intrathoracic organs (S27.-)
- rib fracture (S22.3-, S22.4-)
- spinal cord injury (S24.Ø-, S24.1-)
- traumatic hemopneumothorax (S27.3)
- traumatic hemothorax (S27.1)
- traumatic pneumothorax (S27.Ø)
- wound infection

EXCLUDES 1 *traumatic amputation (partial) of thorax (S28.1)*

The appropriate 7th character is to be added to each code from category S21.
- A initial encounter
- D subsequent encounter
- S sequela

5th **S21.Ø Open wound of breast**
- 6th **S21.ØØ Unspecified open wound of breast**
  - 7th **S21.ØØ1 Unspecified open wound of right breast**
  - 7th **S21.ØØ2 Unspecified open wound of left breast**
  - 7th **S21.ØØ9 Unspecified open wound of unspecified breast**
- 6th **S21.Ø1 Laceration without foreign body of breast**
  - 7th **S21.Ø11 Laceration without foreign body of right breast**
  - 7th **S21.Ø12 Laceration without foreign body of left breast**
  - 7th **S21.Ø19 Laceration without foreign body of unspecified breast**
- 6th **S21.Ø2 Laceration with foreign body of breast**
  - 7th **S21.Ø21 Laceration with foreign body of right breast**
  - 7th **S21.Ø22 Laceration with foreign body of left breast**
  - 7th **S21.Ø29 Laceration with foreign body of unspecified breast**
- 6th **S21.Ø3 Puncture wound without foreign body of breast**
  - 7th **S21.Ø31 Puncture wound without foreign body of right breast**
  - 7th **S21.Ø32 Puncture wound without foreign body of left breast**
  - 7th **S21.Ø39 Puncture wound without foreign body of unspecified breast**
- 6th **S21.Ø4 Puncture wound with foreign body of breast**
  - 7th **S21.Ø41 Puncture wound with foreign body of right breast**
  - 7th **S21.Ø42 Puncture wound with foreign body of left breast**
  - 7th **S21.Ø49 Puncture wound with foreign body of unspecified breast**
- 6th **S21.Ø5 Open bite of breast**

  Bite of breast NOS

  EXCLUDES 1 *superficial bite of breast (S2Ø.17)*
  - 7th **S21.Ø51 Open bite of right breast**
  - 7th **S21.Ø52 Open bite of left breast**
  - 7th **S21.Ø59 Open bite of unspecified breast**

5th **S21.1 Open wound of front wall of thorax without penetration into thoracic cavity**

Open wound of chest without penetration into thoracic cavity
- 6th **S21.1Ø Unspecified open wound of front wall of thorax without penetration into thoracic cavity**
  - 7th **S21.1Ø1 Unspecified open wound of right front wall of thorax without penetration into thoracic cavity**
  - 7th **S21.1Ø2 Unspecified open wound of left front wall of thorax without penetration into thoracic cavity**
  - 7th **S21.1Ø9 Unspecified open wound of unspecified front wall of thorax without penetration into thoracic cavity**
- 6th **S21.11 Laceration without foreign body of front wall of thorax without penetration into thoracic cavity**
  - 7th **S21.111 Laceration without foreign body of right front wall of thorax without penetration into thoracic cavity**
  - 7th **S21.112 Laceration without foreign body of left front wall of thorax without penetration into thoracic cavity**
  - 7th **S21.119 Laceration without foreign body of unspecified front wall of thorax without penetration into thoracic cavity**
- 6th **S21.12 Laceration with foreign body of front wall of thorax without penetration into thoracic cavity**
  - 7th **S21.121 Laceration with foreign body of right front wall of thorax without penetration into thoracic cavity**
  - 7th **S21.122 Laceration with foreign body of left front wall of thorax without penetration into thoracic cavity**
  - 7th **S21.129 Laceration with foreign body of unspecified front wall of thorax without penetration into thoracic cavity**
- 6th **S21.13 Puncture wound without foreign body of front wall of thorax without penetration into thoracic cavity**
  - 7th **S21.131 Puncture wound without foreign body of right front wall of thorax without penetration into thoracic cavity**
  - 7th **S21.132 Puncture wound without foreign body of left front wall of thorax without penetration into thoracic cavity**
  - 7th **S21.139 Puncture wound without foreign body of unspecified front wall of thorax without penetration into thoracic cavity**
- 6th **S21.14 Puncture wound with foreign body of front wall of thorax without penetration into thoracic cavity**
  - 7th **S21.141 Puncture wound with foreign body of right front wall of thorax without penetration into thoracic cavity**
  - 7th **S21.142 Puncture wound with foreign body of left front wall of thorax without penetration into thoracic cavity**
  - 7th **S21.149 Puncture wound with foreign body of unspecified front wall of thorax without penetration into thoracic cavity**
- 6th **S21.15 Open bite of front wall of thorax without penetration into thoracic cavity**

  Bite of front wall of thorax NOS

  EXCLUDES 1 *superficial bite of front wall of thorax (S2Ø.37)*
  - 7th **S21.151 Open bite of right front wall of thorax without penetration into thoracic cavity**
  - 7th **S21.152 Open bite of left front wall of thorax without penetration into thoracic cavity**
  - 7th **S21.159 Open bite of unspecified front wall of thorax without penetration into thoracic cavity**

5th **S21.2 Open wound of back wall of thorax without penetration into thoracic cavity**
- 6th **S21.2Ø Unspecified open wound of back wall of thorax without penetration into thoracic cavity**
  - 7th **S21.2Ø1 Unspecified open wound of right back wall of thorax without penetration into thoracic cavity**
  - 7th **S21.2Ø2 Unspecified open wound of left back wall of thorax without penetration into thoracic cavity**
  - 7th **S21.2Ø9 Unspecified open wound of unspecified back wall of thorax without penetration into thoracic cavity**
- 6th **S21.21 Laceration without foreign body of back wall of thorax without penetration into thoracic cavity**
  - 7th **S21.211 Laceration without foreign body of right back wall of thorax without penetration into thoracic cavity**
  - 7th **S21.212 Laceration without foreign body of left back wall of thorax without penetration into thoracic cavity**
  - 7th **S21.219 Laceration without foreign body of unspecified back wall of thorax without penetration into thoracic cavity**
- 6th **S21.22 Laceration with foreign body of back wall of thorax without penetration into thoracic cavity**
  - 7th **S21.221 Laceration with foreign body of right back wall of thorax without penetration into thoracic cavity**
  - 7th **S21.222 Laceration with foreign body of left back wall of thorax without penetration into thoracic cavity**
  - 7th **S21.229 Laceration with foreign body of unspecified back wall of thorax without penetration into thoracic cavity**

✓6th S21.23 Puncture wound without foreign body of back wall of thorax without penetration into thoracic cavity
- ✓7th S21.231 Puncture wound without foreign body of right back wall of thorax without penetration into thoracic cavity
- ✓7th S21.232 Puncture wound without foreign body of left back wall of thorax without penetration into thoracic cavity
- ✓7th S21.239 Puncture wound without foreign body of unspecified back wall of thorax without penetration into thoracic cavity

✓6th S21.24 Puncture wound with foreign body of back wall of thorax without penetration into thoracic cavity
- ✓7th S21.241 Puncture wound with foreign body of right back wall of thorax without penetration into thoracic cavity
- ✓7th S21.242 Puncture wound with foreign body of left back wall of thorax without penetration into thoracic cavity
- ✓7th S21.249 Puncture wound with foreign body of unspecified back wall of thorax without penetration into thoracic cavity

✓6th S21.25 Open bite of back wall of thorax without penetration into thoracic cavity

Bite of back wall of thorax NOS

EXCLUDES 1 *superficial bite of back wall of thorax (S20.47)*
- ✓7th S21.251 Open bite of right back wall of thorax without penetration into thoracic cavity
- ✓7th S21.252 Open bite of left back wall of thorax without penetration into thoracic cavity
- ✓7th S21.259 Open bite of unspecified back wall of thorax without penetration into thoracic cavity

✓5th S21.3 Open wound of front wall of thorax with penetration into thoracic cavity

Open wound of chest with penetration into thoracic cavity

✓6th S21.30 Unspecified open wound of front wall of thorax with penetration into thoracic cavity
- ✓7th S21.301 Unspecified open wound of right front wall of thorax with penetration into thoracic cavity
- ✓7th S21.302 Unspecified open wound of left front wall of thorax with penetration into thoracic cavity
- ✓7th S21.309 Unspecified open wound of unspecified front wall of thorax with penetration into thoracic cavity

✓6th S21.31 Laceration without foreign body of front wall of thorax with penetration into thoracic cavity
- ✓7th S21.311 Laceration without foreign body of right front wall of thorax with penetration into thoracic cavity
- ✓7th S21.312 Laceration without foreign body of left front wall of thorax with penetration into thoracic cavity
- ✓7th S21.319 Laceration without foreign body of unspecified front wall of thorax with penetration into thoracic cavity

✓6th S21.32 Laceration with foreign body of front wall of thorax with penetration into thoracic cavity
- ✓7th S21.321 Laceration with foreign body of right front wall of thorax with penetration into thoracic cavity
- ✓7th S21.322 Laceration with foreign body of left front wall of thorax with penetration into thoracic cavity
- ✓7th S21.329 Laceration with foreign body of unspecified front wall of thorax with penetration into thoracic cavity

✓6th S21.33 Puncture wound without foreign body of front wall of thorax with penetration into thoracic cavity
- ✓7th S21.331 Puncture wound without foreign body of right front wall of thorax with penetration into thoracic cavity
- ✓7th S21.332 Puncture wound without foreign body of left front wall of thorax with penetration into thoracic cavity
- ✓7th S21.339 Puncture wound without foreign body of unspecified front wall of thorax with penetration into thoracic cavity

✓6th S21.34 Puncture wound with foreign body of front wall of thorax with penetration into thoracic cavity
- ✓7th S21.341 Puncture wound with foreign body of right front wall of thorax with penetration into thoracic cavity
- ✓7th S21.342 Puncture wound with foreign body of left front wall of thorax with penetration into thoracic cavity
- ✓7th S21.349 Puncture wound with foreign body of unspecified front wall of thorax with penetration into thoracic cavity

✓6th S21.35 Open bite of front wall of thorax with penetration into thoracic cavity

EXCLUDES 1 *superficial bite of front wall of thorax (S20.37)*
- ✓7th S21.351 Open bite of right front wall of thorax with penetration into thoracic cavity
- ✓7th S21.352 Open bite of left front wall of thorax with penetration into thoracic cavity
- ✓7th S21.359 Open bite of unspecified front wall of thorax with penetration into thoracic cavity

✓5th S21.4 Open wound of back wall of thorax with penetration into thoracic cavity

✓6th S21.40 Unspecified open wound of back wall of thorax with penetration into thoracic cavity
- ✓7th S21.401 Unspecified open wound of right back wall of thorax with penetration into thoracic cavity
- ✓7th S21.402 Unspecified open wound of left back wall of thorax with penetration into thoracic cavity
- ✓7th S21.409 Unspecified open wound of unspecified back wall of thorax with penetration into thoracic cavity

✓6th S21.41 Laceration without foreign body of back wall of thorax with penetration into thoracic cavity
- ✓7th S21.411 Laceration without foreign body of right back wall of thorax with penetration into thoracic cavity
- ✓7th S21.412 Laceration without foreign body of left back wall of thorax with penetration into thoracic cavity
- ✓7th S21.419 Laceration without foreign body of unspecified back wall of thorax with penetration into thoracic cavity

✓6th S21.42 Laceration with foreign body of back wall of thorax with penetration into thoracic cavity
- ✓7th S21.421 Laceration with foreign body of right back wall of thorax with penetration into thoracic cavity
- ✓7th S21.422 Laceration with foreign body of left back wall of thorax with penetration into thoracic cavity
- ✓7th S21.429 Laceration with foreign body of unspecified back wall of thorax with penetration into thoracic cavity

✓6th S21.43 Puncture wound without foreign body of back wall of thorax with penetration into thoracic cavity
- ✓7th S21.431 Puncture wound without foreign body of right back wall of thorax with penetration into thoracic cavity
- ✓7th S21.432 Puncture wound without foreign body of left back wall of thorax with penetration into thoracic cavity
- ✓7th S21.439 Puncture wound without foreign body of unspecified back wall of thorax with penetration into thoracic cavity

✓6th S21.44 Puncture wound with foreign body of back wall of thorax with penetration into thoracic cavity
- ✓7th S21.441 Puncture wound with foreign body of right back wall of thorax with penetration into thoracic cavity
- ✓7th S21.442 Puncture wound with foreign body of left back wall of thorax with penetration into thoracic cavity
- ✓7th S21.449 Puncture wound with foreign body of unspecified back wall of thorax with penetration into thoracic cavity

√6th **S21.45 Open bite of back wall of thorax with penetration into thoracic cavity**
Bite of back wall of thorax NOS
EXCLUDES 1 *superficial bite of back wall of thorax (S20.47)*
√7th **S21.451 Open bite of right back wall of thorax with penetration into thoracic cavity**
√7th **S21.452 Open bite of left back wall of thorax with penetration into thoracic cavity**
√7th **S21.459 Open bite of unspecified back wall of thorax with penetration into thoracic cavity**

√5th **S21.9 Open wound of unspecified part of thorax**
Open wound of thoracic wall NOS
√x7th **S21.90 Unspecified open wound of unspecified part of thorax**
√x7th **S21.91 Laceration without foreign body of unspecified part of thorax**
√x7th **S21.92 Laceration with foreign body of unspecified part of thorax**
√x7th **S21.93 Puncture wound without foreign body of unspecified part of thorax**
√x7th **S21.94 Puncture wound with foreign body of unspecified part of thorax**
√x7th **S21.95 Open bite of unspecified part of thorax**
EXCLUDES 1 *superficial bite of thorax (S20.97)*

√4th **S22 Fracture of rib(s), sternum and thoracic spine**
NOTE A fracture not indicated as displaced or nondisplaced should be coded to displaced
A fracture not indicated as open or closed should be coded to closed
INCLUDES fracture of thoracic neural arch
fracture of thoracic spinous process
fracture of thoracic transverse process
fracture of thoracic vertebra
fracture of thoracic vertebral arch
▶Code first, if applicable, spinal cord injury (S24.0-, S24.1-)◀
Code also, if applicable, any associated condition such as:
~~spinal cord injury (S24.0-, S24.1-)~~
injury of intrathoracic organ (S27.-)
traumatic hemopneumothorax (S27.2)
traumatic hemothorax (S27.1-)
traumatic pneumothorax (S27.0)
EXCLUDES 1 *transection of thorax (S28.1)*
EXCLUDES 2 *fracture of clavicle (S42.0-)*
*fracture of scapula (S42.1-)*
**AHA:** 2021,1Q,6; 2018,2Q,12; 2015,3Q,37-39

The appropriate 7th character is to be added to each code from category S22.
A initial encounter for closed fracture
B initial encounter for open fracture
D subsequent encounter for fracture with routine healing
G subsequent encounter for fracture with delayed healing
K subsequent encounter for fracture with nonunion
S sequela

√5th **S22.0 Fracture of thoracic vertebra**
√6th **S22.00 Fracture of unspecified thoracic vertebra**
√7th **S22.000 Wedge compression fracture of unspecified thoracic vertebra** HCC ESR COM Q
√7th **S22.001 Stable burst fracture of unspecified thoracic vertebra** HCC ESR COM Q
√7th **S22.002 Unstable burst fracture of unspecified thoracic vertebra** HCC ESR COM Q
√7th **S22.008 Other fracture of unspecified thoracic vertebra** HCC ESR COM Q
√7th **S22.009 Unspecified fracture of unspecified thoracic vertebra** HCC ESR COM Q
√6th **S22.01 Fracture of first thoracic vertebra**
√7th **S22.010 Wedge compression fracture of first thoracic vertebra** HCC ESR COM Q
√7th **S22.011 Stable burst fracture of first thoracic vertebra** HCC ESR COM Q
√7th **S22.012 Unstable burst fracture of first thoracic vertebra** HCC ESR COM Q
√7th **S22.018 Other fracture of first thoracic vertebra** HCC ESR COM Q
√7th **S22.019 Unspecified fracture of first thoracic vertebra** HCC ESR COM Q
√6th **S22.02 Fracture of second thoracic vertebra**
√7th **S22.020 Wedge compression fracture of second thoracic vertebra** HCC ESR COM Q
√7th **S22.021 Stable burst fracture of second thoracic vertebra** HCC ESR COM Q
√7th **S22.022 Unstable burst fracture of second thoracic vertebra** HCC ESR COM Q
√7th **S22.028 Other fracture of second thoracic vertebra** HCC ESR COM Q
√7th **S22.029 Unspecified fracture of second thoracic vertebra** HCC ESR COM Q
√6th **S22.03 Fracture of third thoracic vertebra**
√7th **S22.030 Wedge compression fracture of third thoracic vertebra** HCC ESR COM Q
√7th **S22.031 Stable burst fracture of third thoracic vertebra** HCC ESR COM Q
√7th **S22.032 Unstable burst fracture of third thoracic vertebra** HCC ESR COM Q
√7th **S22.038 Other fracture of third thoracic vertebra** HCC ESR COM Q
√7th **S22.039 Unspecified fracture of third thoracic vertebra** HCC ESR COM Q
√6th **S22.04 Fracture of fourth thoracic vertebra**
√7th **S22.040 Wedge compression fracture of fourth thoracic vertebra** HCC ESR COM Q
√7th **S22.041 Stable burst fracture of fourth thoracic vertebra** HCC ESR COM Q
√7th **S22.042 Unstable burst fracture of fourth thoracic vertebra** HCC ESR COM Q
√7th **S22.048 Other fracture of fourth thoracic vertebra** HCC ESR COM Q
√7th **S22.049 Unspecified fracture of fourth thoracic vertebra** HCC ESR COM Q
√6th **S22.05 Fracture of T5-T6 vertebra**
√7th **S22.050 Wedge compression fracture of T5-T6 vertebra** HCC ESR COM Q
√7th **S22.051 Stable burst fracture of T5-T6 vertebra** HCC ESR COM Q
√7th **S22.052 Unstable burst fracture of T5-T6 vertebra** HCC ESR COM Q
√7th **S22.058 Other fracture of T5-T6 vertebra** HCC ESR COM Q
√7th **S22.059 Unspecified fracture of T5-T6 vertebra** HCC ESR COM Q
√6th **S22.06 Fracture of T7-T8 vertebra**
√7th **S22.060 Wedge compression fracture of T7-T8 vertebra** HCC ESR COM Q
√7th **S22.061 Stable burst fracture of T7-T8 vertebra** HCC ESR COM Q
√7th **S22.062 Unstable burst fracture of T7-T8 vertebra** HCC ESR COM Q
√7th **S22.068 Other fracture of T7-T8 thoracic vertebra** HCC ESR COM Q
√7th **S22.069 Unspecified fracture of T7-T8 vertebra** HCC ESR COM Q
√6th **S22.07 Fracture of T9-T10 vertebra**
√7th **S22.070 Wedge compression fracture of T9-T10 vertebra** HCC ESR COM Q
√7th **S22.071 Stable burst fracture of T9-T10 vertebra** HCC ESR COM Q
√7th **S22.072 Unstable burst fracture of T9-T10 vertebra** HCC ESR COM Q
√7th **S22.078 Other fracture of T9-T10 vertebra** HCC ESR COM Q
√7th **S22.079 Unspecified fracture of T9-T10 vertebra** HCC ESR COM Q
√6th **S22.08 Fracture of T11-T12 vertebra**
√7th **S22.080 Wedge compression fracture of T11-T12 vertebra** HCC ESR COM Q
√7th **S22.081 Stable burst fracture of T11-T12 vertebra** HCC ESR COM Q
√7th **S22.082 Unstable burst fracture of T11-T12 vertebra** HCC ESR COM Q
√7th **S22.088 Other fracture of T11-T12 vertebra** HCC ESR COM Q

✓7th **S22.089** Unspecified fracture of T11-T12 vertebra HCC ESR COM Q
AHA: 2024,4Q,19

✓5th **S22.2** Fracture of sternum
DEF: Break in flat bone (breast bone) in the anterior thorax caused by blunt trauma to the anterior chest.

✓x7th **S22.20** Unspecified fracture of sternum Q
✓x7th **S22.21** Fracture of manubrium Q
✓x7th **S22.22** Fracture of body of sternum Q
✓x7th **S22.23** Sternal manubrial dissociation Q
✓x7th **S22.24** Fracture of xiphoid process Q

✓5th **S22.3** Fracture of one rib
AHA: 2021,1Q,5

✓x7th **S22.31** Fracture of one rib, right side Q
✓x7th **S22.32** Fracture of one rib, left side Q
✓x7th **S22.39** Fracture of one rib, unspecified side Q

✓5th **S22.4** Multiple fractures of ribs
Fractures of two or more ribs
EXCLUDES 1 *flail chest (S22.5-)*
AHA: 2021,1Q,5

✓x7th **S22.41** Multiple fractures of ribs, right side Q
✓x7th **S22.42** Multiple fractures of ribs, left side Q
✓x7th **S22.43** Multiple fractures of ribs, bilateral Q
✓x7th **S22.49** Multiple fractures of ribs, unspecified side Q

✓x7th **S22.5** Flail chest Q
✓x7th **S22.9** Fracture of bony thorax, part unspecified Q

✓4th **S23 Dislocation and sprain of joints and ligaments of thorax**
INCLUDES avulsion of joint or ligament of thorax
laceration of cartilage, joint or ligament of thorax
sprain of cartilage, joint or ligament of thorax
traumatic hemarthrosis of joint or ligament of thorax
traumatic rupture of joint or ligament of thorax
traumatic subluxation of joint or ligament of thorax
traumatic tear of joint or ligament of thorax
Code also any associated open wound
EXCLUDES 2 *dislocation, sprain of sternoclavicular joint (S43.2, S43.6)*
*strain of muscle or tendon of thorax (S29.01-)*

The appropriate 7th character is to be added to each code from category S23.
A initial encounter
D subsequent encounter
S sequela

✓x7th **S23.0** Traumatic rupture of thoracic intervertebral disc
EXCLUDES 1 *rupture or displacement (nontraumatic) of thoracic intervertebral disc NOS (M51.- with fifth character 4)*

✓5th **S23.1** Subluxation and dislocation of thoracic vertebra
Code also any associated:
open wound of thorax (S21.-)
spinal cord injury (S24.0-, S24.1-)
EXCLUDES 2 *fracture of thoracic vertebrae (S22.0-)*

✓6th **S23.10** Subluxation and dislocation of unspecified thoracic vertebra
✓7th **S23.100** Subluxation of unspecified thoracic vertebra
✓7th **S23.101** Dislocation of unspecified thoracic vertebra

✓6th **S23.11** Subluxation and dislocation of T1/T2 thoracic vertebra
✓7th **S23.110** Subluxation of T1/T2 thoracic vertebra
✓7th **S23.111** Dislocation of T1/T2 thoracic vertebra

✓6th **S23.12** Subluxation and dislocation of T2/T3-T3/T4 thoracic vertebra
✓7th **S23.120** Subluxation of T2/T3 thoracic vertebra
✓7th **S23.121** Dislocation of T2/T3 thoracic vertebra
✓7th **S23.122** Subluxation of T3/T4 thoracic vertebra
✓7th **S23.123** Dislocation of T3/T4 thoracic vertebra

✓6th **S23.13** Subluxation and dislocation of T4/T5-T5/T6 thoracic vertebra
✓7th **S23.130** Subluxation of T4/T5 thoracic vertebra
✓7th **S23.131** Dislocation of T4/T5 thoracic vertebra
✓7th **S23.132** Subluxation of T5/T6 thoracic vertebra
✓7th **S23.133** Dislocation of T5/T6 thoracic vertebra

✓6th **S23.14** Subluxation and dislocation of T6/T7-T7/T8 thoracic vertebra
✓7th **S23.140** Subluxation of T6/T7 thoracic vertebra
✓7th **S23.141** Dislocation of T6/T7 thoracic vertebra
✓7th **S23.142** Subluxation of T7/T8 thoracic vertebra
✓7th **S23.143** Dislocation of T7/T8 thoracic vertebra

✓6th **S23.15** Subluxation and dislocation of T8/T9-T9/T10 thoracic vertebra
✓7th **S23.150** Subluxation of T8/T9 thoracic vertebra
✓7th **S23.151** Dislocation of T8/T9 thoracic vertebra
✓7th **S23.152** Subluxation of T9/T10 thoracic vertebra
✓7th **S23.153** Dislocation of T9/T10 thoracic vertebra

✓6th **S23.16** Subluxation and dislocation of T10/T11-T11/T12 thoracic vertebra
✓7th **S23.160** Subluxation of T10/T11 thoracic vertebra
✓7th **S23.161** Dislocation of T10/T11 thoracic vertebra
✓7th **S23.162** Subluxation of T11/T12 thoracic vertebra
✓7th **S23.163** Dislocation of T11/T12 thoracic vertebra

✓6th **S23.17** Subluxation and dislocation of T12/L1 thoracic vertebra
✓7th **S23.170** Subluxation of T12/L1 thoracic vertebra
✓7th **S23.171** Dislocation of T12/L1 thoracic vertebra

✓5th **S23.2** Dislocation of other and unspecified parts of thorax
✓x7th **S23.20** Dislocation of unspecified part of thorax
✓x7th **S23.29** Dislocation of other parts of thorax

✓x7th **S23.3** Sprain of ligaments of thoracic spine

✓5th **S23.4** Sprain of ribs and sternum
✓x7th **S23.41** Sprain of ribs
✓6th **S23.42** Sprain of sternum
~~S23.420 Sprain of sternoclavicular (joint) (ligament)~~
✓7th **S23.421** Sprain of chondrosternal joint
✓7th **S23.428** Other sprain of sternum
✓7th **S23.429** Unspecified sprain of sternum

✓x7th **S23.8** Sprain of other specified parts of thorax
✓x7th **S23.9** Sprain of unspecified parts of thorax

✓4th **S24 Injury of nerves and spinal cord at thorax level**
NOTE Code to highest level of thoracic spinal cord injury.
Injuries to the spinal cord (S24.0 and S24.1) refer to the cord level and not bone level injury, and can affect nerve roots at and below the level given.
Code also any associated:
fracture of thoracic vertebra (S22.0-)
open wound of thorax (S21.-)
transient paralysis (R29.5)
EXCLUDES 2 *injury of brachial plexus (S14.3)*

The appropriate 7th character is to be added to each code from category S24.
A initial encounter
D subsequent encounter
S sequela

✓x7th **S24.0** Concussion and edema of thoracic spinal cord HCC ESR COM

✓5th **S24.1** Other and unspecified injuries of thoracic spinal cord
✓6th **S24.10** Unspecified injury of thoracic spinal cord
✓7th **S24.101** Unspecified injury at T1 level of thoracic spinal cord HCC ESR COM
✓7th **S24.102** Unspecified injury at T2-T6 level of thoracic spinal cord HCC ESR COM
✓7th **S24.103** Unspecified injury at T7-T10 level of thoracic spinal cord HCC ESR COM
✓7th **S24.104** Unspecified injury at T11-T12 level of thoracic spinal cord HCC ESR COM
✓7th **S24.109** Unspecified injury at unspecified level of thoracic spinal cord HCC ESR COM
Injury of thoracic spinal cord NOS

✓6th **S24.11** Complete lesion of thoracic spinal cord
✓7th **S24.111** Complete lesion at T1 level of thoracic spinal cord HCC ESR COM
✓7th **S24.112** Complete lesion at T2-T6 level of thoracic spinal cord HCC ESR COM
✓7th **S24.113** Complete lesion at T7-T10 level of thoracic spinal cord HCC ESR COM

√7th **S24.114 Complete lesion at T11-T12 level of thoracic spinal cord** HCC ESR COM

√7th **S24.119 Complete lesion at unspecified level of thoracic spinal cord** HCC ESR COM

√6th **S24.13 Anterior cord syndrome of thoracic spinal cord**

√7th **S24.131 Anterior cord syndrome at T1 level of thoracic spinal cord** HCC ESR COM

√7th **S24.132 Anterior cord syndrome at T2-T6 level of thoracic spinal cord** HCC ESR COM

√7th **S24.133 Anterior cord syndrome at T7-T10 level of thoracic spinal cord** HCC ESR COM

√7th **S24.134 Anterior cord syndrome at T11-T12 level of thoracic spinal cord** HCC ESR COM

√7th **S24.139 Anterior cord syndrome at unspecified level of thoracic spinal cord** HCC ESR COM

√6th **S24.14 Brown-Sequard syndrome of thoracic spinal cord**

√7th **S24.141 Brown-Sequard syndrome at T1 level of thoracic spinal cord** HCC ESR COM

√7th **S24.142 Brown-Sequard syndrome at T2-T6 level of thoracic spinal cord** HCC ESR COM

√7th **S24.143 Brown-Sequard syndrome at T7-T10 level of thoracic spinal cord** HCC ESR COM

√7th **S24.144 Brown-Sequard syndrome at T11-T12 level of thoracic spinal cord** HCC ESR COM

√7th **S24.149 Brown-Sequard syndrome at unspecified level of thoracic spinal cord** HCC ESR COM

√6th **S24.15 Other incomplete lesions of thoracic spinal cord**

Incomplete lesion of thoracic spinal cord NOS
Posterior cord syndrome of thoracic spinal cord

√7th **S24.151 Other incomplete lesion at T1 level of thoracic spinal cord** HCC ESR COM

√7th **S24.152 Other incomplete lesion at T2-T6 level of thoracic spinal cord** HCC ESR COM

√7th **S24.153 Other incomplete lesion at T7-T10 level of thoracic spinal cord** HCC ESR COM

√7th **S24.154 Other incomplete lesion at T11-T12 level of thoracic spinal cord** HCC ESR COM

√7th **S24.159 Other incomplete lesion at unspecified level of thoracic spinal cord** HCC ESR COM

√x7th **S24.2 Injury of nerve root of thoracic spine**

√x7th **S24.3 Injury of peripheral nerves of thorax**

√x7th **S24.4 Injury of thoracic sympathetic nervous system**

Injury of cardiac plexus
Injury of esophageal plexus
Injury of pulmonary plexus
Injury of stellate ganglion
Injury of thoracic sympathetic ganglion

√x7th **S24.8 Injury of other specified nerves of thorax**

√x7th **S24.9 Injury of unspecified nerve of thorax**

√4th **S25 Injury of blood vessels of thorax**

Code also any associated open wound (S21.-)

The appropriate 7th character is to be added to each code from category S25.
A initial encounter
D subsequent encounter
S sequela

√5th **S25.0 Injury of thoracic aorta**

Injury of aorta NOS

√x7th **S25.00 Unspecified injury of thoracic aorta**

√x7th **S25.01 Minor laceration of thoracic aorta**

Incomplete transection of thoracic aorta
Laceration of thoracic aorta NOS
Superficial laceration of thoracic aorta

√x7th **S25.02 Major laceration of thoracic aorta**

Complete transection of thoracic aorta
Traumatic rupture of thoracic aorta

√x7th **S25.09 Other specified injury of thoracic aorta**

√5th **S25.1 Injury of innominate or subclavian artery**

√6th **S25.10 Unspecified injury of innominate or subclavian artery**

√7th **S25.101 Unspecified injury of right innominate or subclavian artery**

√7th **S25.102 Unspecified injury of left innominate or subclavian artery**

√7th **S25.109 Unspecified injury of unspecified innominate or subclavian artery**

√6th **S25.11 Minor laceration of innominate or subclavian artery**

Incomplete transection of innominate or subclavian artery
Laceration of innominate or subclavian artery NOS
Superficial laceration of innominate or subclavian artery

√7th **S25.111 Minor laceration of right innominate or subclavian artery**

√7th **S25.112 Minor laceration of left innominate or subclavian artery**

√7th **S25.119 Minor laceration of unspecified innominate or subclavian artery**

√6th **S25.12 Major laceration of innominate or subclavian artery**

Complete transection of innominate or subclavian artery
Traumatic rupture of innominate or subclavian artery

√7th **S25.121 Major laceration of right innominate or subclavian artery**

√7th **S25.122 Major laceration of left innominate or subclavian artery**

√7th **S25.129 Major laceration of unspecified innominate or subclavian artery**

√6th **S25.19 Other specified injury of innominate or subclavian artery**

√7th **S25.191 Other specified injury of right innominate or subclavian artery**

√7th **S25.192 Other specified injury of left innominate or subclavian artery**

√7th **S25.199 Other specified injury of unspecified innominate or subclavian artery**

√5th **S25.2 Injury of superior vena cava**

Injury of vena cava NOS

√x7th **S25.20 Unspecified injury of superior vena cava**

√x7th **S25.21 Minor laceration of superior vena cava**

Incomplete transection of superior vena cava
Laceration of superior vena cava NOS
Superficial laceration of superior vena cava

√x7th **S25.22 Major laceration of superior vena cava**

Complete transection of superior vena cava
Traumatic rupture of superior vena cava

√x7th **S25.29 Other specified injury of superior vena cava**

√5th **S25.3 Injury of innominate or subclavian vein**

√6th **S25.30 Unspecified injury of innominate or subclavian vein**

√7th **S25.301 Unspecified injury of right innominate or subclavian vein**

√7th **S25.302 Unspecified injury of left innominate or subclavian vein**

√7th **S25.309 Unspecified injury of unspecified innominate or subclavian vein**

√6th **S25.31 Minor laceration of innominate or subclavian vein**

Incomplete transection of innominate or subclavian vein
Laceration of innominate or subclavian vein NOS
Superficial laceration of innominate or subclavian vein

√7th **S25.311 Minor laceration of right innominate or subclavian vein**

√7th **S25.312 Minor laceration of left innominate or subclavian vein**

√7th **S25.319 Minor laceration of unspecified innominate or subclavian vein**

√6th **S25.32 Major laceration of innominate or subclavian vein**

Complete transection of innominate or subclavian vein
Traumatic rupture of innominate or subclavian vein

√7th **S25.321 Major laceration of right innominate or subclavian vein**

√7th **S25.322 Major laceration of left innominate or subclavian vein**

√7th **S25.329 Major laceration of unspecified innominate or subclavian vein**

√6th **S25.39 Other specified injury of innominate or subclavian vein**

√7th **S25.391 Other specified injury of right innominate or subclavian vein**

√7th **S25.392 Other specified injury of left innominate or subclavian vein**

√7th **S25.399 Other specified injury of unspecified innominate or subclavian vein**

√5th **S25.4 Injury of pulmonary blood vessels**

√6th **S25.40 Unspecified injury of pulmonary blood vessels**

√7th **S25.401 Unspecified injury of right pulmonary blood vessels**

√7th **S25.402 Unspecified injury of left pulmonary blood vessels**

√7th **S25.409 Unspecified injury of unspecified pulmonary blood vessels**

√6th **S25.41 Minor laceration of pulmonary blood vessels**

Incomplete transection of pulmonary blood vessels
Laceration of pulmonary blood vessels NOS
Superficial laceration of pulmonary blood vessels

√7th **S25.411 Minor laceration of right pulmonary blood vessels**

√7th **S25.412 Minor laceration of left pulmonary blood vessels**

√7th **S25.419 Minor laceration of unspecified pulmonary blood vessels**

√6th **S25.42 Major laceration of pulmonary blood vessels**

Complete transection of pulmonary blood vessels
Traumatic rupture of pulmonary blood vessels

√7th **S25.421 Major laceration of right pulmonary blood vessels**

√7th **S25.422 Major laceration of left pulmonary blood vessels**

√7th **S25.429 Major laceration of unspecified pulmonary blood vessels**

√6th **S25.49 Other specified injury of pulmonary blood vessels**

√7th **S25.491 Other specified injury of right pulmonary blood vessels**

√7th **S25.492 Other specified injury of left pulmonary blood vessels**

√7th **S25.499 Other specified injury of unspecified pulmonary blood vessels**

√5th **S25.5 Injury of intercostal blood vessels**

√6th **S25.50 Unspecified injury of intercostal blood vessels**

√7th **S25.501 Unspecified injury of intercostal blood vessels, right side**

√7th **S25.502 Unspecified injury of intercostal blood vessels, left side**

√7th **S25.509 Unspecified injury of intercostal blood vessels, unspecified side**

√6th **S25.51 Laceration of intercostal blood vessels**

√7th **S25.511 Laceration of intercostal blood vessels, right side**

√7th **S25.512 Laceration of intercostal blood vessels, left side**

√7th **S25.519 Laceration of intercostal blood vessels, unspecified side**

√6th **S25.59 Other specified injury of intercostal blood vessels**

√7th **S25.591 Other specified injury of intercostal blood vessels, right side**

√7th **S25.592 Other specified injury of intercostal blood vessels, left side**

√7th **S25.599 Other specified injury of intercostal blood vessels, unspecified side**

√5th **S25.8 Injury of other blood vessels of thorax**

Injury of azygos vein
Injury of mammary artery or vein

√6th **S25.80 Unspecified injury of other blood vessels of thorax**

√7th **S25.801 Unspecified injury of other blood vessels of thorax, right side**

√7th **S25.802 Unspecified injury of other blood vessels of thorax, left side**

√7th **S25.809 Unspecified injury of other blood vessels of thorax, unspecified side**

√6th **S25.81 Laceration of other blood vessels of thorax**

√7th **S25.811 Laceration of other blood vessels of thorax, right side**

√7th **S25.812 Laceration of other blood vessels of thorax, left side**

√7th **S25.819 Laceration of other blood vessels of thorax, unspecified side**

√6th **S25.89 Other specified injury of other blood vessels of thorax**

√7th **S25.891 Other specified injury of other blood vessels of thorax, right side**

√7th **S25.892 Other specified injury of other blood vessels of thorax, left side**

√7th **S25.899 Other specified injury of other blood vessels of thorax, unspecified side**

√5th **S25.9 Injury of unspecified blood vessel of thorax**

√x7th **S25.90 Unspecified injury of unspecified blood vessel of thorax**

√x7th **S25.91 Laceration of unspecified blood vessel of thorax**

√x7th **S25.99 Other specified injury of unspecified blood vessel of thorax**

√4th **S26 Injury of heart**

Code also any associated:
open wound of thorax (S21.-)
traumatic hemopneumothorax (S27.2)
traumatic hemothorax (S27.1)
traumatic pneumothorax (S27.Ø)

The appropriate 7th character is to be added to each code from category S26.
A initial encounter
D subsequent encounter
S sequela

√5th **S26.Ø Injury of heart with hemopericardium**

√x7th **S26.ØØ Unspecified injury of heart with hemopericardium**

√x7th **S26.Ø1 Contusion of heart with hemopericardium**

√6th **S26.Ø2 Laceration of heart with hemopericardium**

√7th **S26.Ø2Ø Mild laceration of heart with hemopericardium**

Laceration of heart without penetration of heart chamber

√7th **S26.Ø21 Moderate laceration of heart with hemopericardium**

Laceration of heart with penetration of heart chamber

√7th **S26.Ø22 Major laceration of heart with hemopericardium**

Laceration of heart with penetration of multiple heart chambers

√x7th **S26.Ø9 Other injury of heart with hemopericardium**

√5th **S26.1 Injury of heart without hemopericardium**

√x7th **S26.1Ø Unspecified injury of heart without hemopericardium**

√x7th **S26.11 Contusion of heart without hemopericardium**

√x7th **S26.12 Laceration of heart without hemopericardium**

√x7th **S26.19 Other injury of heart without hemopericardium**

√5th **S26.9 Injury of heart, unspecified with or without hemopericardium**

√x7th **S26.9Ø Unspecified injury of heart, unspecified with or without hemopericardium**

√x7th **S26.91 Contusion of heart, unspecified with or without hemopericardium**

**DEF:** Bruising within the heart muscle, with no mention of an open wound, usually caused by blunt chest trauma in motor vehicle accidents, falling from great heights, or receiving CPR.

√x7th **S26.92 Laceration of heart, unspecified with or without hemopericardium**

Laceration of heart NOS

**AHA:** 2019,2Q,24

√x7th **S26.99 Other injury of heart, unspecified with or without hemopericardium**

√4th **S27 Injury of other and unspecified intrathoracic organs**

Code also any associated open wound of thorax (S21.-)

EXCLUDES 2 *injury of cervical esophagus (S1Ø-S19)*
*injury of trachea (cervical) (S1Ø-S19)*

The appropriate 7th character is to be added to each code from category S27.
A initial encounter
D subsequent encounter
S sequela

√x7th **S27.Ø Traumatic pneumothorax**

EXCLUDES 1 *spontaneous pneumothorax (J93.-)*

√x7th **S27.1 Traumatic hemothorax**

√x7th **S27.2 Traumatic hemopneumothorax**

√5th **S27.3 Other and unspecified injuries of lung**

√6th **S27.3Ø Unspecified injury of lung**

√7th **S27.3Ø1 Unspecified injury of lung, unilateral**

√7th **S27.3Ø2 Unspecified injury of lung, bilateral**

√7th **S27.3Ø9 Unspecified injury of lung, unspecified**

√6th **S27.31 Primary blast injury of lung**

Blast injury of lung NOS

√7th **S27.311 Primary blast injury of lung, unilateral**

√7th **S27.312 Primary blast injury of lung, bilateral**

√7th **S27.319 Primary blast injury of lung, unspecified**

√6th S27.32 Contusion of lung
DEF: Bruising of the lung without mention of an open wound.
√7th S27.321 Contusion of lung, unilateral
√7th S27.322 Contusion of lung, bilateral
√7th S27.329 Contusion of lung, unspecified
√6th S27.33 Laceration of lung
√7th S27.331 Laceration of lung, unilateral
√7th S27.332 Laceration of lung, bilateral
√7th S27.339 Laceration of lung, unspecified
√6th S27.39 Other injuries of lung
Secondary blast injury of lung
√7th S27.391 Other injuries of lung, unilateral
√7th S27.392 Other injuries of lung, bilateral
√7th S27.399 Other injuries of lung, unspecified
√5th S27.4 Injury of bronchus
√6th S27.40 Unspecified injury of bronchus
√7th S27.401 Unspecified injury of bronchus, unilateral
√7th S27.402 Unspecified injury of bronchus, bilateral
√7th S27.409 Unspecified injury of bronchus, unspecified
√6th S27.41 Primary blast injury of bronchus
Blast injury of bronchus NOS
√7th S27.411 Primary blast injury of bronchus, unilateral
√7th S27.412 Primary blast injury of bronchus, bilateral
√7th S27.419 Primary blast injury of bronchus, unspecified
√6th S27.42 Contusion of bronchus
√7th S27.421 Contusion of bronchus, unilateral
√7th S27.422 Contusion of bronchus, bilateral
√7th S27.429 Contusion of bronchus, unspecified
√6th S27.43 Laceration of bronchus
√7th S27.431 Laceration of bronchus, unilateral
√7th S27.432 Laceration of bronchus, bilateral
√7th S27.439 Laceration of bronchus, unspecified
√6th S27.49 Other injury of bronchus
Secondary blast injury of bronchus
√7th S27.491 Other injury of bronchus, unilateral
√7th S27.492 Other injury of bronchus, bilateral
√7th S27.499 Other injury of bronchus, unspecified
√5th S27.5 Injury of thoracic trachea
√x7th S27.50 Unspecified injury of thoracic trachea
√x7th S27.51 Primary blast injury of thoracic trachea
Blast injury of thoracic trachea NOS
√x7th S27.52 Contusion of thoracic trachea
√x7th S27.53 Laceration of thoracic trachea
√x7th S27.59 Other injury of thoracic trachea
Secondary blast injury of thoracic trachea
√5th S27.6 Injury of pleura
√x7th S27.60 Unspecified injury of pleura
√x7th S27.63 Laceration of pleura
√x7th S27.69 Other injury of pleura
√5th S27.8 Injury of other specified intrathoracic organs
√6th S27.80 Injury of diaphragm
√7th S27.802 Contusion of diaphragm
√7th S27.803 Laceration of diaphragm
√7th S27.808 Other injury of diaphragm
√7th S27.809 Unspecified injury of diaphragm
√6th S27.81 Injury of esophagus (thoracic part)
√7th S27.812 Contusion of esophagus (thoracic part)
√7th S27.813 Laceration of esophagus (thoracic part)
√7th S27.818 Other injury of esophagus (thoracic part)
√7th S27.819 Unspecified injury of esophagus (thoracic part)
√6th S27.89 Injury of other specified intrathoracic organs
Injury of lymphatic thoracic duct
Injury of thymus gland
√7th S27.892 Contusion of other specified intrathoracic organs
√7th S27.893 Laceration of other specified intrathoracic organs
√7th S27.898 Other injury of other specified intrathoracic organs
√7th S27.899 Unspecified injury of other specified intrathoracic organs
√x7th S27.9 Injury of unspecified intrathoracic organ

√4th **S28 Crushing injury of thorax, and traumatic amputation of part of thorax**

The appropriate 7th character is to be added to each code from category S28.
A initial encounter
D subsequent encounter
S sequela

√x7th S28.0 Crushed chest
Use additional code for all associated injuries
EXCLUDES 1 *flail chest (S22.5)*
√x7th S28.1 Traumatic amputation (partial) of part of thorax, except breast
√5th S28.2 Traumatic amputation of breast
√6th S28.21 Complete traumatic amputation of breast
Traumatic amputation of breast NOS
√7th S28.211 Complete traumatic amputation of right breast
√7th S28.212 Complete traumatic amputation of left breast
√7th S28.219 Complete traumatic amputation of unspecified breast
√6th S28.22 Partial traumatic amputation of breast
√7th S28.221 Partial traumatic amputation of right breast
√7th S28.222 Partial traumatic amputation of left breast
√7th S28.229 Partial traumatic amputation of unspecified breast

√4th **S29 Other and unspecified injuries of thorax**
Code also any associated open wound (S21.-)

The appropriate 7th character is to be added to each code from category S29.
A initial encounter
D subsequent encounter
S sequela

√5th S29.0 Injury of muscle and tendon at thorax level
√6th S29.00 Unspecified injury of muscle and tendon of thorax
√7th S29.001 Unspecified injury of muscle and tendon of front wall of thorax
√7th S29.002 Unspecified injury of muscle and tendon of back wall of thorax
√7th S29.009 Unspecified injury of muscle and tendon of unspecified wall of thorax
√6th S29.01 Strain of muscle and tendon of thorax
√7th S29.011 Strain of muscle and tendon of front wall of thorax
√7th S29.012 Strain of muscle and tendon of back wall of thorax
√7th S29.019 Strain of muscle and tendon of unspecified wall of thorax
√6th S29.02 Laceration of muscle and tendon of thorax
√7th S29.021 Laceration of muscle and tendon of front wall of thorax
√7th S29.022 Laceration of muscle and tendon of back wall of thorax
√7th S29.029 Laceration of muscle and tendon of unspecified wall of thorax
√6th S29.09 Other injury of muscle and tendon of thorax
√7th S29.091 Other injury of muscle and tendon of front wall of thorax
√7th S29.092 Other injury of muscle and tendon of back wall of thorax
√7th S29.099 Other injury of muscle and tendon of unspecified wall of thorax
√x7th S29.8 Other specified injuries of thorax
√x7th S29.9 Unspecified injury of thorax

## Injuries to the abdomen, lower back, lumbar spine, pelvis and external genitals (S30-S39)

INCLUDES injuries to the abdominal wall
injuries to the anus
injuries to the buttock
injuries to the external genitalia
injuries to the flank
injuries to the groin

EXCLUDES 2 *burns and corrosions (T20-T32)*
*effects of foreign body in anus and rectum (T18.5)*
*effects of foreign body in genitourinary tract (T19.-)*
*effects of foreign body in stomach, small intestine and colon (T18.2-T18.4)*
*frostbite (T33-T34)*
*insect bite or sting, venomous (T63.4)*

**S30 Superficial injury of abdomen, lower back, pelvis and external genitals**
EXCLUDES 2 *superficial injury of hip (S70.-)*

The appropriate 7th character is to be added to each code from category S30.
A initial encounter
D subsequent encounter
S sequela

**S30.0 Contusion of lower back and pelvis**
Contusion of buttock
**S30.1 Contusion of abdominal wall**
**S30.11 Contusion of abdominal wall**
**S30.12 Contusion of groin**
**S30.13 Contusion of flank (latus) region**
**S30.2 Contusion of external genital organs**
**S30.20 Contusion of unspecified external genital organ**
**S30.201 Contusion of unspecified external genital organ, male**
**S30.202 Contusion of unspecified external genital organ, female**
**S30.21 Contusion of penis**
**S30.22 Contusion of scrotum and testes**
**S30.23 Contusion of vagina and vulva**
**S30.3 Contusion of anus**
**S30.8 Other superficial injuries of abdomen, lower back, pelvis and external genitals**
**S30.81 Abrasion of abdomen, lower back, pelvis and external genitals**
**S30.810 Abrasion of lower back and pelvis**
**S30.811 Abrasion of abdominal wall**
**S30.812 Abrasion of penis**
**S30.813 Abrasion of scrotum and testes**
**S30.814 Abrasion of vagina and vulva**
**S30.815 Abrasion of unspecified external genital organs, male**
**S30.816 Abrasion of unspecified external genital organs, female**
**S30.817 Abrasion of anus**
**S30.81A Abrasion of flank**
**S30.82 Blister (nonthermal) of abdomen, lower back, pelvis and external genitals**
**S30.820 Blister (nonthermal) of lower back and pelvis**
**S30.821 Blister (nonthermal) of abdominal wall**
**S30.822 Blister (nonthermal) of penis**
**S30.823 Blister (nonthermal) of scrotum and testes**
**S30.824 Blister (nonthermal) of vagina and vulva**
**S30.825 Blister (nonthermal) of unspecified external genital organs, male**
**S30.826 Blister (nonthermal) of unspecified external genital organs, female**
**S30.827 Blister (nonthermal) of anus**
**S30.82A Blister (nonthermal) of flank**
**S30.84 External constriction of abdomen, lower back, pelvis and external genitals**
**S30.840 External constriction of lower back and pelvis**
**S30.841 External constriction of abdominal wall**
**S30.842 External constriction of penis**
Hair tourniquet syndrome of penis
Use additional cause code to identify the constricting item (W49.0-)
**S30.843 External constriction of scrotum and testes**
**S30.844 External constriction of vagina and vulva**
**S30.845 External constriction of unspecified external genital organs, male**
**S30.846 External constriction of unspecified external genital organs, female**
**S30.84A External constriction of flank**
**S30.85 Superficial foreign body of abdomen, lower back, pelvis and external genitals**
Splinter in the abdomen, lower back, pelvis and external genitals
**S30.850 Superficial foreign body of lower back and pelvis**
**S30.851 Superficial foreign body of abdominal wall**
**S30.852 Superficial foreign body of penis**
**S30.853 Superficial foreign body of scrotum and testes**
**S30.854 Superficial foreign body of vagina and vulva**
**S30.855 Superficial foreign body of unspecified external genital organs, male**
**S30.856 Superficial foreign body of unspecified external genital organs, female**
**S30.857 Superficial foreign body of anus**
**S30.85A Superficial foreign body of flank**
**S30.86 Insect bite (nonvenomous) of abdomen, lower back, pelvis and external genitals**
**S30.860 Insect bite (nonvenomous) of lower back and pelvis**
**S30.861 Insect bite (nonvenomous) of abdominal wall**
**S30.862 Insect bite (nonvenomous) of penis**
**S30.863 Insect bite (nonvenomous) of scrotum and testes**
**S30.864 Insect bite (nonvenomous) of vagina and vulva**
**S30.865 Insect bite (nonvenomous) of unspecified external genital organs, male**
**S30.866 Insect bite (nonvenomous) of unspecified external genital organs, female**
**S30.867 Insect bite (nonvenomous) of anus**
**S30.86A Insect bite (nonvenomous) of flank**
**S30.87 Other superficial bite of abdomen, lower back, pelvis and external genitals**
EXCLUDES 1 *open bite of abdomen, lower back, pelvis and external genitals (S31.05, S31.15, S31.25, S31.35, S31.45, S31.55)*
**S30.870 Other superficial bite of lower back and pelvis**
**S30.871 Other superficial bite of abdominal wall**
**S30.872 Other superficial bite of penis**
**S30.873 Other superficial bite of scrotum and testes**
**S30.874 Other superficial bite of vagina and vulva**
**S30.875 Other superficial bite of unspecified external genital organs, male**
**S30.876 Other superficial bite of unspecified external genital organs, female**
**S30.877 Other superficial bite of anus**
**S30.87A Other superficial bite of flank**
**S30.9 Unspecified superficial injury of abdomen, lower back, pelvis and external genitals**
**S30.91 Unspecified superficial injury of lower back and pelvis**
**S30.92 Unspecified superficial injury of abdominal wall**
**S30.93 Unspecified superficial injury of penis**
**S30.94 Unspecified superficial injury of scrotum and testes**
**S30.95 Unspecified superficial injury of vagina and vulva**
**S30.96 Unspecified superficial injury of unspecified external genital organs, male**
**S30.97 Unspecified superficial injury of unspecified external genital organs, female**
**S30.98 Unspecified superficial injury of anus**
**S30.9A Unspecified superficial injury of flank**

4th **S31 Open wound of abdomen, lower back, pelvis and external genitals**

Code also any associated:
spinal cord injury (S24.Ø, S24.1-, S34.Ø-, S34.1-)
wound infection

EXCLUDES 1 *traumatic amputation of part of abdomen, lower back and pelvis (S38.2-, S38.3)*

EXCLUDES 2 *open fracture of pelvis (S32.1- - S32.9 with 7th character B)*
*open wound of hip (S71.ØØ-S71.Ø2)*

The appropriate 7th character is to be added to each code from category S31.
A initial encounter
D subsequent encounter
S sequela

5th **S31.Ø Open wound of lower back and pelvis**

6th **S31.ØØ Unspecified open wound of lower back and pelvis**

7th **S31.ØØØ Unspecified open wound of lower back and pelvis without penetration into retroperitoneum**
Unspecified open wound of lower back and pelvis NOS

7th **S31.ØØ1 Unspecified open wound of lower back and pelvis with penetration into retroperitoneum**

6th **S31.Ø1 Laceration without foreign body of lower back and pelvis**

7th **S31.Ø1Ø Laceration without foreign body of lower back and pelvis without penetration into retroperitoneum**
Laceration without foreign body of lower back and pelvis NOS

7th **S31.Ø11 Laceration without foreign body of lower back and pelvis with penetration into retroperitoneum**

6th **S31.Ø2 Laceration with foreign body of lower back and pelvis**

7th **S31.Ø2Ø Laceration with foreign body of lower back and pelvis without penetration into retroperitoneum**
Laceration with foreign body of lower back and pelvis NOS

7th **S31.Ø21 Laceration with foreign body of lower back and pelvis with penetration into retroperitoneum**

6th **S31.Ø3 Puncture wound without foreign body of lower back and pelvis**

7th **S31.Ø3Ø Puncture wound without foreign body of lower back and pelvis without penetration into retroperitoneum**
Puncture wound without foreign body of lower back and pelvis NOS

7th **S31.Ø31 Puncture wound without foreign body of lower back and pelvis with penetration into retroperitoneum**

6th **S31.Ø4 Puncture wound with foreign body of lower back and pelvis**

7th **S31.Ø4Ø Puncture wound with foreign body of lower back and pelvis without penetration into retroperitoneum**
Puncture wound with foreign body of lower back and pelvis NOS

7th **S31.Ø41 Puncture wound with foreign body of lower back and pelvis with penetration into retroperitoneum**

6th **S31.Ø5 Open bite of lower back and pelvis**
Bite of lower back and pelvis NOS

EXCLUDES 1 *superficial bite of lower back and pelvis (S3Ø.86Ø, S3Ø.87Ø)*

7th **S31.Ø5Ø Open bite of lower back and pelvis without penetration into retroperitoneum**
Open bite of lower back and pelvis NOS

7th **S31.Ø51 Open bite of lower back and pelvis with penetration into retroperitoneum**

5th **S31.1 Open wound of abdominal wall without penetration into peritoneal cavity**
Open wound of abdominal wall NOS

EXCLUDES 2 *open wound of abdominal wall with penetration into peritoneal cavity (S31.6-)*

6th **S31.1Ø Unspecified open wound of abdominal wall without penetration into peritoneal cavity**

7th **S31.1ØØ Unspecified open wound of abdominal wall, right upper quadrant without penetration into peritoneal cavity**

7th **S31.1Ø1 Unspecified open wound of abdominal wall, left upper quadrant without penetration into peritoneal cavity**

7th **S31.1Ø2 Unspecified open wound of abdominal wall, epigastric region without penetration into peritoneal cavity**

7th **S31.1Ø3 Unspecified open wound of abdominal wall, right lower quadrant without penetration into peritoneal cavity**

7th **S31.1Ø4 Unspecified open wound of abdominal wall, left lower quadrant without penetration into peritoneal cavity**

7th **S31.1Ø5 Unspecified open wound of abdominal wall, periumbilic region without penetration into peritoneal cavity**

7th **S31.1Ø6 Unspecified open wound of abdominal wall, right flank without penetration into peritoneal cavity**

7th **S31.1Ø7 Unspecified open wound of abdominal wall, left flank without penetration into peritoneal cavity**

7th **S31.1Ø9 Unspecified open wound of abdominal wall, unspecified quadrant without penetration into peritoneal cavity**
Unspecified open wound of abdominal wall NOS

7th **S31.1ØA Unspecified open wound of abdominal wall, unspecified flank without penetration into peritoneal cavity**
Open wound of abdominal wall of flank NOS without penetration into peritoneal cavity

6th **S31.11 Laceration without foreign body of abdominal wall without penetration into peritoneal cavity**

7th **S31.11Ø Laceration without foreign body of abdominal wall, right upper quadrant without penetration into peritoneal cavity**

7th **S31.111 Laceration without foreign body of abdominal wall, left upper quadrant without penetration into peritoneal cavity**

7th **S31.112 Laceration without foreign body of abdominal wall, epigastric region without penetration into peritoneal cavity**

7th **S31.113 Laceration without foreign body of abdominal wall, right lower quadrant without penetration into peritoneal cavity**

7th **S31.114 Laceration without foreign body of abdominal wall, left lower quadrant without penetration into peritoneal cavity**

7th **S31.115 Laceration without foreign body of abdominal wall, periumbilic region without penetration into peritoneal cavity**

7th **S31.116 Laceration without foreign body of abdominal wall, right flank without penetration into peritoneal cavity**

7th **S31.117 Laceration without foreign body of abdominal wall, left flank without penetration into peritoneal cavity**

7th **S31.119 Laceration without foreign body of abdominal wall, unspecified quadrant without penetration into peritoneal cavity**

7th **S31.11A Laceration without foreign body of abdominal wall, unspecified flank without penetration into peritoneal cavity**
Laceration without foreign body of flank NOS without penetration into peritoneal cavity

6th **S31.12 Laceration with foreign body of abdominal wall without penetration into peritoneal cavity**

7th **S31.12Ø Laceration of abdominal wall with foreign body, right upper quadrant without penetration into peritoneal cavity**

7th **S31.121 Laceration of abdominal wall with foreign body, left upper quadrant without penetration into peritoneal cavity**

7th **S31.122 Laceration of abdominal wall with foreign body, epigastric region without penetration into peritoneal cavity**

7th **S31.123 Laceration of abdominal wall with foreign body, right lower quadrant without penetration into peritoneal cavity**

7th **S31.124 Laceration of abdominal wall with foreign body, left lower quadrant without penetration into peritoneal cavity**

✓7th S31.125 **Laceration of abdominal wall with foreign body, periumbilic region without penetration into peritoneal cavity**

✓7th S31.126 **Laceration with foreign body of abdominal wall, right flank without penetration into peritoneal cavity**

✓7th S31.127 **Laceration with foreign body of abdominal wall, left flank without penetration into peritoneal cavity**

✓7th S31.129 **Laceration of abdominal wall with foreign body, unspecified quadrant without penetration into peritoneal cavity**

✓7th S31.12A **Laceration with foreign body of abdominal wall unspecified flank without penetration into peritoneal cavity**

Laceration with foreign body of abdominal wall of flank NOS without penetration into peritoneal cavity

✓6th S31.13 **Puncture wound of abdominal wall without foreign body without penetration into peritoneal cavity**

✓7th S31.130 **Puncture wound of abdominal wall without foreign body, right upper quadrant without penetration into peritoneal cavity**

✓7th S31.131 **Puncture wound of abdominal wall without foreign body, left upper quadrant without penetration into peritoneal cavity**

✓7th S31.132 **Puncture wound of abdominal wall without foreign body, epigastric region without penetration into peritoneal cavity**

✓7th S31.133 **Puncture wound of abdominal wall without foreign body, right lower quadrant without penetration into peritoneal cavity**

✓7th S31.134 **Puncture wound of abdominal wall without foreign body, left lower quadrant without penetration into peritoneal cavity**

✓7th S31.135 **Puncture wound of abdominal wall without foreign body, periumbilic region without penetration into peritoneal cavity**

✓7th S31.136 **Puncture wound of abdominal wall without foreign body, right flank without penetration into peritoneal cavity**

✓7th S31.137 **Puncture wound of abdominal wall without foreign body, left flank without penetration into peritoneal cavity**

✓7th S31.139 **Puncture wound of abdominal wall without foreign body, unspecified quadrant without penetration into peritoneal cavity**

✓7th S31.13A **Puncture wound of abdominal wall without foreign body, unspecified flank without penetration into peritoneal cavity**

Puncture wound of abdominal wall of flank NOS without foreign body

✓6th S31.14 **Puncture wound of abdominal wall with foreign body without penetration into peritoneal cavity**

✓7th S31.140 **Puncture wound of abdominal wall with foreign body, right upper quadrant without penetration into peritoneal cavity**

✓7th S31.141 **Puncture wound of abdominal wall with foreign body, left upper quadrant without penetration into peritoneal cavity**

✓7th S31.142 **Puncture wound of abdominal wall with foreign body, epigastric region without penetration into peritoneal cavity**

✓7th S31.143 **Puncture wound of abdominal wall with foreign body, right lower quadrant without penetration into peritoneal cavity**

✓7th S31.144 **Puncture wound of abdominal wall with foreign body, left lower quadrant without penetration into peritoneal cavity**

✓7th S31.145 **Puncture wound of abdominal wall with foreign body, periumbilic region without penetration into peritoneal cavity**

✓7th S31.146 **Puncture wound of abdominal wall with foreign body, right flank without penetration into peritoneal cavity**

✓7th S31.147 **Puncture wound of abdominal wall with foreign body, left flank without penetration into peritoneal cavity**

✓7th S31.149 **Puncture wound of abdominal wall with foreign body, unspecified quadrant without penetration into peritoneal cavity**

✓7th S31.14A **Puncture wound of abdominal wall with foreign body, unspecified flank without penetration into peritoneal cavity**

Puncture wound of abdominal wall with foreign body of flank NOS without penetration into peritoneal cavity

✓6th S31.15 **Open bite of abdominal wall without penetration into peritoneal cavity**

Bite of abdominal wall NOS

EXCLUDES 1 *superficial bite of abdominal wall (S30.871)*

✓7th S31.150 **Open bite of abdominal wall, right upper quadrant without penetration into peritoneal cavity**

✓7th S31.151 **Open bite of abdominal wall, left upper quadrant without penetration into peritoneal cavity**

✓7th S31.152 **Open bite of abdominal wall, epigastric region without penetration into peritoneal cavity**

✓7th S31.153 **Open bite of abdominal wall, right lower quadrant without penetration into peritoneal cavity**

✓7th S31.154 **Open bite of abdominal wall, left lower quadrant without penetration into peritoneal cavity**

✓7th S31.155 **Open bite of abdominal wall, periumbilic region without penetration into peritoneal cavity**

✓7th S31.156 **Open bite of abdominal wall, right flank without penetration into peritoneal cavity**

✓7th S31.157 **Open bite of abdominal wall, left flank without penetration into peritoneal cavity**

✓7th S31.159 **Open bite of abdominal wall, unspecified quadrant without penetration into peritoneal cavity**

✓7th S31.15A **Open bite of abdominal wall, unspecified flank without penetration into peritoneal cavity**

Open bite of abdominal wall of flank NOS without penetration into peritoneal cavity

✓5th S31.2 **Open wound of penis**

✓x7th S31.20 **Unspecified open wound of penis**

✓x7th S31.21 **Laceration without foreign body of penis**

✓x7th S31.22 **Laceration with foreign body of penis**

✓x7th S31.23 **Puncture wound without foreign body of penis**

✓x7th S31.24 **Puncture wound with foreign body of penis**

✓x7th S31.25 **Open bite of penis**

Bite of penis NOS

EXCLUDES 1 *superficial bite of penis (S30.862, S30.872)*

✓5th S31.3 **Open wound of scrotum and testes**

✓x7th S31.30 **Unspecified open wound of scrotum and testes**

✓x7th S31.31 **Laceration without foreign body of scrotum and testes**

✓x7th S31.32 **Laceration with foreign body of scrotum and testes**

✓x7th S31.33 **Puncture wound without foreign body of scrotum and testes**

✓x7th S31.34 **Puncture wound with foreign body of scrotum and testes**

✓x7th S31.35 **Open bite of scrotum and testes**

Bite of scrotum and testes NOS

EXCLUDES 1 *superficial bite of scrotum and testes (S30.863, S30.873)*

✓5th S31.4 **Open wound of vagina and vulva**

EXCLUDES 1 *injury to vagina and vulva during delivery (O70.-, O71.4)*

✓x7th S31.40 **Unspecified open wound of vagina and vulva**

✓x7th S31.41 **Laceration without foreign body of vagina and vulva**

✓x7th S31.42 **Laceration with foreign body of vagina and vulva**

✓x7th S31.43 **Puncture wound without foreign body of vagina and vulva**

✓x7th S31.44 **Puncture wound with foreign body of vagina and vulva**

✓x7th S31.45 **Open bite of vagina and vulva**

Bite of vagina and vulva NOS

EXCLUDES 1 *superficial bite of vagina and vulva (S30.864, S30.874)*

**5th S31.5 Open wound of unspecified external genital organs**

EXCLUDES 1 *traumatic amputation of external genital organs (S38.21, S38.22)*

**6th S31.50 Unspecified open wound of unspecified external genital organs**

**7th S31.501 Unspecified open wound of unspecified external genital organs, male**

**7th S31.502 Unspecified open wound of unspecified external genital organs, female**

**6th S31.51 Laceration without foreign body of unspecified external genital organs**

**7th S31.511 Laceration without foreign body of unspecified external genital organs, male**

**7th S31.512 Laceration without foreign body of unspecified external genital organs, female**

**6th S31.52 Laceration with foreign body of unspecified external genital organs**

**7th S31.521 Laceration with foreign body of unspecified external genital organs, male**

**7th S31.522 Laceration with foreign body of unspecified external genital organs, female**

**6th S31.53 Puncture wound without foreign body of unspecified external genital organs**

**7th S31.531 Puncture wound without foreign body of unspecified external genital organs, male**

**7th S31.532 Puncture wound without foreign body of unspecified external genital organs, female**

**6th S31.54 Puncture wound with foreign body of unspecified external genital organs**

**7th S31.541 Puncture wound with foreign body of unspecified external genital organs, male**

**7th S31.542 Puncture wound with foreign body of unspecified external genital organs, female**

**6th S31.55 Open bite of unspecified external genital organs**

Bite of unspecified external genital organs NOS

EXCLUDES 1 *superficial bite of unspecified external genital organs (S30.865, S30.866, S30.875, S30.876)*

**7th S31.551 Open bite of unspecified external genital organs, male**

**7th S31.552 Open bite of unspecified external genital organs, female**

**5th S31.6 Open wound of abdominal wall with penetration into peritoneal cavity**

AHA: 2023,3Q,8

**6th S31.60 Unspecified open wound of abdominal wall with penetration into peritoneal cavity**

**7th S31.600 Unspecified open wound of abdominal wall, right upper quadrant with penetration into peritoneal cavity**

**7th S31.601 Unspecified open wound of abdominal wall, left upper quadrant with penetration into peritoneal cavity**

**7th S31.602 Unspecified open wound of abdominal wall, epigastric region with penetration into peritoneal cavity**

**7th S31.603 Unspecified open wound of abdominal wall, right lower quadrant with penetration into peritoneal cavity**

**7th S31.604 Unspecified open wound of abdominal wall, left lower quadrant with penetration into peritoneal cavity**

**7th S31.605 Unspecified open wound of abdominal wall, periumbilic region with penetration into peritoneal cavity**

**7th S31.606 Unspecified open wound of abdominal wall, right flank with penetration into peritoneal cavity**

**7th S31.607 Unspecified open wound of abdominal wall, left flank with penetration into peritoneal cavity**

**7th S31.609 Unspecified open wound of abdominal wall, unspecified quadrant with penetration into peritoneal cavity**

**7th S31.60A Unspecified open wound of abdominal wall, unspecified flank with penetration into peritoneal cavity**

Unspecified open wound of abdominal wall of flank NOS, with penetration into peritoneal cavity

**6th S31.61 Laceration without foreign body of abdominal wall with penetration into peritoneal cavity**

**7th S31.610 Laceration without foreign body of abdominal wall, right upper quadrant with penetration into peritoneal cavity**

**7th S31.611 Laceration without foreign body of abdominal wall, left upper quadrant with penetration into peritoneal cavity**

**7th S31.612 Laceration without foreign body of abdominal wall, epigastric region with penetration into peritoneal cavity**

**7th S31.613 Laceration without foreign body of abdominal wall, right lower quadrant with penetration into peritoneal cavity**

**7th S31.614 Laceration without foreign body of abdominal wall, left lower quadrant with penetration into peritoneal cavity**

**7th S31.615 Laceration without foreign body of abdominal wall, periumbilic region with penetration into peritoneal cavity**

**7th S31.616 Laceration without foreign body of abdominal wall, right flank with penetration into peritoneal cavity**

**7th S31.617 Laceration without foreign body of abdominal wall, left flank with penetration into peritoneal cavity**

**7th S31.619 Laceration without foreign body of abdominal wall, unspecified quadrant with penetration into peritoneal cavity**

**7th S31.61A Laceration without foreign body of abdominal wall, unspecified flank with penetration into peritoneal cavity**

Laceration without foreign body of abdominal wall of flank NOS, with penetration into peritoneal cavity

**6th S31.62 Laceration with foreign body of abdominal wall with penetration into peritoneal cavity**

**7th S31.620 Laceration with foreign body of abdominal wall, right upper quadrant with penetration into peritoneal cavity**

**7th S31.621 Laceration with foreign body of abdominal wall, left upper quadrant with penetration into peritoneal cavity**

**7th S31.622 Laceration with foreign body of abdominal wall, epigastric region with penetration into peritoneal cavity**

**7th S31.623 Laceration with foreign body of abdominal wall, right lower quadrant with penetration into peritoneal cavity**

**7th S31.624 Laceration with foreign body of abdominal wall, left lower quadrant with penetration into peritoneal cavity**

**7th S31.625 Laceration with foreign body of abdominal wall, periumbilic region with penetration into peritoneal cavity**

**7th S31.626 Laceration with foreign body of abdominal wall, right flank with penetration into peritoneal cavity**

**7th S31.627 Laceration with foreign body of abdominal wall, left flank with penetration into peritoneal cavity**

**7th S31.629 Laceration with foreign body of abdominal wall, unspecified quadrant with penetration into peritoneal cavity**

**7th S31.62A Laceration with foreign body of abdominal wall, unspecified flank with penetration into peritoneal cavity**

Laceration with foreign body of abdominal wall, flank NOS, with penetration into peritoneal cavity

**6th S31.63 Puncture wound without foreign body of abdominal wall with penetration into peritoneal cavity**

**7th S31.630 Puncture wound without foreign body of abdominal wall, right upper quadrant with penetration into peritoneal cavity**

**7th S31.631 Puncture wound without foreign body of abdominal wall, left upper quadrant with penetration into peritoneal cavity**

√7th S31.632 **Puncture wound without foreign body of abdominal wall, epigastric region with penetration into peritoneal cavity**

√7th S31.633 **Puncture wound without foreign body of abdominal wall, right lower quadrant with penetration into peritoneal cavity**

√7th S31.634 **Puncture wound without foreign body of abdominal wall, left lower quadrant with penetration into peritoneal cavity**

√7th S31.635 **Puncture wound without foreign body of abdominal wall, periumbilic region with penetration into peritoneal cavity**

√7th S31.636 **Puncture wound of abdominal wall without foreign body, right flank with penetration into peritoneal cavity**

√7th S31.637 **Puncture wound of abdominal wall without foreign body, left flank with penetration into peritoneal cavity**

√7th S31.639 **Puncture wound without foreign body of abdominal wall, unspecified quadrant with penetration into peritoneal cavity**

√7th S31.63A **Puncture wound of abdominal wall without foreign body, unspecified flank with penetration into peritoneal cavity**
Puncture wound of abdominal wall without foreign body, flank NOS, with penetration into peritoneal cavity

√6th S31.64 **Puncture wound with foreign body of abdominal wall with penetration into peritoneal cavity**

√7th S31.640 **Puncture wound with foreign body of abdominal wall, right upper quadrant with penetration into peritoneal cavity**

√7th S31.641 **Puncture wound with foreign body of abdominal wall, left upper quadrant with penetration into peritoneal cavity**

√7th S31.642 **Puncture wound with foreign body of abdominal wall, epigastric region with penetration into peritoneal cavity**

√7th S31.643 **Puncture wound with foreign body of abdominal wall, right lower quadrant with penetration into peritoneal cavity**

√7th S31.644 **Puncture wound with foreign body of abdominal wall, left lower quadrant with penetration into peritoneal cavity**

√7th S31.645 **Puncture wound with foreign body of abdominal wall, periumbilic region with penetration into peritoneal cavity**

√7th S31.646 **Puncture wound of abdominal wall with foreign body, right flank with penetration into peritoneal cavity**

√7th S31.647 **Puncture wound of abdominal wall with foreign body, left flank with penetration into peritoneal cavity**

√7th S31.649 **Puncture wound with foreign body of abdominal wall, unspecified quadrant with penetration into peritoneal cavity**

√7th S31.64A **Puncture wound of abdominal wall with foreign body, unspecified flank with penetration into peritoneal cavity**
Puncture wound of abdominal wall with foreign body, flank NOS, with penetration into peritoneal cavity

√6th S31.65 **Open bite of abdominal wall with penetration into peritoneal cavity**
EXCLUDES 1 *superficial bite of abdominal wall (S30.861, S30.871)*

√7th S31.650 **Open bite of abdominal wall, right upper quadrant with penetration into peritoneal cavity**

√7th S31.651 **Open bite of abdominal wall, left upper quadrant with penetration into peritoneal cavity**

√7th S31.652 **Open bite of abdominal wall, epigastric region with penetration into peritoneal cavity**

√7th S31.653 **Open bite of abdominal wall, right lower quadrant with penetration into peritoneal cavity**

√7th S31.654 **Open bite of abdominal wall, left lower quadrant with penetration into peritoneal cavity**

√7th S31.655 **Open bite of abdominal wall, periumbilic region with penetration into peritoneal cavity**

√7th S31.656 **Open bite of abdominal wall, right flank with penetration into peritoneal cavity**

√7th S31.657 **Open bite of abdominal wall, left flank with penetration into peritoneal cavity**

√7th S31.659 **Open bite of abdominal wall, unspecified quadrant with penetration into peritoneal cavity**

√7th S31.65A **Open bite of abdominal wall, unspecified flank with penetration into peritoneal cavity**
Open bite of abdominal wall, flank NOS, with penetration into peritoneal cavity

√5th S31.8 **Open wound of other parts of abdomen, lower back and pelvis**

√6th S31.80 **Open wound of unspecified buttock**

√7th S31.801 **Laceration without foreign body of unspecified buttock**

√7th S31.802 **Laceration with foreign body of unspecified buttock**

√7th S31.803 **Puncture wound without foreign body of unspecified buttock**

√7th S31.804 **Puncture wound with foreign body of unspecified buttock**

√7th S31.805 **Open bite of unspecified buttock**
Bite of buttock NOS
EXCLUDES 1 *superficial bite of buttock (S30.870)*

√7th S31.809 **Unspecified open wound of unspecified buttock**

√6th S31.81 **Open wound of right buttock**

√7th S31.811 **Laceration without foreign body of right buttock**

√7th S31.812 **Laceration with foreign body of right buttock**

√7th S31.813 **Puncture wound without foreign body of right buttock**

√7th S31.814 **Puncture wound with foreign body of right buttock**

√7th S31.815 **Open bite of right buttock**
Bite of right buttock NOS
EXCLUDES 1 *superficial bite of buttock (S30.870)*

√7th S31.819 **Unspecified open wound of right buttock**

√6th S31.82 **Open wound of left buttock**

√7th S31.821 **Laceration without foreign body of left buttock**

√7th S31.822 **Laceration with foreign body of left buttock**

√7th S31.823 **Puncture wound without foreign body of left buttock**

√7th S31.824 **Puncture wound with foreign body of left buttock**

√7th S31.825 **Open bite of left buttock**
Bite of left buttock NOS
EXCLUDES 1 *superficial bite of buttock (S30.870)*

√7th S31.829 **Unspecified open wound of left buttock**

√6th S31.83 **Open wound of anus**

√7th S31.831 **Laceration without foreign body of anus**

√7th S31.832 **Laceration with foreign body of anus**

√7th S31.833 **Puncture wound without foreign body of anus**

√7th S31.834 **Puncture wound with foreign body of anus**

√7th S31.835 **Open bite of anus**
Bite of anus NOS
EXCLUDES 1 *superficial bite of anus (S30.877)*

√7th S31.839 **Unspecified open wound of anus**

Chapter 19. Injury, Poisoning and Certain Other Consequences of External Causes

S31.632–S31.839

✓4th **S32 Fracture of lumbar spine and pelvis**

**NOTE** A fracture not indicated as displaced or nondisplaced should be coded to displaced.

A fracture not indicated as opened or closed should be coded to closed.

**INCLUDES** fracture of lumbosacral neural arch
fracture of lumbosacral spinous process
fracture of lumbosacral transverse process
fracture of lumbosacral vertebra
fracture of lumbosacral vertebral arch

Code first any associated spinal cord and spinal nerve injury (S34.-)

**EXCLUDES 1** *transection of abdomen (S38.3)*

**EXCLUDES 2** *fracture of hip NOS (S72.Ø-)*

**AHA:** 2021,1Q,6; 2018,2Q,12; 2015,3Q,37-39; 2012,4Q,93

The appropriate 7th character is to be added to each code from category S32.
A initial encounter for closed fracture
B initial encounter for open fracture
D subsequent encounter for fracture with routine healing
G subsequent encounter for fracture with delayed healing
K subsequent encounter for fracture with nonunion
S sequela

✓5th **S32.Ø Fracture of lumbar vertebra**
Fracture of lumbar spine NOS

✓6th **S32.ØØ Fracture of unspecified lumbar vertebra**
✓7th **S32.ØØØ Wedge compression fracture of unspecified lumbar vertebra** HCC ESR COM Q
✓7th **S32.ØØ1 Stable burst fracture of unspecified lumbar vertebra** HCC ESR COM Q
✓7th **S32.ØØ2 Unstable burst fracture of unspecified lumbar vertebra** HCC ESR COM Q
✓7th **S32.ØØ8 Other fracture of unspecified lumbar vertebra** HCC ESR COM Q
✓7th **S32.ØØ9 Unspecified fracture of unspecified lumbar vertebra** HCC ESR COM Q

✓6th **S32.Ø1 Fracture of first lumbar vertebra**
✓7th **S32.Ø1Ø Wedge compression fracture of first lumbar vertebra** HCC ESR COM Q
✓7th **S32.Ø11 Stable burst fracture of first lumbar vertebra** HCC ESR COM Q
✓7th **S32.Ø12 Unstable burst fracture of first lumbar vertebra** HCC ESR COM Q
✓7th **S32.Ø18 Other fracture of first lumbar vertebra** HCC ESR COM Q
✓7th **S32.Ø19 Unspecified fracture of first lumbar vertebra** HCC ESR COM Q

✓6th **S32.Ø2 Fracture of second lumbar vertebra**
✓7th **S32.Ø2Ø Wedge compression fracture of second lumbar vertebra** HCC ESR COM Q
✓7th **S32.Ø21 Stable burst fracture of second lumbar vertebra** HCC ESR COM Q
✓7th **S32.Ø22 Unstable burst fracture of second lumbar vertebra** HCC ESR COM Q
✓7th **S32.Ø28 Other fracture of second lumbar vertebra** HCC ESR COM Q
✓7th **S32.Ø29 Unspecified fracture of second lumbar vertebra** HCC ESR COM Q

✓6th **S32.Ø3 Fracture of third lumbar vertebra**
✓7th **S32.Ø3Ø Wedge compression fracture of third lumbar vertebra** HCC ESR COM Q
✓7th **S32.Ø31 Stable burst fracture of third lumbar vertebra** HCC ESR COM Q
✓7th **S32.Ø32 Unstable burst fracture of third lumbar vertebra** HCC ESR COM Q
✓7th **S32.Ø38 Other fracture of third lumbar vertebra** HCC ESR COM Q
✓7th **S32.Ø39 Unspecified fracture of third lumbar vertebra** HCC ESR COM Q

✓6th **S32.Ø4 Fracture of fourth lumbar vertebra**
✓7th **S32.Ø4Ø Wedge compression fracture of fourth lumbar vertebra** HCC ESR COM Q
✓7th **S32.Ø41 Stable burst fracture of fourth lumbar vertebra** HCC ESR COM Q
✓7th **S32.Ø42 Unstable burst fracture of fourth lumbar vertebra** HCC ESR COM Q
✓7th **S32.Ø48 Other fracture of fourth lumbar vertebra** HCC ESR COM Q
✓7th **S32.Ø49 Unspecified fracture of fourth lumbar vertebra** HCC ESR COM Q

✓6th **S32.Ø5 Fracture of fifth lumbar vertebra**
✓7th **S32.Ø5Ø Wedge compression fracture of fifth lumbar vertebra** HCC ESR COM Q
✓7th **S32.Ø51 Stable burst fracture of fifth lumbar vertebra** HCC ESR COM Q
✓7th **S32.Ø52 Unstable burst fracture of fifth lumbar vertebra** HCC ESR COM Q
✓7th **S32.Ø58 Other fracture of fifth lumbar vertebra** HCC ESR COM Q
✓7th **S32.Ø59 Unspecified fracture of fifth lumbar vertebra** HCC ESR COM Q

✓5th **S32.1 Fracture of sacrum**

**NOTE** For vertical fractures, code to most medial fracture extension

Use two codes if both a vertical and transverse fracture are present

Code also any associated fracture of pelvic ring (S32.8-)

✓x7th **S32.1Ø Unspecified fracture of sacrum** HCC ESR COM Q

✓6th **S32.11 Zone I fracture of sacrum**
Vertical sacral ala fracture of sacrum

**Vertical Sacral Fracture Zones**

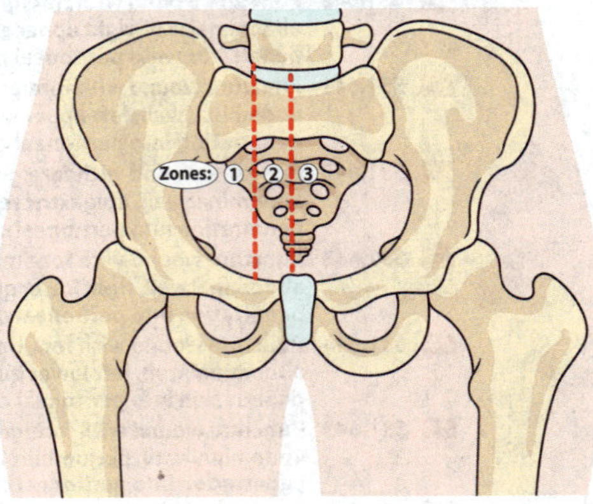


✓7th **S32.11Ø Nondisplaced Zone I fracture of sacrum** HCC ESR COM Q
✓7th **S32.111 Minimally displaced Zone I fracture of sacrum** HCC ESR COM Q
✓7th **S32.112 Severely displaced Zone I fracture of sacrum** HCC ESR COM Q
✓7th **S32.119 Unspecified Zone I fracture of sacrum** HCC ESR COM Q

✓6th **S32.12 Zone II fracture of sacrum**
Vertical foraminal region fracture of sacrum
✓7th **S32.12Ø Nondisplaced Zone II fracture of sacrum** HCC ESR COM Q
✓7th **S32.121 Minimally displaced Zone II fracture of sacrum** HCC ESR COM Q
✓7th **S32.122 Severely displaced Zone II fracture of sacrum** HCC ESR COM Q
✓7th **S32.129 Unspecified Zone II fracture of sacrum** HCC ESR COM Q

✓6th **S32.13 Zone III fracture of sacrum**
Vertical fracture into spinal canal region of sacrum
✓7th **S32.13Ø Nondisplaced Zone III fracture of sacrum** HCC ESR COM Q
✓7th **S32.131 Minimally displaced Zone III fracture of sacrum** HCC ESR COM Q
✓7th **S32.132 Severely displaced Zone III fracture of sacrum** HCC ESR COM Q

✓7th **S32.139** Unspecified Zone III fracture of sacrum HCC ESR COM Q

**Transverse Sacral Fracture Types**

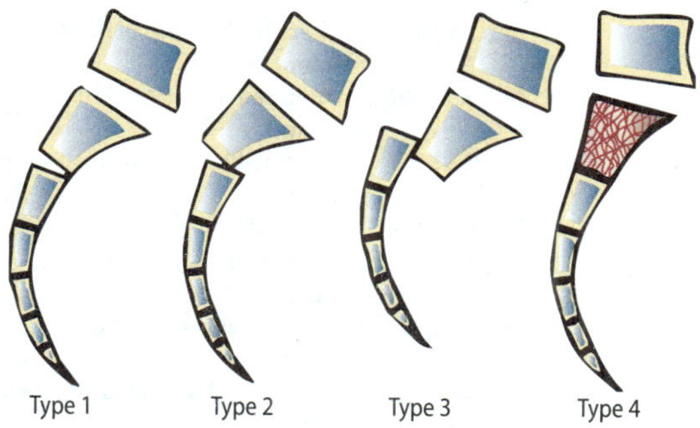


✓x7th **S32.14** Type 1 fracture of sacrum HCC ESR COM Q
- Transverse flexion fracture of sacrum without displacement

✓x7th **S32.15** Type 2 fracture of sacrum HCC ESR COM Q
- Transverse flexion fracture of sacrum with posterior displacement

✓x7th **S32.16** Type 3 fracture of sacrum HCC ESR COM Q
- Transverse extension fracture of sacrum with anterior displacement

✓x7th **S32.17** Type 4 fracture of sacrum HCC ESR COM Q
- Transverse segmental comminution of upper sacrum

✓x7th **S32.19** Other fracture of sacrum HCC ESR COM Q

✓x7th **S32.2** Fracture of coccyx HCC ESR COM Q

✓5th **S32.3** Fracture of ilium
- EXCLUDES 1 *fracture of ilium with associated disruption of pelvic ring (S32.8-)*

✓6th **S32.3Ø** Unspecified fracture of ilium
- ✓7th **S32.3Ø1** Unspecified fracture of right ilium HCC ESR COM Q
- ✓7th **S32.3Ø2** Unspecified fracture of left ilium HCC ESR COM Q
- ✓7th **S32.3Ø9** Unspecified fracture of unspecified ilium HCC ESR COM Q

✓6th **S32.31** Avulsion fracture of ilium
- ✓7th **S32.311** Displaced avulsion fracture of right ilium HCC ESR COM Q
- ✓7th **S32.312** Displaced avulsion fracture of left ilium HCC ESR COM Q
- ✓7th **S32.313** Displaced avulsion fracture of unspecified ilium HCC ESR COM Q
- ✓7th **S32.314** Nondisplaced avulsion fracture of right ilium HCC ESR COM Q
- ✓7th **S32.315** Nondisplaced avulsion fracture of left ilium HCC ESR COM Q
- ✓7th **S32.316** Nondisplaced avulsion fracture of unspecified ilium HCC ESR COM Q

✓6th **S32.39** Other fracture of ilium
- ✓7th **S32.391** Other fracture of right ilium HCC ESR COM Q
- ✓7th **S32.392** Other fracture of left ilium HCC ESR COM Q
- ✓7th **S32.399** Other fracture of unspecified ilium HCC ESR COM Q

✓5th **S32.4** Fracture of acetabulum
- Code also any associated fracture of pelvic ring (S32.8-)
- **AHA:** 2016,3Q,16

✓6th **S32.4Ø** Unspecified fracture of acetabulum
- ✓7th **S32.4Ø1** Unspecified fracture of right acetabulum HCC ESR COM Q
- ✓7th **S32.4Ø2** Unspecified fracture of left acetabulum HCC ESR COM Q
- ✓7th **S32.4Ø9** Unspecified fracture of unspecified acetabulum HCC ESR COM Q

✓6th **S32.41** Fracture of anterior wall of acetabulum
- ✓7th **S32.411** Displaced fracture of anterior wall of right acetabulum HCC ESR COM Q
- ✓7th **S32.412** Displaced fracture of anterior wall of left acetabulum HCC ESR COM Q
- ✓7th **S32.413** Displaced fracture of anterior wall of unspecified acetabulum HCC ESR COM Q
- ✓7th **S32.414** Nondisplaced fracture of anterior wall of right acetabulum HCC ESR COM Q
- ✓7th **S32.415** Nondisplaced fracture of anterior wall of left acetabulum HCC ESR COM Q
- ✓7th **S32.416** Nondisplaced fracture of anterior wall of unspecified acetabulum HCC ESR COM Q

✓6th **S32.42** Fracture of posterior wall of acetabulum
- ✓7th **S32.421** Displaced fracture of posterior wall of right acetabulum HCC ESR COM Q
- ✓7th **S32.422** Displaced fracture of posterior wall of left acetabulum HCC ESR COM Q
- ✓7th **S32.423** Displaced fracture of posterior wall of unspecified acetabulum HCC ESR COM Q
- ✓7th **S32.424** Nondisplaced fracture of posterior wall of right acetabulum HCC ESR COM Q
- ✓7th **S32.425** Nondisplaced fracture of posterior wall of left acetabulum HCC ESR COM Q
- ✓7th **S32.426** Nondisplaced fracture of posterior wall of unspecified acetabulum HCC ESR COM Q

✓6th **S32.43** Fracture of anterior column [iliopubic] of acetabulum
- ✓7th **S32.431** Displaced fracture of anterior column [iliopubic] of right acetabulum HCC ESR COM Q
- ✓7th **S32.432** Displaced fracture of anterior column [iliopubic] of left acetabulum HCC ESR COM Q
- ✓7th **S32.433** Displaced fracture of anterior column [iliopubic] of unspecified acetabulum HCC ESR COM Q
- ✓7th **S32.434** Nondisplaced fracture of anterior column [iliopubic] of right acetabulum HCC ESR COM Q
- ✓7th **S32.435** Nondisplaced fracture of anterior column [iliopubic] of left acetabulum HCC ESR COM Q
- ✓7th **S32.436** Nondisplaced fracture of anterior column [iliopubic] of unspecified acetabulum HCC ESR COM Q

✓6th **S32.44** Fracture of posterior column [ilioischial] of acetabulum
- ✓7th **S32.441** Displaced fracture of posterior column [ilioischial] of right acetabulum HCC ESR COM Q
- ✓7th **S32.442** Displaced fracture of posterior column [ilioischial] of left acetabulum HCC ESR COM Q
- ✓7th **S32.443** Displaced fracture of posterior column [ilioischial] of unspecified acetabulum HCC ESR COM Q
- ✓7th **S32.444** Nondisplaced fracture of posterior column [ilioischial] of right acetabulum HCC ESR COM Q
- ✓7th **S32.445** Nondisplaced fracture of posterior column [ilioischial] of left acetabulum HCC ESR COM Q
- ✓7th **S32.446** Nondisplaced fracture of posterior column [ilioischial] of unspecified acetabulum HCC ESR COM Q

✓6th **S32.45** Transverse fracture of acetabulum
- ✓7th **S32.451** Displaced transverse fracture of right acetabulum HCC ESR COM Q
- ✓7th **S32.452** Displaced transverse fracture of left acetabulum HCC ESR COM Q
- ✓7th **S32.453** Displaced transverse fracture of unspecified acetabulum HCC ESR COM Q
- ✓7th **S32.454** Nondisplaced transverse fracture of right acetabulum HCC ESR COM Q
- ✓7th **S32.455** Nondisplaced transverse fracture of left acetabulum HCC ESR COM Q
- ✓7th **S32.456** Nondisplaced transverse fracture of unspecified acetabulum HCC ESR COM Q

✓6th **S32.46** Associated transverse-posterior fracture of acetabulum
- ✓7th **S32.461** Displaced associated transverse-posterior fracture of right acetabulum HCC ESR COM Q

✓7th **S32.462 Displaced associated transverse-posterior fracture of left acetabulum** HCC ESR COM Q

✓7th **S32.463 Displaced associated transverse-posterior fracture of unspecified acetabulum** HCC ESR COM Q

✓7th **S32.464 Nondisplaced associated transverse-posterior fracture of right acetabulum** HCC ESR COM Q

✓7th **S32.465 Nondisplaced associated transverse-posterior fracture of left acetabulum** HCC ESR COM Q

✓7th **S32.466 Nondisplaced associated transverse-posterior fracture of unspecified acetabulum** HCC ESR COM Q

✓6th **S32.47 Fracture of medial wall of acetabulum**

✓7th **S32.471 Displaced fracture of medial wall of right acetabulum** HCC ESR COM Q

✓7th **S32.472 Displaced fracture of medial wall of left acetabulum** HCC ESR COM Q

✓7th **S32.473 Displaced fracture of medial wall of unspecified acetabulum** HCC ESR COM Q

✓7th **S32.474 Nondisplaced fracture of medial wall of right acetabulum** HCC ESR COM Q

✓7th **S32.475 Nondisplaced fracture of medial wall of left acetabulum** HCC ESR COM Q

✓7th **S32.476 Nondisplaced fracture of medial wall of unspecified acetabulum** HCC ESR COM Q

✓6th **S32.48 Dome fracture of acetabulum**

✓7th **S32.481 Displaced dome fracture of right acetabulum** HCC ESR COM Q

✓7th **S32.482 Displaced dome fracture of left acetabulum** HCC ESR COM Q

✓7th **S32.483 Displaced dome fracture of unspecified acetabulum** HCC ESR COM Q

✓7th **S32.484 Nondisplaced dome fracture of right acetabulum** HCC ESR COM Q

✓7th **S32.485 Nondisplaced dome fracture of left acetabulum** HCC ESR COM Q

✓7th **S32.486 Nondisplaced dome fracture of unspecified acetabulum** HCC ESR COM Q

✓6th **S32.49 Other specified fracture of acetabulum**

✓7th **S32.491 Other specified fracture of right acetabulum** HCC ESR COM Q

✓7th **S32.492 Other specified fracture of left acetabulum** HCC ESR COM Q

✓7th **S32.499 Other specified fracture of unspecified acetabulum** HCC ESR COM Q

✓5th **S32.5 Fracture of pubis**

EXCLUDES 1 *fracture of pubis with associated disruption of pelvic ring (S32.8-)*

✓6th **S32.50 Unspecified fracture of pubis**

✓7th **S32.501 Unspecified fracture of right pubis** HCC ESR COM Q

✓7th **S32.502 Unspecified fracture of left pubis** HCC ESR COM Q

✓7th **S32.509 Unspecified fracture of unspecified pubis** HCC ESR COM Q

✓6th **S32.51 Fracture of superior rim of pubis**

✓7th **S32.511 Fracture of superior rim of right pubis** HCC ESR COM Q

✓7th **S32.512 Fracture of superior rim of left pubis** HCC ESR COM Q

✓7th **S32.519 Fracture of superior rim of unspecified pubis** HCC ESR COM Q

✓6th **S32.59 Other specified fracture of pubis**

✓7th **S32.591 Other specified fracture of right pubis** HCC ESR COM Q

✓7th **S32.592 Other specified fracture of left pubis** HCC ESR COM Q

✓7th **S32.599 Other specified fracture of unspecified pubis** HCC ESR COM Q

✓5th **S32.6 Fracture of ischium**

EXCLUDES 1 *fracture of ischium with associated disruption of pelvic ring (S32.8-)*

✓6th **S32.60 Unspecified fracture of ischium**

✓7th **S32.601 Unspecified fracture of right ischium** HCC ESR COM Q

✓7th **S32.602 Unspecified fracture of left ischium** HCC ESR COM Q

✓7th **S32.609 Unspecified fracture of unspecified ischium** HCC ESR COM Q

✓6th **S32.61 Avulsion fracture of ischium**

✓7th **S32.611 Displaced avulsion fracture of right ischium** HCC ESR COM Q

✓7th **S32.612 Displaced avulsion fracture of left ischium** HCC ESR COM Q

✓7th **S32.613 Displaced avulsion fracture of unspecified ischium** HCC ESR COM Q

✓7th **S32.614 Nondisplaced avulsion fracture of right ischium** HCC ESR COM Q

✓7th **S32.615 Nondisplaced avulsion fracture of left ischium** HCC ESR COM Q

✓7th **S32.616 Nondisplaced avulsion fracture of unspecified ischium** HCC ESR COM Q

✓6th **S32.69 Other specified fracture of ischium**

✓7th **S32.691 Other specified fracture of right ischium** HCC ESR COM Q

✓7th **S32.692 Other specified fracture of left ischium** HCC ESR COM Q

✓7th **S32.699 Other specified fracture of unspecified ischium** HCC ESR COM Q

✓5th **S32.8 Fracture of other parts of pelvis**

Code also any associated:
fracture of acetabulum (S32.4-)
sacral fracture (S32.1-)

**Fractures Disrupting Pelvic Circle**

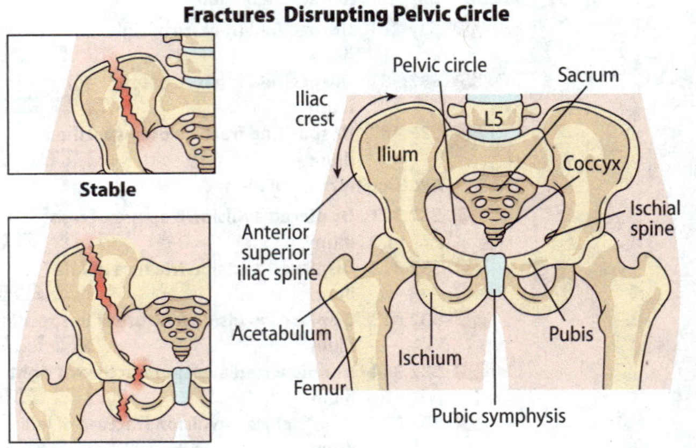


**Unstable** (two-place fracture)

✓6th **S32.81 Multiple fractures of pelvis with disruption of pelvic ring**

Multiple pelvic fractures with disruption of pelvic circle

✓7th **S32.810 Multiple fractures of pelvis with stable disruption of pelvic ring** HCC ESR COM Q

✓7th **S32.811 Multiple fractures of pelvis with unstable disruption of pelvic ring** HCC ESR COM Q

✓x7th **S32.82 Multiple fractures of pelvis without disruption of pelvic ring** HCC ESR COM Q

Multiple pelvic fractures without disruption of pelvic circle

✓x7th **S32.89 Fracture of other parts of pelvis** HCC ESR COM Q

✓x7th **S32.9 Fracture of unspecified parts of lumbosacral spine and pelvis** HCC ESR COM Q

Fracture of lumbosacral spine NOS
Fracture of pelvis NOS

**AHA:** 2012,4Q,93

**S33 Dislocation and sprain of joints and ligaments of lumbar spine and pelvis**

INCLUDES avulsion of joint or ligament of lumbar spine and pelvis
laceration of cartilage, joint or ligament of lumbar spine and pelvis
sprain of cartilage, joint or ligament of lumbar spine and pelvis
traumatic hemarthrosis of joint or ligament of lumbar spine and pelvis
traumatic rupture of joint or ligament of lumbar spine and pelvis
traumatic subluxation of joint or ligament of lumbar spine and pelvis
traumatic tear of joint or ligament of lumbar spine and pelvis

Code also any associated open wound

EXCLUDES 1 *nontraumatic rupture or displacement of lumbar intervertebral disc NOS (M51.-)*
*obstetric damage to pelvic joints and ligaments (O71.6)*

EXCLUDES 2 *dislocation and sprain of joints and ligaments of hip (S73.-)*
*strain of muscle of lower back and pelvis (S39.01-)*

The appropriate 7th character is to be added to each code from category S33.
A initial encounter
D subsequent encounter
S sequela

**S33.0 Traumatic rupture of lumbar intervertebral disc**

EXCLUDES 1 *rupture or displacement (nontraumatic) of lumbar intervertebral disc NOS (M51.- with fifth character 6)*

**S33.1 Subluxation and dislocation of lumbar vertebra**

Code also any associated:
open wound of abdomen, lower back and pelvis (S31)
spinal cord injury (S24.0, S24.1-, S34.0-, S34.1-)

EXCLUDES 2 *fracture of lumbar vertebrae (S32.0-)*

**S33.10 Subluxation and dislocation of unspecified lumbar vertebra**

**S33.100 Subluxation of unspecified lumbar vertebra**

**S33.101 Dislocation of unspecified lumbar vertebra**

**S33.11 Subluxation and dislocation of L1/L2 lumbar vertebra**

**S33.110 Subluxation of L1/L2 lumbar vertebra**

**S33.111 Dislocation of L1/L2 lumbar vertebra**

**S33.12 Subluxation and dislocation of L2/L3 lumbar vertebra**

**S33.120 Subluxation of L2/L3 lumbar vertebra**

**S33.121 Dislocation of L2/L3 lumbar vertebra**

**S33.13 Subluxation and dislocation of L3/L4 lumbar vertebra**

**S33.130 Subluxation of L3/L4 lumbar vertebra**

**S33.131 Dislocation of L3/L4 lumbar vertebra**

**S33.14 Subluxation and dislocation of L4/L5 lumbar vertebra**

**S33.140 Subluxation of L4/L5 lumbar vertebra**

**S33.141 Dislocation of L4/L5 lumbar vertebra**

**S33.2 Dislocation of sacroiliac and sacrococcygeal joint**

**S33.3 Dislocation of other and unspecified parts of lumbar spine and pelvis**

**S33.30 Dislocation of unspecified parts of lumbar spine and pelvis**

**S33.39 Dislocation of other parts of lumbar spine and pelvis**

**S33.4 Traumatic rupture of symphysis pubis**

**S33.5 Sprain of ligaments of lumbar spine**

**S33.6 Sprain of sacroiliac joint**

**S33.8 Sprain of other parts of lumbar spine and pelvis**

**S33.9 Sprain of unspecified parts of lumbar spine and pelvis**

**S34 Injury of lumbar and sacral spinal cord and nerves at abdomen, lower back and pelvis level**

NOTE Code to highest level of lumbar cord injury.
Injuries to the spinal cord (S34.0 and S34.1) refer to the cord level and not bone level injury, and can affect nerve roots at and below the level given.

Code also any associated:
fracture of vertebra (S22.0-, S32.0-)
open wound of abdomen, lower back and pelvis (S31.-)
transient paralysis (R29.5)

The appropriate 7th character is to be added to each code from category S34.
A initial encounter
D subsequent encounter
S sequela

**S34.0 Concussion and edema of lumbar and sacral spinal cord**

**S34.01 Concussion and edema of lumbar spinal cord** HCC ESR COM

**S34.02 Concussion and edema of sacral spinal cord** HCC ESR COM
Concussion and edema of conus medullaris

**S34.1 Other and unspecified injury of lumbar and sacral spinal cord**

**S34.10 Unspecified injury to lumbar spinal cord**

**S34.101 Unspecified injury to L1 level of lumbar spinal cord** HCC ESR COM
Unspecified injury to lumbar spinal cord level 1

**S34.102 Unspecified injury to L2 level of lumbar spinal cord** HCC ESR COM
Unspecified injury to lumbar spinal cord level 2

**S34.103 Unspecified injury to L3 level of lumbar spinal cord** HCC ESR COM
Unspecified injury to lumbar spinal cord level 3

**S34.104 Unspecified injury to L4 level of lumbar spinal cord** HCC ESR COM
Unspecified injury to lumbar spinal cord level 4

**S34.105 Unspecified injury to L5 level of lumbar spinal cord** HCC ESR COM
Unspecified injury to lumbar spinal cord level 5

**S34.109 Unspecified injury to unspecified level of lumbar spinal cord** HCC ESR COM

**S34.11 Complete lesion of lumbar spinal cord**

**S34.111 Complete lesion of L1 level of lumbar spinal cord** HCC ESR COM
Complete lesion of lumbar spinal cord level 1

**S34.112 Complete lesion of L2 level of lumbar spinal cord** HCC ESR COM
Complete lesion of lumbar spinal cord level 2

**S34.113 Complete lesion of L3 level of lumbar spinal cord** HCC ESR COM
Complete lesion of lumbar spinal cord level 3

**S34.114 Complete lesion of L4 level of lumbar spinal cord** HCC ESR COM
Complete lesion of lumbar spinal cord level 4

**S34.115 Complete lesion of L5 level of lumbar spinal cord** HCC ESR COM
Complete lesion of lumbar spinal cord level 5

**S34.119 Complete lesion of unspecified level of lumbar spinal cord** HCC ESR COM

**S34.12 Incomplete lesion of lumbar spinal cord**

**S34.121 Incomplete lesion of L1 level of lumbar spinal cord** HCC ESR COM
Incomplete lesion of lumbar spinal cord level 1

**S34.122 Incomplete lesion of L2 level of lumbar spinal cord** HCC ESR COM
Incomplete lesion of lumbar spinal cord level 2

√7th **S34.123 Incomplete lesion of L3 level of lumbar spinal cord** HCC ESR COM
Incomplete lesion of lumbar spinal cord level 3

√7th **S34.124 Incomplete lesion of L4 level of lumbar spinal cord** HCC ESR COM
Incomplete lesion of lumbar spinal cord level 4

√7th **S34.125 Incomplete lesion of L5 level of lumbar spinal cord** HCC ESR COM
Incomplete lesion of lumbar spinal cord level 5

√7th **S34.129 Incomplete lesion of unspecified level of lumbar spinal cord** HCC ESR COM

√6th **S34.13 Other and unspecified injury to sacral spinal cord**
Other injury to conus medullaris

√7th **S34.131 Complete lesion of sacral spinal cord** HCC ESR COM
Complete lesion of conus medullaris

√7th **S34.132 Incomplete lesion of sacral spinal cord** HCC ESR COM
Incomplete lesion of conus medullaris

√7th **S34.139 Unspecified injury to sacral spinal cord** HCC ESR COM
Unspecified injury of conus medullaris

√5th **S34.2 Injury of nerve root of lumbar and sacral spine**

√x7th **S34.21 Injury of nerve root of lumbar spine**

√x7th **S34.22 Injury of nerve root of sacral spine**

√x7th **S34.3 Injury of cauda equina** HCC ESR COM

√x7th **S34.4 Injury of lumbosacral plexus**

√x7th **S34.5 Injury of lumbar, sacral and pelvic sympathetic nerves**
Injury of celiac ganglion or plexus
Injury of hypogastric plexus
Injury of mesenteric plexus (inferior) (superior)
Injury of splanchnic nerve

√x7th **S34.6 Injury of peripheral nerve(s) at abdomen, lower back and pelvis level**

√x7th **S34.8 Injury of other nerves at abdomen, lower back and pelvis level**

√x7th **S34.9 Injury of unspecified nerves at abdomen, lower back and pelvis level**

√4th **S35 Injury of blood vessels at abdomen, lower back and pelvis level**
Code also any associated open wound (S31.-)

The appropriate 7th character is to be added to each code from category S35.
A initial encounter
D subsequent encounter
S sequela

√5th **S35.Ø Injury of abdominal aorta**
**EXCLUDES 1** *injury of aorta NOS (S25.Ø)*

√x7th **S35.ØØ Unspecified injury of abdominal aorta**

√x7th **S35.Ø1 Minor laceration of abdominal aorta**
Incomplete transection of abdominal aorta
Laceration of abdominal aorta NOS
Superficial laceration of abdominal aorta

√x7th **S35.Ø2 Major laceration of abdominal aorta**
Complete transection of abdominal aorta
Traumatic rupture of abdominal aorta

√x7th **S35.Ø9 Other injury of abdominal aorta**

√5th **S35.1 Injury of inferior vena cava**
Injury of hepatic vein
**EXCLUDES 1** *injury of vena cava NOS (S25.2)*

√x7th **S35.1Ø Unspecified injury of inferior vena cava**

√x7th **S35.11 Minor laceration of inferior vena cava**
Incomplete transection of inferior vena cava
Laceration of inferior vena cava NOS
Superficial laceration of inferior vena cava

√x7th **S35.12 Major laceration of inferior vena cava**
Complete transection of inferior vena cava
Traumatic rupture of inferior vena cava

√x7th **S35.19 Other injury of inferior vena cava**

√5th **S35.2 Injury of celiac or mesenteric artery and branches**

√6th **S35.21 Injury of celiac artery**

√7th **S35.211 Minor laceration of celiac artery**
Incomplete transection of celiac artery
Laceration of celiac artery NOS
Superficial laceration of celiac artery

√7th **S35.212 Major laceration of celiac artery**
Complete transection of celiac artery
Traumatic rupture of celiac artery

√7th **S35.218 Other injury of celiac artery**

√7th **S35.219 Unspecified injury of celiac artery**

√6th **S35.22 Injury of superior mesenteric artery**

√7th **S35.221 Minor laceration of superior mesenteric artery**
Incomplete transection of superior mesenteric artery
Laceration of superior mesenteric artery NOS
Superficial laceration of superior mesenteric artery

√7th **S35.222 Major laceration of superior mesenteric artery**
Complete transection of superior mesenteric artery
Traumatic rupture of superior mesenteric artery

√7th **S35.228 Other injury of superior mesenteric artery**

√7th **S35.229 Unspecified injury of superior mesenteric artery**

√6th **S35.23 Injury of inferior mesenteric artery**

√7th **S35.231 Minor laceration of inferior mesenteric artery**
Incomplete transection of inferior mesenteric artery
Laceration of inferior mesenteric artery NOS
Superficial laceration of inferior mesenteric artery

√7th **S35.232 Major laceration of inferior mesenteric artery**
Complete transection of inferior mesenteric artery
Traumatic rupture of inferior mesenteric artery

√7th **S35.238 Other injury of inferior mesenteric artery**

√7th **S35.239 Unspecified injury of inferior mesenteric artery**

√6th **S35.29 Injury of branches of celiac and mesenteric artery**
Injury of gastric artery
Injury of gastroduodenal artery
Injury of hepatic artery
Injury of splenic artery

√7th **S35.291 Minor laceration of branches of celiac and mesenteric artery**
Incomplete transection of branches of celiac and mesenteric artery
Laceration of branches of celiac and mesenteric artery NOS
Superficial laceration of branches of celiac and mesenteric artery

√7th **S35.292 Major laceration of branches of celiac and mesenteric artery**
Complete transection of branches of celiac and mesenteric artery
Traumatic rupture of branches of celiac and mesenteric artery

√7th **S35.298 Other injury of branches of celiac and mesenteric artery**

√7th **S35.299 Unspecified injury of branches of celiac and mesenteric artery**

√5th **S35.3 Injury of portal or splenic vein and branches**

√6th **S35.31 Injury of portal vein**

√7th **S35.311 Laceration of portal vein**

√7th **S35.318 Other specified injury of portal vein**

√7th **S35.319 Unspecified injury of portal vein**

√6th **S35.32 Injury of splenic vein**

√7th **S35.321 Laceration of splenic vein**

√7th **S35.328 Other specified injury of splenic vein**

√7th **S35.329 Unspecified injury of splenic vein**

S35.33 Injury of superior mesenteric vein
S35.331 Laceration of superior mesenteric vein
S35.338 Other specified injury of superior mesenteric vein
S35.339 Unspecified injury of superior mesenteric vein
S35.34 Injury of inferior mesenteric vein
S35.341 Laceration of inferior mesenteric vein
S35.348 Other specified injury of inferior mesenteric vein
S35.349 Unspecified injury of inferior mesenteric vein
S35.4 Injury of renal blood vessels
S35.40 Unspecified injury of renal blood vessel
S35.401 Unspecified injury of right renal artery
S35.402 Unspecified injury of left renal artery
S35.403 Unspecified injury of unspecified renal artery
S35.404 Unspecified injury of right renal vein
S35.405 Unspecified injury of left renal vein
S35.406 Unspecified injury of unspecified renal vein
S35.41 Laceration of renal blood vessel
S35.411 Laceration of right renal artery
S35.412 Laceration of left renal artery
S35.413 Laceration of unspecified renal artery
S35.414 Laceration of right renal vein
S35.415 Laceration of left renal vein
S35.416 Laceration of unspecified renal vein
S35.49 Other specified injury of renal blood vessel
S35.491 Other specified injury of right renal artery
S35.492 Other specified injury of left renal artery
S35.493 Other specified injury of unspecified renal artery
S35.494 Other specified injury of right renal vein
S35.495 Other specified injury of left renal vein
S35.496 Other specified injury of unspecified renal vein
S35.5 Injury of iliac blood vessels
S35.50 Injury of unspecified iliac blood vessel(s)
S35.51 Injury of iliac artery or vein
Injury of hypogastric artery or vein
S35.511 Injury of right iliac artery
S35.512 Injury of left iliac artery
S35.513 Injury of unspecified iliac artery
S35.514 Injury of right iliac vein
S35.515 Injury of left iliac vein
S35.516 Injury of unspecified iliac vein
S35.53 Injury of uterine artery or vein
S35.531 Injury of right uterine artery
S35.532 Injury of left uterine artery
S35.533 Injury of unspecified uterine artery
S35.534 Injury of right uterine vein
S35.535 Injury of left uterine vein
S35.536 Injury of unspecified uterine vein
S35.59 Injury of other iliac blood vessels
S35.8 Injury of other blood vessels at abdomen, lower back and pelvis level
Injury of ovarian artery or vein
S35.8X Injury of other blood vessels at abdomen, lower back and pelvis level
S35.8X1 Laceration of other blood vessels at abdomen, lower back and pelvis level
S35.8X8 Other specified injury of other blood vessels at abdomen, lower back and pelvis level
S35.8X9 Unspecified injury of other blood vessels at abdomen, lower back and pelvis level
S35.9 Injury of unspecified blood vessel at abdomen, lower back and pelvis level
S35.90 Unspecified injury of unspecified blood vessel at abdomen, lower back and pelvis level
S35.91 Laceration of unspecified blood vessel at abdomen, lower back and pelvis level
S35.99 Other specified injury of unspecified blood vessel at abdomen, lower back and pelvis level

S36 Injury of intra-abdominal organs
Code also any associated open wound (S31.-)

The appropriate 7th character is to be added to each code from category S36.
A initial encounter
D subsequent encounter
S sequela

S36.0 Injury of spleen
AHA: 2015,2Q,36; 2015,1Q,10
S36.00 Unspecified injury of spleen
S36.02 Contusion of spleen
S36.020 Minor contusion of spleen
Contusion of spleen less than 2 cm
S36.021 Major contusion of spleen
Contusion of spleen greater than 2 cm
S36.029 Unspecified contusion of spleen
S36.03 Laceration of spleen
S36.030 Superficial (capsular) laceration of spleen
Laceration of spleen less than 1 cm
Minor laceration of spleen
S36.031 Moderate laceration of spleen
Laceration of spleen 1 to 3 cm
S36.032 Major laceration of spleen
Avulsion of spleen
Laceration of spleen greater than 3 cm
Massive laceration of spleen
Multiple moderate lacerations of spleen
Stellate laceration of spleen
S36.039 Unspecified laceration of spleen
S36.09 Other injury of spleen
S36.1 Injury of liver and gallbladder and bile duct
S36.11 Injury of liver
AHA: 2024,1Q,25
S36.112 Contusion of liver
S36.113 Laceration of liver, unspecified degree
S36.114 Minor laceration of liver
Laceration involving capsule only, or, without significant involvement of hepatic parenchyma [i.e., less than 1 cm deep]
S36.115 Moderate laceration of liver
Laceration involving parenchyma but without major disruption of parenchyma [i.e., less than 10 cm long and less than 3 cm deep]
S36.116 Major laceration of liver
Laceration with significant disruption of hepatic parenchyma [i.e., greater than 10 cm long and 3 cm deep]
Multiple moderate lacerations, with or without hematoma
Stellate laceration of liver
S36.118 Other injury of liver
S36.119 Unspecified injury of liver
S36.12 Injury of gallbladder
S36.122 Contusion of gallbladder
S36.123 Laceration of gallbladder
S36.128 Other injury of gallbladder
S36.129 Unspecified injury of gallbladder
S36.13 Injury of bile duct
S36.2 Injury of pancreas
S36.20 Unspecified injury of pancreas
S36.200 Unspecified injury of head of pancreas
S36.201 Unspecified injury of body of pancreas
S36.202 Unspecified injury of tail of pancreas
S36.209 Unspecified injury of unspecified part of pancreas
S36.22 Contusion of pancreas
S36.220 Contusion of head of pancreas

√7th S36.221 Contusion of body of pancreas
√7th S36.222 Contusion of tail of pancreas
√7th S36.229 Contusion of unspecified part of pancreas
√6th S36.23 Laceration of pancreas, unspecified degree
√7th S36.230 Laceration of head of pancreas, unspecified degree
√7th S36.231 Laceration of body of pancreas, unspecified degree
√7th S36.232 Laceration of tail of pancreas, unspecified degree
√7th S36.239 Laceration of unspecified part of pancreas, unspecified degree
√6th S36.24 Minor laceration of pancreas
√7th S36.240 Minor laceration of head of pancreas
√7th S36.241 Minor laceration of body of pancreas
√7th S36.242 Minor laceration of tail of pancreas
√7th S36.249 Minor laceration of unspecified part of pancreas
√6th S36.25 Moderate laceration of pancreas
√7th S36.250 Moderate laceration of head of pancreas
√7th S36.251 Moderate laceration of body of pancreas
√7th S36.252 Moderate laceration of tail of pancreas
√7th S36.259 Moderate laceration of unspecified part of pancreas
√6th S36.26 Major laceration of pancreas
√7th S36.260 Major laceration of head of pancreas
√7th S36.261 Major laceration of body of pancreas
√7th S36.262 Major laceration of tail of pancreas
√7th S36.269 Major laceration of unspecified part of pancreas
√6th S36.29 Other injury of pancreas
√7th S36.290 Other injury of head of pancreas
√7th S36.291 Other injury of body of pancreas
√7th S36.292 Other injury of tail of pancreas
√7th S36.299 Other injury of unspecified part of pancreas
√5th S36.3 Injury of stomach
√x7th S36.30 Unspecified injury of stomach
√x7th S36.32 Contusion of stomach
√x7th S36.33 Laceration of stomach
√x7th S36.39 Other injury of stomach
√5th S36.4 Injury of small intestine
√6th S36.40 Unspecified injury of small intestine
√7th S36.400 Unspecified injury of duodenum
√7th S36.408 Unspecified injury of other part of small intestine
√7th S36.409 Unspecified injury of unspecified part of small intestine
√6th S36.41 Primary blast injury of small intestine
Blast injury of small intestine NOS
√7th S36.410 Primary blast injury of duodenum
√7th S36.418 Primary blast injury of other part of small intestine
√7th S36.419 Primary blast injury of unspecified part of small intestine
√6th S36.42 Contusion of small intestine
√7th S36.420 Contusion of duodenum
√7th S36.428 Contusion of other part of small intestine
√7th S36.429 Contusion of unspecified part of small intestine
√6th S36.43 Laceration of small intestine
√7th S36.430 Laceration of duodenum
√7th S36.438 Laceration of other part of small intestine
√7th S36.439 Laceration of unspecified part of small intestine
√6th S36.49 Other injury of small intestine
√7th S36.490 Other injury of duodenum
√7th S36.498 Other injury of other part of small intestine
AHA: 2023,3Q,8
√7th S36.499 Other injury of unspecified part of small intestine
√5th S36.5 Injury of colon
EXCLUDES 2 *injury of rectum (S36.6-)*
√6th S36.50 Unspecified injury of colon
√7th S36.500 Unspecified injury of ascending [right] colon
√7th S36.501 Unspecified injury of transverse colon
√7th S36.502 Unspecified injury of descending [left] colon
√7th S36.503 Unspecified injury of sigmoid colon
√7th S36.508 Unspecified injury of other part of colon
√7th S36.509 Unspecified injury of unspecified part of colon
√6th S36.51 Primary blast injury of colon
Blast injury of colon NOS
√7th S36.510 Primary blast injury of ascending [right] colon
√7th S36.511 Primary blast injury of transverse colon
√7th S36.512 Primary blast injury of descending [left] colon
√7th S36.513 Primary blast injury of sigmoid colon
√7th S36.518 Primary blast injury of other part of colon
√7th S36.519 Primary blast injury of unspecified part of colon
√6th S36.52 Contusion of colon
√7th S36.520 Contusion of ascending [right] colon
√7th S36.521 Contusion of transverse colon
√7th S36.522 Contusion of descending [left] colon
√7th S36.523 Contusion of sigmoid colon
√7th S36.528 Contusion of other part of colon
√7th S36.529 Contusion of unspecified part of colon
√6th S36.53 Laceration of colon
√7th S36.530 Laceration of ascending [right] colon
√7th S36.531 Laceration of transverse colon
√7th S36.532 Laceration of descending [left] colon
√7th S36.533 Laceration of sigmoid colon
√7th S36.538 Laceration of other part of colon
√7th S36.539 Laceration of unspecified part of colon
√6th S36.59 Other injury of colon
Secondary blast injury of colon
AHA: 2023,3Q,8
√7th S36.590 Other injury of ascending [right] colon
√7th S36.591 Other injury of transverse colon
√7th S36.592 Other injury of descending [left] colon
√7th S36.593 Other injury of sigmoid colon
√7th S36.598 Other injury of other part of colon
√7th S36.599 Other injury of unspecified part of colon
√5th S36.6 Injury of rectum
√x7th S36.60 Unspecified injury of rectum
√x7th S36.61 Primary blast injury of rectum
Blast injury of rectum NOS
√x7th S36.62 Contusion of rectum
√x7th S36.63 Laceration of rectum
√x7th S36.69 Other injury of rectum
Secondary blast injury of rectum
√5th S36.8 Injury of other intra-abdominal organs
√x7th S36.81 Injury of peritoneum
√6th S36.89 Injury of other intra-abdominal organs
Injury of retroperitoneum
√7th S36.892 Contusion of other intra-abdominal organs
√7th S36.893 Laceration of other intra-abdominal organs
√7th S36.898 Other injury of other intra-abdominal organs
√7th S36.899 Unspecified injury of other intra-abdominal organs
√5th S36.9 Injury of unspecified intra-abdominal organ
√x7th S36.90 Unspecified injury of unspecified intra-abdominal organ
√x7th S36.92 Contusion of unspecified intra-abdominal organ
√x7th S36.93 Laceration of unspecified intra-abdominal organ
√x7th S36.99 Other injury of unspecified intra-abdominal organ

**S37 Injury of urinary and pelvic organs**

Code also any associated open wound (S31.-)

EXCLUDES 1 *obstetric trauma to pelvic organs (O71.-)*

EXCLUDES 2 *injury of peritoneum (S36.81)*
*injury of retroperitoneum (S36.89-)*

The appropriate 7th character is to be added to each code from category S37.
A initial encounter
D subsequent encounter
S sequela

**S37.0 Injury of kidney**

EXCLUDES 2 *acute kidney injury (nontraumatic) (N17.9)*

**S37.00 Unspecified injury of kidney**
- **S37.001 Unspecified injury of right kidney**
- **S37.002 Unspecified injury of left kidney**
- **S37.009 Unspecified injury of unspecified kidney**

**S37.01 Minor contusion of kidney**
Contusion of kidney less than 2 cm
Contusion of kidney NOS
- **S37.011 Minor contusion of right kidney**
- **S37.012 Minor contusion of left kidney**
- **S37.019 Minor contusion of unspecified kidney**

**S37.02 Major contusion of kidney**
Contusion of kidney greater than 2 cm
- **S37.021 Major contusion of right kidney**
- **S37.022 Major contusion of left kidney**
- **S37.029 Major contusion of unspecified kidney**

**S37.03 Laceration of kidney, unspecified degree**
- **S37.031 Laceration of right kidney, unspecified degree**
- **S37.032 Laceration of left kidney, unspecified degree**
- **S37.039 Laceration of unspecified kidney, unspecified degree**

**S37.04 Minor laceration of kidney**
Laceration of kidney less than 1 cm
- **S37.041 Minor laceration of right kidney**
- **S37.042 Minor laceration of left kidney**
- **S37.049 Minor laceration of unspecified kidney**

**S37.05 Moderate laceration of kidney**
Laceration of kidney 1 to 3 cm
- **S37.051 Moderate laceration of right kidney**
- **S37.052 Moderate laceration of left kidney**
- **S37.059 Moderate laceration of unspecified kidney**

**S37.06 Major laceration of kidney**
Avulsion of kidney
Laceration of kidney greater than 3 cm
Massive laceration of kidney
Multiple moderate lacerations of kidney
Stellate laceration of kidney
- **S37.061 Major laceration of right kidney**
- **S37.062 Major laceration of left kidney**
- **S37.069 Major laceration of unspecified kidney**

**S37.09 Other injury of kidney**
- **S37.091 Other injury of right kidney**
- **S37.092 Other injury of left kidney**
- **S37.099 Other injury of unspecified kidney**

**S37.1 Injury of ureter**
- **S37.10 Unspecified injury of ureter**
- **S37.12 Contusion of ureter**
- **S37.13 Laceration of ureter**
- **S37.19 Other injury of ureter**

**S37.2 Injury of bladder**
- **S37.20 Unspecified injury of bladder**
- **S37.22 Contusion of bladder**
- **S37.23 Laceration of bladder**
- **S37.29 Other injury of bladder**

**S37.3 Injury of urethra**
- **S37.30 Unspecified injury of urethra**
- **S37.32 Contusion of urethra**
- **S37.33 Laceration of urethra**
- **S37.39 Other injury of urethra**

**S37.4 Injury of ovary**

**S37.40 Unspecified injury of ovary**
- **S37.401 Unspecified injury of ovary, unilateral**
- **S37.402 Unspecified injury of ovary, bilateral**
- **S37.409 Unspecified injury of ovary, unspecified**

**S37.42 Contusion of ovary**
- **S37.421 Contusion of ovary, unilateral**
- **S37.422 Contusion of ovary, bilateral**
- **S37.429 Contusion of ovary, unspecified**

**S37.43 Laceration of ovary**
- **S37.431 Laceration of ovary, unilateral**
- **S37.432 Laceration of ovary, bilateral**
- **S37.439 Laceration of ovary, unspecified**

**S37.49 Other injury of ovary**
- **S37.491 Other injury of ovary, unilateral**
- **S37.492 Other injury of ovary, bilateral**
- **S37.499 Other injury of ovary, unspecified**

**S37.5 Injury of fallopian tube**

**S37.50 Unspecified injury of fallopian tube**
- **S37.501 Unspecified injury of fallopian tube, unilateral**
- **S37.502 Unspecified injury of fallopian tube, bilateral**
- **S37.509 Unspecified injury of fallopian tube, unspecified**

**S37.51 Primary blast injury of fallopian tube**
Blast injury of fallopian tube NOS
- **S37.511 Primary blast injury of fallopian tube, unilateral**
- **S37.512 Primary blast injury of fallopian tube, bilateral**
- **S37.519 Primary blast injury of fallopian tube, unspecified**

**S37.52 Contusion of fallopian tube**
- **S37.521 Contusion of fallopian tube, unilateral**
- **S37.522 Contusion of fallopian tube, bilateral**
- **S37.529 Contusion of fallopian tube, unspecified**

**S37.53 Laceration of fallopian tube**
- **S37.531 Laceration of fallopian tube, unilateral**
- **S37.532 Laceration of fallopian tube, bilateral**
- **S37.539 Laceration of fallopian tube, unspecified**

**S37.59 Other injury of fallopian tube**
Secondary blast injury of fallopian tube
- **S37.591 Other injury of fallopian tube, unilateral**
- **S37.592 Other injury of fallopian tube, bilateral**
- **S37.599 Other injury of fallopian tube, unspecified**

**S37.6 Injury of uterus**

EXCLUDES 1 *injury to uterus during delivery (O71.-)*
- **S37.60 Unspecified injury of uterus**
- **S37.62 Contusion of uterus**
- **S37.63 Laceration of uterus**
- **S37.69 Other injury of uterus**

**S37.8 Injury of other urinary and pelvic organs**

**S37.81 Injury of adrenal gland**
- **S37.812 Contusion of adrenal gland**
- **S37.813 Laceration of adrenal gland**
- **S37.818 Other injury of adrenal gland**
- **S37.819 Unspecified injury of adrenal gland**

**S37.82 Injury of prostate**
- **S37.822 Contusion of prostate**
- **S37.823 Laceration of prostate**
- **S37.828 Other injury of prostate**
- **S37.829 Unspecified injury of prostate**

**S37.89 Injury of other urinary and pelvic organ**
- **S37.892 Contusion of other urinary and pelvic organ**

√7th S37.893 Laceration of other urinary and pelvic organ

√7th S37.898 Other injury of other urinary and pelvic organ

√7th S37.899 Unspecified injury of other urinary and pelvic organ

√5th S37.9 Injury of unspecified urinary and pelvic organ

√x7th S37.90 Unspecified injury of unspecified urinary and pelvic organ

√x7th S37.92 Contusion of unspecified urinary and pelvic organ

√x7th S37.93 Laceration of unspecified urinary and pelvic organ

√x7th S37.99 Other injury of unspecified urinary and pelvic organ

√4th **S38 Crushing injury and traumatic amputation of abdomen, lower back, pelvis and external genitals**

NOTE An amputation not identified as partial or complete should be coded to complete

The appropriate 7th character is to be added to each code from category S38.
A initial encounter
D subsequent encounter
S sequela

√5th S38.0 Crushing injury of external genital organs

Use additional code for any associated injuries

√6th S38.00 Crushing injury of unspecified external genital organs

√7th S38.001 Crushing injury of unspecified external genital organs, male

√7th S38.002 Crushing injury of unspecified external genital organs, female

√x7th S38.01 Crushing injury of penis

√x7th S38.02 Crushing injury of scrotum and testis

√x7th S38.03 Crushing injury of vulva

√x7th S38.1 Crushing injury of abdomen, lower back, and pelvis

Use additional code for all associated injuries, such as:
fracture of thoracic or lumbar spine and pelvis (S22.0-, S32.-)
injury to intra-abdominal organs (S36.-)
injury to urinary and pelvic organs (S37.-)
open wound of abdominal wall (S31.-)
spinal cord injury (S34.0, S34.1-)

EXCLUDES 2 *crushing injury of external genital organs (S38.0-)*

√5th S38.2 Traumatic amputation of external genital organs

√6th S38.21 Traumatic amputation of female external genital organs

Traumatic amputation of clitoris
Traumatic amputation of labium (majus) (minus)
Traumatic amputation of vulva

√7th S38.211 Complete traumatic amputation of female external genital organs

√7th S38.212 Partial traumatic amputation of female external genital organs

√6th S38.22 Traumatic amputation of penis

√7th S38.221 Complete traumatic amputation of penis

√7th S38.222 Partial traumatic amputation of penis

√6th S38.23 Traumatic amputation of scrotum and testis

√7th S38.231 Complete traumatic amputation of scrotum and testis

√7th S38.232 Partial traumatic amputation of scrotum and testis

√x7th S38.3 Transection (partial) of abdomen

√4th **S39 Other and unspecified injuries of abdomen, lower back, pelvis and external genitals**

Code also any associated open wound (S31.-)

EXCLUDES 2 *sprain of joints and ligaments of lumbar spine and pelvis (S33.-)*

The appropriate 7th character is to be added to each code from category S39.
A initial encounter
D subsequent encounter
S sequela

√5th S39.0 Injury of muscle, fascia and tendon of abdomen, lower back and pelvis

√6th S39.00 Unspecified injury of muscle, fascia and tendon of abdomen, lower back and pelvis

√7th S39.001 Unspecified injury of muscle, fascia and tendon of abdomen

√7th S39.002 Unspecified injury of muscle, fascia and tendon of lower back

√7th S39.003 Unspecified injury of muscle, fascia and tendon of pelvis

√6th S39.01 Strain of muscle, fascia and tendon of abdomen, lower back and pelvis

√7th S39.011 Strain of muscle, fascia and tendon of abdomen

√7th S39.012 Strain of muscle, fascia and tendon of lower back

√7th S39.013 Strain of muscle, fascia and tendon of pelvis

√6th S39.02 Laceration of muscle, fascia and tendon of abdomen, lower back and pelvis

√7th S39.021 Laceration of muscle, fascia and tendon of abdomen

√7th S39.022 Laceration of muscle, fascia and tendon of lower back

√7th S39.023 Laceration of muscle, fascia and tendon of pelvis

√6th S39.09 Other injury of muscle, fascia and tendon of abdomen, lower back and pelvis

√7th S39.091 Other injury of muscle, fascia and tendon of abdomen

√7th S39.092 Other injury of muscle, fascia and tendon of lower back

√7th S39.093 Other injury of muscle, fascia and tendon of pelvis

√5th S39.8 Other specified injuries of abdomen, lower back, pelvis and external genitals

√x7th S39.81 Other specified injuries of abdomen

√x7th S39.82 Other specified injuries of lower back

√x7th S39.83 Other specified injuries of pelvis

√6th S39.84 Other specified injuries of external genitals

√7th S39.840 Fracture of corpus cavernosum penis

√7th S39.848 Other specified injuries of external genitals

√5th S39.9 Unspecified injury of abdomen, lower back, pelvis and external genitals

√x7th S39.91 Unspecified injury of abdomen

√x7th S39.92 Unspecified injury of lower back

√x7th S39.93 Unspecified injury of pelvis

√x7th S39.94 Unspecified injury of external genitals

## Injuries to the shoulder and upper arm (S40-S49)

INCLUDES injuries of axilla
injuries of scapular region

EXCLUDES 2 *burns and corrosions (T20-T32)*
*frostbite (T33-T34)*
*injuries of elbow (S50-S59)*
*insect bite or sting, venomous (T63.4)*

√4th **S40 Superficial injury of shoulder and upper arm**

The appropriate 7th character is to be added to each code from category S40.
A initial encounter
D subsequent encounter
S sequela

√5th S40.0 Contusion of shoulder and upper arm

√6th S40.01 Contusion of shoulder

√7th S40.011 Contusion of right shoulder

√7th S40.012 Contusion of left shoulder

√7th S40.019 Contusion of unspecified shoulder

√6th S40.02 Contusion of upper arm

√7th S40.021 Contusion of right upper arm

√7th S40.022 Contusion of left upper arm

√7th S40.029 Contusion of unspecified upper arm

√5th S40.2 Other superficial injuries of shoulder

√6th S40.21 Abrasion of shoulder

√7th S40.211 Abrasion of right shoulder

√7th S40.212 Abrasion of left shoulder

√7th S40.219 Abrasion of unspecified shoulder

√6th S40.22 Blister (nonthermal) of shoulder

√7th S40.221 Blister (nonthermal) of right shoulder

√7th S40.222 Blister (nonthermal) of left shoulder

√7th S40.229 Blister (nonthermal) of unspecified shoulder

S40.24 External constriction of shoulder
- S40.241 External constriction of right shoulder
- S40.242 External constriction of left shoulder
- S40.249 External constriction of unspecified shoulder

S40.25 Superficial foreign body of shoulder
Splinter in the shoulder
- S40.251 Superficial foreign body of right shoulder
- S40.252 Superficial foreign body of left shoulder
- S40.259 Superficial foreign body of unspecified shoulder

S40.26 Insect bite (nonvenomous) of shoulder
- S40.261 Insect bite (nonvenomous) of right shoulder
- S40.262 Insect bite (nonvenomous) of left shoulder
- S40.269 Insect bite (nonvenomous) of unspecified shoulder

S40.27 Other superficial bite of shoulder
EXCLUDES 1 *open bite of shoulder (S41.05)*
- S40.271 Other superficial bite of right shoulder
- S40.272 Other superficial bite of left shoulder
- S40.279 Other superficial bite of unspecified shoulder

S40.8 Other superficial injuries of upper arm

S40.81 Abrasion of upper arm
- S40.811 Abrasion of right upper arm
- S40.812 Abrasion of left upper arm
- S40.819 Abrasion of unspecified upper arm

S40.82 Blister (nonthermal) of upper arm
- S40.821 Blister (nonthermal) of right upper arm
- S40.822 Blister (nonthermal) of left upper arm
- S40.829 Blister (nonthermal) of unspecified upper arm

S40.84 External constriction of upper arm
- S40.841 External constriction of right upper arm
- S40.842 External constriction of left upper arm
- S40.849 External constriction of unspecified upper arm

S40.85 Superficial foreign body of upper arm
Splinter in the upper arm
- S40.851 Superficial foreign body of right upper arm
- S40.852 Superficial foreign body of left upper arm
- S40.859 Superficial foreign body of unspecified upper arm

S40.86 Insect bite (nonvenomous) of upper arm
- S40.861 Insect bite (nonvenomous) of right upper arm
- S40.862 Insect bite (nonvenomous) of left upper arm
- S40.869 Insect bite (nonvenomous) of unspecified upper arm

S40.87 Other superficial bite of upper arm
EXCLUDES 1 *open bite of upper arm (S41.14)*
EXCLUDES 2 *other superficial bite of shoulder (S40.27-)*
- S40.871 Other superficial bite of right upper arm
- S40.872 Other superficial bite of left upper arm
- S40.879 Other superficial bite of unspecified upper arm

S40.9 Unspecified superficial injury of shoulder and upper arm

S40.91 Unspecified superficial injury of shoulder
- S40.911 Unspecified superficial injury of right shoulder
- S40.912 Unspecified superficial injury of left shoulder
- S40.919 Unspecified superficial injury of unspecified shoulder

S40.92 Unspecified superficial injury of upper arm
- S40.921 Unspecified superficial injury of right upper arm
- S40.922 Unspecified superficial injury of left upper arm
- S40.929 Unspecified superficial injury of unspecified upper arm

## S41 Open wound of shoulder and upper arm

Code also any associated wound infection
EXCLUDES 1 *traumatic amputation of shoulder and upper arm (S48.-)*
EXCLUDES 2 *open fracture of shoulder and upper arm (S42.- with 7th character B or C)*

The appropriate 7th character is to be added to each code from category S41.
- A initial encounter
- D subsequent encounter
- S sequela

S41.0 Open wound of shoulder

S41.00 Unspecified open wound of shoulder
- S41.001 Unspecified open wound of right shoulder
- S41.002 Unspecified open wound of left shoulder
- S41.009 Unspecified open wound of unspecified shoulder

S41.01 Laceration without foreign body of shoulder
- S41.011 Laceration without foreign body of right shoulder
- S41.012 Laceration without foreign body of left shoulder
- S41.019 Laceration without foreign body of unspecified shoulder

S41.02 Laceration with foreign body of shoulder
- S41.021 Laceration with foreign body of right shoulder
- S41.022 Laceration with foreign body of left shoulder
- S41.029 Laceration with foreign body of unspecified shoulder

S41.03 Puncture wound without foreign body of shoulder
- S41.031 Puncture wound without foreign body of right shoulder
- S41.032 Puncture wound without foreign body of left shoulder
- S41.039 Puncture wound without foreign body of unspecified shoulder

S41.04 Puncture wound with foreign body of shoulder
- S41.041 Puncture wound with foreign body of right shoulder
- S41.042 Puncture wound with foreign body of left shoulder
- S41.049 Puncture wound with foreign body of unspecified shoulder

S41.05 Open bite of shoulder
Bite of shoulder NOS
EXCLUDES 1 *superficial bite of shoulder (S40.27)*
- S41.051 Open bite of right shoulder
- S41.052 Open bite of left shoulder
- S41.059 Open bite of unspecified shoulder

S41.1 Open wound of upper arm

S41.10 Unspecified open wound of upper arm
**AHA:** 2016,3Q,24
- S41.101 Unspecified open wound of right upper arm
- S41.102 Unspecified open wound of left upper arm
- S41.109 Unspecified open wound of unspecified upper arm

S41.11 Laceration without foreign body of upper arm
- S41.111 Laceration without foreign body of right upper arm
- S41.112 Laceration without foreign body of left upper arm
- S41.119 Laceration without foreign body of unspecified upper arm

S41.12 Laceration with foreign body of upper arm
- S41.121 Laceration with foreign body of right upper arm
- S41.122 Laceration with foreign body of left upper arm
- S41.129 Laceration with foreign body of unspecified upper arm

S41.13 Puncture wound without foreign body of upper arm
**AHA:** 2016,3Q,24
- S41.131 Puncture wound without foreign body of right upper arm

√7th S41.132 Puncture wound without foreign body of left upper arm

√7th S41.139 Puncture wound without foreign body of unspecified upper arm

√6th S41.14 Puncture wound with foreign body of upper arm

AHA: 2016,3Q,24

√7th S41.141 Puncture wound with foreign body of right upper arm

√7th S41.142 Puncture wound with foreign body of left upper arm

√7th S41.149 Puncture wound with foreign body of unspecified upper arm

√6th S41.15 Open bite of upper arm

Bite of upper arm NOS

EXCLUDES 1 *superficial bite of upper arm (S40.87)*

√7th S41.151 Open bite of right upper arm

√7th S41.152 Open bite of left upper arm

√7th S41.159 Open bite of unspecified upper arm

## √4th S42 Fracture of shoulder and upper arm

NOTE A fracture not indicated as displaced or nondisplaced should be coded to displaced

A fracture not indicated as open or closed should be coded to closed

EXCLUDES 1 *traumatic amputation of shoulder and upper arm (S48.-)*

EXCLUDES 2 *periprosthetic fracture around internal prosthetic shoulder joint (M97.3)*

AHA: 2018,2Q,12; 2015,3Q,37-39

DEF: Diaphysis: Central shaft of a long bone.

DEF: Epiphysis: Proximal and distal rounded ends of a long bone, communicates with the joint.

DEF: Metaphysis: Section of a long bone located between the epiphysis and diaphysis at the proximal and distal ends.

DEF: Physis (growth plate): Narrow zone of cartilaginous tissue between the epiphysis and metaphysis at each end of a long bone. In childhood, proliferation of cells in this zone lengthens the bone. As the bone matures, this area thins, ossification eventually fusing into solid bone and growth stops. ***Synonym(s):*** *Epiphyseal plate.*

The appropriate 7th character is to be added to all codes from category S42 [unless otherwise indicated].
- A initial encounter for closed fracture
- B initial encounter for open fracture
- D subsequent encounter for fracture with routine healing
- G subsequent encounter for fracture with delayed healing
- K subsequent encounter for fracture with nonunion
- P subsequent encounter for fracture with malunion
- S sequela

√5th S42.0 Fracture of clavicle

√6th S42.00 Fracture of unspecified part of clavicle

√7th S42.001 Fracture of unspecified part of right clavicle Q

√7th S42.002 Fracture of unspecified part of left clavicle Q

√7th S42.009 Fracture of unspecified part of unspecified clavicle Q

AHA: 2012,4Q,93

√6th S42.01 Fracture of sternal end of clavicle

√7th S42.011 Anterior displaced fracture of sternal end of right clavicle Q

√7th S42.012 Anterior displaced fracture of sternal end of left clavicle Q

√7th S42.013 Anterior displaced fracture of sternal end of unspecified clavicle Q

Displaced fracture of sternal end of clavicle NOS

√7th S42.014 Posterior displaced fracture of sternal end of right clavicle Q

√7th S42.015 Posterior displaced fracture of sternal end of left clavicle Q

√7th S42.016 Posterior displaced fracture of sternal end of unspecified clavicle Q

√7th S42.017 Nondisplaced fracture of sternal end of right clavicle Q

√7th S42.018 Nondisplaced fracture of sternal end of left clavicle Q

√7th S42.019 Nondisplaced fracture of sternal end of unspecified clavicle Q

√6th S42.02 Fracture of shaft of clavicle

√7th S42.021 Displaced fracture of shaft of right clavicle Q

√7th S42.022 Displaced fracture of shaft of left clavicle Q

√7th S42.023 Displaced fracture of shaft of unspecified clavicle Q

√7th S42.024 Nondisplaced fracture of shaft of right clavicle Q

√7th S42.025 Nondisplaced fracture of shaft of left clavicle Q

√7th S42.026 Nondisplaced fracture of shaft of unspecified clavicle Q

√6th S42.03 Fracture of lateral end of clavicle

Fracture of acromial end of clavicle

√7th S42.031 Displaced fracture of lateral end of right clavicle Q

√7th S42.032 Displaced fracture of lateral end of left clavicle Q

√7th S42.033 Displaced fracture of lateral end of unspecified clavicle Q

√7th S42.034 Nondisplaced fracture of lateral end of right clavicle Q

√7th S42.035 Nondisplaced fracture of lateral end of left clavicle Q

√7th S42.036 Nondisplaced fracture of lateral end of unspecified clavicle Q

√5th S42.1 Fracture of scapula

√6th S42.10 Fracture of unspecified part of scapula

√7th S42.101 Fracture of unspecified part of scapula, right shoulder Q

√7th S42.102 Fracture of unspecified part of scapula, left shoulder Q

√7th S42.109 Fracture of unspecified part of scapula, unspecified shoulder Q

√6th S42.11 Fracture of body of scapula

√7th S42.111 Displaced fracture of body of scapula, right shoulder Q

√7th S42.112 Displaced fracture of body of scapula, left shoulder Q

√7th S42.113 Displaced fracture of body of scapula, unspecified shoulder Q

√7th S42.114 Nondisplaced fracture of body of scapula, right shoulder Q

√7th S42.115 Nondisplaced fracture of body of scapula, left shoulder Q

√7th S42.116 Nondisplaced fracture of body of scapula, unspecified shoulder Q

√6th S42.12 Fracture of acromial process

√7th S42.121 Displaced fracture of acromial process, right shoulder Q

√7th S42.122 Displaced fracture of acromial process, left shoulder Q

√7th S42.123 Displaced fracture of acromial process, unspecified shoulder Q

√7th S42.124 Nondisplaced fracture of acromial process, right shoulder Q

√7th S42.125 Nondisplaced fracture of acromial process, left shoulder Q

√7th S42.126 Nondisplaced fracture of acromial process, unspecified shoulder Q

√6th S42.13 Fracture of coracoid process

√7th S42.131 Displaced fracture of coracoid process, right shoulder Q

√7th S42.132 Displaced fracture of coracoid process, left shoulder Q

√7th S42.133 Displaced fracture of coracoid process, unspecified shoulder Q

√7th S42.134 Nondisplaced fracture of coracoid process, right shoulder Q

√7th S42.135 Nondisplaced fracture of coracoid process, left shoulder Q

√7th S42.136 Nondisplaced fracture of coracoid process, unspecified shoulder Q

√6th S42.14 Fracture of glenoid cavity of scapula

√7th S42.141 Displaced fracture of glenoid cavity of scapula, right shoulder Q

√7th S42.142 Displaced fracture of glenoid cavity of scapula, left shoulder Q
√7th S42.143 Displaced fracture of glenoid cavity of scapula, unspecified shoulder Q
√7th S42.144 Nondisplaced fracture of glenoid cavity of scapula, right shoulder Q
√7th S42.145 Nondisplaced fracture of glenoid cavity of scapula, left shoulder Q
√7th S42.146 Nondisplaced fracture of glenoid cavity of scapula, unspecified shoulder Q

√6th S42.15 Fracture of neck of scapula
√7th S42.151 Displaced fracture of neck of scapula, right shoulder Q
√7th S42.152 Displaced fracture of neck of scapula, left shoulder Q
√7th S42.153 Displaced fracture of neck of scapula, unspecified shoulder Q
√7th S42.154 Nondisplaced fracture of neck of scapula, right shoulder Q
√7th S42.155 Nondisplaced fracture of neck of scapula, left shoulder Q
√7th S42.156 Nondisplaced fracture of neck of scapula, unspecified shoulder Q

√6th S42.19 Fracture of other part of scapula
√7th S42.191 Fracture of other part of scapula, right shoulder Q
√7th S42.192 Fracture of other part of scapula, left shoulder Q
√7th S42.199 Fracture of other part of scapula, unspecified shoulder Q

√5th S42.2 Fracture of upper end of humerus
Fracture of proximal end of humerus
EXCLUDES 2 *fracture of shaft of humerus (S42.3-)*
*physeal fracture of upper end of humerus (S49.Ø-)*

√6th S42.2Ø Unspecified fracture of upper end of humerus
√7th S42.2Ø1 Unspecified fracture of upper end of right humerus Q
√7th S42.2Ø2 Unspecified fracture of upper end of left humerus Q
√7th S42.2Ø9 Unspecified fracture of upper end of unspecified humerus Q

√6th S42.21 Unspecified fracture of surgical neck of humerus
Fracture of neck of humerus NOS
√7th S42.211 Unspecified displaced fracture of surgical neck of right humerus Q
√7th S42.212 Unspecified displaced fracture of surgical neck of left humerus Q
√7th S42.213 Unspecified displaced fracture of surgical neck of unspecified humerus Q
√7th S42.214 Unspecified nondisplaced fracture of surgical neck of right humerus Q
√7th S42.215 Unspecified nondisplaced fracture of surgical neck of left humerus Q
√7th S42.216 Unspecified nondisplaced fracture of surgical neck of unspecified humerus Q

√6th S42.22 2-part fracture of surgical neck of humerus
√7th S42.221 2-part displaced fracture of surgical neck of right humerus Q
√7th S42.222 2-part displaced fracture of surgical neck of left humerus Q
√7th S42.223 2-part displaced fracture of surgical neck of unspecified humerus Q
√7th S42.224 2-part nondisplaced fracture of surgical neck of right humerus Q
√7th S42.225 2-part nondisplaced fracture of surgical neck of left humerus Q
√7th S42.226 2-part nondisplaced fracture of surgical neck of unspecified humerus Q

√6th S42.23 3-part fracture of surgical neck of humerus
√7th S42.231 3-part fracture of surgical neck of right humerus Q
√7th S42.232 3-part fracture of surgical neck of left humerus Q
√7th S42.239 3-part fracture of surgical neck of unspecified humerus Q

√6th S42.24 4-part fracture of surgical neck of humerus
√7th S42.241 4-part fracture of surgical neck of right humerus Q
√7th S42.242 4-part fracture of surgical neck of left humerus Q
√7th S42.249 4-part fracture of surgical neck of unspecified humerus Q

√6th S42.25 Fracture of greater tuberosity of humerus
√7th S42.251 Displaced fracture of greater tuberosity of right humerus Q
√7th S42.252 Displaced fracture of greater tuberosity of left humerus Q
√7th S42.253 Displaced fracture of greater tuberosity of unspecified humerus Q
√7th S42.254 Nondisplaced fracture of greater tuberosity of right humerus Q
√7th S42.255 Nondisplaced fracture of greater tuberosity of left humerus Q
√7th S42.256 Nondisplaced fracture of greater tuberosity of unspecified humerus Q

√6th S42.26 Fracture of lesser tuberosity of humerus
√7th S42.261 Displaced fracture of lesser tuberosity of right humerus Q
√7th S42.262 Displaced fracture of lesser tuberosity of left humerus Q
√7th S42.263 Displaced fracture of lesser tuberosity of unspecified humerus Q
√7th S42.264 Nondisplaced fracture of lesser tuberosity of right humerus Q
√7th S42.265 Nondisplaced fracture of lesser tuberosity of left humerus Q
√7th S42.266 Nondisplaced fracture of lesser tuberosity of unspecified humerus Q

√6th S42.27 Torus fracture of upper end of humerus

The appropriate 7th character is to be added to all codes in subcategory S42.27
A initial encounter for closed fracture
D subsequent encounter for fracture with routine healing
G subsequent encounter for fracture with delayed healing
K subsequent encounter for fracture with nonunion
P subsequent encounter for fracture with malunion
S sequela

√7th S42.271 Torus fracture of upper end of right humerus Q
√7th S42.272 Torus fracture of upper end of left humerus Q
√7th S42.279 Torus fracture of upper end of unspecified humerus Q

√6th S42.29 Other fracture of upper end of humerus
Fracture of anatomical neck of humerus
Fracture of articular head of humerus
**AHA:** 2024,2Q,24; 2019,1Q,18
√7th S42.291 Other displaced fracture of upper end of right humerus Q
√7th S42.292 Other displaced fracture of upper end of left humerus Q
√7th S42.293 Other displaced fracture of upper end of unspecified humerus Q
√7th S42.294 Other nondisplaced fracture of upper end of right humerus Q
√7th S42.295 Other nondisplaced fracture of upper end of left humerus Q
√7th S42.296 Other nondisplaced fracture of upper end of unspecified humerus Q

√5th S42.3 Fracture of shaft of humerus
Fracture of humerus NOS
Fracture of upper arm NOS
EXCLUDES 2 *physeal fractures of upper end of humerus (S49.Ø-)*
*physeal fractures of lower end of humerus (S49.1-)*

√6th S42.3Ø Unspecified fracture of shaft of humerus
√7th S42.3Ø1 Unspecified fracture of shaft of humerus, right arm Q
√7th S42.3Ø2 Unspecified fracture of shaft of humerus, left arm Q
√7th S42.3Ø9 Unspecified fracture of shaft of humerus, unspecified arm Q

6th S42.31 Greenstick fracture of shaft of humerus

The appropriate 7th character is to be added to all codes in subcategory S42.31
A initial encounter for closed fracture
D subsequent encounter for fracture with routine healing
G subsequent encounter for fracture with delayed healing
K subsequent encounter for fracture with nonunion
P subsequent encounter for fracture with malunion
S sequela

7th S42.311 Greenstick fracture of shaft of humerus, right arm Q
7th S42.312 Greenstick fracture of shaft of humerus, left arm Q
7th S42.319 Greenstick fracture of shaft of humerus, unspecified arm Q

6th S42.32 Transverse fracture of shaft of humerus
7th S42.321 Displaced transverse fracture of shaft of humerus, right arm Q
7th S42.322 Displaced transverse fracture of shaft of humerus, left arm Q
7th S42.323 Displaced transverse fracture of shaft of humerus, unspecified arm Q
7th S42.324 Nondisplaced transverse fracture of shaft of humerus, right arm Q
7th S42.325 Nondisplaced transverse fracture of shaft of humerus, left arm Q
7th S42.326 Nondisplaced transverse fracture of shaft of humerus, unspecified arm Q

6th S42.33 Oblique fracture of shaft of humerus
7th S42.331 Displaced oblique fracture of shaft of humerus, right arm Q
7th S42.332 Displaced oblique fracture of shaft of humerus, left arm Q
7th S42.333 Displaced oblique fracture of shaft of humerus, unspecified arm Q
7th S42.334 Nondisplaced oblique fracture of shaft of humerus, right arm Q
7th S42.335 Nondisplaced oblique fracture of shaft of humerus, left arm Q
7th S42.336 Nondisplaced oblique fracture of shaft of humerus, unspecified arm Q

6th S42.34 Spiral fracture of shaft of humerus
7th S42.341 Displaced spiral fracture of shaft of humerus, right arm Q
7th S42.342 Displaced spiral fracture of shaft of humerus, left arm Q
7th S42.343 Displaced spiral fracture of shaft of humerus, unspecified arm Q
7th S42.344 Nondisplaced spiral fracture of shaft of humerus, right arm Q
7th S42.345 Nondisplaced spiral fracture of shaft of humerus, left arm Q
7th S42.346 Nondisplaced spiral fracture of shaft of humerus, unspecified arm Q

6th S42.35 Comminuted fracture of shaft of humerus
7th S42.351 Displaced comminuted fracture of shaft of humerus, right arm Q
7th S42.352 Displaced comminuted fracture of shaft of humerus, left arm Q
7th S42.353 Displaced comminuted fracture of shaft of humerus, unspecified arm Q
7th S42.354 Nondisplaced comminuted fracture of shaft of humerus, right arm Q
7th S42.355 Nondisplaced comminuted fracture of shaft of humerus, left arm Q
7th S42.356 Nondisplaced comminuted fracture of shaft of humerus, unspecified arm Q

6th S42.36 Segmental fracture of shaft of humerus
7th S42.361 Displaced segmental fracture of shaft of humerus, right arm Q
7th S42.362 Displaced segmental fracture of shaft of humerus, left arm Q
7th S42.363 Displaced segmental fracture of shaft of humerus, unspecified arm Q
7th S42.364 Nondisplaced segmental fracture of shaft of humerus, right arm Q
7th S42.365 Nondisplaced segmental fracture of shaft of humerus, left arm Q
7th S42.366 Nondisplaced segmental fracture of shaft of humerus, unspecified arm Q

6th S42.39 Other fracture of shaft of humerus
7th S42.391 Other fracture of shaft of right humerus Q
7th S42.392 Other fracture of shaft of left humerus Q
7th S42.399 Other fracture of shaft of unspecified humerus Q

5th S42.4 Fracture of lower end of humerus

Fracture of distal end of humerus

EXCLUDES 2 *fracture of shaft of humerus (S42.3-)*
*physeal fracture of lower end of humerus (S49.1-)*

6th S42.40 Unspecified fracture of lower end of humerus

Fracture of elbow NOS

7th S42.401 Unspecified fracture of lower end of right humerus Q
7th S42.402 Unspecified fracture of lower end of left humerus Q
7th S42.409 Unspecified fracture of lower end of unspecified humerus Q

6th S42.41 Simple supracondylar fracture without intercondylar fracture of humerus
7th S42.411 Displaced simple supracondylar fracture without intercondylar fracture of right humerus Q
7th S42.412 Displaced simple supracondylar fracture without intercondylar fracture of left humerus Q
7th S42.413 Displaced simple supracondylar fracture without intercondylar fracture of unspecified humerus Q
7th S42.414 Nondisplaced simple supracondylar fracture without intercondylar fracture of right humerus Q
7th S42.415 Nondisplaced simple supracondylar fracture without intercondylar fracture of left humerus Q
7th S42.416 Nondisplaced simple supracondylar fracture without intercondylar fracture of unspecified humerus Q

6th S42.42 Comminuted supracondylar fracture without intercondylar fracture of humerus
7th S42.421 Displaced comminuted supracondylar fracture without intercondylar fracture of right humerus Q
7th S42.422 Displaced comminuted supracondylar fracture without intercondylar fracture of left humerus Q
7th S42.423 Displaced comminuted supracondylar fracture without intercondylar fracture of unspecified humerus Q
7th S42.424 Nondisplaced comminuted supracondylar fracture without intercondylar fracture of right humerus Q
7th S42.425 Nondisplaced comminuted supracondylar fracture without intercondylar fracture of left humerus Q
7th S42.426 Nondisplaced comminuted supracondylar fracture without intercondylar fracture of unspecified humerus Q

6th S42.43 Fracture (avulsion) of lateral epicondyle of humerus
7th S42.431 Displaced fracture (avulsion) of lateral epicondyle of right humerus Q
7th S42.432 Displaced fracture (avulsion) of lateral epicondyle of left humerus Q
7th S42.433 Displaced fracture (avulsion) of lateral epicondyle of unspecified humerus Q
7th S42.434 Nondisplaced fracture (avulsion) of lateral epicondyle of right humerus Q
7th S42.435 Nondisplaced fracture (avulsion) of lateral epicondyle of left humerus Q
7th S42.436 Nondisplaced fracture (avulsion) of lateral epicondyle of unspecified humerus Q

6th S42.44 Fracture (avulsion) of medial epicondyle of humerus
7th S42.441 Displaced fracture (avulsion) of medial epicondyle of right humerus Q

S42.442 Displaced fracture (avulsion) of medial epicondyle of left humerus Q
S42.443 Displaced fracture (avulsion) of medial epicondyle of unspecified humerus Q
S42.444 Nondisplaced fracture (avulsion) of medial epicondyle of right humerus Q
S42.445 Nondisplaced fracture (avulsion) of medial epicondyle of left humerus Q
S42.446 Nondisplaced fracture (avulsion) of medial epicondyle of unspecified humerus Q
S42.447 Incarcerated fracture (avulsion) of medial epicondyle of right humerus Q
S42.448 Incarcerated fracture (avulsion) of medial epicondyle of left humerus Q
S42.449 Incarcerated fracture (avulsion) of medial epicondyle of unspecified humerus Q

S42.45 Fracture of lateral condyle of humerus
Fracture of capitellum of humerus
S42.451 Displaced fracture of lateral condyle of right humerus Q
S42.452 Displaced fracture of lateral condyle of left humerus Q
S42.453 Displaced fracture of lateral condyle of unspecified humerus Q
S42.454 Nondisplaced fracture of lateral condyle of right humerus Q
S42.455 Nondisplaced fracture of lateral condyle of left humerus Q
S42.456 Nondisplaced fracture of lateral condyle of unspecified humerus Q

S42.46 Fracture of medial condyle of humerus
Trochlea fracture of humerus
S42.461 Displaced fracture of medial condyle of right humerus Q
S42.462 Displaced fracture of medial condyle of left humerus Q
S42.463 Displaced fracture of medial condyle of unspecified humerus Q
S42.464 Nondisplaced fracture of medial condyle of right humerus Q
S42.465 Nondisplaced fracture of medial condyle of left humerus Q
S42.466 Nondisplaced fracture of medial condyle of unspecified humerus Q

S42.47 Transcondylar fracture of humerus
S42.471 Displaced transcondylar fracture of right humerus Q
S42.472 Displaced transcondylar fracture of left humerus Q
S42.473 Displaced transcondylar fracture of unspecified humerus Q
S42.474 Nondisplaced transcondylar fracture of right humerus Q
S42.475 Nondisplaced transcondylar fracture of left humerus Q
S42.476 Nondisplaced transcondylar fracture of unspecified humerus Q

S42.48 Torus fracture of lower end of humerus

The appropriate 7th character is to be added to all codes in subcategory S42.48.
A initial encounter for closed fracture
D subsequent encounter for fracture with routine healing
G subsequent encounter for fracture with delayed healing
K subsequent encounter for fracture with nonunion
P subsequent encounter for fracture with malunion
S sequela

S42.481 Torus fracture of lower end of right humerus Q
S42.482 Torus fracture of lower end of left humerus Q
S42.489 Torus fracture of lower end of unspecified humerus Q

S42.49 Other fracture of lower end of humerus
S42.491 Other displaced fracture of lower end of right humerus Q
S42.492 Other displaced fracture of lower end of left humerus Q
S42.493 Other displaced fracture of lower end of unspecified humerus Q
S42.494 Other nondisplaced fracture of lower end of right humerus Q
S42.495 Other nondisplaced fracture of lower end of left humerus Q
S42.496 Other nondisplaced fracture of lower end of unspecified humerus Q

S42.9 Fracture of shoulder girdle, part unspecified
Fracture of shoulder NOS
S42.9Ø Fracture of unspecified shoulder girdle, part unspecified Q
S42.91 Fracture of right shoulder girdle, part unspecified Q
S42.92 Fracture of left shoulder girdle, part unspecified Q

## S43 Dislocation and sprain of joints and ligaments of shoulder girdle

INCLUDES avulsion of joint or ligament of shoulder girdle
laceration of cartilage, joint or ligament of shoulder girdle
sprain of cartilage, joint or ligament of shoulder girdle
traumatic hemarthrosis of joint or ligament of shoulder girdle
traumatic rupture of joint or ligament of shoulder girdle
traumatic subluxation of joint or ligament of shoulder girdle
traumatic tear of joint or ligament of shoulder girdle

Code also any associated open wound

EXCLUDES 2 *strain of muscle, fascia and tendon of shoulder and upper arm (S46.-)*

The appropriate 7th character is to be added to each code from category S43.
A initial encounter
D subsequent encounter
S sequela

S43.Ø Subluxation and dislocation of shoulder joint
Dislocation of glenohumeral joint
Subluxation of glenohumeral joint

S43.ØØ Unspecified subluxation and dislocation of shoulder joint
Dislocation of humerus NOS
Subluxation of humerus NOS
S43.ØØ1 Unspecified subluxation of right shoulder joint
S43.ØØ2 Unspecified subluxation of left shoulder joint
S43.ØØ3 Unspecified subluxation of unspecified shoulder joint
S43.ØØ4 Unspecified dislocation of right shoulder joint
S43.ØØ5 Unspecified dislocation of left shoulder joint
S43.ØØ6 Unspecified dislocation of unspecified shoulder joint

S43.Ø1 Anterior subluxation and dislocation of humerus
S43.Ø11 Anterior subluxation of right humerus
S43.Ø12 Anterior subluxation of left humerus
S43.Ø13 Anterior subluxation of unspecified humerus
S43.Ø14 Anterior dislocation of right humerus
S43.Ø15 Anterior dislocation of left humerus
S43.Ø16 Anterior dislocation of unspecified humerus

S43.Ø2 Posterior subluxation and dislocation of humerus
S43.Ø21 Posterior subluxation of right humerus
S43.Ø22 Posterior subluxation of left humerus
S43.Ø23 Posterior subluxation of unspecified humerus
S43.Ø24 Posterior dislocation of right humerus
S43.Ø25 Posterior dislocation of left humerus
S43.Ø26 Posterior dislocation of unspecified humerus

S43.Ø3 Inferior subluxation and dislocation of humerus
S43.Ø31 Inferior subluxation of right humerus
S43.Ø32 Inferior subluxation of left humerus
S43.Ø33 Inferior subluxation of unspecified humerus
S43.Ø34 Inferior dislocation of right humerus

7th S43.035 Inferior dislocation of left humerus
7th S43.036 Inferior dislocation of unspecified humerus
6th S43.08 Other subluxation and dislocation of shoulder joint
7th S43.081 Other subluxation of right shoulder joint
7th S43.082 Other subluxation of left shoulder joint
7th S43.083 Other subluxation of unspecified shoulder joint
7th S43.084 Other dislocation of right shoulder joint
7th S43.085 Other dislocation of left shoulder joint
7th S43.086 Other dislocation of unspecified shoulder joint
5th S43.1 Subluxation and dislocation of acromioclavicular joint
6th S43.10 Unspecified dislocation of acromioclavicular joint
7th S43.101 Unspecified dislocation of right acromioclavicular joint
7th S43.102 Unspecified dislocation of left acromioclavicular joint
7th S43.109 Unspecified dislocation of unspecified acromioclavicular joint
6th S43.11 Subluxation of acromioclavicular joint
7th S43.111 Subluxation of right acromioclavicular joint
7th S43.112 Subluxation of left acromioclavicular joint
7th S43.119 Subluxation of unspecified acromioclavicular joint
6th S43.12 Dislocation of acromioclavicular joint, 100%-200% displacement
7th S43.121 Dislocation of right acromioclavicular joint, 100%-200% displacement
7th S43.122 Dislocation of left acromioclavicular joint, 100%-200% displacement
7th S43.129 Dislocation of unspecified acromioclavicular joint, 100%-200% displacement
6th S43.13 Dislocation of acromioclavicular joint, greater than 200% displacement
7th S43.131 Dislocation of right acromioclavicular joint, greater than 200% displacement
7th S43.132 Dislocation of left acromioclavicular joint, greater than 200% displacement
7th S43.139 Dislocation of unspecified acromioclavicular joint, greater than 200% displacement
6th S43.14 Inferior dislocation of acromioclavicular joint
7th S43.141 Inferior dislocation of right acromioclavicular joint
7th S43.142 Inferior dislocation of left acromioclavicular joint
7th S43.149 Inferior dislocation of unspecified acromioclavicular joint
6th S43.15 Posterior dislocation of acromioclavicular joint
7th S43.151 Posterior dislocation of right acromioclavicular joint
7th S43.152 Posterior dislocation of left acromioclavicular joint
7th S43.159 Posterior dislocation of unspecified acromioclavicular joint
5th S43.2 Subluxation and dislocation of sternoclavicular joint
6th S43.20 Unspecified subluxation and dislocation of sternoclavicular joint
7th S43.201 Unspecified subluxation of right sternoclavicular joint
7th S43.202 Unspecified subluxation of left sternoclavicular joint
7th S43.203 Unspecified subluxation of unspecified sternoclavicular joint
7th S43.204 Unspecified dislocation of right sternoclavicular joint
7th S43.205 Unspecified dislocation of left sternoclavicular joint
7th S43.206 Unspecified dislocation of unspecified sternoclavicular joint
6th S43.21 Anterior subluxation and dislocation of sternoclavicular joint
7th S43.211 Anterior subluxation of right sternoclavicular joint
7th S43.212 Anterior subluxation of left sternoclavicular joint
7th S43.213 Anterior subluxation of unspecified sternoclavicular joint
7th S43.214 Anterior dislocation of right sternoclavicular joint
7th S43.215 Anterior dislocation of left sternoclavicular joint
7th S43.216 Anterior dislocation of unspecified sternoclavicular joint
6th S43.22 Posterior subluxation and dislocation of sternoclavicular joint
7th S43.221 Posterior subluxation of right sternoclavicular joint
7th S43.222 Posterior subluxation of left sternoclavicular joint
7th S43.223 Posterior subluxation of unspecified sternoclavicular joint
7th S43.224 Posterior dislocation of right sternoclavicular joint
7th S43.225 Posterior dislocation of left sternoclavicular joint
7th S43.226 Posterior dislocation of unspecified sternoclavicular joint
5th S43.3 Subluxation and dislocation of other and unspecified parts of shoulder girdle
6th S43.30 Subluxation and dislocation of unspecified parts of shoulder girdle
Dislocation of shoulder girdle NOS
Subluxation of shoulder girdle NOS
7th S43.301 Subluxation of unspecified parts of right shoulder girdle
7th S43.302 Subluxation of unspecified parts of left shoulder girdle
7th S43.303 Subluxation of unspecified parts of unspecified shoulder girdle
7th S43.304 Dislocation of unspecified parts of right shoulder girdle
7th S43.305 Dislocation of unspecified parts of left shoulder girdle
7th S43.306 Dislocation of unspecified parts of unspecified shoulder girdle
6th S43.31 Subluxation and dislocation of scapula
7th S43.311 Subluxation of right scapula
7th S43.312 Subluxation of left scapula
7th S43.313 Subluxation of unspecified scapula
7th S43.314 Dislocation of right scapula
7th S43.315 Dislocation of left scapula
7th S43.316 Dislocation of unspecified scapula
6th S43.39 Subluxation and dislocation of other parts of shoulder girdle
7th S43.391 Subluxation of other parts of right shoulder girdle
7th S43.392 Subluxation of other parts of left shoulder girdle
7th S43.393 Subluxation of other parts of unspecified shoulder girdle
7th S43.394 Dislocation of other parts of right shoulder girdle
7th S43.395 Dislocation of other parts of left shoulder girdle
7th S43.396 Dislocation of other parts of unspecified shoulder girdle
5th S43.4 Sprain of shoulder joint
6th S43.40 Unspecified sprain of shoulder joint
7th S43.401 Unspecified sprain of right shoulder joint
7th S43.402 Unspecified sprain of left shoulder joint
7th S43.409 Unspecified sprain of unspecified shoulder joint
6th S43.41 Sprain of coracohumeral (ligament)
7th S43.411 Sprain of right coracohumeral (ligament)
7th S43.412 Sprain of left coracohumeral (ligament)
7th S43.419 Sprain of unspecified coracohumeral (ligament)
6th S43.42 Sprain of rotator cuff capsule
EXCLUDES 1 *rotator cuff syndrome (complete) (incomplete), not specified as traumatic (M75.1-)*
EXCLUDES 2 *injury of tendon of rotator cuff (S46.0-)*
7th S43.421 Sprain of right rotator cuff capsule
7th S43.422 Sprain of left rotator cuff capsule
7th S43.429 Sprain of unspecified rotator cuff capsule

S43.43 **Superior glenoid labrum lesion**
SLAP lesion
**AHA:** 2024,2Q,24; 2019,2Q,26
**DEF:** Detachment injury of the superior aspect of the glenoid labrum, which is the ring of fibrocartilage attached to the rim of the glenoid cavity of the scapula.
S43.431 **Superior glenoid labrum lesion of right shoulder**
S43.432 **Superior glenoid labrum lesion of left shoulder**
S43.439 **Superior glenoid labrum lesion of unspecified shoulder**
S43.49 **Other sprain of shoulder joint**
S43.491 **Other sprain of right shoulder joint**
S43.492 **Other sprain of left shoulder joint**
S43.499 **Other sprain of unspecified shoulder joint**
S43.5 **Sprain of acromioclavicular joint**
Sprain of acromioclavicular ligament
S43.50 **Sprain of unspecified acromioclavicular joint**
S43.51 **Sprain of right acromioclavicular joint**
S43.52 **Sprain of left acromioclavicular joint**
S43.6 **Sprain of sternoclavicular joint**
S43.60 **Sprain of unspecified sternoclavicular joint**
S43.61 **Sprain of right sternoclavicular joint**
S43.62 **Sprain of left sternoclavicular joint**
S43.8 **Sprain of other specified parts of shoulder girdle**
S43.80 **Sprain of other specified parts of unspecified shoulder girdle**
S43.81 **Sprain of other specified parts of right shoulder girdle**
S43.82 **Sprain of other specified parts of left shoulder girdle**
S43.9 **Sprain of unspecified parts of shoulder girdle**
S43.90 **Sprain of unspecified parts of unspecified shoulder girdle**
Sprain of shoulder girdle NOS
S43.91 **Sprain of unspecified parts of right shoulder girdle**
S43.92 **Sprain of unspecified parts of left shoulder girdle**

**S44 Injury of nerves at shoulder and upper arm level**
Code also any associated open wound (S41.-)
EXCLUDES 2 *injury of brachial plexus (S14.3-)*

The appropriate 7th character is to be added to each code from category S44.
A initial encounter
D subsequent encounter
S sequela

S44.0 **Injury of ulnar nerve at upper arm level**
EXCLUDES 1 *ulnar nerve NOS (S54.0)*
S44.00 **Injury of ulnar nerve at upper arm level, unspecified arm**
S44.01 **Injury of ulnar nerve at upper arm level, right arm**
S44.02 **Injury of ulnar nerve at upper arm level, left arm**
S44.1 **Injury of median nerve at upper arm level**
EXCLUDES 1 *median nerve NOS (S54.1)*
S44.10 **Injury of median nerve at upper arm level, unspecified arm**
S44.11 **Injury of median nerve at upper arm level, right arm**
S44.12 **Injury of median nerve at upper arm level, left arm**
S44.2 **Injury of radial nerve at upper arm level**
EXCLUDES 1 *radial nerve NOS (S54.2)*
S44.20 **Injury of radial nerve at upper arm level, unspecified arm**
S44.21 **Injury of radial nerve at upper arm level, right arm**
S44.22 **Injury of radial nerve at upper arm level, left arm**
S44.3 **Injury of axillary nerve**
S44.30 **Injury of axillary nerve, unspecified arm**
S44.31 **Injury of axillary nerve, right arm**
S44.32 **Injury of axillary nerve, left arm**
S44.4 **Injury of musculocutaneous nerve**
S44.40 **Injury of musculocutaneous nerve, unspecified arm**
S44.41 **Injury of musculocutaneous nerve, right arm**
S44.42 **Injury of musculocutaneous nerve, left arm**
S44.5 **Injury of cutaneous sensory nerve at shoulder and upper arm level**
S44.50 **Injury of cutaneous sensory nerve at shoulder and upper arm level, unspecified arm**
S44.51 **Injury of cutaneous sensory nerve at shoulder and upper arm level, right arm**
S44.52 **Injury of cutaneous sensory nerve at shoulder and upper arm level, left arm**
S44.8 **Injury of other nerves at shoulder and upper arm level**
S44.8X **Injury of other nerves at shoulder and upper arm level**
S44.8X1 **Injury of other nerves at shoulder and upper arm level, right arm**
S44.8X2 **Injury of other nerves at shoulder and upper arm level, left arm**
S44.8X9 **Injury of other nerves at shoulder and upper arm level, unspecified arm**
S44.9 **Injury of unspecified nerve at shoulder and upper arm level**
S44.90 **Injury of unspecified nerve at shoulder and upper arm level, unspecified arm**
S44.91 **Injury of unspecified nerve at shoulder and upper arm level, right arm**
S44.92 **Injury of unspecified nerve at shoulder and upper arm level, left arm**

**S45 Injury of blood vessels at shoulder and upper arm level**
Code also any associated open wound (S41.-)
EXCLUDES 2 *injury of subclavian artery (S25.1)*
*injury of subclavian vein (S25.3)*

The appropriate 7th character is to be added to each code from category S45.
A initial encounter
D subsequent encounter
S sequela

S45.0 **Injury of axillary artery**
S45.00 **Unspecified injury of axillary artery**
S45.001 **Unspecified injury of axillary artery, right side**
S45.002 **Unspecified injury of axillary artery, left side**
S45.009 **Unspecified injury of axillary artery, unspecified side**
S45.01 **Laceration of axillary artery**
S45.011 **Laceration of axillary artery, right side**
S45.012 **Laceration of axillary artery, left side**
S45.019 **Laceration of axillary artery, unspecified side**
S45.09 **Other specified injury of axillary artery**
S45.091 **Other specified injury of axillary artery, right side**
S45.092 **Other specified injury of axillary artery, left side**
S45.099 **Other specified injury of axillary artery, unspecified side**
S45.1 **Injury of brachial artery**
S45.10 **Unspecified injury of brachial artery**
S45.101 **Unspecified injury of brachial artery, right side**
S45.102 **Unspecified injury of brachial artery, left side**
S45.109 **Unspecified injury of brachial artery, unspecified side**
S45.11 **Laceration of brachial artery**
S45.111 **Laceration of brachial artery, right side**
S45.112 **Laceration of brachial artery, left side**
S45.119 **Laceration of brachial artery, unspecified side**
S45.19 **Other specified injury of brachial artery**
S45.191 **Other specified injury of brachial artery, right side**
S45.192 **Other specified injury of brachial artery, left side**
S45.199 **Other specified injury of brachial artery, unspecified side**
S45.2 **Injury of axillary or brachial vein**
S45.20 **Unspecified injury of axillary or brachial vein**
S45.201 **Unspecified injury of axillary or brachial vein, right side**

- 7th S45.202 Unspecified injury of axillary or brachial vein, left side
- 7th S45.209 Unspecified injury of axillary or brachial vein, unspecified side
- 6th S45.21 Laceration of axillary or brachial vein
  - 7th S45.211 Laceration of axillary or brachial vein, right side
  - 7th S45.212 Laceration of axillary or brachial vein, left side
  - 7th S45.219 Laceration of axillary or brachial vein, unspecified side
- 6th S45.29 Other specified injury of axillary or brachial vein
  - 7th S45.291 Other specified injury of axillary or brachial vein, right side
  - 7th S45.292 Other specified injury of axillary or brachial vein, left side
  - 7th S45.299 Other specified injury of axillary or brachial vein, unspecified side

5th S45.3 Injury of superficial vein at shoulder and upper arm level
- 6th S45.30 Unspecified injury of superficial vein at shoulder and upper arm level
  - 7th S45.301 Unspecified injury of superficial vein at shoulder and upper arm level, right arm
  - 7th S45.302 Unspecified injury of superficial vein at shoulder and upper arm level, left arm
  - 7th S45.309 Unspecified injury of superficial vein at shoulder and upper arm level, unspecified arm
- 6th S45.31 Laceration of superficial vein at shoulder and upper arm level
  - 7th S45.311 Laceration of superficial vein at shoulder and upper arm level, right arm
  - 7th S45.312 Laceration of superficial vein at shoulder and upper arm level, left arm
  - 7th S45.319 Laceration of superficial vein at shoulder and upper arm level, unspecified arm
- 6th S45.39 Other specified injury of superficial vein at shoulder and upper arm level
  - 7th S45.391 Other specified injury of superficial vein at shoulder and upper arm level, right arm
  - 7th S45.392 Other specified injury of superficial vein at shoulder and upper arm level, left arm
  - 7th S45.399 Other specified injury of superficial vein at shoulder and upper arm level, unspecified arm

5th S45.8 Injury of other specified blood vessels at shoulder and upper arm level
- 6th S45.80 Unspecified injury of other specified blood vessels at shoulder and upper arm level
  - 7th S45.801 Unspecified injury of other specified blood vessels at shoulder and upper arm level, right arm
  - 7th S45.802 Unspecified injury of other specified blood vessels at shoulder and upper arm level, left arm
  - 7th S45.809 Unspecified injury of other specified blood vessels at shoulder and upper arm level, unspecified arm
- 6th S45.81 Laceration of other specified blood vessels at shoulder and upper arm level
  - 7th S45.811 Laceration of other specified blood vessels at shoulder and upper arm level, right arm
  - 7th S45.812 Laceration of other specified blood vessels at shoulder and upper arm level, left arm
  - 7th S45.819 Laceration of other specified blood vessels at shoulder and upper arm level, unspecified arm
- 6th S45.89 Other specified injury of other specified blood vessels at shoulder and upper arm level
  - 7th S45.891 Other specified injury of other specified blood vessels at shoulder and upper arm level, right arm
  - 7th S45.892 Other specified injury of other specified blood vessels at shoulder and upper arm level, left arm
  - 7th S45.899 Other specified injury of other specified blood vessels at shoulder and upper arm level, unspecified arm

5th S45.9 Injury of unspecified blood vessel at shoulder and upper arm level
- 6th S45.90 Unspecified injury of unspecified blood vessel at shoulder and upper arm level
  - 7th S45.901 Unspecified injury of unspecified blood vessel at shoulder and upper arm level, right arm
  - 7th S45.902 Unspecified injury of unspecified blood vessel at shoulder and upper arm level, left arm
  - 7th S45.909 Unspecified injury of unspecified blood vessel at shoulder and upper arm level, unspecified arm
- 6th S45.91 Laceration of unspecified blood vessel at shoulder and upper arm level
  - 7th S45.911 Laceration of unspecified blood vessel at shoulder and upper arm level, right arm
  - 7th S45.912 Laceration of unspecified blood vessel at shoulder and upper arm level, left arm
  - 7th S45.919 Laceration of unspecified blood vessel at shoulder and upper arm level, unspecified arm
- 6th S45.99 Other specified injury of unspecified blood vessel at shoulder and upper arm level
  - 7th S45.991 Other specified injury of unspecified blood vessel at shoulder and upper arm level, right arm
  - 7th S45.992 Other specified injury of unspecified blood vessel at shoulder and upper arm level, left arm
  - 7th S45.999 Other specified injury of unspecified blood vessel at shoulder and upper arm level, unspecified arm

## 4th S46 Injury of muscle, fascia and tendon at shoulder and upper arm level

Code also any associated open wound (S41.-)

EXCLUDES 2 *injury of muscle, fascia and tendon at elbow (S56.-)*
*sprain of joints and ligaments of shoulder girdle (S43.9)*

**TIP:** Refer to the Muscle/Tendon table at the beginning of this chapter.

> The appropriate 7th character is to be added to each code from category S46.
> A initial encounter
> D subsequent encounter
> S sequela

5th S46.0 Injury of muscle(s) and tendon(s) of the rotator cuff of shoulder
- 6th S46.00 Unspecified injury of muscle(s) and tendon(s) of the rotator cuff of shoulder
  - 7th S46.001 Unspecified injury of muscle(s) and tendon(s) of the rotator cuff of right shoulder
  - 7th S46.002 Unspecified injury of muscle(s) and tendon(s) of the rotator cuff of left shoulder
  - 7th S46.009 Unspecified injury of muscle(s) and tendon(s) of the rotator cuff of unspecified shoulder
- 6th S46.01 Strain of muscle(s) and tendon(s) of the rotator cuff of shoulder
  - 7th S46.011 Strain of muscle(s) and tendon(s) of the rotator cuff of right shoulder
  - 7th S46.012 Strain of muscle(s) and tendon(s) of the rotator cuff of left shoulder
  - 7th S46.019 Strain of muscle(s) and tendon(s) of the rotator cuff of unspecified shoulder
- 6th S46.02 Laceration of muscle(s) and tendon(s) of the rotator cuff of shoulder
  - 7th S46.021 Laceration of muscle(s) and tendon(s) of the rotator cuff of right shoulder
  - 7th S46.022 Laceration of muscle(s) and tendon(s) of the rotator cuff of left shoulder
  - 7th S46.029 Laceration of muscle(s) and tendon(s) of the rotator cuff of unspecified shoulder
- 6th S46.09 Other injury of muscle(s) and tendon(s) of the rotator cuff of shoulder
  - 7th S46.091 Other injury of muscle(s) and tendon(s) of the rotator cuff of right shoulder
  - 7th S46.092 Other injury of muscle(s) and tendon(s) of the rotator cuff of left shoulder
  - 7th S46.099 Other injury of muscle(s) and tendon(s) of the rotator cuff of unspecified shoulder

S46.1 Injury of muscle, fascia and tendon of long head of biceps
- S46.10 Unspecified injury of muscle, fascia and tendon of long head of biceps
  - S46.101 Unspecified injury of muscle, fascia and tendon of long head of biceps, right arm
  - S46.102 Unspecified injury of muscle, fascia and tendon of long head of biceps, left arm
  - S46.109 Unspecified injury of muscle, fascia and tendon of long head of biceps, unspecified arm
- S46.11 Strain of muscle, fascia and tendon of long head of biceps
  AHA: 2020,1Q,38; 2019,2Q,27
  - S46.111 Strain of muscle, fascia and tendon of long head of biceps, right arm
  - S46.112 Strain of muscle, fascia and tendon of long head of biceps, left arm
  - S46.119 Strain of muscle, fascia and tendon of long head of biceps, unspecified arm
- S46.12 Laceration of muscle, fascia and tendon of long head of biceps
  - S46.121 Laceration of muscle, fascia and tendon of long head of biceps, right arm
  - S46.122 Laceration of muscle, fascia and tendon of long head of biceps, left arm
  - S46.129 Laceration of muscle, fascia and tendon of long head of biceps, unspecified arm
- S46.19 Other injury of muscle, fascia and tendon of long head of biceps
  - S46.191 Other injury of muscle, fascia and tendon of long head of biceps, right arm
  - S46.192 Other injury of muscle, fascia and tendon of long head of biceps, left arm
  - S46.199 Other injury of muscle, fascia and tendon of long head of biceps, unspecified arm

S46.2 Injury of muscle, fascia and tendon of other parts of biceps
- S46.20 Unspecified injury of muscle, fascia and tendon of other parts of biceps
  - S46.201 Unspecified injury of muscle, fascia and tendon of other parts of biceps, right arm
  - S46.202 Unspecified injury of muscle, fascia and tendon of other parts of biceps, left arm
  - S46.209 Unspecified injury of muscle, fascia and tendon of other parts of biceps, unspecified arm
- S46.21 Strain of muscle, fascia and tendon of other parts of biceps
  - S46.211 Strain of muscle, fascia and tendon of other parts of biceps, right arm
  - S46.212 Strain of muscle, fascia and tendon of other parts of biceps, left arm
  - S46.219 Strain of muscle, fascia and tendon of other parts of biceps, unspecified arm
- S46.22 Laceration of muscle, fascia and tendon of other parts of biceps
  - S46.221 Laceration of muscle, fascia and tendon of other parts of biceps, right arm
  - S46.222 Laceration of muscle, fascia and tendon of other parts of biceps, left arm
  - S46.229 Laceration of muscle, fascia and tendon of other parts of biceps, unspecified arm
- S46.29 Other injury of muscle, fascia and tendon of other parts of biceps
  - S46.291 Other injury of muscle, fascia and tendon of other parts of biceps, right arm
  - S46.292 Other injury of muscle, fascia and tendon of other parts of biceps, left arm
  - S46.299 Other injury of muscle, fascia and tendon of other parts of biceps, unspecified arm

S46.3 Injury of muscle, fascia and tendon of triceps
- S46.30 Unspecified injury of muscle, fascia and tendon of triceps
  - S46.301 Unspecified injury of muscle, fascia and tendon of triceps, right arm
  - S46.302 Unspecified injury of muscle, fascia and tendon of triceps, left arm
  - S46.309 Unspecified injury of muscle, fascia and tendon of triceps, unspecified arm
- S46.31 Strain of muscle, fascia and tendon of triceps
  - S46.311 Strain of muscle, fascia and tendon of triceps, right arm
  - S46.312 Strain of muscle, fascia and tendon of triceps, left arm
  - S46.319 Strain of muscle, fascia and tendon of triceps, unspecified arm
- S46.32 Laceration of muscle, fascia and tendon of triceps
  - S46.321 Laceration of muscle, fascia and tendon of triceps, right arm
  - S46.322 Laceration of muscle, fascia and tendon of triceps, left arm
  - S46.329 Laceration of muscle, fascia and tendon of triceps, unspecified arm
- S46.39 Other injury of muscle, fascia and tendon of triceps
  - S46.391 Other injury of muscle, fascia and tendon of triceps, right arm
  - S46.392 Other injury of muscle, fascia and tendon of triceps, left arm
  - S46.399 Other injury of muscle, fascia and tendon of triceps, unspecified arm

S46.8 Injury of other muscles, fascia and tendons at shoulder and upper arm level
- S46.80 Unspecified injury of other muscles, fascia and tendons at shoulder and upper arm level
  - S46.801 Unspecified injury of other muscles, fascia and tendons at shoulder and upper arm level, right arm
  - S46.802 Unspecified injury of other muscles, fascia and tendons at shoulder and upper arm level, left arm
  - S46.809 Unspecified injury of other muscles, fascia and tendons at shoulder and upper arm level, unspecified arm
- S46.81 Strain of other muscles, fascia and tendons at shoulder and upper arm level
  - S46.811 Strain of other muscles, fascia and tendons at shoulder and upper arm level, right arm
  - S46.812 Strain of other muscles, fascia and tendons at shoulder and upper arm level, left arm
  - S46.819 Strain of other muscles, fascia and tendons at shoulder and upper arm level, unspecified arm
- S46.82 Laceration of other muscles, fascia and tendons at shoulder and upper arm level
  - S46.821 Laceration of other muscles, fascia and tendons at shoulder and upper arm level, right arm
  - S46.822 Laceration of other muscles, fascia and tendons at shoulder and upper arm level, left arm
  - S46.829 Laceration of other muscles, fascia and tendons at shoulder and upper arm level, unspecified arm
- S46.89 Other injury of other muscles, fascia and tendons at shoulder and upper arm level
  - S46.891 Other injury of other muscles, fascia and tendons at shoulder and upper arm level, right arm
  - S46.892 Other injury of other muscles, fascia and tendons at shoulder and upper arm level, left arm
  - S46.899 Other injury of other muscles, fascia and tendons at shoulder and upper arm level, unspecified arm

S46.9 Injury of unspecified muscle, fascia and tendon at shoulder and upper arm level
- S46.90 Unspecified injury of unspecified muscle, fascia and tendon at shoulder and upper arm level
  - S46.901 Unspecified injury of unspecified muscle, fascia and tendon at shoulder and upper arm level, right arm
  - S46.902 Unspecified injury of unspecified muscle, fascia and tendon at shoulder and upper arm level, left arm
  - S46.909 Unspecified injury of unspecified muscle, fascia and tendon at shoulder and upper arm level, unspecified arm
- S46.91 Strain of unspecified muscle, fascia and tendon at shoulder and upper arm level
  - S46.911 Strain of unspecified muscle, fascia and tendon at shoulder and upper arm level, right arm
  - S46.912 Strain of unspecified muscle, fascia and tendon at shoulder and upper arm level, left arm

✓7th **S46.919** Strain of unspecified muscle, fascia and tendon at shoulder and upper arm level, unspecified arm

✓6th **S46.92** Laceration of unspecified muscle, fascia and tendon at shoulder and upper arm level

✓7th **S46.921** Laceration of unspecified muscle, fascia and tendon at shoulder and upper arm level, right arm

✓7th **S46.922** Laceration of unspecified muscle, fascia and tendon at shoulder and upper arm level, left arm

✓7th **S46.929** Laceration of unspecified muscle, fascia and tendon at shoulder and upper arm level, unspecified arm

✓6th **S46.99** Other injury of unspecified muscle, fascia and tendon at shoulder and upper arm level

✓7th **S46.991** Other injury of unspecified muscle, fascia and tendon at shoulder and upper arm level, right arm

✓7th **S46.992** Other injury of unspecified muscle, fascia and tendon at shoulder and upper arm level, left arm

✓7th **S46.999** Other injury of unspecified muscle, fascia and tendon at shoulder and upper arm level, unspecified arm

✓4th **S47 Crushing injury of shoulder and upper arm**

Use additional code for all associated injuries

EXCLUDES 2 *crushing injury of elbow (S57.Ø-)*

The appropriate 7th character is to be added to each code from category S47.
- A initial encounter
- D subsequent encounter
- S sequela

✓x7th **S47.1** Crushing injury of right shoulder and upper arm

✓x7th **S47.2** Crushing injury of left shoulder and upper arm

✓x7th **S47.9** Crushing injury of shoulder and upper arm, unspecified arm

✓4th **S48 Traumatic amputation of shoulder and upper arm**

An amputation not identified as partial or complete should be coded to complete

EXCLUDES 1 *traumatic amputation at elbow level (S58.Ø)*

The appropriate 7th character is to be added to each code from category S48.
- A initial encounter
- D subsequent encounter
- S sequela

✓5th **S48.Ø** Traumatic amputation at shoulder joint

✓6th **S48.Ø1** Complete traumatic amputation at shoulder joint

✓7th **S48.Ø11** Complete traumatic amputation at right shoulder joint HCC ESR COM

✓7th **S48.Ø12** Complete traumatic amputation at left shoulder joint HCC ESR COM

✓7th **S48.Ø19** Complete traumatic amputation at unspecified shoulder joint HCC ESR COM

✓6th **S48.Ø2** Partial traumatic amputation at shoulder joint

✓7th **S48.Ø21** Partial traumatic amputation at right shoulder joint HCC ESR COM

✓7th **S48.Ø22** Partial traumatic amputation at left shoulder joint HCC ESR COM

✓7th **S48.Ø29** Partial traumatic amputation at unspecified shoulder joint HCC ESR COM

✓5th **S48.1** Traumatic amputation at level between shoulder and elbow

✓6th **S48.11** Complete traumatic amputation at level between shoulder and elbow

✓7th **S48.111** Complete traumatic amputation at level between right shoulder and elbow HCC ESR COM

✓7th **S48.112** Complete traumatic amputation at level between left shoulder and elbow HCC ESR COM

✓7th **S48.119** Complete traumatic amputation at level between unspecified shoulder and elbow HCC ESR COM

✓6th **S48.12** Partial traumatic amputation at level between shoulder and elbow

✓7th **S48.121** Partial traumatic amputation at level between right shoulder and elbow HCC ESR COM

✓7th **S48.122** Partial traumatic amputation at level between left shoulder and elbow HCC ESR COM

✓7th **S48.129** Partial traumatic amputation at level between unspecified shoulder and elbow HCC ESR COM

✓5th **S48.9** Traumatic amputation of shoulder and upper arm, level unspecified

✓6th **S48.91** Complete traumatic amputation of shoulder and upper arm, level unspecified

✓7th **S48.911** Complete traumatic amputation of right shoulder and upper arm, level unspecified HCC ESR COM

✓7th **S48.912** Complete traumatic amputation of left shoulder and upper arm, level unspecified HCC ESR COM

✓7th **S48.919** Complete traumatic amputation of unspecified shoulder and upper arm, level unspecified HCC ESR COM

✓6th **S48.92** Partial traumatic amputation of shoulder and upper arm, level unspecified

✓7th **S48.921** Partial traumatic amputation of right shoulder and upper arm, level unspecified HCC ESR COM

✓7th **S48.922** Partial traumatic amputation of left shoulder and upper arm, level unspecified HCC ESR COM

✓7th **S48.929** Partial traumatic amputation of unspecified shoulder and upper arm, level unspecified HCC ESR COM

✓4th **S49 Other and unspecified injuries of shoulder and upper arm**

AHA: 2018,2Q,12; 2018,1Q,3

The appropriate 7th character is to be added to each code from subcategories S49.Ø and S49.1.
- A initial encounter for closed fracture
- D subsequent encounter for fracture with routine healing
- G subsequent encounter for fracture with delayed healing
- K subsequent encounter for fracture with nonunion
- P subsequent encounter for fracture with malunion
- S sequela

✓5th **S49.Ø** Physeal fracture of upper end of humerus

AHA: 2019,4Q,56

✓6th **S49.ØØ** Unspecified physeal fracture of upper end of humerus

✓7th **S49.ØØ1** Unspecified physeal fracture of upper end of humerus, right arm P

✓7th **S49.ØØ2** Unspecified physeal fracture of upper end of humerus, left arm P

✓7th **S49.ØØ9** Unspecified physeal fracture of upper end of humerus, unspecified arm P

✓6th **S49.Ø1** Salter-Harris Type I physeal fracture of upper end of humerus

✓7th **S49.Ø11** Salter-Harris Type I physeal fracture of upper end of humerus, right arm P

✓7th **S49.Ø12** Salter-Harris Type I physeal fracture of upper end of humerus, left arm P

✓7th **S49.Ø19** Salter-Harris Type I physeal fracture of upper end of humerus, unspecified arm P

✓6th **S49.Ø2** Salter-Harris Type II physeal fracture of upper end of humerus

✓7th **S49.Ø21** Salter-Harris Type II physeal fracture of upper end of humerus, right arm P

✓7th **S49.Ø22** Salter-Harris Type II physeal fracture of upper end of humerus, left arm P

✓7th **S49.Ø29** Salter-Harris Type II physeal fracture of upper end of humerus, unspecified arm P

✓6th **S49.Ø3** Salter-Harris Type III physeal fracture of upper end of humerus

✓7th **S49.Ø31** Salter-Harris Type III physeal fracture of upper end of humerus, right arm P

✓7th **S49.Ø32** Salter-Harris Type III physeal fracture of upper end of humerus, left arm P

✓7th **S49.Ø39** Salter-Harris Type III physeal fracture of upper end of humerus, unspecified arm P

✓6th **S49.Ø4** Salter-Harris Type IV physeal fracture of upper end of humerus

✓7th **S49.Ø41** Salter-Harris Type IV physeal fracture of upper end of humerus, right arm P

√7th **S49.Ø42 Salter-Harris Type IV physeal fracture of upper end of humerus, left arm** Q

√7th **S49.Ø49 Salter-Harris Type IV physeal fracture of upper end of humerus, unspecified arm** Q

√6th **S49.Ø9 Other physeal fracture of upper end of humerus**

√7th **S49.Ø91 Other physeal fracture of upper end of humerus, right arm** Q

√7th **S49.Ø92 Other physeal fracture of upper end of humerus, left arm** Q

√7th **S49.Ø99 Other physeal fracture of upper end of humerus, unspecified arm** Q

√5th **S49.1 Physeal fracture of lower end of humerus**

**AHA:** 2019,4Q,56

√6th **S49.1Ø Unspecified physeal fracture of lower end of humerus**

√7th **S49.1Ø1 Unspecified physeal fracture of lower end of humerus, right arm** Q

√7th **S49.1Ø2 Unspecified physeal fracture of lower end of humerus, left arm** Q

√7th **S49.1Ø9 Unspecified physeal fracture of lower end of humerus, unspecified arm** Q

√6th **S49.11 Salter-Harris Type I physeal fracture of lower end of humerus**

√7th **S49.111 Salter-Harris Type I physeal fracture of lower end of humerus, right arm** Q

√7th **S49.112 Salter-Harris Type I physeal fracture of lower end of humerus, left arm** Q

√7th **S49.119 Salter-Harris Type I physeal fracture of lower end of humerus, unspecified arm** Q

√6th **S49.12 Salter-Harris Type II physeal fracture of lower end of humerus**

√7th **S49.121 Salter-Harris Type II physeal fracture of lower end of humerus, right arm** Q

√7th **S49.122 Salter-Harris Type II physeal fracture of lower end of humerus, left arm** Q

√7th **S49.129 Salter-Harris Type II physeal fracture of lower end of humerus, unspecified arm** Q

√6th **S49.13 Salter-Harris Type III physeal fracture of lower end of humerus**

√7th **S49.131 Salter-Harris Type III physeal fracture of lower end of humerus, right arm** Q

√7th **S49.132 Salter-Harris Type III physeal fracture of lower end of humerus, left arm** Q

√7th **S49.139 Salter-Harris Type III physeal fracture of lower end of humerus, unspecified arm** Q

√6th **S49.14 Salter-Harris Type IV physeal fracture of lower end of humerus**

√7th **S49.141 Salter-Harris Type IV physeal fracture of lower end of humerus, right arm** Q

√7th **S49.142 Salter-Harris Type IV physeal fracture of lower end of humerus, left arm** Q

√7th **S49.149 Salter-Harris Type IV physeal fracture of lower end of humerus, unspecified arm** Q

√6th **S49.19 Other physeal fracture of lower end of humerus**

√7th **S49.191 Other physeal fracture of lower end of humerus, right arm** Q

√7th **S49.192 Other physeal fracture of lower end of humerus, left arm** Q

√7th **S49.199 Other physeal fracture of lower end of humerus, unspecified arm** Q

√5th **S49.8 Other specified injuries of shoulder and upper arm**

The appropriate 7th character is to be added to each code in subcategory S49.8.
A initial encounter
D subsequent encounter
S sequela

√x7th **S49.8Ø Other specified injuries of shoulder and upper arm, unspecified arm**

√x7th **S49.81 Other specified injuries of right shoulder and upper arm**

√x7th **S49.82 Other specified injuries of left shoulder and upper arm**

√5th **S49.9 Unspecified injury of shoulder and upper arm**

The appropriate 7th character is to be added to each code in subcategory S49.9.
A initial encounter
D subsequent encounter
S sequela

√x7th **S49.9Ø Unspecified injury of shoulder and upper arm, unspecified arm**

√x7th **S49.91 Unspecified injury of right shoulder and upper arm**

√x7th **S49.92 Unspecified injury of left shoulder and upper arm**

## Injuries to the elbow and forearm (S5Ø-S59)

EXCLUDES 2 *burns and corrosions (T2Ø-T32)*
*frostbite (T33-T34)*
*injuries of wrist and hand (S6Ø-S69)*
*insect bite or sting, venomous (T63.4)*

√4th **S5Ø Superficial injury of elbow and forearm**

EXCLUDES 2 *superficial injury of wrist and hand (S6Ø.-)*

The appropriate 7th character is to be added to each code from category S5Ø.
A initial encounter
D subsequent encounter
S sequela

√5th **S5Ø.Ø Contusion of elbow**

√x7th **S5Ø.ØØ Contusion of unspecified elbow**

√x7th **S5Ø.Ø1 Contusion of right elbow**

√x7th **S5Ø.Ø2 Contusion of left elbow**

√5th **S5Ø.1 Contusion of forearm**

√x7th **S5Ø.1Ø Contusion of unspecified forearm**

√x7th **S5Ø.11 Contusion of right forearm**

√x7th **S5Ø.12 Contusion of left forearm**

√5th **S5Ø.3 Other superficial injuries of elbow**

√6th **S5Ø.31 Abrasion of elbow**

√7th **S5Ø.311 Abrasion of right elbow**

√7th **S5Ø.312 Abrasion of left elbow**

√7th **S5Ø.319 Abrasion of unspecified elbow**

√6th **S5Ø.32 Blister (nonthermal) of elbow**

√7th **S5Ø.321 Blister (nonthermal) of right elbow**

√7th **S5Ø.322 Blister (nonthermal) of left elbow**

√7th **S5Ø.329 Blister (nonthermal) of unspecified elbow**

√6th **S5Ø.34 External constriction of elbow**

√7th **S5Ø.341 External constriction of right elbow**

√7th **S5Ø.342 External constriction of left elbow**

√7th **S5Ø.349 External constriction of unspecified elbow**

√6th **S5Ø.35 Superficial foreign body of elbow**

Splinter in the elbow

√7th **S5Ø.351 Superficial foreign body of right elbow**

√7th **S5Ø.352 Superficial foreign body of left elbow**

√7th **S5Ø.359 Superficial foreign body of unspecified elbow**

√6th **S5Ø.36 Insect bite (nonvenomous) of elbow**

√7th **S5Ø.361 Insect bite (nonvenomous) of right elbow**

√7th **S5Ø.362 Insect bite (nonvenomous) of left elbow**

√7th **S5Ø.369 Insect bite (nonvenomous) of unspecified elbow**

√6th **S5Ø.37 Other superficial bite of elbow**

EXCLUDES 1 *open bite of elbow (S51.Ø5)*

√7th **S5Ø.371 Other superficial bite of right elbow**

√7th **S5Ø.372 Other superficial bite of left elbow**

√7th **S5Ø.379 Other superficial bite of unspecified elbow**

√5th **S5Ø.8 Other superficial injuries of forearm**

√6th **S5Ø.81 Abrasion of forearm**

√7th **S5Ø.811 Abrasion of right forearm**

√7th **S5Ø.812 Abrasion of left forearm**

√7th **S5Ø.819 Abrasion of unspecified forearm**

√6th **S5Ø.82 Blister (nonthermal) of forearm**

√7th **S5Ø.821 Blister (nonthermal) of right forearm**

√7th **S5Ø.822 Blister (nonthermal) of left forearm**

Chapter 19. Injury, Poisoning and Certain Other Consequences of External Causes
S49.Ø42–S5Ø.822

✓7th **S5Ø.829** Blister (nonthermal) of unspecified forearm

✓6th **S5Ø.84** External constriction of forearm

✓7th **S5Ø.841** External constriction of right forearm

✓7th **S5Ø.842** External constriction of left forearm

✓7th **S5Ø.849** External constriction of unspecified forearm

✓6th **S5Ø.85** Superficial foreign body of forearm

Splinter in the forearm

✓7th **S5Ø.851** Superficial foreign body of right forearm

✓7th **S5Ø.852** Superficial foreign body of left forearm

✓7th **S5Ø.859** Superficial foreign body of unspecified forearm

✓6th **S5Ø.86** Insect bite (nonvenomous) of forearm

✓7th **S5Ø.861** Insect bite (nonvenomous) of right forearm

✓7th **S5Ø.862** Insect bite (nonvenomous) of left forearm

✓7th **S5Ø.869** Insect bite (nonvenomous) of unspecified forearm

✓6th **S5Ø.87** Other superficial bite of forearm

EXCLUDES 1 *open bite of forearm (S51.85)*

✓7th **S5Ø.871** Other superficial bite of right forearm

✓7th **S5Ø.872** Other superficial bite of left forearm

✓7th **S5Ø.879** Other superficial bite of unspecified forearm

✓5th **S5Ø.9** Unspecified superficial injury of elbow and forearm

✓6th **S5Ø.9Ø** Unspecified superficial injury of elbow

✓7th **S5Ø.9Ø1** Unspecified superficial injury of right elbow

✓7th **S5Ø.9Ø2** Unspecified superficial injury of left elbow

✓7th **S5Ø.9Ø9** Unspecified superficial injury of unspecified elbow

✓6th **S5Ø.91** Unspecified superficial injury of forearm

✓7th **S5Ø.911** Unspecified superficial injury of right forearm

✓7th **S5Ø.912** Unspecified superficial injury of left forearm

✓7th **S5Ø.919** Unspecified superficial injury of unspecified forearm

## ✓4th S51 Open wound of elbow and forearm

Code also any associated wound infection

EXCLUDES 1 *open fracture of elbow and forearm (S52.- with open fracture 7th character)*
*traumatic amputation of elbow and forearm (S58.-)*

EXCLUDES 2 *open wound of wrist and hand (S61.-)*

The appropriate 7th character is to be added to each code from category S51.
A initial encounter
D subsequent encounter
S sequela

✓5th **S51.Ø** Open wound of elbow

✓6th **S51.ØØ** Unspecified open wound of elbow

✓7th **S51.ØØ1** Unspecified open wound of right elbow
AHA: 2012,4Q,108

✓7th **S51.ØØ2** Unspecified open wound of left elbow

✓7th **S51.ØØ9** Unspecified open wound of unspecified elbow
Open wound of elbow NOS

✓6th **S51.Ø1** Laceration without foreign body of elbow

✓7th **S51.Ø11** Laceration without foreign body of right elbow

✓7th **S51.Ø12** Laceration without foreign body of left elbow

✓7th **S51.Ø19** Laceration without foreign body of unspecified elbow

✓6th **S51.Ø2** Laceration with foreign body of elbow

✓7th **S51.Ø21** Laceration with foreign body of right elbow

✓7th **S51.Ø22** Laceration with foreign body of left elbow

✓7th **S51.Ø29** Laceration with foreign body of unspecified elbow

✓6th **S51.Ø3** Puncture wound without foreign body of elbow

✓7th **S51.Ø31** Puncture wound without foreign body of right elbow

✓7th **S51.Ø32** Puncture wound without foreign body of left elbow

✓7th **S51.Ø39** Puncture wound without foreign body of unspecified elbow

✓6th **S51.Ø4** Puncture wound with foreign body of elbow

✓7th **S51.Ø41** Puncture wound with foreign body of right elbow

✓7th **S51.Ø42** Puncture wound with foreign body of left elbow

✓7th **S51.Ø49** Puncture wound with foreign body of unspecified elbow

✓6th **S51.Ø5** Open bite of elbow

Bite of elbow NOS

EXCLUDES 1 *superficial bite of elbow (S5Ø.36, S5Ø.37)*

✓7th **S51.Ø51** Open bite, right elbow

✓7th **S51.Ø52** Open bite, left elbow

✓7th **S51.Ø59** Open bite, unspecified elbow

✓5th **S51.8** Open wound of forearm

EXCLUDES 2 *open wound of elbow (S51.Ø-)*

✓6th **S51.8Ø** Unspecified open wound of forearm
AHA: 2016,3Q,24

✓7th **S51.8Ø1** Unspecified open wound of right forearm

✓7th **S51.8Ø2** Unspecified open wound of left forearm

✓7th **S51.8Ø9** Unspecified open wound of unspecified forearm
Open wound of forearm NOS

✓6th **S51.81** Laceration without foreign body of forearm

✓7th **S51.811** Laceration without foreign body of right forearm

✓7th **S51.812** Laceration without foreign body of left forearm

✓7th **S51.819** Laceration without foreign body of unspecified forearm

✓6th **S51.82** Laceration with foreign body of forearm

✓7th **S51.821** Laceration with foreign body of right forearm

✓7th **S51.822** Laceration with foreign body of left forearm

✓7th **S51.829** Laceration with foreign body of unspecified forearm

✓6th **S51.83** Puncture wound without foreign body of forearm
AHA: 2016,3Q,24

✓7th **S51.831** Puncture wound without foreign body of right forearm

✓7th **S51.832** Puncture wound without foreign body of left forearm

✓7th **S51.839** Puncture wound without foreign body of unspecified forearm

✓6th **S51.84** Puncture wound with foreign body of forearm
AHA: 2016,3Q,24

✓7th **S51.841** Puncture wound with foreign body of right forearm

✓7th **S51.842** Puncture wound with foreign body of left forearm

✓7th **S51.849** Puncture wound with foreign body of unspecified forearm

✓6th **S51.85** Open bite of forearm

Bite of forearm NOS

EXCLUDES 1 *superficial bite of forearm (S5Ø.86, S5Ø.87)*

✓7th **S51.851** Open bite of right forearm

✓7th **S51.852** Open bite of left forearm

✓7th **S51.859** Open bite of unspecified forearm

**S52 Fracture of forearm**

NOTE A fracture not indicated as displaced or nondisplaced should be coded to displaced.

A fracture not indicated as open or closed should be coded to closed.

The open fracture designations are based on the Gustilo open fracture classification.

EXCLUDES 1 *traumatic amputation of forearm (S58.-)*

EXCLUDES 2 *fracture at wrist and hand level (S62.-)*

*periprosthetic fracture around internal prosthetic elbow joint (M97.4)*

**AHA:** 2018,2Q,12; 2016,1Q,33; 2015,3Q,37-39

**DEF:** Diaphysis: Central shaft of a long bone.

**DEF:** Epiphysis: Proximal and distal rounded ends of a long bone, communicates with the joint.

**DEF:** Metaphysis: Section of a long bone located between the epiphysis and diaphysis at the proximal and distal ends.

**DEF:** Physis (growth plate): Narrow zone of cartilaginous tissue between the epiphysis and metaphysis at each end of a long bone. In childhood, proliferation of cells in this zone lengthens the bone. As the bone matures, this area thins, ossification eventually fusing into solid bone and growth stops. ***Synonym(s):*** *Epiphyseal plate.*

The appropriate 7th character is to be added to all codes from category S52 [unless otherwise indicated].

initial encounter for open fracture NOS

- A initial encounter for closed fracture
- B initial encounter for open fracture type I or II
- C initial encounter for open fracture type IIIA, IIIB, or IIIC
- D subsequent encounter for closed fracture with routine healing
- E subsequent encounter for open fracture type I or II with routine healing
- F subsequent encounter for open fracture type IIIA, IIIB, or IIIC with routine healing
- G subsequent encounter for closed fracture with delayed healing
- H subsequent encounter for open fracture type I or II with delayed healing
- J subsequent encounter for open fracture type IIIA, IIIB, or IIIC with delayed healing
- K subsequent encounter for closed fracture with nonunion
- M subsequent encounter for open fracture type I or II with nonunion
- N subsequent encounter for open fracture type IIIA, IIIB, or IIIC with nonunion
- P subsequent encounter for closed fracture with malunion
- Q subsequent encounter for open fracture type I or II with malunion
- R subsequent encounter for open fracture type IIIA, IIIB, or IIIC with malunion
- S sequela

**S52.0 Fracture of upper end of ulna**

Fracture of proximal end of ulna

EXCLUDES 2 *fracture of elbow NOS (S42.40-)*

*fractures of shaft of ulna (S52.2-)*

**S52.00 Unspecified fracture of upper end of ulna**

**S52.001 Unspecified fracture of upper end of right ulna** Q

**S52.002 Unspecified fracture of upper end of left ulna** Q

**S52.009 Unspecified fracture of upper end of unspecified ulna** Q

**S52.01 Torus fracture of upper end of ulna**

The appropriate 7th character is to be added to all codes in subcategory S52.01

- A initial encounter for closed fracture
- D subsequent encounter for fracture with routine healing
- G subsequent encounter for fracture with delayed healing
- K subsequent encounter for fracture with nonunion
- P subsequent encounter for fracture with malunion
- S sequela

**S52.011 Torus fracture of upper end of right ulna** Q

**S52.012 Torus fracture of upper end of left ulna** Q

**S52.019 Torus fracture of upper end of unspecified ulna** Q

**S52.02 Fracture of olecranon process without intraarticular extension of ulna**

**S52.021 Displaced fracture of olecranon process without intraarticular extension of right ulna** Q

**S52.022 Displaced fracture of olecranon process without intraarticular extension of left ulna** Q

**S52.023 Displaced fracture of olecranon process without intraarticular extension of unspecified ulna** Q

**S52.024 Nondisplaced fracture of olecranon process without intraarticular extension of right ulna** Q

**S52.025 Nondisplaced fracture of olecranon process without intraarticular extension of left ulna** Q

**S52.026 Nondisplaced fracture of olecranon process without intraarticular extension of unspecified ulna** Q

**S52.03 Fracture of olecranon process with intraarticular extension of ulna**

**S52.031 Displaced fracture of olecranon process with intraarticular extension of right ulna** Q

**S52.032 Displaced fracture of olecranon process with intraarticular extension of left ulna** Q

**S52.033 Displaced fracture of olecranon process with intraarticular extension of unspecified ulna** Q

**S52.034 Nondisplaced fracture of olecranon process with intraarticular extension of right ulna** Q

**S52.035 Nondisplaced fracture of olecranon process with intraarticular extension of left ulna** Q

**S52.036 Nondisplaced fracture of olecranon process with intraarticular extension of unspecified ulna** Q

**S52.04 Fracture of coronoid process of ulna**

**S52.041 Displaced fracture of coronoid process of right ulna** Q

**S52.042 Displaced fracture of coronoid process of left ulna** Q

**S52.043 Displaced fracture of coronoid process of unspecified ulna** Q

**S52.044 Nondisplaced fracture of coronoid process of right ulna** Q

**S52.045 Nondisplaced fracture of coronoid process of left ulna** Q

**S52.046 Nondisplaced fracture of coronoid process of unspecified ulna** Q

**S52.09 Other fracture of upper end of ulna**

**S52.091 Other fracture of upper end of right ulna** Q

**S52.092 Other fracture of upper end of left ulna** Q

**S52.099 Other fracture of upper end of unspecified ulna** Q

**S52.1 Fracture of upper end of radius**

Fracture of proximal end of radius

EXCLUDES 2 *fracture of shaft of radius (S52.3-)*

*physeal fractures of upper end of radius (S59.2-)*

**S52.10 Unspecified fracture of upper end of radius**

**S52.101 Unspecified fracture of upper end of right radius** Q

**S52.102 Unspecified fracture of upper end of left radius** Q

**S52.109 Unspecified fracture of upper end of unspecified radius** Q

√6th S52.11 Torus fracture of upper end of radius

The appropriate 7th character is to be added to all codes in subcategory S52.11
A initial encounter for closed fracture
D subsequent encounter for fracture with routine healing
G subsequent encounter for fracture with delayed healing
K subsequent encounter for fracture with nonunion
P subsequent encounter for fracture with malunion
S sequela

√7th S52.111 Torus fracture of upper end of right radius Q
√7th S52.112 Torus fracture of upper end of left radius Q
√7th S52.119 Torus fracture of upper end of unspecified radius Q

√6th S52.12 Fracture of head of radius
√7th S52.121 Displaced fracture of head of right radius Q
√7th S52.122 Displaced fracture of head of left radius Q
√7th S52.123 Displaced fracture of head of unspecified radius Q
√7th S52.124 Nondisplaced fracture of head of right radius Q
√7th S52.125 Nondisplaced fracture of head of left radius Q
√7th S52.126 Nondisplaced fracture of head of unspecified radius Q

√6th S52.13 Fracture of neck of radius
√7th S52.131 Displaced fracture of neck of right radius Q
√7th S52.132 Displaced fracture of neck of left radius Q
√7th S52.133 Displaced fracture of neck of unspecified radius Q
√7th S52.134 Nondisplaced fracture of neck of right radius Q
√7th S52.135 Nondisplaced fracture of neck of left radius Q
√7th S52.136 Nondisplaced fracture of neck of unspecified radius Q

√6th S52.18 Other fracture of upper end of radius
√7th S52.181 Other fracture of upper end of right radius Q
√7th S52.182 Other fracture of upper end of left radius Q
√7th S52.189 Other fracture of upper end of unspecified radius Q

√5th S52.2 Fracture of shaft of ulna

√6th S52.20 Unspecified fracture of shaft of ulna
Fracture of ulna NOS
√7th S52.201 Unspecified fracture of shaft of right ulna Q
√7th S52.202 Unspecified fracture of shaft of left ulna Q
√7th S52.209 Unspecified fracture of shaft of unspecified ulna Q

√6th S52.21 Greenstick fracture of shaft of ulna

The appropriate 7th character is to be added to all codes in subcategory S52.21
A initial encounter for closed fracture
D subsequent encounter for fracture with routine healing
G subsequent encounter for fracture with delayed healing
K subsequent encounter for fracture with nonunion
P subsequent encounter for fracture with malunion
S sequela

√7th S52.211 Greenstick fracture of shaft of right ulna Q
√7th S52.212 Greenstick fracture of shaft of left ulna Q
√7th S52.219 Greenstick fracture of shaft of unspecified ulna Q

√6th S52.22 Transverse fracture of shaft of ulna
√7th S52.221 Displaced transverse fracture of shaft of right ulna Q
√7th S52.222 Displaced transverse fracture of shaft of left ulna Q
√7th S52.223 Displaced transverse fracture of shaft of unspecified ulna Q
√7th S52.224 Nondisplaced transverse fracture of shaft of right ulna Q
√7th S52.225 Nondisplaced transverse fracture of shaft of left ulna Q
√7th S52.226 Nondisplaced transverse fracture of shaft of unspecified ulna Q

√6th S52.23 Oblique fracture of shaft of ulna
√7th S52.231 Displaced oblique fracture of shaft of right ulna Q
√7th S52.232 Displaced oblique fracture of shaft of left ulna Q
√7th S52.233 Displaced oblique fracture of shaft of unspecified ulna Q
√7th S52.234 Nondisplaced oblique fracture of shaft of right ulna Q
√7th S52.235 Nondisplaced oblique fracture of shaft of left ulna Q
√7th S52.236 Nondisplaced oblique fracture of shaft of unspecified ulna Q

√6th S52.24 Spiral fracture of shaft of ulna
√7th S52.241 Displaced spiral fracture of shaft of ulna, right arm Q
√7th S52.242 Displaced spiral fracture of shaft of ulna, left arm Q
√7th S52.243 Displaced spiral fracture of shaft of ulna, unspecified arm Q
√7th S52.244 Nondisplaced spiral fracture of shaft of ulna, right arm Q
√7th S52.245 Nondisplaced spiral fracture of shaft of ulna, left arm Q
√7th S52.246 Nondisplaced spiral fracture of shaft of ulna, unspecified arm Q

√6th S52.25 Comminuted fracture of shaft of ulna
√7th S52.251 Displaced comminuted fracture of shaft of ulna, right arm Q
√7th S52.252 Displaced comminuted fracture of shaft of ulna, left arm Q
√7th S52.253 Displaced comminuted fracture of shaft of ulna, unspecified arm Q
√7th S52.254 Nondisplaced comminuted fracture of shaft of ulna, right arm Q
√7th S52.255 Nondisplaced comminuted fracture of shaft of ulna, left arm Q
√7th S52.256 Nondisplaced comminuted fracture of shaft of ulna, unspecified arm Q

√6th S52.26 Segmental fracture of shaft of ulna
√7th S52.261 Displaced segmental fracture of shaft of ulna, right arm Q
√7th S52.262 Displaced segmental fracture of shaft of ulna, left arm Q
√7th S52.263 Displaced segmental fracture of shaft of ulna, unspecified arm Q
√7th S52.264 Nondisplaced segmental fracture of shaft of ulna, right arm Q
√7th S52.265 Nondisplaced segmental fracture of shaft of ulna, left arm Q
√7th S52.266 Nondisplaced segmental fracture of shaft of ulna, unspecified arm Q

√6th S52.27 Monteggia's fracture of ulna
Fracture of upper shaft of ulna with dislocation of radial head
√7th S52.271 Monteggia's fracture of right ulna Q
√7th S52.272 Monteggia's fracture of left ulna Q
√7th S52.279 Monteggia's fracture of unspecified ulna Q

√6th S52.28 Bent bone of ulna
√7th S52.281 Bent bone of right ulna Q
√7th S52.282 Bent bone of left ulna Q
√7th S52.283 Bent bone of unspecified ulna Q

S52.29 Other fracture of shaft of ulna
S52.291 Other fracture of shaft of right ulna Q
S52.292 Other fracture of shaft of left ulna Q
S52.299 Other fracture of shaft of unspecified ulna Q

S52.3 Fracture of shaft of radius
S52.30 Unspecified fracture of shaft of radius
S52.301 Unspecified fracture of shaft of right radius Q
S52.302 Unspecified fracture of shaft of left radius Q
S52.309 Unspecified fracture of shaft of unspecified radius Q

S52.31 Greenstick fracture of shaft of radius

The appropriate 7th character is to be added to all codes in subcategory S52.31.
A initial encounter for closed fracture
D subsequent encounter for fracture with routine healing
G subsequent encounter for fracture with delayed healing
K subsequent encounter for fracture with nonunion
P subsequent encounter for fracture with malunion
S sequela

S52.311 Greenstick fracture of shaft of radius, right arm Q
S52.312 Greenstick fracture of shaft of radius, left arm Q
S52.319 Greenstick fracture of shaft of radius, unspecified arm Q

S52.32 Transverse fracture of shaft of radius
S52.321 Displaced transverse fracture of shaft of right radius Q
S52.322 Displaced transverse fracture of shaft of left radius Q
S52.323 Displaced transverse fracture of shaft of unspecified radius Q
S52.324 Nondisplaced transverse fracture of shaft of right radius Q
S52.325 Nondisplaced transverse fracture of shaft of left radius Q
S52.326 Nondisplaced transverse fracture of shaft of unspecified radius Q

S52.33 Oblique fracture of shaft of radius
S52.331 Displaced oblique fracture of shaft of right radius Q
S52.332 Displaced oblique fracture of shaft of left radius Q
S52.333 Displaced oblique fracture of shaft of unspecified radius Q
S52.334 Nondisplaced oblique fracture of shaft of right radius Q
S52.335 Nondisplaced oblique fracture of shaft of left radius Q
S52.336 Nondisplaced oblique fracture of shaft of unspecified radius Q

S52.34 Spiral fracture of shaft of radius
S52.341 Displaced spiral fracture of shaft of radius, right arm Q
S52.342 Displaced spiral fracture of shaft of radius, left arm Q
S52.343 Displaced spiral fracture of shaft of radius, unspecified arm Q
S52.344 Nondisplaced spiral fracture of shaft of radius, right arm Q
S52.345 Nondisplaced spiral fracture of shaft of radius, left arm Q
S52.346 Nondisplaced spiral fracture of shaft of radius, unspecified arm Q

S52.35 Comminuted fracture of shaft of radius
S52.351 Displaced comminuted fracture of shaft of radius, right arm Q
S52.352 Displaced comminuted fracture of shaft of radius, left arm Q
S52.353 Displaced comminuted fracture of shaft of radius, unspecified arm Q
S52.354 Nondisplaced comminuted fracture of shaft of radius, right arm Q
S52.355 Nondisplaced comminuted fracture of shaft of radius, left arm Q
S52.356 Nondisplaced comminuted fracture of shaft of radius, unspecified arm Q

S52.36 Segmental fracture of shaft of radius
S52.361 Displaced segmental fracture of shaft of radius, right arm Q
S52.362 Displaced segmental fracture of shaft of radius, left arm Q
S52.363 Displaced segmental fracture of shaft of radius, unspecified arm Q
S52.364 Nondisplaced segmental fracture of shaft of radius, right arm Q
S52.365 Nondisplaced segmental fracture of shaft of radius, left arm Q
S52.366 Nondisplaced segmental fracture of shaft of radius, unspecified arm Q

S52.37 Galeazzi's fracture
Fracture of lower shaft of radius with radioulnar joint dislocation
S52.371 Galeazzi's fracture of right radius Q
S52.372 Galeazzi's fracture of left radius Q
S52.379 Galeazzi's fracture of unspecified radius Q

S52.38 Bent bone of radius
S52.381 Bent bone of right radius Q
S52.382 Bent bone of left radius Q
S52.389 Bent bone of unspecified radius Q

S52.39 Other fracture of shaft of radius
S52.391 Other fracture of shaft of radius, right arm Q
S52.392 Other fracture of shaft of radius, left arm Q
S52.399 Other fracture of shaft of radius, unspecified arm Q

S52.5 Fracture of lower end of radius
Fracture of distal end of radius
EXCLUDES 2 *physeal fractures of lower end of radius (S59.2-)*
DEF: Fracture of the distal end of the radius above the wrist, most commonly caused by a fall onto an outstretched hand.

S52.50 Unspecified fracture of the lower end of radius
S52.501 Unspecified fracture of the lower end of right radius Q
S52.502 Unspecified fracture of the lower end of left radius Q
S52.509 Unspecified fracture of the lower end of unspecified radius Q

S52.51 Fracture of radial styloid process
S52.511 Displaced fracture of right radial styloid process Q
S52.512 Displaced fracture of left radial styloid process Q
S52.513 Displaced fracture of unspecified radial styloid process Q
S52.514 Nondisplaced fracture of right radial styloid process Q
S52.515 Nondisplaced fracture of left radial styloid process Q
S52.516 Nondisplaced fracture of unspecified radial styloid process Q

S52.52 Torus fracture of lower end of radius

The appropriate 7th character is to be added to all codes in subcategory S52.52.
A initial encounter for closed fracture
D subsequent encounter for fracture with routine healing
G subsequent encounter for fracture with delayed healing
K subsequent encounter for fracture with nonunion
P subsequent encounter for fracture with malunion
S sequela

S52.521 Torus fracture of lower end of right radius Q
S52.522 Torus fracture of lower end of left radius Q

Chapter 19. Injury, Poisoning and Certain Other Consequences of External Causes

S52.29–S52.522

√7th S52.529 Torus fracture of lower end of unspecified radius Q

√6th S52.53 Colles' fracture

AHA: 2016,2Q,4

DEF: Fracture of the radius at the wrist in which the distal fragment is pushed posteriorly. The dorsal angulation of the fragment results in the wrist cocking up.

√7th S52.531 Colles' fracture of right radius Q

√7th S52.532 Colles' fracture of left radius Q

√7th S52.539 Colles' fracture of unspecified radius Q

√6th S52.54 Smith's fracture

√7th S52.541 Smith's fracture of right radius Q

√7th S52.542 Smith's fracture of left radius Q

√7th S52.549 Smith's fracture of unspecified radius Q

√6th S52.55 Other extraarticular fracture of lower end of radius

√7th S52.551 Other extraarticular fracture of lower end of right radius Q

√7th S52.552 Other extraarticular fracture of lower end of left radius Q

√7th S52.559 Other extraarticular fracture of lower end of unspecified radius Q

√6th S52.56 Barton's fracture

√7th S52.561 Barton's fracture of right radius Q

√7th S52.562 Barton's fracture of left radius Q

√7th S52.569 Barton's fracture of unspecified radius Q

√6th S52.57 Other intraarticular fracture of lower end of radius

AHA: 2025,3Q,14

√7th S52.571 Other intraarticular fracture of lower end of right radius Q

√7th S52.572 Other intraarticular fracture of lower end of left radius Q

√7th S52.579 Other intraarticular fracture of lower end of unspecified radius Q

√6th S52.59 Other fractures of lower end of radius

AHA: 2019,3Q,9

√7th S52.591 Other fractures of lower end of right radius Q

√7th S52.592 Other fractures of lower end of left radius Q

√7th S52.599 Other fractures of lower end of unspecified radius Q

√5th S52.6 Fracture of lower end of ulna

√6th S52.60 Unspecified fracture of lower end of ulna

√7th S52.601 Unspecified fracture of lower end of right ulna Q

√7th S52.602 Unspecified fracture of lower end of left ulna Q

√7th S52.609 Unspecified fracture of lower end of unspecified ulna Q

√6th S52.61 Fracture of ulna styloid process

√7th S52.611 Displaced fracture of right ulna styloid process Q

√7th S52.612 Displaced fracture of left ulna styloid process Q

√7th S52.613 Displaced fracture of unspecified ulna styloid process Q

√7th S52.614 Nondisplaced fracture of right ulna styloid process Q

√7th S52.615 Nondisplaced fracture of left ulna styloid process Q

√7th S52.616 Nondisplaced fracture of unspecified ulna styloid process Q

√6th S52.62 Torus fracture of lower end of ulna

The appropriate 7th character is to be added to all codes in subcategory S52.62.
- A initial encounter for closed fracture
- D subsequent encounter for fracture with routine healing
- G subsequent encounter for fracture with delayed healing
- K subsequent encounter for fracture with nonunion
- P subsequent encounter for fracture with malunion
- S sequela

√7th S52.621 Torus fracture of lower end of right ulna Q

√7th S52.622 Torus fracture of lower end of left ulna Q

√7th S52.629 Torus fracture of lower end of unspecified ulna Q

√6th S52.69 Other fracture of lower end of ulna

AHA: 2019,3Q,9

√7th S52.691 Other fracture of lower end of right ulna Q

√7th S52.692 Other fracture of lower end of left ulna Q

√7th S52.699 Other fracture of lower end of unspecified ulna Q

√5th S52.9 Unspecified fracture of forearm

√x7th S52.90 Unspecified fracture of unspecified forearm Q

√x7th S52.91 Unspecified fracture of right forearm Q

√x7th S52.92 Unspecified fracture of left forearm Q

√4th S53 Dislocation and sprain of joints and ligaments of elbow

INCLUDES avulsion of joint or ligament of elbow
laceration of cartilage, joint or ligament of elbow
sprain of cartilage, joint or ligament of elbow
traumatic hemarthrosis of joint or ligament of elbow
traumatic rupture of joint or ligament of elbow
traumatic subluxation of joint or ligament of elbow
traumatic tear of joint or ligament of elbow

Code also any associated open wound

EXCLUDES 2 *strain of muscle, fascia and tendon at forearm level (S56.-)*

The appropriate 7th character is to be added to each code from category S53.
- A initial encounter
- D subsequent encounter
- S sequela

√5th S53.0 Subluxation and dislocation of radial head

Dislocation of radiohumeral joint
Subluxation of radiohumeral joint

EXCLUDES 1 *Monteggia's fracture-dislocation (S52.27-)*

√6th S53.00 Unspecified subluxation and dislocation of radial head

√7th S53.001 Unspecified subluxation of right radial head

√7th S53.002 Unspecified subluxation of left radial head

√7th S53.003 Unspecified subluxation of unspecified radial head

√7th S53.004 Unspecified dislocation of right radial head

√7th S53.005 Unspecified dislocation of left radial head

√7th S53.006 Unspecified dislocation of unspecified radial head

√6th S53.01 Anterior subluxation and dislocation of radial head

Anteriomedial subluxation and dislocation of radial head

√7th S53.011 Anterior subluxation of right radial head

√7th S53.012 Anterior subluxation of left radial head

√7th S53.013 Anterior subluxation of unspecified radial head

√7th S53.014 Anterior dislocation of right radial head

√7th S53.015 Anterior dislocation of left radial head

√7th S53.016 Anterior dislocation of unspecified radial head

√6th S53.02 Posterior subluxation and dislocation of radial head

Posteriolateral subluxation and dislocation of radial head

√7th S53.021 Posterior subluxation of right radial head

√7th S53.022 Posterior subluxation of left radial head

- ✓7th **S53.023** Posterior subluxation of unspecified radial head
- ✓7th **S53.024** Posterior dislocation of right radial head
- ✓7th **S53.025** Posterior dislocation of left radial head
- ✓7th **S53.026** Posterior dislocation of unspecified radial head

✓6th **S53.03** Nursemaid's elbow
- ✓7th **S53.031** Nursemaid's elbow, right elbow
- ✓7th **S53.032** Nursemaid's elbow, left elbow
- ✓7th **S53.033** Nursemaid's elbow, unspecified elbow

✓6th **S53.09** Other subluxation and dislocation of radial head
- ✓7th **S53.091** Other subluxation of right radial head
- ✓7th **S53.092** Other subluxation of left radial head
- ✓7th **S53.093** Other subluxation of unspecified radial head
- ✓7th **S53.094** Other dislocation of right radial head
- ✓7th **S53.095** Other dislocation of left radial head
- ✓7th **S53.096** Other dislocation of unspecified radial head

✓5th **S53.1** **Subluxation and dislocation of ulnohumeral joint**

Subluxation and dislocation of elbow NOS

EXCLUDES 1 *dislocation of radial head alone (S53.0-)*

✓6th **S53.10** Unspecified subluxation and dislocation of ulnohumeral joint
- ✓7th **S53.101** Unspecified subluxation of right ulnohumeral joint
- ✓7th **S53.102** Unspecified subluxation of left ulnohumeral joint
- ✓7th **S53.103** Unspecified subluxation of unspecified ulnohumeral joint
- ✓7th **S53.104** Unspecified dislocation of right ulnohumeral joint
- ✓7th **S53.105** Unspecified dislocation of left ulnohumeral joint
- ✓7th **S53.106** Unspecified dislocation of unspecified ulnohumeral joint

✓6th **S53.11** Anterior subluxation and dislocation of ulnohumeral joint
- ✓7th **S53.111** Anterior subluxation of right ulnohumeral joint
- ✓7th **S53.112** Anterior subluxation of left ulnohumeral joint
- ✓7th **S53.113** Anterior subluxation of unspecified ulnohumeral joint
- ✓7th **S53.114** Anterior dislocation of right ulnohumeral joint
  AHA: 2012,4Q,108
- ✓7th **S53.115** Anterior dislocation of left ulnohumeral joint
- ✓7th **S53.116** Anterior dislocation of unspecified ulnohumeral joint

✓6th **S53.12** Posterior subluxation and dislocation of ulnohumeral joint
- ✓7th **S53.121** Posterior subluxation of right ulnohumeral joint
- ✓7th **S53.122** Posterior subluxation of left ulnohumeral joint
- ✓7th **S53.123** Posterior subluxation of unspecified ulnohumeral joint
- ✓7th **S53.124** Posterior dislocation of right ulnohumeral joint
- ✓7th **S53.125** Posterior dislocation of left ulnohumeral joint
- ✓7th **S53.126** Posterior dislocation of unspecified ulnohumeral joint

✓6th **S53.13** Medial subluxation and dislocation of ulnohumeral joint
- ✓7th **S53.131** Medial subluxation of right ulnohumeral joint
- ✓7th **S53.132** Medial subluxation of left ulnohumeral joint
- ✓7th **S53.133** Medial subluxation of unspecified ulnohumeral joint
- ✓7th **S53.134** Medial dislocation of right ulnohumeral joint
- ✓7th **S53.135** Medial dislocation of left ulnohumeral joint
- ✓7th **S53.136** Medial dislocation of unspecified ulnohumeral joint

✓6th **S53.14** Lateral subluxation and dislocation of ulnohumeral joint
- ✓7th **S53.141** Lateral subluxation of right ulnohumeral joint
- ✓7th **S53.142** Lateral subluxation of left ulnohumeral joint
- ✓7th **S53.143** Lateral subluxation of unspecified ulnohumeral joint
- ✓7th **S53.144** Lateral dislocation of right ulnohumeral joint
- ✓7th **S53.145** Lateral dislocation of left ulnohumeral joint
- ✓7th **S53.146** Lateral dislocation of unspecified ulnohumeral joint

✓6th **S53.19** Other subluxation and dislocation of ulnohumeral joint
- ✓7th **S53.191** Other subluxation of right ulnohumeral joint
- ✓7th **S53.192** Other subluxation of left ulnohumeral joint
- ✓7th **S53.193** Other subluxation of unspecified ulnohumeral joint
- ✓7th **S53.194** Other dislocation of right ulnohumeral joint
- ✓7th **S53.195** Other dislocation of left ulnohumeral joint
- ✓7th **S53.196** Other dislocation of unspecified ulnohumeral joint

✓5th **S53.2** **Traumatic rupture of radial collateral ligament**

EXCLUDES 1 *sprain of radial collateral ligament NOS (S53.43-)*

- ✓x7th **S53.20** Traumatic rupture of unspecified radial collateral ligament
- ✓x7th **S53.21** Traumatic rupture of right radial collateral ligament
- ✓x7th **S53.22** Traumatic rupture of left radial collateral ligament

✓5th **S53.3** **Traumatic rupture of ulnar collateral ligament**

EXCLUDES 1 *sprain of ulnar collateral ligament (S53.44-)*

- ✓x7th **S53.30** Traumatic rupture of unspecified ulnar collateral ligament
- ✓x7th **S53.31** Traumatic rupture of right ulnar collateral ligament
- ✓x7th **S53.32** Traumatic rupture of left ulnar collateral ligament

✓5th **S53.4** **Sprain of elbow**

EXCLUDES 2 *traumatic rupture of radial collateral ligament (S53.2-)*
*traumatic rupture of ulnar collateral ligament (S53.3-)*

✓6th **S53.40** Unspecified sprain of elbow
- ✓7th **S53.401** Unspecified sprain of right elbow
- ✓7th **S53.402** Unspecified sprain of left elbow
- ✓7th **S53.409** Unspecified sprain of unspecified elbow
  Sprain of elbow NOS

✓6th **S53.41** Radiohumeral (joint) sprain
- ✓7th **S53.411** Radiohumeral (joint) sprain of right elbow
- ✓7th **S53.412** Radiohumeral (joint) sprain of left elbow
- ✓7th **S53.419** Radiohumeral (joint) sprain of unspecified elbow

✓6th **S53.42** Ulnohumeral (joint) sprain
- ✓7th **S53.421** Ulnohumeral (joint) sprain of right elbow
- ✓7th **S53.422** Ulnohumeral (joint) sprain of left elbow
- ✓7th **S53.429** Ulnohumeral (joint) sprain of unspecified elbow

✓6th **S53.43** Radial collateral ligament sprain
- ✓7th **S53.431** Radial collateral ligament sprain of right elbow
- ✓7th **S53.432** Radial collateral ligament sprain of left elbow
- ✓7th **S53.439** Radial collateral ligament sprain of unspecified elbow

✓6th **S53.44** Ulnar collateral ligament sprain
- ✓7th **S53.441** Ulnar collateral ligament sprain of right elbow
- ✓7th **S53.442** Ulnar collateral ligament sprain of left elbow
- ✓7th **S53.449** Ulnar collateral ligament sprain of unspecified elbow

✓6th **S53.49** Other sprain of elbow
- ✓7th **S53.491** Other sprain of right elbow
- ✓7th **S53.492** Other sprain of left elbow
- ✓7th **S53.499** Other sprain of unspecified elbow

**S54 Injury of nerves at forearm level**

Code also any associated open wound (S51.-)

EXCLUDES 2 *injury of nerves at wrist and hand level (S64.-)*

The appropriate 7th character is to be added to each code from category S54.

A initial encounter
D subsequent encounter
S sequela

**S54.0 Injury of ulnar nerve at forearm level**

Injury of ulnar nerve NOS

**S54.00 Injury of ulnar nerve at forearm level, unspecified arm**

**S54.01 Injury of ulnar nerve at forearm level, right arm**

**S54.02 Injury of ulnar nerve at forearm level, left arm**

**S54.1 Injury of median nerve at forearm level**

Injury of median nerve NOS

**S54.10 Injury of median nerve at forearm level, unspecified arm**

**S54.11 Injury of median nerve at forearm level, right arm**

**S54.12 Injury of median nerve at forearm level, left arm**

**S54.2 Injury of radial nerve at forearm level**

Injury of radial nerve NOS

**S54.20 Injury of radial nerve at forearm level, unspecified arm**

**S54.21 Injury of radial nerve at forearm level, right arm**

**S54.22 Injury of radial nerve at forearm level, left arm**

**S54.3 Injury of cutaneous sensory nerve at forearm level**

**S54.30 Injury of cutaneous sensory nerve at forearm level, unspecified arm**

**S54.31 Injury of cutaneous sensory nerve at forearm level, right arm**

**S54.32 Injury of cutaneous sensory nerve at forearm level, left arm**

**S54.8 Injury of other nerves at forearm level**

**S54.8X Injury of other nerves at forearm level**

**S54.8X1 Injury of other nerves at forearm level, right arm**

**S54.8X2 Injury of other nerves at forearm level, left arm**

**S54.8X9 Injury of other nerves at forearm level, unspecified arm**

**S54.9 Injury of unspecified nerve at forearm level**

**S54.90 Injury of unspecified nerve at forearm level, unspecified arm**

**S54.91 Injury of unspecified nerve at forearm level, right arm**

**S54.92 Injury of unspecified nerve at forearm level, left arm**

**S55 Injury of blood vessels at forearm level**

Code also any associated open wound (S51.-)

EXCLUDES 2 *injury of blood vessels at wrist and hand level (S65.-)*
*injury of brachial vessels (S45.1-S45.2)*

The appropriate 7th character is to be added to each code from category S55.

A initial encounter
D subsequent encounter
S sequela

**S55.0 Injury of ulnar artery at forearm level**

**S55.00 Unspecified injury of ulnar artery at forearm level**

**S55.001 Unspecified injury of ulnar artery at forearm level, right arm**

**S55.002 Unspecified injury of ulnar artery at forearm level, left arm**

**S55.009 Unspecified injury of ulnar artery at forearm level, unspecified arm**

**S55.01 Laceration of ulnar artery at forearm level**

**S55.011 Laceration of ulnar artery at forearm level, right arm**

**S55.012 Laceration of ulnar artery at forearm level, left arm**

**S55.019 Laceration of ulnar artery at forearm level, unspecified arm**

**S55.09 Other specified injury of ulnar artery at forearm level**

**S55.091 Other specified injury of ulnar artery at forearm level, right arm**

**S55.092 Other specified injury of ulnar artery at forearm level, left arm**

**S55.099 Other specified injury of ulnar artery at forearm level, unspecified arm**

**S55.1 Injury of radial artery at forearm level**

**S55.10 Unspecified injury of radial artery at forearm level**

**S55.101 Unspecified injury of radial artery at forearm level, right arm**

**S55.102 Unspecified injury of radial artery at forearm level, left arm**

**S55.109 Unspecified injury of radial artery at forearm level, unspecified arm**

**S55.11 Laceration of radial artery at forearm level**

**S55.111 Laceration of radial artery at forearm level, right arm**

**S55.112 Laceration of radial artery at forearm level, left arm**

**S55.119 Laceration of radial artery at forearm level, unspecified arm**

**S55.19 Other specified injury of radial artery at forearm level**

**S55.191 Other specified injury of radial artery at forearm level, right arm**

**S55.192 Other specified injury of radial artery at forearm level, left arm**

**S55.199 Other specified injury of radial artery at forearm level, unspecified arm**

**S55.2 Injury of vein at forearm level**

**S55.20 Unspecified injury of vein at forearm level**

**S55.201 Unspecified injury of vein at forearm level, right arm**

**S55.202 Unspecified injury of vein at forearm level, left arm**

**S55.209 Unspecified injury of vein at forearm level, unspecified arm**

**S55.21 Laceration of vein at forearm level**

**S55.211 Laceration of vein at forearm level, right arm**

**S55.212 Laceration of vein at forearm level, left arm**

**S55.219 Laceration of vein at forearm level, unspecified arm**

**S55.29 Other specified injury of vein at forearm level**

**S55.291 Other specified injury of vein at forearm level, right arm**

**S55.292 Other specified injury of vein at forearm level, left arm**

**S55.299 Other specified injury of vein at forearm level, unspecified arm**

**S55.8 Injury of other blood vessels at forearm level**

**S55.80 Unspecified injury of other blood vessels at forearm level**

**S55.801 Unspecified injury of other blood vessels at forearm level, right arm**

**S55.802 Unspecified injury of other blood vessels at forearm level, left arm**

**S55.809 Unspecified injury of other blood vessels at forearm level, unspecified arm**

**S55.81 Laceration of other blood vessels at forearm level**

**S55.811 Laceration of other blood vessels at forearm level, right arm**

**S55.812 Laceration of other blood vessels at forearm level, left arm**

**S55.819 Laceration of other blood vessels at forearm level, unspecified arm**

**S55.89 Other specified injury of other blood vessels at forearm level**

**S55.891 Other specified injury of other blood vessels at forearm level, right arm**

**S55.892 Other specified injury of other blood vessels at forearm level, left arm**

**S55.899 Other specified injury of other blood vessels at forearm level, unspecified arm**

**S55.9 Injury of unspecified blood vessel at forearm level**

**S55.90 Unspecified injury of unspecified blood vessel at forearm level**

**S55.901 Unspecified injury of unspecified blood vessel at forearm level, right arm**

**S55.902 Unspecified injury of unspecified blood vessel at forearm level, left arm**

**S55.909 Unspecified injury of unspecified blood vessel at forearm level, unspecified arm**

S55.91 Laceration of unspecified blood vessel at forearm level
S55.911 Laceration of unspecified blood vessel at forearm level, right arm
S55.912 Laceration of unspecified blood vessel at forearm level, left arm
S55.919 Laceration of unspecified blood vessel at forearm level, unspecified arm
S55.99 Other specified injury of unspecified blood vessel at forearm level
S55.991 Other specified injury of unspecified blood vessel at forearm level, right arm
S55.992 Other specified injury of unspecified blood vessel at forearm level, left arm
S55.999 Other specified injury of unspecified blood vessel at forearm level, unspecified arm

**S56 Injury of muscle, fascia and tendon at forearm level**

Code also any associated open wound (S51.-)

EXCLUDES 2 *injury of muscle, fascia and tendon at or below wrist (S66.-)*
*sprain of joints and ligaments of elbow (S53.4-)*

**TIP:** Refer to the Muscle/Tendon table at the beginning of this chapter

The appropriate 7th character is to be added to each code from category S56.
A initial encounter
D subsequent encounter
S sequela

S56.0 Injury of flexor muscle, fascia and tendon of thumb at forearm level
S56.00 Unspecified injury of flexor muscle, fascia and tendon of thumb at forearm level
S56.001 Unspecified injury of flexor muscle, fascia and tendon of right thumb at forearm level
S56.002 Unspecified injury of flexor muscle, fascia and tendon of left thumb at forearm level
S56.009 Unspecified injury of flexor muscle, fascia and tendon of unspecified thumb at forearm level
S56.01 Strain of flexor muscle, fascia and tendon of thumb at forearm level
S56.011 Strain of flexor muscle, fascia and tendon of right thumb at forearm level
S56.012 Strain of flexor muscle, fascia and tendon of left thumb at forearm level
S56.019 Strain of flexor muscle, fascia and tendon of unspecified thumb at forearm level
S56.02 Laceration of flexor muscle, fascia and tendon of thumb at forearm level
S56.021 Laceration of flexor muscle, fascia and tendon of right thumb at forearm level
S56.022 Laceration of flexor muscle, fascia and tendon of left thumb at forearm level
S56.029 Laceration of flexor muscle, fascia and tendon of unspecified thumb at forearm level
S56.09 Other injury of flexor muscle, fascia and tendon of thumb at forearm level
S56.091 Other injury of flexor muscle, fascia and tendon of right thumb at forearm level
S56.092 Other injury of flexor muscle, fascia and tendon of left thumb at forearm level
S56.099 Other injury of flexor muscle, fascia and tendon of unspecified thumb at forearm level
S56.1 Injury of flexor muscle, fascia and tendon of other and unspecified finger at forearm level
S56.10 Unspecified injury of flexor muscle, fascia and tendon of other and unspecified finger at forearm level
S56.101 Unspecified injury of flexor muscle, fascia and tendon of right index finger at forearm level
S56.102 Unspecified injury of flexor muscle, fascia and tendon of left index finger at forearm level
S56.103 Unspecified injury of flexor muscle, fascia and tendon of right middle finger at forearm level
S56.104 Unspecified injury of flexor muscle, fascia and tendon of left middle finger at forearm level
S56.105 Unspecified injury of flexor muscle, fascia and tendon of right ring finger at forearm level
S56.106 Unspecified injury of flexor muscle, fascia and tendon of left ring finger at forearm level
S56.107 Unspecified injury of flexor muscle, fascia and tendon of right little finger at forearm level
S56.108 Unspecified injury of flexor muscle, fascia and tendon of left little finger at forearm level
S56.109 Unspecified injury of flexor muscle, fascia and tendon of unspecified finger at forearm level
S56.11 Strain of flexor muscle, fascia and tendon of other and unspecified finger at forearm level
S56.111 Strain of flexor muscle, fascia and tendon of right index finger at forearm level
S56.112 Strain of flexor muscle, fascia and tendon of left index finger at forearm level
S56.113 Strain of flexor muscle, fascia and tendon of right middle finger at forearm level
S56.114 Strain of flexor muscle, fascia and tendon of left middle finger at forearm level
S56.115 Strain of flexor muscle, fascia and tendon of right ring finger at forearm level
S56.116 Strain of flexor muscle, fascia and tendon of left ring finger at forearm level
S56.117 Strain of flexor muscle, fascia and tendon of right little finger at forearm level
S56.118 Strain of flexor muscle, fascia and tendon of left little finger at forearm level
S56.119 Strain of flexor muscle, fascia and tendon of finger of unspecified finger at forearm level
S56.12 Laceration of flexor muscle, fascia and tendon of other and unspecified finger at forearm level
S56.121 Laceration of flexor muscle, fascia and tendon of right index finger at forearm level
S56.122 Laceration of flexor muscle, fascia and tendon of left index finger at forearm level
S56.123 Laceration of flexor muscle, fascia and tendon of right middle finger at forearm level
S56.124 Laceration of flexor muscle, fascia and tendon of left middle finger at forearm level
S56.125 Laceration of flexor muscle, fascia and tendon of right ring finger at forearm level
S56.126 Laceration of flexor muscle, fascia and tendon of left ring finger at forearm level
S56.127 Laceration of flexor muscle, fascia and tendon of right little finger at forearm level
S56.128 Laceration of flexor muscle, fascia and tendon of left little finger at forearm level
S56.129 Laceration of flexor muscle, fascia and tendon of unspecified finger at forearm level
S56.19 Other injury of flexor muscle, fascia and tendon of other and unspecified finger at forearm level
S56.191 Other injury of flexor muscle, fascia and tendon of right index finger at forearm level
S56.192 Other injury of flexor muscle, fascia and tendon of left index finger at forearm level
S56.193 Other injury of flexor muscle, fascia and tendon of right middle finger at forearm level
S56.194 Other injury of flexor muscle, fascia and tendon of left middle finger at forearm level
S56.195 Other injury of flexor muscle, fascia and tendon of right ring finger at forearm level
S56.196 Other injury of flexor muscle, fascia and tendon of left ring finger at forearm level
S56.197 Other injury of flexor muscle, fascia and tendon of right little finger at forearm level
S56.198 Other injury of flexor muscle, fascia and tendon of left little finger at forearm level
S56.199 Other injury of flexor muscle, fascia and tendon of unspecified finger at forearm level

√5th **S56.2 Injury of other flexor muscle, fascia and tendon at forearm level**

√6th **S56.20 Unspecified injury of other flexor muscle, fascia and tendon at forearm level**

√7th **S56.201 Unspecified injury of other flexor muscle, fascia and tendon at forearm level, right arm**

√7th **S56.202 Unspecified injury of other flexor muscle, fascia and tendon at forearm level, left arm**

√7th **S56.209 Unspecified injury of other flexor muscle, fascia and tendon at forearm level, unspecified arm**

√6th **S56.21 Strain of other flexor muscle, fascia and tendon at forearm level**

√7th **S56.211 Strain of other flexor muscle, fascia and tendon at forearm level, right arm**

√7th **S56.212 Strain of other flexor muscle, fascia and tendon at forearm level, left arm**

√7th **S56.219 Strain of other flexor muscle, fascia and tendon at forearm level, unspecified arm**

√6th **S56.22 Laceration of other flexor muscle, fascia and tendon at forearm level**

√7th **S56.221 Laceration of other flexor muscle, fascia and tendon at forearm level, right arm**

√7th **S56.222 Laceration of other flexor muscle, fascia and tendon at forearm level, left arm**

√7th **S56.229 Laceration of other flexor muscle, fascia and tendon at forearm level, unspecified arm**

√6th **S56.29 Other injury of other flexor muscle, fascia and tendon at forearm level**

√7th **S56.291 Other injury of other flexor muscle, fascia and tendon at forearm level, right arm**

√7th **S56.292 Other injury of other flexor muscle, fascia and tendon at forearm level, left arm**

√7th **S56.299 Other injury of other flexor muscle, fascia and tendon at forearm level, unspecified arm**

√5th **S56.3 Injury of extensor or abductor muscles, fascia and tendons of thumb at forearm level**

√6th **S56.30 Unspecified injury of extensor or abductor muscles, fascia and tendons of thumb at forearm level**

√7th **S56.301 Unspecified injury of extensor or abductor muscles, fascia and tendons of right thumb at forearm level**

√7th **S56.302 Unspecified injury of extensor or abductor muscles, fascia and tendons of left thumb at forearm level**

√7th **S56.309 Unspecified injury of extensor or abductor muscles, fascia and tendons of unspecified thumb at forearm level**

√6th **S56.31 Strain of extensor or abductor muscles, fascia and tendons of thumb at forearm level**

√7th **S56.311 Strain of extensor or abductor muscles, fascia and tendons of right thumb at forearm level**

√7th **S56.312 Strain of extensor or abductor muscles, fascia and tendons of left thumb at forearm level**

√7th **S56.319 Strain of extensor or abductor muscles, fascia and tendons of unspecified thumb at forearm level**

√6th **S56.32 Laceration of extensor or abductor muscles, fascia and tendons of thumb at forearm level**

√7th **S56.321 Laceration of extensor or abductor muscles, fascia and tendons of right thumb at forearm level**

√7th **S56.322 Laceration of extensor or abductor muscles, fascia and tendons of left thumb at forearm level**

√7th **S56.329 Laceration of extensor or abductor muscles, fascia and tendons of unspecified thumb at forearm level**

√6th **S56.39 Other injury of extensor or abductor muscles, fascia and tendons of thumb at forearm level**

√7th **S56.391 Other injury of extensor or abductor muscles, fascia and tendons of right thumb at forearm level**

√7th **S56.392 Other injury of extensor or abductor muscles, fascia and tendons of left thumb at forearm level**

√7th **S56.399 Other injury of extensor or abductor muscles, fascia and tendons of unspecified thumb at forearm level**

√5th **S56.4 Injury of extensor muscle, fascia and tendon of other and unspecified finger at forearm level**

√6th **S56.40 Unspecified injury of extensor muscle, fascia and tendon of other and unspecified finger at forearm level**

√7th **S56.401 Unspecified injury of extensor muscle, fascia and tendon of right index finger at forearm level**

√7th **S56.402 Unspecified injury of extensor muscle, fascia and tendon of left index finger at forearm level**

√7th **S56.403 Unspecified injury of extensor muscle, fascia and tendon of right middle finger at forearm level**

√7th **S56.404 Unspecified injury of extensor muscle, fascia and tendon of left middle finger at forearm level**

√7th **S56.405 Unspecified injury of extensor muscle, fascia and tendon of right ring finger at forearm level**

√7th **S56.406 Unspecified injury of extensor muscle, fascia and tendon of left ring finger at forearm level**

√7th **S56.407 Unspecified injury of extensor muscle, fascia and tendon of right little finger at forearm level**

√7th **S56.408 Unspecified injury of extensor muscle, fascia and tendon of left little finger at forearm level**

√7th **S56.409 Unspecified injury of extensor muscle, fascia and tendon of unspecified finger at forearm level**

√6th **S56.41 Strain of extensor muscle, fascia and tendon of other and unspecified finger at forearm level**

√7th **S56.411 Strain of extensor muscle, fascia and tendon of right index finger at forearm level**

√7th **S56.412 Strain of extensor muscle, fascia and tendon of left index finger at forearm level**

√7th **S56.413 Strain of extensor muscle, fascia and tendon of right middle finger at forearm level**

√7th **S56.414 Strain of extensor muscle, fascia and tendon of left middle finger at forearm level**

√7th **S56.415 Strain of extensor muscle, fascia and tendon of right ring finger at forearm level**

√7th **S56.416 Strain of extensor muscle, fascia and tendon of left ring finger at forearm level**

√7th **S56.417 Strain of extensor muscle, fascia and tendon of right little finger at forearm level**

√7th **S56.418 Strain of extensor muscle, fascia and tendon of left little finger at forearm level**

√7th **S56.419 Strain of extensor muscle, fascia and tendon of finger, unspecified finger at forearm level**

√6th **S56.42 Laceration of extensor muscle, fascia and tendon of other and unspecified finger at forearm level**

√7th **S56.421 Laceration of extensor muscle, fascia and tendon of right index finger at forearm level**

√7th **S56.422 Laceration of extensor muscle, fascia and tendon of left index finger at forearm level**

√7th **S56.423 Laceration of extensor muscle, fascia and tendon of right middle finger at forearm level**

√7th **S56.424 Laceration of extensor muscle, fascia and tendon of left middle finger at forearm level**

√7th **S56.425 Laceration of extensor muscle, fascia and tendon of right ring finger at forearm level**

√7th **S56.426 Laceration of extensor muscle, fascia and tendon of left ring finger at forearm level**

√7th **S56.427 Laceration of extensor muscle, fascia and tendon of right little finger at forearm level**

√7th **S56.428 Laceration of extensor muscle, fascia and tendon of left little finger at forearm level**

√7th **S56.429 Laceration of extensor muscle, fascia and tendon of unspecified finger at forearm level**

√6th **S56.49 Other injury of extensor muscle, fascia and tendon of other and unspecified finger at forearm level**

√7th **S56.491 Other injury of extensor muscle, fascia and tendon of right index finger at forearm level**

✓7th S56.492 Other injury of extensor muscle, fascia and tendon of left index finger at forearm level
✓7th S56.493 Other injury of extensor muscle, fascia and tendon of right middle finger at forearm level
✓7th S56.494 Other injury of extensor muscle, fascia and tendon of left middle finger at forearm level
✓7th S56.495 Other injury of extensor muscle, fascia and tendon of right ring finger at forearm level
✓7th S56.496 Other injury of extensor muscle, fascia and tendon of left ring finger at forearm level
✓7th S56.497 Other injury of extensor muscle, fascia and tendon of right little finger at forearm level
✓7th S56.498 Other injury of extensor muscle, fascia and tendon of left little finger at forearm level
✓7th S56.499 Other injury of extensor muscle, fascia and tendon of unspecified finger at forearm level

✓5th S56.5 Injury of other extensor muscle, fascia and tendon at forearm level
✓6th S56.5Ø Unspecified injury of other extensor muscle, fascia and tendon at forearm level
✓7th S56.5Ø1 Unspecified injury of other extensor muscle, fascia and tendon at forearm level, right arm
✓7th S56.5Ø2 Unspecified injury of other extensor muscle, fascia and tendon at forearm level, left arm
✓7th S56.5Ø9 Unspecified injury of other extensor muscle, fascia and tendon at forearm level, unspecified arm
✓6th S56.51 Strain of other extensor muscle, fascia and tendon at forearm level
✓7th S56.511 Strain of other extensor muscle, fascia and tendon at forearm level, right arm
✓7th S56.512 Strain of other extensor muscle, fascia and tendon at forearm level, left arm
✓7th S56.519 Strain of other extensor muscle, fascia and tendon at forearm level, unspecified arm
✓6th S56.52 Laceration of other extensor muscle, fascia and tendon at forearm level
✓7th S56.521 Laceration of other extensor muscle, fascia and tendon at forearm level, right arm
✓7th S56.522 Laceration of other extensor muscle, fascia and tendon at forearm level, left arm
✓7th S56.529 Laceration of other extensor muscle, fascia and tendon at forearm level, unspecified arm
✓6th S56.59 Other injury of other extensor muscle, fascia and tendon at forearm level
✓7th S56.591 Other injury of other extensor muscle, fascia and tendon at forearm level, right arm
✓7th S56.592 Other injury of other extensor muscle, fascia and tendon at forearm level, left arm
✓7th S56.599 Other injury of other extensor muscle, fascia and tendon at forearm level, unspecified arm

✓5th S56.8 Injury of other muscles, fascia and tendons at forearm level
✓6th S56.8Ø Unspecified injury of other muscles, fascia and tendons at forearm level
✓7th S56.8Ø1 Unspecified injury of other muscles, fascia and tendons at forearm level, right arm
✓7th S56.8Ø2 Unspecified injury of other muscles, fascia and tendons at forearm level, left arm
✓7th S56.8Ø9 Unspecified injury of other muscles, fascia and tendons at forearm level, unspecified arm
✓6th S56.81 Strain of other muscles, fascia and tendons at forearm level
✓7th S56.811 Strain of other muscles, fascia and tendons at forearm level, right arm
✓7th S56.812 Strain of other muscles, fascia and tendons at forearm level, left arm
✓7th S56.819 Strain of other muscles, fascia and tendons at forearm level, unspecified arm
✓6th S56.82 Laceration of other muscles, fascia and tendons at forearm level
✓7th S56.821 Laceration of other muscles, fascia and tendons at forearm level, right arm
✓7th S56.822 Laceration of other muscles, fascia and tendons at forearm level, left arm
✓7th S56.829 Laceration of other muscles, fascia and tendons at forearm level, unspecified arm
✓6th S56.89 Other injury of other muscles, fascia and tendons at forearm level
✓7th S56.891 Other injury of other muscles, fascia and tendons at forearm level, right arm
✓7th S56.892 Other injury of other muscles, fascia and tendons at forearm level, left arm
✓7th S56.899 Other injury of other muscles, fascia and tendons at forearm level, unspecified arm

✓5th S56.9 Injury of unspecified muscles, fascia and tendons at forearm level
✓6th S56.9Ø Unspecified injury of unspecified muscles, fascia and tendons at forearm level
✓7th S56.9Ø1 Unspecified injury of unspecified muscles, fascia and tendons at forearm level, right arm
✓7th S56.9Ø2 Unspecified injury of unspecified muscles, fascia and tendons at forearm level, left arm
✓7th S56.9Ø9 Unspecified injury of unspecified muscles, fascia and tendons at forearm level, unspecified arm
✓6th S56.91 Strain of unspecified muscles, fascia and tendons at forearm level
✓7th S56.911 Strain of unspecified muscles, fascia and tendons at forearm level, right arm
✓7th S56.912 Strain of unspecified muscles, fascia and tendons at forearm level, left arm
✓7th S56.919 Strain of unspecified muscles, fascia and tendons at forearm level, unspecified arm
✓6th S56.92 Laceration of unspecified muscles, fascia and tendons at forearm level
✓7th S56.921 Laceration of unspecified muscles, fascia and tendons at forearm level, right arm
✓7th S56.922 Laceration of unspecified muscles, fascia and tendons at forearm level, left arm
✓7th S56.929 Laceration of unspecified muscles, fascia and tendons at forearm level, unspecified arm
✓6th S56.99 Other injury of unspecified muscles, fascia and tendons at forearm level
✓7th S56.991 Other injury of unspecified muscles, fascia and tendons at forearm level, right arm
✓7th S56.992 Other injury of unspecified muscles, fascia and tendons at forearm level, left arm
✓7th S56.999 Other injury of unspecified muscles, fascia and tendons at forearm level, unspecified arm

✓4th **S57 Crushing injury of elbow and forearm**

Use additional code(s) for all associated injuries

EXCLUDES 2 *crushing injury of wrist and hand (S67.-)*

The appropriate 7th character is to be added to each code from category S57.
A initial encounter
D subsequent encounter
S sequela

✓5th S57.Ø Crushing injury of elbow
✓x7th S57.ØØ Crushing injury of unspecified elbow
✓x7th S57.Ø1 Crushing injury of right elbow
✓x7th S57.Ø2 Crushing injury of left elbow
✓5th S57.8 Crushing injury of forearm
✓x7th S57.8Ø Crushing injury of unspecified forearm
✓x7th S57.81 Crushing injury of right forearm
✓x7th S57.82 Crushing injury of left forearm

✓4th **S58 Traumatic amputation of elbow and forearm**

An amputation not identified as partial or complete should be coded to complete

EXCLUDES 1 *traumatic amputation of wrist and hand (S68.-)*

The appropriate 7th character is to be added to each code from category S58.
A initial encounter
D subsequent encounter
S sequela

✓5th S58.Ø Traumatic amputation at elbow level
✓6th S58.Ø1 Complete traumatic amputation at elbow level
✓7th S58.Ø11 Complete traumatic amputation at elbow level, right arm HCC ESR COM

S58.012 Complete traumatic amputation at elbow level, left arm HCC ESR COM

S58.019 Complete traumatic amputation at elbow level, unspecified arm HCC ESR COM

S58.02 Partial traumatic amputation at elbow level

S58.021 Partial traumatic amputation at elbow level, right arm HCC ESR COM

S58.022 Partial traumatic amputation at elbow level, left arm HCC ESR COM

S58.029 Partial traumatic amputation at elbow level, unspecified arm HCC ESR COM

S58.1 Traumatic amputation at level between elbow and wrist

S58.11 Complete traumatic amputation at level between elbow and wrist

S58.111 Complete traumatic amputation at level between elbow and wrist, right arm HCC ESR COM

S58.112 Complete traumatic amputation at level between elbow and wrist, left arm HCC ESR COM

S58.119 Complete traumatic amputation at level between elbow and wrist, unspecified arm HCC ESR COM

S58.12 Partial traumatic amputation at level between elbow and wrist

S58.121 Partial traumatic amputation at level between elbow and wrist, right arm HCC ESR COM

S58.122 Partial traumatic amputation at level between elbow and wrist, left arm HCC ESR COM

S58.129 Partial traumatic amputation at level between elbow and wrist, unspecified arm HCC ESR COM

S58.9 Traumatic amputation of forearm, level unspecified

EXCLUDES 1 *traumatic amputation of wrist (S68.-)*

S58.91 Complete traumatic amputation of forearm, level unspecified

S58.911 Complete traumatic amputation of right forearm, level unspecified HCC ESR COM

S58.912 Complete traumatic amputation of left forearm, level unspecified HCC ESR COM

S58.919 Complete traumatic amputation of unspecified forearm, level unspecified HCC ESR COM

S58.92 Partial traumatic amputation of forearm, level unspecified

S58.921 Partial traumatic amputation of right forearm, level unspecified HCC ESR COM

S58.922 Partial traumatic amputation of left forearm, level unspecified HCC ESR COM

S58.929 Partial traumatic amputation of unspecified forearm, level unspecified HCC ESR COM

S59 Other and unspecified injuries of elbow and forearm

EXCLUDES 2 *other and unspecified injuries of wrist and hand (S69.-)*

AHA: 2018,2Q,12; 2018,1Q,3; 2015,3Q,37-39

The appropriate 7th character is to be added to each code from subcategories S59.0, S59.1, and S59.2.
- A initial encounter for closed fracture
- D subsequent encounter for fracture with routine healing
- G subsequent encounter for fracture with delayed healing
- K subsequent encounter for fracture with nonunion
- P subsequent encounter for fracture with malunion
- S sequela

S59.0 Physeal fracture of lower end of ulna

AHA: 2019,4Q,56

S59.00 Unspecified physeal fracture of lower end of ulna

S59.001 Unspecified physeal fracture of lower end of ulna, right arm P

S59.002 Unspecified physeal fracture of lower end of ulna, left arm P

S59.009 Unspecified physeal fracture of lower end of ulna, unspecified arm P

S59.01 Salter-Harris Type I physeal fracture of lower end of ulna

S59.011 Salter-Harris Type I physeal fracture of lower end of ulna, right arm P

S59.012 Salter-Harris Type I physeal fracture of lower end of ulna, left arm P

S59.019 Salter-Harris Type I physeal fracture of lower end of ulna, unspecified arm P

S59.02 Salter-Harris Type II physeal fracture of lower end of ulna

S59.021 Salter-Harris Type II physeal fracture of lower end of ulna, right arm P

S59.022 Salter-Harris Type II physeal fracture of lower end of ulna, left arm P

S59.029 Salter-Harris Type II physeal fracture of lower end of ulna, unspecified arm P

S59.03 Salter-Harris Type III physeal fracture of lower end of ulna

S59.031 Salter-Harris Type III physeal fracture of lower end of ulna, right arm P

S59.032 Salter-Harris Type III physeal fracture of lower end of ulna, left arm P

S59.039 Salter-Harris Type III physeal fracture of lower end of ulna, unspecified arm P

S59.04 Salter-Harris Type IV physeal fracture of lower end of ulna

S59.041 Salter-Harris Type IV physeal fracture of lower end of ulna, right arm P

S59.042 Salter-Harris Type IV physeal fracture of lower end of ulna, left arm P

S59.049 Salter-Harris Type IV physeal fracture of lower end of ulna, unspecified arm P

S59.09 Other physeal fracture of lower end of ulna

S59.091 Other physeal fracture of lower end of ulna, right arm P

S59.092 Other physeal fracture of lower end of ulna, left arm P

S59.099 Other physeal fracture of lower end of ulna, unspecified arm P

S59.1 Physeal fracture of upper end of radius

AHA: 2019,4Q,56

S59.10 Unspecified physeal fracture of upper end of radius

S59.101 Unspecified physeal fracture of upper end of radius, right arm P

S59.102 Unspecified physeal fracture of upper end of radius, left arm P

S59.109 Unspecified physeal fracture of upper end of radius, unspecified arm P

S59.11 Salter-Harris Type I physeal fracture of upper end of radius

S59.111 Salter-Harris Type I physeal fracture of upper end of radius, right arm P

S59.112 Salter-Harris Type I physeal fracture of upper end of radius, left arm P

S59.119 Salter-Harris Type I physeal fracture of upper end of radius, unspecified arm P

S59.12 Salter-Harris Type II physeal fracture of upper end of radius

S59.121 Salter-Harris Type II physeal fracture of upper end of radius, right arm P

S59.122 Salter-Harris Type II physeal fracture of upper end of radius, left arm P

S59.129 Salter-Harris Type II physeal fracture of upper end of radius, unspecified arm P

S59.13 Salter-Harris Type III physeal fracture of upper end of radius

S59.131 Salter-Harris Type III physeal fracture of upper end of radius, right arm P

S59.132 Salter-Harris Type III physeal fracture of upper end of radius, left arm P

S59.139 Salter-Harris Type III physeal fracture of upper end of radius, unspecified arm P

S59.14 Salter-Harris Type IV physeal fracture of upper end of radius

S59.141 Salter-Harris Type IV physeal fracture of upper end of radius, right arm P

S59.142 Salter-Harris Type IV physeal fracture of upper end of radius, left arm P

S59.149 Salter-Harris Type IV physeal fracture of upper end of radius, unspecified arm P

S59.19 Other physeal fracture of upper end of radius

S59.191 Other physeal fracture of upper end of radius, right arm P

S59.192 Other physeal fracture of upper end of radius, left arm

S59.199 Other physeal fracture of upper end of radius, unspecified arm

S59.2 Physeal fracture of lower end of radius

AHA: 2019,4Q,56

S59.20 Unspecified physeal fracture of lower end of radius

S59.201 Unspecified physeal fracture of lower end of radius, right arm

S59.202 Unspecified physeal fracture of lower end of radius, left arm

S59.209 Unspecified physeal fracture of lower end of radius, unspecified arm

S59.21 Salter-Harris Type I physeal fracture of lower end of radius

S59.211 Salter-Harris Type I physeal fracture of lower end of radius, right arm

S59.212 Salter-Harris Type I physeal fracture of lower end of radius, left arm

S59.219 Salter-Harris Type I physeal fracture of lower end of radius, unspecified arm

S59.22 Salter-Harris Type II physeal fracture of lower end of radius

S59.221 Salter-Harris Type II physeal fracture of lower end of radius, right arm

S59.222 Salter-Harris Type II physeal fracture of lower end of radius, left arm

S59.229 Salter-Harris Type II physeal fracture of lower end of radius, unspecified arm

S59.23 Salter-Harris Type III physeal fracture of lower end of radius

S59.231 Salter-Harris Type III physeal fracture of lower end of radius, right arm

S59.232 Salter-Harris Type III physeal fracture of lower end of radius, left arm

S59.239 Salter-Harris Type III physeal fracture of lower end of radius, unspecified arm

S59.24 Salter-Harris Type IV physeal fracture of lower end of radius

S59.241 Salter-Harris Type IV physeal fracture of lower end of radius, right arm

S59.242 Salter-Harris Type IV physeal fracture of lower end of radius, left arm

S59.249 Salter-Harris Type IV physeal fracture of lower end of radius, unspecified arm

S59.29 Other physeal fracture of lower end of radius

S59.291 Other physeal fracture of lower end of radius, right arm

S59.292 Other physeal fracture of lower end of radius, left arm

S59.299 Other physeal fracture of lower end of radius, unspecified arm

S59.8 Other specified injuries of elbow and forearm

The appropriate 7th character is to be added to each code in subcategory S59.8.
A initial encounter
D subsequent encounter
S sequela

S59.80 Other specified injuries of elbow

S59.801 Other specified injuries of right elbow

S59.802 Other specified injuries of left elbow

S59.809 Other specified injuries of unspecified elbow

S59.81 Other specified injuries of forearm

S59.811 Other specified injuries right forearm

S59.812 Other specified injuries left forearm

S59.819 Other specified injuries unspecified forearm

S59.9 Unspecified injury of elbow and forearm

The appropriate 7th character is to be added to each code in subcategory S59.9.
A initial encounter
D subsequent encounter
S sequela

S59.90 Unspecified injury of elbow

S59.901 Unspecified injury of right elbow

S59.902 Unspecified injury of left elbow

S59.909 Unspecified injury of unspecified elbow

S59.91 Unspecified injury of forearm

S59.911 Unspecified injury of right forearm

S59.912 Unspecified injury of left forearm

S59.919 Unspecified injury of unspecified forearm

## Injuries to the wrist, hand and fingers (S60-S69)

EXCLUDES 2 *burns and corrosions (T20-T32)*
*frostbite (T33-T34)*
*insect bite or sting, venomous (T63.4)*

**S60 Superficial injury of wrist, hand and fingers**

The appropriate 7th character is to be added to each code from category S60.
A initial encounter
D subsequent encounter
S sequela

S60.0 Contusion of finger without damage to nail

EXCLUDES 1 *contusion involving nail (matrix) (S60.1)*

S60.00 Contusion of unspecified finger without damage to nail

Contusion of finger(s) NOS

S60.01 Contusion of thumb without damage to nail

S60.011 Contusion of right thumb without damage to nail

S60.012 Contusion of left thumb without damage to nail

S60.019 Contusion of unspecified thumb without damage to nail

S60.02 Contusion of index finger without damage to nail

S60.021 Contusion of right index finger without damage to nail

S60.022 Contusion of left index finger without damage to nail

S60.029 Contusion of unspecified index finger without damage to nail

S60.03 Contusion of middle finger without damage to nail

S60.031 Contusion of right middle finger without damage to nail

S60.032 Contusion of left middle finger without damage to nail

S60.039 Contusion of unspecified middle finger without damage to nail

S60.04 Contusion of ring finger without damage to nail

S60.041 Contusion of right ring finger without damage to nail

S60.042 Contusion of left ring finger without damage to nail

S60.049 Contusion of unspecified ring finger without damage to nail

S60.05 Contusion of little finger without damage to nail

S60.051 Contusion of right little finger without damage to nail

S60.052 Contusion of left little finger without damage to nail

S60.059 Contusion of unspecified little finger without damage to nail

S60.1 Contusion of finger with damage to nail

S60.10 Contusion of unspecified finger with damage to nail

S60.11 Contusion of thumb with damage to nail

S60.111 Contusion of right thumb with damage to nail

S60.112 Contusion of left thumb with damage to nail

S60.119 Contusion of unspecified thumb with damage to nail

S60.12 Contusion of index finger with damage to nail

S60.121 Contusion of right index finger with damage to nail

S60.122 Contusion of left index finger with damage to nail

S60.129 Contusion of unspecified index finger with damage to nail

S60.13 Contusion of middle finger with damage to nail

S60.131 Contusion of right middle finger with damage to nail

7th S60.132 Contusion of left middle finger with damage to nail
7th S60.139 Contusion of unspecified middle finger with damage to nail
6th S60.14 Contusion of ring finger with damage to nail
7th S60.141 Contusion of right ring finger with damage to nail
7th S60.142 Contusion of left ring finger with damage to nail
7th S60.149 Contusion of unspecified ring finger with damage to nail
6th S60.15 Contusion of little finger with damage to nail
7th S60.151 Contusion of right little finger with damage to nail
7th S60.152 Contusion of left little finger with damage to nail
7th S60.159 Contusion of unspecified little finger with damage to nail
5th S60.2 Contusion of wrist and hand
EXCLUDES 2 *contusion of fingers (S60.0-, S60.1-)*
6th S60.21 Contusion of wrist
7th S60.211 Contusion of right wrist
7th S60.212 Contusion of left wrist
7th S60.219 Contusion of unspecified wrist
6th S60.22 Contusion of hand
7th S60.221 Contusion of right hand
7th S60.222 Contusion of left hand
7th S60.229 Contusion of unspecified hand
5th S60.3 Other superficial injuries of thumb
6th S60.31 Abrasion of thumb
7th S60.311 Abrasion of right thumb
7th S60.312 Abrasion of left thumb
7th S60.319 Abrasion of unspecified thumb
6th S60.32 Blister (nonthermal) of thumb
7th S60.321 Blister (nonthermal) of right thumb
7th S60.322 Blister (nonthermal) of left thumb
7th S60.329 Blister (nonthermal) of unspecified thumb
6th S60.34 External constriction of thumb
Hair tourniquet syndrome of thumb
Use additional cause code to identify the constricting item (W49.0-)
7th S60.341 External constriction of right thumb
7th S60.342 External constriction of left thumb
7th S60.349 External constriction of unspecified thumb
6th S60.35 Superficial foreign body of thumb
Splinter in the thumb
7th S60.351 Superficial foreign body of right thumb
7th S60.352 Superficial foreign body of left thumb
7th S60.359 Superficial foreign body of unspecified thumb
6th S60.36 Insect bite (nonvenomous) of thumb
7th S60.361 Insect bite (nonvenomous) of right thumb
7th S60.362 Insect bite (nonvenomous) of left thumb
7th S60.369 Insect bite (nonvenomous) of unspecified thumb
6th S60.37 Other superficial bite of thumb
EXCLUDES 1 *open bite of thumb (S61.05-, S61.15-)*
7th S60.371 Other superficial bite of right thumb
7th S60.372 Other superficial bite of left thumb
7th S60.379 Other superficial bite of unspecified thumb
6th S60.39 Other superficial injuries of thumb
7th S60.391 Other superficial injuries of right thumb
7th S60.392 Other superficial injuries of left thumb
7th S60.399 Other superficial injuries of unspecified thumb
5th S60.4 Other superficial injuries of other fingers
6th S60.41 Abrasion of fingers
7th S60.410 Abrasion of right index finger
7th S60.411 Abrasion of left index finger
7th S60.412 Abrasion of right middle finger
7th S60.413 Abrasion of left middle finger
7th S60.414 Abrasion of right ring finger
7th S60.415 Abrasion of left ring finger
7th S60.416 Abrasion of right little finger
7th S60.417 Abrasion of left little finger
7th S60.418 Abrasion of other finger
Abrasion of specified finger with unspecified laterality
7th S60.419 Abrasion of unspecified finger
6th S60.42 Blister (nonthermal) of fingers
7th S60.420 Blister (nonthermal) of right index finger
7th S60.421 Blister (nonthermal) of left index finger
7th S60.422 Blister (nonthermal) of right middle finger
7th S60.423 Blister (nonthermal) of left middle finger
7th S60.424 Blister (nonthermal) of right ring finger
7th S60.425 Blister (nonthermal) of left ring finger
7th S60.426 Blister (nonthermal) of right little finger
7th S60.427 Blister (nonthermal) of left little finger
7th S60.428 Blister (nonthermal) of other finger
Blister (nonthermal) of specified finger with unspecified laterality
7th S60.429 Blister (nonthermal) of unspecified finger
6th S60.44 External constriction of fingers
Hair tourniquet syndrome of finger
Use additional cause code to identify the constricting item (W49.0-)
7th S60.440 External constriction of right index finger
7th S60.441 External constriction of left index finger
7th S60.442 External constriction of right middle finger
7th S60.443 External constriction of left middle finger
7th S60.444 External constriction of right ring finger
7th S60.445 External constriction of left ring finger
7th S60.446 External constriction of right little finger
7th S60.447 External constriction of left little finger
7th S60.448 External constriction of other finger
External constriction of specified finger with unspecified laterality
7th S60.449 External constriction of unspecified finger
6th S60.45 Superficial foreign body of fingers
Splinter in the finger(s)
7th S60.450 Superficial foreign body of right index finger
7th S60.451 Superficial foreign body of left index finger
7th S60.452 Superficial foreign body of right middle finger
7th S60.453 Superficial foreign body of left middle finger
7th S60.454 Superficial foreign body of right ring finger
7th S60.455 Superficial foreign body of left ring finger
7th S60.456 Superficial foreign body of right little finger
7th S60.457 Superficial foreign body of left little finger
7th S60.458 Superficial foreign body of other finger
Superficial foreign body of specified finger with unspecified laterality
7th S60.459 Superficial foreign body of unspecified finger
6th S60.46 Insect bite (nonvenomous) of fingers
7th S60.460 Insect bite (nonvenomous) of right index finger
7th S60.461 Insect bite (nonvenomous) of left index finger
7th S60.462 Insect bite (nonvenomous) of right middle finger
7th S60.463 Insect bite (nonvenomous) of left middle finger
7th S60.464 Insect bite (nonvenomous) of right ring finger
7th S60.465 Insect bite (nonvenomous) of left ring finger
7th S60.466 Insect bite (nonvenomous) of right little finger
7th S60.467 Insect bite (nonvenomous) of left little finger

S60.468 Insect bite (nonvenomous) of other finger
Insect bite (nonvenomous) of specified finger with unspecified laterality
S60.469 Insect bite (nonvenomous) of unspecified finger
S60.47 Other superficial bite of fingers
EXCLUDES 1 *open bite of fingers (S61.25-, S61.35-)*
S60.470 Other superficial bite of right index finger
S60.471 Other superficial bite of left index finger
S60.472 Other superficial bite of right middle finger
S60.473 Other superficial bite of left middle finger
S60.474 Other superficial bite of right ring finger
S60.475 Other superficial bite of left ring finger
S60.476 Other superficial bite of right little finger
S60.477 Other superficial bite of left little finger
S60.478 Other superficial bite of other finger
Other superficial bite of specified finger with unspecified laterality
S60.479 Other superficial bite of unspecified finger
S60.5 Other superficial injuries of hand
EXCLUDES 2 *superficial injuries of fingers (S60.3-, S60.4-)*
S60.51 Abrasion of hand
S60.511 Abrasion of right hand
S60.512 Abrasion of left hand
S60.519 Abrasion of unspecified hand
S60.52 Blister (nonthermal) of hand
S60.521 Blister (nonthermal) of right hand
S60.522 Blister (nonthermal) of left hand
S60.529 Blister (nonthermal) of unspecified hand
S60.54 External constriction of hand
S60.541 External constriction of right hand
S60.542 External constriction of left hand
S60.549 External constriction of unspecified hand
S60.55 Superficial foreign body of hand
Splinter in the hand
S60.551 Superficial foreign body of right hand
S60.552 Superficial foreign body of left hand
S60.559 Superficial foreign body of unspecified hand
S60.56 Insect bite (nonvenomous) of hand
S60.561 Insect bite (nonvenomous) of right hand
S60.562 Insect bite (nonvenomous) of left hand
S60.569 Insect bite (nonvenomous) of unspecified hand
S60.57 Other superficial bite of hand
EXCLUDES 1 *open bite of hand (S61.45-)*
S60.571 Other superficial bite of hand of right hand
S60.572 Other superficial bite of hand of left hand
S60.579 Other superficial bite of hand of unspecified hand
S60.8 Other superficial injuries of wrist
S60.81 Abrasion of wrist
S60.811 Abrasion of right wrist
S60.812 Abrasion of left wrist
S60.819 Abrasion of unspecified wrist
S60.82 Blister (nonthermal) of wrist
S60.821 Blister (nonthermal) of right wrist
S60.822 Blister (nonthermal) of left wrist
S60.829 Blister (nonthermal) of unspecified wrist
S60.84 External constriction of wrist
S60.841 External constriction of right wrist
S60.842 External constriction of left wrist
S60.849 External constriction of unspecified wrist
S60.85 Superficial foreign body of wrist
Splinter in the wrist
S60.851 Superficial foreign body of right wrist
S60.852 Superficial foreign body of left wrist
S60.859 Superficial foreign body of unspecified wrist
S60.86 Insect bite (nonvenomous) of wrist
S60.861 Insect bite (nonvenomous) of right wrist
S60.862 Insect bite (nonvenomous) of left wrist
S60.869 Insect bite (nonvenomous) of unspecified wrist
S60.87 Other superficial bite of wrist
EXCLUDES 1 *open bite of wrist (S61.55)*
S60.871 Other superficial bite of right wrist
S60.872 Other superficial bite of left wrist
S60.879 Other superficial bite of unspecified wrist
S60.9 Unspecified superficial injury of wrist, hand and fingers
S60.91 Unspecified superficial injury of wrist
S60.911 Unspecified superficial injury of right wrist
S60.912 Unspecified superficial injury of left wrist
S60.919 Unspecified superficial injury of unspecified wrist
S60.92 Unspecified superficial injury of hand
S60.921 Unspecified superficial injury of right hand
S60.922 Unspecified superficial injury of left hand
S60.929 Unspecified superficial injury of unspecified hand
S60.93 Unspecified superficial injury of thumb
S60.931 Unspecified superficial injury of right thumb
S60.932 Unspecified superficial injury of left thumb
S60.939 Unspecified superficial injury of unspecified thumb
S60.94 Unspecified superficial injury of other fingers
S60.940 Unspecified superficial injury of right index finger
S60.941 Unspecified superficial injury of left index finger
S60.942 Unspecified superficial injury of right middle finger
S60.943 Unspecified superficial injury of left middle finger
S60.944 Unspecified superficial injury of right ring finger
S60.945 Unspecified superficial injury of left ring finger
S60.946 Unspecified superficial injury of right little finger
S60.947 Unspecified superficial injury of left little finger
S60.948 Unspecified superficial injury of other finger
Unspecified superficial injury of specified finger with unspecified laterality
S60.949 Unspecified superficial injury of unspecified finger

**S61 Open wound of wrist, hand and fingers**
Code also any associated wound infection
EXCLUDES 1 *open fracture of wrist, hand and finger (S62.- with 7th character B)*
*traumatic amputation of wrist and hand (S68.-)*

The appropriate 7th character is to be added to each code from category S61.
A initial encounter
D subsequent encounter
S sequela

S61.0 Open wound of thumb without damage to nail
EXCLUDES 1 *open wound of thumb with damage to nail (S61.1-)*
S61.00 Unspecified open wound of thumb without damage to nail
S61.001 Unspecified open wound of right thumb without damage to nail
S61.002 Unspecified open wound of left thumb without damage to nail
S61.009 Unspecified open wound of unspecified thumb without damage to nail
S61.01 Laceration without foreign body of thumb without damage to nail
S61.011 Laceration without foreign body of right thumb without damage to nail
S61.012 Laceration without foreign body of left thumb without damage to nail

√7th S61.019 Laceration without foreign body of unspecified thumb without damage to nail

√6th S61.02 Laceration with foreign body of thumb without damage to nail

√7th S61.021 Laceration with foreign body of right thumb without damage to nail

√7th S61.022 Laceration with foreign body of left thumb without damage to nail

√7th S61.029 Laceration with foreign body of unspecified thumb without damage to nail

√6th S61.03 Puncture wound without foreign body of thumb without damage to nail

√7th S61.031 Puncture wound without foreign body of right thumb without damage to nail

√7th S61.032 Puncture wound without foreign body of left thumb without damage to nail

√7th S61.039 Puncture wound without foreign body of unspecified thumb without damage to nail

√6th S61.04 Puncture wound with foreign body of thumb without damage to nail

√7th S61.041 Puncture wound with foreign body of right thumb without damage to nail

√7th S61.042 Puncture wound with foreign body of left thumb without damage to nail

√7th S61.049 Puncture wound with foreign body of unspecified thumb without damage to nail

√6th S61.05 Open bite of thumb without damage to nail

Bite of thumb NOS

EXCLUDES 1 *superficial bite of thumb (S60.36-, S60.37-)*

√7th S61.051 Open bite of right thumb without damage to nail

√7th S61.052 Open bite of left thumb without damage to nail

√7th S61.059 Open bite of unspecified thumb without damage to nail

√5th S61.1 Open wound of thumb with damage to nail

√6th S61.10 Unspecified open wound of thumb with damage to nail

√7th S61.101 Unspecified open wound of right thumb with damage to nail

√7th S61.102 Unspecified open wound of left thumb with damage to nail

√7th S61.109 Unspecified open wound of unspecified thumb with damage to nail

√6th S61.11 Laceration without foreign body of thumb with damage to nail

√7th S61.111 Laceration without foreign body of right thumb with damage to nail

√7th S61.112 Laceration without foreign body of left thumb with damage to nail

√7th S61.119 Laceration without foreign body of unspecified thumb with damage to nail

√6th S61.12 Laceration with foreign body of thumb with damage to nail

√7th S61.121 Laceration with foreign body of right thumb with damage to nail

√7th S61.122 Laceration with foreign body of left thumb with damage to nail

√7th S61.129 Laceration with foreign body of unspecified thumb with damage to nail

√6th S61.13 Puncture wound without foreign body of thumb with damage to nail

√7th S61.131 Puncture wound without foreign body of right thumb with damage to nail

√7th S61.132 Puncture wound without foreign body of left thumb with damage to nail

√7th S61.139 Puncture wound without foreign body of unspecified thumb with damage to nail

√6th S61.14 Puncture wound with foreign body of thumb with damage to nail

√7th S61.141 Puncture wound with foreign body of right thumb with damage to nail

√7th S61.142 Puncture wound with foreign body of left thumb with damage to nail

√7th S61.149 Puncture wound with foreign body of unspecified thumb with damage to nail

√6th S61.15 Open bite of thumb with damage to nail

Bite of thumb with damage to nail NOS

EXCLUDES 1 *superficial bite of thumb (S60.36-, S60.37-)*

√7th S61.151 Open bite of right thumb with damage to nail

√7th S61.152 Open bite of left thumb with damage to nail

√7th S61.159 Open bite of unspecified thumb with damage to nail

√5th S61.2 Open wound of other finger without damage to nail

EXCLUDES 1 *open wound of finger involving nail (matrix) (S61.3-)*

EXCLUDES 2 *open wound of thumb without damage to nail (S61.0-)*

√6th S61.20 Unspecified open wound of other finger without damage to nail

√7th S61.200 Unspecified open wound of right index finger without damage to nail

√7th S61.201 Unspecified open wound of left index finger without damage to nail

√7th S61.202 Unspecified open wound of right middle finger without damage to nail

√7th S61.203 Unspecified open wound of left middle finger without damage to nail

√7th S61.204 Unspecified open wound of right ring finger without damage to nail

√7th S61.205 Unspecified open wound of left ring finger without damage to nail

√7th S61.206 Unspecified open wound of right little finger without damage to nail

√7th S61.207 Unspecified open wound of left little finger without damage to nail

√7th S61.208 Unspecified open wound of other finger without damage to nail

Unspecified open wound of specified finger with unspecified laterality without damage to nail

√7th S61.209 Unspecified open wound of unspecified finger without damage to nail

√6th S61.21 Laceration without foreign body of finger without damage to nail

√7th S61.210 Laceration without foreign body of right index finger without damage to nail

√7th S61.211 Laceration without foreign body of left index finger without damage to nail

√7th S61.212 Laceration without foreign body of right middle finger without damage to nail

√7th S61.213 Laceration without foreign body of left middle finger without damage to nail

√7th S61.214 Laceration without foreign body of right ring finger without damage to nail

√7th S61.215 Laceration without foreign body of left ring finger without damage to nail

√7th S61.216 Laceration without foreign body of right little finger without damage to nail

√7th S61.217 Laceration without foreign body of left little finger without damage to nail

√7th S61.218 Laceration without foreign body of other finger without damage to nail

Laceration without foreign body of specified finger with unspecified laterality without damage to nail

√7th S61.219 Laceration without foreign body of unspecified finger without damage to nail

√6th S61.22 Laceration with foreign body of finger without damage to nail

√7th S61.220 Laceration with foreign body of right index finger without damage to nail

√7th S61.221 Laceration with foreign body of left index finger without damage to nail

√7th S61.222 Laceration with foreign body of right middle finger without damage to nail

√7th S61.223 Laceration with foreign body of left middle finger without damage to nail

√7th S61.224 Laceration with foreign body of right ring finger without damage to nail

√7th S61.225 Laceration with foreign body of left ring finger without damage to nail

√7th S61.226 Laceration with foreign body of right little finger without damage to nail

√7th S61.227 Laceration with foreign body of left little finger without damage to nail

√7th S61.228 Laceration with foreign body of other finger without damage to nail

Laceration with foreign body of specified finger with unspecified laterality without damage to nail

√7th S61.229 Laceration with foreign body of unspecified finger without damage to nail

S61.23 Puncture wound without foreign body of finger without damage to nail
- S61.230 Puncture wound without foreign body of right index finger without damage to nail
- S61.231 Puncture wound without foreign body of left index finger without damage to nail
- S61.232 Puncture wound without foreign body of right middle finger without damage to nail
- S61.233 Puncture wound without foreign body of left middle finger without damage to nail
- S61.234 Puncture wound without foreign body of right ring finger without damage to nail
- S61.235 Puncture wound without foreign body of left ring finger without damage to nail
- S61.236 Puncture wound without foreign body of right little finger without damage to nail
- S61.237 Puncture wound without foreign body of left little finger without damage to nail
- S61.238 Puncture wound without foreign body of other finger without damage to nail
  Puncture wound without foreign body of specified finger with unspecified laterality without damage to nail
- S61.239 Puncture wound without foreign body of unspecified finger without damage to nail

S61.24 Puncture wound with foreign body of finger without damage to nail
- S61.240 Puncture wound with foreign body of right index finger without damage to nail
- S61.241 Puncture wound with foreign body of left index finger without damage to nail
- S61.242 Puncture wound with foreign body of right middle finger without damage to nail
- S61.243 Puncture wound with foreign body of left middle finger without damage to nail
- S61.244 Puncture wound with foreign body of right ring finger without damage to nail
- S61.245 Puncture wound with foreign body of left ring finger without damage to nail
- S61.246 Puncture wound with foreign body of right little finger without damage to nail
- S61.247 Puncture wound with foreign body of left little finger without damage to nail
- S61.248 Puncture wound with foreign body of other finger without damage to nail
  Puncture wound with foreign body of specified finger with unspecified laterality without damage to nail
- S61.249 Puncture wound with foreign body of unspecified finger without damage to nail

S61.25 Open bite of finger without damage to nail
Bite of finger without damage to nail NOS
EXCLUDES 1 *superficial bite of finger (S60.46-, S60.47-)*
- S61.250 Open bite of right index finger without damage to nail
- S61.251 Open bite of left index finger without damage to nail
- S61.252 Open bite of right middle finger without damage to nail
- S61.253 Open bite of left middle finger without damage to nail
- S61.254 Open bite of right ring finger without damage to nail
- S61.255 Open bite of left ring finger without damage to nail
- S61.256 Open bite of right little finger without damage to nail
- S61.257 Open bite of left little finger without damage to nail
- S61.258 Open bite of other finger without damage to nail
  Open bite of specified finger with unspecified laterality without damage to nail
- S61.259 Open bite of unspecified finger without damage to nail

S61.3 Open wound of other finger with damage to nail

S61.30 Unspecified open wound of finger with damage to nail
- S61.300 Unspecified open wound of right index finger with damage to nail
- S61.301 Unspecified open wound of left index finger with damage to nail
- S61.302 Unspecified open wound of right middle finger with damage to nail
- S61.303 Unspecified open wound of left middle finger with damage to nail
- S61.304 Unspecified open wound of right ring finger with damage to nail
- S61.305 Unspecified open wound of left ring finger with damage to nail
- S61.306 Unspecified open wound of right little finger with damage to nail
- S61.307 Unspecified open wound of left little finger with damage to nail
- S61.308 Unspecified open wound of other finger with damage to nail
  Unspecified open wound of specified finger with unspecified laterality with damage to nail
- S61.309 Unspecified open wound of unspecified finger with damage to nail

S61.31 Laceration without foreign body of finger with damage to nail
- S61.310 Laceration without foreign body of right index finger with damage to nail
- S61.311 Laceration without foreign body of left index finger with damage to nail
- S61.312 Laceration without foreign body of right middle finger with damage to nail
- S61.313 Laceration without foreign body of left middle finger with damage to nail
- S61.314 Laceration without foreign body of right ring finger with damage to nail
- S61.315 Laceration without foreign body of left ring finger with damage to nail
- S61.316 Laceration without foreign body of right little finger with damage to nail
- S61.317 Laceration without foreign body of left little finger with damage to nail
- S61.318 Laceration without foreign body of other finger with damage to nail
  Laceration without foreign body of specified finger with unspecified laterality with damage to nail
- S61.319 Laceration without foreign body of unspecified finger with damage to nail

S61.32 Laceration with foreign body of finger with damage to nail
- S61.320 Laceration with foreign body of right index finger with damage to nail
- S61.321 Laceration with foreign body of left index finger with damage to nail
- S61.322 Laceration with foreign body of right middle finger with damage to nail
- S61.323 Laceration with foreign body of left middle finger with damage to nail
- S61.324 Laceration with foreign body of right ring finger with damage to nail
- S61.325 Laceration with foreign body of left ring finger with damage to nail
- S61.326 Laceration with foreign body of right little finger with damage to nail
- S61.327 Laceration with foreign body of left little finger with damage to nail
- S61.328 Laceration with foreign body of other finger with damage to nail
  Laceration with foreign body of specified finger with unspecified laterality with damage to nail
- S61.329 Laceration with foreign body of unspecified finger with damage to nail

S61.33 Puncture wound without foreign body of finger with damage to nail
- S61.330 Puncture wound without foreign body of right index finger with damage to nail
- S61.331 Puncture wound without foreign body of left index finger with damage to nail
- S61.332 Puncture wound without foreign body of right middle finger with damage to nail
- S61.333 Puncture wound without foreign body of left middle finger with damage to nail
- S61.334 Puncture wound without foreign body of right ring finger with damage to nail
- S61.335 Puncture wound without foreign body of left ring finger with damage to nail

√7th S61.336 Puncture wound without foreign body of right little finger with damage to nail
√7th S61.337 Puncture wound without foreign body of left little finger with damage to nail
√7th S61.338 Puncture wound without foreign body of other finger with damage to nail
Puncture wound without foreign body of specified finger with unspecified laterality with damage to nail
√7th S61.339 Puncture wound without foreign body of unspecified finger with damage to nail
√6th S61.34 Puncture wound with foreign body of finger with damage to nail
√7th S61.340 Puncture wound with foreign body of right index finger with damage to nail
√7th S61.341 Puncture wound with foreign body of left index finger with damage to nail
√7th S61.342 Puncture wound with foreign body of right middle finger with damage to nail
√7th S61.343 Puncture wound with foreign body of left middle finger with damage to nail
√7th S61.344 Puncture wound with foreign body of right ring finger with damage to nail
√7th S61.345 Puncture wound with foreign body of left ring finger with damage to nail
√7th S61.346 Puncture wound with foreign body of right little finger with damage to nail
√7th S61.347 Puncture wound with foreign body of left little finger with damage to nail
√7th S61.348 Puncture wound with foreign body of other finger with damage to nail
Puncture wound with foreign body of specified finger with unspecified laterality with damage to nail
√7th S61.349 Puncture wound with foreign body of unspecified finger with damage to nail
√6th S61.35 Open bite of finger with damage to nail
Bite of finger with damage to nail NOS
EXCLUDES 1 *superficial bite of finger (S60.46-, S60.47-)*
√7th S61.350 Open bite of right index finger with damage to nail
√7th S61.351 Open bite of left index finger with damage to nail
√7th S61.352 Open bite of right middle finger with damage to nail
√7th S61.353 Open bite of left middle finger with damage to nail
√7th S61.354 Open bite of right ring finger with damage to nail
√7th S61.355 Open bite of left ring finger with damage to nail
√7th S61.356 Open bite of right little finger with damage to nail
√7th S61.357 Open bite of left little finger with damage to nail
√7th S61.358 Open bite of other finger with damage to nail
Open bite of specified finger with unspecified laterality with damage to nail
√7th S61.359 Open bite of unspecified finger with damage to nail
√5th S61.4 Open wound of hand
√6th S61.40 Unspecified open wound of hand
√7th S61.401 Unspecified open wound of right hand
√7th S61.402 Unspecified open wound of left hand
√7th S61.409 Unspecified open wound of unspecified hand
√6th S61.41 Laceration without foreign body of hand
√7th S61.411 Laceration without foreign body of right hand
√7th S61.412 Laceration without foreign body of left hand
√7th S61.419 Laceration without foreign body of unspecified hand
√6th S61.42 Laceration with foreign body of hand
√7th S61.421 Laceration with foreign body of right hand
√7th S61.422 Laceration with foreign body of left hand
√7th S61.429 Laceration with foreign body of unspecified hand
√6th S61.43 Puncture wound without foreign body of hand
√7th S61.431 Puncture wound without foreign body of right hand
√7th S61.432 Puncture wound without foreign body of left hand
√7th S61.439 Puncture wound without foreign body of unspecified hand
√6th S61.44 Puncture wound with foreign body of hand
√7th S61.441 Puncture wound with foreign body of right hand
√7th S61.442 Puncture wound with foreign body of left hand
√7th S61.449 Puncture wound with foreign body of unspecified hand
√6th S61.45 Open bite of hand
Bite of hand NOS
EXCLUDES 1 *superficial bite of hand (S60.56-, S60.57-)*
√7th S61.451 Open bite of right hand
√7th S61.452 Open bite of left hand
√7th S61.459 Open bite of unspecified hand
√5th S61.5 Open wound of wrist
√6th S61.50 Unspecified open wound of wrist
√7th S61.501 Unspecified open wound of right wrist
√7th S61.502 Unspecified open wound of left wrist
√7th S61.509 Unspecified open wound of unspecified wrist
√6th S61.51 Laceration without foreign body of wrist
√7th S61.511 Laceration without foreign body of right wrist
√7th S61.512 Laceration without foreign body of left wrist
√7th S61.519 Laceration without foreign body of unspecified wrist
√6th S61.52 Laceration with foreign body of wrist
√7th S61.521 Laceration with foreign body of right wrist
√7th S61.522 Laceration with foreign body of left wrist
√7th S61.529 Laceration with foreign body of unspecified wrist
√6th S61.53 Puncture wound without foreign body of wrist
√7th S61.531 Puncture wound without foreign body of right wrist
√7th S61.532 Puncture wound without foreign body of left wrist
√7th S61.539 Puncture wound without foreign body of unspecified wrist
√6th S61.54 Puncture wound with foreign body of wrist
√7th S61.541 Puncture wound with foreign body of right wrist
√7th S61.542 Puncture wound with foreign body of left wrist
√7th S61.549 Puncture wound with foreign body of unspecified wrist
√6th S61.55 Open bite of wrist
Bite of wrist NOS
EXCLUDES 1 *superficial bite of wrist (S60.86-, S60.87-)*
√7th S61.551 Open bite of right wrist
√7th S61.552 Open bite of left wrist
√7th S61.559 Open bite of unspecified wrist

**S62 Fracture at wrist and hand level**

NOTE A fracture not indicated as displaced or nondisplaced should be coded to displaced

A fracture not indicated as open or closed should be coded to closed

EXCLUDES 1 *traumatic amputation of wrist and hand (S68.-)*

EXCLUDES 2 *fracture of distal parts of ulna and radius (S52.-)*

AHA: 2018,2Q,12; 2015,3Q,37-39

The appropriate 7th character is to be added to each code from category S62.
- A initial encounter for closed fracture
- B initial encounter for open fracture
- D subsequent encounter for fracture with routine healing
- G subsequent encounter for fracture with delayed healing
- K subsequent encounter for fracture with nonunion
- P subsequent encounter for fracture with malunion
- S sequela

**S62.0 Fracture of navicular [scaphoid] bone of wrist**

**S62.00 Unspecified fracture of navicular [scaphoid] bone of wrist**

**S62.001 Unspecified fracture of navicular [scaphoid] bone of right wrist** Q

**S62.002 Unspecified fracture of navicular [scaphoid] bone of left wrist** Q

AHA: 2012,4Q,106

**S62.009 Unspecified fracture of navicular [scaphoid] bone of unspecified wrist** Q

**S62.01 Fracture of distal pole of navicular [scaphoid] bone of wrist**

Fracture of volar tuberosity of navicular [scaphoid] bone of wrist

**S62.011 Displaced fracture of distal pole of navicular [scaphoid] bone of right wrist** Q

**S62.012 Displaced fracture of distal pole of navicular [scaphoid] bone of left wrist** Q

**S62.013 Displaced fracture of distal pole of navicular [scaphoid] bone of unspecified wrist** Q

**S62.014 Nondisplaced fracture of distal pole of navicular [scaphoid] bone of right wrist** Q

**S62.015 Nondisplaced fracture of distal pole of navicular [scaphoid] bone of left wrist** Q

**S62.016 Nondisplaced fracture of distal pole of navicular [scaphoid] bone of unspecified wrist** Q

**S62.02 Fracture of middle third of navicular [scaphoid] bone of wrist**

**S62.021 Displaced fracture of middle third of navicular [scaphoid] bone of right wrist** Q

**S62.022 Displaced fracture of middle third of navicular [scaphoid] bone of left wrist** Q

**S62.023 Displaced fracture of middle third of navicular [scaphoid] bone of unspecified wrist** Q

**S62.024 Nondisplaced fracture of middle third of navicular [scaphoid] bone of right wrist** Q

**S62.025 Nondisplaced fracture of middle third of navicular [scaphoid] bone of left wrist** Q

**S62.026 Nondisplaced fracture of middle third of navicular [scaphoid] bone of unspecified wrist** Q

**S62.03 Fracture of proximal third of navicular [scaphoid] bone of wrist**

**S62.031 Displaced fracture of proximal third of navicular [scaphoid] bone of right wrist** Q

**S62.032 Displaced fracture of proximal third of navicular [scaphoid] bone of left wrist** Q

**S62.033 Displaced fracture of proximal third of navicular [scaphoid] bone of unspecified wrist** Q

**S62.034 Nondisplaced fracture of proximal third of navicular [scaphoid] bone of right wrist** Q

**S62.035 Nondisplaced fracture of proximal third of navicular [scaphoid] bone of left wrist** Q

**S62.036 Nondisplaced fracture of proximal third of navicular [scaphoid] bone of unspecified wrist** Q

**S62.1 Fracture of other and unspecified carpal bone(s)**

EXCLUDES 2 *fracture of scaphoid of wrist (S62.0-)*

**S62.10 Fracture of unspecified carpal bone**

Fracture of wrist NOS

**S62.101 Fracture of unspecified carpal bone, right wrist** Q

**S62.102 Fracture of unspecified carpal bone, left wrist** Q

AHA: 2012,4Q,95

**S62.109 Fracture of unspecified carpal bone, unspecified wrist** Q

**S62.11 Fracture of triquetrum [cuneiform] bone of wrist**

**S62.111 Displaced fracture of triquetrum [cuneiform] bone, right wrist** Q

**S62.112 Displaced fracture of triquetrum [cuneiform] bone, left wrist** Q

**S62.113 Displaced fracture of triquetrum [cuneiform] bone, unspecified wrist** Q

**S62.114 Nondisplaced fracture of triquetrum [cuneiform] bone, right wrist** Q

**S62.115 Nondisplaced fracture of triquetrum [cuneiform] bone, left wrist** Q

**S62.116 Nondisplaced fracture of triquetrum [cuneiform] bone, unspecified wrist** Q

**S62.12 Fracture of lunate [semilunar]**

**S62.121 Displaced fracture of lunate [semilunar], right wrist** Q

**S62.122 Displaced fracture of lunate [semilunar], left wrist** Q

**S62.123 Displaced fracture of lunate [semilunar], unspecified wrist** Q

**S62.124 Nondisplaced fracture of lunate [semilunar], right wrist** Q

**S62.125 Nondisplaced fracture of lunate [semilunar], left wrist** Q

**S62.126 Nondisplaced fracture of lunate [semilunar], unspecified wrist** Q

**S62.13 Fracture of capitate [os magnum] bone**

**S62.131 Displaced fracture of capitate [os magnum] bone, right wrist** Q

**S62.132 Displaced fracture of capitate [os magnum] bone, left wrist** Q

**S62.133 Displaced fracture of capitate [os magnum] bone, unspecified wrist** Q

**S62.134 Nondisplaced fracture of capitate [os magnum] bone, right wrist** Q

**S62.135 Nondisplaced fracture of capitate [os magnum] bone, left wrist** Q

**S62.136 Nondisplaced fracture of capitate [os magnum] bone, unspecified wrist** Q

**S62.14 Fracture of body of hamate [unciform] bone**

Fracture of hamate [unciform] bone NOS

**S62.141 Displaced fracture of body of hamate [unciform] bone, right wrist** Q

**S62.142 Displaced fracture of body of hamate [unciform] bone, left wrist** Q

**S62.143 Displaced fracture of body of hamate [unciform] bone, unspecified wrist** Q

**S62.144 Nondisplaced fracture of body of hamate [unciform] bone, right wrist** Q

**S62.145 Nondisplaced fracture of body of hamate [unciform] bone, left wrist** Q

**S62.146 Nondisplaced fracture of body of hamate [unciform] bone, unspecified wrist** Q

**S62.15 Fracture of hook process of hamate [unciform] bone**

Fracture of unciform process of hamate [unciform] bone

**S62.151 Displaced fracture of hook process of hamate [unciform] bone, right wrist** Q

**S62.152 Displaced fracture of hook process of hamate [unciform] bone, left wrist** Q

7th S62.153 Displaced fracture of hook process of hamate [unciform] bone, unspecified wrist Q
7th S62.154 Nondisplaced fracture of hook process of hamate [unciform] bone, right wrist Q
7th S62.155 Nondisplaced fracture of hook process of hamate [unciform] bone, left wrist Q
7th S62.156 Nondisplaced fracture of hook process of hamate [unciform] bone, unspecified wrist Q

6th S62.16 Fracture of pisiform
7th S62.161 Displaced fracture of pisiform, right wrist Q
7th S62.162 Displaced fracture of pisiform, left wrist Q
7th S62.163 Displaced fracture of pisiform, unspecified wrist Q
7th S62.164 Nondisplaced fracture of pisiform, right wrist Q
7th S62.165 Nondisplaced fracture of pisiform, left wrist Q
7th S62.166 Nondisplaced fracture of pisiform, unspecified wrist Q

6th S62.17 Fracture of trapezium [larger multangular]
7th S62.171 Displaced fracture of trapezium [larger multangular], right wrist Q
7th S62.172 Displaced fracture of trapezium [larger multangular], left wrist Q
7th S62.173 Displaced fracture of trapezium [larger multangular], unspecified wrist Q
7th S62.174 Nondisplaced fracture of trapezium [larger multangular], right wrist Q
7th S62.175 Nondisplaced fracture of trapezium [larger multangular], left wrist Q
7th S62.176 Nondisplaced fracture of trapezium [larger multangular], unspecified wrist Q

6th S62.18 Fracture of trapezoid [smaller multangular]
7th S62.181 Displaced fracture of trapezoid [smaller multangular], right wrist Q
7th S62.182 Displaced fracture of trapezoid [smaller multangular], left wrist Q
7th S62.183 Displaced fracture of trapezoid [smaller multangular], unspecified wrist Q
7th S62.184 Nondisplaced fracture of trapezoid [smaller multangular], right wrist Q
7th S62.185 Nondisplaced fracture of trapezoid [smaller multangular], left wrist Q
7th S62.186 Nondisplaced fracture of trapezoid [smaller multangular], unspecified wrist Q

5th S62.2 Fracture of first metacarpal bone

6th S62.20 Unspecified fracture of first metacarpal bone
7th S62.201 Unspecified fracture of first metacarpal bone, right hand Q
7th S62.202 Unspecified fracture of first metacarpal bone, left hand Q
7th S62.209 Unspecified fracture of first metacarpal bone, unspecified hand Q

6th S62.21 Bennett's fracture
DEF: Intra-articular, two-part fracture at the base of the first metacarpal bone (thumb) on the ulnar side at the carpometacarpal (CMC) joint.
7th S62.211 Bennett's fracture, right hand Q
7th S62.212 Bennett's fracture, left hand Q
7th S62.213 Bennett's fracture, unspecified hand Q

6th S62.22 Rolando's fracture
DEF: Comminuted, three part intra-articular fracture at the base of the thumb metacarpal.
7th S62.221 Displaced Rolando's fracture, right hand Q
7th S62.222 Displaced Rolando's fracture, left hand Q
7th S62.223 Displaced Rolando's fracture, unspecified hand Q
7th S62.224 Nondisplaced Rolando's fracture, right hand Q
7th S62.225 Nondisplaced Rolando's fracture, left hand Q
7th S62.226 Nondisplaced Rolando's fracture, unspecified hand Q

6th S62.23 Other fracture of base of first metacarpal bone
7th S62.231 Other displaced fracture of base of first metacarpal bone, right hand Q
7th S62.232 Other displaced fracture of base of first metacarpal bone, left hand Q
7th S62.233 Other displaced fracture of base of first metacarpal bone, unspecified hand Q
7th S62.234 Other nondisplaced fracture of base of first metacarpal bone, right hand Q
7th S62.235 Other nondisplaced fracture of base of first metacarpal bone, left hand Q
7th S62.236 Other nondisplaced fracture of base of first metacarpal bone, unspecified hand Q

6th S62.24 Fracture of shaft of first metacarpal bone
7th S62.241 Displaced fracture of shaft of first metacarpal bone, right hand Q
7th S62.242 Displaced fracture of shaft of first metacarpal bone, left hand Q
7th S62.243 Displaced fracture of shaft of first metacarpal bone, unspecified hand Q
7th S62.244 Nondisplaced fracture of shaft of first metacarpal bone, right hand Q
7th S62.245 Nondisplaced fracture of shaft of first metacarpal bone, left hand Q
7th S62.246 Nondisplaced fracture of shaft of first metacarpal bone, unspecified hand Q

6th S62.25 Fracture of neck of first metacarpal bone
7th S62.251 Displaced fracture of neck of first metacarpal bone, right hand Q
7th S62.252 Displaced fracture of neck of first metacarpal bone, left hand Q
7th S62.253 Displaced fracture of neck of first metacarpal bone, unspecified hand Q
7th S62.254 Nondisplaced fracture of neck of first metacarpal bone, right hand Q
7th S62.255 Nondisplaced fracture of neck of first metacarpal bone, left hand Q
7th S62.256 Nondisplaced fracture of neck of first metacarpal bone, unspecified hand Q

6th S62.29 Other fracture of first metacarpal bone
7th S62.291 Other fracture of first metacarpal bone, right hand Q
7th S62.292 Other fracture of first metacarpal bone, left hand Q
7th S62.299 Other fracture of first metacarpal bone, unspecified hand Q

5th S62.3 Fracture of other and unspecified metacarpal bone
EXCLUDES 2 *fracture of first metacarpal bone (S62.2-)*

6th S62.30 Unspecified fracture of other metacarpal bone
7th S62.300 Unspecified fracture of second metacarpal bone, right hand Q
7th S62.301 Unspecified fracture of second metacarpal bone, left hand Q
7th S62.302 Unspecified fracture of third metacarpal bone, right hand Q
7th S62.303 Unspecified fracture of third metacarpal bone, left hand Q
7th S62.304 Unspecified fracture of fourth metacarpal bone, right hand Q
7th S62.305 Unspecified fracture of fourth metacarpal bone, left hand Q
7th S62.306 Unspecified fracture of fifth metacarpal bone, right hand Q
7th S62.307 Unspecified fracture of fifth metacarpal bone, left hand Q
7th S62.308 Unspecified fracture of other metacarpal bone Q
Unspecified fracture of specified metacarpal bone with unspecified laterality
7th S62.309 Unspecified fracture of unspecified metacarpal bone Q

6th S62.31 Displaced fracture of base of other metacarpal bone
7th S62.310 Displaced fracture of base of second metacarpal bone, right hand Q
7th S62.311 Displaced fracture of base of second metacarpal bone, left hand Q

✓7th S62.312 Displaced fracture of base of third metacarpal bone, right hand Q
✓7th S62.313 Displaced fracture of base of third metacarpal bone, left hand Q
✓7th S62.314 Displaced fracture of base of fourth metacarpal bone, right hand Q
✓7th S62.315 Displaced fracture of base of fourth metacarpal bone, left hand Q
✓7th S62.316 Displaced fracture of base of fifth metacarpal bone, right hand Q
✓7th S62.317 Displaced fracture of base of fifth metacarpal bone, left hand Q
✓7th S62.318 Displaced fracture of base of other metacarpal bone Q
Displaced fracture of base of specified metacarpal bone with unspecified laterality
✓7th S62.319 Displaced fracture of base of unspecified metacarpal bone Q

✓6th S62.32 Displaced fracture of shaft of other metacarpal bone
✓7th S62.320 Displaced fracture of shaft of second metacarpal bone, right hand Q
✓7th S62.321 Displaced fracture of shaft of second metacarpal bone, left hand Q
✓7th S62.322 Displaced fracture of shaft of third metacarpal bone, right hand Q
✓7th S62.323 Displaced fracture of shaft of third metacarpal bone, left hand Q
✓7th S62.324 Displaced fracture of shaft of fourth metacarpal bone, right hand Q
✓7th S62.325 Displaced fracture of shaft of fourth metacarpal bone, left hand Q
✓7th S62.326 Displaced fracture of shaft of fifth metacarpal bone, right hand Q
✓7th S62.327 Displaced fracture of shaft of fifth metacarpal bone, left hand Q
✓7th S62.328 Displaced fracture of shaft of other metacarpal bone Q
Displaced fracture of shaft of specified metacarpal bone with unspecified laterality
✓7th S62.329 Displaced fracture of shaft of unspecified metacarpal bone Q

✓6th S62.33 Displaced fracture of neck of other metacarpal bone
✓7th S62.330 Displaced fracture of neck of second metacarpal bone, right hand Q
✓7th S62.331 Displaced fracture of neck of second metacarpal bone, left hand Q
✓7th S62.332 Displaced fracture of neck of third metacarpal bone, right hand Q
✓7th S62.333 Displaced fracture of neck of third metacarpal bone, left hand Q
✓7th S62.334 Displaced fracture of neck of fourth metacarpal bone, right hand Q
✓7th S62.335 Displaced fracture of neck of fourth metacarpal bone, left hand Q
✓7th S62.336 Displaced fracture of neck of fifth metacarpal bone, right hand Q
✓7th S62.337 Displaced fracture of neck of fifth metacarpal bone, left hand Q
✓7th S62.338 Displaced fracture of neck of other metacarpal bone Q
Displaced fracture of neck of specified metacarpal bone with unspecified laterality
✓7th S62.339 Displaced fracture of neck of unspecified metacarpal bone Q

✓6th S62.34 Nondisplaced fracture of base of other metacarpal bone
✓7th S62.340 Nondisplaced fracture of base of second metacarpal bone, right hand Q
✓7th S62.341 Nondisplaced fracture of base of second metacarpal bone, left hand Q
✓7th S62.342 Nondisplaced fracture of base of third metacarpal bone, right hand Q
✓7th S62.343 Nondisplaced fracture of base of third metacarpal bone, left hand Q
✓7th S62.344 Nondisplaced fracture of base of fourth metacarpal bone, right hand Q
✓7th S62.345 Nondisplaced fracture of base of fourth metacarpal bone, left hand Q
✓7th S62.346 Nondisplaced fracture of base of fifth metacarpal bone, right hand Q
✓7th S62.347 Nondisplaced fracture of base of fifth metacarpal bone, left hand Q
✓7th S62.348 Nondisplaced fracture of base of other metacarpal bone Q
Nondisplaced fracture of base of specified metacarpal bone with unspecified laterality
✓7th S62.349 Nondisplaced fracture of base of unspecified metacarpal bone Q

✓6th S62.35 Nondisplaced fracture of shaft of other metacarpal bone
✓7th S62.350 Nondisplaced fracture of shaft of second metacarpal bone, right hand Q
✓7th S62.351 Nondisplaced fracture of shaft of second metacarpal bone, left hand Q
✓7th S62.352 Nondisplaced fracture of shaft of third metacarpal bone, right hand Q
✓7th S62.353 Nondisplaced fracture of shaft of third metacarpal bone, left hand Q
✓7th S62.354 Nondisplaced fracture of shaft of fourth metacarpal bone, right hand Q
✓7th S62.355 Nondisplaced fracture of shaft of fourth metacarpal bone, left hand Q
✓7th S62.356 Nondisplaced fracture of shaft of fifth metacarpal bone, right hand Q
✓7th S62.357 Nondisplaced fracture of shaft of fifth metacarpal bone, left hand Q
✓7th S62.358 Nondisplaced fracture of shaft of other metacarpal bone Q
Nondisplaced fracture of shaft of specified metacarpal bone with unspecified laterality
✓7th S62.359 Nondisplaced fracture of shaft of unspecified metacarpal bone Q

✓6th S62.36 Nondisplaced fracture of neck of other metacarpal bone
✓7th S62.360 Nondisplaced fracture of neck of second metacarpal bone, right hand Q
✓7th S62.361 Nondisplaced fracture of neck of second metacarpal bone, left hand Q
✓7th S62.362 Nondisplaced fracture of neck of third metacarpal bone, right hand Q
✓7th S62.363 Nondisplaced fracture of neck of third metacarpal bone, left hand Q
✓7th S62.364 Nondisplaced fracture of neck of fourth metacarpal bone, right hand Q
✓7th S62.365 Nondisplaced fracture of neck of fourth metacarpal bone, left hand Q
✓7th S62.366 Nondisplaced fracture of neck of fifth metacarpal bone, right hand Q
✓7th S62.367 Nondisplaced fracture of neck of fifth metacarpal bone, left hand Q
✓7th S62.368 Nondisplaced fracture of neck of other metacarpal bone Q
Nondisplaced fracture of neck of specified metacarpal bone with unspecified laterality
✓7th S62.369 Nondisplaced fracture of neck of unspecified metacarpal bone Q

✓6th S62.39 Other fracture of other metacarpal bone
✓7th S62.390 Other fracture of second metacarpal bone, right hand Q
✓7th S62.391 Other fracture of second metacarpal bone, left hand Q
✓7th S62.392 Other fracture of third metacarpal bone, right hand Q
✓7th S62.393 Other fracture of third metacarpal bone, left hand Q
✓7th S62.394 Other fracture of fourth metacarpal bone, right hand Q
✓7th S62.395 Other fracture of fourth metacarpal bone, left hand Q
✓7th S62.396 Other fracture of fifth metacarpal bone, right hand Q
✓7th S62.397 Other fracture of fifth metacarpal bone, left hand Q

7th S62.398 Other fracture of other metacarpal bone Q
Other fracture of specified metacarpal bone with unspecified laterality

7th S62.399 Other fracture of unspecified metacarpal bone Q

5th S62.5 Fracture of thumb

6th S62.50 Fracture of unspecified phalanx of thumb

7th S62.501 Fracture of unspecified phalanx of right thumb

7th S62.502 Fracture of unspecified phalanx of left thumb

7th S62.509 Fracture of unspecified phalanx of unspecified thumb

6th S62.51 Fracture of proximal phalanx of thumb

7th S62.511 Displaced fracture of proximal phalanx of right thumb

7th S62.512 Displaced fracture of proximal phalanx of left thumb

7th S62.513 Displaced fracture of proximal phalanx of unspecified thumb

7th S62.514 Nondisplaced fracture of proximal phalanx of right thumb

7th S62.515 Nondisplaced fracture of proximal phalanx of left thumb

7th S62.516 Nondisplaced fracture of proximal phalanx of unspecified thumb

6th S62.52 Fracture of distal phalanx of thumb

7th S62.521 Displaced fracture of distal phalanx of right thumb

7th S62.522 Displaced fracture of distal phalanx of left thumb

7th S62.523 Displaced fracture of distal phalanx of unspecified thumb

7th S62.524 Nondisplaced fracture of distal phalanx of right thumb

7th S62.525 Nondisplaced fracture of distal phalanx of left thumb

7th S62.526 Nondisplaced fracture of distal phalanx of unspecified thumb

5th S62.6 Fracture of other and unspecified finger(s)

EXCLUDES 2 *fracture of thumb (S62.5-)*

6th S62.60 Fracture of unspecified phalanx of finger

7th S62.600 Fracture of unspecified phalanx of right index finger

7th S62.601 Fracture of unspecified phalanx of left index finger

7th S62.602 Fracture of unspecified phalanx of right middle finger

7th S62.603 Fracture of unspecified phalanx of left middle finger

7th S62.604 Fracture of unspecified phalanx of right ring finger

7th S62.605 Fracture of unspecified phalanx of left ring finger

7th S62.606 Fracture of unspecified phalanx of right little finger

7th S62.607 Fracture of unspecified phalanx of left little finger

7th S62.608 Fracture of unspecified phalanx of other finger
Fracture of unspecified phalanx of specified finger with unspecified laterality

7th S62.609 Fracture of unspecified phalanx of unspecified finger

6th S62.61 Displaced fracture of proximal phalanx of finger

7th S62.610 Displaced fracture of proximal phalanx of right index finger

7th S62.611 Displaced fracture of proximal phalanx of left index finger

7th S62.612 Displaced fracture of proximal phalanx of right middle finger

7th S62.613 Displaced fracture of proximal phalanx of left middle finger

7th S62.614 Displaced fracture of proximal phalanx of right ring finger

7th S62.615 Displaced fracture of proximal phalanx of left ring finger

7th S62.616 Displaced fracture of proximal phalanx of right little finger

7th S62.617 Displaced fracture of proximal phalanx of left little finger

7th S62.618 Displaced fracture of proximal phalanx of other finger
Displaced fracture of proximal phalanx of specified finger with unspecified laterality

7th S62.619 Displaced fracture of proximal phalanx of unspecified finger

6th S62.62 Displaced fracture of middle phalanx of finger

7th S62.620 Displaced fracture of middle phalanx of right index finger

7th S62.621 Displaced fracture of middle phalanx of left index finger

7th S62.622 Displaced fracture of middle phalanx of right middle finger

7th S62.623 Displaced fracture of middle phalanx of left middle finger

7th S62.624 Displaced fracture of middle phalanx of right ring finger

7th S62.625 Displaced fracture of middle phalanx of left ring finger

7th S62.626 Displaced fracture of middle phalanx of right little finger

7th S62.627 Displaced fracture of middle phalanx of left little finger

7th S62.628 Displaced fracture of middle phalanx of other finger
Displaced fracture of middle phalanx of specified finger with unspecified laterality

7th S62.629 Displaced fracture of middle phalanx of unspecified finger

6th S62.63 Displaced fracture of distal phalanx of finger

7th S62.630 Displaced fracture of distal phalanx of right index finger

7th S62.631 Displaced fracture of distal phalanx of left index finger

7th S62.632 Displaced fracture of distal phalanx of right middle finger

7th S62.633 Displaced fracture of distal phalanx of left middle finger

7th S62.634 Displaced fracture of distal phalanx of right ring finger

7th S62.635 Displaced fracture of distal phalanx of left ring finger

7th S62.636 Displaced fracture of distal phalanx of right little finger

7th S62.637 Displaced fracture of distal phalanx of left little finger

7th S62.638 Displaced fracture of distal phalanx of other finger
Displaced fracture of distal phalanx of specified finger with unspecified laterality

7th S62.639 Displaced fracture of distal phalanx of unspecified finger

6th S62.64 Nondisplaced fracture of proximal phalanx of finger

7th S62.640 Nondisplaced fracture of proximal phalanx of right index finger

7th S62.641 Nondisplaced fracture of proximal phalanx of left index finger

7th S62.642 Nondisplaced fracture of proximal phalanx of right middle finger

7th S62.643 Nondisplaced fracture of proximal phalanx of left middle finger

7th S62.644 Nondisplaced fracture of proximal phalanx of right ring finger

7th S62.645 Nondisplaced fracture of proximal phalanx of left ring finger

7th S62.646 Nondisplaced fracture of proximal phalanx of right little finger

7th S62.647 Nondisplaced fracture of proximal phalanx of left little finger

7th S62.648 Nondisplaced fracture of proximal phalanx of other finger
Nondisplaced fracture of proximal phalanx of specified finger with unspecified laterality

7th S62.649 Nondisplaced fracture of proximal phalanx of unspecified finger

√6th S62.65 Nondisplaced fracture of middle phalanx of finger
√7th S62.650 Nondisplaced fracture of middle phalanx of right index finger
√7th S62.651 Nondisplaced fracture of middle phalanx of left index finger
√7th S62.652 Nondisplaced fracture of middle phalanx of right middle finger
√7th S62.653 Nondisplaced fracture of middle phalanx of left middle finger
√7th S62.654 Nondisplaced fracture of middle phalanx of right ring finger
√7th S62.655 Nondisplaced fracture of middle phalanx of left ring finger
√7th S62.656 Nondisplaced fracture of middle phalanx of right little finger
√7th S62.657 Nondisplaced fracture of middle phalanx of left little finger
√7th S62.658 Nondisplaced fracture of middle phalanx of other finger
Nondisplaced fracture of middle phalanx of specified finger with unspecified laterality
√7th S62.659 Nondisplaced fracture of middle phalanx of unspecified finger
√6th S62.66 Nondisplaced fracture of distal phalanx of finger
√7th S62.660 Nondisplaced fracture of distal phalanx of right index finger
√7th S62.661 Nondisplaced fracture of distal phalanx of left index finger
√7th S62.662 Nondisplaced fracture of distal phalanx of right middle finger
√7th S62.663 Nondisplaced fracture of distal phalanx of left middle finger
√7th S62.664 Nondisplaced fracture of distal phalanx of right ring finger
√7th S62.665 Nondisplaced fracture of distal phalanx of left ring finger
√7th S62.666 Nondisplaced fracture of distal phalanx of right little finger
√7th S62.667 Nondisplaced fracture of distal phalanx of left little finger
√7th S62.668 Nondisplaced fracture of distal phalanx of other finger
Nondisplaced fracture of distal phalanx of specified finger with unspecified laterality
√7th S62.669 Nondisplaced fracture of distal phalanx of unspecified finger
√5th S62.9 Unspecified fracture of hand
√x7th S62.90 Unspecified fracture of unspecified hand Q
√x7th S62.91 Unspecified fracture of right hand Q
√x7th S62.92 Unspecified fracture of left hand Q

√4th **S63 Dislocation and sprain of joints and ligaments at wrist and hand level**

INCLUDES avulsion of joint or ligament at wrist and hand level
laceration of cartilage, joint or ligament at wrist and hand level
sprain of cartilage, joint or ligament at wrist and hand level
traumatic hemarthrosis of joint or ligament at wrist and hand level
traumatic rupture of joint or ligament at wrist and hand level
traumatic subluxation of joint or ligament at wrist and hand level
traumatic tear of joint or ligament at wrist and hand level

Code also any associated open wound

EXCLUDES 2 *strain of muscle, fascia and tendon of wrist and hand (S66.-)*

AHA: 2025,3Q,14

The appropriate 7th character is to be added to each code from category S63.
A initial encounter
D subsequent encounter
S sequela

√5th S63.0 Subluxation and dislocation of wrist and hand joints
√6th S63.00 Unspecified subluxation and dislocation of wrist and hand
Dislocation of carpal bone NOS
Dislocation of distal end of radius NOS
Subluxation of carpal bone NOS
Subluxation of distal end of radius NOS
√7th S63.001 Unspecified subluxation of right wrist and hand
√7th S63.002 Unspecified subluxation of left wrist and hand
√7th S63.003 Unspecified subluxation of unspecified wrist and hand
√7th S63.004 Unspecified dislocation of right wrist and hand
√7th S63.005 Unspecified dislocation of left wrist and hand
√7th S63.006 Unspecified dislocation of unspecified wrist and hand
√6th S63.01 Subluxation and dislocation of distal radioulnar joint
√7th S63.011 Subluxation of distal radioulnar joint of right wrist
√7th S63.012 Subluxation of distal radioulnar joint of left wrist
√7th S63.013 Subluxation of distal radioulnar joint of unspecified wrist
√7th S63.014 Dislocation of distal radioulnar joint of right wrist
√7th S63.015 Dislocation of distal radioulnar joint of left wrist
√7th S63.016 Dislocation of distal radioulnar joint of unspecified wrist
√6th S63.02 Subluxation and dislocation of radiocarpal joint
√7th S63.021 Subluxation of radiocarpal joint of right wrist
√7th S63.022 Subluxation of radiocarpal joint of left wrist
√7th S63.023 Subluxation of radiocarpal joint of unspecified wrist
√7th S63.024 Dislocation of radiocarpal joint of right wrist
√7th S63.025 Dislocation of radiocarpal joint of left wrist
√7th S63.026 Dislocation of radiocarpal joint of unspecified wrist
√6th S63.03 Subluxation and dislocation of midcarpal joint
√7th S63.031 Subluxation of midcarpal joint of right wrist
√7th S63.032 Subluxation of midcarpal joint of left wrist
√7th S63.033 Subluxation of midcarpal joint of unspecified wrist
√7th S63.034 Dislocation of midcarpal joint of right wrist
√7th S63.035 Dislocation of midcarpal joint of left wrist
√7th S63.036 Dislocation of midcarpal joint of unspecified wrist
√6th S63.04 Subluxation and dislocation of carpometacarpal joint of thumb
EXCLUDES 2 *interphalangeal subluxation and dislocation of thumb (S63.1-)*
√7th S63.041 Subluxation of carpometacarpal joint of right thumb

- ✓7th S63.042 Subluxation of carpometacarpal joint of left thumb
- ✓7th S63.043 Subluxation of carpometacarpal joint of unspecified thumb
- ✓7th S63.044 Dislocation of carpometacarpal joint of right thumb
- ✓7th S63.045 Dislocation of carpometacarpal joint of left thumb
- ✓7th S63.046 Dislocation of carpometacarpal joint of unspecified thumb

✓6th S63.05 Subluxation and dislocation of other carpometacarpal joint

EXCLUDES 2 *subluxation and dislocation of carpometacarpal joint of thumb (S63.04-)*

- ✓7th S63.051 Subluxation of other carpometacarpal joint of right hand
- ✓7th S63.052 Subluxation of other carpometacarpal joint of left hand
- ✓7th S63.053 Subluxation of other carpometacarpal joint of unspecified hand
- ✓7th S63.054 Dislocation of other carpometacarpal joint of right hand
- ✓7th S63.055 Dislocation of other carpometacarpal joint of left hand
- ✓7th S63.056 Dislocation of other carpometacarpal joint of unspecified hand

✓6th S63.06 Subluxation and dislocation of metacarpal (bone), proximal end

- ✓7th S63.061 Subluxation of metacarpal (bone), proximal end of right hand
- ✓7th S63.062 Subluxation of metacarpal (bone), proximal end of left hand
- ✓7th S63.063 Subluxation of metacarpal (bone), proximal end of unspecified hand
- ✓7th S63.064 Dislocation of metacarpal (bone), proximal end of right hand
- ✓7th S63.065 Dislocation of metacarpal (bone), proximal end of left hand
- ✓7th S63.066 Dislocation of metacarpal (bone), proximal end of unspecified hand

✓6th S63.07 Subluxation and dislocation of distal end of ulna

- ✓7th S63.071 Subluxation of distal end of right ulna
- ✓7th S63.072 Subluxation of distal end of left ulna
- ✓7th S63.073 Subluxation of distal end of unspecified ulna
- ✓7th S63.074 Dislocation of distal end of right ulna
- ✓7th S63.075 Dislocation of distal end of left ulna
- ✓7th S63.076 Dislocation of distal end of unspecified ulna

✓6th S63.09 Other subluxation and dislocation of wrist and hand

- ✓7th S63.091 Other subluxation of right wrist and hand
- ✓7th S63.092 Other subluxation of left wrist and hand
- ✓7th S63.093 Other subluxation of unspecified wrist and hand
- ✓7th S63.094 Other dislocation of right wrist and hand
- ✓7th S63.095 Other dislocation of left wrist and hand
- ✓7th S63.096 Other dislocation of unspecified wrist and hand

✓5th S63.1 Subluxation and dislocation of thumb

✓6th S63.10 Unspecified subluxation and dislocation of thumb

- ✓7th S63.101 Unspecified subluxation of right thumb
- ✓7th S63.102 Unspecified subluxation of left thumb
- ✓7th S63.103 Unspecified subluxation of unspecified thumb
- ✓7th S63.104 Unspecified dislocation of right thumb
- ✓7th S63.105 Unspecified dislocation of left thumb
- ✓7th S63.106 Unspecified dislocation of unspecified thumb

✓6th S63.11 Subluxation and dislocation of metacarpophalangeal joint of thumb

- ✓7th S63.111 Subluxation of metacarpophalangeal joint of right thumb
- ✓7th S63.112 Subluxation of metacarpophalangeal joint of left thumb
- ✓7th S63.113 Subluxation of metacarpophalangeal joint of unspecified thumb
- ✓7th S63.114 Dislocation of metacarpophalangeal joint of right thumb
- ✓7th S63.115 Dislocation of metacarpophalangeal joint of left thumb
- ✓7th S63.116 Dislocation of metacarpophalangeal joint of unspecified thumb

✓6th S63.12 Subluxation and dislocation of interphalangeal joint of thumb

- ✓7th S63.121 Subluxation of interphalangeal joint of right thumb
- ✓7th S63.122 Subluxation of interphalangeal joint of left thumb
- ✓7th S63.123 Subluxation of interphalangeal joint of unspecified thumb
- ✓7th S63.124 Dislocation of interphalangeal joint of right thumb
- ✓7th S63.125 Dislocation of interphalangeal joint of left thumb
- ✓7th S63.126 Dislocation of interphalangeal joint of unspecified thumb

✓5th S63.2 Subluxation and dislocation of other finger(s)

EXCLUDES 2 *subluxation and dislocation of thumb (S63.1-)*

✓6th S63.20 Unspecified subluxation of other finger

- ✓7th S63.200 Unspecified subluxation of right index finger
- ✓7th S63.201 Unspecified subluxation of left index finger
- ✓7th S63.202 Unspecified subluxation of right middle finger
- ✓7th S63.203 Unspecified subluxation of left middle finger
- ✓7th S63.204 Unspecified subluxation of right ring finger
- ✓7th S63.205 Unspecified subluxation of left ring finger
- ✓7th S63.206 Unspecified subluxation of right little finger
- ✓7th S63.207 Unspecified subluxation of left little finger
- ✓7th S63.208 Unspecified subluxation of other finger
  Unspecified subluxation of specified finger with unspecified laterality
- ✓7th S63.209 Unspecified subluxation of unspecified finger

✓6th S63.21 Subluxation of metacarpophalangeal joint of finger

- ✓7th S63.210 Subluxation of metacarpophalangeal joint of right index finger
- ✓7th S63.211 Subluxation of metacarpophalangeal joint of left index finger
- ✓7th S63.212 Subluxation of metacarpophalangeal joint of right middle finger
- ✓7th S63.213 Subluxation of metacarpophalangeal joint of left middle finger
- ✓7th S63.214 Subluxation of metacarpophalangeal joint of right ring finger
- ✓7th S63.215 Subluxation of metacarpophalangeal joint of left ring finger
- ✓7th S63.216 Subluxation of metacarpophalangeal joint of right little finger
- ✓7th S63.217 Subluxation of metacarpophalangeal joint of left little finger
- ✓7th S63.218 Subluxation of metacarpophalangeal joint of other finger
  Subluxation of metacarpophalangeal joint of specified finger with unspecified laterality
- ✓7th S63.219 Subluxation of metacarpophalangeal joint of unspecified finger

✓6th S63.22 Subluxation of unspecified interphalangeal joint of finger

- ✓7th S63.220 Subluxation of unspecified interphalangeal joint of right index finger
- ✓7th S63.221 Subluxation of unspecified interphalangeal joint of left index finger
- ✓7th S63.222 Subluxation of unspecified interphalangeal joint of right middle finger
- ✓7th S63.223 Subluxation of unspecified interphalangeal joint of left middle finger
- ✓7th S63.224 Subluxation of unspecified interphalangeal joint of right ring finger
- ✓7th S63.225 Subluxation of unspecified interphalangeal joint of left ring finger
- ✓7th S63.226 Subluxation of unspecified interphalangeal joint of right little finger
- ✓7th S63.227 Subluxation of unspecified interphalangeal joint of left little finger

S63.228 Subluxation of unspecified interphalangeal joint of other finger
Subluxation of unspecified interphalangeal joint of specified finger with unspecified laterality
S63.229 Subluxation of unspecified interphalangeal joint of unspecified finger
S63.23 Subluxation of proximal interphalangeal joint of finger
S63.230 Subluxation of proximal interphalangeal joint of right index finger
S63.231 Subluxation of proximal interphalangeal joint of left index finger
S63.232 Subluxation of proximal interphalangeal joint of right middle finger
S63.233 Subluxation of proximal interphalangeal joint of left middle finger
S63.234 Subluxation of proximal interphalangeal joint of right ring finger
S63.235 Subluxation of proximal interphalangeal joint of left ring finger
S63.236 Subluxation of proximal interphalangeal joint of right little finger
S63.237 Subluxation of proximal interphalangeal joint of left little finger
S63.238 Subluxation of proximal interphalangeal joint of other finger
Subluxation of proximal interphalangeal joint of specified finger with unspecified laterality
S63.239 Subluxation of proximal interphalangeal joint of unspecified finger
S63.24 Subluxation of distal interphalangeal joint of finger
S63.240 Subluxation of distal interphalangeal joint of right index finger
S63.241 Subluxation of distal interphalangeal joint of left index finger
S63.242 Subluxation of distal interphalangeal joint of right middle finger
S63.243 Subluxation of distal interphalangeal joint of left middle finger
S63.244 Subluxation of distal interphalangeal joint of right ring finger
S63.245 Subluxation of distal interphalangeal joint of left ring finger
S63.246 Subluxation of distal interphalangeal joint of right little finger
S63.247 Subluxation of distal interphalangeal joint of left little finger
S63.248 Subluxation of distal interphalangeal joint of other finger
Subluxation of distal interphalangeal joint of specified finger with unspecified laterality
S63.249 Subluxation of distal interphalangeal joint of unspecified finger
S63.25 Unspecified dislocation of other finger
S63.250 Unspecified dislocation of right index finger
S63.251 Unspecified dislocation of left index finger
S63.252 Unspecified dislocation of right middle finger
S63.253 Unspecified dislocation of left middle finger
S63.254 Unspecified dislocation of right ring finger
S63.255 Unspecified dislocation of left ring finger
S63.256 Unspecified dislocation of right little finger
S63.257 Unspecified dislocation of left little finger
S63.258 Unspecified dislocation of other finger
Unspecified dislocation of specified finger with unspecified laterality
S63.259 Unspecified dislocation of unspecified finger
Unspecified dislocation of unspecified finger with unspecified laterality
S63.26 Dislocation of metacarpophalangeal joint of finger
S63.260 Dislocation of metacarpophalangeal joint of right index finger
S63.261 Dislocation of metacarpophalangeal joint of left index finger
S63.262 Dislocation of metacarpophalangeal joint of right middle finger
S63.263 Dislocation of metacarpophalangeal joint of left middle finger
S63.264 Dislocation of metacarpophalangeal joint of right ring finger
S63.265 Dislocation of metacarpophalangeal joint of left ring finger
S63.266 Dislocation of metacarpophalangeal joint of right little finger
S63.267 Dislocation of metacarpophalangeal joint of left little finger
S63.268 Dislocation of metacarpophalangeal joint of other finger
Dislocation of metacarpophalangeal joint of specified finger with unspecified laterality
S63.269 Dislocation of metacarpophalangeal joint of unspecified finger
S63.27 Dislocation of unspecified interphalangeal joint of finger
S63.270 Dislocation of unspecified interphalangeal joint of right index finger
S63.271 Dislocation of unspecified interphalangeal joint of left index finger
S63.272 Dislocation of unspecified interphalangeal joint of right middle finger
S63.273 Dislocation of unspecified interphalangeal joint of left middle finger
S63.274 Dislocation of unspecified interphalangeal joint of right ring finger
S63.275 Dislocation of unspecified interphalangeal joint of left ring finger
S63.276 Dislocation of unspecified interphalangeal joint of right little finger
S63.277 Dislocation of unspecified interphalangeal joint of left little finger
S63.278 Dislocation of unspecified interphalangeal joint of other finger
Dislocation of unspecified interphalangeal joint of specified finger with unspecified laterality
S63.279 Dislocation of unspecified interphalangeal joint of unspecified finger
Dislocation of unspecified interphalangeal joint of unspecified finger without specified laterality
S63.28 Dislocation of proximal interphalangeal joint of finger
S63.280 Dislocation of proximal interphalangeal joint of right index finger
S63.281 Dislocation of proximal interphalangeal joint of left index finger
S63.282 Dislocation of proximal interphalangeal joint of right middle finger
S63.283 Dislocation of proximal interphalangeal joint of left middle finger
S63.284 Dislocation of proximal interphalangeal joint of right ring finger
S63.285 Dislocation of proximal interphalangeal joint of left ring finger
S63.286 Dislocation of proximal interphalangeal joint of right little finger
S63.287 Dislocation of proximal interphalangeal joint of left little finger
S63.288 Dislocation of proximal interphalangeal joint of other finger
Dislocation of proximal interphalangeal joint of specified finger with unspecified laterality
S63.289 Dislocation of proximal interphalangeal joint of unspecified finger
S63.29 Dislocation of distal interphalangeal joint of finger
S63.290 Dislocation of distal interphalangeal joint of right index finger
S63.291 Dislocation of distal interphalangeal joint of left index finger
S63.292 Dislocation of distal interphalangeal joint of right middle finger
S63.293 Dislocation of distal interphalangeal joint of left middle finger
S63.294 Dislocation of distal interphalangeal joint of right ring finger

√7th S63.295 Dislocation of distal interphalangeal joint of left ring finger

√7th S63.296 Dislocation of distal interphalangeal joint of right little finger

√7th S63.297 Dislocation of distal interphalangeal joint of left little finger

√7th S63.298 Dislocation of distal interphalangeal joint of other finger
Dislocation of distal interphalangeal joint of specified finger with unspecified laterality

√7th S63.299 Dislocation of distal interphalangeal joint of unspecified finger

√5th S63.3 Traumatic rupture of ligament of wrist

√6th S63.30 Traumatic rupture of unspecified ligament of wrist

√7th S63.301 Traumatic rupture of unspecified ligament of right wrist

√7th S63.302 Traumatic rupture of unspecified ligament of left wrist

√7th S63.309 Traumatic rupture of unspecified ligament of unspecified wrist

√6th S63.31 Traumatic rupture of collateral ligament of wrist

√7th S63.311 Traumatic rupture of collateral ligament of right wrist

√7th S63.312 Traumatic rupture of collateral ligament of left wrist

√7th S63.319 Traumatic rupture of collateral ligament of unspecified wrist

√6th S63.32 Traumatic rupture of radiocarpal ligament

√7th S63.321 Traumatic rupture of right radiocarpal ligament

√7th S63.322 Traumatic rupture of left radiocarpal ligament

√7th S63.329 Traumatic rupture of unspecified radiocarpal ligament

√6th S63.33 Traumatic rupture of ulnocarpal (palmar) ligament

√7th S63.331 Traumatic rupture of right ulnocarpal (palmar) ligament

√7th S63.332 Traumatic rupture of left ulnocarpal (palmar) ligament

√7th S63.339 Traumatic rupture of unspecified ulnocarpal (palmar) ligament

√6th S63.39 Traumatic rupture of other ligament of wrist

√7th S63.391 Traumatic rupture of other ligament of right wrist

√7th S63.392 Traumatic rupture of other ligament of left wrist

√7th S63.399 Traumatic rupture of other ligament of unspecified wrist

√5th S63.4 Traumatic rupture of ligament of finger at metacarpophalangeal and interphalangeal joint(s)

√6th S63.40 Traumatic rupture of unspecified ligament of finger at metacarpophalangeal and interphalangeal joint

√7th S63.400 Traumatic rupture of unspecified ligament of right index finger at metacarpophalangeal and interphalangeal joint

√7th S63.401 Traumatic rupture of unspecified ligament of left index finger at metacarpophalangeal and interphalangeal joint

√7th S63.402 Traumatic rupture of unspecified ligament of right middle finger at metacarpophalangeal and interphalangeal joint

√7th S63.403 Traumatic rupture of unspecified ligament of left middle finger at metacarpophalangeal and interphalangeal joint

√7th S63.404 Traumatic rupture of unspecified ligament of right ring finger at metacarpophalangeal and interphalangeal joint

√7th S63.405 Traumatic rupture of unspecified ligament of left ring finger at metacarpophalangeal and interphalangeal joint

√7th S63.406 Traumatic rupture of unspecified ligament of right little finger at metacarpophalangeal and interphalangeal joint

√7th S63.407 Traumatic rupture of unspecified ligament of left little finger at metacarpophalangeal and interphalangeal joint

√7th S63.408 Traumatic rupture of unspecified ligament of other finger at metacarpophalangeal and interphalangeal joint
Traumatic rupture of unspecified ligament of specified finger with unspecified laterality at metacarpophalangeal and interphalangeal joint

√7th S63.409 Traumatic rupture of unspecified ligament of unspecified finger at metacarpophalangeal and interphalangeal joint

√6th S63.41 Traumatic rupture of collateral ligament of finger at metacarpophalangeal and interphalangeal joint

√7th S63.410 Traumatic rupture of collateral ligament of right index finger at metacarpophalangeal and interphalangeal joint

√7th S63.411 Traumatic rupture of collateral ligament of left index finger at metacarpophalangeal and interphalangeal joint

√7th S63.412 Traumatic rupture of collateral ligament of right middle finger at metacarpophalangeal and interphalangeal joint

√7th S63.413 Traumatic rupture of collateral ligament of left middle finger at metacarpophalangeal and interphalangeal joint

√7th S63.414 Traumatic rupture of collateral ligament of right ring finger at metacarpophalangeal and interphalangeal joint

√7th S63.415 Traumatic rupture of collateral ligament of left ring finger at metacarpophalangeal and interphalangeal joint

√7th S63.416 Traumatic rupture of collateral ligament of right little finger at metacarpophalangeal and interphalangeal joint

√7th S63.417 Traumatic rupture of collateral ligament of left little finger at metacarpophalangeal and interphalangeal joint

√7th S63.418 Traumatic rupture of collateral ligament of other finger at metacarpophalangeal and interphalangeal joint
Traumatic rupture of collateral ligament of specified finger with unspecified laterality at metacarpophalangeal and interphalangeal joint

√7th S63.419 Traumatic rupture of collateral ligament of unspecified finger at metacarpophalangeal and interphalangeal joint

√6th S63.42 Traumatic rupture of palmar ligament of finger at metacarpophalangeal and interphalangeal joint

√7th S63.420 Traumatic rupture of palmar ligament of right index finger at metacarpophalangeal and interphalangeal joint

√7th S63.421 Traumatic rupture of palmar ligament of left index finger at metacarpophalangeal and interphalangeal joint

√7th S63.422 Traumatic rupture of palmar ligament of right middle finger at metacarpophalangeal and interphalangeal joint

√7th S63.423 Traumatic rupture of palmar ligament of left middle finger at metacarpophalangeal and interphalangeal joint

√7th S63.424 Traumatic rupture of palmar ligament of right ring finger at metacarpophalangeal and interphalangeal joint

√7th S63.425 Traumatic rupture of palmar ligament of left ring finger at metacarpophalangeal and interphalangeal joint

√7th S63.426 Traumatic rupture of palmar ligament of right little finger at metacarpophalangeal and interphalangeal joint

√7th S63.427 Traumatic rupture of palmar ligament of left little finger at metacarpophalangeal and interphalangeal joint

√7th S63.428 **Traumatic rupture of palmar ligament of other finger at metacarpophalangeal and interphalangeal joint**
Traumatic rupture of palmar ligament of specified finger with unspecified laterality at metacarpophalangeal and interphalangeal joint

√7th S63.429 **Traumatic rupture of palmar ligament of unspecified finger at metacarpophalangeal and interphalangeal joint**

√6th S63.43 **Traumatic rupture of volar plate of finger at metacarpophalangeal and interphalangeal joint**

√7th S63.430 **Traumatic rupture of volar plate of right index finger at metacarpophalangeal and interphalangeal joint**

√7th S63.431 **Traumatic rupture of volar plate of left index finger at metacarpophalangeal and interphalangeal joint**

√7th S63.432 **Traumatic rupture of volar plate of right middle finger at metacarpophalangeal and interphalangeal joint**

√7th S63.433 **Traumatic rupture of volar plate of left middle finger at metacarpophalangeal and interphalangeal joint**

√7th S63.434 **Traumatic rupture of volar plate of right ring finger at metacarpophalangeal and interphalangeal joint**

√7th S63.435 **Traumatic rupture of volar plate of left ring finger at metacarpophalangeal and interphalangeal joint**

√7th S63.436 **Traumatic rupture of volar plate of right little finger at metacarpophalangeal and interphalangeal joint**

√7th S63.437 **Traumatic rupture of volar plate of left little finger at metacarpophalangeal and interphalangeal joint**

√7th S63.438 **Traumatic rupture of volar plate of other finger at metacarpophalangeal and interphalangeal joint**
Traumatic rupture of volar plate of specified finger with unspecified laterality at metacarpophalangeal and interphalangeal joint

√7th S63.439 **Traumatic rupture of volar plate of unspecified finger at metacarpophalangeal and interphalangeal joint**

√6th S63.49 **Traumatic rupture of other ligament of finger at metacarpophalangeal and interphalangeal joint**

√7th S63.490 **Traumatic rupture of other ligament of right index finger at metacarpophalangeal and interphalangeal joint**

√7th S63.491 **Traumatic rupture of other ligament of left index finger at metacarpophalangeal and interphalangeal joint**

√7th S63.492 **Traumatic rupture of other ligament of right middle finger at metacarpophalangeal and interphalangeal joint**

√7th S63.493 **Traumatic rupture of other ligament of left middle finger at metacarpophalangeal and interphalangeal joint**

√7th S63.494 **Traumatic rupture of other ligament of right ring finger at metacarpophalangeal and interphalangeal joint**

√7th S63.495 **Traumatic rupture of other ligament of left ring finger at metacarpophalangeal and interphalangeal joint**

√7th S63.496 **Traumatic rupture of other ligament of right little finger at metacarpophalangeal and interphalangeal joint**

√7th S63.497 **Traumatic rupture of other ligament of left little finger at metacarpophalangeal and interphalangeal joint**

√7th S63.498 **Traumatic rupture of other ligament of other finger at metacarpophalangeal and interphalangeal joint**
Traumatic rupture of ligament of specified finger with unspecified laterality at metacarpophalangeal and interphalangeal joint

√7th S63.499 **Traumatic rupture of other ligament of unspecified finger at metacarpophalangeal and interphalangeal joint**

√5th S63.5 **Other and unspecified sprain of wrist**

√6th S63.50 **Unspecified sprain of wrist**

√7th S63.501 **Unspecified sprain of right wrist**

√7th S63.502 **Unspecified sprain of left wrist**

√7th S63.509 **Unspecified sprain of unspecified wrist**

√6th S63.51 **Sprain of carpal (joint)**

√7th S63.511 **Sprain of carpal joint of right wrist**

√7th S63.512 **Sprain of carpal joint of left wrist**

√7th S63.519 **Sprain of carpal joint of unspecified wrist**

√6th S63.52 **Sprain of radiocarpal joint**
EXCLUDES 1 *traumatic rupture of radiocarpal ligament (S63.32-)*

√7th S63.521 **Sprain of radiocarpal joint of right wrist**

√7th S63.522 **Sprain of radiocarpal joint of left wrist**

√7th S63.529 **Sprain of radiocarpal joint of unspecified wrist**

√6th S63.59 **Other specified sprain of wrist**

√7th S63.591 **Other specified sprain of right wrist**

√7th S63.592 **Other specified sprain of left wrist**

√7th S63.599 **Other specified sprain of unspecified wrist**

√5th S63.6 **Other and unspecified sprain of finger(s)**
EXCLUDES 1 *traumatic rupture of ligament of finger at metacarpophalangeal and interphalangeal joint(s) (S63.4-)*

√6th S63.60 **Unspecified sprain of thumb**

√7th S63.601 **Unspecified sprain of right thumb**

√7th S63.602 **Unspecified sprain of left thumb**

√7th S63.609 **Unspecified sprain of unspecified thumb**

√6th S63.61 **Unspecified sprain of other and unspecified finger(s)**

√7th S63.610 **Unspecified sprain of right index finger**

√7th S63.611 **Unspecified sprain of left index finger**

√7th S63.612 **Unspecified sprain of right middle finger**

√7th S63.613 **Unspecified sprain of left middle finger**

√7th S63.614 **Unspecified sprain of right ring finger**

√7th S63.615 **Unspecified sprain of left ring finger**

√7th S63.616 **Unspecified sprain of right little finger**

√7th S63.617 **Unspecified sprain of left little finger**

√7th S63.618 **Unspecified sprain of other finger**
Unspecified sprain of specified finger with unspecified laterality

√7th S63.619 **Unspecified sprain of unspecified finger**

√6th S63.62 **Sprain of interphalangeal joint of thumb**

√7th S63.621 **Sprain of interphalangeal joint of right thumb**

√7th S63.622 **Sprain of interphalangeal joint of left thumb**

√7th S63.629 **Sprain of interphalangeal joint of unspecified thumb**

√6th S63.63 **Sprain of interphalangeal joint of other and unspecified finger(s)**

√7th S63.630 **Sprain of interphalangeal joint of right index finger**

√7th S63.631 **Sprain of interphalangeal joint of left index finger**

√7th S63.632 **Sprain of interphalangeal joint of right middle finger**

√7th S63.633 **Sprain of interphalangeal joint of left middle finger**

√7th S63.634 **Sprain of interphalangeal joint of right ring finger**

√7th S63.635 **Sprain of interphalangeal joint of left ring finger**

√7th S63.636 **Sprain of interphalangeal joint of right little finger**

√7th S63.637 **Sprain of interphalangeal joint of left little finger**

√7th S63.638 **Sprain of interphalangeal joint of other finger**

√7th S63.639 **Sprain of interphalangeal joint of unspecified finger**

√6th S63.64 **Sprain of metacarpophalangeal joint of thumb**

√7th S63.641 **Sprain of metacarpophalangeal joint of right thumb**

√7th S63.642 Sprain of metacarpophalangeal joint of left thumb
√7th S63.649 Sprain of metacarpophalangeal joint of unspecified thumb
√6th S63.65 Sprain of metacarpophalangeal joint of other and unspecified finger(s)
√7th S63.650 Sprain of metacarpophalangeal joint of right index finger
√7th S63.651 Sprain of metacarpophalangeal joint of left index finger
√7th S63.652 Sprain of metacarpophalangeal joint of right middle finger
√7th S63.653 Sprain of metacarpophalangeal joint of left middle finger
√7th S63.654 Sprain of metacarpophalangeal joint of right ring finger
√7th S63.655 Sprain of metacarpophalangeal joint of left ring finger
√7th S63.656 Sprain of metacarpophalangeal joint of right little finger
√7th S63.657 Sprain of metacarpophalangeal joint of left little finger
√7th S63.658 Sprain of metacarpophalangeal joint of other finger
Sprain of metacarpophalangeal joint of specified finger with unspecified laterality
√7th S63.659 Sprain of metacarpophalangeal joint of unspecified finger
√6th S63.68 Other sprain of thumb
√7th S63.681 Other sprain of right thumb
√7th S63.682 Other sprain of left thumb
√7th S63.689 Other sprain of unspecified thumb
√6th S63.69 Other sprain of other and unspecified finger(s)
√7th S63.690 Other sprain of right index finger
√7th S63.691 Other sprain of left index finger
√7th S63.692 Other sprain of right middle finger
√7th S63.693 Other sprain of left middle finger
√7th S63.694 Other sprain of right ring finger
√7th S63.695 Other sprain of left ring finger
√7th S63.696 Other sprain of right little finger
√7th S63.697 Other sprain of left little finger
√7th S63.698 Other sprain of other finger
Other sprain of specified finger with unspecified laterality
√7th S63.699 Other sprain of unspecified finger
√5th S63.8 Sprain of other part of wrist and hand
√6th S63.8X Sprain of other part of wrist and hand
√7th S63.8X1 Sprain of other part of right wrist and hand
√7th S63.8X2 Sprain of other part of left wrist and hand
√7th S63.8X9 Sprain of other part of unspecified wrist and hand
√5th S63.9 Sprain of unspecified part of wrist and hand
√x7th S63.90 Sprain of unspecified part of unspecified wrist and hand
√x7th S63.91 Sprain of unspecified part of right wrist and hand
√x7th S63.92 Sprain of unspecified part of left wrist and hand

√4th **S64 Injury of nerves at wrist and hand level**

Code also any associated open wound (S61.-)

The appropriate 7th character is to be added to each code from category S64.
A initial encounter
D subsequent encounter
S sequela

√5th S64.0 Injury of ulnar nerve at wrist and hand level
√x7th S64.00 Injury of ulnar nerve at wrist and hand level of unspecified arm
√x7th S64.01 Injury of ulnar nerve at wrist and hand level of right arm
√x7th S64.02 Injury of ulnar nerve at wrist and hand level of left arm
√5th S64.1 Injury of median nerve at wrist and hand level
√x7th S64.10 Injury of median nerve at wrist and hand level of unspecified arm
√x7th S64.11 Injury of median nerve at wrist and hand level of right arm
√x7th S64.12 Injury of median nerve at wrist and hand level of left arm
√5th S64.2 Injury of radial nerve at wrist and hand level
√x7th S64.20 Injury of radial nerve at wrist and hand level of unspecified arm
√x7th S64.21 Injury of radial nerve at wrist and hand level of right arm
√x7th S64.22 Injury of radial nerve at wrist and hand level of left arm
√5th S64.3 Injury of digital nerve of thumb
√x7th S64.30 Injury of digital nerve of unspecified thumb
√x7th S64.31 Injury of digital nerve of right thumb
√x7th S64.32 Injury of digital nerve of left thumb
√5th S64.4 Injury of digital nerve of other and unspecified finger
√x7th S64.40 Injury of digital nerve of unspecified finger
√6th S64.49 Injury of digital nerve of other finger
√7th S64.490 Injury of digital nerve of right index finger
√7th S64.491 Injury of digital nerve of left index finger
√7th S64.492 Injury of digital nerve of right middle finger
√7th S64.493 Injury of digital nerve of left middle finger
√7th S64.494 Injury of digital nerve of right ring finger
√7th S64.495 Injury of digital nerve of left ring finger
√7th S64.496 Injury of digital nerve of right little finger
√7th S64.497 Injury of digital nerve of left little finger
√7th S64.498 Injury of digital nerve of other finger
Injury of digital nerve of specified finger with unspecified laterality
√5th S64.8 Injury of other nerves at wrist and hand level
√6th S64.8X Injury of other nerves at wrist and hand level
√7th S64.8X1 Injury of other nerves at wrist and hand level of right arm
√7th S64.8X2 Injury of other nerves at wrist and hand level of left arm
√7th S64.8X9 Injury of other nerves at wrist and hand level of unspecified arm
√5th S64.9 Injury of unspecified nerve at wrist and hand level
√x7th S64.90 Injury of unspecified nerve at wrist and hand level of unspecified arm
√x7th S64.91 Injury of unspecified nerve at wrist and hand level of right arm
√x7th S64.92 Injury of unspecified nerve at wrist and hand level of left arm

√4th **S65 Injury of blood vessels at wrist and hand level**

Code also any associated open wound (S61.-)

The appropriate 7th character is to be added to each code from category S65.
A initial encounter
D subsequent encounter
S sequela

√5th S65.0 Injury of ulnar artery at wrist and hand level
√6th S65.00 Unspecified injury of ulnar artery at wrist and hand level
√7th S65.001 Unspecified injury of ulnar artery at wrist and hand level of right arm
√7th S65.002 Unspecified injury of ulnar artery at wrist and hand level of left arm
√7th S65.009 Unspecified injury of ulnar artery at wrist and hand level of unspecified arm
√6th S65.01 Laceration of ulnar artery at wrist and hand level
√7th S65.011 Laceration of ulnar artery at wrist and hand level of right arm
√7th S65.012 Laceration of ulnar artery at wrist and hand level of left arm
√7th S65.019 Laceration of ulnar artery at wrist and hand level of unspecified arm
√6th S65.09 Other specified injury of ulnar artery at wrist and hand level
√7th S65.091 Other specified injury of ulnar artery at wrist and hand level of right arm
√7th S65.092 Other specified injury of ulnar artery at wrist and hand level of left arm
√7th S65.099 Other specified injury of ulnar artery at wrist and hand level of unspecified arm

S65.1 Injury of radial artery at wrist and hand level
S65.10 Unspecified injury of radial artery at wrist and hand level
S65.101 Unspecified injury of radial artery at wrist and hand level of right arm
S65.102 Unspecified injury of radial artery at wrist and hand level of left arm
S65.109 Unspecified injury of radial artery at wrist and hand level of unspecified arm
S65.11 Laceration of radial artery at wrist and hand level
S65.111 Laceration of radial artery at wrist and hand level of right arm
S65.112 Laceration of radial artery at wrist and hand level of left arm
S65.119 Laceration of radial artery at wrist and hand level of unspecified arm
S65.19 Other specified injury of radial artery at wrist and hand level
S65.191 Other specified injury of radial artery at wrist and hand level of right arm
S65.192 Other specified injury of radial artery at wrist and hand level of left arm
S65.199 Other specified injury of radial artery at wrist and hand level of unspecified arm
S65.2 Injury of superficial palmar arch
S65.20 Unspecified injury of superficial palmar arch
S65.201 Unspecified injury of superficial palmar arch of right hand
S65.202 Unspecified injury of superficial palmar arch of left hand
S65.209 Unspecified injury of superficial palmar arch of unspecified hand
S65.21 Laceration of superficial palmar arch
S65.211 Laceration of superficial palmar arch of right hand
S65.212 Laceration of superficial palmar arch of left hand
S65.219 Laceration of superficial palmar arch of unspecified hand
S65.29 Other specified injury of superficial palmar arch
S65.291 Other specified injury of superficial palmar arch of right hand
S65.292 Other specified injury of superficial palmar arch of left hand
S65.299 Other specified injury of superficial palmar arch of unspecified hand
S65.3 Injury of deep palmar arch
S65.30 Unspecified injury of deep palmar arch
S65.301 Unspecified injury of deep palmar arch of right hand
S65.302 Unspecified injury of deep palmar arch of left hand
S65.309 Unspecified injury of deep palmar arch of unspecified hand
S65.31 Laceration of deep palmar arch
S65.311 Laceration of deep palmar arch of right hand
S65.312 Laceration of deep palmar arch of left hand
S65.319 Laceration of deep palmar arch of unspecified hand
S65.39 Other specified injury of deep palmar arch
S65.391 Other specified injury of deep palmar arch of right hand
S65.392 Other specified injury of deep palmar arch of left hand
S65.399 Other specified injury of deep palmar arch of unspecified hand
S65.4 Injury of blood vessel of thumb
S65.40 Unspecified injury of blood vessel of thumb
S65.401 Unspecified injury of blood vessel of right thumb
S65.402 Unspecified injury of blood vessel of left thumb
S65.409 Unspecified injury of blood vessel of unspecified thumb
S65.41 Laceration of blood vessel of thumb
S65.411 Laceration of blood vessel of right thumb
S65.412 Laceration of blood vessel of left thumb
S65.419 Laceration of blood vessel of unspecified thumb
S65.49 Other specified injury of blood vessel of thumb
S65.491 Other specified injury of blood vessel of right thumb
S65.492 Other specified injury of blood vessel of left thumb
S65.499 Other specified injury of blood vessel of unspecified thumb
S65.5 Injury of blood vessel of other and unspecified finger
S65.50 Unspecified injury of blood vessel of other and unspecified finger
S65.500 Unspecified injury of blood vessel of right index finger
S65.501 Unspecified injury of blood vessel of left index finger
S65.502 Unspecified injury of blood vessel of right middle finger
S65.503 Unspecified injury of blood vessel of left middle finger
S65.504 Unspecified injury of blood vessel of right ring finger
S65.505 Unspecified injury of blood vessel of left ring finger
S65.506 Unspecified injury of blood vessel of right little finger
S65.507 Unspecified injury of blood vessel of left little finger
S65.508 Unspecified injury of blood vessel of other finger
Unspecified injury of blood vessel of specified finger with unspecified laterality
S65.509 Unspecified injury of blood vessel of unspecified finger
S65.51 Laceration of blood vessel of other and unspecified finger
S65.510 Laceration of blood vessel of right index finger
S65.511 Laceration of blood vessel of left index finger
S65.512 Laceration of blood vessel of right middle finger
S65.513 Laceration of blood vessel of left middle finger
S65.514 Laceration of blood vessel of right ring finger
S65.515 Laceration of blood vessel of left ring finger
S65.516 Laceration of blood vessel of right little finger
S65.517 Laceration of blood vessel of left little finger
S65.518 Laceration of blood vessel of other finger
Laceration of blood vessel of specified finger with unspecified laterality
S65.519 Laceration of blood vessel of unspecified finger
S65.59 Other specified injury of blood vessel of other and unspecified finger
S65.590 Other specified injury of blood vessel of right index finger
S65.591 Other specified injury of blood vessel of left index finger
S65.592 Other specified injury of blood vessel of right middle finger
S65.593 Other specified injury of blood vessel of left middle finger
S65.594 Other specified injury of blood vessel of right ring finger
S65.595 Other specified injury of blood vessel of left ring finger
S65.596 Other specified injury of blood vessel of right little finger
S65.597 Other specified injury of blood vessel of left little finger
S65.598 Other specified injury of blood vessel of other finger
Other specified injury of blood vessel of specified finger with unspecified laterality
S65.599 Other specified injury of blood vessel of unspecified finger

5th **S65.8 Injury of other blood vessels at wrist and hand level**

6th **S65.80 Unspecified injury of other blood vessels at wrist and hand level**

7th **S65.801 Unspecified injury of other blood vessels at wrist and hand level of right arm**

7th **S65.802 Unspecified injury of other blood vessels at wrist and hand level of left arm**

7th **S65.809 Unspecified injury of other blood vessels at wrist and hand level of unspecified arm**

6th **S65.81 Laceration of other blood vessels at wrist and hand level**

7th **S65.811 Laceration of other blood vessels at wrist and hand level of right arm**

7th **S65.812 Laceration of other blood vessels at wrist and hand level of left arm**

7th **S65.819 Laceration of other blood vessels at wrist and hand level of unspecified arm**

6th **S65.89 Other specified injury of other blood vessels at wrist and hand level**

7th **S65.891 Other specified injury of other blood vessels at wrist and hand level of right arm**

7th **S65.892 Other specified injury of other blood vessels at wrist and hand level of left arm**

7th **S65.899 Other specified injury of other blood vessels at wrist and hand level of unspecified arm**

5th **S65.9 Injury of unspecified blood vessel at wrist and hand level**

6th **S65.90 Unspecified injury of unspecified blood vessel at wrist and hand level**

7th **S65.901 Unspecified injury of unspecified blood vessel at wrist and hand level of right arm**

7th **S65.902 Unspecified injury of unspecified blood vessel at wrist and hand level of left arm**

7th **S65.909 Unspecified injury of unspecified blood vessel at wrist and hand level of unspecified arm**

6th **S65.91 Laceration of unspecified blood vessel at wrist and hand level**

7th **S65.911 Laceration of unspecified blood vessel at wrist and hand level of right arm**

7th **S65.912 Laceration of unspecified blood vessel at wrist and hand level of left arm**

7th **S65.919 Laceration of unspecified blood vessel at wrist and hand level of unspecified arm**

6th **S65.99 Other specified injury of unspecified blood vessel at wrist and hand level**

7th **S65.991 Other specified injury of unspecified blood vessel at wrist and hand of right arm**

7th **S65.992 Other specified injury of unspecified blood vessel at wrist and hand of left arm**

7th **S65.999 Other specified injury of unspecified blood vessel at wrist and hand of unspecified arm**

4th **S66 Injury of muscle, fascia and tendon at wrist and hand level**

Code also any associated open wound (S61.-)

EXCLUDES 2 *sprain of joints and ligaments of wrist and hand (S63.-)*

**TIP:** Refer to the Muscle/Tendon table at the beginning of this chapter.

The appropriate 7th character is to be added to each code from category S66.

- A initial encounter
- D subsequent encounter
- S sequela

5th **S66.0 Injury of long flexor muscle, fascia and tendon of thumb at wrist and hand level**

6th **S66.00 Unspecified injury of long flexor muscle, fascia and tendon of thumb at wrist and hand level**

7th **S66.001 Unspecified injury of long flexor muscle, fascia and tendon of right thumb at wrist and hand level**

7th **S66.002 Unspecified injury of long flexor muscle, fascia and tendon of left thumb at wrist and hand level**

7th **S66.009 Unspecified injury of long flexor muscle, fascia and tendon of unspecified thumb at wrist and hand level**

6th **S66.01 Strain of long flexor muscle, fascia and tendon of thumb at wrist and hand level**

7th **S66.011 Strain of long flexor muscle, fascia and tendon of right thumb at wrist and hand level**

7th **S66.012 Strain of long flexor muscle, fascia and tendon of left thumb at wrist and hand level**

7th **S66.019 Strain of long flexor muscle, fascia and tendon of unspecified thumb at wrist and hand level**

6th **S66.02 Laceration of long flexor muscle, fascia and tendon of thumb at wrist and hand level**

7th **S66.021 Laceration of long flexor muscle, fascia and tendon of right thumb at wrist and hand level**

7th **S66.022 Laceration of long flexor muscle, fascia and tendon of left thumb at wrist and hand level**

7th **S66.029 Laceration of long flexor muscle, fascia and tendon of unspecified thumb at wrist and hand level**

6th **S66.09 Other specified injury of long flexor muscle, fascia and tendon of thumb at wrist and hand level**

7th **S66.091 Other specified injury of long flexor muscle, fascia and tendon of right thumb at wrist and hand level**

7th **S66.092 Other specified injury of long flexor muscle, fascia and tendon of left thumb at wrist and hand level**

7th **S66.099 Other specified injury of long flexor muscle, fascia and tendon of unspecified thumb at wrist and hand level**

5th **S66.1 Injury of flexor muscle, fascia and tendon of other and unspecified finger at wrist and hand level**

EXCLUDES 2 *injury of long flexor muscle, fascia and tendon of thumb at wrist and hand level (S66.0-)*

6th **S66.10 Unspecified injury of flexor muscle, fascia and tendon of other and unspecified finger at wrist and hand level**

7th **S66.100 Unspecified injury of flexor muscle, fascia and tendon of right index finger at wrist and hand level**

7th **S66.101 Unspecified injury of flexor muscle, fascia and tendon of left index finger at wrist and hand level**

7th **S66.102 Unspecified injury of flexor muscle, fascia and tendon of right middle finger at wrist and hand level**

7th **S66.103 Unspecified injury of flexor muscle, fascia and tendon of left middle finger at wrist and hand level**

7th **S66.104 Unspecified injury of flexor muscle, fascia and tendon of right ring finger at wrist and hand level**

7th **S66.105 Unspecified injury of flexor muscle, fascia and tendon of left ring finger at wrist and hand level**

7th **S66.106 Unspecified injury of flexor muscle, fascia and tendon of right little finger at wrist and hand level**

7th **S66.107 Unspecified injury of flexor muscle, fascia and tendon of left little finger at wrist and hand level**

7th **S66.108 Unspecified injury of flexor muscle, fascia and tendon of other finger at wrist and hand level**

Unspecified injury of flexor muscle, fascia and tendon of specified finger with unspecified laterality at wrist and hand level

7th **S66.109 Unspecified injury of flexor muscle, fascia and tendon of unspecified finger at wrist and hand level**

6th **S66.11 Strain of flexor muscle, fascia and tendon of other and unspecified finger at wrist and hand level**

7th **S66.110 Strain of flexor muscle, fascia and tendon of right index finger at wrist and hand level**

7th **S66.111 Strain of flexor muscle, fascia and tendon of left index finger at wrist and hand level**

7th **S66.112 Strain of flexor muscle, fascia and tendon of right middle finger at wrist and hand level**

7th **S66.113 Strain of flexor muscle, fascia and tendon of left middle finger at wrist and hand level**

7th **S66.114 Strain of flexor muscle, fascia and tendon of right ring finger at wrist and hand level**

7th **S66.115 Strain of flexor muscle, fascia and tendon of left ring finger at wrist and hand level**

7th **S66.116 Strain of flexor muscle, fascia and tendon of right little finger at wrist and hand level**

7th **S66.117 Strain of flexor muscle, fascia and tendon of left little finger at wrist and hand level**

√7th **S66.118 Strain of flexor muscle, fascia and tendon of other finger at wrist and hand level**
Strain of flexor muscle, fascia and tendon of specified finger with unspecified laterality at wrist and hand level

√7th **S66.119 Strain of flexor muscle, fascia and tendon of unspecified finger at wrist and hand level**

√6th **S66.12 Laceration of flexor muscle, fascia and tendon of other and unspecified finger at wrist and hand level**

√7th **S66.120 Laceration of flexor muscle, fascia and tendon of right index finger at wrist and hand level**

√7th **S66.121 Laceration of flexor muscle, fascia and tendon of left index finger at wrist and hand level**

√7th **S66.122 Laceration of flexor muscle, fascia and tendon of right middle finger at wrist and hand level**

√7th **S66.123 Laceration of flexor muscle, fascia and tendon of left middle finger at wrist and hand level**

√7th **S66.124 Laceration of flexor muscle, fascia and tendon of right ring finger at wrist and hand level**

√7th **S66.125 Laceration of flexor muscle, fascia and tendon of left ring finger at wrist and hand level**

√7th **S66.126 Laceration of flexor muscle, fascia and tendon of right little finger at wrist and hand level**

√7th **S66.127 Laceration of flexor muscle, fascia and tendon of left little finger at wrist and hand level**

√7th **S66.128 Laceration of flexor muscle, fascia and tendon of other finger at wrist and hand level**
Laceration of flexor muscle, fascia and tendon of specified finger with unspecified laterality at wrist and hand level

√7th **S66.129 Laceration of flexor muscle, fascia and tendon of unspecified finger at wrist and hand level**

√6th **S66.19 Other injury of flexor muscle, fascia and tendon of other and unspecified finger at wrist and hand level**

√7th **S66.190 Other injury of flexor muscle, fascia and tendon of right index finger at wrist and hand level**

√7th **S66.191 Other injury of flexor muscle, fascia and tendon of left index finger at wrist and hand level**

√7th **S66.192 Other injury of flexor muscle, fascia and tendon of right middle finger at wrist and hand level**

√7th **S66.193 Other injury of flexor muscle, fascia and tendon of left middle finger at wrist and hand level**

√7th **S66.194 Other injury of flexor muscle, fascia and tendon of right ring finger at wrist and hand level**

√7th **S66.195 Other injury of flexor muscle, fascia and tendon of left ring finger at wrist and hand level**

√7th **S66.196 Other injury of flexor muscle, fascia and tendon of right little finger at wrist and hand level**

√7th **S66.197 Other injury of flexor muscle, fascia and tendon of left little finger at wrist and hand level**

√7th **S66.198 Other injury of flexor muscle, fascia and tendon of other finger at wrist and hand level**
Other injury of flexor muscle, fascia and tendon of specified finger with unspecified laterality at wrist and hand level

√7th **S66.199 Other injury of flexor muscle, fascia and tendon of unspecified finger at wrist and hand level**

√5th **S66.2 Injury of extensor muscle, fascia and tendon of thumb at wrist and hand level**

√6th **S66.20 Unspecified injury of extensor muscle, fascia and tendon of thumb at wrist and hand level**

√7th **S66.201 Unspecified injury of extensor muscle, fascia and tendon of right thumb at wrist and hand level**

√7th **S66.202 Unspecified injury of extensor muscle, fascia and tendon of left thumb at wrist and hand level**

√7th **S66.209 Unspecified injury of extensor muscle, fascia and tendon of unspecified thumb at wrist and hand level**

√6th **S66.21 Strain of extensor muscle, fascia and tendon of thumb at wrist and hand level**

√7th **S66.211 Strain of extensor muscle, fascia and tendon of right thumb at wrist and hand level**

√7th **S66.212 Strain of extensor muscle, fascia and tendon of left thumb at wrist and hand level**

√7th **S66.219 Strain of extensor muscle, fascia and tendon of unspecified thumb at wrist and hand level**

√6th **S66.22 Laceration of extensor muscle, fascia and tendon of thumb at wrist and hand level**

√7th **S66.221 Laceration of extensor muscle, fascia and tendon of right thumb at wrist and hand level**

√7th **S66.222 Laceration of extensor muscle, fascia and tendon of left thumb at wrist and hand level**

√7th **S66.229 Laceration of extensor muscle, fascia and tendon of unspecified thumb at wrist and hand level**

√6th **S66.29 Other specified injury of extensor muscle, fascia and tendon of thumb at wrist and hand level**

√7th **S66.291 Other specified injury of extensor muscle, fascia and tendon of right thumb at wrist and hand level**

√7th **S66.292 Other specified injury of extensor muscle, fascia and tendon of left thumb at wrist and hand level**

√7th **S66.299 Other specified injury of extensor muscle, fascia and tendon of unspecified thumb at wrist and hand level**

√5th **S66.3 Injury of extensor muscle, fascia and tendon of other and unspecified finger at wrist and hand level**
EXCLUDES 2 *injury of extensor muscle, fascia and tendon of thumb at wrist and hand level (S66.2-)*

√6th **S66.30 Unspecified injury of extensor muscle, fascia and tendon of other and unspecified finger at wrist and hand level**

√7th **S66.300 Unspecified injury of extensor muscle, fascia and tendon of right index finger at wrist and hand level**

√7th **S66.301 Unspecified injury of extensor muscle, fascia and tendon of left index finger at wrist and hand level**

√7th **S66.302 Unspecified injury of extensor muscle, fascia and tendon of right middle finger at wrist and hand level**

√7th **S66.303 Unspecified injury of extensor muscle, fascia and tendon of left middle finger at wrist and hand level**

√7th **S66.304 Unspecified injury of extensor muscle, fascia and tendon of right ring finger at wrist and hand level**

√7th **S66.305 Unspecified injury of extensor muscle, fascia and tendon of left ring finger at wrist and hand level**

√7th **S66.306 Unspecified injury of extensor muscle, fascia and tendon of right little finger at wrist and hand level**

√7th **S66.307 Unspecified injury of extensor muscle, fascia and tendon of left little finger at wrist and hand level**

√7th **S66.308 Unspecified injury of extensor muscle, fascia and tendon of other finger at wrist and hand level**
Unspecified injury of extensor muscle, fascia and tendon of specified finger with unspecified laterality at wrist and hand level

✓7th **S66.309** Unspecified injury of extensor muscle, fascia and tendon of unspecified finger at wrist and hand level

✓6th **S66.31** Strain of extensor muscle, fascia and tendon of other and unspecified finger at wrist and hand level

✓7th **S66.310** Strain of extensor muscle, fascia and tendon of right index finger at wrist and hand level

✓7th **S66.311** Strain of extensor muscle, fascia and tendon of left index finger at wrist and hand level

✓7th **S66.312** Strain of extensor muscle, fascia and tendon of right middle finger at wrist and hand level

✓7th **S66.313** Strain of extensor muscle, fascia and tendon of left middle finger at wrist and hand level

✓7th **S66.314** Strain of extensor muscle, fascia and tendon of right ring finger at wrist and hand level

✓7th **S66.315** Strain of extensor muscle, fascia and tendon of left ring finger at wrist and hand level

✓7th **S66.316** Strain of extensor muscle, fascia and tendon of right little finger at wrist and hand level

✓7th **S66.317** Strain of extensor muscle, fascia and tendon of left little finger at wrist and hand level

✓7th **S66.318** Strain of extensor muscle, fascia and tendon of other finger at wrist and hand level

Strain of extensor muscle, fascia and tendon of specified finger with unspecified laterality at wrist and hand level

✓7th **S66.319** Strain of extensor muscle, fascia and tendon of unspecified finger at wrist and hand level

✓6th **S66.32** Laceration of extensor muscle, fascia and tendon of other and unspecified finger at wrist and hand level

✓7th **S66.320** Laceration of extensor muscle, fascia and tendon of right index finger at wrist and hand level

✓7th **S66.321** Laceration of extensor muscle, fascia and tendon of left index finger at wrist and hand level

✓7th **S66.322** Laceration of extensor muscle, fascia and tendon of right middle finger at wrist and hand level

✓7th **S66.323** Laceration of extensor muscle, fascia and tendon of left middle finger at wrist and hand level

✓7th **S66.324** Laceration of extensor muscle, fascia and tendon of right ring finger at wrist and hand level

✓7th **S66.325** Laceration of extensor muscle, fascia and tendon of left ring finger at wrist and hand level

✓7th **S66.326** Laceration of extensor muscle, fascia and tendon of right little finger at wrist and hand level

✓7th **S66.327** Laceration of extensor muscle, fascia and tendon of left little finger at wrist and hand level

✓7th **S66.328** Laceration of extensor muscle, fascia and tendon of other finger at wrist and hand level

Laceration of extensor muscle, fascia and tendon of specified finger with unspecified laterality at wrist and hand level

✓7th **S66.329** Laceration of extensor muscle, fascia and tendon of unspecified finger at wrist and hand level

✓6th **S66.39** Other injury of extensor muscle, fascia and tendon of other and unspecified finger at wrist and hand level

✓7th **S66.390** Other injury of extensor muscle, fascia and tendon of right index finger at wrist and hand level

✓7th **S66.391** Other injury of extensor muscle, fascia and tendon of left index finger at wrist and hand level

✓7th **S66.392** Other injury of extensor muscle, fascia and tendon of right middle finger at wrist and hand level

✓7th **S66.393** Other injury of extensor muscle, fascia and tendon of left middle finger at wrist and hand level

✓7th **S66.394** Other injury of extensor muscle, fascia and tendon of right ring finger at wrist and hand level

✓7th **S66.395** Other injury of extensor muscle, fascia and tendon of left ring finger at wrist and hand level

✓7th **S66.396** Other injury of extensor muscle, fascia and tendon of right little finger at wrist and hand level

✓7th **S66.397** Other injury of extensor muscle, fascia and tendon of left little finger at wrist and hand level

✓7th **S66.398** Other injury of extensor muscle, fascia and tendon of other finger at wrist and hand level

Other injury of extensor muscle, fascia and tendon of specified finger with unspecified laterality at wrist and hand level

✓7th **S66.399** Other injury of extensor muscle, fascia and tendon of unspecified finger at wrist and hand level

✓5th **S66.4** Injury of intrinsic muscle, fascia and tendon of thumb at wrist and hand level

✓6th **S66.40** Unspecified injury of intrinsic muscle, fascia and tendon of thumb at wrist and hand level

✓7th **S66.401** Unspecified injury of intrinsic muscle, fascia and tendon of right thumb at wrist and hand level

✓7th **S66.402** Unspecified injury of intrinsic muscle, fascia and tendon of left thumb at wrist and hand level

✓7th **S66.409** Unspecified injury of intrinsic muscle, fascia and tendon of unspecified thumb at wrist and hand level

✓6th **S66.41** Strain of intrinsic muscle, fascia and tendon of thumb at wrist and hand level

✓7th **S66.411** Strain of intrinsic muscle, fascia and tendon of right thumb at wrist and hand level

✓7th **S66.412** Strain of intrinsic muscle, fascia and tendon of left thumb at wrist and hand level

✓7th **S66.419** Strain of intrinsic muscle, fascia and tendon of unspecified thumb at wrist and hand level

✓6th **S66.42** Laceration of intrinsic muscle, fascia and tendon of thumb at wrist and hand level

✓7th **S66.421** Laceration of intrinsic muscle, fascia and tendon of right thumb at wrist and hand level

✓7th **S66.422** Laceration of intrinsic muscle, fascia and tendon of left thumb at wrist and hand level

✓7th **S66.429** Laceration of intrinsic muscle, fascia and tendon of unspecified thumb at wrist and hand level

✓6th **S66.49** Other specified injury of intrinsic muscle, fascia and tendon of thumb at wrist and hand level

✓7th **S66.491** Other specified injury of intrinsic muscle, fascia and tendon of right thumb at wrist and hand level

✓7th **S66.492** Other specified injury of intrinsic muscle, fascia and tendon of left thumb at wrist and hand level

✓7th **S66.499** Other specified injury of intrinsic muscle, fascia and tendon of unspecified thumb at wrist and hand level

✓5th **S66.5** Injury of intrinsic muscle, fascia and tendon of other and unspecified finger at wrist and hand level

EXCLUDES 2 *injury of intrinsic muscle, fascia and tendon of thumb at wrist and hand level (S66.4-)*

✓6th **S66.50** Unspecified injury of intrinsic muscle, fascia and tendon of other and unspecified finger at wrist and hand level

✓7th **S66.500** Unspecified injury of intrinsic muscle, fascia and tendon of right index finger at wrist and hand level

√7th **S66.501 Unspecified injury of intrinsic muscle, fascia and tendon of left index finger at wrist and hand level**

√7th **S66.502 Unspecified injury of intrinsic muscle, fascia and tendon of right middle finger at wrist and hand level**

√7th **S66.503 Unspecified injury of intrinsic muscle, fascia and tendon of left middle finger at wrist and hand level**

√7th **S66.504 Unspecified injury of intrinsic muscle, fascia and tendon of right ring finger at wrist and hand level**

√7th **S66.505 Unspecified injury of intrinsic muscle, fascia and tendon of left ring finger at wrist and hand level**

√7th **S66.506 Unspecified injury of intrinsic muscle, fascia and tendon of right little finger at wrist and hand level**

√7th **S66.507 Unspecified injury of intrinsic muscle, fascia and tendon of left little finger at wrist and hand level**

√7th **S66.508 Unspecified injury of intrinsic muscle, fascia and tendon of other finger at wrist and hand level**

Unspecified injury of intrinsic muscle, fascia and tendon of specified finger with unspecified laterality at wrist and hand level

√7th **S66.509 Unspecified injury of intrinsic muscle, fascia and tendon of unspecified finger at wrist and hand level**

√6th **S66.51 Strain of intrinsic muscle, fascia and tendon of other and unspecified finger at wrist and hand level**

√7th **S66.510 Strain of intrinsic muscle, fascia and tendon of right index finger at wrist and hand level**

√7th **S66.511 Strain of intrinsic muscle, fascia and tendon of left index finger at wrist and hand level**

√7th **S66.512 Strain of intrinsic muscle, fascia and tendon of right middle finger at wrist and hand level**

√7th **S66.513 Strain of intrinsic muscle, fascia and tendon of left middle finger at wrist and hand level**

√7th **S66.514 Strain of intrinsic muscle, fascia and tendon of right ring finger at wrist and hand level**

√7th **S66.515 Strain of intrinsic muscle, fascia and tendon of left ring finger at wrist and hand level**

√7th **S66.516 Strain of intrinsic muscle, fascia and tendon of right little finger at wrist and hand level**

√7th **S66.517 Strain of intrinsic muscle, fascia and tendon of left little finger at wrist and hand level**

√7th **S66.518 Strain of intrinsic muscle, fascia and tendon of other finger at wrist and hand level**

Strain of intrinsic muscle, fascia and tendon of specified finger with unspecified laterality at wrist and hand level

√7th **S66.519 Strain of intrinsic muscle, fascia and tendon of unspecified finger at wrist and hand level**

√6th **S66.52 Laceration of intrinsic muscle, fascia and tendon of other and unspecified finger at wrist and hand level**

√7th **S66.520 Laceration of intrinsic muscle, fascia and tendon of right index finger at wrist and hand level**

√7th **S66.521 Laceration of intrinsic muscle, fascia and tendon of left index finger at wrist and hand level**

√7th **S66.522 Laceration of intrinsic muscle, fascia and tendon of right middle finger at wrist and hand level**

√7th **S66.523 Laceration of intrinsic muscle, fascia and tendon of left middle finger at wrist and hand level**

√7th **S66.524 Laceration of intrinsic muscle, fascia and tendon of right ring finger at wrist and hand level**

√7th **S66.525 Laceration of intrinsic muscle, fascia and tendon of left ring finger at wrist and hand level**

√7th **S66.526 Laceration of intrinsic muscle, fascia and tendon of right little finger at wrist and hand level**

√7th **S66.527 Laceration of intrinsic muscle, fascia and tendon of left little finger at wrist and hand level**

√7th **S66.528 Laceration of intrinsic muscle, fascia and tendon of other finger at wrist and hand level**

Laceration of intrinsic muscle, fascia and tendon of specified finger with unspecified laterality at wrist and hand level

√7th **S66.529 Laceration of intrinsic muscle, fascia and tendon of unspecified finger at wrist and hand level**

√6th **S66.59 Other injury of intrinsic muscle, fascia and tendon of other and unspecified finger at wrist and hand level**

√7th **S66.590 Other injury of intrinsic muscle, fascia and tendon of right index finger at wrist and hand level**

√7th **S66.591 Other injury of intrinsic muscle, fascia and tendon of left index finger at wrist and hand level**

√7th **S66.592 Other injury of intrinsic muscle, fascia and tendon of right middle finger at wrist and hand level**

√7th **S66.593 Other injury of intrinsic muscle, fascia and tendon of left middle finger at wrist and hand level**

√7th **S66.594 Other injury of intrinsic muscle, fascia and tendon of right ring finger at wrist and hand level**

√7th **S66.595 Other injury of intrinsic muscle, fascia and tendon of left ring finger at wrist and hand level**

√7th **S66.596 Other injury of intrinsic muscle, fascia and tendon of right little finger at wrist and hand level**

√7th **S66.597 Other injury of intrinsic muscle, fascia and tendon of left little finger at wrist and hand level**

√7th **S66.598 Other injury of intrinsic muscle, fascia and tendon of other finger at wrist and hand level**

Other injury of intrinsic muscle, fascia and tendon of specified finger with unspecified laterality at wrist and hand level

√7th **S66.599 Other injury of intrinsic muscle, fascia and tendon of unspecified finger at wrist and hand level**

√5th **S66.8 Injury of other specified muscles, fascia and tendons at wrist and hand level**

√6th **S66.80 Unspecified injury of other specified muscles, fascia and tendons at wrist and hand level**

√7th **S66.801 Unspecified injury of other specified muscles, fascia and tendons at wrist and hand level, right hand**

√7th **S66.802 Unspecified injury of other specified muscles, fascia and tendons at wrist and hand level, left hand**

√7th **S66.809 Unspecified injury of other specified muscles, fascia and tendons at wrist and hand level, unspecified hand**

√6th **S66.81 Strain of other specified muscles, fascia and tendons at wrist and hand level**

√7th **S66.811 Strain of other specified muscles, fascia and tendons at wrist and hand level, right hand**

√7th **S66.812 Strain of other specified muscles, fascia and tendons at wrist and hand level, left hand**

√7th **S66.819 Strain of other specified muscles, fascia and tendons at wrist and hand level, unspecified hand**

√6th **S66.82 Laceration of other specified muscles, fascia and tendons at wrist and hand level**

√7th **S66.821 Laceration of other specified muscles, fascia and tendons at wrist and hand level, right hand**

√7th S66.822 Laceration of other specified muscles, fascia and tendons at wrist and hand level, left hand

√7th S66.829 Laceration of other specified muscles, fascia and tendons at wrist and hand level, unspecified hand

√6th S66.89 Other injury of other specified muscles, fascia and tendons at wrist and hand level

√7th S66.891 Other injury of other specified muscles, fascia and tendons at wrist and hand level, right hand

√7th S66.892 Other injury of other specified muscles, fascia and tendons at wrist and hand level, left hand

√7th S66.899 Other injury of other specified muscles, fascia and tendons at wrist and hand level, unspecified hand

√5th S66.9 Injury of unspecified muscle, fascia and tendon at wrist and hand level

√6th S66.90 Unspecified injury of unspecified muscle, fascia and tendon at wrist and hand level

√7th S66.901 Unspecified injury of unspecified muscle, fascia and tendon at wrist and hand level, right hand

√7th S66.902 Unspecified injury of unspecified muscle, fascia and tendon at wrist and hand level, left hand

√7th S66.909 Unspecified injury of unspecified muscle, fascia and tendon at wrist and hand level, unspecified hand

√6th S66.91 Strain of unspecified muscle, fascia and tendon at wrist and hand level

√7th S66.911 Strain of unspecified muscle, fascia and tendon at wrist and hand level, right hand

√7th S66.912 Strain of unspecified muscle, fascia and tendon at wrist and hand level, left hand

√7th S66.919 Strain of unspecified muscle, fascia and tendon at wrist and hand level, unspecified hand

√6th S66.92 Laceration of unspecified muscle, fascia and tendon at wrist and hand level

√7th S66.921 Laceration of unspecified muscle, fascia and tendon at wrist and hand level, right hand

√7th S66.922 Laceration of unspecified muscle, fascia and tendon at wrist and hand level, left hand

√7th S66.929 Laceration of unspecified muscle, fascia and tendon at wrist and hand level, unspecified hand

√6th S66.99 Other injury of unspecified muscle, fascia and tendon at wrist and hand level

√7th S66.991 Other injury of unspecified muscle, fascia and tendon at wrist and hand level, right hand

√7th S66.992 Other injury of unspecified muscle, fascia and tendon at wrist and hand level, left hand

√7th S66.999 Other injury of unspecified muscle, fascia and tendon at wrist and hand level, unspecified hand

√4th **S67 Crushing injury of wrist, hand and fingers**

Use additional code for all associated injuries, such as:
fracture of wrist and hand (S62.-)
open wound of wrist and hand (S61.-)

The appropriate 7th character is to be added to each code from category S67.
A initial encounter
D subsequent encounter
S sequela

√5th S67.0 Crushing injury of thumb

√x7th S67.00 Crushing injury of unspecified thumb

√x7th S67.01 Crushing injury of right thumb

√x7th S67.02 Crushing injury of left thumb

√5th S67.1 Crushing injury of other and unspecified finger(s)

EXCLUDES 2 *crushing injury of thumb (S67.0-)*

√x7th S67.10 Crushing injury of unspecified finger(s)

√6th S67.19 Crushing injury of other finger(s)

√7th S67.190 Crushing injury of right index finger

√7th S67.191 Crushing injury of left index finger

√7th S67.192 Crushing injury of right middle finger

√7th S67.193 Crushing injury of left middle finger

√7th S67.194 Crushing injury of right ring finger

√7th S67.195 Crushing injury of left ring finger

√7th S67.196 Crushing injury of right little finger

√7th S67.197 Crushing injury of left little finger

√7th S67.198 Crushing injury of other finger

Crushing injury of specified finger with unspecified laterality

√5th S67.2 Crushing injury of hand

EXCLUDES 2 *crushing injury of fingers (S67.1-)*
*crushing injury of thumb (S67.0-)*

√x7th S67.20 Crushing injury of unspecified hand

√x7th S67.21 Crushing injury of right hand

√x7th S67.22 Crushing injury of left hand

√5th S67.3 Crushing injury of wrist

√x7th S67.30 Crushing injury of unspecified wrist

√x7th S67.31 Crushing injury of right wrist

√x7th S67.32 Crushing injury of left wrist

√5th S67.4 Crushing injury of wrist and hand

EXCLUDES 1 *crushing injury of hand alone (S67.2-)*
*crushing injury of wrist alone (S67.3-)*

EXCLUDES 2 *crushing injury of fingers (S67.1-)*
*crushing injury of thumb (S67.0-)*

√x7th S67.40 Crushing injury of unspecified wrist and hand

√x7th S67.41 Crushing injury of right wrist and hand

√x7th S67.42 Crushing injury of left wrist and hand

√5th S67.9 Crushing injury of unspecified part(s) of wrist, hand and fingers

√x7th S67.90 Crushing injury of unspecified part(s) of unspecified wrist, hand and fingers

√x7th S67.91 Crushing injury of unspecified part(s) of right wrist, hand and fingers

√x7th S67.92 Crushing injury of unspecified part(s) of left wrist, hand and fingers

√4th **S68 Traumatic amputation of wrist, hand and fingers**

An amputation not identified as partial or complete should be coded to complete.

The appropriate 7th character is to be added to each code from category S68.
A initial encounter
D subsequent encounter
S sequela

√5th S68.0 Traumatic metacarpophalangeal amputation of thumb

Traumatic amputation of thumb NOS

√6th S68.01 Complete traumatic metacarpophalangeal amputation of thumb

√7th S68.011 Complete traumatic metacarpophalangeal amputation of right thumb ESR

√7th S68.012 Complete traumatic metacarpophalangeal amputation of left thumb ESR

√7th S68.019 Complete traumatic metacarpophalangeal amputation of unspecified thumb ESR

√6th S68.02 Partial traumatic metacarpophalangeal amputation of thumb

√7th S68.021 Partial traumatic metacarpophalangeal amputation of right thumb ESR

√7th S68.022 Partial traumatic metacarpophalangeal amputation of left thumb ESR

√7th S68.029 Partial traumatic metacarpophalangeal amputation of unspecified thumb ESR

√5th S68.1 Traumatic metacarpophalangeal amputation of other and unspecified finger

Traumatic amputation of finger NOS

EXCLUDES 2 *traumatic metacarpophalangeal amputation of thumb (S68.0-)*

√6th S68.11 Complete traumatic metacarpophalangeal amputation of other and unspecified finger

√7th S68.110 Complete traumatic metacarpophalangeal amputation of right index finger ESR

√7th S68.111 Complete traumatic metacarpophalangeal amputation of left index finger ESR

√7th S68.112 Complete traumatic metacarpophalangeal amputation of right middle finger ESR

√7th S68.113 Complete traumatic metacarpophalangeal amputation of left middle finger ESR
√7th S68.114 Complete traumatic metacarpophalangeal amputation of right ring finger ESR
√7th S68.115 Complete traumatic metacarpophalangeal amputation of left ring finger ESR
√7th S68.116 Complete traumatic metacarpophalangeal amputation of right little finger ESR
√7th S68.117 Complete traumatic metacarpophalangeal amputation of left little finger ESR
√7th S68.118 Complete traumatic metacarpophalangeal amputation of other finger ESR
Complete traumatic metacarpophalangeal amputation of specified finger with unspecified laterality
√7th S68.119 Complete traumatic metacarpophalangeal amputation of unspecified finger ESR

√6th S68.12 Partial traumatic metacarpophalangeal amputation of other and unspecified finger
√7th S68.120 Partial traumatic metacarpophalangeal amputation of right index finger ESR
√7th S68.121 Partial traumatic metacarpophalangeal amputation of left index finger ESR
√7th S68.122 Partial traumatic metacarpophalangeal amputation of right middle finger ESR
√7th S68.123 Partial traumatic metacarpophalangeal amputation of left middle finger ESR
√7th S68.124 Partial traumatic metacarpophalangeal amputation of right ring finger ESR
√7th S68.125 Partial traumatic metacarpophalangeal amputation of left ring finger ESR
√7th S68.126 Partial traumatic metacarpophalangeal amputation of right little finger ESR
√7th S68.127 Partial traumatic metacarpophalangeal amputation of left little finger ESR
√7th S68.128 Partial traumatic metacarpophalangeal amputation of other finger ESR
Partial traumatic metacarpophalangeal amputation of specified finger with unspecified laterality
√7th S68.129 Partial traumatic metacarpophalangeal amputation of unspecified finger ESR

√5th S68.4 Traumatic amputation of hand at wrist level
Traumatic amputation of hand NOS
Traumatic amputation of wrist
√6th S68.41 Complete traumatic amputation of hand at wrist level
√7th S68.411 Complete traumatic amputation of right hand at wrist level HCC ESR COM
√7th S68.412 Complete traumatic amputation of left hand at wrist level HCC ESR COM
√7th S68.419 Complete traumatic amputation of unspecified hand at wrist level HCC ESR COM
√6th S68.42 Partial traumatic amputation of hand at wrist level
√7th S68.421 Partial traumatic amputation of right hand at wrist level HCC ESR COM
√7th S68.422 Partial traumatic amputation of left hand at wrist level HCC ESR COM
√7th S68.429 Partial traumatic amputation of unspecified hand at wrist level HCC ESR COM

√5th S68.5 Traumatic transphalangeal amputation of thumb
Traumatic interphalangeal joint amputation of thumb
√6th S68.51 Complete traumatic transphalangeal amputation of thumb
√7th S68.511 Complete traumatic transphalangeal amputation of right thumb ESR
√7th S68.512 Complete traumatic transphalangeal amputation of left thumb ESR
√7th S68.519 Complete traumatic transphalangeal amputation of unspecified thumb ESR
√6th S68.52 Partial traumatic transphalangeal amputation of thumb
√7th S68.521 Partial traumatic transphalangeal amputation of right thumb ESR
√7th S68.522 Partial traumatic transphalangeal amputation of left thumb ESR
√7th S68.529 Partial traumatic transphalangeal amputation of unspecified thumb ESR

√5th S68.6 Traumatic transphalangeal amputation of other and unspecified finger
√6th S68.61 Complete traumatic transphalangeal amputation of other and unspecified finger(s)
√7th S68.610 Complete traumatic transphalangeal amputation of right index finger ESR
√7th S68.611 Complete traumatic transphalangeal amputation of left index finger ESR
√7th S68.612 Complete traumatic transphalangeal amputation of right middle finger ESR
√7th S68.613 Complete traumatic transphalangeal amputation of left middle finger ESR
√7th S68.614 Complete traumatic transphalangeal amputation of right ring finger ESR
√7th S68.615 Complete traumatic transphalangeal amputation of left ring finger ESR
√7th S68.616 Complete traumatic transphalangeal amputation of right little finger ESR
√7th S68.617 Complete traumatic transphalangeal amputation of left little finger ESR
√7th S68.618 Complete traumatic transphalangeal amputation of other finger ESR
Complete traumatic transphalangeal amputation of specified finger with unspecified laterality
√7th S68.619 Complete traumatic transphalangeal amputation of unspecified finger ESR
√6th S68.62 Partial traumatic transphalangeal amputation of other and unspecified finger
√7th S68.620 Partial traumatic transphalangeal amputation of right index finger ESR
√7th S68.621 Partial traumatic transphalangeal amputation of left index finger ESR
√7th S68.622 Partial traumatic transphalangeal amputation of right middle finger ESR
√7th S68.623 Partial traumatic transphalangeal amputation of left middle finger ESR
√7th S68.624 Partial traumatic transphalangeal amputation of right ring finger ESR
√7th S68.625 Partial traumatic transphalangeal amputation of left ring finger ESR
√7th S68.626 Partial traumatic transphalangeal amputation of right little finger ESR
√7th S68.627 Partial traumatic transphalangeal amputation of left little finger ESR
√7th S68.628 Partial traumatic transphalangeal amputation of other finger ESR
Partial traumatic transphalangeal amputation of specified finger with unspecified laterality
√7th S68.629 Partial traumatic transphalangeal amputation of unspecified finger ESR

√5th S68.7 Traumatic transmetacarpal amputation of hand
√6th S68.71 Complete traumatic transmetacarpal amputation of hand
√7th S68.711 Complete traumatic transmetacarpal amputation of right hand HCC ESR COM
√7th S68.712 Complete traumatic transmetacarpal amputation of left hand HCC ESR COM
√7th S68.719 Complete traumatic transmetacarpal amputation of unspecified hand HCC ESR COM
√6th S68.72 Partial traumatic transmetacarpal amputation of hand
√7th S68.721 Partial traumatic transmetacarpal amputation of right hand HCC ESR COM
√7th S68.722 Partial traumatic transmetacarpal amputation of left hand HCC ESR COM
√7th S68.729 Partial traumatic transmetacarpal amputation of unspecified hand HCC ESR COM

**S69 Other and unspecified injuries of wrist, hand and finger(s)**

The appropriate 7th character is to be added to each code from category S69.
A initial encounter
D subsequent encounter
S sequela

**S69.8 Other specified injuries of wrist, hand and finger(s)**
- **S69.8Ø** Other specified injuries of unspecified wrist, hand and finger(s)
- **S69.81** Other specified injuries of right wrist, hand and finger(s)
- **S69.82** Other specified injuries of left wrist, hand and finger(s)

**S69.9 Unspecified injury of wrist, hand and finger(s)**
- **S69.9Ø** Unspecified injury of unspecified wrist, hand and finger(s)
- **S69.91** Unspecified injury of right wrist, hand and finger(s)
- **S69.92** Unspecified injury of left wrist, hand and finger(s)

## Injuries to the hip and thigh (S7Ø-S79)

EXCLUDES 2 *burns and corrosions (T2Ø-T32)*
*frostbite (T33-T34)*
*snake bite (T63.Ø-)*
*venomous insect bite or sting (T63.4-)*

**S7Ø Superficial injury of hip and thigh**

The appropriate 7th character is to be added to each code from category S7Ø.
A initial encounter
D subsequent encounter
S sequela

**S7Ø.Ø Contusion of hip**
- **S7Ø.ØØ** Contusion of unspecified hip
- **S7Ø.Ø1** Contusion of right hip
- **S7Ø.Ø2** Contusion of left hip

**S7Ø.1 Contusion of thigh**
- **S7Ø.1Ø** Contusion of unspecified thigh
- **S7Ø.11** Contusion of right thigh
- **S7Ø.12** Contusion of left thigh

**S7Ø.2 Other superficial injuries of hip**

**S7Ø.21 Abrasion of hip**
- **S7Ø.211** Abrasion, right hip
- **S7Ø.212** Abrasion, left hip
- **S7Ø.219** Abrasion, unspecified hip

**S7Ø.22 Blister (nonthermal) of hip**
- **S7Ø.221** Blister (nonthermal), right hip
- **S7Ø.222** Blister (nonthermal), left hip
- **S7Ø.229** Blister (nonthermal), unspecified hip

**S7Ø.24 External constriction of hip**
- **S7Ø.241** External constriction, right hip
- **S7Ø.242** External constriction, left hip
- **S7Ø.249** External constriction, unspecified hip

**S7Ø.25 Superficial foreign body of hip**
Splinter in the hip
- **S7Ø.251** Superficial foreign body, right hip
- **S7Ø.252** Superficial foreign body, left hip
- **S7Ø.259** Superficial foreign body, unspecified hip

**S7Ø.26 Insect bite (nonvenomous) of hip**
- **S7Ø.261** Insect bite (nonvenomous), right hip
- **S7Ø.262** Insect bite (nonvenomous), left hip
- **S7Ø.269** Insect bite (nonvenomous), unspecified hip

**S7Ø.27 Other superficial bite of hip**
EXCLUDES 1 *open bite of hip (S71.Ø5-)*
- **S7Ø.271** Other superficial bite of hip, right hip
- **S7Ø.272** Other superficial bite of hip, left hip
- **S7Ø.279** Other superficial bite of hip, unspecified hip

**S7Ø.3 Other superficial injuries of thigh**

**S7Ø.31 Abrasion of thigh**
- **S7Ø.311** Abrasion, right thigh
- **S7Ø.312** Abrasion, left thigh
- **S7Ø.319** Abrasion, unspecified thigh

**S7Ø.32 Blister (nonthermal) of thigh**
- **S7Ø.321** Blister (nonthermal), right thigh
- **S7Ø.322** Blister (nonthermal), left thigh
- **S7Ø.329** Blister (nonthermal), unspecified thigh

**S7Ø.34 External constriction of thigh**
- **S7Ø.341** External constriction, right thigh
- **S7Ø.342** External constriction, left thigh
- **S7Ø.349** External constriction, unspecified thigh

**S7Ø.35 Superficial foreign body of thigh**
Splinter in the thigh
- **S7Ø.351** Superficial foreign body, right thigh
- **S7Ø.352** Superficial foreign body, left thigh
- **S7Ø.359** Superficial foreign body, unspecified thigh

**S7Ø.36 Insect bite (nonvenomous) of thigh**
- **S7Ø.361** Insect bite (nonvenomous), right thigh
- **S7Ø.362** Insect bite (nonvenomous), left thigh
- **S7Ø.369** Insect bite (nonvenomous), unspecified thigh

**S7Ø.37 Other superficial bite of thigh**
EXCLUDES 1 *open bite of thigh (S71.15)*
- **S7Ø.371** Other superficial bite of right thigh
- **S7Ø.372** Other superficial bite of left thigh
- **S7Ø.379** Other superficial bite of unspecified thigh

**S7Ø.9 Unspecified superficial injury of hip and thigh**

**S7Ø.91 Unspecified superficial injury of hip**
- **S7Ø.911** Unspecified superficial injury of right hip
- **S7Ø.912** Unspecified superficial injury of left hip
- **S7Ø.919** Unspecified superficial injury of unspecified hip

**S7Ø.92 Unspecified superficial injury of thigh**
- **S7Ø.921** Unspecified superficial injury of right thigh
- **S7Ø.922** Unspecified superficial injury of left thigh
- **S7Ø.929** Unspecified superficial injury of unspecified thigh

**S71 Open wound of hip and thigh**

Code also any associated wound infection

EXCLUDES 1 *open fracture of hip and thigh (S72.-)*
*traumatic amputation of hip and thigh (S78.-)*

EXCLUDES 2 *bite of venomous animal (T63.-)*
*open wound of ankle, foot and toes (S91.-)*
*open wound of knee and lower leg (S81.-)*

The appropriate 7th character is to be added to each code from category S71.
A initial encounter
D subsequent encounter
S sequela

**S71.Ø Open wound of hip**

**S71.ØØ Unspecified open wound of hip**
- **S71.ØØ1** Unspecified open wound, right hip
- **S71.ØØ2** Unspecified open wound, left hip
- **S71.ØØ9** Unspecified open wound, unspecified hip

**S71.Ø1 Laceration without foreign body of hip**
- **S71.Ø11** Laceration without foreign body, right hip
- **S71.Ø12** Laceration without foreign body, left hip
- **S71.Ø19** Laceration without foreign body, unspecified hip

**S71.Ø2 Laceration with foreign body of hip**
- **S71.Ø21** Laceration with foreign body, right hip
- **S71.Ø22** Laceration with foreign body, left hip
- **S71.Ø29** Laceration with foreign body, unspecified hip

**S71.Ø3 Puncture wound without foreign body of hip**
- **S71.Ø31** Puncture wound without foreign body, right hip
- **S71.Ø32** Puncture wound without foreign body, left hip
- **S71.Ø39** Puncture wound without foreign body, unspecified hip

S71.04 Puncture wound with foreign body of hip
S71.041 Puncture wound with foreign body, right hip
S71.042 Puncture wound with foreign body, left hip
S71.049 Puncture wound with foreign body, unspecified hip
S71.05 Open bite of hip
Bite of hip NOS
EXCLUDES 1 *superficial bite of hip (S70.26, S70.27)*
S71.051 Open bite, right hip
S71.052 Open bite, left hip
S71.059 Open bite, unspecified hip
S71.1 Open wound of thigh
S71.10 Unspecified open wound of thigh
**AHA:** 2016,3Q,24
S71.101 Unspecified open wound, right thigh
S71.102 Unspecified open wound, left thigh
S71.109 Unspecified open wound, unspecified thigh
S71.11 Laceration without foreign body of thigh
S71.111 Laceration without foreign body, right thigh
S71.112 Laceration without foreign body, left thigh
S71.119 Laceration without foreign body, unspecified thigh
S71.12 Laceration with foreign body of thigh
S71.121 Laceration with foreign body, right thigh
S71.122 Laceration with foreign body, left thigh
S71.129 Laceration with foreign body, unspecified thigh
S71.13 Puncture wound without foreign body of thigh
**AHA:** 2023,3Q,12; 2016,3Q,24
S71.131 Puncture wound without foreign body, right thigh
S71.132 Puncture wound without foreign body, left thigh
S71.139 Puncture wound without foreign body, unspecified thigh
S71.14 Puncture wound with foreign body of thigh
**AHA:** 2016,3Q,24
S71.141 Puncture wound with foreign body, right thigh
S71.142 Puncture wound with foreign body, left thigh
S71.149 Puncture wound with foreign body, unspecified thigh
S71.15 Open bite of thigh
Bite of thigh NOS
EXCLUDES 1 *superficial bite of thigh (S70.37-)*
S71.151 Open bite, right thigh
S71.152 Open bite, left thigh
S71.159 Open bite, unspecified thigh

**S72 Fracture of femur**

NOTE A fracture not indicated as displaced or nondisplaced should be coded to displaced.
A fracture not indicated as open or closed should be coded to closed.
The open fracture designations are based on the Gustilo open fracture classification.

EXCLUDES 1 *traumatic amputation of hip and thigh (S78.-)*
EXCLUDES 2 *fracture of foot (S92.-)*
*fracture of lower leg and ankle (S82.-)*
*periprosthetic fracture of prosthetic implant of hip (M97.0-)*

**AHA:** 2023,3Q,12; 2018,2Q,12; 2016,1Q,33; 2015,3Q,37-39; 2015,1Q,17; 2013,4Q,128
**DEF:** Diaphysis: Central shaft of a long bone.
**DEF:** Epiphysis: Proximal and distal rounded ends of a long bone communicates with the joint.
**DEF:** Metaphysis: Section of a long bone located between the epiphysis and diaphysis at the proximal and distal ends.
**DEF:** Physis (growth plate): Narrow zone of cartilaginous tissue between the epiphysis and metaphysis at each end of a long bone. In childhood, proliferation of cells in this zone lengthens the bone. As the bone matures, this area thins, ossification eventually fusing into solid bone and growth stops. ***Synonym(s):*** *Epiphyseal plate.*

The appropriate 7th character is to be added to all codes from category S72 [unless otherwise indicated].
initial encounter for open fracture NOS
A initial encounter for closed fracture
B initial encounter for open fracture type I or II
C initial encounter for open fracture type IIIA, IIIB, or IIIC
D subsequent encounter for closed fracture with routine healing
E subsequent encounter for open fracture type I or II with routine healing
F subsequent encounter for open fracture type IIIA, IIIB, or IIIC with routine healing
G subsequent encounter for closed fracture with delayed healing
H subsequent encounter for open fracture type I or II with delayed healing
J subsequent encounter for open fracture type IIIA, IIIB, or IIIC with delayed healing
K subsequent encounter for closed fracture with nonunion
M subsequent encounter for open fracture type I or II with nonunion
N subsequent encounter for open fracture type IIIA, IIIB, or IIIC with nonunion
P subsequent encounter for closed fracture with malunion
Q subsequent encounter for open fracture type I or II with malunion
R subsequent encounter for open fracture type IIIA, IIIB, or IIIC with malunion
S sequela

S72.0 Fracture of head and neck of femur
EXCLUDES 2 *physeal fracture of lower end of femur (S79.1-)*
*physeal fracture of upper end of femur (S79.0-)*
**AHA:** 2016,3Q,16
S72.00 Fracture of unspecified part of neck of femur
Fracture of hip NOS
Fracture of neck of femur NOS
S72.001 Fracture of unspecified part of neck of right femur HCC ESR COM Q
S72.002 Fracture of unspecified part of neck of left femur HCC ESR COM Q
S72.009 Fracture of unspecified part of neck of unspecified femur HCC ESR COM Q
S72.01 Unspecified intracapsular fracture of femur
Subcapital fracture of femur
S72.011 Unspecified intracapsular fracture of right femur HCC ESR COM Q
S72.012 Unspecified intracapsular fracture of left femur HCC ESR COM Q
S72.019 Unspecified intracapsular fracture of unspecified femur HCC ESR COM Q

6th **S72.02 Fracture of epiphysis (separation) (upper) of femur**
Transepiphyseal fracture of femur
EXCLUDES 1 *capital femoral epiphyseal fracture (pediatric) of femur (S79.01-)*
*Salter-Harris Type I physeal fracture of upper end of femur (S79.01-)*

7th **S72.021 Displaced fracture of epiphysis (separation) (upper) of right femur** HCC ESR COM Q
7th **S72.022 Displaced fracture of epiphysis (separation) (upper) of left femur** HCC ESR COM Q
7th **S72.023 Displaced fracture of epiphysis (separation) (upper) of unspecified femur** HCC ESR COM Q
7th **S72.024 Nondisplaced fracture of epiphysis (separation) (upper) of right femur** HCC ESR COM Q
7th **S72.025 Nondisplaced fracture of epiphysis (separation) (upper) of left femur** HCC ESR COM Q
7th **S72.026 Nondisplaced fracture of epiphysis (separation) (upper) of unspecified femur** HCC ESR COM Q

6th **S72.03 Midcervical fracture of femur**
Transcervical fracture of femur NOS

7th **S72.031 Displaced midcervical fracture of right femur** HCC ESR COM Q
7th **S72.032 Displaced midcervical fracture of left femur** HCC ESR COM Q
7th **S72.033 Displaced midcervical fracture of unspecified femur** HCC ESR COM Q
7th **S72.034 Nondisplaced midcervical fracture of right femur** HCC ESR COM Q
7th **S72.035 Nondisplaced midcervical fracture of left femur** HCC ESR COM Q
7th **S72.036 Nondisplaced midcervical fracture of unspecified femur** HCC ESR COM Q

6th **S72.04 Fracture of base of neck of femur**
Cervicotrochanteric fracture of femur

7th **S72.041 Displaced fracture of base of neck of right femur** HCC ESR COM Q
7th **S72.042 Displaced fracture of base of neck of left femur** HCC ESR COM Q
7th **S72.043 Displaced fracture of base of neck of unspecified femur** HCC ESR COM Q
7th **S72.044 Nondisplaced fracture of base of neck of right femur** HCC ESR COM Q
7th **S72.045 Nondisplaced fracture of base of neck of left femur** HCC ESR COM Q
7th **S72.046 Nondisplaced fracture of base of neck of unspecified femur** HCC ESR COM Q

6th **S72.05 Unspecified fracture of head of femur**
Fracture of head of femur NOS

7th **S72.051 Unspecified fracture of head of right femur** HCC ESR COM Q
7th **S72.052 Unspecified fracture of head of left femur** HCC ESR COM Q
7th **S72.059 Unspecified fracture of head of unspecified femur** HCC ESR COM Q

6th **S72.06 Articular fracture of head of femur**

7th **S72.061 Displaced articular fracture of head of right femur** HCC ESR COM Q
7th **S72.062 Displaced articular fracture of head of left femur** HCC ESR COM Q
7th **S72.063 Displaced articular fracture of head of unspecified femur** HCC ESR COM Q
7th **S72.064 Nondisplaced articular fracture of head of right femur** HCC ESR COM Q
7th **S72.065 Nondisplaced articular fracture of head of left femur** HCC ESR COM Q
7th **S72.066 Nondisplaced articular fracture of head of unspecified femur** HCC ESR COM Q

6th **S72.09 Other fracture of head and neck of femur**

7th **S72.091 Other fracture of head and neck of right femur** HCC ESR COM Q
7th **S72.092 Other fracture of head and neck of left femur** HCC ESR COM Q
7th **S72.099 Other fracture of head and neck of unspecified femur** HCC ESR COM Q

5th **S72.1 Pertrochanteric fracture**
**AHA:** 2016,3Q,16

6th **S72.10 Unspecified trochanteric fracture of femur**
Fracture of trochanter NOS

7th **S72.101 Unspecified trochanteric fracture of right femur** HCC ESR COM Q
7th **S72.102 Unspecified trochanteric fracture of left femur** HCC ESR COM Q
7th **S72.109 Unspecified trochanteric fracture of unspecified femur** HCC ESR COM Q

6th **S72.11 Fracture of greater trochanter of femur**

7th **S72.111 Displaced fracture of greater trochanter of right femur** HCC ESR COM Q
7th **S72.112 Displaced fracture of greater trochanter of left femur** HCC ESR COM Q
7th **S72.113 Displaced fracture of greater trochanter of unspecified femur** HCC ESR COM Q
7th **S72.114 Nondisplaced fracture of greater trochanter of right femur** HCC ESR COM Q
7th **S72.115 Nondisplaced fracture of greater trochanter of left femur** HCC ESR COM Q
7th **S72.116 Nondisplaced fracture of greater trochanter of unspecified femur** HCC ESR COM Q

6th **S72.12 Fracture of lesser trochanter of femur**

7th **S72.121 Displaced fracture of lesser trochanter of right femur** HCC ESR COM Q
7th **S72.122 Displaced fracture of lesser trochanter of left femur** HCC ESR COM Q
7th **S72.123 Displaced fracture of lesser trochanter of unspecified femur** HCC ESR COM Q
7th **S72.124 Nondisplaced fracture of lesser trochanter of right femur** HCC ESR COM Q
7th **S72.125 Nondisplaced fracture of lesser trochanter of left femur** HCC ESR COM Q
7th **S72.126 Nondisplaced fracture of lesser trochanter of unspecified femur** HCC ESR COM Q

6th **S72.13 Apophyseal fracture of femur**
EXCLUDES 1 *chronic (nontraumatic) slipped upper femoral epiphysis (M93.0-)*

7th **S72.131 Displaced apophyseal fracture of right femur** HCC ESR COM Q
7th **S72.132 Displaced apophyseal fracture of left femur** HCC ESR COM Q
7th **S72.133 Displaced apophyseal fracture of unspecified femur** HCC ESR COM Q
7th **S72.134 Nondisplaced apophyseal fracture of right femur** HCC ESR COM Q
7th **S72.135 Nondisplaced apophyseal fracture of left femur** HCC ESR COM Q
7th **S72.136 Nondisplaced apophyseal fracture of unspecified femur** HCC ESR COM Q

6th **S72.14 Intertrochanteric fracture of femur**

7th **S72.141 Displaced intertrochanteric fracture of right femur** HCC ESR COM Q
7th **S72.142 Displaced intertrochanteric fracture of left femur** HCC ESR COM Q
7th **S72.143 Displaced intertrochanteric fracture of unspecified femur** HCC ESR COM Q
7th **S72.144 Nondisplaced intertrochanteric fracture of right femur** HCC ESR COM Q
7th **S72.145 Nondisplaced intertrochanteric fracture of left femur** HCC ESR COM Q
7th **S72.146 Nondisplaced intertrochanteric fracture of unspecified femur** HCC ESR COM Q

5th **S72.2 Subtrochanteric fracture of femur**

x7th **S72.21 Displaced subtrochanteric fracture of right femur** HCC ESR COM Q
x7th **S72.22 Displaced subtrochanteric fracture of left femur** HCC ESR COM Q
x7th **S72.23 Displaced subtrochanteric fracture of unspecified femur** HCC ESR COM Q
x7th **S72.24 Nondisplaced subtrochanteric fracture of right femur** HCC ESR COM Q

S72.25 Nondisplaced subtrochanteric fracture of left femur HCC ESR COM Q

S72.26 Nondisplaced subtrochanteric fracture of unspecified femur HCC ESR COM Q

S72.3 Fracture of shaft of femur

S72.30 Unspecified fracture of shaft of femur

S72.301 Unspecified fracture of shaft of right femur HCC ESR Q

S72.302 Unspecified fracture of shaft of left femur HCC ESR Q

S72.309 Unspecified fracture of shaft of unspecified femur HCC ESR Q

S72.32 Transverse fracture of shaft of femur

S72.321 Displaced transverse fracture of shaft of right femur HCC ESR Q

S72.322 Displaced transverse fracture of shaft of left femur HCC ESR Q

S72.323 Displaced transverse fracture of shaft of unspecified femur HCC ESR Q

S72.324 Nondisplaced transverse fracture of shaft of right femur HCC ESR Q

S72.325 Nondisplaced transverse fracture of shaft of left femur HCC ESR Q

S72.326 Nondisplaced transverse fracture of shaft of unspecified femur HCC ESR Q

S72.33 Oblique fracture of shaft of femur

S72.331 Displaced oblique fracture of shaft of right femur HCC ESR Q

S72.332 Displaced oblique fracture of shaft of left femur HCC ESR Q

S72.333 Displaced oblique fracture of shaft of unspecified femur HCC ESR Q

S72.334 Nondisplaced oblique fracture of shaft of right femur HCC ESR Q

S72.335 Nondisplaced oblique fracture of shaft of left femur HCC ESR Q

S72.336 Nondisplaced oblique fracture of shaft of unspecified femur HCC ESR Q

S72.34 Spiral fracture of shaft of femur

S72.341 Displaced spiral fracture of shaft of right femur HCC ESR Q

S72.342 Displaced spiral fracture of shaft of left femur HCC ESR Q

S72.343 Displaced spiral fracture of shaft of unspecified femur HCC ESR Q

S72.344 Nondisplaced spiral fracture of shaft of right femur HCC ESR Q

S72.345 Nondisplaced spiral fracture of shaft of left femur HCC ESR Q

S72.346 Nondisplaced spiral fracture of shaft of unspecified femur HCC ESR Q

S72.35 Comminuted fracture of shaft of femur

S72.351 Displaced comminuted fracture of shaft of right femur HCC ESR Q

S72.352 Displaced comminuted fracture of shaft of left femur HCC ESR Q

S72.353 Displaced comminuted fracture of shaft of unspecified femur HCC ESR Q

S72.354 Nondisplaced comminuted fracture of shaft of right femur HCC ESR Q

S72.355 Nondisplaced comminuted fracture of shaft of left femur HCC ESR Q

S72.356 Nondisplaced comminuted fracture of shaft of unspecified femur HCC ESR Q

S72.36 Segmental fracture of shaft of femur

S72.361 Displaced segmental fracture of shaft of right femur HCC ESR Q

S72.362 Displaced segmental fracture of shaft of left femur HCC ESR Q

S72.363 Displaced segmental fracture of shaft of unspecified femur HCC ESR Q

S72.364 Nondisplaced segmental fracture of shaft of right femur HCC ESR Q

S72.365 Nondisplaced segmental fracture of shaft of left femur HCC ESR Q

S72.366 Nondisplaced segmental fracture of shaft of unspecified femur HCC ESR Q

S72.39 Other fracture of shaft of femur

S72.391 Other fracture of shaft of right femur HCC ESR Q

S72.392 Other fracture of shaft of left femur HCC ESR Q

S72.399 Other fracture of shaft of unspecified femur HCC ESR Q

S72.4 Fracture of lower end of femur

Fracture of distal end of femur

EXCLUDES 2 *fracture of shaft of femur (S72.3-)*
*physeal fracture of lower end of femur (S79.1-)*

AHA: 2016,4Q,42

S72.40 Unspecified fracture of lower end of femur

AHA: 2018,1Q,21; 2016,4Q,42

S72.401 Unspecified fracture of lower end of right femur HCC ESR Q

S72.402 Unspecified fracture of lower end of left femur HCC ESR Q

S72.409 Unspecified fracture of lower end of unspecified femur HCC ESR Q

S72.41 Unspecified condyle fracture of lower end of femur

Condyle fracture of femur NOS

S72.411 Displaced unspecified condyle fracture of lower end of right femur HCC ESR Q

S72.412 Displaced unspecified condyle fracture of lower end of left femur HCC ESR Q

S72.413 Displaced unspecified condyle fracture of lower end of unspecified femur HCC ESR Q

S72.414 Nondisplaced unspecified condyle fracture of lower end of right femur HCC ESR Q

S72.415 Nondisplaced unspecified condyle fracture of lower end of left femur HCC ESR Q

S72.416 Nondisplaced unspecified condyle fracture of lower end of unspecified femur HCC ESR Q

S72.42 Fracture of lateral condyle of femur

S72.421 Displaced fracture of lateral condyle of right femur HCC ESR Q

S72.422 Displaced fracture of lateral condyle of left femur HCC ESR Q

S72.423 Displaced fracture of lateral condyle of unspecified femur HCC ESR Q

S72.424 Nondisplaced fracture of lateral condyle of right femur HCC ESR Q

S72.425 Nondisplaced fracture of lateral condyle of left femur HCC ESR Q

S72.426 Nondisplaced fracture of lateral condyle of unspecified femur HCC ESR Q

S72.43 Fracture of medial condyle of femur

S72.431 Displaced fracture of medial condyle of right femur HCC ESR Q

S72.432 Displaced fracture of medial condyle of left femur HCC ESR Q

S72.433 Displaced fracture of medial condyle of unspecified femur HCC ESR Q

S72.434 Nondisplaced fracture of medial condyle of right femur HCC ESR Q

S72.435 Nondisplaced fracture of medial condyle of left femur HCC ESR Q

S72.436 Nondisplaced fracture of medial condyle of unspecified femur HCC ESR Q

S72.44 Fracture of lower epiphysis (separation) of femur

EXCLUDES 1 *Salter-Harris Type I physeal fracture of lower end of femur (S79.11-)*

S72.441 Displaced fracture of lower epiphysis (separation) of right femur HCC ESR Q

S72.442 Displaced fracture of lower epiphysis (separation) of left femur HCC ESR Q

S72.443 Displaced fracture of lower epiphysis (separation) of unspecified femur HCC ESR Q

S72.444 Nondisplaced fracture of lower epiphysis (separation) of right femur HCC ESR Q

S72.445 Nondisplaced fracture of lower epiphysis (separation) of left femur HCC ESR Q

√7th **S72.446 Nondisplaced fracture of lower epiphysis (separation) of unspecified femur** HCC ESR Q

√6th **S72.45 Supracondylar fracture without intracondylar extension of lower end of femur**
Supracondylar fracture of lower end of femur NOS
EXCLUDES 1 *supracondylar fracture with intracondylar extension of lower end of femur (S72.46-)*

√7th **S72.451 Displaced supracondylar fracture without intracondylar extension of lower end of right femur** HCC ESR Q
√7th **S72.452 Displaced supracondylar fracture without intracondylar extension of lower end of left femur** HCC ESR Q
√7th **S72.453 Displaced supracondylar fracture without intracondylar extension of lower end of unspecified femur** HCC ESR Q
√7th **S72.454 Nondisplaced supracondylar fracture without intracondylar extension of lower end of right femur** HCC ESR Q
√7th **S72.455 Nondisplaced supracondylar fracture without intracondylar extension of lower end of left femur** HCC ESR Q
√7th **S72.456 Nondisplaced supracondylar fracture without intracondylar extension of lower end of unspecified femur** HCC ESR Q

√6th **S72.46 Supracondylar fracture with intracondylar extension of lower end of femur**
EXCLUDES 1 *supracondylar fracture without intracondylar extension of lower end of femur (S72.45-)*

√7th **S72.461 Displaced supracondylar fracture with intracondylar extension of lower end of right femur** HCC ESR Q
√7th **S72.462 Displaced supracondylar fracture with intracondylar extension of lower end of left femur** HCC ESR Q
√7th **S72.463 Displaced supracondylar fracture with intracondylar extension of lower end of unspecified femur** HCC ESR Q
√7th **S72.464 Nondisplaced supracondylar fracture with intracondylar extension of lower end of right femur** HCC ESR Q
√7th **S72.465 Nondisplaced supracondylar fracture with intracondylar extension of lower end of left femur** HCC ESR Q
√7th **S72.466 Nondisplaced supracondylar fracture with intracondylar extension of lower end of unspecified femur** HCC ESR Q

√6th **S72.47 Torus fracture of lower end of femur**

The appropriate 7th character is to be added to all codes in subcategory S72.47.
A initial encounter for closed fracture
D subsequent encounter for fracture with routine healing
G subsequent encounter for fracture with delayed healing
K subsequent encounter for fracture with nonunion
P subsequent encounter for fracture with malunion
S sequela

√7th **S72.471 Torus fracture of lower end of right femur** HCC ESR Q
√7th **S72.472 Torus fracture of lower end of left femur** HCC ESR Q
√7th **S72.479 Torus fracture of lower end of unspecified femur** HCC ESR Q

√6th **S72.49 Other fracture of lower end of femur**
√7th **S72.491 Other fracture of lower end of right femur** HCC ESR Q
√7th **S72.492 Other fracture of lower end of left femur** HCC ESR Q
√7th **S72.499 Other fracture of lower end of unspecified femur** HCC ESR Q

√5th **S72.8 Other fracture of femur**
√6th **S72.8X Other fracture of femur**
√7th **S72.8X1 Other fracture of right femur** HCC ESR Q
√7th **S72.8X2 Other fracture of left femur** HCC ESR Q
√7th **S72.8X9 Other fracture of unspecified femur** HCC ESR Q

√5th **S72.9 Unspecified fracture of femur**
Fracture of thigh NOS
Fracture of upper leg NOS
EXCLUDES 1 *fracture of hip NOS (S72.00-, S72.01-)*

√x7th **S72.90 Unspecified fracture of unspecified femur** HCC ESR Q
**AHA:** 2012,4Q,93
√x7th **S72.91 Unspecified fracture of right femur** HCC ESR Q
√x7th **S72.92 Unspecified fracture of left femur** HCC ESR Q

√4th **S73 Dislocation and sprain of joint and ligaments of hip**
INCLUDES avulsion of joint or ligament of hip
laceration of cartilage, joint or ligament of hip
sprain of cartilage, joint or ligament of hip
traumatic hemarthrosis of joint or ligament of hip
traumatic rupture of joint or ligament of hip
traumatic subluxation of joint or ligament of hip
traumatic tear of joint or ligament of hip

Code also any associated open wound
EXCLUDES 2 *strain of muscle, fascia and tendon of hip and thigh (S76.-)*

The appropriate 7th character is to be added to each code from category S73.
A initial encounter
D subsequent encounter
S sequela

√5th **S73.0 Subluxation and dislocation of hip**
EXCLUDES 2 *dislocation and subluxation of hip prosthesis (T84.020, T84.021)*

√6th **S73.00 Unspecified subluxation and dislocation of hip**
Dislocation of hip NOS
Subluxation of hip NOS
√7th **S73.001 Unspecified subluxation of right hip** HCC ESR
√7th **S73.002 Unspecified subluxation of left hip** HCC ESR
√7th **S73.003 Unspecified subluxation of unspecified hip** HCC ESR
√7th **S73.004 Unspecified dislocation of right hip** HCC ESR
√7th **S73.005 Unspecified dislocation of left hip** HCC ESR
√7th **S73.006 Unspecified dislocation of unspecified hip** HCC ESR

√6th **S73.01 Posterior subluxation and dislocation of hip**
√7th **S73.011 Posterior subluxation of right hip** HCC ESR
√7th **S73.012 Posterior subluxation of left hip** HCC ESR
√7th **S73.013 Posterior subluxation of unspecified hip** HCC ESR
√7th **S73.014 Posterior dislocation of right hip** HCC ESR
√7th **S73.015 Posterior dislocation of left hip** HCC ESR
√7th **S73.016 Posterior dislocation of unspecified hip** HCC ESR

√6th **S73.02 Obturator subluxation and dislocation of hip**
√7th **S73.021 Obturator subluxation of right hip** HCC ESR
√7th **S73.022 Obturator subluxation of left hip** HCC ESR
√7th **S73.023 Obturator subluxation of unspecified hip** HCC ESR
√7th **S73.024 Obturator dislocation of right hip** HCC ESR
√7th **S73.025 Obturator dislocation of left hip** HCC ESR
√7th **S73.026 Obturator dislocation of unspecified hip** HCC ESR

√6th **S73.03 Other anterior subluxation and dislocation of hip**
√7th **S73.031 Other anterior subluxation of right hip** HCC ESR
√7th **S73.032 Other anterior subluxation of left hip** HCC ESR
√7th **S73.033 Other anterior subluxation of unspecified hip** HCC ESR

S73.034 Other anterior dislocation of right hip HCC ESR
S73.035 Other anterior dislocation of left hip HCC ESR
S73.036 Other anterior dislocation of unspecified hip HCC ESR
S73.04 Central subluxation and dislocation of hip
S73.041 Central subluxation of right hip HCC ESR
S73.042 Central subluxation of left hip HCC ESR
S73.043 Central subluxation of unspecified hip HCC ESR
S73.044 Central dislocation of right hip HCC ESR
S73.045 Central dislocation of left hip HCC ESR
S73.046 Central dislocation of unspecified hip HCC ESR

S73.1 Sprain of hip
AHA: 2014,4Q,25
S73.10 Unspecified sprain of hip
S73.101 Unspecified sprain of right hip
S73.102 Unspecified sprain of left hip
S73.109 Unspecified sprain of unspecified hip
S73.11 Iliofemoral ligament sprain of hip
S73.111 Iliofemoral ligament sprain of right hip
S73.112 Iliofemoral ligament sprain of left hip
S73.119 Iliofemoral ligament sprain of unspecified hip
S73.12 Ischiocapsular (ligament) sprain of hip
S73.121 Ischiocapsular ligament sprain of right hip
S73.122 Ischiocapsular ligament sprain of left hip
S73.129 Ischiocapsular ligament sprain of unspecified hip
S73.19 Other sprain of hip
S73.191 Other sprain of right hip
S73.192 Other sprain of left hip
S73.199 Other sprain of unspecified hip

## S74 Injury of nerves at hip and thigh level

Code also any associated open wound (S71.-)

EXCLUDES 2 *injury of nerves at ankle and foot level (S94.-)*
*injury of nerves at lower leg level (S84.-)*

The appropriate 7th character is to be added to each code from category S74.
A initial encounter
D subsequent encounter
S sequela

S74.0 Injury of sciatic nerve at hip and thigh level
S74.00 Injury of sciatic nerve at hip and thigh level, unspecified leg
S74.01 Injury of sciatic nerve at hip and thigh level, right leg
S74.02 Injury of sciatic nerve at hip and thigh level, left leg
S74.1 Injury of femoral nerve at hip and thigh level
S74.10 Injury of femoral nerve at hip and thigh level, unspecified leg
S74.11 Injury of femoral nerve at hip and thigh level, right leg
S74.12 Injury of femoral nerve at hip and thigh level, left leg
S74.2 Injury of cutaneous sensory nerve at hip and thigh level
S74.20 Injury of cutaneous sensory nerve at hip and thigh level, unspecified leg
S74.21 Injury of cutaneous sensory nerve at hip and thigh level, right leg
S74.22 Injury of cutaneous sensory nerve at hip and thigh level, left leg
S74.8 Injury of other nerves at hip and thigh level
S74.8X Injury of other nerves at hip and thigh level
S74.8X1 Injury of other nerves at hip and thigh level, right leg
S74.8X2 Injury of other nerves at hip and thigh level, left leg
S74.8X9 Injury of other nerves at hip and thigh level, unspecified leg
S74.9 Injury of unspecified nerve at hip and thigh level
S74.90 Injury of unspecified nerve at hip and thigh level, unspecified leg
S74.91 Injury of unspecified nerve at hip and thigh level, right leg
S74.92 Injury of unspecified nerve at hip and thigh level, left leg

## S75 Injury of blood vessels at hip and thigh level

Code also any associated open wound (S71.-)

EXCLUDES 2 *injury of blood vessels at lower leg level (S85.-)*
*injury of popliteal artery (S85.0)*

The appropriate 7th character is to be added to each code from category S75.
A initial encounter
D subsequent encounter
S sequela

S75.0 Injury of femoral artery
S75.00 Unspecified injury of femoral artery
S75.001 Unspecified injury of femoral artery, right leg
S75.002 Unspecified injury of femoral artery, left leg
S75.009 Unspecified injury of femoral artery, unspecified leg
S75.01 Minor laceration of femoral artery
Incomplete transection of femoral artery
Laceration of femoral artery NOS
Superficial laceration of femoral artery
S75.011 Minor laceration of femoral artery, right leg
S75.012 Minor laceration of femoral artery, left leg
S75.019 Minor laceration of femoral artery, unspecified leg
S75.02 Major laceration of femoral artery
Complete transection of femoral artery
Traumatic rupture of femoral artery
AHA: 2023,3Q,12
S75.021 Major laceration of femoral artery, right leg
S75.022 Major laceration of femoral artery, left leg
S75.029 Major laceration of femoral artery, unspecified leg
S75.09 Other specified injury of femoral artery
S75.091 Other specified injury of femoral artery, right leg
S75.092 Other specified injury of femoral artery, left leg
S75.099 Other specified injury of femoral artery, unspecified leg
S75.1 Injury of femoral vein at hip and thigh level
S75.10 Unspecified injury of femoral vein at hip and thigh level
S75.101 Unspecified injury of femoral vein at hip and thigh level, right leg
S75.102 Unspecified injury of femoral vein at hip and thigh level, left leg
S75.109 Unspecified injury of femoral vein at hip and thigh level, unspecified leg
S75.11 Minor laceration of femoral vein at hip and thigh level
Incomplete transection of femoral vein at hip and thigh level
Laceration of femoral vein at hip and thigh level NOS
Superficial laceration of femoral vein at hip and thigh level
S75.111 Minor laceration of femoral vein at hip and thigh level, right leg
S75.112 Minor laceration of femoral vein at hip and thigh level, left leg
S75.119 Minor laceration of femoral vein at hip and thigh level, unspecified leg
S75.12 Major laceration of femoral vein at hip and thigh level
Complete transection of femoral vein at hip and thigh level
Traumatic rupture of femoral vein at hip and thigh level
AHA: 2023,3Q,12
S75.121 Major laceration of femoral vein at hip and thigh level, right leg
S75.122 Major laceration of femoral vein at hip and thigh level, left leg
S75.129 Major laceration of femoral vein at hip and thigh level, unspecified leg

✓6th S75.19 Other specified injury of femoral vein at hip and thigh level
- ✓7th S75.191 Other specified injury of femoral vein at hip and thigh level, right leg
- ✓7th S75.192 Other specified injury of femoral vein at hip and thigh level, left leg
- ✓7th S75.199 Other specified injury of femoral vein at hip and thigh level, unspecified leg

✓5th S75.2 Injury of greater saphenous vein at hip and thigh level

EXCLUDES 1 *greater saphenous vein NOS (S85.3)*

✓6th S75.20 Unspecified injury of greater saphenous vein at hip and thigh level
- ✓7th S75.201 Unspecified injury of greater saphenous vein at hip and thigh level, right leg
- ✓7th S75.202 Unspecified injury of greater saphenous vein at hip and thigh level, left leg
- ✓7th S75.209 Unspecified injury of greater saphenous vein at hip and thigh level, unspecified leg

✓6th S75.21 Minor laceration of greater saphenous vein at hip and thigh level

Incomplete transection of greater saphenous vein at hip and thigh level

Laceration of greater saphenous vein at hip and thigh level NOS

Superficial laceration of greater saphenous vein at hip and thigh level
- ✓7th S75.211 Minor laceration of greater saphenous vein at hip and thigh level, right leg
- ✓7th S75.212 Minor laceration of greater saphenous vein at hip and thigh level, left leg
- ✓7th S75.219 Minor laceration of greater saphenous vein at hip and thigh level, unspecified leg

✓6th S75.22 Major laceration of greater saphenous vein at hip and thigh level

Complete transection of greater saphenous vein at hip and thigh level

Traumatic rupture of greater saphenous vein at hip and thigh level
- ✓7th S75.221 Major laceration of greater saphenous vein at hip and thigh level, right leg
- ✓7th S75.222 Major laceration of greater saphenous vein at hip and thigh level, left leg
- ✓7th S75.229 Major laceration of greater saphenous vein at hip and thigh level, unspecified leg

✓6th S75.29 Other specified injury of greater saphenous vein at hip and thigh level
- ✓7th S75.291 Other specified injury of greater saphenous vein at hip and thigh level, right leg
- ✓7th S75.292 Other specified injury of greater saphenous vein at hip and thigh level, left leg
- ✓7th S75.299 Other specified injury of greater saphenous vein at hip and thigh level, unspecified leg

✓5th S75.8 Injury of other blood vessels at hip and thigh level

✓6th S75.80 Unspecified injury of other blood vessels at hip and thigh level
- ✓7th S75.801 Unspecified injury of other blood vessels at hip and thigh level, right leg
- ✓7th S75.802 Unspecified injury of other blood vessels at hip and thigh level, left leg
- ✓7th S75.809 Unspecified injury of other blood vessels at hip and thigh level, unspecified leg

✓6th S75.81 Laceration of other blood vessels at hip and thigh level
- ✓7th S75.811 Laceration of other blood vessels at hip and thigh level, right leg
- ✓7th S75.812 Laceration of other blood vessels at hip and thigh level, left leg
- ✓7th S75.819 Laceration of other blood vessels at hip and thigh level, unspecified leg

✓6th S75.89 Other specified injury of other blood vessels at hip and thigh level
- ✓7th S75.891 Other specified injury of other blood vessels at hip and thigh level, right leg
- ✓7th S75.892 Other specified injury of other blood vessels at hip and thigh level, left leg
- ✓7th S75.899 Other specified injury of other blood vessels at hip and thigh level, unspecified leg

✓5th S75.9 Injury of unspecified blood vessel at hip and thigh level

✓6th S75.90 Unspecified injury of unspecified blood vessel at hip and thigh level
- ✓7th S75.901 Unspecified injury of unspecified blood vessel at hip and thigh level, right leg
- ✓7th S75.902 Unspecified injury of unspecified blood vessel at hip and thigh level, left leg
- ✓7th S75.909 Unspecified injury of unspecified blood vessel at hip and thigh level, unspecified leg

✓6th S75.91 Laceration of unspecified blood vessel at hip and thigh level
- ✓7th S75.911 Laceration of unspecified blood vessel at hip and thigh level, right leg
- ✓7th S75.912 Laceration of unspecified blood vessel at hip and thigh level, left leg
- ✓7th S75.919 Laceration of unspecified blood vessel at hip and thigh level, unspecified leg

✓6th S75.99 Other specified injury of unspecified blood vessel at hip and thigh level
- ✓7th S75.991 Other specified injury of unspecified blood vessel at hip and thigh level, right leg
- ✓7th S75.992 Other specified injury of unspecified blood vessel at hip and thigh level, left leg
- ✓7th S75.999 Other specified injury of unspecified blood vessel at hip and thigh level, unspecified leg

## ✓4th S76 Injury of muscle, fascia and tendon at hip and thigh level

Code also any associated open wound (S71.-)

EXCLUDES 2 *injury of muscle, fascia and tendon at lower leg level (S86)*
*sprain of joint and ligament of hip (S73.1)*

**TIP:** Refer to the Muscle/Tendon table at the beginning of this chapter.

The appropriate 7th character is to be added to each code from category S76.
- A initial encounter
- D subsequent encounter
- S sequela

✓5th S76.0 Injury of muscle, fascia and tendon of hip

✓6th S76.00 Unspecified injury of muscle, fascia and tendon of hip
- ✓7th S76.001 Unspecified injury of muscle, fascia and tendon of right hip
- ✓7th S76.002 Unspecified injury of muscle, fascia and tendon of left hip
- ✓7th S76.009 Unspecified injury of muscle, fascia and tendon of unspecified hip

✓6th S76.01 Strain of muscle, fascia and tendon of hip
- ✓7th S76.011 Strain of muscle, fascia and tendon of right hip
- ✓7th S76.012 Strain of muscle, fascia and tendon of left hip
- ✓7th S76.019 Strain of muscle, fascia and tendon of unspecified hip

✓6th S76.02 Laceration of muscle, fascia and tendon of hip
- ✓7th S76.021 Laceration of muscle, fascia and tendon of right hip
- ✓7th S76.022 Laceration of muscle, fascia and tendon of left hip
- ✓7th S76.029 Laceration of muscle, fascia and tendon of unspecified hip

✓6th S76.09 Other specified injury of muscle, fascia and tendon of hip
- ✓7th S76.091 Other specified injury of muscle, fascia and tendon of right hip
- ✓7th S76.092 Other specified injury of muscle, fascia and tendon of left hip
- ✓7th S76.099 Other specified injury of muscle, fascia and tendon of unspecified hip

✓5th S76.1 Injury of quadriceps muscle, fascia and tendon

Injury of patellar ligament (tendon)

✓6th S76.10 Unspecified injury of quadriceps muscle, fascia and tendon
- ✓7th S76.101 Unspecified injury of right quadriceps muscle, fascia and tendon
- ✓7th S76.102 Unspecified injury of left quadriceps muscle, fascia and tendon
- ✓7th S76.109 Unspecified injury of unspecified quadriceps muscle, fascia and tendon

√6th S76.11 Strain of quadriceps muscle, fascia and tendon
√7th S76.111 Strain of right quadriceps muscle, fascia and tendon
√7th S76.112 Strain of left quadriceps muscle, fascia and tendon
√7th S76.119 Strain of unspecified quadriceps muscle, fascia and tendon
√6th S76.12 Laceration of quadriceps muscle, fascia and tendon
√7th S76.121 Laceration of right quadriceps muscle, fascia and tendon
√7th S76.122 Laceration of left quadriceps muscle, fascia and tendon
√7th S76.129 Laceration of unspecified quadriceps muscle, fascia and tendon
√6th S76.19 Other specified injury of quadriceps muscle, fascia and tendon
√7th S76.191 Other specified injury of right quadriceps muscle, fascia and tendon
√7th S76.192 Other specified injury of left quadriceps muscle, fascia and tendon
√7th S76.199 Other specified injury of unspecified quadriceps muscle, fascia and tendon
√5th S76.2 Injury of adductor muscle, fascia and tendon of thigh
√6th S76.20 Unspecified injury of adductor muscle, fascia and tendon of thigh
√7th S76.201 Unspecified injury of adductor muscle, fascia and tendon of right thigh
√7th S76.202 Unspecified injury of adductor muscle, fascia and tendon of left thigh
√7th S76.209 Unspecified injury of adductor muscle, fascia and tendon of unspecified thigh
√6th S76.21 Strain of adductor muscle, fascia and tendon of thigh
√7th S76.211 Strain of adductor muscle, fascia and tendon of right thigh
√7th S76.212 Strain of adductor muscle, fascia and tendon of left thigh
√7th S76.219 Strain of adductor muscle, fascia and tendon of unspecified thigh
√6th S76.22 Laceration of adductor muscle, fascia and tendon of thigh
√7th S76.221 Laceration of adductor muscle, fascia and tendon of right thigh
√7th S76.222 Laceration of adductor muscle, fascia and tendon of left thigh
√7th S76.229 Laceration of adductor muscle, fascia and tendon of unspecified thigh
√6th S76.29 Other injury of adductor muscle, fascia and tendon of thigh
√7th S76.291 Other injury of adductor muscle, fascia and tendon of right thigh
√7th S76.292 Other injury of adductor muscle, fascia and tendon of left thigh
√7th S76.299 Other injury of adductor muscle, fascia and tendon of unspecified thigh
√5th S76.3 Injury of muscle, fascia and tendon of the posterior muscle group at thigh level
√6th S76.30 Unspecified injury of muscle, fascia and tendon of the posterior muscle group at thigh level
√7th S76.301 Unspecified injury of muscle, fascia and tendon of the posterior muscle group at thigh level, right thigh
√7th S76.302 Unspecified injury of muscle, fascia and tendon of the posterior muscle group at thigh level, left thigh
√7th S76.309 Unspecified injury of muscle, fascia and tendon of the posterior muscle group at thigh level, unspecified thigh
√6th S76.31 Strain of muscle, fascia and tendon of the posterior muscle group at thigh level
√7th S76.311 Strain of muscle, fascia and tendon of the posterior muscle group at thigh level, right thigh
√7th S76.312 Strain of muscle, fascia and tendon of the posterior muscle group at thigh level, left thigh
√7th S76.319 Strain of muscle, fascia and tendon of the posterior muscle group at thigh level, unspecified thigh
√6th S76.32 Laceration of muscle, fascia and tendon of the posterior muscle group at thigh level
√7th S76.321 Laceration of muscle, fascia and tendon of the posterior muscle group at thigh level, right thigh
√7th S76.322 Laceration of muscle, fascia and tendon of the posterior muscle group at thigh level, left thigh
√7th S76.329 Laceration of muscle, fascia and tendon of the posterior muscle group at thigh level, unspecified thigh
√6th S76.39 Other specified injury of muscle, fascia and tendon of the posterior muscle group at thigh level
√7th S76.391 Other specified injury of muscle, fascia and tendon of the posterior muscle group at thigh level, right thigh
√7th S76.392 Other specified injury of muscle, fascia and tendon of the posterior muscle group at thigh level, left thigh
√7th S76.399 Other specified injury of muscle, fascia and tendon of the posterior muscle group at thigh level, unspecified thigh
√5th S76.8 Injury of other specified muscles, fascia and tendons at thigh level
√6th S76.80 Unspecified injury of other specified muscles, fascia and tendons at thigh level
√7th S76.801 Unspecified injury of other specified muscles, fascia and tendons at thigh level, right thigh
√7th S76.802 Unspecified injury of other specified muscles, fascia and tendons at thigh level, left thigh
√7th S76.809 Unspecified injury of other specified muscles, fascia and tendons at thigh level, unspecified thigh
√6th S76.81 Strain of other specified muscles, fascia and tendons at thigh level
√7th S76.811 Strain of other specified muscles, fascia and tendons at thigh level, right thigh
√7th S76.812 Strain of other specified muscles, fascia and tendons at thigh level, left thigh
√7th S76.819 Strain of other specified muscles, fascia and tendons at thigh level, unspecified thigh
√6th S76.82 Laceration of other specified muscles, fascia and tendons at thigh level
√7th S76.821 Laceration of other specified muscles, fascia and tendons at thigh level, right thigh
√7th S76.822 Laceration of other specified muscles, fascia and tendons at thigh level, left thigh
√7th S76.829 Laceration of other specified muscles, fascia and tendons at thigh level, unspecified thigh
√6th S76.89 Other injury of other specified muscles, fascia and tendons at thigh level
√7th S76.891 Other injury of other specified muscles, fascia and tendons at thigh level, right thigh
√7th S76.892 Other injury of other specified muscles, fascia and tendons at thigh level, left thigh
√7th S76.899 Other injury of other specified muscles, fascia and tendons at thigh level, unspecified thigh
√5th S76.9 Injury of unspecified muscles, fascia and tendons at thigh level
√6th S76.90 Unspecified injury of unspecified muscles, fascia and tendons at thigh level
√7th S76.901 Unspecified injury of unspecified muscles, fascia and tendons at thigh level, right thigh
√7th S76.902 Unspecified injury of unspecified muscles, fascia and tendons at thigh level, left thigh
√7th S76.909 Unspecified injury of unspecified muscles, fascia and tendons at thigh level, unspecified thigh
√6th S76.91 Strain of unspecified muscles, fascia and tendons at thigh level
√7th S76.911 Strain of unspecified muscles, fascia and tendons at thigh level, right thigh
√7th S76.912 Strain of unspecified muscles, fascia and tendons at thigh level, left thigh
√7th S76.919 Strain of unspecified muscles, fascia and tendons at thigh level, unspecified thigh
√6th S76.92 Laceration of unspecified muscles, fascia and tendons at thigh level
√7th S76.921 Laceration of unspecified muscles, fascia and tendons at thigh level, right thigh
√7th S76.922 Laceration of unspecified muscles, fascia and tendons at thigh level, left thigh

√7th S76.929 Laceration of unspecified muscles, fascia and tendons at thigh level, unspecified thigh

√6th S76.99 Other specified injury of unspecified muscles, fascia and tendons at thigh level

√7th S76.991 Other specified injury of unspecified muscles, fascia and tendons at thigh level, right thigh

√7th S76.992 Other specified injury of unspecified muscles, fascia and tendons at thigh level, left thigh

√7th S76.999 Other specified injury of unspecified muscles, fascia and tendons at thigh level, unspecified thigh

√4th **S77 Crushing injury of hip and thigh**

Use additional code(s) for all associated injuries

EXCLUDES 2 *crushing injury of ankle and foot (S97.-)*
*crushing injury of lower leg (S87.-)*

The appropriate 7th character is to be added to each code from category S77.
A initial encounter
D subsequent encounter
S sequela

√5th S77.Ø Crushing injury of hip

√x7th S77.ØØ Crushing injury of unspecified hip

√x7th S77.Ø1 Crushing injury of right hip

√x7th S77.Ø2 Crushing injury of left hip

√5th S77.1 Crushing injury of thigh

√x7th S77.1Ø Crushing injury of unspecified thigh

√x7th S77.11 Crushing injury of right thigh

√x7th S77.12 Crushing injury of left thigh

√5th S77.2 Crushing injury of hip with thigh

√x7th S77.2Ø Crushing injury of unspecified hip with thigh

√x7th S77.21 Crushing injury of right hip with thigh

√x7th S77.22 Crushing injury of left hip with thigh

√4th **S78 Traumatic amputation of hip and thigh**

An amputation not identified as partial or complete should be coded to complete

EXCLUDES 1 *traumatic amputation of knee (S88.Ø-)*

The appropriate 7th character is to be added to each code from category S78.
A initial encounter
D subsequent encounter
S sequela

√5th S78.Ø Traumatic amputation at hip joint

√6th S78.Ø1 Complete traumatic amputation at hip joint

√7th S78.Ø11 Complete traumatic amputation at right hip joint HCC ESR COM

√7th S78.Ø12 Complete traumatic amputation at left hip joint HCC ESR COM

√7th S78.Ø19 Complete traumatic amputation at unspecified hip joint HCC ESR COM

√6th S78.Ø2 Partial traumatic amputation at hip joint

√7th S78.Ø21 Partial traumatic amputation at right hip joint HCC ESR COM

√7th S78.Ø22 Partial traumatic amputation at left hip joint HCC ESR COM

√7th S78.Ø29 Partial traumatic amputation at unspecified hip joint HCC ESR COM

√5th S78.1 Traumatic amputation at level between hip and knee

EXCLUDES 1 *traumatic amputation of knee (S88.Ø-)*

√6th S78.11 Complete traumatic amputation at level between hip and knee

√7th S78.111 Complete traumatic amputation at level between right hip and knee HCC ESR COM

√7th S78.112 Complete traumatic amputation at level between left hip and knee HCC ESR COM

√7th S78.119 Complete traumatic amputation at level between unspecified hip and knee HCC ESR COM

√6th S78.12 Partial traumatic amputation at level between hip and knee

√7th S78.121 Partial traumatic amputation at level between right hip and knee HCC ESR COM

√7th S78.122 Partial traumatic amputation at level between left hip and knee HCC ESR COM

√7th S78.129 Partial traumatic amputation at level between unspecified hip and knee HCC ESR COM

√5th S78.9 Traumatic amputation of hip and thigh, level unspecified

√6th S78.91 Complete traumatic amputation of hip and thigh, level unspecified

√7th S78.911 Complete traumatic amputation of right hip and thigh, level unspecified HCC ESR COM

√7th S78.912 Complete traumatic amputation of left hip and thigh, level unspecified HCC ESR COM

√7th S78.919 Complete traumatic amputation of unspecified hip and thigh, level unspecified HCC ESR COM

√6th S78.92 Partial traumatic amputation of hip and thigh, level unspecified

√7th S78.921 Partial traumatic amputation of right hip and thigh, level unspecified HCC ESR COM

√7th S78.922 Partial traumatic amputation of left hip and thigh, level unspecified HCC ESR COM

√7th S78.929 Partial traumatic amputation of unspecified hip and thigh, level unspecified HCC ESR COM

√4th **S79 Other and unspecified injuries of hip and thigh**

NOTE A fracture not indicated as open or closed should be coded to closed

AHA: 2018,2Q,12; 2018,1Q,3; 2015,3Q,37-39

The appropriate 7th character is to be added to each code from subcategories S79.Ø and S79.1.
A initial encounter for closed fracture
D subsequent encounter for fracture with routine healing
G subsequent encounter for fracture with delayed healing
K subsequent encounter for fracture with nonunion
P subsequent encounter for fracture with malunion
S sequela

√5th S79.Ø Physeal fracture of upper end of femur

EXCLUDES 1 *apophyseal fracture of upper end of femur (S72.13-)*
*nontraumatic slipped upper femoral epiphysis (M93.Ø-)*

AHA: 2019,4Q,56

√6th S79.ØØ Unspecified physeal fracture of upper end of femur

√7th S79.ØØ1 Unspecified physeal fracture of upper end of right femur HCC ESR COM P

√7th S79.ØØ2 Unspecified physeal fracture of upper end of left femur HCC ESR COM P

√7th S79.ØØ9 Unspecified physeal fracture of upper end of unspecified femur HCC ESR COM P

√6th S79.Ø1 Salter-Harris Type I physeal fracture of upper end of femur

Acute on chronic slipped capital femoral epiphysis (traumatic)
Acute slipped capital femoral epiphysis (traumatic)
Capital femoral epiphyseal fracture

EXCLUDES 1 *chronic slipped upper femoral epiphysis (nontraumatic) (M93.Ø2-)*

√7th S79.Ø11 Salter-Harris Type I physeal fracture of upper end of right femur HCC ESR COM P

√7th S79.Ø12 Salter-Harris Type I physeal fracture of upper end of left femur HCC ESR COM P

√7th S79.Ø19 Salter-Harris Type I physeal fracture of upper end of unspecified femur HCC ESR COM P

√6th S79.Ø9 Other physeal fracture of upper end of femur

√7th S79.Ø91 Other physeal fracture of upper end of right femur HCC ESR COM P

√7th S79.Ø92 Other physeal fracture of upper end of left femur HCC ESR COM P

√7th S79.Ø99 Other physeal fracture of upper end of unspecified femur HCC ESR COM P

S79.1 Physeal fracture of lower end of femur
AHA: 2019,4Q,56
S79.10 Unspecified physeal fracture of lower end of femur
S79.101 Unspecified physeal fracture of lower end of right femur HCC ESR Q
S79.102 Unspecified physeal fracture of lower end of left femur HCC ESR Q
S79.109 Unspecified physeal fracture of lower end of unspecified femur HCC ESR Q
S79.11 Salter-Harris Type I physeal fracture of lower end of femur
S79.111 Salter-Harris Type I physeal fracture of lower end of right femur HCC ESR Q
S79.112 Salter-Harris Type I physeal fracture of lower end of left femur HCC ESR Q
S79.119 Salter-Harris Type I physeal fracture of lower end of unspecified femur HCC ESR Q
S79.12 Salter-Harris Type II physeal fracture of lower end of femur
S79.121 Salter-Harris Type II physeal fracture of lower end of right femur HCC ESR Q
S79.122 Salter-Harris Type II physeal fracture of lower end of left femur HCC ESR Q
S79.129 Salter-Harris Type II physeal fracture of lower end of unspecified femur HCC ESR Q
S79.13 Salter-Harris Type III physeal fracture of lower end of femur
S79.131 Salter-Harris Type III physeal fracture of lower end of right femur HCC ESR Q
S79.132 Salter-Harris Type III physeal fracture of lower end of left femur HCC ESR Q
S79.139 Salter-Harris Type III physeal fracture of lower end of unspecified femur HCC ESR Q
S79.14 Salter-Harris Type IV physeal fracture of lower end of femur
S79.141 Salter-Harris Type IV physeal fracture of lower end of right femur HCC ESR Q
S79.142 Salter-Harris Type IV physeal fracture of lower end of left femur HCC ESR Q
S79.149 Salter-Harris Type IV physeal fracture of lower end of unspecified femur HCC ESR Q
S79.19 Other physeal fracture of lower end of femur
S79.191 Other physeal fracture of lower end of right femur HCC ESR Q
S79.192 Other physeal fracture of lower end of left femur HCC ESR Q
S79.199 Other physeal fracture of lower end of unspecified femur HCC ESR Q
S79.8 Other specified injuries of hip and thigh

The appropriate 7th character is to be added to each code in subcategory S79.8.
A initial encounter
D subsequent encounter
S sequela

S79.81 Other specified injuries of hip
S79.811 Other specified injuries of right hip
S79.812 Other specified injuries of left hip
S79.819 Other specified injuries of unspecified hip
S79.82 Other specified injuries of thigh
S79.821 Other specified injuries of right thigh
S79.822 Other specified injuries of left thigh
S79.829 Other specified injuries of unspecified thigh
S79.9 Unspecified injury of hip and thigh

The appropriate 7th character is to be added to each code in subcategory S79.9.
A initial encounter
D subsequent encounter
S sequela

S79.91 Unspecified injury of hip
S79.911 Unspecified injury of right hip
S79.912 Unspecified injury of left hip
S79.919 Unspecified injury of unspecified hip
S79.92 Unspecified injury of thigh
S79.921 Unspecified injury of right thigh
S79.922 Unspecified injury of left thigh
S79.929 Unspecified injury of unspecified thigh

## Injuries to the knee and lower leg (S80-S89)

EXCLUDES 2 *burns and corrosions (T20-T32)*
*frostbite (T33-T34)*
*injuries of ankle and foot, except fracture of ankle and malleolus (S90-S99)*
*insect bite or sting, venomous (T63.4)*

**S80 Superficial injury of knee and lower leg**
EXCLUDES 2 *superficial injury of ankle and foot (S90.-)*

The appropriate 7th character is to be added to each code from category S80.
A initial encounter
D subsequent encounter
S sequela

S80.0 Contusion of knee
S80.00 Contusion of unspecified knee
S80.01 Contusion of right knee
S80.02 Contusion of left knee
S80.1 Contusion of lower leg
S80.10 Contusion of unspecified lower leg
S80.11 Contusion of right lower leg
S80.12 Contusion of left lower leg
S80.2 Other superficial injuries of knee
S80.21 Abrasion of knee
S80.211 Abrasion, right knee
S80.212 Abrasion, left knee
S80.219 Abrasion, unspecified knee
S80.22 Blister (nonthermal) of knee
S80.221 Blister (nonthermal), right knee
S80.222 Blister (nonthermal), left knee
S80.229 Blister (nonthermal), unspecified knee
S80.24 External constriction of knee
S80.241 External constriction, right knee
S80.242 External constriction, left knee
S80.249 External constriction, unspecified knee
S80.25 Superficial foreign body of knee
Splinter in the knee
S80.251 Superficial foreign body, right knee
S80.252 Superficial foreign body, left knee
S80.259 Superficial foreign body, unspecified knee
S80.26 Insect bite (nonvenomous) of knee
S80.261 Insect bite (nonvenomous), right knee
S80.262 Insect bite (nonvenomous), left knee
S80.269 Insect bite (nonvenomous), unspecified knee
S80.27 Other superficial bite of knee
EXCLUDES 1 *open bite of knee (S81.05-)*
S80.271 Other superficial bite of right knee
S80.272 Other superficial bite of left knee
S80.279 Other superficial bite of unspecified knee
S80.8 Other superficial injuries of lower leg
S80.81 Abrasion of lower leg
S80.811 Abrasion, right lower leg
S80.812 Abrasion, left lower leg
S80.819 Abrasion, unspecified lower leg
S80.82 Blister (nonthermal) of lower leg
S80.821 Blister (nonthermal), right lower leg
S80.822 Blister (nonthermal), left lower leg
S80.829 Blister (nonthermal), unspecified lower leg
S80.84 External constriction of lower leg
S80.841 External constriction, right lower leg
S80.842 External constriction, left lower leg
S80.849 External constriction, unspecified lower leg

√6th **S80.85 Superficial foreign body of lower leg**
Splinter in the lower leg
√7th **S80.851 Superficial foreign body, right lower leg**
√7th **S80.852 Superficial foreign body, left lower leg**
√7th **S80.859 Superficial foreign body, unspecified lower leg**
√6th **S80.86 Insect bite (nonvenomous) of lower leg**
√7th **S80.861 Insect bite (nonvenomous), right lower leg**
√7th **S80.862 Insect bite (nonvenomous), left lower leg**
√7th **S80.869 Insect bite (nonvenomous), unspecified lower leg**
√6th **S80.87 Other superficial bite of lower leg**
EXCLUDES 1 *open bite of lower leg (S81.85-)*
√7th **S80.871 Other superficial bite, right lower leg**
√7th **S80.872 Other superficial bite, left lower leg**
√7th **S80.879 Other superficial bite, unspecified lower leg**
√5th **S80.9 Unspecified superficial injury of knee and lower leg**
√6th **S80.91 Unspecified superficial injury of knee**
√7th **S80.911 Unspecified superficial injury of right knee**
√7th **S80.912 Unspecified superficial injury of left knee**
√7th **S80.919 Unspecified superficial injury of unspecified knee**
√6th **S80.92 Unspecified superficial injury of lower leg**
√7th **S80.921 Unspecified superficial injury of right lower leg**
√7th **S80.922 Unspecified superficial injury of left lower leg**
√7th **S80.929 Unspecified superficial injury of unspecified lower leg**

√4th **S81 Open wound of knee and lower leg**
Code also any associated wound infection
EXCLUDES 1 *open fracture of knee and lower leg (S82.-)*
*traumatic amputation of lower leg (S88.-)*
EXCLUDES 2 *open wound of ankle and foot (S91.-)*

The appropriate 7th character is to be added to each code from category S81.
A initial encounter
D subsequent encounter
S sequela

√5th **S81.0 Open wound of knee**
√6th **S81.00 Unspecified open wound of knee**
√7th **S81.001 Unspecified open wound, right knee**
√7th **S81.002 Unspecified open wound, left knee**
√7th **S81.009 Unspecified open wound, unspecified knee**
√6th **S81.01 Laceration without foreign body of knee**
√7th **S81.011 Laceration without foreign body, right knee**
√7th **S81.012 Laceration without foreign body, left knee**
√7th **S81.019 Laceration without foreign body, unspecified knee**
√6th **S81.02 Laceration with foreign body of knee**
√7th **S81.021 Laceration with foreign body, right knee**
√7th **S81.022 Laceration with foreign body, left knee**
√7th **S81.029 Laceration with foreign body, unspecified knee**
√6th **S81.03 Puncture wound without foreign body of knee**
**AHA:** 2025,1Q,31
√7th **S81.031 Puncture wound without foreign body, right knee**
√7th **S81.032 Puncture wound without foreign body, left knee**
√7th **S81.039 Puncture wound without foreign body, unspecified knee**
√6th **S81.04 Puncture wound with foreign body of knee**
√7th **S81.041 Puncture wound with foreign body, right knee**
√7th **S81.042 Puncture wound with foreign body, left knee**
√7th **S81.049 Puncture wound with foreign body, unspecified knee**
√6th **S81.05 Open bite of knee**
Bite of knee NOS
EXCLUDES 1 *superficial bite of knee (S80.27-)*
√7th **S81.051 Open bite, right knee**
√7th **S81.052 Open bite, left knee**
√7th **S81.059 Open bite, unspecified knee**
√5th **S81.8 Open wound of lower leg**
√6th **S81.80 Unspecified open wound of lower leg**
**AHA:** 2016,3Q,24
√7th **S81.801 Unspecified open wound, right lower leg**
√7th **S81.802 Unspecified open wound, left lower leg**
√7th **S81.809 Unspecified open wound, unspecified lower leg**
√6th **S81.81 Laceration without foreign body of lower leg**
√7th **S81.811 Laceration without foreign body, right lower leg**
√7th **S81.812 Laceration without foreign body, left lower leg**
√7th **S81.819 Laceration without foreign body, unspecified lower leg**
√6th **S81.82 Laceration with foreign body of lower leg**
√7th **S81.821 Laceration with foreign body, right lower leg**
√7th **S81.822 Laceration with foreign body, left lower leg**
√7th **S81.829 Laceration with foreign body, unspecified lower leg**
√6th **S81.83 Puncture wound without foreign body of lower leg**
**AHA:** 2016,3Q,24
√7th **S81.831 Puncture wound without foreign body, right lower leg**
√7th **S81.832 Puncture wound without foreign body, left lower leg**
√7th **S81.839 Puncture wound without foreign body, unspecified lower leg**
√6th **S81.84 Puncture wound with foreign body of lower leg**
**AHA:** 2016,3Q,24
√7th **S81.841 Puncture wound with foreign body, right lower leg**
√7th **S81.842 Puncture wound with foreign body, left lower leg**
√7th **S81.849 Puncture wound with foreign body, unspecified lower leg**
√6th **S81.85 Open bite of lower leg**
Bite of lower leg NOS
EXCLUDES 1 *superficial bite of lower leg (S80.86-, S80.87-)*
√7th **S81.851 Open bite, right lower leg**
√7th **S81.852 Open bite, left lower leg**
√7th **S81.859 Open bite, unspecified lower leg**

**S82 Fracture of lower leg, including ankle**

NOTE A fracture not indicated as displaced or nondisplaced should be coded to displaced

A fracture not indicated as open or closed should be coded to closed

The open fracture designations are based on the Gustilo open fracture classification.

INCLUDES fracture of malleolus

EXCLUDES 1 *traumatic amputation of lower leg (S88.-)*

EXCLUDES 2 *fracture of foot, except ankle (S92.-)*

*periprosthetic fracture around internal prosthetic ankle joint (M97.2)*

*periprosthetic fracture around internal prosthetic implant of knee joint (M97.1-)*

**AHA:** 2018,2Q,12; 2016,1Q,33; 2015,3Q,37-39

**DEF:** Diaphysis: Central shaft of a long bone.

**DEF:** Epiphysis: Proximal and distal rounded ends of a long bone, communicates with the joint.

**DEF:** Metaphysis: Section of a long bone located between the epiphysis and diaphysis at the proximal and distal ends.

**DEF:** Physis (growth plate): Narrow zone of cartilaginous tissue between the epiphysis and metaphysis at each end of a long bone. In childhood, proliferation of cells in this zone lengthens the bone. As the bone matures, this area thins, ossification eventually fusing into solid bone and growth stops. ***Synonym(s):*** *Epiphyseal plate.*

The appropriate 7th character is to be added to all codes from category S82 [unless otherwise indicated].

initial encounter for open fracture NOS
- A initial encounter for closed fracture
- B initial encounter for open fracture type I or II
- C initial encounter for open fracture type IIIA, IIIB, or IIIC
- D subsequent encounter for closed fracture with routine healing
- E subsequent encounter for open fracture type I or II with routine healing
- F subsequent encounter for open fracture type IIIA, IIIB, or IIIC with routine healing
- G subsequent encounter for closed fracture with delayed healing
- H subsequent encounter for open fracture type I or II with delayed healing
- J subsequent encounter for open fracture type IIIA, IIIB, or IIIC with delayed healing
- K subsequent encounter for closed fracture with nonunion
- M subsequent encounter for open fracture type I or II with nonunion
- N subsequent encounter for open fracture type IIIA, IIIB, or IIIC with nonunion
- P subsequent encounter for closed fracture with malunion
- Q subsequent encounter for open fracture type I or II with malunion
- R subsequent encounter for open fracture type IIIA, IIIB, or IIIC with malunion
- S sequela

**S82.0 Fracture of patella**

Knee cap

**S82.00 Unspecified fracture of patella**
- **S82.001 Unspecified fracture of right patella** Q
- **S82.002 Unspecified fracture of left patella** Q
- **S82.009 Unspecified fracture of unspecified patella** Q

**S82.01 Osteochondral fracture of patella**
- **S82.011 Displaced osteochondral fracture of right patella** Q
- **S82.012 Displaced osteochondral fracture of left patella** Q
- **S82.013 Displaced osteochondral fracture of unspecified patella** Q
- **S82.014 Nondisplaced osteochondral fracture of right patella** Q
- **S82.015 Nondisplaced osteochondral fracture of left patella** Q
- **S82.016 Nondisplaced osteochondral fracture of unspecified patella** Q

**S82.02 Longitudinal fracture of patella**
- **S82.021 Displaced longitudinal fracture of right patella** Q
- **S82.022 Displaced longitudinal fracture of left patella** Q
- **S82.023 Displaced longitudinal fracture of unspecified patella** Q
- **S82.024 Nondisplaced longitudinal fracture of right patella** Q
- **S82.025 Nondisplaced longitudinal fracture of left patella** Q
- **S82.026 Nondisplaced longitudinal fracture of unspecified patella** Q

**S82.03 Transverse fracture of patella**
- **S82.031 Displaced transverse fracture of right patella** Q
- **S82.032 Displaced transverse fracture of left patella** Q
- **S82.033 Displaced transverse fracture of unspecified patella** Q
- **S82.034 Nondisplaced transverse fracture of right patella** Q
- **S82.035 Nondisplaced transverse fracture of left patella** Q
- **S82.036 Nondisplaced transverse fracture of unspecified patella** Q

**S82.04 Comminuted fracture of patella**
- **S82.041 Displaced comminuted fracture of right patella** Q
- **S82.042 Displaced comminuted fracture of left patella** Q
- **S82.043 Displaced comminuted fracture of unspecified patella** Q
- **S82.044 Nondisplaced comminuted fracture of right patella** Q
- **S82.045 Nondisplaced comminuted fracture of left patella** Q
- **S82.046 Nondisplaced comminuted fracture of unspecified patella** Q

**S82.09 Other fracture of patella**
- **S82.091 Other fracture of right patella** Q
- **S82.092 Other fracture of left patella** Q
- **S82.099 Other fracture of unspecified patella** Q

**S82.1 Fracture of upper end of tibia**

Fracture of proximal end of tibia

EXCLUDES 2 *fracture of shaft of tibia (S82.2-)*

*physeal fracture of upper end of tibia (S89.0-)*

**S82.10 Unspecified fracture of upper end of tibia**
- **S82.101 Unspecified fracture of upper end of right tibia** Q
- **S82.102 Unspecified fracture of upper end of left tibia** Q
- **S82.109 Unspecified fracture of upper end of unspecified tibia** Q

**S82.11 Fracture of tibial spine**
- **S82.111 Displaced fracture of right tibial spine** Q
- **S82.112 Displaced fracture of left tibial spine** Q
- **S82.113 Displaced fracture of unspecified tibial spine** Q
- **S82.114 Nondisplaced fracture of right tibial spine** Q
- **S82.115 Nondisplaced fracture of left tibial spine** Q
- **S82.116 Nondisplaced fracture of unspecified tibial spine** Q

**S82.12 Fracture of lateral condyle of tibia**
- **S82.121 Displaced fracture of lateral condyle of right tibia** Q
- **S82.122 Displaced fracture of lateral condyle of left tibia** Q
- **S82.123 Displaced fracture of lateral condyle of unspecified tibia** Q
- **S82.124 Nondisplaced fracture of lateral condyle of right tibia** Q
- **S82.125 Nondisplaced fracture of lateral condyle of left tibia** Q
- **S82.126 Nondisplaced fracture of lateral condyle of unspecified tibia** Q

**S82.13 Fracture of medial condyle of tibia**
- **S82.131 Displaced fracture of medial condyle of right tibia** Q

Chapter 19. Injury, Poisoning and Certain Other Consequences of External Causes

S82–S82.131

S82.132 Displaced fracture of medial condyle of left tibia
S82.133 Displaced fracture of medial condyle of unspecified tibia
S82.134 Nondisplaced fracture of medial condyle of right tibia
S82.135 Nondisplaced fracture of medial condyle of left tibia
S82.136 Nondisplaced fracture of medial condyle of unspecified tibia

S82.14 Bicondylar fracture of tibia
Fracture of tibial plateau NOS
S82.141 Displaced bicondylar fracture of right tibia
S82.142 Displaced bicondylar fracture of left tibia
S82.143 Displaced bicondylar fracture of unspecified tibia
S82.144 Nondisplaced bicondylar fracture of right tibia
S82.145 Nondisplaced bicondylar fracture of left tibia
S82.146 Nondisplaced bicondylar fracture of unspecified tibia

S82.15 Fracture of tibial tuberosity
S82.151 Displaced fracture of right tibial tuberosity
S82.152 Displaced fracture of left tibial tuberosity
S82.153 Displaced fracture of unspecified tibial tuberosity
S82.154 Nondisplaced fracture of right tibial tuberosity
S82.155 Nondisplaced fracture of left tibial tuberosity
S82.156 Nondisplaced fracture of unspecified tibial tuberosity

S82.16 Torus fracture of upper end of tibia

The appropriate 7th character is to be added to all codes in subcategory S82.16.
- A initial encounter for closed fracture
- D subsequent encounter for fracture with routine healing
- G subsequent encounter for fracture with delayed healing
- K subsequent encounter for fracture with nonunion
- P subsequent encounter for fracture with malunion
- S sequela

S82.161 Torus fracture of upper end of right tibia
S82.162 Torus fracture of upper end of left tibia
S82.169 Torus fracture of upper end of unspecified tibia

S82.19 Other fracture of upper end of tibia
S82.191 Other fracture of upper end of right tibia
S82.192 Other fracture of upper end of left tibia
S82.199 Other fracture of upper end of unspecified tibia

S82.2 Fracture of shaft of tibia

S82.20 Unspecified fracture of shaft of tibia
Fracture of tibia NOS
S82.201 Unspecified fracture of shaft of right tibia
S82.202 Unspecified fracture of shaft of left tibia
S82.209 Unspecified fracture of shaft of unspecified tibia

S82.22 Transverse fracture of shaft of tibia
S82.221 Displaced transverse fracture of shaft of right tibia
S82.222 Displaced transverse fracture of shaft of left tibia
S82.223 Displaced transverse fracture of shaft of unspecified tibia
S82.224 Nondisplaced transverse fracture of shaft of right tibia
S82.225 Nondisplaced transverse fracture of shaft of left tibia
S82.226 Nondisplaced transverse fracture of shaft of unspecified tibia

S82.23 Oblique fracture of shaft of tibia
S82.231 Displaced oblique fracture of shaft of right tibia
S82.232 Displaced oblique fracture of shaft of left tibia
S82.233 Displaced oblique fracture of shaft of unspecified tibia
S82.234 Nondisplaced oblique fracture of shaft of right tibia
S82.235 Nondisplaced oblique fracture of shaft of left tibia
S82.236 Nondisplaced oblique fracture of shaft of unspecified tibia

S82.24 Spiral fracture of shaft of tibia
Toddler fracture
S82.241 Displaced spiral fracture of shaft of right tibia
S82.242 Displaced spiral fracture of shaft of left tibia
S82.243 Displaced spiral fracture of shaft of unspecified tibia
S82.244 Nondisplaced spiral fracture of shaft of right tibia
S82.245 Nondisplaced spiral fracture of shaft of left tibia
S82.246 Nondisplaced spiral fracture of shaft of unspecified tibia

S82.25 Comminuted fracture of shaft of tibia
S82.251 Displaced comminuted fracture of shaft of right tibia
S82.252 Displaced comminuted fracture of shaft of left tibia
S82.253 Displaced comminuted fracture of shaft of unspecified tibia
S82.254 Nondisplaced comminuted fracture of shaft of right tibia
S82.255 Nondisplaced comminuted fracture of shaft of left tibia
S82.256 Nondisplaced comminuted fracture of shaft of unspecified tibia

S82.26 Segmental fracture of shaft of tibia
S82.261 Displaced segmental fracture of shaft of right tibia
S82.262 Displaced segmental fracture of shaft of left tibia
S82.263 Displaced segmental fracture of shaft of unspecified tibia
S82.264 Nondisplaced segmental fracture of shaft of right tibia
S82.265 Nondisplaced segmental fracture of shaft of left tibia
S82.266 Nondisplaced segmental fracture of shaft of unspecified tibia

S82.29 Other fracture of shaft of tibia
S82.291 Other fracture of shaft of right tibia
S82.292 Other fracture of shaft of left tibia
S82.299 Other fracture of shaft of unspecified tibia

S82.3 Fracture of lower end of tibia

EXCLUDES 1 *bimalleolar fracture of lower leg (S82.84-)*
*fracture of medial malleolus alone (S82.5-)*
*Maisonneuve's fracture (S82.86-)*
*pilon fracture of distal tibia (S82.87-)*
*trimalleolar fractures of lower leg (S82.85-)*

S82.30 Unspecified fracture of lower end of tibia
S82.301 Unspecified fracture of lower end of right tibia
S82.302 Unspecified fracture of lower end of left tibia
S82.309 Unspecified fracture of lower end of unspecified tibia

✓6th S82.31 Torus fracture of lower end of tibia

The appropriate 7th character is to be added to all codes in subcategory S82.31.
A initial encounter for closed fracture
D subsequent encounter for fracture with routine healing
G subsequent encounter for fracture with delayed healing
K subsequent encounter for fracture with nonunion
P subsequent encounter for fracture with malunion
S sequela

✓7th S82.311 Torus fracture of lower end of right tibia Q
✓7th S82.312 Torus fracture of lower end of left tibia Q
✓7th S82.319 Torus fracture of lower end of unspecified tibia Q

✓6th S82.39 Other fracture of lower end of tibia
AHA: 2015,1Q,25
✓7th S82.391 Other fracture of lower end of right tibia Q
✓7th S82.392 Other fracture of lower end of left tibia Q
✓7th S82.399 Other fracture of lower end of unspecified tibia Q

✓5th S82.4 Fracture of shaft of fibula
EXCLUDES 2 *fracture of lateral malleolus alone (S82.6-)*

✓6th S82.40 Unspecified fracture of shaft of fibula
✓7th S82.401 Unspecified fracture of shaft of right fibula Q
✓7th S82.402 Unspecified fracture of shaft of left fibula Q
✓7th S82.409 Unspecified fracture of shaft of unspecified fibula Q

✓6th S82.42 Transverse fracture of shaft of fibula
✓7th S82.421 Displaced transverse fracture of shaft of right fibula Q
✓7th S82.422 Displaced transverse fracture of shaft of left fibula Q
✓7th S82.423 Displaced transverse fracture of shaft of unspecified fibula Q
✓7th S82.424 Nondisplaced transverse fracture of shaft of right fibula Q
✓7th S82.425 Nondisplaced transverse fracture of shaft of left fibula Q
✓7th S82.426 Nondisplaced transverse fracture of shaft of unspecified fibula Q

✓6th S82.43 Oblique fracture of shaft of fibula
✓7th S82.431 Displaced oblique fracture of shaft of right fibula Q
✓7th S82.432 Displaced oblique fracture of shaft of left fibula Q
✓7th S82.433 Displaced oblique fracture of shaft of unspecified fibula Q
✓7th S82.434 Nondisplaced oblique fracture of shaft of right fibula Q
✓7th S82.435 Nondisplaced oblique fracture of shaft of left fibula Q
✓7th S82.436 Nondisplaced oblique fracture of shaft of unspecified fibula Q

✓6th S82.44 Spiral fracture of shaft of fibula
✓7th S82.441 Displaced spiral fracture of shaft of right fibula Q
✓7th S82.442 Displaced spiral fracture of shaft of left fibula Q
✓7th S82.443 Displaced spiral fracture of shaft of unspecified fibula Q
✓7th S82.444 Nondisplaced spiral fracture of shaft of right fibula Q
✓7th S82.445 Nondisplaced spiral fracture of shaft of left fibula Q
✓7th S82.446 Nondisplaced spiral fracture of shaft of unspecified fibula Q

✓6th S82.45 Comminuted fracture of shaft of fibula
✓7th S82.451 Displaced comminuted fracture of shaft of right fibula Q
✓7th S82.452 Displaced comminuted fracture of shaft of left fibula Q
✓7th S82.453 Displaced comminuted fracture of shaft of unspecified fibula Q
✓7th S82.454 Nondisplaced comminuted fracture of shaft of right fibula Q
✓7th S82.455 Nondisplaced comminuted fracture of shaft of left fibula Q
✓7th S82.456 Nondisplaced comminuted fracture of shaft of unspecified fibula Q

✓6th S82.46 Segmental fracture of shaft of fibula
✓7th S82.461 Displaced segmental fracture of shaft of right fibula Q
✓7th S82.462 Displaced segmental fracture of shaft of left fibula Q
✓7th S82.463 Displaced segmental fracture of shaft of unspecified fibula Q
✓7th S82.464 Nondisplaced segmental fracture of shaft of right fibula Q
✓7th S82.465 Nondisplaced segmental fracture of shaft of left fibula Q
✓7th S82.466 Nondisplaced segmental fracture of shaft of unspecified fibula Q

✓6th S82.49 Other fracture of shaft of fibula
✓7th S82.491 Other fracture of shaft of right fibula Q
✓7th S82.492 Other fracture of shaft of left fibula Q
✓7th S82.499 Other fracture of shaft of unspecified fibula Q

✓5th S82.5 Fracture of medial malleolus
EXCLUDES 1 *pilon fracture of distal tibia (S82.87-)*
*Salter-Harris type III of lower end of tibia (S89.13-)*
*Salter-Harris type IV of lower end of tibia (S89.14-)*

✓x7th S82.51 Displaced fracture of medial malleolus of right tibia Q
✓x7th S82.52 Displaced fracture of medial malleolus of left tibia Q
✓x7th S82.53 Displaced fracture of medial malleolus of unspecified tibia Q
✓x7th S82.54 Nondisplaced fracture of medial malleolus of right tibia Q
✓x7th S82.55 Nondisplaced fracture of medial malleolus of left tibia Q
✓x7th S82.56 Nondisplaced fracture of medial malleolus of unspecified tibia Q

✓5th S82.6 Fracture of lateral malleolus
EXCLUDES 1 *pilon fracture of distal tibia (S82.87-)*

✓x7th S82.61 Displaced fracture of lateral malleolus of right fibula Q
✓x7th S82.62 Displaced fracture of lateral malleolus of left fibula Q
✓x7th S82.63 Displaced fracture of lateral malleolus of unspecified fibula Q
✓x7th S82.64 Nondisplaced fracture of lateral malleolus of right fibula Q
✓x7th S82.65 Nondisplaced fracture of lateral malleolus of left fibula Q
✓x7th S82.66 Nondisplaced fracture of lateral malleolus of unspecified fibula Q

✓5th S82.8 Other fractures of lower leg

✓6th S82.81 Torus fracture of upper end of fibula

The appropriate 7th character is to be added to all codes in subcategory S82.81
A initial encounter for closed fracture
D subsequent encounter for fracture with routine healing
G subsequent encounter for fracture with delayed healing
K subsequent encounter for fracture with nonunion
P subsequent encounter for fracture with malunion
S sequela

✓7th S82.811 Torus fracture of upper end of right fibula Q
✓7th S82.812 Torus fracture of upper end of left fibula Q
✓7th S82.819 Torus fracture of upper end of unspecified fibula Q

✓6th **S82.82 Torus fracture of lower end of fibula**

The appropriate 7th character is to be added to all codes in subcategory S82.82.
- A initial encounter for closed fracture
- D subsequent encounter for fracture with routine healing
- G subsequent encounter for fracture with delayed healing
- K subsequent encounter for fracture with nonunion
- P subsequent encounter for fracture with malunion
- S sequela

✓7th **S82.821 Torus fracture of lower end of right fibula** Q
✓7th **S82.822 Torus fracture of lower end of left fibula** Q
✓7th **S82.829 Torus fracture of lower end of unspecified fibula** Q

✓6th **S82.83 Other fracture of upper and lower end of fibula**

AHA: 2015,1Q,25

✓7th **S82.831 Other fracture of upper and lower end of right fibula** Q
✓7th **S82.832 Other fracture of upper and lower end of left fibula** Q
✓7th **S82.839 Other fracture of upper and lower end of unspecified fibula** Q

✓6th **S82.84 Bimalleolar fracture of lower leg**

**Right Bimalleolar Fracture**

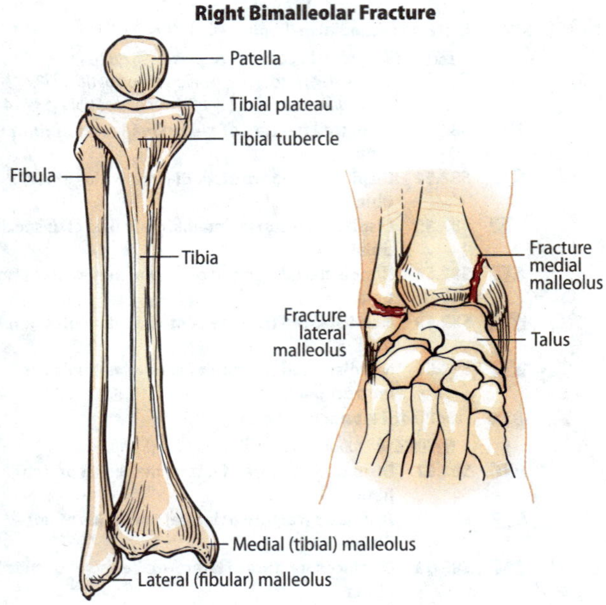


✓7th **S82.841 Displaced bimalleolar fracture of right lower leg** Q
✓7th **S82.842 Displaced bimalleolar fracture of left lower leg** Q
✓7th **S82.843 Displaced bimalleolar fracture of unspecified lower leg** Q
✓7th **S82.844 Nondisplaced bimalleolar fracture of right lower leg** Q
✓7th **S82.845 Nondisplaced bimalleolar fracture of left lower leg** Q
✓7th **S82.846 Nondisplaced bimalleolar fracture of unspecified lower leg** Q

✓6th **S82.85 Trimalleolar fracture of lower leg**

✓7th **S82.851 Displaced trimalleolar fracture of right lower leg** Q
✓7th **S82.852 Displaced trimalleolar fracture of left lower leg** Q
✓7th **S82.853 Displaced trimalleolar fracture of unspecified lower leg** Q
✓7th **S82.854 Nondisplaced trimalleolar fracture of right lower leg** Q
✓7th **S82.855 Nondisplaced trimalleolar fracture of left lower leg** Q
✓7th **S82.856 Nondisplaced trimalleolar fracture of unspecified lower leg** Q

✓6th **S82.86 Maisonneuve's fracture**

✓7th **S82.861 Displaced Maisonneuve's fracture of right leg** Q
✓7th **S82.862 Displaced Maisonneuve's fracture of left leg** Q
✓7th **S82.863 Displaced Maisonneuve's fracture of unspecified leg** Q
✓7th **S82.864 Nondisplaced Maisonneuve's fracture of right leg** Q
✓7th **S82.865 Nondisplaced Maisonneuve's fracture of left leg** Q
✓7th **S82.866 Nondisplaced Maisonneuve's fracture of unspecified leg** Q

✓6th **S82.87 Pilon fracture of tibia**

✓7th **S82.871 Displaced pilon fracture of right tibia** Q
✓7th **S82.872 Displaced pilon fracture of left tibia** Q
✓7th **S82.873 Displaced pilon fracture of unspecified tibia** Q
✓7th **S82.874 Nondisplaced pilon fracture of right tibia** Q
✓7th **S82.875 Nondisplaced pilon fracture of left tibia** Q
✓7th **S82.876 Nondisplaced pilon fracture of unspecified tibia** Q

✓6th **S82.89 Other fractures of lower leg**

Fracture of ankle NOS

✓7th **S82.891 Other fracture of right lower leg** Q
✓7th **S82.892 Other fracture of left lower leg** Q
✓7th **S82.899 Other fracture of unspecified lower leg** Q

✓5th **S82.9 Unspecified fracture of lower leg**

✓x7th **S82.9Ø Unspecified fracture of unspecified lower leg** Q
✓x7th **S82.91 Unspecified fracture of right lower leg** Q
✓x7th **S82.92 Unspecified fracture of left lower leg** Q

✓4th **S83 Dislocation and sprain of joints and ligaments of knee**

INCLUDES avulsion of joint or ligament of knee
laceration of cartilage, joint or ligament of knee
sprain of cartilage, joint or ligament of knee
traumatic hemarthrosis of joint or ligament of knee
traumatic rupture of joint or ligament of knee
traumatic subluxation of joint or ligament of knee
traumatic tear of joint or ligament of knee

Code also any associated open wound

EXCLUDES 2 *derangement of patella (M22.Ø-M22.3)*
*injury of patellar ligament (tendon) (S76.1-)*
*internal derangement of knee (M23.-)*
*old dislocation of knee (M24.36)*
*pathological dislocation of knee (M24.36)*
*recurrent dislocation of knee (M22.Ø)*
*strain of muscle, fascia and tendon of lower leg (S86.-)*

The appropriate 7th character is to be added to each code from category S83.
- A initial encounter
- D subsequent encounter
- S sequela

✓5th **S83.Ø Subluxation and dislocation of patella**

✓6th **S83.ØØ Unspecified subluxation and dislocation of patella**

✓7th **S83.ØØ1 Unspecified subluxation of right patella**
✓7th **S83.ØØ2 Unspecified subluxation of left patella**
✓7th **S83.ØØ3 Unspecified subluxation of unspecified patella**
✓7th **S83.ØØ4 Unspecified dislocation of right patella**
✓7th **S83.ØØ5 Unspecified dislocation of left patella**
✓7th **S83.ØØ6 Unspecified dislocation of unspecified patella**

✓6th **S83.Ø1 Lateral subluxation and dislocation of patella**

✓7th **S83.Ø11 Lateral subluxation of right patella**
✓7th **S83.Ø12 Lateral subluxation of left patella**
✓7th **S83.Ø13 Lateral subluxation of unspecified patella**
✓7th **S83.Ø14 Lateral dislocation of right patella**
✓7th **S83.Ø15 Lateral dislocation of left patella**
✓7th **S83.Ø16 Lateral dislocation of unspecified patella**

✓6th **S83.Ø9 Other subluxation and dislocation of patella**

✓7th **S83.Ø91 Other subluxation of right patella**

S83.092 Other subluxation of left patella
S83.093 Other subluxation of unspecified patella
S83.094 Other dislocation of right patella
S83.095 Other dislocation of left patella
S83.096 Other dislocation of unspecified patella

S83.1 Subluxation and dislocation of knee
EXCLUDES 2 *instability of knee prosthesis (T84.022, T84.023)*

S83.10 Unspecified subluxation and dislocation of knee
S83.101 Unspecified subluxation of right knee
S83.102 Unspecified subluxation of left knee
S83.103 Unspecified subluxation of unspecified knee
S83.104 Unspecified dislocation of right knee
S83.105 Unspecified dislocation of left knee
S83.106 Unspecified dislocation of unspecified knee

S83.11 Anterior subluxation and dislocation of proximal end of tibia
Posterior subluxation and dislocation of distal end of femur
S83.111 Anterior subluxation of proximal end of tibia, right knee
S83.112 Anterior subluxation of proximal end of tibia, left knee
S83.113 Anterior subluxation of proximal end of tibia, unspecified knee
S83.114 Anterior dislocation of proximal end of tibia, right knee
S83.115 Anterior dislocation of proximal end of tibia, left knee
S83.116 Anterior dislocation of proximal end of tibia, unspecified knee

S83.12 Posterior subluxation and dislocation of proximal end of tibia
Anterior dislocation of distal end of femur
S83.121 Posterior subluxation of proximal end of tibia, right knee
S83.122 Posterior subluxation of proximal end of tibia, left knee
S83.123 Posterior subluxation of proximal end of tibia, unspecified knee
S83.124 Posterior dislocation of proximal end of tibia, right knee
S83.125 Posterior dislocation of proximal end of tibia, left knee
S83.126 Posterior dislocation of proximal end of tibia, unspecified knee

S83.13 Medial subluxation and dislocation of proximal end of tibia
S83.131 Medial subluxation of proximal end of tibia, right knee
S83.132 Medial subluxation of proximal end of tibia, left knee
S83.133 Medial subluxation of proximal end of tibia, unspecified knee
S83.134 Medial dislocation of proximal end of tibia, right knee
S83.135 Medial dislocation of proximal end of tibia, left knee
S83.136 Medial dislocation of proximal end of tibia, unspecified knee

S83.14 Lateral subluxation and dislocation of proximal end of tibia
S83.141 Lateral subluxation of proximal end of tibia, right knee
S83.142 Lateral subluxation of proximal end of tibia, left knee
S83.143 Lateral subluxation of proximal end of tibia, unspecified knee
S83.144 Lateral dislocation of proximal end of tibia, right knee
S83.145 Lateral dislocation of proximal end of tibia, left knee
S83.146 Lateral dislocation of proximal end of tibia, unspecified knee

S83.19 Other subluxation and dislocation of knee
S83.191 Other subluxation of right knee
S83.192 Other subluxation of left knee
S83.193 Other subluxation of unspecified knee
S83.194 Other dislocation of right knee
S83.195 Other dislocation of left knee
S83.196 Other dislocation of unspecified knee

S83.2 Tear of meniscus, current injury
EXCLUDES 1 *old bucket-handle tear (M23.2)*
AHA: 2019,2Q,26

S83.20 Tear of unspecified meniscus, current injury
Tear of meniscus of knee NOS
S83.200 Bucket-handle tear of unspecified meniscus, current injury, right knee
S83.201 Bucket-handle tear of unspecified meniscus, current injury, left knee
S83.202 Bucket-handle tear of unspecified meniscus, current injury, unspecified knee
S83.203 Other tear of unspecified meniscus, current injury, right knee
S83.204 Other tear of unspecified meniscus, current injury, left knee
S83.205 Other tear of unspecified meniscus, current injury, unspecified knee
S83.206 Unspecified tear of unspecified meniscus, current injury, right knee
S83.207 Unspecified tear of unspecified meniscus, current injury, left knee
S83.209 Unspecified tear of unspecified meniscus, current injury, unspecified knee

S83.21 Bucket-handle tear of medial meniscus, current injury
S83.211 Bucket-handle tear of medial meniscus, current injury, right knee
S83.212 Bucket-handle tear of medial meniscus, current injury, left knee
S83.219 Bucket-handle tear of medial meniscus, current injury, unspecified knee

S83.22 Peripheral tear of medial meniscus, current injury
S83.221 Peripheral tear of medial meniscus, current injury, right knee
S83.222 Peripheral tear of medial meniscus, current injury, left knee
S83.229 Peripheral tear of medial meniscus, current injury, unspecified knee

S83.23 Complex tear of medial meniscus, current injury
S83.231 Complex tear of medial meniscus, current injury, right knee
S83.232 Complex tear of medial meniscus, current injury, left knee
S83.239 Complex tear of medial meniscus, current injury, unspecified knee

S83.24 Other tear of medial meniscus, current injury
S83.241 Other tear of medial meniscus, current injury, right knee
S83.242 Other tear of medial meniscus, current injury, left knee
S83.249 Other tear of medial meniscus, current injury, unspecified knee

S83.25 Bucket-handle tear of lateral meniscus, current injury
S83.251 Bucket-handle tear of lateral meniscus, current injury, right knee
S83.252 Bucket-handle tear of lateral meniscus, current injury, left knee
S83.259 Bucket-handle tear of lateral meniscus, current injury, unspecified knee

S83.26 Peripheral tear of lateral meniscus, current injury
S83.261 Peripheral tear of lateral meniscus, current injury, right knee
S83.262 Peripheral tear of lateral meniscus, current injury, left knee
S83.269 Peripheral tear of lateral meniscus, current injury, unspecified knee

S83.27 Complex tear of lateral meniscus, current injury
S83.271 Complex tear of lateral meniscus, current injury, right knee
S83.272 Complex tear of lateral meniscus, current injury, left knee
S83.279 Complex tear of lateral meniscus, current injury, unspecified knee

S83.28 Other tear of lateral meniscus, current injury
S83.281 Other tear of lateral meniscus, current injury, right knee
S83.282 Other tear of lateral meniscus, current injury, left knee

7th S83.289 Other tear of lateral meniscus, current injury, unspecified knee

5th S83.3 Tear of articular cartilage of knee, current

x7th S83.30 Tear of articular cartilage of unspecified knee, current
x7th S83.31 Tear of articular cartilage of right knee, current
x7th S83.32 Tear of articular cartilage of left knee, current

5th S83.4 Sprain of collateral ligament of knee

6th S83.40 Sprain of unspecified collateral ligament of knee
7th S83.401 Sprain of unspecified collateral ligament of right knee
7th S83.402 Sprain of unspecified collateral ligament of left knee
7th S83.409 Sprain of unspecified collateral ligament of unspecified knee

6th S83.41 Sprain of medial collateral ligament of knee
Sprain of tibial collateral ligament
7th S83.411 Sprain of medial collateral ligament of right knee
7th S83.412 Sprain of medial collateral ligament of left knee
7th S83.419 Sprain of medial collateral ligament of unspecified knee

6th S83.42 Sprain of lateral collateral ligament of knee
Sprain of fibular collateral ligament
7th S83.421 Sprain of lateral collateral ligament of right knee
7th S83.422 Sprain of lateral collateral ligament of left knee
7th S83.429 Sprain of lateral collateral ligament of unspecified knee

5th S83.5 Sprain of cruciate ligament of knee
AHA: 2016,2Q,3

6th S83.50 Sprain of unspecified cruciate ligament of knee
7th S83.501 Sprain of unspecified cruciate ligament of right knee
7th S83.502 Sprain of unspecified cruciate ligament of left knee
7th S83.509 Sprain of unspecified cruciate ligament of unspecified knee

6th S83.51 Sprain of anterior cruciate ligament of knee
7th S83.511 Sprain of anterior cruciate ligament of right knee
7th S83.512 Sprain of anterior cruciate ligament of left knee
7th S83.519 Sprain of anterior cruciate ligament of unspecified knee

6th S83.52 Sprain of posterior cruciate ligament of knee
7th S83.521 Sprain of posterior cruciate ligament of right knee
7th S83.522 Sprain of posterior cruciate ligament of left knee
7th S83.529 Sprain of posterior cruciate ligament of unspecified knee

5th S83.6 Sprain of the superior tibiofibular joint and ligament

x7th S83.60 Sprain of the superior tibiofibular joint and ligament, unspecified knee
x7th S83.61 Sprain of the superior tibiofibular joint and ligament, right knee
x7th S83.62 Sprain of the superior tibiofibular joint and ligament, left knee

5th S83.8 Sprain of other specified parts of knee

6th S83.8X Sprain of other specified parts of knee
7th S83.8X1 Sprain of other specified parts of right knee
7th S83.8X2 Sprain of other specified parts of left knee
7th S83.8X9 Sprain of other specified parts of unspecified knee

5th S83.9 Sprain of unspecified site of knee

x7th S83.90 Sprain of unspecified site of unspecified knee
x7th S83.91 Sprain of unspecified site of right knee
x7th S83.92 Sprain of unspecified site of left knee

4th S84 Injury of nerves at lower leg level

Code also any associated open wound (S81.-)

EXCLUDES 2 *injury of nerves at ankle and foot level (S94.-)*

The appropriate 7th character is to be added to each code from category S84.
A initial encounter
D subsequent encounter
S sequela

5th S84.0 Injury of tibial nerve at lower leg level

x7th S84.00 Injury of tibial nerve at lower leg level, unspecified leg
x7th S84.01 Injury of tibial nerve at lower leg level, right leg
x7th S84.02 Injury of tibial nerve at lower leg level, left leg

5th S84.1 Injury of peroneal nerve at lower leg level

x7th S84.10 Injury of peroneal nerve at lower leg level, unspecified leg
x7th S84.11 Injury of peroneal nerve at lower leg level, right leg
x7th S84.12 Injury of peroneal nerve at lower leg level, left leg

5th S84.2 Injury of cutaneous sensory nerve at lower leg level

x7th S84.20 Injury of cutaneous sensory nerve at lower leg level, unspecified leg
x7th S84.21 Injury of cutaneous sensory nerve at lower leg level, right leg
x7th S84.22 Injury of cutaneous sensory nerve at lower leg level, left leg

5th S84.8 Injury of other nerves at lower leg level

6th S84.80 Injury of other nerves at lower leg level
7th S84.801 Injury of other nerves at lower leg level, right leg
7th S84.802 Injury of other nerves at lower leg level, left leg
7th S84.809 Injury of other nerves at lower leg level, unspecified leg

5th S84.9 Injury of unspecified nerve at lower leg level

x7th S84.90 Injury of unspecified nerve at lower leg level, unspecified leg
x7th S84.91 Injury of unspecified nerve at lower leg level, right leg
x7th S84.92 Injury of unspecified nerve at lower leg level, left leg

4th S85 Injury of blood vessels at lower leg level

Code also any associated open wound (S81.-)

EXCLUDES 2 *injury of blood vessels at ankle and foot level (S95.-)*

The appropriate 7th character is to be added to each code from category S85.
A initial encounter
D subsequent encounter
S sequela

5th S85.0 Injury of popliteal artery

6th S85.00 Unspecified injury of popliteal artery
7th S85.001 Unspecified injury of popliteal artery, right leg
7th S85.002 Unspecified injury of popliteal artery, left leg
7th S85.009 Unspecified injury of popliteal artery, unspecified leg

6th S85.01 Laceration of popliteal artery
7th S85.011 Laceration of popliteal artery, right leg
7th S85.012 Laceration of popliteal artery, left leg
7th S85.019 Laceration of popliteal artery, unspecified leg

6th S85.09 Other specified injury of popliteal artery
7th S85.091 Other specified injury of popliteal artery, right leg
7th S85.092 Other specified injury of popliteal artery, left leg
7th S85.099 Other specified injury of popliteal artery, unspecified leg

5th S85.1 Injury of tibial artery

6th S85.10 Unspecified injury of unspecified tibial artery
Injury of tibial artery NOS
7th S85.101 Unspecified injury of unspecified tibial artery, right leg
7th S85.102 Unspecified injury of unspecified tibial artery, left leg

S85.109 Unspecified injury of unspecified tibial artery, unspecified leg

S85.11 Laceration of unspecified tibial artery

S85.111 Laceration of unspecified tibial artery, right leg

S85.112 Laceration of unspecified tibial artery, left leg

S85.119 Laceration of unspecified tibial artery, unspecified leg

S85.12 Other specified injury of unspecified tibial artery

S85.121 Other specified injury of unspecified tibial artery, right leg

S85.122 Other specified injury of unspecified tibial artery, left leg

S85.129 Other specified injury of unspecified tibial artery, unspecified leg

S85.13 Unspecified injury of anterior tibial artery

S85.131 Unspecified injury of anterior tibial artery, right leg

S85.132 Unspecified injury of anterior tibial artery, left leg

S85.139 Unspecified injury of anterior tibial artery, unspecified leg

S85.14 Laceration of anterior tibial artery

S85.141 Laceration of anterior tibial artery, right leg

S85.142 Laceration of anterior tibial artery, left leg

S85.149 Laceration of anterior tibial artery, unspecified leg

S85.15 Other specified injury of anterior tibial artery

S85.151 Other specified injury of anterior tibial artery, right leg

S85.152 Other specified injury of anterior tibial artery, left leg

S85.159 Other specified injury of anterior tibial artery, unspecified leg

S85.16 Unspecified injury of posterior tibial artery

S85.161 Unspecified injury of posterior tibial artery, right leg

S85.162 Unspecified injury of posterior tibial artery, left leg

S85.169 Unspecified injury of posterior tibial artery, unspecified leg

S85.17 Laceration of posterior tibial artery

S85.171 Laceration of posterior tibial artery, right leg

S85.172 Laceration of posterior tibial artery, left leg

S85.179 Laceration of posterior tibial artery, unspecified leg

S85.18 Other specified injury of posterior tibial artery

S85.181 Other specified injury of posterior tibial artery, right leg

S85.182 Other specified injury of posterior tibial artery, left leg

S85.189 Other specified injury of posterior tibial artery, unspecified leg

S85.2 Injury of peroneal artery

S85.20 Unspecified injury of peroneal artery

S85.201 Unspecified injury of peroneal artery, right leg

S85.202 Unspecified injury of peroneal artery, left leg

S85.209 Unspecified injury of peroneal artery, unspecified leg

S85.21 Laceration of peroneal artery

S85.211 Laceration of peroneal artery, right leg

S85.212 Laceration of peroneal artery, left leg

S85.219 Laceration of peroneal artery, unspecified leg

S85.29 Other specified injury of peroneal artery

S85.291 Other specified injury of peroneal artery, right leg

S85.292 Other specified injury of peroneal artery, left leg

S85.299 Other specified injury of peroneal artery, unspecified leg

S85.3 Injury of greater saphenous vein at lower leg level

Injury of greater saphenous vein NOS

Injury of saphenous vein NOS

S85.30 Unspecified injury of greater saphenous vein at lower leg level

S85.301 Unspecified injury of greater saphenous vein at lower leg level, right leg

S85.302 Unspecified injury of greater saphenous vein at lower leg level, left leg

S85.309 Unspecified injury of greater saphenous vein at lower leg level, unspecified leg

S85.31 Laceration of greater saphenous vein at lower leg level

S85.311 Laceration of greater saphenous vein at lower leg level, right leg

S85.312 Laceration of greater saphenous vein at lower leg level, left leg

S85.319 Laceration of greater saphenous vein at lower leg level, unspecified leg

S85.39 Other specified injury of greater saphenous vein at lower leg level

S85.391 Other specified injury of greater saphenous vein at lower leg level, right leg

S85.392 Other specified injury of greater saphenous vein at lower leg level, left leg

S85.399 Other specified injury of greater saphenous vein at lower leg level, unspecified leg

S85.4 Injury of lesser saphenous vein at lower leg level

S85.40 Unspecified injury of lesser saphenous vein at lower leg level

S85.401 Unspecified injury of lesser saphenous vein at lower leg level, right leg

S85.402 Unspecified injury of lesser saphenous vein at lower leg level, left leg

S85.409 Unspecified injury of lesser saphenous vein at lower leg level, unspecified leg

S85.41 Laceration of lesser saphenous vein at lower leg level

S85.411 Laceration of lesser saphenous vein at lower leg level, right leg

S85.412 Laceration of lesser saphenous vein at lower leg level, left leg

S85.419 Laceration of lesser saphenous vein at lower leg level, unspecified leg

S85.49 Other specified injury of lesser saphenous vein at lower leg level

S85.491 Other specified injury of lesser saphenous vein at lower leg level, right leg

S85.492 Other specified injury of lesser saphenous vein at lower leg level, left leg

S85.499 Other specified injury of lesser saphenous vein at lower leg level, unspecified leg

S85.5 Injury of popliteal vein

S85.50 Unspecified injury of popliteal vein

S85.501 Unspecified injury of popliteal vein, right leg

S85.502 Unspecified injury of popliteal vein, left leg

S85.509 Unspecified injury of popliteal vein, unspecified leg

S85.51 Laceration of popliteal vein

S85.511 Laceration of popliteal vein, right leg

S85.512 Laceration of popliteal vein, left leg

S85.519 Laceration of popliteal vein, unspecified leg

S85.59 Other specified injury of popliteal vein

S85.591 Other specified injury of popliteal vein, right leg

S85.592 Other specified injury of popliteal vein, left leg

S85.599 Other specified injury of popliteal vein, unspecified leg

S85.8 Injury of other blood vessels at lower leg level

S85.80 Unspecified injury of other blood vessels at lower leg level

S85.801 Unspecified injury of other blood vessels at lower leg level, right leg

S85.802 Unspecified injury of other blood vessels at lower leg level, left leg

S85.809 Unspecified injury of other blood vessels at lower leg level, unspecified leg

√6th S85.81 Laceration of other blood vessels at lower leg level
√7th S85.811 Laceration of other blood vessels at lower leg level, right leg
√7th S85.812 Laceration of other blood vessels at lower leg level, left leg
√7th S85.819 Laceration of other blood vessels at lower leg level, unspecified leg
√6th S85.89 Other specified injury of other blood vessels at lower leg level
√7th S85.891 Other specified injury of other blood vessels at lower leg level, right leg
√7th S85.892 Other specified injury of other blood vessels at lower leg level, left leg
√7th S85.899 Other specified injury of other blood vessels at lower leg level, unspecified leg
√5th S85.9 Injury of unspecified blood vessel at lower leg level
√6th S85.90 Unspecified injury of unspecified blood vessel at lower leg level
√7th S85.901 Unspecified injury of unspecified blood vessel at lower leg level, right leg
√7th S85.902 Unspecified injury of unspecified blood vessel at lower leg level, left leg
√7th S85.909 Unspecified injury of unspecified blood vessel at lower leg level, unspecified leg
√6th S85.91 Laceration of unspecified blood vessel at lower leg level
√7th S85.911 Laceration of unspecified blood vessel at lower leg level, right leg
√7th S85.912 Laceration of unspecified blood vessel at lower leg level, left leg
√7th S85.919 Laceration of unspecified blood vessel at lower leg level, unspecified leg
√6th S85.99 Other specified injury of unspecified blood vessel at lower leg level
√7th S85.991 Other specified injury of unspecified blood vessel at lower leg level, right leg
√7th S85.992 Other specified injury of unspecified blood vessel at lower leg level, left leg
√7th S85.999 Other specified injury of unspecified blood vessel at lower leg level, unspecified leg

√4th **S86 Injury of muscle, fascia and tendon at lower leg level**

Code also any associated open wound (S81.-)

EXCLUDES 2 *injury of muscle, fascia and tendon at ankle (S96.-)*
*injury of patellar ligament (tendon) (S76.1-)*
*sprain of joints and ligaments of knee (S83.-)*

**TIP:** Refer to the Muscle/Tendon table at the beginning of this chapter.

The appropriate 7th character is to be added to each code from category S86.
A initial encounter
D subsequent encounter
S sequela

√5th S86.0 Injury of Achilles tendon
√6th S86.00 Unspecified injury of Achilles tendon
√7th S86.001 Unspecified injury of right Achilles tendon
√7th S86.002 Unspecified injury of left Achilles tendon
√7th S86.009 Unspecified injury of unspecified Achilles tendon
√6th S86.01 Strain of Achilles tendon
√7th S86.011 Strain of right Achilles tendon
√7th S86.012 Strain of left Achilles tendon
√7th S86.019 Strain of unspecified Achilles tendon
√6th S86.02 Laceration of Achilles tendon
√7th S86.021 Laceration of right Achilles tendon
√7th S86.022 Laceration of left Achilles tendon
√7th S86.029 Laceration of unspecified Achilles tendon
√6th S86.09 Other specified injury of Achilles tendon
√7th S86.091 Other specified injury of right Achilles tendon
√7th S86.092 Other specified injury of left Achilles tendon
√7th S86.099 Other specified injury of unspecified Achilles tendon

√5th S86.1 Injury of other muscle(s) and tendon(s) of posterior muscle group at lower leg level
√6th S86.10 Unspecified injury of other muscle(s) and tendon(s) of posterior muscle group at lower leg level
√7th S86.101 Unspecified injury of other muscle(s) and tendon(s) of posterior muscle group at lower leg level, right leg
√7th S86.102 Unspecified injury of other muscle(s) and tendon(s) of posterior muscle group at lower leg level, left leg
√7th S86.109 Unspecified injury of other muscle(s) and tendon(s) of posterior muscle group at lower leg level, unspecified leg
√6th S86.11 Strain of other muscle(s) and tendon(s) of posterior muscle group at lower leg level
√7th S86.111 Strain of other muscle(s) and tendon(s) of posterior muscle group at lower leg level, right leg
√7th S86.112 Strain of other muscle(s) and tendon(s) of posterior muscle group at lower leg level, left leg
√7th S86.119 Strain of other muscle(s) and tendon(s) of posterior muscle group at lower leg level, unspecified leg
√6th S86.12 Laceration of other muscle(s) and tendon(s) of posterior muscle group at lower leg level
√7th S86.121 Laceration of other muscle(s) and tendon(s) of posterior muscle group at lower leg level, right leg
√7th S86.122 Laceration of other muscle(s) and tendon(s) of posterior muscle group at lower leg level, left leg
√7th S86.129 Laceration of other muscle(s) and tendon(s) of posterior muscle group at lower leg level, unspecified leg
√6th S86.19 Other injury of other muscle(s) and tendon(s) of posterior muscle group at lower leg level
√7th S86.191 Other injury of other muscle(s) and tendon(s) of posterior muscle group at lower leg level, right leg
√7th S86.192 Other injury of other muscle(s) and tendon(s) of posterior muscle group at lower leg level, left leg
√7th S86.199 Other injury of other muscle(s) and tendon(s) of posterior muscle group at lower leg level, unspecified leg
√5th S86.2 Injury of muscle(s) and tendon(s) of anterior muscle group at lower leg level
√6th S86.20 Unspecified injury of muscle(s) and tendon(s) of anterior muscle group at lower leg level
√7th S86.201 Unspecified injury of muscle(s) and tendon(s) of anterior muscle group at lower leg level, right leg
√7th S86.202 Unspecified injury of muscle(s) and tendon(s) of anterior muscle group at lower leg level, left leg
√7th S86.209 Unspecified injury of muscle(s) and tendon(s) of anterior muscle group at lower leg level, unspecified leg
√6th S86.21 Strain of muscle(s) and tendon(s) of anterior muscle group at lower leg level
√7th S86.211 Strain of muscle(s) and tendon(s) of anterior muscle group at lower leg level, right leg
√7th S86.212 Strain of muscle(s) and tendon(s) of anterior muscle group at lower leg level, left leg
√7th S86.219 Strain of muscle(s) and tendon(s) of anterior muscle group at lower leg level, unspecified leg
√6th S86.22 Laceration of muscle(s) and tendon(s) of anterior muscle group at lower leg level
√7th S86.221 Laceration of muscle(s) and tendon(s) of anterior muscle group at lower leg level, right leg
√7th S86.222 Laceration of muscle(s) and tendon(s) of anterior muscle group at lower leg level, left leg
√7th S86.229 Laceration of muscle(s) and tendon(s) of anterior muscle group at lower leg level, unspecified leg

√6th S86.29 Other injury of muscle(s) and tendon(s) of anterior muscle group at lower leg level
√7th S86.291 Other injury of muscle(s) and tendon(s) of anterior muscle group at lower leg level, right leg
√7th S86.292 Other injury of muscle(s) and tendon(s) of anterior muscle group at lower leg level, left leg
√7th S86.299 Other injury of muscle(s) and tendon(s) of anterior muscle group at lower leg level, unspecified leg
√5th S86.3 Injury of muscle(s) and tendon(s) of peroneal muscle group at lower leg level
√6th S86.3Ø Unspecified injury of muscle(s) and tendon(s) of peroneal muscle group at lower leg level
√7th S86.3Ø1 Unspecified injury of muscle(s) and tendon(s) of peroneal muscle group at lower leg level, right leg
√7th S86.3Ø2 Unspecified injury of muscle(s) and tendon(s) of peroneal muscle group at lower leg level, left leg
√7th S86.3Ø9 Unspecified injury of muscle(s) and tendon(s) of peroneal muscle group at lower leg level, unspecified leg
√6th S86.31 Strain of muscle(s) and tendon(s) of peroneal muscle group at lower leg level
√7th S86.311 Strain of muscle(s) and tendon(s) of peroneal muscle group at lower leg level, right leg
√7th S86.312 Strain of muscle(s) and tendon(s) of peroneal muscle group at lower leg level, left leg
√7th S86.319 Strain of muscle(s) and tendon(s) of peroneal muscle group at lower leg level, unspecified leg
√6th S86.32 Laceration of muscle(s) and tendon(s) of peroneal muscle group at lower leg level
√7th S86.321 Laceration of muscle(s) and tendon(s) of peroneal muscle group at lower leg level, right leg
√7th S86.322 Laceration of muscle(s) and tendon(s) of peroneal muscle group at lower leg level, left leg
√7th S86.329 Laceration of muscle(s) and tendon(s) of peroneal muscle group at lower leg level, unspecified leg
√6th S86.39 Other injury of muscle(s) and tendon(s) of peroneal muscle group at lower leg level
√7th S86.391 Other injury of muscle(s) and tendon(s) of peroneal muscle group at lower leg level, right leg
√7th S86.392 Other injury of muscle(s) and tendon(s) of peroneal muscle group at lower leg level, left leg
√7th S86.399 Other injury of muscle(s) and tendon(s) of peroneal muscle group at lower leg level, unspecified leg
√5th S86.8 Injury of other muscles and tendons at lower leg level
√6th S86.8Ø Unspecified injury of other muscles and tendons at lower leg level
√7th S86.8Ø1 Unspecified injury of other muscle(s) and tendon(s) at lower leg level, right leg
√7th S86.8Ø2 Unspecified injury of other muscle(s) and tendon(s) at lower leg level, left leg
√7th S86.8Ø9 Unspecified injury of other muscle(s) and tendon(s) at lower leg level, unspecified leg
√6th S86.81 Strain of other muscles and tendons at lower leg level
√7th S86.811 Strain of other muscle(s) and tendon(s) at lower leg level, right leg
√7th S86.812 Strain of other muscle(s) and tendon(s) at lower leg level, left leg
√7th S86.819 Strain of other muscle(s) and tendon(s) at lower leg level, unspecified leg
√6th S86.82 Laceration of other muscles and tendons at lower leg level
√7th S86.821 Laceration of other muscle(s) and tendon(s) at lower leg level, right leg
√7th S86.822 Laceration of other muscle(s) and tendon(s) at lower leg level, left leg
√7th S86.829 Laceration of other muscle(s) and tendon(s) at lower leg level, unspecified leg
√6th S86.89 Other injury of other muscles and tendons at lower leg level
√7th S86.891 Other injury of other muscle(s) and tendon(s) at lower leg level, right leg
√7th S86.892 Other injury of other muscle(s) and tendon(s) at lower leg level, left leg
√7th S86.899 Other injury of other muscle(s) and tendon(s) at lower leg level, unspecified leg
√5th S86.9 Injury of unspecified muscle and tendon at lower leg level
√6th S86.9Ø Unspecified injury of unspecified muscle and tendon at lower leg level
√7th S86.9Ø1 Unspecified injury of unspecified muscle(s) and tendon(s) at lower leg level, right leg
√7th S86.9Ø2 Unspecified injury of unspecified muscle(s) and tendon(s) at lower leg level, left leg
√7th S86.9Ø9 Unspecified injury of unspecified muscle(s) and tendon(s) at lower leg level, unspecified leg
√6th S86.91 Strain of unspecified muscle and tendon at lower leg level
√7th S86.911 Strain of unspecified muscle(s) and tendon(s) at lower leg level, right leg
√7th S86.912 Strain of unspecified muscle(s) and tendon(s) at lower leg level, left leg
√7th S86.919 Strain of unspecified muscle(s) and tendon(s) at lower leg level, unspecified leg
√6th S86.92 Laceration of unspecified muscle and tendon at lower leg level
√7th S86.921 Laceration of unspecified muscle(s) and tendon(s) at lower leg level, right leg
√7th S86.922 Laceration of unspecified muscle(s) and tendon(s) at lower leg level, left leg
√7th S86.929 Laceration of unspecified muscle(s) and tendon(s) at lower leg level, unspecified leg
√6th S86.99 Other injury of unspecified muscle and tendon at lower leg level
√7th S86.991 Other injury of unspecified muscle(s) and tendon(s) at lower leg level, right leg
√7th S86.992 Other injury of unspecified muscle(s) and tendon(s) at lower leg level, left leg
√7th S86.999 Other injury of unspecified muscle(s) and tendon(s) at lower leg level, unspecified leg

√4th **S87 Crushing injury of lower leg**
Use additional code(s) for all associated injuries
EXCLUDES 2 *crushing injury of ankle and foot (S97.-)*

The appropriate 7th character is to be added to each code from category S87.
A initial encounter
D subsequent encounter
S sequela

√5th S87.Ø Crushing injury of knee
√x7th S87.ØØ Crushing injury of unspecified knee
√x7th S87.Ø1 Crushing injury of right knee
√x7th S87.Ø2 Crushing injury of left knee
√5th S87.8 Crushing injury of lower leg
√x7th S87.8Ø Crushing injury of unspecified lower leg
√x7th S87.81 Crushing injury of right lower leg
√x7th S87.82 Crushing injury of left lower leg

√4th **S88 Traumatic amputation of lower leg**
An amputation not identified as partial or complete should be coded to complete
EXCLUDES 1 *traumatic amputation of ankle and foot (S98.-)*

The appropriate 7th character is to be added to each code from category S88.
A initial encounter
D subsequent encounter
S sequela

√5th S88.Ø Traumatic amputation at knee level
√6th S88.Ø1 Complete traumatic amputation at knee level
AHA: 2023,1Q,27,29
√7th S88.Ø11 Complete traumatic amputation at knee level, right lower leg HCC ESR COM

7th S88.012 Complete traumatic amputation at knee level, left lower leg HCC ESR COM
7th S88.019 Complete traumatic amputation at knee level, unspecified lower leg HCC ESR COM
6th S88.02 Partial traumatic amputation at knee level
7th S88.021 Partial traumatic amputation at knee level, right lower leg HCC ESR COM
7th S88.022 Partial traumatic amputation at knee level, left lower leg HCC ESR COM
7th S88.029 Partial traumatic amputation at knee level, unspecified lower leg HCC ESR COM
5th S88.1 Traumatic amputation at level between knee and ankle
6th S88.11 Complete traumatic amputation at level between knee and ankle
7th S88.111 Complete traumatic amputation at level between knee and ankle, right lower leg HCC ESR COM
7th S88.112 Complete traumatic amputation at level between knee and ankle, left lower leg HCC ESR COM
7th S88.119 Complete traumatic amputation at level between knee and ankle, unspecified lower leg HCC ESR COM
6th S88.12 Partial traumatic amputation at level between knee and ankle
7th S88.121 Partial traumatic amputation at level between knee and ankle, right lower leg HCC ESR COM
7th S88.122 Partial traumatic amputation at level between knee and ankle, left lower leg HCC ESR COM
7th S88.129 Partial traumatic amputation at level between knee and ankle, unspecified lower leg HCC ESR COM
5th S88.9 Traumatic amputation of lower leg, level unspecified
6th S88.91 Complete traumatic amputation of lower leg, level unspecified
7th S88.911 Complete traumatic amputation of right lower leg, level unspecified HCC ESR COM
7th S88.912 Complete traumatic amputation of left lower leg, level unspecified HCC ESR COM
7th S88.919 Complete traumatic amputation of unspecified lower leg, level unspecified HCC ESR COM
6th S88.92 Partial traumatic amputation of lower leg, level unspecified
7th S88.921 Partial traumatic amputation of right lower leg, level unspecified HCC ESR COM
7th S88.922 Partial traumatic amputation of left lower leg, level unspecified HCC ESR COM
7th S88.929 Partial traumatic amputation of unspecified lower leg, level unspecified HCC ESR COM

4th **S89 Other and unspecified injuries of lower leg**

NOTE A fracture not indicated as open or closed should be coded to closed.

EXCLUDES 2 *other and unspecified injuries of ankle and foot (S99.-)*

AHA: 2018,2Q,12; 2018,1Q,3; 2015,3Q,37-39

The appropriate 7th character is to be added to each code from subcategories S89.0, S89.1, S89.2, and S89.3.
- A initial encounter for closed fracture
- D subsequent encounter for fracture with routine healing
- G subsequent encounter for fracture with delayed healing
- K subsequent encounter for fracture with nonunion
- P subsequent encounter for fracture with malunion
- S sequela

5th S89.0 Physeal fracture of upper end of tibia
AHA: 2019,4Q,56
6th S89.00 Unspecified physeal fracture of upper end of tibia
7th S89.001 Unspecified physeal fracture of upper end of right tibia P
7th S89.002 Unspecified physeal fracture of upper end of left tibia P
7th S89.009 Unspecified physeal fracture of upper end of unspecified tibia P
6th S89.01 Salter-Harris Type I physeal fracture of upper end of tibia
7th S89.011 Salter-Harris Type I physeal fracture of upper end of right tibia P
7th S89.012 Salter-Harris Type I physeal fracture of upper end of left tibia P
7th S89.019 Salter-Harris Type I physeal fracture of upper end of unspecified tibia P
6th S89.02 Salter-Harris Type II physeal fracture of upper end of tibia
7th S89.021 Salter-Harris Type II physeal fracture of upper end of right tibia P
7th S89.022 Salter-Harris Type II physeal fracture of upper end of left tibia P
7th S89.029 Salter-Harris Type II physeal fracture of upper end of unspecified tibia P
6th S89.03 Salter-Harris Type III physeal fracture of upper end of tibia
7th S89.031 Salter-Harris Type III physeal fracture of upper end of right tibia P
7th S89.032 Salter-Harris Type III physeal fracture of upper end of left tibia P
7th S89.039 Salter-Harris Type III physeal fracture of upper end of unspecified tibia P
6th S89.04 Salter-Harris Type IV physeal fracture of upper end of tibia
7th S89.041 Salter-Harris Type IV physeal fracture of upper end of right tibia P
7th S89.042 Salter-Harris Type IV physeal fracture of upper end of left tibia P
7th S89.049 Salter-Harris Type IV physeal fracture of upper end of unspecified tibia P
6th S89.09 Other physeal fracture of upper end of tibia
7th S89.091 Other physeal fracture of upper end of right tibia P
7th S89.092 Other physeal fracture of upper end of left tibia P
7th S89.099 Other physeal fracture of upper end of unspecified tibia P
5th S89.1 Physeal fracture of lower end of tibia
AHA: 2019,4Q,56
6th S89.10 Unspecified physeal fracture of lower end of tibia
7th S89.101 Unspecified physeal fracture of lower end of right tibia P
7th S89.102 Unspecified physeal fracture of lower end of left tibia P
7th S89.109 Unspecified physeal fracture of lower end of unspecified tibia P
6th S89.11 Salter-Harris Type I physeal fracture of lower end of tibia
7th S89.111 Salter-Harris Type I physeal fracture of lower end of right tibia P
7th S89.112 Salter-Harris Type I physeal fracture of lower end of left tibia P
7th S89.119 Salter-Harris Type I physeal fracture of lower end of unspecified tibia P
6th S89.12 Salter-Harris Type II physeal fracture of lower end of tibia
7th S89.121 Salter-Harris Type II physeal fracture of lower end of right tibia P
7th S89.122 Salter-Harris Type II physeal fracture of lower end of left tibia P
7th S89.129 Salter-Harris Type II physeal fracture of lower end of unspecified tibia P
6th S89.13 Salter-Harris Type III physeal fracture of lower end of tibia
EXCLUDES 1 *fracture of medial malleolus (adult) (S82.5-)*
7th S89.131 Salter-Harris Type III physeal fracture of lower end of right tibia P
7th S89.132 Salter-Harris Type III physeal fracture of lower end of left tibia P
7th S89.139 Salter-Harris Type III physeal fracture of lower end of unspecified tibia P
6th S89.14 Salter-Harris Type IV physeal fracture of lower end of tibia
EXCLUDES 1 *fracture of medial malleolus (adult) (S82.5-)*
7th S89.141 Salter-Harris Type IV physeal fracture of lower end of right tibia P
7th S89.142 Salter-Harris Type IV physeal fracture of lower end of left tibia P

S89.149 Salter-Harris Type IV physeal fracture of lower end of unspecified tibia Q

S89.19 Other physeal fracture of lower end of tibia

S89.191 Other physeal fracture of lower end of right tibia Q

S89.192 Other physeal fracture of lower end of left tibia Q

S89.199 Other physeal fracture of lower end of unspecified tibia Q

S89.2 Physeal fracture of upper end of fibula

AHA: 2019,4Q,56

S89.20 Unspecified physeal fracture of upper end of fibula

S89.201 Unspecified physeal fracture of upper end of right fibula Q

S89.202 Unspecified physeal fracture of upper end of left fibula Q

S89.209 Unspecified physeal fracture of upper end of unspecified fibula Q

S89.21 Salter-Harris Type I physeal fracture of upper end of fibula

S89.211 Salter-Harris Type I physeal fracture of upper end of right fibula Q

S89.212 Salter-Harris Type I physeal fracture of upper end of left fibula Q

S89.219 Salter-Harris Type I physeal fracture of upper end of unspecified fibula Q

S89.22 Salter-Harris Type II physeal fracture of upper end of fibula

S89.221 Salter-Harris Type II physeal fracture of upper end of right fibula Q

S89.222 Salter-Harris Type II physeal fracture of upper end of left fibula Q

S89.229 Salter-Harris Type II physeal fracture of upper end of unspecified fibula Q

S89.29 Other physeal fracture of upper end of fibula

S89.291 Other physeal fracture of upper end of right fibula Q

S89.292 Other physeal fracture of upper end of left fibula Q

S89.299 Other physeal fracture of upper end of unspecified fibula Q

S89.3 Physeal fracture of lower end of fibula

AHA: 2019,4Q,56

S89.30 Unspecified physeal fracture of lower end of fibula

S89.301 Unspecified physeal fracture of lower end of right fibula Q

S89.302 Unspecified physeal fracture of lower end of left fibula Q

S89.309 Unspecified physeal fracture of lower end of unspecified fibula Q

S89.31 Salter-Harris Type I physeal fracture of lower end of fibula

S89.311 Salter-Harris Type I physeal fracture of lower end of right fibula Q

S89.312 Salter-Harris Type I physeal fracture of lower end of left fibula Q

S89.319 Salter-Harris Type I physeal fracture of lower end of unspecified fibula Q

S89.32 Salter-Harris Type II physeal fracture of lower end of fibula

S89.321 Salter-Harris Type II physeal fracture of lower end of right fibula Q

S89.322 Salter-Harris Type II physeal fracture of lower end of left fibula Q

S89.329 Salter-Harris Type II physeal fracture of lower end of unspecified fibula Q

S89.39 Other physeal fracture of lower end of fibula

S89.391 Other physeal fracture of lower end of right fibula Q

S89.392 Other physeal fracture of lower end of left fibula Q

S89.399 Other physeal fracture of lower end of unspecified fibula Q

S89.8 Other specified injuries of lower leg

The appropriate 7th character is to be added to each code in subcategory S89.8.
A initial encounter
D subsequent encounter
S sequela

S89.80 Other specified injuries of unspecified lower leg

S89.81 Other specified injuries of right lower leg

S89.82 Other specified injuries of left lower leg

S89.9 Unspecified injury of lower leg

The appropriate 7th character is to be added to each code in subcategory S89.9.
A initial encounter
D subsequent encounter
S sequela

S89.90 Unspecified injury of unspecified lower leg

S89.91 Unspecified injury of right lower leg

S89.92 Unspecified injury of left lower leg

## Injuries to the ankle and foot (S90-S99)

EXCLUDES 2 *burns and corrosions (T20-T32)*
*fracture of ankle and malleolus (S82.-)*
*frostbite (T33-T34)*
*insect bite or sting, venomous (T63.4)*

**S90 Superficial injury of ankle, foot and toes**

The appropriate 7th character is to be added to each code from category S90.
A initial encounter
D subsequent encounter
S sequela

S90.0 Contusion of ankle

S90.00 Contusion of unspecified ankle

S90.01 Contusion of right ankle

S90.02 Contusion of left ankle

S90.1 Contusion of toe without damage to nail

S90.11 Contusion of great toe without damage to nail

S90.111 Contusion of right great toe without damage to nail

S90.112 Contusion of left great toe without damage to nail

S90.119 Contusion of unspecified great toe without damage to nail

S90.12 Contusion of lesser toe without damage to nail

S90.121 Contusion of right lesser toe(s) without damage to nail

S90.122 Contusion of left lesser toe(s) without damage to nail

S90.129 Contusion of unspecified lesser toe(s) without damage to nail
Contusion of toe NOS

S90.2 Contusion of toe with damage to nail

S90.21 Contusion of great toe with damage to nail

S90.211 Contusion of right great toe with damage to nail

S90.212 Contusion of left great toe with damage to nail

S90.219 Contusion of unspecified great toe with damage to nail

S90.22 Contusion of lesser toe with damage to nail

S90.221 Contusion of right lesser toe(s) with damage to nail

S90.222 Contusion of left lesser toe(s) with damage to nail

S90.229 Contusion of unspecified lesser toe(s) with damage to nail

S90.3 Contusion of foot

EXCLUDES 2 *contusion of toes (S90.1-, S90.2-)*

S90.30 Contusion of unspecified foot
Contusion of foot NOS

S90.31 Contusion of right foot

S90.32 Contusion of left foot

✓5th S90.4 Other superficial injuries of toe
- ✓6th S90.41 Abrasion of toe
  - ✓7th S90.411 Abrasion, right great toe
  - ✓7th S90.412 Abrasion, left great toe
  - ✓7th S90.413 Abrasion, unspecified great toe
  - ✓7th S90.414 Abrasion, right lesser toe(s)
  - ✓7th S90.415 Abrasion, left lesser toe(s)
  - ✓7th S90.416 Abrasion, unspecified lesser toe(s)
- ✓6th S90.42 Blister (nonthermal) of toe
  - ✓7th S90.421 Blister (nonthermal), right great toe
  - ✓7th S90.422 Blister (nonthermal), left great toe
  - ✓7th S90.423 Blister (nonthermal), unspecified great toe
  - ✓7th S90.424 Blister (nonthermal), right lesser toe(s)
  - ✓7th S90.425 Blister (nonthermal), left lesser toe(s)
  - ✓7th S90.426 Blister (nonthermal), unspecified lesser toe(s)
- ✓6th S90.44 External constriction of toe
  - Hair tourniquet syndrome of toe
  - ✓7th S90.441 External constriction, right great toe
  - ✓7th S90.442 External constriction, left great toe
  - ✓7th S90.443 External constriction, unspecified great toe
  - ✓7th S90.444 External constriction, right lesser toe(s)
  - ✓7th S90.445 External constriction, left lesser toe(s)
  - ✓7th S90.446 External constriction, unspecified lesser toe(s)
- ✓6th S90.45 Superficial foreign body of toe
  - Splinter in the toe
  - ✓7th S90.451 Superficial foreign body, right great toe
  - ✓7th S90.452 Superficial foreign body, left great toe
  - ✓7th S90.453 Superficial foreign body, unspecified great toe
  - ✓7th S90.454 Superficial foreign body, right lesser toe(s)
  - ✓7th S90.455 Superficial foreign body, left lesser toe(s)
  - ✓7th S90.456 Superficial foreign body, unspecified lesser toe(s)
- ✓6th S90.46 Insect bite (nonvenomous) of toe
  - ✓7th S90.461 Insect bite (nonvenomous), right great toe
  - ✓7th S90.462 Insect bite (nonvenomous), left great toe
  - ✓7th S90.463 Insect bite (nonvenomous), unspecified great toe
  - ✓7th S90.464 Insect bite (nonvenomous), right lesser toe(s)
  - ✓7th S90.465 Insect bite (nonvenomous), left lesser toe(s)
  - ✓7th S90.466 Insect bite (nonvenomous), unspecified lesser toe(s)
- ✓6th S90.47 Other superficial bite of toe
  - EXCLUDES 1 *open bite of toe (S91.15-, S91.25-)*
  - ✓7th S90.471 Other superficial bite of right great toe
  - ✓7th S90.472 Other superficial bite of left great toe
  - ✓7th S90.473 Other superficial bite of unspecified great toe
  - ✓7th S90.474 Other superficial bite of right lesser toe(s)
  - ✓7th S90.475 Other superficial bite of left lesser toe(s)
  - ✓7th S90.476 Other superficial bite of unspecified lesser toe(s)

✓5th S90.5 Other superficial injuries of ankle
- ✓6th S90.51 Abrasion of ankle
  - ✓7th S90.511 Abrasion, right ankle
  - ✓7th S90.512 Abrasion, left ankle
  - ✓7th S90.519 Abrasion, unspecified ankle
- ✓6th S90.52 Blister (nonthermal) of ankle
  - ✓7th S90.521 Blister (nonthermal), right ankle
  - ✓7th S90.522 Blister (nonthermal), left ankle
  - ✓7th S90.529 Blister (nonthermal), unspecified ankle
- ✓6th S90.54 External constriction of ankle
  - ✓7th S90.541 External constriction, right ankle
  - ✓7th S90.542 External constriction, left ankle
  - ✓7th S90.549 External constriction, unspecified ankle
- ✓6th S90.55 Superficial foreign body of ankle
  - Splinter in the ankle
  - ✓7th S90.551 Superficial foreign body, right ankle
  - ✓7th S90.552 Superficial foreign body, left ankle
  - ✓7th S90.559 Superficial foreign body, unspecified ankle
- ✓6th S90.56 Insect bite (nonvenomous) of ankle
  - ✓7th S90.561 Insect bite (nonvenomous), right ankle
  - ✓7th S90.562 Insect bite (nonvenomous), left ankle
  - ✓7th S90.569 Insect bite (nonvenomous), unspecified ankle
- ✓6th S90.57 Other superficial bite of ankle
  - EXCLUDES 1 *open bite of ankle (S91.05-)*
  - ✓7th S90.571 Other superficial bite of ankle, right ankle
  - ✓7th S90.572 Other superficial bite of ankle, left ankle
  - ✓7th S90.579 Other superficial bite of ankle, unspecified ankle

✓5th S90.8 Other superficial injuries of foot
- ✓6th S90.81 Abrasion of foot
  - ✓7th S90.811 Abrasion, right foot
  - ✓7th S90.812 Abrasion, left foot
  - ✓7th S90.819 Abrasion, unspecified foot
- ✓6th S90.82 Blister (nonthermal) of foot
  - ✓7th S90.821 Blister (nonthermal), right foot
  - ✓7th S90.822 Blister (nonthermal), left foot
  - ✓7th S90.829 Blister (nonthermal), unspecified foot
- ✓6th S90.84 External constriction of foot
  - ✓7th S90.841 External constriction, right foot
  - ✓7th S90.842 External constriction, left foot
  - ✓7th S90.849 External constriction, unspecified foot
- ✓6th S90.85 Superficial foreign body of foot
  - Splinter in the foot
  - ✓7th S90.851 Superficial foreign body, right foot
  - ✓7th S90.852 Superficial foreign body, left foot
  - ✓7th S90.859 Superficial foreign body, unspecified foot
- ✓6th S90.86 Insect bite (nonvenomous) of foot
  - ✓7th S90.861 Insect bite (nonvenomous), right foot
  - ✓7th S90.862 Insect bite (nonvenomous), left foot
  - ✓7th S90.869 Insect bite (nonvenomous), unspecified foot
- ✓6th S90.87 Other superficial bite of foot
  - EXCLUDES 1 *open bite of foot (S91.35-)*
  - ✓7th S90.871 Other superficial bite of right foot
  - ✓7th S90.872 Other superficial bite of left foot
  - ✓7th S90.879 Other superficial bite of unspecified foot

✓5th S90.9 Unspecified superficial injury of ankle, foot and toe
- ✓6th S90.91 Unspecified superficial injury of ankle
  - ✓7th S90.911 Unspecified superficial injury of right ankle
  - ✓7th S90.912 Unspecified superficial injury of left ankle
  - ✓7th S90.919 Unspecified superficial injury of unspecified ankle
- ✓6th S90.92 Unspecified superficial injury of foot
  - ✓7th S90.921 Unspecified superficial injury of right foot
  - ✓7th S90.922 Unspecified superficial injury of left foot
  - ✓7th S90.929 Unspecified superficial injury of unspecified foot
- ✓6th S90.93 Unspecified superficial injury of toes
  - ✓7th S90.931 Unspecified superficial injury of right great toe
  - ✓7th S90.932 Unspecified superficial injury of left great toe
  - ✓7th S90.933 Unspecified superficial injury of unspecified great toe
  - ✓7th S90.934 Unspecified superficial injury of right lesser toe(s)
  - ✓7th S90.935 Unspecified superficial injury of left lesser toe(s)
  - ✓7th S90.936 Unspecified superficial injury of unspecified lesser toe(s)

**S91 Open wound of ankle, foot and toes**

Code also any associated wound infection

EXCLUDES 1 *open fracture of ankle, foot and toes (S92.- with 7th character B)*
*traumatic amputation of ankle and foot (S98.-)*

AHA: 2021,1Q,7

The appropriate 7th character is to be added to each code from category S91.
A initial encounter
D subsequent encounter
S sequela

**S91.0 Open wound of ankle**

S91.00 Unspecified open wound of ankle
- S91.001 Unspecified open wound, right ankle
- S91.002 Unspecified open wound, left ankle
- S91.009 Unspecified open wound, unspecified ankle

S91.01 Laceration without foreign body of ankle
- S91.011 Laceration without foreign body, right ankle
- S91.012 Laceration without foreign body, left ankle
- S91.019 Laceration without foreign body, unspecified ankle

S91.02 Laceration with foreign body of ankle
- S91.021 Laceration with foreign body, right ankle
- S91.022 Laceration with foreign body, left ankle
- S91.029 Laceration with foreign body, unspecified ankle

S91.03 Puncture wound without foreign body of ankle
- S91.031 Puncture wound without foreign body, right ankle
- S91.032 Puncture wound without foreign body, left ankle
- S91.039 Puncture wound without foreign body, unspecified ankle

S91.04 Puncture wound with foreign body of ankle
- S91.041 Puncture wound with foreign body, right ankle
- S91.042 Puncture wound with foreign body, left ankle
- S91.049 Puncture wound with foreign body, unspecified ankle

S91.05 Open bite of ankle

EXCLUDES 1 *superficial bite of ankle (S90.56-, S90.57-)*

- S91.051 Open bite, right ankle
- S91.052 Open bite, left ankle
- S91.059 Open bite, unspecified ankle

**S91.1 Open wound of toe without damage to nail**

S91.10 Unspecified open wound of toe without damage to nail
- S91.101 Unspecified open wound of right great toe without damage to nail
- S91.102 Unspecified open wound of left great toe without damage to nail
- S91.103 Unspecified open wound of unspecified great toe without damage to nail
- S91.104 Unspecified open wound of right lesser toe(s) without damage to nail
- S91.105 Unspecified open wound of left lesser toe(s) without damage to nail
- S91.106 Unspecified open wound of unspecified lesser toe(s) without damage to nail
- S91.109 Unspecified open wound of unspecified toe(s) without damage to nail

S91.11 Laceration without foreign body of toe without damage to nail
- S91.111 Laceration without foreign body of right great toe without damage to nail
- S91.112 Laceration without foreign body of left great toe without damage to nail
- S91.113 Laceration without foreign body of unspecified great toe without damage to nail
- S91.114 Laceration without foreign body of right lesser toe(s) without damage to nail
- S91.115 Laceration without foreign body of left lesser toe(s) without damage to nail
- S91.116 Laceration without foreign body of unspecified lesser toe(s) without damage to nail
- S91.119 Laceration without foreign body of unspecified toe without damage to nail

S91.12 Laceration with foreign body of toe without damage to nail
- S91.121 Laceration with foreign body of right great toe without damage to nail
- S91.122 Laceration with foreign body of left great toe without damage to nail
- S91.123 Laceration with foreign body of unspecified great toe without damage to nail
- S91.124 Laceration with foreign body of right lesser toe(s) without damage to nail
- S91.125 Laceration with foreign body of left lesser toe(s) without damage to nail
- S91.126 Laceration with foreign body of unspecified lesser toe(s) without damage to nail
- S91.129 Laceration with foreign body of unspecified toe(s) without damage to nail

S91.13 Puncture wound without foreign body of toe without damage to nail
- S91.131 Puncture wound without foreign body of right great toe without damage to nail
- S91.132 Puncture wound without foreign body of left great toe without damage to nail
- S91.133 Puncture wound without foreign body of unspecified great toe without damage to nail
- S91.134 Puncture wound without foreign body of right lesser toe(s) without damage to nail
- S91.135 Puncture wound without foreign body of left lesser toe(s) without damage to nail
- S91.136 Puncture wound without foreign body of unspecified lesser toe(s) without damage to nail
- S91.139 Puncture wound without foreign body of unspecified toe(s) without damage to nail

S91.14 Puncture wound with foreign body of toe without damage to nail
- S91.141 Puncture wound with foreign body of right great toe without damage to nail
- S91.142 Puncture wound with foreign body of left great toe without damage to nail
- S91.143 Puncture wound with foreign body of unspecified great toe without damage to nail
- S91.144 Puncture wound with foreign body of right lesser toe(s) without damage to nail
- S91.145 Puncture wound with foreign body of left lesser toe(s) without damage to nail
- S91.146 Puncture wound with foreign body of unspecified lesser toe(s) without damage to nail
- S91.149 Puncture wound with foreign body of unspecified toe(s) without damage to nail

S91.15 Open bite of toe without damage to nail

Bite of toe NOS

EXCLUDES 1 *superficial bite of toe (S90.46-, S90.47-)*

- S91.151 Open bite of right great toe without damage to nail
- S91.152 Open bite of left great toe without damage to nail
- S91.153 Open bite of unspecified great toe without damage to nail
- S91.154 Open bite of right lesser toe(s) without damage to nail
- S91.155 Open bite of left lesser toe(s) without damage to nail
- S91.156 Open bite of unspecified lesser toe(s) without damage to nail
- S91.159 Open bite of unspecified toe(s) without damage to nail

**S91.2 Open wound of toe with damage to nail**

S91.20 Unspecified open wound of toe with damage to nail
- S91.201 Unspecified open wound of right great toe with damage to nail
- S91.202 Unspecified open wound of left great toe with damage to nail

- ✓7th **S91.2Ø3** Unspecified open wound of unspecified great toe with damage to nail
- ✓7th **S91.2Ø4** Unspecified open wound of right lesser toe(s) with damage to nail
- ✓7th **S91.2Ø5** Unspecified open wound of left lesser toe(s) with damage to nail
- ✓7th **S91.2Ø6** Unspecified open wound of unspecified lesser toe(s) with damage to nail
- ✓7th **S91.2Ø9** Unspecified open wound of unspecified toe(s) with damage to nail

✓6th **S91.21** Laceration without foreign body of toe with damage to nail
- ✓7th **S91.211** Laceration without foreign body of right great toe with damage to nail
- ✓7th **S91.212** Laceration without foreign body of left great toe with damage to nail
- ✓7th **S91.213** Laceration without foreign body of unspecified great toe with damage to nail
- ✓7th **S91.214** Laceration without foreign body of right lesser toe(s) with damage to nail
- ✓7th **S91.215** Laceration without foreign body of left lesser toe(s) with damage to nail
- ✓7th **S91.216** Laceration without foreign body of unspecified lesser toe(s) with damage to nail
- ✓7th **S91.219** Laceration without foreign body of unspecified toe(s) with damage to nail

✓6th **S91.22** Laceration with foreign body of toe with damage to nail
- ✓7th **S91.221** Laceration with foreign body of right great toe with damage to nail
- ✓7th **S91.222** Laceration with foreign body of left great toe with damage to nail
- ✓7th **S91.223** Laceration with foreign body of unspecified great toe with damage to nail
- ✓7th **S91.224** Laceration with foreign body of right lesser toe(s) with damage to nail
- ✓7th **S91.225** Laceration with foreign body of left lesser toe(s) with damage to nail
- ✓7th **S91.226** Laceration with foreign body of unspecified lesser toe(s) with damage to nail
- ✓7th **S91.229** Laceration with foreign body of unspecified toe(s) with damage to nail

✓6th **S91.23** Puncture wound without foreign body of toe with damage to nail
- ✓7th **S91.231** Puncture wound without foreign body of right great toe with damage to nail
- ✓7th **S91.232** Puncture wound without foreign body of left great toe with damage to nail
- ✓7th **S91.233** Puncture wound without foreign body of unspecified great toe with damage to nail
- ✓7th **S91.234** Puncture wound without foreign body of right lesser toe(s) with damage to nail
- ✓7th **S91.235** Puncture wound without foreign body of left lesser toe(s) with damage to nail
- ✓7th **S91.236** Puncture wound without foreign body of unspecified lesser toe(s) with damage to nail
- ✓7th **S91.239** Puncture wound without foreign body of unspecified toe(s) with damage to nail

✓6th **S91.24** Puncture wound with foreign body of toe with damage to nail
- ✓7th **S91.241** Puncture wound with foreign body of right great toe with damage to nail
- ✓7th **S91.242** Puncture wound with foreign body of left great toe with damage to nail
- ✓7th **S91.243** Puncture wound with foreign body of unspecified great toe with damage to nail
- ✓7th **S91.244** Puncture wound with foreign body of right lesser toe(s) with damage to nail
- ✓7th **S91.245** Puncture wound with foreign body of left lesser toe(s) with damage to nail
- ✓7th **S91.246** Puncture wound with foreign body of unspecified lesser toe(s) with damage to nail
- ✓7th **S91.249** Puncture wound with foreign body of unspecified toe(s) with damage to nail

✓6th **S91.25** Open bite of toe with damage to nail

Bite of toe with damage to nail NOS

EXCLUDES 1 *superficial bite of toe (S9Ø.46-, S9Ø.47-)*
- ✓7th **S91.251** Open bite of right great toe with damage to nail
- ✓7th **S91.252** Open bite of left great toe with damage to nail
- ✓7th **S91.253** Open bite of unspecified great toe with damage to nail
- ✓7th **S91.254** Open bite of right lesser toe(s) with damage to nail
- ✓7th **S91.255** Open bite of left lesser toe(s) with damage to nail
- ✓7th **S91.256** Open bite of unspecified lesser toe(s) with damage to nail
- ✓7th **S91.259** Open bite of unspecified toe(s) with damage to nail

✓5th **S91.3** Open wound of foot

✓6th **S91.3Ø** Unspecified open wound of foot
- ✓7th **S91.3Ø1** Unspecified open wound, right foot
- ✓7th **S91.3Ø2** Unspecified open wound, left foot
- ✓7th **S91.3Ø9** Unspecified open wound, unspecified foot

✓6th **S91.31** Laceration without foreign body of foot
- ✓7th **S91.311** Laceration without foreign body, right foot
- ✓7th **S91.312** Laceration without foreign body, left foot
- ✓7th **S91.319** Laceration without foreign body, unspecified foot

✓6th **S91.32** Laceration with foreign body of foot
- ✓7th **S91.321** Laceration with foreign body, right foot
- ✓7th **S91.322** Laceration with foreign body, left foot
- ✓7th **S91.329** Laceration with foreign body, unspecified foot

✓6th **S91.33** Puncture wound without foreign body of foot
- ✓7th **S91.331** Puncture wound without foreign body, right foot
- ✓7th **S91.332** Puncture wound without foreign body, left foot
- ✓7th **S91.339** Puncture wound without foreign body, unspecified foot

✓6th **S91.34** Puncture wound with foreign body of foot
- ✓7th **S91.341** Puncture wound with foreign body, right foot
- ✓7th **S91.342** Puncture wound with foreign body, left foot
- ✓7th **S91.349** Puncture wound with foreign body, unspecified foot

✓6th **S91.35** Open bite of foot

EXCLUDES 1 *superficial bite of foot (S9Ø.86-, S9Ø.87-)*
- ✓7th **S91.351** Open bite, right foot
- ✓7th **S91.352** Open bite, left foot
- ✓7th **S91.359** Open bite, unspecified foot

## ✓4th S92 Fracture of foot and toe, except ankle

**NOTE** A fracture not indicated as displaced or nondisplaced should be coded to displaced

A fracture not indicated as open or closed should be coded to closed.

EXCLUDES 2 *fracture of ankle (S82.-)*
*fracture of malleolus (S82.-)*
*traumatic amputation of ankle and foot (S98.-)*

**AHA:** 2018,2Q,12; 2015,3Q,37-39

The appropriate 7th character is to be added to each code from category S92.

- A initial encounter for closed fracture
- B initial encounter for open fracture
- D subsequent encounter for fracture with routine healing
- G subsequent encounter for fracture with delayed healing
- K subsequent encounter for fracture with nonunion
- P subsequent encounter for fracture with malunion
- S sequela

✓5th **S92.Ø** Fracture of calcaneus

Heel bone
Os calcis

EXCLUDES 2 *physeal fracture of calcaneus (S99.Ø-)*

✓6th **S92.ØØ** Unspecified fracture of calcaneus
- ✓7th **S92.ØØ1** Unspecified fracture of right calcaneus Q
- ✓7th **S92.ØØ2** Unspecified fracture of left calcaneus Q
- ✓7th **S92.ØØ9** Unspecified fracture of unspecified calcaneus Q

S92.01 Fracture of body of calcaneus
- S92.011 Displaced fracture of body of right calcaneus Q
- S92.012 Displaced fracture of body of left calcaneus Q
- S92.013 Displaced fracture of body of unspecified calcaneus Q
- S92.014 Nondisplaced fracture of body of right calcaneus Q
- S92.015 Nondisplaced fracture of body of left calcaneus Q
- S92.016 Nondisplaced fracture of body of unspecified calcaneus Q

S92.02 Fracture of anterior process of calcaneus
- S92.021 Displaced fracture of anterior process of right calcaneus Q
- S92.022 Displaced fracture of anterior process of left calcaneus Q
- S92.023 Displaced fracture of anterior process of unspecified calcaneus Q
- S92.024 Nondisplaced fracture of anterior process of right calcaneus Q
- S92.025 Nondisplaced fracture of anterior process of left calcaneus Q
- S92.026 Nondisplaced fracture of anterior process of unspecified calcaneus Q

S92.03 Avulsion fracture of tuberosity of calcaneus
- S92.031 Displaced avulsion fracture of tuberosity of right calcaneus Q
- S92.032 Displaced avulsion fracture of tuberosity of left calcaneus Q
- S92.033 Displaced avulsion fracture of tuberosity of unspecified calcaneus Q
- S92.034 Nondisplaced avulsion fracture of tuberosity of right calcaneus Q
- S92.035 Nondisplaced avulsion fracture of tuberosity of left calcaneus Q
- S92.036 Nondisplaced avulsion fracture of tuberosity of unspecified calcaneus Q

S92.04 Other fracture of tuberosity of calcaneus
- S92.041 Displaced other fracture of tuberosity of right calcaneus Q
- S92.042 Displaced other fracture of tuberosity of left calcaneus Q
- S92.043 Displaced other fracture of tuberosity of unspecified calcaneus Q
- S92.044 Nondisplaced other fracture of tuberosity of right calcaneus Q
- S92.045 Nondisplaced other fracture of tuberosity of left calcaneus Q
- S92.046 Nondisplaced other fracture of tuberosity of unspecified calcaneus Q

S92.05 Other extraarticular fracture of calcaneus
- S92.051 Displaced other extraarticular fracture of right calcaneus Q
- S92.052 Displaced other extraarticular fracture of left calcaneus Q
- S92.053 Displaced other extraarticular fracture of unspecified calcaneus Q
- S92.054 Nondisplaced other extraarticular fracture of right calcaneus Q
- S92.055 Nondisplaced other extraarticular fracture of left calcaneus Q
- S92.056 Nondisplaced other extraarticular fracture of unspecified calcaneus Q

S92.06 Intraarticular fracture of calcaneus
- S92.061 Displaced intraarticular fracture of right calcaneus Q
- S92.062 Displaced intraarticular fracture of left calcaneus Q
- S92.063 Displaced intraarticular fracture of unspecified calcaneus Q
- S92.064 Nondisplaced intraarticular fracture of right calcaneus Q
- S92.065 Nondisplaced intraarticular fracture of left calcaneus Q
- S92.066 Nondisplaced intraarticular fracture of unspecified calcaneus Q

S92.1 Fracture of talus

Astragalus

S92.10 Unspecified fracture of talus
- S92.101 Unspecified fracture of right talus Q
- S92.102 Unspecified fracture of left talus Q
- S92.109 Unspecified fracture of unspecified talus Q

S92.11 Fracture of neck of talus
- S92.111 Displaced fracture of neck of right talus Q
- S92.112 Displaced fracture of neck of left talus Q
- S92.113 Displaced fracture of neck of unspecified talus Q
- S92.114 Nondisplaced fracture of neck of right talus Q
- S92.115 Nondisplaced fracture of neck of left talus Q
- S92.116 Nondisplaced fracture of neck of unspecified talus Q

S92.12 Fracture of body of talus
- S92.121 Displaced fracture of body of right talus Q
- S92.122 Displaced fracture of body of left talus Q
- S92.123 Displaced fracture of body of unspecified talus Q
- S92.124 Nondisplaced fracture of body of right talus Q
- S92.125 Nondisplaced fracture of body of left talus Q
- S92.126 Nondisplaced fracture of body of unspecified talus Q

S92.13 Fracture of posterior process of talus
- S92.131 Displaced fracture of posterior process of right talus Q
- S92.132 Displaced fracture of posterior process of left talus Q
- S92.133 Displaced fracture of posterior process of unspecified talus Q
- S92.134 Nondisplaced fracture of posterior process of right talus Q
- S92.135 Nondisplaced fracture of posterior process of left talus Q
- S92.136 Nondisplaced fracture of posterior process of unspecified talus Q

S92.14 Dome fracture of talus

EXCLUDES 1 *osteochondritis dissecans (M93.2)*
- S92.141 Displaced dome fracture of right talus Q
- S92.142 Displaced dome fracture of left talus Q
- S92.143 Displaced dome fracture of unspecified talus Q
- S92.144 Nondisplaced dome fracture of right talus Q
- S92.145 Nondisplaced dome fracture of left talus Q
- S92.146 Nondisplaced dome fracture of unspecified talus Q

S92.15 Avulsion fracture (chip fracture) of talus
- S92.151 Displaced avulsion fracture (chip fracture) of right talus Q
- S92.152 Displaced avulsion fracture (chip fracture) of left talus Q
- S92.153 Displaced avulsion fracture (chip fracture) of unspecified talus Q
- S92.154 Nondisplaced avulsion fracture (chip fracture) of right talus Q
- S92.155 Nondisplaced avulsion fracture (chip fracture) of left talus Q
- S92.156 Nondisplaced avulsion fracture (chip fracture) of unspecified talus Q

S92.19 Other fracture of talus
- S92.191 Other fracture of right talus Q
- S92.192 Other fracture of left talus Q
- S92.199 Other fracture of unspecified talus Q

√5th **S92.2 Fracture of other and unspecified tarsal bone(s)**

√6th **S92.20 Fracture of unspecified tarsal bone(s)**

√7th **S92.201** Fracture of unspecified tarsal bone(s) of right foot Q

√7th **S92.202** Fracture of unspecified tarsal bone(s) of left foot Q

√7th **S92.209** Fracture of unspecified tarsal bone(s) of unspecified foot Q

√6th **S92.21 Fracture of cuboid bone**

√7th **S92.211** Displaced fracture of cuboid bone of right foot Q

√7th **S92.212** Displaced fracture of cuboid bone of left foot Q

√7th **S92.213** Displaced fracture of cuboid bone of unspecified foot Q

√7th **S92.214** Nondisplaced fracture of cuboid bone of right foot Q

√7th **S92.215** Nondisplaced fracture of cuboid bone of left foot Q

√7th **S92.216** Nondisplaced fracture of cuboid bone of unspecified foot Q

√6th **S92.22 Fracture of lateral cuneiform**

√7th **S92.221** Displaced fracture of lateral cuneiform of right foot Q

√7th **S92.222** Displaced fracture of lateral cuneiform of left foot Q

√7th **S92.223** Displaced fracture of lateral cuneiform of unspecified foot Q

√7th **S92.224** Nondisplaced fracture of lateral cuneiform of right foot Q

√7th **S92.225** Nondisplaced fracture of lateral cuneiform of left foot Q

√7th **S92.226** Nondisplaced fracture of lateral cuneiform of unspecified foot Q

√6th **S92.23 Fracture of intermediate cuneiform**

√7th **S92.231** Displaced fracture of intermediate cuneiform of right foot Q

√7th **S92.232** Displaced fracture of intermediate cuneiform of left foot Q

√7th **S92.233** Displaced fracture of intermediate cuneiform of unspecified foot Q

√7th **S92.234** Nondisplaced fracture of intermediate cuneiform of right foot Q

√7th **S92.235** Nondisplaced fracture of intermediate cuneiform of left foot Q

√7th **S92.236** Nondisplaced fracture of intermediate cuneiform of unspecified foot Q

√6th **S92.24 Fracture of medial cuneiform**

√7th **S92.241** Displaced fracture of medial cuneiform of right foot Q

√7th **S92.242** Displaced fracture of medial cuneiform of left foot Q

√7th **S92.243** Displaced fracture of medial cuneiform of unspecified foot Q

√7th **S92.244** Nondisplaced fracture of medial cuneiform of right foot Q

√7th **S92.245** Nondisplaced fracture of medial cuneiform of left foot Q

√7th **S92.246** Nondisplaced fracture of medial cuneiform of unspecified foot Q

√6th **S92.25 Fracture of navicular [scaphoid] of foot**

√7th **S92.251** Displaced fracture of navicular [scaphoid] of right foot Q

√7th **S92.252** Displaced fracture of navicular [scaphoid] of left foot Q

√7th **S92.253** Displaced fracture of navicular [scaphoid] of unspecified foot Q

√7th **S92.254** Nondisplaced fracture of navicular [scaphoid] of right foot Q

√7th **S92.255** Nondisplaced fracture of navicular [scaphoid] of left foot Q

√7th **S92.256** Nondisplaced fracture of navicular [scaphoid] of unspecified foot Q

√5th **S92.3 Fracture of metatarsal bone(s)**

EXCLUDES 2 *physeal fracture of metatarsal (S99.1-)*

AHA: 2018,1Q,3

√6th **S92.30 Fracture of unspecified metatarsal bone(s)**

√7th **S92.301** Fracture of unspecified metatarsal bone(s), right foot Q

√7th **S92.302** Fracture of unspecified metatarsal bone(s), left foot Q

√7th **S92.309** Fracture of unspecified metatarsal bone(s), unspecified foot Q

√6th **S92.31 Fracture of first metatarsal bone**

√7th **S92.311** Displaced fracture of first metatarsal bone, right foot Q

√7th **S92.312** Displaced fracture of first metatarsal bone, left foot Q

√7th **S92.313** Displaced fracture of first metatarsal bone, unspecified foot Q

√7th **S92.314** Nondisplaced fracture of first metatarsal bone, right foot Q

√7th **S92.315** Nondisplaced fracture of first metatarsal bone, left foot Q

√7th **S92.316** Nondisplaced fracture of first metatarsal bone, unspecified foot Q

√6th **S92.32 Fracture of second metatarsal bone**

√7th **S92.321** Displaced fracture of second metatarsal bone, right foot Q

√7th **S92.322** Displaced fracture of second metatarsal bone, left foot Q

√7th **S92.323** Displaced fracture of second metatarsal bone, unspecified foot Q

√7th **S92.324** Nondisplaced fracture of second metatarsal bone, right foot Q

√7th **S92.325** Nondisplaced fracture of second metatarsal bone, left foot Q

√7th **S92.326** Nondisplaced fracture of second metatarsal bone, unspecified foot Q

√6th **S92.33 Fracture of third metatarsal bone**

√7th **S92.331** Displaced fracture of third metatarsal bone, right foot Q

√7th **S92.332** Displaced fracture of third metatarsal bone, left foot Q

√7th **S92.333** Displaced fracture of third metatarsal bone, unspecified foot Q

√7th **S92.334** Nondisplaced fracture of third metatarsal bone, right foot Q

√7th **S92.335** Nondisplaced fracture of third metatarsal bone, left foot Q

√7th **S92.336** Nondisplaced fracture of third metatarsal bone, unspecified foot Q

√6th **S92.34 Fracture of fourth metatarsal bone**

√7th **S92.341** Displaced fracture of fourth metatarsal bone, right foot Q

√7th **S92.342** Displaced fracture of fourth metatarsal bone, left foot Q

√7th **S92.343** Displaced fracture of fourth metatarsal bone, unspecified foot Q

√7th **S92.344** Nondisplaced fracture of fourth metatarsal bone, right foot Q

√7th **S92.345** Nondisplaced fracture of fourth metatarsal bone, left foot Q

√7th **S92.346** Nondisplaced fracture of fourth metatarsal bone, unspecified foot Q

√6th **S92.35 Fracture of fifth metatarsal bone**

√7th **S92.351** Displaced fracture of fifth metatarsal bone, right foot Q

√7th **S92.352** Displaced fracture of fifth metatarsal bone, left foot Q

√7th **S92.353** Displaced fracture of fifth metatarsal bone, unspecified foot Q

√7th **S92.354** Nondisplaced fracture of fifth metatarsal bone, right foot Q

√7th **S92.355** Nondisplaced fracture of fifth metatarsal bone, left foot Q

√7th **S92.356** Nondisplaced fracture of fifth metatarsal bone, unspecified foot Q

✓5th **S92.4 Fracture of great toe**

EXCLUDES 2 *physeal fracture of phalanx of toe (S99.2-)*

✓6th **S92.40 Unspecified fracture of great toe**

✓7th **S92.401 Displaced unspecified fracture of right great toe**

✓7th **S92.402 Displaced unspecified fracture of left great toe**

✓7th **S92.403 Displaced unspecified fracture of unspecified great toe**

✓7th **S92.404 Nondisplaced unspecified fracture of right great toe**

✓7th **S92.405 Nondisplaced unspecified fracture of left great toe**

✓7th **S92.406 Nondisplaced unspecified fracture of unspecified great toe**

✓6th **S92.41 Fracture of proximal phalanx of great toe**

✓7th **S92.411 Displaced fracture of proximal phalanx of right great toe**

✓7th **S92.412 Displaced fracture of proximal phalanx of left great toe**

✓7th **S92.413 Displaced fracture of proximal phalanx of unspecified great toe**

✓7th **S92.414 Nondisplaced fracture of proximal phalanx of right great toe**

✓7th **S92.415 Nondisplaced fracture of proximal phalanx of left great toe**

✓7th **S92.416 Nondisplaced fracture of proximal phalanx of unspecified great toe**

✓6th **S92.42 Fracture of distal phalanx of great toe**

✓7th **S92.421 Displaced fracture of distal phalanx of right great toe**

✓7th **S92.422 Displaced fracture of distal phalanx of left great toe**

✓7th **S92.423 Displaced fracture of distal phalanx of unspecified great toe**

✓7th **S92.424 Nondisplaced fracture of distal phalanx of right great toe**

✓7th **S92.425 Nondisplaced fracture of distal phalanx of left great toe**

✓7th **S92.426 Nondisplaced fracture of distal phalanx of unspecified great toe**

✓6th **S92.49 Other fracture of great toe**

✓7th **S92.491 Other fracture of right great toe**

✓7th **S92.492 Other fracture of left great toe**

✓7th **S92.499 Other fracture of unspecified great toe**

✓5th **S92.5 Fracture of lesser toe(s)**

EXCLUDES 2 *physeal fracture of phalanx of toe (S99.2-)*

✓6th **S92.50 Unspecified fracture of lesser toe(s)**

✓7th **S92.501 Displaced unspecified fracture of right lesser toe(s)**

✓7th **S92.502 Displaced unspecified fracture of left lesser toe(s)**

✓7th **S92.503 Displaced unspecified fracture of unspecified lesser toe(s)**

✓7th **S92.504 Nondisplaced unspecified fracture of right lesser toe(s)**

✓7th **S92.505 Nondisplaced unspecified fracture of left lesser toe(s)**

✓7th **S92.506 Nondisplaced unspecified fracture of unspecified lesser toe(s)**

✓6th **S92.51 Fracture of proximal phalanx of lesser toe(s)**

✓7th **S92.511 Displaced fracture of proximal phalanx of right lesser toe(s)**

✓7th **S92.512 Displaced fracture of proximal phalanx of left lesser toe(s)**

✓7th **S92.513 Displaced fracture of proximal phalanx of unspecified lesser toe(s)**

✓7th **S92.514 Nondisplaced fracture of proximal phalanx of right lesser toe(s)**

✓7th **S92.515 Nondisplaced fracture of proximal phalanx of left lesser toe(s)**

✓7th **S92.516 Nondisplaced fracture of proximal phalanx of unspecified lesser toe(s)**

✓6th **S92.52 Fracture of middle phalanx of lesser toe(s)**

✓7th **S92.521 Displaced fracture of middle phalanx of right lesser toe(s)**

✓7th **S92.522 Displaced fracture of middle phalanx of left lesser toe(s)**

✓7th **S92.523 Displaced fracture of middle phalanx of unspecified lesser toe(s)**

✓7th **S92.524 Nondisplaced fracture of middle phalanx of right lesser toe(s)**

✓7th **S92.525 Nondisplaced fracture of middle phalanx of left lesser toe(s)**

✓7th **S92.526 Nondisplaced fracture of middle phalanx of unspecified lesser toe(s)**

✓6th **S92.53 Fracture of distal phalanx of lesser toe(s)**

✓7th **S92.531 Displaced fracture of distal phalanx of right lesser toe(s)**

✓7th **S92.532 Displaced fracture of distal phalanx of left lesser toe(s)**

✓7th **S92.533 Displaced fracture of distal phalanx of unspecified lesser toe(s)**

✓7th **S92.534 Nondisplaced fracture of distal phalanx of right lesser toe(s)**

✓7th **S92.535 Nondisplaced fracture of distal phalanx of left lesser toe(s)**

✓7th **S92.536 Nondisplaced fracture of distal phalanx of unspecified lesser toe(s)**

✓6th **S92.59 Other fracture of lesser toe(s)**

✓7th **S92.591 Other fracture of right lesser toe(s)**

✓7th **S92.592 Other fracture of left lesser toe(s)**

✓7th **S92.599 Other fracture of unspecified lesser toe(s)**

✓5th **S92.8 Other fracture of foot, except ankle**

✓6th **S92.81 Other fracture of foot**

Sesamoid fracture of foot

**AHA:** 2016,4Q,68

✓7th **S92.811 Other fracture of right foot** Q

✓7th **S92.812 Other fracture of left foot** Q

✓7th **S92.819 Other fracture of unspecified foot** Q

✓5th **S92.9 Unspecified fracture of foot and toe**

✓6th **S92.90 Unspecified fracture of foot**

✓7th **S92.901 Unspecified fracture of right foot** Q

✓7th **S92.902 Unspecified fracture of left foot** Q

✓7th **S92.909 Unspecified fracture of unspecified foot** Q

✓6th **S92.91 Unspecified fracture of toe**

✓7th **S92.911 Unspecified fracture of right toe(s)**

✓7th **S92.912 Unspecified fracture of left toe(s)**

✓7th **S92.919 Unspecified fracture of unspecified toe(s)**

✓4th **S93 Dislocation and sprain of joints and ligaments at ankle, foot and toe level**

INCLUDES avulsion of joint or ligament of ankle, foot and toe
laceration of cartilage, joint or ligament of ankle, foot and toe
sprain of cartilage, joint or ligament of ankle, foot and toe
traumatic hemarthrosis of joint or ligament of ankle, foot and toe
traumatic rupture of joint or ligament of ankle, foot and toe
traumatic subluxation of joint or ligament of ankle, foot and toe
traumatic tear of joint or ligament of ankle, foot and toe

Code also any associated open wound

EXCLUDES 2 *strain of muscle and tendon of ankle and foot (S96.-)*

The appropriate 7th character is to be added to each code from category S93.
A initial encounter
D subsequent encounter
S sequela

✓5th **S93.0 Subluxation and dislocation of ankle joint**

Subluxation and dislocation of astragalus
Subluxation and dislocation of fibula, lower end
Subluxation and dislocation of talus
Subluxation and dislocation of tibia, lower end

√x7th **S93.01 Subluxation of right ankle joint**

√x7th **S93.02 Subluxation of left ankle joint**

√x7th **S93.03 Subluxation of unspecified ankle joint**

√x7th **S93.04 Dislocation of right ankle joint**

√x7th **S93.05 Dislocation of left ankle joint**

√x7th **S93.06 Dislocation of unspecified ankle joint**

√5th S93.1 Subluxation and dislocation of toe

√6th S93.10 Unspecified subluxation and dislocation of toe
Dislocation of toe NOS
Subluxation of toe NOS

√7th S93.101 Unspecified subluxation of right toe(s)
√7th S93.102 Unspecified subluxation of left toe(s)
√7th S93.103 Unspecified subluxation of unspecified toe(s)
√7th S93.104 Unspecified dislocation of right toe(s)
√7th S93.105 Unspecified dislocation of left toe(s)
√7th S93.106 Unspecified dislocation of unspecified toe(s)

√6th S93.11 Dislocation of interphalangeal joint

√7th S93.111 Dislocation of interphalangeal joint of right great toe
√7th S93.112 Dislocation of interphalangeal joint of left great toe
√7th S93.113 Dislocation of interphalangeal joint of unspecified great toe
√7th S93.114 Dislocation of interphalangeal joint of right lesser toe(s)
√7th S93.115 Dislocation of interphalangeal joint of left lesser toe(s)
√7th S93.116 Dislocation of interphalangeal joint of unspecified lesser toe(s)
√7th S93.119 Dislocation of interphalangeal joint of unspecified toe(s)

√6th S93.12 Dislocation of metatarsophalangeal joint

√7th S93.121 Dislocation of metatarsophalangeal joint of right great toe
√7th S93.122 Dislocation of metatarsophalangeal joint of left great toe
√7th S93.123 Dislocation of metatarsophalangeal joint of unspecified great toe
√7th S93.124 Dislocation of metatarsophalangeal joint of right lesser toe(s)
√7th S93.125 Dislocation of metatarsophalangeal joint of left lesser toe(s)
√7th S93.126 Dislocation of metatarsophalangeal joint of unspecified lesser toe(s)
√7th S93.129 Dislocation of metatarsophalangeal joint of unspecified toe(s)

√6th S93.13 Subluxation of interphalangeal joint

√7th S93.131 Subluxation of interphalangeal joint of right great toe
√7th S93.132 Subluxation of interphalangeal joint of left great toe
√7th S93.133 Subluxation of interphalangeal joint of unspecified great toe
√7th S93.134 Subluxation of interphalangeal joint of right lesser toe(s)
√7th S93.135 Subluxation of interphalangeal joint of left lesser toe(s)
√7th S93.136 Subluxation of interphalangeal joint of unspecified lesser toe(s)
√7th S93.139 Subluxation of interphalangeal joint of unspecified toe(s)

√6th S93.14 Subluxation of metatarsophalangeal joint

√7th S93.141 Subluxation of metatarsophalangeal joint of right great toe
√7th S93.142 Subluxation of metatarsophalangeal joint of left great toe
√7th S93.143 Subluxation of metatarsophalangeal joint of unspecified great toe
√7th S93.144 Subluxation of metatarsophalangeal joint of right lesser toe(s)
√7th S93.145 Subluxation of metatarsophalangeal joint of left lesser toe(s)
√7th S93.146 Subluxation of metatarsophalangeal joint of unspecified lesser toe(s)
√7th S93.149 Subluxation of metatarsophalangeal joint of unspecified toe(s)

√5th S93.3 Subluxation and dislocation of foot

EXCLUDES 2 *dislocation of toe (S93.1-)*

√6th S93.30 Unspecified subluxation and dislocation of foot
Dislocation of foot NOS
Subluxation of foot NOS

√7th S93.301 Unspecified subluxation of right foot
√7th S93.302 Unspecified subluxation of left foot
√7th S93.303 Unspecified subluxation of unspecified foot
√7th S93.304 Unspecified dislocation of right foot
√7th S93.305 Unspecified dislocation of left foot
√7th S93.306 Unspecified dislocation of unspecified foot

√6th S93.31 Subluxation and dislocation of tarsal joint

√7th S93.311 Subluxation of tarsal joint of right foot
√7th S93.312 Subluxation of tarsal joint of left foot
√7th S93.313 Subluxation of tarsal joint of unspecified foot
√7th S93.314 Dislocation of tarsal joint of right foot
√7th S93.315 Dislocation of tarsal joint of left foot
√7th S93.316 Dislocation of tarsal joint of unspecified foot

√6th S93.32 Subluxation and dislocation of tarsometatarsal joint

√7th S93.321 Subluxation of tarsometatarsal joint of right foot
√7th S93.322 Subluxation of tarsometatarsal joint of left foot
√7th S93.323 Subluxation of tarsometatarsal joint of unspecified foot
√7th S93.324 Dislocation of tarsometatarsal joint of right foot
√7th S93.325 Dislocation of tarsometatarsal joint of left foot
√7th S93.326 Dislocation of tarsometatarsal joint of unspecified foot

√6th S93.33 Other subluxation and dislocation of foot

√7th S93.331 Other subluxation of right foot
√7th S93.332 Other subluxation of left foot
√7th S93.333 Other subluxation of unspecified foot
√7th S93.334 Other dislocation of right foot
√7th S93.335 Other dislocation of left foot
√7th S93.336 Other dislocation of unspecified foot

√5th S93.4 Sprain of ankle

EXCLUDES 2 *injury of Achilles tendon (S86.0-)*

√6th S93.40 Sprain of unspecified ligament of ankle
Sprain of ankle NOS
Sprained ankle NOS

√7th S93.401 Sprain of unspecified ligament of right ankle
√7th S93.402 Sprain of unspecified ligament of left ankle
√7th S93.409 Sprain of unspecified ligament of unspecified ankle

√6th S93.41 Sprain of calcaneofibular ligament

√7th S93.411 Sprain of calcaneofibular ligament of right ankle
√7th S93.412 Sprain of calcaneofibular ligament of left ankle
√7th S93.419 Sprain of calcaneofibular ligament of unspecified ankle

√6th S93.42 Sprain of deltoid ligament

√7th S93.421 Sprain of deltoid ligament of right ankle
√7th S93.422 Sprain of deltoid ligament of left ankle
√7th S93.429 Sprain of deltoid ligament of unspecified ankle

√6th S93.43 Sprain of tibiofibular ligament

√7th S93.431 Sprain of tibiofibular ligament of right ankle
√7th S93.432 Sprain of tibiofibular ligament of left ankle
√7th S93.439 Sprain of tibiofibular ligament of unspecified ankle

√6th S93.49 Sprain of other ligament of ankle
Sprain of internal collateral ligament
Sprain of talofibular ligament

√7th S93.491 Sprain of other ligament of right ankle
√7th S93.492 Sprain of other ligament of left ankle
√7th S93.499 Sprain of other ligament of unspecified ankle

√5th S93.5 Sprain of toe

√6th S93.50 Unspecified sprain of toe

√7th S93.501 Unspecified sprain of right great toe
√7th S93.502 Unspecified sprain of left great toe
√7th S93.503 Unspecified sprain of unspecified great toe

S93.504 Unspecified sprain of right lesser toe(s)
S93.505 Unspecified sprain of left lesser toe(s)
S93.506 Unspecified sprain of unspecified lesser toe(s)
S93.509 Unspecified sprain of unspecified toe(s)
S93.51 Sprain of interphalangeal joint of toe
S93.511 Sprain of interphalangeal joint of right great toe
S93.512 Sprain of interphalangeal joint of left great toe
S93.513 Sprain of interphalangeal joint of unspecified great toe
S93.514 Sprain of interphalangeal joint of right lesser toe(s)
S93.515 Sprain of interphalangeal joint of left lesser toe(s)
S93.516 Sprain of interphalangeal joint of unspecified lesser toe(s)
S93.519 Sprain of interphalangeal joint of unspecified toe(s)
S93.52 Sprain of metatarsophalangeal joint of toe
S93.521 Sprain of metatarsophalangeal joint of right great toe
S93.522 Sprain of metatarsophalangeal joint of left great toe
S93.523 Sprain of metatarsophalangeal joint of unspecified great toe
S93.524 Sprain of metatarsophalangeal joint of right lesser toe(s)
S93.525 Sprain of metatarsophalangeal joint of left lesser toe(s)
S93.526 Sprain of metatarsophalangeal joint of unspecified lesser toe(s)
S93.529 Sprain of metatarsophalangeal joint of unspecified toe(s)
S93.6 Sprain of foot
EXCLUDES 2 *sprain of metatarsophalangeal joint of toe (S93.52-)*
*sprain of toe (S93.5-)*
S93.60 Unspecified sprain of foot
S93.601 Unspecified sprain of right foot
S93.602 Unspecified sprain of left foot
S93.609 Unspecified sprain of unspecified foot
S93.61 Sprain of tarsal ligament of foot
S93.611 Sprain of tarsal ligament of right foot
S93.612 Sprain of tarsal ligament of left foot
S93.619 Sprain of tarsal ligament of unspecified foot
S93.62 Sprain of tarsometatarsal ligament of foot
S93.621 Sprain of tarsometatarsal ligament of right foot
S93.622 Sprain of tarsometatarsal ligament of left foot
S93.629 Sprain of tarsometatarsal ligament of unspecified foot
S93.69 Other sprain of foot
S93.691 Other sprain of right foot
S93.692 Other sprain of left foot
S93.699 Other sprain of unspecified foot

**S94 Injury of nerves at ankle and foot level**
Code also any associated open wound (S91.-)
The appropriate 7th character is to be added to each code from category S94.
A initial encounter
D subsequent encounter
S sequela

S94.0 Injury of lateral plantar nerve
S94.00 Injury of lateral plantar nerve, unspecified leg
S94.01 Injury of lateral plantar nerve, right leg
S94.02 Injury of lateral plantar nerve, left leg
S94.1 Injury of medial plantar nerve
S94.10 Injury of medial plantar nerve, unspecified leg
S94.11 Injury of medial plantar nerve, right leg
S94.12 Injury of medial plantar nerve, left leg
S94.2 Injury of deep peroneal nerve at ankle and foot level
Injury of terminal, lateral branch of deep peroneal nerve
S94.20 Injury of deep peroneal nerve at ankle and foot level, unspecified leg
S94.21 Injury of deep peroneal nerve at ankle and foot level, right leg
S94.22 Injury of deep peroneal nerve at ankle and foot level, left leg
S94.3 Injury of cutaneous sensory nerve at ankle and foot level
S94.30 Injury of cutaneous sensory nerve at ankle and foot level, unspecified leg
S94.31 Injury of cutaneous sensory nerve at ankle and foot level, right leg
S94.32 Injury of cutaneous sensory nerve at ankle and foot level, left leg
S94.8 Injury of other nerves at ankle and foot level
S94.8X Injury of other nerves at ankle and foot level
S94.8X1 Injury of other nerves at ankle and foot level, right leg
S94.8X2 Injury of other nerves at ankle and foot level, left leg
S94.8X9 Injury of other nerves at ankle and foot level, unspecified leg
S94.9 Injury of unspecified nerve at ankle and foot level
S94.90 Injury of unspecified nerve at ankle and foot level, unspecified leg
S94.91 Injury of unspecified nerve at ankle and foot level, right leg
S94.92 Injury of unspecified nerve at ankle and foot level, left leg

**S95 Injury of blood vessels at ankle and foot level**
Code also any associated open wound (S91.-)
EXCLUDES 2 *injury of posterior tibial artery and vein (S85.1-, S85.8-)*
The appropriate 7th character is to be added to each code from category S95.
A initial encounter
D subsequent encounter
S sequela

S95.0 Injury of dorsal artery of foot
S95.00 Unspecified injury of dorsal artery of foot
S95.001 Unspecified injury of dorsal artery of right foot
S95.002 Unspecified injury of dorsal artery of left foot
S95.009 Unspecified injury of dorsal artery of unspecified foot
S95.01 Laceration of dorsal artery of foot
S95.011 Laceration of dorsal artery of right foot
S95.012 Laceration of dorsal artery of left foot
S95.019 Laceration of dorsal artery of unspecified foot
S95.09 Other specified injury of dorsal artery of foot
S95.091 Other specified injury of dorsal artery of right foot
S95.092 Other specified injury of dorsal artery of left foot
S95.099 Other specified injury of dorsal artery of unspecified foot
S95.1 Injury of plantar artery of foot
S95.10 Unspecified injury of plantar artery of foot
S95.101 Unspecified injury of plantar artery of right foot
S95.102 Unspecified injury of plantar artery of left foot
S95.109 Unspecified injury of plantar artery of unspecified foot
S95.11 Laceration of plantar artery of foot
S95.111 Laceration of plantar artery of right foot
S95.112 Laceration of plantar artery of left foot
S95.119 Laceration of plantar artery of unspecified foot
S95.19 Other specified injury of plantar artery of foot
S95.191 Other specified injury of plantar artery of right foot
S95.192 Other specified injury of plantar artery of left foot

√7th S95.199 Other specified injury of plantar artery of unspecified foot

√5th S95.2 Injury of dorsal vein of foot

√6th S95.20 Unspecified injury of dorsal vein of foot

√7th S95.201 Unspecified injury of dorsal vein of right foot

√7th S95.202 Unspecified injury of dorsal vein of left foot

√7th S95.209 Unspecified injury of dorsal vein of unspecified foot

√6th S95.21 Laceration of dorsal vein of foot

√7th S95.211 Laceration of dorsal vein of right foot

√7th S95.212 Laceration of dorsal vein of left foot

√7th S95.219 Laceration of dorsal vein of unspecified foot

√6th S95.29 Other specified injury of dorsal vein of foot

√7th S95.291 Other specified injury of dorsal vein of right foot

√7th S95.292 Other specified injury of dorsal vein of left foot

√7th S95.299 Other specified injury of dorsal vein of unspecified foot

√5th S95.8 Injury of other blood vessels at ankle and foot level

√6th S95.80 Unspecified injury of other blood vessels at ankle and foot level

√7th S95.801 Unspecified injury of other blood vessels at ankle and foot level, right leg

√7th S95.802 Unspecified injury of other blood vessels at ankle and foot level, left leg

√7th S95.809 Unspecified injury of other blood vessels at ankle and foot level, unspecified leg

√6th S95.81 Laceration of other blood vessels at ankle and foot level

√7th S95.811 Laceration of other blood vessels at ankle and foot level, right leg

√7th S95.812 Laceration of other blood vessels at ankle and foot level, left leg

√7th S95.819 Laceration of other blood vessels at ankle and foot level, unspecified leg

√6th S95.89 Other specified injury of other blood vessels at ankle and foot level

√7th S95.891 Other specified injury of other blood vessels at ankle and foot level, right leg

√7th S95.892 Other specified injury of other blood vessels at ankle and foot level, left leg

√7th S95.899 Other specified injury of other blood vessels at ankle and foot level, unspecified leg

√5th S95.9 Injury of unspecified blood vessel at ankle and foot level

√6th S95.90 Unspecified injury of unspecified blood vessel at ankle and foot level

√7th S95.901 Unspecified injury of unspecified blood vessel at ankle and foot level, right leg

√7th S95.902 Unspecified injury of unspecified blood vessel at ankle and foot level, left leg

√7th S95.909 Unspecified injury of unspecified blood vessel at ankle and foot level, unspecified leg

√6th S95.91 Laceration of unspecified blood vessel at ankle and foot level

√7th S95.911 Laceration of unspecified blood vessel at ankle and foot level, right leg

√7th S95.912 Laceration of unspecified blood vessel at ankle and foot level, left leg

√7th S95.919 Laceration of unspecified blood vessel at ankle and foot level, unspecified leg

√6th S95.99 Other specified injury of unspecified blood vessel at ankle and foot level

√7th S95.991 Other specified injury of unspecified blood vessel at ankle and foot level, right leg

√7th S95.992 Other specified injury of unspecified blood vessel at ankle and foot level, left leg

√7th S95.999 Other specified injury of unspecified blood vessel at ankle and foot level, unspecified leg

√4th **S96 Injury of muscle and tendon at ankle and foot level**

Code also any associated open wound (S91.-)

EXCLUDES 2 *injury of Achilles tendon (S86.0-)*
*sprain of joints and ligaments of ankle and foot (S93.-)*

**TIP:** Refer to the Muscle/Tendon table at the beginning of this chapter.

The appropriate 7th character is to be added to each code from category S96.
A initial encounter
D subsequent encounter
S sequela

√5th S96.0 Injury of muscle and tendon of long flexor muscle of toe at ankle and foot level

√6th S96.00 Unspecified injury of muscle and tendon of long flexor muscle of toe at ankle and foot level

√7th S96.001 Unspecified injury of muscle and tendon of long flexor muscle of toe at ankle and foot level, right foot

√7th S96.002 Unspecified injury of muscle and tendon of long flexor muscle of toe at ankle and foot level, left foot

√7th S96.009 Unspecified injury of muscle and tendon of long flexor muscle of toe at ankle and foot level, unspecified foot

√6th S96.01 Strain of muscle and tendon of long flexor muscle of toe at ankle and foot level

√7th S96.011 Strain of muscle and tendon of long flexor muscle of toe at ankle and foot level, right foot

√7th S96.012 Strain of muscle and tendon of long flexor muscle of toe at ankle and foot level, left foot

√7th S96.019 Strain of muscle and tendon of long flexor muscle of toe at ankle and foot level, unspecified foot

√6th S96.02 Laceration of muscle and tendon of long flexor muscle of toe at ankle and foot level

√7th S96.021 Laceration of muscle and tendon of long flexor muscle of toe at ankle and foot level, right foot

√7th S96.022 Laceration of muscle and tendon of long flexor muscle of toe at ankle and foot level, left foot

√7th S96.029 Laceration of muscle and tendon of long flexor muscle of toe at ankle and foot level, unspecified foot

√6th S96.09 Other injury of muscle and tendon of long flexor muscle of toe at ankle and foot level

√7th S96.091 Other injury of muscle and tendon of long flexor muscle of toe at ankle and foot level, right foot

√7th S96.092 Other injury of muscle and tendon of long flexor muscle of toe at ankle and foot level, left foot

√7th S96.099 Other injury of muscle and tendon of long flexor muscle of toe at ankle and foot level, unspecified foot

√5th S96.1 Injury of muscle and tendon of long extensor muscle of toe at ankle and foot level

√6th S96.10 Unspecified injury of muscle and tendon of long extensor muscle of toe at ankle and foot level

√7th S96.101 Unspecified injury of muscle and tendon of long extensor muscle of toe at ankle and foot level, right foot

√7th S96.102 Unspecified injury of muscle and tendon of long extensor muscle of toe at ankle and foot level, left foot

√7th S96.109 Unspecified injury of muscle and tendon of long extensor muscle of toe at ankle and foot level, unspecified foot

√6th S96.11 Strain of muscle and tendon of long extensor muscle of toe at ankle and foot level

√7th S96.111 Strain of muscle and tendon of long extensor muscle of toe at ankle and foot level, right foot

√7th S96.112 Strain of muscle and tendon of long extensor muscle of toe at ankle and foot level, left foot

√7th S96.119 Strain of muscle and tendon of long extensor muscle of toe at ankle and foot level, unspecified foot

√6th S96.12 Laceration of muscle and tendon of long extensor muscle of toe at ankle and foot level
√7th S96.121 Laceration of muscle and tendon of long extensor muscle of toe at ankle and foot level, right foot
√7th S96.122 Laceration of muscle and tendon of long extensor muscle of toe at ankle and foot level, left foot
√7th S96.129 Laceration of muscle and tendon of long extensor muscle of toe at ankle and foot level, unspecified foot
√6th S96.19 Other specified injury of muscle and tendon of long extensor muscle of toe at ankle and foot level
√7th S96.191 Other specified injury of muscle and tendon of long extensor muscle of toe at ankle and foot level, right foot
√7th S96.192 Other specified injury of muscle and tendon of long extensor muscle of toe at ankle and foot level, left foot
√7th S96.199 Other specified injury of muscle and tendon of long extensor muscle of toe at ankle and foot level, unspecified foot
√5th S96.2 Injury of intrinsic muscle and tendon at ankle and foot level
√6th S96.20 Unspecified injury of intrinsic muscle and tendon at ankle and foot level
√7th S96.201 Unspecified injury of intrinsic muscle and tendon at ankle and foot level, right foot
√7th S96.202 Unspecified injury of intrinsic muscle and tendon at ankle and foot level, left foot
√7th S96.209 Unspecified injury of intrinsic muscle and tendon at ankle and foot level, unspecified foot
√6th S96.21 Strain of intrinsic muscle and tendon at ankle and foot level
√7th S96.211 Strain of intrinsic muscle and tendon at ankle and foot level, right foot
√7th S96.212 Strain of intrinsic muscle and tendon at ankle and foot level, left foot
√7th S96.219 Strain of intrinsic muscle and tendon at ankle and foot level, unspecified foot
√6th S96.22 Laceration of intrinsic muscle and tendon at ankle and foot level
√7th S96.221 Laceration of intrinsic muscle and tendon at ankle and foot level, right foot
√7th S96.222 Laceration of intrinsic muscle and tendon at ankle and foot level, left foot
√7th S96.229 Laceration of intrinsic muscle and tendon at ankle and foot level, unspecified foot
√6th S96.29 Other specified injury of intrinsic muscle and tendon at ankle and foot level
√7th S96.291 Other specified injury of intrinsic muscle and tendon at ankle and foot level, right foot
√7th S96.292 Other specified injury of intrinsic muscle and tendon at ankle and foot level, left foot
√7th S96.299 Other specified injury of intrinsic muscle and tendon at ankle and foot level, unspecified foot
√5th S96.8 Injury of other specified muscles and tendons at ankle and foot level
√6th S96.80 Unspecified injury of other specified muscles and tendons at ankle and foot level
√7th S96.801 Unspecified injury of other specified muscles and tendons at ankle and foot level, right foot
√7th S96.802 Unspecified injury of other specified muscles and tendons at ankle and foot level, left foot
√7th S96.809 Unspecified injury of other specified muscles and tendons at ankle and foot level, unspecified foot
√6th S96.81 Strain of other specified muscles and tendons at ankle and foot level
√7th S96.811 Strain of other specified muscles and tendons at ankle and foot level, right foot
√7th S96.812 Strain of other specified muscles and tendons at ankle and foot level, left foot
√7th S96.819 Strain of other specified muscles and tendons at ankle and foot level, unspecified foot
√6th S96.82 Laceration of other specified muscles and tendons at ankle and foot level
√7th S96.821 Laceration of other specified muscles and tendons at ankle and foot level, right foot
√7th S96.822 Laceration of other specified muscles and tendons at ankle and foot level, left foot
√7th S96.829 Laceration of other specified muscles and tendons at ankle and foot level, unspecified foot
√6th S96.89 Other specified injury of other specified muscles and tendons at ankle and foot level
√7th S96.891 Other specified injury of other specified muscles and tendons at ankle and foot level, right foot
√7th S96.892 Other specified injury of other specified muscles and tendons at ankle and foot level, left foot
√7th S96.899 Other specified injury of other specified muscles and tendons at ankle and foot level, unspecified foot
√5th S96.9 Injury of unspecified muscle and tendon at ankle and foot level
√6th S96.90 Unspecified injury of unspecified muscle and tendon at ankle and foot level
√7th S96.901 Unspecified injury of unspecified muscle and tendon at ankle and foot level, right foot
√7th S96.902 Unspecified injury of unspecified muscle and tendon at ankle and foot level, left foot
√7th S96.909 Unspecified injury of unspecified muscle and tendon at ankle and foot level, unspecified foot
√6th S96.91 Strain of unspecified muscle and tendon at ankle and foot level
√7th S96.911 Strain of unspecified muscle and tendon at ankle and foot level, right foot
√7th S96.912 Strain of unspecified muscle and tendon at ankle and foot level, left foot
√7th S96.919 Strain of unspecified muscle and tendon at ankle and foot level, unspecified foot
√6th S96.92 Laceration of unspecified muscle and tendon at ankle and foot level
√7th S96.921 Laceration of unspecified muscle and tendon at ankle and foot level, right foot
√7th S96.922 Laceration of unspecified muscle and tendon at ankle and foot level, left foot
√7th S96.929 Laceration of unspecified muscle and tendon at ankle and foot level, unspecified foot
√6th S96.99 Other specified injury of unspecified muscle and tendon at ankle and foot level
√7th S96.991 Other specified injury of unspecified muscle and tendon at ankle and foot level, right foot
√7th S96.992 Other specified injury of unspecified muscle and tendon at ankle and foot level, left foot
√7th S96.999 Other specified injury of unspecified muscle and tendon at ankle and foot level, unspecified foot

√4th **S97 Crushing injury of ankle and foot**

Use additional code(s) for all associated injuries

The appropriate 7th character is to be added to each code from category S97.
A initial encounter
D subsequent encounter
S sequela

√5th S97.0 Crushing injury of ankle
√x7th S97.00 Crushing injury of unspecified ankle
√x7th S97.01 Crushing injury of right ankle
√x7th S97.02 Crushing injury of left ankle
√5th S97.1 Crushing injury of toe
√6th S97.10 Crushing injury of unspecified toe(s)
√7th S97.101 Crushing injury of unspecified right toe(s)
√7th S97.102 Crushing injury of unspecified left toe(s)
√7th S97.109 Crushing injury of unspecified toe(s)
Crushing injury of toe NOS
√6th S97.11 Crushing injury of great toe
√7th S97.111 Crushing injury of right great toe

√7th S97.112 Crushing injury of left great toe
√7th S97.119 Crushing injury of unspecified great toe
√6th S97.12 Crushing injury of lesser toe(s)
√7th S97.121 Crushing injury of right lesser toe(s)
√7th S97.122 Crushing injury of left lesser toe(s)
√7th S97.129 Crushing injury of unspecified lesser toe(s)
√5th S97.8 Crushing injury of foot
√x7th S97.8Ø Crushing injury of unspecified foot
Crushing injury of foot NOS
√x7th S97.81 Crushing injury of right foot
√x7th S97.82 Crushing injury of left foot

√4th **S98 Traumatic amputation of ankle and foot**
An amputation not identified as partial or complete should be coded to complete

The appropriate 7th character is to be added to each code from category S98.
A initial encounter
D subsequent encounter
S sequela

√5th S98.Ø Traumatic amputation of foot at ankle level
√6th S98.Ø1 Complete traumatic amputation of foot at ankle level
√7th S98.Ø11 Complete traumatic amputation of right foot at ankle level HCC ESR COM
√7th S98.Ø12 Complete traumatic amputation of left foot at ankle level HCC ESR COM
√7th S98.Ø19 Complete traumatic amputation of unspecified foot at ankle level HCC ESR COM
√6th S98.Ø2 Partial traumatic amputation of foot at ankle level
√7th S98.Ø21 Partial traumatic amputation of right foot at ankle level HCC ESR COM
√7th S98.Ø22 Partial traumatic amputation of left foot at ankle level HCC ESR COM
√7th S98.Ø29 Partial traumatic amputation of unspecified foot at ankle level HCC ESR COM
√5th S98.1 Traumatic amputation of one toe
√6th S98.11 Complete traumatic amputation of great toe
√7th S98.111 Complete traumatic amputation of right great toe ESR
√7th S98.112 Complete traumatic amputation of left great toe ESR
√7th S98.119 Complete traumatic amputation of unspecified great toe ESR
√6th S98.12 Partial traumatic amputation of great toe
√7th S98.121 Partial traumatic amputation of right great toe ESR
√7th S98.122 Partial traumatic amputation of left great toe ESR
√7th S98.129 Partial traumatic amputation of unspecified great toe ESR
√6th S98.13 Complete traumatic amputation of one lesser toe
Traumatic amputation of toe NOS
√7th S98.131 Complete traumatic amputation of one right lesser toe ESR
√7th S98.132 Complete traumatic amputation of one left lesser toe ESR
√7th S98.139 Complete traumatic amputation of one unspecified lesser toe ESR
√6th S98.14 Partial traumatic amputation of one lesser toe
√7th S98.141 Partial traumatic amputation of one right lesser toe ESR
√7th S98.142 Partial traumatic amputation of one left lesser toe ESR
√7th S98.149 Partial traumatic amputation of one unspecified lesser toe ESR
√5th S98.2 Traumatic amputation of two or more lesser toes
√6th S98.21 Complete traumatic amputation of two or more lesser toes
√7th S98.211 Complete traumatic amputation of two or more right lesser toes ESR
√7th S98.212 Complete traumatic amputation of two or more left lesser toes ESR
√7th S98.219 Complete traumatic amputation of two or more unspecified lesser toes ESR
√6th S98.22 Partial traumatic amputation of two or more lesser toes
√7th S98.221 Partial traumatic amputation of two or more right lesser toes ESR
√7th S98.222 Partial traumatic amputation of two or more left lesser toes ESR
√7th S98.229 Partial traumatic amputation of two or more unspecified lesser toes ESR
√5th S98.3 Traumatic amputation of midfoot
√6th S98.31 Complete traumatic amputation of midfoot
√7th S98.311 Complete traumatic amputation of right midfoot HCC ESR COM
√7th S98.312 Complete traumatic amputation of left midfoot HCC ESR COM
√7th S98.319 Complete traumatic amputation of unspecified midfoot HCC ESR COM
√6th S98.32 Partial traumatic amputation of midfoot
√7th S98.321 Partial traumatic amputation of right midfoot HCC ESR COM
√7th S98.322 Partial traumatic amputation of left midfoot HCC ESR COM
√7th S98.329 Partial traumatic amputation of unspecified midfoot HCC ESR COM
√5th S98.9 Traumatic amputation of foot, level unspecified
√6th S98.91 Complete traumatic amputation of foot, level unspecified
√7th S98.911 Complete traumatic amputation of right foot, level unspecified HCC ESR COM
√7th S98.912 Complete traumatic amputation of left foot, level unspecified HCC ESR COM
√7th S98.919 Complete traumatic amputation of unspecified foot, level unspecified HCC ESR COM
√6th S98.92 Partial traumatic amputation of foot, level unspecified
√7th S98.921 Partial traumatic amputation of right foot, level unspecified HCC ESR COM
√7th S98.922 Partial traumatic amputation of left foot, level unspecified HCC ESR COM
√7th S98.929 Partial traumatic amputation of unspecified foot, level unspecified HCC ESR COM

√4th **S99 Other and unspecified injuries of ankle and foot**
AHA: 2018,2Q,12; 2018,1Q,3; 2016,4Q,68-69
√5th S99.Ø Physeal fracture of calcaneus
AHA: 2019,4Q,56

The appropriate 7th character is to be added to each code from subcategory S99.Ø.
A initial encounter for closed fracture
B initial encounter for open fracture
D subsequent encounter for fracture with routine healing
G subsequent encounter for fracture with delayed healing
K subsequent encounter for fracture with nonunion
P subsequent encounter for fracture with malunion
S sequela

√6th S99.ØØ Unspecified physeal fracture of calcaneus
√7th S99.ØØ1 Unspecified physeal fracture of right calcaneus P
√7th S99.ØØ2 Unspecified physeal fracture of left calcaneus P
√7th S99.ØØ9 Unspecified physeal fracture of unspecified calcaneus P
√6th S99.Ø1 Salter-Harris Type I physeal fracture of calcaneus
√7th S99.Ø11 Salter-Harris Type I physeal fracture of right calcaneus P
√7th S99.Ø12 Salter-Harris Type I physeal fracture of left calcaneus P
√7th S99.Ø19 Salter-Harris Type I physeal fracture of unspecified calcaneus P
√6th S99.Ø2 Salter-Harris Type II physeal fracture of calcaneus
√7th S99.Ø21 Salter-Harris Type II physeal fracture of right calcaneus P
√7th S99.Ø22 Salter-Harris Type II physeal fracture of left calcaneus P

✓7th S99.029 Salter-Harris Type II physeal fracture of unspecified calcaneus Q

✓6th S99.03 Salter-Harris Type III physeal fracture of calcaneus

✓7th S99.031 Salter-Harris Type III physeal fracture of right calcaneus Q

✓7th S99.032 Salter-Harris Type III physeal fracture of left calcaneus Q

✓7th S99.039 Salter-Harris Type III physeal fracture of unspecified calcaneus Q

✓6th S99.04 Salter-Harris Type IV physeal fracture of calcaneus

✓7th S99.041 Salter-Harris Type IV physeal fracture of right calcaneus Q

✓7th S99.042 Salter-Harris Type IV physeal fracture of left calcaneus Q

✓7th S99.049 Salter-Harris Type IV physeal fracture of unspecified calcaneus Q

✓6th S99.09 Other physeal fracture of calcaneus

✓7th S99.091 Other physeal fracture of right calcaneus Q

✓7th S99.092 Other physeal fracture of left calcaneus Q

✓7th S99.099 Other physeal fracture of unspecified calcaneus Q

✓5th S99.1 Physeal fracture of metatarsal

AHA: 2019,4Q,56

The appropriate 7th character is to be added to each code from subcategory S99.1
A initial encounter for closed fracture
B initial encounter for open fracture
D subsequent encounter for fracture with routine healing
G subsequent encounter for fracture with delayed healing
K subsequent encounter for fracture with nonunion
P subsequent encounter for fracture with malunion
S sequela

✓6th S99.10 Unspecified physeal fracture of metatarsal

✓7th S99.101 Unspecified physeal fracture of right metatarsal Q

✓7th S99.102 Unspecified physeal fracture of left metatarsal Q

✓7th S99.109 Unspecified physeal fracture of unspecified metatarsal Q

✓6th S99.11 Salter-Harris Type I physeal fracture of metatarsal

✓7th S99.111 Salter-Harris Type I physeal fracture of right metatarsal Q

✓7th S99.112 Salter-Harris Type I physeal fracture of left metatarsal Q

✓7th S99.119 Salter-Harris Type I physeal fracture of unspecified metatarsal Q

✓6th S99.12 Salter-Harris Type II physeal fracture of metatarsal

✓7th S99.121 Salter-Harris Type II physeal fracture of right metatarsal Q

✓7th S99.122 Salter-Harris Type II physeal fracture of left metatarsal Q

✓7th S99.129 Salter-Harris Type II physeal fracture of unspecified metatarsal Q

✓6th S99.13 Salter-Harris Type III physeal fracture of metatarsal

✓7th S99.131 Salter-Harris Type III physeal fracture of right metatarsal Q

✓7th S99.132 Salter-Harris Type III physeal fracture of left metatarsal Q

✓7th S99.139 Salter-Harris Type III physeal fracture of unspecified metatarsal Q

✓6th S99.14 Salter-Harris Type IV physeal fracture of metatarsal

✓7th S99.141 Salter-Harris Type IV physeal fracture of right metatarsal Q

✓7th S99.142 Salter-Harris Type IV physeal fracture of left metatarsal Q

✓7th S99.149 Salter-Harris Type IV physeal fracture of unspecified metatarsal Q

✓6th S99.19 Other physeal fracture of metatarsal

✓7th S99.191 Other physeal fracture of right metatarsal Q

✓7th S99.192 Other physeal fracture of left metatarsal Q

✓7th S99.199 Other physeal fracture of unspecified metatarsal Q

✓5th S99.2 Physeal fracture of phalanx of toe

AHA: 2019,4Q,56

The appropriate 7th character is to be added to each code from subcategories S99.2.
A initial encounter for closed fracture
B initial encounter for open fracture
D subsequent encounter for fracture with routine healing
G subsequent encounter for fracture with delayed healing
K subsequent encounter for fracture with nonunion
P subsequent encounter for fracture with malunion
S sequela

✓6th S99.20 Unspecified physeal fracture of phalanx of toe

✓7th S99.201 Unspecified physeal fracture of phalanx of right toe

✓7th S99.202 Unspecified physeal fracture of phalanx of left toe

✓7th S99.209 Unspecified physeal fracture of phalanx of unspecified toe

✓6th S99.21 Salter-Harris Type I physeal fracture of phalanx of toe

✓7th S99.211 Salter-Harris Type I physeal fracture of phalanx of right toe

✓7th S99.212 Salter-Harris Type I physeal fracture of phalanx of left toe

✓7th S99.219 Salter-Harris Type I physeal fracture of phalanx of unspecified toe

✓6th S99.22 Salter-Harris Type II physeal fracture of phalanx of toe

✓7th S99.221 Salter-Harris Type II physeal fracture of phalanx of right toe

✓7th S99.222 Salter-Harris Type II physeal fracture of phalanx of left toe

✓7th S99.229 Salter-Harris Type II physeal fracture of phalanx of unspecified toe

✓6th S99.23 Salter-Harris Type III physeal fracture of phalanx of toe

✓7th S99.231 Salter-Harris Type III physeal fracture of phalanx of right toe

✓7th S99.232 Salter-Harris Type III physeal fracture of phalanx of left toe

✓7th S99.239 Salter-Harris Type III physeal fracture of phalanx of unspecified toe

✓6th S99.24 Salter-Harris Type IV physeal fracture of phalanx of toe

✓7th S99.241 Salter-Harris Type IV physeal fracture of phalanx of right toe

✓7th S99.242 Salter-Harris Type IV physeal fracture of phalanx of left toe

✓7th S99.249 Salter-Harris Type IV physeal fracture of phalanx of unspecified toe

✓6th S99.29 Other physeal fracture of phalanx of toe

✓7th S99.291 Other physeal fracture of phalanx of right toe

✓7th S99.292 Other physeal fracture of phalanx of left toe

✓7th S99.299 Other physeal fracture of phalanx of unspecified toe

✓5th S99.8 Other specified injuries of ankle and foot

The appropriate 7th character is to be added to each code from subcategory S99.8.
A initial encounter
D subsequent encounter
S sequela

✓6th S99.81 Other specified injuries of ankle

✓7th S99.811 Other specified injuries of right ankle

✓7th S99.812 Other specified injuries of left ankle

✓7th S99.819 Other specified injuries of unspecified ankle

✓6th S99.82 Other specified injuries of foot

✓7th S99.821 Other specified injuries of right foot

✓7th S99.822 Other specified injuries of left foot

✓7th S99.829 Other specified injuries of unspecified foot

√5th **S99.9 Unspecified injury of ankle and foot**

The appropriate 7th character is to be added to each code from subcategory S99.9.
A initial encounter
D subsequent encounter
S sequela

√6th **S99.91 Unspecified injury of ankle**

√7th **S99.911 Unspecified injury of right ankle**

√7th **S99.912 Unspecified injury of left ankle**

√7th **S99.919 Unspecified injury of unspecified ankle**

√6th **S99.92 Unspecified injury of foot**

√7th **S99.921 Unspecified injury of right foot**

√7th **S99.922 Unspecified injury of left foot**

√7th **S99.929 Unspecified injury of unspecified foot**

## INJURY, POISONING AND CERTAIN OTHER CONSEQUENCES OF EXTERNAL CAUSES (TØ7-T88)

### Injuries involving multiple body regions (TØ7)

EXCLUDES 1 *burns and corrosions (T2Ø-T32)*
*frostbite (T33-T34)*
*insect bite or sting, venomous (T63.4)*
*sunburn (L55.-)*

√x7th **TØ7 Unspecified multiple injuries**

EXCLUDES 1 *injury NOS (T14.9Ø)*

**AHA:** 2017,4Q,26

The appropriate 7th character is to be added to code TØ7.
A initial encounter
D subsequent encounter
S sequela

### Injury of unspecified body region (T14)

√4th **T14 Injury of unspecified body region**

EXCLUDES 1 *multiple unspecified injuries (TØ7)*

**AHA:** 2017,4Q,26

The appropriate 7th character is to be added to each code from category T14.
A initial encounter
D subsequent encounter
S sequela

√x7th **T14.8 Other injury of unspecified body region**

Abrasion NOS
Contusion NOS
Crush injury NOS
Fracture NOS
Skin injury NOS
Vascular injury NOS
Wound NOS

√5th **T14.9 Unspecified injury**

√x7th **T14.9Ø Injury, unspecified**

Injury NOS

√x7th **T14.91 Suicide attempt** HCC Rx ESR COM

Attempted suicide NOS

### Effects of foreign body entering through natural orifice (T15-T19)

Use additional code, if known, for foreign body entering into or through a natural orifice (W44.-)

EXCLUDES 2 *foreign body accidentally left in operation wound (T81.5-)*
*foreign body in penetrating wound - see open wound by body region*
*residual foreign body in soft tissue (M79.5)*
*splinter, without open wound - see superficial injury by body region*

√4th **T15 Foreign body on external eye**

EXCLUDES 2 *foreign body in penetrating wound of orbit and eye ball (SØ5.4-, SØ5.5-)*
*open wound of eyelid and periocular area (SØ1.1-)*
*retained (old) foreign body in penetrating wound of orbit and eye ball (HØ5.5-, H44.6-, H44.7-)*
*retained foreign body in eyelid (HØ2.8-)*
*superficial foreign body of eyelid and periocular area (SØØ.25-)*

The appropriate 7th character is to be added to each code from category T15.
A initial encounter
D subsequent encounter
S sequela

√5th **T15.Ø Foreign body in cornea**

√x7th **T15.ØØ Foreign body in cornea, unspecified eye**

√x7th **T15.Ø1 Foreign body in cornea, right eye**

√x7th **T15.Ø2 Foreign body in cornea, left eye**

√5th **T15.1 Foreign body in conjunctival sac**

√x7th **T15.1Ø Foreign body in conjunctival sac, unspecified eye**

√x7th **T15.11 Foreign body in conjunctival sac, right eye**

√x7th **T15.12 Foreign body in conjunctival sac, left eye**

√5th **T15.8 Foreign body in other and multiple parts of external eye**

Foreign body in lacrimal punctum

√x7th **T15.8Ø Foreign body in other and multiple parts of external eye, unspecified eye**

√x7th **T15.81 Foreign body in other and multiple parts of external eye, right eye**

√x7th **T15.82 Foreign body in other and multiple parts of external eye, left eye**

√5th **T15.9 Foreign body on external eye, part unspecified**

√x7th **T15.9Ø Foreign body on external eye, part unspecified, unspecified eye**

√x7th **T15.91 Foreign body on external eye, part unspecified, right eye**

√x7th **T15.92 Foreign body on external eye, part unspecified, left eye**

√4th **T16 Foreign body in ear**

INCLUDES foreign body in auditory canal

The appropriate 7th character is to be added to each code from category T16.
A initial encounter
D subsequent encounter
S sequela

√x7th **T16.1 Foreign body in right ear**

√x7th **T16.2 Foreign body in left ear**

√x7th **T16.9 Foreign body in ear, unspecified ear**

√4th **T17 Foreign body in respiratory tract**

The appropriate 7th character is to be added to each code from category T17.
A initial encounter
D subsequent encounter
S sequela

√x7th **T17.Ø Foreign body in nasal sinus**

√x7th **T17.1 Foreign body in nostril**

Foreign body in nose NOS

√5th **T17.2 Foreign body in pharynx**

Foreign body in nasopharynx
Foreign body in throat NOS

√6th **T17.2Ø Unspecified foreign body in pharynx**

√7th **T17.2ØØ Unspecified foreign body in pharynx causing asphyxiation**

√7th **T17.2Ø8 Unspecified foreign body in pharynx causing other injury**

√6th T17.21 Gastric contents in pharynx
Aspiration of gastric contents into pharynx
Vomitus in pharynx
√7th T17.210 Gastric contents in pharynx causing asphyxiation
√7th T17.218 Gastric contents in pharynx causing other injury
√6th T17.22 Food in pharynx
Bones in pharynx
Seeds in pharynx
√7th T17.220 Food in pharynx causing asphyxiation
√7th T17.228 Food in pharynx causing other injury
√6th T17.29 Other foreign object in pharynx
√7th T17.290 Other foreign object in pharynx causing asphyxiation
√7th T17.298 Other foreign object in pharynx causing other injury
√5th T17.3 Foreign body in larynx
√6th T17.30 Unspecified foreign body in larynx
√7th T17.300 Unspecified foreign body in larynx causing asphyxiation
√7th T17.308 Unspecified foreign body in larynx causing other injury
√6th T17.31 Gastric contents in larynx
Aspiration of gastric contents into larynx
Vomitus in larynx
√7th T17.310 Gastric contents in larynx causing asphyxiation
√7th T17.318 Gastric contents in larynx causing other injury
√6th T17.32 Food in larynx
Bones in larynx
Seeds in larynx
√7th T17.320 Food in larynx causing asphyxiation
√7th T17.328 Food in larynx causing other injury
√6th T17.39 Other foreign object in larynx
√7th T17.390 Other foreign object in larynx causing asphyxiation
√7th T17.398 Other foreign object in larynx causing other injury
√5th T17.4 Foreign body in trachea
√6th T17.40 Unspecified foreign body in trachea
√7th T17.400 Unspecified foreign body in trachea causing asphyxiation
√7th T17.408 Unspecified foreign body in trachea causing other injury
√6th T17.41 Gastric contents in trachea
Aspiration of gastric contents into trachea
Vomitus in trachea
√7th T17.410 Gastric contents in trachea causing asphyxiation
√7th T17.418 Gastric contents in trachea causing other injury
√6th T17.42 Food in trachea
Bones in trachea
Seeds in trachea
√7th T17.420 Food in trachea causing asphyxiation
√7th T17.428 Food in trachea causing other injury
√6th T17.49 Other foreign object in trachea
√7th T17.490 Other foreign object in trachea causing asphyxiation
√7th T17.498 Other foreign object in trachea causing other injury
√5th T17.5 Foreign body in bronchus
√6th T17.50 Unspecified foreign body in bronchus
√7th T17.500 Unspecified foreign body in bronchus causing asphyxiation
√7th T17.508 Unspecified foreign body in bronchus causing other injury
√6th T17.51 Gastric contents in bronchus
Aspiration of gastric contents into bronchus
Vomitus in bronchus
√7th T17.510 Gastric contents in bronchus causing asphyxiation
√7th T17.518 Gastric contents in bronchus causing other injury
√6th T17.52 Food in bronchus
Bones in bronchus
Seeds in bronchus
√7th T17.520 Food in bronchus causing asphyxiation
√7th T17.528 Food in bronchus causing other injury
√6th T17.59 Other foreign object in bronchus
√7th T17.590 Other foreign object in bronchus causing asphyxiation
√7th T17.598 Other foreign object in bronchus causing other injury
√5th T17.8 Foreign body in other parts of respiratory tract
Foreign body in bronchioles
Foreign body in lung
√6th T17.80 Unspecified foreign body in other parts of respiratory tract
√7th T17.800 Unspecified foreign body in other parts of respiratory tract causing asphyxiation
√7th T17.808 Unspecified foreign body in other parts of respiratory tract causing other injury
√6th T17.81 Gastric contents in other parts of respiratory tract
Aspiration of gastric contents into other parts of respiratory tract
Vomitus in other parts of respiratory tract
√7th T17.810 Gastric contents in other parts of respiratory tract causing asphyxiation
√7th T17.818 Gastric contents in other parts of respiratory tract causing other injury
√6th T17.82 Food in other parts of respiratory tract
Bones in other parts of respiratory tract
Seeds in other parts of respiratory tract
√7th T17.820 Food in other parts of respiratory tract causing asphyxiation
√7th T17.828 Food in other parts of respiratory tract causing other injury
√6th T17.89 Other foreign object in other parts of respiratory tract
√7th T17.890 Other foreign object in other parts of respiratory tract causing asphyxiation
√7th T17.898 Other foreign object in other parts of respiratory tract causing other injury
√5th T17.9 Foreign body in respiratory tract, part unspecified
√6th T17.90 Unspecified foreign body in respiratory tract, part unspecified
√7th T17.900 Unspecified foreign body in respiratory tract, part unspecified causing asphyxiation
√7th T17.908 Unspecified foreign body in respiratory tract, part unspecified causing other injury
√6th T17.91 Gastric contents in respiratory tract, part unspecified
Aspiration of gastric contents into respiratory tract, part unspecified
Vomitus in trachea respiratory tract, part unspecified
√7th T17.910 Gastric contents in respiratory tract, part unspecified causing asphyxiation
√7th T17.918 Gastric contents in respiratory tract, part unspecified causing other injury
√6th T17.92 Food in respiratory tract, part unspecified
Bones in respiratory tract, part unspecified
Seeds in respiratory tract, part unspecified
√7th T17.920 Food in respiratory tract, part unspecified causing asphyxiation
√7th T17.928 Food in respiratory tract, part unspecified causing other injury
√6th T17.99 Other foreign object in respiratory tract, part unspecified
√7th T17.990 Other foreign object in respiratory tract, part unspecified in causing asphyxiation
AHA: 2019,3Q,15
√7th T17.998 Other foreign object in respiratory tract, part unspecified causing other injury

√4th **T18 Foreign body in alimentary tract**

EXCLUDES 2 *foreign body in pharynx (T17.2-)*

The appropriate 7th character is to be added to each code from category T18.
A initial encounter
D subsequent encounter
S sequela

√x7th T18.0 Foreign body in mouth

√5th **T18.1 Foreign body in esophagus**

EXCLUDES 2 *foreign body in respiratory tract (T17.-)*

√6th **T18.10 Unspecified foreign body in esophagus**

√7th **T18.100 Unspecified foreign body in esophagus causing compression of trachea**

Unspecified foreign body in esophagus causing obstruction of respiration

√7th **T18.108 Unspecified foreign body in esophagus causing other injury**

√6th **T18.11 Gastric contents in esophagus**

Vomitus in esophagus

√7th **T18.110 Gastric contents in esophagus causing compression of trachea**

Gastric contents in esophagus causing obstruction of respiration

√7th **T18.118 Gastric contents in esophagus causing other injury**

√6th **T18.12 Food in esophagus**

Bones in esophagus
Seeds in esophagus

√7th **T18.120 Food in esophagus causing compression of trachea**

Food in esophagus causing obstruction of respiration

√7th **T18.128 Food in esophagus causing other injury**

√6th **T18.19 Other foreign object in esophagus**

**AHA:** 2022,1Q,27; 2015,1Q,23

√7th **T18.190 Other foreign object in esophagus causing compression of trachea**

Other foreign body in esophagus causing obstruction of respiration

**TIP:** Any foreign object lodged in the esophagus requires immediate treatment and is considered an injury. Assign this code when there is respiratory compromise or compression. If no respiratory compromise or compression is documented, assign code T18.198-.

√7th **T18.198 Other foreign object in esophagus causing other injury**

**TIP:** Any foreign object lodged in the esophagus requires immediate treatment and is considered an injury. Assign this code when there is no respiratory compromise or compression. If respiratory compromise or compression is documented, assign code T18.190-.

√x7th **T18.2 Foreign body in stomach**

√x7th **T18.3 Foreign body in small intestine**

√x7th **T18.4 Foreign body in colon**

√x7th **T18.5 Foreign body in anus and rectum**

Foreign body in rectosigmoid (junction)

√x7th **T18.8 Foreign body in other parts of alimentary tract**

√x7th **T18.9 Foreign body of alimentary tract, part unspecified**

Foreign body in digestive system NOS
Swallowed foreign body NOS

√4th **T19 Foreign body in genitourinary tract**

EXCLUDES 2 *complications due to implanted mesh (T83.7-)*
*mechanical complications of contraceptive device (intrauterine) (vaginal) (T83.3-)*
*presence of contraceptive device (intrauterine) (vaginal) (Z97.5)*

The appropriate 7th character is to be added to each code from category T19.
A initial encounter
D subsequent encounter
S sequela

√x7th **T19.0 Foreign body in urethra**

√x7th **T19.1 Foreign body in bladder**

√x7th **T19.2 Foreign body in vulva and vagina**

√x7th **T19.3 Foreign body in uterus**

√x7th **T19.4 Foreign body in penis**

√x7th **T19.8 Foreign body in other parts of genitourinary tract**

√x7th **T19.9 Foreign body in genitourinary tract, part unspecified**

## BURNS AND CORROSIONS (T20-T32)

INCLUDES burns (thermal) from electrical heating appliances
burns (thermal) from electricity
burns (thermal) from flame
burns (thermal) from friction
burns (thermal) from hot air and hot gases
burns (thermal) from hot objects
burns (thermal) from lightning
burns (thermal) from radiation
chemical burn [corrosion] (external) (internal)
scalds

EXCLUDES 2 *erythema [dermatitis] ab igne (L59.0)*
*radiation-related disorders of the skin and subcutaneous tissue (L55-L59)*
*sunburn (L55.-)*

**AHA:** 2016,2Q,4

### Burns and corrosions of external body surface, specified by site (T20-T25)

INCLUDES burns and corrosions of first degree [erythema]
burns and corrosions of second degree [blisters] [epidermal loss]
burns and corrosions of third degree [deep necrosis of underlying tissue] [full-thickness skin loss]

Use additional code from category T31 or T32 to identify extent of body surface involved

√4th **T20 Burn and corrosion of head, face, and neck**

EXCLUDES 2 *burn and corrosion of ear drum (T28.41, T28.91)*
*burn and corrosion of eye and adnexa (T26.-)*
*burn and corrosion of mouth and pharynx (T28.0)*

**AHA:** 2015,1Q,18-19

The appropriate 7th character is to be added to each code from category T20.
A initial encounter
D subsequent encounter
S sequela

√5th **T20.0 Burn of unspecified degree of head, face, and neck**

Use additional external cause code to identify the source, place and intent of the burn (X00-X19, X75-X77, X96-X98, Y92)

√x7th **T20.00 Burn of unspecified degree of head, face, and neck, unspecified site**

√6th **T20.01 Burn of unspecified degree of ear [any part, except ear drum]**

EXCLUDES 2 *burn of ear drum (T28.41-)*

√7th **T20.011 Burn of unspecified degree of right ear [any part, except ear drum]**

√7th **T20.012 Burn of unspecified degree of left ear [any part, except ear drum]**

√7th **T20.019 Burn of unspecified degree of unspecified ear [any part, except ear drum]**

√x7th **T20.02 Burn of unspecified degree of lip(s)**

√x7th **T20.03 Burn of unspecified degree of chin**

√x7th **T20.04 Burn of unspecified degree of nose (septum)**

√x7th **T20.05 Burn of unspecified degree of scalp [any part]**

√x7th **T20.06 Burn of unspecified degree of forehead and cheek**

√x7th **T20.07 Burn of unspecified degree of neck**

√x7th **T20.09 Burn of unspecified degree of multiple sites of head, face, and neck**

√5th **T20.1 Burn of first degree of head, face, and neck**

Use additional external cause code to identify the source, place and intent of the burn (X00-X19, X75-X77, X96-X98, Y92)

√x7th **T20.10 Burn of first degree of head, face, and neck, unspecified site**

√6th **T20.11 Burn of first degree of ear [any part, except ear drum]**

EXCLUDES 2 *burn of ear drum (T28.41-)*

√7th **T20.111 Burn of first degree of right ear [any part, except ear drum]**

√7th **T20.112 Burn of first degree of left ear [any part, except ear drum]**

√7th **T20.119 Burn of first degree of unspecified ear [any part, except ear drum]**

√x7th **T20.12 Burn of first degree of lip(s)**

√x7th **T20.13 Burn of first degree of chin**

√x7th **T20.14 Burn of first degree of nose (septum)**

√x7th **T20.15 Burn of first degree of scalp [any part]**

√x7th **T20.16 Burn of first degree of forehead and cheek**

√x7th **T20.17 Burn of first degree of neck**

√x 7th **T2Ø.19** Burn of first degree of multiple sites of head, face, and neck

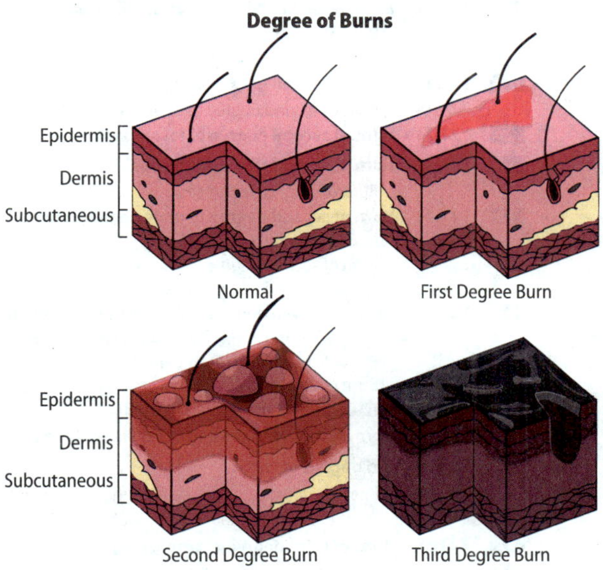


√5th **T2Ø.2** **Burn of second degree of head, face, and neck**
Use additional external cause code to identify the source, place and intent of the burn (XØØ-X19, X75-X77, X96-X98, Y92)

√x 7th **T2Ø.2Ø** Burn of second degree of head, face, and neck, unspecified site

√6th **T2Ø.21** Burn of second degree of ear [any part, except ear drum]
EXCLUDES 2 *burn of ear drum (T28.41-)*

√7th **T2Ø.211** Burn of second degree of right ear [any part, except ear drum]

√7th **T2Ø.212** Burn of second degree of left ear [any part, except ear drum]

√7th **T2Ø.219** Burn of second degree of unspecified ear [any part, except ear drum]

√x 7th **T2Ø.22** Burn of second degree of lip(s)

√x 7th **T2Ø.23** Burn of second degree of chin

√x 7th **T2Ø.24** Burn of second degree of nose (septum)

√x 7th **T2Ø.25** Burn of second degree of scalp [any part]

√x 7th **T2Ø.26** Burn of second degree of forehead and cheek

√x 7th **T2Ø.27** Burn of second degree of neck

√x 7th **T2Ø.29** Burn of second degree of multiple sites of head, face, and neck

√5th **T2Ø.3** **Burn of third degree of head, face, and neck**
Use additional external cause code to identify the source, place and intent of the burn (XØØ-X19, X75-X77, X96-X98, Y92)

√x 7th **T2Ø.3Ø** Burn of third degree of head, face, and neck, unspecified site COM

√6th **T2Ø.31** Burn of third degree of ear [any part, except ear drum]
EXCLUDES 2 *burn of ear drum (T28.41-)*
AHA: 2015,1Q,18

√7th **T2Ø.311** Burn of third degree of right ear [any part, except ear drum] COM

√7th **T2Ø.312** Burn of third degree of left ear [any part, except ear drum] COM

√7th **T2Ø.319** Burn of third degree of unspecified ear [any part, except ear drum] COM

√x 7th **T2Ø.32** Burn of third degree of lip(s) COM

√x 7th **T2Ø.33** Burn of third degree of chin COM

√x 7th **T2Ø.34** Burn of third degree of nose (septum) COM

√x 7th **T2Ø.35** Burn of third degree of scalp [any part] COM

√x 7th **T2Ø.36** Burn of third degree of forehead and cheek COM

√x 7th **T2Ø.37** Burn of third degree of neck COM

√x 7th **T2Ø.39** Burn of third degree of multiple sites of head, face, and neck COM

√5th **T2Ø.4** **Corrosion of unspecified degree of head, face, and neck**
Code first (T51-T65) to identify chemical and intent
Use additional external cause code to identify place (Y92)

√x 7th **T2Ø.4Ø** Corrosion of unspecified degree of head, face, and neck, unspecified site

√6th **T2Ø.41** Corrosion of unspecified degree of ear [any part, except ear drum]
EXCLUDES 2 *corrosion of ear drum (T28.91-)*

√7th **T2Ø.411** Corrosion of unspecified degree of right ear [any part, except ear drum]

√7th **T2Ø.412** Corrosion of unspecified degree of left ear [any part, except ear drum]

√7th **T2Ø.419** Corrosion of unspecified degree of unspecified ear [any part, except ear drum]

√x 7th **T2Ø.42** Corrosion of unspecified degree of lip(s)

√x 7th **T2Ø.43** Corrosion of unspecified degree of chin

√x 7th **T2Ø.44** Corrosion of unspecified degree of nose (septum)

√x 7th **T2Ø.45** Corrosion of unspecified degree of scalp [any part]

√x 7th **T2Ø.46** Corrosion of unspecified degree of forehead and cheek

√x 7th **T2Ø.47** Corrosion of unspecified degree of neck

√x 7th **T2Ø.49** Corrosion of unspecified degree of multiple sites of head, face, and neck

√5th **T2Ø.5** **Corrosion of first degree of head, face, and neck**
Code first (T51-T65) to identify chemical and intent
Use additional external cause code to identify place (Y92)

√x 7th **T2Ø.5Ø** Corrosion of first degree of head, face, and neck, unspecified site

√6th **T2Ø.51** Corrosion of first degree of ear [any part, except ear drum]
EXCLUDES 2 *corrosion of ear drum (T28.91-)*

√7th **T2Ø.511** Corrosion of first degree of right ear [any part, except ear drum]

√7th **T2Ø.512** Corrosion of first degree of left ear [any part, except ear drum]

√7th **T2Ø.519** Corrosion of first degree of unspecified ear [any part, except ear drum]

√x 7th **T2Ø.52** Corrosion of first degree of lip(s)

√x 7th **T2Ø.53** Corrosion of first degree of chin

√x 7th **T2Ø.54** Corrosion of first degree of nose (septum)

√x 7th **T2Ø.55** Corrosion of first degree of scalp [any part]

√x 7th **T2Ø.56** Corrosion of first degree of forehead and cheek

√x 7th **T2Ø.57** Corrosion of first degree of neck

√x 7th **T2Ø.59** Corrosion of first degree of multiple sites of head, face, and neck

√5th **T2Ø.6** **Corrosion of second degree of head, face, and neck**
Code first (T51-T65) to identify chemical and intent
Use additional external cause code to identify place (Y92)

√x 7th **T2Ø.6Ø** Corrosion of second degree of head, face, and neck, unspecified site

√6th **T2Ø.61** Corrosion of second degree of ear [any part, except ear drum]
EXCLUDES 2 *corrosion of ear drum (T28.91-)*

√7th **T2Ø.611** Corrosion of second degree of right ear [any part, except ear drum]

√7th **T2Ø.612** Corrosion of second degree of left ear [any part, except ear drum]

√7th **T2Ø.619** Corrosion of second degree of unspecified ear [any part, except ear drum]

√x 7th **T2Ø.62** Corrosion of second degree of lip(s)

√x 7th **T2Ø.63** Corrosion of second degree of chin

√x 7th **T2Ø.64** Corrosion of second degree of nose (septum)

√x 7th **T2Ø.65** Corrosion of second degree of scalp [any part]

√x 7th **T2Ø.66** Corrosion of second degree of forehead and cheek

√x 7th **T2Ø.67** Corrosion of second degree of neck

√x 7th **T2Ø.69** Corrosion of second degree of multiple sites of head, face, and neck

√5th **T2Ø.7** **Corrosion of third degree of head, face, and neck**
Code first (T51-T65) to identify chemical and intent
Use additional external cause code to identify place (Y92)

√x 7th **T2Ø.7Ø** Corrosion of third degree of head, face, and neck, unspecified site COM

√6th **T2Ø.71** Corrosion of third degree of ear [any part, except ear drum]
EXCLUDES 2 *corrosion of ear drum (T28.91-)*

√7th **T2Ø.711** Corrosion of third degree of right ear [any part, except ear drum] COM

√7th **T2Ø.712** Corrosion of third degree of left ear [any part, except ear drum] COM

√7th **T2Ø.719** Corrosion of third degree of unspecified ear [any part, except ear drum] COM

√x7th T20.72 **Corrosion of third degree of lip(s)** COM

√x7th T20.73 **Corrosion of third degree of chin** COM

√x7th T20.74 **Corrosion of third degree of nose (septum)** COM

√x7th T20.75 **Corrosion of third degree of scalp [any part]** COM

√x7th T20.76 **Corrosion of third degree of forehead and cheek** COM

√x7th T20.77 **Corrosion of third degree of neck** COM

√x7th T20.79 **Corrosion of third degree of multiple sites of head, face, and neck** COM

√4th **T21 Burn and corrosion of trunk**

INCLUDES burns and corrosion of hip region

EXCLUDES 2 *burns and corrosion of axilla (T22.- with fifth character 4)*
*burns and corrosion of scapular region (T22.- with fifth character 6)*
*burns and corrosion of shoulder (T22.- with fifth character 5)*

The appropriate 7th character is to be added to each code from category T21.
A initial encounter
D subsequent encounter
S sequela

√5th **T21.0 Burn of unspecified degree of trunk**

Use additional external cause code to identify the source, place and intent of the burn (X00-X19, X75-X77, X96-X98, Y92)

√x7th T21.00 **Burn of unspecified degree of trunk, unspecified site**

√x7th T21.01 **Burn of unspecified degree of chest wall**
Burn of unspecified degree of breast

√x7th T21.02 **Burn of unspecified degree of abdominal wall**
Burn of unspecified degree of flank
Burn of unspecified degree of groin

√x7th T21.03 **Burn of unspecified degree of upper back**
Burn of unspecified degree of interscapular region

√x7th T21.04 **Burn of unspecified degree of lower back**

√x7th T21.05 **Burn of unspecified degree of buttock**
Burn of unspecified degree of anus

√x7th T21.06 **Burn of unspecified degree of male genital region**
Burn of unspecified degree of penis
Burn of unspecified degree of scrotum
Burn of unspecified degree of testis

√x7th T21.07 **Burn of unspecified degree of female genital region**
Burn of unspecified degree of labium (majus) (minus)
Burn of unspecified degree of perineum
Burn of unspecified degree of vulva
EXCLUDES 2 *burn of vagina (T28.3)*

√x7th T21.09 **Burn of unspecified degree of other site of trunk**

√5th **T21.1 Burn of first degree of trunk**

Use additional external cause code to identify the source, place and intent of the burn (X00-X19, X75-X77, X96-X98, Y92)

√x7th T21.10 **Burn of first degree of trunk, unspecified site**

√x7th T21.11 **Burn of first degree of chest wall**
Burn of first degree of breast

√x7th T21.12 **Burn of first degree of abdominal wall**
Burn of first degree of flank
Burn of first degree of groin

√x7th T21.13 **Burn of first degree of upper back**
Burn of first degree of interscapular region

√x7th T21.14 **Burn of first degree of lower back**

√x7th T21.15 **Burn of first degree of buttock**
Burn of first degree of anus

√x7th T21.16 **Burn of first degree of male genital region**
Burn of first degree of penis
Burn of first degree of scrotum
Burn of first degree of testis

√x7th T21.17 **Burn of first degree of female genital region**
Burn of first degree of labium (majus) (minus)
Burn of first degree of perineum
Burn of first degree of vulva
EXCLUDES 2 *burn of vagina (T28.3)*

√x7th T21.19 **Burn of first degree of other site of trunk**

√5th **T21.2 Burn of second degree of trunk**

Use additional external cause code to identify the source, place and intent of the burn (X00-X19, X75-X77, X96-X98, Y92)

√x7th T21.20 **Burn of second degree of trunk, unspecified site**

√x7th T21.21 **Burn of second degree of chest wall**
Burn of second degree of breast

√x7th T21.22 **Burn of second degree of abdominal wall**
Burn of second degree of flank
Burn of second degree of groin

√x7th T21.23 **Burn of second degree of upper back**
Burn of second degree of interscapular region

√x7th T21.24 **Burn of second degree of lower back**

√x7th T21.25 **Burn of second degree of buttock**
Burn of second degree of anus

√x7th T21.26 **Burn of second degree of male genital region**
Burn of second degree of penis
Burn of second degree of scrotum
Burn of second degree of testis

√x7th T21.27 **Burn of second degree of female genital region**
Burn of second degree of labium (majus) (minus)
Burn of second degree of perineum
Burn of second degree of vulva
EXCLUDES 2 *burn of vagina (T28.3)*

√x7th T21.29 **Burn of second degree of other site of trunk**

√5th **T21.3 Burn of third degree of trunk**

Use additional external cause code to identify the source, place and intent of the burn (X00-X19, X75-X77, X96-X98, Y92)

√x7th T21.30 **Burn of third degree of trunk, unspecified site** COM

√x7th T21.31 **Burn of third degree of chest wall** COM
Burn of third degree of breast
AHA: 2016,2Q,5

√x7th T21.32 **Burn of third degree of abdominal wall** COM
Burn of third degree of flank
Burn of third degree of groin

√x7th T21.33 **Burn of third degree of upper back** COM
Burn of third degree of interscapular region

√x7th T21.34 **Burn of third degree of lower back** COM

√x7th T21.35 **Burn of third degree of buttock** COM
Burn of third degree of anus

√x7th T21.36 **Burn of third degree of male genital region** COM
Burn of third degree of penis
Burn of third degree of scrotum
Burn of third degree of testis

√x7th T21.37 **Burn of third degree of female genital region** COM
Burn of third degree of labium (majus) (minus)
Burn of third degree of perineum
Burn of third degree of vulva
EXCLUDES 2 *burn of vagina (T28.3)*

√x7th T21.39 **Burn of third degree of other site of trunk** COM

√5th **T21.4 Corrosion of unspecified degree of trunk**

Code first (T51-T65) to identify chemical and intent
Use additional external cause code to identify place (Y92)

√x7th T21.40 **Corrosion of unspecified degree of trunk, unspecified site**

√x7th T21.41 **Corrosion of unspecified degree of chest wall**
Corrosion of unspecified degree of breast

√x7th T21.42 **Corrosion of unspecified degree of abdominal wall**
Corrosion of unspecified degree of flank
Corrosion of unspecified degree of groin

√x7th T21.43 **Corrosion of unspecified degree of upper back**
Corrosion of unspecified degree of interscapular region

√x7th T21.44 **Corrosion of unspecified degree of lower back**

√x7th T21.45 **Corrosion of unspecified degree of buttock**
Corrosion of unspecified degree of anus

√x7th T21.46 **Corrosion of unspecified degree of male genital region**
Corrosion of unspecified degree of penis
Corrosion of unspecified degree of scrotum
Corrosion of unspecified degree of testis

√x7th T21.47 **Corrosion of unspecified degree of female genital region**
Corrosion of unspecified degree of labium (majus) (minus)
Corrosion of unspecified degree of perineum
Corrosion of unspecified degree of vulva
EXCLUDES 2 *corrosion of vagina (T28.8)*

√x7th T21.49 **Corrosion of unspecified degree of other site of trunk**

HCC CMS-HCC Rx Rx HCC ESR ESRD HCC COM Commercial HCC N Newborn: 0 P Pediatric: 0-17 M Maternity: 9-64 A Adult: 15-124

**T21.5 Corrosion of first degree of trunk**
Code first (T51-T65) to identify chemical and intent
Use additional external cause code to identify place (Y92)

- **T21.50 Corrosion of first degree of trunk, unspecified site**
- **T21.51 Corrosion of first degree of chest wall**
  Corrosion of first degree of breast
- **T21.52 Corrosion of first degree of abdominal wall**
  Corrosion of first degree of flank
  Corrosion of first degree of groin
- **T21.53 Corrosion of first degree of upper back**
  Corrosion of first degree of interscapular region
- **T21.54 Corrosion of first degree of lower back**
- **T21.55 Corrosion of first degree of buttock**
  Corrosion of first degree of anus
- **T21.56 Corrosion of first degree of male genital region**
  Corrosion of first degree of penis
  Corrosion of first degree of scrotum
  Corrosion of first degree of testis
- **T21.57 Corrosion of first degree of female genital region**
  Corrosion of first degree of labium (majus) (minus)
  Corrosion of first degree of perineum
  Corrosion of first degree of vulva
  EXCLUDES 2 *corrosion of vagina (T28.8)*
- **T21.59 Corrosion of first degree of other site of trunk**

**T21.6 Corrosion of second degree of trunk**
Code first (T51-T65) to identify chemical and intent
Use additional external cause code to identify place (Y92)

- **T21.60 Corrosion of second degree of trunk, unspecified site**
- **T21.61 Corrosion of second degree of chest wall**
  Corrosion of second degree of breast
- **T21.62 Corrosion of second degree of abdominal wall**
  Corrosion of second degree of flank
  Corrosion of second degree of groin
- **T21.63 Corrosion of second degree of upper back**
  Corrosion of second degree of interscapular region
- **T21.64 Corrosion of second degree of lower back**
- **T21.65 Corrosion of second degree of buttock**
  Corrosion of second degree of anus
- **T21.66 Corrosion of second degree of male genital region**
  Corrosion of second degree of penis
  Corrosion of second degree of scrotum
  Corrosion of second degree of testis
- **T21.67 Corrosion of second degree of female genital region**
  Corrosion of second degree of labium (majus) (minus)
  Corrosion of second degree of perineum
  Corrosion of second degree of vulva
  EXCLUDES 2 *corrosion of vagina (T28.8)*
- **T21.69 Corrosion of second degree of other site of trunk**

**T21.7 Corrosion of third degree of trunk**
Code first (T51-T65) to identify chemical and intent
Use additional external cause code to identify place (Y92)

- **T21.70 Corrosion of third degree of trunk, unspecified site** COM
- **T21.71 Corrosion of third degree of chest wall** COM
  Corrosion of third degree of breast
- **T21.72 Corrosion of third degree of abdominal wall** COM
  Corrosion of third degree of flank
  Corrosion of third degree of groin
- **T21.73 Corrosion of third degree of upper back** COM
  Corrosion of third degree of interscapular region
- **T21.74 Corrosion of third degree of lower back** COM
- **T21.75 Corrosion of third degree of buttock** COM
  Corrosion of third degree of anus
- **T21.76 Corrosion of third degree of male genital region** COM
  Corrosion of third degree of penis
  Corrosion of third degree of scrotum
  Corrosion of third degree of testis
- **T21.77 Corrosion of third degree of female genital region** COM
  Corrosion of third degree of labium (majus) (minus)
  Corrosion of third degree of perineum
  Corrosion of third degree of vulva
  EXCLUDES 2 *corrosion of vagina (T28.8)*
- **T21.79 Corrosion of third degree of other site of trunk** COM

## T22 Burn and corrosion of shoulder and upper limb, except wrist and hand

EXCLUDES 2 *burn and corrosion of interscapular region (T21.-)*
*burn and corrosion of wrist and hand (T23.-)*

The appropriate 7th character is to be added to each code from category T22.
A initial encounter
D subsequent encounter
S sequela

**T22.0 Burn of unspecified degree of shoulder and upper limb, except wrist and hand**
Use additional external cause code to identify the source, place and intent of the burn (X00-X19, X75-X77, X96-X98, Y92)

- **T22.00 Burn of unspecified degree of shoulder and upper limb, except wrist and hand, unspecified site**
- **T22.01 Burn of unspecified degree of forearm**
  - **T22.011 Burn of unspecified degree of right forearm**
  - **T22.012 Burn of unspecified degree of left forearm**
  - **T22.019 Burn of unspecified degree of unspecified forearm**
- **T22.02 Burn of unspecified degree of elbow**
  - **T22.021 Burn of unspecified degree of right elbow**
  - **T22.022 Burn of unspecified degree of left elbow**
  - **T22.029 Burn of unspecified degree of unspecified elbow**
- **T22.03 Burn of unspecified degree of upper arm**
  - **T22.031 Burn of unspecified degree of right upper arm**
  - **T22.032 Burn of unspecified degree of left upper arm**
  - **T22.039 Burn of unspecified degree of unspecified upper arm**
- **T22.04 Burn of unspecified degree of axilla**
  - **T22.041 Burn of unspecified degree of right axilla**
  - **T22.042 Burn of unspecified degree of left axilla**
  - **T22.049 Burn of unspecified degree of unspecified axilla**
- **T22.05 Burn of unspecified degree of shoulder**
  - **T22.051 Burn of unspecified degree of right shoulder**
  - **T22.052 Burn of unspecified degree of left shoulder**
  - **T22.059 Burn of unspecified degree of unspecified shoulder**
- **T22.06 Burn of unspecified degree of scapular region**
  - **T22.061 Burn of unspecified degree of right scapular region**
  - **T22.062 Burn of unspecified degree of left scapular region**
  - **T22.069 Burn of unspecified degree of unspecified scapular region**
- **T22.09 Burn of unspecified degree of multiple sites of shoulder and upper limb, except wrist and hand**
  - **T22.091 Burn of unspecified degree of multiple sites of right shoulder and upper limb, except wrist and hand**
  - **T22.092 Burn of unspecified degree of multiple sites of left shoulder and upper limb, except wrist and hand**
  - **T22.099 Burn of unspecified degree of multiple sites of unspecified shoulder and upper limb, except wrist and hand**

**T22.1 Burn of first degree of shoulder and upper limb, except wrist and hand**
Use additional external cause code to identify the source, place and intent of the burn (X00-X19, X75-X77, X96-X98, Y92)

- **T22.10 Burn of first degree of shoulder and upper limb, except wrist and hand, unspecified site**
- **T22.11 Burn of first degree of forearm**
  - **T22.111 Burn of first degree of right forearm**
  - **T22.112 Burn of first degree of left forearm**
  - **T22.119 Burn of first degree of unspecified forearm**
- **T22.12 Burn of first degree of elbow**
  - **T22.121 Burn of first degree of right elbow**
  - **T22.122 Burn of first degree of left elbow**
  - **T22.129 Burn of first degree of unspecified elbow**

- ✓6th **T22.13** Burn of first degree of upper arm
  - ✓7th **T22.131** Burn of first degree of right upper arm
  - ✓7th **T22.132** Burn of first degree of left upper arm
  - ✓7th **T22.139** Burn of first degree of unspecified upper arm
- ✓6th **T22.14** Burn of first degree of axilla
  - ✓7th **T22.141** Burn of first degree of right axilla
  - ✓7th **T22.142** Burn of first degree of left axilla
  - ✓7th **T22.149** Burn of first degree of unspecified axilla
- ✓6th **T22.15** Burn of first degree of shoulder
  - ✓7th **T22.151** Burn of first degree of right shoulder
  - ✓7th **T22.152** Burn of first degree of left shoulder
  - ✓7th **T22.159** Burn of first degree of unspecified shoulder
- ✓6th **T22.16** Burn of first degree of scapular region
  - ✓7th **T22.161** Burn of first degree of right scapular region
  - ✓7th **T22.162** Burn of first degree of left scapular region
  - ✓7th **T22.169** Burn of first degree of unspecified scapular region
- ✓6th **T22.19** Burn of first degree of multiple sites of shoulder and upper limb, except wrist and hand
  - ✓7th **T22.191** Burn of first degree of multiple sites of right shoulder and upper limb, except wrist and hand
  - ✓7th **T22.192** Burn of first degree of multiple sites of left shoulder and upper limb, except wrist and hand
  - ✓7th **T22.199** Burn of first degree of multiple sites of unspecified shoulder and upper limb, except wrist and hand

✓5th **T22.2** Burn of second degree of shoulder and upper limb, except wrist and hand
Use additional external cause code to identify the source, place and intent of the burn (X00-X19, X75-X77, X96-X98, Y92)

- ✓x7th **T22.20** Burn of second degree of shoulder and upper limb, except wrist and hand, unspecified site
- ✓6th **T22.21** Burn of second degree of forearm
  - ✓7th **T22.211** Burn of second degree of right forearm
  - ✓7th **T22.212** Burn of second degree of left forearm
  - ✓7th **T22.219** Burn of second degree of unspecified forearm
- ✓6th **T22.22** Burn of second degree of elbow
  - ✓7th **T22.221** Burn of second degree of right elbow
  - ✓7th **T22.222** Burn of second degree of left elbow
  - ✓7th **T22.229** Burn of second degree of unspecified elbow
- ✓6th **T22.23** Burn of second degree of upper arm
  - ✓7th **T22.231** Burn of second degree of right upper arm
  - ✓7th **T22.232** Burn of second degree of left upper arm
  - ✓7th **T22.239** Burn of second degree of unspecified upper arm
- ✓6th **T22.24** Burn of second degree of axilla
  - ✓7th **T22.241** Burn of second degree of right axilla
  - ✓7th **T22.242** Burn of second degree of left axilla
  - ✓7th **T22.249** Burn of second degree of unspecified axilla
- ✓6th **T22.25** Burn of second degree of shoulder
  - ✓7th **T22.251** Burn of second degree of right shoulder
  - ✓7th **T22.252** Burn of second degree of left shoulder
  - ✓7th **T22.259** Burn of second degree of unspecified shoulder
- ✓6th **T22.26** Burn of second degree of scapular region
  - ✓7th **T22.261** Burn of second degree of right scapular region
  - ✓7th **T22.262** Burn of second degree of left scapular region
  - ✓7th **T22.269** Burn of second degree of unspecified scapular region
- ✓6th **T22.29** Burn of second degree of multiple sites of shoulder and upper limb, except wrist and hand
  - ✓7th **T22.291** Burn of second degree of multiple sites of right shoulder and upper limb, except wrist and hand
  - ✓7th **T22.292** Burn of second degree of multiple sites of left shoulder and upper limb, except wrist and hand
  - ✓7th **T22.299** Burn of second degree of multiple sites of unspecified shoulder and upper limb, except wrist and hand

✓5th **T22.3** Burn of third degree of shoulder and upper limb, except wrist and hand
Use additional external cause code to identify the source, place and intent of the burn (X00-X19, X75-X77, X96-X98, Y92)

- ✓x7th **T22.30** Burn of third degree of shoulder and upper limb, except wrist and hand, unspecified site COM
- ✓6th **T22.31** Burn of third degree of forearm
  - ✓7th **T22.311** Burn of third degree of right forearm COM
  - ✓7th **T22.312** Burn of third degree of left forearm COM
  - ✓7th **T22.319** Burn of third degree of unspecified forearm COM
- ✓6th **T22.32** Burn of third degree of elbow
  - ✓7th **T22.321** Burn of third degree of right elbow COM
  - ✓7th **T22.322** Burn of third degree of left elbow COM
  - ✓7th **T22.329** Burn of third degree of unspecified elbow COM
- ✓6th **T22.33** Burn of third degree of upper arm
  - ✓7th **T22.331** Burn of third degree of right upper arm COM
  - ✓7th **T22.332** Burn of third degree of left upper arm COM
  - ✓7th **T22.339** Burn of third degree of unspecified upper arm COM
- ✓6th **T22.34** Burn of third degree of axilla
  - ✓7th **T22.341** Burn of third degree of right axilla COM
  - ✓7th **T22.342** Burn of third degree of left axilla COM
  - ✓7th **T22.349** Burn of third degree of unspecified axilla COM
- ✓6th **T22.35** Burn of third degree of shoulder
  - ✓7th **T22.351** Burn of third degree of right shoulder COM
  - ✓7th **T22.352** Burn of third degree of left shoulder COM
  - ✓7th **T22.359** Burn of third degree of unspecified shoulder COM
- ✓6th **T22.36** Burn of third degree of scapular region
  - ✓7th **T22.361** Burn of third degree of right scapular region COM
  - ✓7th **T22.362** Burn of third degree of left scapular region COM
  - ✓7th **T22.369** Burn of third degree of unspecified scapular region COM
- ✓6th **T22.39** Burn of third degree of multiple sites of shoulder and upper limb, except wrist and hand
  - ✓7th **T22.391** Burn of third degree of multiple sites of right shoulder and upper limb, except wrist and hand COM
  - ✓7th **T22.392** Burn of third degree of multiple sites of left shoulder and upper limb, except wrist and hand COM
  - ✓7th **T22.399** Burn of third degree of multiple sites of unspecified shoulder and upper limb, except wrist and hand COM

✓5th **T22.4** Corrosion of unspecified degree of shoulder and upper limb, except wrist and hand
Code first (T51-T65) to identify chemical and intent
Use additional external cause code to identify place (Y92)

- ✓x7th **T22.40** Corrosion of unspecified degree of shoulder and upper limb, except wrist and hand, unspecified site
- ✓6th **T22.41** Corrosion of unspecified degree of forearm
  - ✓7th **T22.411** Corrosion of unspecified degree of right forearm
  - ✓7th **T22.412** Corrosion of unspecified degree of left forearm
  - ✓7th **T22.419** Corrosion of unspecified degree of unspecified forearm
- ✓6th **T22.42** Corrosion of unspecified degree of elbow
  - ✓7th **T22.421** Corrosion of unspecified degree of right elbow
  - ✓7th **T22.422** Corrosion of unspecified degree of left elbow
  - ✓7th **T22.429** Corrosion of unspecified degree of unspecified elbow

√6th T22.43 Corrosion of unspecified degree of upper arm
√7th T22.431 Corrosion of unspecified degree of right upper arm
√7th T22.432 Corrosion of unspecified degree of left upper arm
√7th T22.439 Corrosion of unspecified degree of unspecified upper arm
√6th T22.44 Corrosion of unspecified degree of axilla
√7th T22.441 Corrosion of unspecified degree of right axilla
√7th T22.442 Corrosion of unspecified degree of left axilla
√7th T22.449 Corrosion of unspecified degree of unspecified axilla
√6th T22.45 Corrosion of unspecified degree of shoulder
√7th T22.451 Corrosion of unspecified degree of right shoulder
√7th T22.452 Corrosion of unspecified degree of left shoulder
√7th T22.459 Corrosion of unspecified degree of unspecified shoulder
√6th T22.46 Corrosion of unspecified degree of scapular region
√7th T22.461 Corrosion of unspecified degree of right scapular region
√7th T22.462 Corrosion of unspecified degree of left scapular region
√7th T22.469 Corrosion of unspecified degree of unspecified scapular region
√6th T22.49 Corrosion of unspecified degree of multiple sites of shoulder and upper limb, except wrist and hand
√7th T22.491 Corrosion of unspecified degree of multiple sites of right shoulder and upper limb, except wrist and hand
√7th T22.492 Corrosion of unspecified degree of multiple sites of left shoulder and upper limb, except wrist and hand
√7th T22.499 Corrosion of unspecified degree of multiple sites of unspecified shoulder and upper limb, except wrist and hand
√5th T22.5 Corrosion of first degree of shoulder and upper limb, except wrist and hand
Code first (T51-T65) to identify chemical and intent
Use additional external cause code to identify place (Y92)
√x7th T22.50 Corrosion of first degree of shoulder and upper limb, except wrist and hand unspecified site
√6th T22.51 Corrosion of first degree of forearm
√7th T22.511 Corrosion of first degree of right forearm
√7th T22.512 Corrosion of first degree of left forearm
√7th T22.519 Corrosion of first degree of unspecified forearm
√6th T22.52 Corrosion of first degree of elbow
√7th T22.521 Corrosion of first degree of right elbow
√7th T22.522 Corrosion of first degree of left elbow
√7th T22.529 Corrosion of first degree of unspecified elbow
√6th T22.53 Corrosion of first degree of upper arm
√7th T22.531 Corrosion of first degree of right upper arm
√7th T22.532 Corrosion of first degree of left upper arm
√7th T22.539 Corrosion of first degree of unspecified upper arm
√6th T22.54 Corrosion of first degree of axilla
√7th T22.541 Corrosion of first degree of right axilla
√7th T22.542 Corrosion of first degree of left axilla
√7th T22.549 Corrosion of first degree of unspecified axilla
√6th T22.55 Corrosion of first degree of shoulder
√7th T22.551 Corrosion of first degree of right shoulder
√7th T22.552 Corrosion of first degree of left shoulder
√7th T22.559 Corrosion of first degree of unspecified shoulder
√6th T22.56 Corrosion of first degree of scapular region
√7th T22.561 Corrosion of first degree of right scapular region
√7th T22.562 Corrosion of first degree of left scapular region
√7th T22.569 Corrosion of first degree of unspecified scapular region
√6th T22.59 Corrosion of first degree of multiple sites of shoulder and upper limb, except wrist and hand
√7th T22.591 Corrosion of first degree of multiple sites of right shoulder and upper limb, except wrist and hand
√7th T22.592 Corrosion of first degree of multiple sites of left shoulder and upper limb, except wrist and hand
√7th T22.599 Corrosion of first degree of multiple sites of unspecified shoulder and upper limb, except wrist and hand
√5th T22.6 Corrosion of second degree of shoulder and upper limb, except wrist and hand
Code first (T51-T65) to identify chemical and intent
Use additional external cause code to identify place (Y92)
√x7th T22.60 Corrosion of second degree of shoulder and upper limb, except wrist and hand, unspecified site
√6th T22.61 Corrosion of second degree of forearm
√7th T22.611 Corrosion of second degree of right forearm
√7th T22.612 Corrosion of second degree of left forearm
√7th T22.619 Corrosion of second degree of unspecified forearm
√6th T22.62 Corrosion of second degree of elbow
√7th T22.621 Corrosion of second degree of right elbow
√7th T22.622 Corrosion of second degree of left elbow
√7th T22.629 Corrosion of second degree of unspecified elbow
√6th T22.63 Corrosion of second degree of upper arm
√7th T22.631 Corrosion of second degree of right upper arm
√7th T22.632 Corrosion of second degree of left upper arm
√7th T22.639 Corrosion of second degree of unspecified upper arm
√6th T22.64 Corrosion of second degree of axilla
√7th T22.641 Corrosion of second degree of right axilla
√7th T22.642 Corrosion of second degree of left axilla
√7th T22.649 Corrosion of second degree of unspecified axilla
√6th T22.65 Corrosion of second degree of shoulder
√7th T22.651 Corrosion of second degree of right shoulder
√7th T22.652 Corrosion of second degree of left shoulder
√7th T22.659 Corrosion of second degree of unspecified shoulder
√6th T22.66 Corrosion of second degree of scapular region
√7th T22.661 Corrosion of second degree of right scapular region
√7th T22.662 Corrosion of second degree of left scapular region
√7th T22.669 Corrosion of second degree of unspecified scapular region
√6th T22.69 Corrosion of second degree of multiple sites of shoulder and upper limb, except wrist and hand
√7th T22.691 Corrosion of second degree of multiple sites of right shoulder and upper limb, except wrist and hand
√7th T22.692 Corrosion of second degree of multiple sites of left shoulder and upper limb, except wrist and hand
√7th T22.699 Corrosion of second degree of multiple sites of unspecified shoulder and upper limb, except wrist and hand
√5th T22.7 Corrosion of third degree of shoulder and upper limb, except wrist and hand
Code first (T51-T65) to identify chemical and intent
Use additional external cause code to identify place (Y92)
√x7th T22.70 Corrosion of third degree of shoulder and upper limb, except wrist and hand, unspecified site COM
√6th T22.71 Corrosion of third degree of forearm
√7th T22.711 Corrosion of third degree of right forearm COM
√7th T22.712 Corrosion of third degree of left forearm COM
√7th T22.719 Corrosion of third degree of unspecified forearm COM

- 6th **T22.72 Corrosion of third degree of elbow**
  - 7th T22.721 Corrosion of third degree of right elbow COM
  - 7th T22.722 Corrosion of third degree of left elbow COM
  - 7th T22.729 Corrosion of third degree of unspecified elbow COM
- 6th **T22.73 Corrosion of third degree of upper arm**
  - 7th T22.731 Corrosion of third degree of right upper arm COM
  - 7th T22.732 Corrosion of third degree of left upper arm COM
  - 7th T22.739 Corrosion of third degree of unspecified upper arm COM
- 6th **T22.74 Corrosion of third degree of axilla**
  - 7th T22.741 Corrosion of third degree of right axilla COM
  - 7th T22.742 Corrosion of third degree of left axilla COM
  - 7th T22.749 Corrosion of third degree of unspecified axilla COM
- 6th **T22.75 Corrosion of third degree of shoulder**
  - 7th T22.751 Corrosion of third degree of right shoulder COM
  - 7th T22.752 Corrosion of third degree of left shoulder COM
  - 7th T22.759 Corrosion of third degree of unspecified shoulder COM
- 6th **T22.76 Corrosion of third degree of scapular region**
  - 7th T22.761 Corrosion of third degree of right scapular region COM
  - 7th T22.762 Corrosion of third degree of left scapular region COM
  - 7th T22.769 Corrosion of third degree of unspecified scapular region COM
- 6th **T22.79 Corrosion of third degree of multiple sites of shoulder and upper limb, except wrist and hand**
  - 7th T22.791 Corrosion of third degree of multiple sites of right shoulder and upper limb, except wrist and hand COM
  - 7th T22.792 Corrosion of third degree of multiple sites of left shoulder and upper limb, except wrist and hand COM
  - 7th T22.799 Corrosion of third degree of multiple sites of unspecified shoulder and upper limb, except wrist and hand COM

## 4th T23 Burn and corrosion of wrist and hand

**AHA:** 2015,1Q,19

The appropriate 7th character is to be added to each code from category T23.
A initial encounter
D subsequent encounter
S sequela

### 5th T23.Ø Burn of unspecified degree of wrist and hand

Use additional external cause code to identify the source, place and intent of the burn (XØØ-X19, X75-X77, X96-X98, Y92)

- 6th **T23.ØØ Burn of unspecified degree of hand, unspecified site**
  - 7th T23.ØØ1 Burn of unspecified degree of right hand, unspecified site
  - 7th T23.ØØ2 Burn of unspecified degree of left hand, unspecified site
  - 7th T23.ØØ9 Burn of unspecified degree of unspecified hand, unspecified site
- 6th **T23.Ø1 Burn of unspecified degree of thumb (nail)**
  - 7th T23.Ø11 Burn of unspecified degree of right thumb (nail)
  - 7th T23.Ø12 Burn of unspecified degree of left thumb (nail)
  - 7th T23.Ø19 Burn of unspecified degree of unspecified thumb (nail)
- 6th **T23.Ø2 Burn of unspecified degree of single finger (nail) except thumb**
  - 7th T23.Ø21 Burn of unspecified degree of single right finger (nail) except thumb
  - 7th T23.Ø22 Burn of unspecified degree of single left finger (nail) except thumb
  - 7th T23.Ø29 Burn of unspecified degree of unspecified single finger (nail) except thumb
- 6th **T23.Ø3 Burn of unspecified degree of multiple fingers (nail), not including thumb**
  - 7th T23.Ø31 Burn of unspecified degree of multiple right fingers (nail), not including thumb
  - 7th T23.Ø32 Burn of unspecified degree of multiple left fingers (nail), not including thumb
  - 7th T23.Ø39 Burn of unspecified degree of unspecified multiple fingers (nail), not including thumb
- 6th **T23.Ø4 Burn of unspecified degree of multiple fingers (nail), including thumb**
  - 7th T23.Ø41 Burn of unspecified degree of multiple right fingers (nail), including thumb
  - 7th T23.Ø42 Burn of unspecified degree of multiple left fingers (nail), including thumb
  - 7th T23.Ø49 Burn of unspecified degree of unspecified multiple fingers (nail), including thumb
- 6th **T23.Ø5 Burn of unspecified degree of palm**
  - 7th T23.Ø51 Burn of unspecified degree of right palm
  - 7th T23.Ø52 Burn of unspecified degree of left palm
  - 7th T23.Ø59 Burn of unspecified degree of unspecified palm
- 6th **T23.Ø6 Burn of unspecified degree of back of hand**
  - 7th T23.Ø61 Burn of unspecified degree of back of right hand
  - 7th T23.Ø62 Burn of unspecified degree of back of left hand
  - 7th T23.Ø69 Burn of unspecified degree of back of unspecified hand
- 6th **T23.Ø7 Burn of unspecified degree of wrist**
  - 7th T23.Ø71 Burn of unspecified degree of right wrist
  - 7th T23.Ø72 Burn of unspecified degree of left wrist
  - 7th T23.Ø79 Burn of unspecified degree of unspecified wrist
- 6th **T23.Ø9 Burn of unspecified degree of multiple sites of wrist and hand**
  - 7th T23.Ø91 Burn of unspecified degree of multiple sites of right wrist and hand
  - 7th T23.Ø92 Burn of unspecified degree of multiple sites of left wrist and hand
  - 7th T23.Ø99 Burn of unspecified degree of multiple sites of unspecified wrist and hand

### 5th T23.1 Burn of first degree of wrist and hand

Use additional external cause code to identify the source, place and intent of the burn (XØØ-X19, X75-X77, X96-X98, Y92)

- 6th **T23.1Ø Burn of first degree of hand, unspecified site**
  - 7th T23.1Ø1 Burn of first degree of right hand, unspecified site
  - 7th T23.1Ø2 Burn of first degree of left hand, unspecified site
  - 7th T23.1Ø9 Burn of first degree of unspecified hand, unspecified site
- 6th **T23.11 Burn of first degree of thumb (nail)**
  - 7th T23.111 Burn of first degree of right thumb (nail)
  - 7th T23.112 Burn of first degree of left thumb (nail)
  - 7th T23.119 Burn of first degree of unspecified thumb (nail)
- 6th **T23.12 Burn of first degree of single finger (nail) except thumb**
  - 7th T23.121 Burn of first degree of single right finger (nail) except thumb
  - 7th T23.122 Burn of first degree of single left finger (nail) except thumb
  - 7th T23.129 Burn of first degree of unspecified single finger (nail) except thumb
- 6th **T23.13 Burn of first degree of multiple fingers (nail), not including thumb**
  - 7th T23.131 Burn of first degree of multiple right fingers (nail), not including thumb
  - 7th T23.132 Burn of first degree of multiple left fingers (nail), not including thumb
  - 7th T23.139 Burn of first degree of unspecified multiple fingers (nail), not including thumb
- 6th **T23.14 Burn of first degree of multiple fingers (nail), including thumb**
  - 7th T23.141 Burn of first degree of multiple right fingers (nail), including thumb
  - 7th T23.142 Burn of first degree of multiple left fingers (nail), including thumb
  - 7th T23.149 Burn of first degree of unspecified multiple fingers (nail), including thumb

- T23.15 Burn of first degree of palm
  - T23.151 Burn of first degree of right palm
  - T23.152 Burn of first degree of left palm
  - T23.159 Burn of first degree of unspecified palm
- T23.16 Burn of first degree of back of hand
  - T23.161 Burn of first degree of back of right hand
  - T23.162 Burn of first degree of back of left hand
  - T23.169 Burn of first degree of back of unspecified hand
- T23.17 Burn of first degree of wrist
  - T23.171 Burn of first degree of right wrist
  - T23.172 Burn of first degree of left wrist
  - T23.179 Burn of first degree of unspecified wrist
- T23.19 Burn of first degree of multiple sites of wrist and hand
  - T23.191 Burn of first degree of multiple sites of right wrist and hand
  - T23.192 Burn of first degree of multiple sites of left wrist and hand
  - T23.199 Burn of first degree of multiple sites of unspecified wrist and hand

**T23.2 Burn of second degree of wrist and hand**

Use additional external cause code to identify the source, place and intent of the burn (X00-X19, X75-X77, X96-X98, Y92)

- T23.20 Burn of second degree of hand, unspecified site
  - T23.201 Burn of second degree of right hand, unspecified site
  - T23.202 Burn of second degree of left hand, unspecified site
  - T23.209 Burn of second degree of unspecified hand, unspecified site
- T23.21 Burn of second degree of thumb (nail)
  - T23.211 Burn of second degree of right thumb (nail)
  - T23.212 Burn of second degree of left thumb (nail)
  - T23.219 Burn of second degree of unspecified thumb (nail)
- T23.22 Burn of second degree of single finger (nail) except thumb
  - T23.221 Burn of second degree of single right finger (nail) except thumb
  - T23.222 Burn of second degree of single left finger (nail) except thumb
  - T23.229 Burn of second degree of unspecified single finger (nail) except thumb
- T23.23 Burn of second degree of multiple fingers (nail), not including thumb
  - T23.231 Burn of second degree of multiple right fingers (nail), not including thumb
  - T23.232 Burn of second degree of multiple left fingers (nail), not including thumb
  - T23.239 Burn of second degree of unspecified multiple fingers (nail), not including thumb
- T23.24 Burn of second degree of multiple fingers (nail), including thumb
  - T23.241 Burn of second degree of multiple right fingers (nail), including thumb
  - T23.242 Burn of second degree of multiple left fingers (nail), including thumb
  - T23.249 Burn of second degree of unspecified multiple fingers (nail), including thumb
- T23.25 Burn of second degree of palm
  - T23.251 Burn of second degree of right palm
  - T23.252 Burn of second degree of left palm
  - T23.259 Burn of second degree of unspecified palm
- T23.26 Burn of second degree of back of hand
  - T23.261 Burn of second degree of back of right hand
  - T23.262 Burn of second degree of back of left hand
  - T23.269 Burn of second degree of back of unspecified hand
- T23.27 Burn of second degree of wrist
  - T23.271 Burn of second degree of right wrist
  - T23.272 Burn of second degree of left wrist
  - T23.279 Burn of second degree of unspecified wrist
- T23.29 Burn of second degree of multiple sites of wrist and hand
  - T23.291 Burn of second degree of multiple sites of right wrist and hand
  - T23.292 Burn of second degree of multiple sites of left wrist and hand
  - T23.299 Burn of second degree of multiple sites of unspecified wrist and hand

**T23.3 Burn of third degree of wrist and hand**

Use additional external cause code to identify the source, place and intent of the burn (X00-X19, X75-X77, X96-X98, Y92)

- T23.30 Burn of third degree of hand, unspecified site
  - AHA: 2016,2Q,5
  - T23.301 Burn of third degree of right hand, unspecified site COM
  - T23.302 Burn of third degree of left hand, unspecified site COM
  - T23.309 Burn of third degree of unspecified hand, unspecified site COM
- T23.31 Burn of third degree of thumb (nail)
  - T23.311 Burn of third degree of right thumb (nail) COM
  - T23.312 Burn of third degree of left thumb (nail) COM
  - T23.319 Burn of third degree of unspecified thumb (nail) COM
- T23.32 Burn of third degree of single finger (nail) except thumb
  - T23.321 Burn of third degree of single right finger (nail) except thumb COM
  - T23.322 Burn of third degree of single left finger (nail) except thumb COM
  - T23.329 Burn of third degree of unspecified single finger (nail) except thumb COM
- T23.33 Burn of third degree of multiple fingers (nail), not including thumb
  - T23.331 Burn of third degree of multiple right fingers (nail), not including thumb COM
  - T23.332 Burn of third degree of multiple left fingers (nail), not including thumb COM
  - T23.339 Burn of third degree of unspecified multiple fingers (nail), not including thumb COM
- T23.34 Burn of third degree of multiple fingers (nail), including thumb
  - T23.341 Burn of third degree of multiple right fingers (nail), including thumb COM
  - T23.342 Burn of third degree of multiple left fingers (nail), including thumb COM
  - T23.349 Burn of third degree of unspecified multiple fingers (nail), including thumb COM
- T23.35 Burn of third degree of palm
  - T23.351 Burn of third degree of right palm COM
  - T23.352 Burn of third degree of left palm COM
  - T23.359 Burn of third degree of unspecified palm COM
- T23.36 Burn of third degree of back of hand
  - T23.361 Burn of third degree of back of right hand COM
  - T23.362 Burn of third degree of back of left hand COM
  - T23.369 Burn of third degree of back of unspecified hand COM
- T23.37 Burn of third degree of wrist
  - T23.371 Burn of third degree of right wrist COM
  - T23.372 Burn of third degree of left wrist COM
  - T23.379 Burn of third degree of unspecified wrist COM
- T23.39 Burn of third degree of multiple sites of wrist and hand
  - T23.391 Burn of third degree of multiple sites of right wrist and hand COM
  - T23.392 Burn of third degree of multiple sites of left wrist and hand COM
  - T23.399 Burn of third degree of multiple sites of unspecified wrist and hand COM

**5th T23.4 Corrosion of unspecified degree of wrist and hand**
Code first (T51-T65) to identify chemical and intent
Use additional external cause code to identify place (Y92)

- 6th **T23.40** Corrosion of unspecified degree of hand, unspecified site
  - 7th **T23.401** Corrosion of unspecified degree of right hand, unspecified site
  - 7th **T23.402** Corrosion of unspecified degree of left hand, unspecified site
  - 7th **T23.409** Corrosion of unspecified degree of unspecified hand, unspecified site
- 6th **T23.41** Corrosion of unspecified degree of thumb (nail)
  - 7th **T23.411** Corrosion of unspecified degree of right thumb (nail)
  - 7th **T23.412** Corrosion of unspecified degree of left thumb (nail)
  - 7th **T23.419** Corrosion of unspecified degree of unspecified thumb (nail)
- 6th **T23.42** Corrosion of unspecified degree of single finger (nail) except thumb
  - 7th **T23.421** Corrosion of unspecified degree of single right finger (nail) except thumb
  - 7th **T23.422** Corrosion of unspecified degree of single left finger (nail) except thumb
  - 7th **T23.429** Corrosion of unspecified degree of unspecified single finger (nail) except thumb
- 6th **T23.43** Corrosion of unspecified degree of multiple fingers (nail), not including thumb
  - 7th **T23.431** Corrosion of unspecified degree of multiple right fingers (nail), not including thumb
  - 7th **T23.432** Corrosion of unspecified degree of multiple left fingers (nail), not including thumb
  - 7th **T23.439** Corrosion of unspecified degree of unspecified multiple fingers (nail), not including thumb
- 6th **T23.44** Corrosion of unspecified degree of multiple fingers (nail), including thumb
  - 7th **T23.441** Corrosion of unspecified degree of multiple right fingers (nail), including thumb
  - 7th **T23.442** Corrosion of unspecified degree of multiple left fingers (nail), including thumb
  - 7th **T23.449** Corrosion of unspecified degree of unspecified multiple fingers (nail), including thumb
- 6th **T23.45** Corrosion of unspecified degree of palm
  - 7th **T23.451** Corrosion of unspecified degree of right palm
  - 7th **T23.452** Corrosion of unspecified degree of left palm
  - 7th **T23.459** Corrosion of unspecified degree of unspecified palm
- 6th **T23.46** Corrosion of unspecified degree of back of hand
  - 7th **T23.461** Corrosion of unspecified degree of back of right hand
  - 7th **T23.462** Corrosion of unspecified degree of back of left hand
  - 7th **T23.469** Corrosion of unspecified degree of back of unspecified hand
- 6th **T23.47** Corrosion of unspecified degree of wrist
  - 7th **T23.471** Corrosion of unspecified degree of right wrist
  - 7th **T23.472** Corrosion of unspecified degree of left wrist
  - 7th **T23.479** Corrosion of unspecified degree of unspecified wrist
- 6th **T23.49** Corrosion of unspecified degree of multiple sites of wrist and hand
  - 7th **T23.491** Corrosion of unspecified degree of multiple sites of right wrist and hand
  - 7th **T23.492** Corrosion of unspecified degree of multiple sites of left wrist and hand
  - 7th **T23.499** Corrosion of unspecified degree of multiple sites of unspecified wrist and hand

**5th T23.5 Corrosion of first degree of wrist and hand**
Code first (T51-T65) to identify chemical and intent
Use additional external cause code to identify place (Y92)

- 6th **T23.50** Corrosion of first degree of hand, unspecified site
  - 7th **T23.501** Corrosion of first degree of right hand, unspecified site
  - 7th **T23.502** Corrosion of first degree of left hand, unspecified site
  - 7th **T23.509** Corrosion of first degree of unspecified hand, unspecified site
- 6th **T23.51** Corrosion of first degree of thumb (nail)
  - 7th **T23.511** Corrosion of first degree of right thumb (nail)
  - 7th **T23.512** Corrosion of first degree of left thumb (nail)
  - 7th **T23.519** Corrosion of first degree of unspecified thumb (nail)
- 6th **T23.52** Corrosion of first degree of single finger (nail) except thumb
  - 7th **T23.521** Corrosion of first degree of single right finger (nail) except thumb
  - 7th **T23.522** Corrosion of first degree of single left finger (nail) except thumb
  - 7th **T23.529** Corrosion of first degree of unspecified single finger (nail) except thumb
- 6th **T23.53** Corrosion of first degree of multiple fingers (nail), not including thumb
  - 7th **T23.531** Corrosion of first degree of multiple right fingers (nail), not including thumb
  - 7th **T23.532** Corrosion of first degree of multiple left fingers (nail), not including thumb
  - 7th **T23.539** Corrosion of first degree of unspecified multiple fingers (nail), not including thumb
- 6th **T23.54** Corrosion of first degree of multiple fingers (nail), including thumb
  - 7th **T23.541** Corrosion of first degree of multiple right fingers (nail), including thumb
  - 7th **T23.542** Corrosion of first degree of multiple left fingers (nail), including thumb
  - 7th **T23.549** Corrosion of first degree of unspecified multiple fingers (nail), including thumb
- 6th **T23.55** Corrosion of first degree of palm
  - 7th **T23.551** Corrosion of first degree of right palm
  - 7th **T23.552** Corrosion of first degree of left palm
  - 7th **T23.559** Corrosion of first degree of unspecified palm
- 6th **T23.56** Corrosion of first degree of back of hand
  - 7th **T23.561** Corrosion of first degree of back of right hand
  - 7th **T23.562** Corrosion of first degree of back of left hand
  - 7th **T23.569** Corrosion of first degree of back of unspecified hand
- 6th **T23.57** Corrosion of first degree of wrist
  - 7th **T23.571** Corrosion of first degree of right wrist
  - 7th **T23.572** Corrosion of first degree of left wrist
  - 7th **T23.579** Corrosion of first degree of unspecified wrist
- 6th **T23.59** Corrosion of first degree of multiple sites of wrist and hand
  - 7th **T23.591** Corrosion of first degree of multiple sites of right wrist and hand
  - 7th **T23.592** Corrosion of first degree of multiple sites of left wrist and hand
  - 7th **T23.599** Corrosion of first degree of multiple sites of unspecified wrist and hand

**5th T23.6 Corrosion of second degree of wrist and hand**
Code first (T51-T65) to identify chemical and intent
Use additional external cause code to identify place (Y92)

- 6th **T23.60** Corrosion of second degree of hand, unspecified site
  - 7th **T23.601** Corrosion of second degree of right hand, unspecified site
  - 7th **T23.602** Corrosion of second degree of left hand, unspecified site
  - 7th **T23.609** Corrosion of second degree of unspecified hand, unspecified site
- 6th **T23.61** Corrosion of second degree of thumb (nail)
  - 7th **T23.611** Corrosion of second degree of right thumb (nail)

√7th T23.612 Corrosion of second degree of left thumb (nail)
√7th T23.619 Corrosion of second degree of unspecified thumb (nail)
√6th T23.62 Corrosion of second degree of single finger (nail) except thumb
√7th T23.621 Corrosion of second degree of single right finger (nail) except thumb
√7th T23.622 Corrosion of second degree of single left finger (nail) except thumb
√7th T23.629 Corrosion of second degree of unspecified single finger (nail) except thumb
√6th T23.63 Corrosion of second degree of multiple fingers (nail), not including thumb
√7th T23.631 Corrosion of second degree of multiple right fingers (nail), not including thumb
√7th T23.632 Corrosion of second degree of multiple left fingers (nail), not including thumb
√7th T23.639 Corrosion of second degree of unspecified multiple fingers (nail), not including thumb
√6th T23.64 Corrosion of second degree of multiple fingers (nail), including thumb
√7th T23.641 Corrosion of second degree of multiple right fingers (nail), including thumb
√7th T23.642 Corrosion of second degree of multiple left fingers (nail), including thumb
√7th T23.649 Corrosion of second degree of unspecified multiple fingers (nail), including thumb
√6th T23.65 Corrosion of second degree of palm
√7th T23.651 Corrosion of second degree of right palm
√7th T23.652 Corrosion of second degree of left palm
√7th T23.659 Corrosion of second degree of unspecified palm
√6th T23.66 Corrosion of second degree of back of hand
√7th T23.661 Corrosion of second degree back of right hand
√7th T23.662 Corrosion of second degree back of left hand
√7th T23.669 Corrosion of second degree back of unspecified hand
√6th T23.67 Corrosion of second degree of wrist
√7th T23.671 Corrosion of second degree of right wrist
√7th T23.672 Corrosion of second degree of left wrist
√7th T23.679 Corrosion of second degree of unspecified wrist
√6th T23.69 Corrosion of second degree of multiple sites of wrist and hand
√7th T23.691 Corrosion of second degree of multiple sites of right wrist and hand
√7th T23.692 Corrosion of second degree of multiple sites of left wrist and hand
√7th T23.699 Corrosion of second degree of multiple sites of unspecified wrist and hand
√5th T23.7 Corrosion of third degree of wrist and hand
Code first (T51-T65) to identify chemical and intent
Use additional external cause code to identify place (Y92)
√6th T23.7Ø Corrosion of third degree of hand, unspecified site
√7th T23.7Ø1 Corrosion of third degree of right hand, unspecified site COM
√7th T23.7Ø2 Corrosion of third degree of left hand, unspecified site COM
√7th T23.7Ø9 Corrosion of third degree of unspecified hand, unspecified site COM
√6th T23.71 Corrosion of third degree of thumb (nail)
√7th T23.711 Corrosion of third degree of right thumb (nail) COM
√7th T23.712 Corrosion of third degree of left thumb (nail) COM
√7th T23.719 Corrosion of third degree of unspecified thumb (nail) COM
√6th T23.72 Corrosion of third degree of single finger (nail) except thumb
√7th T23.721 Corrosion of third degree of single right finger (nail) except thumb COM
√7th T23.722 Corrosion of third degree of single left finger (nail) except thumb COM
√7th T23.729 Corrosion of third degree of unspecified single finger (nail) except thumb COM
√6th T23.73 Corrosion of third degree of multiple fingers (nail), not including thumb
√7th T23.731 Corrosion of third degree of multiple right fingers (nail), not including thumb COM
√7th T23.732 Corrosion of third degree of multiple left fingers (nail), not including thumb COM
√7th T23.739 Corrosion of third degree of unspecified multiple fingers (nail), not including thumb COM
√6th T23.74 Corrosion of third degree of multiple fingers (nail), including thumb
√7th T23.741 Corrosion of third degree of multiple right fingers (nail), including thumb COM
√7th T23.742 Corrosion of third degree of multiple left fingers (nail), including thumb COM
√7th T23.749 Corrosion of third degree of unspecified multiple fingers (nail), including thumb COM
√6th T23.75 Corrosion of third degree of palm
√7th T23.751 Corrosion of third degree of right palm COM
√7th T23.752 Corrosion of third degree of left palm COM
√7th T23.759 Corrosion of third degree of unspecified palm COM
√6th T23.76 Corrosion of third degree of back of hand
√7th T23.761 Corrosion of third degree of back of right hand COM
√7th T23.762 Corrosion of third degree of back of left hand COM
√7th T23.769 Corrosion of third degree back of unspecified hand COM
√6th T23.77 Corrosion of third degree of wrist
√7th T23.771 Corrosion of third degree of right wrist COM
√7th T23.772 Corrosion of third degree of left wrist COM
√7th T23.779 Corrosion of third degree of unspecified wrist COM
√6th T23.79 Corrosion of third degree of multiple sites of wrist and hand
√7th T23.791 Corrosion of third degree of multiple sites of right wrist and hand COM
√7th T23.792 Corrosion of third degree of multiple sites of left wrist and hand COM
√7th T23.799 Corrosion of third degree of multiple sites of unspecified wrist and hand COM

√4th **T24 Burn and corrosion of lower limb, except ankle and foot**
EXCLUDES 2 *burn and corrosion of ankle and foot (T25.-)*
*burn and corrosion of hip region (T21.-)*

The appropriate 7th character is to be added to each code from category T24.
A initial encounter
D subsequent encounter
S sequela

√5th T24.Ø Burn of unspecified degree of lower limb, except ankle and foot
Use additional external cause code to identify the source, place and intent of the burn (XØØ-X19, X75-X77, X96-X98, Y92)
√6th T24.ØØ Burn of unspecified degree of unspecified site of lower limb, except ankle and foot
√7th T24.ØØ1 Burn of unspecified degree of unspecified site of right lower limb, except ankle and foot
√7th T24.ØØ2 Burn of unspecified degree of unspecified site of left lower limb, except ankle and foot
√7th T24.ØØ9 Burn of unspecified degree of unspecified site of unspecified lower limb, except ankle and foot
√6th T24.Ø1 Burn of unspecified degree of thigh
√7th T24.Ø11 Burn of unspecified degree of right thigh
√7th T24.Ø12 Burn of unspecified degree of left thigh
√7th T24.Ø19 Burn of unspecified degree of unspecified thigh
√6th T24.Ø2 Burn of unspecified degree of knee
√7th T24.Ø21 Burn of unspecified degree of right knee
√7th T24.Ø22 Burn of unspecified degree of left knee

7th T24.029 Burn of unspecified degree of unspecified knee
6th T24.03 Burn of unspecified degree of lower leg
7th T24.031 Burn of unspecified degree of right lower leg
7th T24.032 Burn of unspecified degree of left lower leg
7th T24.039 Burn of unspecified degree of unspecified lower leg
6th T24.09 Burn of unspecified degree of multiple sites of lower limb, except ankle and foot
7th T24.091 Burn of unspecified degree of multiple sites of right lower limb, except ankle and foot
7th T24.092 Burn of unspecified degree of multiple sites of left lower limb, except ankle and foot
7th T24.099 Burn of unspecified degree of multiple sites of unspecified lower limb, except ankle and foot
5th T24.1 Burn of first degree of lower limb, except ankle and foot
Use additional external cause code to identify the source, place and intent of the burn (X00-X19, X75-X77, X96-X98, Y92)
6th T24.10 Burn of first degree of unspecified site of lower limb, except ankle and foot
7th T24.101 Burn of first degree of unspecified site of right lower limb, except ankle and foot
7th T24.102 Burn of first degree of unspecified site of left lower limb, except ankle and foot
7th T24.109 Burn of first degree of unspecified site of unspecified lower limb, except ankle and foot
6th T24.11 Burn of first degree of thigh
7th T24.111 Burn of first degree of right thigh
7th T24.112 Burn of first degree of left thigh
7th T24.119 Burn of first degree of unspecified thigh
6th T24.12 Burn of first degree of knee
7th T24.121 Burn of first degree of right knee
7th T24.122 Burn of first degree of left knee
7th T24.129 Burn of first degree of unspecified knee
6th T24.13 Burn of first degree of lower leg
7th T24.131 Burn of first degree of right lower leg
7th T24.132 Burn of first degree of left lower leg
7th T24.139 Burn of first degree of unspecified lower leg
6th T24.19 Burn of first degree of multiple sites of lower limb, except ankle and foot
7th T24.191 Burn of first degree of multiple sites of right lower limb, except ankle and foot
7th T24.192 Burn of first degree of multiple sites of left lower limb, except ankle and foot
7th T24.199 Burn of first degree of multiple sites of unspecified lower limb, except ankle and foot
5th T24.2 Burn of second degree of lower limb, except ankle and foot
Use additional external cause code to identify the source, place and intent of the burn (X00-X19, X75-X77, X96-X98, Y92)
6th T24.20 Burn of second degree of unspecified site of lower limb, except ankle and foot
7th T24.201 Burn of second degree of unspecified site of right lower limb, except ankle and foot
7th T24.202 Burn of second degree of unspecified site of left lower limb, except ankle and foot
7th T24.209 Burn of second degree of unspecified site of unspecified lower limb, except ankle and foot
6th T24.21 Burn of second degree of thigh
7th T24.211 Burn of second degree of right thigh
7th T24.212 Burn of second degree of left thigh
7th T24.219 Burn of second degree of unspecified thigh
6th T24.22 Burn of second degree of knee
7th T24.221 Burn of second degree of right knee
7th T24.222 Burn of second degree of left knee
7th T24.229 Burn of second degree of unspecified knee
6th T24.23 Burn of second degree of lower leg
7th T24.231 Burn of second degree of right lower leg
7th T24.232 Burn of second degree of left lower leg
7th T24.239 Burn of second degree of unspecified lower leg
6th T24.29 Burn of second degree of multiple sites of lower limb, except ankle and foot
7th T24.291 Burn of second degree of multiple sites of right lower limb, except ankle and foot
7th T24.292 Burn of second degree of multiple sites of left lower limb, except ankle and foot
7th T24.299 Burn of second degree of multiple sites of unspecified lower limb, except ankle and foot
5th T24.3 Burn of third degree of lower limb, except ankle and foot
Use additional external cause code to identify the source, place and intent of the burn (X00-X19, X75-X77, X96-X98, Y92)
6th T24.30 Burn of third degree of unspecified site of lower limb, except ankle and foot
7th T24.301 Burn of third degree of unspecified site of right lower limb, except ankle and foot COM
7th T24.302 Burn of third degree of unspecified site of left lower limb, except ankle and foot COM
7th T24.309 Burn of third degree of unspecified site of unspecified lower limb, except ankle and foot COM
6th T24.31 Burn of third degree of thigh
7th T24.311 Burn of third degree of right thigh COM
7th T24.312 Burn of third degree of left thigh COM
7th T24.319 Burn of third degree of unspecified thigh COM
6th T24.32 Burn of third degree of knee
7th T24.321 Burn of third degree of right knee COM
7th T24.322 Burn of third degree of left knee COM
7th T24.329 Burn of third degree of unspecified knee COM
6th T24.33 Burn of third degree of lower leg
7th T24.331 Burn of third degree of right lower leg COM
7th T24.332 Burn of third degree of left lower leg COM
7th T24.339 Burn of third degree of unspecified lower leg COM
6th T24.39 Burn of third degree of multiple sites of lower limb, except ankle and foot
AHA: 2016,2Q,4
7th T24.391 Burn of third degree of multiple sites of right lower limb, except ankle and foot COM
7th T24.392 Burn of third degree of multiple sites of left lower limb, except ankle and foot COM
7th T24.399 Burn of third degree of multiple sites of unspecified lower limb, except ankle and foot COM
5th T24.4 Corrosion of unspecified degree of lower limb, except ankle and foot
Code first (T51-T65) to identify chemical and intent
Use additional external cause code to identify place (Y92)
6th T24.40 Corrosion of unspecified degree of unspecified site of lower limb, except ankle and foot
7th T24.401 Corrosion of unspecified degree of unspecified site of right lower limb, except ankle and foot
7th T24.402 Corrosion of unspecified degree of unspecified site of left lower limb, except ankle and foot
7th T24.409 Corrosion of unspecified degree of unspecified site of unspecified lower limb, except ankle and foot
6th T24.41 Corrosion of unspecified degree of thigh
7th T24.411 Corrosion of unspecified degree of right thigh
7th T24.412 Corrosion of unspecified degree of left thigh
7th T24.419 Corrosion of unspecified degree of unspecified thigh
6th T24.42 Corrosion of unspecified degree of knee
7th T24.421 Corrosion of unspecified degree of right knee

T24.422 Corrosion of unspecified degree of left knee
T24.429 Corrosion of unspecified degree of unspecified knee
T24.43 Corrosion of unspecified degree of lower leg
T24.431 Corrosion of unspecified degree of right lower leg
T24.432 Corrosion of unspecified degree of left lower leg
T24.439 Corrosion of unspecified degree of unspecified lower leg
T24.49 Corrosion of unspecified degree of multiple sites of lower limb, except ankle and foot
T24.491 Corrosion of unspecified degree of multiple sites of right lower limb, except ankle and foot
T24.492 Corrosion of unspecified degree of multiple sites of left lower limb, except ankle and foot
T24.499 Corrosion of unspecified degree of multiple sites of unspecified lower limb, except ankle and foot

T24.5 Corrosion of first degree of lower limb, except ankle and foot
Code first (T51-T65) to identify chemical and intent
Use additional external cause code to identify place (Y92)
T24.50 Corrosion of first degree of unspecified site of lower limb, except ankle and foot
T24.501 Corrosion of first degree of unspecified site of right lower limb, except ankle and foot
T24.502 Corrosion of first degree of unspecified site of left lower limb, except ankle and foot
T24.509 Corrosion of first degree of unspecified site of unspecified lower limb, except ankle and foot
T24.51 Corrosion of first degree of thigh
T24.511 Corrosion of first degree of right thigh
T24.512 Corrosion of first degree of left thigh
T24.519 Corrosion of first degree of unspecified thigh
T24.52 Corrosion of first degree of knee
T24.521 Corrosion of first degree of right knee
T24.522 Corrosion of first degree of left knee
T24.529 Corrosion of first degree of unspecified knee
T24.53 Corrosion of first degree of lower leg
T24.531 Corrosion of first degree of right lower leg
T24.532 Corrosion of first degree of left lower leg
T24.539 Corrosion of first degree of unspecified lower leg
T24.59 Corrosion of first degree of multiple sites of lower limb, except ankle and foot
T24.591 Corrosion of first degree of multiple sites of right lower limb, except ankle and foot
T24.592 Corrosion of first degree of multiple sites of left lower limb, except ankle and foot
T24.599 Corrosion of first degree of multiple sites of unspecified lower limb, except ankle and foot

T24.6 Corrosion of second degree of lower limb, except ankle and foot
Code first (T51-T65) to identify chemical and intent
Use additional external cause code to identify place (Y92)
T24.60 Corrosion of second degree of unspecified site of lower limb, except ankle and foot
T24.601 Corrosion of second degree of unspecified site of right lower limb, except ankle and foot
T24.602 Corrosion of second degree of unspecified site of left lower limb, except ankle and foot
T24.609 Corrosion of second degree of unspecified site of unspecified lower limb, except ankle and foot
T24.61 Corrosion of second degree of thigh
T24.611 Corrosion of second degree of right thigh
T24.612 Corrosion of second degree of left thigh
T24.619 Corrosion of second degree of unspecified thigh
T24.62 Corrosion of second degree of knee
T24.621 Corrosion of second degree of right knee
T24.622 Corrosion of second degree of left knee
T24.629 Corrosion of second degree of unspecified knee
T24.63 Corrosion of second degree of lower leg
T24.631 Corrosion of second degree of right lower leg
T24.632 Corrosion of second degree of left lower leg
T24.639 Corrosion of second degree of unspecified lower leg
T24.69 Corrosion of second degree of multiple sites of lower limb, except ankle and foot
T24.691 Corrosion of second degree of multiple sites of right lower limb, except ankle and foot
T24.692 Corrosion of second degree of multiple sites of left lower limb, except ankle and foot
T24.699 Corrosion of second degree of multiple sites of unspecified lower limb, except ankle and foot

T24.7 Corrosion of third degree of lower limb, except ankle and foot
Code first (T51-T65) to identify chemical and intent
Use additional external cause code to identify place (Y92)
T24.70 Corrosion of third degree of unspecified site of lower limb, except ankle and foot
T24.701 Corrosion of third degree of unspecified site of right lower limb, except ankle and foot COM
T24.702 Corrosion of third degree of unspecified site of left lower limb, except ankle and foot COM
T24.709 Corrosion of third degree of unspecified site of unspecified lower limb, except ankle and foot COM
T24.71 Corrosion of third degree of thigh
T24.711 Corrosion of third degree of right thigh COM
T24.712 Corrosion of third degree of left thigh COM
T24.719 Corrosion of third degree of unspecified thigh COM
T24.72 Corrosion of third degree of knee
T24.721 Corrosion of third degree of right knee COM
T24.722 Corrosion of third degree of left knee COM
T24.729 Corrosion of third degree of unspecified knee COM
T24.73 Corrosion of third degree of lower leg
T24.731 Corrosion of third degree of right lower leg COM
T24.732 Corrosion of third degree of left lower leg COM
T24.739 Corrosion of third degree of unspecified lower leg COM
T24.79 Corrosion of third degree of multiple sites of lower limb, except ankle and foot
T24.791 Corrosion of third degree of multiple sites of right lower limb, except ankle and foot COM
T24.792 Corrosion of third degree of multiple sites of left lower limb, except ankle and foot COM
T24.799 Corrosion of third degree of multiple sites of unspecified lower limb, except ankle and foot COM

**✓4th T25 Burn and corrosion of ankle and foot**

The appropriate 7th character is to be added to each code from category T25.
A initial encounter
D subsequent encounter
S sequela

✓5th **T25.0 Burn of unspecified degree of ankle and foot**
Use additional external cause code to identify the source, place and intent of the burn (X00-X19, X75-X77, X96-X98, Y92)
✓6th **T25.01 Burn of unspecified degree of ankle**
✓7th **T25.011 Burn of unspecified degree of right ankle**
✓7th **T25.012 Burn of unspecified degree of left ankle**
✓7th **T25.019 Burn of unspecified degree of unspecified ankle**
✓6th **T25.02 Burn of unspecified degree of foot**
EXCLUDES 2 *burn of unspecified degree of toe(s) (nail) (T25.03-)*
✓7th **T25.021 Burn of unspecified degree of right foot**
✓7th **T25.022 Burn of unspecified degree of left foot**
✓7th **T25.029 Burn of unspecified degree of unspecified foot**
✓6th **T25.03 Burn of unspecified degree of toe(s) (nail)**
✓7th **T25.031 Burn of unspecified degree of right toe(s) (nail)**
✓7th **T25.032 Burn of unspecified degree of left toe(s) (nail)**
✓7th **T25.039 Burn of unspecified degree of unspecified toe(s) (nail)**
✓6th **T25.09 Burn of unspecified degree of multiple sites of ankle and foot**
✓7th **T25.091 Burn of unspecified degree of multiple sites of right ankle and foot**
✓7th **T25.092 Burn of unspecified degree of multiple sites of left ankle and foot**
✓7th **T25.099 Burn of unspecified degree of multiple sites of unspecified ankle and foot**
✓5th **T25.1 Burn of first degree of ankle and foot**
Use additional external cause code to identify the source, place and intent of the burn (X00-X19, X75-X77, X96-X98, Y92)
✓6th **T25.11 Burn of first degree of ankle**
✓7th **T25.111 Burn of first degree of right ankle**
✓7th **T25.112 Burn of first degree of left ankle**
✓7th **T25.119 Burn of first degree of unspecified ankle**
✓6th **T25.12 Burn of first degree of foot**
EXCLUDES 2 *burn of first degree of toe(s) (nail) (T25.13-)*
✓7th **T25.121 Burn of first degree of right foot**
✓7th **T25.122 Burn of first degree of left foot**
✓7th **T25.129 Burn of first degree of unspecified foot**
✓6th **T25.13 Burn of first degree of toe(s) (nail)**
✓7th **T25.131 Burn of first degree of right toe(s) (nail)**
✓7th **T25.132 Burn of first degree of left toe(s) (nail)**
✓7th **T25.139 Burn of first degree of unspecified toe(s) (nail)**
✓6th **T25.19 Burn of first degree of multiple sites of ankle and foot**
✓7th **T25.191 Burn of first degree of multiple sites of right ankle and foot**
✓7th **T25.192 Burn of first degree of multiple sites of left ankle and foot**
✓7th **T25.199 Burn of first degree of multiple sites of unspecified ankle and foot**
✓5th **T25.2 Burn of second degree of ankle and foot**
Use additional external cause code to identify the source, place and intent of the burn (X00-X19, X75-X77, X96-X98, Y92)
✓6th **T25.21 Burn of second degree of ankle**
✓7th **T25.211 Burn of second degree of right ankle**
✓7th **T25.212 Burn of second degree of left ankle**
✓7th **T25.219 Burn of second degree of unspecified ankle**
✓6th **T25.22 Burn of second degree of foot**
EXCLUDES 2 *burn of second degree of toe(s) (nail) (T25.23-)*
✓7th **T25.221 Burn of second degree of right foot**
✓7th **T25.222 Burn of second degree of left foot**
✓7th **T25.229 Burn of second degree of unspecified foot**
✓6th **T25.23 Burn of second degree of toe(s) (nail)**
✓7th **T25.231 Burn of second degree of right toe(s) (nail)**
✓7th **T25.232 Burn of second degree of left toe(s) (nail)**
✓7th **T25.239 Burn of second degree of unspecified toe(s) (nail)**
✓6th **T25.29 Burn of second degree of multiple sites of ankle and foot**
✓7th **T25.291 Burn of second degree of multiple sites of right ankle and foot**
✓7th **T25.292 Burn of second degree of multiple sites of left ankle and foot**
✓7th **T25.299 Burn of second degree of multiple sites of unspecified ankle and foot**
✓5th **T25.3 Burn of third degree of ankle and foot**
Use additional external cause code to identify the source, place and intent of the burn (X00-X19, X75-X77, X96-X98, Y92)
✓6th **T25.31 Burn of third degree of ankle**
✓7th **T25.311 Burn of third degree of right ankle** COM
✓7th **T25.312 Burn of third degree of left ankle** COM
✓7th **T25.319 Burn of third degree of unspecified ankle** COM
✓6th **T25.32 Burn of third degree of foot**
EXCLUDES 2 *burn of third degree of toe(s) (nail) (T25.33-)*
✓7th **T25.321 Burn of third degree of right foot** COM
✓7th **T25.322 Burn of third degree of left foot** COM
✓7th **T25.329 Burn of third degree of unspecified foot** COM
✓6th **T25.33 Burn of third degree of toe(s) (nail)**
✓7th **T25.331 Burn of third degree of right toe(s) (nail)** COM
✓7th **T25.332 Burn of third degree of left toe(s) (nail)** COM
✓7th **T25.339 Burn of third degree of unspecified toe(s) (nail)** COM
✓6th **T25.39 Burn of third degree of multiple sites of ankle and foot**
✓7th **T25.391 Burn of third degree of multiple sites of right ankle and foot** COM
✓7th **T25.392 Burn of third degree of multiple sites of left ankle and foot** COM
✓7th **T25.399 Burn of third degree of multiple sites of unspecified ankle and foot** COM
✓5th **T25.4 Corrosion of unspecified degree of ankle and foot**
Code first (T51-T65) to identify chemical and intent
Use additional external cause code to identify place (Y92)
✓6th **T25.41 Corrosion of unspecified degree of ankle**
✓7th **T25.411 Corrosion of unspecified degree of right ankle**
✓7th **T25.412 Corrosion of unspecified degree of left ankle**
✓7th **T25.419 Corrosion of unspecified degree of unspecified ankle**
✓6th **T25.42 Corrosion of unspecified degree of foot**
EXCLUDES 2 *corrosion of unspecified degree of toe(s) (nail) (T25.43-)*
✓7th **T25.421 Corrosion of unspecified degree of right foot**
✓7th **T25.422 Corrosion of unspecified degree of left foot**
✓7th **T25.429 Corrosion of unspecified degree of unspecified foot**
✓6th **T25.43 Corrosion of unspecified degree of toe(s) (nail)**
✓7th **T25.431 Corrosion of unspecified degree of right toe(s) (nail)**
✓7th **T25.432 Corrosion of unspecified degree of left toe(s) (nail)**
✓7th **T25.439 Corrosion of unspecified degree of unspecified toe(s) (nail)**
✓6th **T25.49 Corrosion of unspecified degree of multiple sites of ankle and foot**
✓7th **T25.491 Corrosion of unspecified degree of multiple sites of right ankle and foot**
✓7th **T25.492 Corrosion of unspecified degree of multiple sites of left ankle and foot**
✓7th **T25.499 Corrosion of unspecified degree of multiple sites of unspecified ankle and foot**

T25.5 Corrosion of first degree of ankle and foot
Code first (T51-T65) to identify chemical and intent
Use additional external cause code to identify place (Y92)
T25.51 Corrosion of first degree of ankle
T25.511 Corrosion of first degree of right ankle
T25.512 Corrosion of first degree of left ankle
T25.519 Corrosion of first degree of unspecified ankle
T25.52 Corrosion of first degree of foot
EXCLUDES 2 *corrosion of first degree of toe(s) (nail) (T25.53-)*
T25.521 Corrosion of first degree of right foot
T25.522 Corrosion of first degree of left foot
T25.529 Corrosion of first degree of unspecified foot
T25.53 Corrosion of first degree of toe(s) (nail)
T25.531 Corrosion of first degree of right toe(s) (nail)
T25.532 Corrosion of first degree of left toe(s) (nail)
T25.539 Corrosion of first degree of unspecified toe(s) (nail)
T25.59 Corrosion of first degree of multiple sites of ankle and foot
T25.591 Corrosion of first degree of multiple sites of right ankle and foot
T25.592 Corrosion of first degree of multiple sites of left ankle and foot
T25.599 Corrosion of first degree of multiple sites of unspecified ankle and foot
T25.6 Corrosion of second degree of ankle and foot
Code first (T51-T65) to identify chemical and intent
Use additional external cause code to identify place (Y92)
T25.61 Corrosion of second degree of ankle
T25.611 Corrosion of second degree of right ankle
T25.612 Corrosion of second degree of left ankle
T25.619 Corrosion of second degree of unspecified ankle
T25.62 Corrosion of second degree of foot
EXCLUDES 2 *corrosion of second degree of toe(s) (nail) (T25.63-)*
T25.621 Corrosion of second degree of right foot
T25.622 Corrosion of second degree of left foot
T25.629 Corrosion of second degree of unspecified foot
T25.63 Corrosion of second degree of toe(s) (nail)
T25.631 Corrosion of second degree of right toe(s) (nail)
T25.632 Corrosion of second degree of left toe(s) (nail)
T25.639 Corrosion of second degree of unspecified toe(s) (nail)
T25.69 Corrosion of second degree of multiple sites of ankle and foot
T25.691 Corrosion of second degree of right ankle and foot
T25.692 Corrosion of second degree of left ankle and foot
T25.699 Corrosion of second degree of unspecified ankle and foot
T25.7 Corrosion of third degree of ankle and foot
Code first (T51-T65) to identify chemical and intent
Use additional external cause code to identify place (Y92)
T25.71 Corrosion of third degree of ankle
T25.711 Corrosion of third degree of right ankle COM
T25.712 Corrosion of third degree of left ankle COM
T25.719 Corrosion of third degree of unspecified ankle COM
T25.72 Corrosion of third degree of foot
EXCLUDES 2 *corrosion of third degree of toe(s) (nail) (T25.73-)*
T25.721 Corrosion of third degree of right foot COM
T25.722 Corrosion of third degree of left foot COM
T25.729 Corrosion of third degree of unspecified foot COM
T25.73 Corrosion of third degree of toe(s) (nail)
T25.731 Corrosion of third degree of right toe(s) (nail) COM
T25.732 Corrosion of third degree of left toe(s) (nail) COM
T25.739 Corrosion of third degree of unspecified toe(s) (nail) COM
T25.79 Corrosion of third degree of multiple sites of ankle and foot
T25.791 Corrosion of third degree of multiple sites of right ankle and foot COM
T25.792 Corrosion of third degree of multiple sites of left ankle and foot COM
T25.799 Corrosion of third degree of multiple sites of unspecified ankle and foot COM

## Burns and corrosions confined to eye and internal organs (T26-T28)

T26 Burn and corrosion confined to eye and adnexa

The appropriate 7th character is to be added to each code from category T26.
A initial encounter
D subsequent encounter
S sequela

T26.Ø Burn of eyelid and periocular area
Use additional external cause code to identify the source, place and intent of the burn (XØØ-X19, X75-X77, X96-X98, Y92)
T26.ØØ Burn of unspecified eyelid and periocular area
T26.Ø1 Burn of right eyelid and periocular area
T26.Ø2 Burn of left eyelid and periocular area
T26.1 Burn of cornea and conjunctival sac
Use additional external cause code to identify the source, place and intent of the burn (XØØ-X19, X75-X77, X96-X98, Y92)
T26.1Ø Burn of cornea and conjunctival sac, unspecified eye
T26.11 Burn of cornea and conjunctival sac, right eye
T26.12 Burn of cornea and conjunctival sac, left eye
T26.2 Burn with resulting rupture and destruction of eyeball
Use additional external cause code to identify the source, place and intent of the burn (XØØ-X19, X75-X77, X96-X98, Y92)
T26.2Ø Burn with resulting rupture and destruction of unspecified eyeball
T26.21 Burn with resulting rupture and destruction of right eyeball
T26.22 Burn with resulting rupture and destruction of left eyeball
T26.3 Burns of other specified parts of eye and adnexa
Use additional external cause code to identify the source, place and intent of the burn (XØØ-X19, X75-X77, X96-X98, Y92)
T26.3Ø Burns of other specified parts of unspecified eye and adnexa
T26.31 Burns of other specified parts of right eye and adnexa
T26.32 Burns of other specified parts of left eye and adnexa
T26.4 Burn of eye and adnexa, part unspecified
Use additional external cause code to identify the source, place and intent of the burn (XØØ-X19, X75-X77, X96-X98, Y92)
T26.4Ø Burn of unspecified eye and adnexa, part unspecified
T26.41 Burn of right eye and adnexa, part unspecified
T26.42 Burn of left eye and adnexa, part unspecified
T26.5 Corrosion of eyelid and periocular area
Code first (T51-T65) to identify chemical and intent
Use additional external cause code to identify place (Y92)
T26.5Ø Corrosion of unspecified eyelid and periocular area
T26.51 Corrosion of right eyelid and periocular area
T26.52 Corrosion of left eyelid and periocular area
T26.6 Corrosion of cornea and conjunctival sac
Code first (T51-T65) to identify chemical and intent
Use additional external cause code to identify place (Y92)
T26.6Ø Corrosion of cornea and conjunctival sac, unspecified eye
T26.61 Corrosion of cornea and conjunctival sac, right eye
T26.62 Corrosion of cornea and conjunctival sac, left eye

✓5th T26.7 **Corrosion with resulting rupture and destruction of eyeball**
Code first (T51-T65) to identify chemical and intent
Use additional external cause code to identify place (Y92)
✓x7th T26.70 **Corrosion with resulting rupture and destruction of unspecified eyeball**
✓x7th T26.71 **Corrosion with resulting rupture and destruction of right eyeball**
✓x7th T26.72 **Corrosion with resulting rupture and destruction of left eyeball**

✓5th T26.8 **Corrosions of other specified parts of eye and adnexa**
Code first (T51-T65) to identify chemical and intent
Use additional external cause code to identify place (Y92)
✓x7th T26.80 **Corrosions of other specified parts of unspecified eye and adnexa**
✓x7th T26.81 **Corrosions of other specified parts of right eye and adnexa**
✓x7th T26.82 **Corrosions of other specified parts of left eye and adnexa**

✓5th T26.9 **Corrosion of eye and adnexa, part unspecified**
Code first (T51-T65) to identify chemical and intent
Use additional external cause code to identify place (Y92)
✓x7th T26.90 **Corrosion of unspecified eye and adnexa, part unspecified**
✓x7th T26.91 **Corrosion of right eye and adnexa, part unspecified**
✓x7th T26.92 **Corrosion of left eye and adnexa, part unspecified**

✓4th **T27 Burn and corrosion of respiratory tract**
Use additional external cause code to identify place (Y92)
Use additional external cause code to identify the source and intent of the burn (XØØ-X19, X75-X77, X96-X98)

The appropriate 7th character is to be added to each code from category T27.
A initial encounter
D subsequent encounter
S sequela

✓x7th T27.Ø **Burn of larynx and trachea**
✓x7th T27.1 **Burn involving larynx and trachea with lung**
✓x7th T27.2 **Burn of other parts of respiratory tract**
Burn of thoracic cavity
✓x7th T27.3 **Burn of respiratory tract, part unspecified**
✓x7th T27.4 **Corrosion of larynx and trachea**
Code first (T51-T65) to identify chemical and intent
✓x7th T27.5 **Corrosion involving larynx and trachea with lung**
Code first (T51-T65) to identify chemical and intent
✓x7th T27.6 **Corrosion of other parts of respiratory tract**
Code first (T51-T65) to identify chemical and intent
✓x7th T27.7 **Corrosion of respiratory tract, part unspecified**
Code first (T51-T65) to identify chemical and intent

✓4th **T28 Burn and corrosion of other internal organs**
Use additional external cause code to identify place (Y92)
Use additional external cause code to identify the source and intent of the burn (XØØ-X19, X75-X77, X96-X98)

The appropriate 7th character is to be added to each code from category T28.
A initial encounter
D subsequent encounter
S sequela

✓x7th T28.Ø **Burn of mouth and pharynx**
✓x7th T28.1 **Burn of esophagus**
✓x7th T28.2 **Burn of other parts of alimentary tract**
✓x7th T28.3 **Burn of internal genitourinary organs**
✓5th T28.4 **Burns of other and unspecified internal organs**
✓x7th T28.40 **Burn of unspecified internal organ**
✓6th T28.41 **Burn of ear drum**
✓7th T28.411 **Burn of right ear drum**
✓7th T28.412 **Burn of left ear drum**
✓7th T28.419 **Burn of unspecified ear drum**
✓x7th T28.49 **Burn of other internal organ**
✓x7th T28.5 **Corrosion of mouth and pharynx**
Code first (T51-T65) to identify chemical and intent
✓x7th T28.6 **Corrosion of esophagus**
Code first (T51-T65) to identify chemical and intent
✓x7th T28.7 **Corrosion of other parts of alimentary tract**
Code first (T51-T65) to identify chemical and intent
✓x7th T28.8 **Corrosion of internal genitourinary organs**
Code first (T51-T65) to identify chemical and intent
✓5th T28.9 **Corrosions of other and unspecified internal organs**
Code first (T51-T65) to identify chemical and intent
✓x7th T28.90 **Corrosions of unspecified internal organs**
✓6th T28.91 **Corrosions of ear drum**
✓7th T28.911 **Corrosions of right ear drum**
✓7th T28.912 **Corrosions of left ear drum**
✓7th T28.919 **Corrosions of unspecified ear drum**
✓x7th T28.99 **Corrosions of other internal organs**

## Burns and corrosions of multiple and unspecified body regions (T3Ø-T32)

✓4th **T3Ø Burn and corrosion, body region unspecified**
T3Ø.Ø **Burn of unspecified body region, unspecified degree**
Burn NOS
Multiple burns NOS
This code is not for inpatient use. Code to specified site and degree of burns
T3Ø.4 **Corrosion of unspecified body region, unspecified degree**
Corrosion NOS
Multiple corrosion NOS
This code is not for inpatient use. Code to specified site and degree of corrosion

✓4th **T31 Burns classified according to extent of body surface involved**
NOTE This category is to be used as the primary code only when the site of the burn is unspecified. It should be used as a supplementary code with categories T2Ø-T25 when the site is specified.

T31.Ø **Burns involving less than 1Ø% of body surface**
✓5th T31.1 **Burns involving 1Ø-19% of body surface**
T31.1Ø **Burns involving 1Ø-19% of body surface with Ø% to 9% third degree burns** COM
Burns involving 1Ø-19% of body surface NOS
T31.11 **Burns involving 1Ø-19% of body surface with 1Ø-19% third degree burns** HCC ESR COM
✓5th T31.2 **Burns involving 2Ø-29% of body surface**
T31.2Ø **Burns involving 2Ø-29% of body surface with Ø% to 9% third degree burns** COM
Burns involving 2Ø-29% of body surface NOS
T31.21 **Burns involving 2Ø-29% of body surface with 1Ø-19% third degree burns** HCC ESR COM
T31.22 **Burns involving 2Ø-29% of body surface with 2Ø-29% third degree burns** HCC ESR COM
✓5th T31.3 **Burns involving 3Ø-39% of body surface**
T31.3Ø **Burns involving 3Ø-39% of body surface with Ø% to 9% third degree burns** COM
Burns involving 3Ø-39% of body surface NOS
T31.31 **Burns involving 3Ø-39% of body surface with 1Ø-19% third degree burns** HCC ESR COM
T31.32 **Burns involving 3Ø-39% of body surface with 2Ø-29% third degree burns** HCC ESR COM
T31.33 **Burns involving 3Ø-39% of body surface with 3Ø-39% third degree burns** HCC ESR COM
✓5th T31.4 **Burns involving 4Ø-49% of body surface**
T31.4Ø **Burns involving 4Ø-49% of body surface with Ø% to 9% third degree burns** COM
Burns involving 4Ø-49% of body surface NOS
T31.41 **Burns involving 4Ø-49% of body surface with 1Ø-19% third degree burns** HCC ESR COM
T31.42 **Burns involving 4Ø-49% of body surface with 2Ø-29% third degree burns** HCC ESR COM
T31.43 **Burns involving 4Ø-49% of body surface with 3Ø-39% third degree burns** HCC ESR COM
T31.44 **Burns involving 4Ø-49% of body surface with 4Ø-49% third degree burns** HCC ESR COM
✓5th T31.5 **Burns involving 5Ø-59% of body surface**
T31.5Ø **Burns involving 5Ø-59% of body surface with Ø% to 9% third degree burns** COM
Burns involving 5Ø-59% of body surface NOS
T31.51 **Burns involving 5Ø-59% of body surface with 1Ø-19% third degree burns** HCC ESR COM

T31.52 **Burns involving 50-59% of body surface with 20-29% third degree burns** HCC ESR COM

T31.53 **Burns involving 50-59% of body surface with 30-39% third degree burns** HCC ESR COM

T31.54 **Burns involving 50-59% of body surface with 40-49% third degree burns** HCC ESR COM

T31.55 **Burns involving 50-59% of body surface with 50-59% third degree burns** HCC ESR COM

✓5th **T31.6 Burns involving 60-69% of body surface**

T31.60 **Burns involving 60-69% of body surface with 0% to 9% third degree burns** COM
Burns involving 60-69% of body surface NOS

T31.61 **Burns involving 60-69% of body surface with 10-19% third degree burns** HCC ESR COM

T31.62 **Burns involving 60-69% of body surface with 20-29% third degree burns** HCC ESR COM

T31.63 **Burns involving 60-69% of body surface with 30-39% third degree burns** HCC ESR COM

T31.64 **Burns involving 60-69% of body surface with 40-49% third degree burns** HCC ESR COM

T31.65 **Burns involving 60-69% of body surface with 50-59% third degree burns** HCC ESR COM

T31.66 **Burns involving 60-69% of body surface with 60-69% third degree burns** HCC ESR COM

✓5th **T31.7 Burns involving 70-79% of body surface**

T31.70 **Burns involving 70-79% of body surface with 0% to 9% third degree burns** COM
Burns involving 70-79% of body surface NOS

T31.71 **Burns involving 70-79% of body surface with 10-19% third degree burns** HCC ESR COM

T31.72 **Burns involving 70-79% of body surface with 20-29% third degree burns** HCC ESR COM

T31.73 **Burns involving 70-79% of body surface with 30-39% third degree burns** HCC ESR COM

T31.74 **Burns involving 70-79% of body surface with 40-49% third degree burns** HCC ESR COM

T31.75 **Burns involving 70-79% of body surface with 50-59% third degree burns** HCC ESR COM

T31.76 **Burns involving 70-79% of body surface with 60-69% third degree burns** HCC ESR COM

T31.77 **Burns involving 70-79% of body surface with 70-79% third degree burns** HCC ESR COM

✓5th **T31.8 Burns involving 80-89% of body surface**

T31.80 **Burns involving 80-89% of body surface with 0% to 9% third degree burns** COM
Burns involving 80-89% of body surface NOS

T31.81 **Burns involving 80-89% of body surface with 10-19% third degree burns** HCC ESR COM

T31.82 **Burns involving 80-89% of body surface with 20-29% third degree burns** HCC ESR COM

T31.83 **Burns involving 80-89% of body surface with 30-39% third degree burns** HCC ESR COM

T31.84 **Burns involving 80-89% of body surface with 40-49% third degree burns** HCC ESR COM

T31.85 **Burns involving 80-89% of body surface with 50-59% third degree burns** HCC ESR COM

T31.86 **Burns involving 80-89% of body surface with 60-69% third degree burns** HCC ESR COM

T31.87 **Burns involving 80-89% of body surface with 70-79% third degree burns** HCC ESR COM

T31.88 **Burns involving 80-89% of body surface with 80-89% third degree burns** HCC ESR COM

✓5th **T31.9 Burns involving 90% or more of body surface**

T31.90 **Burns involving 90% or more of body surface with 0% to 9% third degree burns** COM
Burns involving 90% or more of body surface NOS

T31.91 **Burns involving 90% or more of body surface with 10-19% third degree burns** HCC ESR COM

T31.92 **Burns involving 90% or more of body surface with 20-29% third degree burns** HCC ESR COM

T31.93 **Burns involving 90% or more of body surface with 30-39% third degree burns** HCC ESR COM

T31.94 **Burns involving 90% or more of body surface with 40-49% third degree burns** HCC ESR COM

T31.95 **Burns involving 90% or more of body surface with 50-59% third degree burns** HCC ESR COM

T31.96 **Burns involving 90% or more of body surface with 60-69% third degree burns** HCC ESR COM

T31.97 **Burns involving 90% or more of body surface with 70-79% third degree burns** HCC ESR COM

T31.98 **Burns involving 90% or more of body surface with 80-89% third degree burns** HCC ESR COM

T31.99 **Burns involving 90% or more of body surface with 90% or more third degree burns** HCC ESR COM

**Rule of Nines Estimation of Total Body Surface Burned**

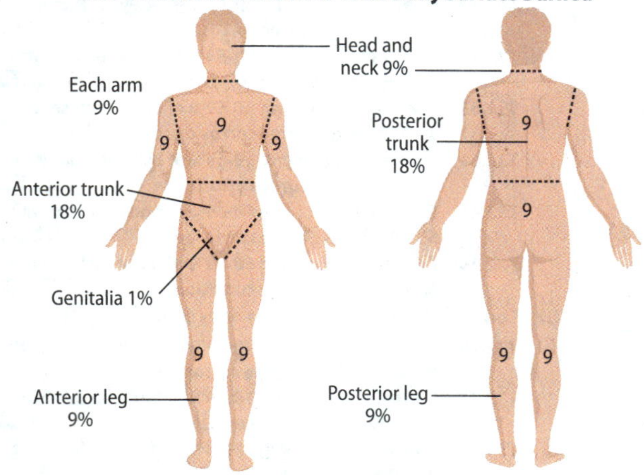


✓4th **T32 Corrosions classified according to extent of body surface involved**

NOTE This category is to be used as the primary code only when the site of the corrosion is unspecified. It may be used as a supplementary code with categories T20-T25 when the site is specified.

**T32.0 Corrosions involving less than 10% of body surface**

✓5th **T32.1 Corrosions involving 10-19% of body surface**

T32.10 **Corrosions involving 10-19% of body surface with 0% to 9% third degree corrosion** COM
Corrosions involving 10-19% of body surface NOS

T32.11 **Corrosions involving 10-19% of body surface with 10-19% third degree corrosion** HCC ESR COM

✓5th **T32.2 Corrosions involving 20-29% of body surface**

T32.20 **Corrosions involving 20-29% of body surface with 0% to 9% third degree corrosion** COM

T32.21 **Corrosions involving 20-29% of body surface with 10-19% third degree corrosion** HCC ESR COM

T32.22 **Corrosions involving 20-29% of body surface with 20-29% third degree corrosion** HCC ESR COM

✓5th **T32.3 Corrosions involving 30-39% of body surface**

T32.30 **Corrosions involving 30-39% of body surface with 0% to 9% third degree corrosion** COM

T32.31 **Corrosions involving 30-39% of body surface with 10-19% third degree corrosion** HCC ESR COM

T32.32 **Corrosions involving 30-39% of body surface with 20-29% third degree corrosion** HCC ESR COM

T32.33 **Corrosions involving 30-39% of body surface with 30-39% third degree corrosion** HCC ESR COM

✓5th **T32.4 Corrosions involving 40-49% of body surface**

T32.40 **Corrosions involving 40-49% of body surface with 0% to 9% third degree corrosion** COM

T32.41 **Corrosions involving 40-49% of body surface with 10-19% third degree corrosion** HCC ESR COM

T32.42 **Corrosions involving 40-49% of body surface with 20-29% third degree corrosion** HCC ESR COM

T32.43 **Corrosions involving 40-49% of body surface with 30-39% third degree corrosion** HCC ESR COM

T32.44 **Corrosions involving 40-49% of body surface with 40-49% third degree corrosion** HCC ESR COM

✓5th **T32.5 Corrosions involving 50-59% of body surface**

T32.50 **Corrosions involving 50-59% of body surface with 0% to 9% third degree corrosion** COM

T32.51 **Corrosions involving 50-59% of body surface with 10-19% third degree corrosion** HCC ESR COM

T32.52 **Corrosions involving 50-59% of body surface with 20-29% third degree corrosion** HCC ESR COM

T32.53 Corrosions involving 50-59% of body surface with 30-39% third degree corrosion HCC ESR COM
T32.54 Corrosions involving 50-59% of body surface with 40-49% third degree corrosion HCC ESR COM
T32.55 Corrosions involving 50-59% of body surface with 50-59% third degree corrosion HCC ESR COM
√5th T32.6 Corrosions involving 60-69% of body surface
T32.60 Corrosions involving 60-69% of body surface with 0% to 9% third degree corrosion COM
T32.61 Corrosions involving 60-69% of body surface with 10-19% third degree corrosion HCC ESR COM
T32.62 Corrosions involving 60-69% of body surface with 20-29% third degree corrosion HCC ESR COM
T32.63 Corrosions involving 60-69% of body surface with 30-39% third degree corrosion HCC ESR COM
T32.64 Corrosions involving 60-69% of body surface with 40-49% third degree corrosion HCC ESR COM
T32.65 Corrosions involving 60-69% of body surface with 50-59% third degree corrosion HCC ESR COM
T32.66 Corrosions involving 60-69% of body surface with 60-69% third degree corrosion HCC ESR COM
√5th T32.7 Corrosions involving 70-79% of body surface
T32.70 Corrosions involving 70-79% of body surface with 0% to 9% third degree corrosion COM
T32.71 Corrosions involving 70-79% of body surface with 10-19% third degree corrosion HCC ESR COM
T32.72 Corrosions involving 70-79% of body surface with 20-29% third degree corrosion HCC ESR COM
T32.73 Corrosions involving 70-79% of body surface with 30-39% third degree corrosion HCC ESR COM
T32.74 Corrosions involving 70-79% of body surface with 40-49% third degree corrosion HCC ESR COM
T32.75 Corrosions involving 70-79% of body surface with 50-59% third degree corrosion HCC ESR COM
T32.76 Corrosions involving 70-79% of body surface with 60-69% third degree corrosion HCC ESR COM
T32.77 Corrosions involving 70-79% of body surface with 70-79% third degree corrosion HCC ESR COM
√5th T32.8 Corrosions involving 80-89% of body surface
T32.80 Corrosions involving 80-89% of body surface with 0% to 9% third degree corrosion COM
T32.81 Corrosions involving 80-89% of body surface with 10-19% third degree corrosion HCC ESR COM
T32.82 Corrosions involving 80-89% of body surface with 20-29% third degree corrosion HCC ESR COM
T32.83 Corrosions involving 80-89% of body surface with 30-39% third degree corrosion HCC ESR COM
T32.84 Corrosions involving 80-89% of body surface with 40-49% third degree corrosion HCC ESR COM
T32.85 Corrosions involving 80-89% of body surface with 50-59% third degree corrosion HCC ESR COM
T32.86 Corrosions involving 80-89% of body surface with 60-69% third degree corrosion HCC ESR COM
T32.87 Corrosions involving 80-89% of body surface with 70-79% third degree corrosion HCC ESR COM
T32.88 Corrosions involving 80-89% of body surface with 80-89% third degree corrosion HCC ESR COM
√5th T32.9 Corrosions involving 90% or more of body surface
T32.90 Corrosions involving 90% or more of body surface with 0% to 9% third degree corrosion COM
T32.91 Corrosions involving 90% or more of body surface with 10-19% third degree corrosion HCC ESR COM
T32.92 Corrosions involving 90% or more of body surface with 20-29% third degree corrosion HCC ESR COM
T32.93 Corrosions involving 90% or more of body surface with 30-39% third degree corrosion HCC ESR COM
T32.94 Corrosions involving 90% or more of body surface with 40-49% third degree corrosion HCC ESR COM
T32.95 Corrosions involving 90% or more of body surface with 50-59% third degree corrosion HCC ESR COM
T32.96 Corrosions involving 90% or more of body surface with 60-69% third degree corrosion HCC ESR COM
T32.97 Corrosions involving 90% or more of body surface with 70-79% third degree corrosion HCC ESR COM
T32.98 Corrosions involving 90% or more of body surface with 80-89% third degree corrosion HCC ESR COM
T32.99 Corrosions involving 90% or more of body surface with 90% or more third degree corrosion HCC ESR COM

## Frostbite (T33-T34)

EXCLUDES 2 *hypothermia and other effects of reduced temperature (T68, T69.-)*

√4th **T33 Superficial frostbite**

INCLUDES frostbite with partial thickness skin loss

The appropriate 7th character is to be added to each code from category T33.
A initial encounter
D subsequent encounter
S sequela

√5th T33.0 Superficial frostbite of head
√6th T33.01 Superficial frostbite of ear
√7th T33.011 Superficial frostbite of right ear
√7th T33.012 Superficial frostbite of left ear
√7th T33.019 Superficial frostbite of unspecified ear
√x7th T33.02 Superficial frostbite of nose
√x7th T33.09 Superficial frostbite of other part of head
√x7th T33.1 Superficial frostbite of neck
√x7th T33.2 Superficial frostbite of thorax
√x7th T33.3 Superficial frostbite of abdominal wall, lower back and pelvis
√5th T33.4 Superficial frostbite of arm
EXCLUDES 2 *superficial frostbite of wrist and hand (T33.5-)*
√x7th T33.40 Superficial frostbite of unspecified arm
√x7th T33.41 Superficial frostbite of right arm
√x7th T33.42 Superficial frostbite of left arm
√5th T33.5 Superficial frostbite of wrist, hand, and fingers
√6th T33.51 Superficial frostbite of wrist
√7th T33.511 Superficial frostbite of right wrist
√7th T33.512 Superficial frostbite of left wrist
√7th T33.519 Superficial frostbite of unspecified wrist
√6th T33.52 Superficial frostbite of hand
EXCLUDES 2 *superficial frostbite of fingers (T33.53-)*
√7th T33.521 Superficial frostbite of right hand
√7th T33.522 Superficial frostbite of left hand
√7th T33.529 Superficial frostbite of unspecified hand
√6th T33.53 Superficial frostbite of finger(s)
√7th T33.531 Superficial frostbite of right finger(s)
√7th T33.532 Superficial frostbite of left finger(s)
√7th T33.539 Superficial frostbite of unspecified finger(s)
√5th T33.6 Superficial frostbite of hip and thigh
√x7th T33.60 Superficial frostbite of unspecified hip and thigh
√x7th T33.61 Superficial frostbite of right hip and thigh
√x7th T33.62 Superficial frostbite of left hip and thigh
√5th T33.7 Superficial frostbite of knee and lower leg
EXCLUDES 2 *superficial frostbite of ankle and foot (T33.8-)*
√x7th T33.70 Superficial frostbite of unspecified knee and lower leg
√x7th T33.71 Superficial frostbite of right knee and lower leg
√x7th T33.72 Superficial frostbite of left knee and lower leg
√5th T33.8 Superficial frostbite of ankle, foot, and toe(s)
√6th T33.81 Superficial frostbite of ankle
√7th T33.811 Superficial frostbite of right ankle
√7th T33.812 Superficial frostbite of left ankle
√7th T33.819 Superficial frostbite of unspecified ankle
√6th T33.82 Superficial frostbite of foot
√7th T33.821 Superficial frostbite of right foot
√7th T33.822 Superficial frostbite of left foot
√7th T33.829 Superficial frostbite of unspecified foot
√6th T33.83 Superficial frostbite of toe(s)
√7th T33.831 Superficial frostbite of right toe(s)
√7th T33.832 Superficial frostbite of left toe(s)
√7th T33.839 Superficial frostbite of unspecified toe(s)

- T33.9 **Superficial frostbite of other and unspecified sites**
  - T33.9Ø **Superficial frostbite of unspecified sites**
    - Superficial frostbite NOS
  - T33.99 **Superficial frostbite of other sites**
    - Superficial frostbite of leg NOS
    - Superficial frostbite of trunk NOS

**T34 Frostbite with tissue necrosis**

The appropriate 7th character is to be added to each code from category T34.
A initial encounter
D subsequent encounter
S sequela

- T34.Ø **Frostbite with tissue necrosis of head**
  - T34.Ø1 **Frostbite with tissue necrosis of ear**
    - T34.Ø11 **Frostbite with tissue necrosis of right ear** COM
    - T34.Ø12 **Frostbite with tissue necrosis of left ear** COM
    - T34.Ø19 **Frostbite with tissue necrosis of unspecified ear** COM
  - T34.Ø2 **Frostbite with tissue necrosis of nose** COM
  - T34.Ø9 **Frostbite with tissue necrosis of other part of head** COM
- T34.1 **Frostbite with tissue necrosis of neck** COM
- T34.2 **Frostbite with tissue necrosis of thorax** COM
- T34.3 **Frostbite with tissue necrosis of abdominal wall, lower back and pelvis** COM
- T34.4 **Frostbite with tissue necrosis of arm**
  - EXCLUDES 2 *frostbite with tissue necrosis of wrist and hand (T34.5-)*
  - T34.4Ø **Frostbite with tissue necrosis of unspecified arm** COM
  - T34.41 **Frostbite with tissue necrosis of right arm** COM
  - T34.42 **Frostbite with tissue necrosis of left arm** COM
- T34.5 **Frostbite with tissue necrosis of wrist, hand, and finger(s)**
  - T34.51 **Frostbite with tissue necrosis of wrist**
    - T34.511 **Frostbite with tissue necrosis of right wrist** COM
    - T34.512 **Frostbite with tissue necrosis of left wrist** COM
    - T34.519 **Frostbite with tissue necrosis of unspecified wrist** COM
  - T34.52 **Frostbite with tissue necrosis of hand**
    - EXCLUDES 2 *frostbite with tissue necrosis of finger(s) (T34.53-)*
    - T34.521 **Frostbite with tissue necrosis of right hand** COM
    - T34.522 **Frostbite with tissue necrosis of left hand** COM
    - T34.529 **Frostbite with tissue necrosis of unspecified hand** COM
  - T34.53 **Frostbite with tissue necrosis of finger(s)**
    - T34.531 **Frostbite with tissue necrosis of right finger(s)** COM
    - T34.532 **Frostbite with tissue necrosis of left finger(s)** COM
    - T34.539 **Frostbite with tissue necrosis of unspecified finger(s)** COM
- T34.6 **Frostbite with tissue necrosis of hip and thigh**
  - T34.6Ø **Frostbite with tissue necrosis of unspecified hip and thigh**
  - T34.61 **Frostbite with tissue necrosis of right hip and thigh**
  - T34.62 **Frostbite with tissue necrosis of left hip and thigh** COM
- T34.7 **Frostbite with tissue necrosis of knee and lower leg**
  - EXCLUDES 2 *frostbite with tissue necrosis of ankle and foot (T34.8-)*
  - T34.7Ø **Frostbite with tissue necrosis of unspecified knee and lower leg** COM
  - T34.71 **Frostbite with tissue necrosis of right knee and lower leg** COM
  - T34.72 **Frostbite with tissue necrosis of left knee and lower leg** COM
- T34.8 **Frostbite with tissue necrosis of ankle, foot, and toe(s)**
  - T34.81 **Frostbite with tissue necrosis of ankle**
    - T34.811 **Frostbite with tissue necrosis of right ankle** COM
    - T34.812 **Frostbite with tissue necrosis of left ankle** COM
    - T34.819 **Frostbite with tissue necrosis of unspecified ankle** COM
  - T34.82 **Frostbite with tissue necrosis of foot**
    - T34.821 **Frostbite with tissue necrosis of right foot**
    - T34.822 **Frostbite with tissue necrosis of left foot**
    - T34.829 **Frostbite with tissue necrosis of unspecified foot**
  - T34.83 **Frostbite with tissue necrosis of toe(s)**
    - T34.831 **Frostbite with tissue necrosis of right toe(s)**
    - T34.832 **Frostbite with tissue necrosis of left toe(s)**
    - T34.839 **Frostbite with tissue necrosis of unspecified toe(s)**
- T34.9 **Frostbite with tissue necrosis of other and unspecified sites**
  - T34.9Ø **Frostbite with tissue necrosis of unspecified sites**
    - Frostbite with tissue necrosis NOS
  - T34.99 **Frostbite with tissue necrosis of other sites**
    - Frostbite with tissue necrosis of leg NOS
    - Frostbite with tissue necrosis of trunk NOS

## Poisoning by, adverse effects of and underdosing of drugs, medicaments and biological substances (T36-T5Ø)

INCLUDES adverse effect of correct substance properly administered
poisoning by overdose of substance
poisoning by wrong substance given or taken in error
underdosing by (inadvertently) (deliberately) taking less substance than prescribed or instructed

Code first, for adverse effects, the nature of the adverse effect, such as:
- adverse effect NOS (T88.7)
- aspirin gastritis (K29.-)
- blood disorders (D56-D76)
- contact dermatitis (L23-L25)
- dermatitis due to substances taken internally (L27.-)
- nephropathy (N14.Ø-N14.2)

NOTE The drug giving rise to the adverse effect should be identified by use of codes from categories T36-T5Ø with fifth or sixth character 5.

Use additional code(s) to specify:
- manifestations of poisoning
- underdosing or failure in dosage during medical and surgical care (Y63.6, Y63.8-Y63.9)
- underdosing of medication regimen (Z91.12-, Z91.13-)

EXCLUDES 1 *toxic reaction to local anesthesia in pregnancy (O29.3-)*
EXCLUDES 2 *abuse and dependence of psychoactive substances (F1Ø-F19)*
*abuse of non-dependence-producing substances (F55.-)*
*drug reaction and poisoning affecting newborn (PØØ-P96)*
*immunodeficiency due to drugs (D84.821)*
*pathological drug intoxication (inebriation) (F1Ø-F19)*

**AHA:** 2018,4Q,71; 2016,2Q,8; 2015,3Q,22

**T36 Poisoning by, adverse effect of and underdosing of systemic antibiotics**

EXCLUDES 1 *antineoplastic antibiotics (T45.1-)*
*locally applied antibiotic NEC (T49.Ø)*
*topically used antibiotic for ear, nose and throat (T49.6)*
*topically used antibiotic for eye (T49.5)*

The appropriate 7th character is to be added to each code from category T36.
A initial encounter
D subsequent encounter
S sequela

- T36.Ø **Poisoning by, adverse effect of and underdosing of penicillins**
  - T36.ØX **Poisoning by, adverse effect of and underdosing of penicillins**
    - T36.ØX1 **Poisoning by penicillins, accidental (unintentional)**
      - Poisoning by penicillins NOS
    - T36.ØX2 **Poisoning by penicillins, intentional self-harm** HCC Rx ESR COM
    - T36.ØX3 **Poisoning by penicillins, assault**
    - T36.ØX4 **Poisoning by penicillins, undetermined**
    - T36.ØX5 **Adverse effect of penicillins** UPD
    - T36.ØX6 **Underdosing of penicillins** UPD

√5th **T36.1 Poisoning by, adverse effect of and underdosing of cephalosporins and other beta-lactam antibiotics**

√6th **T36.1X Poisoning by, adverse effect of and underdosing of cephalosporins and other beta-lactam antibiotics**

√7th **T36.1X1 Poisoning by cephalosporins and other beta-lactam antibiotics, accidental (unintentional)**
Poisoning by cephalosporins and other beta-lactam antibiotics NOS

√7th **T36.1X2 Poisoning by cephalosporins and other beta-lactam antibiotics, intentional self-harm** HCC Rx ESR COM

√7th **T36.1X3 Poisoning by cephalosporins and other beta-lactam antibiotics, assault**

√7th **T36.1X4 Poisoning by cephalosporins and other beta-lactam antibiotics, undetermined**

√7th **T36.1X5 Adverse effect of cephalosporins and other beta-lactam antibiotics** UPD

√7th **T36.1X6 Underdosing of cephalosporins and other beta-lactam antibiotics** UPD

√5th **T36.2 Poisoning by, adverse effect of and underdosing of chloramphenicol group**

√6th **T36.2X Poisoning by, adverse effect of and underdosing of chloramphenicol group**

√7th **T36.2X1 Poisoning by chloramphenicol group, accidental (unintentional)**
Poisoning by chloramphenicol group NOS

√7th **T36.2X2 Poisoning by chloramphenicol group, intentional self-harm** HCC Rx ESR COM

√7th **T36.2X3 Poisoning by chloramphenicol group, assault**

√7th **T36.2X4 Poisoning by chloramphenicol group, undetermined**

√7th **T36.2X5 Adverse effect of chloramphenicol group** UPD

√7th **T36.2X6 Underdosing of chloramphenicol group** UPD

√5th **T36.3 Poisoning by, adverse effect of and underdosing of macrolides**

√6th **T36.3X Poisoning by, adverse effect of and underdosing of macrolides**

√7th **T36.3X1 Poisoning by macrolides, accidental (unintentional)**
Poisoning by macrolides NOS

√7th **T36.3X2 Poisoning by macrolides, intentional self-harm** HCC Rx ESR COM

√7th **T36.3X3 Poisoning by macrolides, assault**

√7th **T36.3X4 Poisoning by macrolides, undetermined**

√7th **T36.3X5 Adverse effect of macrolides** UPD

√7th **T36.3X6 Underdosing of macrolides** UPD

√5th **T36.4 Poisoning by, adverse effect of and underdosing of tetracyclines**

√6th **T36.4X Poisoning by, adverse effect of and underdosing of tetracyclines**

√7th **T36.4X1 Poisoning by tetracyclines, accidental (unintentional)**
Poisoning by tetracyclines NOS

√7th **T36.4X2 Poisoning by tetracyclines, intentional self-harm** HCC Rx ESR COM

√7th **T36.4X3 Poisoning by tetracyclines, assault**

√7th **T36.4X4 Poisoning by tetracyclines, undetermined**

√7th **T36.4X5 Adverse effect of tetracyclines** UPD

√7th **T36.4X6 Underdosing of tetracyclines** UPD

√5th **T36.5 Poisoning by, adverse effect of and underdosing of aminoglycosides**
Poisoning by, adverse effect of and underdosing of streptomycin

√6th **T36.5X Poisoning by, adverse effect of and underdosing of aminoglycosides**

√7th **T36.5X1 Poisoning by aminoglycosides, accidental (unintentional)**
Poisoning by aminoglycosides NOS

√7th **T36.5X2 Poisoning by aminoglycosides, intentional self-harm** HCC Rx ESR COM

√7th **T36.5X3 Poisoning by aminoglycosides, assault**

√7th **T36.5X4 Poisoning by aminoglycosides, undetermined**

√7th **T36.5X5 Adverse effect of aminoglycosides** UPD

√7th **T36.5X6 Underdosing of aminoglycosides** UPD

√5th **T36.6 Poisoning by, adverse effect of and underdosing of rifampicins**

√6th **T36.6X Poisoning by, adverse effect of and underdosing of rifampicins**

√7th **T36.6X1 Poisoning by rifampicins, accidental (unintentional)**
Poisoning by rifampicins NOS

√7th **T36.6X2 Poisoning by rifampicins, intentional self-harm** HCC Rx ESR COM

√7th **T36.6X3 Poisoning by rifampicins, assault**

√7th **T36.6X4 Poisoning by rifampicins, undetermined**

√7th **T36.6X5 Adverse effect of rifampicins** UPD

√7th **T36.6X6 Underdosing of rifampicins** UPD

√5th **T36.7 Poisoning by, adverse effect of and underdosing of antifungal antibiotics, systemically used**

√6th **T36.7X Poisoning by, adverse effect of and underdosing of antifungal antibiotics, systemically used**

√7th **T36.7X1 Poisoning by antifungal antibiotics, systemically used, accidental (unintentional)**
Poisoning by antifungal antibiotics, systemically used NOS

√7th **T36.7X2 Poisoning by antifungal antibiotics, systemically used, intentional self-harm** HCC Rx ESR COM

√7th **T36.7X3 Poisoning by antifungal antibiotics, systemically used, assault**

√7th **T36.7X4 Poisoning by antifungal antibiotics, systemically used, undetermined**

√7th **T36.7X5 Adverse effect of antifungal antibiotics, systemically used** UPD

√7th **T36.7X6 Underdosing of antifungal antibiotics, systemically used** UPD

√5th **T36.8 Poisoning by, adverse effect of and underdosing of other systemic antibiotics**

√6th **T36.8X Poisoning by, adverse effect of and underdosing of other systemic antibiotics**
**AHA:** 2017,1Q,39

√7th **T36.8X1 Poisoning by other systemic antibiotics, accidental (unintentional)**
Poisoning by other systemic antibiotics NOS

√7th **T36.8X2 Poisoning by other systemic antibiotics, intentional self-harm** HCC Rx ESR COM

√7th **T36.8X3 Poisoning by other systemic antibiotics, assault**

√7th **T36.8X4 Poisoning by other systemic antibiotics, undetermined**

√7th **T36.8X5 Adverse effect of other systemic antibiotics** UPD

√7th **T36.8X6 Underdosing of other systemic antibiotics** UPD

√5th **T36.9 Poisoning by, adverse effect of and underdosing of unspecified systemic antibiotic**

√x7th **T36.91 Poisoning by unspecified systemic antibiotic, accidental (unintentional)**
Poisoning by systemic antibiotic NOS

√x7th **T36.92 Poisoning by unspecified systemic antibiotic, intentional self-harm** HCC Rx ESR COM

√x7th **T36.93 Poisoning by unspecified systemic antibiotic, assault**

√x7th **T36.94 Poisoning by unspecified systemic antibiotic, undetermined**

√x7th **T36.95 Adverse effect of unspecified systemic antibiotic** UPD

√x7th **T36.96 Underdosing of unspecified systemic antibiotic** UPD

√5th **T36.A Poisoning by, adverse effect of and underdosing of fluoroquinolone antibiotics**

√6th **T36.AX Poisoning by, adverse effect of and underdosing of fluoroquinolone antibiotics**

√7th **T36.AX1 Poisoning by fluoroquinolone antibiotics, accidental (unintentional)**
Poisoning by fluoroquinolone antibiotics NOS

√7th **T36.AX2 Poisoning by fluoroquinolone antibiotics, intentional self-harm** HCC Rx ESR

√7th **T36.AX3 Poisoning by fluoroquinolone antibiotics, assault**

√7th **T36.AX4 Poisoning by fluoroquinolone antibiotics, undetermined**

√7th **T36.AX5 Adverse effect of fluoroquinolone antibiotics**

√7th T36.AX6 Underdosing of fluoroquinolone antibiotics

√4th **T37 Poisoning by, adverse effect of and underdosing of other systemic anti-infectives and antiparasitics**

EXCLUDES 1 *anti-infectives topically used for ear, nose and throat (T49.6-)*
*anti-infectives topically used for eye (T49.5-)*
*locally applied anti-infectives NEC (T49.Ø-)*

The appropriate 7th character is to be added to each code from category T37.
A initial encounter
D subsequent encounter
S sequela

√5th **T37.Ø Poisoning by, adverse effect of and underdosing of sulfonamides**

√6th T37.ØX Poisoning by, adverse effect of and underdosing of sulfonamides

√7th T37.ØX1 Poisoning by sulfonamides, accidental (unintentional)
Poisoning by sulfonamides NOS

√7th T37.ØX2 Poisoning by sulfonamides, intentional self-harm HCC Rx ESR COM

√7th T37.ØX3 Poisoning by sulfonamides, assault

√7th T37.ØX4 Poisoning by sulfonamides, undetermined

√7th T37.ØX5 Adverse effect of sulfonamides UPD

√7th T37.ØX6 Underdosing of sulfonamides UPD

√5th **T37.1 Poisoning by, adverse effect of and underdosing of antimycobacterial drugs**

EXCLUDES 1 *rifampicins (T36.6-)*
*streptomycin (T36.5-)*

√6th T37.1X Poisoning by, adverse effect of and underdosing of antimycobacterial drugs

√7th T37.1X1 Poisoning by antimycobacterial drugs, accidental (unintentional)
Poisoning by antimycobacterial drugs NOS

√7th T37.1X2 Poisoning by antimycobacterial drugs, intentional self-harm HCC Rx ESR COM

√7th T37.1X3 Poisoning by antimycobacterial drugs, assault

√7th T37.1X4 Poisoning by antimycobacterial drugs, undetermined

√7th T37.1X5 Adverse effect of antimycobacterial drugs UPD

√7th T37.1X6 Underdosing of antimycobacterial drugs UPD

√5th **T37.2 Poisoning by, adverse effect of and underdosing of antimalarials and drugs acting on other blood protozoa**

EXCLUDES 1 *hydroxyquinoline derivatives (T37.8-)*

√6th T37.2X Poisoning by, adverse effect of and underdosing of antimalarials and drugs acting on other blood protozoa

√7th T37.2X1 Poisoning by antimalarials and drugs acting on other blood protozoa, accidental (unintentional)
Poisoning by antimalarials and drugs acting on other blood protozoa NOS

√7th T37.2X2 Poisoning by antimalarials and drugs acting on other blood protozoa, intentional self-harm HCC Rx ESR COM

√7th T37.2X3 Poisoning by antimalarials and drugs acting on other blood protozoa, assault

√7th T37.2X4 Poisoning by antimalarials and drugs acting on other blood protozoa, undetermined

√7th T37.2X5 Adverse effect of antimalarials and drugs acting on other blood protozoa UPD

√7th T37.2X6 Underdosing of antimalarials and drugs acting on other blood protozoa UPD

√5th **T37.3 Poisoning by, adverse effect of and underdosing of other antiprotozoal drugs**

√6th T37.3X Poisoning by, adverse effect of and underdosing of other antiprotozoal drugs

√7th T37.3X1 Poisoning by other antiprotozoal drugs, accidental (unintentional)
Poisoning by other antiprotozoal drugs NOS

√7th T37.3X2 Poisoning by other antiprotozoal drugs, intentional self-harm HCC Rx ESR COM

√7th T37.3X3 Poisoning by other antiprotozoal drugs, assault

√7th T37.3X4 Poisoning by other antiprotozoal drugs, undetermined

√7th T37.3X5 Adverse effect of other antiprotozoal drugs UPD

√7th T37.3X6 Underdosing of other antiprotozoal drugs UPD

√5th **T37.4 Poisoning by, adverse effect of and underdosing of anthelminthics**

√6th T37.4X Poisoning by, adverse effect of and underdosing of anthelminthics

√7th T37.4X1 Poisoning by anthelminthics, accidental (unintentional)
Poisoning by anthelminthics NOS

√7th T37.4X2 Poisoning by anthelminthics, intentional self-harm HCC Rx ESR COM

√7th T37.4X3 Poisoning by anthelminthics, assault

√7th T37.4X4 Poisoning by anthelminthics, undetermined

√7th T37.4X5 Adverse effect of anthelminthics UPD

√7th T37.4X6 Underdosing of anthelminthics UPD

√5th **T37.5 Poisoning by, adverse effect of and underdosing of antiviral drugs**

EXCLUDES 1 *amantadine (T42.8-)*
*cytarabine (T45.1-)*

√6th T37.5X Poisoning by, adverse effect of and underdosing of antiviral drugs

√7th T37.5X1 Poisoning by antiviral drugs, accidental (unintentional)
Poisoning by antiviral drugs NOS

√7th T37.5X2 Poisoning by antiviral drugs, intentional self-harm HCC Rx ESR COM

√7th T37.5X3 Poisoning by antiviral drugs, assault

√7th T37.5X4 Poisoning by antiviral drugs, undetermined

√7th T37.5X5 Adverse effect of antiviral drugs UPD

√7th T37.5X6 Underdosing of antiviral drugs UPD

√5th **T37.8 Poisoning by, adverse effect of and underdosing of other specified systemic anti-infectives and antiparasitics**

Poisoning by, adverse effect of and underdosing of hydroxyquinoline derivatives

EXCLUDES 1 *antimalarial drugs (T37.2-)*

√6th T37.8X Poisoning by, adverse effect of and underdosing of other specified systemic anti-infectives and antiparasitics

√7th T37.8X1 Poisoning by other specified systemic anti-infectives and antiparasitics, accidental (unintentional)
Poisoning by other specified systemic anti-infectives and antiparasitics NOS

√7th T37.8X2 Poisoning by other specified systemic anti-infectives and antiparasitics, intentional self-harm HCC Rx ESR COM

√7th T37.8X3 Poisoning by other specified systemic anti-infectives and antiparasitics, assault

√7th T37.8X4 Poisoning by other specified systemic anti-infectives and antiparasitics, undetermined

√7th T37.8X5 Adverse effect of other specified systemic anti-infectives and antiparasitics UPD

√7th T37.8X6 Underdosing of other specified systemic anti-infectives and antiparasitics UPD

√5th **T37.9 Poisoning by, adverse effect of and underdosing of unspecified systemic anti-infective and antiparasitics**

√x7th T37.91 Poisoning by unspecified systemic anti-infective and antiparasitics, accidental (unintentional)
Poisoning by, adverse effect of and underdosing of systemic anti-infective and antiparasitics NOS

√x7th T37.92 Poisoning by unspecified systemic anti-infective and antiparasitics, intentional self-harm HCC Rx ESR COM

√x7th T37.93 Poisoning by unspecified systemic anti-infective and antiparasitics, assault

√x7th T37.94 Poisoning by unspecified systemic anti-infective and antiparasitics, undetermined

√x7th T37.95 Adverse effect of unspecified systemic anti-infective and antiparasitic UPD

√x7th T37.96 Underdosing of unspecified systemic anti-infectives and antiparasitics UPD

**T38 Poisoning by, adverse effect of and underdosing of hormones and their synthetic substitutes and antagonists, not elsewhere classified**

EXCLUDES 1 *mineralocorticoids and their antagonists (T50.0-)*
*oxytocic hormones (T48.0-)*
*parathyroid hormones and derivatives (T50.9-)*

The appropriate 7th character is to be added to each code from category T38.
A initial encounter
D subsequent encounter
S sequela

**T38.0 Poisoning by, adverse effect of and underdosing of glucocorticoids and synthetic analogues**

EXCLUDES 1 *glucocorticoids, topically used (T49.-)*

**T38.0X Poisoning by, adverse effect of and underdosing of glucocorticoids and synthetic analogues**

**T38.0X1 Poisoning by glucocorticoids and synthetic analogues, accidental (unintentional)**
Poisoning by glucocorticoids and synthetic analogues NOS

**T38.0X2 Poisoning by glucocorticoids and synthetic analogues, intentional self-harm** HCC Rx ESR COM

**T38.0X3 Poisoning by glucocorticoids and synthetic analogues, assault**

**T38.0X4 Poisoning by glucocorticoids and synthetic analogues, undetermined**

**T38.0X5 Adverse effect of glucocorticoids and synthetic analogues** UPD

**T38.0X6 Underdosing of glucocorticoids and synthetic analogues** UPD

**T38.1 Poisoning by, adverse effect of and underdosing of thyroid hormones and substitutes**

**T38.1X Poisoning by, adverse effect of and underdosing of thyroid hormones and substitutes**

**T38.1X1 Poisoning by thyroid hormones and substitutes, accidental (unintentional)**
Poisoning by thyroid hormones and substitutes NOS

**T38.1X2 Poisoning by thyroid hormones and substitutes, intentional self-harm** HCC Rx ESR COM

**T38.1X3 Poisoning by thyroid hormones and substitutes, assault**

**T38.1X4 Poisoning by thyroid hormones and substitutes, undetermined**

**T38.1X5 Adverse effect of thyroid hormones and substitutes** UPD

**T38.1X6 Underdosing of thyroid hormones and substitutes** UPD

**T38.2 Poisoning by, adverse effect of and underdosing of antithyroid drugs**

**T38.2X Poisoning by, adverse effect of and underdosing of antithyroid drugs**

**T38.2X1 Poisoning by antithyroid drugs, accidental (unintentional)**
Poisoning by antithyroid drugs NOS

**T38.2X2 Poisoning by antithyroid drugs, intentional self-harm** HCC Rx ESR COM

**T38.2X3 Poisoning by antithyroid drugs, assault**

**T38.2X4 Poisoning by antithyroid drugs, undetermined**

**T38.2X5 Adverse effect of antithyroid drugs** UPD

**T38.2X6 Underdosing of antithyroid drugs** UPD

**T38.3 Poisoning by, adverse effect of and underdosing of insulin and oral hypoglycemic [antidiabetic] drugs**

**T38.3X Poisoning by, adverse effect of and underdosing of insulin and oral hypoglycemic [antidiabetic] drugs**
AHA: 2026,1Q,24

**T38.3X1 Poisoning by insulin and oral hypoglycemic [antidiabetic] drugs, accidental (unintentional)**
Poisoning by insulin and oral hypoglycemic [antidiabetic] drugs NOS

**T38.3X2 Poisoning by insulin and oral hypoglycemic [antidiabetic] drugs, intentional self-harm** HCC Rx ESR COM

**T38.3X3 Poisoning by insulin and oral hypoglycemic [antidiabetic] drugs, assault**

**T38.3X4 Poisoning by insulin and oral hypoglycemic [antidiabetic] drugs, undetermined**

**T38.3X5 Adverse effect of insulin and oral hypoglycemic [antidiabetic] drugs** UPD

**T38.3X6 Underdosing of insulin and oral hypoglycemic [antidiabetic] drugs** UPD

**T38.4 Poisoning by, adverse effect of and underdosing of oral contraceptives**
Poisoning by, adverse effect of and underdosing of multiple- and single-ingredient oral contraceptive preparations

**T38.4X Poisoning by, adverse effect of and underdosing of oral contraceptives**

**T38.4X1 Poisoning by oral contraceptives, accidental (unintentional)**
Poisoning by oral contraceptives NOS

**T38.4X2 Poisoning by oral contraceptives, intentional self-harm** HCC Rx ESR COM

**T38.4X3 Poisoning by oral contraceptives, assault**

**T38.4X4 Poisoning by oral contraceptives, undetermined**

**T38.4X5 Adverse effect of oral contraceptives** UPD

**T38.4X6 Underdosing of oral contraceptives** UPD

**T38.5 Poisoning by, adverse effect of and underdosing of other estrogens and progestogens**
Poisoning by, adverse effect of and underdosing of estrogens and progestogens mixtures and substitutes

**T38.5X Poisoning by, adverse effect of and underdosing of other estrogens and progestogens**

**T38.5X1 Poisoning by other estrogens and progestogens, accidental (unintentional)**
Poisoning by other estrogens and progestogens NOS

**T38.5X2 Poisoning by other estrogens and progestogens, intentional self-harm** HCC Rx ESR COM

**T38.5X3 Poisoning by other estrogens and progestogens, assault**

**T38.5X4 Poisoning by other estrogens and progestogens, undetermined**

**T38.5X5 Adverse effect of other estrogens and progestogens** UPD

**T38.5X6 Underdosing of other estrogens and progestogens** UPD

**T38.6 Poisoning by, adverse effect of and underdosing of antigonadotrophins, antiestrogens, antiandrogens, not elsewhere classified**
Poisoning by, adverse effect of and underdosing of tamoxifen

**T38.6X Poisoning by, adverse effect of and underdosing of antigonadotrophins, antiestrogens, antiandrogens, not elsewhere classified**

**T38.6X1 Poisoning by antigonadotrophins, antiestrogens, antiandrogens, not elsewhere classified, accidental (unintentional)**
Poisoning by antigonadotrophins, antiestrogens, antiandrogens, not elsewhere classified NOS

**T38.6X2 Poisoning by antigonadotrophins, antiestrogens, antiandrogens, not elsewhere classified, intentional self-harm** HCC Rx ESR COM

**T38.6X3 Poisoning by antigonadotrophins, antiestrogens, antiandrogens, not elsewhere classified, assault**

**T38.6X4 Poisoning by antigonadotrophins, antiestrogens, antiandrogens, not elsewhere classified, undetermined**

**T38.6X5 Adverse effect of antigonadotrophins, antiestrogens, antiandrogens, not elsewhere classified** UPD

**T38.6X6 Underdosing of antigonadotrophins, antiestrogens, antiandrogens, not elsewhere classified** UPD

**T38.7 Poisoning by, adverse effect of and underdosing of androgens and anabolic congeners**

**T38.7X Poisoning by, adverse effect of and underdosing of androgens and anabolic congeners**

**T38.7X1 Poisoning by androgens and anabolic congeners, accidental (unintentional)**
Poisoning by androgens and anabolic congeners NOS

**T38.7X2 Poisoning by androgens and anabolic congeners, intentional self-harm** HCC Rx ESR COM

T38.7X3 Poisoning by androgens and anabolic congeners, assault
T38.7X4 Poisoning by androgens and anabolic congeners, undetermined
T38.7X5 Adverse effect of androgens and anabolic congeners UPD
T38.7X6 Underdosing of androgens and anabolic congeners UPD

T38.8 Poisoning by, adverse effect of and underdosing of other and unspecified hormones and synthetic substitutes

T38.80 Poisoning by, adverse effect of and underdosing of unspecified hormones and synthetic substitutes
T38.801 Poisoning by unspecified hormones and synthetic substitutes, accidental (unintentional)
Poisoning by unspecified hormones and synthetic substitutes NOS
T38.802 Poisoning by unspecified hormones and synthetic substitutes, intentional self-harm HCC Rx ESR COM
T38.803 Poisoning by unspecified hormones and synthetic substitutes, assault
T38.804 Poisoning by unspecified hormones and synthetic substitutes, undetermined
T38.805 Adverse effect of unspecified hormones and synthetic substitutes UPD
T38.806 Underdosing of unspecified hormones and synthetic substitutes UPD

T38.81 Poisoning by, adverse effect of and underdosing of anterior pituitary [adenohypophyseal] hormones
T38.811 Poisoning by anterior pituitary [adenohypophyseal] hormones, accidental (unintentional)
Poisoning by anterior pituitary [adenohypophyseal] hormones NOS
T38.812 Poisoning by anterior pituitary [adenohypophyseal] hormones, intentional self-harm HCC Rx ESR COM
T38.813 Poisoning by anterior pituitary [adenohypophyseal] hormones, assault
T38.814 Poisoning by anterior pituitary [adenohypophyseal] hormones, undetermined
T38.815 Adverse effect of anterior pituitary [adenohypophyseal] hormones UPD
T38.816 Underdosing of anterior pituitary [adenohypophyseal] hormones UPD

T38.89 Poisoning by, adverse effect of and underdosing of other hormones and synthetic substitutes
AHA: 2026,1Q,24,25
TIP: Use this subcategory when the poisoning is caused by injectable GLP-1 medications.
T38.891 Poisoning by other hormones and synthetic substitutes, accidental (unintentional)
Poisoning by other hormones and synthetic substitutes NOS
T38.892 Poisoning by other hormones and synthetic substitutes, intentional self-harm HCC Rx ESR COM
T38.893 Poisoning by other hormones and synthetic substitutes, assault
T38.894 Poisoning by other hormones and synthetic substitutes, undetermined
T38.895 Adverse effect of other hormones and synthetic substitutes UPD
T38.896 Underdosing of other hormones and synthetic substitutes UPD

T38.9 Poisoning by, adverse effect of and underdosing of other and unspecified hormone antagonists

T38.90 Poisoning by, adverse effect of and underdosing of unspecified hormone antagonists
T38.901 Poisoning by unspecified hormone antagonists, accidental (unintentional)
Poisoning by unspecified hormone antagonists NOS
T38.902 Poisoning by unspecified hormone antagonists, intentional self-harm HCC Rx ESR COM
T38.903 Poisoning by unspecified hormone antagonists, assault
T38.904 Poisoning by unspecified hormone antagonists, undetermined
T38.905 Adverse effect of unspecified hormone antagonists UPD
T38.906 Underdosing of unspecified hormone antagonists UPD

T38.99 Poisoning by, adverse effect of and underdosing of other hormone antagonists
T38.991 Poisoning by other hormone antagonists, accidental (unintentional)
Poisoning by other hormone antagonists NOS
T38.992 Poisoning by other hormone antagonists, intentional self-harm HCC Rx ESR COM
T38.993 Poisoning by other hormone antagonists, assault
T38.994 Poisoning by other hormone antagonists, undetermined
T38.995 Adverse effect of other hormone antagonists UPD
T38.996 Underdosing of other hormone antagonists UPD

T39 Poisoning by, adverse effect of and underdosing of nonopioid analgesics, antipyretics and antirheumatics

The appropriate 7th character is to be added to each code from category T39.
A initial encounter
D subsequent encounter
S sequela

T39.0 Poisoning by, adverse effect of and underdosing of salicylates

T39.01 Poisoning by, adverse effect of and underdosing of aspirin
Poisoning by, adverse effect of and underdosing of acetylsalicylic acid
T39.011 Poisoning by aspirin, accidental (unintentional)
T39.012 Poisoning by aspirin, intentional self-harm HCC Rx ESR COM
T39.013 Poisoning by aspirin, assault
T39.014 Poisoning by aspirin, undetermined
T39.015 Adverse effect of aspirin UPD
AHA: 2016,1Q,15
T39.016 Underdosing of aspirin UPD

T39.09 Poisoning by, adverse effect of and underdosing of other salicylates
T39.091 Poisoning by salicylates, accidental (unintentional)
Poisoning by salicylates NOS
T39.092 Poisoning by salicylates, intentional self-harm HCC Rx ESR COM
T39.093 Poisoning by salicylates, assault
T39.094 Poisoning by salicylates, undetermined
T39.095 Adverse effect of salicylates UPD
T39.096 Underdosing of salicylates UPD

T39.1 Poisoning by, adverse effect of and underdosing of 4-Aminophenol derivatives

T39.1X Poisoning by, adverse effect of and underdosing of 4-Aminophenol derivatives
T39.1X1 Poisoning by 4-Aminophenol derivatives, accidental (unintentional)
Poisoning by 4-Aminophenol derivatives NOS
T39.1X2 Poisoning by 4-Aminophenol derivatives, intentional self-harm HCC Rx ESR COM
T39.1X3 Poisoning by 4-Aminophenol derivatives, assault
T39.1X4 Poisoning by 4-Aminophenol derivatives, undetermined
T39.1X5 Adverse effect of 4-Aminophenol derivatives UPD
T39.1X6 Underdosing of 4-Aminophenol derivatives UPD

T39.2 Poisoning by, adverse effect of and underdosing of pyrazolone derivatives

T39.2X Poisoning by, adverse effect of and underdosing of pyrazolone derivatives
T39.2X1 Poisoning by pyrazolone derivatives, accidental (unintentional)
Poisoning by pyrazolone derivatives NOS
T39.2X2 Poisoning by pyrazolone derivatives, intentional self-harm HCC Rx ESR COM

√7th **T39.2X3 Poisoning by pyrazolone derivatives, assault**

√7th **T39.2X4 Poisoning by pyrazolone derivatives, undetermined**

√7th **T39.2X5 Adverse effect of pyrazolone derivatives** UPD

√7th **T39.2X6 Underdosing of pyrazolone derivatives** UPD

√5th **T39.3 Poisoning by, adverse effect of and underdosing of other nonsteroidal anti-inflammatory drugs [NSAID]**

√6th **T39.31 Poisoning by, adverse effect of and underdosing of propionic acid derivatives**

Poisoning by, adverse effect of and underdosing of fenoprofen

Poisoning by, adverse effect of and underdosing of flurbiprofen

Poisoning by, adverse effect of and underdosing of ibuprofen

Poisoning by, adverse effect of and underdosing of ketoprofen

Poisoning by, adverse effect of and underdosing of naproxen

Poisoning by, adverse effect of and underdosing of oxaprozin

√7th **T39.311 Poisoning by propionic acid derivatives, accidental (unintentional)**

√7th **T39.312 Poisoning by propionic acid derivatives, intentional self-harm** HCC Rx ESR COM

√7th **T39.313 Poisoning by propionic acid derivatives, assault**

√7th **T39.314 Poisoning by propionic acid derivatives, undetermined**

√7th **T39.315 Adverse effect of propionic acid derivatives** UPD

√7th **T39.316 Underdosing of propionic acid derivatives** UPD

√6th **T39.39 Poisoning by, adverse effect of and underdosing of other nonsteroidal anti-inflammatory drugs [NSAID]**

√7th **T39.391 Poisoning by other nonsteroidal anti-inflammatory drugs [NSAID], accidental (unintentional)**

Poisoning by other nonsteroidal anti-inflammatory drugs NOS

√7th **T39.392 Poisoning by other nonsteroidal anti-inflammatory drugs [NSAID], intentional self-harm** HCC Rx ESR COM

√7th **T39.393 Poisoning by other nonsteroidal anti-inflammatory drugs [NSAID], assault**

√7th **T39.394 Poisoning by other nonsteroidal anti-inflammatory drugs [NSAID], undetermined**

√7th **T39.395 Adverse effect of other nonsteroidal anti-inflammatory drugs [NSAID]** UPD

√7th **T39.396 Underdosing of other nonsteroidal anti-inflammatory drugs [NSAID]** UPD

√5th **T39.4 Poisoning by, adverse effect of and underdosing of antirheumatics, not elsewhere classified**

EXCLUDES 1 *poisoning by, adverse effect of and underdosing of glucocorticoids (T38.Ø-)*
*poisoning by, adverse effect of and underdosing of salicylates (T39.Ø-)*

√6th **T39.4X Poisoning by, adverse effect of and underdosing of antirheumatics, not elsewhere classified**

√7th **T39.4X1 Poisoning by antirheumatics, not elsewhere classified, accidental (unintentional)**

Poisoning by antirheumatics, not elsewhere classified NOS

√7th **T39.4X2 Poisoning by antirheumatics, not elsewhere classified, intentional self-harm** HCC Rx ESR COM

√7th **T39.4X3 Poisoning by antirheumatics, not elsewhere classified, assault**

√7th **T39.4X4 Poisoning by antirheumatics, not elsewhere classified, undetermined**

√7th **T39.4X5 Adverse effect of antirheumatics, not elsewhere classified** UPD

√7th **T39.4X6 Underdosing of antirheumatics, not elsewhere classified** UPD

√5th **T39.8 Poisoning by, adverse effect of and underdosing of other nonopioid analgesics and antipyretics, not elsewhere classified**

√6th **T39.8X Poisoning by, adverse effect of and underdosing of other nonopioid analgesics and antipyretics, not elsewhere classified**

√7th **T39.8X1 Poisoning by other nonopioid analgesics and antipyretics, not elsewhere classified, accidental (unintentional)**

Poisoning by other nonopioid analgesics and antipyretics, not elsewhere classified NOS

√7th **T39.8X2 Poisoning by other nonopioid analgesics and antipyretics, not elsewhere classified, intentional self-harm** HCC Rx ESR COM

√7th **T39.8X3 Poisoning by other nonopioid analgesics and antipyretics, not elsewhere classified, assault**

√7th **T39.8X4 Poisoning by other nonopioid analgesics and antipyretics, not elsewhere classified, undetermined**

√7th **T39.8X5 Adverse effect of other nonopioid analgesics and antipyretics, not elsewhere classified** UPD

√7th **T39.8X6 Underdosing of other nonopioid analgesics and antipyretics, not elsewhere classified** UPD

√5th **T39.9 Poisoning by, adverse effect of and underdosing of unspecified nonopioid analgesic, antipyretic and antirheumatic**

√x7th **T39.91 Poisoning by unspecified nonopioid analgesic, antipyretic and antirheumatic, accidental (unintentional)**

Poisoning by nonopioid analgesic, antipyretic and antirheumatic NOS

√x7th **T39.92 Poisoning by unspecified nonopioid analgesic, antipyretic and antirheumatic, intentional self-harm** HCC Rx ESR COM

√x7th **T39.93 Poisoning by unspecified nonopioid analgesic, antipyretic and antirheumatic, assault**

√x7th **T39.94 Poisoning by unspecified nonopioid analgesic, antipyretic and antirheumatic, undetermined**

√x7th **T39.95 Adverse effect of unspecified nonopioid analgesic, antipyretic and antirheumatic** UPD

√x7th **T39.96 Underdosing of unspecified nonopioid analgesic, antipyretic and antirheumatic** UPD

√4th **T4Ø Poisoning by, adverse effect of and underdosing of narcotics and psychodysleptics [hallucinogens]**

EXCLUDES 2 *drug dependence and related mental and behavioral disorders due to psychoactive substance use (F1Ø.-F19.-)*

The appropriate 7th character is to be added to each code from category T4Ø.
A initial encounter
D subsequent encounter
S sequela

√5th **T4Ø.Ø Poisoning by, adverse effect of and underdosing of opium**

√6th **T4Ø.ØX Poisoning by, adverse effect of and underdosing of opium**

√7th **T4Ø.ØX1 Poisoning by opium, accidental (unintentional)** HCC ESR COM

Poisoning by opium NOS

√7th **T4Ø.ØX2 Poisoning by opium, intentional self-harm** HCC Rx ESR COM

√7th **T4Ø.ØX3 Poisoning by opium, assault**

√7th **T4Ø.ØX4 Poisoning by opium, undetermined** HCC ESR COM

√7th **T4Ø.ØX5 Adverse effect of opium** UPD

√7th **T4Ø.ØX6 Underdosing of opium** UPD

√5th **T4Ø.1 Poisoning by and adverse effect of heroin**

√6th **T4Ø.1X Poisoning by and adverse effect of heroin**

√7th **T4Ø.1X1 Poisoning by heroin, accidental (unintentional)** HCC ESR COM

Poisoning by heroin NOS

√7th **T4Ø.1X2 Poisoning by heroin, intentional self-harm** HCC Rx ESR COM

√7th **T4Ø.1X3 Poisoning by heroin, assault**

√7th **T4Ø.1X4 Poisoning by heroin, undetermined** HCC ESR COM

✓5th **T40.2** Poisoning by, adverse effect of and underdosing of other opioids
- ✓6th **T40.2X** Poisoning by, adverse effect of and underdosing of other opioids
  - ✓7th **T40.2X1** Poisoning by other opioids, accidental (unintentional) HCC ESR COM
    - Poisoning by other opioids NOS
  - ✓7th **T40.2X2** Poisoning by other opioids, intentional self-harm HCC Rx ESR COM
  - ✓7th **T40.2X3** Poisoning by other opioids, assault
  - ✓7th **T40.2X4** Poisoning by other opioids, undetermined HCC ESR COM
  - ✓7th **T40.2X5** Adverse effect of other opioids UPD
    - AHA: 2020,2Q,24
  - ✓7th **T40.2X6** Underdosing of other opioids UPD

✓5th **T40.3** Poisoning by, adverse effect of and underdosing of methadone
- ✓6th **T40.3X** Poisoning by, adverse effect of and underdosing of methadone
  - ✓7th **T40.3X1** Poisoning by methadone, accidental (unintentional) HCC ESR COM
    - Poisoning by methadone NOS
  - ✓7th **T40.3X2** Poisoning by methadone, intentional self-harm HCC Rx ESR COM
  - ✓7th **T40.3X3** Poisoning by methadone, assault
  - ✓7th **T40.3X4** Poisoning by methadone, undetermined HCC ESR COM
  - ✓7th **T40.3X5** Adverse effect of methadone UPD
  - ✓7th **T40.3X6** Underdosing of methadone UPD

✓5th **T40.4** Poisoning by, adverse effect of and underdosing of other synthetic narcotics
- AHA: 2025,4Q,38; 2020,4Q,40
- ✓6th **T40.41** Poisoning by, adverse effect of and underdosing of fentanyl or fentanyl analogs
  - ✓7th **T40.411** Poisoning by fentanyl or fentanyl analogs, accidental (unintentional) HCC ESR COM
  - ✓7th **T40.412** Poisoning by fentanyl or fentanyl analogs, intentional self-harm HCC Rx ESR COM
  - ✓7th **T40.413** Poisoning by fentanyl or fentanyl analogs, assault
  - ✓7th **T40.414** Poisoning by fentanyl or fentanyl analogs, undetermined HCC ESR COM
  - ✓7th **T40.415** Adverse effect of fentanyl or fentanyl analogs UPD
  - ✓7th **T40.416** Underdosing of fentanyl or fentanyl analogs UPD
- ✓6th **T40.42** Poisoning by, adverse effect of and underdosing of tramadol
  - ✓7th **T40.421** Poisoning by tramadol, accidental (unintentional) HCC ESR COM
  - ✓7th **T40.422** Poisoning by tramadol, intentional self-harm HCC Rx ESR COM
  - ✓7th **T40.423** Poisoning by tramadol, assault
  - ✓7th **T40.424** Poisoning by tramadol, undetermined HCC ESR COM
  - ✓7th **T40.425** Adverse effect of tramadol UPD
  - ✓7th **T40.426** Underdosing of tramadol UPD
- ✓6th **T40.49** Poisoning by, adverse effect of and underdosing of other synthetic narcotics
  - ✓7th **T40.491** Poisoning by other synthetic narcotics, accidental (unintentional) HCC ESR COM
  - ✓7th **T40.492** Poisoning by other synthetic narcotics, intentional self-harm HCC Rx ESR COM
  - ✓7th **T40.493** Poisoning by other synthetic narcotics, assault
  - ✓7th **T40.494** Poisoning by other synthetic narcotics, undetermined HCC ESR COM
  - ✓7th **T40.495** Adverse effect of other synthetic narcotics UPD
  - ✓7th **T40.496** Underdosing of other synthetic narcotics UPD

✓5th **T40.5** Poisoning by, adverse effect of and underdosing of cocaine
- ✓6th **T40.5X** Poisoning by, adverse effect of and underdosing of cocaine
  - ✓7th **T40.5X1** Poisoning by cocaine, accidental (unintentional) HCC ESR COM
    - Poisoning by cocaine NOS
    - AHA: 2016,2Q,8
  - ✓7th **T40.5X2** Poisoning by cocaine, intentional self-harm HCC Rx ESR COM
  - ✓7th **T40.5X3** Poisoning by cocaine, assault
  - ✓7th **T40.5X4** Poisoning by cocaine, undetermined HCC ESR COM
  - ✓7th **T40.5X5** Adverse effect of cocaine UPD
  - ✓7th **T40.5X6** Underdosing of cocaine UPD

✓5th **T40.6** Poisoning by, adverse effect of and underdosing of other and unspecified narcotics
- ✓6th **T40.60** Poisoning by, adverse effect of and underdosing of unspecified narcotics
  - ✓7th **T40.601** Poisoning by unspecified narcotics, accidental (unintentional) HCC ESR COM
    - Poisoning by narcotics NOS
  - ✓7th **T40.602** Poisoning by unspecified narcotics, intentional self-harm HCC Rx ESR COM
  - ✓7th **T40.603** Poisoning by unspecified narcotics, assault
  - ✓7th **T40.604** Poisoning by unspecified narcotics, undetermined HCC ESR COM
  - ✓7th **T40.605** Adverse effect of unspecified narcotics UPD
  - ✓7th **T40.606** Underdosing of unspecified narcotics UPD
- ✓6th **T40.69** Poisoning by, adverse effect of and underdosing of other narcotics
  - ✓7th **T40.691** Poisoning by other narcotics, accidental (unintentional) HCC ESR COM
    - Poisoning by other narcotics NOS
  - ✓7th **T40.692** Poisoning by other narcotics, intentional self-harm HCC Rx ESR COM
  - ✓7th **T40.693** Poisoning by other narcotics, assault
  - ✓7th **T40.694** Poisoning by other narcotics, undetermined HCC ESR COM
  - ✓7th **T40.695** Adverse effect of other narcotics UPD
  - ✓7th **T40.696** Underdosing of other narcotics UPD

✓5th **T40.7** Poisoning by, adverse effect of and underdosing of cannabis (derivatives)
- ✓6th **T40.71** Poisoning by, adverse effect of and underdosing of cannabis (derivatives)
  - AHA: 2021,4Q,30
  - ✓7th **T40.711** Poisoning by cannabis, accidental (unintentional)
  - ✓7th **T40.712** Poisoning by cannabis, intentional self-harm HCC Rx ESR COM
  - ✓7th **T40.713** Poisoning by cannabis, assault
  - ✓7th **T40.714** Poisoning by cannabis, undetermined
  - ✓7th **T40.715** Adverse effect of cannabis UPD
  - ✓7th **T40.716** Underdosing of cannabis UPD
- ✓6th **T40.72** Poisoning by, adverse effect of and underdosing of synthetic cannabinoids
  - AHA: 2021,4Q,30
  - ✓7th **T40.721** Poisoning by synthetic cannabinoids, accidental (unintentional)
  - ✓7th **T40.722** Poisoning by synthetic cannabinoids, intentional self-harm HCC Rx ESR COM
  - ✓7th **T40.723** Poisoning by synthetic cannabinoids, assault
  - ✓7th **T40.724** Poisoning by synthetic cannabinoids, undetermined
  - ✓7th **T40.725** Adverse effect of synthetic cannabinoids UPD
  - ✓7th **T40.726** Underdosing of synthetic cannabinoids UPD

✓5th **T40.8** Poisoning by and adverse effect of lysergide [LSD]
- ✓6th **T40.8X** Poisoning by and adverse effect of lysergide [LSD]
  - ✓7th **T40.8X1** Poisoning by lysergide [LSD], accidental (unintentional) HCC ESR COM
    - Poisoning by lysergide [LSD] NOS
  - ✓7th **T40.8X2** Poisoning by lysergide [LSD], intentional self-harm HCC Rx ESR COM
  - ✓7th **T40.8X3** Poisoning by lysergide [LSD], assault
  - ✓7th **T40.8X4** Poisoning by lysergide [LSD], undetermined HCC ESR COM

√5th **T40.9 Poisoning by, adverse effect of and underdosing of other and unspecified psychodysleptics [hallucinogens]**

√6th **T40.90 Poisoning by, adverse effect of and underdosing of unspecified psychodysleptics [hallucinogens]**

√7th **T40.901 Poisoning by unspecified psychodysleptics [hallucinogens], accidental (unintentional)** HCC ESR COM

√7th **T40.902 Poisoning by unspecified psychodysleptics [hallucinogens], intentional self-harm** HCC Rx ESR COM

√7th **T40.903 Poisoning by unspecified psychodysleptics [hallucinogens], assault**

√7th **T40.904 Poisoning by unspecified psychodysleptics [hallucinogens], undetermined** HCC ESR COM

√7th **T40.905 Adverse effect of unspecified psychodysleptics [hallucinogens]** UPD

√7th **T40.906 Underdosing of unspecified psychodysleptics [hallucinogens]** UPD

√6th **T40.99 Poisoning by, adverse effect of and underdosing of other psychodysleptics [hallucinogens]**

√7th **T40.991 Poisoning by other psychodysleptics [hallucinogens], accidental (unintentional)** HCC ESR COM

Poisoning by other psychodysleptics [hallucinogens] NOS

√7th **T40.992 Poisoning by other psychodysleptics [hallucinogens], intentional self-harm** HCC Rx ESR COM

√7th **T40.993 Poisoning by other psychodysleptics [hallucinogens], assault**

√7th **T40.994 Poisoning by other psychodysleptics [hallucinogens], undetermined** HCC ESR COM

√7th **T40.995 Adverse effect of other psychodysleptics [hallucinogens]** UPD

√7th **T40.996 Underdosing of other psychodysleptics [hallucinogens]** UPD

√4th **T41 Poisoning by, adverse effect of and underdosing of anesthetics and therapeutic gases**

EXCLUDES 1 *benzodiazepines (T42.4-)*
*cocaine (T40.5-)*
*complications of anesthesia during labor and delivery (O74.-)*
*complications of anesthesia during pregnancy (O29.-)*
*complications of anesthesia during the puerperium (O89.-)*
*opioids (T40.0-T40.2-)*

The appropriate 7th character is to be added to each code from category T41.
A initial encounter
D subsequent encounter
S sequela

√5th **T41.0 Poisoning by, adverse effect of and underdosing of inhaled anesthetics**

EXCLUDES 1 *oxygen (T41.5-)*

√6th **T41.0X Poisoning by, adverse effect of and underdosing of inhaled anesthetics**

√7th **T41.0X1 Poisoning by inhaled anesthetics, accidental (unintentional)**

Poisoning by inhaled anesthetics NOS

√7th **T41.0X2 Poisoning by inhaled anesthetics, intentional self-harm** HCC Rx ESR COM

√7th **T41.0X3 Poisoning by inhaled anesthetics, assault**

√7th **T41.0X4 Poisoning by inhaled anesthetics, undetermined**

√7th **T41.0X5 Adverse effect of inhaled anesthetics** UPD

√7th **T41.0X6 Underdosing of inhaled anesthetics** UPD

√5th **T41.1 Poisoning by, adverse effect of and underdosing of intravenous anesthetics**

Poisoning by, adverse effect of and underdosing of thiobarbiturates

√6th **T41.1X Poisoning by, adverse effect of and underdosing of intravenous anesthetics**

√7th **T41.1X1 Poisoning by intravenous anesthetics, accidental (unintentional)**

Poisoning by intravenous anesthetics NOS

√7th **T41.1X2 Poisoning by intravenous anesthetics, intentional self-harm** HCC Rx ESR COM

√7th **T41.1X3 Poisoning by intravenous anesthetics, assault**

√7th **T41.1X4 Poisoning by intravenous anesthetics, undetermined**

√7th **T41.1X5 Adverse effect of intravenous anesthetics** UPD

√7th **T41.1X6 Underdosing of intravenous anesthetics** UPD

√5th **T41.2 Poisoning by, adverse effect of and underdosing of other and unspecified general anesthetics**

√6th **T41.20 Poisoning by, adverse effect of and underdosing of unspecified general anesthetics**

√7th **T41.201 Poisoning by unspecified general anesthetics, accidental (unintentional)**

Poisoning by general anesthetics NOS

√7th **T41.202 Poisoning by unspecified general anesthetics, intentional self-harm** HCC Rx ESR COM

√7th **T41.203 Poisoning by unspecified general anesthetics, assault**

√7th **T41.204 Poisoning by unspecified general anesthetics, undetermined**

√7th **T41.205 Adverse effect of unspecified general anesthetics** UPD

**AHA:** 2016,4Q,73

√7th **T41.206 Underdosing of unspecified general anesthetics** UPD

√6th **T41.29 Poisoning by, adverse effect of and underdosing of other general anesthetics**

√7th **T41.291 Poisoning by other general anesthetics, accidental (unintentional)**

Poisoning by other general anesthetics NOS

√7th **T41.292 Poisoning by other general anesthetics, intentional self-harm** HCC Rx ESR COM

√7th **T41.293 Poisoning by other general anesthetics, assault**

√7th **T41.294 Poisoning by other general anesthetics, undetermined**

√7th **T41.295 Adverse effect of other general anesthetics** UPD

√7th **T41.296 Underdosing of other general anesthetics** UPD

√5th **T41.3 Poisoning by, adverse effect of and underdosing of local anesthetics**

Cocaine (topical)

EXCLUDES 2 *poisoning by cocaine used as a central nervous system stimulant (T40.5X1-T40.5X4)*

√6th **T41.3X Poisoning by, adverse effect of and underdosing of local anesthetics**

√7th **T41.3X1 Poisoning by local anesthetics, accidental (unintentional)**

Poisoning by local anesthetics NOS

√7th **T41.3X2 Poisoning by local anesthetics, intentional self-harm** HCC Rx ESR COM

√7th **T41.3X3 Poisoning by local anesthetics, assault**

√7th **T41.3X4 Poisoning by local anesthetics, undetermined**

√7th **T41.3X5 Adverse effect of local anesthetics** UPD

√7th **T41.3X6 Underdosing of local anesthetics** UPD

√5th **T41.4 Poisoning by, adverse effect of and underdosing of unspecified anesthetic**

√x7th **T41.41 Poisoning by unspecified anesthetic, accidental (unintentional)**

Poisoning by anesthetic NOS

√x7th **T41.42 Poisoning by unspecified anesthetic, intentional self-harm** HCC Rx ESR COM

√x7th **T41.43 Poisoning by unspecified anesthetic, assault**

√x7th **T41.44 Poisoning by unspecified anesthetic, undetermined**

√x7th **T41.45 Adverse effect of unspecified anesthetic** UPD

√x7th **T41.46 Underdosing of unspecified anesthetics** UPD

√5th **T41.5 Poisoning by, adverse effect of and underdosing of therapeutic gases**

√6th **T41.5X Poisoning by, adverse effect of and underdosing of therapeutic gases**

√7th **T41.5X1 Poisoning by therapeutic gases, accidental (unintentional)**

Poisoning by therapeutic gases NOS

√7th **T41.5X2 Poisoning by therapeutic gases, intentional self-harm** HCC Rx ESR COM

√7th **T41.5X3 Poisoning by therapeutic gases, assault**

√7th **T41.5X4 Poisoning by therapeutic gases, undetermined**

T41.5X5 Adverse effect of therapeutic gases UPD

T41.5X6 Underdosing of therapeutic gases UPD

**T42 Poisoning by, adverse effect of and underdosing of antiepileptic, sedative- hypnotic and antiparkinsonism drugs**

EXCLUDES 2 *drug dependence and related mental and behavioral disorders due to psychoactive substance use (F10.- - F19.-)*

The appropriate 7th character is to be added to each code from category T42.
A initial encounter
D subsequent encounter
S sequela

**T42.0 Poisoning by, adverse effect of and underdosing of hydantoin derivatives**

**T42.0X Poisoning by, adverse effect of and underdosing of hydantoin derivatives**

T42.0X1 Poisoning by hydantoin derivatives, accidental (unintentional)
Poisoning by hydantoin derivatives NOS

T42.0X2 Poisoning by hydantoin derivatives, intentional self-harm HCC Rx ESR COM

T42.0X3 Poisoning by hydantoin derivatives, assault

T42.0X4 Poisoning by hydantoin derivatives, undetermined

T42.0X5 Adverse effect of hydantoin derivatives UPD

T42.0X6 Underdosing of hydantoin derivatives UPD

**T42.1 Poisoning by, adverse effect of and underdosing of iminostilbenes**
Poisoning by, adverse effect of and underdosing of carbamazepine

**T42.1X Poisoning by, adverse effect of and underdosing of iminostilbenes**

T42.1X1 Poisoning by iminostilbenes, accidental (unintentional)
Poisoning by iminostilbenes NOS

T42.1X2 Poisoning by iminostilbenes, intentional self-harm HCC Rx ESR COM

T42.1X3 Poisoning by iminostilbenes, assault

T42.1X4 Poisoning by iminostilbenes, undetermined

T42.1X5 Adverse effect of iminostilbenes UPD

T42.1X6 Underdosing of iminostilbenes UPD

**T42.2 Poisoning by, adverse effect of and underdosing of succinimides and oxazolidinediones**

**T42.2X Poisoning by, adverse effect of and underdosing of succinimides and oxazolidinediones**

T42.2X1 Poisoning by succinimides and oxazolidinediones, accidental (unintentional)
Poisoning by succinimides and oxazolidinediones NOS

T42.2X2 Poisoning by succinimides and oxazolidinediones, intentional self-harm HCC Rx ESR COM

T42.2X3 Poisoning by succinimides and oxazolidinediones, assault

T42.2X4 Poisoning by succinimides and oxazolidinediones, undetermined

T42.2X5 Adverse effect of succinimides and oxazolidinediones UPD

T42.2X6 Underdosing of succinimides and oxazolidinediones UPD

**T42.3 Poisoning by, adverse effect of and underdosing of barbiturates**

EXCLUDES 1 *poisoning by, adverse effect of and underdosing of thiobarbiturates (T41.1-)*

**T42.3X Poisoning by, adverse effect of and underdosing of barbiturates**

T42.3X1 Poisoning by barbiturates, accidental (unintentional)
Poisoning by barbiturates NOS

T42.3X2 Poisoning by barbiturates, intentional self-harm HCC Rx ESR COM

T42.3X3 Poisoning by barbiturates, assault

T42.3X4 Poisoning by barbiturates, undetermined

T42.3X5 Adverse effect of barbiturates UPD

T42.3X6 Underdosing of barbiturates UPD

**T42.4 Poisoning by, adverse effect of and underdosing of benzodiazepines**

**T42.4X Poisoning by, adverse effect of and underdosing of benzodiazepines**

T42.4X1 Poisoning by benzodiazepines, accidental (unintentional)
Poisoning by benzodiazepines NOS

T42.4X2 Poisoning by benzodiazepines, intentional self-harm HCC Rx ESR COM

T42.4X3 Poisoning by benzodiazepines, assault

T42.4X4 Poisoning by benzodiazepines, undetermined

T42.4X5 Adverse effect of benzodiazepines UPD

T42.4X6 Underdosing of benzodiazepines UPD

**T42.5 Poisoning by, adverse effect of and underdosing of mixed antiepileptics**

**T42.5X Poisoning by, adverse effect of and underdosing of antiepileptics**

T42.5X1 Poisoning by mixed antiepileptics, accidental (unintentional)
Poisoning by mixed antiepileptics NOS

T42.5X2 Poisoning by mixed antiepileptics, intentional self-harm HCC Rx ESR COM

T42.5X3 Poisoning by mixed antiepileptics, assault

T42.5X4 Poisoning by mixed antiepileptics, undetermined

T42.5X5 Adverse effect of mixed antiepileptics UPD

T42.5X6 Underdosing of mixed antiepileptics UPD

**T42.6 Poisoning by, adverse effect of and underdosing of other antiepileptic and sedative-hypnotic drugs**
Poisoning by, adverse effect of and underdosing of methaqualone
Poisoning by, adverse effect of and underdosing of valproic acid

EXCLUDES 1 *poisoning by, adverse effect of and underdosing of carbamazepine (T42.1-)*

**T42.6X Poisoning by, adverse effect of and underdosing of other antiepileptic and sedative-hypnotic drugs**

T42.6X1 Poisoning by other antiepileptic and sedative-hypnotic drugs, accidental (unintentional)
Poisoning by other antiepileptic and sedative-hypnotic drugs NOS

T42.6X2 Poisoning by other antiepileptic and sedative-hypnotic drugs, intentional self-harm HCC Rx ESR COM

T42.6X3 Poisoning by other antiepileptic and sedative-hypnotic drugs, assault

T42.6X4 Poisoning by other antiepileptic and sedative-hypnotic drugs, undetermined

T42.6X5 Adverse effect of other antiepileptic and sedative-hypnotic drugs UPD

T42.6X6 Underdosing of other antiepileptic and sedative-hypnotic drugs UPD

**T42.7 Poisoning by, adverse effect of and underdosing of unspecified antiepileptic and sedative-hypnotic drugs**

T42.71 Poisoning by unspecified antiepileptic and sedative-hypnotic drugs, accidental (unintentional)
Poisoning by antiepileptic and sedative-hypnotic drugs NOS

T42.72 Poisoning by unspecified antiepileptic and sedative-hypnotic drugs, intentional self-harm HCC Rx ESR COM

T42.73 Poisoning by unspecified antiepileptic and sedative-hypnotic drugs, assault

T42.74 Poisoning by unspecified antiepileptic and sedative-hypnotic drugs, undetermined

T42.75 Adverse effect of unspecified antiepileptic and sedative-hypnotic drugs UPD

T42.76 Underdosing of unspecified antiepileptic and sedative-hypnotic drugs UPD

√5th **T42.8 Poisoning by, adverse effect of and underdosing of antiparkinsonism drugs and other central muscle-tone depressants**
Poisoning by, adverse effect of and underdosing of amantadine

√6th **T42.8X Poisoning by, adverse effect of and underdosing of antiparkinsonism drugs and other central muscle-tone depressants**

√7th **T42.8X1 Poisoning by antiparkinsonism drugs and other central muscle-tone depressants, accidental (unintentional)**
Poisoning by antiparkinsonism drugs and other central muscle-tone depressants NOS

√7th **T42.8X2 Poisoning by antiparkinsonism drugs and other central muscle-tone depressants, intentional self-harm** HCC Rx ESR COM

√7th **T42.8X3 Poisoning by antiparkinsonism drugs and other central muscle-tone depressants, assault**

√7th **T42.8X4 Poisoning by antiparkinsonism drugs and other central muscle-tone depressants, undetermined**

√7th **T42.8X5 Adverse effect of antiparkinsonism drugs and other central muscle-tone depressants** UPD

√7th **T42.8X6 Underdosing of antiparkinsonism drugs and other central muscle-tone depressants** UPD

√4th **T43 Poisoning by, adverse effect of and underdosing of psychotropic drugs, not elsewhere classified**

EXCLUDES 1 ~~*appetite depressants (T50.5-)*~~
~~*barbiturates (T42.3-)*~~
~~*benzodiazepines (T42.4-)*~~
~~*methaqualone (T42.6-)*~~
~~*psychodysleptics [hallucinogens] (T40.7-T40.9-)*~~

EXCLUDES 2 ▶*appetite depressants (T50.5-)*◀
▶*barbiturates (T42.3-)*◀
▶*benzodiazepines (T42.4-)*◀
*drug dependence and related mental and behavioral disorders due to psychoactive substance use (F10.- – F19.-)*
▶*methaqualone (T42.6-)*◀
▶*psychodysleptics [hallucinogens] (T40.7-T40.9-)*◀

The appropriate 7th character is to be added to each code from category T43.
A initial encounter
D subsequent encounter
S sequela

√5th **T43.0 Poisoning by, adverse effect of and underdosing of tricyclic and tetracyclic antidepressants**

√6th **T43.01 Poisoning by, adverse effect of and underdosing of tricyclic antidepressants**

√7th **T43.011 Poisoning by tricyclic antidepressants, accidental (unintentional)**
Poisoning by tricyclic antidepressants NOS

√7th **T43.012 Poisoning by tricyclic antidepressants, intentional self-harm** HCC Rx ESR COM

√7th **T43.013 Poisoning by tricyclic antidepressants, assault**

√7th **T43.014 Poisoning by tricyclic antidepressants, undetermined**

√7th **T43.015 Adverse effect of tricyclic antidepressants** UPD

√7th **T43.016 Underdosing of tricyclic antidepressants** UPD

√6th **T43.02 Poisoning by, adverse effect of and underdosing of tetracyclic antidepressants**

√7th **T43.021 Poisoning by tetracyclic antidepressants, accidental (unintentional)**
Poisoning by tetracyclic antidepressants NOS

√7th **T43.022 Poisoning by tetracyclic antidepressants, intentional self-harm** HCC Rx ESR COM

√7th **T43.023 Poisoning by tetracyclic antidepressants, assault**

√7th **T43.024 Poisoning by tetracyclic antidepressants, undetermined**

√7th **T43.025 Adverse effect of tetracyclic antidepressants** UPD

√7th **T43.026 Underdosing of tetracyclic antidepressants** UPD

√5th **T43.1 Poisoning by, adverse effect of and underdosing of monoamine-oxidase-inhibitor antidepressants**

√6th **T43.1X Poisoning by, adverse effect of and underdosing of monoamine-oxidase-inhibitor antidepressants**

√7th **T43.1X1 Poisoning by monoamine-oxidase-inhibitor antidepressants, accidental (unintentional)**
Poisoning by monoamine-oxidase- inhibitor antidepressants NOS

√7th **T43.1X2 Poisoning by monoamine-oxidase-inhibitor antidepressants, intentional self-harm** HCC Rx ESR COM

√7th **T43.1X3 Poisoning by monoamine-oxidase-inhibitor antidepressants, assault**

√7th **T43.1X4 Poisoning by monoamine-oxidase-inhibitor antidepressants, undetermined**

√7th **T43.1X5 Adverse effect of monoamine-oxidase-inhibitor antidepressants** UPD

√7th **T43.1X6 Underdosing of monoamine-oxidase-inhibitor antidepressants** UPD

√5th **T43.2 Poisoning by, adverse effect of and underdosing of other and unspecified antidepressants**

√6th **T43.20 Poisoning by, adverse effect of and underdosing of unspecified antidepressants**

√7th **T43.201 Poisoning by unspecified antidepressants, accidental (unintentional)**
Poisoning by antidepressants NOS

√7th **T43.202 Poisoning by unspecified antidepressants, intentional self-harm** HCC Rx ESR COM

√7th **T43.203 Poisoning by unspecified antidepressants, assault**

√7th **T43.204 Poisoning by unspecified antidepressants, undetermined**

√7th **T43.205 Adverse effect of unspecified antidepressants** UPD
Antidepressant discontinuation syndrome

√7th **T43.206 Underdosing of unspecified antidepressants** UPD

√6th **T43.21 Poisoning by, adverse effect of and underdosing of selective serotonin and norepinephrine reuptake inhibitors**
Poisoning by, adverse effect of and underdosing of SSNRI antidepressants

√7th **T43.211 Poisoning by selective serotonin and norepinephrine reuptake inhibitors, accidental (unintentional)**

√7th **T43.212 Poisoning by selective serotonin and norepinephrine reuptake inhibitors, intentional self-harm** HCC Rx ESR COM

√7th **T43.213 Poisoning by selective serotonin and norepinephrine reuptake inhibitors, assault**

√7th **T43.214 Poisoning by selective serotonin and norepinephrine reuptake inhibitors, undetermined**

√7th **T43.215 Adverse effect of selective serotonin and norepinephrine reuptake inhibitors** UPD

√7th **T43.216 Underdosing of selective serotonin and norepinephrine reuptake inhibitors** UPD

√6th **T43.22 Poisoning by, adverse effect of and underdosing of selective serotonin reuptake inhibitors**
Poisoning by, adverse effect of and underdosing of SSRI antidepressants

√7th **T43.221 Poisoning by selective serotonin reuptake inhibitors, accidental (unintentional)**

√7th **T43.222 Poisoning by selective serotonin reuptake inhibitors, intentional self-harm** HCC Rx ESR COM

√7th **T43.223 Poisoning by selective serotonin reuptake inhibitors, assault**

√7th **T43.224 Poisoning by selective serotonin reuptake inhibitors, undetermined**

√7th **T43.225 Adverse effect of selective serotonin reuptake inhibitors** UPD
**AHA:** 2024,4Q,16; 2022,2Q,11

T43.226 Underdosing of selective serotonin reuptake inhibitors UPD

T43.29 Poisoning by, adverse effect of and underdosing of other antidepressants

T43.291 Poisoning by other antidepressants, accidental (unintentional)
Poisoning by other antidepressants NOS

T43.292 Poisoning by other antidepressants, intentional self-harm HCC Rx ESR COM

T43.293 Poisoning by other antidepressants, assault

T43.294 Poisoning by other antidepressants, undetermined

T43.295 Adverse effect of other antidepressants UPD

T43.296 Underdosing of other antidepressants UPD

T43.3 Poisoning by, adverse effect of and underdosing of phenothiazine antipsychotics and neuroleptics

T43.3X Poisoning by, adverse effect of and underdosing of phenothiazine antipsychotics and neuroleptics

T43.3X1 Poisoning by phenothiazine antipsychotics and neuroleptics, accidental (unintentional)
Poisoning by phenothiazine antipsychotics and neuroleptics NOS

T43.3X2 Poisoning by phenothiazine antipsychotics and neuroleptics, intentional self-harm HCC Rx ESR COM

T43.3X3 Poisoning by phenothiazine antipsychotics and neuroleptics, assault

T43.3X4 Poisoning by phenothiazine antipsychotics and neuroleptics, undetermined

T43.3X5 Adverse effect of phenothiazine antipsychotics and neuroleptics UPD

T43.3X6 Underdosing of phenothiazine antipsychotics and neuroleptics UPD

T43.4 Poisoning by, adverse effect of and underdosing of butyrophenone and thiothixene neuroleptics

T43.4X Poisoning by, adverse effect of and underdosing of butyrophenone and thiothixene neuroleptics

T43.4X1 Poisoning by butyrophenone and thiothixene neuroleptics, accidental (unintentional)
Poisoning by butyrophenone and thiothixene neuroleptics NOS

T43.4X2 Poisoning by butyrophenone and thiothixene neuroleptics, intentional self-harm HCC Rx ESR COM

T43.4X3 Poisoning by butyrophenone and thiothixene neuroleptics, assault

T43.4X4 Poisoning by butyrophenone and thiothixene neuroleptics, undetermined

T43.4X5 Adverse effect of butyrophenone and thiothixene neuroleptics UPD

T43.4X6 Underdosing of butyrophenone and thiothixene neuroleptics UPD

T43.5 Poisoning by, adverse effect of and underdosing of other and unspecified antipsychotics and neuroleptics
EXCLUDES 1 *poisoning by, adverse effect of and underdosing of rauwolfia (T46.5-)*

T43.50 Poisoning by, adverse effect of and underdosing of unspecified antipsychotics and neuroleptics

T43.501 Poisoning by unspecified antipsychotics and neuroleptics, accidental (unintentional)
Poisoning by antipsychotics and neuroleptics NOS

T43.502 Poisoning by unspecified antipsychotics and neuroleptics, intentional self-harm HCC Rx ESR COM

T43.503 Poisoning by unspecified antipsychotics and neuroleptics, assault

T43.504 Poisoning by unspecified antipsychotics and neuroleptics, undetermined

T43.505 Adverse effect of unspecified antipsychotics and neuroleptics UPD
AHA: 2022,4Q,24

T43.506 Underdosing of unspecified antipsychotics and neuroleptics UPD

T43.59 Poisoning by, adverse effect of and underdosing of other antipsychotics and neuroleptics
AHA: 2017,1Q,40

T43.591 Poisoning by other antipsychotics and neuroleptics, accidental (unintentional)
Poisoning by other antipsychotics and neuroleptics NOS

T43.592 Poisoning by other antipsychotics and neuroleptics, intentional self-harm HCC Rx ESR COM

T43.593 Poisoning by other antipsychotics and neuroleptics, assault

T43.594 Poisoning by other antipsychotics and neuroleptics, undetermined

T43.595 Adverse effect of other antipsychotics and neuroleptics UPD
AHA: 2022,2Q,11

T43.596 Underdosing of other antipsychotics and neuroleptics UPD

T43.6 Poisoning by, adverse effect of and underdosing of psychostimulants
EXCLUDES 1 *poisoning by, adverse effect of and underdosing of cocaine (T40.5-)*

T43.60 Poisoning by, adverse effect of and underdosing of unspecified psychostimulant

T43.601 Poisoning by unspecified psychostimulants, accidental (unintentional) HCC ESR COM
Poisoning by psychostimulants NOS

T43.602 Poisoning by unspecified psychostimulants, intentional self-harm HCC Rx ESR COM

T43.603 Poisoning by unspecified psychostimulants, assault

T43.604 Poisoning by unspecified psychostimulants, undetermined HCC ESR COM

T43.605 Adverse effect of unspecified psychostimulants UPD

T43.606 Underdosing of unspecified psychostimulants UPD

T43.61 Poisoning by, adverse effect of and underdosing of caffeine

T43.611 Poisoning by caffeine, accidental (unintentional) HCC ESR COM
Poisoning by caffeine NOS

T43.612 Poisoning by caffeine, intentional self-harm HCC Rx ESR COM

T43.613 Poisoning by caffeine, assault

T43.614 Poisoning by caffeine, undetermined HCC ESR COM

T43.615 Adverse effect of caffeine UPD

T43.616 Underdosing of caffeine UPD

T43.62 Poisoning by, adverse effect of and underdosing of amphetamines

T43.621 Poisoning by amphetamines, accidental (unintentional) HCC ESR COM
Poisoning by amphetamines NOS
AHA: 2021,3Q,8

T43.622 Poisoning by amphetamines, intentional self-harm HCC Rx ESR COM

T43.623 Poisoning by amphetamines, assault

T43.624 Poisoning by amphetamines, undetermined HCC ESR COM

T43.625 Adverse effect of amphetamines UPD

T43.626 Underdosing of amphetamines UPD

T43.63 Poisoning by, adverse effect of and underdosing of methylphenidate

T43.631 Poisoning by methylphenidate, accidental (unintentional) HCC ESR COM
Poisoning by methylphenidate NOS

T43.632 Poisoning by methylphenidate, intentional self-harm HCC Rx ESR COM

T43.633 Poisoning by methylphenidate, assault

T43.634 Poisoning by methylphenidate, undetermined HCC ESR COM

T43.635 Adverse effect of methylphenidate UPD

T43.636 Underdosing of methylphenidate UPD

√6th T43.64 **Poisoning by ecstasy**
Poisoning by 3,4-methylenedioxymethamphetamine
Poisoning by MDMA
**AHA:** 2018,4Q,30-31

√7th T43.641 **Poisoning by ecstasy, accidental (unintentional)** HCC ESR COM
Poisoning by ecstasy NOS

√7th T43.642 **Poisoning by ecstasy, intentional self-harm** HCC Rx ESR COM

√7th T43.643 **Poisoning by ecstasy, assault**

√7th T43.644 **Poisoning by ecstasy, undetermined** HCC ESR COM

√6th T43.65 **Poisoning by, adverse effect of and underdosing of methamphetamines**
**AHA:** 2022,4Q,45-47

√7th T43.651 **Poisoning by methamphetamines accidental (unintentional)** HCC ESR COM
Poisoning by methamphetamines NOS
**AHA:** 2022,4Q,46

√7th T43.652 **Poisoning by methamphetamines intentional self-harm** HCC Rx ESR COM

√7th T43.653 **Poisoning by methamphetamines, assault**

√7th T43.654 **Poisoning by methamphetamines, undetermined** HCC ESR COM

√7th T43.655 **Adverse effect of methamphetamines** UPD
**AHA:** 2022,4Q,46

√7th T43.656 **Underdosing of methamphetamines** UPD

√6th T43.69 **Poisoning by, adverse effect of and underdosing of other psychostimulants**

√7th T43.691 **Poisoning by other psychostimulants, accidental (unintentional)** HCC ESR COM
Poisoning by other psychostimulants NOS

√7th T43.692 **Poisoning by other psychostimulants, intentional self-harm** HCC Rx ESR COM

√7th T43.693 **Poisoning by other psychostimulants, assault**

√7th T43.694 **Poisoning by other psychostimulants, undetermined** HCC ESR COM

√7th T43.695 **Adverse effect of other psychostimulants** UPD

√7th T43.696 **Underdosing of other psychostimulants** UPD

√5th T43.8 **Poisoning by, adverse effect of and underdosing of other psychotropic drugs**

√6th T43.8X **Poisoning by, adverse effect of and underdosing of other psychotropic drugs**

√7th T43.8X1 **Poisoning by other psychotropic drugs, accidental (unintentional)**
Poisoning by other psychotropic drugs NOS

√7th T43.8X2 **Poisoning by other psychotropic drugs, intentional self-harm** HCC Rx ESR COM

√7th T43.8X3 **Poisoning by other psychotropic drugs, assault**

√7th T43.8X4 **Poisoning by other psychotropic drugs, undetermined**

√7th T43.8X5 **Adverse effect of other psychotropic drugs** UPD

√7th T43.8X6 **Underdosing of other psychotropic drugs** UPD

√5th T43.9 **Poisoning by, adverse effect of and underdosing of unspecified psychotropic drug**

√x7th T43.91 **Poisoning by unspecified psychotropic drug, accidental (unintentional)**
Poisoning by psychotropic drug NOS

√x7th T43.92 **Poisoning by unspecified psychotropic drug, intentional self-harm** HCC Rx ESR COM

√x7th T43.93 **Poisoning by unspecified psychotropic drug, assault**

√x7th T43.94 **Poisoning by unspecified psychotropic drug, undetermined**

√x7th T43.95 **Adverse effect of unspecified psychotropic drug** UPD

√x7th T43.96 **Underdosing of unspecified psychotropic drug** UPD

√4th **T44 Poisoning by, adverse effect of and underdosing of drugs primarily affecting the autonomic nervous system**

The appropriate 7th character is to be added to each code from category T44.
A initial encounter
D subsequent encounter
S sequela

√5th T44.Ø **Poisoning by, adverse effect of and underdosing of anticholinesterase agents**

√6th T44.ØX **Poisoning by, adverse effect of and underdosing of anticholinesterase agents**

√7th T44.ØX1 **Poisoning by anticholinesterase agents, accidental (unintentional)**
Poisoning by anticholinesterase agents NOS

√7th T44.ØX2 **Poisoning by anticholinesterase agents, intentional self-harm** HCC Rx ESR COM

√7th T44.ØX3 **Poisoning by anticholinesterase agents, assault**

√7th T44.ØX4 **Poisoning by anticholinesterase agents, undetermined**

√7th T44.ØX5 **Adverse effect of anticholinesterase agents** UPD

√7th T44.ØX6 **Underdosing of anticholinesterase agents** UPD

√5th T44.1 **Poisoning by, adverse effect of and underdosing of other parasympathomimetics [cholinergics]**

√6th T44.1X **Poisoning by, adverse effect of and underdosing of other parasympathomimetics [cholinergics]**

√7th T44.1X1 **Poisoning by other parasympathomimetics [cholinergics], accidental (unintentional)**
Poisoning by other parasympathomimetics [cholinergics] NOS

√7th T44.1X2 **Poisoning by other parasympathomimetics [cholinergics], intentional self-harm** HCC Rx ESR COM

√7th T44.1X3 **Poisoning by other parasympathomimetics [cholinergics], assault**

√7th T44.1X4 **Poisoning by other parasympathomimetics [cholinergics], undetermined**

√7th T44.1X5 **Adverse effect of other parasympathomimetics [cholinergics]** UPD

√7th T44.1X6 **Underdosing of other parasympathomimetics [cholinergics]** UPD

√5th T44.2 **Poisoning by, adverse effect of and underdosing of ganglionic blocking drugs**

√6th T44.2X **Poisoning by, adverse effect of and underdosing of ganglionic blocking drugs**

√7th T44.2X1 **Poisoning by ganglionic blocking drugs, accidental (unintentional)**
Poisoning by ganglionic blocking drugs NOS

√7th T44.2X2 **Poisoning by ganglionic blocking drugs, intentional self-harm** HCC Rx ESR COM

√7th T44.2X3 **Poisoning by ganglionic blocking drugs, assault**

√7th T44.2X4 **Poisoning by ganglionic blocking drugs, undetermined**

√7th T44.2X5 **Adverse effect of ganglionic blocking drugs** UPD

√7th T44.2X6 **Underdosing of ganglionic blocking drugs** UPD

√5th T44.3 **Poisoning by, adverse effect of and underdosing of other parasympatholytics [anticholinergics and antimuscarinics] and spasmolytics**
Poisoning by, adverse effect of and underdosing of papaverine

√6th T44.3X **Poisoning by, adverse effect of and underdosing of other parasympatholytics [anticholinergics and antimuscarinics] and spasmolytics**

√7th T44.3X1 **Poisoning by other parasympatholytics [anticholinergics and antimuscarinics] and spasmolytics, accidental (unintentional)**
Poisoning by other parasympatholytics [anticholinergics and antimuscarinics] and spasmolytics NOS

√7th T44.3X2 **Poisoning by other parasympatholytics [anticholinergics and antimuscarinics] and spasmolytics, intentional self-harm** HCC Rx ESR COM

√7th T44.3X3 **Poisoning by other parasympatholytics [anticholinergics and antimuscarinics] and spasmolytics, assault**

√7th T44.3X4 **Poisoning by other parasympatholytics [anticholinergics and antimuscarinics] and spasmolytics, undetermined**

√7th T44.3X5 **Adverse effect of other parasympatholytics [anticholinergics and antimuscarinics] and spasmolytics** UPD

√7th T44.3X6 **Underdosing of other parasympatholytics [anticholinergics and antimuscarinics] and spasmolytics** UPD

√5th T44.4 **Poisoning by, adverse effect of and underdosing of predominantly alpha-adrenoreceptor agonists**
Poisoning by, adverse effect of and underdosing of metaraminol

√6th T44.4X **Poisoning by, adverse effect of and underdosing of predominantly alpha-adrenoreceptor agonists**

√7th T44.4X1 **Poisoning by predominantly alpha-adrenoreceptor agonists, accidental (unintentional)**
Poisoning by predominantly alpha-adrenoreceptor agonists NOS

√7th T44.4X2 **Poisoning by predominantly alpha-adrenoreceptor agonists, intentional self-harm** HCC Rx ESR COM

√7th T44.4X3 **Poisoning by predominantly alpha-adrenoreceptor agonists, assault**

√7th T44.4X4 **Poisoning by predominantly alpha-adrenoreceptor agonists, undetermined**

√7th T44.4X5 **Adverse effect of predominantly alpha-adrenoreceptor agonists** UPD

√7th T44.4X6 **Underdosing of predominantly alpha-adrenoreceptor agonists** UPD

√5th T44.5 **Poisoning by, adverse effect of and underdosing of predominantly beta-adrenoreceptor agonists**
EXCLUDES 1 *poisoning by, adverse effect of and underdosing of beta-adrenoreceptor agonists used in asthma therapy (T48.6-)*

√6th T44.5X **Poisoning by, adverse effect of and underdosing of predominantly beta-adrenoreceptor agonists**

√7th T44.5X1 **Poisoning by predominantly beta-adrenoreceptor agonists, accidental (unintentional)**
Poisoning by predominantly beta-adrenoreceptor agonists NOS

√7th T44.5X2 **Poisoning by predominantly beta-adrenoreceptor agonists, intentional self-harm** HCC Rx ESR COM

√7th T44.5X3 **Poisoning by predominantly beta-adrenoreceptor agonists, assault**

√7th T44.5X4 **Poisoning by predominantly beta-adrenoreceptor agonists, undetermined**

√7th T44.5X5 **Adverse effect of predominantly beta-adrenoreceptor agonists** UPD

√7th T44.5X6 **Underdosing of predominantly beta-adrenoreceptor agonists** UPD

√5th T44.6 **Poisoning by, adverse effect of and underdosing of alpha-adrenoreceptor antagonists**
EXCLUDES 1 *poisoning by, adverse effect of and underdosing of ergot alkaloids (T48.0)*

√6th T44.6X **Poisoning by, adverse effect of and underdosing of alpha-adrenoreceptor antagonists**

√7th T44.6X1 **Poisoning by alpha-adrenoreceptor antagonists, accidental (unintentional)**
Poisoning by alpha-adrenoreceptor antagonists NOS

√7th T44.6X2 **Poisoning by alpha-adrenoreceptor antagonists, intentional self-harm** HCC Rx ESR COM

√7th T44.6X3 **Poisoning by alpha-adrenoreceptor antagonists, assault**

√7th T44.6X4 **Poisoning by alpha-adrenoreceptor antagonists, undetermined**

√7th T44.6X5 **Adverse effect of alpha-adrenoreceptor antagonists** UPD

√7th T44.6X6 **Underdosing of alpha-adrenoreceptor antagonists** UPD

√5th T44.7 **Poisoning by, adverse effect of and underdosing of beta-adrenoreceptor antagonists**

√6th T44.7X **Poisoning by, adverse effect of and underdosing of beta-adrenoreceptor antagonists**

√7th T44.7X1 **Poisoning by beta-adrenoreceptor antagonists, accidental (unintentional)**
Poisoning by beta-adrenoreceptor antagonists NOS

√7th T44.7X2 **Poisoning by beta-adrenoreceptor antagonists, intentional self-harm** HCC Rx ESR COM

√7th T44.7X3 **Poisoning by beta-adrenoreceptor antagonists, assault**

√7th T44.7X4 **Poisoning by beta-adrenoreceptor antagonists, undetermined**

√7th T44.7X5 **Adverse effect of beta-adrenoreceptor antagonists** UPD

√7th T44.7X6 **Underdosing of beta-adrenoreceptor antagonists** UPD

√5th T44.8 **Poisoning by, adverse effect of and underdosing of centrally-acting and adrenergic-neuron- blocking agents**
EXCLUDES 2 *poisoning by, adverse effect of and underdosing of clonidine (T46.5)*
*poisoning by, adverse effect of and underdosing of guanethidine (T46.5)*

√6th T44.8X **Poisoning by, adverse effect of and underdosing of centrally-acting and adrenergic- neuron-blocking agents**

√7th T44.8X1 **Poisoning by centrally-acting and adrenergic-neuron-blocking agents, accidental (unintentional)**
Poisoning by centrally-acting and adrenergic-neuron-blocking agents NOS

√7th T44.8X2 **Poisoning by centrally-acting and adrenergic-neuron-blocking agents, intentional self-harm** HCC Rx ESR COM

√7th T44.8X3 **Poisoning by centrally-acting and adrenergic-neuron-blocking agents, assault**

√7th T44.8X4 **Poisoning by centrally-acting and adrenergic-neuron-blocking agents, undetermined**

√7th T44.8X5 **Adverse effect of centrally-acting and adrenergic-neuron-blocking agents** UPD

√7th T44.8X6 **Underdosing of centrally-acting and adrenergic-neuron-blocking agents** UPD

√5th T44.9 **Poisoning by, adverse effect of and underdosing of other and unspecified drugs primarily affecting the autonomic nervous system**
Poisoning by, adverse effect of and underdosing of drug stimulating both alpha and beta-adrenoreceptors

√6th T44.90 **Poisoning by, adverse effect of and underdosing of unspecified drugs primarily affecting the autonomic nervous system**

√7th T44.901 **Poisoning by unspecified drugs primarily affecting the autonomic nervous system, accidental (unintentional)**
Poisoning by unspecified drugs primarily affecting the autonomic nervous system NOS

√7th T44.902 **Poisoning by unspecified drugs primarily affecting the autonomic nervous system, intentional self-harm** HCC Rx ESR COM

√7th T44.903 **Poisoning by unspecified drugs primarily affecting the autonomic nervous system, assault**

√7th T44.904 **Poisoning by unspecified drugs primarily affecting the autonomic nervous system, undetermined**

√7th T44.905 **Adverse effect of unspecified drugs primarily affecting the autonomic nervous system** UPD

√7th T44.906 **Underdosing of unspecified drugs primarily affecting the autonomic nervous system** UPD

6th **T44.99 Poisoning by, adverse effect of and underdosing of other drugs primarily affecting the autonomic nervous system**

7th **T44.991 Poisoning by other drug primarily affecting the autonomic nervous system, accidental (unintentional)**
Poisoning by other drugs primarily affecting the autonomic nervous system NOS

7th **T44.992 Poisoning by other drug primarily affecting the autonomic nervous system, intentional self-harm** HCC Rx ESR COM

7th **T44.993 Poisoning by other drug primarily affecting the autonomic nervous system, assault**

7th **T44.994 Poisoning by other drug primarily affecting the autonomic nervous system, undetermined**

7th **T44.995 Adverse effect of other drug primarily affecting the autonomic nervous system** UPD

7th **T44.996 Underdosing of other drug primarily affecting the autonomic nervous system** UPD

4th **T45 Poisoning by, adverse effect of and underdosing of primarily systemic and hematological agents, not elsewhere classified**

The appropriate 7th character is to be added to each code from category T45.
A initial encounter
D subsequent encounter
S sequela

5th **T45.Ø Poisoning by, adverse effect of and underdosing of antiallergic and antiemetic drugs**
EXCLUDES 1 *poisoning by, adverse effect of and underdosing of phenothiazine-based neuroleptics (T43.3)*

6th **T45.ØX Poisoning by, adverse effect of and underdosing of antiallergic and antiemetic drugs**

7th **T45.ØX1 Poisoning by antiallergic and antiemetic drugs, accidental (unintentional)**
Poisoning by antiallergic and antiemetic drugs NOS

7th **T45.ØX2 Poisoning by antiallergic and antiemetic drugs, intentional self-harm** HCC Rx ESR COM

7th **T45.ØX3 Poisoning by antiallergic and antiemetic drugs, assault**

7th **T45.ØX4 Poisoning by antiallergic and antiemetic drugs, undetermined**

7th **T45.ØX5 Adverse effect of antiallergic and antiemetic drugs** UPD

7th **T45.ØX6 Underdosing of antiallergic and antiemetic drugs** UPD

5th **T45.1 Poisoning by, adverse effect of and underdosing of antineoplastic and immunosuppressive drugs**
EXCLUDES 1 *poisoning by, adverse effect of and underdosing of immune checkpoint inhibitors and immunostimulant drugs (T45.A)*
*poisoning by, adverse effect of and underdosing of tamoxifen (T38.6)*

**AHA:** 2019,1Q,17,20; 2014,4Q,22

6th **T45.1X Poisoning by, adverse effect of and underdosing of antineoplastic and immunosuppressive drugs**

7th **T45.1X1 Poisoning by antineoplastic and immunosuppressive drugs, accidental (unintentional)**
Poisoning by antineoplastic and immunosuppressive drugs NOS

7th **T45.1X2 Poisoning by antineoplastic and immunosuppressive drugs, intentional self-harm** HCC Rx ESR COM

7th **T45.1X3 Poisoning by antineoplastic and immunosuppressive drugs, assault**

7th **T45.1X4 Poisoning by antineoplastic and immunosuppressive drugs, undetermined**

7th **T45.1X5 Adverse effect of antineoplastic and immunosuppressive drugs** UPD
**AHA:** 2024,1Q,25; 2023,2Q,10; 2021,3Q,4; 2020,4Q,11; 2020,3Q,22; 2019,2Q,24,28

7th **T45.1X6 Underdosing of antineoplastic and immunosuppressive drugs** UPD

5th **T45.2 Poisoning by, adverse effect of and underdosing of vitamins**
EXCLUDES 2 *poisoning by, adverse effect of and underdosing of iron (T45.4)*
*poisoning by, adverse effect of and underdosing of nicotinic acid (derivatives) (T46.7)*
*poisoning by, adverse effect of and underdosing of vitamin K (T45.7)*

6th **T45.2X Poisoning by, adverse effect of and underdosing of vitamins**

7th **T45.2X1 Poisoning by vitamins, accidental (unintentional)**
Poisoning by vitamins NOS

7th **T45.2X2 Poisoning by vitamins, intentional self-harm** HCC Rx ESR COM

7th **T45.2X3 Poisoning by vitamins, assault**

7th **T45.2X4 Poisoning by vitamins, undetermined**

7th **T45.2X5 Adverse effect of vitamins** UPD

7th **T45.2X6 Underdosing of vitamins** UPD
EXCLUDES 1 *vitamin deficiencies (E5Ø-E56)*

5th **T45.3 Poisoning by, adverse effect of and underdosing of enzymes**

6th **T45.3X Poisoning by, adverse effect of and underdosing of enzymes**

7th **T45.3X1 Poisoning by enzymes, accidental (unintentional)**
Poisoning by enzymes NOS

7th **T45.3X2 Poisoning by enzymes, intentional self-harm** HCC Rx ESR COM

7th **T45.3X3 Poisoning by enzymes, assault**

7th **T45.3X4 Poisoning by enzymes, undetermined**

7th **T45.3X5 Adverse effect of enzymes** UPD

7th **T45.3X6 Underdosing of enzymes** UPD

5th **T45.4 Poisoning by, adverse effect of and underdosing of iron and its compounds**

6th **T45.4X Poisoning by, adverse effect of and underdosing of iron and its compounds**

7th **T45.4X1 Poisoning by iron and its compounds, accidental (unintentional)**
Poisoning by iron and its compounds NOS

7th **T45.4X2 Poisoning by iron and its compounds, intentional self-harm** HCC Rx ESR COM

7th **T45.4X3 Poisoning by iron and its compounds, assault**

7th **T45.4X4 Poisoning by iron and its compounds, undetermined**

7th **T45.4X5 Adverse effect of iron and its compounds** UPD

7th **T45.4X6 Underdosing of iron and its compounds** UPD
EXCLUDES 1 *iron deficiency (E61.1)*

5th **T45.5 Poisoning by, adverse effect of and underdosing of anticoagulants and antithrombotic drugs**

6th **T45.51 Poisoning by, adverse effect of and underdosing of anticoagulants**

7th **T45.511 Poisoning by anticoagulants, accidental (unintentional)**
Poisoning by anticoagulants NOS

7th **T45.512 Poisoning by anticoagulants, intentional self-harm** HCC Rx ESR COM

7th **T45.513 Poisoning by anticoagulants, assault**

7th **T45.514 Poisoning by anticoagulants, undetermined**

7th **T45.515 Adverse effect of anticoagulants** UPD
**AHA:** 2021,1Q,4; 2016,1Q,14; 2013,2Q,34

7th **T45.516 Underdosing of anticoagulants** UPD

6th **T45.52 Poisoning by, adverse effect of and underdosing of antithrombotic drugs**
Poisoning by, adverse effect of and underdosing of antiplatelet drugs
EXCLUDES 2 *poisoning by, adverse effect of and underdosing of acetylsalicylic acid (T39.Ø1-)*
*poisoning by, adverse effect of and underdosing of aspirin (T39.Ø1-)*

7th **T45.521 Poisoning by antithrombotic drugs, accidental (unintentional)**
Poisoning by antithrombotic drug NOS

7th **T45.522 Poisoning by antithrombotic drugs, intentional self-harm** HCC Rx ESR COM

T45.523 Poisoning by antithrombotic drugs, assault

T45.524 Poisoning by antithrombotic drugs, undetermined

T45.525 Adverse effect of antithrombotic drugs UPD
AHA: 2016,1Q,15

T45.526 Underdosing of antithrombotic drugs UPD

T45.6 Poisoning by, adverse effect of and underdosing of fibrinolysis-affecting drugs

T45.60 Poisoning by, adverse effect of and underdosing of unspecified fibrinolysis-affecting drugs

T45.601 Poisoning by unspecified fibrinolysis-affecting drugs, accidental (unintentional)
Poisoning by fibrinolysis-affecting drug NOS

T45.602 Poisoning by unspecified fibrinolysis-affecting drugs, intentional self-harm HCC Rx ESR COM

T45.603 Poisoning by unspecified fibrinolysis-affecting drugs, assault

T45.604 Poisoning by unspecified fibrinolysis-affecting drugs, undetermined

T45.605 Adverse effect of unspecified fibrinolysis-affecting drugs UPD

T45.606 Underdosing of unspecified fibrinolysis-affecting drugs UPD

T45.61 Poisoning by, adverse effect of and underdosing of thrombolytic drugs

T45.611 Poisoning by thrombolytic drug, accidental (unintentional)
Poisoning by thrombolytic drug NOS

T45.612 Poisoning by thrombolytic drug, intentional self-harm HCC Rx ESR COM

T45.613 Poisoning by thrombolytic drug, assault

T45.614 Poisoning by thrombolytic drug, undetermined

T45.615 Adverse effect of thrombolytic drugs UPD
AHA: 2017,2Q,9

T45.616 Underdosing of thrombolytic drugs UPD

T45.62 Poisoning by, adverse effect of and underdosing of hemostatic drugs

T45.621 Poisoning by hemostatic drug, accidental (unintentional)
Poisoning by hemostatic drug NOS

T45.622 Poisoning by hemostatic drug, intentional self-harm HCC Rx ESR COM

T45.623 Poisoning by hemostatic drug, assault

T45.624 Poisoning by hemostatic drug, undetermined

T45.625 Adverse effect of hemostatic drug UPD

T45.626 Underdosing of hemostatic drugs UPD

T45.69 Poisoning by, adverse effect of and underdosing of other fibrinolysis-affecting drugs

T45.691 Poisoning by other fibrinolysis-affecting drugs, accidental (unintentional)
Poisoning by other fibrinolysis-affecting drug NOS

T45.692 Poisoning by other fibrinolysis-affecting drugs, intentional self-harm HCC Rx ESR COM

T45.693 Poisoning by other fibrinolysis-affecting drugs, assault

T45.694 Poisoning by other fibrinolysis-affecting drugs, undetermined

T45.695 Adverse effect of other fibrinolysis-affecting drugs UPD

T45.696 Underdosing of other fibrinolysis-affecting drugs UPD

T45.7 Poisoning by, adverse effect of and underdosing of anticoagulant antagonists, vitamin K and other coagulants

T45.7X Poisoning by, adverse effect of and underdosing of anticoagulant antagonists, vitamin K and other coagulants

T45.7X1 Poisoning by anticoagulant antagonists, vitamin K and other coagulants, accidental (unintentional)
Poisoning by anticoagulant antagonists, vitamin K and other coagulants NOS

T45.7X2 Poisoning by anticoagulant antagonists, vitamin K and other coagulants, intentional self-harm HCC Rx ESR COM

T45.7X3 Poisoning by anticoagulant antagonists, vitamin K and other coagulants, assault

T45.7X4 Poisoning by anticoagulant antagonists, vitamin K and other coagulants, undetermined

T45.7X5 Adverse effect of anticoagulant antagonists, vitamin K and other coagulants UPD

T45.7X6 Underdosing of anticoagulant antagonist, vitamin K and other coagulants UPD
EXCLUDES 1 *vitamin K deficiency (E56.1)*

T45.8 Poisoning by, adverse effect of and underdosing of other primarily systemic and hematological agents
Poisoning by, adverse effect of and underdosing of liver preparations and other antianemic agents
Poisoning by, adverse effect of and underdosing of natural blood and blood products
Poisoning by, adverse effect of and underdosing of plasma substitute
EXCLUDES 2 *poisoning by, adverse effect of and underdosing of immunoglobulin (T50.Z1)*
*poisoning by, adverse effect of and underdosing of iron (T45.4)*
*transfusion reactions (T80.-)*

T45.8X Poisoning by, adverse effect of and underdosing of other primarily systemic and hematological agents

T45.8X1 Poisoning by other primarily systemic and hematological agents, accidental (unintentional)
Poisoning by other primarily systemic and hematological agents NOS

T45.8X2 Poisoning by other primarily systemic and hematological agents, intentional self-harm HCC Rx ESR COM

T45.8X3 Poisoning by other primarily systemic and hematological agents, assault

T45.8X4 Poisoning by other primarily systemic and hematological agents, undetermined

T45.8X5 Adverse effect of other primarily systemic and hematological agents UPD
AHA: 2016,4Q,42

T45.8X6 Underdosing of other primarily systemic and hematological agents UPD

T45.9 Poisoning by, adverse effect of and underdosing of unspecified primarily systemic and hematological agent

T45.91 Poisoning by unspecified primarily systemic and hematological agent, accidental (unintentional)
Poisoning by primarily systemic and hematological agent NOS

T45.92 Poisoning by unspecified primarily systemic and hematological agent, intentional self-harm HCC Rx ESR COM

T45.93 Poisoning by unspecified primarily systemic and hematological agent, assault

T45.94 Poisoning by unspecified primarily systemic and hematological agent, undetermined

T45.95 Adverse effect of unspecified primarily systemic and hematological agent UPD

T45.96 Underdosing of unspecified primarily systemic and hematological agent UPD

T45.A Poisoning by, adverse effect of and underdosing of immune checkpoint inhibitors and immunostimulant drugs
EXCLUDES 1 *poisoning by, adverse effect of and underdosing of antineoplastic and immunosuppressive drug (T45.1)*
AHA: 2024,4Q,28

T45.AX Poisoning by, adverse effect of and underdosing of immune checkpoint inhibitors and immunostimulant drugs

T45.AX1 Poisoning by immune checkpoint inhibitors and immunostimulant drugs, accidental (unintentional)
▶Poisoning by immune checkpoint inhibitors and immunostimulant drugs NOS◀

T45.AX2 Poisoning by immune checkpoint inhibitors and immunostimulant drugs, intentional self-harm HCC Rx ESR COM

√7th **T45.AX3 Poisoning by immune checkpoint inhibitors and immunostimulant drugs, assault**

√7th **T45.AX4 Poisoning by immune checkpoint inhibitors and immunostimulant drugs, undetermined**

√7th **T45.AX5 Adverse effect of immune checkpoint inhibitors and immunostimulant drugs**

√7th **T45.AX6 Underdosing of immune checkpoint inhibitors and immunostimulant drugs**

√4th **T46 Poisoning by, adverse effect of and underdosing of agents primarily affecting the cardiovascular system**

EXCLUDES 1 *poisoning by, adverse effect of and underdosing of metaraminol (T44.4)*

The appropriate 7th character is to be added to each code from category T46.
A initial encounter
D subsequent encounter
S sequela

√5th **T46.Ø Poisoning by, adverse effect of and underdosing of cardiac-stimulant glycosides and drugs of similar action**

√6th **T46.ØX Poisoning by, adverse effect of and underdosing of cardiac-stimulant glycosides and drugs of similar action**

√7th **T46.ØX1 Poisoning by cardiac-stimulant glycosides and drugs of similar action, accidental (unintentional)**
Poisoning by cardiac-stimulant glycosides and drugs of similar action NOS

√7th **T46.ØX2 Poisoning by cardiac-stimulant glycosides and drugs of similar action, intentional self-harm** HCC Rx ESR COM

√7th **T46.ØX3 Poisoning by cardiac-stimulant glycosides and drugs of similar action, assault**

√7th **T46.ØX4 Poisoning by cardiac-stimulant glycosides and drugs of similar action, undetermined**

√7th **T46.ØX5 Adverse effect of cardiac-stimulant glycosides and drugs of similar action** UPD

√7th **T46.ØX6 Underdosing of cardiac-stimulant glycosides and drugs of similar action** UPD

√5th **T46.1 Poisoning by, adverse effect of and underdosing of calcium-channel blockers**

√6th **T46.1X Poisoning by, adverse effect of and underdosing of calcium-channel blockers**

√7th **T46.1X1 Poisoning by calcium-channel blockers, accidental (unintentional)**
Poisoning by calcium-channel blockers NOS

√7th **T46.1X2 Poisoning by calcium-channel blockers, intentional self-harm** HCC Rx ESR COM

√7th **T46.1X3 Poisoning by calcium-channel blockers, assault**

√7th **T46.1X4 Poisoning by calcium-channel blockers, undetermined**

√7th **T46.1X5 Adverse effect of calcium-channel blockers** UPD

√7th **T46.1X6 Underdosing of calcium-channel blockers** UPD
**AHA:** 2023,1Q,39

√5th **T46.2 Poisoning by, adverse effect of and underdosing of other antidysrhythmic drugs, not elsewhere classified**

EXCLUDES 1 *poisoning by, adverse effect of and underdosing of beta-adrenoreceptor antagonists (T44.7-)*

√6th **T46.2X Poisoning by, adverse effect of and underdosing of other antidysrhythmic drugs**

√7th **T46.2X1 Poisoning by other antidysrhythmic drugs, accidental (unintentional)**
Poisoning by other antidysrhythmic drugs NOS

√7th **T46.2X2 Poisoning by other antidysrhythmic drugs, intentional self-harm** HCC Rx ESR COM

√7th **T46.2X3 Poisoning by other antidysrhythmic drugs, assault**

√7th **T46.2X4 Poisoning by other antidysrhythmic drugs, undetermined**

√7th **T46.2X5 Adverse effect of other antidysrhythmic drugs** UPD

√7th **T46.2X6 Underdosing of other antidysrhythmic drugs** UPD

√5th **T46.3 Poisoning by, adverse effect of and underdosing of coronary vasodilators**
Poisoning by, adverse effect of and underdosing of dipyridamole

EXCLUDES 1 *poisoning by, adverse effect of and underdosing of calcium-channel blockers (T46.1)*

√6th **T46.3X Poisoning by, adverse effect of and underdosing of coronary vasodilators**

√7th **T46.3X1 Poisoning by coronary vasodilators, accidental (unintentional)**
Poisoning by coronary vasodilators NOS

√7th **T46.3X2 Poisoning by coronary vasodilators, intentional self-harm** HCC Rx ESR COM

√7th **T46.3X3 Poisoning by coronary vasodilators, assault**

√7th **T46.3X4 Poisoning by coronary vasodilators, undetermined**

√7th **T46.3X5 Adverse effect of coronary vasodilators** UPD

√7th **T46.3X6 Underdosing of coronary vasodilators** UPD

√5th **T46.4 Poisoning by, adverse effect of and underdosing of angiotensin-converting-enzyme inhibitors**

√6th **T46.4X Poisoning by, adverse effect of and underdosing of angiotensin-converting-enzyme inhibitors**

√7th **T46.4X1 Poisoning by angiotensin-converting-enzyme inhibitors, accidental (unintentional)**
Poisoning by angiotensin-converting-enzyme inhibitors NOS

√7th **T46.4X2 Poisoning by angiotensin-converting-enzyme inhibitors, intentional self-harm** HCC Rx ESR COM

√7th **T46.4X3 Poisoning by angiotensin-converting-enzyme inhibitors, assault**

√7th **T46.4X4 Poisoning by angiotensin-converting-enzyme inhibitors, undetermined**

√7th **T46.4X5 Adverse effect of angiotensin-converting-enzyme inhibitors** UPD

√7th **T46.4X6 Underdosing of angiotensin-converting-enzyme inhibitors** UPD

√5th **T46.5 Poisoning by, adverse effect of and underdosing of other antihypertensive drugs**

EXCLUDES 2 *poisoning by, adverse effect of and underdosing of beta-adrenoreceptor antagonists (T44.7)*
*poisoning by, adverse effect of and underdosing of calcium-channel blockers (T46.1)*
*poisoning by, adverse effect of and underdosing of diuretics (T5Ø.Ø-T5Ø.2)*

√6th **T46.5X Poisoning by, adverse effect of and underdosing of other antihypertensive drugs**

√7th **T46.5X1 Poisoning by other antihypertensive drugs, accidental (unintentional)**
Poisoning by other antihypertensive drugs NOS

√7th **T46.5X2 Poisoning by other antihypertensive drugs, intentional self-harm** HCC Rx ESR COM

√7th **T46.5X3 Poisoning by other antihypertensive drugs, assault**

√7th **T46.5X4 Poisoning by other antihypertensive drugs, undetermined**

√7th **T46.5X5 Adverse effect of other antihypertensive drugs** UPD

√7th **T46.5X6 Underdosing of other antihypertensive drugs** UPD
**AHA:** 2023,1Q,39; 2022,1Q,36

√5th **T46.6 Poisoning by, adverse effect of and underdosing of antihyperlipidemic and antiarteriosclerotic drugs**

√6th **T46.6X Poisoning by, adverse effect of and underdosing of antihyperlipidemic and antiarteriosclerotic drugs**

√7th **T46.6X1 Poisoning by antihyperlipidemic and antiarteriosclerotic drugs, accidental (unintentional)**
Poisoning by antihyperlipidemic and antiarteriosclerotic drugs NOS

√7th **T46.6X2 Poisoning by antihyperlipidemic and antiarteriosclerotic drugs, intentional self-harm** HCC Rx ESR COM



T45.AX3–T46.6X2

T46.6X3 Poisoning by antihyperlipidemic and antiarteriosclerotic drugs, assault

T46.6X4 Poisoning by antihyperlipidemic and antiarteriosclerotic drugs, undetermined

T46.6X5 Adverse effect of antihyperlipidemic and antiarteriosclerotic drugs UPD

T46.6X6 Underdosing of antihyperlipidemic and antiarteriosclerotic drugs UPD

**T46.7 Poisoning by, adverse effect of and underdosing of peripheral vasodilators**

Poisoning by, adverse effect of and underdosing of nicotinic acid (derivatives)

EXCLUDES 1 *poisoning by, adverse effect of and underdosing of papaverine (T44.3)*

T46.7X Poisoning by, adverse effect of and underdosing of peripheral vasodilators

T46.7X1 Poisoning by peripheral vasodilators, accidental (unintentional)

Poisoning by peripheral vasodilators NOS

T46.7X2 Poisoning by peripheral vasodilators, intentional self-harm HCC Rx ESR COM

T46.7X3 Poisoning by peripheral vasodilators, assault

T46.7X4 Poisoning by peripheral vasodilators, undetermined

T46.7X5 Adverse effect of peripheral vasodilators UPD

T46.7X6 Underdosing of peripheral vasodilators UPD

**T46.8 Poisoning by, adverse effect of and underdosing of antivaricose drugs, including sclerosing agents**

T46.8X Poisoning by, adverse effect of and underdosing of antivaricose drugs, including sclerosing agents

T46.8X1 Poisoning by antivaricose drugs, including sclerosing agents, accidental (unintentional)

Poisoning by antivaricose drugs, including sclerosing agents NOS

T46.8X2 Poisoning by antivaricose drugs, including sclerosing agents, intentional self-harm HCC Rx ESR COM

T46.8X3 Poisoning by antivaricose drugs, including sclerosing agents, assault

T46.8X4 Poisoning by antivaricose drugs, including sclerosing agents, undetermined

T46.8X5 Adverse effect of antivaricose drugs, including sclerosing agents UPD

T46.8X6 Underdosing of antivaricose drugs, including sclerosing agents UPD

**T46.9 Poisoning by, adverse effect of and underdosing of other and unspecified agents primarily affecting the cardiovascular system**

T46.90 Poisoning by, adverse effect of and underdosing of unspecified agents primarily affecting the cardiovascular system

T46.901 Poisoning by unspecified agents primarily affecting the cardiovascular system, accidental (unintentional)

T46.902 Poisoning by unspecified agents primarily affecting the cardiovascular system, intentional self-harm HCC Rx ESR COM

T46.903 Poisoning by unspecified agents primarily affecting the cardiovascular system, assault

T46.904 Poisoning by unspecified agents primarily affecting the cardiovascular system, undetermined

T46.905 Adverse effect of unspecified agents primarily affecting the cardiovascular system UPD

T46.906 Underdosing of unspecified agents primarily affecting the cardiovascular system UPD

T46.99 Poisoning by, adverse effect of and underdosing of other agents primarily affecting the cardiovascular system

T46.991 Poisoning by other agents primarily affecting the cardiovascular system, accidental (unintentional)

T46.992 Poisoning by other agents primarily affecting the cardiovascular system, intentional self-harm HCC Rx ESR COM

T46.993 Poisoning by other agents primarily affecting the cardiovascular system, assault

T46.994 Poisoning by other agents primarily affecting the cardiovascular system, undetermined

T46.995 Adverse effect of other agents primarily affecting the cardiovascular system UPD

T46.996 Underdosing of other agents primarily affecting the cardiovascular system UPD

**T47 Poisoning by, adverse effect of and underdosing of agents primarily affecting the gastrointestinal system**

The appropriate 7th character is to be added to each code from category T47.
- A initial encounter
- D subsequent encounter
- S sequela

**T47.Ø Poisoning by, adverse effect of and underdosing of histamine H2-receptor blockers**

T47.ØX Poisoning by, adverse effect of and underdosing of histamine H2-receptor blockers

T47.ØX1 Poisoning by histamine H2-receptor blockers, accidental (unintentional)

Poisoning by histamine H2-receptor blockers NOS

T47.ØX2 Poisoning by histamine H2-receptor blockers, intentional self-harm HCC Rx ESR COM

T47.ØX3 Poisoning by histamine H2-receptor blockers, assault

T47.ØX4 Poisoning by histamine H2-receptor blockers, undetermined

T47.ØX5 Adverse effect of histamine H2-receptor blockers UPD

T47.ØX6 Underdosing of histamine H2-receptor blockers UPD

**T47.1 Poisoning by, adverse effect of and underdosing of other antacids and anti-gastric-secretion drugs**

T47.1X Poisoning by, adverse effect of and underdosing of other antacids and anti-gastric-secretion drugs

T47.1X1 Poisoning by other antacids and anti-gastric-secretion drugs, accidental (unintentional)

Poisoning by other antacids and anti-gastric-secretion drugs NOS

T47.1X2 Poisoning by other antacids and anti-gastric-secretion drugs, intentional self-harm HCC Rx ESR COM

T47.1X3 Poisoning by other antacids and anti-gastric-secretion drugs, assault

T47.1X4 Poisoning by other antacids and anti-gastric-secretion drugs, undetermined

T47.1X5 Adverse effect of other antacids and anti-gastric-secretion drugs UPD

T47.1X6 Underdosing of other antacids and anti-gastric-secretion drugs UPD

**T47.2 Poisoning by, adverse effect of and underdosing of stimulant laxatives**

T47.2X Poisoning by, adverse effect of and underdosing of stimulant laxatives

T47.2X1 Poisoning by stimulant laxatives, accidental (unintentional)

Poisoning by stimulant laxatives NOS

T47.2X2 Poisoning by stimulant laxatives, intentional self-harm HCC Rx ESR COM

T47.2X3 Poisoning by stimulant laxatives, assault

T47.2X4 Poisoning by stimulant laxatives, undetermined

T47.2X5 Adverse effect of stimulant laxatives UPD

T47.2X6 Underdosing of stimulant laxatives UPD

**T47.3 Poisoning by, adverse effect of and underdosing of saline and osmotic laxatives**

T47.3X Poisoning by and adverse effect of saline and osmotic laxatives

T47.3X1 Poisoning by saline and osmotic laxatives, accidental (unintentional)

Poisoning by saline and osmotic laxatives NOS

T47.3X2 Poisoning by saline and osmotic laxatives, intentional self-harm HCC Rx ESR COM

√7th T47.3X3 **Poisoning by saline and osmotic laxatives, assault**

√7th T47.3X4 **Poisoning by saline and osmotic laxatives, undetermined**

√7th T47.3X5 **Adverse effect of saline and osmotic laxatives** UPD

√7th T47.3X6 **Underdosing of saline and osmotic laxatives** UPD

√5th T47.4 **Poisoning by, adverse effect of and underdosing of other laxatives**

√6th T47.4X **Poisoning by, adverse effect of and underdosing of other laxatives**

√7th T47.4X1 **Poisoning by other laxatives, accidental (unintentional)**

Poisoning by other laxatives NOS

√7th T47.4X2 **Poisoning by other laxatives, intentional self-harm** HCC Rx ESR COM

√7th T47.4X3 **Poisoning by other laxatives, assault**

√7th T47.4X4 **Poisoning by other laxatives, undetermined**

√7th T47.4X5 **Adverse effect of other laxatives** UPD

√7th T47.4X6 **Underdosing of other laxatives** UPD

√5th T47.5 **Poisoning by, adverse effect of and underdosing of digestants**

√6th T47.5X **Poisoning by, adverse effect of and underdosing of digestants**

√7th T47.5X1 **Poisoning by digestants, accidental (unintentional)**

Poisoning by digestants NOS

√7th T47.5X2 **Poisoning by digestants, intentional self-harm** HCC Rx ESR COM

√7th T47.5X3 **Poisoning by digestants, assault**

√7th T47.5X4 **Poisoning by digestants, undetermined**

√7th T47.5X5 **Adverse effect of digestants** UPD

√7th T47.5X6 **Underdosing of digestants** UPD

√5th T47.6 **Poisoning by, adverse effect of and underdosing of antidiarrheal drugs**

EXCLUDES 2 *poisoning by, adverse effect of and underdosing of systemic antibiotics and other anti-infectives (T36-T37)*

√6th T47.6X **Poisoning by, adverse effect of and underdosing of antidiarrheal drugs**

√7th T47.6X1 **Poisoning by antidiarrheal drugs, accidental (unintentional)**

Poisoning by antidiarrheal drugs NOS

√7th T47.6X2 **Poisoning by antidiarrheal drugs, intentional self-harm** HCC Rx ESR COM

√7th T47.6X3 **Poisoning by antidiarrheal drugs, assault**

√7th T47.6X4 **Poisoning by antidiarrheal drugs, undetermined**

√7th T47.6X5 **Adverse effect of antidiarrheal drugs** UPD

√7th T47.6X6 **Underdosing of antidiarrheal drugs** UPD

√5th T47.7 **Poisoning by, adverse effect of and underdosing of emetics**

√6th T47.7X **Poisoning by, adverse effect of and underdosing of emetics**

√7th T47.7X1 **Poisoning by emetics, accidental (unintentional)**

Poisoning by emetics NOS

√7th T47.7X2 **Poisoning by emetics, intentional self-harm** HCC Rx ESR COM

√7th T47.7X3 **Poisoning by emetics, assault**

√7th T47.7X4 **Poisoning by emetics, undetermined**

√7th T47.7X5 **Adverse effect of emetics** UPD

√7th T47.7X6 **Underdosing of emetics** UPD

√5th T47.8 **Poisoning by, adverse effect of and underdosing of other agents primarily affecting gastrointestinal system**

√6th T47.8X **Poisoning by, adverse effect of and underdosing of other agents primarily affecting gastrointestinal system**

√7th T47.8X1 **Poisoning by other agents primarily affecting gastrointestinal system, accidental (unintentional)**

Poisoning by other agents primarily affecting gastrointestinal system NOS

√7th T47.8X2 **Poisoning by other agents primarily affecting gastrointestinal system, intentional self-harm** HCC Rx ESR COM

√7th T47.8X3 **Poisoning by other agents primarily affecting gastrointestinal system, assault**

√7th T47.8X4 **Poisoning by other agents primarily affecting gastrointestinal system, undetermined**

√7th T47.8X5 **Adverse effect of other agents primarily affecting gastrointestinal system** UPD

√7th T47.8X6 **Underdosing of other agents primarily affecting gastrointestinal system** UPD

√5th T47.9 **Poisoning by, adverse effect of and underdosing of unspecified agents primarily affecting the gastrointestinal system**

√x7th T47.91 **Poisoning by unspecified agents primarily affecting the gastrointestinal system, accidental (unintentional)**

Poisoning by agents primarily affecting the gastrointestinal system NOS

√x7th T47.92 **Poisoning by unspecified agents primarily affecting the gastrointestinal system, intentional self-harm** HCC Rx ESR COM

√x7th T47.93 **Poisoning by unspecified agents primarily affecting the gastrointestinal system, assault**

√x7th T47.94 **Poisoning by unspecified agents primarily affecting the gastrointestinal system, undetermined**

√x7th T47.95 **Adverse effect of unspecified agents primarily affecting the gastrointestinal system** UPD

√x7th T47.96 **Underdosing of unspecified agents primarily affecting the gastrointestinal system** UPD

√4th T48 **Poisoning by, adverse effect of and underdosing of agents primarily acting on smooth and skeletal muscles and the respiratory system**

The appropriate 7th character is to be added to each code from category T48.
A initial encounter
D subsequent encounter
S sequela

√5th T48.Ø **Poisoning by, adverse effect of and underdosing of oxytocic drugs**

EXCLUDES 1 *poisoning by, adverse effect of and underdosing of estrogens, progestogens and antagonists (T38.4-T38.6)*

√6th T48.ØX **Poisoning by, adverse effect of and underdosing of oxytocic drugs**

√7th T48.ØX1 **Poisoning by oxytocic drugs, accidental (unintentional)**

Poisoning by oxytocic drugs NOS

√7th T48.ØX2 **Poisoning by oxytocic drugs, intentional self-harm** HCC Rx ESR COM

√7th T48.ØX3 **Poisoning by oxytocic drugs, assault**

√7th T48.ØX4 **Poisoning by oxytocic drugs, undetermined**

√7th T48.ØX5 **Adverse effect of oxytocic drugs** UPD

√7th T48.ØX6 **Underdosing of oxytocic drugs** UPD

√5th T48.1 **Poisoning by, adverse effect of and underdosing of skeletal muscle relaxants [neuromuscular blocking agents]**

√6th T48.1X **Poisoning by, adverse effect of and underdosing of skeletal muscle relaxants [neuromuscular blocking agents]**

√7th T48.1X1 **Poisoning by skeletal muscle relaxants [neuromuscular blocking agents], accidental (unintentional)**

Poisoning by skeletal muscle relaxants [neuromuscular blocking agents] NOS

√7th T48.1X2 **Poisoning by skeletal muscle relaxants [neuromuscular blocking agents], intentional self-harm** HCC Rx ESR COM

√7th T48.1X3 **Poisoning by skeletal muscle relaxants [neuromuscular blocking agents], assault**

√7th T48.1X4 **Poisoning by skeletal muscle relaxants [neuromuscular blocking agents], undetermined**

√7th T48.1X5 **Adverse effect of skeletal muscle relaxants [neuromuscular blocking agents]** UPD

√7th T48.1X6 **Underdosing of skeletal muscle relaxants [neuromuscular blocking agents]** UPD

**T48.2 Poisoning by, adverse effect of and underdosing of other and unspecified drugs acting on muscles**

**T48.20 Poisoning by, adverse effect of and underdosing of unspecified drugs acting on muscles**

**T48.201 Poisoning by unspecified drugs acting on muscles, accidental (unintentional)**
Poisoning by unspecified drugs acting on muscles NOS

**T48.202 Poisoning by unspecified drugs acting on muscles, intentional self-harm** HCC Rx ESR COM

**T48.203 Poisoning by unspecified drugs acting on muscles, assault**

**T48.204 Poisoning by unspecified drugs acting on muscles, undetermined**

**T48.205 Adverse effect of unspecified drugs acting on muscles** UPD

**T48.206 Underdosing of unspecified drugs acting on muscles** UPD

**T48.29 Poisoning by, adverse effect of and underdosing of other drugs acting on muscles**

**T48.291 Poisoning by other drugs acting on muscles, accidental (unintentional)**
Poisoning by other drugs acting on muscles NOS

**T48.292 Poisoning by other drugs acting on muscles, intentional self-harm** HCC Rx ESR COM

**T48.293 Poisoning by other drugs acting on muscles, assault**

**T48.294 Poisoning by other drugs acting on muscles, undetermined**

**T48.295 Adverse effect of other drugs acting on muscles** UPD

**T48.296 Underdosing of other drugs acting on muscles** UPD

**T48.3 Poisoning by, adverse effect of and underdosing of antitussives**

**T48.3X Poisoning by, adverse effect of and underdosing of antitussives**

**T48.3X1 Poisoning by antitussives, accidental (unintentional)**
Poisoning by antitussives NOS

**T48.3X2 Poisoning by antitussives, intentional self-harm** HCC Rx ESR COM

**T48.3X3 Poisoning by antitussives, assault**

**T48.3X4 Poisoning by antitussives, undetermined**

**T48.3X5 Adverse effect of antitussives** UPD

**T48.3X6 Underdosing of antitussives** UPD

**T48.4 Poisoning by, adverse effect of and underdosing of expectorants**

**T48.4X Poisoning by, adverse effect of and underdosing of expectorants**

**T48.4X1 Poisoning by expectorants, accidental (unintentional)**
Poisoning by expectorants NOS

**T48.4X2 Poisoning by expectorants, intentional self-harm** HCC Rx ESR COM

**T48.4X3 Poisoning by expectorants, assault**

**T48.4X4 Poisoning by expectorants, undetermined**

**T48.4X5 Adverse effect of expectorants** UPD

**T48.4X6 Underdosing of expectorants** UPD

**T48.5 Poisoning by, adverse effect of and underdosing of other anti-common-cold drugs**
Poisoning by, adverse effect of and underdosing of decongestants
EXCLUDES 2 *poisoning by, adverse effect of and underdosing of antipyretics, NEC (T39.9-)*
*poisoning by, adverse effect of and underdosing of non-steroidal antiinflammatory drugs (T39.3-)*
*poisoning by, adverse effect of and underdosing of salicylates (T39.0-)*

**T48.5X Poisoning by, adverse effect of and underdosing of other anti-common-cold drugs**

**T48.5X1 Poisoning by other anti-common-cold drugs, accidental (unintentional)**
Poisoning by other anti-common-cold drugs NOS

**T48.5X2 Poisoning by other anti-common-cold drugs, intentional self-harm** HCC Rx ESR COM

**T48.5X3 Poisoning by other anti-common-cold drugs, assault**

**T48.5X4 Poisoning by other anti-common-cold drugs, undetermined**

**T48.5X5 Adverse effect of other anti-common-cold drugs** UPD

**T48.5X6 Underdosing of other anti-common-cold drugs** UPD

**T48.6 Poisoning by, adverse effect of and underdosing of antiasthmatics, not elsewhere classified**
Poisoning by, adverse effect of and underdosing of beta-adrenoreceptor agonists used in asthma therapy
EXCLUDES 1 *poisoning by, adverse effect of and underdosing of anterior pituitary [adenohypophyseal] hormones (T38.8)*
*poisoning by, adverse effect of and underdosing of beta-adrenoreceptor agonists not used in asthma therapy (T44.5)*

**T48.6X Poisoning by, adverse effect of and underdosing of antiasthmatics**

**T48.6X1 Poisoning by antiasthmatics, accidental (unintentional)**
Poisoning by antiasthmatics NOS

**T48.6X2 Poisoning by antiasthmatics, intentional self-harm** HCC Rx ESR COM

**T48.6X3 Poisoning by antiasthmatics, assault**

**T48.6X4 Poisoning by antiasthmatics, undetermined**

**T48.6X5 Adverse effect of antiasthmatics** UPD

**T48.6X6 Underdosing of antiasthmatics** UPD
AHA: 2024,1Q,23

**T48.9 Poisoning by, adverse effect of and underdosing of other and unspecified agents primarily acting on the respiratory system**

**T48.90 Poisoning by, adverse effect of and underdosing of unspecified agents primarily acting on the respiratory system**

**T48.901 Poisoning by unspecified agents primarily acting on the respiratory system, accidental (unintentional)**

**T48.902 Poisoning by unspecified agents primarily acting on the respiratory system, intentional self-harm** HCC Rx ESR COM

**T48.903 Poisoning by unspecified agents primarily acting on the respiratory system, assault**

**T48.904 Poisoning by unspecified agents primarily acting on the respiratory system, undetermined**

**T48.905 Adverse effect of unspecified agents primarily acting on the respiratory system** UPD

**T48.906 Underdosing of unspecified agents primarily acting on the respiratory system** UPD

**T48.99 Poisoning by, adverse effect of and underdosing of other agents primarily acting on the respiratory system**

**T48.991 Poisoning by other agents primarily acting on the respiratory system, accidental (unintentional)**

**T48.992 Poisoning by other agents primarily acting on the respiratory system, intentional self-harm** HCC Rx ESR COM

**T48.993 Poisoning by other agents primarily acting on the respiratory system, assault**

**T48.994 Poisoning by other agents primarily acting on the respiratory system, undetermined**

**T48.995 Adverse effect of other agents primarily acting on the respiratory system** UPD

**T48.996 Underdosing of other agents primarily acting on the respiratory system** UPD

**T49 Poisoning by, adverse effect of and underdosing of topical agents primarily affecting skin and mucous membrane and by ophthalmological, otorhinorlaryngological and dental drugs** (4th)

INCLUDES poisoning by, adverse effect of and underdosing of glucocorticoids, topically used

The appropriate 7th character is to be added to each code from category T49.
- A initial encounter
- D subsequent encounter
- S sequela

**T49.Ø Poisoning by, adverse effect of and underdosing of local antifungal, anti-infective and anti-inflammatory drugs** (5th)

**T49.ØX Poisoning by, adverse effect of and underdosing of local antifungal, anti-infective and anti-inflammatory drugs** (6th)

- (7th) **T49.ØX1 Poisoning by local antifungal, anti-infective and anti-inflammatory drugs, accidental (unintentional)**
  Poisoning by local antifungal, anti-infective and anti-inflammatory drugs NOS
- (7th) **T49.ØX2 Poisoning by local antifungal, anti-infective and anti-inflammatory drugs, intentional self-harm** HCC Rx ESR COM
- (7th) **T49.ØX3 Poisoning by local antifungal, anti-infective and anti-inflammatory drugs, assault**
- (7th) **T49.ØX4 Poisoning by local antifungal, anti-infective and anti-inflammatory drugs, undetermined**
- (7th) **T49.ØX5 Adverse effect of local antifungal, anti-infective and anti-inflammatory drugs** UPD
- (7th) **T49.ØX6 Underdosing of local antifungal, anti-infective and anti-inflammatory drugs** UPD

**T49.1 Poisoning by, adverse effect of and underdosing of antipruritics** (5th)

**T49.1X Poisoning by, adverse effect of and underdosing of antipruritics** (6th)

- (7th) **T49.1X1 Poisoning by antipruritics, accidental (unintentional)**
  Poisoning by antipruritics NOS
- (7th) **T49.1X2 Poisoning by antipruritics, intentional self-harm** HCC Rx ESR COM
- (7th) **T49.1X3 Poisoning by antipruritics, assault**
- (7th) **T49.1X4 Poisoning by antipruritics, undetermined**
- (7th) **T49.1X5 Adverse effect of antipruritics** UPD
- (7th) **T49.1X6 Underdosing of antipruritics** UPD

**T49.2 Poisoning by, adverse effect of and underdosing of local astringents and local detergents** (5th)

**T49.2X Poisoning by, adverse effect of and underdosing of local astringents and local detergents** (6th)

- (7th) **T49.2X1 Poisoning by local astringents and local detergents, accidental (unintentional)**
  Poisoning by local astringents and local detergents NOS
- (7th) **T49.2X2 Poisoning by local astringents and local detergents, intentional self-harm** HCC Rx ESR COM
- (7th) **T49.2X3 Poisoning by local astringents and local detergents, assault**
- (7th) **T49.2X4 Poisoning by local astringents and local detergents, undetermined**
- (7th) **T49.2X5 Adverse effect of local astringents and local detergents** UPD
- (7th) **T49.2X6 Underdosing of local astringents and local detergents** UPD

**T49.3 Poisoning by, adverse effect of and underdosing of emollients, demulcents and protectants** (5th)

**T49.3X Poisoning by, adverse effect of and underdosing of emollients, demulcents and protectants** (6th)

- (7th) **T49.3X1 Poisoning by emollients, demulcents and protectants, accidental (unintentional)**
  Poisoning by emollients, demulcents and protectants NOS
- (7th) **T49.3X2 Poisoning by emollients, demulcents and protectants, intentional self-harm** HCC Rx ESR COM
- (7th) **T49.3X3 Poisoning by emollients, demulcents and protectants, assault**
- (7th) **T49.3X4 Poisoning by emollients, demulcents and protectants, undetermined**
- (7th) **T49.3X5 Adverse effect of emollients, demulcents and protectants** UPD
- (7th) **T49.3X6 Underdosing of emollients, demulcents and protectants** UPD

**T49.4 Poisoning by, adverse effect of and underdosing of keratolytics, keratoplastics, and other hair treatment drugs and preparations** (5th)

**T49.4X Poisoning by, adverse effect of and underdosing of keratolytics, keratoplastics, and other hair treatment drugs and preparations** (6th)

- (7th) **T49.4X1 Poisoning by keratolytics, keratoplastics, and other hair treatment drugs and preparations, accidental (unintentional)**
  Poisoning by keratolytics, keratoplastics, and other hair treatment drugs and preparations NOS
- (7th) **T49.4X2 Poisoning by keratolytics, keratoplastics, and other hair treatment drugs and preparations, intentional self-harm** HCC Rx ESR COM
- (7th) **T49.4X3 Poisoning by keratolytics, keratoplastics, and other hair treatment drugs and preparations, assault**
- (7th) **T49.4X4 Poisoning by keratolytics, keratoplastics, and other hair treatment drugs and preparations, undetermined**
- (7th) **T49.4X5 Adverse effect of keratolytics, keratoplastics, and other hair treatment drugs and preparations** UPD
- (7th) **T49.4X6 Underdosing of keratolytics, keratoplastics, and other hair treatment drugs and preparations** UPD

**T49.5 Poisoning by, adverse effect of and underdosing of ophthalmological drugs and preparations** (5th)

**T49.5X Poisoning by, adverse effect of and underdosing of ophthalmological drugs and preparations** (6th)

- (7th) **T49.5X1 Poisoning by ophthalmological drugs and preparations, accidental (unintentional)**
  Poisoning by ophthalmological drugs and preparations NOS
- (7th) **T49.5X2 Poisoning by ophthalmological drugs and preparations, intentional self-harm** HCC Rx ESR COM
- (7th) **T49.5X3 Poisoning by ophthalmological drugs and preparations, assault**
- (7th) **T49.5X4 Poisoning by ophthalmological drugs and preparations, undetermined**
- (7th) **T49.5X5 Adverse effect of ophthalmological drugs and preparations** UPD
- (7th) **T49.5X6 Underdosing of ophthalmological drugs and preparations** UPD

**T49.6 Poisoning by, adverse effect of and underdosing of otorhinolaryngological drugs and preparations** (5th)

**T49.6X Poisoning by, adverse effect of and underdosing of otorhinolaryngological drugs and preparations** (6th)

- (7th) **T49.6X1 Poisoning by otorhinolaryngological drugs and preparations, accidental (unintentional)**
  Poisoning by otorhinolaryngological drugs and preparations NOS
- (7th) **T49.6X2 Poisoning by otorhinolaryngological drugs and preparations, intentional self-harm** HCC Rx ESR COM
- (7th) **T49.6X3 Poisoning by otorhinolaryngological drugs and preparations, assault**
- (7th) **T49.6X4 Poisoning by otorhinolaryngological drugs and preparations, undetermined**
- (7th) **T49.6X5 Adverse effect of otorhinolaryngological drugs and preparations** UPD
- (7th) **T49.6X6 Underdosing of otorhinolaryngological drugs and preparations** UPD

**T49.7 Poisoning by, adverse effect of and underdosing of dental drugs, topically applied** (5th)

**T49.7X Poisoning by, adverse effect of and underdosing of dental drugs, topically applied** (6th)

- (7th) **T49.7X1 Poisoning by dental drugs, topically applied, accidental (unintentional)**
  Poisoning by dental drugs, topically applied NOS

√7th T49.7X2 Poisoning by dental drugs, topically applied, intentional self-harm HCC Rx ESR COM

√7th T49.7X3 Poisoning by dental drugs, topically applied, assault

√7th T49.7X4 Poisoning by dental drugs, topically applied, undetermined

√7th T49.7X5 Adverse effect of dental drugs, topically applied UPD

√7th T49.7X6 Underdosing of dental drugs, topically applied UPD

√5th T49.8 Poisoning by, adverse effect of and underdosing of other topical agents

Poisoning by, adverse effect of and underdosing of spermicides

√6th T49.8X Poisoning by, adverse effect of and underdosing of other topical agents

√7th T49.8X1 Poisoning by other topical agents, accidental (unintentional)

Poisoning by other topical agents NOS

√7th T49.8X2 Poisoning by other topical agents, intentional self-harm HCC Rx ESR COM

√7th T49.8X3 Poisoning by other topical agents, assault

√7th T49.8X4 Poisoning by other topical agents, undetermined

√7th T49.8X5 Adverse effect of other topical agents UPD

√7th T49.8X6 Underdosing of other topical agents UPD

√5th T49.9 Poisoning by, adverse effect of and underdosing of unspecified topical agent

√x7th T49.91 Poisoning by unspecified topical agent, accidental (unintentional)

√x7th T49.92 Poisoning by unspecified topical agent, intentional self-harm HCC Rx ESR COM

√x7th T49.93 Poisoning by unspecified topical agent, assault

√x7th T49.94 Poisoning by unspecified topical agent, undetermined

√x7th T49.95 Adverse effect of unspecified topical agent UPD

√x7th T49.96 Underdosing of unspecified topical agent UPD

√4th T50 Poisoning by, adverse effect of and underdosing of diuretics and other and unspecified drugs, medicaments and biological substances

The appropriate 7th character is to be added to each code from category T50.
A initial encounter
D subsequent encounter
S sequela

√5th T50.0 Poisoning by, adverse effect of and underdosing of mineralocorticoids and their antagonists

√6th T50.0X Poisoning by, adverse effect of and underdosing of mineralocorticoids and their antagonists

√7th T50.0X1 Poisoning by mineralocorticoids and their antagonists, accidental (unintentional)

Poisoning by mineralocorticoids and their antagonists NOS

√7th T50.0X2 Poisoning by mineralocorticoids and their antagonists, intentional self-harm HCC Rx ESR COM

√7th T50.0X3 Poisoning by mineralocorticoids and their antagonists, assault

√7th T50.0X4 Poisoning by mineralocorticoids and their antagonists, undetermined

√7th T50.0X5 Adverse effect of mineralocorticoids and their antagonists UPD

√7th T50.0X6 Underdosing of mineralocorticoids and their antagonists UPD

√5th T50.1 Poisoning by, adverse effect of and underdosing of loop [high-ceiling] diuretics

√6th T50.1X Poisoning by, adverse effect of and underdosing of loop [high-ceiling] diuretics

√7th T50.1X1 Poisoning by loop [high-ceiling] diuretics, accidental (unintentional)

Poisoning by loop [high-ceiling] diuretics NOS

√7th T50.1X2 Poisoning by loop [high-ceiling] diuretics, intentional self-harm HCC Rx ESR COM

√7th T50.1X3 Poisoning by loop [high-ceiling] diuretics, assault

√7th T50.1X4 Poisoning by loop [high-ceiling] diuretics, undetermined

√7th T50.1X5 Adverse effect of loop [high-ceiling] diuretics UPD

√7th T50.1X6 Underdosing of loop [high-ceiling] diuretics UPD

√5th T50.2 Poisoning by, adverse effect of and underdosing of carbonic-anhydrase inhibitors, benzothiadiazides and other diuretics

Poisoning by, adverse effect of and underdosing of acetazolamide

√6th T50.2X Poisoning by, adverse effect of and underdosing of carbonic-anhydrase inhibitors, benzothiadiazides and other diuretics

√7th T50.2X1 Poisoning by carbonic-anhydrase inhibitors, benzothiadiazides and other diuretics, accidental (unintentional)

Poisoning by carbonic-anhydrase inhibitors, benzothiadiazides and other diuretics NOS

√7th T50.2X2 Poisoning by carbonic-anhydrase inhibitors, benzothiadiazides and other diuretics, intentional self-harm HCC Rx ESR COM

√7th T50.2X3 Poisoning by carbonic-anhydrase inhibitors, benzothiadiazides and other diuretics, assault

√7th T50.2X4 Poisoning by carbonic-anhydrase inhibitors, benzothiadiazides and other diuretics, undetermined

√7th T50.2X5 Adverse effect of carbonic-anhydrase inhibitors, benzothiadiazides and other diuretics UPD

√7th T50.2X6 Underdosing of carbonic-anhydrase inhibitors, benzothiadiazides and other diuretics UPD

√5th T50.3 Poisoning by, adverse effect of and underdosing of electrolytic, caloric and water-balance agents

Poisoning by, adverse effect of and underdosing of oral rehydration salts

√6th T50.3X Poisoning by, adverse effect of and underdosing of electrolytic, caloric and water-balance agents

√7th T50.3X1 Poisoning by electrolytic, caloric and water-balance agents, accidental (unintentional)

Poisoning by electrolytic, caloric and water-balance agents NOS

√7th T50.3X2 Poisoning by electrolytic, caloric and water-balance agents, intentional self-harm HCC Rx ESR COM

√7th T50.3X3 Poisoning by electrolytic, caloric and water-balance agents, assault

√7th T50.3X4 Poisoning by electrolytic, caloric and water-balance agents, undetermined

√7th T50.3X5 Adverse effect of electrolytic, caloric and water-balance agents UPD

AHA: 2022,2Q,10

√7th T50.3X6 Underdosing of electrolytic, caloric and water-balance agents UPD

√5th T50.4 Poisoning by, adverse effect of and underdosing of drugs affecting uric acid metabolism

√6th T50.4X Poisoning by, adverse effect of and underdosing of drugs affecting uric acid metabolism

√7th T50.4X1 Poisoning by drugs affecting uric acid metabolism, accidental (unintentional)

Poisoning by drugs affecting uric acid metabolism NOS

√7th T50.4X2 Poisoning by drugs affecting uric acid metabolism, intentional self-harm HCC Rx ESR COM

√7th T50.4X3 Poisoning by drugs affecting uric acid metabolism, assault

√7th T50.4X4 Poisoning by drugs affecting uric acid metabolism, undetermined

√7th T50.4X5 Adverse effect of drugs affecting uric acid metabolism UPD

√7th T50.4X6 Underdosing of drugs affecting uric acid metabolism UPD

√5th T50.5 Poisoning by, adverse effect of and underdosing of appetite depressants

√6th T50.5X Poisoning by, adverse effect of and underdosing of appetite depressants

√7th T50.5X1 Poisoning by appetite depressants, accidental (unintentional)

Poisoning by appetite depressants NOS

7th T50.5X2 Poisoning by appetite depressants, intentional self-harm HCC Rx ESR COM
7th T50.5X3 Poisoning by appetite depressants, assault
7th T50.5X4 Poisoning by appetite depressants, undetermined
7th T50.5X5 Adverse effect of appetite depressants UPD
7th T50.5X6 Underdosing of appetite depressants UPD
5th T50.6 Poisoning by, adverse effect of and underdosing of antidotes and chelating agents
Poisoning by, adverse effect of and underdosing of alcohol deterrents
6th T50.6X Poisoning by, adverse effect of and underdosing of antidotes and chelating agents
7th T50.6X1 Poisoning by antidotes and chelating agents, accidental (unintentional)
Poisoning by antidotes and chelating agents NOS
7th T50.6X2 Poisoning by antidotes and chelating agents, intentional self-harm HCC Rx ESR COM
7th T50.6X3 Poisoning by antidotes and chelating agents, assault
7th T50.6X4 Poisoning by antidotes and chelating agents, undetermined
7th T50.6X5 Adverse effect of antidotes and chelating agents UPD
7th T50.6X6 Underdosing of antidotes and chelating agents UPD
5th T50.7 Poisoning by, adverse effect of and underdosing of analeptics and opioid receptor antagonists
6th T50.7X Poisoning by, adverse effect of and underdosing of analeptics and opioid receptor antagonists
7th T50.7X1 Poisoning by analeptics and opioid receptor antagonists, accidental (unintentional)
Poisoning by analeptics and opioid receptor antagonists NOS
7th T50.7X2 Poisoning by analeptics and opioid receptor antagonists, intentional self-harm HCC Rx ESR COM
7th T50.7X3 Poisoning by analeptics and opioid receptor antagonists, assault
7th T50.7X4 Poisoning by analeptics and opioid receptor antagonists, undetermined
7th T50.7X5 Adverse effect of analeptics and opioid receptor antagonists UPD
7th T50.7X6 Underdosing of analeptics and opioid receptor antagonists UPD
5th T50.8 Poisoning by, adverse effect of and underdosing of diagnostic agents
6th T50.8X Poisoning by, adverse effect of and underdosing of diagnostic agents
7th T50.8X1 Poisoning by diagnostic agents, accidental (unintentional)
Poisoning by diagnostic agents NOS
7th T50.8X2 Poisoning by diagnostic agents, intentional self-harm HCC Rx ESR COM
7th T50.8X3 Poisoning by diagnostic agents, assault
7th T50.8X4 Poisoning by diagnostic agents, undetermined
7th T50.8X5 Adverse effect of diagnostic agents UPD
AHA: 2023,3Q,4; 2022,4Q,33; 2021,3Q,9-10
7th T50.8X6 Underdosing of diagnostic agents UPD
5th T50.A Poisoning by, adverse effect of and underdosing of bacterial vaccines
6th T50.A1 Poisoning by, adverse effect of and underdosing of pertussis vaccine, including combinations with a pertussis component
7th T50.A11 Poisoning by pertussis vaccine, including combinations with a pertussis component, accidental (unintentional)
7th T50.A12 Poisoning by pertussis vaccine, including combinations with a pertussis component, intentional self-harm HCC Rx ESR COM
7th T50.A13 Poisoning by pertussis vaccine, including combinations with a pertussis component, assault
7th T50.A14 Poisoning by pertussis vaccine, including combinations with a pertussis component, undetermined
7th T50.A15 Adverse effect of pertussis vaccine, including combinations with a pertussis component UPD
7th T50.A16 Underdosing of pertussis vaccine, including combinations with a pertussis component UPD
6th T50.A2 Poisoning by, adverse effect of and underdosing of mixed bacterial vaccines without a pertussis component
7th T50.A21 Poisoning by mixed bacterial vaccines without a pertussis component, accidental (unintentional)
7th T50.A22 Poisoning by mixed bacterial vaccines without a pertussis component, intentional self-harm HCC Rx ESR COM
7th T50.A23 Poisoning by mixed bacterial vaccines without a pertussis component, assault
7th T50.A24 Poisoning by mixed bacterial vaccines without a pertussis component, undetermined
7th T50.A25 Adverse effect of mixed bacterial vaccines without a pertussis component UPD
7th T50.A26 Underdosing of mixed bacterial vaccines without a pertussis component UPD
6th T50.A9 Poisoning by, adverse effect of and underdosing of other bacterial vaccines
7th T50.A91 Poisoning by other bacterial vaccines, accidental (unintentional)
7th T50.A92 Poisoning by other bacterial vaccines, intentional self-harm HCC Rx ESR COM
7th T50.A93 Poisoning by other bacterial vaccines, assault
7th T50.A94 Poisoning by other bacterial vaccines, undetermined
7th T50.A95 Adverse effect of other bacterial vaccines UPD
7th T50.A96 Underdosing of other bacterial vaccines UPD
5th T50.B Poisoning by, adverse effect of and underdosing of viral vaccines
6th T50.B1 Poisoning by, adverse effect of and underdosing of smallpox vaccines
7th T50.B11 Poisoning by smallpox vaccines, accidental (unintentional)
7th T50.B12 Poisoning by smallpox vaccines, intentional self-harm HCC Rx ESR COM
7th T50.B13 Poisoning by smallpox vaccines, assault
7th T50.B14 Poisoning by smallpox vaccines, undetermined
7th T50.B15 Adverse effect of smallpox vaccines UPD
7th T50.B16 Underdosing of smallpox vaccines UPD
6th T50.B9 Poisoning by, adverse effect of and underdosing of other viral vaccines
7th T50.B91 Poisoning by other viral vaccines, accidental (unintentional)
7th T50.B92 Poisoning by other viral vaccines, intentional self-harm HCC Rx ESR COM
7th T50.B93 Poisoning by other viral vaccines, assault
7th T50.B94 Poisoning by other viral vaccines, undetermined
7th T50.B95 Adverse effect of other viral vaccines UPD
AHA: 2021,1Q,43
7th T50.B96 Underdosing of other viral vaccines UPD
5th T50.Z Poisoning by, adverse effect of and underdosing of other vaccines and biological substances
6th T50.Z1 Poisoning by, adverse effect of and underdosing of immunoglobulin
7th T50.Z11 Poisoning by immunoglobulin, accidental (unintentional)
7th T50.Z12 Poisoning by immunoglobulin, intentional self-harm HCC Rx ESR COM
7th T50.Z13 Poisoning by immunoglobulin, assault
7th T50.Z14 Poisoning by immunoglobulin, undetermined
7th T50.Z15 Adverse effect of immunoglobulin UPD
7th T50.Z16 Underdosing of immunoglobulin UPD

√6th T5Ø.Z9 Poisoning by, adverse effect of and underdosing of other vaccines and biological substances
- √7th T5Ø.Z91 Poisoning by other vaccines and biological substances, accidental (unintentional)
- √7th T5Ø.Z92 Poisoning by other vaccines and biological substances, intentional self-harm HCC Rx ESR COM
- √7th T5Ø.Z93 Poisoning by other vaccines and biological substances, assault
- √7th T5Ø.Z94 Poisoning by other vaccines and biological substances, undetermined
- √7th T5Ø.Z95 Adverse effect of other vaccines and biological substances UPD
  - AHA: 2020,1Q,18
- √7th T5Ø.Z96 Underdosing of other vaccines and biological substances UPD

√5th T5Ø.9 Poisoning by, adverse effect of and underdosing of other and unspecified drugs, medicaments and biological substances

√6th T5Ø.9Ø Poisoning by, adverse effect of and underdosing of unspecified drugs, medicaments and biological substances
- √7th T5Ø.9Ø1 Poisoning by unspecified drugs, medicaments and biological substances, accidental (unintentional)
- √7th T5Ø.9Ø2 Poisoning by unspecified drugs, medicaments and biological substances, intentional self-harm HCC Rx ESR COM
- √7th T5Ø.9Ø3 Poisoning by unspecified drugs, medicaments and biological substances, assault
- √7th T5Ø.9Ø4 Poisoning by unspecified drugs, medicaments and biological substances, undetermined
- √7th T5Ø.9Ø5 Adverse effect of unspecified drugs, medicaments and biological substances
- √7th T5Ø.9Ø6 Underdosing of unspecified drugs, medicaments and biological substances

√6th T5Ø.91 Poisoning by, adverse effect of and underdosing of multiple unspecified drugs, medicaments and biological substances

Multiple drug ingestion NOS

Code also any specific drugs, medicaments and biological substances
- √7th T5Ø.911 Poisoning by multiple unspecified drugs, medicaments and biological substances, accidental (unintentional)
- √7th T5Ø.912 Poisoning by multiple unspecified drugs, medicaments and biological substances, intentional self-harm HCC Rx ESR COM
- √7th T5Ø.913 Poisoning by multiple unspecified drugs, medicaments and biological substances, assault
- √7th T5Ø.914 Poisoning by multiple unspecified drugs, medicaments and biological substances, undetermined
- √7th T5Ø.915 Adverse effect of multiple unspecified drugs, medicaments and biological substances UPD
- √7th T5Ø.916 Underdosing of multiple unspecified drugs, medicaments and biological substances UPD

√6th T5Ø.99 Poisoning by, adverse effect of and underdosing of other drugs, medicaments and biological substances
- √7th T5Ø.991 Poisoning by other drugs, medicaments and biological substances, accidental (unintentional)
- √7th T5Ø.992 Poisoning by other drugs, medicaments and biological substances, intentional self-harm HCC Rx ESR COM
- √7th T5Ø.993 Poisoning by other drugs, medicaments and biological substances, assault
- √7th T5Ø.994 Poisoning by other drugs, medicaments and biological substances, undetermined
- √7th T5Ø.995 Adverse effect of other drugs, medicaments and biological substances
  - AHA: 2023,3Q,4
- √7th T5Ø.996 Underdosing of other drugs, medicaments and biological substances

## Toxic effects of substances chiefly nonmedicinal as to source (T51-T65)

NOTE When no intent is indicated code to accidental. Undetermined intent is only for use when there is specific documentation in the record that the intent of the toxic effect cannot be determined.

Use additional code(s) for all associated manifestations of toxic effect, such as:
- personal history of foreign body fully removed (Z87.821)
- respiratory conditions due to external agents (J6Ø-J7Ø)
- to identify any retained foreign body, if applicable (Z18.-)

EXCLUDES 1 *contact with and (suspected) exposure to toxic substances (Z77.-)*

AHA: 2017,1Q,39-40

√4th **T51 Toxic effect of alcohol**

The appropriate 7th character is to be added to each code from category T51.
- A initial encounter
- D subsequent encounter
- S sequela

√5th T51.Ø Toxic effect of ethanol

Toxic effect of ethyl alcohol

EXCLUDES 2 *acute alcohol intoxication or "hangover" effects (F1Ø.129, F1Ø.229, F1Ø.929)*
*drunkenness (F1Ø.129, F1Ø.229, F1Ø.929)*
*pathological alcohol intoxication (F1Ø.129, F1Ø.229, F1Ø.929)*

√6th T51.ØX Toxic effect of ethanol
- √7th T51.ØX1 Toxic effect of ethanol, accidental (unintentional) ESR
  - Toxic effect of ethanol NOS
- √7th T51.ØX2 Toxic effect of ethanol, intentional self-harm HCC Rx ESR COM
- √7th T51.ØX3 Toxic effect of ethanol, assault
- √7th T51.ØX4 Toxic effect of ethanol, undetermined ESR

√5th T51.1 Toxic effect of methanol

Toxic effect of methyl alcohol

√6th T51.1X Toxic effect of methanol
- √7th T51.1X1 Toxic effect of methanol, accidental (unintentional)
  - Toxic effect of methanol NOS
- √7th T51.1X2 Toxic effect of methanol, intentional self-harm HCC Rx ESR COM
- √7th T51.1X3 Toxic effect of methanol, assault
- √7th T51.1X4 Toxic effect of methanol, undetermined

√5th T51.2 Toxic effect of 2-Propanol

Toxic effect of isopropyl alcohol

√6th T51.2X Toxic effect of 2-Propanol
- √7th T51.2X1 Toxic effect of 2-Propanol, accidental (unintentional)
  - Toxic effect of 2-Propanol NOS
- √7th T51.2X2 Toxic effect of 2-Propanol, intentional self-harm HCC Rx ESR COM
- √7th T51.2X3 Toxic effect of 2-Propanol, assault
- √7th T51.2X4 Toxic effect of 2-Propanol, undetermined

√5th T51.3 Toxic effect of fusel oil

Toxic effect of amyl alcohol
Toxic effect of butyl [1-butanol] alcohol
Toxic effect of propyl [1-propanol] alcohol

√6th T51.3X Toxic effect of fusel oil
- √7th T51.3X1 Toxic effect of fusel oil, accidental (unintentional)
  - Toxic effect of fusel oil NOS
- √7th T51.3X2 Toxic effect of fusel oil, intentional self-harm HCC Rx ESR COM
- √7th T51.3X3 Toxic effect of fusel oil, assault
- √7th T51.3X4 Toxic effect of fusel oil, undetermined

√5th T51.8 Toxic effect of other alcohols

√6th T51.8X Toxic effect of other alcohols
- √7th T51.8X1 Toxic effect of other alcohols, accidental (unintentional)
  - Toxic effect of other alcohols NOS
- √7th T51.8X2 Toxic effect of other alcohols, intentional self-harm HCC Rx ESR COM
- √7th T51.8X3 Toxic effect of other alcohols, assault
- √7th T51.8X4 Toxic effect of other alcohols, undetermined

√5th **T51.9 Toxic effect of unspecified alcohol**

√x7th **T51.91 Toxic effect of unspecified alcohol, accidental (unintentional)**

√x7th **T51.92 Toxic effect of unspecified alcohol, intentional self-harm** HCC Rx ESR COM

√x7th **T51.93 Toxic effect of unspecified alcohol, assault**

√x7th **T51.94 Toxic effect of unspecified alcohol, undetermined**

√4th **T52 Toxic effect of organic solvents**

EXCLUDES 1 *halogen derivatives of aliphatic and aromatic hydrocarbons (T53.-)*

The appropriate 7th character is to be added to each code from category T52.
A initial encounter
D subsequent encounter
S sequela

√5th **T52.Ø Toxic effects of petroleum products**

Toxic effects of ether petroleum
Toxic effects of gasoline [petrol]
Toxic effects of kerosene [paraffin oil]
Toxic effects of naphtha petroleum
Toxic effects of paraffin wax
Toxic effects of spirit petroleum

√6th **T52.ØX Toxic effects of petroleum products**

√7th **T52.ØX1 Toxic effect of petroleum products, accidental (unintentional)**
Toxic effects of petroleum products NOS

√7th **T52.ØX2 Toxic effect of petroleum products, intentional self-harm** HCC Rx ESR COM

√7th **T52.ØX3 Toxic effect of petroleum products, assault**

√7th **T52.ØX4 Toxic effect of petroleum products, undetermined**

√5th **T52.1 Toxic effects of benzene**

EXCLUDES 1 *homologues of benzene (T52.2)*
*nitroderivatives and aminoderivatives of benzene and its homologues (T65.3)*

√6th **T52.1X Toxic effects of benzene**

√7th **T52.1X1 Toxic effect of benzene, accidental (unintentional)**
Toxic effects of benzene NOS

√7th **T52.1X2 Toxic effect of benzene, intentional self-harm** HCC Rx ESR COM

√7th **T52.1X3 Toxic effect of benzene, assault**

√7th **T52.1X4 Toxic effect of benzene, undetermined**

√5th **T52.2 Toxic effects of homologues of benzene**

Toxic effects of toluene [methylbenzene]
Toxic effects of xylene [dimethylbenzene]

√6th **T52.2X Toxic effects of homologues of benzene**

√7th **T52.2X1 Toxic effect of homologues of benzene, accidental (unintentional)**
Toxic effects of homologues of benzene NOS

√7th **T52.2X2 Toxic effect of homologues of benzene, intentional self-harm** HCC Rx ESR COM

√7th **T52.2X3 Toxic effect of homologues of benzene, assault**

√7th **T52.2X4 Toxic effect of homologues of benzene, undetermined**

√5th **T52.3 Toxic effects of glycols**

√6th **T52.3X Toxic effects of glycols**

√7th **T52.3X1 Toxic effect of glycols, accidental (unintentional)**
Toxic effects of glycols NOS

√7th **T52.3X2 Toxic effect of glycols, intentional self-harm** HCC Rx ESR COM

√7th **T52.3X3 Toxic effect of glycols, assault**

√7th **T52.3X4 Toxic effect of glycols, undetermined**

√5th **T52.4 Toxic effects of ketones**

√6th **T52.4X Toxic effects of ketones**

√7th **T52.4X1 Toxic effect of ketones, accidental (unintentional)**
Toxic effects of ketones NOS

√7th **T52.4X2 Toxic effect of ketones, intentional self-harm** HCC Rx ESR COM

√7th **T52.4X3 Toxic effect of ketones, assault**

√7th **T52.4X4 Toxic effect of ketones, undetermined**

√5th **T52.8 Toxic effects of other organic solvents**

● √6th **T52.81 Toxic effects of alkenes**

● √7th **T52.811 Toxic effect of alkenes, accidental (unintentional)**
Toxic effects of alkenes NOS

● √7th **T52.812 Toxic effect of alkenes, intentional self-harm**

● √7th **T52.813 Toxic effect of alkenes, assault**

● √7th **T52.814 Toxic effect of alkenes, undetermined**

● √6th **T52.82 Toxic effects of cycloparaffins**

Toxic effects of cycloalkanes
Toxic effects of naphthenes

● √7th **T52.821 Toxic effect of cycloparaffins, accidental (unintentional)**
Toxic effects of cycloparaffins NOS

● √7th **T52.822 Toxic effect of cycloparaffins, intentional self-harm**

● √7th **T52.823 Toxic effect of cycloparaffins, assault**

● √7th **T52.824 Toxic effect of cycloparaffins, undetermined**

● √6th **T52.89 Toxic effects of other organic solvents**

● √7th **T52.891 Toxic effect of other organic solvents, accidental (unintentional)**
Toxic effects of other organic solvents NOS

● √7th **T52.892 Toxic effect of other organic solvents, intentional self-harm**

● √7th **T52.893 Toxic effect of other organic solvents, assault**

● √7th **T52.894 Toxic effect of other organic solvents, undetermined**

~~**T52.8X Toxic effects of other organic solvents**~~

~~**T52.8X1 Toxic effect of other organic solvents, accidental (unintentional)**~~

~~**T52.8X2 Toxic effect of other organic solvents, intentional self-harm**~~

~~**T52.8X3 Toxic effect of other organic solvents, assault**~~

~~**T52.8X4 Toxic effect of other organic solvents, undetermined**~~

√5th **T52.9 Toxic effects of unspecified organic solvent**

√x7th **T52.91 Toxic effect of unspecified organic solvent, accidental (unintentional)**

√x7th **T52.92 Toxic effect of unspecified organic solvent, intentional self-harm** HCC Rx ESR COM

√x7th **T52.93 Toxic effect of unspecified organic solvent, assault**

√x7th **T52.94 Toxic effect of unspecified organic solvent, undetermined**

√4th **T53 Toxic effect of halogen derivatives of aliphatic and aromatic hydrocarbons**

The appropriate 7th character is to be added to each code from category T53.
A initial encounter
D subsequent encounter
S sequela

√5th **T53.Ø Toxic effects of carbon tetrachloride**

Toxic effects of tetrachloromethane

√6th **T53.ØX Toxic effects of carbon tetrachloride**

√7th **T53.ØX1 Toxic effect of carbon tetrachloride, accidental (unintentional)**
Toxic effects of carbon tetrachloride NOS

√7th **T53.ØX2 Toxic effect of carbon tetrachloride, intentional self-harm** HCC Rx ESR COM

√7th **T53.ØX3 Toxic effect of carbon tetrachloride, assault**

√7th **T53.ØX4 Toxic effect of carbon tetrachloride, undetermined**

√5th **T53.1 Toxic effects of chloroform**

Toxic effects of trichloromethane

√6th **T53.1X Toxic effects of chloroform**

√7th **T53.1X1 Toxic effect of chloroform, accidental (unintentional)**
Toxic effects of chloroform NOS

√7th **T53.1X2 Toxic effect of chloroform, intentional self-harm** HCC Rx ESR COM

√7th **T53.1X3 Toxic effect of chloroform, assault**

√7th **T53.1X4 Toxic effect of chloroform, undetermined**

√5th **T53.2 Toxic effects of trichloroethylene**
Toxic effects of trichloroethene
√6th **T53.2X Toxic effects of trichloroethylene**
√7th **T53.2X1 Toxic effect of trichloroethylene, accidental (unintentional)**
Toxic effects of trichloroethylene NOS
√7th **T53.2X2 Toxic effect of trichloroethylene, intentional self-harm** HCC Rx ESR COM
√7th **T53.2X3 Toxic effect of trichloroethylene, assault**
√7th **T53.2X4 Toxic effect of trichloroethylene, undetermined**

√5th **T53.3 Toxic effects of tetrachloroethylene**
Toxic effect of tetrachloroethene
Toxic effects of perchloroethylene
√6th **T53.3X Toxic effects of tetrachloroethylene**
√7th **T53.3X1 Toxic effect of tetrachloroethylene, accidental (unintentional)**
Toxic effects of tetrachloroethylene NOS
√7th **T53.3X2 Toxic effect of tetrachloroethylene, intentional self-harm** HCC Rx ESR COM
√7th **T53.3X3 Toxic effect of tetrachloroethylene, assault**
√7th **T53.3X4 Toxic effect of tetrachloroethylene, undetermined**

√5th **T53.4 Toxic effects of dichloromethane**
Toxic effects of methylene chloride
√6th **T53.4X Toxic effects of dichloromethane**
√7th **T53.4X1 Toxic effect of dichloromethane, accidental (unintentional)**
Toxic effects of dichloromethane NOS
√7th **T53.4X2 Toxic effect of dichloromethane, intentional self-harm** HCC Rx ESR COM
√7th **T53.4X3 Toxic effect of dichloromethane, assault**
√7th **T53.4X4 Toxic effect of dichloromethane, undetermined**

√5th **T53.5 Toxic effects of chlorofluorocarbons**
√6th **T53.5X Toxic effects of chlorofluorocarbons**
√7th **T53.5X1 Toxic effect of chlorofluorocarbons, accidental (unintentional)**
Toxic effects of chlorofluorocarbons NOS
√7th **T53.5X2 Toxic effect of chlorofluorocarbons, intentional self-harm** HCC Rx ESR COM
√7th **T53.5X3 Toxic effect of chlorofluorocarbons, assault**
√7th **T53.5X4 Toxic effect of chlorofluorocarbons, undetermined**

√5th **T53.6 Toxic effects of other halogen derivatives of aliphatic hydrocarbons**
√6th **T53.6X Toxic effects of other halogen derivatives of aliphatic hydrocarbons**
√7th **T53.6X1 Toxic effect of other halogen derivatives of aliphatic hydrocarbons, accidental (unintentional)**
Toxic effects of other halogen derivatives of aliphatic hydrocarbons NOS
√7th **T53.6X2 Toxic effect of other halogen derivatives of aliphatic hydrocarbons, intentional self-harm** HCC Rx ESR COM
√7th **T53.6X3 Toxic effect of other halogen derivatives of aliphatic hydrocarbons, assault**
√7th **T53.6X4 Toxic effect of other halogen derivatives of aliphatic hydrocarbons, undetermined**

√5th **T53.7 Toxic effects of other halogen derivatives of aromatic hydrocarbons**
√6th **T53.7X Toxic effects of other halogen derivatives of aromatic hydrocarbons**
√7th **T53.7X1 Toxic effect of other halogen derivatives of aromatic hydrocarbons, accidental (unintentional)**
Toxic effects of other halogen derivatives of aromatic hydrocarbons NOS
√7th **T53.7X2 Toxic effect of other halogen derivatives of aromatic hydrocarbons, intentional self-harm** HCC Rx ESR COM
√7th **T53.7X3 Toxic effect of other halogen derivatives of aromatic hydrocarbons, assault**
√7th **T53.7X4 Toxic effect of other halogen derivatives of aromatic hydrocarbons, undetermined**

√5th **T53.9 Toxic effects of unspecified halogen derivatives of aliphatic and aromatic hydrocarbons**
√x7th **T53.91 Toxic effect of unspecified halogen derivatives of aliphatic and aromatic hydrocarbons, accidental (unintentional)**
√x7th **T53.92 Toxic effect of unspecified halogen derivatives of aliphatic and aromatic hydrocarbons, intentional self-harm** HCC Rx ESR COM
√x7th **T53.93 Toxic effect of unspecified halogen derivatives of aliphatic and aromatic hydrocarbons, assault**
√x7th **T53.94 Toxic effect of unspecified halogen derivatives of aliphatic and aromatic hydrocarbons, undetermined**

√4th **T54 Toxic effect of corrosive substances**

The appropriate 7th character is to be added to each code from category T54.
A initial encounter
D subsequent encounter
S sequela

√5th **T54.Ø Toxic effects of phenol and phenol homologues**
√6th **T54.ØX Toxic effects of phenol and phenol homologues**
√7th **T54.ØX1 Toxic effect of phenol and phenol homologues, accidental (unintentional)**
Toxic effects of phenol and phenol homologues NOS
√7th **T54.ØX2 Toxic effect of phenol and phenol homologues, intentional self-harm** HCC Rx ESR COM
√7th **T54.ØX3 Toxic effect of phenol and phenol homologues, assault**
√7th **T54.ØX4 Toxic effect of phenol and phenol homologues, undetermined**

√5th **T54.1 Toxic effects of other corrosive organic compounds**
√6th **T54.1X Toxic effects of other corrosive organic compounds**
√7th **T54.1X1 Toxic effect of other corrosive organic compounds, accidental (unintentional)**
Toxic effects of other corrosive organic compounds NOS
√7th **T54.1X2 Toxic effect of other corrosive organic compounds, intentional self-harm** HCC Rx ESR COM
√7th **T54.1X3 Toxic effect of other corrosive organic compounds, assault**
√7th **T54.1X4 Toxic effect of other corrosive organic compounds, undetermined**

√5th **T54.2 Toxic effects of corrosive acids and acid-like substances**
Toxic effects of hydrochloric acid
Toxic effects of sulfuric acid
√6th **T54.2X Toxic effects of corrosive acids and acid-like substances**
√7th **T54.2X1 Toxic effect of corrosive acids and acid-like substances, accidental (unintentional)**
Toxic effects of corrosive acids and acid-like substances NOS
√7th **T54.2X2 Toxic effect of corrosive acids and acid-like substances, intentional self-harm** HCC Rx ESR COM
√7th **T54.2X3 Toxic effect of corrosive acids and acid-like substances, assault**
√7th **T54.2X4 Toxic effect of corrosive acids and acid-like substances, undetermined**

√5th **T54.3 Toxic effects of corrosive alkalis and alkali-like substances**
Toxic effects of potassium hydroxide
Toxic effects of sodium hydroxide
√6th **T54.3X Toxic effects of corrosive alkalis and alkali-like substances**
√7th **T54.3X1 Toxic effect of corrosive alkalis and alkali-like substances, accidental (unintentional)**
Toxic effects of corrosive alkalis and alkali-like substances NOS
√7th **T54.3X2 Toxic effect of corrosive alkalis and alkali-like substances, intentional self-harm** HCC Rx ESR COM
√7th **T54.3X3 Toxic effect of corrosive alkalis and alkali-like substances, assault**
√7th **T54.3X4 Toxic effect of corrosive alkalis and alkali-like substances, undetermined**

√5th **T54.9 Toxic effects of unspecified corrosive substance**
√x7th **T54.91 Toxic effect of unspecified corrosive substance, accidental (unintentional)**

√x7th **T54.92** Toxic effect of unspecified corrosive substance, intentional self-harm HCC Rx ESR COM

√x7th **T54.93** Toxic effect of unspecified corrosive substance, assault

√x7th **T54.94** Toxic effect of unspecified corrosive substance, undetermined

√4th **T55 Toxic effect of soaps and detergents**

The appropriate 7th character is to be added to each code from category T55.
A initial encounter
D subsequent encounter
S sequela

√5th **T55.Ø** Toxic effect of soaps

√6th **T55.ØX** Toxic effect of soaps

√7th **T55.ØX1** Toxic effect of soaps, accidental (unintentional)
Toxic effect of soaps NOS

√7th **T55.ØX2** Toxic effect of soaps, intentional self-harm HCC Rx ESR COM

√7th **T55.ØX3** Toxic effect of soaps, assault

√7th **T55.ØX4** Toxic effect of soaps, undetermined

√5th **T55.1** Toxic effect of detergents

√6th **T55.1X** Toxic effect of detergents

√7th **T55.1X1** Toxic effect of detergents, accidental (unintentional)
Toxic effect of detergents NOS

√7th **T55.1X2** Toxic effect of detergents, intentional self-harm HCC Rx ESR COM

√7th **T55.1X3** Toxic effect of detergents, assault

√7th **T55.1X4** Toxic effect of detergents, undetermined

√4th **T56 Toxic effect of metals**

INCLUDES toxic effects of fumes and vapors of metals
toxic effects of metals from all sources, except medicinal substances

Use additional code to identify any retained metal foreign body, if applicable (Z18.Ø-, T18.1-)

EXCLUDES 1 *arsenic and its compounds (T57.Ø)*
*manganese and its compounds (T57.2)*

The appropriate 7th character is to be added to each code from category T56.
A initial encounter
D subsequent encounter
S sequela

√5th **T56.Ø** Toxic effects of lead and its compounds

√6th **T56.ØX** Toxic effects of lead and its compounds

√7th **T56.ØX1** Toxic effect of lead and its compounds, accidental (unintentional)
Toxic effects of lead and its compounds NOS

√7th **T56.ØX2** Toxic effect of lead and its compounds, intentional self-harm HCC Rx ESR COM

√7th **T56.ØX3** Toxic effect of lead and its compounds, assault

√7th **T56.ØX4** Toxic effect of lead and its compounds, undetermined

√5th **T56.1** Toxic effects of mercury and its compounds

√6th **T56.1X** Toxic effects of mercury and its compounds

√7th **T56.1X1** Toxic effect of mercury and its compounds, accidental (unintentional)
Toxic effects of mercury and its compounds NOS

√7th **T56.1X2** Toxic effect of mercury and its compounds, intentional self-harm HCC Rx ESR COM

√7th **T56.1X3** Toxic effect of mercury and its compounds, assault

√7th **T56.1X4** Toxic effect of mercury and its compounds, undetermined

√5th **T56.2** Toxic effects of chromium and its compounds

√6th **T56.2X** Toxic effects of chromium and its compounds

√7th **T56.2X1** Toxic effect of chromium and its compounds, accidental (unintentional)
Toxic effects of chromium and its compounds NOS

√7th **T56.2X2** Toxic effect of chromium and its compounds, intentional self-harm HCC Rx ESR COM

√7th **T56.2X3** Toxic effect of chromium and its compounds, assault

√7th **T56.2X4** Toxic effect of chromium and its compounds, undetermined

√5th **T56.3** Toxic effects of cadmium and its compounds

√6th **T56.3X** Toxic effects of cadmium and its compounds

√7th **T56.3X1** Toxic effect of cadmium and its compounds, accidental (unintentional)
Toxic effects of cadmium and its compounds NOS

√7th **T56.3X2** Toxic effect of cadmium and its compounds, intentional self-harm HCC Rx ESR COM

√7th **T56.3X3** Toxic effect of cadmium and its compounds, assault

√7th **T56.3X4** Toxic effect of cadmium and its compounds, undetermined

√5th **T56.4** Toxic effects of copper and its compounds

√6th **T56.4X** Toxic effects of copper and its compounds

√7th **T56.4X1** Toxic effect of copper and its compounds, accidental (unintentional)
Toxic effects of copper and its compounds NOS

√7th **T56.4X2** Toxic effect of copper and its compounds, intentional self-harm HCC Rx ESR COM

√7th **T56.4X3** Toxic effect of copper and its compounds, assault

√7th **T56.4X4** Toxic effect of copper and its compounds, undetermined

√5th **T56.5** Toxic effects of zinc and its compounds

√6th **T56.5X** Toxic effects of zinc and its compounds

√7th **T56.5X1** Toxic effect of zinc and its compounds, accidental (unintentional)
Toxic effects of zinc and its compounds NOS

√7th **T56.5X2** Toxic effect of zinc and its compounds, intentional self-harm HCC Rx ESR COM

√7th **T56.5X3** Toxic effect of zinc and its compounds, assault

√7th **T56.5X4** Toxic effect of zinc and its compounds, undetermined

√5th **T56.6** Toxic effects of tin and its compounds

√6th **T56.6X** Toxic effects of tin and its compounds

√7th **T56.6X1** Toxic effect of tin and its compounds, accidental (unintentional)
Toxic effects of tin and its compounds NOS

√7th **T56.6X2** Toxic effect of tin and its compounds, intentional self-harm HCC Rx ESR COM

√7th **T56.6X3** Toxic effect of tin and its compounds, assault

√7th **T56.6X4** Toxic effect of tin and its compounds, undetermined

√5th **T56.7** Toxic effects of beryllium and its compounds

√6th **T56.7X** Toxic effects of beryllium and its compounds

√7th **T56.7X1** Toxic effect of beryllium and its compounds, accidental (unintentional)
Toxic effects of beryllium and its compounds NOS

√7th **T56.7X2** Toxic effect of beryllium and its compounds, intentional self-harm HCC Rx ESR COM

√7th **T56.7X3** Toxic effect of beryllium and its compounds, assault

√7th **T56.7X4** Toxic effect of beryllium and its compounds, undetermined

√5th **T56.8** Toxic effects of other metals

√6th **T56.81** Toxic effect of thallium

√7th **T56.811** Toxic effect of thallium, accidental (unintentional)
Toxic effect of thallium NOS

√7th **T56.812** Toxic effect of thallium, intentional self-harm HCC Rx ESR COM

√7th **T56.813** Toxic effect of thallium, assault

√7th **T56.814** Toxic effect of thallium, undetermined

T56.82 Toxic effect of gadolinium
EXCLUDES 1 *adverse effect of diagnostic agents (T50.8X5-)*
AHA: 2023,4Q,44-45
T56.821 Toxic effect of gadolinium, accidental (unintentional)
Toxic effect of gadolinium NOS
T56.822 Toxic effect of gadolinium, intentional self-harm HCC Rx ESR COM
T56.823 Toxic effect of gadolinium, assault
T56.824 Toxic effect of gadolinium, undetermined
T56.89 Toxic effects of other metals
T56.891 Toxic effect of other metals, accidental (unintentional)
Toxic effects of other metals NOS
T56.892 Toxic effect of other metals, intentional self-harm HCC Rx ESR COM
T56.893 Toxic effect of other metals, assault
T56.894 Toxic effect of other metals, undetermined
T56.9 Toxic effects of unspecified metal
T56.91 Toxic effect of unspecified metal, accidental (unintentional)
T56.92 Toxic effect of unspecified metal, intentional self-harm HCC Rx ESR COM
T56.93 Toxic effect of unspecified metal, assault
T56.94 Toxic effect of unspecified metal, undetermined

## T57 Toxic effect of other inorganic substances

The appropriate 7th character is to be added to each code from category T57.
A initial encounter
D subsequent encounter
S sequela

T57.0 Toxic effect of arsenic and its compounds
T57.0X Toxic effect of arsenic and its compounds
T57.0X1 Toxic effect of arsenic and its compounds, accidental (unintentional)
Toxic effect of arsenic and its compounds NOS
T57.0X2 Toxic effect of arsenic and its compounds, intentional self-harm HCC Rx ESR COM
T57.0X3 Toxic effect of arsenic and its compounds, assault
T57.0X4 Toxic effect of arsenic and its compounds, undetermined
T57.1 Toxic effect of phosphorus and its compounds
EXCLUDES 1 *organophosphate insecticides (T60.0)*
T57.1X Toxic effect of phosphorus and its compounds
T57.1X1 Toxic effect of phosphorus and its compounds, accidental (unintentional)
Toxic effect of phosphorus and its compounds NOS
T57.1X2 Toxic effect of phosphorus and its compounds, intentional self-harm HCC Rx ESR COM
T57.1X3 Toxic effect of phosphorus and its compounds, assault
T57.1X4 Toxic effect of phosphorus and its compounds, undetermined
T57.2 Toxic effect of manganese and its compounds
T57.2X Toxic effect of manganese and its compounds
T57.2X1 Toxic effect of manganese and its compounds, accidental (unintentional)
Toxic effect of manganese and its compounds NOS
T57.2X2 Toxic effect of manganese and its compounds, intentional self-harm HCC Rx ESR COM
T57.2X3 Toxic effect of manganese and its compounds, assault
T57.2X4 Toxic effect of manganese and its compounds, undetermined
T57.3 Toxic effect of hydrogen cyanide
T57.3X Toxic effect of hydrogen cyanide
T57.3X1 Toxic effect of hydrogen cyanide, accidental (unintentional)
Toxic effect of hydrogen cyanide NOS
T57.3X2 Toxic effect of hydrogen cyanide, intentional self-harm HCC Rx ESR COM
T57.3X3 Toxic effect of hydrogen cyanide, assault
T57.3X4 Toxic effect of hydrogen cyanide, undetermined
T57.8 Toxic effect of other specified inorganic substances
T57.8X Toxic effect of other specified inorganic substances
T57.8X1 Toxic effect of other specified inorganic substances, accidental (unintentional)
Toxic effect of other specified inorganic substances NOS
T57.8X2 Toxic effect of other specified inorganic substances, intentional self-harm HCC Rx ESR COM
T57.8X3 Toxic effect of other specified inorganic substances, assault
T57.8X4 Toxic effect of other specified inorganic substances, undetermined
T57.9 Toxic effect of unspecified inorganic substance
T57.91 Toxic effect of unspecified inorganic substance, accidental (unintentional)
T57.92 Toxic effect of unspecified inorganic substance, intentional self-harm HCC Rx ESR COM
T57.93 Toxic effect of unspecified inorganic substance, assault
T57.94 Toxic effect of unspecified inorganic substance, undetermined

## T58 Toxic effect of carbon monoxide

INCLUDES asphyxiation from carbon monoxide
toxic effect of carbon monoxide from all sources

The appropriate 7th character is to be added to each code from category T58.
A initial encounter
D subsequent encounter
S sequela

T58.0 Toxic effect of carbon monoxide from motor vehicle exhaust
Toxic effect of exhaust gas from gas engine
Toxic effect of exhaust gas from motor pump
T58.01 Toxic effect of carbon monoxide from motor vehicle exhaust, accidental (unintentional)
T58.02 Toxic effect of carbon monoxide from motor vehicle exhaust, intentional self-harm HCC Rx ESR COM
T58.03 Toxic effect of carbon monoxide from motor vehicle exhaust, assault
T58.04 Toxic effect of carbon monoxide from motor vehicle exhaust, undetermined
T58.1 Toxic effect of carbon monoxide from utility gas
Toxic effect of acetylene
Toxic effect of gas NOS used for lighting, heating, cooking
Toxic effect of water gas
T58.11 Toxic effect of carbon monoxide from utility gas, accidental (unintentional)
T58.12 Toxic effect of carbon monoxide from utility gas, intentional self-harm HCC Rx ESR COM
T58.13 Toxic effect of carbon monoxide from utility gas, assault
T58.14 Toxic effect of carbon monoxide from utility gas, undetermined
T58.2 Toxic effect of carbon monoxide from incomplete combustion of other domestic fuels
Toxic effect of carbon monoxide from incomplete combustion of coal, coke, kerosene, wood
T58.2X Toxic effect of carbon monoxide from incomplete combustion of other domestic fuels
T58.2X1 Toxic effect of carbon monoxide from incomplete combustion of other domestic fuels, accidental (unintentional)
T58.2X2 Toxic effect of carbon monoxide from incomplete combustion of other domestic fuels, intentional self-harm HCC Rx ESR COM
T58.2X3 Toxic effect of carbon monoxide from incomplete combustion of other domestic fuels, assault

✓7th T58.2X4 **Toxic effect of carbon monoxide from incomplete combustion of other domestic fuels, undetermined**

✓5th T58.8 **Toxic effect of carbon monoxide from other source**
Toxic effect of carbon monoxide from blast furnace gas
Toxic effect of carbon monoxide from fuels in industrial use
Toxic effect of carbon monoxide from kiln vapor

✓6th T58.8X **Toxic effect of carbon monoxide from other source**

✓7th T58.8X1 **Toxic effect of carbon monoxide from other source, accidental (unintentional)**

✓7th T58.8X2 **Toxic effect of carbon monoxide from other source, intentional self-harm** HCC Rx ESR COM

✓7th T58.8X3 **Toxic effect of carbon monoxide from other source, assault**

✓7th T58.8X4 **Toxic effect of carbon monoxide from other source, undetermined**

✓5th T58.9 **Toxic effect of carbon monoxide from unspecified source**

✓x7th T58.91 **Toxic effect of carbon monoxide from unspecified source, accidental (unintentional)**

✓x7th T58.92 **Toxic effect of carbon monoxide from unspecified source, intentional self-harm** HCC Rx ESR COM

✓x7th T58.93 **Toxic effect of carbon monoxide from unspecified source, assault**

✓x7th T58.94 **Toxic effect of carbon monoxide from unspecified source, undetermined**

✓4th T59 **Toxic effect of other gases, fumes and vapors**

INCLUDES aerosol propellants

EXCLUDES 1 *chlorofluorocarbons (T53.5)*

The appropriate 7th character is to be added to each code from category T59.
A initial encounter
D subsequent encounter
S sequela

✓5th T59.Ø **Toxic effect of nitrogen oxides**

✓6th T59.ØX **Toxic effect of nitrogen oxides**

✓7th T59.ØX1 **Toxic effect of nitrogen oxides, accidental (unintentional)**
Toxic effect of nitrogen oxides NOS

✓7th T59.ØX2 **Toxic effect of nitrogen oxides, intentional self-harm** HCC Rx ESR COM

✓7th T59.ØX3 **Toxic effect of nitrogen oxides, assault**

✓7th T59.ØX4 **Toxic effect of nitrogen oxides, undetermined**

✓5th T59.1 **Toxic effect of sulfur dioxide**

✓6th T59.1X **Toxic effect of sulfur dioxide**

✓7th T59.1X1 **Toxic effect of sulfur dioxide, accidental (unintentional)**
Toxic effect of sulfur dioxide NOS

✓7th T59.1X2 **Toxic effect of sulfur dioxide, intentional self-harm** HCC Rx ESR COM

✓7th T59.1X3 **Toxic effect of sulfur dioxide, assault**

✓7th T59.1X4 **Toxic effect of sulfur dioxide, undetermined**

✓5th T59.2 **Toxic effect of formaldehyde**

✓6th T59.2X **Toxic effect of formaldehyde**

✓7th T59.2X1 **Toxic effect of formaldehyde, accidental (unintentional)**
Toxic effect of formaldehyde NOS

✓7th T59.2X2 **Toxic effect of formaldehyde, intentional self-harm** HCC Rx ESR COM

✓7th T59.2X3 **Toxic effect of formaldehyde, assault**

✓7th T59.2X4 **Toxic effect of formaldehyde, undetermined**

✓5th T59.3 **Toxic effect of lacrimogenic gas**
Toxic effect of tear gas

✓6th T59.3X **Toxic effect of lacrimogenic gas**

✓7th T59.3X1 **Toxic effect of lacrimogenic gas, accidental (unintentional)**
Toxic effect of lacrimogenic gas NOS

✓7th T59.3X2 **Toxic effect of lacrimogenic gas, intentional self-harm** HCC Rx ESR COM

✓7th T59.3X3 **Toxic effect of lacrimogenic gas, assault**

✓7th T59.3X4 **Toxic effect of lacrimogenic gas, undetermined**

✓5th T59.4 **Toxic effect of chlorine gas**

✓6th T59.4X **Toxic effect of chlorine gas**

✓7th T59.4X1 **Toxic effect of chlorine gas, accidental (unintentional)**
Toxic effect of chlorine gas NOS

✓7th T59.4X2 **Toxic effect of chlorine gas, intentional self-harm** HCC Rx ESR COM

✓7th T59.4X3 **Toxic effect of chlorine gas, assault**

✓7th T59.4X4 **Toxic effect of chlorine gas, undetermined**

✓5th T59.5 **Toxic effect of fluorine gas and hydrogen fluoride**

✓6th T59.5X **Toxic effect of fluorine gas and hydrogen fluoride**

✓7th T59.5X1 **Toxic effect of fluorine gas and hydrogen fluoride, accidental (unintentional)**
Toxic effect of fluorine gas and hydrogen fluoride NOS

✓7th T59.5X2 **Toxic effect of fluorine gas and hydrogen fluoride, intentional self-harm** HCC Rx ESR COM

✓7th T59.5X3 **Toxic effect of fluorine gas and hydrogen fluoride, assault**

✓7th T59.5X4 **Toxic effect of fluorine gas and hydrogen fluoride, undetermined**

✓5th T59.6 **Toxic effect of hydrogen sulfide**

✓6th T59.6X **Toxic effect of hydrogen sulfide**

✓7th T59.6X1 **Toxic effect of hydrogen sulfide, accidental (unintentional)**
Toxic effect of hydrogen sulfide NOS

✓7th T59.6X2 **Toxic effect of hydrogen sulfide, intentional self-harm** HCC Rx ESR COM

✓7th T59.6X3 **Toxic effect of hydrogen sulfide, assault**

✓7th T59.6X4 **Toxic effect of hydrogen sulfide, undetermined**

✓5th T59.7 **Toxic effect of carbon dioxide**

✓6th T59.7X **Toxic effect of carbon dioxide**

✓7th T59.7X1 **Toxic effect of carbon dioxide, accidental (unintentional)**
Toxic effect of carbon dioxide NOS

✓7th T59.7X2 **Toxic effect of carbon dioxide, intentional self-harm** HCC Rx ESR COM

✓7th T59.7X3 **Toxic effect of carbon dioxide, assault**

✓7th T59.7X4 **Toxic effect of carbon dioxide, undetermined**

✓5th T59.8 **Toxic effect of other specified gases, fumes and vapors**

✓6th T59.81 **Toxic effect of smoke**
Smoke inhalation

EXCLUDES 2 *toxic effect of cigarette (tobacco) smoke (T65.22-)*

✓7th T59.811 **Toxic effect of smoke, accidental (unintentional)**
Toxic effect of smoke NOS
**AHA:** 2013,4Q,121

✓7th T59.812 **Toxic effect of smoke, intentional self-harm** HCC Rx ESR COM

✓7th T59.813 **Toxic effect of smoke, assault**

✓7th T59.814 **Toxic effect of smoke, undetermined**

● ✓6th T59.82 **Toxic effects of hexamethylene diisocyanate**

● ✓7th T59.821 **Toxic effect of hexamethylene diisocyanate, accidental (unintentional)**
Toxic effects of hexamethylene diisocyanate NOS

● ✓7th T59.822 **Toxic effect of hexamethylene diisocyanate, intentional self-harm**

● ✓7th T59.823 **Toxic effect of hexamethylene diisocyanate, assault**

● ✓7th T59.824 **Toxic effect of hexamethylene diisocyanate, undetermined**

✓6th T59.89 **Toxic effect of other specified gases, fumes and vapors**

✓7th T59.891 **Toxic effect of other specified gases, fumes and vapors, accidental (unintentional)**

✓7th T59.892 **Toxic effect of other specified gases, fumes and vapors, intentional self-harm** HCC Rx ESR COM

✓7th T59.893 **Toxic effect of other specified gases, fumes and vapors, assault**

✓7th T59.894 **Toxic effect of other specified gases, fumes and vapors, undetermined**

√5th **T59.9 Toxic effect of unspecified gases, fumes and vapors**

√x7th **T59.91 Toxic effect of unspecified gases, fumes and vapors, accidental (unintentional)**

√x7th **T59.92 Toxic effect of unspecified gases, fumes and vapors, intentional self-harm** HCC Rx ESR COM

√x7th **T59.93 Toxic effect of unspecified gases, fumes and vapors, assault**

√x7th **T59.94 Toxic effect of unspecified gases, fumes and vapors, undetermined**

√4th **T6Ø Toxic effect of pesticides**

INCLUDES toxic effect of wood preservatives

The appropriate 7th character is to be added to each code from category T6Ø.
A initial encounter
D subsequent encounter
S sequela

√5th **T6Ø.Ø Toxic effect of organophosphate and carbamate insecticides**

√6th **T6Ø.ØX Toxic effect of organophosphate and carbamate insecticides**

√7th **T6Ø.ØX1 Toxic effect of organophosphate and carbamate insecticides, accidental (unintentional)**
Toxic effect of organophosphate and carbamate insecticides NOS

√7th **T6Ø.ØX2 Toxic effect of organophosphate and carbamate insecticides, intentional self-harm** HCC Rx ESR COM

√7th **T6Ø.ØX3 Toxic effect of organophosphate and carbamate insecticides, assault**

√7th **T6Ø.ØX4 Toxic effect of organophosphate and carbamate insecticides, undetermined**

√5th **T6Ø.1 Toxic effect of halogenated insecticides**

EXCLUDES 1 *chlorinated hydrocarbon (T53.-)*

√6th **T6Ø.1X Toxic effect of halogenated insecticides**

√7th **T6Ø.1X1 Toxic effect of halogenated insecticides, accidental (unintentional)**
Toxic effect of halogenated insecticides NOS

√7th **T6Ø.1X2 Toxic effect of halogenated insecticides, intentional self-harm** HCC Rx ESR COM

√7th **T6Ø.1X3 Toxic effect of halogenated insecticides, assault**

√7th **T6Ø.1X4 Toxic effect of halogenated insecticides, undetermined**

√5th **T6Ø.2 Toxic effect of other insecticides**

√6th **T6Ø.2X Toxic effect of other insecticides**

√7th **T6Ø.2X1 Toxic effect of other insecticides, accidental (unintentional)**
Toxic effect of other insecticides NOS

√7th **T6Ø.2X2 Toxic effect of other insecticides, intentional self-harm** HCC Rx ESR COM

√7th **T6Ø.2X3 Toxic effect of other insecticides, assault**

√7th **T6Ø.2X4 Toxic effect of other insecticides, undetermined**

√5th **T6Ø.3 Toxic effect of herbicides and fungicides**

√6th **T6Ø.3X Toxic effect of herbicides and fungicides**

√7th **T6Ø.3X1 Toxic effect of herbicides and fungicides, accidental (unintentional)**
Toxic effect of herbicides and fungicides NOS

√7th **T6Ø.3X2 Toxic effect of herbicides and fungicides, intentional self-harm** HCC Rx ESR COM

√7th **T6Ø.3X3 Toxic effect of herbicides and fungicides, assault**

√7th **T6Ø.3X4 Toxic effect of herbicides and fungicides, undetermined**

√5th **T6Ø.4 Toxic effect of rodenticides**

EXCLUDES 1 *strychnine and its salts (T65.1)*
*thallium (T56.81-)*

√6th **T6Ø.4X Toxic effect of rodenticides**

√7th **T6Ø.4X1 Toxic effect of rodenticides, accidental (unintentional)**
Toxic effect of rodenticides NOS

√7th **T6Ø.4X2 Toxic effect of rodenticides, intentional self-harm** HCC Rx ESR COM

√7th **T6Ø.4X3 Toxic effect of rodenticides, assault**

√7th **T6Ø.4X4 Toxic effect of rodenticides, undetermined**

√5th **T6Ø.8 Toxic effect of other pesticides**

√6th **T6Ø.8X Toxic effect of other pesticides**

√7th **T6Ø.8X1 Toxic effect of other pesticides, accidental (unintentional)**
Toxic effect of other pesticides NOS

√7th **T6Ø.8X2 Toxic effect of other pesticides, intentional self-harm** HCC Rx ESR COM

√7th **T6Ø.8X3 Toxic effect of other pesticides, assault**

√7th **T6Ø.8X4 Toxic effect of other pesticides, undetermined**

√5th **T6Ø.9 Toxic effect of unspecified pesticide**

√x7th **T6Ø.91 Toxic effect of unspecified pesticide, accidental (unintentional)**

√x7th **T6Ø.92 Toxic effect of unspecified pesticide, intentional self-harm** HCC Rx ESR COM

√x7th **T6Ø.93 Toxic effect of unspecified pesticide, assault**

√x7th **T6Ø.94 Toxic effect of unspecified pesticide, undetermined**

√4th **T61 Toxic effect of noxious substances eaten as seafood**

EXCLUDES 1 *allergic reaction to food, such as:*
*toxic effect of aflatoxin and other mycotoxins (T64)*
*toxic effect of cyanides (T65.Ø-)*
*toxic effect of harmful algae bloom (T65.82-)*
*toxic effect of hydrogen cyanide (T57.3-)*
*toxic effect of mercury (T56.1-)*
*toxic effect of red tide (T65.82-)*
*anaphylactic reaction or shock due to adverse food reaction (T78.Ø-)*
*bacterial foodborne intoxications (AØ5.-)*
*dermatitis (L23.6, L25.4, L27.2)*
*food protein-induced enterocolitis syndrome (K52.21)*
*food protein-induced enteropathy (K52.22)*
*gastroenteritis (noninfective) (K52.29)*

The appropriate 7th character is to be added to each code from category T61.
A initial encounter
D subsequent encounter
S sequela

√5th **T61.Ø Ciguatera fish poisoning**

√x7th **T61.Ø1 Ciguatera fish poisoning, accidental (unintentional)**

√x7th **T61.Ø2 Ciguatera fish poisoning, intentional self-harm** HCC Rx ESR COM

√x7th **T61.Ø3 Ciguatera fish poisoning, assault**

√x7th **T61.Ø4 Ciguatera fish poisoning, undetermined**

√5th **T61.1 Scombroid fish poisoning**
Histamine-like syndrome

√x7th **T61.11 Scombroid fish poisoning, accidental (unintentional)**

√x7th **T61.12 Scombroid fish poisoning, intentional self-harm** HCC Rx ESR COM

√x7th **T61.13 Scombroid fish poisoning, assault**

√x7th **T61.14 Scombroid fish poisoning, undetermined**

√5th **T61.7 Other fish and shellfish poisoning**

√6th **T61.77 Other fish poisoning**

√7th **T61.771 Other fish poisoning, accidental (unintentional)**

√7th **T61.772 Other fish poisoning, intentional self-harm** HCC Rx ESR COM

√7th **T61.773 Other fish poisoning, assault**

√7th **T61.774 Other fish poisoning, undetermined**

√6th **T61.78 Other shellfish poisoning**

√7th **T61.781 Other shellfish poisoning, accidental (unintentional)**

√7th **T61.782 Other shellfish poisoning, intentional self-harm** HCC Rx ESR COM

√7th **T61.783 Other shellfish poisoning, assault**

√7th **T61.784 Other shellfish poisoning, undetermined**

√5th **T61.8 Toxic effect of other seafood**

√6th **T61.8X Toxic effect of other seafood**

√7th **T61.8X1 Toxic effect of other seafood, accidental (unintentional)**

√7th **T61.8X2 Toxic effect of other seafood, intentional self-harm** HCC Rx ESR COM

√7th **T61.8X3 Toxic effect of other seafood, assault**

√7th **T61.8X4 Toxic effect of other seafood, undetermined**

√5th **T61.9 Toxic effect of unspecified seafood**

√x7th **T61.91 Toxic effect of unspecified seafood, accidental (unintentional)**

√x7th **T61.92 Toxic effect of unspecified seafood, intentional self-harm** HCC Rx ESR COM

√x7th **T61.93 Toxic effect of unspecified seafood, assault**

√x7th **T61.94 Toxic effect of unspecified seafood, undetermined**

√4th **T62 Toxic effect of other noxious substances eaten as food**

EXCLUDES 1 *allergic reaction to food, such as:*
*toxic effect of aflatoxin and other mycotoxins (T64)*
*toxic effect of cyanides (T65.Ø-)*
*toxic effect of hydrogen cyanide (T57.3-)*
*toxic effect of mercury (T56.1-)*
*anaphylactic shock (reaction) due to adverse food reaction (T78.Ø-)*
*bacterial food borne intoxications (AØ5.-)*
*dermatitis (L23.6, L25.4, L27.2)*
*food protein-induced enterocolitis syndrome (K52.21)*
*food protein-induced enteropathy (K52.22)*
*gastroenteritis (noninfective) (K52.29)*

The appropriate 7th character is to be added to each code from category T62.
A initial encounter
D subsequent encounter
S sequela

√5th **T62.Ø Toxic effect of ingested mushrooms**

√6th **T62.ØX Toxic effect of ingested mushrooms**

√7th **T62.ØX1 Toxic effect of ingested mushrooms, accidental (unintentional)**
Toxic effect of ingested mushrooms NOS

√7th **T62.ØX2 Toxic effect of ingested mushrooms, intentional self-harm** HCC Rx ESR COM

√7th **T62.ØX3 Toxic effect of ingested mushrooms, assault**

√7th **T62.ØX4 Toxic effect of ingested mushrooms, undetermined**

√5th **T62.1 Toxic effect of ingested berries**

√6th **T62.1X Toxic effect of ingested berries**

√7th **T62.1X1 Toxic effect of ingested berries, accidental (unintentional)**
Toxic effect of ingested berries NOS

√7th **T62.1X2 Toxic effect of ingested berries, intentional self-harm** HCC Rx ESR COM

√7th **T62.1X3 Toxic effect of ingested berries, assault**

√7th **T62.1X4 Toxic effect of ingested berries, undetermined**

√5th **T62.2 Toxic effect of other ingested (parts of) plant(s)**

√6th **T62.2X Toxic effect of other ingested (parts of) plant(s)**

√7th **T62.2X1 Toxic effect of other ingested (parts of) plant(s), accidental (unintentional)**
Toxic effect of other ingested (parts of) plant(s) NOS

√7th **T62.2X2 Toxic effect of other ingested (parts of) plant(s), intentional self-harm** HCC Rx ESR COM

√7th **T62.2X3 Toxic effect of other ingested (parts of) plant(s), assault**

√7th **T62.2X4 Toxic effect of other ingested (parts of) plant(s), undetermined**

√5th **T62.8 Toxic effect of other specified noxious substances eaten as food**

√6th **T62.8X Toxic effect of other specified noxious substances eaten as food**

√7th **T62.8X1 Toxic effect of other specified noxious substances eaten as food, accidental (unintentional)**
Toxic effect of other specified noxious substances eaten as food NOS

√7th **T62.8X2 Toxic effect of other specified noxious substances eaten as food, intentional self-harm** HCC Rx ESR COM

√7th **T62.8X3 Toxic effect of other specified noxious substances eaten as food, assault**

√7th **T62.8X4 Toxic effect of other specified noxious substances eaten as food, undetermined**

√5th **T62.9 Toxic effect of unspecified noxious substance eaten as food**

√x7th **T62.91 Toxic effect of unspecified noxious substance eaten as food, accidental (unintentional)**
Toxic effect of unspecified noxious substance eaten as food NOS

√x7th **T62.92 Toxic effect of unspecified noxious substance eaten as food, intentional self-harm** HCC Rx ESR COM

√x7th **T62.93 Toxic effect of unspecified noxious substance eaten as food, assault**

√x7th **T62.94 Toxic effect of unspecified noxious substance eaten as food, undetermined**

√4th **T63 Toxic effect of contact with venomous animals and plants**

INCLUDES bite or touch of venomous animal
pricked or stuck by thorn or leaf

EXCLUDES 2 *ingestion of toxic animal or plant (T61.-, T62.-)*

The appropriate 7th character is to be added to each code from category T63.
A initial encounter
D subsequent encounter
S sequela

√5th **T63.Ø Toxic effect of snake venom**

√6th **T63.ØØ Toxic effect of unspecified snake venom**

√7th **T63.ØØ1 Toxic effect of unspecified snake venom, accidental (unintentional)**
Toxic effect of unspecified snake venom NOS

√7th **T63.ØØ2 Toxic effect of unspecified snake venom, intentional self-harm** HCC Rx ESR COM

√7th **T63.ØØ3 Toxic effect of unspecified snake venom, assault**

√7th **T63.ØØ4 Toxic effect of unspecified snake venom, undetermined**

√6th **T63.Ø1 Toxic effect of rattlesnake venom**

√7th **T63.Ø11 Toxic effect of rattlesnake venom, accidental (unintentional)**
Toxic effect of rattlesnake venom NOS

√7th **T63.Ø12 Toxic effect of rattlesnake venom, intentional self-harm** HCC Rx ESR COM

√7th **T63.Ø13 Toxic effect of rattlesnake venom, assault**

√7th **T63.Ø14 Toxic effect of rattlesnake venom, undetermined**

√6th **T63.Ø2 Toxic effect of coral snake venom**

√7th **T63.Ø21 Toxic effect of coral snake venom, accidental (unintentional)**
Toxic effect of coral snake venom NOS

√7th **T63.Ø22 Toxic effect of coral snake venom, intentional self-harm** HCC Rx ESR COM

√7th **T63.Ø23 Toxic effect of coral snake venom, assault**

√7th **T63.Ø24 Toxic effect of coral snake venom, undetermined**

√6th **T63.Ø3 Toxic effect of taipan venom**

√7th **T63.Ø31 Toxic effect of taipan venom, accidental (unintentional)**
Toxic effect of taipan venom NOS

√7th **T63.Ø32 Toxic effect of taipan venom, intentional self-harm** HCC Rx ESR COM

√7th **T63.Ø33 Toxic effect of taipan venom, assault**

√7th **T63.Ø34 Toxic effect of taipan venom, undetermined**

√6th **T63.Ø4 Toxic effect of cobra venom**

√7th **T63.Ø41 Toxic effect of cobra venom, accidental (unintentional)**
Toxic effect of cobra venom NOS

√7th **T63.Ø42 Toxic effect of cobra venom, intentional self-harm** HCC Rx ESR COM

√7th **T63.Ø43 Toxic effect of cobra venom, assault**

√7th **T63.Ø44 Toxic effect of cobra venom, undetermined**

√6th **T63.Ø6 Toxic effect of venom of other North and South American snake**

√7th **T63.Ø61 Toxic effect of venom of other North and South American snake, accidental (unintentional)**
Toxic effect of venom of other North and South American snake NOS

√7th **T63.Ø62 Toxic effect of venom of other North and South American snake, intentional self-harm** HCC Rx ESR COM

√7th **T63.Ø63 Toxic effect of venom of other North and South American snake, assault**

√7th T63.064 Toxic effect of venom of other North and South American snake, undetermined

√6th T63.07 Toxic effect of venom of other Australian snake

√7th T63.071 Toxic effect of venom of other Australian snake, accidental (unintentional)
Toxic effect of venom of other Australian snake NOS

√7th T63.072 Toxic effect of venom of other Australian snake, intentional self-harm HCC Rx ESR COM

√7th T63.073 Toxic effect of venom of other Australian snake, assault

√7th T63.074 Toxic effect of venom of other Australian snake, undetermined

√6th T63.08 Toxic effect of venom of other African and Asian snake

√7th T63.081 Toxic effect of venom of other African and Asian snake, accidental (unintentional)
Toxic effect of venom of other African and Asian snake NOS

√7th T63.082 Toxic effect of venom of other African and Asian snake, intentional self-harm HCC Rx ESR COM

√7th T63.083 Toxic effect of venom of other African and Asian snake, assault

√7th T63.084 Toxic effect of venom of other African and Asian snake, undetermined

√6th T63.09 Toxic effect of venom of other snake

√7th T63.091 Toxic effect of venom of other snake, accidental (unintentional)
Toxic effect of venom of other snake NOS

√7th T63.092 Toxic effect of venom of other snake, intentional self-harm HCC Rx ESR COM

√7th T63.093 Toxic effect of venom of other snake, assault

√7th T63.094 Toxic effect of venom of other snake, undetermined

√5th T63.1 Toxic effect of venom of other reptiles

√6th T63.11 Toxic effect of venom of gila monster

√7th T63.111 Toxic effect of venom of gila monster, accidental (unintentional)
Toxic effect of venom of gila monster NOS

√7th T63.112 Toxic effect of venom of gila monster, intentional self-harm HCC Rx ESR COM

√7th T63.113 Toxic effect of venom of gila monster, assault

√7th T63.114 Toxic effect of venom of gila monster, undetermined

√6th T63.12 Toxic effect of venom of other venomous lizard

√7th T63.121 Toxic effect of venom of other venomous lizard, accidental (unintentional)
Toxic effect of venom of other venomous lizard NOS

√7th T63.122 Toxic effect of venom of other venomous lizard, intentional self-harm HCC Rx ESR COM

√7th T63.123 Toxic effect of venom of other venomous lizard, assault

√7th T63.124 Toxic effect of venom of other venomous lizard, undetermined

√6th T63.19 Toxic effect of venom of other reptiles

√7th T63.191 Toxic effect of venom of other reptiles, accidental (unintentional)
Toxic effect of venom of other reptiles NOS

√7th T63.192 Toxic effect of venom of other reptiles, intentional self-harm HCC Rx ESR COM

√7th T63.193 Toxic effect of venom of other reptiles, assault

√7th T63.194 Toxic effect of venom of other reptiles, undetermined

√5th T63.2 Toxic effect of venom of scorpion

√6th T63.2X Toxic effect of venom of scorpion

√7th T63.2X1 Toxic effect of venom of scorpion, accidental (unintentional)
Toxic effect of venom of scorpion NOS

√7th T63.2X2 Toxic effect of venom of scorpion, intentional self-harm HCC Rx ESR COM

√7th T63.2X3 Toxic effect of venom of scorpion, assault

√7th T63.2X4 Toxic effect of venom of scorpion, undetermined

√5th T63.3 Toxic effect of venom of spider

√6th T63.30 Toxic effect of unspecified spider venom

√7th T63.301 Toxic effect of unspecified spider venom, accidental (unintentional)

√7th T63.302 Toxic effect of unspecified spider venom, intentional self-harm HCC Rx ESR COM

√7th T63.303 Toxic effect of unspecified spider venom, assault

√7th T63.304 Toxic effect of unspecified spider venom, undetermined

√6th T63.31 Toxic effect of venom of black widow spider

√7th T63.311 Toxic effect of venom of black widow spider, accidental (unintentional)

√7th T63.312 Toxic effect of venom of black widow spider, intentional self-harm HCC Rx ESR COM

√7th T63.313 Toxic effect of venom of black widow spider, assault

√7th T63.314 Toxic effect of venom of black widow spider, undetermined

√6th T63.32 Toxic effect of venom of tarantula

√7th T63.321 Toxic effect of venom of tarantula, accidental (unintentional)

√7th T63.322 Toxic effect of venom of tarantula, intentional self-harm HCC Rx ESR COM

√7th T63.323 Toxic effect of venom of tarantula, assault

√7th T63.324 Toxic effect of venom of tarantula, undetermined

√6th T63.33 Toxic effect of venom of brown recluse spider

√7th T63.331 Toxic effect of venom of brown recluse spider, accidental (unintentional)

√7th T63.332 Toxic effect of venom of brown recluse spider, intentional self-harm HCC Rx ESR COM

√7th T63.333 Toxic effect of venom of brown recluse spider, assault

√7th T63.334 Toxic effect of venom of brown recluse spider, undetermined

√6th T63.39 Toxic effect of venom of other spider

√7th T63.391 Toxic effect of venom of other spider, accidental (unintentional)

√7th T63.392 Toxic effect of venom of other spider, intentional self-harm HCC Rx ESR COM

√7th T63.393 Toxic effect of venom of other spider, assault

√7th T63.394 Toxic effect of venom of other spider, undetermined

√5th T63.4 Toxic effect of venom of other arthropods

Use additional code, if applicable, for anaphylactic shock (T78.2)

√6th T63.41 Toxic effect of venom of centipedes and venomous millipedes

√7th T63.411 Toxic effect of venom of centipedes and venomous millipedes, accidental (unintentional)

√7th T63.412 Toxic effect of venom of centipedes and venomous millipedes, intentional self-harm HCC Rx ESR COM

√7th T63.413 Toxic effect of venom of centipedes and venomous millipedes, assault

√7th T63.414 Toxic effect of venom of centipedes and venomous millipedes, undetermined

√6th T63.42 Toxic effect of venom of ants

√7th T63.421 Toxic effect of venom of ants, accidental (unintentional)

√7th T63.422 Toxic effect of venom of ants, intentional self-harm HCC Rx ESR COM

√7th T63.423 Toxic effect of venom of ants, assault

√7th T63.424 Toxic effect of venom of ants, undetermined

√6th T63.43 Toxic effect of venom of caterpillars

√7th T63.431 Toxic effect of venom of caterpillars, accidental (unintentional)

√7th T63.432 Toxic effect of venom of caterpillars, intentional self-harm HCC Rx ESR COM

√7th T63.433 Toxic effect of venom of caterpillars, assault

√7th T63.434 Toxic effect of venom of caterpillars, undetermined

√6th **T63.44 Toxic effect of venom of bees**

√7th **T63.441 Toxic effect of venom of bees, accidental (unintentional)**

√7th **T63.442 Toxic effect of venom of bees, intentional self-harm** HCC Rx ESR COM

√7th **T63.443 Toxic effect of venom of bees, assault**

√7th **T63.444 Toxic effect of venom of bees, undetermined**

√6th **T63.45 Toxic effect of venom of hornets**

√7th **T63.451 Toxic effect of venom of hornets, accidental (unintentional)**

√7th **T63.452 Toxic effect of venom of hornets, intentional self-harm** HCC Rx ESR COM

√7th **T63.453 Toxic effect of venom of hornets, assault**

√7th **T63.454 Toxic effect of venom of hornets, undetermined**

√6th **T63.46 Toxic effect of venom of wasps**

Toxic effect of yellow jacket

√7th **T63.461 Toxic effect of venom of wasps, accidental (unintentional)**

√7th **T63.462 Toxic effect of venom of wasps, intentional self-harm** HCC Rx ESR COM

√7th **T63.463 Toxic effect of venom of wasps, assault**

√7th **T63.464 Toxic effect of venom of wasps, undetermined**

√6th **T63.48 Toxic effect of venom of other arthropod**

√7th **T63.481 Toxic effect of venom of other arthropod, accidental (unintentional)**

√7th **T63.482 Toxic effect of venom of other arthropod, intentional self-harm** HCC Rx ESR COM

√7th **T63.483 Toxic effect of venom of other arthropod, assault**

√7th **T63.484 Toxic effect of venom of other arthropod, undetermined**

√5th **T63.5 Toxic effect of contact with venomous fish**

EXCLUDES 2 *poisoning by ingestion of fish (T61.-)*

√6th **T63.51 Toxic effect of contact with stingray**

√7th **T63.511 Toxic effect of contact with stingray, accidental (unintentional)**

√7th **T63.512 Toxic effect of contact with stingray, intentional self-harm** HCC Rx ESR COM

√7th **T63.513 Toxic effect of contact with stingray, assault**

√7th **T63.514 Toxic effect of contact with stingray, undetermined**

√6th **T63.59 Toxic effect of contact with other venomous fish**

√7th **T63.591 Toxic effect of contact with other venomous fish, accidental (unintentional)**

√7th **T63.592 Toxic effect of contact with other venomous fish, intentional self-harm** HCC Rx ESR COM

√7th **T63.593 Toxic effect of contact with other venomous fish, assault**

√7th **T63.594 Toxic effect of contact with other venomous fish, undetermined**

√5th **T63.6 Toxic effect of contact with other venomous marine animals**

EXCLUDES 1 *sea-snake venom (T63.Ø9)*

EXCLUDES 2 *poisoning by ingestion of shellfish (T61.78-)*

√6th **T63.61 Toxic effect of contact with Portuguese Man-o-war**

Toxic effect of contact with bluebottle

√7th **T63.611 Toxic effect of contact with Portuguese Man-o-war, accidental (unintentional)**

√7th **T63.612 Toxic effect of contact with Portuguese Man-o-war, intentional self-harm** HCC Rx ESR COM

√7th **T63.613 Toxic effect of contact with Portuguese Man-o-war, assault**

√7th **T63.614 Toxic effect of contact with Portuguese Man-o-war, undetermined**

√6th **T63.62 Toxic effect of contact with other jellyfish**

√7th **T63.621 Toxic effect of contact with other jellyfish, accidental (unintentional)**

√7th **T63.622 Toxic effect of contact with other jellyfish, intentional self-harm** HCC Rx ESR COM

√7th **T63.623 Toxic effect of contact with other jellyfish, assault**

√7th **T63.624 Toxic effect of contact with other jellyfish, undetermined**

√6th **T63.63 Toxic effect of contact with sea anemone**

√7th **T63.631 Toxic effect of contact with sea anemone, accidental (unintentional)**

√7th **T63.632 Toxic effect of contact with sea anemone, intentional self-harm** HCC Rx ESR COM

√7th **T63.633 Toxic effect of contact with sea anemone, assault**

√7th **T63.634 Toxic effect of contact with sea anemone, undetermined**

√6th **T63.69 Toxic effect of contact with other venomous marine animals**

√7th **T63.691 Toxic effect of contact with other venomous marine animals, accidental (unintentional)**

√7th **T63.692 Toxic effect of contact with other venomous marine animals, intentional self-harm** HCC Rx ESR COM

√7th **T63.693 Toxic effect of contact with other venomous marine animals, assault**

√7th **T63.694 Toxic effect of contact with other venomous marine animals, undetermined**

√5th **T63.7 Toxic effect of contact with venomous plant**

√6th **T63.71 Toxic effect of contact with venomous marine plant**

√7th **T63.711 Toxic effect of contact with venomous marine plant, accidental (unintentional)**

√7th **T63.712 Toxic effect of contact with venomous marine plant, intentional self-harm** HCC Rx ESR COM

√7th **T63.713 Toxic effect of contact with venomous marine plant, assault**

√7th **T63.714 Toxic effect of contact with venomous marine plant, undetermined**

√6th **T63.79 Toxic effect of contact with other venomous plant**

√7th **T63.791 Toxic effect of contact with other venomous plant, accidental (unintentional)**

√7th **T63.792 Toxic effect of contact with other venomous plant, intentional self-harm** HCC Rx ESR COM

√7th **T63.793 Toxic effect of contact with other venomous plant, assault**

√7th **T63.794 Toxic effect of contact with other venomous plant, undetermined**

√5th **T63.8 Toxic effect of contact with other venomous animals**

√6th **T63.81 Toxic effect of contact with venomous frog**

EXCLUDES 1 *contact with nonvenomous frog (W62.Ø)*

√7th **T63.811 Toxic effect of contact with venomous frog, accidental (unintentional)**

√7th **T63.812 Toxic effect of contact with venomous frog, intentional self-harm** HCC Rx ESR COM

√7th **T63.813 Toxic effect of contact with venomous frog, assault**

√7th **T63.814 Toxic effect of contact with venomous frog, undetermined**

√6th **T63.82 Toxic effect of contact with venomous toad**

EXCLUDES 1 *contact with nonvenomous toad (W62.1)*

√7th **T63.821 Toxic effect of contact with venomous toad, accidental (unintentional)**

√7th **T63.822 Toxic effect of contact with venomous toad, intentional self-harm** HCC Rx ESR COM

√7th **T63.823 Toxic effect of contact with venomous toad, assault**

√7th **T63.824 Toxic effect of contact with venomous toad, undetermined**

√6th **T63.83 Toxic effect of contact with other venomous amphibian**

EXCLUDES 1 *contact with nonvenomous amphibian (W62.9)*

√7th **T63.831 Toxic effect of contact with other venomous amphibian, accidental (unintentional)**

√7th **T63.832 Toxic effect of contact with other venomous amphibian, intentional self-harm** HCC Rx ESR COM

√7th **T63.833 Toxic effect of contact with other venomous amphibian, assault**

√7th **T63.834 Toxic effect of contact with other venomous amphibian, undetermined**

√6th T63.89 Toxic effect of contact with other venomous animals
√7th T63.891 Toxic effect of contact with other venomous animals, accidental (unintentional)
√7th T63.892 Toxic effect of contact with other venomous animals, intentional self-harm HCC Rx ESR COM
√7th T63.893 Toxic effect of contact with other venomous animals, assault
√7th T63.894 Toxic effect of contact with other venomous animals, undetermined

√5th T63.9 Toxic effect of contact with unspecified venomous animal
√x7th T63.91 Toxic effect of contact with unspecified venomous animal, accidental (unintentional)
√x7th T63.92 Toxic effect of contact with unspecified venomous animal, intentional self-harm HCC Rx ESR COM
√x7th T63.93 Toxic effect of contact with unspecified venomous animal, assault
√x7th T63.94 Toxic effect of contact with unspecified venomous animal, undetermined

√4th **T64 Toxic effect of aflatoxin and other mycotoxin food contaminants**

The appropriate 7th character is to be added to each code from category T64.
A initial encounter
D subsequent encounter
S sequela

√5th T64.0 Toxic effect of aflatoxin
√x7th T64.01 Toxic effect of aflatoxin, accidental (unintentional)
√x7th T64.02 Toxic effect of aflatoxin, intentional self-harm HCC Rx ESR COM
√x7th T64.03 Toxic effect of aflatoxin, assault
√x7th T64.04 Toxic effect of aflatoxin, undetermined

√5th T64.8 Toxic effect of other mycotoxin food contaminants
√x7th T64.81 Toxic effect of other mycotoxin food contaminants, accidental (unintentional)
√x7th T64.82 Toxic effect of other mycotoxin food contaminants, intentional self-harm HCC Rx ESR COM
√x7th T64.83 Toxic effect of other mycotoxin food contaminants, assault
√x7th T64.84 Toxic effect of other mycotoxin food contaminants, undetermined

√4th **T65 Toxic effect of other and unspecified substances**

The appropriate 7th character is to be added to each code from category T65.
A initial encounter
D subsequent encounter
S sequela

√5th T65.0 Toxic effect of cyanides
EXCLUDES 1 *hydrogen cyanide (T57.3-)*
√6th T65.0X Toxic effect of cyanides
√7th T65.0X1 Toxic effect of cyanides, accidental (unintentional)
Toxic effect of cyanides NOS
√7th T65.0X2 Toxic effect of cyanides, intentional self-harm HCC Rx ESR COM
√7th T65.0X3 Toxic effect of cyanides, assault
√7th T65.0X4 Toxic effect of cyanides, undetermined

√5th T65.1 Toxic effect of strychnine and its salts
√6th T65.1X Toxic effect of strychnine and its salts
√7th T65.1X1 Toxic effect of strychnine and its salts, accidental (unintentional)
Toxic effect of strychnine and its salts NOS
√7th T65.1X2 Toxic effect of strychnine and its salts, intentional self-harm HCC Rx ESR COM
√7th T65.1X3 Toxic effect of strychnine and its salts, assault
√7th T65.1X4 Toxic effect of strychnine and its salts, undetermined

√5th T65.2 Toxic effect of tobacco and nicotine
EXCLUDES 2 *nicotine dependence (F17.-)*
√6th T65.21 Toxic effect of chewing tobacco
√7th T65.211 Toxic effect of chewing tobacco, accidental (unintentional)
Toxic effect of chewing tobacco NOS
√7th T65.212 Toxic effect of chewing tobacco, intentional self-harm HCC Rx ESR COM
√7th T65.213 Toxic effect of chewing tobacco, assault
√7th T65.214 Toxic effect of chewing tobacco, undetermined
√6th T65.22 Toxic effect of tobacco cigarettes
Toxic effect of tobacco smoke
Use additional code for exposure to second hand tobacco smoke (Z57.31, Z77.22)
√7th T65.221 Toxic effect of tobacco cigarettes, accidental (unintentional)
Toxic effect of tobacco cigarettes NOS
√7th T65.222 Toxic effect of tobacco cigarettes, intentional self-harm HCC Rx ESR COM
√7th T65.223 Toxic effect of tobacco cigarettes, assault
√7th T65.224 Toxic effect of tobacco cigarettes, undetermined
√6th T65.29 Toxic effect of other tobacco and nicotine
√7th T65.291 Toxic effect of other tobacco and nicotine, accidental (unintentional)
Toxic effect of other tobacco and nicotine NOS
√7th T65.292 Toxic effect of other tobacco and nicotine, intentional self-harm HCC Rx ESR COM
√7th T65.293 Toxic effect of other tobacco and nicotine, assault
√7th T65.294 Toxic effect of other tobacco and nicotine, undetermined

√5th T65.3 Toxic effect of nitroderivatives and aminoderivatives of benzene and its homologues
Toxic effect of aniline [benzenamine]
Toxic effect of nitrobenzene
Toxic effect of trinitrotoluene
√6th T65.3X Toxic effect of nitroderivatives and aminoderivatives of benzene and its homologues
√7th T65.3X1 Toxic effect of nitroderivatives and aminoderivatives of benzene and its homologues, accidental (unintentional)
Toxic effect of nitroderivatives and aminoderivatives of benzene and its homologues NOS
√7th T65.3X2 Toxic effect of nitroderivatives and aminoderivatives of benzene and its homologues, intentional self-harm HCC Rx ESR COM
√7th T65.3X3 Toxic effect of nitroderivatives and aminoderivatives of benzene and its homologues, assault
√7th T65.3X4 Toxic effect of nitroderivatives and aminoderivatives of benzene and its homologues, undetermined

√5th T65.4 Toxic effect of carbon disulfide
√6th T65.4X Toxic effect of carbon disulfide
√7th T65.4X1 Toxic effect of carbon disulfide, accidental (unintentional)
Toxic effect of carbon disulfide NOS
√7th T65.4X2 Toxic effect of carbon disulfide, intentional self-harm HCC Rx ESR COM
√7th T65.4X3 Toxic effect of carbon disulfide, assault
√7th T65.4X4 Toxic effect of carbon disulfide, undetermined

√5th T65.5 Toxic effect of nitroglycerin and other nitric acids and esters
Toxic effect of 1,2,3-Propanetriol trinitrate
√6th T65.5X Toxic effect of nitroglycerin and other nitric acids and esters
√7th T65.5X1 Toxic effect of nitroglycerin and other nitric acids and esters, accidental (unintentional)
Toxic effect of nitroglycerin and other nitric acids and esters NOS
√7th T65.5X2 Toxic effect of nitroglycerin and other nitric acids and esters, intentional self-harm HCC Rx ESR COM
√7th T65.5X3 Toxic effect of nitroglycerin and other nitric acids and esters, assault
√7th T65.5X4 Toxic effect of nitroglycerin and other nitric acids and esters, undetermined

✓5th **T65.6 Toxic effect of paints and dyes, not elsewhere classified**

✓6th **T65.6X Toxic effect of paints and dyes, not elsewhere classified**

✓7th **T65.6X1 Toxic effect of paints and dyes, not elsewhere classified, accidental (unintentional)**
Toxic effect of paints and dyes NOS

✓7th **T65.6X2 Toxic effect of paints and dyes, not elsewhere classified, intentional self-harm** HCC Rx ESR COM

✓7th **T65.6X3 Toxic effect of paints and dyes, not elsewhere classified, assault**

✓7th **T65.6X4 Toxic effect of paints and dyes, not elsewhere classified, undetermined**

✓5th **T65.8 Toxic effect of other specified substances**

✓6th **T65.81 Toxic effect of latex**

✓7th **T65.811 Toxic effect of latex, accidental (unintentional)**
Toxic effect of latex NOS

✓7th **T65.812 Toxic effect of latex, intentional self-harm** HCC Rx ESR COM

✓7th **T65.813 Toxic effect of latex, assault**

✓7th **T65.814 Toxic effect of latex, undetermined**

✓6th **T65.82 Toxic effect of harmful algae and algae toxins**
Toxic effect of blue-green algae bloom
Toxic effect of (harmful) algae bloom NOS
Toxic effect of brown tide
Toxic effect of cyanobacteria bloom
Toxic effect of Florida red tide
Toxic effect of pfiesteria piscicida
Toxic effect of red tide

✓7th **T65.821 Toxic effect of harmful algae and algae toxins, accidental (unintentional)**
Toxic effect of harmful algae and algae toxins NOS

✓7th **T65.822 Toxic effect of harmful algae and algae toxins, intentional self-harm** HCC Rx ESR COM

✓7th **T65.823 Toxic effect of harmful algae and algae toxins, assault**

✓7th **T65.824 Toxic effect of harmful algae and algae toxins, undetermined**

✓6th **T65.83 Toxic effect of fiberglass**

✓7th **T65.831 Toxic effect of fiberglass, accidental (unintentional)**
Toxic effect of fiberglass NOS

✓7th **T65.832 Toxic effect of fiberglass, intentional self-harm** HCC Rx ESR COM

✓7th **T65.833 Toxic effect of fiberglass, assault**

✓7th **T65.834 Toxic effect of fiberglass, undetermined**

✓6th **T65.84 Toxic effect of xylazine**
Use additional code(s) for all associated manifestations, such as:
cellulitis and acute lymphangitis (LØ3.-)
cutaneous abscess, furuncle and carbuncle (LØ2.-)
non-pressure chronic ulcer of lower limb, not elsewhere classified (L97.-)
non-pressure chronic ulcer of skin, not elsewhere classified (L98.4-)
**AHA:** 2025,4Q,38

✓7th **T65.841 Toxic effect of xylazine, accidental (unintentional)**
Toxic effect of xylazine NOS

✓7th **T65.842 Toxic effect of xylazine, intentional self-harm** HCC Rx ESR

✓7th **T65.843 Toxic effect of xylazine, assault**

✓7th **T65.844 Toxic effect of xylazine, undetermined**

● ✓6th **T65.85 Toxic effect of medetomidine**
Use additional code to identify associated manifestations, such as:
bradycardia NOS (RØØ.1)
somnolence, stupor and coma (R4Ø.-)

● ✓7th **T65.851 Toxic effect of medetomidine, accidental (unintentional)**
Toxic effect of medetomidine NOS

● ✓7th **T65.852 Toxic effect of medetomidine, intentional self-harm**

● ✓7th **T65.853 Toxic effect of medetomidine, assault**

● ✓7th **T65.854 Toxic effect of medetomidine, undetermined**

✓6th **T65.89 Toxic effect of other specified substances**

✓7th **T65.891 Toxic effect of other specified substances, accidental (unintentional)**
Toxic effect of other specified substances NOS
**AHA:** 2018,1Q,5

✓7th **T65.892 Toxic effect of other specified substances, intentional self-harm** HCC Rx ESR COM

✓7th **T65.893 Toxic effect of other specified substances, assault**

✓7th **T65.894 Toxic effect of other specified substances, undetermined**

✓5th **T65.9 Toxic effect of unspecified substance**

✓x7th **T65.91 Toxic effect of unspecified substance, accidental (unintentional)**
Poisoning NOS

✓x7th **T65.92 Toxic effect of unspecified substance, intentional self-harm** HCC Rx ESR COM

✓x7th **T65.93 Toxic effect of unspecified substance, assault**

✓x7th **T65.94 Toxic effect of unspecified substance, undetermined**

## Other and unspecified effects of external causes (T66-T78)

▶Code also, if applicable, place of occurrence, such as:◀
▶highway rest stop (Y92.523)◀
▶school (private) (public) (state) as the place of occurrence of the external cause (Y92.21-)◀
▶service areas as the place of occurrence of the external cause (Y92.52-)◀
▶single-family non-institutional (private) house as the place of occurrence of the external cause (Y92.Ø1-)◀
▶transport vehicle as the place of occurrence of the external cause (Y92.81-)◀

✓x7th **T66 Radiation sickness, unspecified**

EXCLUDES 1 *specified adverse effects of radiation, such as:*
*radiation gastroenteritis and colitis (K52.Ø)*
*radiation pneumonitis (J7Ø.Ø)*
*radiation related disorders of the skin and subcutaneous tissue (L55-L59)*
*radiation sunburn (L55.-)*
*burns (T2Ø-T31)*
*leukemia (C91-C95)*

The appropriate 7th character is to be added to code T66.
A initial encounter
D subsequent encounter
S sequela

✓4th **T67 Effects of heat and light**

EXCLUDES 1 *erythema [dermatitis] ab igne (L59.Ø)*
*malignant hyperpyrexia due to anesthesia (T88.3)*
*radiation-related disorders of the skin and subcutaneous tissue (L55-L59)*

EXCLUDES 2 *burns (T2Ø-T31)*
*sunburn (L55.-)*
*sweat disorder due to heat (L74-L75)*

The appropriate 7th character is to be added to each code from category T67.
A initial encounter
D subsequent encounter
S sequela

✓5th **T67.Ø Heatstroke and sunstroke**
Use additional code(s) to identify any associated complications of heatstroke, such as:
coma and stupor (R4Ø.-)
rhabdomyolysis (M62.82)
systemic inflammatory response syndrome (R65.1-)
**AHA:** 2019,4Q,17-18
**DEF:** Headache, vertigo, cramps, and elevated body temperature due to prolonged exposure to high environmental temperatures that requires emergency intervention.

✓x7th **T67.Ø1 Heatstroke and sunstroke**
Heat apoplexy
Heat pyrexia
Siriasis
Thermoplegia

✓x7th **T67.Ø2 Exertional heatstroke**

✓x7th **T67.Ø9 Other heatstroke and sunstroke**

√x7th **T67.1 Heat syncope**
Heat collapse

√x7th **T67.2 Heat cramp**

√x7th **T67.3 Heat exhaustion, anhydrotic**
Heat prostration due to water depletion
EXCLUDES 1 *heat exhaustion due to salt depletion (T67.4)*

√x7th **T67.4 Heat exhaustion due to salt depletion**
Heat prostration due to salt (and water) depletion

√x7th **T67.5 Heat exhaustion, unspecified**
Heat prostration NOS

√x7th **T67.6 Heat fatigue, transient**

√x7th **T67.7 Heat edema**

√x7th **T67.8 Other effects of heat and light**

√x7th **T67.9 Effect of heat and light, unspecified**

√x7th **T68 Hypothermia**
Accidental hypothermia
Hypothermia NOS
Use additional code to identify source of exposure:
exposure to excessive cold of man-made origin (W93)
exposure to excessive cold of natural origin (X31)
EXCLUDES 1 *hypothermia following anesthesia (T88.51)*
*hypothermia of newborn (P80.-)*
*hypothermia not associated with low environmental temperature (R68.0)*
EXCLUDES 2 *frostbite (T33-T34)*

The appropriate 7th character is to be added to code T68.
A initial encounter
D subsequent encounter
S sequela

√4th **T69 Other effects of reduced temperature**
Use additional code to identify source of exposure:
exposure to excessive cold of man-made origin (W93)
exposure to excessive cold of natural origin (X31)
EXCLUDES 2 *frostbite (T33-T34)*

The appropriate 7th character is to be added to each code from category T69.
A initial encounter
D subsequent encounter
S sequela

√5th **T69.0 Immersion hand and foot**

√6th **T69.01 Immersion hand**

√7th **T69.011 Immersion hand, right hand**

√7th **T69.012 Immersion hand, left hand**

√7th **T69.019 Immersion hand, unspecified hand**

√6th **T69.02 Immersion foot**
Trench foot

√7th **T69.021 Immersion foot, right foot**

√7th **T69.022 Immersion foot, left foot**

√7th **T69.029 Immersion foot, unspecified foot**

√x7th **T69.1 Chilblains**
**DEF:** Red, swollen, itchy skin primarily affecting the fingers and toes, nose and ears, and legs. Chilblains follows damp-cold exposure, and can also be associated with pruritus and a burning feeling.

√x7th **T69.8 Other specified effects of reduced temperature**

√x7th **T69.9 Effect of reduced temperature, unspecified**

√4th **T70 Effects of air pressure and water pressure**

The appropriate 7th character is to be added to each code from category T70.
A initial encounter
D subsequent encounter
S sequela

√x7th **T70.0 Otitic barotrauma**
Aero-otitis media
Effects of change in ambient atmospheric pressure or water pressure on ears

√x7th **T70.1 Sinus barotrauma**
Aerosinusitis
Effects of change in ambient atmospheric pressure on sinuses

√5th **T70.2 Other and unspecified effects of high altitude**
EXCLUDES 2 *polycythemia due to high altitude (D75.1)*

√x7th **T70.20 Unspecified effects of high altitude**

√x7th **T70.29 Other effects of high altitude**
Alpine sickness
Anoxia due to high altitude
Barotrauma NOS
Hypobaropathy
Mountain sickness

√x7th **T70.3 Caisson disease [decompression sickness]**
Compressed-air disease
Diver's palsy or paralysis
**DEF:** Rapid reduction in air pressure while breathing compressed air. Symptoms include skin lesions, joint pains, and respiratory and neurological problems.

√x7th **T70.4 Effects of high-pressure fluids**
Hydraulic jet injection (industrial)
Pneumatic jet injection (industrial)
Traumatic jet injection (industrial)

√x7th **T70.8 Other effects of air pressure and water pressure**

√x7th **T70.9 Effect of air pressure and water pressure, unspecified**

√4th **T71 Asphyxiation**
Mechanical suffocation
Traumatic suffocation
EXCLUDES 1 *acute respiratory distress (syndrome) (J80)*
*anoxia due to high altitude (T70.2)*
*asphyxia from carbon monoxide (T58.-)*
*asphyxia from inhalation of food or foreign body (T17.-)*
*asphyxia from other gases, fumes and vapors (T59.-)*
*asphyxia NOS (R09.01)*
*respiratory distress (syndrome) in newborn (P22.-)*

The appropriate 7th character is to be added to each code from category T71.
A initial encounter
D subsequent encounter
S sequela

√5th **T71.1 Asphyxiation due to mechanical threat to breathing**
Suffocation due to mechanical threat to breathing

√6th **T71.11 Asphyxiation due to smothering under pillow**

√7th **T71.111 Asphyxiation due to smothering under pillow, accidental**
Asphyxiation due to smothering under pillow NOS

√7th **T71.112 Asphyxiation due to smothering under pillow, intentional self-harm** HCC Rx ESR COM

√7th **T71.113 Asphyxiation due to smothering under pillow, assault**

√7th **T71.114 Asphyxiation due to smothering under pillow, undetermined**

√6th **T71.12 Asphyxiation due to plastic bag**

√7th **T71.121 Asphyxiation due to plastic bag, accidental**
Asphyxiation due to plastic bag NOS

√7th **T71.122 Asphyxiation due to plastic bag, intentional self-harm** HCC Rx ESR COM

√7th **T71.123 Asphyxiation due to plastic bag, assault**

√7th **T71.124 Asphyxiation due to plastic bag, undetermined**

√6th **T71.13 Asphyxiation due to being trapped in bed linens**

√7th **T71.131 Asphyxiation due to being trapped in bed linens, accidental**
Asphyxiation due to being trapped in bed linens NOS

√7th **T71.132 Asphyxiation due to being trapped in bed linens, intentional self-harm** HCC Rx ESR COM

√7th **T71.133 Asphyxiation due to being trapped in bed linens, assault**

√7th **T71.134 Asphyxiation due to being trapped in bed linens, undetermined**

√6th **T71.14 Asphyxiation due to smothering under another person's body (in bed)**

√7th **T71.141 Asphyxiation due to smothering under another person's body (in bed), accidental**
Asphyxiation due to smothering under another person's body (in bed) NOS

√7th **T71.143 Asphyxiation due to smothering under another person's body (in bed), assault**

√7th **T71.144 Asphyxiation due to smothering under another person's body (in bed), undetermined**

- ✓6th **T71.15 Asphyxiation due to smothering in furniture**
  - ✓7th **T71.151 Asphyxiation due to smothering in furniture, accidental**
    Asphyxiation due to smothering in furniture NOS
  - ✓7th **T71.152 Asphyxiation due to smothering in furniture, intentional self-harm** HCC Rx ESR COM
  - ✓7th **T71.153 Asphyxiation due to smothering in furniture, assault**
  - ✓7th **T71.154 Asphyxiation due to smothering in furniture, undetermined**
- ✓6th **T71.16 Asphyxiation due to hanging**
  Hanging by window shade cord
  Use additional code for any associated injuries, such as:
  crushing injury of neck (S17.-)
  fracture of cervical vertebrae (S12.Ø-S12.2-)
  open wound of neck (S11.-)
  - ✓7th **T71.161 Asphyxiation due to hanging, accidental**
    Asphyxiation due to hanging NOS
    Hanging NOS
  - ✓7th **T71.162 Asphyxiation due to hanging, intentional self-harm** HCC Rx ESR COM
  - ✓7th **T71.163 Asphyxiation due to hanging, assault**
  - ✓7th **T71.164 Asphyxiation due to hanging, undetermined**
- ✓6th **T71.19 Asphyxiation due to mechanical threat to breathing due to other causes**
  - ✓7th **T71.191 Asphyxiation due to mechanical threat to breathing due to other causes, accidental**
    Asphyxiation due to other causes NOS
  - ✓7th **T71.192 Asphyxiation due to mechanical threat to breathing due to other causes, intentional self-harm** HCC Rx ESR COM
  - ✓7th **T71.193 Asphyxiation due to mechanical threat to breathing due to other causes, assault**
  - ✓7th **T71.194 Asphyxiation due to mechanical threat to breathing due to other causes, undetermined**

✓5th **T71.2 Asphyxiation due to systemic oxygen deficiency due to low oxygen content in ambient air**
Suffocation due to systemic oxygen deficiency due to low oxygen content in ambient air

- ✓x7th **T71.2Ø Asphyxiation due to systemic oxygen deficiency due to low oxygen content in ambient air due to unspecified cause**
- ✓x7th **T71.21 Asphyxiation due to cave-in or falling earth**
  Use additional code for any associated cataclysm (X34-X38)
- ✓6th **T71.22 Asphyxiation due to being trapped in a car trunk**
  - ✓7th **T71.221 Asphyxiation due to being trapped in a car trunk, accidental**
  - ✓7th **T71.222 Asphyxiation due to being trapped in a car trunk, intentional self-harm** HCC Rx ESR COM
  - ✓7th **T71.223 Asphyxiation due to being trapped in a car trunk, assault**
  - ✓7th **T71.224 Asphyxiation due to being trapped in a car trunk, undetermined**
- ✓6th **T71.23 Asphyxiation due to being trapped in a (discarded) refrigerator**
  - ✓7th **T71.231 Asphyxiation due to being trapped in a (discarded) refrigerator, accidental**
  - ✓7th **T71.232 Asphyxiation due to being trapped in a (discarded) refrigerator, intentional self-harm** HCC Rx ESR COM
  - ✓7th **T71.233 Asphyxiation due to being trapped in a (discarded) refrigerator, assault**
  - ✓7th **T71.234 Asphyxiation due to being trapped in a (discarded) refrigerator, undetermined**
- ✓x7th **T71.29 Asphyxiation due to being trapped in other low oxygen environment**

✓x7th **T71.9 Asphyxiation due to unspecified cause**
Suffocation (by strangulation) due to unspecified cause
Suffocation NOS
Systemic oxygen deficiency due to low oxygen content in ambient air due to unspecified cause
Systemic oxygen deficiency due to mechanical threat to breathing due to unspecified cause
Traumatic asphyxia NOS

✓4th **T73 Effects of other deprivation**

The appropriate 7th character is to be added to each code from category T73.
A initial encounter
D subsequent encounter
S sequela

- ✓x7th **T73.Ø Starvation**
  Deprivation of food
  AHA: 2026,1Q,27
- ✓x7th **T73.1 Deprivation of water**
- ✓x7th **T73.2 Exhaustion due to exposure**
- ✓x7th **T73.3 Exhaustion due to excessive exertion**
  Exhaustion due to overexertion
- ✓x7th **T73.8 Other effects of deprivation**
- ✓x7th **T73.9 Effect of deprivation, unspecified**

✓4th **T74 Adult and child abuse, neglect and other maltreatment, confirmed**
Use additional code, if applicable, to identify any associated current injury
Use additional external cause code to identify perpetrator, if known (YØ7.-)
EXCLUDES 1 *abuse and maltreatment in pregnancy (O9A.3-, O9A.4-, O9A.5-)*
*adult and child maltreatment, suspected (T76.-)*

The appropriate 7th character is to be added to each code from category T74.
A initial encounter
D subsequent encounter
S sequela

- ✓5th **T74.Ø Neglect or abandonment, confirmed**
  - ✓x7th **T74.Ø1 Adult neglect or abandonment, confirmed** A
  - ✓x7th **T74.Ø2 Child neglect or abandonment, confirmed** P
- ✓5th **T74.1 Physical abuse, confirmed**
  EXCLUDES 2 *sexual abuse (T74.2-)*
  - ✓x7th **T74.11 Adult physical abuse, confirmed** A
  - ✓x7th **T74.12 Child physical abuse, confirmed** P
    EXCLUDES 2 *shaken infant syndrome (T74.4)*
- ✓5th **T74.2 Sexual abuse, confirmed**
  Rape, confirmed
  Sexual assault, confirmed
  - ✓x7th **T74.21 Adult sexual abuse, confirmed** A
  - ✓x7th **T74.22 Child sexual abuse, confirmed** P
- ✓5th **T74.3 Psychological abuse, confirmed**
  Bullying and intimidation, confirmed
  Intimidation through social media, confirmed
  Target of threatened harm, confirmed
  Target of threatened physical violence, confirmed
  Target of threatened sexual abuse, confirmed
  - ✓x7th **T74.31 Adult psychological abuse, confirmed** A
  - ✓x7th **T74.32 Child psychological abuse, confirmed** P
- ✓x7th **T74.4 Shaken infant syndrome** P
- ✓5th **T74.5 Forced sexual exploitation, confirmed**
  AHA: 2018,4Q,32-33,65
  - ✓x7th **T74.51 Adult forced sexual exploitation, confirmed** A
  - ✓x7th **T74.52 Child sexual exploitation, confirmed** P
- ✓5th **T74.6 Forced labor exploitation, confirmed**
  AHA: 2018,4Q,32-33,65
  - ✓x7th **T74.61 Adult forced labor exploitation, confirmed** A
  - ✓x7th **T74.62 Child forced labor exploitation, confirmed** P
- ✓5th **T74.9 Unspecified maltreatment, confirmed**
  - ✓x7th **T74.91 Unspecified adult maltreatment, confirmed** A
  - ✓x7th **T74.92 Unspecified child maltreatment, confirmed** P
- ✓5th **T74.A Financial abuse, confirmed**
  AHA: 2023,1Q,4
  - ✓x7th **T74.A1 Adult financial abuse, confirmed** A
  - ✓x7th **T74.A2 Child financial abuse, confirmed** P

**T75 Other and unspecified effects of other external causes**
EXCLUDES 1 *adverse effects NEC (T78.-)*
EXCLUDES 2 *burns (electric) (T20-T31)*
The appropriate 7th character is to be added to each code from category T75.
A initial encounter
D subsequent encounter
S sequela

**T75.0 Effects of lightning**
Struck by lightning
**T75.00 Unspecified effects of lightning**
Struck by lightning NOS
**T75.01 Shock due to being struck by lightning**
**T75.09 Other effects of lightning**
Use additional code for other effects of lightning

**T75.1 Unspecified effects of drowning and nonfatal submersion**
Immersion
EXCLUDES 1 *specified effects of drowning - code to effects*
AHA: 2023,1Q,25

**T75.2 Effects of vibration**
**T75.20 Unspecified effects of vibration**
**T75.21 Pneumatic hammer syndrome**
**T75.22 Traumatic vasospastic syndrome**
**T75.23 Vertigo from infrasound**
EXCLUDES 1 *vertigo NOS (R42)*
**T75.29 Other effects of vibration**

**T75.3 Motion sickness**
Airsickness
Seasickness
Travel sickness
Use additional external cause code to identify vehicle or type of motion (Y92.81-)

**T75.4 Electrocution**
Shock from electric current
Shock from electroshock gun (taser)

**T75.8 Other specified effects of external causes**
**T75.81 Effects of abnormal gravitation [G] forces**
**T75.82 Effects of weightlessness**
**T75.83 Effects of war theater**
Use additional code to identify associated manifestations
**T75.830 Gulf war illness**
Gulf war syndrome
**T75.838 Effects of other war theater**
**T75.89 Other specified effects of external causes**

**T76 Adult and child abuse, neglect and other maltreatment, suspected**
Use additional code, if applicable, to identify any associated current injury
EXCLUDES 1 *adult and child maltreatment, confirmed (T74.-)*
*suspected abuse and maltreatment in pregnancy (O9A.3-, O9A.4-, O9A.5-)*
*suspected adult physical abuse, ruled out (Z04.71)*
*suspected adult sexual abuse, ruled out (Z04.41)*
*suspected child physical abuse, ruled out (Z04.72)*
*suspected child sexual abuse, ruled out (Z04.42)*
AHA: 2018,4Q,72
The appropriate 7th character is to be added to each code from category T76.
A initial encounter
D subsequent encounter
S sequela

**T76.0 Neglect or abandonment, suspected**
**T76.01 Adult neglect or abandonment, suspected** A
**T76.02 Child neglect or abandonment, suspected** P

**T76.1 Physical abuse, suspected**
**T76.11 Adult physical abuse, suspected** A
**T76.12 Child physical abuse, suspected** P
AHA: 2019,2Q,12

**T76.2 Sexual abuse, suspected**
Rape, suspected
EXCLUDES 1 *alleged abuse, ruled out (Z04.7)*
**T76.21 Adult sexual abuse, suspected** A
**T76.22 Child sexual abuse, suspected** P

**T76.3 Psychological abuse, suspected**
Bullying and intimidation, suspected
Intimidation through social media, suspected
Target of threatened harm, suspected
Target of threatened physical violence, suspected
Target of threatened sexual abuse, suspected
**T76.31 Adult psychological abuse, suspected** A
**T76.32 Child psychological abuse, suspected** P

**T76.5 Forced sexual exploitation, suspected**
AHA: 2018,4Q,32-33,65
**T76.51 Adult forced sexual exploitation, suspected** A
**T76.52 Child sexual exploitation, suspected** P

**T76.6 Forced labor exploitation, suspected**
AHA: 2018,4Q,32-33,65
**T76.61 Adult forced labor exploitation, suspected** A
**T76.62 Child forced labor exploitation, suspected** P

**T76.9 Unspecified maltreatment, suspected**
**T76.91 Unspecified adult maltreatment, suspected** A
**T76.92 Unspecified child maltreatment, suspected** P

**T76.A Financial abuse, suspected**
AHA: 2023,1Q,4
**T76.A1 Adult financial abuse, suspected** A
**T76.A2 Child financial abuse, suspected** P

**T78 Adverse effects, not elsewhere classified**
EXCLUDES 2 *complications of surgical and medical care NEC (T80-T88)*
The appropriate 7th character is to be added to each code from category T78.
A initial encounter
D subsequent encounter
S sequela

**T78.0 Anaphylactic reaction due to food**
Anaphylactic reaction due to adverse food reaction
Anaphylactic shock or reaction due to nonpoisonous foods
Anaphylactoid reaction due to food
**T78.00 Anaphylactic reaction due to unspecified food**
**T78.01 Anaphylactic reaction due to peanuts**
**T78.02 Anaphylactic reaction due to shellfish (crustaceans)**
**T78.03 Anaphylactic reaction due to other fish**
**T78.04 Anaphylactic reaction due to fruits and vegetables**
**T78.05 Anaphylactic reaction due to tree nuts and seeds**
EXCLUDES 2 *anaphylactic reaction due to peanuts (T78.01)*
**T78.06 Anaphylactic reaction due to food additives**
**T78.07 Anaphylactic reaction due to milk and dairy products**
**T78.070 Anaphylactic reaction due to milk and dairy products with tolerance to baked milk**
EXCLUDES 1 *Anaphylactic reaction due to milk and dairy products with reactivity to baked milk (T78.071)*
**T78.071 Anaphylactic reaction due to milk and dairy products with reactivity to baked milk**
EXCLUDES 1 *Anaphylactic reaction due to milk and dairy products with tolerance to baked milk (T78.070)*
**T78.079 Anaphylactic reaction due to milk and dairy products, unspecified**
**T78.08 Anaphylactic reaction due to eggs**
**T78.080 Anaphylactic reaction due to egg with tolerance to baked egg**
EXCLUDES 1 *Anaphylactic reaction due to egg with reactivity to baked egg (T78.081)*
**T78.081 Anaphylactic reaction due to egg with reactivity to baked egg**
EXCLUDES 1 *Anaphylactic reaction due to egg with tolerance to baked egg (T78.080)*
**T78.089 Anaphylactic reaction due to eggs, unspecified**

√x7th **T78.Ø9 Anaphylactic reaction due to other food products**

√5th **T78.1 Other adverse food reactions, not elsewhere classified**

Use additional code to identify the type of reaction, if applicable

EXCLUDES 1 *anaphylactic reaction or shock due to adverse food reaction (T78.Ø-)*
*anaphylactic reaction due to food (T78.Ø-)*
*bacterial food borne intoxications (AØ5.-)*

EXCLUDES 2 *allergic and dietetic gastroenteritis and colitis (K52.29)*
*allergic rhinitis due to food (J3Ø.5)*
*dermatitis due to food in contact with skin (L23.6, L24.6, L25.4)*
*dermatitis due to ingested food (L27.2)*
*food protein-induced enterocolitis syndrome (K52.21)*
*food protein-induced enteropathy (K52.22)*

√6th **T78.11 Other adverse food reactions due to milk and dairy products**

√7th **T78.11Ø Other adverse food reactions due to milk and dairy products with tolerance to baked milk**

EXCLUDES 1 *Other adverse food reaction due to milk and dairy products with reactivity to baked milk (T78.111)*

√7th **T78.111 Other adverse food reaction due to milk and dairy products with reactivity to baked milk**

EXCLUDES 1 *Other adverse food reaction due to milk and dairy products with tolerance to baked milk (T78.11Ø)*

√7th **T78.119 Other adverse food reaction due to milk and dairy products with baked milk tolerance/reactivity, unspecified**

√6th **T78.12 Other adverse food reaction due to eggs**

√7th **T78.12Ø Other adverse food reaction due to egg with tolerance to baked egg**

EXCLUDES 1 *Other adverse food reaction due to egg with reactivity to baked egg (T78.121)*

√7th **T78.121 Other adverse food reaction due to egg with reactivity to baked egg**

EXCLUDES 1 *Other adverse food reaction due to egg with tolerance to baked egg (T78.12Ø)*

√7th **T78.129 Other adverse food reaction due to egg with baked egg tolerance/reactivity, unspecified**

√x7th **T78.19 Other adverse food reactions, not elsewhere classified**

√x7th **T78.2 Anaphylactic shock, unspecified**

Allergic shock
Anaphylactic reaction
Anaphylaxis

EXCLUDES 1 *anaphylactic reaction or shock due to adverse effect of correct medicinal substance properly administered (T88.6)*
*anaphylactic reaction or shock due to adverse food reaction (T78.Ø-)*
*anaphylactic reaction or shock due to serum (T8Ø.5-)*

√x7th **T78.3 Angioneurotic edema**

Allergic angioedema
Giant urticaria
Quincke's edema

EXCLUDES 1 *serum urticaria (T8Ø.6-)*
*urticaria (L5Ø.-)*

√5th **T78.4 Other and unspecified allergy**

EXCLUDES 1 *specified types of allergic reaction such as:*
*allergic diarrhea (K52.29)*
*allergic gastroenteritis and colitis (K52.29)*
*dermatitis (L23-L25, L27.-)*
*food protein-induced enterocolitis syndrome (K52.21)*
*food protein-induced enteropathy (K52.22)*
*hay fever (J3Ø.1)*

√x7th **T78.4Ø Allergy, unspecified**

Allergic reaction NOS
Hypersensitivity NOS

√x7th **T78.41 Arthus phenomenon**

Arthus reaction

√x7th **T78.49 Other allergy**

**AHA:** 2021,1Q,42

√x7th **T78.8 Other adverse effects, not elsewhere classified**

## Certain early complications of trauma (T79)

√4th **T79 Certain early complications of trauma, not elsewhere classified**

EXCLUDES 2 *acute respiratory distress syndrome (J8Ø)*
*complications occurring during or following medical procedures (T8Ø-T88)*
*complications of surgical and medical care NEC (T8Ø-T88)*
*newborn respiratory distress syndrome (P22.Ø)*

The appropriate 7th character is to be added to each code from category T79.
A initial encounter
D subsequent encounter
S sequela

√x7th **T79.Ø Air embolism (traumatic)** HCC ESR COM

EXCLUDES 1 *air embolism complicating abortion or ectopic or molar pregnancy (OØØ-OØ7, OØ8.2)*
*air embolism complicating pregnancy, childbirth and the puerperium (O88.Ø)*
*air embolism following infusion, transfusion, and therapeutic injection (T8Ø.Ø)*
*air embolism following procedure NEC (T81.7-)*

**DEF:** Arterial or venous obstruction due to the introduction of air bubbles into the blood vessels following surgery or trauma.

√x7th **T79.1 Fat embolism (traumatic)** HCC ESR COM

EXCLUDES 1 *fat embolism complicating:*
*abortion or ectopic or molar pregnancy (OØØ-OØ7, OØ8.2)*
*pregnancy, childbirth and the puerperium (O88.8)*

**DEF:** Arterial blockage due to the entrance of fat into the circulatory system after a fracture of the large bones or administration of corticosteroids.

√x7th **T79.2 Traumatic secondary and recurrent hemorrhage and seroma** ESR

√x7th **T79.4 Traumatic shock** HCC ESR COM

Shock (immediate) (delayed) following injury

EXCLUDES 1 *anaphylactic shock due to adverse food reaction (T78.Ø-)*
*anaphylactic shock due to correct medicinal substance properly administered (T88.6)*
*anaphylactic shock due to serum (T8Ø.5-)*
*anaphylactic shock NOS (T78.2)*
*electric shock (T75.4)*
*nontraumatic shock NEC (R57.-)*
*obstetric shock (O75.1)*
*postprocedural shock (T81.1-)*
*septic shock (R65.21)*
*shock complicating abortion or ectopic or molar pregnancy (OØØ-OØ7, OØ8.3)*
*shock due to anesthesia (T88.2)*
*shock due to lightning (T75.Ø1)*
*shock NOS (R57.9)*

√x7th **T79.5 Traumatic anuria** ESR

Crush syndrome
Renal failure following crushing

√x7th **T79.6 Traumatic ischemia of muscle** ESR

Traumatic rhabdomyolysis
Volkmann's ischemic contracture

EXCLUDES 2 *anterior tibial syndrome (M76.8)*
*compartment syndrome (traumatic) (T79.A-)*
*nontraumatic ischemia of muscle (M62.2-)*

**AHA:** 2019,2Q,12

√x7th **T79.7 Traumatic subcutaneous emphysema** ESR

EXCLUDES 2 *emphysema NOS (J43)*
*emphysema (subcutaneous) resulting from a procedure (T81.82)*

√5th **T79.A Traumatic compartment syndrome**

EXCLUDES 1 *fibromyalgia (M79.7)*
*nontraumatic compartment syndrome (M79.A-)*

EXCLUDES 2 *traumatic ischemic infarction of muscle (T79.6)*

**DEF:** Compression of nerves and blood vessels within an enclosed muscle space due to previous trauma, which leads to impaired blood flow and muscle and nerve damage.

√x7th **T79.AØ Compartment syndrome, unspecified** ESR
Compartment syndrome NOS

√6th **T79.A1 Traumatic compartment syndrome of upper extremity**
Traumatic compartment syndrome of shoulder, arm, forearm, wrist, hand, and fingers

√7th **T79.A11 Traumatic compartment syndrome of right upper extremity** ESR

√7th **T79.A12 Traumatic compartment syndrome of left upper extremity** ESR

√7th **T79.A19 Traumatic compartment syndrome of unspecified upper extremity** ESR

√6th **T79.A2 Traumatic compartment syndrome of lower extremity**
Traumatic compartment syndrome of hip, buttock, thigh, leg, foot, and toes

√7th **T79.A21 Traumatic compartment syndrome of right lower extremity** ESR

√7th **T79.A22 Traumatic compartment syndrome of left lower extremity** ESR

√7th **T79.A29 Traumatic compartment syndrome of unspecified lower extremity** ESR

√x7th **T79.A3 Traumatic compartment syndrome of abdomen** ESR

√x7th **T79.A9 Traumatic compartment syndrome of other sites** ESR

√x7th **T79.8 Other early complications of trauma** ESR

√x7th **T79.9 Unspecified early complication of trauma** ESR

## Complications of surgical and medical care, not elsewhere classified (T8Ø-T88)

Use additional code for adverse effect, if applicable, to identify drug (T36-T5Ø with fifth or sixth character 5)
Use additional code(s) to identify the specified condition resulting from the complication
Use additional code to identify devices involved and details of circumstances (Y62-Y82)

EXCLUDES 2 *any encounters with medical care for postprocedural conditions in which no complications are present, such as:*
*artificial opening status (Z93.-)*
*closure of external stoma (Z43.-)*
*fitting and adjustment of external prosthetic device (Z44.-)*
*burns and corrosions from local applications and irradiation (T2Ø-T32)*
*complications of surgical procedures during pregnancy, childbirth and the puerperium (OØØ-O9A)*
*mechanical complication of respirator [ventilator] (J95.85Ø)*
*poisoning and toxic effects of drugs and chemicals (T36-T65 with fifth or sixth character 1-4 or 6)*
*postprocedural fever (R5Ø.82)*
*specified complications classified elsewhere, such as:*
*cerebrospinal fluid leak from spinal puncture (G97.Ø)*
*colostomy malfunction (K94.Ø-)*
*disorders of fluid and electrolyte imbalance (E86-E87)*
*functional disturbances following cardiac surgery (I97.Ø-I97.1)*
*intraoperative and postprocedural complications of specified body systems (D78.-, E36.-, E89.-, G97.3-, G97.4, H59.3-, H59.-, H95.2-, H95.3, I97.4-, I97.5, J95.6-, J95.7, K91.6-, L76.-, M96.-, N99.-)*
*ostomy complications (J95.Ø-, K94.-, N99.5-)*
*postgastric surgery syndromes (K91.1)*
*postlaminectomy syndrome NEC (M96.1)*
*postmastectomy lymphedema syndrome (I97.2)*
*postsurgical blind-loop syndrome (K91.2)*
*ventilator associated pneumonia (J95.851)*

**AHA:** 2015,1Q,15

√4th **T8Ø Complications following infusion, transfusion and therapeutic injection**

INCLUDES complications following perfusion

EXCLUDES 2 *bone marrow transplant rejection (T86.Ø1)*
*febrile nonhemolytic transfusion reaction (R5Ø.84)*
*fluid overload due to transfusion (E87.71)*
*posttransfusion purpura (D69.51)*
*transfusion (red blood cell) associated hemochromatosis (E83.111)*
*transfusion associated circulatory overload (TACO) (E87.71)*
*transfusion related acute lung injury (TRALI) (J95.84)*

The appropriate 7th character is to be added to each code from category T8Ø.
A initial encounter
D subsequent encounter
S sequela

√x7th **T8Ø.Ø Air embolism following infusion, transfusion and therapeutic injection**

√x7th **T8Ø.1 Vascular complications following infusion, transfusion and therapeutic injection**
Use additional code to identify the vascular complication

EXCLUDES 2 *extravasation of vesicant agent (T8Ø.81-)*
*infiltration of vesicant agent (T8Ø.81-)*
*postprocedural vascular complications (T81.7-)*
*vascular complications specified as due to prosthetic devices, implants and grafts (T82.8-, T83.8-, T84.8-, T85.8-)*



Chapter 19. Injury, Poisoning and Certain Other Consequences of External Causes
T79.A–T8Ø.1

√5th **T80.2 Infections following infusion, transfusion and therapeutic injection**

Use additional code (R65.2-) to identify severe sepsis, if applicable
Use additional code to identify the specific infection, such as:
sepsis (A41.9)

EXCLUDES 2 *infections specified as due to prosthetic devices, implants and grafts (T82.6-T82.7, T83.5-T83.6, T84.5-T84.7, T85.7)*
*postprocedural infections (T81.4-)*

**AHA:** 2018,4Q,62

√6th **T80.21 Infection due to central venous catheter**

Infection due to pulmonary artery catheter (Swan-Ganz catheter)

**AHA:** 2019,1Q,13-14

**DEF:** Central venous catheter: Catheter positioned in the superior vena cava or right atrium and introduced through a large vein, such as the jugular or subclavian, and used to measure venous pressure or administer fluids or medication.

**TIP:** Code assignment is based on the location of the catheter and not how the catheter is being used; for example, for hemodialysis. Infections resulting from catheters that are not central lines should be coded to T82.7-.

√7th **T80.211 Bloodstream infection due to central venous catheter**

Bloodstream infection due to Hickman catheter
Bloodstream infection due to peripherally inserted central catheter (PICC)
Bloodstream infection due to portacath (port-a-cath)
Bloodstream infection due to pulmonary artery catheter
Bloodstream infection due to triple lumen catheter
Bloodstream infection due to umbilical venous catheter
Catheter-related bloodstream infection (CRBSI) NOS
Central line-associated bloodstream infection (CLABSI)

**AHA:** 2019,1Q,13,14; 2018,4Q,89

√7th **T80.212 Local infection due to central venous catheter**

Exit or insertion site infection
Local infection due to Hickman catheter
Local infection due to peripherally inserted central catheter (PICC)
Local infection due to portacath (port-a-cath)
Local infection due to pulmonary artery catheter
Local infection due to triple lumen catheter
Local infection due to umbilical venous catheter
Port or reservoir infection
Tunnel infection

√7th **T80.218 Other infection due to central venous catheter**

Other central line-associated infection
Other infection due to Hickman catheter
Other infection due to peripherally inserted central catheter (PICC)
Other infection due to portacath (port-a-cath)
Other infection due to pulmonary artery catheter
Other infection due to triple lumen catheter
Other infection due to umbilical venous catheter

√7th **T80.219 Unspecified infection due to central venous catheter**

Central line-associated infection NOS
Unspecified infection due to Hickman catheter
Unspecified infection due to peripherally inserted central catheter (PICC)
Unspecified infection due to portacath (port-a-cath)
Unspecified infection due to pulmonary artery catheter
Unspecified infection due to triple lumen catheter
Unspecified infection due to umbilical venous catheter

√x7th **T80.22 Acute infection following transfusion, infusion, or injection of blood and blood products**

√x7th **T80.29 Infection following other infusion, transfusion and therapeutic injection**

√5th **T80.3 ABO incompatibility reaction due to transfusion of blood or blood products**

EXCLUDES 1 *minor blood group antigens reactions (Duffy) (E) (K) (Kell) (Kidd) (Lewis) (M) (N) (P) (S) (T80.A-)*

√x7th **T80.30 ABO incompatibility reaction due to transfusion of blood or blood products, unspecified**

ABO incompatibility blood transfusion NOS
Reaction to ABO incompatibility from transfusion NOS

√6th **T80.31 ABO incompatibility with hemolytic transfusion reaction**

√7th **T80.310 ABO incompatibility with acute hemolytic transfusion reaction**

ABO incompatibility with hemolytic transfusion reaction less than 24 hours after transfusion
Acute hemolytic transfusion reaction (AHTR) due to ABO incompatibility

√7th **T80.311 ABO incompatibility with delayed hemolytic transfusion reaction**

ABO incompatibility with hemolytic transfusion reaction 24 hours or more after transfusion
Delayed hemolytic transfusion reaction (DHTR) due to ABO incompatibility

√7th **T80.319 ABO incompatibility with hemolytic transfusion reaction, unspecified**

ABO incompatibility with hemolytic transfusion reaction at unspecified time after transfusion
Hemolytic transfusion reaction (HTR) due to ABO incompatibility NOS

√x7th **T80.39 Other ABO incompatibility reaction due to transfusion of blood or blood products**

Delayed serologic transfusion reaction (DSTR) from ABO incompatibility
Other ABO incompatible blood transfusion
Other reaction to ABO incompatible blood transfusion

√5th **T80.4 Rh incompatibility reaction due to transfusion of blood or blood products**

Reaction due to incompatibility of Rh antigens (C) (c) (D) (E) (e)

√x7th **T80.40 Rh incompatibility reaction due to transfusion of blood or blood products, unspecified**

Reaction due to Rh factor in transfusion NOS
Rh incompatible blood transfusion NOS

√6th **T80.41 Rh incompatibility with hemolytic transfusion reaction**

√7th **T80.410 Rh incompatibility with acute hemolytic transfusion reaction**

Acute hemolytic transfusion reaction (AHTR) due to Rh incompatibility
Rh incompatibility with hemolytic transfusion reaction less than 24 hours after transfusion

√7th **T80.411 Rh incompatibility with delayed hemolytic transfusion reaction**

Delayed hemolytic transfusion reaction (DHTR) due to Rh incompatibility
Rh incompatibility with hemolytic transfusion reaction 24 hours or more after transfusion

√7th **T80.419 Rh incompatibility with hemolytic transfusion reaction, unspecified**
Hemolytic transfusion reaction (HTR) due to Rh incompatibility NOS
Rh incompatibility with hemolytic transfusion reaction at unspecified time after transfusion

√x7th **T80.49 Other Rh incompatibility reaction due to transfusion of blood or blood products**
Delayed serologic transfusion reaction (DSTR) from Rh incompatibility
Other reaction to Rh incompatible blood transfusion

√5th **T80.A Non-ABO incompatibility reaction due to transfusion of blood or blood products**
Reaction due to incompatibility of minor antigens (Duffy) (Kell) (Kidd) (Lewis) (M) (N) (P) (S)

√x7th **T80.A0 Non-ABO incompatibility reaction due to transfusion of blood or blood products, unspecified**
Non-ABO antigen incompatibility reaction from transfusion NOS

√6th **T80.A1 Non-ABO incompatibility with hemolytic transfusion reaction**

√7th **T80.A10 Non-ABO incompatibility with acute hemolytic transfusion reaction**
Acute hemolytic transfusion reaction (AHTR) due to non-ABO incompatibility
Non-ABO incompatibility with hemolytic transfusion reaction less than 24 hours after transfusion

√7th **T80.A11 Non-ABO incompatibility with delayed hemolytic transfusion reaction**
Delayed hemolytic transfusion reaction (DHTR) due to non-ABO incompatibility
Non-ABO incompatibility with hemolytic transfusion reaction 24 or more hours after transfusion

√7th **T80.A19 Non-ABO incompatibility with hemolytic transfusion reaction, unspecified**
Hemolytic transfusion reaction (HTR) due to non-ABO incompatibility NOS
Non-ABO incompatibility with hemolytic transfusion reaction at unspecified time after transfusion

√x7th **T80.A9 Other non-ABO incompatibility reaction due to transfusion of blood or blood products**
Delayed serologic transfusion reaction (DSTR) from non-ABO incompatibility
Other reaction to non-ABO incompatible blood transfusion

√5th **T80.5 Anaphylactic reaction due to serum**
Allergic shock due to serum
Anaphylactic shock due to serum
Anaphylactoid reaction due to serum
Anaphylaxis due to serum
EXCLUDES 1 *ABO incompatibility reaction due to transfusion of blood or blood products (T80.3-)*
*allergic reaction or shock NOS (T78.2)*
*anaphylactic reaction or shock due to adverse effect of correct medicinal substance properly administered (T88.6)*
*anaphylactic reaction or shock NOS (T78.2)*
*other serum reaction (T80.6-)*
**DEF:** Life-threatening hypersensitivity to a foreign serum causing respiratory distress, vascular collapse, and shock.

√x7th **T80.51 Anaphylactic reaction due to administration of blood and blood products**

√x7th **T80.52 Anaphylactic reaction due to vaccination**
**AHA:** 2021,1Q,43

√x7th **T80.59 Anaphylactic reaction due to other serum**

√5th **T80.6 Other serum reactions**
Intoxication by serum
Protein sickness
Serum rash
Serum sickness
Serum urticaria
EXCLUDES 2 *serum hepatitis (B16-B19)*
**DEF:** Serum sickness: Hypersensitivity to a foreign serum that causes fever, hives, swelling, and lymphadenopathy.

√x7th **T80.61 Other serum reaction due to administration of blood and blood products**

√x7th **T80.62 Other serum reaction due to vaccination**
**AHA:** 2021,1Q,42

√x7th **T80.69 Other serum reaction due to other serum**
Code also, if applicable, arthropathy in hypersensitivity reactions classified elsewhere (M36.4)

√5th **T80.8 Other complications following infusion, transfusion and therapeutic injection**

√6th **T80.81 Extravasation of vesicant agent**
Infiltration of vesicant agent

√7th **T80.810 Extravasation of vesicant antineoplastic chemotherapy**
Infiltration of vesicant antineoplastic chemotherapy

√7th **T80.818 Extravasation of other vesicant agent**
Infiltration of other vesicant agent

√x7th **T80.82 Complication of immune effector cellular therapy**
Complication of chimeric antigen receptor (CAR-T) cell therapy
Complication of IEC therapy
Use additional code to identify the specific complication, such as:
cytokine release syndrome (D89.83-)
immune effector cell-associated neurotoxicity syndrome (G92.0-)
EXCLUDES 2 *adverse effect of immune checkpoint inhibitors and immunostimulant drugs (T45.AX5)*
*complication of bone marrow transplant (T86.0)*
*complication of stem cell transplant (T86.5)*
**AHA:** 2025,3Q,21; 2021,4Q,31

√x7th **T80.89 Other complications following infusion, transfusion and therapeutic injection**
Delayed serologic transfusion reaction (DSTR), unspecified incompatibility
Use additional code to identify graft-versus-host reaction, if applicable, (D89.81-)
**AHA:** 2020,4Q,14

√5th **T80.9 Unspecified complication following infusion, transfusion and therapeutic injection**

√x7th **T80.90 Unspecified complication following infusion and therapeutic injection**

√6th **T80.91 Hemolytic transfusion reaction, unspecified incompatibility**
EXCLUDES 1 *ABO incompatibility with hemolytic transfusion reaction (T80.31-)*
*non-ABO incompatibility with hemolytic transfusion reaction (T80.A1-)*
*Rh incompatibility with hemolytic transfusion reaction (T80.41-)*

√7th **T80.910 Acute hemolytic transfusion reaction, unspecified incompatibility**

√7th **T80.911 Delayed hemolytic transfusion reaction, unspecified incompatibility**

√7th **T80.919 Hemolytic transfusion reaction, unspecified incompatibility, unspecified as acute or delayed**
Hemolytic transfusion reaction NOS

√x7th **T80.92 Unspecified transfusion reaction**
Transfusion reaction NOS

✓4th **T81 Complications of procedures, not elsewhere classified**

Use additional code for adverse effect, if applicable, to identify drug (T36-T5Ø with fifth or sixth character 5)

EXCLUDES 2 *complications following immunization (T88.Ø-T88.1)*
*complications following infusion, transfusion and therapeutic injection (T8Ø.-)*
*complications of transplanted organs and tissue (T86.-)*
*specified complications classified elsewhere, such as:*
*complication of prosthetic devices, implants and grafts (T82-T85)*
*dermatitis due to drugs and medicaments (L23.3, L24.4, L25.1, L27.Ø-L27.1)*
*endosseous dental implant failure (M27.6-)*
*floppy iris syndrome (IFIS) (intraoperative) (H21.81)*
*intraoperative and postprocedural complications of specific body system (D78.-, E36.-, E89.-, G97.3-, G97.4, H59.3-, H59.-, H95.2-, H95.3, I97.4-, I97.5, J95, K91.-, L76.-, M96.-, N99.-)*
*ostomy complications (J95.Ø-, K94.-, N99.5-)*
*plateau iris syndrome (post-iridectomy) (postprocedural) H21.82*
*poisoning and toxic effects of drugs and chemicals (T36-T65 with fifth or sixth character 1-4)*

**AHA:** 2019,2Q,21

The appropriate 7th character is to be added to each code from category T81.
A initial encounter
D subsequent encounter
S sequela

✓5th **T81.1 Postprocedural shock**

Shock during or resulting from a procedure, not elsewhere classified

EXCLUDES 1 *anaphylactic shock NOS (T78.2)*
*anaphylactic shock due to correct substance properly administered (T88.6)*
*anaphylactic shock due to serum (T8Ø.5-)*
*electric shock (T75.4)*
*obstetric shock (O75.1)*
*shock due to anesthesia (T88.2)*
*shock following abortion or ectopic or molar pregnancy (OØØ-OØ7, OØ8.3)*
*traumatic shock (T79.4)*

**AHA:** 2021,1Q,13

✓x7th **T81.1Ø Postprocedural shock unspecified**
Collapse NOS during or resulting from a procedure, not elsewhere classified
Postprocedural failure of peripheral circulation
Postprocedural shock NOS

✓x7th **T81.11 Postprocedural cardiogenic shock** ESR

✓x7th **T81.12 Postprocedural septic shock** ESR UPD
Postprocedural endotoxic shock resulting from a procedure, not elsewhere classified
Postprocedural gram-negative shock resulting from a procedure, not elsewhere classified
Code first underlying infection
Use additional code, to identify any associated acute organ dysfunction, if applicable
**AHA:** 2018,4Q,63

✓x7th **T81.19 Other postprocedural shock**
Postprocedural hypovolemic shock

✓5th **T81.3 Disruption of wound, not elsewhere classified**

Disruption of any suture materials or other closure methods

EXCLUDES 1 *breakdown (mechanical) of permanent sutures (T85.612)*
*displacement of permanent sutures (T85.622)*
*disruption of cesarean delivery wound (O9Ø.Ø)*
*disruption of perineal obstetric wound (O9Ø.1)*
*mechanical complication of permanent sutures NEC (T85.692)*

**AHA:** 2014,1Q,23

✓x7th **T81.3Ø Disruption of wound, unspecified**
Disruption of wound NOS

✓x7th **T81.31 Disruption of external operation (surgical) wound, not elsewhere classified**
Dehiscence of operation wound NOS
Disruption of operation wound NOS
Disruption or dehiscence of closure of cornea
Disruption or dehiscence of closure of mucosa
Disruption or dehiscence of closure of skin and subcutaneous tissue
Full-thickness skin disruption or dehiscence
Superficial disruption or dehiscence of operation wound
EXCLUDES 1 *dehiscence of amputation stump (T87.81)*

✓6th **T81.32 Disruption of internal operation (surgical) wound, not elsewhere classified**
**AHA:** 2024,4Q,29-30; 2020,2Q,22; 2017,3Q,4

✓7th **T81.32Ø Disruption or dehiscence of gastrointestinal tract anastomosis, repair, or closure**

✓7th **T81.321 Disruption or dehiscence of closure of internal operation (surgical) wound of abdominal wall muscle or fascia**

✓7th **T81.328 Disruption or dehiscence of closure of other specified internal operation (surgical) wound**
Disruption or dehiscence of closure of muscle or muscle flap (other than abdominal wall muscle)
Disruption or dehiscence of closure of ribs or rib cage
Disruption or dehiscence of closure of skull or craniotomy
Disruption or dehiscence of closure of sternum or sternotomy
Disruption or dehiscence of closure of superficial or muscular fascia (other than abdominal wall fascia)
Disruption or dehiscence of closure of tendon or ligament

✓7th **T81.329 Deep disruption or dehiscence of operation wound, unspecified**
Deep disruption or dehiscence of operation wound NOS

✓x7th **T81.33 Disruption of traumatic injury wound repair**
Disruption or dehiscence of closure of traumatic laceration (external) (internal)

✓5th **T81.4 Infection following a procedure**

Wound abscess following a procedure
Code also, if applicable, disruption of internal operation (surgical) wound (T81.32-)
Use additional code (R65.2-) to identify severe sepsis, if applicable
Use additional code to identify infection

EXCLUDES 2 *bleb associated endophthalmitis (H59.4-)*
*infection due to infusion, transfusion and therapeutic injection (T8Ø.2-)*
*infection due to prosthetic devices, implants and grafts (T82.6-T82.7, T83.5-T83.6, T84.5-T84.7, T85.7)*
*obstetric surgical wound infection (O86.Ø-)*
*postprocedural fever NOS (R5Ø.82)*
*postprocedural retroperitoneal abscess (K68.11)*

**AHA:** 2024,1Q,19; 2018,4Q,33-34,62; 2014,1Q,23

✓x7th **T81.4Ø Infection following a procedure, unspecified**

✓x7th **T81.41 Infection following a procedure, superficial incisional surgical site**
Stitch abscess following a procedure
Subcutaneous abscess following a procedure

✓x7th **T81.42 Infection following a procedure, deep incisional surgical site**
Intra-muscular abscess following a procedure

✓x7th **T81.43 Infection following a procedure, organ and space surgical site**
Intra-abdominal abscess following a procedure
Subphrenic abscess following a procedure

✓x7th **T81.44 Sepsis following a procedure** ESR COM
Use additional code to identify the sepsis

✓x7th **T81.49 Infection following a procedure, other surgical site**

✓5th **T81.5 Complications of foreign body accidentally left in body following procedure**

**AHA:** 2014,4Q,24

✓6th **T81.5Ø Unspecified complication of foreign body accidentally left in body following procedure**

✓7th **T81.5ØØ Unspecified complication of foreign body accidentally left in body following surgical operation**

√7th **T81.501** Unspecified complication of foreign body accidentally left in body following infusion or transfusion

√7th **T81.502** Unspecified complication of foreign body accidentally left in body following kidney dialysis Rx ESR

√7th **T81.503** Unspecified complication of foreign body accidentally left in body following injection or immunization

√7th **T81.504** Unspecified complication of foreign body accidentally left in body following endoscopic examination

√7th **T81.505** Unspecified complication of foreign body accidentally left in body following heart catheterization

√7th **T81.506** Unspecified complication of foreign body accidentally left in body following aspiration, puncture or other catheterization

√7th **T81.507** Unspecified complication of foreign body accidentally left in body following removal of catheter or packing

√7th **T81.508** Unspecified complication of foreign body accidentally left in body following other procedure

√7th **T81.509** Unspecified complication of foreign body accidentally left in body following unspecified procedure

√6th **T81.51** Adhesions due to foreign body accidentally left in body following procedure

√7th **T81.510** Adhesions due to foreign body accidentally left in body following surgical operation

√7th **T81.511** Adhesions due to foreign body accidentally left in body following infusion or transfusion

√7th **T81.512** Adhesions due to foreign body accidentally left in body following kidney dialysis Rx ESR

√7th **T81.513** Adhesions due to foreign body accidentally left in body following injection or immunization

√7th **T81.514** Adhesions due to foreign body accidentally left in body following endoscopic examination

√7th **T81.515** Adhesions due to foreign body accidentally left in body following heart catheterization

√7th **T81.516** Adhesions due to foreign body accidentally left in body following aspiration, puncture or other catheterization

√7th **T81.517** Adhesions due to foreign body accidentally left in body following removal of catheter or packing

√7th **T81.518** Adhesions due to foreign body accidentally left in body following other procedure

√7th **T81.519** Adhesions due to foreign body accidentally left in body following unspecified procedure

√6th **T81.52** Obstruction due to foreign body accidentally left in body following procedure

√7th **T81.520** Obstruction due to foreign body accidentally left in body following surgical operation

√7th **T81.521** Obstruction due to foreign body accidentally left in body following infusion or transfusion

√7th **T81.522** Obstruction due to foreign body accidentally left in body following kidney dialysis Rx ESR

√7th **T81.523** Obstruction due to foreign body accidentally left in body following injection or immunization

√7th **T81.524** Obstruction due to foreign body accidentally left in body following endoscopic examination

√7th **T81.525** Obstruction due to foreign body accidentally left in body following heart catheterization

√7th **T81.526** Obstruction due to foreign body accidentally left in body following aspiration, puncture or other catheterization

√7th **T81.527** Obstruction due to foreign body accidentally left in body following removal of catheter or packing

√7th **T81.528** Obstruction due to foreign body accidentally left in body following other procedure

√7th **T81.529** Obstruction due to foreign body accidentally left in body following unspecified procedure

√6th **T81.53** Perforation due to foreign body accidentally left in body following procedure

√7th **T81.530** Perforation due to foreign body accidentally left in body following surgical operation

√7th **T81.531** Perforation due to foreign body accidentally left in body following infusion or transfusion

√7th **T81.532** Perforation due to foreign body accidentally left in body following kidney dialysis Rx ESR

√7th **T81.533** Perforation due to foreign body accidentally left in body following injection or immunization

√7th **T81.534** Perforation due to foreign body accidentally left in body following endoscopic examination

√7th **T81.535** Perforation due to foreign body accidentally left in body following heart catheterization

√7th **T81.536** Perforation due to foreign body accidentally left in body following aspiration, puncture or other catheterization

√7th **T81.537** Perforation due to foreign body accidentally left in body following removal of catheter or packing

√7th **T81.538** Perforation due to foreign body accidentally left in body following other procedure

√7th **T81.539** Perforation due to foreign body accidentally left in body following unspecified procedure

√6th **T81.59** Other complications of foreign body accidentally left in body following procedure

EXCLUDES 2 *obstruction or perforation due to prosthetic devices and implants intentionally left in body (T82.0-T82.5, T83.0-T83.4, T83.7, T84.0-T84.4, T85.0-T85.6)*

√7th **T81.590** Other complications of foreign body accidentally left in body following surgical operation

AHA: 2025,2Q,10

√7th **T81.591** Other complications of foreign body accidentally left in body following infusion or transfusion

√7th **T81.592** Other complications of foreign body accidentally left in body following kidney dialysis Rx ESR

√7th **T81.593** Other complications of foreign body accidentally left in body following injection or immunization

√7th **T81.594** Other complications of foreign body accidentally left in body following endoscopic examination

√7th **T81.595** Other complications of foreign body accidentally left in body following heart catheterization

√7th **T81.596** Other complications of foreign body accidentally left in body following aspiration, puncture or other catheterization

√7th **T81.597** Other complications of foreign body accidentally left in body following removal of catheter or packing

√7th **T81.598** Other complications of foreign body accidentally left in body following other procedure

√7th **T81.599** Other complications of foreign body accidentally left in body following unspecified procedure

√5th **T81.6** Acute reaction to foreign substance accidentally left during a procedure

EXCLUDES 2 *complications of foreign body accidentally left in body cavity or operation wound following procedure (T81.5-)*

√x7th **T81.60** Unspecified acute reaction to foreign substance accidentally left during a procedure

√x7th **T81.61 Aseptic peritonitis due to foreign substance accidentally left during a procedure**
Chemical peritonitis

√x7th **T81.69 Other acute reaction to foreign substance accidentally left during a procedure**

√5th **T81.7 Vascular complications following a procedure, not elsewhere classified**
Air embolism following procedure NEC
Phlebitis or thrombophlebitis resulting from a procedure
EXCLUDES 1 *embolism complicating abortion or ectopic or molar pregnancy (O00-O07, O08.2)*
*embolism complicating pregnancy, childbirth and the puerperium (O88.-)*
*traumatic embolism (T79.0)*
EXCLUDES 2 *embolism due to prosthetic devices, implants and grafts (T82.8-, T83.81, T84.8-, T85.81-)*
*embolism following infusion, transfusion and therapeutic injection (T80.0)*
**AHA:** 2019,2Q,22

√6th **T81.71 Complication of artery following a procedure, not elsewhere classified**

√7th **T81.710 Complication of mesenteric artery following a procedure, not elsewhere classified**

√7th **T81.711 Complication of renal artery following a procedure, not elsewhere classified**

√7th **T81.718 Complication of other artery following a procedure, not elsewhere classified**
**AHA:** 2024,4Q,19; 2019,2Q,21-22

√7th **T81.719 Complication of unspecified artery following a procedure, not elsewhere classified**

√x7th **T81.72 Complication of vein following a procedure, not elsewhere classified**

√5th **T81.8 Other complications of procedures, not elsewhere classified**
EXCLUDES 2 *hypothermia following anesthesia (T88.51)*
*malignant hyperpyrexia due to anesthesia (T88.3)*

√x7th **T81.81 Complication of inhalation therapy**

√x7th **T81.82 Emphysema (subcutaneous) resulting from a procedure**

√x7th **T81.83 Persistent postprocedural fistula**
Code also, if applicable, disruption of internal operation (surgical) wound (T81.32-)
Use additional code, if known, for site of fistula such as:
anal fistula (K60.3-)
anorectal fistula (K60.5-)
bladder fistula (N32.2)
other female intestinal-genital tract fistulae (N82.4)
**AHA:** 2024,3Q,4; 2023,1Q,30; 2017,3Q,3-4

√x7th **T81.89 Other complications of procedures, not elsewhere classified**
Use additional code to specify complication, such as:
postprocedural delirium (F05)
**AHA:** 2026,1Q,28; 2014,1Q,23

√x7th **T81.9 Unspecified complication of procedure**

√4th **T82 Complications of cardiac and vascular prosthetic devices, implants and grafts**
EXCLUDES 2 *failure and rejection of transplanted organs and tissue (T86.-)*
**AHA:** 2020,3Q,36-37

The appropriate 7th character is to be added to each code from category T82.
A initial encounter
D subsequent encounter
S sequela

√5th **T82.0 Mechanical complication of heart valve prosthesis**
Mechanical complication of artificial heart valve
EXCLUDES 1 *mechanical complication of biological heart valve graft (T82.22-)*

√x7th **T82.01 Breakdown (mechanical) of heart valve prosthesis**

√x7th **T82.02 Displacement of heart valve prosthesis**
Malposition of heart valve prosthesis

√x7th **T82.03 Leakage of heart valve prosthesis**

√x7th **T82.09 Other mechanical complication of heart valve prosthesis**
Obstruction (mechanical) of heart valve prosthesis
Perforation of heart valve prosthesis
Protrusion of heart valve prosthesis

√5th **T82.1 Mechanical complication of cardiac electronic device**

√6th **T82.11 Breakdown (mechanical) of cardiac electronic device**

√7th **T82.110 Breakdown (mechanical) of cardiac electrode**

√7th **T82.111 Breakdown (mechanical) of cardiac pulse generator (battery)**

√7th **T82.118 Breakdown (mechanical) of other cardiac electronic device**

√7th **T82.119 Breakdown (mechanical) of unspecified cardiac electronic device**

√6th **T82.12 Displacement of cardiac electronic device**
Malposition of cardiac electronic device

√7th **T82.120 Displacement of cardiac electrode**

√7th **T82.121 Displacement of cardiac pulse generator (battery)**

√7th **T82.128 Displacement of other cardiac electronic device**

√7th **T82.129 Displacement of unspecified cardiac electronic device**

√6th **T82.19 Other mechanical complication of cardiac electronic device**
Leakage of cardiac electronic device
Obstruction of cardiac electronic device
Perforation of cardiac electronic device
Protrusion of cardiac electronic device

√7th **T82.190 Other mechanical complication of cardiac electrode**

√7th **T82.191 Other mechanical complication of cardiac pulse generator (battery)**

√7th **T82.198 Other mechanical complication of other cardiac electronic device**

√7th **T82.199 Other mechanical complication of unspecified cardiac device**

√5th **T82.2 Mechanical complication of coronary artery bypass graft and biological heart valve graft**
EXCLUDES 1 *mechanical complication of artificial heart valve prosthesis (T82.0-)*

√6th **T82.21 Mechanical complication of coronary artery bypass graft**

√7th **T82.211 Breakdown (mechanical) of coronary artery bypass graft**

√7th **T82.212 Displacement of coronary artery bypass graft**
Malposition of coronary artery bypass graft

√7th **T82.213 Leakage of coronary artery bypass graft**

√7th **T82.218 Other mechanical complication of coronary artery bypass graft**
Obstruction, mechanical of coronary artery bypass graft
Perforation of coronary artery bypass graft
Protrusion of coronary artery bypass graft

√6th **T82.22 Mechanical complication of biological heart valve graft**

√7th **T82.221 Breakdown (mechanical) of biological heart valve graft**

√7th **T82.222 Displacement of biological heart valve graft**
Malposition of biological heart valve graft

√7th **T82.223 Leakage of biological heart valve graft**

√7th **T82.228 Other mechanical complication of biological heart valve graft**
Obstruction of biological heart valve graft
Perforation of biological heart valve graft
Protrusion of biological heart valve graft

√5th **T82.3 Mechanical complication of other vascular grafts**

√6th **T82.31 Breakdown (mechanical) of other vascular grafts**

√7th **T82.310 Breakdown (mechanical) of aortic (bifurcation) graft (replacement)** ESR
**AHA:** 2020,3Q,3-8

√7th **T82.311 Breakdown (mechanical) of carotid arterial graft (bypass)** ESR

√7th **T82.312 Breakdown (mechanical) of femoral arterial graft (bypass)** ESR

√7th **T82.318 Breakdown (mechanical) of other vascular grafts** ESR

√7th **T82.319 Breakdown (mechanical) of unspecified vascular grafts** ESR

T82.32 Displacement of other vascular grafts
Malposition of other vascular grafts
T82.320 Displacement of aortic (bifurcation) graft (replacement) ESR
T82.321 Displacement of carotid arterial graft (bypass) ESR
T82.322 Displacement of femoral arterial graft (bypass) ESR
T82.328 Displacement of other vascular grafts ESR
T82.329 Displacement of unspecified vascular grafts ESR
T82.33 Leakage of other vascular grafts
T82.330 Leakage of aortic (bifurcation) graft (replacement) ESR
AHA: 2020,3Q,3-8
T82.331 Leakage of carotid arterial graft (bypass) ESR
T82.332 Leakage of femoral arterial graft (bypass) ESR
T82.338 Leakage of other vascular grafts ESR
T82.339 Leakage of unspecified vascular graft ESR
T82.39 Other mechanical complication of other vascular grafts
Obstruction (mechanical) of other vascular grafts
Perforation of other vascular grafts
Protrusion of other vascular grafts
T82.390 Other mechanical complication of aortic (bifurcation) graft (replacement) ESR
AHA: 2020,3Q,3-5
T82.391 Other mechanical complication of carotid arterial graft (bypass) ESR
T82.392 Other mechanical complication of femoral arterial graft (bypass) ESR
T82.398 Other mechanical complication of other vascular grafts ESR
T82.399 Other mechanical complication of unspecified vascular grafts ESR

T82.4 Mechanical complication of vascular dialysis catheter
Mechanical complication of hemodialysis catheter
EXCLUDES 1 *mechanical complication of intraperitoneal dialysis catheter (T85.62)*
T82.41 Breakdown (mechanical) of vascular dialysis catheter Rx ESR
T82.42 Displacement of vascular dialysis catheter Rx ESR
Malposition of vascular dialysis catheter
T82.43 Leakage of vascular dialysis catheter Rx ESR
T82.49 Other complication of vascular dialysis catheter Rx ESR
Obstruction (mechanical) of vascular dialysis catheter
Perforation of vascular dialysis catheter
Protrusion of vascular dialysis catheter

T82.5 Mechanical complication of other cardiac and vascular devices and implants
EXCLUDES 2 *mechanical complication of epidural and subdural infusion catheter (T85.61)*
T82.51 Breakdown (mechanical) of other cardiac and vascular devices and implants
T82.510 Breakdown (mechanical) of surgically created arteriovenous fistula ESR
AHA: 2020,3Q,36
T82.511 Breakdown (mechanical) of surgically created arteriovenous shunt ESR
AHA: 2020,3Q,37
T82.512 Breakdown (mechanical) of artificial heart HCC
T82.513 Breakdown (mechanical) of balloon (counterpulsation) device ESR
T82.514 Breakdown (mechanical) of infusion catheter ESR
T82.515 Breakdown (mechanical) of umbrella device ESR
T82.518 Breakdown (mechanical) of other cardiac and vascular devices and implants ESR
T82.519 Breakdown (mechanical) of unspecified cardiac and vascular devices and implants
T82.52 Displacement of other cardiac and vascular devices and implants
Malposition of other cardiac and vascular devices and implants
T82.520 Displacement of surgically created arteriovenous fistula ESR
AHA: 2020,3Q,36
T82.521 Displacement of surgically created arteriovenous shunt ESR
T82.522 Displacement of artificial heart HCC
T82.523 Displacement of balloon (counterpulsation) device ESR
T82.524 Displacement of infusion catheter ESR
AHA: 2020,2Q,21; 2019,3Q,15
T82.525 Displacement of umbrella device ESR
T82.528 Displacement of other cardiac and vascular devices and implants ESR
T82.529 Displacement of unspecified cardiac and vascular devices and implants
T82.53 Leakage of other cardiac and vascular devices and implants
T82.530 Leakage of surgically created arteriovenous fistula ESR
AHA: 2020,3Q,36
T82.531 Leakage of surgically created arteriovenous shunt ESR
T82.532 Leakage of artificial heart HCC
T82.533 Leakage of balloon (counterpulsation) device ESR
T82.534 Leakage of infusion catheter ESR
T82.535 Leakage of umbrella device ESR
T82.538 Leakage of other cardiac and vascular devices and implants ESR
T82.539 Leakage of unspecified cardiac and vascular devices and implants
T82.59 Other mechanical complication of other cardiac and vascular devices and implants
Obstruction (mechanical) of other cardiac and vascular devices and implants
Perforation of other cardiac and vascular devices and implants
Protrusion of other cardiac and vascular devices and implants
T82.590 Other mechanical complication of surgically created arteriovenous fistula ESR
AHA: 2020,3Q,36
T82.591 Other mechanical complication of surgically created arteriovenous shunt ESR
T82.592 Other mechanical complication of artificial heart HCC
T82.593 Other mechanical complication of balloon (counterpulsation) device ESR
T82.594 Other mechanical complication of infusion catheter ESR
T82.595 Other mechanical complication of umbrella device ESR
T82.598 Other mechanical complication of other cardiac and vascular devices and implants ESR
T82.599 Other mechanical complication of unspecified cardiac and vascular devices and implants

T82.6 Infection and inflammatory reaction due to cardiac valve prosthesis ESR
Use additional code to identify infection
AHA: 2025,1Q,19,20

**T82.7 Infection and inflammatory reaction due to other cardiac and vascular devices, implants and grafts** ESR
Use additional code to identify infection
**AHA:** 2019,1Q,13-14
**DEF:** Midline catheter: Long peripheral catheter introduced via the cephalic, basilic, brachial, or median cubital veins in the upper arm and positioned so that the tip is level or near the level of the axilla and distal to the shoulder. Midline catheters are typically used for IV access, fluid replacement, and medication administration.
**TIP:** Assign this code for infections and/or cellulitis resulting from catheters that are not centrally placed (e.g., midline catheters).

**T82.8 Other specified complications of cardiac and vascular prosthetic devices, implants and grafts**
**AHA:** 2016,4Q,70

**T82.81 Embolism due to cardiac and vascular prosthetic devices, implants and grafts**
**T82.817 Embolism due to cardiac prosthetic devices, implants and grafts**
**T82.818 Embolism due to vascular prosthetic devices, implants and grafts** ESR

**T82.82 Fibrosis due to cardiac and vascular prosthetic devices, implants and grafts**
**T82.827 Fibrosis due to cardiac prosthetic devices, implants and grafts**
**T82.828 Fibrosis due vascular prosthetic devices, implants and grafts** ESR

**T82.83 Hemorrhage due to cardiac and vascular prosthetic devices, implants and grafts**
**T82.837 Hemorrhage due to cardiac prosthetic devices, implants and grafts**
**T82.838 Hemorrhage due to vascular prosthetic devices, implants and grafts** ESR
**AHA:** 2020,3Q,36-37

**T82.84 Pain due to cardiac and vascular prosthetic devices, implants and grafts**
**T82.847 Pain due to cardiac prosthetic devices, implants and grafts**
**T82.848 Pain due to vascular prosthetic devices, implants and grafts** ESR

**T82.85 Stenosis due to cardiac and vascular prosthetic devices, implants and grafts**
**T82.855 Stenosis of coronary artery stent**
In-stent stenosis (restenosis) of coronary artery stent
Restenosis of coronary artery stent
**AHA:** 2026,1Q,35; 2025,2Q,26; 2025,1Q,20; 2021,3Q,6-7
**T82.856 Stenosis of peripheral vascular stent** ESR
In-stent stenosis (restenosis) of peripheral vascular stent
Restenosis of peripheral vascular stent
**T82.857 Stenosis of other cardiac prosthetic devices, implants and grafts**
**AHA:** 2026,1Q,35; 2025,1Q,19
**T82.858 Stenosis of other vascular prosthetic devices, implants and grafts** ESR

**T82.86 Thrombosis of cardiac and vascular prosthetic devices, implants and grafts**
**AHA:** 2023,2Q,7
**T82.867 Thrombosis due to cardiac prosthetic devices, implants and grafts**
**AHA:** 2026,1Q,35
**T82.868 Thrombosis due to vascular prosthetic devices, implants and grafts** ESR

**T82.89 Other specified complication of cardiac and vascular prosthetic devices, implants and grafts**
**T82.897 Other specified complication of cardiac prosthetic devices, implants and grafts**
**AHA:** 2019,2Q,33
**T82.898 Other specified complication of vascular prosthetic devices, implants and grafts** ESR
**AHA:** 2020,3Q,3-5

**T82.9 Unspecified complication of cardiac and vascular prosthetic device, implant and graft**

**T83 Complications of genitourinary prosthetic devices, implants and grafts**
EXCLUDES 2 *failure and rejection of transplanted organs and tissue (T86.-)*
**AHA:** 2016,4Q,70-71

The appropriate 7th character is to be added to each code from category T83.
A initial encounter
D subsequent encounter
S sequela

**T83.0 Mechanical complication of urinary catheter**
EXCLUDES 2 *complications of stoma of urinary tract (N99.5-)*

**T83.01 Breakdown (mechanical) of urinary catheter**
**T83.010 Breakdown (mechanical) of cystostomy catheter** ESR
**T83.011 Breakdown (mechanical) of indwelling urethral catheter** ESR
**T83.012 Breakdown (mechanical) of nephrostomy catheter** ESR
**T83.018 Breakdown (mechanical) of other urinary catheter** ESR
Breakdown (mechanical) of Hopkins catheter
Breakdown (mechanical) of ileostomy catheter
Breakdown (mechanical) urostomy catheter

**T83.02 Displacement of urinary catheter**
Malposition of urinary catheter
**T83.020 Displacement of cystostomy catheter** ESR
**T83.021 Displacement of indwelling urethral catheter** ESR
**T83.022 Displacement of nephrostomy catheter** ESR
**T83.028 Displacement of other urinary catheter** ESR
Displacement of Hopkins catheter
Displacement of ileostomy catheter
Displacement of urostomy catheter

**T83.03 Leakage of urinary catheter**
**T83.030 Leakage of cystostomy catheter** ESR
**AHA:** 2021,4Q,18
**T83.031 Leakage of indwelling urethral catheter** ESR
**T83.032 Leakage of nephrostomy catheter** ESR
**T83.038 Leakage of other urinary catheter** ESR
Leakage of Hopkins catheter
Leakage of ileostomy catheter
Leakage of urostomy catheter

**T83.09 Other mechanical complication of urinary catheter**
Obstruction (mechanical) of urinary catheter
Perforation of urinary catheter
Protrusion of urinary catheter
**T83.090 Other mechanical complication of cystostomy catheter** ESR
**T83.091 Other mechanical complication of indwelling urethral catheter** ESR
**T83.092 Other mechanical complication of nephrostomy catheter** ESR
**T83.098 Other mechanical complication of other urinary catheter** ESR
Other mechanical complication of Hopkins catheter
Other mechanical complication of ileostomy catheter
Other mechanical complication of urostomy catheter

√5th **T83.1 Mechanical complication of other urinary devices and implants**

√6th **T83.11 Breakdown (mechanical) of other urinary devices and implants**

√7th **T83.110 Breakdown (mechanical) of urinary electronic stimulator device** ESR

EXCLUDES 2 *breakdown (mechanical) of electrode (lead) for sacral nerve neurostimulator (T85.111)*
*breakdown (mechanical) of implanted electronic sacral neurostimulator, pulse generator or receiver (T85.113)*

√7th **T83.111 Breakdown (mechanical) of implanted urinary sphincter** ESR

√7th **T83.112 Breakdown (mechanical) of indwelling ureteral stent** ESR

√7th **T83.113 Breakdown (mechanical) of other urinary stents** ESR

Breakdown (mechanical) of ileal conduit stent
Breakdown (mechanical) of nephroureteral stent

√7th **T83.118 Breakdown (mechanical) of other urinary devices and implants** ESR

√6th **T83.12 Displacement of other urinary devices and implants**

Malposition of other urinary devices and implants

√7th **T83.120 Displacement of urinary electronic stimulator device** ESR

EXCLUDES 2 *displacement of electrode (lead) for sacral nerve neurostimulator (T85.121)*
*displacement of implanted electronic sacral neurostimulator, pulse generator or receiver (T85.123)*

√7th **T83.121 Displacement of implanted urinary sphincter** ESR

√7th **T83.122 Displacement of indwelling ureteral stent** ESR

√7th **T83.123 Displacement of other urinary stents** ESR

Displacement of ileal conduit stent
Displacement of nephroureteral stent

√7th **T83.128 Displacement of other urinary devices and implants** ESR

√6th **T83.19 Other mechanical complication of other urinary devices and implants**

Leakage of other urinary devices and implants
Obstruction (mechanical) of other urinary devices and implants
Perforation of other urinary devices and implants
Protrusion of other urinary devices and implants

√7th **T83.190 Other mechanical complication of urinary electronic stimulator device** ESR

EXCLUDES 2 *other mechanical complication of electrode (lead) for sacral nerve neurostimulator (T85.191)*
*other mechanical complication of implanted electronic sacral neurostimulator, pulse generator or receiver (T85.193)*

√7th **T83.191 Other mechanical complication of implanted urinary sphincter** ESR

√7th **T83.192 Other mechanical complication of indwelling ureteral stent** ESR

√7th **T83.193 Other mechanical complication of other urinary stent** ESR

Other mechanical complication of ileal conduit stent
Other mechanical complication of nephroureteral stent

√7th **T83.198 Other mechanical complication of other urinary devices and implants** ESR

√5th **T83.2 Mechanical complication of graft of urinary organ**

√x7th **T83.21 Breakdown (mechanical) of graft of urinary organ** ESR

√x7th **T83.22 Displacement of graft of urinary organ** ESR

Malposition of graft of urinary organ

√x7th **T83.23 Leakage of graft of urinary organ** ESR

√x7th **T83.24 Erosion of graft of urinary organ** ESR

√x7th **T83.25 Exposure of graft of urinary organ** ESR

√x7th **T83.29 Other mechanical complication of graft of urinary organ** ESR

Obstruction (mechanical) of graft of urinary organ
Perforation of graft of urinary organ
Protrusion of graft of urinary organ

√5th **T83.3 Mechanical complication of intrauterine contraceptive device**

√x7th **T83.31 Breakdown (mechanical) of intrauterine contraceptive device**

√x7th **T83.32 Displacement of intrauterine contraceptive device**

Malposition of intrauterine contraceptive device
Missing string of intrauterine contraceptive device
**AHA:** 2018,1Q,5

√x7th **T83.39 Other mechanical complication of intrauterine contraceptive device**

Leakage of intrauterine contraceptive device
Obstruction (mechanical) of intrauterine contraceptive device
Perforation of intrauterine contraceptive device
Protrusion of intrauterine contraceptive device

√5th **T83.4 Mechanical complication of other prosthetic devices, implants and grafts of genital tract**

√6th **T83.41 Breakdown (mechanical) of other prosthetic devices, implants and grafts of genital tract**

√7th **T83.410 Breakdown (mechanical) of implanted penile prosthesis** ESR

Breakdown (mechanical) of penile prosthesis cylinder
Breakdown (mechanical) of penile prosthesis pump
Breakdown (mechanical) of penile prosthesis reservoir

√7th **T83.411 Breakdown (mechanical) of implanted testicular prosthesis** ESR

√7th **T83.418 Breakdown (mechanical) of other prosthetic devices, implants and grafts of genital tract** ESR

√6th **T83.42 Displacement of other prosthetic devices, implants and grafts of genital tract**

Malposition of other prosthetic devices, implants and grafts of genital tract

√7th **T83.420 Displacement of implanted penile prosthesis** ESR

Displacement of penile prosthesis cylinder
Displacement of penile prosthesis pump
Displacement of penile prosthesis reservoir

√7th **T83.421 Displacement of implanted testicular prosthesis** ESR

√7th **T83.428 Displacement of other prosthetic devices, implants and grafts of genital tract** ESR

**AHA:** 2018,1Q,5

√6th **T83.49 Other mechanical complication of other prosthetic devices, implants and grafts of genital tract**

Leakage of other prosthetic devices, implants and grafts of genital tract
Obstruction, mechanical of other prosthetic devices, implants and grafts of genital tract
Perforation of other prosthetic devices, implants and grafts of genital tract
Protrusion of other prosthetic devices, implants and grafts of genital tract

√7th **T83.490 Other mechanical complication of implanted penile prosthesis** ESR

Other mechanical complication of penile prosthesis cylinder
Other mechanical complication of penile prosthesis pump
Other mechanical complication of penile prosthesis reservoir

√7th **T83.491 Other mechanical complication of implanted testicular prosthesis** ESR

√7th **T83.498 Other mechanical complication of other prosthetic devices, implants and grafts of genital tract** ESR

✓5th **T83.5 Infection and inflammatory reaction due to prosthetic device, implant and graft in urinary system**
Use additional code to identify infection

✓6th **T83.51 Infection and inflammatory reaction due to urinary catheter**
EXCLUDES 2 *complications of stoma of urinary tract (N99.5-)*
**AHA:** 2019,3Q,17

✓7th **T83.51Ø Infection and inflammatory reaction due to cystostomy catheter** ESR

✓7th **T83.511 Infection and inflammatory reaction due to indwelling urethral catheter** ESR
**AHA:** 2022,2Q,7

✓7th **T83.512 Infection and inflammatory reaction due to nephrostomy catheter** ESR

✓7th **T83.518 Infection and inflammatory reaction due to other urinary catheter** ESR
Infection and inflammatory reaction due to Hopkins catheter
Infection and inflammatory reaction due to ileostomy catheter
Infection and inflammatory reaction due to urostomy catheter

✓6th **T83.59 Infection and inflammatory reaction due to prosthetic device, implant and graft in urinary system**

✓7th **T83.59Ø Infection and inflammatory reaction due to implanted urinary neurostimulation device** ESR
EXCLUDES 2 *infection and inflammatory reaction due to electrode lead of sacral nerve neurostimulator (T85.732)*
*infection and inflammatory reaction due to pulse generator or receiver of sacral nerve neurostimulator (T85.734)*

✓7th **T83.591 Infection and inflammatory reaction due to implanted urinary sphincter** ESR

✓7th **T83.592 Infection and inflammatory reaction due to indwelling ureteral stent** ESR

✓7th **T83.593 Infection and inflammatory reaction due to other urinary stents** ESR
Infection and inflammatory reaction due to ileal conduit stents
Infection and inflammatory reaction due to nephroureteral stent

✓7th **T83.598 Infection and inflammatory reaction due to other prosthetic device, implant and graft in urinary system** ESR
**AHA:** 2020,3Q,25

✓5th **T83.6 Infection and inflammatory reaction due to prosthetic device, implant and graft in genital tract**
Use additional code to identify infection

✓x7th **T83.61 Infection and inflammatory reaction due to implanted penile prosthesis** ESR
Infection and inflammatory reaction due to penile prosthesis cylinder
Infection and inflammatory reaction due to penile prosthesis pump
Infection and inflammatory reaction due to penile prosthesis reservoir

✓x7th **T83.62 Infection and inflammatory reaction due to implanted testicular prosthesis** ESR

✓x7th **T83.69 Infection and inflammatory reaction due to other prosthetic device, implant and graft in genital tract** ESR

✓5th **T83.7 Complications due to implanted mesh and other prosthetic materials**

✓6th **T83.71 Erosion of implanted mesh and other prosthetic materials**

✓7th **T83.711 Erosion of implanted vaginal mesh to surrounding organ or tissue** ESR
Erosion of implanted vaginal mesh into pelvic floor muscles

✓7th **T83.712 Erosion of implanted urethral mesh to surrounding organ or tissue** ESR
Erosion of implanted female urethral sling
Erosion of implanted male urethral sling
Erosion of implanted urethral mesh into pelvic floor muscles

✓7th **T83.713 Erosion of implanted urethral bulking agent to surrounding organ or tissue** ESR

✓7th **T83.714 Erosion of implanted ureteral bulking agent to surrounding organ or tissue** ESR

✓7th **T83.718 Erosion of other implanted mesh to organ or tissue** ESR

✓7th **T83.719 Erosion of other prosthetic materials to surrounding organ or tissue** ESR

✓6th **T83.72 Exposure of implanted mesh and other prosthetic materials into surrounding organ or tissue**
Extrusion of implanted mesh

✓7th **T83.721 Exposure of implanted vaginal mesh into vagina** ESR
Exposure of implanted vaginal mesh through vaginal wall

✓7th **T83.722 Exposure of implanted urethral mesh into urethra** ESR
Exposure of implanted female urethral sling
Exposure of implanted male urethral sling
Exposure of implanted urethral mesh through urethral wall

✓7th **T83.723 Exposure of implanted urethral bulking agent into urethra** ESR

✓7th **T83.724 Exposure of implanted ureteral bulking agent into ureter** ESR

✓7th **T83.728 Exposure of other implanted mesh into organ or tissue** ESR

✓7th **T83.729 Exposure of other prosthetic materials into organ or tissue** ESR

✓x7th **T83.79 Other specified complications due to other genitourinary prosthetic materials** ESR

✓5th **T83.8 Other specified complications of genitourinary prosthetic devices, implants and grafts**

✓x7th **T83.81 Embolism due to genitourinary prosthetic devices, implants and grafts** ESR

✓x7th **T83.82 Fibrosis due to genitourinary prosthetic devices, implants and grafts** ESR

✓x7th **T83.83 Hemorrhage due to genitourinary prosthetic devices, implants and grafts** ESR
**AHA:** 2025,2Q,21

✓x7th **T83.84 Pain due to genitourinary prosthetic devices, implants and grafts** ESR

✓x7th **T83.85 Stenosis due to genitourinary prosthetic devices, implants and grafts** ESR

✓x7th **T83.86 Thrombosis due to genitourinary prosthetic devices, implants and grafts** ESR
**AHA:** 2024,3Q,6

✓x7th **T83.89 Other specified complication of genitourinary prosthetic devices, implants and grafts** ESR
**AHA:** 2022,3Q,13; 2016,1Q,19

✓x7th **T83.9 Unspecified complication of genitourinary prosthetic device, implant and graft** ESR

✓4th **T84 Complications of internal orthopedic prosthetic devices, implants and grafts**
EXCLUDES 2 *failure and rejection of transplanted organs and tissues (T86.-)*
*fracture of bone following insertion of orthopedic implant, joint prosthesis or bone plate (M96.6)*

The appropriate 7th character is to be added to each code from category T84.
A initial encounter
D subsequent encounter
S sequela

✓5th **T84.Ø Mechanical complication of internal joint prosthesis**

✓6th **T84.Ø1 Broken internal joint prosthesis**
Breakage (fracture) of prosthetic joint
Broken prosthetic joint implant
EXCLUDES 1 *periprosthetic joint implant fracture (M97.-)*
**AHA:** 2016,4Q,42

✓7th **T84.Ø1Ø Broken internal right hip prosthesis** ESR

✓7th **T84.Ø11 Broken internal left hip prosthesis** ESR

√7th T84.012 **Broken internal right knee prosthesis** ESR

√7th T84.013 **Broken internal left knee prosthesis** ESR

√7th T84.018 **Broken internal joint prosthesis, other site** ESR
Use additional code to identify the joint (Z96.6-)

√7th T84.019 **Broken internal joint prosthesis, unspecified site** ESR

√6th T84.02 **Dislocation of internal joint prosthesis**
Instability of internal joint prosthesis
Subluxation of internal joint prosthesis
**AHA:** 2026,2Q,3; 2019,2Q,27

√7th T84.020 **Dislocation of internal right hip prosthesis** ESR

√7th T84.021 **Dislocation of internal left hip prosthesis** ESR

√7th T84.022 **Instability of internal right knee prosthesis** ESR

√7th T84.023 **Instability of internal left knee prosthesis** ESR

√7th T84.028 **Dislocation of other internal joint prosthesis** ESR
Use additional code to identify the joint (Z96.6-)

√7th T84.029 **Dislocation of unspecified internal joint prosthesis** ESR

√6th T84.03 **Mechanical loosening of internal prosthetic joint**
Aseptic loosening of prosthetic joint

√7th T84.030 **Mechanical loosening of internal right hip prosthetic joint** ESR

√7th T84.031 **Mechanical loosening of internal left hip prosthetic joint** ESR

√7th T84.032 **Mechanical loosening of internal right knee prosthetic joint** ESR

√7th T84.033 **Mechanical loosening of internal left knee prosthetic joint** ESR

√7th T84.038 **Mechanical loosening of other internal prosthetic joint** ESR
Use additional code to identify the joint (Z96.6-)

√7th T84.039 **Mechanical loosening of unspecified internal prosthetic joint** ESR

√6th T84.05 **Periprosthetic osteolysis of internal prosthetic joint**
Use additional code to identify major osseous defect, if applicable (M89.7-)

√7th T84.050 **Periprosthetic osteolysis of internal prosthetic right hip joint** ESR

√7th T84.051 **Periprosthetic osteolysis of internal prosthetic left hip joint** ESR

√7th T84.052 **Periprosthetic osteolysis of internal prosthetic right knee joint** ESR

√7th T84.053 **Periprosthetic osteolysis of internal prosthetic left knee joint** ESR

√7th T84.058 **Periprosthetic osteolysis of other internal prosthetic joint** ESR
Use additional code to identify the joint (Z96.6-)

√7th T84.059 **Periprosthetic osteolysis of unspecified internal prosthetic joint** ESR

√6th T84.06 **Wear of articular bearing surface of internal prosthetic joint**

√7th T84.060 **Wear of articular bearing surface of internal prosthetic right hip joint** ESR

√7th T84.061 **Wear of articular bearing surface of internal prosthetic left hip joint** ESR

√7th T84.062 **Wear of articular bearing surface of internal prosthetic right knee joint** ESR

√7th T84.063 **Wear of articular bearing surface of internal prosthetic left knee joint** ESR

√7th T84.068 **Wear of articular bearing surface of other internal prosthetic joint** ESR
Use additional code to identify the joint (Z96.6-)

√7th T84.069 **Wear of articular bearing surface of unspecified internal prosthetic joint** ESR

√6th T84.09 **Other mechanical complication of internal joint prosthesis**
Prosthetic joint implant failure NOS
**AHA:** 2026,2Q,3; 2019,1Q,20

√7th T84.090 **Other mechanical complication of internal right hip prosthesis** ESR

√7th T84.091 **Other mechanical complication of internal left hip prosthesis** ESR

√7th T84.092 **Other mechanical complication of internal right knee prosthesis** ESR

√7th T84.093 **Other mechanical complication of internal left knee prosthesis** ESR

√7th T84.098 **Other mechanical complication of other internal joint prosthesis** ESR
Use additional code to identify the joint (Z96.6-)

√7th T84.099 **Other mechanical complication of unspecified internal joint prosthesis** ESR

√5th T84.1 **Mechanical complication of internal fixation device of bones of limb**
EXCLUDES 2 *mechanical complication of internal fixation device of bones of feet (T84.2-)*
*mechanical complication of internal fixation device of bones of fingers (T84.2-)*
*mechanical complication of internal fixation device of bones of hands (T84.2-)*
*mechanical complication of internal fixation device of bones of toes (T84.2-)*

√6th T84.11 **Breakdown (mechanical) of internal fixation device of bones of limb**

√7th T84.110 **Breakdown (mechanical) of internal fixation device of right humerus** ESR

√7th T84.111 **Breakdown (mechanical) of internal fixation device of left humerus** ESR

√7th T84.112 **Breakdown (mechanical) of internal fixation device of bone of right forearm** ESR

√7th T84.113 **Breakdown (mechanical) of internal fixation device of bone of left forearm** ESR

√7th T84.114 **Breakdown (mechanical) of internal fixation device of right femur** ESR

√7th T84.115 **Breakdown (mechanical) of internal fixation device of left femur** ESR

√7th T84.116 **Breakdown (mechanical) of internal fixation device of bone of right lower leg** ESR

√7th T84.117 **Breakdown (mechanical) of internal fixation device of bone of left lower leg** ESR

√7th T84.119 **Breakdown (mechanical) of internal fixation device of unspecified bone of limb** ESR

√6th T84.12 **Displacement of internal fixation device of bones of limb**
Malposition of internal fixation device of bones of limb

√7th T84.120 **Displacement of internal fixation device of right humerus** ESR

√7th T84.121 **Displacement of internal fixation device of left humerus** ESR

√7th T84.122 **Displacement of internal fixation device of bone of right forearm** ESR

√7th T84.123 **Displacement of internal fixation device of bone of left forearm** ESR

√7th T84.124 **Displacement of internal fixation device of right femur** ESR

√7th T84.125 **Displacement of internal fixation device of left femur** ESR

√7th T84.126 **Displacement of internal fixation device of bone of right lower leg** ESR

√7th T84.127 **Displacement of internal fixation device of bone of left lower leg** ESR

√7th T84.129 **Displacement of internal fixation device of unspecified bone of limb** ESR

√6th **T84.19 Other mechanical complication of internal fixation device of bones of limb**
Obstruction (mechanical) of internal fixation device of bones of limb
Perforation of internal fixation device of bones of limb
Protrusion of internal fixation device of bones of limb

√7th **T84.190 Other mechanical complication of internal fixation device of right humerus** ESR

√7th **T84.191 Other mechanical complication of internal fixation device of left humerus** ESR

√7th **T84.192 Other mechanical complication of internal fixation device of bone of right forearm** ESR

√7th **T84.193 Other mechanical complication of internal fixation device of bone of left forearm** ESR

√7th **T84.194 Other mechanical complication of internal fixation device of right femur** ESR

√7th **T84.195 Other mechanical complication of internal fixation device of left femur** ESR

√7th **T84.196 Other mechanical complication of internal fixation device of bone of right lower leg** ESR

√7th **T84.197 Other mechanical complication of internal fixation device of bone of left lower leg** ESR

√7th **T84.199 Other mechanical complication of internal fixation device of unspecified bone of limb** ESR

√5th **T84.2 Mechanical complication of internal fixation device of other bones**

√6th **T84.21 Breakdown (mechanical) of internal fixation device of other bones**

√7th **T84.210 Breakdown (mechanical) of internal fixation device of bones of hand and fingers** ESR

√7th **T84.213 Breakdown (mechanical) of internal fixation device of bones of foot and toes** ESR

√7th **T84.216 Breakdown (mechanical) of internal fixation device of vertebrae** ESR

√7th **T84.218 Breakdown (mechanical) of internal fixation device of other bones** ESR

√6th **T84.22 Displacement of internal fixation device of other bones**
Malposition of internal fixation device of other bones

√7th **T84.220 Displacement of internal fixation device of bones of hand and fingers** ESR

√7th **T84.223 Displacement of internal fixation device of bones of foot and toes** ESR

√7th **T84.226 Displacement of internal fixation device of vertebrae** ESR

√7th **T84.228 Displacement of internal fixation device of other bones** ESR

√6th **T84.29 Other mechanical complication of internal fixation device of other bones**
Obstruction (mechanical) of internal fixation device of other bones
Perforation of internal fixation device of other bones
Protrusion of internal fixation device of other bones

√7th **T84.290 Other mechanical complication of internal fixation device of bones of hand and fingers** ESR

√7th **T84.293 Other mechanical complication of internal fixation device of bones of foot and toes** ESR

√7th **T84.296 Other mechanical complication of internal fixation device of vertebrae** ESR
**AHA:** 2024,2Q,12

√7th **T84.298 Other mechanical complication of internal fixation device of other bones** ESR

√5th **T84.3 Mechanical complication of other bone devices, implants and grafts**
EXCLUDES 2 *other complications of bone graft (T86.83-)*

√6th **T84.31 Breakdown (mechanical) of other bone devices, implants and grafts**

√7th **T84.310 Breakdown (mechanical) of electronic bone stimulator** ESR

√7th **T84.318 Breakdown (mechanical) of other bone devices, implants and grafts** ESR

√6th **T84.32 Displacement of other bone devices, implants and grafts**
Malposition of other bone devices, implants and grafts

√7th **T84.320 Displacement of electronic bone stimulator** ESR

√7th **T84.328 Displacement of other bone devices, implants and grafts** ESR
**AHA:** 2014,4Q,28

√6th **T84.39 Other mechanical complication of other bone devices, implants and grafts**
Obstruction (mechanical) of other bone devices, implants and grafts
Perforation of other bone devices, implants and grafts
Protrusion of other bone devices, implants and grafts

√7th **T84.390 Other mechanical complication of electronic bone stimulator** ESR

√7th **T84.398 Other mechanical complication of other bone devices, implants and grafts** ESR

√5th **T84.4 Mechanical complication of other internal orthopedic devices, implants and grafts**

√6th **T84.41 Breakdown (mechanical) of other internal orthopedic devices, implants and grafts**

√7th **T84.410 Breakdown (mechanical) of muscle and tendon graft** ESR

√7th **T84.418 Breakdown (mechanical) of other internal orthopedic devices, implants and grafts** ESR

√6th **T84.42 Displacement of other internal orthopedic devices, implants and grafts**
Malposition of other internal orthopedic devices, implants and grafts

√7th **T84.420 Displacement of muscle and tendon graft** ESR

√7th **T84.428 Displacement of other internal orthopedic devices, implants and grafts** ESR

√6th **T84.49 Other mechanical complication of other internal orthopedic devices, implants and grafts**
Mechanical complication of other internal orthopedic devices, implants and grafts NOS
Obstruction (mechanical) of other internal orthopedic devices, implants and grafts
Perforation of other internal orthopedic devices, implants and grafts
Protrusion of other internal orthopedic devices, implants and grafts

√7th **T84.490 Other mechanical complication of muscle and tendon graft** ESR

√7th **T84.498 Other mechanical complication of other internal orthopedic devices, implants and grafts** ESR

√5th **T84.5 Infection and inflammatory reaction due to internal joint prosthesis**
Use additional code to identify infection
**AHA:** 2019,3Q,16; 2015,1Q,16

√x7th **T84.50 Infection and inflammatory reaction due to unspecified internal joint prosthesis** ESR

√x7th **T84.51 Infection and inflammatory reaction due to internal right hip prosthesis** ESR

√x7th **T84.52 Infection and inflammatory reaction due to internal left hip prosthesis** ESR

√x7th **T84.53 Infection and inflammatory reaction due to internal right knee prosthesis** ESR

√x7th **T84.54 Infection and inflammatory reaction due to internal left knee prosthesis** ESR

√x7th **T84.59 Infection and inflammatory reaction due to other internal joint prosthesis** ESR

√5th **T84.6 Infection and inflammatory reaction due to internal fixation device**
Use additional code to identify infection

√x7th **T84.60 Infection and inflammatory reaction due to internal fixation device of unspecified site** ESR

√6th **T84.61 Infection and inflammatory reaction due to internal fixation device of arm**

√7th **T84.610 Infection and inflammatory reaction due to internal fixation device of right humerus** ESR

√7th **T84.611 Infection and inflammatory reaction due to internal fixation device of left humerus** ESR

T84.612 **Infection and inflammatory reaction due to internal fixation device of right radius** ESR

T84.613 **Infection and inflammatory reaction due to internal fixation device of left radius** ESR

T84.614 **Infection and inflammatory reaction due to internal fixation device of right ulna** ESR

T84.615 **Infection and inflammatory reaction due to internal fixation device of left ulna** ESR

T84.619 **Infection and inflammatory reaction due to internal fixation device of unspecified bone of arm** ESR

T84.62 **Infection and inflammatory reaction due to internal fixation device of leg**

T84.620 **Infection and inflammatory reaction due to internal fixation device of right femur** ESR

T84.621 **Infection and inflammatory reaction due to internal fixation device of left femur** ESR

T84.622 **Infection and inflammatory reaction due to internal fixation device of right tibia** ESR

T84.623 **Infection and inflammatory reaction due to internal fixation device of left tibia** ESR

T84.624 **Infection and inflammatory reaction due to internal fixation device of right fibula** ESR

T84.625 **Infection and inflammatory reaction due to internal fixation device of left fibula** ESR

T84.629 **Infection and inflammatory reaction due to internal fixation device of unspecified bone of leg** ESR

T84.63 **Infection and inflammatory reaction due to internal fixation device of spine** ESR

T84.69 **Infection and inflammatory reaction due to internal fixation device of other site** ESR

T84.7 **Infection and inflammatory reaction due to other internal orthopedic prosthetic devices, implants and grafts** ESR

Use additional code to identify infection

T84.8 **Other specified complications of internal orthopedic prosthetic devices, implants and grafts**

T84.81 **Embolism due to internal orthopedic prosthetic devices, implants and grafts** ESR

T84.82 **Fibrosis due to internal orthopedic prosthetic devices, implants and grafts** ESR

**AHA:** 2025,1Q,25

T84.83 **Hemorrhage due to internal orthopedic prosthetic devices, implants and grafts** ESR

T84.84 **Pain due to internal orthopedic prosthetic devices, implants and grafts** ESR

**AHA:** 2024,2Q,12

T84.85 **Stenosis due to internal orthopedic prosthetic devices, implants and grafts** ESR

T84.86 **Thrombosis due to internal orthopedic prosthetic devices, implants and grafts** ESR

T84.89 **Other specified complication of internal orthopedic prosthetic devices, implants and grafts** ESR

T84.9 **Unspecified complication of internal orthopedic prosthetic device, implant and graft** ESR

**T85 Complications of other internal prosthetic devices, implants and grafts**

EXCLUDES 2 *failure and rejection of transplanted organs and tissue (T86.-)*

**AHA:** 2023,2Q,7; 2016,4Q,71-72

The appropriate 7th character is to be added to each code from category T85.
A initial encounter
D subsequent encounter
S sequela

T85.0 **Mechanical complication of ventricular intracranial (communicating) shunt**

T85.01 **Breakdown (mechanical) of ventricular intracranial (communicating) shunt** ESR

T85.02 **Displacement of ventricular intracranial (communicating) shunt** ESR

Malposition of ventricular intracranial (communicating) shunt

T85.03 **Leakage of ventricular intracranial (communicating) shunt** ESR

T85.09 **Other mechanical complication of ventricular intracranial (communicating) shunt** ESR

Obstruction (mechanical) of ventricular intracranial (communicating) shunt
Perforation of ventricular intracranial (communicating) shunt
Protrusion of ventricular intracranial (communicating) shunt

T85.1 **Mechanical complication of implanted electronic stimulator of nervous system**

T85.11 **Breakdown (mechanical) of implanted electronic stimulator of nervous system**

T85.110 **Breakdown (mechanical) of implanted electronic neurostimulator of brain electrode (lead)** ESR

T85.111 **Breakdown (mechanical) of implanted electronic neurostimulator of peripheral nerve electrode (lead)** ESR

Breakdown of electrode (lead) for cranial nerve neurostimulators
Breakdown of electrode (lead) for gastric neurostimulator
Breakdown of electrode (lead) for sacral nerve neurostimulator
Breakdown of electrode (lead) for vagal nerve neurostimulators

T85.112 **Breakdown (mechanical) of implanted electronic neurostimulator of spinal cord electrode (lead)** ESR

T85.113 **Breakdown (mechanical) of implanted electronic neurostimulator, generator** ESR

Breakdown (mechanical) of implanted electronic neurostimulator generator, brain, peripheral, gastric, spinal
Breakdown (mechanical) of implanted electronic sacral neurostimulator, pulse generator or receiver

T85.118 **Breakdown (mechanical) of other implanted electronic stimulator of nervous system** ESR

T85.12 **Displacement of implanted electronic stimulator of nervous system**

Malposition of implanted electronic stimulator of nervous system

T85.120 **Displacement of implanted electronic neurostimulator of brain electrode (lead)** ESR

T85.121 **Displacement of implanted electronic neurostimulator of peripheral nerve electrode (lead)** ESR

Displacement of electrode (lead) for cranial nerve neurostimulators
Displacement of electrode (lead) for gastric neurostimulator
Displacement of electrode (lead) for sacral nerve neurostimulator
Displacement of electrode (lead) for vagal nerve neurostimulators

T85.122 **Displacement of implanted electronic neurostimulator of spinal cord electrode (lead)** ESR

T85.123 **Displacement of implanted electronic neurostimulator, generator** ESR

Displacement of implanted electronic neurostimulator generator, brain, peripheral, gastric, spinal
Displacement of implanted electronic sacral neurostimulator, pulse generator or receiver

T85.128 **Displacement of other implanted electronic stimulator of nervous system** ESR

Chapter 19. Injury, Poisoning and Certain Other Consequences of External Causes

T84.612–T85.128

√6th **T85.19 Other mechanical complication of implanted electronic stimulator of nervous system**
Leakage of implanted electronic stimulator of nervous system
Obstruction (mechanical) of implanted electronic stimulator of nervous system
Perforation of implanted electronic stimulator of nervous system
Protrusion of implanted electronic stimulator of nervous system

√7th **T85.190 Other mechanical complication of implanted electronic neurostimulator of brain electrode (lead)** ESR

√7th **T85.191 Other mechanical complication of implanted electronic neurostimulator of peripheral nerve electrode (lead)** ESR
Other mechanical complication of electrode (lead) for cranial nerve neurostimulators
Other mechanical complication of electrode (lead) for gastric neurostimulator
Other mechanical complication of electrode (lead) for sacral nerve neurostimulator
Other mechanical complication of electrode (lead) for vagal nerve neurostimulators

√7th **T85.192 Other mechanical complication of implanted electronic neurostimulator of spinal cord electrode (lead)** ESR

√7th **T85.193 Other mechanical complication of implanted electronic neurostimulator, generator** ESR
Other mechanical complication of implanted electronic neurostimulator generator, brain, peripheral, gastric, spinal
Other mechanical complication of implanted electronic sacral neurostimulator, pulse generator or receiver

√7th **T85.199 Other mechanical complication of other implanted electronic stimulator of nervous system** ESR

√5th **T85.2 Mechanical complication of intraocular lens**

√x7th **T85.21 Breakdown (mechanical) of intraocular lens**

√x7th **T85.22 Displacement of intraocular lens**
Malposition of intraocular lens

√x7th **T85.29 Other mechanical complication of intraocular lens**
Obstruction (mechanical) of intraocular lens
Perforation of intraocular lens
Protrusion of intraocular lens

√5th **T85.3 Mechanical complication of other ocular prosthetic devices, implants and grafts**
EXCLUDES 2 *other complications of corneal graft (T86.84-)*

√6th **T85.31 Breakdown (mechanical) of other ocular prosthetic devices, implants and grafts**

√7th **T85.310 Breakdown (mechanical) of prosthetic orbit of right eye**

√7th **T85.311 Breakdown (mechanical) of prosthetic orbit of left eye**

√7th **T85.318 Breakdown (mechanical) of other ocular prosthetic devices, implants and grafts**

√6th **T85.32 Displacement of other ocular prosthetic devices, implants and grafts**
Malposition of other ocular prosthetic devices, implants and grafts

√7th **T85.320 Displacement of prosthetic orbit of right eye**

√7th **T85.321 Displacement of prosthetic orbit of left eye**

√7th **T85.328 Displacement of other ocular prosthetic devices, implants and grafts**

√6th **T85.39 Other mechanical complication of other ocular prosthetic devices, implants and grafts**
Obstruction (mechanical) of other ocular prosthetic devices, implants and grafts
Perforation of other ocular prosthetic devices, implants and grafts
Protrusion of other ocular prosthetic devices, implants and grafts

√7th **T85.390 Other mechanical complication of prosthetic orbit of right eye**

√7th **T85.391 Other mechanical complication of prosthetic orbit of left eye**

√7th **T85.398 Other mechanical complication of other ocular prosthetic devices, implants and grafts**

√5th **T85.4 Mechanical complication of breast prosthesis and implant**

√x7th **T85.41 Breakdown (mechanical) of breast prosthesis and implant**

√x7th **T85.42 Displacement of breast prosthesis and implant**
Malposition of breast prosthesis and implant

√x7th **T85.43 Leakage of breast prosthesis and implant**

√x7th **T85.44 Capsular contracture of breast implant**

√x7th **T85.49 Other mechanical complication of breast prosthesis and implant**
Obstruction (mechanical) of breast prosthesis and implant
Perforation of breast prosthesis and implant
Protrusion of breast prosthesis and implant

√5th **T85.5 Mechanical complication of gastrointestinal prosthetic devices, implants and grafts**

√6th **T85.51 Breakdown (mechanical) of gastrointestinal prosthetic devices, implants and grafts**

√7th **T85.510 Breakdown (mechanical) of bile duct prosthesis**

√7th **T85.511 Breakdown (mechanical) of esophageal anti-reflux device**

√7th **T85.518 Breakdown (mechanical) of other gastrointestinal prosthetic devices, implants and grafts**

√6th **T85.52 Displacement of gastrointestinal prosthetic devices, implants and grafts**
Malposition of gastrointestinal prosthetic devices, implants and grafts

√7th **T85.520 Displacement of bile duct prosthesis**

√7th **T85.521 Displacement of esophageal anti-reflux device**

√7th **T85.528 Displacement of other gastrointestinal prosthetic devices, implants and grafts**

√6th **T85.59 Other mechanical complication of gastrointestinal prosthetic devices, implants and**
Obstruction, mechanical of gastrointestinal prosthetic devices, implants and grafts
Perforation of gastrointestinal prosthetic devices, implants and grafts
Protrusion of gastrointestinal prosthetic devices, implants and grafts

√7th **T85.590 Other mechanical complication of bile duct prosthesis**

√7th **T85.591 Other mechanical complication of esophageal anti-reflux device**

√7th **T85.598 Other mechanical complication of other gastrointestinal prosthetic devices, implants and grafts**

√5th **T85.6 Mechanical complication of other specified internal and external prosthetic devices, implants and grafts**

√6th **T85.61 Breakdown (mechanical) of other specified internal prosthetic devices, implants and grafts**

√7th **T85.610 Breakdown (mechanical) of cranial or spinal infusion catheter**
Breakdown (mechanical) of epidural infusion catheter
Breakdown (mechanical) of intrathecal infusion catheter
Breakdown (mechanical) of subarachnoid infusion catheter
Breakdown (mechanical) of subdural infusion catheter

√7th **T85.611 Breakdown (mechanical) of intraperitoneal dialysis catheter** Rx ESR
EXCLUDES 1 *mechanical complication of vascular dialysis catheter (T82.4-)*

√7th **T85.612 Breakdown (mechanical) of permanent sutures**
EXCLUDES 1 *mechanical complication of permanent (wire) suture used in bone repair (T84.1-T84.2)*

√7th **T85.613 Breakdown (mechanical) of artificial skin graft and decellularized allodermis**
Failure of artificial skin graft and decellularized allodermis
Non-adherence of artificial skin graft and decellularized allodermis
Poor incorporation of artificial skin graft and decellularized allodermis
Shearing of artificial skin graft and decellularized allodermis

√7th **T85.614 Breakdown (mechanical) of insulin pump**

√7th **T85.615 Breakdown (mechanical) of other nervous system device, implant or graft** ESR
Breakdown (mechanical) of intrathecal infusion pump

√7th **T85.618 Breakdown (mechanical) of other specified internal prosthetic devices, implants and grafts**

√6th **T85.62 Displacement of other specified internal prosthetic devices, implants and grafts**
Malposition of other specified internal prosthetic devices, implants and grafts

√7th **T85.620 Displacement of cranial or spinal infusion catheter**
Displacement of epidural infusion catheter
Displacement of intrathecal infusion catheter
Displacement of subarachnoid infusion catheter
Displacement of subdural infusion catheter

√7th **T85.621 Displacement of intraperitoneal dialysis catheter** Rx ESR
EXCLUDES 1 *mechanical complication of vascular dialysis catheter (T82.4-)*

√7th **T85.622 Displacement of permanent sutures**
EXCLUDES 1 *mechanical complication of permanent (wire) suture used in bone repair (T84.1-T84.2)*

√7th **T85.623 Displacement of artificial skin graft and decellularized allodermis**
Dislodgement of artificial skin graft and decellularized allodermis

√7th **T85.624 Displacement of insulin pump**

√7th **T85.625 Displacement of other nervous system device, implant or graft** ESR
Displacement of intrathecal infusion pump

√7th **T85.628 Displacement of other specified internal prosthetic devices, implants and grafts**

√6th **T85.63 Leakage of other specified internal prosthetic devices, implants and grafts**

√7th **T85.630 Leakage of cranial or spinal infusion catheter**
Leakage of epidural infusion catheter
Leakage of intrathecal infusion catheter infusion catheter
Leakage of subarachnoid infusion catheter
Leakage of subdural infusion catheter
**AHA:** 2022,3Q,24

√7th **T85.631 Leakage of intraperitoneal dialysis catheter** Rx ESR
EXCLUDES 1 *mechanical complication of vascular dialysis catheter (T82.4)*

√7th **T85.633 Leakage of insulin pump**

√7th **T85.635 Leakage of other nervous system device, implant or graft** ESR
Leakage of intrathecal infusion pump

√7th **T85.638 Leakage of other specified internal prosthetic devices, implants and grafts**

√6th **T85.69 Other mechanical complication of other specified internal prosthetic devices, implants and grafts**
Obstruction, mechanical of other specified internal prosthetic devices, implants and grafts
Perforation of other specified internal prosthetic devices, implants and grafts
Protrusion of other specified internal prosthetic devices, implants and grafts

√7th **T85.690 Other mechanical complication of cranial or spinal infusion catheter**
Other mechanical complication of epidural infusion catheter
Other mechanical complication of intrathecal infusion catheter
Other mechanical complication of subarachnoid infusion catheter
Other mechanical complication of subdural infusion catheter

√7th **T85.691 Other mechanical complication of intraperitoneal dialysis catheter** Rx ESR
EXCLUDES 1 *mechanical complication of vascular dialysis catheter (T82.4)*

√7th **T85.692 Other mechanical complication of permanent sutures**
EXCLUDES 1 *mechanical complication of permanent (wire) suture used in bone repair (T84.1-T84.2)*

√7th **T85.693 Other mechanical complication of artificial skin graft and decellularized allodermis**

√7th **T85.694 Other mechanical complication of insulin pump**

√7th **T85.695 Other mechanical complication of other nervous system device, implant or graft** ESR
Other mechanical complication of intrathecal infusion pump

√7th **T85.698 Other mechanical complication of other specified internal prosthetic devices, implants and grafts**
Mechanical complication of nonabsorbable surgical material NOS

√5th **T85.7 Infection and inflammatory reaction due to other internal prosthetic devices, implants and grafts**
Use additional code to identify infection

√x7th **T85.71 Infection and inflammatory reaction due to peritoneal dialysis catheter** Rx ESR

√x7th **T85.72 Infection and inflammatory reaction due to insulin pump** ESR

√6th **T85.73 Infection and inflammatory reaction due to nervous system devices, implants and graft**

√7th **T85.730 Infection and inflammatory reaction due to ventricular intracranial (communicating) shunt** ESR

√7th **T85.731 Infection and inflammatory reaction due to implanted electronic neurostimulator of brain, electrode (lead)** ESR

√7th **T85.732 Infection and inflammatory reaction due to implanted electronic neurostimulator of peripheral nerve, electrode (lead)** ESR
Infection and inflammatory reaction due to electrode (lead) for cranial nerve neurostimulators
Infection and inflammatory reaction due to electrode (lead) for gastric neurostimulator
Infection and inflammatory reaction due to electrode (lead) for sacral nerve neurostimulator
Infection and inflammatory reaction due to electrode (lead) for vagal nerve neurostimulators

√7th **T85.733 Infection and inflammatory reaction due to implanted electronic neurostimulator of spinal cord, electrode (lead)** ESR

√7th **T85.734 Infection and inflammatory reaction due to implanted electronic neurostimulator, generator** ESR
Generator pocket infection

√7th **T85.735 Infection and inflammatory reaction due to cranial or spinal infusion catheter** ESR
Infection and inflammatory reaction due to epidural catheter
Infection and inflammatory reaction due to intrathecal infusion catheter
Infection and inflammatory reaction due to subarachnoid catheter
Infection and inflammatory reaction due to subdural catheter

√7th **T85.738 Infection and inflammatory reaction due to other nervous system device, implant or graft** ESR
Infection and inflammatory reaction due to intrathecal infusion pump

√x7th **T85.79 Infection and inflammatory reaction due to other internal prosthetic devices, implants and grafts** ESR
**AHA:** 2023,2Q,27; 2022,2Q,7

√5th **T85.8 Other specified complications of internal prosthetic devices, implants and grafts, not elsewhere classified**

√6th **T85.81 Embolism due to internal prosthetic devices, implants and grafts, not elsewhere classified**

√7th **T85.810 Embolism due to nervous system prosthetic devices, implants and grafts** ESR

√7th **T85.818 Embolism due to other internal prosthetic devices, implants and grafts**

√6th **T85.82 Fibrosis due to internal prosthetic devices, implants and grafts, not elsewhere classified**

√7th **T85.820 Fibrosis due to nervous system prosthetic devices, implants and grafts** ESR

√7th **T85.828 Fibrosis due to other internal prosthetic devices, implants and grafts**

√6th **T85.83 Hemorrhage due to internal prosthetic devices, implants and grafts, not elsewhere classified**

√7th **T85.830 Hemorrhage due to nervous system prosthetic devices, implants and grafts** ESR

√7th **T85.838 Hemorrhage due to other internal prosthetic devices, implants and grafts**

√6th **T85.84 Pain due to internal prosthetic devices, implants and grafts, not elsewhere classified**

√7th **T85.840 Pain due to nervous system prosthetic devices, implants and grafts** ESR

√7th **T85.848 Pain due to other internal prosthetic devices, implants and grafts**

√6th **T85.85 Stenosis due to internal prosthetic devices, implants and grafts, not elsewhere classified**

√7th **T85.850 Stenosis due to nervous system prosthetic devices, implants and grafts** ESR

√7th **T85.858 Stenosis due to other internal prosthetic devices, implants and grafts**

√6th **T85.86 Thrombosis due to internal prosthetic devices, implants and grafts, not elsewhere classified**
**AHA:** 2024,2Q,7

√7th **T85.860 Thrombosis due to nervous system prosthetic devices, implants and grafts** ESR

√7th **T85.868 Thrombosis due to other internal prosthetic devices, implants and grafts**

√6th **T85.89 Other specified complication of internal prosthetic devices, implants and grafts, not elsewhere classified**
Erosion or breakdown of subcutaneous device pocket
**AHA:** 2024,2Q,8

√7th **T85.890 Other specified complication of nervous system prosthetic devices, implants and grafts** ESR

√7th **T85.898 Other specified complication of other internal prosthetic devices, implants and grafts**

√x7th **T85.9 Unspecified complication of internal prosthetic device, implant and graft**
Complication of internal prosthetic device, implant and graft NOS

√4th **T86 Complications of transplanted organs and tissue**
Use additional code to identify other transplant complications, such as:
graft-versus-host disease (D89.81-)
malignancy associated with organ transplant (C80.2)
post-transplant lymphoproliferative disorders (PTLD) (D47.Z1)
**AHA:** 2020,1Q,18

√5th **T86.0 Complications of bone marrow transplant**

**T86.00 Unspecified complication of bone marrow transplant** HCC Rx ESR COM

**T86.01 Bone marrow transplant rejection** HCC Rx ESR COM

**T86.02 Bone marrow transplant failure** HCC Rx ESR COM

**T86.03 Bone marrow transplant infection** HCC Rx ESR COM

**T86.09 Other complications of bone marrow transplant** HCC Rx ESR COM
**AHA:** 2023,3Q,19

√5th **T86.1 Complications of kidney transplant**

**T86.10 Unspecified complication of kidney transplant** Rx COM

**T86.11 Kidney transplant rejection** Rx COM

**T86.12 Kidney transplant failure** Rx COM
**AHA:** 2013,1Q,24

**T86.13 Kidney transplant infection** Rx COM
Use additional code to specify infection

**T86.19 Other complication of kidney transplant** Rx COM
**AHA:** 2019,2Q,7

√5th **T86.2 Complications of heart transplant**
**EXCLUDES 1** *complication of:*
*artificial heart device (T82.5-)*
*heart-lung transplant (T86.3-)*

**T86.20 Unspecified complication of heart transplant** HCC Rx ESR COM

**T86.21 Heart transplant rejection** HCC Rx ESR COM

**T86.22 Heart transplant failure** HCC Rx ESR COM

**T86.23 Heart transplant infection** HCC Rx ESR COM
Use additional code to specify infection

√6th **T86.29 Other complications of heart transplant**

**T86.290 Cardiac allograft vasculopathy** HCC Rx ESR COM
**EXCLUDES 1** *atherosclerosis of coronary arteries (I25.75-, I25.76-, I25.81-)*

**T86.298 Other complications of heart transplant** HCC Rx ESR COM

√5th **T86.3 Complications of heart-lung transplant**

**T86.30 Unspecified complication of heart-lung transplant** HCC Rx ESR COM

**T86.31 Heart-lung transplant rejection** HCC Rx ESR COM

**T86.32 Heart-lung transplant failure** HCC Rx ESR COM

**T86.33 Heart-lung transplant infection** HCC Rx ESR COM
Use additional code to specify infection

**T86.39 Other complications of heart-lung transplant** HCC Rx ESR COM

√5th **T86.4 Complications of liver transplant**

**T86.40 Unspecified complication of liver transplant** HCC Rx ESR COM

**T86.41 Liver transplant rejection** HCC Rx ESR COM

**T86.42 Liver transplant failure** HCC Rx ESR COM

**T86.43 Liver transplant infection** HCC Rx ESR COM
Use additional code to identify infection, such as:
cytomegalovirus (CMV) infection (B25.-)

**T86.49 Other complications of liver transplant** HCC Rx ESR COM

**T86.5 Complications of stem cell transplant** HCC Rx ESR COM
Complications from stem cells from peripheral blood
Complications from stem cells from umbilical cord
**AHA:** 2020,4Q,14

√5th **T86.8 Complications of other transplanted organs and tissues**

√6th **T86.81 Complications of lung transplant**
**EXCLUDES 1** *complication of heart-lung transplant (T86.3-)*

**T86.810 Lung transplant rejection** HCC Rx ESR COM

**T86.811 Lung transplant failure** HCC Rx ESR COM

T86.812 Lung transplant infection HCC Rx ESR COM
Use additional code to specify infection

T86.818 Other complications of lung transplant HCC Rx ESR COM
AHA: 2019,2Q,6

T86.819 Unspecified complication of lung transplant HCC Rx ESR COM

✓6th T86.82 Complications of skin graft (allograft) (autograft)
EXCLUDES 2 *complication of artificial skin graft (T85.693)*

T86.820 Skin graft (allograft) rejection
T86.821 Skin graft (allograft) (autograft) failure
T86.822 Skin graft (allograft) (autograft) infection
Use additional code to specify infection
T86.828 Other complications of skin graft (allograft) (autograft)
T86.829 Unspecified complication of skin graft (allograft) (autograft)

✓6th T86.83 Complications of bone graft
EXCLUDES 2 *mechanical complications of bone graft (T84.3-)*

T86.830 Bone graft rejection
T86.831 Bone graft failure
T86.832 Bone graft infection
Use additional code to specify infection
T86.838 Other complications of bone graft
AHA: 2023,1Q,30
T86.839 Unspecified complication of bone graft

✓6th T86.84 Complications of corneal transplant
EXCLUDES 2 *mechanical complications of corneal graft (T85.3-)*
AHA: 2020,4Q,40

✓7th T86.840 Corneal transplant rejection
T86.8401 Corneal transplant rejection, right eye
T86.8402 Corneal transplant rejection, left eye
T86.8403 Corneal transplant rejection, bilateral
T86.8409 Corneal transplant rejection, unspecified eye

✓7th T86.841 Corneal transplant failure
T86.8411 Corneal transplant failure, right eye
T86.8412 Corneal transplant failure, left eye
T86.8413 Corneal transplant failure, bilateral
T86.8419 Corneal transplant failure, unspecified eye

✓7th T86.842 Corneal transplant infection
Use additional code to specify infection
T86.8421 Corneal transplant infection, right eye ESR
T86.8422 Corneal transplant infection, left eye ESR
T86.8423 Corneal transplant infection, bilateral ESR
T86.8429 Corneal transplant infection, unspecified eye ESR

✓7th T86.848 Other complications of corneal transplant
T86.8481 Other complications of corneal transplant, right eye
T86.8482 Other complications of corneal transplant, left eye
T86.8483 Other complications of corneal transplant, bilateral
T86.8489 Other complications of corneal transplant, unspecified eye

✓7th T86.849 Unspecified complication of corneal transplant
T86.8491 Unspecified complication of corneal transplant, right eye
T86.8492 Unspecified complication of corneal transplant, left eye
T86.8493 Unspecified complication of corneal transplant, bilateral
T86.8499 Unspecified complication of corneal transplant, unspecified eye

✓6th T86.85 Complication of intestine transplant
T86.850 Intestine transplant rejection HCC Rx ESR COM
T86.851 Intestine transplant failure HCC Rx ESR COM
T86.852 Intestine transplant infection HCC Rx ESR COM
Use additional code to specify infection
T86.858 Other complications of intestine transplant HCC Rx ESR COM
T86.859 Unspecified complication of intestine transplant HCC Rx ESR COM

✓6th T86.89 Complications of other transplanted tissue
Transplant failure or rejection of pancreas
AHA: 2020,1Q,18
T86.890 Other transplanted tissue rejection
T86.891 Other transplanted tissue failure
T86.892 Other transplanted tissue infection
Use additional code to specify infection
T86.898 Other complications of other transplanted tissue
T86.899 Unspecified complication of other transplanted tissue

✓5th T86.9 Complication of unspecified transplanted organ and tissue
T86.90 Unspecified complication of unspecified transplanted organ and tissue
T86.91 Unspecified transplanted organ and tissue rejection
T86.92 Unspecified transplanted organ and tissue failure
T86.93 Unspecified transplanted organ and tissue infection
Use additional code to specify infection
T86.99 Other complications of unspecified transplanted organ and tissue

## ✓4th T87 Complications peculiar to reattachment and amputation

✓5th T87.0 Complications of reattached (part of) upper extremity
✓6th T87.0X Complications of reattached (part of) upper extremity
T87.0X1 Complications of reattached (part of) right upper extremity HCC ESR COM
T87.0X2 Complications of reattached (part of) left upper extremity HCC ESR COM
T87.0X9 Complications of reattached (part of) unspecified upper extremity HCC ESR COM

✓5th T87.1 Complications of reattached (part of) lower extremity
✓6th T87.1X Complications of reattached (part of) lower extremity
T87.1X1 Complications of reattached (part of) right lower extremity HCC ESR COM
T87.1X2 Complications of reattached (part of) left lower extremity HCC ESR COM
T87.1X9 Complications of reattached (part of) unspecified lower extremity HCC ESR COM

T87.2 Complications of other reattached body part ESR

✓5th T87.3 Neuroma of amputation stump
DEF: Non-neoplastic tumor generated at the proximal end of severed, partially transected, or injured nerve following amputation.
T87.30 Neuroma of amputation stump, unspecified extremity HCC ESR COM
T87.31 Neuroma of amputation stump, right upper extremity HCC ESR COM
T87.32 Neuroma of amputation stump, left upper extremity HCC ESR COM
T87.33 Neuroma of amputation stump, right lower extremity HCC ESR COM
T87.34 Neuroma of amputation stump, left lower extremity HCC ESR COM

✓5th T87.4 Infection of amputation stump
T87.40 Infection of amputation stump, unspecified extremity HCC ESR COM
T87.41 Infection of amputation stump, right upper extremity HCC ESR COM
T87.42 Infection of amputation stump, left upper extremity HCC ESR COM
T87.43 Infection of amputation stump, right lower extremity HCC ESR COM
T87.44 Infection of amputation stump, left lower extremity HCC ESR COM

√5th **T87.5 Necrosis of amputation stump**

**T87.50 Necrosis of amputation stump, unspecified extremity** HCC ESR COM

**T87.51 Necrosis of amputation stump, right upper extremity** HCC ESR COM

**T87.52 Necrosis of amputation stump, left upper extremity** HCC ESR COM

**T87.53 Necrosis of amputation stump, right lower extremity** HCC ESR COM

**T87.54 Necrosis of amputation stump, left lower extremity** HCC ESR COM

√5th **T87.8 Other complications of amputation stump**

**T87.81 Dehiscence of amputation stump** HCC ESR COM

**T87.89 Other complications of amputation stump** HCC ESR COM

Amputation stump contracture
Amputation stump contracture of next proximal joint
Amputation stump edema
Amputation stump flexion
Amputation stump hematoma

EXCLUDES 2 *phantom limb syndrome (G54.6-G54.7)*

**AHA:** 2022,3Q,11

**T87.9 Unspecified complications of amputation stump** HCC ESR COM

√4th **T88 Other complications of surgical and medical care, not elsewhere classified**

EXCLUDES 2 *complication following infusion, transfusion and therapeutic injection (T8Ø.-)*
*complication following procedure NEC (T81.-)*
*complications of anesthesia in labor and delivery (O74.-)*
*complications of anesthesia in pregnancy (O29.-)*
*complications of anesthesia in puerperium (O89.-)*
*complications of devices, implants and grafts (T82-T85)*
*complications of obstetric surgery and procedure (O75.4)*
*dermatitis due to drugs and medicaments (L23.3, L24.4, L25.1, L27.Ø-L27.1)*
*poisoning and toxic effects of drugs and chemicals (T36-T65 with fifth or sixth character 1-4)*
*specified complications classified elsewhere*

The appropriate 7th character is to be added to each code from category T88.
A initial encounter
D subsequent encounter
S sequela

√x7th **T88.Ø Infection following immunization**

Sepsis following immunization

**AHA:** 2018,4Q,62-63

√x7th **T88.1 Other complications following immunization, not elsewhere classified**

Generalized vaccinia
Rash following immunization

EXCLUDES 1 *vaccinia not from vaccine (BØ8.Ø11)*

EXCLUDES 2 *anaphylactic shock due to serum (T8Ø.5-)*
*other serum reactions (T8Ø.6-)*
*postimmunization arthropathy (MØ2.2)*
*postimmunization encephalitis (GØ4.Ø2)*
*postimmunization fever (R5Ø.83)*

√x7th **T88.2 Shock due to anesthesia**

Use additional code for adverse effect, if applicable, to identify drug (T41.- with fifth or sixth character 5)

EXCLUDES 1 *complications of anesthesia (in):*
*labor and delivery (O74.-)*
*postprocedural shock NOS (T81.1-)*
*pregnancy (O29.-)*
*puerperium (O89.-)*

√x7th **T88.3 Malignant hyperthermia due to anesthesia**

Use additional code for adverse effect, if applicable, to identify drug (T41.- with fifth or sixth character 5)

√x7th **T88.4 Failed or difficult intubation**

√5th **T88.5 Other complications of anesthesia**

Use additional code for adverse effect, if applicable, to identify drug (T41.- with fifth or sixth character 5)

√x7th **T88.51 Hypothermia following anesthesia**

√x7th **T88.52 Failed moderate sedation during procedure**

Failed conscious sedation during procedure

EXCLUDES 2 *personal history of failed moderate sedation (Z92.83)*

√x7th **T88.53 Unintended awareness under general anesthesia during procedure**

EXCLUDES 2 *personal history of unintended awareness under general anesthesia (Z92.84)*

**AHA:** 2016,4Q,72-73

√x7th **T88.59 Other complications of anesthesia**

√x7th **T88.6 Anaphylactic reaction due to adverse effect of correct drug or medicament properly administered**

Anaphylactic shock due to adverse effect of correct drug or medicament properly administered
Anaphylactoid reaction NOS

Use additional code for adverse effect, if applicable, to identify drug (T36-T5Ø with fifth or sixth character 5)

EXCLUDES 1 *anaphylactic reaction due to serum (T8Ø.5-)*
*anaphylactic shock or reaction due to adverse food reaction (T78.Ø-)*

**AHA:** 2020,1Q,18

√x7th **T88.7 Unspecified adverse effect of drug or medicament**

Drug hypersensitivity NOS
Drug reaction NOS

Use additional code for adverse effect, if applicable, to identify drug (T36-T5Ø with fifth or sixth character 5)

EXCLUDES 1 *specified adverse effects of drugs and medicaments (AØØ-R94 and T8Ø-T88.6, T88.8)*

√x7th **T88.8 Other specified complications of surgical and medical care, not elsewhere classified**

Use additional code to identify the complication

**AHA:** 2022,2Q,7

√x7th **T88.9 Complication of surgical and medical care, unspecified**

# Chapter 20. External Causes of Morbidity (VØØ–Y99)



## Chapter-specific Guidelines with Coding Examples

The chapter-specific guidelines from the ICD-10-CM Official Guidelines for Coding and Reporting have been provided below. Along with these guidelines are coding examples, contained in the shaded boxes, that have been developed to help illustrate the coding and/or sequencing guidance found in these guidelines.

The external causes of morbidity codes should never be sequenced as the first-listed or principal diagnosis.

External cause codes are intended to provide data for injury research and evaluation of injury prevention strategies. These codes capture how the injury or health condition happened (cause), the intent (unintentional or accidental; or intentional, such as suicide or assault), the place where the event occurred the activity of the patient at the time of the event, and the person's status (e.g., civilian, military).

There is no national requirement for mandatory ICD-10-CM external cause code reporting. Unless a provider is subject to a state-based external cause code reporting mandate or these codes are required by a particular payer, reporting of ICD-10-CM codes in Chapter 20, External Causes of Morbidity, is not required. In the absence of a mandatory reporting requirement, providers are encouraged to voluntarily report external cause codes, as they provide valuable data for injury research and evaluation of injury prevention strategies.

**a. General external cause coding guidelines**

**1) Used with any code in the range of A00.0–T88.9, Z00–Z99**

An external cause code may be used with any code in the range of AØØ.Ø-T88.9, ZØØ-Z99, classification that represents a health condition due to an external cause. Though they are most applicable to injuries, they are also valid for use with such things as infections or diseases due to an external source, and other health conditions, such as a heart attack that occurs during strenuous physical activity.

> Actinic reticuloid due to tanning bed use
>
> **L57.1** **Actinic reticuloid**
>
> **W89.1XXA** **Exposure to tanning bed, initial encounter**
>
> *Explanation:* An external cause code may be used with any code in the range of AØØ.Ø–T88.9, ZØØ–Z99, classifications that describe health conditions due to an external cause. Code W89.1 Exposure to tanning bed requires a seventh character of A to report this initial encounter, with a placeholder X for the fifth and sixth characters.

**2) External cause code used for length of treatment**

Assign the external cause code, with the appropriate 7th character (initial encounter, subsequent encounter or sequela) for each encounter for which the injury or condition is being treated.

Most categories in chapter 20 have a 7th character requirement for each applicable code. Most categories in this chapter have three 7th character values: A, initial encounter, D, subsequent encounter and S, sequela. While the patient may be seen by a new or different provider over the course of treatment for an injury or condition, assignment of the 7th character for external cause should match the 7th character of the code assigned for the associated injury or condition for the encounter.

**3) Use the full range of external cause codes**

Use the full range of external cause codes to completely describe the cause, the intent, the place of occurrence, and if applicable, the activity of the patient at the time of the event, and the patient's status, for all injuries, and other health conditions due to an external cause.

**4) Assign as many external cause codes as necessary**

Assign as many external cause codes as necessary to fully explain each cause. If only one external code can be recorded, assign the code most related to the principal diagnosis.

**5) The selection of the appropriate external cause code**

The selection of the appropriate external cause code is guided by the Alphabetic Index of External Causes and by Inclusion and Exclusion notes in the Tabular List.

**6) External cause code can never be a principal diagnosis**

An external cause code can never be a principal (first-listed) diagnosis.

**7) Combination external cause codes**

Certain of the external cause codes are combination codes that identify sequential events that result in an injury, such as a fall which results in striking against an object. The injury may be due to either event or both. The combination external cause code used should correspond to the sequence of events regardless of which caused the most serious injury.

> Toddler tripped and fell while walking and struck his head on an end table, sustaining a scalp contusion
>
> **SØØ.Ø3XA** **Contusion of scalp, initial encounter**
>
> **WØ1.19ØA** **Fall on same level from slipping, tripping and stumbling with subsequent striking against furniture, initial encounter**
>
> *Explanation:* Combination external cause codes identify sequential events that result in an injury, such as a fall resulting in striking against an object. The injury may be due to either or both events.

**8) No external cause code needed in certain circumstances**

No external cause code from Chapter 20 is needed if the external cause and intent are included in a code from another chapter (e.g., T36.ØX1-, Poisoning by penicillins, accidental (unintentional)).

**b. Place of occurrence guideline**

Codes from category Y92, Place of occurrence of the external cause, are secondary codes for use after other external cause codes to identify the location of the patient at the time of injury or other condition.

Generally, a place of occurrence code is assigned only once, at the initial encounter for treatment. However, in the rare instance that a new injury occurs during hospitalization, an additional place of occurrence code may be assigned. No 7th characters are used for Y92.

Do not use place of occurrence code Y92.9 if the place is not stated or is not applicable.

> A farmer was working in his barn and sustained a foot contusion when the horse stepped on his left foot
>
> **S9Ø.32XA** **Contusion of left foot, initial encounter**
>
> **W55.19XA** **Other contact with horse, initial encounter**
>
> **Y92.71** **Barn as the place of occurrence of the external cause**
>
> *Explanation:* A place-of-occurrence code from category Y92 is assigned at the initial encounter to identify the location of the patient at the time the injury occurred.

**c. Activity code**

Assign a code from category Y93, Activity code, to describe the activity of the patient at the time the injury or other health condition occurred.

An activity code is used only once, at the initial encounter for treatment. Only one code from Y93 should be recorded on a medical record.

The activity codes are not applicable to poisonings, adverse effects, misadventures or sequela.

Do not assign Y93.9, Unspecified activity, if the activity is not stated.

A code from category Y93 is appropriate for use with external cause and intent codes if identifying the activity provides additional information about the event.

> Ranch hand who was grooming a horse sustained a foot contusion when the horse stepped on his left foot
>
> **S9Ø.32XA** **Contusion of left foot, initial encounter**
>
> **W55.19XA** **Other contact with horse, initial encounter**
>
> **Y93.K3** **Activity, grooming and shearing an animal**
>
> *Explanation:* One activity code from category Y93 is assigned at the initial encounter only to describe the activity of the patient at the time the injury occurred.

**d. Place of occurrence, activity, and status codes used with other external cause code**

When applicable, place of occurrence, activity, and external cause status codes are sequenced after the main external cause code(s). Regardless of the number of external cause codes assigned, generally there should be only one place of occurrence code, one activity code, and one external cause status code assigned to an encounter. However, in the rare instance that a new injury occurs during hospitalization, an additional place of occurrence code may be assigned.

**e. If the reporting format limits the number of external cause codes**

If the reporting format limits the number of external cause codes that can be used in reporting clinical data, report the code for the cause/intent most related to the principal diagnosis. If the format permits capture of additional external cause codes, the cause/intent, including medical misadventures, of the additional events should be reported rather than the codes for place, activity, or external status.

**f. Multiple external cause coding guidelines**

More than one external cause code is required to fully describe the external cause of an illness or injury. The assignment of external cause codes should be sequenced in the following priority:

If two or more events cause separate injuries, an external cause code should be assigned for each cause. The first-listed external cause code will be selected in the following order:

External codes for child and adult abuse take priority over all other external cause codes.

*See Section I.C.19., Child and Adult abuse guidelines.*

External cause codes for terrorism events take priority over all other external cause codes except child and adult abuse.

External cause codes for cataclysmic events take priority over all other external cause codes except child and adult abuse and terrorism.

External cause codes for transport accidents take priority over all other external cause codes except cataclysmic events, child and adult abuse and terrorism.

Activity and external cause status codes are assigned following all causal (intent) external cause codes.

The first-listed external cause code should correspond to the cause of the most serious diagnosis due to an assault, accident, or self-harm, following the order of hierarchy listed above..

30-year-old man accidentally discharged his hunting rifle, sustaining an open gunshot wound, with no retained bullet fragments, to the right thigh, which caused him to fall down the stairs, resulting in closed displaced comminuted fracture of his left radial shaft

| | |
|---|---|
| **S71.131A** | **Puncture wound without foreign body, right thigh, initial encounter** |
| **W33.Ø2XA** | **Accidental discharge of hunting rifle, initial encounter** |
| **S52.352A** | **Displaced comminuted fracture of shaft of radius, left arm, initial encounter for closed fracture** |
| **W1Ø.9XXA** | **Fall (on) (from) unspecified stairs and steps, initial encounter** |

*Explanation:* If two or more events cause separate injuries, an external cause code should be assigned for each cause.

**g. Child and adult abuse guideline**

Adult and child abuse, neglect and maltreatment are classified as assault. Any of the assault codes may be used to indicate the external cause of any injury resulting from the confirmed abuse.

For confirmed cases of abuse, neglect and maltreatment, when the perpetrator is known, a code from YØ7, Perpetrator of maltreatment and neglect, should accompany any other assault codes.

*See Section I.C.19. Adult and child abuse, neglect and other maltreatment*

**h. Unknown or undetermined intent guideline**

If the intent (accident, self-harm, assault) of the cause of an injury or other condition is unknown or unspecified, code the intent as accidental intent. All transport accident categories assume accidental intent.

**1) Use of undetermined intent**

External cause codes for events of undetermined intent are only for use if the documentation in the record specifies that the intent cannot be determined.

**i. Sequelae (late effects) of external cause guidelines**

**1) Sequelae external cause codes**

Sequela are reported using the external cause code with the 7th character "S" for sequela. These codes should be used with any report of a late effect or sequela resulting from a previous injury.

*See Section I.B.10. Sequela (Late Effects)*

**2) Sequela external cause code with a related current injury**

A sequela external cause code should never be used with a related current nature of injury code.

**3) Use of sequela external cause codes for subsequent visits**

Use a late effect external cause code for subsequent visits when a late effect of the initial injury is being treated. Do not use a late effect external cause code for subsequent visits for follow-up care (e.g., to assess healing, to receive rehabilitative therapy) of the injury when no late effect of the injury has been documented.

**j. Terrorism guidelines**

**1) Cause of injury identified by the Federal Government (FBI) as terrorism**

When the cause of an injury is identified by the Federal Government (FBI) as terrorism, the first-listed external cause code should be a code from category Y38, Terrorism. The definition of terrorism employed by the FBI is found at the inclusion note at the beginning of category Y38. Use additional code for place of occurrence (Y92.-). More than one Y38 code may be assigned if the injury is the result of more than one mechanism of terrorism.

**2) Cause of an injury is suspected to be the result of terrorism**

When the cause of an injury is suspected to be the result of terrorism a code from category Y38 should not be assigned. Suspected cases should be classified as assault.

**3) Code Y38.9, Terrorism, secondary effects**

Assign code Y38.9, Terrorism, secondary effects, for conditions occurring subsequent to the terrorist event. This code should not be assigned for conditions that are due to the initial terrorist act.

It is acceptable to assign code Y38.9 with another code from Y38 if there is an injury due to the initial terrorist event and an injury that is a subsequent result of the terrorist event.

**k. External cause status**

A code from category Y99, External cause status, should be assigned whenever any other external cause code is assigned for an encounter, including an Activity code, except for the events noted below. Assign a code from category Y99, External cause status, to indicate the work status of the person at the time the event occurred. The status code indicates whether the event occurred during military activity, whether a non-military person was at work, whether an individual including a student or volunteer was involved in a non-work activity at the time of the causal event.

A code from Y99, External cause status, should be assigned, when applicable, with other external cause codes, such as transport accidents and falls. The external cause status codes are not applicable to poisonings, adverse effects, misadventures or late effects.

Do not assign a code from category Y99 if no other external cause codes (cause, activity) are applicable for the encounter.

An external cause status code is used only once, at the initial encounter for treatment. Only one code from Y99 should be recorded on a medical record.

Do not assign code Y99.9, Unspecified external cause status, if the status is not stated.

# Chapter 20. External Causes of Morbidity (VØØ-Y99)

**NOTE** This chapter permits the classification of environmental events and circumstances as the cause of injury, and other adverse effects. Where a code from this section is applicable, it is intended that it shall be used secondary to a code from another chapter of the Classification indicating the nature of the condition. Most often, the condition will be classifiable to Chapter 19, Injury, poisoning and certain other consequences of external causes (SØØ-T88). Other conditions that may be stated to be due to external causes are classified in Chapters I to XVIII. For these conditions, codes from Chapter 20 should be used to provide additional information as to the cause of the condition.

**AHA:** 2018,4Q,58-60

This chapter contains the following blocks:

VØØ-VØ9 Pedestrian injured in transport accident
VØØ-V99 Transport accidents
VØØ-X58 Accidents
V1Ø-V19 Pedal cycle rider injured in transport accident
V2Ø-V29 Motorcycle rider injured in transport accident
V3Ø-V39 Occupant of three-wheeled motor vehicle injured in transport accident
V4Ø-V49 Car occupant injured in transport accident
V5Ø-V59 Occupant of pick-up truck or van injured in transport accident
V6Ø-V69 Occupant of heavy transport vehicle injured in transport accident
V7Ø-V79 Bus occupant injured in transport accident
V8Ø-V89 Other land transport accidents
V9Ø-V94 Water transport accidents
V95-V97 Air and space transport accidents
V98-V99 Other and unspecified transport accidents
WØØ-W19 Slipping, tripping, stumbling and falls
WØØ-X58 Other external causes of accidental injury
W2Ø-W49 Exposure to inanimate mechanical forces
W5Ø-W64 Exposure to animate mechanical forces
W65-W74 Accidental non-transport drowning and submersion
W85-W99 Exposure to electric current, radiation and extreme ambient air temperature and pressure
XØØ-XØ8 Exposure to smoke, fire and flames
X1Ø-X19 Contact with heat and hot substances
X3Ø-X39 Exposure to forces of nature
X5Ø Overexertion and strenuous or repetitive movements
X52-X58 Accidental exposure to other specified factors
X71-X83 Intentional self-harm
X92-YØ8 Assault
Y21-Y33 Event of undetermined intent
Y35-Y38 Legal intervention, operations of war, military operations, and terrorism
Y62-Y69 Misadventures to patients during surgical and medical care
Y62-Y84 Complications of medical and surgical care
Y7Ø-Y82 Medical devices associated with adverse incidents in diagnostic and therapeutic use
Y83-Y84 Surgical and other medical procedures as the cause of abnormal reaction of the patient, or of later complication, without mention of misadventure at the time of the procedure
Y9Ø-Y99 Supplementary factors related to causes of morbidity classified elsewhere

## ACCIDENTS (VØØ-X58)

**AHA:** 2018,2Q,7-8

### Transport accidents (VØØ-V99)

**NOTE** This section is structured in 12 groups. Those relating to land transport accidents (VØØ-V89) reflect the victim's mode of transport and are subdivided to identify the victim's 'counterpart' or the type of event. The vehicle of which the injured person is an occupant is identified in the first two characters since it is seen as the most important factor to identify for prevention purposes. A transport accident is one in which the vehicle involved must be moving or running or in use for transport purposes at the time of the accident.

Use additional code to identify:
airbag injury (W22.1)
type of street or road (Y92.4-)
use of cellular telephone and other electronic equipment at the time of the transport accident (Y93.C-)

**EXCLUDES 1** *agricultural vehicles in stationary use or maintenance (W31.-)*
*assault by crashing of motor vehicle (YØ3.-)*
*automobile or motor cycle in stationary use or maintenance - code to type of accident*
*crashing of motor vehicle, undetermined intent (Y32)*
*intentional self-harm by crashing of motor vehicle (X82)*

**EXCLUDES 2** *transport accidents due to cataclysm (X34-X38)*

**NOTE** Definitions related to transport accidents:

(a) A transport accident (VØØ-V99) is any accident involving a device designed primarily for, or used at the time primarily for, conveying persons or good from one place to another.

(b) A public highway [trafficway] or street is the entire width between property lines (or other boundary lines) of land open to the public as a matter of right or custom for purposes of moving persons or property from one place to another. A roadway is that part of the public highway designed, improved and customarily used for vehicular traffic.

(c) A traffic accident is any vehicle accident occurring on the public highway [i.e. originating on, terminating on, or involving a vehicle partially on the highway]. A vehicle accident is assumed to have occurred on the public highway unless another place is specified, except in the case of accidents involving only off-road motor vehicles, which are classified as nontraffic accidents unless the contrary is stated.

(d) A nontraffic accident is any vehicle accident that occurs entirely in any place other than a public highway.

(e) A pedestrian is any person involved in an accident who was not at the time of the accident riding in or on a motor vehicle, railway train, streetcar or animal-drawn or other vehicle, or on a pedal cycle or animal. This includes, a person changing a tire, working on a parked car, or a person on foot. It also includes the user of a pedestrian conveyance such as a baby stroller, ice-skates, skis, sled, roller skates, a skateboard, nonmotorized or motorized wheelchair, motorized mobility scooter, or nonmotorized scooter.

(f) A driver is an occupant of a transport vehicle who is operating or intending to operate it.

(g) A passenger is any occupant of a transport vehicle other than the driver, except a person traveling on the outside of the vehicle.

(h) A person on the outside of a vehicle is any person being transported by a vehicle but not occupying the space normally reserved for the driver or passengers, or the space intended for the transport of property. This includes a person travelling on the bodywork, bumper, fender, roof, running board or step of a vehicle, as well as, hanging on the outside of the vehicle.

(i) A pedal cycle is any land transport vehicle operated solely by nonmotorized pedals including a bicycle or tricycle.

(j) A pedal cyclist is any person riding a pedal cycle or in a sidecar or trailer attached to a pedal cycle.

(k) A motorcycle is a two-wheeled motor vehicle with one or two riding saddles and sometimes with a third wheel for the support of a sidecar. The sidecar is considered part of the motorcycle. This includes a moped, motor scooter, or motorized bicycle.

(l) A motorcycle rider is any person riding a motorcycle or in a sidecar or trailer attached to the motorcycle.

(m) A three-wheeled motor vehicle is a motorized tricycle designed primarily for on-road use. This includes a motor-driven tricycle, a motorized rickshaw, or a three-wheeled motor car.

(n) A car [automobile] is a four-wheeled motor vehicle designed primarily for carrying up to 7 persons. A trailer being towed by the car is considered part of the car. It does not include a van or minivan — see definition (o).

(o) A pick-up truck or van is a four or six-wheeled motor vehicle designed for carrying passengers as well as property or cargo weighing less than the local limit for classification as a heavy goods vehicle, and not requiring a special driver's license. This includes a minivan and a sport-utility vehicle (SUV).

(p) A heavy transport vehicle is a motor vehicle designed primarily for carrying property, meeting local criteria for classification as a heavy goods vehicle in terms of weight and requiring a special driver's license.

(q) A bus (coach) is a motor vehicle designed or adapted primarily for carrying more than 1Ø passengers, and requiring a special driver's license.

(r) A railway train or railway vehicle is any device, with or without freight or passenger cars couple to it, designed for traffic on a railway track. This includes subterranean (subways) or elevated trains.

(s) A streetcar, is a device designed and used primarily for transporting passengers within a municipality, running on rails, usually subject to normal traffic control signals, and operated principally on a right-of-way that forms part of the roadway. This includes a tram or trolley that runs on rails. A trailer being towed by a streetcar is considered part of the streetcar.

(t) A special vehicle mainly used on industrial premises is a motor vehicle designed primarily for use within the buildings and premises of industrial or commercial establishments. This includes battery-powered airport passenger vehicles or baggage/mail trucks, forklifts, coal-cars in a coal mine, logging cars and trucks used in mines or quarries.

(u) A special vehicle mainly used in agriculture is a motor vehicle designed specifically for use in farming and agriculture (horticulture), to work the land, tend and harvest crops and transport materials on the farm. This includes harvesters, farm machinery and tractor and trailers.

(v) A special construction vehicle is a motor vehicle designed specifically for use on construction and demolition sites. This includes bulldozers, diggers, earth levellers, dump trucks. backhoes, front-end loaders, pavers, and mechanical shovels.

(w) A special all-terrain vehicle is a motor vehicle of special design to enable it to negotiate over rough or soft terrain, snow or sand. Examples of special design are high construction, special wheels and tires, tracks, and support on a cushion of air. This includes snow mobiles, All-terrain vehicles (ATV), and dune buggies. It does not include passenger vehicle designated as Sport Utility Vehicles. (SUV)

(x) A watercraft is any device designed for transporting passengers or goods on water. This includes motor or sailboats, ships, and hovercraft.

(y) An aircraft is any device for transporting passengers or goods in the air. This includes hot-air balloons, gliders, helicopters and airplanes.

(z) A military vehicle is any motorized vehicle operating on a public roadway owned by the military and being operated by a member of the military.

## Pedestrian injured in transport accident (VØØ-VØ9)

INCLUDES person changing tire on transport vehicle
person examining engine of vehicle broken down in (on side of) road

EXCLUDES 1 *fall due to non-transport collision with other person (WØ3)*
*pedestrian on foot falling (slipping) on ice and snow (WØØ.-)*
*struck or bumped by another person (W51)*

The appropriate 7th character is to be added to each code from categories VØØ-VØ9.
A initial encounter
D subsequent encounter
S sequela

✓4th **VØØ Pedestrian conveyance accident**

Use additional place of occurrence and activity external cause codes, if known (Y92.-, Y93.-)

EXCLUDES 1 *collision with another person without fall (W51)*
*fall due to person on foot colliding with another person on foot (WØ3)*
*fall from non-moving wheelchair, nonmotorized scooter and motorized mobility scooter without collision (WØ5.-)*
*pedestrian (conveyance) collision with other land transport vehicle (VØ1-VØ9)*
*pedestrian on foot falling (slipping) on ice and snow (WØØ.-)*

✓5th **VØØ.Ø Pedestrian on foot injured in collision with pedestrian conveyance**

✓x7th **VØØ.Ø1 Pedestrian on foot injured in collision with roller-skater**

✓x7th **VØØ.Ø2 Pedestrian on foot injured in collision with skateboarder**

✓6th **VØØ.Ø3 Pedestrian on foot injured in collision with standing micro-mobility pedestrian conveyance**

✓7th **VØØ.Ø31 Pedestrian on foot injured in collision with rider of standing electric scooter**

✓7th **VØØ.Ø38 Pedestrian on foot injured in collision with rider of other standing micro-mobility pedestrian conveyance**
Pedestrian on foot injured in collision with rider of hoverboard
Pedestrian on foot injured in collision with rider of segway

✓x7th **VØØ.Ø9 Pedestrian on foot injured in collision with other pedestrian conveyance**

✓5th **VØØ.1 Rolling-type pedestrian conveyance accident**

EXCLUDES 1 *accident with baby stroller (VØØ.82-)*
*accident with motorized mobility scooter (VØØ.83-)*
*accident with wheelchair (powered) (VØØ.81-)*

✓6th **VØØ.11 In-line roller-skate accident**

✓7th **VØØ.111 Fall from in-line roller-skates**

✓7th **VØØ.112 In-line roller-skater colliding with stationary object**

✓7th **VØØ.118 Other in-line roller-skate accident**

EXCLUDES 1 *roller-skater collision with other land transport vehicle (VØ1-VØ9 with 5th character 1)*

✓6th **VØØ.12 Non-in-line roller-skate accident**

✓7th **VØØ.121 Fall from non-in-line roller-skates**

✓7th **VØØ.122 Non-in-line roller-skater colliding with stationary object**

✓7th **VØØ.128 Other non-in-line roller-skating accident**

EXCLUDES 1 *roller-skater collision with other land transport vehicle (VØ1-VØ9 with 5th character 1)*

✓6th **VØØ.13 Skateboard accident**

✓7th **VØØ.131 Fall from skateboard**

✓7th **VØØ.132 Skateboarder colliding with stationary object**

✓7th **VØØ.138 Other skateboard accident**

EXCLUDES 1 *skateboarder collision with other land transport vehicle (VØ1-VØ9 with 5th character 2)*

✓6th **VØØ.14 Scooter (nonmotorized) accident**

EXCLUDES 1 *motor scooter accident (V2Ø-V29)*

✓7th **VØØ.141 Fall from scooter (nonmotorized)**

✓7th **VØØ.142 Scooter (nonmotorized) colliding with stationary object**

✓7th **VØØ.148 Other scooter (nonmotorized) accident**

EXCLUDES 1 *scooter (nonmotorized) collision with other land transport vehicle (VØ1-VØ9 with fifth character 9)*

✓6th **VØØ.15 Heelies accident**
Rolling shoe
Wheeled shoe
Wheelies accident

✓7th **VØØ.151 Fall from heelies**

✓7th **VØØ.152 Heelies colliding with stationary object**

✓7th **VØØ.158 Other heelies accident**

✓6th **VØØ.18 Accident on other rolling-type pedestrian conveyance**

✓7th **VØØ.181 Fall from other rolling-type pedestrian conveyance**

✓7th **VØØ.182 Pedestrian on other rolling-type pedestrian conveyance colliding with stationary object**

✓7th **VØØ.188 Other accident on other rolling-type pedestrian conveyance**

✓5th **VØØ.2 Gliding-type pedestrian conveyance accident**

✓6th **VØØ.21 Ice-skates accident**

✓7th **VØØ.211 Fall from ice-skates**

✓7th **VØØ.212 Ice-skater colliding with stationary object**

✓7th **VØØ.218 Other ice-skates accident**

EXCLUDES 1 *ice-skater collision with other land transport vehicle (VØ1-VØ9 with 5th character 9)*

✓6th **VØØ.22 Sled accident**

✓7th **VØØ.221 Fall from sled**

✓7th **VØØ.222 Sledder colliding with stationary object**

✓7th **VØØ.228 Other sled accident**

EXCLUDES 1 *sled collision with other land transport vehicle (VØ1-VØ9 with 5th character 9)*

✓6th **VØØ.28 Other gliding-type pedestrian conveyance accident**

✓7th **VØØ.281 Fall from other gliding-type pedestrian conveyance**

✓7th **VØØ.282 Pedestrian on other gliding-type pedestrian conveyance colliding with stationary object**

✓7th **VØØ.288 Other accident on other gliding-type pedestrian conveyance**

EXCLUDES 1 *gliding-type pedestrian conveyance collision with other land transport vehicle (VØ1-VØ9 with 5th character 9)*

✓5th **VØØ.3 Flat-bottomed pedestrian conveyance accident**

✓6th **VØØ.31 Snowboard accident**

✓7th **VØØ.311 Fall from snowboard**

✓7th **VØØ.312 Snowboarder colliding with stationary object**

√7th **V00.318 Other snowboard accident**

EXCLUDES 1 *snowboarder collision with other land transport vehicle (V01-V09 with 5th character 9)*

√6th **V00.32 Snow-ski accident**

√7th **V00.321 Fall from snow-skis**

√7th **V00.322 Snow-skier colliding with stationary object**

√7th **V00.328 Other snow-ski accident**

EXCLUDES 1 *snow-skier collision with other land transport vehicle (V01-V09 with 5th character 9)*

√6th **V00.38 Other flat-bottomed pedestrian conveyance accident**

√7th **V00.381 Fall from other flat-bottomed pedestrian conveyance**

√7th **V00.382 Pedestrian on other flat-bottomed pedestrian conveyance colliding with stationary object**

√7th **V00.388 Other accident on other flat-bottomed pedestrian conveyance**

√5th **V00.8 Accident on other pedestrian conveyance**

√6th **V00.81 Accident with wheelchair (powered)**

√7th **V00.811 Fall from moving wheelchair (powered)**

EXCLUDES 1 *fall from non-moving wheelchair (W05.0)*

√7th **V00.812 Wheelchair (powered) colliding with stationary object**

√7th **V00.818 Other accident with wheelchair (powered)**

√6th **V00.82 Accident with baby stroller**

√7th **V00.821 Fall from baby stroller**

√7th **V00.822 Baby stroller colliding with stationary object**

√7th **V00.828 Other accident with baby stroller**

√6th **V00.83 Accident with motorized mobility scooter**

√7th **V00.831 Fall from motorized mobility scooter**

EXCLUDES 1 *fall from non-moving motorized mobility scooter (W05.2)*

√7th **V00.832 Motorized mobility scooter colliding with stationary object**

√7th **V00.838 Other accident with motorized mobility scooter**

√6th **V00.84 Accident with standing micro-mobility pedestrian conveyance**

√7th **V00.841 Fall from standing electric scooter**

√7th **V00.842 Pedestrian on standing electric scooter colliding with stationary object**

√7th **V00.848 Other accident with standing micro-mobility pedestrian conveyance**
Accident with hoverboard
Accident with segway

√6th **V00.89 Accident on other pedestrian conveyance**

√7th **V00.891 Fall from other pedestrian conveyance**

√7th **V00.892 Pedestrian on other pedestrian conveyance colliding with stationary object**

√7th **V00.898 Other accident on other pedestrian conveyance**

EXCLUDES 1 *other pedestrian (conveyance) collision with other land transport vehicle (V01-V09 with 5th character 9)*

√4th **V01 Pedestrian injured in collision with pedal cycle**

√5th **V01.0 Pedestrian injured in collision with pedal cycle in nontraffic accident**

√x7th **V01.00 Pedestrian on foot injured in collision with pedal cycle in nontraffic accident**
Pedestrian NOS injured in collision with pedal cycle in nontraffic accident

√x7th **V01.01 Pedestrian on roller-skates injured in collision with pedal cycle in nontraffic accident**

√x7th **V01.02 Pedestrian on skateboard injured in collision with pedal cycle in nontraffic accident**

√6th **V01.03 Pedestrian on standing micro-mobility pedestrian conveyance injured in collision with pedal cycle in nontraffic accident**

√7th **V01.031 Pedestrian on standing electric scooter injured in collision with pedal cycle in nontraffic accident**

√7th **V01.038 Pedestrian on other standing micro-mobility pedestrian conveyance injured in collision with pedal cycle in nontraffic accident**
Pedestrian on hoverboard injured in collision with pedal cycle in nontraffic accident
Pedestrian on segway injured in collision with pedal cycle in nontraffic accident

√x7th **V01.09 Pedestrian with other conveyance injured in collision with pedal cycle in nontraffic accident**
Pedestrian in motorized mobility scooter injured in collision with pedal cycle in nontraffic accident
Pedestrian in wheelchair (powered) injured in collision with pedal cycle in nontraffic accident
Pedestrian on ice-skates injured in collision with pedal cycle in nontraffic accident
Pedestrian on nonmotorized scooter injured in collision with pedal cycle in nontraffic accident
Pedestrian on sled injured in collision with pedal cycle in nontraffic accident
Pedestrian on snowboard injured in collision with pedal cycle in nontraffic accident
Pedestrian on snow-skis injured in collision with pedal cycle in nontraffic accident
Pedestrian with baby stroller injured in collision with pedal cycle in nontraffic accident

√5th **V01.1 Pedestrian injured in collision with pedal cycle in traffic accident**

√x7th **V01.10 Pedestrian on foot injured in collision with pedal cycle in traffic accident**
Pedestrian NOS injured in collision with pedal cycle in traffic accident

√x7th **V01.11 Pedestrian on roller-skates injured in collision with pedal cycle in traffic accident**

√x7th **V01.12 Pedestrian on skateboard injured in collision with pedal cycle in traffic accident**

√6th **V01.13 Pedestrian on standing micro-mobility pedestrian conveyance injured in collision with pedal cycle in traffic accident**

√7th **V01.131 Pedestrian on standing electric scooter injured in collision with pedal cycle in traffic accident**

√7th **V01.138 Pedestrian on other standing micro-mobility pedestrian conveyance injured in collision with pedal cycle in traffic accident**
Pedestrian on hoverboard injured in collision with pedal cycle in traffic accident
Pedestrian on segway injured in collision with pedal cycle in traffic accident

√x7th **V01.19 Pedestrian with other conveyance injured in collision with pedal cycle in traffic accident**
Pedestrian in motorized mobility scooter injured in collision with pedal cycle in traffic accident
Pedestrian in wheelchair (powered) injured in collision with pedal cycle in traffic accident
Pedestrian on ice-skates injured in collision with pedal cycle in traffic accident
Pedestrian on nonmotorized scooter injured in collision with pedal cycle in traffic accident
Pedestrian on sled injured in collision with pedal cycle in traffic accident
Pedestrian on snowboard injured in collision with pedal cycle in traffic accident
Pedestrian on snow-skis injured in collision with pedal cycle in traffic accident
Pedestrian with baby stroller injured in collision with pedal cycle in traffic accident

√5th **V01.9 Pedestrian injured in collision with pedal cycle, unspecified whether traffic or nontraffic accident**

√x7th **V01.90 Pedestrian on foot injured in collision with pedal cycle, unspecified whether traffic or nontraffic accident**
Pedestrian NOS injured in collision with pedal cycle, unspecified whether traffic or nontraffic accident

✓x7th **V01.91 Pedestrian on roller-skates injured in collision with pedal cycle, unspecified whether traffic or nontraffic accident**

✓x7th **V01.92 Pedestrian on skateboard injured in collision with pedal cycle, unspecified whether traffic or nontraffic accident**

✓6th **V01.93 Pedestrian on standing micro-mobility pedestrian conveyance injured in collision with pedal cycle, unspecified whether traffic or nontraffic accident**

✓7th **V01.931 Pedestrian on standing electric scooter injured in collision with pedal cycle, unspecified whether traffic or nontraffic accident**

✓7th **V01.938 Pedestrian on other standing micro-mobility pedestrian conveyance injured in collision with pedal cycle, unspecified whether traffic or nontraffic accident**

Pedestrian on hoverboard injured in collision with pedal cycle, unspecified whether traffic or nontraffic accident

Pedestrian on segway injured in collision with pedal cycle, unspecified whether traffic or nontraffic accident

✓x7th **V01.99 Pedestrian with other conveyance injured in collision with pedal cycle, unspecified whether traffic or nontraffic accident**

Pedestrian in motorized mobility scooter injured in collision with pedal cycle, unspecified whether traffic or nontraffic accident

Pedestrian in wheelchair (powered) injured in collision with pedal cycle, unspecified whether traffic or nontraffic accident

Pedestrian on ice-skates injured in collision with pedal cycle unspecified, whether traffic or nontraffic accident

Pedestrian on nonmotorized scooter injured in collision with pedal cycle, unspecified whether traffic or nontraffic accident

Pedestrian on sled injured in collision with pedal cycle unspecified, whether traffic or nontraffic accident

Pedestrian on snowboard injured in collision with pedal cycle, unspecified whether traffic or nontraffic accident

Pedestrian on snow-skis injured in collision with pedal cycle, unspecified whether traffic or nontraffic accident

Pedestrian with baby stroller injured in collision with pedal cycle, unspecified whether traffic or nontraffic accident

✓4th **V02 Pedestrian injured in collision with two- or three-wheeled motor vehicle**

✓5th **V02.0 Pedestrian injured in collision with two- or three-wheeled motor vehicle in nontraffic accident**

✓x7th **V02.00 Pedestrian on foot injured in collision with two- or three-wheeled motor vehicle in nontraffic accident**

Pedestrian NOS injured in collision with two- or three-wheeled motor vehicle in nontraffic accident

✓x7th **V02.01 Pedestrian on roller-skates injured in collision with two- or three-wheeled motor vehicle in nontraffic accident**

✓x7th **V02.02 Pedestrian on skateboard injured in collision with two- or three-wheeled motor vehicle in nontraffic accident**

✓6th **V02.03 Pedestrian on standing micro-mobility pedestrian conveyance injured in collision with two- or three-wheeled motor vehicle in nontraffic accident**

✓7th **V02.031 Pedestrian on standing electric scooter injured in collision with two- or three-wheeled motor vehicle in nontraffic accident**

✓7th **V02.038 Pedestrian on other standing micro-mobility pedestrian conveyance injured in collision with two- or three-wheeled motor vehicle in nontraffic accident**

Pedestrian on hoverboard injured in collision with two-or three wheeled motor vehicle in nontraffic accident

Pedestrian on segway injured in collision with two- or three-wheeled motor vehicle in nontraffic accident

✓x7th **V02.09 Pedestrian with other conveyance injured in collision with two- or three-wheeled motor vehicle in nontraffic accident**

Pedestrian in motorized mobility scooter injured in collision with two- or three-wheeled motor vehicle in nontraffic accident

Pedestrian in wheelchair (powered) injured in collision with two- or three-wheeled motor vehicle in nontraffic accident

Pedestrian on ice-skates injured in collision with two- or three-wheeled motor vehicle in nontraffic accident

Pedestrian on nonmotorized scooter injured in collision with two- or three-wheeled motor vehicle in nontraffic accident

Pedestrian on sled injured in collision with two- or three-wheeled motor vehicle in nontraffic accident

Pedestrian on snowboard injured in collision with two- or three-wheeled motor vehicle in nontraffic accident

Pedestrian on snow-skis injured in collision with two- or three-wheeled motor vehicle in nontraffic accident

Pedestrian with baby stroller injured in collision with two- or three-wheeled motor vehicle in nontraffic accident

✓5th **V02.1 Pedestrian injured in collision with two- or three-wheeled motor vehicle in traffic accident**

✓x7th **V02.10 Pedestrian on foot injured in collision with two- or three-wheeled motor vehicle in traffic accident**

Pedestrian NOS injured in collision with two- or three-wheeled motor vehicle in traffic accident

✓x7th **V02.11 Pedestrian on roller-skates injured in collision with two- or three-wheeled motor vehicle in traffic accident**

✓x7th **V02.12 Pedestrian on skateboard injured in collision with two- or three-wheeled motor vehicle in traffic accident**

✓6th **V02.13 Pedestrian on standing micro-mobility pedestrian conveyance injured in collision with two- or three-wheeled motor vehicle in traffic accident**

✓7th **V02.131 Pedestrian on standing electric scooter injured in collision with two- or three-wheeled motor vehicle in traffic accident**

✓7th **V02.138 Pedestrian on other standing micro-mobility pedestrian conveyance injured in collision with two- or three-wheeled motor vehicle in traffic accident**

Pedestrian on hoverboard injured in collision with two-or three wheeled motor vehicle in traffic accident

Pedestrian on segway injured in collision with two- or three-wheeled motor vehicle in traffic accident

✓x7th **V02.19 Pedestrian with other conveyance injured in collision with two- or three-wheeled motor vehicle in traffic accident**

Pedestrian in motorized mobility scooter injued in collision with two- or three-wheeled motor vehicle in traffic accident

Pedestrian in wheelchair (powered) injured in collision with two- or three-wheeled motor vehicle in traffic accident

Pedestrian on ice-skates injured in collision with two- or three-wheeled motor vehicle in traffic accident

Pedestrian on nonmotorized scooter injured in collision with two- or three-wheeled motor vehicle in traffic accident

Pedestrian on sled injured in collision with two- or three-wheeled motor vehicle in traffic accident

Pedestrian on snowboard injured in collision with two- or three-wheeled motor vehicle in traffic accident

Pedestrian on snow-skis injured in collision with two- or three-wheeled motor vehicle in traffic accident

Pedestrian with baby stroller injured in collision with two- or three-wheeled motor vehicle in traffic accident

V02.9 **Pedestrian injured in collision with two- or three-wheeled motor vehicle, unspecified whether traffic or nontraffic accident**

V02.90 **Pedestrian on foot injured in collision with two- or three-wheeled motor vehicle, unspecified whether traffic or nontraffic accident**
Pedestrian NOS injured in collision with two- or three-wheeled motor vehicle, unspecified whether traffic or nontraffic accident

V02.91 **Pedestrian on roller-skates injured in collision with two- or three-wheeled motor vehicle, unspecified whether traffic or nontraffic accident**

V02.92 **Pedestrian on skateboard injured in collision with two- or three-wheeled motor vehicle, unspecified whether traffic or nontraffic accident**

V02.93 **Pedestrian on standing micro-mobility pedestrian conveyance injured in collision with two- or three-wheeled motor vehicle, unspecified whether traffic or nontraffic accident**

V02.931 **Pedestrian on standing electric scooter injured in collision with two- or three wheeled motor vehicle, unspecified whether traffic or nontraffic accident**

V02.938 **Pedestrian on other standing micro-mobility pedestrian conveyance injured in collision with two- or three wheeled motor vehicle, unspecified whether traffic or nontraffic accident**
Pedestrian on hoverboard injured in collision with two-three-wheeled motor vehicle, unspecified whether traffic or nontraffic accident
Pedestrian on segway injured in collision with two- or three wheeled motor vehicle, unspecified whether traffic or nontraffic accident

V02.99 **Pedestrian with other conveyance injured in collision with two- or three-wheeled motor vehicle, unspecified whether traffic or nontraffic accident**
Pedestrian in motorized mobility scooter injured in collision with two- or three wheeled motor vehicle, unspecified whether traffic or nontraffic accident
Pedestrian in wheelchair (powered) injured in collision with two- or three-wheeled motor vehicle, unspecified whether traffic or nontraffic accident
Pedestrian on ice-skates injured in collision with two- or three-wheeled motor vehicle, unspecified whether traffic or nontraffic accident
Pedestrian on nonmotorized scooter injured in collision with two- or three-wheeled motor vehicle, unspecified whether traffic or nontraffic accident
Pedestrian on sled injured in collision with two- or three-wheeled motor vehicle, unspecified whether traffic or nontraffic accident
Pedestrian on snowboard injured in collision with two- or three-wheeled motor vehicle, unspecified whether traffic or nontraffic accident
Pedestrian on snow-skis injured in collision with two- or three-wheeled motor vehicle, unspecified whether traffic or nontraffic accident
Pedestrian with baby stroller injured in collision with two- or three-wheeled motor vehicle, unspecified whether traffic or nontraffic accident

## V03 Pedestrian injured in collision with car, pick-up truck or van

V03.0 **Pedestrian injured in collision with car, pick-up truck or van in nontraffic accident**

V03.00 **Pedestrian on foot injured in collision with car, pick-up truck or van in nontraffic accident**
Pedestrian NOS injured in collision with car, pick-up truck or van in nontraffic accident

V03.01 **Pedestrian on roller-skates injured in collision with car, pick-up truck or van in nontraffic accident**

V03.02 **Pedestrian on skateboard injured in collision with car, pick-up truck or van in nontraffic accident**

V03.03 **Pedestrian on standing micro-mobility pedestrian conveyance injured in collision with car, pick-up or van in nontraffic accident**

V03.031 **Pedestrian on standing electric scooter injured in collision with car, pick-up or van in nontraffic accident**

V03.038 **Pedestrian on other standing micro-mobility pedestrian conveyance injured in collision with car, pick-up or van in nontraffic accident**
Pedestrian on hoverboard injured in collision with car, pick-up or van in nontraffic accident
Pedestrian on segway injured in collision with car, pick-up or van in nontraffic accident

V03.09 **Pedestrian with other conveyance injured in collision with car, pick-up truck or van in nontraffic accident**
Pedestrian in motorized mobility scooter injured in collision with car, pick-up truck or van in nontraffic accident
Pedestrian in wheelchair (powered) injured in collision with car, pick-up truck or van in nontraffic accident
Pedestrian on ice-skates injured in collision with car, pick-up truck or van in nontraffic accident
Pedestrian on nonmotorized scooter injured in collision with car, pick-up truck or van in nontraffic accident
Pedestrian on sled injured in collision with car, pick-up truck or van in nontraffic accident
Pedestrian on snowboard injured in collision with car, pick-up truck or van in nontraffic accident
Pedestrian on snow-skis injured in collision with car, pick-up truck or van in nontraffic accident
Pedestrian with baby stroller injured in collision with car, pick-up truck or van in nontraffic accident

V03.1 **Pedestrian injured in collision with car, pick-up truck or van in traffic accident**

V03.10 **Pedestrian on foot injured in collision with car, pick-up truck or van in traffic accident**
Pedestrian NOS injured in collision with car, pick-up truck or van in traffic accident

V03.11 **Pedestrian on roller-skates injured in collision with car, pick-up truck or van in traffic accident**

V03.12 **Pedestrian on skateboard injured in collision with car, pick-up truck or van in traffic accident**

V03.13 **Pedestrian on standing micro-mobility pedestrian conveyance injured in collision with car, pick-up or van in traffic accident**

V03.131 **Pedestrian on standing electric scooter injured in collision with car, pick-up or van in traffic accident**

V03.138 **Pedestrian on other standing micro-mobility pedestrian conveyance injured in collision with car, pick-up or van in traffic accident**
Pedestrian on hoverboard injured in collision with car, pick-up or van in traffic accident
Pedestrian on segway injured in collision with car, pick-up or van in traffic accident

V03.19 **Pedestrian with other conveyance injured in collision with car, pick-up truck or van in traffic accident**
Pedestrian in motorized mobility scooter injured in collision with car, pick-up truck or van in nontraffic accident
Pedestrian in wheelchair (powered) injured in collision with car, pick-up truck or van in traffic accident
Pedestrian on ice-skates injured in collision with car, pick-up truck or van in traffic accident
Pedestrian on nonmotorized scooter injured in collision with car, pick-up truck or van in nontraffic accident
Pedestrian on sled injured in collision with car, pick-up truck or van in traffic accident
Pedestrian on snowboard injured in collision with car, pick-up truck or van in traffic accident
Pedestrian on snow-skis injured in collision with car, pick-up truck or van in traffic accident
Pedestrian with baby stroller injured in collision with car, pick-up truck or van in traffic accident

V03.9 **Pedestrian injured in collision with car, pick-up truck or van, unspecified whether traffic or nontraffic accident**

V03.90 **Pedestrian on foot injured in collision with car, pick-up truck or van, unspecified whether traffic or nontraffic accident**
Pedestrian NOS injured in collision with car, pick-up truck or van, unspecified whether traffic or nontraffic accident

V03.91 **Pedestrian on roller-skates injured in collision with car, pick-up truck or van, unspecified whether traffic or nontraffic accident**

√x7th **V03.92 Pedestrian on skateboard injured in collision with car, pick-up truck or van, unspecified whether traffic or nontraffic accident**

√6th **V03.93 Pedestrian on standing micro-mobility pedestrian conveyance injured in collision with car, pick-up or van, unspecified whether traffic or nontraffic accident**

√7th **V03.931 Pedestrian on standing electric scooter injured in collision with car, pick-up or van, unspecified whether traffic or nontraffic accident**

√7th **V03.938 Pedestrian on other standing micro-mobility pedestrian conveyance injured in collision with car, pick-up or van, unspecified whether traffic or nontraffic accident**
Pedestrian on hoverboard injured in collision with car, pick-up or van, unspecified whether traffic or nontraffic accident
Pedestrian on segway injured in collision with car, pick-up or van, unspecified whether traffic or nontraffic accident

√x7th **V03.99 Pedestrian with other conveyance injured in collision with car, pick-up truck or van, unspecified whether traffic or nontraffic accident**
Pedestrian in motorized mobility scooter injured in collision with car, pick-up truck or van, unspecified whether traffic or nontraffic accident
Pedestrian in wheelchair (powered) injured in collision with car, pick-up truck or van, unspecified whether traffic or nontraffic accident
Pedestrian on ice-skates injured in collision with car, pick-up truck or van, unspecified whether traffic or nontraffic accident
Pedestrian on nonmotorized scooter injured in collision with car, pick-up truck or van, unspecified whether traffic or nontraffic accident
Pedestrian on sled injured in collision with car, pick-up truck or van in nontraffic accident
Pedestrian on snowboard injured in collision with car, pick-up truck or van, unspecified whether traffic or nontraffic accident
Pedestrian on snow-skis injured in collision with car, pick-up truck or van, unspecified whether traffic or nontraffic accident
Pedestrian with baby stroller injured in collision with car, pick-up truck or van, unspecified whether traffic or nontraffic accident

√4th **V04 Pedestrian injured in collision with heavy transport vehicle or bus**

EXCLUDES 1 *pedestrian injured in collision with military vehicle (V09.01, V09.21)*

√5th **V04.0 Pedestrian injured in collision with heavy transport vehicle or bus in nontraffic accident**

√x7th **V04.00 Pedestrian on foot injured in collision with heavy transport vehicle or bus in nontraffic accident**
Pedestrian NOS injured in collision with heavy transport vehicle or bus in nontraffic accident

√x7th **V04.01 Pedestrian on roller-skates injured in collision with heavy transport vehicle or bus in nontraffic accident**

√x7th **V04.02 Pedestrian on skateboard injured in collision with heavy transport vehicle or bus in nontraffic accident**

√6th **V04.03 Pedestrian on standing micro-mobility pedestrian conveyance injured in collision with heavy transport vehicle or bus in nontraffic accident**

√7th **V04.031 Pedestrian on standing electric scooter injured in collision with heavy transport vehicle or bus in nontraffic accident**

√7th **V04.038 Pedestrian on other standing micro-mobility pedestrian conveyance injured in collision with heavy transport vehicle or bus in nontraffic accident**
Pedestrian on hoverboard injured in collision with heavy transport vehicle or bus in nontraffic accident
Pedestrian on segway injured in collision with heavy transport vehicle or bus in nontraffic accident

√x7th **V04.09 Pedestrian with other conveyance injured in collision with heavy transport vehicle or bus in nontraffic accident**
Pedestrian in motorized mobility scooter injured in collision with heavy transport vehicle or bus in nontraffic accident
Pedestrian in wheelchair (powered) injured in collision with heavy transport vehicle or bus in nontraffic accident
Pedestrian on ice-skates injured in collision with heavy transport vehicle or bus in nontraffic accident
Pedestrian on nonmotorized scooter injured in collision with heavy transport vehicle or bus in nontraffic accident
Pedestrian on sled injured in collision with heavy transport vehicle or bus in nontraffic accident
Pedestrian on snowboard injured in collision with heavy transport vehicle or bus in nontraffic accident
Pedestrian on snow-skis injured in collision with heavy transport vehicle or bus in nontraffic accident
Pedestrian with baby stroller injured in collision with heavy transport vehicle or bus in nontraffic accident

√5th **V04.1 Pedestrian injured in collision with heavy transport vehicle or bus in traffic accident**

√x7th **V04.10 Pedestrian on foot injured in collision with heavy transport vehicle or bus in traffic accident**
Pedestrian NOS injured in collision with heavy transport vehicle or bus in traffic accident

√x7th **V04.11 Pedestrian on roller-skates injured in collision with heavy transport vehicle or bus in traffic accident**

√x7th **V04.12 Pedestrian on skateboard injured in collision with heavy transport vehicle or bus in traffic accident**

√6th **V04.13 Pedestrian on standing micro-mobility pedestrian conveyance injured in collision with heavy transport vehicle or bus in traffic accident**

√7th **V04.131 Pedestrian on standing electric scooter injured in collision with heavy transport vehicle or bus in traffic accident**

√7th **V04.138 Pedestrian on other standing micro-mobility pedestrian conveyance injured in collision with heavy transport vehicle or bus in traffic accident**
Pedestrian on hoverboard injured in collision with heavy transport vehicle or bus in traffic accident
Pedestrian on segway injured in collision with heavy transport vehicle or bus in traffic accident

√x7th **V04.19 Pedestrian with other conveyance injured in collision with heavy transport vehicle or bus in traffic accident**
Pedestrian in motorized mobility scooter injured in collision with heavy transport vehicle or bus in traffic accident
Pedestrian in wheelchair (powered) injured in collision with heavy transport vehicle or bus in traffic accident
Pedestrian on ice-skates injured in collision with heavy transport vehicle or bus in traffic accident
Pedestrian on nonmotorized scooter injured in collision with heavy transport vehicle or bus in traffic accident
Pedestrian on sled injured in collision with heavy transport vehicle or bus in traffic accident
Pedestrian on snowboard injured in collision with heavy transport vehicle or bus in traffic accident
Pedestrian on snow-skis injured in collision with heavy transport vehicle or bus in traffic accident
Pedestrian with baby stroller injured in collision with heavy transport vehicle or bus in traffic accident

√5th **V04.9 Pedestrian injured in collision with heavy transport vehicle or bus, unspecified whether traffic or nontraffic accident**

√x7th **V04.90 Pedestrian on foot injured in collision with heavy transport vehicle or bus, unspecified whether traffic or nontraffic accident**
Pedestrian NOS injured in collision with heavy transport vehicle or bus, unspecified whether traffic or nontraffic accident

√x7th **V04.91 Pedestrian on roller-skates injured in collision with heavy transport vehicle or bus, unspecified whether traffic or nontraffic accident**

√x7th **V04.92 Pedestrian on skateboard injured in collision with heavy transport vehicle or bus, unspecified whether traffic or nontraffic accident**

6th **V04.93 Pedestrian on standing micro-mobility pedestrian conveyance injured in collision with heavy transport vehicle or bus, unspecified whether traffic or nontraffic accident**

7th **V04.931 Pedestrian on standing electric scooter injured in collision with heavy transport vehicle or bus, unspecified whether traffic or nontraffic accident**

7th **V04.938 Pedestrian on other standing micro-mobility pedestrian conveyance injured in collision with heavy transport vehicle or bus, unspecified whether traffic or nontraffic accident**

Pedestrian on hoverboard injured in collision with heavy transport vehicle or bus, unspecified whether traffic or nontraffic accident

Pedestrian on segway injured in collision with heavy transport vehicle or bus, unspecified whether traffic or nontraffic accident

x7th **V04.99 Pedestrian with other conveyance injured in collision with heavy transport vehicle or bus, unspecified whether traffic or nontraffic accident**

Pedestrian in motorized mobility scooter injured in collision with heavy transport vehicle or bus, unspecified whether traffic or nontraffic accident

Pedestrian in wheelchair (powered) injured in collision with heavy transport vehicle or bus, unspecified whether traffic or nontraffic accident

Pedestrian on ice-skates injured in collision with heavy transport vehicle or bus, unspecified whether traffic or nontraffic accident

Pedestrian on nonmotorized scooter injured in collision with heavy transport vehicle or bus, unspecified whether traffic or nontraffic accident

Pedestrian on sled injured in collision with heavy transport vehicle or bus, unspecified whether traffic or nontraffic accident

Pedestrian on snowboard injured in collision with heavy transport vehicle or bus, unspecified whether traffic or nontraffic accident

Pedestrian on snow-skis injured in collision with heavy transport vehicle or bus, unspecified whether traffic or nontraffic accident

Pedestrian with baby stroller injured in collision with heavy transport vehicle or bus, unspecified whether traffic or nontraffic accident

4th **V05 Pedestrian injured in collision with railway train or railway vehicle**

5th **V05.0 Pedestrian injured in collision with railway train or railway vehicle in nontraffic accident**

x7th **V05.00 Pedestrian on foot injured in collision with railway train or railway vehicle in nontraffic accident**

Pedestrian NOS injured in collision with railway train or railway vehicle in nontraffic accident

x7th **V05.01 Pedestrian on roller-skates injured in collision with railway train or railway vehicle in nontraffic accident**

x7th **V05.02 Pedestrian on skateboard injured in collision with railway train or railway vehicle in nontraffic accident**

6th **V05.03 Pedestrian on standing micro-mobility pedestrian conveyance injured in collision with railway train or railway vehicle in nontraffic accident**

7th **V05.031 Pedestrian on standing electric scooter injured in collision with railway train or railway vehicle in nontraffic accident**

7th **V05.038 Pedestrian on other standing micro-mobility pedestrian conveyance injured in collision with railway train or railway vehicle in nontraffic accident**

Pedestrian on hoverboard injured in collision with railway train or railway vehicle in nontraffic accident

Pedestrian on segway injured in collision with railway train or railway vehicle in nontraffic accident

x7th **V05.09 Pedestrian with other conveyance injured in collision with railway train or railway vehicle in nontraffic accident**

Pedestrian in motorized mobility scooter injured in collision with railway train or railway vehicle in nontraffic accident

Pedestrian in wheelchair (powered) injured in collision with railway train or railway vehicle in nontraffic accident

Pedestrian on ice-skates injured in collision with railway train or railway vehicle in nontraffic accident

Pedestrian on nonmotorized scooter injured in collision with railway train or railway vehicle in nontraffic accident

Pedestrian on sled injured in collision with railway train or railway vehicle in nontraffic accident

Pedestrian on snowboard injured in collision with railway train or railway vehicle in nontraffic accident

Pedestrian on snow-skis injured in collision with railway train or railway vehicle in nontraffic accident

Pedestrian with baby stroller injured in collision with railway train or railway vehicle in nontraffic accident

5th **V05.1 Pedestrian injured in collision with railway train or railway vehicle in traffic accident**

x7th **V05.10 Pedestrian on foot injured in collision with railway train or railway vehicle in traffic accident**

Pedestrian NOS injured in collision with railway train or railway vehicle in traffic accident

x7th **V05.11 Pedestrian on roller-skates injured in collision with railway train or railway vehicle in traffic accident**

x7th **V05.12 Pedestrian on skateboard injured in collision with railway train or railway vehicle in traffic accident**

6th **V05.13 Pedestrian on standing micro-mobility pedestrian conveyance injured in collision with railway train or railway vehicle in traffic accident**

7th **V05.131 Pedestrian on standing electric scooter injured in collision with railway train or railway vehicle in traffic accident**

7th **V05.138 Pedestrian on other standing micro-mobility pedestrian conveyance injured in collision with railway train or railway vehicle in traffic accident**

Pedestrian on hoverboard injured in collision with railway train or railway vehicle in traffic accident

Pedestrian on segway injured in collision with railway train or railway vehicle in traffic accident

x7th **V05.19 Pedestrian with other conveyance injured in collision with railway train or railway vehicle in traffic accident**

Pedestrian in motorized mobility scooter injured in collision with railway train or railway vehicle in traffic accident

Pedestrian in wheelchair (powered) injured in collision with railway train or railway vehicle in traffic accident

Pedestrian on ice-skates injured in collision with railway train or railway vehicle in traffic accident

Pedestrian on nonmotorized scooter injured in collision with railway train or railway vehicle in traffic accident

Pedestrian on sled injured in collision with railway train or railway vehicle in traffic accident

Pedestrian on snowboard injured in collision with railway train or railway vehicle in traffic accident

Pedestrian on snow-skis injured in collision with railway train or railway vehicle in traffic accident

Pedestrian with baby stroller injured in collision with railway train or railway vehicle in traffic accident

5th **V05.9 Pedestrian injured in collision with railway train or railway vehicle, unspecified whether traffic or nontraffic accident**

x7th **V05.90 Pedestrian on foot injured in collision with railway train or railway vehicle, unspecified whether traffic or nontraffic accident**

Pedestrian NOS injured in collision with railway train or railway vehicle, unspecified whether traffic or nontraffic accident

x7th **V05.91 Pedestrian on roller-skates injured in collision with railway train or railway vehicle, unspecified whether traffic or nontraffic accident**

x7th **V05.92 Pedestrian on skateboard injured in collision with railway train or railway vehicle, unspecified whether traffic or nontraffic accident**

✓6th **V05.93 Pedestrian on standing micro-mobility pedestrian conveyance injured in collision with railway train or railway vehicle, unspecified whether traffic or nontraffic accident**

✓7th **V05.931 Pedestrian on standing electric scooter injured in collision with railway train or railway vehicle, unspecified whether traffic or nontraffic accident**

✓7th **V05.938 Pedestrian on other standing micro-mobility pedestrian conveyance injured in collision with railway train or railway vehicle, unspecified whether traffic or nontraffic accident**

Pedestrian on hoverboard injured in collision with railway train or railway vehicle, unspecified whether traffic or nontraffic accident

Pedestrian on segway injured in collision with railway train or railway vehicle, unspecified whether traffic or nontraffic accident

✓x7th **V05.99 Pedestrian with other conveyance injured in collision with railway train or railway vehicle, unspecified whether traffic or nontraffic accident**

Pedestrian in motorized mobility scooter injured in collision with railway train or railway vehicle, unspecified whether traffic or nontraffic

Pedestrian in wheelchair (powered) injured in collision with railway train or railway vehicle, unspecified whether traffic or nontraffic

Pedestrian on ice-skates injured in collision with railway train or railway vehicle, unspecified whether traffic or nontraffic

Pedestrian on nonmotorized scooter injured in collision with railway train or railway vehicle, unspecified whether traffic or nontraffic

Pedestrian on sled injured in collision with railway train or railway vehicle, unspecified whether traffic or nontraffic

Pedestrian on snowboard injured in collision with railway train or railway vehicle, unspecified whether traffic or nontraffic

Pedestrian on snow-skis injured in collision with railway train or railway vehicle, unspecified whether traffic or nontraffic

Pedestrian with baby stroller injured in collision with railway train or railway vehicle, unspecified whether traffic or nontraffic

✓4th **V06 Pedestrian injured in collision with other nonmotor vehicle**

INCLUDES collision with animal-drawn vehicle, animal being ridden, nonpowered streetcar

EXCLUDES 1 *pedestrian injured in collision with pedestrian conveyance (V00.0-)*

✓5th **V06.0 Pedestrian injured in collision with other nonmotor vehicle in nontraffic accident**

✓x7th **V06.00 Pedestrian on foot injured in collision with other nonmotor vehicle in nontraffic accident**

Pedestrian NOS injured in collision with other nonmotor vehicle in nontraffic accident

✓x7th **V06.01 Pedestrian on roller-skates injured in collision with other nonmotor vehicle in nontraffic accident**

✓x7th **V06.02 Pedestrian on skateboard injured in collision with other nonmotor vehicle in nontraffic accident**

✓6th **V06.03 Pedestrian on standing micro-mobility pedestrian conveyance injured in collision with other nonmotor vehicle in nontraffic accident**

✓7th **V06.031 Pedestrian on standing electric scooter injured in collision with other nonmotor vehicle in nontraffic accident**

✓7th **V06.038 Pedestrian on other standing micro-mobility pedestrian conveyance injured in collision with other nonmotor vehicle in nontraffic accident**

Pedestrian on hoverboard injured in collision with other nonmotor vehicle in nontraffic accident

Pedestrian on segway injured in collision with other nonmotor vehicle in nontraffic accident

✓x7th **V06.09 Pedestrian with other conveyance injured in collision with other nonmotor vehicle in nontraffic accident**

Pedestrian in motorized mobility scooter injured in collision with other nonmotor vehicle in nontraffic accident

Pedestrian in wheelchair (powered) injured in collision with other nonmotor vehicle in nontraffic accident

Pedestrian on ice-skates injured in collision with other nonmotor vehicle in nontraffic accident

Pedestrian on nonmotorized scooter injured in collision with other nonmotor vehicle in nontraffic accident

Pedestrian on sled injured in collision with other nonmotor vehicle in nontraffic accident

Pedestrian on snowboard injured in collision with other nonmotor vehicle in nontraffic accident

Pedestrian on snow-skis injured in collision with other nonmotor vehicle in nontraffic accident

Pedestrian with baby stroller injured in collision with other nonmotor vehicle in nontraffic accident

✓5th **V06.1 Pedestrian injured in collision with other nonmotor vehicle in traffic accident**

✓x7th **V06.10 Pedestrian on foot injured in collision with other nonmotor vehicle in traffic accident**

Pedestrian NOS injured in collision with other nonmotor vehicle in traffic accident

✓x7th **V06.11 Pedestrian on roller-skates injured in collision with other nonmotor vehicle in traffic accident**

✓x7th **V06.12 Pedestrian on skateboard injured in collision with other nonmotor vehicle in traffic accident**

✓6th **V06.13 Pedestrian on standing micro-mobility pedestrian conveyance injured in collision with other nonmotor vehicle in traffic accident**

✓7th **V06.131 Pedestrian on standing electric scooter injured in collision with other nonmotor vehicle in traffic accident**

✓7th **V06.138 Pedestrian on other standing micro-mobility pedestrian conveyance injured in collision with other nonmotor vehicle in traffic accident**

Pedestrian on hoverboard injured in collision with other nonmotor vehicle in traffic accident

Pedestrian on segway injured in collision with other nonmotor vehicle in traffic accident

✓x7th **V06.19 Pedestrian with other conveyance injured in collision with other nonmotor vehicle in traffic accident**

Pedestrian in motorized mobility scooter injured in collision with other nonmotor vehicle in traffic accident

Pedestrian in wheelchair (powered) injured in collision with other nonmotor vehicle in traffic accident

Pedestrian on ice-skates injured in collision with other nonmotor vehicle in traffic accident

Pedestrian on nonmotorized scooter injured in collision with other nonmotor vehicle in traffic accident

Pedestrian on sled injured in collision with other nonmotor vehicle in traffic accident

Pedestrian on snowboard injured in collision with other nonmotor vehicle in traffic accident

Pedestrian on snow-skis injured in collision with other nonmotor vehicle in traffic accident

Pedestrian with baby stroller injured in collision with other nonmotor vehicle in nontraffic accident

✓5th **V06.9 Pedestrian injured in collision with other nonmotor vehicle, unspecified whether traffic or nontraffic accident**

✓x7th **V06.90 Pedestrian on foot injured in collision with other nonmotor vehicle, unspecified whether traffic or nontraffic accident**

Pedestrian NOS injured in collision with other nonmotor vehicle, unspecified whether traffic or nontraffic accident

✓x7th **V06.91 Pedestrian on roller-skates injured in collision with other nonmotor vehicle, unspecified whether traffic or nontraffic accident**

✓x7th **V06.92 Pedestrian on skateboard injured in collision with other nonmotor vehicle, unspecified whether traffic or nontraffic accident**

√6th V06.93 **Pedestrian on standing micro-mobility pedestrian conveyance injured in collision with other nonmotor vehicle, unspecified whether traffic or nontraffic accident**

√7th V06.931 **Pedestrian on standing electric scooter injured in collision with other nonmotor vehicle, unspecified whether traffic or nontraffic accident**

√7th V06.938 **Pedestrian on other standing micro-mobility pedestrian conveyance injured in collision with other nonmotor vehicle, unspecified whether traffic or nontraffic accident**

Pedestrian on hoverboard injured in collision with other nonmotor vehicle, unspecified whether traffic or nontraffic accident

Pedestrian on segway injured in collision with other nonmotor vehicle, unspecified whether traffic or nontraffic accident

√x7th V06.99 **Pedestrian with other conveyance injured in collision with other nonmotor vehicle, unspecified whether traffic or nontraffic accident**

Pedestrian in motorized mobility scooter injured in collision with other nonmotorized vehicle, unspecified whether traffic or nontraffic accident

Pedestrian in wheelchair (powered) injured in collision with other nonmotor vehicle, unspecified whether traffic or nontraffic accident

Pedestrian on ice-skates injured in collision with other nonmotor vehicle, unspecified whether traffic or nontraffic accident

Pedestrian on nonmotorized scooter injured in collision with other nonmotor vehicle, unspecified whether traffic or nontraffic accident

Pedestrian on sled injured in collision with other nonmotor vehicle, unspecified whether traffic or nontraffic accident

Pedestrian on snowboard injured in collision with other nonmotor vehicle, unspecified whether traffic or nontraffic accident

Pedestrian on snow-skis injured in collision with other nonmotor vehicle, unspecified whether traffic or nontraffic accident

Pedestrian with baby stroller injured in collision with other nonmotor vehicle, unspecified whether traffic or nontraffic accident

√4th V09 **Pedestrian injured in other and unspecified transport accidents**

√5th V09.0 **Pedestrian injured in nontraffic accident involving other and unspecified motor vehicles**

√x7th V09.00 **Pedestrian injured in nontraffic accident involving unspecified motor vehicles**

√x7th V09.01 **Pedestrian injured in nontraffic accident involving military vehicle**

√x7th V09.09 **Pedestrian injured in nontraffic accident involving other motor vehicles**

Pedestrian injured in nontraffic accident by special vehicle

√x7th V09.1 **Pedestrian injured in unspecified nontraffic accident**

√5th V09.2 **Pedestrian injured in traffic accident involving other and unspecified motor vehicles**

√x7th V09.20 **Pedestrian injured in traffic accident involving unspecified motor vehicles**

√x7th V09.21 **Pedestrian injured in traffic accident involving military vehicle**

√x7th V09.29 **Pedestrian injured in traffic accident involving other motor vehicles**

√x7th V09.3 **Pedestrian injured in unspecified traffic accident**

√x7th V09.9 **Pedestrian injured in unspecified transport accident**

## Pedal cycle rider injured in transport accident (V10-V19)

INCLUDES any non-motorized vehicle, excluding an animal-drawn vehicle, or a sidecar or trailer attached to the pedal cycle

EXCLUDES 2 *rupture of pedal cycle tire (W37.0)*

The appropriate 7th character is to be added to each code from categories V10-V19.
A initial encounter
D subsequent encounter
S sequela

√4th V10 **Pedal cycle rider injured in collision with pedestrian or animal**

EXCLUDES 1 *pedal cycle rider collision with animal-drawn vehicle or animal being ridden (V16.-)*

√x7th V10.0 **Pedal cycle driver injured in collision with pedestrian or animal in nontraffic accident**

√x7th V10.1 **Pedal cycle passenger injured in collision with pedestrian or animal in nontraffic accident**

√x7th V10.2 **Unspecified pedal cyclist injured in collision with pedestrian or animal in nontraffic accident**

√x7th V10.3 **Person boarding or alighting a pedal cycle injured in collision with pedestrian or animal**

√x7th V10.4 **Pedal cycle driver injured in collision with pedestrian or animal in traffic accident**

√x7th V10.5 **Pedal cycle passenger injured in collision with pedestrian or animal in traffic accident**

√x7th V10.9 **Unspecified pedal cyclist injured in collision with pedestrian or animal in traffic accident**

√4th V11 **Pedal cycle rider injured in collision with other pedal cycle**

√x7th V11.0 **Pedal cycle driver injured in collision with other pedal cycle in nontraffic accident**

√x7th V11.1 **Pedal cycle passenger injured in collision with other pedal cycle in nontraffic accident**

√x7th V11.2 **Unspecified pedal cyclist injured in collision with other pedal cycle in nontraffic accident**

√x7th V11.3 **Person boarding or alighting a pedal cycle injured in collision with other pedal cycle**

√x7th V11.4 **Pedal cycle driver injured in collision with other pedal cycle in traffic accident**

√x7th V11.5 **Pedal cycle passenger injured in collision with other pedal cycle in traffic accident**

√x7th V11.9 **Unspecified pedal cyclist injured in collision with other pedal cycle in traffic accident**

√4th V12 **Pedal cycle rider injured in collision with two- or three-wheeled motor vehicle**

√x7th V12.0 **Pedal cycle driver injured in collision with two- or three-wheeled motor vehicle in nontraffic accident**

√x7th V12.1 **Pedal cycle passenger injured in collision with two- or three-wheeled motor vehicle in nontraffic accident**

√x7th V12.2 **Unspecified pedal cyclist injured in collision with two- or three-wheeled motor vehicle in nontraffic accident**

√x7th V12.3 **Person boarding or alighting a pedal cycle injured in collision with two- or three-wheeled motor vehicle**

√x7th V12.4 **Pedal cycle driver injured in collision with two- or three-wheeled motor vehicle in traffic accident**

√x7th V12.5 **Pedal cycle passenger injured in collision with two- or three-wheeled motor vehicle in traffic accident**

√x7th V12.9 **Unspecified pedal cyclist injured in collision with two- or three-wheeled motor vehicle in traffic accident**

√4th V13 **Pedal cycle rider injured in collision with car, pick-up truck or van**

√x7th V13.0 **Pedal cycle driver injured in collision with car, pick-up truck or van in nontraffic accident**

√x7th V13.1 **Pedal cycle passenger injured in collision with car, pick-up truck or van in nontraffic accident**

√x7th V13.2 **Unspecified pedal cyclist injured in collision with car, pick-up truck or van in nontraffic accident**

√x7th V13.3 **Person boarding or alighting a pedal cycle injured in collision with car, pick-up truck or van**

√x7th V13.4 **Pedal cycle driver injured in collision with car, pick-up truck or van in traffic accident**

√x7th V13.5 **Pedal cycle passenger injured in collision with car, pick-up truck or van in traffic accident**

√x7th V13.9 **Unspecified pedal cyclist injured in collision with car, pick-up truck or van in traffic accident**

√4th V14 **Pedal cycle rider injured in collision with heavy transport vehicle or bus**

EXCLUDES 1 *pedal cycle rider injured in collision with military vehicle (V19.81)*

√x7th V14.0 **Pedal cycle driver injured in collision with heavy transport vehicle or bus in nontraffic accident**

✓x7th **V14.1 Pedal cycle passenger injured in collision with heavy transport vehicle or bus in nontraffic accident**

✓x7th **V14.2 Unspecified pedal cyclist injured in collision with heavy transport vehicle or bus in nontraffic accident**

✓x7th **V14.3 Person boarding or alighting a pedal cycle injured in collision with heavy transport vehicle or bus**

✓x7th **V14.4 Pedal cycle driver injured in collision with heavy transport vehicle or bus in traffic accident**

✓x7th **V14.5 Pedal cycle passenger injured in collision with heavy transport vehicle or bus in traffic accident**

✓x7th **V14.9 Unspecified pedal cyclist injured in collision with heavy transport vehicle or bus in traffic accident**

✓4th **V15 Pedal cycle rider injured in collision with railway train or railway vehicle**

✓x7th **V15.Ø Pedal cycle driver injured in collision with railway train or railway vehicle in nontraffic accident**

✓x7th **V15.1 Pedal cycle passenger injured in collision with railway train or railway vehicle in nontraffic accident**

✓x7th **V15.2 Unspecified pedal cyclist injured in collision with railway train or railway vehicle in nontraffic accident**

✓x7th **V15.3 Person boarding or alighting a pedal cycle injured in collision with railway train or railway vehicle**

✓x7th **V15.4 Pedal cycle driver injured in collision with railway train or railway vehicle in traffic accident**

✓x7th **V15.5 Pedal cycle passenger injured in collision with railway train or railway vehicle in traffic accident**

✓x7th **V15.9 Unspecified pedal cyclist injured in collision with railway train or railway vehicle in traffic accident**

✓4th **V16 Pedal cycle rider injured in collision with other nonmotor vehicle**

INCLUDES collision with animal-drawn vehicle, animal being ridden, streetcar

✓x7th **V16.Ø Pedal cycle driver injured in collision with other nonmotor vehicle in nontraffic accident**

✓x7th **V16.1 Pedal cycle passenger injured in collision with other nonmotor vehicle in nontraffic accident**

✓x7th **V16.2 Unspecified pedal cyclist injured in collision with other nonmotor vehicle in nontraffic accident**

✓x7th **V16.3 Person boarding or alighting a pedal cycle injured in collision with other nonmotor vehicle in nontraffic accident**

✓x7th **V16.4 Pedal cycle driver injured in collision with other nonmotor vehicle in traffic accident**

✓x7th **V16.5 Pedal cycle passenger injured in collision with other nonmotor vehicle in traffic accident**

✓x7th **V16.9 Unspecified pedal cyclist injured in collision with other nonmotor vehicle in traffic accident**

✓4th **V17 Pedal cycle rider injured in collision with fixed or stationary object**

✓x7th **V17.Ø Pedal cycle driver injured in collision with fixed or stationary object in nontraffic accident**

✓x7th **V17.1 Pedal cycle passenger injured in collision with fixed or stationary object in nontraffic accident**

✓x7th **V17.2 Unspecified pedal cyclist injured in collision with fixed or stationary object in nontraffic accident**

✓x7th **V17.3 Person boarding or alighting a pedal cycle injured in collision with fixed or stationary object**

✓x7th **V17.4 Pedal cycle driver injured in collision with fixed or stationary object in traffic accident**

✓x7th **V17.5 Pedal cycle passenger injured in collision with fixed or stationary object in traffic accident**

✓x7th **V17.9 Unspecified pedal cyclist injured in collision with fixed or stationary object in traffic accident**

✓4th **V18 Pedal cycle rider injured in noncollision transport accident**

INCLUDES fall or thrown from pedal cycle (without antecedent collision)
overturning pedal cycle NOS
overturning pedal cycle without collision

✓x7th **V18.Ø Pedal cycle driver injured in noncollision transport accident in nontraffic accident**

✓x7th **V18.1 Pedal cycle passenger injured in noncollision transport accident in nontraffic accident**

✓x7th **V18.2 Unspecified pedal cyclist injured in noncollision transport accident in nontraffic accident**

✓x7th **V18.3 Person boarding or alighting a pedal cycle injured in noncollision transport accident**

✓x7th **V18.4 Pedal cycle driver injured in noncollision transport accident in traffic accident**

✓x7th **V18.5 Pedal cycle passenger injured in noncollision transport accident in traffic accident**

✓x7th **V18.9 Unspecified pedal cyclist injured in noncollision transport accident in traffic accident**

✓4th **V19 Pedal cycle rider injured in other and unspecified transport accidents**

✓5th **V19.Ø Pedal cycle driver injured in collision with other and unspecified motor vehicles in nontraffic accident**

✓x7th **V19.ØØ Pedal cycle driver injured in collision with unspecified motor vehicles in nontraffic accident**

✓x7th **V19.Ø9 Pedal cycle driver injured in collision with other motor vehicles in nontraffic accident**

✓5th **V19.1 Pedal cycle passenger injured in collision with other and unspecified motor vehicles in nontraffic accident**

✓x7th **V19.1Ø Pedal cycle passenger injured in collision with unspecified motor vehicles in nontraffic accident**

✓x7th **V19.19 Pedal cycle passenger injured in collision with other motor vehicles in nontraffic accident**

✓5th **V19.2 Unspecified pedal cyclist injured in collision with other and unspecified motor vehicles in nontraffic accident**

✓x7th **V19.2Ø Unspecified pedal cyclist injured in collision with unspecified motor vehicles in nontraffic accident**
Pedal cycle collision NOS, nontraffic

✓x7th **V19.29 Unspecified pedal cyclist injured in collision with other motor vehicles in nontraffic accident**

✓x7th **V19.3 Pedal cyclist (driver) (passenger) injured in unspecified nontraffic accident**
Pedal cycle accident NOS, nontraffic
Pedal cyclist injured in nontraffic accident NOS

✓5th **V19.4 Pedal cycle driver injured in collision with other and unspecified motor vehicles in traffic accident**

✓x7th **V19.4Ø Pedal cycle driver injured in collision with unspecified motor vehicles in traffic accident**

✓x7th **V19.49 Pedal cycle driver injured in collision with other motor vehicles in traffic accident**

✓5th **V19.5 Pedal cycle passenger injured in collision with other and unspecified motor vehicles in traffic accident**

✓x7th **V19.5Ø Pedal cycle passenger injured in collision with unspecified motor vehicles in traffic accident**

✓x7th **V19.59 Pedal cycle passenger injured in collision with other motor vehicles in traffic accident**

✓5th **V19.6 Unspecified pedal cyclist injured in collision with other and unspecified motor vehicles in traffic accident**

✓x7th **V19.6Ø Unspecified pedal cyclist injured in collision with unspecified motor vehicles in traffic accident**
Pedal cycle collision NOS (traffic)

✓x7th **V19.69 Unspecified pedal cyclist injured in collision with other motor vehicles in traffic accident**

✓5th **V19.8 Pedal cyclist (driver) (passenger) injured in other specified transport accidents**

✓x7th **V19.81 Pedal cyclist (driver) (passenger) injured in transport accident with military vehicle**

✓x7th **V19.88 Pedal cyclist (driver) (passenger) injured in other specified transport accidents**

✓x7th **V19.9 Pedal cyclist (driver) (passenger) injured in unspecified traffic accident**
Pedal cycle accident NOS

## Motorcycle rider injured in transport accident (V2Ø-V29)

INCLUDES electric bicycle
e-bike
e-bicycle
moped
motorcycle with sidecar
motorized bicycle
motor scooter

EXCLUDES 1 *three-wheeled motor vehicle (V3Ø-V39)*

**AHA:** 2022,4Q,47

The appropriate 7th character is to be added to each code from categories V2Ø-V29.
A initial encounter
D subsequent encounter
S sequela

✓4th **V2Ø Motorcycle rider injured in collision with pedestrian or animal**

EXCLUDES 1 *motorcycle rider collision with animal-drawn vehicle or animal being ridden (V26.-)*

✓5th **V2Ø.Ø Motorcycle driver injured in collision with pedestrian or animal in nontraffic accident**

✓x7th **V2Ø.Ø1 Electric (assisted) bicycle driver injured in collision with pedestrian or animal in nontraffic accident**

✓x7th **V2Ø.Ø9 Other motorcycle driver injured in collision with pedestrian or animal in nontraffic accident**

✓5th **V2Ø.1 Motorcycle passenger injured in collision with pedestrian or animal in nontraffic accident**

✓x7th **V2Ø.11 Electric (assisted) bicycle passenger injured in collision with pedestrian or animal in nontraffic accident**

V20.19 Other motorcycle passenger injured in collision with pedestrian or animal in nontraffic accident

V20.2 Unspecified motorcycle rider injured in collision with pedestrian or animal in nontraffic accident

V20.21 Unspecified electric (assisted) bicycle rider injured in collision with pedestrian or animal in nontraffic accident

V20.29 Unspecified rider of other motorcycle injured in collision with pedestrian or animal in nontraffic accident

V20.3 Person boarding or alighting a motorcycle injured in collision with pedestrian or animal

V20.31 Person boarding or alighting an electric (assisted) bicycle injured in collision with pedestrian or animal

V20.39 Person boarding or alighting other motorcycle injured in collision with pedestrian or animal

V20.4 Motorcycle driver injured in collision with pedestrian or animal in traffic accident

V20.41 Electric (assisted) bicycle driver injured in collision with pedestrian or animal in traffic accident

V20.49 Other motorcycle driver injured in collision with pedestrian or animal in traffic accident

V20.5 Motorcycle passenger injured in collision with pedestrian or animal in traffic accident

V20.51 Electric (assisted) bicycle passenger injured in collision with pedestrian or animal in traffic accident

V20.59 Other motorcycle passenger injured in collision with pedestrian or animal in traffic accident

V20.9 Unspecified motorcycle rider injured in collision with pedestrian or animal in traffic accident

V20.91 Unspecified electric (assisted) bicycle rider injured in collision with pedestrian or animal in traffic accident

V20.99 Unspecified rider of other motorcycle injured in collision with pedestrian or animal in traffic accident

**V21 Motorcycle rider injured in collision with pedal cycle**

V21.0 Motorcycle driver injured in collision with pedal cycle in nontraffic accident

V21.01 Electric (assisted) bicycle driver injured in collision with pedal cycle in nontraffic accident

V21.09 Other motorcycle driver injured in collision with pedal cycle in nontraffic accident

V21.1 Motorcycle passenger injured in collision with pedal cycle in nontraffic accident

V21.11 Electric (assisted) bicycle passenger injured in collision with pedal cycle in nontraffic accident

V21.19 Other motorcycle passenger injured in collision with pedal cycle in nontraffic accident

V21.2 Unspecified motorcycle rider injured in collision with pedal cycle in nontraffic accident

V21.21 Unspecified electric (assisted) bicycle rider injured in collision with pedal cycle in nontraffic accident

V21.29 Unspecified rider of other motorcycle injured in collision with pedal cycle in nontraffic accident

V21.3 Person boarding or alighting a motorcycle injured in collision with pedal cycle

V21.31 Person boarding or alighting an electric (assisted) bicycle injured in collision with pedal cycle

V21.39 Person boarding or alighting other motorcycle injured in collision with pedal cycle

V21.4 Motorcycle driver injured in collision with pedal cycle in traffic accident

V21.41 Electric (assisted) bicycle driver injured in collision with pedal cycle in traffic accident

V21.49 Other motorcycle driver injured in collision with pedal cycle in traffic accident

V21.5 Motorcycle passenger injured in collision with pedal cycle in traffic accident

V21.51 Electric (assisted) bicycle passenger injured in collision with pedal cycle in traffic accident

V21.59 Other motorcycle passenger injured in collision with pedal cycle in traffic accident

V21.9 Unspecified motorcycle rider injured in collision with pedal cycle in traffic accident

V21.91 Unspecified electric (assisted) bicycle rider injured in collision with pedal cycle in traffic accident

V21.99 Unspecified rider of other motorcycle injured in collision with pedal cycle in traffic accident

**V22 Motorcycle rider injured in collision with two- or three-wheeled motor vehicle**

V22.0 Motorcycle driver injured in collision with two- or three-wheeled motor vehicle in nontraffic accident

V22.01 Electric (assisted) bicycle driver injured in collision with two- or three-wheeled motor vehicle in nontraffic accident

V22.09 Other motorcycle driver injured in collision with two- or three-wheeled motor vehicle in nontraffic accident

V22.1 Motorcycle passenger injured in collision with two- or three-wheeled motor vehicle in nontraffic accident

V22.11 Electric (assisted) bicycle passenger injured in collision with two- or three-wheeled motor vehicle in nontraffic accident

V22.19 Other motorcycle passenger injured in collision with two- or three-wheeled motor vehicle in nontraffic accident

V22.2 Unspecified motorcycle rider injured in collision with two- or three-wheeled motor vehicle in nontraffic accident

V22.21 Unspecified electric (assisted) bicycle rider injured in collision with two- or three-wheeled motor vehicle in nontraffic accident

V22.29 Unspecified rider of other motorcycle injured in collision with two- or three-wheeled motor vehicle in nontraffic accident

V22.3 Person boarding or alighting a motorcycle injured in collision with two- or three-wheeled motor vehicle

V22.31 Person boarding or alighting an electric (assisted) bicycle injured in collision with two- or three-wheeled motor vehicle

V22.39 Person boarding or alighting other motorcycle injured in collision with two- or three-wheeled motor vehicle

V22.4 Motorcycle driver injured in collision with two- or three-wheeled motor vehicle in traffic accident

V22.41 Electric (assisted) bicycle driver injured in collision with two- or three-wheeled motor vehicle in traffic accident

V22.49 Other motorcycle driver injured in collision with two- or three-wheeled motor vehicle in traffic accident

V22.5 Motorcycle passenger injured in collision with two- or three-wheeled motor vehicle in traffic accident

V22.51 Electric (assisted) bicycle passenger injured in collision with two- or three-wheeled motor vehicle in traffic accident

V22.59 Other motorcycle passenger injured in collision with two- or three-wheeled motor vehicle in traffic accident

V22.9 Unspecified motorcycle rider injured in collision with two- or three-wheeled motor vehicle in traffic accident

V22.91 Unspecified electric (assisted) bicycle rider injured in collision with two- or three-wheeled motor vehicle in traffic accident

V22.99 Unspecified rider of other motorcycle injured in collision with two- or three-wheeled motor vehicle in traffic accident

**V23 Motorcycle rider injured in collision with car, pick-up truck or van**

V23.0 Motorcycle driver injured in collision with car, pick-up truck or van in nontraffic accident

V23.01 Electric (assisted) bicycle driver injured in collision with car, pick-up truck or van in nontraffic accident

V23.09 Other motorcycle driver injured in collision with car, pick-up truck or van in nontraffic accident

V23.1 Motorcycle passenger injured in collision with car, pick-up truck or van in nontraffic accident

V23.11 Electric (assisted) bicycle passenger injured in collision with car, pick-up truck or van in nontraffic accident

V23.19 Other motorcycle passenger injured in collision with car, pick-up truck or van in nontraffic accident

V23.2 Unspecified motorcycle rider injured in collision with car, pick-up truck or van in nontraffic accident

V23.21 Unspecified electric (assisted) bicycle rider injured in collision with car, pick-up truck or van in nontraffic accident

V23.29 Unspecified rider of other motorcycle injured in collision with car, pick-up truck or van in nontraffic accident

V23.3 Person boarding or alighting a motorcycle injured in collision with car, pick-up truck or van

V23.31 Person boarding or alighting an electric (assisted) bicycle injured in collision with car, pick-up truck or van

√x7th **V23.39** Person boarding or alighting other motorcycle injured in collision with car, pick-up truck or van

√5th **V23.4** Motorcycle driver injured in collision with car, pick-up truck or van in traffic accident

√x7th **V23.41** Electric (assisted) bicycle driver injured in collision with car, pick-up truck or van in traffic accident

√x7th **V23.49** Other motorcycle driver injured in collision with car, pick-up truck or van in traffic accident

√5th **V23.5** Motorcycle passenger injured in collision with car, pick-up truck or van in traffic accident

√x7th **V23.51** Electric (assisted) bicycle passenger injured in collision with car, pick-up truck or van in traffic accident

√x7th **V23.59** Other motorcycle passenger injured in collision with car, pick-up truck or van in traffic accident

√5th **V23.9** Unspecified motorcycle rider injured in collision with car, pick-up truck or van in traffic accident

√x7th **V23.91** Unspecified electric (assisted) bicycle rider injured in collision with car, pick-up truck or van in traffic accident

√x7th **V23.99** Unspecified rider of other motorcycle injured in collision with car, pick-up truck or van in traffic accident

√4th **V24 Motorcycle rider injured in collision with heavy transport vehicle or bus**

EXCLUDES 1 *motorcycle rider injured in collision with military vehicle (V29.818)*

√5th **V24.0** Motorcycle driver injured in collision with heavy transport vehicle or bus in nontraffic accident

√x7th **V24.01** Electric (assisted) bicycle driver injured in collision with heavy transport vehicle or bus in nontraffic accident

√x7th **V24.09** Other motorcycle driver injured in collision with heavy transport vehicle or bus in nontraffic accident

√5th **V24.1** Motorcycle passenger injured in collision with heavy transport vehicle or bus in nontraffic accident

√x7th **V24.11** Electric (assisted) bicycle passenger injured in collision with heavy transport vehicle or bus in nontraffic accident

√x7th **V24.19** Other motorcycle passenger injured in collision with heavy transport vehicle or bus in nontraffic accident

√5th **V24.2** Unspecified motorcycle rider injured in collision with heavy transport vehicle or bus in nontraffic accident

√x7th **V24.21** Unspecified electric (assisted) bicycle rider injured in collision with heavy transport vehicle or bus in nontraffic accident

√x7th **V24.29** Unspecified rider of other motorcycle injured in collision with heavy transport vehicle or bus in nontraffic accident

√5th **V24.3** Person boarding or alighting a motorcycle injured in collision with heavy transport vehicle or bus

√x7th **V24.31** Person boarding or alighting an electric (assisted) bicycle injured in collision with heavy transport vehicle or bus

√x7th **V24.39** Person boarding or alighting other motorcycle injured in collision with heavy transport vehicle or bus

√5th **V24.4** Motorcycle driver injured in collision with heavy transport vehicle or bus in traffic accident

√x7th **V24.41** Electric (assisted) bicycle driver injured in collision with heavy transport vehicle or bus in traffic accident

√x7th **V24.49** Other motorcycle driver injured in collision with heavy transport vehicle or bus in traffic accident

√5th **V24.5** Motorcycle passenger injured in collision with heavy transport vehicle or bus in traffic accident

√x7th **V24.51** Electric (assisted) bicycle passenger injured in collision with heavy transport vehicle or bus in traffic accident

√x7th **V24.59** Other motorcycle passenger injured in collision with heavy transport vehicle or bus in traffic accident

√5th **V24.9** Unspecified motorcycle rider injured in collision with heavy transport vehicle or bus in traffic accident

√x7th **V24.91** Unspecified electric (assisted) bicycle rider injured in collision with heavy transport vehicle or bus in traffic accident

√x7th **V24.99** Unspecified rider of other motorcycle injured in collision with heavy transport vehicle or bus in traffic accident

√4th **V25 Motorcycle rider injured in collision with railway train or railway vehicle**

√5th **V25.0** Motorcycle driver injured in collision with railway train or railway vehicle in nontraffic accident

√x7th **V25.01** Electric (assisted) bicycle driver injured in collision with railway train or railway vehicle in nontraffic accident

√x7th **V25.09** Other motorcycle driver injured in collision with railway train or railway vehicle in nontraffic accident

√5th **V25.1** Motorcycle passenger injured in collision with railway train or railway vehicle in nontraffic accident

√x7th **V25.11** Electric (assisted) bicycle passenger injured in collision with railway train or railway vehicle in nontraffic accident

√x7th **V25.19** Other motorcycle passenger injured in collision with railway train or railway vehicle in nontraffic accident

√5th **V25.2** Unspecified motorcycle rider injured in collision with railway train or railway vehicle in nontraffic accident

√x7th **V25.21** Unspecified electric (assisted) bicycle rider injured in collision with railway train or railway vehicle in nontraffic accident

√x7th **V25.29** Unspecified rider of other motorcycle injured in collision with railway train or railway vehicle in nontraffic accident

√5th **V25.3** Person boarding or alighting a motorcycle injured in collision with railway train or railway vehicle

√x7th **V25.31** Person boarding or alighting an electric (assisted) bicycle injured in collision with railway train or railway vehicle

√x7th **V25.39** Person boarding or alighting other motorcycle injured in collision with railway train or railway vehicle

√5th **V25.4** Motorcycle driver injured in collision with railway train or railway vehicle in traffic accident

√x7th **V25.41** Electric (assisted) bicycle driver injured in collision with railway train or railway vehicle in traffic accident

√x7th **V25.49** Other motorcycle driver injured in collision with railway train or railway vehicle in traffic accident

√5th **V25.5** Motorcycle passenger injured in collision with railway train or railway vehicle in traffic accident

√x7th **V25.51** Electric (assisted) bicycle passenger injured in collision with railway train or railway vehicle in traffic accident

√x7th **V25.59** Other motorcycle passenger injured in collision with railway train or railway vehicle in traffic accident

√5th **V25.9** Unspecified motorcycle rider injured in collision with railway train or railway vehicle in traffic accident

√x7th **V25.91** Unspecified electric (assisted) bicycle rider injured in collision with railway train or railway vehicle in traffic accident

√x7th **V25.99** Unspecified rider of other motorcycle injured in collision with railway train or railway vehicle in traffic accident

√4th **V26 Motorcycle rider injured in collision with other nonmotor vehicle**

INCLUDES collision with animal-drawn vehicle, animal being ridden, streetcar

√5th **V26.0** Motorcycle driver injured in collision with other nonmotor vehicle in nontraffic accident

√x7th **V26.01** Electric (assisted) bicycle driver injured in collision with other nonmotor vehicle in nontraffic accident

√x7th **V26.09** Other motorcycle driver injured in collision with other nonmotor vehicle in nontraffic accident

√5th **V26.1** Motorcycle passenger injured in collision with other nonmotor vehicle in nontraffic accident

√x7th **V26.11** Electric (assisted) bicycle passenger injured in collision with other nonmotor vehicle in nontraffic accident

√x7th **V26.19** Other motorcycle passenger injured in collision with other nonmotor vehicle in nontraffic accident

√5th **V26.2** Unspecified motorcycle rider injured in collision with other nonmotor vehicle in nontraffic accident

√x7th **V26.21** Unspecified electric (assisted) bicycle rider injured in collision with other nonmotor vehicle in nontraffic accident

√x7th **V26.29** Unspecified rider of other motorcycle injured in collision with other nonmotor vehicle in nontraffic accident

√5th **V26.3** Person boarding or alighting a motorcycle injured in collision with other nonmotor vehicle

√x7th **V26.31** Person boarding or alighting an electric (assisted) bicycle injured in collision with other nonmotor vehicle

√x7th V26.39 Person boarding or alighting other motorcycle injured in collision with other nonmotor vehicle

√5th V26.4 Motorcycle driver injured in collision with other nonmotor vehicle in traffic accident

√x7th V26.41 Electric (assisted) bicycle driver injured in collision with other nonmotor vehicle in traffic accident

√x7th V26.49 Other motorcycle driver injured in collision with other nonmotor vehicle in traffic accident

√5th V26.5 Motorcycle passenger injured in collision with other nonmotor vehicle in traffic accident

√x7th V26.51 Electric (assisted) bicycle passenger injured in collision with other nonmotor vehicle in traffic accident

√x7th V26.59 Other motorcycle passenger injured in collision with other nonmotor vehicle in traffic accident

√5th V26.9 Unspecified motorcycle rider injured in collision with other nonmotor vehicle in traffic accident

√x7th V26.91 Unspecified electric (assisted) bicycle rider injured in collision with other nonmotor vehicle in traffic accident

√x7th V26.99 Unspecified rider of other motorcycle injured in collision with other nonmotor vehicle in traffic accident

√4th **V27 Motorcycle rider injured in collision with fixed or stationary object**

√5th V27.0 Motorcycle driver injured in collision with fixed or stationary object in nontraffic accident

√x7th V27.01 Electric (assisted) bicycle driver injured in collision with fixed or stationary object in nontraffic accident

√x7th V27.09 Other motorcycle driver injured in collision with fixed or stationary object in nontraffic accident

√5th V27.1 Motorcycle passenger injured in collision with fixed or stationary object in nontraffic accident

√x7th V27.11 Electric (assisted) bicycle passenger injured in collision with fixed or stationary object in nontraffic accident

√x7th V27.19 Other motorcycle passenger injured in collision with fixed or stationary object in nontraffic accident

√5th V27.2 Unspecified motorcycle rider injured in collision with fixed or stationary object in nontraffic accident

√x7th V27.21 Unspecified electric (assisted) bicycle rider injured in collision with fixed or stationary object in nontraffic accident

√x7th V27.29 Unspecified rider of other motorcycle injured in collision with fixed or stationary object in nontraffic accident

√5th V27.3 Person boarding or alighting a motorcycle injured in collision with fixed or stationary object

√x7th V27.31 Person boarding or alighting an electric (assisted) bicycle injured in collision with fixed or stationary object

√x7th V27.39 Person boarding or alighting other motorcycle injured in collision with fixed or stationary object

√5th V27.4 Motorcycle driver injured in collision with fixed or stationary object in traffic accident

√x7th V27.41 Electric (assisted) bicycle driver injured in collision with fixed or stationary object in traffic accident

√x7th V27.49 Other motorcycle driver injured in collision with fixed or stationary object in traffic accident

√5th V27.5 Motorcycle passenger injured in collision with fixed or stationary object in traffic accident

√x7th V27.51 Electric (assisted) bicycle passenger injured in collision with fixed or stationary object in traffic accident

√x7th V27.59 Other motorcycle passenger injured in collision with fixed or stationary object in traffic accident

√5th V27.9 Unspecified motorcycle rider injured in collision with fixed or stationary object in traffic accident

√x7th V27.91 Unspecified electric (assisted) bicycle rider injured in collision with fixed or stationary object in traffic accident

√x7th V27.99 Unspecified rider of other motorcycle injured in collision with fixed or stationary object in traffic accident

√4th **V28 Motorcycle rider injured in noncollision transport accident**

INCLUDES fall or thrown from motorcycle (without antecedent collision)
overturning motorcycle NOS
overturning motorcycle without collision

√5th V28.0 Motorcycle driver injured in noncollision transport accident in nontraffic accident

√x7th V28.01 Electric (assisted) bicycle driver injured in noncollision transport accident in nontraffic accident

√x7th V28.09 Other motorcycle driver injured in noncollision transport accident in nontraffic accident

√5th V28.1 Motorcycle passenger injured in noncollision transport accident in nontraffic accident

√x7th V28.11 Electric (assisted) bicycle passenger injured in noncollision transport accident in nontraffic accident

√x7th V28.19 Other motorcycle passenger injured in noncollision transport accident in nontraffic accident

√5th V28.2 Unspecified motorcycle rider injured in noncollision transport accident in nontraffic accident

√x7th V28.21 Unspecified electric (assisted) bicycle rider injured in noncollision transport accident in nontraffic accident

√x7th V28.29 Unspecified rider of other motorcycle injured in noncollision transport accident in nontraffic accident

√5th V28.3 Person boarding or alighting a motorcycle injured in noncollision transport accident

√x7th V28.31 Person boarding or alighting an electric (assisted) bicycle injured in noncollision transport accident

√x7th V28.39 Person boarding or alighting other motorcycle injured in noncollision transport accident

√5th V28.4 Motorcycle driver injured in noncollision transport accident in traffic accident

√x7th V28.41 Electric (assisted) bicycle driver injured in noncollision transport accident in traffic accident

√x7th V28.49 Other motorcycle driver injured in noncollision transport accident in traffic accident

√5th V28.5 Motorcycle passenger injured in noncollision transport accident in traffic accident

√x7th V28.51 Electric (assisted) bicycle passenger injured in noncollision transport accident in traffic accident

√x7th V28.59 Other motorcycle passenger injured in noncollision transport accident in traffic accident

√5th V28.9 Unspecified motorcycle rider injured in noncollision transport accident in traffic accident

√x7th V28.91 Unspecified electric (assisted) bicycle rider injured in noncollision transport accident in traffic accident

√x7th V28.99 Unspecified rider of other motorcycle injured in noncollision transport accident in traffic accident

√4th **V29 Motorcycle rider injured in other and unspecified transport accidents**

√5th V29.0 Motorcycle driver injured in collision with other and unspecified motor vehicles in nontraffic accident

√6th V29.00 Motorcycle driver injured in collision with unspecified motor vehicles in nontraffic accident

√7th V29.001 Electric (assisted) bicycle driver injured in collision with unspecified motor vehicles in nontraffic accident

√7th V29.008 Other motorcycle driver injured in collision with unspecified motor vehicles in nontraffic accident

√6th V29.09 Motorcycle driver injured in collision with other motor vehicles in nontraffic accident

√7th V29.091 Electric (assisted) bicycle driver injured in collision with other motor vehicles in nontraffic accident

√7th V29.098 Other motorcycle driver injured in collision with other motor vehicles in nontraffic accident

√5th V29.1 Motorcycle passenger injured in collision with other and unspecified motor vehicles in nontraffic accident

√6th V29.10 Motorcycle passenger injured in collision with unspecified motor vehicles in nontraffic accident

√7th V29.101 Electric (assisted) bicycle passenger injured in collision with unspecified motor vehicles in nontraffic accident

√7th V29.108 Other motorcycle passenger injured in collision with unspecified motor vehicles in nontraffic accident

√6th V29.19 Motorcycle passenger injured in collision with other motor vehicles in nontraffic accident

√7th V29.191 Electric (assisted) bicycle passenger injured in collision with other motor vehicles in nontraffic accident

√7th V29.198 Other motorcycle passenger injured in collision with other motor vehicles in nontraffic accident

√5th V29.2 Unspecified motorcycle rider injured in collision with other and unspecified motor vehicles in nontraffic accident

√6th V29.20 Unspecified motorcycle rider injured in collision with unspecified motor vehicles in nontraffic accident

√7th V29.201 Unspecified electric (assisted) bicycle rider injured in collision with unspecified motor vehicles in nontraffic accident

√7th **V29.208 Unspecified rider of other motorcycle injured in collision with unspecified motor vehicles in nontraffic accident**
Motorcycle collision NOS, nontraffic

√6th **V29.29 Unspecified motorcycle rider injured in collision with other motor vehicles in nontraffic accident**

√7th **V29.291 Unspecified electric (assisted) bicycle rider injured in collision with other motor vehicles in nontraffic accident**

√7th **V29.298 Unspecified rider of other motorcycle injured in collision with other motor vehicles in nontraffic accident**

√5th **V29.3 Motorcycle rider (driver) (passenger) injured in unspecified nontraffic accident**

√x7th **V29.31 Electric (assisted) bicycle (driver) (passenger) injured in unspecified nontraffic accident**

√x7th **V29.39 Other motorcycle (driver) (passenger) injured in unspecified nontraffic accident**
Motorcycle accident NOS, nontraffic
Motorcycle rider injured in nontraffic accident NOS

√5th **V29.4 Motorcycle driver injured in collision with other and unspecified motor vehicles in traffic accident**

√6th **V29.40 Motorcycle driver injured in collision with unspecified motor vehicles in traffic accident**

√7th **V29.401 Electric (assisted) bicycle driver injured in collision with unspecified motor vehicles in traffic accident**

√7th **V29.408 Other motorcycle driver injured in collision with unspecified motor vehicles in traffic accident**

√6th **V29.49 Motorcycle driver injured in collision with other motor vehicles in traffic accident**

√7th **V29.491 Electric (assisted) bicycle driver injured in collision with other motor vehicles in traffic accident**

√7th **V29.498 Other motorcycle driver injured in collision with other motor vehicles in traffic accident**

√5th **V29.5 Motorcycle passenger injured in collision with other and unspecified motor vehicles in traffic accident**

√6th **V29.50 Motorcycle passenger injured in collision with unspecified motor vehicles in traffic accident**

√7th **V29.501 Electric (assisted) bicycle passenger injured in collision with unspecified motor vehicles in traffic accident**

√7th **V29.508 Other motorcycle passenger injured in collision with unspecified motor vehicles in traffic accident**

√6th **V29.59 Motorcycle passenger injured in collision with other motor vehicles in traffic accident**

√7th **V29.591 Electric (assisted) bicycle passenger injured in collision with other motor vehicles in traffic accident**

√7th **V29.598 Other motorcycle passenger injured in collision with other motor vehicles in traffic accident**

√5th **V29.6 Unspecified motorcycle rider injured in collision with other and unspecified motor vehicles in traffic accident**

√6th **V29.60 Unspecified motorcycle rider injured in collision with unspecified motor vehicles in traffic accident**

√7th **V29.601 Unspecified electric (assisted) bicycle rider injured in collision with unspecified motor vehicles in traffic accident**

√7th **V29.608 Unspecified rider of other motorcycle injured in collision with unspecified motor vehicles in traffic accident**
Motorcycle collision NOS (traffic)

√6th **V29.69 Unspecified motorcycle rider injured in collision with other motor vehicles in traffic accident**

√7th **V29.691 Unspecified electric (assisted) bicycle rider injured in collision with other motor vehicles in traffic accident**

√7th **V29.698 Unspecified rider of other motorcycle injured in collision with other motor vehicles in traffic accident**

√5th **V29.8 Motorcycle rider (driver) (passenger) injured in other specified transport accidents**

√6th **V29.81 Motorcycle rider (driver) (passenger) injured in transport accident with military vehicle**

√7th **V29.811 Electric (assisted) bicycle rider (driver) (passenger) injured in transport accident with military vehicle**

√7th **V29.818 Rider (driver) (passenger) of other motorcycle injured in transport accident with military vehicle**

√6th **V29.88 Motorcycle rider (driver) (passenger) injured in other specified transport accidents**

√7th **V29.881 Electric (assisted) bicycle rider (driver) (passenger) injured in other specified transport accidents**

√7th **V29.888 Rider (driver) (passenger) of other motorcycle injured in other specified transport accidents**

√5th **V29.9 Motorcycle rider (driver) (passenger) injured in unspecified traffic accident**

√x7th **V29.91 Electric (assisted) bicycle rider (driver) (passenger) injured in unspecified traffic accident**

√x7th **V29.99 Rider (driver) (passenger) of other motorcycle injured in unspecified traffic accident**
Motorcycle accident NOS

## Occupant of three-wheeled motor vehicle injured in transport accident (V30-V39)

INCLUDES motorized tricycle
motorized rickshaw
three-wheeled motor car

EXCLUDES 1 *all-terrain vehicles (V86.-)*
*motorcycle with sidecar (V20-V29)*
*vehicle designed primarily for off-road use (V86.-)*

The appropriate 7th character is to be added to each code from categories V30-V39.
A initial encounter
D subsequent encounter
S sequela

√4th **V30 Occupant of three-wheeled motor vehicle injured in collision with pedestrian or animal**
EXCLUDES 1 *three-wheeled motor vehicle collision with animal-drawn vehicle or animal being ridden (V36.-)*

√x7th **V30.0 Driver of three-wheeled motor vehicle injured in collision with pedestrian or animal in nontraffic accident**

√x7th **V30.1 Passenger in three-wheeled motor vehicle injured in collision with pedestrian or animal in nontraffic accident**

√x7th **V30.2 Person on outside of three-wheeled motor vehicle injured in collision with pedestrian or animal in nontraffic accident**

√x7th **V30.3 Unspecified occupant of three-wheeled motor vehicle injured in collision with pedestrian or animal in nontraffic accident**

√x7th **V30.4 Person boarding or alighting a three-wheeled motor vehicle injured in collision with pedestrian or animal**

√x7th **V30.5 Driver of three-wheeled motor vehicle injured in collision with pedestrian or animal in traffic accident**

√x7th **V30.6 Passenger in three-wheeled motor vehicle injured in collision with pedestrian or animal in traffic accident**

√x7th **V30.7 Person on outside of three-wheeled motor vehicle injured in collision with pedestrian or animal in traffic accident**

√x7th **V30.9 Unspecified occupant of three-wheeled motor vehicle injured in collision with pedestrian or animal in traffic accident**

√4th **V31 Occupant of three-wheeled motor vehicle injured in collision with pedal cycle**

√x7th **V31.0 Driver of three-wheeled motor vehicle injured in collision with pedal cycle in nontraffic accident**

√x7th **V31.1 Passenger in three-wheeled motor vehicle injured in collision with pedal cycle in nontraffic accident**

√x7th **V31.2 Person on outside of three-wheeled motor vehicle injured in collision with pedal cycle in nontraffic accident**

√x7th **V31.3 Unspecified occupant of three-wheeled motor vehicle injured in collision with pedal cycle in nontraffic accident**

√x7th **V31.4 Person boarding or alighting a three-wheeled motor vehicle injured in collision with pedal cycle**

√x7th **V31.5 Driver of three-wheeled motor vehicle injured in collision with pedal cycle in traffic accident**

√x7th **V31.6 Passenger in three-wheeled motor vehicle injured in collision with pedal cycle in traffic accident**

√x7th **V31.7 Person on outside of three-wheeled motor vehicle injured in collision with pedal cycle in traffic accident**

√x7th **V31.9 Unspecified occupant of three-wheeled motor vehicle injured in collision with pedal cycle in traffic accident**

√4th **V32 Occupant of three-wheeled motor vehicle injured in collision with two- or three-wheeled motor vehicle**

√x7th **V32.0 Driver of three-wheeled motor vehicle injured in collision with two- or three-wheeled motor vehicle in nontraffic accident**

√x7th **V32.1 Passenger in three-wheeled motor vehicle injured in collision with two- or three-wheeled motor vehicle in nontraffic accident**

√x 7th V32.2 Person on outside of three-wheeled motor vehicle injured in collision with two- or three-wheeled motor vehicle in nontraffic accident

√x 7th V32.3 Unspecified occupant of three-wheeled motor vehicle injured in collision with two- or three-wheeled motor vehicle in nontraffic accident

√x 7th V32.4 Person boarding or alighting a three-wheeled motor vehicle injured in collision with two- or three-wheeled motor vehicle

√x 7th V32.5 Driver of three-wheeled motor vehicle injured in collision with two- or three-wheeled motor vehicle in traffic accident

√x 7th V32.6 Passenger in three-wheeled motor vehicle injured in collision with two- or three-wheeled motor vehicle in traffic accident

√x 7th V32.7 Person on outside of three-wheeled motor vehicle injured in collision with two- or three-wheeled motor vehicle in traffic accident

√x 7th V32.9 Unspecified occupant of three-wheeled motor vehicle injured in collision with two- or three-wheeled motor vehicle in traffic accident

√4th **V33 Occupant of three-wheeled motor vehicle injured in collision with car, pick-up truck or van**

√x 7th V33.0 Driver of three-wheeled motor vehicle injured in collision with car, pick-up truck or van in nontraffic accident

√x 7th V33.1 Passenger in three-wheeled motor vehicle injured in collision with car, pick-up truck or van in nontraffic accident

√x 7th V33.2 Person on outside of three-wheeled motor vehicle injured in collision with car, pick-up truck or van in nontraffic accident

√x 7th V33.3 Unspecified occupant of three-wheeled motor vehicle injured in collision with car, pick-up truck or van in nontraffic accident

√x 7th V33.4 Person boarding or alighting a three-wheeled motor vehicle injured in collision with car, pick-up truck or van

√x 7th V33.5 Driver of three-wheeled motor vehicle injured in collision with car, pick-up truck or van in traffic accident

√x 7th V33.6 Passenger in three-wheeled motor vehicle injured in collision with car, pick-up truck or van in traffic accident

√x 7th V33.7 Person on outside of three-wheeled motor vehicle injured in collision with car, pick-up truck or van in traffic accident

√x 7th V33.9 Unspecified occupant of three-wheeled motor vehicle injured in collision with car, pick-up truck or van in traffic accident

√4th **V34 Occupant of three-wheeled motor vehicle injured in collision with heavy transport vehicle or bus**

EXCLUDES 1 *occupant of three-wheeled motor vehicle injured in collision with military vehicle (V39.81)*

√x 7th V34.0 Driver of three-wheeled motor vehicle injured in collision with heavy transport vehicle or bus in nontraffic accident

√x 7th V34.1 Passenger in three-wheeled motor vehicle injured in collision with heavy transport vehicle or bus in nontraffic accident

√x 7th V34.2 Person on outside of three-wheeled motor vehicle injured in collision with heavy transport vehicle or bus in nontraffic accident

√x 7th V34.3 Unspecified occupant of three-wheeled motor vehicle injured in collision with heavy transport vehicle or bus in nontraffic accident

√x 7th V34.4 Person boarding or alighting a three-wheeled motor vehicle injured in collision with heavy transport vehicle or bus

√x 7th V34.5 Driver of three-wheeled motor vehicle injured in collision with heavy transport vehicle or bus in traffic accident

√x 7th V34.6 Passenger in three-wheeled motor vehicle injured in collision with heavy transport vehicle or bus in traffic accident

√x 7th V34.7 Person on outside of three-wheeled motor vehicle injured in collision with heavy transport vehicle or bus in traffic accident

√x 7th V34.9 Unspecified occupant of three-wheeled motor vehicle injured in collision with heavy transport vehicle or bus in traffic accident

√4th **V35 Occupant of three-wheeled motor vehicle injured in collision with railway train or railway vehicle**

√x 7th V35.0 Driver of three-wheeled motor vehicle injured in collision with railway train or railway vehicle in nontraffic accident

√x 7th V35.1 Passenger in three-wheeled motor vehicle injured in collision with railway train or railway vehicle in nontraffic accident

√x 7th V35.2 Person on outside of three-wheeled motor vehicle injured in collision with railway train or railway vehicle in nontraffic accident

√x 7th V35.3 Unspecified occupant of three-wheeled motor vehicle injured in collision with railway train or railway vehicle in nontraffic accident

√x 7th V35.4 Person boarding or alighting a three-wheeled motor vehicle injured in collision with railway train or railway vehicle

√x 7th V35.5 Driver of three-wheeled motor vehicle injured in collision with railway train or railway vehicle in traffic accident

√x 7th V35.6 Passenger in three-wheeled motor vehicle injured in collision with railway train or railway vehicle in traffic accident

√x 7th V35.7 Person on outside of three-wheeled motor vehicle injured in collision with railway train or railway vehicle in traffic accident

√x 7th V35.9 Unspecified occupant of three-wheeled motor vehicle injured in collision with railway train or railway vehicle in traffic accident

√4th **V36 Occupant of three-wheeled motor vehicle injured in collision with other nonmotor vehicle**

INCLUDES collision with animal-drawn vehicle, animal being ridden, streetcar

√x 7th V36.0 Driver of three-wheeled motor vehicle injured in collision with other nonmotor vehicle in nontraffic accident

√x 7th V36.1 Passenger in three-wheeled motor vehicle injured in collision with other nonmotor vehicle in nontraffic accident

√x 7th V36.2 Person on outside of three-wheeled motor vehicle injured in collision with other nonmotor vehicle in nontraffic accident

√x 7th V36.3 Unspecified occupant of three-wheeled motor vehicle injured in collision with other nonmotor vehicle in nontraffic accident

√x 7th V36.4 Person boarding or alighting a three-wheeled motor vehicle injured in collision with other nonmotor vehicle

√x 7th V36.5 Driver of three-wheeled motor vehicle injured in collision with other nonmotor vehicle in traffic accident

√x 7th V36.6 Passenger in three-wheeled motor vehicle injured in collision with other nonmotor vehicle in traffic accident

√x 7th V36.7 Person on outside of three-wheeled motor vehicle injured in collision with other nonmotor vehicle in traffic accident

√x 7th V36.9 Unspecified occupant of three-wheeled motor vehicle injured in collision with other nonmotor vehicle in traffic accident

√4th **V37 Occupant of three-wheeled motor vehicle injured in collision with fixed or stationary object**

√x 7th V37.0 Driver of three-wheeled motor vehicle injured in collision with fixed or stationary object in nontraffic accident

√x 7th V37.1 Passenger in three-wheeled motor vehicle injured in collision with fixed or stationary object in nontraffic accident

√x 7th V37.2 Person on outside of three-wheeled motor vehicle injured in collision with fixed or stationary object in nontraffic accident

√x 7th V37.3 Unspecified occupant of three-wheeled motor vehicle injured in collision with fixed or stationary object in nontraffic accident

√x 7th V37.4 Person boarding or alighting a three-wheeled motor vehicle injured in collision with fixed or stationary object

√x 7th V37.5 Driver of three-wheeled motor vehicle injured in collision with fixed or stationary object in traffic accident

√x 7th V37.6 Passenger in three-wheeled motor vehicle injured in collision with fixed or stationary object in traffic accident

√x 7th V37.7 Person on outside of three-wheeled motor vehicle injured in collision with fixed or stationary object in traffic accident

√x 7th V37.9 Unspecified occupant of three-wheeled motor vehicle injured in collision with fixed or stationary object in traffic accident

√4th **V38 Occupant of three-wheeled motor vehicle injured in noncollision transport accident**

INCLUDES fall or thrown from three-wheeled motor vehicle
overturning of three-wheeled motor vehicle NOS
overturning of three-wheeled motor vehicle without collision

√x 7th V38.0 Driver of three-wheeled motor vehicle injured in noncollision transport accident in nontraffic accident

√x 7th V38.1 Passenger in three-wheeled motor vehicle injured in noncollision transport accident in nontraffic accident

√x 7th V38.2 Person on outside of three-wheeled motor vehicle injured in noncollision transport accident in nontraffic accident

√x 7th V38.3 Unspecified occupant of three-wheeled motor vehicle injured in noncollision transport accident in nontraffic accident

√x 7th V38.4 Person boarding or alighting a three-wheeled motor vehicle injured in noncollision transport accident

√x 7th V38.5 Driver of three-wheeled motor vehicle injured in noncollision transport accident in traffic accident

√x 7th V38.6 Passenger in three-wheeled motor vehicle injured in noncollision transport accident in traffic accident

√x 7th V38.7 Person on outside of three-wheeled motor vehicle injured in noncollision transport accident in traffic accident

√x 7th V38.9 Unspecified occupant of three-wheeled motor vehicle injured in noncollision transport accident in traffic accident

√4th **V39 Occupant of three-wheeled motor vehicle injured in other and unspecified transport accidents**

√5th V39.0 Driver of three-wheeled motor vehicle injured in collision with other and unspecified motor vehicles in nontraffic accident

√x 7th V39.00 Driver of three-wheeled motor vehicle injured in collision with unspecified motor vehicles in nontraffic accident

√x 7th V39.09 Driver of three-wheeled motor vehicle injured in collision with other motor vehicles in nontraffic accident

5th V39.1 **Passenger in three-wheeled motor vehicle injured in collision with other and unspecified motor vehicles in nontraffic accident**

x7th **V39.10** **Passenger in three-wheeled motor vehicle injured in collision with unspecified motor vehicles in nontraffic accident**

x7th **V39.19** **Passenger in three-wheeled motor vehicle injured in collision with other motor vehicles in nontraffic accident**

5th V39.2 **Unspecified occupant of three-wheeled motor vehicle injured in collision with other and unspecified motor vehicles in nontraffic accident**

x7th **V39.20** **Unspecified occupant of three-wheeled motor vehicle injured in collision with unspecified motor vehicles in nontraffic accident**
Collision NOS involving three-wheeled motor vehicle, nontraffic

x7th **V39.29** **Unspecified occupant of three-wheeled motor vehicle injured in collision with other motor vehicles in nontraffic accident**

x7th **V39.3** **Occupant (driver) (passenger) of three-wheeled motor vehicle injured in unspecified nontraffic accident**
Accident NOS involving three-wheeled motor vehicle, nontraffic
Occupant of three-wheeled motor vehicle injured in nontraffic accident NOS

5th V39.4 **Driver of three-wheeled motor vehicle injured in collision with other and unspecified motor vehicles in traffic accident**

x7th **V39.40** **Driver of three-wheeled motor vehicle injured in collision with unspecified motor vehicles in traffic accident**

x7th **V39.49** **Driver of three-wheeled motor vehicle injured in collision with other motor vehicles in traffic accident**

5th V39.5 **Passenger in three-wheeled motor vehicle injured in collision with other and unspecified motor vehicles in traffic accident**

x7th **V39.50** **Passenger in three-wheeled motor vehicle injured in collision with unspecified motor vehicles in traffic accident**

x7th **V39.59** **Passenger in three-wheeled motor vehicle injured in collision with other motor vehicles in traffic accident**

5th V39.6 **Unspecified occupant of three-wheeled motor vehicle injured in collision with other and unspecified motor vehicles in traffic accident**

x7th **V39.60** **Unspecified occupant of three-wheeled motor vehicle injured in collision with unspecified motor vehicles in traffic accident**
Collision NOS involving three-wheeled motor vehicle (traffic)

x7th **V39.69** **Unspecified occupant of three-wheeled motor vehicle injured in collision with other motor vehicles in traffic accident**

5th V39.8 **Occupant (driver) (passenger) of three-wheeled motor vehicle injured in other specified transport accidents**

x7th **V39.81** **Occupant (driver) (passenger) of three-wheeled motor vehicle injured in transport accident with military vehicle**

x7th **V39.89** **Occupant (driver) (passenger) of three-wheeled motor vehicle injured in other specified transport accidents**

x7th **V39.9** **Occupant (driver) (passenger) of three-wheeled motor vehicle injured in unspecified traffic accident**
Accident NOS involving three-wheeled motor vehicle

## Car occupant injured in transport accident (V40-V49)

INCLUDES a four-wheeled motor vehicle designed primarily for carrying passengers
automobile (pulling a trailer or camper)

EXCLUDES 1 *bus (V50-V59)*
*minibus (V50-V59)*
*minivan (V50-V59)*
*motorcoach (V70-V79)*
*pick-up truck (V50-V59)*
*sport utility vehicle (SUV) (V50-V59)*

The appropriate 7th character is to be added to each code from categories V40-V49.
A initial encounter
D subsequent encounter
S sequela

4th **V40 Car occupant injured in collision with pedestrian or animal**

EXCLUDES 1 *car collision with animal-drawn vehicle or animal being ridden (V46.-)*

x7th **V40.0** **Car driver injured in collision with pedestrian or animal in nontraffic accident**

x7th **V40.1** **Car passenger injured in collision with pedestrian or animal in nontraffic accident**

x7th **V40.2** **Person on outside of car injured in collision with pedestrian or animal in nontraffic accident**

x7th **V40.3** **Unspecified car occupant injured in collision with pedestrian or animal in nontraffic accident**

x7th **V40.4** **Person boarding or alighting a car injured in collision with pedestrian or animal**

x7th **V40.5** **Car driver injured in collision with pedestrian or animal in traffic accident**

x7th **V40.6** **Car passenger injured in collision with pedestrian or animal in traffic accident**

x7th **V40.7** **Person on outside of car injured in collision with pedestrian or animal in traffic accident**

x7th **V40.9** **Unspecified car occupant injured in collision with pedestrian or animal in traffic accident**

4th **V41 Car occupant injured in collision with pedal cycle**

x7th **V41.0** **Car driver injured in collision with pedal cycle in nontraffic accident**

x7th **V41.1** **Car passenger injured in collision with pedal cycle in nontraffic accident**

x7th **V41.2** **Person on outside of car injured in collision with pedal cycle in nontraffic accident**

x7th **V41.3** **Unspecified car occupant injured in collision with pedal cycle in nontraffic accident**

x7th **V41.4** **Person boarding or alighting a car injured in collision with pedal cycle**

x7th **V41.5** **Car driver injured in collision with pedal cycle in traffic accident**

x7th **V41.6** **Car passenger injured in collision with pedal cycle in traffic accident**

x7th **V41.7** **Person on outside of car injured in collision with pedal cycle in traffic accident**

x7th **V41.9** **Unspecified car occupant injured in collision with pedal cycle in traffic accident**

4th **V42 Car occupant injured in collision with two- or three-wheeled motor vehicle**

x7th **V42.0** **Car driver injured in collision with two- or three-wheeled motor vehicle in nontraffic accident**

x7th **V42.1** **Car passenger injured in collision with two- or three-wheeled motor vehicle in nontraffic accident**

x7th **V42.2** **Person on outside of car injured in collision with two- or three-wheeled motor vehicle in nontraffic accident**

x7th **V42.3** **Unspecified car occupant injured in collision with two- or three-wheeled motor vehicle in nontraffic accident**

x7th **V42.4** **Person boarding or alighting a car injured in collision with two- or three-wheeled motor vehicle**

x7th **V42.5** **Car driver injured in collision with two- or three-wheeled motor vehicle in traffic accident**

x7th **V42.6** **Car passenger injured in collision with two- or three-wheeled motor vehicle in traffic accident**

x7th **V42.7** **Person on outside of car injured in collision with two- or three-wheeled motor vehicle in traffic accident**

x7th **V42.9** **Unspecified car occupant injured in collision with two- or three-wheeled motor vehicle in traffic accident**

4th **V43 Car occupant injured in collision with car, pick-up truck or van**

5th **V43.0** **Car driver injured in collision with car, pick-up truck or van in nontraffic accident**

x7th **V43.01** **Car driver injured in collision with sport utility vehicle in nontraffic accident**

x7th **V43.02** **Car driver injured in collision with other type car in nontraffic accident**

x7th **V43.03** **Car driver injured in collision with pick-up truck in nontraffic accident**

x7th **V43.04** **Car driver injured in collision with van in nontraffic accident**

5th **V43.1** **Car passenger injured in collision with car, pick-up truck or van in nontraffic accident**

x7th **V43.11** **Car passenger injured in collision with sport utility vehicle in nontraffic accident**

x7th **V43.12** **Car passenger injured in collision with other type car in nontraffic accident**

x7th **V43.13** **Car passenger injured in collision with pick-up truck in nontraffic accident**

x7th **V43.14** **Car passenger injured in collision with van in nontraffic accident**

5th **V43.2** **Person on outside of car injured in collision with car, pick-up truck or van in nontraffic accident**

x7th **V43.21** **Person on outside of car injured in collision with sport utility vehicle in nontraffic accident**

V43.22 Person on outside of car injured in collision with other type car in nontraffic accident
V43.23 Person on outside of car injured in collision with pick-up truck in nontraffic accident
V43.24 Person on outside of car injured in collision with van in nontraffic accident

V43.3 Unspecified car occupant injured in collision with car, pick-up truck or van in nontraffic accident
V43.31 Unspecified car occupant injured in collision with sport utility vehicle in nontraffic accident
V43.32 Unspecified car occupant injured in collision with other type car in nontraffic accident
V43.33 Unspecified car occupant injured in collision with pick-up truck in nontraffic accident
V43.34 Unspecified car occupant injured in collision with van in nontraffic accident

V43.4 Person boarding or alighting a car injured in collision with car, pick-up truck or van
V43.41 Person boarding or alighting a car injured in collision with sport utility vehicle
V43.42 Person boarding or alighting a car injured in collision with other type car
V43.43 Person boarding or alighting a car injured in collision with pick-up truck
V43.44 Person boarding or alighting a car injured in collision with van

V43.5 Car driver injured in collision with car, pick-up truck or van in traffic accident
V43.51 Car driver injured in collision with sport utility vehicle in traffic accident
V43.52 Car driver injured in collision with other type car in traffic accident
V43.53 Car driver injured in collision with pick-up truck in traffic accident
V43.54 Car driver injured in collision with van in traffic accident

V43.6 Car passenger injured in collision with car, pick-up truck or van in traffic accident
V43.61 Car passenger injured in collision with sport utility vehicle in traffic accident
V43.62 Car passenger injured in collision with other type car in traffic accident
V43.63 Car passenger injured in collision with pick-up truck in traffic accident
V43.64 Car passenger injured in collision with van in traffic accident

V43.7 Person on outside of car injured in collision with car, pick-up truck or van in traffic accident
V43.71 Person on outside of car injured in collision with sport utility vehicle in traffic accident
V43.72 Person on outside of car injured in collision with other type car in traffic accident
V43.73 Person on outside of car injured in collision with pick-up truck in traffic accident
V43.74 Person on outside of car injured in collision with van in traffic accident

V43.9 Unspecified car occupant injured in collision with car, pick-up truck or van in traffic accident
V43.91 Unspecified car occupant injured in collision with sport utility vehicle in traffic accident
V43.92 Unspecified car occupant injured in collision with other type car in traffic accident
V43.93 Unspecified car occupant injured in collision with pick-up truck in traffic accident
V43.94 Unspecified car occupant injured in collision with van in traffic accident

**V44 Car occupant injured in collision with heavy transport vehicle or bus**

EXCLUDES 1 *car occupant injured in collision with military vehicle (V49.81)*

V44.0 Car driver injured in collision with heavy transport vehicle or bus in nontraffic accident
V44.1 Car passenger injured in collision with heavy transport vehicle or bus in nontraffic accident
V44.2 Person on outside of car injured in collision with heavy transport vehicle or bus in nontraffic accident
V44.3 Unspecified car occupant injured in collision with heavy transport vehicle or bus in nontraffic accident
V44.4 Person boarding or alighting a car injured in collision with heavy transport vehicle or bus
V44.5 Car driver injured in collision with heavy transport vehicle or bus in traffic accident
V44.6 Car passenger injured in collision with heavy transport vehicle or bus in traffic accident
V44.7 Person on outside of car injured in collision with heavy transport vehicle or bus in traffic accident
V44.9 Unspecified car occupant injured in collision with heavy transport vehicle or bus in traffic accident

**V45 Car occupant injured in collision with railway train or railway vehicle**

V45.0 Car driver injured in collision with railway train or railway vehicle in nontraffic accident
V45.1 Car passenger injured in collision with railway train or railway vehicle in nontraffic accident
V45.2 Person on outside of car injured in collision with railway train or railway vehicle in nontraffic accident
V45.3 Unspecified car occupant injured in collision with railway train or railway vehicle in nontraffic accident
V45.4 Person boarding or alighting a car injured in collision with railway train or railway vehicle
V45.5 Car driver injured in collision with railway train or railway vehicle in traffic accident
V45.6 Car passenger injured in collision with railway train or railway vehicle in traffic accident
V45.7 Person on outside of car injured in collision with railway train or railway vehicle in traffic accident
V45.9 Unspecified car occupant injured in collision with railway train or railway vehicle in traffic accident

**V46 Car occupant injured in collision with other nonmotor vehicle**

INCLUDES collision with animal-drawn vehicle, animal being ridden, streetcar

V46.0 Car driver injured in collision with other nonmotor vehicle in nontraffic accident
V46.1 Car passenger injured in collision with other nonmotor vehicle in nontraffic accident
V46.2 Person on outside of car injured in collision with other nonmotor vehicle in nontraffic accident
V46.3 Unspecified car occupant injured in collision with other nonmotor vehicle in nontraffic accident
V46.4 Person boarding or alighting a car injured in collision with other nonmotor vehicle
V46.5 Car driver injured in collision with other nonmotor vehicle in traffic accident
V46.6 Car passenger injured in collision with other nonmotor vehicle in traffic accident
V46.7 Person on outside of car injured in collision with other nonmotor vehicle in traffic accident
V46.9 Unspecified car occupant injured in collision with other nonmotor vehicle in traffic accident

**V47 Car occupant injured in collision with fixed or stationary object**

AHA: 2016,4Q,73

V47.0 Car driver injured in collision with fixed or stationary object in nontraffic accident
V47.1 Car passenger injured in collision with fixed or stationary object in nontraffic accident
V47.2 Person on outside of car injured in collision with fixed or stationary object in nontraffic accident
V47.3 Unspecified car occupant injured in collision with fixed or stationary object in nontraffic accident
V47.4 Person boarding or alighting a car injured in collision with fixed or stationary object
V47.5 Car driver injured in collision with fixed or stationary object in traffic accident
V47.6 Car passenger injured in collision with fixed or stationary object in traffic accident
V47.7 Person on outside of car injured in collision with fixed or stationary object in traffic accident
V47.9 Unspecified car occupant injured in collision with fixed or stationary object in traffic accident

**V48 Car occupant injured in noncollision transport accident**

INCLUDES overturning car NOS
overturning car without collision

V48.0 Car driver injured in noncollision transport accident in nontraffic accident
V48.1 Car passenger injured in noncollision transport accident in nontraffic accident
V48.2 Person on outside of car injured in noncollision transport accident in nontraffic accident
V48.3 Unspecified car occupant injured in noncollision transport accident in nontraffic accident
V48.4 Person boarding or alighting a car injured in noncollision transport accident

√x7th V48.5 **Car driver injured in noncollision transport accident in traffic accident**

√x7th V48.6 **Car passenger injured in noncollision transport accident in traffic accident**

√x7th V48.7 **Person on outside of car injured in noncollision transport accident in traffic accident**

√x7th V48.9 **Unspecified car occupant injured in noncollision transport accident in traffic accident**

√4th **V49 Car occupant injured in other and unspecified transport accidents**

√5th V49.0 **Driver injured in collision with other and unspecified motor vehicles in nontraffic accident**

√x7th V49.00 **Driver injured in collision with unspecified motor vehicles in nontraffic accident**

√x7th V49.09 **Driver injured in collision with other motor vehicles in nontraffic accident**

√5th V49.1 **Passenger injured in collision with other and unspecified motor vehicles in nontraffic accident**

√x7th V49.10 **Passenger injured in collision with unspecified motor vehicles in nontraffic accident**

√x7th V49.19 **Passenger injured in collision with other motor vehicles in nontraffic accident**

√5th V49.2 **Unspecified car occupant injured in collision with other and unspecified motor vehicles in nontraffic accident**

√x7th V49.20 **Unspecified car occupant injured in collision with unspecified motor vehicles in nontraffic accident**
Car collision NOS, nontraffic

√x7th V49.29 **Unspecified car occupant injured in collision with other motor vehicles in nontraffic accident**

√x7th V49.3 **Car occupant (driver) (passenger) injured in unspecified nontraffic accident**
Car accident NOS, nontraffic
Car occupant injured in nontraffic accident NOS

√5th V49.4 **Driver injured in collision with other and unspecified motor vehicles in traffic accident**

√x7th V49.40 **Driver injured in collision with unspecified motor vehicles in traffic accident**

√x7th V49.49 **Driver injured in collision with other motor vehicles in traffic accident**

√5th V49.5 **Passenger injured in collision with other and unspecified motor vehicles in traffic accident**

√x7th V49.50 **Passenger injured in collision with unspecified motor vehicles in traffic accident**

√x7th V49.59 **Passenger injured in collision with other motor vehicles in traffic accident**

√5th V49.6 **Unspecified car occupant injured in collision with other and unspecified motor vehicles in traffic accident**

√x7th V49.60 **Unspecified car occupant injured in collision with unspecified motor vehicles in traffic accident**
Car collision NOS (traffic)

√x7th V49.69 **Unspecified car occupant injured in collision with other motor vehicles in traffic accident**

√5th V49.8 **Car occupant (driver) (passenger) injured in other specified transport accidents**

√x7th V49.81 **Car occupant (driver) (passenger) injured in transport accident with military vehicle**

√x7th V49.88 **Car occupant (driver) (passenger) injured in other specified transport accidents**

√x7th V49.9 **Car occupant (driver) (passenger) injured in unspecified traffic accident**
Car accident NOS

## Occupant of pick-up truck or van injured in transport accident (V50-V59)

INCLUDES a four or six wheel motor vehicle designed primarily for carrying passengers and property but weighing less than the local limit for classification as a heavy goods vehicle
minibus
minivan
sport utility vehicle (SUV)
truck
van

EXCLUDES 1 *heavy transport vehicle (V60-V69)*

The appropriate 7th character is to be added to each code from categories V50-V59.
A initial encounter
D subsequent encounter
S sequela

√4th **V50 Occupant of pick-up truck or van injured in collision with pedestrian or animal**

EXCLUDES 1 *pick-up truck or van collision with animal-drawn vehicle or animal being ridden (V56.-)*

√x7th V50.0 **Driver of pick-up truck or van injured in collision with pedestrian or animal in nontraffic accident**

√x7th V50.1 **Passenger in pick-up truck or van injured in collision with pedestrian or animal in nontraffic accident**

√x7th V50.2 **Person on outside of pick-up truck or van injured in collision with pedestrian or animal in nontraffic accident**

√x7th V50.3 **Unspecified occupant of pick-up truck or van injured in collision with pedestrian or animal in nontraffic accident**

√x7th V50.4 **Person boarding or alighting a pick-up truck or van injured in collision with pedestrian or animal**

√x7th V50.5 **Driver of pick-up truck or van injured in collision with pedestrian or animal in traffic accident**

√x7th V50.6 **Passenger in pick-up truck or van injured in collision with pedestrian or animal in traffic accident**

√x7th V50.7 **Person on outside of pick-up truck or van injured in collision with pedestrian or animal in traffic accident**

√x7th V50.9 **Unspecified occupant of pick-up truck or van injured in collision with pedestrian or animal in traffic accident**

√4th **V51 Occupant of pick-up truck or van injured in collision with pedal cycle**

√x7th V51.0 **Driver of pick-up truck or van injured in collision with pedal cycle in nontraffic accident**

√x7th V51.1 **Passenger in pick-up truck or van injured in collision with pedal cycle in nontraffic accident**

√x7th V51.2 **Person on outside of pick-up truck or van injured in collision with pedal cycle in nontraffic accident**

√x7th V51.3 **Unspecified occupant of pick-up truck or van injured in collision with pedal cycle in nontraffic accident**

√x7th V51.4 **Person boarding or alighting a pick-up truck or van injured in collision with pedal cycle**

√x7th V51.5 **Driver of pick-up truck or van injured in collision with pedal cycle in traffic accident**

√x7th V51.6 **Passenger in pick-up truck or van injured in collision with pedal cycle in traffic accident**

√x7th V51.7 **Person on outside of pick-up truck or van injured in collision with pedal cycle in traffic accident**

√x7th V51.9 **Unspecified occupant of pick-up truck or van injured in collision with pedal cycle in traffic accident**

√4th **V52 Occupant of pick-up truck or van injured in collision with two- or three-wheeled motor vehicle**

√x7th V52.0 **Driver of pick-up truck or van injured in collision with two- or three-wheeled motor vehicle in nontraffic accident**

√x7th V52.1 **Passenger in pick-up truck or van injured in collision with two- or three-wheeled motor vehicle in nontraffic accident**

√x7th V52.2 **Person on outside of pick-up truck or van injured in collision with two- or three-wheeled motor vehicle in nontraffic accident**

√x7th V52.3 **Unspecified occupant of pick-up truck or van injured in collision with two- or three-wheeled motor vehicle in nontraffic accident**

√x7th V52.4 **Person boarding or alighting a pick-up truck or van injured in collision with two- or three-wheeled motor vehicle**

√x7th V52.5 **Driver of pick-up truck or van injured in collision with two- or three-wheeled motor vehicle in traffic accident**

√x7th V52.6 **Passenger in pick-up truck or van injured in collision with two- or three-wheeled motor vehicle in traffic accident**

√x7th V52.7 **Person on outside of pick-up truck or van injured in collision with two- or three-wheeled motor vehicle in traffic accident**

√x7th V52.9 **Unspecified occupant of pick-up truck or van injured in collision with two- or three-wheeled motor vehicle in traffic accident**

**V53 Occupant of pick-up truck or van injured in collision with car, pick-up truck or van**

- V53.0 Driver of pick-up truck or van injured in collision with car, pick-up truck or van in nontraffic accident
- V53.1 Passenger in pick-up truck or van injured in collision with car, pick-up truck or van in nontraffic accident
- V53.2 Person on outside of pick-up truck or van injured in collision with car, pick-up truck or van in nontraffic accident
- V53.3 Unspecified occupant of pick-up truck or van injured in collision with car, pick-up truck or van in nontraffic accident
- V53.4 Person boarding or alighting a pick-up truck or van injured in collision with car, pick-up truck or van
- V53.5 Driver of pick-up truck or van injured in collision with car, pick-up truck or van in traffic accident
- V53.6 Passenger in pick-up truck or van injured in collision with car, pick-up truck or van in traffic accident
- V53.7 Person on outside of pick-up truck or van injured in collision with car, pick-up truck or van in traffic accident
- V53.9 Unspecified occupant of pick-up truck or van injured in collision with car, pick-up truck or van in traffic accident

**V54 Occupant of pick-up truck or van injured in collision with heavy transport vehicle or bus**

EXCLUDES 1 *occupant of pick-up truck or van injured in collision with military vehicle (V59.81)*

- V54.0 Driver of pick-up truck or van injured in collision with heavy transport vehicle or bus in nontraffic accident
- V54.1 Passenger in pick-up truck or van injured in collision with heavy transport vehicle or bus in nontraffic accident
- V54.2 Person on outside of pick-up truck or van injured in collision with heavy transport vehicle or bus in nontraffic accident
- V54.3 Unspecified occupant of pick-up truck or van injured in collision with heavy transport vehicle or bus in nontraffic accident
- V54.4 Person boarding or alighting a pick-up truck or van injured in collision with heavy transport vehicle or bus
- V54.5 Driver of pick-up truck or van injured in collision with heavy transport vehicle or bus in traffic accident
- V54.6 Passenger in pick-up truck or van injured in collision with heavy transport vehicle or bus in traffic accident
- V54.7 Person on outside of pick-up truck or van injured in collision with heavy transport vehicle or bus in traffic accident
- V54.9 Unspecified occupant of pick-up truck or van injured in collision with heavy transport vehicle or bus in traffic accident

**V55 Occupant of pick-up truck or van injured in collision with railway train or railway vehicle**

- V55.0 Driver of pick-up truck or van injured in collision with railway train or railway vehicle in nontraffic accident
- V55.1 Passenger in pick-up truck or van injured in collision with railway train or railway vehicle in nontraffic accident
- V55.2 Person on outside of pick-up truck or van injured in collision with railway train or railway vehicle in nontraffic accident
- V55.3 Unspecified occupant of pick-up truck or van injured in collision with railway train or railway vehicle in nontraffic accident
- V55.4 Person boarding or alighting a pick-up truck or van injured in collision with railway train or railway vehicle
- V55.5 Driver of pick-up truck or van injured in collision with railway train or railway vehicle in traffic accident
- V55.6 Passenger in pick-up truck or van injured in collision with railway train or railway vehicle in traffic accident
- V55.7 Person on outside of pick-up truck or van injured in collision with railway train or railway vehicle in traffic accident
- V55.9 Unspecified occupant of pick-up truck or van injured in collision with railway train or railway vehicle in traffic accident

**V56 Occupant of pick-up truck or van injured in collision with other nonmotor vehicle**

INCLUDES collision with animal-drawn vehicle, animal being ridden, streetcar

- V56.0 Driver of pick-up truck or van injured in collision with other nonmotor vehicle in nontraffic accident
- V56.1 Passenger in pick-up truck or van injured in collision with other nonmotor vehicle in nontraffic accident
- V56.2 Person on outside of pick-up truck or van injured in collision with other nonmotor vehicle in nontraffic accident
- V56.3 Unspecified occupant of pick-up truck or van injured in collision with other nonmotor vehicle in nontraffic accident
- V56.4 Person boarding or alighting a pick-up truck or van injured in collision with other nonmotor vehicle
- V56.5 Driver of pick-up truck or van injured in collision with other nonmotor vehicle in traffic accident
- V56.6 Passenger in pick-up truck or van injured in collision with other nonmotor vehicle in traffic accident
- V56.7 Person on outside of pick-up truck or van injured in collision with other nonmotor vehicle in traffic accident
- V56.9 Unspecified occupant of pick-up truck or van injured in collision with other nonmotor vehicle in traffic accident

**V57 Occupant of pick-up truck or van injured in collision with fixed or stationary object**

- V57.0 Driver of pick-up truck or van injured in collision with fixed or stationary object in nontraffic accident
- V57.1 Passenger in pick-up truck or van injured in collision with fixed or stationary object in nontraffic accident
- V57.2 Person on outside of pick-up truck or van injured in collision with fixed or stationary object in nontraffic accident
- V57.3 Unspecified occupant of pick-up truck or van injured in collision with fixed or stationary object in nontraffic accident
- V57.4 Person boarding or alighting a pick-up truck or van injured in collision with fixed or stationary object
- V57.5 Driver of pick-up truck or van injured in collision with fixed or stationary object in traffic accident
- V57.6 Passenger in pick-up truck or van injured in collision with fixed or stationary object in traffic accident
- V57.7 Person on outside of pick-up truck or van injured in collision with fixed or stationary object in traffic accident
- V57.9 Unspecified occupant of pick-up truck or van injured in collision with fixed or stationary object in traffic accident

**V58 Occupant of pick-up truck or van injured in noncollision transport accident**

INCLUDES overturning pick-up truck or van NOS
overturning pick-up truck or van without collision

- V58.0 Driver of pick-up truck or van injured in noncollision transport accident in nontraffic accident
- V58.1 Passenger in pick-up truck or van injured in noncollision transport accident in nontraffic accident
- V58.2 Person on outside of pick-up truck or van injured in noncollision transport accident in nontraffic accident
- V58.3 Unspecified occupant of pick-up truck or van injured in noncollision transport accident in nontraffic accident
- V58.4 Person boarding or alighting a pick-up truck or van injured in noncollision transport accident
- V58.5 Driver of pick-up truck or van injured in noncollision transport accident in traffic accident
- V58.6 Passenger in pick-up truck or van injured in noncollision transport accident in traffic accident
- V58.7 Person on outside of pick-up truck or van injured in noncollision transport accident in traffic accident
- V58.9 Unspecified occupant of pick-up truck or van injured in noncollision transport accident in traffic accident

**V59 Occupant of pick-up truck or van injured in other and unspecified transport accidents**

- V59.0 Driver of pick-up truck or van injured in collision with other and unspecified motor vehicles in nontraffic accident
  - V59.00 Driver of pick-up truck or van injured in collision with unspecified motor vehicles in nontraffic accident
  - V59.09 Driver of pick-up truck or van injured in collision with other motor vehicles in nontraffic accident
- V59.1 Passenger in pick-up truck or van injured in collision with other and unspecified motor vehicles in nontraffic accident
  - V59.10 Passenger in pick-up truck or van injured in collision with unspecified motor vehicles in nontraffic accident
  - V59.19 Passenger in pick-up truck or van injured in collision with other motor vehicles in nontraffic accident
- V59.2 Unspecified occupant of pick-up truck or van injured in collision with other and unspecified motor vehicles in nontraffic accident
  - V59.20 Unspecified occupant of pick-up truck or van injured in collision with unspecified motor vehicles in nontraffic accident
    Collision NOS involving pick-up truck or van, nontraffic
  - V59.29 Unspecified occupant of pick-up truck or van injured in collision with other motor vehicles in nontraffic accident
- V59.3 Occupant (driver) (passenger) of pick-up truck or van injured in unspecified nontraffic accident
  Accident NOS involving pick-up truck or van, nontraffic
  Occupant of pick-up truck or van injured in nontraffic accident NOS
- V59.4 Driver of pick-up truck or van injured in collision with other and unspecified motor vehicles in traffic accident
  - V59.40 Driver of pick-up truck or van injured in collision with unspecified motor vehicles in traffic accident
  - V59.49 Driver of pick-up truck or van injured in collision with other motor vehicles in traffic accident

Chapter 20. External Causes of Morbidity

√5th **V59.5** **Passenger in pick-up truck or van injured in collision with other and unspecified motor vehicles in traffic accident**

√x7th **V59.50** Passenger in pick-up truck or van injured in collision with unspecified motor vehicles in traffic accident

√x7th **V59.59** Passenger in pick-up truck or van injured in collision with other motor vehicles in traffic accident

√5th **V59.6** **Unspecified occupant of pick-up truck or van injured in collision with other and unspecified motor vehicles in traffic accident**

√x7th **V59.60** Unspecified occupant of pick-up truck or van injured in collision with unspecified motor vehicles in traffic accident

Collision NOS involving pick-up truck or van (traffic)

√x7th **V59.69** Unspecified occupant of pick-up truck or van injured in collision with other motor vehicles in traffic accident

√5th **V59.8** **Occupant (driver) (passenger) of pick-up truck or van injured in other specified transport accidents**

√x7th **V59.81** Occupant (driver) (passenger) of pick-up truck or van injured in transport accident with military vehicle

√x7th **V59.88** Occupant (driver) (passenger) of pick-up truck or van injured in other specified transport accidents

√x7th **V59.9** **Occupant (driver) (passenger) of pick-up truck or van injured in unspecified traffic accident**

Accident NOS involving pick-up truck or van

## Occupant of heavy transport vehicle injured in transport accident (V60-V69)

INCLUDES 18 wheeler
armored car
panel truck

EXCLUDES1 *bus*
*motorcoach*

The appropriate 7th character is to be added to each code from categories V60-V69.
A initial encounter
D subsequent encounter
S sequela

√4th **V60** **Occupant of heavy transport vehicle injured in collision with pedestrian or animal**

EXCLUDES1 *heavy transport vehicle collision with animal-drawn vehicle or animal being ridden (V66.-)*

√x7th **V60.0** Driver of heavy transport vehicle injured in collision with pedestrian or animal in nontraffic accident

√x7th **V60.1** Passenger in heavy transport vehicle injured in collision with pedestrian or animal in nontraffic accident

√x7th **V60.2** Person on outside of heavy transport vehicle injured in collision with pedestrian or animal in nontraffic accident

√x7th **V60.3** Unspecified occupant of heavy transport vehicle injured in collision with pedestrian or animal in nontraffic accident

√x7th **V60.4** Person boarding or alighting a heavy transport vehicle injured in collision with pedestrian or animal

√x7th **V60.5** Driver of heavy transport vehicle injured in collision with pedestrian or animal in traffic accident

√x7th **V60.6** Passenger in heavy transport vehicle injured in collision with pedestrian or animal in traffic accident

√x7th **V60.7** Person on outside of heavy transport vehicle injured in collision with pedestrian or animal in traffic accident

√x7th **V60.9** Unspecified occupant of heavy transport vehicle injured in collision with pedestrian or animal in traffic accident

√4th **V61** **Occupant of heavy transport vehicle injured in collision with pedal cycle**

√x7th **V61.0** Driver of heavy transport vehicle injured in collision with pedal cycle in nontraffic accident

√x7th **V61.1** Passenger in heavy transport vehicle injured in collision with pedal cycle in nontraffic accident

√x7th **V61.2** Person on outside of heavy transport vehicle injured in collision with pedal cycle in nontraffic accident

√x7th **V61.3** Unspecified occupant of heavy transport vehicle injured in collision with pedal cycle in nontraffic accident

√x7th **V61.4** Person boarding or alighting a heavy transport vehicle injured in collision with pedal cycle while boarding or alighting

√x7th **V61.5** Driver of heavy transport vehicle injured in collision with pedal cycle in traffic accident

√x7th **V61.6** Passenger in heavy transport vehicle injured in collision with pedal cycle in traffic accident

√x7th **V61.7** Person on outside of heavy transport vehicle injured in collision with pedal cycle in traffic accident

√x7th **V61.9** Unspecified occupant of heavy transport vehicle injured in collision with pedal cycle in traffic accident

√4th **V62** **Occupant of heavy transport vehicle injured in collision with two- or three-wheeled motor vehicle**

√x7th **V62.0** Driver of heavy transport vehicle injured in collision with two- or three-wheeled motor vehicle in nontraffic accident

√x7th **V62.1** Passenger in heavy transport vehicle injured in collision with two- or three-wheeled motor vehicle in nontraffic accident

√x7th **V62.2** Person on outside of heavy transport vehicle injured in collision with two- or three-wheeled motor vehicle in nontraffic accident

√x7th **V62.3** Unspecified occupant of heavy transport vehicle injured in collision with two- or three-wheeled motor vehicle in nontraffic accident

√x7th **V62.4** Person boarding or alighting a heavy transport vehicle injured in collision with two- or three-wheeled motor vehicle

√x7th **V62.5** Driver of heavy transport vehicle injured in collision with two- or three-wheeled motor vehicle in traffic accident

√x7th **V62.6** Passenger in heavy transport vehicle injured in collision with two- or three-wheeled motor vehicle in traffic accident

√x7th **V62.7** Person on outside of heavy transport vehicle injured in collision with two- or three-wheeled motor vehicle in traffic accident

√x7th **V62.9** Unspecified occupant of heavy transport vehicle injured in collision with two- or three-wheeled motor vehicle in traffic accident

√4th **V63** **Occupant of heavy transport vehicle injured in collision with car, pick-up truck or van**

√x7th **V63.0** Driver of heavy transport vehicle injured in collision with car, pick-up truck or van in nontraffic accident

√x7th **V63.1** Passenger in heavy transport vehicle injured in collision with car, pick-up truck or van in nontraffic accident

√x7th **V63.2** Person on outside of heavy transport vehicle injured in collision with car, pick-up truck or van in nontraffic accident

√x7th **V63.3** Unspecified occupant of heavy transport vehicle injured in collision with car, pick-up truck or van in nontraffic accident

√x7th **V63.4** Person boarding or alighting a heavy transport vehicle injured in collision with car, pick-up truck or van

√x7th **V63.5** Driver of heavy transport vehicle injured in collision with car, pick-up truck or van in traffic accident

√x7th **V63.6** Passenger in heavy transport vehicle injured in collision with car, pick-up truck or van in traffic accident

√x7th **V63.7** Person on outside of heavy transport vehicle injured in collision with car, pick-up truck or van in traffic accident

√x7th **V63.9** Unspecified occupant of heavy transport vehicle injured in collision with car, pick-up truck or van in traffic accident

√4th **V64** **Occupant of heavy transport vehicle injured in collision with heavy transport vehicle or bus**

EXCLUDES1 *occupant of heavy transport vehicle injured in collision with military vehicle (V69.81)*

√x7th **V64.0** Driver of heavy transport vehicle injured in collision with heavy transport vehicle or bus in nontraffic accident

√x7th **V64.1** Passenger in heavy transport vehicle injured in collision with heavy transport vehicle or bus in nontraffic accident

√x7th **V64.2** Person on outside of heavy transport vehicle injured in collision with heavy transport vehicle or bus in nontraffic accident

√x7th **V64.3** Unspecified occupant of heavy transport vehicle injured in collision with heavy transport vehicle or bus in nontraffic accident

√x7th **V64.4** Person boarding or alighting a heavy transport vehicle injured in collision with heavy transport vehicle or bus while boarding or alighting

√x7th **V64.5** Driver of heavy transport vehicle injured in collision with heavy transport vehicle or bus in traffic accident

√x7th **V64.6** Passenger in heavy transport vehicle injured in collision with heavy transport vehicle or bus in traffic accident

√x7th **V64.7** Person on outside of heavy transport vehicle injured in collision with heavy transport vehicle or bus in traffic accident

√x7th **V64.9** Unspecified occupant of heavy transport vehicle injured in collision with heavy transport vehicle or bus in traffic accident

√4th **V65** **Occupant of heavy transport vehicle injured in collision with railway train or railway vehicle**

√x7th **V65.0** Driver of heavy transport vehicle injured in collision with railway train or railway vehicle in nontraffic accident

√x7th **V65.1** Passenger in heavy transport vehicle injured in collision with railway train or railway vehicle in nontraffic accident

√x7th **V65.2** Person on outside of heavy transport vehicle injured in collision with railway train or railway vehicle in nontraffic accident

√x7th **V65.3** Unspecified occupant of heavy transport vehicle injured in collision with railway train or railway vehicle in nontraffic accident

√x7th **V65.4** Person boarding or alighting a heavy transport vehicle injured in collision with railway train or railway vehicle

√x7th **V65.5** Driver of heavy transport vehicle injured in collision with railway train or railway vehicle in traffic accident

V65.6 Passenger in heavy transport vehicle injured in collision with railway train or railway vehicle in traffic accident

V65.7 Person on outside of heavy transport vehicle injured in collision with railway train or railway vehicle in traffic accident

V65.9 Unspecified occupant of heavy transport vehicle injured in collision with railway train or railway vehicle in traffic accident

**V66 Occupant of heavy transport vehicle injured in collision with other nonmotor vehicle**

INCLUDES collision with animal-drawn vehicle, animal being ridden, streetcar

V66.0 Driver of heavy transport vehicle injured in collision with other nonmotor vehicle in nontraffic accident

V66.1 Passenger in heavy transport vehicle injured in collision with other nonmotor vehicle in nontraffic accident

V66.2 Person on outside of heavy transport vehicle injured in collision with other nonmotor vehicle in nontraffic accident

V66.3 Unspecified occupant of heavy transport vehicle injured in collision with other nonmotor vehicle in nontraffic accident

V66.4 Person boarding or alighting a heavy transport vehicle injured in collision with other nonmotor vehicle

V66.5 Driver of heavy transport vehicle injured in collision with other nonmotor vehicle in traffic accident

V66.6 Passenger in heavy transport vehicle injured in collision with other nonmotor vehicle in traffic accident

V66.7 Person on outside of heavy transport vehicle injured in collision with other nonmotor vehicle in traffic accident

V66.9 Unspecified occupant of heavy transport vehicle injured in collision with other nonmotor vehicle in traffic accident

**V67 Occupant of heavy transport vehicle injured in collision with fixed or stationary object**

V67.0 Driver of heavy transport vehicle injured in collision with fixed or stationary object in nontraffic accident

V67.1 Passenger in heavy transport vehicle injured in collision with fixed or stationary object in nontraffic accident

V67.2 Person on outside of heavy transport vehicle injured in collision with fixed or stationary object in nontraffic accident

V67.3 Unspecified occupant of heavy transport vehicle injured in collision with fixed or stationary object in nontraffic accident

V67.4 Person boarding or alighting a heavy transport vehicle injured in collision with fixed or stationary object

V67.5 Driver of heavy transport vehicle injured in collision with fixed or stationary object in traffic accident

V67.6 Passenger in heavy transport vehicle injured in collision with fixed or stationary object in traffic accident

V67.7 Person on outside of heavy transport vehicle injured in collision with fixed or stationary object in traffic accident

V67.9 Unspecified occupant of heavy transport vehicle injured in collision with fixed or stationary object in traffic accident

**V68 Occupant of heavy transport vehicle injured in noncollision transport accident**

INCLUDES overturning heavy transport vehicle NOS
overturning heavy transport vehicle without collision

V68.0 Driver of heavy transport vehicle injured in noncollision transport accident in nontraffic accident

V68.1 Passenger in heavy transport vehicle injured in noncollision transport accident in nontraffic accident

V68.2 Person on outside of heavy transport vehicle injured in noncollision transport accident in nontraffic accident

V68.3 Unspecified occupant of heavy transport vehicle injured in noncollision transport accident in nontraffic accident

V68.4 Person boarding or alighting a heavy transport vehicle injured in noncollision transport accident

V68.5 Driver of heavy transport vehicle injured in noncollision transport accident in traffic accident

V68.6 Passenger in heavy transport vehicle injured in noncollision transport accident in traffic accident

V68.7 Person on outside of heavy transport vehicle injured in noncollision transport accident in traffic accident

V68.9 Unspecified occupant of heavy transport vehicle injured in noncollision transport accident in traffic accident

**V69 Occupant of heavy transport vehicle injured in other and unspecified transport accidents**

V69.0 Driver of heavy transport vehicle injured in collision with other and unspecified motor vehicles in nontraffic accident

V69.00 Driver of heavy transport vehicle injured in collision with unspecified motor vehicles in nontraffic accident

V69.09 Driver of heavy transport vehicle injured in collision with other motor vehicles in nontraffic accident

V69.1 Passenger in heavy transport vehicle injured in collision with other and unspecified motor vehicles in nontraffic accident

V69.10 Passenger in heavy transport vehicle injured in collision with unspecified motor vehicles in nontraffic accident

V69.19 Passenger in heavy transport vehicle injured in collision with other motor vehicles in nontraffic accident

V69.2 Unspecified occupant of heavy transport vehicle injured in collision with other and unspecified motor vehicles in nontraffic accident

V69.20 Unspecified occupant of heavy transport vehicle injured in collision with unspecified motor vehicles in nontraffic accident
Collision NOS involving heavy transport vehicle, nontraffic

V69.29 Unspecified occupant of heavy transport vehicle injured in collision with other motor vehicles in nontraffic accident

V69.3 Occupant (driver) (passenger) of heavy transport vehicle injured in unspecified nontraffic accident
Accident NOS involving heavy transport vehicle, nontraffic
Occupant of heavy transport vehicle injured in nontraffic accident NOS

V69.4 Driver of heavy transport vehicle injured in collision with other and unspecified motor vehicles in traffic accident

V69.40 Driver of heavy transport vehicle injured in collision with unspecified motor vehicles in traffic accident

V69.49 Driver of heavy transport vehicle injured in collision with other motor vehicles in traffic accident

V69.5 Passenger in heavy transport vehicle injured in collision with other and unspecified motor vehicles in traffic accident

V69.50 Passenger in heavy transport vehicle injured in collision with unspecified motor vehicles in traffic accident

V69.59 Passenger in heavy transport vehicle injured in collision with other motor vehicles in traffic accident

V69.6 Unspecified occupant of heavy transport vehicle injured in collision with other and unspecified motor vehicles in traffic accident

V69.60 Unspecified occupant of heavy transport vehicle injured in collision with unspecified motor vehicles in traffic accident
Collision NOS involving heavy transport vehicle (traffic)

V69.69 Unspecified occupant of heavy transport vehicle injured in collision with other motor vehicles in traffic accident

V69.8 Occupant (driver) (passenger) of heavy transport vehicle injured in other specified transport accidents

V69.81 Occupant (driver) (passenger) of heavy transport vehicle injured in transport accidents with military vehicle

V69.88 Occupant (driver) (passenger) of heavy transport vehicle injured in other specified transport accidents

V69.9 Occupant (driver) (passenger) of heavy transport vehicle injured in unspecified traffic accident
Accident NOS involving heavy transport vehicle

## Bus occupant injured in transport accident (V70-V79)

INCLUDES motorcoach
EXCLUDES 1 *minibus (V50-V59)*

The appropriate 7th character is to be added to each code from categories V70-V79.
A initial encounter
D subsequent encounter
S sequela

**V70 Bus occupant injured in collision with pedestrian or animal**

EXCLUDES 1 *bus collision with animal-drawn vehicle or animal being ridden (V76.-)*

V70.0 Driver of bus injured in collision with pedestrian or animal in nontraffic accident

V70.1 Passenger on bus injured in collision with pedestrian or animal in nontraffic accident

V70.2 Person on outside of bus injured in collision with pedestrian or animal in nontraffic accident

V70.3 Unspecified occupant of bus injured in collision with pedestrian or animal in nontraffic accident

V70.4 Person boarding or alighting from bus injured in collision with pedestrian or animal

V70.5 Driver of bus injured in collision with pedestrian or animal in traffic accident

V70.6 Passenger on bus injured in collision with pedestrian or animal in traffic accident
V70.7 Person on outside of bus injured in collision with pedestrian or animal in traffic accident
V70.9 Unspecified occupant of bus injured in collision with pedestrian or animal in traffic accident

**V71 Bus occupant injured in collision with pedal cycle**
V71.0 Driver of bus injured in collision with pedal cycle in nontraffic accident
V71.1 Passenger on bus injured in collision with pedal cycle in nontraffic accident
V71.2 Person on outside of bus injured in collision with pedal cycle in nontraffic accident
V71.3 Unspecified occupant of bus injured in collision with pedal cycle in nontraffic accident
V71.4 Person boarding or alighting from bus injured in collision with pedal cycle
V71.5 Driver of bus injured in collision with pedal cycle in traffic accident
V71.6 Passenger on bus injured in collision with pedal cycle in traffic accident
V71.7 Person on outside of bus injured in collision with pedal cycle in traffic accident
V71.9 Unspecified occupant of bus injured in collision with pedal cycle in traffic accident

**V72 Bus occupant injured in collision with two- or three-wheeled motor vehicle**
V72.0 Driver of bus injured in collision with two- or three-wheeled motor vehicle in nontraffic accident
V72.1 Passenger on bus injured in collision with two- or three-wheeled motor vehicle in nontraffic accident
V72.2 Person on outside of bus injured in collision with two- or three-wheeled motor vehicle in nontraffic accident
V72.3 Unspecified occupant of bus injured in collision with two- or three-wheeled motor vehicle in nontraffic accident
V72.4 Person boarding or alighting from bus injured in collision with two- or three-wheeled motor vehicle
V72.5 Driver of bus injured in collision with two- or three-wheeled motor vehicle in traffic accident
V72.6 Passenger on bus injured in collision with two- or three-wheeled motor vehicle in traffic accident
V72.7 Person on outside of bus injured in collision with two- or three-wheeled motor vehicle in traffic accident
V72.9 Unspecified occupant of bus injured in collision with two- or three-wheeled motor vehicle in traffic accident

**V73 Bus occupant injured in collision with car, pick-up truck or van**
V73.0 Driver of bus injured in collision with car, pick-up truck or van in nontraffic accident
V73.1 Passenger on bus injured in collision with car, pick-up truck or van in nontraffic accident
V73.2 Person on outside of bus injured in collision with car, pick-up truck or van in nontraffic accident
V73.3 Unspecified occupant of bus injured in collision with car, pick-up truck or van in nontraffic accident
V73.4 Person boarding or alighting from bus injured in collision with car, pick-up truck or van
V73.5 Driver of bus injured in collision with car, pick-up truck or van in traffic accident
V73.6 Passenger on bus injured in collision with car, pick-up truck or van in traffic accident
V73.7 Person on outside of bus injured in collision with car, pick-up truck or van in traffic accident
V73.9 Unspecified occupant of bus injured in collision with car, pick-up truck or van in traffic accident

**V74 Bus occupant injured in collision with heavy transport vehicle or bus**
EXCLUDES 1 *bus occupant injured in collision with military vehicle (V79.81)*
V74.0 Driver of bus injured in collision with heavy transport vehicle or bus in nontraffic accident
V74.1 Passenger on bus injured in collision with heavy transport vehicle or bus in nontraffic accident
V74.2 Person on outside of bus injured in collision with heavy transport vehicle or bus in nontraffic accident
V74.3 Unspecified occupant of bus injured in collision with heavy transport vehicle or bus in nontraffic accident
V74.4 Person boarding or alighting from bus injured in collision with heavy transport vehicle or bus
V74.5 Driver of bus injured in collision with heavy transport vehicle or bus in traffic accident
V74.6 Passenger on bus injured in collision with heavy transport vehicle or bus in traffic accident
V74.7 Person on outside of bus injured in collision with heavy transport vehicle or bus in traffic accident
V74.9 Unspecified occupant of bus injured in collision with heavy transport vehicle or bus in traffic accident

**V75 Bus occupant injured in collision with railway train or railway vehicle**
V75.0 Driver of bus injured in collision with railway train or railway vehicle in nontraffic accident
V75.1 Passenger on bus injured in collision with railway train or railway vehicle in nontraffic accident
V75.2 Person on outside of bus injured in collision with railway train or railway vehicle in nontraffic accident
V75.3 Unspecified occupant of bus injured in collision with railway train or railway vehicle in nontraffic accident
V75.4 Person boarding or alighting from bus injured in collision with railway train or railway vehicle
V75.5 Driver of bus injured in collision with railway train or railway vehicle in traffic accident
V75.6 Passenger on bus injured in collision with railway train or railway vehicle in traffic accident
V75.7 Person on outside of bus injured in collision with railway train or railway vehicle in traffic accident
V75.9 Unspecified occupant of bus injured in collision with railway train or railway vehicle in traffic accident

**V76 Bus occupant injured in collision with other nonmotor vehicle**
INCLUDES collision with animal-drawn vehicle, animal being ridden, streetcar
V76.0 Driver of bus injured in collision with other nonmotor vehicle in nontraffic accident
V76.1 Passenger on bus injured in collision with other nonmotor vehicle in nontraffic accident
V76.2 Person on outside of bus injured in collision with other nonmotor vehicle in nontraffic accident
V76.3 Unspecified occupant of bus injured in collision with other nonmotor vehicle in nontraffic accident
V76.4 Person boarding or alighting from bus injured in collision with other nonmotor vehicle
V76.5 Driver of bus injured in collision with other nonmotor vehicle in traffic accident
V76.6 Passenger on bus injured in collision with other nonmotor vehicle in traffic accident
V76.7 Person on outside of bus injured in collision with other nonmotor vehicle in traffic accident
V76.9 Unspecified occupant of bus injured in collision with other nonmotor vehicle in traffic accident

**V77 Bus occupant injured in collision with fixed or stationary object**
V77.0 Driver of bus injured in collision with fixed or stationary object in nontraffic accident
V77.1 Passenger on bus injured in collision with fixed or stationary object in nontraffic accident
V77.2 Person on outside of bus injured in collision with fixed or stationary object in nontraffic accident
V77.3 Unspecified occupant of bus injured in collision with fixed or stationary object in nontraffic accident
V77.4 Person boarding or alighting from bus injured in collision with fixed or stationary object
V77.5 Driver of bus injured in collision with fixed or stationary object in traffic accident
V77.6 Passenger on bus injured in collision with fixed or stationary object in traffic accident
V77.7 Person on outside of bus injured in collision with fixed or stationary object in traffic accident
V77.9 Unspecified occupant of bus injured in collision with fixed or stationary object in traffic accident

**V78 Bus occupant injured in noncollision transport accident**
INCLUDES overturning bus NOS
overturning bus without collision
V78.0 Driver of bus injured in noncollision transport accident in nontraffic accident
V78.1 Passenger on bus injured in noncollision transport accident in nontraffic accident
V78.2 Person on outside of bus injured in noncollision transport accident in nontraffic accident
V78.3 Unspecified occupant of bus injured in noncollision transport accident in nontraffic accident
V78.4 Person boarding or alighting from bus injured in noncollision transport accident

√x7th **V78.5** Driver of bus injured in noncollision transport accident in traffic accident

√x7th **V78.6** Passenger on bus injured in noncollision transport accident in traffic accident

√x7th **V78.7** Person on outside of bus injured in noncollision transport accident in traffic accident

√x7th **V78.9** Unspecified occupant of bus injured in noncollision transport accident in traffic accident

√4th **V79 Bus occupant injured in other and unspecified transport accidents**

√5th **V79.0** Driver of bus injured in collision with other and unspecified motor vehicles in nontraffic accident

√x7th **V79.00** Driver of bus injured in collision with unspecified motor vehicles in nontraffic accident

√x7th **V79.09** Driver of bus injured in collision with other motor vehicles in nontraffic accident

√5th **V79.1** Passenger on bus injured in collision with other and unspecified motor vehicles in nontraffic accident

√x7th **V79.10** Passenger on bus injured in collision with unspecified motor vehicles in nontraffic accident

√x7th **V79.19** Passenger on bus injured in collision with other motor vehicles in nontraffic accident

√5th **V79.2** Unspecified bus occupant injured in collision with other and unspecified motor vehicles in nontraffic accident

√x7th **V79.20** Unspecified bus occupant injured in collision with unspecified motor vehicles in nontraffic accident
Bus collision NOS, nontraffic

√x7th **V79.29** Unspecified bus occupant injured in collision with other motor vehicles in nontraffic accident

√x7th **V79.3** Bus occupant (driver) (passenger) injured in unspecified nontraffic accident
Bus accident NOS, nontraffic
Bus occupant injured in nontraffic accident NOS

√5th **V79.4** Driver of bus injured in collision with other and unspecified motor vehicles in traffic accident

√x7th **V79.40** Driver of bus injured in collision with unspecified motor vehicles in traffic accident

√x7th **V79.49** Driver of bus injured in collision with other motor vehicles in traffic accident

√5th **V79.5** Passenger on bus injured in collision with other and unspecified motor vehicles in traffic accident

√x7th **V79.50** Passenger on bus injured in collision with unspecified motor vehicles in traffic accident

√x7th **V79.59** Passenger on bus injured in collision with other motor vehicles in traffic accident

√5th **V79.6** Unspecified bus occupant injured in collision with other and unspecified motor vehicles in traffic accident

√x7th **V79.60** Unspecified bus occupant injured in collision with unspecified motor vehicles in traffic accident
Bus collision NOS (traffic)

√x7th **V79.69** Unspecified bus occupant injured in collision with other motor vehicles in traffic accident

√5th **V79.8** Bus occupant (driver) (passenger) injured in other specified transport accidents

√x7th **V79.81** Bus occupant (driver) (passenger) injured in transport accidents with military vehicle

√x7th **V79.88** Bus occupant (driver) (passenger) injured in other specified transport accidents

√x7th **V79.9** Bus occupant (driver) (passenger) injured in unspecified traffic accident
Bus accident NOS

## Other land transport accidents (V80-V89)

The appropriate 7th character is to be added to each code from categories V80-V89.
A initial encounter
D subsequent encounter
S sequela

√4th **V80 Animal-rider or occupant of animal-drawn vehicle injured in transport accident**

√5th **V80.0** Animal-rider or occupant of animal drawn vehicle injured by fall from or being thrown from animal or animal-drawn vehicle in noncollision accident

√6th **V80.01** Animal-rider injured by fall from or being thrown from animal in noncollision accident

√7th **V80.010** Animal-rider injured by fall from or being thrown from horse in noncollision accident

√7th **V80.018** Animal-rider injured by fall from or being thrown from other animal in noncollision accident

√x7th **V80.02** Occupant of animal-drawn vehicle injured by fall from or being thrown from animal-drawn vehicle in noncollision accident
Overturning animal-drawn vehicle NOS
Overturning animal-drawn vehicle without collision

√5th **V80.1** Animal-rider or occupant of animal-drawn vehicle injured in collision with pedestrian or animal
EXCLUDES 1 *animal-rider or animal-drawn vehicle collision with animal-drawn vehicle or animal being ridden (V80.7)*

√x7th **V80.11** Animal-rider injured in collision with pedestrian or animal

√x7th **V80.12** Occupant of animal-drawn vehicle injured in collision with pedestrian or animal

√5th **V80.2** Animal-rider or occupant of animal-drawn vehicle injured in collision with pedal cycle

√x7th **V80.21** Animal-rider injured in collision with pedal cycle

√x7th **V80.22** Occupant of animal-drawn vehicle injured in collision with pedal cycle

√5th **V80.3** Animal-rider or occupant of animal-drawn vehicle injured in collision with two- or three-wheeled motor vehicle

√x7th **V80.31** Animal-rider injured in collision with two- or three-wheeled motor vehicle

√x7th **V80.32** Occupant of animal-drawn vehicle injured in collision with two- or three-wheeled motor vehicle

√5th **V80.4** Animal-rider or occupant of animal-drawn vehicle injured in collision with car, pick-up truck, van, heavy transport vehicle or bus
EXCLUDES 1 *animal-rider injured in collision with military vehicle (V80.910)*
*occupant of animal-drawn vehicle injured in collision with military vehicle (V80.920)*

√x7th **V80.41** Animal-rider injured in collision with car, pick-up truck, van, heavy transport vehicle or bus

√x7th **V80.42** Occupant of animal-drawn vehicle injured in collision with car, pick-up truck, van, heavy transport vehicle or bus

√5th **V80.5** Animal-rider or occupant of animal-drawn vehicle injured in collision with other specified motor vehicle

√x7th **V80.51** Animal-rider injured in collision with other specified motor vehicle

√x7th **V80.52** Occupant of animal-drawn vehicle injured in collision with other specified motor vehicle

√5th **V80.6** Animal-rider or occupant of animal-drawn vehicle injured in collision with railway train or railway vehicle

√x7th **V80.61** Animal-rider injured in collision with railway train or railway vehicle

√x7th **V80.62** Occupant of animal-drawn vehicle injured in collision with railway train or railway vehicle

√5th **V80.7** Animal-rider or occupant of animal-drawn vehicle injured in collision with other nonmotor vehicles

√6th **V80.71** Animal-rider or occupant of animal-drawn vehicle injured in collision with animal being ridden

√7th **V80.710** Animal-rider injured in collision with other animal being ridden

√7th **V80.711** Occupant of animal-drawn vehicle injured in collision with animal being ridden

√6th **V80.72** Animal-rider or occupant of animal-drawn vehicle injured in collision with other animal-drawn vehicle

√7th **V80.720** Animal-rider injured in collision with animal-drawn vehicle

√7th **V80.721** Occupant of animal-drawn vehicle injured in collision with other animal-drawn vehicle

√6th **V80.73** Animal-rider or occupant of animal-drawn vehicle injured in collision with streetcar

√7th **V80.730** Animal-rider injured in collision with streetcar

√7th **V80.731** Occupant of animal-drawn vehicle injured in collision with streetcar

√6th **V80.79** Animal-rider or occupant of animal-drawn vehicle injured in collision with other nonmotor vehicles

√7th **V80.790** Animal-rider injured in collision with other nonmotor vehicles

√7th **V80.791** Occupant of animal-drawn vehicle injured in collision with other nonmotor vehicles

√5th **V80.8** Animal-rider or occupant of animal-drawn vehicle injured in collision with fixed or stationary object

√x7th **V80.81** Animal-rider injured in collision with fixed or stationary object

√x7th **V80.82** Occupant of animal-drawn vehicle injured in collision with fixed or stationary object

√5th **V80.9 Animal-rider or occupant of animal-drawn vehicle injured in other and unspecified transport accidents**

√6th **V80.91 Animal-rider injured in other and unspecified transport accidents**

√7th **V80.910 Animal-rider injured in transport accident with military vehicle**

√7th **V80.918 Animal-rider injured in other transport accident**

√7th **V80.919 Animal-rider injured in unspecified transport accident**
Animal rider accident NOS

√6th **V80.92 Occupant of animal-drawn vehicle injured in other and unspecified transport accidents**

√7th **V80.920 Occupant of animal-drawn vehicle injured in transport accident with military vehicle**

√7th **V80.928 Occupant of animal-drawn vehicle injured in other transport accident**

√7th **V80.929 Occupant of animal-drawn vehicle injured in unspecified transport accident**
Animal-drawn vehicle accident NOS

√4th **V81 Occupant of railway train or railway vehicle injured in transport accident**

INCLUDES derailment of railway train or railway vehicle
person on outside of train

EXCLUDES 1 *streetcar (V82.-)*

√x7th **V81.0 Occupant of railway train or railway vehicle injured in collision with motor vehicle in nontraffic accident**

EXCLUDES 1 *occupant of railway train or railway vehicle injured due to collision with military vehicle (V81.83)*

√x7th **V81.1 Occupant of railway train or railway vehicle injured in collision with motor vehicle in traffic accident**

EXCLUDES 1 *occupant of railway train or railway vehicle injured due to collision with military vehicle (V81.83)*

√x7th **V81.2 Occupant of railway train or railway vehicle injured in collision with or hit by rolling stock**

√x7th **V81.3 Occupant of railway train or railway vehicle injured in collision with other object**
Railway collision NOS

√x7th **V81.4 Person injured while boarding or alighting from railway train or railway vehicle**

√x7th **V81.5 Occupant of railway train or railway vehicle injured by fall in railway train or railway vehicle**

√x7th **V81.6 Occupant of railway train or railway vehicle injured by fall from railway train or railway vehicle**

√x7th **V81.7 Occupant of railway train or railway vehicle injured in derailment without antecedent collision**

√5th **V81.8 Occupant of railway train or railway vehicle injured in other specified railway accidents**

√x7th **V81.81 Occupant of railway train or railway vehicle injured due to explosion or fire on train**

√x7th **V81.82 Occupant of railway train or railway vehicle injured due to object falling onto train**
Occupant of railway train or railway vehicle injured due to falling earth onto train
Occupant of railway train or railway vehicle injured due to falling rocks onto train
Occupant of railway train or railway vehicle injured due to falling snow onto train
Occupant of railway train or railway vehicle injured due to falling trees onto train

√x7th **V81.83 Occupant of railway train or railway vehicle injured due to collision with military vehicle**

√x7th **V81.89 Occupant of railway train or railway vehicle injured due to other specified railway accident**

√x7th **V81.9 Occupant of railway train or railway vehicle injured in unspecified railway accident**
Railway accident NOS

√4th **V82 Occupant of powered streetcar injured in transport accident**

INCLUDES interurban electric car
person on outside of streetcar
tram (car)
trolley (car)

EXCLUDES 1 *bus (V70-V79)*
*motorcoach (V70-V79)*
*nonpowered streetcar (V76.-)*
*train (V81.-)*

√x7th **V82.0 Occupant of streetcar injured in collision with motor vehicle in nontraffic accident**

√x7th **V82.1 Occupant of streetcar injured in collision with motor vehicle in traffic accident**

√x7th **V82.2 Occupant of streetcar injured in collision with or hit by rolling stock**

√x7th **V82.3 Occupant of streetcar injured in collision with other object**

EXCLUDES 1 *collision with animal-drawn vehicle or animal being ridden (V82.8)*

√x7th **V82.4 Person injured while boarding or alighting from streetcar**

√x7th **V82.5 Occupant of streetcar injured by fall in streetcar**

EXCLUDES 1 *fall in streetcar:*
*while boarding or alighting (V82.4)*
*with antecedent collision (V82.0-V82.3)*

√x7th **V82.6 Occupant of streetcar injured by fall from streetcar**

EXCLUDES 1 *fall from streetcar:*
*while boarding or alighting (V82.4)*
*with antecedent collision (V82.0-V82.3)*

√x7th **V82.7 Occupant of streetcar injured in derailment without antecedent collision**

EXCLUDES 1 *occupant of streetcar injured in derailment with antecedent collision (V82.0-V82.3)*

√x7th **V82.8 Occupant of streetcar injured in other specified transport accidents**
Streetcar collision with military vehicle
Streetcar collision with train or nonmotor vehicles

√x7th **V82.9 Occupant of streetcar injured in unspecified traffic accident**
Streetcar accident NOS

√4th **V83 Occupant of special vehicle mainly used on industrial premises injured in transport accident**

INCLUDES battery-powered airport passenger vehicle
battery-powered truck (baggage) (mail)
coal-car in mine
forklift (truck)
logging car
self-propelled industrial truck
station baggage truck (powered)
tram, truck, or tub (powered) in mine or quarry

EXCLUDES 1 *special construction vehicles (V85.-)*
*special industrial vehicle in stationary use or maintenance (W31.-)*

√x7th **V83.0 Driver of special industrial vehicle injured in traffic accident**

√x7th **V83.1 Passenger of special industrial vehicle injured in traffic accident**

√x7th **V83.2 Person on outside of special industrial vehicle injured in traffic accident**

√x7th **V83.3 Unspecified occupant of special industrial vehicle injured in traffic accident**

√x7th **V83.4 Person injured while boarding or alighting from special industrial vehicle**

√x7th **V83.5 Driver of special industrial vehicle injured in nontraffic accident**

√x7th **V83.6 Passenger of special industrial vehicle injured in nontraffic accident**

√x7th **V83.7 Person on outside of special industrial vehicle injured in nontraffic accident**

√x7th **V83.9 Unspecified occupant of special industrial vehicle injured in nontraffic accident**
Special-industrial-vehicle accident NOS

√4th **V84 Occupant of special vehicle mainly used in agriculture injured in transport accident**

INCLUDES self-propelled farm machinery
tractor (and trailer)

EXCLUDES 1 *animal-powered farm machinery accident (W30.8-)*
*contact with combine harvester (W30.0)*
*special agricultural vehicle in stationary use or maintenance (W30.-)*

√x7th **V84.0 Driver of special agricultural vehicle injured in traffic accident**

√x7th **V84.1 Passenger of special agricultural vehicle injured in traffic accident**

√x7th **V84.2 Person on outside of special agricultural vehicle injured in traffic accident**

√x7th **V84.3 Unspecified occupant of special agricultural vehicle injured in traffic accident**

√x7th **V84.4 Person injured while boarding or alighting from special agricultural vehicle**

√x7th **V84.5 Driver of special agricultural vehicle injured in nontraffic accident**

√x7th **V84.6 Passenger of special agricultural vehicle injured in nontraffic accident**

√x7th **V84.7 Person on outside of special agricultural vehicle injured in nontraffic accident**

√x7th **V84.9 Unspecified occupant of special agricultural vehicle injured in nontraffic accident**
Special-agricultural vehicle accident NOS

**V85 Occupant of special construction vehicle injured in transport accident**

INCLUDES bulldozer
digger
dump truck
earth-leveller
mechanical shovel
road-roller

EXCLUDES 1 *special construction vehicle in stationary use or maintenance (W31.-)*
*special industrial vehicle (V83.-)*

- **V85.Ø Driver of special construction vehicle injured in traffic accident**
- **V85.1 Passenger of special construction vehicle injured in traffic accident**
- **V85.2 Person on outside of special construction vehicle injured in traffic accident**
- **V85.3 Unspecified occupant of special construction vehicle injured in traffic accident**
- **V85.4 Person injured while boarding or alighting from special construction vehicle**
- **V85.5 Driver of special construction vehicle injured in nontraffic accident**
- **V85.6 Passenger of special construction vehicle injured in nontraffic accident**
- **V85.7 Person on outside of special construction vehicle injured in nontraffic accident**
- **V85.9 Unspecified occupant of special construction vehicle injured in nontraffic accident**
  Special-construction-vehicle accident NOS

**V86 Occupant of special all-terrain or other off-road motor vehicle, injured in transport accident**

EXCLUDES 1 *special all-terrain vehicle in stationary use or maintenance (W31.-)*
*sport-utility vehicle (V5Ø-V59)*
*three-wheeled motor vehicle designed for on-road use (V3Ø-V39)*

**AHA:** 2017,4Q,26

**V86.Ø Driver of special all-terrain or other off-road motor vehicle injured in traffic accident**
- **V86.Ø1 Driver of ambulance or fire engine injured in traffic accident**
- **V86.Ø2 Driver of snowmobile injured in traffic accident**
- **V86.Ø3 Driver of dune buggy injured in traffic accident**
- **V86.Ø4 Driver of military vehicle injured in traffic accident**
- **V86.Ø5 Driver of 3- or 4- wheeled all-terrain vehicle (ATV) injured in traffic accident**
- **V86.Ø6 Driver of dirt bike or motor/cross bike injured in traffic accident**
- **V86.Ø9 Driver of other special all-terrain or other off-road motor vehicle injured in traffic accident**
  Driver of go cart injured in traffic accident
  Driver of golf cart injured in traffic accident

**V86.1 Passenger of special all-terrain or other off-road motor vehicle injured in traffic accident**
- **V86.11 Passenger of ambulance or fire engine injured in traffic accident**
- **V86.12 Passenger of snowmobile injured in traffic accident**
- **V86.13 Passenger of dune buggy injured in traffic accident**
- **V86.14 Passenger of military vehicle injured in traffic accident**
- **V86.15 Passenger of 3- or 4- wheeled all-terrain vehicle (ATV) injured in traffic accident**
- **V86.16 Passenger of dirt bike or motor/cross bike injured in traffic accident**
- **V86.19 Passenger of other special all-terrain or other off-road motor vehicle injured in traffic accident**
  Passenger of go cart injured in traffic accident
  Passenger of golf cart injured in traffic accident

**V86.2 Person on outside of special all-terrain or other off-road motor vehicle injured in traffic accident**
- **V86.21 Person on outside of ambulance or fire engine injured in traffic accident**
- **V86.22 Person on outside of snowmobile injured in traffic accident**
- **V86.23 Person on outside of dune buggy injured in traffic accident**
- **V86.24 Person on outside of military vehicle injured in traffic accident**
- **V86.25 Person on outside of 3- or 4- wheeled all-terrain vehicle (ATV) injured in traffic accident**
- **V86.26 Person on outside of dirt bike or motor/cross bike injured in traffic accident**
- **V86.29 Person on outside of other special all-terrain or other off-road motor vehicle injured in traffic accident**
  Person on outside of go cart in traffic accident
  Person on outside of golf cart injured in traffic accident

**V86.3 Unspecified occupant of special all-terrain or other off-road motor vehicle injured in traffic accident**
- **V86.31 Unspecified occupant of ambulance or fire engine injured in traffic accident**
- **V86.32 Unspecified occupant of snowmobile injured in traffic accident**
- **V86.33 Unspecified occupant of dune buggy injured in traffic accident**
- **V86.34 Unspecified occupant of military vehicle injured in traffic accident**
- **V86.35 Unspecified occupant of 3- or 4- wheeled all-terrain vehicle (ATV) injured in traffic accident**
- **V86.36 Unspecified occupant of dirt bike or motor/cross bike injured in traffic accident**
- **V86.39 Unspecified occupant of other special all-terrain or other off-road motor vehicle injured in traffic accident**
  Unspecified occupant of go cart injured in traffic accident
  Unspecified occupant of golf cart injured in traffic accident

**V86.4 Person injured while boarding or alighting from special all-terrain or other off-road motor vehicle**
- **V86.41 Person injured while boarding or alighting from ambulance or fire engine**
- **V86.42 Person injured while boarding or alighting from snowmobile**
- **V86.43 Person injured while boarding or alighting from dune buggy**
- **V86.44 Person injured while boarding or alighting from military vehicle**
- **V86.45 Person injured while boarding or alighting from a 3- or 4- wheeled all-terrain vehicle (ATV)**
- **V86.46 Person injured while boarding or alighting from a dirt bike or motor/cross bike**
- **V86.49 Person injured while boarding or alighting from other special all-terrain or other off-road motor vehicle**
  Person injured while boarding or alighting from go cart
  Person injured while boarding or alighting from golf cart

**V86.5 Driver of special all-terrain or other off-road motor vehicle injured in nontraffic accident**
- **V86.51 Driver of ambulance or fire engine injured in nontraffic accident**
- **V86.52 Driver of snowmobile injured in nontraffic accident**
- **V86.53 Driver of dune buggy injured in nontraffic accident**
- **V86.54 Driver of military vehicle injured in nontraffic accident**
- **V86.55 Driver of 3- or 4- wheeled all-terrain vehicle (ATV) injured in nontraffic accident**
- **V86.56 Driver of dirt bike or motor/cross bike injured in nontraffic accident**
- **V86.59 Driver of other special all-terrain or other off-road motor vehicle injured in nontraffic accident**
  Driver of go cart injured in nontraffic accident
  Driver of golf cart injured in nontraffic accident

**V86.6 Passenger of special all-terrain or other off-road motor vehicle injured in nontraffic accident**
- **V86.61 Passenger of ambulance or fire engine injured in nontraffic accident**
- **V86.62 Passenger of snowmobile injured in nontraffic accident**
- **V86.63 Passenger of dune buggy injured in nontraffic accident**
- **V86.64 Passenger of military vehicle injured in nontraffic accident**
- **V86.65 Passenger of 3- or 4- wheeled all-terrain vehicle (ATV) injured in nontraffic accident**
- **V86.66 Passenger of dirt bike or motor/cross bike injured in nontraffic accident**
- **V86.69 Passenger of other special all-terrain or other off-road motor vehicle injured in nontraffic accident**
  Passenger of go cart injured in nontraffic accident
  Passenger of golf cart injured in nontraffic accident

**V86.7 Person on outside of special all-terrain or other off-road motor vehicle injured in nontraffic accident**
- **V86.71 Person on outside of ambulance or fire engine injured in nontraffic accident**

√x7th **V86.72 Person on outside of snowmobile injured in nontraffic accident**

√x7th **V86.73 Person on outside of dune buggy injured in nontraffic accident**

√x7th **V86.74 Person on outside of military vehicle injured in nontraffic accident**

√x7th **V86.75 Person on outside of 3- or 4- wheeled all-terrain vehicle (ATV) injured in nontraffic accident**

√x7th **V86.76 Person on outside of dirt bike or motor/cross bike injured in nontraffic accident**

√x7th **V86.79 Person on outside of other special all-terrain or other off-road motor vehicles injured in nontraffic accident**
Person on outside of go cart injured in nontraffic accident
Person on outside of golf cart injured in nontraffic accident

√5th **V86.9 Unspecified occupant of special all-terrain or other off-road motor vehicle injured in nontraffic accident**

√x7th **V86.91 Unspecified occupant of ambulance or fire engine injured in nontraffic accident**

√x7th **V86.92 Unspecified occupant of snowmobile injured in nontraffic accident**

√x7th **V86.93 Unspecified occupant of dune buggy injured in nontraffic accident**

√x7th **V86.94 Unspecified occupant of military vehicle injured in nontraffic accident**

√x7th **V86.95 Unspecified occupant of 3- or 4- wheeled all-terrain vehicle (ATV) injured in nontraffic accident**

√x7th **V86.96 Unspecified occupant of dirt bike or motor/cross bike injured in nontraffic accident**

√x7th **V86.99 Unspecified occupant of other special all-terrain or other off-road motor vehicle injured in nontraffic accident**
Off-road motor-vehicle accident NOS
Other motor-vehicle accident NOS
Unspecified occupant of go cart injured in nontraffic accident
Unspecified occupant of golf cart injured in nontraffic accident

√4th **V87 Traffic accident of specified type but victim's mode of transport unknown**

EXCLUDES 1 *collision involving:*
*pedal cycle (V1Ø-V19)*
*pedestrian (VØ1-VØ9)*

√x7th **V87.Ø Person injured in collision between car and two- or three-wheeled powered vehicle (traffic)**

√x7th **V87.1 Person injured in collision between other motor vehicle and two- or three-wheeled motor vehicle (traffic)**

√x7th **V87.2 Person injured in collision between car and pick-up truck or van (traffic)**

√x7th **V87.3 Person injured in collision between car and bus (traffic)**

√x7th **V87.4 Person injured in collision between car and heavy transport vehicle (traffic)**

√x7th **V87.5 Person injured in collision between heavy transport vehicle and bus (traffic)**

√x7th **V87.6 Person injured in collision between railway train or railway vehicle and car (traffic)**

√x7th **V87.7 Person injured in collision between other specified motor vehicles (traffic)**

√x7th **V87.8 Person injured in other specified noncollision transport accidents involving motor vehicle (traffic)**

√x7th **V87.9 Person injured in other specified (collision)(noncollision) transport accidents involving nonmotor vehicle (traffic)**

√4th **V88 Nontraffic accident of specified type but victim's mode of transport unknown**

EXCLUDES 1 *collision involving:*
*pedal cycle (V1Ø-V19)*
*pedestrian (VØ1-VØ9)*

√x7th **V88.Ø Person injured in collision between car and two- or three-wheeled motor vehicle, nontraffic**

√x7th **V88.1 Person injured in collision between other motor vehicle and two- or three-wheeled motor vehicle, nontraffic**

√x7th **V88.2 Person injured in collision between car and pick-up truck or van, nontraffic**

√x7th **V88.3 Person injured in collision between car and bus, nontraffic**

√x7th **V88.4 Person injured in collision between car and heavy transport vehicle, nontraffic**

√x7th **V88.5 Person injured in collision between heavy transport vehicle and bus, nontraffic**

√x7th **V88.6 Person injured in collision between railway train or railway vehicle and car, nontraffic**

√x7th **V88.7 Person injured in collision between other specified motor vehicle, nontraffic**

√x7th **V88.8 Person injured in other specified noncollision transport accidents involving motor vehicle, nontraffic**

√x7th **V88.9 Person injured in other specified (collision)(noncollision) transport accidents involving nonmotor vehicle, nontraffic**

√4th **V89 Motor- or nonmotor-vehicle accident, type of vehicle unspecified**

√x7th **V89.Ø Person injured in unspecified motor-vehicle accident, nontraffic**
Motor-vehicle accident NOS, nontraffic

√x7th **V89.1 Person injured in unspecified nonmotor-vehicle accident, nontraffic**
Nonmotor-vehicle accident NOS (nontraffic)

√x7th **V89.2 Person injured in unspecified motor-vehicle accident, traffic**
Motor-vehicle accident [MVA] NOS
Road (traffic) accident [RTA] NOS

√x7th **V89.3 Person injured in unspecified nonmotor-vehicle accident, traffic**
Nonmotor-vehicle traffic accident NOS

√x7th **V89.9 Person injured in unspecified vehicle accident**
Collision NOS

## Water transport accidents (V9Ø-V94)

The appropriate 7th character is to be added to each code from categories V9Ø-V94.
A initial encounter
D subsequent encounter
S sequela

√4th **V9Ø Drowning and submersion due to accident to watercraft**

EXCLUDES 1 *civilian water transport accident involving military watercraft (V94.81-)*
*fall into water not from watercraft (W16.-)*
*military watercraft accident in military or war operations (Y36.Ø-, Y37.Ø-)*
*water-transport-related drowning or submersion without accident to watercraft (V92.-)*

√5th **V9Ø.Ø Drowning and submersion due to watercraft overturning**

√x7th **V9Ø.ØØ Drowning and submersion due to merchant ship overturning**

√x7th **V9Ø.Ø1 Drowning and submersion due to passenger ship overturning**
Drowning and submersion due to Ferry-boat overturning
Drowning and submersion due to Liner overturning

√x7th **V9Ø.Ø2 Drowning and submersion due to fishing boat overturning**

√x7th **V9Ø.Ø3 Drowning and submersion due to other powered watercraft overturning**
Drowning and submersion due to Hovercraft (on open water) overturning
Drowning and submersion due to Jet ski overturning

√x7th **V9Ø.Ø4 Drowning and submersion due to sailboat overturning**

√x7th **V9Ø.Ø5 Drowning and submersion due to canoe or kayak overturning**

√x7th **V9Ø.Ø6 Drowning and submersion due to (nonpowered) inflatable craft overturning**

√x7th **V9Ø.Ø8 Drowning and submersion due to other unpowered watercraft overturning**
Drowning and submersion due to windsurfer overturning

√x7th **V9Ø.Ø9 Drowning and submersion due to unspecified watercraft overturning**
Drowning and submersion due to boat NOS overturning
Drowning and submersion due to ship NOS overturning
Drowning and submersion due to watercraft NOS overturning

√5th **V9Ø.1 Drowning and submersion due to watercraft sinking**

√x7th **V9Ø.1Ø Drowning and submersion due to merchant ship sinking**

√x7th **V9Ø.11 Drowning and submersion due to passenger ship sinking**
Drowning and submersion due to Ferry-boat sinking
Drowning and submersion due to Liner sinking

√x7th **V9Ø.12 Drowning and submersion due to fishing boat sinking**

V90.13 **Drowning and submersion due to other powered watercraft sinking**
Drowning and submersion due to Hovercraft (on open water) sinking
Drowning and submersion due to Jet ski sinking

V90.14 **Drowning and submersion due to sailboat sinking**

V90.15 **Drowning and submersion due to canoe or kayak sinking**

V90.16 **Drowning and submersion due to (nonpowered) inflatable craft sinking**

V90.18 **Drowning and submersion due to other unpowered watercraft sinking**

V90.19 **Drowning and submersion due to unspecified watercraft sinking**
Drowning and submersion due to boat NOS sinking
Drowning and submersion due to ship NOS sinking
Drowning and submersion due to watercraft NOS sinking

V90.2 **Drowning and submersion due to falling or jumping from burning watercraft**

V90.20 **Drowning and submersion due to falling or jumping from burning merchant ship**

V90.21 **Drowning and submersion due to falling or jumping from burning passenger ship**
Drowning and submersion due to falling or jumping from burning Ferry-boat
Drowning and submersion due to falling or jumping from burning Liner

V90.22 **Drowning and submersion due to falling or jumping from burning fishing boat**

V90.23 **Drowning and submersion due to falling or jumping from other burning powered watercraft**
Drowning and submersion due to falling and jumping from burning Hovercraft (on open water)
Drowning and submersion due to falling and jumping from burning Jet ski

V90.24 **Drowning and submersion due to falling or jumping from burning sailboat**

V90.25 **Drowning and submersion due to falling or jumping from burning canoe or kayak**

V90.26 **Drowning and submersion due to falling or jumping from burning (nonpowered) inflatable craft**

V90.27 **Drowning and submersion due to falling or jumping from burning water-skis**

V90.28 **Drowning and submersion due to falling or jumping from other burning unpowered watercraft**
Drowning and submersion due to falling and jumping from burning surf-board
Drowning and submersion due to falling and jumping from burning windsurfer

V90.29 **Drowning and submersion due to falling or jumping from unspecified burning watercraft**
Drowning and submersion due to falling or jumping from burning boat NOS
Drowning and submersion due to falling or jumping from burning ship NOS
Drowning and submersion due to falling or jumping from burning watercraft NOS

V90.3 **Drowning and submersion due to falling or jumping from crushed watercraft**

V90.30 **Drowning and submersion due to falling or jumping from crushed merchant ship**

V90.31 **Drowning and submersion due to falling or jumping from crushed passenger ship**
Drowning and submersion due to falling and jumping from crushed Ferry boat
Drowning and submersion due to falling and jumping from crushed Liner

V90.32 **Drowning and submersion due to falling or jumping from crushed fishing boat**

V90.33 **Drowning and submersion due to falling or jumping from other crushed powered watercraft**
Drowning and submersion due to falling and jumping from crushed Hovercraft
Drowning and submersion due to falling and jumping from crushed Jet ski

V90.34 **Drowning and submersion due to falling or jumping from crushed sailboat**

V90.35 **Drowning and submersion due to falling or jumping from crushed canoe or kayak**

V90.36 **Drowning and submersion due to falling or jumping from crushed (nonpowered) inflatable craft**

V90.37 **Drowning and submersion due to falling or jumping from crushed water-skis**

V90.38 **Drowning and submersion due to falling or jumping from other crushed unpowered watercraft**
Drowning and submersion due to falling and jumping from crushed surf-board
Drowning and submersion due to falling and jumping from crushed windsurfer

V90.39 **Drowning and submersion due to falling or jumping from crushed unspecified watercraft**
Drowning and submersion due to falling and jumping from crushed boat NOS
Drowning and submersion due to falling and jumping from crushed ship NOS
Drowning and submersion due to falling and jumping from crushed watercraft NOS

V90.8 **Drowning and submersion due to other accident to watercraft**

V90.80 **Drowning and submersion due to other accident to merchant ship**

V90.81 **Drowning and submersion due to other accident to passenger ship**
Drowning and submersion due to other accident to Ferry-boat
Drowning and submersion due to other accident to Liner

V90.82 **Drowning and submersion due to other accident to fishing boat**

V90.83 **Drowning and submersion due to other accident to other powered watercraft**
Drowning and submersion due to other accident to Hovercraft (on open water)
Drowning and submersion due to other accident to Jet ski

V90.84 **Drowning and submersion due to other accident to sailboat**

V90.85 **Drowning and submersion due to other accident to canoe or kayak**

V90.86 **Drowning and submersion due to other accident to (nonpowered) inflatable craft**

V90.87 **Drowning and submersion due to other accident to water-skis**

V90.88 **Drowning and submersion due to other accident to other unpowered watercraft**
Drowning and submersion due to other accident to surf-board
Drowning and submersion due to other accident to windsurfer

V90.89 **Drowning and submersion due to other accident to unspecified watercraft**
Drowning and submersion due to other accident to boat NOS
Drowning and submersion due to other accident to ship NOS
Drowning and submersion due to other accident to watercraft NOS

## V91 Other injury due to accident to watercraft

INCLUDES any injury except drowning and submersion as a result of an accident to watercraft

EXCLUDES 1 *civilian water transport accident involving military watercraft (V94.81-)*
*military watercraft accident in military or war operations (Y36, Y37.-)*

EXCLUDES 2 *drowning and submersion due to accident to watercraft (V90.-)*

V91.0 **Burn due to watercraft on fire**

EXCLUDES 1 *burn from localized fire or explosion on board ship without accident to watercraft (V93.-)*

V91.00 **Burn due to merchant ship on fire**

V91.01 **Burn due to passenger ship on fire**
Burn due to Ferry-boat on fire
Burn due to Liner on fire

V91.02 **Burn due to fishing boat on fire**

V91.03 **Burn due to other powered watercraft on fire**
Burn due to Hovercraft (on open water) on fire
Burn due to Jet ski on fire

V91.04 **Burn due to sailboat on fire**

V91.05 **Burn due to canoe or kayak on fire**

V91.06 **Burn due to (nonpowered) inflatable craft on fire**

V91.07 **Burn due to water-skis on fire**

V91.08 **Burn due to other unpowered watercraft on fire**

√x7th **V91.09 Burn due to unspecified watercraft on fire**
Burn due to boat NOS on fire
Burn due to ship NOS on fire
Burn due to watercraft NOS on fire

√5th **V91.1 Crushed between watercraft and other watercraft or other object due to collision**
Crushed by lifeboat after abandoning ship in a collision
NOTE Select the specified type of watercraft that the victim was on at the time of the collision

√x7th **V91.10 Crushed between merchant ship and other watercraft or other object due to collision**

√x7th **V91.11 Crushed between passenger ship and other watercraft or other object due to collision**
Crushed between Ferry-boat and other watercraft or other object due to collision
Crushed between Liner and other watercraft or other object due to collision

√x7th **V91.12 Crushed between fishing boat and other watercraft or other object due to collision**

√x7th **V91.13 Crushed between other powered watercraft and other watercraft or other object due to collision**
Crushed between Hovercraft (on open water) and other watercraft or other object due to collision
Crushed between Jet ski and other watercraft or other object due to collision

√x7th **V91.14 Crushed between sailboat and other watercraft or other object due to collision**

√x7th **V91.15 Crushed between canoe or kayak and other watercraft or other object due to collision**

√x7th **V91.16 Crushed between (nonpowered) inflatable craft and other watercraft or other object due to collision**

√x7th **V91.18 Crushed between other unpowered watercraft and other watercraft or other object due to collision**
Crushed between surfboard and other watercraft or other object due to collision
Crushed between windsurfer and other watercraft or other object due to collision

√x7th **V91.19 Crushed between unspecified watercraft and other watercraft or other object due to collision**
Crushed between boat NOS and other watercraft or other object due to collision
Crushed between ship NOS and other watercraft or other object due to collision
Crushed between watercraft NOS and other watercraft or other object due to collision

√5th **V91.2 Fall due to collision between watercraft and other watercraft or other object**
Fall while remaining on watercraft after collision
NOTE Select the specified type of watercraft that the victim was on at the time of the collision
EXCLUDES 1 *crushed between watercraft and other watercraft and other object due to collision (V91.1-)*
*drowning and submersion due to falling from crushed watercraft (V90.3-)*

√x7th **V91.20 Fall due to collision between merchant ship and other watercraft or other object**

√x7th **V91.21 Fall due to collision between passenger ship and other watercraft or other object**
Fall due to collision between Ferry-boat and other watercraft or other object
Fall due to collision between Liner and other watercraft or other object

√x7th **V91.22 Fall due to collision between fishing boat and other watercraft or other object**

√x7th **V91.23 Fall due to collision between other powered watercraft and other watercraft or other object**
Fall due to collision between Hovercraft (on open water) and other watercraft or other object
Fall due to collision between Jet ski and other watercraft or other object

√x7th **V91.24 Fall due to collision between sailboat and other watercraft or other object**

√x7th **V91.25 Fall due to collision between canoe or kayak and other watercraft or other object**

√x7th **V91.26 Fall due to collision between (nonpowered) inflatable craft and other watercraft or other object**

√x7th **V91.29 Fall due to collision between unspecified watercraft and other watercraft or other object**
Fall due to collision between boat NOS and other watercraft or other object
Fall due to collision between ship NOS and other watercraft or other object
Fall due to collision between watercraft NOS and other watercraft or other object

√5th **V91.3 Hit or struck by falling object due to accident to watercraft**
Hit or struck by falling object (part of damaged watercraft or other object) after falling or jumping from damaged watercraft
EXCLUDES 2 *drowning or submersion due to fall or jumping from damaged watercraft (V90.2-, V90.3-)*

√x7th **V91.30 Hit or struck by falling object due to accident to merchant ship**

√x7th **V91.31 Hit or struck by falling object due to accident to passenger ship**
Hit or struck by falling object due to accident to Ferry-boat
Hit or struck by falling object due to accident to Liner

√x7th **V91.32 Hit or struck by falling object due to accident to fishing boat**

√x7th **V91.33 Hit or struck by falling object due to accident to other powered watercraft**
Hit or struck by falling object due to accident to Hovercraft (on open water)
Hit or struck by falling object due to accident to Jet ski

√x7th **V91.34 Hit or struck by falling object due to accident to sailboat**

√x7th **V91.35 Hit or struck by falling object due to accident to canoe or kayak**

√x7th **V91.36 Hit or struck by falling object due to accident to (nonpowered) inflatable craft**

√x7th **V91.37 Hit or struck by falling object due to accident to water-skis**
Hit by water-skis after jumping off of waterskis

√x7th **V91.38 Hit or struck by falling object due to accident to other unpowered watercraft**
Hit or struck by object after falling off damaged windsurfer
Hit or struck by surf-board after falling off damaged surf-board

√x7th **V91.39 Hit or struck by falling object due to accident to unspecified watercraft**
Hit or struck by falling object due to accident to boat NOS
Hit or struck by falling object due to accident to ship NOS
Hit or struck by falling object due to accident to watercraft NOS

√5th **V91.8 Other injury due to other accident to watercraft**

√x7th **V91.80 Other injury due to other accident to merchant ship**

√x7th **V91.81 Other injury due to other accident to passenger ship**
Other injury due to other accident to Ferry-boat
Other injury due to other accident to Liner

√x7th **V91.82 Other injury due to other accident to fishing boat**

√x7th **V91.83 Other injury due to other accident to other powered watercraft**
Other injury due to other accident to Hovercraft (on open water)
Other injury due to other accident to Jet ski

√x7th **V91.84 Other injury due to other accident to sailboat**

√x7th **V91.85 Other injury due to other accident to canoe or kayak**

√x7th **V91.86 Other injury due to other accident to (nonpowered) inflatable craft**

√x7th **V91.87 Other injury due to other accident to water-skis**

√x7th **V91.88 Other injury due to other accident to other unpowered watercraft**
Other injury due to other accident to surf-board
Other injury due to other accident to windsurfer

√x7th **V91.89 Other injury due to other accident to unspecified watercraft**
Other injury due to other accident to boat NOS
Other injury due to other accident to ship NOS
Other injury due to other accident to watercraft NOS

**V92 Drowning and submersion due to accident on board watercraft, without accident to watercraft**

EXCLUDES 1 *civilian water transport accident involving military watercraft (V94.81-)*
*drowning or submersion of diver who voluntarily jumps from boat not involved in an accident (W16.711, W16.721)*
*drowning or submersion due to accident to watercraft (V9Ø-V91)*
*fall into water without watercraft (W16.-)*
*military watercraft accident in military or war operations (Y36, Y37)*

**V92.Ø Drowning and submersion due to fall off watercraft**
Drowning and submersion due to fall from gangplank of watercraft
Drowning and submersion due to fall overboard watercraft
EXCLUDES 2 *hitting head on object or bottom of body of water due to fall from watercraft (V94.Ø-)*

**V92.ØØ Drowning and submersion due to fall off merchant ship**

**V92.Ø1 Drowning and submersion due to fall off passenger ship**
Drowning and submersion due to fall off Ferry-boat
Drowning and submersion due to fall off Liner

**V92.Ø2 Drowning and submersion due to fall off fishing boat**

**V92.Ø3 Drowning and submersion due to fall off other powered watercraft**
Drowning and submersion due to fall off Hovercraft (on open water)
Drowning and submersion due to fall off Jet ski

**V92.Ø4 Drowning and submersion due to fall off sailboat**

**V92.Ø5 Drowning and submersion due to fall off canoe or kayak**

**V92.Ø6 Drowning and submersion due to fall off (nonpowered) inflatable craft**

**V92.Ø7 Drowning and submersion due to fall off water-skis**
EXCLUDES 1 *drowning and submersion due to falling off burning water-skis (V9Ø.27)*
*drowning and submersion due to falling off crushed water-skis (V9Ø.37)*
*hit by boat while water-skiing NOS (V94.-)*

**V92.Ø8 Drowning and submersion due to fall off other unpowered watercraft**
Drowning and submersion due to fall off surf-board
Drowning and submersion due to fall off windsurfer
EXCLUDES 1 *drowning and submersion due to fall off burning unpowered watercraft (V9Ø.28)*
*drowning and submersion due to fall off crushed unpowered watercraft (V9Ø.38)*
*drowning and submersion due to fall off damaged unpowered watercraft (V9Ø.88)*
*drowning and submersion due to rider of nonpowered watercraft being hit by other watercraft (V94.-)*
*other injury due to rider of nonpowered watercraft being hit by other watercraft (V94.-)*

**V92.Ø9 Drowning and submersion due to fall off unspecified watercraft**
Drowning and submersion due to fall off boat NOS
Drowning and submersion due to fall off ship
Drowning and submersion due to fall off watercraft NOS

**V92.1 Drowning and submersion due to being thrown overboard by motion of watercraft**
EXCLUDES 1 *drowning and submersion due to fall off surf-board (V92.Ø8)*
*drowning and submersion due to fall off water-skis (V92.Ø7)*
*drowning and submersion due to fall off windsurfer (V92.Ø8)*

**V92.1Ø Drowning and submersion due to being thrown overboard by motion of merchant ship**

**V92.11 Drowning and submersion due to being thrown overboard by motion of passenger ship**
Drowning and submersion due to being thrown overboard by motion of Ferry-boat
Drowning and submersion due to being thrown overboard by motion of Liner

**V92.12 Drowning and submersion due to being thrown overboard by motion of fishing boat**

**V92.13 Drowning and submersion due to being thrown overboard by motion of other powered watercraft**
Drowning and submersion due to being thrown overboard by motion of Hovercraft

**V92.14 Drowning and submersion due to being thrown overboard by motion of sailboat**

**V92.15 Drowning and submersion due to being thrown overboard by motion of canoe or kayak**

**V92.16 Drowning and submersion due to being thrown overboard by motion of (nonpowered) inflatable craft**

**V92.19 Drowning and submersion due to being thrown overboard by motion of unspecified watercraft**
Drowning and submersion due to being thrown overboard by motion of boat NOS
Drowning and submersion due to being thrown overboard by motion of ship NOS
Drowning and submersion due to being thrown overboard by motion of watercraft NOS

**V92.2 Drowning and submersion due to being washed overboard from watercraft**
Code first any associated cataclysm (X37.Ø-)

**V92.2Ø Drowning and submersion due to being washed overboard from merchant ship**

**V92.21 Drowning and submersion due to being washed overboard from passenger ship**
Drowning and submersion due to being washed overboard from Ferry-boat
Drowning and submersion due to being washed overboard from Liner

**V92.22 Drowning and submersion due to being washed overboard from fishing boat**

**V92.23 Drowning and submersion due to being washed overboard from other powered watercraft**
Drowning and submersion due to being washed overboard from Hovercraft (on open water)
Drowning and submersion due to being washed overboard from Jet ski

**V92.24 Drowning and submersion due to being washed overboard from sailboat**

**V92.25 Drowning and submersion due to being washed overboard from canoe or kayak**

**V92.26 Drowning and submersion due to being washed overboard from (nonpowered) inflatable craft**

**V92.27 Drowning and submersion due to being washed overboard from water-skis**
EXCLUDES 1 *drowning and submersion due to fall off water-skis (V92.Ø7)*

**V92.28 Drowning and submersion due to being washed overboard from other unpowered watercraft**
Drowning and submersion due to being washed overboard from surf-board
Drowning and submersion due to being washed overboard from windsurfer

**V92.29 Drowning and submersion due to being washed overboard from unspecified watercraft**
Drowning and submersion due to being washed overboard from boat NOS
Drowning and submersion due to being washed overboard from ship NOS
Drowning and submersion due to being washed overboard from watercraft NOS

**V93 Other injury due to accident on board watercraft, without accident to watercraft**

EXCLUDES 1 *civilian water transport accident involving military watercraft (V94.81-)*
*military watercraft accident in military or war operations (Y36, Y37.-)*
*other injury due to accident to watercraft (V91.-)*
EXCLUDES 2 *drowning and submersion due to accident on board watercraft, without accident to watercraft (V92.-)*

**V93.Ø Burn due to localized fire on board watercraft**
EXCLUDES 1 *burn due to watercraft on fire (V91.Ø-)*

**V93.ØØ Burn due to localized fire on board merchant vessel**

**V93.Ø1 Burn due to localized fire on board passenger vessel**
Burn due to localized fire on board Ferry-boat
Burn due to localized fire on board Liner

**V93.Ø2 Burn due to localized fire on board fishing boat**

√x7th **V93.03 Burn due to localized fire on board other powered watercraft**
Burn due to localized fire on board Hovercraft
Burn due to localized fire on board Jet ski

√x7th **V93.04 Burn due to localized fire on board sailboat**

√x7th **V93.09 Burn due to localized fire on board unspecified watercraft**
Burn due to localized fire on board boat NOS
Burn due to localized fire on board ship NOS
Burn due to localized fire on board watercraft NOS

√5th **V93.1 Other burn on board watercraft**
Burn due to source other than fire on board watercraft
EXCLUDES 1 *burn due to watercraft on fire (V91.0-)*

√x7th **V93.10 Other burn on board merchant vessel**

√x7th **V93.11 Other burn on board passenger vessel**
Other burn on board Ferry-boat
Other burn on board Liner

√x7th **V93.12 Other burn on board fishing boat**

√x7th **V93.13 Other burn on board other powered watercraft**
Other burn on board Hovercraft
Other burn on board Jet ski

√x7th **V93.14 Other burn on board sailboat**

√x7th **V93.19 Other burn on board unspecified watercraft**
Other burn on board boat NOS
Other burn on board ship NOS
Other burn on board watercraft NOS

√5th **V93.2 Heat exposure on board watercraft**
EXCLUDES 1 *exposure to man-made heat not aboard watercraft (W92)*
*exposure to natural heat while on board watercraft (X30)*
*exposure to sunlight while on board watercraft (X32)*
EXCLUDES 2 *burn due to fire on board watercraft (V93.0-)*

√x7th **V93.20 Heat exposure on board merchant ship**

√x7th **V93.21 Heat exposure on board passenger ship**
Heat exposure on board Ferry-boat
Heat exposure on board Liner

√x7th **V93.22 Heat exposure on board fishing boat**

√x7th **V93.23 Heat exposure on board other powered watercraft**
Heat exposure on board hovercraft

√x7th **V93.24 Heat exposure on board sailboat**

√x7th **V93.29 Heat exposure on board unspecified watercraft**
Heat exposure on board boat NOS
Heat exposure on board ship NOS
Heat exposure on board watercraft NOS

√5th **V93.3 Fall on board watercraft**
EXCLUDES 1 *fall due to collision of watercraft (V91.2-)*

√x7th **V93.30 Fall on board merchant ship**

√x7th **V93.31 Fall on board passenger ship**
Fall on board Ferry-boat
Fall on board Liner

√x7th **V93.32 Fall on board fishing boat**

√x7th **V93.33 Fall on board other powered watercraft**
Fall on board Hovercraft (on open water)
Fall on board Jet ski

√x7th **V93.34 Fall on board sailboat**

√x7th **V93.35 Fall on board canoe or kayak**

√x7th **V93.36 Fall on board (nonpowered) inflatable craft**

√x7th **V93.38 Fall on board other unpowered watercraft**

√x7th **V93.39 Fall on board unspecified watercraft**
Fall on board boat NOS
Fall on board ship NOS
Fall on board watercraft NOS

√5th **V93.4 Struck by falling object on board watercraft**
Hit by falling object on board watercraft
EXCLUDES 1 *struck by falling object due to accident to watercraft (V91.3)*

√x7th **V93.40 Struck by falling object on merchant ship**

√x7th **V93.41 Struck by falling object on passenger ship**
Struck by falling object on Ferry-boat
Struck by falling object on Liner

√x7th **V93.42 Struck by falling object on fishing boat**

√x7th **V93.43 Struck by falling object on other powered watercraft**
Struck by falling object on Hovercraft

√x7th **V93.44 Struck by falling object on sailboat**

√x7th **V93.48 Struck by falling object on other unpowered watercraft**

√x7th **V93.49 Struck by falling object on unspecified watercraft**

√5th **V93.5 Explosion on board watercraft**
Boiler explosion on steamship
EXCLUDES 2 *fire on board watercraft (V93.0-)*

√x7th **V93.50 Explosion on board merchant ship**

√x7th **V93.51 Explosion on board passenger ship**
Explosion on board Ferry-boat
Explosion on board Liner

√x7th **V93.52 Explosion on board fishing boat**

√x7th **V93.53 Explosion on board other powered watercraft**
Explosion on board Hovercraft
Explosion on board Jet ski

√x7th **V93.54 Explosion on board sailboat**

√x7th **V93.59 Explosion on board unspecified watercraft**
Explosion on board boat NOS
Explosion on board ship NOS
Explosion on board watercraft NOS

√5th **V93.6 Machinery accident on board watercraft**
EXCLUDES 1 *machinery explosion on board watercraft (V93.4-)*
*machinery fire on board watercraft (V93.0-)*

√x7th **V93.60 Machinery accident on board merchant ship**

√x7th **V93.61 Machinery accident on board passenger ship**
Machinery accident on board Ferry-boat
Machinery accident on board Liner

√x7th **V93.62 Machinery accident on board fishing boat**

√x7th **V93.63 Machinery accident on board other powered watercraft**
Machinery accident on board Hovercraft

√x7th **V93.64 Machinery accident on board sailboat**

√x7th **V93.69 Machinery accident on board unspecified watercraft**
Machinery accident on board boat NOS
Machinery accident on board ship NOS
Machinery accident on board watercraft NOS

√5th **V93.8 Other injury due to other accident on board watercraft**
Accidental poisoning by gases or fumes on watercraft

√x7th **V93.80 Other injury due to other accident on board merchant ship**

√x7th **V93.81 Other injury due to other accident on board passenger ship**
Other injury due to other accident on board Ferry-boat
Other injury due to other accident on board Liner

√x7th **V93.82 Other injury due to other accident on board fishing boat**

√x7th **V93.83 Other injury due to other accident on board other powered watercraft**
Other injury due to other accident on board Hovercraft
Other injury due to other accident on board Jet ski

√x7th **V93.84 Other injury due to other accident on board sailboat**

√x7th **V93.85 Other injury due to other accident on board canoe or kayak**

√x7th **V93.86 Other injury due to other accident on board (nonpowered) inflatable craft**

√x7th **V93.87 Other injury due to other accident on board water-skis**
Hit or struck by object while waterskiing

√x7th **V93.88 Other injury due to other accident on board other unpowered watercraft**
Hit or struck by object while on board windsurfer
Hit or struck by object while surfing

√x7th **V93.89 Other injury due to other accident on board unspecified watercraft**
Other injury due to other accident on board boat NOS
Other injury due to other accident on board ship NOS
Other injury due to other accident on board watercraft NOS

√4th **V94 Other and unspecified water transport accidents**
EXCLUDES 1 *military watercraft accidents in military or war operations (Y36, Y37)*

√x7th **V94.0 Hitting object or bottom of body of water due to fall from watercraft**
EXCLUDES 2 *drowning and submersion due to fall from watercraft (V92.0-)*

V94.1 **Bather struck by watercraft**
Swimmer hit by watercraft
V94.11 **Bather struck by powered watercraft**
V94.12 **Bather struck by nonpowered watercraft**
V94.2 **Rider of nonpowered watercraft struck by other watercraft**
V94.21 **Rider of nonpowered watercraft struck by other nonpowered watercraft**
Canoer hit by other nonpowered watercraft
Surfer hit by other nonpowered watercraft
Windsurfer hit by other nonpowered watercraft
V94.22 **Rider of nonpowered watercraft struck by powered watercraft**
Canoer hit by motorboat
Surfer hit by motorboat
Windsurfer hit by motorboat
V94.3 **Injury to rider of (inflatable) watercraft being pulled behind other watercraft**
V94.31 **Injury to rider of (inflatable) recreational watercraft being pulled behind other watercraft**
Injury to rider of inner-tube pulled behind motor boat
V94.32 **Injury to rider of non-recreational watercraft being pulled behind other watercraft**
Injury to occupant of dingy being pulled behind boat or ship
Injury to occupant of life-raft being pulled behind boat or ship
V94.4 **Injury to barefoot water-skier**
Injury to person being pulled behind boat or ship
V94.8 **Other water transport accident**
V94.81 **Water transport accident involving military watercraft**
V94.810 **Civilian watercraft involved in water transport accident with military watercraft**
Passenger on civilian watercraft injured due to accident with military watercraft
V94.811 **Civilian in water injured by military watercraft**
V94.818 **Other water transport accident involving military watercraft**
V94.89 **Other water transport accident**
V94.9 **Unspecified water transport accident**
Water transport accident NOS

## Air and space transport accidents (V95-V97)

EXCLUDES 1 *military aircraft accidents in military or war operations (Y36, Y37)*

The appropriate 7th character is to be added to each code from categories V95-V97.
A initial encounter
D subsequent encounter
S sequela

V95 **Accident to powered aircraft causing injury to occupant**
V95.0 **Helicopter accident injuring occupant**
V95.00 **Unspecified helicopter accident injuring occupant**
V95.01 **Helicopter crash injuring occupant**
V95.02 **Forced landing of helicopter injuring occupant**
V95.03 **Helicopter collision injuring occupant**
Helicopter collision with any object, fixed, movable or moving
V95.04 **Helicopter fire injuring occupant**
V95.05 **Helicopter explosion injuring occupant**
V95.09 **Other helicopter accident injuring occupant**
V95.1 **Ultralight, microlight or powered-glider accident injuring occupant**
V95.10 **Unspecified ultralight, microlight or powered-glider accident injuring occupant**
V95.11 **Ultralight, microlight or powered-glider crash injuring occupant**
V95.12 **Forced landing of ultralight, microlight or powered-glider injuring occupant**
V95.13 **Ultralight, microlight or powered-glider collision injuring occupant**
Ultralight, microlight or powered-glider collision with any object, fixed, movable or moving
V95.14 **Ultralight, microlight or powered-glider fire injuring occupant**
V95.15 **Ultralight, microlight or powered-glider explosion injuring occupant**
V95.19 **Other ultralight, microlight or powered-glider accident injuring occupant**
V95.2 **Other private fixed-wing aircraft accident injuring occupant**
V95.20 **Unspecified accident to other private fixed-wing aircraft, injuring occupant**
V95.21 **Other private fixed-wing aircraft crash injuring occupant**
V95.22 **Forced landing of other private fixed-wing aircraft injuring occupant**
V95.23 **Other private fixed-wing aircraft collision injuring occupant**
Other private fixed-wing aircraft collision with any object, fixed, movable or moving
V95.24 **Other private fixed-wing aircraft fire injuring occupant**
V95.25 **Other private fixed-wing aircraft explosion injuring occupant**
V95.29 **Other accident to other private fixed-wing aircraft injuring occupant**
V95.3 **Commercial fixed-wing aircraft accident injuring occupant**
V95.30 **Unspecified accident to commercial fixed-wing aircraft injuring occupant**
V95.31 **Commercial fixed-wing aircraft crash injuring occupant**
V95.32 **Forced landing of commercial fixed-wing aircraft injuring occupant**
V95.33 **Commercial fixed-wing aircraft collision injuring occupant**
Commercial fixed-wing aircraft collision with any object, fixed, movable or moving
V95.34 **Commercial fixed-wing aircraft fire injuring occupant**
V95.35 **Commercial fixed-wing aircraft explosion injuring occupant**
V95.39 **Other accident to commercial fixed-wing aircraft injuring occupant**
V95.4 **Spacecraft accident injuring occupant**
V95.40 **Unspecified spacecraft accident injuring occupant**
V95.41 **Spacecraft crash injuring occupant**
V95.42 **Forced landing of spacecraft injuring occupant**
V95.43 **Spacecraft collision injuring occupant**
Spacecraft collision with any object, fixed, moveable or moving
V95.44 **Spacecraft fire injuring occupant**
V95.45 **Spacecraft explosion injuring occupant**
V95.49 **Other spacecraft accident injuring occupant**
V95.8 **Other powered aircraft accidents injuring occupant**
V95.9 **Unspecified aircraft accident injuring occupant**
Air transport accident NOS
Aircraft accident NOS

V96 **Accident to nonpowered aircraft causing injury to occupant**
V96.0 **Balloon accident injuring occupant**
V96.00 **Unspecified balloon accident injuring occupant**
V96.01 **Balloon crash injuring occupant**
V96.02 **Forced landing of balloon injuring occupant**
V96.03 **Balloon collision injuring occupant**
Balloon collision with any object, fixed, moveable or moving
V96.04 **Balloon fire injuring occupant**
V96.05 **Balloon explosion injuring occupant**
V96.09 **Other balloon accident injuring occupant**
V96.1 **Hang-glider accident injuring occupant**
V96.10 **Unspecified hang-glider accident injuring occupant**
V96.11 **Hang-glider crash injuring occupant**
V96.12 **Forced landing of hang-glider injuring occupant**
V96.13 **Hang-glider collision injuring occupant**
Hang-glider collision with any object, fixed, moveable or moving
V96.14 **Hang-glider fire injuring occupant**
V96.15 **Hang-glider explosion injuring occupant**
V96.19 **Other hang-glider accident injuring occupant**
V96.2 **Glider (nonpowered) accident injuring occupant**
V96.20 **Unspecified glider (nonpowered) accident injuring occupant**

✓x7th **V96.21 Glider (nonpowered) crash injuring occupant**

✓x7th **V96.22 Forced landing of glider (nonpowered) injuring occupant**

✓x7th **V96.23 Glider (nonpowered) collision injuring occupant**

Glider (nonpowered) collision with any object, fixed, moveable or moving

✓x7th **V96.24 Glider (nonpowered) fire injuring occupant**

✓x7th **V96.25 Glider (nonpowered) explosion injuring occupant**

✓x7th **V96.29 Other glider (nonpowered) accident injuring occupant**

✓x7th **V96.8 Other nonpowered-aircraft accidents injuring occupant**

Kite carrying a person accident injuring occupant

✓x7th **V96.9 Unspecified nonpowered-aircraft accident injuring occupant**

Nonpowered-aircraft accident NOS

✓4th **V97 Other specified air transport accidents**

✓x7th **V97.0 Occupant of aircraft injured in other specified air transport accidents**

Fall in, on or from aircraft in air transport accident

EXCLUDES 1 *accident while boarding or alighting aircraft (V97.1)*

✓x7th **V97.1 Person injured while boarding or alighting from aircraft**

✓5th **V97.2 Parachutist accident**

✓x7th **V97.21 Parachutist entangled in object**

Parachutist landing in tree

✓x7th **V97.22 Parachutist injured on landing**

✓x7th **V97.29 Other parachutist accident**

✓5th **V97.3 Person on ground injured in air transport accident**

✓x7th **V97.31 Hit by object falling from aircraft**

Hit by crashing aircraft
Injured by aircraft hitting car
Injured by aircraft hitting house

✓x7th **V97.32 Injured by rotating propeller**

✓x7th **V97.33 Sucked into jet engine**

✓x7th **V97.39 Other injury to person on ground due to air transport accident**

✓5th **V97.8 Other air transport accidents, not elsewhere classified**

EXCLUDES 1 *aircraft accident NOS (V95.9)*
*exposure to changes in air pressure during ascent or descent (W94.-)*

✓6th **V97.81 Air transport accident involving military aircraft**

✓7th **V97.810 Civilian aircraft involved in air transport accident with military aircraft**

Passenger in civilian aircraft injured due to accident with military aircraft

✓7th **V97.811 Civilian injured by military aircraft**

✓7th **V97.818 Other air transport accident involving military aircraft**

✓x7th **V97.89 Other air transport accidents, not elsewhere classified**

Injury from machinery on aircraft

## Other and unspecified transport accidents (V98-V99)

EXCLUDES 1 *vehicle accident, type of vehicle unspecified (V89.-)*

The appropriate 7th character is to be added to each code from categories V98-V99.
A initial encounter
D subsequent encounter
S sequela

✓4th **V98 Other specified transport accidents**

✓x7th **V98.0 Accident to, on or involving cable-car, not on rails**

Caught or dragged by cable-car, not on rails
Fall or jump from cable-car, not on rails
Object thrown from or in cable-car, not on rails

✓x7th **V98.1 Accident to, on or involving land-yacht**

✓x7th **V98.2 Accident to, on or involving ice yacht**

✓x7th **V98.3 Accident to, on or involving ski lift**

Accident to, on or involving ski chair-lift
Accident to, on or involving ski-lift with gondola

✓x7th **V98.8 Other specified transport accidents**

✓x7th **V99 Unspecified transport accident**

# OTHER EXTERNAL CAUSES OF ACCIDENTAL INJURY (W00-X58)

## Slipping, tripping, stumbling and falls (W00-W19)

EXCLUDES 1 *assault involving a fall (Y01-Y02)*
*fall from animal (V80.-)*
*fall (in) (from) machinery (in operation) (W28-W31)*
*fall (in) (from) transport vehicle (V01-V99)*
*intentional self-harm involving a fall (X80-X81)*

EXCLUDES 2 *at risk for fall (history of fall) Z91.81*
*fall (in) (from) burning building (X00.-)*
*fall into fire (X00-X04, X08)*

The appropriate 7th character is to be added to each code from categories W00-W19.
A initial encounter
D subsequent encounter
S sequela

✓4th **W00 Fall due to ice and snow**

INCLUDES pedestrian on foot falling (slipping) on ice and snow

EXCLUDES 1 *fall on (from) ice and snow involving pedestrian conveyance (V00.-)*
*fall from stairs and steps not due to ice and snow (W10.-)*

**AHA:** 2016,2Q,4

✓x7th **W00.0 Fall on same level due to ice and snow**

✓x7th **W00.1 Fall from stairs and steps due to ice and snow**

✓x7th **W00.2 Other fall from one level to another due to ice and snow**

✓x7th **W00.9 Unspecified fall due to ice and snow**

✓4th **W01 Fall on same level from slipping, tripping and stumbling**

INCLUDES fall on moving sidewalk

EXCLUDES 1 *fall due to bumping (striking) against object (W18.0-)*
*fall in shower or bathtub (W18.2-)*
*fall off or from toilet (W18.1-)*
*fall on same level from slipping, tripping and stumbling due to ice or snow (W00.0)*
*fall on same level NOS (W18.30)*
*slipping, tripping and stumbling NOS (W18.40)*
*slipping, tripping and stumbling without falling (W18.4-)*

✓x7th **W01.0 Fall on same level from slipping, tripping and stumbling without subsequent striking against object**

Falling over animal

✓5th **W01.1 Fall on same level from slipping, tripping and stumbling with subsequent striking against object**

✓x7th **W01.10 Fall on same level from slipping, tripping and stumbling with subsequent striking against unspecified object**

✓6th **W01.11 Fall on same level from slipping, tripping and stumbling with subsequent striking against sharp object**

✓7th **W01.110 Fall on same level from slipping, tripping and stumbling with subsequent striking against sharp glass**

✓7th **W01.111 Fall on same level from slipping, tripping and stumbling with subsequent striking against power tool or machine**

✓7th **W01.118 Fall on same level from slipping, tripping and stumbling with subsequent striking against other sharp object**

✓7th **W01.119 Fall on same level from slipping, tripping and stumbling with subsequent striking against unspecified sharp object**

✓6th **W01.19 Fall on same level from slipping, tripping and stumbling with subsequent striking against other object**

✓7th **W01.190 Fall on same level from slipping, tripping and stumbling with subsequent striking against furniture**

✓7th **W01.198 Fall on same level from slipping, tripping and stumbling with subsequent striking against other object**

✓x7th **W03 Other fall on same level due to collision with another person**

Fall due to non-transport collision with other person

EXCLUDES 1 *collision with another person without fall (W51)*
*crushed or pushed by a crowd or human stampede (W52)*
*fall due to ice or snow (W00)*
*fall involving pedestrian conveyance (V00-V09)*
*fall on same level NOS (W18.30)*

**AHA:** 2012,4Q,108

√x7th **W04 Fall while being carried or supported by other persons**
Accidentally dropped while being carried

√4th **W05 Fall from non-moving wheelchair, nonmotorized scooter and motorized mobility scooter**
EXCLUDES 1 *fall from moving motorized mobility scooter (V00.831)*
*fall from moving wheelchair (powered) (V00.811)*
*fall from nonmotorized scooter (V00.141)*

√x7th **W05.0 Fall from non-moving wheelchair**
AHA: 2019,2Q,27

√x7th **W05.1 Fall from non-moving nonmotorized scooter**

√x7th **W05.2 Fall from non-moving motorized mobility scooter**

√x7th **W06 Fall from bed**

√x7th **W07 Fall from chair**

√x7th **W08 Fall from other furniture**
Fall from stool

√4th **W09 Fall on and from playground equipment**
EXCLUDES 1 *fall involving recreational machinery (W31)*

√x7th **W09.0 Fall on or from playground slide**

√x7th **W09.1 Fall from playground swing**

√x7th **W09.2 Fall on or from jungle gym**

√x7th **W09.8 Fall on or from other playground equipment**

√4th **W10 Fall on and from stairs and steps**
EXCLUDES 1 *Fall from stairs and steps due to ice and snow (W00.1)*

√x7th **W10.0 Fall (on)(from) escalator**

√x7th **W10.1 Fall (on)(from) sidewalk curb**

√x7th **W10.2 Fall (on)(from) incline**
Fall (on) (from) ramp

√x7th **W10.8 Fall (on) (from) other stairs and steps**

√x7th **W10.9 Fall (on) (from) unspecified stairs and steps**

√x7th **W11 Fall on and from ladder**

√x7th **W12 Fall on and from scaffolding**

√4th **W13 Fall from, out of or through building or structure**

√x7th **W13.0 Fall from, out of or through balcony**
Fall from, out of or through railing

√x7th **W13.1 Fall from, out of or through bridge**

√x7th **W13.2 Fall from, out of or through roof**

√x7th **W13.3 Fall through floor**

√x7th **W13.4 Fall from, out of or through window**
EXCLUDES 2 *fall with subsequent striking against sharp glass (W01.110-)*

√x7th **W13.8 Fall from, out of or through other building or structure**
Fall from, out of or through flag-pole
Fall from, out of or through viaduct
Fall from, out of or through wall

√x7th **W13.9 Fall from, out of or through building, not otherwise specified**
EXCLUDES 1 *collapse of a building or structure (W20.-)*
*fall or jump from burning building or structure (X00.-)*

√x7th **W14 Fall from tree**

√x7th **W15 Fall from cliff**

√4th **W16 Fall, jump or diving into water**
EXCLUDES 1 *accidental non-watercraft drowning and submersion not involving fall (W65-W74)*
*effects of air pressure from diving (W94.-)*
*fall into water from watercraft (V90-V94)*
*hitting an object or against bottom when falling from watercraft (V94.0)*
EXCLUDES 2 *striking or hitting diving board (W21.4)*

√5th **W16.0 Fall into swimming pool**
Fall into swimming pool NOS
EXCLUDES 1 *fall into empty swimming pool (W17.3)*

√6th **W16.01 Fall into swimming pool striking water surface**

√7th **W16.011 Fall into swimming pool striking water surface causing drowning and submersion**
EXCLUDES 1 *drowning and submersion while in swimming pool without fall (W67)*

√7th **W16.012 Fall into swimming pool striking water surface causing other injury**

√6th **W16.02 Fall into swimming pool striking bottom**

√7th **W16.021 Fall into swimming pool striking bottom causing drowning and submersion**
EXCLUDES 1 *drowning and submersion while in swimming pool without fall (W67)*

√7th **W16.022 Fall into swimming pool striking bottom causing other injury**

√6th **W16.03 Fall into swimming pool striking wall**

√7th **W16.031 Fall into swimming pool striking wall causing drowning and submersion**
EXCLUDES 1 *drowning and submersion while in swimming pool without fall (W67)*

√7th **W16.032 Fall into swimming pool striking wall causing other injury**

√5th **W16.1 Fall into natural body of water**
Fall into lake
Fall into open sea
Fall into river
Fall into stream

√6th **W16.11 Fall into natural body of water striking water surface**

√7th **W16.111 Fall into natural body of water striking water surface causing drowning and submersion**
EXCLUDES 1 *drowning and submersion while in natural body of water without fall (W69)*

√7th **W16.112 Fall into natural body of water striking water surface causing other injury**

√6th **W16.12 Fall into natural body of water striking bottom**

√7th **W16.121 Fall into natural body of water striking bottom causing drowning and submersion**
EXCLUDES 1 *drowning and submersion while in natural body of water without fall (W69)*

√7th **W16.122 Fall into natural body of water striking bottom causing other injury**

√6th **W16.13 Fall into natural body of water striking side**

√7th **W16.131 Fall into natural body of water striking side causing drowning and submersion**
EXCLUDES 1 *drowning and submersion while in natural body of water without fall (W69)*

√7th **W16.132 Fall into natural body of water striking side causing other injury**

√5th **W16.2 Fall in (into) filled bathtub or bucket of water**

√6th **W16.21 Fall in (into) filled bathtub**
EXCLUDES 1 *fall into empty bathtub (W18.2)*

√7th **W16.211 Fall in (into) filled bathtub causing drowning and submersion**
EXCLUDES 1 *drowning and submersion while in filled bathtub without fall (W65)*

√7th **W16.212 Fall in (into) filled bathtub causing other injury**

√6th **W16.22 Fall in (into) bucket of water**

√7th **W16.221 Fall in (into) bucket of water causing drowning and submersion**

√7th **W16.222 Fall in (into) bucket of water causing other injury**

√5th **W16.3 Fall into other water**
Fall into fountain
Fall into reservoir

√6th **W16.31 Fall into other water striking water surface**

√7th **W16.311 Fall into other water striking water surface causing drowning and submersion**
EXCLUDES 1 *drowning and submersion while in other water without fall (W73)*

√7th **W16.312 Fall into other water striking water surface causing other injury**

√6th **W16.32 Fall into other water striking bottom**

√7th **W16.321 Fall into other water striking bottom causing drowning and submersion**
EXCLUDES 1 *drowning and submersion while in other water without fall (W73)*

7th W16.322 **Fall into other water striking bottom causing other injury**

6th W16.33 **Fall into other water striking wall**

7th W16.331 **Fall into other water striking wall causing drowning and submersion**

EXCLUDES 1 *drowning and submersion while in other water without fall (W73)*

7th W16.332 **Fall into other water striking wall causing other injury**

5th W16.4 **Fall into unspecified water**

x7th W16.41 **Fall into unspecified water causing drowning and submersion**

x7th W16.42 **Fall into unspecified water causing other injury**

5th W16.5 **Jumping or diving into swimming pool**

6th W16.51 **Jumping or diving into swimming pool striking water surface**

7th W16.511 **Jumping or diving into swimming pool striking water surface causing drowning and submersion**

EXCLUDES 1 *drowning and submersion while in swimming pool without jumping or diving (W67)*

7th W16.512 **Jumping or diving into swimming pool striking water surface causing other injury**

6th W16.52 **Jumping or diving into swimming pool striking bottom**

7th W16.521 **Jumping or diving into swimming pool striking bottom causing drowning and submersion**

EXCLUDES 1 *drowning and submersion while in swimming pool without jumping or diving (W67)*

7th W16.522 **Jumping or diving into swimming pool striking bottom causing other injury**

6th W16.53 **Jumping or diving into swimming pool striking wall**

7th W16.531 **Jumping or diving into swimming pool striking wall causing drowning and submersion**

EXCLUDES 1 *drowning and submersion while in swimming pool without jumping or diving (W67)*

7th W16.532 **Jumping or diving into swimming pool striking wall causing other injury**

5th W16.6 **Jumping or diving into natural body of water**

Jumping or diving into lake
Jumping or diving into open sea
Jumping or diving into river
Jumping or diving into stream

6th W16.61 **Jumping or diving into natural body of water striking water surface**

7th W16.611 **Jumping or diving into natural body of water striking water surface causing drowning and submersion**

EXCLUDES 1 *drowning and submersion while in natural body of water without jumping or diving (W69)*

7th W16.612 **Jumping or diving into natural body of water striking water surface causing other injury**

6th W16.62 **Jumping or diving into natural body of water striking bottom**

7th W16.621 **Jumping or diving into natural body of water striking bottom causing drowning and submersion**

EXCLUDES 1 *drowning and submersion while in natural body of water without jumping or diving (W69)*

7th W16.622 **Jumping or diving into natural body of water striking bottom causing other injury**

5th W16.7 **Jumping or diving from boat**

EXCLUDES 1 *fall from boat into water - see watercraft accident (V90-V94)*

6th W16.71 **Jumping or diving from boat striking water surface**

7th W16.711 **Jumping or diving from boat striking water surface causing drowning and submersion**

7th W16.712 **Jumping or diving from boat striking water surface causing other injury**

6th W16.72 **Jumping or diving from boat striking bottom**

7th W16.721 **Jumping or diving from boat striking bottom causing drowning and submersion**

7th W16.722 **Jumping or diving from boat striking bottom causing other injury**

5th W16.8 **Jumping or diving into other water**

Jumping or diving into fountain
Jumping or diving into reservoir

6th W16.81 **Jumping or diving into other water striking water surface**

7th W16.811 **Jumping or diving into other water striking water surface causing drowning and submersion**

EXCLUDES 1 *drowning and submersion while in other water without jumping or diving (W73)*

7th W16.812 **Jumping or diving into other water striking water surface causing other injury**

6th W16.82 **Jumping or diving into other water striking bottom**

7th W16.821 **Jumping or diving into other water striking bottom causing drowning and submersion**

EXCLUDES 1 *drowning and submersion while in other water without jumping or diving (W73)*

7th W16.822 **Jumping or diving into other water striking bottom causing other injury**

6th W16.83 **Jumping or diving into other water striking wall**

7th W16.831 **Jumping or diving into other water striking wall causing drowning and submersion**

EXCLUDES 1 *drowning and submersion while in other water without jumping or diving (W73)*

7th W16.832 **Jumping or diving into other water striking wall causing other injury**

5th W16.9 **Jumping or diving into unspecified water**

x7th W16.91 **Jumping or diving into unspecified water causing drowning and submersion**

x7th W16.92 **Jumping or diving into unspecified water causing other injury**

4th W17 **Other fall from one level to another**

x7th W17.0 **Fall into well**

x7th W17.1 **Fall into storm drain or manhole**

x7th W17.2 **Fall into hole**

Fall into pit

x7th W17.3 **Fall into empty swimming pool**

EXCLUDES 1 *fall into filled swimming pool (W16.0-)*

x7th W17.4 **Fall from dock**

5th W17.8 **Other fall from one level to another**

x7th W17.81 **Fall down embankment (hill)**

x7th W17.82 **Fall from (out of) grocery cart**

Fall due to grocery cart tipping over

x7th W17.89 **Other fall from one level to another**

Fall from cherry picker
Fall from lifting device
Fall from mobile elevated work platform [MEWP]
Fall from sky lift
**AHA:** 2015,2Q,6

4th W18 **Other slipping, tripping and stumbling and falls**

5th W18.0 **Fall due to bumping against object**

Striking against object with subsequent fall

EXCLUDES 1 *fall on same level due to slipping, tripping, or stumbling with subsequent striking against object (W01.1-)*

x7th W18.00 **Striking against unspecified object with subsequent fall**

x7th W18.01 **Striking against sports equipment with subsequent fall**

x7th W18.02 **Striking against glass with subsequent fall**

x7th W18.09 **Striking against other object with subsequent fall**

5th W18.1 **Fall from or off toilet**

x7th W18.11 **Fall from or off toilet without subsequent striking against object**

Fall from (off) toilet NOS

x7th W18.12 **Fall from or off toilet with subsequent striking against object**

√x7th **W18.2 Fall in (into) shower or empty bathtub**
EXCLUDES 1 *fall in full bathtub causing drowning or submersion (W16.21-)*

√5th **W18.3 Other and unspecified fall on same level**
√x7th **W18.30 Fall on same level, unspecified**
√x7th **W18.31 Fall on same level due to stepping on an object**
Fall on same level due to stepping on an animal
EXCLUDES 1 *slipping, tripping and stumbling without fall due to stepping on animal (W18.41)*
√x7th **W18.39 Other fall on same level**

√5th **W18.4 Slipping, tripping and stumbling without falling**
EXCLUDES 1 *collision with another person without fall (W51)*
√x7th **W18.40 Slipping, tripping and stumbling without falling, unspecified**
√x7th **W18.41 Slipping, tripping and stumbling without falling due to stepping on object**
Slipping, tripping and stumbling without falling due to stepping on animal
EXCLUDES 1 *slipping, tripping and stumbling with fall due to stepping on animal (W18.31)*
√x7th **W18.42 Slipping, tripping and stumbling without falling due to stepping into hole or opening**
√x7th **W18.43 Slipping, tripping and stumbling without falling due to stepping from one level to another**
√x7th **W18.49 Other slipping, tripping and stumbling without falling**

√x7th **W19 Unspecified fall**
Accidental fall NOS
**AHA:** 2012,4Q,95

## Exposure to inanimate mechanical forces (W20-W49)

EXCLUDES 1 *assault (X92-Y09)*
*contact or collision with animals or persons (W50-W64)*
*exposure to inanimate mechanical forces involving military or war operations (Y36.-, Y37.-)*
*intentional self-harm (X71-X83)*

The appropriate 7th character is to be added to each code from categories W20-W49.
A initial encounter
D subsequent encounter
S sequela

√4th **W20 Struck by thrown, projected or falling object**
Code first any associated:
cataclysm (X34-X39)
lightning strike (T75.00)
EXCLUDES 1 *falling object in machinery accident (W24, W28-W31)*
*falling object in transport accident (V01-V99)*
*object set in motion by explosion (W35-W40)*
*object set in motion by firearm (W32-W34)*
*struck by thrown sports equipment (W21.-)*
√x7th **W20.0 Struck by falling object in cave-in**
EXCLUDES 2 *asphyxiation due to cave-in (T71.21)*
√x7th **W20.1 Struck by object due to collapse of building**
EXCLUDES 1 *struck by object due to collapse of burning building (X00.2, X02.2)*
√x7th **W20.8 Other cause of strike by thrown, projected or falling object**
EXCLUDES 1 *struck by thrown sports equipment (W21.-)*

√4th **W21 Striking against or struck by sports equipment**
EXCLUDES 1 *assault with sports equipment (Y08.0-)*
*striking against or struck by sports equipment with subsequent fall (W18.01)*
√5th **W21.0 Struck by hit or thrown ball**
√x7th **W21.00 Struck by hit or thrown ball, unspecified type**
√x7th **W21.01 Struck by football**
√x7th **W21.02 Struck by soccer ball**
√x7th **W21.03 Struck by baseball**
√x7th **W21.04 Struck by golf ball**
√x7th **W21.05 Struck by basketball**
√x7th **W21.06 Struck by volleyball**
√x7th **W21.07 Struck by softball**
√x7th **W21.09 Struck by other hit or thrown ball**
√5th **W21.1 Struck by bat, racquet or club**
√x7th **W21.11 Struck by baseball bat**
√x7th **W21.12 Struck by tennis racquet**
√x7th **W21.13 Struck by golf club**
√x7th **W21.19 Struck by other bat, racquet or club**
√5th **W21.2 Struck by hockey stick or puck**
√6th **W21.21 Struck by hockey stick**
√7th **W21.210 Struck by ice hockey stick**
√7th **W21.211 Struck by field hockey stick**
√6th **W21.22 Struck by hockey puck**
√7th **W21.220 Struck by ice hockey puck**
√7th **W21.221 Struck by field hockey puck**
√5th **W21.3 Struck by sports foot wear**
√x7th **W21.31 Struck by shoe cleats**
Stepped on by shoe cleats
√x7th **W21.32 Struck by skate blades**
Skated over by skate blades
√x7th **W21.39 Struck by other sports foot wear**
√x7th **W21.4 Striking against diving board**
Use additional code for subsequent falling into water, if applicable (W16.-)
√5th **W21.8 Striking against or struck by other sports equipment**
√x7th **W21.81 Striking against or struck by football helmet**
√x7th **W21.89 Striking against or struck by other sports equipment**
√x7th **W21.9 Striking against or struck by unspecified sports equipment**

√4th **W22 Striking against or struck by other objects**
EXCLUDES 1 *striking against or struck by object with subsequent fall (W18.09)*
√5th **W22.0 Striking against stationary object**
EXCLUDES 1 *striking against stationary sports equipment (W21.8)*
√x7th **W22.01 Walked into wall**
√x7th **W22.02 Walked into lamppost**
√x7th **W22.03 Walked into furniture**
√6th **W22.04 Striking against wall of swimming pool**
√7th **W22.041 Striking against wall of swimming pool causing drowning and submersion**
EXCLUDES 1 *drowning and submersion while swimming without striking against wall (W67)*
√7th **W22.042 Striking against wall of swimming pool causing other injury**
√x7th **W22.09 Striking against other stationary object**
√5th **W22.1 Striking against or struck by automobile airbag**
√x7th **W22.10 Striking against or struck by unspecified automobile airbag**
√x7th **W22.11 Striking against or struck by driver side automobile airbag**
√x7th **W22.12 Striking against or struck by front passenger side automobile airbag**
√x7th **W22.19 Striking against or struck by other automobile airbag**
√x7th **W22.8 Striking against or struck by other objects**
Striking against or struck by object NOS
EXCLUDES 1 *struck by thrown, projected or falling object (W20.-)*

√4th **W23 Caught, crushed, jammed or pinched in or between objects**
EXCLUDES 1 *injury caused by cutting or piercing instruments (W25-W27)*
*injury caused by firearms malfunction (W32.1, W33.1-, W34.1-)*
*injury caused by lifting and transmission devices (W24.-)*
*injury caused by machinery (W28-W31)*
*injury caused by nonpowered hand tools (W27.-)*
*injury caused by struck by thrown, projected or falling object (W20.-)*
*injury caused by transport vehicle being used as a means of transportation (V01-V99)*
√x7th **W23.0 Caught, crushed, jammed, or pinched between moving objects**
√x7th **W23.1 Caught, crushed, jammed, or pinched between stationary objects**
√x7th **W23.2 Caught, crushed, jammed or pinched between a moving and stationary object**
**AHA:** 2022,4Q,48

**√4th W24 Contact with lifting and transmission devices, not elsewhere classified**

EXCLUDES 1 *transport accidents (V01-V99)*

**√x7th W24.0 Contact with lifting devices, not elsewhere classified**

Contact with chain hoist
Contact with drive belt
Contact with pulley (block)

**√x7th W24.1 Contact with transmission devices, not elsewhere classified**

Contact with transmission belt or cable

**√x7th W25 Contact with sharp glass**

Code first any associated:
injury due to flying glass from explosion or firearm discharge (W32-W40)
transport accident (V00-V99)

EXCLUDES 1 *fall on same level due to slipping, tripping and stumbling with subsequent striking against sharp glass (W01.110-)*
*striking against sharp glass with subsequent fall (W18.02-)*

EXCLUDES 2 *glass embedded in skin (W45.-)*

**√4th W26 Contact with other sharp objects**

EXCLUDES 2 *sharp object(s) embedded in skin (W45.-)*

**AHA:** 2016,4Q,73

**√x7th W26.0 Contact with knife**

EXCLUDES 1 *contact with electric knife (W29.1)*

**√x7th W26.1 Contact with sword or dagger**

**√x7th W26.2 Contact with edge of stiff paper**

Paper cut

**√x7th W26.8 Contact with other sharp object(s), not elsewhere classified**

Contact with tin can lid

**√x7th W26.9 Contact with unspecified sharp object(s)**

**√4th W27 Contact with nonpowered hand tool**

**√x7th W27.0 Contact with workbench tool**

Contact with auger
Contact with axe
Contact with chisel
Contact with handsaw
Contact with screwdriver

**√x7th W27.1 Contact with garden tool**

Contact with hoe
Contact with nonpowered lawn mower
Contact with pitchfork
Contact with rake

**√x7th W27.2 Contact with scissors**

**√x7th W27.3 Contact with needle (sewing)**

EXCLUDES 1 *contact with hypodermic needle (W46.-)*

**√x7th W27.4 Contact with kitchen utensil**

Contact with can-opener NOS
Contact with fork
Contact with ice-pick

**√x7th W27.5 Contact with paper-cutter**

**√x7th W27.8 Contact with other nonpowered hand tool**

Contact with nonpowered sewing machine
Contact with shovel

**√x7th W28 Contact with powered lawn mower**

Powered lawn mower (commercial) (residential)

EXCLUDES 1 *contact with nonpowered lawn mower (W27.1)*

EXCLUDES 2 *exposure to electric current (W86.-)*

**√4th W29 Contact with other powered hand tools and household machinery**

EXCLUDES 1 *contact with commercial machinery (W31.82)*
*contact with hot household appliance (X15)*
*contact with nonpowered hand tool (W27.-)*
*exposure to electric current (W86)*

**√x7th W29.0 Contact with powered kitchen appliance**

Contact with blender
Contact with can-opener
Contact with garbage disposal
Contact with mixer

**√x7th W29.1 Contact with electric knife**

**√x7th W29.2 Contact with other powered household machinery**

Contact with electric fan
Contact with powered dryer (clothes) (powered) (spin)
Contact with sewing machine
Contact with washing-machine

**√x7th W29.3 Contact with powered garden and outdoor hand tools and machinery**

Contact with chainsaw
Contact with edger
Contact with garden cultivator (tiller)
Contact with hedge trimmer
Contact with other powered garden tool

EXCLUDES 1 *contact with powered lawn mower (W28)*

**√x7th W29.4 Contact with nail gun**

**√x7th W29.8 Contact with other powered hand tools and household machinery**

Contact with do-it-yourself tool NOS

**√4th W30 Contact with agricultural machinery**

INCLUDES animal-powered farm machine

EXCLUDES 1 *agricultural transport vehicle accident (V01-V99)*
*explosion of grain store (W40.8)*
*exposure to electric current (W86.-)*

**√x7th W30.0 Contact with combine harvester**

Contact with reaper
Contact with thresher

**√x7th W30.1 Contact with power take-off devices (PTO)**

**√x7th W30.2 Contact with hay derrick**

**√x7th W30.3 Contact with grain storage elevator**

EXCLUDES 1 *explosion of grain store (W40.8)*

**√5th W30.8 Contact with other specified agricultural machinery**

**√x7th W30.81 Contact with agricultural transport vehicle in stationary use**

Contact with agricultural transport vehicle under repair, not on public roadway

EXCLUDES 1 *agricultural transport vehicle accident (V01-V99)*

**√x7th W30.89 Contact with other specified agricultural machinery**

**√x7th W30.9 Contact with unspecified agricultural machinery**

Contact with farm machinery NOS

**√4th W31 Contact with other and unspecified machinery**

EXCLUDES 1 *contact with agricultural machinery (W30.-)*
*contact with machinery in transport under own power or being towed by a vehicle (V01-V99)*
*exposure to electric current (W86)*

**√x7th W31.0 Contact with mining and earth-drilling machinery**

Contact with bore or drill (land) (seabed)
Contact with shaft hoist
Contact with shaft lift
Contact with undercutter

**√x7th W31.1 Contact with metalworking machines**

Contact with abrasive wheel
Contact with forging machine
Contact with lathe
Contact with mechanical shears
Contact with metal drilling machine
Contact with metal sawing machine
Contact with milling machine
Contact with power press
Contact with rolling-mill

**√x7th W31.2 Contact with powered woodworking and forming machines**

Contact with band saw
Contact with bench saw
Contact with circular saw
Contact with molding machine
Contact with overhead plane
Contact with powered saw
Contact with radial saw
Contact with sander

EXCLUDES 1 *nonpowered woodworking tools (W27.0)*

**√x7th W31.3 Contact with prime movers**

Contact with gas turbine
Contact with internal combustion engine
Contact with steam engine
Contact with water driven turbine

**√5th W31.8 Contact with other specified machinery**

**√x7th W31.81 Contact with recreational machinery**

Contact with roller coaster

√x7th **W31.82 Contact with other commercial machinery**
Contact with commercial electric fan
Contact with commercial kitchen appliances
Contact with commercial powered dryer (clothes) (powered) (spin)
Contact with commercial sewing machine
Contact with commercial washing-machine
EXCLUDES 1 *contact with household machinery (W29.-)*
*contact with powered lawn mower (W28)*

√x7th **W31.83 Contact with special construction vehicle in stationary use**
Contact with special construction vehicle under repair, not on public roadway
EXCLUDES 1 *special construction vehicle accident (V01-V99)*

√x7th **W31.89 Contact with other specified machinery**

√x7th **W31.9 Contact with unspecified machinery**
Contact with machinery NOS

√4th **W32 Accidental handgun discharge and malfunction**
INCLUDES accidental discharge and malfunction of gun for single hand use
accidental discharge and malfunction of pistol
accidental discharge and malfunction of revolver
handgun discharge and malfunction NOS
EXCLUDES 1 *accidental airgun discharge and malfunction (W34.010, W34.110)*
*accidental BB gun discharge and malfunction (W34.010, W34.110)*
*accidental pellet gun discharge and malfunction (W34.010, W34.110)*
*accidental shotgun discharge and malfunction (W33.01, W33.11)*
*assault by handgun discharge (X93)*
*handgun discharge involving legal intervention (Y35.0-)*
*handgun discharge involving military or war operations (Y36.4-)*
*intentional self-harm by handgun discharge (X72)*
*Very pistol discharge and malfunction (W34.09, W34.19)*

√x7th **W32.0 Accidental handgun discharge**

√x7th **W32.1 Accidental handgun malfunction**
Injury due to explosion of handgun (parts)
Injury due to malfunction of mechanism or component of handgun
Injury due to recoil of handgun
Powder burn from handgun

√4th **W33 Accidental rifle, shotgun and larger firearm discharge and malfunction**
INCLUDES rifle, shotgun and larger firearm discharge and malfunction NOS
EXCLUDES 1 *accidental airgun discharge and malfunction (W34.010, W34.110)*
*accidental BB gun discharge and malfunction (W34.010, W34.110)*
*accidental handgun discharge and malfunction (W32.-)*
*accidental pellet gun discharge and malfunction (W34.010, W34.110)*
*assault by rifle, shotgun and larger firearm discharge (X94)*
*firearm discharge involving legal intervention (Y35.0-)*
*firearm discharge involving military or war operations (Y36.4-)*
*intentional self-harm by rifle, shotgun and larger firearm discharge (X73)*

√5th **W33.0 Accidental rifle, shotgun and larger firearm discharge**

√x7th **W33.00 Accidental discharge of unspecified larger firearm**
Discharge of unspecified larger firearm NOS

√x7th **W33.01 Accidental discharge of shotgun**
Discharge of shotgun NOS

√x7th **W33.02 Accidental discharge of hunting rifle**
Discharge of hunting rifle NOS

√x7th **W33.03 Accidental discharge of machine gun**
Discharge of machine gun NOS

√x7th **W33.09 Accidental discharge of other larger firearm**
Discharge of other larger firearm NOS

√5th **W33.1 Accidental rifle, shotgun and larger firearm malfunction**
Injury due to explosion of rifle, shotgun and larger firearm (parts)
Injury due to malfunction of mechanism or component of rifle, shotgun and larger firearm
Injury due to piercing, cutting, crushing or pinching due to (by) slide trigger mechanism, scope or other gun part
Injury due to recoil of rifle, shotgun and larger firearm
Powder burn from rifle, shotgun and larger firearm

√x7th **W33.10 Accidental malfunction of unspecified larger firearm**
Malfunction of unspecified larger firearm NOS

√x7th **W33.11 Accidental malfunction of shotgun**
Malfunction of shotgun NOS

√x7th **W33.12 Accidental malfunction of hunting rifle**
Malfunction of hunting rifle NOS

√x7th **W33.13 Accidental malfunction of machine gun**
Malfunction of machine gun NOS

√x7th **W33.19 Accidental malfunction of other larger firearm**
Malfunction of other larger firearm NOS

√4th **W34 Accidental discharge and malfunction from other and unspecified firearms and guns**

√5th **W34.0 Accidental discharge from other and unspecified firearms and guns**

√x7th **W34.00 Accidental discharge from unspecified firearms or gun**
Discharge from firearm NOS
Gunshot wound NOS
Shot NOS

√6th **W34.01 Accidental discharge of gas, air or spring-operated guns**

√7th **W34.010 Accidental discharge of airgun**
Accidental discharge of BB gun
Accidental discharge of pellet gun

√7th **W34.011 Accidental discharge of paintball gun**
Accidental injury due to paintball discharge

√7th **W34.018 Accidental discharge of other gas, air or spring-operated gun**

√x7th **W34.09 Accidental discharge from other specified firearms**
Accidental discharge from Very pistol [flare]

√5th **W34.1 Accidental malfunction from other and unspecified firearms and guns**

√x7th **W34.10 Accidental malfunction from unspecified firearms or gun**
Firearm malfunction NOS

√6th **W34.11 Accidental malfunction of gas, air or spring-operated guns**

√7th **W34.110 Accidental malfunction of airgun**
Accidental malfunction of BB gun
Accidental malfunction of pellet gun

√7th **W34.111 Accidental malfunction of paintball gun**
Accidental injury due to paintball gun malfunction

√7th **W34.118 Accidental malfunction of other gas, air or spring-operated gun**

√x7th **W34.19 Accidental malfunction from other specified firearms**
Accidental malfunction from Very pistol [flare]

√x7th **W35 Explosion and rupture of boiler**
EXCLUDES 1 *explosion and rupture of boiler on watercraft (V93.4)*

√4th **W36 Explosion and rupture of gas cylinder**

√x7th **W36.1 Explosion and rupture of aerosol can**

√x7th **W36.2 Explosion and rupture of air tank**

√x7th **W36.3 Explosion and rupture of pressurized-gas tank**

√x7th **W36.8 Explosion and rupture of other gas cylinder**

√x7th **W36.9 Explosion and rupture of unspecified gas cylinder**

√4th **W37 Explosion and rupture of pressurized tire, pipe or hose**

√x7th **W37.0 Explosion of bicycle tire**

√x7th **W37.8 Explosion and rupture of other pressurized tire, pipe or hose**

√x7th **W38 Explosion and rupture of other specified pressurized devices**

√x7th **W39 Discharge of firework**

**W40 Explosion of other materials**

EXCLUDES 1 *assault by explosive material (X96)*
*explosion involving legal intervention (Y35.1-)*
*explosion involving military or war operations (Y36.0-, Y36.2-)*
*intentional self-harm by explosive material (X75)*

**W40.0 Explosion of blasting material**
Explosion of blasting cap
Explosion of detonator
Explosion of dynamite
Explosion of explosive (any) used in blasting operations

**W40.1 Explosion of explosive gases**
Explosion of acetylene
Explosion of butane
Explosion of coal gas
Explosion of explosive gas
Explosion of fire damp
Explosion of gasoline fumes
Explosion in mine NOS
Explosion of methane
Explosion of propane

**W40.8 Explosion of other specified explosive materials**
Explosion in dump NOS
Explosion in factory NOS
Explosion in grain store
Explosion in munitions
EXCLUDES 1 *explosion involving legal intervention (Y35.1-)*
*explosion involving military or war operations (Y36.0-, Y36.2-)*

**W40.9 Explosion of unspecified explosive materials**
Explosion NOS

**W42 Exposure to noise**

**W42.0 Exposure to supersonic waves**

**W42.9 Exposure to other noise**
Exposure to sound waves NOS

**W44 Foreign body entering into or through a natural orifice**

EXCLUDES 2 *contact with other sharp objects (W26)*
*contact with sharp glass (W25)*
*foreign body or object entering through skin (W45)*

AHA: 2023,4Q,45-46

**W44.A Battery entering into or through a natural orifice**

**W44.A0 Battery unspecified, entering into or through a natural orifice**

**W44.A1 Button battery entering into or through a natural orifice**

**W44.A9 Other batteries entering into or through a natural orifice**
Cylindrical battery entering into or through a natural orifice

**W44.B Plastic entering into or through a natural orifice**

**W44.B0 Plastic object unspecified, entering into or through a natural orifice**

**W44.B1 Plastic bead entering into or through a natural orifice**
EXCLUDES 2 *plastic jewelry entering into or through a natural orifice (W44.B4)*

**W44.B2 Plastic coin entering into or through a natural orifice**

**W44.B3 Plastic toy and toy part entering into or through a natural orifice**

**W44.B4 Plastic jewelry entering into or through a natural orifice**
EXCLUDES 2 *plastic bead entering into or through a natural orifice (W44.B1)*

**W44.B5 Plastic bottle entering into or through a natural orifice**

**W44.B9 Other plastic object entering into or through a natural orifice**

**W44.C Glass entering into or through a natural orifice**

**W44.C0 Glass unspecified, entering into or through a natural orifice**

**W44.C1 Sharp glass entering into or through a natural orifice**
Glass shard entering into or through a natural orifice

**W44.C2 Intact glass entering into or through a natural orifice**
Intact glass bottle entering into or through a natural orifice

**W44.D Magnetic metal entering into or through a natural orifice**

**W44.D0 Magnetic metal object unspecified, entering into or through a natural orifice**

**W44.D1 Magnetic metal bead entering into or through a natural orifice**

**W44.D2 Magnetic metal coin entering into or through a natural orifice**

**W44.D3 Magnetic metal toy entering into or through a natural orifice**

**W44.D4 Magnetic metal jewelry entering into or through a natural orifice**

**W44.D9 Other magnetic metal objects entering into or through a natural orifice**

**W44.E Non-magnetic metal entering into or through a natural orifice**

**W44.E0 Non-magnetic metal object unspecified, entering into or through a natural orifice**

**W44.E1 Non-magnetic metal bead entering into or through a natural orifice**

**W44.E2 Non-magnetic metal coin entering into or through a natural orifice**

**W44.E3 Non-magnetic metal toy entering into or through a natural orifice**

**W44.E4 Non-magnetic metal jewelry entering into or through a natural orifice**

**W44.E9 Other non-magnetic metal objects entering into or through a natural orifice**
Bottle cap entering into or through a natural orifice
Can lid entering into or through a natural orifice
Pull tab entering into or through a natural orifice

**W44.F Objects of natural or organic material entering into or through a natural orifice**

**W44.F0 Objects of natural or organic material unspecified, entering into or through a natural orifice**

**W44.F1 Bezoar entering into or through a natural orifice**

**W44.F2 Rubber band entering into or through a natural orifice**

**W44.F3 Food entering into or through a natural orifice**

**W44.F4 Insect entering into or through a natural orifice**

**W44.F9 Other object of natural or organic material, entering into or through a natural orifice**

**W44.G Other non-organic objects entering into or through a natural orifice**

**W44.G0 Other non-organic objects unspecified, entering into or through a natural orifice**

**W44.G1 Audio device entering into or through a natural orifice**
Ear buds
Hearing aids

**W44.G2 Combination metal and plastic toy and toy part entering into or through natural orifice**

**W44.G3 Combination metal and plastic jewelry entering into or through a natural orifice**

**W44.G9 Other non-organic objects entering into or through a natural orifice**

**W44.H Other sharp object entering into or through a natural orifice**

**W44.H0 Other sharp object unspecified, entering into or through a natural orifice**

**W44.H1 Needle entering into or through a natural orifice**
Dart entering into or through a natural orifice
Hypodermic needle entering into or through a natural orifice
Safety pin entering into or through a natural orifice
Sewing needle entering into or through a natural orifice

**W44.H2 Knife, sword or dagger entering into or through a natural orifice**

**W44.H9 Other sharp object entering into or through a natural orifice**
Shard pottery entering into or through a natural orifice

**W44.8 Other foreign body entering into or through a natural orifice**

**W44.9 Unspecified foreign body entering into or through a natural orifice**
Foreign body NOS entering into or through a natural orifice

**W45 Foreign body or object entering through skin**

INCLUDES foreign body or object embedded in skin
nail embedded in skin

EXCLUDES 2 *contact with hand tools (nonpowered) (powered) (W27-W29)*
*contact with other sharp objects (W26.-)*
*contact with sharp glass (W25.-)*
*struck by objects (W20-W22)*

**W45.0 Nail entering through skin**

**W45.3 Fishing hook entering through skin**

√x7th **W45.8 Other foreign body or object entering through skin**
Splinter in skin NOS

√4th **W46 Contact with hypodermic needle**

√x7th **W46.Ø Contact with hypodermic needle**
Hypodermic needle stick NOS

√x7th **W46.1 Contact with contaminated hypodermic needle**

√4th **W49 Exposure to other inanimate mechanical forces**
INCLUDES exposure to abnormal gravitational [G] forces
exposure to inanimate mechanical forces NEC
EXCLUDES 1 *exposure to inanimate mechanical forces involving military or war operations (Y36.-, Y37.-)*

√5th **W49.Ø Item causing external constriction**

√x7th **W49.Ø1 Hair causing external constriction**

√x7th **W49.Ø2 String or thread causing external constriction**

√x7th **W49.Ø3 Rubber band causing external constriction**

√x7th **W49.Ø4 Ring or other jewelry causing external constriction**

√x7th **W49.Ø9 Other specified item causing external constriction**

√x7th **W49.9 Exposure to other inanimate mechanical forces**

## Exposure to animate mechanical forces (W5Ø-W64)

EXCLUDES 1 *toxic effect of contact with venomous animals and plants (T63.-)*

The appropriate 7th character is to be added to each code from categories W5Ø-W64.
A initial encounter
D subsequent encounter
S sequela

√4th **W5Ø Accidental hit, strike, kick, twist, bite or scratch by another person**
INCLUDES hit, strike, kick, twist, bite, or scratch by another person NOS
EXCLUDES 1 *assault by bodily force (YØ4)*
*struck by objects (W2Ø-W22)*

√x7th **W5Ø.Ø Accidental hit or strike by another person**
Hit or strike by another person NOS

√x7th **W5Ø.1 Accidental kick by another person**
Kick by another person NOS

√x7th **W5Ø.2 Accidental twist by another person**
Twist by another person NOS

√x7th **W5Ø.3 Accidental bite by another person**
Bite by another person NOS
Human bite

√x7th **W5Ø.4 Accidental scratch by another person**
Scratch by another person NOS

√x7th **W51 Accidental striking against or bumped into by another person**
EXCLUDES 1 *assault by striking against or bumping into by another person (YØ4.2)*
*fall due to collision with another person (WØ3)*

√x7th **W52 Crushed, pushed or stepped on by crowd or human stampede**
Crushed, pushed or stepped on by crowd or human stampede with or without fall

√4th **W53 Contact with rodent**
INCLUDES contact with saliva, feces or urine of rodent

√5th **W53.Ø Contact with mouse**

√x7th **W53.Ø1 Bitten by mouse**

√x7th **W53.Ø9 Other contact with mouse**

√5th **W53.1 Contact with rat**

√x7th **W53.11 Bitten by rat**

√x7th **W53.19 Other contact with rat**

√5th **W53.2 Contact with squirrel**

√x7th **W53.21 Bitten by squirrel**

√x7th **W53.29 Other contact with squirrel**

√5th **W53.8 Contact with other rodent**

√x7th **W53.81 Bitten by other rodent**

√x7th **W53.89 Other contact with other rodent**

√4th **W54 Contact with dog**
INCLUDES contact with saliva, feces or urine of dog

√x7th **W54.Ø Bitten by dog**

√x7th **W54.1 Struck by dog**
Knocked over by dog

√x7th **W54.8 Other contact with dog**

√4th **W55 Contact with other mammals**
INCLUDES contact with saliva, feces or urine of mammal
EXCLUDES 1 *animal being ridden - see transport accidents*
*bitten or struck by dog (W54)*
*bitten or struck by rodent (W53.-)*
*contact with marine mammals (W56.-)*

√5th **W55.Ø Contact with cat**

√x7th **W55.Ø1 Bitten by cat**

√x7th **W55.Ø3 Scratched by cat**

√x7th **W55.Ø9 Other contact with cat**

√5th **W55.1 Contact with horse**

√x7th **W55.11 Bitten by horse**

√x7th **W55.12 Struck by horse**

√x7th **W55.19 Other contact with horse**

√5th **W55.2 Contact with cow**
Contact with bull

√x7th **W55.21 Bitten by cow**

√x7th **W55.22 Struck by cow**
Gored by bull

√x7th **W55.29 Other contact with cow**

√5th **W55.3 Contact with other hoof stock**
Contact with goats
Contact with sheep

√x7th **W55.31 Bitten by other hoof stock**

√x7th **W55.32 Struck by other hoof stock**
Gored by goat
Gored by ram

√x7th **W55.39 Other contact with other hoof stock**

√5th **W55.4 Contact with pig**

√x7th **W55.41 Bitten by pig**

√x7th **W55.42 Struck by pig**

√x7th **W55.49 Other contact with pig**

√5th **W55.5 Contact with raccoon**

√x7th **W55.51 Bitten by raccoon**

√x7th **W55.52 Struck by raccoon**

√x7th **W55.59 Other contact with raccoon**

√5th **W55.8 Contact with other mammals**

√x7th **W55.81 Bitten by other mammals**

√x7th **W55.82 Struck by other mammals**

√x7th **W55.89 Other contact with other mammals**

√4th **W56 Contact with nonvenomous marine animal**
EXCLUDES 1 *contact with venomous marine animal (T63.-)*

√5th **W56.Ø Contact with dolphin**

√x7th **W56.Ø1 Bitten by dolphin**

√x7th **W56.Ø2 Struck by dolphin**

√x7th **W56.Ø9 Other contact with dolphin**

√5th **W56.1 Contact with sea lion**

√x7th **W56.11 Bitten by sea lion**

√x7th **W56.12 Struck by sea lion**

√x7th **W56.19 Other contact with sea lion**

√5th **W56.2 Contact with orca**
Contact with killer whale

√x7th **W56.21 Bitten by orca**

√x7th **W56.22 Struck by orca**

√x7th **W56.29 Other contact with orca**

√5th **W56.3 Contact with other marine mammals**

√x7th **W56.31 Bitten by other marine mammals**

√x7th **W56.32 Struck by other marine mammals**

√x7th **W56.39 Other contact with other marine mammals**

√5th **W56.4 Contact with shark**

√x7th **W56.41 Bitten by shark**

√x7th **W56.42 Struck by shark**

√x7th **W56.49 Other contact with shark**

√5th **W56.5 Contact with other fish**

√x7th **W56.51 Bitten by other fish**

√x7th **W56.52 Struck by other fish**

√x7th **W56.59 Other contact with other fish**

5th **W56.8 Contact with other nonvenomous marine animals**
√x7th **W56.81 Bitten by other nonvenomous marine animals**
√x7th **W56.82 Struck by other nonvenomous marine animals**
√x7th **W56.89 Other contact with other nonvenomous marine animals**

√x7th **W57 Bitten or stung by nonvenomous insect and other nonvenomous arthropods**
EXCLUDES 1 *contact with venomous insects and arthropods (T63.2-, T63.3-, T63.4-)*

4th **W58 Contact with crocodile or alligator**
5th **W58.Ø Contact with alligator**
√x7th **W58.Ø1 Bitten by alligator**
√x7th **W58.Ø2 Struck by alligator**
√x7th **W58.Ø3 Crushed by alligator**
√x7th **W58.Ø9 Other contact with alligator**
5th **W58.1 Contact with crocodile**
√x7th **W58.11 Bitten by crocodile**
√x7th **W58.12 Struck by crocodile**
√x7th **W58.13 Crushed by crocodile**
√x7th **W58.19 Other contact with crocodile**

4th **W59 Contact with other nonvenomous reptiles**
EXCLUDES 1 *contact with venomous reptile (T63.Ø-, T63.1-)*
5th **W59.Ø Contact with nonvenomous lizards**
√x7th **W59.Ø1 Bitten by nonvenomous lizards**
√x7th **W59.Ø2 Struck by nonvenomous lizards**
√x7th **W59.Ø9 Other contact with nonvenomous lizards**
Exposure to nonvenomous lizards
5th **W59.1 Contact with nonvenomous snakes**
√x7th **W59.11 Bitten by nonvenomous snake**
√x7th **W59.12 Struck by nonvenomous snake**
√x7th **W59.13 Crushed by nonvenomous snake**
√x7th **W59.19 Other contact with nonvenomous snake**
5th **W59.2 Contact with turtles**
EXCLUDES 1 *contact with tortoises (W59.8-)*
√x7th **W59.21 Bitten by turtle**
√x7th **W59.22 Struck by turtle**
√x7th **W59.29 Other contact with turtle**
Exposure to turtles
5th **W59.8 Contact with other nonvenomous reptiles**
√x7th **W59.81 Bitten by other nonvenomous reptiles**
√x7th **W59.82 Struck by other nonvenomous reptiles**
√x7th **W59.83 Crushed by other nonvenomous reptiles**
√x7th **W59.89 Other contact with other nonvenomous reptiles**

√x7th **W6Ø Contact with nonvenomous plant thorns and spines and sharp leaves**
EXCLUDES 1 *contact with venomous plants (T63.7-)*

4th **W61 Contact with birds (domestic) (wild)**
INCLUDES contact with excreta of birds
5th **W61.Ø Contact with parrot**
√x7th **W61.Ø1 Bitten by parrot**
√x7th **W61.Ø2 Struck by parrot**
√x7th **W61.Ø9 Other contact with parrot**
Exposure to parrots
5th **W61.1 Contact with macaw**
√x7th **W61.11 Bitten by macaw**
√x7th **W61.12 Struck by macaw**
√x7th **W61.19 Other contact with macaw**
Exposure to macaws
5th **W61.2 Contact with other psittacines**
√x7th **W61.21 Bitten by other psittacines**
√x7th **W61.22 Struck by other psittacines**
√x7th **W61.29 Other contact with other psittacines**
Exposure to other psittacines
5th **W61.3 Contact with chicken**
√x7th **W61.32 Struck by chicken**
√x7th **W61.33 Pecked by chicken**
√x7th **W61.39 Other contact with chicken**
Exposure to chickens
5th **W61.4 Contact with turkey**
√x7th **W61.42 Struck by turkey**
√x7th **W61.43 Pecked by turkey**
√x7th **W61.49 Other contact with turkey**
5th **W61.5 Contact with goose**
√x7th **W61.51 Bitten by goose**
√x7th **W61.52 Struck by goose**
√x7th **W61.59 Other contact with goose**
5th **W61.6 Contact with duck**
√x7th **W61.61 Bitten by duck**
√x7th **W61.62 Struck by duck**
√x7th **W61.69 Other contact with duck**
5th **W61.9 Contact with other birds**
√x7th **W61.91 Bitten by other birds**
√x7th **W61.92 Struck by other birds**
√x7th **W61.99 Other contact with other birds**
Contact with bird NOS

4th **W62 Contact with nonvenomous amphibians**
EXCLUDES 1 *contact with venomous amphibians (T63.81-T63.83)*
√x7th **W62.Ø Contact with nonvenomous frogs**
√x7th **W62.1 Contact with nonvenomous toads**
√x7th **W62.9 Contact with other nonvenomous amphibians**

√x7th **W64 Exposure to other animate mechanical forces**
INCLUDES exposure to nonvenomous animal NOS
EXCLUDES 1 *contact with venomous animal (T63.-)*

## Accidental non-transport drowning and submersion (W65-W74)

EXCLUDES 1 *accidental drowning and submersion due to fall into water (W16.-)*
*accidental drowning and submersion due to water transport accident (V9Ø.-, V92.-)*
EXCLUDES 2 *accidental drowning and submersion due to cataclysm (X34-X39)*

The appropriate 7th character is to be added to each code from categories W65-W74.
A initial encounter
D subsequent encounter
S sequela

√x7th **W65 Accidental drowning and submersion while in bath-tub**
EXCLUDES 1 *accidental drowning and submersion due to fall in (into) bathtub (W16.211)*

√x7th **W67 Accidental drowning and submersion while in swimming-pool**
EXCLUDES 1 *accidental drowning and submersion due to fall into swimming pool (W16.Ø11, W16.Ø21, W16.Ø31)*
*accidental drowning and submersion due to striking into wall of swimming pool (W22.Ø41)*
**AHA:** 2023,1Q,25

√x7th **W69 Accidental drowning and submersion while in natural water**
Accidental drowning and submersion while in lake
Accidental drowning and submersion while in open sea
Accidental drowning and submersion while in river
Accidental drowning and submersion while in stream
EXCLUDES 1 *accidental drowning and submersion due to fall into natural body of water (W16.111, W16.121, W16.131)*

√x7th **W73 Other specified cause of accidental non-transport drowning and submersion**
Accidental drowning and submersion while in quenching tank
Accidental drowning and submersion while in reservoir
EXCLUDES 1 *accidental drowning and submersion due to fall into other water (W16.311, W16.321, W16.331)*

√x7th **W74 Unspecified cause of accidental drowning and submersion**
Drowning NOS

## Exposure to electric current, radiation and extreme ambient air temperature and pressure (W85-W99)

EXCLUDES 1 exposure to:
*failure in dosage of radiation or temperature during surgical and medical care (Y63.2-Y63.5)*
*lightning (T75.0-)*
*natural cold (X31)*
*natural heat (X30)*
*natural radiation NOS (X39)*
*radiological procedure and radiotherapy (Y84.2)*
*sunlight (X32)*

AHA: 2018,2Q,7-8

The appropriate 7th character is to be added to each code from categories W85-W99.
A initial encounter
D subsequent encounter
S sequela

**W85 Exposure to electric transmission lines**
Broken power line

**W86 Exposure to other specified electric current**
**W86.0 Exposure to domestic wiring and appliances**
**W86.1 Exposure to industrial wiring, appliances and electrical machinery**
Exposure to conductors
Exposure to control apparatus
Exposure to electrical equipment and machinery
Exposure to transformers
**W86.8 Exposure to other electric current**
Exposure to wiring and appliances in or on farm (not farmhouse)
Exposure to wiring and appliances in or on public building
Exposure to wiring and appliances in or on residential institutions
Exposure to wiring and appliances in or on schools
Exposure to wiring and appliances outdoors

**W88 Exposure to ionizing radiation**
EXCLUDES 1 *exposure to sunlight (X32)*
**W88.0 Exposure to X-rays**
**W88.1 Exposure to radioactive isotopes**
**W88.8 Exposure to other ionizing radiation**

**W89 Exposure to man-made visible and ultraviolet light**
INCLUDES exposure to welding light (arc)
EXCLUDES 2 *exposure to sunlight (X32)*
**W89.0 Exposure to welding light (arc)**
**W89.1 Exposure to tanning bed**
**W89.8 Exposure to other man-made visible and ultraviolet light**
**W89.9 Exposure to unspecified man-made visible and ultraviolet light**

**W90 Exposure to other nonionizing radiation**
EXCLUDES 2 *exposure to sunlight (X32)*
AHA: 2019,1Q,21
**W90.0 Exposure to radiofrequency**
**W90.1 Exposure to infrared radiation**
**W90.2 Exposure to laser radiation**
**W90.8 Exposure to other nonionizing radiation**

**W92 Exposure to excessive heat of man-made origin**

**W93 Exposure to excessive cold of man-made origin**
**W93.0 Contact with or inhalation of dry ice**
**W93.01 Contact with dry ice**
**W93.02 Inhalation of dry ice**
**W93.1 Contact with or inhalation of liquid air**
**W93.11 Contact with liquid air**
Contact with liquid hydrogen
Contact with liquid nitrogen
**W93.12 Inhalation of liquid air**
Inhalation of liquid hydrogen
Inhalation of liquid nitrogen
**W93.2 Prolonged exposure in deep freeze unit or refrigerator**
**W93.8 Exposure to other excessive cold of man-made origin**

**W94 Exposure to high and low air pressure and changes in air pressure**
**W94.0 Exposure to prolonged high air pressure**
**W94.1 Exposure to prolonged low air pressure**
**W94.11 Exposure to residence or prolonged visit at high altitude**
**W94.12 Exposure to other prolonged low air pressure**
**W94.2 Exposure to rapid changes in air pressure during ascent**
**W94.21 Exposure to reduction in atmospheric pressure while surfacing from deep-water diving**
**W94.22 Exposure to reduction in atmospheric pressure while surfacing from underground**
**W94.23 Exposure to sudden change in air pressure in aircraft during ascent**
**W94.29 Exposure to other rapid changes in air pressure during ascent**
**W94.3 Exposure to rapid changes in air pressure during descent**
**W94.31 Exposure to sudden change in air pressure in aircraft during descent**
**W94.32 Exposure to high air pressure from rapid descent in water**
**W94.39 Exposure to other rapid changes in air pressure during descent**

**W99 Exposure to other man-made environmental factors**

## Exposure to smoke, fire and flames (X00-X08)

EXCLUDES 1 *arson (X97)*
EXCLUDES 2 *explosions (W35-W40)*
*lightning (T75.0-)*
*transport accident (V01-V99)*

AHA: 2018,2Q,7-8

The appropriate 7th character is to be added to each code from categories X00-X08.
A initial encounter
D subsequent encounter
S sequela

**X00 Exposure to uncontrolled fire in building or structure**
INCLUDES conflagration in building or structure
Code first any associated cataclysm
EXCLUDES 2 *exposure to ignition or melting of nightwear (X05)*
*exposure to ignition or melting of other clothing and apparel (X06.-)*
*exposure to other specified smoke, fire and flames (X08.-)*
AHA: 2016,2Q,5
**X00.0 Exposure to flames in uncontrolled fire in building or structure**
**X00.1 Exposure to smoke in uncontrolled fire in building or structure**
**X00.2 Injury due to collapse of burning building or structure in uncontrolled fire**
EXCLUDES 1 *injury due to collapse of building not on fire (W20.1)*
**X00.3 Fall from burning building or structure in uncontrolled fire**
**X00.4 Hit by object from burning building or structure in uncontrolled fire**
AHA: 2016,2Q,4
**X00.5 Jump from burning building or structure in uncontrolled fire**
**X00.8 Other exposure to uncontrolled fire in building or structure**

**X01 Exposure to uncontrolled fire, not in building or structure**
INCLUDES exposure to forest fire
**X01.0 Exposure to flames in uncontrolled fire, not in building or structure**
**X01.1 Exposure to smoke in uncontrolled fire, not in building or structure**
**X01.3 Fall due to uncontrolled fire, not in building or structure**
**X01.4 Hit by object due to uncontrolled fire, not in building or structure**
**X01.8 Other exposure to uncontrolled fire, not in building or structure**

**X02 Exposure to controlled fire in building or structure**
INCLUDES exposure to fire in fireplace
exposure to fire in stove
**X02.0 Exposure to flames in controlled fire in building or structure**
**X02.1 Exposure to smoke in controlled fire in building or structure**
**X02.2 Injury due to collapse of burning building or structure in controlled fire**
EXCLUDES 1 *injury due to collapse of building not on fire (W20.1)*
**X02.3 Fall from burning building or structure in controlled fire**
**X02.4 Hit by object from burning building or structure in controlled fire**
**X02.5 Jump from burning building or structure in controlled fire**
**X02.8 Other exposure to controlled fire in building or structure**

**X03 Exposure to controlled fire, not in building or structure**
INCLUDES exposure to bon fire
exposure to camp-fire
exposure to trash fire

**X03.0 Exposure to flames in controlled fire, not in building or structure**

**X03.1 Exposure to smoke in controlled fire, not in building or structure**

**X03.3 Fall due to controlled fire, not in building or structure**

**X03.4 Hit by object due to controlled fire, not in building or structure**

**X03.8 Other exposure to controlled fire, not in building or structure**

**X04 Exposure to ignition of highly flammable material**
Exposure to ignition of gasoline
Exposure to ignition of kerosene
Exposure to ignition of petrol
EXCLUDES 2 *exposure to ignition or melting of nightwear (X05)*
*exposure to ignition or melting of other clothing and apparel (X06)*
AHA: 2016,2Q,4

**X05 Exposure to ignition or melting of nightwear**
EXCLUDES 2 *exposure to uncontrolled fire in building or structure (X00.-)*
*exposure to controlled fire in building or structure (X02.-)*
*exposure to controlled fire, not in building or structure (X03.-)*
*exposure to ignition of highly flammable materials (X04.-)*
*exposure to uncontrolled fire, not in building or structure (X01.-)*

**X06 Exposure to ignition or melting of other clothing and apparel**
EXCLUDES 2 *exposure to uncontrolled fire in building or structure (X00.-)*
*exposure to controlled fire in building or structure (X02.-)*
*exposure to controlled fire, not in building or structure (X03.-)*
*exposure to ignition of highly flammable materials (X04.-)*
*exposure to uncontrolled fire, not in building or structure (X01.-)*

**X06.0 Exposure to ignition of plastic jewelry**

**X06.1 Exposure to melting of plastic jewelry**

**X06.2 Exposure to ignition of other clothing and apparel**

**X06.3 Exposure to melting of other clothing and apparel**

**X08 Exposure to other specified smoke, fire and flames**

**X08.0 Exposure to bed fire**
Exposure to mattress fire

**X08.00 Exposure to bed fire due to unspecified burning material**

**X08.01 Exposure to bed fire due to burning cigarette**

**X08.09 Exposure to bed fire due to other burning material**

**X08.1 Exposure to sofa fire**

**X08.10 Exposure to sofa fire due to unspecified burning material**

**X08.11 Exposure to sofa fire due to burning cigarette**

**X08.19 Exposure to sofa fire due to other burning material**

**X08.2 Exposure to other furniture fire**

**X08.20 Exposure to other furniture fire due to unspecified burning material**

**X08.21 Exposure to other furniture fire due to burning cigarette**

**X08.29 Exposure to other furniture fire due to other burning material**

**X08.8 Exposure to other specified smoke, fire and flames**

## Contact with heat and hot substances (X10-X19)

EXCLUDES 1 *exposure to excessive natural heat (X30)*
*exposure to fire and flames (X00-X08)*
AHA: 2018,2Q,7-8

The appropriate 7th character is to be added to each code from categories X10-X19.
A initial encounter
D subsequent encounter
S sequela

**X10 Contact with hot drinks, food, fats and cooking oils**

**X10.0 Contact with hot drinks**

**X10.1 Contact with hot food**

**X10.2 Contact with fats and cooking oils**

**X11 Contact with hot tap-water**
INCLUDES contact with boiling tap-water
contact with boiling water NOS
EXCLUDES 1 *contact with water heated on stove (X12)*

**X11.0 Contact with hot water in bath or tub**
EXCLUDES 1 *contact with running hot water in bath or tub (X11.1)*

**X11.1 Contact with running hot water**
Contact with hot water running out of hose
Contact with hot water running out of tap

**X11.8 Contact with other hot tap-water**
Contact with hot tap-water NOS
Contact with hot water in bucket

**X12 Contact with other hot fluids**
Contact with water heated on stove
EXCLUDES 1 *hot (liquid) metals (X18)*

**X13 Contact with steam and other hot vapors**

**X13.0 Inhalation of steam and other hot vapors**

**X13.1 Other contact with steam and other hot vapors**

**X14 Contact with hot air and other hot gases**

**X14.0 Inhalation of hot air and gases**

**X14.1 Other contact with hot air and other hot gases**

**X15 Contact with hot household appliances**
EXCLUDES 1 *contact with heating appliances (X16)*
*contact with powered household appliances (W29.-)*
*exposure to controlled fire in building or structure due to household appliance (X02.8)*
*exposure to household appliances electrical current (W86.0)*

**X15.0 Contact with hot stove (kitchen)**

**X15.1 Contact with hot toaster**

**X15.2 Contact with hotplate**

**X15.3 Contact with hot saucepan or skillet**
Contact with hot cooking pan
Contact with hot cooking pot

**X15.8 Contact with other hot household appliances**
Contact with cooker
Contact with kettle
Contact with light bulbs

**X16 Contact with hot heating appliances, radiators and pipes**
EXCLUDES 1 *contact with powered appliances (W29.-)*
*exposure to controlled fire in building or structure due to appliance (X02.8)*
*exposure to industrial appliances electrical current (W86.1)*

**X17 Contact with hot engines, machinery and tools**
EXCLUDES 1 *contact with hot heating appliances, radiators and pipes (X16)*
*contact with hot household appliances (X15)*

**X18 Contact with other hot metals**
Contact with liquid metal

**X19 Contact with other heat and hot substances**
EXCLUDES 1 *objects that are not normally hot, e.g., an object made hot by a house fire (X00-X08)*

## Exposure to forces of nature (X30-X39)

AHA: 2018,2Q,7-8

The appropriate 7th character is to be added to each code from categories X30-X39.
A initial encounter
D subsequent encounter
S sequela

**X30 Exposure to excessive natural heat**
Exposure to excessive heat as the cause of sunstroke
Exposure to heat NOS
EXCLUDES 1 *excessive heat of man-made origin (W92)*
*exposure to man-made radiation (W89)*
*exposure to sunlight (X32)*
*exposure to tanning bed (W89)*

√x7th **X31 Exposure to excessive natural cold**
Excessive cold as the cause of chilblains NOS
Excessive cold as the cause of immersion foot or hand
Exposure to cold NOS
Exposure to weather conditions
EXCLUDES 1 *cold of man-made origin (W93.-)*
*contact with or inhalation of dry ice (W93.-)*
*contact with or inhalation of liquefied gas (W93.-)*

√x7th **X32 Exposure to sunlight**
EXCLUDES 1 *man-made radiation (tanning bed) (W89)*
EXCLUDES 2 *radiation-related disorders of the skin and subcutaneous tissue (L55-L59)*

√x7th **X34 Earthquake**
EXCLUDES 2 *tidal wave (tsunami) due to earthquake (X37.41)*

√x7th **X35 Volcanic eruption**
EXCLUDES 2 *tidal wave (tsunami) due to volcanic eruption (X37.41)*

√4th **X36 Avalanche, landslide and other earth movements**
INCLUDES victim of mudslide of cataclysmic nature
EXCLUDES 1 *earthquake (X34)*
EXCLUDES 2 *transport accident involving collision with avalanche or landslide not in motion (VØ1-V99)*

√x7th **X36.Ø Collapse of dam or man-made structure causing earth movement**

√x7th **X36.1 Avalanche, landslide, or mudslide**

√4th **X37 Cataclysmic storm**

√x7th **X37.Ø Hurricane**
Storm surge
Typhoon

√x7th **X37.1 Tornado**
Cyclone
Twister

√x7th **X37.2 Blizzard (snow)(ice)**

√x7th **X37.3 Dust storm**

√5th **X37.4 Tidalwave**

√x7th **X37.41 Tidal wave due to earthquake or volcanic eruption**
Tidal wave NOS
Tsunami

√x7th **X37.42 Tidal wave due to storm**

√x7th **X37.43 Tidal wave due to landslide**

√x7th **X37.8 Other cataclysmic storms**
Cloudburst
Torrential rain
EXCLUDES 2 *flood (X38)*

√x7th **X37.9 Unspecified cataclysmic storm**
Storm NOS
EXCLUDES 1 *collapse of dam or man-made structure causing earth movement (X36.Ø)*

√x7th **X38 Flood**
Flood arising from remote storm
Flood of cataclysmic nature arising from melting snow
Flood resulting directly from storm
EXCLUDES 1 *collapse of dam or man-made structure causing earth movement (X36.Ø)*
*tidal wave caused by storm (X37.42)*
*tidal wave NOS (X37.41)*

√4th **X39 Exposure to other forces of nature**

√5th **X39.Ø Exposure to natural radiation**
EXCLUDES 1 *contact with and (suspected) exposure to radon and other naturally occurring radiation (Z77.123)*
*exposure to man-made radiation (W88-W9Ø)*
*exposure to sunlight (X32)*

√x7th **X39.Ø1 Exposure to radon**

√x7th **X39.Ø8 Exposure to other natural radiation**

√x7th **X39.8 Other exposure to forces of nature**

## Overexertion and strenuous or repetitive movements (X5Ø)

√4th **X5Ø Overexertion and strenuous or repetitive movements**
**AHA:** 2018,2Q,7-8; 2016,4Q,73-74

The appropriate 7th character is to be added to each code from category X5Ø.
A initial encounter
D subsequent encounter
S sequela

√x7th **X5Ø.Ø Overexertion from strenuous movement or load**
Lifting heavy objects
Lifting weights

√x7th **X5Ø.1 Overexertion from prolonged static or awkward postures**
Prolonged bending
Prolonged kneeling
Prolonged reaching
Prolonged sitting
Prolonged standing
Prolonged twisting
Static bending
Static kneeling
Static reaching
Static sitting
Static standing
Static twisting

√x7th **X5Ø.3 Overexertion from repetitive movements**
Use of hand as hammer
EXCLUDES 2 *overuse from prolonged static or awkward postures (X5Ø.1)*

√x7th **X5Ø.9 Other and unspecified overexertion or strenuous movements or postures**
Contact pressure
Contact stress

## Accidental exposure to other specified factors (X52-X58)

**AHA:** 2018,2Q,7-8

The appropriate 7th character is to be added to each code from categories X52-X58.
A initial encounter
D subsequent encounter
S sequela

√x7th **X52 Prolonged stay in weightless environment**
Weightlessness in spacecraft (simulator)

√x7th **X58 Exposure to other specified factors**
Accident NOS
Exposure NOS

## Intentional self-harm (X71-X83)

Purposely self-inflicted injury
Suicide (attempted)

The appropriate 7th character is to be added to each code from categories X71-X83.
A initial encounter
D subsequent encounter
S sequela

√4th **X71 Intentional self-harm by drowning and submersion**

√x7th **X71.Ø Intentional self-harm by drowning and submersion while in bathtub** HCC Rx ESR COM

√x7th **X71.1 Intentional self-harm by drowning and submersion while in swimming pool** HCC Rx ESR COM

√x7th **X71.2 Intentional self-harm by drowning and submersion after jump into swimming pool** HCC Rx ESR COM

√x7th **X71.3 Intentional self-harm by drowning and submersion in natural water** HCC Rx ESR COM

√x7th **X71.8 Other intentional self-harm by drowning and submersion** HCC Rx ESR COM

√x7th **X71.9 Intentional self-harm by drowning and submersion, unspecified** HCC Rx ESR COM

√x7th **X72 Intentional self-harm by handgun discharge** HCC Rx ESR COM
Intentional self-harm by gun for single hand use
Intentional self-harm by pistol
Intentional self-harm by revolver
EXCLUDES 1 *Very pistol (X74.8)*

√4th **X73 Intentional self-harm by rifle, shotgun and larger firearm discharge**
EXCLUDES 1 *airgun (X74.Ø1)*

√x7th **X73.Ø Intentional self-harm by shotgun discharge** HCC Rx ESR COM

√x7th X73.1 Intentional self-harm by hunting rifle discharge HCC Rx ESR COM

√x7th X73.2 Intentional self-harm by machine gun discharge HCC Rx ESR COM

√x7th X73.8 Intentional self-harm by other larger firearm discharge HCC Rx ESR COM

√x7th X73.9 Intentional self-harm by unspecified larger firearm discharge HCC Rx ESR COM

√4th X74 Intentional self-harm by other and unspecified firearm and gun discharge

√5th X74.Ø Intentional self-harm by gas, air or spring-operated guns

√x7th X74.Ø1 Intentional self-harm by airgun HCC Rx ESR COM
Intentional self-harm by BB gun discharge
Intentional self-harm by pellet gun discharge

√x7th X74.Ø2 Intentional self-harm by paintball gun HCC Rx ESR COM

√x7th X74.Ø9 Intentional self-harm by other gas, air or spring-operated gun HCC Rx ESR COM

√x7th X74.8 Intentional self-harm by other firearm discharge HCC Rx ESR COM
Intentional self-harm by Very pistol [flare] discharge

√x7th X74.9 Intentional self-harm by unspecified firearm discharge HCC Rx ESR COM

√x7th X75 Intentional self-harm by explosive material HCC Rx ESR COM

√x7th X76 Intentional self-harm by smoke, fire and flames HCC Rx ESR COM

√4th X77 Intentional self-harm by steam, hot vapors and hot objects

√x7th X77.Ø Intentional self-harm by steam or hot vapors HCC Rx ESR COM

√x7th X77.1 Intentional self-harm by hot tap water HCC Rx ESR COM

√x7th X77.2 Intentional self-harm by other hot fluids HCC Rx ESR COM

√x7th X77.3 Intentional self-harm by hot household appliances HCC Rx ESR COM

√x7th X77.8 Intentional self-harm by other hot objects HCC Rx ESR COM

√x7th X77.9 Intentional self-harm by unspecified hot objects HCC Rx ESR COM

√4th X78 Intentional self-harm by sharp object

√x7th X78.Ø Intentional self-harm by sharp glass HCC Rx ESR COM

√x7th X78.1 Intentional self-harm by knife HCC Rx ESR COM

√x7th X78.2 Intentional self-harm by sword or dagger HCC Rx ESR COM

√x7th X78.8 Intentional self-harm by other sharp object HCC Rx ESR COM
AHA: 2022,1Q,27

√x7th X78.9 Intentional self-harm by unspecified sharp object HCC Rx ESR COM

√x7th X79 Intentional self-harm by blunt object HCC Rx ESR COM

√x7th X8Ø Intentional self-harm by jumping from a high place HCC Rx ESR COM
Intentional fall from one level to another

√4th X81 Intentional self-harm by jumping or lying in front of moving object

√x7th X81.Ø Intentional self-harm by jumping or lying in front of motor vehicle HCC Rx ESR COM

√x7th X81.1 Intentional self-harm by jumping or lying in front of (subway) train HCC Rx ESR COM

√x7th X81.8 Intentional self-harm by jumping or lying in front of other moving object HCC Rx ESR COM

√4th X82 Intentional self-harm by crashing of motor vehicle

√x7th X82.Ø Intentional collision of motor vehicle with other motor vehicle HCC Rx ESR COM

√x7th X82.1 Intentional collision of motor vehicle with train HCC Rx ESR COM

√x7th X82.2 Intentional collision of motor vehicle with tree HCC Rx ESR COM

√x7th X82.8 Other intentional self-harm by crashing of motor vehicle HCC Rx ESR COM

√4th X83 Intentional self-harm by other specified means

EXCLUDES 1 *intentional self-harm by poisoning or contact with toxic substance - see Table of Drugs and Chemicals*

√x7th X83.Ø Intentional self-harm by crashing of aircraft HCC Rx ESR COM

√x7th X83.1 Intentional self-harm by electrocution HCC Rx ESR COM

√x7th X83.2 Intentional self-harm by exposure to extremes of cold HCC Rx ESR COM

√x7th X83.8 Intentional self-harm by other specified means HCC Rx ESR COM

## Assault (X92-YØ9)

INCLUDES homicide
injuries inflicted by another person with intent to injure or kill, by any means

EXCLUDES 1 *injuries due to legal intervention (Y35.-)*
*injuries due to operations of war (Y36.-)*
*injuries due to terrorism (Y38.-)*

The appropriate 7th character is to be added to each code from categories X92-YØ4 and YØ8.
A initial encounter
D subsequent encounter
S sequela

√4th X92 Assault by drowning and submersion

√x7th X92.Ø Assault by drowning and submersion while in bathtub

√x7th X92.1 Assault by drowning and submersion while in swimming pool

√x7th X92.2 Assault by drowning and submersion after push into swimming pool

√x7th X92.3 Assault by drowning and submersion in natural water

√x7th X92.8 Other assault by drowning and submersion

√x7th X92.9 Assault by drowning and submersion, unspecified

√x7th X93 Assault by handgun discharge
Assault by discharge of gun for single hand use
Assault by discharge of pistol
Assault by discharge of revolver
EXCLUDES 1 *Very pistol (X95.8)*

√4th X94 Assault by rifle, shotgun and larger firearm discharge
EXCLUDES 1 *airgun (X95.Ø1)*

√x7th X94.Ø Assault by shotgun

√x7th X94.1 Assault by hunting rifle

√x7th X94.2 Assault by machine gun

√x7th X94.8 Assault by other larger firearm discharge

√x7th X94.9 Assault by unspecified larger firearm discharge

√4th X95 Assault by other and unspecified firearm and gun discharge

√5th X95.Ø Assault by gas, air or spring-operated guns

√x7th X95.Ø1 Assault by airgun discharge
Assault by BB gun discharge
Assault by pellet gun discharge

√x7th X95.Ø2 Assault by paintball gun discharge

√x7th X95.Ø9 Assault by other gas, air or spring-operated gun

√x7th X95.8 Assault by other firearm discharge
Assault by Very pistol [flare] discharge

√x7th X95.9 Assault by unspecified firearm discharge
AHA: 2025,1Q,31; 2023,3Q,8,12

√4th X96 Assault by explosive material
EXCLUDES 1 *incendiary device (X97)*
*terrorism involving explosive material (Y38.2-)*

√x7th X96.Ø Assault by antipersonnel bomb
EXCLUDES 1 *antipersonnel bomb use in military or war (Y36.2-)*

√x7th X96.1 Assault by gasoline bomb

√x7th X96.2 Assault by letter bomb

√x7th X96.3 Assault by fertilizer bomb

√x7th X96.4 Assault by pipe bomb

√x7th X96.8 Assault by other specified explosive

√x7th X96.9 Assault by unspecified explosive

√x7th X97 Assault by smoke, fire and flames
Assault by arson
Assault by cigarettes
Assault by incendiary device

√4th X98 Assault by steam, hot vapors and hot objects

√x7th X98.Ø Assault by steam or hot vapors

√x7th X98.1 Assault by hot tap water

√x7th X98.2 Assault by hot fluids

√x7th X98.3 Assault by hot household appliances

√x7th X98.8 Assault by other hot objects

√x7th X98.9 Assault by unspecified hot objects

√4th X99 Assault by sharp object
EXCLUDES 1 *assault by strike by sports equipment (YØ8.Ø-)*

√x7th X99.Ø Assault by sharp glass

√x7th **X99.1 Assault by knife**

√x7th **X99.2 Assault by sword or dagger**

√x7th **X99.8 Assault by other sharp object**

√x7th **X99.9 Assault by unspecified sharp object**

Assault by stabbing NOS

√x7th **Y00 Assault by blunt object**

EXCLUDES 1 *assault by strike by sports equipment (Y08.0-)*

√x7th **Y01 Assault by pushing from high place**

√4th **Y02 Assault by pushing or placing victim in front of moving object**

√x7th **Y02.0 Assault by pushing or placing victim in front of motor vehicle**

√x7th **Y02.1 Assault by pushing or placing victim in front of (subway) train**

√x7th **Y02.8 Assault by pushing or placing victim in front of other moving object**

√4th **Y03 Assault by crashing of motor vehicle**

√x7th **Y03.0 Assault by being hit or run over by motor vehicle**

√x7th **Y03.8 Other assault by crashing of motor vehicle**

√4th **Y04 Assault by bodily force**

EXCLUDES 1 *assault by:*
*submersion (X92.-)*
*use of weapon (X93-X95, X99, Y00)*

√x7th **Y04.0 Assault by unarmed brawl or fight**

√x7th **Y04.1 Assault by human bite**

√x7th **Y04.2 Assault by strike against or bumped into by another person**

√x7th **Y04.8 Assault by other bodily force**

Assault by bodily force NOS

√4th **Y07 Perpetrator of assault, maltreatment and neglect**

NOTE Codes from this category are for use only in cases of confirmed abuse (T74.-)

Selection of the correct perpetrator code is based on the relationship between the perpetrator and the victim

INCLUDES perpetrator of abandonment
perpetrator of emotional neglect
perpetrator of mental cruelty
perpetrator of physical abuse
perpetrator of physical neglect
perpetrator of sexual abuse
perpetrator of torture
perpetrator of verbal abuse

√5th **Y07.0 Spouse or partner, perpetrator of maltreatment and neglect**

Spouse or partner, perpetrator of maltreatment and neglect against spouse or partner

AHA: 2023,1Q,5

√6th **Y07.01 Husband, perpetrator of maltreatment and neglect**

**Y07.010 Husband, current, perpetrator of maltreatment and neglect**

**Y07.011 Husband, former, perpetrator of maltreatment and neglect**

√6th **Y07.02 Wife, perpetrator of maltreatment and neglect**

**Y07.020 Wife, current, perpetrator of maltreatment and neglect**

**Y07.021 Wife, former, perpetrator of maltreatment and neglect**

√6th **Y07.03 Male partner, perpetrator of maltreatment and neglect**

Male intimate or dating partner, perpetrator of maltreatment and neglect

**Y07.030 Male partner, current, perpetrator of maltreatment and neglect**

**Y07.031 Male partner, former, perpetrator of maltreatment and neglect**

√6th **Y07.04 Female partner, perpetrator of maltreatment and neglect**

Female intimate or dating partner, perpetrator of maltreatment and neglect

**Y07.040 Female partner, current, perpetrator of maltreatment and neglect**

**Y07.041 Female partner, former, perpetrator of maltreatment and neglect**

√6th **Y07.05 Non-binary partner, perpetrator of maltreatment and neglect**

Gender non-conforming partner, perpetrator of maltreatment and neglect

**Y07.050 Non-binary partner, current, perpetrator of maltreatment and neglect**

**Y07.051 Non-binary partner, former, perpetrator of maltreatment and neglect**

√5th **Y07.1 Parent (adoptive) (biological), perpetrator of maltreatment and neglect**

**Y07.11 Biological father, perpetrator of maltreatment and neglect**

**Y07.12 Biological mother, perpetrator of maltreatment and neglect**

**Y07.13 Adoptive father, perpetrator of maltreatment and neglect**

**Y07.14 Adoptive mother, perpetrator of maltreatment and neglect**

√5th **Y07.4 Other family member, perpetrator of maltreatment and neglect**

AHA: 2023,1Q,5

√6th **Y07.41 Sibling, perpetrator of maltreatment and neglect**

EXCLUDES 1 *stepsibling, perpetrator of maltreatment and neglect (Y07.435, Y07.436)*

**Y07.410 Brother, perpetrator of maltreatment and neglect**

**Y07.411 Sister, perpetrator of maltreatment and neglect**

√6th **Y07.42 Foster parent, perpetrator of maltreatment and neglect**

**Y07.420 Foster father, perpetrator of maltreatment and neglect**

**Y07.421 Foster mother, perpetrator of maltreatment and neglect**

√6th **Y07.43 Stepparent or stepsibling, perpetrator of maltreatment and neglect**

**Y07.430 Stepfather, perpetrator of maltreatment and neglect**

**Y07.432 Male friend of parent (co-residing in household), perpetrator of maltreatment and neglect**

**Y07.433 Stepmother, perpetrator of maltreatment and neglect**

**Y07.434 Female friend of parent (co-residing in household), perpetrator of maltreatment and neglect**

**Y07.435 Stepbrother, perpetrator of maltreatment and neglect**

**Y07.436 Stepsister, perpetrator of maltreatment and neglect**

**Y07.44 Child, perpetrator of maltreatment and neglect**

Adopted child, perpetrator of maltreatment and neglect
Biological child, perpetrator of maltreatment and neglect
Daughter, perpetrator of maltreatment and neglect
Foster child, perpetrator of maltreatment and neglect
In-law child, perpetrator of maltreatment and neglect
Non-binary child, perpetrator of maltreatment and neglect
Son, perpetrator of maltreatment and neglect
Stepchild, perpetrator of maltreatment and neglect

**Y07.45 Grandchild, perpetrator of maltreatment and neglect**

Adopted grandchild, perpetrator of maltreatment and neglect
Biological grandchild, perpetrator of maltreatment and neglect
Foster grandchild, perpetrator of maltreatment and neglect
Granddaughter, perpetrator of maltreatment and neglect
Grandson, perpetrator of maltreatment and neglect
In-law grandchild, perpetrator of maltreatment and neglect
Non-binary grandchild, perpetrator of maltreatment and neglect
Step grandchild, perpetrator of maltreatment and neglect

**Y07.46 Grandparent, perpetrator of maltreatment and neglect**

Grandfather, perpetrator of maltreatment and neglect
Grandmother, perpetrator of maltreatment and neglect
Non-binary grandparent, perpetrator of maltreatment and neglect

**Y07.47 Parental sibling, perpetrator of maltreatment and neglect**

Aunt, perpetrator of maltreatment and neglect
Non-binary parental sibling, perpetrator of maltreatment and neglect
Uncle, perpetrator of maltreatment and neglect

√6th Y07.49 **Other family member, perpetrator of maltreatment and neglect**

Y07.490 **Male cousin, perpetrator of maltreatment and neglect**

Y07.491 **Female cousin, perpetrator of maltreatment and neglect**

Y07.499 **Other family member, perpetrator of maltreatment and neglect**

√5th Y07.5 **Non-family member, perpetrator of maltreatment and neglect**

AHA: 2023,1Q,5

Y07.50 **Unspecified non-family member, perpetrator of maltreatment and neglect**

√6th Y07.51 **Daycare provider, perpetrator of maltreatment and neglect**

Y07.510 **At-home childcare provider, perpetrator of maltreatment and neglect**

Y07.511 **Daycare center childcare provider, perpetrator of maltreatment and neglect**

Y07.512 **At-home adultcare provider, perpetrator of maltreatment and neglect**

Y07.513 **Adultcare center provider, perpetrator of maltreatment and neglect**

Y07.519 **Unspecified daycare provider, perpetrator of maltreatment and neglect**

√6th Y07.52 **Healthcare provider, perpetrator of maltreatment and neglect**

Y07.521 **Mental health provider, perpetrator of maltreatment and neglect**

Y07.528 **Other therapist or healthcare provider, perpetrator of maltreatment and neglect**

Nurse perpetrator of maltreatment and neglect
Occupational therapist perpetrator of maltreatment and neglect
Physical therapist perpetrator of maltreatment and neglect
Speech therapist perpetrator of maltreatment and neglect

Y07.529 **Unspecified healthcare provider, perpetrator of maltreatment and neglect**

Y07.53 **Teacher or instructor, perpetrator of maltreatment and neglect**

Coach, perpetrator of maltreatment and neglect

Y07.54 **Acquaintance or friend, perpetrator of maltreatment and neglect**

Y07.59 **Other non-family member, perpetrator of maltreatment and neglect**

Y07.6 **Multiple perpetrators of maltreatment and neglect**

AHA: 2018,4Q,32

Y07.9 **Unspecified perpetrator of maltreatment and neglect**

√4th **Y08 Assault by other specified means**

√5th Y08.0 **Assault by strike by sport equipment**

√x7th Y08.01 **Assault by strike by hockey stick**

√x7th Y08.02 **Assault by strike by baseball bat**

√x7th Y08.09 **Assault by strike by other specified type of sport equipment**

√5th Y08.8 **Assault by other specified means**

√x7th Y08.81 **Assault by crashing of aircraft**

√x7th Y08.89 **Assault by other specified means**

**Y09 Assault by unspecified means**

Assassination (attempted) NOS
Homicide (attempted) NOS
Manslaughter (attempted) NOS
Murder (attempted) NOS

## Event of undetermined intent (Y21-Y33)

Undetermined intent is only for use when there is specific documentation in the record that the intent of the injury cannot be determined. If no such documentation is present, code to accidental (unintentional).

The appropriate 7th character is to be added to each code from categories Y21-Y33.
A initial encounter
D subsequent encounter
S sequela

√4th **Y21 Drowning and submersion, undetermined intent**

√x7th Y21.0 **Drowning and submersion while in bathtub, undetermined intent**

√x7th Y21.1 **Drowning and submersion after fall into bathtub, undetermined intent**

√x7th Y21.2 **Drowning and submersion while in swimming pool, undetermined intent**

√x7th Y21.3 **Drowning and submersion after fall into swimming pool, undetermined intent**

√x7th Y21.4 **Drowning and submersion in natural water, undetermined intent**

√x7th Y21.8 **Other drowning and submersion, undetermined intent**

√x7th Y21.9 **Unspecified drowning and submersion, undetermined intent**

√x7th **Y22 Handgun discharge, undetermined intent**

Discharge of gun for single hand use, undetermined intent
Discharge of pistol, undetermined intent
Discharge of revolver, undetermined intent

EXCLUDES 2 *Very pistol (Y24.8)*

√4th **Y23 Rifle, shotgun and larger firearm discharge, undetermined intent**

EXCLUDES 2 *airgun (Y24.0)*

√x7th Y23.0 **Shotgun discharge, undetermined intent**

√x7th Y23.1 **Hunting rifle discharge, undetermined intent**

√x7th Y23.2 **Military firearm discharge, undetermined intent**

√x7th Y23.3 **Machine gun discharge, undetermined intent**

√x7th Y23.8 **Other larger firearm discharge, undetermined intent**

√x7th Y23.9 **Unspecified larger firearm discharge, undetermined intent**

√4th **Y24 Other and unspecified firearm discharge, undetermined intent**

√x7th Y24.0 **Airgun discharge, undetermined intent**

BB gun discharge, undetermined intent
Pellet gun discharge, undetermined intent

√x7th Y24.8 **Other firearm discharge, undetermined intent**

Paintball gun discharge, undetermined intent
Very pistol [flare] discharge, undetermined intent

√x7th Y24.9 **Unspecified firearm discharge, undetermined intent**

√x7th **Y25 Contact with explosive material, undetermined intent**

√x7th **Y26 Exposure to smoke, fire and flames, undetermined intent**

√4th **Y27 Contact with steam, hot vapors and hot objects, undetermined intent**

√x7th Y27.0 **Contact with steam and hot vapors, undetermined intent**

√x7th Y27.1 **Contact with hot tap water, undetermined intent**

√x7th Y27.2 **Contact with hot fluids, undetermined intent**

√x7th Y27.3 **Contact with hot household appliance, undetermined intent**

√x7th Y27.8 **Contact with other hot objects, undetermined intent**

√x7th Y27.9 **Contact with unspecified hot objects, undetermined intent**

√4th **Y28 Contact with sharp object, undetermined intent**

√x7th Y28.0 **Contact with sharp glass, undetermined intent**

√x7th Y28.1 **Contact with knife, undetermined intent**

√x7th Y28.2 **Contact with sword or dagger, undetermined intent**

√x7th Y28.8 **Contact with other sharp object, undetermined intent**

√x7th Y28.9 **Contact with unspecified sharp object, undetermined intent**

√x7th **Y29 Contact with blunt object, undetermined intent**

√x7th **Y30 Falling, jumping or pushed from a high place, undetermined intent**

Victim falling from one level to another, undetermined intent

√x7th **Y31 Falling, lying or running before or into moving object, undetermined intent**

√x7th **Y32 Crashing of motor vehicle, undetermined intent**

√x7th **Y33 Other specified events, undetermined intent**

## Legal intervention, operations of war, military operations, and terrorism (Y35-Y38)

The appropriate 7th character is to be added to each code from categories Y35-Y38.
A initial encounter
D subsequent encounter
S sequela

**4th Y35 Legal intervention**

INCLUDES any injury sustained as a result of an encounter with any law enforcement official, serving in any capacity at the time of the encounter, whether on-duty or off-duty. Includes injury to law enforcement official, suspect and bystander

AHA: 2019,4Q,18-19

**5th Y35.0 Legal intervention involving firearm discharge**

**6th Y35.00 Legal intervention involving unspecified firearm discharge**
Legal intervention involving gunshot wound
Legal intervention involving shot NOS

**7th Y35.001 Legal intervention involving unspecified firearm discharge, law enforcement official injured**
**7th Y35.002 Legal intervention involving unspecified firearm discharge, bystander injured**
**7th Y35.003 Legal intervention involving unspecified firearm discharge, suspect injured**
**7th Y35.009 Legal intervention involving unspecified firearm discharge, unspecified person injured**

**6th Y35.01 Legal intervention involving injury by machine gun**
**7th Y35.011 Legal intervention involving injury by machine gun, law enforcement official injured**
**7th Y35.012 Legal intervention involving injury by machine gun, bystander injured**
**7th Y35.013 Legal intervention involving injury by machine gun, suspect injured**
**7th Y35.019 Legal intervention involving injury by machine gun, unspecified person injured**

**6th Y35.02 Legal intervention involving injury by handgun**
**7th Y35.021 Legal intervention involving injury by handgun, law enforcement official injured**
**7th Y35.022 Legal intervention involving injury by handgun, bystander injured**
**7th Y35.023 Legal intervention involving injury by handgun, suspect injured**
**7th Y35.029 Legal intervention involving injury by handgun, unspecified person injured**

**6th Y35.03 Legal intervention involving injury by rifle pellet**
**7th Y35.031 Legal intervention involving injury by rifle pellet, law enforcement official injured**
**7th Y35.032 Legal intervention involving injury by rifle pellet, bystander injured**
**7th Y35.033 Legal intervention involving injury by rifle pellet, suspect injured**
**7th Y35.039 Legal intervention involving injury by rifle pellet, unspecified person injured**

**6th Y35.04 Legal intervention involving injury by rubber bullet**
**7th Y35.041 Legal intervention involving injury by rubber bullet, law enforcement official injured**
**7th Y35.042 Legal intervention involving injury by rubber bullet, bystander injured**
**7th Y35.043 Legal intervention involving injury by rubber bullet, suspect injured**
**7th Y35.049 Legal intervention involving injury by rubber bullet, unspecified person injured**

**6th Y35.09 Legal intervention involving other firearm discharge**
**7th Y35.091 Legal intervention involving other firearm discharge, law enforcement official injured**
**7th Y35.092 Legal intervention involving other firearm discharge, bystander injured**
**7th Y35.093 Legal intervention involving other firearm discharge, suspect injured**
**7th Y35.099 Legal intervention involving other firearm discharge, unspecified person injured**

**5th Y35.1 Legal intervention involving explosives**

**6th Y35.10 Legal intervention involving unspecified explosives**
**7th Y35.101 Legal intervention involving unspecified explosives, law enforcement official injured**
**7th Y35.102 Legal intervention involving unspecified explosives, bystander injured**
**7th Y35.103 Legal intervention involving unspecified explosives, suspect injured**
**7th Y35.109 Legal intervention involving unspecified explosives, unspecified person injured**

**6th Y35.11 Legal intervention involving injury by dynamite**
**7th Y35.111 Legal intervention involving injury by dynamite, law enforcement official injured**
**7th Y35.112 Legal intervention involving injury by dynamite, bystander injured**
**7th Y35.113 Legal intervention involving injury by dynamite, suspect injured**
**7th Y35.119 Legal intervention involving injury by dynamite, unspecified person injured**

**6th Y35.12 Legal intervention involving injury by explosive shell**
**7th Y35.121 Legal intervention involving injury by explosive shell, law enforcement official injured**
**7th Y35.122 Legal intervention involving injury by explosive shell, bystander injured**
**7th Y35.123 Legal intervention involving injury by explosive shell, suspect injured**
**7th Y35.129 Legal intervention involving injury by explosive shell, unspecified person injured**

**6th Y35.19 Legal intervention involving other explosives**
Legal intervention involving injury by grenade
Legal intervention involving injury by mortar bomb

**7th Y35.191 Legal intervention involving other explosives, law enforcement official injured**
**7th Y35.192 Legal intervention involving other explosives, bystander injured**
**7th Y35.193 Legal intervention involving other explosives, suspect injured**
**7th Y35.199 Legal intervention involving other explosives, unspecified person injured**

**5th Y35.2 Legal intervention involving gas**
Legal intervention involving asphyxiation by gas
Legal intervention involving poisoning by gas

**6th Y35.20 Legal intervention involving unspecified gas**
**7th Y35.201 Legal intervention involving unspecified gas, law enforcement official injured**
**7th Y35.202 Legal intervention involving unspecified gas, bystander injured**
**7th Y35.203 Legal intervention involving unspecified gas, suspect injured**
**7th Y35.209 Legal intervention involving unspecified gas, unspecified person injured**

**6th Y35.21 Legal intervention involving injury by tear gas**
**7th Y35.211 Legal intervention involving injury by tear gas, law enforcement official injured**
**7th Y35.212 Legal intervention involving injury by tear gas, bystander injured**
**7th Y35.213 Legal intervention involving injury by tear gas, suspect injured**
**7th Y35.219 Legal intervention involving injury by tear gas, unspecified person injured**

**6th Y35.29 Legal intervention involving other gas**
**7th Y35.291 Legal intervention involving other gas, law enforcement official injured**
**7th Y35.292 Legal intervention involving other gas, bystander injured**
**7th Y35.293 Legal intervention involving other gas, suspect injured**
**7th Y35.299 Legal intervention involving other gas, unspecified person injured**

**5th Y35.3 Legal intervention involving blunt objects**
Legal intervention involving being hit or struck by blunt object

**6th Y35.30 Legal intervention involving unspecified blunt objects**
**7th Y35.301 Legal intervention involving unspecified blunt objects, law enforcement official injured**
**7th Y35.302 Legal intervention involving unspecified blunt objects, bystander injured**

√7th Y35.303 Legal intervention involving unspecified blunt objects, suspect injured
√7th Y35.309 Legal intervention involving unspecified blunt objects, unspecified person injured
√6th Y35.31 Legal intervention involving baton
√7th Y35.311 Legal intervention involving baton, law enforcement official injured
√7th Y35.312 Legal intervention involving baton, bystander injured
√7th Y35.313 Legal intervention involving baton, suspect injured
√7th Y35.319 Legal intervention involving baton, unspecified person injured
√6th Y35.39 Legal intervention involving other blunt objects
√7th Y35.391 Legal intervention involving other blunt objects, law enforcement official injured
√7th Y35.392 Legal intervention involving other blunt objects, bystander injured
√7th Y35.393 Legal intervention involving other blunt objects, suspect injured
√7th Y35.399 Legal intervention involving other blunt objects, unspecified person injured
√5th Y35.4 Legal intervention involving sharp objects
Legal intervention involving being cut by sharp objects
Legal intervention involving being stabbed by sharp objects
√6th Y35.40 Legal intervention involving unspecified sharp objects
√7th Y35.401 Legal intervention involving unspecified sharp objects, law enforcement official injured
√7th Y35.402 Legal intervention involving unspecified sharp objects, bystander injured
√7th Y35.403 Legal intervention involving unspecified sharp objects, suspect injured
√7th Y35.409 Legal intervention involving unspecified sharp objects, unspecified person injured
√6th Y35.41 Legal intervention involving bayonet
√7th Y35.411 Legal intervention involving bayonet, law enforcement official injured
√7th Y35.412 Legal intervention involving bayonet, bystander injured
√7th Y35.413 Legal intervention involving bayonet, suspect injured
√7th Y35.419 Legal intervention involving bayonet, unspecified person injured
√6th Y35.49 Legal intervention involving other sharp objects
√7th Y35.491 Legal intervention involving other sharp objects, law enforcement official injured
√7th Y35.492 Legal intervention involving other sharp objects, bystander injured
√7th Y35.493 Legal intervention involving other sharp objects, suspect injured
√7th Y35.499 Legal intervention involving other sharp objects, unspecified person injured
√5th Y35.8 Legal intervention involving other specified means
AHA: 2019,4Q,19
√6th Y35.81 Legal intervention involving manhandling
√7th Y35.811 Legal intervention involving manhandling, law enforcement official injured
√7th Y35.812 Legal intervention involving manhandling, bystander injured
√7th Y35.813 Legal intervention involving manhandling, suspect injured
√7th Y35.819 Legal intervention involving manhandling, unspecified person injured
√6th Y35.83 Legal intervention involving a conducted energy device
Electroshock device (taser)
Stun gun
√7th Y35.831 Legal intervention involving a conducted energy device, law enforcement official injured
√7th Y35.832 Legal intervention involving a conducted energy device, bystander injured
√7th Y35.833 Legal intervention involving a conducted energy device, suspect injured
√7th Y35.839 Legal intervention involving a conducted energy device, unspecified person injured
√6th Y35.89 Legal intervention involving other specified means
√7th Y35.891 Legal intervention involving other specified means, law enforcement official injured
√7th Y35.892 Legal intervention involving other specified means, bystander injured
√7th Y35.893 Legal intervention involving other specified means, suspect injured
AHA: 2018,1Q,5
√7th Y35.899 Legal intervention involving other specified means, unspecified person injured
√5th Y35.9 Legal intervention, means unspecified
√x7th Y35.91 Legal intervention, means unspecified, law enforcement official injured
√x7th Y35.92 Legal intervention, means unspecified, bystander injured
√x7th Y35.93 Legal intervention, means unspecified, suspect injured
√x7th Y35.99 Legal intervention, means unspecified, unspecified person injured

√4th **Y36 Operations of war**

INCLUDES injuries to military personnel and civilians caused by war, civil insurrection, and peacekeeping missions

EXCLUDES 1 *injury to military personnel occurring during peacetime military operations (Y37.-)*
*military vehicles involved in transport accidents with non-military vehicle during peacetime (V09.01, V09.21, V19.81, V29.818, V39.81, V49.81, V59.81, V69.81, V79.81)*

AHA: 2014,3Q,4

√5th Y36.0 War operations involving explosion of marine weapons
√6th Y36.00 War operations involving explosion of unspecified marine weapon
War operations involving underwater blast NOS
√7th Y36.000 War operations involving explosion of unspecified marine weapon, military personnel
√7th Y36.001 War operations involving explosion of unspecified marine weapon, civilian
√6th Y36.01 War operations involving explosion of depth-charge
√7th Y36.010 War operations involving explosion of depth-charge, military personnel
√7th Y36.011 War operations involving explosion of depth-charge, civilian
√6th Y36.02 War operations involving explosion of marine mine
War operations involving explosion of marine mine, at sea or in harbor
√7th Y36.020 War operations involving explosion of marine mine, military personnel
√7th Y36.021 War operations involving explosion of marine mine, civilian
√6th Y36.03 War operations involving explosion of sea-based artillery shell
√7th Y36.030 War operations involving explosion of sea-based artillery shell, military personnel
√7th Y36.031 War operations involving explosion of sea-based artillery shell, civilian
√6th Y36.04 War operations involving explosion of torpedo
√7th Y36.040 War operations involving explosion of torpedo, military personnel
√7th Y36.041 War operations involving explosion of torpedo, civilian
√6th Y36.05 War operations involving accidental detonation of onboard marine weapons
√7th Y36.050 War operations involving accidental detonation of onboard marine weapons, military personnel
√7th Y36.051 War operations involving accidental detonation of onboard marine weapons, civilian
√6th Y36.09 War operations involving explosion of other marine weapons
√7th Y36.090 War operations involving explosion of other marine weapons, military personnel
√7th Y36.091 War operations involving explosion of other marine weapons, civilian

√5th **Y36.1 War operations involving destruction of aircraft**

√6th **Y36.10 War operations involving unspecified destruction of aircraft**

√7th **Y36.100 War operations involving unspecified destruction of aircraft, military personnel**

√7th **Y36.101 War operations involving unspecified destruction of aircraft, civilian**

√6th **Y36.11 War operations involving destruction of aircraft due to enemy fire or explosives**

War operations involving destruction of aircraft due to air to air missile
War operations involving destruction of aircraft due to explosive placed on aircraft
War operations involving destruction of aircraft due to rocket propelled grenade [RPG]
War operations involving destruction of aircraft due to small arms fire
War operations involving destruction of aircraft due to surface to air missile

√7th **Y36.110 War operations involving destruction of aircraft due to enemy fire or explosives, military personnel**

√7th **Y36.111 War operations involving destruction of aircraft due to enemy fire or explosives, civilian**

√6th **Y36.12 War operations involving destruction of aircraft due to collision with other aircraft**

√7th **Y36.120 War operations involving destruction of aircraft due to collision with other aircraft, military personnel**

√7th **Y36.121 War operations involving destruction of aircraft due to collision with other aircraft, civilian**

√6th **Y36.13 War operations involving destruction of aircraft due to onboard fire**

√7th **Y36.130 War operations involving destruction of aircraft due to onboard fire, military personnel**

√7th **Y36.131 War operations involving destruction of aircraft due to onboard fire, civilian**

√6th **Y36.14 War operations involving destruction of aircraft due to accidental detonation of onboard munitions and explosives**

√7th **Y36.140 War operations involving destruction of aircraft due to accidental detonation of onboard munitions and explosives, military personnel**

√7th **Y36.141 War operations involving destruction of aircraft due to accidental detonation of onboard munitions and explosives, civilian**

√6th **Y36.19 War operations involving other destruction of aircraft**

√7th **Y36.190 War operations involving other destruction of aircraft, military personnel**

√7th **Y36.191 War operations involving other destruction of aircraft, civilian**

√5th **Y36.2 War operations involving other explosions and fragments**

EXCLUDES 1 *war operations involving explosion of aircraft (Y36.1-)*
*war operations involving explosion of marine weapons (Y36.0-)*
*war operations involving explosion of nuclear weapons (Y36.5-)*
*war operations involving explosion occurring after cessation of hostilities (Y36.8-)*

√6th **Y36.20 War operations involving unspecified explosion and fragments**

War operations involving air blast NOS
War operations involving blast fragments NOS
War operations involving blast NOS
War operations involving blast wave NOS
War operations involving blast wind NOS
War operations involving explosion of bomb NOS
War operations involving explosion NOS

√7th **Y36.200 War operations involving unspecified explosion and fragments, military personnel**

√7th **Y36.201 War operations involving unspecified explosion and fragments, civilian**

√6th **Y36.21 War operations involving explosion of aerial bomb**

√7th **Y36.210 War operations involving explosion of aerial bomb, military personnel**

√7th **Y36.211 War operations involving explosion of aerial bomb, civilian**

√6th **Y36.22 War operations involving explosion of guided missile**

√7th **Y36.220 War operations involving explosion of guided missile, military personnel**

√7th **Y36.221 War operations involving explosion of guided missile, civilian**

√6th **Y36.23 War operations involving explosion of improvised explosive device [IED]**

War operations involving explosion of person-borne improvised explosive device [IED]
War operations involving explosion of roadside improvised explosive device [IED]
War operations involving explosion of vehicle-borne improvised explosive device [IED]

√7th **Y36.230 War operations involving explosion of improvised explosive device [IED], military personnel**

√7th **Y36.231 War operations involving explosion of improvised explosive device [IED], civilian**

√6th **Y36.24 War operations involving explosion due to accidental detonation and discharge of own munitions or munitions launch device**

√7th **Y36.240 War operations involving explosion due to accidental detonation and discharge of own munitions or munitions launch device, military personnel**

√7th **Y36.241 War operations involving explosion due to accidental detonation and discharge of own munitions or munitions launch device, civilian**

√6th **Y36.25 War operations involving fragments from munitions**

√7th **Y36.250 War operations involving fragments from munitions, military personnel**

√7th **Y36.251 War operations involving fragments from munitions, civilian**

√6th **Y36.26 War operations involving fragments of improvised explosive device [IED]**

War operations involving fragments of person-borne improvised explosive device [IED]
War operations involving fragments of roadside improvised explosive device [IED]
War operations involving fragments of vehicle-borne improvised explosive device [IED]

√7th **Y36.260 War operations involving fragments of improvised explosive device [IED], military personnel**

√7th **Y36.261 War operations involving fragments of improvised explosive device [IED], civilian**

√6th **Y36.27 War operations involving fragments from weapons**

√7th **Y36.270 War operations involving fragments from weapons, military personnel**

√7th **Y36.271 War operations involving fragments from weapons, civilian**

√6th **Y36.29 War operations involving other explosions and fragments**

War operations involving explosion of grenade
War operations involving explosions of land mine
War operations involving shrapnel NOS

√7th **Y36.290 War operations involving other explosions and fragments, military personnel**

√7th **Y36.291 War operations involving other explosions and fragments, civilian**

√5th **Y36.3 War operations involving fires, conflagrations and hot substances**

War operations involving smoke, fumes, and heat from fires, conflagrations and hot substances

EXCLUDES 1 *war operations involving fires and conflagrations aboard military aircraft (Y36.1-)*
*war operations involving fires and conflagrations aboard military watercraft (Y36.0-)*
*war operations involving fires and conflagrations caused indirectly by conventional weapons (Y36.2-)*
*war operations involving fires and thermal effects of nuclear weapons (Y36.53-)*

√6th **Y36.30 War operations involving unspecified fire, conflagration and hot substance**

√7th **Y36.300 War operations involving unspecified fire, conflagration and hot substance, military personnel**

√7th **Y36.301 War operations involving unspecified fire, conflagration and hot substance, civilian**

√6th **Y36.31 War operations involving gasoline bomb**
War operations involving incendiary bomb
War operations involving petrol bomb
√7th **Y36.31Ø War operations involving gasoline bomb, military personnel**
√7th **Y36.311 War operations involving gasoline bomb, civilian**
√6th **Y36.32 War operations involving incendiary bullet**
√7th **Y36.32Ø War operations involving incendiary bullet, military personnel**
√7th **Y36.321 War operations involving incendiary bullet, civilian**
√6th **Y36.33 War operations involving flamethrower**
√7th **Y36.33Ø War operations involving flamethrower, military personnel**
√7th **Y36.331 War operations involving flamethrower, civilian**
√6th **Y36.39 War operations involving other fires, conflagrations and hot substances**
√7th **Y36.39Ø War operations involving other fires, conflagrations and hot substances, military personnel**
√7th **Y36.391 War operations involving other fires, conflagrations and hot substances, civilian**
√5th **Y36.4 War operations involving firearm discharge and other forms of conventional warfare**
√6th **Y36.41 War operations involving rubber bullets**
√7th **Y36.41Ø War operations involving rubber bullets, military personnel**
√7th **Y36.411 War operations involving rubber bullets, civilian**
√6th **Y36.42 War operations involving firearms pellets**
√7th **Y36.42Ø War operations involving firearms pellets, military personnel**
√7th **Y36.421 War operations involving firearms pellets, civilian**
√6th **Y36.43 War operations involving other firearms discharge**
War operations involving bullets NOS
EXCLUDES 1 *war operations involving munitions fragments (Y36.25-)*
*war operations involving incendiary bullets (Y36.32-)*
√7th **Y36.43Ø War operations involving other firearms discharge, military personnel**
√7th **Y36.431 War operations involving other firearms discharge, civilian**
√6th **Y36.44 War operations involving unarmed hand to hand combat**
EXCLUDES 1 *war operations involving combat using blunt or piercing object (Y36.45-)*
*war operations involving intentional restriction of air and airway (Y36.46-)*
*war operations involving unintentional restriction of air and airway (Y36.47-)*
√7th **Y36.44Ø War operations involving unarmed hand to hand combat, military personnel**
√7th **Y36.441 War operations involving unarmed hand to hand combat, civilian**
√6th **Y36.45 War operations involving combat using blunt or piercing object**
√7th **Y36.45Ø War operations involving combat using blunt or piercing object, military personnel**
√7th **Y36.451 War operations involving combat using blunt or piercing object, civilian**
√6th **Y36.46 War operations involving intentional restriction of air and airway**
√7th **Y36.46Ø War operations involving intentional restriction of air and airway, military personnel**
√7th **Y36.461 War operations involving intentional restriction of air and airway, civilian**
√6th **Y36.47 War operations involving unintentional restriction of air and airway**
√7th **Y36.47Ø War operations involving unintentional restriction of air and airway, military personnel**
√7th **Y36.471 War operations involving unintentional restriction of air and airway, civilian**
√6th **Y36.49 War operations involving other forms of conventional warfare**
√7th **Y36.49Ø War operations involving other forms of conventional warfare, military personnel**
√7th **Y36.491 War operations involving other forms of conventional warfare, civilian**
√5th **Y36.5 War operations involving nuclear weapons**
War operations involving dirty bomb NOS
√6th **Y36.5Ø War operations involving unspecified effect of nuclear weapon**
√7th **Y36.5ØØ War operations involving unspecified effect of nuclear weapon, military personnel**
√7th **Y36.5Ø1 War operations involving unspecified effect of nuclear weapon, civilian**
√6th **Y36.51 War operations involving direct blast effect of nuclear weapon**
War operations involving blast pressure of nuclear weapon
√7th **Y36.51Ø War operations involving direct blast effect of nuclear weapon, military personnel**
√7th **Y36.511 War operations involving direct blast effect of nuclear weapon, civilian**
√6th **Y36.52 War operations involving indirect blast effect of nuclear weapon**
War operations involving being struck or crushed by blast debris of nuclear weapon
War operations involving being thrown by blast of nuclear weapon
√7th **Y36.52Ø War operations involving indirect blast effect of nuclear weapon, military personnel**
√7th **Y36.521 War operations involving indirect blast effect of nuclear weapon, civilian**
√6th **Y36.53 War operations involving thermal radiation effect of nuclear weapon**
War operation involving fireball effects from nuclear weapon
War operations involving direct heat from nuclear weapon
√7th **Y36.53Ø War operations involving thermal radiation effect of nuclear weapon, military personnel**
√7th **Y36.531 War operations involving thermal radiation effect of nuclear weapon, civilian**
√6th **Y36.54 War operation involving nuclear radiation effects of nuclear weapon**
War operation involving acute radiation exposure from nuclear weapon
War operation involving exposure to immediate ionizing radiation from nuclear weapon
War operation involving fallout exposure from nuclear weapon
War operation involving secondary effects of nuclear weapons
√7th **Y36.54Ø War operation involving nuclear radiation effects of nuclear weapon, military personnel**
√7th **Y36.541 War operation involving nuclear radiation effects of nuclear weapon, civilian**
√6th **Y36.59 War operation involving other effects of nuclear weapons**
√7th **Y36.59Ø War operation involving other effects of nuclear weapons, military personnel**
√7th **Y36.591 War operation involving other effects of nuclear weapons, civilian**
√5th **Y36.6 War operations involving biological weapons**
√6th **Y36.6X War operations involving biological weapons**
√7th **Y36.6XØ War operations involving biological weapons, military personnel**
√7th **Y36.6X1 War operations involving biological weapons, civilian**
√5th **Y36.7 War operations involving chemical weapons and other forms of unconventional warfare**
EXCLUDES 1 *war operations involving incendiary devices (Y36.3-, Y36.5-)*
√6th **Y36.7X War operations involving chemical weapons and other forms of unconventional warfare**
√7th **Y36.7XØ War operations involving chemical weapons and other forms of unconventional warfare, military personnel**

Y36.7X1 **War operations involving chemical weapons and other forms of unconventional warfare, civilian**

Y36.8 **War operations occurring after cessation of hostilities**
War operations classifiable to categories Y36.Ø-Y36.8 but occurring after cessation of hostilities

Y36.81 **Explosion of mine placed during war operations but exploding after cessation of hostilities**

Y36.81Ø **Explosion of mine placed during war operations but exploding after cessation of hostilities, military personnel**

Y36.811 **Explosion of mine placed during war operations but exploding after cessation of hostilities, civilian**

Y36.82 **Explosion of bomb placed during war operations but exploding after cessation of hostilities**

Y36.82Ø **Explosion of bomb placed during war operations but exploding after cessation of hostilities, military personnel**

Y36.821 **Explosion of bomb placed during war operations but exploding after cessation of hostilities, civilian**

Y36.88 **Other war operations occurring after cessation of hostilities**

Y36.88Ø **Other war operations occurring after cessation of hostilities, military personnel**

Y36.881 **Other war operations occurring after cessation of hostilities, civilian**

Y36.89 **Unspecified war operations occurring after cessation of hostilities**

Y36.89Ø **Unspecified war operations occurring after cessation of hostilities, military personnel**

Y36.891 **Unspecified war operations occurring after cessation of hostilities, civilian**

Y36.9 **Other and unspecified war operations**

Y36.9Ø **War operations, unspecified**

Y36.91 **War operations involving unspecified weapon of mass destruction [WMD]**

Y36.92 **War operations involving friendly fire**

Y36.A **Blast overpressure in war operations**
Code also type of explosive, if known
accidental detonation of onboard munitions (Y36.14Ø)
explosion of grenade (Y36.29Ø)
explosion of torpedo (Y36.Ø4Ø)
improvised explosive device (Y36.23Ø)

Y36.A1 **Low level blast overpressure in war operations**
LLB overpressure in war operations
Low level blast overpressure due to explosion in war operations

Y36.A2 **High level blast overpressure in war operations**
High level blast overpressure due to explosion in war operations
HLB overpressure in war operations

## Y37 Military operations

INCLUDES injuries to military personnel and civilians occurring during peacetime on military property and during routine military exercises and operations

EXCLUDES 1 *military aircraft involved in aircraft accident with civilian aircraft (V97.81-)*
*military vehicles involved in transport accident with civilian vehicle (VØ9.Ø1, VØ9.21, V19.81, V29.818, V39.81, V49.81, V59.81, V69.81, V79.81)*
*military watercraft involved in water transport accident with civilian watercraft (V94.81-)*
*war operations (Y36.-)*

Y37.Ø **Military operations involving explosion of marine weapons**

Y37.ØØ **Military operations involving explosion of unspecified marine weapon**
Military operations involving underwater blast NOS

Y37.ØØØ **Military operations involving explosion of unspecified marine weapon, military personnel**

Y37.ØØ1 **Military operations involving explosion of unspecified marine weapon, civilian**

Y37.Ø1 **Military operations involving explosion of depth-charge**

Y37.Ø1Ø **Military operations involving explosion of depth-charge, military personnel**

Y37.Ø11 **Military operations involving explosion of depth-charge, civilian**

Y37.Ø2 **Military operations involving explosion of marine mine**
Military operations involving explosion of marine mine, at sea or in harbor

Y37.Ø2Ø **Military operations involving explosion of marine mine, military personnel**

Y37.Ø21 **Military operations involving explosion of marine mine, civilian**

Y37.Ø3 **Military operations involving explosion of sea-based artillery shell**

Y37.Ø3Ø **Military operations involving explosion of sea-based artillery shell, military personnel**

Y37.Ø31 **Military operations involving explosion of sea-based artillery shell, civilian**

Y37.Ø4 **Military operations involving explosion of torpedo**

Y37.Ø4Ø **Military operations involving explosion of torpedo, military personnel**

Y37.Ø41 **Military operations involving explosion of torpedo, civilian**

Y37.Ø5 **Military operations involving accidental detonation of onboard marine weapons**

Y37.Ø5Ø **Military operations involving accidental detonation of onboard marine weapons, military personnel**

Y37.Ø51 **Military operations involving accidental detonation of onboard marine weapons, civilian**

Y37.Ø9 **Military operations involving explosion of other marine weapons**

Y37.Ø9Ø **Military operations involving explosion of other marine weapons, military personnel**

Y37.Ø91 **Military operations involving explosion of other marine weapons, civilian**

Y37.1 **Military operations involving destruction of aircraft**

Y37.1Ø **Military operations involving unspecified destruction of aircraft**

Y37.1ØØ **Military operations involving unspecified destruction of aircraft, military personnel**

Y37.1Ø1 **Military operations involving unspecified destruction of aircraft, civilian**

Y37.11 **Military operations involving destruction of aircraft due to enemy fire or explosives**
Military operations involving destruction of aircraft due to air to air missile
Military operations involving destruction of aircraft due to explosive placed on aircraft
Military operations involving destruction of aircraft due to rocket propelled grenade [RPG]
Military operations involving destruction of aircraft due to small arms fire
Military operations involving destruction of aircraft due to surface to air missile

Y37.11Ø **Military operations involving destruction of aircraft due to enemy fire or explosives, military personnel**

Y37.111 **Military operations involving destruction of aircraft due to enemy fire or explosives, civilian**

Y37.12 **Military operations involving destruction of aircraft due to collision with other aircraft**

Y37.12Ø **Military operations involving destruction of aircraft due to collision with other aircraft, military personnel**

Y37.121 **Military operations involving destruction of aircraft due to collision with other aircraft, civilian**

Y37.13 **Military operations involving destruction of aircraft due to onboard fire**

Y37.13Ø **Military operations involving destruction of aircraft due to onboard fire, military personnel**

Y37.131 **Military operations involving destruction of aircraft due to onboard fire, civilian**

Y37.14 **Military operations involving destruction of aircraft due to accidental detonation of onboard munitions and explosives**

Y37.14Ø **Military operations involving destruction of aircraft due to accidental detonation of onboard munitions and explosives, military personnel**

Y37.141 **Military operations involving destruction of aircraft due to accidental detonation of onboard munitions and explosives, civilian**

**Y37.19 Military operations involving other destruction of aircraft**

**Y37.19Ø Military operations involving other destruction of aircraft, military personnel**

**Y37.191 Military operations involving other destruction of aircraft, civilian**

**Y37.2 Military operations involving other explosions and fragments**

EXCLUDES 1 *military operations involving explosion of aircraft (Y37.1-)*
*military operations involving explosion of marine weapons (Y37.Ø-)*
*military operations involving explosion of nuclear weapons (Y37.5-)*

**Y37.2Ø Military operations involving unspecified explosion and fragments**

Military operations involving air blast NOS
Military operations involving blast fragments NOS
Military operations involving blast NOS
Military operations involving blast wave NOS
Military operations involving blast wind NOS
Military operations involving explosion of bomb NOS
Military operations involving explosion NOS

**Y37.2ØØ Military operations involving unspecified explosion and fragments, military personnel**

**Y37.2Ø1 Military operations involving unspecified explosion and fragments, civilian**

**Y37.21 Military operations involving explosion of aerial bomb**

**Y37.21Ø Military operations involving explosion of aerial bomb, military personnel**

**Y37.211 Military operations involving explosion of aerial bomb, civilian**

**Y37.22 Military operations involving explosion of guided missile**

**Y37.22Ø Military operations involving explosion of guided missile, military personnel**

**Y37.221 Military operations involving explosion of guided missile, civilian**

**Y37.23 Military operations involving explosion of improvised explosive device [IED]**

Military operations involving explosion of person-borne improvised explosive device [IED]
Military operations involving explosion of roadside improvised explosive device [IED]
Military operations involving explosion of vehicle-borne improvised explosive device [IED]

**Y37.23Ø Military operations involving explosion of improvised explosive device [IED], military personnel**

**Y37.231 Military operations involving explosion of improvised explosive device [IED], civilian**

**Y37.24 Military operations involving explosion due to accidental detonation and discharge of own munitions or munitions launch device**

**Y37.24Ø Military operations involving explosion due to accidental detonation and discharge of own munitions or munitions launch device, military personnel**

**Y37.241 Military operations involving explosion due to accidental detonation and discharge of own munitions or munitions launch device, civilian**

**Y37.25 Military operations involving fragments from munitions**

**Y37.25Ø Military operations involving fragments from munitions, military personnel**

**Y37.251 Military operations involving fragments from munitions, civilian**

**Y37.26 Military operations involving fragments of improvised explosive device [IED]**

Military operations involving fragments of person-borne improvised explosive device [IED]
Military operations involving fragments of roadside improvised explosive device [IED]
Military operations involving fragments of vehicle-borne improvised explosive device [IED]

**Y37.26Ø Military operations involving fragments of improvised explosive device [IED], military personnel**

**Y37.261 Military operations involving fragments of improvised explosive device [IED], civilian**

**Y37.27 Military operations involving fragments from weapons**

**Y37.27Ø Military operations involving fragments from weapons, military personnel**

**Y37.271 Military operations involving fragments from weapons, civilian**

**Y37.29 Military operations involving other explosions and fragments**

Military operations involving explosion of grenade
Military operations involving explosions of land mine
Military operations involving shrapnel NOS

**Y37.29Ø Military operations involving other explosions and fragments, military personnel**

**Y37.291 Military operations involving other explosions and fragments, civilian**

**Y37.3 Military operations involving fires, conflagrations and hot substances**

Military operations involving smoke, fumes, and heat from fires, conflagrations and hot substances

EXCLUDES 1 *military operations involving fires and conflagrations aboard military aircraft (Y37.1-)*
*military operations involving fires and conflagrations aboard military watercraft (Y37.Ø-)*
*military operations involving fires and conflagrations caused indirectly by conventional weapons (Y37.2-)*
*military operations involving fires and thermal effects of nuclear weapons (Y36.53-)*

**Y37.3Ø Military operations involving unspecified fire, conflagration and hot substance**

**Y37.3ØØ Military operations involving unspecified fire, conflagration and hot substance, military personnel**

**Y37.3Ø1 Military operations involving unspecified fire, conflagration and hot substance, civilian**

**Y37.31 Military operations involving gasoline bomb**

Military operations involving incendiary bomb
Military operations involving petrol bomb

**Y37.31Ø Military operations involving gasoline bomb, military personnel**

**Y37.311 Military operations involving gasoline bomb, civilian**

**Y37.32 Military operations involving incendiary bullet**

**Y37.32Ø Military operations involving incendiary bullet, military personnel**

**Y37.321 Military operations involving incendiary bullet, civilian**

**Y37.33 Military operations involving flamethrower**

**Y37.33Ø Military operations involving flamethrower, military personnel**

**Y37.331 Military operations involving flamethrower, civilian**

**Y37.39 Military operations involving other fires, conflagrations and hot substances**

**Y37.39Ø Military operations involving other fires, conflagrations and hot substances, military personnel**

**Y37.391 Military operations involving other fires, conflagrations and hot substances, civilian**

**Y37.4 Military operations involving firearm discharge and other forms of conventional warfare**

**Y37.41 Military operations involving rubber bullets**

**Y37.41Ø Military operations involving rubber bullets, military personnel**

**Y37.411 Military operations involving rubber bullets, civilian**

**Y37.42 Military operations involving firearms pellets**

**Y37.42Ø Military operations involving firearms pellets, military personnel**

**Y37.421 Military operations involving firearms pellets, civilian**

**Y37.43 Military operations involving other firearms discharge**

Military operations involving bullets NOS

EXCLUDES 1 *military operations involving munitions fragments (Y37.25-)*
*military operations involving incendiary bullets (Y37.32-)*

**Y37.43Ø Military operations involving other firearms discharge, military personnel**

Y37.431 **Military operations involving other firearms discharge, civilian**

Y37.44 **Military operations involving unarmed hand to hand combat**

EXCLUDES 1 *military operations involving combat using blunt or piercing object (Y37.45-)*
*military operations involving intentional restriction of air and airway (Y37.46-)*
*military operations involving unintentional restriction of air and airway (Y37.47-)*

Y37.44Ø **Military operations involving unarmed hand to hand combat, military personnel**

Y37.441 **Military operations involving unarmed hand to hand combat, civilian**

Y37.45 **Military operations involving combat using blunt or piercing object**

Y37.45Ø **Military operations involving combat using blunt or piercing object, military personnel**

Y37.451 **Military operations involving combat using blunt or piercing object, civilian**

Y37.46 **Military operations involving intentional restriction of air and airway**

Y37.46Ø **Military operations involving intentional restriction of air and airway, military personnel**

Y37.461 **Military operations involving intentional restriction of air and airway, civilian**

Y37.47 **Military operations involving unintentional restriction of air and airway**

Y37.47Ø **Military operations involving unintentional restriction of air and airway, military personnel**

Y37.471 **Military operations involving unintentional restriction of air and airway, civilian**

Y37.49 **Military operations involving other forms of conventional warfare**

Y37.49Ø **Military operations involving other forms of conventional warfare, military personnel**

Y37.491 **Military operations involving other forms of conventional warfare, civilian**

Y37.5 **Military operations involving nuclear weapons**

Military operation involving dirty bomb NOS

Y37.5Ø **Military operations involving unspecified effect of nuclear weapon**

Y37.5ØØ **Military operations involving unspecified effect of nuclear weapon, military personnel**

Y37.5Ø1 **Military operations involving unspecified effect of nuclear weapon, civilian**

Y37.51 **Military operations involving direct blast effect of nuclear weapon**

Military operations involving blast pressure of nuclear weapon

Y37.51Ø **Military operations involving direct blast effect of nuclear weapon, military personnel**

Y37.511 **Military operations involving direct blast effect of nuclear weapon, civilian**

Y37.52 **Military operations involving indirect blast effect of nuclear weapon**

Military operations involving being struck or crushed by blast debris of nuclear weapon
Military operations involving being thrown by blast of nuclear weapon

Y37.52Ø **Military operations involving indirect blast effect of nuclear weapon, military personnel**

Y37.521 **Military operations involving indirect blast effect of nuclear weapon, civilian**

Y37.53 **Military operations involving thermal radiation effect of nuclear weapon**

Military operation involving fireball effects from nuclear weapon
Military operations involving direct heat from nuclear weapon

Y37.53Ø **Military operations involving thermal radiation effect of nuclear weapon, military personnel**

Y37.531 **Military operations involving thermal radiation effect of nuclear weapon, civilian**

Y37.54 **Military operation involving nuclear radiation effects of nuclear weapon**

Military operation involving acute radiation exposure from nuclear weapon
Military operation involving exposure to immediate ionizing radiation from nuclear weapon
Military operation involving fallout exposure from nuclear weapon
Military operation involving secondary effects of nuclear weapons

Y37.54Ø **Military operation involving nuclear radiation effects of nuclear weapon, military personnel**

Y37.541 **Military operation involving nuclear radiation effects of nuclear weapon, civilian**

Y37.59 **Military operation involving other effects of nuclear weapons**

Y37.59Ø **Military operation involving other effects of nuclear weapons, military personnel**

Y37.591 **Military operation involving other effects of nuclear weapons, civilian**

Y37.6 **Military operations involving biological weapons**

Y37.6X **Military operations involving biological weapons**

Y37.6XØ **Military operations involving biological weapons, military personnel**

Y37.6X1 **Military operations involving biological weapons, civilian**

Y37.7 **Military operations involving chemical weapons and other forms of unconventional warfare**

EXCLUDES 1 *military operations involving incendiary devices (Y36.3-, Y36.5-)*

Y37.7X **Military operations involving chemical weapons and other forms of unconventional warfare**

Y37.7XØ **Military operations involving chemical weapons and other forms of unconventional warfare, military personnel**

Y37.7X1 **Military operations involving chemical weapons and other forms of unconventional warfare, civilian**

Y37.9 **Other and unspecified military operations**

Y37.9Ø **Military operations, unspecified**

Y37.91 **Military operations involving unspecified weapon of mass destruction [WMD]**

Y37.92 **Military operations involving friendly fire**

Y37.A **Blast overpressure in military operations**

Code also type of explosive, if known
accidental detonation of onboard munitions (Y37.14Ø)
explosion of grenade (Y37.29Ø)
explosion of torpedo (Y37.Ø4Ø)
improvised explosive device (Y37.23Ø)

Y37.A1 **Low level blast overpressure in military operations**

LLB overpressure in military operations
Low level blast overpressure due to explosion in military operations

Y37.A2 **High level blast overpressure in military operations**

High level blast overpressure due to explosion in military operations
HLB overpressure in military operations

## Y38 Terrorism

NOTE These codes are for use to identify injuries resulting from the unlawful use of force or violence against persons or property to intimidate or coerce a Government, the civilian population, or any segment thereof, in furtherance of political or social objective

Use additional code for place of occurrence (Y92.-)

Y38.Ø **Terrorism involving explosion of marine weapons**

Terrorism involving depth-charge
Terrorism involving marine mine
Terrorism involving mine NOS, at sea or in harbor
Terrorism involving sea-based artillery shell
Terrorism involving torpedo
Terrorism involving underwater blast

Y38.ØX **Terrorism involving explosion of marine weapons**

Y38.ØX1 **Terrorism involving explosion of marine weapons, public safety official injured**

Y38.ØX2 **Terrorism involving explosion of marine weapons, civilian injured**

7th **Y38.ØX3 Terrorism involving explosion of marine weapons, terrorist injured**

5th **Y38.1 Terrorism involving destruction of aircraft**
Terrorism involving aircraft being shot down
Terrorism involving aircraft burned
Terrorism involving aircraft exploded
Terrorism involving aircraft used as a weapon

6th **Y38.1X Terrorism involving destruction of aircraft**

7th **Y38.1X1 Terrorism involving destruction of aircraft, public safety official injured**

7th **Y38.1X2 Terrorism involving destruction of aircraft, civilian injured**

7th **Y38.1X3 Terrorism involving destruction of aircraft, terrorist injured**

5th **Y38.2 Terrorism involving other explosions and fragments**
Terrorism involving antipersonnel (fragments) bomb
Terrorism involving blast NOS
Terrorism involving explosion (fragments) of artillery shell
Terrorism involving explosion (fragments) of bomb
Terrorism involving explosion (fragments) of grenade
Terrorism involving explosion (fragments) of guided missile
Terrorism involving explosion (fragments) of land mine
Terrorism involving explosion (fragments) of rocket
Terrorism involving explosion (fragments) of shell
Terrorism involving explosion of breech block
Terrorism involving explosion of cannon block
Terrorism involving explosion of mortar bomb
Terrorism involving explosion of munitions
Terrorism involving explosion NOS
Terrorism involving mine NOS, on land
Terrorism involving shrapnel

EXCLUDES 1 *terrorism involving explosion of nuclear weapon (Y38.5)*
*terrorism involving suicide bomber (Y38.81)*

6th **Y38.2X Terrorism involving other explosions and fragments**

7th **Y38.2X1 Terrorism involving other explosions and fragments, public safety official injured**

7th **Y38.2X2 Terrorism involving other explosions and fragments, civilian injured**

7th **Y38.2X3 Terrorism involving other explosions and fragments, terrorist injured**

5th **Y38.3 Terrorism involving fires, conflagration and hot substances**
Terrorism involving conflagration NOS
Terrorism involving fire NOS
Terrorism involving petrol bomb

EXCLUDES 1 *terrorism involving fire or heat of nuclear weapon (Y38.5)*

6th **Y38.3X Terrorism involving fires, conflagration and hot substances**

7th **Y38.3X1 Terrorism involving fires, conflagration and hot substances, public safety official injured**

7th **Y38.3X2 Terrorism involving fires, conflagration and hot substances, civilian injured**

7th **Y38.3X3 Terrorism involving fires, conflagration and hot substances, terrorist injured**

5th **Y38.4 Terrorism involving firearms**
Terrorism involving carbine bullet
Terrorism involving machine gun bullet
Terrorism involving pellets (shotgun)
Terrorism involving pistol bullet
Terrorism involving rifle bullet
Terrorism involving rubber (rifle) bullet

6th **Y38.4X Terrorism involving firearms**

7th **Y38.4X1 Terrorism involving firearms, public safety official injured**

7th **Y38.4X2 Terrorism involving firearms, civilian injured**

7th **Y38.4X3 Terrorism involving firearms, terrorist injured**

5th **Y38.5 Terrorism involving nuclear weapons**
Terrorism involving blast effects of nuclear weapon
Terrorism involving exposure to ionizing radiation from nuclear weapon
Terrorism involving fireball effect of nuclear weapon
Terrorism involving heat from nuclear weapon

6th **Y38.5X Terrorism involving nuclear weapons**

7th **Y38.5X1 Terrorism involving nuclear weapons, public safety official injured**

7th **Y38.5X2 Terrorism involving nuclear weapons, civilian injured**

7th **Y38.5X3 Terrorism involving nuclear weapons, terrorist injured**

5th **Y38.6 Terrorism involving biological weapons**
Terrorism involving anthrax
Terrorism involving cholera
Terrorism involving smallpox

6th **Y38.6X Terrorism involving biological weapons**

7th **Y38.6X1 Terrorism involving biological weapons, public safety official injured**

7th **Y38.6X2 Terrorism involving biological weapons, civilian injured**

7th **Y38.6X3 Terrorism involving biological weapons, terrorist injured**

5th **Y38.7 Terrorism involving chemical weapons**
Terrorism involving gases, fumes, chemicals
Terrorism involving hydrogen cyanide
Terrorism involving phosgene
Terrorism involving sarin

6th **Y38.7X Terrorism involving chemical weapons**

7th **Y38.7X1 Terrorism involving chemical weapons, public safety official injured**

7th **Y38.7X2 Terrorism involving chemical weapons, civilian injured**

7th **Y38.7X3 Terrorism involving chemical weapons, terrorist injured**

5th **Y38.8 Terrorism involving other and unspecified means**

x7th **Y38.80 Terrorism involving unspecified means**
Terrorism NOS

6th **Y38.81 Terrorism involving suicide bomber**

7th **Y38.811 Terrorism involving suicide bomber, public safety official injured**

7th **Y38.812 Terrorism involving suicide bomber, civilian injured**

6th **Y38.89 Terrorism involving other means**
Terrorism involving drowning and submersion
Terrorism involving lasers
Terrorism involving piercing or stabbing instruments

7th **Y38.891 Terrorism involving other means, public safety official injured**

7th **Y38.892 Terrorism involving other means, civilian injured**

7th **Y38.893 Terrorism involving other means, terrorist injured**

5th **Y38.9 Terrorism, secondary effects**

NOTE This code is for use to identify conditions occurring subsequent to a terrorist attack not those that are due to the initial terrorist attack

6th **Y38.9X Terrorism, secondary effects**

7th **Y38.9X1 Terrorism, secondary effects, public safety official injured**

7th **Y38.9X2 Terrorism, secondary effects, civilian injured**

## COMPLICATIONS OF MEDICAL AND SURGICAL CARE (Y62-Y84)

INCLUDES complications of medical devices
surgical and medical procedures as the cause of abnormal reaction of the patient, or of later complication, without mention of misadventure at the time of the procedure

### Misadventures to patients during surgical and medical care (Y62-Y69)

EXCLUDES 1 *surgical and medical procedures as the cause of abnormal reaction of the patient, without mention of misadventure at the time of the procedure (Y83-Y84)*

EXCLUDES 2 *breakdown or malfunctioning of medical device (during procedure) (after implantation) (ongoing use) (Y7Ø-Y82)*

4th **Y62 Failure of sterile precautions during surgical and medical care**

**Y62.Ø Failure of sterile precautions during surgical operation**

**Y62.1 Failure of sterile precautions during infusion or transfusion**

**Y62.2 Failure of sterile precautions during kidney dialysis and other perfusion** Rx ESR

**Y62.3 Failure of sterile precautions during injection or immunization**

**Y62.4 Failure of sterile precautions during endoscopic examination**

**Y62.5 Failure of sterile precautions during heart catheterization**

**Y62.6 Failure of sterile precautions during aspiration, puncture and other catheterization**

**Y62.8 Failure of sterile precautions during other surgical and medical care**

**Y62.9** Failure of sterile precautions during unspecified surgical and medical care

**Y63** Failure in dosage during surgical and medical care
EXCLUDES 2 *accidental overdose of drug or wrong drug given in error (T36-T5Ø)*
- **Y63.Ø** Excessive amount of blood or other fluid given during transfusion or infusion
- **Y63.1** Incorrect dilution of fluid used during infusion
- **Y63.2** Overdose of radiation given during therapy
- **Y63.3** Inadvertent exposure of patient to radiation during medical care
- **Y63.4** Failure in dosage in electroshock or insulin-shock therapy
- **Y63.5** Inappropriate temperature in local application and packing
- **Y63.6** Underdosing and nonadministration of necessary drug, medicament or biological substance
  AHA: 2018,4Q,72
- **Y63.8** Failure in dosage during other surgical and medical care
  AHA: 2018,4Q,72
- **Y63.9** Failure in dosage during unspecified surgical and medical care
  AHA: 2018,4Q,72

**Y64** Contaminated medical or biological substances
- **Y64.Ø** Contaminated medical or biological substance, transfused or infused
- **Y64.1** Contaminated medical or biological substance, injected or used for immunization
- **Y64.8** Contaminated medical or biological substance administered by other means
- **Y64.9** Contaminated medical or biological substance administered by unspecified means
  Administered contaminated medical or biological substance NOS

**Y65** Other misadventures during surgical and medical care
- **Y65.Ø** Mismatched blood in transfusion
- **Y65.1** Wrong fluid used in infusion
- **Y65.2** Failure in suture or ligature during surgical operation
- **Y65.3** Endotracheal tube wrongly placed during anesthetic procedure
- **Y65.4** Failure to introduce or to remove other tube or instrument
  AHA: 2025,2Q,10
- **Y65.5** Performance of wrong procedure (operation)
  - **Y65.51** Performance of wrong procedure (operation) on correct patient
    Wrong device implanted into correct surgical site
    EXCLUDES 1 *performance of correct procedure (operation) on wrong side or body part (Y65.53)*
  - **Y65.52** Performance of procedure (operation) on patient not scheduled for surgery
    Performance of procedure (operation) intended for another patient
    Performance of procedure (operation) on wrong patient
  - **Y65.53** Performance of correct procedure (operation) on wrong side or body part
    Performance of correct procedure (operation) on wrong side
    Performance of correct procedure (operation) on wrong site
- **Y65.8** Other specified misadventures during surgical and medical care
  AHA: 2022,1Q,22; 2019,2Q,23-24

**Y66** Nonadministration of surgical and medical care
Premature cessation of surgical and medical care
EXCLUDES 1 *DNR status (Z66)*
*palliative care (Z51.5)*

**Y69** Unspecified misadventure during surgical and medical care

## Medical devices associated with adverse incidents in diagnostic and therapeutic use (Y7Ø-Y82)

INCLUDES breakdown or malfunction of medical devices (during use) (after implantation) (ongoing use)

EXCLUDES 2 *later complications following use of medical devices without breakdown or malfunctioning of device (Y83-Y84)*
*misadventure to patients during surgical and medical care, classifiable to (Y62-Y69)*
*surgical and other medical procedures as the cause of abnormal reaction of the patient, or of later complication, without mention of misadventure at the time of the procedure (Y83-Y84)*

**Y7Ø** Anesthesiology devices associated with adverse incidents
- **Y7Ø.Ø** Diagnostic and monitoring anesthesiology devices associated with adverse incidents
- **Y7Ø.1** Therapeutic (nonsurgical) and rehabilitative anesthesiology devices associated with adverse incidents
- **Y7Ø.2** Prosthetic and other implants, materials and accessory anesthesiology devices associated with adverse incidents
- **Y7Ø.3** Surgical instruments, materials and anesthesiology devices (including sutures) associated with adverse incidents
- **Y7Ø.8** Miscellaneous anesthesiology devices associated with adverse incidents, not elsewhere classified

**Y71** Cardiovascular devices associated with adverse incidents
- **Y71.Ø** Diagnostic and monitoring cardiovascular devices associated with adverse incidents
- **Y71.1** Therapeutic (nonsurgical) and rehabilitative cardiovascular devices associated with adverse incidents
- **Y71.2** Prosthetic and other implants, materials and accessory cardiovascular devices associated with adverse incidents
- **Y71.3** Surgical instruments, materials and cardiovascular devices (including sutures) associated with adverse incidents
- **Y71.8** Miscellaneous cardiovascular devices associated with adverse incidents, not elsewhere classified

**Y72** Otorhinolaryngological devices associated with adverse incidents
- **Y72.Ø** Diagnostic and monitoring otorhinolaryngological devices associated with adverse incidents
- **Y72.1** Therapeutic (nonsurgical) and rehabilitative otorhinolaryngological devices associated with adverse incidents
- **Y72.2** Prosthetic and other implants, materials and accessory otorhinolaryngological devices associated with adverse incidents
- **Y72.3** Surgical instruments, materials and otorhinolaryngological devices (including sutures) associated with adverse incidents
- **Y72.8** Miscellaneous otorhinolaryngological devices associated with adverse incidents, not elsewhere classified

**Y73** Gastroenterology and urology devices associated with adverse incidents
- **Y73.Ø** Diagnostic and monitoring gastroenterology and urology devices associated with adverse incidents
- **Y73.1** Therapeutic (nonsurgical) and rehabilitative gastroenterology and urology devices associated with adverse incidents
- **Y73.2** Prosthetic and other implants, materials and accessory gastroenterology and urology devices associated with adverse incidents
- **Y73.3** Surgical instruments, materials and gastroenterology and urology devices (including sutures) associated with adverse incidents
- **Y73.8** Miscellaneous gastroenterology and urology devices associated with adverse incidents, not elsewhere classified

**Y74** General hospital and personal-use devices associated with adverse incidents
- **Y74.Ø** Diagnostic and monitoring general hospital and personal-use devices associated with adverse incidents
- **Y74.1** Therapeutic (nonsurgical) and rehabilitative general hospital and personal-use devices associated with adverse incidents
- **Y74.2** Prosthetic and other implants, materials and accessory general hospital and personal-use devices associated with adverse incidents
- **Y74.3** Surgical instruments, materials and general hospital and personal-use devices (including sutures) associated with adverse incidents
- **Y74.8** Miscellaneous general hospital and personal-use devices associated with adverse incidents, not elsewhere classified

**Y75** Neurological devices associated with adverse incidents
- **Y75.Ø** Diagnostic and monitoring neurological devices associated with adverse incidents
- **Y75.1** Therapeutic (nonsurgical) and rehabilitative neurological devices associated with adverse incidents
- **Y75.2** Prosthetic and other implants, materials and neurological devices associated with adverse incidents
- **Y75.3** Surgical instruments, materials and neurological devices (including sutures) associated with adverse incidents
- **Y75.8** Miscellaneous neurological devices associated with adverse incidents, not elsewhere classified

**Y76** Obstetric and gynecological devices associated with adverse incidents
- **Y76.Ø** Diagnostic and monitoring obstetric and gynecological devices associated with adverse incidents
- **Y76.1** Therapeutic (nonsurgical) and rehabilitative obstetric and gynecological devices associated with adverse incidents
- **Y76.2** Prosthetic and other implants, materials and accessory obstetric and gynecological devices associated with adverse incidents

**Y76.3** **Surgical instruments, materials and obstetric and gynecological devices (including sutures) associated with adverse incidents**

**Y76.8** **Miscellaneous obstetric and gynecological devices associated with adverse incidents, not elsewhere classified**

4th **Y77** **Ophthalmic devices associated with adverse incidents**

**Y77.Ø** **Diagnostic and monitoring ophthalmic devices associated with adverse incidents**

5th **Y77.1** **Therapeutic (nonsurgical) and rehabilitative ophthalmic devices associated with adverse incidents**

AHA: 2020,4Q,41

**Y77.11** **Contact lens associated with adverse incidents**

Rigid gas permeable contact lens associated with adverse incidents

Soft (hydrophilic) contact lens associated with adverse incidents

**Y77.19** **Other therapeutic (nonsurgical) and rehabilitative ophthalmic devices associated with adverse incidents**

**Y77.2** **Prosthetic and other implants, materials and accessory ophthalmic devices associated with adverse incidents**

**Y77.3** **Surgical instruments, materials and ophthalmic devices (including sutures) associated with adverse incidents**

**Y77.8** **Miscellaneous ophthalmic devices associated with adverse incidents, not elsewhere classified**

4th **Y78** **Radiological devices associated with adverse incidents**

**Y78.Ø** **Diagnostic and monitoring radiological devices associated with adverse incidents**

**Y78.1** **Therapeutic (nonsurgical) and rehabilitative radiological devices associated with adverse incidents**

**Y78.2** **Prosthetic and other implants, materials and accessory radiological devices associated with adverse incidents**

**Y78.3** **Surgical instruments, materials and radiological devices (including sutures) associated with adverse incidents**

**Y78.8** **Miscellaneous radiological devices associated with adverse incidents, not elsewhere classified**

4th **Y79** **Orthopedic devices associated with adverse incidents**

**Y79.Ø** **Diagnostic and monitoring orthopedic devices associated with adverse incidents**

**Y79.1** **Therapeutic (nonsurgical) and rehabilitative orthopedic devices associated with adverse incidents**

**Y79.2** **Prosthetic and other implants, materials and accessory orthopedic devices associated with adverse incidents**

**Y79.3** **Surgical instruments, materials and orthopedic devices (including sutures) associated with adverse incidents**

**Y79.8** **Miscellaneous orthopedic devices associated with adverse incidents, not elsewhere classified**

4th **Y8Ø** **Physical medicine devices associated with adverse incidents**

**Y8Ø.Ø** **Diagnostic and monitoring physical medicine devices associated with adverse incidents**

**Y8Ø.1** **Therapeutic (nonsurgical) and rehabilitative physical medicine devices associated with adverse incidents**

**Y8Ø.2** **Prosthetic and other implants, materials and accessory physical medicine devices associated with adverse incidents**

**Y8Ø.3** **Surgical instruments, materials and physical medicine devices (including sutures) associated with adverse incidents**

**Y8Ø.8** **Miscellaneous physical medicine devices associated with adverse incidents, not elsewhere classified**

4th **Y81** **General- and plastic-surgery devices associated with adverse incidents**

**Y81.Ø** **Diagnostic and monitoring general- and plastic-surgery devices associated with adverse incidents**

**Y81.1** **Therapeutic (nonsurgical) and rehabilitative general- and plastic-surgery devices associated with adverse incidents**

**Y81.2** **Prosthetic and other implants, materials and accessory general- and plastic-surgery devices associated with adverse incidents**

**Y81.3** **Surgical instruments, materials and general- and plastic-surgery devices (including sutures) associated with adverse incidents**

**Y81.8** **Miscellaneous general- and plastic-surgery devices associated with adverse incidents, not elsewhere classified**

4th **Y82** **Other and unspecified medical devices associated with adverse incidents**

**Y82.8** **Other medical devices associated with adverse incidents**

**Y82.9** **Unspecified medical devices associated with adverse incidents**

## Surgical and other medical procedures as the cause of abnormal reaction of the patient, or of later complication, without mention of misadventure at the time of the procedure (Y83-Y84)

EXCLUDES 1 *misadventures to patients during surgical and medical care, classifiable to (Y62-Y69)*

EXCLUDES 2 *breakdown or malfunctioning of medical device (during procedure) (after implantation) (ongoing use) (Y7Ø-Y82)*

4th **Y83** **Surgical operation and other surgical procedures as the cause of abnormal reaction of the patient, or of later complication, without mention of misadventure at the time of the procedure**

**Y83.Ø** **Surgical operation with transplant of whole organ as the cause of abnormal reaction of the patient, or of later complication, without mention of misadventure at the time of the procedure**

**Y83.1** **Surgical operation with implant of artificial internal device as the cause of abnormal reaction of the patient, or of later complication, without mention of misadventure at the time of the procedure**

**Y83.2** **Surgical operation with anastomosis, bypass or graft as the cause of abnormal reaction of the patient, or of later complication, without mention of misadventure at the time of the procedure**

**Y83.3** **Surgical operation with formation of external stoma as the cause of abnormal reaction of the patient, or of later complication, without mention of misadventure at the time of the procedure**

**Y83.4** **Other reconstructive surgery as the cause of abnormal reaction of the patient, or of later complication, without mention of misadventure at the time of the procedure**

**Y83.5** **Amputation of limb(s) as the cause of abnormal reaction of the patient, or of later complication, without mention of misadventure at the time of the procedure**

**Y83.6** **Removal of other organ (partial) (total) as the cause of abnormal reaction of the patient, or of later complication, without mention of misadventure at the time of the procedure**

**Y83.8** **Other surgical procedures as the cause of abnormal reaction of the patient, or of later complication, without mention of misadventure at the time of the procedure**

AHA: 2023,2Q,14

**Y83.9** **Surgical procedure, unspecified as the cause of abnormal reaction of the patient, or of later complication, without mention of misadventure at the time of the procedure**

4th **Y84** **Other medical procedures as the cause of abnormal reaction of the patient, or of later complication, without mention of misadventure at the time of the procedure**

**Y84.Ø** **Cardiac catheterization as the cause of abnormal reaction of the patient, or of later complication, without mention of misadventure at the time of the procedure**

**Y84.1** **Kidney dialysis as the cause of abnormal reaction of the patient, or of later complication, without mention of misadventure at the time of the procedure**

**Y84.2** **Radiological procedure and radiotherapy as the cause of abnormal reaction of the patient, or of later complication, without mention of misadventure at the time of the procedure**

AHA: 2019,1Q,21; 2017,1Q,33

**Y84.3** **Shock therapy as the cause of abnormal reaction of the patient, or of later complication, without mention of misadventure at the time of the procedure**

**Y84.4** **Aspiration of fluid as the cause of abnormal reaction of the patient, or of later complication, without mention of misadventure at the time of the procedure**

**Y84.5** **Insertion of gastric or duodenal sound as the cause of abnormal reaction of the patient, or of later complication, without mention of misadventure at the time of the procedure**

**Y84.6** **Urinary catheterization as the cause of abnormal reaction of the patient, or of later complication, without mention of misadventure at the time of the procedure**

AHA: 2025,2Q,20

**Y84.7** **Blood-sampling as the cause of abnormal reaction of the patient, or of later complication, without mention of misadventure at the time of the procedure**

**Y84.8** **Other medical procedures as the cause of abnormal reaction of the patient, or of later complication, without mention of misadventure at the time of the procedure**

AHA: 2024,1Q,26; 2023,2Q,28; 2021,1Q,5; 2014,4Q,24

**Y84.9** **Medical procedure, unspecified as the cause of abnormal reaction of the patient, or of later complication, without mention of misadventure at the time of the procedure**

## Supplementary factors related to causes of morbidity classified elsewhere (Y90-Y99)

NOTE These categories may be used to provide supplementary information concerning causes of morbidity. They are not to be used for single-condition coding.

**✓4th Y90 Evidence of alcohol involvement determined by blood alcohol level**

Code first any associated alcohol related disorders (F10)

**Y90.0** Blood alcohol level of less than 20 mg/100 ml

**Y90.1** Blood alcohol level of 20-39 mg/100 ml

**Y90.2** Blood alcohol level of 40-59 mg/100 ml

**Y90.3** Blood alcohol level of 60-79 mg/100 ml

**Y90.4** Blood alcohol level of 80-99 mg/100 ml

**Y90.5** Blood alcohol level of 100-119 mg/100 ml

**Y90.6** Blood alcohol level of 120-199 mg/100 ml

**Y90.7** Blood alcohol level of 200-239 mg/100 ml

**Y90.8** Blood alcohol level of 240 mg/100 ml or more

**Y90.9** Presence of alcohol in blood, level not specified

**✓4th Y92 Place of occurrence of the external cause**

Place of occurrence should be recorded only at the initial encounter for treatment

The following category is for use, when relevant, to identify the place of occurrence of the external cause. Use in conjunction with an activity code.

**✓5th Y92.0 Non-institutional (private) residence as the place of occurrence of the external cause**

EXCLUDES 1 *abandoned or derelict house (Y92.89)*
*home under construction but not yet occupied (Y92.6-)*
*institutional place of residence (Y92.1-)*

**✓6th Y92.00 Unspecified non-institutional (private) residence as the place of occurrence of the external cause**

**Y92.000** Kitchen of unspecified non-institutional (private) residence as the place of occurrence of the external cause

**Y92.001** Dining room of unspecified non-institutional (private) residence as the place of occurrence of the external cause

**Y92.002** Bathroom of unspecified non-institutional (private) residence as the place of occurrence of the external cause

**Y92.003** Bedroom of unspecified non-institutional (private) residence as the place of occurrence of the external cause

**Y92.007** Garden or yard of unspecified non-institutional (private) residence as the place of occurrence of the external cause

**Y92.008** Other place in unspecified non-institutional (private) residence as the place of occurrence of the external cause

**Y92.009** Unspecified place in unspecified non-institutional (private) residence as the place of occurrence of the external cause

Home (NOS) as the place of occurrence of the external cause

**✓6th Y92.01 Single-family non-institutional (private) house as the place of occurrence of the external cause**

Farmhouse as the place of occurrence of the external cause

EXCLUDES 1 *barn (Y92.71)*
*chicken coop or hen house (Y92.72)*
*farm field (Y92.73)*
*orchard (Y92.74)*
*single family mobile home or trailer (Y92.02-)*
*slaughter house (Y92.86)*

**Y92.010** Kitchen of single-family (private) house as the place of occurrence of the external cause

**Y92.011** Dining room of single-family (private) house as the place of occurrence of the external cause

**Y92.012** Bathroom of single-family (private) house as the place of occurrence of the external cause

**Y92.013** Bedroom of single-family (private) house as the place of occurrence of the external cause

**Y92.014** Private driveway to single-family (private) house as the place of occurrence of the external cause

**Y92.015** Private garage of single-family (private) house as the place of occurrence of the external cause

**Y92.016** Swimming-pool in single-family (private) house or garden as the place of occurrence of the external cause

AHA: 2023,1Q,25

**Y92.017** Garden or yard in single-family (private) house as the place of occurrence of the external cause

**Y92.018** Other place in single-family (private) house as the place of occurrence of the external cause

**Y92.019** Unspecified place in single-family (private) house as the place of occurrence of the external cause

**✓6th Y92.02 Mobile home as the place of occurrence of the external cause**

**Y92.020** Kitchen in mobile home as the place of occurrence of the external cause

**Y92.021** Dining room in mobile home as the place of occurrence of the external cause

**Y92.022** Bathroom in mobile home as the place of occurrence of the external cause

**Y92.023** Bedroom in mobile home as the place of occurrence of the external cause

**Y92.024** Driveway of mobile home as the place of occurrence of the external cause

**Y92.025** Garage of mobile home as the place of occurrence of the external cause

**Y92.026** Swimming-pool of mobile home as the place of occurrence of the external cause

**Y92.027** Garden or yard of mobile home as the place of occurrence of the external cause

**Y92.028** Other place in mobile home as the place of occurrence of the external cause

**Y92.029** Unspecified place in mobile home as the place of occurrence of the external cause

**✓6th Y92.03 Apartment as the place of occurrence of the external cause**

Condominium as the place of occurrence of the external cause

Co-op apartment as the place of occurrence of the external cause

**Y92.030** Kitchen in apartment as the place of occurrence of the external cause

**Y92.031** Bathroom in apartment as the place of occurrence of the external cause

**Y92.032** Bedroom in apartment as the place of occurrence of the external cause

**Y92.038** Other place in apartment as the place of occurrence of the external cause

**Y92.039** Unspecified place in apartment as the place of occurrence of the external cause

**✓6th Y92.04 Boarding-house as the place of occurrence of the external cause**

**Y92.040** Kitchen in boarding-house as the place of occurrence of the external cause

**Y92.041** Bathroom in boarding-house as the place of occurrence of the external cause

**Y92.042** Bedroom in boarding-house as the place of occurrence of the external cause

**Y92.043** Driveway of boarding-house as the place of occurrence of the external cause

**Y92.044** Garage of boarding-house as the place of occurrence of the external cause

**Y92.045** Swimming-pool of boarding-house as the place of occurrence of the external cause

**Y92.046** Garden or yard of boarding-house as the place of occurrence of the external cause

**Y92.048** Other place in boarding-house as the place of occurrence of the external cause

**Y92.049** Unspecified place in boarding-house as the place of occurrence of the external cause

**✓6th Y92.09 Other non-institutional residence as the place of occurrence of the external cause**

AHA: 2017,2Q,10

**Y92.090** Kitchen in other non-institutional residence as the place of occurrence of the external cause

**Y92.091** Bathroom in other non-institutional residence as the place of occurrence of the external cause

Y92.092 Bedroom in other non-institutional residence as the place of occurrence of the external cause

Y92.093 Driveway of other non-institutional residence as the place of occurrence of the external cause

Y92.094 Garage of other non-institutional residence as the place of occurrence of the external cause

Y92.095 Swimming-pool of other non-institutional residence as the place of occurrence of the external cause

Y92.096 Garden or yard of other non-institutional residence as the place of occurrence of the external cause

Y92.098 Other place in other non-institutional residence as the place of occurrence of the external cause

Y92.099 Unspecified place in other non-institutional residence as the place of occurrence of the external cause

✓5th Y92.1 Institutional (nonprivate) residence as the place of occurrence of the external cause

Y92.10 Unspecified residential institution as the place of occurrence of the external cause

✓6th Y92.11 Children's home and orphanage as the place of occurrence of the external cause

Y92.110 Kitchen in children's home and orphanage as the place of occurrence of the external cause

Y92.111 Bathroom in children's home and orphanage as the place of occurrence of the external cause

Y92.112 Bedroom in children's home and orphanage as the place of occurrence of the external cause

Y92.113 Driveway of children's home and orphanage as the place of occurrence of the external cause

Y92.114 Garage of children's home and orphanage as the place of occurrence of the external cause

Y92.115 Swimming-pool of children's home and orphanage as the place of occurrence of the external cause

Y92.116 Garden or yard of children's home and orphanage as the place of occurrence of the external cause

Y92.118 Other place in children's home and orphanage as the place of occurrence of the external cause

Y92.119 Unspecified place in children's home and orphanage as the place of occurrence of the external cause

✓6th Y92.12 Nursing home as the place of occurrence of the external cause

Home for the sick as the place of occurrence of the external cause

Hospice as the place of occurrence of the external cause

AHA: 2017,2Q,10

Y92.120 Kitchen in nursing home as the place of occurrence of the external cause

Y92.121 Bathroom in nursing home as the place of occurrence of the external cause

Y92.122 Bedroom in nursing home as the place of occurrence of the external cause

Y92.123 Driveway of nursing home as the place of occurrence of the external cause

Y92.124 Garage of nursing home as the place of occurrence of the external cause

Y92.125 Swimming-pool of nursing home as the place of occurrence of the external cause

Y92.126 Garden or yard of nursing home as the place of occurrence of the external cause

Y92.128 Other place in nursing home as the place of occurrence of the external cause

Y92.129 Unspecified place in nursing home as the place of occurrence of the external cause

✓6th Y92.13 Military base as the place of occurrence of the external cause

EXCLUDES 1 *military training grounds (Y92.84)*

Y92.130 Kitchen on military base as the place of occurrence of the external cause

Y92.131 Mess hall on military base as the place of occurrence of the external cause

Y92.133 Barracks on military base as the place of occurrence of the external cause

Y92.135 Garage on military base as the place of occurrence of the external cause

Y92.136 Swimming-pool on military base as the place of occurrence of the external cause

Y92.137 Garden or yard on military base as the place of occurrence of the external cause

Y92.138 Other place on military base as the place of occurrence of the external cause

Y92.139 Unspecified place military base as the place of occurrence of the external cause

✓6th Y92.14 Prison as the place of occurrence of the external cause

Y92.140 Kitchen in prison as the place of occurrence of the external cause

Y92.141 Dining room in prison as the place of occurrence of the external cause

Y92.142 Bathroom in prison as the place of occurrence of the external cause

Y92.143 Cell of prison as the place of occurrence of the external cause

Y92.146 Swimming-pool of prison as the place of occurrence of the external cause

Y92.147 Courtyard of prison as the place of occurrence of the external cause

Y92.148 Other place in prison as the place of occurrence of the external cause

Y92.149 Unspecified place in prison as the place of occurrence of the external cause

✓6th Y92.15 Reform school as the place of occurrence of the external cause

Y92.150 Kitchen in reform school as the place of occurrence of the external cause

Y92.151 Dining room in reform school as the place of occurrence of the external cause

Y92.152 Bathroom in reform school as the place of occurrence of the external cause

Y92.153 Bedroom in reform school as the place of occurrence of the external cause

Y92.154 Driveway of reform school as the place of occurrence of the external cause

Y92.155 Garage of reform school as the place of occurrence of the external cause

Y92.156 Swimming-pool of reform school as the place of occurrence of the external cause

Y92.157 Garden or yard of reform school as the place of occurrence of the external cause

Y92.158 Other place in reform school as the place of occurrence of the external cause

Y92.159 Unspecified place in reform school as the place of occurrence of the external cause

✓6th Y92.16 School dormitory as the place of occurrence of the external cause

EXCLUDES 1 *reform school as the place of occurrence of the external cause (Y92.15-)*
*school buildings and grounds as the place of occurrence of the external cause (Y92.2-)*
*school sports and athletic areas as the place of occurrence of the external cause (Y92.3-)*

Y92.160 Kitchen in school dormitory as the place of occurrence of the external cause

Y92.161 Dining room in school dormitory as the place of occurrence of the external cause

Y92.162 Bathroom in school dormitory as the place of occurrence of the external cause

Y92.163 Bedroom in school dormitory as the place of occurrence of the external cause

Y92.168 Other place in school dormitory as the place of occurrence of the external cause

Y92.169 Unspecified place in school dormitory as the place of occurrence of the external cause

✓6th Y92.19 Other specified residential institution as the place of occurrence of the external cause

AHA: 2017,2Q,10

Y92.190 Kitchen in other specified residential institution as the place of occurrence of the external cause

Y92.191 **Dining room in other specified residential institution as the place of occurrence of the external cause**

Y92.192 **Bathroom in other specified residential institution as the place of occurrence of the external cause**

Y92.193 **Bedroom in other specified residential institution as the place of occurrence of the external cause**

Y92.194 **Driveway of other specified residential institution as the place of occurrence of the external cause**

Y92.195 **Garage of other specified residential institution as the place of occurrence of the external cause**

Y92.196 **Pool of other specified residential institution as the place of occurrence of the external cause**

Y92.197 **Garden or yard of other specified residential institution as the place of occurrence of the external cause**

Y92.198 **Other place in other specified residential institution as the place of occurrence of the external cause**

Y92.199 **Unspecified place in other specified residential institution as the place of occurrence of the external cause**

✓5th Y92.2 **School, other institution and public administrative area as the place of occurrence of the external cause**

Building and adjacent grounds used by the general public or by a particular group of the public

EXCLUDES 1 *building under construction as the place of occurrence of the external cause (Y92.6)*
*residential institution as the place of occurrence of the external cause (Y92.1)*
*school dormitory as the place of occurrence of the external cause (Y92.16-)*
*sports and athletics area of schools as the place of occurrence of the external cause (Y92.3-)*

✓6th Y92.21 **School (private) (public) (state) as the place of occurrence of the external cause**

Y92.210 **Daycare center as the place of occurrence of the external cause**

Y92.211 **Elementary school as the place of occurrence of the external cause**

Kindergarten as the place of occurrence of the external cause

Y92.212 **Middle school as the place of occurrence of the external cause**

Y92.213 **High school as the place of occurrence of the external cause**

**AHA:** 2012,4Q,108

Y92.214 **College as the place of occurrence of the external cause**

University as the place of occurrence of the external cause

Y92.215 **Trade school as the place of occurrence of the external cause**

Y92.218 **Other school as the place of occurrence of the external cause**

Y92.219 **Unspecified school as the place of occurrence of the external cause**

Y92.22 **Religious institution as the place of occurrence of the external cause**

Church as the place of occurrence of the external cause
Mosque as the place of occurrence of the external cause
Synagogue as the place of occurrence of the external cause

✓6th Y92.23 **Hospital as the place of occurrence of the external cause**

EXCLUDES 1 *ambulatory (outpatient) health services establishments (Y92.53-)*
*home for the sick as the place of occurrence of the external cause (Y92.12-)*
*hospice as the place of occurrence of the external cause (Y92.12-)*
*nursing home as the place of occurrence of the external cause (Y92.12-)*

Y92.230 **Patient room in hospital as the place of occurrence of the external cause**

Y92.231 **Patient bathroom in hospital as the place of occurrence of the external cause**

Y92.232 **Corridor of hospital as the place of occurrence of the external cause**

Y92.233 **Cafeteria of hospital as the place of occurrence of the external cause**

Y92.234 **Operating room of hospital as the place of occurrence of the external cause**

Y92.238 **Other place in hospital as the place of occurrence of the external cause**

Y92.239 **Unspecified place in hospital as the place of occurrence of the external cause**

✓6th Y92.24 **Public administrative building as the place of occurrence of the external cause**

Y92.240 **Courthouse as the place of occurrence of the external cause**

Y92.241 **Library as the place of occurrence of the external cause**

Y92.242 **Post office as the place of occurrence of the external cause**

Y92.243 **City hall as the place of occurrence of the external cause**

Y92.248 **Other public administrative building as the place of occurrence of the external cause**

✓6th Y92.25 **Cultural building as the place of occurrence of the external cause**

Y92.250 **Art Gallery as the place of occurrence of the external cause**

Y92.251 **Museum as the place of occurrence of the external cause**

Y92.252 **Music hall as the place of occurrence of the external cause**

Y92.253 **Opera house as the place of occurrence of the external cause**

Y92.254 **Theater (live) as the place of occurrence of the external cause**

Y92.258 **Other cultural public building as the place of occurrence of the external cause**

Y92.26 **Movie house or cinema as the place of occurrence of the external cause**

Y92.29 **Other specified public building as the place of occurrence of the external cause**

Assembly hall as the place of occurrence of the external cause
Clubhouse as the place of occurrence of the external cause

✓5th Y92.3 **Sports and athletics area as the place of occurrence of the external cause**

✓6th Y92.31 **Athletic court as the place of occurrence of the external cause**

EXCLUDES 1 *tennis court in private home or garden (Y92.09)*

Y92.310 **Basketball court as the place of occurrence of the external cause**

Y92.311 **Squash court as the place of occurrence of the external cause**

Y92.312 **Tennis court as the place of occurrence of the external cause**

Y92.318 **Other athletic court as the place of occurrence of the external cause**

✓6th Y92.32 **Athletic field as the place of occurrence of the external cause**

Y92.320 **Baseball field as the place of occurrence of the external cause**

Y92.321 **Football field as the place of occurrence of the external cause**

Y92.322 **Soccer field as the place of occurrence of the external cause**

Y92.328 **Other athletic field as the place of occurrence of the external cause**

Cricket field as the place of occurrence of the external cause
Hockey field as the place of occurrence of the external cause

✓6th Y92.33 **Skating rink as the place of occurrence of the external cause**

Y92.330 **Ice skating rink (indoor) (outdoor) as the place of occurrence of the external cause**

Y92.331 **Roller skating rink as the place of occurrence of the external cause**

Y92.34 **Swimming pool (public) as the place of occurrence of the external cause**

EXCLUDES 1 *swimming pool in private home or garden (Y92.016)*

**Y92.39 Other specified sports and athletic area as the place of occurrence of the external cause**
Golf-course as the place of occurrence of the external cause
Gymnasium as the place of occurrence of the external cause
Riding-school as the place of occurrence of the external cause
Stadium as the place of occurrence of the external cause

√5th **Y92.4 Street, highway and other paved roadways as the place of occurrence of the external cause**
EXCLUDES 1 *private driveway of residence (Y92.014, Y92.024, Y92.043, Y92.093, Y92.113, Y92.123, Y92.154, Y92.194)*

√6th **Y92.41 Street and highway as the place of occurrence of the external cause**
**Y92.410 Unspecified street and highway as the place of occurrence of the external cause**
Road NOS as the place of occurrence of the external cause
**Y92.411 Interstate highway as the place of occurrence of the external cause**
Freeway as the place of occurrence of the external cause
Motorway as the place of occurrence of the external cause
**Y92.412 Parkway as the place of occurrence of the external cause**
**Y92.413 State road as the place of occurrence of the external cause**
**Y92.414 Local residential or business street as the place of occurrence of the external cause**
**Y92.415 Exit ramp or entrance ramp of street or highway as the place of occurrence of the external cause**

√6th **Y92.48 Other paved roadways as the place of occurrence of the external cause**
**Y92.480 Sidewalk as the place of occurrence of the external cause**
**Y92.481 Parking lot as the place of occurrence of the external cause**
**Y92.482 Bike path as the place of occurrence of the external cause**
**Y92.488 Other paved roadways as the place of occurrence of the external cause**

√5th **Y92.5 Trade and service area as the place of occurrence of the external cause**
EXCLUDES 1 *garage in private home (Y92.015)*
*schools and other public administration buildings (Y92.2-)*

√6th **Y92.51 Private commercial establishments as the place of occurrence of the external cause**
**Y92.510 Bank as the place of occurrence of the external cause**
**Y92.511 Restaurant or cafe as the place of occurrence of the external cause**
**Y92.512 Supermarket, store or market as the place of occurrence of the external cause**
**Y92.513 Shop (commercial) as the place of occurrence of the external cause**

√6th **Y92.52 Service areas as the place of occurrence of the external cause**
**Y92.520 Airport as the place of occurrence of the external cause**
**Y92.521 Bus station as the place of occurrence of the external cause**
**Y92.522 Railway station as the place of occurrence of the external cause**
**Y92.523 Highway rest stop as the place of occurrence of the external cause**
**Y92.524 Gas station as the place of occurrence of the external cause**
Petroleum station as the place of occurrence of the external cause
Service station as the place of occurrence of the external cause

√6th **Y92.53 Ambulatory health services establishments as the place of occurrence of the external cause**
**Y92.530 Ambulatory surgery center as the place of occurrence of the external cause**
Outpatient surgery center, including that connected with a hospital as the place of occurrence of the external cause
Same day surgery center, including that connected with a hospital as the place of occurrence of the external cause
**Y92.531 Health care provider office as the place of occurrence of the external cause**
Physician office as the place of occurrence of the external cause
**Y92.532 Urgent care center as the place of occurrence of the external cause**
**Y92.538 Other ambulatory health services establishments as the place of occurrence of the external cause**
AHA: 2019,1Q,21

**Y92.59 Other trade areas as the place of occurrence of the external cause**
Casino as the place of occurrence of the external cause
Garage (commercial) as the place of occurrence of the external cause
Hotel as the place of occurrence of the external cause
Office building as the place of occurrence of the external cause
Radio or television station as the place of occurrence of the external cause
Shopping mall as the place of occurrence of the external cause
Warehouse as the place of occurrence of the external cause

√5th **Y92.6 Industrial and construction area as the place of occurrence of the external cause**
**Y92.61 Building [any] under construction as the place of occurrence of the external cause**
**Y92.62 Dock or shipyard as the place of occurrence of the external cause**
Dockyard as the place of occurrence of the external cause
Dry dock as the place of occurrence of the external cause
Shipyard as the place of occurrence of the external cause
**Y92.63 Factory as the place of occurrence of the external cause**
Factory building as the place of occurrence of the external cause
Factory premises as the place of occurrence of the external cause
Industrial yard as the place of occurrence of the external cause
**Y92.64 Mine or pit as the place of occurrence of the external cause**
Mine as the place of occurrence of the external cause
**Y92.65 Oil rig as the place of occurrence of the external cause**
Pit (coal) (gravel) (sand) as the place of occurrence of the external cause
**Y92.69 Other specified industrial and construction area as the place of occurrence of the external cause**
Gasworks as the place of occurrence of the external cause
Power-station (coal) (nuclear) (oil) as the place of occurrence of the external cause
Tunnel under construction as the place of occurrence of the external cause
Workshop as the place of occurrence of the external cause

√5th **Y92.7 Farm as the place of occurrence of the external cause**
Ranch as the place of occurrence of the external cause
EXCLUDES 1 *farmhouse and home premises of farm (Y92.01-)*
**Y92.71 Barn as the place of occurrence of the external cause**
**Y92.72 Chicken coop as the place of occurrence of the external cause**
Hen house as the place of occurrence of the external cause
**Y92.73 Farm field as the place of occurrence of the external cause**
**Y92.74 Orchard as the place of occurrence of the external cause**
**Y92.79 Other farm location as the place of occurrence of the external cause**

**Y92.8 Other places as the place of occurrence of the external cause**

**Y92.81 Transport vehicle as the place of occurrence of the external cause**

EXCLUDES 1 *transport accidents (VØØ-V99)*

**Y92.81Ø Car as the place of occurrence of the external cause**

**Y92.811 Bus as the place of occurrence of the external cause**

**Y92.812 Truck as the place of occurrence of the external cause**

**Y92.813 Airplane as the place of occurrence of the external cause**

**Y92.814 Boat as the place of occurrence of the external cause**

**Y92.815 Train as the place of occurrence of the external cause**

**Y92.816 Subway car as the place of occurrence of the external cause**

**Y92.818 Other transport vehicle as the place of occurrence of the external cause**

**Y92.82 Wilderness area**

**Y92.82Ø Desert as the place of occurrence of the external cause**

**Y92.821 Forest as the place of occurrence of the external cause**

**Y92.828 Other wilderness area as the place of occurrence of the external cause**

Marsh as the place of occurrence of the external cause

Mountain as the place of occurrence of the external cause

Prairie as the place of occurrence of the external cause

Swamp as the place of occurrence of the external cause

**Y92.83 Recreation area as the place of occurrence of the external cause**

**Y92.83Ø Public park as the place of occurrence of the external cause**

**Y92.831 Amusement park as the place of occurrence of the external cause**

**Y92.832 Beach as the place of occurrence of the external cause**

Seashore as the place of occurrence of the external cause

**Y92.833 Campsite as the place of occurrence of the external cause**

**Y92.834 Zoological garden (Zoo) as the place of occurrence of the external cause**

**Y92.838 Other recreation area as the place of occurrence of the external cause**

**Y92.84 Military training ground as the place of occurrence of the external cause**

**Y92.85 Railroad track as the place of occurrence of the external cause**

**Y92.86 Slaughter house as the place of occurrence of the external cause**

**Y92.89 Other specified places as the place of occurrence of the external cause**

Derelict house as the place of occurrence of the external cause

**Y92.9 Unspecified place or not applicable**

**Y93 Activity codes**

Y93.Ø Activities involving walking and running
Y93.1 Activities involving water and water craft
Y93.2 Activities involving ice and snow
Y93.3 Activities involving climbing, rappelling, and jumping off
Y93.4 Activities involving dancing and other rhythmic movement
Y93.5 Activities involving other sports and athletics played individually
Y93.6 Activities involving other sports and athletics played as a team or group
Y93.7 Activities involving other specified sports and athletics
Y93.8 Activities, other specified
Y93.9 Activity, unspecified
Y93.A Activities involving other cardiorespiratory exercise
Y93.B Activities involving other muscle strengthening exercises
Y93.C Activities involving computer technology and electronic devices
Y93.D Activities involving arts and handcrafts
Y93.E Activities involving personal hygiene and interior property and clothing maintenance
Y93.F Activities involving caregiving
Y93.G Activities involving food preparation, cooking and grilling
Y93.H Activities involving exterior property and land maintenance, building and construction
Y93.I Activities involving roller coasters and other types of external motion
Y93.J Activities involving playing musical instrument
Y93.K Activities involving animal care
Y93.L Other outdoor activity

NOTE Category Y93 is provided for use to indicate the activity of the person seeking healthcare for an injury or health condition, such as a heart attack while shoveling snow, which resulted from, or was contributed to, by the activity. These codes are appropriate for use for both acute injuries, such as those from chapter 19, and conditions that are due to the long-term, cumulative effects of an activity, such as those from chapter 13. They are also appropriate for use with external cause codes for cause and intent if identifying the activity provides additional information on the event. These codes should be used in conjunction with codes for external cause status (Y99) and place of occurrence (Y92).

This section contains the following broad activity categories:

**Y93.Ø Activities involving walking and running**

EXCLUDES 1 *activity, walking an animal (Y93.K1)*
*activity, walking or running on a treadmill (Y93.A1)*

**Y93.Ø1 Activity, walking, marching and hiking**

Activity, walking, marching and hiking on level or elevated terrain

EXCLUDES 1 *activity, mountain climbing (Y93.31)*

**Y93.Ø2 Activity, running**

**Y93.1 Activities involving water and water craft**

EXCLUDES 1 *activities involving ice (Y93.2-)*

**Y93.11 Activity, swimming**

**Y93.12 Activity, springboard and platform diving**

**Y93.13 Activity, water polo**

**Y93.14 Activity, water aerobics and water exercise**

**Y93.15 Activity, underwater diving and snorkeling**

Activity, SCUBA diving

**Y93.16 Activity, rowing, canoeing, kayaking, rafting and tubing**

Activity, canoeing, kayaking, rafting and tubing in calm and turbulent water

**Y93.17 Activity, water skiing and wake boarding**

**Y93.18 Activity, surfing, windsurfing and boogie boarding**

Activity, water sliding

**Y93.19 Activity, other involving water and watercraft**

Activity involving water NOS
Activity, parasailing
Activity, water survival training and testing

**Y93.2 Activities involving ice and snow**

EXCLUDES 1 *activity, shoveling ice and snow (Y93.H1)*

**Y93.21 Activity, ice skating**

Activity, figure skating (singles) (pairs)
Activity, ice dancing

EXCLUDES 1 *activity, ice hockey (Y93.22)*

**Y93.22 Activity, ice hockey**

Y93.23 **Activity, snow (alpine) (downhill) skiing, snowboarding, sledding, tobogganing and snow tubing**
EXCLUDES 1 *activity, cross country skiing (Y93.24)*

Y93.24 **Activity, cross country skiing**
Activity, nordic skiing

Y93.29 **Activity, other involving ice and snow**
Activity involving ice and snow NOS

✓5th Y93.3 **Activities involving climbing, rappelling and jumping off**
EXCLUDES 1 *activity, hiking on level or elevated terrain (Y93.Ø1)*
*activity, jumping rope (Y93.56)*
*activity, trampoline jumping (Y93.44)*

Y93.31 **Activity, mountain climbing, rock climbing and wall climbing**

Y93.32 **Activity, rappelling**

Y93.33 **Activity, BASE jumping**
Activity, Building, Antenna, Span, Earth jumping

Y93.34 **Activity, bungee jumping**

Y93.35 **Activity, hang gliding**

Y93.39 **Activity, other involving climbing, rappelling and jumping off**

✓5th Y93.4 **Activities involving dancing and other rhythmic movement**
EXCLUDES 1 *activity, martial arts (Y93.75)*

Y93.41 **Activity, dancing**
AHA: 2012,4Q,108

Y93.42 **Activity, yoga**

Y93.43 **Activity, gymnastics**
Activity, rhythmic gymnastics
EXCLUDES 1 *activity, trampolining (Y93.44)*

Y93.44 **Activity, trampolining**

Y93.45 **Activity, cheerleading**

Y93.49 **Activity, other involving dancing and other rhythmic movements**

✓5th Y93.5 **Activities involving other sports and athletics played individually**
EXCLUDES 1 *activity, dancing (Y93.41)*
*activity, gymnastic (Y93.43)*
*activity, trampolining (Y93.44)*
*activity, yoga (Y93.42)*

Y93.51 **Activity, roller skating (inline) and skateboarding**

Y93.52 **Activity, horseback riding**

Y93.53 **Activity, golf**

Y93.54 **Activity, bowling**

Y93.55 **Activity, bike riding**

Y93.56 **Activity, jumping rope**

Y93.57 **Activity, non-running track and field events**
EXCLUDES 1 *activity, running (any form) (Y93.Ø2)*

Y93.59 **Activity, other involving other sports and athletics played individually**
EXCLUDES 1 *activities involving climbing, rappelling, and jumping (Y93.3-)*
*activities involving ice and snow (Y93.2-)*
*activities involving walking and running (Y93.Ø-)*
*activities involving water and watercraft (Y93.1-)*

✓5th Y93.6 **Activities involving other sports and athletics played as a team or group**
EXCLUDES 1 *activity, ice hockey (Y93.22)*
*activity, water polo (Y93.13)*

Y93.61 **Activity, American tackle football**
Activity, football NOS

Y93.62 **Activity, American flag or touch football**

Y93.63 **Activity, rugby**

Y93.64 **Activity, baseball**
Activity, softball

Y93.65 **Activity, lacrosse and field hockey**

Y93.66 **Activity, soccer**

Y93.67 **Activity, basketball**

Y93.68 **Activity, volleyball (beach) (court)**

Y93.6A **Activity, physical games generally associated with school recess, summer camp and children**
Activity, capture the flag
Activity, dodge ball
Activity, four square
Activity, kickball

Y93.69 **Activity, other involving other sports and athletics played as a team or group**
Activity, cricket

✓5th Y93.7 **Activities involving other specified sports and athletics**

Y93.71 **Activity, boxing**

Y93.72 **Activity, wrestling**

Y93.73 **Activity, racquet and hand sports**
Activity, handball
Activity, racquetball
Activity, squash
Activity, tennis

Y93.74 **Activity, frisbee**
Activity, ultimate frisbee

Y93.75 **Activity, martial arts**
Activity, combatives

Y93.79 **Activity, other specified sports and athletics**
EXCLUDES 1 *sports and athletics activities specified in categories Y93.Ø-Y93.6*

✓5th Y93.A **Activities involving other cardiorespiratory exercise**
Activities involving physical training

Y93.A1 **Activity, exercise machines primarily for cardiorespiratory conditioning**
Activity, elliptical and stepper machines
Activity, stationary bike
Activity, treadmill

Y93.A2 **Activity, calisthenics**
Activity, jumping jacks
Activity, warm up and cool down

Y93.A3 **Activity, aerobic and step exercise**

Y93.A4 **Activity, circuit training**

Y93.A5 **Activity, obstacle course**
Activity, challenge course
Activity, confidence course

Y93.A6 **Activity, grass drills**
Activity, guerilla drills

Y93.A9 **Activity, other involving cardiorespiratory exercise**
EXCLUDES 1 *activities involving cardiorespiratory exercise specified in categories Y93.Ø-Y93.7*

✓5th Y93.B **Activities involving other muscle strengthening exercises**

Y93.B1 **Activity, exercise machines primarily for muscle strengthening**

Y93.B2 **Activity, push-ups, pull-ups, sit-ups**

Y93.B3 **Activity, free weights**
Activity, barbells
Activity, dumbbells

Y93.B4 **Activity, pilates**

Y93.B9 **Activity, other involving muscle strengthening exercises**
EXCLUDES 1 *activities involving muscle strengthening specified in categories Y93.Ø-Y93.A*

✓5th Y93.C **Activities involving computer technology and electronic devices**
EXCLUDES 1 *activity, electronic musical keyboard or instruments (Y93.J-)*

Y93.C1 **Activity, computer keyboarding**
Activity, electronic game playing using keyboard or other stationary device

Y93.C2 **Activity, hand held interactive electronic device**
Activity, cellular telephone and communication device
Activity, electronic game playing using interactive device
EXCLUDES 1 *activity, electronic game playing using keyboard or other stationary device (Y93.C1)*

Y93.C9 **Activity, other involving computer technology and electronic devices**

✓5th Y93.D **Activities involving arts and handcrafts**
EXCLUDES 1 *activities involving playing musical instrument (Y93.J-)*

Y93.D1 **Activity, knitting and crocheting**

Y93.D2 **Activity, sewing**

Y93.D3 **Activity, furniture building and finishing**
Activity, furniture repair

Y93.D9 **Activity, other involving arts and handcrafts**

✓5th **Y93.E Activities involving personal hygiene and interior property and clothing maintenance**

EXCLUDES 1 *activities involving cooking and grilling (Y93.G-)*
*activities involving caregiving (Y93.F-)*
*activities involving exterior property and land maintenance, building and construction (Y93.H-)*
*activity, dishwashing (Y93.G1)*
*activity, food preparation (Y93.G1)*
*activity, gardening (Y93.H2)*

**Y93.E1 Activity, personal bathing and showering**
**Y93.E2 Activity, laundry**
**Y93.E3 Activity, vacuuming**
**Y93.E4 Activity, ironing**
**Y93.E5 Activity, floor mopping and cleaning**
**Y93.E6 Activity, residential relocation**
Activity, packing up and unpacking involved in moving to a new residence
**Y93.E8 Activity, other personal hygiene**
**Y93.E9 Activity, other interior property and clothing maintenance**

✓5th **Y93.F Activities involving caregiving**

Activity involving the provider of caregiving

**Y93.F1 Activity, caregiving, bathing**
**Y93.F2 Activity, caregiving, lifting**
**Y93.F9 Activity, other caregiving**

✓5th **Y93.G Activities involving food preparation, cooking and grilling**

**Y93.G1 Activity, food preparation and clean up**
Activity, dishwashing
**Y93.G2 Activity, grilling and smoking food**
**Y93.G3 Activity, cooking and baking**
Activity, use of stove, oven and microwave oven
**Y93.G9 Activity, other involving cooking and grilling**

✓5th **Y93.H Activities involving exterior property and land maintenance, building and construction**

**Y93.H1 Activity, digging, shoveling and raking**
Activity, dirt digging
Activity, raking leaves
Activity, snow shoveling
**Y93.H2 Activity, gardening and landscaping**
Activity, pruning, trimming shrubs, weeding
**Y93.H3 Activity, building and construction**
**Y93.H9 Activity, other involving exterior property and land maintenance, building and construction**

✓5th **Y93.I Activities involving roller coasters and other types of external motion**

**Y93.I1 Activity, roller coaster riding**
**Y93.I9 Activity, other involving external motion**

✓5th **Y93.J Activities involving playing musical instrument**

Activity involving playing electric musical instrument

**Y93.J1 Activity, piano playing**
Activity, musical keyboard (electronic) playing
**Y93.J2 Activity, drum and other percussion instrument playing**
**Y93.J3 Activity, string instrument playing**
**Y93.J4 Activity, winds and brass instrument playing**

✓5th **Y93.K Activities involving animal care**

EXCLUDES 1 *activity, horseback riding (Y93.52)*

**Y93.K1 Activity, walking an animal**
**Y93.K2 Activity, milking an animal**
**Y93.K3 Activity, grooming and shearing an animal**
**Y93.K9 Activity, other involving animal care**

✓5th **Y93.L Other outdoor activity**

**Y93.L1 Activity, splitting wood**
**Y93.L9 Activity, other outdoor activity**

✓5th **Y93.8 Activities, other specified**

**Y93.81 Activity, refereeing a sports activity**
**Y93.82 Activity, spectator at an event**
**Y93.83 Activity, rough housing and horseplay**
**Y93.84 Activity, sleeping**
**Y93.85 Activity, choking game**
Activity, blackout game
Activity, fainting game
Activity, pass out game
**AHA:** 2016,4Q,74-76
**Y93.89 Activity, other specified**

**Y93.9 Activity, unspecified**

**Y95 Nosocomial condition**
**AHA:** 2013,4Q,119

✓4th **Y99 External cause status**

NOTE A single code from category Y99 should be used in conjunction with the external cause code(s) assigned to a record to indicate the status of the person at the time the event occurred.

**Y99.Ø Civilian activity done for income or pay**
Civilian activity done for financial or other compensation
EXCLUDES 1 *military activity (Y99.1)*
*volunteer activity (Y99.2)*

**Y99.1 Military activity**
EXCLUDES 1 *activity of off duty military personnel (Y99.8)*

**Y99.2 Volunteer activity**
EXCLUDES 1 *activity of child or other family member assisting in compensated work of other family member (Y99.8)*

**Y99.8 Other external cause status**
Activity of child or other family member assisting in compensated work of other family member
Activity NEC
Hobby not done for income
Leisure activity
Off-duty activity of military personnel
Recreation or sport not for income or while a student
Student activity
EXCLUDES 1 *civilian activity done for income or compensation (Y99.Ø)*
*military activity (Y99.1)*
**AHA:** 2012,4Q,108

**Y99.9 Unspecified external cause status**

# Chapter 21. Factors Influencing Health Status and Contact with Health Services (Z00–Z99)

## Chapter-specific Guidelines with Coding Examples

The chapter-specific guidelines from the d Official Guidelines for Coding and Reporting have been provided below. Along with these guidelines are coding examples, contained in the shaded boxes, that have been developed to help illustrate the coding and/or sequencing guidance found in these guidelines.

**Note:** The chapter-specific guidelines provide additional information about the use of Z codes for specified encounters.

**a. Use of Z Codes in any healthcare setting**

Z codes are for use in any healthcare setting. Z codes may be used as either a first-listed (principal diagnosis code in the inpatient setting) or secondary code, depending on the circumstances of the encounter. Certain Z codes may only be used as first-listed or principal diagnosis.

Patient with middle lobe lung cancer presents for initiation of chemotherapy

**Z51.11** **Encounter for antineoplastic chemotherapy**

**C34.2** **Malignant neoplasm of middle lobe, bronchus or lung**

*Explanation:* A Z code can be used as first-listed in this situation based on guidelines in this chapter as well as chapter 2, "Neoplasms."

Patient has chronic lymphocytic leukemia for which the patient had previous chemotherapy and is now in remission

**C91.11** **Chronic lymphocytic leukemia of B-cell type in remission**

**Z92.21** **Personal history of antineoplastic chemotherapy**

*Explanation:* The personal history Z code is used to describe a secondary (supplementary) diagnosis to identify that this patient has had chemotherapy in the past.

**b. Z Codes indicate a reason for an encounter or provide additional information about a patient encounter**

Z codes are not procedure codes. A corresponding procedure code must accompany a Z code to describe any procedure performed.

**c. Categories of Z Codes**

**1) Contact/exposure**

Category Z20 indicates contact with, and suspected exposure to, communicable diseases. These codes are for patients who are suspected to have been exposed to a disease by close personal contact with an infected individual or are in an area where a disease is epidemic.

Category Z77, Other contact with and (suspected) exposures hazardous to health, indicates contact with and suspected exposures hazardous to health.

Contact/exposure codes may be used as a first-listed code to explain an encounter for testing, or, more commonly, as a secondary code to identify a potential risk.

**2) Inoculations and vaccinations**

Code Z23 is for encounters for inoculations and vaccinations. It indicates that a patient is being seen to receive a prophylactic inoculation against a disease. Procedure codes are required to identify the actual administration of the injection and the type(s) of immunizations given. Code Z23 may be used as a secondary code if the inoculation is given as a routine part of preventive health care, such as a well-baby visit.

**3) Status**

Status codes indicate that a patient is either a carrier of a disease or has the sequelae or residual of a past disease or condition. This includes such things as the presence of prosthetic or mechanical devices resulting from past treatment. A status code is informative, because the status may affect the course of treatment and its outcome. A status code is distinct from a history code. The history code indicates that the patient no longer has the condition.

A status code should not be used with a diagnosis code from one of the body system chapters, if the diagnosis code includes the information provided by the status code. For example, code Z94.1, Heart transplant status, should not be used with a code from subcategory T86.2, Complications of heart transplant. The status code does not provide additional information. The complication code indicates that the patient is a heart transplant patient.

For encounters for weaning from a mechanical ventilator, assign a code from subcategory J96.1, Chronic respiratory failure, followed by code Z99.11, Dependence on respirator [ventilator] status.

The status Z codes/categories are:

Z14 Genetic carrier

Genetic carrier status indicates that a person carries a gene, associated with a particular disease, which may be passed to offspring who may develop that disease. The person does not have the disease and is not at risk of developing the disease.

Z15 Genetic susceptibility to disease

Genetic susceptibility indicates that a person has a gene that increases the risk of that person developing the disease.

Codes from category Z15 should generally not be used as principal or first-listed codes. If the patient has the condition to which he/she is susceptible, and that condition is the reason for the encounter, the code for the current condition should be sequenced first. If the patient is being seen for follow-up after completed treatment for this condition, and the condition no longer exists, a follow-up code should be sequenced first, followed by the appropriate personal history and genetic susceptibility codes. If the purpose of the encounter is genetic counseling associated with procreative management, code Z31.5, Encounter for genetic counseling, should be assigned as the first-listed code, followed by a code from category Z15. Additional codes should be assigned for any applicable family or personal history.

Z16 Resistance to antimicrobial drugs

This category indicates that a patient has a condition that is resistant to antimicrobial drug treatment. Sequence the infection code first.

Z17 Estrogen, and other hormones and factors receptor status

Z18 Retained foreign body fragments

Z19 Hormone sensitivity malignancy status

Z21 Asymptomatic HIV infection status

This code indicates that a patient has tested positive for HIV but has manifested no signs or symptoms of the disease.

Z22 Carrier of infectious disease

Carrier status indicates that a person harbors the specific organisms of a disease without manifest symptoms and is capable of transmitting the infection.

Z28.3 Underimmunization status

*See Section I.B.14. for underimmunization documentation by clinicians other than the patient's provider.*

Z33.1 Pregnant state, incidental

This code is a secondary code only for use when the pregnancy is in no way complicating the reason for visit. Otherwise, a code from the obstetric chapter is required.

Z66 Do not resuscitate

This code may be used when it is documented by the provider that a patient is on do not resuscitate status at any time during the stay.

Z67 Blood type

Z68 Body mass index (BMI)

BMI codes should only be assigned when there is an associated, reportable diagnosis (such as obesity or anorexia) documented by the patient's provider.

Do not assign BMI codes during pregnancy. When the documentation reflects fluctuating BMI values during the current encounter for an associated reportable condition, assign a code for the most severe value.

*See Section I.B.14. for BMI documentation by clinicians other than the patient's provider.*

Z74.01 Bed confinement status

Z76.82 Awaiting organ transplant status

Z78 Other specified health status

Code Z78.1, Physical restraint status, may be used when it is documented by the provider that a patient has been put in restraints during the current encounter. Please note that this code should not be reported when it is documented by the provider that a patient is temporarily restrained during a procedure.

Z79 Long-term (current) drug therapy

Codes from this category indicate a patient's continuous use of a prescribed drug (including such things as aspirin therapy) for the long-term treatment of a condition or for prophylactic use. It is not for use for patients who have addictions to drugs. This subcategory is not for use of medications for detoxification or maintenance programs to prevent withdrawal symptoms (e.g., methadone maintenance for opiate dependence). Assign the appropriate code for the drug use, abuse, or dependence instead.

Assign a code from Z79 if the patient is receiving a medication for an extended period as a prophylactic measure (such as for the prevention of deep vein thrombosis) or as treatment of a chronic condition (such as arthritis) or a disease requiring a lengthy course of treatment (such as cancer). Do not assign a code from category Z79 for medication being administered for a brief period of time to treat an acute illness or injury (such as a course of antibiotics to treat acute bronchitis).

Z88 Allergy status to drugs, medicaments and biological substances

Except: Z88.9, Allergy status to unspecified drugs, medicaments and biological substances status

Z89 Acquired absence of limb

Z9Ø Acquired absence of organs, not elsewhere classified

Z91.Ø- Allergy status, other than to drugs and biological substances

Z92.82 Status post administration of tPA (rtPA) in a different facility within the last 24 hours prior to admission to a current facility

Assign code Z92.82, Status post administration of tPA (rtPA) in a different facility within the last 24 hours prior to admission to current facility, as a secondary diagnosis when a patient is received by transfer into a facility and documentation indicates they were administered tissue plasminogen activator (tPA) within the last 24 hours prior to admission to the current facility.

This guideline applies even if the patient is still receiving the tPA at the time they are received into the current facility.

The appropriate code for the condition for which the tPA was administered (such as cerebrovascular disease or myocardial infarction) should be assigned first.

Code Z92.82 is only applicable to the receiving facility record and not to the transferring facility record.

Z93 Artificial opening status

Z94 Transplanted organ and tissue status

Z95 Presence of cardiac and vascular implants and grafts

Z96 Presence of other functional implants

Z97 Presence of other devices

Z98 Other postprocedural states

Assign code Z98.85, Transplanted organ removal status, to indicate that a transplanted organ has been previously removed. This code should not be assigned for the encounter in which the transplanted organ is removed. The complication necessitating removal of the transplant organ should be assigned for that encounter.

*See section I.C.19. for information on the coding of organ transplant complications.*

Z99 Dependence on enabling machines and devices, not elsewhere classified

Note: Categories Z89-Z9Ø and Z93-Z99 are for use only if there are no complications or malfunctions of the organ or tissue replaced, the amputation site or the equipment on which the patient is dependent.

**4) History (of)**

There are two types of history Z codes, personal and family. Personal history codes explain a patient's past medical condition that no longer exists and is not receiving any treatment, but that has the potential for recurrence, and therefore may require continued monitoring.

Family history codes are for use when a patient has a family member(s) who has had a particular disease that causes the patient to be at higher risk of also contracting the disease.

Personal history codes may be used in conjunction with follow-up codes and family history codes may be used in conjunction with screening codes to explain the need for a test or procedure. History codes are also acceptable on any medical record regardless of the reason for visit. A history of an illness, even if no longer present, is important information that may alter the type of treatment ordered.

The reason for the encounter (for example, screening or counseling) should be sequenced first and the appropriate personal and/or family history code(s) should be assigned as additional diagnos(es).

The history Z code categories are:

Z8Ø Family history of primary malignant neoplasm

Z81 Family history of mental and behavioral disorders

Z82 Family history of certain disabilities and chronic diseases (leading to disablement)

Z83 Family history of other specific disorders

Z84 Family history of other conditions

**Z84.A Family history of exposure to diethylstilbestrol**

**Note: Code Z84.A, Family history of exposure to diethylstilbestrol (DES), is assigned when the patient has a family member that was exposed to DES that could cause the patient to be at a higher risk for a condition related to the exposure. This code is used, for example, when the patient's maternal grandmother was exposed to DES**

Z85 Personal history of malignant neoplasm

Z86 Personal history of certain other diseases

Z87 Personal history of other diseases and conditions

Z91.4- Personal history of psychological trauma, not elsewhere classified

Z91.5- Personal history of self-harm

Z91.81 History of falling

Z91.82 Personal history of military deployment

Z91.85 Personal history of military service

Z92 Personal history of medical treatment

Except: Z92.Ø, Personal history of contraception

Except: Z92.82, Status post administration of tPA (rtPA) in a different facility within the last 24 hours prior to admission to a current facility

**5) Screening**

Screening is the testing for disease or disease precursors in seemingly well individuals so that early detection and treatment can be provided for those who test positive for the disease (e.g., screening mammogram).

The testing of a person to rule out or confirm a suspected diagnosis because the patient has some sign or symptom is a diagnostic examination, not a screening. In these cases, the sign or symptom is used to explain the reason for the test.

A screening code may be a first-listed code if the reason for the visit is specifically the screening exam. It may also be used as an additional code if the screening is done during an office visit for other health problems. A screening code is not necessary if the screening is inherent to a routine examination, such as a pap smear done during a routine pelvic examination.

Should a condition be discovered during the screening then the code for the condition may be assigned as an additional diagnosis.

Prostate screening of healthy 5Ø-year-old male patient; PSA noted to be elevated but normal digital rectal exam

**Z12.5 Encounter for screening for malignant neoplasm of prostate**

**R97.2Ø Elevated prostate specific antigen [PSA]**

*Explanation:* The patient had no signs or symptoms of any prostate-related illness prior to coming in for the screening. The screening code is appropriately used as the first-listed code to signify that this was for routine screening. The elevated PSA is reported as a secondary diagnosis to reflect that an abnormal lab value was found as a result of the screening procedure(s).

The Z code indicates that a screening exam is planned. A procedure code is required to confirm that the screening was performed.

The screening Z codes/categories:

Z11 Encounter for screening for infectious and parasitic diseases

Z12 Encounter for screening for malignant neoplasms

Z13 Encounter for screening for other diseases and disorders

Except: Z13.9, Encounter for screening, unspecified

Z36 Encounter for antenatal screening for mother

**6) Observation**

There are three observation Z code categories. They are for use in very limited circumstances when a person is being observed for a suspected condition that is ruled out. The observation codes are not for use if an injury or illness or any signs or symptoms related to the suspected condition are present. In such cases the diagnosis/symptom code is used with the corresponding external cause code.

The observation codes are primarily to be used as a principal/first-listed diagnosis. An observation code may be assigned as a secondary diagnosis code when the patient is being observed for a condition that is ruled out and is unrelated to the principal/first-listed diagnosis. Also, when the principal diagnosis is required to be a code from category Z38, Liveborn infants according to place of birth and type of delivery. Then a code from category ZØ5, Encounter for observation and evaluation of newborn for suspected diseases and conditions ruled out, is sequenced after the Z38 code. Additional codes may be used in addition to the observation code but only if they are unrelated to the suspected condition being observed.

Codes from subcategory Z03.7, Encounter for suspected maternal and fetal conditions ruled out, may either be used as a first-listed or as an additional code assignment depending on the case. They are for use in very limited circumstances on a maternal record when an encounter is for a suspected maternal or fetal condition that is ruled out during that encounter (for example, a maternal or fetal condition may be suspected due to an abnormal test result). These codes should not be used when the condition is confirmed. In those cases, the confirmed condition should be coded. In addition, these codes are not for use if an illness or any signs or symptoms related to the suspected condition or problem are present. In such cases the diagnosis/symptom code is used.

Additional codes may be used in addition to the code from subcategory Z03.7, but only if they are unrelated to the suspected condition being evaluated.

Codes from subcategory Z03.7 may not be used for encounters for antenatal screening of mother. *See Section I.C.21. Screening.*

For encounters for suspected fetal condition that are inconclusive following testing and evaluation, assign the appropriate code from category O35, O36, O40 or O41.

The observation Z code categories:

| | |
|---|---|
| Z03 | Encounter for medical observation for suspected diseases and conditions ruled out |
| Z04 | Encounter for examination and observation for other reasons<br>Except: Z04.9, Encounter for examination and observation for unspecified reason |
| Z05 | Encounter for observation and evaluation of newborn for suspected diseases and conditions ruled out |

**7) Aftercare**

Aftercare visit codes cover situations when the initial treatment of a disease has been performed and the patient requires continued care during the healing or recovery phase, or for the long-term consequences of the disease. The aftercare Z code should not be used if treatment is directed at a current, acute disease. The diagnosis code is to be used in these cases.

The aftercare Z codes should also not be used for aftercare for injuries. For aftercare of an injury, assign the acute injury code with the appropriate 7th character (for subsequent encounter).

The aftercare codes are generally first listed to explain the specific reason for the encounter. An aftercare code may be reported as an additional code when a specific type of aftercare is provided in addition to the reason for the encounter. An example of this would be the closure of a colostomy during an encounter for treatment of another condition.

Aftercare codes should be used in conjunction with other aftercare codes or diagnosis codes to provide better detail on the specifics of an aftercare encounter visit, unless otherwise directed by the classification. The sequencing of multiple aftercare codes depends on the circumstances of the encounter.

Patient presents for third round of gemcitabine and first dose of antineoplastic radiation therapy for advanced pancreatic carcinoma

| | |
|---|---|
| **Z51.11** | **Encounter for antineoplastic chemotherapy** |
| **Z51.0** | **Encounter for antineoplastic radiation therapy** |
| **C25.9** | **Malignant neoplasm of pancreas, unspecified** |

*Explanation:* Gemcitabine is an antineoplastic chemotherapy. Since the encounter was solely to administer antineoplastic treatment, both forms of treatment are reported and either code can be the first-listed diagnosis, followed by the neoplastic condition code. Aftercare codes are typically not assigned for current treatment of disease; however, Z51.0 and subcategory Z51.1 are an exception to this standard.

Certain aftercare Z code categories need a secondary diagnosis code to describe the resolving condition or sequelae. For others, the condition is included in the code title.

Additional Z code aftercare category terms include fitting and adjustment, and attention to artificial openings.

Status Z codes may be used with aftercare Z codes to indicate the nature of the aftercare. For example code Z95.1, Presence of aortocoronary bypass graft, may be used with code Z48.812, Encounter for surgical aftercare following surgery on the circulatory system, to indicate the surgery for which the aftercare is being performed. A status code should not be used when the aftercare code indicates the type of status, such as using Z43.0, Encounter for attention to tracheostomy, with Z93.0, Tracheostomy status.

The aftercare codes are generally found in the following categories:

| | |
|---|---|
| Z42 | Encounter for plastic and reconstructive surgery following medical procedure or healed injury |
| Z43 | Encounter for attention to artificial openings |
| Z44 | Encounter for fitting and adjustment of external prosthetic device |
| Z45 | Encounter for adjustment and management of implanted device |
| Z46 | Encounter for fitting and adjustment of other devices |
| Z47 | Orthopedic aftercare |
| Z48 | Encounter for other postprocedural aftercare |
| Z49 | Encounter for care involving renal dialysis |
| Z51 | Encounter for other aftercare and medical care |

**8) Follow-up**

The follow-up codes are used to explain continuing surveillance following completed treatment of a disease, condition, or injury. They imply that the condition has been fully treated and no longer exists. They should not be confused with aftercare codes, or injury codes with a 7th character for subsequent encounter, that explain ongoing care of a healing condition or its sequelae. Follow-up codes may be used in conjunction with history codes to provide the full picture of the healed condition and its treatment. The follow-up code is sequenced first, followed by the history code.

A follow-up code may be used to explain multiple visits. Should a condition be found to have recurred on the follow-up visit, then the diagnosis code for the condition should be assigned in place of the follow-up code.

The follow-up Z codes/categories:

| | |
|---|---|
| Z08 | Encounter for follow-up examination after completed treatment for malignant neoplasm |
| Z09 | Encounter for follow-up examination after completed treatment for conditions other than malignant neoplasm |

Codes Z08, Encounter for follow-up examination after completed treatment for malignant neoplasm, and Z09, Encounter for follow up examination after completed treatment for conditions other than malignant neoplasm, may be assigned following any type of completed treatment modality (including both medical and surgical treatments).

| | |
|---|---|
| Z39 | Encounter for maternal postpartum care and examination |

Follow-up for patient several months after completing a regime of IV antibiotics for recurrent pneumonia; lungs are clear and pneumonia is resolved

| | |
|---|---|
| **Z09** | **Encounter for follow-up examination after completed treatment for conditions other than malignant neoplasm** |
| **Z87.01** | **Personal history of pneumonia (recurrent)** |

*Explanation:* Code Z09 identifies the follow-up visit as being unrelated to a malignant neoplasm, and code Z87 describes the condition that has now resolved.

Follow-up for patient several months after completing a regime of IV antibiotics for recurrent pneumonia; pneumonia has recurred, and a new antibiotic regimen has been prescribed

| | |
|---|---|
| **J18.9** | **Pneumonia, unspecified organism** |

*Explanation:* Since the follow-up exam for pneumonia determined that the pneumonia was not resolved or recurred, code Z09 Encounter for follow-up examination after completed treatment for conditions other than malignant neoplasm, no longer applies. Instead the first-listed code describes the pneumonia.

**9) Donor**

Codes in category Z52, Donors of organs and tissues, are used for living individuals who are donating blood or other body tissue. These codes are for individuals donating for others, as well as for self-donations. They are not used to identify cadaveric donations.

**10) Counseling**

Counseling Z codes are used when a patient or family member receives assistance in the aftermath of an illness or injury, or when support is required in coping with family or social problems.

The counseling Z codes/categories:

| | |
|---|---|
| Z30.0- | Encounter for general counseling and advice on contraception |
| Z31.5 | Encounter for procreative genetic counseling |
| Z31.6- | Encounter for general counseling and advice on procreation |
| Z32.2 | Encounter for childbirth instruction |
| Z32.3 | Encounter for childcare instruction |
| Z69 | Encounter for mental health services for victim and perpetrator of abuse |

| | |
|---|---|
| Z70 | Counseling related to sexual attitude, behavior and orientation |
| Z71 | Persons encountering health services for other counseling and medical advice, not elsewhere classified<br>Note: Code Z71.84, Encounter for health counseling related to travel, is to be used for health risk and safety counseling for future travel purposes.<br>Code Z71.85, Encounter for immunization safety counseling, is to be used for counseling of the patient or caregiver regarding the safety of a vaccine. This code should not be used for the provision of general information regarding risks and potential side effects during routine encounters for the administration of vaccines.<br>Code Z71.87, Encounter for pediatric-to-adult transition counseling, should be assigned when pediatric-to-adult transition counseling is the sole reason for the encounter or when this counseling is provided in addition to other services, such as treatment of a chronic condition. If both transition counseling and treatment of a medical condition are provided during the same encounter, the code(s) for the medical condition(s) treated and code Z71.87 should be assigned, with sequencing depending on the circumstances of the encounter. |
| Z76.81 | Expectant mother prebirth pediatrician visit |

**11) Encounters for obstetrical and reproductive services**

*See Section I.C.15. Pregnancy, Childbirth, and the Puerperium, for further instruction on the use of these codes.*

Z codes for pregnancy are for use in those circumstances when none of the problems or complications included in the codes from the Obstetrics chapter exist (a routine prenatal visit or postpartum care). Codes in category Z34, Encounter for supervision of normal pregnancy, are always first-listed and are not to be used with any other code from the OB chapter.

Codes in category Z3A, Weeks of gestation, may be assigned to provide additional information about the pregnancy. Category Z3A codes should not be assigned for pregnancies with abortive outcomes (categories O00-O08), elective termination of pregnancy (code Z33.2), nor for postpartum conditions, as category Z3A is not applicable to these conditions. The date of the admission should be used to determine weeks of gestation for inpatient admissions that encompass more than one gestational week.

The outcome of delivery, category Z37, should be included on all maternal delivery records. It is always a secondary code.

Codes in category Z37 should not be used on the newborn record.

Z codes for family planning (contraceptive) or procreative management and counseling should be included on an obstetric record either during the pregnancy or the postpartum stage, if applicable.

Z codes/categories for obstetrical and reproductive services:

| | |
|---|---|
| Z30 | Encounter for contraceptive management |
| Z31 | Encounter for procreative management |
| Z32.2 | Encounter for childbirth instruction |
| Z32.3 | Encounter for childcare instruction |
| Z33 | Pregnant state |
| Z34 | Encounter for supervision of normal pregnancy |
| Z36 | Encounter for antenatal screening of mother |
| Z3A | Weeks of gestation |
| Z37 | Outcome of delivery |
| Z39 | Encounter for maternal postpartum care and examination |
| Z76.81 | Expectant mother prebirth pediatrician visit |

**12) Routine and administrative examinations**

The Z codes allow for the description of encounters for routine examinations, such as, a general check-up, or, examinations for administrative purposes, such as, a pre-employment physical. The codes are not to be used if the examination is for diagnosis of a suspected condition or for treatment purposes. In such cases the diagnosis code is used. During a routine exam, should a diagnosis or condition be discovered, it should be coded as an additional code. Pre-existing and chronic conditions and history codes may also be included as additional codes as long as the examination is for administrative purposes and not focused on any particular condition.

Some of the codes for routine health examinations distinguish between "with" and "without" abnormal findings. Code assignment depends on the information that is known at the time the encounter is being coded. For example, if no abnormal findings were found during the examination, but the encounter is being coded before test results are back, it is acceptable to assign the code for "without abnormal findings." When assigning a code for "with abnormal findings," additional code(s) should be assigned to identify the specific abnormal finding(s).

12-month-old boy presented for well-child visit; pediatrician notices some eczema on the child's scalp and back of the knees

**Z00.121 Encounter for routine child health examination with abnormal findings**

**L30.9 Dermatitis, unspecified**

*Explanation:* The Z code identifying that this is a routine well-child visit is reported first. Because an abnormal finding (eczema) was documented, a code for this condition may also be appended.

Pre-operative examination and pre-procedural laboratory examination Z codes are for use only in those situations when a patient is being cleared for a procedure or surgery and no treatment is given.

The Z codes/categories for routine and administrative examinations:

| | |
|---|---|
| Z00 | Encounter for general examination without complaint, suspected or reported diagnosis |
| Z01 | Encounter for other special examination without complaint, suspected or reported diagnosis |
| Z02 | Encounter for administrative examination<br>Except: Z02.9, Encounter for administrative examinations, unspecified |
| Z32.0- | Encounter for pregnancy test |

**13) Miscellaneous Z codes**

The miscellaneous Z codes capture a number of other health care encounters that do not fall into one of the other categories. Some of these codes identify the reason for the encounter; others are for use as additional codes that provide useful information on circumstances that may affect a patient's care and treatment.

**Prophylactic organ removal**

For encounters specifically for prophylactic removal of an organ (such as prophylactic removal of breasts due to a genetic susceptibility to cancer or a family history of cancer), the principal or first-listed code should be a code from subcategory Z40.0, Encounter for prophylactic surgery for risk factors related to malignant neoplasms, or subcategory Z40.8, Encounter for other prophylactic surgery. If applicable, assign additional code(s) to identify any associated risk factor (such as genetic susceptibility or family history).

If the patient has a malignancy of one site and is having prophylactic removal at another site to prevent either a new primary malignancy or metastatic disease, a code for the malignancy should also be assigned in addition to a code from subcategory Z40.0, Encounter for prophylactic surgery for risk factors related to malignant neoplasms. A Z40.0 code should not be assigned if the patient is having organ removal for treatment of a malignancy, such as the removal of the testes for the treatment of prostate cancer.

Miscellaneous Z codes/subcategories/categories:

| | |
|---|---|
| Z28 | Immunization not carried out<br>Except: Z28.3-, Underimmunization status |
| Z29 | Encounter for other prophylactic measures |
| Z40 | Encounter for prophylactic surgery |
| Z41 | Encounter for procedures for purposes other than remedying health state<br>Except: Z41.9, Encounter for procedure for purposes other than remedying health state, unspecified |
| Z53 | Persons encountering health services for specific procedures and treatment, not carried out |
| Z72 | Problems related to lifestyle<br>Note: These codes should be assigned only when the documentation specifies that the patient has an associated problem |
| Z73 | Problems related to life management difficulty<br>Note: These codes should be assigned only when the documentation specifies that the patient has an associated problem. |
| Z74 | Problems related to care provider dependency<br>Except: Z74.01, Bed confinement status |
| Z75 | Problems related to medical facilities and other health care |
| Z76.0 | Encounter for issue of repeat prescription |
| Z76.3 | Healthy person accompanying sick person |
| Z76.4 | Other boarder to healthcare facility |
| Z76.5 | Malingerer [conscious simulation] |
| Z91.1- | Patient's noncompliance with medical treatment and regimen |
| Z91.A- | Caregiver's noncompliance with patient's medical treatment and regimen |

Z91.B Personal risk factor of exposure to diethylstilbestrol

**Note: This code is assigned to show the patient was directly exposed to DES in utero (e.g., when the patient's mother was exposed to DES while the patient was in utero).**

Z91.83 Wandering in diseases classified elsewhere

Z91.84- Oral health risk factors

Z91.89 Other specified personal risk factors, not elsewhere classified

*See Section I.B.14. for Z55-Z65 Persons with potential health hazards related to socioeconomic and psychosocial circumstances, documentation by clinicians other than the patient's provider*

**14)Nonspecific Z codes**

Certain Z codes are so non-specific, or potentially redundant with other codes in the classification, that there can be little justification for their use in the inpatient setting. Their use in the outpatient setting should be limited to those instances when there is no further documentation to permit more precise coding. Otherwise, any sign or symptom or any other reason for visit that is captured in another code should be used.

Nonspecific Z codes/categories:

Z02.9 Encounter for administrative examinations, unspecified

Z04.9 Encounter for examination and observation for unspecified reason

Z13.9 Encounter for screening, unspecified

Z41.9 Encounter for procedure for purposes other than remedying health state, unspecified

Z52.9 Donor of unspecified organ or tissue

Z86.59 Personal history of other mental and behavioral disorders

Z88.9 Allergy status to unspecified drugs, medicaments and biological substances status

Z92.Ø Personal history of contraception

**15)Z codes that may only be principal/first-listed diagnosis**

The following Z codes/subcategories/categories may only be reported as the principal/first-listed diagnosis, except when there are multiple encounters on the same day and the medical records for the encounters are combined:

ZØØ Encounter for general examination without complaint, suspected or reported diagnosis
Except: ZØØ.6

ZØ1 Encounter for other special examination without complaint, suspected or reported diagnosis

ZØ2 Encounter for administrative examination

ZØ4 Encounter for examination and observation for other reasons

Z33.2 Encounter for elective termination of pregnancy

Z31.81 Encounter for male factor infertility in female patient

Z31.83 Encounter for assisted reproductive fertility procedure cycle

Z31.84 Encounter for fertility preservation procedure

Z34 Encounter for supervision of normal pregnancy

Z39 Encounter for maternal postpartum care and examination

Z38 Liveborn infants according to place of birth and type of delivery

Z4Ø Encounter for prophylactic surgery

Z42 Encounter for plastic and reconstructive surgery following medical procedure or healed injury

Z51.Ø Encounter for antineoplastic radiation therapy

Z51.1- Encounter for antineoplastic chemotherapy and immunotherapy

Z52 Donors of organs and tissues
Except: Z52.9, Donor of unspecified organ or tissue

Z76.1 Encounter for health supervision and care of foundling

Z76.2 Encounter for health supervision and care of other healthy infant and child

Z99.12 Encounter for respirator [ventilator] dependence during power failure

Female patient seen at 32 weeks' gestation to check the progress of her first pregnancy

**Z34.Ø3 Encounter for supervision of normal first pregnancy, third trimester**

**Z3A.32 32 weeks gestation of pregnancy**

*Explanation:* Category Z34 is appropriate as a first-listed diagnosis. Category Z3A helps to clarify at which point in the pregnancy the patient was provided supervision.

**16)Newborns and infants**

*See Section I.C.16. Newborn (Perinatal) Guidelines, for further instruction on the use of these codes.*

Newborn Z codes/subcategories/categories:

Z76.1 Encounter for health supervision and care of foundling

ZØØ.1- Encounter for routine child health examination

Z38 Liveborn infants according to place of birth and type of delivery

**17)Social determinants of health**

Social determinants of health (SDOH) codes describing social problems, conditions, or risk factors that influence a patient's health should be assigned when this information is documented in the patient's medical record. Assign as many SDOH codes as are necessary to describe all of the social problems, conditions, or risk factors documented during the current episode of care. For example, a patient who lives alone may suffer an acute injury temporarily impacting their ability to perform routine activities of daily living. When documented as such, this would support assignment of code Z6Ø.2, Problems related to living alone. However, merely living alone, without documentation of a risk or unmet need for assistance at home, would not support assignment of code Z6Ø.2. Documentation by a clinician (or patient-reported information that is signed off by a clinician) that the patient expressed concerns with access and availability of food would support assignment of code Z59.41, Food insecurity. Similarly, medical record documentation indicating the patient is experiencing homelessness would support assignment of a code from subcategory Z59.Ø, Homelessness.

For social determinants of health classified to chapter 21, such as information found in categories Z55-Z65, Persons with potential health hazards related to socioeconomic and psychosocial circumstances, code assignment may be based on medical record documentation from clinicians involved in the care of the patient who are not the patient's provider since this information represents social information, rather than medical diagnoses. For example, coding professionals may utilize documentation of social information from social workers, community health workers, case managers, or nurses, if their documentation is included in the official medical record.

Patient self-reported documentation may be used to assign codes for social determinants of health, as long as the patient self-reported information is signed-off by and incorporated into the medical record by either a clinician or provider.

Social determinants of health codes are located primarily in these Z code categories:

Z55 Problems related to education and literacy

Z56 Problems related to employment and unemployment

Z57 Occupational exposure to risk factors

Z58 Problems related to physical environment

Z59 Problems related to housing and economic circumstances

Z6Ø Problems related to social environment

Z62 Problems related to upbringing

Z63 Other problems related to primary support group, including family circumstances

Z64 Problems related to certain psychosocial circumstances

Z65 Problems related to other psychosocial circumstances

*See Section I.B.14. Documentation by Clinicians Other than the Patient's Provider.*

# Chapter 21. Factors Influencing Health Status and Contact With Health Services (Z00-Z99)

NOTE Z codes represent reasons for encounters. A corresponding procedure code must accompany a Z code if a procedure is performed. Categories Z00-Z99 are provided for occasions when circumstances other than a disease, injury or external cause classifiable to categories A00-Y89 are recorded as "diagnoses" or "problems." This can arise in two main ways:

(a) When a person who may or may not be sick encounters the health services for some specific purpose, such as to receive limited care or service for a current condition, to donate an organ or tissue, to receive prophylactic vaccination (immunization), or to discuss a problem which is in itself not a disease or injury.

(b) When some circumstance or problem is present which influences the person's health status but is not in itself a current illness or injury.

**AHA:** 2018,4Q,60-61

This chapter contains the following blocks:

| | |
|---|---|
| Z00-Z13 | Persons encountering health services for examinations |
| Z14-Z15 | Genetic carrier and genetic susceptibility to disease |
| Z16 | Resistance to antimicrobial drugs |
| Z17 | estrogen, and other hormones and factors receptor status |
| Z18 | Retained foreign body fragments |
| Z19 | Hormone sensitivity malignancy status |
| Z20-Z29 | Persons with potential health hazards related to communicable diseases |
| Z30-Z39 | Persons encountering health services in circumstances related to reproduction |
| Z40-Z53 | Encounters for other specific health care |
| Z55-Z65 | Persons with potential health hazards related to socioeconomic and psychosocial circumstances |
| Z66 | Do not resuscitate status |
| Z67 | Blood type |
| Z68 | Body mass index (BMI) |
| Z69-Z76 | Persons encountering health services in other circumstances |
| Z77-Z99 | Persons with potential health hazards related to family and personal history and certain conditions influencing health status |

## Persons encountering health services for examinations (Z00-Z13)

NOTE Nonspecific abnormal findings disclosed at the time of these examinations are classified to categories R70-R94.

EXCLUDES 2 *examinations related to pregnancy and reproduction (Z30-Z36, Z39.-)*

✓4th **Z00 Encounter for general examination without complaint, suspected or reported diagnosis**

EXCLUDES 1 *encounter for examination for administrative purposes (Z02.-)*

EXCLUDES 2 *encounter for pre-procedural examinations (Z01.81-)*
*special screening examinations (Z11-Z13)*

**AHA:** 2017,4Q,95

✓5th **Z00.0 Encounter for general adult medical examination**

Encounter for adult periodic examination (annual) (physical) and any associated laboratory and radiologic examinations

EXCLUDES 1 *encounter for examination of sign or symptom - code to sign or symptom*
*general health check-up of infant or child (Z00.12.-)*

**Z00.00 Encounter for general adult medical examination without abnormal findings** PDx A

Encounter for adult health check-up NOS

**AHA:** 2016,1Q,36

**Z00.01 Encounter for general adult medical examination with abnormal findings** PDx A

Use additional code to identify abnormal findings

**AHA:** 2016,1Q,35-36

✓5th **Z00.1 Encounter for newborn, infant and child health examinations**

✓6th **Z00.11 Newborn health examination**

Health check for child under 29 days old

Use additional code to identify any abnormal findings

EXCLUDES 1 *health check for child over 28 days old (Z00.12-)*

**Z00.110 Health examination for newborn under 8 days old** PDx N

Health check for newborn under 8 days old

**Z00.111 Health examination for newborn 8 to 28 days old** PDx N

Health check for newborn 8 to 28 days old
Newborn weight check

✓6th **Z00.12 Encounter for routine child health examination**

Health check (routine) for child over 28 days old
Immunizations appropriate for age
Routine developmental screening of infant or child
Routine vison and hearing testing

EXCLUDES 1 *health check for child under 29 days old (Z00.11-)*
*health supervision of foundling or other healthy infant or child (Z76.1-Z76.2)*
*newborn health examination (Z00.11-)*

**AHA:** 2018,4Q,36

**Z00.121 Encounter for routine child health examination with abnormal findings** PDx P

Use additional code to identify abnormal findings

**AHA:** 2024,4Q,6; 2016,1Q,34-35

**Z00.129 Encounter for routine child health examination without abnormal findings** PDx P

Encounter for routine child health examination NOS

**AHA:** 2016,1Q,34

**Z00.2 Encounter for examination for period of rapid growth in childhood** PDx P

**Z00.3 Encounter for examination for adolescent development state** PDx P

Encounter for puberty development state

**Z00.5 Encounter for examination of potential donor of organ and tissue** PDx

**Z00.6 Encounter for examination for normal comparison and control in clinical research program**

Examination of participant or control in clinical research program

✓5th **Z00.7 Encounter for examination for period of delayed growth in childhood**

**Z00.70 Encounter for examination for period of delayed growth in childhood without abnormal findings** PDx P

**Z00.71 Encounter for examination for period of delayed growth in childhood with abnormal findings** PDx P

Use additional code to identify abnormal findings

**Z00.8 Encounter for other general examination** PDx

Encounter for health examination in population surveys

✓4th **Z01 Encounter for other special examination without complaint, suspected or reported diagnosis**

INCLUDES routine examination of specific system

NOTE Codes from category Z01 represent the reason for the encounter. A separate procedure code is required to identify any examinations or procedures performed

EXCLUDES 1 *encounter for examination for administrative purposes (Z02.-)*
*encounter for examination for suspected conditions, proven not to exist (Z03.-)*
*encounter for laboratory, radiologic and imaging examinations for sign(s) and symptom(s) - code to the sign(s) or symptom(s)*

EXCLUDES 2 *encounter for laboratory and radiologic examinations as a component of general medical examinations (Z00.0-)*
*screening examinations (Z11-Z13)*

✓5th **Z01.0 Encounter for examination of eyes and vision**

EXCLUDES 1 *examination for driving license (Z02.4)*

**Z01.00 Encounter for examination of eyes and vision without abnormal findings** PDx

Encounter for examination of eyes and vision NOS

**Z01.01 Encounter for examination of eyes and vision with abnormal findings** PDx

Use additional code to identify abnormal findings

**AHA:** 2016,4Q,21

✓6th **Z01.02 Encounter for examination of eyes and vision following failed vision screening**

EXCLUDES 1 *encounter for examination of eyes and vision with abnormal findings (Z01.01)*
*encounter for examination of eyes and vision without abnormal findings (Z01.00)*

**AHA:** 2019,4Q,20

**Z01.020 Encounter for examination of eyes and vision following failed vision screening without abnormal findings** PDx

Z01.021 **Encounter for examination of eyes and vision following failed vision screening with abnormal findings** PDx
Use additional code to identify abnormal findings

✓5th Z01.1 **Encounter for examination of ears and hearing**

Z01.10 **Encounter for examination of ears and hearing without abnormal findings** PDx
Encounter for examination of ears and hearing NOS
AHA: 2016,4Q,24

✓6th Z01.11 **Encounter for examination of ears and hearing with abnormal findings**
AHA: 2016,3Q,17-18

Z01.110 **Encounter for hearing examination following failed hearing screening** PDx

Z01.118 **Encounter for examination of ears and hearing with other abnormal findings** PDx
Use additional code to identify abnormal findings

Z01.12 **Encounter for hearing conservation and treatment** PDx

✓5th Z01.2 **Encounter for dental examination and cleaning**

Z01.20 **Encounter for dental examination and cleaning without abnormal findings** PDx
Encounter for dental examination and cleaning NOS

Z01.21 **Encounter for dental examination and cleaning with abnormal findings** PDx
Use additional code to identify abnormal findings

✓5th Z01.3 **Encounter for examination of blood pressure**

Z01.30 **Encounter for examination of blood pressure without abnormal findings** PDx
Encounter for examination of blood pressure NOS

Z01.31 **Encounter for examination of blood pressure with abnormal findings** PDx
Use additional code to identify abnormal findings

✓5th Z01.4 **Encounter for gynecological examination**
EXCLUDES 2 *pregnancy examination or test (Z32.0-)*
*routine examination for contraceptive maintenance (Z30.4-)*

✓6th Z01.41 **Encounter for routine gynecological examination**
Encounter for general gynecological examination with or without cervical smear
Encounter for gynecological examination (general) (routine) NOS
Encounter for pelvic examination (annual) (periodic)
Use additional code:
for screening for human papillomavirus, if applicable, (Z11.51)
for screening vaginal pap smear, if applicable (Z12.72)
to identify acquired absence of uterus, if applicable (Z90.71-)
EXCLUDES 1 *gynecologic examination status-post hysterectomy for malignant condition (Z08)*
*screening cervical pap smear not a part of a routine gynecological examination (Z12.4)*

Z01.411 **Encounter for gynecological examination (general) (routine) with abnormal findings** PDx
Use additional code to identify abnormal findings

Z01.419 **Encounter for gynecological examination (general) (routine) without abnormal findings** PDx

Z01.42 **Encounter for cervical smear to confirm findings of recent normal smear following initial abnormal smear** PDx

✓5th Z01.8 **Encounter for other specified special examinations**

✓6th Z01.81 **Encounter for preprocedural examinations**
Encounter for preoperative examinations
Encounter for radiological and imaging examinations as part of preprocedural examination
TIP: Assign a code for the condition necessitating surgery and any findings as additional diagnoses.

Z01.810 **Encounter for preprocedural cardiovascular examination** PDx

Z01.811 **Encounter for preprocedural respiratory examination** PDx

Z01.812 **Encounter for preprocedural laboratory examination** PDx
Blood and urine tests prior to treatment or procedure
AHA: 2023,2Q,3; 2020,3Q,14

Z01.818 **Encounter for other preprocedural examination** PDx
Encounter for examinations prior to antineoplastic chemotherapy
Encounter for preprocedural examination NOS

Z01.82 **Encounter for allergy testing** PDx
EXCLUDES 1 *encounter for antibody response examination (Z01.84)*

Z01.83 **Encounter for blood typing** PDx
Encounter for Rh typing

Z01.84 **Encounter for antibody response examination** PDx
Encounter for immunity status testing
EXCLUDES 1 *encounter for allergy testing (Z01.82)*
AHA: 2020,2Q,11

Z01.89 **Encounter for other specified special examinations** PDx

✓4th **Z02 Encounter for administrative examination**

Z02.0 **Encounter for examination for admission to educational institution** PDx
Encounter for examination for admission to preschool (education)
Encounter for examination for re-admission to school following illness or medical treatment

Z02.1 **Encounter for pre-employment examination** PDx

Z02.2 **Encounter for examination for admission to residential institution** PDx
EXCLUDES 1 *examination for admission to prison (Z02.89)*

Z02.3 **Encounter for examination for recruitment to armed forces** PDx

Z02.4 **Encounter for examination for driving license** PDx

Z02.5 **Encounter for examination for participation in sport** PDx
EXCLUDES 1 *blood-alcohol and blood-drug test (Z02.83)*

Z02.6 **Encounter for examination for insurance purposes** PDx

✓5th Z02.7 **Encounter for issue of medical certificate**
EXCLUDES 1 *encounter for general medical examination (Z00-Z01, Z02.0-Z02.6, Z02.8-Z02.9)*

Z02.71 **Encounter for disability determination** PDx
Encounter for issue of medical certificate of incapacity
Encounter for issue of medical certificate of invalidity

Z02.79 **Encounter for issue of other medical certificate** PDx

✓5th Z02.8 **Encounter for other administrative examinations**

Z02.81 **Encounter for paternity testing** PDx

Z02.82 **Encounter for adoption services** PDx

Z02.83 **Encounter for blood-alcohol and blood-drug test** PDx
Use additional code for findings of alcohol or drugs in blood (R78.-)

Z02.84 **Encounter for child welfare exam** P
Encounter for child welfare screening exam
EXCLUDES 2 *encounter for examination and observation for alleged child physical abuse (Z04.72)*
*encounter for examination and observation for alleged child rape (Z04.42)*
AHA: 2023,4Q,49

Z02.89 **Encounter for other administrative examinations** PDx
Encounter for examination for admission to prison
Encounter for examination for admission to summer camp
Encounter for immigration examination
Encounter for naturalization examination
Encounter for premarital examination
EXCLUDES 1 *health supervision of foundling or other healthy infant or child (Z76.1-Z76.2)*

Z02.9 **Encounter for administrative examinations, unspecified** PDx

✓4th **Z03 Encounter for medical observation for suspected diseases and conditions ruled out**

This category is to be used when a person without a diagnosis is suspected of having an abnormal condition, without signs or symptoms, which requires study, but after examination and observation, is ruled out. This category is also for use for administrative and legal observation status.

EXCLUDES 1 *contact with and (suspected) exposures hazardous to health (Z77.-)*
*encounter for observation and evaluation of newborn for suspected diseases and conditions ruled out (Z05.-)*
*person with feared complaint in whom no diagnosis is made (Z71.1)*
*signs or symptoms under study - code to signs or symptoms*

**AHA:** 2020,2Q,8; 2018,2Q,7-8; 2017,4Q,27

**Z03.6 Encounter for observation for suspected toxic effect from ingested substance ruled out**
Encounter for observation for suspected adverse effect from drug
Encounter for observation for suspected poisoning

✓5th **Z03.7 Encounter for suspected maternal and fetal conditions ruled out**
Encounter for suspected maternal and fetal conditions not found
EXCLUDES 1 *known or suspected fetal anomalies affecting management of mother, not ruled out (O26.-, O35.-, O36.-, O40.-, O41.-)*

**Z03.71 Encounter for suspected problem with amniotic cavity and membrane ruled out** M
Encounter for suspected oligohydramnios ruled out
Encounter for suspected polyhydramnios ruled out

**Z03.72 Encounter for suspected placental problem ruled out** M

**Z03.73 Encounter for suspected fetal anomaly ruled out** M

**Z03.74 Encounter for suspected problem with fetal growth ruled out** M

**Z03.75 Encounter for suspected cervical shortening ruled out** M

**Z03.79 Encounter for other suspected maternal and fetal conditions ruled out** M

✓5th **Z03.8 Encounter for observation for other suspected diseases and conditions ruled out**

✓6th **Z03.81 Encounter for observation for suspected exposure to biological agents ruled out**

**Z03.810 Encounter for observation for suspected exposure to anthrax ruled out**

**Z03.818 Encounter for observation for suspected exposure to other biological agents ruled out**
**AHA:** 2020,2Q,8; 2020,1Q,34-36
**TIP:** Possible or actual exposure to COVID-19 should be coded using Z20.822 Contact with and (suspected) exposure to COVID-19, even when the COVID-19 infection has been ruled out.

✓6th **Z03.82 Encounter for observation for suspected foreign body ruled out**
EXCLUDES 1 *retained foreign body (Z18.-)*
*residual foreign body in soft tissue (M79.5)*
*retained foreign body in eyelid (H02.81)*
EXCLUDES 2 *confirmed foreign body ingestion or aspiration including:*
*foreign body in alimentary tract (T18)*
*foreign body in ear (T16)*
*foreign body in respiratory tract (T17)*
*foreign body on external eye (T15)*
**AHA:** 2020,4Q,42

**Z03.821 Encounter for observation for suspected ingested foreign body ruled out**

**Z03.822 Encounter for observation for suspected aspirated (inhaled) foreign body ruled out**

**Z03.823 Encounter for observation for suspected inserted (injected) foreign body ruled out**
Encounter for observation for suspected inserted (injected) foreign body in eye ruled out
Encounter for observation for suspected inserted (injected) foreign body in orifice ruled out
Encounter for observation for suspected inserted (injected) foreign body in skin ruled out

**Z03.83 Encounter for observation for suspected conditions related to home physiologic monitoring device ruled out**
Encounter for observation for apnea alarm without findings
Encounter for observation for bradycardia alarm without findings
Encounter for observation for malfunction of home cardiorespiratory monitor
Encounter for observation for non-specific findings home physiologic monitoring device
Encounter for observation for pulse oximeter alarm without findings
EXCLUDES 1 *apnea NOS (R06.81)*
*neonatal bradycardia (P29.12)*
*newborn apnea (P28.4-)*
*primary sleep apnea of newborn (P28.3-)*
*sleep apnea (G47.3-)*
**AHA:** 2022,4Q,51

**Z03.89 Encounter for observation for other suspected diseases and conditions ruled out**

✓4th **Z04 Encounter for examination and observation for other reasons**

This category is to be used when a person without a diagnosis is suspected of having an abnormal condition, without signs or symptoms, which requires study, but after examination and observation, is ruled-out. This category is also for use for administrative and legal observation status.

INCLUDES encounter for examination for medicolegal reasons

**AHA:** 2018,2Q,7-8

**Z04.1 Encounter for examination and observation following transport accident** PDx
EXCLUDES 1 *encounter for examination and observation following work accident (Z04.2)*
**AHA:** 2019,2Q,11; 2018,2Q,8

**Z04.2 Encounter for examination and observation following work accident** PDx

**Z04.3 Encounter for examination and observation following other accident** PDx

✓5th **Z04.4 Encounter for examination and observation following alleged rape**
Encounter for examination and observation of victim following alleged rape
Encounter for examination and observation of victim following alleged sexual abuse

**Z04.41 Encounter for examination and observation following alleged adult rape** PDx A
Suspected adult rape, ruled out
Suspected adult sexual abuse, ruled out

**Z04.42 Encounter for examination and observation following alleged child rape** PDx P
Suspected child rape, ruled out
Suspected child sexual abuse, ruled out

**Z04.6 Encounter for general psychiatric examination, requested by authority** PDx

✓5th **Z04.7 Encounter for examination and observation following alleged physical abuse**

**Z04.71 Encounter for examination and observation following alleged adult physical abuse** PDx A
Suspected adult physical abuse, ruled out
EXCLUDES 1 *confirmed case of adult physical abuse (T74.-)*
*encounter for examination and observation following alleged adult sexual abuse (Z04.41)*
*suspected case of adult physical abuse, not ruled out (T76.-)*

**Z04.72 Encounter for examination and observation following alleged child physical abuse** PDx P
Suspected child physical abuse, ruled out
EXCLUDES 1 *confirmed case of child physical abuse (T74.-)*
*encounter for examination and observation following alleged child sexual abuse (Z04.42)*
*suspected case of child physical abuse, not ruled out (T76.-)*

✓5th **Z04.8 Encounter for examination and observation for other specified reasons**
Encounter for examination and observation for request for expert evidence
AHA: 2018,4Q,32,35,72

**Z04.81 Encounter for examination and observation of victim following forced sexual exploitation** PDx

**Z04.82 Encounter for examination and observation of victim following forced labor exploitation** PDx

**Z04.89 Encounter for examination and observation for other specified reasons** PDx

**Z04.9 Encounter for examination and observation for unspecified reason** PDx
Encounter for observation NOS

✓4th **Z05 Encounter for observation and evaluation of newborn for suspected diseases and conditions ruled out**
This category is to be used for newborns, within the neonatal period (the first 28 days of life), who are suspected of having an abnormal condition, but without signs or symptoms, and which, after examination and observation, is ruled out.
AHA: 2022,1Q,17-18; 2017,4Q,27; 2016,4Q,77

**Z05.0 Observation and evaluation of newborn for suspected cardiac condition ruled out** N

**Z05.1 Observation and evaluation of newborn for suspected infectious condition ruled out** N
AHA: 2019,2Q,10

**Z05.2 Observation and evaluation of newborn for suspected neurological condition ruled out** N

**Z05.3 Observation and evaluation of newborn for suspected respiratory condition ruled out** N

✓5th **Z05.4 Observation and evaluation of newborn for suspected genetic, metabolic or immunologic condition ruled out**

**Z05.41 Observation and evaluation of newborn for suspected genetic condition ruled out** N
AHA: 2016,4Q,55

**Z05.42 Observation and evaluation of newborn for suspected metabolic condition ruled out** N

**Z05.43 Observation and evaluation of newborn for suspected immunologic condition ruled out** N

**Z05.5 Observation and evaluation of newborn for suspected gastrointestinal condition ruled out** N

**Z05.6 Observation and evaluation of newborn for suspected genitourinary condition ruled out** N

✓5th **Z05.7 Observation and evaluation of newborn for suspected skin, subcutaneous, musculoskeletal and connective tissue condition ruled out**

**Z05.71 Observation and evaluation of newborn for suspected skin and subcutaneous tissue condition ruled out** N

**Z05.72 Observation and evaluation of newborn for suspected musculoskeletal condition ruled out** N

**Z05.73 Observation and evaluation of newborn for suspected connective tissue condition ruled out** N

✓5th **Z05.8 Observation and evaluation of newborn for other specified suspected condition ruled out**
AHA: 2023,4Q,48; 2022,1Q,17-18

**Z05.81 Observation and evaluation of newborn for suspected condition related to home physiologic monitoring device ruled out** N
Encounter for observation of newborn for apnea alarm without findings
Encounter for observation of newborn for bradycardia alarm without findings
Encounter for observation of newborn for malfunction of home cardiorespiratory monitor
Encounter for observation of newborn for non-specific findings home physiologic monitoring device
Encounter for observation of newborn for pulse oximeter alarm without findings
EXCLUDES 1 *encounter for observation for suspected conditions related to home physiologic monitoring device ruled out (Z03.83)*
*neonatal bradycardia (P29.12)*
*other newborn apnea (P28.4-)*
*primary sleep apnea of newborn (P28.3-)*

**Z05.89 Observation and evaluation of newborn for other specified suspected condition ruled out** N

**Z05.9 Observation and evaluation of newborn for unspecified suspected condition ruled out** N

**Z08 Encounter for follow-up examination after completed treatment for malignant neoplasm**
Medical surveillance following completed treatment
Use additional code to identify any acquired absence of organs (Z90.-)
Use additional code to identify the personal history of malignant neoplasm (Z85.-)
EXCLUDES 1 *aftercare following medical care (Z43-Z49, Z51)*
AHA: 2020,3Q,30

**Z09 Encounter for follow-up examination after completed treatment for conditions other than malignant neoplasm**
Medical surveillance following completed treatment
Use additional code to identify any applicable history of disease code (Z86.-, Z87.-)
EXCLUDES 1 *aftercare following medical care (Z43-Z49, Z51)*
*surveillance of contraception (Z30.4-)*
*surveillance of prosthetic and other medical devices (Z44-Z46)*
AHA: 2022,3Q,4; 2021,1Q,33; 2020,2Q,10; 2017,1Q,9; 2015,1Q,8

✓4th **Z11 Encounter for screening for infectious and parasitic diseases**
Screening is the testing for disease or disease precursors in asymptomatic individuals so that early detection and treatment can be provided for those who test positive for the disease.
EXCLUDES 1 *encounter for diagnostic examination - code to sign or symptom*

**Z11.0 Encounter for screening for intestinal infectious diseases**

**Z11.1 Encounter for screening for respiratory tuberculosis**
Encounter for screening for active tuberculosis disease

**Z11.2 Encounter for screening for other bacterial diseases**

**Z11.3 Encounter for screening for infections with a predominantly sexual mode of transmission**
EXCLUDES 2 *encounter for screening for human immunodeficiency virus [HIV] (Z11.4)*
*encounter for screening for human papillomavirus (Z11.51)*

**Z11.4 Encounter for screening for human immunodeficiency virus [HIV]**

✓5th **Z11.5 Encounter for screening for other viral diseases**
EXCLUDES 2 *encounter for screening for viral intestinal disease (Z11.0)*

**Z11.51 Encounter for screening for human papillomavirus (HPV)**

**Z11.52 Encounter for screening for COVID-19**
AHA: 2023,2Q,3; 2021,1Q,27,37,41

**Z11.59 Encounter for screening for other viral diseases**
AHA: 2020,3Q,14

**Z11.6 Encounter for screening for other protozoal diseases and helminthiases**
EXCLUDES 2 *encounter for screening for protozoal intestinal disease (Z11.0)*

**Z11.7 Encounter for testing for latent tuberculosis infection**
AHA: 2019,4Q,20

**Z11.8 Encounter for screening for other infectious and parasitic diseases**
Encounter for screening for chlamydia
Encounter for screening for mycoses
Encounter for screening for rickettsial
Encounter for screening for spirochetal

**Z11.9 Encounter for screening for infectious and parasitic diseases, unspecified**

✓4th **Z12 Encounter for screening for malignant neoplasms**
Screening is the testing for disease or disease precursors in asymptomatic individuals so that early detection and treatment can be provided for those who test positive for the disease.
Use additional code to identify any family history of malignant neoplasm (Z80.-)
EXCLUDES 1 *encounter for diagnostic examination - code to sign or symptom*

**Z12.0 Encounter for screening for malignant neoplasm of stomach**

✓5th **Z12.1 Encounter for screening for malignant neoplasm of intestinal tract**
AHA: 2017,1Q,8,9

**Z12.10 Encounter for screening for malignant neoplasm of intestinal tract, unspecified**

**Z12.11 Encounter for screening for malignant neoplasm of colon** Q
Encounter for screening colonoscopy NOS
**AHA:** 2019,1Q,32-33; 2018,1Q,6
**TIP:** Surveillance colonoscopies are a type of screening exam used to screen for malignancies in those patients with history of polyps and/or cancer (previously removed). If polyps or cancer are removed during the colonoscopy, code the appropriate neoplasm code instead of Z12.11.

**Z12.12 Encounter for screening for malignant neoplasm of rectum**
**AHA:** 2018,1Q,6

**Z12.13 Encounter for screening for malignant neoplasm of small intestine**

**Z12.2 Encounter for screening for malignant neoplasm of respiratory organs**

✓5th **Z12.3 Encounter for screening for malignant neoplasm of breast**

**Z12.31 Encounter for screening mammogram for malignant neoplasm of breast**
EXCLUDES 1 *inconclusive mammogram (R92.2)*
**AHA:** 2023,4Q,44; 2015,1Q,24

**Z12.39 Encounter for other screening for malignant neoplasm of breast**

**Z12.4 Encounter for screening for malignant neoplasm of cervix**
Encounter for screening pap smear for malignant neoplasm of cervix
EXCLUDES 1 *when screening is part of general gynecological examination (Z01.4-)*
EXCLUDES 2 *encounter for screening for human papillomavirus (Z11.51)*

**Z12.5 Encounter for screening for malignant neoplasm of prostate**

**Z12.6 Encounter for screening for malignant neoplasm of bladder**

✓5th **Z12.7 Encounter for screening for malignant neoplasm of other genitourinary organs**

**Z12.71 Encounter for screening for malignant neoplasm of testis**

**Z12.72 Encounter for screening for malignant neoplasm of vagina**
Vaginal pap smear status-post hysterectomy for non-malignant condition
Use additional code to identify acquired absence of uterus (Z90.71-)
EXCLUDES 1 *vaginal pap smear status-post hysterectomy for malignant conditions (Z08)*

**Z12.73 Encounter for screening for malignant neoplasm of ovary**

**Z12.79 Encounter for screening for malignant neoplasm of other genitourinary organs**

✓5th **Z12.8 Encounter for screening for malignant neoplasm of other sites**

**Z12.81 Encounter for screening for malignant neoplasm of oral cavity**

**Z12.82 Encounter for screening for malignant neoplasm of nervous system**

**Z12.83 Encounter for screening for malignant neoplasm of skin**

**Z12.89 Encounter for screening for malignant neoplasm of other sites**
**AHA:** 2021,1Q,14

**Z12.9 Encounter for screening for malignant neoplasm, site unspecified**

✓4th **Z13 Encounter for screening for other diseases and disorders**
Screening is the testing for disease or disease precursors in asymptomatic individuals so that early detection and treatment can be provided for those who test positive for the disease.
EXCLUDES 1 *encounter for diagnostic examination - code to sign or symptom*

**Z13.0 Encounter for screening for diseases of the blood and blood-forming organs and certain disorders involving the immune mechanism**

**Z13.1 Encounter for screening for diabetes mellitus**

✓5th **Z13.2 Encounter for screening for nutritional, metabolic and other endocrine disorders**

**Z13.21 Encounter for screening for nutritional disorder**

✓6th **Z13.22 Encounter for screening for metabolic disorder**

**Z13.220 Encounter for screening for lipoid disorders**
Encounter for screening for cholesterol level
Encounter for screening for hypercholesterolemia
Encounter for screening for hyperlipidemia

**Z13.228 Encounter for screening for other metabolic disorders**

**Z13.29 Encounter for screening for other suspected endocrine disorder**
EXCLUDES 2 *encounter for screening for diabetes mellitus (Z13.1)*

✓5th **Z13.3 Encounter for screening examination for mental health and behavioral disorders**
**AHA:** 2018,4Q,35-36

**Z13.30 Encounter for screening examination for mental health and behavioral disorders, unspecified**

**Z13.31 Encounter for screening for depression**
Encounter for screening for depression for child or adolescent
Encounter for screening for depression, adult

**Z13.32 Encounter for screening for maternal depression** M
Encounter for screening for perinatal depression

**Z13.39 Encounter for screening examination for other mental health and behavioral disorders**
Encounter for screening for alcoholism
Encounter for screening for intellectual disabilities

✓5th **Z13.4 Encounter for screening for certain developmental disorders in childhood**
Encounter for development testing of infant or child
Encounter for screening for developmental handicaps in early childhood
EXCLUDES 2 *encounter for routine child health examination (Z00.12-)*
**AHA:** 2018,4Q,36

**Z13.40 Encounter for screening for unspecified developmental delays**

**Z13.41 Encounter for autism screening**

**Z13.42 Encounter for screening for global developmental delays (milestones)**
Encounter for screening for developmental handicaps in early childhood

**Z13.49 Encounter for screening for other developmental delays**

**Z13.5 Encounter for screening for eye and ear disorders**
EXCLUDES 2 *encounter for general hearing examination (Z01.1-)*
*encounter for general vision examination (Z01.0-)*
**AHA:** 2016,3Q,17

**Z13.6 Encounter for screening for cardiovascular disorders**

✓5th **Z13.7 Encounter for screening for genetic and chromosomal anomalies**
EXCLUDES 1 *genetic testing for procreative management (Z31.4-)*

**Z13.71 Encounter for nonprocreative screening for genetic disease carrier status**

**Z13.79 Encounter for other screening for genetic and chromosomal anomalies**

✓5th **Z13.8 Encounter for screening for other specified diseases and disorders**
EXCLUDES 2 *screening for malignant neoplasms (Z12.-)*

✓6th **Z13.81 Encounter for screening for digestive system disorders**

**Z13.810 Encounter for screening for upper gastrointestinal disorder**

**Z13.811 Encounter for screening for lower gastrointestinal disorder**
EXCLUDES 1 *encounter for screening for intestinal infectious disease (Z11.0)*

**Z13.818 Encounter for screening for other digestive system disorders**

✓6th **Z13.82 Encounter for screening for musculoskeletal disorder**

**Z13.820 Encounter for screening for osteoporosis**

**Z13.828 Encounter for screening for other musculoskeletal disorder**

**Z13.83 Encounter for screening for respiratory disorder NEC**
EXCLUDES 1 *encounter for screening for respiratory tuberculosis (Z11.1)*

**Z13.84 Encounter for screening for dental disorders**

✓6th **Z13.85 Encounter for screening for nervous system disorders**
**Z13.850 Encounter for screening for traumatic brain injury**
**Z13.858 Encounter for screening for other nervous system disorders**
**Z13.88 Encounter for screening for disorder due to exposure to contaminants**
EXCLUDES 1 *those exposed to contaminants without suspected disorders (Z57.-, Z77.-)*
**Z13.89 Encounter for screening for other disorder**
Encounter for screening for genitourinary disorders
**Z13.9 Encounter for screening, unspecified**

## Genetic carrier and genetic susceptibility to disease (Z14-Z15)

✓4th **Z14 Genetic carrier**
**DEF:** Individuals carrying a gene mutation associated with a certain disease that typically do not develop the disease but are able to pass the mutated genes to offspring.
✓5th **Z14.0 Hemophilia A carrier**
**Z14.01 Asymptomatic hemophilia A carrier**
**Z14.02 Symptomatic hemophilia A carrier**
**Z14.1 Cystic fibrosis carrier**
**Z14.8 Genetic carrier of other disease**

✓4th **Z15 Genetic susceptibility to disease**
INCLUDES confirmed abnormal gene
Use additional code, if applicable, for any associated family history of the disease (Z80-Z84)
EXCLUDES 1 *chromosomal anomalies (Q90-Q99)*
✓5th **Z15.0 Genetic susceptibility to malignant neoplasm**
Code first, if applicable, any current malignant neoplasm (C00-C75, C81-C96)
Use additional code, if applicable, for any personal history of malignant neoplasm (Z85.-)
**Z15.01 Genetic susceptibility to malignant neoplasm of breast**
**Z15.02 Genetic susceptibility to malignant neoplasm of ovary**
**Z15.03 Genetic susceptibility to malignant neoplasm of prostate**
**Z15.04 Genetic susceptibility to malignant neoplasm of endometrium**
**Z15.05 Genetic susceptibility to malignant neoplasm of fallopian tube(s)**
✓6th **Z15.06 Genetic susceptibility to malignant neoplasm of digestive system**
**Z15.060 Genetic susceptibility to colorectal cancer**
**Z15.068 Genetic susceptibility to other malignant neoplasm of digestive system**
Genetic susceptibility to biliary tract cancer
Genetic susceptibility to gastric cancer
Genetic susceptibility to pancreatic cancer
Genetic susceptibility to small bowel cancer
**Z15.07 Genetic susceptibility to malignant neoplasm of urinary tract**
**Z15.09 Genetic susceptibility to other malignant neoplasm**
**AHA:** 2021,1Q,14
**Z15.1 Genetic susceptibility to epilepsy and neurodevelopmental disorders**
Code also, if applicable, related disorders such as:
developmental and epileptic encephalopathy (G93.45)
developmental disorder of speech and language (F80.-)
developmental disorders of scholastic skills (F81.-)
epilepsy, by specific type (G40.-)
intellectual disabilities (F70-F79)
other neurodevelopmental disorder (F88)
pervasive developmental disorders (F84.-)
**AHA:** 2024,4Q,31
**Z15.2 Genetic susceptibility to obesity**
Code also, if applicable, any associated manifestations, such as:
other obesity (E66.8-)
polyphagia (R63.2)
Use additional code to identify body mass index (BMI), if known (Z68.-)
**AHA:** 2024,4Q,31
**Z15.3 Genetic susceptibility to kidney disease**
Code also, if applicable, hypertension (I10-I1A)
✓5th **Z15.8 Genetic susceptibility to other disease**
**Z15.81 Genetic susceptibility to multiple endocrine neoplasia [MEN]**
EXCLUDES 1 *multiple endocrine neoplasia [MEN] syndromes (E31.2-)*
**DEF:** Group of conditions in which several endocrine glands grow excessively (such as in adenomatous hyperplasia) and/or develop benign or malignant tumors. Tumors and hyperplasia associated with MEN often produce excess hormones, which impede normal physiology. There is no comprehensive cure known for MEN syndrome. Treatment is directed at the hyperplasia or tumors in each individual gland. Tumors are usually surgically removed and oral medications or hormonal injections are used to correct hormone imbalances.
**Z15.89 Genetic susceptibility to other disease**

## Resistance to antimicrobial drugs (Z16)

✓4th **Z16 Resistance to antimicrobial drugs**
NOTE The codes in this category are provided for use as additional codes to identify the resistance and non-responsiveness of a condition to antimicrobial drugs.
Code first the infection
EXCLUDES 1 *Methicillin resistant Staphylococcus aureus infection (A49.02)*
*Methicillin resistant Staphylococcus aureus pneumonia (J15.212)*
*sepsis due to Methicillin resistant Staphylococcus aureus (A41.02)*
✓5th **Z16.1 Resistance to beta lactam antibiotics**
**Z16.10 Resistance to unspecified beta lactam antibiotics** UPD
**Z16.11 Resistance to penicillins** UPD
Resistance to amoxicillin
Resistance to ampicillin
**Z16.12 Extended spectrum beta lactamase (ESBL) resistance** UPD
EXCLUDES 2 *Methicillin resistant Staphylococcus aureus infection in diseases classified elsewhere (B95.62)*
**Z16.13 Resistance to carbapenem** UPD
**AHA:** 2023,4Q,47
**Z16.19 Resistance to other specified beta lactam antibiotics** UPD
Resistance to cephalosporins
✓5th **Z16.2 Resistance to other antibiotics**
**Z16.20 Resistance to unspecified antibiotic** UPD
Resistance to antibiotics NOS
**Z16.21 Resistance to vancomycin** UPD
**Z16.22 Resistance to vancomycin related antibiotics** UPD
**Z16.23 Resistance to quinolones and fluoroquinolones** UPD
**Z16.24 Resistance to multiple antibiotics** UPD
**Z16.29 Resistance to other single specified antibiotic** UPD
Resistance to aminoglycosides
Resistance to macrolides
Resistance to sulfonamides
Resistance to tetracyclines
✓5th **Z16.3 Resistance to other antimicrobial drugs**
EXCLUDES 1 *resistance to antibiotics (Z16.1-, Z16.2-)*
**Z16.30 Resistance to unspecified antimicrobial drugs** UPD
Drug resistance NOS
**Z16.31 Resistance to antiparasitic drug(s)** UPD
Resistance to quinine and related compounds
**Z16.32 Resistance to antifungal drug(s)** UPD
**Z16.33 Resistance to antiviral drug(s)** UPD
✓6th **Z16.34 Resistance to antimycobacterial drug(s)**
Resistance to tuberculostatics
**Z16.341 Resistance to single antimycobacterial drug** UPD
Resistance to antimycobacterial drug NOS
**Z16.342 Resistance to multiple antimycobacterial drugs** UPD
**Z16.35 Resistance to multiple antimicrobial drugs** UPD
EXCLUDES 1 *resistance to multiple antibiotics only (Z16.24)*
**Z16.39 Resistance to other specified antimicrobial drug** UPD

## Estrogen, and other hormones and factors receptor status (Z17)

✓4th **Z17 Estrogen, and other hormones and factors receptor status**

NOTE Use one code, as available, for each receptor: Z17.0, Z17.1, Z17.2-, Z17.3-

Code first malignant neoplasm, such as:
malignant neoplasm of breast (C50.-)
malignant neoplasm of ovary (C56.-)

**AHA:** 2022,3Q,14

**DEF:** Receptor status of breast cancer cells for the hormone estrogen that is used to help determine treatment and evaluate prognosis. ER+ breast cancer responds to hormone therapies while ER- breast cancer does not.

**Z17.0 Estrogen receptor positive status [ER+]** UPD

**Z17.1 Estrogen receptor negative status [ER-]** UPD

✓5th **Z17.2 Progesterone receptor status**

**AHA:** 2024,4Q,31

**Z17.21 Progesterone receptor positive status** UPD
PR+

**Z17.22 Progesterone receptor negative status** UPD
PR-

✓5th **Z17.3 Human epidermal growth factor 2 receptor**

**AHA:** 2024,4Q,31

**Z17.31 Human epidermal growth factor receptor 2 positive status**
HER2+

**Z17.32 Human epidermal growth factor receptor 2 negative status**
HER2-

✓5th **Z17.4 Combined receptor status**

NOTE Assign a code from subcategory Z17.4- when only a combined receptor status is documented

**AHA:** 2024,4Q,31

✓6th **Z17.41 Hormone receptor positive**
HR+

**Z17.410 Hormone receptor positive with human epidermal growth factor receptor 2 positive status**
HR+ with HER2+

**Z17.411 Hormone receptor positive with human epidermal growth factor receptor 2 negative status**
HR+ with HER2-

✓6th **Z17.42 Hormone receptor negative**
HR-

**Z17.420 Hormone receptor negative with human epidermal growth factor receptor 2 positive status**
HR- with HER2+

**Z17.421 Hormone receptor negative with human epidermal growth factor receptor 2 negative status**
HR- with HER2-
TNBC
Triple negative breast cancer

## Retained foreign body fragments (Z18)

✓4th **Z18 Retained foreign body fragments**

INCLUDES embedded fragment (status)
embedded splinter (status)
retained foreign body status

EXCLUDES 1 *artificial joint prosthesis status (Z96.6-)*
*foreign body accidentally left during a procedure (T81.5-)*
*foreign body entering through orifice (T15-T19)*
*in situ cardiac device (Z95.-)*
*organ or tissue replaced by means other than transplant (Z96.-, Z97.-)*
*organ or tissue replaced by transplant (Z94.-)*
*personal history of retained foreign body fully removed Z87.821*
*superficial foreign body (non-embedded splinter) - code to superficial foreign body, by site*

**AHA:** 2023,2Q,27

**DEF:** Embedded or retained fragment, splinter, or foreign body, natural or synthetic that can cause infection.

✓5th **Z18.0 Retained radioactive fragments**

**Z18.01 Retained depleted uranium fragments**

**Z18.09 Other retained radioactive fragments**
Other retained depleted isotope fragments
Retained nontherapeutic radioactive fragments

✓5th **Z18.1 Retained metal fragments**

EXCLUDES 1 *retained radioactive metal fragments (Z18.01-Z18.09)*

**Z18.10 Retained metal fragments, unspecified**
Retained metal fragment NOS

**Z18.11 Retained magnetic metal fragments**

**Z18.12 Retained nonmagnetic metal fragments**

**Z18.2 Retained plastic fragments**
Acrylics fragments
Diethylhexyl phthalates fragments
Isocyanate fragments

✓5th **Z18.3 Retained organic fragments**

**Z18.31 Retained animal quills or spines**

**Z18.32 Retained tooth**

**Z18.33 Retained wood fragments**

**Z18.39 Other retained organic fragments**

✓5th **Z18.8 Other specified retained foreign body**

**Z18.81 Retained glass fragments**

**Z18.83 Retained stone or crystalline fragments**
Retained concrete or cement fragments

**Z18.89 Other specified retained foreign body fragments**

**Z18.9 Retained foreign body fragments, unspecified material**

## Hormone sensitivity malignancy status (Z19)

✓4th **Z19 Hormone sensitivity malignancy status**

Code first malignant neoplasm — see Table of Neoplasms, by site, malignant

**AHA:** 2016,4Q,76

**Z19.1 Hormone sensitive malignancy status** UPD

**Z19.2 Hormone resistant malignancy status** UPD
Castrate resistant prostate malignancy status

## Persons with potential health hazards related to communicable diseases (Z20-Z29)

✓4th **Z20 Contact with and (suspected) exposure to communicable diseases**

EXCLUDES 1 *carrier of infectious disease (Z22.-)*
*diagnosed current infectious or parasitic disease - see Alphabetic Index*

EXCLUDES 2 *personal history of infectious and parasitic diseases (Z86.1-)*

✓5th **Z20.0 Contact with and (suspected) exposure to intestinal infectious diseases**

**Z20.01 Contact with and (suspected) exposure to intestinal infectious diseases due to Escherichia coli (E. coli)**

**Z20.09 Contact with and (suspected) exposure to other intestinal infectious diseases**

**Z20.1 Contact with and (suspected) exposure to tuberculosis**

**Z20.2 Contact with and (suspected) exposure to infections with a predominantly sexual mode of transmission**

**Z20.3 Contact with and (suspected) exposure to rabies**

**Z20.4 Contact with and (suspected) exposure to rubella**

**Z20.5 Contact with and (suspected) exposure to viral hepatitis**

**Z20.6 Contact with and (suspected) exposure to human immunodeficiency virus [HIV]**

EXCLUDES 1 *asymptomatic human immunodeficiency virus [HIV] HIV infection status (Z21)*

**Z20.7 Contact with and (suspected) exposure to pediculosis, acariasis and other infestations**

✓5th **Z20.8 Contact with and (suspected) exposure to other communicable diseases**

✓6th **Z20.81 Contact with and (suspected) exposure to other bacterial communicable diseases**

**Z20.810 Contact with and (suspected) exposure to anthrax**

**Z20.811 Contact with and (suspected) exposure to meningococcus**

**Z20.818 Contact with and (suspected) exposure to other bacterial communicable diseases**

**AHA:** 2019,2Q,10

✓6th **Z20.82 Contact with and (suspected) exposure to other viral communicable diseases**

**Z20.820 Contact with and (suspected) exposure to varicella**

**Z20.821 Contact with and (suspected) exposure to Zika virus**
AHA: 2018,4Q,35,64

**Z20.822 Contact with and (suspected) exposure to COVID-19**
Contact with and (suspected) exposure to SARS-CoV-2
AHA: 2023,2Q,3; 2022,2Q,28-29; 2021,4Q,109; 2021,1Q,27-29,37-38,41

**Z20.828 Contact with and (suspected) exposure to other viral communicable diseases**
AHA: 2022,3Q,4; 2021,1Q,37-38; 2020,4Q,99; 2020,3Q,14-15; 2020,2Q,4,8; 2020,1Q,34-36

**Z20.89 Contact with and (suspected) exposure to other communicable diseases**

**Z20.9 Contact with and (suspected) exposure to unspecified communicable disease**

**Z21 Asymptomatic human immunodeficiency virus [HIV] infection status** HCC Rx ESR COM
HIV positive NOS
Code first human immunodeficiency virus [HIV] disease complicating pregnancy, childbirth and the puerperium, if applicable (O98.7-)
EXCLUDES 1 *acquired immunodeficiency syndrome (B20)*
*contact with human immunodeficiency virus [HIV] (Z20.6)*
*exposure to human immunodeficiency virus [HIV] (Z20.6)*
*human immunodeficiency virus [HIV] disease (B20)*
*inconclusive laboratory evidence of human immunodeficiency virus [HIV] (R75)*
AHA: 2022,1Q,36; 2019,1Q,8-11
DEF: Phase of human immunodeficiency virus (HIV) infection with no clinical symptoms. This phase may last for 10 years or more.

√4th **Z22 Carrier of infectious disease**
INCLUDES colonization status
suspected carrier
EXCLUDES 2 *carrier of viral hepatitis (B18.-)*

**Z22.0 Carrier of typhoid**

**Z22.1 Carrier of other intestinal infectious diseases**

**Z22.2 Carrier of diphtheria**

√5th **Z22.3 Carrier of other specified bacterial diseases**

**Z22.31 Carrier of bacterial disease due to meningococci**

√6th **Z22.32 Carrier of bacterial disease due to staphylococci**

**Z22.321 Carrier or suspected carrier of Methicillin susceptible Staphylococcus aureus**
MSSA colonization

**Z22.322 Carrier or suspected carrier of Methicillin resistant Staphylococcus aureus**
MRSA colonization
DEF: Carriers (colonization) of methicillin resistant *Staphylococcus aureus* (MRSA) have MRSA on their skin or in their body but do not exhibit signs of infection. These individuals are able to pass MRSA on to others who may develop an infection.

√6th **Z22.33 Carrier of bacterial disease due to streptococci**

**Z22.330 Carrier of Group B streptococcus**
EXCLUDES 1 *carrier of streptococcus group B (GBS) complicating pregnancy, childbirth and the puerperium (O99.82-)*

**Z22.338 Carrier of other streptococcus**

√6th **Z22.34 Carrier of Acinetobacter baumannii**
AHA: 2023,4Q,47

**Z22.340 Carrier of carbapenem-resistant Acinetobacter baumannii**

**Z22.341 Carrier of carbapenem-sensitive Acinetobacter baumannii**

**Z22.349 Carrier of Acinetobacter baumannii, unspecified**

√6th **Z22.35 Carrier of Enterobacterales**
Carrier of E. coli
Carrier of K. pneumoniae
AHA: 2023,4Q,47

**Z22.350 Carrier of carbapenem-resistant Enterobacterales**

**Z22.358 Carrier of other Enterobacterales**
Carrier of carbapenem-sensitive Enterobacterales
Carrier of ESBL-producing Enterobacterales
Carrier of extended-spectrum beta-lactamase producing Enterobacterales

**Z22.359 Carrier of Enterobacterales, unspecified**

**Z22.39 Carrier of other specified bacterial diseases**

**Z22.4 Carrier of infections with a predominantly sexual mode of transmission**

**Z22.6 Carrier of human T-lymphotropic virus type-1 [HTLV-1] infection**

**Z22.7 Latent tuberculosis**
Latent tuberculosis infection (LTBI)
EXCLUDES 1 *nonspecific reaction to cell mediated immunity measurement of gamma interferon antigen response without active tuberculosis (R76.12)*
*nonspecific reaction to tuberculin skin test without active tuberculosis (R76.11)*
AHA: 2019,4Q,19

**Z22.8 Carrier of other infectious diseases**

**Z22.9 Carrier of infectious disease, unspecified**

**Z23 Encounter for immunization**
NOTE Procedure codes are required to identify the types of immunizations given
Code first any routine childhood examination
Code also, if applicable, encounter for immunization safety counseling (Z71.85)

√4th **Z28 Immunization not carried out and underimmunization status**
INCLUDES vaccination not carried out
Code also, if applicable, encounter for immunization safety counseling (Z71.85)

√5th **Z28.0 Immunization not carried out because of contraindication**
DEF: Contraindication: Situation where a drug, surgery, or other procedure may negatively affect or cause harm to a patient.

**Z28.01 Immunization not carried out because of acute illness of patient**

**Z28.02 Immunization not carried out because of chronic illness or condition of patient**

**Z28.03 Immunization not carried out because of immune compromised state of patient**

**Z28.04 Immunization not carried out because of patient allergy to vaccine or component**

**Z28.09 Immunization not carried out because of other contraindication**

**Z28.1 Immunization not carried out because of patient decision for reasons of belief or group pressure**
Immunization not carried out because of religious belief

√5th **Z28.2 Immunization not carried out because of patient decision for other and unspecified reason**

**Z28.20 Immunization not carried out because of patient decision for unspecified reason**

**Z28.21 Immunization not carried out because of patient refusal**

**Z28.29 Immunization not carried out because of patient decision for other reason**

√5th **Z28.3 Underimmunization status**
Use additional code, if applicable, to identify:
immunization not carried out because of contraindication (Z28.0-)
immunization not carried out because of patient decision for other and unspecified reason (Z28.2-)
immunization not carried out because of patient decision for reasons of belief or group pressure (Z28.1)
immunization not carried out for other reason (Z28.8-)
AHA: 2022,1Q,4-5

√6th **Z28.31 Underimmunization for COVID-19 status**
NOTE These codes should not be used for individuals who are not eligible for the COVID-19 vaccines, as determined by the healthcare provider.

**Z28.310 Unvaccinated for COVID-19** UPD

**Z28.311 Partially vaccinated for COVID-19** UPD

**Z28.39 Other underimmunization status** UPD
Delinquent immunization status
Lapsed immunization schedule status

√5th **Z28.8 Immunization not carried out for other reason**

**Z28.81 Immunization not carried out due to patient having had the disease**

**Z28.82 Immunization not carried out because of caregiver refusal**

Immunization not carried out because of guardian refusal

Immunization not carried out because of parent refusal

EXCLUDES 1 *immunization not carried out because of caregiver refusal because of religious belief (Z28.1)*

**Z28.83 Immunization not carried out due to unavailability of vaccine**

Delay in delivery of vaccine

Lack of availability of vaccine

Manufacturer delay of vaccine

**AHA:** 2018,4Q,36

**Z28.89 Immunization not carried out for other reason**

**Z28.9 Immunization not carried out for unspecified reason**

√4th **Z29 Encounter for other prophylactic measures**

EXCLUDES 1 *desensitization to allergens (Z51.6)*
*prophylactic surgery (Z40.-)*

**AHA:** 2016,4Q,78-79

√5th **Z29.1 Encounter for prophylactic immunotherapy**

Encounter for administration of immunoglobulin

**Z29.11 Encounter for prophylactic immunotherapy for respiratory syncytial virus (RSV)**

**AHA:** 2025,3Q,10

**Z29.12 Encounter for prophylactic antivenin**

**Z29.13 Encounter for prophylactic Rho(D) immune globulin**

**AHA:** 2019,3Q,5

▲ **Z29.14 Encounter for prophylactic rabies immune globin**

**Z29.3 Encounter for prophylactic fluoride administration**

√5th **Z29.8 Encounter for other specified prophylactic measures**

**AHA:** 2023,4Q,49; 2022,2Q,27

**Z29.81 Encounter for HIV pre-exposure prophylaxis**

Code also, if applicable, risk factors for HIV, such as:
contact with and (suspected) exposure to human immunodeficiency virus [HIV] (Z20.6)
high risk sexual behavior (Z72.5-)

**Z29.89 Encounter for other specified prophylactic measures**

**Z29.9 Encounter for prophylactic measures, unspecified**

## Persons encountering health services in circumstances related to reproduction (Z30-Z39)

√4th **Z30 Encounter for contraceptive management**

**AHA:** 2016,4Q,78

**DEF:** Contraceptive management to prevent pregnancy. Methods include oral medications, intrauterine devices, and surgical procedures for males and females (sterilization).

√5th **Z30.0 Encounter for general counseling and advice on contraception**

√6th **Z30.01 Encounter for initial prescription of contraceptives**

EXCLUDES 1 *encounter for surveillance of contraceptives (Z30.4-)*

**Z30.011 Encounter for initial prescription of contraceptive pills**

**Z30.012 Encounter for prescription of emergency contraception**

Encounter for postcoital contraception

**Z30.013 Encounter for initial prescription of injectable contraceptive**

**Z30.014 Encounter for initial prescription of intrauterine contraceptive device**

EXCLUDES 1 *encounter for insertion of intrauterine contraceptive device (Z30.430, Z30.432)*

**Z30.015 Encounter for initial prescription of vaginal ring hormonal contraceptive**

**Z30.016 Encounter for initial prescription of transdermal patch hormonal contraceptive device**

**Z30.017 Encounter for initial prescription of implantable subdermal contraceptive**

**Z30.018 Encounter for initial prescription of other contraceptives**

Encounter for initial prescription of barrier contraception

Encounter for initial prescription of diaphragm

**Z30.019 Encounter for initial prescription of contraceptives, unspecified**

**Z30.02 Counseling and instruction in natural family planning to avoid pregnancy**

**Z30.09 Encounter for other general counseling and advice on contraception**

Encounter for family planning advice NOS

**Z30.2 Encounter for sterilization**

**AHA:** 2021,3Q,13

√5th **Z30.4 Encounter for surveillance of contraceptives**

**Z30.40 Encounter for surveillance of contraceptives, unspecified**

**Z30.41 Encounter for surveillance of contraceptive pills**

Encounter for repeat prescription for contraceptive pill

**Z30.42 Encounter for surveillance of injectable contraceptive**

√6th **Z30.43 Encounter for surveillance of intrauterine contraceptive device**

**Z30.430 Encounter for insertion of intrauterine contraceptive device**

**Z30.431 Encounter for routine checking of intrauterine contraceptive device**

**Z30.432 Encounter for removal of intrauterine contraceptive device**

**Z30.433 Encounter for removal and reinsertion of intrauterine contraceptive device**

Encounter for replacement of intrauterine contraceptive device

**Z30.44 Encounter for surveillance of vaginal ring hormonal contraceptive device**

**Z30.45 Encounter for surveillance of transdermal patch hormonal contraceptive device**

**Z30.46 Encounter for surveillance of implantable subdermal contraceptive**

Encounter for checking, reinsertion or removal of implantable subdermal contraceptive

**Z30.49 Encounter for surveillance of other contraceptives**

Encounter for surveillance of barrier contraception

Encounter for surveillance of diaphragm

**Z30.8 Encounter for other contraceptive management**

Encounter for postvasectomy sperm count

Encounter for routine examination for contraceptive maintenance

EXCLUDES 1 *sperm count following sterilization reversal (Z31.42)*
*sperm count for fertility testing (Z31.41)*

**Z30.9 Encounter for contraceptive management, unspecified**

√4th **Z31 Encounter for procreative management**

EXCLUDES 2 *complications associated with artificial fertilization (N98.-)*
*female infertility (N97.-)*
*male infertility (N46.-)*

**Z31.0 Encounter for reversal of previous sterilization**

√5th **Z31.4 Encounter for procreative investigation and testing**

EXCLUDES 1 *postvasectomy sperm count (Z30.8)*

**Z31.41 Encounter for fertility testing**

Encounter for fallopian tube patency testing

Encounter for sperm count for fertility testing

**Z31.42 Aftercare following sterilization reversal**

Sperm count following sterilization reversal

√6th **Z31.43 Encounter for genetic testing of female for procreative management**

Use additional code for recurrent pregnancy loss, if applicable (N96, O26.2-)

EXCLUDES 1 *nonprocreative genetic testing (Z13.7-)*

**Z31.430 Encounter of female for testing for genetic disease carrier status for procreative management**

**Z31.438 Encounter for other genetic testing of female for procreative management**

√6th **Z31.44 Encounter for genetic testing of male for procreative management**

EXCLUDES 1 *nonprocreative genetic testing (Z13.7-)*

**Z31.440 Encounter of male for testing for genetic disease carrier status for procreative management**

**Z31.441 Encounter for testing of male partner of patient with recurrent pregnancy loss** A

Z31.448 Encounter for other genetic testing of male for procreative management A

Z31.49 Encounter for other procreative investigation and testing

Z31.5 Encounter for procreative genetic counseling
AHA: 2017,4Q,27

√5th Z31.6 Encounter for general counseling and advice on procreation

Z31.61 Procreative counseling and advice using natural family planning

Z31.62 Encounter for fertility preservation counseling
Encounter for fertility preservation counseling prior to cancer therapy
Encounter for fertility preservation counseling prior to surgical removal of gonads

Z31.69 Encounter for other general counseling and advice on procreation

Z31.7 Encounter for procreative management and counseling for gestational carrier
EXCLUDES 1 *pregnant state, gestational carrier (Z33.3)*
AHA: 2016,4Q,78

√5th Z31.8 Encounter for other procreative management

Z31.81 Encounter for male factor infertility in female patient PDx

Z31.82 Encounter for Rh incompatibility status
AHA: 2015,3Q,40; 2014,4Q,17

Z31.83 Encounter for assisted reproductive fertility procedure cycle PDx
Patient undergoing in vitro fertilization cycle
Use additional code to identify the type of infertility
EXCLUDES 1 *pre-cycle diagnosis and testing - code to reason for encounter*
AHA: 2022,2Q,15-16

Z31.84 Encounter for fertility preservation procedure PDx
Encounter for fertility preservation procedure prior to cancer therapy
Encounter for fertility preservation procedure prior to surgical removal of gonads

Z31.89 Encounter for other procreative management

Z31.9 Encounter for procreative management, unspecified

√4th Z32 Encounter for pregnancy test and childbirth and childcare instruction

√5th Z32.0 Encounter for pregnancy test

Z32.00 Encounter for pregnancy test, result unknown
Encounter for pregnancy test NOS

Z32.01 Encounter for pregnancy test, result positive COM M

Z32.02 Encounter for pregnancy test, result negative

Z32.2 Encounter for childbirth instruction

Z32.3 Encounter for childcare instruction
Encounter for prenatal or postpartum childcare instruction

√4th Z33 Pregnant state

Z33.1 Pregnant state, incidental COM M
Pregnancy NOS
Pregnant state NOS
EXCLUDES 1 *complications of pregnancy (O00-O9A)*
*pregnant state, gestational carrier (Z33.3)*

Z33.2 Encounter for elective termination of pregnancy PDx M
EXCLUDES 1 *early fetal death with retention of dead fetus (O02.1)*
*late fetal death (O36.4)*
*spontaneous abortion (O03)*
AHA: 2024,3Q,9; 2023,2Q,15; 2022,1Q,20
TIP: Do not assign a code from category Z3A with this code.

Z33.3 Pregnant state, gestational carrier COM M
EXCLUDES 1 *encounter for procreative management and counseling for gestational carrier (Z31.7)*
AHA: 2016,4Q,78

√4th Z34 Encounter for supervision of normal pregnancy
EXCLUDES 1 *any complication of pregnancy (O00-O9A)*
*encounter for pregnancy test (Z32.0-)*
*encounter for supervision of high risk pregnancy (O09.-)*
AHA: 2019,3Q,5; 2014,4Q,17

√5th Z34.0 Encounter for supervision of normal first pregnancy

Z34.00 Encounter for supervision of normal first pregnancy, unspecified trimester COM PDx M

Z34.01 Encounter for supervision of normal first pregnancy, first trimester COM PDx M

Z34.02 Encounter for supervision of normal first pregnancy, second trimester COM PDx M

Z34.03 Encounter for supervision of normal first pregnancy, third trimester COM PDx M

√5th Z34.8 Encounter for supervision of other normal pregnancy

Z34.80 Encounter for supervision of other normal pregnancy, unspecified trimester COM PDx M

Z34.81 Encounter for supervision of other normal pregnancy, first trimester COM PDx M

Z34.82 Encounter for supervision of other normal pregnancy, second trimester COM PDx M

Z34.83 Encounter for supervision of other normal pregnancy, third trimester COM PDx M

√5th Z34.9 Encounter for supervision of normal pregnancy, unspecified

Z34.90 Encounter for supervision of normal pregnancy, unspecified, unspecified trimester COM PDx M

Z34.91 Encounter for supervision of normal pregnancy, unspecified, first trimester COM PDx M

Z34.92 Encounter for supervision of normal pregnancy, unspecified, second trimester COM PDx M

Z34.93 Encounter for supervision of normal pregnancy, unspecified, third trimester COM PDx M

√4th Z36 Encounter for antenatal screening of mother
INCLUDES encounter for placental sample (taken vaginally)
screening is the testing for disease or disease precursors in asymptomatic individuals so that early detection and treatment can be provided for those who test positive for the disease.
EXCLUDES 1 *diagnostic examination - code to sign or symptom*
*encounter for suspected maternal and fetal conditions ruled out (Z03.7-)*
*suspected fetal condition affecting management of pregnancy - code to condition in Chapter 15*
EXCLUDES 2 *abnormal findings on antenatal screening of mother (O28.-)*
*genetic counseling and testing (Z31.43-, Z31.5)*
*routine prenatal care (Z34)*
AHA: 2017,4Q,28

Z36.0 Encounter for antenatal screening for chromosomal anomalies COM M
▶Encounter for antenatal screening for Down syndrome◀
▶Encounter for antenatal screening for fetal aneuploidy◀
▶Encounter for antenatal screening for Patau syndrome◀
▶Encounter for antenatal screening for Trisomy 13◀
▶Encounter for antenatal screening for Trisomy 21◀

Z36.1 Encounter for antenatal screening for raised alphafetoprotein level COM M
Encounter for antenatal screening for elevated maternal serum alphafetoprotein level
DEF: High levels of alpha-fetoprotein (AFP) that may indicate a possibility of spina bifida and other neural tube defects, anencephaly, or omphalocele in the fetus.

Z36.2 Encounter for other antenatal screening follow-up COM M
Non-visualized anatomy on a previous scan

Z36.3 Encounter for antenatal screening for malformations COM M
Screening for a suspected anomaly

Z36.4 Encounter for antenatal screening for fetal growth retardation COM M
Intrauterine growth restriction (IUGR)/small-for-dates

Z36.5 Encounter for antenatal screening for isoimmunization COM M

√5th Z36.8 Encounter for other antenatal screening

Z36.81 Encounter for antenatal screening for hydrops fetalis COM M
DEF: Hydrops fetalis: Abnormal accumulation of fluid in two or more parts of the fetus, such as ascites, effusion of the pleural or pericardial tissues, or edema.

Z36.82 Encounter for antenatal screening for nuchal translucency COM M

Z36.83 Encounter for fetal screening for congenital cardiac abnormalities COM M

Z36.84 Encounter for antenatal screening for fetal lung maturity COM M

Z36.85 Encounter for antenatal screening for Streptococcus B COM M

Z36.86 Encounter for antenatal screening for cervical length COM M
Screening for risk of pre-term labor

Z36.87 Encounter for antenatal screening for uncertain dates COM M

Z36.88 **Encounter for antenatal screening for fetal macrosomia** COM M
Screening for large-for-dates

Z36.89 **Encounter for other specified antenatal screening** COM M

Z36.8A **Encounter for antenatal screening for other genetic defects** COM M

Z36.9 **Encounter for antenatal screening, unspecified** COM M

✓4th **Z3A Weeks of gestation**

NOTE Codes from category Z3A are for use, only on the maternal record, to indicate the weeks of gestation of the pregnancy, if known.

Code first obstetric condition or encounter for delivery (O09-O60, O80-O82, O94-O9A)

**AHA:** 2022,2Q,3; 2019,2Q,11; 2016,2Q,34; 2014,3Q,17; 2014,2Q,9; 2013,2Q,33

**TIP:** Do not assign a code from this category with codes from categories O00-O08 or code Z33.2.

✓5th Z3A.Ø **Weeks of gestation of pregnancy, unspecified or less than 1Ø weeks**

Z3A.ØØ **Weeks of gestation of pregnancy not specified** COM UPD M
Z3A.Ø1 **Less than 8 weeks gestation of pregnancy** COM UPD M
Z3A.Ø8 **8 weeks gestation of pregnancy** COM UPD M
Z3A.Ø9 **9 weeks gestation of pregnancy** COM UPD M

✓5th Z3A.1 **Weeks of gestation of pregnancy, weeks 1Ø-19**

Z3A.1Ø **1Ø weeks gestation of pregnancy** COM UPD M
Z3A.11 **11 weeks gestation of pregnancy** COM UPD M
Z3A.12 **12 weeks gestation of pregnancy** COM UPD M
Z3A.13 **13 weeks gestation of pregnancy** COM UPD M
Z3A.14 **14 weeks gestation of pregnancy** COM UPD M
Z3A.15 **15 weeks gestation of pregnancy** COM UPD M
Z3A.16 **16 weeks gestation of pregnancy** COM UPD M
Z3A.17 **17 weeks gestation of pregnancy** COM UPD M
Z3A.18 **18 weeks gestation of pregnancy** COM UPD M
Z3A.19 **19 weeks gestation of pregnancy** COM UPD M

✓5th Z3A.2 **Weeks of gestation of pregnancy, weeks 2Ø-29**

Z3A.2Ø **2Ø weeks gestation of pregnancy** COM UPD M
Z3A.21 **21 weeks gestation of pregnancy** COM UPD M
Z3A.22 **22 weeks gestation of pregnancy** COM UPD M
Z3A.23 **23 weeks gestation of pregnancy** COM UPD M
Z3A.24 **24 weeks gestation of pregnancy** COM UPD M
Z3A.25 **25 weeks gestation of pregnancy** COM UPD M
Z3A.26 **26 weeks gestation of pregnancy** COM UPD M
Z3A.27 **27 weeks gestation of pregnancy** COM UPD M
Z3A.28 **28 weeks gestation of pregnancy** COM UPD M
Z3A.29 **29 weeks gestation of pregnancy** COM UPD M

✓5th Z3A.3 **Weeks of gestation of pregnancy, weeks 3Ø-39**

Z3A.3Ø **3Ø weeks gestation of pregnancy** COM UPD M
Z3A.31 **31 weeks gestation of pregnancy** COM UPD M
Z3A.32 **32 weeks gestation of pregnancy** COM UPD M
Z3A.33 **33 weeks gestation of pregnancy** COM UPD M
Z3A.34 **34 weeks gestation of pregnancy** COM UPD M
Z3A.35 **35 weeks gestation of pregnancy** COM UPD M
Z3A.36 **36 weeks gestation of pregnancy** COM UPD M
Z3A.37 **37 weeks gestation of pregnancy** COM UPD M
Z3A.38 **38 weeks gestation of pregnancy** COM UPD M
Z3A.39 **39 weeks gestation of pregnancy** COM UPD M

✓5th Z3A.4 **Weeks of gestation of pregnancy, weeks 4Ø or greater**

**AHA:** 2014,4Q,23

Z3A.4Ø **4Ø weeks gestation of pregnancy** COM UPD M
Z3A.41 **41 weeks gestation of pregnancy** COM UPD M
Z3A.42 **42 weeks gestation of pregnancy** COM UPD M
Z3A.49 **Greater than 42 weeks gestation of pregnancy** COM UPD M

✓4th **Z37 Outcome of delivery**

This category is intended for use as an additional code to identify the outcome of delivery on the mother's record. It is not for use on the newborn record.

EXCLUDES 1 *stillbirth (P95)*

Z37.Ø **Single live birth** COM UPD M
**AHA:** 2024,3Q,9; 2016,2Q,34; 2014,2Q,9

Z37.1 **Single stillbirth** COM UPD M
Z37.2 **Twins, both liveborn** COM UPD M
Z37.3 **Twins, one liveborn and one stillborn** COM UPD M
Z37.4 **Twins, both stillborn** COM UPD M

✓5th Z37.5 **Other multiple births, all liveborn**

Z37.5Ø **Multiple births, unspecified, all liveborn** COM UPD M
Z37.51 **Triplets, all liveborn** COM UPD M
Z37.52 **Quadruplets, all liveborn** COM UPD M
Z37.53 **Quintuplets, all liveborn** COM UPD M
Z37.54 **Sextuplets, all liveborn** COM UPD M
Z37.59 **Other multiple births, all liveborn** COM UPD M

✓5th Z37.6 **Other multiple births, some liveborn**

Z37.6Ø **Multiple births, unspecified, some liveborn** COM UPD M
Z37.61 **Triplets, some liveborn** COM UPD M
Z37.62 **Quadruplets, some liveborn** COM UPD M
Z37.63 **Quintuplets, some liveborn** COM UPD M
Z37.64 **Sextuplets, some liveborn** COM UPD M
Z37.69 **Other multiple births, some liveborn** COM UPD M

Z37.7 **Other multiple births, all stillborn** COM UPD M

Z37.9 **Outcome of delivery, unspecified** COM UPD M
Multiple birth NOS
Single birth NOS

✓4th **Z38 Liveborn infants according to place of birth and type of delivery**

This category is for use as the principal code on the initial record of a newborn baby. It is to be used for the initial birth record only. It is not to be used on the mother's record.

**AHA:** 2020,2Q,13; 2017,2Q,5-7; 2016,3Q,18; 2015,2Q,15

**TIP:** For attending physician services, a code from this category can be reported as first listed every time the physician visits the newborn during the birth admission.

✓5th Z38.Ø **Single liveborn infant, born in hospital**
Single liveborn infant, born in birthing center or other health care facility

Z38.ØØ **Single liveborn infant, delivered vaginally** COM PDx N
Z38.Ø1 **Single liveborn infant, delivered by cesarean** COM PDx N

Z38.1 **Single liveborn infant, born outside hospital** COM PDx N

Z38.2 **Single liveborn infant, unspecified as to place of birth** COM PDx N
Single liveborn infant NOS

✓5th Z38.3 **Twin liveborn infant, born in hospital**

Z38.3Ø **Twin liveborn infant, delivered vaginally** COM PDx N
Z38.31 **Twin liveborn infant, delivered by cesarean** COM PDx N

Z38.4 **Twin liveborn infant, born outside hospital** COM PDx N

Z38.5 **Twin liveborn infant, unspecified as to place of birth** COM PDx N

✓5th Z38.6 **Other multiple liveborn infant, born in hospital**

Z38.61 **Triplet liveborn infant, delivered vaginally** COM PDx N
Z38.62 **Triplet liveborn infant, delivered by cesarean** COM PDx N
Z38.63 **Quadruplet liveborn infant, delivered vaginally** COM PDx N
Z38.64 **Quadruplet liveborn infant, delivered by cesarean** COM PDx N
Z38.65 **Quintuplet liveborn infant, delivered vaginally** COM PDx N
Z38.66 **Quintuplet liveborn infant, delivered by cesarean** COM PDx N
Z38.68 **Other multiple liveborn infant, delivered vaginally** COM PDx N
Z38.69 **Other multiple liveborn infant, delivered by cesarean** COM PDx N

Z38.7 Other multiple liveborn infant, born outside hospital COM PDx N

Z38.8 Other multiple liveborn infant, unspecified as to place of birth COM PDx N

Z39 Encounter for maternal postpartum care and examination

Z39.0 Encounter for care and examination of mother immediately after delivery COM PDx M
Care and observation in uncomplicated cases when the delivery occurs outside a healthcare facility
EXCLUDES 1 *care for postpartum complication - see Alphabetic Index*
AHA: 2021,3Q,13

Z39.1 Encounter for care and examination of lactating mother PDx M
Encounter for supervision of lactation
EXCLUDES 1 *disorders of lactation (O92.-)*

Z39.2 Encounter for routine postpartum follow-up COM PDx M

## Encounters for other specific health care (Z40-Z53)

Categories Z40-Z53 are intended for use to indicate a reason for care. They may be used for patients who have already been treated for a disease or injury, but who are receiving aftercare or prophylactic care, or care to consolidate the treatment, or to deal with a residual state

EXCLUDES 2 *follow-up examination for medical surveillance after treatment (Z08-Z09)*

Z40 Encounter for prophylactic surgery
EXCLUDES 1 *organ donations (Z52.-)*
*therapeutic organ removal - code to condition*
DEF: Treatment measure intended to prevent or ward off a disease or condition.

Z40.0 Encounter for prophylactic surgery for risk factors related to malignant neoplasms
Admission for prophylactic organ removal
Use additional code to identify risk factor, such as genetic susceptibility to malignant neoplasm (Z15.-)
AHA: 2017,4Q,28-29

Z40.00 Encounter for prophylactic removal of unspecified organ PDx

Z40.01 Encounter for prophylactic removal of breast PDx

Z40.02 Encounter for prophylactic removal of ovary(s) PDx

Z40.03 Encounter for prophylactic removal of fallopian tube(s) PDx

Z40.09 Encounter for prophylactic removal of other organ PDx

Z40.8 Encounter for other prophylactic surgery

Z40.81 Encounter for prophylactic surgery for removal of ovary(s) for persons without known genetic/familial risk factors
Encounter for prophylactic oophorectomy for persons without known genetic/ familial risk factors

Z40.82 Encounter for prophylactic surgery for removal of fallopian tube(s) for persons without known genetic/familial risk factors
Encounter for prophylactic salpingectomy for persons without known genetic/familial risk factors
Opportunistic salpingectomy

Z40.89 Encounter for other prophylactic surgery

Z40.9 Encounter for prophylactic surgery, unspecified PDx

Z41 Encounter for procedures for purposes other than remedying health state

Z41.1 Encounter for cosmetic surgery
Encounter for cosmetic breast implant
Encounter for cosmetic procedure
EXCLUDES 1 *encounter for plastic and reconstructive surgery following medical procedure or healed injury (Z42.-)*
*encounter for post-mastectomy breast implantation (Z42.1)*

Z41.2 Encounter for routine and ritual male circumcision
AHA: 2018,3Q,15
TIP: This code should only be reported when the circumcision is elective (unrelated to a specific diagnosis) and was not performed during the birth admission.

Z41.3 Encounter for ear piercing

Z41.8 Encounter for other procedures for purposes other than remedying health state

Z41.9 Encounter for procedure for purposes other than remedying health state, unspecified

Z42 Encounter for plastic and reconstructive surgery following medical procedure or healed injury
EXCLUDES 1 *encounter for cosmetic plastic surgery (Z41.1)*
*encounter for plastic surgery for treatment of current injury - code to relevent injury*

Z42.1 Encounter for breast reconstruction following mastectomy PDx A
EXCLUDES 1 *deformity and disproportion of reconstructed breast (N65.1-)*

Z42.8 Encounter for other plastic and reconstructive surgery following medical procedure or healed injury PDx
AHA: 2017,1Q,42

Z43 Encounter for attention to artificial openings
INCLUDES closure of artificial openings
passage of sounds or bougies through artificial openings
reforming artificial openings
removal of catheter from artificial openings
toilet or cleansing of artificial openings
EXCLUDES 1 *complications of external stoma (J95.0-, K94.-, N99.5-)*
EXCLUDES 2 *fitting and adjustment of prosthetic and other devices (Z44-Z46)*
AHA: 2019,2Q,33

Z43.0 Encounter for attention to tracheostomy HCC ESR COM

Z43.1 Encounter for attention to gastrostomy HCC ESR COM
EXCLUDES 2 *artificial opening status only, without need for care (Z93.-)*

Z43.2 Encounter for attention to ileostomy HCC ESR COM

Z43.3 Encounter for attention to colostomy HCC ESR COM

Z43.4 Encounter for attention to other artificial openings of digestive tract HCC ESR COM

Z43.5 Encounter for attention to cystostomy HCC ESR COM

Z43.6 Encounter for attention to other artificial openings of urinary tract HCC ESR COM
Encounter for attention to nephrostomy
Encounter for attention to ureterostomy
Encounter for attention to urethrostomy

Z43.7 Encounter for attention to artificial vagina

Z43.8 Encounter for attention to other artificial openings HCC ESR COM

Z43.9 Encounter for attention to unspecified artificial opening HCC ESR COM

Z44 Encounter for fitting and adjustment of external prosthetic device
INCLUDES removal or replacement of external prosthetic device
EXCLUDES 1 *malfunction or other complications of device - see Alphabetical Index*
*presence of prosthetic device (Z97.-)*

Z44.0 Encounter for fitting and adjustment of artificial arm

Z44.00 Encounter for fitting and adjustment of unspecified artificial arm

Z44.001 Encounter for fitting and adjustment of unspecified right artificial arm COM

Z44.002 Encounter for fitting and adjustment of unspecified left artificial arm COM

Z44.009 Encounter for fitting and adjustment of unspecified artificial arm, unspecified arm COM

Z44.01 Encounter for fitting and adjustment of complete artificial arm

Z44.011 Encounter for fitting and adjustment of complete right artificial arm COM

Z44.012 Encounter for fitting and adjustment of complete left artificial arm COM

Z44.019 Encounter for fitting and adjustment of complete artificial arm, unspecified arm COM

Z44.02 Encounter for fitting and adjustment of partial artificial arm

Z44.021 Encounter for fitting and adjustment of partial artificial right arm COM

Z44.022 Encounter for fitting and adjustment of partial artificial left arm COM

Z44.029 Encounter for fitting and adjustment of partial artificial arm, unspecified arm COM

√5th **Z44.1 Encounter for fitting and adjustment of artificial leg**

√6th **Z44.10 Encounter for fitting and adjustment of unspecified artificial leg**

**Z44.101 Encounter for fitting and adjustment of unspecified right artificial leg** HCC ESR COM

**Z44.102 Encounter for fitting and adjustment of unspecified left artificial leg** HCC ESR COM

**Z44.109 Encounter for fitting and adjustment of unspecified artificial leg, unspecified leg** HCC ESR COM

√6th **Z44.11 Encounter for fitting and adjustment of complete artificial leg**

**Z44.111 Encounter for fitting and adjustment of complete right artificial leg** HCC ESR COM

**Z44.112 Encounter for fitting and adjustment of complete left artificial leg** HCC ESR COM

**Z44.119 Encounter for fitting and adjustment of complete artificial leg, unspecified leg** HCC ESR COM

√6th **Z44.12 Encounter for fitting and adjustment of partial artificial leg**

**Z44.121 Encounter for fitting and adjustment of partial artificial right leg** HCC ESR COM

**Z44.122 Encounter for fitting and adjustment of partial artificial left leg** HCC ESR COM

**Z44.129 Encounter for fitting and adjustment of partial artificial leg, unspecified leg** HCC ESR COM

√5th **Z44.2 Encounter for fitting and adjustment of artificial eye**

EXCLUDES 1 *mechanical complication of ocular prosthesis (T85.3)*

**Z44.20 Encounter for fitting and adjustment of artificial eye, unspecified**

**Z44.21 Encounter for fitting and adjustment of artificial right eye**

**Z44.22 Encounter for fitting and adjustment of artificial left eye**

√5th **Z44.3 Encounter for fitting and adjustment of external breast prosthesis**

EXCLUDES 1 *complications of breast implant (T85.4-)*
*encounter for adjustment or removal of breast implant (Z45.81-)*
*encounter for breast reconstruction following mastectomy (Z42.1)*
*encounter for initial breast implant insertion for cosmetic breast augmentation (Z41.1)*

**Z44.30 Encounter for fitting and adjustment of external breast prosthesis, unspecified breast**

**Z44.31 Encounter for fitting and adjustment of external right breast prosthesis**

**Z44.32 Encounter for fitting and adjustment of external left breast prosthesis**

**Z44.8 Encounter for fitting and adjustment of other external prosthetic devices**

**Z44.9 Encounter for fitting and adjustment of unspecified external prosthetic device**

√4th **Z45 Encounter for adjustment and management of implanted device**

INCLUDES removal or replacement of implanted device

EXCLUDES 1 *malfunction or other complications of device - see Alphabetical Index*

EXCLUDES 2 *encounter for fitting and adjustment of non-implanted device (Z46.-)*

√5th **Z45.0 Encounter for adjustment and management of cardiac device**

**TIP:** Assign an additional code for the associated condition if that condition requires constant intervention from the device, as in cases of sick sinus syndrome. For conditions that do not require constant intervention from the device, as in cases of ventricular fibrillation, an additional code for the associated condition should be assigned only if the patient is experiencing the condition and the device is firing during the current admission.

√6th **Z45.01 Encounter for adjustment and management of cardiac pacemaker**

Encounter for adjustment and management of cardiac resynchronization therapy pacemaker (CRT-P)

EXCLUDES 1 *encounter for adjustment and management of automatic implantable cardiac defibrillator with synchronous cardiac pacemaker (Z45.02)*

**Z45.010 Encounter for checking and testing of cardiac pacemaker pulse generator [battery]**

Encounter for replacing cardiac pacemaker pulse generator [battery]

**Z45.018 Encounter for adjustment and management of other part of cardiac pacemaker**

EXCLUDES 1 *presence of other part of cardiac pacemaker (Z95.0)*

EXCLUDES 2 *presence of prosthetic and other devices (Z95.1-Z95.5, Z95.811-Z97)*

**Z45.02 Encounter for adjustment and management of automatic implantable cardiac defibrillator**

Encounter for adjustment and management of automatic implantable cardiac defibrillator with synchronous cardiac pacemaker

Encounter for adjustment and management of cardiac resynchronization therapy defibrillator (CRT-D)

**AHA:** 2024,1Q,21-22

**Z45.09 Encounter for adjustment and management of other cardiac device**

**Z45.1 Encounter for adjustment and management of infusion pump**

**Z45.2 Encounter for adjustment and management of vascular access device**

Encounter for adjustment and management of vascular catheters

EXCLUDES 1 *encounter for adjustment and management of renal dialysis catheter (Z49.01)*

**AHA:** 2020,2Q,21; 2018,3Q,20

√5th **Z45.3 Encounter for adjustment and management of implanted devices of the special senses**

**Z45.31 Encounter for adjustment and management of implanted visual substitution device**

√6th **Z45.32 Encounter for adjustment and management of implanted hearing device**

EXCLUDES 1 *encounter for fitting and adjustment of hearing aid (Z46.1)*

**Z45.320 Encounter for adjustment and management of bone conduction device**

**Z45.321 Encounter for adjustment and management of cochlear device**

**Z45.328 Encounter for adjustment and management of other implanted hearing device**

√5th **Z45.4 Encounter for adjustment and management of implanted nervous system device**

**Z45.41 Encounter for adjustment and management of cerebrospinal fluid drainage device**

Encounter for adjustment and management of cerebral ventricular (communicating) shunt

**Z45.42 Encounter for adjustment and management of neurostimulator**
Encounter for adjustment and management of brain neurostimulator
Encounter for adjustment and management of gastric neurostimulator
Encounter for adjustment and management of peripheral nerve neurostimulator
Encounter for adjustment and management of sacral nerve neurostimulator
Encounter for adjustment and management of spinal cord neurostimulator
Encounter for adjustment and management of vagus nerve neurostimulator

**Z45.49 Encounter for adjustment and management of other implanted nervous system device**
**AHA:** 2014,3Q,19

√5th **Z45.8 Encounter for adjustment and management of other implanted devices**

√6th **Z45.81 Encounter for adjustment or removal of breast implant**
Encounter for elective implant exchange (different material) (different size)
Encounter for removal of tissue expander with or without synchronous insertion of permanent implant
EXCLUDES 1 *complications of breast implant (T85.4-)*
*encounter for breast reconstruction following mastectomy (Z42.1)*
*encounter for initial breast implant insertion for cosmetic breast augmentation (Z41.1)*

**Z45.811 Encounter for adjustment or removal of right breast implant**

**Z45.812 Encounter for adjustment or removal of left breast implant**

**Z45.819 Encounter for adjustment or removal of unspecified breast implant**

**Z45.82 Encounter for adjustment or removal of myringotomy device (stent) (tube)**

**Z45.89 Encounter for adjustment and management of other implanted devices**
**AHA:** 2014,4Q,26-28

**Z45.9 Encounter for adjustment and management of unspecified implanted device**

√4th **Z46 Encounter for fitting and adjustment of other devices**
INCLUDES removal or replacement of other device
EXCLUDES 1 *malfunction or other complications of device - see Alphabetical Index*
EXCLUDES 2 *encounter for fitting and management of implanted devices (Z45.-)*
*issue of repeat prescription only (Z76.Ø)*
*presence of prosthetic and other devices (Z95-Z97)*

**Z46.Ø Encounter for fitting and adjustment of spectacles and contact lenses**

**Z46.1 Encounter for fitting and adjustment of hearing aid**
EXCLUDES 1 *encounter for adjustment and management of implanted hearing device (Z45.32-)*

**Z46.2 Encounter for fitting and adjustment of other devices related to nervous system and special senses**
EXCLUDES 2 *encounter for adjustment and management of implanted nervous system device (Z45.4-)*
*encounter for adjustment and management of implanted visual substitution device (Z45.31)*

**Z46.3 Encounter for fitting and adjustment of dental prosthetic device**
Encounter for fitting and adjustment of dentures

**Z46.4 Encounter for fitting and adjustment of orthodontic device**

√5th **Z46.5 Encounter for fitting and adjustment of other gastrointestinal appliance and device**
EXCLUDES 1 *encounter for attention to artificial openings of digestive tract (Z43.1-Z43.4)*

**Z46.51 Encounter for fitting and adjustment of gastric lap band**

**Z46.59 Encounter for fitting and adjustment of other gastrointestinal appliance and device**

**Z46.6 Encounter for fitting and adjustment of urinary device**
EXCLUDES 2 *attention to artificial openings of urinary tract (Z43.5, Z43.6)*

√5th **Z46.8 Encounter for fitting and adjustment of other specified devices**

**Z46.81 Encounter for fitting and adjustment of insulin pump**
Encounter for insulin pump instruction and training
Encounter for insulin pump titration

**Z46.82 Encounter for fitting and adjustment of non-vascular catheter**

**Z46.89 Encounter for fitting and adjustment of other specified devices**
Encounter for fitting and adjustment of wheelchair

**Z46.9 Encounter for fitting and adjustment of unspecified device**

√4th **Z47 Orthopedic aftercare**
EXCLUDES 1 *aftercare for healing fracture - code to fracture with 7th character D*

**Z47.1 Aftercare following joint replacement surgery**
Use additional code to identify the joint (Z96.6-)
**AHA:** 2020,1Q,23

**Z47.2 Encounter for removal of internal fixation device**
EXCLUDES 1 *encounter for adjustment of internal fixation device for fracture treatment - code to fracture with appropriate 7th character*
*encounter for removal of external fixation device - code to fracture with 7th character D*
*infection or inflammatory reaction to internal fixation device (T84.6-)*
*mechanical complication of internal fixation device (T84.1-)*

√5th **Z47.3 Aftercare following explantation of joint prosthesis**
Aftercare following explantation of joint prosthesis, staged procedure
Encounter for joint prosthesis insertion following prior explantation of joint prosthesis
**AHA:** 2020,1Q,23; 2015,1Q,16
**TIP:** For staged removal of elbow joint prosthesis, assign code Z47.1.

**Z47.31 Aftercare following explantation of shoulder joint prosthesis**
EXCLUDES 1 *acquired absence of shoulder joint following prior explantation of shoulder joint prosthesis (Z89.23-)*
*shoulder joint prosthesis explantation status (Z89.23-)*

**Z47.32 Aftercare following explantation of hip joint prosthesis**
EXCLUDES 1 *acquired absence of hip joint following prior explantation of hip joint prosthesis (Z89.62-)*
*hip joint prosthesis explantation status (Z89.62-)*

**Z47.33 Aftercare following explantation of knee joint prosthesis**
EXCLUDES 1 *acquired absence of knee joint following prior explantation of knee prosthesis (Z89.52-)*
*knee joint prosthesis explantation status (Z89.52-)*

√5th **Z47.8 Encounter for other orthopedic aftercare**

**Z47.81 Encounter for orthopedic aftercare following surgical amputation**
Use additional code to identify the limb amputated (Z89.-)

**Z47.82 Encounter for orthopedic aftercare following scoliosis surgery**

**Z47.89 Encounter for other orthopedic aftercare**
**AHA:** 2015,1Q,8

**Z48 Encounter for other postprocedural aftercare**

EXCLUDES 1 *encounter for aftercare following injury - code to Injury, by site, with appropriate 7th character for subsequent encounter*
*encounter for follow-up examination after completed treatment (Z08-Z09)*

EXCLUDES 2 *encounter for attention to artificial openings (Z43.-)*
*encounter for fitting and adjustment of prosthetic and other devices (Z44-Z46)*

**AHA:** 2015,4Q,38; 2015,1Q,6-7

**Z48.0 Encounter for attention to dressings, sutures and drains**

EXCLUDES 1 *encounter for planned postprocedural wound closure (Z48.1)*

**Z48.00 Encounter for change or removal of nonsurgical wound dressing**
Encounter for change or removal of wound dressing NOS

**Z48.01 Encounter for change or removal of surgical wound dressing**
**AHA:** 2019,2Q,33

**Z48.02 Encounter for removal of sutures**
Encounter for removal of staples

**Z48.03 Encounter for change or removal of drains**
**AHA:** 2019,2Q,33

**Z48.1 Encounter for planned postprocedural wound closure**

EXCLUDES 1 *encounter for attention to dressings and sutures (Z48.0-)*

**Z48.2 Encounter for aftercare following organ transplant**

**Z48.21 Encounter for aftercare following heart transplant** HCC Rx ESR COM

**Z48.22 Encounter for aftercare following kidney transplant** Rx COM

**Z48.23 Encounter for aftercare following liver transplant** HCC Rx ESR COM

**Z48.24 Encounter for aftercare following lung transplant** HCC Rx ESR COM

**Z48.28 Encounter for aftercare following multiple organ transplant**

**Z48.280 Encounter for aftercare following heart-lung transplant** HCC Rx ESR COM

**Z48.288 Encounter for aftercare following multiple organ transplant**

**Z48.29 Encounter for aftercare following other organ transplant**

**Z48.290 Encounter for aftercare following bone marrow transplant** HCC Rx ESR COM

**Z48.298 Encounter for aftercare following other organ transplant**

**Z48.3 Aftercare following surgery for neoplasm**
Use additional code to identify the neoplasm

**Z48.8 Encounter for other specified postprocedural aftercare**

**Z48.81 Encounter for surgical aftercare following surgery on specified body systems**
These codes identify the body system requiring aftercare. They are for use in conjunction with other aftercare codes to fully explain the aftercare encounter. The condition treated should also be coded if still present.

EXCLUDES 1 *aftercare for injury - code the injury with 7th character D*
*aftercare following surgery for neoplasm (Z48.3)*

EXCLUDES 2 *aftercare following organ transplant (Z48.2-)*
*orthopedic aftercare (Z47.-)*

**AHA:** 2015,4Q,38

**Z48.810 Encounter for surgical aftercare following surgery on the sense organs**

**Z48.811 Encounter for surgical aftercare following surgery on the nervous system**

EXCLUDES 2 *encounter for surgical aftercare following surgery on the sense organs (Z48.810)*

**Z48.812 Encounter for surgical aftercare following surgery on the circulatory system**
**AHA:** 2012,4Q,96

**Z48.813 Encounter for surgical aftercare following surgery on the respiratory system**
**AHA:** 2019,2Q,33

**Z48.814 Encounter for surgical aftercare following surgery on the teeth or oral cavity**

**Z48.815 Encounter for surgical aftercare following surgery on the digestive system**

**Z48.816 Encounter for surgical aftercare following surgery on the genitourinary system**

EXCLUDES 1 *encounter for aftercare following sterilization reversal (Z31.42)*

**Z48.817 Encounter for surgical aftercare following surgery on the skin and subcutaneous tissue**

**Z48.89 Encounter for other specified surgical aftercare**

**Z49 Encounter for care involving renal dialysis**
Code also associated end stage renal disease (N18.6)

**Z49.0 Preparatory care for renal dialysis**
Encounter for dialysis instruction and training

**Z49.01 Encounter for fitting and adjustment of extracorporeal dialysis catheter** Rx ESR
Removal or replacement of renal dialysis catheter
Toilet or cleansing of renal dialysis catheter

**Z49.02 Encounter for fitting and adjustment of peritoneal dialysis catheter** Rx ESR

**Z49.3 Encounter for adequacy testing for dialysis**

**Z49.31 Encounter for adequacy testing for hemodialysis** Rx ESR

**Z49.32 Encounter for adequacy testing for peritoneal dialysis** Rx ESR
Encounter for peritoneal equilibration test

**Z51 Encounter for other aftercare and medical care**
Code also condition requiring care

EXCLUDES 1 *follow-up examination after treatment (Z08-Z09)*

**Z51.0 Encounter for antineoplastic radiation therapy** PDx
**AHA:** 2025,4Q,5; 2017,4Q,103
**TIP:** Do not assign when admission is for insertion/implantation of radioactive elements. Assign a code for the malignancy instead. Any complications related to the radioactive elements should be assigned as secondary diagnoses.

**Z51.1 Encounter for antineoplastic chemotherapy and immunotherapy**

EXCLUDES 2 *encounter for chemotherapy and immunotherapy for nonneoplastic condition - code to condition*

**Z51.11 Encounter for antineoplastic chemotherapy** PDx
**AHA:** 2025,2Q,16; 2022,1Q,16; 2015,3Q,19

**Z51.12 Encounter for antineoplastic immunotherapy** PDx
**AHA:** 2024,1Q,24

**Z51.5 Encounter for palliative care**
▶Encounter for comfort care◀
▶Encounter for hospice care◀
**AHA:** 2022,1Q,18; 2020,4Q,98; 2017,1Q,48

**Z51.6 Encounter for desensitization to allergens**
**AHA:** 2025,2Q,16; 2016,4Q,77

**Z51.8 Encounter for other specified aftercare**

EXCLUDES 1 *holiday relief care (Z75.5)*

**Z51.81 Encounter for therapeutic drug level monitoring**
Code also any long-term (current) drug therapy (Z79.-)

EXCLUDES 1 *encounter for blood-drug test for administrative or medicolegal reasons (Z02.83)*

**DEF:** Drug monitoring: Measurement of the level of a specific drug in the body or measurement of a specific function to assess effectiveness of a drug.

**Z51.89 Encounter for other specified aftercare**
**AHA:** 2012,4Q,95-97

**Z51.A Encounter for sepsis aftercare**
**AHA:** 2024,4Q,34

**Z52 Donors of organs and tissues**

INCLUDES autologous and other living donors

EXCLUDES 1 *cadaveric donor - omit code*
*examination of potential donor (Z00.5)*

**AHA:** 2012,4Q,99

**Z52.0 Blood donor**

**Z52.00 Unspecified blood donor**

**Z52.000 Unspecified donor, whole blood** PDx

**Z52.001 Unspecified donor, stem cells** PDx

**Z52.008 Unspecified donor, other blood** PDx

**Z52.01 Autologous blood donor**

**Z52.010 Autologous donor, whole blood** PDx

Z52.011 Autologous donor, stem cells PDx
Z52.018 Autologous donor, other blood PDx
✓6th Z52.09 Other blood donor
Volunteer donor
Z52.090 Other blood donor, whole blood PDx
Z52.091 Other blood donor, stem cells PDx
Z52.098 Other blood donor, other blood PDx
✓5th Z52.1 Skin donor
Z52.10 Skin donor, unspecified PDx
Z52.11 Skin donor, autologous PDx
Z52.19 Skin donor, other PDx
✓5th Z52.2 Bone donor
Z52.20 Bone donor, unspecified PDx
Z52.21 Bone donor, autologous PDx
Z52.29 Bone donor, other PDx
Z52.3 Bone marrow donor PDx
Z52.4 Kidney donor PDx
Z52.5 Cornea donor PDx
Z52.6 Liver donor PDx
✓5th Z52.8 Donor of other specified organs or tissues
✓6th Z52.81 Egg (Oocyte) donor
Z52.810 Egg (Oocyte) donor under age 35, anonymous recipient PDx
Egg donor under age 35 NOS
Z52.811 Egg (Oocyte) donor under age 35, designated recipient PDx
Z52.812 Egg (Oocyte) donor age 35 and over, anonymous recipient PDx
Egg donor age 35 and over NOS
Z52.813 Egg (Oocyte) donor age 35 and over, designated recipient PDx
Z52.819 Egg (Oocyte) donor, unspecified PDx
Z52.89 Donor of other specified organs or tissues PDx
Z52.9 Donor of unspecified organ or tissue
Donor NOS

✓4th **Z53 Persons encountering health services for specific procedures and treatment, not carried out**
✓5th Z53.0 Procedure and treatment not carried out because of contraindication
Z53.01 Procedure and treatment not carried out due to patient smoking
Z53.09 Procedure and treatment not carried out because of other contraindication
Z53.1 Procedure and treatment not carried out because of patient's decision for reasons of belief and group pressure
✓5th Z53.2 Procedure and treatment not carried out because of patient's decision for other and unspecified reasons
Z53.20 Procedure and treatment not carried out because of patient's decision for unspecified reasons
Z53.21 Procedure and treatment not carried out due to patient leaving prior to being seen by health care provider
Z53.29 Procedure and treatment not carried out because of patient's decision for other reasons
✓5th Z53.3 Procedure converted to open procedure
AHA: 2016,4Q,79
Z53.31 Laparoscopic surgical procedure converted to open procedure UPD
Z53.32 Thoracoscopic surgical procedure converted to open procedure UPD
Z53.33 Arthroscopic surgical procedure converted to open procedure UPD
Z53.39 Other specified procedure converted to open procedure UPD
Z53.8 Procedure and treatment not carried out for other reasons
Z53.9 Procedure and treatment not carried out, unspecified reason

## Persons with potential health hazards related to socioeconomic and psychosocial circumstances (Z55-Z65)

**AHA:** 2021,4Q,34-37; 2019,4Q,66; 2018,4Q,58,73; 2018,1Q,18
**DEF:** Social determinants of health: Socioeconomic factors that can affect a person's health, including both environmental and societal conditions such as education and literacy, employment, health behaviors, housing, lack of adequate food or water, occupational exposure to risk factors, social support, transportation, and violence. Tracking social needs that impact patients allows providers to identify population health trends and to promote the personalized care that addresses the medical and social needs of individual patients. ***Synonym(s):*** *SDOH.*
**TIP:** Because codes in these categories represent social information rather than medical diagnoses, they can be assigned based on documentation by nonphysician clinicians involved in the care of these patients as well as self-reported documentation from the patient, as long as the information is approved and incorporated into the medical record by a clinician or provider.

✓4th **Z55 Problems related to education and literacy**
EXCLUDES 1 *disorders of psychological development (F80-F89)*
Z55.0 Illiteracy and low-level literacy
Z55.1 Schooling unavailable and unattainable
Z55.2 Failed school examinations
Z55.3 Underachievement in school
Z55.4 Educational maladjustment and discord with teachers and classmates
Z55.5 Less than a high school diploma UPD
No general equivalence degree (GED)
Z55.6 Problems related to health literacy UPD
Difficulty understanding health related information
Difficulty understanding medication instructions
Problem completing medical forms
AHA: 2023,1Q,6
Z55.8 Other problems related to education and literacy
Problems related to inadequate teaching
Z55.9 Problems related to education and literacy, unspecified
Academic problems NOS

✓4th **Z56 Problems related to employment and unemployment**
EXCLUDES 2 *occupational exposure to risk factors (Z57.-)*
*problems related to housing and economic circumstances (Z59.-)*
Z56.0 Unemployment, unspecified
Z56.1 Change of job A
Z56.2 Threat of job loss
Z56.3 Stressful work schedule
Z56.4 Discord with boss and workmates
Z56.5 Uncongenial work environment
Difficult conditions at work
Z56.6 Other physical and mental strain related to work
Workplace stress
✓5th Z56.8 Other problems related to employment
Z56.81 Sexual harassment on the job
Z56.82 Military deployment status
Individual (civilian or military) currently deployed in theater or in support of military war, peacekeeping and humanitarian operations
Z56.89 Other problems related to employment
Furloughed
Underemployed
Z56.9 Unspecified problems related to employment
Occupational problems NOS

✓4th **Z57 Occupational exposure to risk factors**
Z57.0 Occupational exposure to noise
Z57.1 Occupational exposure to radiation
Z57.2 Occupational exposure to dust
✓5th Z57.3 Occupational exposure to other air contaminants
Z57.31 Occupational exposure to environmental tobacco smoke
EXCLUDES 2 *exposure to environmental tobacco smoke (Z77.22)*
Z57.39 Occupational exposure to other air contaminants
Z57.4 Occupational exposure to toxic agents in agriculture
Occupational exposure to solids, liquids, gases or vapors in agriculture
Z57.5 Occupational exposure to toxic agents in other industries
Occupational exposure to solids, liquids, gases or vapors in other industries
Z57.6 Occupational exposure to extreme temperature
Z57.7 Occupational exposure to vibration
Z57.8 Occupational exposure to other risk factors

**Z57.9 Occupational exposure to unspecified risk factor**

**Z58 Problems related to physical environment**
EXCLUDES 2 *occupational exposure (Z57.-)*

**Z58.6 Inadequate drinking-water supply** UPD
Lack of safe drinking water
EXCLUDES 2 *deprivation of water (T73.1)*

**Z58.8 Other problems related to physical environment**
AHA: 2023,1Q,6

**Z58.81 Basic services unavailable in physical environment** UPD
Unable to obtain internet service, due to unavailability in geographic area
Unable to obtain telephone service, due to unavailability in geographic area
Unable to obtain utilities, due to inadequate physical environment

**Z58.89 Other problems related to physical environment** UPD

**Z59 Problems related to housing and economic circumstances**
EXCLUDES 2 *problems related to upbringing (Z62.-)*

**Z59.Ø Homelessness**

**Z59.ØØ Homelessness unspecified** UPD

**Z59.Ø1 Sheltered homelessness** UPD
Doubled up
Living in a shelter such as: motel, scattered site housing, temporary or transitional living situation

**Z59.Ø2 Unsheltered homelessness** UPD
Lives in a homeless encampment
Residing in place not meant for human habitation such as: abandoned buildings, cars, parks, sidewalk
Residing on the street

**Z59.1 Inadequate housing**
EXCLUDES 2 *problems related to the natural and physical environment (Z77.1-)*
AHA: 2023,1Q,6

**Z59.1Ø Inadequate housing, unspecified** UPD
Inadequate housing NOS

**Z59.11 Inadequate housing environmental temperature** UPD
Lack of air conditioning
Lack of heating

**Z59.12 Inadequate housing utilities** UPD
Lack of electricity services
Lack of gas services
Lack of oil services
Lack of water services
EXCLUDES 2 *basic services unavailable in physical environment (Z58.81)*
*financial insecurity, difficulty paying for utilities (Z59.861)*
*lack of adequate food (Z59.4-)*
*other problems related to housing and economic circumstances (Z59.8-)*

**Z59.19 Other inadequate housing** UPD
Pest infestation
Poor housing weatherization
Restriction of space
Technical defects in home preventing adequate care
Unsatisfactory surroundings

**Z59.2 Discord with neighbors, lodgers and landlord**

**Z59.3 Problems related to living in residential institution**
Boarding-school resident
EXCLUDES 1 *institutional upbringing (Z62.22)*

**Z59.4 Lack of adequate food**
EXCLUDES 2 *deprivation of food (T73.Ø)*
*effects of hunger (T73.Ø)*
*inappropriate diet or eating habits (Z72.4)*
*malnutrition (E4Ø-E46)*

**Z59.41 Food insecurity** UPD

**Z59.48 Other specified lack of adequate food** UPD
Inadequate food
Lack of food

**Z59.5 Extreme poverty**

**Z59.6 Low income**

**Z59.7 Insufficient social insurance and welfare support**
Insufficient social and welfare insurance
AHA: 2024,4Q,34

**Z59.71 Insufficient health insurance coverage** UPD
Inadequate social insurance
Insufficient social insurance
No health insurance coverage

**Z59.72 Insufficient welfare support** UPD
Inadequate welfare support

**Z59.8 Other problems related to housing and economic circumstances**
AHA: 2022,4Q,52

**Z59.81 Housing instability, housed**
Foreclosure on home loan
Past due on rent or mortgage
Unwanted multiple moves in the last 12 months

**Z59.811 Housing instability, housed, with risk of homelessness** UPD
Imminent risk of homelessness

**Z59.812 Housing instability, housed, homelessness in past 12 months** UPD

**Z59.819 Housing instability, housed unspecified** UPD
EXCLUDES 2 *extreme poverty (Z59.5)*
*financial insecurity (Z59.86-)*
*low income (Z59.6)*
*material hardship due to limited financial resources, not elsewhere classified (Z59.87)*

**Z59.82 Transportation insecurity** UPD
Excessive transportation time
Inaccessible transportation
Inadequate transportation
Lack of transportation
Unaffordable transportation
Unreliable transportation
Unsafe transportation
EXCLUDES 2 *unavailability and inaccessibility of healthcare facilities (Z75.3)*

**Z59.86 Financial insecurity**
Burdensome debt
Economic strain
Financial strain
Money problems
Running out of money
Unable to make ends meet
EXCLUDES 2 *extreme poverty (Z59.5)*
*low income (Z59.6)*
*material hardship, not elsewhere classified (Z59.87)*

**Z59.861 Financial insecurity, difficulty paying for utilities** UPD
Difficulty paying for electricity
Difficulty paying for heat
Difficulty paying for oil
Difficulty paying water bill
Utility disconnect notice due to inability to pay
EXCLUDES 2 *inadequate housing utilities (Z59.12)*

**Z59.868 Other specified financial insecurity** UPD
Bankruptcy

**Z59.869 Financial insecurity, unspecified** UPD

**Z59.87 Material hardship due to limited financial resources, not elsewhere classified** UPD
Material deprivation due to limited financial resources
Unable to obtain adequate childcare due to limited financial resources
Unable to obtain adequate clothing due to limited financial resources
Unable to obtain basic needs due to limited financial resources
EXCLUDES 2 *extreme poverty (Z59.5)*
*financial insecurity, not elsewhere classified (Z59.86-)*
*low income (Z59.6)*

Z59.89 **Other problems related to housing and economic circumstances** UPD
Foreclosure on loan
Isolated dwelling
Problems with creditors

Z59.9 **Problem related to housing and economic circumstances, unspecified**

√4th Z60 **Problems related to social environment**

Z60.0 **Problems of adjustment to life-cycle transitions**
Empty nest syndrome
Phase of life problem
Problem with adjustment to retirement [pension]

Z60.2 **Problems related to living alone**

Z60.3 **Acculturation difficulty**
Problem with migration
Problem with social transplantation
**DEF:** Problem adapting to a different culture or environment not based on any coexisting mental disorder.

Z60.4 **Social exclusion and rejection**
Exclusion and rejection on the basis of personal characteristics, such as unusual physical appearance, illness or behavior.
Social isolation
EXCLUDES 1 *target of adverse discrimination such as for racial or religious reasons (Z60.5)*

Z60.5 **Target of (perceived) adverse discrimination and persecution**
EXCLUDES 1 *social exclusion and rejection (Z60.4)*

Z60.8 **Other problems related to social environment**
Inadequate social support
Lack of emotional support

Z60.9 **Problem related to social environment, unspecified**

√4th Z62 **Problems related to upbringing**
INCLUDES current and past negative life events in childhood
current and past problems of a child related to upbringing
EXCLUDES 2 *maltreatment syndrome (T74.-)*
*problems related to housing and economic circumstances (Z59.-)*

Z62.0 **Inadequate parental supervision and control**

Z62.1 **Parental overprotection**

√5th Z62.2 **Upbringing away from parents**
EXCLUDES 1 *problems with boarding school (Z59.3)*
**AHA:** 2023,4Q,49

Z62.21 **Child in welfare custody** P
Child in foster care
Child in welfare guardianship

Z62.22 **Institutional upbringing**
Child living in group home
Child living in orphanage
Code also, if applicable, child in welfare custody (Z62.21)

Z62.23 **Child in custody of non-parental relative** UPD P
Child in care of non-parental family member
Child in custody of grandparent
Child in kinship care
Guardianship by non-parental relative
Code also, if applicable, child in welfare custody (Z62.21)

Z62.24 **Child in custody of non-relative guardian** UPD P
Code also, if applicable, child in welfare custody (Z62.21)

Z62.29 **Other upbringing away from parents**

Z62.3 **Hostility towards and scapegoating of child** P

Z62.6 **Inappropriate (excessive) parental pressure**

√5th Z62.8 **Other specified problems related to upbringing**
Code also, if applicable:
absence of family member (Z63.3-)
disappearance and death of family member (Z63.4)
disruption of family by separation and divorce (Z63.5)
other specified problems related to primary support group (Z63.8)
other stressful life events affecting family and household (Z63.7-)

√6th Z62.81 **Personal history of abuse in childhood**
Personal history of abuse in adolescence
**AHA:** 2023,1Q,6

Z62.810 **Personal history of physical and sexual abuse in childhood**
EXCLUDES 1 *current child physical abuse (T74.12, T76.12)*
*current child sexual abuse (T74.22, T76.22)*

Z62.811 **Personal history of psychological abuse in childhood**
EXCLUDES 1 *current child psychological abuse (T74.32, T76.32)*

Z62.812 **Personal history of neglect in childhood**
EXCLUDES 1 *current child neglect (T74.02, T76.02)*

Z62.813 **Personal history of forced labor or sexual exploitation in childhood**
**AHA:** 2018,4Q,32,35

Z62.814 **Personal history of child financial abuse** UPD
EXCLUDES 1 *current child financial abuse (T74.A2)*

Z62.815 **Personal history of intimate partner abuse in childhood** UPD
EXCLUDES 2 *adult and child abuse, neglect and other maltreatment, confirmed (T74.-)*

Z62.819 **Personal history of unspecified abuse in childhood**
EXCLUDES 1 *current child abuse NOS (T74.92, T76.92)*

√6th Z62.82 **Parent-child conflict**
**AHA:** 2023,4Q,49

Z62.820 **Parent-biological child conflict**
Parent-child problem NOS

Z62.821 **Parent-adopted child conflict**

Z62.822 **Parent-foster child conflict**

Z62.823 **Parent-step child conflict** UPD

√6th Z62.83 **Non-parental relative or guardian-child conflict**
**AHA:** 2023,4Q,50

Z62.831 **Non-parental relative-child conflict** UPD
Grandparent-child conflict
Kinship-care child conflict
Non-parental relative legal guardian-child conflict
Other relative-child conflict
EXCLUDES 1 *group home staff-child conflict (Z62.833)*

Z62.832 **Non-relative guardian-child conflict** UPD
EXCLUDES 1 *group home staff-child conflict (Z62.833)*

Z62.833 **Group home staff-child conflict** UPD

√6th Z62.89 **Other specified problems related to upbringing**

Z62.890 **Parent-child estrangement NEC**

Z62.891 **Sibling rivalry**

Z62.892 **Runaway [from current living environment]** UPD
Child leaving living situation without permission
**AHA:** 2023,4Q,50

Z62.898 **Other specified problems related to upbringing**

Z62.9 **Problem related to upbringing, unspecified**

**Z63 Other problems related to primary support group, including family circumstances**
EXCLUDES 2 *maltreatment syndrome (T74.-, T76)*
*parent-child problems (Z62.-)*
*problems related to negative life events in childhood (Z62.-)*
*problems related to upbringing (Z62.-)*

**Z63.0 Problems in relationship with spouse or partner**
Relationship distress with spouse or intimate partner
EXCLUDES 1 *counseling for spousal or partner abuse problems (Z69.1)*
*counseling related to sexual attitude, behavior, and orientation (Z70.-)*

**Z63.1 Problems in relationship with in-laws**

**Z63.3 Absence of family member**
EXCLUDES 1 *absence of family member due to disappearance and death (Z63.4)*
*absence of family member due to separation and divorce (Z63.5)*

**Z63.31 Absence of family member due to military deployment**
Individual or family affected by other family member being on military deployment
EXCLUDES 1 *family disruption due to return of family member from military deployment (Z63.71)*

**Z63.32 Other absence of family member**

**Z63.4 Disappearance and death of family member**
Assumed death of family member
Bereavement
**AHA:** 2014,1Q,25

**Z63.5 Disruption of family by separation and divorce**
Marital estrangement

**Z63.6 Dependent relative needing care at home**

**Z63.7 Other stressful life events affecting family and household**

**Z63.71 Stress on family due to return of family member from military deployment**
Individual or family affected by family member having returned from military deployment (current or past conflict)

**Z63.72 Alcoholism and drug addiction in family**

**Z63.79 Other stressful life events affecting family and household**
Anxiety (normal) about sick person in family
Health problems within family
Ill or disturbed family member
Isolated family

**Z63.8 Other specified problems related to primary support group**
Family discord NOS
Family estrangement NOS
High expressed emotional level within family
Inadequate family support NOS
Inadequate or distorted communication within family

**Z63.9 Problem related to primary support group, unspecified**
Relationship disorder NOS

**Z64 Problems related to certain psychosocial circumstances**

**Z64.0 Problems related to unwanted pregnancy**

**Z64.1 Problems related to multiparity**

**Z64.4 Discord with counselors**
Discord with probation officer
Discord with social worker

**Z65 Problems related to other psychosocial circumstances**

**Z65.0 Conviction in civil and criminal proceedings without imprisonment**

**Z65.1 Imprisonment and other incarceration**

**Z65.2 Problems related to release from prison**

**Z65.3 Problems related to other legal circumstances**
Arrest
Child custody or support proceedings
Litigation
Prosecution

**Z65.4 Victim of crime and terrorism**
Victim of torture

**Z65.5 Exposure to disaster, war and other hostilities**
EXCLUDES 1 *target of perceived discrimination or persecution (Z60.5)*

**Z65.8 Other specified problems related to psychosocial circumstances**
At risk for feeling loneliness
Religious or spiritual problem

**Z65.9 Problem related to unspecified psychosocial circumstances**

## Do not resuscitate status (Z66)

**Z66 Do not resuscitate**
DNR status
**DEF:** Medical order written by a physician that instructs others not to perform cardiopulmonary resuscitation (CPR), intubation, or advanced cardiac life support (ACLS). It prevents unnecessary invasive treatment to prolong life should breathing stop or cardiac arrest occur.

## Blood type (Z67)

**Z67 Blood type**
**AHA:** 2015,3Q,40

**Z67.1 Type A blood**
**Z67.10 Type A blood, Rh positive**
**Z67.11 Type A blood, Rh negative**

**Z67.2 Type B blood**
**Z67.20 Type B blood, Rh positive**
**Z67.21 Type B blood, Rh negative**

**Z67.3 Type AB blood**
**Z67.30 Type AB blood, Rh positive**
**Z67.31 Type AB blood, Rh negative**

**Z67.4 Type O blood**
**Z67.40 Type O blood, Rh positive**
**Z67.41 Type O blood, Rh negative**

**Z67.9 Unspecified blood type**
**Z67.90 Unspecified blood type, Rh positive**
**Z67.91 Unspecified blood type, Rh negative**

**Z67.A Duffy phenotype**
**AHA:** 2024,4Q,32

**Z67.A1 Duffy null**
Duffy phenotype Fy(a-b-)

**Z67.A2 Duffy a positive**
Duffy phenotype Fy(a+b-)

**Z67.A3 Duffy b positive**
Duffy phenotype Fy(a-b+)

**Z67.A4 Duffy a and b positive**
Duffy phenotype Fy(a+b+)

## Body mass index [BMI] (Z68)

**Z68 Body mass index [BMI]**
Kilograms per meters squared

NOTE BMI adult codes are for use for persons 20 years of age or older

BMI pediatric codes are for use for persons 2-19 years of age.

These percentiles are based on the growth charts published by the Centers for Disease Control and Prevention (CDC)

**AHA:** 2022,3Q,6; 2019,4Q,19,57; 2018,4Q,73,77-83; 2017,1Q,39
**DEF:** Index used to help determine whether an individual is underweight, a healthy weight, overweight, or obese.
**TIP:** A BMI code may be assigned based on medical record documentation from clinicians who are not the patient's provider. However, the BMI must be associated with a condition that meets the definition of a reportable diagnosis, per the ICD-10-CM Official Guidelines for Coding and Reporting, and that condition can only be reported when documented by the patient's provider.

▲ **Z68.1 Body mass index [BMI] 19.9 or less, adult**
**AHA:** 2024,4Q,13

● **Z68.18 Body mass index [BMI] 18.4 or less, adult**
● **Z68.19 Body mass index [BMI] 18.5-19.9, adult**

**Z68.2 Body mass index [BMI] 20-29, adult**
**Z68.20 Body mass index [BMI] 20.0-20.9, adult** UPD A
**Z68.21 Body mass index [BMI] 21.0-21.9, adult** UPD A
**Z68.22 Body mass index [BMI] 22.0-22.9, adult** UPD A
**Z68.23 Body mass index [BMI] 23.0-23.9, adult** UPD A
**Z68.24 Body mass index [BMI] 24.0-24.9, adult** UPD A
**Z68.25 Body mass index [BMI] 25.0-25.9, adult** UPD A
**Z68.26 Body mass index [BMI] 26.0-26.9, adult** UPD A
**Z68.27 Body mass index [BMI] 27.0-27.9, adult** UPD A
**Z68.28 Body mass index [BMI] 28.0-28.9, adult** UPD A
**Z68.29 Body mass index [BMI] 29.0-29.9, adult** UPD A

**Z68.3 Body mass index [BMI] 30-39, adult**
**Z68.30 Body mass index [BMI] 30.0-30.9, adult** UPD A

Z68.31 Body mass index [BMI] 31.0-31.9, adult UPD A
Z68.32 Body mass index [BMI] 32.0-32.9, adult UPD A
Z68.33 Body mass index [BMI] 33.0-33.9, adult UPD A
Z68.34 Body mass index [BMI] 34.0-34.9, adult UPD A
Z68.35 Body mass index [BMI] 35.0-35.9, adult UPD A
Z68.36 Body mass index [BMI] 36.0-36.9, adult UPD A
Z68.37 Body mass index [BMI] 37.0-37.9, adult UPD A
Z68.38 Body mass index [BMI] 38.0-38.9, adult UPD A
Z68.39 Body mass index [BMI] 39.0-39.9, adult UPD A

✓5th **Z68.4 Body mass index [BMI] 40 or greater, adult**
Z68.41 Body mass index [BMI] 40.0-44.9, adult HCC ESR UPD A
Z68.42 Body mass index [BMI] 45.0-49.9, adult HCC ESR UPD A
Z68.43 Body mass index [BMI] 50.0-59.9, adult HCC ESR UPD A
Z68.44 Body mass index [BMI] 60.0-69.9, adult HCC ESR UPD A
Z68.45 Body mass index [BMI] 70 or greater, adult HCC ESR UPD A

✓5th **Z68.5 Body mass index [BMI] pediatric**
AHA: 2024,4Q,33; 2018,4Q,81-82
Z68.51 Body mass index [BMI] pediatric, less than 5th percentile for age UPD
Z68.52 Body mass index [BMI] pediatric, 5th percentile to less than 85th percentile for age UPD
Z68.53 Body mass index [BMI] pediatric, 85th percentile to less than 95th percentile for age UPD
Z68.54 Body mass index [BMI] pediatric, 95th percentile for age to less than 120% of the 95th percentile for age UPD
Z68.55 Body mass index [BMI] pediatric, 120% of the 95th percentile for age to less than 140% of the 95th percentile for age UPD
Z68.56 Body mass index [BMI] pediatric, greater than or equal to 140% of the 95th percentile for age HCC ESR UPD

## Persons encountering health services in other circumstances (Z69-Z76)

✓4th **Z69 Encounter for mental health services for victim and perpetrator of abuse**
INCLUDES counseling for victims and perpetrators of abuse

✓5th **Z69.0 Encounter for mental health services for child abuse problems**

✓6th **Z69.01 Encounter for mental health services for parental child abuse**

Z69.010 Encounter for mental health services for victim of parental child abuse P
- Encounter for mental health services for victim of child abuse by parent
- Encounter for mental health services for victim of child neglect by parent
- Encounter for mental health services for victim of child psychological abuse by parent
- Encounter for mental health services for victim of child sexual abuse by parent

Z69.011 Encounter for mental health services for perpetrator of parental child abuse
- Encounter for mental health services for perpetrator of parental child neglect
- Encounter for mental health services for perpetrator of parental child psychological abuse
- Encounter for mental health services for perpetrator of parental child sexual abuse

EXCLUDES 1 *encounter for mental health services for non-parental child abuse (Z69.02-)*

✓6th **Z69.02 Encounter for mental health services for non-parental child abuse**

Z69.020 Encounter for mental health services for victim of non-parental child abuse P
- Encounter for mental health services for victim of non-parental child neglect
- Encounter for mental health services for victim of non-parental child psychological abuse
- Encounter for mental health services for victim of non-parental child sexual abuse

Z69.021 Encounter for mental health services for perpetrator of non-parental child abuse
- Encounter for mental health services for perpetrator of non-parental child neglect
- Encounter for mental health services for perpetrator of non-parental child psychological abuse
- Encounter for mental health services for perpetrator of non-parental child sexual abuse

✓5th **Z69.1 Encounter for mental health services for spousal or partner abuse problems**

Z69.11 Encounter for mental health services for victim of spousal or partner abuse
- Encounter for mental health services for victim of spouse or partner neglect
- Encounter for mental health services for victim of spouse or partner psychological abuse
- Encounter for mental health services for victim of spouse or partner violence, physical

Z69.12 Encounter for mental health services for perpetrator of spousal or partner abuse
- Encounter for mental health services for perpetrator of spouse or partner neglect
- Encounter for mental health services for perpetrator of spouse or partner psychological abuse
- Encounter for mental health services for perpetrator of spouse or partner violence, physical
- Encounter for mental health services for perpetrator of spouse or partner violence, sexual

✓5th **Z69.8 Encounter for mental health services for victim or perpetrator of other abuse**

Z69.81 Encounter for mental health services for victim of other abuse
- Encounter for mental health services for victim of non-spousal adult abuse
- Encounter for mental health services for victim of spouse or partner violence, sexual
- Encounter for rape victim counseling

Z69.82 Encounter for mental health services for perpetrator of other abuse
- Encounter for mental health services for perpetrator of non-spousal adult abuse

✓4th **Z70 Counseling related to sexual attitude, behavior and orientation**
INCLUDES encounter for mental health services for sexual attitude, behavior and orientation
EXCLUDES 2 *contraceptive or procreative counseling (Z30-Z31)*

Z70.0 Counseling related to sexual attitude

Z70.1 Counseling related to patient's sexual behavior and orientation
- Patient concerned regarding impotence
- Patient concerned regarding non-responsiveness
- Patient concerned regarding promiscuity
- Patient concerned regarding sexual orientation

Z70.2 Counseling related to sexual behavior and orientation of third party
- Advice sought regarding sexual behavior and orientation of child
- Advice sought regarding sexual behavior and orientation of partner
- Advice sought regarding sexual behavior and orientation of spouse

Z70.3 Counseling related to combined concerns regarding sexual attitude, behavior and orientation

Z70.8 Other sex counseling
- Encounter for sex education

Z70.9 Sex counseling, unspecified

Chapter 21. Factors Influencing Health Status and Contact With Health Services

Z68.31–Z70.9

**4th Z71 Persons encountering health services for other counseling and medical advice, not elsewhere classified**

EXCLUDES 2 *contraceptive or procreation counseling (Z3Ø-Z31)*
*sex counseling (Z7Ø.-)*

**Z71.Ø Person encountering health services to consult on behalf of another person**

Person encountering health services to seek advice or treatment for non-attending third party

EXCLUDES 2 *anxiety (normal) about sick person in family (Z63.7)*
*expectant (adoptive) parent(s) pre-birth pediatrician visit (Z76.81)*

**Z71.1 Person with feared health complaint in whom no diagnosis is made**

"Worried well"
Person encountering health services in which problem was normal state
Person encountering health services with feared condition which was not demonstrated

EXCLUDES 1 *medical observation for suspected diseases and conditions proven not to exist (ZØ3.-)*

**Z71.2 Person consulting for explanation of examination or test findings**

**Z71.3 Dietary counseling and surveillance**

Use additional code for any associated underlying medical condition
Use additional code to identify body mass index (BMI), if known (Z68.-)

**5th Z71.4 Alcohol abuse counseling and surveillance**

Use additional code for alcohol abuse or dependence (F1Ø.-)

**Z71.41 Alcohol abuse counseling and surveillance of alcoholic**

**Z71.42 Counseling for family member of alcoholic**

Counseling for significant other, partner, or friend of alcoholic

**5th Z71.5 Drug abuse counseling and surveillance**

Use additional code for drug abuse or dependence (F11-F16, F18-F19)

**Z71.51 Drug abuse counseling and surveillance of drug abuser**

**Z71.52 Counseling for family member of drug abuser**

Counseling for significant other, partner, or friend of drug abuser

**Z71.6 Tobacco abuse counseling**

Use additional code for nicotine dependence (F17.-)

**Z71.7 Human immunodeficiency virus [HIV] counseling**

**AHA:** 2026,1Q,27

**5th Z71.8 Other specified counseling**

EXCLUDES 2 *counseling for contraception (Z3Ø.Ø-)*

**AHA:** 2017,4Q,27

**Z71.81 Spiritual or religious counseling**

**Z71.82 Exercise counseling**

**Z71.83 Encounter for nonprocreative genetic counseling**

EXCLUDES 1 *counseling for procreative genetics (Z31.5)*
*counseling for procreative management (Z31.6)*

**Z71.84 Encounter for health counseling related to travel**

Encounter for health risk and safety counseling for (international) travel
Code also, if applicable, encounter for immunization (Z23)

EXCLUDES 2 *encounter for administrative examination (ZØ2.-)*
*encounter for other special examination without complaint, suspected or reported diagnosis (ZØ1.-)*

**AHA:** 2019,4Q,20,57

**Z71.85 Encounter for immunization safety counseling**

Encounter for vaccine product safety counseling
Code also, if applicable, encounter for immunization (Z23)
Code also, if applicable, immunization not carried out (Z28.-)

EXCLUDES 1 *encounter for health counseling related to travel (Z71.84)*

**AHA:** 2021,4Q,34

**Z71.87 Encounter for pediatric-to-adult transition counseling**

Code also chronic condition, if applicable, such as:
autism spectrum disorder (F84.Ø)
congenital malformations of the circulatory system (Q2Ø-Q28)
cystic fibrosis (E84-)
sickle-cell disorder (D57-)

**AHA:** 2022,4Q,51

**Z71.88 Encounter for counseling for socioeconomic factors**

**AHA:** 2022,4Q,51

**Z71.89 Other specified counseling**

**Z71.9 Counseling, unspecified**

Encounter for medical advice NOS

**4th Z72 Problems related to lifestyle**

EXCLUDES 2 *problems related to life-management difficulty (Z73.-)*
*problems related to socioeconomic and psychosocial circumstances (Z55-Z65)*

**Z72.Ø Tobacco use**

Tobacco use NOS

EXCLUDES 1 *history of tobacco dependence (Z87.891)*
*nicotine dependence (F17.2-)*
*tobacco dependence (F17.2-)*
*tobacco use during pregnancy (O99.33-)*

**Z72.3 Lack of physical exercise**

**Z72.4 Inappropriate diet and eating habits**

EXCLUDES 1 *behavioral eating disorders of infancy or childhood (F98.2-F98.3)*
*eating disorders (F5Ø.-)*
*lack of adequate food (Z59.48)*
*malnutrition and other nutritional deficiencies (E4Ø-E64)*

**5th Z72.5 High risk sexual behavior**

Promiscuity

EXCLUDES 1 *paraphilias (F65)*

**Z72.51 High risk heterosexual behavior**

**Z72.52 High risk homosexual behavior**

**Z72.53 High risk bisexual behavior**

**Z72.6 Gambling and betting**

EXCLUDES 1 *compulsive or pathological gambling (F63.Ø)*

**5th Z72.8 Other problems related to lifestyle**

**6th Z72.81 Antisocial behavior**

EXCLUDES 1 *conduct disorders (F91.-)*

**Z72.81Ø Child and adolescent antisocial behavior** P

Antisocial behavior (child) (adolescent) without manifest psychiatric disorder
Delinquency NOS
Group delinquency
Offenses in the context of gang membership
Stealing in company with others
Truancy from school

**Z72.811 Adult antisocial behavior** A

Adult antisocial behavior without manifest psychiatric disorder

**6th Z72.82 Problems related to sleep**

**Z72.82Ø Sleep deprivation**

Lack of adequate sleep

EXCLUDES 1 *insomnia (G47.Ø-)*

**Z72.821 Inadequate sleep hygiene**

Bad sleep habits
Irregular sleep habits
Unhealthy sleep wake schedule

EXCLUDES 1 *insomnia (F51.Ø-, G47.Ø-)*

**Z72.823 Risk of suffocation (smothering) under another while sleeping** UPD

Child-caregiver co-sleeping
Infant bed-sharing

**AHA:** 2022,4Q,51

**Z72.89 Other problems related to lifestyle**

Self-damaging behavior

**Z72.9 Problem related to lifestyle, unspecified**

**4th Z73 Problems related to life management difficulty**

EXCLUDES 2 *problems related to socioeconomic and psychosocial circumstances (Z55-Z65)*

**DEF:** State of emotional, mental, and physical exhaustion causing difficulties in managing personal, school, or work circumstances. It is usually due to prolonged stress or poor interpersonal relationship skills or parenting skills.

**Z73.Ø Burn-out**

**Z73.1 Type A behavior pattern**

**Z73.2 Lack of relaxation and leisure**

**Z73.3 Stress, not elsewhere classified**
Physical and mental strain NOS
EXCLUDES 1 *stress related to employment or unemployment (Z56.-)*

**Z73.4 Inadequate social skills, not elsewhere classified**

**Z73.5 Social role conflict, not elsewhere classified**

**Z73.6 Limitation of activities due to disability**
EXCLUDES 1 *care-provider dependency (Z74.-)*

✓5th **Z73.8 Other problems related to life management difficulty**

✓6th **Z73.81 Behavioral insomnia of childhood**
**DEF:** Behaviors on the part of the child or caregivers that cause negative compliance with a child's sleep schedule resulting in lack of adequate sleep.

**Z73.810 Behavioral insomnia of childhood, sleep-onset association type** P

**Z73.811 Behavioral insomnia of childhood, limit setting type** P

**Z73.812 Behavioral insomnia of childhood, combined type** P

**Z73.819 Behavioral insomnia of childhood, unspecified type** P

**Z73.82 Dual sensory impairment**

**Z73.89 Other problems related to life management difficulty**

**Z73.9 Problem related to life management difficulty, unspecified**

✓4th **Z74 Problems related to care provider dependency**
EXCLUDES 2 *dependence on enabling machines or devices NEC (Z99.-)*

✓5th **Z74.0 Reduced mobility**

**Z74.01 Bed confinement status**
Bedridden

**Z74.09 Other reduced mobility**
Chair ridden
Reduced mobility NOS
EXCLUDES 2 *wheelchair dependence (Z99.3)*

**Z74.1 Need for assistance with personal care**

**Z74.2 Need for assistance at home and no other household member able to render care**

**Z74.3 Need for continuous supervision**

**Z74.8 Other problems related to care provider dependency**

**Z74.9 Problem related to care provider dependency, unspecified**

✓4th **Z75 Problems related to medical facilities and other health care**

**Z75.0 Medical services not available in home**
EXCLUDES 1 *no other household member able to render care (Z74.2)*

**Z75.1 Person awaiting admission to adequate facility elsewhere**

**Z75.2 Other waiting period for investigation and treatment**

**Z75.3 Unavailability and inaccessibility of health-care facilities**
EXCLUDES 1 *bed unavailable (Z75.1)*

**Z75.4 Unavailability and inaccessibility of other helping agencies**

**Z75.5 Holiday relief care**

**Z75.8 Other problems related to medical facilities and other health care**

**Z75.9 Unspecified problem related to medical facilities and other health care**

✓4th **Z76 Persons encountering health services in other circumstances**

**Z76.0 Encounter for issue of repeat prescription**
Encounter for issue of repeat prescription for appliance
Encounter for issue of repeat prescription for medicaments
Encounter for issue of repeat prescription for spectacles
EXCLUDES 2 *issue of medical certificate (Z02.7)*
*repeat prescription for contraceptive (Z30.4-)*

**Z76.1 Encounter for health supervision and care of foundling** PDx

**Z76.2 Encounter for health supervision and care of other healthy infant and child** PDx P
Encounter for medical or nursing care or supervision of healthy infant under circumstances such as adverse socioeconomic conditions at home
Encounter for medical or nursing care or supervision of healthy infant under circumstances such as awaiting foster or adoptive placement
Encounter for medical or nursing care or supervision of healthy infant under circumstances such as maternal illness
Encounter for medical or nursing care or supervision of healthy infant under circumstances such as number of children at home preventing or interfering with normal care

**Z76.3 Healthy person accompanying sick person**

**Z76.4 Other boarder to healthcare facility**
EXCLUDES 1 *homelessness (Z59.0-)*

**Z76.5 Malingerer [conscious simulation]**
Person feigning illness (with obvious motivation)
EXCLUDES 1 *factitious disorder (F68.1-, F68.A)*
*peregrinating patient (F68.1-)*
**DEF:** Act of intentionally exaggerating an illness or disability in order to receive personal gain or to avoid punishment or responsibility.

✓5th **Z76.8 Persons encountering health services in other specified circumstances**

**Z76.81 Expectant parent(s) prebirth pediatrician visit**
Pre-adoption pediatrician visit for adoptive parent(s)

**Z76.82 Awaiting organ transplant status**
Patient waiting for organ availability

**Z76.89 Persons encountering health services in other specified circumstances**
Persons encountering health services NOS
**AHA:** 2014,2Q,10

## Persons with potential health hazards related to family and personal history and certain conditions influencing health status (Z77-Z99)

Code also any follow-up examination (Z08-Z09)

✓4th **Z77 Other contact with and (suspected) exposures hazardous to health**
INCLUDES contact with and (suspected) exposures to potential hazards to health
EXCLUDES 2 *contact with and (suspected) exposure to communicable diseases (Z20.-)*
*exposure to (parental) (environmental) tobacco smoke in the perinatal period (P96.81)*
*newborn affected by noxious substances transmitted via placenta or breast milk (P04.-)*
*occupational exposure to risk factors (Z57.-)*
*retained foreign body (Z18.-)*
*retained foreign body fully removed (Z87.821)*
*toxic effects of substances chiefly nonmedicinal as to source (T51-T65)*

✓5th **Z77.0 Contact with and (suspected) exposure to hazardous, chiefly nonmedicinal, chemicals**

✓6th **Z77.01 Contact with and (suspected) exposure to hazardous metals**

**Z77.010 Contact with and (suspected) exposure to arsenic**

**Z77.011 Contact with and (suspected) exposure to lead**

**Z77.012 Contact with and (suspected) exposure to uranium**
EXCLUDES 1 *retained depleted uranium fragments (Z18.01)*

● **Z77.013 Contact with and (suspected) exposure to gadolinium**

**Z77.018 Contact with and (suspected) exposure to other hazardous metals**
Contact with and (suspected) exposure to chromium compounds
Contact with and (suspected) exposure to nickel dust

✓6th **Z77.02 Contact with and (suspected) exposure to hazardous aromatic compounds**

**Z77.020 Contact with and (suspected) exposure to aromatic amines**

**Z77.021 Contact with and (suspected) exposure to benzene**

**Z77.028 Contact with and (suspected) exposure to other hazardous aromatic compounds**
Aromatic dyes NOS
Polycyclic aromatic hydrocarbons

✓6th **Z77.09 Contact with and (suspected) exposure to other hazardous, chiefly nonmedicinal, chemicals**

**Z77.090 Contact with and (suspected) exposure to asbestos**

**Z77.098 Contact with and (suspected) exposure to other hazardous, chiefly nonmedicinal, chemicals**
Dyes NOS

✓5th **Z77.1 Contact with and (suspected) exposure to environmental pollution and hazards in the physical environment**

✓6th **Z77.11 Contact with and (suspected) exposure to environmental pollution**

**Z77.110 Contact with and (suspected) exposure to air pollution**

Z77.111 **Contact with and (suspected) exposure to water pollution**

Z77.112 **Contact with and (suspected) exposure to soil pollution**

Z77.118 **Contact with and (suspected) exposure to other environmental pollution**

√6th Z77.12 **Contact with and (suspected) exposure to hazards in the physical environment**

Z77.120 **Contact with and (suspected) exposure to mold (toxic)**

Z77.121 **Contact with and (suspected) exposure to harmful algae and algae toxins**

Contact with and (suspected) exposure to (harmful) algae bloom NOS

Contact with and (suspected) exposure to blue-green algae bloom

Contact with and (suspected) exposure to brown tide

Contact with and (suspected) exposure to cyanobacteria bloom

Contact with and (suspected) exposure to Florida red tide

Contact with and (suspected) exposure to pfiesteria piscicida

Contact with and (suspected) exposure to red tide

Z77.122 **Contact with and (suspected) exposure to noise**

Z77.123 **Contact with and (suspected) exposure to radon and other naturally occurring radiation**

EXCLUDES 2 *radiation exposure as the cause of a confirmed condition (W88-W90, X39.0-)*
*radiation sickness NOS (T66)*

Z77.128 **Contact with and (suspected) exposure to other hazards in the physical environment**

√5th Z77.2 **Contact with and (suspected) exposure to other hazardous substances**

Z77.21 **Contact with and (suspected) exposure to potentially hazardous body fluids**

Z77.22 **Contact with and (suspected) exposure to environmental tobacco smoke (acute) (chronic)**

Exposure to second hand tobacco smoke (acute) (chronic)

Passive smoking (acute) (chronic)

EXCLUDES 1 *nicotine dependence (F17.-)*
*tobacco use (Z72.0)*

EXCLUDES 2 *occupational exposure to environmental tobacco smoke (Z57.31)*

Z77.29 **Contact with and (suspected) exposure to other hazardous substances**

**AHA:** 2025,3Q,11; 2016,2Q,33

√5th Z77.3 **Contact with and (suspected) exposure to war theater**

Z77.31 **Contact with and (suspected) exposure to Gulf War theater**

Contact with and (suspected) exposure to Persian Gulf War theater

● Z77.32 **Contact with and (suspected) exposure to burn pits in war theater**

● Z77.33 **Contact with and (suspected) exposure to Agent Orange**

Z77.39 **Contact with and (suspected) exposure to other war theater**

~~Agent Orange exposure~~

● √5th Z77.4 **Contact with and (suspected) exposure to blast overpressure**

● Z77.40 **Contact with and (suspected) exposure to unspecified blast overpressure**

Contact with and (suspected) exposure to blast overpressure NOS

● Z77.41 **Contact with and (suspected) exposure to low-level blast overpressure**

Contact with and (suspected) exposure to LLB overpressure

● Z77.42 **Contact with and (suspected) exposure to high-level blast overpressure**

Contact with and (suspected) exposure to HLB overpressure

● Z77.49 **Contact with and (suspected) exposure to other blast overpressure**

Z77.9 **Other contact with and (suspected) exposures hazardous to health**

√4th **Z78 Other specified health status**

EXCLUDES 2 *asymptomatic human immunodeficiency virus [HIV] infection status (Z21)*
*postprocedural status (Z93-Z99)*
*sex reassignment status ►(Z87.890-)◄*

Z78.0 **Asymptomatic menopausal state** A

Menopausal state NOS

Postmenopausal status NOS

EXCLUDES 2 *symptomatic menopausal state (N95.1)*

Z78.1 **Physical restraint status**

EXCLUDES 1 *physical restraint due to a procedure - omit code*

**DEF:** Application of mechanical restraining devices or manual restraints to limit physical mobility of a patient.

Z78.9 **Other specified health status**

√4th **Z79 Long term (current) drug therapy**

INCLUDES long term (current) drug use for prophylactic purposes

Code also any therapeutic drug level monitoring (Z51.81)

EXCLUDES 2 *drug abuse and dependence (F11-F19)*
*drug use complicating pregnancy, childbirth, and the puerperium (O99.32-)*

**AHA:** 2024,2Q,26; 2021,1Q,12

√5th Z79.0 **Long term (current) use of anticoagulants and antithrombotics/antiplatelets**

EXCLUDES 2 *long term (current) use of aspirin (Z79.82)*

Z79.01 **Long term (current) use of anticoagulants**

**AHA:** 2023,2Q,28; 2022,2Q,17; 2021,1Q,4; 2020,2Q,20

Z79.02 **Long term (current) use of antithrombotics/antiplatelets** UPD

Z79.1 **Long term (current) use of non-steroidal anti-inflammatories (NSAID)** UPD

EXCLUDES 2 *long term (current) use of aspirin (Z79.82)*

Z79.2 **Long term (current) use of antibiotics** UPD

Z79.3 **Long term (current) use of hormonal contraceptives**

Long term (current) use of birth control pill or patch

Z79.4 **Long term (current) use of insulin** HCC Rx ESR COM

EXCLUDES 2 *long-term (current) use of injectable non-insulin antidiabetic drugs (Z79.85)*
*long term (current) use of oral antidiabetic drugs (Z79.84)*
*long term (current) use of oral hypoglycemic drugs (Z79.84)*

**AHA:** 2020,3Q,31

√5th Z79.5 **Long term (current) use of steroids**

Z79.51 **Long term (current) use of inhaled steroids** UPD

Z79.52 **Long term (current) use of systemic steroids** UPD

**AHA:** 2024,3Q,14

√5th Z79.6 **Long term (current) use of immunomodulators and immunosuppressants**

EXCLUDES 2 *long term (current) use of steroids (Z79.5-)*
*long term (current) use of agents affecting estrogen receptors and estrogen levels (Z79.81-)*

**AHA:** 2022,4Q,50

Z79.60 **Long term (current) use of unspecified immunomodulators and immunosuppressants** UPD

Z79.61 **Long term (current) use of immunomodulator** UPD

Long term (current) use of apremilast

Long term (current) use of immunomodulatory imide drug

Long term (current) use of lenalidomide

Long term (current) use of pomalidomide

√6th Z79.62 **Long term (current) use of immunosuppressant**

Z79.620 **Long term (current) use of immunosuppressive biologic** UPD

Long term (current) use of adalimumab

Long term (current) use of etanercept

Long term (current) use of infliximab

Long term (current) use of monoclonal antibodies

Z79.621 **Long term (current) use of calcineurin inhibitor** UPD

Long term (current) use of cyclosporine

Long term (current) use of tacrolimus

Z79.622 **Long term (current) use of Janus kinase inhibitor** UPD

Long term (current) use of tofacitinib

Z79.623 **Long term (current) use of mammalian target of rapamycin (mTOR) inhibitor** UPD
Long term (current) use of sirolimus

Z79.624 **Long term (current) use of inhibitors of nucleotide synthesis** UPD
Long term (current) use of azathioprine
Long term (current) use of mycophenolate
Long term (current) use of purine synthesis (IMDH) inhibitors

✓6th Z79.63 **Long term (current) use of chemotherapeutic agent**

Z79.630 **Long term (current) use of alkylating agent** UPD
Long term (current) use of chlorambucil
Long term (current) use of cisplatin
Long term (current) use of cyclophosphamide

Z79.631 **Long term (current) use of antimetabolite agent** UPD
Long term (current) use of 5-fluorouracil
Long term (current) use of 6-mercaptopurine
Long term (current) use of cytarabine
Long term (current) use of methotrexate

Z79.632 **Long term (current) use of antitumor antibiotic** UPD
Long term (current) use of bleomycin
Long term (current) use of doxorubicin
Long term (current) use of mitomycin C

Z79.633 **Long term (current) use of mitotic inhibitor** UPD
Long term (current) use of paclitaxel
Long term (current) use of plant alkaloids
Long term (current) use of vinblastine
Long term (current) use of vincristine

Z79.634 **Long term (current) use of topoisomerase inhibitor** UPD
Long term (current) use of etoposide
Long term (current) use of irinotecan
Long term (current) use of topotecan

Z79.64 **Long term (current) use of myelosuppressive agent** UPD
Long term (current) use of hydroxyurea

Z79.69 **Long term (current) use of other immunomodulators and immunosuppressants** UPD

✓5th Z79.8 **Other long term (current) drug therapy**

✓6th Z79.81 **Long term (current) use of agents affecting estrogen receptors and estrogen levels**
Code first, if applicable:
malignant neoplasm of breast (C50.-)
malignant neoplasm of prostate (C61)
Use additional code, if applicable, to identify:
estrogen receptor positive status (Z17.0)
family history of breast cancer (Z80.3)
genetic susceptibility to malignant neoplasm (cancer) (Z15.0-)
personal history of breast cancer (Z85.3)
personal history of prostate cancer (Z85.46)
postmenopausal status (Z78.0)
EXCLUDES 1 *hormone replacement therapy (Z79.890)*
**AHA:** 2022,3Q,14

Z79.810 **Long term (current) use of selective estrogen receptor modulators (SERMs)** UPD
Long term (current) use of toremifene (Fareston)
Long term (current) use of raloxifene (Evista)
Long term (current) use of tamoxifen (Nolvadex)

Z79.811 **Long term (current) use of aromatase inhibitors** UPD
Long term (current) use of anastrozole (Arimidex)
Long term (current) use of exemestane (Aromasin)
Long term (current) use of letrozole (Femara)

Z79.818 **Long term (current) use of other agents affecting estrogen receptors and estrogen levels** UPD
Long term (current) use of estrogen receptor downregulators
Long term (current) use of fulvestrant (Faslodex)
Long term (current) use of gonadotropin-releasing hormone (GnRH) agonist
Long term (current) use of goserelin acetate (Zoladex)
Long term (current) use of leuprolide acetate (leuprorelin) (Lupron)
Long term (current) use of megestrol acetate (Megace)

Z79.82 **Long term (current) use of aspirin**

Z79.83 **Long term (current) use of bisphosphonates** UPD
**AHA:** 2016,4Q,42

Z79.84 **Long term (current) use of oral hypoglycemic drugs** UPD
Long term (current) use of oral antidiabetic drugs
EXCLUDES 2 *long-term (current) use of injectable non-insulin antidiabetic drugs (Z79.85)*
*long term (current) use of insulin (Z79.4)*
**AHA:** 2020,3Q,31; 2016,4Q,76

Z79.85 **Long-term (current) use of injectable non-insulin antidiabetic drugs** UPD
EXCLUDES 2 *long term (current) use of insulin (Z79.4)*
*long term (current) use of oral hypoglycemic drugs (Z79.84)*
**AHA:** 2022,4Q,50

✓5th Z79.89 **Other long term (current) drug therapy**

Z79.890 **Hormone replacement therapy** UPD

Z79.891 **Long term (current) use of opiate analgesic**
Long term (current) use of methadone for pain management
EXCLUDES 1 ~~*methadone use NOS (F11.9-)*~~
~~*use of methadone for treatment of heroin addiction (F11.2-)*~~
EXCLUDES 2 ▶*methadone use NOS (F11.9-)*◀
▶*use of methadone for treatment of heroin addiction (F11.2-)*◀

Z79.899 **Other long term (current) drug therapy**
**AHA:** 2026,1Q,25; 2023,3Q,17-18; 2020,4Q,11; 2020,3Q,31; 2020,2Q,14; 2015,4Q,34; 2015,3Q,21

✓4th **Z80 Family history of primary malignant neoplasm**

Z80.0 **Family history of malignant neoplasm of digestive organs** UPD
Conditions classifiable to C15-C26
**AHA:** 2018,1Q,6

Z80.1 **Family history of malignant neoplasm of trachea, bronchus and lung** UPD
Conditions classifiable to C33-C34

Z80.2 **Family history of malignant neoplasm of other respiratory and intrathoracic organs** UPD
Conditions classifiable to C30-C32, C37-C39

Z80.3 **Family history of malignant neoplasm of breast** UPD
Conditions classifiable to C50.-

✓5th Z80.4 **Family history of malignant neoplasm of genital organs**
Conditions classifiable to C51-C63

Z80.41 **Family history of malignant neoplasm of ovary** UPD

Z80.42 **Family history of malignant neoplasm of prostate** UPD

Z80.43 **Family history of malignant neoplasm of testis** UPD

Z80.44 **Family history of malignant neoplasm of fallopian tube(s)** UPD

Z80.49 **Family history of malignant neoplasm of other genital organs** UPD

✓5th Z80.5 **Family history of malignant neoplasm of urinary tract**
Conditions classifiable to C64-C68

Z80.51 **Family history of malignant neoplasm of kidney** UPD

Z80.52 **Family history of malignant neoplasm of bladder** UPD

Z80.59 **Family history of malignant neoplasm of other urinary tract organ** UPD

Z80.6 **Family history of leukemia** UPD
Conditions classifiable to C91-C95

Z80.7 **Family history of other malignant neoplasms of lymphoid, hematopoietic and related tissues** UPD
Conditions classifiable to C81-C90, C96.-

Z80.8 **Family history of malignant neoplasm of other organs or systems** UPD
Conditions classifiable to C00-C14, C40-C49, C69-C79

Z80.9 **Family history of malignant neoplasm, unspecified** UPD
Conditions classifiable to C80.1

✓4th **Z81 Family history of mental and behavioral disorders**

Z81.0 **Family history of intellectual disabilities**
Conditions classifiable to F70-F79

Z81.1 **Family history of alcohol abuse and dependence**
Conditions classifiable to F10.-

Z81.2 **Family history of tobacco abuse and dependence**
Conditions classifiable to F17.-

Z81.3 **Family history of other psychoactive substance abuse and dependence**
Conditions classifiable to F11-F16, F18-F19

Z81.4 **Family history of other substance abuse and dependence**
Conditions classifiable to F55

Z81.8 **Family history of other mental and behavioral disorders**
Conditions classifiable elsewhere in F01-F99

✓4th **Z82 Family history of certain disabilities and chronic diseases (leading to disablement)**

Z82.0 **Family history of epilepsy and other diseases of the nervous system** UPD
Conditions classifiable to G00-G99

Z82.1 **Family history of blindness and visual loss** UPD
Conditions classifiable to H54.-

Z82.2 **Family history of deafness and hearing loss** UPD
Conditions classifiable to H90-H91

Z82.3 **Family history of stroke** UPD
Conditions classifiable to I60-I64

✓5th Z82.4 **Family history of ischemic heart disease and other diseases of the circulatory system**
Conditions classifiable to I00-I5A, I65-I99

Z82.41 **Family history of sudden cardiac death** UPD

Z82.49 **Family history of ischemic heart disease and other diseases of the circulatory system** UPD

Z82.5 **Family history of asthma and other chronic lower respiratory diseases** UPD
Conditions classifiable to J40-J47
EXCLUDES 2 *family history of other diseases of the respiratory system (Z83.6)*

✓5th Z82.6 **Family history of arthritis and other diseases of the musculoskeletal system and connective tissue**
Conditions classifiable to M00-M99

Z82.61 **Family history of arthritis** UPD

Z82.62 **Family history of osteoporosis** UPD

Z82.69 **Family history of other diseases of the musculoskeletal system and connective tissue** UPD

✓5th Z82.7 **Family history of congenital malformations, deformations and chromosomal abnormalities**
Conditions classifiable to Q00-Q99

Z82.71 **Family history of polycystic kidney** UPD

Z82.79 **Family history of other congenital malformations, deformations and chromosomal abnormalities** UPD

Z82.8 **Family history of other disabilities and chronic diseases leading to disablement, not elsewhere classified** UPD

✓4th **Z83 Family history of other specific disorders**
EXCLUDES 2 *contact with and (suspected) exposure to communicable disease in the family (Z20.-)*

Z83.0 **Family history of human immunodeficiency virus [HIV] disease** UPD
Conditions classifiable to B20

Z83.1 **Family history of other infectious and parasitic diseases** UPD
Conditions classifiable to A00-B19, B25-B94, B99

Z83.2 **Family history of diseases of the blood and blood-forming organs and certain disorders involving the immune mechanism** UPD
Conditions classifiable to D50-D89

Z83.3 **Family history of diabetes mellitus** UPD
Conditions classifiable to E08-E13

✓5th Z83.4 **Family history of other endocrine, nutritional and metabolic diseases**
Conditions classifiable to E00-E07, E15-E88

Z83.41 **Family history of multiple endocrine neoplasia [MEN] syndrome** UPD

Z83.42 **Family history of familial hypercholesterolemia** UPD
AHA: 2016,4Q,77

✓6th Z83.43 **Family history of other disorder of lipoprotein metabolism and other lipidemias**
AHA: 2018,4Q,6,35

Z83.430 **Family history of elevated lipoprotein(a)** UPD
Family history of elevated Lp(a)

Z83.438 **Family history of other disorder of lipoprotein metabolism and other lipidemia** UPD
Family history of familial combined hyperlipidemia

Z83.49 **Family history of other endocrine, nutritional and metabolic diseases** UPD

✓5th Z83.5 **Family history of eye and ear disorders**

✓6th Z83.51 **Family history of eye disorders**
Conditions classifiable to H00-H53, H55-H59
EXCLUDES 2 *family history of blindness and visual loss (Z82.1)*

Z83.511 **Family history of glaucoma** UPD

Z83.518 **Family history of other specified eye disorder** UPD

Z83.52 **Family history of ear disorders** UPD
Conditions classifiable to H60-H83, H92-H95
EXCLUDES 2 *family history of deafness and hearing loss (Z82.2)*

Z83.6 **Family history of other diseases of the respiratory system** UPD
Conditions classifiable to J00-J39, J60-J99
EXCLUDES 2 *family history of asthma and other chronic lower respiratory diseases (Z82.5)*

✓5th Z83.7 **Family history of diseases of the digestive system**
Conditions classifiable to D12, K00-K93

✓6th Z83.71 **Family history of colonic polyps**
EXCLUDES 2 *family history of malignant neoplasm of digestive organs (Z80.0)*
AHA: 2023,4Q,47-48; 2021,1Q,14

Z83.710 **Family history of adenomatous and serrated polyps** UPD
Conditions classifiable to D12.-
Family history of tubular adenoma polyps
Family history of tubulovillous adenoma polyps
Family history of villous adenoma polyps

Z83.711 **Family history of hyperplastic colon polyps** UPD

Z83.718 **Family history of other colon polyps** UPD
Family history of inflammatory colon polyps

Z83.719 **Family history of colon polyps, unspecified** UPD
Family history of colon polyps NOS

Z83.72 **Family history of familial adenomatous polyposis** UPD
AHA: 2024,4Q,33

Z83.79 **Family history of other diseases of the digestive system** UPD

✓4th **Z84 Family history of other conditions**

Z84.0 **Family history of diseases of the skin and subcutaneous tissue** UPD
Conditions classifiable to L00-L99

✓5th Z84.1 **Family history of disorders of kidney and ureter**
Conditions classifiable to N00-N29

Z84.11 **Family history of APOL1-mediated kidney disease [AMKD]** UPD

Z84.19 **Family history of other disorders of kidney and ureter** UPD

**Z84.2** **Family history of other diseases of the genitourinary system** UPD
Conditions classifiable to N30-N99

**Z84.3** **Family history of consanguinity** UPD

**Z84.8** **Family history of other specified conditions**

**Z84.81** **Family history of carrier of genetic disease** UPD
AHA: 2021,1Q,14

**Z84.82** **Family history of sudden infant death syndrome** UPD
Family history of SIDS
AHA: 2016,4Q,77

**Z84.89** **Family history of other specified conditions** UPD

**Z84.A** **Family history of exposure to diethylstilbestrol** UPD
DES granddaughter or grandson
Family history of DES exposure
Third generation DES exposure

**Z85 Personal history of malignant neoplasm**

Code first any follow-up examination after treatment of malignant neoplasm (Z08)

Use additional code to identify:
- alcohol use and dependence (F10.-)
- exposure to environmental tobacco smoke (Z77.22)
- history of tobacco dependence (Z87.891)
- occupational exposure to environmental tobacco smoke (Z57.31)
- tobacco dependence (F17.-)
- tobacco use (Z72.0)

EXCLUDES 2 *personal history of benign neoplasm (Z86.01-)*
*personal history of carcinoma-in-situ (Z86.00-)*

AHA: 2022,3Q,28; 2020,3Q,30; 2018,4Q,64

**Z85.0** **Personal history of malignant neoplasm of digestive organs**
AHA: 2017,1Q,9

**Z85.00** **Personal history of malignant neoplasm of unspecified digestive organ**

**Z85.01** **Personal history of malignant neoplasm of esophagus**
Conditions classifiable to C15

**Z85.02** **Personal history of malignant neoplasm of stomach**

**Z85.020** **Personal history of malignant carcinoid tumor of stomach**
Conditions classifiable to C7A.092

**Z85.028** **Personal history of other malignant neoplasm of stomach**
Conditions classifiable to C16

**Z85.03** **Personal history of malignant neoplasm of large intestine**

**Z85.030** **Personal history of malignant carcinoid tumor of large intestine**
Conditions classifiable to C7A.022-C7A.025, C7A.029

**Z85.038** **Personal history of other malignant neoplasm of large intestine**
Conditions classifiable to C18

**Z85.04** **Personal history of malignant neoplasm of rectum, rectosigmoid junction, and anus**

**Z85.040** **Personal history of malignant carcinoid tumor of rectum**
Conditions classifiable to C7A.026

**Z85.048** **Personal history of other malignant neoplasm of rectum, rectosigmoid junction, and anus**
Conditions classifiable to C19-C21

**Z85.05** **Personal history of malignant neoplasm of liver**
Conditions classifiable to C22

**Z85.06** **Personal history of malignant neoplasm of small intestine**

**Z85.060** **Personal history of malignant carcinoid tumor of small intestine**
Conditions classifiable to C7A.01-

**Z85.068** **Personal history of other malignant neoplasm of small intestine**
Conditions classifiable to C17

**Z85.07** **Personal history of malignant neoplasm of pancreas**
Conditions classifiable to C25

**Z85.09** **Personal history of malignant neoplasm of other digestive organs**

**Z85.1** **Personal history of malignant neoplasm of trachea, bronchus and lung**

**Z85.11** **Personal history of malignant neoplasm of bronchus and lung**

**Z85.110** **Personal history of malignant carcinoid tumor of bronchus and lung**
Conditions classifiable to C7A.090

**Z85.118** **Personal history of other malignant neoplasm of bronchus and lung**
Conditions classifiable to C34

**Z85.12** **Personal history of malignant neoplasm of trachea**
Conditions classifiable to C33

**Z85.2** **Personal history of malignant neoplasm of other respiratory and intrathoracic organs**

**Z85.20** **Personal history of malignant neoplasm of unspecified respiratory organ**

**Z85.21** **Personal history of malignant neoplasm of larynx**
Conditions classifiable to C32

**Z85.22** **Personal history of malignant neoplasm of nasal cavities, middle ear, and accessory sinuses**
Conditions classifiable to C30-C31

**Z85.23** **Personal history of malignant neoplasm of thymus**

**Z85.230** **Personal history of malignant carcinoid tumor of thymus**
Conditions classifiable to C7A.091

**Z85.238** **Personal history of other malignant neoplasm of thymus**
Conditions classifiable to C37

**Z85.29** **Personal history of malignant neoplasm of other respiratory and intrathoracic organs**

**Z85.3** **Personal history of malignant neoplasm of breast**
Conditions classifiable to C50.-

**Z85.4** **Personal history of malignant neoplasm of genital organs**
Conditions classifiable to C51-C63

**Z85.40** **Personal history of malignant neoplasm of unspecified female genital organ**

**Z85.41** **Personal history of malignant neoplasm of cervix uteri**

**Z85.42** **Personal history of malignant neoplasm of other parts of uterus**

**Z85.43** **Personal history of malignant neoplasm of ovary**

**Z85.44** **Personal history of malignant neoplasm of other female genital organs**
AHA: 2024,2Q,11

**Z85.45** **Personal history of malignant neoplasm of unspecified male genital organ**

**Z85.46** **Personal history of malignant neoplasm of prostate**
AHA: 2023,2Q,5

**Z85.47** **Personal history of malignant neoplasm of testis**

**Z85.48** **Personal history of malignant neoplasm of epididymis**

**Z85.49** **Personal history of malignant neoplasm of other male genital organs**

**Z85.4A** **Personal history of malignant neoplasm of fallopian tube(s)**

**Z85.5** **Personal history of malignant neoplasm of urinary tract**
Conditions classifiable to C64-C68

**Z85.50** **Personal history of malignant neoplasm of unspecified urinary tract organ**

**Z85.51** **Personal history of malignant neoplasm of bladder**

**Z85.52** **Personal history of malignant neoplasm of kidney**

EXCLUDES 1 *personal history of malignant neoplasm of renal pelvis (Z85.53)*

**Z85.520** **Personal history of malignant carcinoid tumor of kidney**
Conditions classifiable to C7A.093

**Z85.528** **Personal history of other malignant neoplasm of kidney**
Conditions classifiable to C64

**Z85.53** **Personal history of malignant neoplasm of renal pelvis**

**Z85.54** **Personal history of malignant neoplasm of ureter**

**Z85.59** **Personal history of malignant neoplasm of other urinary tract organ**

**Z85.6** **Personal history of leukemia**
Conditions classifiable to C91-C95

EXCLUDES 1 *leukemia in remission C91.0-C95.9 with 5th character 1*

✓5th **Z85.7 Personal history of other malignant neoplasms of lymphoid, hematopoietic and related tissues**

**Z85.71 Personal history of Hodgkin lymphoma**
Conditions classifiable to C81

**Z85.72 Personal history of non-Hodgkin lymphomas**
Conditions classifiable to C82-C85
**AHA:** 2022,3Q,28

**Z85.79 Personal history of other malignant neoplasms of lymphoid, hematopoietic and related tissues**
Conditions classifiable to C88-C9Ø, C96
EXCLUDES 1 *multiple myeloma in remission (C9Ø.Ø1)*
*plasma cell leukemia in remission (C9Ø.11)*
*plasmacytoma in remission (C9Ø.21)*

✓5th **Z85.8 Personal history of malignant neoplasms of other organs and systems**
Conditions classifiable to CØØ-C14, C4Ø-C49, C69-C75, C7A.Ø98, C76-C79

✓6th **Z85.81 Personal history of malignant neoplasm of lip, oral cavity, and pharynx**
Conditions classifiable to CØØ-C14

**Z85.81Ø Personal history of malignant neoplasm of tongue**

**Z85.818 Personal history of malignant neoplasm of other sites of lip, oral cavity, and pharynx**

**Z85.819 Personal history of malignant neoplasm of unspecified site of lip, oral cavity, and pharynx**

✓6th **Z85.82 Personal history of malignant neoplasm of skin**

**Z85.82Ø Personal history of malignant melanoma of skin**
Conditions classifiable to C43
**AHA:** 2022,3Q,9

**Z85.821 Personal history of Merkel cell carcinoma**
Conditions classifiable to C4A

**Z85.828 Personal history of other malignant neoplasm of skin**
Conditions classifiable to C44

✓6th **Z85.83 Personal history of malignant neoplasm of bone and soft tissue**
Conditions classifiable to C4Ø-C41; C45-C49

**Z85.83Ø Personal history of malignant neoplasm of bone**

**Z85.831 Personal history of malignant neoplasm of soft tissue**
EXCLUDES 2 *personal history of malignant neoplasm of skin (Z85.82-)*

✓6th **Z85.84 Personal history of malignant neoplasm of eye and nervous tissue**
Conditions classifiable to C69-C72

**Z85.84Ø Personal history of malignant neoplasm of eye**

**Z85.841 Personal history of malignant neoplasm of brain**

**Z85.848 Personal history of malignant neoplasm of other parts of nervous tissue**

✓6th **Z85.85 Personal history of malignant neoplasm of endocrine glands**
Conditions classifiable to C73-C75

**Z85.85Ø Personal history of malignant neoplasm of thyroid**

**Z85.858 Personal history of malignant neoplasm of other endocrine glands**
**AHA:** 2024,2Q,10

**Z85.89 Personal history of malignant neoplasm of other organs and systems**
Conditions classifiable to C7A.Ø98, C76, C77-C79

**Z85.9 Personal history of malignant neoplasm, unspecified**
Conditions classifiable to C7A.ØØ, C8Ø.1

✓4th **Z86 Personal history of certain other diseases**
Code first any follow-up examination after treatment (ZØ9)

✓5th **Z86.Ø Personal history of in-situ and benign neoplasms and neoplasms of uncertain behavior**
EXCLUDES 2 *personal history of malignant neoplasms (Z85.-)*
**AHA:** 2017,1Q,9

✓6th **Z86.ØØ Personal history of in-situ neoplasm**
Conditions classifiable to DØØ-DØ9
**AHA:** 2019,4Q,20

**Z86.ØØØ Personal history of in-situ neoplasm of breast**
Conditions classifiable to DØ5

**Z86.ØØ1 Personal history of in-situ neoplasm of cervix uteri**
Conditions classifiable to DØ6
Personal history of cervical intraepithelial neoplasia III [CIN III]

**Z86.ØØ2 Personal history of in-situ neoplasm of other and unspecified genital organs**
Conditions classifiable to DØ7
Personal history of high-grade prostatic intraepithelial neoplasia III [HGPIN III]
Personal history of vaginal intraepithelial neoplasia III [VAIN III]
Personal history of vulvar intraepithelial neoplasia III [VIN III]

**Z86.ØØ3 Personal history of in-situ neoplasm of oral cavity, esophagus and stomach**
Conditions classifiable to DØØ

**Z86.ØØ4 Personal history of in-situ neoplasm of other and unspecified digestive organs**
Conditions classifiable to DØ1
Personal history of anal intraepithelial neoplasia (AIN III)

**Z86.ØØ5 Personal history of in-situ neoplasm of middle ear and respiratory system**
Conditions classifiable to DØ2

**Z86.ØØ6 Personal history of melanoma in-situ**
Conditions classifiable to DØ3
EXCLUDES 2 *sites other than skin - code to personal history of in-situ neoplasm of the site*

**Z86.ØØ7 Personal history of in-situ neoplasm of skin**
Conditions classifiable to DØ4
Personal history of carcinoma in situ of skin

**Z86.ØØ8 Personal history of in-situ neoplasm of other site**
Conditions classifiable to DØ9

**Z86.ØØA Personal history of in-situ neoplasm of the fallopian tube(s)**

✓6th **Z86.Ø1 Personal history of benign neoplasm**

✓7th **Z86.Ø1Ø Personal history of colon polyps**
Personal history of colorectal polyps
Personal history of rectal polyps
**AHA:** 2024,4Q,33; 2021,1Q,14; 2017,1Q,14

**Z86.Ø1ØØ Personal history of colon polyps, unspecified** UPD
Personal history of colon polyps NOS

**Z86.Ø1Ø1 Personal history of adenomatous and serrated colon polyps** UPD
Personal history of sessile adenomatous colon polyp
Personal history of sessile serrated colon polyp
Personal history of traditional serrated adenoma polyps
Personal history of tubular adenoma polyps
Personal history of tubulovillous adenoma polyps
Personal history of villous adenoma polyps

**Z86.Ø1Ø2 Personal history of hyperplastic colon polyps** UPD

**Z86.Ø1Ø9 Personal history of other colon polyps** UPD

**Z86.Ø11 Personal history of benign neoplasm of the brain**

**Z86.Ø12 Personal history of benign carcinoid tumor**

**Z86.Ø18 Personal history of other benign neoplasm**
AHA: 2017,1Q,14

**Z86.Ø3 Personal history of neoplasm of uncertain behavior**

**Z86.1 Personal history of infectious and parasitic diseases**
Conditions classifiable to AØØ-B89, B99
EXCLUDES 1 *personal history of infectious diseases specific to a body system*
*sequelae of infectious and parasitic diseases (B9Ø-B94)*

**Z86.11 Personal history of tuberculosis**

**Z86.12 Personal history of poliomyelitis**

**Z86.13 Personal history of malaria**

**Z86.14 Personal history of Methicillin resistant Staphylococcus aureus infection**
Personal history of MRSA infection

**Z86.15 Personal history of latent tuberculosis infection**

**Z86.16 Personal history of COVID-19** UPD
EXCLUDES 1 *post COVID-19 condition (UØ9.9)*
AHA: 2021,4Q,107-108; 2021,1Q,28-29,33-35,40-41,44-45

● **Z86.17 Personal history of Clostridioides difficile infection**
Personal history of Clostridium difficile colitis (fulminant) (nonfulminant)
Personal history of foodborne intoxication by Clostridium difficile
Personal history of Pseudomembraneous colitis
EXCLUDES 1 *enterocolitis due to Clostridium difficile, recurrent (AØ4.71)*

**Z86.19 Personal history of other infectious and parasitic diseases**
AHA: 2022,3Q,4; 2021,1Q,33-34,40; 2020,3Q,13; 2020,2Q,10,12

**Z86.2 Personal history of diseases of the blood and blood-forming organs and certain disorders involving the immune mechanism**
Conditions classifiable to D5Ø-D89

**Z86.3 Personal history of endocrine, nutritional and metabolic diseases**
Conditions classifiable to EØØ-E88

**Z86.31 Personal history of diabetic foot ulcer**
EXCLUDES 2 *current diabetic foot ulcer (EØ8.621, EØ9.621, E1Ø.621, E11.621, E13.621)*

**Z86.32 Personal history of gestational diabetes**
Personal history of conditions classifiable to O24.4-
EXCLUDES 1 *gestational diabetes mellitus in current pregnancy (O24.4-)*

**Z86.39 Personal history of other endocrine, nutritional and metabolic disease**
AHA: 2020,1Q,12

**Z86.5 Personal history of mental and behavioral disorders**
Conditions classifiable to F4Ø-F59

**Z86.51 Personal history of combat and operational stress reaction** A

**Z86.59 Personal history of other mental and behavioral disorders**

**Z86.6 Personal history of diseases of the nervous system and sense organs**
Conditions classifiable to GØØ-G99, HØØ-H95

**Z86.61 Personal history of infections of the central nervous system**
Personal history of encephalitis
Personal history of meningitis

**Z86.69 Personal history of other diseases of the nervous system and sense organs**
AHA: 2016,4Q,24

**Z86.7 Personal history of diseases of the circulatory system**
Conditions classifiable to IØØ-I99
EXCLUDES 2 *old myocardial infarction (I25.2)*
*personal history of anaphylactic shock (Z87.892)*
*postmyocardial infarction syndrome (I24.1)*

**Z86.71 Personal history of venous thrombosis and embolism**

**Z86.711 Personal history of pulmonary embolism**

**Z86.718 Personal history of other venous thrombosis and embolism**
AHA: 2020,2Q,20

**Z86.72 Personal history of thrombophlebitis**

**Z86.73 Personal history of transient ischemic attack (TIA), and cerebral infarction without residual deficits**
Personal history of prolonged reversible ischemic neurological deficit (PRIND)
Personal history of stroke NOS without residual deficits
EXCLUDES 1 *personal history of traumatic brain injury (Z87.82Ø)*
*sequelae of cerebrovascular disease (I69.-)*
AHA: 2023,1Q,37; 2012,4Q,92

**Z86.74 Personal history of sudden cardiac arrest**
Personal history of sudden cardiac death successfully resuscitated
AHA: 2024,1Q,27

**Z86.79 Personal history of other diseases of the circulatory system**
AHA: 2022,2Q,14; 2020,1Q,12

**Z87 Personal history of other diseases and conditions**
Code first any follow-up examination after treatment (ZØ9)
AHA: 2022,4Q,50-51

**Z87.Ø Personal history of diseases of the respiratory system**
Conditions classifiable to JØØ-J99

**Z87.Ø1 Personal history of pneumonia (recurrent)**

**Z87.Ø9 Personal history of other diseases of the respiratory system**

**Z87.1 Personal history of diseases of the digestive system**
Conditions classifiable to KØØ-K93

**Z87.11 Personal history of peptic ulcer disease**

**Z87.19 Personal history of other diseases of the digestive system**
AHA: 2017,1Q,14

**Z87.2 Personal history of diseases of the skin and subcutaneous tissue**
Conditions classifiable to LØØ-L99
EXCLUDES 2 *personal history of diabetic foot ulcer (Z86.31)*

**Z87.3 Personal history of diseases of the musculoskeletal system and connective tissue**
Conditions classifiable to MØØ-M99
EXCLUDES 2 *personal history of (healed) traumatic fracture (Z87.81)*

**Z87.31 Personal history of (healed) nontraumatic fracture**

**Z87.31Ø Personal history of (healed) osteoporosis fracture**
Personal history of (healed) collapsed vertebra due to osteoporosis
Personal history of (healed) fragility fracture
TIP: Assign for history of osteoporosis fractures that have resolved, even when a code from category M80 indicating current osteoporosis fracture is also reported.

**Z87.311 Personal history of (healed) other pathological fracture**
Personal history of (healed) collapsed vertebra NOS
EXCLUDES 2 *personal history of osteoporosis fracture (Z87.31Ø)*

**Z87.312 Personal history of (healed) stress fracture**
Personal history of (healed) fatigue fracture

**Z87.39 Personal history of other diseases of the musculoskeletal system and connective tissue**

**Z87.4 Personal history of diseases of the genitourinary system**
Conditions classifiable to NØØ-N99

**Z87.41 Personal history of dysplasia of the female genital tract**
EXCLUDES 1 *personal history of intraepithelial neoplasia III of female genital tract (Z86.ØØ1, Z86.ØØ8, Z86.ØØA)*
*personal history of malignant neoplasm of female genital tract (Z85.4Ø-Z85.44, Z85.4A)*

**Z87.41Ø Personal history of cervical dysplasia**

**Z87.411 Personal history of vaginal dysplasia**

**Z87.412 Personal history of vulvar dysplasia**

**Z87.42 Personal history of other diseases of the female genital tract**

**Z87.43 Personal history of diseases of the male genital organs**

**Z87.43Ø Personal history of prostatic dysplasia**
EXCLUDES 1 *personal history of malignant neoplasm of prostate (Z85.46)*

Z87.438 Personal history of other diseases of male genital organs

Z87.44 Personal history of diseases of the urinary system

EXCLUDES 1 *personal history of malignant neoplasm of cervix uteri (Z85.41)*

Z87.440 Personal history of urinary (tract) infections

Z87.441 Personal history of nephrotic syndrome

Z87.442 Personal history of urinary calculi

Personal history of kidney stones

Z87.448 Personal history of other diseases of urinary system

Z87.5 Personal history of complications of pregnancy, childbirth and the puerperium

Conditions classifiable to O00-O9A

EXCLUDES 2 *recurrent pregnancy loss (N96)*

Z87.51 Personal history of pre-term labor

EXCLUDES 1 *current pregnancy with history of pre-term labor (O09.21-)*

Z87.59 Personal history of other complications of pregnancy, childbirth and the puerperium

Personal history of trophoblastic disease

AHA: 2026,1Q,28

Z87.6 Personal history of certain (corrected) conditions arising in the perinatal period

Conditions classifiable to P00-P96

EXCLUDES 1 *personal history of (corrected) congenital malformations (Z87.7-)*

Z87.61 Personal history of (corrected) necrotizing enterocolitis of newborn UPD

Z87.68 Personal history of other (corrected) conditions arising in the perinatal period UPD

Z87.7 Personal history of (corrected) congenital malformations

Conditions classifiable to Q00-Q89 that have been repaired or corrected

EXCLUDES 2 *congenital malformations that have been partially corrected or repaired but which still require medical treatment - code to condition*
*other postprocedural states (Z98.-)*
*personal history of medical treatment (Z92.-)*
*presence of cardiac and vascular implants and grafts (Z95.-)*
*presence of other devices (Z97.-)*
*presence of other functional implants (Z96.-)*
*transplanted organ and tissue status (Z94.-)*

Z87.71 Personal history of (corrected) congenital malformations of genitourinary system

Z87.710 Personal history of (corrected) hypospadias

Z87.718 Personal history of other specified (corrected) congenital malformations of genitourinary system

Z87.72 Personal history of (corrected) congenital malformations of nervous system and sense organs

Z87.720 Personal history of (corrected) congenital malformations of eye

Z87.721 Personal history of (corrected) congenital malformations of ear

Z87.728 Personal history of other specified (corrected) congenital malformations of nervous system and sense organs

Z87.73 Personal history of (corrected) congenital malformations of digestive system

Z87.730 Personal history of (corrected) cleft lip and palate

Z87.731 Personal history of (corrected) tracheoesophageal fistula or atresia UPD

Z87.732 Personal history of (corrected) persistent cloaca or cloacal malformations UPD

Z87.738 Personal history of other specified (corrected) congenital malformations of digestive system

Z87.74 Personal history of (corrected) congenital malformations of heart and circulatory system

Z87.75 Personal history of (corrected) congenital malformations of respiratory system

Z87.76 Personal history of (corrected) congenital malformations of integument, limbs and musculoskeletal system

Z87.760 Personal history of (corrected) congenital diaphragmatic hernia or other congenital diaphragm malformations UPD

Z87.761 Personal history of (corrected) gastroschisis UPD

Z87.762 Personal history of (corrected) prune belly malformation UPD

Z87.763 Personal history of other (corrected) congenital abdominal wall malformations UPD

Z87.768 Personal history of other specified (corrected) congenital malformations of integument, limbs and musculoskeletal system UPD

Z87.79 Personal history of other (corrected) congenital malformations

Z87.790 Personal history of (corrected) congenital malformations of face and neck

Z87.798 Personal history of other (corrected) congenital malformations

Z87.8 Personal history of other specified conditions

EXCLUDES 2 *personal history of self harm (Z91.5-)*

Z87.81 Personal history of (healed) traumatic fracture

EXCLUDES 2 *personal history of (healed) nontraumatic fracture (Z87.31-)*

Z87.82 Personal history of other (healed) physical injury and trauma

Conditions classifiable to S00-T88, except traumatic fractures

Z87.820 Personal history of traumatic brain injury

EXCLUDES 1 *personal history of transient ischemic attack (TIA), and cerebral infarction without residual deficits (Z86.73)*

Z87.821 Personal history of retained foreign body fully removed

Z87.828 Personal history of other (healed) physical injury and trauma

Z87.89 Personal history of other specified conditions

▲ Z87.890 Personal history of sex reassignment

▶Personal history of gender transition◀

● Z87.8901 Personal history of social gender transition

● Z87.8902 Personal history of medical gender transition

Personal history of pharmacological (hormonal) gender transition

● Z87.8903 Personal history of surgical gender transition

● Z87.8904 Personal history of intersex surgery

● Z87.8909 Personal history of unspecified gender transition

Z87.891 Personal history of nicotine dependence

EXCLUDES 1 *current nicotine dependence (F17.2-)*

AHA: 2017,2Q,27

Z87.892 Personal history of anaphylaxis

Code also allergy status such as:
allergy status to drugs, medicaments and biological substances (Z88.-)
allergy status, other than to drugs and biological substances (Z91.0-)

AHA: 2025,2Q,16

● Z87.893 Personal history of gender detransition

Code also personal history of sex reassignment (Z87.890-)

Z87.898 Personal history of other specified conditions

AHA: 2013,1Q,21

Z88 Allergy status to drugs, medicaments and biological substances

EXCLUDES 2 *allergy status, other than to drugs and biological substances (Z91.0-)*

AHA: 2025,2Q,16; 2015,3Q,23

Z88.0 Allergy status to penicillin

Z88.1 Allergy status to other antibiotic agents

Z88.2 Allergy status to sulfonamides

Z88.3 Allergy status to other anti-infective agents

Z88.4 Allergy status to anesthetic agent

Z88.5 Allergy status to narcotic agent

**Z88.6** Allergy status to analgesic agent
**Z88.7** Allergy status to serum and vaccine
**Z88.8** Allergy status to other drugs, medicaments and biological substances
**Z88.9** Allergy status to unspecified drugs, medicaments and biological substances

**Z89 Acquired absence of limb** (4th)
INCLUDES amputation status
postprocedural loss of limb
post-traumatic loss of limb
EXCLUDES 1 *acquired deformities of limbs (M20-M21)*
*congenital absence of limbs (Q71-Q73)*

**Z89.0** Acquired absence of thumb and other finger(s) (5th)
**Z89.01** Acquired absence of thumb (6th)
**Z89.011** Acquired absence of right thumb
**Z89.012** Acquired absence of left thumb
**Z89.019** Acquired absence of unspecified thumb
**Z89.02** Acquired absence of other finger(s) (6th)
EXCLUDES 2 *acquired absence of thumb (Z89.01-)*
**Z89.021** Acquired absence of right finger(s)
**Z89.022** Acquired absence of left finger(s)
**Z89.029** Acquired absence of unspecified finger(s)

**Z89.1** Acquired absence of hand and wrist (5th)
**Z89.11** Acquired absence of hand (6th)
**Z89.111** Acquired absence of right hand COM
**Z89.112** Acquired absence of left hand COM
**Z89.119** Acquired absence of unspecified hand COM
**Z89.12** Acquired absence of wrist (6th)
Disarticulation at wrist
**Z89.121** Acquired absence of right wrist COM
**Z89.122** Acquired absence of left wrist COM
**Z89.129** Acquired absence of unspecified wrist COM

**Z89.2** Acquired absence of upper limb above wrist (5th)
**Z89.20** Acquired absence of upper limb, unspecified level (6th)
**Z89.201** Acquired absence of right upper limb, unspecified level COM
**Z89.202** Acquired absence of left upper limb, unspecified level COM
**Z89.209** Acquired absence of unspecified upper limb, unspecified level COM
Acquired absence of arm NOS
**Z89.21** Acquired absence of upper limb below elbow (6th)
**Z89.211** Acquired absence of right upper limb below elbow COM
**Z89.212** Acquired absence of left upper limb below elbow COM
**Z89.219** Acquired absence of unspecified upper limb below elbow COM
**Z89.22** Acquired absence of upper limb above elbow (6th)
Disarticulation at elbow
**Z89.221** Acquired absence of right upper limb above elbow COM
**Z89.222** Acquired absence of left upper limb above elbow COM
**Z89.229** Acquired absence of unspecified upper limb above elbow COM
**Z89.23** Acquired absence of shoulder (6th)
Acquired absence of shoulder joint following explantation of shoulder joint prosthesis, with or without presence of antibiotic-impregnated cement spacer
**Z89.231** Acquired absence of right shoulder
**Z89.232** Acquired absence of left shoulder
**Z89.239** Acquired absence of unspecified shoulder

**Z89.4** Acquired absence of toe(s), foot, and ankle (5th)
**Z89.41** Acquired absence of great toe (6th)
**Z89.411** Acquired absence of right great toe ESR
**Z89.412** Acquired absence of left great toe ESR
**Z89.419** Acquired absence of unspecified great toe ESR
**Z89.42** Acquired absence of other toe(s) (6th)
EXCLUDES 2 *acquired absence of great toe (Z89.41-)*
**Z89.421** Acquired absence of other right toe(s) ESR
**Z89.422** Acquired absence of other left toe(s) ESR
**Z89.429** Acquired absence of other toe(s), unspecified side ESR
**Z89.43** Acquired absence of foot (6th)
**Z89.431** Acquired absence of right foot HCC ESR COM
**Z89.432** Acquired absence of left foot HCC ESR COM
**Z89.439** Acquired absence of unspecified foot HCC ESR COM
**Z89.44** Acquired absence of ankle (6th)
Disarticulation of ankle
**Z89.441** Acquired absence of right ankle HCC ESR COM
**Z89.442** Acquired absence of left ankle HCC ESR COM
**Z89.449** Acquired absence of unspecified ankle HCC ESR COM

**Z89.5** Acquired absence of leg below knee (5th)
**Z89.51** Acquired absence of leg below knee (6th)
**Z89.511** Acquired absence of right leg below knee HCC ESR COM
**Z89.512** Acquired absence of left leg below knee HCC ESR COM
**Z89.519** Acquired absence of unspecified leg below knee HCC ESR COM
**Z89.52** Acquired absence of knee (6th)
Acquired absence of knee joint following explantation of knee joint prosthesis, with or without presence of antibiotic-impregnated cement spacer
**Z89.521** Acquired absence of right knee
**Z89.522** Acquired absence of left knee
**Z89.529** Acquired absence of unspecified knee

**Z89.6** Acquired absence of leg above knee (5th)
**Z89.61** Acquired absence of leg above knee (6th)
Acquired absence of leg NOS
Disarticulation at knee
**Z89.611** Acquired absence of right leg above knee HCC ESR COM
**Z89.612** Acquired absence of left leg above knee HCC ESR COM
**Z89.619** Acquired absence of unspecified leg above knee HCC ESR COM
**Z89.62** Acquired absence of hip (6th)
Acquired absence of hip joint following explantation of hip joint prosthesis, with or without presence of antibiotic-impregnated cement spacer
Disarticulation at hip
**Z89.621** Acquired absence of right hip joint
**Z89.622** Acquired absence of left hip joint
**Z89.629** Acquired absence of unspecified hip joint

**Z89.9** Acquired absence of limb, unspecified COM

**Z90 Acquired absence of organs, not elsewhere classified** (4th)
INCLUDES postprocedural or post-traumatic loss of body part NEC
EXCLUDES 1 *congenital absence - see Alphabetical Index*
EXCLUDES 2 *postprocedural absence of endocrine glands (E89.-)*

**Z90.0** Acquired absence of part of head and neck (5th)
**Z90.01** Acquired absence of eye
**Z90.02** Acquired absence of larynx
**Z90.09** Acquired absence of other part of head and neck
Acquired absence of nose
EXCLUDES 2 *teeth (K08.1)*

**Z90.1** Acquired absence of breast and nipple (5th)
AHA: 2022,3Q,8
**Z90.10** Acquired absence of unspecified breast and nipple
**Z90.11** Acquired absence of right breast and nipple
**Z90.12** Acquired absence of left breast and nipple
**Z90.13** Acquired absence of bilateral breasts and nipples
**Z90.2** Acquired absence of lung [part of]
**Z90.3** Acquired absence of stomach [part of]

Chapter 21. Factors Influencing Health Status and Contact With Health Services
Z88.6–Z90.3

√5th **Z90.4 Acquired absence of other specified parts of digestive tract**

√6th **Z90.41 Acquired absence of pancreas**

Code also exocrine pancreatic insufficiency (K86.81)
Use additional code to identify any associated:
diabetes mellitus, postpancreatectomy (E13.-)
insulin use (Z79.4)
AHA: 2024,2Q,10

**Z90.410 Acquired total absence of pancreas**
Acquired absence of pancreas NOS

**Z90.411 Acquired partial absence of pancreas**

**Z90.49 Acquired absence of other specified parts of digestive tract**

**Z90.5 Acquired absence of kidney**

**Z90.6 Acquired absence of other parts of urinary tract**
Acquired absence of bladder

√5th **Z90.7 Acquired absence of genital organ(s)**

EXCLUDES 1 *personal history of sex reassignment ▶(Z87.890-)◀*

EXCLUDES 2 *female genital mutilation status (N90.81-)*

√6th **Z90.71 Acquired absence of cervix and uterus**

**Z90.710 Acquired absence of both cervix and uterus**
Acquired absence of uterus NOS
Status post total hysterectomy

**Z90.711 Acquired absence of uterus with remaining cervical stump**
Status post partial hysterectomy with remaining cervical stump

**Z90.712 Acquired absence of cervix with remaining uterus**

√6th **Z90.72 Acquired absence of ovaries**

**Z90.721 Acquired absence of ovaries, unilateral**

**Z90.722 Acquired absence of ovaries, bilateral**

**Z90.79 Acquired absence of other genital organ(s)**
AHA: 2023,2Q,5

√5th **Z90.8 Acquired absence of other organs**

**Z90.81 Acquired absence of spleen**

**Z90.89 Acquired absence of other organs**
AHA: 2023,3Q,13

√4th **Z91 Personal risk factors, not elsewhere classified**

EXCLUDES 2 *contact with and (suspected) exposures hazardous to health (Z77.-)*
*exposure to pollution and other problems related to physical environment (Z77.1-)*
*female genital mutilation status (N90.81-)*
*occupational exposure to risk factors (Z57.-)*
*personal history of physical injury and trauma (Z87.81, Z87.82-)*

√5th **Z91.0 Allergy status, other than to drugs and biological substances**

EXCLUDES 2 *allergy status to drugs, medicaments, and biological substances (Z88.-)*

√6th **Z91.01 Food allergy status**

EXCLUDES 2 *food additives allergy status (Z91.02)*

**Z91.010 Allergy to peanuts**

√7th **Z91.011 Allergy to milk products**

EXCLUDES 1 *lactose intolerance (E73.-)*

**Z91.0110 Allergy to milk products, unspecified** UPD

**Z91.0111 Allergy to milk products with tolerance to baked milk** UPD

EXCLUDES 1 *allergy to milk products with reactivity to baked milk (Z91.0112)*

**Z91.0112 Allergy to milk products with reactivity to baked milk** UPD

EXCLUDES 1 *allergy to milk products with tolerance to baked milk (Z91.0111)*

√7th **Z91.012 Allergy to eggs**

**Z91.0120 Allergy to eggs, unspecified** UPD

**Z91.0121 Allergy to eggs with tolerance to baked egg** UPD

EXCLUDES 1 *allergy to eggs with reactivity to baked egg (Z91.0122)*

**Z91.0122 Allergy to eggs with reactivity to baked egg** UPD

EXCLUDES 1 *allergy to egg with tolerance to baked egg (Z91.0121)*

**Z91.013 Allergy to seafood**
Allergy to octopus or squid ink
Allergy to shellfish

**Z91.014 Allergy to mammalian meats**
Allergy to beef
Allergy to lamb
Allergy to pork
Allergy to red meats
▶Alpha-gal syndrome (AGS)◀
AHA: 2021,4Q,33

**Z91.018 Allergy to other foods**
Allergy to nuts other than peanuts

**Z91.02 Food additives allergy status**

√6th **Z91.03 Insect allergy status**

**Z91.030 Bee allergy status**

**Z91.038 Other insect allergy status**

√6th **Z91.04 Nonmedicinal substance allergy status**

**Z91.040 Latex allergy status**
Latex sensitivity status

**Z91.041 Radiographic dye allergy status**
Allergy status to contrast media used for diagnostic X-ray procedure

**Z91.048 Other nonmedicinal substance allergy status**

**Z91.09 Other allergy status, other than to drugs and biological substances**

√5th **Z91.1 Patient's noncompliance with medical treatment and regimen**

Code also, if applicable, to identify underdosing of specific drug (T36-T50 with final character 6)

EXCLUDES 2 *caregiver noncompliance with patient's medical treatment and regimen (Z91.A-)*

AHA: 2022,4Q,49

√6th **Z91.11 Patient's noncompliance with dietary regimen**

Code also, if applicable, food insecurity (Z59.4-)

**Z91.110 Patient's noncompliance with dietary regimen due to financial hardship** UPD

**Z91.118 Patient's noncompliance with dietary regimen for other reason** UPD
Inability to comply with dietary regimen

**Z91.119 Patient's noncompliance with dietary regimen due to unspecified reason** UPD

√6th **Z91.12 Patient's intentional underdosing of medication regimen**

Code first underdosing of medication (T36-T50) with fifth or sixth character 6
AHA: 2018,4Q,72

**Z91.120 Patient's intentional underdosing of medication regimen due to financial hardship**

**Z91.128 Patient's intentional underdosing of medication regimen for other reason**

√6th **Z91.13 Patient's unintentional underdosing of medication regimen**

Code first underdosing of medication (T36-T50) with fifth or sixth character 6
AHA: 2018,4Q,72

**Z91.130 Patient's unintentional underdosing of medication regimen due to age-related debility**

**Z91.138 Patient's unintentional underdosing of medication regimen for other reason**

√6th **Z91.14 Patient's other noncompliance with medication regimen**
Patient's underdosing of medication NOS
Code first, if applicable, adverse effect of underdosing (T36-T5Ø)
**AHA:** 2023,1Q,7; 2022,1Q,36; 2018,4Q,72
**Z91.141 Patient's other noncompliance with medication regimen due to financial hardship** UPD
**Z91.148 Patient's other noncompliance with medication regimen for other reason** UPD

√6th **Z91.15 Patient's noncompliance with renal dialysis**
**AHA:** 2023,1Q,7
**Z91.151 Patient's noncompliance with renal dialysis due to financial hardship** Rx ESR UPD
**Z91.158 Patient's noncompliance with renal dialysis for other reason** Rx ESR UPD

√6th **Z91.19 Patient's noncompliance with other medical treatment and regimen**
Patient's nonadherence to medical treatment
**Z91.19Ø Patient's noncompliance with other medical treatment and regimen due to financial hardship** UPD
**Z91.198 Patient's noncompliance with other medical treatment and regimen for other reason** UPD
**AHA:** 2024,1Q,23
**Z91.199 Patient's noncompliance with other medical treatment and regimen due to unspecified reason** UPD

√5th **Z91.A Caregiver's noncompliance with patient's medical treatment and regimen**
**AHA:** 2023,4Q,48; 2022,4Q,49

√6th **Z91.A1 Caregiver's noncompliance with patient's dietary regimen**
Caregiver's inability to comply with patient's dietary regimen
Code also, if applicable, food insecurity (Z59.4-)
**Z91.A1Ø Caregiver's noncompliance with patient's dietary regimen due to financial hardship** UPD
**Z91.A18 Caregiver's noncompliance with patient's dietary regimen for other reason** UPD

√6th **Z91.A2 Caregiver's intentional underdosing of patient's medication regimen**
Code first underdosing of medication (T36-T5Ø) with fifth or sixth character 6
**Z91.A2Ø Caregiver's intentional underdosing of patient's medication regimen due to financial hardship** UPD
**Z91.A28 Caregiver's intentional underdosing of medication regimen for other reason** UPD

**Z91.A3 Caregiver's unintentional underdosing of patient's medication regimen** UPD
Code first underdosing of medication (T36-T5Ø) with fifth or sixth character 6

√6th **Z91.A4 Caregiver's other noncompliance with patient's medication regimen**
Caregiver's underdosing of patient's medication NOS
Caregiver's underdosing with patient's medication NOS
**Z91.A41 Caregiver's other noncompliance with patient's medication regimen due to financial hardship** UPD
**Z91.A48 Caregiver's other noncompliance with patient's medication regimen for other reason** UPD

√6th **Z91.A5 Caregiver's noncompliance with patient's renal dialysis**
**Z91.A51 Caregiver's noncompliance with patient's renal dialysis due to financial hardship** Rx ESR UPD
**Z91.A58 Caregiver's noncompliance with patient's renal dialysis for other reason** Rx ESR UPD

√6th **Z91.A9 Caregiver's noncompliance with patient's other medical treatment and regimen**
Caregiver's nonadherence to patient's medical treatment
**Z91.A91 Caregiver's noncompliance with patient's other medical treatment and regimen due to financial hardship** UPD
**Z91.A98 Caregiver's noncompliance with patient's other medical treatment and regimen for other reason** UPD

√5th **Z91.4 Personal history of psychological trauma, not elsewhere classified**
**AHA:** 2023,1Q,7

√6th **Z91.41 Personal history of adult abuse**
EXCLUDES 2 *personal history of abuse in childhood (Z62.81-)*
**Z91.41Ø Personal history of adult physical and sexual abuse** A
EXCLUDES 1 *current adult physical abuse (T74.11, T76.11)*
*current adult sexual abuse (T74.21, T76.11)*
**Z91.411 Personal history of adult psychological abuse** A
**Z91.412 Personal history of adult neglect** A
EXCLUDES 1 *current adult neglect (T74.Ø1, T76.Ø1)*
**Z91.413 Personal history of adult financial abuse** UPD
**Z91.414 Personal history of adult intimate partner abuse** UPD
**Z91.419 Personal history of unspecified adult abuse** A

**Z91.42 Personal history of forced labor or sexual exploitation**
**AHA:** 2018,4Q,32,35
**Z91.49 Other personal history of psychological trauma, not elsewhere classified**

√5th **Z91.5 Personal history of self-harm**
Code also mental health disorder, if known
**AHA:** 2021,4Q,33
**Z91.51 Personal history of suicidal behavior** UPD
Personal history of parasuicide
Personal history of self-poisoning
Personal history of suicide attempt
**Z91.52 Personal history of nonsuicidal self-harm** UPD
Personal history of nonsuicidal self-injury
Personal history of self-inflicted injury without suicidal intent
Personal history of self-mutilation

√5th **Z91.8 Other specified personal risk factors, not elsewhere classified**
**Z91.81 History of falling**
At risk for falling
**Z91.82 Personal history of military deployment** A
Individual (civilian or military) with past history of military war, peacekeeping and humanitarian deployment (current or past conflict)
Returned from military deployment
EXCLUDES 2 *personal history of military service (Z91.85)*
***Z91.83 Wandering in diseases classified elsewhere***
Code first underlying disorder such as:
Alzheimer's disease (G3Ø.-)
autism or pervasive developmental disorder (F84.-)
intellectual disabilities (F7Ø-F79)
unspecified dementia with behavioral disturbance (FØ3.9-, FØ3.A-, FØ3.B-, FØ3.C-)

√6th **Z91.84 Oral health risk factors**
**AHA:** 2017,4Q,29
**Z91.841 Risk for dental caries, low**
**Z91.842 Risk for dental caries, moderate**
**Z91.843 Risk for dental caries, high**
**Z91.849 Unspecified risk for dental caries**

**Z91.85 Personal history of military service** UPD
Personal history of serving in the armed forces
Personal history of veteran
EXCLUDES 2 *personal history of military deployment (Z91.82)*
**AHA:** 2023,4Q,48

Z91.89 **Other specified personal risk factors, not elsewhere classified**
Increased risk for social isolation
**AHA:** 2017,1Q,45

Z91.B **Personal risk factor of exposure to diethylstilbestrol**
DES daughter or son
Personal risk factor of exposure to DES
Personal risk factor of exposure to DES in utero
Second generation DES exposure
Code also, associated conditions, such as:
conditions classifiable to C5Ø.-
osteoporosis (M8Ø.-)
premature menopause (E28.31-)

√4th **Z92 Personal history of medical treatment**
EXCLUDES 2 *postprocedural states (Z98.-)*

Z92.Ø **Personal history of contraception**
EXCLUDES 1 *counseling or management of current contraceptive practices (Z3Ø.-)*
*long term (current) use of contraception (Z79.3)*
*presence of (intrauterine) contraceptive device (Z97.5)*

√5th Z92.2 **Personal history of drug therapy**
EXCLUDES 2 *long term (current) drug therapy (Z79.-)*

Z92.21 **Personal history of antineoplastic chemotherapy**

Z92.22 **Personal history of monoclonal drug therapy**
EXCLUDES 2 *personal history of immune checkpoint inhibitor therapy (Z92.26)*

Z92.23 **Personal history of estrogen therapy**

√6th Z92.24 **Personal history of steroid therapy**

Z92.24Ø **Personal history of inhaled steroid therapy**

Z92.241 **Personal history of systemic steroid therapy**
Personal history of steroid therapy NOS

Z92.25 **Personal history of immunosuppression therapy**
EXCLUDES 2 *personal history of steroid therapy (Z92.24)*

Z92.26 **Personal history of immune checkpoint inhibitor therapy**
Personal history of ICI drug therapy
**AHA:** 2024,4Q,34

Z92.29 **Personal history of other drug therapy**

Z92.3 **Personal history of irradiation**
Personal history of exposure to therapeutic radiation
EXCLUDES 1 *exposure to radiation in the physical environment (Z77.12)*
*occupational exposure to radiation (Z57.1)*

√5th Z92.8 **Personal history of other medical treatment**

Z92.81 **Personal history of extracorporeal membrane oxygenation (ECMO)**

Z92.82 **Status post administration of tPA (rtPA) in a different facility within the last 24 hours prior to admission to current facility** UPD
Code first condition requiring tPA administration, such as:
acute cerebral infarction (I63.-)
acute myocardial infarction (I21.-, I22.-)
**AHA:** 2013,4Q,124

Z92.83 **Personal history of failed moderate sedation**
Personal history of failed conscious sedation
EXCLUDES 2 *failed moderate sedation during procedure (T88.52)*

Z92.84 **Personal history of unintended awareness under general anesthesia**
EXCLUDES 2 *unintended awareness under general anesthesia during procedure (T88.53)*
**AHA:** 2016,4Q,72-73,77

√6th Z92.85 **Personal history of cellular therapy**
EXCLUDES 2 *personal history of immune checkpoint inhibitor therapy (Z92.26)*
**AHA:** 2021,4Q,33-34

Z92.85Ø **Personal history of Chimeric Antigen Receptor T-cell therapy** UPD
Personal history of CAR T-cell therapy

Z92.858 **Personal history of other cellular therapy** UPD

Z92.859 **Personal history of cellular therapy, unspecified** UPD

Z92.86 **Personal history of gene therapy** UPD
**AHA:** 2021,4Q,33-34

Z92.89 **Personal history of other medical treatment**
**AHA:** 2020,1Q,18

√4th **Z93 Artificial opening status**
EXCLUDES 1 *artificial openings requiring attention or management (Z43.-)*
*complications of external stoma (J95.Ø-, K94.-, N99.5-)*

Z93.Ø **Tracheostomy status** HCC ESR COM
**AHA:** 2013,4Q,129

Z93.1 **Gastrostomy status** HCC ESR COM

Z93.2 **Ileostomy status** HCC ESR COM
Ileal pouch status
Kock pouch status

Z93.3 **Colostomy status** HCC ESR COM

Z93.4 **Other artificial openings of gastrointestinal tract status** HCC ESR COM

√5th Z93.5 **Cystostomy status**

Z93.5Ø **Unspecified cystostomy status** HCC ESR COM

Z93.51 **Cutaneous-vesicostomy status** HCC ESR COM

Z93.52 **Appendico-vesicostomy status** HCC ESR COM

Z93.59 **Other cystostomy status** HCC ESR COM

Z93.6 **Other artificial openings of urinary tract status** HCC ESR COM
Nephrostomy status
Ureterostomy status
Urethrostomy status

Z93.8 **Other artificial opening status** HCC ESR COM

Z93.9 **Artificial opening status, unspecified** HCC ESR COM

√4th **Z94 Transplanted organ and tissue status**
INCLUDES organ or tissue replaced by heterogenous or homogenous transplant
EXCLUDES 1 *complications of transplanted organ or tissue - see Alphabetical Index*
EXCLUDES 2 *presence of vascular grafts (Z95.-)*

Z94.Ø **Kidney transplant status** Rx COM

Z94.1 **Heart transplant status** HCC Rx ESR COM
EXCLUDES 1 *artificial heart status (Z95.812)*
*heart-valve replacement status (Z95.2-Z95.4)*

Z94.2 **Lung transplant status** HCC Rx ESR COM

Z94.3 **Heart and lungs transplant status** HCC Rx ESR COM

Z94.4 **Liver transplant status** HCC Rx ESR COM

Z94.5 **Skin transplant status**
Autogenous skin transplant status

Z94.6 **Bone transplant status**

Z94.7 **Corneal transplant status**

√5th Z94.8 **Other transplanted organ and tissue status**

Z94.81 **Bone marrow transplant status** HCC Rx ESR COM

Z94.82 **Intestine transplant status** HCC Rx ESR COM

Z94.83 **Pancreas transplant status** HCC Rx ESR COM

Z94.84 **Stem cells transplant status** HCC Rx ESR COM

Z94.89 **Other transplanted organ and tissue status**

Z94.9 **Transplanted organ and tissue status, unspecified**

√4th **Z95 Presence of cardiac and vascular implants and grafts**
EXCLUDES 2 *complications of cardiac and vascular devices, implants and grafts (T82.-)*

Z95.Ø **Presence of cardiac pacemaker**
Presence of cardiac resynchronization therapy (CRT-P) pacemaker
EXCLUDES 1 *adjustment or management of cardiac device (Z45.Ø-)*
*adjustment or management of cardiac pacemaker (Z45.Ø)*
*presence of automatic (implantable) cardiac defibrillator with synchronous cardiac pacemaker (Z95.81Ø)*
**AHA:** 2022,2Q,14; 2019,1Q,33
**TIP:** Assign an additional code for the associated condition if that condition requires constant intervention from the device, as in cases of sick sinus syndrome. For conditions that do not require constant intervention from the device, as in cases of ventricular fibrillation, an additional code for the associated condition should be assigned only if the patient is experiencing the condition and the device is firing during the current admission.

Z95.1 **Presence of aortocoronary bypass graft**
Presence of coronary artery bypass graft

Z95.2 **Presence of prosthetic heart valve**
Presence of heart valve NOS

Z95.3 **Presence of xenogenic heart valve**

Z95.4 **Presence of other heart-valve replacement**



HCC CMS-HCC Rx Rx HCC ESR ESRD HCC COM Commercial HCC PDx Primary Dx Only N Newborn: 0 P Pediatric: 0-17 M Maternity: 9-64 A Adult: 15-124

Z95.5 Presence of coronary angioplasty implant and graft
EXCLUDES 1 *coronary angioplasty status without implant and graft (Z98.61)*

✓5th Z95.8 Presence of other cardiac and vascular implants and grafts

✓6th Z95.81 Presence of other cardiac implants and grafts

Z95.810 Presence of automatic (implantable) cardiac defibrillator
Presence of automatic (implantable) cardiac defibrillator with synchronous cardiac pacemaker
Presence of cardiac resynchronization therapy defibrillator (CRT-D)
Presence of cardioverter-defibrillator (ICD)
AHA: 2022,2Q,14; 2019,1Q,33
TIP: Assign an additional code for the associated condition if that condition requires constant intervention from the device, as in cases of sick sinus syndrome. For conditions that do not require constant intervention from the device, as in cases of ventricular fibrillation, an additional code for the associated condition should be assigned only if the patient is experiencing the condition and the device is firing during the current admission.

Z95.811 Presence of heart assist device HCC ESR COM

Z95.812 Presence of fully implantable artificial heart HCC ESR COM

Z95.818 Presence of other cardiac implants and grafts

✓6th Z95.82 Presence of other vascular implants and grafts

Z95.820 Peripheral vascular angioplasty status with implants and grafts
EXCLUDES 1 *peripheral vascular angioplasty without implant and graft (Z98.62)*

Z95.828 Presence of other vascular implants and grafts
Presence of intravascular prosthesis NEC
AHA: 2026,2Q,14

Z95.9 Presence of cardiac and vascular implant and graft, unspecified

✓4th Z96 Presence of other functional implants
EXCLUDES 2 *complications of internal prosthetic devices, implants and grafts (T82-T85)*
*fitting and adjustment of prosthetic and other devices (Z44-Z46)*

Z96.0 Presence of urogenital implants

Z96.1 Presence of intraocular lens
Presence of pseudophakia

✓5th Z96.2 Presence of otological and audiological implants

Z96.20 Presence of otological and audiological implant, unspecified

Z96.21 Cochlear implant status

Z96.22 Myringotomy tube(s) status

Z96.29 Presence of other otological and audiological implants
Presence of bone-conduction hearing device
Presence of eustachian tube stent
Stapes replacement

Z96.3 Presence of artificial larynx

✓5th Z96.4 Presence of endocrine implants

Z96.41 Presence of insulin pump (external) (internal)

Z96.49 Presence of other endocrine implants

Z96.5 Presence of tooth-root and mandibular implants

✓5th Z96.6 Presence of orthopedic joint implants
AHA: 2019,3Q,16

Z96.60 Presence of unspecified orthopedic joint implant

✓6th Z96.61 Presence of artificial shoulder joint

Z96.611 Presence of right artificial shoulder joint

Z96.612 Presence of left artificial shoulder joint

Z96.619 Presence of unspecified artificial shoulder joint

✓6th Z96.62 Presence of artificial elbow joint

Z96.621 Presence of right artificial elbow joint

Z96.622 Presence of left artificial elbow joint

Z96.629 Presence of unspecified artificial elbow joint

✓6th Z96.63 Presence of artificial wrist joint

Z96.631 Presence of right artificial wrist joint

Z96.632 Presence of left artificial wrist joint

Z96.639 Presence of unspecified artificial wrist joint

✓6th Z96.64 Presence of artificial hip joint
Hip-joint replacement (partial) (total)

Z96.641 Presence of right artificial hip joint

Z96.642 Presence of left artificial hip joint

Z96.643 Presence of artificial hip joint, bilateral

Z96.649 Presence of unspecified artificial hip joint

✓6th Z96.65 Presence of artificial knee joint

Z96.651 Presence of right artificial knee joint

Z96.652 Presence of left artificial knee joint

Z96.653 Presence of artificial knee joint, bilateral

Z96.659 Presence of unspecified artificial knee joint

✓6th Z96.66 Presence of artificial ankle joint

Z96.661 Presence of right artificial ankle joint

Z96.662 Presence of left artificial ankle joint

Z96.669 Presence of unspecified artificial ankle joint

✓6th Z96.69 Presence of other orthopedic joint implants

Z96.691 Finger-joint replacement of right hand

Z96.692 Finger-joint replacement of left hand

Z96.693 Finger-joint replacement, bilateral

Z96.698 Presence of other orthopedic joint implants

Z96.7 Presence of other bone and tendon implants
Presence of skull plate

✓5th Z96.8 Presence of other specified functional implants

Z96.81 Presence of artificial skin

Z96.82 Presence of neurostimulator
Presence of brain neurostimulator
Presence of gastric neurostimulator
Presence of peripheral nerve neurostimulator
Presence of sacral nerve neurostimulator
Presence of spinal cord neurostimulator
Presence of vagus nerve neurostimulator
AHA: 2019,4Q,19

Z96.89 Presence of other specified functional implants

Z96.9 Presence of functional implant, unspecified

✓4th Z97 Presence of other devices
EXCLUDES 1 *complications of internal prosthetic devices, implants and grafts (T82-T85)*
EXCLUDES 2 *fitting and adjustment of prosthetic and other devices (Z44-Z46)*
*presence of cerebrospinal fluid drainage device (Z98.2)*

Z97.0 Presence of artificial eye

✓5th Z97.1 Presence of artificial limb (complete) (partial)

Z97.10 Presence of artificial limb (complete) (partial), unspecified COM

Z97.11 Presence of artificial right arm (complete) (partial) COM

Z97.12 Presence of artificial left arm (complete) (partial) COM

Z97.13 Presence of artificial right leg (complete) (partial) HCC COM

Z97.14 Presence of artificial left leg (complete) (partial) HCC COM

Z97.15 Presence of artificial arms, bilateral (complete) (partial) COM

Z97.16 Presence of artificial legs, bilateral (complete) (partial) HCC COM

Z97.2 Presence of dental prosthetic device (complete) (partial)
Presence of dentures (complete) (partial)

Z97.3 Presence of spectacles and contact lenses

Z97.4 Presence of external hearing-aid

Z97.5 Presence of (intrauterine) contraceptive device
EXCLUDES 1 *checking, reinsertion or removal of implantable subdermal contraceptive (Z30.46)*
*checking, reinsertion or removal of intrauterine contraceptive device (Z30.43-)*

Z97.8 Presence of other specified devices

**Z98 Other postprocedural states**
EXCLUDES 2 *aftercare (Z43-Z49, Z51)*
*follow-up medical care (ZØ8-ZØ9)*
*Fontan related circulation (I27.84-)*
*postprocedural complication - see Alphabetical Index*

**Z98.Ø Intestinal bypass and anastomosis status**
EXCLUDES 2 *bariatric surgery status (Z98.84)*
*gastric bypass status (Z98.84)*
*obesity surgery status (Z98.84)*

**Z98.1 Arthrodesis status**
AHA: 2024,1Q,23

**Z98.2 Presence of cerebrospinal fluid drainage device**
Presence of CSF shunt

**Z98.3 Post therapeutic collapse of lung status** UPD
Code first underlying disease

**Z98.4 Cataract extraction status**
Use additional code to identify intraocular lens implant status (Z96.1)
EXCLUDES 1 *aphakia (H27.Ø)*

**Z98.41 Cataract extraction status, right eye**
**Z98.42 Cataract extraction status, left eye**
**Z98.49 Cataract extraction status, unspecified eye**

**Z98.5 Sterilization status**
EXCLUDES 1 *female infertility (N97.-)*
*male infertility (N46.-)*

**Z98.51 Tubal ligation status**
**Z98.52 Vasectomy status** A

**Z98.6 Angioplasty status**
**Z98.61 Coronary angioplasty status**
EXCLUDES 1 *coronary angioplasty status with implant and graft (Z95.5)*

**Z98.62 Peripheral vascular angioplasty status**
EXCLUDES 1 *peripheral vascular angioplasty status with implant and graft (Z95.82Ø)*

**Z98.8 Other specified postprocedural states**
**Z98.81 Dental procedure status**
**Z98.81Ø Dental sealant status**
**Z98.811 Dental restoration status**
Dental crown status
Dental fillings status
**Z98.818 Other dental procedure status**

**Z98.82 Breast implant status**
EXCLUDES 1 *breast implant removal status (Z98.86)*
AHA: 2022,3Q,8

**Z98.83 Filtering (vitreous) bleb after glaucoma surgery status**
EXCLUDES 1 *inflammation (infection) of postprocedural bleb (H59.4-)*
AHA: 2020,3Q,29

**Z98.84 Bariatric surgery status**
Gastric banding status
Gastric bypass status for obesity
Obesity surgery status
EXCLUDES 1 *bariatric surgery status complicating pregnancy, childbirth, or the puerperium (O99.84)*
EXCLUDES 2 *intestinal bypass and anastomosis status (Z98.Ø)*
AHA: 2025,4Q,7-8; 2020,1Q,12

**Z98.85 Transplanted organ removal status**
Transplanted organ previously removed due to complication, failure, rejection or infection
EXCLUDES 1 *encounter for removal of transplanted organ - code to complication of transplanted organ (T86.-)*

**Z98.86 Personal history of breast implant removal**
**Z98.87 Personal history of in utero procedure**
**Z98.87Ø Personal history of in utero procedure during pregnancy**
EXCLUDES 2 *complications from in utero procedure for current pregnancy (O35.7)*
*supervision of current pregnancy with history of in utero procedure during previous pregnancy (OØ9.82-)*

**Z98.871 Personal history of in utero procedure while a fetus**

**Z98.89 Other specified postprocedural states**
**Z98.89Ø Other specified postprocedural states**
Personal history of surgery, not elsewhere classified
AHA: 2023,3Q,13
**Z98.891 History of uterine scar from previous surgery**
EXCLUDES 1 *maternal care due to uterine scar from previous surgery (O34.2-)*
AHA: 2016,4Q,51-52,76

**Z99 Dependence on enabling machines and devices, not elsewhere classified**
AHA: 2020,1Q,11

**Z99.Ø Dependence on aspirator**
**Z99.1 Dependence on respirator**
Dependence on ventilator
**Z99.11 Dependence on respirator [ventilator] status** HCC ESR COM
Ventilator status
AHA: 2015,1Q,21
**Z99.12 Encounter for respirator [ventilator] dependence during power failure** HCC ESR COM PDx
EXCLUDES 1 *mechanical complication of respirator [ventilator] (J95.85Ø)*

**Z99.2 Dependence on renal dialysis** Rx ESR
Hemodialysis status
Peritoneal dialysis status
Presence of arteriovenous shunt for dialysis
Renal dialysis status NOS
EXCLUDES 1 *encounter for fitting and adjustment of dialysis catheter (Z49.Ø-)*
EXCLUDES 2 *noncompliance with renal dialysis (Z91.15-)*
AHA: 2026,2Q,14; 2022,3Q,15; 2016,1Q,12; 2013,4Q,125

**Z99.3 Dependence on wheelchair**
Wheelchair confinement status
Code first cause of dependence, such as:
muscular dystrophy (G71.Ø-)
obesity (E66.-)

**Z99.8 Dependence on other enabling machines and devices**
**Z99.81 Dependence on supplemental oxygen**
Dependence on long-term oxygen
AHA: 2013,4Q,129
**Z99.89 Dependence on other enabling machines and devices**
Dependence on machine or device NOS
AHA: 2020,1Q,11

# Chapter 22. Codes for Special Purposes (UØØ–U85)

## Chapter-specific Guidelines

UØ7.Ø Vaping-related disorder (see Section I.C.10.e., Vaping-related disorders)

UØ7.1 COVID-19 (see Section I.C.1.g.1., COVID-19 infection)

UØ9.9 Post COVID-19 condition, unspecified (see Section I.C.1.g.1.m.)

# Chapter 22. Codes for Special Purposes (U00-U85)

This chapter contains the following blocks:

U00-U49 Provisional assignment of new diseases of uncertain etiology or emergency use

## Provisional assignment of new diseases of uncertain etiology or emergency use (U00-U49)

✓4th **U07 Emergency use of U07**

**U07.0 Vaping-related disorder**

Dabbing related lung damage
Dabbing related lung injury
E-cigarette, or vaping, product use associated lung injury [EVALI]
Electronic cigarette related lung damage
Electronic cigarette related lung injury
Use additional code, to identify manifestations, such as:
abdominal pain (R10.84)
acute respiratory distress syndrome (J80)
diarrhea (R19.7)
drug-induced interstitial lung disorder (J70.4)
lipoid pneumonia (J69.1)
weight loss (R63.4)

**AHA:** 2025,3Q,11

**DEF:** Respiratory illness or injury caused by harmful aerosolized substances and chemicals produced by electronic cigarettes, vapes, e-pipes, and other battery-powered vaping devices. Symptoms may include shortness of breath and fever, while some patients experience severe, sometimes fatal, lung damage. ***Synonym(s):*** *e-cigarette and vaping product use-associated lung injury, EVALI.*

**U07.1 COVID-19**

Use additional code to identify pneumonia or other manifestations, such as:
Use additional code, if applicable, for associated conditions such as:
COVID-19 associated coagulopathy (D68.8)
disseminated intravascular coagulation (D65)
hypercoagulable states (D68.69)
pneumonia due to COVID-19 (J12.82)
thrombophilia (D68.69)

EXCLUDES 2 *coronavirus as the cause of diseases classified elsewhere (B97.2-)*
*pneumonia due to SARS-associated coronavirus (J12.81)*

**AHA:** 2025,1Q,3,34; 2022,2Q,28; 2021,4Q,101,107-108; 2021,1Q,25-30,31-49; 2020,4Q,14,99; 2020,3Q,9-16; 2020,2Q,3-13

**DEF:** First diagnosed in December 2019 in China, coronavirus disease 2019 (COVID-19) is a respiratory infection caused by a newly identified (novel) virus not previously seen in humans, known as severe acute respiratory syndrome coronavirus 2 (SARS-CoV-2). Symptoms of this lower respiratory illness include fever, dry cough, and tiredness that may progress to include difficulty breathing. Older patients and those with high blood pressure, heart problems, and diabetes are more likely to develop serious symptoms of the illness. ***Synonym(s):*** *SARS-CoV-2, coronavirus disease 2019.*

**TIP:** Code U07.1 should not be assigned based solely on a positive COVID-19 blood test. A confirmed diagnosis of COVID-19 must be documented by the provider. If the diagnosis is unclear, a query should be submitted to the provider for clarification.

✓4th **U09 Post COVID-19 condition**

**U09.9 Post COVID-19 condition, unspecified**

NOTE This code enables establishment of a link with COVID-19.

This code is not to be used in cases that are still presenting with active COVID-19. However, an exception is made in cases of re-infection with COVID-19, occurring with a condition related to prior COVID-19.

Post-acute sequela of COVID-19
Code first the specific condition related to COVID-19 if known, such as:
chronic respiratory failure (J96.1-)
loss of smell (R43.8)
loss of taste (R43.8)
multisystem inflammatory syndrome (M35.81)
pulmonary embolism (I26.-)
pulmonary fibrosis (J84.10)

**AHA:** 2021,4Q,31-32,102-106

# Appendixes

## Appendix A: Valid 3-character ICD-10-CM Codes

| | |
|---|---|
| A09 | Infectious gastroenteritis and colitis, unspecified |
| A33 | Tetanus neonatorum |
| A34 | Obstetrical tetanus |
| A35 | Other tetanus |
| A46 | Erysipelas |
| A55 | Chlamydial lymphogranuloma (venereum) |
| A57 | Chancroid |
| A58 | Granuloma inguinale |
| A64 | Unspecified sexually transmitted disease |
| A65 | Nonvenereal syphilis |
| A70 | Chlamydia psittaci infections |
| A78 | Q fever |
| A86 | Unspecified viral encephalitis |
| A89 | Unspecified viral infection of central nervous system |
| A90 | Dengue fever [classical dengue] |
| A91 | Dengue hemorrhagic fever |
| A94 | Unspecified arthropod-borne viral fever |
| A99 | Unspecified viral hemorrhagic fever |
| B03 | Smallpox |
| B04 | Monkeypox |
| B09 | Unspecified viral infection characterized by skin and mucous membrane lesions |
| B20 | Human immunodeficiency virus [HIV] disease |
| B49 | Unspecified mycosis |
| B54 | Unspecified malaria |
| B59 | Pneumocystosis |
| B64 | Unspecified protozoal disease |
| B72 | Dracunculiasis |
| B75 | Trichinellosis |
| B79 | Trichuriasis |
| B80 | Enterobiasis |
| B86 | Scabies |
| B89 | Unspecified parasitic disease |
| B91 | Sequelae of poliomyelitis |
| B92 | Sequelae of leprosy |
| C01 | Malignant neoplasm of base of tongue |
| C07 | Malignant neoplasm of parotid gland |
| C12 | Malignant neoplasm of pyriform sinus |
| C19 | Malignant neoplasm of rectosigmoid junction |
| C20 | Malignant neoplasm of rectum |
| C23 | Malignant neoplasm of gallbladder |
| C33 | Malignant neoplasm of trachea |
| C37 | Malignant neoplasm of thymus |
| C52 | Malignant neoplasm of vagina |
| C55 | Malignant neoplasm of uterus, part unspecified |
| C58 | Malignant neoplasm of placenta |
| C61 | Malignant neoplasm of prostate |
| C73 | Malignant neoplasm of thyroid gland |
| D34 | Benign neoplasm of thyroid gland |
| D45 | Polycythemia vera |
| D62 | Acute posthemorrhagic anemia |
| D65 | Disseminated intravascular coagulation [defibrination syndrome] |
| D66 | Hereditary factor VIII deficiency |
| D67 | Hereditary factor IX deficiency |
| D77 | Other disorders of blood and blood-forming organs in diseases classified elsewhere |
| E02 | Subclinical iodine-deficiency hypothyroidism |
| E15 | Nondiabetic hypoglycemic coma |
| E35 | Disorders of endocrine glands in diseases classified elsewhere |
| E40 | Kwashiorkor |
| E41 | Nutritional marasmus |
| E42 | Marasmic kwashiorkor |
| E43 | Unspecified severe protein-calorie malnutrition |
| E45 | Retarded development following protein-calorie malnutrition |
| E46 | Unspecified protein-calorie malnutrition |
| E52 | Niacin deficiency [pellagra] |
| E54 | Ascorbic acid deficiency |
| E58 | Dietary calcium deficiency |
| E59 | Dietary selenium deficiency |
| E60 | Dietary zinc deficiency |
| E65 | Localized adiposity |
| E68 | Sequelae of hyperalimentation |
| F04 | Amnestic disorder due to known physiological condition |
| F05 | Delirium due to known physiological condition |
| F09 | Unspecified mental disorder due to known physiological condition |
| F21 | Schizotypal disorder |
| F22 | Delusional disorders |
| F23 | Brief psychotic disorder |
| F24 | Shared psychotic disorder |
| F28 | Other psychotic disorder not due to a substance or known physiological condition |
| F29 | Unspecified psychosis not due to a substance or known physiological condition |
| F39 | Unspecified mood [affective] disorder |
| F42 | Obsessive-compulsive disorder |
| F54 | Psychological and behavioral factors associated with disorders or diseases classified elsewhere |
| F59 | Unspecified behavioral syndromes associated with physiological disturbances and physical factors |
| F66 | Other sexual disorders |
| F69 | Unspecified disorder of adult personality and behavior |
| F70 | Mild intellectual disabilities |
| F71 | Moderate intellectual disabilities |
| F72 | Severe intellectual disabilities |
| F73 | Profound intellectual disabilities |
| F79 | Unspecified intellectual disabilities |
| F82 | Specific developmental disorder of motor function |
| F88 | Other disorders of psychological development |
| F89 | Unspecified disorder of psychological development |
| F99 | Mental disorder, not otherwise specified |
| G01 | Meningitis in bacterial diseases classified elsewhere |
| G02 | Meningitis in other infectious and parasitic diseases classified elsewhere |
| G07 | Intracranial and intraspinal abscess and granuloma in diseases classified elsewhere |
| G08 | Intracranial and intraspinal phlebitis and thrombophlebitis |
| G09 | Sequelae of inflammatory diseases of central nervous system |
| G10 | Huntington's disease |
| G14 | Postpolio syndrome |
| G26 | Extrapyramidal and movement disorders in diseases classified elsewhere |
| G53 | Cranial nerve disorders in diseases classified elsewhere |
| G55 | Nerve root and plexus compressions in diseases classified elsewhere |
| G59 | Mononeuropathy in diseases classified elsewhere |
| G63 | Polyneuropathy in diseases classified elsewhere |
| G64 | Other disorders of peripheral nervous system |
| G94 | Other disorders of brain in diseases classified elsewhere |
| H22 | Disorders of iris and ciliary body in diseases classified elsewhere |
| H28 | Cataract in diseases classified elsewhere |
| H32 | Chorioretinal disorders in diseases classified elsewhere |
| H42 | Glaucoma in diseases classified elsewhere |
| I00 | Rheumatic fever without heart involvement |
| I10 | Essential (primary) hypertension |
| I32 | Pericarditis in diseases classified elsewhere |
| I38 | Endocarditis, valve unspecified |
| I39 | Endocarditis and heart valve disorders in diseases classified elsewhere |
| I41 | Myocarditis in diseases classified elsewhere |
| I43 | Cardiomyopathy in diseases classified elsewhere |
| I52 | Other heart disorders in diseases classified elsewhere |
| I5A | Non-ischemic myocardial injury (non-traumatic) |
| I76 | Septic arterial embolism |
| I81 | Portal vein thrombosis |
| I96 | Gangrene, not elsewhere classified |
| J00 | Acute nasopharyngitis (common cold) |
| J13 | Pneumonia due to Streptococcus pneumoniae |
| J14 | Pneumonia due to Hemophilus influenzae |

| | |
|---|---|
| J17 | Pneumonia in diseases classified elsewhere |
| J22 | Unspecified acute lower respiratory infection |
| J36 | Peritonsillar abscess |
| J40 | Bronchitis, not specified as acute or chronic |
| J42 | Unspecified chronic bronchitis |
| J4B | Pulmonary mycetoma |
| J60 | Coalworker's pneumoconiosis |
| J61 | Pneumoconiosis due to asbestos and other mineral fibers |
| J64 | Unspecified pneumoconiosis |
| J65 | Pneumoconiosis associated with tuberculosis |
| J80 | Acute respiratory distress syndrome |
| J90 | Pleural effusion, not elsewhere classified |
| J99 | Respiratory disorders in diseases classified elsewhere |
| K23 | Disorders of esophagus in diseases classified elsewhere |
| K30 | Functional dyspepsia |
| K36 | Other appendicitis |
| K37 | Unspecified appendicitis |
| K67 | Disorders of peritoneum in infectious diseases classified elsewhere |
| K77 | Liver disorders in diseases classified elsewhere |
| K87 | Disorders of gallbladder, biliary tract and pancreas in diseases classified elsewhere |
| L00 | Staphylococcal scalded skin syndrome |
| L14 | Bullous disorders in diseases classified elsewhere |
| L22 | Diaper dermatitis |
| L26 | Exfoliative dermatitis |
| L42 | Pityriasis rosea |
| L45 | Papulosquamous disorders in diseases classified elsewhere |
| L52 | Erythema nodosum |
| L54 | Erythema in diseases classified elsewhere |
| L62 | Nail disorders in diseases classified elsewhere |
| L80 | Vitiligo |
| L83 | Acanthosis nigricans |
| L84 | Corns and callosities |
| L86 | Keratoderma in diseases classified elsewhere |
| L88 | Pyoderma gangrenosum |
| L99 | Other disorders of skin and subcutaneous tissue in diseases classified elsewhere |
| N08 | Glomerular disorders in diseases classified elsewhere |
| N10 | Acute tubulo-interstitial nephritis |
| N12 | Tubulo-interstitial nephritis, not specified as acute or chronic |
| N16 | Renal tubulo-interstitial disorders in diseases classified elsewhere |
| N19 | Unspecified kidney failure |
| N22 | Calculus of urinary tract in diseases classified elsewhere |
| N23 | Unspecified renal colic |
| N29 | Other disorders of kidney and ureter in diseases classified elsewhere |
| N33 | Bladder disorders in diseases classified elsewhere |
| N37 | Urethral disorders in diseases classified elsewhere |
| N51 | Disorders of male genital organs in diseases classified elsewhere |
| N61 | Inflammatory disorders of breast |
| N62 | Hypertrophy of breast |
| N72 | Inflammatory disease of cervix uteri |
| N74 | Female pelvic inflammatory disorders in diseases classified elsewhere |
| N86 | Erosion and ectropion of cervix uteri |
| N96 | Recurrent pregnancy loss |
| O68 | Labor and delivery complicated by abnormality of fetal acid-base balance |
| O76 | Abnormality in fetal heart rate and rhythm complicating labor and delivery |
| O80 | Encounter for full-term uncomplicated delivery |
| O82 | Encounter for cesarean delivery without indication |
| O85 | Puerperal sepsis |
| O94 | Sequelae of complication of pregnancy, childbirth, and the puerperium |
| P53 | Hemorrhagic disease of newborn |
| P60 | Disseminated intravascular coagulation of newborn |
| P84 | Other problems with newborn |
| P90 | Convulsions of newborn |
| P95 | Stillbirth |
| Q02 | Microcephaly |
| R12 | Heartburn |
| R17 | Unspecified jaundice |
| R21 | Rash and other nonspecific skin eruption |
| R32 | Unspecified urinary incontinence |
| R34 | Anuria and oliguria |
| R37 | Sexual dysfunction, unspecified |
| R42 | Dizziness and giddiness |
| R52 | Pain, unspecified |
| R54 | Age-related physical debility |
| R55 | Syncope and collapse |
| R58 | Hemorrhage, not elsewhere classified |
| R61 | Generalized hyperhidrosis |
| R64 | Cachexia |
| R69 | Illness, unspecified |
| R75 | Inconclusive laboratory evidence of human immunodeficiency virus [HIV] |
| R81 | Glycosuria |
| R99 | Ill-defined and unknown cause of mortality |
| Y09 | Assault by unspecified means |
| Y66 | Nonadministration of surgical and medical care |
| Y69 | Unspecified misadventure during surgical and medical care |
| Y95 | Nosocomial condition |
| Z08 | Encounter for follow-up examination after completed treatment for malignant neoplasm |
| Z09 | Encounter for follow-up examination after completed treatment for conditions other than malignant neoplasm |
| Z21 | Asymptomatic human immunodeficiency virus [HIV] infection status |
| Z23 | Encounter for immunization |
| Z66 | Do not resuscitate |

# Appendix B: Pharmacology List 2027

This section enables the coder to quickly review drugs, drug actions, and indications that are often associated with overlooked or undocumented diagnoses. The coder should review the patient's medication record and know what condition the physician is treating with the prescribed medication based on documentation in the medical record. When documentation is lacking, the coder can reference this section to locate the drug, determine the drug action, confirm drug indications, and when necessary query the physician. When applicable, some of the drugs provided in this resource have also been mapped to their appropriate Z code for long-term drug use.

| Drug | Z Code | Drug Action/Classification | Indications |
|---|---|---|---|
| 5-fluorouracil (5-FU) [fluorouracil] | Z79.631 | Antimetabolite agent | Skin, colorectal, breast, stomach, and pancreas cancer |
| 6-mercaptopurine (6-MP) [mercaptopurine] | Z79.631 | Antimetabolite agent | Acute lymphoblastic leukemia |
| Abilify [aripiprazole] | | Antipsychotic | Depression; bipolar I disorder; schizophrenia; autism symptoms |
| Acarbose [acarbose] | Z79.84 | Oral hypoglycemic | Diabetes mellitus |
| Acetaminophen with codeine [acetaminophen/codeine phosphate] | Z79.891 | Analgesic, narcotic | Moderate to severe pain |
| Aclasta [zoledronic acid] | Z79.83 | Bisphosphonate | Osteoporosis in postmenopausal women; Paget's disease |
| Actemra [tocilizumab] | Z79.620 | Immunosuppressive biologic/monoclonal antibody | Rheumatoid arthritis; systemic sclerosis-associated interstitial lung disease; giant cell arteritis; polyarticular or systemic juvenile idiopathic arthritis; cytokine release syndrome; COVID-19 for certain pediatric and adult populations |
| Actimmune [interferon gamma-1b] | Z79.69 | Other immunosuppressant/ immunomodulator | Chronic granulomatous disease; malignant osteopetrosis |
| Activella [estradiol/norethindrone acetate] | Z79.890 | Estrogen therapy | Menopause symptoms; vaginal and vulvar atrophy; osteoporosis prevention |
| Actonel [risedronate sodium] | Z79.83 | Bisphosphonate | Osteoporosis; Paget's disease |
| Actoplus Met [metformin hydrochloride/ pioglitazone hydrochloride] | Z79.84 | Oral hypoglycemic | Diabetes mellitus |
| Actos [pioglitazone hydrochloride] | Z79.84 | Oral hypoglycemic | Diabetes mellitus |
| Aczone [dapsone] | | Acne agent, topical | Acne vulgaris |
| Adderall XR [amphetamine aspartate and sulfate/dextroamphetamine saccharate and sulfate] | | CNS stimulant | Attention deficit hyperactivity disorder (ADHD) |
| Adlarity [donepezil hydrochloride] | | Acetylcholinesterase/cholinesterase inhibitors | Dementia due to Alzheimer's |
| Admelog [insulin lispro] | Z79.4 | Insulin | Diabetes mellitus |
| Advair [fluticasone propionate/salmeterol xinafoate] | Z79.51 | Corticosteroid – inhaled/antiasthmatic | Prophylaxis and treatment of asthma and COPD |
| Advil [ibuprofen] | Z79.1 | Nonsteroidal anti-inflammatory drug (NSAID) | Pain or fever relief |
| Afrezza [human insulin recombinant] | | Insulin – inhaled | Diabetes mellitus |
| Agamree [vamorolone] | Z79.52 | Corticosteroid | Duchenne muscular dystrophy |
| Aggrastat [tirofiban hydrochloride] | Z79.02 | Antiplatelet | Unstable angina; heart attacks |
| Aimovig [erenumab-aooe] | Z79.620 | Immunosuppressive biologic/monoclonal antibody | Migraine headache prevention |
| AirDuo RespiClick [fluticasone propionate/ salmeterol xinafoate] | Z79.51 | Corticosteroid – inhaled/antiasthmatic | Asthma |
| Aklief [trifarotene] | | Acne agent, topical | Acne vulgaris |
| Aldactone [spironolactone] | | Cardiovascular agent; antihypertensive agent; diuretic; electrolytic and renal agent | Severe heart failure; ascites associated with cirrhosis; hypokalemia; hypertension; fluid retention in heart failure, cirrhosis, and nephrotic syndrome |
| Aleve [naproxen sodium] | Z79.1 | Nonsteroidal anti-inflammatory drug (NSAID) | Reduction of temporary aches and pains |
| Allegra allergy [fexofenadine hydrochloride] | | Antihistamine | Seasonal allergic rhinitis |
| Allopurinol [allopurinol] | | Antigout | Gouty arthritis; renal calculus; hyperuricemia; hyperuricemia secondary to leukemia; hyperuricemia secondary to lymphoma |
| Alora [estradiol] | Z79.890 | Estrogen therapy | Menopause symptoms |
| Alphagan P [brimonidine tartrate] | | Antiglaucoma agent (ophthalmic); antihypertensive, ocular | Open angle glaucoma or another condition in which pressure in the eye is too high (ocular hypertension) |
| Alprazolam [alprazolam] | | Antianxiety; sedative/hypnotic | Anxiety and panic disorders |
| Altabax [retapamulin] | Z79.2 | Antibiotic, topical | Skin infections |
| Altace [ramipril] | | ACE inhibitor | Congestive heart failure; hypertension |
| Alvesco [ciclesonide] | Z79.51 | Corticosteroid – inhaled; antiasthmatic | Prophylaxis and treatment of asthma |
| Amaryl [glimepiride] | Z79.84 | Oral hypoglycemic | Diabetes mellitus |
| Ambien [zolpidem tartrate] | | CNS depressant; anxiolytic/sedative/hypnotic | Insomnia |
| Amikacin [amikacin sulfate] | Z79.2 | Antibiotic | Gram-negative bacterial infections such as Pseudomonas, Escherichia coli (E. coli), Proteus, Klebsiella-Enterobacter-Serratia |

| Drug | Z Code | Drug Action/Classification | Indications |
|---|---|---|---|
| Amitriptyline HCl [amitriptyline hydrochloride] | | Antidepressant | Depression |
| Amoxicillin [amoxicillin] | Z79.2 | Antibiotic | Treatment of infections with a broad spectrum of bactericidal activity against many gram-positive and gram-negative microorganisms; otitis media, gonorrhea, skin, respiratory, gastrointestinal, and genitourinary infections |
| Ampicillin [ampicillin sodium] | Z79.2 | Antibiotic | Bacterial infections |
| Ampyra [dalfampridine] | | Potassium channel blocker | Improvement in walking in patients with multiple sclerosis |
| Amrix [cyclobenzaprine hydrochloride] | | | Adjunct to rest and physical therapy for muscle spasms |
| Anaprox DS [naproxen sodium] | Z79.1 | Nonsteroidal anti-inflammatory drug (NSAID) | Pain, inflammation or fever relief |
| Anastrozole [anastrozole] | Z79.811 | Aromatase inhibitor | Postmenopausal breast cancer |
| Androderm [testosterone] | Z79.890 | Testosterone therapy – topical | Primary hypogonadism; hypogonadotropic hypogonadism |
| AndroGel [testosterone] | Z79.890 | Testosterone therapy – topical | Primary hypogonadism; hypogonadotropic hypogonadism |
| Angeliq [drospirenone/estradiol] | Z79.890 | Estrogen therapy | Menopause symptoms |
| Angiomax [bivalirudin] | Z79.02 | Antithrombotic | Prevention of blood clots |
| Antineoplastic/chemotherapy | | Antineoplastic | Cancer |
| Aphexda [motixafortide] | | Immunostimulant | Multiple myeloma |
| Apidra [insulin glulisine recombinant] | Z79.4 | Insulin | Diabetes mellitus |
| Aranelle [ethinyl estradiol/norethindrone] | Z79.3 | Contraceptive | Prevention of pregnancy; acne |
| Aranesp [darbepoetin alfa] | | Erythropoiesis-stimulating agent (ESA) | Treatment of anemia in disorders such as CKD and neoplasms |
| Aredia [pamidronate disodium] | Z79.83 | Bisphosphonate | Osteoporosis |
| Argatroban [argatroban] | Z79.02 | Antithrombotic | Prophylaxis and treatment of venous thrombosis in thrombocytopenia patients |
| Aricept [donepezil hydrochloride] | | Acetylcholinesterase/cholinesterase inhibitors | Dementia due to Alzheimer's |
| Arimidex [anastrozole] | Z79.811 | Aromatase inhibitor; antineoplastic | Postmenopausal breast cancer |
| Arixtra [fondaparinux sodium] | Z79.01 | Anticoagulant | Venous thrombosis and pulmonary embolism |
| Arnuity Ellipta [fluticasone furoate] | Z79.51 | Corticosteroid – inhaled; antiasthmatic | Prophylaxis and treatment of asthma |
| Aromasin [exemestane] | Z79.811 | Aromatase inhibitor | Postmenopausal breast cancer |
| Arthrotec [diclofenac sodium/misoprostol] | Z79.1 | Nonsteroidal anti-inflammatory drug (NSAID)-prostaglandin combo | Treatment of patients with osteoarthritis or rheumatoid arthritis who may develop stomach ulcers from taking nonsteroidal anti-inflammatory drugs (NSAIDs) alone |
| Asmanex [mometasone furoate] | Z79.51 | Corticosteroid – inhaled; antiasthmatic | Prophylaxis and treatment of asthma |
| Astagraf XL [tacrolimus] | Z79.621 | Calcineurin inhibitor; immunosuppressant | Prophylaxis of organ transplant rejection |
| Atelvia [risedronate sodium] | Z79.83 | Bisphosphonate | Osteoporosis |
| Atenolol [atenolol] | | Beta blocker | Angina pectoris; hypertension; acute myocardial infarction |
| Ativan [lorazepam] | | Antianxiety; sedative/hypnotic | Anxiety disorder associated with depressive symptoms; controls tension, agitation, irritability, and insomnia |
| Atripla [efavirenz/emtricitabine/tenofovir disoproxil fumarate] | | Antiretroviral | HIV |
| Atrovent HFA [ipratropium bromide] | | Antiasthmatic/bronchodilator | Chronic bronchitis, emphysema; bronchial asthma |
| Augmentin [amoxicillin/clavulanate potassium] | Z79.2 | Antibiotic | Bacterial infections of the middle ear, lower respiratory, sinus, skin and skin structures; urinary tract infections |
| Augtyro [repotrectinib] | | Kinase inhibitor | ROS1-Positive non-small cell lung cancer |
| Avapro [irbesartan] | | Antihypertensive | Hypertension |
| Avelox [moxifloxacin hydrochloride] | Z79.2 | Antibiotic | Bacterial infections of the skin, sinuses, lungs, or stomach; plague |
| Aviane-28 [ethinyl estradiol/levonorgestrel] | Z79.3 | Contraceptive | Prevention of pregnancy |
| Avonex [interferon beta-1a] | Z79.69 | Other immunosuppressant/ immunomodulator | Treatment of relapsing multiple sclerosis |
| Axid AR [nizatidine] | | Histamine H2-receptor antagonist | Acid/peptic disorder; gastroesophageal reflux; duodenal, gastric, and peptic ulcers |
| Ayvakit [avapritinib] | | Multikinase inhibitor | Unresectable or metastatic gastrointestinal stromal tumor (GIST); advanced systemic mastocytosis |
| Azactam [aztreonam] | Z79.2 | Antibiotic | Severe bacterial infections |
| Azithromycin [azithromycin] | Z79.2 | Antibiotic | Bacterial infections |
| Azstarys [serdexmethylphenidate and dexmethylphenidate] | | CNS stimulant | Attention deficit hyperactivity disorder (ADHD) |
| Bactrim [sulfamethoxazole/trimethoprim] | Z79.2 | Antibiotic | Urinary tract infections; acute otitis media; acute exacerbation of chronic bronchitis; shigellosis; Pneumocystis carinii infections |
| Basaglar [insulin glargine] | Z79.4 | Insulin | Diabetes mellitus |

| Drug | Z Code | Drug Action/Classification | Indications |
|---|---|---|---|
| Bayer [acetylsalicylic acid] | Z79.82 | Aspirin | Prophylaxis and treatment of heart attacks, angina or strokes; reduction of fever, pain, and inflammation |
| Benztropine mesylate [benztropine mesylate] | | Anticholinergic antiparkinson agent | Parkinson's disease |
| Betaseron [interferon beta-1b] | Z79.69 | Other immunosuppressant/ immunomodulator | Treatment of relapsing multiple sclerosis |
| Betoptic [betaxolol hydrochloride] | | Beta blocker; ophthalmic glaucoma agent | Lowering of intraocular pressure; also used for treatment of ocular hypertension and chronic open-angle glaucoma |
| Beyaz [drospirenone/ethinyl estradiol/ levomefolate calcium] | Z79.3 | Contraceptive | Prevention of pregnancy; acne vulgaris |
| Beyfortus [nirsevimab-alip] | Z79.620 | Immunostimulant; monoclonal antibody | Lower respiratory tract disease (LRTD) caused by RSV |
| Biaxin XL [clarithromycin] | Z79.2 | Antibiotic | Acid/peptic disorder or ulcer; acute exacerbation chronic bronchitis; human immunodeficiency virus; lower and upper respiratory tract infection; sinus infection; prophylaxis mycobacterium avium complex; pharyngitis; pneumonia; tonsillitis |
| Bijuva [estradiol/progesterone] | Z79.890 | Estrogen/progesterone therapy | Menopausal symptoms |
| Biktarvy [bictegravir sodium/emtricitabine/ tenofovir alafenamide fumarate] | | Antiretroviral | HIV |
| Biltricide [praziquantel] | | Antiparasitic | Infections from Schistosoma species and liver flukes |
| Bimzelx [bimekizumab] | Z79.69 | Other immunosuppressant/ immunomodulator | Plaque psoriasis |
| Binosto [alendronate sodium] | Z79.83 | Bisphosphonate | Osteoporosis |
| Bleomycin [bleomycin] | Z79.632 | Antitumor antibiotic | Squamous cell carcinoma; Hodgkin's disease; non-Hodgkin's lymphoma; malignant pleural effusion; testicular cancer |
| Brenzavvy [bexagliflozin] | Z79.84 | Oral hypoglycemic | Diabetes mellitus |
| Breo Ellipta [fluticasone furoate/vilanterol trifenatate] | Z79.51 | Corticosteroid – inhaled; antiasthmatic | Asthma and COPD |
| Brexafemme [ibrexafungerp] | | Antifungal | Vulvovaginal candidiasis |
| Briellyn [ethinyl estradiol/norethindrone] | Z79.3 | Contraceptive | Prevention of pregnancy |
| Brilinta [ticagrelor] | Z79.02 | Antiplatelet | Unstable angina; heart attacks; prevention of blood clots |
| Brisdelle [paroxetine mesylate] | | Selective serotonin reuptake inhibitor (SSRI) | Vasomotor symptoms related to menopause |
| Briumvi [ublituximab-xiiy] | Z79.620 | Immunosuppressive biologic; monoclonal antibody | Multiple sclerosis |
| Bufferin [aspirin] | Z79.82 | Aspirin | Pain, reduce fever or inflammation; prophylaxis and treatment of heart attack, stroke, angina |
| Buprenorphine HCl and Naloxone HCl [buprenorphine hydrochloride/naloxone hydrochloride] | Z79.891 | Analgesic, narcotic | Opioid addiction |
| Buspirone HCl [buspirone hydrochloride] | | Antianxiety | Generalized anxiety disorder |
| Busulfex [busulfan] | Z79.630 | Chemotherapeutic alkylating agent | Chronic myelogenous leukemia |
| Butrans [buprenorphine] | Z79.891 | Analgesic, narcotic | Chronic pain |
| Bydureon bcise [exenatide] | Z79.85 | Antidiabetic – non-insulin injectable | Diabetes mellitus |
| Byetta [exenatide] | Z79.85 | Antidiabetic – non-insulin injectable | Diabetes mellitus |
| Caldolor [ibuprofen] | Z79.1 | Nonsteroidal anti-inflammatory drug (NSAID) | Pain or fever relief |
| Cambia [diclofenac potassium] | Z79.1 | Nonsteroidal anti-inflammatory drug (NSAID) | Migraine headache |
| Camila [norethindrone] | Z79.3 | Contraceptive | Prevention of pregnancy; menstrual disorders |
| Camptosar [irinotecan] | Z79.634 | Topoisomerase inhibitor | Metastatic colon or rectal cancer |
| Camzyos [mavacamten] | | Cardiovascular agent | Symptomatic obstructive hypertrophic cardiomyopathy (HCM) |
| Caplyta [lumateperone] | | Antipsychotic | Schizophrenia |
| Cardizem CD [diltiazem hydrochloride] | | Calcium channel blocker | Chronic stable angina; angina due to coronary artery spasm; hypertension |
| Cardura [doxazosin mesylate] | | Antiadrenergic; antihypertensive | Benign prostatic hyperplasia; hypertension |
| Carmustine [carmustine] | Z79.630 | Chemotherapeutic alkylating agent | Brain tumors; Hodgkin's disease; multiple myeloma; non-Hodgkin's lymphoma |
| Cefazolin sodium [cefazolin sodium] | Z79.2 | Antibiotic | Bacterial infections |
| Cefepime hydrochloride [cefepime hydrochloride] | Z79.2 | Antibiotic | Bacterial infections |
| Cefprozil [cefprozil] | Z79.2 | Antibiotic | Bacterial infections |
| Ceftriaxone [ceftriaxone sodium] | Z79.2 | Antibiotic | Bacterial infections |
| Cefuroxime sodium [cefuroxime sodium] | Z79.2 | Antibiotic | Bacterial infections |

Appendix B: Pharmacology List 2027

| Drug | Z Code | Drug Action/Classification | Indications |
|---|---|---|---|
| Celebrex [celecoxib] | Z79.1 | Nonsteroidal anti-inflammatory drug (NSAID) | Osteoarthritis; rheumatoid arthritis; juvenile rheumatoid arthritis; ankylosing spondylitis; acute pain; primary dysmenorrhea |
| Celestone Soluspan [betamethasone acetate/betamethasone sodium phosphate] | Z79.52 | Corticosteroid; antiasthmatic | Asthma; severe inflammation |
| Celexa [citalopram hydrobromide] | | Antidepressant | Depression |
| CellCept [mycophenolate mofetil] | Z79.624 | Inhibitors of nucleotide synthesis; immunosuppressant | Prophylaxis of organ transplant rejection |
| Centany [mupirocin] | Z79.2 | Antibiotic, topical | Bacterial skin infections |
| Cephalexin [cephalexin] | Z79.2 | Antibiotic | Bacterial infections |
| Cerubidine [daunorubicin hydrochloride] | Z79.632 | Antitumor antibiotic | Leukemia |
| Chlorambucil [chlorambucil] | Z79.630 | Chemotherapeutic alkylating agent | Chronic lymphocytic leukemia; malignant lymphoma |
| Cibinqo [abrocitinib] | Z79.622 | Janus kinase (JAK) inhibitor | Atopic dermatitis |
| Cimduo [lamivudine/tenofovir disoproxil fumarate] | | Antiretroviral | HIV |
| Cipro [ciprofloxacin hydrochloride] | Z79.2 | Antibiotic | Cystitis; infectious diarrhea; gonorrhea; bone and joint infection; gastrointestinal tract infection; lower and upper respiratory tract infection; sinus infection; urinary tract infection; nosocomial pneumonia; chronic prostatitis |
| Ciprofloxacin [ciprofloxacin] | Z79.2 | Antibiotic | Bacterial infections |
| Cisplatin [cisplatin] | Z79.630 | Chemotherapeutic alkylating agent | Cancer |
| Clarithromycin [clarithromycin] | Z79.2 | Antibiotic | Skin and respiratory bacterial infections; stomach ulcers caused by Helicobacter pylori |
| Claritin [loratadine] | | Antihistamine | Seasonal allergic rhinitis; chronic idiopathic urticaria |
| Cleocin [clindamycin phosphate] | Z79.2 | Antibiotic | Bacterial infections |
| Climara [estradiol] | Z79.890 | Estrogen therapy | Osteoporosis; menopausal symptoms; vaginal and vulvar atrophy; hypoestrogenism; ovarian failure |
| Clindamycin [clindamycin phosphate] | Z79.2 | Antibiotic | Bacterial infections |
| Clonazepam [clonazepam] | | Anticonvulsant | Absence, akinetic, and myoclonic epilepsy; Lennox-Gastaut syndrome; panic disorders |
| Clonidine HCl [clonidine hydrochloride] | | Antihypertensive | Hypertension |
| Clopidogrel bisulfate [clopidogrel bisulfate] | Z79.02 | Antiplatelet | Unstable angina; heart attacks; prevention of blood clots |
| Codeine [codeine sulfate] | Z79.891 | Analgesic, narcotic | Mild to moderate pain |
| Colace [docusate sodium] | | Gastrointestinal agent; laxative, stool softener | Constipation |
| Colazal [balsalazide] | | Anti-inflammatory | Ulcerative colitis |
| Colocort [hydrocortisone] | Z79.52 | Corticosteroid | Inflammation of the colon |
| Columvi [glofitamab-gxbm] | Z79.620 | Monoclonal antibody | Large B-cell lymphoma |
| CombiPatch [ethinyl estradiol/norethindrone acetate] | Z79.890 | Estrogen therapy | Menopause symptoms; vaginal and vulvar atrophy; osteoporosis prevention |
| Combivent Respimat [ipratropium bromide/ albuterol sulfate] | | Antiasthmatic/bronchodilator | Chronic bronchitis, emphysema; bronchial asthma |
| Compro [prochlorperazine] | | Antiemetic; antipsychotic | Nausea and vomiting; manic phase of bipolar syndrome or schizophrenia |
| Copaxone [glatiramer acetate] | Z79.69 | Other immunosuppressant/ immunomodulator | Multiple sclerosis |
| Coreg [carvedilol] | | Beta blocker | Hypertension; chronic heart failure; left ventricular dysfunction following myocardial infarction |
| Coreg CR [carvedilol phosphate] | | Beta blocker | Hypertension; chronic heart failure; left ventricular dysfunction following myocardial infarction |
| Cortef [hydrocortisone] | Z79.52 | Corticosteroid | Severe inflammation |
| Cortenema [hydrocortisone] | Z79.52 | Corticosteroid | Inflammation of the colon |
| Cortifoam [hydrocortisone acetate] | Z79.52 | Corticosteroid | Colon and rectum inflammation |
| Cosentyx [secukinumab] | Z79.620 | Immunosuppressive biologic; monoclonal antibody | Plaque psoriasis; psoriatic arthritis; ankylosing spondylitis |
| Cozaar [losartan potassium] | | Antihypertensive | Hypertension |
| Crestor [rosuvastatin calcium] | | HMG-CoA reductase inhibitor (statin) | Hypercholesterolemia; hyperlipidemia; hyperproteinemia |
| Cyclosporine [cyclosporine] | Z79.621 | Calcineurin inhibitor | Prophylaxis of organ transplant rejection |
| Cyltezo [adalimumab-abdm] | Z79.620 | Immunosuppressive biologic; monoclonal antibody | Rheumatoid arthritis; juvenile idiopathic arthritis; psoriatic arthritis; Crohn's disease; ulcerative colitis; plaque psoriasis |
| Cymbalta [duloxetine hydrochloride] | | Antidepressant, serotonin and norepinephrine reuptake inhibitor (SNRI) | Major depressive disorder; general anxiety disorder; fibromyalgia; diabetic peripheral neuropathy; chronic musculoskeletal pain |

| Drug | Z Code | Drug Action/Classification | Indications |
|---|---|---|---|
| Cytarabine [cytarabine] | Z79.631 | Antimetabolite agent | Leukemia |
| Cytomel [liothyronine sodium] | | Thyroid hormone | Hypothyroidism or prevention of euthyroid goiters |
| Cytoxan [cyclophosphamide] | Z79.630 | Chemotherapeutic alkylating agent | Cancer |
| Daptomycin [daptomycin] | Z79.2 | Antibiotic | Bacterial infections of the skin, underlying tissues, and bloodstream |
| Daybue [trofinetide] | | CNS agent | Rett syndrome |
| Daypro [oxaprozin] | Z79.1 | Nonsteroidal anti-inflammatory drug (NSAID) | Osteoarthritis; rheumatoid arthritis; juvenile rheumatoid arthritis |
| Daysee [ethinyl estradiol/levonorgestrel] | Z79.3 | Contraceptive | Prevention of pregnancy |
| Defencath [taurolidine, heparin] | Z79.01 | Antimicrobial; anticoagulant | Catheter-related bloodstream infections |
| Delestrogen [estradiol valerate] | Z79.890 | Estrogen therapy | Menopause symptoms |
| Demerol [meperidine hydrochloride] | Z79.891 | Analgesic, narcotic | Moderate to severe pain |
| Depakote [divalproex sodium] | | Anticonvulsant | Bipolar affective disorder; complex absence, complex partial and mixed pattern epilepsy; migraine headache |
| Depo-Medrol [methylprednisolone acetate] | Z79.52 | Corticosteroid | Arthritis; joint disorders |
| Depo-Provera [medroxyprogesterone acetate] | Z79.3 | Contraceptive | Prevention of pregnancy |
| Depo-SubQ Provera [medroxyprogesterone acetate] | Z79.3 | Contraceptive | Prevention of pregnancy; menstrual disorder pain |
| Descovy [emtricitabine/tenofovir alafenamide] | | Antiretroviral | HIV |
| Desogestrel/ethinyl estradiol [desogestrel/ethinyl estradiol] | Z79.3 | Contraceptive | Prevention of pregnancy |
| Detrol [tolterodine tartrate] | | Muscarinic receptor antagonist | Overactive bladders in patients with urinary frequency, urgency, or urge incontinence |
| Dexamethasone Intensol [dexamethasone] | Z79.52 | Corticosteroid | Arthritis; allergic disorders; breathing disorders; inflammation; lupus |
| Dexilant [dexlansoprazole] | | Proton pump inhibitor | Erosive esophagitis; heartburn; nonerosive gastroesophageal reflux disease |
| DiaBeta [glyburide] | Z79.84 | Oral hypoglycemic | Diabetes mellitus |
| Diclegis [doxylamine succinate/pyridoxine hydrochloride] | | Antiemetic | Nausea/vomiting in pregnancy |
| Dificid [fidaxomicin] | Z79.2 | Antibiotic | Clostridium difficile |
| Diflucan [fluconazole] | | Antifungal | Oropharyngeal and esophageal candidiasis; cryptococcal meningitis in AIDS patients; vaginal candidiasis |
| Digoxin [digoxin] | | Antiarrhythmic; inotropic agent | Heart failure; atrial flutter; atrial fibrillation; supraventricular tachycardia |
| Dilantin [phenytoin sodium] | | Anticonvulsant | Grand mal and psychomotor seizures |
| Dilaudid [hydromorphone hydrochloride] | Z79.891 | Analgesic, narcotic | Moderate to severe pain |
| Diovan [valsartan] | | Antihypertensive | Hypertension; heart failure; post-myocardial infarction |
| Diskets [methadone hydrochloride] | | Opioid agonist | Treatment of opioid addiction |
| Disulfiram [disulfiram] | | Alcohol treatment | Alcoholism |
| Divigel [estradiol] | Z79.890 | Estrogen therapy – topical | Menopause symptoms |
| Dovato [dolutegravir sodium/lamivudine] | | Antiretroviral | HIV |
| Doxorubicin [doxorubicin] | Z79.632 | Antitumor antibiotic | Hodgkin lymphoma; non-Hodgkin lymphoma; specific types of cancers and leukemias |
| Doxycycline [doxycycline] | Z79.2 | Antibiotic | Bacterial infections; acne |
| Duavee [bazedoxifene acetate/conjugated estrogens] | Z79.890 | Estrogen therapy | Menopause symptoms; osteoporosis |
| Duetact [glimepiride/pioglitazone hydrochloride] | Z79.84 | Oral hypoglycemic | Diabetes mellitus |
| Duexis [famotidine/ibuprofen] | Z79.1 | Nonsteroidal anti-inflammatory drug (NSAID) | Osteoarthritis and rheumatoid arthritis; reduce risk of upper gastrointestinal ulcers |
| Dulera [formoterol fumarate/mometasone furoate] | Z79.51 | Corticosteroid – inhaled; antiasthmatic | Asthma |
| Dupixent [dupilumab] | Z79.620 | Immunosuppressive biologic; monoclonal antibody | Atopic dermatitis; asthma; chronic rhinosinusitis with nasal polys; eosinophilic esophagitis; prurigo nodularis |
| Duramorph PF [morphine sulfate] | Z79.891 | Analgesic, narcotic | Moderate to severe pain |
| Durlaza [aspirin] | Z79.82 | Aspirin | Pain; inflammation; prevention of heart attack, stroke, angina |
| Dymista [azelastine/fluticasone] | | Corticosteroid – intranasal | Seasonal allergies |
| E.E.S. [erythromycin ethylsuccinate] | Z79.2 | Antibiotic | Bacterial infections |
| Efavirenz (efavirenz) | | Antiretroviral | HIV |

| Drug | Z Code | Drug Action/Classification | Indications |
|---|---|---|---|
| Effexor XR [venlafaxine hydrochloride] | | Antidepressant, serotonin and norepinephrine reuptake inhibitors (SNRIs) | Major depressive disorder; social anxiety disorder; panic disorder |
| Effient [prasugrel hydrochloride] | Z79.Ø2 | Antiplatelet | Reduce risk of heart attack or stroke |
| Elestrin [estradiol] | Z79.89Ø | Estrogen therapy | Menopause symptoms |
| Elfabrio [pegunigalsidase alfa-iwxj] | | Enzyme replacement therapy | Fabry disease |
| Eligard [leuprolide acetate] | Z79.818 | Agents affecting estrogen receptors and estrogen levels | Palliative treatment of prostate cancer symptoms |
| Eliquis [apixaban] | Z79.Ø1 | Anticoagulant | Venous thrombosis |
| Elrexfio [elranatamab-bcmm] | Z79.62Ø | Monoclonal antibody | Multiple myeloma |
| Enbrel [etanercept] | Z79.62Ø | Immunosuppressive biologic; antirheumatic | Rheumatoid arthritis; polyarticular juvenile idiopathic arthritis; psoriatic arthritis; ankylosing spondylitis; plaque psoriasis |
| Enjaymo [sutimlimab-jome] | Z79.69 | Other immunosuppressant/ immunomodulator | Decreases need for red blood cell transfusion due to breakdown of red blood cells (hemolysis) in adults with cold agglutinin disease (CAD) |
| Enpresse-28 [ethinyl estradiol/ levonorgestrel] | Z79.3 | Contraceptive | Prevention of pregnancy |
| Entocort EC [budesonide] | Z79.52 | Corticosteroid | Crohn's disease; ulcerative colitis |
| Entresto [sacubitril/valsartan] | | Angiotensin II receptor blocker; neprilysin inhibitor | Chronic heart failure |
| Entyvio [vedolizumab] | Z79.62Ø | Immunosuppressive biologic; monoclonal antibody | Crohn's disease; ulcerative colitis |
| Envarsus XR [tacrolimus] | Z79.621 | Calcineurin inhibitor | Prophylaxis of organ transplant rejection |
| Epinephrine [epinephrine] | | Bronchodilator, cardiotonic | Hypotension associated with septic shock; anaphylaxis |
| Epivir, Epivir-HBV [lamivudine] | | Antiretroviral | HIV; chronic hepatitis B |
| Epkinly [epcoritamab-bysp] | Z79.62Ø | Monoclonal antibody | Large B-cell lymphoma; high-grade B-cell lymphoma |
| Eptifibatide [eptifibatide] | Z79.Ø2 | Antiplatelet | Unstable angina; heart attacks; prevention of blood clots |
| Erelzi [etanercept-szzs] | Z79.62Ø | Immunosuppressive biologic | Rheumatoid arthritis; polyarticular juvenile idiopathic arthritis; psoriatic arthritis; ankylosing spondylitis |
| Ertapenem [ertapenem sodium] | Z79.2 | Antibiotic | Bacterial infections of the stomach, urinary tract, pelvis, skin, and lung |
| ERYC [erythromycin] | Z79.2 | Antibiotic | Respiratory tract infections |
| Erygel [erythromycin] | Z79.2 | Antibiotic, topical | Bacterial skin infections |
| EryPed [erythromycin ethylsuccinate] | Z79.2 | Antibiotic | Bacterial infections; rheumatic fever attacks |
| Ery-Tab [erythromycin] | Z79.2 | Antibiotic | Bacterial infections |
| Erythrocin [erythromycin lactobionate] | Z79.2 | Antibiotic | Bacterial infections |
| Erythromycin [erythromycin] | Z79.2 | Antibiotic | Respiratory tract infections |
| Estrace [estradiol] | Z79.89Ø | Estrogen therapy | Vaginal cream for treatment of vaginal and vulvar atrophy |
| EstroGel [estradiol] | Z79.89Ø | Estrogen therapy – topical | Menopause symptoms |
| Etoposide [etoposide] | Z79.634 | Topoisomerase inhibitor | Small cell lung cancer |
| Evista [raloxifene hydrochloride] | Z79.81Ø | Selective estrogen receptor modulator (SERM) | Osteoporosis in postmenopausal women |
| Exemestane [exemestane] | Z79.811 | Aromatase inhibitor | Postmenopausal breast cancer |
| Exxua [gepirone] | | Antidepressant | Major depressive disorder |
| Fareston [toremifene citrate] | Z79.81Ø | Selective estrogen receptor modulator (SERM) | Postmenopausal breast cancer |
| Farxiga [dapagliflozin propanediol] | Z79.84 | Oral hypoglycemic | Diabetes mellitus |
| Faslodex [fulvestrant] | Z79.818 | Agents affecting estrogen receptors and estrogen levels | Hormone-related breast cancer; metastatic breast cancer |
| Feldene [piroxicam] | Z79.1 | Nonsteroidal anti-inflammatory drug (NSAID) | Treatment of pain and inflammation due to arthritis |
| Femara [letrozole] | Z79.811 | Aromatase inhibitor | Postmenopausal breast cancer |
| Femhrt [ethinyl estradiol/norethindrone acetate] | Z79.3, Z79.89Ø | Contraceptive; estrogen therapy | Prevention of pregnancy; menopause symptoms; osteoporosis prevention |
| Femring [estradiol acetate] | Z79.89Ø | Estrogen therapy | Osteoporosis prevention; menopausal symptoms; hypoestrogenism; ovarian failure |
| Fentanyl citrate [fentanyl citrate] | Z79.891 | Analgesic, narcotic | Postprocedural or chronic pain |
| Fentora [fentanyl citrate] | Z79.891 | Analgesic, narcotic | Breakthrough cancer pain |
| Fetroja [cefiderocol] | Z79.2 | Antibiotic | Complicated urinary tract infections; hospital-acquired bacterial pneumonia; ventilator-associated bacterial pneumonia |
| Fiasp [insulin aspart] | Z79.4 | Insulin | Diabetes mellitus |
| Filspari [sparsentan] | | Endothelin and angiotensin II receptor antagonist | Primary immunoglobulin A nephropathy (IgAN) |

| Drug | Z Code | Drug Action/Classification | Indications |
|---|---|---|---|
| Fioricet with codeine [acetaminophen/ butalbital/caffeine/codeine phosphate] | Z79.891 | Analgesic, narcotic | Tension headaches |
| Firmagon [degarelix] | Z79.89Ø | Hormone therapy | Prostate cancer |
| Flagyl [metronidazole] | Z79.2 | Antibiotic | Bacterial infections |
| Flavoxate HCl [flavoxate hydrochloride] | | Urinary antispasmodic | Relief of dysuria, urgency, nocturia, suprapubic pain, frequency, and incontinence associated with cystitis, prostatitis, urethritis, and urethrocystitis/urethrotrigonitis |
| Flomax [tamsulosin hydrochloride] | | Antiadrenergic | Benign prostatic hyperplasia |
| Flonase allergy relief [fluticasone propionate] | | Corticosteroid – intranasal | Perennial and seasonal allergic rhinitis |
| Flovent HFA [fluticasone propionate] | Z79.51 | Corticosteroid – inhaled; antiasthmatic | Asthma |
| Fosamax [alendronate sodium] | Z79.83 | Bisphosphonate | Osteoporosis; Paget's disease |
| Fosinopril sodium [fosinopril sodium] | | ACE inhibitor | Hypertension; heart failure |
| Fosrenol [lanthanum carbonate] | | Phosphate binder | End-stage renal disease (ESRD) |
| Fragmin [dalteparin sodium] | Z79.Ø1 | Anticoagulant | Venous thrombosis |
| Fruzaqla [fruquintinib] | | Kinase inhibitor | Colorectal cancer |
| Gengraf [cyclosporine] | Z79.621 | Calcineurin inhibitor | Prophylaxis of organ transplant rejection |
| Gentamicin sulfate [gentamicin sulfate] | Z79.2 | Antibiotic | Severe bacterial infections |
| Gildagia [ethinyl estradiol/norethindrone] | Z79.3 | Contraceptive | Prevention of pregnancy |
| Gildess 24 FE [ethinyl estradiol/ norethindrone acetate] | Z79.3 | Contraceptive | Prevention of pregnancy |
| Glimepiride [glimepiride] | Z79.84 | Oral hypoglycemic | Diabetes mellitus |
| Glucotrol XL [glipizide] | Z79.84 | Oral hypoglycemic | Diabetes mellitus |
| Glumetza [metformin hydrochloride] | Z79.84 | Oral hypoglycemic | Diabetes mellitus |
| Glyburide (micronized) [glyburide] | Z79.84 | Oral hypoglycemic | Diabetes mellitus |
| Glynase [glyburide] | Z79.84 | Oral hypoglycemic | Diabetes mellitus |
| Glyset [miglitol] | Z79.84 | Oral hypoglycemic | Diabetes mellitus |
| Harvoni [ledipasvir/sofosbuvir] | | Antiviral | Chronic hepatitis C |
| Heparin sodium [heparin sodium] | Z79.Ø1 | Anticoagulant | Prophylaxis and treatment of venous thrombosis, pulmonary embolism; prevention of cerebral thrombosis; treatment of consumptive coagulopathies |
| Hiprex [methenamine] | Z79.2 | Antibiotic | Recurring bladder infection |
| Humalog [insulin lispro recombinant] | Z79.4 | Insulin | Diabetes mellitus |
| Humira [adalimumab] | Z79.62Ø | Immunosuppressive biologic; monoclonal antibody | Rheumatoid arthritis; juvenile idiopathic arthritis; psoriatic arthritis; Crohn's disease; ulcerative colitis; plaque psoriasis; hidradenitis suppurativa; uveitis |
| Humulin R [insulin recombinant] | Z79.4 | Insulin | Diabetes mellitus |
| Hycamtin [topotecan hydrochloride] | Z79.634 | Topoisomerase inhibitor | Ovarian cancer; small cell lung cancer; cervical cancer |
| Hydrocodone [acetaminophen/hydrocodone bitartrate] | Z79.891 | Analgesic, narcotic | Moderate to severe pain |
| Hydrocodone bitartrate and acetaminophen [acetaminophen/ hydrocodone bitartrate] | Z79.891 | Analgesic, narcotic | Moderate to severe pain |
| Hydrocortisone [hydrocortisone] | Z79.52 | Corticosteroid | Addison's disease; arthritis; immune disorders; allergies; breathing problems |
| Hydromorphone HCl [hydromorphone hydrochloride] | Z79.891 | Analgesic, narcotic | Moderate to severe pain |
| Hydroxyurea [hydroxyurea] | Z79.64 | Myelosuppressive agent | Pain related to sickle cell disease; chronic myeloid leukemia; ovarian cancer; skin cancer |
| Hyrimoz [adalimumab-adaz] | Z79.62Ø | Immunosuppressive biologic; monoclonal antibody | Rheumatoid arthritis; juvenile idiopathic arthritis; psoriatic arthritis; Crohn's disease; ulcerative colitis; plaque psoriasis; ankylosing spondylitis |
| Hyzaar [hydrochlorothiazide/ losartan potassium] | | Antihypertensive | Hypertension |
| Ibsrela [tenapanor hydrochloride] | | NHE-3 inhibitor | Irritable bowel syndrome with constipation (IBS-C) |
| Ibuprofen [ibuprofen] | Z79.1 | Nonsteroidal anti-inflammatory drug (NSAID) | Pain or fever relief |
| Imitrex [sumatriptan succinate] | | Antimigraine | Migraine headache |
| Imjudo [tremelimumab] | Z79.62Ø | Immunosuppressive biologic; monoclonal antibody | Unresectable hepatocellular carcinoma |
| Imuran [azathioprine] | Z79.624 | Inhibitors of nucleotide synthesis; antirheumatic; immunosuppressant | Rheumatoid arthritis; prophylaxis of organ transplant rejection |
| Indocin [indomethacin] | Z79.1 | Nonsteroidal anti-inflammatory drug (NSAID) | Treatment of pain and inflammation |
| Inpefa [sotagliflozin] | | Cardiovascular agent | Heart failure |

| Drug | Z Code | Drug Action/Classification | Indications |
|---|---|---|---|
| Intron A [interferon alfa 2-b] | Z79.69 | Other immunosuppressant/ immunomodulator | Cancer; hepatitis |
| Invanz [ertapenem sodium] | Z79.2 | Antibiotic | Bacterial infections of the stomach, urinary tract, pelvis, skin, and lung |
| Invokamet [canagliflozin/metformin hydrochloride] | Z79.84 | Oral hypoglycemic | Diabetes mellitus |
| Invokana [canagliflozin] | Z79.84 | Oral hypoglycemic | Diabetes mellitus |
| Isoniazid [isoniazid] | Z79.2 | Antibiotic | Tuberculosis |
| Isoproterenol hydrochloride [isoproterenol hydrochloride] | | Adrenergic agent/catecholamine | Shock; cardiac arrest; heart failure; bronchospasm |
| Isopto Carpine [pilocarpine hydrochloride] | | Cholinergic parasympathomimetic agent | Reduction of intraocular pressure in open-angle glaucoma or ocular hypertension; management of acute angle-closure glaucoma |
| Isordil Titradose [isosorbide dinitrate] | | Smooth muscle relaxant | Acute anginal attacks |
| Isturisa [osilodrostat] | | Cortisol synthesis inhibitor | Cushing's disease in adults |
| Ixempra [ixabepilone] | Z79.633 | Mitotic inhibitor | Advanced breast cancer |
| Izervay [avacincaptad pegol] | | Anti-angiogenic ophthalmic agent | Geographic atrophy due to age-related macular degeneration |
| Jantoven [warfarin sodium] | Z79.Ø1 | Anticoagulant | Venous thrombosis, pulmonary embolism; prevention of cerebral thrombosis; treatment of consumptive coagulopathies |
| Janumet [metformin hydrochloride/ sitagliptin phosphate] | Z79.84 | Oral hypoglycemic | Diabetes mellitus |
| Januvia [sitagliptin phosphate] | Z79.84 | Oral hypoglycemic | Diabetes mellitus |
| Jaypirca [pirtobrutinib] | | Kinase inhibitor | Mantle cell lymphoma |
| Jentadueto [linagliptin/metformin hydrochloride]] | Z79.84 | Oral hypoglycemic | Diabetes mellitus |
| Jesduvroq [daprodustat] | | Erythropoiesis-stimulating agent (ESA) | Treatment of anemia in CKD patients on dialysis |
| Junel [ethinyl estradiol/norethindrone acetate] | Z79.3 | Contraceptive | Prevention of pregnancy |
| Katerzia [amlodipine benzoate] | | Antihypertensive | Hypertension; coronary artery disease (CAD); chronic stable angina; prinzmetal's angina; variant angina |
| Kazano [alogliptin benzoate/metformin hydrochloride] | Z79.84 | Oral hypoglycemic | Diabetes mellitus |
| Kenalog-10; Kenalog-40 [triamcinolone acetonide] | Z79.52 | Corticosteroid | Gouty arthritis; bursitis; tenosynovitis; epicondylitis; rheumatoid arthritis; synovitis; osteoarthritis |
| Keytruda [pembrolizumab] | Z79.62Ø | Immunosuppressive biologic; monoclonal antibody | Unresectable or metastatic melanoma |
| Kimmtrak [tebentafusp-tebn] | | Antineoplastic | Uveal melanoma |
| Klaron [sulfacetamide sodium] | Z79.2 | Antibiotic, topical | Acne vulgaris |
| Klonopin [clonazepam] | | Anticonvulsant; CNS depressant | Epilepsy; seizures; panic disorder |
| Klor-Con [potassium chloride] | | Mineral; electrolyte | Hypokalemia |
| Kombiglyze [metformin hydrochloride/ saxagliptin hydrochloride] | Z79.84 | Oral hypoglycemic | Diabetes mellitus |
| K-Tab [potassium chloride] | | Mineral; electrolyte | Hypokalemia |
| Lamisil [terbinafine hydrochloride] | | Antifungal | Tinea cruris (jock itch); T. pedis (athlete's foot); T. corporis (ringworm) |
| Lanoxin [digoxin] | | Antiarrhythmic; inotropic agent | Congestive heart failure; chronic atrial fibrillation |
| Lantus [insulin glargine recombinant] | Z79.4 | Insulin | Diabetes mellitus |
| Lasix [furosemide] | | Antihypertensive; diuretic | Hypertension; edema associated with heart failure and renal disease |
| Leqembi [lecanemab-irmb] | | Amyloid beta-directed antibody | Dementia due to Alzheimer's |
| Lescol XL [fluvastatin sodium] | | HMG-CoA reductase inhibitor (statin) | Hypercholesterolemia; hyperlipidemia; hyperlipoproteinemia |
| Letrozole [letrozole] | Z79.811 | Aromatase inhibitor; antineoplastic | Postmenopausal breast cancer |
| Leukeran [chlorambucil] | Z79.63Ø | Chemotherapeutic alkylating agent | Cancer |
| Levemir [insulin detemir recombinant] | Z79.4 | Insulin | Diabetes mellitus |
| Levonest [levonorgestrel/ethinyl estradiol] | Z79.3 | Contraceptive | Prevention of pregnancy; menstrual disorders; acne |
| Levoxyl [levothyroxine sodium] | Z79.89Ø | Thyroid hormone | Hypothyroidism; pituitary thyrotropin suppression |
| Lexapro [escitalopram oxalate] | | Antidepressant, selective serotonin reuptake inhibitor (SSRI) | Depression; anxiety |
| Lialda [mesalamine] | | Anti-inflammatory | Ulcerative colitis |
| Lidocaine HCl [lidocaine hydrochloride] | | Antiarrhythmic | Management of ventricular arrhythmias or during cardiac manipulation, such as cardiac surgery |
| Liletta [levonorgestrel] | Z79.3 | Contraceptive | Intrauterine device to prevent pregnancy |

| Drug | Z Code | Drug Action/Classification | Indications |
|---|---|---|---|
| Lincocin [lincocin hydrochloride] | Z79.2 | Antibiotic | Severe bacterial infections |
| Lipitor [atorvastatin calcium] | | HMG-CoA reductase inhibitor (statin) | Hypercholesterolemia; hyperlipidemia; hyperproteinemia |
| Lisinopril [lisinopril] | | ACE inhibitor | Congestive heart failure; hypertension |
| Litfulo [ritlecitinib] | | Multikinase inhibitor | Alopecia areata |
| Lithium carbonate [lithium carbonate] | | Antimanic | Control of manic episodes in bipolar disorders |
| Livtencity [maribavir] | | Antiviral | Post-transplant CMV infection/disease |
| Lo Loestrin Fe [ethinyl estradiol/ norethindrone acetate] | Z79.3 | Contraceptive | Prevention of pregnancy |
| Locoid [hydrocortisone butyrate] | Z79.52 | Corticosteroid – topical | Atopic dermatitis; other dermatoses |
| Lomotil [diphenoxylate hydrochloride/ atropine sulfate] | | Antidiarrheal | Symptoms of chronic and functional diarrhea |
| Lopid [gemfibrozil] | | Lipid regulating agent | Hypercholesterolemia; hyperlipidemia; hyperlipoproteinemia; hypertriglyceridemia |
| Lopressor [metoprolol tartrate] | | Beta blocker | Angina pectoris; hypertension; acute myocardial infarction |
| Loqtorzi [toripalimab-tpzi] | Z79.620 | Monoclonal antibody | Nasopharyngeal carcinoma |
| Lorazepam [lorazepam] | | Antianxiety; sedative/hypnotic; anticonvulsant; antiemetic | Anxiety disorder associated with depressive symptoms; controls tension, agitation, irritability, and insomnia |
| Loryna [drospirenone/ethinyl estradiol] | Z79.3 | Contraceptive | Prevention of pregnancy |
| LoSeasonique [ethinyl estradiol/ levonorgestrel] | Z79.3 | Contraceptive | Prevention of pregnancy |
| Lotensin [benazepril hydrochloride] | | ACE inhibitor | Hypertension |
| Lotrel [amlodipine besylate/benazepril hydrochloride] | | Antihypertensive | Hypertension |
| Lovastatin [lovastatin] | | HMG-CoA reductase inhibitor (statin) | Hypercholesterolemia; hyperlipidemia; hyperlipoproteinemia |
| Lovenox [enoxaparin sodium] | Z79.01 | Anticoagulant | Venous thrombosis and pulmonary embolism |
| Low-Ogestrel-28 [norgestrel/ethinyl estradiol] | Z79.3 | Contraceptive | Prevention of pregnancy |
| Lupkynis [voclosporin] | Z79.621 | Calcineurin inhibitor; immunosuppressant | Lupus nephritis |
| Lupron Depot [leuprolide acetate] | Z79.818 | Agents affecting estrogen receptors and estrogen levels; antineoplastic | Endometriosis symptoms; uterine fibroids; symptoms of prostate cancer |
| Macrobid [nitrofurantoin] | Z79.2 | Antibiotic | Urinary tract infections |
| Macrodantin [nitrofurantoin] | Z79.2 | Antibiotic | Urinary tract infections |
| Meclizine hydrochloride [meclizine hydrochloride] | | Antihistamine; antiemetic | Nausea, vomiting, and dizziness associated with motion sickness; symptoms of vertigo |
| Medrol [methylprednisolone] | Z79.52 | Corticosteroid | Allergic and edematous states; collagen disorders |
| Megace ES [megestrol acetate] | Z79.818 | Agents affecting estrogen receptors and estrogen levels; progestin; antineoplastic | Endometrial or advanced breast cancers; weight loss due to AIDS |
| Menest [esterified estrogens] | Z79.890 | Estrogen therapy | Menopause symptoms; ovarian failure |
| Menostar [estradiol] | Z79.890 | Estrogen therapy | Menopause symptoms; osteoporosis prevention |
| Mepron [atovaquone] | Z79.2 | Antibiotic | Pneumonia due to Pneumocystis jirovecii |
| Merrem [meropenem] | Z79.2 | Antibiotic | Bacterial infections of skin or stomach; bacterial meningitis |
| Mesalamine [mesalamine] | | Anti-inflammatory | Ulcerative colitis |
| Metformin [metformin hydrochloride] | Z79.84 | Oral hypoglycemic | Diabetes mellitus |
| Methadone HCl [methadone hydrochloride] | Z79.891 | Analgesic, narcotic; opioid agonist | Pain; treatment of opioid addiction |
| Methadose [methadone hydrochloride] | Z79.891 | Analgesic, narcotic; opioid agonist | Acute and chronic pain |
| Methergine [methylergonovine maleate] | | Oxytocic agent | Routine management of postpartum hemorrhage after delivery of placenta |
| Methotrexate sodium [methotrexate sodium] | Z79.631 | Antimetabolite agent | Cancer |
| Methylprednisolone [methylprednisolone] | Z79.52 | Corticosteroid | Inflammatory disorders |
| Metronidazole [metronidazole] | Z79.2 | Antibiotic | Bacterial infections |
| Miacalcin [calcitonin salmon] | | Calcitonin | Hypercalcemia; osteoporosis; Paget's disease |
| Miebo [perfluorhexyloctane] | | Ophthalmic anti-inflammatory agent | Dry eye disease |
| Minivelle [estradiol] | Z79.890 | Estrogen therapy | Menopause symptoms; osteoporosis prevention |
| Minocin [minocycline hydrochloride] | Z79.2 | Antibiotic | Bacterial infections; acne |
| Mirena [levonorgestrel] | Z79.3 | Contraceptive | Intrauterine device for prevention of pregnancy; menstrual disorders |
| Mitomycin [mitomycin] | Z79.632 | Antitumor antibiotic; antineoplastic | Stomach and pancreas cancer |
| Mobic [meloxicam] | Z79.1 | Nonsteroidal anti-inflammatory drug (NSAID) | Treatment of pain and inflammation due to osteoarthritis and rheumatoid arthritis |

| Drug | Z Code | Drug Action/Classification | Indications |
|---|---|---|---|
| Monoclonal antibodies | Z79.620 | Immunosuppressive biologic | Cancer; prophylaxis of organ transplant rejection |
| Monodox [doxycycline] | Z79.2 | Antibiotic | Bacterial infections; acne |
| Mono-Linyah [norgestimate/ethinyl estradiol] | Z79.3 | Contraceptive | Prevention of pregnancy; menstrual disorders; acne |
| Monurol [fosfomycin tromethamine] | Z79.2 | Antibiotic | Bacterial bladder infections |
| Morphine sulfate [morphine sulfate] | Z79.891 | Analgesic, narcotic | Moderate to severe pain |
| Motrin IB [ibuprofen] | Z79.1 | Nonsteroidal anti-inflammatory drug (NSAID) | Pain or fever relief |
| Mounjaro [tirzepatide] | Z79.85 | Antidiabetic – non-insulin injectable | Diabetes mellitus |
| MS Contin [morphine sulfate] | Z79.891 | Analgesic, narcotic | Moderate to severe pain |
| Multaq [dronedarone hydrochloride] | | Antiarrhythmic | Atrial fibrillation; atrial flutter |
| Mycobutin [rifabutin] | Z79.2 | Antibiotic | Mycobacterium avium complex (MAC) prophylactic in HIV patients |
| Mytesi [crofelemer] | | Antidiarrheal | Diarrhea occurring in HIV/AIDs patient's on anti-retroviral therapy |
| Nabumetone [nabumetone] | Z79.1 | Nonsteroidal anti-inflammatory drug (NSAID) | Osteoarthritis and rheumatoid arthritis |
| Nalfon [fenoprofen calcium] | Z79.1 | Nonsteroidal anti-inflammatory drug (NSAID) | Pain or inflammation relief; osteoarthritis; rheumatoid arthritis |
| Namzaric [memantine/donepezil hydrochlorides] | | Acetylcholinesterase/cholinesterase inhibitors | Dementia due to Alzheimer's |
| Naprelan [naproxen sodium] | Z79.1 | Nonsteroidal anti-inflammatory drug (NSAID) | Pain or inflammation relief |
| Naprosyn [naproxen] | Z79.1 | Nonsteroidal anti-inflammatory drug (NSAID) | Rheumatoid, gouty arthritis and osteoarthritis; ankylosing spondylitis; bursitis; dysmenorrhea; pain, mild to moderate; tendonitis |
| Natazia [estradiol valerate/dienogest] | Z79.3 | Contraceptive | Prevention of pregnancy; menstrual disorders |
| Nebupent [pentamidine isethionate] | Z79.2 | Antibiotic; antifungal | Fungal infections; Pneumocystis jirovecii (carinii) pneumonia in HIV patients |
| Nefazodone HCl [nefazodone hydrochloride] | | Antidepressant | Depression |
| Nembutal sodium [pentobarbital sodium] | | Sedative/hypnotic | Insomnia; adjunct medication in diagnostic procedures or for emergency use with convulsive disorders |
| NeoProfen [ibuprofen lysine] | Z79.1 | Nonsteroidal anti-inflammatory drug (NSAID) | Pain or fever relief in premature infants |
| Neoral [cyclosporine] | Z79.621 | Calcineurin inhibitor | Prophylaxis of organ transplant rejection; rheumatoid arthritis; psoriasis |
| Neosporin [bacitracin, neomycin] | Z79.2 | Antibiotic, topical | Bacterial skin infections |
| Neurontin [gabapentin] | | Anticonvulsant | Postherpetic neuralgia; partial onset seizures |
| Nexium [esomeprazole magnesium] | | Proton pump inhibitor | Gastroesophageal reflux disease (GERD); erosive esophagitis |
| Nexletol [bempedoic acid] | | Antihyperlipidemic | Heterozygous familial hypercholesterolemia; established atherosclerotic cardiovascular disease requiring additional lowering of LDL-C |
| Nexplanon [etonogestrel] | Z79.3 | Contraceptive | Implantable device used for prevention of pregnancy |
| Ngenla [somatrogon-ghla] | | Growth hormone | Growth failure |
| Nitrofurantoin [nitrofurantoin] | Z79.2 | Antibiotic | Bacterial urinary tract infections |
| Nitrostat [nitroglycerin] | | Muscle relaxant; antianginal; antihypertensive; coronary vasodilator | Angina pectoris; heart failure associated with myocardial infarction; hypertension, perioperative; surgery, adjunct |
| Norpace [disopyramide phosphate] | | Antiarrhythmic | Coronary artery disease; prevention, recurrence, and control of unifocal, multifocal, and paired PVCs |
| Norvasc [amlodipine besylate] | | Antihypertensive | Hypertension; coronary artery disease (CAD); chronic stable angina; prinzmetal's angina; variant angina |
| Novolin [insulin recombinant] | Z79.4 | Insulin | Diabetes mellitus |
| Novolog [insulin aspart recombinant] | Z79.4 | Insulin | Diabetes mellitus |
| Nucynta [tapentadol hydrochloride] | Z79.891 | Analgesic, narcotic | Moderate to severe pain |
| NuvaRing [etonogestrel/ethinyl estradiol] | Z79.3 | Contraceptive | Vaginal ring to prevent pregnancy |
| Ogsiveo [nirogacestat] | | Antineoplastic | Desmoid tumors |
| Ojjaara [momelotinib] | Z79.622 | Janus kinase (JAK) inhibitor | Myelofibrosis |
| Olumiant [baricitinib] | Z79.622 | Janus kinase (JAK) inhibitor | Rheumatoid arthritis |
| Omvoh [mirikizumab-mrkz] | Z79.620 | Monoclonal antibody | Ulcerative colitis |
| Opdualag [nivolumab and relatlimab-rmbw] | | Antineoplastic combination | Unresectable or metastatic melanoma |
| Oracea [doxycycline] | Z79.2 | Antibiotic | Rosacea |
| Orapred ODT [prednisolone sodium phosphate] | Z79.52 | Corticosteroid | Inflammatory disorders |
| Orbactiv [oritavancin diphosphate] | Z79.2 | Antibiotic | Bacterial skin infections |

| Drug | Z Code | Drug Action/Classification | Indications |
|---|---|---|---|
| Orencia [abatacept] | Z79.69 | Other immunosuppressant/ immunomodulator | Rheumatoid arthritis; polyarticular juvenile idiopathic arthritis; psoriatic arthritis; prophylaxis of acute graft versus host disease (aGVHD) |
| Orilissa [elagolix] | Z79.890 | Hormone therapy | Pain associated with endometriosis |
| Orphenadrine citrate [orphenadrine citrate] | | Muscle relaxant | Acute spasms, tension, and post-trauma cases |
| Orserdu [elacestrant] | Z79.818 | Agents affecting estrogen receptors and estrogen levels | Advanced or metastatic breast cancer |
| Oseni [alogliptin benzoate/pioglitazone hydrochloride] | Z79.84 | Oral hypoglycemic | Diabetes mellitus |
| Osphena [ospemifene] | Z79.810 | Selective estrogen receptor modulator (SERM) | Postmenopausal dyspareunia due to vaginal atrophy; osteoporosis; menopausal symptoms |
| Otezla [apremilast] | Z79.61 | Immunomodulator; antirheumatic | Psoriatic arthritis; plaque psoriasis; oral ulcers associated with Behcet's disease |
| Oxazepam [oxazepam] | | Antianxiety | Anxiety, tension, and withdrawal from alcohol |
| Oxbryta [voxelotor] | | Hemoglobin S polymerization inhibitor | Sickle cell disease |
| Oxycodone HCl [oxycodone hydrochloride] | Z79.891 | Analgesic, narcotic | Moderate to severe pain |
| OxyContin [oxycodone hydrochloride] | Z79.891 | Analgesic, narcotic | Moderate to severe pain |
| Ozempic [semaglutide] | Z79.85 | Antidiabetic – non-insulin injectable | Diabetes mellitus |
| Paclitaxel [paclitaxel] | Z79.633 | Mitotic inhibitor | Cancer of the breast, ovaries, and lung; AIDS-related Kaposi's sarcoma |
| Paxil [paroxetine hydrochloride] | | Antidepressant; selective serotonin reuptake inhibitor (SSRI) | Obsessive-compulsive disorder; major depressive disorder; panic disorder; social anxiety disorder; generalized anxiety disorder; posttraumatic stress disorder |
| Paxlovid [nirmatrelvir, ritonavir] | | Antiviral | COVID-19 |
| PediaPred [prednisolone sodium phosphate] | Z79.52 | Corticosteroid | Inflammatory disorders |
| PegIntron [peginterferon alfa-2b] | Z79.69 | Other immunosuppressant/ immunomodulator; antiviral | Hepatitis C |
| Penicillin-VK [penicillin V potassium] | Z79.2 | Antibiotic | Chorea, prevention; endocarditis, prevention, secondary to tooth extraction; erysipelas; infections of the skin, skin structures, and upper respiratory tract; rheumatic fever, prophylaxis; scarlet fever; Vincent's gingivitis; Vincent's pharyngitis |
| Pentam [pentamidine isethionate] | Z79.2 | Antibiotic; antifungal | Severe bacterial lung infections; fungal infections; Pneumocystis jirovecii (carinii) pneumonia |
| Pentasa [mesalamine] | | Anti-inflammatory | Crohn's disease; ulcerative colitis |
| Pepcid AC [famotidine] | | Histamine H2-receptor inhibitor | Acid/peptic disorder; adenoma, secretory; gastroesophageal reflux; duodenal and gastric ulcer; Zollinger-Ellison syndrome |
| Percocet [oxycodone hydrochloride/ acetaminophen] | Z79.891 | Analgesic, narcotic | Moderate to severe pain |
| Persantine [dipyridamole] | Z79.02 | Antiplatelet | Prevention of blood clots after heart valve surgery |
| Pfizerpen [penicillin g potassium] | Z79.2 | Antibiotic | Severe bacterial infections |
| Phenobarbital [phenobarbital sodium] | | Anticonvulsant | Grand mal epilepsy; sedative |
| Piqray [alpelisib] | | Kinase inhibitor | Postmenopausal advanced or metastatic breast cancer |
| Pitocin [oxytocin] | | Uterotonic | Induction or stimulation of labor at term; control of bleeding after childbirth |
| Plan B One-Step [levonorgestrel] | Z79.3 | Contraceptive | Prevention of pregnancy |
| Plavix [clopidogrel bisulfate] | Z79.02 | Antiplatelet | Lessening of the chance of heart attack or stroke |
| Pluvicto [lutetium Lu 177 vipivotide tetraxetan] | | Radioligand therapeutic agent | Metastatic castration-resistant prostate cancer (mCRPC) |
| Pomalyst [pomalidomide] | Z79.61 | Immunomodulator; antineoplastic | Multiple myeloma; Kaposi sarcoma |
| Pombiliti [cipaglucosidase alfa-atga] | | Lysosomal enzyme | Pompe disease |
| Ponstel [mefenamic acid] | Z79.1 | Nonsteroidal anti-inflammatory drug (NSAID) | Mild to moderate pain; primary dysmenorrhea |
| Ponvory [ponesimod] | Z79.69 | Other immunosuppressant/ immunomodulator | Relapsing forms of multiple sclerosis (MS) |
| Pradaxa [dabigatran etexilate mesylate] | Z79.01 | Anticoagulant | Prophylaxis and treatment of blood clots in patients with atrial fibrillation |
| Prasugrel [prasugrel hydrochloride] | Z79.02 | Antiplatelet | Lessening the chance of heart attack or stroke |
| Pravastatin sodium [pravastatin sodium] | | HMG-CoA reductase inhibitor (statin) | Hypercholesterolemia; hyperlipidemia; hyperlipoproteinemia |
| Prednisolone [prednisolone] | Z79.52 | Corticosteroid | Inflammatory disorders |
| Prednisone [prednisone] | Z79.52 | Corticosteroid | Immunosuppressant effects; relief of inflammation; used in arthritis, polymyositis and other systemic diseases |
| Pregnyl [chorionic gonadotropin] | | Gonadotropic hormone | Prepubertal cryptorchidism; hypogonadism; corpus luteum insufficiency and infertility |

| Drug | Z Code | Drug Action/Classification | Indications |
|---|---|---|---|
| Prempro [conjugated estrogens/ medroxyprogesterone acetate] | Z79.890 | Estrogen/progesterone therapy | Menopause symptoms; osteoporosis; atrophic vaginitis |
| Prevacid [lansoprazole] | | Proton pump inhibitor | Acid/peptic disorder; erosive esophagitis; duodenal ulcer; Zollinger-Ellison syndrome |
| Prezcobix [darunavir/cobicistat] | | Antiretroviral | HIV |
| Prezista [darunavir] | | Antiretroviral | HIV |
| Priftin [rifapentine] | Z79.2 | Antibiotic | Tuberculosis |
| Prilosec [omeprazole magnesium] | | Proton pump inhibitor | Acid/peptic disorder; endocrine adenoma; erosive esophagitis; systemic mastocytosis; gastroesophageal reflux; duodenal, peptic and gastric ulcer; Zollinger-Ellison syndrome |
| Primaxin [cilastatin sodium/imipenem] | Z79.2 | Antibiotic | Bacterial septicemia; endocarditis; bacterial infections of the skin, lower respiratory tract, intra-abdomen, bones, and joints |
| Pristiq [desvenlafaxine] | | Antidepressant; serotonin and norepinephrine reuptake inhibitor (SNRI) | Major depressive disorder |
| Procardia [nifedipine] | | Calcium channel blocker | Vasospastic angina; chronic stable angina; hypertension |
| Prograf [tacrolimus] | Z79.621 | Calcineurin inhibitor | Prophylaxis of organ transplant rejection |
| Prolia [denosumab] | Z79.620 | Immunosuppressive biologic; monoclonal antibody | Osteoporosis |
| Promethazine hydrochloride [promethazine hydrochloride] | | Anesthesia, adjunct to; antiemetic; antihistamine; antitussive/expectorant; sedative/hypnotic; vertigo/motion sickness/ vomiting | Anesthesia; adjunct; angioedema; conjunctivitis; dermographism; hypersensitivity, motion sickness; pain; perennial, seasonal, and allergic rhinitis; sedation, obstetrical; urticaria |
| Propranolol hydrochloride [propranolol hydrochloride] | | Beta blocker | Angina pectoris; hypertension; cardiac arrhythmias |
| Protonix [pantoprazole sodium] | | Proton pump inhibitor | Short-term treatment and maintenance therapy of erosive esophagitis associated with gastroesophageal reflux disease (GERD) |
| Protopic [tacrolimus] | Z79.621 | Calcineurin inhibitor | Atomic dermatitis (eczema) |
| Proventil-HFA [albuterol sulfate] | | Antiasthmatic/bronchodilator | Asthma |
| Provera [medroxyprogesterone acetate] | Z79.3, Z79.890 | Contraceptive; progestin; antineoplastic | Prevention of pregnancy; amenorrhea; carcinoma, endometrium, adjunct; carcinoma, renal; hemorrhage |
| Prozac [fluoxetine hydrochloride] | | Selective serotonin reuptake inhibitor (SSRI) | Bulimia nervosa; depression; obsessive-compulsive disorder |
| Pulmicort [budesonide] | Z79.51 | Corticosteroid – inhaled; antiasthmatic | Prophylaxis and treatment of asthma |
| Qalsody [tofersen] | | CNS agent | Amyotrophic lateral sclerosis |
| Qelbree [viloxazine hydrochloride] | | Selective norepinephrine reuptake inhibitor | Attention deficit hyperactivity disorder (ADHD) |
| Qnasl [beclomethasone dipropionate] | | Corticosteroid – intranasal | Perennial and seasonal allergies; vasomotor rhinitis |
| Qtern [dapagliflozin/saxagliptin] | Z79.84 | Oral hypoglycemic | Diabetes mellitus |
| Quinapril hydrochloride [quinapril hydrochloride] | | ACE inhibitor | Hypertension; heart failure |
| Qulipta [atogepant] | | Calcitonin gene-related peptide inhibitor | Migraine headache prevention |
| Quviviq [daridorexant hydrochloride] | | CNS depressant | Insomnia |
| Qvar Redihaler [beclomethasone dipropionate] | Z79.51 | Corticosteroid – inhaled; antiasthmatic | Prophylaxis and treatment of asthma |
| Raloxifene HCl [raloxifene hydrochloride] | Z79.810 | Selective estrogen receptor modulator (SERM) | Osteoporosis in postmenopausal women |
| Rapaflo [silodosin] | | Antiadrenergic | Benign prostatic hyperplasia |
| Rapamune [sirolimus] | Z79.623 | Mammalian target of rapamycin (mTOR) inhibitor | Prophylaxis of organ transplant rejection |
| Rayos [prednisone] | Z79.52 | Corticosteroid; antiasthmatic | Arthritis; blood disorders; allergies; asthma |
| Rebif [interferon beta-1a] | Z79.69 | Other immunosuppressant/ immunomodulator | Treatment of relapsing multiple sclerosis |
| Reclast [zoledronic acid] | Z79.83 | Bisphosphonate | Osteoporosis; Paget's disease; bone cancer |
| Relenza [zanamivir] | | Antiviral | Treat and prevent influenza A and B |
| Relyvrio [sodium phenylbutyrate/ taurursodiol] | | Central nervous system agent | Amyotrophic lateral sclerosis (ALS) |
| Remicade [infliximab] | Z79.620 | Immunosuppressive biologic; monoclonal antibody | Ankylosing spondylitis; psoriatic arthritis; rheumatoid arthritis; Crohn's disease; ulcerative colitis |
| Renvela [sevelamer carbonate] | | Phosphate binder | Chronic kidney disease (CKD) on dialysis |
| Repaglinide [repaglinide] | Z79.84 | Oral hypoglycemic | Diabetes mellitus |
| Restasis [cyclosporine ophthalmic emulsion] | Z79.621 | Calcineurin inhibitor | Ocular inflammation due to keratoconjunctivitis sicca |
| Restoril [temazepam] | | Sedative/hypnotic | Insomnia |
| Retrovir [zidovudine] | | Antiretroviral | HIV |

| Drug | Z Code | Drug Action/Classification | Indications |
|---|---|---|---|
| Revlimid [lenalidomide] | Z79.61 | Immunomodulator; antineoplastic | Multiple myeloma following autologous stem cell transplant; myelodysplastic syndromes; mantle cell lymphoma |
| Reyvow [lasmiditan] | | Antimigraine | Migraine headache |
| Rezzayo [rezafungin] | | Antifungal | Candidemia; invasive candidiasis |
| Rifadin [rifampin] | Z79.2 | Antibiotic | Tuberculosis |
| Rimactane [rifampin] | Z79.2 | Antibiotic | Tuberculosis |
| Rinvoq [upadacitinib] | Z79.622 | Janus kinase (JAK) inhibitor | Rheumatoid arthritis; psoriatic arthritis; ankylosing spondylitis; ulcerative colitis |
| Risperdal [risperidone] | | Antipsychotic/antimanic | Schizophrenia; bipolar I disorder |
| Ritalin [methylphenidate hydrochloride] | | CNS stimulant | Attention deficit hyperactivity disorder (ADHD); narcolepsy |
| Rituxan [rituximab] | Z79.620 | Immunosuppressive biologic; monoclonal antibody | Non-Hodgkin's lymphoma; chronic lymphocytic leukemia; rheumatoid arthritis; granulomatosis with polyangiitis; pemphigus vulgaris |
| Roxicodone [oxycodone hydrochloride] | Z79.891 | Analgesic, narcotic | Pain relief |
| Rukobia [fostemsavir tromethamine] | | Antiretroviral | HIV |
| Rybelsus [semaglutide] | Z79.84 | Oral hypoglycemic | Diabetes mellitus |
| Rystiggo [rozanolixizumab-noli] | | Antineoplastic | Myasthenia gravis |
| Ryzneuta [efbemalenograstim alfa-vuxw] | | Immunostimulant | Neutropenia |
| Sabril [vigabatrin] | | Anticonvulsant | Refractory complex partial seizures |
| Sandimmune [cyclosporine] | Z79.621 | Calcineurin inhibitor | Prophylaxis of organ transplant rejection |
| Savaysa [edoxaban tosylate] | Z79.01 | Anticoagulant | Prophylaxis and treatment of venous thrombosis, pulmonary embolism; prevention of blood clots due to atrial fibrillation |
| Scemblix [asciminib hydrochloride] | | Kinase inhibitor | Philadelphia chromosome-positive chronic myeloid leukemia |
| Seasonale [levonorgestrel/ethinyl estradiol] | Z79.3 | Contraceptive | Prevention of pregnancy |
| Seasonique [ethinyl estradiol/levonorgestrel] | Z79.3 | Contraceptive | Prevention of pregnancy |
| Septra [sulfamethoxazole trimethoprim] | Z79.2 | Antibiotic | Urinary tract infections; acute otitis media; acute exacerbations of chronic bronchitis; shigellosis |
| Serevent [salmeterol xinafoate] | | Bronchodilator | Asthma |
| Seromycin [cycloserine] | Z79.2 | Antibiotic | Tuberculosis; urinary tract infections |
| Seroquel XR [quetiapine fumarate] | | Antipsychotic | Schizophrenia; bipolar disorder; major depressive disorder |
| Silvadene [silver sulfadiazine] | Z79.2 | Antibiotic, topical | Wound sepsis due to second/third degree burns |
| Simulect [basiliximab] | Z79.620 | Immunosuppressive biologic; monoclonal antibody | Prophylaxis of organ transplant rejection |
| Sinemet [carbidopa/levodopa] | | Antiparkinsonism | Parkinson's disease |
| Singulair [montelukast sodium] | | Antiasthmatic | Asthma; exercise-induced bronchoconstriction; perennial and seasonal allergic rhinitis |
| Sirolimus [sirolimus] | Z79.623 | Mammalian target of rapamycin (mTOR) inhibitor | Prophylaxis of organ transplant rejection |
| Sitagliptin [sitagliptin/metformin hydrochloride] | Z79.84 | Oral hypoglycemic | Diabetes mellitus |
| Sivextro [tedizolid phosphate] | Z79.2 | Antibiotic | Skin infections including MRSA |
| Skyclarys [omaveloxolone] | | CNS stimulant | Friedrich's ataxia |
| Skyla [levonorgestrel] | Z79.3 | Contraceptive | Intrauterine device to prevent pregnancy |
| Skyrizi [risankizumab] | Z79.620 | Immunosuppressive biologic; monoclonal antibody | Plaque psoriasis |
| Sodium nitroprusside [sodium nitroprusside] | | Vasodilator | Hypertensive crisis; control surgical bleeding; acute congestive heart failure |
| Soliqua [insulin glargine/lixisenatide] | Z79.4 | Insulin | Diabetes mellitus |
| Solodyn [minocycline hydrochloride] | Z79.2 | Antibiotic | Bacterial infections |
| Solosec [secnidazole] | Z79.2 | Antibiotic | Bacterial vaginal inflammation; trichomoniasis |
| Soltamox [tamoxifen citrate] | Z79.810 | Selective estrogen receptor modulator (SERM) | Breast cancer |
| Solu-Cortef [hydrocortisone sodium succinate] | Z79.52 | Corticosteroid; antiasthmatic | Asthma; severe inflammation; allergic reactions |
| Solu-Medrol [methylprednisolone sodium succinate] | Z79.52 | Corticosteroid | Anti-inflammatory and antiallergenic for shock and ulcerative colitis |
| Sotyktu [deucravacitinib] | | Multikinase inhibitor | Plaque psoriasis |
| Spiriva [tiotropium bromide] | | Antiasthmatic/bronchodilator | Chronic obstructive pulmonary disease (COPD); asthma |
| Sprintec [norgestimate/ethinyl estradiol] | Z79.3 | Contraceptive | Prevention of pregnancy |
| Stelara [ustekinumab] | Z79.620 | Immunosuppressive biologic; monoclonal antibody | Plaque psoriasis; psoriatic arthritis; Crohn's disease; ulcerative colitis |

| Drug | Z Code | Drug Action/Classification | Indications |
|---|---|---|---|
| Strattera [atomoxetine hydrochloride] | | CNS stimulant | Attention deficit hyperactivity disorder (ADHD) |
| Streptomycin sulfate [streptomycin sulfate] | Z79.2 | Antibiotic | Severe bacterial infections |
| Suboxone [buprenorphine/naloxone] | | Opioid agonist | Treatment of opioid addiction |
| Sunlenca [lenacapavir] | | Antiretroviral | HIV |
| Supprelin LA [histrelin acetate] | Z79.818 | Agents affecting estrogen receptors and estrogen levels | Precocious puberty |
| Suprax [cefixime] | Z79.2 | Antibiotic | Bacterial infections |
| Sylatron [peginterferon alfa-2b] | Z79.69 | Other immunosuppressant/ immunomodulator | Prevention of recurrent malignant melanoma |
| Symbicort [budesonide/formoterol fumarate dihydrate] | Z79.51 | Corticosteroid – inhaled; antiasthmatic | Prophylaxis and treatment of asthma and COPD |
| Symbyax [olanzapine/fluoxetine] | | Antidepressant | Acute depressive episodes associated with bipolar I disorder; treatment-resistant depression |
| Symlin [pramlintide] | Z79.85 | Antidiabetic – non-insulin injectable | Diabetes mellitus |
| Symtuza [darunavir/cobicistat/emtricitabine/ tenofovir alafenamide] | | Antiretroviral | HIV |
| Synarel [nafarelin acetate] | Z79.818 | Agents affecting estrogen receptors and estrogen levels | Endometriosis symptoms; precocious puberty |
| Synercid [dalfopristin/quinupristin] | Z79.2 | Antibiotic | Severe blood infections |
| Synjardy [empagliflozin/metformin hydrochloride] | Z79.84 | Oral hypoglycemic | Diabetes mellitus |
| Synthroid [levothyroxine sodium] | Z79.890 | Thyroid hormone | Hypothyroidism |
| Tacrolimus [tacrolimus] | Z79.621 | Calcineurin inhibitor | Prophylaxis of organ transplant rejection |
| Talicia [omeprazole magnesium/ amoxicillin/ rifabutin] | Z79.2 | Combination antibiotic | Helicobacter pylori |
| Taltz [ixekizumab] | Z79.620 | Immunosuppressive biologic; monoclonal antibody | Plaque psoriasis; psoriatic arthritis; ankylosing spondylitis; axial spondyloarthritis |
| Talvey [talquetamab-tgvs] | | Antineoplastic | Multiple myeloma |
| Tamiflu [oseltamivir phosphate] | | Antiviral | Treatment and prevention of influenza A and B |
| Tamoxifen citrate [tamoxifen citrate] | Z79.810 | Selective estrogen receptor modulator (SERM) | Metastatic breast cancer in postmenopausal women |
| Tavneos [avacopan] | Z79.69 | Other immunosuppressant/ immunomodulator | ANCA-associated vasculitis |
| Taxotere [docetaxel] | Z79.633 | Mitotic inhibitor | Cancer |
| Tazicef [ceftazidime] | Z79.2 | Antibiotic | Confirmed or suspected bacterial infections |
| Teflaro [ceftaroline fosamil] | Z79.2 | Antibiotic | Bacterial skin infections; pneumonia |
| Tegretol [carbamazepine] | | Anticonvulsant; analgesic | Epilepsy, especially with complex symptomatology; specific analgesic for trigeminal neuralgia |
| Temozolomide [temozolomide] | Z79.630 | Chemotherapeutic alkylating agent | Chronic myelogenous leukemia |
| Tenormin [atenolol] | | Beta blocker | Angina pectoris; hypertension; acute myocardial infarction |
| Terazosin HCl [terazosin hydrochloride] | | Antiadrenergic | Benign prostatic hypertrophy; hypertension |
| Terlivaz [terlipressin] | | Antidiuretic hormone | Kidney function in hepatorenal syndrome |
| Testim [testosterone] | Z79.890 | Testosterone therapy – topical | Primary hypogonadism |
| Tetracycline [tetracycline] | Z79.2 | Antibiotic | Bacterial infections |
| Thalomid [thalidomide] | Z79.61 | Immunomodulator | Multiple myeloma; erythema nodosum leprosum |
| Tiazac [diltiazem hydrochloride] | | Calcium channel blocker | Chronic stable angina; atrial fibrillation; atrial flutter; hypertension; paroxysmal supraventricular tachycardia |
| Tobradex [tobramycin/dexamethasone] | | Aminoglycoside ocular anti-infective; anti-inflammatory | Infectious conjunctivitis; dermatosis, corticosteroid-responsive with secondary infection; foreign body in eye; corneal inflammation; uveitis |
| Tobramycin [dexamethasone/tobramycin] | Z79.2 | Antibiotic | Bacterial eye infections |
| Topamax [topiramate] | | Anticonvulsant | Epilepsy; primary generalized tonic-clonic seizures; seizures associated with Lennox-Gastaut syndrome; migraine headache |
| Toprol-XL [metoprolol succinate] | | Beta blocker | Angina pectoris; hypertension |
| Toremifene citrate [toremifene citrate] | Z79.810 | Selective estrogen receptor modulator (SERM) | Metastatic breast cancer in postmenopausal women |
| Torisel [temsirolimus] | Z79.623 | Mammalian target of rapamycin (mTOR) inhibitor | Renal cell carcinoma |
| Toujeo Solostar [insulin glargine recombinant] | Z79.4 | Insulin | Diabetes mellitus |
| Tradjenta [linagliptin] | Z79.84 | Oral hypoglycemic | Diabetes mellitus |
| Trazodone HCl [trazodone hydrochloride] | | Antidepressant | Depression |

| Drug | Z Code | Drug Action/Classification | Indications |
|---|---|---|---|
| Trelegy Ellipta [fluticasone furoate/umeclidinium bromide/vilanterol trifenatate] | Z79.51 | Corticosteroid – inhaled; antiasthmatic | COPD |
| Trelstar [triptorelin pamoate] | Z79.818 | Agents affecting estrogen receptors and estrogen levels | Palliative treatment of prostate cancer symptoms |
| Tremfya [guselkumab] | Z79.620 | Immunosuppressive biologic; monoclonal antibody | Plaque psoriasis |
| Tresiba [insulin degludec] | Z79.4 | Insulin | Diabetes mellitus |
| Triamterene and hydrochlorothiazide [triamterene/ hydrochlorothiazide] | | Antihypertensive; diuretic | Edema; hypertension |
| Trijardy XR [empagliflozin/linagliptin/metformin hydrochloride] | Z79.84 | Oral hypoglycemic | Diabetes mellitus |
| Tri-Lo-Estarylla [ethinyl estradiol/norgestimate] | Z79.3 | Contraceptive | Prevention of pregnancy |
| Tri-Lo-Sprintec [ethinyl estradiol/norgestimate] | Z79.3 | Contraceptive | Prevention of pregnancy |
| Trimethoprim [trimethoprim] | Z79.2 | Antibiotic | Acute exacerbation chronic bronchitis; travelers' diarrhea; infections of the middle, lower respiratory tract, and urinary tract; pneumonia, pneumocystis; shigellosis |
| Triptodur [triptorelin] | Z79.818 | Agents affecting estrogen receptors and estrogen levels | Precocious puberty |
| Tri-Sprintec [ethinyl estradiol/norgestimate] | Z79.3 | Contraceptive | Prevention of pregnancy; acne |
| Trokendi XR [topiramate] | | Anticonvulsant | Epilepsy; primary generalized tonic-clonic seizures; seizures associated with Lennox-Gastaut syndrome; migraine headache |
| Trulicity [dulaglutide] | Z79.85 | Antidiabetic – non-insulin injectable | Diabetes mellitus |
| Truqap [capivasertib] | | Antineoplastic; kinase inhibitor | Breast cancer |
| Truvada [emtricitabine/tenofovir disoproxil fumarate] | | Antiretroviral | HIV |
| Turalio [pexidartinib] | | Kinase inhibitor | Symptomatic tenosynovial giant cell tumor |
| Tygacil [tigecycline] | Z79.2 | Antibiotic | Bacterial skin or digestive system infections; pneumonia |
| Tzield [teplizumab-mzwv] | Z79.85 | Antidiabetic – non-insulin injectable | Delay onset of stage 3 type 1 diabetes |
| Ubrelvy [ubrogepant] | | Calcitonin gene-related peptide inhibitor | Migraine headache |
| Unasyn [ampicillin sodium/sulbactam sodium] | Z79.2 | Antibiotic | Bacterial infections |
| Vabomere [meropenem; vaborbactam] | Z79.2 | Antibiotic | Complicated urinary tract infections; pyelonephritis |
| Vabysmo [faricimab-svoa] | | Anti-angiogenic ophthalmic agent | Neovascular age-related macular degeneration; diabetic macular edema |
| Vagifem [estradiol] | Z79.890 | Estrogen therapy | Menopause symptoms |
| Valium [diazepam] | | Antianxiety; muscle relaxant; anticonvulsant | Anxiety, tension, withdrawal from alcohol; muscle spasms and anticonvulsant therapy; epilepsy, generalized tonic-clonic; status epilepticus; stiff-person syndrome; tetanus |
| Vancocin HCl [vancomycin hydrochloride] | Z79.2 | Antibiotic | Severe bacterial infections |
| Vancomycin HCl [vancomycin hydrochloride] | Z79.2 | Antibiotic | Severe bacterial infections |
| Vanflyta [quizartinib] | | Kinase inhibitor | Acute myeloid leukemia |
| Varenicline tartrate [varenicline tartrate] | | Smoking cessation aid | Nicotine addiction; smoking |
| Vasotec [enalaprilat maleate] | | ACE inhibitor | Congestive heart failure; hypertension |
| Velivet [desogestrel/ethinyl estradiol] | Z79.3 | Contraceptive | Prevention of pregnancy |
| Velsipity [etrasimod] | | Anti-inflammatory | Ulcerative colitis |
| Venlafaxine HCl [venlafaxine hydrochloride] | | Antidepressant, serotonin and norepinephrine reuptake inhibitor (SNRI) | Major depressive disorder; social anxiety disorder; panic disorder |
| Ventolin HFA [albuterol sulfate] | | Antiasthmatic/bronchodilator | Asthma |
| Veozah [fezolinetant] | | CNS agent | Menopause symptoms |
| Verapamil HCL [verapamil hydrochloride] | | Calcium channel blocker | Angina pectoris; chronic stable angina; atrial fibrillation; atrial flutter; paroxysmal supraventricular tachycardia; ventricular arrhythmia; hypertension |
| Viagra [sildenafil citrate] | | Phosphodiesterase-5 (PDE5) inhibitor | Erectile dysfunction |
| Vibativ [telavancin hydrochloride] | Z79.2 | Antibiotic | Pneumonia; severe bacterial skin infections |
| Vibramycin [doxycycline calcium] | Z79.2 | Antibiotic | Bacterial infections |
| Victoza [liraglutide] | Z79.85 | Antidiabetic – non-insulin injectable | Diabetes mellitus |
| Vinblastine sulfate [vinblastine sulfate] | Z79.633 | Mitotic inhibitor | Cancer |
| Vincristine sulfate PFS [vincristine sulfate] | Z79.633 | Mitotic inhibitor | Cancer |
| Virazole [ribavirin] | | Antiviral | Respiratory syncytial virus (RSV) |
| Viread [tenofovir disoproxil fumarate] | | Antiretroviral | HIV; chronic hepatitis B |

| Drug | Z Code | Drug Action/Classification | Indications |
|---|---|---|---|
| Voltaren Arthritis Pain [diclofenac sodium] | Z79.1 | Nonsteroidal anti-inflammatory drug (NSAID) | Treatment of pain, inflammation, and joint stiffness due to arthritis |
| Vonjo [pacritinib] | | Multikinase inhibitor | Treats intermediate or high-risk primary or secondary myelofibrosis in adults with low platelets |
| Voquezna [vonoprazan, amoxicillin, and clarithromycin] | Z79.2 | Antibiotic, antimicrobial; potassium-competitive acid blocker | Helicobacter pylori |
| Vtama [tapinarof] | | Topical antipsoriatic | Plaque psoriasis |
| Vumerity [diroximel fumarate] | Z79.69 | Other immunosuppressant/ immunomodulator | Relapsing forms of multiple sclerosis (MS) |
| Vytorin [ezetimibe/simvastatin] | | HMG-CoA reductase inhibitor (statin); cholesterol absorption inhibitor | Hyperlipidemia; hypercholesterolemia |
| Wakix [pitolisant hydrochloride] | | CNS stimulant | Narcolepsy |
| Warfarin sodium [warfarin sodium] | Z79.01 | Anticoagulant | Prophylaxis and treatment of venous thrombosis; treatment of atrial fibrillation with embolization (pulmonary embolism), arrhythmias, myocardial infarction, and stroke prevention |
| Wellbutrin SR, Wellbutrin XL [bupropion hydrochloride] | | Antidepressant | Depression |
| Xacduro [sulbactam, durlobactam] | Z79.2 | Antibiotic | Hospital-acquired bacterial pneumonia and ventilator-associated bacterial pneumonia caused by Acinetobacter baumannii-calcoaceticus complex |
| Xalatan [latanoprost] | | Prostaglandin F2? analogue | Glaucoma, open-angle; ocular hypertension |
| Xanax, Xanax XR [alprazolam] | | Antianxiety; sedative/hypnotic | Anxiety disorders with panic disorder and depression |
| Xarelto [rivaroxaban] | Z79.01 | Anticoagulant | Prophylaxis and treatment of venous thrombosis, pulmonary embolism; prevention of blood clots due to atrial fibrillation |
| Xdemvy [lotilaner] | | Antiparasitic | Demodex blepharitis |
| Xeljanz, Xeljanz XR [tofacitinib citrate] | Z79.622 | Janus kinase (JAK) inhibitor | Rheumatoid arthritis; psoriatic arthritis |
| Xeloda [capecitabine] | Z79.631 | Antimetabolite agent | Cancer of the breast, colon, colorectal |
| Xelstrym [dextroamphetamine] | | CNS stimulant | Attention deficit hyperactivity disorder (ADHD) |
| Xenleta [lefamulin acetate] | Z79.2 | Antibiotic | Community-acquired bacterial pneumonia |
| Xgeva [denosumab] | Z79.620 | Immunosuppressive biologic; monoclonal antibody | Treatment and prevention of bone resorption and prevention of bone fracture |
| Xifaxan [rifaximin] | Z79.2 | Antibiotic | E. coli diarrhea |
| Xigduo XR [dapagliflozin/metformin hydrochloride] | Z79.84 | Oral hypoglycemic | Diabetes mellitus |
| Xpovio [selinexor] | | Antineoplastic | Multiple myeloma in adults |
| Xulane [ethinyl estradiol/norelgestromin] | Z79.3 | Contraceptive | Prevention of pregnancy |
| Xultophy 100/3.6 [insulin degludec/ liraglutide] | Z79.4 | Insulin | Diabetes mellitus |
| Xyrem [sodium oxybate] | | CNS depressant; anxiolytic/sedative/hypnotic | Cataplexy and/or excessive daytime sleepiness in narcolepsy |
| Xyzal Allergy 24Hr [levocetirizine dihydrochloride] | | Antihistamine | Perennial allergic rhinitis; chronic idiopathic urticaria |
| Yasmin [drospirenone/ethinyl estradiol] | Z79.3 | Contraceptive | Prevention of pregnancy |
| Yaz [drospirenone/ethinyl estradiol] | Z79.3 | Contraceptive | Prevention of pregnancy; menstrual disorders |
| Zavzpret [zavegepant] | | Calcitonin gene-related peptide inhibitor | Migraine headache |
| Zerbaxa [ceftolozane sulfate/tazobactam sodium] | Z79.2 | Antibiotic | Complicated urinary tract and intra-abdominal infections |
| Zestoretic [lisinopril/hydrochlorothiazide] | | ACE inhibitor | Congestive heart failure; hypertension |
| Zestril [lisinopril] | | ACE inhibitor | Congestive heart failure; hypertension |
| Zetia [ezetimibe] | | Antihyperlipidemic | Hypercholesterolemia; sitosterolemia |
| Ziac [bisoprolol fumarate/ hydrochlorothiazide] | | Antihypertensive | Hypertension |
| Zilbrysq [zilucoplan] | Z79.69 | Other immunosuppressant/ immunomodulator | Myasthenia gravis |
| Zipsor [diclofenac potassium] | Z79.1 | Nonsteroidal anti-inflammatory drug (NSAID) | Pain and inflammation relief |
| Zithromax [azithromycin] | Z79.2 | Antibiotic | Infections of the cervix, lower respiratory tract, skin and skin structures, urethra, nongonococcal; mycobacterium avium complex; pharyngitis, streptococcal pneumonia; tonsillitis |
| Zocor [simvastatin] | | HMG-CoA reductase inhibitor (statin) | Hypercholesterolemia; hyperlipidemia; hyperlipoproteinemia; hypertriglyceridemia |
| Zoladex [goserelin acetate] | Z79.818 | Agents affecting estrogen receptors and estrogen levels | Palliative treatment of prostate cancer and breast cancer symptoms; endometriosis |
| Zoloft [sertraline hydrochloride] | | Antidepressant | Anxiety with panic disorder and depression; obsessive-compulsive disorder |

| Drug | Z Code | Drug Action/Classification | Indications |
|---|---|---|---|
| Zometa [zoledronic acid] | Z79.83 | Bisphosphonate | Multiple myeloma; Paget's disease |
| Zortress [everolimus] | Z79.623 | Mammalian target of rapamycin (mTOR) inhibitor | Prophylaxis of organ transplant rejection |
| Zovia 1/50E-28 [ethinyl estradiol/ethynodiol diacetate] | Z79.3 | Contraceptive | Prevention of pregnancy |
| Zovirax [acyclovir] | | Antiviral | Genital herpes and herpes zoster infections |
| Zubsolv [buprenorphine/naloxone] | | Opioid agonist | Treatment of opioid addiction |
| Zurzuvae [zuranolone] | | CNS agent | Postpartum depression |
| Zyloprim [allopurinol] | | Antigout | Gouty arthritis; renal calculus; hyperuricemia; hyperuricemia secondary to leukemia; hyperuricemia secondary to lymphoma |
| Zynyz [retifanlimab-dlwr] | Z79.60 | Immune checkpoint inhibitor; immunosuppressant | Merkel cell carcinoma |
| Zyprexa [olanzapine] | | Antipsychotic/antimanic | Psychotic disorders; schizophrenia |
| Zyrtec allergy [cetirizine hydrochloride] | | Antihistamine | Perennial and seasonal allergic rhinitis; chronic urticaria |
| Zyvox [linezolid] | Z79.2 | Antibiotic | Severe bacterial infections |

# Appendix C: Z Codes for Long-Term Drug Use with Associated Drugs

This resource correlates the Z codes that are used to identify current long-term drug use with a list of drugs that are typically categorized to that class of drug. These lists are not all-inclusive, providing only the more commonly used drugs.

**Z79.Ø1 Long term (current) use of anticoagulants**
Arixtra
Defencath
Eliquis
Fragmin
Heparin
Jantoven
Lovenox
Pradaxa
Savaysa
Warfarin
Xarelto

**Z79.Ø2 Long term (current) use of antithrombotics/antiplatelets**
Aggrastat
Angiomax
Argatroban
Brilinta
Clopidogrel bisulfate
Effient
Eptifibatide
Persantine
Plavix
Prasugrel

**Z79.1 Long term (current) use of non-steroidal anti-inflammatories (NSAID)**
Advil
Aleve
Anaprox DS
Arthrotec
Caldolor
Cambia
Celebrex
Daypro
Duexis
Feldene
Ibuprofen
Indocin
Mobic
Motrin IB
Nabumetone
Nalfon
Naprelan
Naprosyn
NeoProfen
Ponstel
Voltaren Arthritis Pain
Zipsor

**Z79.2 Long term (current) use of antibiotics**
Altabax
Amikacin
Amoxicillin
Ampicillin
Augmentin
Avelox
Azactam
Azithromycin
Bactrim
Biaxin XL
Cefazolin sodium
Cefepime hydrochloride
Cefprozil
Ceftriaxone
Cefuroxime sodium
Centany
Cephalexin
Cipro
Ciprofloxacin
Clarithromycin
Cleocin
Clindamycin
Daptomycin
Dificid
Doxycycline
E.E.S.
Ertapenem
ERYC
Erygel
EryPed
Ery-Tab
Erythrocin
Erythromycin
Fetroja
Flagyl
Gentamicin sulfate
Hiprex
Invanz
Isoniazid
Klaron
Lincocin
Macrobid
Macrodantin
Mepron
Merrem
Metronidazole
Minocin
Monodox
Monurol
Mycobutin
Nebupent
Neosporin
Nitrofurantoin
Oracea
Orbactiv
Penicillin-VK
Pentam
Pfizerpen
Priftin
Primaxin
Rifadin
Rimactane
Septra
Seromycin
Silvadene
Sivextro
Solodyn
Solosec
Streptomycin sulfate
Suprax
Synercid
Talicia
Tazicef
Teflaro
Tetracycline
Tobramycin
Trimethoprim
Tygacil
Unasyn
Vabomere
Vancocin HCl
Vancomycin HCl
Vibativ
Vibramycin
Voquezna
Xacduro
Xenleta
Xifaxan
Zerbaxa
Zithromax
Zyvox

**Z79.3 Long term (current) use of hormonal contraceptives**
Aranelle
Aviane-28
Beyaz
Briellyn
Camila
Daysee
Depo-Provera
Depo-SubQ Provera
Desogestrel/ethinyl estradiol
Enpresse-28
Femhrt
Gildagia
Gildess 24 FE
Junel
Levonest
Liletta
Lo Loestrin Fe
Loryna
LoSeasonique
Low-Ogestrel-28
Mirena
Mono-Linyah
Natazia
Nexplanon
NuvaRing
Plan B One-Step
Provera
Seasonale
Seasonique
Skyla
Sprintec
Tri-Lo-Estarylla
Tri-Lo-Sprintec
Tri-Sprintec
Velivet
Xulane
Yasmin
Yaz
Zovia 1/50E-28

**Z79.4 Long term (current) use of insulin**
Admelog
Apidra
Basaglar
Fiasp
Humalog
Humulin R
Lantus
Levemir
Novolin
Novolog
Soliqua
Toujeo Solostar
Tresiba
Xultophy 100/3.6

**Z79.51 Long term (current) use of inhaled steroids**
Advair
AirDuo RespiClick
Alvesco
Arnuity Ellipta
Asmanex
Breo Ellipta
Dulera
Flovent HFA
Pulmicort
Qvar Redihaler
Symbicort
Trelegy Ellipta

**Z79.52 Long term (current) use of systemic steroids**
Agamree
Celestone Soluspan
Colocort
Cortef
Cortenema
Cortifoam
Depo-Medrol
Dexamethasone Intensol
Entocort EC
Hydrocortisone
Kenalog-10
Kenalog-40
Locoid
Medrol
Methylprednisolone
Orapred ODT
PediaPred
Prednisolone
Prednisone
Rayos
Solu-Cortef
Solu-Medrol

**Z79.61 Long term (current) use of immunomodulator**
Otezla
Pomalyst
Revlimid
Thalomid

**Z79.62Ø Long term (current) use of immunosuppressive biologic**
Actemra
Aimovig
Beyfortus
Briumvi
Columvi
Cosentyx
Cyltezo
Dupixent
Elrexfio
Enbrel
Entyvio
Epkinly
Humira
Hyrimoz
Imjudo
Keytruda
Loqtorzi
Monoclonal antibodies
Omvoh
Prolia
Remicade
Rituxan
Simulect
Skyrizi
Stelara
Taltz
Tremfya
Xgeva

**Z79.621 Long term (current) use of calcineurin inhibitor**
Astagraf XL
Cyclosporine
Envarsus XR
Gengraf
Lupkynis
Neoral
Prograf
Protopic
Restasis
Sandimmune
Tacrolimus

**Z79.622 Long term (current) use of Janus kinase inhibitor**
Cibinqo
Ojjaara
Olumiant
Rinvoq
Xeljanz
Xeljanz XR

**Z79.623 Long term (current) use of mammalian target of rapamycin (mTOR) inhibitor**
Rapamune
Sirolimus
Torisel
Zortress

**Z79.624 Long term (current) use of inhibitors of nucleotide synthesis**
CellCept
Imuran

**Z79.630 Long term (current) use of alkylating agent**
Busulfex
Carmustine
Chlorambucil
Cisplatin
Cytoxan
Leukeran
Temozolomide

**Z79.631 Long term (current) use of antimetabolite agent**
5-fluorouracil (5-FU)
6-mercaptopurine (6-MP)
Cytarabine
Methotrexate sodium
Xeloda

**Z79.632 Long term (current) use of antitumor antibiotic**
Bleomycin
Cerubidine
Doxorubicin
Mitomycin

**Z79.633 Long term (current) use of mitotic inhibitor**
Ixempra
Paclitaxel
Taxotere
Vinblastine sulfate
Vincristine sulfate PFS

**Z79.634 Long term (current) use of topoisomerase inhibitor**
Camptosar
Etoposide
Hycamtin

**Z79.64 Long term (current) use of myelosuppressive agent**
Hydroxyurea

**Z79.69 Long term (current) use of other immunomodulators and immunosuppressants**
Actimmune
Avonex
Betaseron
Bimzelx-bkzx
Copaxone
Enjaymo
Intron A
Orencia
PegIntron
Ponvory
Rebif
Sylatron
Tavneos
Vumerity
Zilbrysq
Zynyz

**Z79.810 Long term (current) use of selective estrogen receptor modulators (SERMs)**
Evista
Fareston
Osphena
Raloxifene HCl
Soltamox
Tamoxifen citrate
Toremifene citrate

**Z79.811 Long term (current) use of aromatase inhibitors**
Anastrozole
Arimidex
Aromasin
Exemestane
Femara
Letrozole

**Z79.818 Long term (current) use of other agents affecting estrogen receptors and estrogen levels**
Eligard
Faslodex
Lupron Depot
Megace ES
Orserdu
Supprelin LA
Synarel
Trelstar
Triptodur
Zoladex

**Z79.82 Long term (current) use of aspirin**
Bayer
Bufferin
Durlaza

**Z79.83 Long term (current) use of bisphosphonates**
Aclasta
Actonel
Aredia
Atelvia
Binosto
Fosamax
Reclast
Zometa

**Z79.84 Long term (current) use of oral hypoglycemic drugs**
Acarbose
Actoplus Met
Actos
Amaryl
Brenzavvy
DiaBeta
Duetact
Farxiga
Glimepiride
Glucotrol XL
Glumetza
Glyburide
Glynase
Glyset
Invokamet
Invokana
Janumet
Januvia
Jentadueto
Kazano
Kombiglyze
Metformin
Oseni
Qtern
Repaglinide
Rybelsus
Sitagliptin
Synjardy
Tradjenta
Trijardy XR
Xigduo XR

**Z79.85 Long-term (current) use of injectable non-insulin antidiabetic drugs**
Bydureon bcise
Byetta
Mounjaro
Ozempic
Symlin
Trulicity
Tzield
Victoza

**Z79.890 Hormone replacement therapy**
Activella
Alora
Androderm
AndroGel
Angeliq
Bijuva
Climara
CombiPatch
Delestrogen
Divigel
Duavee
Elestrin
Estrace
EstroGel
Femhrt
Femring
Firmagon
Levoxyl
Menest
Menostar
Minivelle
Orilissa
Prempro
Provera
Synthroid
Testim
Vagifem

**Z79.891 Long term (current) use of opiate analgesic**
Acetaminophen with codeine
Buprenorphine HCl and Naloxone HCl
Butrans
Codeine
Demerol
Dilaudid
Duramorph PF
Fentanyl citrate
Fentora
Fioricet with codeine
Hydrocodone
Hydrocodone bitartrate and acetaminophen
Hydromorphone HCl
Methadone HCl
Methadose
Morphine sulfate
MS Contin
Nucynta
Oxycodone HCl
OxyContin
Percocet
Roxicodone

# Appendix D: Z Codes Only as Principal/First-Listed Diagnosis

ZØØ.ØØ
ZØØ.Ø1
ZØØ.11Ø
ZØØ.111
ZØØ.121
ZØØ.129
ZØØ.2
ZØØ.3
ZØØ.5
ZØØ.7Ø
ZØØ.71
ZØØ.8
ZØ1.ØØ
ZØ1.Ø1
ZØ1.Ø2Ø
ZØ1.Ø21
ZØ1.1Ø
ZØ1.11Ø
ZØ1.118
ZØ1.12
ZØ1.2Ø
ZØ1.21
ZØ1.3Ø
ZØ1.31
ZØ1.411
ZØ1.419
ZØ1.42
ZØ1.81Ø
ZØ1.811
ZØ1.812
ZØ1.818
ZØ1.82
ZØ1.83
ZØ1.84
ZØ1.89
ZØ2.Ø
ZØ2.1
ZØ2.2
ZØ2.3
ZØ2.4
ZØ2.5
ZØ2.6
ZØ2.71
ZØ2.79
ZØ2.81
ZØ2.82
ZØ2.83
ZØ2.84
ZØ2.89
ZØ2.9
ZØ4.1
ZØ4.2
ZØ4.3
ZØ4.41
ZØ4.42
ZØ4.6
ZØ4.71
ZØ4.72
ZØ4.81
ZØ4.82
ZØ4.89
ZØ4.9
Z31.81
Z31.83
Z31.84
Z33.2
Z34.ØØ
Z34.Ø1
Z34.Ø2
Z34.Ø3
Z34.8Ø
Z34.81
Z34.82
Z34.83
Z34.9Ø
Z34.91
Z34.92
Z34.93
Z38.ØØ
Z38.Ø1
Z38.1
Z38.2
Z38.3Ø
Z38.31
Z38.4
Z38.5
Z38.61
Z38.62
Z38.63
Z38.64
Z38.65
Z38.66
Z38.68
Z38.69
Z38.7
Z38.8
Z39.Ø
Z39.1
Z39.2
Z4Ø.ØØ
Z4Ø.Ø1
Z4Ø.Ø2
Z4Ø.Ø3
Z4Ø.Ø9
Z4Ø.81
Z4Ø.82
Z4Ø.89
Z4Ø.9
Z42.1
Z42.8
Z51.Ø
Z51.11
Z51.12
Z52.ØØØ
Z52.ØØ1
Z52.ØØ8
Z52.Ø1Ø
Z52.Ø11
Z52.Ø18
Z52.Ø9Ø
Z52.Ø91
Z52.Ø98
Z52.1Ø
Z52.11
Z52.19
Z52.2Ø
Z52.21
Z52.29
Z52.3
Z52.4
Z52.5
Z52.6
Z52.81Ø
Z52.811
Z52.812
Z52.813
Z52.819
Z52.89
Z76.1
Z76.2
Z99.12

Appendix D: Z Codes Only as Principal/First-Listed Diagnosis

# Appendix E: Centers for Medicare & Medicaid Services Hierarchical Condition Categories (CMS-HCC)

In the 1970s, Medicare began demonstration projects that contracted with health maintenance organizations (HMOs) to provide care for Medicare beneficiaries in exchange for prospective payments. In 1985, this project changed from demonstration status to a regular part of the Medicare program, Medicare Part C. The Balanced Budget Act (BBA) of 1997 named Medicare's Part C managed care program Medicare+Choice, and the Medicare Modernization Act (MMA) of 2003 again renamed it to Medicare Advantage (MA).

Medicare is one of the world's largest health insurance programs, and about one-third of the beneficiaries on Medicare are enrolled in an MA private health care plan. Due to the great variance in the health status of Medicare beneficiaries, risk adjustment provides a means of adequately compensating those plans with large numbers of seriously ill patients while not overburdening other plans that have healthier individuals. Medicare Advantage (MA) plans have been using the Hierarchical Condition Category (HCC) risk adjustment model since 2004.

## The Risk Adjustment Model

The primary purpose of a risk adjustment model is to predict (on average) the future health care costs for specific consortiums enrolled in Medicare Advantage (MA) health plans. CMS is then able to provide capitation payments to these private health plans. Capitation payments are an incentive for health plans to enroll not only healthier individuals but those with chronic conditions or who are more seriously ill by removing some of the financial burden.

The MA risk adjustment model uses HCCs to assess the disease burden of its enrollees. HCC diagnostic groupings were created after examining claims data so that enrollees with similar disease processes, and consequently similar health care expenditures, could be pooled into a larger data set in which an average expenditure rate could be determined. The medical conditions included in HCC categories are those that were determined to most predictably affect the health status and health care costs of any individual. Several important principles to the risk adjustment model and the development of the HCC categories include but are not limited to:

1. The HCC diagnostic categories should be clinically meaningful.
   - Diagnostic categories are well-defined.
   - Clinically specific diseases or medical conditions are grouped to each category.
2. The HCC diagnostic categories should predict medical expenditures.
   - The diagnoses grouped to a specific category should have as close to the same cost burden not only in the current year but also in the future.
3. The HCC diagnostic categories should have adequate sample sizes and discretionary categories excluded to be as accurate and stable in their estimate of costs as possible.
   - A diagnostic category that groups extremely rare diseases or conditions would not be reliably effective in determining current or future costs.
   - Codes that are not credible as cost predictors or may be subject to coding variation should be excluded, when possible.
4. The HCC diagnostic categories should be both hierarchical and additive.
   - Hierarchical measurement is used within a specific disease process.
   - Disease processes that are unrelated to each other are measured additively.
5. The diagnostic classification should encourage specificity and should not reward coding proliferation.
   - More diagnosis codes and vague diagnosis codes do not equal greater disease burden.

Beginning in CY 2024, CMS finalized implementing a revised version of the CMS-HCC risk-adjustment model. This model was phased-in with completion in CY2026 and incorporates all of the following:

- Updated data years used for model calibration
- Updated denominator year used in determining the average per capita predicted expenditures to create relative factors in the model
- A clinical reclassification of the hierarchical condition categories (HCCs) using ICD-10-CM codes

The CMS-HCC v28 model has 115 payment HCCs resulting in more appropriate relative weights because they reflect more recent utilization, coding, and expenditure patterns. Beneficiary risk scores or plan average risk scores may change depending on each individual beneficiary's combination of diagnoses or the clinical profile of a plan's enrollee population.

## Risk Adjustment Factors

The CMS-HCC risk adjustment model uses "risk adjustment factors" to calculate a risk score for each member. This score summarizes that particular patient's expected cost of care relative to other members'. Each member's risk score is based on demographic and health status information and is calculated as the sum of these demographic and health factors weighted by their estimated marginal contributions to total risk. The model also takes into account where the patient resides (community or institutional), Medicaid eligibility (full or partial benefits), the patient's Medicare enrollment status (new or established), age, disability status, whether the patient is frail or has end-stage renal disease (ESRD), and even prescription drug use.

No procedure codes, ICD-10-PCS or CPT, are included in the MA risk adjustment model. The model relies solely on diagnostic and demographic data. Not all ICD-10-CM diagnoses map to an HCC, and there is no specific code sequencing involved. The CMS-HCC model is additive as well as hierarchical. The additive functionality allows a patient to have more than one HCC category assigned, providing a more complete clinical picture and prediction of resource consumption. The hierarchical aspect of the model provides a means of ranking diagnoses that are similar in disease process, by severity. The hierarchy of the condition categories ensures the patient's conditions are classified to the most severe condition within the related group. Less severe conditions within a particular hierarchy are superseded by more severe diagnoses within the same group. The hierarchy and additive relationship permits this model to characterize the person's illness level within each disease process, while still allowing the effects of unrelated disease processes to be counted in the patient's overall score.

Certain combinations of coexisting diagnoses for an individual can increase medical costs. The CMS-HCC model adjusts for these higher costs by the addition of "disease interaction" factors. For each patient, multiple HCCs assigned, along with demographic and disease interaction factors, are used to calculate a single, combined risk adjustment factor (RAF). The RAF score for an individual member represents all of the HCCs that have been submitted from all sources for that member to CMS during the course of an entire calendar year.

There are separate CMS-HCC models for new enrollees and continuing enrollees. The new enrollee model uses demographic factors only, such as age, sex, and disability status, and is used when the enrollee has less than 12 months of medical history. The community model accounts for age, sex, original reason for Medicare entitlement (age or disability), Medicaid eligibility, and clinical conditions as measured by HCCs. In the second step, expected costs are adjusted for outliers based on the member's risk score and whether the patient has ESRD.

Demographic data (age, sex, eligibility) as well as health status (diagnoses codes submitted on claims to CMS) of an MA population are used to determine the reimbursement to the health plan to care for their members.

CMS considers a RAF score of 1.0 as the benchmark to indicate the score of the average healthy patient with the same demographic and diagnostic factors. These patients are expected to use average or lower-than-average resources. When the RAF score is higher than 1.0, CMS considers the patient to be sicker than the average patient with the same criteria and expects greater-than-average resource utilization. Beginning in PY2026 100% of the RAF score will be based on the 2024 CMS-HCC model.

A low RAF score may accurately indicate a healthier patient, but it may also falsely indicate a healthier patient due to incomplete or inaccurate coding, incomplete or insufficient record documentation, or patients who fail to complete an annual assessment.

A high RAF score may accurately indicate a sicker patient, or it may be falsely inflated from overcoding due to diagnoses that are reported but not documented, or from copying and pasting from previous encounters or problem lists of resolved conditions.

## Documentation Requirements

Payment is made per HCC category (not per diagnosis code). No matter how many times in the year the diagnosis codes are reported, a single payment is made to the MA plan each year. Each year the list of HCCs and the RAF for each patient is "reset." This means the annual health assessment is extremely important, and adequate documentation is critical. Accurate risk adjustment payment relies on complete medical record documentation and diagnosis coding. CMS requires that all applicable diagnosis codes be reported and that all diagnoses be reported to the highest level of specificity and that these be substantiated by the medical record.

> CMS's Guiding Principle:
> The risk adjustment diagnosis must be based on clinical medical record documentation from a face-to-face encounter, coded according to the *ICD-10-CM Guidelines for Coding and Reporting*; assigned based on dates of service within the data collection period, submitted to the MA organization from an appropriate risk adjustment provider type and an appropriate risk adjustment physician data source.

A "face-to-face" health service encounter between a patient and healthcare provider describes an encounter between the patient and the provider (MD, DO), including qualified nonphysician practitioners (NPP) (e.g., nurse practitioner or physician's assistant), which is face-to-face with the patient. CMS provides a current listing of acceptable physician specialty types for risk adjustment data submission within the 2012 Regional Technical Assistance Participant Guide. The only exception to the face-to-face encounter requirement is pathology services (professional component only). Due to the 2019 Coronavirus Disease (COVID-19) pandemic, CMS is allowing MA organizations to submit diagnoses from telehealth services that meet the risk adjustment face-to-face requirement when the services are provided using interactive audio and video telecommunications systems that permit real-time interactive communication. Currently, CMS does not provide a listing of all services that are considered face-to-face visits for risk adjustment data, but does provide guidance on what types of services are not acceptable for risk adjustment in the Participant Guide. For example, diagnostic radiology does not qualify because diagnostic radiologists typically do not document confirmed diagnoses. Other examples of services that are not acceptable include diagnostic reports that have not been interpreted, such as laboratory reports. Beginning in CY 2027, CMS finalized the proposal to exclude diagnoses identified as audio-only services using modifier "93" or "FQ". These services do not meet the face-to-face requirement for risk adjustment reporting.

It is essential that the medical record documentation show evidence by provider authentication that the direct face-to-face service was personally furnished by the physician or qualified NPP. Examples of these services include office visits, hospital visits, preoperative anesthesia assessment, and surgical and invasive procedures.

Risk adjustment relies on annual health information. Each enrollee is assigned an individual risk score based on the health status information obtained from the diagnosis codes on the claims. The CMS-HCC model relies on ICD-10-CM coding specificity for accurate risk adjustment by using the most specific code available that is substantiated by the documentation in the medical record. Providers should fully document and accurately code the evaluation and management of all severe and chronic conditions to ensure a full, complete, and accurate clinical record of the patient's condition and reflect the work involved in caring for the patient, particularly those with complex and challenging health issues. All conditions affecting the treatment or management of the patient's health should be documented at least once a year, as applicable to care provided, to accurately describe the true complexity and severity of the patient's health. If the diagnosis coding on the claim is not accurate or complete, the claim may indicate that the provider did much less medical decision-making, evaluation, and management than was actually performed.

Documentation to support or validate risk adjustment conditions may be found anywhere in the note for the face-to-face encounter. It is important to ensure that the note accurately reflects all chronic conditions that affect the health and care of the patient. Each encounter must be unique and reflect only that visit as it occurred. Insufficient documentation influences the assignment of diagnosis codes and directly affects the patient's risk score.

Documentation should properly validate all reported conditions. Each page of progress notes should be properly authenticated and include the patient's name and the date.

Providers should document each clinical diagnosis to the highest degree of specificity per encounter, including all complications and/or manifestations, including clear links to causal conditions. Only confirmed conditions should be documented—no rule-out conditions or abnormal findings without clinical significance. All known conditions, including chronic conditions, that affect the care and treatment of the patient at least once per year should be noted.

Providers should specifically document the condition and clinical significance, and any pertinent changes, using terminology such as decreased, increased, worsening, improving, or unchanged, or abnormal findings.

### Documentation Tips

- Document all cause-and-effect relationships.
- Report the most specific diagnosis code available that is supported by the documentation.
- Include all current diagnoses as part of the current medical decision-making, and document for every visit.
- Identify diagnoses that are current or chronic problems rather than a past medical history or previous resolved condition.
- Document history of heart attack, status codes, etc., that affect the patient's care as "history of" or "PMH" when they no longer exist or are not current conditions.
- Ensure medical record documentation for each encounter includes the date, signature, and credentials/specialty.
- Document the thought processes used to assess each condition.
- Know high weighted HCCs that are often undiagnosed or undercoded.
- Avoid "unspecified" codes.
- Ensure the codes reported are accurate.
- Ensure each encounter is billed.
- Review rejection reports, and audit reports to assess risks.

## Audits

Because reimbursement is by patient, rather than based on an average of the entire population, and is based upon documentation, there is the potential for upcoding. Audits are conducted by the MA plan and CMS recovery auditors.

### Initial Validation Audit (IVA)

CMS requires that the MA plan validate HCCs. This is usually performed by an independent auditor working with the plan or a contracted vendor to validate the MA plan's data submitted to CMS.

The MA plan submits the one best medical record that supports each HCC identified for the beneficiary.

### Risk Adjustment Data Validation Audit

Risk adjustment data validation (RADV) audits are performed by CMS to validate the integrity and accuracy of risk-adjusted payments by verifying that the diagnosis codes the MA plans submit are supported by the medical record documentation for a member. Beginning March 2026, CMS has six RADV audits scheduled through April 2027.

MA plans can be selected by CMS for RADV audits annually and if chosen are required to submit their members' medical records to CMS. Providers are required to assist the MA plan by providing the medical record documentation included in the audit. Even though each diagnosis needs to be reported only once in a calendar year, during a RADV audit up to five dates of service may be submitted to support any one HCC.

To be validated, medical record documentation must meet certain criteria and standards. Even if the diagnosis is documented and coded correctly, any deficiency in the documentation can make the encounter and the HCC invalid. Diagnoses that cannot be validated are considered payment errors. The results of the audit are communicated to the MA plan, which then communicates these results to the provider. Under- and overpayments are subject to payment adjustment. The results of RADV audits can be extrapolated over the MA plan population to calculate potential payment errors and overpayments/recoupments. Regulations include a RADV appeal process, a document dispute process, and a procedure for obtaining physician-signature attestations.

CMS published a checklist available to provide guidance on how to ensure that medical records will validate the conditions submitted for risk adjustment by an MA plan. This checklist instructs that records should be reviewed to ensure:

- The record is for the correct patient with sufficient patient identifiers on each page of the medical record.
- The record is legible.
- The service is from a face-to-face visit with a valid provider type.
- The diagnosis is found and supported within the medical record.
- The record contains an acceptable provider signature, which includes the credentials of the provider.

Mitigate audit risk by coding each reportable diagnosis each time it meets reporting guidelines. Audit regularly to assess areas of risk and in need of improvement and to capture conditions documented but not coded. Check for additional qualifying HCCs. Ensure claims are submitted and that corrected claims are submitted when indicated. There are three claims submission deadlines: January, March, and September. CMS adjusts each member's risk score twice a year, with the final reconciliation in August of the year after the plan year.

If providers emphasize correct coding and documentation and perform internal audits to determine where the risks are and prepare for audits, incorrect payment is less likely.

For additional information on risk adjustment coding, see Optum's *Risk Adjustment Coding and HCC Guide*.

# Appendix F: Centers for Medicare & Medicaid Services Quality Payment Program

In 2015, in an effort to repeal the faulty Medicare sustainable growth rate (SGR), focus on quality of patient outcomes, and control Medicare spending, Congress passed the Medicare Access and CHIP Reauthorization Act (MACRA), which included sweeping changes for practitioners who provide services reimbursed under the Medicare physician fee schedule (MPFS). MACRA repealed the Medicare SGR methodology used for updating the MPFS and replaced it with the Quality Payment Program (QPP).

Under the QPP, providers who demonstrate success at controlling costs while providing high-quality care to their patients are eligible to earn increased payments. Clinicians who successfully report on determined criteria receive a larger payment. Beginning with the 2022 payment year and beyond, the maximum negative payment adjustment for those who do not participate or do not fulfill the defined requirements during each performance year will be up to 9 percent of Medicare Part B reimbursements. Payment adjustments (positive, neutral, or negative) received for the 2028 payment year will be based on the MIPS final score for the 2026 performance year.

## Passage of the Medicare Access and CHIP Reauthorization Act of 2015

The final rule for implementing MACRA was published November 4, 2016. The final rule primarily provided details on how the QPP was to be implemented, including requiring the secretary of Health and Human Services (HHS) to sunset the value-based (VM) modifier incentive program, the Medicare electronic health record (EHR) incentive program, and the Physician Quality Reporting System (PQRS), and incorporated these incentive programs into the QPP.

## Replacement of the Sustainable Growth Rate

Under the SGR, if overall physician costs were higher than a targeted Medicare expenditure, payments were reduced across the board. With the SGR method, payments to clinicians would have resulted in substantial cuts.

Because the QPP replaces the SGR methodology, the following revisions were detailed in MACRA:

- Established conversion factor updates:
  - a Medicare physician fee schedule conversion factor adjustment of 0.5 percent in 2016–2019 and a conversion factor adjustment of 0.00 percent for 2020–2026
  - the qualifying participant (QP) alternative payment models (APM) conversion factor of 0.75 percent and a nonqualifying provider APM conversion factor of 0.25 percent for 2026 and each subsequent year

Under the QPP, the Centers for Medicare and Medicaid Services (CMS) aims to:

- Support quality of patient care improvement by focusing on better outcomes for patients, decreasing provider burden, and preserving the independent clinical practice
- Promote the adoption of APMs, which align incentives across healthcare stakeholders
- Advance existing efforts of delivery system reform, including ensuring a smooth transition to a new system that promotes high-quality, efficient care through unification of CMS legacy programs such as the EHR incentive program

## Quality Payment Program Established

The MACRA final rule established the Quality Payment Program (QPP) effective January 1, 2017. Within the QPP there are two interrelated pathways: Advanced Alternative Payment Models (APM) and the Merit-based Incentive Payment System (MIPS).

Eligible clinicians (EC) select the track/pathway—MIPS or advanced APMs—they wish to participate in based on the practice size, specialty, location, and patient population. Unlike previous quality initiatives, a provider does not have to enroll in the QPP. However, groups wishing to participate in the MIPS program via the Consumer Assessment of Healthcare Providers and Systems (CAHPS) for MIPS survey measures or CMS Web Interface (WI) must register by June 30 each year. Note that beginning with the 2022 performance period, the CMS WI will no longer be available as a submission or collection type. The CAHPS for MIPS survey is an optional quality measure that groups participating in MIPS can elect to administer.

In the 2020 Physician Fee Schedule Final Rule, CMS finalized a new participation framework to begin in 2021 known as MIPS Value Pathways (MVPs). The MVPs allow for a more cohesive participation experience by connecting activities and measures that are relevant to a specialty, medical condition, or a particular population. Due to the 2019 Coronavirus public health emergency (PHE), CMS postponed the implementation of MVPs as a reporting option for MIPS measures and activities until 2023. CMS finalized proposed updates for the criteria, process, and MVP implementation and finalized 12 MVPs for the 2023 performance year. For the 2026 performance year, there are 27 finalized MVPs. Twenty-one existing MVPs have all been modified and there are six new MVPs for reporting in the CY 2026 performance period. For additional and updated information on MVPs, see https://qpp.cms.gov/mips/mips-value-pathways.

## Merit-based Incentive Payment System

MIPS is the track for clinicians who opt to participate in traditional Medicare as opposed to participating through an advanced APM. In doing so, clinicians may earn a payment adjustment related to evidence-based and practice-specific quality data. As a result, depending on the degree and success of performance in all four categories, clinicians receive one of the following:

- Positive payment adjustment in which additional compensation is received
- Neutral payment adjustment that neither increases nor reduces Medicare payments
- Negative payment adjustment of up to 9 percent of Medicare payment furnished in calendar year (CY) 2026

Participation in the MIPS track is determined based on the amount billed to Medicare and the number of beneficiaries seen per year. The following provider types are eligible for participation if they meet or exceed at least one of the following criteria:

- Medicare billings are greater than $90,000.
- More than 200 covered services are provided to Medicare Part B patients.
- Care is provided to more than 200 Medicare patients each year.

The following clinician types are considered ECs:

- Physicians (MD, DO, DDS, DMD, DPM, OD)
- Physician assistants (PA)
- Nurse practitioners (NP)
- Clinical nurse specialists (CNS)
- Certified registered nurse anesthetists (CRNA)
- Physical therapists (PT)
- Occupational therapists (OT)
- Qualified speech-language pathologists
- Qualified audiologists
- Clinical psychologists
- Osteopathic practitioners
- Chiropractor
- Registered dieticians or nutrition professionals
- Clinical social workers
- Certified nurse midwives

## Anatomy of MIPS

A measurement-based regime creates a single reporting framework for physicians that comprise four performance categories:

- Quality
- Improvement Activities (IA)
- Promoting Interoperability
- Cost

MIPS eligible clinicians may participate in the program as an individual clinician, group, virtual group, or APM entity. Each of the four performance categories has been weighted, with greatest emphasis placed on the Quality category. Performance category weights for individuals, groups, and virtual groups placed the Quality category at 30 percent, Promoting Interoperability is second at 25 percent, IA at 15 percent, and Cost at 30 percent. Performance category weights for APM entities reporting traditional MIPS are weighted differently than these participation levels. The emphasis is still on the Quality category at 50 percent, Promoting Interoperability is second at 30 percent, Improvement Activities is third at 20 percent, and Cost is at 0 percent. Beginning with the 2022 performance period regardless of participation level (e.g., individual, group, etc.) the quality and cost performance categories will be equally weighted at 30%.

The 2026 MIPS performance threshold equates to 75 points out of a possible 100 points. Simply put, eligible clinicians are required to score 75 points to avoid up to a negative 9 percent payment adjustment.

### Quality Performance

Under the MIPS Quality performance category, ECs and groups must select six measures from a listing of almost 200 measures, with at least one of the six measures being an outcome measure, high-priority measure (in absences of outcome measure), or complete specialty measure set. Patient outcomes such as mortality, whether a patient is readmitted to the hospital, and the patient's experience are areas that CMS and the healthcare industry seek to improve. An outcome measure is the way CMS can quantify changes in the health of an individual, groups of individuals, and even certain populations that they can attribute back to a specific intervention or series of interventions.

Quality measures are tools for quantifying, or measuring, healthcare processes and patient outcomes and perceptions, as well as organizational structure and/or systems linked to the ability to provide high-quality healthcare. These measures play an important role under the MIPS. Reporting should be done on a minimum of half of the EC's or group practice's Medicare Part B patients. Performance data is reported for 75 percent of the patients who qualify for each measure. This threshold will remain at 75% through the 2028 performance period.

### Improvement Activities

The IA category assesses to what degree a clinician participates in activities designed to improve clinical practices. ECs are required to attest that they have participated in two high-weighted activities, one high-weighted activity and two medium-weighted activities, or four medium-weighted activities. The activities may be selected from an inventory of over 95 activities across eight subcategories for 90 consecutive days. These eight subcategories include:

- Expanded practice access
- Population management
- Care coordination
- Beneficiary engagement
- Patient safety and practice assessment
- Advancing health and wellness
- Behavioral and mental health
- Emergency preparedness and response

This category was created with some inherent flexibility; for example, for groups with 15 or fewer participants, nonpatient-facing clinicians (e.g., pathologists), or those ECs in a rural or health professional shortage area (HPSA) receive two times the points when they report activities for at least 90 consecutive days.

### Promoting Interoperability

CMS wants to encourage and promote the use of certified EHR technology (CEHRT) among providers and, in particular, the use of interoperability and sharing of information among clinicians and between providers and patients. In response to the 21st Century Cures Act Final Rule, CMS updated the CEHRT requirements to include technology certified to the 2015 Edition Cures Update certification criteria, the current 2015 Edition certification criteria, or a combination of both criteria to collect and report PI data.

Successful reporting of measures in this category require the EC to report measures from the four objectives and measures based exclusively on the 2015 edition of CEHRT and, as applicable, claim an exclusion. Exclusions are reported by submitting a "0" in addition to the exclusion type that applies to the EC because some measures may be associated with more than one exclusion.

The PI performance category contains five objectives:

- E-Prescribing
- Health Information Exchange
- Provider to Patient Exchange
- Public Health and Clinical Data Exchange
- Protecting Patient Health Information

Data collected for each of the five objectives must be submitted for the same minimum continuous 180 days (unless an exclusion is applicable).

### Cost

In this performance category, CMS determines an EC or group practice's cost score by calculating data from two measures previously included in the value-based payment modifier that involves the total cost of care for attributed beneficiaries and what Medicare spends per beneficiary. This amount is the total of both Medicare Part A and B payments from three days before through 30 days after a beneficiary has had an inpatient hospitalization episode. CMS then determines which ECs and practices have an adequate number of beneficiaries and hospitalizations associated with them. This number is compared with national benchmarks established for the performance period.

There are a total of 35 cost measures:

- Episode-based cost measures based on a range of procedures, acute inpatient medical conditions, and chronic conditions
- Population-based cost measures focused more broadly on primary and inpatient care.

For procedure episodes, the case minimum established is 10 with credit for the episodes going to the clinician who performs the procedure. For acute inpatient medical condition episodes, the case minimum is set at 20, and credit is assigned to each clinician who bills the inpatient evaluation and management (E/M) claim lines during a triggered inpatient hospitalization under a TIN that furnishes at least 30 percent of the inpatient E/M claim lines during that particular hospitalization.

Clinicians have no additional submission responsibilities associated with this category as the score is determined from Medicare administrative claims data.

The category also has separate benchmarks. The Cost score is determined and compared with those benchmarks with points assigned based on the decile system in a similar manner to the Quality performance category with some differences such as:

- Benchmarks for performance are for the *same* year versus prior year performance.
- Scores are determined once case minimum requirements for each of the two measures in this category have been met.

Starting with the 2026 performance period, for new cost measures there will be a 2-year information-only feedback period. During this time clinicians will receive feedback on their measure performance, but these will not count toward their cost category score. Note: There are no new cost measures for 2026.

## MIPS Scoring

CMS uses scoring to determine an EC's successful participation in the QPP and thereby determine if the clinician's reimbursement will be negative, neutral, or positive.

The scoring methodology is a unified approach across all performance categories, allowing eligible clinicians to understand what is expected so they can perform successfully in the MIPS. For more information and details on QPP, see https:/ qpp.cms.gov.

## Notes

## Notes

## Chapter 3. Diseases of the Blood and Blood-forming Organs and Certain Disorders Involving the Immune Mechanism (D5Ø–D89)

**Red Blood Cells**

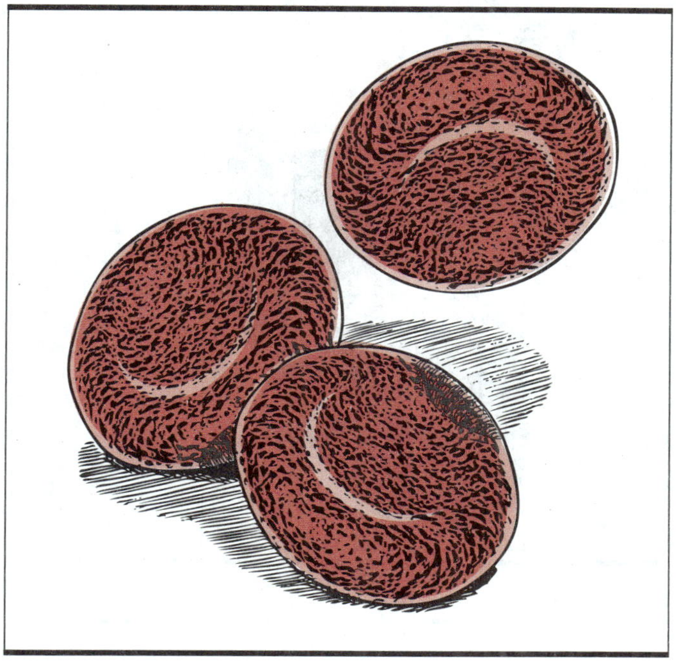

**White Blood Cell**

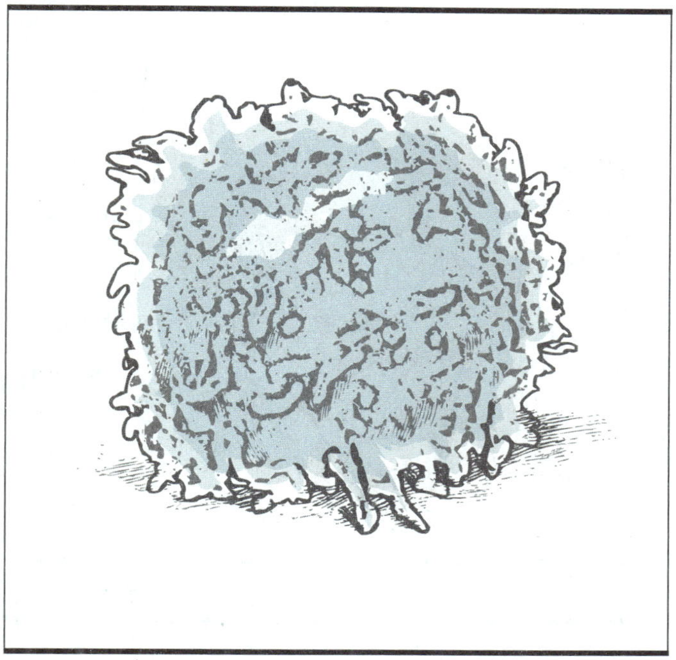

**Platelet**

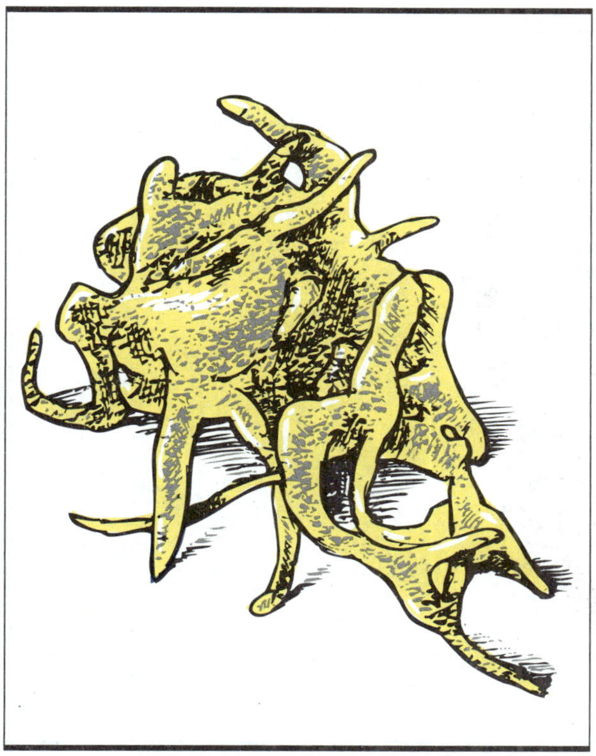

**Coagulation**

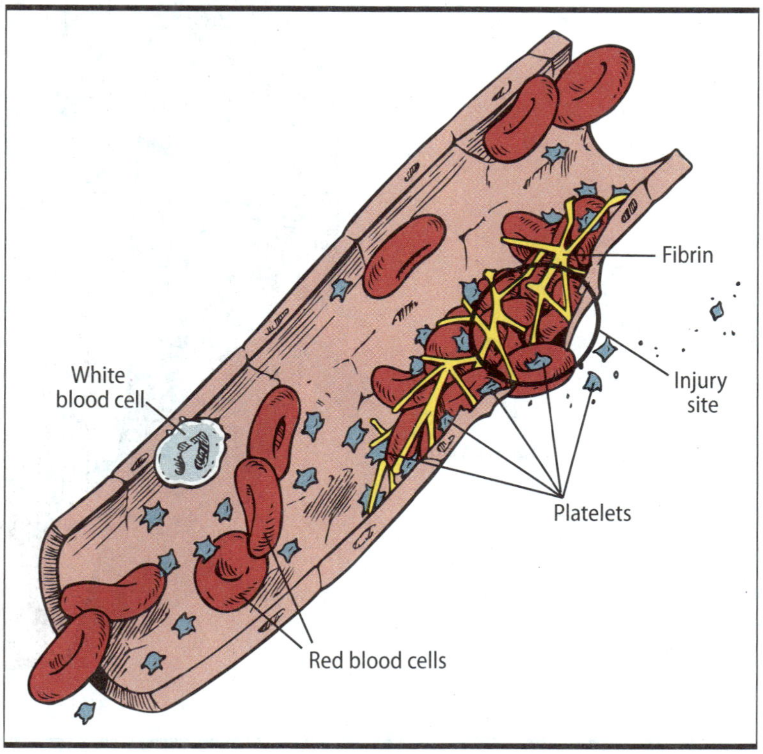

## Spleen Anatomical Location and External Structures

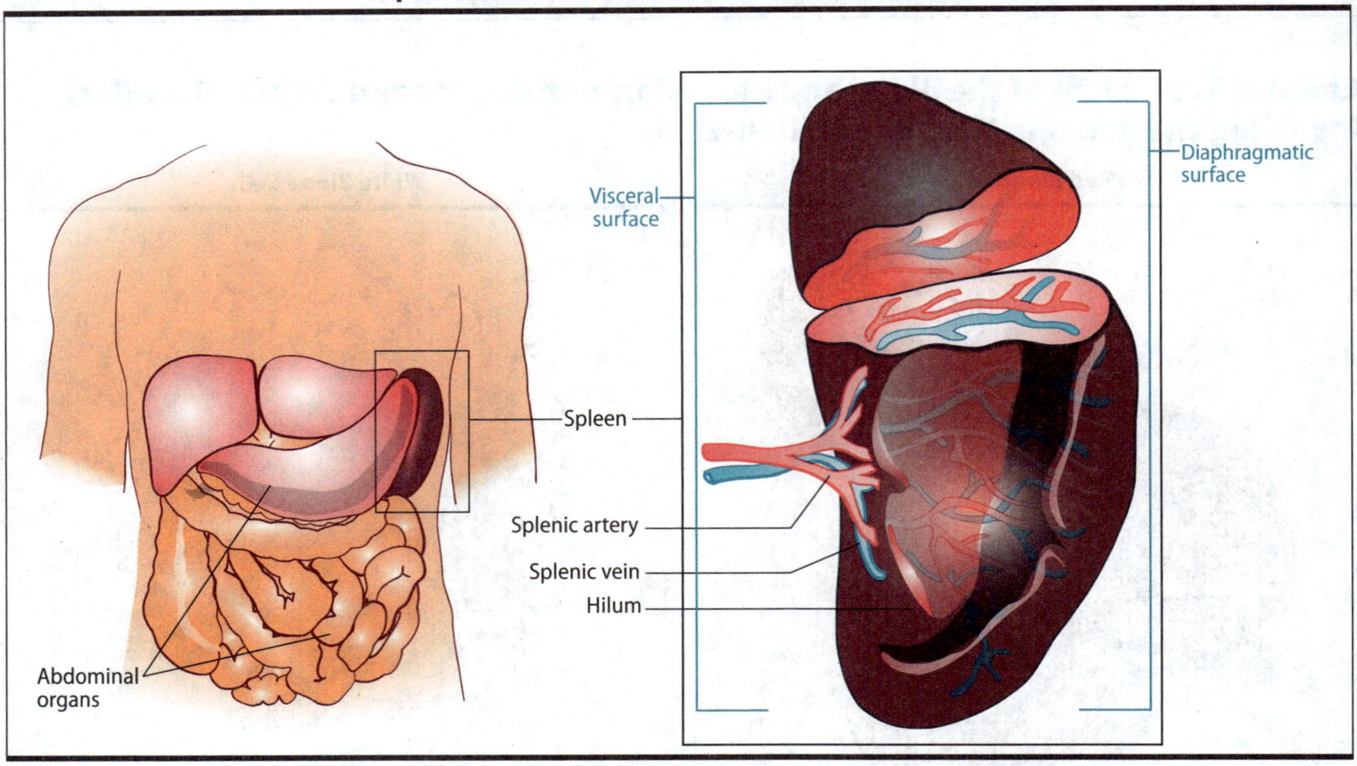


## Spleen Interior Structures

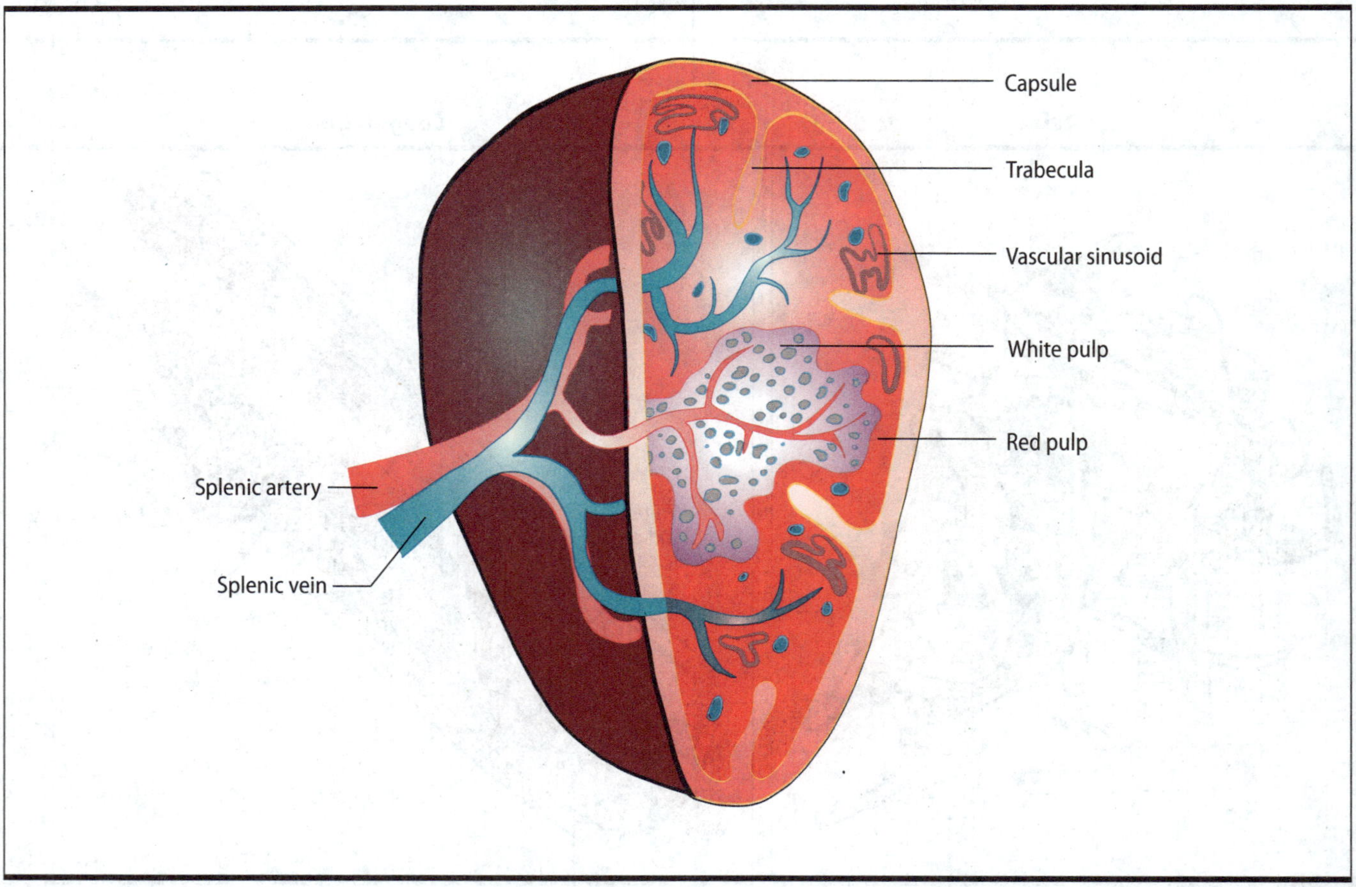

# Chapter 4. Endocrine, Nutritional and Metabolic Diseases (EØØ–E89)

## Endocrine System

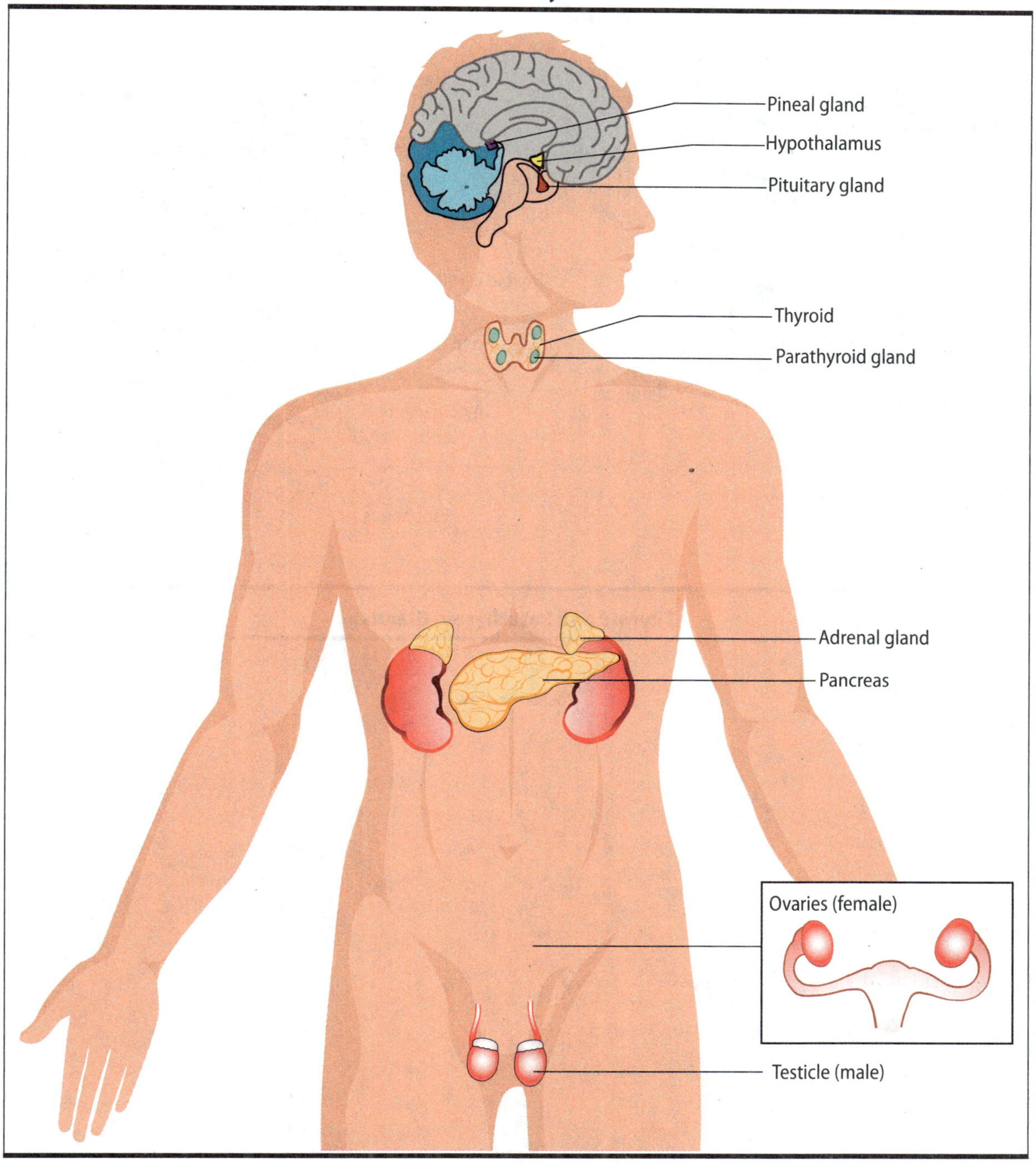

## Thyroid

### Anterior view

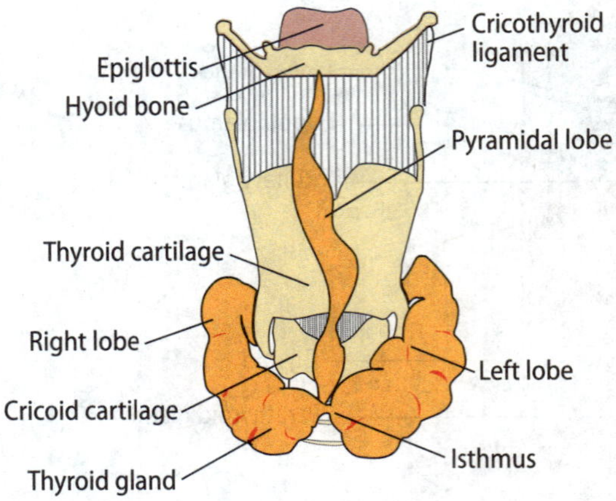


### Lateral view

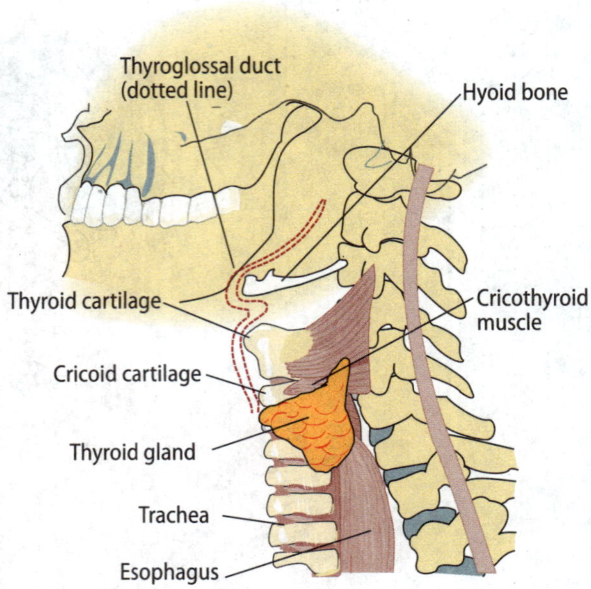


## Thyroid and Parathyroid Glands

### Posterior view

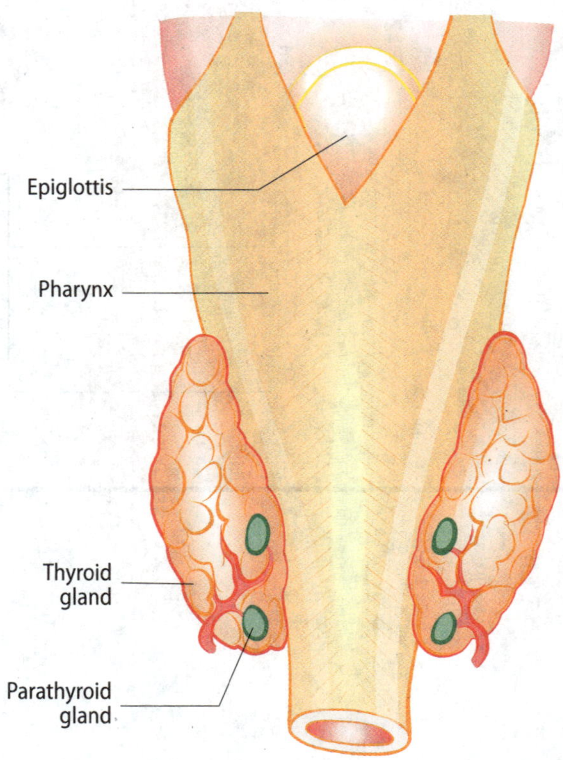

## Pancreas

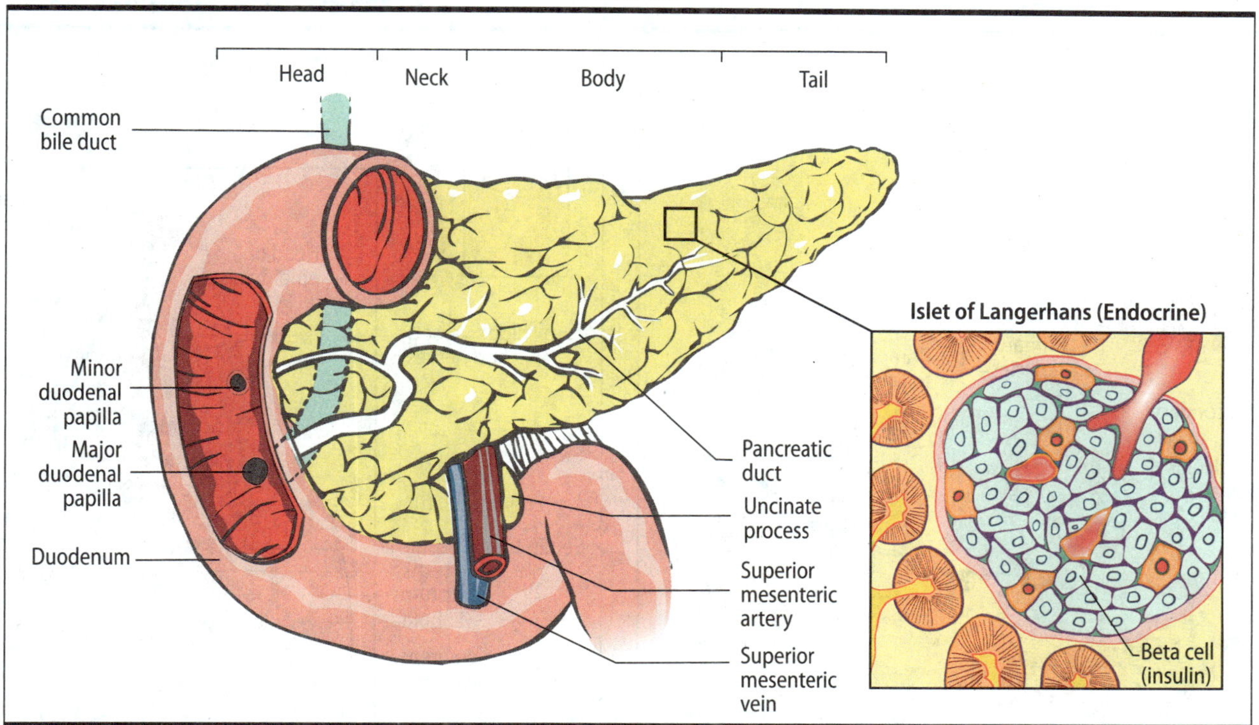


## Anatomy of the Adrenal Gland

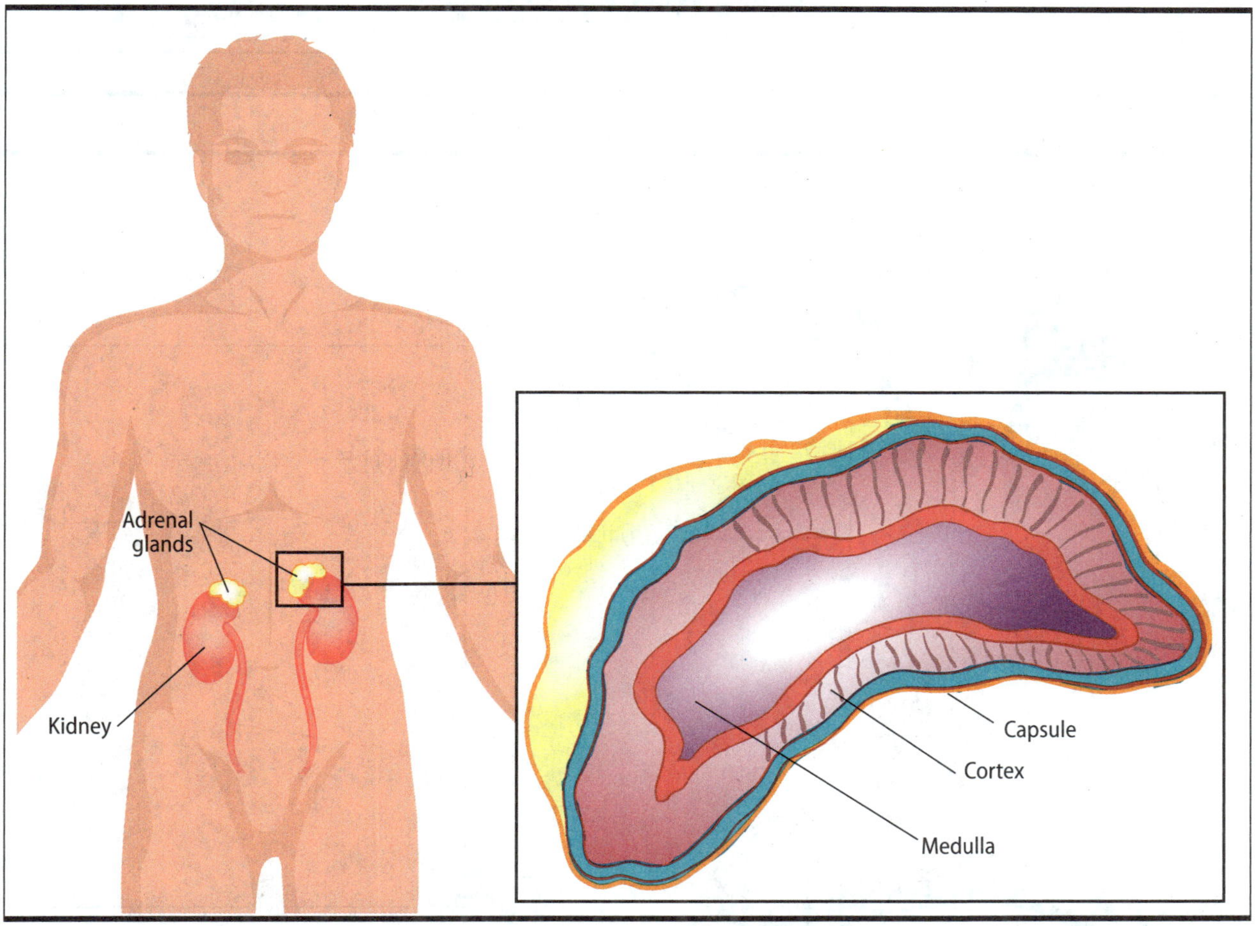

## Structure of an Ovary

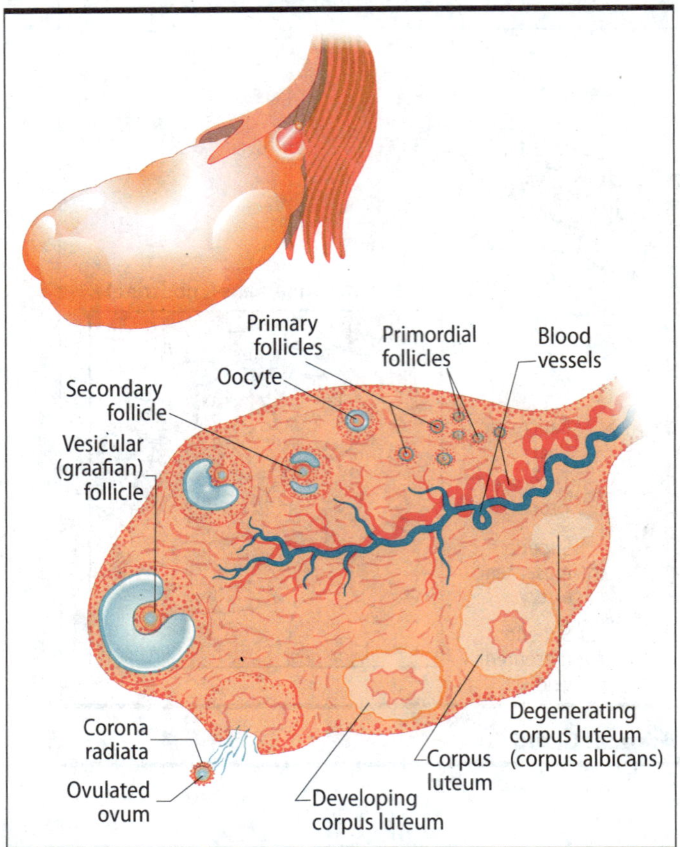


## Testis and Associated Structures

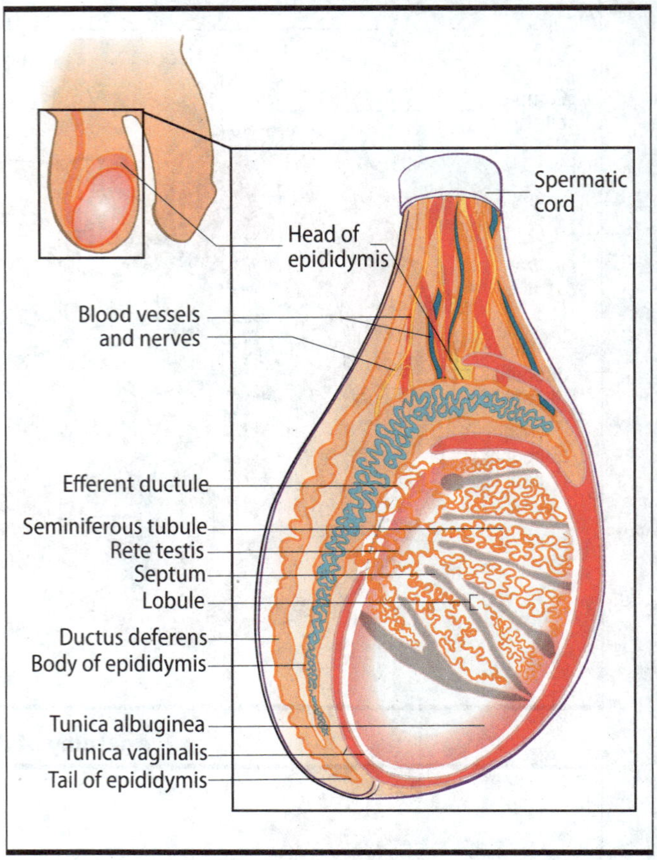


## Thymus

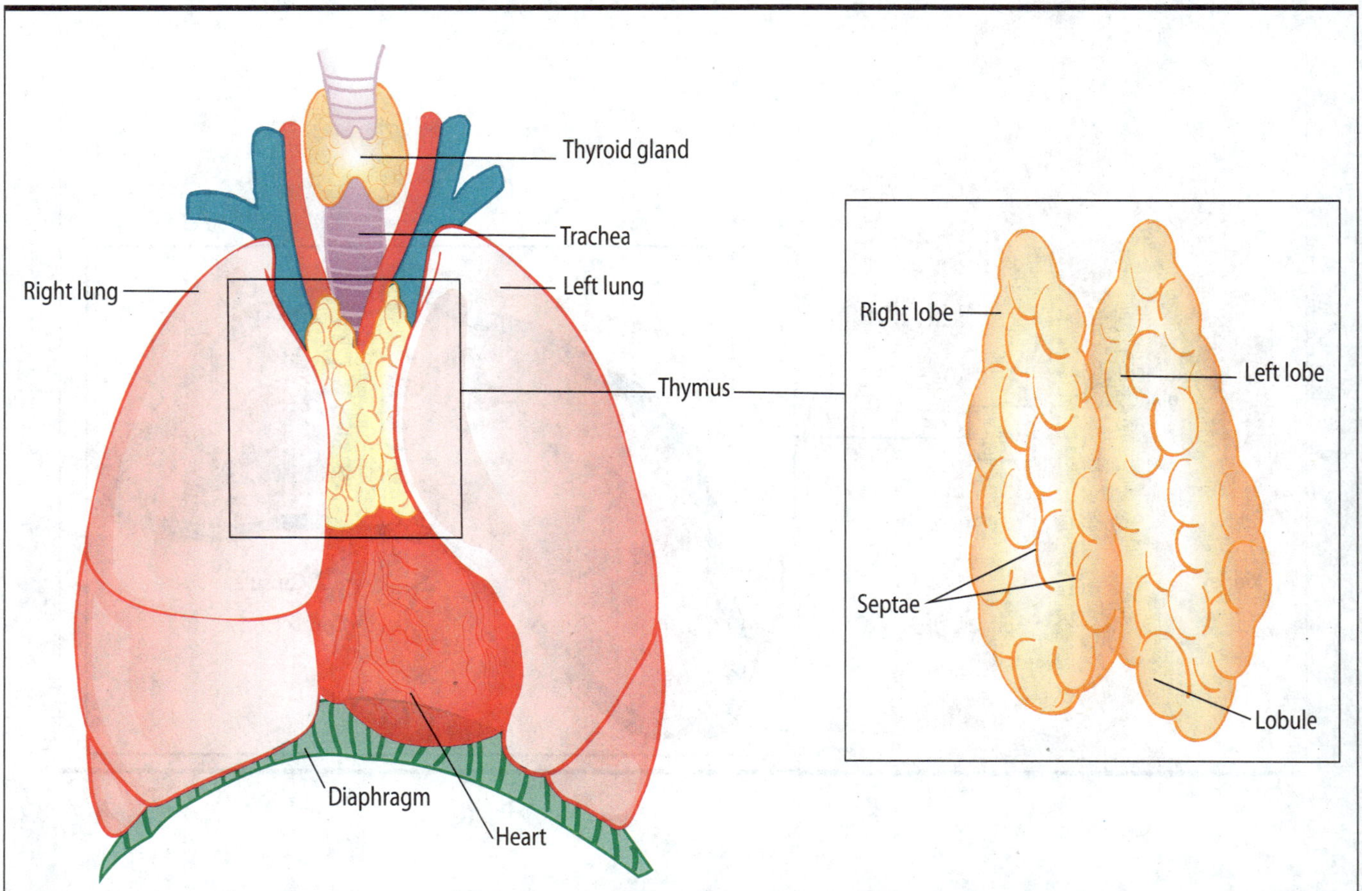

# Chapter 6. Diseases of the Nervous System (GØØ–G99)

## Brain

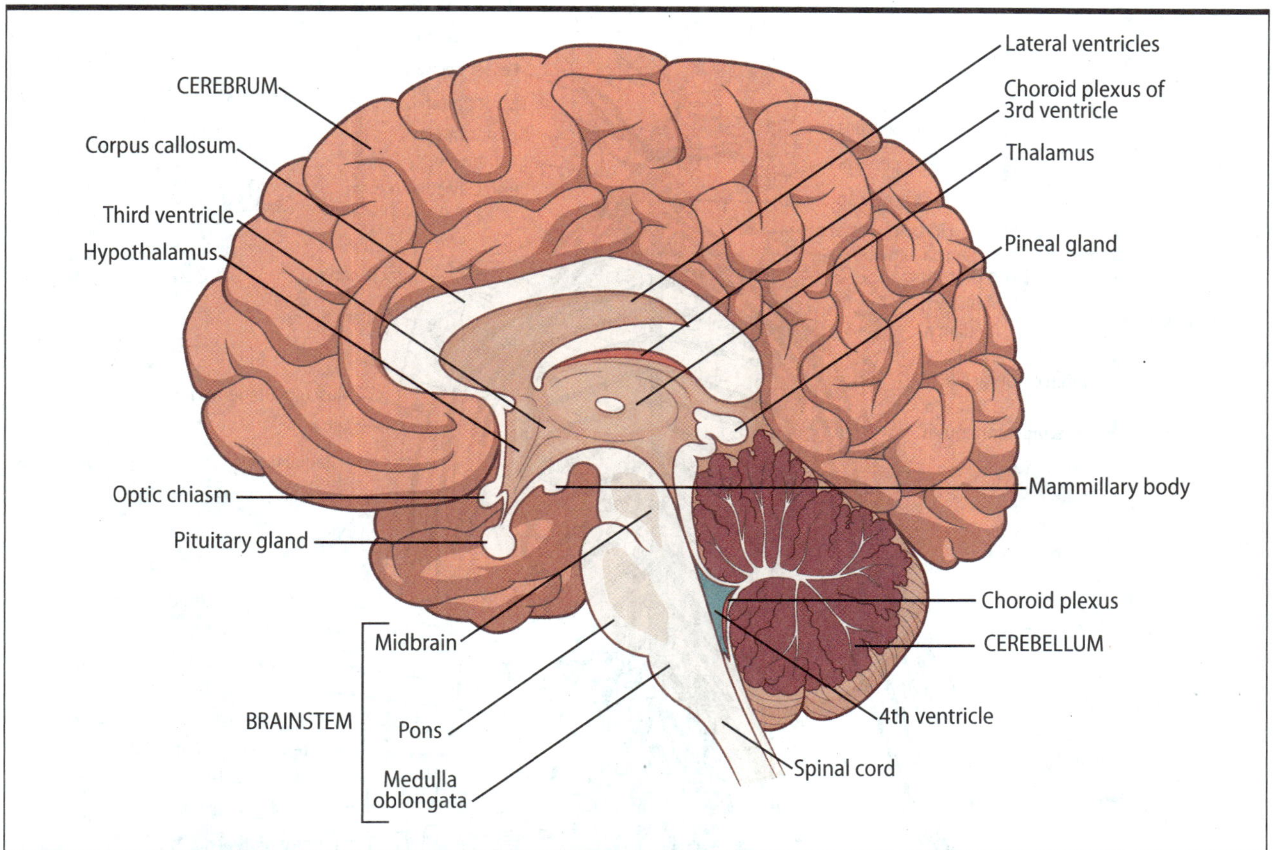


## Cranial Nerves

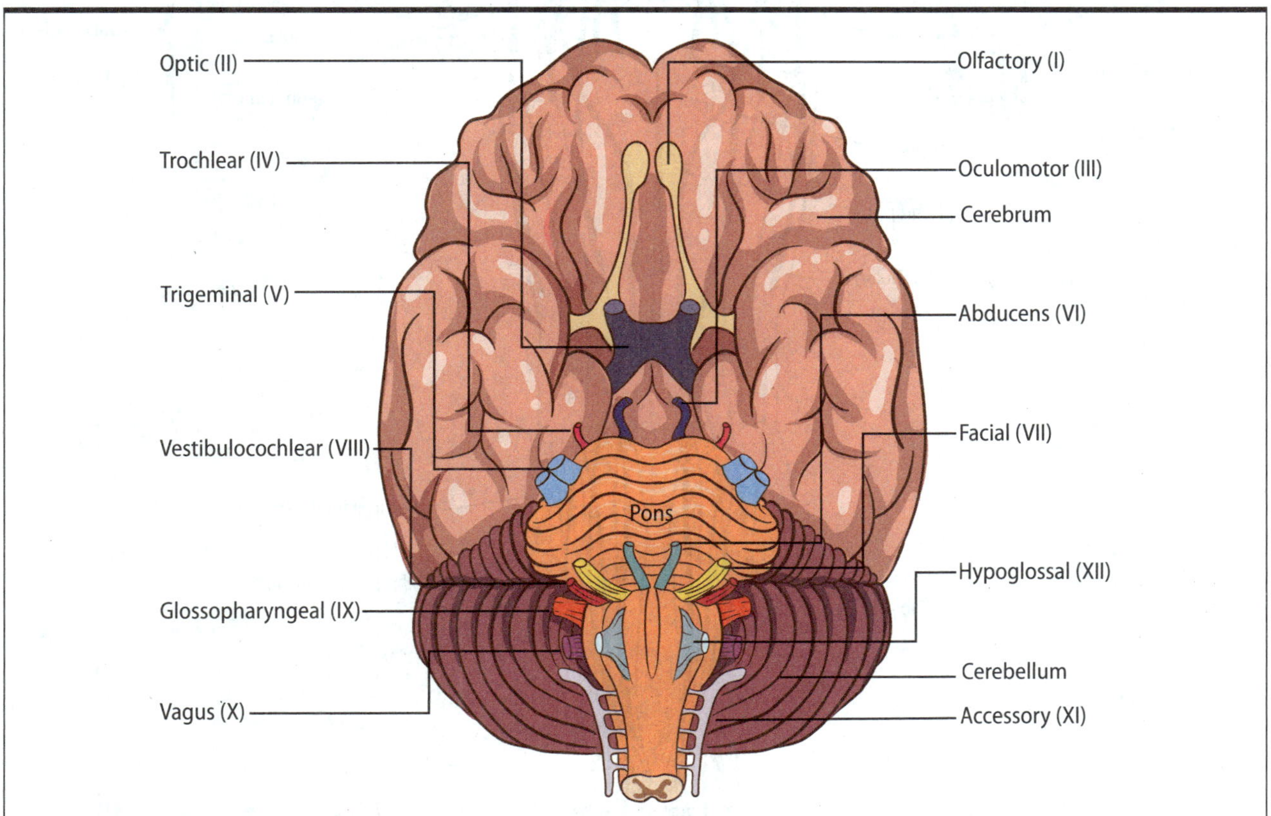

## Peripheral Nervous System

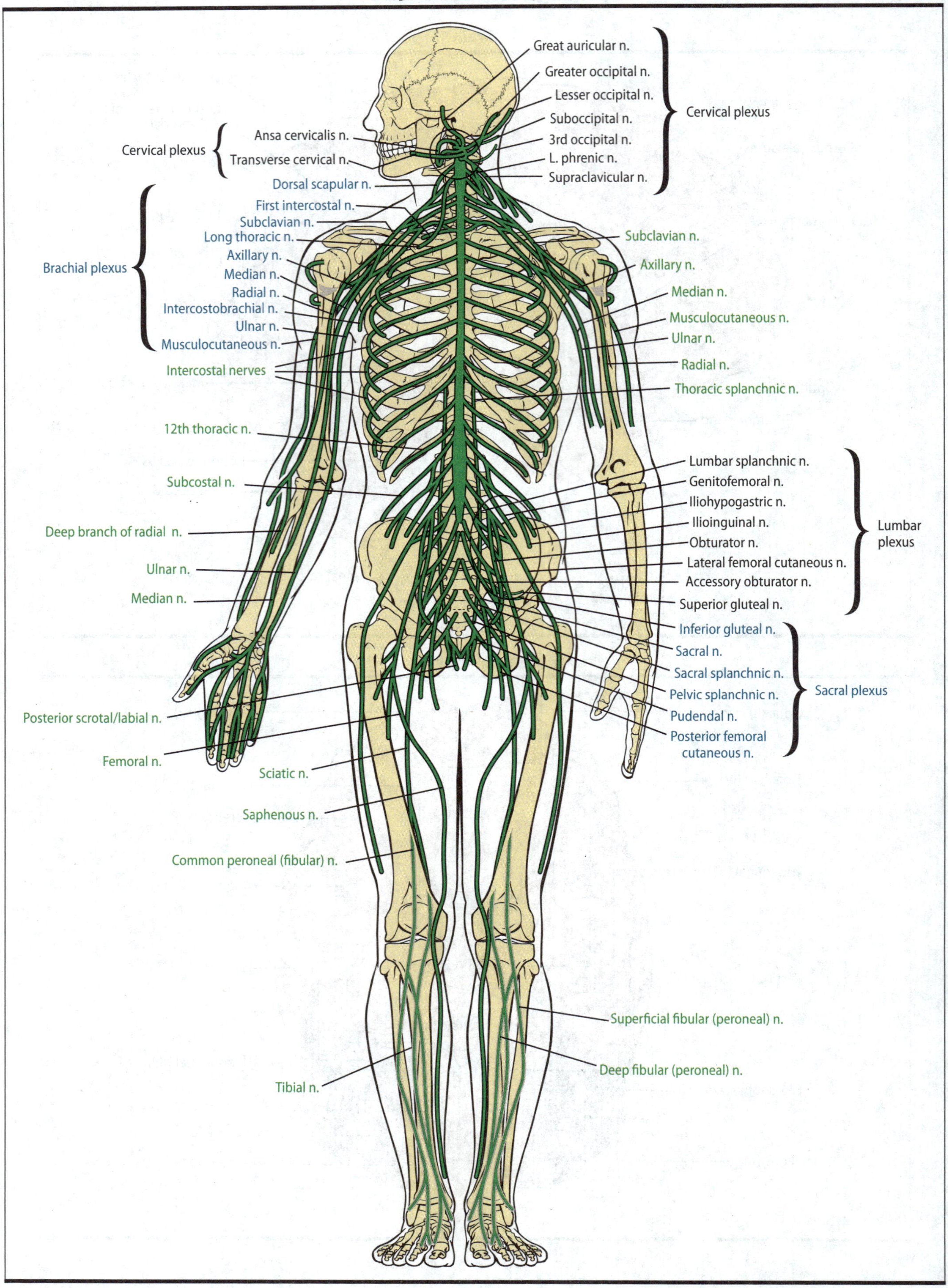

## Spinal Cord and Spinal Nerves

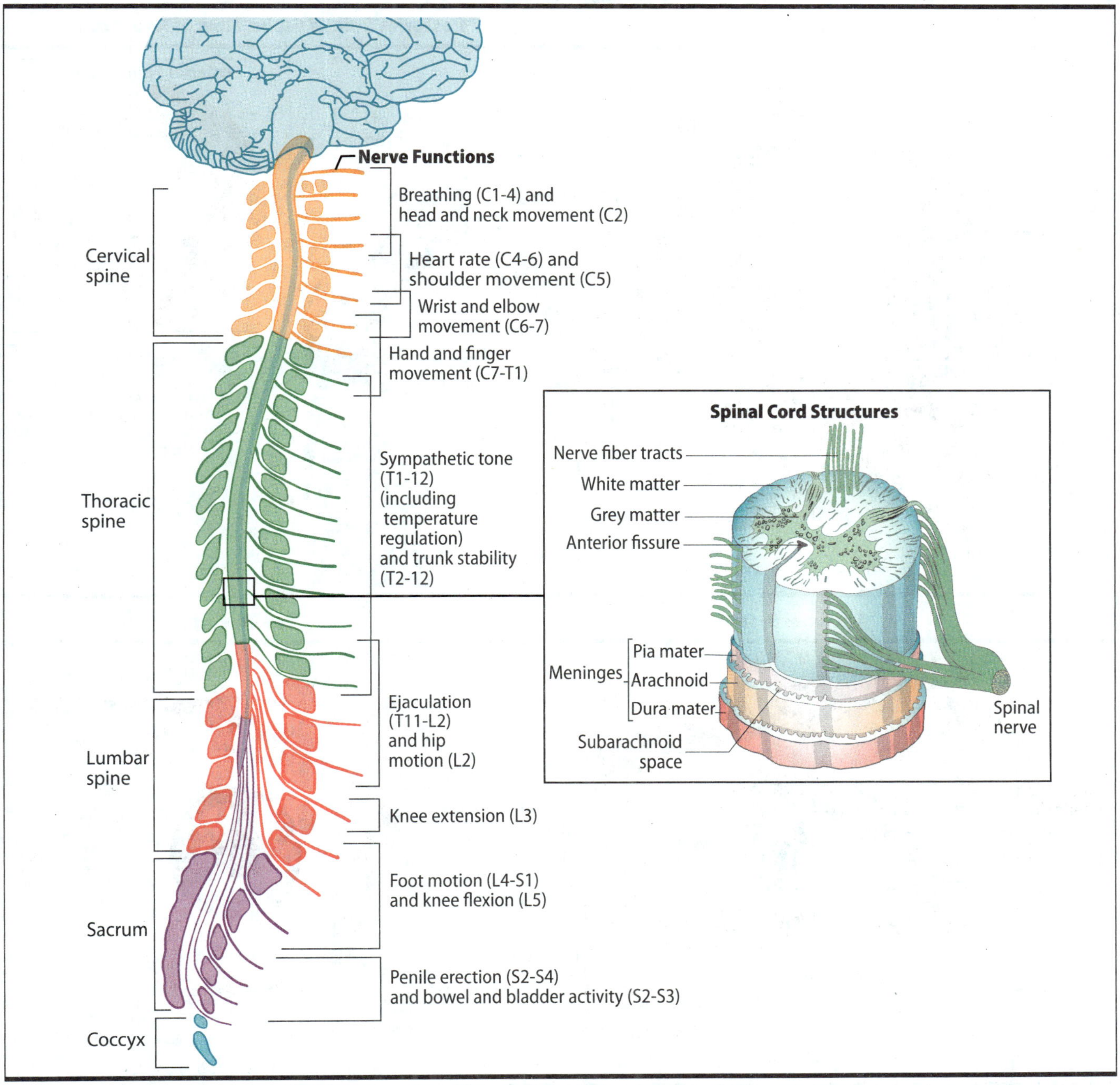


## Nerve Cell

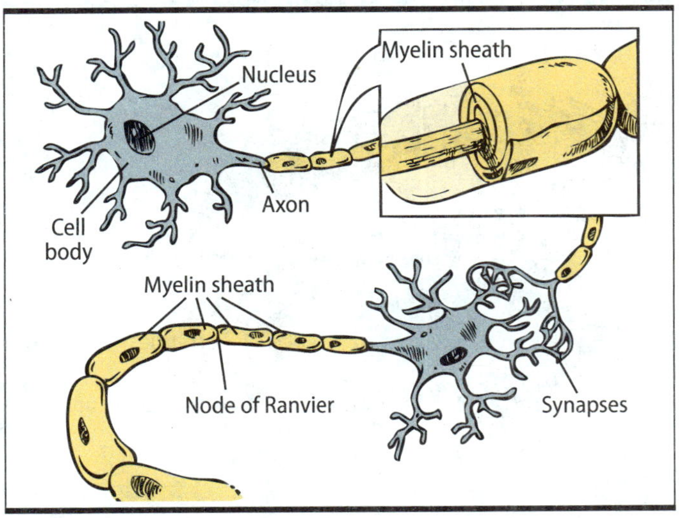


## Trigeminal and Facial Nerve Branches

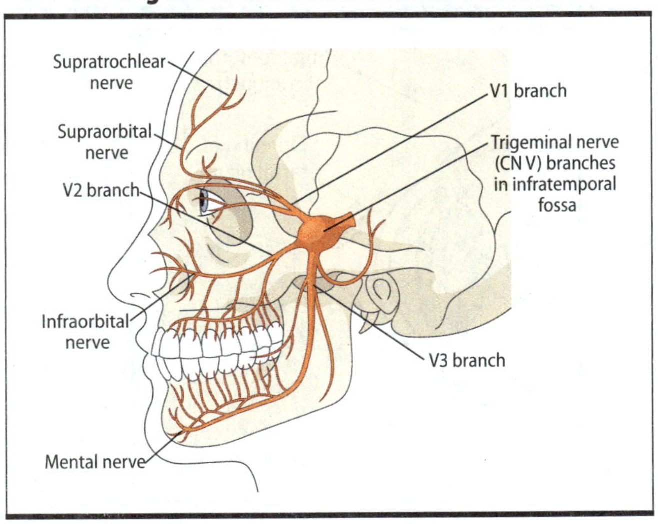

# Chapter 7. Diseases of the Eye and Adnexa (HØØ–H59)

## Eye

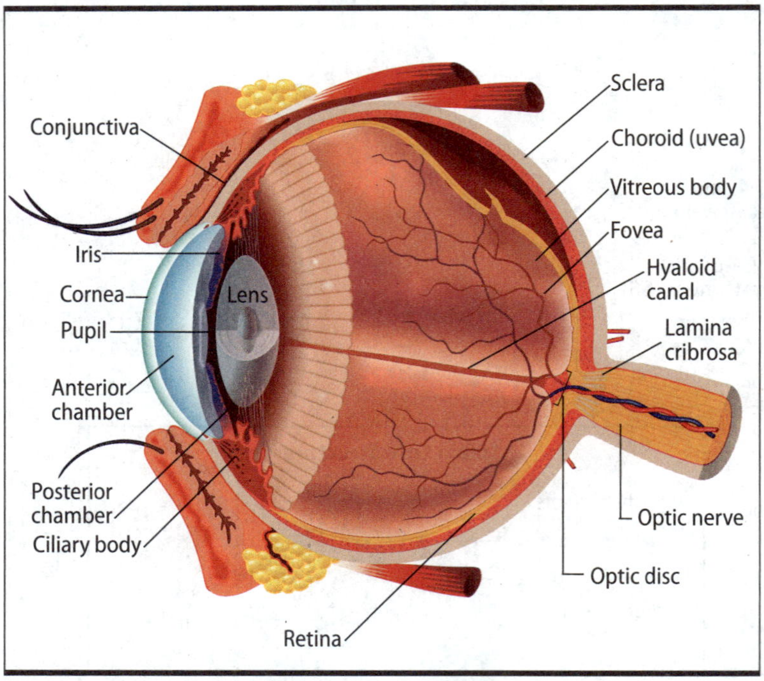


## Posterior Pole of Globe/Flow of Aqueous Humor

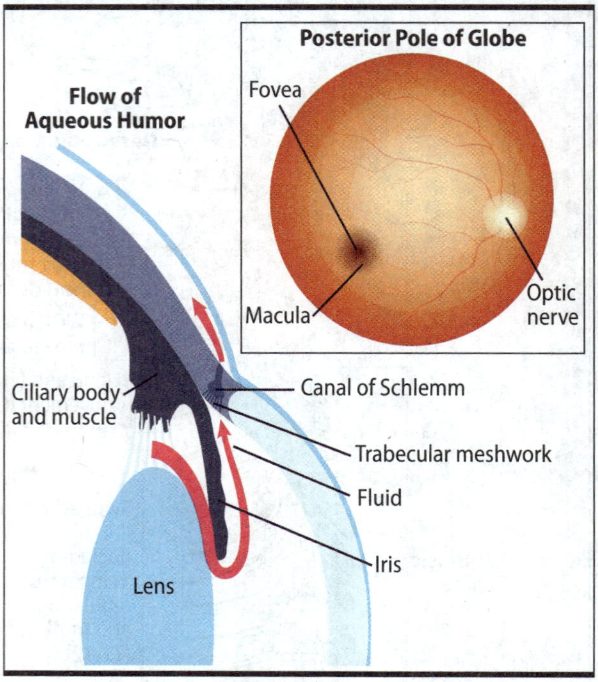


## Lacrimal System

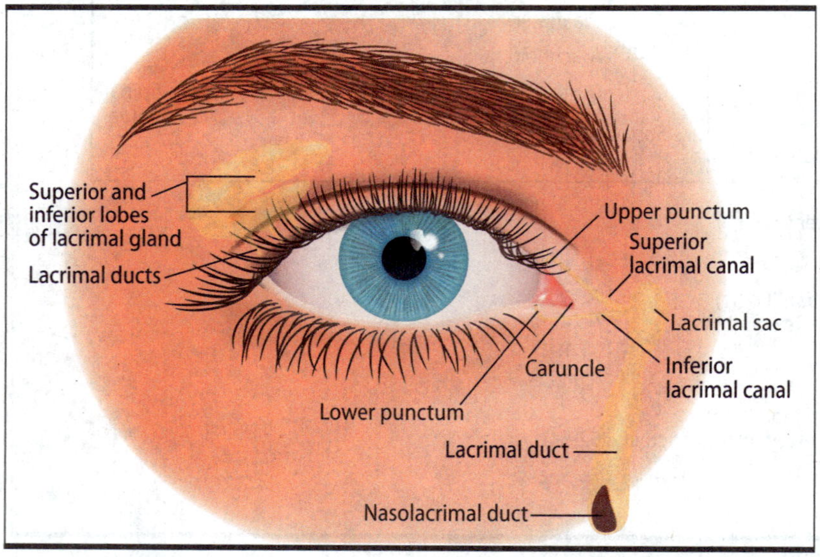


## Eye Musculature

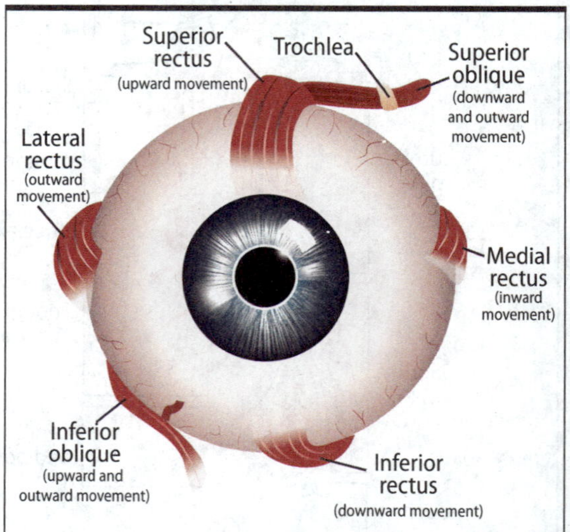


Muscles and actions of eye

## Eyelid Structures

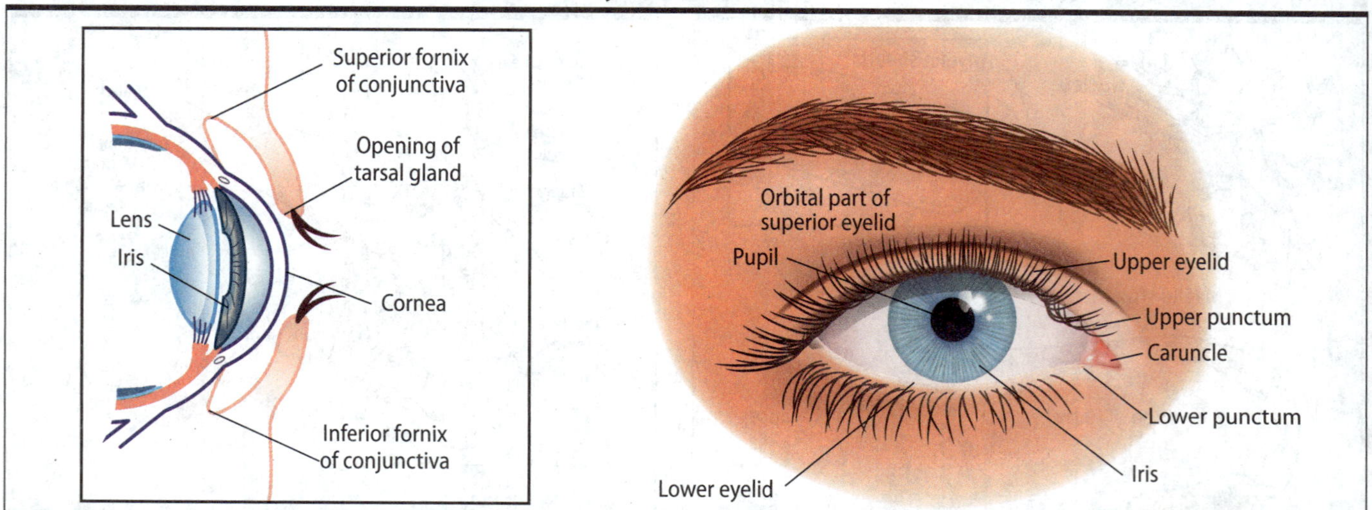

# Chapter 8. Diseases of the Ear and Mastoid Process (H6Ø–H95)

**Ear Anatomy**

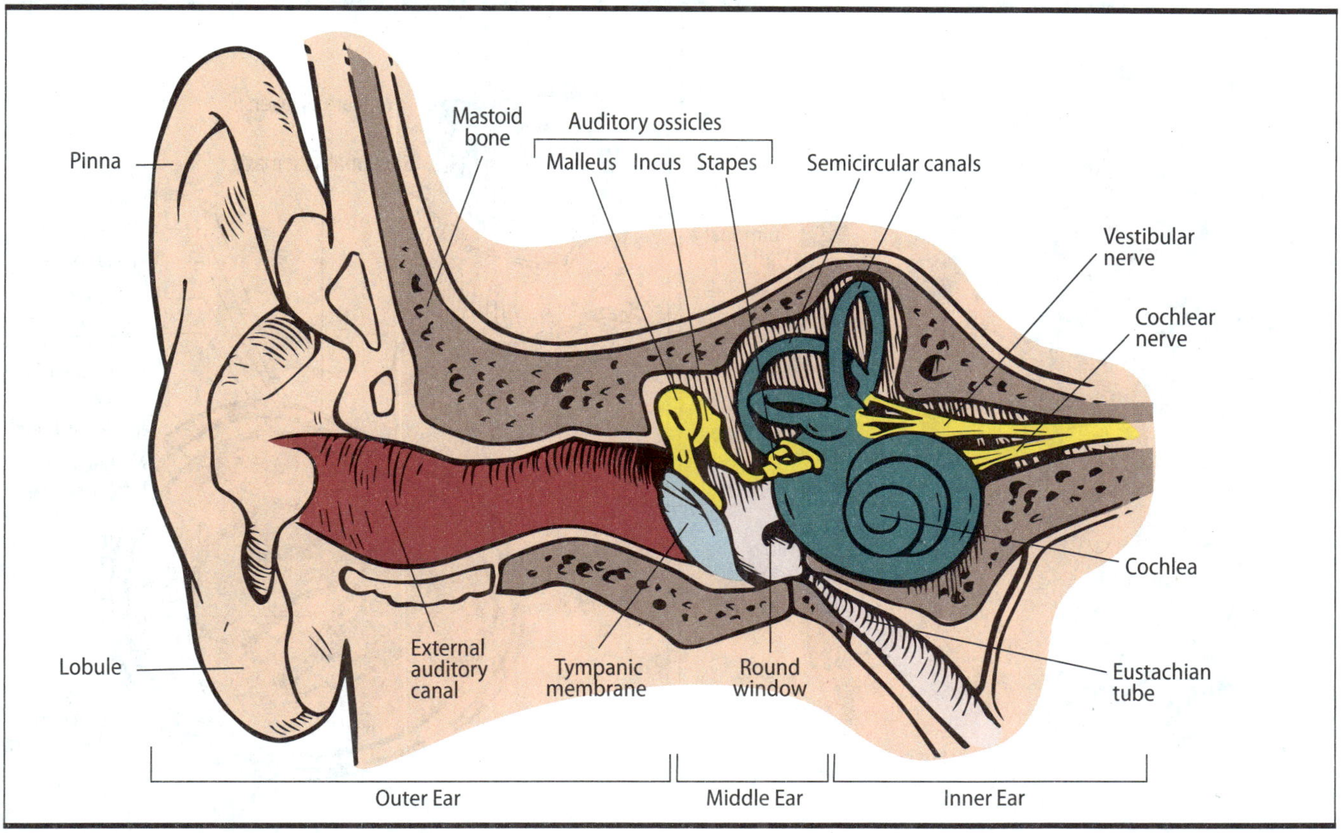

# Chapter 9. Diseases of the Circulatory System (I00–I99)

## Anatomy of the Heart

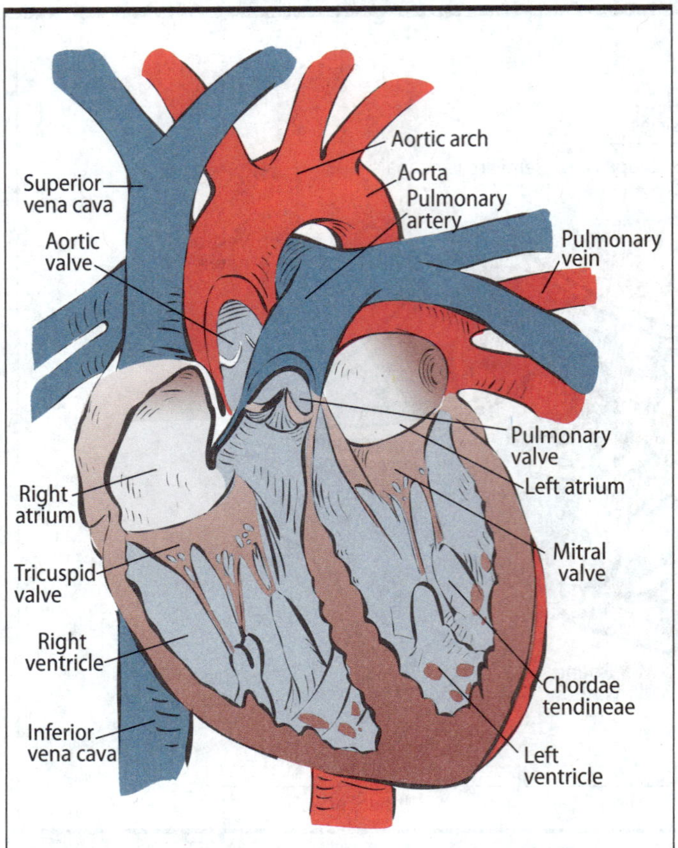


## Heart Cross Section

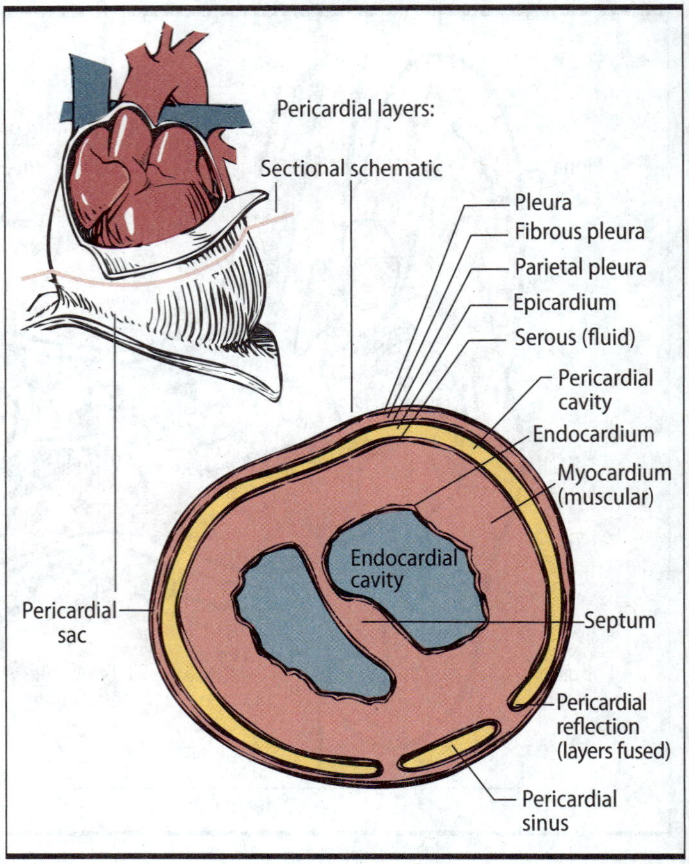


## Heart Valves

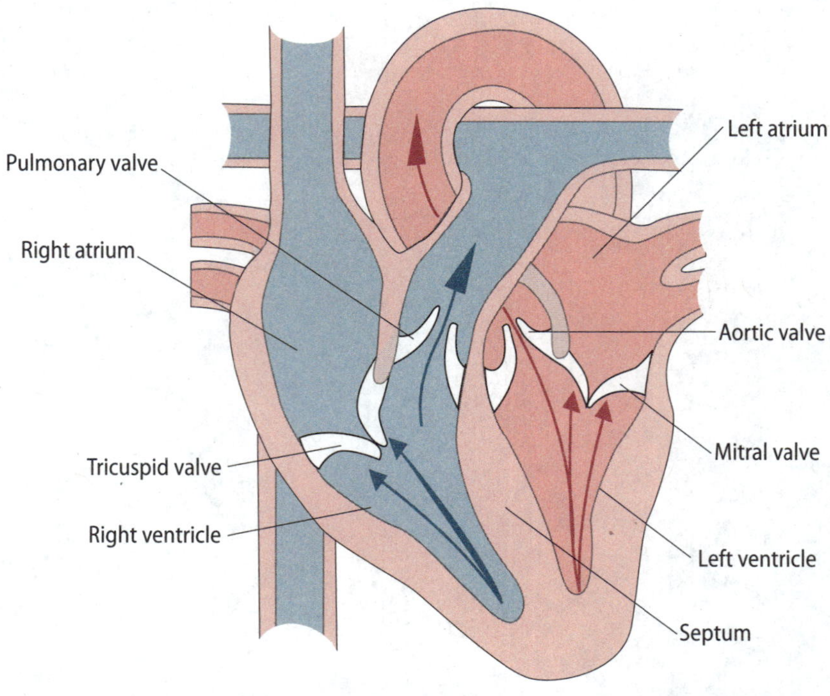


Schematic shows valves of the heart as blood is pumped out. The septum is the wall dividing the left and right ventricles. The papillary muscles and chordae tendineae (above right) function to open and close the atrioventricular valves

## Heart Conduction System

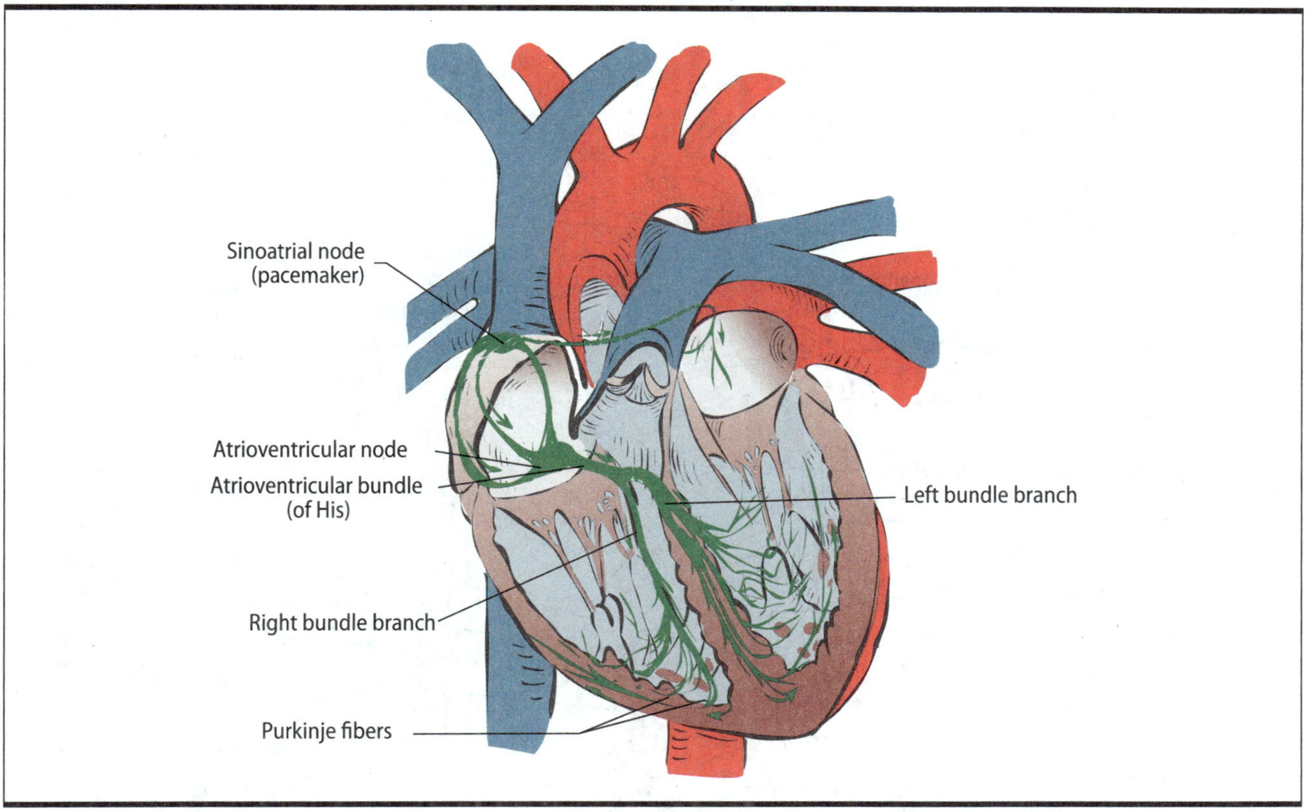


## Coronary Arteries

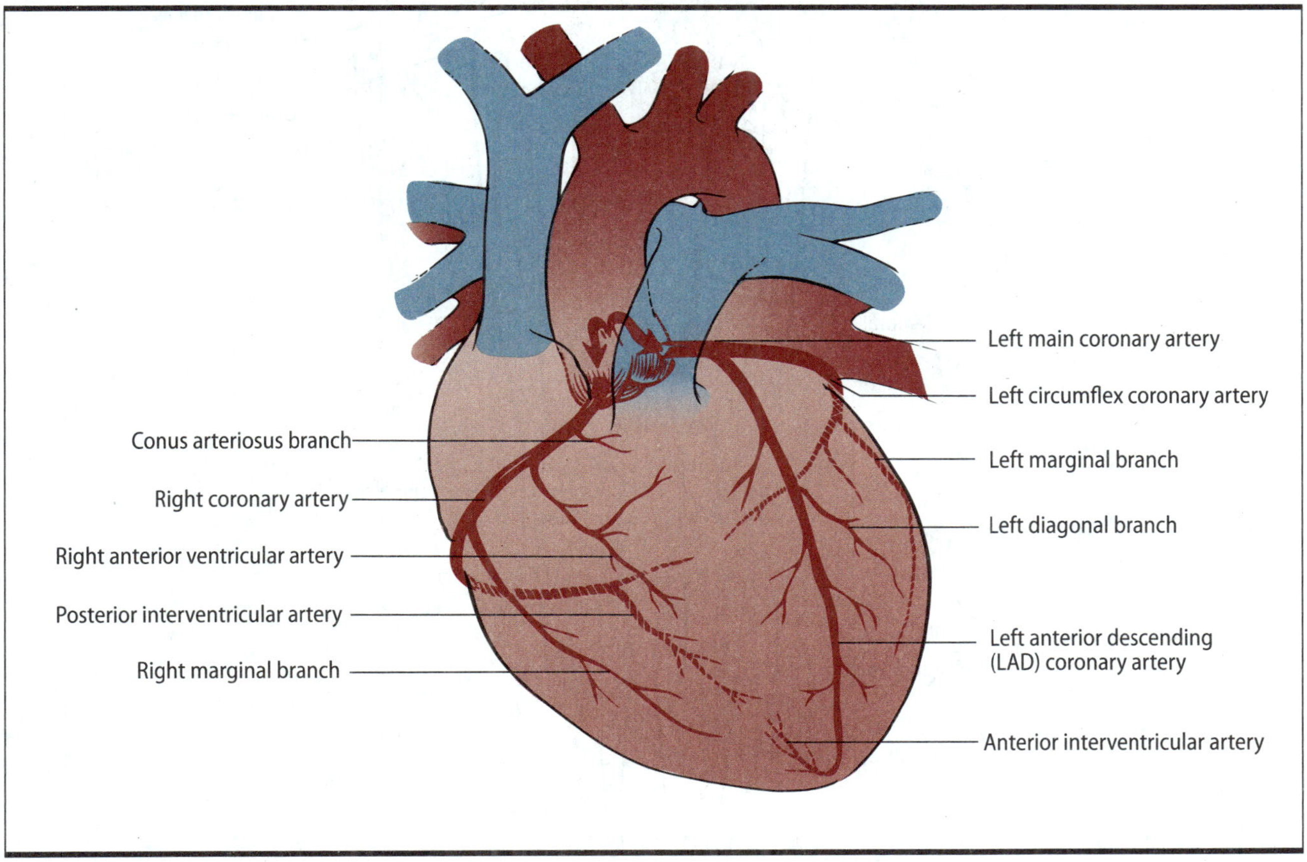

## Arteries

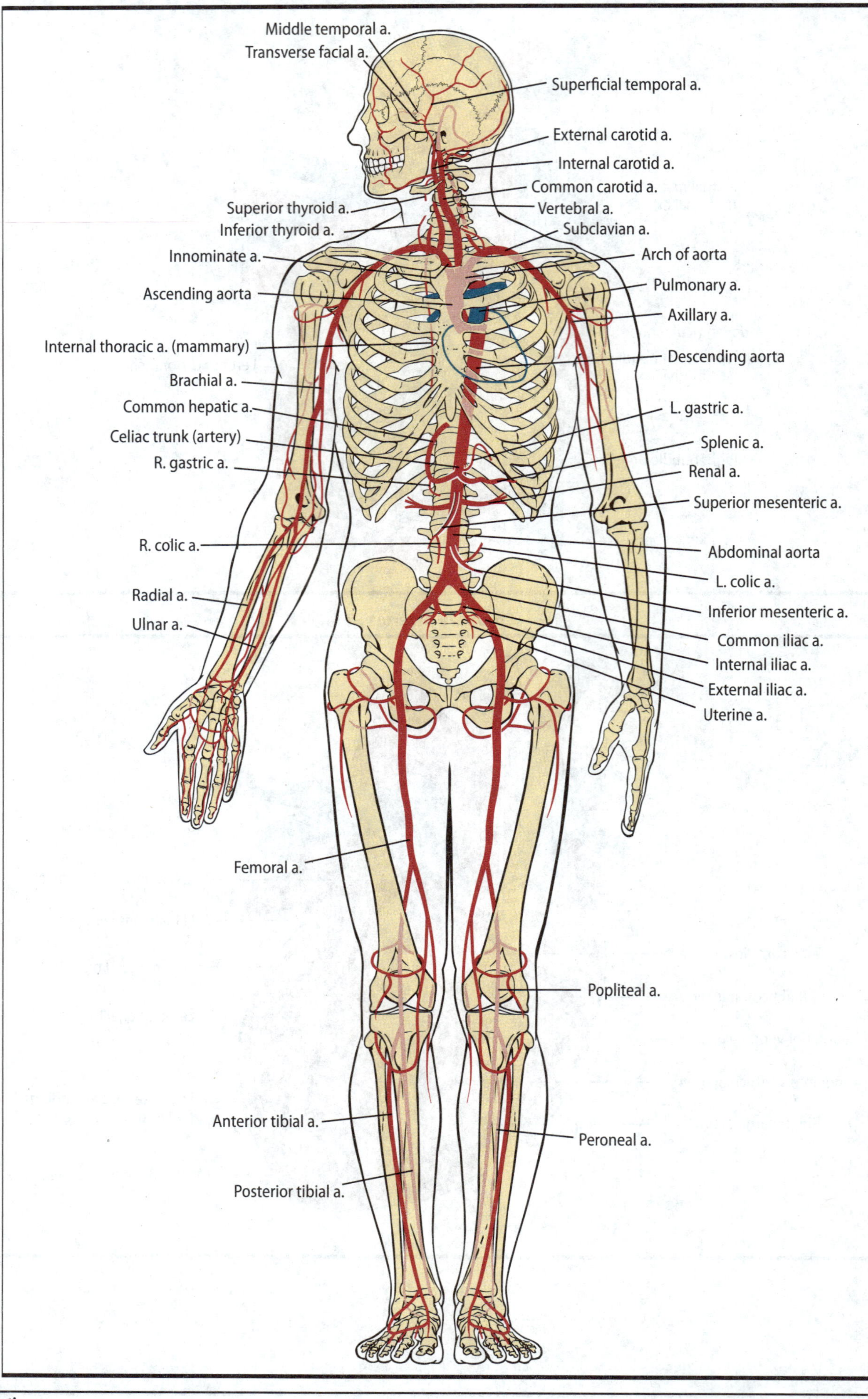
Middle temporal a.
Transverse facial a.
Superficial temporal a.
External carotid a.
Internal carotid a.
Common carotid a.
Superior thyroid a.
Vertebral a.
Inferior thyroid a.
Subclavian a.
Innominate a.
Arch of aorta
Pulmonary a.
Ascending aorta
Axillary a.
Internal thoracic a. (mammary)
Descending aorta
Brachial a.
Common hepatic a.
L. gastric a.
Celiac trunk (artery)
Splenic a.
R. gastric a.
Renal a.
Superior mesenteric a.
R. colic a.
Abdominal aorta
L. colic a.
Radial a.
Inferior mesenteric a.
Ulnar a.
Common iliac a.
Internal iliac a.
External iliac a.
Uterine a.
Femoral a.
Popliteal a.
Anterior tibial a.
Peroneal a.
Posterior tibial a.

## Veins

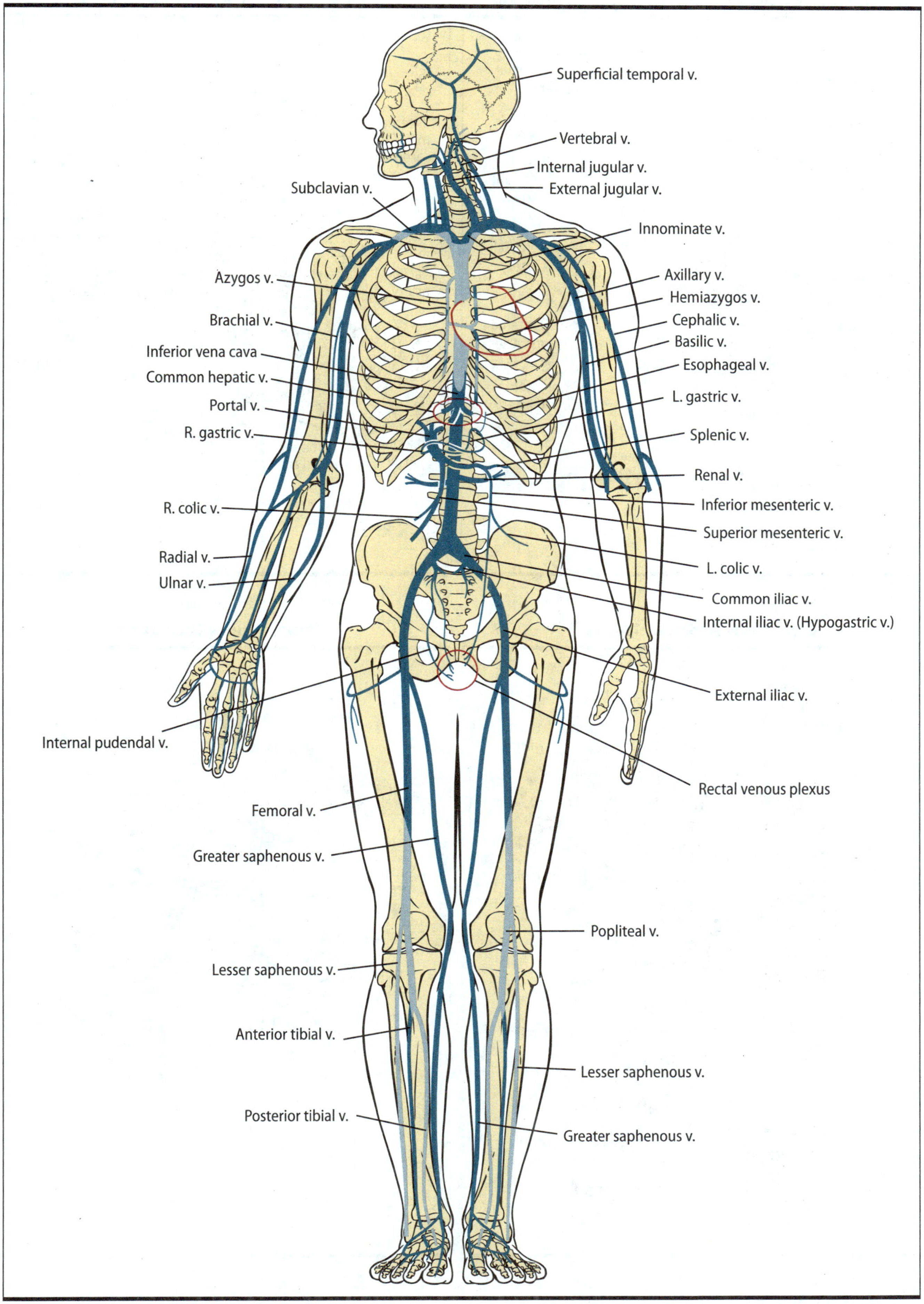
Superficial temporal v.
Vertebral v.
Internal jugular v.
External jugular v.
Subclavian v.
Innominate v.
Azygos v.
Axillary v.
Hemiazygos v.
Brachial v.
Cephalic v.
Basilic v.
Inferior vena cava
Common hepatic v.
Esophageal v.
Portal v.
L. gastric v.
R. gastric v.
Splenic v.
Renal v.
R. colic v.
Inferior mesenteric v.
Superior mesenteric v.
Radial v.
L. colic v.
Ulnar v.
Common iliac v.
Internal iliac v. (Hypogastric v.)
External iliac v.
Internal pudendal v.
Rectal venous plexus
Femoral v.
Greater saphenous v.
Popliteal v.
Lesser saphenous v.
Anterior tibial v.
Lesser saphenous v.
Posterior tibial v.
Greater saphenous v.

## Internal Carotid and Vertebral Arteries and Branches

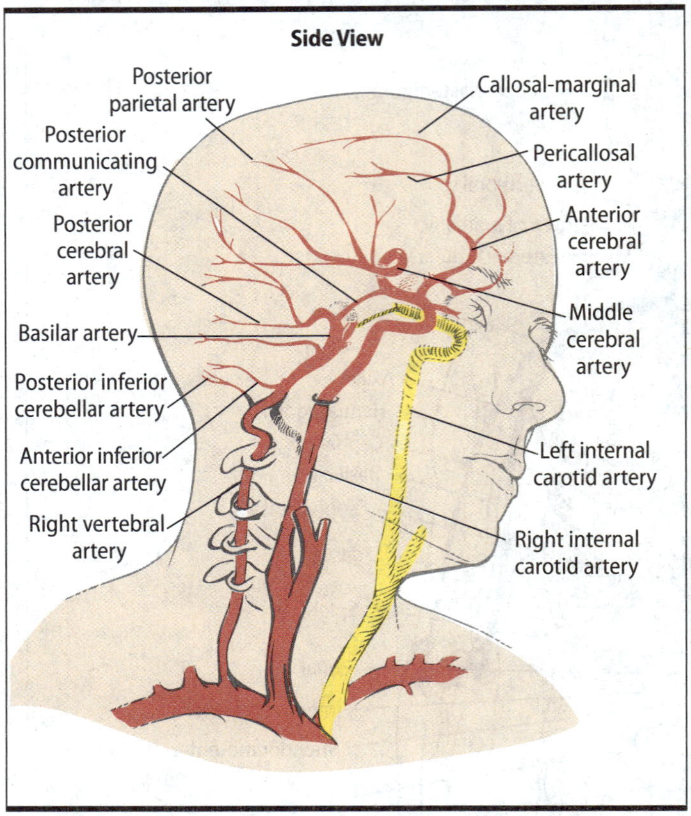


## External Carotid Artery and Branches

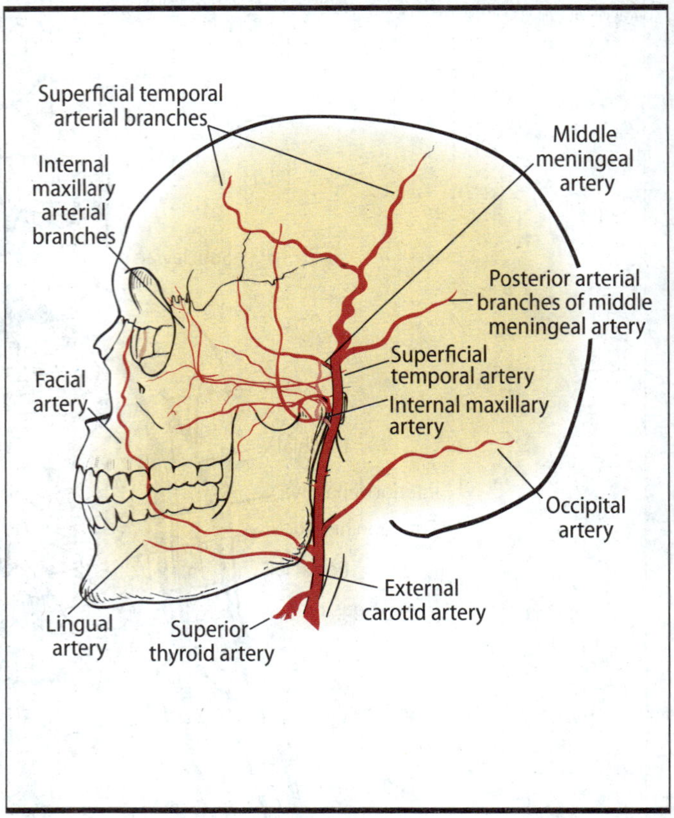


## Branches of Abdominal Aorta

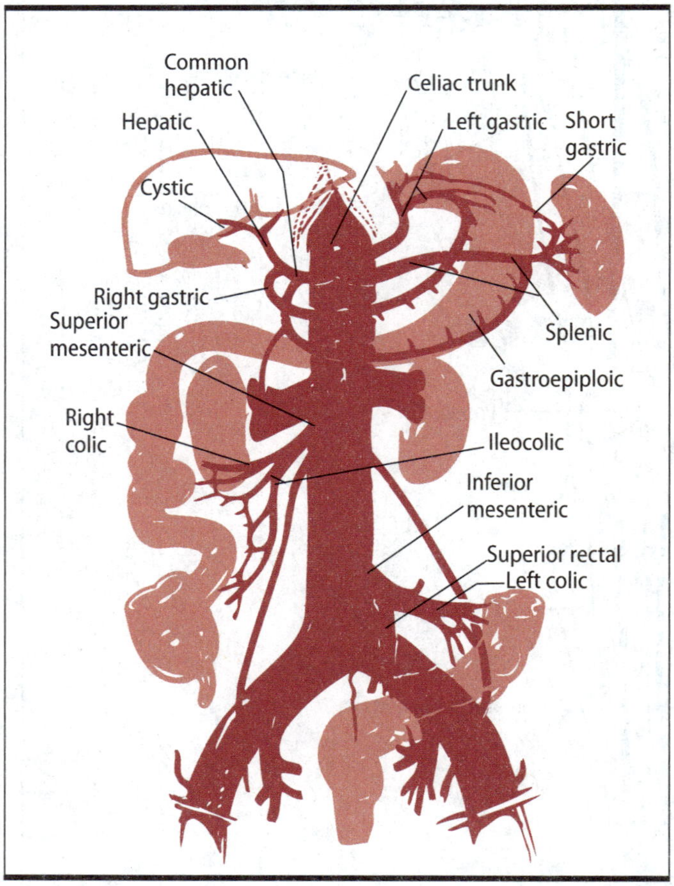


## Portal Venous Circulation

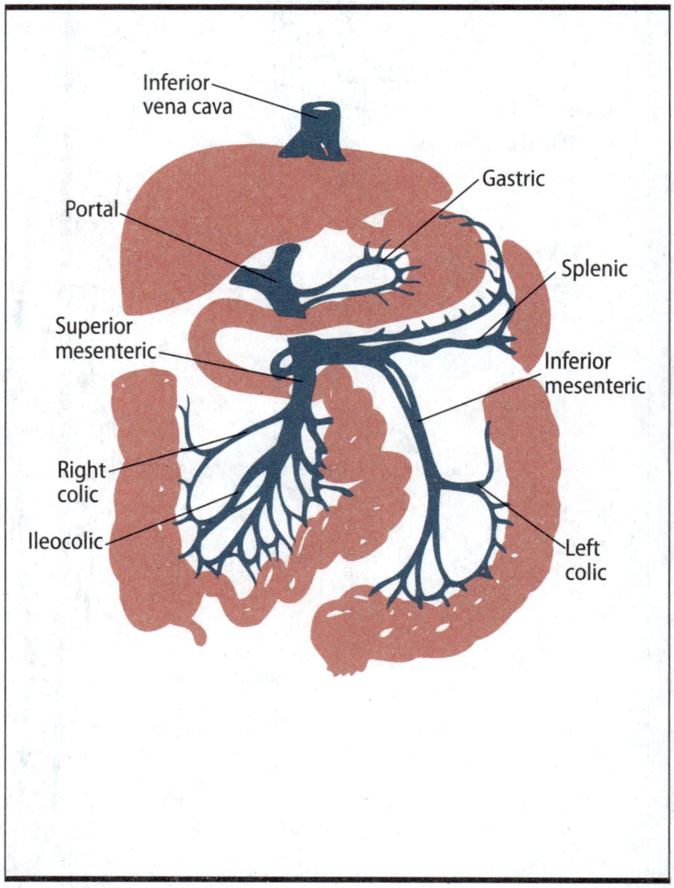

## Lymphatic System

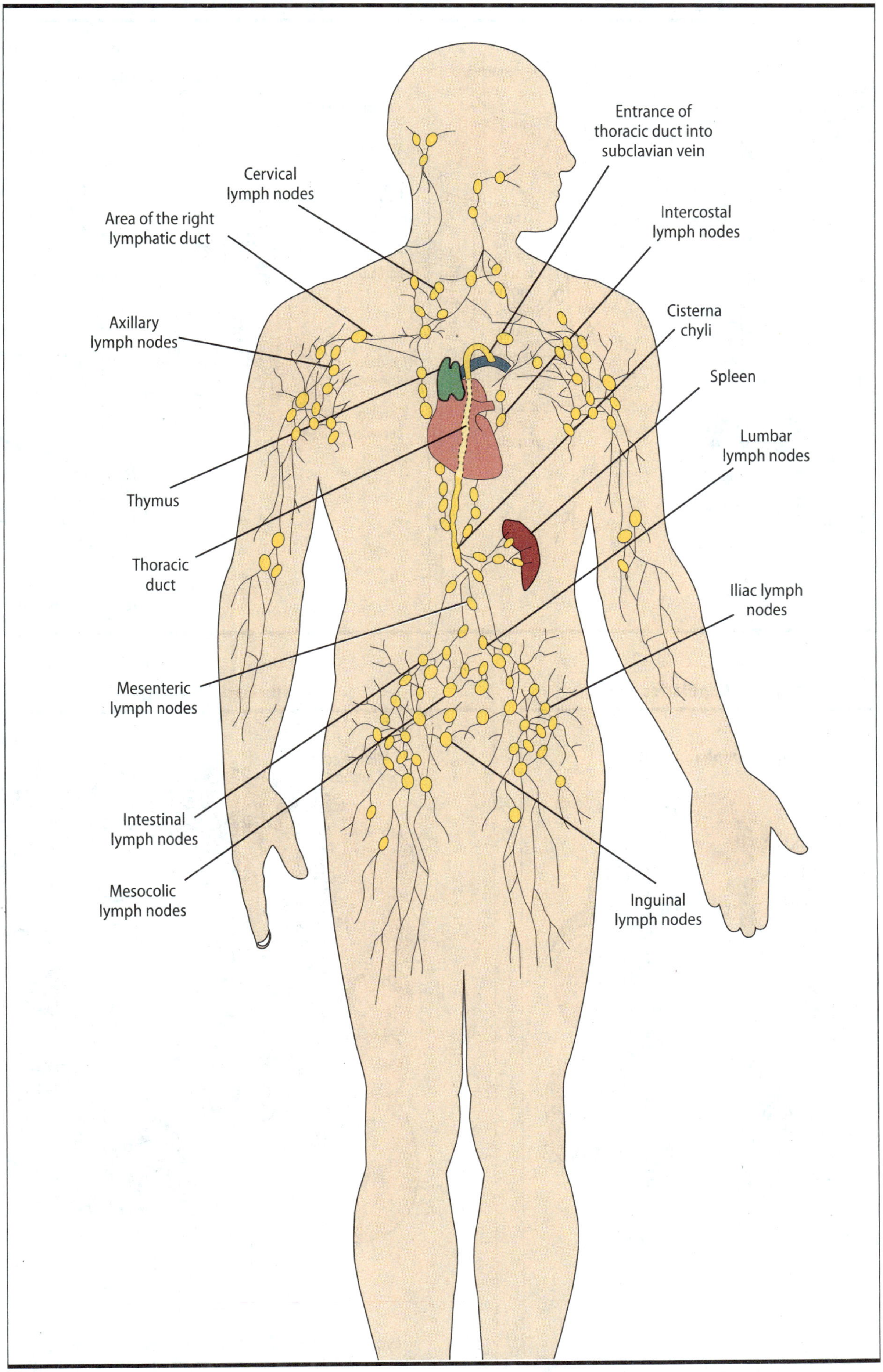

## Axillary Lymph Nodes

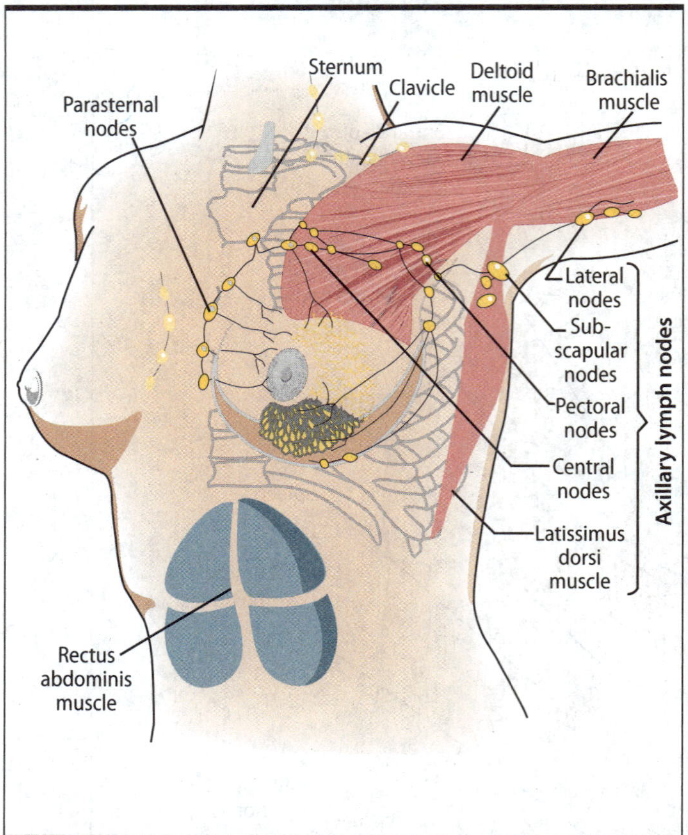


## Lymphatic System of Head and Neck

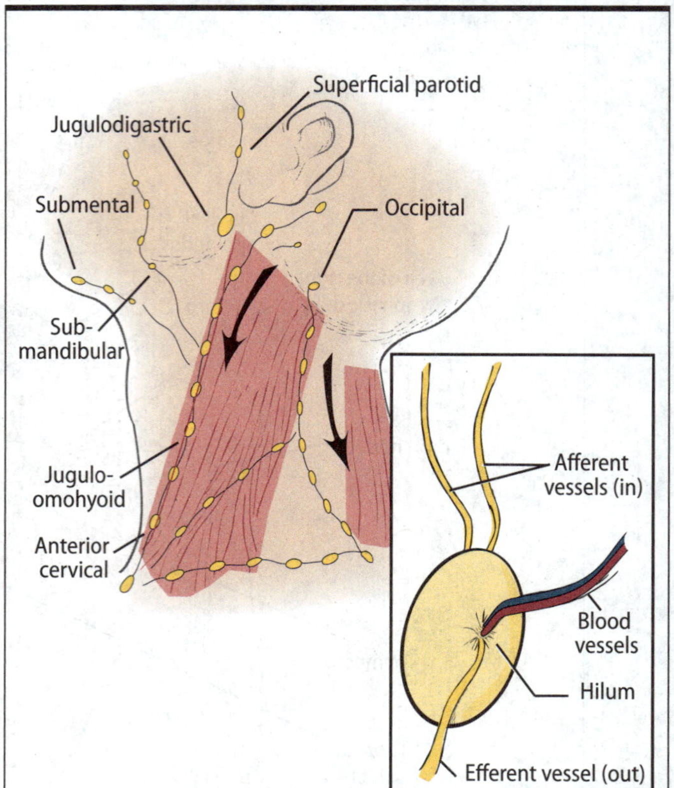


Schematic of lymph node

## Lymphatic Capillaries

Schematic of lymphatic capillaries

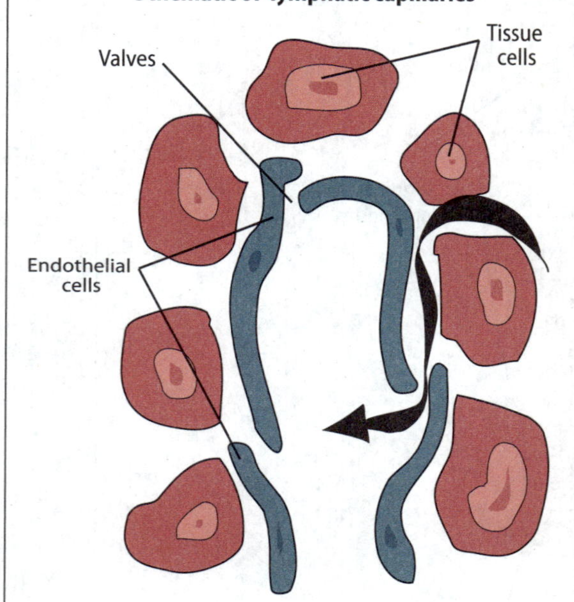


Fluids and particles can enter the capillary through overlapping valves

## Lymphatic Drainage

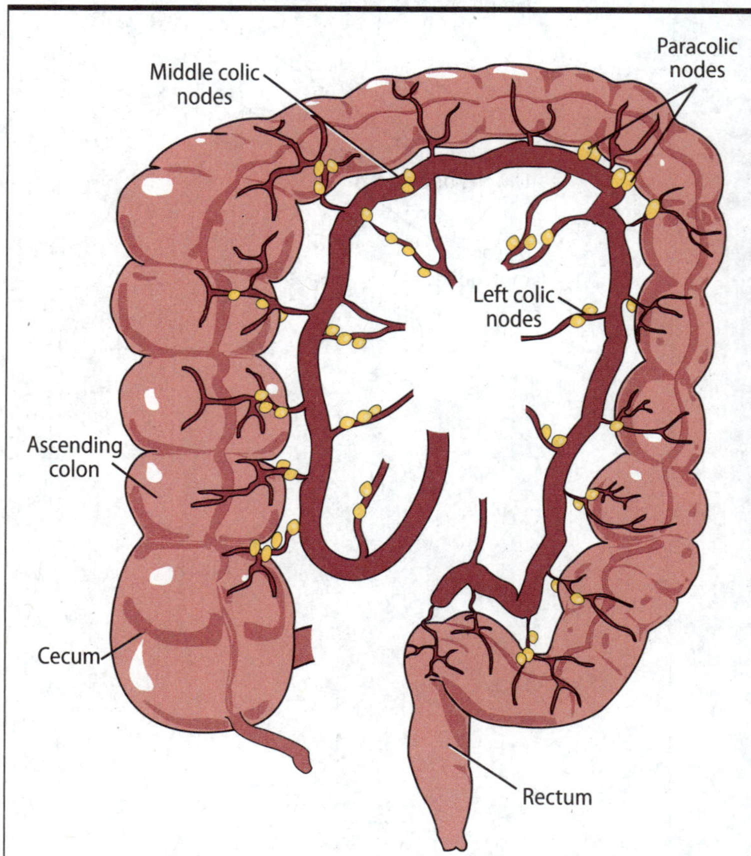


Lymphatic drainage of the colon follows blood supply

# Chapter 10. Diseases of the Respiratory System (JØØ-J99, UØ7.Ø)

## Respiratory System

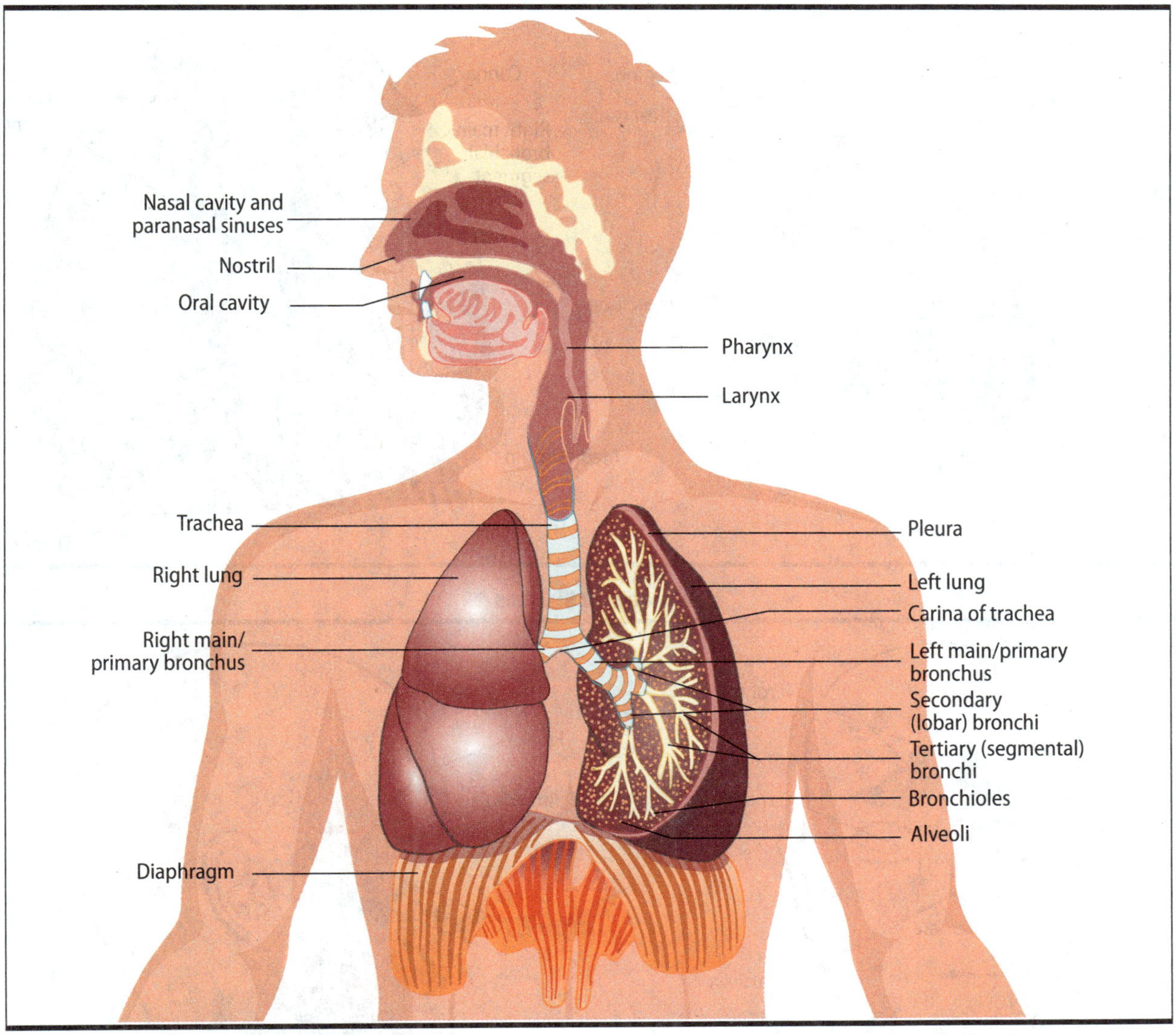


## Upper Respiratory System

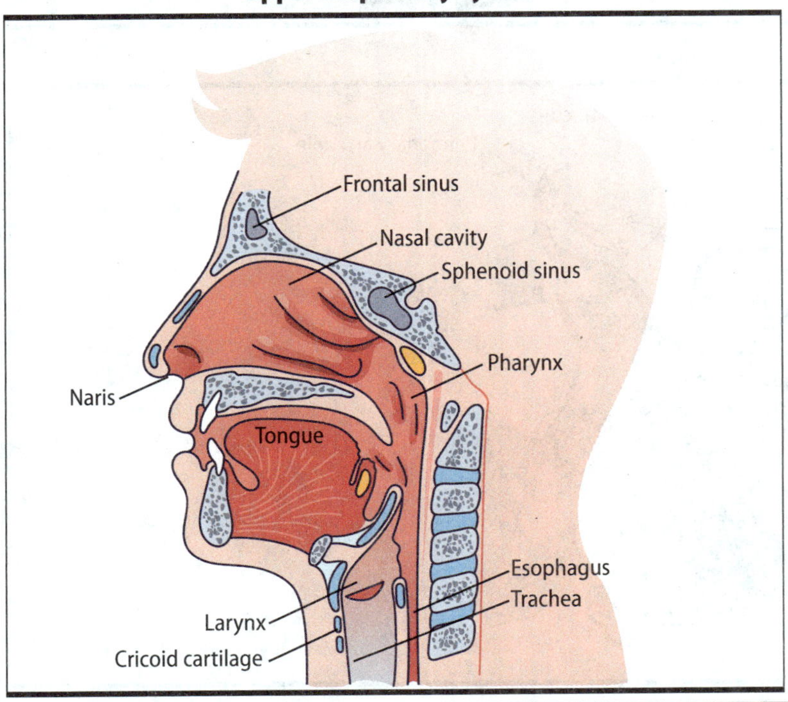


## Nasal Cavity

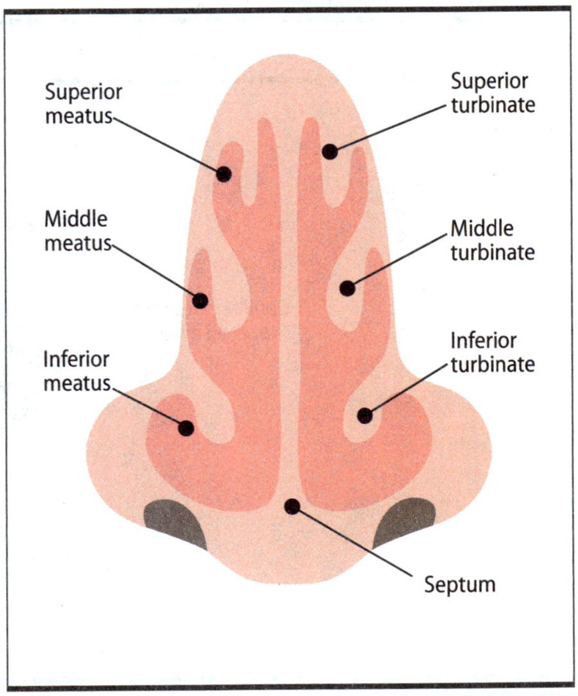

## Lower Respiratory System

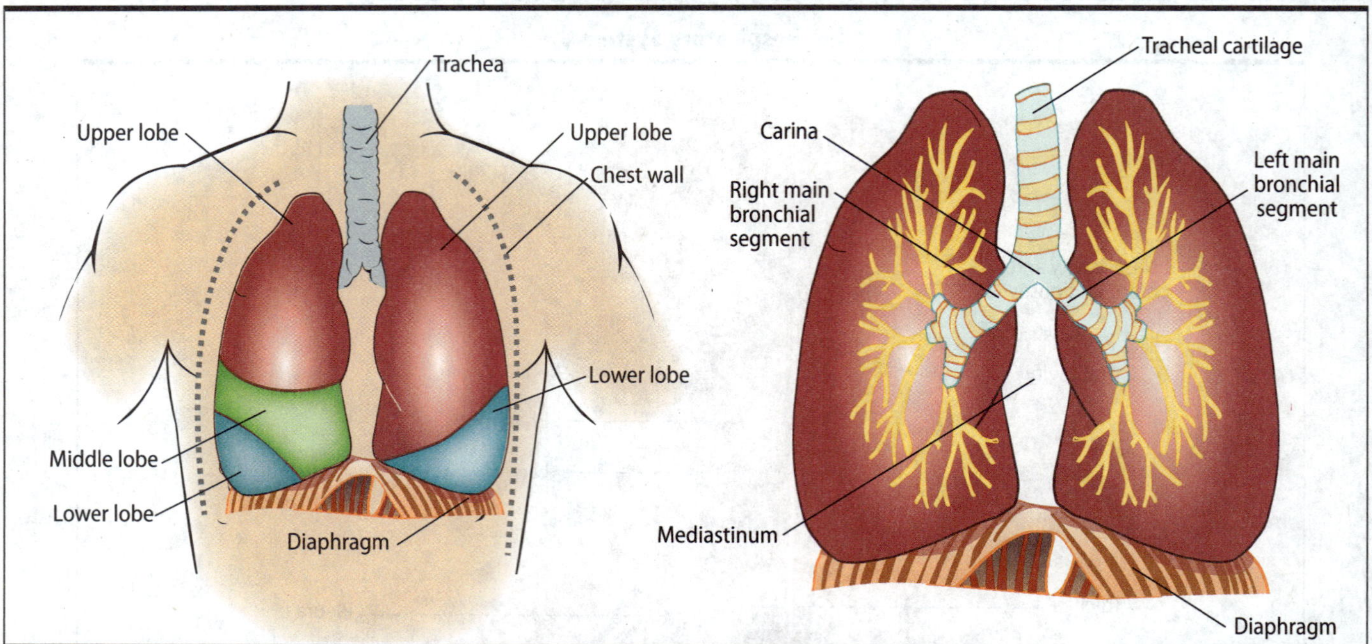


## Paranasal Sinuses

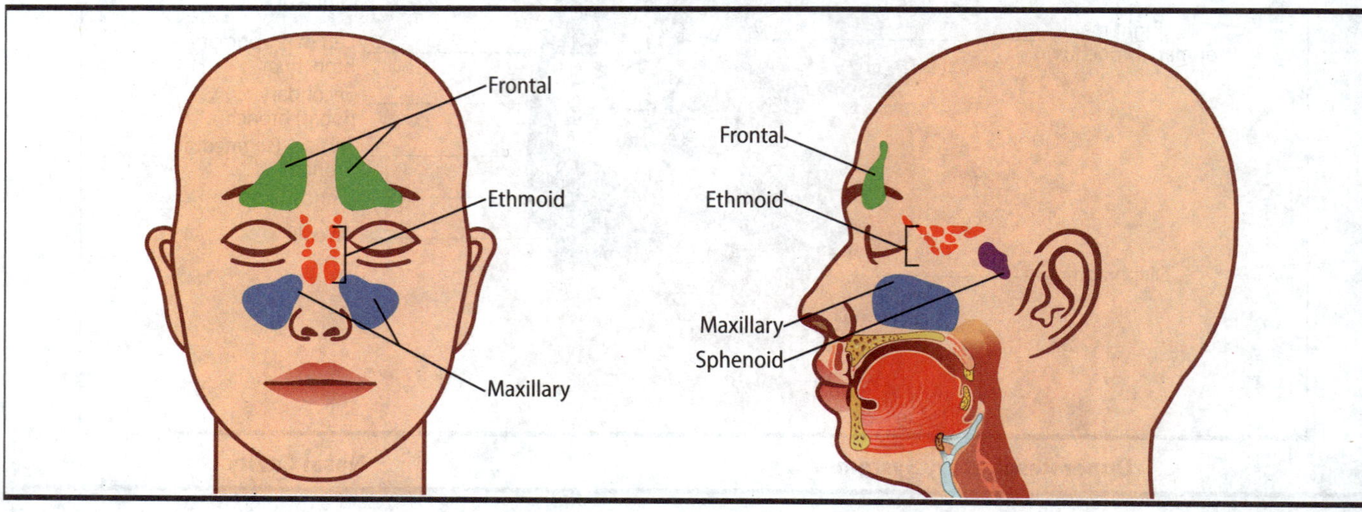


## Alveoli

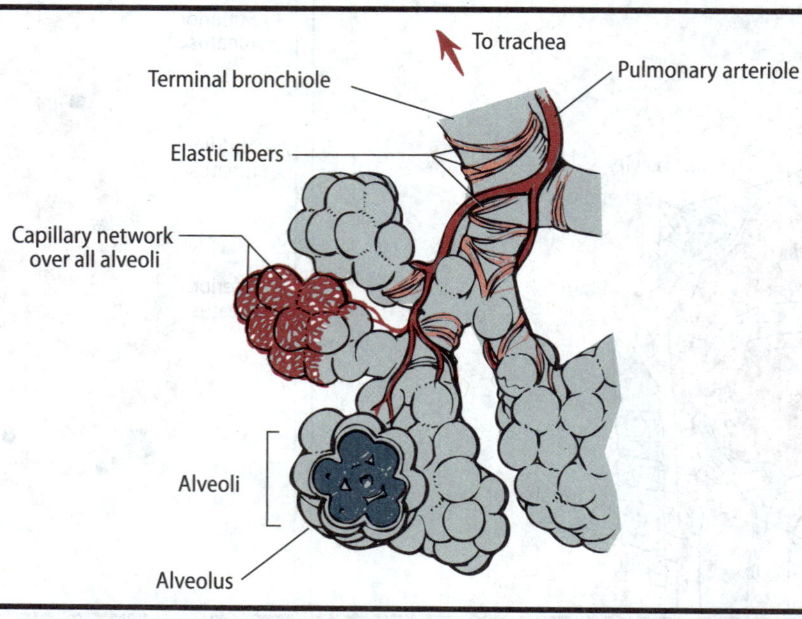

## Lung Segments

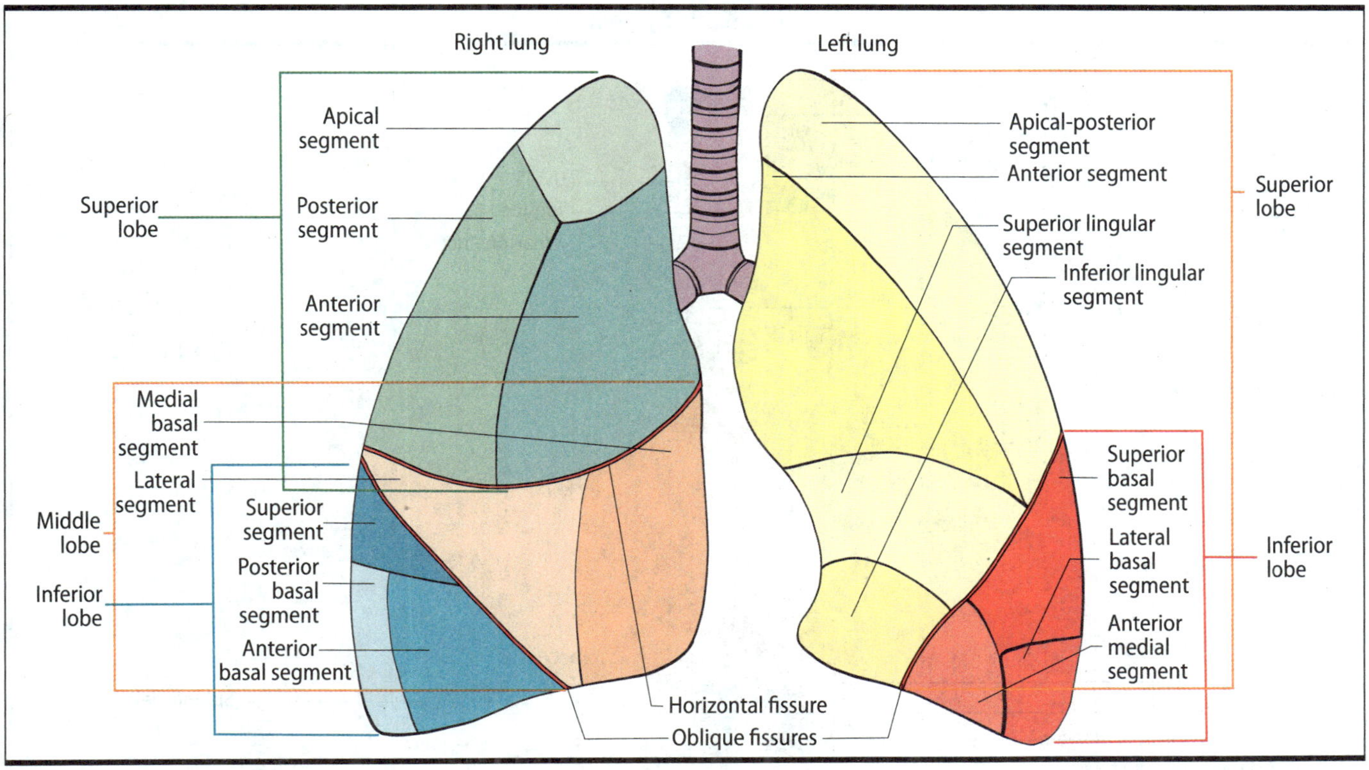

# Chapter 11. Diseases of the Digestive System (KØØ–K95)

## Digestive System

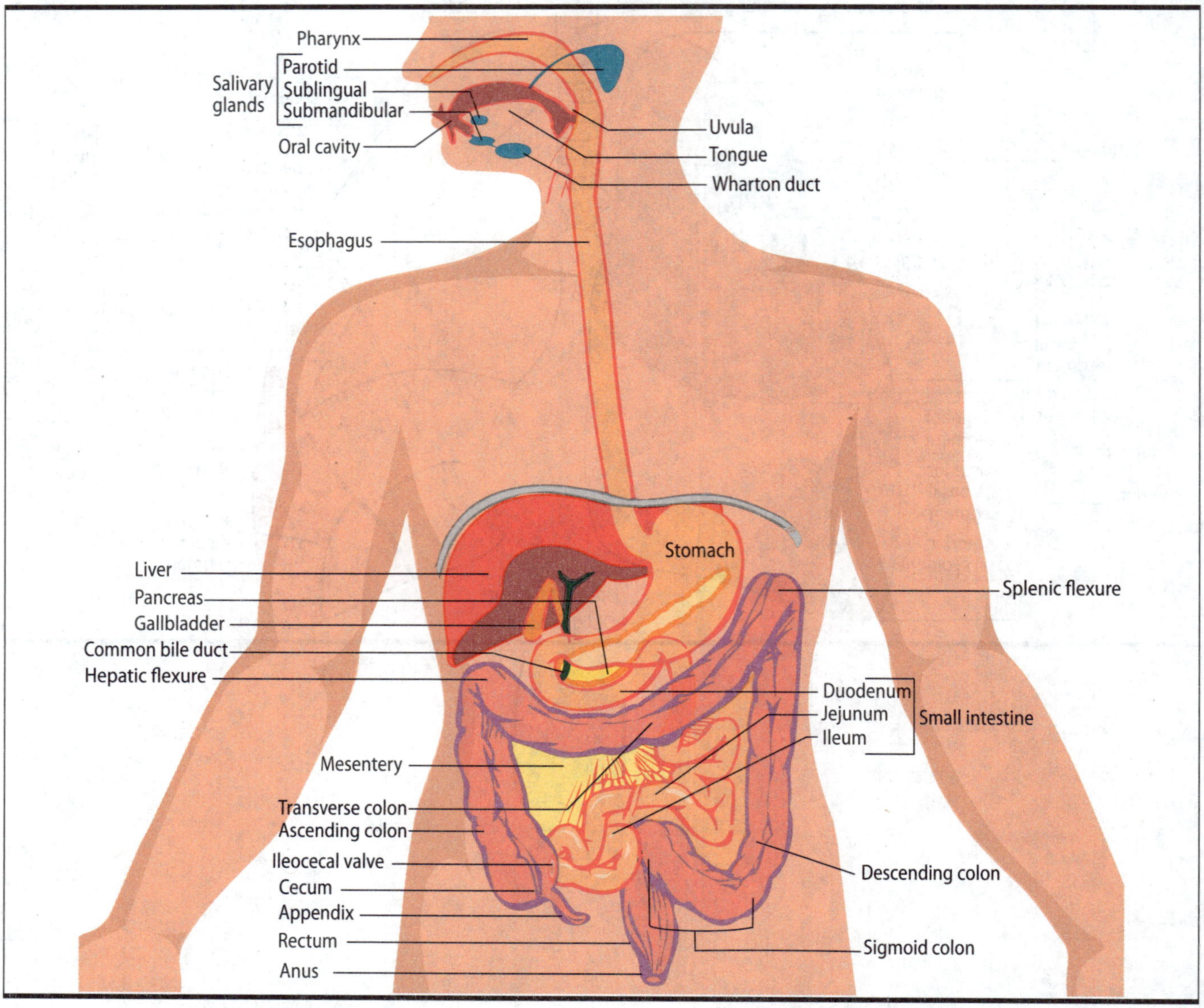


## Omentum and Mesentery

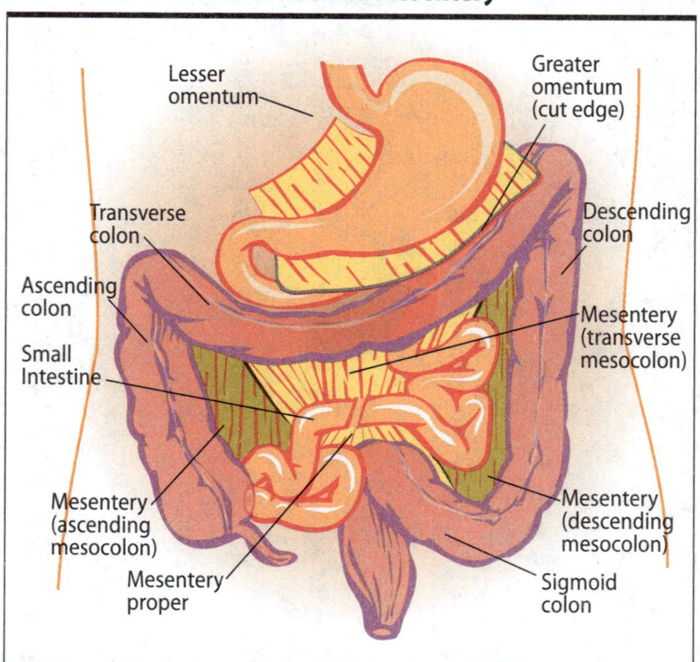


## Peritoneum and Retroperitoneum

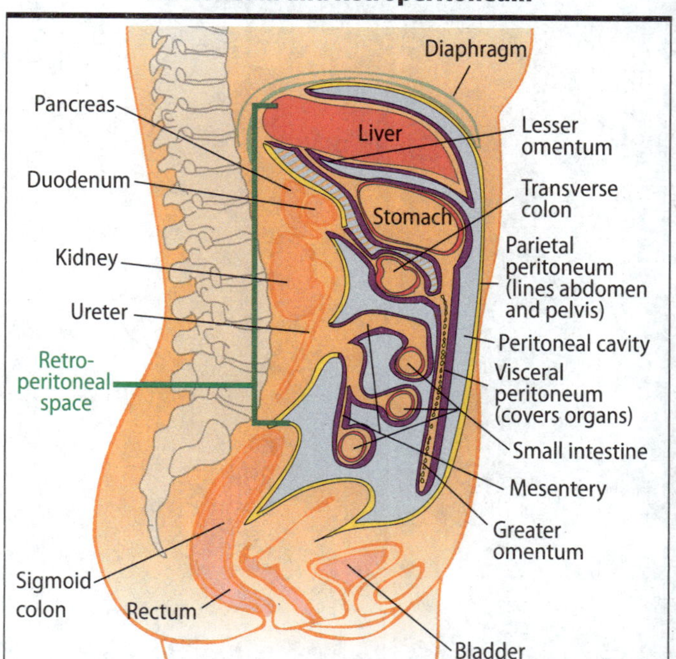

# Chapter 12. Diseases of the Skin and Subcutaneous Tissue (LØØ–L99)

**Nail Anatomy**

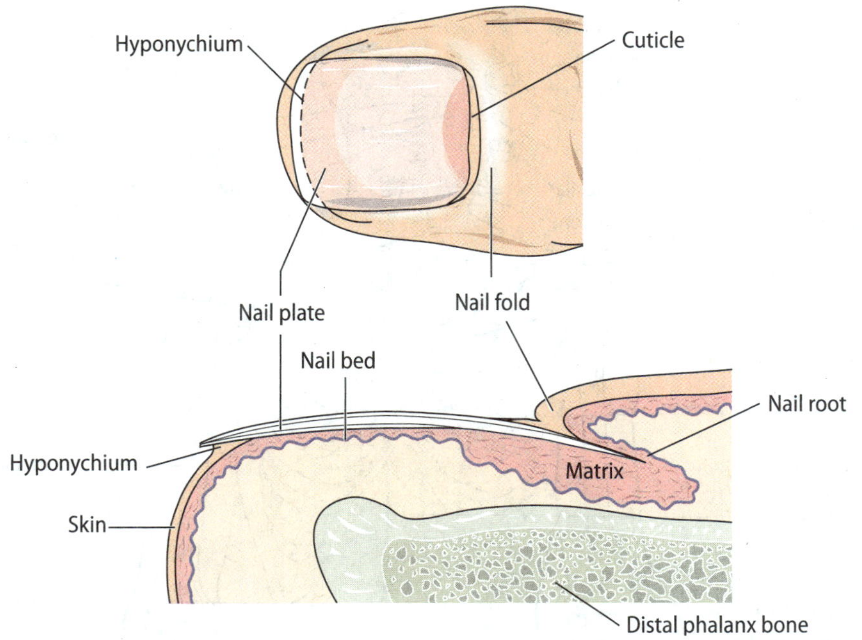


**Skin and Subcutaneous Tissue**

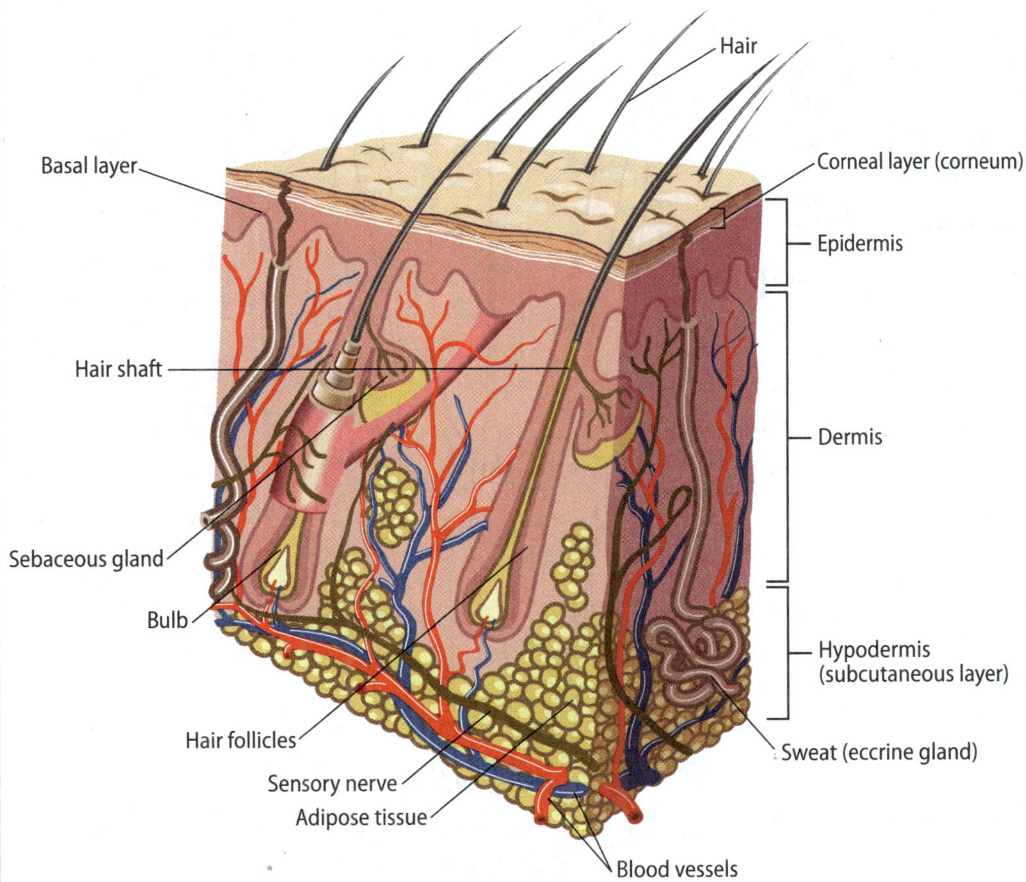

# Chapter 13. Diseases of the Musculoskeletal System and Connective Tissue (MØØ–M99)

## Bones and Joints

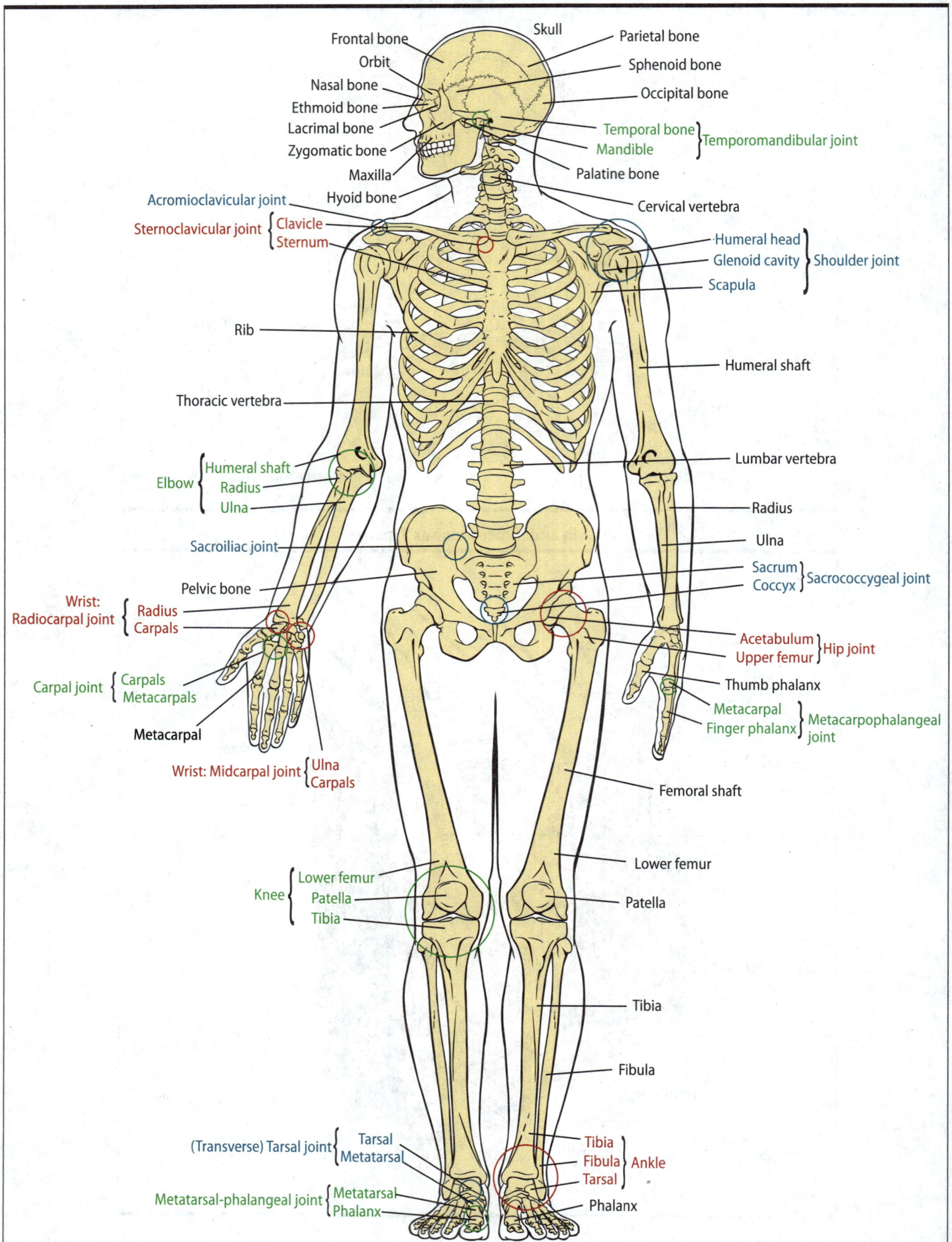

## Shoulder Anterior View

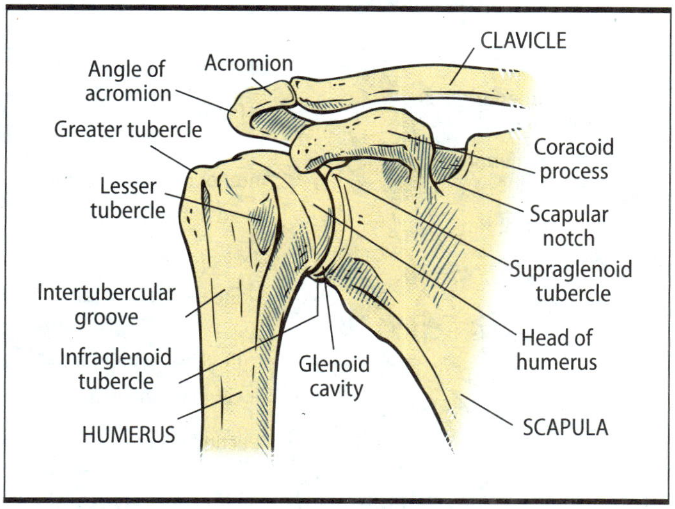


## Shoulder Posterior View

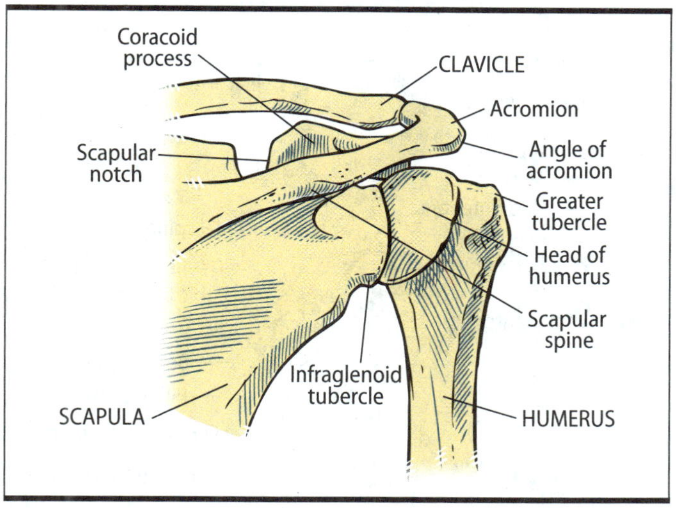


## Elbow Anterior View

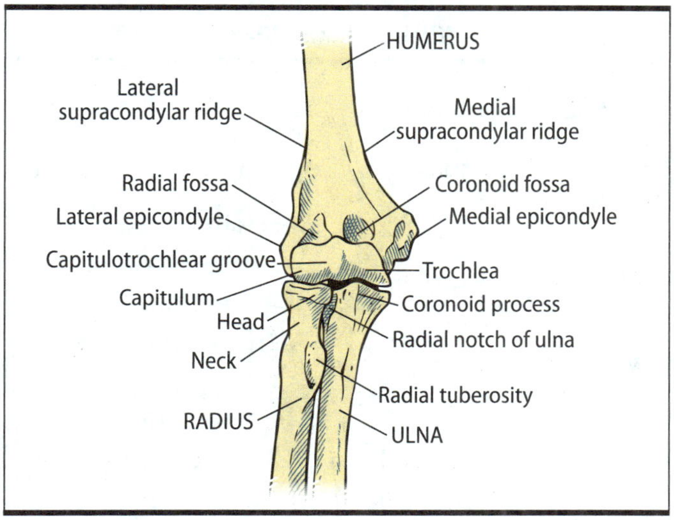


## Elbow Posterior View

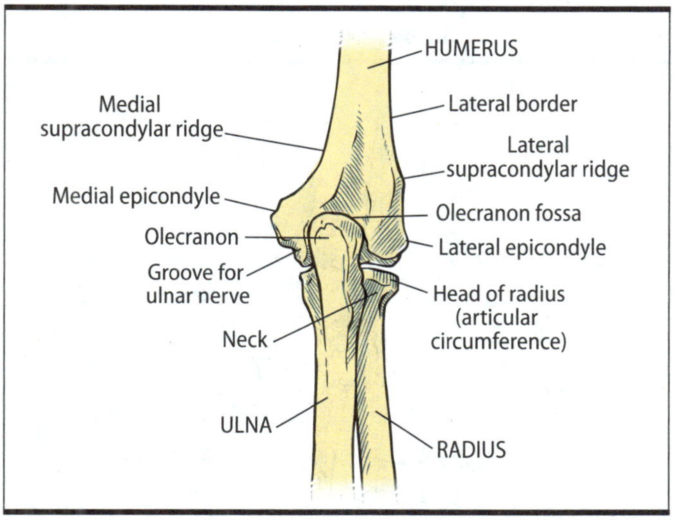


## Hand

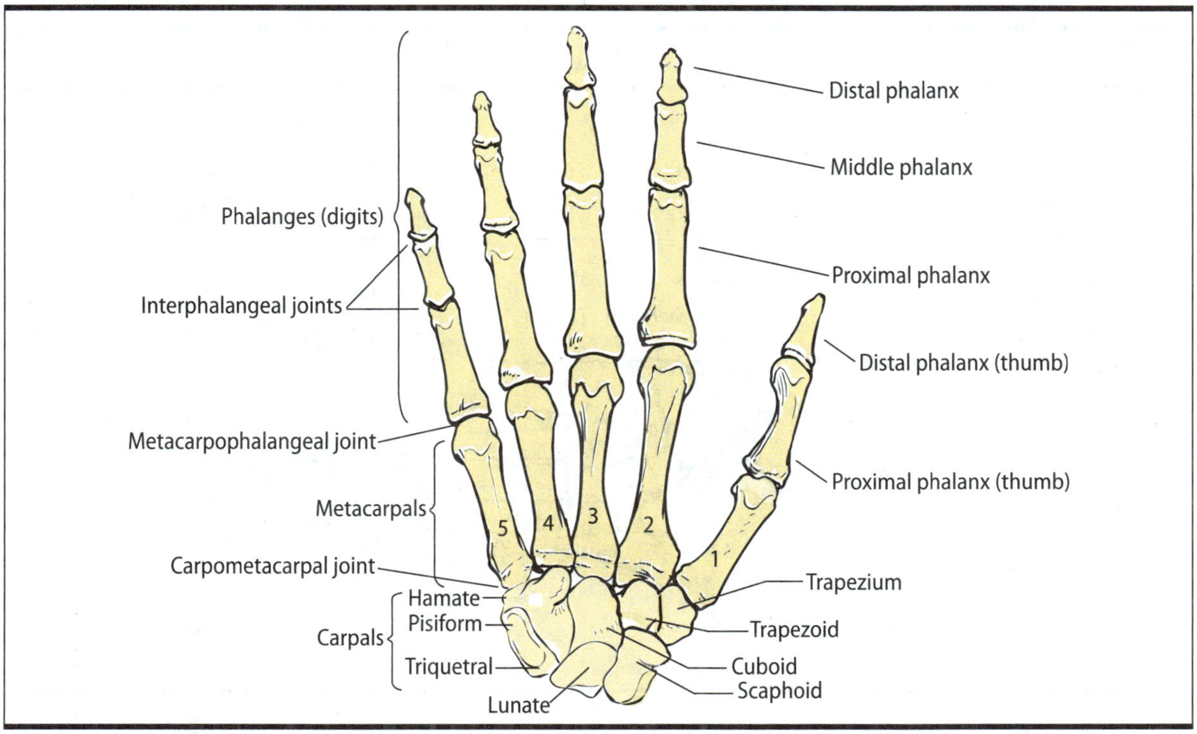

## Hip Anterior View

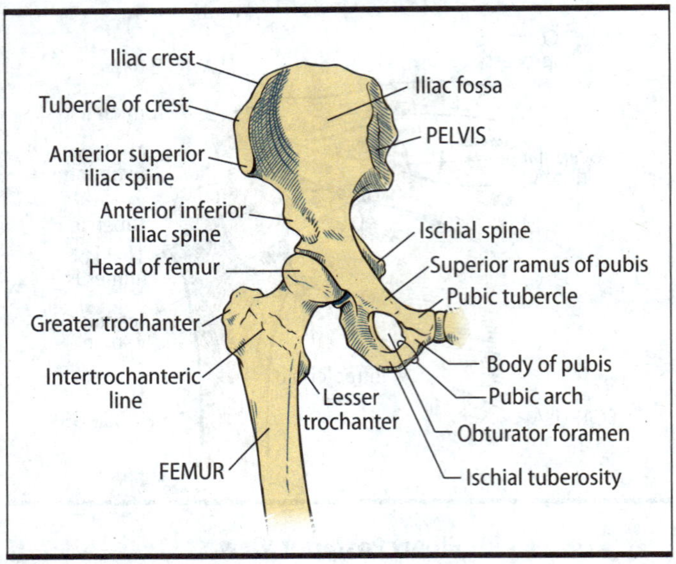


## Hip Posterior View

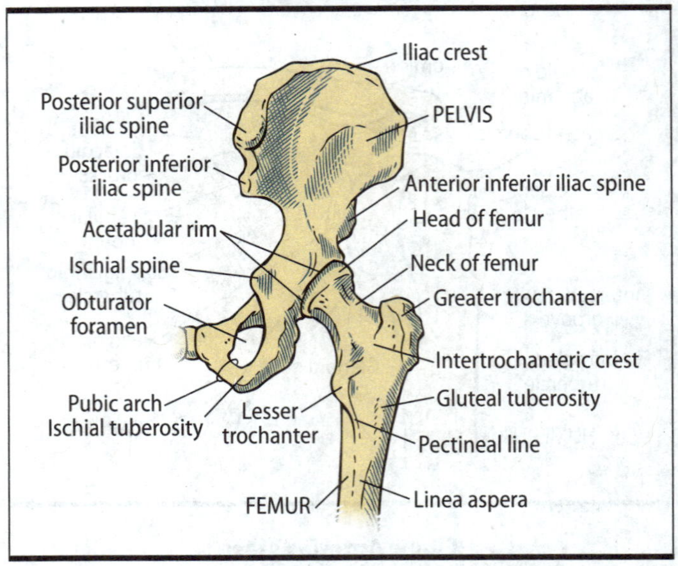


## Knee Anterior View

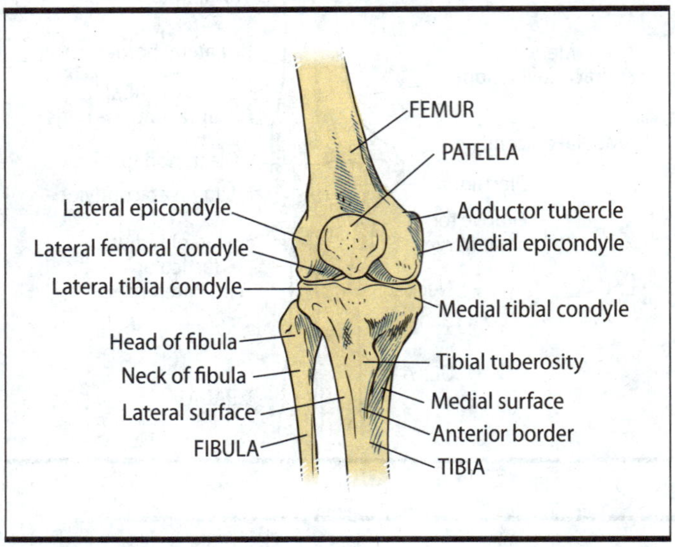


## Knee Posterior View

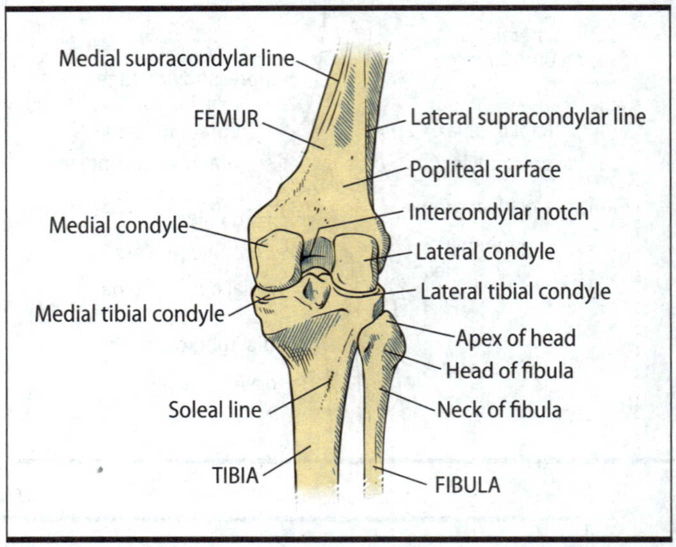


## Foot

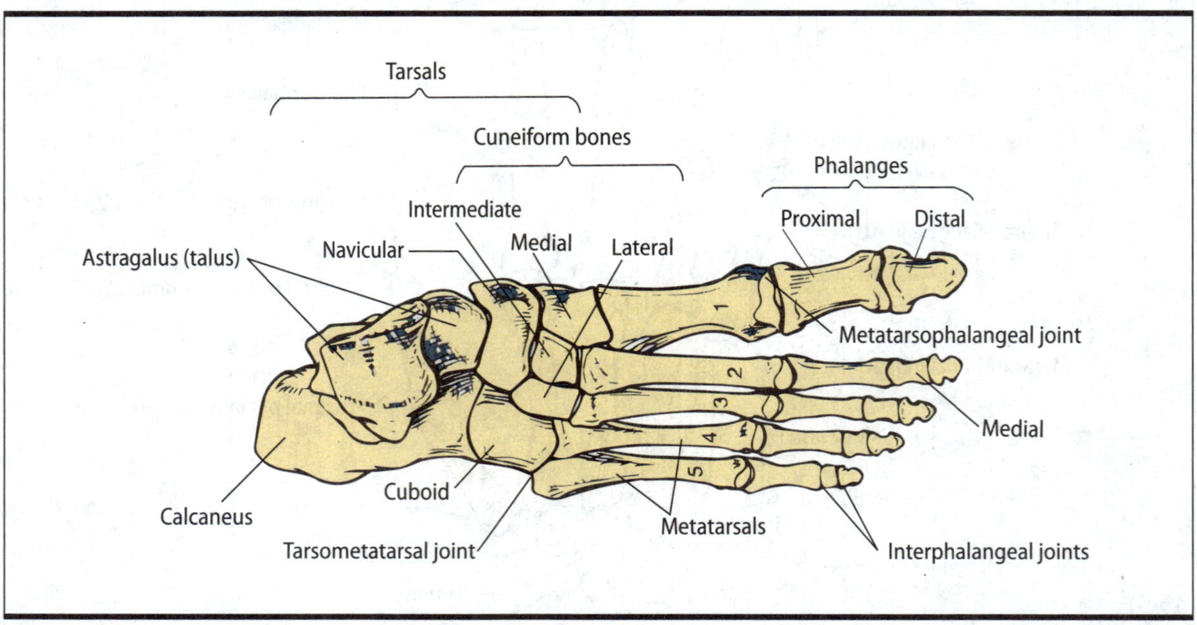

## Muscles

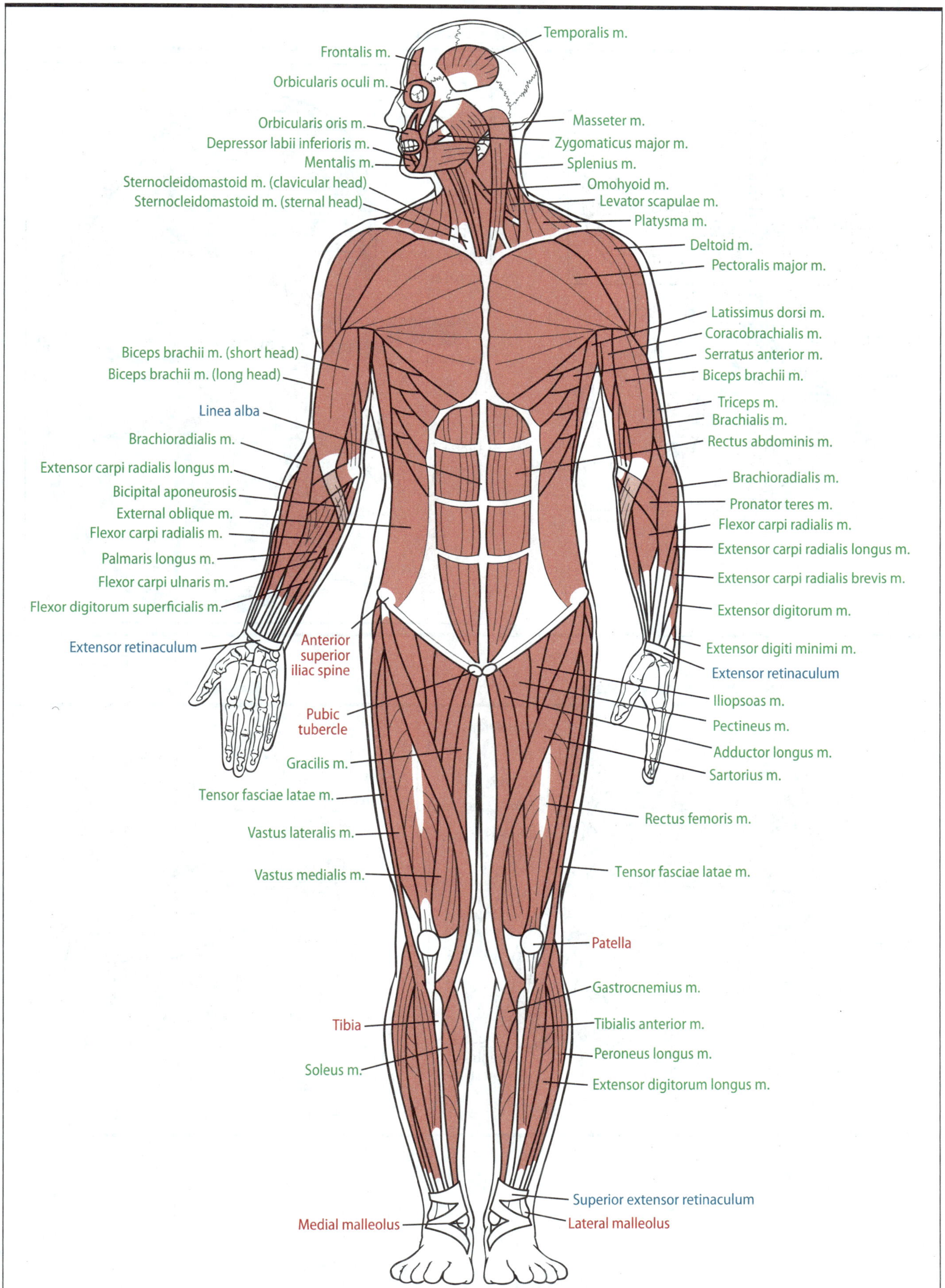

Temporalis m.
Frontalis m.
Orbicularis oculi m.
Orbicularis oris m.
Depressor labii inferioris m.
Mentalis m.
Sternocleidomastoid m. (clavicular head)
Sternocleidomastoid m. (sternal head)
Masseter m.
Zygomaticus major m.
Splenius m.
Omohyoid m.
Levator scapulae m.
Platysma m.
Deltoid m.
Pectoralis major m.
Latissimus dorsi m.
Coracobrachialis m.
Serratus anterior m.
Biceps brachii m.
Biceps brachii m. (short head)
Biceps brachii m. (long head)
Linea alba
Triceps m.
Brachialis m.
Rectus abdominis m.
Brachioradialis m.
Extensor carpi radialis longus m.
Bicipital aponeurosis
External oblique m.
Flexor carpi radialis m.
Palmaris longus m.
Flexor carpi ulnaris m.
Flexor digitorum superficialis m.
Brachioradialis m.
Pronator teres m.
Flexor carpi radialis m.
Extensor carpi radialis longus m.
Extensor carpi radialis brevis m.
Extensor digitorum m.
Extensor retinaculum
Anterior superior iliac spine
Extensor digiti minimi m.
Extensor retinaculum
Iliopsoas m.
Pectineus m.
Adductor longus m.
Sartorius m.
Pubic tubercle
Gracilis m.
Tensor fasciae latae m.
Vastus lateralis m.
Vastus medialis m.
Rectus femoris m.
Tensor fasciae latae m.
Patella
Gastrocnemius m.
Tibia
Tibialis anterior m.
Peroneus longus m.
Soleus m.
Extensor digitorum longus m.
Superior extensor retinaculum
Medial malleolus
Lateral malleolus

# Chapter 14. Diseases of the Genitourinary System (NØØ–N99)

**Urinary System**

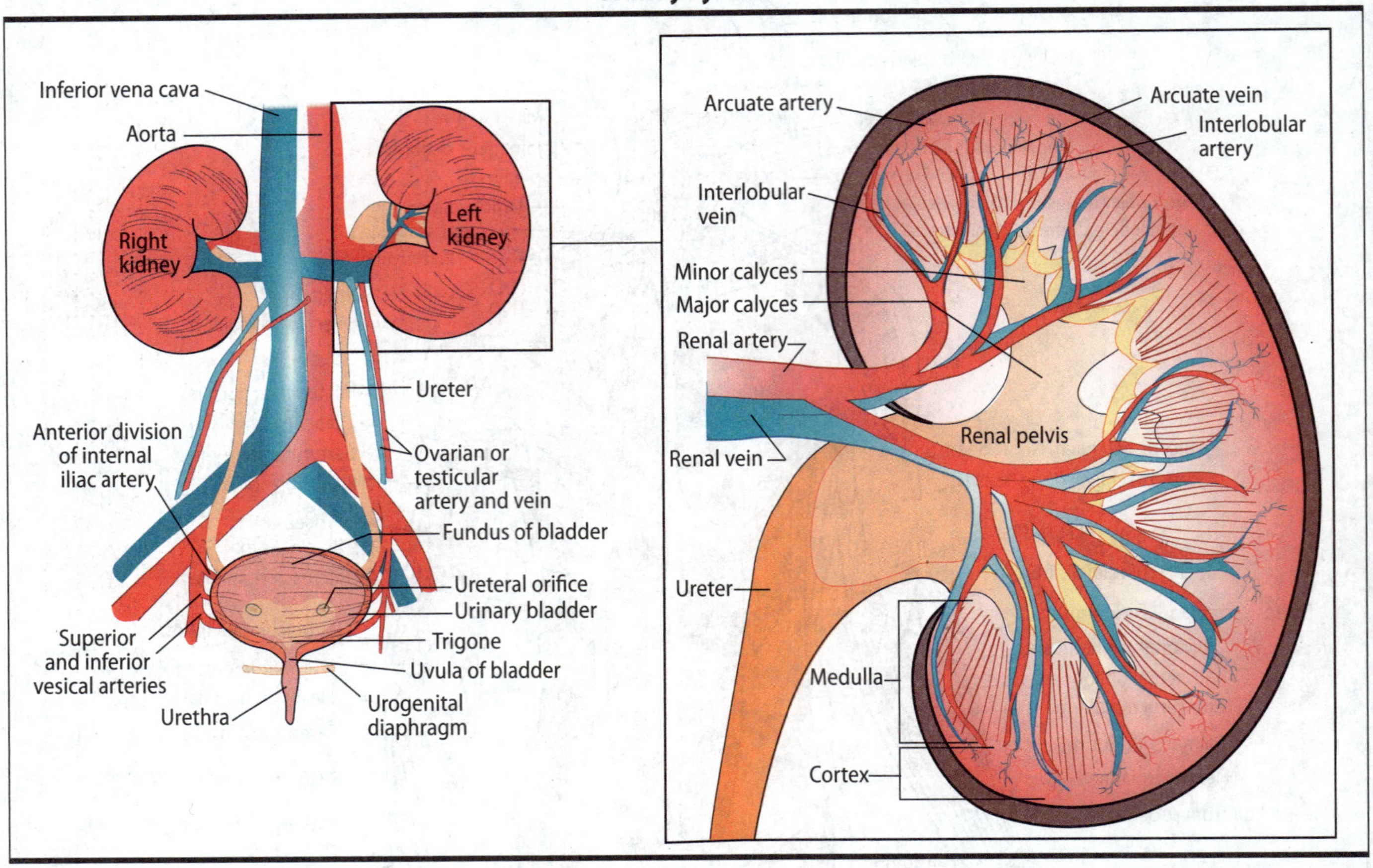


**Male Genitourinary System**

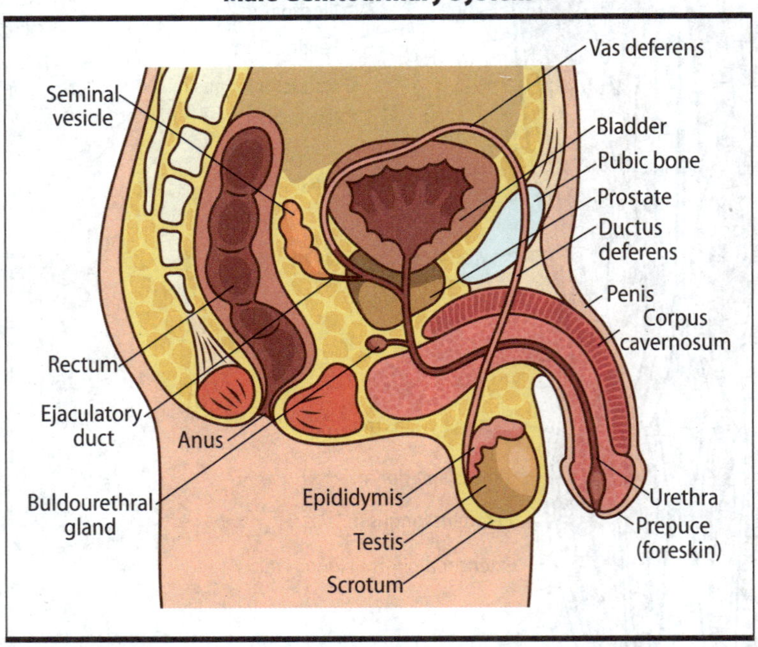


**Male Bladder**

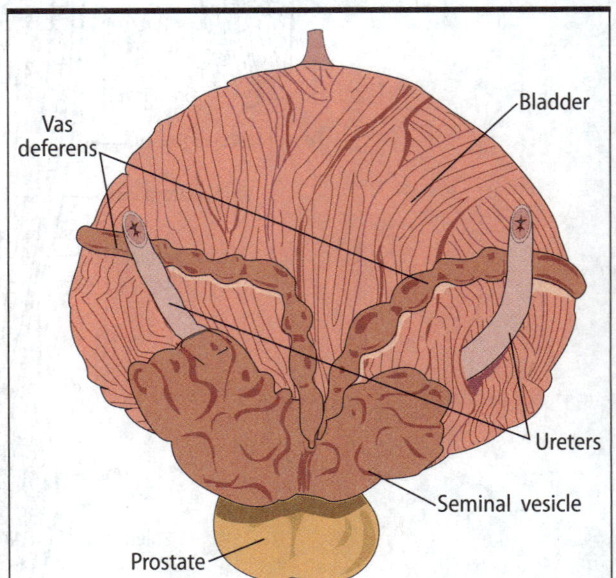


Posterior view of male bladder and prostate

## Female Genitourinary System

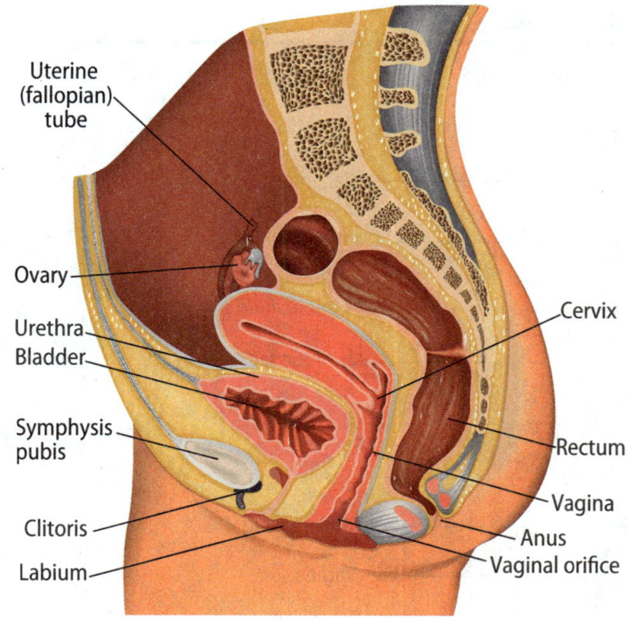


## Female Bladder

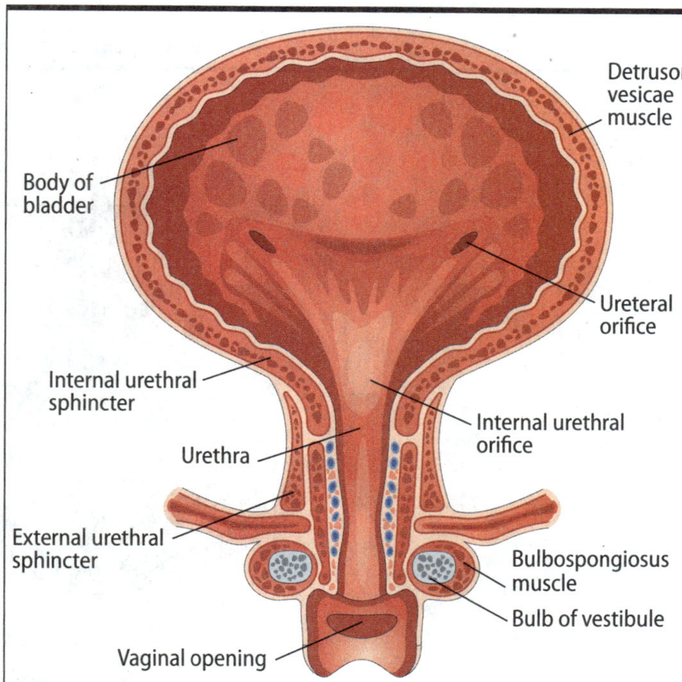


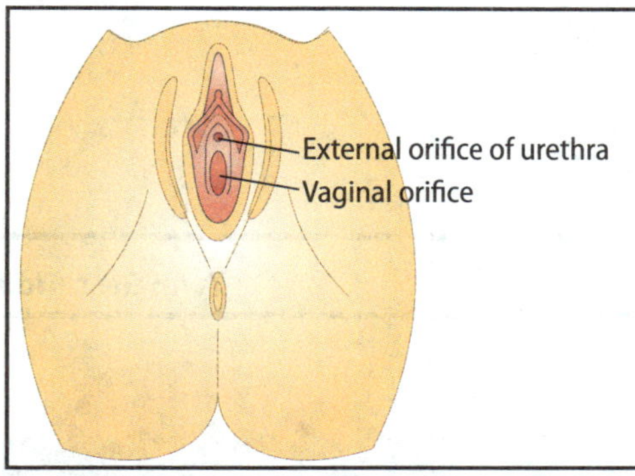


## Female Internal Genitalia

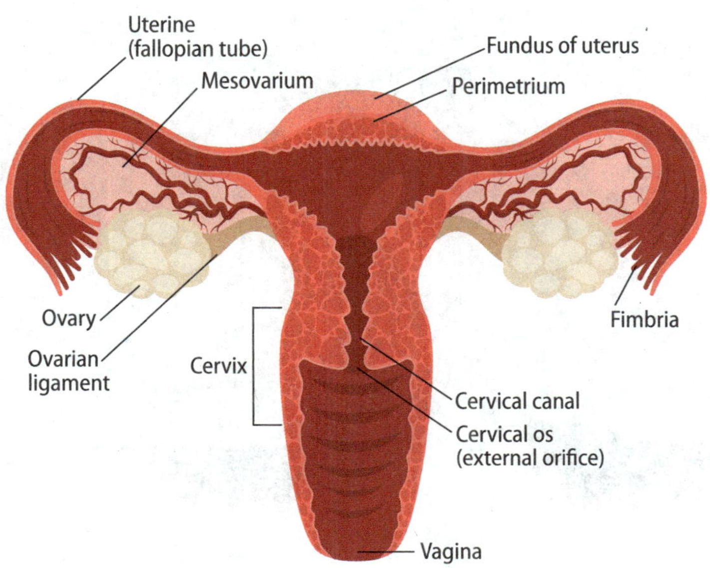

# Chapter 15. Pregnancy, Childbirth and the Puerperium (OØØ–O9A)

## Term Pregnancy – Single Gestation

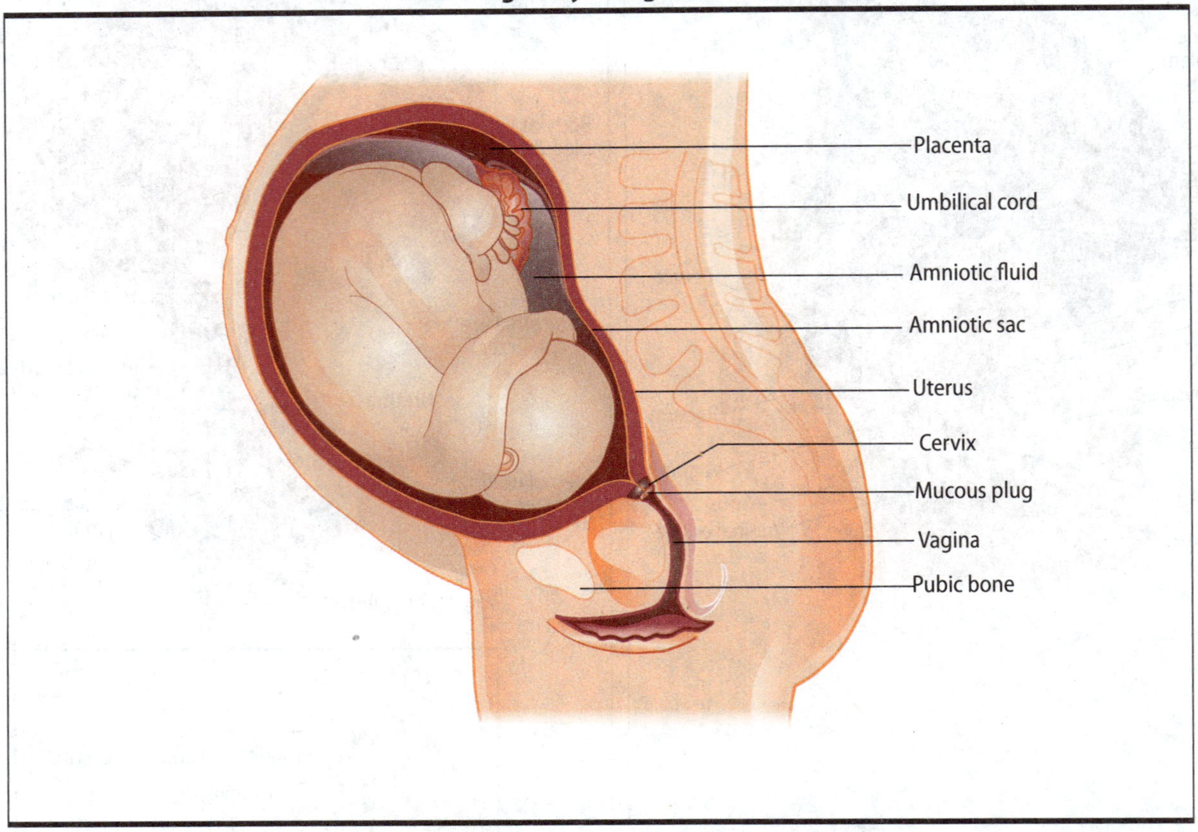


## Twin Gestation–Dichorionic–Diamniotic (DI-DI)

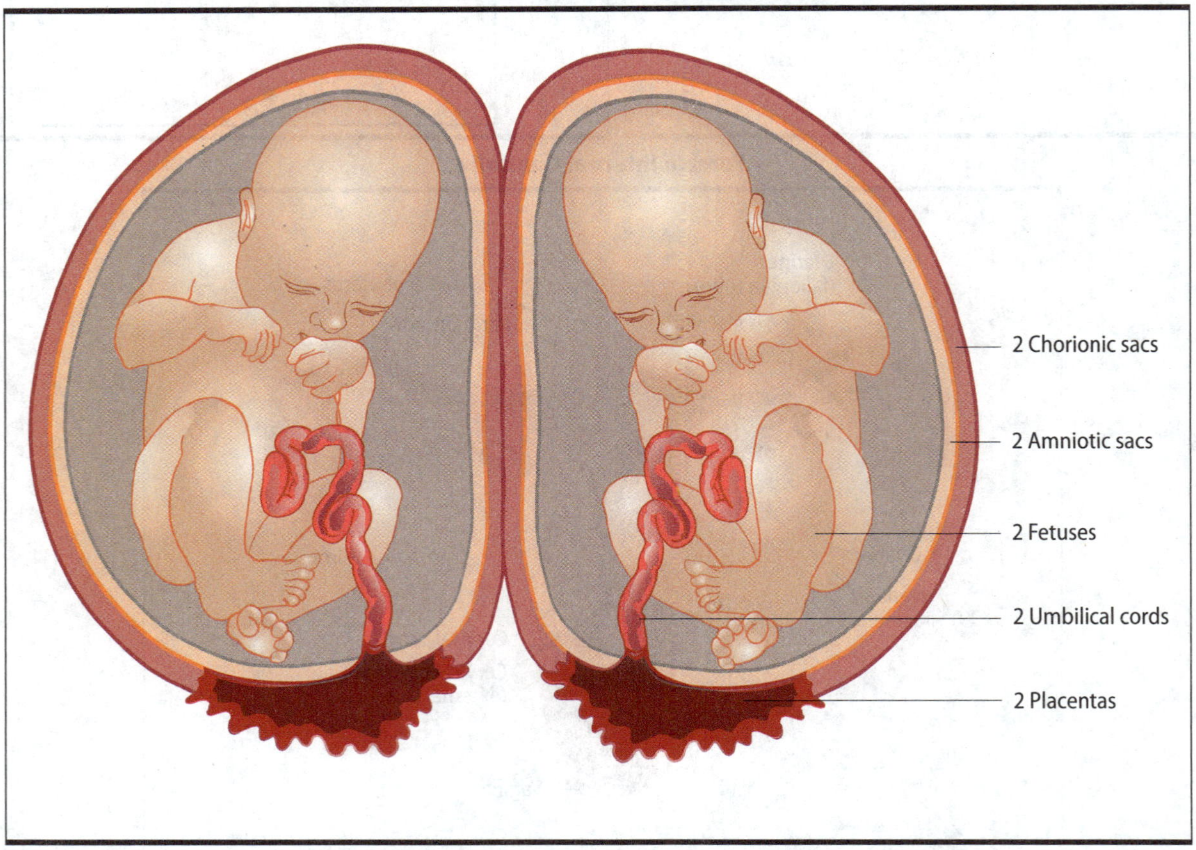

**Twin Gestation–Monochorionic–Diamniotic (MO-DI)**

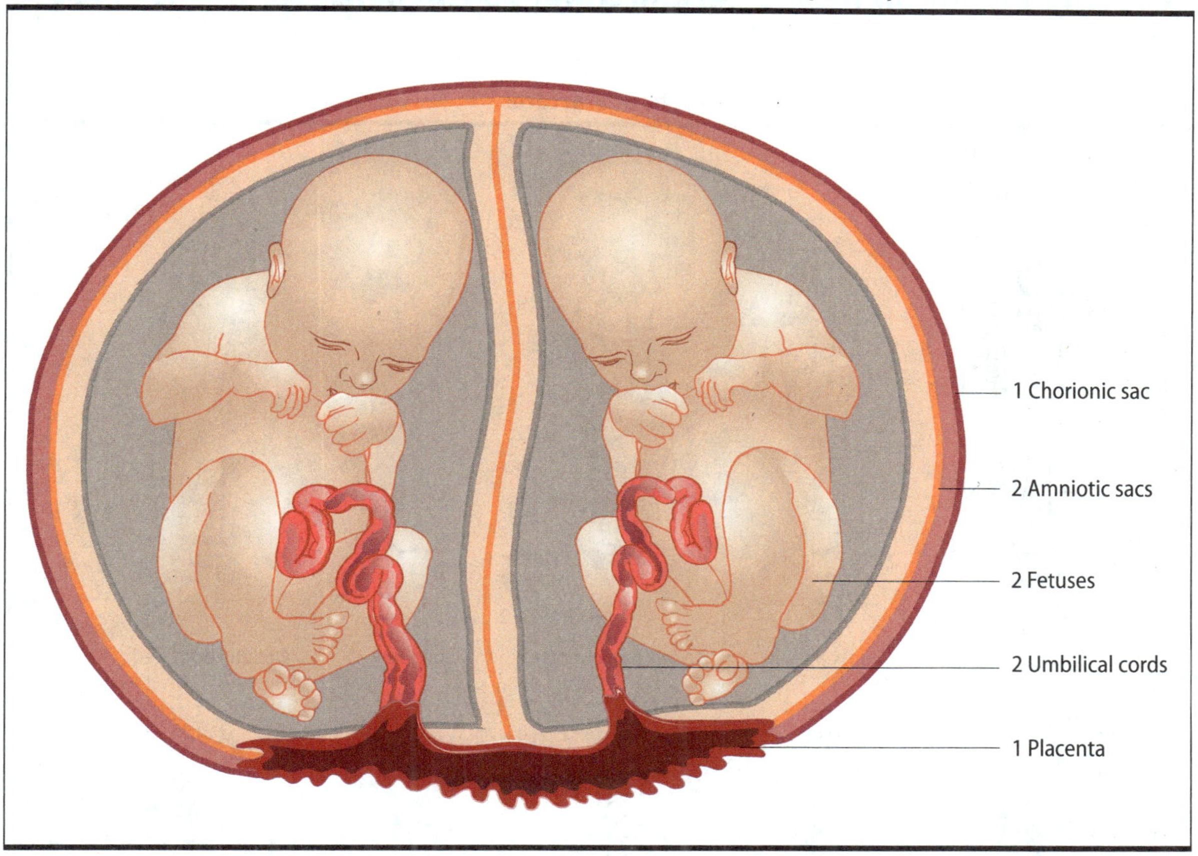


**Twin Gestation–Monochorionic–Monoamniotic (MO-MO)**

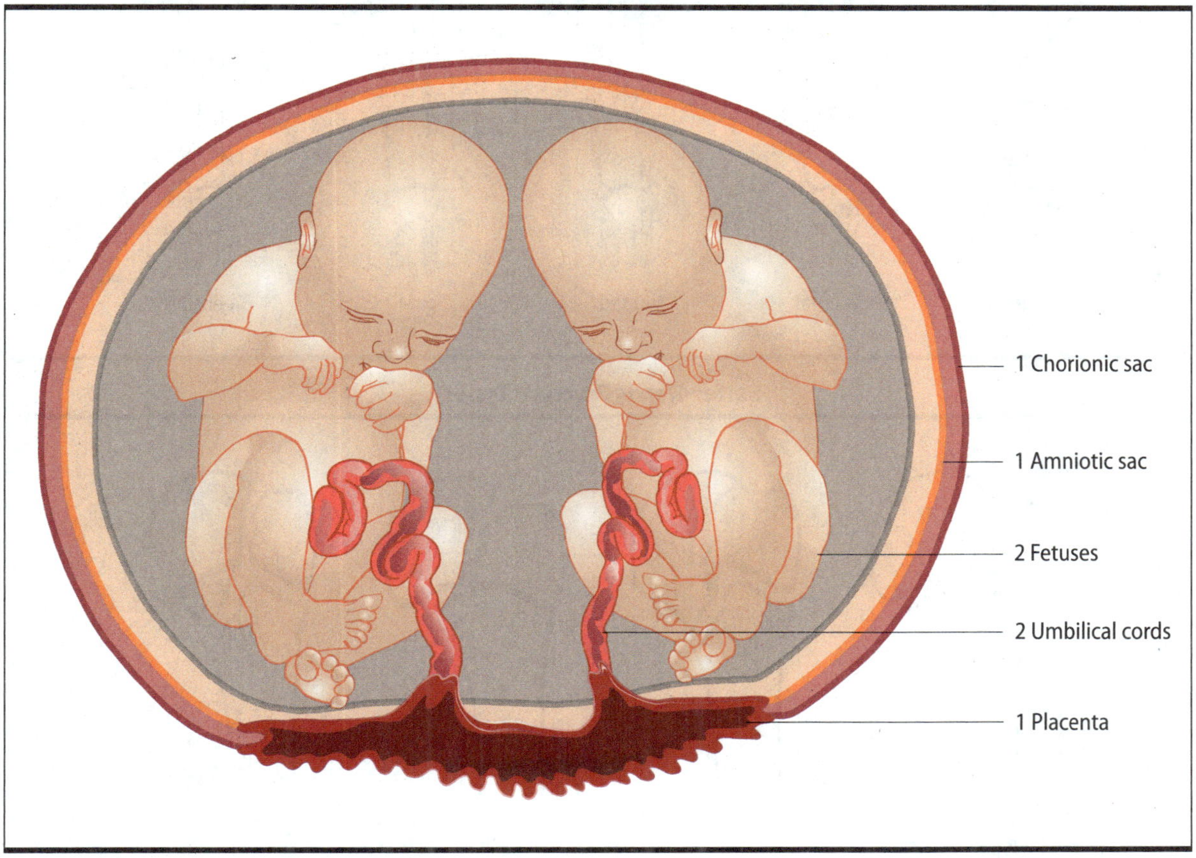

# Chapter 19. Injury, Poisoning and Certain Other Consequences of External Causes (SØØ–T88)

**Types of Fractures**

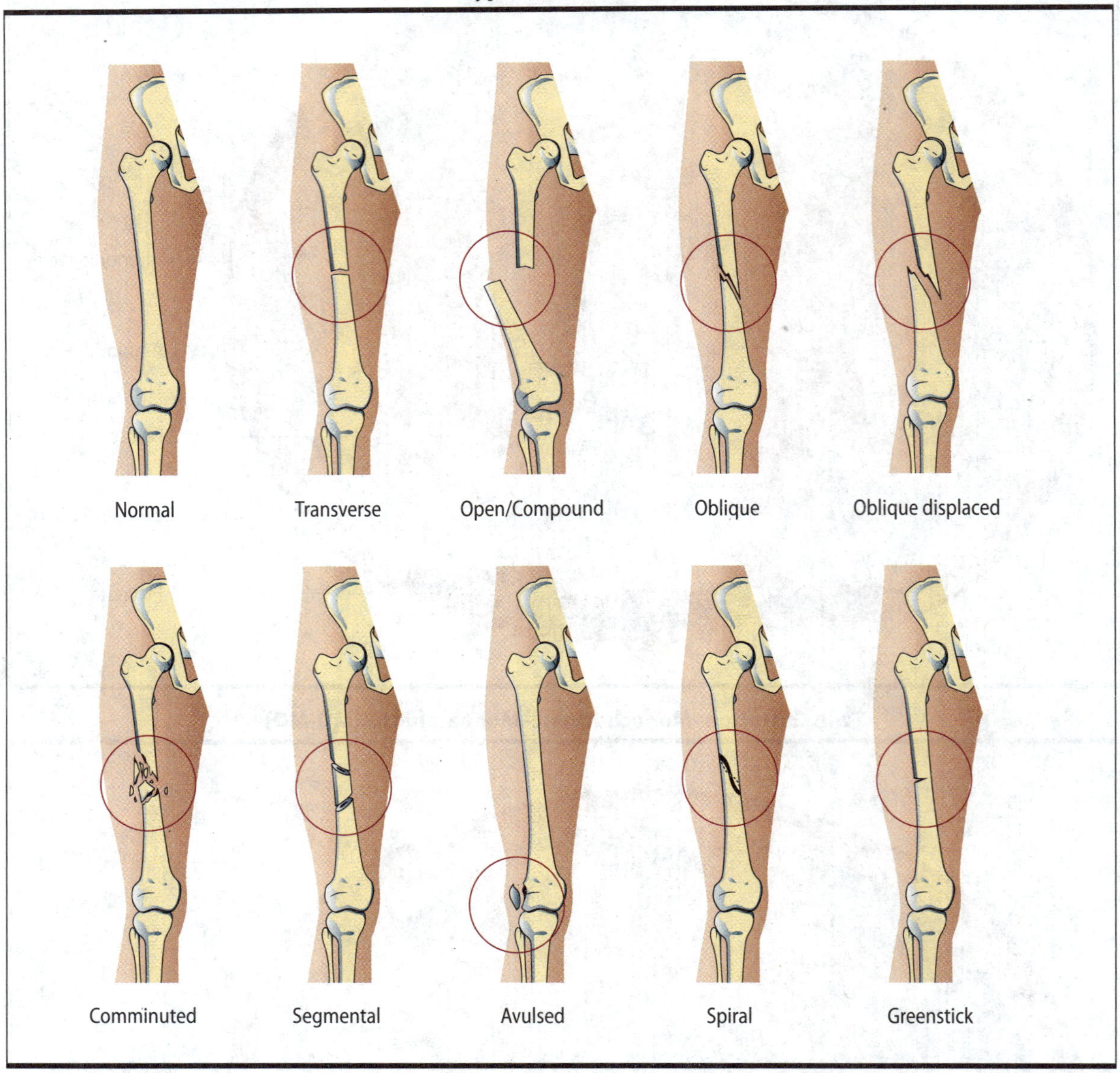


**Salter-Harris Fracture Types**

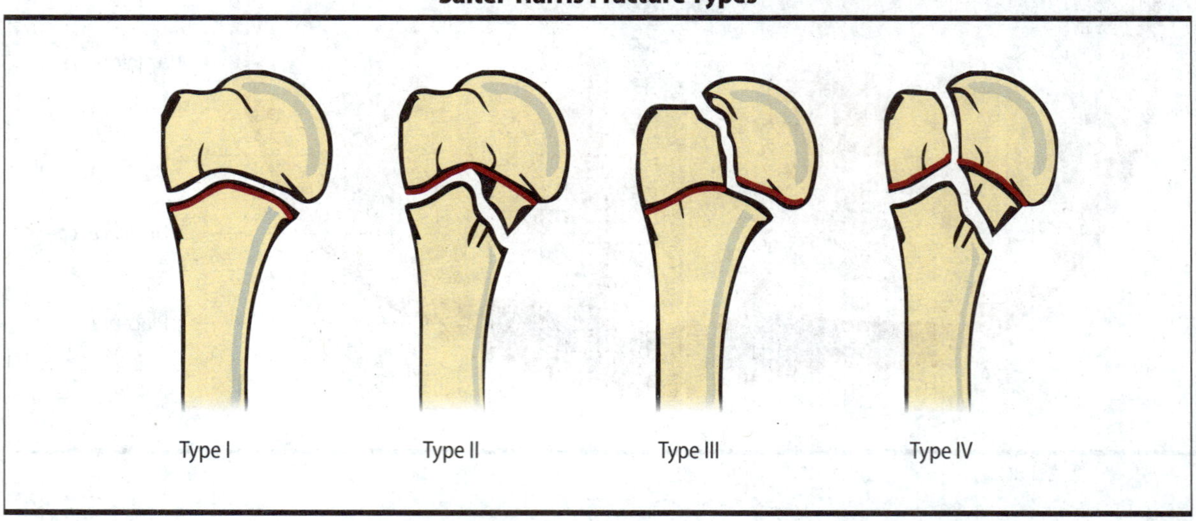